KU-474-678

Immunologic Renal Diseases

Immunologic Renal Diseases

Editors

Eric G. Neilson, M.D.
C. Mahlon Kline Professor of Medicine and Pediatrics
Chief, Renal-Electrolyte and Hypertension Division
Department of Medicine
University of Pennsylvania
Philadelphia, Pennsylvania

William G. Couser, M.D.
Belding H. Scribner Professor of Medicine
Head, Division of Nephrology
Department of Medicine
University of Washington
School of Medicine
Seattle, Washington

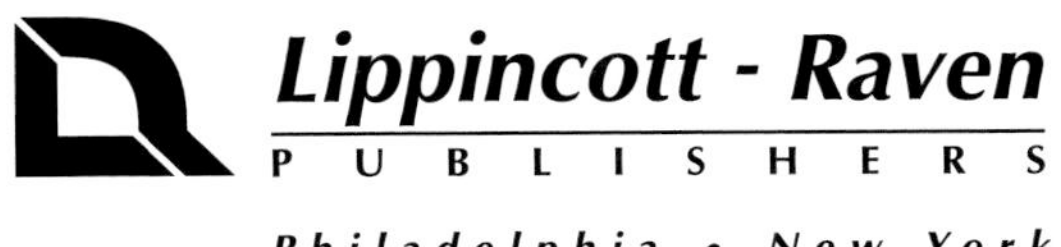

Lippincott - Raven
PUBLISHERS
Philadelphia • New York

Acquisitions Editor: Mark Placito
Developmental Editor: Rhoda Dunn
Manufacturing Manager: Dennis Teston
Production Manager: Lawrence Bernstein
Production Editor: Daniel Kulkosky
Cover Designer: Ede Dreikers
Indexer: Mary Kidd
Compositor: Lippincott-Raven
Printer: Kingsport Press

Printed in the United States of America

9 8 7 6 5 4 3 2 1

Library of Congress Cataloging-in-Publication Data

Immunologic renal diseases / editors, Eric G. Neilson, William G. Couser.
p. cm.
Includes bibliographical references and index.
ISBN 0-397-51671-1
1. Kidneys—Pathophysiology. 2. Kidneys—Immunology.
3. Immunopathology. I. Neilson, Eric G. II. Couser, William G.
[DNLM:1. Kidney Diseases—immunology. 2. Kidney Diseases—complications. 3. Immunologic Diseases—complications. WJ 300 I334 1996]
RC903.9.I456 1996
616.6′1079—dc20
DNLM/DLC
for Library of Congress 96-26842
CIP

To my former fellows and students who have helped me better understand the work we have done together, to Laurence E. Earley and Edward W. Holmes, who have always made me feel welcome at the University of Pennsylvania, and to S. Michael Phillips, who let me join his laboratory many years ago when I knew absolutely nothing about research. And to my wife Linda and children Tinsley and Sigrid, for the many happy hours away from the laboratory.

E.G.N.

To Edmund J. Lewis, who introduced me to the area of immune renal disease and first suggested ways in which it could be studied in the laboratory, to the many fellows who have continuously stimulated and sustained me in these efforts over the years (particularly David Salant, Steve Adler, and Rick Johnson), to the technicians who have made so many of the experiments work (particularly Chris Darby, Pam Pritzl, Kathy Gordon, and Jeff Pippin), and to my many patients, whose diseases have always provided the most important insights. And to my wife Linda and children Grif and Tommy, who have so gracefully endured the many hours I have had to flee intimacy in order to pursue my own dreams, including this book.

W.G.C.

Contents

IV. Response to Immune Injury

V. Animal Models of Immunologic Renal Diseases

VI. Clinical Aspects of Immunologic Renal Diseases

A. Patient Evaluation and General Considerations

B. Primary Glomerular Diseases

Contributors

Dale R. Abrahamson, Ph.D.
Professor of Cell Biology
Department of Cell Biology
University of Alabama at Birmingham
Birmingham, Alabama 35294

Christine K. Abrass, M.D.
Professor of Medicine
Department of Medicine
Department of Veterans Affairs
Puget Sound Health Care System and
University of Washington School of Medicine
1660 South Columbian Way
Seattle, Washington 98108

Stephen Adler, M.D.
Professor of Medicine
Division of Nephrology
Department of Medicine
New York Medical College
Renal Center, Westchester Medical Center
Valhalla, New York 10514

Charles E. Alpers, M.D.
Associate Professor of Pathology
Department of Pathology
University of Washington Medical Center
1959 Northeast Pacific Street
Seattle, Washington 98195

Gerald B. Appel, M.D.
Clinical Professor of Medicine
Division of Nephrology
Columbia-Presbyterian Medical Center
622 West 168th Street
New York, New York 10032

Robert C. Atkins, D.Sc., F.R.A.C.P.
Professor of Medicine
Department of Nephrology
Monash Medical Centre
246 Clayton Road
Clayton, Victoria 3168
Australia

Ellis D. Avner, M.D.
Gertrude Lee Chandler Tucker Professor
Chairman, Department of Pediatrics
Rainbow Babies and Children's Hospital
Case Western Reserve University
11100 Euclid Avenue
Cleveland, Ohio 44106

Barbara J. Ballermann, M.D.
Associate Professor of Medicine
Department of Medicine
Johns Hopkins University School of Medicine
Ross Research Building, Room 954
720 Rutland Avenue
Baltimore, Maryland 21205

Jeffrey L. Barnes, Ph.D.
Associate Professor of Medicine
Department of Medicine
Division of Nephrology
University of Texas Health Science Center at San Antonio
7703 Floyd Curl Drive
San Antonio, Texas 78284

William M. Bennett, M.D.
Professor of Medicine and Pharmacology
Division of Nephrology, Hypertension, and Clinical Pharmacology
Oregon Health Sciences University
3314 Southwest U.S. Veterans Hospital Road, PP262
Portland, Oregon 97201

J. Andrew Bertolatus, M.D.
Associate Professor of Medicine
Department of Internal Medicine
University of Iowa
200 Hawkins Drive
Iowa City, Iowa 52242

Daniel J. Birmingham, Ph.D.
Assistant Professor of Medicine
Department of Medicine
Ohio State University
1654 Upham Drive, Room N-210
Columbus, Ohio 43210

Roland C. Blantz, M.D.
Professor of Medicine
Department of Medicine
University of California, San Diego
Veterans Affairs Medical Center (111H)
San Diego, California 92161

Warren Kline Bolton, M.D.
Professor of Medicine
Chief, Division of Nephrology
Department of Internal Medicine
University of Virginia Health Sciences Center
Box 133, Jefferson Park Avenue
Charlottesville, Virginia 22908

Hugh R. Brady, M.D., Ph.D., F.R.C.P.I.
Professor of Medicine and Therapeutics
Department of Medicine and Therapeutics
Mater Miseracordiae Hospital
University College Dublin
41 Eccles Street
Dublin 7, Ireland

John R. Brandt, M.D.
Clinical Instructor of Medicine
Division of Nephrology
Children's Hospital Medical Center
4800 Sandpoint Way NE
Seattle, Washington 98105

Barbara A. Burke, M.D.
Professor Emeritus of Pathology
Departments of Laboratory Medicine and Pathology
University of Minnesota Hospital
Box 491 UMHC
420 Delaware Street SE
Minneapolis, Minnesota 55455

J. Stewart Cameron, M.D., F.R.C.P.
Emeritus Professor of Renal Medicine
Renal Unit
United Medical and Dental Schools of Guy's and St. Thomas Hospitals
London Bridge
London SE1 9RT
United Kingdom

Yi Pu Chen, M.D.
Professor of Medicine
Institute of Nephrology
Beijing Medical University
No. 8 Xishiku Street
Beijing 100034
People's Republic of China

William L. Clapp, M.D.
Assistant Professor of Pathology
Department of Pathology and Laboratory Medicine
University of Florida College of Medicine
Veterans Affairs Medical Center
Gainesville, Florida 32610

Fernando G. Cosio, M.D.
Professor of Medicine
Department of Medicine
Ohio State University
1654 Upham Drive
Room N-210
Columbus, Ohio 43210

William G. Couser, M.D.
Belding H. Scribner Professor of Medicine
Head, Division of Nephrology
Department of Medicine
University of Washington School of Medicine
Health Sciences Building BB-1265
1959 Northeast Pacific, Box 356521
Seattle, Washington 98195

Theodore M. Danoff, M.D., Ph.D.
Assistant Professor of Medicine
Renal Electrolyte and Hypertension Division
University of Pennsylvania
700 Clinical Research Building
415 Curie Boulevard
Philadelphia, Pennsylvania 19104

Angelo M. de Mattos, M.D.
Assistant Professor of Medicine
Department of Medicine
Division of Nephrology
Oregon Health Sciences University
3181 Southwest Sam Jackson Park Road, MQ360
Portland, Oregon 97201

Michael J. Dunn, M.D.
Dean and Executive Vice President
Medical College of Wisconsin
8701 Watertown Plank Road
Milwaukee, Wisconsin 53226

Marlies Elger, Dr.Phil.
Department of Anatomy and Cell Biology
University of Heidelberg
Im Neuenheimer Feld 307
Heidelberg 69120
Germany

Ronald J. Falk, M.D.
Professor of Medicine
Director
Division of Nephrology and Hypertension
University of North Carolina
3034 Old Clinic Building
Chapel Hill, North Carolina 27599

Jürgen Floege, M.D.
Associate Professor of Medicine
Division of Nephrology
University Medical School
Konstanty-Gutschow-Str. 8
Hannover 30625
Germany

Agnes B. Fogo, M.D.
Associate Professor of Pathology and Pediatrics
Department of Pathology
Vanderbilt University Medical Center
21st and Garland
Nashville, Tennessee 37232

Mary H. Foster, M.D.
Assistant Professor of Medicine
Department of Medicine
University of Pennsylvania
700 Clinical Research Building
415 Curie Boulevard
Philadelphia, Pennsylvania 19104

Francis B. Gabbai, M.D.
Associate Professor of Medicine
Department of Medicine
University of California, San Diego
Veterans Affairs Medical Center (111H)
3550 La Jolla Village Drive
San Diego, California 92161

Richard J. Glassock, M.D.
Professor and Chairman
Department of Internal Medicine
University of Kentucky College of Medicine
Kentucky Clinic J-525
Lexington, Kentucky 40536

Tom Greene, Ph.D.
Associate Staff in Biostatistics
Department of Biostatistics and Epidemiology
Cleveland Clinic Foundation
9500 Euclid Avenue
Cleveland, Ohio 44195

Philip F. Halloran, M.D., Ph.D.
Professor of Medicine and Immunology
Division of Nephrology
Department of Medicine
University of Alberta
8249 114th Street, #205
Edmonton, Alberta T6G 2R8
Canada

Lee A. Hebert, M.D.
Professor of Medicine
Director, Division of Nephrology
Department of Internal Medicine
Ohio State University Medical Center
1654 Upham Drive
Means Hall, Room N-210
Columbus, Ohio 43210

Marie-Josée Hébert, M.D., F.R.C.P.(C).
Renal Division
Brigham and Women's Hospital
Harvard Medical School
Boston, Massachusetts 02115

Peter S. Heeger, M.D.
Assistant Professor of Medicine
Department of Medicine
Case Western Reserve University
Cleveland Veterans Affairs Medical Center
10701 East Boulevard, 111-K(W)
Cleveland, Ohio 44106

Lawrence B. Holtzmann
Department of Internal Medicine, Nephrology
University of Michigan Medical Center
3914 Taubman Center
1500 East Medical Center Drive
Ann Arbor, Michigan 48109

Jeremy Hughes, M.A., M.R.C.P.
Lecturer in Medicine
Division of Renal and Inflammatory Disease
University Hospital
Nottingham NG7 2UH
United Kingdom

Lawrence G. Hunsicker, M.D.
Professor of Medicine
Department of Internal Medicine
University of Iowa Hospitals
200 Hawkins Drive
Iowa City, Iowa 52242

Iekuni Ichikawa, M.D.
Professor of Pediatrics
Head, Division of Pediatric Nephrology
Vanderbilt University
1161 21st Avenue South
C-4204 Medical Center North
Nashville, Tennessee 37232

J. Charles Jennette, M.D.
Professor and Vice Chairman
Department of Pathology and Laboratory Medicine
Director, Nephrology Laboratory
University of North Carolina
3034 Old Clinic Building
Chapel Hill, North Carolina 27559

Richard J. Johnson, M.D., F.A.C.P.
Professor of Medicine
Department of Medicine
Division of Nephrology
University of Washington Medical Center
1959 Pacific Street NE
Seattle, Washington 98195

Brigitte K. Kaissling, M.D.
Professor of Anatomy
Anatomical Department
University of Zürich
Winterthurerstr. 190
Zürich 8057
Switzerland

Raghulam Kalluri, Ph.D.
Research Associate
Department of Medicine
Renal-Electrolyte and Hypertension Division
University of Pennsylvania
700 Clinical Research Building
415 Curie Boulevard
Philadelphia, Pennsylvania 19104

Bernard S. Kaplan, M.B., B.Ch.
Professor of Pediatrics and Medicine
Division of Nephrology
The Children's Hospital of Philadelphia
University of Pennsylvania
34th Street and Civic Center Boulevard
Philadelphia, Pennsylvania 19104

Michael Kashgarian, M.D.
Professor of Pathology and Biology
Department of Pathology
Yale University School of Medicine
310 Cedar Street
New Haven, Connecticut 06510

Clifford E. Kashtan, M.D.
Associate Professor of Pediatrics
Department of Pediatrics
University of Minnesota
Box 491 UMHC
13-242 Moos Tower
420 Delaware Street SE
Minneapolis, Minnesota 55455

Gur P. Kaushal, Ph.D.
Assistant Professor of Medicine and Biochemistry
Department of Medicine
University of Arkansas for Medical Sciences
4301 West Markham Street, Slot 501
Little Rock, Arkansas 72205

Carolyn J. Kelly, M.D.
Associate Professor of Medicine
Division of Nephrology - Hypertension
University of California at San Diego
Veterans Affairs Medical Center, San Diego
3550 La Jolla Village Drive, 111H
San Diego, California 92161

Vicki R. Kelley, Ph.D.
Associate Professor of Medicine
Department of Medicine
Brigham and Women's Hospital
Harvard Medical School
75 Francis Street
Boston, Massachusetts 02115

Dontscho Kerjaschki, M.D.
Professor of Medicine
Institute of Clinical Pathology
University of Vienna - General Hospital
Währinger Gürtel 18-20
Vienna A 1090
Austria

Youngki Kim, M.D.
Professor of Pediatrics
Departments of Pediatrics, Laboratory Medicine, and Pathology
University of Minnesota Hospital
Box 491 UMHC
420 Delaware Street SE
Minneapolis, Minnesota 55455

Paul L. Kimmel, M.D.
Professor of Medicine
Department of Medicine
George Washington University Medical Center
2150 Pennsylvania Avenue NW
Washington, D.C. 20037

Seymour J. Klebanoff, M.D., Ph.D.
Professor of Medicine
Division of Infectious Diseases
Box 357185
University of Washington
Seattle, Washington 98195

Karl G. Koenig, M.D.
Assistant Professor of Medicine
Department of Internal Medicine
Division of Nephrology
University of Virginia Health Sciences Center
Box 133, Jefferson Park Avenue
Charlottesville, Virginia 22908

Valentina Kon, M.D.
Associate Professor of Pediatrics
Division of Pediatric Nephrology
Vanderbilt University Medical Center
1161 21st Avenue South
C-4204 Medical Center North
Nashville, Tennessee 37232

Stephen M. Korbet, M.D., F.A.C.P.
Professor of Medicine
Section of Nephrology
Department of Medicine
Rush Medical College
Rush Presbyterian - St. Luke's Medical Center
1653 West Congress Parkway
Chicago, Illinois 60612

Alan M. Krensky, M.D.
Shelagh Galligan Professor
Department of Pediatrics
Stanford University
300 Pasteur Drive
Stanford, California 94305

Wilhelm Kriz, M.D.
Professor of Anatomy
Department of Anatomy and Cell Biology I
University of Heidelberg
Im Neuenheimer Feld 307
Heidelberg 6120
Germany

Dean A. Kujubu
Assistant Professor
Department of Medicine
Renal-Electrolyte and Hypertension Division
University of Pennsylvania and
The Veteran's Memorial Hospital
700 Clinical Research Building
415 Curie Boulevard
Philadelphia, Pennsylvania 19104

Hui Y. Lan, M.D., Ph.D.
Senior Lecturer of Medicine
Department of Nephrology
Monash Medical Centre
246 Clayton Road
Clayton, Victoria 3168
Australia

Joseph Lau, M.D.
Associate Professor of Medicine
Department of Medicine
Division of Clinical Care Research
New England Medical Center
750 Washington Street, Box 63
Boston, Massachusetts 02111

Michel Le Hir, Dr.Phil.
Anatomical Department
University of Zürich
Winterthurerstr. 190
Zürich 8057
Switzerland

Daniel J. Legault, M.D.
Nephrology Division
Department of Internal Medicine
University of Michigan,
Ann Arbor, Michigan 48109

Andrew S. Levey, M.D.
Professor of Medicine
Tufts University School of Medicine
Director, Nephrology Clinical Research Center
New England Medical Center
750 Washington Street, Box 784
Boston, Massachusetts 02111

Michael P. Madaio, M.D.
Associate Professor of Medicine
Department of Medicine
University of Pennsylvania
700 Clinical Research Building
415 Curie Boulevard
Philadelphia, Pennsylvania 19010

Tobias A. Marsen, M.D.
Doctor of Internal Medicine
Klinik IV für Innere Medizin
University of Cologne
Joseph-Stelmann-Str. 9
Cologne 50924
Germany

Katsuyiki Matsui, M.D.
Assistant Professor of Medicine
Institute of Clincial Pathology
University of Vienna
General Hospital
Währinger Gürtel 18-20
A 1090 Vienna
Austria

Catherine M. Meyers, M.D.
Assistant Professor of Medicine
Department of Medicine
Renal Electrolyte and Hypertension Division
University of Pennsylvania
700 Clinical Research Building
415 Curie Boulevard
Philadelphia, Pennsylvania 19104

Kevin E. C. Meyers M.B., Ch.
Division of Nephrology
The Children's Hospital of Pennsylvania
University of Pennsylvania
34th Street and Civic Center Boulevard
Philadelphia, Pennsylvania 19104

Robert B. Miller, M.D.
Senior Fellow, Pediatric Nephrology
Department of Pediatrics
University of Minnesota
Box 491 UMHC
420 Delaware Street SE
Minneapolis, Minnesota 55455

Andrew F. Mooney, B.Med.Sci (Hons), B.M., B.S., M.R.C.P.
MRC Training Fellow
Honorary Senior Registrar
Division of Renal and Inflammatory Disease
Department of Medicine
University of Nottingham Hospital
Nottingham NG7 2UH
United Kingdom

Gerhard A. Müller, M.D.
Professor of Medicine
Center of Internal Medicine, Nephrology, and Rheumatology
Georg-August-University
Robert-Koch-Str. 40
Göttingen 37075
Germany

Yasuhiro Natori, Ph.D.
Division Head
Division of Pathophysiology
Research Institute
International Medical Center of Japan
1-21-1 Toyama, Shinjuku-ku
Tokyo 162
Japan

Eric G. Neilson, M.D.
C. Mahlon Kline Professor of Medicine and Pediatrics
Chief, Renal-Electrolyte and Hypertension Division
Department of Medicine
University of Pennsylvania
700 Clinical Research Building
415 Curie Boulevard
Philadelphia, Pennsylvania 19104

David J. Nikolic-Paterson, B.Sc., D.Phil.
Senior Research Officer
Department of Nephrology
Monash Medical Center
246 Clayton Road
Clayton, Victoria 3168
Australia

Ali J. Olyaei, Pharm.D.
Assistant Professor of Medicine
Division of Nephrology and Hypertension
Oregon Health Sciences University
3181 SW Sam Jackson Park Road
Portland, Oregon 97201

James M. Pattison, B.M., B.Ch., M.R.C.P.
Senior Registrar in Renal Medicine
Guy s Hosptial
London SE1 9RT
United Kingdom

Andrew J. Rees, M.Sc., F.R.C.P.
Regius Professor of Medicine
Department of Medicine and Therapeutics
University of Aberdeen
Polwarth Building
Foresterhill
Aberdeen AB9 2ZD
United Kingdom

Giuseppe Remuzzi, M.D.
Associate Professor
Mario Negri Institute for Pharmacological Research
Division of Nephrology and Dialysis
Ospedali Riuniti Di Bergamo
Via Gavazzeni 11
24125 Bergamo
Italy

Harald D. Rupprecht, M.D.
Instructor in Medicine
Medizinische Klinik IV
Universität Erlangen-Nürnberg
Krankenhausstr. 12
Erlangen 91054
Germany

David J. Salant, M.B., B.Ch.
Professor of Medicine, Pathology, and Laboratory Medicine
Department of Medicine
Boston University Medical Center
88 East Newton Street
Boston, Massachusetts 02118

John S. Savill, B.A., M.B., CH.B., Ph.D., F.R.C.P.
Professor of Medicine
Division of Renal and Inflammatory Disease
Department of Medicine
University Hospital
Nottingham NG7 2UH
United Kingdom

H. William Schnaper, M.D.
Associate Professor of Pediatrics
Department of Pediatrics
Northwestern University Medical School
Attending Physician
Children's Memorial Hospital
303 East Chicago Avenue, Peds W-140
Chicago, Illinois 60611

Melvin M. Schwartz, M.D.
Professor of Pathology
Rush Presbyterian St. Luke's Medical Center
1753 West Congress Parkway
Chicago, Illinois 60612

Sudhir V. Shah, M.D.
Director, Division of Nephrology
Professor of Medicine
Department of Medicine
University of Arkansas for Medical Sciences
4301 West Markham Street, Slot 501
Little Rock, Arkansas 72205

Fujio Shimizu, M.D., Ph.D.
Professor of Immunology and Chief
Institute of Nephrology
Department of Immunology
Niigata University School of Medicine
Asahimachi-dori 1-757
Niigata 951
Japan

Richard K. Sibley, M.D.
Professor of Pathology
Department of Pathology
Stanford University Medical Center
300 Pasteur Drive
Stanford, California 94305

Gary G. Singer, M.D.
Assistant Professor of Internal Medicine
Associate Director of Transplant Nephrology
Renal Division
Washington University School of Medicine
St. Louis, Missouri 63110

Rolf A. K. Stahl, M.D.
Professor of Medicine
Medizinische Klinik
Universitäts-Krankenhaus Eppendorf
Martinistrasse 52
Hamburg 20246
Germany

R. Bernd Sterzel, M.D.
Professor of Internal Medicine
Medizinische Klinik IV
University of Erlangen-Nürnberg
Krankenhausstrasse 52
Erlangen 91054
Germany

Frank Strutz, M.D.
Georg-August-Universität Göttingen
Zentrum Innere Medizin und Poliklinik
Abteilung Nephrolgie und Rheumatologie
Robert-Koch-Str. 40
Göttingen 37075
Germany

Laurence A. Turka, M.D.
Associate Professor of Medicine
Department of Medicine
University of Pennsylvania
409 Clinical Research Building
422 Curie Boulevard
Philadelphia, Pennsylvania 19104

Gregory B. Vanden Heuvel, Ph.D.
Postdoctoral Associate
Section of Nephrology
Department of Medicine
Yale University School of Medicine
333 Cedar Street
New Haven, Connecticut 06510

Leendert A. Van Es, M.D.
Department of Nephrology
University Hospital
Rynsburgerweg 10
Leiden 2333-AA
The Netherlands

Hai Yan Wang, M.D.
Professor of Medicine
Institute of Nephrology
Beijing Medical University
No. 8 Xishiku Street
Beijing 100034
People's Republic of China

Roger C. Wiggins, M.B., B.Chir.
Professor of Medicine
Department of Internal Medicine, Nephrology
University of Michigan Medical Center
3914 Taubman Center
1500 East Medical Center Drive
Ann Arbor, Michigan 48109

Curtis B. Wilson, M.D.
Senior Member
The Scripps Research Institute
10666 North Torrey Pines Road IMM5
La Jolla, California 92037

Rudolf P. Wüthrich, M.D.
Associate Professor of Medicine
Division of Nephrology
University Hospital
Zürich 8091
Switzerland

Norishige Yoshikawa, M.D., Ph.D.
Professor of Health Science
Department of Health Science
Kobe University School of Medicine
7-10-2 Tomogaoka, Suma-ku
Kobe City 654-01
Japan

Carla Zoja
Institute Member
Mario Negri Institute for Pharmacological Research
Via Govasseni 11
24125 Bergamo
Italy

Preface

The discipline of immune renal disease has grown enormously over the past several decades. Today we are surrounded by rapidly expanding scientific information related to disease mechanisms on the one hand and difficult treatment decisions for patients afflicted with these diseases on the other. There is no single source which provides the investigator and the clinician with an integrated view of this discipline or that brings the science of the subject to the bedside. Better health is intuitively rooted in the science of medicine and its application to clinical practice. This book was conceived to fill that need in the area of immunologic renal disease.

Both of us became fascinated by immune diseases of the kidney at stages of our training when career decisions are made. We have each worked in this field as both investigators and clinicians and contributed to its evolution since that time. We began our work in the era of renal immunopathology in the 60's and 70's with its focus on the antibody and humoral mediators of injury, progressed through the rapid expansion of immunology with an emphasis on antigen presentation and the cellular immune system in the 1980's and have now evolved in the current era of molecular biology with its accompanying techniques of in situ hybridization, polymerase chain reaction, gene cloning and mapping and gene transfer therapy. Cell biology has evolved as well over this interval from the time when the study of the isolated glomerulus was thought to be novel to an era where we now have immortalized clones of each of the glomerular and interstitial cell types and have developed a rapidly expanding list of growth factors and cytokines that communicate with circulating and resident cells to modulate function in disease and repair. Each era has built on, rather than supplanted, the ones which preceded it. The study of the kidney, long dominated by individuals with expertise primarily in renal physiology, is now being pursued aggressively by an army of nephrologists and renal pathologists with skills in basic immunology, cell biology and molecular biology.

However, the study of mechanisms of immune renal disease long preceded our entry into this field, and we owe a profound debt to generations of earlier investigators who not only identified most of these diseases as ones with an immunologic basis, but founded the discipline which has so fascinated us and many other students of these diseases. To put the modern era into perspective, the highlights in the evolution of our understanding of mechanisms of immune renal disease through 1984 are reviewed by Glassock in the first chapter of this book.

With the above background in mind, it is our conviction that the subject of immunologic renal injury now warrants more attention than can be provided by a single chapter or section in a general textbook on renal disease. Our book was designed to provide comprehensive information to a physician with a patient with immune renal injury to the kidney. Chapters 2–34 contain what is currently known or suspected of the immunologic mechanisms which underly human renal injury and their consequences on renal structure and function. Chapters 37–56 cover the clinical manifestations and recognized disease entities that result from those processes, including discussions of the pathogenesis, pathology, clinical presentation and current treatment of each of them. The two sections of the book are joined by Chapters 35 and 36 which review the animal models that have been so useful in defining much of what we know about this subject.

In all cases, the chapters are authored by leading investigators and clinicians in the field who have been charged with providing comprehensive views of their topics without focusing solely on their own work. In this first edition we have also attempted to tie these chapters together through an organization in which the reader may move easily back and forth from basic science to clinical applications.

We believe this textbook will contribute in two ways. First, by facilitating and clarifying the application of basic science to the understanding of immunologic renal disease in man, thereby stimulating new discoveries and more progress in this area. And second, by improving the care and treatment of sick patients because of a better appreciation for the mechanisms of disease. It is our fond hope that our readers will join the editors and contributors in striving to achieve both of these goals.

Finally, our warm wishes to Mark Placito and Rhoda Gail Dunn at Lippincott-Raven for their help and guidance in preparing this book.

Eric G. Neilson, M.D.
William G. Couser, M.D.

Immunologic Renal Diseases

Immunologic Renal Diseases,
edited by E. G. Neilson and W. G. Couser.
Lippincott-Raven Publishers, Philadelphia © 1997

CHAPTER 1

Introduction

The History of Renal Immunopathology

Richard J. Glassock

IN THE BEGINNING

Although renal immunopathology has only recently evolved into a discrete scientific discipline, it has its roots in the broad field of immunology, which dates to antiquity. The first recorded document that embraced the concept of protective immunity was in the diary of Thucydides, a Greek Philosopher, who stated in 430 B.C. in reference to a plague that was threatening Athens, "no one caught the disease twice or if he did, the second attack was never fatal."(1,2)

Recognition that prior exposure to a disease seemed to provide a measure of protection led to a variety of practices in many cultures over succeeding centuries. However, great attention was focused on intentional exposure to disease as a method of affording protection by the famous "Royal Experiment," conducted in 1721 under the urging of Lady Mary Wortley Montagu, the wife of the British Ambassador to Turkey. In this experiment, two royal princes were successfully protected from an epidemic of smallpox by the practice "variolation" (3,4) where material from healing smallpox blisters were inoculated into healthy individuals. It is noteworthy that this successful experiment involving the two royal princes was preceded by a pilot experiment involving six condemned criminals from Neugate Prison, all of whom survived the experiment and were subsequently pardoned (3). The concept of protective immunity was firmly established when Edward Jenner inoculated Sarah Niemes with material from a cowpox pustule on May 14, 1796. This immunization (subsequently called *vaccination*) established immunology as an experimental science, in this case by an uncontrolled clinical trial. It is also noteworthy that Jenner's manuscripts describing his experiments were rejected by the Royal Society and published privately in 1798 (5).

Many theories were subsequently expounded to explain "acquired immunity," but the debate ultimately centered on humoral versus cellular mechanisms. Elie Metchnikoff in 1884 postulated that the defense against infection (principally Anthrax) was vested in phagocytes (6,7). His contemporary, Louis Pasteur, was the champion of the humoral theory of acquired immunity (8,9). In 1890, Von Behring and Kitasato (10) showed unequivocally that serum from animals immunized with diphtheria and tetanus contained substances that inhibited the exotoxins elaborated by these organisms. This experiment, coupled with the fame and influence of Pasteur, caused the cellular theory to rapidly decline. Von Behring was awarded the first Nobel Prize in 1901 for these seminal studies on the humoral aspects of acquired immunity. Subsequently, Jules Bordet demonstrated that erythrocytes could be lysed in the absence of cells, which further reinforced the position of the humoral theory (11). Paul Ehrlich's (12) classic work on diphtheria antitoxins in 1897 clearly established that acquired immunity was due to the presence of antibodies in

R. J. Glassock: Department of Internal Medicine, University of Kentucky College of Medicine, Lexington, Kentucky 40536.

[1]This review will primarily consider historical events and seminal discoveries in the field of renal immunopathology and related areas through 1976, the year of publication of the first edition of *The Kidney*, edited by B.M. Brenner and F.C. Rector, Jr. and published by WB Saunders, Philadelphia, in 1976. The reader is referred to the first through the fifth editions of *The Kidney* for developments in the field of renal immunopathology occurring since 1976. The chapters on The Renal Response to Immunologic Injury by Curtis B. Wilson and Frank J. Dixon found in these editions of *The Kidney* are particularly useful sources of historical references since 1976.

immune serum. These findings resulted in the nearly exclusive focus of the field of immunology on the protective effects of antibody. Despite the fact that Metchnikoff shared the Nobel Prize with Ehrlich in 1908, research on the cellular aspects of immunity lay largely dormant for another 50 years.

Thus, the prevailing view at the beginning of the twentieth century was that immunologic responses were largely protective in nature and that this protection was mediated almost exclusively by antibody. So pervasive was this attitude that Paul Erlich proclaimed in 1901 that "the immunity reaction . . . is prevented from acting against the organisms own elements and so giving rise to autotoxins . . . so that we might be justified in speaking of a 'horror autotoxicus of the organism.'" Therefore, the often-quoted "horror autotoxicus" postulate did not claim that autoantibodies may not be formed, but only that they are prevented from acting on the organism (13).

A TURNING POINT

Shortly after Erlich proclaimed his postulate of "horror autotoxicus," a remarkable series of observations overturned prevailing dogma regarding the exclusively protective role for immunity, and the new science of immunopathology was born. In 1902, Paul Portier and Charles Richet of Paris (14) discovered anaphylaxis; in 1903 Maurice Arthus of Freiburg (15) discovered the phenomena bearing his name; in 1904 Julius Donath and Karl Landsteiner of Vienna (16) discovered the cold-reacting autoantibody mediating paroxysmal nocturnal hemoglobinuria; and in 1906 Clemens Von Pirquet and Bela Schick (17) described and analyzed serum sickness. Charles Richet was awarded the Nobel prize in 1913 for his studies of anaphylaxis, which, in an interesting footnote on history, were carried out aboard the yacht of the Prince of Monaco. The terms *allergy*, or *altered reactivity*, were coined by Von Pirquet to signify this paradigm shift in thinking about immunity (17,18) (Figure 1).

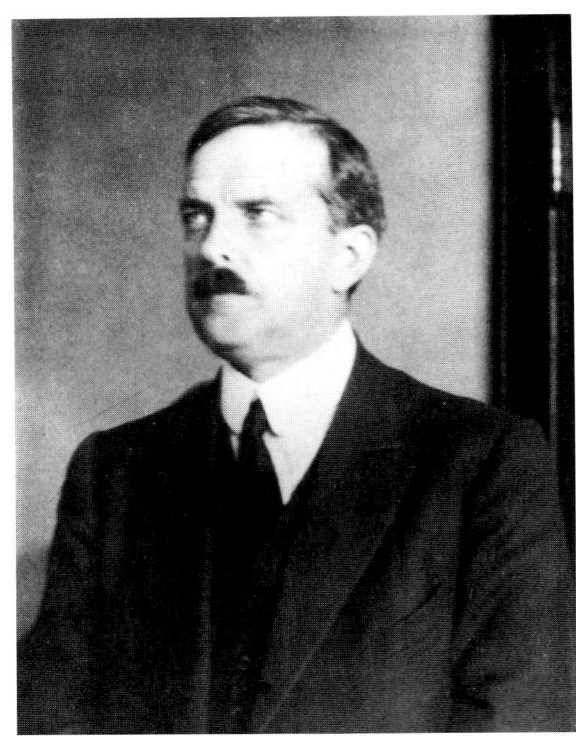

FIG. 1. Clemens Von Pirquet (circa 1911). From the Library of Medicine.

The description of serum sickness was to presage later interest in immune complexes as phlogistic elements in disease. The work on anaphylaxis and autoantibody-mediated hemolysis clearly set the stage for studies of organ-specific autoimmunity (19). Nevertheless, little occurred immediately following these seminal observations to advance the field of autoimmunity and immunopathology. Indeed, there was a dearth of observation in these fields for another 30 years, perhaps because of World War I and the death of leading investigators such as Ehrlich, Pasteur, and Metchnikoff. Nevertheless, the fundamental science of immunology continued to advance, particularly in the area of immunochemistry, led by the research of Landsteiner, Heidelberg, Pauling, Boyd, and Marrack (19).

In these early years, the renal aspects of immunopathology languished in back waters of science, with most of the earlier attention being focused on hemolytic disease, sperm and testicular autoimmunity, encephalomyelitis, sympathetic ophthalmia, anaphylaxis, and autoimmune thyroid disease. Lindemann's (20) pioneering work on the nephrotoxicity of heterologous antikidney sera, conducted in 1900, was largely neglected, although Wilson and Oliver (21) identified the glomerulus as the target of antikidney sera in 1920. Von Pirquet clearly delineated that the glomerulonephritis that accompanied serum sickness was related to "toxic bodies" appearing in the circulation as antigen was being cleared from the circulation by newly formed antibody (18) (Figure 2). These "toxic bodies" were later identified by Germuth, Dixon, and others as immune complexes (22–24).

EXPERIMENTAL RENAL DISEASE REDISCOVERED

The field of renal immunopathology was reinvigorated by the now classic studies of Matozo Masugi, carried out between 1929 and 1935, on the experimental disease induced by heterologous antikidney antibodies (now known as *nephrotoxic serum nephritis* or *Masugi nephri-*

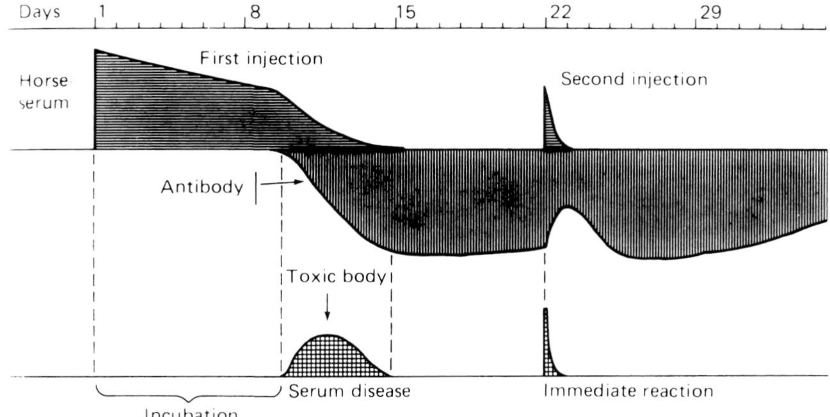

FIG. 2. Events occurring in serum sickness from the original studies of von Pirquet and Schick (circa 1906). Reproduced from Silverstein, ref. 1, with permission.

tis) (25–27). Masugi, a student of Aschoff, as Professor of Pathology at Chiba Medical College in Japan, clearly established that this form of experimental glomerulonephritis was due to interaction of heterologous antibody with antigenic targets in the kidney. In follow-up studies carried out between 1936 and 1939, Smadel, Farr, and co-workers studied the acute and chronic stages of nephrotoxic serum nephritis and the influence of strain, sex, and diet (28–31). Kay in 1940 and 1942 conducted a novel series of experiments that clearly demonstrated that nephrotoxic serum nephritis consisted of two phases: an initial or heterologous phase that was due the effect of the initial injection of heterologous antiserum; and a second or autologous phase that was due to the binding of endogenously synthesized host (autologous) antibody direct to the deposits of heterologous antibody and the glomeruli. This crucial experiment illustrated that a host-derived response to an altered or "planted" antigen could induce disease (32,33).

THE MODERN ERA OF RENAL IMMUNOPATHOLOGY

Thus, with the onset of World War II, the science of renal immunopathology had progressed only modestly since the seminal discoveries of Richet, Arthus, Donath, Landsteiner, Von Pirquet and Schick, and the original studies of Lindemann and Masugi. However, the pace of discovery was soon to quicken, in part because of renewed interest in serum sickness. Arnold Rich and his co-workers initiated this with a series of studies carried out between 1943 and 1946 on classic "one-shot" acute serum sickness (34,36). They characterized the renal lesions that resulted from a single large injection of heterologous serum protein. The response to purified serum proteins was subsequently studied by Hawn and Janeway in 1947 (37) and by Germuth in 1953 (22).

The atomic era that developed after 1945 also made available radioisotopes for tagging these purified serum proteins and stimulated research on the quantitative aspects of serum sickness. The experiments of Pressman, Talmage, Germuth, Dixon, and co-workers, carried out between 1949 and 1953, placed experimental serum sickness on firm quantitative grounds (22,38–40). The phase where antigen excess was replaced with antibody excess and where circulating immune complexes were formed was defined as the period when renal lesions occurred. Thus, the "toxic bodies" identified by Von Pirquet some 50 years earlier were clearly identified as complexes of antigen and antibody (immune complexes).

The studies of Germuth and co-workers, and of Dixon and colleagues carried out between 1951 and 1957 can justifiably be cited at the beginning of the modern era of renal immunopathology (22–24,40). At nearly the same time, others were investigating the nature of the antigen responsible for nephrotoxic serum nephritis and beginning to exploit the effect of intentional immunization of animals with extracts of homologous or heterologous kidney (Cavelti, Frick, and Heymann) (41–43).

The laboratory group headed by Frank Dixon, both in Pittsburgh and La Jolla, became a Mecca for investigation of the harmful effects of immune responses, with significant emphasis on kidney disease (40). Weigle, Cochrane, Vasquez, Feldman, Hammer, and Unanue were early members of this extremely productive and influential group (44–49). Indeed, Dixon inherited the mantle of his predecessor, Von Pirquet, who had carried out seminal studies that overturned the paradigm of an exclusively protective role for immunity (Figure 3).

The introduction of immunofluorescence techniques by Coons and Kaplan in 1950 (50), electron microscopic techniques for the study of human renal tissue in 1957 (51,52), and improvements in methods for the application of protein isolation and characterization added significantly to the scope and sophistication of experimental

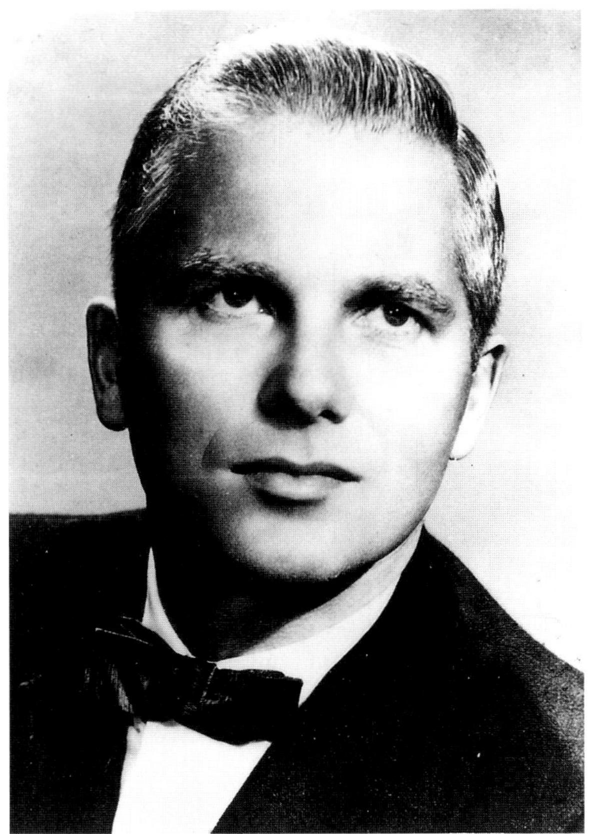

FIG. 3. Frank J. Dixon (circa 1967).

design (53,54). In particular, the technique of immunofluorescence, as applied to renal pathology, afforded an entirely new dimension to the study of kidney disease. The pictures of green (or red) deposits of immunoglobulins brought a brilliant new reality to renal immunology.

The effects of chronic and repeated administration of foreign serum proteins (chronic serum sickness) were elegantly and diligently pursued by Dixon and co-workers (24,40,49,55,57). Simultaneously, the fine pathogenic details of the course of both the heterologous and autologous phases of nephrotoxic serum nephritis were described by Unanue, Hammer, and Dixon and co-workers (47–49). With the emergence of better understanding of the pathogenic events underlying nephrotoxic serum nephritis and acute and chronic serum sickness, attention began to turn to the factors involved in mediating the injury induced by direct binding of antibody or by the deposition of immune complexes from the circulation. Studies of complement, platelets, and polymorphonuclear-leukocytes and vasoactive amines were the focus of initial inquiries. Cellular immunity, at least as mediated by sensitized lymphoid cells, was largely a neglected field during this first phase of the modern era of renal pathology.

By 1966, the field of experimental immunologic renal disease was dominated by three areas of investigation: disease mediated by the administration of heterologous antibodies to renal tissue (nephrotoxic serum nephritis), disease mediated by circulating immune complexes (serum sickness), and disease mediated by the active immunization with extracts of kidney tissue ("autoimmune" or autologous immune complex experimental nephritis). This latter area consisted of two areas of interest, one led by Raymond Steblay, involving immunization of animals with heterologous glomerular-rich antigens in which an autologous (autoimmune) response to glomerular basement membrane (GBM) antigens was involved in the pathogenesis (58); the other involving immunization of animals with homologous or heterologous tubular-rich extracts in which an autologous response to nonglomerular basement membrane antigens appeared to be involved (Heymann nephritis) (43). The literature and the number of laboratories engaged in experimental studies of renal immunopathology had expanded greatly, and in the elegant review published by Unanue and Dixon in 1967, a total of 442 references could be cited (49).

Advances in fundamental immunology, including transplantation biology, immunochemistry, complement, and cellular immunity were also occurring at a rapid rate. Stimulated by these advances and eager to explore the relevance of experimental immunopathology to human disease, numerous studies of human immune mediated renal disease began to be reported. By 1967 the first report of a human prototype of antiglomerular basement membrane antibody disease was reported (59). Human surrogates of the experimental disease induced by active immunization of animals with homologous tubular-rich extracts were also described. Human kidney transplantation afforded a new and unique opportunity to explore immune mediated renal disease through studies of recurrence of glomerulonephritis in kidney isografts and allografts (60,61). Studies of human renal isografts clearly demonstrated that recurrence of glomerulonephritis, probably by immune mechanisms, was a common event when prolonged survival of a kidney graft was likely and the genetic barrier to successful transplantation was absent (61).

Studies of human renal tissue obtained by renal biopsy through the new techniques of immunofluorescence and electron microscopy allow direct comparisons of patterns of experimental disease and their putative animal counterparts (53,54,62–64). Morphology was related to pathogenesis in what now appears to be an overly simplistic manner. Thus, "granular" or "lumpy-bumpy" deposits of immune reactants were equated with circulating immune complex disease through comparison to acute and chronic serum sickness and "linear" deposits of immune reactants were equated with antibodies to glomerular basement membrane through comparison with nephrotoxic serum nephritis. Whereas these analogies were correct in a limited way, future experiments were to prove that morphologic appearance often provided only a clue to underlying pathogenetic heterogeneity. The discovery that a "granular pattern" of immunofluorescence and electron-dense deposits could be formed when a circulating antibody reacted to a discontinuously distributed antigen present in the subepithelial space sealed the fate of the direct linkage of morphologic appearance to specific pathogenic mechanisms (65–68). Nevertheless, the statement by Unanue and Dixon in the initial paragraphs of their 1967 review remains true today (49):

> On theoretical and experimental grounds, it now appears that immunologic renal injury can be produced by two means: first, by antibodies capable of reacting with an antigen fixed in the kidneys as in the case of anti-kidney sera and, second, by circulating antigen–antibody complexes themselves immunologically unrelated to the kidney, which accumulate in glomeruli as in the case of serum sickness.

What was missing in 1967 and has evolved subsequently is the extraordinary diversity of the antigens "fixed in the kidney" and the variety of antigen–antibody systems unrelated to the kidney that can evoke tissue injury (69). In addition, although not well appreciated in 1967, it subsequently became very clear that immune complexes could form in situ and have an appearance very similar to immune complexes deposited from the circulation (65,68).

BROADENING CONCEPTS: CELLS, MEDIATORS, AND MODELS

The role of cell-mediated hypersensitivity in pathogenesis was one of the neglected areas of research in immunologic renal disease, except in the field of renal allotransplantation. Sporadic studies in the earlier 1970s indicated that in vitro tests frequently demonstrated evidence of a lymphocyte response to renal antigens (for example) (70). The relevance of these findings to the pathogenesis of glomerular disease was challenged in a powerfully worded editorial by Frank Dixon published in 1970 (71). He emphasized that such in vitro reactivity is an expected accompaniment of a humoral response, that such in vitro tests could have diagnostic utility, but that the role of sensitized lymphocytes in pathogenesis "remains to be established." Much later, as the fine details of the cellular aspects of humoral immunity were unraveled and better ways of detecting better subsets of lymphocytes in diseased tissues were developed, it became very clear that various immunologically competent cells play direct roles in the mediation of tissue injury. Experiments involving short-term culture of isolated glomeruli were among the first to reemphasize the pathogenetic role of mononuclear cells in glomerular disease, particularly those of the monocyte/macrophage lineage (72). In addition, the development of models of experimentally induced interstitial nephritis, particularly the studies of Neilson and colleagues, greatly advanced the position of cell-mediated immunity as an important aspect of the pathogenesis of renal disease (73).

As mentioned earlier, the emergence of renal transplantation as an experimental form of renal replacement therapy in the early 1960s profoundly stimulated investigation of the mechanisms underlying renal allograft rejection (60). Fundamental studies of chemical suppression of immune responses were extremely important in triggering this focus on transplantation biology. Because of the paucity of evidence for the involvement of humoral processes in renal allograft rejection, except for the hyperacute rejection that occurred when renal allografts were place in previously sensitized individuals, and because of the abundant presence of lymphocytes and "immunoblasts" in the parenchyma of the rejected graft and the demonstrated sensitivity of rejection crises to glucocorticoids, most investigators initially focused on how the antigens contained within the foreign graft evoked a cell-mediated response (74). With the definition of the Mac antigen by Dausset (75) and the 4a and 4b system by Van Rood (76), the field of human histocompatibility was begun. In a series of workshops, beginning at Duke University in 1964 (72), the immunogenetics of the human histocompatibility locus, subsequently designated *human leukocyte antigen* or *HLA system*, was progressively defined. The development of assays using lymphocytotoxicity and polyclonal antibodies by Terasaki and McClelland (78) permitted reproducible testing of the antigenic specificities of the human HLA system on a large scale. Within a short period of time, the gene loci responsible for determining the HLA specificities were identified. Whereas many hoped that "tissue typing" would ultimately prevent breach of the allograft barrier, it quickly became apparent that the extraordinary complexity and diversity of the HLA system would make this an unlikely possibility. Nevertheless, progress in the understanding of the genetic basis of tissue compatibility and the cellular mechanisms underlying graft rejections came quickly and dramatically. A side benefit of the enormous efforts directed to understanding the human major histocompatibility complex (MHC) was the determination that genes at these loci were related to susceptibility for a variety of human renal diseases (79,80).

The period between 1965 and 1975 was also characterized by an explosion of interest in the mediator systems involved in models of disease. The initial focus was on complement and polymorphonuclear leukocytes (81,82) but interest quickly spread to other factors, including coagulation, monocytes, platelets, peptides, and lipids (83,84). The availability of reproducible models of glomerular injury and new techniques for examining physiologic perturbations (e.g., micropuncture) reawakened interest in the pathophysiologic aspects of experimental renal disease, a field that had been briefly explored by Smadel and Farr in 1939 and then neglected. These studies yielded significant insights into the physiologic mechanisms of some of the manifestations of experimental glomerular injury, specifically, proteinuria, altered glomerular filtration rate, and abnormalities of sodium chloride homeostasis (85,86). The joining of experimental renal immunopathology and physiology proved extraordinarily fruitful, and the application of the newly acquired knowledge to human disease has provided a rationale for newer approaches to therapy.

In addition to studies that greatly expanded knowledge regarding the role of cells (lymphocytes, platelets, monocytes, and neutrophils) and soluble mediator systems (coagulation proteins, complement, vasoactive peptide, amines, lipids, cytokines, and growth factors) (87,88) in renal injury, a plethora of new models of renal injury were described. These included ones that were experimentally induced and those that developed spontaneously in inbred or outbred strains. Renal lesions were produced experimentally by chemical compounds, lectins, charged proteins, bacteria and viruses, aggregated plasma proteins, renal extracts, and heterologous antibodies to non-basement-membrane antigens (87). Few of these experimental models had any known direct counterpart to human disease, but each proved extremely useful in demonstrating the variety of ways by which renal injury could be initiated and propagated. Even more importantly, these new models provided powerful new tools to explore how mediator systems, such as complement and polymorphonuclear leukocytes, interacted to produce injury. The seminal observations of Couser, Salant, and co-workers (88) clarified this field considerably.

Spontaneous occurrence of immune-mediated renal disease in animals afforded many opportunities to study disease perhaps more akin to the human disease. The discovery of the development of a lupuslike disease, including glomerulonephritis, in strains of New Zealand mice by Helyer and Howie in 1963 (89) represented a major event. Studies continue today on this interesting model that has shed much light on the fundamental mechanisms of autoimmunity.

One experimentally induced model, in particular, has an interesting history and has had a profound impact on how we think about the immunopathogenesis of renal disease. As mentioned earlier, studies carried by Cavelti, Frick, and Heymann reported on the induction of renal lesions in rats by repeated immunization of homologous or heterologous renal extracts (enriched for tubular antigens) (41–43). Only the model described by Heymann and co-workers was reproducible enough for further investigation. The lesions produced were of the membranous glomerulonephritis type, with heavy granular deposits of immunoglobulin G and subepithelial electron-dense deposits accompanied by severe nephrotic syndrome. Thus, the model resembled spontaneous glomerulonephritis in humans. The antigen responsible for the induction of disease appeared to be derived from brush border of the proximal tubule (90). Early attempts to transfer disease with lymphoid cells suggested an autoimmune etiology, but these could not be regularly reproduced. With the identification of an endogenous renal tubular epithelial cell antigen in glomerular deposits by Edgington and co-workers (90,91), it appeared that circulating immune complexes composed of autoantibodies and a renal tubular epithelial cell antigen were depositing in the kidneys [autologous immune complex nephritis (AICN)] (91). However, the experiments of Van Damme, Hoedemaker, Vernier, Couser, and Wilson (67–69) changed the paradigm by directly demonstrating that an antigen immunologically very closely related, if not identical, to the proximal renal tubular antigen could also be found on the surface of glomerular visceral epithelial cells. Thus, the autoantibodies evoked by immunization with renal extracts (Fraction IA) could bind with glomerular antigens *in situ* and cause the formation of subepithelial electron-dense and granular immunoglobulin deposits due to the discontinuous nature of the distribution of the glomerular antigen (92). Subsequently, the responsible antigen has been isolated and very well characterized by Kerjaschki and Farquahar (93) and the mechanism of formation of immune deposits demonstrated in detail. Unfortunately, the model still has not been found to recapitulate the events in human disease, except in rare circumstances. However, its relevance to understanding membrane nephropathy in man is reviewed by Couser and Alpers in Chapter 47. Nevertheless, studies of this model have proven very powerful in exploring the pathophysiology of proteinuria, edema, nephrotic syndrome, and in examining the formation of immune complexes in situ and the role of complement in proteinuria.

The field of cellular immunity in human renal disease was largely left to transplantation biology, where clear evidence had accumulated that the pathologic manifestations of acute rejection were mediated by sensitized infiltrating lymphoid cells.

EXPLORATION OF HUMAN RENAL DISEASE

Although immune mechanisms had been suspected in the pathogenesis of human renal disease since the studies of Masugi in the 1930s, the immune basis of renal disease was nothing more than a vague hypothesis until renal tissue obtained by the newly described technique of percutaneous renal biopsy in the prone position (94) began to be studied by immunofluorescence and electron microscopic techniques (53,62–64). These studies provided much more direct evidence of an immune basis for renal disease because of the deposits of immunoglobulins in renal tissue. Indeed, only a few years later, progress in defining a possible immune basis of human renal disease was well enough developed for an extensive review by Peters and Freedman, published in three issues of the New England Journal of Medicine in 1959 (95). Between

1960 and 1965, numerous reports of the immunopathology of human renal disease appeared (69). At first, reagents were crude and the specificity of the finding suspect. The lack of availability of reliable commercial reagents and the need to freeze and ship specimens to central locations for immunopathologic study hampered collaborative research. Nevertheless, by 1967, studies by immunofluorescence utilizing renal biopsy-obtained tissue began to define new entities. More noteworthy among these new entities was the description of mesangial IgA/IgG deposits by Berger and Hinglais in 1968 (96). Lerner, Glassock, and Dixon in 1967 described for the first time the passive transfer of a human antiglomerular basement membrane antibody-mediated disease to an experimental animal and defined the recurrence of this disease in a human renal allograft (59). Thus, human antiglomerular basement membrane antibody-mediated disease represented the first, and thus far only, disease in which all of Koch's postulates for defining the etiopathogenesis of a disease have been fulfilled. Subsequent application of electron microscopy, immunofluorescence, and immunochemical analytical techniques was to define a number of new clinical pathologic entities, such as C1q nephropathy (97), dense deposit disease (98), IgM nephropathy (99), fibrillary and immunotactoid glomerulonephritis (100), and thin basement membrane nephropathy (101). As mentioned earlier, the field of transplantation was to contribute further information through studies of the recurrent disease (61).

THE FIELD MATURES

In the first quarter century of its modern existence (1950–1975), the field of renal immunopathology had evolved from a few experimentally induced models (nephrotoxic serum nephritis and serum sickness) and narrowly focused rudimentary concepts of pathogenesis (antiglomerular basement membrane antibody-induced disease and circulating immune complex-associated injury) to a wide variety of experimental models of both induced and spontaneous categories and a broad array of potential pathways for injury. The separation of basic pathogenic events and mediator systems was blurred as new scenarios emerged (102–106).

Thus, revised immunopathogenetic classification schema required incorporation of information concerning the source of the antibody or cellular vector of disease (heterologous, autologous; endogenous or exogenous); the nature of the antigen (soluble, insoluble, circulating, native, tissue-bound, replicating, nonreplicating, charged, noncharged); tissue localization of the immune reaction (basement membrane, mesangial cell, tubular cell, visceral epithelial cell); and mediator system involvement (leukocyte-dependent, complement-dependent, lymphocyte cell-mediated response). Great progress had been made in identifying the biochemical nature of the antigens and antibodies involved in the pathogenesis of experimental renal disease. Reagents for the identification of specific effector cells and/or antibodies became increasingly refined. Techniques for the direct measurement of the circulating "toxic bodies" of Von Pirquet became readily available (105). In vitro tests of cell-mediated hypersensitivity were widely applied to studies of human renal disease. Cell culture techniques generated new insights into the cellular participants in disease (see Chapters 29–31). The roles of coagulation (83–84) (Chapter 23), complement (108) (Chapter 18), leukocytes (81) (Chapters 26,28), and platelets (109) (Chapter 27) in renal disease were extensively studied. New mediator systems including prostaglandins, thromboxanes, leukotrienes and lipoxins (Chapter 22), and toxic oxygen radicals (Chapter 19) were identified and extensively explored (110). New immunologic markers of previously poorly understood disease were discovered; most noteworthy was the recognition of a role for anti-neutrophil cytoplasmic antibodies in human vasculitis (111) (see Chapter 49).

Thus, by 1975, the comprehensive review of the field by Wilson and Dixon contained over 1,000 references (69). Renal immunopathology was now firmly established as a research discipline in many laboratories throughout the world. A new generation of investigators, attracted by the excitement and potential for discovery, were trained by scientists who had joined the field early in its development. The trainees of Dixon, Feldman, Cochrane, Andres, McCluskey, Peters, Cameron, Berger, Hamburger, Heptinstall, Pirani, Kark, Kincaid-Smith, and other pioneers began to spread the gospel of renal immunopathology. The parent disciplines of immunology and pathology were also progressing rapidly with the description of immunoglobulin structure, chemical isolation and characterization of mediators, and definitions of the role of T and B cells in the immune response. The field of renal physiology that had dominated the discipline of nephrology for over 40 years began to give way to the new and emerging field of renal immunology.

Yet, despite the enormous expansion of knowledge in basic sciences, progress in unraveling the complexities of human disease proceeded slowly. Although new "entities" had been described, precious little was known about etiology, and many disorders simply had no plausible theory to explain their pathogenesis. Nevertheless, pathways potentially responsible for superimposed lesions of glomerular disease (e.g., crescents and sclerosis) were being defined with greater precision.

THE DAWN OF THE MOLECULAR AND CELL BIOLOGY ERA

The cloning of DNA in the development of recombinant DNA technology and the emergence of basic knowledge regarding cell–cell and intracellular communication brought about a slow revolution in renal immunopathology. The description of the role of cytokines and growth factors in disease (see Chapter 20), the delineation of cell-adhesion molecule interactions in renal inflammation (see Chapter 25), and the unraveling of the complex interactions between lipid, peptide, and amine mediators began to demonstrate possible new approaches to therapy (110). Analysis of the genetic factors involved in the immune responsiveness began to clear the path for a new understanding of susceptibility to disease based on molecular events (see Chapter 5).

The evolution of our understanding of antibasement membrane antibody disease is a paradigm of progress in this molecular and cell biology era and is reviewed by Neilson and colleagues in Chapter 43. Thirty years ago, our understanding of anti–glomerular-based membrane antibody disease was elementary. Immunoglobulin autoantibodies to an undefined antigen arose in the circulation by poorly delineated mechanisms (59,112). Binding of autoantibody to the basement membrane induced injury and led to the production of glomerular crescents in renal failure—again, by unknown mechanisms. Today, we know that the antigen is a small peptide epitope on a larger globular domain of the α_3 chain of type IV collagen (113,114). The genetic locus determining this antigen has been mapped to chromosome 2 and cloned (113,114). The genetic susceptibility to disease has been localized to the HLA DRB1*15 alleles of the class II region of the MHC (115). Presumably, the endogenous basement membrane peptide or some exogenous peptide possessing a very similar motif binds to the groove in the MHC peptide receptor and, with involvement of accessory signals and in collaboration with a T-cell receptor on a T-helper cell, leads to the production of autoantibodies in large amounts from B-cells programmed to produce such IgG upon stimulation by T-helper cells. Early removal of this autoantibody with plasma exchange greatly ameliorates disease (116). The autoantibodies bind to the native basement membrane antigen, uniformly distributed along all capillary walls, leading to the local activation of cell adhesion molecules and immobilization and emigration of leukocytes (polymorphonuclear leukocytes and monocytes). Local release of enzymes and generation of toxic oxygen radicals cause degradation of basement membrane and "gaps" in the integrity of the capillary wall (117). Emigration of circulating monocytes, entrapment of extravasated leukocytes, and activation of resident monocytes leads to the elaboration of cytokines and causes the synthesis of cell-associated prothrombotic factors, which leads directly to polymerization of fibrinogen that had escaped into Bowman's space as a result of the large gaps in the capillary wall (118). Cellular infiltrates and cytokine release begets local proliferation and "crescent" formation (see Chapter 32). Promotion of fibrosis is generated via transforming growth factor β1 release and invasion of Bowman's space by periglomerular myofibroblasts (119).

Thus, except for the initial events that cause the production of auto-antibasement membrane antibodies, 30 years of progress has led to a fairly comprehensive understanding of at least one of the "models" of immune-mediated glomerular injury. From the historical perspective, progress in the understanding of "fibrosis" has also been equally spectacular. We now have a beginning understanding of how the glomeruli scar in response to diverse immune injury. Specifically, we are now beginning to understand how cell-derived molecules, such as platelet-derived growth factor, basic fibroblast growth factor, and transforming growth factor β1, act to cause scarring as one pathway in the resolution of glomerular and tubular interstitial injury (120,120) (see Chapter 34).

From the broadest perspective, the field of renal immunopathology is returning to its roots in fundamental immunobiology and cellular pathology. It has adopted the tools of the fundamental molecular and cellular investigator and applied them to models of immune injury, much as Dixon and his colleagues did 40 years earlier in applying the newly developed techniques and tools of radioisotope tagging and immunofluorescence to models of renal disease that had been developed much earlier by Lindemann, Von Pirquet, and Masugi. The cycle of discovery by applying technical developments to existing laboratory-based models of disease has been largely responsible for the ever-progressive maturation of the field of immunopathology (see Chapters 35,36).

A BRIGHT FUTURE

The decade of the 1960s represented a turning point in the history of the study of immune-mediated renal disease, and it appears likely with the turn of this century that the long-promised benefits of study of experimental immune renal disease to the understanding and therapy of human immune renal disease will finally occur.

First, identification of the amino acid sequences in the peptide groove of the MHC molecules responsible for associating peptide antigen motifs with T-cell receptors will likely lead to a more precise definition of the molecular basis susceptibility and offer new approaches to limiting the activation of the autoimmune and alloimmune response, perhaps involving simple, relatively nontoxic, orally administered chemicals.

Second, recognition and delineation of the early signals and effectors involved in immune-mediated inflammation, including allograft rejection, will lead to more specific modulators that can limit damaging inflammation while leaving protective responses undisturbed.

Third, understanding of the pathways for healing and resolution of immune-mediated renal diseases, with and without fibrosis, will lead to more refined approaches to progressive disease.

Fourth, discovery of new potential pathogenetic pathways will be quickly evaluated in vitro and in vivo by exploitation of induced alterations in gene transcription or by site-directed mutations. New experimental models derived from such genomic transformations will provide powerful research tools.

Fifth, application of new techniques in renal biopsy (such as quantitative polymerase chain reaction and in situ hybridization) will uncover nuances of renal immunopathology not readily appreciated by application of the now standard techniques of immunofluorescence, electron microscopy, and light microscopy.

As a result of these developments, diseases currently believed to be homogenous with respect to pathogenesis will likely be further subdivided and reclassified. Newer, noninvasive methods to diagnose and evaluate human immune renal disease will likely be developed and applied. Renal biopsy may be transformed from a "diagnostic" procedure to a method of assessing prognosis. As our understanding of the mechanisms of progression becomes more complete, a renewed focus on early detection of disease will almost certainly evolve.

CONCLUDING REMARKS: HISTORICAL PERSPECTIVE

What lessons or insights can one glean from this brief history of some of the major events that have contributed to the evolution of renal immunology as a vital discipline? One common thread present throughout this development has been the application of new techniques to the study of models of disease. The use of immunofluorescence and radioisotope tagging in the study of nephrotoxic serum nephritis and acute and chronic sickness are early examples; tissue culture of explanted glomeruli and transgenic methodology are more modern versions. However, one should be careful to remember that models of disease in experimental animals can illustrate only the possibility that similar processes are operative in humans. Too often in the history of renal immunology, the translation of results from experimental disease to man has been too direct. In the final analysis, the proper study of human disease is in humans. Unfortunately, in the past it has been difficult to carry out critical studies of pathogenesis and mediation in human subjects. Nevertheless, from time to time, studies of rare "experiments of nature" have provided new insights. Perhaps the new techniques of molecular biology will afford a new opportunity to explore the mysteries of human disease in a more direct manner. Despite these caveats, it is very clear that renal immunology has developed to a point where major pathogenetic mechanisms have been delineated, and a broad array of overlapping and sometimes redundant mediator pathways have been described. Investigators of immunologically mediated renal disease are increasingly focusing on basic mechanisms of tissue injury and repair, common to many organ systems.

Increasingly, pathways of damage that have roots in very fundamental protective mechanisms are being found. This phenomenon represents completion of a cycle begun when Charles Richet overturned the paradigm that all immunologic processes were protective in nature. Indeed, all of renal immunology rests on the notion that processes that evolved to protect the organism from harm can be turned toward the organism in a harmful way.

Along the way, we have learned a great deal about antibody and cells, complement and coagulation, cytokines and growth factors, peptides, lipids, amines, and toxic oxygen radicals, and each of these is reviewed separately in individual chapters of this book. One cannot help but be impressed with the wondrous array of processes that nature has at her disposal to deal with disease and how perturbations in one system can lead to such marked effects in another system.

Many have contributed to this enlightenment, but this brief review of the history of renal immunology cannot do justice to all those who have made it such an inspirational, vital, and dynamic field. The personalities who have shaped the enterprise are rich and varied, and only a few have been specifically mentioned. This should not be taken as a sign that they are of lesser importance to the evolving story of renal immunology. However, one of them, Frank Dixon, was a charismatic force who led a field into a new era of biology with his forceful intellect and his incisive approach to experimental pathology. His contemporaries and colleagues, including Andres, Cochrane, Feldman, Germuth, Good, McCluskey, and Unanue ignited interest in an area of science that was to blossom well beyond their original concepts. This book is a testimony to the maturation of a field of inquiry whose modern era began less than 50 years ago.

My own path through this era has been immensely gratifying. It has brought me in close contact with innumerable clinicians and scientists throughout the world, including four Nobel laureates. Having been present in the early days of the founding of both modern renal immunology and organ transplantation was a stroke of good fortune. This history of renal immunology is as much a personal recollection of events as it is a recitation of facts. Hopefully, it illustrates the intellectual roots for many of the elegant presentations that follow. Of course, as we all know, the most exciting chapters have not yet been written.

Acknowledgment

This contribution is dedicated to my mentor, Frank J. Dixon, M.D., Emeritus Director, Scripps Research Institute. Dr. Dixon is regarded by many as the father of modern renal immunopathology. I am deeply indebted to him for introducing me to the field in 1965 and for giving me the opportunity to share in the excitement of discovery.

REFERENCES

1. Silverstein AM. *A History of Immunology*. New York: Academic Press, 1989;2.

2. Thucydides. *The Peloponnesian War*. Translated by Crawley. New York: Modern Library, 1934;112.
3. Silverstein AM. *A History of Immunology* New York: Academic Press, 1989;28–30.
4. Sloane H. An account of inoculation. *Philos Trans R Soc (Lond)* 1756;49:56.
5. Jenner E. *An inquiry into the causes and effects of the vareolae vaccine*. London: Sampson Low, 1798.
6. Metchinkoff E. Üeber eine sprosspilz krankheit der Daphnein: Bertiag zur lehre Üeber den kampf der phagocyten gegen krankheitserregen. *Virchows Arch* 1884;96:177.
7. Metchnikoff O. *The Life of Eli Metchnikoff*. Boston: Houghton, Mifflin,1921.
8. Pasteur L. Sur les malades virulentes, et en particulier sur la maladies vulgairement cholera des poules. *CR Hebd Seances Acad Sci* 1880; 90:239.
9. Vallery-Radot R. *The Life of Pasteur*. New York: Dover, 1960.
10. Von Behring E, Kitasato S. Üeber das zustandekommen der diphtheria-immunitat and der tetanus-immunitat bei theiren. *Dtsch Med Wochenschr* 1890;16:113.
11. Bordet, J. Sur l'agglutination et la dissolution des globules rouges par le serum d'animaux injects de sange defibrinat. *Ann Inst Pasteur Paris* 1899;12:688.
12. Ehrlich P. Die wertbe messung des diphtherie-heilserums und deren theoretische grundlagen. *Klin Jahrb* 1899:6:299.
13. Ehrlich P, Morgenroth J. Üeber hämolysis, funfte mitt heilung. *Berl Klin Wochenschr* 1901;28:251.
14. Portier P, Richet C. De l'action anaphylactique de certains venins. *CR Seances Soc Biol Sis Fil* 1902;54:170.
15. Arthus M. Lesions cutanees produites par les injections de serum de cheval chez le lapin anaphylactise par et pour ce-serum. *CR Seances Soc Biol Sis Fil* 1903;55:817.
16. Donath J, Landsteiner K. Üeber paroxysmal hamoglobinurie. *Muench Med Wochenschr* 1904;521:1590.
17. Von Pirquet C, Schick B. *Die Serum Krankheit*. Vienna: Deuticke, 1906.
18. Von Pirquet C. Allergy. *Munchen Med. Wochenschr* 53:1457, 1906 and *Arch Intern Med* 1911;7:259–288. (Translation)
19. Silverstein AM. *A History of Immunology*. New York: Academic Press, 1989;214–251.
20. Lindemann W. Sur la mode dÆaction de certain poisons renaux. *Ann Inst Pasteur* 1900;14:49–59.
21. Wilson G, Oliver J. Experiments on production of specific antisera for infections of unknown cause. III Nephrotoxins: their specificity as demonstrated by the method of selective absorption. *J Exp Med* 1920; 32:183.
22. Germuth F. Comparative histologic and immunologic study in rabbits of induced hypersensitivity of serum sickness type. *J Exp Med* 1953; 97:257.
23. Weigle W, Dixon F. Relationship of circulating antigen-antibody complexes, antigen elimination and complement fixation in serum sickness. *Proc Soc Exp Biol Med* 1958;99:226.
24. Dixon FJ. *Harvey Lecture* 1963:58:21.
25. Masugi M, Tomizuka Y. Uiber die spezifischen zytotoxishen veranderungen der niere und der leber durch das spezifische antiserum. Zieglieech ein beitrag zur pathogenese dei glomerulonephritis. *Tr Jpn Path Soc* 1931;21:329–341.
26. Masugi M, Sato Y, Murasawa S, Tomizuka Y. Uber die experimentelle glomerulonephritis durch das spezifische anti-nierenserum. *Tr Jpn Path Soc* 1932;22:614–628.
27. Okabayashi A, Kondo Y. *Masugi Nephritis and Its Immunopathologic Implication*. Tokyo: Igaku-Shoin, 1980.
28. Smadel J. Experimental nephritis in rats induced by injection of anti-kidney serum: preparation and immunological studies of nephrotoxin. *J Exp Med* 1936;64:921.
29. Smadel, J. Experimental nephritis in rats produced by injection of anti-kidney serum III. Pathological studies of the acute and chronic disease. *J Exp Med* 1937;65:541–555.
30. Smadel J, Farr L. Experimental nephritis in rats inuduced by injection of anti-kidney serum: clinical and functional studies. *J Exp Med* 1937;65:527.
31. Smadel J, Farr L. Effect of dietary protein on course of nephrotoxic serum nephritis. *Am J Pathol* 1939;15–199.
32. Kay C. Mechanism by which experimental nephritis is produced in rabbits injected with nephrotoxic duck serum. *J Exp Med* 1940;72:559.
33. Kay C. Mechanism of forms of glomerulonephritis nephrotoxic nephritis in rabbits. *Am J Med Sci* 1942;204:483.
34. Rich A, Gregory J. Expeimental demonstration that periarteritis nodosa is manifestation of hypersensitivity. *Bull Johns Hopkins Hosp* 1943;72:65.
35. Rich A, Gregory J. Experimental evidence that lesions with basic characteristics of rheumatic carditis can result from anaphylactic hypersensitivity. *Bull Johns Hopkins Hosp* 1943;73:239.
36. Gregory J, Rich A. Role of hypersensitivity in periarteritis nodosa as indicated by 7 cases developing during serum sickness and sulfonamide therapy. *Bull Johns Hopkins Hosp* 1943;73:239.
37. Hawn CVZ, Janeway L. Histological and serological sequences in experimental hypersensitivity. *J Exp Med* 1947;86:571.
38. Pressman D. The zone of localization of antibodies III. The specific localization of antibodies to rat kidney. *Cancer* 1949;2:697–700.
39. Talmage D, Dixon F, Bukantz S, Dammin G. Antigen elimination from blood as early manifestation of immune response. *J Immunol* 1951;67:243.
40. Dixon F, Wilson C. The development of immunopathologic investigations of kidney disease. *Am J Kidney Dis* 1990;6:574–578.
41. Cavelti PA, Cavelti ES. Studies on pathogenesis of glomerulonephritis; production of glomerulonephritis in rats by means of autoantibodies in kidney. *Arch Pathol* 1945;39:148.
42. Frick V. Nephritis durch nieren auto-anti kroner. *Z Immunitats/Osschung* 1950;107:411–417.
43. Heymann W, Hackel D, Harwood J, et al. Production of the nephrotic syndrome in rats by Freunds adjuvant and rat kidney suspension. *Proc Soc Exp Biol Med* 1959;100:660–664.
44. Dixon FJ. Use of I131 in immunologic investigation. *J Allergy* 1953; 24:548.
45. Cochrane CG, Weigle W, Dixon F. The role of polymorphonuclear leukocytes in the initiation and cessation of the arthus vasculitis. *J Exp Med* 1959;110:481.
46. Dixon F, Feldman J, Vasquez J. Experimental glomerulonephritis. The pathogenesis of a laboratory model resembling the spectrum of human glomerulonephritis. *J Exp Med* 1961;113:899.
47. Hammer D, Dixon F. Experimental glomerulonephritis. II. Immunologic events in the pathogenesis of nephrotoxic serum nephritis in the rat. *J Exp Med* 1963;117:1019.
48. Unanue E, Dixon F. Experimental glomerulonephritis. IV. Participation of complement in nephrotoxic nephritis. *J Exp Med* 1964;119:865.
49. Unanue E, Dixon FJ. Experimental glomerulonephritis: immunological events and pathogenetic mechanism. *Adv Immunol* "67;6:1–89.
50. Coons A, Kaplan M. Localization of antigen in tissue cells II. Improvements in method for the detection of antigen by means of fluorescent antibody. *J Exp Med* 1950;91:1–13.
51. Farquhar M, Verner R, Good R. Studies on familial nephrosis II. Glomerular changes observed by the electron microscope. *Am J Pathol* 1957;33:791–817.
52. Folli G, Pollack V, Reed R, Pirani C, Kark R. Electromicroscopic studies of reversible renal lesions in the adult nephrotic syndrome. *Ann Intern Med* 1958;49:775–795.
53. Mellors RC. Histochemical demonstration of the in-vivo localization of antibodies, antigenic components of the kidney and the pathogenesis of glomerulonephritis. *J Histochem Cytochem* 1955;3:284.
54. Lange K, Treser G, Segal I, Ty A, Wasserman E. Routine immunohistology in renal diseases. *Ann Intern Med* 1966;64:25.
55. Unanue E, Dixon F. *J Exp Med* 1965;121:715.
56. Unanue E, Dixon F. Experimental glomerulonephritis. VI. The autologous phase of nephrotoxic serum nephritis. *J Exp Med* 1965;121:695.
57. Unanue E, Dixon F. Experimental allergic glomerulonephritis induced in the rabbit with heterologous renal antigens. *J Exp Med* 1967;125:149.
58. Steblay, R. Glomerulonephritis induced in sheep by injections of heterologous glomerular basement membrane and Freund's complete adjuvant. *J Exp Med* 1962;116:253–272.
59. Lerner R, Glassock R, Dixon F. The role of anti-glomerular basement membrane antibody in the pathogenesis of human glomerulonephritis. *J Exp Med* 1967;126:989–1001.
60. Terasaki P, ed. *History of Transplantation. Thirty-Five Recollections*. Los Angeles: UCLA Tissue Typing Laboratory, 1991.
61. Glassock R, Feldman D, Reynolds E, Dammin G, Merrill J. Human renal isografts. A clinical and pathologic analysis. *Medicine (Baltimore)* 1968;47:411.
62. Freedman R, Markowitz P. Immunological studies in nephritis. *Lancet* 1959;2:45–46.

63. Koffler D, Paronetto F. Immunofluorescent localization of immunoglobulin, complement and fibrinogen in human diseases. II. Acute, subacute and chronic glomerulonephritis. *J Clin Invest* 1965;44 1665.
64. Michael AF, Drummond K, Good R, Vernier R. Acute post-streptococcal glomerulonephritis: immune deposit disease. *J Clin Invest* 1966;45:237.
65. Sugisaki T, Klassen J, Andres G, Milgrom F, McCluskey R. Passive transfer of Heymann nephritis with serum. *Kidney Int* 1973:3:66.
66. Barabas AZ, Lannigan R. Induction of an autologous immune complex glomerulonephritis in the rat by the intravenous injection of heterologous anti-rat kidney tubular antibody. I. Production of a chrome progressive immune complex glomerulonephritis. *Pr J Exp Pathol* 1974;55:47.
67. VanDamme BJC, Fleuren GT, Bakker WW, Vernier R, Hoedemaker PhJ. Experimental glomerulonephritis in the rat induced by antibodies directed against tubular antigens. V. Fixed glomerular antigens in the pathogenesis of heterologous immune complex glomerulonephritis. *Lab Invest* 1978;38:502.
68. Couser W, Steimuller D, Stillmant M, Salant D, Lowenstein L. Experimental glomerulonephritis in the isolated perfused rat kidney. *J Clin Invest* 1978;62:1275.
69. Wilson C, Dixon FJ. The renal response to immunological injury. In: B Brenner, F Rector, eds. *The Kidney*. Philadelphia: WB Saunders, 1976;838–940.
70. Rocklin R, Lewis E, David J. In vitro evidence for cellular hypersensitivity to glomerular basement membrane antigens in human glomerulonephritis. *N Engl J Med* 1970;283:497–501.
71. Dixon FJ. What are sensitized cells doing in glomerulonephritis? *N Engl J Med* 1970;283:536–537.
72. Holdsworth S, Thomson N, Glasgow E, Dowling J, Atkins R. Tissue culture of isolated glomeruli in experimental crescent glomerulonephritis. *J Exp Med* 1978;147:98.
73. Neilson E, Phillips S. Cell-mediated immunity in interstitial nephritis. I. T-lymphocyte systems in nephritic guinea pigs: the natural history and diversity of the immune response. *J Immunol* 1979;123:2373–2380.
74. Moore FD. *Give and Take. The Development of Tissue Transplantation*. Philadelphia: WB Saunders, 1964.
75. Dausset J. Leuko-agglutinins. IV. Leucoagglutinins and blood transfusion. *Vox Sang* 1954;4:190.
76. Van Rood JJ, van Leevwen A. Leukocyte grouping. A method and its application. *J Clin Invest* 1963;42:1382.
77. Amos DB. *1st Histocompatibility Testing Workshop*, Duke University, 1964.
78. Terasaki P, McClelland JD. Microdroplet assay of human serum cytotoxins. *Nature* 1964:204:988.
79. Rees A, Peters D, Compston D, Batchelor J. Strong association with HLA DRw-2 and antibody mediated goodpasture's syndrome. *Lancet* 1978;1:966.
80. Klouda PJ, Manor J, Acheson E, Dyer P, Golby F, Harris R, Lawler W, Mallick N, Williams, G. Strong association between idiopathic membranous nephropathy and HLA-DRw-3. *Lancet* 1979;2:770.
81. Cochrane CG, Unanue ER, Dixon FJ. A role of polymorphonuclear leukocytes and complement in Nephrotoxic nephritis. *J Exp Med* 1965;122:99.
82. Cochrane CG. Immunologic tissue injury by neutrophilic leukocytes. *Adv Immunol* 1968;9:97.
83. Vassali P, McCluskey R. The pathogenetic role of the coagulation process in glomerular disease of immunological origin. *Adv Nephrol* 1971;1:47.
84. Kincaid-Smith P. Participation of Intravascular coagulation in the pathogenesis of glomerular and vascular lesion. *Kidney Int* 1975;2:85.
85. Maddox D, Bennett I, Deen W, Glassock R, Brenner B. Control of proximal fluid reabsorption in experimental glomerulonephritis. *J Clin Invest* 1975:55:1315.
86. Chang R, Deen W, Robertson L, Bennett C, Glassock R, Brenner B. Permselectivity of the glomerular capillary wall. Studies of experimental glomerulonephritis in the rat using neutral dextran. *J Clin Invest* 1976;57:1272.
87. Wilson CB, Dixon FJ. The renal response to immunological injury. In: B Brenner, F Rector, eds. *The Kidney*, 1st ed. Philadelphia: WB Saunders, 1976;838–940.
88. Couser WG. Mediation of glomerular injury. *J Clin Invest* 1993;71: 808–811.
89. Helyer B, Howie, JB. Renal disease associated with positive lupus erythematosus tests in an inbred strain of mice. *Nature* 1963;197:197.
90. Edgington T, Glassock R, Dixon F. Autologous immune complex nephritis induced with renal tubular antigen. I: Identification and isolation of the pathogenic antigen. *J Exp Med* 1968;127:555.
91. Glassock T, Edgington T, Dixon F. Autologous immune complex nephritis induced with renal tubular antigen. II. The pathogenetic mechanism. *J Exp Med* 1968;127:573.
92. Couser W, Salant D. In-situ immune complex formation and glomerular injury. *Kidney Int* 1980;17:1.
93. Kerjaschki D. Molecular pathogenesis of membranous nephropathy. *Kidney Int* 1992;41:1090–1105.
94. Kark RM, Muehrcke R. Biopsy of the kidney in the prone position. *Lancet* 1954;1:1047–1049.
95. Peters JH, Freedman P. Immunological aspects of renal disease. *N Engl J Med* 1959;261:1166–1175;1225–1235;1275–1281.
96. Berger J, Hinglais N. Les depots intercapillaries d'IgA-IgG, *J Urol Nephrol (Paris)* 1968;74:694.
97. Jennette J, Falk RJ, C1q Nephropathy. In: S Massry, R Glassock, eds. *Textbook of Nephrology*, 3rd ed. Baltimore: Williams and Wilkins, 1995;749–752.
98. Berger J, Galle P. Depots' deuses au sein des membranes basales due rein. Etude en microscope optique et electronque. *Press Med* 1965; 49:2351.
99. Cohen AH, Border W, Glassock R. Nephrotic syndrome with mesangial IgM deposits. *Lab Invest* 1978;39:21–27.
100. Korbet S, Schwartz M, Lewis E. Immunotactoid glomerulopathy. *Am J Kidney Dis* 1991;17:247–257.
101. Dische F, Weston M, Parsons N. Abnormally thin basement membranes associated with hematuria, proteinuria or renal failure in adults. *Am J Nephrol* 1985;5:103.
102. Germuth FG, Rodriquez E. *Immunopathology of the Renal Glomerulus*. Boston: Little, Brown, 1973.
103. McCluskey R, Klassen T. Immunologically-mediated glomerular, tubular and interstitial renal disease. *N Engl J Med* 1973;288:564.
104. Andres F, Brentjens J, Caldwell PRB. Formation of immune deposits and disease. *Lab Invest* 1986;55:510–520.
105. Wilson LB, Dixon F. Immunopathology and glomerulonephritis. *Annu Rev Med* 1974;25:83.
106. Hoedemaeker, PhJ, Aton J, Hogendom PC. Pathogenesis of glomerulonephritis: experimental models revisited. *Adv Nephrol* 1991;20:73–90.
107. Border W. Immune complex detection in glomerular diseases. *Nephron* 1979;24:106.
108. Thomson NM, Naish P, Simpson I, Peters D. The Role of C3 in the autologous phase of nephrotoxic nephritis. *Clin Exp Immunol* 1976;24:464.
109. Cameron JS. Platelets and glomerulonephritis. *Nephron*. 1977;18:233.
110. Wilson CB. Renal response to immunological glomerular injury. In: BM Brenner, ed. *The Kidney*, 5th ed. Philadelphia: WB Saunders,1996;1258–1284.
111. Van der Woude FJ, Rasmussen N, Lobatto S. Auto-antibodies against neutrophils and monocytes: tool in diagnosis and marker of disease activity in WegenerÆs Granulomatosis. *Lancet* 1985;1:425.
112. Wilson C, Dixon F. Anti-glomerular basement membrane antibody induced glomerulonephritis. *Kidney Int* 1973;3:74.
113. Weislander J, Bygrene P, Hernegard D. Isolation of the specific glomerular basement membrane antigen involved in goodpastureÆs syndrome. *Proc Natl Acad Sci USA* 1984;81:1544–1548.
114. Turner N, Mason P, Brown R. Molecular cloning of the goodpasture antigen demonstrates it to be the α3 chain of type IV collagen. *J Clin Invest* 1992;89:592–601.
115. Huey B, McCormach K, Capper J, Ratliff C, Colonibe B, Garovory M, Wilum CB. Association of HLA-DR and HLA-DQ types with anti-GBM nephritis by sequence specific oligonucleotide probe hybridization. *Kidney Int* 1993;44:307–312.
116. Lockwood CM, Boulton-Jones J, Lowenthal R, Simpson I, Peters DK, Wilson CB. Recovery from goodpasture's syndrome after immunosuppressive treatment and plasmapheresis. *Br Med J* 1975;2:252.
117. Salant, D. Immunopathogenesis of crescentic glomerulonephritis and lung purpura. *Kidney Int* 1987;32:408.
118. Atkins RC, Holdsworth SG, Glasgow EF, Matthew F. The macrophage in human rapidly progressive glomerulonephritis. *Lancet* 1976;1:8–30.
119. Border W, Brees D, Noble N. Transforming growth factor-b and extracellular matrix deposition in the kidney. *Contrib Nephrol* 1994; 107:140–145.
120. Couser WG, Johnson RJ. Mechanisms of progressive renal disease in glomerulonephritis. *Am J Kidney Dis* 1994;23:193–198.
121. Border W, Noble N. Transforming growth factor-b in tissue fibrosis. *N Engl J Med* 1994;331:1286–1292.

PART I

Normal Pathophysiology

Immunologic Renal Diseases,
edited by E. G. Neilson and W. G. Couser.
Lippincott-Raven Publishers, Philadelphia © 1997

CHAPTER 2

Microanatomy of the Kidney: Vessels, Interstitium, and Glomerulus

Marlies Elger, Brigitte Kaissling, Michel Le Hir, Wilhelm Kriz

It has become impossible to summarize the anatomy of the kidney on a few pages. Therefore, this chapter will deal in some detail only with certain aspects of kidney organization—the renal vasculature, the interstitium, and the glomerulus—thus, the topics most relevant for the general goal of this book. A short description of the general microscopic anatomy of the kidney (hardly more than the terminology) in advance is thought to provide a framework for the selected topics.

NEPHRONS AND COLLECTING DUCTS

The specific structural units of the kidney are the nephrons. In humans each kidney has an estimated one million nephrons (1). This number is established during prenatal development; after birth, new nephrons cannot be developed and lost nephrons cannot be replaced.

The nephron consists of a renal corpuscle (glomerulus) connected to a complicated and twisted tubule that finally drains into a collecting duct. Based on the location of renal corpuscles within the cortex, three types of nephrons can be distinguished: superficial, midcortical, and juxtamedullary. The tubular part of the nephron consists of a proximal tubule and a distal tubule connected by a loop of Henle. For details of subdivision, see Figure 1 and Table 1.

According to the length of the loops of Henle, two types of nephrons can be distinguished: those with long loops and those with short loops (including those with cortical loops). Short loops turn back in the outer medulla or even in the cortex (cortical loops). Long loops turn back at successive levels of the inner medulla, many already in the beginning of the inner medulla, others reach the intermediate level, and only a few reach the tip of the papilla.

The collecting ducts are formed in the renal cortex when several nephrons join (Fig. 1 and Table 1). A connecting tubule is interposed between a nephron and a cortical collecting duct. Connecting tubules of deep and superficial nephrons differ. The connecting tubules of deep nephrons generally form arcades that ascend within the renal cortex before draining into a collecting duct (Fig. 2). Superficial nephrons drain via an individual connecting tubule. Compared with rats, rabbits, and pigs, arcades are rarely encountered in the human kidney. Cortical collecting ducts descend within the medullary rays of the cortex. They traverse the outer medulla as unbranched tubes. On entering the inner medulla, they fuse successively and ultimately open as papillary ducts into the renal pelvis.

The uriniferous tubules (nephrons and collecting ducts) are lined by single-layered transporting epithelia, showing characteristic cytological features in each portion (2, 3). The proximal tubule is characterized by a relatively high number of cells that extensively interdigitate with each other by lateral cell processes. The apical surface is tremendously increased in area by a well-developed brush border. This increase in luminal area is paralleled by an increase in basolateral cell membrane area due to the extensive lateral interdigitation. The interdigitating processes are filled with rod-shaped mitochondria closely associated with lateral cell membranes. The cells are interconnected by leaky tight junctions.

The subsequent descending thin limbs of Henle's loop differ in cellular character. In addition to differences between short and long descending thin limbs, the long descending limbs change in organization as they descend into the inner medulla. Proximal tubules and descending thin limbs are nephron segments that are permeable to

M. Elger and Wilhelm Kriz: Institut für Anatomie und Zellbiologie I, Universität Heidelberg, Heidelberg, Germany.
B. Kaissling and M. Le Hir: Anatomisches Institut, Universität Zürich-Irchel, Zurich, Switzerland.

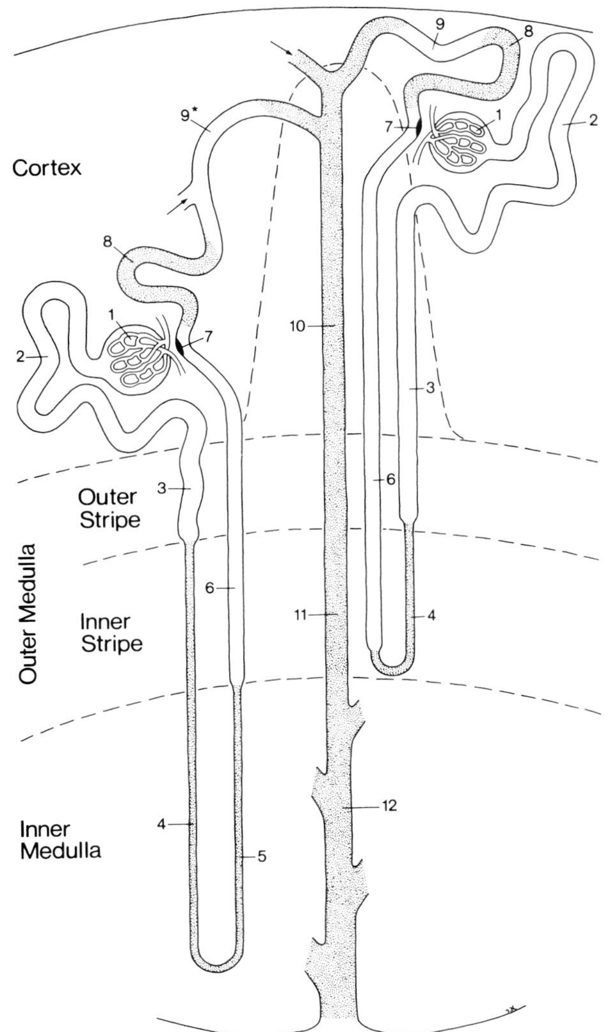

FIG. 1. Nephrons and collecting duct system. Shown are a short-looped and a long-looped nephron, together with a collecting duct (not drawn to scale). Within the cortex a medullary ray is delineated by a dashed line. 1, Renal corpuscle including Bowman's capsule and the glomerulus (glomerular tuft); 2, proximal convoluted tubule; 3, proximal straight tubule; 4, descending thin limb; 5, ascending thin limb; 6, distal straight tubule (thick ascending limb); 7, macula densa located within the final portion of the thick ascending limb; 8, distal convoluted tubule; 9, connecting tubule of the juxtamedullary nephron that forms an arcade; 10, cortical collecting duct; 11, outer medullary connecting duct; 12, inner medullary collecting duct.

TABLE 1. *Subdivisions of the nephron and collecting duct system*

- I. Nephron
  - A. Renal corpuscle
    - 1. Glomerulus (the most frequently used term to refer to the entire renal corpuscle)
    - 2. Bowman's capsule
  - B. Tubule
    - 1. Proximal tubule
      - a. Convoluted part
      - b. Straight part (pars recta) or descending thick limb of Henle's loop
    - 2. Intermediate tubule
      - a. Descending part or thin descending limb of Henle's loop
      - b. Ascending part or thin ascending limb of Henle's loop
    - 3. Distal tubule
      - a. Straight part or thick ascending limb of Henle's loop, subdivided into a medullary and a cortical part; the latter contains in its terminal portion the macula densa
      - b. Convoluted part
- II. Collecting duct system
  - A. Connecting tubule (including the arcades in most species)
  - B. Collecting duct
    - 1. Cortical collecting duct
    - 2. Outer medullary collecting duct subdivided into an outer- and inner-stripe portion
    - 3. Inner medullary collecting duct subdivided into a basal, middle, and papillary portion

Modified with permission (130).

water. Their cell membranes are stuffed with the channel protein aquaporin 1 (chip 28) (4).

Thin ascending limbs are only found in long loops being established by a highly interdigitating epithelium. The thick ascending limbs of Henle's loops generally start at the border between inner and outer medulla and ascend into the cortex to terminate shortly after their affixation to their parent glomerulus at the macula densa. The subsequent distal convoluted tubule is a comparably high epithelium with extensive lateral interdigitation and a dense armament of mitochondria. The ascending nephron segments (thin and thick limbs) as well as the distal convoluted tubule totally lack water-channel proteins in their cell membrane; thus, these nephron segments are fairly impermeable to water (4).

By definition, the collecting duct system starts with the connecting tubules. Along this tubular portion, confluences of nephrons occur, i.e., the identity of an individual nephron is no longer maintained (at least in those nephrons that drain by arcades). Beginning with the connecting tubule, the epithelium is heterogenously composed of at least two cell types. In addition to the specific cell type (connecting tubule cell; collecting duct cell), intercalated cells are found interspersed between the specific cells of each tubular portion (2,3). There are at least two types of intercalated cells: the type A intercalated cell is responsible for proton secretion and the type B intercalated cell is responsible for bicarbonate secretion. Intercalated cells are found in connecting tubules as well as in all parts of the collecting duct (with the exception of the very last portions of the inner medullary collecting duct, which consistently lack intercalated cells). Connecting tubule cells as well as the collecting duct cells in the various portions of the collecting duct differ considerably in their

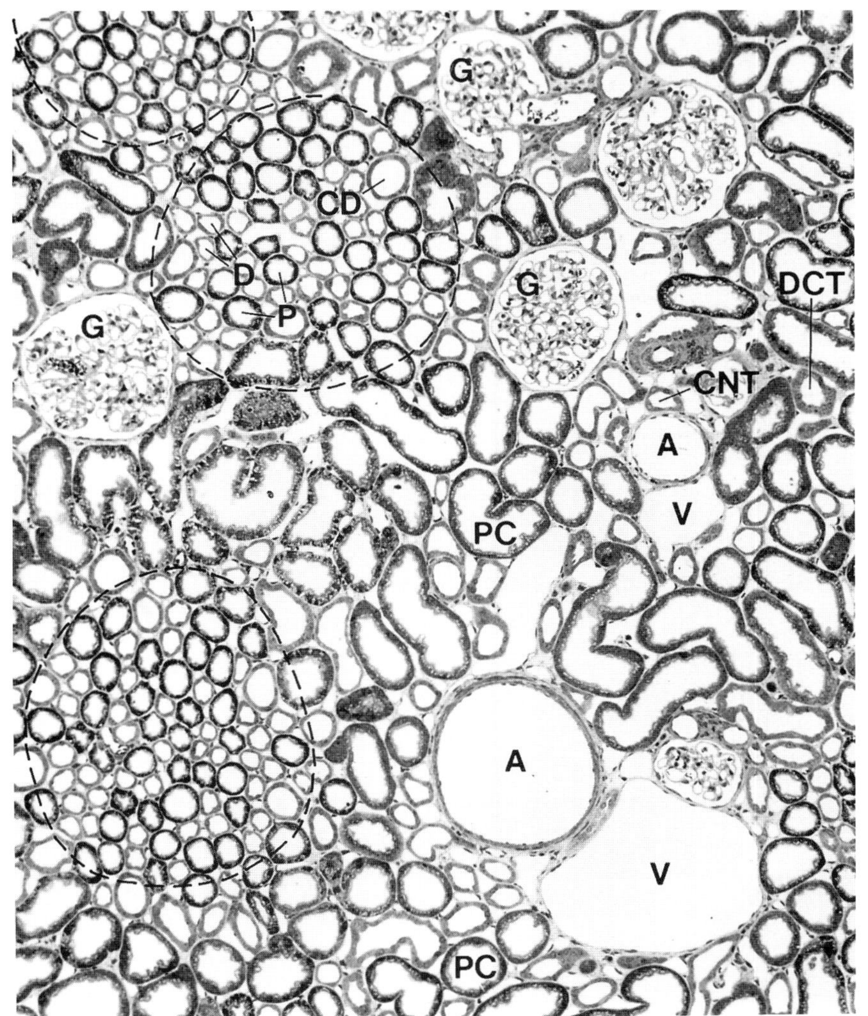

FIG. 2. Renal cortex (human). Section of a plane perpendicular to the corticopapillary axis showing medullary rays (delineated by dotted lines) and cortical radial (interlobular) vessels (A, artery; V, vein) in cross section. In addition to cortical radial vessels, the cortical labyrinth contains glomeruli (G) and convoluted proximal (PC) and distal (DCT) tubules embedded into the interstitial tissue. Connecting tubules (CNT) may ascend as arcades along the cortical radial vessels. In the medullary rays, straight proximal tubules (P) and collecting tubules descend to the outer medulla, and straight distal tubules (D, thick ascending limb) ascend. 1-µm Epon section, light microscopy. Magnification ×120.

armament of transporters and channels and thus differ considerably in their contributions to the final adjustment of the urine. However, they are specific in that their permeability to water can be regulated by antidiuretic hormone (ADH). In the absence of ADH, these tubular portions are impermeable to water; in response to ADH, these tubular portions become highly permeable to water. As has been shown recently (4), a water-channel protein (aquaporin 2), which is normally stored membrane bound in vesicles in the apical plasma of those cells, can be inserted into the apical plasma membrane in reponse to ADH, making this tubular segment permeable to water. This mechanism is subject to the change in excretion of a hypo- or isotonic urine to a hypertonic concentrated urine.

The subdivision of the renal parenchyma into various regions is underlain by a fairly strict distribution of the various nephron and collecting duct segments. The renal cortex (Fig. 2) is subdivided into a cortical labyrinth and the medullary rays of the cortex. The cortical labyrinth contains the glomeruli and the proximal convoluted as well as distal convoluted tubules and most of the collecting tubules. The medullary rays of the cortex contain the straight tubular portions (i.e., the cortical pars recta of the proximal tubule, the cortical thick ascending limb, and the cortical collecting ducts).

The medulla is divided into an outer medulla (subdivided into an outer stripe and inner stripe) and an inner medulla. The outer medulla has a similar tubular composition as the medullary rays of the cortex. The prominent tubular portion is the pars recta of the proximal tubule. Because the pars recta of proximal tubules of juxtamedullary nephrons in contrast to their name do not take a straight course but have more the shape of a corkscrew, most of the tubular portions in the outer stripe are proximal tubules. The inner stripe contains the descending thin limbs of short and long loops and the thick ascending limbs, as well as the collecting ducts, which are unbranched tubes along the entire outer medulla. The inner medulla contains the thin descending and thin ascending limbs of long loops of Henle. The inner medullary collecting ducts characteristically join successively to ultimately establish the papillary ducts (2,5).

MICROVASCULATURE OF THE KIDNEY

The microvascular pattern of the kidney is similarly organized in all mammalian species. Therefore it seems possible to describe what may be called a basic mammalian pattern of the intrarenal microvasculature (2,6–8) (Figs. 3 and 4). The description may begin with the interlobar arteries, which enter the kidney substance roughly between adjacent renal lobes. They extend toward the cortex on either side of a renal pyramid in the space between the wall of the pelvis (or calyx) and the adjacent cortical tissue. At the junction of the cortex and medulla, they divide and pass over into the arcuate arteries, which also undergo several divisions. They give rise to the cortical radial arteries (interlobular arteries), which ascend radially through the cortex. No arteries penetrate the medulla.

Most afferent arterioles arise from cortical radial arteries, but others may arise from arcuate or even interlobar arteries (supplying a small proportion of juxtamedullary glomeruli). Afferent arterioles supply the glomerular tufts. Aglomerular tributaries to the capillary plexus are rarely found; it is generally agreed that these vessels result from degeneration of the associated glomeruli. Thus, the blood supply of the peritubular capillaries of the cortex and the medulla is exclusively postglomerular.

Glomeruli are drained by efferent arterioles. Two basic types can be distinguished: cortical and juxtamedullary efferent arterioles. Cortical efferent arterioles, which derive from superficial and midcortical glomeruli, supply the capillary plexus of the cortex, which consists of the long-meshed capillary plexus of the medullary rays and the more dense and round-meshed plexus of the cortical labyrinth. Both plexus receive blood directly from efferent arterioles. However, the venous drainage of the medullary rays has to pass through the capillaries of the cortical labyrinth to gain access to interlobular veins. The functional significance of this arrangement is not known.

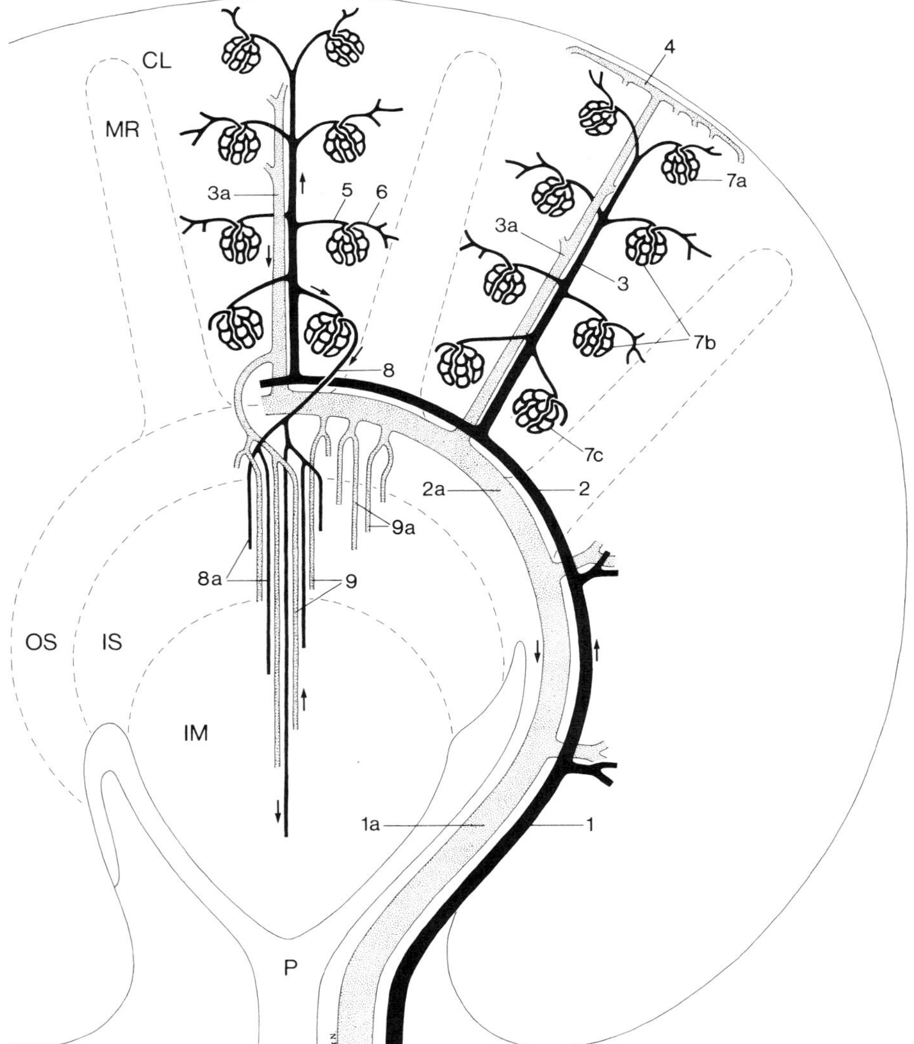

FIG. 3. Intrarenal vessels in a unipapillary kidney (rat). The section plane is parallel to the corticomedullary axis. Arterial and venous vessels are shown in black and gray, respectively; peritubular capillaries and lymphatics are not included (not drawn to scale). The medullary rays (MR) in the cortex, which contain descending and ascending tubule segments, are delineated from the cortical labyrinth (CL) by a dashed line; OS, IS, outer and inner stripes of the outer medulla; IM, inner medulla; P, renal pelvis; 1/1a, interlobar artery and vein; 2/2a, arcuate artery and vein; 3/3a cortical radial (interlobular) artery and vein; 4, stellate vein; 5, afferent arteriole; 6, efferent arteriole; 6a, juxtamedullary efferent arteriole; 7a/7b/7c, superficial, midcortical, and juxtamedullary glomeruli; and 8/8a, descending vasa recta and ascending vasa recta in vascular bundle.

This pattern would provide the basis for a cortical recycling system. Substances reabsorbed from straight tubules in the medullary rays could, via this capillary bridge, be reoffered to proximal convoluted tubules.

The efferent arterioles of juxtamedullary glomeruli represent the supplying vessels of the renal medulla. Immediately after leaving the glomerulus, these vessels turn toward the medulla and divide into the descending vasa recta. The trunk of the efferent arteriole as well as its first divisions give rise to small side branches that supply the sparse capillary plexus of the outer stripe of the outer medulla. The descending vasa recta then penetrate the inner stripe of the outer medulla in cone-shaped vascular bundles. At intervals individual vasa recta leave the bundles to supply the capillary plexus at the adjacent medullary level. Most descending vasa recta leave the bundle within the inner stripe and only a small proportion enters the inner medulla and even less reach the tip of the papilla.

The vessels that drain the peritubular capillaries of the renal medulla are the ascending vasa recta. In the inner medulla they arise at every level, ascending as unbranched vessels toward the border between inner and outer medulla. Afterward they traverse the inner stripe within the vascular bundles. The ascending vasa recta that drain the inner stripe may either join the vascular bundles (from the lowest portion of the inner stripe) or may ascend directly to the outer stripe between the bundles.

In the outer stripe, the entirety of ascending vasa recta arising from deeper parts of the medulla traverse the outer stripe as individual wavy vessels, with wide lumina interspersed among the tubules. They contact the tubules (mostly descending proximal tubules) like true capillaries. Because true capillaries derived from direct branches of efferent arterioles are relatively scarce, it is the ascending vasa recta that form the capillary plexus of the outer stripe. Finally, the ascending vasa recta empty into arcuate veins or into basal portions of cortical radial veins (interlobular veins).

The organization of the vascular bundles results in a separation of the blood flow to the inner stripe from that to the inner medulla. Descending vasa recta supplying the inner medulla traverse the inner stripe within the vascular bundles. Therefore, blood flowing to the inner medulla has not been exposed previously to tubules of the inner or outer stripe. All ascending vasa recta originating from the inner medulla traverse the inner stripe within the vascular bundles. Thus, blood that has perfused tubules of the inner medulla does not subsequently perfuse tubules of the inner stripe. However, the blood returning from either the inner medulla or the inner stripe does perfuse the tubules of the outer stripe. It has been suggested that this arrangement in the outer stripe functions as the ultimate trap to prevent solute loss from the medulla by establishing a countercurrent relationship between all the ascending vasa recta and the descending proximal straight tubules and collecting ducts.

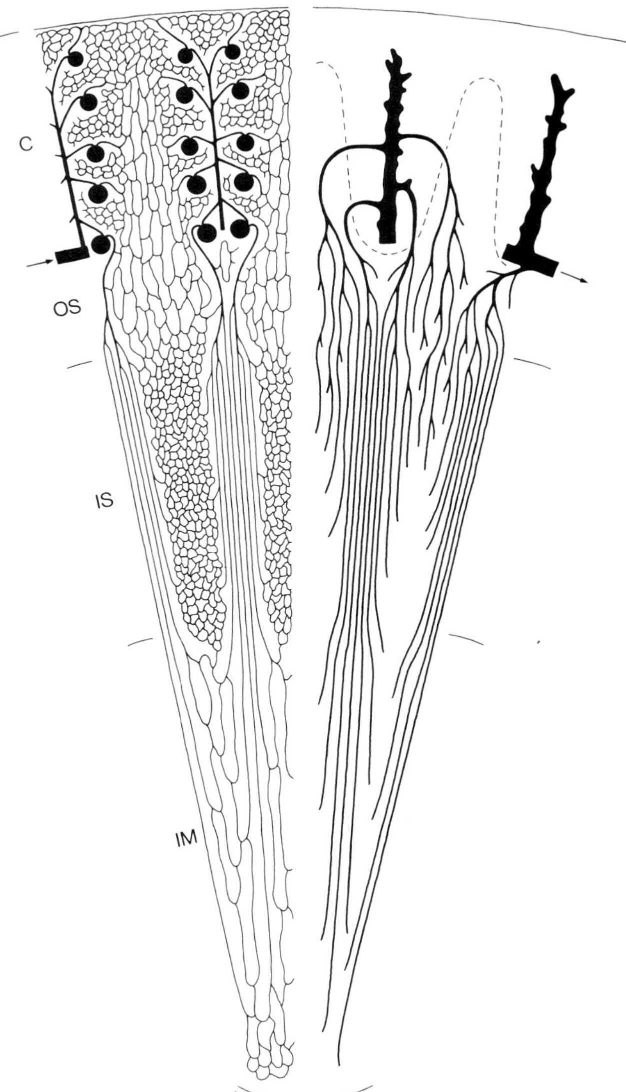

FIG. 4. Microvasculature of the rat kidney: C, cortex; OS, IS, outer and inner stripes of the outer medulla; IM, inner medulla. **Left:** Arterial vessels and capillaries. An arcuate artery *(arrows)* gives rise to a cortical radial (interlobular) artery, from which afferent arterioles originate to supply the glomeruli. The efferent arterioles of the juxtamedullary glomeruli descend into the medulla and divide into the decending vasa recta, which, together with the ascending vasa recta, form the vascular bundles of the renal medulla. At intervals, descending vasa recta leave the bundles and form the interbundle capillary plexus. **Right:** Venous vessels. The interlobular veins start in the superficial cortex. In the inner cortex, they, together with the arcuate veins, receive the ascending vasa recta from the medulla. The vasa recta ascending from the inner medulla all traverse the inner stripe within the vascular bundles, whereas most of the vasa recta from the inner stripe ascend outside the bundles. Both of these types of ascending vasa recta traverse the outer stripe as wide, tortuous channels. Modified with permission (7).

The intrarenal veins accompany the arteries. Central to the renal drainage of the kidney are the arcuate veins, which, in contrast to arcuate arteries, do form real anastomosing arches at the corticomedullary border. They accept the veins from the cortex (cortical radial veins, which in humans may begin as stellate veins on the renal surface) and from the renal medulla. The arcuate veins join to form interlobar veins, which course beside the corresponding arteries. They unite in variable patterns, finally establishing a single renal vein.

Intrarenal Nerves

The efferent nerves of the kidney consist of sympathetic nerves and terminal axons, which course beside the intrarenal arteries and afferent and efferent arterioles (2, 8). The descending vasa recta within the medulla are also innervated by adrenergic nerve terminals as far as they are enveloped by smooth muscle cells. In the rat this corresponds to the border between outer and inner stripes. A particularly dense assembly of nerve terminals is found around the juxtaglomerular apparatus.

Tubules have direct contact to terminal axons only when they are located around the arteries or the arterioles. As stated by Barajas (9), "the tubular innervation consists of occasional fibres adjacent to perivascular tubules." The density of nerve contacts to convoluted proximal tubules is low; contacts to straight proximal tubules, straight distal tubules, and collecting ducts (located in the medullary rays and the outer medulla) have never been encountered. The overwhelming majority of tubular portions have no direct relationships to nerve terminals.

Little is known about afferent nerves of the kidney; they are commonly believed to be sparse, but the issue remains unresolved.

INTERSTITIUM

The cellular constituents of the interstitium are resident fibroblasts, which establish the scaffolding frame for tubules, renal corpuscles and blood vessels, and varying amounts of migrating cells of the immune system (10). The space between the cells is filled with extracellular matrix: ground substance (proteoglycans, glycoproteins), fibrils, and interstitial fluid (11,12).

Fibroblasts

The most evident function of fibroblasts is the production and modeling of extracellular material, such as collagenous and noncollagenous fibers and ground substance (12). The modulation of this synthetic function by cytokines, secreted by immune cells, epithelial cells, and endothelial cells in the local environment of fibroblasts, accounts in part for the increase in deposition of matrix during inflammatory processes (12–15).

From a morphological point of view, fibroblasts are the central cells in the renal interstitium (16,17). They are interconnected by morphologically specialized contacts (11), and they adhere by specific attachment to the basement membranes surrounding the tubules, the renal cor-

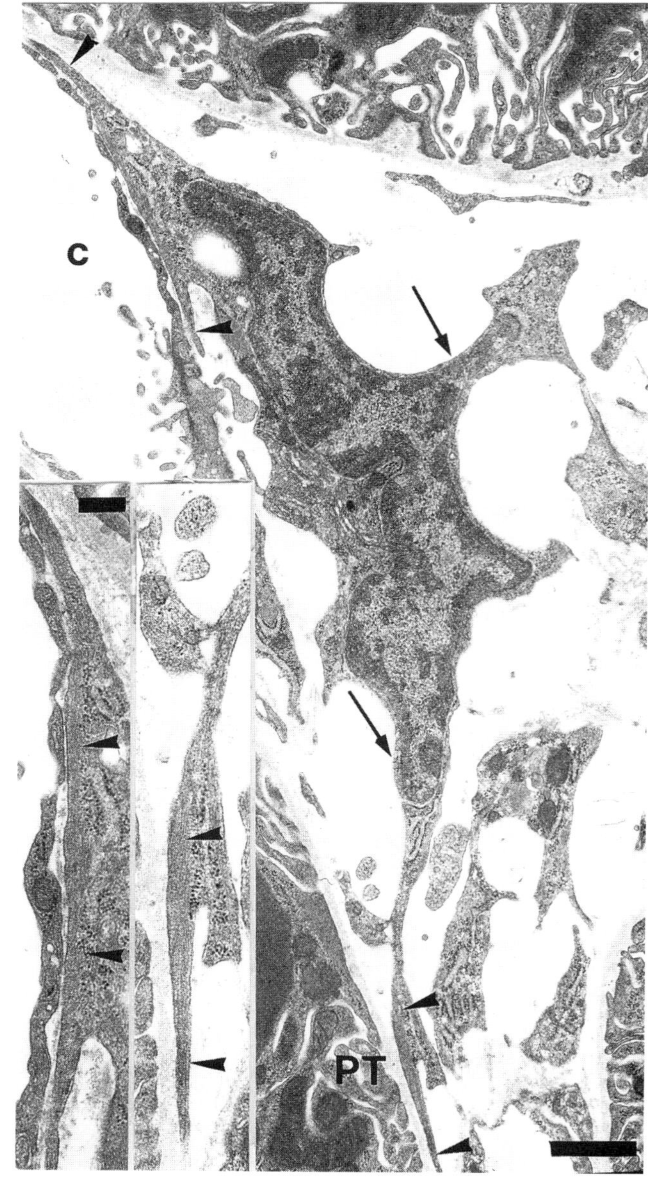

FIG. 5. Fibroblast in the cortical peritubular interstitium of a healthy rat. Stellate pericaryon with broad concavities are shown. The nucleus extends into the cytoplasmic processes (arrows), and adhesion of fibroblast processes to the basement membrane of a capillary (c) and proximal tubule (PT) by pediclelike "attachment plaques" (arrowheads and inserts) may be seen. Transmission electron microscopy (TEM). Magnification ×10,500; bar, ~1 μm. Inserts: Magnification ×20,600; bar, 0.5 μm. Reprinted with permission (17).

puscles, and capillaries. They are in close touch with lymphatics, nerve terminals, and all types of migrating interstitial cells.

Renal fibroblasts are similar in shape and ultrastructure to fibroblasts in the interstitium of other organs (18–20). Their nuclear profiles are often stellate (Fig. 5), surrounded by a thin rim of cytoplasm devoid of cell organelles. The attenuated cytoplasmic processes extend far from the pericaryon and often penetrate the narrow space between adjacent basement membranes of tubules, and capillaries. Characteristic of fibroblasts is the extensive protein synthesis apparatus, represented by abundant anastomosing profiles of rough endoplasmic reticulum (ER) and free ribosomes (Fig. 5). The presence of Golgi fields in the processes points to the release of procollagen into the extracellular space at these sites (12). Lysosomal elements are rarely observed under control conditions.

Components of the cytoskeleton are particularly apparent in fibroblasts. In electron micrographs, a thin dark layer consisting of actin filaments is visible under the plasma membrane of the pericaryon and of the cytoplasmic processes (21) (Figs. 5 and 6). Actin filaments are especially prominent in attachment plaques, by which the fibroblasts establish connection to the basement membranes of tubules and capillaries (Figs. 5 and 6). Alpha-smooth muscle actin is occasionally detected by immu-

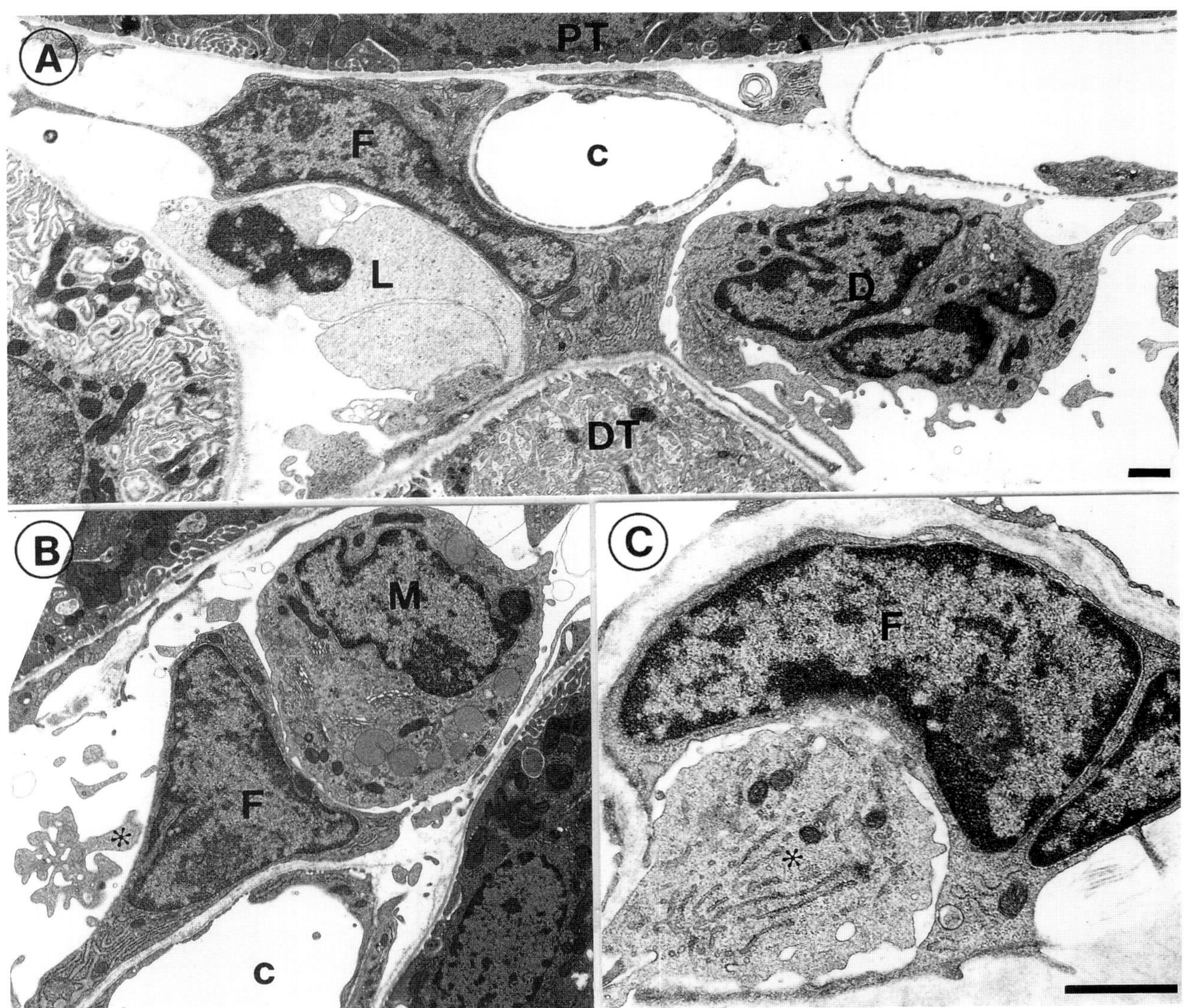

FIG. 6. Association of fibroblasts to renal structures and cells in the cortical peritubular interstitium. **A:** Fibroblast (F) extending between a distal (DT) and a proximal tubule (PT), partly enclosing a capillary (c), a lymphocyte (L), and the pericaryon of a dendritic cell (D) in focal interstitial nephritis. **B:** Fibroblast (F) adjacent to an inactive macrophage (M) with numerous primary lysosomes. C, capillary; *, process of a dendritic cell. **C:** Fibroblast pericaryon, enclosing a large portion of a dendritic cell (*). TEM. Magnification: ×5,700 (**A** and **B**); ×16,000 (**C**). Bar, ~1 µm. Reprinted with permission (A,B [10]; C [17]).

nohistochemistry in fibroblast pedicles of healthy kidneys of humans (22). In junctional complexes between fibroblasts, actin filaments are seen in close association with the plasma membrane. These junctions resemble intermediate junctions that also have been observed between tendon fibroblasts (23). Tight and gap junctions are present between medullary fibroblasts (24).

Phenotypical modulations of fibroblasts, which are likely to be reversible, occur in vivo under the influence of environmental factors, such as extracellular matrix composition, cytokines, and growth factors (12,19,25–27). Myofibroblasts abound under pathological conditions, e.g., in inflammations and interstitial fibrosis (12, 22). Myofibroblasts display an increase in alpha-smooth muscle actin, a nucleus with numerous indentations and an enlarged pericaryon, containing many cell organelles (26); they are coupled by gap junctions (19). It is still a subject of debate as to whether myofibroblasts represent

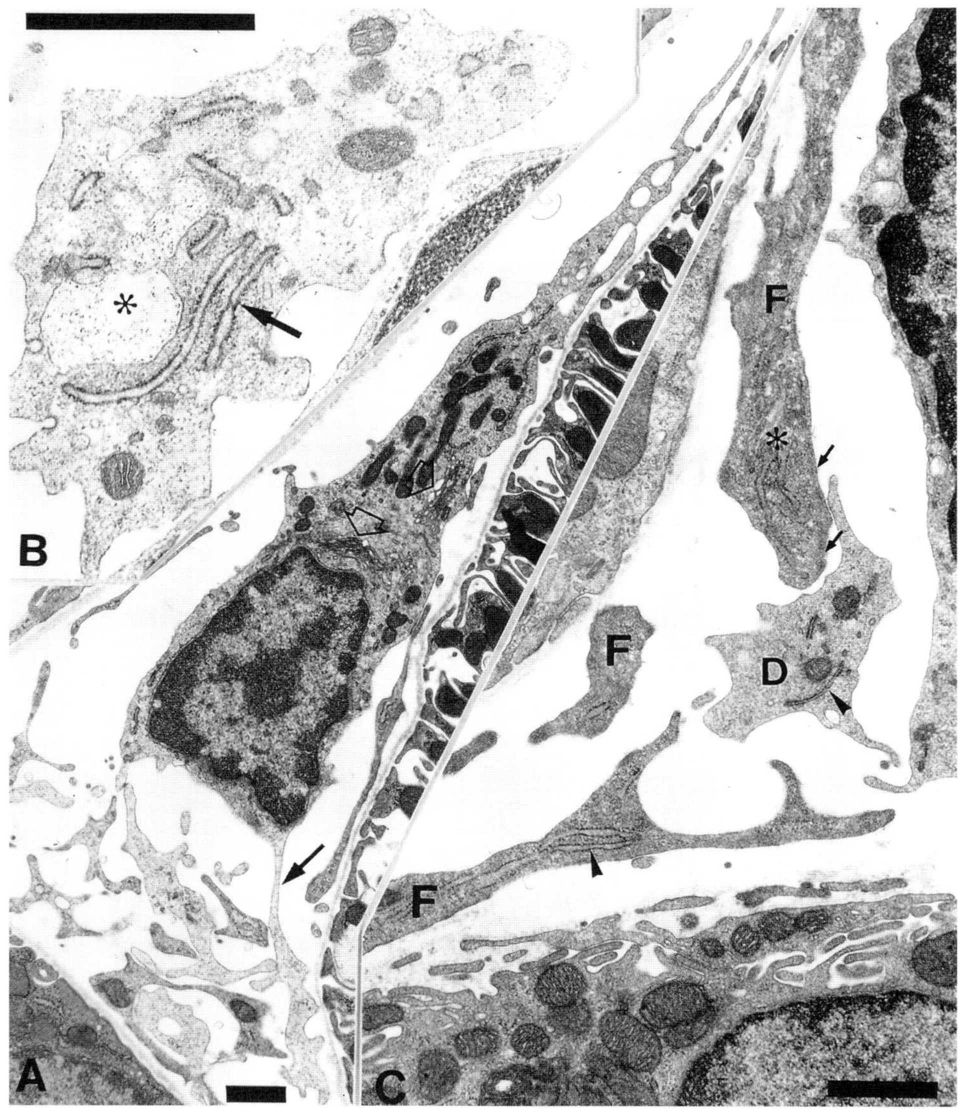

FIG. 7. Dendritic cell in the cortical peritubular interstitium of a healthy rat. **A:** Pericaryon with the rounded nucleus, Golgi apparatus *(open arrows)*, mitochondria, and profiles of rough endoplasmic reticulum. Cytoplasmic extensions of the pericaryon display characteristic holes, and the dendritiform processes *(arrow)* lack cell organelles and show a less dense cytoplasm than do the adjacent processes of fibroblasts. **B:** A few narrow profiles of rough endoplasmic reticulum *(arrow)*, short profiles of mitochondria, and a macropinosome *(asterisk)* in a dendritic cell. **C:** Comparison of processes of dendritic cells (D) and of fibroblasts (F); in the latter Golgi apparatus *(asterisk)*, wide profiles of rough endoplasmic reticulum *(arrowheads)* and actin filaments *(small arrows)* under the plasmalemma are visible. TEM. Magnification: ×7,800 (**A**); ×30,000 (**B**); ×14,000 (**C**). Bars, 1 μm. Reprinted with permission (10).

a modulation of fibroblasts (26–29) or derive from a different cell lineage (14).

Cells of the Immune System

Monocytes/macrophages and lymphocytes have long been described to reside in the interstitium of healthy kidneys (21,30–32). More recently, a distinction between macrophages and dendritic cells has been made (17, 33,34).

Macrophages have the capacity for phagocytosis. This is the basis for their most important and most specific functions: antimicrobial activity, clearance of damaged host cells, and tumoricidal activity. Major histocompatibility complex (MHC) class II, which is not constitutively expressed by macrophages, may be upregulated by proinflammatory cytokines. Macrophages (Fig. 6) have a large cell body with large, plump, but rather short processes and numerous surface folds in an activated status. Their prominent lysosomal apparatus distinguishes them from other immune cells.

Dendritic cells share several functional characteristics with macrophages. However, they constitute a distinct cell lineage of bone marrow origin (35–38). They are "professional" antigen-presenting cells and can take up antigens and process them to short peptides, which can be presented to T cells in the context of MHC class II. Their constitutively high expression of MHC class II, their supply with costimulatory molecules, and their tropism to lymphatic organs explain how dendritic cells display by far the highest potency in the stimulation of naive T cells (35,36). As in other peripheral tissues, dendritic cells turn over rapidly in the kidney (37,38). They exit the organs mainly via lymphatics and enter lymphatic organs where antigen presentation takes place (35,36).

In the healthy kidney there are usually many more dendritic cells than macrophages (17). In marked contrast to the latter, dendritic cells in healthy renal interstitium lack the prominent lysosomal apparatus. Renal dendritic cells and fibroblasts are difficult to distinguish on a morphological basis because both may show a stellate cellular shape and both display substantial amounts of mitochondria and ER. The nucleus of dendritic cells (Fig. 7) is rounded, often with deep indentations. In contrast to fibroblasts, the major cell organelles in dendritic cells are confined to the pericaryon, and the cell processes are often ramified like dendrites (Figs. 6 and 7). Moreover, in ultrathin sections the processes as well as the pericaryon often have "holes," which may represent macropinosomes described in cultured dendritic cells (39). The most distinctive morphological difference to fibroblasts is the absence of the subplasmalemmal layer of actin filaments (Figs. 6 and 7). They also lack structurally defined attachments to the basement membranes of tubules and vessels and lack junctional complexes. However, circumscribed contacts to fibroblasts and other interstitial cells exist. Intermediate filaments may be abundant in the pericaryon of dendritic cells.

Lymphocytes comprise several functionally well-defined classes, such as cytotoxic killer cells, T-helper cells, etc. In the interstitium of healthy kidneys, lymphocytes are rare. They can generally be distinguished on the basis of their usually round nucleus, displaying extensive heterochromatin condensations, and their low number of cell organelles (Fig. 6). In inflamed areas, focal contacts between lymphocytes and fibroblasts are particularly frequent.

Cortical Interstitium and Lymphatics

The fractional volume of the cortical interstitium in human kidneys has been calculated to range from 5% to 37%, with a tendency to increase with age (30). A subdivision is generally made between the peritubular interstitium surrounding the tubules and capillaries (Fig. 8) and

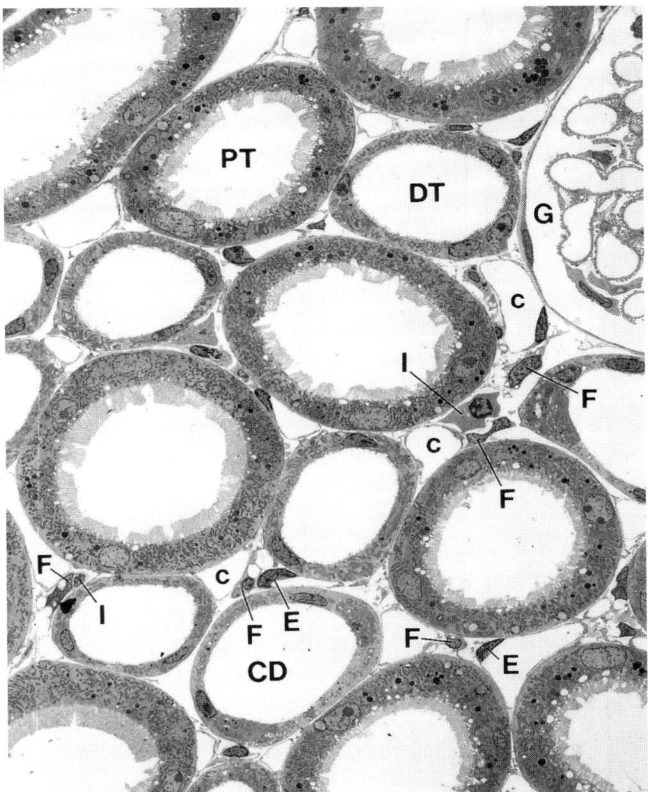

FIG. 8. Peritubular interstitium in rat renal cortex. The peritubular interstitium occupies the space between the nephrons and peritubular capillaries (c) and contains different types of interstitial cells: F, resident fibroblasts; I, migrating cells of the immune system; E, endothelial cells; P, proximal tubule; D, distal tubule; CD, collecting duct. TEM. Magnification ×740.

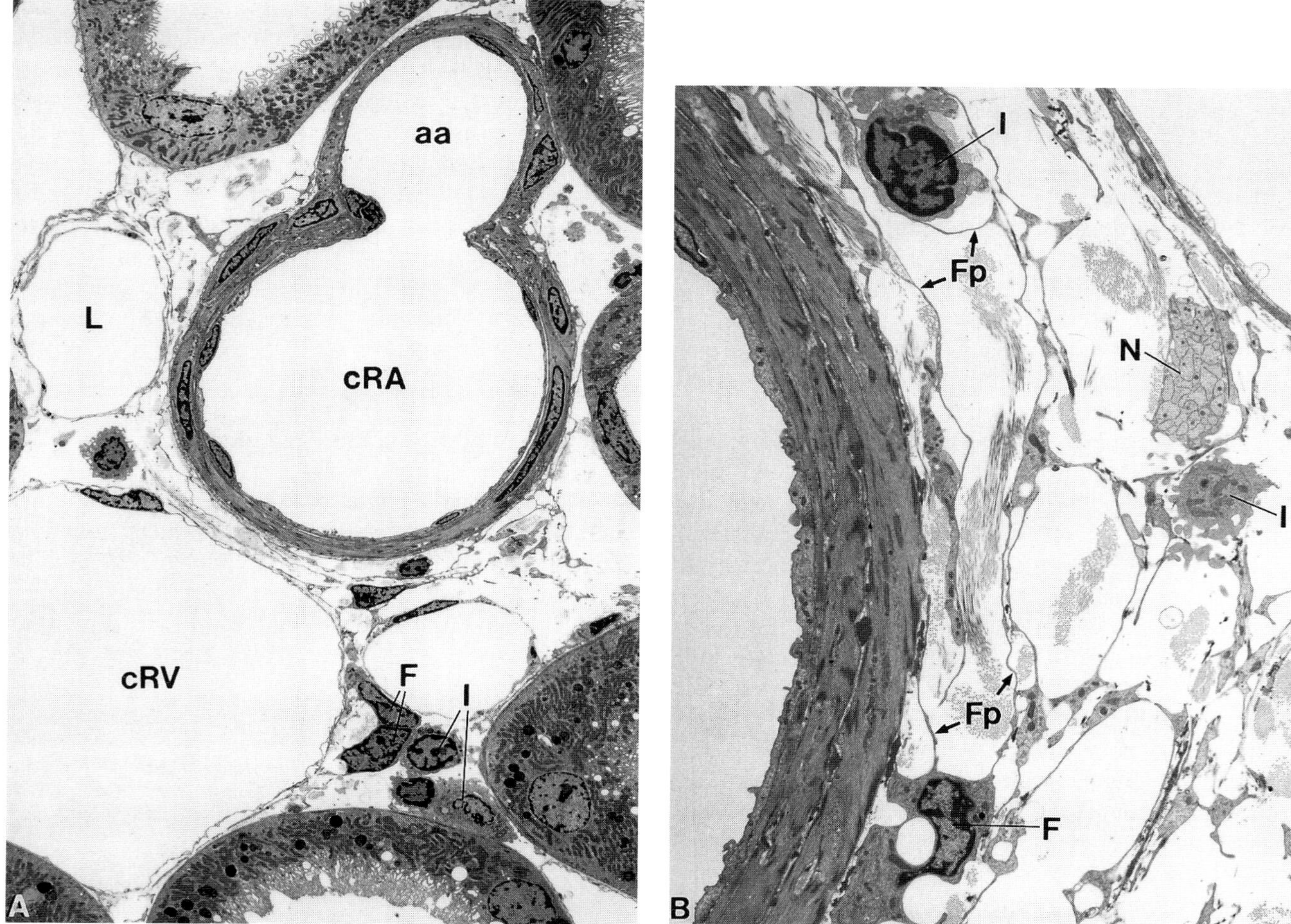

FIG. 9. Periarterial interstitium in rat renal cortex. **A:** Cross section through a cortical radial artery (cRA) and origin of an afferent arteriole (aa); the vessels are surrounded by loose connective tissue, which also contains lymphatic capillaries (L). cRV, cortical radial vein; F, fibroblast; I, immune cell. **B:** The periarterial connective tissue sheath consists of fibroblasts (F) with extremely attenuated cell processes *(arrows)* that form meshes enclosing bundles of collagen fibers and abundant ground substance. Immune cells (I) are usually present in the periarterial interstitium. N, nerve. TEM. Magnification: ×1,100 (**A**); ×1,900 (**B**).

the periarterial interstitium, which accompanies the intrarenal arteries and contains the lymphatics (Fig. 9). Both are continuous with each other.

In the cortical peritubular interstitium of healthy kidneys, the majority of interstitial cells are fibroblasts and dendritic cells. However, macrophages, identified by morphology and by immunostaining [in rats using the macrophage-specific marker ED2 (17,40,41)], and lymphocytes are almost absent.

The close spatial association of fibroblasts and dendritic cells is striking. Portions of dendritic cells may be almost completely enclosed by fibroblasts (Figs. 6, 8, and 10). At light microscopic levels immunocytochemistry facilitates it to distinguish between both cell types. Cortical (peritubular) fibroblasts exhibit the enzyme ecto-5′-nucleotidase (5′NT), demonstrated so far in rats (17,42–44) and mice, whereas dendritic cells have a high expression of MHC class II (34–36).

The activity of 5′NT in cortical fibroblasts shows some regional variation. Normally, the activity of the enzyme is highest in fibroblasts in the deep cortical labyrinth (42,44). However, under anemic conditions the activity of the enzyme is also strongly upregulated in fibroblasts in the superficial cortex and to a lower extent in the medullary rays (45–47). This suggests a link between the expression of 5′NT and the synthesis of erythropoietin (48,49). Indeed, colocalization of 5′NT and erythropoietin–messenger RNA demonstrated that 5′NT-positive fibroblasts synthesize renal erythropoietin (50,51). The enzyme 5′NT is a source of extracellular adenosine. Known targets for extracellular adenosine are the cortical radial vessels, the glomerular arterioles, the renin-con-

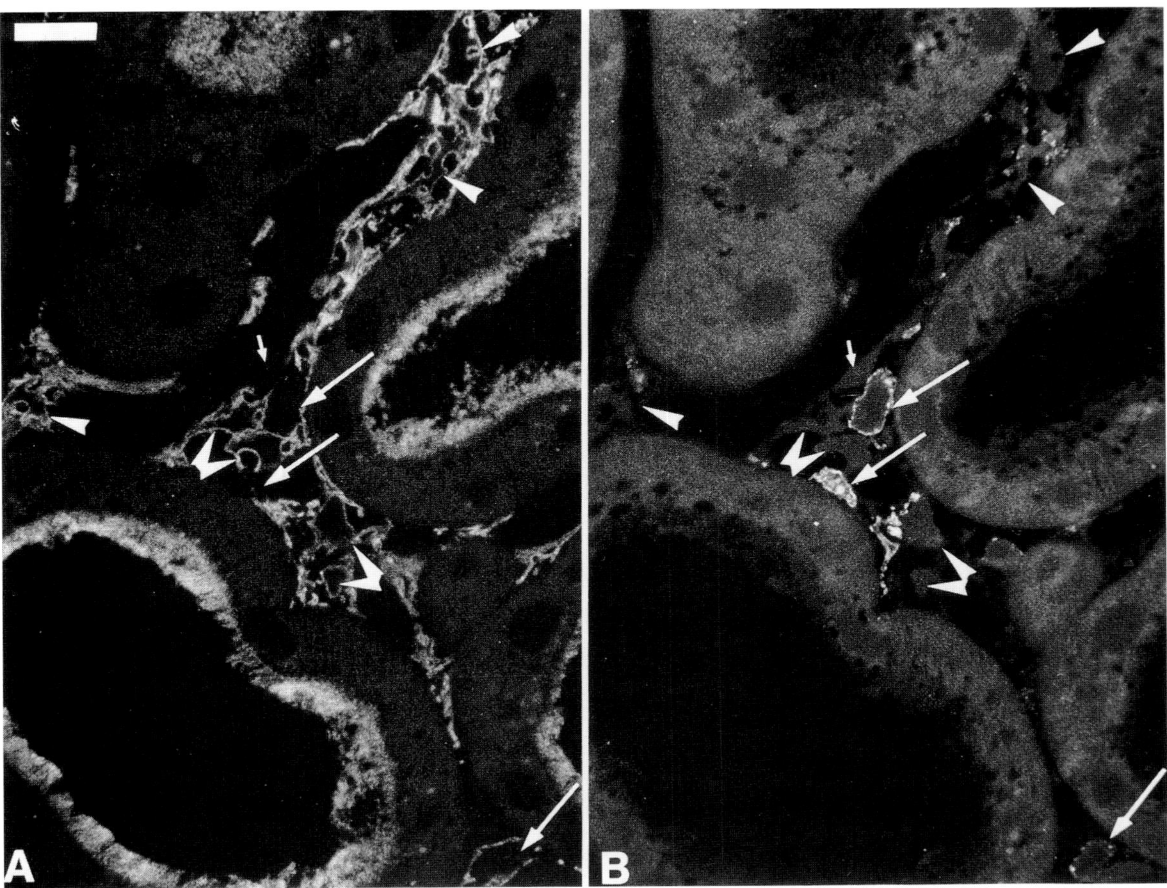

FIG. 10. Immunofluorescent double labeling with anti–ecto-5′-nucleotidase and anti–MHC class II (OX 6) in rat kidney cortex (1-μm cryostat section). **A:** Ecto-5′-nucleotidase–related fluorescence. **B:** MHC class II–related fluorescence. Ecto-5′-nucleotidase–positive interstitial cells *(arrowheads)* show the characteristic profiles of fibroblasts. They are closely intermingled with MHC class II–positive cells *(arrows)*. Capillary endothelia *(short arrow)* are negative with both antibodies. LM. Reprinted with permission (10). Magnification ×1,100; bar, ~10 μm.

taining granular cells, and the nerve endings along the arterioles and tubules (49,52).

The periarterial interstitium is a loose layer of connective tissue surrounding the intrarenal arteries and terminates along the afferent arterioles at the glomerulus (Figs. 9 and 11). The renal veins are in apposition to this sheath but not included in it (53). The scaffold of the periarterial connective tissue sheath is constituted of fibroblasts with extremely attenuated cell processes that form large, loose meshes filled with prominent bundles of collagenous fibers and large quantities of ground substance. The periarterial fibroblasts regularly display alpha-smooth muscle actin and intermediate filaments of the vimentin type (40), but they lack 5′NT (17).

In addition to dendritic cells and a few lymphocytes, numerous macrophages are regularly found (17,40). The relatively great number of macrophages around the intrarenal arteries may result from the fact that the periarterial interstitium is linked to the connective tissue of the pelvic wall. This continuity establishes a pathway for retrograde infection of the renal cortex. Under conditions of inflammation, huge accumulations of lymphocytes can be seen, restricted to the periarterial connective tissue sheath.

Intrarenal nerve fibers and lymphatics are embedded in the periarterial tissue (Figs. 9 and 11) (53–55). Lymphatics start in the vicinity of the afferent arteriole (56) and leave the kidney running within the periarterial tissue sheath toward the hilum. In addition to the lymphatics, the periarterial tissue itself constitutes a pathway for interstitial fluid drainage, as shown by injection of tracers (53). A pathway toward lymphatics via the peritubular and periarterial interstitium may be important for the systemic distribution of substances that are released into the peritubular interstitium. This suggestion has been made for renin (53) and may also apply to other protein hormones such as erythropoietin, as well as to a variety of vasoactive substances.

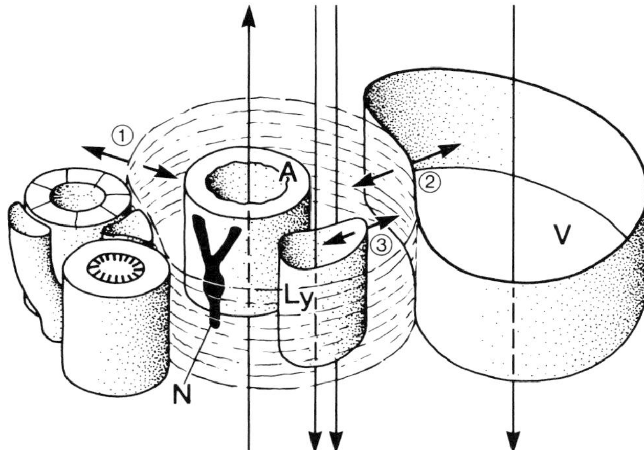

FIG. 11. A schematic of a transverse section of a cortical radial artery, showing the relations~hips between the periarterial sheath and the neighboring structures as well as a possible exchange of interstitial fluid in the periarterial sheath with (1) the peritubular interstitium, (2) the accompanying vein, and (3) lymphatics (LY). The *long arrows* indicate the flow in the respective vessels. N, nerve running along the artery. Modified with permission (53).

Medullary Interstitium

The medullary interstitial volume increases from the corticomedullary border toward the tip of the papilla. The peritubular (interbundle) interstitium of the outer stripe is extremely sparse (fractional volume ~3–5%), like the interstitium within the vascular bundle of the entire outer medulla. In rats the fractional interstitial volume in the interbundle compartment of the inner stripe amounts to about 10% and increases to about 30% in the papillary tip (57,58). The cellular composition of the medullary interstitium is similar to that in the cortex. The incidence of dendritic cells expressing MHC class II shows some regional variations. From all renal zones, it is the highest in the inner stripe (Fig. 12). In lower levels of the inner medulla, immune cells are no longer detectable.

Fibroblasts in the entire medulla show the same basic characteristics as in the renal cortex, namely attachment of their processes to the basement membrane of tubules and vessels, interconnections by specific junctions (24), high quantities of rough ER, bundles of actin filaments (alpha-smooth muscle actin) under the plasma membrane, and intermediate filaments. However, the phenotype of fibroblasts shows progressive variation from the outer toward the inner medulla (Fig. 13). In contrast to cortical peritubular fibroblasts, medullary fibroblasts do not display 5′NT. Within the inner stripe and the inner medulla, actin and vimentin filaments in fibroblasts become increasingly prominent. The cisterns of the rough ER and the perinuclear cisterns become strikingly widened and densely filled with flocculent material. Focally, ER membranes are apposed to the plasmalemma

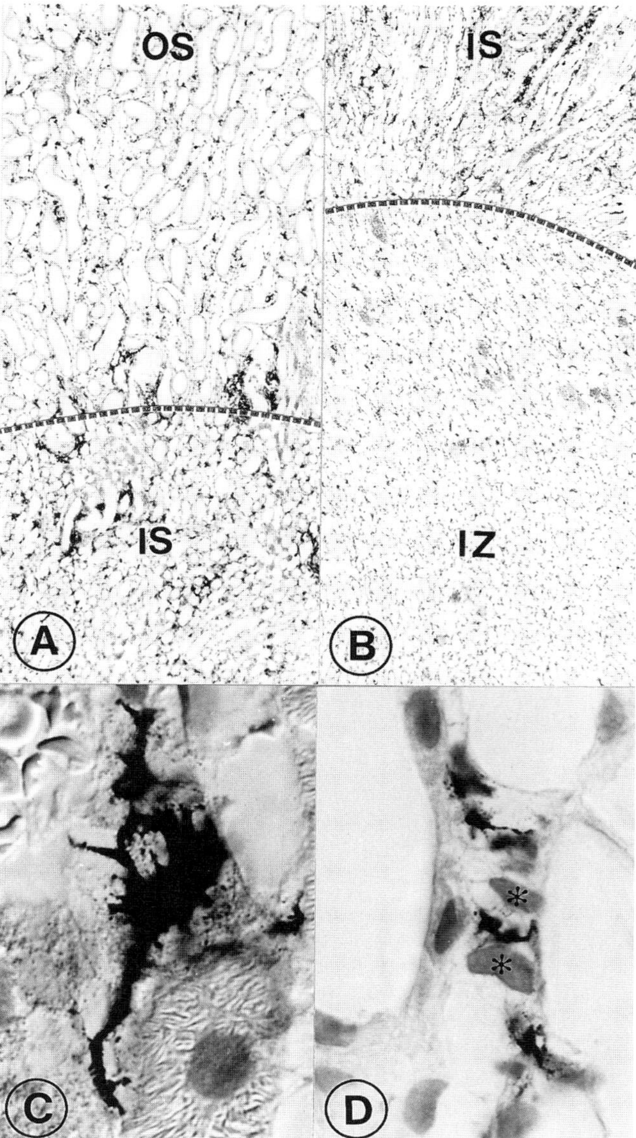

FIG. 12. Distribution and shapes of MHC class II–positive cells throughout the medullary renal zones (rat; antibody OX 6, immunogold technique with silver enhancement; cryostat sections). **A and B:** In cortex and outer stripe (OS), MHC class II–positive cells are evenly distributed throughout the interstitium; their frequency is highest in the inner stripe (IS) and decreases in the upper third of the inner zone (IZ). In deeper levels they are no longer detected. Shapes of MHC class II–positive cells suggest their identification as dendritic cells in inner stripe (**C**) and in inner zone (**D**). In the latter, processes of these cells suggest their identification between ladder runglike oriented lipid-laden fibroblasts (*). LM. Magnification: ×56, bar 100 μm (**A**); ×1,500, bar ~10 μm (**C–D**). Reprinted with permission (17).

(Fig. 13) (21). These features seem to be associated with specific yet unknown functional conditions.

Within the inner medulla, the interstitial cells are oriented strictly perpendicularly toward the longitudinal axis of the tubules and vessels, all running in parallel

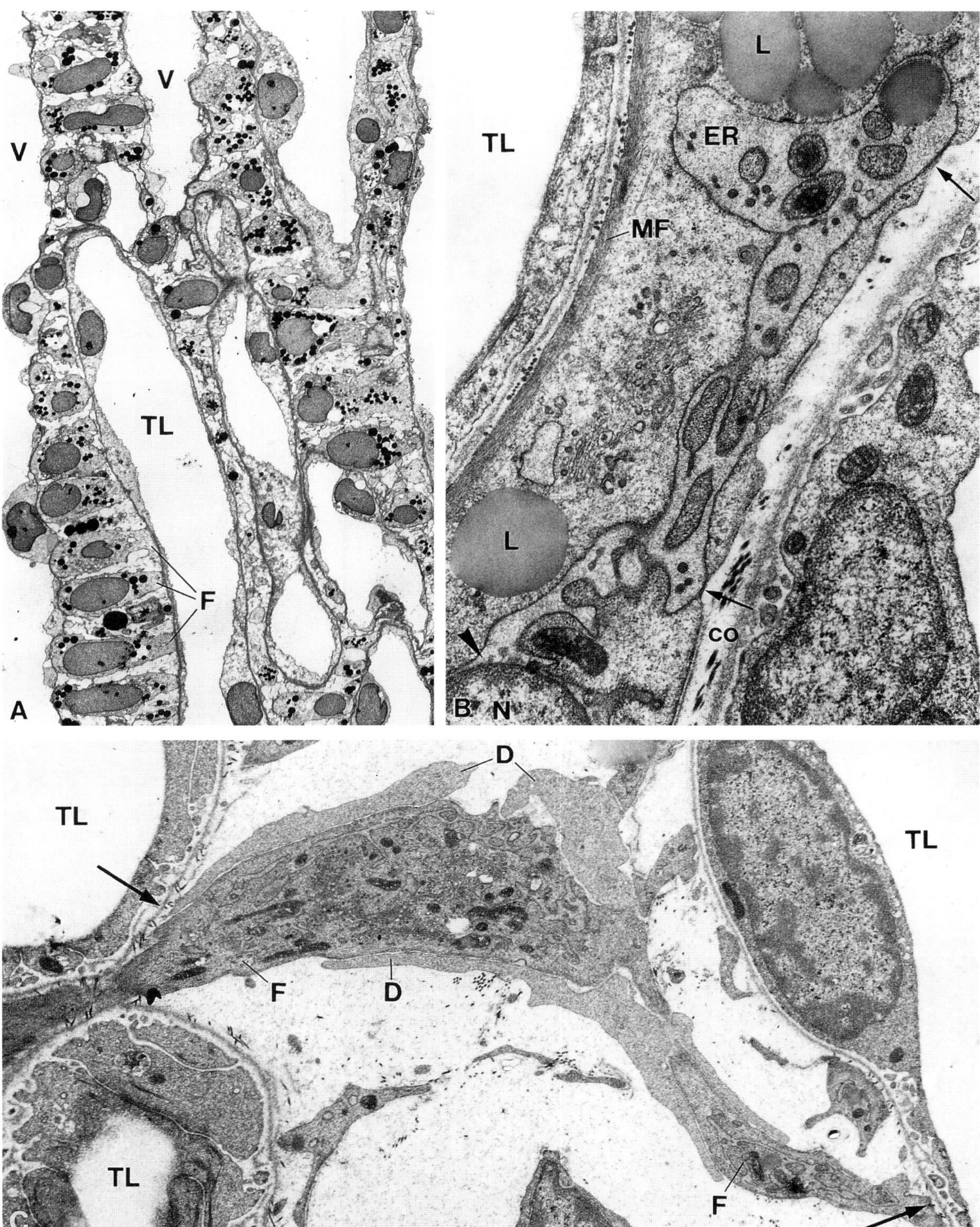

FIG. 13. Medullary interstitium. **A:** Longitudinal section of the inner medulla. The interstitial cells (F) are arranged perpendicularly to the longitudinally running renal tubules (TL, thin limb) and/or vasa recta (V). Fibroblasts may be especially rich in lipid droplets; hence, their designation as lipid-laden interstitial cells. **B:** Part of an inner medullary fibroblast. Lipid droplets (L) are accumulated in the cytoplasm. The rough endoplasmatic reticulum (ER) has widened cisternae that are in close connection to the plasmalemma *(large arrows)*. The *arrowhead* marks the transition of ER to dilated perinuclear cistern (N, nucleus). Note the subplasmalemmal layer of actin filaments (MF). co, collagenous fibers; TL, thin limb of Henle. **C:** Narrow spatial association of a fibroblast (F) and processes of dendritic cells (D) at the transition to the inner medulla. Fibroblast processes are connected *(arrows)* with the basement membranes of renal tubules (TL). TEM. Magnification: ×1,000 (**A**); ×18,600 (**B**); ×8,550 (**C**).

(Figs. 12D and 13A). They anchor to the basement membrane of loops of Henle and vasa recta. Because of their conspicuous amounts of lipid droplets, the inner medullary interstitial cells can usually be distinguished from the interstitial fibroblasts in the other renal zones, as so-called lipid-laden interstitial cells (2,11,31,59). In agreement with other investigators (30,60,61), we believe that these cells are a specific population of fibroblasts.

Furthermore, fibroblasts in the inner medulla produce large amounts of glycosaminoglycans, which are particularly abundant in the inner medullary interstitium (11). Finally, they produce vasoactive lipids, particularly prostaglandin E_2 (62–64). These may affect not only the renomedullary hemodynamics, but also, in an autocrine pathway, the contractile tone of the interstitial cells themselves, possibly acting on the volume of the interstitium (65).

GLOMERULUS (RENAL CORPUSCLE)

The glomerulus (Figs. 14 and 15) is composed of a tuft of specialized capillaries attached to the mesangium, both of which are enclosed in a pouchlike blind extension of

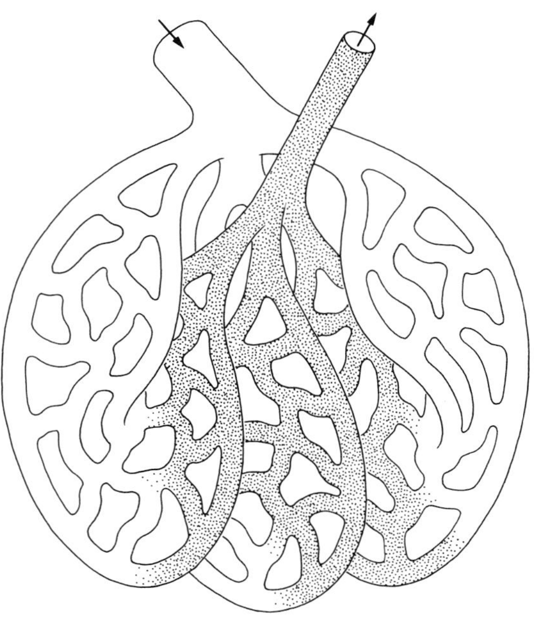

FIG. 14. Branching pattern of the glomerular tuft. Immediately after its entrance into the tuft, the afferent arteriole splits into large superficially located capillaries that are the supplying vessels of glomerular lobules (three are shown). The capillaries run toward the urinary pole. After turning back, they unite to establish the efferent arteriole still inside the glomerular tuft. Thus, in contrast to the afferent arteriole, the efferent arteriole has an intraglomerular segment. An afferent and efferent capillary domain are distinguished. The efferent capillary domain occupies roughly a quarter sector of the tuft (stippled). It is partly covered by the afferent domain. Modified with permission (66).

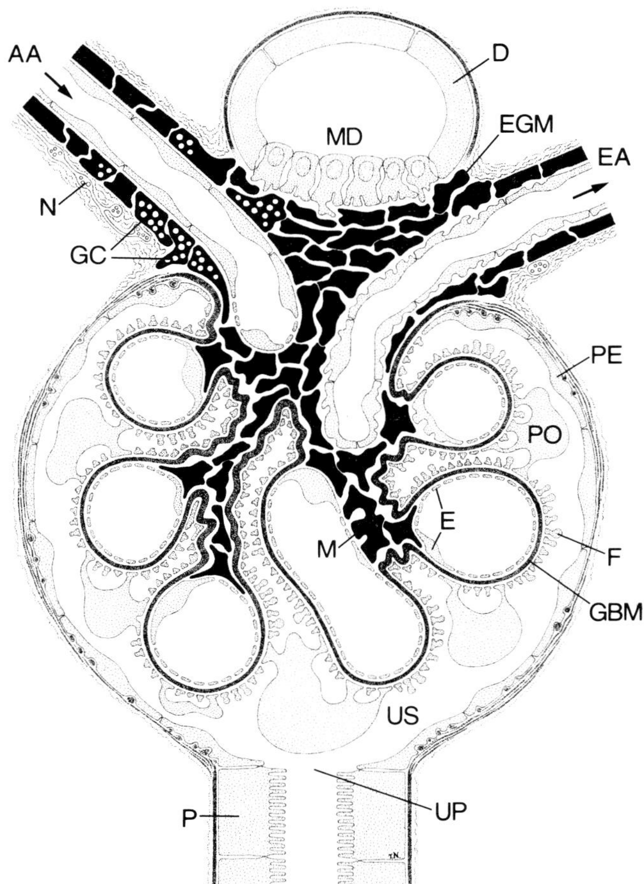

FIG. 15. Diagram of a longitudinal section of a renal corpuscle and the juxtaglomerular apparatus (JGA). The capillary tuft consists of a network of specialized capillaries, which are outlined by a fenestrated endothelium (E). At the vascular pole an afferent arteriole (AA) enters and an efferent arteriole (EA) leaves the tuft. The capillary network is surrounded by Bowman's capsule, comprising two different epithelia. The visceral epithelium, consisting of highly branched podocytes (PO) directly follows (together with the GBM) the surface of the capillaries and the mesangium (M). At the vascular pole, the visceral epithelium and GBM are reflected into the parietal epithelium (PE) of Bowman's capsule (and its basement membrane), which passes over into the epithelium of the proximal tubule (P) at the urinary pole. Mesangial cells (M) are situated in the axes of glomerular lobules. At the vascular pole the glomerular mesangium is continuous with the extraglomerular mesangium (EGM), consisting of cells and matrix. The EGM together with the terminal portion of the afferent arteriole (containing the granular cells, GC), the efferent arteriole, and the macula densa (MD) of the distal tubule establish the JGA. All cells that are suggested to be of smooth muscle origin are shown in a dark color. F, foot processes; N, sympathetic nerve terminals; US, urinary space. Modified with permission (131).

the tubule, i.e., Bowman's capsule. The capillaries and mesangium are covered by epithelial cells, forming the visceral epithelium of Bowman's capsule (podocytes), which at the vascular pole is reflected to become the parietal epithelium of Bowman's capsule. At the interface between the glomerular capillaries and the mesangium on one side and the podocyte layer on the other side the glomerular basement membrane (GBM) is developed. The space between both layers of Bowman's capsule represents the urinary space that at the urinary pole is continuing as the tubule lumen (Fig. 15).

The reflection of the parietal epithelium of Bowman's capsule into the visceral epithelium creates an oval opening in the glomerulus through which the glomerular arterioles, together with the glomerular mesangium, enter the glomerular tuft. This opening may be called the glomerular hilum and represents the glomerular vascular pole.

At the entrance level the afferent arteriole divides into several (two to five) primary capillary branches (Fig. 14). Each of these branches gives rise to an anastomosing capillary network that courses toward the urinary pole and after turning back courses toward the vascular pole. The initial branching of the afferent arteriole underlies the subdivision of the glomerular tuft into several lobules (which are not strictly separated from each other).

In contrast to the afferent arteriole, the efferent arteriole is established inside the glomerular tuft by confluence of tributaries from each lobule (66,67) (Figs. 14–17). The efferent arteriole has a significant intraglomerular segment that leaves the glomerulus through the glomerular stalk. Outside the glomerulus, it is first associated with the extraglomerular mesangium, which fills the space between the afferent and the efferent arteriole. Along the course through the extraglomerular mesangium, the surrounding mesangial and/or extraglomerular mesangial

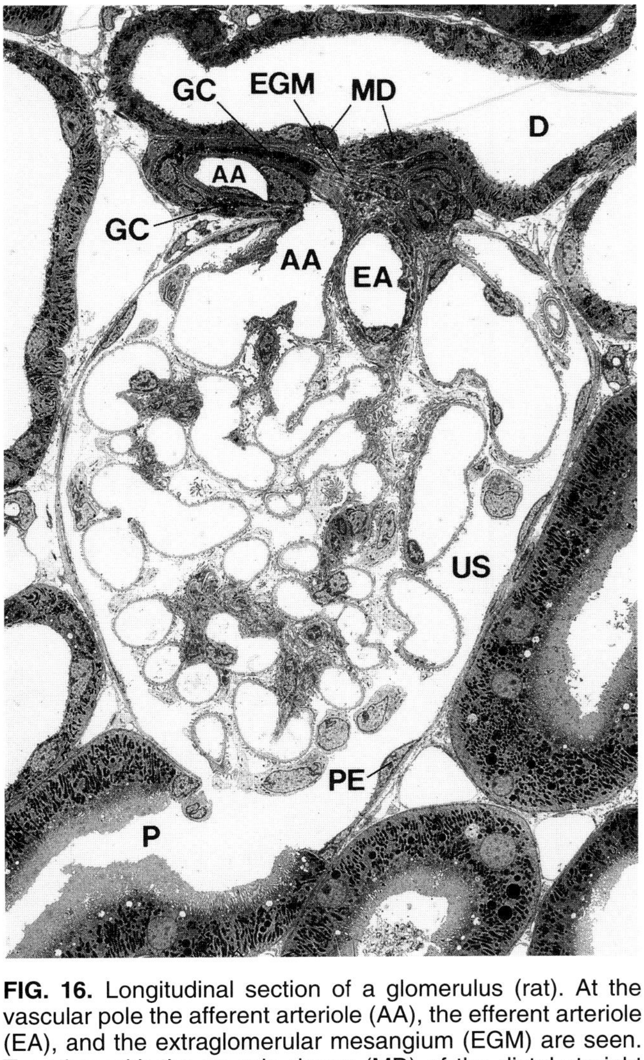

FIG. 16. Longitudinal section of a glomerulus (rat). At the vascular pole the afferent arteriole (AA), the efferent arteriole (EA), and the extraglomerular mesangium (EGM) are seen. Together with the macula densa (MD) of the distal straight tubule (D), the arterioles (with the granulated cells, GC) and the EGM are part of the juxtaglomerular apparatus. At the urinary pole, the parietal epithelium (PE) of Bowman's capsule transforms into the epithelium of the proximal tubule (P). US, urinary space. TEM. Magnification ×750.

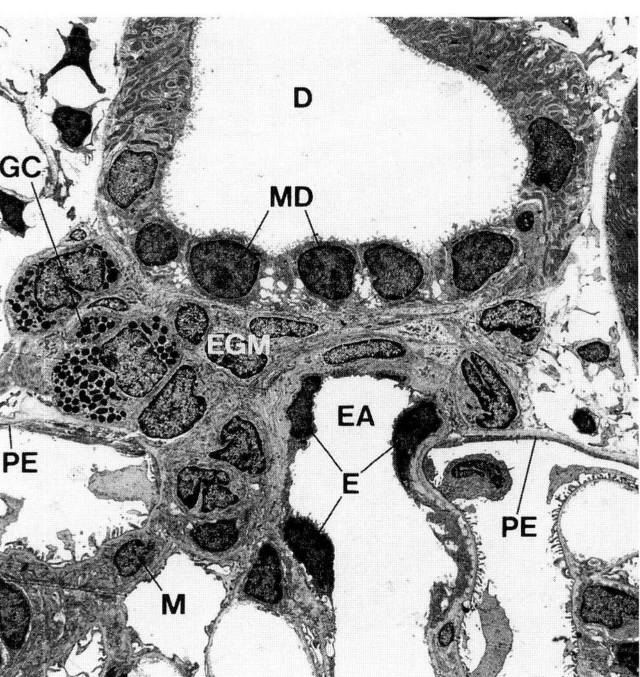

FIG. 17. Longitudinal section of the vascular pole showing the constituents of the juxtaglomerular apparatus. The macula densa (MD) of the straight distal tubule (D) is attached to the extraglomerular mesangium (EGM), which is situated in the angle between the afferent arteriole and efferent arteriole (EA). Note the dilated intercellular spaces between the macula densa cells. The terminal portion of the afferent arteriole (which in this figure is hit in a tangential section plane) is characterized by the abundance of granulated cells (GC, compare with Fig. 27). The outflow segment of the EA is marked by the thick wall and the high number of endothelial cell bodies (E). Within the glomerular stalk the EGM continues into the mesangium (M). PE, parietal epithelium of Bowman's capsule. TEM. Magnification ×1,500.

cells are gradually replaced by smooth muscle cells. Thus, after leaving the extraglomerular mesangium, the efferent vessel is established as a proper arteriole.

Glomerular capillaries (Figs. 18 and 19 are a unique type of blood vessel made up of nothing but an endothelial tube. A small stripe of the outer aspect of this tube is in touch with the mesangium; a major part bulges toward the urinary space and is covered by the GBM and the podocyte layer. This peripheral portion of the capillary wall represents the filtration area. The small portion of the capillary wall facing the mesangium is not underlain by a basement membrane but directly abuts the mesangium.

The glomerular mesangium represents the axis of a glomerular lobule, to which the glomerular capillaries are attached. Apart from this attachment site, the mesangium

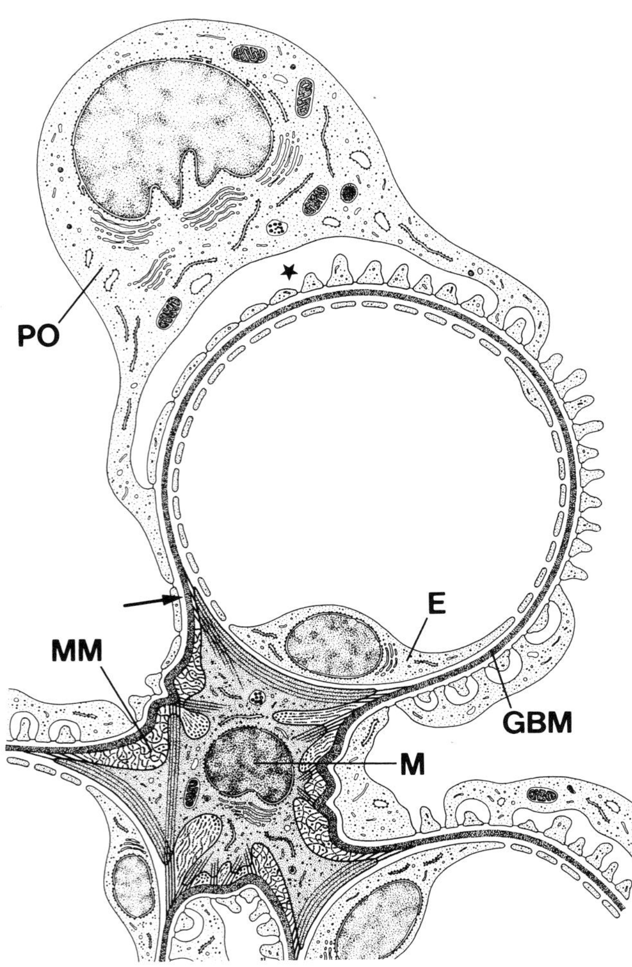

FIG. 18. Spatial relationships of a glomerular capillary to the visceral epithelium (podocytes, PO) and the GBM as well as to the mesangium. The glomerular capillary consists of a fenestrated endothelium (E). The peripheral portion of the capillary is surrounded by the GBM, which, at the mesangial angles *(arrow)*, deviates from the pericapillary course and covers the mesangium. The interdigitating system of the podocyte foot processes forms the distal layer of the filtration barrier. Note the subcellular space (*). Connections between mesangial cell processes and the GBM are prominent at mesangial angles and are also numerous along the perimesangial GBM. Many of these connections are mediated by microfibrils, which are a major constituent of the mesangial matrix (MM). Thus, a mechanical firm linkage of the perimesangial GBM to the contractile apparatus of the mesangial cells (M) is established. Modified with permission (2).

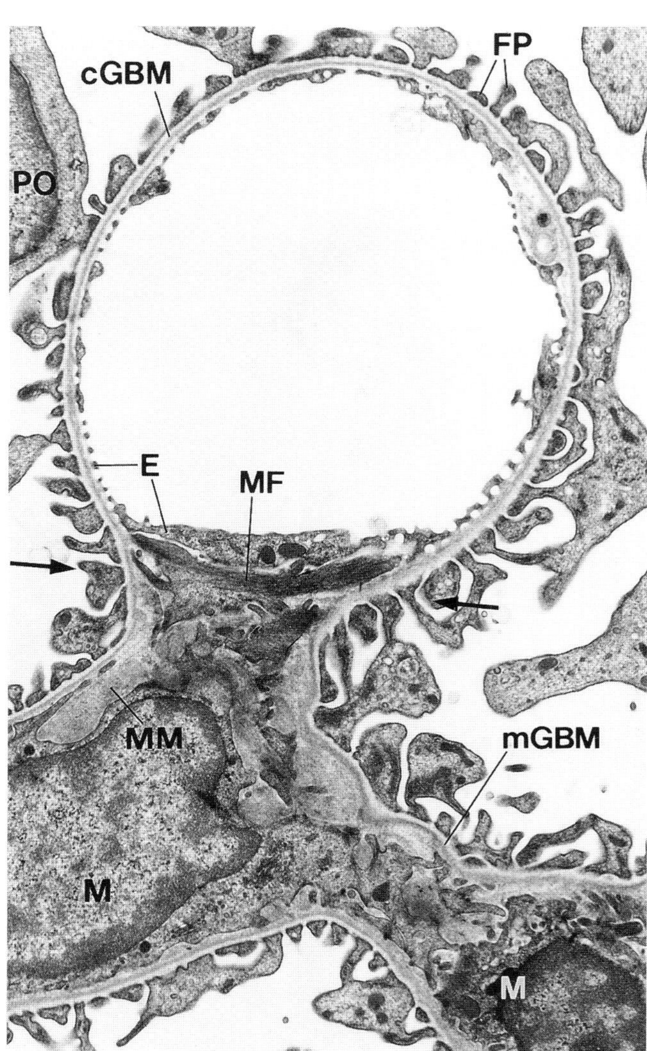

FIG. 19. Glomerular capillary (cross section). The capillary (C) is outlined by a flat fenestrated endothelium (E). The podocyte layer (PO) and the GBM do not encircle the capillary completely. Two subdomains of the GBM are delineated from each other by mesangial angles *(arrows)*: the pericapillary GBM (cGBM) and perimesangial GBM (mGBM). Two mesangial cells (M) with their nuclei and their cell processes are seen embedded in the mesangial matrix (MM). At the capillary–mesangial interface, mesangial cell processes containing dense bundles of microfilaments (MF) interconnect the GBM portions of two mesangial angles (*arrows*) on either side of the mesangium. Both the pGBM and mGBM are lined by the foot processes (FP) and filtration slits of the podocyte layer. TEM. Magnification ×9,700.

is bounded by the perimesangial part of the GBM, which is covered by a layer of podocytes.

Glomerular Basement Membrane

The GBM serves as the skeleton of the glomerular tuft (Figs. 15 and 18–20). It represents a complexly folded sack whose opening is the glomerular hilum. The outer aspect of this GBM sack is completely covered with podocytes. The interior of the sack is filled with the capillaries and mesangium. Thus, on its inner aspect the GBM is in touch either with capillaries or with the mesangium; these subdivisions are called the peripheral (pericapillary) and perimesangial parts, respectively. At the transition of the pericapillary to the perimesangial part, the GBM changes from a convex pericapillary into a concave perimesangial course; the turning points are called mesangial angles.

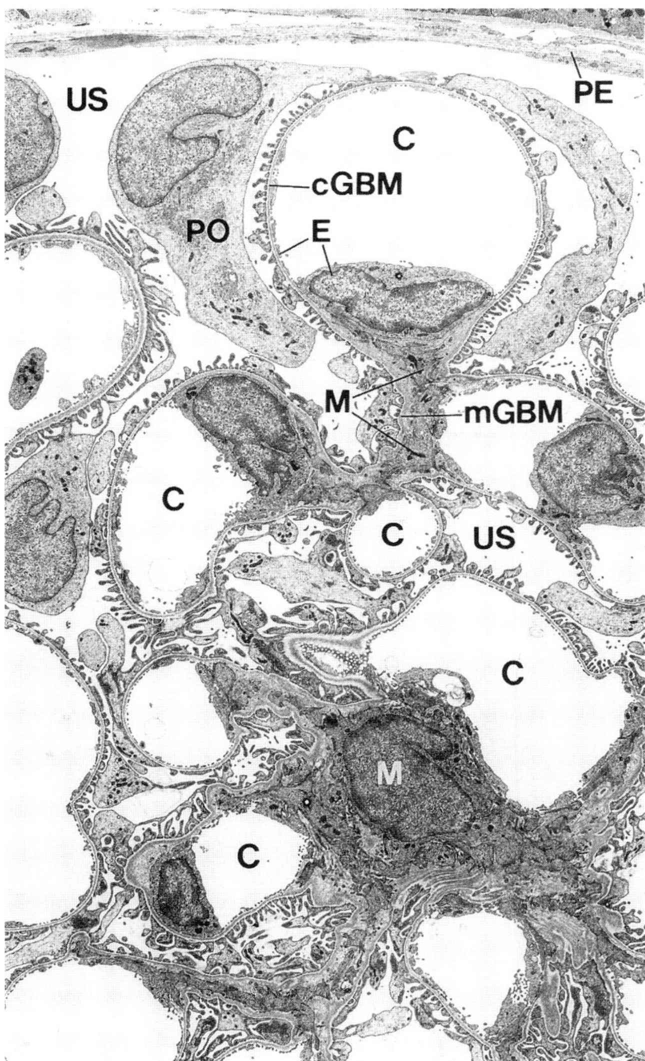

FIG. 20. Section of a glomerular lobule, showing several capillaries (C), the axial position of the mesangium (M), and the visceral epithelium (PO, podocytes). The GBM and the visceral epithelium follow the outer surface of the capillaries and the mesangium as a common cover, except for the capillary–mesangial interface, where the capillary endothelium (E) directly abuts the mesangium. Thus, two subdomains of the GBM (and of the podocyte layer) can be distinguished: the pericapillary (peripheral) GBM (cGBM; faced by podocytes and endothelium) and the perimesangial GBM (mGBM; bordered by podocytes and the mesangium) (see also Fig. 19). The peripheral part of the capillary establishes the site of filtration. PE, parietal epithelium of Bowman's capsule; US, urinary space. TEM. Magnification ×2,500.

In electron micrographs of traditionally fixed tissue, the GBM appears as a trilaminar structure made up of a lamina densa bounded by two less dense layers: the lamina rara interna and externa (Fig. 21). Recent studies using freeze techniques show only one dense layer directly attached to the bases of the epithelium and endothelium (68,69).

The major components of the GBM include type IV collagen, heparan sulfate proteoglycans, and laminin in accordance with basement membranes at other sites (70). Type V and VI collagen and entactin also have been demonstrated. On the other hand, the GBM has several unique properties, notably a distinct spectrum of type IV collagen and laminin isoforms (71).

At least six different type IV collagen genes have been cloned that encode the $\alpha1$ to $\alpha6$ chains, respectively, of type IV collagen. The $\alpha3$(IV) and $\alpha4$(IV) chains are located in the lamina densa of the GBM, whereas the classical $\alpha1$(IV) and $\alpha2$(IV) are found in the subendothelial space (corresponding to the lamina rara interna) and in the mesangium. This suggests that $\alpha3$ and $\alpha4$, along with $\alpha5$, form a network that is separate from that consisting of $\alpha1$ and $\alpha2$ chains (72). The functional importance of the recently described chains becomes evident when looking at their involvement in glomerular diseases: Goodpasture syndrome is mediated by pathogenic antibodies that are targeted to the $\alpha3$(IV) chain; Alport syndrome is caused by mutations in the gene encoding the $\alpha5$(IV) chain (73).

Current models depict the basic structure of the basement membrane as a three-dimensional network of collagen type IV. Monomers of type IV collagen consist of a triple helix 400 nm in length that, at its carboxy-terminal end, has a large noncollagenous globular domain, called NC1. At the amino-terminus the helix possesses a triple helical rod 60 nm in length, the 7S domain. Interactions between the 7S domains of two triple helices or the NC1 domains of four triple helices allow collagen type IV monomers to form dimers and tetramers. In addition, triple helical strands interconnect by lateral associations via binding of NC1 domains to sites along the collagenous region (70). These interactions between type IV collagen triple helices result in a flexible, nonfibrillar polygonal assembly that is considered to provide mechanical strength to the basement membrane and to serve as a scaffold for alignment of other matrix components.

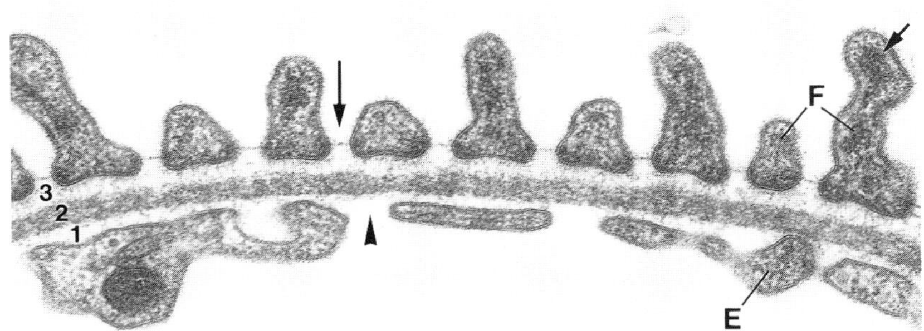

FIG. 21. Filtration barrier. The glomerular capillary wall is cut perpendicularly to the long axis of interdigitating foot processes. The peripheral part of the glomerular capillary wall comprises the fenestrated endothelial layer (E), the GBM, and the interdigitating foot processes (F). *Arrowheads* point to the open endothelial pores. The glomerular basement membrane shows a lamina densa (2) bounded by the lamina rara interna (1) and the lamina rara externa (3). The foot processes are separated by an intercellular space (filtration slit) and derive from two podocytes. Every other foot process belongs to one cell, and the others belong to the neighboring cell. The filtration slits are bridged by thin diaphragms (long arrows). Note the dense assemblies of microfilaments (*short arrow*). C, capillary lumen. TEM. Magnification ×45,000.

The major glycoproteins of the GBM are fibronectin, laminin, and entactin. Laminin is the most prominent noncollagenous component found in basement membranes. It consists of three polypeptide chains (A, B1, and B2), two of which are glycosylated and cross-linked by disulfide bridges (70). In the GBM the B1 chain is probably replaced by the highly homologous S-laminin (72). Laminin is thought to bind directly or via entactin (74) to type IV collagen as well as to integrin and nonintegrin cell surface receptors of endothelial and epithelial cells. An important factor for the adhesion of the glomerular endothelial cells to collagen is the integrin α3β1, and α5β1 is the major fibronectin receptor on these cells. In rat podocytes, α3β1 integrin is responsible for the attachment to type 4 collagen and laminin (75,76).

The electronegative charge of the GBM is mainly due to polyanionic proteoglycans. The major proteoglycan of the GBM is a large heparan sulfate proteoglycan called perlecan, which is composed of a core protein (400 kDa) and usually three heparan sulfate side chains (glycosaminoglycans) (71,77,78). In addition, heparan sulfate proteoglycans with smaller core proteins are present in the GBM (79). Proteoglycan molecules aggregate to form a meshwork that is kept highly hydrated by water molecules trapped in the interstices of the matrix. Within the GBM, heparan sulfate proteoglycans may act as an anticlogging agent to prevent hydrogen bonding and adsorption of anionic plasma proteins and maintain an efficient flow of water through the membrane (77).

Mesangium

Within the glomerular tuft, three cell types occur, all of which are in close contact with the GBM: mesangial cells, endothelial cells, and podocytes. The numerical ratio in the rat has been calculated to be 2:3:1.

Mesangial cells together with the mesangial matrix establish the glomerular mesangium. The mesangium occupies the axial region of a glomerular lobule, around which the glomerular capillaries pursue a tortuous course. Together with the capillaries, the mesangium occupies the space inside the GBM (Figs. 15 and 18–20).

Mesangial cells are irregular in shape, with many processes extending from the cell body toward the GBM. In these processes (and to a lesser extent in cell bodies) dense assemblies of microfilaments are found that have been shown to contain actin, myosin, and alpha-actinin (80).

The processes of mesangial cells course toward the GBM to which they are attached, either directly or mediated by the interposition of microfibrils. The GBM represents the effector structure of mesangial contractility (81,82). Mesangial cell–GBM connections are especially prominent beside the capillaries. At these sites mesangial cell processes (densely stuffed with microfilament bundles) extend underneath the capillary endothelium toward the mesangial angles of the GBM where they are anchored. Generally, two processes interconnect the GBM from two opposing mesangial angles (Fig. 19). Functionally the microfilament bundles bridge the entire distance between both mesangial angles. In the axial mesangial region, as well, microfilament bundles within mesangial processes generally bridge opposing parts of the GBM (Fig. 22).

The mesangial matrix fills the highly irregular spaces between the mesangial cells and the perimesangial GBM (Figs. 19 and 22) (71,83). The ultrastructural organization of this matrix is incompletely understood. A large number of common extracellular matrix proteins have been demonstrated within the mesangial matrix, includ-

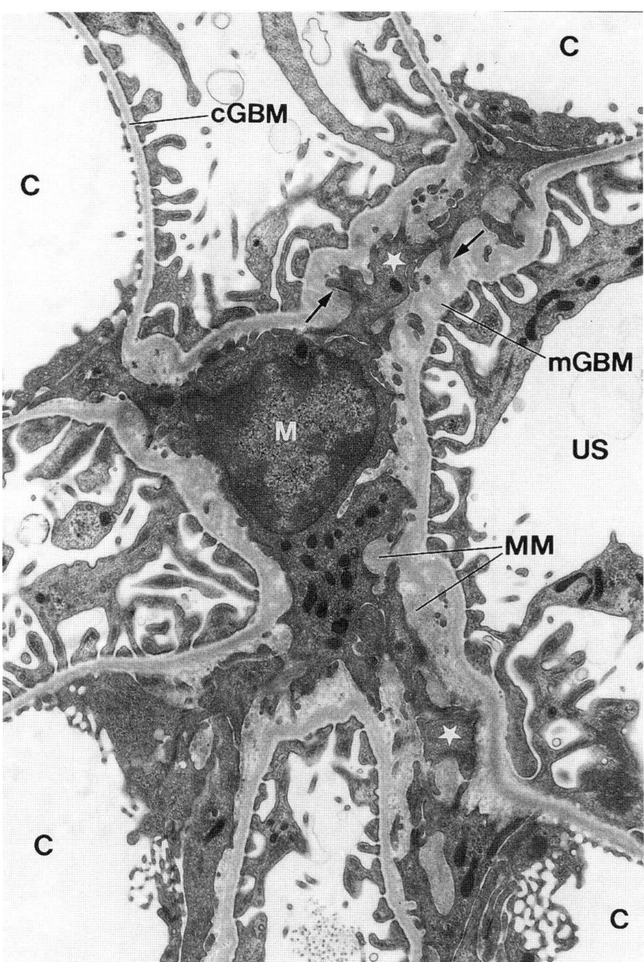

FIG. 22. Center of a glomerular lobule showing the axial position of a mesangial cell. The mesangial cell body (M) gives rise to several large processes (stars), which extend toward the peripherally located capillaries (C). Small finger-like processes are directed and attached to the perimesangial GBM (mGBM); they contain dense bundles of microfilaments (arrows). In contrast to the pericapillary GBM (cGBM), the mGBM is folded in many places. Note the mesangial matrix (MM). US, urinary space. TEM. Magnification ×8,800.

ing several types of collagens (III, IV, V, and VI), as well as several components of microfibrillar proteins (fibrillin, MAGP, MP78, MP340). The matrix also contains several glycoproteins (fibronectin is most densely accumulated) as well as several types of proteoglycans, including the small protoglycans biglycan and decorin.

The basic ultrastructural organization of the matrix is a network of microfibrils. In specimens prepared for transmission electron microscopy (TEM) by routine methods, a fine filamentous network is seen that possibly corresponds to the collagenous microfibrils. In specimens prepared by a technique that avoids osmium tetroxide and uses tannic acid for staining, the mesangial matrix has been observed to contain a dense network of elastic microfibrils. These structures are unbranched, noncollagenous, tubular structures that have an indefinite length and are of a diameter of about 15 nm. This dense three-dimensional network of microfibrils establishes a functionally continuous medium anchoring the mesangial cells to the GBM (83).

Endothelium

Glomerular endothelial cells consist of cell bodies (generally located close to the mesangial axis) and peripherally located attenuated and highly fenestrated cytoplasmic sheets (Figs. 15 and 18–20). Unlike fenestrated endothelia at other sites of the body, glomerular endothelial pores lack a diaphragm and are virtually open (Figs. 21 and 23). Pores bridged by diaphragms in glomerular capillaries are only found along the outflow segment of the efferent arteriole (67). The round to oval pores have a diameter of 50–100 nm. The luminal membrane of endothelial cells is negatively charged due to its cell coat of several polyanionic glycoproteins, including podocalyxin (84).

Endothelial cells are active participants in the processes controlling coagulation, inflammation, and immune processes. Renal endothelial cells share an antigen system with cells of the monocyte/macrophage lineage; they express surface antigens of the class II histocompatibility antigens. Glomerular endothelial cells synthesize and release endothelin-1 and endothelium-derived relaxing factor (85–87).

Visceral Epithelium

The visceral epithelium of Bowman's capsule consists of highly differentiated cells, the podocytes (Figs. 15, 18, 20, and 23). In the developing glomerulus, podocytes are of a simple polygonal shape. In rats, mitotic activity of these cells is completed soon after birth, along with the cessation of the formation of new nephron anlagen. In humans this point is reached during prenatal life (88). Differentiated podocytes appear to be unable to replicate; thus, in the adult, degenerated podocytes cannot be replaced. In response to an extreme mitogenic stimulation (e.g., by a basic fibroblast growth factor, FGF-2), the nucleus of these cells may undergo mitotic division; however, the cells are unable to complete cell division, resulting in bi- or multinucleated cells (89). Those multinucleated cells may be regarded as extreme forms of cell hypertrophy; they generally exhibit maladaptive changes.

Podocytes have a voluminous cell body, which bulges into the urinary space (Figs. 18, 23, and 24). The cells give rise to long primary processes that extend toward the capillaries to which they attach by numerous foot processes (including the most distal portions of primary processes). The foot processes of neighboring podocytes

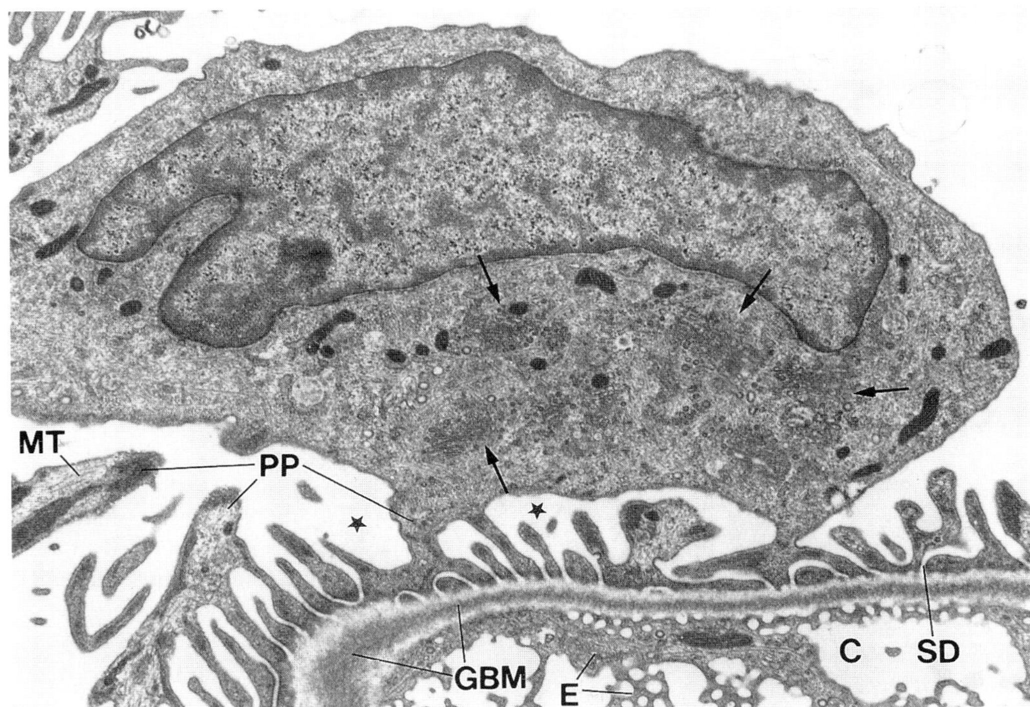

FIG. 23. Section of a podocyte and the filtration barrier. The major cell body is elevated from the GBM. The base of the epithelium consists of the interdigitating pattern of cell processes, which are attached to the GBM. Note the sub–cell body space *(stars)*. The cell body contains a large nucleus with indentations and a well-developed Golgi apparatus *(arrows)*. Numerous microtubules (MT) extend from the cell body into the primary processes (PP). Due to the slightly oblique section plane, the slit diaphragms (SD) between the foot processes are difficult to see. The slit diaphragm represents the border between the apical membrane domain (encircling the cell body and upper parts of the processes) and the basal membrane domain (restricted to the sole plates of the foot processes). C, capillary lumen; E, oblique section of the fenestrated endothelium. TEM. Magnification ×13,000.

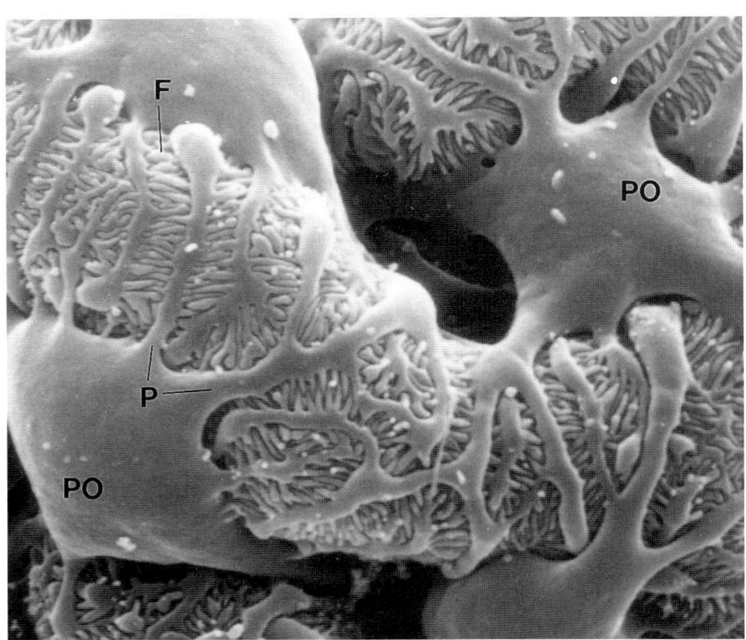

FIG. 24. Scanning electron micrograph of rat glomerular capillaries. The urinary side of the capillary is covered by the highly branched cells (podocytes, PO) of the visceral layer. The interdigitating system of primary (P) and secondary (F) processes lines the entire surface of the tuft and also proceeds beneath the cell bodies (see Fig. 23). The foot processes (F) of neighboring cells interdigitate regularly, sparing the filtration slits in between. Magnification ×7,000.

regularly interdigitate whith each other, leaving between them meandering slits (filtration slits), that are bridged by an extracellular structure, the so-called slit diaphragm (Figs. 21, 23, and 24).

Podocytes are polarized epithelial cells with a luminal and a basal cell membrane domain; the latter corresponds to the sole plates of the foot processes, which are embedded in the GBM. The border between basal and luminal membrane is represented by the slit diaphragm.

The luminal membrane and the slit diaphragm are covered by a thick surface coat rich in sialoglycoproteins (including podocalyxin, podoendin, and others), which are responsible for the highly negative surface charge of the podocytes (84,88,90). At variance to the luminal membrane, the abluminal membrane contains N-acetyl-D-galactosamine residues of glycoconjugates (91) and two podocyte-specific proteins (92,93). Other membrane proteins, such as the C3b-receptor (94) and glycoprotein 330/megalin (95), are present on the entire surface of podocytes. Megalin, a glycoprotein of 330 kDa (96), is a major podocyte antigen of rat Heymann nephritis. It is associated with the endoplasmic reticulum and Golgi apparatus and, at the cell surface, with coated pits.

The cell body contains a prominent nucleus, a well-developed Golgi system, abundant rough and smooth endoplasmic reticulum, prominent lysosomes, and many mitochondria (Fig. 23). In contrast to the cell body, the cell processes contain only a few organelles. The density of organelles in the cell body indicates a high level of anabolic as well as catabolic activity. In addition to the work necessary to sustain structural integrity of these specialized cells, most if not all components of the GBM are synthesized by podocytes (97).

A well-developed cytoskeleton accounts for the complex shape of the cells. In the cell body and the primary processes, microtubules and intermediate filaments (vimentin, desmin) dominate, whereas microfilaments are densely accumulated in the foot processes (80) (Figs. 21, 23, and 25). In the cell body and the primary processes, actin-containing microfilaments are seen as a thin layer underlying the apical cell membrane. In the foot processes the prominent bundles of microfilaments are arranged in the longitudinal axis of foot processes. At the transition to the primary processes, the microfilament bundles form loops roughly parallel to the turning point of the slit and extend into the adjacent process of the same cell. Peripherally they appear to anchor in the dense cytoplasm associated with the basal cell membrane of podocytes, i.e., the sole plates of foot processes (Figs. 21 and 25) (98). Anchoring of the sole plates to the GBM is achieved by a specific $\alpha3\beta1$ integrin (rat) (75,76). Within the cytoplasm, integrins interact with the cytoskeletal proteins talin and vinculin.

The filtration slits are the sites of convective fluid flow through the visceral epithelium. They have the constant width of about 30 to 40 nm. The structure and biochemical composition of the slit membrane is unknown. Chemically fixed and tannic acid–treated tissue show a zipperlike structure with a row of pores of approximately 4×14 nm on either side of a central bar (99). Little is known about proteins making up this structure. In addition to a 51-kDa protein localized in the slit membrane (100,101), the ZO-1 protein was found at the insertion sites of the slit membrane to the cell membrane (102).

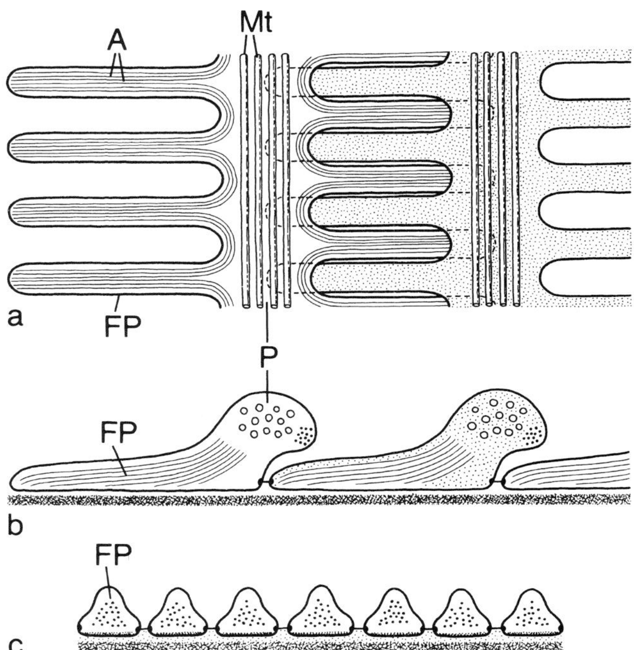

FIG. 25. Arrangement of cytoskeletal elements in podocyte processes. View from above (**a**) and section of foot processes parallel (**b**) and perpendicular to (**c**) the longitudinal axis of foot processes. Two major processes (one stippled, one blank) with their foot processes are shown. The actin filaments (A) of foot processes form continuous loops that end in the foot process sole plates. At their bend they are in close association with microtubules (MT) that run longitudinally in the major processes. Modified with permission (98).

The surface charge of podocytes contributes to the maintenance of the interdigitating pattern of the foot processes. In response to neutralization of the surface charge by cationic substances (e.g., protamin sulfate), the foot processes retract, and tight junctions may be formed between adjacent foot processes (103).

Parietal Epithelium

The parietal layer of Bowman's capsule consists of squamous epithelial cells resting on a basement membrane (Figs. 15–17 and 20). The flat cells are polygonal, with a central cilium and few microvilli. Parietal cells are filled with bundles of actin filaments coursing in all directions around the glomerulus (104).

The basement membrane is, at variance to the GBM, composed of several dense layers that are separated by translucent layers and contain bundles of fibrils (microligaments) (105). Recent studies suggest a role of type XIV collagen in the organization of the multilayered basement membrane of Bowman's capsule (106). In contrast to the GBM, the predominant proteoglycan of this basement membrane is a chondroitin sulfate proteoglycan (71).

The transition from the GBM to the basement membrane of Bowman's capsule borders the glomerular entrance. This transitional region is mechanically connected to the smooth muscle cells of the afferent and efferent arterioles as well as to extraglomerular mesangial cells.

Filtration Barrier

Filtration through the glomerular capillary wall occurs along an extracellular pathway including the endothelial pores, the GBM, and the slit diaphragms between the podocyte foot processes (Fig. 21). All of these components may be quite permeable for water; thus, the high permeability for water, small solutes, and ions is based on the fact that no cell membranes are interposed. The hydraulic conductance of the individual layers of the filtration barrier is difficult to study. In a mathematical model of glomerular filtration, the hydraulic resistance of the endothelium was predicted to be small, whereas the GBM and filtration slits contribute roughly one half each to the total hydraulic resistance of the capillary wall (107).

The barrier function of the glomerular capillary wall for macromolecules is selective for size, shape, and charge (108,109). The charge selectivity of the barrier is based on the dense accumulation of negatively charged molecules throughout the entire depth of the filtration barrier, including the surface coat of endothelial and epithelial cells and the high content of negatively charged heparan sulfate proteoglycans in the GBM. Polyanionic macromolecules, such as plasma proteins, are repelled by the electronegative shield originating from the dense assemblies of negative charges. Removal or blocking of the negative charge in experimental models results in proteinuria (79).

The size selectivity of the filtration barrier is in part established by the dense network of the GBM. However, the most restrictive part appears to be the slit diaphragm. Uncharged macromolecules up to an effective radius of 1.8 nm pass freely through the filter. Larger components are more and more restricted (indicated by their fractional clearances, which progressively decrease) and are totally restricted at effective radii of more than 4.0 nm. Effective radius is an empirical value measured in artificial membranes that takes into account the shape of macromolecules and attributes a radius to nonspherical molecules. Plasma albumin has an effective radius of 3.6 nm; without the repulsion due to the negative charge, plasma albumin would pass through the filter in considerable amounts (110).

The crucial importance of the slit diaphragm for size selectivity has been proven by means of experiments with feritin. Although native anionic ferritin particles accumulate at the level of endothelial fenestrae and within the subendothelial space, the cationized form of ferritin penetrates the lamina densa and accumulates beneath the slit diaphragm. Thus, the more proximal parts of the barrier are more responsible for charge selectivity, whereas the terminal slit diaphragm is the most important part for size selectivity (107).

Stability of the Glomerular Tuft

The main challenge to glomerular capillaries is to combine selective leakiness with stability. The walls of glomerular capillaries do not look as if they could resist high transmural pressure gradients. It appears that several structures/mechanisms are involved in counteracting the distending forces to which the capillary wall is constantly exposed. The locus of action of all these forces is the GBM, a tough collagenous mat that fulfills a skeletal function in the glomerulus.

Two systems appear to be responsible for the development of stabilizing forces (83,111). A basic system consists of the GBM and the mesangium. Cylinders of the GBM in fact largely define the shape of glomerular capillaries. However, these cylinders do not completely encircle the capillary tube; they are open toward the mesangium. Mechanically, they are completed by contractile mesangial cell processes that bridge the gaps of the GBM by interconnecting opposing mesangial angles (Figs. 18, 19). Moreover, throughout the mesangium, opposing portions of the GBM are bridged by contractile mesangial cell processes generating inwardly directed forces that balance the expansile forces resulting from pressure gradients across the GBM (83,111).

Podocytes act as a second structure-stabilizing system superimposed on the mesangium–GBM system. Two mechanisms appear to be involved. First, podocytes stabilize the folding pattern of glomerular capillaries by fixing the turning points of the GBM between neighboring capillaries. Podocytes are generally attached to several capillaries via their foot and primary processes. However, cytoskeletal elements passing from one major process through the cell body into other major processes are not a prominent feature. Thus, the arrangement of the cytoskeleton in the podocyte as a whole does not suggest that a single podocyte would be able to establish a strong mechanical linkage among the group of capillaries to

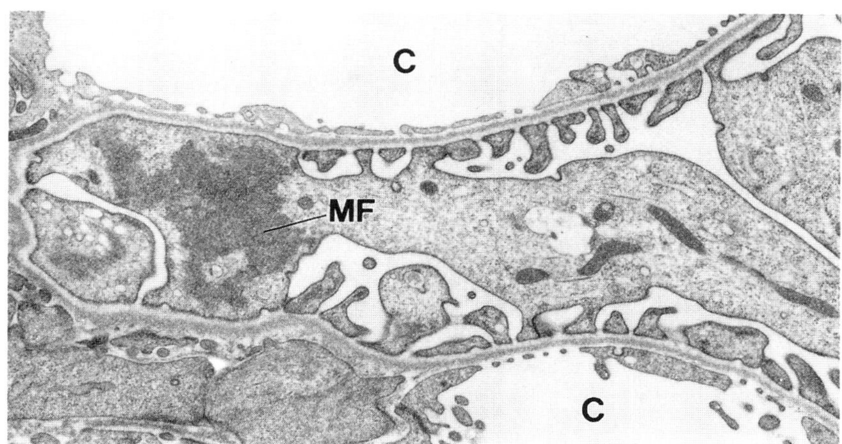

FIG. 26. Part of a podocyte process in the rat filling the angle between two adjacent capillary loops (C). The cytoplasm is densely filled with actin filaments (MF). By interconnecting opposing parts of the GBM, such process portions appear to stabilize the folding pattern of the capillary network. TEM. Magnification ×13,100.

which its processes attach. On the other hand, the narrow angles between neighboring capillaries are frequently filled out by terminal portions attaching to the GBM, when the latter passes over from one capillary to the neighboring capillary. These terminal process portions contain a densely developed cytoskeleton of microfilaments (Fig. 26). Thus, by interconnection of the opposing parts of the GBM at such niches, they may effectively contribute to the maintenance of the GBM folding pattern and thus to the capillary pattern (88).

Secondly, podocytes may contribute to structural stability of glomerular capillaries by a mechanism comparable with that of pericytes elsewhere in the body. Podocytes are attached to the GBM by foot processes that cover almost entirely the outer aspect of the GBM (Figs. 15, 19, and 23). Podocyte foot processes possess a well developed contractile system (actin, alpha-actinin, myosin) arranged longitudinally in each foot process (80,89, 112) (Fig. 21). By way of intermediate proteins (vinculin, talin) and membrane-spanning integrins ($\alpha3\beta1$ integrin has specifically been localized at this site), this system attaches tightly to collagen IV, fibronectin, and laminin of the GBM (75,113). Because podocyte foot processes are attached in various angles on the GBM, they may function as numerous small, stabilizing patches on the GBM, counteracting locally the elastic distension of the GBM. To illustrate the possible effect of such a system, imagine a simple air balloon on the outer surface of which stripes of a less expandable material are firmly fixed. When the balloon is blown up, the distension of just the areas covered with the stripes will be delayed. Thus, the mechanical relevance of podocyte foot processes might simply be that the GBM will never approach its tensile strength limit (114,115). However, because the rigidity of podocyte foot processes is based on a contractile system, the actual tone of this system may be subject to regulation and might influence the strength of the total elastic restoring forces of the capillary wall.

JUXTAGLOMERULAR APPARATUS

The juxtaglomerular apparatus is situated at the vascular pole of the glomerulus. It comprises (a) the macula densa, (b) the extraglomerular mesangium, and (c) the terminal portion of the afferent arteriole with its renin-producing granular cells as well as the beginning of the efferent arteriole (Figs. 15–17).

The macula densa is a plaque of specialized cells in the wall of the thick ascending limb at the site where it is affixed to the extraglomerular mesangium of the parent glomerulus. The most obvious structural feature are the large narrowly packed cell nuclei, which accounts for the name macula densa (116).

In contrast to other parts of the thick ascending limb, the macula densa cells do not interdigitate with each other but have a polygonal outline. The luminal cell membrane is densely studded by stubby microvilli and bears one cilium. At the basis, the cells display numerous infoldings of the plasma membrane. Narrow basal plasma membrane folds are anchored to the underlying basement membrane, blending with the matrix of the extraglomerular mesangium (2). The lateral membrane of macula densa cells bears folds and microvilli that are frequently connected to those of neighboring cells by desmosomes. Near the apex the cells are joined by tight junctions consisting of several parallel junctional strands, similar to those in other parts of the thick ascending limb. The cells contain the usual cytoplasmic organelles, comprising some small mitochondria, Golgi apparatus, and smooth endoplasmic reticulum; free ribosomes are abundant, but rough endoplasmic reticulum is rare. Few small lysosomes may be encountered in the apical cell portion.

The lateral intercellular spaces are a prominent feature of the macula densa. Electron microscopic studies and studies on isolated macula densa segments in vitro have shown that the width of the lateral intercellular spaces varies under different functional conditions (117,118). In agreement with the suggestion that water flow through the macula densa epithelium is secondary to active sodium reabsorption, compounds such as furosemide, which blocks sodium transport, as well as high osmolalities of impermeable solutes such as mannitol, are associated with narrowing of the intercellular spaces (117,119). The spaces are apparently dilated under most physiological conditions, usually regarded as normal control conditions. The most conspicuous immunocytochemical difference of macula densa cells to any other epithelial cell of the nephron is the high content of nitric oxide synthase I (120).

At the vascular pole of the glomerulus, the mesangium passes through the opening of Bowman's capsule and continues into the extraglomerular mesangium (121), also called lacis cells or the Goormaghtigh cell field (Figs. 15–17). The extraglomerular mesangium represents a solid complex of cells and matrix that is neither penetrated by blood vessels nor lymphatic capillaries.

The extraglomerular mesangium is located in the cone-shaped space between the two glomerular arterioles and the macula densa cells of the thick ascending limb and, laterally, faces the renal interstitium. Extraglomerular mesangial cells are flat and elongated, separating into bunches of long cell processes at their poles (122). The cells are embedded in extraglomerular mesangial matrix. At variance to the intraglomerular mesangial matrix, microfibrils are only rarely found. Affixation of macula densa cells to the extraglomerular mesangium appears to be mediated by β6-integrin, which is known to associate with av to form the fibronectin binding heterodimer αvβ6 (123).

Although direct evidence is lacking, extraglomerular mesangial cells can be expected to be contractile for several reasons. First, in their processes, they contain prominent bundles of microfilaments containing F-actin. Second, like intraglomerular mesangial cells, they have strong structural similarities with arteriolar smooth muscle cells and granular cells, suggesting that they are all of the same origin. Third, these cells are all extensively coupled by gap junctions (124,125).

The contractile processes of extraglomerular mesangial cells are connected to the basement membrane of Bowman's capsule and to the walls of both glomerular arterioles. As a whole, the extraglomerular mesangium interconnects all structures of the glomerular entrance. The extraglomerular mesangium can be regarded as a closure device of the glomerular entrance, maintaining its structural integrity against the distending forces exerted to the entrance by the high intraarteriolar and intraglomerular pressure.

The granular cells are assembled in clusters within the terminal portion of the afferent arteriole, replacing ordinary smooth muscle cells (Figs. 16, 17, and 27). Their name refers to the specific cytoplasmic granules, which are dark, membrane-bound, and irregular in size and shape. Renin, the major secretion product, is stored in the

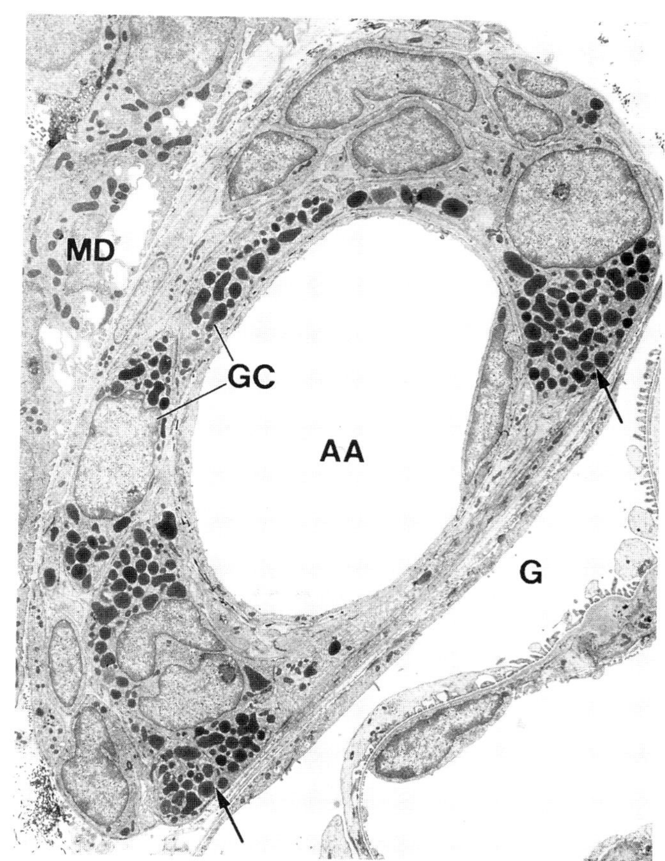

FIG. 27. Afferent arteriole near the vascular pole. In the end portion of the afferent arteriole (AA) several smooth muscle cells (SMC) are replaced by granular cells (GC) containing noticeable accumulations of renin granules *(arrows)*. G, glomerulus; MD, cells of the macula densa. TEM. Magnification ×2,700.

dark amorphous granules. Small granules with crystalline substructure represent protogranules containing both renin prosegment and mature renin. Renin release occurs by exocytosis into the surrounding interstitium (126).

Granular cells are modified smooth muscle cells. Under conditions requiring enhanced renin synthesis (e.g., volume depletion or stenosis of the renal artery), additional smooth muscle cells located upstream in the wall of the afferent arteriole (and of the cortical radial artery) may transform into granular cells (126,127). Granular cells are connected to the extraglomerular mesangial cells, to adjacent smooth muscle cells, and to endothelial cells by gap junctions, and are densely innervated by sympathetic nerve terminals (126).

The structural organization of the juxtaglomerular apparatus suggests a regulatory function. Goormaghtigh (128) was the first to propose that some component of the distal urine is sensed by the macula densa, and this information is used to adjust the tonus of the glomerular arterioles, thereby producing a change in glomerular blood flow and filtration rate. Even if many details of this mechanism are still subject to debate, the essence of this hypothesis has been verified by many studies and is known as the tubular glomerular feedback mechanism (129). In addition, the juxtaglomerular apparatus seems to be the main site of regulation of renin secretion; this is not only of local but apparently also of systemic relevance. It is widely believed that the extraglomerular mesangium receives signals from the macula densa, modulating and transferring them to the renin-producing granular cells and the smooth muscle cells of the glomerular arterioles.

REFERENCES

1. Smith HW. *The kidney: structure and function in health and disease.* New York: Oxford University Press; 1951.
2. Kriz W, Kaissling B. Structural organization of the mammalian kidney. In: Seldin DW, Giebisch G, eds. *The kidney: physiology and pathophysiology*. New York: Raven; 1992:707–777.
3. Kaissling B, Kriz W. Morphology of the loop of Henle, distal tubule and collecting duct. In: Windhager EE, ed. *Handbook of physiology: section on renal physiology*. New York: Oxford University Press; 1992:109–167.
4. Sabolic J, Brown D. Water channels in renal and nonrenal tissues. *News Physiol Sci* 1995;10:12–17.
5. Tisher CC, Brenner BM. Structure and function of the glomerulus. In: Tisher CC, Brenner BM, eds. *Renal pathology*. Philadelphia: JB Lippincott; 1989:92–110.
6. Fourman J, Moffat DB. *The blood vessels of the kidney*. Oxford: Blackwell Scientific, 1971.
7. Rollhäuser H, Kriz W, Heinke W. Das Gefässsystem der Rattenniere. *Z Zellforsch* 1964;64:381–403.
8. Lemley KV, Kriz W. Structure and function of the renal vasculature. In: Tisher CC, Brenner BM, eds. *Renal pathology*. Philadelphia: JB Lippincott; 1989:926–964.
9. Barajas L. Innervation of the renal cortex. *Fed Proc* 1978;37:1192–1201.
10. Kaissling B, Hegyi I, Loffing J, Le Hir M. Morphology of interstitial cells in the healthy kidney—review. *Anat Embryol* 1996;193:303–318.
11. Lemley KV, Kriz W. Anatomy of the renal interstitium. *Kidney Int* 1991;39:370–381.
12. Postlethwaite AE, Kang AH. Fibroblasts and matrix proteins. In: Gallin JI, Goldstein IM, Snyderman R, eds. *Inflammation: basic principles and clinical correlates*. New York: Raven; 1992:747–773.
13. Kuncio GS, Neilson EG, Haverty T. Mechanisms of tubulointerstitial fibrosis. *Kidney Int* 1991;39:550–556.
14. Strutz F, Okada H, Lo CW, et al. Identification and characterization of a fibroblast marker: FSP1. *J Cell Biol* 1995;130:393–405.
15. Fine LG, Norman JT, Ong A. Cell–cell cross-talk in the pathogenesis of renal interstitial fibrosis. *Kidney Int* 1995;47(suppl 49):S48–S50.
16. Takashi-Iwanaga H. The three-dimensional cytoarchitecture of the interstitial tissue in the rat kidney. *Cell Tissue Res* 1991;264:269–281.
17. Kaissling B, Le Hir M. Characterization and distribution of interstitial cell types in the renal cortex of rat. *Kidney Int* 1994;45:709–720.
18. Hashizume T, Imayama S, Hori Y. Scanning electron microscopic study on dendritic cells and fibroblasts in connective tissue. *J Electron Microsc* 1993;41:434–437.
19. Sappino AP, Schürch W, Gabbiani G. Different repertoire of fibroblastic cells: expression of cytoskeletal proteins as markers of phenotypic modulations. *Lab Invest* 1990;63:144–161.
20. Brouwer A, Wisse E, Knook DL. Sinusoidal endothelial cells and perisinusoidal fat-storing cells. In: Arias IM, Jakoby WB, Popper H, Schachter D, Shafritz DA, eds. *The liver: biology and pathobiology*. New York: Raven; 1988:665–682.
21. Bulger RE, Nagle RB. Ultrastructure of the interstitium in the rabbit kidney. *Am J Anat* 1973;136:183–204.
22. Alpers CE, Hudkins KL, Floege J, Johnson RJ. Human renal cortical interstitial cells with some features of smooth muscle cells participate in tubulointerstitial and crescentic glomerular injury. *J Am Soc Nephrol* 1994;5:201–210.
23. Squier CA, Bausch WH. Three-dimensional organization of fibroblasts and collagen fibrils in rat tail tendon. *Cell Tissue Res* 1984;238:319–327.
24. Schiller A, Taugner R. Junctions between interstitial cells of the renal medulla: A freeze-fracture study. *Cell Tissue Res* 1979;203:231–240.
25. Vyalov S, Desmouliere A, Gabbiani G. GM-CSF–induced granulation tissue formation: relationships between macrophage and myofibroblast accumulation. *Virchows Arch [B]* 1995;63:231–239.
26. Desmouliere A, Gabbiani G. Myofibroblast differentiation during fibrosis. *Exp Nephrol* 1995;3:134–139.
27. Diamond JR, Van Goor H, Ding G, Engelmyer E. Myofibroblasts in experimental hydronephrosis. *Am J Pathol* 1995;146:121–129.
28. Bellows CG, Melcher AH, Bhargava U, Aubin JE. Fibroblasts contracting three-dimensional collagen gels exhibit ultrastructure consistent with either contraction or protein secretion. *J Ultrastruct Res* 1982;78:178–192.
29. Rodemann HP, Müller GA, Knecht A, Norman JT, Fine LG. Fibroblasts of rabbit kidney in culture. I. Characterization and identification of cell-specific marker. *Am J Physiol* 1991;261:F283–F291.
30. Tisher CC, Madsen KM. Anatomy of the renal interstitium. In: Davison AM, Briggs JD, Green R, et al, eds. *Nephrology. Vol. 1. Proceedings of the Xth International Congress of Nephrology*. London: Bailliere Tindall; 1988:587–598.
31. Bohman S-O. The ultrastructure of the renal medulla and the interstitial cells. In: Mandal AK, Bohman S-O, eds. *The renal papilla and hypertension*. New York: Plenum; 1980:7–33.
32. Romen W, Thoenes W. Histiocytäre und fibrocytäre Eigenschaften der interstitiellen Zellen der Nierenrinde. *Virchows Arch [B]* 1970;5:365–375.
33. Austyn JM, Hankins DF, Larsen CP, Morris PJ, Rao AS, Roake JA. Isolation and characterization of dendritic cells from mouse heart and kidney. *J Histochem Cytochem* 1993;41:335–341.
34. Hart DNJ, Fabre JW. Major histocompatibility complex antigens in rat kidney, ureter, and bladder. *Transplantation* 1981;31:318–325.
35. Steinman RM. The dendritic cell system and its role in immunogenicity. *Ann Rev Immunol* 1991;9:271–296.
36. Knight SC, Stagg AJ. Antigen-presenting cell types. *Curr Opin Immunol* 1993;5:374–382.
37. Leczynsky D, Renkonen R, Häyry P. Localization and turnover rate of renal dendritic cells. *Am J Anat* 1985;21:355–360.
38. Stein-Oakley AN, Jablonski P, Kraft N, et al. Differential irradiation effects on rat interstitial dendritic cells. *Transplant Proc* 1991;23:632–634.
39. Steinman RM, Swanson J. The endocytic activity of dendritic cells. *J Exp Med* 1995;182:283–288.
40. Yamate J, Tatsumi M, Nakatsuji S, Kuwamura M, Kotani T, Sakuma S. Immunohistochemical observations on the kinetics of macrophages and myofibroblasts in rat renal interstitial fibrosis induced by cis-diamminedichloroplatinum. *J Comp Pathol* 1995;112:27–39.
41. Dijkstra CD, Döpp EA, Joling P, Kraal G. The heterogeneity of mononuclear phagocytes in lymphoid organs: distinct macrophage subpopulations in the rat recognized by mononuclear antibodies ED1, ED2, ED3. *Immunology* 1985;54:589–599.
42. Dawson TP, Gandhi R, Le Hir M, Kaissling B. Ecto-58-nucleotidase: Localization in rat kidney by light microscopic histochemical methods. *J Histochem Cytochem* 1989;37:39–47.
43. Gandhi R, Le Hir M, Kaissling B. Immunolocalization of ecto-58-nucleotidase in the kidney by a monoclonal antibody. *Histochemistry* 1990;95:165–174.
44. Le Hir M, Kaissling B. Distribution of 58-nucleotidase in the renal interstitium of the rat. *Cell Tissue Res* 1989;258:177–182.
45. Kurtz A, Eckhardt K-U, Neumann R, Kaissling B, Le Hir M, Bauer C. Site of erythropoietin formation. *Contrib Nephrol* 1989;76:14–23.
46. Kaissling B, Spiess S, Rinne B, Le Hir M. Effects of anemia on the morphology of the renal cortex of rats. *Am J Physiol* 1993;264:F608–F617.
47. Le Hir M, Kaissling B. Distribution of 5' nucleotidase in fibroblasts of cortical labyrinth of rat kidney. *Renal Physiol Biochem* 1989;12:313–319.
48. Le Hir M, Eckardt KU, Kaissling B, Koury ST, Kurtz A. Structure–function correlations in erythropoietin formation and oxygen sensing in the kidney. *Klin Wochenschr* 1991;69:567–575.

49. Le Hir M, Kaissling B. Distribution and regulation of renal ecto-5' nucleotidase: implications for physiological functions of adenosine. *Am J Physiol* 1993;264:F377–F387.
50. Bachmann S, Le Hir M, Eckardt K-U. Co-localization of erythropoietin mRNA and ecto-58-nucleotidase immunoreactivity in peritubular cells of rat renal cortex indicates that fibroblasts produce erythropoietin. *J Histochem Cytochem* 1993;41:335–341.
51. Maxwell PH, Osmond MK, Pugh CW, et al. Identification of the renal erythropoietin-producing cells using transgenic mice. *Kidney Int* 1993;44:1149–1162.
52. Spielman WS, Arend LJ. Adenosine receptors and signaling in the kidney. *Hypertension* 1991;17:117–130.
53. Kriz W. A periarterial pathway for intrarenal distribution of renin. *Kidney Int* 1987;31, Suppl 20:S–51–S–56.
54. Gorgas K. Structure and innervation of the juxtaglomerular apparatus of the rat. *Adv Anat Embryol Cell Biol* 1978;54:5–84.
55. Fourman J. The adrenergic innervation of the efferent arterioles and the vasa recta in the mammalian kidney. *Experientia* 1970;26: 293–294.
56. Kriz W, Dieterich HJ. Das Lymphgefäss system der Niere bei einigen Säugetieren. Licht-und elektronenmikroskopische Untersuchungen. *Z Anat Entwicklungsgesch* 1970;131:111–147.
57. Pfaller W. Structure function correlation in rat kidney. Quantitative correlation of structure and function in the normal and injured rat kidney. *Adv Anat Embryol Cell Biol* 1982;70:1–106.
58. Knepper MA, Danielson RA, Saidel GM, Post RS. Quantitative analysis of renal medullary anatomy in rats and rabbits. *Kidney Int* 1977;12:313–323.
59. Bulger RE, Trump BF. Fine structure of the rat renal papilla. *Am J Anat* 1966;118:685–722.
60. Nagano M, Ishimura K, Fujita H. Fine structural study on the development of the renal medullary interstitial cells (known to secrete antihypertensive factors) of Wistar Kyoto as well as spontaneously hypertensive rats. *J Electron Microsc* 1988;21:223–233.
61. Sundelin B, Bohmann S-O. Postnatal development of the interstitial tissue of the rat kidney. *Anat Embryol* 1990;182:307–317.
62. Muirhead EE. The medullipin system of blood pressure control. *Am J Hypertens* 1991;4(suppl):S556–S568.
63. Zusman RM, Keiser HR. Prostaglandin biosynthesis by rabbit renomedullary interstitial cells in tissue culture. *J Clin Invest* 1977; 60:215–223.
64. Vernace MA, Mento PF, Maita ME, et al. Osmolar regulation of endothelin signaling in rat medullary interstitial cells. *J Clin Invest* 1995;96:183–191.
65. Hughes AK, Barry WH, Kohan DE. Identification of a contractile function for renal medullary interstitial cells. *J Clin Invest* 1995;96: 411–416.
66. Winkler D, Elger M, Sakai T, Kriz W. Branching and confluence pattern of glomerular arterioles in the rat. *Kidney Int* 1991;39(suppl 32): S2–S8.
67. Elger M, Sakai T, Winkler D, Kriz W. Structure of the outflow segment of the efferent arteriole in rat superficial glomeruli. *Contrib Nephrol* 1991;95:22–33.
68. Reale E, Luciano L. The laminae rarae of the glomerular basement membrane. *Contr Nephrol* 1990;80:32–40.
69. Inoue S. Ultrastructural architecture of basement membranes. *Contrib Nephrol* 1994;107:21–28.
70. Timpl R, Dziadek M. Structure, development, and molecular pathology of basement membranes. *Int Rev Exp Pathol* 1986;29:1–112.
71. Couchman JR, Beavan LA, McCarthy KJ. Glomerular matrix: synthesis, turnover and role in mesangial expansion. *Kidney Int* 1994;45: 328–335.
72. Sanes JR, Engvall E, Butkowski R, Hunter DD. Molecular heterogeneity of basal laminae: isoforms of laminin and type IV collagen at the neuromuscular junction and elsewhere. *J Cell Biol* 1990;111: 1685–1699.
73. Tryggvason K. Molecular properties and diseases of collagens. *Kidney Int* 1995;47(suppl 49):24–28.
74. Katz A, Fish A, Kleppel MM, Hagen SG, Michael AF, Butkowski RJ. Renal entactin (nidogen): isolation, characterization and tissue distribution. *Kidney Int* 1991;40:643–652.
75. Adler S. Characterization of glomerular epithelial cell matrix receptors. *Am J Pathol* 1992;141:571–578.
76. Cybulsky AV, Carbonetto S, Huang Q, McTavish AJ, Cyr M-D. Adhesion of rat glomerular epithelial cells to extracellular matrices: role of β1 integrins. *Kidney Int* 1992;42:1099–1106.
77. Kanwar YS. Biology of disease. Biophysiology of glomerular filtration and proteinuria. *Lab Invest* 1984;51:7–21.
78. Noonan DM, Fulle A, Valente P, et al. The complete sequence of perlecan, a basement membrane heparan sulfate proteoglycan, reveals extensive similarity with laminin a chain, low density lipoprotein-receptor, and the neural cell adhesion molecule. *J Biol Chem* 1991;266: 22939–22947.
79. Farquhar MG. The glomerular basement membrane: a selective macromolecular filter. *Matrix*. New York: Plenum Press, 365–418.
80. Drenckhahn D, Franke RP. Ultrastructural organization of contractile and cytoskeletal proteins in glomerular podocytes of chicken, rat, and man. *Lab Invest* 1988;59:673–682.
81. Sakai T, Kriz W. The structural relationship between mesangial cells and basement membrane of the renal glomerulus. *Anat Embryol* 1987;176:373–386.
82. Kriz W, Elger M, Lemley KV, Sakai T. Mesangial cell–glomerular basement membrane connections counteract glomerular capillary and mesangium expansion. *Am J Nephrol* 1990;10(suppl 1):4–13.
83. Kriz W, Elger M, Mundel P, Lemley KV. Structure-stabilizing forces in the glomerular tuft. *J Am Soc Nephrol* 1995;5:1731–1739.
84. Sawada H, Stukenbrok H, Kerjaschki D, Farquhar MG. Epithelial polyanion (podocalyxin) is found on the sides but not the soles of the foot processes of the glomerular epithelium. *Am J Pathol* 1986;125: 309–318.
85. Ott MJ, Olson JL, Ballermann BJ. Phenotypic differences between glomerular capillary (GE) and aortic (AE) endothelial cells in vitro [Abstract]. *J Am Soc Nephrol* 1993;4:564.
86. Wiggins RC, Fantone J, Phan SH. Mechanisms of vascular injury. In: Tisher CC, Brenner BM, eds. *Renal pathology*. Philadelphia: JB Lippincott; 1989:965–993.
87. Savage COS. The biology of the glomerulus: endothelial cells. *Kidney Int* 1994;45:314–319.
88. Mundel P, Kriz W. Structure and function of podocytes: an update. *Anat Embryol* 1995;192:385–397.
89. Kriz W, Hähnel B, Rösener S, Elger M. Long-term treatment of rats with FGF-2 results in focal segmental glomerulosclerosis. *Kidney Int* 1995;48:1435–1450.
90. Huang TW, Langlois JC. Podoendin. A new cell surface protein of the podocyte and endothelium. *J Exp Med* 1985;162:245–267.
91. Roth J, Brown D, Orci L. Regional distribution of N-acetyl-D-galactosamine residues in the glycocalyx of glomerular podocytes. *J Cell Biol* 1983;96:1189–1196.
92. Cittanova ML, Chatelet F, Ardaillou N, Galceran M, Verroust P, Ronco R. Identification of a 135 kD protein expressed at the sole of human podocyte foot processes and on the human podocyte clonal cell line HGVEC.SV1A4. *J Am Soc Nephrol* 1992;3:579.
93. Tissari J, Holthöfer H, Miettinen A. Novel 13 a antigen is an integral protein of the basolateral membrane of rat glomerular podocytes [Abstract]. *Lab Invest* 1994;71:519–527.
94. Kazatchkine MD, Fearon DT, Appay MD, Mandet C, Bariety J. Immunohistochemical study of the human glomerular C3b receptor in normal kidney and in seventy-five cases of renal diseases. *J Clin Invest* 1982;69:900–912.
95. Kerjaschki D, Farquhar MG. Immunocytochemical localization of the Heymann antigen (gp 330) in glomerular epithelial cells of normal Lewis rats. *J Exp Med* 1983;157:667–686.
96. Saito A, Pietromonaco S, Loo AK-C, Farquhar MG. Complete cloning and sequencing of rat gp330/"megalin," a distinctive member of the low density lipoprotein receptor gene family. *Proc Natl Acad Sci U S A* 1994;91:9725–9729.
97. Abrahamson DR. Structure and development of the glomerular capillary wall and basement membrane. *Am J Physiol* 1987;253:F783–F794.
98. Kriz W, Mundel P, Elger M. The contractile apparatus of podocytes is arranged to counteract GBM expansion. *Contrib Nephrol* 1994;107: 1–9.
99. Rodewald R, Karnovsky MJ. Porous substructure of the glomerular slit diophragm in the rat and mouse. *J Cell Biol* 1974;60:423–433.
100. Orikasa M, Matsui K, Oite T, Shimizu F. Massive proteinuria induced in rats by a single intravenous injection of a monoclonal antibody. *J Immunol* 1988;141:807–815.
101. Kawachi H, Abrahamson DR, St. John PL, et al. Developmental

expression of the nephritogenetic antigen of monoclonal antibody 5-1-6. *Am J Physiol* 1995;147:823–833.

102. Schnabel E, Anderson JM, Farquhar MG. The tight junction protein ZO-1 is concentrated along slit diaphragms of the glomerular epithelium. *J Cell Biol* 1990;111:1255–1263.
103. Andrews PM. Morphological alterations of the glomerular (visceral) epithelium in response to pathological and experimental situations. *J Electr Microsc Tech* 1988;9:115–144.
104. Pease DC. Myoid features of renal corpuscles and tubules. *J Ultrastruct Res* 1968;23:304–320.
105. Mbassa G, Elger M, Kriz W. The ultrastructural organization of the basement membrane of Bowman's capsule in the rat renal corpuscle. *Cell Tissue Res* 1988;253:151–163.
106. Lethias C, Aubert-Foucher E, Dublet B, et al. Structure, molecular assembly and tissue distribution of facit collagen molecules. *Contrib Nephrol* 1994;107:57–63.
107. Drumond MC, Deen WM. Structural determinants of glomerular hydraulic permeability. *Am J Physiol* 1994;266:F1–F12.
108. Daniels BS. The role of the glomerular epithelial cell in the maintenance of the glomerular filtration barrier. *Am J Nephrol* 1993;13: 318–323.
109. Daniels BS, Deen WM, Mayer G, Meyer T, Hostetter TH. Glomerular permeability barrier in the rat. *J Clin Invest* 1993;92:929–936.
110. Deen WM, Bohrer MP, Brenner BM. Macromolecule transport across glomerular capillaries: application of pore theory. *Kidney Int* 1979; 16:353–365.
111. Lemley KV, Elger M, Koeppen-Hagemann I, et al. The glomerular mesangium: capillary support function and its failure under experimental conditions. *Clin Invest* 1992;70:843–856.
112. Vasmant D, Maurice M, Feldmann G. Cytoskeleton ultrastructure of podocytes and glomerular endothelial cells in man and in the rat. *Anat Rec* 1984;210:17–24.
113. Kerjaschki D, Ojha PP, Susani M, et al. A β1-integrin receptor for fibronectin in human kidney glomeruli. *Am J Pathol* 1989;134: 481–489.
114. Welling LW, Grantham JJ. Physical properties of isolated perfused renal tubules and tubular basement membranes. *J Clin Invest* 1972; 51:1063–1075.
115. Welling LW, Zupka MT, Welling DJ. Mechanical properties of basement membrane. *News Physiol Sci* 1995;10:30–35.
116. Zimmermann KW. Ueber den Bau des Glomerulus der Saeugerniere. *Z Mikrosc Anat Forsch* 1933;32:176–278.
117. Kaissling B, Kriz W. Variability of intercellular spaces between macula densa cells: a transmission electron microscopic study in rabbits and rats. *Kidney Int* 1982;22(suppl 12):S9–S17.
118. Kirk KL, Bell PD, Barfuss DW, Ribadeneira M. Direct visualization of the isolated and perfused macula densa. *Am J Physiol* 1985;248: F890–F894.
119. Alcorn D, Anderson WP, Ryan GB. Morphological changes in the renal macula densa during natriuresis and diuresis. *Renal Physiol* 1986;9:335–347.
120. Mundel P, Bachmann S, Bader M, et al. Expression of nitric oxide synthase in kidney macula densa cells. *Kidney Int* 1992;42:1017–1019.
121. Barajas L, Salido EC, Smolens P, Hart D, Stein JH. Pathology of the juxtaglomerular apparatus including Bartter's syndrome. In: Tisher CC, Brenner BM, eds. *Renal pathology*. Philadelphia: JB Lippincott; 1989:877–912.
122. Spanidis A, Wunsch H. *Rekonstruktion einer Goormaghtigh'schen und einer Epitheloiden Zelle der Kaninchenniere* [Dissertation]. Heidelberg Universität; 1979.
123. Breuss JM, Gillett N, Lu L, Sheppard D, Pytela R. Restricted distribution of integrin 6 mRNA in primate epithelial tissue. *J Histochem Cytochem* 1993;41:1521–1527.
124. Pricam C, Humbert F, Perrelet A, Orci L. Gap junctions in mesangial and lacis cells. *J Cell Biol* 1974;63:349–354.
125. Taugner R, Schiller A, Kaissling B, Kriz W. Gap junctional coupling between the JGA and the glomerular tuft. *Cell Tissue Res* 1978;186: 279–285.
126. Taugner R, Hackenthal E. *The juxtaglomerular apparatus*. Berlin: Springer-Verlag, 1989.
127. Gomez RA, Chevalier RL, Everett AD, et al. Recruitment of renin gene-expressing cells in adult rat kidneys. *Am J Physiol* 1990;259: F660–F665.
128. Goormaghtigh N. L'appareil neuro-myo-artériel juxta-glomérulaire du rein: ses réactions en pathologie et ses rapports avec le tube urinifère. *C R Soc Biol* 1937;124:293–296.
129. Schnermann J, Briggs JP. The role of adenosine in cell-to-cell signaling in the juxtagomerular apparatus. *Semin Nephrol* 1993;13:236–245.
130. Beck FX, Dörge A, Rick R, Schramm M, Thurau K. The distribution of potassium, sodium and chloride across the apical membrane of renal tubular cells. Effects of acute metabolic alkalosis. *Pfluegers Arch* 1988;411:259–270.
131. Elger M, Kriz W. The renal glomerulus—the structural basis of ultrafiltration. In: Cameron S, Davison AM, Grünfeld J-P, Kerr D, Ritz E, eds. *Oxford textbook of clinical nephrology*. Oxford, England: Oxford University Press; 1992:129–141.

Immunologic Renal Diseases,
edited by E. G. Neilson and W. G. Couser.
Lippincott-Raven Publishers, Philadelphia © 1997

CHAPTER 3

Glomerular Filtration

Valentina Kon and Iekuni Ichikawa

The essential function of the kidney is to preserve constancy of body fluids by removing water and potentially harmful metabolic end-products, such as urea, uric acid, sulfates, and phosphates. The kidneys also maintain constancy of the internal environment by preserving blood pressure and the essential solutes, including sodium, chloride, bicarbonate, sugars, and amino acids. This process begins at the glomerulus, where plasma is ultrafiltered under pressure through the semipermeable glomerular capillary wall. The ultrafiltration separates plasma water and crystalloids from blood cells and protein macromolecules, which remain in the circulation. The magnitude of this process is enormous. Thus, glomerular filtration processes some 180 L, or about four to five times the total body water, each day. Assessment of glomerular filtration rate (GFR) is the single most important measurement of renal function.

WHOLE KIDNEY GFR

Number of Nephrons

The whole kidney GFR is determined by the number of individual filtering nephrons in both kidneys and the level of filtration in individual nephron units. Previous estimates were 1,000,000 nephrons in each adult kidney, but recent careful, unbiased stereologic methods indicate that this number is, on average, 617,000 glomeruli (1). In the absence of disease, this number is expected to remain constant until late in life. In humans, new nephron formation is complete by about 36 weeks of gestation. Thereafter, there is no reactivation of nephronogenesis, even after extensive loss of renal parenchyma. Therefore, an increase in the total GFR reflects enhanced filtration in individual glomeruli. Conversely, unless there is surgical or traumatic loss of nephrons, a decrease in total GFR reflects a reduction in the rate of filtration in individual glomeruli. An important exception occurs during the normal aging process, in which glomeruli are lost due to scarring (see below). It is also important to recognize the specific situation in kidneys undergoing chronic disease processes. In this setting, nephrons are characterized by extreme heterogeneity in both structure and function, with some glomeruli having no filtration and other glomeruli having compensatory hyperfiltration. On the whole kidney level, the GFR in this setting reflects the sum of highly variable levels of single-nephron GFR (SNGFR) and does not represent a uniform or even directionally similar change in function in any specific population of glomeruli.

V. Kon and I. Ichikawa: Division of Pediatric Nephrology, Department of Pediatrics, Vanderbilt University, Nashville, Tennessee 37232.

Determinants of SNGFR

Glomerular ultrafiltration proceeds under hydraulic pressure through a semipermeable glomerular capillary wall. Qualitatively, the forces are identical to those occurring in other systemic capillary beds. However, quantitatively, the glomerular ultrafiltration forces are different and ensure the stunning magnitude of plasma ultrafiltration. The rate of fluid flux across a unit capillary wall (J_v) is described by the following equation:

$$\begin{aligned} J_v &= k\,(\Delta P - \Delta\pi) \\ &= k\,[(P_{GC} - P_{BS}) - (p_{GC} - \pi_{BS})], \end{aligned}$$

where k represents the permeability coefficient of the glomerular capillary wall and ΔP is the transcapillary hydraulic pressure difference, i.e., the difference between glomerular capillary hydraulic pressure (P_{GC}) and Bowman's space hydraulic pressure (P_{BS}). $\Delta\pi$ is the transcapillary oncotic pressure difference, or the difference between glomerular capillary oncotic pressure (π_{GC}) and Bowman's space oncotic pressure (π_{BS}).

The mathematical model, developed to define the hemodynamics within the glomerular capillary bed, is based in part on experimental observations and in part on certain assumptions enumerated below (2–5). Because of its simplicity and applicability, the model is widely accepted. Thus:

1. Relative to the plasma protein concentration and, therefore, the oncotic pressure of glomerular capillary plasma, the corresponding values of glomerular filtrates are extremely small and taken to be zero, i.e., $\pi_{BS} = 0$.
2. Permeability of the glomerular capillary to water is constant along the length of the glomerular capillary.
3. The hydraulic pressure decrease along the glomerular capillary is negligible.
4. Oncotic pressure of the glomerular plasma can be calculated from the protein concentration using the Landis-Pappenheimer equation (least-square fit).

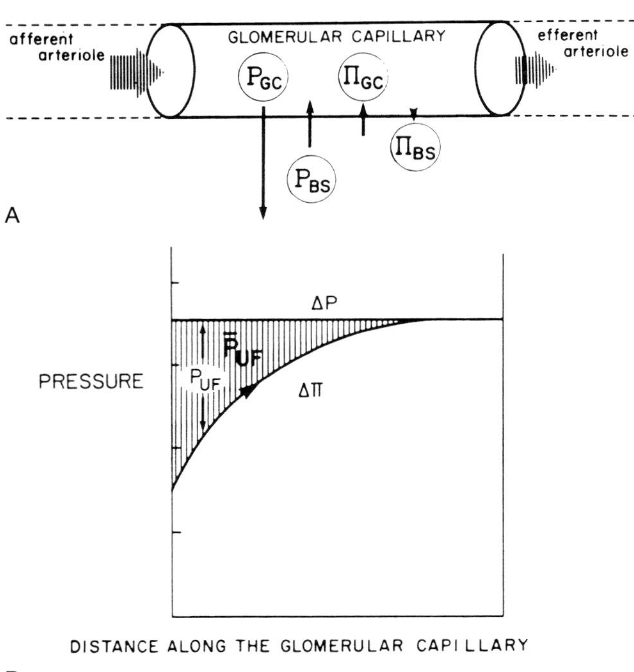

FIG. 1. Schema of glomerular filtration process. **A:** Idealized glomerular capillary. Fluid movement is determined by hydraulic pressure within the glomerular capillary (P_{GC}) and Bowman space (P_{BS}) and oncotic pressure within the glomerular capillary (II_{GC}) and Bowman space (II_{BS}). **B:** Transcapillary hydraulic pressure difference $DP = P_{GC} - P_{BS}$; transcapillary oncotic pressure difference $DII = II_{GC} - II_{BS}$. Because ultrafiltrate in the Bowman space is colloid free, $II_{BS} = 0$, II_{GC} (hence DII) increases progressively, so that P_{UF} decreases along the glomerular capillary. P_{UF}, mean net ultrafiltration pressure. [Reprinted with permission (201).]

The glomerular capillary network is modeled as the idealized form of a cylindrical tube extending from the afferent to efferent ends (Fig. 1). Across this network, a large colloid-free portion of the glomerular plasma is lost by filtration. The profiles of forces acting along the glomerular capillaries are shown in the lower part of this figure (6). The ΔP is constant from the afferent to efferent ends. By contrast, $\Delta\pi$ increases progressively from the afferent to efferent ends. $\Delta\pi$ is regarded as equal to π_{GC} because of the colloid-free nature of Bowman's space fluid; i.e., $\pi_{BS} = 0$. Because of the loss of this colloid-free solution as filtrate, $\Delta\pi$ (or π_{GC}) increases progressively along the capillary. The net ultrafiltration pressure (P_{UF}) at any point along the glomerular capillary is given by the difference between ΔP and $\Delta\pi$ and decreases progressively toward the efferent end. Therefore, the P_{UF} will be equal to the difference between ΔP and $\Delta\pi$ integrated over the entire length of the capillary. It is not known precisely at what point along the capillary ΔP balances $\Delta\pi$ or attains so-called filtration pressure equilibrium. In some species such as the rodent, filtration pressure equilibrium is reached, and the pattern for the increase in plasma oncotic pressure becomes a function of the capillary length and the point at which the filtration pressure equilibrium is attained. This equilibration point can vary. For example, an increase in the plasma flow rate can change the net ultrafiltration pressure (i.e., the shaded area in Fig. 1). When the various forces are expressed as average values over the entire length of the capillary, SNGFR is given by the following equation:

$$\begin{aligned} \text{SNGFR} &= K_f \times P_{UF} \\ &= K_f \times (\Delta P - \Delta\pi) \\ &= (k \times s) \times [(P_{GC} - P_{BS}) \times (\pi_{GC} - \pi_{BS})] \end{aligned}$$

where K_f is the glomerular capillary ultrafiltration coefficient and encompasses s, which is the total surface area available for filtration, and k, which is the hydraulic permeability of the capillary; P_{UF} is the net ultrafiltration pressure and encompasses ΔP and $\Delta\pi$, which are the mean glomerular transcapillary hydraulic and colloid osmotic pressure differences, respectively; P_{GC} and P_{BS} are the mean hydraulic pressures in the glomerular capillary and Bowman's space, respectively; and π_{GC} and π_{BS} are the mean oncotic pressures in the glomerular capillary and Bowman's space, respectively. π_{BS} is regarded as 0 and SNGFR changes in accordance with changes in P_{UF} and K_f. In summary, therefore, the determinants of SNGFR are as follows:

1. Mean glomerular transcapillary hydraulic pressure difference, $\Delta P = (P_{GC} - P_{BS})$
2. Systemic plasma colloid osmotic pressure, $\Delta\pi$
3. Glomerular plasma flow rate, Q_A
4. Glomerular capillary ultrafiltration coefficient, K_f, where $\Delta\pi$ and Q_A affect SNGFR through modulation of π_{GC} and hence $\Delta\pi$

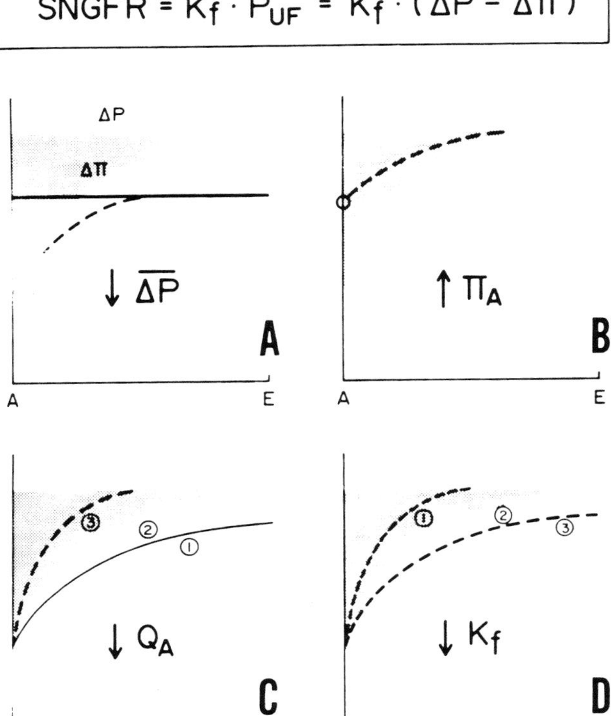

FIG. 2. Schematic representation of the process of glomerular ultrafiltration with reduced mean transcapillary hydraulic pressure difference $\overline{\Delta P}$ (**A**) with increased systemic colloid osmotic pressure (π_A) (**B**); with reduced glomerular plasma flow rate (Q_A) (**C**); and with reduced ultrafiltration pressure ($\bar{P}_{UF}$) (**D**), determined by the normal profiles of hydraulic (ΔP) and oncotic (π_A) pressure differences. The altered ΔP profile as a consequence of each of the above changes is given by an interrupted curve in each panel. Curve 1 in **C** and curve 3 in **D** represent disequilibrium. The Starling equation (top panel) describes the determinants for SNGFR.

Each of these determinants can affect SNGFR (Fig. 2). These functional determinants are in turn modulated by specific loci within the glomerulus, including the afferent and efferent arterioles and the glomerular capillaries. These structures possess an extensive array of receptors for a variety of hormones and cytokines. In addition, the glomerulus is itself capable of biosynthesis of many vasoactive substances, including angiotensin II (Ang II), endothelin, and prostaglandins.

Heterogeneity Among Nephrons (Structure/Function)

Even in the absence of disease, the GFR is not uniform among the nephrons. Filtration in juxtamedullary glomeruli is estimated to be twice as high as in cortical glomeruli (7). The differences parallel differences in the architecture between these two populations. Juxtamedullary glomeruli are larger, have a larger filtering area, and have longer tubular components than the cortical counterparts (7). Although the functional significance of these differences is not yet certain, it has been postulated to involve regulation of fluid balance. For example, redistribution of flow toward the deeper nephrons occurs in salt- and fluid-retaining states such as congestive heart failure and nephrotic syndrome. The longer loops of these nephrons in turn contribute to the enhanced salt reabsorption in such circumstances. Conversely, SNGFR increases in the outer cortical nephrons with increased sodium intake. This adaptation facilitates excretion of extra fluid by the shorter loops (7). Differences in the microvasculature between juxtamedullary and cortical glomeruli are being uncovered. Juxtamedullary arterioles are more responsive than cortical arterioles to vasoactive stimuli such as adrenergic stimulation (8). However, although autoregulatory blood flow is efficient in these juxtamedullary glomeruli under normal physiologic conditions, juxtamedullary microvascular dysfunction has been observed in several disease states. For example, in the rat model of diabetes mellitus, juxtamedullary afferent arterioles appear to be maximally dilated but have a blunted response to norepinephrine. These changes may contribute to the hyperfiltration that characterizes diabetes. Efferent arteriolar responsiveness appears unchanged (9). Differences in glomerular size impacts SNGFR. Although juxtamedullary glomeruli in children are larger than in the cortical zone, recent data indicate that there is little difference in these glomerular areas in normal young adults (10). Altered glomerular size in this population may therefore reflect adaptation to injury. Indeed, the presence of glomerular hypertrophy in the juxtamedullary region in adults may be taken to reflect loss of glomeruli elsewhere in the kidney, such as in obsolescence associated with aging or existence of destructive disease.

MODULATION OF FILTRATION BY GLOMERULAR EFFECTOR LOCI

Afferent Arteriole

The afferent arteriole affects glomerular filtration by regulating the rate of plasma flow into the glomerular capillary network and also by regulating the intraglomerular pressure. In general, changes in the glomerular capillary plasma flow rate are more likely to influence GFR than are changes in the glomerular capillary pressure. This is because the renal microvasculature has sensitive pressure and not flow sensors that autoregulate P_{GC}. In addition, changes in the glomerular pressure lead to directionally similar changes in the opposing oncotic pressure so that the net effect on SNGFR is minimal (Fig. 2A). As noted above, the filtration process removes essentially protein-free fluid into Bowman's space and causes a progressive increase in intracapillary protein concentration and therefore the oncotic pressure. Because the glomerular capillary hydraulic pressure is constant, the transcapillary fluid transfer dissipates the net ultrafiltration pressure along the glomerular capillary length (Fig. 1).

Moreover, glomerular pressure remains stable over a wide range of systemic blood pressures (11). In response to decreased systemic blood pressures, this adaptation reflects afferent arteriolar dilation, as well as efferent arteriolar constriction (11–13). Conversely, the spontaneously hypertensive rat, which is characterized by high systemic blood pressure, has glomerular capillary pressure in the normal range. This adaptation reflects the afferent arteriolar vasoconstriction that prevents direct transmission of systemic hypertension (14,15). Clinically, GFR is preserved over a wide range of systemic blood pressures. For example, humans with mild to moderate systemic hypertension usually have normal GFR levels (16). Only when there is profound or prolonged hypotension or in certain disease states is a decrease in systemic blood pressure accompanied by a decrease in GFR (see Defense of GFR).

Glomerular plasma flow rate is another determinant of SNGFR that is modulated by afferent arteriolar tone. Although the impact of changes in glomerular pressure in regulating GFR is subtle, changes in glomerular plasma flow are more likely to affect GFR. For any given change in glomerular plasma flow rate, effects on GFR depend on the cause of the change in plasma flow rate and, importantly, whether other determinants of SNGFR also have been modified. Changes in the plasma flow rate are most influential under the condition of filtration pressure equilibrium (Fig. 1). This means that GFR is most dependent on the rate of plasma flow at the lower plasma flow rates and less so as the plasma flow rate increases. Although filtration pressure equilibrium is known to prevail in normal Munich-Wistar rats, it is not known whether it characterizes glomerular filtration in humans. Nevertheless, even in humans, dependency of GFR on renal blood flow is most apparent at the lowest levels of blood flow.

Efferent Arteriole

Like the afferent arteriole, the efferent arteriole also can modulate the plasma flow rate. However, its most prominent role is linked to regulation of glomerular capillary pressure. A selective increase in the efferent arteriolar resistance predicts a decline in glomerular plasma flow rate similar to that expected from increased afferent arteriolar resistance. However, the SNGFR remains constant. This occurs because the glomerular capillary pressure upstream to the vasoconstriction increases and preserves glomerular filtration. This mechanism is pivotal in preserving GFR in many conditions, such as volume depletion, congestive heart failure, renal artery stenosis, and other settings characterized by renal hypoperfusion (13,17,18). An important factor in these settings is activation of the renin–angiotensin system. Ang II has a prominent role in maintaining efferent arteriolar tone, which in turn maintains or increases intraglomerular pressure and preserves the rate of glomerular filtration. Although the effects of a Ang II on efferent arterioles have been most extensively studied, a host of other hormones and cytokines modulate vascular resistance at this site. These include endothelin, vasopressin, bradykinin, platelet activating factor, atrial natriuretic factor, insulin-like growth factor, and leukotrienes, among others (19–25).

Recently, studies have exposed the structural complexity of the outflow tract of the efferent arteriole. Thus, the efferent arteriole is already formed while it is inside the glomerulus by the consolidation of capillary tributaries. This intraglomerular segment is surrounded by mesangial cells, their processes, and extracellular matrix. After leaving the glomerulus, the segment enters the extraglomerular matrix and is surrounded by smooth muscle cell processes and several layers of the extraglomerular mesangial cells (26–28). This anatomic arrangement causes the lumen of the efferent arteriole to be conspicuously narrower than the afferent arteriole. Narrowing of the extraglomerular segment has been previously recognized but was ascribed to endothelial cell prominence and therefore believed unlikely to modulate dynamic changes in efferent arteriolar tone. Moreover, in contrast to the lengthy and muscular afferent arteriole, the relatively short efferent arteriole has an apparent paucity of contractile elements. As such, the vigorous changes in efferent arteriolar resistance long appreciated in micropuncture studies were somewhat perplexing. However, this anatomic arrangement suggests that mesangial cells that have contractile properties regulate the efferent arteriolar tone. Thus, it is postulated that intraglomerular and extraglomerular mesangial cells synchronously, or independently, provide the dynamic modulation of efferent arteriolar tone (26). Some of the pressure decrease occurs within the intraglomerular segment. The layered structure of the extraglomerular segment appears particularly suited for allowing the gradual dissipation of the 30 mm Hg drop from inside to outside the glomerulus. In addition to active modulation of the efferent arteriolar tone, the anatomical arrangement whereby the glomerular basement membrane encases the glomerular capillaries, mesangium, and afferent and efferent arterioles within the vascular pole also suggests passive regulation of the efferent arteriolar tone (Fig. 3). It has been proposed that the glomerular basement membrane, which provides its own structural stability and resilience, is tethered either directly or by extracellular microfibrils to mesangial cells and thus maintains structural stability (28). In this scenario, therefore, an increase in afferent arteriolar pressure

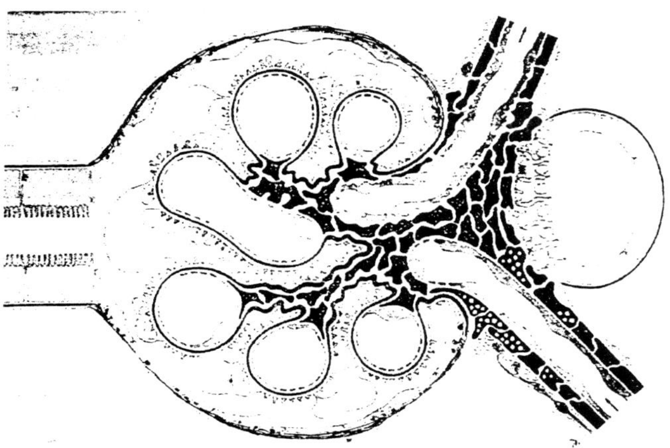

FIG. 3. Schema of glomerulus. Blood enters the glomerular capillary through the afferent arteriole, courses through the capillary tuft, and exits through the efferent arteriole. Filtration takes place across the capillary wall into Bowman's space. The mesangial cells (black) are strategically located to control the filtration surface area. Reproduced with permission from Dr. W. Kriz. (See also Chapter 2).

may be expected by acting on the other components enclosed in the vascular compartment to increase efferent arteriolar resistance even without active contraction of the muscle layer surrounding the efferent arteriole.

Glomerular Capillaries

Another locus for regulation of GFR resides within the glomerular capillary bed itself and is represented by the glomerular capillary ultrafiltration coefficient, K_f (Fig. 3). This parameter encompasses the hydraulic conductivity to water and the surface area available for filtration. Each of these variables can be altered independently by a variety of physiologic and pathophysiologic processes. The mathematical model predicts that changes in K_f will lead to similar changes in $\Delta\pi$ (Fig. 2D), which limit the impact of K_f on SNGFR under normal physiologic conditions. For example, an increase in the value of K_f will rather permit achievement of filtration pressure equilibrium when $\Delta P = \Delta\pi$, at which point any further increase in the value of K_f would allow filtration to cease closer to the afferent arteriole. Thus, because K_f modulates SNGFR only under conditions of disequilibrium, once filtration pressure equilibrium ensues, experimental data and the mathematical model predict that SNGFR will not respond to alterations in K_f. Nevertheless, a large decrease in the value of K_f can induce filtration pressure disequilibrium. This has been shown in response to a variety of hormones and cytokines as well as several animal models of disease, including glomerulonephritis (29–31), acute renal failure (32), chronic ureteral obstruction (33), puromycin aminonucleoside-induced nephrosis (34), and chronic protein malnutrition (35). Recent studies indicate the need for some modifications from the original mathematical model of glomerular ultrafiltration (4,36). Recent reevaluation of distribution of blood flow and local filtration has been performed in a mathematical model based on three-dimensional reconstructed glomerular capillary segments by morphometric techniques (36). These studies reiterated the long-appreciated complexity of the glomerular capillary organization but also documented heterogeneity of capillary dimension (37–43). Reconstitution of hemodynamics in this model reaffirmed that the total capillary network axial pressure drop (ΔP) is only about 3 mm Hg and thus corresponds to the value estimated by the homogeneous capillary model. However, the reconstructed glomerulus also indicates that the filtration process is heterogeneous within the glomerular capillary tuft. Some capillary segments are predicted to operate at or near filtration pressure equilibrium, whereas others are far from reaching equilibrium (36,44). These findings imply that K_f values obtained from the homogeneous model systematically underestimate K_f values; moreover, this underestimation becomes greatest as filtration equilibrium is approached. The new considerations also suggest that previous calculations of K_f may have been somewhat insensitive. Nevertheless, as discussed above, micropuncture experiments indicate that values of K_f indeed change in response to various hormones and cytokines as well as in several animal models of disease even in the absence of structural glomerular disease. However, the decrease in K_f must be profound (>50%) in order for it to result in a change in SNGFR.

Mesangial cells have been implicated in the regulation of surface area. Morphologically, the glomerular mesangial cells are well suited to this function. Like smooth muscle cells, mesangial cells possess cytoskeletal scaffolding, actin, and myosin; have receptors for a variety of vasoactive substances; and have the ability to contract (see Chapter 29). A biochemical parameter of mesangial cell contraction, myosin light chain phosphorylation, has been shown to increase dramatically in response to Ang II, arginine vasopressin, endothelin, and pathophysiologic conditions such as exposure to cyclosporine or increase in osmolality (45–48).

Decrease in K_f reflects changes in available filtration surface area and has been linked to decrease in the filtration area as a result of mesangial cell contraction (Fig. 4) or the more chronic circumstance where decrease in the number and/or caliber of open capillary loops occurs as the result of glomerulosclerosis. However, increase in the value of K_f has not been extensively studied. New information regarding the changes in glomerular filtration area in more chronic settings has been obtained through morphologic studies. In chronic disorders, such as renal ablation and diabetes, hyperfiltration is accompanied by glomerular hypertrophy. The increase of total surface area in these settings can reflect a change in total capillary length or increase in capillary diameter, or both.

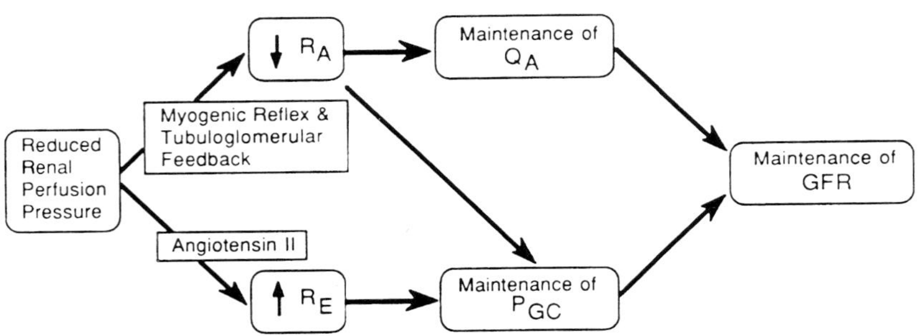

FIG. 4. Mechanisms contributing to the autoregulatory maintenance of renal blood flow and GFRs in the face of a reduction in renal perfusion pressure. R_A (afferent) and R_E (efferent) arteriolar resistance; Q_A, glomerular plasma flow rate; P_{GC}, glomerular capillary hydraulic pressure; GFR, glomerular filtration rate. [Reprinted with permission (18).]

In rats with acute diabetes there is lengthening of glomerular capillaries, which is followed by branching of the glomerular capillaries (43). After weeks of diabetes, the branching seemingly balances the total length increase. Capillary proliferation also has been documented in hypertrophied glomeruli in lithium nephropathy (49) and following nephrectomy (42). The implication of these studies is that after certain types of injury an increase in surface area is predicted to increase the value of K_f and thus preserve or increase the level of SNGFR.

DEFENSE OF GFR

Adjustment in GFR When Blood Pressure Changes

Many nonmammalian vertebrate species have effective homeostatic mechanisms to drastically alter GFR (50). This capacity to alter GFR is a critically important part of the mechanisms that maintain hydration in these species. They can afford to markedly alter GFR because toxic nitrogenous wastes are excreted through nonrenal organs such as gills, skin, and cloaca. In contrast, mammals, with their highly variable fluid intake, have developed an even greater capability to conserve and eliminate water from the body, largely through an expanded and highly regulated reabsorptive capacity of the renal tubules. However, because glomeruli are the only route for elimination of metabolic wastes and toxins, the GFR in mammals is constant, and high relative to other species. Furthermore, specific mechanisms are recognized that maintain GFR stable over a wide range of blood pressure and extracellular fluid (ECF) volume, which ensure an effective removal of large amounts of nitrogenous waste that are constantly produced. The mechanisms that maintain GFR stable depend on adjustments at the glomerular loci, namely the afferent and efferent arterioles, and likely also in the glomerular capillary bed itself (Fig. 4). Two mechanisms, namely the myogenic reflex and tubuloglomerular feedback, are important for the autoregulation of GFR during changes in blood pressure.

Myogenic Reflex

The myogenic reflex describes the theory that an increase in transmural pressure increases vascular tone. In the renal circulation this is particularly important in the afferent arteriole. This reflex is independent of renal nerves or macula densa mechanisms and reflects the inherent characteristics of the vessel (51,52). This response has been demonstrated in isolated perfused renal vessels, in which a change in vasomotor tone occurs in response to changes in the perfusion pressure. This response was blocked by a smooth muscle relaxant, papavarine (53). The observation that calcium-channel blockers prevented spontaneous action potentials and vascular contraction implied that vascular stretch depolarizes cells, which leads to increase in Ca^{2+} influx and contraction (54). Recent studies also have implicated that the cytochrome P-450 metabolites of arachidonic acid participate in the myogenic response in renal afferent arterioles (55). The cytochrome P-450 inhibitors were shown to attenuate the vasoconstrictive response in afferent arterioles in the perfused rat juxtamedullary microvascular preparation over renal perfusion pressures that range from 80 to 160 mm Hg. Attenuation of this response was associated with significant impairment in autoregulation in the glomerular capillary pressure, although the resultant SNGFR was not measured. Each of the primary cytochrome P-450 products of arachidonic acid formed in the kidney are considered as candidates for this effect, including 11-, 12-, 14-, 15-, epoxyeicosatrienoic acids-, 20-, and hydroxyeicosatetraenoic acid, because each of these substances has been shown to regulate vasomotor tone in various vessels. However, definitive identification of which metabolite is responsible in the renal circulation awaits further studies.

Tubuloglomerular Feedback

Constancy of GFR is also determined by the tubuloglomerular feedback system, which describes the coupling of the distal nephron flow and SNGFR. In each nephron, the distal tubule returns to the parent glomerulus and contributes to the formation of the juxtaglomerular apparatus, which consists of specialized cells of the macula densa located between the afferent and efferent arterioles and the glomerulus. In this system, the stimulus is related to the rate of distal flow and also to the composition of the tubular fluid, particularly chloride concentration and osmolality (56–60). The signal is perceived in the macula densa and transmitted to the vascular structures of the nephron, particularly the afferent arteriole, but also to the efferent arteriole and the glomerular capillary, which in turn adjust the rate of filtration. This feedback is well suited to adjust the rate of filtration, as well as to maintaining constancy of salt and water delivery to the distal nephron, where tubular reabsorption is precisely regulated. Thus, an inverse relationship between filtration and tubular flow is established such that a decrease in tubular flow is anticipated to increase the rate of SNGFR and vice versa.

The vascular response has been linked to several substances, including adenosine (61), thromboxane A2 (62), and particularly Ang II, which is synthesized in the macula densa as well as in the glomerulus (62–64). Recently, convincing evidence has accumulated that nitric oxide (NO) has an important role in regulating glomerular hemodynamics through the glomerular feedback mechanism (see Chapter 21). Ito et al. used an in vitro preparation in which both the afferent arteriole and the attached macula densa were simultaneously perfused to show that inhibition of NO synthesis NG-nitro-L-arginine methyl ester (by L-NAME) only in the macula densa perfusate constricted the afferent arteriole. Importantly, this effect was observed with high but not low sodium chloride (NaCl) perfusate, indicating that NO produced within the macula densa modulates afferent arteriolar constriction induced by high NaCl concentrations (65,66). Micropuncture studies performed by Wilcox et al. also demonstrated that perfusion of the loop of Henle with inhibitors of NO lowers stop flow glomerular pressure in vivo. This effect was reversed by L-arginine, which amplifies NO synthesis (67). Further support for an important role of NO in tubuloglomerular feedback comes from immunohistochemical studies that show distinct isoforms of NO synthase (NOS) in the juxtaglomerular apparatus in the rat. Inducible NOS was demonstrated in the terminal afferent arteriole, occasionally in the initial efferent arterioles, as well as in the distal tubule. By contrast, constitutive NOS was localized throughout the cytoplasm of the macula densa cells, where it appeared to be associated with small vesicles, clearly lending support to a pivotal role for NO in the response arm of tubuloglomerular feedback (68). (The NO system is discussed in more detail in Chapter 2).

Adjustment in GFR When Volume Changes

Classically, the term GFR autoregulation has been described only in the context of preservation of GFR during acute changes in renal perfusion pressure. However, threat to GFR homeostasis comes when ECF volume changes even without changes in renal perfusion pressure. Many nonmammalian vertebral species markedly modify GFR during alteration in ECF volume by intermittent glomerular perfusion. In these species, GFR serves primarily as a volume regulator. They can afford to have intermittent glomerular perfusion because toxic nitrogenous wastes are eliminated through circulatory systems independent of glomerular perfusion, including cloaca and gills. By contrast, in mammals nitrogenous wastes are eliminated almost exclusively through the glomerulus, and almost all the blood entering the kidney must pass through the glomerulus. Therefore, mammals, unlike other vertebrates, must maintain constant high GFR. This is achieved through the four mechanisms described below.

Preservation of Blood Pressure

When the body faces a reduction in plasma or circulating volume, extremely powerful neurohumoral systems become activated to prevent reduction in blood pressure. The chronotropic and innotropic effects directed by the adrenergic system, by acting on the heart, mimimize the otherwise inevitable reduction in cardiac output. Although Ohm's law predicts that a decrease in cardiac output leads to a decrease in blood pressure, activation of the adrenergic nervous and humoral systems, particularly angiotensin and vasopressin, by raising the peripheral vascular resistance, nullify the reduction in cardiac output to maintain normal blood pressure. This response is protected by multiple compensatory systems, i.e., experimental inhibition of one system leads to further activation of others. The net effect of these compensations is that, experimentally, it is difficult to reduce blood pressure (69). Teleologically, maintenance of blood pressure is geared to the homeostasis of the circulation of the brain and the heart, which on a minute-to-minute basis are most critical for life. Thus, the precapillary sphincter (or vascular beds) of these two organs escape from (or are insensitive to) the constrictive action of the adrenergic, angiotensin, or vasopressin system. Due to this lack of changes in the vascular resistance, together with maintained perfusion pressure, blood flow to these organs is preserved, as predicted by Ohm's law. Thus, during ECF volume contraction, the vascular beds in the heart and brain do not contribute to increase in peripheral vascular resistance.

Fractional Renal Blood Flow

Although preservation of blood flow to the heart and brain is paramount and these vascular beds do not participate in adaptation to ECV changes, nevertheless, in relative terms, the contribution of the renal vascular beds to the increase in total peripheral vascular resistance during ECF volume contraction is substantially less than other circulation such as skeletal muscles and gastrointestinal tract. Indeed, when ECF volume decreases, the fraction of the renal vascular resistance contributing to the total systemic vascular resistance decreases, although in absolute terms the renal vascular resistance increases (70). Thus, during reduced cardiac output or ECF volume contraction, a relatively higher fraction goes to the kidney when compared with steady-state euhydration conditions. This study also showed that this relative renal vasodilation during ECF volume contraction is attributed largely to the kidney's unique ability to generate vasodilative prostaglandins, which balance vasoconstrictors, such as vasopressin and angiotensin.

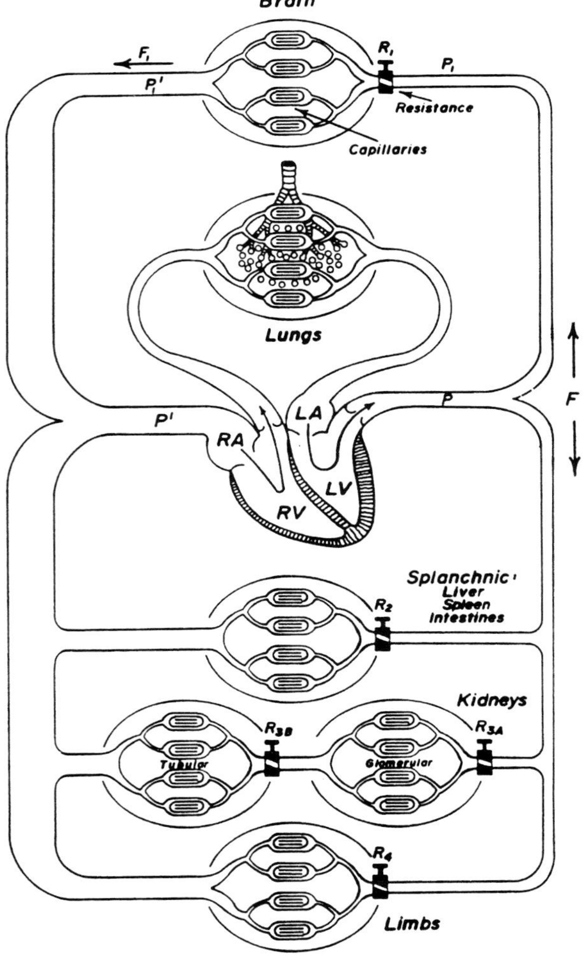

FIG. 5. Interdependence of pressure, flow, and resistance. Systemic circulatory pressure (P) is a function of the cardiac output (F) and the resistance to flow (R) offered by the various vascular beds, which are arranged in parallel ($1/R = 1/R_1 + 1/R_2 + 1/R_3 + 1/R_4 + \ldots 1/R_x$). Exception occurs in the kidney, where two resistances are arranged in series such that the total resistance is the sum of preglomerular and pretubular resistances. Constancy of systemic blood pressure reflects flow through individual beds and is inversely proportional to the resistance they offer, which in turn is determined by their arterioles. [Reprinted with permission (202).]

Efferent Arteriolar Vasomotor Tone

The third rescue mechanism for preservation of GFR during ECF volume reduction comes from the unique arrangement of sphinctors within the renal circulatory system (see below). Thus, although both glomeruli and tubules have, like other organs, a precapillary sphincter, the precapillary sphincter upstream to the tubule-perfusing system also functions as a postcapillary sphincter for the glomerulus (Fig. 5). This arrangement allows the renal vasculature to contribute to the increase in peripheral vascular resistance during ECF volume reduction without sacrificing GFR. Thus, during volume contraction, not only the afferent arteriole but also the efferent arteriole constrict, thereby contributing to the increase in peripheral vascular resistance. However, constriction of the latter preserves the glomerular pressure. This response contrasts with the state of other organ beds, in which the constriction of their precapillary sphincters automatically leads to a reduction in intracapillary pressure. A micropuncture study measuring glomerular pressure showed that during physiologic volume contraction, the glomerular pressure is substantially raised above normal levels due to the potent constrictive action of Ang II on the efferent arteriole (71).

Preservation of Glomerular Size

The fourth mechanism for GFR protection during ECF volume changes lies in the homeostatic mechanism to maintain the structural integrity of the glomerulus. This again reiterates differences between mammalian and nonmammalian vertebrates. Morphologic investigations of fish kidneys show that their glomeruli are larger during volume expansion and smaller during volume contraction. In several euryhaline species, in adaptation to their changing habitat during their life cycle, marked alterations in size and structure of glomeruli occur (69). The adrenocortical–hypophysial axis (i.e., vasopressin, prolactin, somatostatin) is believed to be involved in this (hydration-dependent) change in glomerular size (72). As discussed above, although such changes in glomerular size appear highly pertinent in nonmammalian species to maintain volume homeostasis, they are detrimental in mammalian species, which are committed to eliminating toxic nitrogenous wastes through the glomerulus. A recent study (70,73) demonstrated that mammals have an effective mechanism to abrogate this potent effect of circulating ECF volume on the glomerular size, effectively preventing the occurrence of glomerular atrophy during volume contraction through angiotensin actions.

Autoregulatory Derangements

Although both myogenic reflex and tubular glomerular feedback function to preserve a stable GFR, the relative contribution of each of these mechanisms is uncertain and likely depends on the particular circumstance. Compensation offered by both of these mechanisms can be overcome when disturbance in the systemic circulation is directly transmitted to the kidney and the filtration rate is affected. Normally, the afferent and efferent arterioles are efficient in adjusting the vascular resistance to maintain a constant level of glomerular pressure, glomerular plasma flow rate, and GFR. However, an extreme decrease in renal perfusion pressure, as might occur in circulatory collapse, can overwhelm the compensatory afferent arteriolar dilation and efferent arteriolar constrictions. Even a modest decrease in renal perfusion pressure may, in certain settings, precipitate hypoperfusion and hypofiltration. This has been shown during acute administration of vasodilators, which induced systemic and renal vasodilation (74,75). Impairment in autoregulation also has been documented in several animal models of common clinical entities, including volume depletion, congestive heart failure, and glomerulonephritis (76) during the recovery phase of postischemic acute renal failure and during hyperglycemia (77). All of these settings involved impaired autoregulation in response to a modest reduction in renal perfusion pressure, which had little or no effect on euvolemic animals. Thus, a decrease in renal perfusion pressure from 120 to 180 torr in the setting of volume depletion or congestive heart failure caused a somewhat curtailed dilation of the afferent arteriole (Fig. 6). This afferent arteriolar dilation led to relative maintenance of the renal plasma flow rate. On the other hand, a strikingly blunted response was observed in the efferent arteriole, which, instead of normal constriction, underwent paradoxical vasodilation in the setting of volume depletion and congestive heart failure. Noteworthy, these studies also showed that the efferent arteriole appears to be insensitive to the constrictive effects of exogenous Ang II. Taken together, these observations explain the predisposition of volume depletion and heart failure to have severe reduction in GFR with only a modest decrease in systemic blood pressure. Furthermore, this disrupted autoregulation is specifically linked to an abnormal response of the efferent arteriole. An abnormal response of the afferent arteriole in aberrant autoregulation also has been observed. Micropuncture studies 24 hr after 75% nephrectomy found that impairment in glomerular capillary pressure reflected vasodilation of the afferent arteriole, rendering it unresponsive to subsequent perturbation in renal perfusion pressure (76,78,79). These observations suggest that damaged kidneys have impairment in autoregulation of renal blood flow, which underlies their predisposition to reduction in GFR with additional or superimposed injury.

Although systemic vasodilation predisposes to autoregulatory decompensation, this is not always the case. For example, normal pregnancy is characterized by a decrease in systemic blood pressure and renal vasodilation (80–85). During elevation in blood pressure induced by bilateral carotid occlusion, autoregulation of the blood flow was maintained in pregnant rats. Conversely, graded aortic occlusion showed that the autoregulatory threshold below which renal blood flow decreased was between 90 and 100 mm Hg for mid-term and virgin rats but was only slightly lower at 88 mm Hg for late pregnancy. Thus, renal autoregulation, at least for blood flow, is maintained during pregnancy with a slight shift in the renal autoregulatory threshold in late pregnancy, which has

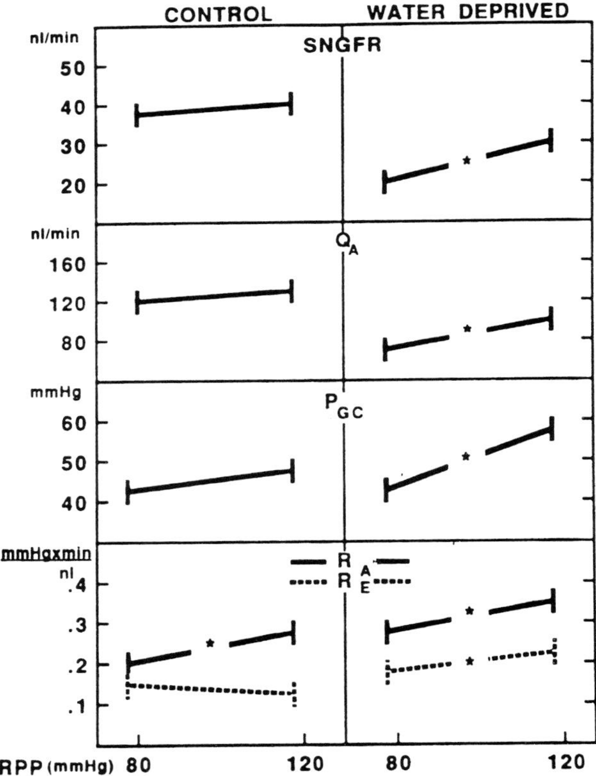

FIG. 6. Effect of graded reduction in renal perfusion pressure (from 120 to 80 mm Hg) on glomerular parameters in volume-deprived rats. Q_A, glomerular capillary plasma flow rate: P_{GC}, mean glomerular capillary hydraulic pressure; R_A and R_E, afferent and efferent arteriolar resistance. Note the impaired autoregulation of SNGFR in water-deprived animals, due to inability to maintain both Q_A and P_{GC}; the latter, in turn, is due to inability to appropriately increase R_E in response to the lowered perfusion pressure. (Reprinted with permission (13).]

been postulated to prevent the kidney from hypoperfusion during late gestational hypotension (83).

GLOMERULAR SIEVING OF MACROMOLECULES

The enormity of the quantity of filtrate generated by the glomerulus underscores specific features of the glomerular capillary bed, which allows high permeability to water and small molecules while at the same time providing efficient selectivity that bars cells, proteins larger than albumin, and charged molecules (86,87). This barrier function of the glomerular capillaries is influenced by the size, shape, and charge of the macromolecules. Micropuncture studies and urinary clearance analyses that compare concentration of a given macromolecule in Bowman's space/urine to plasma have been used to obtain a sieving coefficient for a variety of macromolecules. Sieving coefficients inversely correlated with the effective radius of the protein. Thus, clearance of the largest proteins, such as albumin and γ-globulin, is markedly less than that of smaller proteins such as monomeric immunoglobulin light chains (88,89). Molecules without charge, including dextran and polyvinylpyrolidone, which are neither reabsorbed nor secreted (unlike proteins), have been extensively used to study glomerular capillary permeability both in experimental settings as well as in human diseases (88–98). In addition, however, greater restriction of anionic than of neutral or cationic molecules suggests an electrostatic barrier that is charge selective. The observation that for a given chromatographic radius and charge density protein sieving coefficient is smaller than that of neutral dextrans also suggests the existence of glomerular shape selectivity. Thus, proteins are believed to behave as rigid spheres, whereas dextrans are more compliant and so have smaller effective radii (89).

Based on these observations, the filtration barrier of the glomerular capillary has been modeled as a membrane punctuated with pores. Initially, the isoporous model assumed cylindrical pores of uniform size (88). However, behavior of large test molecules redefined the model to postulate two distinct populations of pores (89). The majority of pores have a mean radius of ~5.0 Å, whereas only a small fraction has been estimated to have radii ~of 7.0 nm, in effect providing a so-called shunt pathway (89). Although ~1% of filtrate is believed to traverse through the shunt pathway, this is sufficient to account for the increased transport of large molecules as well as albumin in several experimental models and diseases characterized by proteinuria. Thus, increased fractional clearance of large-sized dextran was observed in nephrotoxic serum nephritis (90) and puromycin aminonucleoside nephritis (99), as well as in minimal change nephrotic syndrome (89), diabetic nephropathy (92), and immunoglobulin A nephropathy (94). Moreover, the antiproteinuric effects of angiotensin-converting enzyme (ACEI) have been postulated to be due in part to reduction in this shunt pathway (93,94). In addition, depletion of anionic glycoprotein components such as heparan sulfate proteoglycans has been postulated to contribute to loss of the electrostatic barrier function. Thus, infusion of polycations, which neutralizes glomerular anionic sites, is associated with proteinuria and impairment of barrier size selectivity (100). This has been offered as an alternative mechanism for proteinuria, whereby albumin with a radius of 3.6 nm can pass through the 5.0-nm pores, even without changes in the barrier size selectivity. Nevertheless, recent studies claim that the anionic charge of glomeruli is insufficient to affect clearance based on charge repulsion (101). Moreover, other studies fail to show a substantive difference between albumin and dextran (102). Taken together, charge selectivity may not be the primary determinant of sieving, but together with size and shape selectivity underlie the selective hindrance for macromolecular movement across the glomerular capillary.

It appears that each of the three major components of the glomerular capillary wall provide impedance to macromolecular filtration. Thus, permeability of isolated glomerular basement membrane was much higher than in intact glomeruli, implying that endothelial and epithelial cells are important in this barrier function (103). In this regard, native anionic ferritin particles accumulate in endothelial fenestrae and in the lamina rara interna of the basement membrane. By contrast, cationic form of ferritin traverse the endothelium and basement membrane and accumulate in the lamina rara externa under the slit diaphragm of epithelial cells, indicating that the innermost components of the glomerular capillary provide electrostatic impedance, whereas the outer components, which include the epithelial cell slit diaphragm, furnish the restrictive size selection (104). Indeed, epithelial cells appear to provide a most significant element in glomerular permeability (see Chapter 31). Thus, significant proteinuria is typically accompanied by dissolution of normal interdigitation of epithelial podocytes. Notably, infusion of exogenous polycations, which causes proteinuria, also results in this structural lesion in epithelial cells (100). In some animal models of proteinuria, complete detachment of epithelial cell podocytes from the underlying basement membrane is seen (105–108), although such denudation of the basement membrane is observed only infrequently in human disease (107). Even without such obvious or extensive damage, it is clear that epithelial cells play an important role in permselectivity. Thus, injection of antibodies to renal tubule brush border antigen (Fx1A), which cross-reacts with glomerular epithelial cells, results in an experimental model of membranous nephropathy (109,110). A recent study showed that anti-Fx1A antibody contains activity to b1-integrin and inhibits adhesion and growth of cultured glomerular epithelial cells (111). These findings suggest that altered cytoskeleton–integrin matrix interaction perturbs the slit diaphragm and thus leads to loss of normal filtration function (112) (see also Chapters 17, 31).

It is important to underscore that the above-described determinants of SNGFR also impact filtration of macromolecules. Glomerular capillary flow rate, but particularly the glomerular capillary pressure, modulates membrane pore structure such that increase in glomerular pressure amplifies the shunt pathway and augments proteinuria. The mechanism for this effect can be attributed to Ang II. Thus, infusion of Ang II, or endogenous stimulation of Ang II activity, increases the fractional excretion of protein, whereas decreasing the pressure has the opposite effect (113,114). In humans, infusion of hyperoncotic albumin, which increased blood volume, renal blood flow, and GFR was associated with a selective increase in clearance of large, but not small, dextran molecules (115). These studies underscore that glomerular hemodynamic changes, through increasing the large, nonselective pores in the glomerular membrane, can allow macromolecules to escape into the urinary space (Fig. 7). It is of interest that acute exercise-induced proteinuria, in which the sieving defect is believed to be linked to increased intraglomerular pressure, is lessened by pretreatment with ACEI (116). In chronic disease states, antagonism of Ang II actions also lessens proteinuria (117–120). The mechanism for this antiproteinuric effect is in part related to decreased efferent arteriolar resistance and therefore glomerular capillary pressure (121). Although this effect occurs at least in part because of a decrease in Ang II, it also occurs because of an increase in bradykinin, which is also elevated during ACEI, and can be abolished by bradykinin antagonism (120). Although hemodynamic effects are important in modulating proteinuria, it is likely that more chronic antagonism of Ang II activity by ACEI or Ang II antagonist also preserves glomerular structure and so lessens proteinuria. Although ACEI lowered proteinuria in nondiabetic, normotensive proteinuric patients (120,122), acute injection of Ang II did not re-establish proteinuria, despite the return of the filtration fraction to pre-ACEI levels (123).

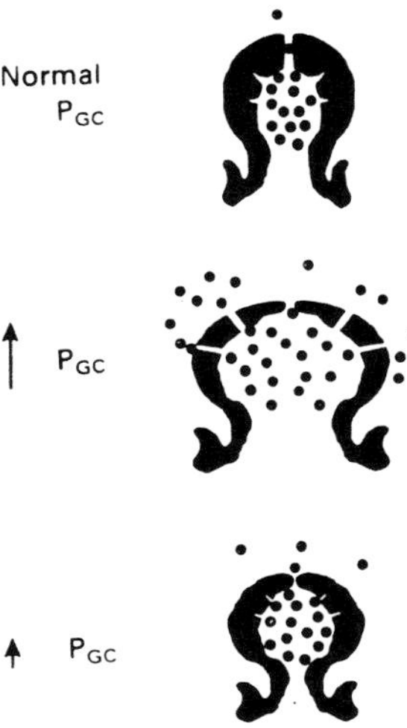

FIG. 7. Schematic presentation of the relationship among glomerular capillary pressure (P_{GC}), functional pores in the glomerular capillary wall, and glomerular macromolecular sieving, postulated on the basis of experimental data and calculations. In contrast to normal steady-state condition (top), the high local level of endogenous Ang II (middle) drastically raises P_{GC}, which in turn increases non–size-selective pores on the capillary wall, thereby allowing the bulk of macromolecules to escape into the Bowman's space and into the urine. When the high P_{GC} is largely attenuated (bottom), the abnormal presence of a large number of nonselective pores and the sieving defect are largely corrected. [Reprinted with permission (203).]

CLINICAL ASSESSMENT OF GFR

Normal Levels and Physiologic Variability in GFR (see also Chapter 37)

Normal GFR is 120 ml/min/1.73 m^2. The mean values for men and women 20–40 years of age are 127–130 ml/min/1.73 m^2 and 118–120 ml/min/1.73 m^2, respectively (124,125,125a). Normalization for body surface area gives smaller variation within the population than normalizing for weight (126). As noted in the previous section, the level of GFR is remarkably constant and reflects efficient homeostatic mechanisms that preserve the rate of filtration over a range of systemic circulatory derangements. Physiologic factors affect GFR. First is age (Table 1). At birth, GFR, even when corrected for body surface area, is lower than in adults. Maturational increase in GFR continues through the first 2 years of life and reaches normal adult levels, corrected for surface area, at about 2 years of age (127). At the other end of the spectrum, a decrease in GFR begins at approximately 40 years of age, at which time there is a linear decrease by 0.8–1.0 ml/min/year. Thus, GFR in men 80–89 years of age is about half the value of levels in individuals 20–29 years of age (Table 1) (128).

Diurnal variation is another physiologic factor that influences the level of GFR. The total amplitude of the variance may be as much as 20–30% of the mean value. The levels of GFR are lowest during the night, then increase rapidly after awakening, peaking at mid-day (129), regardless of diet/protein intake (130). The circadian rhythm in GFR variability occurs not only in normal individuals but also has been observed in patients with nephrotic syndrome and varying degrees of renal functional impairment (130). These observations suggest that if the duration of urine collection for assessment of GFR

TABLE 1. *Average reported plasma creatinine and creatinine clearance at different ages*

Age (yr)	Serum creatinine (mg/dl)	Creatinine clearance (ml/min/1.73 m^2)
Term infants	0.3–1.0	25
2–10	0.2	76
10–20	0.5	95
20–29	0.95	103
30–39	1.03	100
40–49	1.05	84
50–59	1.08	78
60–69	1.06	68
70–79	1.03	59
80–89	1.06	47
90–99	1.06	37

Higher GFR values have been estimated from inulin clearances, on average by 20% above values reported for creatinine clearance (124,125,125a).

is less than 24 hr, the time of day of specimen collection should be taken into account.

Diet affects GFR. In the dog, one protein feeding can double GFR for a period of 4–6 hr. Repeated protein meals cause an even more sustained elevation in GFR (124,131,132). In humans, protein feedings have a similar effect, particularly after a meat meal (133). Furthermore, a mixture of essential and nonessential amino acids has a more pronounced effect on GFR than branched-chain amino acids (134). The mechanisms for these physiologic effects on GFR are likely linked to increases in renal blood flow, which in turn are modulated by vasoactive substances, including Ang II, vasopressin, prostaglandin, and glucagon (134–136). Taken together, these observations indicate that care must be exercised in interpreting the level of GFR measurement in a particular patient and circumstance.

Inulin Clearance

Substances reaching the kidney may undergo one of several processes, i.e., glomerular filtration, tubule reabsorption, tubule secretion, and intrarenal metabolism. These considerations necessitated the search for an "ideal GFR marker." Among various substances considered, inulin emerged and has remained the standard against which all other techniques of measuring GFR are compared to validate their accuracy. Polyfructosan S also has been used as a GFR marker (137). This substance offers the advantage of higher water solubility, and its preparation does not require heating. Inulin is a polymer of fructose, containing, on average, 32 fructose residues and has a molecular weight of about 5,700 daltons. Natural inulin is derived from plant tubers such as dahlias, chicory, and Jerusalem artichokes. Although the molecular configuration of inulin varies depending on the source, the Stokes-Einstein radius that affects filtration is constant at about 5.0 nm. Inulin fulfills the following criteria:

1. It is freely and completely filterable at the glomerulus.
2. It is neither secreted nor reabsorbed by tubules.
3. It is neither metabolized nor synthesized by the kidney.
4. It is not bound to plasma proteins, or if it is, the free unbound as well as the bound components can be measured separately.
5. It is physiologically inert.

Because of these characteristics of inulin, the rate of inulin filtered into Bowman's space equals the urinary excretion of inulin. Moreover, inulin concentration in Bowman's space equals that of plasma. Thus, the flow rate of the fluid filtered into Bowman's space: GFR = C_{inulin} = $U_{inulin} \cdot V/P_{inulin}$. For example, if P = 0.5 mg/ml, U = 50 mg/ml, and V = 1.1 ml/min, C_{inulin} = GFR = 110 ml/min. Although this is a straightforward relationship, there are several points worth emphasizing. It is plasma, not urine, that is being cleared of inulin. In the above example, all inulin is removed from 110 ml of plasma each minute. The inulin clearance is independent of the rate of urinary flow rate; thus, the concentration of inulin in the urine increases as the volume decreases and vice versa at a given GFR. The inulin clearance is also independent of the concentration of inulin in the plasma; thus, as plasma inulin concentration increases, its appearance in the urine increases as more is filtered.

Numerous human and micropuncture studies have reaffirmed inulin clearance as an ideal marker of GFR (138–140). 99.3% of inulin injected into an early portion of the proximal tubule was recovered from the distal nephron (as well as from the ureteral urine), indicating that inulin is not absorbed (141). Moreover, secretion by the tubule was ruled out by the observation that loading the peritubular capillary with inulin did not change the amount of inulin recovered from the distal nephron. Clearance of inulin also has been found to be accurate and reproducible, having an intratest and intertest precision of about 2% and 6%, respectively. To obtain a C_{inulin} measurement, the patient must have an intravenous line for injection and must be capable of reliable urine collection. A priming dose of 20 ml/m^2 of 10% inulin in normal saline is given intravenously, followed by a sustaining infusion of 1% inulin given intravenously at a rate of 85 ml/m^2/hr. The accuracy of the test is facilitated by ensuring diuresis, which minimizes the error in the measurement of urinary flow rate. After an equilibration time of about 30 min, two or three consecutively timed urine specimens are obtained over 30–60 min each, and blood samples for inulin determination are obtained midpoint in each urine collection.

Although inulin clearance remains the most accurate method of determining GFR, at the time of its original appraisal as a GFR marker, Homer Smith cautioned that in certain circumstances inulin may fail as a GFR marker. He considered circumstances in which inulin's free filtration across the glomerular basement membrane is impaired or a tubule backleak is present (142). Recently, Rosenbaum et al. (143) suggested that inulin is not freely filtered in kidney donors or in kidney transplant recipients. The C_{creat}/C_{inulin} ratio was about 1.5 compared with 1.0 in normal patients with two kidneys. The onus was on altered handling of the inulin, and not creatinine, in this circumstance because C_{urea}/C_{inulin} and $C_{iothalomate}/C_{inulin}$ ratios were also increased. These observations were further supported by the findings that C_{creat}/C_{inulin} ratio is also increased in the uninephrectomized dog, where no confounding tubular handling of creatinine occurs. In this regard, the dog is unique, in that creatinine is neither secreted nor reabsorbed by the tubules and therefore equal to the inulin clearance (144). However, the abnormality in inulin handling appears transient as the ratio normalized within 6 months of nephrectomy. Moreover, in a recent study of children with renal transplants, no difference in ratios in the clearances of creatinine, iothalomate, and inulin was observed (145), leaving uncertain whether the solitary-transplanted kidneys indeed have impairment in inulin handling. Homer Smith's other concern that substantial tubular leakage back into the bloodstream affects inulin as a GFR marker has been demonstrated in experimental models including postischemic acute renal failure (142). However, although tubular leakage back into the bloodstream is believed to occur in humans with extensive tubular damage (146, 147), the extent to which this lowers the apparent GFR is not quantitative and likely varies, depending on the lesion. These considerations notwithstanding, inulin clearance as the most accurate measure of GFR remains unchallenged. Its major drawback is that it is cumbersome for routine clinical use, including the preparation of the inulin itself, and requires continuous intravenous infusion. Moreover, measurements of inulin levels are not routinely available in hospital clinical laboratories. These drawbacks have led to the development of other methods to estimate GFR.

Creatinine

Serum Creatinine

In clinical practice, GFR is most often estimated from measurements of serum creatinine concentrations and the clearance of endogenously produced creatinine (see also Chapter 37). These require only collections of urine and/or blood samples. Most commonly, renal function is estimated simply by obtaining a serum creatinine measurement that often is used as the initial screening assessment, as well as in the monitoring of the rate of deterioration of renal function. In the steady state, when $U_{creat} \cdot V$ = creatinine excretion rate = creatinine production rate = constant, GFR is inversely proportional to plasma creatinine concentration because GFR = $(U_{creat} \cdot V)/P_{creat}$ = constant GFR. Thus, an increase of plasma creatinine from 1 to 2 mg/dl or from 4 to 8 mg/dl represents a functional loss of half of GFR between measurements, although the absolute decline in function is less in the latter as is the fractional residual function. The utility of this measurement stems from the relatively constant production of daily creatinine, which is independent of diet, protein catabolism, and physical activity. Also at steady state, i.e., when P_{creat} remains stable, the rate of production equals the rate of excretion (= $U_{creat} \cdot V$). Creatinine is produced from the metabolism of endogenous creatinine and phosphocreatine and is a function of muscle mass. In individuals of average build, creatinine production is 15–20 mg/kg/day in men and 15 mg/kg/day in women (148). This quantity of creatinine produced daily is expected to be entirely excreted in a 24-hr period and is used to check the completeness of a 24-hr urine collection. Thus, complete urinary collection in a 60-kg woman is expected to yield approximately 900 mg creatinine. Although constant in most circumstances, certain conditions do affect creatinine production: athletic build, obesity (149), rheumatoid arthritis (150), and spinal cord injury (151). It is also important to adjust for muscle mass in patients with malnutrition due to anorexia (152), as well as the elderly, particularly debilitated nursing home patients (153).

Although reasonable as a screening test for renal dysfunction, serum creatinine does not accurately estimate GFR (154) . A decrease in creatinine clearance (C_{creat}) by some 40–50% of normal may be accompanied by only a subtle increase in plasma creatinine (Fig. 8). This error is further heightened when GFR decreases (155–158). As noted above, the reciprocal of P_{creat} changes in the same direction as GFR and is roughly proportional to the change. The $1/P_{creat}$ values, measured at multiple time points, have been used to follow the progressive reduction in GFR in chronic renal failure and to predict the time for renal replacement therapy based on a linear regression line over time (159). However, recent studies document variability in creatinine metabolism during progressive renal disease, so caution in interpreting this measurement is suggested. Additionally, concern has been raised regarding the statistical fitting of straight lines of $1/P_{creat}$ data (160,161).

Creatinine Clearance

GFR estimates are frequently obtained by endogenous creatinine clearances, although creatinine is not an ideal marker of GFR. In addition to the above-noted circumstances in which creatinine production is altered, creati-

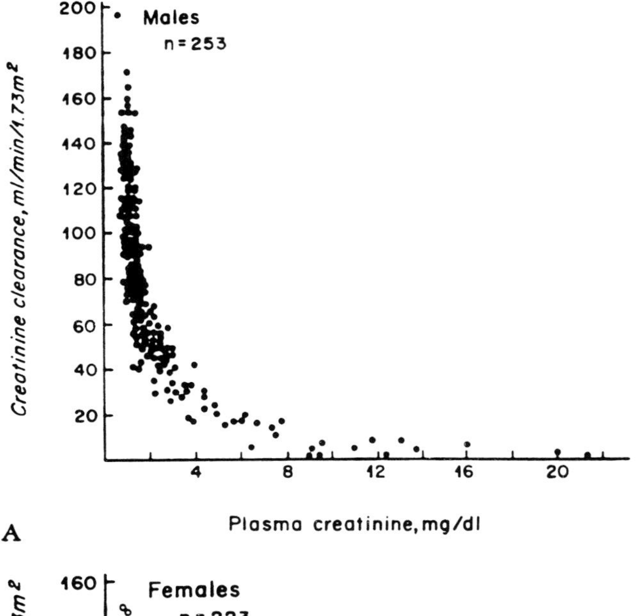

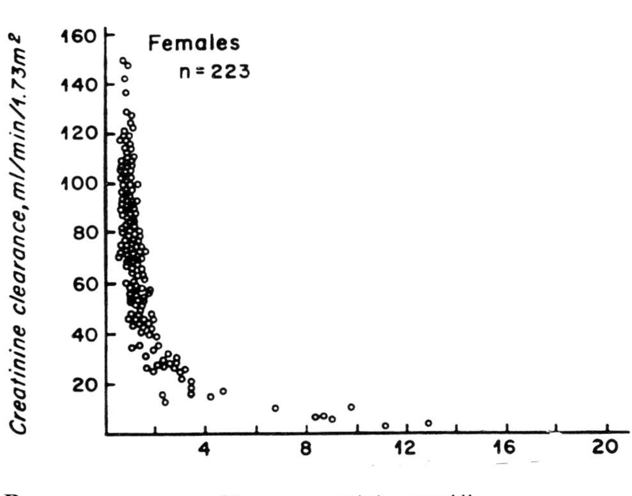

FIG. 8. Correlation between creatinine clearance and plasma creatinine in men (**A**) and women (**B**). [Reprinted with permission (154).]

nine is also secreted by the renal tubules and undergoes extrarenal excretion. Consequently, creatinine clearances overestimate GFR. At normal levels of renal function, creatinine clearances overestimate clearance of inulin by about 10%; at GFR levels of 40–70 ml/min, the overestimation is about 50%; at GFR levels less than 40 ml/min, the overestimation may be greater than 100% (124). This overestimation relates to the fact that as the GFR decreases, the portion of creatinine secreted by the tubule increases and there is greater urinary excretion of creatinine; i.e., increase in the numerator of the creatinine equation (U · V/P). A second reason for the overestimation relates to the measurement of plasma creatinine. If this is done by the Jaffe reaction (alkaline picrate), the method detects not only creatinine but also noncreatinine chromogens, elevating plasma creatinine assessment by ~0.2 mg/dl compared with creatinine measurements by high-performance liquid chromatography (HPLC). Because urine has but negligible amounts of noncreatinine chromogens, only the denominator of the creatinine clearance equation is increased. At normal GFR levels, the rate in tubule secretion of creatinine is roughly offset by the noncreatinine chromogen overestimation of plasma creatinine, and the creatinine clearance predicts the actual GFR. However, as GFR decreases, the offsetting effects diverge, and the overestimation is rather exacerbated. Finally, the third reason for overestimation of GFR by creatinine clearance relates to interference by several medications, including cimetidine, trimethoprim, triamterene, spironolactone, and amiloride, which inhibit tubular secretion of creatinine. Interestingly, one of these medications, cimetidine, has been used precisely because it inhibits tubular secretion to obtain a more "accurate" creatinine clearance (162,163).

GFR Measured by Radiolabeled Clearances

Radionucleotide markers have been used to circumvent some of the technical problems and measuring inaccuracies in plasma creatinine and creatinine clearances as estimates of GFR. Nuclides of inulin, including ^{14}C- and ^{3}H-inulin have been used in experimental animals. In humans, other isotopes that are handled by the kidney in a manner much like inulin have been used (although a small amount of tubular secretion and reabsorption occurs). These include ^{125}I-iothalomate, "cold" (nonradioactive) iothalomate (Conray), ^{51}Cr-labeled ethylenediaminetetraacetic acid (^{51}Cr-EDTA), and ^{99m}Tc-labeled diethylenetriaminepentaacetic acid (^{99m}Tc-DTPA). These radionucleotides are easily measured in plasma and urine samples and have good correlation with C_{inulin}. For example, ^{125}I-iothalomate and DTPA overestimate C-inulin by about 10% over a range of GFR between 10 and 80 ml/min (164–166). ^{51}Cr-EDTA underestimates C_{inulin} by a similar degree. Because exposure to radioactive substances is undesirable, these compounds are used only as single injections.

In the United States, ^{125}I-iothalomate has gained popularity. This is an isotopically tagged tri-iodinated derivative of benzoic acid. The test is straightforward. After oral water-loading (5–10 ml/kg), a subcutaneous injection of ^{125}I (30–50 μCi) and epinephrine (to slow its absorption) is administered and produces constant plasma concentrations. After 45–60 min of equilibration, three to four timed urine collections together with plasma samples are obtained. The calculation of GFR is units (cpm) V/P(cpm). This method yields highly reproducible measurements of GFR and has a degree of experimental variability similar to that of inulin clearances (167). The entire test takes fewer than 3 hr and can be performed in the office or outpatient setting. Another advantage is that same-day assessment and calculation of GFR are easily obtained. The isotope's long half-life permits flexibility regarding when the samples are processed. One disadvantage is the need for simultaneous oral Lugol's iodine to block thyroid uptake of the isotope, and the related disadvantage of exclusion of certain patients, including children and pregnant women. These concerns notwithstanding, this particular radioactive marker of GFR is increasingly used due to its simplicity and accuracy. Recently, constant infusion of nonradioactive iothalamate was delivered by subcutaneous route in children and shown to yield an accurate GFR over a wide range of values (165). The advantage of this method includes a nonradioactive marker that can be infused over a long period of time to ensure achievement of a steady state. Once this is achieved, only one blood sample is necessary. Disadvantages include the longer duration of the test and requirement for access to HPLC for measurement of iothalomate.

Plasma Disappearance

The need for continuous infusion of a marker for glomerular filtration with the above methods and collection of complete, precisely timed urine samples has led to the development of simplified methods for estimating GFR after a single injection of a suitable marker. After an initial period of distribution within the body, the plasma concentration will decline over time as a result of renal excretion. Analysis of the plasma disappearance then is taken as an estimate of GFR. ^{51}Cr-EDTA, DTPA, ^{125}I-iothalomate, sodium iothalomate, exogenous creatinine, and inulin have all been used in this assay. Of these, ^{51}Cr-EDTA and labeled and nonradioactive iothalomate are currently in use. Five to six samples are taken, two to three in the first 20 min, then at longer intervals up to 3 to 4 hr. These tests have several prerequisites: precision in dosage of the marker, sufficient number of blood samples that document the rate of disappearance of the marker, and analysis that gives the best fit model. There are three models: the integral Nosslin model, the two-compartment model, and the one-compartment slope intercept model (168,169). Recently, a modified plasma clearance technique using nonradioactive iothalamate was used (170, 171). Blood samples were obtained at 60, 90, and 120 min after iothalomate injection. The study was conducted in 24 patients with various renal diseases whose inulin clearances ranged between 10 and 130 ml/min, as well as in normal subjects. Excellent correlation was observed between this modified plasma clearance method and standard renal inulin clearance ($C_{Iot}/C_{inulin} = 1.05$). Correlation with standard renal clearance of iothalomate was also high, with a ratio of 0.99 over the entire spectrum of renal function, including in those with nephrotic syndrome or polycystic kidney disease (172).

AMBULATORY RENAL MONITORING (ARM)

A novel approach to the measurement of GFR is a noninvasive external radionucleotide counting system used to determine the minute-to-minute rate of disappearance from the extracellular space of a radiolabeled marker of GFR after a single injection (173–175). The radiolabeled pharmaceutical agent is ^{99m}Tc-DTPA. The components of ARM include a detector that perceives the radioactivity and a shield to insulate it from interference, enclosed in a cuff the size of that used in measuring blood pressure. Once wrapped around the arm, the cuff forms a shielded cylinder with the detector unit inside, facing the arm. The extremity is used because it can be isolated from the rest of the extracellular space sensed by the detector and because it can be relatively isolated from radioactivity emanating from other organs. Collection of data is achieved via a pocket-sized computer.

This is the newest of methods for evaluation of GFR and offers the distinct advantage of providing noninvasive, real-time assessment of GFR. Monitoring of radioactivity is attained over a 5- to 10-min period in patients with normal renal function and 10- to 15-min duration in patients with more impaired renal function (GFR <30 ml/min). Excellent correlation between ARM and ^{125}I-iothalomate was shown in 59 patients with various degrees of renal dysfunction (Fig. 8). The reproducibility of GFR values by ARM within an individual is superior to even iothalamate GFR measurements (coefficient of variance 3.8% vs. 6.0–7.5% by standard clearance techniques) as is the reproducibility (coefficient of variance 5% vs. 15%). This methodology therefore has the potential not only for rapid documentation of GFR but also for monitoring of patients who are predictably at risk for developing renal failure (e.g., after cardiac surgery, renal revascularization, contrast media-induced nephropathy, nephrotoxic drug administration, etc.).

CLINICAL CORRELATES OF EXPERIMENTAL DATA

Aging (Decrease in Number of Glomeruli)

Aging reduces every aspect of renal function (176). Tubular function is lessened (e.g., reabsorption of glucose decreases) and regulation of water is compromised (177). The glomerular capillary wall selectivity properties are diminished, with a resulting increase in appearance of proteinuria (178). As noted above, GFR decreases by about 0.8 to 1.0 ml/min with every year of life after 40 years of age (179,180). Although the age-related decrease in GFR by itself does not cause problems, the older kidney is more vulnerable to superimposed injury. Importantly, serum creatinine remains constant, in part because up to 50% of filtration can be lost without a noticeable change in this parameter and in part due to reduction in muscle mass with aging, which causes reduction in creatinine production (181).

The mechanism for the reduction in GFR reflects the dropout of a number of filtering glomeruli. Glomerulosclerosis has long been known to accompany normal aging (182). Newer studies with unbiased morphometry support that a significant proportion of these glomeruli become totally resorbed. Furthermore, atubular glomeruli have been observed during aging, which may further contribute to decreased levels of GFR. Micropuncture studies confirm that the decrease in whole-kidney GFR in aged rats is not because of a decrease in filtration in individual glomeruli. Indeed, SNGFR has been shown to be only slightly decreased, unchanged, or increased in old rats (14,183). It is possible that the older rats showed hyperfiltration and increased glomerular pressure, reflecting a compensatory response to a more extensive glomerular damage/glomerular resorption and maximal recruitment of function from the remaining nephrons. Although hyperfiltration and decreased renal reserve have been documented in older rats, this function may not be impaired in older humans. Patients 60 to 85 years of age were found to have baseline GFRs of ~70 ml/min/1.73 m^2 and had normal renal reserves (184). Because animals develop glomerulosclerosis much faster than do humans, hyperfiltration and decreased recruitment of function from the remaining nephrons may not be relevant to humans until loss of nephrons reaches an advanced stage.

Age-dependent decline in renal function is not the same in men and women. Women are relatively protected against age-dependent deterioration in GFR and also have a delay in the appearance of structural injury. Men are more likely to develop progressive renal disease associated with diabetes, hypertension (185,186), and autosomal-dominant polycystic disease (187). Proteinuria and hypertension are more common in men than women kidney donors at long-term follow-up (188). The mechanism for this gender-based difference in renal scarring has been investigated in animal models. As in humans, male rats are more susceptible to glomerulosclerosis (37,189), both spontaneously in some strains and after renal ablation (190). Baylis studied intact and castrated aging male and female rats. Intact males developed glomerular injury and proteinuria, whereas females, both intact and ovariectomized, and castrated males were protected from injury. Thus, the presence of androgens, rather than the absence of estrogen, is implicated in the increased susceptibility to age-dependent glomerular damage. In this connection, Remuzzi et al. observed that mesangial matrix accumulation correlated with gender-related differences in glomerular filtration and proteinuria in rats (191). Thus, androgens appear to confer additional susceptibility to loss of glomeruli, possibly by enhancing accumulation of matrix material.

Renal Vasodilation (Decreased R_A, R_E, and K_f)

It has long been appreciated that infusion of potent vasodilators such as prostaglandins, bradykinin, acetylcholine, and histamine increase renal blood flow (75, 192,193). However, the increase in renal blood flow in these as well as numerous other settings is regularly unaccompanied by elevation in GFR. Micropuncture measurements during infusion of several of the above vasodilators showed that elevated plasma flow occurs and reflects a reduction in the afferent and efferent arteriolar resistances, particularly the former. Furthermore, although glomerular capillary pressure is not affected by vasodilator infusion, K_f decreases markedly. The net result of these two opposing forces is a stable GFR. These findings are relevant to clinical settings in which pharmacologically induced or spontaneous increase in renal blood (plasma) flow does not increase the level of GFR (e.g., lack of improvement in GFR with an increase in renal blood flow in the setting of acute renal failure).

Congestive Heart Failure (Decreased R_A and Increased R_E)

In congestive heart failure, glomerular filtration is under the opposing influences of low plasma flow rate and high glomerular capillary hydraulic pressure, which promote high filtration fraction. These prevailing hemodynamics predict the preservation of GFR in compensated heart failure, despite relative hypoperfusion of the glomerulus (17,18). The use of vasodilating agents (such as ACEI) is common in this setting but can result in apparent divergent effects on the GFR (18). Thus, GFR can increase or decrease or remain unaffected after ACEI use. Increase in GFR reflects improved renal perfusion due to decreased arteriolar resistance (preferentially afferent arteriolar resistance). Furthermore, inhibition of Ang II actions increases the glomerular capillary ultrafiltration coefficient, which is otherwise low in congestive heart failure. Pivotal to an increase in GFR after ACEI use is preservation of intraglomerular pressure, which reflects a lack of a deleterious dilation of the efferent arteriole (13). On the other hand, when GFR decreases with ACEI treatment, the underlying mechanism is a preferential decrease in the efferent arteriolar tone. This decreased arteriolar resistance may increase renal plasma flow. However, due to the profound reduction in the efferent arteriolar tone, the intraglomerular pressure decreases, which in turn lowers GFR.

The effects of ACEI to lower GFR are mediated in part by accumulation of bradykinin because ACE not only converts angiotensin I to Ang II, but also mediates the degradation of the vasodilating bradykinin. Thus, ACEI treatment not only decreases Ang II but also increases bradykinin levels. Bradykinin has a preferential dilating effect on the efferent arteriole. Thus, the mechanism of ACEI-induced decompensation in GFR in the setting of congestive heart failure, or any other condition where the glomerular pressure and filtration are dependent on Ang II–induced constriction of the efferent arteriole, is bradykinin mediated dilatation of the efferent arteriole. Of note, animal experiments show that antagonism of Ang II actions by another method, namely, Ang II receptor antagonists, is devoid of this efferent arteriolar dilation because the receptor antagonists do not affect Ang converting enzyme and therefore do not increase bradykinin.

Nephrotic Syndrome (Decreased K_f)

Isolated change in the plasma protein concentration, such as the hypoalbuminemia associated with nephrotic syndrome, predicts a reciprocal change in GFR. However, animal models as well as human conditions characterized by hypoalbuminemia do not follow the predicted change. Micropuncture studies confirm that concomitant changes in other determinants of GFR offset the predicted effect (194). Thus, despite a reduced plasma protein concentration, and hence lower oncotic pressure which should increase ultrafiltration, GFR is typically normal or even low in humans with nephrotic syndrome as well as in animal models. Importantly, the hypofiltration occurs in the face of little or no glomerular sclerosis, implying a functional basis for the prevailing GFR. An increase in the glomerular capillary hydraulic pressure also has been observed in experimental models of nephrotic syndrome (97,195–197). Similar changes have been extrapolated in humans with membranous and minimal change nephrotic syndromes (97). This increased glomerular hydraulic pressure together with lower glomerular oncotic pressure is expected to further augment filtration. Instead, these forces are offset by a profound decrease in the glomerular capillary ultrafiltration coefficient, K_f. Indeed, micropuncture studies in animal models with proteinuria (34,95, 196,197) confirm that K_f is reduced (34,95,196–198). Of interest, protein malnutrition, which was associated with only a modest decrease in plasma oncotic pressure, also caused a decrease in K_f. Conversely, elevation in plasma protein by infusion of hyperoncotic albumin into normal rats was accompanied by an increase in the ultrafiltration coefficient (199). These observations suggest that protein/oncotic pressure may directly or indirectly modulate K_f, although the mechanisms are not clear and may involve actions of vasoactive substances

K_f is defined by the surface area available for filtration and the hydraulic permeability of the capillary wall. Thus, either or both may be decreased in nephrotic syndrome and contribute to the low K_f in this setting. However, assessment of the precise contribution of each is difficult because these factors cannot be easily quantitated and because the structural counterparts to these functional parameters are not clearly defined. Nevertheless, morphologic assessment of glomeruli suggests an increase in the surface area available for filtration, implicating a decrease in the hydraulic conductivity component, k. Structural changes of the capillary wall were documented in nephrotic syndrome with a dramatic reduction in filtration slit frequency (95,98,200). Although these changes are proposed to underlie a defect in glomerular capillary sieving function and the resultant proteinuria that characterize nephrotic syndrome, it is not known whether this changes the filtration capacity. Children with kwashiorkor have foot process broadening and effacement but no proteinuria. Rather, these changes predict decreased K_f and are associated with decreased GFR, supporting a role of decreased hydraulic conductivity in lowering filtration.

REFERENCES

1. Nyengaard JR, Bendtsen TF. Glomerular number and size in relation to age, kidney weight, and body surface in normal man. *Anat Rec* 1992;232:194–201.
2. Ichikawa I, Maddox DA, Cogan MG, Brenner BM. Dynamics of glomerular ultrafiltration in euvolemic Munich-Wistar rats. *Renal Physiol* 1978;1:121.
3. Brenner BM,Troy JL, Daugharty TM. The dynamics of glomerular ultrafiltration in the rat. *J Clin Invest* 1971;50:1776.
4. Deen WM, Robertson CR, Brenner BM. A model of glomerular ultrafiltration in the rat. *Am J Physiol* 1972;223:1178–83.
5. Maddox DA, Deen WM, Brenner BM. Dynamics of glomerular ultrafiltration. VI. Studies in the primate. *Kidney Int* 1974;5:271.
6. Kon V, Ichikawa I. Hormonal regulation of glomerular filtration. *Annu Rev Med* 1985;36:515–31.
7. Valtin H. Renal hemodynamics and oxygen consumption. In: Valtin H, ed. *Renal function: mechanisms preserving fluid and solute balance in health.* Boston: Little, Brown; 1983:101–18.
8. Chen J, Fleming JT. Juxtamedullary afferent and efferent arterioles constrict to renal nerve stimulation. *Kidney Int* 1993;44:684–91.
9. Ohishi K, Okwueze MI, Vari RC, Carmines PK. Juxtamedullary microvascular dysfunction during the hyperfiltration stage of diabetes mellitus. *Am J Physiol* 1994;267:F99–105.
10. Newbold KM, Sandison A, Howie AJ. Comparison of size of juxtamedullary and outer cortical glomeruli in normal adult kidney. *Virchows Arch [A]* 1992;420:127–9.
11. Robertson CR, Deen WM, Troy JL, Brenner BM. Dynamics of glomerular ultrafiltration in the rat. III. Hemodynamics and autoregulation. *Am J Physiol* 1972;223:1191–200.
12. Osswald H, Haas JA, Marchand GR, Knox FG. Glomerular dynamics in dogs at reduced renal artery pressure. *Am J Physiol* 1979;236:F25.
13. Yoshioka T, Yared A, Kon V, Ichikawa I. Impaired preservation of GFR during hypotension in preexistent renal hypoperfusion. *Am J Physiol* 1989;256:F314–20.
14. Anderson S, Rennke HG, Zatz R. Glomerular adaptations with normal aging and with long-term converting enzyme inhibition in rats. *Am J Physiol* 1994;267:F35–43.
15. Arendshorst WJ, Beierwaltes WH. Renal and nephron hemodynamics in spontaneously hypertensive rats. *Am J Physiol* 1979;236:F246–51.
16. London GM, Safar ME, Levenson JA, Simon AC, Temmar MA. Renal filtration fraction, effective vascular compliance and partition of fluid volumes in sustained essential hypertension. *Kidney Int* 1981; 20:99–103.
17. Ichikawa I, Pfeffer JM, Hostetter TH, Brenner BM. Role of angiotensin II in the altered renal function of congestive heart failure. *Circ Res* 1984;55:669.
18. Badr KF, Ichikawa I. Prerenal failure: a deleterious shift from renal compensation to decompensation. *N Engl J Med* 1988;319:623–9.
19. Ballermann BJ, Skorecki KL, Brenner BM. Reduced glomerular angiotensin II receptor density in early untreated diabetes mellitus in the rat. *Am J Physiol* 1984;247:F110.

20. Bianchi C, Gutkowska J, Thibault G, et al. Distinct localization of atrial natriuretic factor and angiotensin II binding sites in the glomerulus. *Am J Physiol* 1986;251:F594.
21. Abboud HE, Dousa TP. Action of adenosine on cyclic 3858-nucleotides in glomeruli. *Am J Physiol* 1983;244:F633.
22. Martin ER, Brenner BM, Ballermann BJ. Identification of specific, high affinity endothelin (EN) binding sites in rat renal papillary (P) and glomerular (G) membranes. *Kidney Int* 1989;35:316.
23. Ballermann BJ, Lewis RA, Corey EJ, et al. Identification and characterization of leukotriene C4 receptors in isolated rat renal glomeruli. *Circ Res* 1985;56:324.
24. Schlondorff D, Yoo P, Alpert BE. Stimulation of adenylate cyclase in isolated rat glomeruli by prostaglandins. *Am J Physiol* 1978;235: F458.
25. Scharschmidt LA, Dunn MJ. Prostaglandin synthesis by rat glomerular mesangial cells in culture. *J Clin Invest* 1983;71:1756.
26. Winkler D, Elger M, Sakai T, Kriz W. Branching and confluence pattern of glomerular arterioles in the rat. *Kidney Int* 1991;39(suppl):2–8.
27. Elger M, Sakai T, Winkler D, Kriz W. Structure of the outflow segment of the efferent arteriole in rat superficial glomeruli. *Contrib Nephrol* 1991;95:22–33.
28. Kriz W, Elger M, Mundel P, Lemley KV. Structure-stabilizing forces in the glomerular tuft. *J Am Soc Nephrol* 1995;5:1731–9.
29. Maddox DA, Bennett CM, Deen WM, et al. Determinants of glomerular filtration in experimental glomerulonephritis in the rat. *J Clin Invest* 1975;55:305.
30. Blantz RC, Tucker BJ, Wilson CB. The acute effects of antiglomerular basement membrane antibody upon glomerular filtration in the rat. *J Clin Invest* 1978;61:910.
31. Chang RLS, Deen WM, Robertson CR, et al. Permselectivity of the glomerular capillary wall: studies of experimental glomerulonephritis in the rat. *J Clin Invest* 1976;57:1272.
32. Daugharty TM, Ueki IF, Mercer PF, Brenner BM. Dynamics of glomerular ultrafiltration in the rat. V. Response to ischemic injury. *J Clin Invest* 1974;53:105.
33. Ichikawa I, Brenner BM. Local intrarenal vasocontrictor–vasodilation interactions in mild partial ureteral obstruction. *Am J Physiol* 1979;236:F131.
34. Bohrer MP. Mechanisms of the puromycin-induced defects in the transglomerular passage of water and macromolecules. *J Clin Invest* 1977;60:152.
35. Ichikawa I, Purkerson ML, Klahr S, et al. Mechanism of reduced glomerular filtration rate in chronic malnutrition. *J Clin Invest* 1980;65:982.
36. Remuzzi A, Brenner BM, Pata V, et al. Three-dimensional reconstructed glomerular capillary network: blood flow distribution and local filtration. *Am J Physiol* 1992;263:F562–72.
37. Lambert PP, Aeikens B, Bohle A, Hanus F, Pegoff S, Van Damme M. A network model of glomerular function. *Microcvasc Res* 1982;23: 99–128.
38. Shea SM. Glomerular hemodynamics and vascular structure. The pattern and dimensions of a single rat glomerular capillary network reconstructed from ultra thin sections. *Microvasc Res* 1979;18: 129–43.
39. Shea SM, Raskowa J. Glomerular hemodynamics and vascular structure in uremia: a network analysis of glomerular path lengths and maximal blood transit times computed for a microvascular model reconstructed from subserial ultrathin sections. *Microvasc Res* 1984; 28:37–50.
40. Marcussen N. Biology of disease. Atubular glomeruli and the structural basis for chronic renal failure. *Lab Invest* 1992;66:265–84.
41. Nyengaard JR. The quantitative development of glomerular capillaries in rats with special reference to unbiased stereological estimates of their number and sizes. *Microvasc Res* 1993;45:243–61.
42. Nyengaard JR. Number and dimensions of rat glomerular capillaries in normal development and after nephrectomy. *Kidney Int* 1993;43: 1049–57.
43. Nyengaard JR, Rasch R. The impact of experimental diabetes mellitus in rats on glomerular capillary number and sizes. *Diabetologia* 1993;36:189–94.
44. Iordache BE, Remuzzi A. Numerical analysis of blood flow in reconstructed glomerular capillary segments. *Micro Vasc Res* 1995;49: 1–11.
45. Kreisberg JI, Venkatachalam MA, Radnik RA, Patel PY. Role of myosin light-chain phosphorylation and microtubules in stress fiber morphology in cultured mesangial cells. *Am J Physiol* 1985;249: F227–35.
46. Hiraoka-Yoshimoto M, Higashida K, Takeda M, Kawamoto S, Ichikawa I, Hoover RL. Characterization of mysin heavy and light chains in cultured mesangial cells. *Kidney Int* 1991;40:1013–9.
47. Takeda M, Breyer MD, Noland TD, et al. Endothelin-1 receptor antagonist: effects on endothelin- and cyclosporine-treated mesangial cells. *Kidney Int* 1992;42:1713–9.
48. Takeda M, Homma T, Breyer M, et al. Volume and agonist-induced regulation of myosin light-chain phosphorylation in glomerular mesangial cells. *Am J Physiol* 1993;264:F421–6.
49. Christensen S, Ottosen PD. Lithium-induced uremia in rats—a new model of chronic renal failure. *Pflugers Arch* 1983;399:208–12.
50. Dantzler WH. Comparative physiology of the vertebrate kidney. In: Dantzler WH, ed. *Zoolphysiology*. Vol. 22. Berlin: Springer-Verlag; 1989.
51. Bayliss WM. On the local reaction of the arterial to changes of internal pressure. *J Physiol Lond* 1902;28:220–31.
52. Harder DR, Kauser K, Roman RJ, Lombard JH. Mechanism of pressure-induced myogenic activation of cerebral and renal arteries: role of endothelium. *J Hypertens* 1989;7(suppl):11–5.
53. Edwards RM. Segmental effects of norepinephrine and angiotensin II on isolated renal microvessels. *Am J Physiol* 1983;244:F526.
54. Harder DR, Gibert R, Lombard JH. Vascular muscle cell depolarization and activation in renal arteries on elevation of transmural pressure. *Am J Physiol* 1987;253:F778.
55. Imig JD, Zou A-P, Ortiz de Montellano PR, Sui Z, Roman RJ. Cytochrome P-450 inhibitors alter afferent arteriolar responses to elevations in pressure. *Am J Physiol* 1994;266:H1879–85.
56. Bell PD, McLean CB, Navar LG. Dissociation of tubuloglomerular feedback responses from distal tubular chloride concentration in the rat. *Am J Physiol* 1981;240:F111.
57. Schnermann J, Persson AEG, Agerup B. Tubuloglomerular feedback: nonlinear relation between glomerular hydrostatic pressure and loop of henle perfusion rate. *J Clin Invest* 1973;52:862.
58. Schnermann J, Ploth DW, Hermle M. Activation of tubulo-glomerular feedback by chloride transport. *Pflugers Arch* 1976;362:229.
59. Bell Pd, Reddinton M. Intracellular calcium in the transmission of tubuloglomerular feedback signals. *Am J Physiol* 1983;245:F295.
60. Bell PD,Reddington M,Ploth D, Navar LG. Tubuloglomerular feedback-mediated decreases in glomerular pressure in Munich-Wistar rats. *Am J Physiol* 1984;247:F877.
61. Schnermann J, Briggs JP. Interaction between loop of Henle flow and arterial pressure as determinants of glomerular pressure. *Am J Physiol* 1989;256:F421–9.
62. Welch WJ, Wilcox CS. Modulating role for thromboxane in the tubuloglomerular feedback response in the rat. *J Clin Invest* 1988;81: 1843–9.
63. Weihprecht H, Lorenz JN, Briggs JP, Schnermann J. Vasoconstrictor effect of angiotensin and vasopressin in isolated rabbit afferent arterioles. *Am J Physiol* 1991;261:F273–82.
64. Mitchell KD, Navar LG. Enhanced tubuloglomerular feedback during peritubular infusions of angiotensins I and II. *Am J Physiol* 1988;255: F383–90.
65. Ito S, Arima S, Ren YL, Juncos LA, Carretero OA. Endothelium-derived relaxing factor/nitric oxide modulates angiotenin II action in the isolated microperfuled rabbit afferent but not efferent arteriole. *J Clin Invest* 1993;91:2012–9.
66. Ito S, Ren YL. Evidence for the role of nitric oxide in macula densa control of glomerular hemodynamics. *J Clin Invest* 1993;92:1093–8.
67. Wilcox CS, Welch WJ, Murad F, et al. Nitric oxide synthase in macula densa regulates glomerular capillary pressure. *Proc Natl Acad Sci U S A* 1992;89:11993–7.
68. Tojo A, Gross SS, Zhang L, et al. Immunocytochemical localization of distinct isoforms of nitric oxide synthase in the juxtaglomerular apparatus of normal rat kidney. *J Am Soc Nephrol* 1994;4:1438–47.
69. Andrews CEJ, Brenner BM. Relative contributions of arginine vasopressin and angiotensin II to maintenance of systemic arterial pressure in the anesthetized water-deprived rat. *Circ Res* 1981;48:254–8.
70. Yared A, Kon V, Ichikawa I. Mechanism of preservation of glomerular perfusion and filtration during acute extracellular fluid volume depletion. *J Clin Invest* 1985;75:1447–87.
71. Kon V, Yared A, Ichikawa I. Role of renal sympathetic nerves in mediating hypoperfusion of renal cortical microcirculation in experi-

mental congestive heart failure and acute fluid volume depletion. *J Clin Invest* 1985;76:1913–20.
72. Elger M, Hentschel H. The glomerulus of a stenohaline fresh-water teleost carassius awiatus gibelio, adapted to saline water. A scanning and transmission electron-microscopic. *Cell Tissue Res* 1981;220: 73–85.
73. Okubo S, Niimura F, Matsusaka T, Fogo A, Inagami T, Hogan BLM, Ichikawa I. Evidence from a gene targeting study that glomerular size is autoregulated during alteration in ECF volume in mammals due to angiotensin. *J Am Soc Nephrol* (Abstr). In press.
74. Baer PG, Navar LG. Renal vasodilation and uncoupling of blood flow and filtration rate autoregulation. *Kidney Int* 1973;4:12–21.
75. Baer PG, Navar LG, Guyton AC. Renal autoregulation, filtration rate, and electrolyte excretion during vasodilation. *Am J Physiol* 1970;219: 619.
76. Pelayo JC, Westcott JY. Impaired autoregulation of glomerular capillary hydrostatic pressure in the rat remnant nephron. *J Clin Invest* 1991;88:101–5.
77. Woods LL, Mizelle HL, Hall JE. Control of renal hemodynamics in hyperglycemia: possible role of tubuloglomerular feedback. *Am J Physiol* 1987;252:F65–73.
78. Bidani AK, Schwartz MM, Lewis EJ. Renal autoregulation and vulnerability to hypertensive injury in remnant kidney. *Am J Physiol* 1987;252:F1003–10.
79. Iversen BM, Ofstad J. Loss of renal blood flow autoregulation in chronic glomerulonephritic rats. *Am J Physiol* 1988;254:F284–90.
80. Baylis C. Renal effects of cyclooxgenase inhibition in the pregnant rat. *Am J Physiol* 1987;253:F158–63.
81. Baylis C, Collins RC. Angiotensin II inhibition on blood pressure and renal hemodynamics in pregnant rats. *Am J Physiol* 1986;250:F308–14.
82. Baylis C. Effect of amino acid infusion as an index of renal vasodilatory capacity in pregnant rats. *Am J Physiol* 1988;23:F650–6.
83. Baylis C, Blantz RC. Tubuloglomerular feedback in virgin and 12-day–pregnant rats. *Am J Physiol* 1985;249:F169–73.
84. Lindheimer MD, Katz AI. Renal physiology and disease in pregnancy. In: Seldin DW, Giebisch G, eds. *The kidney; physiology and pathophysiology.* New York: Raven; 1992:3371–432.
85. Woods LL, Mizelle HL, Hall JE. Autoregulation of renal blood flow and glomerular filtration rate in the pregnancy rabbit. *Am J Physiol* 1987;252:R69–72.
86. Deen WM, Satvat B, Jamieson JM. Theoretical model for glomerular filtration of charged solutes. *Am J Physiol* 1980;238:F126–39.
87. Deen WM, Myers BD, Brenner BM. The glomerular barrier to macromolecules: theoretical and experimental considerations. In: Brenner BM, ed. *Contemporary issues in nephrology.* Vol. 9. New York: Churchill-Livingstone; 1982:1–29.
88. Deen WM, Bohrer MP, Brenner BM. Macromolecular transport across glomerular ccapillaries; application of pore theory. *Kidney Int* 1979;16:353–65.
89. Deen WM, Bridges CR, Brenner BM, Myers BD. Heteroporous model of glomerular size-selectivity: application to normal and nephrotic humans. *Am J Physiol* 1985;249:F374–89.
90. Alfino PA, Neugarten J, Shacht RG, Dworkin LD, Baldwin DS. Glomerular size selective barrier dysfunction in nephrotoxic serum nephritis. *Kidney Int* 1988;34:151–5.
91. Olson JL. Role of heparin as a protective agent following reduction of renal mass. *Kidney Int* 1984;25:376–82.
92. Myers BD, Winetz JA, Chui F, Michaels AS. Mechanisms of proteinuria in diabetic nephropathy: a study of glomerular barrier function. *Kidney Int* 1982;21:96–105.
93. Morelli E, Loon N, Meyer T, Peters W, Myers BD. Effects of converting-enzyme inhibition on barrier function in diabetic glomerulopathy. *Diabetes* 1990;39:76–82.
94. Remuzzi A, Perticucci E, Ruggenenti P, Mosconi L, Limonta M, Remuzzi G. Antiotensin converting enzyme inhibition improves glomerular size-selectivity in IgA nephropathy. *Kidney Int* 1991;39: 1267–73.
95. Guasch A, Deen WM, Myers BD. Charge selectivity of the glomerular filtration barrier in healthy and nephrotic humans. *J Clin Invest* 1993;92:2274–82.
96. Guasch A, Myers BD. Determinants of glomerular hypofiltration in nephrotic patients with minimal change nephropathy. *J Am Soc Nephrol* 1994;4:1571–81.
97. Ting RH, Kristal B, Myers BD. The biophysical basis of hypofiltration in nephrotic humans with membranous nephropathy. *Kidney Int* 1994;45:390–7.
98. Drummond MC, Kristal B, Myers BD, Deen WM. Structural basis for reduced glomerular filtration capacity in nephrotic humans. *J Clin Invest* 1994;94:1187–95.
99. Olson JS, Rennke HG, Venkatachalam MA. Alteration in the charge and size selectivity barrier of the glomerular filter in aminonucleoside nephrosis in rats. *Lab Invest* 1981;44:271–9.
100. Hunsicker LG, Shearer TP, Shaffer SJ. Acute reversible proteinuria induced by infusion of the polycation hexadimetheine. *Kidney Int* 1981;20:7–17.
101. Comper WD, Lee ASN, Tay M, Adal Y. Anionic charge concentration of rat kidney glomeruli and glomerular basement membrane. *Biochem J* 1993;289:647–52.
102. Robinson GB, Walton HA. Glomerular basement membrane as a compressible filter. *Microvasc Res* 1989;38:36–48.
103. Daniels BS, Hauser EB, Deen WM, Hostetter TH. Glomerular basement membrane: in vitro studies of water and protein permeability. *Am J Physiol* 1992;262:F919–26.
104. Rennke HG, Vankatachalam MA. Glomerular permeability: in vivo tracer studies with polyanionic polyanionic and poly cationic ferritins. *Kidney Int* 1977;11:44.
105. Fries JWU, Sandstrom DJ, Meyer TW, Rennke HG. Glomerular hypertrophy and epithelial cell injury modulate progressive glomerulosclerosis in the rat. *Lab Invest* 1989;60:205–18.
106. Schwartz MM, Bidani AK, Lewis EJ. Glomerular epithelial cell function and pathology following extreme ablation of renal mass. *Am J Pathol* 1987;126:315–24.
107. Schwartz MM, Korbet SM. Primary focal segmental glomerulosclerosis: pathology, histological variants, and pathogenesis. *Am J Kidney Dis* 1993;22:874–83.
108. Nagata M, Schärer K, Kriz W. Glomerular damage after uninephrectomy in young rats. I. Hypertrophy and distortion of capillary architecture. *Kidney Int* 1992;42:136–47.
109. Salant DJ, Madaio MP, Adler S, Stilmant MM, Couser WG. Altered glomerular permeability induced by F(ab8)2 and Fab8 antibodies to rat renal tubular epithelial antigen. *Kidney Int* 1981;21:36–43.
110. Mendrick DL, Rennke HG. Induction of proteinuria in the rats by a monoclonal antibody against SGP-115/107. *Kidney Int* 1988;33:818–30.
111. Adler S, Chen X. Anti-Fx1A antibody recognizes a b1-integrin on glomerular epithelial cells and inhibits adhesion and growth. *Am J Physiol* 1992;31:F770–6.
112. Salant DJ. The structural biology of glomerular epithelial cells in proteinuric diseases. *Curr Opin Nephrol Hypertens* 1994;3:569–74.
113. Yoshioka T, Mitarai T, Kon V, Deen WM, Rennke HG, Ichikawa I. Role of angiotensin II in an overt functional proteinuria. *Kidney Int* 1986;30:538–45.
114. Eisenbach GM, Van Liew JB, Boylan JW. Effect of angiotensin on the filtration of protein in the rat kidney: a micropuncture study. *Kidney Int* 1975;8:80–7.
115. Shemesh O, Deen WM, McNeely E, Myers BD. Effect of colloid volume expansion on glomerular barrier size selectivity in humans. *Kidney Int* 1986;29:916–23.
116. Cosenzi A, Carraro M, Sacerdote A, et al. Involvement of renin angiotensin system in the patholgenesis of postexercise proteinuria. *Scand J Urol* 1993;27:301–4.
117. Maschio G, Cagnoli L, Claroni F, et al. ACE inhibition reduces proteinuria in normotensive patients with IgA nephropathy: a multicentre, randomized, placebo-controlled study. *Nephrol Dial Transplant* 1994;9:265–9.
118. Ruilope LM, Alcazar JM, Hernandez E, Praga M, Lahera V, Rodicio JL. Long-term influences of antihypertensive therapy on microalbuminuria in essential hypertension. *Kidney Int* 1994;45(suppl):171–3.
119. Anderson S, Rennke HG, Brenner BM. Therapeutic advantage of converting enzyme inhibitors in arresting progressive renal disease associated with systemic hypertension in the rat. *J Clin Invest* 1986; 77:1993–2000.
120. Tanaka R, Kon V, Yoshioka T, Ichikawa I, Fogo A. Angiotensin converting enzyme inhibitor modulates glomerular function and structure by distinct mechanisms. *Kidney Int* 1994;45:537–43.
121. Kon V, Fogo A, Ichikawa I. Bradykinin causes selective efferent arteriolar dilation during angiotensin I converting enzyme inhibition. *Kidney Int* 1993;44:545–50.

122. Yoshida Y,Kawamura T,Ikoma M,Fogo A, Ichikawa I. Effects of antihypertensive drugs on glomerular morphology. *Kidney Int* 1989; 36:626–35.
123. Heeg JE, deJong PE, van der Hem GK, de Zeeuw D. Angiotensin II does not acutely reverse the reduction of proteinuria by long-term ACE inhibition. *Kidney Int* 1991;40:734–41.
124. Smith HW. *The kidney:* structure and function in health and disease. New York: Oxford University Press; 1951:182–94.
125. Wesson LG. *Physiology of the human kidney.* New York: Grune & Stratton; 1969.
125a. Kampmann J, Siersbaek-Nielsen K, Kristensen M, Molholm Hansen J. Rapid evaluation of creatinine clearance. *Acta Med Scand* 1974; 196:517–20.
126. McIntosh JF, Moller E, Van Slyke DD. Studies of urea excretion. III. The influence of body size on urea output. *J Clin Invest* 1928;6:467–82.
127. Black DAK, Cameron JS. Renal Function. *Chemical diagnosis of disease.* New York: Elsevier; 1979:453–524.
128. Bosch JP, Lew S, Glabman S, Lauer A. Renal hemodynamic changes in humans. Response to protein loading in normal and diseased kidneys. *Am J Med* 1986;81:809–15.
129. Wesson LG, Lauler DP. Diurnal cycle of glomerular filtration rate and sodium and chloride excretion during responses to altered salt and water balance in man. *J Clin Invest* 1961;40:1967–77.
130. Van Acker BAC, Koomen GCM, Koopman MG, Krediet RT, Arisz L. Discrepancy between circadian rhythms of inulin and creatinine clearance. *J Lab Clin Med* 1992;120:400–10.
131. Shannon JA, Joliffe N, Smith HW. The excretion of urine in the dog. IV. The effect of maintenance diet, feeding, etc. upon the quantity of glomerular filtrate. *Am J Physiol* 1932;101:625–37.
132. Pitts RF. The effect of protein and amino acids metabolism on the urea and xylose clearance. *J Nutr* 1935;9:657–65.
133. Jones MG, Lee K, Swaminathan R. The effect of dietary protein on glomerular filtration rate in normal subjects. *Clin Nephrol* 1987;27:71–5.
134. Claris-Appiano A, Assael BM, Tirelli AS, Marra B, Cavanna G. Lack of glomerular hemodynamic stimulation after infusion of branched chain amino acids. *Kidney Int* 1988;33:91–4.
135. Hirschberg RR, Zipser RD, Slomowitz LA, Kopple JD. Glucagon and prostaglandins are the mediators of amino acid–induced rise in renal hemodynamics. *Kidney Int* 1988;33:1147–55.
136. Hostetter TH. Human renal response to a meat meal. *Am J Physiol* 1986;19:F613–8.
137. Hart O. Ein neues inulinahnliches Polygructosesaccharid. *Klin Wochenschr* 1963;41:769–70.
138. Smith HW. *Principles of renal physiology.* New York: Oxford University Press; 1956.
139. Gutman Y, Gottschalk CW, Lassiter WE. Micropuncture study of inulin absorption in the rat kidney. *Science* 1965;147:753–4.
140. Harris CA, Baer PG, Chirito E, Dirks JH. Composition of mammalian glomerular filtrate. *Am J Physiol* 1974;227:972–6.
141. Marsh D, Frasier C. Reliability of inulin for determining volume flow in rat renal cortical tubules. *Am J Physiol* 1965;209:283–6.
142. Smith HW. Note on the interpretation of clearance methods in the diseased kidney. *J Clin Invest* 1941;20:631–5.
143. Rosenbaum RW, Hruska KA. Inulin: an inadequate marker of glomerular filtration rate in kidney donors and transplant recipients? *Kidney Int* 1979;16:179–86.
144. Heller J, Horacek V, Hollyova J. Comparison of inulin and creatinine and clearance in dogs after unilateral nephrectomy. *Nephron* 1980;25: 299.
145. Mak RHK, Dahhan JA, Azzopardi D, Bosque M, Chantler C, Haycock GB. Measurements of glomerular filtration rate in children after renal transplantation. *Kidney Int* 1983;23:410–3.
146. Carrie BJ, Golbetz HV, Michaels AS, Myers BD. Creatinine: an inadequate filtration marker in glomerular diseases. *Am J Med* 1980;69: 177–82.
147. Myers BM, Chui F, Hilberman M, Michaels AS. Trans-tubular leakage of glomerular filtrate in human acute renal failure. *Am J Physiol* 1979;237:F319–25.
148. Graystone JE. Creatinine excretion during growth. In: Cheek DB, ed. *Human growth.* Philadelphia: Lea & Febiger; 1968:182–97.
149. Salazar DE, Corcoran GD. Predicting creatinine clearance and renal drug clearance in obese patients from estimated fat free body mass. *Am J Med* 1988;84:1053–60.
150. Boers M, Dijkmans DA, Dreedveld FC, Mattie H. Errors in the prediction of creatinine clearance in patients with rheumatoid arthritis. *Br J Rheumatol* 1988;27:233–5.
151. Mohler JL, Ellison MF, Flanigan RC. Creatinine clearance prediction in spinal cord injury patients: comparison of 6 prediction equations. *J Urol* 1988;139:706–9.
152. Brion LP, Boeck MA, Gauthier B, Nussbaum MP, Schwartz GJ. Estimation of glomerular filtration rate in anorectic adolescents. *Pediatr Nephrol* 1989;3:16–21.
153. Goldberg TH, Finkelstein MS. Difficulties in estimating glomerular filtration rate in the elderly. *Arch Intern Med* 1987;147:1430–3.
154. Duarte CG. Renal function tests—clinical laboratory procedures and diagnosis. In: Duarte CG, ed. *Pediatric textbook of fluids and electrolytes.* Boston: Little, Brown; 1980:14.
155. Mitch WE, Collier VU, Walser M. Creatinine metabolism in chronic renal failure. *Clin Sci* 1980;58:327.
156. Shemesh O, Golbetz H, Kriss JP, Myers BD. Limitations of creatinine as a filtration marker in glomerulopathic patients. *Kidney Int* 1985;28: 830–8.
157. Cook JGH. Factors influencing the assay of creatinine. *Ann Clin Biochem* 1975;24:85–97.
158. Perrone RD, Madias NE, Levey AS. Serum creatinine as an index of renal function: new insighs into old concepts. *Clin Chem* 1992;38: 1933–53.
159. Mitch WE, Walser M, Buffington GA, Lemann J. A simple method of estimating progression of chronic renal failure. *Lancet* 1976;2: 1326–8.
160. Walser M, Drew I, LaFrance ND. Creatinine measurements often yielded false estimates of progression in chronic renal failure. *Kidney Int* 1988;34:412–8.
161. Levey AS, Berg RL, Gassman JJ, Hall PM, Walker WG. Creatinine filtration, secretion, and excretion during progressive renal disease. *Kidney Int* 1989;27:S73–80.
162. Hilbrands LB, Artz MA, Wetzels JFM, Koene AP. Cimetidine improves the reliability of creatinine as a marker of glomerular filtration. *Kidney Int* 1991;40:1171–6.
163. van Acker B, Koomen GCM, Koopman MG, de Waart DR, Arisz L. Creatinine clearance during cimetidine administration for measurement of glomerular filtration rate. *Lancet* 1992;340:1326–9.
164. Dalmeida W, Suki WN. Measurement of GFR with non-radioisotopic radio contrast agents. *Kidney Int* 1988;34:725–8.
165. Sigman EM, Elwood CM, Knox F. The measurement of glomerular filtration rate in man with sodium iothalamate (131 I-Conray). *J Nucl Med* 1966;7:60–8.
166. Barbour GL, Crumb CK, Boyd CM, Reeves RD, Rastogi SP, Patterson RM. Comparison of inulin, iothalamate and ^{99m}Tc-DTPA for measurement of glomerular filtration rate. *J Nucl Med* 1976;17:317–20.
167. Israelit AH, Long DL, White MG, Hull AR. Measurement of glomerular filtration rate utilizing a single subcutaneous injection of ^{125}I-iothalamate. *Kidney Int* 1973;4:346–9.
168. Schuster VL, Seldin DW. Renal clearance. In: Seldin DW, Giebisch G, eds. *The kidney: physiology and patholphysiology.* New York: Raven; 1985:365–95.
169. Nosslin B. Determination of clearance and distribution volume with a single injection technique. *Acta Med Scand* 1965;442:97–101.
170. Isaka Y, Fujiwara Y, Yamamoto S, et al. Modified plasma clearance technique using nonradioactive iothalamate for measuring GFR. *Kidney Int* 1992;42:1006–11.
171. Gaspari F, Mosconi L, Vigano G, et al. Measurement of GFR with a single intravenous injection of nonradioactive iothalamate. *Kidney Int* 1992;41:1081–4.
172. Hall JE, Guyton AC, Farr BM. A single-injection method for measuring glomerular filtration rate. *Am J Physiol* 1977;232:F72–6.
173. Rabito CA, Moore RH, Bougas C, Dragotakes SC. Noninvasive, real-time monitoring of renal function: the ambulatory renal monitor. *J Nucl Med* 1993;34:199–207.
174. Rabito CA, Fang LST, Waltman AC. Renal function in patients at risk of contrast material–induced acute renal failure: noninvasive, real-time monitoring. *Radiol* 1993;186:851–4.
175. Rabito CA, Panico F, Rubin R, Tolkoff-Rubin N, Teplick R. Noninvasive, real-time monitoring of renal function during critical care. *J Am Soc Nephrol* 1994;4:1421–8.
176. Meyer BR. Renal function in aging. *J Am Geriatr Soc* 1989;37:791.
177. Solomon LR, Lye M. Hypernatraemia in the elderly patient. *Gerontology* 1990;36:171.

178. Corman B, Chami Khazraji S, Schaeverbeke J, Michel JB. Effect of feeding on glomerular filtration rate and proteinuria in conscious aging rats. *Am J Physiol* 1988;255:F250.
179. Davies DF, Shock NW. Age changes in glomerular filtration rate, effective renal plasma flow and tubular excretory capacity in adult males. *J Clin Invest* 1950;29:496.
180. Cockroft DW, Gault MH. Prediction of creatinine clearance from serum creatinine. *Nephron* 1976;16:31.
181. Rowe J, Andres R, Tobin JD, Norris AH, Shock NW. The effect of age on creatinine clearance in men: a cross-sectional and longitudinal study. *J Gerontol* 1976;31:155.
182. Kaplan C, Pasternack B, Shah H, Gallo G. Age-related incidence of sclerotic glomeruli in human kidneys. *Am J Physiol* 1975;80:227.
183. Baylis C. Age-dependent glomerular damage in the rat. *J Clin Invest* 1994;94:1823–9.
184. Bohler J, Gloer D, Reetze-Bonorden P, Keller E, Schollmeyer PJ. Renal functional reserve in elderly patients. *Clin Nephrol* 1993;39: 145–50.
185. Wesson LG Jr. Renal hemodynamics in physiological states. In: Wesson LG Jr, ed. *Physiology of the human kidney*. New York: Grune & Stratton; 1969:96–108.
186. Hollenberg NK, Adams DF, Solomon HS, Rashid A, Abrams HL, Merrill JP. Senescence and the renal vasculature in normal man. *Circ Res* 1974;34:309–16.
187. Gretz N, Zeier M, Geberth S, Strauch M, Ritz E. Is gender a determinant for evolution of renal failure? A study of autosomal dominant polycystic kidney disease. *Am J Kidney Dis* 1989;14:178–83.
188. Hakim RM, Goldser RC, Brenner BM. Hypertension and proteinuria: long-term sequelae of uninephrectomy in humans. *Kidney Int* 1984; 25:930–6.
189. Baylis C, Wilson CB. Sex and the single kidney. *Am J Kidney Dis* 1989;13:290–8.
190. Remuzzi A, Puntorieri S, Alfano M, et al. Pathophysiologic implications of proteinuria in a rat model of progressive glomerular injury. *Lab Invest* 1992;67:572–9.
191. Remuzzi A, Puntorieri S, Mazzoleni A, Remuzzi G. Sex related differences in glomerular ultrafiltration and proteinuria in Munich Wistar rats. *Kidney Int* 1988;34:481–6.
192. Baylis C, Deen WM, Myers BD, Brenner BM. Effects of some vasodilator drugs on transcapillary fluid exchange in renal cortex. *Am J Physiol* 1976;230:1148.
193. Yoshioka T, Yared A, Miyazawa H, Ichikawa I. In vivo influence of prostaglandin I2 on systemic and renal circulation in the rat. *Hypertension* 1985;7:867.
194. Ichikawa I, Rennke HG, Hoyer JR, et al. Role for intrarenal mechanisms in the impaired salt excretion of experimental nephrotic syndrome. *J Clin Invest* 1983;71:91–103.
195. Allison MEM, Wilson CB, Gottschalk CW. Pathophysiology of experimental glomerulonephritis in rats. *J Clin Invest* 1974;53:1402–23.
196. Ichikawa I, Hoyer JR, Seiler WM, Brenner BM. Mechanisms of glomerulotubular balance in the setting of heterogeneous glomerular injury. *J Clin Invest* 1982;69:185–98.
197. Yoshioka T, Rennke HG, Salant dJ, Deen WM, Ichikawa I. Role of abnormally high transmural pressure in the permselectivity defect of glomerular capillary wall: a study in early passive Heymann nephritis. *Circ Res* 1987;61:531–8.
198. Bennett CM, Glassock RJ, Chang RLS, Deen WS, Robertson CR, Brenner BM. Permselectivity of the glomerular capillary wall: studies of experimental glomerulonephritis in the rat using dextran sulfate. *J Clin Invest* 1976;57:1287–94.
199. Baylis C, Ichikawa I, Willis WT, Wilson CB, Brenner BM. Dynamics of glomerular ultrafiltration. IX. Effects of plasma protein concentration. *Am J Physiol* 1977;232:F58–71.
200. Guasch A, Hashimoto H, Sibley RK, Deen WM, Myers BD. Glomerular dysfunction in nephrotic humans with minimal changes or focal glomerosclerosis. *Am J Physiol* 1991;260:F728–37.
201. Kon V, Ichikawa I. Research Seminar: Physiology of acute renal failure. *J Pediatr* 1984;105:351–7.
202. Shepherd JT, Vanhoutte PM. *The human cardiovascular system: facts and concepts*. New York: Raven Press; 1979.
203. Ichikawa I, Harris RC. Angiotensin actions in the kidney. Renewed insight into the old hormone. *Kidney Int* 1991;40:583–96.

Immunologic Renal Diseases,
edited by E. G. Neilson and W. G. Couser.
Lippincott-Raven Publishers, Philadelphia © 1997

CHAPTER 4

Normal Immune Responses

Laurence A. Turka

OVERVIEW: ROLE OF THE IMMUNE SYSTEM IN NORMAL HOMEOSTASIS

Over centuries of evolution, the immune system developed a highly specialized and tightly regulated series of responses, the primary function of which is traditionally described as discriminating between self and nonself. Based on the concept that immune responses can be primarily provoked by tissue destruction, it also has been proposed that the immune system senses tissue damage/danger, a distinction which, to a large extent, may be primarily semantic. In either case, activation of cells of the immune system provokes both local and systemic responses. When the kidney is the primary site inciting the immune response, it follows that it is likely to be the local target of the response as well. A classic example of this is allograft rejection, in which the entire kidney is perceived as "nonself" by the immune system. Thus, it initiates the response and becomes its target. However, the kidney may also be a secondary, or promiscuous, target of an immune response initiated at a distant site. This might occur either because of cross-reactivity between the initial target and an antigen located within the kidney (postulated to contribute to post-streptococcal glomerulonephritis), or because the kidney is an innocent bystander adversely affected by an immune response (for example, immune-complex-mediated glomerulonephritis secondary to any of a number of causes). Thus, immunologically mediated renal disease can occur in a wide variety of clinical circumstances and, depending on the nature of the evoked response, can take any of several forms. This chapter is designed to provide an overview of the physiology of normal immune responses that will serve as a foundation the understanding the pathophysiology of immune-mediated renal disease. To do so, we review immune system development, then the mechanisms that initiate an immune response, and finally, the mechanisms that regulate, and ultimately terminate, a response.

L. A. Turka: Department of Medicine, University of Pennsylvania, Philadelphia, Pennsylvania 19104.

CELLS AND DEVELOPMENTAL ASPECTS OF THE IMMUNE SYSTEM

Immune responses involved coordinate interactions between a variety of cell types (Fig. 1). Cells such as T cells, B cells, natural killer (NK) cells, macrophages, and dendritic cells are of hematopoietic origin and play the primary roles in immune homeostasis.

T cells, B cells, and NK cells are thought to all arise from a common precursor stem cell (1). These cells show many similarities in antigen recognition and intracellular signaling, but have distinct immune functions. T cells account for what is termed cellular immunity. This includes delayed-type hypersensitivity reactions, cell-mediated lympholysis, and most forms of transplantation reactions (such as allograft rejection and graft-versus-host disease) that can be seen as a combination of the first two responses. The hallmark of cellular responses is that lymphocytes act either directly on the target cell, in which instance cell–cell contact is required (such as in cell-mediated lympholysis) or locally through elaborated cytokines in which case the target cell/antigen must be nearby (such as in delayed-type hypersensitivity). B cells form the humoral arm of the immune system. Antibodies produced by B cells circulate throughout the body and are present in secreted fluids and mucosal surfaces. These antibodies can act independently of lymphocytes by fixing complement or targeting cells for phagocytosis (a process termed opsonization). Antibody binding to cells can also serve as a stimulus for cell-mediated lympholysis (antibody-dependent cellular cytotoxicity). NK cells appeared early in the evolution of the vertebrate

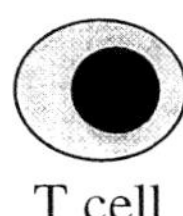

Subdivided into helper cells which initiate immune responses through the production of cytokines, and cytotoxic cells which lyse targets cells expressing foreign proteins

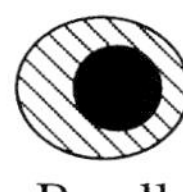

Differentiates into plasma cells which produce antibodies. Also serves to present antigen to helper T cells.

A primitive immune effector which kills target cells that fail to express self proteins.

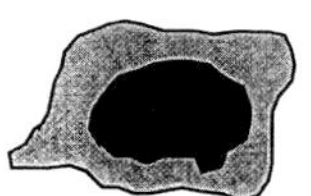

Mediates non-specific inflammation and tissue destruction when activated by T cell-derived cytokines. Also presents antigen to helper T cells.

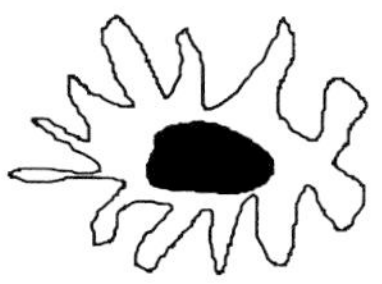

Specialized type antigen-presenting cell which is particularly potent at capturing and presenting antigens.

A

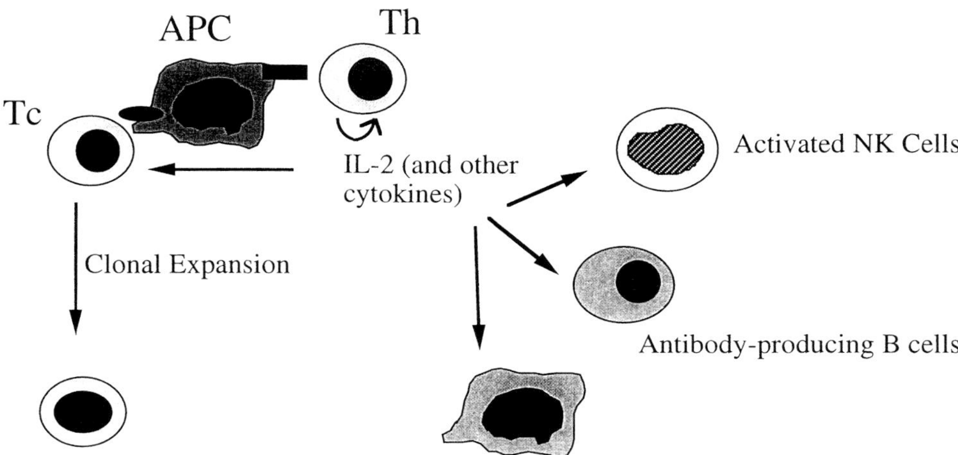

B

FIG. 1. The immune system: cells and responses. **A:** Cells of the immune system. There are five basic types of immunologically active effector cells: T and B lymphocytes, NK cells, macrophages, and dendritic cells. **B:** Overview of the immune response. MHC class-II-restricted CD4+ T helper cells (Th) initiate immune responses by secreting cytokines such as IL-2. These cytokines are used in an autocrine fashion by the Th cells themselves and in a paracrine fashion by the other major subset of T cells, MHC class-I-restricted CD8+ cytotoxic T cells (Tc). The latter require activation by antigen in order to respond to cytokines. Since antigen-presenting cells (APCs) bear class I and class II antigens on their surface, they are able to stimulate Th and Tc simultaneously in a three-cell complex. This is an efficient way to sustain a response since cytokines act in local microenvironments. Other immune effector cells present locally such as NK cells, B cells, and macrophages will be activated as well.

immune system and form part of the cellular immune response. Rather than recognizing and reacting to non-self antigens (as do T cells), they appear to lyse cells that *fail* to express self-antigens (see below). This relatively primitive form of immunity is ineffective against certain types of pathogens such as viruses, but probably contributes to transplantation responses and tumor surveillance.

Macrophages and dendritic cells are nonlymphoid cells of hematopoietic origin that play a crucial role in initiating immune responses by presenting foreign antigens to T cells, a function that can be performed by B cells as well. In addition to these specialized antigen-presenting cells (APCs), under certain circumstances nonhematopoietic cells such as endothelial cells and renal epithelial cells may present antigens as well.

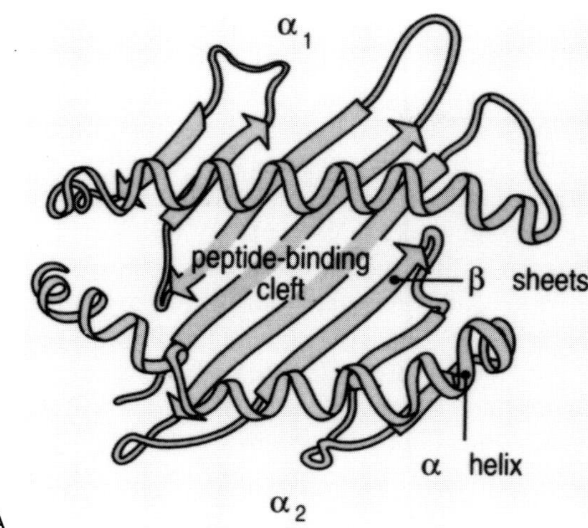

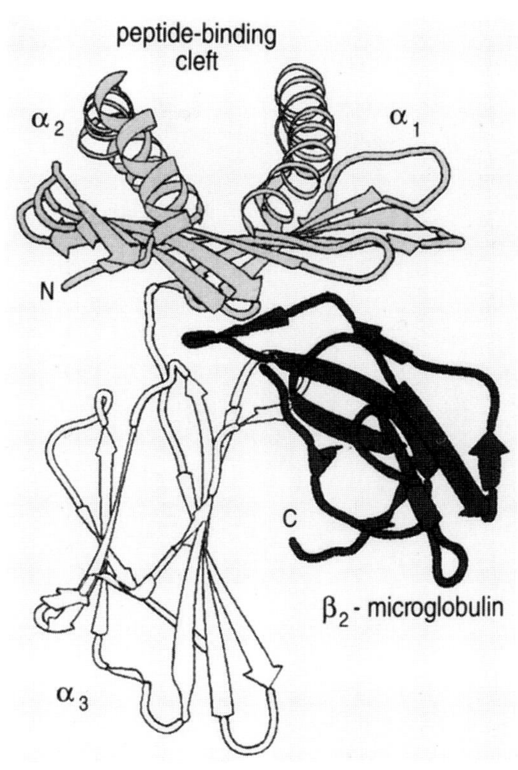

FIG. 2. Structure of an MHC molecule. The crystal structure of an MHC class I molecule, as solved by X-ray crystallography, reveals a peptide-binding groove with sides formed by two α-helices and a floor consisting of a β-pleated sheet: an overhead view of the peptide-binding groove **(A)** and a view from the side of the entire molecule **(B)**. Reprinted with permission from C. A. Janeway and P. Travers, *Immunobiology*, Current Biology Ltd., London.

T Cells

T cells, through their antigens receptors, recognize foreign proteins in the form of short peptide fragments (9–15 amino acids) presented in the antigen-binding groove of major histocompatibility complex (MHC) molecules (Fig. 2) (2–4). Peptide binding to MHC is absolutely required, as unbound peptides will not activate T cells. Two other important features are that the MHC loci are highly polymorphic (see below), and the immune response is self-MHC restricted (5). The latter means that, in general, T cells are only activated by peptides bound to self-MHC molecules. This is a consequence of T-cell development in the thymus, where appropriate signals for maturation are delivered only to T cells that bind MHC (see below). Since only self-MHC molecules are available, it follows that only self-MHC-restricted T cells will mature. Thus, a given T cell that responds to a peptide antigen presented by self-MHC will not respond to that same peptide antigen presented by a foreign MHC molecule.

The T-Cell Receptor

One of the hallmarks identifying T cells is the T-cell receptor for antigen (TCR) itself (Fig. 3). The receptor is a heterodimer formed using two of four possible molecules, the α, β, γ, or δ chain. To form the heterodimer, α pairs with β, and γ with δ (6,7). Most T cells formed in the thymus use the αβ heterodimer, and these constitute most cells found in the blood and in peripheral lymphoid organs such as lymph nodes and spleen. TCR γδ cells are particularly prominent in the skin and in mucosal surfaces such as the tongue, the vagina, and the intestinal epithelium.

The genes encoding the TCR chains are members of the immunoglobulin (Ig) supergene family (8,9). This is a large family of genes, many of which are found on B, T, and NK cells. Although all members of this family share certain features of structural similarity, the TCR genes are most closely related to their B-cell homologues, the Ig genes. Although soluble Ig is familiar to us as antibodies, surface Igs form the B-cell antigen receptor, and thus the similarity between the TCR and Ig genes is not surprising.

The universe of antigens is enormous, and therefore a diverse repertoire of TCRs and Igs is needed to mount an appropriate response. In theory, this could be accomplished by having a large number of intact TCR and Ig genes contained within the genome, with each T or B cell then selectively activating and transcribing a different one. However, given the numbers of lymphocytes that are generated in humans (well over 10^{10}), this would require more space than exists in the genome. The solution that has evolved uses a limited number of gene elements to create a relatively limitless repertoire, in large part through a process of genetic rearrangement known as V(D)J recombination (10). Thus, both TCR and Ig genes are formed through the rearrangement of genetic loci

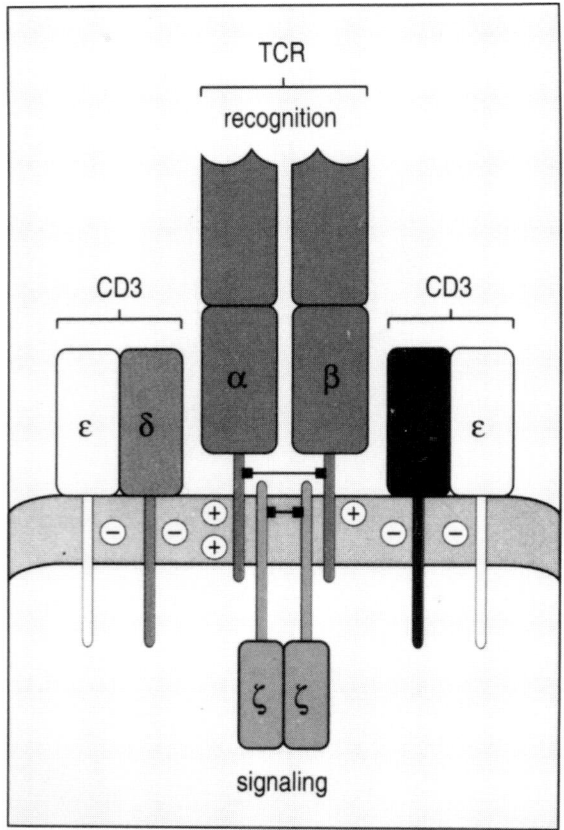

FIG. 3. Schematic diagram of the T-cell receptor (TCR)–CD3 complex. The TCR–CD3 complex consists of the TCR itself, which binds antigen, and associated chains that are collectively called CD3. These chains, whose precise stoichiometry is believed to be as shown here, serve to transduce signals from the TCR itself into the cell interior, leading to T-cell activation. Reprinted with permission from C. A. Janeway and P. Travers, *Immunobiology,* Current Biology Ltd., London.

from their germline configuration. The process of rearrangement is cell and lineage specific, such that TCR loci only rearrange in T cells and Ig loci only in B cells. This process is illustrated for the TCR α and β loci in Fig. 4. Considering the TCRβ chain, we see that the mature TCRβ-chain gene contains four regions, a variable or V region, a diversity or D region, a joining or J region, and a constant or C region. (The TCR δ locus and the Ig heavy-chain locus also have V, D, and J regions. The TCR α and γ loci and the Ig light-chain loci lack a D region). In mice, the genomic β locus contains ~20 different Vβ regions, 2 Dβ regions, and 12 Jβ regions. To create the gene encoding a β chain, the genomic locus rearranges to place end to end one Vβ, one Dβ, and one Jβ. The Cβ region is, as named, constant, and thus is not thought to contribute to repertoire diversity. It also does not become directly joined to the V, D, and J DNA segments. Rather, following transcription into RNA, the intron between the Jβ and Cβ regions, as well as any intervening nonutilized Jβ, segments are removed during RNA editing. The final transcript thus places V, D, J, and C contiguously.

V(D)J recombination generates repertoire diversity by at least three distinct mechanisms. The first and perhaps most important is combinatorial diversity. As indicated, random recombination can generate ~500 different β-chain genes. At the TCR α locus, the 100 V and 50 J elements can give rise to 5,000 distinct α-chain genes. The second mechanism is junctional diversity (11). During V(D)J recombination, junctional nucleotides (those at the termini of the germline genetic element) can be deleted, or alternatively, nucleotides not encoded in the germline can be added at the junctional sites, a process known as N-nucleotide addition. Assuming the number of nucleotides deleted or added is a multiple of 3 (so as not to alter the reading frame), this will alter the length, sequence, and functional specificity of the final protein. Thus, two TCR β chains using the same V, D, and J regions can differ in specificity based on N-nucleotide addition. Finally, because antigen specificity is dictated by a heterodimer, antigen specificity for any given β chain will vary depending upon which a chain it is paired with. Similar considerations exist for TCR γ and δ, as well as for Ig heavy and light chains. Thus, combinatorial associations contribute to diversity.

This system is extraordinarily powerful in generating diversity. In mice, combinatorial diversity can produce 500 distinct β chains and 5,000 distinct α chains. Thus, 2.5 million different TCRαβ heterodimers can be formed through V(D)J recombination and differential pairing. When deletion of junctional nucleotides and N-nucleotide addition are also considered, the number of unique TCRαβ heterodimers that can be produced is seen to be quite large.

Thymic Development–T-Cell Selection

T cells are so named because, in most instances, their development depends on the thymus, an organ whose stromal cells are embryologically derived from pharyngeal pouches (12). In the absence of a thymus, such as in the nude mice strain, T cells are either absent, or extremely rare, and animals are grossly immunodeficient. Once mature T cells are formed, however, they no longer need a thymus, as evidenced by the ability of T cells adoptively transferred to syngeneic nude mice to colonize the animals and function. Similarly, incidental thymectomy during corrective cardiac surgery in children does not lead to immunodeficiency. By adulthood, the thymus involutes, producing few if any new T cells. While it was once thought that all T cells developed in the thymus, there is increasing evidence for extrathymic development of at least some T cells (see below), although the degree to which these cells are required for normal immune function is not clear (13).

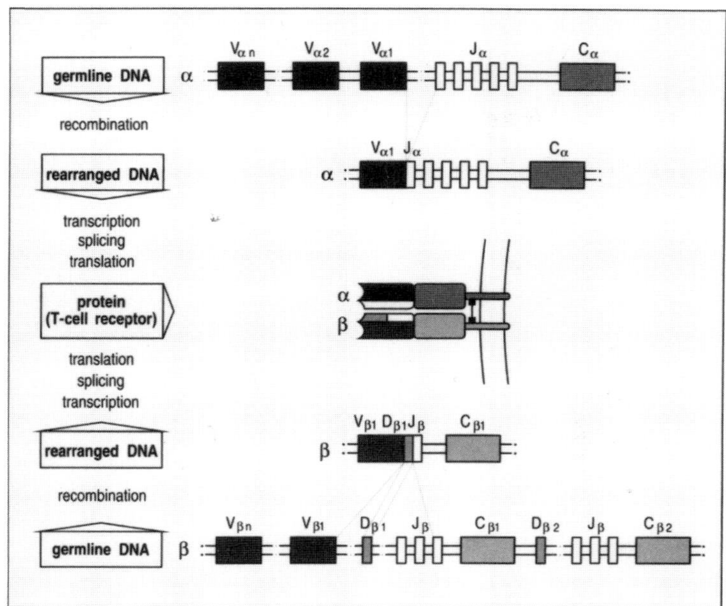

FIG. 4. T-cell receptor (TCR) α and β gene rearrangement. The mature TCR α and β genes are formed by recombination of segments of DNA from their germline configuration. For the α chain *(top)*, a Vα segment rearranges to be placed in juxtaposition to a Jα segment, creating a functional exon. The Cα gene segment is not rearranged, but is transcribed along with VJ and then subsequently spliced to VJ during mRNA editing. The β chain *(bottom)*, like the immunoglobulin heavy chains, uses a D region. Reprinted with permission from C. A. Janeway and P. Travers, *Immunobiology*, Current Biology Ltd., London.

Early in fetal development, T-cell precursors, residing in the fetal liver and the yolk sac migrate to and colonize the thymus (14). Once in the thymus, these cells undergo TCR gene rearrangement via V(D)J recombination. This is a random process, and the TCRs created will fall into one of three categories (Fig. 5). First, the TCR may have no affinity for self-MHC molecules. While not directly harmful, such a T cell is of no inherent value to the organism either, since the immune response is self-MHC restricted and, except in the special case of transplantation, only self-MHC molecules are available for antigen presentation. A second type of TCR that can be created directly recognizes self-MHC or, more likely, a self-peptide bound to self-MHC (in the absence of foreign peptides, MHC molecules "present" self-peptides as part of normal immune surveillance). A T cell bearing this type of TCR is potentially autoreactive and, as is discussed below, is either deleted or inactivated. The third type of TCR has substantial intrinsic affinity for self-MHC, but not enough to be activated in the absence of foreign protein. Thymocytes bearing these TCRs are beneficial and should mature into T cells.

Although it is difficult to know what percentage of thymocytes bear TCRs from each of the three categories, only 1–5% of all thymocytes complete maturation (15). Thus, 95–99% of thymocytes suffer an intrathymic death. Since thymocytes falling into categories 1 and 2 do not mature, and only those in category 3 survive, it also follows that the fate of any given thymocyte is determined by the specificity of its antigen receptor. The process by which thymocytes survive or die based on their TCR specificity is known as thymic selection.

A fundamental concept underlying thymic selection is that selection occurs in both a positive and a negative sense (16–18). Thymocytes will not complete maturation unless they receive a positive signal (through a process called positive selection) (19). This mechanism provides a way to selectively "promote" a desirable population of cells, such as those that have affinity for self-MHC, and therefore could mediate an MHC-restricted immune response. The positive signal that is required for maturation is delivered when the TCR on the developing thymocyte binds to an MHC molecule present on a thymic epithelial cell. Thymic epithelial cells are a unique type of cell located throughout the thymic cortex and thus are well situated to encounter developing thymocytes migrating through the cortex. Thymocytes whose TCRs do not engage MHC molecules on thymic epithelial cells fail to be positively selected and die through a poorly understood process of "benign neglect." In the scheme outlined above (Fig. 5), this is the fate of cells whose TCRs fall in category 1.

Referring again to Fig. 5, thymocytes with TCRs of type 2 or 3 will be positively selected. However, those in the former group are potentially autoreactive. The process of negative selection (also called clonal deletion) eliminates these cells. As with positive selection, the signal for negative selection is delivered through the TCR, since this is the only means to identify autoreactive cells. In general, thymocytes undergo negative selection when their TCRs bind to MHC molecules present on bone-marrow-derived macrophages, a population of hematopoietic cells that have taken up residence within the thymus. Thus, while both positive and negative selection occur through the TCR engagement, in most cases they are mediated by distinct cell types (thymic epithelial cells versus bone-marrow-derived macrophages). For the purposes of explanation, it has been assumed that positive

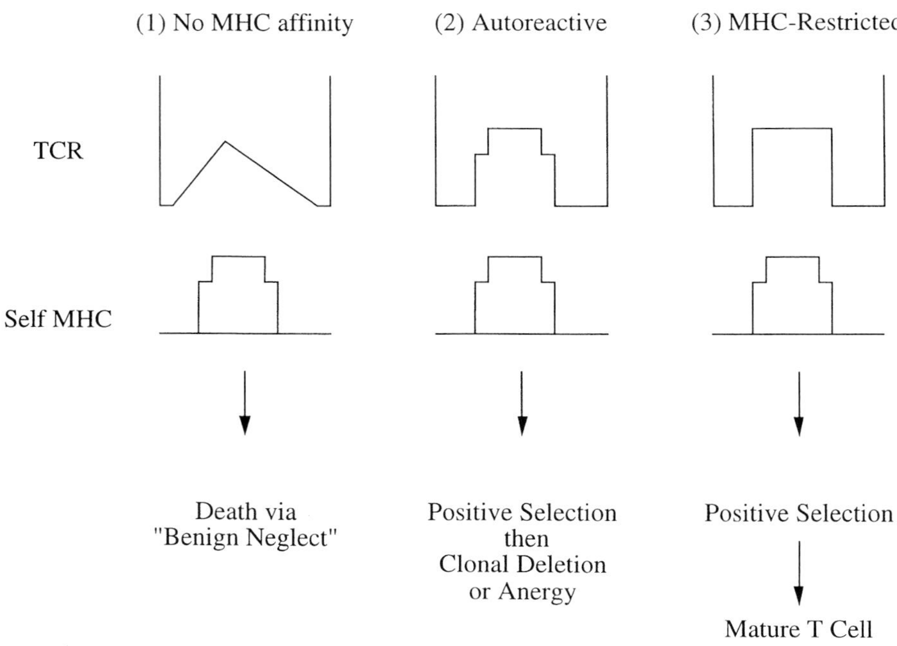

FIG. 5. T-cell receptor (TCR) selection. The processes of V(D)J recombination, imprecise joining, and N-nucleotide addition that create T-cell receptor genes are random and, in theory, three types of TCRs are generated. Those with no intrinsic MHC affinity fail to be positively selected and die via "benign neglect" *(left)*. Those with excessive MHC affinity are potentially autoreactive *(middle)*. They may be positively selected, but then are also eliminated by clonal deletion (negative selection) or, in some cases, escape death, but are anergized. Those with intermediate MHC affinity are still able to undergo positive selection, but escape clonal deletion, eventually becoming mature T cells. Parallel processes act during B-cell development to eliminate autoreactive cells. There is no analogous process of positive selection during B-cell development, but survival of B cells following affinity maturation (see the text) has some parallels.

selection occurs first. That is, that cells of TCR type 2 are positively selected and then subsequently eliminated by clonal deletion. In most models examined to date, this appears to be the case, but there are well-described instances in which autoreactive cells are eliminated by clonal deletion prior to positive selection of a fraction of the survivors (20).

The events occurring during negative selection have been the subject of intensive investigation. It appears that TCR engagement leading to clonal deletion induces the affected cell to undergo programmed cell death via a process known as apoptosis (21). This process is characterized by the activation of an endogenous "suicide program." A characteristic finding of cells induced to undergo apoptosis is the fragmentation of chromosomal DNA into a ladder of 200 base-pair increments, consistent with breakage at nucleosomal sites. This, and other features, distinguish apoptosis from necrosis. Apoptotic cell death is by no means a unique feature of thymocytes, but is a "normal" feature of a variety of mature and immature cells. Indeed, as will be seen later, apoptosis is an important mechanism for the effector and termination phases of immune responses.

In contrast to negative selection, the events occurring during positive selection are less well understood. TCR ligation during positive selection results in thymocyte activation as evidenced by upregulation of certain activation antigens (including the TCR itself) (16), yet the intracellular events by which surface signaling conveys longevity to the cell, allowing it to avoid death by benign neglect, are unknown

When the above schema is considered in detail, an apparent paradox arises. Even though positive selection occurs following the engagement of an MHC molecule on a thymic epithelial cell, and negative selection through binding to an MHC molecule on a bone-marrow-derived macrophage, in both instances binding occurs through the TCR. How then does the thymocyte receive a signal leading to cell "promotion" in the first instance and cell death in the latter? At least three models have been proposed to explain this phenomenon: the affinity hypothesis, the second signal hypothesis, and the maturation hypothesis (16).

The affinity hypothesis proposes that "strong" interactions between the TCR and MHC+peptide lead to clonal deletion, whereas weaker interactions provide sufficient stimulation for positive selection (22). A strong interaction might be one characterized by high avidity between the TCR and its ligand. Alternatively (but not exclusively), it might be one in which many TCR molecules on the surface of a thymocyte are ligated, rather than just a few.

Another proposed hypothesis whereby TCR interactions can lead alternatively to negative or positive selection is that the provision of an additional, "second," signal differentiates the two and determines the fate of the cell. Several candidate second-signaling pathways have been proposed, in particular that mediated through the T-cell surface molecule CD28. In vitro, CD28 stimulation has been shown to synergize with TCR stimulation to lead to programmed cell death of immature thymocytes (23). Whether this is a physiologically relevant in vivo pathway remains to be determined.

The third proposed explanation for thymic selection is the maturational hypothesis. This holds that there are no intrinsic differences in cell surface events that mediate positive versus negative selection, but that the different results seen reflect the maturational state of the thymocyte. Since, in most instances, positive selection appears to precede clonal deletion, such an explanation is plausible. Indeed, there are known differences in TCR composition, TCR signaling, and thymocyte responses based on maturational state.

These three models are not mutually exclusive and may all operate at some level although, at present, most experimental evidence supports the affinity model.

It is important to recognize that thymic tolerance is not mediated solely by clonal deletion. After the initial studies demonstrating clonal deletion of cells bearing TCRs reacting to autoantigens, it was appreciated that deletion was not universal for all self-antigens. In some instances, it was shown that potentially autoreactive cells matured normally and were found in the peripheral lymphoid compartment. However, close examination of these cells showed that they were anergic (that is, nonresponsive to antigen). The reasons why these cells were anergic was unclear, but several distinct mechanisms may be involved, including downregulation of the TCR or of the CD4 or CD8 coreceptors (see below), as well as intrinsic alterations in cell signal transduction. In any event, clonal anergy appears to be an alternative to clonal deletion in the development of tolerance within the thymus.

Regardless as to how tolerance is induced in the thymus, it can only work for antigens that are found there. The question arises then whether all self-antigens are present in the thymus. These could be brought in by circulating macrophages or captured from the circulation by resident macrophages. Although formally possible, in reality this seems improbable. More likely, in addition to thymic (central) tolerance, there are mechanisms that induce and maintain peripheral tolerance. These might include restricted delivery of costimulatory signals or induction of regulatory cytokines or of suppressor cells (see below).

TCR αβ Versus γδ Cells

As noted above, there are four TCR loci: α, β, γ, and δ. In general, TCRs are expressed on the surface of T cells as α-β or γ-δ heterodimers. The vast majority of T cells present in the thymus, peripheral blood, lymph nodes, and spleen are TCRαβ cells. TCRγδ cells are a distinct minority in those tissues, but are found in significantly higher proportions in mucosal tissues such as skin, gut, tongue, and vagina. The ontogeny of TCRγδ cells is not as well understood as that of TCRαβ cells, but appears to follow the same rules with regard to gene recombination and selection. One important difference is that most γ-δ T cells are both CD4- and CD8-.

The function of TCRγδ cells has not been fully elucidated. Their distribution suggests a role in the defense against bacterial and/or parasitic pathogens. Observations that γ-δ T cells recognize mycobacterial antigens and heat-shock proteins support this hypothesis (7,24). Whatever the target antigens of γ-δ T cells are, we do not understand how those antigens are seen. It is not even known whether antigen is presented to γ-δ T cells by MHC molecules, with some studies indicating that a class-I-like molecule known as CD1 may present to γ-δ T cells (24). Recent work demonstrating that γ-δ T cells can recognize nonpeptide organic phosphates as antigens suggests yet other alternative systems for antigen presentation (25).

Extrathymic T-Cell Development

The gut is rich in lymphoid tissue (gut-associated lymphoid tissue) that is divided into three anatomic locations. The first is Peyer patches, which are lymphoid aggregates found in the terminal ileum. These can be thought of as lymph nodes in that they serve as the induction site for immune responses to antigens in the intestinal lumen. A second lymphoid population is the lamina propria lymphocytes, a mixture of T and B cells whose functions are unknown. The third population of cells are the intestinal epithelial lymphocytes (IELs) present in the epithelial layer of the small bowel, averaging 1 IEL per 5–10 epithelial cells. The predominant cells in the IEL population are T cells and consist of both TCRαβ and TCRγδ cells. Many IELs, both αβ and γδ cells, express an aberrant CD8 homodimer that is not found in T cells maturing in the thymus. Irradiation-reconstitution experiments to analyze the origin of these cells by using T-cell deficient mice and athymic mice indicate that they are of extrathymic origin (26). As with lamina propria lymphocytes, the function of IELs is uncertain.

B Cells

Although their immunologic functions are quite distinct, there are an extraordinary number of parallels between T cells and B cells, including development, receptor structure, tolerogenic mechanisms, and signaling. One of the most important similarities is apparent from the nomenclature of the gene family to which the TCR belongs, that is, the Ig supergene family. Ig genes, expressed exclusively in B cells, are the prototype for a large number of immunologically important genes, including the TCR. Secreted Ig gene products are antibodies, the basis for humoral immunity. Membrane-bound Ig gene products are B-cell receptors for antigen (BCRs), the B-cell "equivalent" of the TCRs.

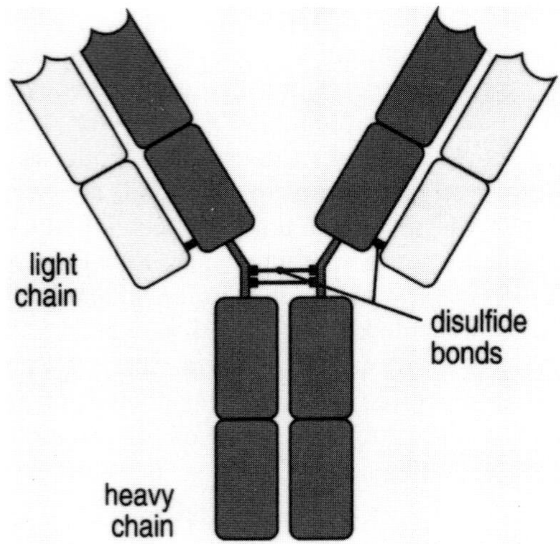

FIG. 6. Schematic diagram of an immunoglobulin (Ig) molecule. The Ig molecule consists of two light chains and two heavy chains. Disulfide bonds link each light chain to a heavy chain and the heavy chains to each other. The distal ends of each light-chain–heavy-chain pair form an antigen-binding site. The proximal ends of the heavy chain bind to Fc receptors on phagocytic cells. Reprinted with permission from C. A. Janeway and P. Travers, *Immunobiology*, Current Biology Ltd., London.

Immunoglobulins

A single Ig, either surface bound or secreted, actually consists of four separate molecules, two light chains and two heavy chains (Fig. 6). Alternative RNA splicing of the heavy-chain transcripts determines whether the Ig molecule is secreted or membrane bound (27). As shown in Fig. 6, each light chain pairs with a heavy chain to form an antigen-binding site. Thus, the mature Ig monomer binds two antigenic epitopes. As with the TCR, the genes encoding these chains are created by V(D)J recombination of germline alleles, and similar considerations apply as to generating diversity by this means. There are a few important differences between TCRs and BCRs that should be noted. First, in the case of the heavy chain of secreted Ig molecules, the choice of the constant (C) region that is used has important functional implications for the Ig itself, as Ig isotypes differ in their ability to multimerize, target to different compartments, fix complement, and so on. Second, an individual B cell has the ability to switch isotypes (and hence C-region usage) during its life span. Both of these distinctions between T and B cells involve the selection and function of the isotype. A third difference between TCRs and Igs is that Ig genes can undergo further changes following B-cell encounter with antigen. This process, known as somatic mutation, promotes the development of high-affinity antibodies (see below).

B-Cell Development/Deletion of Autoreactive Cells

In birds, B cells develop in a discrete organ known as the bursa of Fabricius. Mammals do not have a bursa, however, and there is no single discrete organ of B-cell development that functions as a homologue to the thymus for T cells. Instead, B cells develop at multiple sites including the liver, bone marrow, and spleen. The processes of B-cell development, selection, and elimination or inactivation of autoreactive cells are very similar to those for T cells and will not be elaborated upon further. There are, however, two important processes that are unique to B cells: isotype switching and affinity maturation.

Isotype Switching

There are five primary classes (isotypes) of Ig—IgM, IgD, IgG, IgE, and IgA—as determined by which constant region the heavy chain uses, the μ, δ, γ, ε, or α segments, respectively (Table 1) (28). The μ and δ segments are close together on the chromosome and far upstream of the others. Mature naive B cells express both IgM and IgD on their surface, the only instance in which B cells express more than one Ig isotype. Both IgM and IgD function as BCRs for antigen. After activation, the B cell undergoes a process of isotype switching to either IgG (which has several subclasses, IgG1, IgG2a, IgG2b, and IgG3), IgE, or IgA as part of further differentiation and

TABLE 1. *General properties of immunoglobulins*

Property	IgM	IgG	IgA	IgE	IgD
Usual Form	Pentamer or hexamer	Monomer	Monomer or dimer	Monomer	Monomer
Valence	10,12	2	2,4	2	2
Half-life(days)	10	21	6	2	3
Complement activation					
Classic pathway	Yes	Yes	No	No	No
Alternate pathway	No	No	Yes	No	No
Binds to phagocytes through Fc receptors	Yes	No	No	No	No
Binds to mast cells through Fc receptors	No	No	No	Yes	No

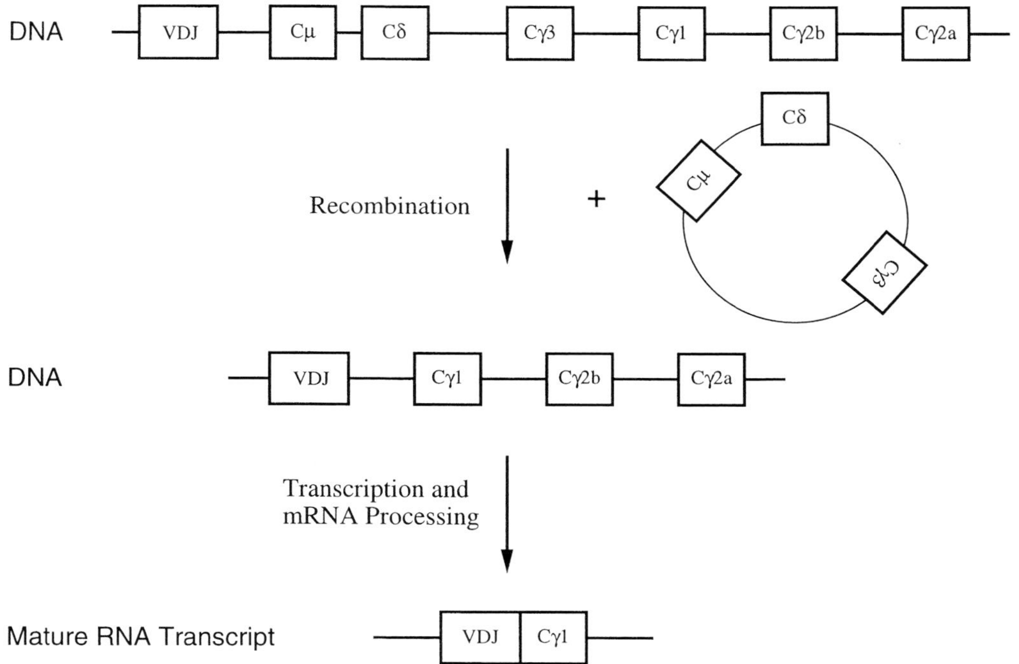

FIG. 7. Isotype switching. During maturation and differentiation, B cells can switch the isotype of immunoglobulin (Ig) that they make by changing the constant (C) region of the Ig that is transcribed. Since, except in the case of the C locus, only the C region immediately downstream of the VDJ cassette is transcribed, isotype switching involves genetic recombination through a specialized "switch recombinase." During this recombination, intervening segments of DNA are excised out, while downstream DNA remains unaltered. In the example shown here, a B cell switches from IgM to IgG1.

expansion (Fig. 7) (29,30). This process is mediated via a so-called "switch recombinase." Since the C region used in the mature mRNA is the one most 5′ to the rearranged V(D)J segment, isotype switching is accomplished by deletion of intervening C regions that are upstream of the new one to be expressed.

Somatic Mutation and Affinity Maturation

Following immunization with an antigen, B cells are able to undergo somatic mutation in their Ig genes (31). In humans and mice, somatic mutation is primarily the result of point mutations. In other species, notably chickens, it is the result of gene conversion, a process in which blocks of sequence are copied from a donor pseudogene into the functional Ig gene. Both types of somatic mutation occur following B-cell activation and expansion, and their purpose is to refine the Ig repertoire further. The mutation process itself is essentially random; therefore, some mutated Ig genes will have unchanged antigen affinity and some will have higher antigen affinity, whereas others will have lower. Since B-cell expansion, maturation, and survival depend upon continued antigen stimulation, those B cells whose somatic mutations have led to high-affinity Ig genes will have a selective survival advantage. The result is affinity maturation during the immune response.

Natural Killer Cells

NK cells are capable of lysing a variety of viral-infected and tumor cells in vitro. They are variably classified as lymphocytes and are clearly distinct from either T or B cells, but their precise lineage is not known. It is hypothesized that they represent the remnant of a primitive form of immunity—one that arose prior to the development of the TCR. This is consistent with the finding that athymic mice, as well as mice that are defective in V(D)J recombination, all have NK cells (32). Regulation of NK cytotoxicity has been the subject of intense investigation. One of the most interesting aspects of NK-mediated cytotoxicity is that, unlike cytotoxic T lymphocytes, which are activated to kill upon specific recognition of antigen, NK cells seem constitutively able to kill many cell types, but are *inactivated* if the target expresses self-MHC class I molecules (33). Thus, this is a form of self–nonself recognition. At least two families of receptors that inactivate NK cells have been identified. In the mouse, the Ly-49 family of lectins are expressed on NK cells, can bind self-class I and, in doing so, inactivate the cell (34). No human homologue for Ly-49 is known to date, but the search for one has revealed instead new Ig superfamily members expressed on human NK cells that serve the same function (35). Thus, at least two discrete mechanisms exist to regulate NK cytotoxicity.

Specialized Antigen-Presenting Cells

For reasons that will be detailed later in the chapter, immune responses are initiated most effectively (perhaps even exclusively) when antigen is presented to T cells by specialized, or "professional," APCs. Monocytes/macrophages, dendritic cells, and activated (but not resting) B cells are all professional APCs and have certain shared characteristics, including hematopoietic origin, expression of class II MHC molecules (see below), and ability to provide costimulatory signals to T cells (see below). Professional APCs are also highly efficient at capturing antigen for subsequent presentation to T cells. Macrophages and dendritic cells do this through phagocytosis. B cells capture foreign antigen through their surface Ig molecules that serve as their antigen receptors. Once antigen binds to surface Ig, the Ig–antigen complex is internalized. All three cell types are able to degrade internalized antigens by proteolysis and process them into peptide fragments that are capable of being recognized by T cells. The efficiency of these three types of professional APCs differs, with dendritic cells being the most potent and activated B cells the least. For example, a "concentration" of dendritic cells of <1% is still sufficient to present antigen effectively to T cells, whereas substantially higher APC–T-cell ratios are required for macrophages and B cells (36). Some of the factors responsible for differential antigen-presenting capacity include the density of MHC molecules and costimulatory molecules on the APC. Physical factors such as the shape of the APC may be important as well. For example, dendritic cells have many dendrites (hence their name) that project out from the cell surface. This gives these cells a very high surface area to volume ratio and means that many T cells can simultaneously bind to a single dendritic cell.

Anatomically, these cells are well situated to capture and subsequently present antigens. Both dendritic cells and macrophages are widely distributed throughout body organs and tissues. In particular, dendritic cells are thought to be sentinel cells of the immune system and, in some instances, have acquired distinct names when located within distinct tissues. For example, dendritic cells in the epidermal layer of the skin are known as Langerhans cells. As is discussed in detail later, it is thought that these cells are responsible for initiating many immune responses. In the case of transplantation, for example, depletion of dendritic cells from tissue or organ grafts such as thyroid cell, pancreatic islet cells, or kidneys can greatly prolong graft survival in animal models, in some instances leading to antigen-specific tolerance (37). B cells are more restricted in their distribution, found primarily in the blood, lymphatics, and peripheral lymphoid organs such as lymph nodes, spleen, and bone marrow. As these are the same sites where T cells are located, B cells are well situated to present antigens to T cells.

Nonhematopoietic Cells with Immune Function

A variety of cells whose primary functions are nonimmunologic may be active participants in immune responses as well. This may occur through the induction of cell surface proteins that are required to initiate immune responses such as MHC class II molecules (see below), or through the elaboration of cytokines that support the initiation and perpetuation of responses. Recently, a great deal of attention has been focused on endothelial cells. In studies using human endothelial cells isolated from umbilical cords, as well as with porcine endothelial cells, it appears that these cells are capable of supporting immune responses in many of the same ways as professional APCs, including the expression of MHC class II molecules, costimulatory molecules, and secretion of proinflammatory cytokines (38). This would seem to be a physiologically adaptive response to promote recruitment of lymphoid and myeloid cells to sites of infection and/or tissue damage. In the absence of an endothelial response, the immune cells might be blinded to pathogens in tissue parenchyma with the exception of certain tissues, such as the liver, with nonendothelialized sinusoids. In the case of transplantation, this feature of endothelial cells contributes to the high relative immunogenicity of vascularized organ allografts compared with tissue grafts. It also promotes the endothelium as a target for rejection. Selected epithelial cells appear to have immunologic functions as well. For example, renal proximal tubular cells can be induced to express MHC class II molecules (39). This is not a unique feature of this organ, but has been described for several other epithelial cells types.

INITIATING THE RESPONSE TO FOREIGN ANTIGEN

To respond to a foreign antigen, the immune system, especially T cells, must first "see" the antigen. As noted above, T cells, through their antigen receptors (TCRs) recognize foreign peptides in the antigen-binding groove of MHC molecules. It is an historical curiosity of interest to nephrologists that these genes, which are critically important for immune responses in general, were discovered because the ability of inbred strains of mice to reject organ and tissue transplants segregated primarily with this genetic locus; hence its role in histocompatibility. In humans, the MHC genes lie on the short arm of chromosome 6 (Fig. 8). There are several well-characterized loci

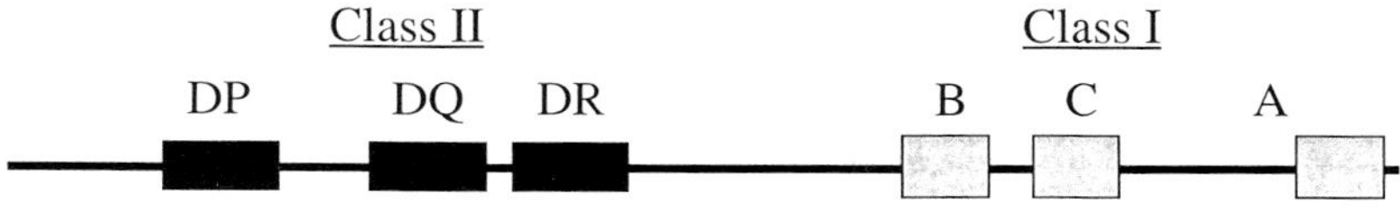

Expression Pattern:

Class II	Class I
Macrophages Dendritic cells B cells Activated T cells Activated endothelium	All nucleated cells

FIG. 8. Genomic organization of the HLA region: schematic diagram of the HLA region and the pattern of expression of class I and class II gene products. The HLA region is found on the short arm of chromosome 6 with the class II loci being centromeric. Each of the class II regions shown actually consist of an α and a β locus, but are grouped together for illustrative purposes. The genes are expressed codominantly; therefore, the products of both the maternal and paternal alleles can be found on the appropriate cell surfaces. Loci not shown that are important in antigen presentation are the LMP and TAP genes located between DP and DQ, and the DM locus that is placed between DP and LMP/TAP (see the text for details).

in this region, which broadly subdivide into class I and class II genes. In humans, the MHC class I genes expressed on the cell surface consist of HLA-A, -B, and -C loci, and cell surface class II genes are the HLA-DR, -DP, and -DQ loci. In mice, the MHC locus is called H-2. Here, the class I loci are K (for example, H-2K), D, and L, and the class II loci are A and E (usually referred to as I-A and I-E). I-A appears to be the homologue of the human class II locus HLA-DQ, and I-E is the homologue of HLA-DR. Differences during the evolution of the human and murine class I genes make similar homology assignments impossible.

Alleles at all these loci are codominantly expressed and thus, barring homozygosity, humans can express 12 distinct HLA proteins on a given cell. The loci are highly polymorphic, as shown in Table 2, which indicates the number of known alleles at each locus. In particular, the HLA-B and DR loci are among the most polymorphic in the human genome. This extensive polymorphism plus codominant expression means that two randomly chosen individuals will always have at least one (and usually multiple) HLA disparities. The ability of T cells to react to foreign HLA molecules (see below) is the major stimulus for transplant rejection.

TABLE 2. *HLA polymorphism*

	Class I loci			Class II loci		
	A	B	C	DR	DQ	DP
Alleles known	41	62	18	100	22	51
Alleles serologically detectable	23	39	8	18	7	6

Alleles known refers to the number of genetic variants known at this locus based on DNA typing. *Alleles serologically detectable* refers to the subset of the known alleles that can be detected using allele-specific monoclonal antibodies.

Antigen Presentation

MHC genes are subdivided into two classes, I and II, based on genetic and structural homology. These two classes have distinct functions in immune homeostasis with class I molecules presenting endogenous antigens and class II molecules presenting exogenous antigens. The teleologic reasons for this compartmentalization have been debated. In any event, class II molecules are important for initiating immune responses to foreign proteins. As such, it is appropriate that they are found primarily on APCs (see below). Class I molecules are found on all cells and primarily present endogenous (that is, cytosolic) antigens. They are important for immune surveillance against cells that have been infected or altered in some way that leads to the production of novel/foreign proteins (for example, by a virus or by malignant transformation).

MHC Class II Genes

Structure

A class II molecule is a heterodimer consisting of two noncovalently linked glycoproteins, the α and β chains (40,41). In general, the α chains show little allelic variation, with most of the polymorphisms in class II being attributable to the β chain, although both chains are encoded in the MHC. For example the murine I-A region actually consists of two loci, Ab and Aa. In the case of human MHC class II genes, the situation can be somewhat more complex. The DQ region genes consist of two α-chain genes, DQA1 and DQA2, and three β-chain genes, DQB1-3. However, only DQA1 and DQB1 are expressed, the remainder being pseudogenes. Pseudogenes are present throughout the MHC, presumably arising as gene duplication events. A proposed reason for evolutionary conservation of these pseudogenes is that they function as sequence donors through gene conversion, thus serving as a source of new polymorphisms. The evolutionary value of MHC polymorphism itself has been debated quite extensively, yet remains unsettled. The most popular hypothesis is that polymorphisms for genes that present antigens to the immune system are strongly adaptive for species survival, making it more difficult for pathogens to evade immune recognition (42).

Expression

Unlike class I genes, which are ubiquitously expressed, the pattern of class II expression is much more restricted (Fig. 8) (41). Protein products of these genes are found primarily on APCs (that is, dendritic cells, macrophages, and B cells). Even though these cells constitutively express class II molecules, expression increases with activation of the APC, either by encounter with antigen or by cytokines such as interferon (IFN)-γ. Although non-APCs do not express class II molecules in their basal state, stimulation with IFN-γ induces class II expression on selected cell types such as endothelium, renal proximal tubules, and keratinocytes. In humans, activated T cells express class II molecules as well; in mice, however, T cells clearly are class II negative. As is discussed below, the role of class II molecules is in initiating immune responses. The relative inability of non-APCs to provide additional stimuli that are needed to initiate responses calls into question the role of class II molecules on these cells.

Function

In general, MHC class II molecules serve to present exogenous antigens to T cells (Fig. 9). Thus, their expression on APCs is logical, since these cells capture foreign proteins (either through phagocytosis in the case of macrophages and dendritic cells or through surface Igs in the case of B cells). As with all rules, however, there are exceptions, as shown in isolated reports demonstrating class II presentation of endogenous (that is, intracellular) antigens.

Mature T cells are subdivided based on reciprocal expression of either the CD4 or CD8 glycoproteins. CD4+ T cells have MHC class-II-restricted TCRs, and CD8+ T cells are MHC class I restricted in their antigen recognition (43,44). This means that recognition of exogenous antigens processed by APCs is almost entirely dependent on CD4+ cells. One can think then of MHC class II molecules and CD4+ T cells as being of primary importance in the response to extracellular antigens. This includes parasites, many bacteria, and intact virus particles. As is shown below, the response of CD4+ cells may be to produce cytokines that support the expansion and differentiation of B cells into antibody-producing plasma cells (humoral immunity), or to produce proinflammatory cytokines that activate macrophages and CD8+ cytotoxic T lymphocytes (cellular immunity). In the former case, antibodies can serve to neutralize and/or opsonize extracellular pathogens. In the latter case, cytotoxic T lymphocyte (CTL) function also will require recognition of intracellular antigens presented on MHC class I molecules (see below).

Invariant Chain and DM: Other Genes Required for Class II Antigen Presentation

Class II molecules present peptides derived from exogenous antigens, whereas class I molecules present endogenous antigens. Specialized peptide transporters exist to mobilize endogenous peptides into the endoplasmic reticulum (ER) to associate with nascent class I molecules (see below). Class II molecules must be kept "free," however, until they are translocated into the endosome, where they can bind to exogenous antigens, that is, peptides derived from phagocytosed proteins. To prevent class II molecules from binding endogenous peptides transported into the ER, a specialized mechanism has evolved that utilizes two additional gene products: invariant chain and DM.

Invariant Chain. The invariant chain (frequently abbreviated as Ii) is so named because it was discovered as a nonpolymorphic (that is, invariant) molecule associated with the otherwise highly polymorphic MHC class II α-β heterodimer. One function of Ii is to prevent premature loading of peptides onto class II molecules (45). If this were the only function of Ii, then, in the absence of invariant chain, T-cell maturation and MHC class II expression should be normal, but the types of peptides found on class II molecules differ. In fact, Ii knockout mice have defects in class II antigen expression/presentation and CD4+ T-cell maturation, suggesting a more involved role for Ii (46). Therefore, the invariant chain probably serves several functions in class II antigen presentation, including protein folding, prevention of premature peptide loading, targeting of class II molecules through the Golgi and into the endosomal compartment, and retention in the endosomes for loading with exogenous peptide.

DM. The DM locus was discovered based on the analysis of mutant cell lines defective in class II antigen presentation, but without defects in known class II genes themselves or in Ii. Eventually, the genetic defect was mapped to a segment of the MHC containing the nonclassic class II genes encoding DM (47). Like classic MHC class II genes, DM is an α-β heterodimer. However, unlike the classic genes, it has very limited polymorphism. The function(s) of the DM protein are not totally clear. A consensus model proposes that DM is required for the efficient dissociation of Ii from the MHC class II

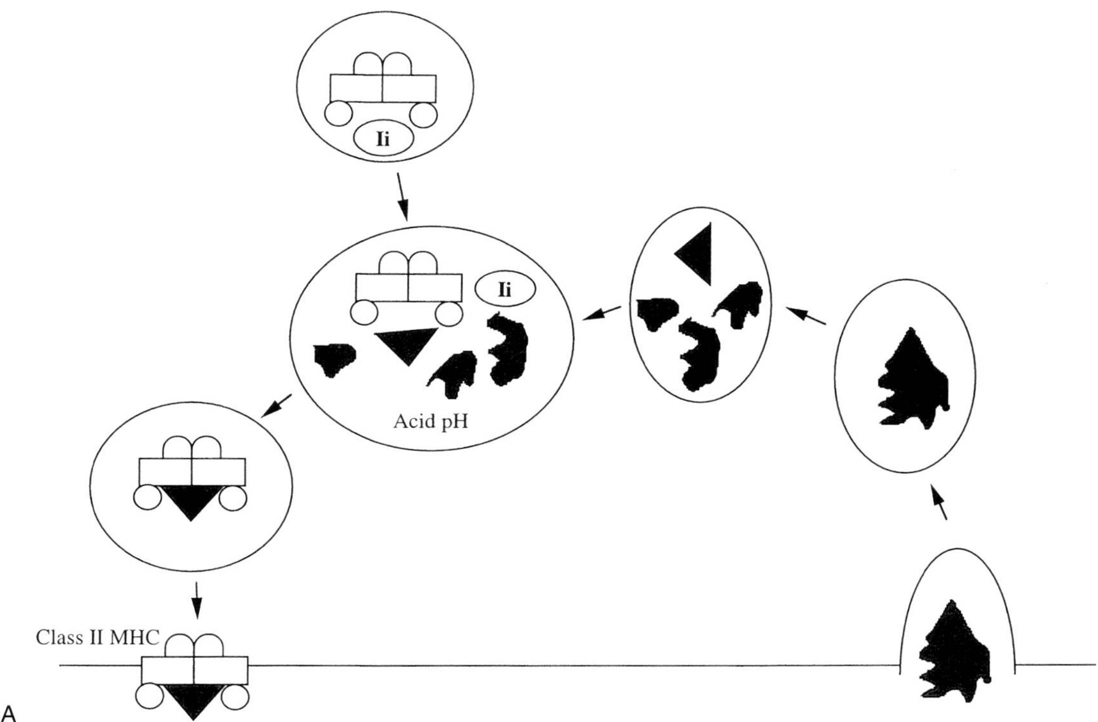

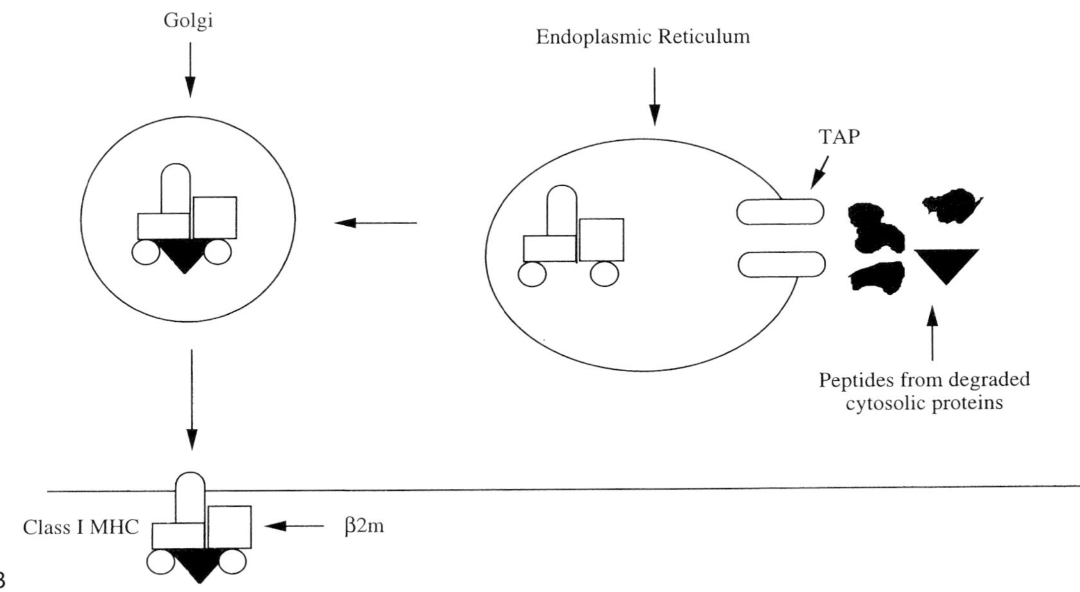

FIG. 9. Two routes of antigen presentation. **A:** Class II antigen presentation. Exogenous antigen is internalized into acidified endosomes. In the acid milieu, proteases degrade the protein into peptide fragments. These proteases also release the invariant chain (Ii) from MHC class II, allowing it to bind peptides. Release of Ii allows the class II molecules loaded with peptides to move to the cell surface. **B:** Class I antigen presentation. Peptides derived from degraded cytosolic proteins are transported into the endoplasmic reticulum by TAP proteins (see the text). There, the peptides associate with class I molecules. This releases the chaperone protein calnexin (not shown), allowing the class I–peptide complex to move to the Golgi and from there to the cell surface.

heterodimer. According to this model, in the absence of DM, Ii remains coupled to the heterodimer, and a peptide derived from Ii termed CLIP (class-II-associated invariant-chain peptide) is found in the antigen-binding groove of cell surface MHC class II molecules (48).

MHC Class I Genes

Structure

The protein products of MHC class I genes are expressed on the surface of cells as part of a heterodimer, the other molecule being β_2-microglobulin (β_2m), a gene that is not part of the MHC (41). The class I gene product is larger (sometimes called the heavy chain) and spans the cellular membrane, whereas the smaller β_2m (sometimes called the light chain) is entirely extracellular. These two chains are noncovalently associated.

As noted above, all of the class I loci are extremely polymorphic (41). In contrast, although the structure of β_2m differs from species to species, within a given species it exhibits little if any meaningful polymorphism. Nonetheless, it is important in immune responses, because efficient expression of the MHC class I gene product on the cell surface depends on β_2m. Studies in mice made deficient in β_2m via gene targeting (β_2m "knockout" mice) show essentially no class I gene product on the cell surface as measured serologically (that is, with antibodies) (49), although some conformationally altered class I gene products may get to the cell surface in the absence of β_2m.

Expression

In contrast to class II molecules whose pattern of distribution is relatively restrictive, MHC class I molecules are found on virtually all cells. Expression of class I molecules is usually upregulated in inflammatory states, primarily through the effects of IFN-γ and tumor necrosis factor.

Function

Although isolated exceptions exists, MHC class I molecules generally present endogenous peptides, that is, those that are produced in the endoplasmic reticulum. Therefore, they are often thought of as critical to immune surveillance against intracellular pathogens that utilize the host protein-producing apparatus such as viruses. The constitutive presence of class I molecules on the surface of virtually all cells enables class-I-restricted CD8+ T cells to survey these cells continually for the presence of foreign proteins. If found, this could mean that the cell has become infected and is producing viral proteins. Alternatively, neoantigens produced as a result of malignant transformation may be recognized as foreign, and this can trigger or facilitate an antitumor immune response. A by-product of this system is that the presence of foreign MHC class I molecules on cells of transplanted organs and tissues will mean that those cells are perceived as foreign by the immune system.

Nonclassic MHC Class I Molecules

In addition to the class I loci described above, in both mice and humans, there are so-called "nonclassic" class I genes encoded in the MHC (41). In mice, examples are the TL and Qa antigens. In humans, examples are HLA-E, -F, and -G. It should be noted that these murine and human nonclassic genes are not homologues of one another. Some of these genes do not appear to be expressed as protein products. In other cases, the proteins are much more restricted in their patterns of expression than classic class I molecules. Furthermore, polymorphism is minor or absent. The role of these genes in immune responses has not been elucidated, and the lack of evolutionary conservation of these loci has called into question whether they serve an important function at all.

LMP and TAP: Other Genes with a Role in Class I Presentation

Since class I molecules present endogenous antigens, we need to consider how the peptides derived from those antigens actually get loaded onto class I molecules.

LMP. The peptides themselves are derived from proteolytic cleavage of cytosolic proteins. One of the primary proteases responsible for this is the multi-unit cytosolic protease called the proteosome (50). Two subunits of the proteosome, LMP2 and LMP7, are encoded within the MHC and therefore have been the focus of much attention. Their inclusion in the proteosome complex led to speculation that they would be absolutely required for class I antigen processing. This turns out not to be true, as cells lacking both LMP2 and LMP7 can present antigens in association with class I. However, LMP2 and LMP7 do affect class I antigen presentation by altering the specificity of protein cleavage by the proteosome, favoring cleavages generating positively charged or hydrophobic carboxyterminal peptides.

TAP. Following proteolytic cleavage of proteins to generate "loadable" peptides, those peptides need to access the compartment where the newly synthesized class I molecules reside. This is accomplished by an ATP-binding transporter known as TAP (for transporter associated with antigen processing), which transports cytosolic peptides into the endoplasmic reticulum. There, the peptides are loaded onto class I molecules, releasing class I from its chaperones and allowing it to be ex-

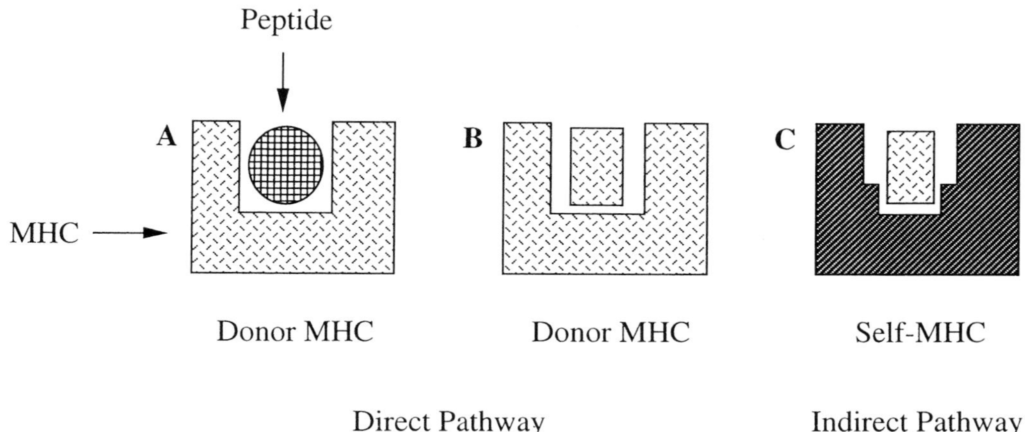

FIG. 10. Two pathways of allorecognition. In the direct pathway of allorecognition, T cells recognize an intact allogeneic MHC molecule (here labeled "donor MHC") that can have either an extraneous peptide **(A)** or a peptide derived from the MHC molecule itself **(B)** in its antigen-binding groove. In the indirect pathway, a self-MHC molecule presents an immunogenic peptide derived from an allogeneic MHC molecule **(C)**.

pressed on the cell surface. The complex providing TAP function is encoded by two genes, TAP1 and TAP2, both of which are located within the MHC. As expected, cells defective in TAP1 or TAP2 are deficient in class I antigen presentation and have severely reduced levels of surface class I and CD8+ T cells (51).

Alloantigens

Although most antigenic proteins can only be recognized as processed peptide fragments in the antigen-binding groove of MHC molecules, there are two notable exceptions: alloantigens and superantigens. Alloantigens are allogeneic (that is, foreign or "nonself") MHC antigens. Since the MHC loci are highly polymorphic, any two given individuals are likely to have different alleles at most, if not all, loci. Alloantigens can of course be processed and presented like any other foreign protein, and this pathway is usually called "indirect" allorecognition, to denote the fact that the alloantigen is recognized in the context of a self-MHC molecule (Fig. 10). However, TCRs also can bind and respond to intact foreign MHC molecules. Since the alloantigen is, in this instance, recognized in toto on the surface of the allogeneic cell, this pathway is referred to as "direct" allorecognition. It is believed that T cells can respond directly to alloantigens since TCRs have intrinsic MHC affinity, and the degree of similarity between distinct MHC alleles far outweighs the differences. Thus, it is postulated that the physical structure of foreign MHC probably mimics that of self-MHC plus foreign peptide. The intrinsic affinity of the TCR for MHC may also serve to explain why such a high fraction of T cells are alloreactive ($1/10–1/10^2$, compared with a frequency of $1/10^4–1/10^5$ for a nominal antigen, see Table 3) (52).

Superantigens

Bacterial Superantigens

Certain bacterial proteins have several unusual features (Table 3) (53). Separate regions of the intact protein have the capacity to bind to MHC molecules and TCRs directly, without prior processing into antigenic peptides

TABLE 3. *Distinguishing characteristics of different types of antigens*

Feature	Nominal antigen	Alloantigen (direct pathway)	Superantigen
Frequency of T cells that respond	0.0001–0.00001%	0.01–1%	1–30%
MHC restriction	Yes	Not applicable	No
Antigen processed into peptide fragments	Yes	No	No
TCR-chain binding	αβHeterodimer	αβHeterodimer	β Chain alone

MHC, major histocompatibility complex; TCR, T-cell receptor.

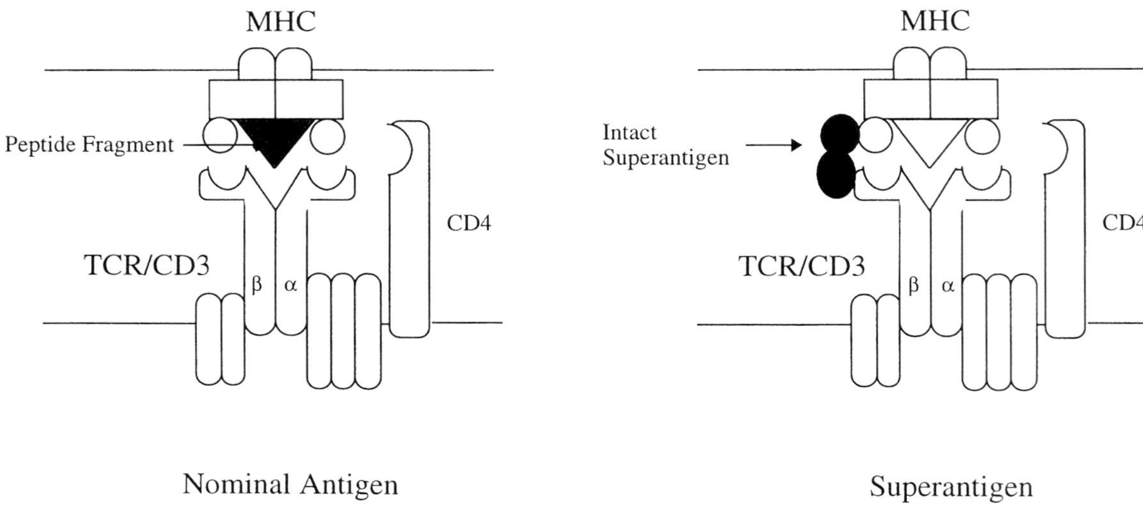

FIG. 11. Different types of antigen presentation. Antigenic peptide fragments are presented to T cells in the antigen-binding groove of an MHC molecule *(left)*. In contrast, superantigens *(right)* have to ability to bind directly to the TCRβ chain and to MHC class II molecules without any prior processing.

(Fig. 11). Since they bind directly to the TCR, they stimulate T cells in an MHC-unrestricted manner. Binding to the TCR occurs almost exclusively through the TCRVβ chain, the TCRα chain being in general irrelevant. Finally, any given protein of this class will usually bind to each of several TCRVβ chains and virtually all MHC molecules (although with varying affinity). As a consequence of these latter characteristics, these proteins bind to and hence activate an enormous percentage of T cells (10–30%). This is a 3- to 4-log higher percentage of T cells than is activated by nominal antigens. In recognitions of these characteristics, these proteins have been termed superantigens. Examples of superantigens are the staphylococcal exotoxins and certain streptococcal cell wall toxins, including the one responsible for toxic shock-syndrome (TSS). Interestingly, the pathogenesis of TSS appears to be the result of massive polyclonal T-cell activation, not of direct injury by the toxin.

Viral Superantigens

In 1976, Festenstein described a phenomenon wherein cells from one mouse mounted in vitro and in vivo immune responses against cells from an MHC-matched animal, yet the responses only worked in one direction, that is, the "stimulator" cells did not react to the "responder" cells, a situation quite unlike MHC alloreactivity (54). Classic genetics demonstrated that the phenomenon segregated to a series of independent loci where apparent alleles were dominantly expressed. These loci were termed mls (minor lymphocyte stimulating). Mice were defined as expressing or not expressing a gene product at a given locus. Thus, a mouse that was mls^{a-} would react to one that was mls^{a+} but otherwise genetically identical, whereas the converse was not true. After many years, further studies revealed that mls gene products were superantigens, thus accounting for their ability to provoke strong immune responses. Finally, in 1991, several groups simultaneously reported that the mls loci were retroviral genes that had already been identified as mouse mammary tumor viruses (MMTVs) [reviewed by Marrack et al. (55)]. "Infection" with these retroviruses was either endogenous (that is, inherited in the genome) or exogenous (transmitted through lactation). Several explanations of evolutionary adaptability have been put forward to explain their persistence in mice, but none have yet been proven. One of the leading hypotheses builds on the observation that mice infected with MMTV delete large numbers of T cells with certain TCRVβs, since the retroviral genes are seen as self, and therefore those T cells would be self-reactive. It is proposed that TCR deletion will protect against diseases caused by bacterial superantigens. Although this hypothesis is attractive, it remains unproven.

With the discovery of the existence of retrovirally encoded superantigens in the murine genome either as a result of endogenous carriage or exogenous infection, the question arises as to whether the human genome carries similar endogenous retroviruses. While studies with an outbred human population are by necessity more difficult than with an inbred mouse population, there is as of yet no evidence for endogenous retroviral-encoded superantigens in the human genome. Of interest, there has been at least one report suggesting that HIV may encode one or more superantigens, based on the TCRVß response of infected individuals (56). Other human pathogens for which evidence of a superantigenlike effect has been found include rabies virus and mycoplasma arthriditis, a possible causative agent in rheumatoid arthritis.

Anatomic Sites of Antigen Encounter and Sensitization

In considering immune responses, it is often useful to separate the response into two phases: the initiation phase and the effector phase. Most antigens are encountered first in nonimmune tissues. Thus, although the bulk of lymphocytes are in the spleen and lymph nodes, it is unusual for a foreign antigen to make its first entrance into the body at that site. More typically, initial sites of encounter are the skin, respiratory tract, or gastrointestinal tract. Using the skin as a typical site, let us examine antigen encounter. Upon first exposure to the antigen, resident APCs of dendritic lineage (which in the skin are called Langerhans cells) take up and process the protein into antigenic peptides for display on MHC class II molecules. The dendritic cells also upregulate and/or newly express a variety of activation markers and cell surface proteins important to support the activation of T cells. These include MHC class II molecules themselves, adhesion molecules such as ICAM-1, and costimulatory molecules of the B7 family (see below). Most importantly, dendritic cells leave the skin and migrate to regional lymph nodes where they can present the antigen to T cells (57). The importance of this phenomenon is illustrated by the fact that depletion of dendritic cells from the skin markedly blunts (sometimes completely) the response to applied antigens. As is outlined in greater detail below, it is in the peripheral lymphoid tissue that CD4+ (helper) T cells first respond to antigen by elaborating a variety of cytokines, thus completing the initiation phase of the immune response. Following this, activated effector cells, both T and B lymphocytes, as well as macrophages and NK cells, migrate out of the lymph nodes to the site of antigen where they actually effect their response. Thus, one can think of immune responses being initiated within the lymphoid tissue, but being effected at a distal site. An exception to this is the response to alloantigens, where to some extent the presence of large numbers of donor-type APCs can lead to the recruitment and activation of T cells within the graft itself.

T-Cell Activation

As recently as 15 years ago, T cells, like many other cells, were essentially "black boxes" in that we knew very little about their surface receptors, and even less about the signaling pathways that coupled activation of the surface receptors to intracellular responses. Although our knowledge is not complete, the picture is much clearer today.

Engagement by Antigen, Intracellular Signaling Pathways

The T-cell receptor for antigen (TCR) is a heterodimer of two closely related members of the Ig gene superfamily (58). Both the α and β chains are transmembrane proteins with short cytoplasmic tails. Consistent with this, it appears that they do not transmit intracellular signals themselves, but rather they rely on an associated group of proteins known as CD3, with which they form the TCR–CD3 complex (Fig. 3). There are five different CD3 chains: γ, δ, ε, ζ, and η. Recent reports suggest that the stoichiometry of the TCR–CD3 complex is 1 TCR α-β heterodimer, 2 ε chains, 2 ζ chains, 1 γ chain, and 1 δ chain. The η chain is derived from alternate splicing of the gene encoding ζ. While most TCR–CD3 complexes have 2 ζ chains, apparently some have 1 ζ and 1 η, or even 2 η chains. The significance of this is unclear, although it has been suggested that T cells using the η-η homodimer in their TCR–CD3 complexes may respond to antigen differently, perhaps even undergoing cell death rather than proliferating (59). If so, this could be the structural basis for differential T-cell responses observed in a variety of in vitro and in vivo models. The pivotal role of the ζ chain in T-cell signaling makes this a plausible theory.

Once the TCR binds antigen, a cascade of pathways are activated (Fig. 12) (58). Many of the most proximal signals are transduced through cytosolic protein tyrosine kinases. One of the most important events in this cascade is tyrosine phosphorylation, and hence activation, of the CD3ζ chain. This appears to be a pivotal event in T-cell activation. In vitro, when a fusion protein construct with the CD8 extracellular domain and the ζ intracellular domain is expressed in T cells, the cells become fully activated upon stimulation with anti-CD8 monoclonal antibody. Thus, many of the earlier events following TCR stimulation are directed toward ζ-chain activation, and

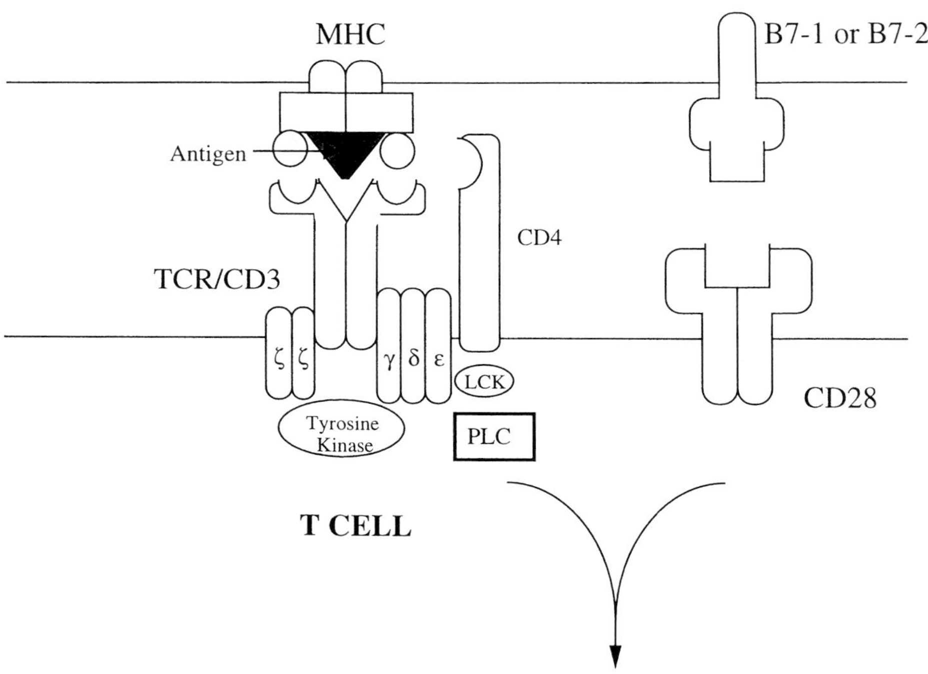

FIG. 12. T-cell activation. T cells require two signals for complete activation. The first signal, shown on the *left*, is antigen-specific and is delivered through T-cell receptor (TCR) engagement of antigen bound to MHC. TCR signals are transduced to the cell interior through associated chains (the γ, δ, ε, and ζ chains are shown here) of the CD3 complex. Through intracellular tyrosine kinases, this links the TCR to activation of phospholipase C (PLC), a second messenger system used in a variety of cells. In the case of a CD4+ T cell (as shown here), CD4 binds to nonpolymorphic regions of MHC class II molecules. This leads to increased adhesion as well as signal transduction through the tyrosine kinase p56lck (lck), thus assisting in T-cell activation through signal 1. The second signal is antigen nonspecific and is often termed a costimulatory signal. One such signal is delivered through the T-cell accessory molecule CD28 binding to either of its ligands B7-1 or B7-2.

phosphorylation of this chain seems to be sufficient to replicate T-cell responses following antigen encounter. Phosphorylation of the ζ chain ultimately leads to tyrosine phosphorylation, and hence activation, of phospholipase Cγ1. It is believed that activation of this enzyme is primarily responsible for initiation of inositol phospholipid hydrolysis, a central event in the activation of many eukaryotic cells. Through intermediaries, this leads to a rise in intracellular calcium and activation of protein kinase C. These signals are by themselves sufficient to allow a resting T cells to exit G0 phase of the cell cycle and enter G1. Many new proteins are expressed as a result, including the nuclear protooncogene c-myc, and the β chain of the interleukin 2 (IL-2) receptor. However, studies over the last decade have established that this is not sufficient to enable cells to traverse the cell cycle, proliferate, and produce cytokines. A second, costimulatory signal, is needed.

Costimulatory Signals

Early studies on T-cell stimulatory requirements by necessity used transformed T-cell lines (hybridomas), as lack of knowledge of T-cell growth requirements and the identity of T-cell growth factors precluded the use of normal T cells [reviewed by Janeway and Bottomly (60)]. These studies showed that stimulation of the TCR was sufficient to lead to full activation of the hybridoma. With the identification and cloning of T-cell growth factors such as IL-2, studies on normal T cells became feasible. These studies showed that TCR stimulation (signal 1) alone did not by itself support T-cell activation, proliferation, and cytokine production. A costimulatory signal (signal 2) was needed as well (Fig. 12). The pathway(s) that provided costimulation were initially unclear, except it was recognized that APCs could deliver the signal through a cell–cell interaction with the T cells. Subsequent work has identified several pathways that, to varying degrees, may provide costimulatory signals, depending in part upon the precise definition of costimulation used.

A liberal definition of costimulatory signals might be those that synergize with TCR stimulation leading to completion of the cell cycle and proliferation. Such signals by necessity would lead to cytokine production as well, since the failure of signal 1 alone to lead to proliferation is largely related to the absence of IL-2 production. However, important studies of T-cell activation requirements over the past 10 years have demonstrated that TCR stimulation by itself not only fails to lead to proliferation, but in the absence of signal 2 actually induces anergy in the T cell (Fig. 13), a state in which the cell is nonresponsive, even to appropriate stimuli (that is, signals 1 plus 2) (61,62). Furthermore, anergy persists for at least several weeks. Interestingly, proliferation and avoidance of anergy are distinct events, as some "costimulatory" signals that support T-cell proliferation do not prevent anergy induction (63). Therefore a more stringent definition of costimulation would exclude these signals, including only those that prevent anergy as well.

With the recognition of the requirement for costimulation, a large number of molecules have been demonstrated to some degree to mediate costimulatory pathways, at least the liberal definition of synergism with TCR stimulation for proliferation. Most prominent in this list would be the T-cell surface molecule LFA-1 (CD11a/CD18) (64). This is a member of the integrin family whose counter-receptors, ICAM-1, -2, and -3 are widely distributed on a variety of cell types. Signals through LFA-1 appear to be mediated by the same pathways as those through the TCR, and thus ligation of this receptor might be seen to augment TCR-mediated signals. Several other molecules meeting this definition of costimulation include the ligand for CD40 (termed CD40 ligand), heat-stable antigen (whose ligand is unknown), CD27, CD7, and CD5. However, none of these pathways have been shown to prevent anergy induction in T cells. The only pathway that satisfies that more stringent definition of costimulation is that mediated by the CD28 surface receptor.

CD28 is a member of the Ig gene superfamily expressed on 80% of human T cells and all murine T cells (65). This pathway delivers intracellular signals distinct from those of the TCR, including activation of PI-3-kinase. Activation of the CD28 pathway provides costimulation for proliferation and cytokine production as well as prevents anergy induction. Augmentation of cytokine production occurs both via activation of cytokine gene transcription as well as by stabilization of cytokine mRNAs, allowing far greater degrees of translation into protein production than would otherwise occur. CD28 has at least two natural ligands that have been cloned: B7-1 (CD80) and B7-2 (CD86). Both are expressed almost exclusively on activated APCs. Their presence on APCs is crucial for full T-cell activation. Their absence on non-APCs may be an important mechanism to maintain peripheral tolerance, in that potentially autoreactive T cells with TCRs directed against self-antigens would be anergized by contact with those antigens on non-APCs,

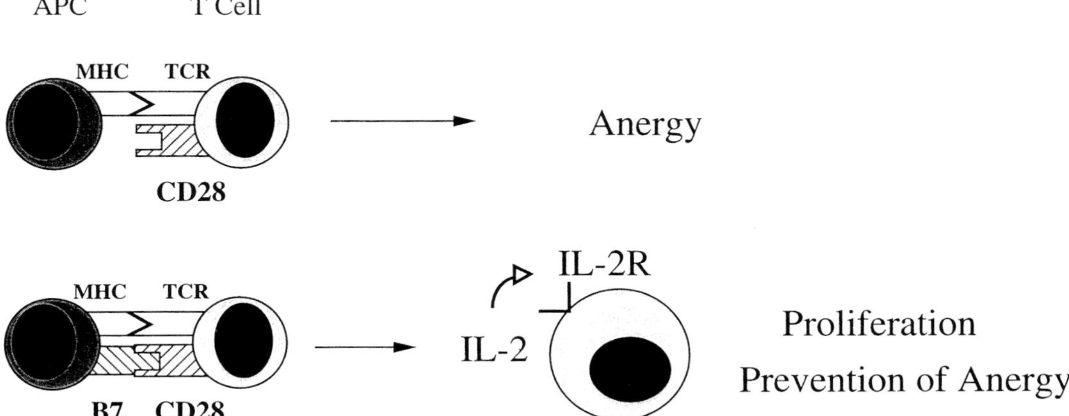

FIG. 13. Anergy induction in mature T cells. Stimulation through the T-cell receptor alone induces anergy in T cells *(top)* (see the text for details). A second (costimulatory) signal, such as that delivered through the CD28–B7 interaction, is required for induction of cytokine gene expression, proliferation, and prevention of anergy *(bottom)*.

rather than activated by them. Consistent with this, mice expressing B7-1 as a transgene can, under appropriate circumstances, develop autoimmune reactions against the tissue expressing B7-1 (66). It is not known why CD28 has two ligands, although recent evidence suggests that stimulation of CD28 through B7-1 may lead to a qualitatively different type of T-cell response (Th1, see below) versus stimulation with B7-2 (Th2). In addition, B7-2 is expressed earlier in the immune response, suggesting that it may serve to stimulate CD28 to avoid T-cell anergy, whereas B7-1, expressed later, may be more important in amplifying the response. It should also be noted that activated T cells express a CD28 homologue called CTLA4. Studies in CD28-knockout mice demonstrate that, unlike CD28, CTLA4 does not transduce a stimulatory signal to the cell interior, and suggest that the signal is instead a negative one, which may be important in terminating immune responses (see below).

TABLE 4. *Selected cytokines and their effects*[a]

Cytokine	Cell of origin	Action(s)
IL-1α and IL-1β	Macrophages, epithelial cells	Proinflammatory[b]
IL-2	T cells	T- and B-cell growth factor
IL-3	T cells	Hematopoiesis
IL-4	T cells, mast cells, basophils	B-cell activation, induces Th2 responses
IL-5	T cells, mast cells	Eosinophil growth factor
IL-6	T cells, macrophages	Proinflammatory
IL-7	Stromal cells in thymus and marrow	Growth/maintenance factor for immature T and B cells
IL-8[c]	Macrophages	Leukocyte chemotaxis
IL-10	T cells, macrophages	Suppresses macrophage functions
IL-12	APCs	NK cell growth/activation factor, induces Th 1 responses
IL-15	T cells	Same as IL-2
IFN-γ	T cells, NK cells	Activates macrophages, increases MHC expression, induces IL-12 production
TNF	T cells, macrophages, NK cells	Proinflammatory
TGF-β	Macrophages, T cells	Anti-inflammatory

[a] APC, antigen-presenting cell; IL, interleukin; IFN, interferon; MHC, major histocompatibility complex; NK, natural killer; TNF, tumor necrosis factor; TGF, transforming growth factor.

[b] Proinflammatory and anti-inflammatory actions include effects on vasodilatation, leukocyte recruitment, antigen presentation, and so on.

[c] IL-8 is a part of the chemokine family, other members of which, including MIP-1α, MIP-1β, MCP-1, and RANTES, also are strong chemoattractants for leukocytes.

T-Cell Effector Function

Cytokines

The ability of activated T cells to direct immune responses depends to a large extent on the cytokines they produce. These exert effects directly upon other immune effector cells, inducing their activation and growth, as well as in some cases leading them to produce their own cytokines. The list of cytokines is large and growing. Table 4 outlines selected known cytokines, their source, and their effects. What follows below is a consideration of three important effects of cytokines, listed by the target cell rather than the cytokine itself.

Cytotoxic Lymphocyte Differentiation and Function

With a few minor exceptions, virtually all CTLs are MHC class-I-restricted CD8+ cells. Unlike CD4+ T cells, which make large amounts of cytokines, CD8+ T cells make far less, and therefore they often are dependent on cytokines produced locally by CD4+ cells (67). IL-2 seems to be their most important growth factor, and provision of exogenous recombinant IL-2 to isolated CD8+ T cells can make up for much the deficit seen by removal of the CD4+ population. Other cytokines that exert effects on this cell population include IFN-γ and IL-6, both of which promote activation more than expansion.

Activated CTLs possess two mechanisms to kill their targets, both of which require cell–cell contact (68). The first mechanism is through perforin, a protein found in most CTLs and NK cells. Perforin is related to C6–C9, components of the membrane attack complex of complement. Perforin, like complement components, has the capacity to induce transmembrane pores in the target cell, leading to target cell lysis. Although it was originally thought that membrane lysis by perforin was the sole mediator of CTL killing, several inconsistencies with that model were evident, including the ability of CTLs to kill in the absence of calcium (perforin killing requires calcium) and the refractoriness of CTLs to their own killing while retaining susceptibility to lysis by other cells. These inconsistencies have begun to be explained with the elucidation of the second mechanism of CTL killing, the Fas pathway. Fas (CD95) is a member of the tumor necrosis factor (TNF) receptor family and is the surface mediator of a pathway that, when activated, induces the cell to undergo programmed cell death through apoptosis (69). Many cells express Fas, and activated CTLs express Fas ligand. Killing of target cells via Fas accounts for most of unexplained phenomenon in the "perforin only" model. It is currently believed that both mechanisms of killing are available to CTLs in vivo.

B-Cell Help

The B-cell response to most protein antigens requires T-cell help. The stimulatory requirements for B cells and the ways in which B and T cells interact are discussed in detail in the section on B-cell activation. The only point to be made here is that T cells can provide B-cell help both through secreted cytokines (in particular, IL-2, IL-4, and IL-5) that act as growth and differentiation factors for T cells, and through T-cell surface proteins that bind to receptors on activated B cells upon cell–cell contact. T-cell help is critical to promote B-cell proliferation and maturation into high-affinity antibody-secreting plasma cells.

Macrophage Activation

The activated macrophage is one of the most important mediators of many types of immune responses, especially delayed-type hypersensitivity (DTH) and related cellular immune reactions. Resting macrophages must be activated in order to exert their full inflammatory and cytopathic effects. Two types of cytokines produced by T cells are important in this process: IFN-γ and the colony-stimulating factors GM-CSF (granylocyte-macrophage colony-stimulating factor) and IL-3. The ways in which IFN-γ does this are numerous (70). To note some of the important ones, it enhances phagocytosis, stimulates macrophage secretion of the proinflammatory agents TNF and IL-1, stimulates production and secretion of reactive oxygen products (such as superoxide and nitric oxide) that are important mechanisms for the cytopathic effect of macrophages, and upregulates MHC expression on macrophages. The effects of GM-CSF and IL-3 are exerted primarily indirectly through the bone marrow, as these hemopoietins regulate the production and release of macrophages (and granulocytes).

Implications of the Class I/Class II Dichotomy

One of the implications of the fact that the majority of cytokines come from CD4+ cells is that, in general, these cells are critical to initiate most immune responses. Since CD4+ cells bear MHC class-II-restricted TCRs, a corollary of this is that immune responses require MHC class II+ cells. This fits well with the known distribution of class II molecules, being found primarily on APCs that would be the same cells capturing and presenting foreign proteins to begin with. What has remained somewhat less clear is how these cytokines get where they are needed. Cytokines have short biologic half-lives and, in general, should be thought of as paracrine, not endocrine, agents. That is, they act locally. Therefore, a coordinated immune response requires class-I- and class-II-restricted antigen presentation in the same microenvironment to stimulate both CD4+ and CD8+ cells locally. In the case of allograft rejection, a single cell, the donor APC, can provide both class-I- and class-II-restricted foreign antigens. For other antigens, one way this requirement can be met is through tissue macrophages/dendritic cells that are present in most parenchymal organs providing stimulation to CD4+ T cells. These will produce cytokines that can be used by locally activated CTLs. Alternatively, antigens captured by APCs can be brought to regional lymph nodes. Cytokines produced there can activate CD8+ cells that migrated there following activation in tissue, or that were activated in the node itself.

B-Cell Activation

As with aspects of development, the parallels between B-cell activation and T-cell activation are numerous. This section summarizes these and highlights the distinctions.

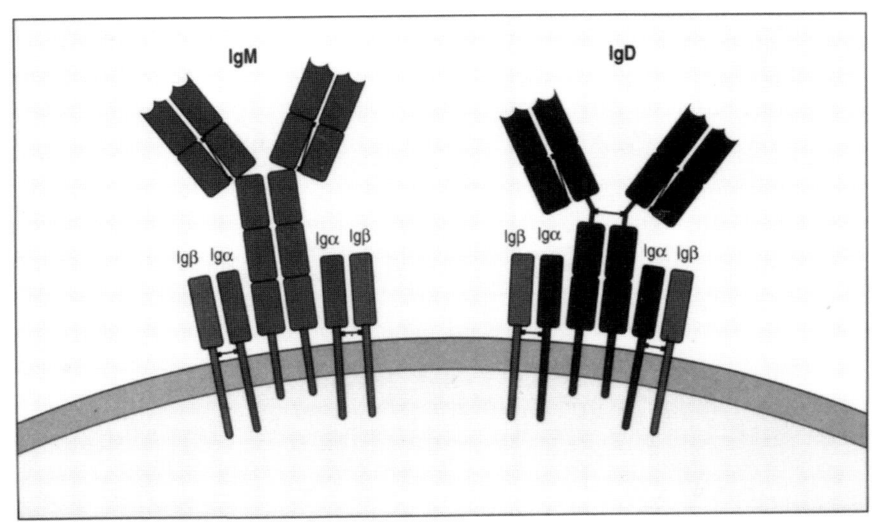

FIG. 14. Surface immunoglobulin is of the B-cell receptor for antigen. Transmembrane immunoglobulins (either IgM or IgD) form the antigen-binding portion of the B-cell receptor. Nonpolymorphic proteins known as Igα and Igβ form part of the signaling complex. Reprinted with permission from C. A. Janeway and P. Travers, *Immunobiology*, Current Biology Ltd., London.

Engagement by Antigen, Intracellular Signaling Pathways

The BCR complex (Fig. 14) contains an Ig molecule that serves an antigen-recognition function, noncovalently linked to a heterodimer comprised of two chains called Ig-α and Ig-β (recently named CD79a and CD79b) (71). A stoichiometry of 1 Ig molecule associated with two Ig-α–Ig-β heterodimers has been suggested. The Ig-α–Ig-β dimer is believed to be the signal transducing element of the BCR complex, linking it to an activation cascade of tyrosine kinases, some of which are shared with T cells, others of which are B cell specific. The downstream marker of signal transduction in B cells is the same as that in T cells, inositol phospholipid hydrolysis.

T-Independent Antigens

B-cell activation through the Ig receptor requires cross-linking of surface Ig molecules (Fig. 15) (72). The same is true of the TCR; however, the TCR ligands, MHC molecules, are cell surface molecules, and their relative immobilization in a membrane appears to provide sufficient cross-linking for T cells. In the case of B cells whose receptors are binding soluble molecules, only cer-

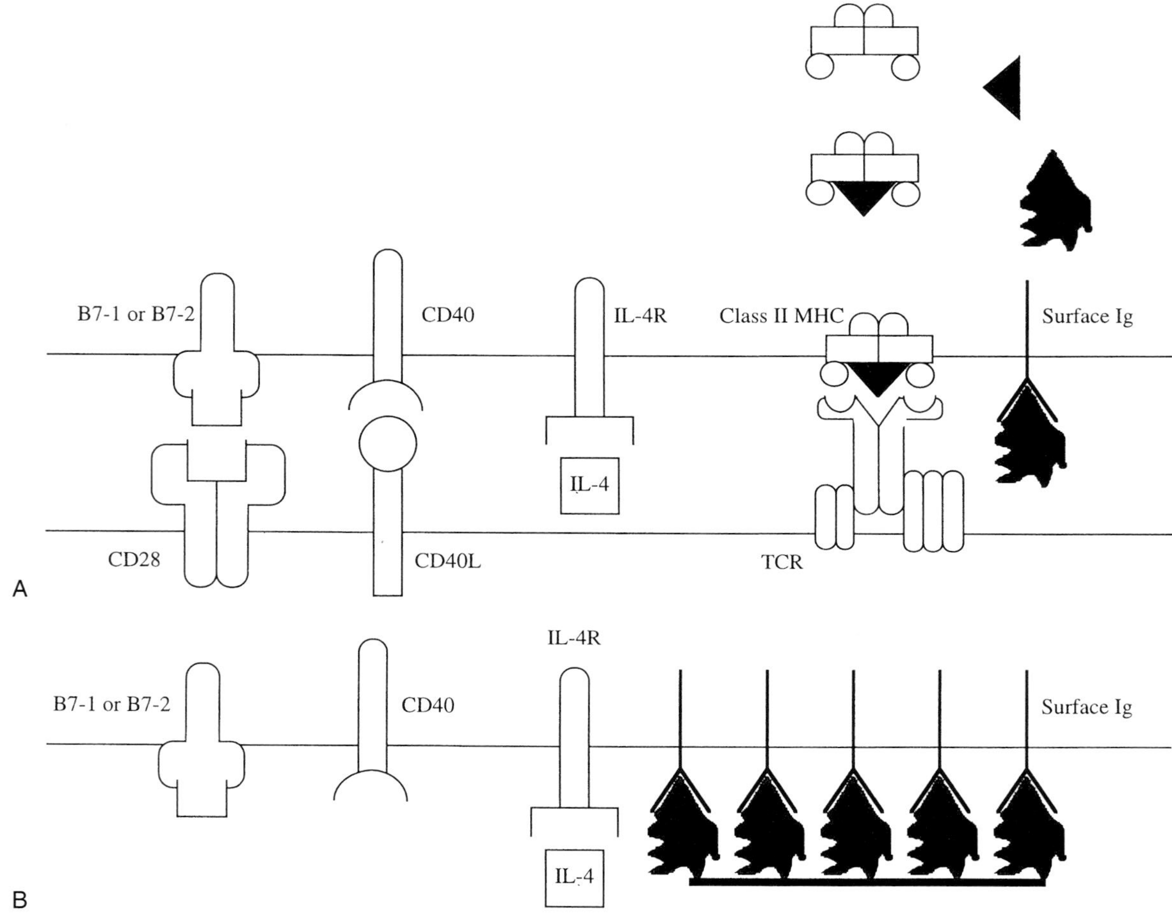

FIG. 15. Two types of B-cell activation. **A:** Cognate T-cell–B-cell help. B cells capture antigens through their surface immunoglobulin (Ig) receptors, process them, and present peptide fragments on MHC class II molecules. T cells specific for that peptide antigen–class II complex will become activated, as a result of which they express CD40 ligand (CD40L) on their surface. This binds to CD40 on the B cell, rescuing the B cell from apoptosis and providing additional signals needed for activation as well. T cells also receive signals from this interaction. T cells also secrete lymphokines such as IL-4 and IL-2 (not shown) that can provide help and differentiative signals to the B cell as well. B-cell activation through MHC class II, CD40, and IL-4 each lead to upregulation of B7 molecules that provide costimulatory signals to the T cell through CD28. **B:** T independent antigens. When the antigen that binds the B-cell surface Ig receptor has multiple repetitive epitopes, it can cross-link Ig extensively. This by itself is sufficient to initiate B-cell activation that requires additional help only in the form of IL-4. The source of IL-4 is this type of B-cell activation is undetermined.

tain types of antigen containing repetitive epitopes will meet this requirement. Most antigens in this category are polysaccharides—in particular bacterial capsular polysaccharides. The capacity of these antigens to cross-link surface Ig means that T cells themselves are not required for the B-cell response. Thus, T-cell-deficient animals such as athymic nude mice will have normal antibody responses to these antigens. In recognition of this, and to distinguish these antigens from those that require T-cell–B-cell contact in order to elicit a B-cell response, they are called T-independent antigens.

Cognate Interactions: Costimulatory Signals

Most B-cell antigens are probably not able to cross-link Ig extensively and therefore are unable by themselves to activate B cells. They depend on a process known as T-cell–B cell cognate help (Fig. 15) (73,74). In this instance, the non-cross-linking antigen that binds to the B-cell surface Ig is internalized and presented to CD4+ T cells on B-cell MHC class II molecules. The T-cell–B-cell contact initiated in this way also allows the B-cell surface receptor CD40 to bind to its ligand on the T cell (known as CD40 ligand). Signals through CD40 act in concert with T-cell-derived cytokines to activate the B cell. Although MHC class II molecules, upon engaging TCRs, can transmit certain signals to the B-cell interior, it is unclear at present what role, if any, they play in B-cell activation to T-dependent antigens.

One important aspect of cognate help is that is it reciprocal. CD40-activated B cells upregulate a number of molecules, including both the known CD28 ligands, B7-1 and B7-2 (Fig. 15). Therefore, at the same time that B cells are receiving help from T cells (through CD40 ligand), they are also providing help to T cells through B7 (75). Thus, cognate interactions between T and B cells are symbiotic in that each cell both receives and delivers a critical signal.

Antibody Secretion

Following appropriate activation and signaling, previously naive B cells secrete IgM and proceed through one of two fates: development into memory cells (see below) or differentiation into antibody-secreting plasma cells (76,77). The latter fate frequently is accompanied by somatic mutation (see above) and isotype switching to IgA, IgG, or IgE, although some plasma cells do not class switch and secrete IgM. This process occurs over a period of 2–3 weeks, so that the initial antibody response in a naive animal is IgM, with subsequent maturation to IgG and IgA. Some of the distinctions between Ig isotypes are outlined in Table 1. IgM antibodies are markers of a primary immune response, since isotype switching has not yet occurred. These antibodies have a relatively short half-life (6 days) and exist in multivalent forms as pentamers and hexamers. This multivalency increases affinity, which is useful since somatic mutation and selection of high-affinity clones has not yet occurred. IgG antibodies are the serum secondary antibodies for most pathogens. They have a long half-life (23 days) and are transferred across the placenta. IgA antibodies exits both as monomers and dimers and are secretory Igs that are transferred across mucosal surfaces and provide mucosal humoral immunity. IgE exists in very low levels in the blood, but is efficiently captured onto the surface of mast cells and basophils, which engagement by antigen triggers degranulation of the cell, leading to allergic and anaphylactic responses.

Antibodies can function in several different ways, varying by isotype. These mechanisms include fixation of complement, opsonization for phagocytosis by FcR+ cells, opsonization for lysis by cells capable of antibody-dependent cellular cytotoxicity, and induction of eosinophil degranulation.

REGULATING THE RESPONSE TO FOREIGN ANTIGEN

Migration and Adhesion of Immune Cells

As sophisticated as the mechanisms of immunologic recognition may be, they will of little avail unless lymphocytes and other immune effector cells have access to the inflammatory site. It is exceedingly rare for foreign antigens to be located primarily and initially in peripheral lymphoid tissue. Almost always, they are introduced into the body elsewhere (for example, skin, or mucosal surfaces). While a few lymphocytes are normally resident in most parenchymal organs and tissues, clearly during an immune response the number of cells that become localized to the site of inflammation increases by several logs. It is through the expression and regulation of adhesion molecules that this process takes place.

The molecules that regulate adhesion fall into three primary families: selectins, integrins, and Ig superfamily proteins. Members of each family play a distinct role in coordinating adhesion and migration of lymphocytes [reviewed by Imhof and Dunon (78)].

Selectins and "Rolling/Tethering"

When an inflammatory process occurs, leukocytes (by which is meant cells of lymphoid and myeloid lineage) need to get to the inflammatory site (Fig. 16). They are, however, unable to access that site directly, as it is hidden behind endothelium. Although normally leukocytes are rushing through the bloodstream, local vasodilation in response to inflammation increases the volume of blood flow and at the same time decreases the flow rate. As

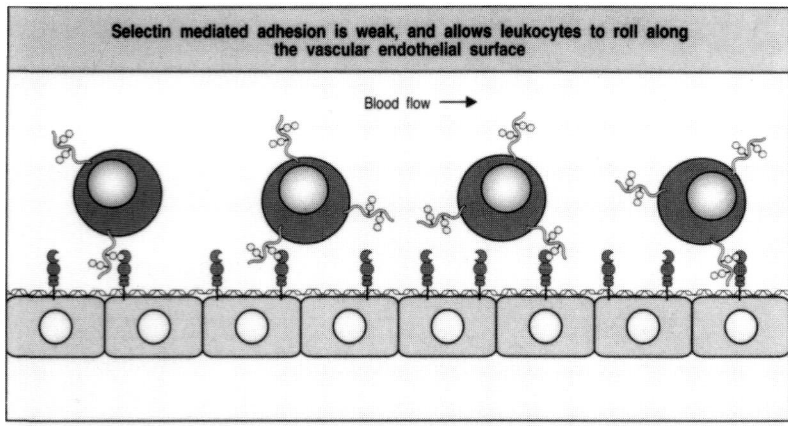

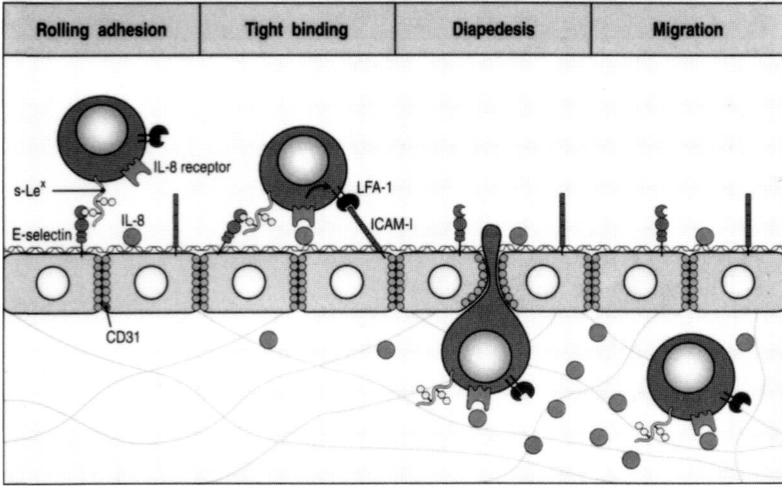

FIG. 16. A model for cell adhesion and migration. Inflammatory mediators such as tumor necrosis factor induce the expression of selectins on endothelial cells. The relatively weak interaction of selectins with their ligands such as sialyl Lewis X (s-Le^x) is sufficient for transient adhesion of the leukocyte. This adhesion, however, is broken by shear forces of blood flow, reestablished distally, broken again, and so on, so that the leukocyte rolls along the endothelium. Triggering of the cell through chemokines such as IL-8 induces high affinity in the integrin LFA-1 for its ligand ICAM-1. This is a strong adhesive interaction that withstands shear forces of the bloodstream. Subsequently, the leukocyte migrates through the endothelium. Reprinted with permission from C. A. Janeway and P. Travers, *Immunobiology*, Current Biology Ltd., London.

cells flow slower, they have a greater chance of reacting with the endothelium and adhering to it. Nonetheless, leukocytes adhere poorly to resting endothelial cells. However, in response to inflammatory stimuli such as the macrophage products TNF and IL-1, both lymphocytes and endothelial cells upregulate selectins on their cell surface (79). The selectin family of molecules share a common structural backbone that includes a lectin (sugar-binding) domain. As a result of the lectin domain, the ligands for the selectins are sugars, such as sialated or sulfated Lewis blood group antigens X and A (sialyl Lewis X and sialyl Lewis A). These sugars can be found on any one of a number of proteins expressed by lymphocytes and endothelia, and thus each cell type bears both selectins and selectin ligands. Selectins mediate transient adhesion of the lymphocyte to the endothelium so that the cell appears to roll along the surface of the blood vessel, a phenomenon that also has been termed "tethering."

Chemokines and Triggering

Lymphocytes slowed down by selectin interactions come into more prolonged contact with the endothelium. As a result, lymphocytes are stimulated by chemokines, a group of small proinflammatory molecules produced by endothelia, fibroblasts, platelets, and monocytes. Once secreted, chemokines such as IL-8 associate with cell surface proteoglycans on endothelial cells (such as CD44) through their heparin-binding domains. This retains the chemokines locally, enabling them to activate lymphocytes and neutrophils as they roll by. When the chemokines bind to their receptors on leukocytes, they trigger the adhesive function of integrins (80).

Adhesion

The integrin family of molecules are α-β heterodimers formed by noncovalent association (81). There are 15 known α chains and eight known β chains, and at least 21 different α-β combinations have been described. Depending on the specific integrin, the ligand may be an extracellular matrix molecule or a cell surface protein. The ligands for one of the first known and best characterized integrins, LFA-1, are the Ig superfamily gene members ICAM-1, -2, and -3. LFA-1 is expressed on most leukocytes. ICAM-1 is weakly expressed on resting endothelium, but induced by activation with IL-1 and TNF. Thus, they form a potential adhesion pair to enable leukocytes to adhere to endothelia at the sites of inflammation. An important property of integrins such as LFA-1 is that their baseline state is one of low affinity for their ligands. This prevents unneeded adhesion of leukocytes to normal endothelium. Activation of the LFA-1-bearing cell (such as by chemokines) triggers the transition of LFA-1 to a high-affinity state for ICAM-1, leading to tight adhesion of the leukocyte to the endothelial cell (80).

Transmigration

This is the final step required to get the leukocyte to the site of inflammation and occurs rapidly after adhesion. Both the transient nature of integrin triggering as well as shedding of cell surface selectin molecules assist in detaching the leukocyte from the vessel wall. The events that take place during actual locomotion/transmigration remain poorly characterized (78).

Th1 and Th2 Responses

Generation of Th1 and Th2 Cells

During the 1980s, an increasing number of cytokines secreted by T cells and macrophages were identified. In studies examining cytokine production by T-cell clones, Mosmann and colleagues made the surprising discovery that many murine CD4+ T-cell clones could be subdivided into one of two categories based on the cytokines they produced (82). So-called Th1 (for T helper-type 1) clones produced IL-2 and IFN-γ, while Th2 clones produced IL-4, IL-5, and IL-10 (Fig. 17). As the effects of these cytokines became known, it was apparent that the subdivision of production correlated with a categorization of function; namely, that the cytokines produced by Th1 clones provided help for cellular immune responses while Th2-derived cytokines provided help for humoral responses (83–85). Thus, the Th1-derived cytokines were growth and maturation/activation factors for cytotoxic T lymphocytes and NK cells (especially IL-2) and macro-

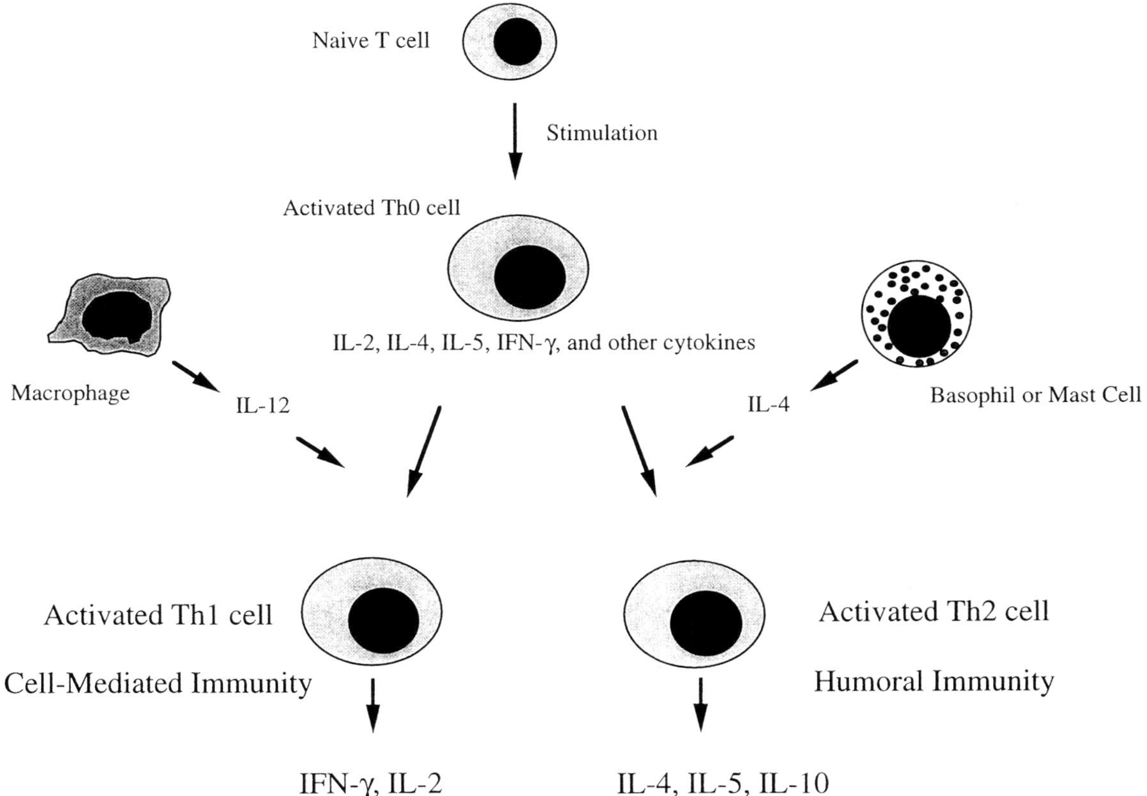

FIG. 17. Two types of T-helper cells. When previously unactivated ("naive") T cells are stimulated, they secrete low levels of virtually all T-cell-derived cytokines. They are frequently referred to as Th0 cells. Further differentiation is largely under the control of exogenous cytokines. IL-12, produced by activated antigen-presenting cells, strongly directs T cells toward the Th1 phenotype. These cells produce interferon-γ and IL-2 and direct cell-mediated immunity. IL-4, believed to be initially produced by basophils and/or mast cells, directs T cells toward the Th2 phenotype. Th2 cells, responsible for providing B-cell help for humoral immunity, secrete IL-4, IL-5, and IL-10.

phages (particularly IFN-γ). In contrast, Th2 cytokines performed similar functions for B cells. Interestingly, Th1 cytokines not only promote cellular responses, but they tend to inhibit humoral responses, and the reciprocal is true of Th2 cytokines so that these seem to be mutually antagonistic pathways, although as expected there are exceptions. The original findings arose out of the murine system, but most researchers report similar findings with human T cells and rat T cells as well, so it is likely that this dichotomy applies to most species.

Since the original observations of Th1 and Th2 cells were with T-cell clones, it was a matter of some contention as to whether these findings were an in vitro culture artifact as a result of the way in which clones are generated by repetitive antigen stimulation: that is, did Th1 and Th2 cells exist in vivo? The evidence is abundant now that Th1 and Th2 cells do indeed exist in physiologic situations. It appears that undifferentiated "naive" T cells that have not been previously exposed to antigen mature and differentiate roughly according to the following schema (Fig. 17). Following antigen encounter, the cells secrete a pattern of so-called Th0 cytokines, which consists of low levels of most Th1 *and* Th2 cytokines. The subsequent fate of the cell is then determined largely by its external milieu. At present, the primary known factors that influence the cytokine-differentiation profile of a T cell are other cytokines themselves, namely, IL-4 and IL-12 (86,87). When T cells are stimulated in the presence of IL-4 they develop into Th2 cells, whereas in the presence of IL-12 they become Th1 cells. Under the competing influence of both cytokines, the effects of IL-4 appear to predominate. What then are the sources of IL-4 and IL-12 that act upon the T cells? The primary producers of IL-12 are APCs themselves, which secrete IL-12 following activation (such as by antigen) particularly when stimulated by small amounts of IFN-γ, the initial source of which may be NK cells. Since the main sources of IL-4 are T cells themselves, it has been problematic to explain where the initial IL-4 could come from to drive T cells subsequently toward IL-4 production. The recent discovery that mast cells and basophils make IL-4 has led to the hypothesis that they are the initial source early in the immune response. One other possible parameter that may influence the type of Th cell that develops is the type of costimulatory signal the T cell receives, as studies have suggested that one of the CD28 ligands, B7-1, promotes a Th1 response, whereas the other, B7-2, promotes a Th2 response (88). This will doubtless require further investigation.

Role of Th1 and Th2 Cytokines in the Response to Pathogens

It is easy to see how this system might be manipulated in vaccine strategies to elicit particular types of immune responses by targeting antigen toward or away from macrophages to elicit Th1 (cellular) or Th2 (humoral) responses, respectively. The emerging different types of immune responses are not merely immunologic nuances, but have important consequences for the organism. The response of mice to *Leishmania major* offers one of the best examples (83,84). *Leishmania* are protozoal organisms that are intracellular parasites of macrophages. In humans, the spectrum of disease that is seen varies from a self-contained cutaneous form to a disseminated visceral form that is usually fatal. In mice, animals of the C3H strain heal their infection locally and develop cell-mediated immunity to *Leishmania.* On the other hand, mice of the BALB/c strain develop chronic disseminated fatal infections. Resistant C3H mice make a Th1 response to *Leishmania* whereas susceptible BALB/c mice make a Th2 response. This is not just an association, but appears to be causal as external manipulation of the response alters the course of the disease. For example, when normally resistant C3H mice are treated with an anti-IFN-γ antibody, they develop disseminated infections. Neutralization of IL-4 in BALB/c mice confers disease resistance. Thus, the immune response dictates the type of the disease seen. This is not to imply that Th1 responses are all good and Th2 bad as, in the case of other pathogens such as certain helminths, the Th2 responses are often protective.

Emergence of Memory Cells

Development of Memory

Although we have only a patchy understanding of how immunologic memory is generated or maintained, we utilize this phenomenon frequently as it forms the basis for vaccination. The principle of immunologic memory is that the immune response to a previously seen antigen is both faster and more effective than the response to a new antigen (76). There are probably several reasons for this. First, lymphocytes can be subdivided based on their cell surface phenotype into naive and memory cells. Naive cells are those that have never encountered their target antigens and therefore have never been stimulated, and memory cells are those that have been stimulated, survived (see below), and maturated into a memory phenotype. The signals that instruct a lymphocyte to become a memory cell are not known. As might be expected, newborn mammals have predominantly naive cells, with the proportion of memory cells increasing with age. One of the reasons that a recall response to antigen is more robust than an initial response is that memory cells seem to be more easily activated than naive cells and make more cytokines than do activated naive cells (89). A second basis for immunologic memory is precursor frequency. Sensitive limiting dilution assays have shown an increase in the frequency of antigen-reactive cells following exposure to an antigen. A third mechanism for immunologic memory is utilized only by the B-cell compartment, namely, affinity maturation. As detailed above, exposure to antigen leads to refinement of the antibody repertoire with selection of high-affinity antibody-producing B cells. Thus, antibody production in a memory response is significantly more effective than in a primary response.

Mechanisms for Maintenance of Memory

Immunologists have been unable to agree as to how immunologic memory is maintained [reviewed by Sprent (76)]. One of the main difficulties is uncertainty regarding the life span of memory T and B cells. If, as some studies indicate, memory cells are long-lived, then immunologic memory is self-explanatory based on the principles above. However, a sizable number of studies indicate that memory T cells are not long-lasting. If this is true, then other explanations must be invoked. Several have been proposed, including stimulation by cross-reactive antigens and persistence of antigen. In the latter instance, this could take the form of chronic subclinical infection. Another possibility is that antigen in the form of antigen–antibody complexes persists and serves as a reservoir of antigen for repetitive stimulation of lymphocytes. There is abundant evidence that this does occur in some model systems, where antigen–antibody complexes have been shown to persist for at least 1 year on the surface of follicular dendritic cells located within lymph nodes and spleen.

Terminating the Immune Response

For the organism to survive, it is as important to terminate the immune response when appropriate as it was to initiate it. In retrospect, this seems obvious. For example, since antigen stimulation triggers lymphoid proliferation, in the absence of cell death repeated encounter with pathogens would lead to massive continued expansion of the lymphoid pool, turning us into giant lymph nodes. Nonetheless, until recently, the mechanisms by which immune responses are terminated have been sorely neglected. Interest in this area, however, has been rekindled recently. As we now understand it, lymphocytes are constantly dying during the course of an immune response, only to be replaced by new ones (Fig. 18). When antigen is gone, normally no new ones are generated and the response is ended. Failure to eliminate cells normally means the response may continue even in the absence of antigen, and this can have serious adverse consequences.

When and How?

The fact that withdrawl of antigen ends a response means that the immune response is not inherently self-sustaining, but requires continued "initiation" through encounter with antigen. The first step therefore to ending an immune response is to destroy the source of antigen. Depending on the nature of the pathogen, this might be through engulfment and digestion of bacteria by macrophages and neutrophils, lysis of virally infected cells by CTLs, or antibody-mediated destruction of target organisms. In any event, when the inciting antigen is gone, there will be no more initiating stimulus to induce growth factor production, cell proliferation, and cell activation.

However, what about the expanded and activated effector cell population that already exists? At first glance, it might seem that these cells are irrelevant, since in the absence of antigen they will do little harm. In fact, this is not the case. A significant amount of immune-mediated tissue injury is promiscuous, that is, antigen nonspecific. There are several reasons for this. First, some mediators

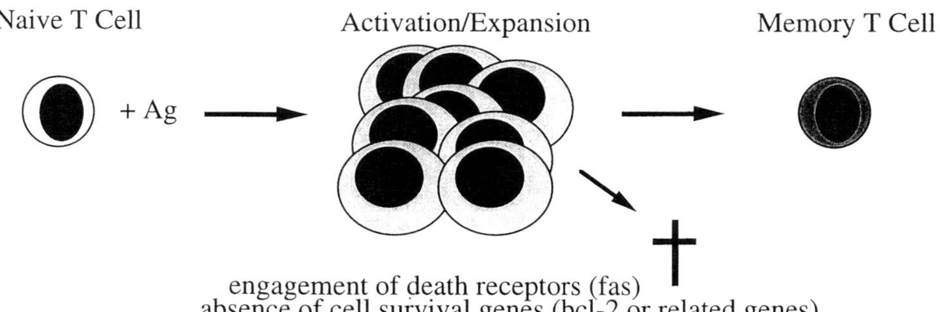

FIG. 18. Life and death in the immune response. Following challenge with antigen, a small number of antigen-specific T cells undergo clonal expansion and activation, becoming a large population of effector cells (both helper and cytotoxic T cells). After a period of time, the majority of these cells undergo programmed cell death through a variety of mechanisms, leaving behind a small number of antigen-specific memory cells. Under conditions of antigen persistence, this scenario is continually repeated and a dynamic equilibrium is reached. When the antigen is no longer present, the stimulus for expansion is removed, and the T-cell population returns to roughly its baseline level. Similar processes and considerations apply to B-cell stimulation and B-cell memory.

of injury, such as macrophages, do not have antigen receptors and act relatively indiscriminately to destroy local tissues. Second, high cytokine levels can activate some T and NK cells even in the absence of antigen stimulation. Therefore, in a mixed population of lymphocytes at an inflammatory site, high levels of cytokines produced by cells responding to an antigen can trigger activation in some cells that are not antigen specific. If some of these cells are actually self-reactive (see above), an autoimmune response will ensue. Third, antibodies can cause disease by being nonspecifically trapped in certain target tissues that are prone to this, such as synovia and glomeruli, leading to immune-complex-mediated arthritis and glomerulonephritis. This latter phenomenon is reminiscent of lupus both in humans and in animal models.

It should be evident, then, that elimination or inactivation of immune-response cells once they are no longer needed is both desirable and necessary. This is accomplished largely through induction of programmed cell death in the responding cells. Over the past 3 years, many new genes have been identified that regulate cell death pathways in lymphocytes and other cells (90). Some of these appear to convey resistance to programmed cell death and can be thought of as cell survival genes, whereas others are ligands for, or surface receptors of, pathways that induce cell death.

At present, we have only a limited understanding as to how most of these pathways are coordinated and regulated. Two of the most prominent cell survival genes are *bcl-2* and *bcl-x* (90–92). These are related genes that are members of a larger family. Both are expressed in lymphocytes and convey resistance to certain stimuli of programmed cell death. Knockout mice with targeted deletions of these genes demonstrate markedly impaired T-cell maturation (*bcl-x*) or normal maturation with grossly diminished survival of mature cells (*bcl-2*), suggesting that they are required for the survival of developing or mature T and B cells. The regulation of intracellular levels of cell survival genes such as *bcl-2* or *bcl-x* following T-cell and B-cell activation seems likely to be a mechanism for controlling life or death of the lymphocyte.

Some of the most exciting insights into how immune responses are terminated comes from the convergence of work in programmed cell death and autoimmune mice. Several years ago, two interesting antibodies were reported. The first antibody was in the murine system, directed at a cell surface antigen that was called fas (93 and see above). The second antibody, in the human system, bound to a protein called APO-1 (94). Ligation of either fas or APO-1 with the appropriate antibody induced programmed cell death (apoptosis) in the target cell. The nature of the target antigens was unknown at that time, nor was it clear what their relevance might be to normal immune homeostasis. Concurrent with this work, intensive investigations were under way to clone the genes whose mutant alleles were responsible for two interesting autoimmune mouse strains: lpr (lymphoproliferative) and gld (generalized lymphadenopathy). As the names imply, mice homozygous for mutant alleles at these loci exhibited profound lymphadenopathy with accumulation of abnormal T cells. Both lpr and gld mice developed autoimmune disease reminiscent of lupus, with autoimmune arthritis and immune-complex-mediated glomerulonephritis that led to eventual death by uremia. When the lpr and gld genes were identified, it was shown that the lpr gene was fas and the gld gene was its ligand (termed fas ligand) [reviewed by Nagata and Golstein (93) and Yakahashi et al. (95)]. It was also shown that APO-1 was the human homologue of fas. Based on these and other studies of the expression patterns of fas and fas ligand, it is clear that much of the phenotype of lpr and gld mice comes not from abnormal proliferation of T cells, but from failure of the cells to die normally. Subsequent studies have shown that activated T cells express both fas and fas ligand on their surface (96). This means that elimination of fas+ cells can be through "fratricide" or "suicide." In any event, fas represents a normal pathway for the elimination of lymphocytes after they are no longer needed. Importantly, expression of fas does not indicate susceptibility to fas-mediated cell death. Intracellular proteins associated with fas are necessary to activate the "death" machinery. Thus, fas+ T cells resist anti-fas killing 1 day after activation, but are sensitive by day 6 (97). As has so often been the case in immunology, these naturally occurring mutant mice have helped uncover an important principle, the need for cell death.

SUMMARY

This chapter has provided a brief overview of normal immune responses, particularly the development and function of immune effector cells, as a background to more specific aspects of immune perturbations that cause, or occur as a result of, renal disease. Improved understanding of these areas is critical to designing rational strategies to prevent and treat immunologically mediated renal diseases. As increasing numbers of clinical syndromes are found to have immune etiologies, advances in this area likely will have a major impact on the future treatment of renal diseases.

REFERENCES

1. Kincade PW, Gimble JM. B Lymphocytes. In: Paul WE, ed. *Fundamental immunology*. 3rd ed. New York: Raven, 1993:43–73.
2. Davis MM, Bjorkman PJ. T-cell antigen receptor genes and T-cell recognition. *Nature* 1988;334:395–402.
3. Buus S, Sette A, Colon SM, Miles C, Grey HM. The relation between major histocompatibility complex (MHC) restriction and the capacity of Ia to bind immunogenic peptides. *Science* 1987;235:1353–8.
4. Falk K, Rotzsche O, Stevanovic S, Jung G, Rammensee HG. Allele-specific motifs revealed by sequencing of self peptides eluted from MHC molecules. *Nature* 1991;351:290–6.

5. Zinkernagel RM, Doherty PC. Restriction of in vitro T cell-mediated cytotoxicity in lymphocytic choriomeningitis within a syngeneic or semiallogeneic system. *Nature* 1974;248:701–2.
6. Matis LA. The molecular basis of T-cell specificity. *Annu Rev Immunol* 1990;8:65–82.
7. Brenner MB, Strominger JL, Krangel MS. The gamma delta T cell receptor. *Adv Immunol* 1988;43:133–92.
8. Hedrick SM, Cohen DI, Nielsen EA, Davis MM. Isolation of cDNA clones encoding T cell-specific membrane-associated proteins. *Nature* 1984;308:149–53.
9. Loh EY, Lanier LL, Turck CW, et al. Identification and sequence of a fourth human T cell antigen receptor chain. *Nature* 1987;330:569–72.
10. Shatz DG, Oettiger MA, Schlissel MS. V(D)J recombination: molecular biology and regulation. *Annu Rev Immunol* 1993;10:359–380.
11. Alt F, Baltimore D. Joining of immunoglobulin heavy chain gene segments: implications from a chromosome with evidence of three D-JH fusions. *Proc Natl Acad Science USA* 1982;79:4118–22.
12. Pritchard H, Micklem HS. Haemopoeitic stem cells and progenitors of functional T lymphocytes in the bone marrow of nude mice. *Clin Exp Immonol* 1973;14:597–607.
13. Rocha B, Vassali P, Guy-Grand D. The V beta repertoire of mouse gut homodimeric alpha CD3+ intra-epithelial T cell receptor alpha/beta+ lymphocytes reveals a major extra-thymic pathway of T cell differentiation. *J Exp Med* 1991;173:483–6.
14. Owen JJT, Jenkinson EJ. Embryology of the immune system. *Prog Allergy* 1981;29:1–34.
15. Scollay RG, Butcher EC, Weissman IL. Thymus cell migration: quantitative aspects of cellular traffic from the thymus to the periphery in mice. *Eur J Immunol* 1980;10:210–8.
16. Blackman M, Kappler J, Marrack P. The role of the T cell receptor in positive and negative selection of developing T cells. *Science* 1990; 248:1335–41.
17. Sprent J, Gao EK, Webb SR. T cell reactivity to MHC molecules: immunity versus tolerance. *Science* 1990;248:1357–63.
18. von Boehmer H, Kisielow P. Self–nonself discrimination by T cells. *Science* 1990;248:1369–72.
19. Teh HS, Kisielow P, Scott B, et al. Thymic major histocompatibility complex antigens and the alpha beta T cell receptor determine the CD4/CD8 phenotype of cells. *Nature* 1988;335:229–33.
20. Pircher H, Burki K, Lang R, Hengarter H, Zinkernagel RM. Tolerance induction on double specific T-cell receptor transgenic mice varies with antigen. *Nature* 1989;342:559–61.
21. Smith CA, Williams GT, Kingston R, Jenkinson EJ, Owen JJT. Antibodies to CD3/T-cell receptor complex induce death by apoptosis in immature T cells in thymic cultures. *Nature* 1989;337:181–3.
22. Ashton-Rickardt PG, Banderia A, Delaney JR, et al. Evidence for a differential avidity model of T cell selection in the thymus. *Cell* 1994; 76:651–63.
23. Punt JA, Osborne BA, Takahama Y, Sharrow SO, Singer A. Negative selection of CD4+CD8+ thymocytes by T cell receptor-induced apoptosis requires a costimulatory signal that can be provided by CD28. *J Exp Med* 1994;179:709–13.
24. Porcelli S, Morita CT, Brenner MB. CD1b restricts the response of human CD4-8- T lymphocytes to a microbial antigen. *Nature* 1992; 360:593–7.
25. Tanaka T, Sano S, Nieves E, et al. Nonpeptide ligands for human gamma delta T cells. *Proc Natl Acad Sci USA* 1994;91:8175–9.
26. Rocha B, Vassalli P, Guy-Grand D. Thymic and extrathymic origins of gut intraepithelial lymphocyte populations in mice. *J Exp Med* 1994;180:681–6.
27. Rogers J, Early P, Carter C, et al. Two mRNAs with different 3′ ends encode membrane-bound and secreted forms of immunoglobulin micro chain. *Cell* 1980;20:303–12.
28. Davies DR, Metzger H. Structural basis of antibody function. *Rev Immunol* 1983;1:87–117.
29. Wabl MR, Forni L, Loor F. Switch in immunoglobulin class production observed in single clones of committed lymphocytes. *Science* 1978;199:1078–80.
30. Honjo T, Kataoka T. Organization of immunoglobulin heavy chain genes and allelic deletion model. *Proc Natl Acad Sci USA* 1978;75: 2140–4.
31. Kim S, Davis M, Sinn E, Patten P, Hood L. Antibody diversity: somatic hypermutation of rearranged Vh genes. *Cell* 1981;27:573–81.
32. Dorshkind K, Pollack SB, Bosma MJ, Phillips RA. Natural killer (NK) cells are present in mice with severe combined immunodeficiency (SCID). *J Immunol* 1985;134:3798–801.
33. Ohlen C, Kling G, Hoglund P, et al. Prevention of allogeneic bone marrow graft rejection by H-2 transgene in donor mice. *Science* 1989; 246:666–8.
34. Yokoyama WM, Seaman WE. The Ly-49 and NKR-P1 gene families encoding lectin-like receptors on natural killer cells. *Annu Rev Immunol* 1993;11:613–35.
35. Colonna M, Samaridis J. Cloning of immunoglobulin-superfamily members associated with HLA-C and HLA-B recognition by human natural killer cells. *Science* 1995;268:405–8.
36. Steinman RM. The dendritic cell system and its role in immunogenicity. *Annu Rev Immunol* 1991;9:271–96.
37. Lafferty K, Prowse S, Simeonovic C, Warren HS. Immunobiology of tissue transplantation: a return to the passenger leucocyte concept. In: Paul WE, Fatham CG, Metzgar H, eds. *Annual review of immunology*. Palo Alto, CA: Annual Reviews, 1983:143–73.
38. Pober JS, Cotran RS. Immunologic interactions of T lymphocytes with vascular endothelium. *Adv Immunol* 1991;50:261–302.
39. Rubin-Kelley VE, Jevnikar AM. Antigen presentation by renal tubular epithelial cells. *J Am Soc Nephrol* 1991;2:13–26.
40. Brown JH, Jardetsky TS, Gorga JC, et al. The three-dimensional structure of the human class II histocompatibility antigen HLA-DR1. *Nature* 1993;364:33–9.
41. Hansen TH, Carreno BM, Sachs DH. The major histocompatibility complex. In: Paul WE, ed. *Fundamental immunology*. 3rd ed. New York: Raven, 1993:577–628.
42. Hill AV, Elvin J, Willis AC, et al. Molecular analysis of the association of B53 and resistance to severe malaria. *Nature* 1992;360:434–40.
43. Salter RD, Benjamin RJ, Wesley PK. A binding site for the T-cell co-receptor CD8 on the $alpha_3$ domain of HLA-A2. *Nature* 1990;345: 41–6.
44. Cammarota G, Scheirle A, Takacs B. Identification of a CD4 binding site on the $beta_2$ domain of HLA-DR molecules. *Nature* 1992;356: 799–801.
45. Roche PA, Marks MS, Cresswell P. Formation of a nine subunit complex by HLA class II glycoproteins and the invariant chain. *Nature* 1991;354:392–4.
46. Viville S, Neefjes J, Dierich A, et al. Mice lacking the MHC class II-associated invariant chain. *Cell* 1993;72:635–48.
47. Mellins E, Kempin S, Smith L, Monji T, Pious D. A gene required for class II-restricted antigen presentation maps to the major histocompatibility complex. *J Exp Med* 1991;174:1607–15.
48. Morris P, Shaman J, Attaya M, et al. An essential role for HLA-DM in antigen presentation by class II major histocompatibility molecules. *Nature* 1994;368:551–4.
49. Zijlstra M, Bix M, Simister NE, Loring JM, Raulet DH, Jaenisch R. Beta 2-microglobulin deficient mice lack CD4-8+ cytolytic T cells. *Nature* 1990;344:742–6.
50. Monaco JJ. Molecular mechanisms of antigen processing. In: Hames BC, Glover DM, eds. *Molecular immunology*. 2nd ed. Oxford: Oxford University Press, 1996 (in press).
51. Van Kaer L, Ashton-Rickardt PG, Ploegh HL, Tonegawa S. TAP1 mutant mice are deficient in antigen presentation, surface class I molecules, and CD4-8+ T cells. *Cell* 1992;71:1205–14.
52. Fischer Lindahl K, Wilson DB. Histocompatibility antigen-activated cytotoxic T lymphocytes. II. Estimates of frequency and specificity of precursors. *J Exp Med* 1977;145:508–22.
53. Marrack P, Kappler J. The staphylococcal enterotoxins and their relatives. *Science* 1990;248:705–11.
54. Festenstein H. The Mls system. *Transplant Proc* 1976;8:339–42.
55. Marrack P, Winslow GM, Choi Y, et al. The bacterial and mouse mammary tumor virus superantigens: two different families of proteins with the same functions. *Immunol Rev* 1993;131:79–92.
56. Imberti L, Sottini A, Bettinardi A, Puoti M, Primi D. Selective depletion in HIV infection of T cells that bear specific T cell receptor B beta sequences. *Science* 1991;254:860–2.
57. Austyn JM, Kupiec-Weglinski JW, Hankins DF, Morris PJ. Migration pattern of dendritic cells in the mouse. *J Exp Med* 1988;167: 646–651.
58. Weiss A, Littman DR. Signal transduction by lymphocyte antigen receptors. *Cell* 1994;76:263–74.
59. Mercep M, Weissman AM, Frank SJ, Klausner RD, Ashwell JD.

Activation-driven programmed cell death and T cell receptor zeta eta expression. *Science* 1989;246:1162–5.
60. Janeway CH, Bottomly K. Signals and signs for lymphocyte responses. *Cell* 1994;76:275–85.
61. Scwartz RH. A cell culture model for T lymphocyte clonal anergy. *Science* 1990;248:1349–56.
62. Linsley PS, Ledbetter JA. The role of the CD28 receptor during T cell responses to antigen. *Annu Rev Immunol* 1993;11:191–221.
63. Boussiotis VA, Barber DL, Nakarai T, et al. Prevention of T cell anergy by signaling through the gamma c chain of the IL-2 receptor. *Science* 1994;266:1039–42.
64. Van Seventer GA, Shimizu Y, Horgan KJ, Shaw S. The LFA-1 ligand ICAM-1 provides an important costimulatory signal for T cell receptor-mediated activation of resting T cells. *J Immunol* 1990;144:4579–86.
65. June CH, Bluestone JA, Nadler LM, Thompson CB. The B7 and CD28 receptor families. *Immunol Today* 1994;15:321–31.
66. Harlan DM, Hangarter H, Huang ML, et al. Mice expressing both B7-1 and viral glycoprotein on pancreatic beta cells along with glycoprotein-specific transgenic T cells develop diabetes due to a breakdown of T-lymphocyte unresponsiveness. *Proc Natl Acad Sci USA* 1994; 91:3137–41.
67. Keene JA, Forman J. Helper activity is required for the in vivo generation of cytotoxic T lymphocytes. *J Exp Med* 1982;155:768–82.
68. Lowin B, Hahne M, Mattmann C, Tschopp J. Cytolytic T-cell cytotoxicity is mediated through perforin and Fas lytic pathways. *Nature* 1994;370:650–2.
69. Watanabe-Fukunaga R, Branna CI, Copeland NG, Jenkins NA, Nagata S. Lymphoproliferation disorder in mice explained by defects in Fas antigen that mediates apoptosis. *Nature* 1992;356:314–7.
70. Perussia B, Kobayashi M, Rossi ME, Anegon I, Trinchieri G. Immune interferon enhances functional properties of human granulocytes: role of Fc receptors and effect of lymphotoxin, tumor necrosis factor, and granulocyte-macrophage colony-stimulating factor. *J Immunol* 1987;138:765–74.
71. Pleiman CM, D'Ambrosio D, Cambier JC. The B-cell antigen receptor complex: structure and signal transduction. *Immunol Today* 1994; 15:393–9.
72. Pecanha L, Snapper C, Finkelman F, Mond J. Dextran-conjugated anti-Ig antibodies as a model for T-cell independent type 2 antigen-mediated stimulation of Ig secretion in vitro. *J Immunol* 1991;146: 833–9.
73. Parker DC. T cell-dependent cell activation. *Annu Rev Immunol* 1993; 11:331–40.
74. Noelle RJ, Roy M, Shephard DM, Stamekovic I, Ledbetter JA, Aruffo A. A 39-kDa protein in activated helper T cells binds CD40 and transduces the signal for cognate activation of B cells. *Proc Natl Acad Sci USA* 1992;89:6550–4.
75. Caux C, Massacrier C, Vanbervliet B, et al. Activation of human dendritic cells through CD40 cross-linking. *J Exp Med* 1994;180:1263–72.
76. Sprent J. T and B memory cells. *Cell* 1994;76:315–22.
77. MacLennan IC, Liu YJ, Johnson GD. Maturation and dispersal of B-cell clones during T cell-dependent antibody responses. *Immunol Rev* 1992;126:143–61.
78. Imhof BA, Dunon D. Leukocyte migration and adhesion. *Adv Immunol* 1995;58:345–416.
79. Bevilacqua M, Butcher E, Furie B, et al. Selectins: a family of adhesion receptors. *Cell* 1991;67:233.
80. Lawrence MB, Springer TA. Leukocytes role on a selectin at physiologic flow rate: distinction from and prerequisite for adhesion through integrins. *Cell* 1991;65:859–73.
81. Hynes R. Integrins, versatility, modulation, and signaling in cell adhesion. *Cell* 1992;69:11–25.
82. Mosmann TR, Cherwinski H, Bond MW, Giedlin MA, Coffman RL. Two types of murine helper T cell clones. I. Definition according to profiles of lymphokine activities and secreted proteins. *J Immunol* 1986;136:2348–57.
83. Heinzel FP, Sadick MD, Holaday BJ, Coffman RL, Locksley RM. Reciprocal expression of interferon gamma or interleukin 4 during the resolution or progression of murine leishmaniasis. *J Exp Med* 1989; 169:59–72.
84. Sher A, Gazzinelli RT, Oswald IP, et al. Role of T-cell derived cytokines in the down regulation of immune responses in parasitic and retroviral infection. *Immunol Rev* 1992;127:182–204.
85. Yamamura M, Uyemura K, Deans RJ, et al. Defining protective responses to pathogens: cytokine profiles in leprosy lesions. *Science* 1991;254:277–9.
86. Hsieh CS, Macatonia SE, Tripp CS, Wolf SF, O'Garra A, Murphy KM. Development of T_H1 CD4+ T cells through IL-12 produced by listeria-induced macrophages. *Science* 1993;260:496–7.
87. Le Gros G, Ben-Sasson SZ, Seder R, Finkelman FD, Paul WE. Generation of interleukin 4 (IL-4)-producing cells in vivo and in vitro: IL-2 and IL-4 are required for in vitro generation of IL-4 producing cells. *J Exp Med* 1990;172:921–9.
88. Kuchroo VK, Das DP, Brown JA, et al. B7-1 and B7-2 costimulatory molecules activate differentially the Th1/Th2 development pathways: application to autoimmune disease therapy. *Cell* 1995;80:707–18.
89. Cerottini JC, MacDonald HR. The cellular basis of T-cell memory. *Annu Rev Immunol* 1989;7:77–89.
90. Thompson CB. Apoptosis in the pathogenesis and treatment of disease. *Science* 1995;267:1456–62.
91. Hockenbery D, Nunez G, Milliman C, Schreiber RD, Korsmeyer SJ. Bcl-2 is an inner mitochondrial membrane protein that blocks programmed cell death. *Nature* 1990;348:334–6.
92. Boise LH, Gonzalez-Garcia M, Postema CE, et al. Bcl-x, a bcl-2-related gene that functions as a dominant regulator of apoptotic cell death. *Cell* 1993;74:597–608.
93. Nagata S, Golstein P. The Fas death factor. *Science* 1995;267:1449–56.
94. Trauth BC, Klas C, Peters AM, et al. Monoclonal antibody-mediated tumor regression by induction of apoptosis. *Science* 1989;245:301–5.
95. Takahashi T, Tanaka M, Brannan CI, et al. Generalized lyphoproliferative disease in mice, caused by a point mutation in the Fas ligand. *Cell* 1994;76:969–76.
96. Dhien J, Walczak H, Baumler C, Debatin KM, Krammer PH. Autocrine T-cell suicide mediated by APO-1/(Fas/CD95). *Nature* 1995;373:438–41.
97. Klas C, Debatin KM, Jonker RR, Krammer PH. Activation interferes with the APO-1 pathway in mature human T cells. *Int Immunol* 1993; 5:625–30.

PART II

The Immune Response in Renal Injury

A. Induction of the Nephritogenic Immune Response

Immunologic Renal Diseases,
edited by E. G. Neilson and W. G. Couser.
Lippincott-Raven Publishers, Philadelphia © 1997

CHAPTER 5

Immunogenetics of Renal Disease

Andrew J. Rees

INTRODUCTION

Since the earliest attempts to understand the pathogenesis of nephritis, there has been considerable interest in the possibility that inheritance might contribute to susceptibility. This was expressed first by Wells (1) in 1812, who observed that the siblings of a child who developed nephritis after scarlet fever were much more likely to develop nephritis than were the siblings of children who developed scarlet without nephritis. He attributed this "in part to a similarity of constitution derived from both parents." The familial predisposition to poststreptococcal nephritis has been confirmed many times since and extended to other types of glomerular disease—most notably, mesangial IgA disease (2). Unfortunately, attempts to identify the genes responsible have generally been unsatisfactory.

The pathogenesis of glomerular and tubulointerstitial nephritis is discussed extensively in other chapters. Most, if not all, types are caused by local immune responses within the glomerulus or interstitium. Some of the antigens involved are self-proteins subjected to autoimmune attack; others are extrinsic, having been planted in the kidney either because they have a particular affinity for the glomerulus or because they have been deposited as an immune complex. Experimental models of nephritis suggest that chronic glomerular inflammation requires a persistent immune response. This implies that most types of clinical nephritis are caused by autoimmunity or are the result of persistent antigenic challenge.

The results from studies of experimental models of nephritis suggest that specific binding of antibody (and possibly T cells) within the kidney is relatively innocuous but that it causes the cellular and humoral mediators responsible for injury to localize there. The intensity of the inflammation that results is tightly regulated and may resolve completely or persist and eventually destroy the kidney by progressive scarring. The processes responsible are beginning to be understood at the molecular and cellular levels—at least in outline. They are discussed extensively elsewhere in the book, but it is important to describe the principles here to grasp the way in which heredity may distort the normal responses and predispose to disease:

1. Immune responses are initiated after antigen is taken up by antigen-presenting cells (APC), which digest it to peptides in a specialized endosomal compartment, where it binds to nascent major histocompatibility complex (MHC) molecules; the MHC–peptide complexes are then expressed on the cell surface.
2. The interaction of T cell receptors (TCR) with MHC–peptide complexes determines the nature of the subsequent immune response, in particular whether T helper (Th) cells are switched off (anergized), develop into Th1 cells, Th2 cells, or regulatory T cells. The fate of Th cells is determined by the strength of the interaction between MHC–peptide and TCR, by costimulatory signals from the APC, and by the ambient concentrations of cytokines.
3. The intensity and duration of the inflammation that follows are amplified by proinflammatory cytokines that activate leukocytes and endothelial cells, and are damped down by antiinflammatory cytokines that reverse these changes.

Both immune and inflammatory responses are dynamic processes whose efficiency varies markedly in different inbred strains of mice and rats, and it is not surprising that the variation has a profound influence on host resistance to infection (3) and susceptibility to immunologically mediated disorders, including autoimmune disease (4) and nephritis (5). Classical breeding studies first showed the power of heredity on immune responses and the extent it contributes to the susceptibility to inflamma-

A. J. Rees: Department of Medicine and Therapeutics, University of Aberdeen, Aberdeen AB9 2ZD, Scotland.

tory disease (6–8). Identification of the genes responsible is a formidable task that had to start with an analysis of candidate genes. Early studies showed that MHC class II alleles acted as immune response genes that determined the ability of an individual to respond to a specific epitope and, coincidentally, that they determined susceptibility to autoimmune disease (9). Nevertheless, understanding the contribution of specific genetic loci to the dynamic control of the immune response calls for a more subtle approach to the genetic analysis. Molecular techniques for studying complex disease processes resulted in the development of genome wide maps (10–12), enabling multiple loci responsible for a particular trait to be mapped to a chromosomal segment. This is important because mutations in control regions of genes, as well as coding sequences, can now be studied and because genome wide search screening can now be performed to identify chromosomal segments linked to (or associated with) particular diseases. These techniques often involve multiple comparisons between test and control samples, and rigorous new statistical techniques have had to be developed (13–15).

With this chapter, the author proposes to (a) review the inherited variations in immune responses and their role in susceptibility to disease; (b) discuss the techniques available for the genetic analysis of complex traits; (c) describe the contribution of heredity to experimental models of immunologically mediated renal disease; and (d) analyze the data on inherited susceptibility to glomerulonephritis in man, most of which pertains to the HLA complex.

GENETICS OF IMMUNE RESPONSES

Background

Selective breeding of experimental animals has been the standard way to analyze complex genetic traits and has been used to great effect to dissect the immunologic and inflammatory responses. Various types of unbred strain can be produced for specific purposes (Table 1). *Recombinant inbred strains* are produced by repeated brother-sister mating and enable experiments to be performed on genetically identical stock. Numerous inbred strains of mice and rats are available, each with different characteristics. They were crucial to the identification of immune response gene effects of the MHC and its role in the development of experimental autoimmune disease. Inbred strains have also been essential for demonstrating the consequences of inherited biases to Th1 or Th2 immune responses when mice are exposed to specific pathogens (3,16,17) and, more recently, to the development for autoimmune disease (4). However, additional breeding strategies or molecular techniques are usually needed to identify which genes are responsible for a given trait.

TABLE 1. *Inbred strains of mice*

Strain	Description
Inbred Strains	Strains maintained by strict brother sister mating to provide a uniform genetic stock
Congenic strains	Strains in which a chromosomal segment carrying a gene of interest is transferred from one inbred strain to another through repeated backcrossing and selection. It usually takes 2.5-3 years at 3-4 generations per year to raise congenic strains. The length of chromosomal segment transferred is the principal limitation.
Recombinant inbred strains	Inbred strains resulting from crossing two selected inbred strains followed by repeated brother sister mating for 20 or more generations. This results in a set of strains each of which is homozygous a particular gene from one or other of the original strains.
Recombinant congenic strains	Inbred strains in which brother sister matings are introduced only after a predetermined number of backcrosses.
Consomic strains	An inbred strain in which a single chromosome from one strain is replaced by that of another

Congenic mice are strains in which a chromosomal segment carrying a gene of interest is transferred from one inbred strain to another. They are raised by crossing inbred mice from one strain with mice bearing the gene to be introduced. F1 mice are then backcrossed with the original strain, and the progeny who inherited the gene of interest are selected for further breeding. Repeated cycles of backcrossing and selection for at least 20 generations should provide enough recombinations to ensure that the only "foreign gene" is the one of interest. Thereafter, brother-sister matings are performed to maintain the unbred line. Congenic strains have been used extensively to study the role of specific loci within the MHC (18,19), but the principal limitations of raising new strains are the time involved (typically at least 2.5–3 years) and the length of the chromosomal segment transferred.

Recombinant inbred strains result from crossing two inbred strains followed by repeated brother-sister mating to produce a set of new inbred strains homozygous for an assortment of the genes from the original parental strains. They have been used to study the genes responsible for severe renal disease in lupus-prone NZB/NZW mice (20–22) and are a powerful resource for more detailed genome searching techniques (see later). The same principles apply to *recombinant congenic strains*, in which brother-sister mating is introduced only after backcrossing for a defined number of generations. The strains that result are inbred mice in which a proportion of genes are derived from one of the potential strains. They are especially useful for analyzing phenotypes produced by the interaction of several different genes (23). Finally, *consomic strains* have been produced in which a single chromosome from a parental strain is introduced (7). Few of these are available yet, but they are sure to be important in the future.

The development of inbred strains relies on techniques introduced nearly a hundred years ago and have been supplemented recently by two additional approaches: "knock out" mice in which an individual gene is deleted and "transgenic" mice in which a particular gene is introduced. The two techniques can, of course, be combined so that a deleted gene can be replaced with a different or a mutated gene to investigate allele-specific effects on the immune system in mice with otherwise identical genetic backgrounds. This approach has been used to great effect for studying the role of MHC molecules, using specific murine (H-2) alleles (8,24) and by transfer of human genes encoding DR molecules into mice (25,26). The recent improvements in technique of gene transfer enabling yeast artificial chromosomes containing 20 kb DNA will now enable polymorphisms of regulatory elements to be studied in this way (27).

Segregation Analysis

Genome wide searches are now being applied regularly to identify loci responsible for complex genetic traits, including the susceptibility to autoimmune and inflammatory disease experimentally in both rodents and in man. The mass of results obtained from single experiments emphasizes the need for appropriate statistical analysis because linkage of a complex trait to a specific chromosomal region is only the first step in the process of identifying the responsible gene.

The first stage is a program of selective breeding between the susceptible strain and a selected nonsusceptible strain. The choice of the combination has major effects on the results because loci from some nonsusceptible strains interact with genes in susceptible strains to aggravate disease (8,28). The cumulative frequency of the disease is ascertained in both parental strains and their F1 generation. The process is then repeated for F2 hybrids and for F1 mice backcrossed with one of the parental strains. This enables the chromosomal regions bearing disease susceptibility genes to be identified by segregation analysis using probes for polymorphic candidate genes in which the parental strains are known to be different (MHC, etc.) or by using anonymous "microsatellite markers" distributed throughout the genome (10,11).

In principle, the approach is not new and is well illustrated by early studies on the role of the MHC (H-2 complex in mice) that demonstrated linkage between inheritance of certain H-2 alleles and susceptibility to particular autoimmune diseases (9). Druet's (29) early studies of susceptibility to antiglomerular basement membrane disease in Brown-Norway (BN) rats treated with mercuric chloride provide an excellent example. Brown-Norway rats develop anti-GBM (laminin) antibodies and nephritis when injected with mercuric chloride, whereas Lewis rats do not. Selective breeding studies between BN and Lewis rats showed that all animals in the F1 generation develop the disease. Analysis of the F2 generation and F1 animals backcrossed with Lewis rats showed that the disease phenotype was linked to the BN MHC (RT1-n), but that only half the F2 and F1 backcrossed rats with RT1-n developed the disease, demonstrating that genes unlinked the MHC were also essential for susceptibility; standard genetic formulas suggested that another two to three genes were involved. In fact, it has become a general rule that experimental autoimmune diseases are linked to MHC class II genes and that other unlinked genes are also critical for susceptibility (8,30,31). The challenge posed by these studies is to identify the nature and function of the modifying genes.

Originally, the only approach to this problem was to study polymorphisms of small numbers of candidate genes from the many thousands of those that might be involved. However, the situation has now been transformed by the availability of easy-to-use maps of markers covering entire mouse and rat genomes (10,11). These maps are constructed from microsatellites consisting of short dinucleotide repeats that occur at intervals of about 105 bp and vary allelically between inbred strains of mice. Microsatellite markers can be amplified from small quantities of DNA using unique flanking sequences in the polymerase chain reaction (PCR). Size differences of the various alleles can be identified easily on gels and used to construct maps (32). This approach has been pioneered in studies of non-obese diabetic (NOD) mice (33) and has already led to the identification of 13 separate loci in, addition to the MHC, that confer susceptibility to diabetes (8). The same approach has since been applied to a number of different autoimmune diseases (28,31), including murine models of lupus nephritis (see later). Comparison of studies in different models suggests that certain genes confer an increased-risk autoimmunity generally, whereas others are unique to a particular model. The nature of these genes is of critical importance and currently under intense investigation, and some colocalize with genes known to influence apoptosis (22), T and B cell function, macrophage activation (3,7), and T cell responses to IL-12 (34).

Once a trait has been mapped to a chromosomal segment, more concentrated sets of markers can be used to position the susceptibility locus more precisely until the segment is short enough to be cloned directly into yeast artificial chromosomes (YACs) and eventually into contigs so that it can be sequenced: a process known as *posi-*

tional cloning. An alternative approach is to study candidate genes already localized to the relevant chromosome segment. Most commonly, however, a combination of the two approaches is used.

The presence of multiple genetic loci that influence susceptibility raises the question of how they interact. Two types of genetic model should be considered: epistatic models, i.e., models based on interaction between different susceptibility genes, and heterogeneity models, in which the genes act independently. The data on all the autoimmune and inflammatory diseases studied to date favor epistatic models (28). Thus, no single gene is sufficient (or even necessary) to cause the disease; the more susceptibility alleles at unlinked loci, the greater the risk of developing the disease; and different combinations of susceptibility alleles can have the same effect.

Thus, genome wide searches involve multiple comparisons within a single experiment and uncertainties about the model of inheritance. Necessarily, the experiments require rigorous statistical approaches to avoid spurious linkage due purely to chance. The methods available for this have been reviewed recently (13–15).

Evidence that heredity has a powerful influence on immunologic and inflammatory responses derives from four sources: (a) selective breeding studies in which animals were bred for extremes of immune or inflammatory responsiveness; (b) surveys of the susceptibility of different inbred strains of mice and rats to microbial and viral pathogens; (c) analysis of susceptibility to spontaneous and provoked autoimmune disease in inbred strains of mice and rats; and (d) transgenic and knock out mice, which provide evidence of a role for specific genes.

GENETICS OF IMMUNE RESPONSES

The Major Histocompatibility Complex

All discussions about immunogenetics have to start with the MHC. It is central to recognition of antigen by T cells, and plays a crucial role in shaping the T cell repertoire during ontogeny and in maintaining tolerance to self-proteins during adult life (35). The normal functions of the MHC are described in detail in other chapters, but brief mention must be made of it here before emphasizing the role of polymorphism at MHC loci on the development of autoimmune and inflammatory conditions.

Major histocompatibility complex molecules are heterodimeric transmembrane proteins that are expressed at the cell surface. Class I molecules are expressed on all cells. Typically, they present peptides derived from intracellular proteins to CD8 T cells, though recently they have also been shown to bind some exogenously derived peptides (36). Class II molecules are expressed constitutively on professional antigen presenting cells, including dendritic cells and some macrophages, but can be induced on many cell types by interferon-γ. They present peptides from exogenous proteins to CD4 T helper cells.

Crystallographic studies have shown that class I and II molecules have remarkably similar three-dimensional structures (37). Both have an antigen binding groove comprised of a beta pleated floor and bounded by alpha helical sides. They differ, in that the class I groove has closed ends and is now known to bind peptides 8 or 9 amino acids in length, whereas the class II groove is open at both ends and binds peptides 12–25 or more residues in length. The polymorphisms that distinguish MHC types cause substitutions of amino acid residues that line the peptide binding groove. This influences its shape and charge and so constrains the range of peptides that can be accommodated. This provides an explanation for the differential responses of different inbred mouse strains to chemically defined antigens.

Considerable progress has been made in determining the rules that govern peptide binding to a variety of MHC class I and class II molecules (38). Peptides are bound in an extended linear conformation stabilized by multiple interactions between the peptide backbone and relatively conserved MHC residues. In this conformation, approximately 2 of every 3 peptide side chains are orientated into the groove, and stable binding depends upon their accommodation in reciprocal "pockets" in the groove. Major histocompatibility complex types differ substantially at the polymorphic residues that line pockets and, thus, in the range of peptide side chains accepted. These constraints on the structure of peptides forming stable MHC complexes may be described with motifs (39). The combination of restrictions on peptide length and the presence of 2–3 type-specific pockets capable of accepting only a limited range of side chains means that class I molecules are able to bind a limited set of motifs. In contrast, motifs for class II molecules have been more difficult to identify because interactions at most of the 11 amino acids lying within the groove can influence binding. Techniques have been developed that accurately predict binding by summing the measured contribution of each possible amino acid at each position in the bound peptide; but so far, only a few class II types have been analyzed in this exhaustive way (40,41). For most class II types, current motifs identify only peptide side chains particularly important for binding—so-called anchor residues—and take no account of other residues.

Processing of whole antigen into peptides is a crucial step in antigen presentation as there is increasing evidence that it is influenced by heredity. Endogenous proteins are broken down in the cytoplasm, principally by the ubiquitin-proteosome pathway, which is highly conserved in eukaryotic cells (42), and cells use this pathway for MHC class I processing (43). Proteins bind to ubiquitins that target them to the proteosome, a 700-kD multicomponent cylindrical particle that catalyzes proteins in peptides with 5–11 residues (36). The peptides are then transported into the endoplasmic reticulum by ATP-dependent peptide transporters comprised of two chains—TAP-1 and TAP-2. TAP transporters bind peptides of between five and twelve amino acids (44), especially those with hydrophobic or basic amino acids at their C-termini (45), i.e., those most suitable for binding to class I molecules. TAP molecules also associate directly with nascent class I heavy chains, which presumably increases the efficiency of peptide loading, and there are allele-specific differences in the efficiency with which this occurs (46). The TAP genes are located within the MHC class II region and are polymorphic. In the rat, the polymorphism has functional consequences and TAP molecules selectively transport peptides that bind class I molecules with which they are in linkage disequilibrium (45,47). However, polymorphism of the TAP genes in mice and man do not appear to have functional consequences (48), and early studies describing associations between TAP gene polymorphisms with disease in man are better explained by linkage disequilibrium with HLA-DQ alleles (49). Once loaded with peptide, class I molecules are transported to the cell surface for presentation to CD8 positive T cells.

Processing of exogenous proteins utilizes the endosomal pathway, and binding to class II molecules takes place in a specialized late endosomal compartment (35). Nascent class II molecules are targeted to this compartment bound to invariant chain (Ii), which is also important for preventing class II molecules from binding peptides prematurely in the endoplasmic reticulum. Once in the peptide compartment, Ii is released, probably through the action of the HLA-DM, a nonpolymorphic class II-like molecule encoded by a gene located between the DQ and DP loci in the HLA class II region (50). The emptied class II molecules then bind appropriate peptides and are transported to the cell surface for presentation to CD4 positive T cells. There are differences in the the degree of DM dependence of different class II alleles, at least in mice. H2-Ak (51,52) and H2-Ad (53) cells are both almost fully functional in DM-deficient antigen presenting cells, and in vitro the Ii derived peptide (CLIP) dissociates rapidly from H2-Ak class II, but not from H2-A2 (54). The reasons for the differences are uncertain, but have clear implications for the efficiency of peptide presentation by class II molecules. Thus, polymorphism in the pressing pathway for class I and class II influence peptide lowering of MHC molecules. The effects of the polymorphism or susceptibility to disease has yet to be studied.

Characterization of allele-specific differences in class II-associated peptides presented to T helper cells has considerable importance in the search for T cell epitopes responsible for susceptibility to autoimmune disease. This has been done by sequencing of pools of naturally processed peptides eluted from class II molecules (55, 56) and through various types of peptide binding study (40,41). In principle, it should be possible to use these approaches to identify autoantigen-derived peptides presented in an allele-specific manner to T cells in patients with autoimmune disease, especially where both positive and negative HLA associations are known (57,58). However, at present, accurate algorithms for predicting HLA class II binding are available for only a limited set of DR types; T cell epitope predictions depend solely on relative predicted binding affinities and take no account of processing, which is bound to constrain which peptides are available for binding to class II molecules. Furthermore, the relationship between antigen presentation and the immune response to it is known. It is frequently assumed that autoimmunity is directed at autoantigen-derived peptides particularly well presented by disease-associated alleles. This assumption may be wrong, and it is likely that tolerance is most securely established to better presented self-peptides.

Interestingly, the disease-associated peptide in one animal model of autoimmunity binds the restricting class II with very low affinity to its restricting class II molecule (59). It would be illuminating to compare the immune response to a clinically relevant self-antigen with its presentation by disease-associated and protective class II alleles, but this has yet to be done. Unfortunately, while T cell responses have been well characterized (60–62) in several autoimmune diseases, the natural presentation of the relevant self-antigen has been characterized in only one. We have recently discovered that the autoantigen attacked in Goodpasture's disease is presented by the disease-associated DR2 molecule as two nested sets of peptides (63), using a biochemical approach developed from that described by Nelson et al. (64,65). Unfortunately, the peptide specificity of patients' T cells is not yet well characterized in this disease.

Quantitative Differences in Immune Responses

Antibody Titre

Biozzi and his colleagues (6) pioneered the approach of selective inbreeding of strains of mice that produce high (H) or low (L) antibody responses when immunized with a variety of antigens (6). High and low strains have a greater than 200-fold difference in antibody responses to a wide range of soluble and cellular antigens. The two strains differ in their susceptibility to infection, with the low antibody producing strain having more resistance to *Salmonella typhimurium, Yersinia*, and *Leishmania*. This pattern of resistance might suggest that H strain mice have a predominantly Th2 phenotype, but the strains have similar delayed type hypersensitivity responses, at least to *Yersinia* (6). The H strain is also susceptible to experimental autoimmune encephalomyelitis (EAE) (66) and collagen arthritis, (67) diseases mediated by Th1 responses. Neither strain has been used to study susceptibility to experimental nephritis.

Classical genetic analysis (6) and more recent genome wide comparisons of H and L antibody producing strains have linked to quantitative differences in antibody response to the MHC on chromosome 17. The immunoglobulin heavy chain locus in chromosome 12 has important effects on the magnitude of antibody synthesis (68), which is interesting in light of the associations between Ig G(m) allotypes and susceptibility to human diseases, including nephritis. Additional loci that influence antibody production have been identified on chromosomes 4, 8, and 18, but none corresponds to loci identified as determining susceptibility to autoimmune disease (28). However, some high responder strains have a deletion of 73 amino acids of the intracytoplasmic chain of the high-affinity Fc gamma receptor (CD64), which is identical to the deletion found in NOD mice (68,69); unfortunately, the deletion is not linked to immunoglobulin synthesis as to diabetes.

Antibody Affinity

Selective breeding has been used to raise strains of mice that differ in their ability to produce high-affinity antibody (70). The genes responsible have not been characterized, but the strains show markedly different responses to chronic serum sickness (71). High-affinity producers develop mild injury and mesangial IgG deposits, whereas the low-affinity strain had more severe injury with deposition of immunoglobulin in capillary loops.

Qualitative Differences in Immune Responses

Inheritance also influences the type of immune responses in other ways, notably, the balance between different subsets of T helper cells. This is influenced in part by MHC genes and in part by genes at other loci.

Th1/Th2 Balance

Systematic analysis of response to infection revealed marked differences in susceptibility to a wide variety of intracellular parasites, including toxoplasmosis, *Leishmania*, and mycobacterial disease (3). It is now clear that qualitative differences in the immune response to the pathogens have a substantial influence on these processes. Thus, strains of mice resistant to Leishmaniasis develop strongly polarized Th1 responses to the pathogen, with Th cells secreting dependent on secretion of large amounts of interleukin-12 and interferon-γ, whereas susceptible strains have Th2 responses dependent on IL-4 (3,72).

Susceptibility to autoimmune disease is also influenced the nature of the Th response. Thus, both EAE and diabetes are dependent on the development of Th1 responses (30). The importance of this genetically determined dichotomy for the spontaneous development of autoimmune disease has been demonstrated recently using doubly transgenic mice whose T cells express receptors for a target antigen expressed in the pancreas (73). Expression of these genes in B10.D2 mice (which mount Th1 responses) resulted in insulitis with the development of diabetes, whereas similar expression in Balb/c (Th2) mice caused no disease, even though they have the same MHC type. The genetic basis for the difference in response of B10.D2 and Balb/c mice to *Leishmania* has been localized to a gene on chromosome 11 and correlates with differences in responsiveness of lymphocytes to interleukin-12 (34). Thus, Balb/c mice are able to respond to IL-12 only transiently, whereas B10.D2 mice have sustained responses. This provides an extremely elegant explanation for their respective phenotypes. Notably, this locus is linked to the development of insulitis and diabetes in NOD mice (28).

There may be other pathways through which inheritance biases Th responses toward Th1 or Th2 phenotypes. Mason and his colleagues (74) showed that inherited differences in the corticosterone response to stress correlates with the Th phenotype and susceptibility to autoimmune disease. Thus, mice (C57/BL) and rat (Lewis) strains with low corticosterone responses develop Th1 responses and are susceptible to EAE, whereas high-responding strains (BALB/c mice, PVG rats) produce Th2 responses and are resistant to EAE. It should also be noted that the MHC class II alleles on which a particular peptide is presented determines whether a T cell clone develops into a Th1 or a Th2 cell (75,76).

CD4/CD8 Ratio

The Th1/Th2 paradigm is equally applicable to the control of immune responses in man but has yet to be subjected to genetic analysis. However, a recent family study examined that another aspect of immune regulation, the ratio of CD4/CD8 positive T cells, was under genetic control and most probably inherited in recessive fashion but modified by background genes (77).

Inflammation

Inbred strains of mice selected for high or low inflammatory responses to subcutaneous polyacrylamide microbreds have been bred (78). This produced lines that differed markedly in the inflammatory response in which roughly 25% were controlled by heredity. It would be of great interest to study insusceptibility to nephritis in these mice and to identify the genes responsible for the phenotype.

Macrophage Activation

Inherited difference in macrophage activation is one of the principal reasons that different inbred mouse strains show marked differences in susceptibility to intracellular parasites such as mycobacteria, *Leishmania*, and *Salmonella typhimurium* (3,7). The trait has been mapped to chromosome 1 in mice, and the gene responsible has now been cloned and termed *Nramp-1* (79,80). It encodes an 548 amino acid transmembrane protein, the characteristics of a signaling molecule. As yet with no clear function (81,82), macrophages from resistant strains produce more oxygen radicals and unstable nitrogen intermediates when stimulated in vitro and release more proinflammatory cytokines (3). The gene encoding the human NRAMP has been cloned, shown to be polymorphic (83) and linked to a polymorphism or IL-8 receptor gene (84). As in mice, Nramp polymorphism is functionally distinct but has yet to be studied in patients with renal disease (84).

Cytokines

Cytokines play a crucial role in the control of all aspects of the inflammatory response and are obvious candidates for mediating genetically determined differences in inflammation. Considerable efforts are being made to define functional polymorphisms of cytokine genes and their associations with disease. Polymorphisms have now been described in many of the genes, and functional effects have been reported for some of them. A polymorphism in the first intron of the IL-I receptor antagonist gene, IL-IRN, does this. Thus, monocytes from individuals homozygous for the IL-1RN2 allele have been reported to release more IL-I receptor antagonist and less IL-1α when stimulated (85). This allele has also been associated with rheumatoid arthritis and other inflammatory diseases (reviewed in 86). The genes encoding human TNFα and TNFβ are located in the HLA class III region and show extensive polymorphism (87). There is a polymorphism into 5 untranslated region at position 308 that has two alleles (TNF1 and TNF2). The TNF1 allele is commonly found in HLA-A1, B8, and DR3 haplotypes and has been reported to be associated with high TNF production (88), but this conclusion has been challenged recently (89). Similarly, a restriction fragment length polymorphism (RFLP) caused by a base charge in the first section is in linkage disequilibrium with HLA—B7 (87) and may be associated with reduced TNF synthesis (90). Other cytokine genes that are polymorphic include IL-1α (91), IL-1β (92), and IL-8 (93), and tandem repeats have been linked to many others (94).

In summary, there are strong genetic influences on the type and magnitude of immunologic and inflammatory responses. Some of the genes responsible have been identified, and loci encoding others have been assigned to particular chromosomal segments, many of which are known to encode potential candidate genes, for example, the MHC and various cytokines. Localization involving the use of genome wide searches demands the application of special statistical techniques in addition to those of molecular biology; these will now be reviewed.

EXPERIMENTAL MODELS OF NEPHRITIS

Experimental nephritis has been used extensively to provide an insight into the pathogenesis of their human counterparts, including attempts to identify genes that confer susceptibility. The models can be separated into those in which the immune response is directed solely against the kidney and those in which the renal disease is part of a more general loss of immunologic tolerance. Experimental allergic glomerulonephritis (EAG) and antitubular basement membrane disease are examples of the former group, and mercuric chloride-induced glomerulonephritis and murine models of lupus are examples of the latter.

Models Restricted of the Kidney

Experimental Allergic Glomerulonephritis

Anti-GBM antibody-mediated nephritis has been described in many species, including horses, sheep, rabbits, rats, and mice, but analysis of the genetics of susceptibility has been restricted to rodents. The disease can be induced in various rat strains by injection of heterologous, homologous, or even isologous GBM (95–97), and the trait is linked to the MHC (95). The resultant injury was relatively mild in the earliest experiments using BN rats, but has been more severe in recent descriptions: the reasons for this are not known. Susceptible rat strains with severe glomerular injury include BN (RT1-n) and WKY (RT1-k); PVG (RT1-c) and DA (RT1-a) rats develop anti-GBM antibody responses without injury, and Lewis (RT1-E) and WAG (RT1-u) rats are resistant. However, it is of interest that a subline of WKY rats, which is RT1-l, is susceptible but gets much milder disease, which demonstrates that the RT1-l haplotype is not the only reason that Lewis rats fail to develop EAG (98). The host factors responsible for the differences in the severity of injury have not been defined, but Bolton and his colleagues (99) correlated injury with the development of delayed type hypersensitivity. WKY rats tend to produce a Th1 phenotype but BN rats do not. The specificity of the autoantibody response is probably the same in different strains and, as in the human disease, is probably an NC1 domain of type IV collagen (100).

Heymann Nephritis

Heymann nephritis is caused by autoimmunity to megalin, a protein expressed in the clatherin-coated pits of podocytes, as well as in tubular epithelial cells. Susceptibility is linked to MHC (101): Lewis and AS strain rats (both RT1-e) are both susceptible to the disease, whereas BN rats are not. BDV (RT1-d) and Lewis AVN (RT1-a) rats have shown intermediate responses, and AVN (RT1-a) and DA (RT1-a) rats are resistant (102). Again, the results demonstrate the influence of background genes in rats that inherit susceptible MHC.

Anti-TBM Nephritis in Rats

Rats, mice, and guinea pigs all develop tubulointerstitial nephritis when injected with TBM. Susceptible strains of rats injected with bovine TBM include: AVN (RT1-a), DA (RT1-a), BDV (RT1-a), and BN (RT1-n), whereas Lewis (RT1-e) are resistant. Careful breeding studies showed that differences between the strains was not determined by the MHC but was dependent on expression of the relevant antigen in the TBM. Thus, sera from susceptible BN rats did not bind to kidneys from Lewis rats, whereas sera from Lewis rats bound to BN tubular basement membrane (103–105). Breeding studies showed that the disease was linked to expression of the target antigen in (BN x Lewis) F2 animals. F344 and Agus were the only two strains to express the TBM antigen but be resistant to the disease because they failed to mount the autoantibody response (103–105).

Anti-TBM disease in Mice

The mechanism of injury in anti-TBM disease in mice has been extensively investigated by Neilson and his colleagues (see chapter 36). They showed that the disease is caused by cell-mediated immunity, despite the presence of anti-TBM antibodies, and that susceptibility is linked to MHC (106). Strains of mice bearing H-2s (SJL, A.SW, and B10.S) are all susceptible and, in fact, an s allele at the K locus is sufficient. The disease is caused by H-2k restricted cytotoxic T cells in these mice. Anti-TBM disease in guinea pigs is also linked to the MHC; strain XIII animals are susceptible, whereas strain II animals are not (107).

kdkd Mice

Brief mention should be made of the interstitial nephritis that develops spontaneously in kdkd mice. This is an autosomal recessive disorder with complete penetrance. The gene responsible has not been identified (108), but susceptibility tracks with the source of bone marrow in kdkd ⇔ CBA/Ca bone marrow chimeras. This suggests that the defective gene controls an aspect of immunity (109).

The main conclusion to be drawn from these experimental studies is that the MHC is central to the development of these renal-specific models of autoimmunity, but the influence of background genes is also important. This is most apparent in anti-TBM nephritis in rats but clearly operates in EAG. Studies have yet to be performed to localize the responsible genes.

Models Involving Generalized Loss of Tolerance

Severe glomerulonephritis develops in two different settings in which there is generalized loss of tolerance: (a) in rodents with polyclonal B cell activation, either provoked in rats and mice by a variety of stimuli including parasitic infection, graft-versus-host disease and exposure to mercury, gold, or penicillamine and (b) in spontaneous models of lupus in mice.

Polyclonal B Cell Activation

Polyclonal activation occurs in a variety of settings in which B cells are stimulated directly by allogenic or autoreactive T cells (reviewed in 110,111). This results in synthesis of autoantibodies, which, in selected strains, include anti-laminin antibodies that bind to the GBM and cause nephritis. This can occur in chronic graft-versus-host disease induced by parent to F1 grafts [e.g., DBA/2 ⇒ (C 57 BL/10 x DBA 12) F1]; host-versus-graft disease in BALB/c mice injected at birth with spleen cells (C57BL/6 x BALB/c) F1; or, most notably, by exposure of susceptible strains of rats and mice to mercuric chloride [gold salts and penicillamine have the same effect (see 110,111)]. Disease in each of these cases in thought to selectively involve the development of Th2 cells, as evidenced by high-circulating IgE concentrations, and increased synthesis of IL 4 and IL-5 (112). The immunogenetics of these diseases have been investigated most extensively in rats and mice injected with mercuric chloride, and the remainder of the discussion will be restricted to them. As described earlier, the disease is linked to the MHC in rats but it also involves at least two to three other genes (29). Susceptible strains carry the RT1-n haplotype and include MAXX and DZB rats, as well as BN. Rats with RT-1 c, a, k, f have intermediate susceptibility, and Lewis rats (RT1-l) are resistant. H 2-s mouse strains are susceptible and H2-2d resistant. As are the other models with polyclonal B cell activation, susceptible strains have clear evidence of a polarized Th2 response, whereas resistant strains do not.

Recent work has centered on the reasons for the difference between BN and Lewis strains. Oliveira and colleagues (113) showed that mercuric chloride stimulated mast cells from BN rats to release IL-4, whereas mast cells from Lewis rats showed no response. Prigent et al. (114) demonstrated that lymphocytes from both strains proliferate when incubated with mercuric chloride, and that lymphocytes from BN rats synthesized IL-4 and IFN-γ, whereas those from Lewis rats released only IFN-γ. This suggests there is a genetically determined difference in IL-4 response to mercury, but its nature and the location of the gene responsible have not been identified.

MURINE MODELS OF LUPUS

A variety of strains of lupus-prone mice have been developed, of which NZB/NZW and MRL/*lpr* have been studied most thoroughly (31). The NZB/NZW strain was raised in the 1950s and has many of the familiar features of lupus. There is polyclonal B cell activation, which results in hyperglobulinemia and synthesis of a range of autoantibodies, including those to single- and double-stranded DNA. Clinically, the mice have a high incidence of autoimmune hemolytic anemia and develop severe progressive glomerulonephritis, which is morphologically similar to lupus nephritis; over 85% of female NZB/NZW mice die from renal failure (114). There is a small phenocopy rate in NZB mice, up to 10% of which develop a lupus-like syndrome. Furthermore, the lupus genes are not fully penetrant in NZB/NZW mice, and 10–15% do not develop severe renal disease in some colonies (115). MRL/*lpr* mice also develop a polyclonal B cell activation with antibodies to DNA and nephritis. The *lpr* mutation, however, results in widespread lymphadenopathy, which is associated with lupus only in mice with the MRL background. The genetics of both strains have been analyzed in detail using a mixture of classical and molecular techniques, including genome wide screening (31,115).

NZB/NZW Lupus-Prone Mice

The development of severe renal disease in NZB/NZW mice requires a genetic contribution from both parental strains, and MHC genes from both strains play a major role (31,115–118). Backcross analysis using NZB x (NZBxNZW) F1 mice demonstrate a strong but imperfect correlation between the NZB MHC haplotype $H2^z$ and the presence of autoantibodies and renal disease (116); subsequent studies have shown that the results cannot be explained by linkage to genes at adjacent loci (117). Similar data have been presented for NZB x SWR mice, which also develop lupus (119). Thus, it seems likely that NZW MHC class II molecules ($I\text{-}A^z$ or $I\text{-}E^z$) contribute strongly to the development of lupus nephritis in this model. Studies with congenic mice demonstrate that NZB MHC class II genes are also important for susceptibility. NZB mice congenic for the $H2^b$ haplotype (which expresses only I-A because of a mutation in the promoter region of the I-E α chain) do not develop lupus when crossed with NZW mice, whereas mice congenic for $H2^{bm12}$ behave like normal NZB mice in that they develop anti-DNA antibodies and severe renal disease when crossed with NZW (119). The sole difference between the $H2^b$ and the $H2^{bm12}$ haplotypes lies in the β chain of the MHC class II I-A molecule, which has amino acid substitutions at three critical residues (120,121). These studies clearly implicate the NZB I-A locus in the disease and suggest a role for heterozygosity of the MHC. The effect of heterozygosity is not unique to the $H2^{d/z}$. Recent studies have shown that b and v alleles also increase the effect of the z allele (20).

The reasons for the heterozygosity effect have been discussed in detail by Nygard et al. (122), who suggest that the critical event is the formation of a hybrid class II molecule with an α-chain from one of the parental strains coupled with a β-chain from the other. Alternative explanations include the potential for two different class II molecules to present a wider range of self-peptides, and an influence of heterozygosity on decreasing expression of I-A or I-E, as compared with the homozygous state. It should be emphasized that heterozygosity is not essential because a proportion of homozygous $H2^{z/z}$ NZB/NZW F2 mice develop the disease (123). Furthermore, New Zealand mixed strains of mice produced by Rudofsky et al. (21,22) from brother-sister matings from F2 NZB/NZW mice were bred for the severity of the nephritis. The incidence of nephritis varied from 0% to 89% in twelve of these strains studied in detail, and all the nephritic strains were homozygous for the $H2^z$; tantalizingly, most were also deficient in C5 component of complement.

Contribution of Other Genes

NZB mice have a major deletion in the genes that encode the T cell receptor (124–126). The deletion spans the region from the Cβ1 to the Jβ2 loci and has functionally important consequences, but does not influence susceptibility to lupus. Three groups have now used genome screening approaches to map genes responsible for lupus nephritis with remarkably similar results (20,22,123). They all identified recessive disease susceptibility loci on chromosomes 1, 4, and 7 (see Table 2) in addition to the MHC on chromosome 17. Kono et al. (123) also identified additional loci on chromosomes 5, 6, and 11 and Drake et al. (20) found loci on chromosomes 10, 13, and 19. Of particular interest is the observation by all three groups that the loci on chromosomes 1, 4, and 7 were all linked to the severity of nephritis independently of the magnitude of autoantibody responses or of other aspects

TABLE 2. *Chromosomal Locations of loci mapped to susceptibility in NZB/NZW mice*

Chromosome	(NZBxNZW) F2	NZMxC57BL/6	(NZBxSJ/M)xNXW	Candidate Genes
1	LBW-7	sle-1	+ +	Fas ligand, CD40 ligand, E,P and L Selectin
4	LBW-2	sle-2	+ +	TNFR2 (CD120b), IFN α/β, leuk assoc gene (lag), Lympho specific tyrosine kinase
5	LBW-3			
6	LBW-4			
7	LBW-5	sle-3	+ +	Lmrd, bcl-3, oct-1, TGFb1
10	LBW-8			
13			+ +	
17	LBW-1	sle-4	+ +	MHC Class II
18	LBW-6			
19			+ +	

Lbw loci 1-8 from Konon et al (123), sle loci 1-4 from Morel et al (22), and + + loci from Drake et al (20) who did not assign names to the loci they identified. Loci shown in bold are those associated with the severity of glomerulonephritis.

NB. The candidate gene Lmrd in the renal disease modifying locus identified by Watson et al in MRL/lpr lupus prone mice.

of lupus. Furthermore, the chromosome 7 markers mapped the same region as the previously described renal disease modifying locus-1 (*Lmrd-1*) identified in MRL/*lpr* lupus-prone mice (127). The identity of the genes responsible is not known, but candidates include apoptosis-related genes, including TNF receptor II (CD120b); *Fas* ligand and OX 40 ligand; E, P, and L selectins; α/β interferons, and poorly characterized genes involved in lymphocyte proliferation (20,22,123).

*MRL/*lpr *Lupus-Prone Mice*

Much of the recent analysis of this strain has focused on the nature of the *lpr* mutation because of its role in producing the lupus syndrome. Watanabe-Fukanaga et al. (128) showed that the *lpr* phenotype is caused by a mutation in the second intron of the *Fas* gene and that it limits its expression. *Fas* is a surface receptor found on T cells, B cells, and macrophages, which initiates apoptosis and could be crucial for the negative selection of T cells in the thymus during otongeny (that is, for editing the T cell repertoire). The importance of this mutation for the development of autoimmunity in MRL mice has been demonstrated by linkage studies (127) and by proof of its pathogenetic role by correction of the phenotype by expression of the normal gene on a T cell specific promoter in transgenic mice (129). Further evidence that inappropriate control of apoptosis predisposes to the lupus syndrome comes from other sources: a point mutation of the *Fas* gene (*lpr cg*) causes a single amino acid substitution in the *Fas* protein and is associated with lupus (131). Overexpression of Bcl-2, a protein that confers resistance to apoptosis, is also associated with lupus (132). Thus, it appears that failure to eliminate potentially autoreactive T cells and B cells by apoptosis causes lupus in MRL mice, but it is apparent that full expression of the syndrome requires contributions of other genes from the MRL background. More subtle differences in the *Fas/Fas* ligand interaction also influence immune responsiveness (23); it will be of interest to know whether they also contribute to susceptibility to nephritis.

Linkage studies by Watson et al. (127) have identified genes on chromosome 7 and chromosome 12 that are strongly associated with a predisposition to severe nephritis in MRL/*lpr* mice (Table 1). As described earlier, the locus on chromosome 7 maps to the same segment as do genes responsible for nephritis in NZB/NZW mice. Kinjoh, Kyogoku, and Good (133) have provided further evidence for an inherited susceptibility to glomerulonephritis in the MRL background. They developed strains of mice derived from brother-sister matings of MRL/*lpr* and BXSB/*lpr* mice that spontaneously develop severe crescentic nephritis with scanty immune deposits. These mice develop autoantibodies to neutrophil cytoplasmic antigens (ANCA) but not anti-DNA antibodies (134). Kinjo mice shows are homozygous for the MRL MHC, but other loci responsible for the phenotype have yet to be mapped. Thus, it appears that the interactions of genes at a number of different loci are responsible for the susceptibility to autoimmunity and to the development of nephritis in MRL/*lpr* in mice.

GENETIC ANALYSIS AND COMPLEX TRAITS

Identifying Susceptibility Genes in Humans

Identifying susceptibility genes in outbred populations such as man is an even more formidable task, but not impossible, especially if searches can be restricted to relatively discrete areas of the genome (Table 3). It is possi-

TABLE 3. *Methods for identifying susceptibility genes*

Method	Description
Linkage Analysis	Family studies of large kindreds Assumes a model of inheritance Efficient for monogenic disorders Relatively ineffective for complex diseases
Allele Sharing	Family studies of kindreds with 2 or more affected members No assumptions about mode of inheritance Can be used for quantitative traits Can be applied to complex disorders More robust than linkage studies
Population Associations	No need for multiplex families Can be applied to rare disorders Problems of control population resolved by using parental alleles Can be used to identify relative predispositional effects

ble to use the results from studies in mice to focus studies in humans because of the considerable similarity (synteny) between chromosome segments in the two species. However, genome wide linkage studies in multiplex families are already being performed for many autoimmune diseases, again most notably in diabetes (28).

There are special statistical problems inherent in studies of autoimmune disease, including glomerulonephritis. They are complex disorders and often rare, which means that it is difficult to collect sufficient kindreds with more than one affected member, even though the relative risk to a sibling is highly increased. Disease definition also presents a problem familiar to nephrologists; for example: membranous nephropathy occurs in many clinical contexts, including systemic lupus and as an adverse reaction to drugs. Inheritance could influence the severity and persistence of disease rather than the underlying susceptibility, which means that care must be taken to ensure that patients are a uniform group with regard to the stage of their disease. There are data to suggest that this occurs in many types of nephritis (5). This means that great care must be taken in selecting patient groups before attempting to find susceptibility genes. Three types of approaches have been used to do this: linkage analysis, allele sharing methods, and association studies (Table 3) (13–15).

Family Studies

Linkage Analysis

Linkage analysis is the traditional genetic approach to identifying genes that cause disease and remains the method of choice in single gene disorders. It relies on demonstration of significant deviation from the expected Mendelian ratio of inheritance of the candidate gene in family members with the disease. The mode of inheritance has to be specified (e.g., dominant or recessive with various degrees of penetrance), and the method is critically dependent on correct assignment of family members to diseased or nondiseased groups. These conditions cause problems when analyzing complex disorders and linkage analyses. It is not likely to be useful to examining the inheritance of nephritis generally, but could be applied to mesangial IgA disease, in which a familial incidence is sufficiently common (2), or to exceptional outbreaks of nephritis in geographically remote areas such as that described by Scolari et al. (135).

Allele Sharing Methods

Allele sharing methods are now used much more commonly than are linkage studies for analyzing complex disorders. They seek merely to prove that the inheritance pattern of a chromosomal region is inconsistent random Mendelian inheritance by showing that affected relatives inherit identical copies of the region more often than expected by chance. They use no assumptions about specific models of inheritance, so they are more robust than linkage analyses. This means that they are less affected by the problems of incomplete penetrance, phenocopy, and heterogeneity.

It is simplest to analyze affected sibling pairs, but the method can be extended to cover other relationships (13). Ideally, the parents are studied together with the affected sibling pairs, as this enables the origin of alleles at each locus to be identified, and the affected siblings to be assigned identical by descent (IBD) for 0, 1, or 2 copies of an allele at a given locus. The combined results of sets of affected sibling pairs can then be compared with the expected Mendelian ratios of 25%, 50%, 25%, for 0, 1,and 2 shared alleles; significance is assessed by χ^2 test (136). It is not always possible to identify the chromosomal origin of a particular shared allele, either because the parents could not be studied or because they both had similar copies of the given marker. In this circumstance, affected siblings who share the same chromosomal segment (or alternatively, the same allele at the particular locus) are referred to as being identical by state (IBS). In some instances, the chromosomal origins can be inferred from the data, but methods for analyzing IBS data have been developed that do not rely on this assumption. Affected sibling pair methods can also be applied to quantitative traits loci (QTL), such as the magnitude of antibody responses (137). These methods have been used successfully in immunogenetic studies to demonstrate linkage of HLA to insulin dependent diabetes melitis (IDDM) and to show that IgE levels are limited to a segment of chromosome containing the gene for IL-4, but analytical methods are complex (see 13). Undoubtedly, this approach will be used extensively over the next few years to identify genes responsible for important aspects of the immune and inflammatory responses.

Population Association Studies

Nephrologists are familiar with association studies from countless studies of HLA alleles in various types of nephritis (5). The frequencies of the marker (for example, HLA allele, cytokine gene polymorphism, or a microsatellite marker) are estimated in disease and control samples, and the significance of associations is calculated from contingency tables after appropriate correction for multiple comparisons: for example, by multiplying the probability value obtained by the number of comparisons made. This should always be done on the initial studies but is unnecessary on later studies to confirm the original association. The strength of the association is usually assessed by the "odds ratio" (OR), which is obtained simply by multiplying diagonally opposite cells in a 2 X 2 table. The OR is greatly influenced by the frequency of the marker in the control population; thus, a marker that is rare in the controls will tend to have a much greater OR. The etiologic fraction is an alternative measure of the strength of association that is unaffected by the frequency in the marker population and so can be used to compare the strengths of association of different markers (138).

Relative Predispositional Effects

When an allele at a highly polymorphic locus has a very strong association with a given disease, it is very difficult to ascertain whether other alleles at the same locus also have effects, either by contributing to susceptibility or by protecting against it. This is often the case with HLA alleles and immunologically mediated diseases such as nephritis. These are termed *relative predispositional effects*, and a method has been devised to analyze them (139). It relies on the fact that relative frequencies of neutral alleles should be the same in disease and control samples under all circumstances. This allows the relative frequencies of the remaining alleles to be compared for differences using the X^2 test after alleles showing the strongest associations are removed sequentially from the analysis. The method is used to study the relative effects of different HLA class II alleles in IDDM (140), and its application to Goodpasture's disease will be discussed later.

Affected Family-Based Controls

Three major pitfalls devalue the results of population association studies: (a) chance associations caused by failure to correct appropriately for multiple comparisons or through using sample sizes that are too small; (b) failure to ensure that the disease sample is homogeneous in terms of pathogenesis, stage of disease, and the population from which the subjects are drawn; and (c) inappropriateness of the control sample. The last of these can present enormous problems in populations where there has been recent admixture in the frequencies of HLA alleles and other polymorphic markers because of racial differences. One way to circumvent the problem is to derive a control sample from the parental alleles, an approach called the affected-family-based controls (AFBC) method. The method is based on the assumption that parental alleles not transmitted to the affected child should not be associated with the disease, so their frequencies ought to provide the perfect ethnically matched sample of control alleles. A statistic, termed the *haplotype relative risk*, can be calculated from contingency tables in the same way as the OR and tested for significance by X^2. The confidence in associations identified by the AFBC method can be further strengthened by assessing the results obtained with the transmission disequilibrium test (142) to confirm that parents heterozygous for susceptibility and nonsusceptibility alleles transmit the susceptibility allele to affected offspring significantly more often than expected by chance. These are now considered to be the methods of choice for population association studies, but there is need for a word of caution because both tests rest on the assumption that alleles are either associated or not associated with a disease, and this is not always the case (e.g., in the case of the HLA complex). Nevertheless, they do circumvent some of the most serious problems with population association studies and should certainly be applied more widely; they are discussed in detail by Thomson (143).

THE HLA COMPLEX

The genes that encode the HLA lie on the short arm of chromosome 6 in the distal portion of the 6p21.3 band (Fig. 1) and have been segregated into three regions, designated classes II, III, and I, in order from the centromere. Class I and II genetic loci are highly polymorphic, the class III locus less so. The products of these classes have been characterized serologically and biochemically.

The class I region consists of HLA-A, B, and C loci, as well as a large number of less well characterized genes. There are at least 24 different HLA-A, 50 HLA-B, and 11 HLA-C alleles whose products are expressed on all cells. Class I molecules consist of two polypeptide chains. The 44-kD heavy chain spans the plasma membrane and has an extracellular portion divided into three domains (α1, α2, α3), each of about 90 amino acids encoded by separate exons. The heavy chain bound covalently to β2 microglobulin ($\beta 2_m$) is relatively conserved, while the α1 and α2 domains are highly polymorphic.

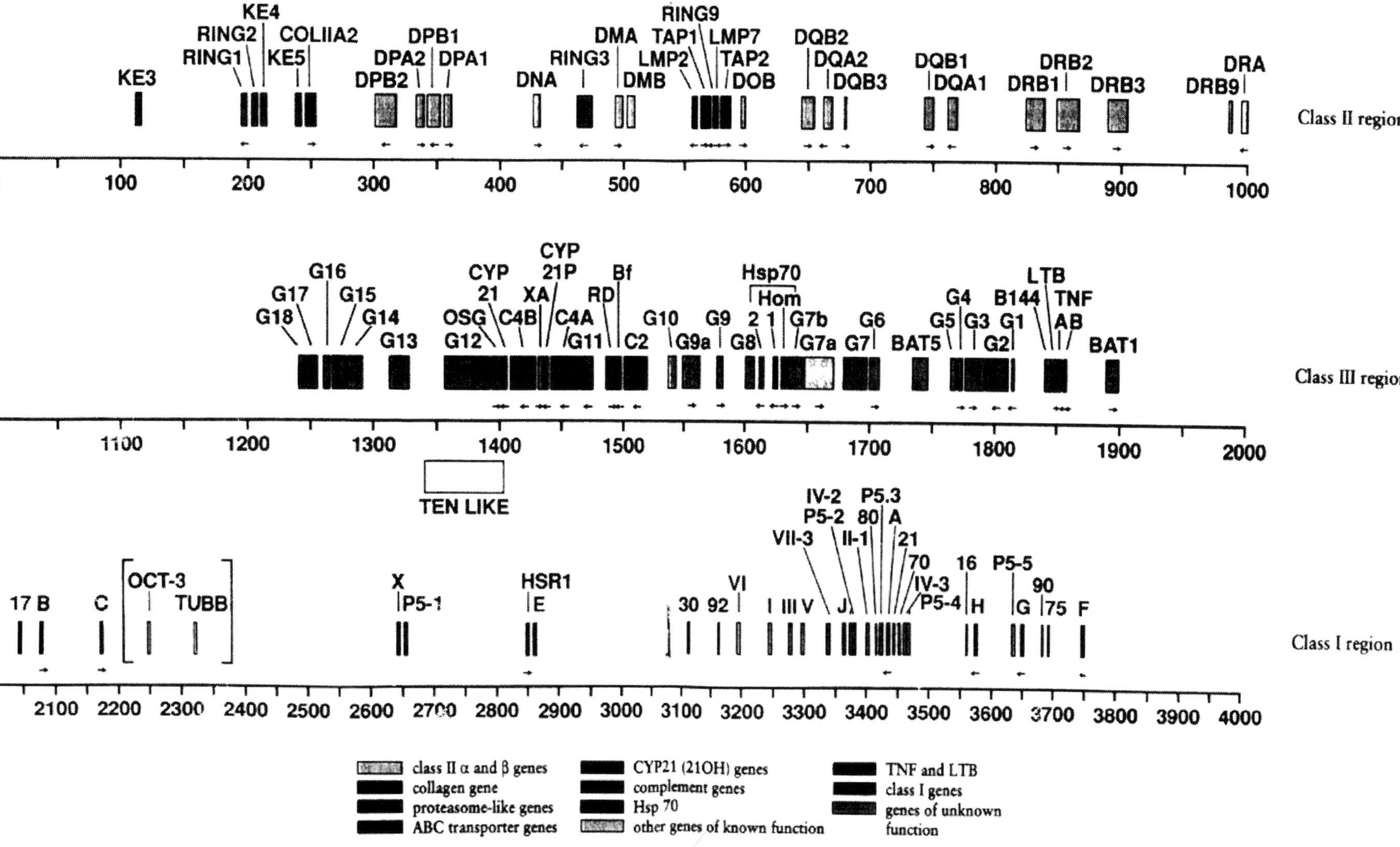

FIG. 1. Map of the human major histocompatibility complex. From Campbell and Trowsdale, ref. 144, with permission.

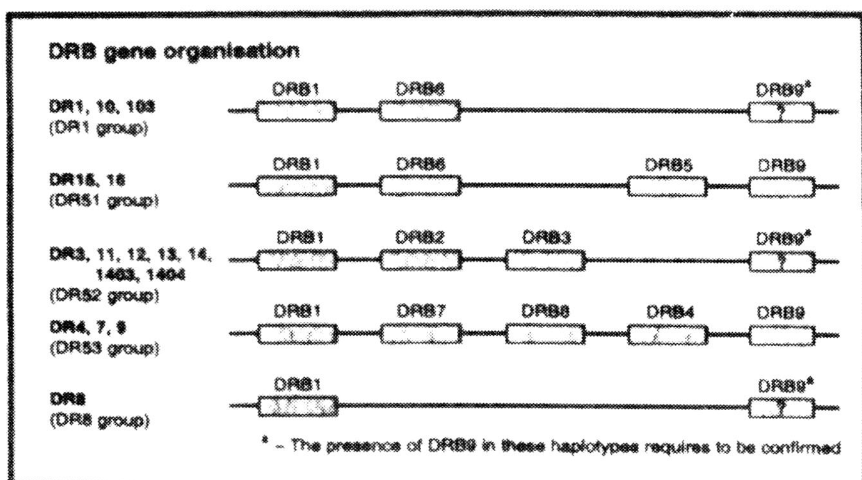

FIG. 2. HLA-DR B loci showing which genes are expressed on which haplotype.

The MHC class II region contains genes encoding at least three years expressed class II molecules DR, DQ, and DP (Fig. 2). Each of these is a heterodimer consisting of heavy (α) and light chains (β), with molecular weights of 30–34 and 26–29 kD. The α chains are encoded by single functional genes (DPA1, DQαA, and DRA), but the β chains are more complicated. DP and DQ β chains are also encoded by single functional genes (DPB1, DQB), but the DRA gene products can combine with products of at least two β chain genes (DRB1 and DRB3, DRB4 or DRB5). The combination α1 and β1 chains is responsible for DR specificities 1-w18, whereas binding of a1 to the β3 or β4 chain is responsible for DRw52 and DRw53 specificities, and combination with β5 forms the unique second DR molecule expressed on all DR2-bearing haplotypes. There are at least eight other genes in this region that are not expressed, referred to as pseudogenes. Finally, as discussed earlier, the class II region also contains genes whose products are essential for processing antigens for presentation by class I molecules (LMP 2 and LMP 7, and TAP 1 and TAP 2) and by class II molecules (HLA DM).

All the expressed class II B genes are polymorphic. There are at least 18 DRβ alleles, 10 DQβ alleles, and 14 DPβ alleles. There is much less polymorphism of the a chain genes. Only DQA is extensively polymorphic, and it has at least eight alleles. There is extensive linkage disequilibrium between genes in the HLA complex, with particular haplotypes found in different populations (Table 4); this complicates interpretation of HLA associations with disease, and it is often impossible to decide which genetic locus is primarily associated with a given disease.

The class III region is very diverse, spans 120 kb between class I and class II, and is less well characterized. It contains an undetermined number of apparently unrelated genes, including those encoding complement components C4, C2, and factor B, tumor necrosis factor α and β, heat shock proteins of the HSP60 family, collagen type XI and adrenal steroid 21-hydroxylase enzymes, and many other unidentified genes (145).

The genes for C2 and factor B lie about 400 bp apart, and both are polymorphic, though much less so than are class I and II genes. Endonucleases have been used to define RFLPs of the C2 and BF genes (144). At least five DNA polymorphisms have been defined in a 20-kb segment of DNA encompassing the C2 and BF loci. These reflect polymorphisms of the complement components and are usually detected serologically on the basis of electrophoretic mobility. C2 has three variants, C2A, C2B, and C2C; C2C is the most common, with a gene

TABLE 4. *Selected DR and DQ haplotypes found commonly in Caucasoid populations, showing alleles at DRB1, DQA1 and DQB1 loci.*

Haplotype	DRB1	DQA1	DQB1
DR1	0101	0101	0501
DR2	1501	0102	0602
	1502	0103	0601
	1601	0102	0502
DR3	0301	0501	0201
DR4	0401	0301	0301
	0401	0301	0302
	0404	0301	0302
	0403	0301	0301
	0402	0301	0302
	0405	0301	0401
DR5	1101	0501	0301
DR6	1401	0101	0503
	1301	0103	0603
	1302	0102	0604
DR7	0701	0201	0201
	0701	0201	0303
DR8	0801	0401	0402
	0803	0103	0601
DR9	0901	0301	0303
DR10	1001	0301	0501

Adapted from Nepom and Erlich (146).

frequency of 0.97, whereas C2A and C2B are much rarer. There are patients who are C2-deficient, with a C2Q0 gene (Q0: quantity zero). Polymorphisms of BF have been detected by agrose gel electrophoresis. The two major variants are BFF (fast gene product) and BFS (slow gene product). There are two major variants and up to 14 rarer variants. In Caucasoids, the BFS allele is the most common, with a gene frequency of 0, 7, and no factor B deficiency has been identified.

C4 is a serum glycoprotein that occurs in two forms, C4A and C4B. C4A and C4B are both extensively polymorphic in man, with 13 alleles at the C4A locus and 22 at the C4B locus, identified by protein electrophoresis. Null alleles are characterized by the absence of any bands and are designated *Q0* (e.g., C45AQ0 and C4BQ0). Null alleles of either C4A or C4B are relatively common and are found in about 25% of Caucasoids. Complete deficiency of C4, i.e., an individual with two null alleles at both loci, is found in less than 5% of people. C4B is more active than C4A in hemolytic assays; although it is the subject of considerable interest, there is no information about the relative activities if allelic variants.

Recombination between C2, BF, C4A, and C4B loci has not been observed in man, so genes in this region display very strong linkage disequilibrium. This means that identifying the allele at a particular locus allows one to predict those that will be present at other loci; for this reason, combinations of alleles at C2, BF, C4A, and C4B are often referred to as complotypes (145). Only 15 of these complotypes are observed in Caucasians, the most common being BFS, C2C, C4A3, C4B1, and abbreviated SC31, which has a gene frequency of about 40%. In many cases this linkage disequilibrium extends to neighboring HLA-B and HLA-DR loci; when this occurs, they are termed *extended haplotypes* (146). It is interesting that the three most common extended haplotypes, namely, B8, SCO1, DR3 and B7, SC31, DR2 and B44, SC30, and DR4 have all been associated with autoimmunity.

ASSOCIATION WITH DISEASE

MHC in Human Glomerulonephritis

The data from the studies of experimental glomerulonephritis suggest that MHC is involved in both organ-specific and generalized autoimmunity. This provides strong justification for the detailed examination of the HLA complex in humans with glomerular disease. Early studies using serologic techniques to examine the HLA class II region showed strong positive associations between particular HLA molecules and various types of nephritis in Caucasoid populations [e.g., anti-GBM disease, membranous nephropathy, and minimal change nephrotic syndrome (MCNS) in children] (5,146,147).

TABLE 5. *HLA Class II associations with glomerulonephritis, established by serologic techniques.*

	Caucasoids		Japanese	
	Specificity	RR	Specificity	RR
Goodpasture Syndrome	DR2(w15)	10.5		
Membranous nephropathy	DR3	5.6	DR2(w15)	6.8
Mesangial IgA disease	None		DR4	2.6
Minimal chage nephrotic syndrome	DR7	5.8	DR8	10.1

See text for full data.

Similar studies in Japanese populations revealed equally strong but different associations (Table 5). This provides strong evidence for the involvement of HLA genes in nephritis, but there are huge problems in interpreting the data. The original methods lacked precision and identified broad HLA specificities rather than individual DR alleles. They were unable to distinguish between effects at the different class II loci (DR, DP, and DQ). Furthermore, they were conducted against a background of uncertainty of the structural functional relationships of HLA molecules and profound ignorance of the immunopathogenesis of nephritis.

The development of molecular techniques for examining the HLA complex has enabled more recent studies to be conducted with much greater precision and, as discussed earlier, there is now a broad understanding of how HLA molecules present peptides to T cells, based on the definition of HLA class I and class II molecules to atomic resolution by crystallography and a knowledge of the characteristics of naturally processed peptides that can be eluted from them.

Goodpasture's Disease

Goodpasture's disease is the one type of clinical nephritis whose pathogenesis is understood. It is caused by autoimmunity to the GBM and characterized pathogenic antibodies to the NC1 domain of the α3 chain of type IV collagen [α3(IV)NC1] (148). The anti-GBM antibodies have highly restricted specificity, and antibodies from different patients cross-inhibit each other. Genetic factors undoubtedly play a role in susceptibility to this disease. A familial incidence has been described, and the disease has been reported in four sibling pairs (149,150), including two set of identical twins (151). However, the importance of nongenetic factors is emphasized by two sets of individual twins in our series who are discordant for the disease and another set reported by others (152).

Goodpasture's disease was originally associated with DR2-bearing haplotypes in a study of 17 British Caucasoid patients diagnosed by immunohistology and radioimmunoassay (153). The strength of the association (OR 16) meant that the association was statistically significant, despite the small numbers. A subsequent study extended the series to 38 patients, 34 of whom (88%) had DR2, compared with 19% of 153 controls (154). There was also a weaker association with HLA-7 but no more than would have been expected from the known linkage disequilibrium between DR2 and B7 (154): Confirmation of these associations came from small studies from Australia (155) and the US (156).

The DR2 specificity has been split into DR15 and DR16. Together, they are comprised of at least 11 alleles at the DRB1 locus (DRB1*1501–1505 and DRB1*1601–1606) and 1 at the DRB5 locus (DRB5*0101), which is expressed at relatively low levels on all DR2 haplotypes. The DRB1*1501 allele is overwhelmingly the most common allele in North European Caucasoids and accounts for 90% of DR2 specificity in them. There is strong linkage disequilibrium between DR alleles and DQ6. Consequently, the DR2 association with Goodpasture's could have been due to primary associations with any of these alleles or even with alleles at other, more distant though still linked loci. These issues have now been resolved using sequence-specific oligonucleotides to identify alleles at DR and DQ loci. Studies from the US (157), Australia (158), and France (159), as well as our laboratory (160), have shown that almost all the patients with Goodpasture's inherit the haplotype defined by DRB1*1501, DRB5*0101, and DQB1*0602 alleles. But in each case the number of patients studied was insufficient to distinguish between DR and DQ effects or to ascertain whether the less common alleles also increased susceptibility.

Recently, we have addressed issues in a new cohort of 82 patients (161). The results again confined the strong associations with DRB1*1501 and DQB1*0602 (present in 74% and 79% of cases, compared with 28% and 27% of controls). There was also an excess of DRB1*1502 alleles, and the relative proportions of B1*1501 and 1502 alleles were the same as in controls, suggesting that both alleles confer susceptibility. None of the patients had BRB1*16 alleles, and, in fact, no DR16 alleles have been recorded in 153 patients from four series assessed by molecular typing, whereas at least 6 would have been expected, based on the minimum number of DR2 positive gametes. This provides strong evidence that DR15 and DR16 alleles differ in their ability to cause Goodpasture's disease: DR15 and DR16 are also differently associated with IDDM.

Relative predispositional analysis reveals less strong associations with DR alleles (but not with DQ). There was a positive association with DR4 alleles and a significant negative association with DR7 and, possibly, with DR1 (161). These findings appear remarkably constant across the different series (Table 6), which provides a rationale comparing the amino acid sequences of alleles that confer susceptibility with those associated with resistance. This comparison shows a progressive increase in the number of nonconservative substitutions in the polymorphic residues that make up the second peptide binding pocket using the nomenclature of Brown (see 37) (Table 7). These data raise the question of whether allele-specific differences in Goodpasture antigen-derived peptides underly the different associations; specifically, whether expression of DR7 or DR1 influence the peptides presented by DR15 when both are expressed by an APC. The naturally processed Goodpasture antigen-derived peptides expressed on the surface of APCs will have to be characterized if these questions are to be

TABLE 6. *Summary of reported HLA-DRB1 associations with Goodpasture's disease*

			DRB1 allele frequencies (phenotype)				
Country	No. of Patients	Year	DRB1 *15	*04	*16	*01	*07
UK	82	1996	.79[a]	.43	0	.1[c]	.05[b]
USA	23	1993	.91[a]	.35	0	.13	.04
France	12	1992	.92[a]	.58	0	0	0
Australia	36	1991	.64[a]	.58	0	.06	.03[d]

[a]p<0.0001
[b]p=0.0002
[c]p=0.0005
[d]p=0.05
See references 158, 159, 160 and 161.

TABLE 7. *Amino acid at polymorphic residues of HLA-DR alleles ordered on the basis of their association with Goodpasture's Disease. Single letter amino acid code is used.*

		Amino acid position					
Strength of Association	DRB1	β13	β26	β28	β70	β71	β74
+ + +	1501	R	F	D	Q	A	A
	1502	–	–	–	–	–	–
	1503	–	–	–	–	–	–
+	0401	H	–	–	–	K	–
	0403	H	–	–	–	R	E
	0404	H	–	–	–	R	–
	0405	H	–	–	–	R	–
	0406	H	–	–	–	R	E
	0407	H	–	–	–	R	E
	0410	H	–	–	–	R	–
Neutral	0301	S	Y	–	–	K	R
	1601/2	–	–	–	D	R	–
–	0101	F	L	E	–	R	–
	0102	F	L	E	–	R	–
	0103	F	L	E	D	E	–
– –	07	Y	–	E	D	R	Q
	DRB5* 0101	Y	–	H	D	R	–

answered. We have recently characterized two nested sets from homozygous DRB1*1501 APC and shown that they have intermediate affinity for DR15 (63); comparisons with other alleles are also being made.

Analogies with experimental models suggest that HLA class II alleles are etiologically involved in Goodpasture's disease, but that genes at other loci will also be important. A significant association with Gm (IgG) allotypes has been described (162), but other candidate genes have not been examined systematically. The rationale for such studies will become increasingly strong if human genes are identified that predispose to autoimmunity (28).

The data on Goodpasture's disease illustrate the power of the genetic approach in an autoimmune disease caused by loss of tolerance to a single antigen. The results are remarkably clear-cut and reproducible, and they provide insight into pathogenesis. Unfortunately, no other type of nephritis is sufficiently characterized to allow this approach.

Idiopathic Membranous Nephropathy

Idiopathic membranous nephropathy (IMN) is a frequent cause of nephrotic syndrome in adults characterized by diffuse thickening of the glomerular capillary wall. There is granular deposition of immunoglobulins and complement visible on immunofluorescence; subepithelial electron-dense deposits are also evident on electron microscopy. There is little doubt that IMN is an immunologically mediated disease, although the mechanism is uncertain. Identical appearances can be produced experimentally, either by autoantibodies to glomerular epithelial cells in rats with Heymann nephritis or by serum sickness after injection of cationic antigens into rabbits. In humans, there is tentative evidence for the presence of autoantibodies to glomerular structures (see Chapter 9).

Familial membranous nephropathy has been described in siblings (163, 164), including two pairs of monozygotic twins. Results from population association studies also show the importance of heredity for susceptibility. IMN has been repeatedly associated with certain HLA antigens (Tables 8,9). Between 55% and 78% of North European Caucasoids who develop IMN have the DR3 allele, compared with 20–25% of controls (165–176), and similarly high frequencies have been recorded in Spain (166) and in Italy (171). By contrast, Vaughan et al. (175) observed a much lower frequency of DR3 in Greek patients with IMN and a slightly lower frequency in controls (33% and 15%), and Garovoy (166) had previously reported a relatively low frequency in North American patients. IMN also has a strong HLA association in Japanese patients, but with DR2 (B1*1501) rather than DR3 (177-180). HLA-DR3 is very uncommon in the Japanese but, even so, the difference is

TABLE 8. *Idiopathic membranous nephropathy:HLA-DR3 antigen frequency in Caucasians*

Author (year)	Ref	Country	Patients %(n)	Controls %9(n)	OR* >1
Klouda (1979)	165	UK	75(32)	20(60	12
Garovoy (1980)	166	UK	73(55)	21(3184)	8.7
Garovoy (1980)	166	Spain	67(39)	21(3184)	7.5
Garovoy (1980)	166	USA	33(33)	21(3184)	1.9
Muller (1981)	167	Germany	76(21)	23(122)	10.7
Le Petit (1982)	168	France	65(26)	20(74)	7.42
Rashid) (1983	169	UK	53(35)	27(325)	3.05
Papiha) (1987	170	UK	52(55)	23(70)	3.64
Zucchelli (1987)	171	Italy	55(55)	25(65)	3.67
Roccatello (1987)	172	Italy	61(18)	17(526)	7.6
Vaughan (1989)	173	UK	65(31)	37(55)	2.9
Cameron (1990)	174	UK	78(78)	–	–
Vaughan (1995)	175	UK	80(52)	27(100)	10.6
Vaughan (1995)	175	Greek	33(29)	15(92)	3.0

*Odds Ratio

striking because the frequency of DR2 is reduced in Caucasoids with IMN. There are at least three possible explanations: both DR molecules share the properties needed to confer susceptibility to the disease; the DR molecules themselves do not confer susceptibility but are in linkage disequilibrium with the single true susceptibility gene; or the pathogenesis of MGN is different in different populations.

Most attention has focused on the second of these ideas. Vaughan et al. (173) had already suggested in an

TABLE 9. *Idiopathic membranous nephropathy:HLA-DR2 antigen frequency in Japanese*

Author (year)	Ref	Country	Patients %(n)	Controls %9(n)	OR* >1
Hiki (1984)	177	Japan	80(50)	36(884)	7.12
Tomura (1984)	178	Japan	74(50)	30(158)	6.5
Naito (1987)	179	Japan	80(15)	39(100)	6.3
Ogahata) (1992	180	Japan	80(30)	30(50)	9.3

R = Odds Ratio

earlier study of British patients that the primary association was with a DQA1 allele, which is inherited exclusively with DR3 and DR5, rather than with DR3 itself. Using data from two other published studies, they made an indirect estimate of the likely frequency of this allele in the two groups of IMN patients and found them to be remarkably similar to their own findings. A common DQ association could also explain the differences between the Greek and British patients, as the frequency of DQA1*0501 was significantly increased in both groups (British, 85% versus 45%; OR 7.4; p=.00007: Greek - 96% versus 66%; OR 9.7; p=.0009). Ogahara et al. (180) also concluded that the HLA association in their Japanese patients was best explained by a DQ association, even though the frequency of DR2 was greatly increased (80% versus 30% for controls, OR 9.3). This conclusion was based on the observation that a 6.2-kb RFLP detected with a DQA probe was present in 87% patients and 14% of random controls (OR 39.9, $p=1.7\times10^{-10}$). Furthermore, the 6.2-kb RFLP was not found in any of a group of local controls matched for DR2. However, when the patients' DQA alleles were identified by sequence-specific oligonucleotide typing, 22 were DQA1*01 alleles and none were DQA1*0501, so the reasons for racial differences remain to be explained. C4A null alleles are commonly found in Caucasoids with IMN as part of the DR3 B8 A3 extended haplotype, but Japanese DR2-bearing haplotypes do not have null alleles at this locus (181). Demaine et al. (181a) reported that there was an increased incidence of heterozygosity using probes for a human T cell receptor gene, but studies with probes have been very difficult to reproduce.

Minimal Change Nephrotic Syndrome

Minimal change nephrotic syndrome is the most common form of nephrotic syndrome in childhood but can occur at any age. There are plenty of clues to suggest that MCNS is an immunologic disease, but the exact pathogenesis is unknown. There have been a large number of studies to look for associations with MCNS. In 1976, Thompson et al. (182) reported an association with HLA-B12 of 71 affected children, 54% inherited HLA-B12, compared with 15% of 39 controls (relative risk 6.3; etiology fraction, 0.45). Trompeter et al. (183) confirmed this association in a larger group of patients from the same institution, but the results were less striking. Since then, at least seven other studies of Caucasian children from various European countries and from Australia have failed to show a convincing association with HLA-B12 (184–191), but almost all have demonstrated an association with the class II specificity HLA-DR7 (Table 10) (186,187,190,192). It is notable that HLA-DR7 is in linkage disequilibrium with B12, which probably accounts for the original suggestion of a B12 association. However, the association of MCNS with DR7 does not extend to other racial groups, and Japanese children suffering from MCNS appear to inherit the class II antigen DR8 more frequently than do controls (13/28 compared with 9/114; relative risk, 10.1; etiology fraction, 0.42) (192). Clearly, studies of the DQ loci will be needed in both populations before these differences can be interpreted.

TABLE 10. *Minimal-change nephrotic syndrome:HLA Class II antigen frequencies*

Author (year)	Ref	Country	Patients %(n)	Controls %(n)	OR >1
HLA-DR7					
Alfiler (1980)	[186]	Australia	71(42)	30(121)	5.9
Mouzon-Cambon (1981)	[187]	France	74(38)	30(91)	6.3
Ruder (1982)	[190]	Germany	59(54)	18(100)	6.3
Nunez-Rolden (1982)	[140]	Spain	72(50)	38(179)	4.2
Komori (1983)	[192]	Japan	3.6(28)	2.6(114)	NS
HLA-DRw8					
Komori (1983)	[192]	Japan	46(28)	8(114)	10.1

OR Odds Ratio

Mesangial IgA Nephropathy

Mesangial IgA nephropathy (IgAN) is probably the most common chronic glomerulonephritis in the world, and a significant proportion of affected patients develop end-stage renal failure. Patients with IgA nephropathy have a generalized disease of cellular and humoral immunity (2). An autoimmune model has been postulated for the disease recently because IgG autoantibodies against specific determinants on mesangial cells have been found in sera from some patients, but the findings have been difficult to reproduce. (See Chapter 42)

The familial incident of IgAN is well described in both Caucasians and Japanese populations, and there are reports of disease in HLA identical siblings and in twins. A number of studies, though not all, have linked familial IgAN to particular alleles. Levy and Lesavre (2) analyzed data from all reported families, including ten affected sibs they had studied. There was a significant deviation from the expected Mendelian pattern of inheritance for HLA haplotypes, but as the authors emphasize, the use of reported families could have biased the results in favor of sharing based on the stage of the disease or its tendency to progress to end-stage renal failure. In 1978, Berthoux et al. (193) reported IgA nephropathy to be associated with HLA-Bw35, but only two of sixteen subsequent studies have supported this (194–209).

Faucet (200) in 1980 reported that the frequency of DR4 was significantly increased in a group of 45 French patients with IgA disease but, again, other studies have not confirmed this (194,199,203–211) (Table 11). The sit-

TABLE 11. *Mesangial IgA nephropathy: HLA DR4 antigen frequency in Caucasians*

Author (year)	Ref	Country	Patients %(n)	Controls %(n)	OR >1
Brettle (1978)	[194]	UK	24(17)	33(208)	0.62
Mouzan-Cambon (1980)	[210]	France	0(11)	12(90)	
Bignon (1980)	[199]	France	14(35)	21(56)	0.61
Faucet (1980)	[200]	France	49(45)*	19(113)	3.96
Rambausek) (1982	[203]	FRG	17(36)	26(248)	0.56
Le Petit (1982)	[204]	France	22(49)	34(74)	0.57
Berger (1984)	[211]	France	43(30)*	13(106)	5.02
Feehally (1984)	[206]	UK	37(46)	32(385)	1.01
Hanly (1984)	[207]	Ireland	30(46)	33(212)	0.88
Waldo (1986)	[208]	USA	40(27)	28	
Berthoux (1988)	[209]	France	25(1985)	32(124)	0.69

*Significant result
OR Odds Ratio

uation is quite different in the Japanese, where separate studies have shown an increased prevalence on HLA-DR4, with an incidence of about 60% in patients, compared with 32–44% in healthy controls (179,212–219) (Table 12). It was hoped that the advent of the molecular approach to typing, together with studies of the DQ and DP loci, would resolve these differences but, unfortunately, this has not turned out to be the case. Moore et al. (220) and Li et al. (221) both reported significant though different DQ associations (with the undefined RFLPs T2 and T6, and with DQw7, respectively). Subsequently, Moore confirmed his findings in a second set of British Caucasoids, but could not demonstrate the association in Italian or Finnish patients (222). There were no DR or DQ associations in groups of German and American patients (223,224); nor were DP associations identified (225).

No clear conclusions can be drawn from the data on European Caucasoids, but the HLA complex appears to confer susceptibility for the disease in other populations. This is certainly the case in the Japanese, though the locus primarily associated with the disease has not been defined. The sibling pair analysis of family data provides some evidence for HLA involvement in Caucasoids, but ascertainment bias remains to be excluded. Above all, the data emphasize the need for well-designed studies, with regard to both the uniformity of the disease group and the appropriateness of the control sample. This could be achieved using family-based association methodology.

TABLE 12. *Mesangial IgA nephropathy: HLA DR4 antigen frequency in Japanese*

Author (year)	Ref	Patients %(n)	Controls %(n)	OR >1
Kashiwabara (1982)	[212]	66(42)*	39(158)	3.1
Kasahara (1982)	[215]	60(104)*	36(147)	2.6
Hiki (1982)	[216]	66(80)*	41(884)	2.78
Komori (1983)	[213]	55(51)	44(114)	1.6
Kohara (1985)	[217]	58(41)	32(63)	3.03
Naito (1987)	[179]	58(70)*	34(100)	2.7
Hiki (1990)**	[218]	60(130)*	42(472)	2.1
Abe (1993)	[219]	66(32)	42(124)	2.6

*Significant result
OR Odds Ratio
**80 patients included in Hiki (1982) study

A number of other immunogenetic markers have been studied in IgA disease, and the results have been reviewed by Levy and Lesavre (2) and by Rambausek (223). A study of German patients suggested an association with immunoglobulin Cα switch region polymorphism, significantly more patients being homozygous for the 7.4-kb allele (226). This finding was not confirmed in British, Finnish, or Italian patients (227). However, an increased frequency of rare switch region alleles were reported in French patients (2). Again, these results reinforce the difficulties of using population association studies to investigate diseases of uncertain pathogenesis and etiology. Similar comments can be applied to the studies of IgA complement allotypes in IgA nephropathy (reviewed in 2,223).

ANCA Associated Vasculitis

Small vessel vasculitis associated with ANCA frequently presents with focal necrotizing glomerulonephritis, extensive crescent formation, and scanty immune deposits. Clinically, many of the patients are diagnosed clinically as having microscopic polyangiitis or Wegener's granulomatosis, but some present with predominantly glomerular disease (see chapter 49). Over 90% of untreated patients with active disease have detectable ANCA, usually directed against myeloperoxidase (MPO) or proteinase-3 (Pr-3). The recognition that autoimmunity to neutrophil cytoplasmic antigens might be involved in the pathogenesis (228) has led to a reexamination of the possible involvement of the HLA complex in these disorders.

These diseases have been reported in siblings, but identical twins discordant for the disease have also been observed (228). Early studies were performed before ANCA could be assayed and so are subject to some uncertainty. Nevertheless, Muller et al. (229) in 1984 reported that idiopathic RPGN was associated with HLA-DR2, MT3, and the complement allotype BfF, especially when inherited together as an extended haplotype. No patient was said to have had evidence of systemic disease, which is surprising in view of the high incidence of systemic symptoms in most series of RPGN. The 45 patients studied by Elkon et al. (230), all presented with vasculitis, and most had crescentic nephritis. The frequency of DR2 was significantly increased in patients diagnosed as having Wegener's granulomatosis (65% for the 17 patients versus 21% for 113 controls, x^2-12.1), but not in the group as a whole. The hope for more precise definition of the patients by the specificity of their autoantibodies has proved over-optimistic. We reported that the frequency of HLA DQB1*0301 was significantly increased in a group of 59 patients (231), especially when found on a DR4-bearing haplotype. This association was independent of the clinical diagnosis and of the ANCA specificity. Zhang et al. (232) did not confirm these findings in another study of British Caucasoids and did not identify any significant associations. A third study, this time of Dutch patients, failed to find any positive associations but did report a significant negative association with HLA-DR6 (233). Each of these studies was relatively small, and the results probably say more about ascribing statistical significance than about the nature of small vessel vasculitis.

The α1 antitrypsin locus is the one susceptibility locus identified with certainty. Wegener's granulomatosis and patients with anti-Pr-3 antibodies more generally are associated inheritance of one of the relative deficiency alleles (Table 13). The association was first described in a group of French patients in which the Z allele was significantly more common (234). This result has been confirmed by all five subsequent studies (235–239). α-1 Antitrypsin is the main physiologic inhibitor of Pr-3 (but not of MPO), so loss of this inhibition provides a natural explanation for the findings, although rather an unconvincing one, given the small reduction in enzymic activity. There is a single study describing the association of the C3 allele C3F and vasculitis that gave an OR of 2.6 for heterozygotes and 5.1 for homozygotes, compared with individually homozygous for the C3S allele (240).

TABLE 13. *α1 Anti-trypsin phenotypes in patients with ANCA positive vasculitis*

Author [reference]	ANCA specificity (no. of subjects)	Severe Deficiency (ZZ)	Moderate Deficiency (MZ,SZ,SS)	Sufficient (others)
Esnault	αPR3 (8)	.375	.25	.375
[234]	αMPO (6)	0	.167	.833
Llotta [236]	cANCA (32) (includes 25aPR3)	.0625	.094	.844
Savidge	αPR3 (31)	.032	.097	.821
[237]	αMPO (29)	0	0	100
Ezouki [238]	αPR3 (105)	.009	.162	.748
Griffiths	cANCA (99)	.010	.090	.910
[239]	pANCA (99)	0	.06	.940

The frequencies of sufficient, moderately deficient and deficient phenotypes in normal European caucasoid populations are in the region of .96, .04, and <.05 respectively. cANCA positive patients in all six studies had significant increase in the frequency of severe or moderately deficient α1 anti trypsin phenotypes.

Systemic Lupus Erythematosus

Systemic lupus erythematosus (SLE) is the prototype of a non-organ-specific autoimmune disease with immune complexes deposited in all pathologic lesions and antibody-mediated damage occurring in both lymphoid and nonlymphoid tissues. The occurrence of familial cases suggests a role for genetic factors that predispose to SLE. As many as 5% of patients with SLE have a relative with the same disease, and 57% of monozygotic twins are concordant for SLE. The occurrence of SLE in dizygotic twins is similar to that of other first-degree relatives. Thus, both genetic and environmental factors play a significant role in susceptibility to SLE.

Clinically detectable evidence of renal involvement in SLE is seen in about 50% of patients, though electron-microscopically detectable abnormalities are ubiquitous, even when renal function and sediment are entirely normal. Thus, when considering the immunogenetics of lupus nephritis, one must necessarily consider the genetic aspects of SLE in general and the wide variety of autoimmune systems involved (241).

Initial studies of class II antigens demonstrated a raised prevalence of HLA-DR2 and HLA-DR3 in Caucasian SLE patients (242,243). Subsequent studies have, in general, only confirmed the DR3 association, though Woodrow (242), combining the data from eight published reports, found that the presence of DR2 and DR3 is associated with an increased risk of developing SLE of 2 and 2.4. TheDR2 association has also been seen in a study of SLE in southern Chinese (relative risk, 2.64) (244).

The strongest disease susceptibility genes to be identified in humans to date are those responsible for deficiencies of the proteins of the classical pathway of complement, encoded within (C2 and C4) and without (Clq) the MHC. Inherited complete deficiencies of those proteins account for only a tiny minority of patients suffering from SLE, and the prevalence of SLE in patients with hereditary deficiencies of the proteins of the classical pathway of complement is 68–88%. Recognition of these facts have stimulated detailed studies of complement proteins to look for partial deficiencies (reviewed in 246).

The complement components C4 and C2 are encoded within the MHC, and it has been suggested that the association of SLE with deficiency of these components occurs as a result of genetic linkage with other immune response genes, perhaps located within the class II region. This does not seem likely to be the explanation, as patients with complete deficiencies of these proteins have a variety of MHC haplotypes (245). Many workers have looked for evidence of partial complement deficiency in patients with SLE. The C4A and C4B proteins exhibit extensive polymorphism, as discussed earlier in this chapter, and a number of groups have shown a markedly raised prevalence of C4AQ0 genes in patients with lupus nephritis (246). However, the majority of these C4AQ0 alleles were on DR3-bearing haplotypes (245,246). The relative contributions of each of these alleles to disease susceptibility is difficult to assess, though Bachelor et al. have found an increased prevalence of the C4A1Q allele in DR3-negative lupus patients (247). Indeed, the C4AQ0 allele appears to occur more commonly in lupus patients from other racial groups, compared with nonlupus individuals of similar descent.

The recent discovery that the genes for tumor necrosis factor are encoded within the MHC has led to the search for polymorphisms of these genes. Jacob et al. (248) have found reduced TNFα production in the offspring of lupus-susceptible (NZW) mice crossed with nonsusceptible mice (NZB), and regular injections of TNFα reduced the severity of nephritis and prolonged survival in these mice. Recently, they have described analogous observations in patients with SLE (248). These observations imply that inherited variation in TNF expression may be another disease susceptibility gene for SLE.

Thus, the causes of SLE in humans are likely to be multifactorial. Genetic factors certainly exist which, taken alone, are relatively weak but may act in consort to determine disease susceptibility. Alternatively, they may merely represent linkage to another true susceptibility gene.

Poststreptococcal Glomerulonephritis

The familial incidence is well recognized in epidemic outbreaks and is likely to reflect the presence of genetically determined susceptibility. However, there is no real evidence about the genes involved. Layrisse et al. (249) were unable to find evidence of linkage to the HLA complex in 18 affected Venezuelan families, but did report a weak association of HLA-DR4 in 42 unrelated patients. Given the problems of small sample sizes, this suggestion must be confirmed before being accepted. Two small studies from Japan of class II associations are unconvincing (250,251). Taken together, these results provide no evidence of association.

HLA Alleles and the Severity of Disease

Thus far, this chapter has been concerned only with the effects of HLA alleles on susceptibility to nephritis. There is also evidence that the HLA complex influences the severity of nephritis and its tendency to relapse or to progress to end-stage renal failure, though this is even more difficult to interpret. Reported associations with severity have often been with haplotypes rather than alleles, and there are even fewer precedents from experimental studies to guide interpretation of such associations. Nevertheless, the existence of extended haplotypes and of functional polymorphisms of genes encoding complement and TNF within the class III region provide a basis for the results. Ascertainment biases present enormous difficulties that can be avoided only by prospective studies: Surveys of patients entering end-stage renal failure programs may provide a prima facie case (252,253) but strictly are uninterpretable.

The severity of anti-GBM disease has been reported to be influenced by whether HLA-B7 is inherited together with DR2 in the study of 38 patients by Rees et al. (154). They reported that those with B7 had significantly higher serum creatinine concentrations at presentation and a worse outlook in patients with B7, even though anti-GBM antibody titres were similar. Analysis of these data showed that these effects could not be explained by the known linkage disequilibrium between B7 and DR2, which suggests that B7-bearing haplotypes have independent effects on the severity of the disease.

In children with MCNS, Trompeter et al. (183) reported that inheritance of HLA-B12 was associated with relapse within 3 years of standard doses of cyclophosphamide therapy.

Although there are no definite associations between HLA antigens and susceptibility to mesangiocapillary nephritis, Welch et al. (254) have suggested that, despite treatment with steroids, patients with the extended haplotype HLA-B8 DR3 are significantly more likely to develop renal failure than are patients with other haplotypes.

The data on membranous nephropathy are also contradictory. Zucchelli et al. (171) have suggested that patients with the HLA-DR3, B8 haplotype have a worse prognosis, whereas Short et al. (176) reported that patients with HLA-DR3, BfF1, B18 did worse than did patients with other DR3-bearing haplotypes, including those bearing B8. Short et al. (174) could not detect any effect of the HLA complex on prognosis, which is probably the correct answer.

CONCLUSION

The approach to the genetic analysis of complex disorders has been transformed over the past decade, mainly because of developments in molecular genetics, but also through much more rigorous mathematical treatments of the results obtained. In some respects, nephritis is relatively rare, which presents difficulties in assembling families with more than one affected individual. Groups of patients will have to be assembled from a wide area, which increases the problem of obtaining appropriately matched control groups. Finally, the disease entities may not be homogeneous. However, there are now methods to deal with each of these difficulties, and the precedents from experimental models of nephritis and from other immunologically mediated diseases provide more than enough justification for future studies. The rate at which the genetic approach to immunologic disease provides new insights into pathogenesis is likely to continue to increase.

REFERENCES

1. Wells WC. Observations on the dropsy which succeeds scarlet fever. *Trans Soc Improve Med Chir Know* 1812;13:167–186.
2. Levy M, Lesavre P. Genetic factors in IgA nephropathy (Berger's Disease). *Adv Nephrol* 1992;21:23–51.
3. McLeod R, Buschman E, Arbuckle LD, Skamene E. Immunogenetics in the analysis of resistance to intracellular pathogens. *Curr Opin Immunol* 1995;7:539–592.
4. Charlton B, Lafferty KJ. The Th1/Th2 balance and autoimmunity. *Curr Opin Immunol* 1995;7:793–798.
5. Rees AJ. Immunogenetics of glomerulonephritis. *Kidney Int* 1994;45: 377–383.
6. Biozzi G, Mouton G, Sant' Anna OA, Passos HC, Cennari M, Reis MH. Genetics of immunoresponsiveness to natural antigens in the mouse. *Curr Top Microbiol Immunol* 1980;85:31–98.
7. Nadeau JH, Arbuckle LD, Skamene E. Genetic dissection of inflammatory responses. *J Inflam* 1995;45:27–48.
8. Wicker LS, Todd JA, Peterson LB. Genetic control of autoimmune diabetes in the NOD mouse. *Ann Rev Immunol* 1995;13:179–200.
9. Benacerraf B. Role of MHC gene products in immune regulation. *Science* 1981;212:1229–1238.
10. Dietrich W, Miller J, Steen R, Merchant M, Damron D, Nahf R, Joyce D, Wessel M, Dredge R, Marquis A, Stein L, Goodman L, Page D, Lander ES. A genetic map of the mouse with 4006 simple sequence length polymorphisms. *Nature Genet* 1994;7:220–245.
11. Jacob HJ, Brown DM, Bunker RK, et al. A genetic linkage map of the laboratory rat, *Rattus norvegicus*. *Nature Genet* 1995;9:63–69.
12. Gyapay G, Morissette J, Vignal A, Dib C, Fizames C, Marc S, Bernadi G, Lathrop GM. 1996–1994 Genethon-human genetic linkage map. *Nature Genet* 1994;7:246–339.
13. Lander ES, Schork NJ. Genetic Dissection of complex traits. *Science* 1994;265:2037–2049.
14. Weeks DE, Lathrop M. Polygenic disease: methods for mapping complex traits. *Trends Genet* 1995;513–519.
15. Jorde LB. Linkage disequilibrium as a gene-mapping tool. *Am J Hum Genet* 1995;56:11–14.
16. Krco CJ, David CS. Genetics of Immune Response. *CRC Crit Rev Immunol* 1981;1:211–257.
17. Pearce EJ, Reiner SL. Induction of Th2 responses in infectious diseases. *Curr Opin Immunol* 1995;7:497–504.
18. Chiang BL, Bearer E, Ansari A, Dorshkind K, Gershwin ME. BM12 mutation and autoantibodies to dsDNA in NZB.H-2^{bm12} mice. *J Immunol* 1990;145:94–101.
19. Wicker LS, Appel MC, Dotta F, Pressey A, Miller BJ, DeLarato LH, Fischer PA, Boltz RC Jr, Peterson LB. Autoimmune syndromes in major histocompatability (MHC) congenic strains of nonobese diabetic (NOD) mice. The NOD MHC is dominant for insulitis and cyclophosphamide-induced diabetes. *J Exp Med* 1992;176:67–77.
20. Drake CG, Rozzo SJ, Hirschfeld HF, Swarnworawong NP, Palmer E, Kotzin BL. Analysis of New Zealand contribution to Lupus-like renal disease. *J Immunol* 1995;154:2441–2447.
21. Rudofsky UH, Evans BD, Balaban SL, Mottironi VD, Gabgielstien AE. Differences in expression of lupus in New Zealand mixes H-2^z homozygous inbred strains of mice derived from New Zealand black and New Zealand white mice. *Lab Invest* 1993;68:419–426.
22. Morel L, Rudofsky UH, Longmate JA, Schiffenbauer J, Wakeland EK. Polygenic control of susceptibility to murine systemic lupus erythematosus. *Immunity* 1994;219–229.
23. Groot PC, Moen CJA, Dietrich W, Stoye JP, Lander ES, Demant P. The recombinant congenic strains for the analysis of multigenic traits: genetic composition. *FASEB J* 1992;6:2826–2835.
24. Yamamura K, Miyazaki T, Uno M, Toyanaga T, Miyazaki J. Nonobese diabetes transgenic mouse. *Springer Semin Immunopathol* 1992;114:115–125.
25. Woods A, Chen HY, Trumbauer ME, Sirotina A, Cummings R, Zaller DM. Human major histocompatibility complex class II-restricted T cell responses in transgenic mice. *J Exp Med* 1994;180: 173–181.
26. Altmann DM, Douek DC, Frater AJ, Hetherington CM, Inoko H, Elliot JI. The T cell response of HLA-transgenic mice to human myelin basic protein and other antigens in the presence and absence of human CD4. *J Exp Med* 1995;181:867–876.
27. Larsson SH, Charlieu JP, Miyagawa K, Engelkamp D, Rassoulzadegan M, Cuzin F, van Heyningen V, Hastie ND. Subnuclear localization of WT1 in splining or transcription factor domains is regulated by alternative splicing. *Cell* 1995;81:391–401.
28. Vyse TJ, Todd JA. Genetic analysis of autoimmune disease. *Cell* 1996;85:311–318.
29. Druet E,Sapin C, Gunther E, Feingold N, Druet P. Mercuric chloride-induced anti-glomerular basement membrane antibodies in the rat: genetic studies. *Eur J Immunol* 1977;7:348–351.
30. Liblau RS, Singer SM, McDevitt HO. Th1 and Th2 CD4 - T cells in the pathogenesis of organ-specific autoimmune diseases. *Immunol Today* 1995;16:34–38.
31. Theofilopoulos AN. The basis of autoimmunity: part II genetic predisposition. *Immunol Today* 1995;16:150–158.
32. Hearne CM, Ghosh S, Todd JA. Microsatellites for linkage analysis to genetic traits. *Trends Genet* 1992;8:288–294.
33. Todd JA, Aitman TJ, Cornall RJ, Ghosh S, Hall JRS, Hearne CM, Knight AM, McAleer MA, Prins J-b, Rodrigues N, Lathrop M, Pressey A, DeLarato NH, Peterson LB, Wicker LS. The genetic analysis of autoimmune type I diabetes in mice. *Nature* 1991;351: 542–547.
34. Guler ML, Gorham JD, Hsieh C-S, Mackey AJ, Steen RG, Dietrich WF, Murphy KM. Genetic susceptibility to Leishmania in Th1 cell development. *Science* 1996;271:984–987.
35. Germain RN. MHC dependent antigen processing and presentation: providing ligands for T cell activation. *Cell* 1994;76:287–299.
36. York IA, Rock KL. Antigen processing and presentation by the class I major histocompatibility complex. *Ann Rev Immunol* 1996;14: 369–396.
37. Madden DR. The three dimensional structure of peptide MHC complexes. *Ann Rev Immunol* 1995;13:587–622.
38. Rammensee HG. Chemistry of peptides associated with MHC class I and class II molecules. *Curr Opin Immunol* 1995;7:85–96.
39. Rammensee HG, Friede T, Stevanovic S. MHC ligands and peptide motifs: first listing. *Immunogenetics* 1995;41:178–228.
40. Hammer J, Bono E, Gallazzi F, Belunis C, Nagy Z, Sinigaglia F. Precise prediction of major histocompatibility complex class II-peptide interactions based on peptide side chain scanning. *J Exp Med* 1994; 180:2353–2358.
41. Marshall K, Wilson K, Zaller D, Rothbard J. Prediction of peptide affinity to HLA-DR molecules. *Biomed Pept Prot Nucl Acids* 1995;1: 157–162.
42. Goldberg AL, St John AC. Intracellular protein degradation in mammalian and bacterial cells: part II. *Ann Rev Biochem* 45:747–803.
43. Lehner PJ, Cresswell P. Processing and delivery of peptides presented by MHC class I molecules. *Curr Opin Immunol* 1996;8:59–67.
44. Momburg F, Roelse J, Hammerling GJ, Neefjes JJ. Peptide size selection by the major histocompatibility complex-encoded peptide transporter. *J Exp Med* 1994;179:1613–1623.
45. Momberg F, Roelse J, Howard JC, Butcher GW, Hammerling GJ, Neefjes JJ. *Nature* 1994;367:648–651.
46. Neefjes JJ, Ploegh HL. Allele and locus specific differences in cell surface expression and the association of HLA class I heavy chain with beta-2 microglobulin. *Eur J Immunol* 1988;18:801–810.
47. Heemels M-T, Ploegh HL. Substrate specificity of the allelic variants of the TAP peptide transporter. *Immunity* 1994;I:775–784.
48. Schumacher TN, Kantesaria DV, Roopenian DC, Ploegh HL. Transporters from H-2 b,H-2 k and H-2 g7 (NOD/Lt) haplotype transport similar sets of peptides. *Proc Natl Acad Sci USA* 1994;92: 13004–13008.
49. Jackson DG, Capra JD. TAP-2 association with insulin-dependent diabetes mellitus is secondary to HLA-DQB1. *Hum Immunol* 1995; 43:57–65.
50. Denzin LK, Cresswell P. HLA-DM induces CLIP dissociation from MHC class II alpha beta dimers and facilitates peptide loading. *Cell* 1995;82:155–165.
51. Brooks AG, Campbell PL, Reynolds P, Gautam AM, McCluskey J. Antigen presentation and assembly by mouse I-Ak class II molecules

in APC containing deleted or mutated HLA-DM genes. *J Immunol* 1994;153:5382–5392.

52. Diment S, Shinde S. Selective processing of exogenous antigens by antigen-presenting cells with deleted MHC genes. *J Immunol* 1995;154:530–535.
53. Stebbins CC, Loss GE Jr, Elias CG, Chervonsky A, Sant AJ. The requirement for DM in class II restricted antigen presentation and stable dimer formation is allele and species specific. *J Exp Med* 1995; 181:223–234.
54. Sette A, Southwood S, Miller J, Appella E. Binding of major histocompatibility complex class II to the invariant chain derived peptide, CLIP, is regulated by allelic polymorphism in the class II. *J Exp Med* 1995;181:677–683.
55. Rudensky A, Preston-Hurlburt P, Hong S, Barlow A, Janeway CA. Sequence analysis of peptides bound to MHC class II molecules. *Nature* 1991;353:622–627.
56. Chicz RM, Urban RG, Gorga JC, Vignali DA, Lane WS, Strominger JL. Specificity and promiscuity among naturally processed peptides bound to HLA DR molecules. *J Exp Med* 1993;178:27–47.
57. Wucherpfennig KW, Bei Y, Bhol K etc. Structural basis for major histocompatibility complex (MHC)-linked susceptibility to autoimmunity: charged residues of a single MHC pocket confer selective presentation of self-peptides in pemphigus vulgaris. *Proc Natl Acad Sci USA* 1995;181:1847–1855.
58. Hammer J, Gallazzi F, Bono E, et al. Peptide binding specificity of HLA-DR4 molecules: correlation with rheumatoid arthritis association. *J Exp Med* 1995;181:1847–1855.
59. Fairchild P, Wildgoose R, Atherton E, Webb S, Wraith D. An autoantigenic T cell epitope forms unstable complexes with class II MHC: a novel route of escape from tolerance induction. *Int Immunol* 1993;5:1151–1158.
60. Valli A, Sette A, Kappos L, et al. Binding of myelin basic protein peptides I human histcompatibility leukocyte antigen class II molecules and their recognition by T cells from multiple sclerosis patients. *J Clin Invest* 1993;91:616–628.
61. Matsuo H, Battocchi A-P, Hawke S, etc . Peptide selected T cell lines from patients and controls recognise peptides that are not processed from whole acetylcholine receptor. *J Immunol* 1995;155:3683–3692.
62. Siliman M, Kaplan E, Yanagawa T, Hidaka Y, Fisfalen ME, DeGroot LJ. T cells recognise multiple epitopes in the human thyrotropin receptor extracellular domain. *J Clin Endocrin Metab* 1995;80;905–914.
63. Phelps RG, Turner AN, Rees AJ. Direct identification of naturally processed peptides bound to HLA-DR 15. *J Biol Chem* 1996;271: 18549–18553.
64. Nelson CA, Roof RW, McCourt DW, Unanue ER. Identification of naturally processed peptide from hen egg lysozyme bound to the murine major histocompatibility complex class II molecule I-Ak. *Proc Nat Acad Sci USA* 1992;89:7380–7383.
65. Nelson CA, Viner N, Young S, Petzold S, Benoist C, Mathis D, Unanue ER. Amino acid residues on the I-Ak alpha-chain required for binding and stability of two antigenic peptides. *J Immunol* 1996;156: 176–182.
66. Baker D, Rosenwasser OA, O'Neill JK, Turk JL. Genetic analysis of experimental allergic encephalomyelitis in mice. *J Immunol* 1995;155: 4046–4051.
67. De Franco M, Gille-Perramant MF, Mevel JC, Couderc J. T helper subset involvement in two high antibody responder lines of mice (Biozzi): HI (susceptible) and HII (resistant) to collagen-induced arthritis. *Eur J Immunol* 1995;25:132–136.
68. Puel A, Groot PC, Lathrop MG, Demant P, Mouton D. Mapping genes controlling antibody production in Biozzi mice. *J Immunol* 1995;154:5799–5805.
69. Prins JB, Todd JA, Rodrigues ND, Gosh S, Hogarth PM, Wicker LS, Gaffney E, Podolin PL, Fischer PA, Sirotina A, Peterson LB. Linkage on chromosome 3 of autoimmune diabetes and defective Fc receptor for IgG in NOD mice. *Science* 1993;260:695–698.
70. Stewart MR, Reinhardt MC, Staines NA. The genetic control of antibody affinity. Evidence from breeding studies with mice selectively bred for either high or low antibody affinity antibody production. *Immunology* 1979;37:697–702.
71. Devey ME, Stewart MR. The induction of chronic antigen–antibody complex disease in selectively bred mice producing either high or low affinity antibody to protein antigens. *Immunology* 1980;41: 303–311.
72. Paul WE, Seder RA. Lymphocyte responses and cytokines. *Cell* 1994;76:241–251.
73. Scott B, Liblau RS, Degermann S, Marconi LA, Ogata L, Caton AJ, McDevitt HO, Lo D. A role for non-MHC genetic polymorphism in susceptibility to spontaneous autoimmunity. *Immunity* 1994;1:73–82.
74. Mason D. Genetic variation in the stress response: susceptibility to experimental allergic encephalomyelitis and implications for human inflammatory disease. *Immunol Today* 1991;12:57–60.
75. Murray JS, Pfeiffer C, Madri J, Bottomley K. Major histocompatibility complex (MHC) control of CD4 T cell subset activation, II. A single peptide induces either humoral or cell mediated responses in mice of distinct MHC genotype. *Eur J Immunol* 1992;22:559–565.
76. Murray JS, Madri J, Pasqualini T, Bottomley K. Functional CD4 subset interplay in an intact immune system. *J Immunol* 1993;150: 4270–4276.
77. Amadori A, Zamarchi R, De Silvestro G, Forza G, Cavatton G, Danieli GA, Clementi M, Chieco-Bianchi L. Genetic control of the CD4/CD8 T-cell ratio in humans. *Nature Med* 1995;1:1279–1283.
78. Ibanez OM, Stiffel C, Ribeiro OG, Cabrera WK, Massa S, de Franco M, Sant' Anna OA, Decreusefond C, Mouton D, Siqueira M. Genetics of nonspecific immunity: I. Bidirectional selective breeding of lines of mice endowed with maximal and minimal inflammatory responsiveness. *Eur J Immunol* 1992;22:2555–2563.
79. Blackwell JM, Barton White JK, Roach TIA, Shaw MA, Whitehead TA, Mock BA, Searle S, Williams H, Baker AM. Genetic regulation of leishmanial and mycobacterial infection: the Lsh/Ity/Bcg story continues. *Immunol Lett* 1994;43:99–107.
80. Vidal SM, Malo D, Vogan K, Skemene E, Gros P. Natural resistance gene to infection with intracellular parasites: identification for a candidate gene for Bcg. *Cell* 1993;73:1–20.
81. Malo D, Vogan K, Vidal S, Hu J, Cellier M, Schurr E, Fuks A, Bumstead N, Morgan K, Gros G. Haplotype mapping and sequence analysis of the mouse *Nramp* gene which predicts susceptibility to infection with intracellular parasites. *Genomics* 1994;23:51–61.
82. Buschman E, Taniyama T, Nakamura R, Skamene E. Functional expression of the Bcg gene in macrophages. *Res Immunol* 1989;140: 793–797.
83. Cellier M, Govoni G, Vidal S, Groulx N, Liu J, Sanchez F, Skamena E, Schurr E, Gros P. The human NRAMP gene: cDNA cloning, chromosomal mapping, genomic organisation and tissue specific expression. *J Exp Med* 1994;180:1741–1752.
84. White JK, Shaw MA, Barton CH, Cerretti DP, Williams H, Mock BA, Carter NP, Peacock CS, Blackwell JM. Genetic and physical mapping of 2q35 in the region of the NRAMP and IL8R genes: identification of a polymorphic repeat in exon 2 of NRAMP. *Genomics* 1994;295–302.
85. Danis VA, Millington M, Hyland VJ, Grennan D, Cytokine production by normal human monocytes: inter-subject variation and relationship to an IL-1 receptor antagonist gene polymorphism. *Clin Exp Immunol* 1995;99:303–310.
86. Lennard AC. Interleukin-1 receptor antagonist. *CRC Crit Rev Immunol* 1995;15:77–105.
87. Wilson AG, di Giovine FS, Duff GW. Genetics of tumour necrosis factor-α in autoimmune, infectious, and neoplastic diseases. *J Inflam* 1995;45:1–12.
88. Wilson AG, de Vries N, Pociot F, di Giovine F, van der Putte LBA, Duff GW. An allelic polymorphism within the human tumour necrosis promoter region is strongly associated with HLA A1, B8, DR3 alleles. *J Exp Med* 1993;177:567–560.
89. Stuber F, Udalova IA, Book M, Drutskaya N, Kruprash DV, Turetskaya RL, Schrade FU, Nedospasov SA. -308 tumour necrosis factor (TNF) polymorphism is not associated with survival in severe sepsis and is unrelated to lipopolysaccharide inducibility of the human promoter. *J Inflam* 1996;46:42–50.
90. Bendtzen K, Morling N, Fomsgaard A, Svenson M, Jakobsen B, Odum N Svejgaard A. Association between hla-dr2 and production of tumour necrosis factor and interleukin -1 a by mononuclear cells activated by lipopolysaccharide. *Scand J Immunol* 1988;28: 599–606.
91. Bailly S, di Giovine FS, Blakemore AI, Duff GW. Genetic polymorphism of human interleukin-1 α. *Eur J Immunol* 1993;23:1240–1245.
92. Pociot F, Molvig J, Wogensen, Worsae H, Nerup J. A taq I polymorphism in the human interleukin gene correlates with IL-1 β secretion in vitro. *Eur J Clin Invest* 1992;22:396–402.

93. Fey MF, Tobler A. An interleukin-8 (IL-8) cDNA clone identifies a frequent HindIII polymorphism. *Human Genet* 1993;91:298.
94. Jacob CO, Mykytyn K, Tashman N. DNA polymorphism in cytokine genes based on length variation in simple-sequence tandem repeats. *Immunogenetics* 1993;38:251–257.
95. Stuffers-Heimann, M., Günther, E. And Van Es. L.A. Induction of autoimmunity to antigens of the glomerular basement membrane in inbred Brown-Norway rats. *Immunology* 1979;36:759–767.
96. Sado Y, Naito I, Akita M, Okigaki T. Strain specific responses of inbred rats on the severity of experimental autoimmune glomerulonephritis. *J Clin Lab Immunol* 1986;19:193–199.
97. Pusey CD, Holland MJ, Cashman SJ, et al. Experimental autoimmune glomerulonephritis induced by homologous and isologous glomerular basement membrane in Brown-Norway rats. *Nephrol Dial Transplant* 1991;6:457–465.
98. Mavronmatidis K, Reynolds J, Cashman SJ, Evans DJ, Pusey CD. Experimental autoimmune glomerulonephritis (EAG) in the WKY rat. *J Pathol* 1993;169:125A.
99. Bolton WK, May WJ, Sturgill BC. Proliferative autoimmune glomerulonephritis in rats: a model of autoimmune glomerulonephritis in humans. *Kidney Int* 1993;44(2):294–306.
100. Sado Y, Kagawa M, Naito I, Ogikaki T. Properties of bovine nephrotogenic antigen that induces anti-GBM nephritis in rats and its similarity to the Goodpasture antigen. *Virchows Archiv B Cell Pathol* 1991;60:3345–351.
101. Stenglein B, Thoenes GH, Günther E. Genetically controlled autologous immune complex glomerulonephritis in rats. *J Immunol* 1975; 115(4):895–897.
102. Stenglein B, Thoenes GH, Günther E. Genetic control of susceptibility to autologous immune complex glomerulonephritis in inbred rat strains. *Clin Exp Immunol* 1978;33:88–94.
103. Lehman DH, Curtis B, Wilson, Dixon FJ. Interstitial nephritis in rats immunised with heterologous tubular basement membrane. *Kidney Int* 1974;5:187–195.
104. Krieger A, Thoenes GH, Günther E. Genetic control of autoimmune tubulointerstitial nephritis in rats. *Clin Immunol Immunopathol* 1981; 21:301–308.
105. Andres GA, McCluskey T. Tubular and interstitial renal disease due to immunologic mechanisms. *Kidney Int* 1975;7:271–289.
106. Neilson EG, Phillips SM. Murine interstitial nephritis. I. Analysis of disease susceptibility and its relationship to pleomorphic gene products defining both immune-response genes and a restrictive requirement for cytotoxic T cells at H-2K. *J Exp Med* 1982;155: 1075–1085.
107. Hyman LR, Steinberg AD, Colvin RB, Bernard EF. Immunopathogenesis of autoimmune tubulointerstitial nephritis II. Role of an immune response gene linked to the major histocompatibility complex. *J Immunol* 1976;117(5-2):1894–1897.
108. Smoyer WE, Kelly CJ. Inherited interstitial nephritis in kdkd mice. *Int Rev Immunol* 1994;11:245–251.
109. Neilson EG, McCafferry E, Feldman A, Clayman MD, Zakheim B, Korngold R. Spontaneous interstitial nephritis in kd/kd mice. I. An experimental model of autoimmune renal disease. *J Immunol* 1984; 133(5):2560–2565.
110. Goldman M, Druet P. The Thl/Th2 concept and its relevance to renal disorder and transplantation immunity. *Nephrol Dial Transplant* 1995;10:1282–1284.
111. Goldman M, Druet P, Gleichmann E. T_H2 cells in systematic autoimmunity: insights from allogeneic diseases and chemically-induced autoimmunity. *Immunol Today* 1991;12:223–227.
112. Goldman M, Druet P. The Thl/Th2 concept and its relevance to renal disorder and transplantation immunity. *Nephrol Dial Transplant* 1995;10:1282–1284.
113. Oliveira DB, Gillespie K, Wolfreys K, Mathieson PW, Quasim F, Coleman JW. Compounds that induce autoimmunity in the brown Norway rat sensitise mast cells for mediator release and interleukin-4 expression. *Eur J Immunol* 1995;25:2259–2264.
114. Prigent P, Saoudi A, Pannetier C, Graber P, Bonnefoy JY, Druet P, Hirsch F. Mercuric chloride, a chemical responsible for T helper cell (Th)2-mediated autoimmunity in brown Norway rats, directly triggers T cells to produce interleukin-4. *J Clin Invest* 1995;96:1484–1489.
115. Howie and Heyler 1968,116. Drake CG, Rozzo SJ, Vyse TJ, Palmer E, Kotzin BL. Genetic contribution to lupus like disease in (NZB x NZW) F1 mice. *Immunol Rev* 1995;144:51–73.
116. Hirose S, Ueda G, Noguchi K, Okada T, Sekigawa I, Stao H, Shirai T. Requirement of H-2 heterozygosity for autoimmunity in (NZBx NZW)F1 hybrid mice. *Eur J Immunol* 1986;16:1631–1633.
117. Kotzin BL, Palmer E. The contribution of NZW genes to lupus-like disease in (NZBxNZW)F1 mice. *J Exp Med* 1987;165:1237–1251.
118. Babcock SK, Appel VB, Schieff M, Palmer E, Kotzin BL. Genetic analysis of the imperfect association of H-2 haplotype with lupus-like autoimmune disease. *Proc Natl Acad Sci USA* 1989;86:7552–7555.
119. Ghatak S, Sainis K, Owen FL, Datta SK. T cell receptor beta and I-A beta chain genes of normal SWR mice are linked with the development of lupus nephritis in NZBxSWR crosses. *Proc Natl Acad Sci USA* 1987;84:6850–6853.
120. Chiang BL, Bearer E, Ansari A, Dorshkind K, Gershwin ME. The BM12 mutation and autoantibodies of dsDNA in NZB.H-2bm12 mice. *J Immunol* 1990;145:94–101.
121. Mengle-gaw L, Conners S, McDevitt HO, Fathman CG. Gene conversion between murine class II major histocompatibility complex loci. Functions and molecular evidence from bm12 mutant. *J Exp Med* 1984;160:1184–1194.
122. Nygard NR, McCarthy DM, Schiffenbauer J, Schwartz BD. Mixed haplotypes and autoimmunity. *Immunol Today* 1993;14:53–56.
123. Kono DH, Burlingame RW, Owens DG, Kuramochi A, Balderas RS, Balomenos D, Theofilopoulos AN. Lupus susceptibility loci in New Zealand mice. *Proc Natl Acad Sci USA* 1994;10168–10172.
124. Kotzin BL, Barr VL, Palmer E. A large deletion within the T-cell receptor beta-chain gene complex in New Zealand white mice. *Science* 1985;229:167–171.
125. Noonan DJ, Kofler R, Singer PA, Cardenas G, Dixon FJ, Theophilopoulos AN. Delineation of a defect in T cell receptor β genes of NZW mice predisposed to autoimmunity. *J Exp Med* 1986;163: 644–653.
126. Behkle MA, Chou HS, Huppik Loh DY. Murine T cell receptor Vβ deletion mutants with deletions of β chain variable region genes. *Proc Natl Acad ScI USA* 1986;83:767–771.
127. Watson ML, Rao JK, Gikeson GS, Ruiz P, Eicher EM, Pesetsky DS, Matsuzawa A, Rochell JM, Seldin MF. Genetic analysis of MRL-*lpr* mice: relationship of the *Fas* apoptosis gene to disease manifestation and renal disease-modifying loci. *J Exp Med* 1992;176: 1645–1656.
128. Watanabe-Fugunaka R, Brannan CI, Copeland NG, Jenkins NA, Nagata S. Lymphoproliferation disorder in mice explained by defects in *Fas* antigen that medicates apoptosis. *Nature* 1992;356: 314–317.
129. Wu J, Zhou T, Zhang J, Gause WC, Mountz JD. Correction of accelerated autoimmune disease by early replacement of the mutated *lpr* gene with the normal *Fas* apoptosis gene in the T cells of transgenic MRL-*lpr/lpr* mice. *Proc Natl Acad Sci USA* 1995;91: 2344–2348.
130. Matsuzawa A, Moriyama T, Kaneko T, Tanaka M, Kimura M, Ikeda H, Katagiri T. A new allele of the *lpr* locus, *lprg*, that complements the gld gene in induction of lymphadenopathy in the mouse. *J Exp Med* 1990;171:519–531.
131. Davidson WF, Dumont FJ, Bedigian HG, Fowlkes BJ, Morse HC. Phenotypic, functional, and molecular genetic comparisons of the abnormal lymphoid cells of C3H-*lpr.lrp* and C3H-*gld/gld* mice. *J Immunol* 1987;136:4075–4084.
132. Strasser A, Whittingham S, Vaux DL, Bath ML, Adams JM, Cory S, Harris AW. Enforced BCL2 expression in B lymphoid cells prolongs antibody responses and elicits autoimmune disease. *Proc Natl Acad Sci USA* 1991;88:8661–8665.
133. Kinjoh K, Kyogoku M, Good RA. Genetic selection for crescent formation yields mouse strain with rapidly progressive glomerulonephritis and small vessel vasculitis. *Proc Natl Acad Sci USA* 1993;90: 3413–3417.
134. Kettitz R, Yang JJ, Kinjo K, Jenette JC, Falk RJ. Animal models in ANCA vasculitis. *Clin Exp Immunol* 1995;101(Suppl):12–15.
135. Scolari F, Amoroso A, Savoldi S, Prati E, Scaini P, Manganoni A, Borelli I, Mazzola G, Canale L, Sacchi G. Familial occurrences of primary glomerulonephritis: evidence for a role for genetic factors. *Nephrol Dial Transplant* 1992;7:587–596.
136. Suarez BK, Rice J, Reich T. The generalized sib pair IBD distribution: its use in detection of linkage. *Ann Hum Genet* 1978;42:87–94.
137. Lander ES, Botstein D. Mapping Mendelian factors underlying quantitative traits using RFLP linkage maps. *Genetics* 1989;121:185–199.

138. Green A. The epidemiologic approach to studies of the association between HLA and disease II: estimation of absolute risks etiologic and preventative fraction. *Tissue Antigens* 1982;19:259–268.
139. Payami H, Joe S, Farid NR, Stenszky V, Chan SH, Yeo PPB, Cheah JS, Thomson G. Relative predispositional effects (RPEs) of marker alleles with disease: HLA DR alleles and Graves Disease. *Am J Hum Genet* 1989;45:541–556.
140. Thomson G, Robinson WP, Kuhner MK, et al. Genetic heterogeneity, modes of inheritance and risk estimates for a joint study of Caucasians with insulin dependent diabetes mellitus. *Am J Hum Genet* 1988;43:799–816.
141. Thomson G. Mapping disease genes: family-based association studies. *Am J Hum Genet* 1995;57:487–498.
142. Hodge SE. Linkage analysis versus association analysis: distinguishing between two models that explain disease-marker associations. *Am J Hum Genet* 1993;53:367–384.
143. Thomson G. HLA disease associations: models for the study of complex human genetic disorders. *CRC Crit Rev Clin Lab Sci* 1995;32: 183–219.
144. Campbell RD, Trowsdale J. Map of the Human MHC. *Immunol Today* 1993;14:349–352.
145. Campbell DR, Low SKA, Reid KBM, Sim RB. Structure organisation and regulation of the complement genes. *Ann Rev Immunol* 1988;6: 161–195.
146. Nepom GT, Erlich H. MHC class II molecules and autoimmunity. *Ann Rev Immunol* 1991;9:493–525.
147. Burns A, Li P, Rees AJ. Immunogenetics of nephritis. In: Pusey CD, ed. *Immunology of Renal Diseases*. Dordrecht: Kluwer Academic Publishers, 1991.
148. Turner AN, Lockwood CM, Rees AJ. Goodpasture's disease. In: RW Shrier, CW Gottschalk, eds. *Diseases of the Kidney*, 5th ed. Boston: Little, Brown & Co, 1993;1865–1894.
149. Gossain V, Gerstein AR, Janes AW Goodpasture's syndrome: a familial occurrence. *Am Rev Respir Dis* 1972;105:621–624.
150. Simonsen H, Brun C, Thomsen OF, Larsen S, Ladefoged J. Goodpasture's syndrome in twins. *Acta Med Scand* 1982;212:425–428.
151. d'Apice AJ, Kincaid Smith P, Becker GH, Loughhead MG, Freeman JW, Sands JM. Goodpasture's syndrome in identical twins. *Ann Intern Med* 1978;88:61–62.
152. Almkuist R D, Buckalew VM Jr, Hirszel P, Maher JF, James PM, Wilson, CB. Recurrence of anti-glomerular basement membrane antibody mediated glomerulonephritis in an isograft. *Clin Immunol Immunopathol* 1981;18:54–60.
153. Rees AJ, Peters DK, Compston DA, Batchelor JR. Strong association between HLA-DRW2 and antibody-mediated Goodpasture's syndrome. *Lancet* 1978;1:966–968.
154. Rees AJ, Peters DK, Amos N, Welsh KI, Batchelor JR. The influence of HLA-linked genes on the severity of anti-GBM antibody-mediated nephritis. *Kidney Int* 1984;26:445–450.
155. Perl SI, Pussell BA, Charlsworth JA, MacDonald GJ, Wolnizer M. Goodpasture's (anti-GBM) disease and HLA-DRw2. *N Engl J Med* 1981;305:463–464.
156. Garovoy MR. Immunogenetic associations in nephrotic states. *Contemp Issues Nephrol* 1982;9:259–282.
157. Huey B, McCormick K, Capper J, Ratliff C, Colombe BW, Garovoy MR, Wilson CB. Associations of HLA-DR and HLA-DQ types with anti-GBM nephritis by sequence-specific oligonucleotide probe hybridization. *Kidney Int* 1993;44:307–312.
158. Dunckley H, Chapman JR, Burke J, Charlesworth J, Hayes J, Harwood E, Hutchison B, Ibels L, Kalowski S, Kinkaid-Smith P, Lawrence S, Lewis D, Moran J, Pussell BA, Restifo A, Stewart J, Thacher G, Walker R, Waugh D, Wilson D, Wyndham R. HLA-DR and DQ genotyping in anti-GBM disease. *Dis Markers* 1991;9: 249–296.
159. Mercier B, Bourbigot O Raguenes O, Rondeau E, Simon P, Legrendre C, Hurault de Ligny B, Lang P, Mourad G, Legrand D, Coville P, Ferec C. HLA class II typing of Goodpasture's syndrome affected patients. *JASN* 1992;3:658(abs).
160. Burns AP, Fisher M, Pusey CD, Rees AJ. Molecular analysis of HLA class II genes in Goodpasture's disease. *Quart J Med* 1995;88: 93–100.
161. Fisher M, Pusey CD, Vaughan RW, Rees AJ. Susceptibility to Goodpasture's is strongly associated with HLA-DRB1 genes. *Kidney Int*, in press.
162. Rees AJ, Demaine AG, Welsh KI. Association of immunoglobulin Gm allotypes with antiglomerular basement membrane antibodies and their titer. *Hum Immunol* 1984;10:213–220.
163. Short CD, Feehally J, Gokal R, Mallick NP. Familial membranous nephropathy. *Brit Med J* 1984;289:1500.
164. Vangelista A, Tazzari R, Banomini V. Idiopathic membranous nephropathy in 2 twin brothers. *Nephron* 1988;50:79–80.
165. Klouda PT, Manos J, Acheson EJ, Dyer PA, Goldby FS, Harris R, Lawler W, Mallick NP, Williams G. Strong association between idiopathic membranous nephropathy and HLA-DRW3. *Lancet* 1979;2: 770–771.
166. Garovoy MR. Idiopathic membranous glomerulonephritis (IMGN): an HLA associated disease. In: Terasaki P, ed *Histocompatibility workshop 1980*. Los Angeles: Los Angeles University Press, 1980;673–680.
167. Muller GA, Muller CA, Liebau G, Kompf J, Ising H, Wernet P. Strong association of idiopathic membranous nephropathy (IMN) with HLA-DR3 and MT-2 without involvement of HLA-b18 and no association to BfF1. *Tissue Antigens* 1981;17:332–337.
168. Le Petit JC, Laurent B, Berthoux FC. HLA-DR3 and idiopathic membranous nephritis (IMN) association. *Tissue Antigens* 1982;20: 227–228.
169. Rashid HU, Papiha SS, Agroyannis B, Morley AR, Ward MK, Kerr DN. The associations of HLA and other genetic markers with glomerulonephritis. *Hum Genet* 1983;63:38–44.
170. Papiha SS, Pareek SK, Rodger RS, Morley AR, Wilkinson R, Roberts DF, Kerr DN. HLA-A,B,DR and Bf allotypes in patients with idiopathic membranous nephropathy (IMN). *Kidney Int* 1987;31:130–134.
171. Zucchelli P, Ponticelli C, Cagnoli L, Aroldi A, Tabacchi P. Genetic factors in the outcome of idiopathic membranous nephropathy [letter]. *Nephrol Dial Transplant* 1987;1:265–266.
172. Roccatello D, Coppo R, Amoroso A, Curtoni ES, Martina ES, Basolo B, Amore A, Rollino C, Picciotto G. Failure to relate mononuclear phagocyte system function to HLA-A,B,C, DR, DQ antigens in membranous nephropathy. *Am J Kidney Dis* 1987;31:130–134.
173. Vaughan RW, Demaine AG, Welsh KI. A DQA1 allele is strongly associated with idiopathic membranous nephropathy. *Tissue Antigens* 1989;34:261–269.
174. Cameron JS, Healy MJR, Adu D. The Medical Research Council trial of short-term high-dose alternate day prednisolone in idiopathic membranous nephropathy with nephrotic syndrome in adults. *Quart J Med* 1990;74:133–156.
175. Vaughan RW, Tighe MR, Boki, Alexopoulos S, Papadakis J, Lanchbury JS, Welsh KI, Williams DG. An analysis of HLA class II gene polymorphism in British and Greek idiopathic membranous nephropathy patients. *Eur J Immunogenet* 1995;22:179–186.
176. Short CD, Dyer PA, Cairns SA, Manost J, Waltons C, Harris R, Mallick NP. A major histocompatibility system halotype associated with poor prognosis in idiopathic membranous nephropathy. *Dis Markers* 1983;1:189–196.
177. Hiki Y, Kobayashi Y, Itoh I, Kashiwagi N. Strong association of HLA-DR2 and MT1 with idiopathic membranous nephropathy in Japan. *Kidney Int* 1984;25:953–957.
178. Tomura S, Kashiwabara H, Tuchida H, Shishido H, Sakurai S, Tsuji K, Takeuchi J. Strong association of idiopathic membranous nephropathy with HLA-DR2 and MT1 in Japanese. *Nephron* 1984; 36:242–245.
179. Naito S, Kohara M, Arakawa A. Association of class II antigens of HLA with primary glomerulopathies. *Nephron* 1987;45:111–114.
180. Ogahara S, Naito S, Abe K, Michinaga I, Arakawa A. Analysis of HLA class II genes in Japanese patients with membranous nephropathy. *Kidney Int* 1992;41:175–182.
181. Sacks SH, Nomura S, Warner C, Naito S, Ogahara S, Vaughan R, Briggs D. Analysis of complement C4 loci in Caucasoids and Japanese with idiopathic membranous nephropathy. *Kidney Int* 1992;42: 882–887.
181a. Demaine AG, Vaughan RW, Taube DH, Welsh KI. Association of membranous nephropathy with T-cell receptor switch region polymorphisms. *Immunogenetics* 1988;27:19–23.
182. Thompson PD, Barratt TM, Stokes CR, Turner MW. HLA antigens and atopic features in steroid-responsive childhood nephrotic syndrome. *Lancet* 1976;2:765–768.
183. Trompeter PD, Barratt TM, Kay R, Turner MW, Soothill JF. HLA atopy and cyclophosphamide in steroid responsive childhood nephrotic syndrome. *Kidney Int* 1980;17:113–117.

184. O'Regan D, O'Callaghan U, Dundon S, Reen DJ. HLA antigens and steroid responsive nephrotic syndrome in childhood. *Tissue Antigens* 1980;16:147–151.
185. Lenhard V, Dippel J, Muller Wiefel DE, Schroder D, Seidl S, Scharer K. HLA antigens in children with idiopathic nephrotic syndrome. *Proc EDTA* 1980;17:673–677.
186. Alfiler CA, Roy LP, Doran T, Sheldon A, Bashir H. HLA-DRw7 and steroid responsive-nephrotic syndrome in childhood. *Clin Nephrol* 1980;14:71–74.
187. Mouzon-Cambon A, Bouissou F, Dutau G, Barthe P, Parra MT, Sevin A, Ohayon E. HLA-DR7 in children with idiopathic nephrotic syndrome. Correlation with atopy. *Tissue Antigens* 1981;17:518–524.
188. Noss G, Bachmann HJ, Obling H. Association of minimal change nephrotic syndrome (MCNS) with HLA-B8 and B13. *Clin Nephrol* 1981;15:172–174.
189. Meadow SR, Sarsfield JK, Scott DG, Rajah SM. Steroid responsive nephrotic syndrome and allergy:Immunological studies. *Arch Dis Child* 1981;56:517–524.
190. Ruder H, Scharer K, Lenhard V, Wingen AM, Oplez G. HLA phenotypes and idiopathic nephrotic syndrome in children. *Proc EDTA* 1982;19:602–606.
191. Rashid HU, Papiha SS, Agroyannis B, Morley AR, Ward MK, Kerr DN. The associations of HLA and other genetic markers with glomerulonephritis. *Hum Genet* 1983;63:38–44.
192. Komori K, Nose Y, Inouye H, Tsuji K, Nomoto Y, Tomino Y, Sakai H, Iwagaki H, Itoh H, Hasegawa O. Immunogenetic study in patients with chronic glomerulonephritis. *Tokai J Exp Clin Med* 1983;8: 135–148.
193. Berthoux, Gagne A, Sabatier JC, et al. HLA Bw35 antigen and mesangial IgA glomerulonephritis. *N Engl J Med* 1978;298: 1035–1035.
194. Brettle R, Peters DK, Batchelor JR. Mesangial IgA glomerulonephritis and HLA antigens. *N Engl J Med* 1978;299:200–201.
195. Noel LH, Descamps B, Jungers P, Bach JF, Busson M, Suet C, Hors J, Dausset J. HLA antigens in three types of glomerulonephritis Clin Immunol. *Immunopathol* 1978;10:19–23.
196. Nagy J, Hamorl A, Ambrus M, Nernadi E. More on IgA glomerulonephritis and HLA antigens. *N Engl J Med* 1979;300:92.
197. Savi M, Neri TM, Silvestri MG, Allegri L, Migone L. HLA antigens and IgA mesangial glomerulonephritis. *Clin Nephrol* 1979;12:45–46.
198. Macdonald IM, Dumble LJ, Kincaid Smith PS. HLA Bw35, circulating immune complexes and IgA deposits in mesangial proliferative glomerulonephritis. *Aust N Z J Med* 1980;10:480–481.
199. Bignon JD, Houssin A, Soulillou J, Denis J, Guimbretiere J, Guenel J. HLA antigens and Berger's disease. *Tissue Antigens* 1980;16: 108–111.
200. Faucet R, Le Pogamp P, Genetet B, Chevet D, Gueguen M, Simon P, Ramee MP, Cartier F. HLA-DR4 antigen and IgA nephropathy. *Tissue Antigens* 1980;16:405–410.
201. Moutonen J, Paternack A, Helin H, Rilva A, Penttinen K, Wager O, Harmoinen A. Circulating immune complexes, the concentration of serum IgA and the distribution of HLA antigens in IgA nephropathy. *Nephron* 1981;29:170–175.
202. Arnaiz-Villena A, Gonzalo A, Mampaso F, Teruel JL, Ortunno J. HLA and IgA nephropathy in Spanish population. *Tissue Antigens* 1981;17:549–550.
203. Rambausek M, Seelig HP, Andressy K, Waldherr R, Lenhard V, Ritz E. Clinical and serological features of mesangial IgA glomerulonephritis. *Proc EDTA* 1982;19:663–668.
204. Le Petit JC, Cazes MH, Berthoux JC, Van Loghem E, Goguen J, Seger J, Chapuis-Cellier C, Marcellin M, De Lange G, Garovoy MR, Serre JL, Brizard CP, Carpenter CD. Genetic investigation in mesangial IgA nephropathy. *Tissue Antigens* 1982;19:108–114.
205. Julian BA, Wyatt RJ, McMorrow RG, Galla JH. Serum complement proteins in IgA nephropathy. *Clin Nephrol* 1983;20:251–258.
206. Feehally J, Dyer PA, Davidson JA, Harris R, Mallick NP. Immunogenetics of IgA nephropathy: experience in a UK centre. *Dis Markers* 1984;2:493–500.
207. Hanly P, Garrett P, Spencer S, O'Dwyer WF. HLA-A,-B, and -DR antigens in IgA nephropathy. *Tissue Antigens* 1984;23:270–273.
208. Waldo BF, Beischel L, West CD. IgA synthesis by lymphocytes from patients with IgA nephropathy and their relatives. *Kidney Int* 1986; 29:1229–1232.
209. Berthoux FC, Alamartine E, Pommier G, Le Petit JC. HLA and IgA nephritis revisited 10 years later : HLA B35 antigen as a prognostic factor. *N Engl J Med* 1988;319:1609–1610.
210. Mouzon-Cambon A, Ohayon E, Bouissou F, Barthe P. HLA-DR typing in children with glomerular disease. *Lancet* 1980;2:868.
211. Berger J. IgA mesangial nephropathy. 1968 -1983 *Contrib Nephrol* 1984;40:4–6.
212. Kashiwabara H, Shishido H, Tomura S, Tuchida H, Miyajima T. Strong association between IgA nephropathy and HLA-DR4 antigen. *Kidney Int* 1982;22:377–382.
213. Komori K, Nose Y, Inouye H, Tsuji K, Nomoto Y, Tomino Y, Sakai H, Iwagaki H, Itoh H, Hasegawa O. Immunogenetic study in patients with chronic glomerulonephritis. *Tokai J Exp Clin Med* 1983;8: 135–148.
214. Komori K, Nose Y, Inouye H, Tsuji K, Nomoto Y, Sakai H. Study of HLA system in IgA nephropathy. *Tissue Antigens* 1979;14:32–36.215.
215. Kasahara M, Hamada K, Okuyama T, Ishikawa N, Ogasawara K, Ikeda H, Takenouchi T, Wakisaka A, Aizawa M, Kataoka Y, Miyamoto R, Kohara M, Naito S, Kashiwagi N, Hiki Y. Role of HLA in IgA nephropathy. *Clin Immunol Immunopathol* 1982;25: 189–195.
216. Hiki Y, Kobayashi Y, Tateno S, Sada M, Kashiwagi N. Strong association of HLA-DR4 with benign IgA nephropathy. *Nephron* 1982;32: 222–226.
217. Kohara M, Naito S, Arakawa K, Miyata J, Chihara J, Taguchi T, Takebayashi S. The strong association of HLA-DR4 with spherical mesangial dense deposits in IgA nephropathy. *J Clin Lab Immunol* 1985;18:157–160.
218. Hiki Y, Kobayashi Y, Ookubo M, Kashiwagi N. The role of HLA-DR4 in long-term prognosis of IgA nephropathy. *Nephron* 1990;54: 264–265.
219. Abe J, Kohsaka T, Tanaka M, Kobayashi N. Genetic study of HLA class II and class III region in the disease associated with IgA nephropathy. *Nephron* 1993;65:17–22.
220. Moore RH, Hitman GA, Lucas FY, Richards NT, Venning MC, Papiha S, Goodship THJ, Fidler A, Awad J, Festenstein H, Cunningham J, Marsh FP. HLA DQ gene polymorphism associated with primary IgA nephropathy. *Kidney Int* 1990;37:991–995.
221. Li KTP, Burns AP, So AKL, Pusey CD, Feehally J, Rees AJ. The DQ W& allele at the HLA DQB locus is associated with susceptibility to IgA nephropathy in Caucasians. *Kidney Int* 1991;39:961–965.
222. Moore RH, Medcraft J, Sinico RA, Mustonen J, Venning MC, Richards NT, D'Amico G, Hitman GA. Association of HLA DQ gene polymorphism in European IgA nephropathy. *Nephrol Dial Transplant* 1990;5:581–581.
223. Rambausek MH, Waldherr R, Ritz E. Immunogenetic findings in glomerulonephritis. *Kidney Int* 1993;43 suppl 39:S3–S8.
224. Luger AM, Komathireddy G, Walker RE, Pandey JP, Hoffman RW. Molecular and serological analysis of HLA genes and immunoglobulin allotypes in IgA nephropathy. *Autoimmunity* 1994;19:1–5.
225. Moore RH, Hitman GA, Medcraft J, Sinico RA, Mustonen J, Lucas EY, D'Amico G. HLA-DP gene polymorphism in primary IgA nephropathy: no association. *Nephrol Dial Transplant* 1992;7: 200–204.
226. Demaine AG, Rambausek MH, Knight JF, Williams DG, Welsh KI, Ritz E. Relation of IgA glomerulonephritis to polymorphism of the immunoglobulin heavy chain switch region. *J Clin Invest* 1988; 81:611–614.
227. Moore RH, Hitman GA, Sinico RA, Mustonen J, Medcraft J, Lucas EY, Richards NT, Venning MC, Cunningham J, Marsh FP, D'Amico G. Immunoglobulin heavy chain switch region gene polymorphisms in glomerulonephritis. *Kidney Int* 1990;38:332–336.
228. Rees AJ. Vasculitis and the kidney. *Curr Opin Nephrol Hypertens* 1996;5:274–281.
229. Muller GA, Gebhardt M, Kompf J, Baldwin WM: Association between rapidly progressive glomerulonephritis and the properdin factor BfF and different HLA-D region products. *Kidney Int* 1984;25: 115–8.
230. Elkon KB, Sutherland DC, Rees AJ, Hughes GRV, Batchelor JR. HLA frequencies in systemic vasculitis: increase in HLA DR2 in Wegeners Granulomatosis. *Arthritis Rheum* 1983;26:98–101.
231. Spencer SJW, Burns A, Gaskin G, Pusey CD, Rees AJ: HLA class II specificities in vasculitis with antibodies to neutrophil cytoplasmic antigens. *Kidney Int* 1992;41:1059–1063.
232. Zhang L, Jayne DR, Zhao MH, Lockwood CM, Oliveira DB: Distrib-

ution of MHC class II alleles in primary systematic vasculitis. *Kidney Int* 1995;47:294–298.

233. Hagen EC, Stegeman CA, D'Amaro J, Shrender GMT, Lems SPM, Cohen Tervaert JW, DeJong GMTh, Hene RJ, Kallenberg CGM, Daha MR. Decreased frequency of HLA DR6 in Wegeners Granulomatosis. *Kidney Int* 1995;48;801–805.
234. Esnault VLM, Testa A, Audrain M, et al. Alpha l-antitrypsin genetic polymorphism in ANCA-positive systemic vasculitis. *Kidney Int* 1993;43:1329–32.
235. O'Donoghue DJ, Guickian M, Blundell G, Winney RJ. Alpha-1-proteinase inhibitor and pulmonary haemorrhage in systemic vasculitis. In: Gross WL, ed. *ANCA-Associated Vasculitides: Immunological and Clinical Aspects*. New York: Plenum Press, 1993;331–335.
236. Lhotta K, Vogel W, Meisl T, Buxbaum M, Neyer U, Sandholzer C, Konig P. Alpha 1-antitrypsin in patients with anti-neutrophil cytoplasmic antibody-positive vasculitis. *Clin Sci* 1994;87:693–695.
237. Savige JA, Chang L, Cook L, Burdon J, Daskalakis M, Doery J. Alpha 1-antitrypsin deficiency and anti-proteinase 3 antibodies in anti-neutrophil cytoplasmic antibody (ANCA)-associated systematic vasculitis. *Clin Exp Immunol* 1995;100:194–197.
238. Elzouki AN, Segelmark M, Wieslander J, Eriksson S. Strong link between the alpha 1-antitrypsin PiZ allele and Wegender's granulomatosis. *J Intern Med* 1994;236:543–548.
239. Griffith ME, Lovegrove JU, Gaskin G, Whitehouse DB, et al. C-antineutrophil cytoplasmic antibody positivity in vasculitis patients is associated with the Z allele of alpha-1-antitrypsin, and P-antineutrophil cytoplasmic antibody positivity with the S allele. *Nephrol Dial Transplant* 1996;11:438–443.
240. Finn JE, Zhang L, Agrawal S, Jayne DRW, et al. Molecular analysis of C3 allotypes in patients with systemic vasculitis. *Nephrol Dial Transplant* 1994;9:1564–1567.
241. Lewkonia RM. The clinical genetics of lupus. *Lupus* 1992;1:55–62.
242. Woodrow JC. Immunogenetics of systemic lupus erythematosus. *J Rheumatol* 1988;15:197–199.
243. Fronek Z, Timmerman LA, Alper CA, et al. Major histocompatibility genes and susceptibility to systemic lupus erythematosus. *Arthritis Rheum* 1990;33:1542–1553.
244. Hawkins BR, Wong KL, Chan KH, Dunckley H Serjeantson SW. Strong association between the major histocompatibility complex and systemic lupus erythematosus in southern Chinese. *J Rheumatol* 1987;15:197–199.
245. Hartnung K, Bauer Mp, Coldwey R, Fricke M, Kalden JR, Lakomek HJ, Peter JH, Schrendel D, Schneider PM, Seuchter SA, Stangel W, Deichter HRT. Major histocompatibility haplotypes and complement C4 alleles in systemic lupus erythematosus. *J Clin Invest* 1992;90: 1346–1351.
246. Davies KA, Schifferli JA, Walport MJ. Complement deficiency and immune complex disease. *Springer Semin Immunopathol* 1994;15: 397–416.
247. Batchelor JR, Fielder AHL, Walport MJ. Family study of the major histocompatibility complex in HLa-DR3 negative patients with systemic lupus erythematosus. *Clin Exp Immunol* 1987;70:364–371.
248. Jacob CO, Fronek Z, Lewis GD, Koo M, Hansen JA, McDevitt HO. Heritable major histocompatibility complex class-II associated differences in production of tumor necrosis factor a: relevance to the genetic predisposition to systemic lupus erythematosus. *Proc Natl Acad Sci USA* 1990;87:1233–1237.
249. Layrisse Z, Rodriguez-Iturbe B, Garcia Ramirez R, Rodriguez A, Tiwari J. Family studies of the HLA system in acute post streptococcal glomerulonephritis. *Hum Immunol* 1983;7:177–185.
250. Sasazuki T, Hayase R, Iwanoto I, Tsuchida H. HLA and acute post streptococcal glomerulonephritis. *N Eng J Med* 1979;301:1184–1185.
251. Naito S, Kohara M, Arakawa K. Associations of class II antigens with primary glomerulopathies. *Nephron* 1987;45:111–114.
252. Freedman BI, Spray BJ, Heise ER. HLA associations in IgA nephropathy and focal segmental glomerulosclerosis. *Am J Kidney Dis* 1994;23;352–357.
253. Freedman BI, Spray BJ, Dunston GM, Heise ER. HLA associations in end-stage renal disease due to membranous glomerulonephritis: HLA-DR3 associations with progressive renal failure. *Am J Kidney Dis* 1994;23:797–782.
254. Welch TR, Beischel L, Balakrishnan K, Quinlan M, West CD. Major-histocompatibility complex extended haplotypes in membranoproliferative glomerulonephritis. *N Engl J Med* 1986;314:1476–1481.

Immunologic Renal Diseases,
edited by E. G. Neilson and W. G. Couser.
Lippincott-Raven Publishers, Philadelphia © 1997

CHAPTER 6

Immunologic Tolerance and the Induction of Autoimmunity

Peter S. Heeger and Eric G. Neilson

INTRODUCTION

Immunologic tolerance has fascinated immunologists and clinicians for well over a century. The initial scientific interest in this field, published in the late 19th century, is attributed to Erlich and Morgenroth (1). These investigators noted that goats readily made anti–red blood cell (anti-RBC) antibodies in response to injected foreign red blood cells, but did not respond to their own cells (1). Based on this observation, they coined the term "horror atoxicus," which was meant to imply that the immune system has an abhorrence to the production of antibodies with autoreactive potential. This concept was later supported by Owen's observations of blood cell chimeric, dizygotic cattle twins: although each twin's blood contained a mixture of cells derived from both animals (due to shared placental circulations), no alloantibodies were produced (2). Several years later, Burnet and Fenner interpreted Owen's observations as meaning that recognition of self (as opposed to nonself) is a process learned during fetal development (3). It was not until 1953, however, that Billingham, Brent, and Medawar experimentally confirmed the acquired nature of "self-tolerance" by showing that transfer of allogeneic cells into a fetal mouse induced tolerance to the alloantigens (as measured by skin graft acceptance) once the animal matured (4).

These seminal descriptions of immunologic tolerance to self-antigens have since begged the question of mechanism, with much of the emphasis placed on the understanding of the following: How can the immune system recognize and destroy, potentially, any "foreign" antigen, and yet not respond to parenchymal self? A corollary question additionally arises: How, and under what circumstances, is immunologic tolerance to self overcome, thus resulting in autoimmune responses? Much basic research in immunology over the last 50 years has focused on these issues. It is the goal of this chapter to review our present understanding of immunologic tolerance and to explore how the failure of normal tolerogenic mechanisms can result in the development of autoimmune responses.

ORGANIZATION OF THE IMMUNE SYSTEM

As discussed in Chapter 4, the mammalian immune system has evolved in response to attack from foreign invaders of many sorts and can be thought of as being comprised of two broad subdivisions. The central component of the humoral arm of the immune system is the antibody-secreting B lymphocyte. Antibodies produced by B cells bind to native, soluble, foreign antigens and stimulate a number of effector functions. The huge potential immunologic variability of the antibody response is determined by site-specific recombination events splicing one of a number of V_H, D_H, and J_H genes to a C_H gene segment, to form the heavy-chain gene, and a kappa (κ) or lambda (λ) V_L gene segment to a C_L chain to form the light-chain gene (5). Functional antibodies consisting of two heavy chains and two light chains are then secreted by the B cell [reviewed by Carayannopoulos and Capra (6)]. Crystal structures of immunoglobulins (Igs) have determined that the antigen-binding site consists of the highly variable VDJ_H and VJ_L junction of the antibody

P. S. Heeger: Nephrology Section, Department of Medicine, Cleveland VA Medical Center, Case Western Reserve School of Medicine, Cleveland, Ohio 44106.

E. G. Neilson: Penn Center for Molecular Studies of Kidney Diseases, Renal-Electrolyte and Hypertension Division of the Department of Medicine, Graduate Groups in Immunology and Cell Biology, University of Pennsylvania, Philadelphia, Pennsylvania 19104.

molecule, also known as CDR3 (complementarity determining region 3) region (6).

Partially in response to the ability of foreign invaders to elude the antibody response by "hiding" intracellularly, the immune system has evolved to include the T-cell arm of the immune system (see Chapter 4). Since the function of γδ-expressing T cells is not clearly established, this review focuses on the more abundant αβ-expressing T cells. T lymphocytes do not recognize native antigens, but instead recognize processed peptides expressed on antigen-presenting cells (APCs) in the context of major histocompatibility complex (MHC) molecules, through the use of heterodimeric αβ T-cell receptors (TCRs) (7–9). In an analogous situation to B cells, the ability of T lymphocytes to recognize a diverse array of antigens is determined by site-specific recombination events that occur in individual T cells during ontogeny, which splice together variable (V), junctional (J), diversity (D), and constant (C) region β gene segments, and V, J, and Cα gene segments, to form productively rearranged TCR α and β genes [reviewed by Hedrick and Eidelman (7)]. This is a largely stochastic process, implying that the organism will rearrange functional TCRs capable of recognizing foreign as well as self-antigens.

Studies of TCR sequence homology to Igs (10), and mutational analysis of TCR residues in the region of the VDJβ junction and the VJα junction, have determined that these regions, known as TCR CDR3 regions, interact directly with the peptide/MHC complex, while other portions of the TCR interact with nonpolymorphic regions of the MHC (11,12). T-cell recognition of peptide MHC is strengthened, and partially defined, by the cobinding of T-cell-expressed CD4 or CD8 to nonpolymorphic regions of the MHC (12). T cells coexpressing an αβ TCR and CD4 recognize antigen in the context of MHC II and primarily exhibit "helper" (cytokine production) functions, whereas T cells coexpressing CD8 recognize antigen in the context of MHC I and primarily exhibit "effector" functions (12).

T-CELL TOLERANCE

Development of the Functional T-Cell Repertoire

Present immunologic dogma conceptualizes T-cell ontogeny as a highly controlled developmental process that can be arbitrarily divided into three parts [reviewed by von Boehmer (13)]. During the initial maturation stage, early thymocyte precursors are induced to express αβ TCRs on their surface (13). The largely stochastic nature of TCR gene rearrangement during this process leads to the expression of TCRs that potentially recognize both foreign and self-antigens, in addition to expressing TCRs that may be useless to the organism because they do not recognize peptides in the context of self-MHC. Subsequently, those T cells that can recognize foreign peptides in the context of self-MHC are positively selected by internal ligands in order to be useful for the individual organism (13). Finally, those T cells that recognize self-antigens are eliminated from the T-cell repertoire by a process known as negative selection (14).

Initial Maturation of the Pre-T Cell

Immature CD4–CD8– (double negative) thymocyte precursors initially migrate into the thymus between developmental days 11 and 14 of the mouse and at an analogous time in humans (15) (Fig. 1). These double-negative thymocyte precursors are destined to die by apoptosis unless induced to mature further (13,16). Once in the thymus, CD4–CD8–TCR– precursors first rearrange their TCR β-chain genes in order to produce a TCR β-chain protein (13,16). Successful expression of TCR β on the surface of thymocytes has three important consequences: (a) It leads to proliferation and expansion of the thymocyte and maturation into the CD4+CD8+ (double positive) stage. Those cells incapable of expressing a functional TCR β chain are, on the other hand, eliminated by programmed cell death (17,18). (b) It prevents rearrangement of the second TCR β-chain gene (if the first rearrangement is successful), a process called allelic exclusion (thus preventing the expression of two TCR β chains on one T cell) (13). (c) Finally, successful rearrangement and expression of the TCR β chain enhances rearrangement and expression of the TCR α-chain gene, resulting in a CD4+CD8+TCR^{lo} phenotype (13,19) (Fig. 1). There is no allelic exclusion of the TCR α-chain rearrangement process, however, and single mature T cells expressing two different α chains have been demonstrated (13,20). The exact nature of the positively selecting signal leading to the maturation from a double-negative to a dou-

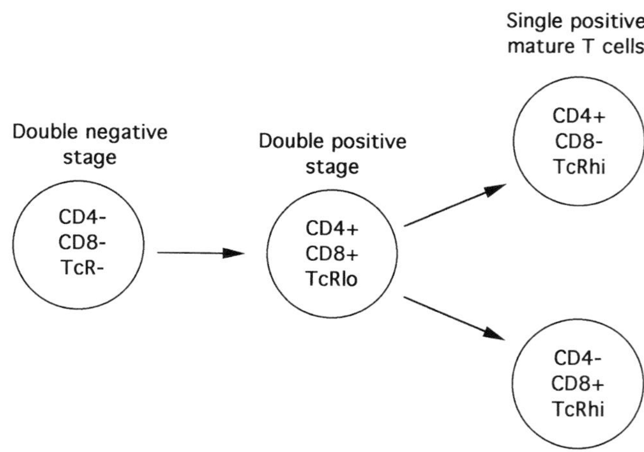

FIG. 1. T-cell development proceeds through developmentally distinct stages.

ble-positive stage has not yet been fully elucidated, although progress is being made in this area (13,21).

Positive Selection of Immature CD4+CD8+TCR^{lo} Thymocytes into Mature CD4+CD8–TCR^{hi} or CD4–CD8+TCR^{hi} T Cells

The ensuing step in T-cell ontogeny is the positive selection of double-positive thymocyte precursors expressing low levels of TCR on their surface (CD4+CD8+ TCR^{lo}) into mature CD4+CD8–TCR^{hi} or CD4–CD8+ TCR^{hi} T cells, functionally capable of recognizing antigen in the context of self-MHC (13). The modern concepts about positive selection initially arose from a series of experimental observations made in reconstituted, lethally irradiated bone marrow chimeric mice (22,23) and from experiments showing that antibodies to MHC I prevented development of CD8+ T cells, while antibodies to MHC II prevented the development of CD4+ T cells (24). More definitive evidence for positive selection arose out of the technologic advances in the 1980s. The most elegant system employed a TCR transgenic mouse, in which all of the T cells were genetically engineered to express a TCR that recognizes a male-specific antigen, H-Y, in the context of MHC class I D^b (25–27). The CD8+ T lymphocytes from female D^b animals (that do not express H-Y) made transgenic for this TCR, all expressed the anti–H-Y receptor on their surface, as would be predicted by positive selection (25–27). On the other hand, if the transgenic anti–H-Y thymocytes were transferred into an irradiated female mouse lacking the D^b MHC molecule, no CD8+ T cells were found (26,27). Further experiments using genetically crossed strains of mice confirmed that a positively selecting MHC background was necessary for CD8+ T-cell development (25–27). Similar experiments have been performed using an MHC class II–restricted TCR transgenic mouse, with analogous results (28). Finally, positive selection has been confirmed using the knockout approach: MHC class I knockout mice (in which MHC class I molecules were removed by site-specific recombination) were shown to develop without CD8+ T cells (29), whereas MHC II knockouts were shown to lack CD4+ T cells (30,31).

The positive selection process also results in double-positive TCR^{lo} cells maturing to either CD4+CD8–TCR^{hi} or CD4–CD8+TCR^{hi}, but not both (the single-positive stage; Fig. 1). How this occurs is not yet clear, although two theoretical possibilities have been proposed. A detailed explanation of this topic is beyond the scope of this chapter and can be obtained elsewhere (13).

The nature of the positively selecting signal within the thymus has been an area of intensive investigation over the last several years, with the most recent data suggesting that complexes of self-peptide plus self-MHC molecules are the positively selecting ligands. As will be discussed shortly, these seem to be the same ligands that lead to the elimination of self-reactive T cells through negative selection. How similar ligands can lead to both positive and negative selection of thymocytes has also been a heavily debated topic and is discussed after a more detailed review of negative selection.

Negative Selection of T Cells in the Thymus

The theoretical framework for negative selection grew out of Owen's observations (2), and experimental demonstration by Billingham et al. (4), that immunologic tolerance could be acquired during fetal development. Based on these findings, Burnet developed his clonal selection theory, which stated that T cells expressing receptors specific for molecules present during development of an organism were eliminated from the repertoire (32). Lederberg expanded on these thoughts by suggesting that immune cells pass through a developmental stage of tolerizability, after which time an encounter with antigen would induce a response (33).

It has taken more than 30 years, and required two important technical discoveries, to show experimentally that negative selection is an important tolerogenic process. One finding was that certain antigens, encoded by endogenous tumor viruses (that is, Mls), could react with all T cells expressing certain TCR Vβ gene products, thus acting as superantigens [reviewed by Janeway (34)]. The availability of monoclonal antibodies to individual Vβ regions allowed investigators to follow the fate of T cells expressing these particular Vβ genes (35). These experiments showed that T cells with Vβ-gene products reacting with a given endogenous superantigen could be found within the thymus at the immature double-positive TCR^{lo} stage (35). However, single-positive thymocytes expressing the given Vβ-gene product were markedly depleted, thus indicating elimination prior to full maturation (35).

The second discovery that helped to define negative selection as a prominent tolerogenic process was the production of TCR αβ transgenic mice, specifically, the transgenic anti–H-Y in the context of D^b, as discussed in the previous section on positive selection (36). In transgenic female D^b animals lacking the H-Y antigen, the overwhelming majority of T cells are CD8+ and express the transgenic anti–H-Y TCR (37). In male mice expressing the H-Y antigen, however, massive deletion of double-positive T cells occurs within the thymus, resulting in a thymus weighing 5–10% of normal (37). Similar results have been described in several different transgenic models using both CD4- and CD8-restricted TCRs, thus generalizing the relevance of the phenomenon (38,39).

Considerable discussion has revolved around which antigens are presented to thymocytes in order to mediate negative selection. It has become clear from transgenic mouse studies that very low concentrations of antigens

($\leq 10^{-10}$ M) can cause thymic deletion (40). In fact, thymic negative selection can be mediated by an antigen levels undetectable by standard methods, but present when assayed by the polymerase chain reaction (41,42). Most antigens intrinsically found in the thymus are likely available to induce negative selection, and experimental data suggest that the high thymic blood flow allows many circulating antigens access to the negative selection process (14). On the other hand, one recent report revealed that a proportion of T cells reactive to the complement component, C5, escaped thymic deletion, despite significant serum levels (43). Additionally, there are certainly many antigens that are organ specific and do not circulate, and are thus not readily accessible to thymic negative selection. T cells reactive to these antigens will therefore not be eliminated during ontogeny and pose an autoreactive threat to the organism. The immune system must control these autoreactive cells in other ways.

Although initial work implied that only thymic dendritic cells were capable of eliminating autoreactive T cells (44), it is now clear thymic negative selection is not a function of a particular APC, but instead is an inherent property of the thymocyte and/or its microenvironment (45–47). Additionally, experimental data using superantigen and transgenic models of negative selection have revealed that intrathymic deletion can occur in immature (just prior to becoming double positive) (48), double-positive (35) or single-positive thymocytes (49), as long as they express TCR αβ heterodimers. The actual stage of central deletion in normal (nontransgenic) mice, in response to standard self-antigens, is not yet known.

Mechanistically, present data imply that negative selection is mediated via apoptotic deletion of thymocytes after recognition of high-affinity self-antigens (50). Work in other systems has implicated the fas antigen as an important mediator of apoptosis [reviewed by Singer et al. (51)]. Interestingly, however, thymic elimination of thymoctyes proceeds normally in MRL *lpr/lpr* mice, which contain a mutation in the fas antigen (52), indicating that this apoptotic deletion of self-reactive thymocytes proceeds via a pathway unrelated to fas. The specific nature of thymic apoptosis is presently unknown, but there is some evidence that the process is mediated by endogenous glucocorticoids (53).

The Thymic Paradox

The previous discussions of positive and negative selection pointed out that both processes occur within the thymus, and that both processes are mediated by thymocyte TCR recognition of peptide/MHC. How the same interaction can lead to diametrically opposed outcomes has been a hotly debated issue by many members of the immunologic community and has been appropriately named the thymic paradox. Several potential solutions to this paradox exist, and are outlined below.

Positive Selection Does Not Exist

Matzinger has proposed that the development of the T-cell repertoire does not require an intrathymic positive selection step, and that only negative selection of high-affinity self-reactive T cells occurs in the thymus, thus obviating the thymic paradox (23). This author points out that not all of the transgenic animal studies support positive selection, and that many of the experiments implicating thymic positive selection could be potentially interpreted as simply a lack of negative selection (23). Although this theory is certainly controversial and goes against the current immunologic dogma, the arguments are well thought out, persuasive, and theoretically testable, and thus should not be discarded.

Differential Expression of Ligands by Differing Cell Types

Assuming that positive selection does occur, one theory to explain how peptide/MHC complexes can potentially lead to both positive and negative selection hypothesizes that positive selection occurs on specialized thymic epithelial cells (TECs), whereas negative selection occurs on bone-marrow-derived thymic dendritic cells. This hypothesis presupposes that the thymic dendritic cells express peptides representative of those found in the periphery that are used to eliminate self-reactive T cells, whereas TECs express a set of peptides unique to the thymus and are used to mediate a positive selection response. The model has recently come under criticism due to experiments showing a) that peptides eluted from TECs are not unique (54), and (b) that various cell types can induce both positive and negative selection (45–47).

Maturational Stage Hypothesis

This explanation assumes that thymocytes at different maturational stages respond differently to similar ligands. The theory states that at some point during ontogeny, thymocytes are subject to negative selecting signals, while at other points during ontogeny, the same ligands expressed on the same cells induce a positive selection response in the thymocyte. Findings showing that negative selection can occur at many developmental stages (35,48,49) make this hypothesis less appealing, although a role for maturational stage cannot yet be fully ruled out.

Differential Avidity Hypothesis

Much of the recent experimental data suggest that the response of a given thymocyte to a given peptide/MHC complex depends on the strength of the recognition event. The most meaningful data come from several experiments performed using fetal thymic organ cultures

(FTOCs) and TCR transgenic mice and will be reviewed in some detail. Fetal thymus tissue can be excised on developmental day 16 and grown in vitro (55). At this time, the thymic lobes contain mainly double-negative cells that mature normally, mimicking normal thymocyte development (55). To study the role of peptides in positive selection, investigators used an FTOC from a beta-2-microglobulin (β_2m)-deficient mouse (56) (created as a β_2 knockout) or a Tap-1-deficient mouse (Tap 1 is required to transport peptides into the endoplasmic reticulum to combine with MHC I prior to expression on the cell surface) (57). In FTOCs from both of these animals, no MHC I and no peptides are expressed by thymic tissue, and no CD8+ T cells develop in the culture (56,57). Exogenous addition of β_2m and a single peptide, however, leads to low but detectable thymic expression of MHC I and allows development of a population of CD8+ T cells (56,57). Interestingly, exogenous addition of several different peptides led to the development of more CD8+ T cells than addition of a single peptide (56,57).

The system was then made more elegant through the crossing of a β_2m-deficient mouse expressing MHC I K^b, with a TCR transgenic mouse expressing a TCR specific for an ovalbumin (ova) peptide in the context of K^b (58). Since all of the thymocytes in these cultures express the same TCR, it became easily possible to analyze the affect of different exogenous peptides on T-cell development. The presence or absence of ova-specific CD8+ T cells in the FTOCs could be determined by fluorescence-activated cell sorter (FACS) analysis after the addition of ova, or after the addition of mutated ova peptides (with single amino acid substitutions) (58). Without the addition of exogenous peptide, CD8+ T-cell development occurred normally in the β_2m-deficient heterozygote (β_2m+/–), but no CD8+ T cells developed in the β_2m-deficient homozygote (β_2m–/–) (58). Addition of one of several substituted ova peptides, shown to bind well to K^b, led to positive selection of CD8+ ova-specific T cells in the β_2m homozygote (although the native ova peptide was unable to do so) (58). One of these peptides led to positive selection of ova-specific CD8+ T cells when expressed at a low ligand density in the β_2m homozygote FTOCs, but mediated negative selection of ova-specific CD8+ T cells when expressed at a high ligand density in the β_2m heterozygote FTOCs (58). The same peptides could not activate mature CD8+ ova-specific T cells, however (58). Using other double transgenic models—MHC-I-deficient animals with T cells specific for viral peptides—additional experimental evidence revealed that single peptides could induce positive selection if added to the FTOC at a low dose, but would result in deletion if given at a much higher dose (59,60).

The experiments demonstrate that the process of positive selection is both peptide dependent and highly specific (61). They also suggest that the fate of a thymocyte is determined by the avidity of the interaction between the TCRs on the thymocytes and the peptide/MHC complexes expressed on the thymic stromal cells (Fig. 2) (62, 63). In this model, avidity is determined by both the strength of the individual TCR/peptide/MHC interactions (affinity) and by their number (62,63). In essence, the thymocyte is programmed to die unless rescued by a positive selecting signal above a given threshold. However, if the strength of the interaction is much higher, and above a second threshold, the thymocyte receives a different signal resulting in apoptosis (62,63). As a consequence, a thymocyte that either interacts with many low-affinity peptide/self-MHC molecules or interacts with a rare high-affinity ligand will be positively selected to differentiate further (62,63). On the other hand, a thymocyte that receives no signal or one that recognizes a high density of high-affinity ligands will be deleted (62,63). Importantly, using a unique in vivo system, Hsu et al. have recently shown that the differential avidity model of T-cell development seems to be relevant in vivo, as well as in the FTOC systems (64).

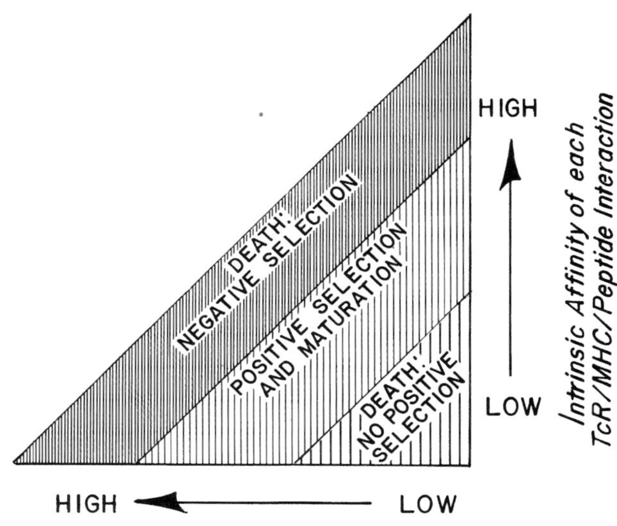

FIG. 2. Differential avidity hypothesis of T-cell selection in the thymus. See the text for details.

Although the differential avidity model of thymic selection provides a plausible solution to the thymic paradox, it would be premature to state that our knowledge of the developing T-cell repertoire is complete. The theoretical framework just outlined needs to be further tested experimentally in order to better define the process of T-cell differentiation.

T-CELL ACTIVATION

Once a thymocyte has progressed through positive selection and has survived negative selection, it emerges from the thymus as a mature, virgin CD4+ or CD8+ T cell, poised to recognize and respond to foreign antigens

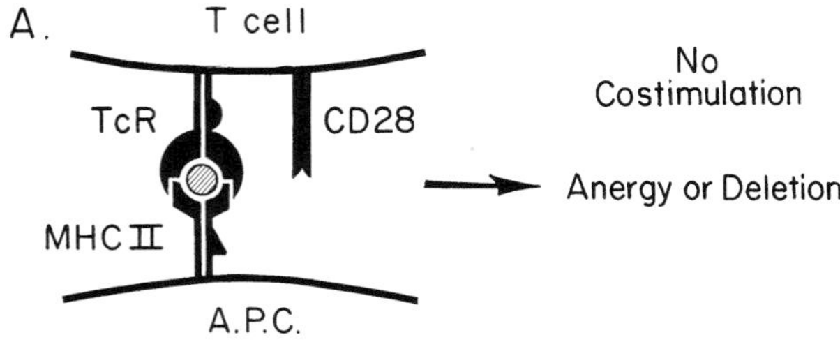

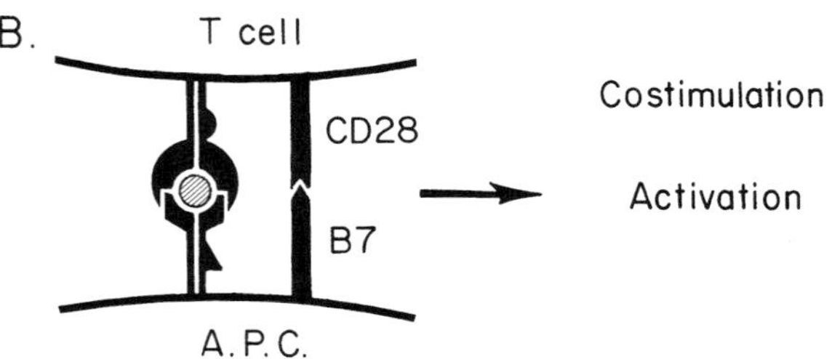

FIG. 3. The role of costimulation in T-cell activation. **A:** T-cell recognition of peptide/MHC without costimulation leads to anergy or deletion. **B:** T-cell recognition of peptide/MHC with appropriate costimulation leads to activation. *TCR,* T-cell receptor; *APC,* antigen-presenting cell.

presented in the context of self-MHC. TCR interaction with peptide/MHC alone (known as "signal 1"), however, is not enough to initiate immune activation. As originally proposed by Bretscher and Cohn (for B-cell activation) (65) and later expounded upon by Lafferty and Cunningham (66), full T-cell activation requires a second "costimulatory" signal (67,68). In fact, recent evidence suggests that delivery of signal 1, without the second costimulatory signal, results in a T-cell deletion (47), or a form of T-cell unresponsiveness called anergy (67,69) (Figure 3). Anergized T cells in culture do not proliferate, and make little interleukin 2 (IL-2) when rechallenged with antigen, but will divide in response to the application of exogenous IL-2 (69). The mechanisms responsible for these inhibitory effects are not yet fully characterized, but may involve the expression of specific repressor proteins that inhibit IL-2 transcription (68). A detailed review of costimulatory signals and T-cell activation can be found in Chapters 4 and 8; only selected issues will be discussed here.

Full activation of CD4+ T cells can be induced via costimulatory signals delivered through T-cell-expressed CD28 or CTLA-4 (68,70), and the recently characterized APC-expressed CD80 (B7) and CD86 (B7-2) (68,71,72). This type of costimulation can prevent the anergy or cell death response noted upon stimulation of the TCR alone (68,70). Additional or adjunctive costimulatory signals can be delivered through heat-stable antigen (HSA), lymphocyte function-associated antigen 3 (LFA-3), intracellular adhesion molecules 1 and 2 (ICAM-1 and ICAM-2), and vascular cell adhesion molecule 1 (VCAM-1) (73–75). Both VCAM-1 and ICAM-1 are inducible with a variety of stimuli and can thus have potentially varying effects depending on the level of expression (75). Interestingly, renal proximal tubular cells express both ICAM-

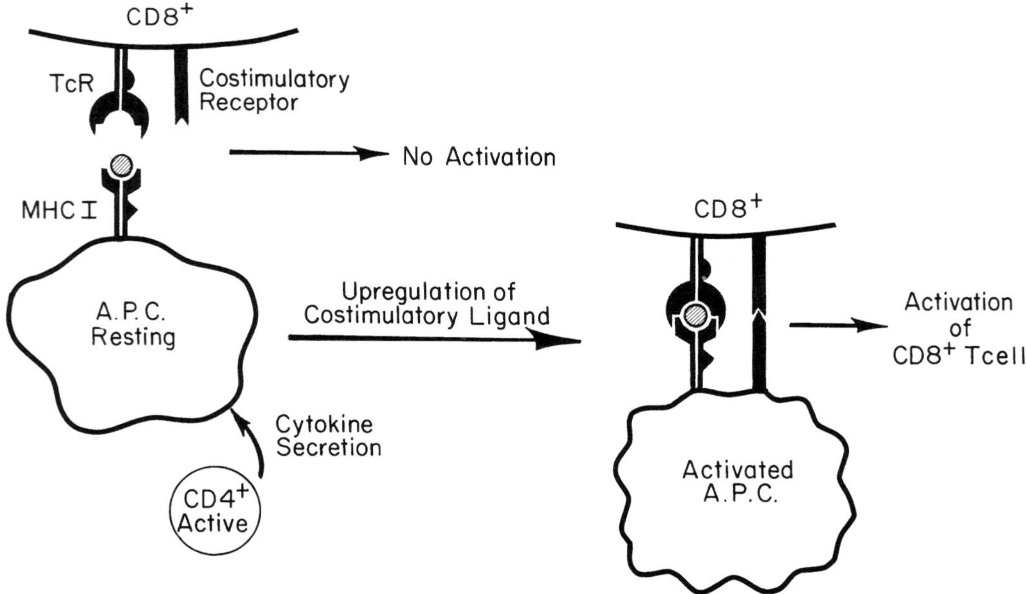

FIG. 4. Proposed mechanism of CD8+ T-cell activation. A resting antigen-presenting cell *(APC)* cannot activate a CD8+ T cell because it lacks expression of costimulatory molecules. Activated CD4+ T cells secrete cytokines that lead to surface expression of costimulatory molecules on the APC, thus resulting in activation of the CD8+ T cell.

1 (76) and VCAM-1 (77) in a cytokine-regulated manner. Anti-ICAM-1 antibodies can prevent proximal tubular cells from presenting antigen to T-cell hybridomas (76), while VCAM-1 expression is increased in lupus nephritis (77), suggesting a role for both molecules in autoimmune renal disease.

CD8+ T cells generally require a costimulatory signal for complete activation as well. The exact nature of the second signal for CD8+ cytotoxic T-cell activation is not yet clearly defined, but seems to be delivered by CD4+ helper T cells [reviewed by Matzinger (47)]. The simplest explanation is that signal 1 (CD8+ T-cell recognition of MHC I plus peptide) leads to a state of activation that requires additional IL-2, or else the CD8+ cell dies (68, 78). The additional IL-2 could be provided by a CD4+ helper cell in close proximity and perhaps recognizing the same APC as the CD8+ cell (68,78). As an alternative model, Matzinger has suggested that resting APCs may not express costimulatory signals for cytotoxic T-cell responses, but could be induced to do so by helper T cells (47). Thus, a CD8+ T-cell interacting with an unstimulated APC would be tolerized (signal 1 without signal 2), while a CD8+ T cell interacting with a stimulated APC (from a previous interaction with a CD4+ cell) would receive appropriate costimulation and become activated (Fig. 4) (47). This interesting hypothesis awaits experimental verification and the molecular characterization of the specific costimulatory signals involved.

PERIPHERAL MECHANISMS OF T-CELL TOLERANCE

The Need for Peripheral Mechanisms of T-Cell Tolerance

Many studies have demonstrated the presence of autoreactive T cells in normal individuals, indicating that intrathymic tolerogenic processes are insufficient to prevent some autoreactive T cells from escaping into the periphery. This may, in part, be due to the expression of some antigens only on peripheral tissues, thus avoiding thymic negative selection of T cells reactive to these antigens. Other antigens, such as those related to lactation in females, are not initially expressed in the organism. Mature T cells developing prior to the expression of such antigens will also escape thymic deletion. Perhaps more importantly, the central negative selection process is envisioned to be a threshold phenomenon; that is, only a thymocyte recognizing a self-antigen with an avidity above a given threshold will be deleted. This inherently implies that some thymocytes will fall just below the threshold, thus escaping negative selection. Such thymocytes, once released into the periphery as mature T cells, may be able to recognize autoantigens if seen under appropriate circumstances (that is, high antigen concentrations or increased costimulation). Finally, one study has suggested that TCRs of mature T cells undergo somatic mutation during antigenic activation (in an analogous manner to that which occurs routinely in B cells), thus potentially evolving into autoreactive cells in the periphery (79). To control these potentially destructive autoreactive T cells, the immune system has developed several peripheral tolerance mechanisms.

Clonal Ignorance

CD4+ T cells are notably ignorant of antigens that are not expressed in the context of MHC II [reviewed by Rubin-Kelley and Jevnikar (80)]. Since MHC II has a limited constitutive tissue distribution (although it can be induced in additional tissues under certain circumstances), there are many antigens ignored by self-reactive CD4+ T cells (80). Indirect evidence for this phenomenon comes from experiments in murine lupus, in which MHC II blockade with anti-MHC antibodies prevented T-cell-mediated renal disease (81), and in autoimmune interstitial nephritis, in which cytokine induction of renal tubular MHC II expression correlated with the induced susceptibility to CD4+ T-cell-mediated renal disease in otherwise resistant animals (80,82).

Additionally, work in the last several years has demonstrated that naive (not previously stimulated), mature T cells generally do not circulate to peripheral tissues, but remain in the bloodstream or within the secondary lymph organs, where they are most likely to encounter foreign antigen [reviewed by Springer (83) and Mackay (84)]. This relative exclusion from peripheral tissues is partially explained by the high cell surface expression of L-selectin, a lymph node homing receptor (83,84). Once a T cell becomes activated, however, the surface expression of L-selectin (among many other surface antigens) is downregulated, and the T cell can circulate more widely (83,84). Such an exclusion from nonlymphoid organs provides a partial explanation for how self-reactive T cells (that have escaped thymic deletion) may not recognize and respond to tissue-specific antigens.

Experimental evidence implicating T-cell ignorance as a form of peripheral tolerance comes from a number of elegant studies using organ-specific expression of antigens in transgenic mice [reviewed by Miller and Morahan (85)]. In one example, a transgenic mouse expressing the lymphocytic choriomeningitis virus (LCMV) glycoprotein (GP) in pancreatic β cells was produced (86,87). These mice were mated with a CD8+ TCR transgenic mouse, whose T cells recognized a GP epitope in the context of the appropriate MHC I (87). In this double-transgenic animal, the anti-GP T cells were not deleted centrally, and normal levels of CD8 and TCR were found on their surface (87). Despite this, there was no pancreatic β-cell infiltration or diabetes. If the mice were first infected with LCMV, however, they developed selective destruction of β-cells leading to diabetes (87). These findings suggest that autoreactive cells can be present peripherally, but not "see" their ligand unless activated first. Similar findings in other systems are consistent with this phenomenon (85).

The existence of ignorance to self-antigens is also illustrated by the recent description of cryptic antigenic determinants (see cryptic and dominant antigens, below) (88). In several experimental systems, immunization with an intact self-antigen does not result in an autoimmune T-cell response. However, if immunization is performed with a peptide derived from the intact protein antigen, the animal develops an autoimmune response directed at that antigen (88). These types of studies reveal that the self-reactive T cells can be ignorant to a given antigen because they rarely, if ever, encounter it. The presence of T cells reactive to such cryptic antigens, normally hidden from the immune system, has been demonstrated to be important in the development of certain autoimmune reactions (89,90).

As illustrated by these examples, nonreactivity to peripheral antigens presents a precarious situation for the organism, allowing the potential for autoimmune reactions. Since autoimmunity is a rare event, other fail-safe tolerogenic mechanisms must, and do, exist.

Exhaustion and Peripheral Deletion

Under normal circumstances, antigen-specific T cells initially proliferate markedly in response to foreign antigenic stimuli and subsequently clear the inciting antigen from the organism [reviewed by Sprent (91)]. At this point, since there is no further need for these antigen-specific T cells, it might be predicted that they should be widely eliminated (leaving only a small number of memory cells for future use). In fact, experimental studies have demonstrated that elimination of T cells after a strong antigen-specific proliferative response does occur (91). Direct evidence for T-cell elimination through this mechanism of so-called T cell "exhaustion" has derived from studies with superantigens (92,93), but similar findings were also noted in selected TCR transgenic mice after exposure to their relevant peptides (94–97). A precise explanation for T-cell elimination under these circumstances is not yet available. Cell death may occur as a result of prolonged TCR stimulation leading to apoptosis (93) or may reflect lack of contact with essential growth-requiring stimuli such as IL-2 (98). Other authors have suggested that this elimination of T cells occurs as the antigen is presented by nonprofessional APCs that are incapable of providing costimulation (47,99) and thus induce deletion (that is, they deliver signal 1 without signal 2). Further work is required to verify any or all of these hypotheses.

Irrespective of the mechanism, it has long been postulated that T-cell elimination through "exhaustion" of an immune response could theoretically result in tolerance to the original antigen (100). Work using superantigens, and following the fate of specific Vβ-gene-expressing T cells with monoclonal antibodies, has revealed that tolerance can be induced in this manner [reviewed by Sprent (91)]. Further evidence for T-cell exhaustion as a form of tolerance comes from studies using LCMV-reactive, TCR transgenic mice. These experiments have revealed that exposure to LCMV can result in T-cell proliferation followed by elimination, with subsequent tolerance and perisistence of the viral infection (96).

On the other hand, multiple analyses have shown that peripheral T-cell deletion can occur without an initial proliferation step (101,102). In fact, peripheral deletion without prior proliferation may be a more important tolerogenic mechanism than exhaustion under most circumstances (91,102).

Several experiments have suggested that peripheral deletion in these situations may occur through apoptosis after high-affinity interactions of T cells with their ligands (103). Additionally, the finding that MLR *lpr/lpr* mice (which lack the fas apoptosis antigen) are unable to delete autoreactive T cells peripherally (52,103) implicates a role for fas in this process.

T-Cell Anergy in Vivo

In some in vivo experimental systems, peripheral recognition of autoantigens seems to result in a form of T-cell unresponsiveness, or anergy, analogous to that defined in vitro (69). In one study, T cells from a female TCR transgenic mouse reactive to H-Y (a male-specific antigen) were transferred to male nude mice (which lack their own T cells) (97). The transferred cells downregulated their TCRs and CD8 molecules and were subsequently unable to respond to their appropriate ligands in vitro (97). Interestingly, removing the cells from the "anergizing" environment, and secondarily transferring them to a female nude mouse, enabled eventual recovery of reactivity (97).

In another elegant experiment, the MHC I K^b was used as a transgenic antigen linked to an inducible promoter and expressed solely in the liver (104). These mice were crossed with a T-cell transgenic mouse with a specificity against K^b. Since the investigators demonstrated that the mice had no thymic expression of K^b, any tolerogenic effect could be attributed directly to peripheral mechanisms alone. Interestingly, the resultant mice did not reject K^b skin grafts, indicating specific tolerance to the foreign antigen (104). FACS of the T cells from the mice revealed downregulation of TCR expression, as well as decreased numbers of transgenic CD8+ T cells (104). As hepatic levels of K^b were increased, through the use of the inducible promoter, TCR expression was downregulated even further (104).

Additional in vivo evidence for anergy comes from a recently published experiment using chimeric mice. These investigators nicely demonstrated that the outcome of a T-cell interaction with its peptide/MHC ligand, activation, anergy, or deletion can be determined solely by the level of antigen expression (105).

An emerging consensus derived from all of these analyses suggests that the distinction between anergy and peripheral deletion is blurred, and that peripheral tolerance may be a multistep process (14,106). Self-reactive T cells escaping central deletion, but encountering their ligands peripherally, may downregulate TCR (or CD8) expression and become unable to respond to antigen (14, 106). If exposed to higher concentrations of antigen, they can further downregulate TCR expression and can eventually be deleted (14,106).

The molecular mechanisms involved in mediating peripheral deletion or anergy in vivo are not entirely understood. The in vitro studies on T-cell activation described previously have, however, led investigators to hypothesize that high-affinity recognition of antigen without costimulation may cause deletion in vivo. To study this question, mice were made transgenic for the pancreatic β-cell expression of either MHC I-E (thus acting as a foreign antigen), B7 (CD80), or both (107). Mice transgenic for both I-E and B7 developed pancreatic infiltration and diabetes, while those expressing I-E alone did not. Additionally, the mice expressing I-E alone were tolerant to subsequent engraftment of pancreatic islets expressing both B7 and I-E, suggesting that antigen expression without costimulation can induce tolerance (107).

Finally, although the data implicating peripheral deletion as a tolerogenic mechanism are quite strong, as alluded above, the data implicating anergy are subject to a number of criticisms. From a teleologic standpoint, it does not entirely make sense for an organism to maintain, but inactivate, a T cell that it will never use and that presents an autoimmune risk (47). Experimentally, it is difficult to truly separate anergy from deletion as in vivo processes—perhaps the detection of anergy is an interim state on the way to cell death—that is, a single encounter with self-antigen could lead to deletion, but, during the apoptotic process, surface expression of TCR and CD8 is decreased, and the cells do not respond normally to antigenic stimuli. The final word is not yet in, but if T-cell anergy is going to emerge as an expected protective mechanism of peripheral tolerance against autoimmunity, then more in vivo experiments will be needed to show its application toward true structural antigens that reflect normal parenchymal self.

Cytokine-Mediated Diversion

Many studies in both rodents and humans have demonstrated that CD4+ T lymphocytes can be subdivided into functionally distinct subgroups based on cytokine profiles [reviewed by Paul and Seder (108)] (Fig. 5). Th1 cells, which predominantly produce interferon-γ (IFN-γ) and IL-2 are proinflammatory and provide help for cell-mediated immune responses (108–110). Th2 cells, on the other hand, which produce IL-4, IL-5, IL-6, IL-10, and IL-13, can inhibit Th1 cells and provide help for the induction of humoral immune responses (108–110). Both Th1 and

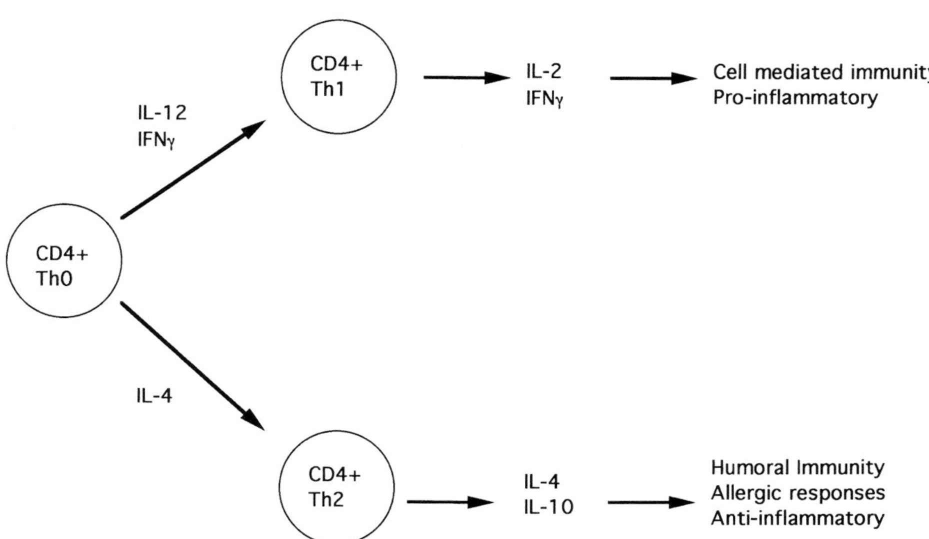

FIG. 5. Development and differential effects of Th1 and Th2 T-cell subsets. *IFN-γ,* interferon gamma; *IL,* interleukin.

Th2 cells are thought to develop from a common undifferentiated precursor capable of producing cytokines of both subtypes: the Th0 cell (108). Factors leading to differentiation into one subtype or the other are being heavily investigated, but it is clear that the cytokines themselves, often under the control of a genetic predisposition, are essential in the differentiation process (108). IFN-γ and IL-12 induce Th1 cells and inhibit the production of Th2 cells (108,111), whereas IL-4 and IL-10 induce Th2 cells and prevent the production of Th1 cells (108,112). Although the majority of data derive from studies on CD4+ cells, there is some evidence for the existence of similar subtypes in CD8+ T cells as well (113).

The functional importance of the Th1/Th2 paradigm, as it applies to peripheral tolerance, is underscored by several observations made in murine *Leishmania* infections (108). Mice that are genetically predisposed to develop a Th1, cell-mediated immune response upon infection with *Leishmania* (an obligate intracellular parasite) can effectively contain the infection and cure the disease (114). On the other hand, mice that develop a Th2 response upon infection are unable to contain the disease and die of disseminated leishmaniasis (114). Interestingly, a susceptible animal can be converted to a resistant one by blocking the development of the Th2 response, either by using antibodies to IL-4 (115) or by treating the animal with IL-12 (116). Thus, although the animal contains a T-cell repertoire capable of curing the infection, cytokine-mediated "diversion" of the immune response can induce tolerance to the invading organism. Analogously, a resistant animal can be converted to a susceptible one through appropriate cytokine manipulation, revealing that tolerance can be overcome through cytokine-mediated diversion, as well (108). Work performed in other models of parasitic infections has confirmed the relevance of these findings (117). As is discussed later, in the section on autoimmunity, recent work has additionally suggested that cytokine-mediated diversion may play an important role in the induction of autoimmune responses.

Anti-idiotypic Networks

The recognition of the huge potential diversity of the immune system led to the hypothesis that the highly variable binding regions of antibodies may themselves be immunogenic. Initial experiments revealed that antibodies could be produced that specifically recognized distinct epitopes, or idiotypes, on other antibodies. The discovery of these anti-idiotypic antibodies led Jerne to propose the network theory of antibody regulation in 1974 (118). He suggested that antibodies could regulate immune responses by interacting with idiotypic determinants in the variable (V) regions of other antibodies (118). Thus, an anti-idiotypic antibody would recognize an epitope on the primary antibody and regulate its production or function (118). The evidence for the presence of idiotypic networks within the B-cell repertoire discussed further in the section on B-cell tolerance. The subsequent discovery of αβ TCRs made the existence of a similar regulatory network of T-cell idiotypes and anti-idiotypic T cells theoretically plausible.

Studies in the rodent model of multiple sclerosis, experimental allergic encephalomyelitis (EAE), suggest that anti-idiotypic T cells do exist and can regulate immune responses. A series of elegant studies by Vandenbark, Offner, and colleagues showed that immunization with peptides derived from TCRs of disease-producing T-cell clones (TCR peptide vaccines) could both prevent disease and rapidly reverse disease symptoms (119,120). The authors hypothesized that the expansion of disease-mediating T-cell clones induced a counterregulatory T-cell response capable of modulating disease, and that TCR peptide vaccines boost this regulatory response, thus stopping disease progression (119,120). Consistent with this hypothesis is the finding that T cells isolated from animals immunized with myelin basic protein to get EAE proliferated strongly to TCR peptides derived from pathogenic T cells, despite never being vaccinated with these peptides (119,120). Further work by a number of investigators led to the conclusion that the TCR pep-

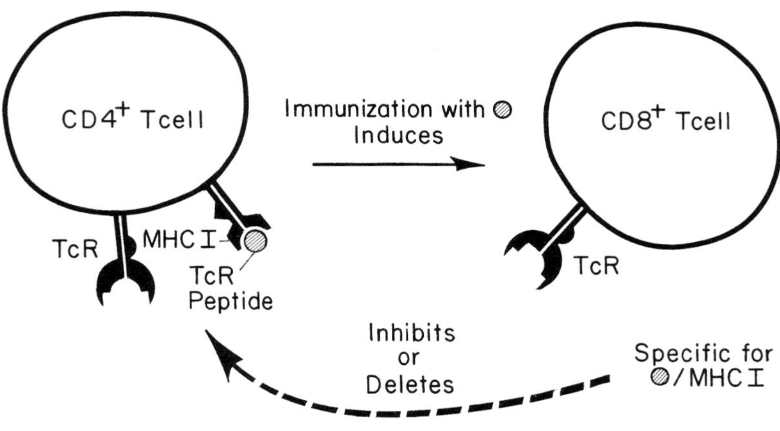

FIG. 6. Proposed mechanism of action of T-cell receptor peptide vaccines. CD4+ T cells express peptides derived from their T-cell receptors *(TCRs)* on their cell surface in the context of MHC I. Immunization with such a TCR-derived peptide induces a regulatory CD8+ T cell with specificity for the TCR peptide/MHC I complex and inhibits or deletes the CD4+ T cell.

tide vaccinations resulted in the emergence of anti-idiotypic CD8+ T cells (121,122). These regulatory cells were, in turn, shown to inactivate the disease-producing T cells via anergy induction or deletion (121,122). Presumably, the disease-producing T cells process and present various endogenous antigenic peptides on their cell surface in the context of MHC I, including peptides derived from their own unique TCR (Fig. 6). Immunization with peptides derived from these TCRs then primes the immune system to produce anti-idiotypic T cells capable of recognizing these unique TCR peptide/MHC complexes, thus allowing a regulatory immune response. Related studies have been performed in other systems, including studies in experimental models of renal disease [reviewed by Neilson (123)], and have generally reached similar conclusions, although some dissenting studies have been published [reviewed by Ridgeway et al. (124)]. Many questions remain about such regulatory networks, including what regulates the anti-idiotypic cells (that is, anti-anti-idiotypic T cells), and under what circumstances anti-idiotypic regulation of immunity is an important tolerogenic mechanism.

Suppression

The phenomenon of cell-mediated immune suppression can be defined as the failure to respond to a given antigen in the presence of suppressor cells, while removal of the suppressor cells restores immune responsiveness. Gershon and Kondo initially demonstrated the suppressor phenomenon by using antibody responses to sheep red blood cells (SRBCs) in irradiated, reconstituted mice (125). Later work by many investigators clearly demonstrated the presence of suppressor T-cell responses to exogenous antigens (126), and self-antigens (127), in a variety of experimental systems [reviewed by Sercarz et al. (128) and Nossal (129)].

Although these findings implicate T-cell-mediated suppression as a mechanism of peripheral tolerance, many immunologists have become skeptical of its existence. This skepticism is a result of several observations that have come to light within the past decade [reviewed by Bloom et al. (130)]. One problem is that suppressor cells do not have a distinct phenotype (129,130). Both CD4+ and CD8+ cells, some with "suppressor inducer" activity, some with anti-idiotypic specificity, and some with antigen specificity but without MHC restriction, have been implicated as suppressors in various systems. Additionally, various surface markers have been associated with suppressor cell function, but no consensus identifying markers has emerged (129,130). In some systems, suppressor cell networks or cascades have been deduced and include a number of diverse soluble suppressor factors (129–131). The presence of these soluble suppressor factors, although active functionally, has thus far eluded molecular confirmation. The disparity and inconsistency of all of these reports have cast some doubts about the veracity of specific suppressor cells.

Perhaps more damaging to the reputation of suppressor cells, however, is the mystery of I-J determinants. In the mid 1970s, certain antimurine MHC antisera were found to react with a subset of T cells with suppressor activity (132). The determinants defined by this antisera mapped to the MHC region of murine chromosome 17, between I-Eα and I-Eβ, and were named I-J (132). The findings were confirmed by a number of laboratories, and I-J became a recognized marker of suppression (133). To the surprise of many, however, DNA sequence analysis from the putative I-J region on chromosome 17 did not reveal any evidence for a gene encoding an I-J polypeptide (134) and, despite much effort, no molecular characterization of an I-J cDNA, or protein, has been performed (133).

Despite all of these criticisms, the presence of T-cell-mediated suppression as a phenomenon is difficult to dispute. It should be emphasized that simply because suppression is not fully understood does not mean that suppression is a fallacy. Importantly, within the last several years, investigators have begun to reexamine suppression and to put a slightly altered twist on the interpretation of the older observations (133). As just noted, several investigators have provided evidence for the existence of an anti-idiotypic CD8+ T cell that prevents T-cell-induced experimental autoallergic encephalomyelitis, a rodent model of multiple sclerosis (133). This is clearly one form of a suppressor T cell. Additionally, a panel of isolated CD4+ suppressor T-cell clones capable of preventing EAE was recently shown to recognize the same antigenic determinants and express similar TCRs as their disease-mediating CD4+ counterparts (135). The different functional phenotypes correlated with differential expression of certain cytokines: the suppressor clones expressed high levels of IL-10 and transforming growth factor β, while the pathogenic clones produced high levels of IFN-γ (135).

Thus, suppression may not be distinct from the other mechanisms of peripheral tolerance already mentioned (133). In some cases, T cells that are not phenotypically different from helper or effector cells may exert their suppressive effects via the preferential secretion of certain cytokine profiles. In other situations, suppressor cells may be anti-idiotypic T cells capable of killing or inhibiting (via anergy induction) their target T cells that exhibit the given idiotype. Whether or not these new hypotheses regarding T-cell suppression are correct awaits experimental verification. Suffice it to say that the evidence for suppression as a tolerogenic phenomenon is quite compelling, and ongoing investigative analysis is likely to clarify many of the unanswered questions.

Veto Cells

One additional form of immune regulation related to suppression, as originally described in an in vitro allogeneic cytotoxic lymphocyte response (CTL), is the veto phenomenon. In this system, responder splenocytes of MHC haplotype A were primed in vitro with irradiated MHC-disparate stimulator cells (haplotype B) and then tested for their ability to kill target cells of the B haplotype (136). Miller and Derry showed that the addition of splenocytes from nude mice expressing the B haplotype suppressed the ability of A cells to kill B targets. They suggested that the responder A cells were "vetoed" by the additional cells (136). Later work has shown that precultured T cells and CD8+ T-cell lines exhibit this same property (137,138). These T cells notably have other primary functions and do not require engagement of their own TCR to cause veto inhibition (137,138). Instead, it has become clear that the responding cells recognize a cell surface antigen on the veto cells, which subsequently leads to inactivation. Several experiments have implicated the CD8 glycoprotein as one such cell surface antigen capable of mediating the veto effect (139–141). The following model has been hypothesized to explain adequately the varied experimental findings associated with veto inhibition (Fig. 7): the veto signal is transmitted through the interaction of CD8 on the veto cell with MHC I on the responding cell, while the responding cell is also being activated by the interaction of its TCR with peptide/MHC on the veto cell. The TCR on the veto cell does not participate. The exact mechanism of veto inactivation is unknown, although some experiments implicate deletion by apoptosis (141,142). Finally, although the veto phenomenon has been well established as an in vitro finding, its relevance to in vivo tolerance has yet to be proven definitively. There are a number of experiments suggesting that the veto effect may occur in vivo, but additional mechanisms of tolerance could not be excluded as operating under these circumstances (143,144) and further work is required.

Summary of T-Cell Tolerogenic Mechanisms

As can be seen in Fig. 8, it is possible to envision T-cell tolerance as the sum of several multilayered mechanisms that act in concert to prevent autoreactivity. The primary event is likely to be central thymic deletion of high-affinity autoreactive T cells. Those self-reactive T lymphocytes escaping thymic deletion may not be able to "see" their ligands, either because the antigens are se-

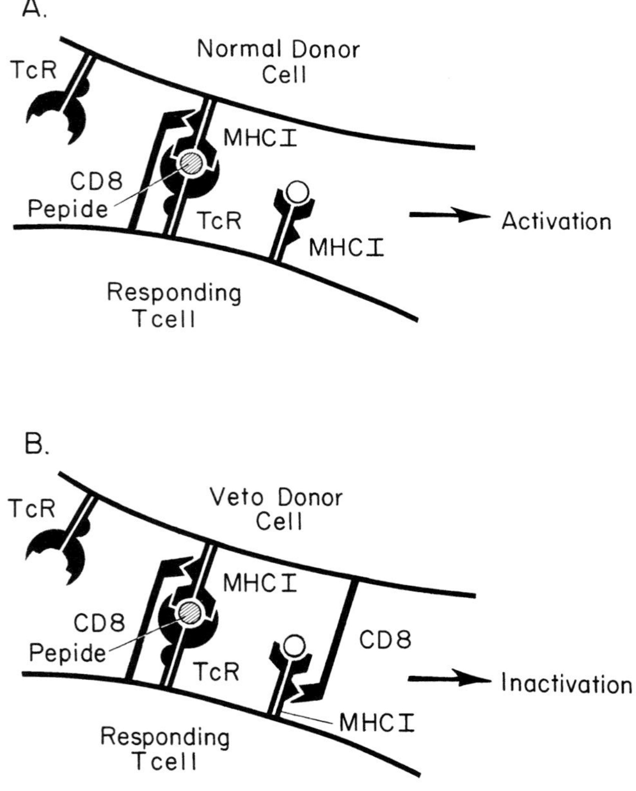

FIG. 7. Proposed mechanism of the veto effect in alloimmune responses. **A:** Alloactivation: a recipient T cell becomes activated upon recognition of a donor cell. **B:** Veto inhibition: veto donor cells express CD8, which delivers an inhibitory signal to the T cell through interaction with T-cell-expressed MHC I.

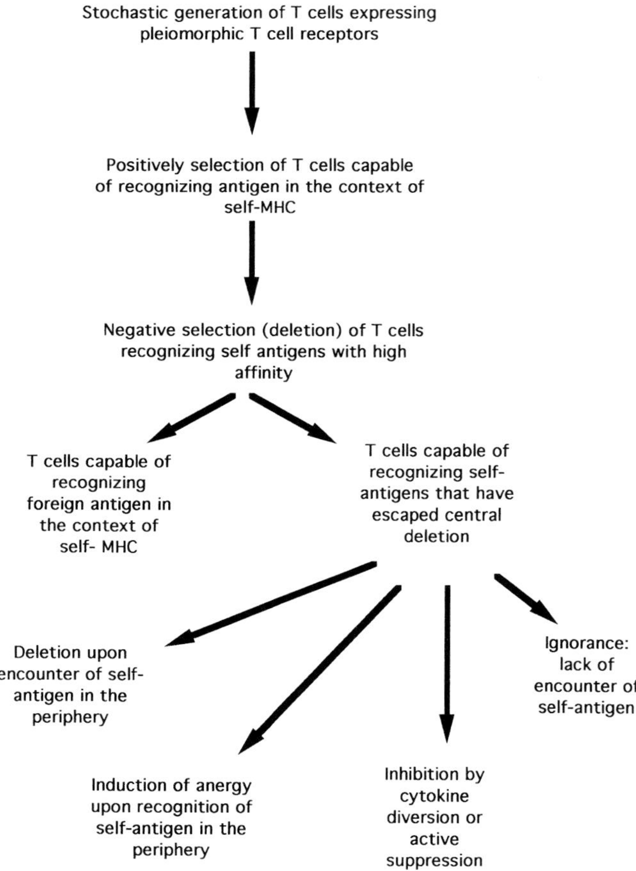

FIG. 8. Summary of the mechanisms of T-cell tolerance.

questered, the antigens are not expressed in the context of self-MHC, or the naive T cells are unable to circulate into peripheral organs. Other mature self-reactive T cells are controlled through peripheral deletion, through the down-regulation of TCR (and/or CD8) surface expression or through the induction of clonal anergy. The effects of Th2-like cytokines, such as IL-4, IL-10, and possibly transforming growth factor β, can additionally divert the autoreactive response to one that is not pathogenic, despite clonal expansion. Finally, active suppression, mediated by antigen-specific T cells, or veto cells, may provide additional levels of control. As is discussed later in this chapter, the development of autoimmune reactions requires overcoming all of these tolerogenic mechanisms.

B-CELL TOLERANCE

B-Cell Development

Through the identification of several B-cell surface markers and the use of a number of targeted gene disruption experiments, some of the mystery of B-cell development has become unraveled. A brief overview is presented here, and the reader is referred to one of several recent reviews for a more detailed discussion (13,145).

The initial event in B-cell development in the bone marrow is VDJ rearrangement of the μ heavy chain (146). The rearranged V_HDJ_H μ chain is then initially expressed on the cell surface in association with a surrogate light chain, λ5 (147). Data from knockout mice suggest that expression of this pre-B-cell receptor stimulates further B-cell differentiation (and is thus a form of positive selection), leads to allelic exclusion of the second μ chain, and probably stimulates light-chain rearrangement (148). The ligand for this pre-B-cell receptor is not known. Light-chain rearrangement then proceeds with the κ-chain recombination generally occurring prior to a λ-chain rearrangement (145). Once both the heavy and light chains have been rearranged, an immunoglobulin-M (IgM) heteromer is expressed on the immature B-cell surface, and the B cell is first able to recognize the antigenic universe. Rearrangement of the δ_H-chain gene then ensues, with the subsequent coexpression of IgM and IgD on the cell surface (13,145). Much progress has been made in understanding some of the essential inducing agents and signal transduction molecules involved in regulating this developmental process, but the reader is referred elsewhere for a discussion of these issues [reviewed by Hagman and Grosschedl (149) and Rosenberg and Kincade (150)].

Once the mature B cell is released from the bone marrow, it circulates in the blood and then migrates across high endothelial venules to the secondary lymphoid organs: the lymph nodes, spleen, tonsils, and Peyer patches [reviewed by Picker and Butcher (151)]. Within these organs, the B cells become activated after receiving T-cell help and interacting with antigens in specialized B-cell follicles (152,153). The activated B cells form germinal centers and then undergo somatic mutation of their V-region genes in order to form higher-affinity antibodies (affinity maturation) (153,154).

The Need for B-Cell Tolerance

If, as just outlined, an antigen-specific T cell is required to provide help for B-cell activation, can T-cell tolerance alone prevent the production of autoreactive B cells? Clearly the answer is no. Without B-cell tolerogenic mechanisms, an organism would be at great risk for the production of autoantibodies directed at foreign antigens that cross-react with self-determinants. T-cell-independent polyclonal activation of B cells could additionally result in autoimmune phenomena. Finally, somatic mutation in germinal centers allows for the development of a higher-affinity antibody response, but could potentially produce plasma cells with antibodies capable of recognizing self-constituents. For these reasons, it is imperative that an organism be able to tolerize its B cells to self-antigens.

Tolerogenic Mechanisms for B Cells

The major tolerogenic mechanisms for T cells, including clonal ignorance, clonal deletion, and anergy, also apply to B cells, although some differences do exist. Note, however, that the distinction between central and peripheral mechanisms of B-cell tolerance, based on current experimental data, is not as clear as that found in the T-cell compartment.

Clonal Ignorance

Analogous to clonal ignorance in T cells, the presence of a self-antigen has been demonstrated to have no effect occasionally on the B-cell repertoire. Many normal individuals have autoantibodies (that is, anti-DNA antibodies) without clinical evidence of autoimmune disease (155). The study of Ig-transgenic animal systems has been useful in understanding the persistence of these autoreactive B cells. In a double-transgenic animal expressing antilysozyme antibodies and very low concentrations of lysozyme (only 5% of the antigen receptors were estimated to be occupied by the antigen), the transgenic B cells were phenotypically normal and capable of producing antibodies in vivo (156). Other examples of clonal ignorance have been documented when the autoantibody's affinity for its autoantigen is low (157,158). It therefore seems most likely that B cells reactive to antigens sequestered from the immune system (that is, found only intracellularly), B cells recognizing antigens found in very low quantities, or B cells recognizing self-antigens below some threshold affinity level can remain ignorant to the immune stimulus.

Clonal Deletion and Receptor Editing

Analogous to the T-cell tolerogenic process, negative selection in the bone marrow has emerged as the predominant mechanism of B-cell tolerance. Initial data implicating clonal deletion of B cells as a tolerogenic process showed that B cells failed to develop in mice treated from birth with goat antisera directed at IgM (159). Once again, however, definitive evidence for clonal deletion came out of studies using transgenic animals.

The first example employed an Ig-transgenic mouse system expressing an IgM antibody with specificity toward both MHC I K^k and K^b. In comparison to control strains, expression of the transgene in a K^b- or K^k-expressing strain led to a marked reduction in the number of peripheral B cells and an absence of the specific IgM antibody (160). Although this experiment suggested that the deletion process occurred centrally (that is, in the bone marrow), later studies using double-transgenic mice, expressing K^b only in the liver, and anti-K^b antibody, revealed that deletion could occur peripherally as well (161).

Further evidence for deletion came from a double-transgenic system in which either an antilysozyme IgM or IgD transgenic mouse was mated with another transgenic mouse expressing a membrane-bound form of lysozyme (162). No mature lysozyme-binding B cells were detected in the lymph nodes or spleen of either the IgM or IgD transgenic animals, although some self-reactive, immature B cells were found in the bone marrow (162,163). These immature B cells could be rescued to develop into mature antilysozyme B cells in an in vitro lysozyme-free environment, however (163). Interestingly, if the same antilysozyme B cells were also made transgenic for an anti-apoptosis gene, *bcl-2*, enormous numbers of the maturationally arrested B-cell precursors could be found in the bone marrow, spleen, and peripheral blood (164). These findings suggested that maturational arrest, upon recognition of self-antigens, could be separated from intiation of cell death (presumably apoptosis).

Clarification of these observations came from the discovery of "receptor editing," using the Ig-transgenic mouse expressing IgM reactive to MHC I $K^{b,k}$ (165). Tiegs et al. showed that immature B cells recognizing their ligand first undergo a maturational arrest and then reactivate their machinery for Ig V-region gene arrangement (165). Some of the B cells from these mice were able to replace the transgenic κ chain with an endogenously produced λ chain, thus giving the B cell a new, nonself, specificity (165). These cells were then detected peripherally and behaved like normal virgin B cells (165). Other workers have confirmed receptor editing as an important tolerogenic mechanism, although some discussion remains about the exact timing of the editing event (166,167).

A composite model based on these studies is illustrated in Fig. 9 (14). An immature B cell expressing an IgM or IgD receptor reactive to a self-antigen (presumably above some affinity threshold) initially undergoes a maturational arrest. At this time, an attempt is made by the B cell to produce a nonself-reactive antigen receptor via receptor editing. If such an attempt is successful, then B-cell development continues and the mature B cell is

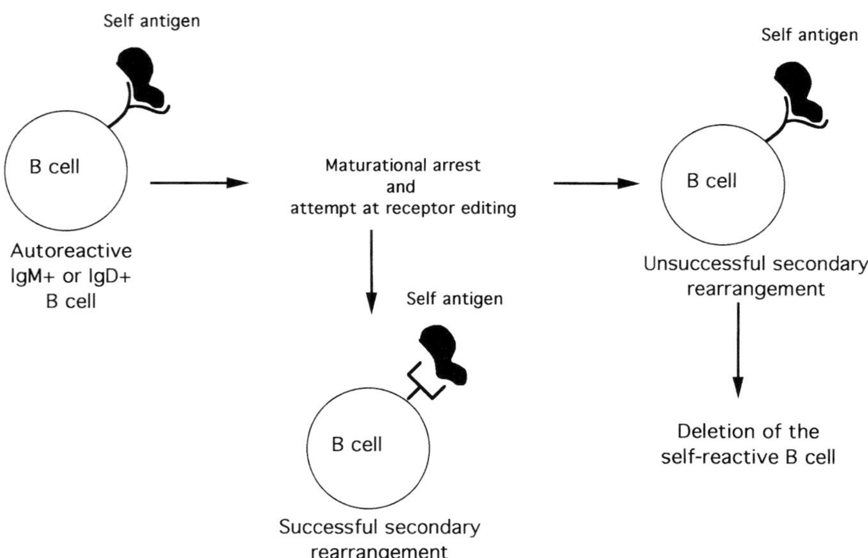

FIG. 9. B-cell receptor editing. See the text for details.

released into the periphery. If a newly rearranged, non-self-reactive V chain cannot be produced, the immature B cell undergoes apoptotic death.

Clonal Anergy of B Cells

The term clonal anergy was coined by Nossal and Pike to describe in tolerant mice the persistence of receptor-positive B cells (or in in vitro systems) that were functionally inactive (168). In this original work, splenic cells were assayed for their ability to recognize fluorescein bound to the protein flagellen (168). In untreated control mice, 1.4–2.7% of the splenocytes specifically responded to the antigen (168). Tolerance induction did not change the phenotype of the splenic B cells, but the number of antigen-responsive B cells dropped to <0.6% (168). These classic experiments were initially interpreted as inducing anergy because (a) there was no notable phenotypic change in the B-cell population and (b) there was a detectable decrease in antigen-specific responses (168). The extremely low number of antigen-specific cells at baseline presents a problem for this interpretation, however. All of the antigen-specific B cells could have been deleted (as opposed to anergized), but because of the low number of cells to begin with, it would be difficult to detect such change (47).

More recent work implicating B-cell anergy as a tolerogenic process used an Ig-transgenic mouse system in which it was much easier to follow the fate of the given antigen-specific B cell. Goodnow and colleagues produced a doubly transgenic mouse expressing both an antilysozyme antibody and a soluble form (as opposed to a membrane-bound form) of lysozyme (169). No antilysozyme antibody production was noted in these mice despite the continued ability to detect the B cells in the spleen, lymph nodes, and Peyer patches, thus defining a population of anergic B cells (169). Further work showed that the anergy could be induced either centrally or peripherally (156).

The cellular processes involved in silencing anergized B cells are only partially understood. The anergic antilysozyme B cells from Goodnow's model had a profound inability to respond to appropriate signals in vitro, had significantly downregulated the expression of IgM receptors on their surface, and had a marked defect in their ability to differentiate into antibody-secreting plasma cells (169): that is, upon transfer to an antigen-free environment (a syngeneic mouse lacking the lysozyme transgene), they recovered normal expression of IgM, but were unable to produce antibodies unless they remained in the antigen-free environment for a prolonged period of time (169). More recent studies have additionally noted that these anergic B cells have a specific defect in their antigen presentation ability (170). Further work is required to decipher better the basis of this unresponsive state.

Despite the fact that B-cell anergy has been described in a number of systems, it has also come under a number of criticisms (47). Notably, the antilysozyme B cells in Goodnow's model system are barely capable of responding to any stimulus, and recent work has revealed that these anergic cells only survive for 3–4 days (171), compared with the normal 4- to 5-week life span of mature B cells. As is the case for anergic T cells, the differentiation between anergy and cell death is not clearly distinct. For the moment, however, the predominant thinking in immunologic circles is that B-cell anergy does occur in some experimental systems. Whether it will emerge as a preeminent tolerogenic process for B cells in vivo awaits further research.

Positive Selection of the Secondary B-Cell Response in Germinal Centers

As just noted, the ability of B cells to undergo affinity maturation within germinal centers presents a unique problem for immune tolerance. The extensive hypermutation of heavy-chain and light-chain genes during the somatic mutation process could potentially result in antibodies with lower affinity to the antigen than the original B cell and could lead to antibodies reactive to self-constituents. How the immune system selects for only those B cells recognizing foreign antigen with high affinity is only partially understood. It is known that B cells proliferating in germinal centers downregulate their Ig receptors and become extremely short-lived (13,172,173). Upon reemergence of the newly mutated receptor, the B cell is programmed to undergo apoptotic death, unless rescued (that is, positively selected) by antigen recognition on follicular dendritic cells (13,172,173). Ligation of the B-cell surface molecule CD40 seems to be important in this regard (13,172,173). The end result is that B cells with low-affinity receptors die from apoptosis, while those with high-affinity receptors are positively selected to become plasma cells or memory cells (13,172–174).

It remains unclear, however, why self-reactive B cells are not selected in this process. An interesting report recently showed, however, that self-reactive B cells are somehow denied access to the germinal centers as long as foreign antigen-reactive B cells are present in sufficient quantity (175). The antiself B cells seem to pile up outside of the follicle and then die of apoptosis (175). The molecular and cellular basis of this poorly understood process, known as "competitive exclusion," is presently under intensive investigative scrutiny.

Idiotypic B-Cell Networks

As alluded to earlier, an idiotype is an antigenic determinant derived from the variable region of a given antibody (123,176): that is, determinants on the antibody

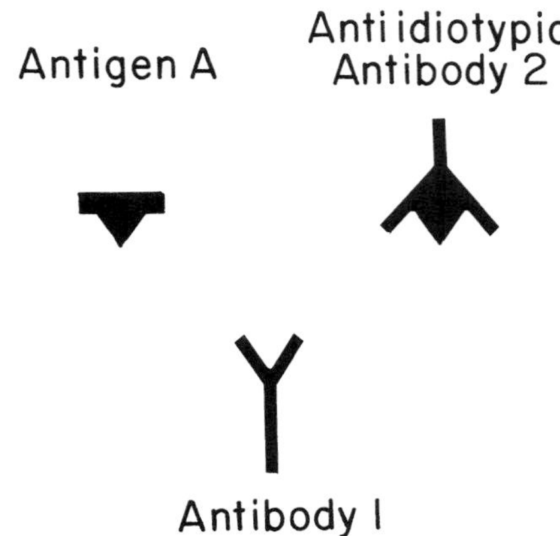

FIG. 10. Anti-idiotypic antibodies mimic antigenic structure. Antibody 1 recognizes antigen A. Anti-idiotypic antibody 2 recognizes the unique antigen combining site of antibody 1 and mimics the internal structure of antigen A.

itself can act as antigens. Such idiotypes can be defined serologically through recognition by anti-idiotypic antibodies (176). The existence of idiotypes and anti-idiotypic antibodies led Jerne to propose the network theory of immune regulation (118). His theory had two important implications (118,176). First, every antibody expresses at least one (and usually many) idiotype(s), thus allowing for the development of antibodies directed at that idiotype (Fig. 10) and defining a network of interrelated antibodies. Such an anti-idiotypic network could regulate the levels of antibody produced, by either stimulating B cells through their idiotype-expressing receptors or by directly blocking the secreted idiotype-expressing antibody itself (123,176). The second implication of the theory follows from an understanding of the antibody relationships in the network and reveals that an anti-idiotypic antibody can mimic the three-dimensional structure of the original antigen. To illustrate, Fig. 10 depicts two antibodies, the first of which, antibody 1, recognizes antigen A. The second, anti-idiotypic, antibody 2 recognizes the antigen-combining site of antibody 1. Since both the anti-idiotypic antibody 2 and the original antigen A can be bound by antibody 1, antibody 2 could represent an internal image of antigen A (118,123,176).

Work in several experimental systems has demonstrated the existence of anti-idiotypic antibodies both in vivo and in vitro (123,176,177). Additionally, there have been a number of reports showing that anti-idiotypic antibodies can mimic antigens (176). For example, anti-idiotypic antibodies (antibody 2 in Fig. 10) directed at specific determinants on anti-insulin antibodies (antibody 1 in Fig. 10) have been isolated (178). These anti-idiotypic antibodies were shown to bind to insulin receptors and to stimulate glycolysis, thus mimicking the structure and function of insulin (178). Numerous other examples have been demonstrated as well (176). In most of these studies, however, demonstration of the idiotype–anti-idiotype interaction required a nonphysiologic external intervention. What remains unclear is what physiologic role idiotypic networks play in the normal development and regulation of B-cell repertoires.

The Nature of the Tolerizing Signal for B Cells

The factors determining how a B cell will respond to a given stimulus, be they ignorance, activation, receptor editing/deletion, or anergy, are areas of ongoing investigation, and only partial answers are known. Clearly, some of these factors relate to specific characteristics of the antigen–antigen receptor interaction, as illustrated by Goodnow's antilysozyme Ig-transgenic mouse system (156,157). This model and others (158,179) have elegantly demonstrated that the level of antigen expression, the intrinsic affinity of the antigen receptor for its ligand, and the degree of antigen receptor cross-linking all can affect the outcome of the interaction.

The presence or absence of appropriate costimulation, as originally hypothesized by Bretscher and Cohn (65), also appears to influence significantly the outcome of a B-cell interaction with its specific ligand. Recent in vitro work has demonstrated that extensive cross-linking of mature B-cell antigen receptors by specific antigen induces B-cell unresponsiveness followed by apoptosis (180). This phenomenon can be entirely prevented (in fact, the cells are activated instead) through ligation of CD40 and addition of IL-4 to the culture system, presumably through supplying appropriate costimulatory signals (180). Whether these findings are reflective of in vivo tolerance mechanisms remains to be seen.

Although it is clear that both mature and immature B cells can be tolerized, some data suggest that immature B cells, and B cells undergoing affinity maturation in germinal centers, are uniquely susceptible to signals leading to anergy or deletion (157,161,162,172,181). Whether these findings simply reflect differences in experimental design, or B cells truly pass through stages of tolerizability (where, for example, the presence or absence of costimulation is irrelevant), remains to be established.

Based on these experimental findings, a model of B-cell response to antigen recognition can be hypothesized (Fig. 11). Analogous to the findings in T cells, the B-cell response to antigen is partially determined by avidity of the receptor–antigen interaction, where avidity is comprised of intrinsic affinity, quantity of antigen, and valence of the antigen (increased valence leads to extensive cross-linking). Low-affinity interactions (or those where the antigen concentrations are extremely low) are ignored by B cells, while higher-affinity interactions, especially those with extensive receptor cross-linking, lead to aner-

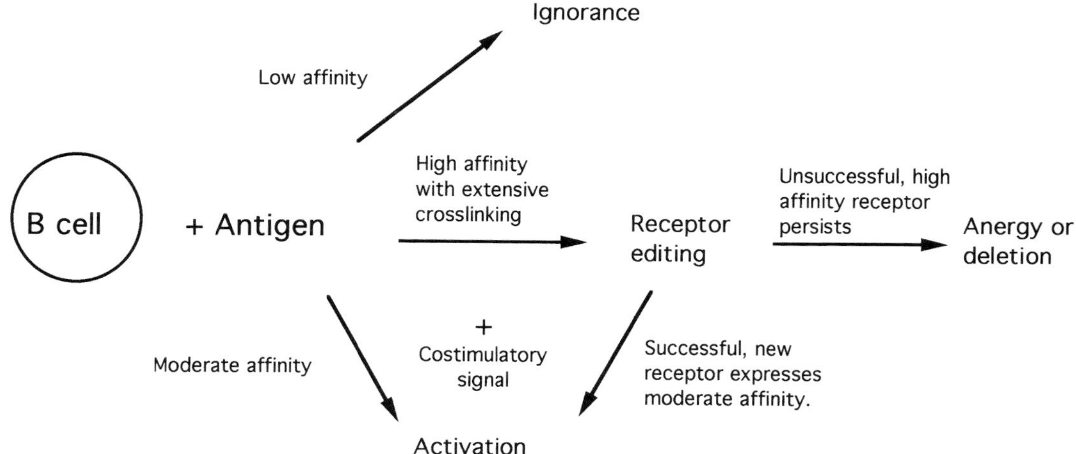

FIG. 11. Summary of the potential outcomes of a B-cell interaction with antigen.

gy or receptor editing/deletion. Negative selection of this sort may occur at any developmental stage, but in mature B cells, it is likely to be mediated by antigen recognition without appropriate costimulatory signals. Activation of mature B cells, on the other hand, seems to require a moderate- to high-affinity antigen recognition in the presence of appropriate costimulatory signals. Ongoing studies will help to verify this model.

AUTOIMMUNITY

Evolutionary pressures have led to the development of a mammalian immune system capable of recognizing and destroying a huge variety of invading pathogens. This diversity necessarily results in the random development of some immune cells that will recognize self-antigens and are thus potentially dangerous to the host organism. As outlined in the previous sections, the immune system has evolved a number of redundant tolerogenic processes to prevent these autoreactive cells from causing damage. Thus, the mechanisms of immunologic tolerance, and the tendency to react to self-antigens (through autoreactive T and B cells) can be envisioned as occupying opposite sides of a traditional scale. Normally, the scales are heavily weighted toward tolerance, but under unusual circumstances the tolerogenic mechanisms can be circumvented, and the scales tip toward autoimmunity. It is the goal of this section to establish a theoretical framework for how tolerance can be overcome, and under what circumstances autoimmunity prevails. It is important to realize that the overwhelming majority of the data derive from studies in controlled mammalian animal systems, so that extrapolation to human autoimmune disease does not necessarily follow. However, many of the experimental findings in animals are supported by circumstantial evidence in human diseases, thus partially validating the concepts.

T and B Cells Reactive to Self-Antigens Are Found in Normal Hosts

It has been repeatedly demonstrated that normal hosts contain T cells and B cells that are capable of recognizing self-antigens. Antibodies that bind to cytoskeletal proteins, DNA, membrane antigens, Igs, and peptide hormones can be detected in individuals without any evidence of autoimmunity [reviewed by Avrameas (155)]. When tested in vitro, most of these autoantibodies are cross-reactive to foreign antigens, are of the IgM isotype, and have low avidity to their autoantigens (155). Some of them are produced by a subtype of B cells expressing the CD5 antigen. CD5+ B cells may develop from a separate lineage from other B cells, are preferentially abundant in the relatively protected peritoneal cavity, and in contrast to the short-lived nature of CD5– B cells, are long-lived and capable of self-renewal (182,183). Whether this unusual subset of B lymphocytes preferentially contributes to autoimmunity is discussed below.

T lymphocytes reactive to autoantigens are also present in normal hosts. It has been clearly documented that autoreactive T cells can be detected in nondiseased animals (184) and in normal human peripheral blood (185).

These autoreactive T and B lymphocytes likely exist in the periphery of normal individuals because central deletion mechanisms are incomplete. As just outlined, the experimental evidence suggests that central deletion functions to eliminate high-avidity autoreactive cells, but those cells expressing receptors with avidity to self-antigens just below the threshold will continue to develop and thus be released into the periphery. The additional mechanisms of ignorance, anergy, suppression in its various forms, and cytokine diversion contribute to controlling these autoreactive cells. When such tolerogenic mechanisms fail, the normally quiescent autoreactive cells become capable mediators of autoimmune injury.

Genetic Issues

Autoimmunity depends on the activation of autoreactive T cells upon recognition of their specific peptide/MHC ligand and/or activation of an autoreactive B cell upon recognition of its particular antigen. Certain inherited genes might preferentially predispose individuals to these autorecognition events. Recent work in molecular immunology has focused on evaluating whether the expression of specific TCR genes, Ig genes, and MHC alleles predispose individuals to the development of autoimmunity.

T-Cell Receptor Genes

It has been hypothesized that the presence or absence of particular TCR genes, or allelic variants of those genes, predisposes an individual organism to develop autoimmune disease. Initial studies of EAE in rodents revealed that the overwhelming majority of pathogenic T cells expressed TCR Vβ8 and that elimination of the Vβ8-expressing T cells with specific antibodies effectively ameliorated symptoms of the disease (186,187). Initial data from humans with multiple sclerosis also revealed a preference for Vβ8 expression in myelin basic protein reactive T lymphocytes [reviewed by Gold (188)]. This so-called "TCR Vβ-gene restriction" in autoimmune disease has generated much interest for two reasons: (a) the preferential expression of limited Vβ genes in disease could be indicative of a genetic predisposition to disease susceptibility (that is, perhaps susceptible individuals contain a high percentage of Vβ8-expressing T cells in their peripheral T-cell repertoire or express an unusual allelic variant of Vβ8), and (b) restricted Vβ-gene expression could allow for specific immunotherapy targeting autoreactive cells that express the pathogenic Vβ gene (that is, with anti-Vβ antibodies).

Since the initial reports, TCR V-region gene restriction has been evaluated in a number of autoimmune disease models (including renal diseases), as well as in several human autoimmune diseases (188–190). In many cases a restriction of TCR V genes has been documented, while in other situations the autoreactive T-cell response seems to be more diverse (188–190). Additionally, there are no experimental data linking particular TCR V-region allelic variants to specific autoimmune diseases in animals or humans. Current thinking in most immunologic circles is that specific TCR V-region gene expression does not genetically predispose individuals to autoimmune disease. Instead, any detected restriction of TCR V-region gene expression more likely reflects antigen-driven clonal expansion of T cells expressing structurally related TCRs.

Immunoglobulin Genes

Similar questions have been raised about the association of individual Ig genes with autoreactive immune responses. Animal models of antibody-mediated hemolytic anemia (191) and systemic lupus erythematosis (SLE) (192) have provided useful systems for the evaluation of these questions. NZB mice develop hemolytic anemia secondary to autoreactive antibodies recognizing unknown epitopes on intact RBCs (191). Molecular analysis of these antibodies has revealed a wide range of V_H and V_K genes that do not differ from the repertoire of genes used for the recognition of foreign antigens (193, 194): that is, there is no particular set of Ig V-region genes associated with the development of disease (193, 194). Additionally, although Ig haplotypic variants can be defined, work in murine models of lupus has not revealed any association between individual haplotypes and a predisposition to autoimmune responses (192). On the other hand, the structure of anti-DNA antibodies seems to be highly conserved in many different strains of mice (192,195). Although these data suggest that most anti-DNA antibodies are encoded by structurally similar genes in germline configurations, the findings do not support an Ig genetic basis for the autoreactive response. Instead, the findings are once again best interpreted as being consistent with an antigen-driven clonal expansion of autoreactive B cells that express structurally similar receptors (192,195).

MHC Alleles

Although there does not seem to be a genetic link between TCR gene expression or Ig gene expression and the development of autoimmune disease, there is a strong association between the expression of certain MHC alleles and autoimmune phenomena, in both animal models and in human diseases. For example, the susceptibility to EAE (186,196), murine interstitial nephritis (197,198), collagen-induced arthritis (199–201), and murine diabetes (200,202), among many others, has been definitively linked to the expression of certain MHC alleles. Table 1 lists a number of human diseases that are linked to individual MHC gene polymorphisms. Many potential explanations for these associations have been hypothesized, although a general consensus has not yet been reached.

Studies of the development of diabetes in NOD mice have provided some insight into how MHC alleles can

TABLE 1. *HLA associations with selected human autoimmune diseases (288–290)*

Type 1 diabetes mellitus	DR4, DR3
Rheumatoid arthritis	DR1, DRw6, DR4
Celiac disease	DQw2
Pemphigus vulgaris	DR4/Dw10, DR6/Dw9
Multiple sclerosis	DR2/Dw2
Systemic lupus erythematosis	DR2, DR3
Graves disease	DR3
Sjogren syndrome	DR3
Ankylosing spondylitis	B27

influence the predisposition to autoimmunity. These animals develop pancreatic T-cell infiltrates directed at islet cell antigens beginning at an early age, which eventually results in β-cell destruction and diabetes (202). Susceptibility to disease is partially determined by the presence of an unusual MHC II haplotype, H-2^{g7} (202). NOD mice that are homozygous for H-2^{g7} develop diabetes, but heterozygotes do not (203). Additionally, NOD mice only express MHC II I-A molecules (as opposed to expressing both I-A and I-E alleles in most mice) and, if made transgenic for any I-E molecule, they become resistant to the development of disease (204). These data imply that there is some reduced ability of H-2^{g7} molecules to mediate central deletion or peripheral tolerance, which can be complemented with a normal MHC allele. The specific defect has not been defined, but defective in vitro antigen-presenting functions by H-2^{g7}-expressing cells have been documented (205).

Molecular analysis of the H-2^{g7} allele has provided further clues into understanding its association with diabetes. The I-Aβ chain of the H-2^{g7} molecule contains a His-Ser motif at positions 56 and 57, within the antigen-binding site, as opposed to a Pro-Asp motif found in most other animal strains (206). This allows binding of negatively charged carboxy-terminal peptides not bound by other MHC alleles (207). Therefore, the presence of the H-2^{g7} molecule allows for the presentation of a different set of autoantigenic peptides than other MHC alleles, providing a potential molecular explanation for the expansion of autoreactive T cells not seen in other strains of mice. Interestingly, the same His-Ser motif is found in the analogous position of the human DQb allele: one that has been associated with a high risk of developing diabetes in humans (200).

The complexities of MHC associations with disease are partially illustrated by the finding that expression of MHC I is also important in the development of diabetes in NOD mice. NOD mice without MHC I, through targeted disruption of the $β_2$m gene, do not get diabetes (208,209). Remarkably, the expression of diabetes is also diminished in congenic NOD mice expressing H-2^{g7}, but with different class I alleles (210). These findings suggest that, in addition to the initial recognition and expansion of autoreactive CD4+ T cells, the islet cells must express an appropriate MHC I molecule in order to be destroyed by an autoreactive CD8+ effector cell population.

The linkage of a particular MHC allele to a given autoimmune disease may be due to factors other than its ability to bind or present autoantigens. Some authors have postulated that particular MHC haplotypes can influence the strength of a given immune response (211), independent of their ability to bind antigenic peptides: that is, some MHC haplotypes are associated with strong responses, whereas others are associated with weaker responses. The molecular basis for such a response is not clearly understood, although it has been hypothesized that non-MHC genes encoded within the region of the MHC could modulate immune responses. Potential examples are tumor necrosis factor or complement proteins, both of which could influence an immune response and are encoded by genes found within the MHC. Whether or not allelic variants of these (or other) genes lead to quantitative or qualitative differences in immune responses remains to be established.

It also be should be pointed out that many strong associations between MHC alleles and autoimmune diseases have not yet been explained. Despite an intensive investigative effort, for example, there is no clear molecular or functional explanation for the association of HLA-B27 with ankylosing spondylitis. Suffice it to say that the associations between MHC alleles and autoimmune disease implicate a genetic link in some situations, but that the specific mechanisms are yet to be fully defined.

Autoantigens and Autoantigenic Determinants

Further understanding of the pathophysiologic basis for autoimmunity has come from the identification and analysis of autoantigens and their disease-relevant epitopes. Some of these autoantigens, as originally identified in animal systems and later confirmed to be relevant to selected human autoimmune diseases, are shown in Table 2.

TABLE 2. *Representative examples of known autoantigens*

Disease	Antigen	Ref.
Heyman nephritis	Brush border gp 330	(291)
Antitubular basement membrane disease	3M-1 glycoprotein	(292)
Diabetes mellitus	Glutamic acid decarboxylase	(293)
Experimental allergic encephalomyelitis	Myelin basic protein Proteolipid protein	(288, 294)
Myasthenia gravis	Acetylcholine receptor	(295)
Graves disease	TSH receptor	(288)
Collagen arthritis	Type II collagen	(288)

TSH, thyroid-stimulating hormone.

Molecular Mimicry and Cross-Reactivity

One hypothesis broadly speculated to play a role in initiating autoimmune responses is that infectious agents may contain antigenic epitopes that closely resemble self-proteins, thus triggering a cross-reactive autoimmune response (212). Such cross-reactivity could be a random event or could have been evolutionarily selected to engender a selective advantage to the invading organism, a process called molecular mimicry (212). Most of the evidence for molecular mimicry is circumstantial, however, and is derived from protein sequence homologies determined from data-base searches. Many of these homologies do not have any epidemiologic basis; for example, a rabies virus epitope shares homology with the insulin receptor, but rabies has no known link to diabetes (212).

In other instances, epidemiologic links have bolstered the significance of such findings. Streptococcal M proteins, for example, share epitopes with myocardial proteins (including myosin), and certain streptococcal species are linked to the development of rheumatic carditis (213,214). Despite this, there is no evidence that these infectious antigens directly induce autoimmune injury.

More definitive data implicating molecular mimicry have been published in a few cases. T cells reactive to a synthetic peptide of hepatitis-B-virus polymerase (which is homologous to myelin basic protein) have been shown to induce experimental allergic encephalomyelitis, and immunization with a yeast histone (which is homologous to a retinal binding protein) was demonstrated to induce autoimmune uveitis (215,216). In another recently described study, T cells reactive to glutamate decarboxylase, a known target antigen of diabetes in NOD mice (90), also recognized a cross-reactive epitope from a coxsackievirus protein (217). Interestingly, the cross-reactivity only occurred in NOD mice and not in the context of nine other MHC alleles tested (217), further strengthening the previously described link between diabetes and certain MHC haplotypes. These findings are potentially of great interest to human diabetes in that an association with coxsackievirus and diabetes has been described (218), and the MHC allele of the NOD mouse strongly resembles its human counterpart (206).

Cross-reactive T-cell responses have also been documented in protein antigens that are evolutionarily highly conserved (219). The best example is that of mycobacterial tuberculosis (MTB) and heat-shock proteins (219). T-cell clones obtained from an arthritic joint of a rat with adjuvant arthritis were shown to recognize MTB antigens, HSP 65, and human arthritic joint fluid, establishing a potential link between tuberculosis and human autoimmune arthritis (220–223).

The molecular basis for these antigenic cross-reactions is being actively investigated because it had been originally assumed that TCR recognition of antigen/MHC was highly specific and cross-reactivity extremely unlikely. One possibility to account for cross-reactive priming of T-cell responses is that T cells may express more than one distinct TCR. The lack of α-chain allelic exclusion has been shown to result occasionally in the surface expression of more than one functional αβ heterodimer on a given T cell (20). These recent findings suggest a novel pathogenic mechanism for the development of autoimmune responses. If a single T cell has one receptor that recognizes foreign peptide in the context of MHC, while the other is specific for a self-antigen (and has escaped central deletion), stimulation by the foreign peptide could lead to the expansion of an autoreactive T-cell repertoire (Fig. 12). The induction of autoimmunity by this mechanism awaits experimental confirmation.

Data obtained from in vitro model systems have also revealed that some T cells (presumably expressing a single unique TCR) will respond to peptides unrelated to their original known specificity, as long as they are presented in the context of the appropriate MHC molecule (224). Although such degeneracy of recognition is demonstrable, it is not a generalizable phenomenon. Further systematic substitution analysis of peptide epitopes has shown that some peptide residues are important for binding to the MHC molecule, some are essential for T-cell recognition of the peptide, and others can be radically changed without altering T-cell recognition (225). Which residues have what function needs to be determined for each individual peptide/MHC complex. Clearly, however, single T-cell clones can respond to more than one peptide antigen, thus providing a molecular basis for cross-reactive responses.

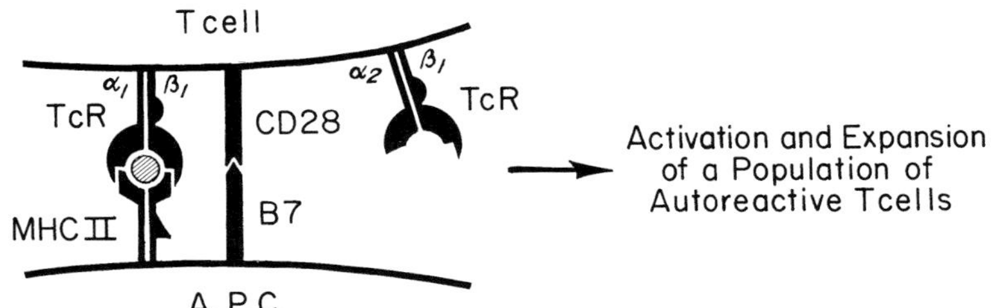

FIG. 12. A T cell expressing two distinct α chains could become an autoreactive threat. The T-cell receptor *(TCR)* α1β1 recognizes foreign peptide and self-MHC, whereas the TCR α2β1 recognizes self-peptide and self-MHC. Appropriate activation of the T cell through α1β1 can thus additionally prime an autoreactive T-cell response.

Finally, viruses have been implicated in directly initiating autoimmune responses in selected cases. Viruses have been demonstrated to induce diabetes directly in one animal model (226) and are strongly implicated as etiologic agents in several cases of human diabetes (218,227,228). The detection of measles virus genome in a case of human chronic autoimmune hepatitis suggests that the persistence of viral integration can elicit a response that is perceived by the immune system as foreign (229).

Superantigens

Superantigens stimulate a high proportion of CD4+ T cells (between 5% and 50%) through cross-linking of the outer portion of certain Vβ-expressing TCRs and MHC molecules on APCs (Fig. 13) (230). Members of one family of exogenous superantigens, consisting of toxic bacterial proteins, have been hypothesized to participate in autoimmune responses. Staphylococcal enterotoxin B (SEB) predominantly affects Vβ8-expressing T cells (124, 231), the dominant mediators of the autoimmune response in some rodent models of EAE (186). SEB treatment of animals in remission from EAE was shown to exacerbate the disease via expansion of Vβ8+ T cells (232). Additionally, some animals immunized with myelin basic protein (MBP), but that did not become symptomatic, developed full-blown EAE after treatment with SEB (232).

Other indirect evidence supporting superantigens as mediators of autoimmune responses come from studies revealing limited TCR Vβ-gene expression in human joints afflicted with rheumatoid arthritis (233,234). The finding of a high deduced amino acid homology among all of the TCR β chains in the CDR4 region of superantigen binding (233,234) suggests that the autoreactive response could have been initiated by a superantigen. Superantigens have also been demonstrated to induce inflammatory cytokine gene expression in synovial cells (235) and to induce polyclonal B-cell responses (236), further establishing a potential link between these molecules and autoimmunity. Despite these intriguing findings, there has not, as yet, been any definitive proof that superantigens participate in the initiation or propagation of autoimmune responses in humans.

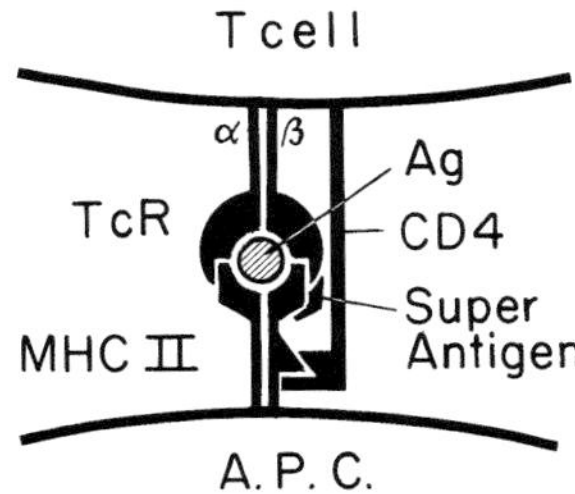

FIG. 13. Superantigens activate CD4+ T cells through cross-linking of MHC II and the β chain of certain T-cell receptors.

Autoimmunity May be a Primary Abnormality in the Target Organ

Much of the previous discussion has focused on exogenous factors as initiators or mediators of autoimmune diseases. In contrast, several authors have suggested that autoimmunity could result from abnormal antigenic expression by a target organ (47,211). In this scenario, the immune system would be responding normally to otherwise hidden antigenic determinants, and no outside stimulating processes or abnormalities in immune regulation need be invoked. This is mostly a theoretical argument in that there exist few experimental data to corroborate it. One piece of evidence favoring this hypothesis comes out of studies of myasthenia gravis, in which autoantibodies directed at acetylcholine receptors result in muscle weakness (237). Clinical studies in myasthenia have strongly suggested that the thymus is partially responsible for the manifestations of disease—in many cases, thymectomies are curative (238). Interestingly, the thymus of patients with myasthenia contains abnormal expression of fetal acetylcholine receptors (239). This finding raises the possibility that an appropriate immune response directed at an abnormally expressed antigen (the fetal acetylcholine receptor) causes disease by cross-reacting with normal acetylcholine receptors (47). Whether this theory can be generalized as an important pathogenic mechanism for induction of autoimmune responses is yet to be established.

Immunodominant and Cryptic Antigenic Determinants

Studies over the last 15 years have noted that T-cell responses are focused toward restricted antigenic determinants derived from individual proteins [reviewed by Sercarz et al. (88)]: that is, only certain immunodominant epitopes derived from an intact antigenic protein are seen by the immune system. Immunodominant epitopes have been defined for both model antigens, such as hen-egg lysozyme (88), and disease-relevant autoantigens, such as myelin basic protein (240) and 3M-1, the target antigen of murine interstitial nephritis (190). Why one epitope is selected in an immune response, while others are neglected, is not fully understood, although important factors include (a) the binding ability of the peptide determinant for the MHC molecule, (b) the number of MHC/peptide complexes available for interaction with T cells, (c) the number and affinity of T cells within the repertoire capable of interacting with the given peptide/MHC complex, (d) the structural characteristics of the native antigen that may place constraints upon uptake and enzymatic processing by APCs, and (e) the specific enzymatic processing characteristics of the APC itself [reviewed by Sercarz et al. (88)].

Multiple investigators have also demonstrated in vitro T-cell responses to peptide determinants derived from the known sequence of a native antigen, in which the same T cells are unable to respond to the native protein itself (241–243). Presumably, these "cryptic determinants" are not readily presented to the immune system in vivo, but can be selected for, using in vitro T-cell culture systems. It would be expected that potentially autoreactive T cells recognizing such cryptic epitopes would normally exist in ignorance within the organism (243).

Recent work, however, has shown that cryptic peptides can become unmasked under certain conditions. Elegant studies in both EAE and murine diabetes have established that initial autoimmune responses are directed at a few immunodominant epitopes derived from single autoantigens (89,90). As the disease progresses, though, T-cell reactivity toward previously cryptic determinants within the original target protein can be demonstrated (89,90). In fact, disease progression is associated with the detection of reactivity toward epitopes derived from other antigens (that is, heat-shock proteins) as well (89,90).

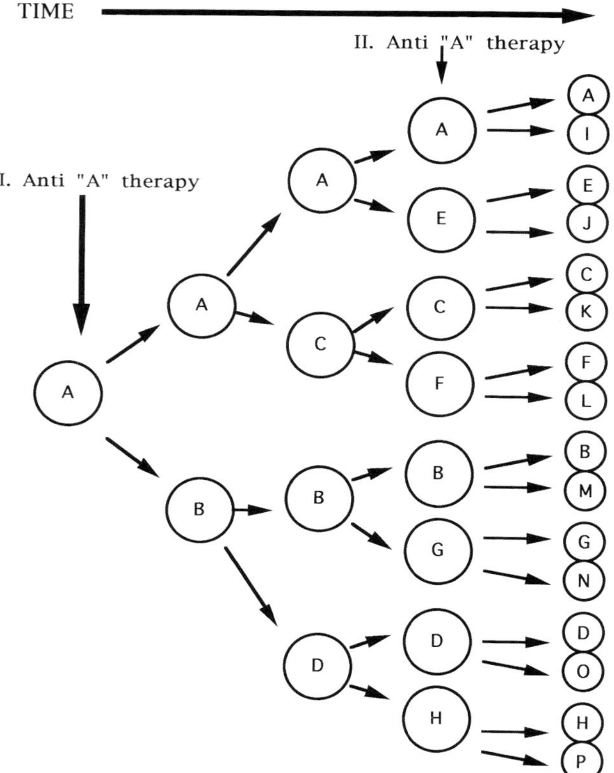

FIG. 14. Epitope spreading of the autoimmune response. The initial autoimmune response is directed at *epitope A*, but spreads to additional epitopes *(B–P)* as the immune response progresses. Intervention at time point I with therapy aimed at epitope A is likely to be efficacious. The same intervention at time point II is unlikely to be effective because the autoreactive immune response is no longer focused on a single epitope.

Such findings have resulted in the theory of "determinant spreading" in autoimmunity (Fig. 14), which suggests that autoimmune diseases may be initiated by T cells reactive to single epitopes, but later spread to additional epitopes, both within the original target antigen (intramolecular) and in additional proteins (intermolecular), as the disease progresses (88–90). The theory has obvious implications for antigen-based therapeutic strategies for autoimmune diseases. As illustrated in Fig. 14, therapy targeting T cells reactive to the original inciting autoantigenic epitope would be expected to treat the disease process effectively only if implemented before the immune response has spread to other epitopes. Studies in EAE and murine diabetes have thus far been entirely consistent with such a theoretical framework (89,90). Whether epitope spreading participates in the pathogenesis of other models of autoimmune diseases, or in human autoimmunity, is presently under investigation.

The operative mechanisms of emerging autoreactivity directed at cryptic epitopes during autoimmune responses are not yet fully elucidated, but are likely to be multifactorial in nature [reviewed by Sercarz et al. (88)]. Activation of APCs by inflammatory mediators, particularly IFN-γ, has been shown to alter proteolytic processing of antigen (when compared with unstimulated APCs) (244–246). T-cell infiltration and release of IFN-γ during an autoimmune response can thus potentially lead to the presentation of cryptic epitopes through APC activation and altered antigenic processing. Antigenic processing by cells of different cell lineages can differ as well (88). During organ-specific autoimmune responses, autoantigens could thus be presented by a variety of APCs, including endothelial and epithelial cells expressing MHC II, and capable of presenting different peptides than professional APCs. This would provide another potential mechanism for inducing immune responses to cryptic determinants.

Endogenously synthesized antigens are degraded by different proteolytic pathways (with different resultant peptide determinants) than exogenous antigens taken up by APCs (247). Tissue destruction during autoimmune responses could result in the extracellular release of antigens that are normally processed through endogenous pathways, with subsequent uptake and degradation by APCs. This altered processing pathway could once again result in appropriate presentation of previously cryptic epitopes and thus permit activation of otherwise ignorant bystander T cells.

Finally, it should be noted that epitope spreading seems to occur in B-cell-mediated autoimmune diseases as well. The progressive spreading of autoantibody specificity from a single antigen to multiple antigens has been well documented in several model systems, including murine lupus (248) and an autoimmune disease of the ovary (249). Mechanisms of epitope spreading in B-cell-mediated responses are presently unknown.

Antigen Presentation and Autoimmune Responses

As discussed in detail in the earlier section on tolerance, activation of a CD4+ T cell occurs when the T-cell recognizes antigen expressed in the context of MHC II and receives a second costimulatory signal. Many immunologists have hypothesized that alterations in the expression of MHC II or costimulation could contribute to the pathogenesis of autoimmune responses.

Expression of MHC II

The cellular distribution of MHC II is limited to a small subset of cells, in contrast to the ubiquitous expression of MHC I. One hypothesis to account for avoidance of autoimmunity is that most cells do not express MHC II and are therefore unable to present antigen to T cells. Could induced expression of MHC II, that is, during viral infections, lead to the induction of autoimmune responses? Initial excitement for this idea derived from the finding that thyroid epithelial cells and renal epithelial cells upregulated MHC II and acquired APC properties after exposure to IFN-γ or viral infections (250). Additional data derived from murine interstitial nephritis suggest that IFN-γ induction of MHC II on renal epithelial cell contributed to the induction of autoimmune renal disease in an otherwise resistant strain of mice (82). Interestingly, studies on the pancreas of a child who died 24 h after the diagnosis of diabetes mellitus revealed pancreatic β-cell expression of MHC II, with both CD4 and CD8 T-cell infiltrates, also suggesting that increased expression of MHC II could contribute to autoimmune responses (251).

On the other hand, increased expression of MHC II on nonprofessional APCs would allow CD4+ T cells to receive signal 1 via TCR interaction of peptide/MHC. Without a concomitant costimulatory signal, however, the expected outcome would be tolerance, not activation. Studies in keratinocytes experimentally confirm this prediction (252,253). Additionally, when mice were made transgenic for MHC II antigens in pancreatic β cells, they did not develop diabetes unless huge quantities of MHC II caused a direct toxic effect on the β cells themselves—there was no immunologically mediated β-cell destruction (254,255). It therefore seems unlikely that increased expression of MHC II on nonprofessional APCs solely leads to autoimmune responses. However, induced expression of MHC II antigens could contribute as an aggravating process in inflammatory tissue destruction.

Costimulatory Signals and Autoimmune Responses

Addition of costimulatory molecules to cells that normally do not express them has been demonstrated to induce immune responses. Tumor cells that are not immunogenic, for example, can be made immunogenic by fusion with B cells (thus providing costimulatory molecules) (256) or by transfection with B7 (257). The need for costimulatory signals as important mediators of autoimmune responses has been more indirect, as illustrated by an interesting series of experiments by Governman et al. (258), who developed a TCR transgenic mouse with specificity for an immunodominant epitope of EAE. The autoreactive transgenic T cells escaped central deletion and could be found in the periphery. Mice raised under sterile conditions did not develop autoimmune disease, but EAE was easy to induce with immunization and occasionally occurred spontaneously in nonsterile facilities (258). These experiments suggest a role for external stimuli as coinducers of autoimmune responses, perhaps by inducing costimulatory signals.

Direct experimental evidence for a role for costimulatory signals in autoimmunity comes from the experiments in which mice expressing foreign MHC on pancreatic β cells were crossed with TCR transgenics specific for the foreign MHC (259). These mice did not develop autoimmune responses against the β cells and did not develop diabetes. If made a triple transgenic, however, by crossing with a mouse expressing IL-2 in pancreatic islets, florid immune responses directed at the β cells resulted in diabetes (259). IL-2 clearly provided a costimulatory role in these experiments, although the molecular nature of the costimulatory signal remains conjectural.

Abnormalities in Immune Regulation

As described earlier in this chapter, multiple overlapping mechanisms contribute to maintaining tolerance to antigenic self. Autoimmune disease can be envisioned as developing when one or more of these tolerogenic mechanism fail, and the other mechanisms are unable to compensate adequately. Failure of individual tolerogenic mechanisms has been documented in some experimental systems, although the etiology of the failure is not always so clear.

Abnormalities in Deletion: Lessons from fas and bcl-2

Central and peripheral deletion of autoreactive T cells are important tolerogenic mechanisms. Recent work in several model systems has implicated abnormalities in this deletion process as pathogenic for autoimmune disease.

MRL-*lpr*/*lpr* mice develop lymphadenopathy due to expansion of CD4–CD8– T cells and have large numbers of autoreactive CD4+ T cells capable of proving help for the production of autoantibodies (51,260). These abnormalities result in immune-complex nephritis and vasculitis that resemble human systemic lupus erythematosis. The central role played by the autoreactive CD4+ T cells in this disease process is illustrated by the fact that administration of anti-CD4 antibodies retards the progression of disease (261), MHC II knockout mice bred into *lpr* backgrounds do not develop the disease (81) and, apparently, CD4 knockouts bred into *lpr* backgrounds do not develop the disease either (51).

The defect in the *lpr* locus has been shown to be a mutation in the fas apoptosis gene (262). This finding implicates a failure to delete autoreactive CD4+ T cells as pathogenic process in MRL-*lpr/lpr* mice. Central deletion, however, as induced by superantigens, appears to occur normally in these animals (263). Recently published work using a TCR transgenic mouse system has determined that the *lpr* mutation results in deficient peripheral deletion, although central deletion remains intact (52). Interestingly, there is some evidence that blockade of fas antigen-mediated apoptosis occurs in some human forms of lupus as well (264). Similarly, *gld* mice exhibit an analogous lupuslike phenotype and have been shown to have a mutation in the fas ligand (265), again implicating a failure of apoptosis as important in the development of autoimmunity.

In corroborative experiments, Strasser et al. targeted the apoptosis-preventing bcl-2 gene to B cells by using an Ig promoter (164). These mice developed high circulating levels of Igs, developed anti-DNA antibodies, and died of severe immune-complex glomerulonephritis (164). Additionally, defective B-cell apoptosis likely plays a role in the development pathogenic autoantibodies in NZB mice, although this abnormality is bcl-2 independent (266).

In another set of experiments, a transgenic mouse was constructed expressing an autoreactive anti–red blood cell antibody. Although most of the pathogenic B cells were deleted, some mice still developed anemia (183). Further work revealed that a subpopulation of transgenic antibody-producing, CD5+ B cells escaped the tolerogenic process and proliferated within the relatively protected peritoneal cavity (183). How these cells escaped peripheral deletion is not known, although there is some evidence that bcl-2 expression plays a role (267).

It is important to note that most autoantibodies are not produced by CD5+ B cells, suggesting that other mechanisms of avoiding tolerogenesis are operative in other situations. In one set of experiments, pre-B-cell clones from NZB×NZW F_1 mice (that develop a lupuslike syndrome), but not from normal mice, were able to differentiate in severe-combined-immunodeficiency mice lacking T cells (268). Despite the lack of T-cell help, these pre-B cells produced high titers of anti-DNA antibodies and, in some cases, developed autoimmune disease (268). This intriguing finding suggests that B cells from NZB× NZW F_1 mice are less susceptible to normal tolerogenic processes. The causative mechanism for this defect is presently unknown.

As outlined earlier, one mechanism of B-cell tolerance is receptor editing. Many B cells expressing high-affinity receptors for self-antigens attempt to rearrange a new light-chain gene in order to alter their antigenic specificity. It has been hypothesized that failure to edit successfully an autoreactive B-cell receptor results in apoptosis. In one interesting genetic analysis of κ-encoded pathogenic human anti-DNA light chains in patients with SLE, it was found that all of the Vκ/Jκ rearrangements were likely to be primary rearrangements (269). The authors suggested that the failure of tolerogenesis for these autoantibody-producing B cells may thus be secondary to an inability to perform receptor editing appropriately. A number of additional explanations could account for the findings, but the hypothesis remains an intriguing one.

Idiotypic Networks and Induction of Autoimmune Responses

Although a physiologic role for idiotypic networks in tolerogenesis remains to be formally defined (see previous sections on T-cell and B-cell tolerance), anti-idiotypic B-cell responses have occasionally been implicated in the development of autoimmune diseases. BisQ is an organic compound that is known to bind specifically to acetylcholine receptors (the target antigen of myasthenia gravis) (270). Rabbits immunized with BisQ developed anti-BisQ antibodies, as well as anti-idiotypic [anti-(anti-BisQ)] antibodies (270). Additionally, many of the mice developed symptoms of myasthenia gravis (270). Apparently, the anti-BisQ antibodies mimicked the internal structure of the acetylcholine receptor (that is, antibody 2 in Fig. 10), and the anti-idiotypic antibody was able to bind to the receptor itself and thus cause disease (Fig. 10) (270). In another experimental system, an anti-idiotypic antibody light chain from an MRL-*lpr/lpr* mouse with shared structural homology to the U1 snRNP autoantigen was able to induce an autoimmune response in normal mice (271). Whether anti-idiotypic antibodies play similar roles in the development of human autoimmune disease is presently unknown.

Cytokine-Mediated Diversion and Autoimmune Responses

As stated earlier in this chapter, CD4+ T cells can be divided into two distinct functional subsets based on their production of cytokines (108): Th1 cells produce IFN-γ, IL-2, and tumor necrosis factor, are proinflammatory, and provide help for cell-mediated immune responses (108–110), whereas Th2 cells produce IL-4, IL-5, IL-6, IL-10, and IL-13, can inhibit Th1 cells, and provide help for the induction of humoral immune responses (108–110). Recent work suggests that the development of T-cell subsets in a given host can play a role in the development of autoimmunity. Experimental evidence from several autoimmune disease models, including murine interstitial nephritis, suggests that the autoreactive T-cell response is mediated by Th1 CD4+ T cells (190,272–275). Additionally, administration of IL-4 to mice with EAE led to an expansion of Th2 cells and effectively ameliorated the course of the clinical disease (276). Under these circumstances, autoreactive Th2 T cells can be detected in the mouse, but the cells are not pathogenic. Other investigators have demonstrated that administration of recombinant IL-12 [an inducer of Th1 cells (277)] can worsen the course of EAE, whereas therapy with anti-IL-12 antibodies can prevent or ameliorate the disease (278).

Further evidence for a tolerogenic effect of Th2 versus Th1 cells comes from transgenic mouse models of autoimmune disease. A TCR transgenic mouse, in which the majority of CD4+ T cells were directed at a hemaglutinin (HA)-specific peptide in the context of I-A^d, was crossed with one of two I-A^d transgenics expressing HA in pancreatic islet cells, one mouse with a genetic Th1 predisposition and the other with a genetic Th2 predisposition (279). Interestingly, the double transgenic on the Th2 background did not develop diabetes or insulitis (279). T cells from this transgenic mouse were not deleted and were producing high levels of IL-4. In contrast, the double transgenic with the Th1 background developed early spontaneous diabetes and insulitis, and its T cells produced high levels of IFN-γ but minimal IL-4 (279). In another system, the MHC I-A^{g7} haplotype found in NOD mice was found to lead preferentially to the expansion of autoreactive Th1 cells and diabetes (280). Transgenic mice expressing a mutated I-A^{g7}, however, do not develop diabetes and contain autoreactive T cells that are functionally consistent with a Th2 phenotype (280). In total, these results implicate the preferential expansion of Th subtypes as important determinants of tolerance versus autoreactivity in selected animals models of autoimmunity (274). Whether cytokine-induced immune diversion is an relevant pathogenic mechanism for the development of other autoimmune disease models, or for human autoimmunity, is presently under investigation.

Immunologic Suppression and Autoimmune Disease

As stated in the section on peripheral tolerance, T-cell-mediated suppression is a well-documented immunologic observation, although the molecular mechanisms responsible for the suppressive phenotype are still being elucidated. As demonstrated by a number of studies in interstitial nephritis in rodents, suppression can play an important role in the development of autoimmune responses (see Chapter 12). Antitubular basement membrane disease in rats is induced in susceptible strains through immunization with tubular basement membrane (TBM) antigens (281,282). The brown Norway (BN) rat and the LEW.IN rat (MHC identical to BN and neonatally tolerized to BN alloantigens), however, do not develop interstitial injury after immunization with self-TBM (281–284). In the case of the LEW.IN rat, this is because the animals do not express the autoantigen in their kidneys (281–284). In response to immunization with BN TBM (a therefore foreign antigen), however, LEW.IN rats develop an anti-TBM T-cell response that can be reproducibly assayed using a delayed-type hypersensitivity response (283). Interestingly, when MHC-compatible BN rat T cells were added to the LEW.IN cells, anti-TBM delayed-type hypersensitivity response was prevented (283). These findings suggest that the BN rat contains antigen-specific suppressor cells that normally prevent autoreactivity to TBM (283).

Similar results came out of studies on spontaneous interstitial nephritis in kdkd mice, a strain mutated from the MHC identical CBA/Ca strain (285,286). The kdkd mice develop interstitial nephritis with 100% penetrance, beginning at 8–10 weeks of age, whereas the CBA/Ca mice do not develop renal disease (285,286). Transfer of CD8+ splenic T cells from CBA/Ca mice into kdkd mice prevents the expression of disease in the kdkd mice (287), once again suggesting that abnormalities in suppression can permit autoreactivity to a self-antigen and thus result in an autoimmune disease. Whether analogous abnormalities in T-cell immunoregulation are pathogenic in human autoimmune responses is presently unknown.

Development of Autoimmune Diseases: A Theoretical Framework

Our present understanding of immunologic tolerance, and our knowledge of the multiple abnormalities associated with experimental autoimmune responses, suggest the following model to describe the development of autoimmune diseases (Fig. 15). This model is not meant to be regarded as fact, but is simply meant to serve as a theoretical framework for conceptualizing autoimmunity. It is hoped that ongoing experimental work will test and refine this model in an effort to improve our comprehension of the pathogenesis of autoimmunity.

As a starting point, each individual is bestowed a genetic background of MHC molecules that partially determine the specific antigenic epitopes recognized by that individual's immune system and may additionally influence the magnitude of the immune response toward a given antigen. Based on the expression of certain MHC haplotypes, some individuals will therefore be born with an inherited predisposition to certain autoimmune diseases.

During the normal course of immunologic development, both T and B cells go through a period of negative selection (in the thymus and bone marrow, respectively), in which those lymphocytes recognizing self-determi-

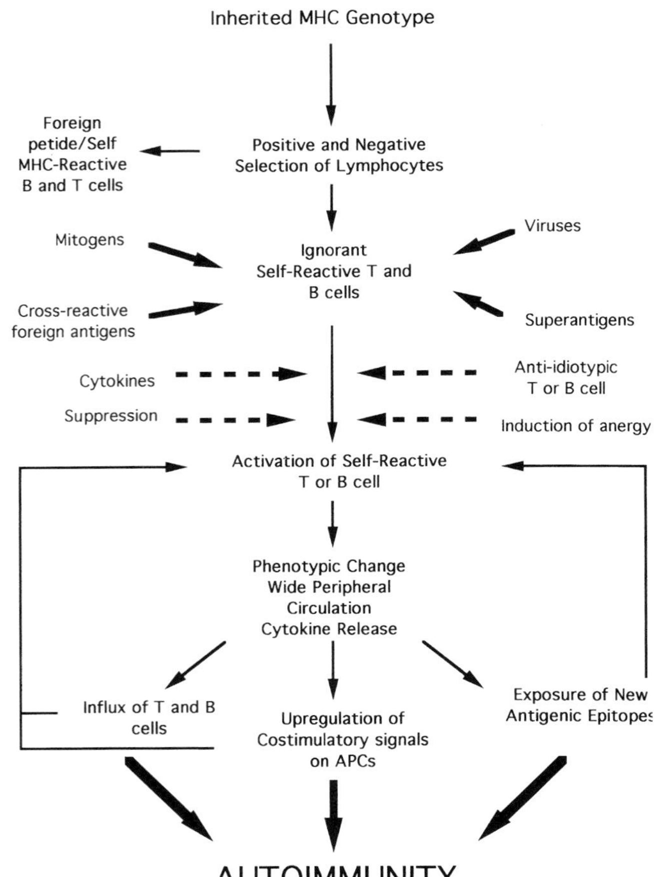

FIG. 15. Model of the development of autoimmune responses *(solid arrows)* positive effects and *(dashed arrows)* inhibitory effects.

nants with high affinity are eliminated from the immunologic repertoire. It is possible that an inherited or acquired inability to mediate this central deletion process could result in the peripheral release of a population of polyclonal autoreactive lymphocytes, although no such abnormality has been clearly described. However, assuming central deletion occurs normally, a proportion of the remaining lymphocytes released into the periphery will still be reactive to self-antigens (albeit at a lower affinity than those deleted centrally). These remaining self-reactive lymphocytes will then be kept in abeyance via clonal ignorance, that is, sequestration of antigens in immunologically privileged sites, antigenic expression at levels below thresholds required for recognition/activation, or expression of antigens without appropriate MHC molecules or without appropriate costimulatory signals.

Occasionally, however, these self-reactive lymphocytes may become activated. Such activation may be caused by cross-reactivity to an epitope from an invading infectious organism, exposure to an abnormally expressed self-determinant that is otherwise sequestered from the immune system, exposure to a superantigen or other mitogen that leads to polyclonal T-cell or B-cell activation, in direct response to a viral infection, or by other undescribed mechanisms. Additionally, it remains theoretically possible that a given autoreactive T or B cell may somehow acquire a mutation that engenders it with the ability to become activated without the usual stringent costimulatory requirements.

Generally, when such activation occurs, the potentially pathogenic self-reactive lymphocyte is prevented from causing any damage due to the redundancy of the other peripheral tolerogenic mechanisms, which include peripheral deletion or receptor editing (for B cells), the induction of anergy, cytokine-mediated diversion, anti-idiotypic immune responses, and other modes of active suppression. Under rare circumstances, however, and for reasons that are not inherently obvious, all of these various layers of protection from autoimmunity can fail, thus resulting in activation and clonal expansion of the autoreactive lymphocytes.

Subsequent B-cell activation and autoantibody production, if uncontrolled, can result in autoimmune disease via a number of well-described effector mechanisms (reviewed elsewhere in this volume). T-cell activation leads to phenotypic changes in the expression of surface molecules, and the production and secretion of cytokines, which subsequently allow the lymphocytes to circulate more widely—throughout the parenchymal organs. T-cell recognition of its self-determinant within the parenchymal organ can then lead to clonal expansion, further cytokine release, and tissue destruction via known effector mechanisms. One result of cytokine release from activated T cells is the chemoattraction of other inflammatory cells into the region (via chemokines, reviewed in Chapter 24). Additionally, the release of a number of cytokines can cause upregulation of MHC and other costimulatory molecules, allowing expression of cryptic epitopes and activation of T cells that were otherwise ignorant to parenchymal antigens. Thus, a vicious cycle of T-cell activation, chemoattraction, new antigen exposure and presentation, and further T-cell activation is set up, resulting in organ-specific autoimmune injury. One important consequence of this vicious cycle is that the initial pathogenic autoreactive immune response may have been directed toward a single (or a few) antigenic epitopes, but the resulting autoimmune disease may involve a polyclonal response directed at multiple antigens. Whether the ensuing disease is short-lived or chronic will then depend on a number of factors, including (but not limited to) whether the source of antigenic stimulus is ongoing or transient, and whether the known peripheral mechanisms of tolerance can be induced to control the autoimmune response.

CONCLUDING REMARKS

In summary, it can be appreciated that the immune system is designed such that tolerance to self is overwhelmingly likely and that many layers of tolerogenic mechanisms must be surmounted in order enable autoimmune reactions to occur. In selected rare instances, however, tolerance in its many forms can be overcome, resulting in autoimmune disease. It is hoped that ongoing research efforts will help to determine better how tolerance is normally maintained and how it is overcome in specific instances of human autoimmune disease. A thorough understanding of these pathophysiologic mechanisms may then lead to the development of more specific, and less toxic therapies.

Acknowledgments

P.S.H. is a recipient of a Clinical Investigator's Award (K08 DK-02125-01) from the National Institutes of Health. Special thanks to Nancy Burgard for her work on the illustrations.

REFERENCES

1. Ehrlich P, Morgenroth J. On hemolysins: third communication. In: *The collected papers of Paul Ehrlich*; vol 2. London: Pergamon, 1957:205–12.
2. Owen R. Immunogenetic consequences of vascular anastomoses between bovine twins. *Science* 1945;102:400–1.
3. Burnet F, Fenner F. *The production of antibodies*. Melbourne: Macmillan, 1949.
4. Billingham R, Brent L, Medawar PB. Actively acquired tolerance to foreign cells. *Nature* 1953;172:603–6.
5. Tonegawa S. Somatic generation of antibody diversity. *Nature* 1983; 302:575.
6. Carayannopoulos L, Capra J. Immunoglobulins. In: Paul WE, ed. *Fundamental immunology*. 3rd ed. New York: Raven, 1993:283–314.
7. Hedrick S, Eidelman F. T lymphocyte antigen receptors. In: Paul WE, ed. *Fundamental immunology*. 3rd ed. New York: Raven, 1993:383–420.
8. Davis MM, Bjorkman PJ. T-cell antigen receptor genes and T-cell recognition. *Nature* 1988;334:395.
9. Buus S, Sette A, Colon SM, Miles C, Grey HM. The relation between major histocompatibility complex (MHC) restriction and the capacity of Ia to bind immunogenic peptides. *Science* 1987;235:1353–8.
10. Chothia C, Bosswell D, Lesk A. The outline structure of the T-cell αβ receptor. *EMBO J* 1988;7:3745–55.
11. Danska JS, Livingstone AM, Paragras V, Ishihara T, Fathman CG. The presumptive CDR3 regions of both T cell receptor alpha and beta chains determine T cell specificity for myoglobin peptides. *J Exp Med* 1990;172:27–34.
12. Jorgensen J, Reay P, Ehrich E, Davis M. Molecular components of T-cell recognition. *Annu Rev Immunol* 1992;10:835–73.
13. von Boehmer H. Positive selection of lymphocytes. *Cell* 1994;70: 219–28.
14. Nossal G. Negative selection of lymphocytes. *Cell* 1994;76:229–39.
15. Ikuta K, Uchida N, Friedman J, Weissman I. Lymphocyte development from stem cells. *Annu Rev Immunol* 1992;10:759–83.
16. Mombaerts P, Clarke A, Rudnicki M, et al. Mutations in T cell antigen receptor genes α and β block thymocyte development at different stages. *Nature* 1992;360:225–31.
17. Mombaerts P, Iacomini J, Johnson R, Herrup K, Tonegawa S, Papaioannou V. RAG-1-deficient mice have no mature B and T lymphocytes. *Cell* 1992;68:869–77.
18. Shinkai Y, Rathbun G, Lam K-P, et al. RAG-2-deficient mice lack mature lymphocytes owing to inability to initiate V(D)J rearrangement. *Cell* 1992;68:855–67.
19. Kishi H, Borgulya P, Scott B, et al. Surface expression of the β T cell receptor (TCR) chain in the absence of other TCR or CD3 proteins on immature T cells. *EMBO J* 1991;10:93–100.
20. Padocan E, Casorati G, Dellabona P, Meyer S, Brockhaus M, Lanzacchia A. Expression of two T cell receptor alpha chains: dual receptor T cells. *Science* 1993;262:422–4.
21. Groettrup M, von Boehmer H. *Cell surface expression of the T cell receptor β chain on pre-T cells* [PhD dissertation]. Basil, Switzerland: University of Basil, 1993.
22. Bevan M. In radiation chimaera, host H-2 antigens determine immune responsiveness of donor cytotoxic cells. *Nature* 1977;269:417–8.
23. Matzinger P. Why positive selection? *Immunol Rev* 1993;135:81–117.
24. Zuniga-Pflucker J, McCarthy S, Weston M, Longo D, Singer A, Kruisbeek A. Positive selection of CD4–/CD8+ T cells in the thymus of normal mice. *Nature* 1988;338:76–78.
25. Scott B, Bluthman H, Teh H, von Boehmer H. The generation of mature T cells requires interaction of the αβ T-cell receptor with major histocompatibility antigens. *Nature* 1989;338:591–3.
26. Teh H, Kisielow P, Scott B, et al. Thymic major histocompatibility complex antigens and the αβ T-cell receptor determine the CD4/CD8 phenotype of T cells. *Nature* 1988;335:229–33.
27. Kisielow P, Teh H, Bluthmann H, von Boehmer H. Positive selection of antigen-specific T cells in thymus by restricting MHC molecules. *Nature* 1988;335:730–3.
28. Kaye J, Hsu M, Sauron M, Jameson J, Gascoigne R, Hedrick S. Selective development of CD4+ T cells in transgenic mice expressing a class II MHC-restricted antigen receptor. *Nature* 1989;341:746–9.
29. Zijlstra M, Bix M, Simister N, Loring J, Raulet D, Jaenisch R. Beta 2-microglobulin deficient mice lack CD4–CD8+ cytolytic T cells. *Nature* 1990;344:742.
30. Cosgrove D, Gray D, Dierich A, et al. Mice lacking MHC II molecules. *Cell* 1991;66:1051–66.
31. Grusby M, Hohnson R, Papaioannou V, Glimcher L. Depletion of CD4+ T cells in major histocompatibility complex, class II-deficient mice. *Science* 1991;253:1417.
32. Burnet F. A modification of Jerne's theory of antibody production using the concept of clonal selection. *Aust J Sci* 1957;20:67–9.
33. Lederberg J. Genes and antibodies: do antigens bear instructions for antibody specificity or do they select cell lines that arise by mutation? *Science* 1959;129:1649–53.
34. Janeway C. Self superantigens? *Cell* 1990;63:659–61.
35. Kappler J, Roehm N, Marrack P. T cell tolerance by clonal elimination in the thymus. *Cell* 1987;49:273–80.
36. Bluthman H, Kisielow P, Uematsu Y, et al. T cell specific deletion of T cell receptor transgenes allows functional rearrangement of endogenous α and β genes. *Nature* 1988;334:156.
37. Kisielow P, Bluthman H, Staerz U, Steinmetz M, von Boehmer H. Tolerance in T cell receptor transgenic mice involves deletion of nonmature CD4+8+ thymocytes. *Nature* 1988;333.
38. von Boehmer H. Developmental biology of T cells in T cell receptor transgenic mice. *Annu Rev Immunol* 1990;8:531–56.
39. Sha W, Nelson C, Newberry R, Kranz D, Russell J, Loh D. Positive and negative selection of an antigen receptor on T cells in transgenic mice. *Nature* 1988;336:73–6.
40. Adelstein S, Pritchard-Briscoe H, Anderson T, et al. Induction of self-tolerance in T cells but not in B cells of transgenic mice expressing little self antigen. *Science* 1991;251:1223–5.
41. Jolicoeur C, Hanahan D, Smith K. T cell tolerance toward a transgenic β-cell antigen and transcription of endogenous pancreatic genes in thymus. *Proc Natl Acad Sci USA* 1994;91:6707–11.
42. Heath W, Allison J, Hoffman M, et al. Autoimmune diabetes as a consequence of locally produced interleukin-2. *Nature* 1992;359: 547–9.
43. Zal T, Volkman A, Stockinger B. Mechanisms of tolerance induction in major histocompatibility complex class II-restricted T cells specific for a blood-borne self-antigen. *J Exp Med* 1994;180:2089–99.
44. Kyeski B, Fathman C, Rouse R. Intrathymic presentation of circulating non-MHC antigens by medullary dendritic cells: an antigen-dependent microenvironment for T cell differentiation. *J Exp Med* 1986; 163:231–46.
45. Pircher H, Brduscha K, Steinhoff U, et al. Tolerance induction by clonal deletion of CD4+8+ thymocytes in vitro does not require dedicated antigen-presenting cells. *Eur J Immunol* 1993;23:669–74.
46. Matzinger P, Guerder S. Does T-cell tolerance require a dedicated antigen-presenting cell? *Nature* 1989;338:74–6.
47. Matzinger P. Tolerance, danger, and the extended family. *Annu Rev Immunol* 1994;12:991–1045.
48. Zinkernagel R, Pircher H, Ohashi P, et al. T and B cell tolerance and responses to viral antigens in transgenic mice: implications for the

pathogenesis of autoimmune versus immunopathological disease. *Immunol Rev* 1991;122:133–71.
49. Guidos C, Danska J, Fathman C, Weissman I. T cell receptor-mediated negative selection of autoreactive T lymphocyte precursors occurs after commitment to the CD4 or CD8 lineages. *J Exp Med* 1990;172:835–45.
50. Murphy K, Heimberger A, Loh D. Induction by antigen of intrathymic apoptosis of CD4+CD8+ TCRlo thymocytes in vivo. *Science* 1990;250:1720–2.
51. Singer G, Carrera A, Marshak-Rothstein A, Martinez-AC, Abbas A. Apoptosis, Fas and systemic autoimmunity: the MRL-lpr/lpr model. *Curr Opin Immunol* 1994;6:913–20.
52. Singer G, Abbas A. The Fas antigen is involved in peripheral but not thymic deletion of T lymphocytes in T cell receptor transgenic mice. *Immunity* 1994;1:365–371.
53. Geenen V, Kroemer G. Multiple ways to cellular immune tolerance. *Immunol Today* 1993;14:573–5.
54. Marrack P, Ignatowicz L, Lappler J, Boymel J, Freed J. Comparison of peptides bound to spleen and thymus class II. *J Exp Med* 1993;178: 2173–82.
55. Jenkinson E, Owen J. T-cell differentiation in thymus organ cultures. *Semin Immunol* 1990;2:51–8.
56. Hogquist K, Gavin M, Bevin M. Positive selection of CD8+ T cells induced by major histocompatibility complex binding peptides in fetal thymic organ culture. *J Exp Med* 1993;177:1469–73.
57. Ashton-Rickardt P, van Kaer L, Schumacher T, Pleogh H, Tonegawa S. Peptide contributes to the specificity of positive selection of CD8+ T cells in the thymus. *Cell* 1993;73:1041–9.
58. Hogquist K, Jameson S, Heath W, Howard J, Bevan M, Carbone F. T cell receptor antiagonist peptides induce positive selection. *Cell* 1994; 76:17–27.
59. Sebzda E, Wallace V, Mayer J, Yeung R, Mak T, Ohashi P. Positive and negative thymocyte selection induced by different concentrations of a single peptide. *Science* 1994;263:1615–8.
60. Ashton-Rickardt P, Bandeira A, Delaney J, et al. Evidence for a differential avidity model of T cell selection in the thymus. *Cell* 1994; 76:651–63.
61. Hogquist K, Jameson S, Bevan M. The ligand for positive selection of T lymphocytes in the thymus. *Curr Opin Immunol* 1994;6:273–8.
62. Janeway C Jr. Thymic selection: two pathways to life and two to death. *Immunity* 1994;1:3–6.
63. Ashton-Rickardt P, Tonegawa S. A differential avidity model for T cell selection. *Immunol Today* 1994;15:262–6.
64. Hsu B, Evavold B, Allen P. Modulation of T cell development by an endogenous altered peptide ligand. *J Exp Med* 1995;181:805–10.
65. Bretscher P, Cohn M. A theory of self–nonself discrimination. *Science* 1970;169:1042–9.
66. Lafferty K, Cunningham A. A new analysis of allogeneic interactions. *Aust J Exp Biol Med Sci* 1975;53:27–42.
67. Liu Y, Linsley P. Costimulation of T-cell growth. *Curr Opin Immunol* 1992;4:265–70.
68. Schwartz R. Costimulation of T lymphocytes: the role of CD28, CTLA-4, and B7/BB1 in interleukin-2 production and immunotherapy. *Cell* 1992;71:1065–8.
69. Schwartz R. A cell culture model for T lymphocyte clonal anergy. *Science* 1990;248:1349–56.
70. Harding F, McArthur J, Gross J, Raulet D, Allison J. CD28-mediated signalling co-stimulates murine T cells and prevents induction of anergy in T-cell clones. *Nature* 1992;356:607–9.
71. Azuma M, Ito D, Yagita H, et al. B70 antigen is a second ligand for CTLA-4 and CD28. *Nature* 1993;366:76.
72. Freeman G, Borriello F, Hodes R, et al. Murine B7-2, an alternative CTLA4 counterreceptor that costimulates T cell proliferation and interleukin 2 production. *J Exp Med* 1993;178:2185.
73. Liu Y, Jones B, Aruffo A, Sullivan K, Lonsley P, Janeway J, CA. Heat-stable antigen is a costimulatory molecule for CD4 T cell growth. *J Exp Med* 1992;175:437–45.
74. Kuhlman P, Moy V, Lollo B, Brian A. The accessory function of murine intracellular adhesion molecule-1 in T lymphocyte activation: contribution of adhesion and co-activation. *J Immunol* 1991;146: 1773–82.
75. Springer TA. Adhesion receptors of the immune system. *Nature* 1990;346:425–34.
76. Jevnikar A, Wuthrich R, Takei F, et al. Differing regulation and function of ICAM-1 and class II antigens on renal tubular cells. *Kidney Int* 1990;38:417–25.
77. Wulthrich R. Vascular cell adhesion molecule-1 (VCAM-1) expression in murine lupus nephritis. *Kidney Int* 1992;42:903–14.
78. Keene J, Forman J. Helper activity is required for the in vivo generation of cytotoxic T lymphocytes. *J Exp Med* 1982;155:768–82.
79. Zheng B, Xue W, Kelsoe G. Locus-specific somatic hypermutation in germinal centre T cells. *Nature* 1994;372:556–9.
80. Rubin-Kelley V, Jevnikar A. Antigen presentation by renal tubular epithelial cells. *JASN* 1991;2:13–26.
81. Jevnikar A, Brusby M, Glimcher L. Prevention of nephritis in MHC class II-deficient MRL-lpr mice. *J Exp Med* 1994;179:1137–43.
82. Haverty TP, Watanabe M, Neilson EG, Kelly CJ. Protective modulation of class II MHC gene expression in tubular epithelium by target antigen-specific antibodies: cell-surface directed down-regulation of transcription can influence susceptibility to murine tubulointerstitial nephritis. *J Immunol* 1989;143:1133–41.
83. Springer T. Traffic signals for lymphocyte recirculation and leukocyte emigration: the multistep paradigm. *Cell* 1994;76:301–14.
84. Mackay C. Homing of naive, memory and effector lymphocytes. *Curr Opin Immunol* 1993;5:423–7.
85. Miller J, Morahan G. Peripheral T cell tolerance. *Annu Rev Immunol* 1992;10:51–69.
86. Oldstone M, Nerenberg M, Southern P, Price J, Lewicki H. Virus infection triggers insulin-dependent diabetes mellitus in a transgenic model: role of anti-self (virus) immune response. *Cell* 1991;65:319–31.
87. Ohashi P, Oehen S, Buerki K, et al. Ablation of "tolerance" and induction of diabetes by virus infection in viral antigen transgenic mice. *Cell* 1991;65:305–17.
88. Sercarz E, Lehman P, Ametani A, Benichou G, Miller A, Moudgil K. Dominance and crypticity of T cell antigenic determinants. *Annu Rev Immunol* 1993;11:729–66.
89. Lehmann P, Forsthuber T, Miller A, Sercarz E. Spreading of T cell autoimmunity to cryptic determinants of an autoantigen. *Nature* 1992;358:155–7.
90. Kaufman D, Claire-Salzier M, Tian J, et al. Spontaneous loss of T-cell tolerance to glutamic acid decarboxylase in murine insulin-dependent diabetes. *Nature* 1993;366:69–72.
91. Sprent J. T and B memory cells. *Cell* 1994;76:315–22.
92. Huang L, Crispe I. Superantigen-driven peripheral deletion of T cells. Apoptosis occurs in cells that have lost the alpha/beta T cell receptor. *J Immunol* 1993;151:1844–51.
93. Webb S, Morris C, Sprent J. Extrathymic tolerance of mature T cells: clonal elimination as a consequence of immunity. *Cell* 1990;63: 1249–56.
94. Fink P, Fang C, Turk G. The induction of peripheral tolerance by the chronic activation and deletion of CD4+Vβ5+cells. *J Immunol* 1994; 152:4270–81.
95. Carlow D, Teh S, van Oers N, Miller R, Teh H. Peripheral tolerance throgh clonal deletion of mature CD4–CD8+ T cells. *Int Immunol* 1992;4:599–610.
96. Moskophidis D, Lechner F, Pircher H, Zinkernagel R. Virus persistence in acutely infected immunocompetent mice exhaustion of antiviral cytotoxic effector T cells. *Nature* 1993;362:758–61.
97. Rocha S, von Boehmer H. Peripheral selection of the T cell repertoire. *Science* 1991;251:1225–8.
98. Cohen J, Duke R, Sellins K. Stimulation by superantigen. *Nature* 1991;352:199–200.
99. Miller J, Flavell R. T-cell tolerance and autoimmunity in transgenic models of central and peripheral tolerance. *Curr Opin Immunol* 1994; 6:892–9.
100. Simonsen M. Graft versus host reactions: their natural history and applicability as tools of research. *Prog Allergy* 1962;6:349–467.
101. Jones L, Chin L, Longo D, Kruisbeek A. Peripheral clonal elimination functional T cells. *Science* 1990;250:1726–9.
102. Critchfield J, Racke M, Zuniga-Pflucker J, Cannella B, Goverman J, Lenardo M. T cell deletion in high antigen dose therapy of autoimmune encephalomyelitis. *Science* 1994;263:1139–43.
103. Nagata S, Golstein P. The fas death factor. *Science* 1995;267:1449–56.
104. Ferber I, Schonrich G, Schenkel J, Mellor A, Hammerling G, Arold B. Levels of peripheral T cell tolerance induced by different doses of tolerogen. *Science* 1994;263:674–6.

105. Rocha B, Grandien A, Freitas A. Anergy and exhaustion are independent mechanisms of peripheral T cell tolerance. *J Exp Med* 1995;181:993–1003.
106. Arnold B, Schonrich G, Hammerling G. Multiple levels of peripheral tolerance. *Immunol Today* 1993;14:12–4.
107. Guerder S, Meyerhoff J, Flavell R. The role of the T cell costimulator B7-1 in autoimmunity and the induction and maintenance of tolerance to peripheral antigen. *Immunity* 1994;1:155–66.
108. Paul W, Seder R. Lymphocyte responses and cytokines. *Cell* 1994;76:241–51.
109. Mosmann T, Cherwinski H, Bond M, Giedlin M, Coffman R. Two types of murine helper T cell clone. I. Definition according to lymphokine activities and secreted proteins. *J Immunol* 1986;136:2348–57.
110. Cherwinski HM, Schumacher JH, Brown KD, Mosmann TR. Two types of mouse helper T cell clone. III. Further differences in lymphokine synthesis between Th1 and Th2 clones revealed by RNA hybridization, functionally monospecific bioassays, and monoclonal antibodies. *J Exp Med* 1987;166:1229–44.
111. Manetti R, Parronchi P, Grazia Giudizi M, et al. Natural killer cell stimulatory factor (interleukin 12) induces T helper type 1-specific immune responses and inhibits the development of IL-4-producing Th cells. *J Exp Med* 1993;177:1199–204.
112. Seder R, Paul W, Davis M, Fazekas de St Groth B. The presence of interleukin 4 during in vitro priming determines the lymphokine-producing potential of CD4+ T cells from T cell receptor transgenic mice. *J Exp Med* 1992;176:1091–8.
113. Erard F, Wild M-T, Garcia-Sanz J, Gros L. Switch of CD8 T cells to noncytolytic CD8–CD4– cells that make Th2 cytokines and helper B cells. *Science* 1993;260:1802–5.
114. Heinzel F, Sadick M, Holaday B, Coffman R, Locksley R. Reciprocal expression of interferon γ or interleukin 4 during the resolution or progression of murine leishmaniasis: evidence for expansion of distinct helper T cell subsets. *J Exp Med* 1989;169:59.
115. Sadick M, Heinzel F, Holaday B, Pu R, Dawkins R, Locksley R. Cure of murine leishmaniasis with anti-interleukin 4 monoclonal antibody. *J Exp Med* 1990;171:115–27.
116. Heinzel F, Schoenhaut D, Rerko R, Rosser L, Gately M. Recombinant interleukin 12 cures mice infected with Leishmania major. *J Exp Med* 1993;177:1505–9.
117. Sher A, Coffman R. Regulation of immunity to parasites by T cells and T cell-derived cytokines. *Annu Rev Immunol* 1992;10:385–409.
118. Jerne N. Toward a network theory of the immune system. *Ann Immunol (Paris)* 1974;125C:373–89.
119. Offner H, Hashim G, Vandenbark A. T cell receptor peptide therapy triggers autoregulation of experimental encephalomyelitis. *Science* 1991;251:430–2.
120. Vandenbark A, Hashim G, Offner H. Immunization with a synthetic T-cell receptor V-region peptide protects against experimental autoimmune encephalomyelitis. *Nature* 1989;341:541–4.
121. Kuhrober A, Schirmbeck R, Reimann J. Vaccination with T cell receptor peptides primes anti-receptor cytotoxic T lymphocytes (CTL) and anergizes T cells specifically recognized by these CTL. *Eur J Immunol* 1994;24:1172–80.
122. Gaur A, Ruberti G, Haspel R, Mayer J, Fathman C. Requirement for CD8+ cells in T cell receptor peptide-induced clonal unresponsiveness. *Science* 1993;259:91–4.
123. Neilson E. T cell regulation, anti-idiotypic immunity, and the nephritogenic immune response. *Kidney Int* 1983;24:289–302.
124. Ridgeway W, Weiner H, Fathman C. Regulation of autoimmune response. *Curr Opin Immunol* 1994;6:946–55.
125. Gershon R, Kondo K. Cell interaction in the induction of tolerance: the role of thymic lymphocytes. *Immunology* 1970;18:723.
126. Weigle W, Siekman O, Soyle M, Chiller J. Possible roles of suppressor cells in immunologic tolerance. *Transplant Rev* 1975;26:186.
127. Pierres M, Germain R. Antigen-specific T cell mediated suppression. IV. Role of macrophages in generation of L-glutamic acid–L-alanine–L-tyrosine (GAT) responder mice by nonresponder-derived GAT-suppressor factor. *J Immunol* 1978;121:1306.
128. Sercarz E, Oki A, Gammon G. Central versus peripheral tolerance: clonal inactivation versus suppressor T cells, the second half of the "Thirty Years War." *Immunology* 1989;2(Suppl):9–14.
129. Nossal G. Immunologic tolerance. In: Paul WE, ed. *Fundamental immunology*. 2nd ed. New York: Raven, 1989:571–86.
130. Bloom B, Salgame P, Diamond B. Revisiting and revising suppressor T cells. *Immunol Today* 1992;13:131–5.
131. Neilson E, Kelly C, Clayman M, et al. Murine interstitial nephritis. VII. Suppression of renal injury after treatment with soluble suppressor factor TsF1. *J Immunol* 1987;139:1518–24.
132. Murphy D, Erzenberg L, Okumura K, Herzenberg L, McDevitt H. A new I-subregion (I-J) marked by a locus (Ia-4) controlling surface determinants on suppressor T lymphocytes. *J Exp Med* 1976;144:699.
133. Bloom B, Modlin R, Salgame P. Stigma variations: observations on suppressor T cells and leprosy. *Annu Rev Immunol* 1992;10:453–88.
134. Kronenberg M, Steinmetz M, Kobori J, et al. RNA transcripts for I-J polypeptides are apparently not encoded between the I-A and I-E subregions of the murine major histocompatibility complex. *Proc Natl Acad Sci USA* 1983;80:5704.
135. Chen Y, Kuchroo V, Inobe J, Hafler D, Weiner H. Regulatory T cell clones induced by oral tolerance: suppression of autoimmune encephalomyelitis. *Science* 1994;265:1237–40.
136. Miller R, Derry H. A cell population in vv spleen can prevent generation of cytotoxic lymphocytes by normal spleen cells against self antigens of the nu/nu spleen. *J Immunol* 1979;122:1502–9.
137. Claesson M, Miller R. Functional heterogeneity in allospecific cytotoxic T lymphocyte clones. I. CTL clones express strong anti-self suppressive activity. *J Exp Med* 1984;160:1702–16.
138. Muraoka S, Ehman D, Miller R. Irreversible inactivation of activated cytotoxic T lymphocyte precursor cells by "anti-self" suppressor cells present in murine bone marrow T cell colonies. *Eur J Immunol* 1984;14:1010–6.
139. Kaplan D, Hambor J, Tykocinski M. An immunoregulatory function for the CD8 molecule. *Proc Natl Acad Sci USA* 1989;86:8512–5.
140. Hambor J, Weber M, Tykocinski M, Kaplan D. Regulation of allogeneic responses by expression of CD8 alpha chain on stimulator cells. *Int Immunol* 1990;9:879–83.
141. Sambhara S, Miller R. Programmed cell death of T cells signaled by the T cell receptor and $\alpha3$ domain of class I MHC. *Science* 1991;252:1424–7.
142. Zhang L, Martin D, Fung-Leung W-P, Teh H-S, Miller R. Peripheral deletion of mature CD8+ antigen-specific T cells after in vivo exposure to male antigen. *J Immunol* 1992;148:3740–5.
143. Fink P, Weissman I, Bevan M. Haplotype specific suppression of cytotoxic T cell induction by antigen inappropriately presented on T cells. *J Exp Med* 1983;157:141–54.
144. Rammensee H, Fink P, Bevan M. Functional clonal deletion of class I-specific cytotoxic T lymphocytes by veto cells that express antigen. *J Immunol* 1984;133:2390–6.
145. Pfeffer K, Mak T. Lymphocyte ontogeny and activation in gene targeted mutant mice. *Annu Rev Immunol* 1994;12:367–412.
146. Yancopoulos G, Alt R. Developmentally controlled and tissue-specific expression of unrearranged Vh gene segments. *Cell* 1985;40:271–81.
147. Pillai S, Baltimore D. Formation of disulfide-linked $\mu_2\omega_2$ tetramers in pre-B cells by the 18 Kd ω-immunoglobulin light chain. *Nature* 1987;329:172–4.
148. Kitamura D, Kudo A, Schaal S, Muller W, Melchers F, Rajewsky K. A critical role for the $\lambda5$ protein in B cell development. *Cell* 1992;69:823–31.
149. Hagman J, Grosschedl R. Regulation of gene expression at early stages of B-cell differentiation. *Curr Opin Immunol* 1994;6:222–30.
150. Rosenberg N, Kincade P. B-lineage differentiation in normal and transformed cells and the microenvironment that supports it. *Curr Opin Immunol* 1994;6:203–11.
151. Picker L, Butcher E. Physiological and molecular mechanisms of lymphocyte homing. *Annu Rev Immunol* 1992;10:561–91.
152. Szakal A, Holmes K, Tew J. Transport of immune complexes from the subcapsular sinus to lymph node follicles on the surface of nonphagocytic cells, including cells with dendritic morphology. *J Immunol* 1983;131:1714.
153. Jacob J, Kelsoe G, Rajewsky K, Weiss U. Intraclonal generation of antibody mutants in germinal centers. *Nature* 1991;354:389–92.
154. Berek C, Berger A, Apel M. Maturation of the immune response in germinal centers. *Cell* 1991;67:1121–9.
155. Avrameas S. Natural autoantibodies: from horror autotoxicus to gnothi seauton. *Immunol Today* 1991;12:154–9.
156. Goodnow C, Crosbie J, Jorgensen H, Brink R, Basten A. Induction of self-tolerance in mature peripheral B lymphocytes. *Nature* 1989;343:385–91.

157. Goodnow G. Transgenic mice and analysis of B-cell tolerance. *Annu Rev Immunol* 1992;10:489–518.
158. Nemazee D, Russell D, Arnold B, et al. Clonal deletion of autospecific B lymphocytes. *Immunol Rev* 1991;122:117–32.
159. Lawton A, Cooper M. Modification of B lymphocyte differentiation by anti-immunoglobulins. *Contemp Top Immunobiol* 1974;3:193–255.
160. Nemazee D, Burki K. Clonal deletion of B lymphocytes in a transgenic mouse bearing anti-MHC class I antibody genes. *Nature* 1989;337:562–6.
161. Russell D, Dembic Z, Morahan G, Miller J, Burki K, Nemazee D. Peripheral deletion of self-reactive B cells. *Nature* 1991;354:308–11.
162. Hartley S, Crosbie J, Brink R, Kantor A, Basten A, Goodnow C. Elimination from peripheral lymphoid tissues of self-reactive B lymphocytes recognizing membrane-bound antigens. *Nature* 1991;353:765–9.
163. Hartley S, Cooke M, Fulcher D, et al. Elimination of self-reactive B lymphocytes proceeds in two stages: arrested development and cell death. *Cell* 1993;72:325–35.
164. Strasser A, Whittingham S, Vaux D, et al. Enforced bcl-2 expression in B lymphoid cell prolongs antibody responses and elicits autoimmune disease. *Proc Natl Acad Sci USA* 1991;88:8661–5.
165. Tiegs S, Russel D, Nemazee D. Receptor editing in self-reactive bone marrow B cells. *J Exp Med* 1993;177:1009–20.
166. Gay D, Saunders T, Camper S, Weigert M. Receptor editing: an approach by autoreactive B cells to escape tolerance. *J Exp Med* 1993;177:999–1008.
167. Radic M, Erikson J, Litwin S, Weigert M. B lymphocytes may escape tolerance by revising their antigen receptors. *J Exp Med* 1993;177.
168. Nossal G, Pike B. Clonal anergy: persistence in tolerant mice of antigen-binding B lymphocytes incapable of responding to antigen or mitogen. *Proc Natl Acad Sci USA* 1980;77:1602–6.
169. Goodnow C, Crosbie J, Adelstein S, et al. Altered immunoglobulin expression and functional silencing of self-reactive B lymphocytes in transgenic mice. *Nature* 1989;334:676–82.
170. Eris J, Basten A, Kehry M, Hodgkin P. Anergic self-reactive B cells present self antigen and respond normally to CD40 dependent T-cell signals but are defective in antigen-receptor-mediated antigen presentation. *Proc Natl Acad Sci USA* 1994;91:4392–4396.
171. Fulcher D, Basten A. Reduced life span of anergic self-reactive B cells in double-transgenic model. *J Exp Med* 1994;179:125–34.
172. Linton P, Rudie A, Nr K. Tolerance susceptibility of newly generating memory B cells. *J Immunol* 1991;146:4099–104.
173. Liu Y, Joshua D, Williams G, Smith C, Gordan J, MacLennan I. Mechanism of antigen driven selection in germinal centers. *Nature* 1989;342:929–31.
174. Weiss U, Zoebelein R, Rajewsky K. Accumulation of somatic mutants in the B cell compartment after primary immunization with a T cell-dependent antigen. *Eur J Immunol* 1992;22:511–7.
175. Cyster J, Hartley S, Goodnow C. Competition for follicular niches excludes self-reactive cells from the recirculating B cell repertoire. *Nature* 1994;371:389–95.
176. Burdette S, Schwartz R. Idiotypes and idiotypic networks. *N Engl J Med* 1987;314:219–24.
177. Kearney J. Idiotypic networks. In: Paul WE, eds. *Fundamental immunology*. 3rd ed. New York: Raven, 1993:887–902.
178. Sege K, Peterson P. Use of anti-idiotypic antibodies as cell surface receptor probes. *Proc Natl Acad Sci USA* 1978;75:2443–7.
179. Erikson J, Radic M, Camper S, Hardy R, Carmack C, Weigert M. Expression of anti-DNA immunoglobulin transgene in non-autoimmune mice. *Nature* 1991;349:331–4.
180. Parry S, Hasbold J, Holman M, Klaus G. Hypercross-linking surface IgM or IgD receptors on mature B cells induces apoptosis that is reversed by costimulation with IL-4 and anti-CD40. *J Immunol* 1994;152:2821–9.
181. Chen C, Nagy Z, Radic M, et al. The site and stage of anti-DNA B-cell deletion. *Nature* 1995;373:252–5.
182. Kantor A. The development and repertoire of B-1 cells. *Immunol Today* 1991;12:389–91.
183. Murakami M, Tsubata T, Okamoto M, et al. Antigen induced apoptotic death of Ly-1 B cells responsible for autoimmune disease in transgenic mice. *Nature* 1992;357:77–80.
184. Mann R, Kelly CJ, Hines WH, et al. Effector T cell differentiation in experimental interstitial nephritis. I. The development and modulation of effector lymphocyte maturation by I-J+ regulatory T cells. *J Immunol* 1987;138:4200–8.
185. Burns J, Rosenzweig A, Zweiman B, Lisak R. Isolation of myelin basic protein-reactive T cell lines from normal human blood. *Cell Immunol* 1983;81:435–40.
186. Acha-Orbea H, Mitchell DJ, Timmermann L, et al. Limited heterogeneity of T cell receptors from lymphocytes mediating autoimmune encephalomyelitis allows specific immune intervention. *Cell* 1988;54:263–73.
187. Urban JL, Kumar V, Kono DH, et al. Restricted use of T cell receptor V genes in murine autoimmune encephalomyelitis raises possibilities for antibody therapy. *Cell* 1988;54:577–92.
188. Gold D. TCR V gene usage in autoimmunity. *Curr Opin Immunol* 1994;6:907–12.
189. Capra J, Jb N. Is there V region restriction in autoimmune diseases? *Immunologist* 1993;1:1.
190. Heeger PS, Smoyer WE, Saad T, Albert S, Kelly CJ, Neilson EG. Molecular analysis of the helper T cell response in murine interstitial nephritis. *J Clin Invest* 1994;94:2084–92.
191. Izui S. Autoimmune hemolytic anemia. *Curr Opin Immunol* 1994;6:926–30.
192. Logtenberg T. How unique are pathogenic anti-DNA autoantibody V regions? *Curr Opin Immunol* 1994;6:921–5.
193. Reininger L, Shibata T, Ozaki S, Shirai T, Jaton J-C, Izui S. Variable region sequences of pathogenic anti-mouse red blood cell autoantibodies from autoimmune NZB mice. *Eur J Immunol* 1990;20:771–7.
194. Scott B, Sadigh S, Stow M, Mageed R, Andrew E, Maini R. Molecular mechanisms resulting in pathogenic anti-mouse erythrocyte antibodies in New Zealand black mice. *Clin Exp Immunol* 1993;93:26–33.
195. Marion R, Tillman S, Jou N, Hill R. Selection of immunoglobulin variable regions in autoimmunity to DNA. *Immunol Rev* 1992;218:123–49.
196. Wisniewsky H, Keith A. Chronic relapsing experimental allergic encephalomyelitis: an experimental model for multiple sclerosis. *Ann Neurol* 1977;1:144–8.
197. Kelly C, Korngold R, Mann R, Clayman M, Haverty T, Neilson E. Spontaneous interstitial nephritis in kdkd mice. II. Characterization of a tubular antigen-specific, H2K-restricted Lyt2+ effector T cell that mediates destructive tubulointerstitial injury. *J Immunol* 1986;136:526–31.
198. Neilson EG, Phillips SM. Murine interstitial nephritis. I. Analysis of disease susceptibility and its relationship of pleiomorphic gene products defining both immune-response genes and a restrictive requirement for cytotoxic T cells at H-2K. *J Exp Med* 1982;155:1075–85.
199. Courtenay J, Dallman M, Dayan A, Martin A, Mosedale B. Immunization against heterologous type II collagen induces arthritis in mice. *Nature* 1980;283:665.
200. Todd J, Acha-Orbea H, Bell J, et al. A molecular basis for MHC II-associated autoimmunity. *Science* 1988;240:1003–9.
201. Trentham D, Townes A, Kang A. Autoimmunity to type II collagen: experimental model of arthritis. *J Exp Med* 1977;146:857.
202. Serreze D, Leiter E. Genetic and pathogenic basis of autoimmune diabetes in NOD mice. *Curr Opin Immunol* 1994;6:900–6.
203. Prochazka M, Serreze D, Worthen S, Leiter E. Genetic control of diabetogenesis in NOD/Lt mice: development and analysis of congenic stocks. *Diabetes* 1989;38:1446–55.
204. Lund T, O'Reilly L, Hutchings P, et al. Prevention of insulin-dependent diabetes mellitus in non-obese diabetic mice by transgenes encoding modified I-A β chain or normal I-E α chain. *Nature* 1990;345:727–9.
205. Serreze D. Autoimmune diabetes results from genetic defects manifest by antigen presenting cells. *FASEB J* 1993;7:1092–6.
206. Acha-Orbea H, McDevitt H. The first external domain of the nonobese diabetic mouse class II I-Aβ chain is unique. *Proc Natl Acad Sci USA* 1987;84:2435–9.
207. Reich E, von Grafenstein H, Barlow A, Swenson K, Williams K, Janeway C. Self peptides isolated from MHC glycoproteins of nonobese diabetic mice. *J Immunol* 1994;152:2279–88.
208. Wicker L, Leiter E, Todd J, et al. β_2-Microglobulin-deficient NOD mice do not develop insulitis or diabetes. *Diabetes* 1994;43:500–4.
209. Serreze D, Leiter E, Christianson G, Greiner D, Roopenian D. MHC class I deficient NOD-β_2m^{null} mice are diabetes and insulitis resistant. *Diabetes* 1994;43:505–9.

210. Ikegami H, Kawaguchi Y, Ueda H, et al. MHC-linked diabetogenic gene of the NOD mouse: molecular mapping of the 3′ boundary of the diabetogenic region. *Biochem Biophys Res Commun* 1993;192:677–82.
211. Wilkin T. Pro: evidence for a primary lesion in the target organ in autoimmune disease. *Int Arch Allergy Immunol* 1994;103:323–7.
212. Oldstone M. Molecular mimicry and autoimmune disease. *Cell* 1987; 50:819–20.
213. Dale J, Beachley E. Multiple heart-crossreactive epitopes of streptococcal M proteins. *J Exp Med* 1985;161:113.
214. Krishner K, Cunningham M. Myosin: a link between streptococci and the heart. *Science* 1985;227:413.
215. Singh V, Kalra H, Yamaki K, Abe T, Donoso L, Shinohara T. Molecular mimicry between a uveitopathic site of S-antigen and viral peptides. *J Immunol* 1990;144:1282.
216. Fujinami R, Oldstone M. Amino acid homology between the encephalitogenic site of myelin basic protein and virus: mechanism for autoimmunity. *Science* 1985;230:1043.
217. Tian J, Lehmann P, Kaufman D. T cell cross-reactivity between coxsackievirus and glutamate decarboxylase is associated with a murine diabetes susceptibility allele. *J Exp Med* 1994;180:1979–84.
218. D'Alessio D. A case–control study of group B coxsackievirus immunoglobin M antibody prevalence and HLA-DR antigens in newly diagnosed cases of insulin-dependent diabetes mellitus. *Am J Epidemiol* 1992;135:1331.
219. Cohen I. Autoimmunity to the chaperonins in the pathogenesis of arthritis and diabetes. *Annu Rev Immunol* 1991;9:567.
220. Gaston J, Life P, Jenner P, Colston M, Bacon P. Recognition of a mycobacteria-specific epitope in the 65-Kd heat-shock protein by synovial fluid-derived T-cell clones. *J Exp Med* 1990;171:339.
221. van Eden W, Holoshitz J, Nevo Z, Frenkel A, Klajman A, Cohen I. Arthritis induce by a T-lymphocyte clone that responds to *Mycobacterium tuberculosis* and to cartilage proteoglycans. *Proc Natl Acad Sci USA* 1982;82:5117.
222. van Eden W, Thole J, van der Zee R, Noordzij A. Cloning of the mycobacterial epitope recognized by T lymphocytes in adjuvant arthritis. *Nature* 1988;331:171.
223. van Eden W. Heat shock proteins as immunogenic bacterial antigens with the potential to induce and regulate autoimmune arthritis. *Immunol Rev* 1991;121:5.
224. Bhardwaj V, Kumar V, Geysen H, Sercarz E. Degenerate recognition of a dissimilar antigenic peptide by myelin basic protein-reactive T cells. *J Immunol* 1993;151:5000–10.
225. Sette A, Alexander J, Ruppert J, et al. Antigen analogs/MHC complexes as specific T cell receptor antagonists. *Annu Rev Immunol* 1994;12:413–32.
226. Gubersky D, Thomas V, Shek W, et al. Induction of type I diabetes by Kilham's rat virus in diabetes-resistant BB/Wor rats. *Science* 1991; 254:1010.
227. Frisk G, Fohlman J, Kobbah M, Al E. High frequency of Coxsackie-B virus-specific IgM in children developing type I diabetes during a period of high diabetes morbidity. *J Med Virol* 1985;17:219.
228. Yoon J, Austin M, Onodera T, Notkins A. Virus induced diabetes mellitus. *N Engl J Med* 1979;300:1173.
229. Robertson D, Guy EC, Zhang S, Wright R. Persistent measles virus genome in autoimmune chronic active hepatitis. *Lancet* 1987;2:9–11.
230. Marrack P, Kaappler J. The staphylococcal enterotoxins and their relatives. *Science* 1990;248:705–11.
231. Rellahan B, Jones L, Kruisbeck A, Fry A, Matis L. In vivo induction of anergy in peripheral Vβ8 + T cells by staphylococcal enterotoxin B. *J Exp Med* 1990;172:1091–100.
232. Brocke S, Gaur A, Piercy C, et al. Induction of relapsing paralysis in experimental autoimmune encephalomyelitis by bacterial superantigen. *Nature* 1993;365:642–4.
233. Howell M, Dively J, Lundeen K, et al. Limited T-cell receptor β-chain heterogeneity among interleukin-2 receptor-positive synovial T-cells suggests a role for superantigen in rheumatoid arthritis. *Proc Natl Acad Sci USA* 1991;88:10921.
234. Paliard X, West S, Lafferty J, et al. Evidence for the effects of a superantigen in rheumatoid arthritis. *Science* 1991;253:325–9.
235. Mourad W, Mehindate K, Schall T, McColl S. Engagement of major histocompatibility complex class-II molecules by superantigen induces inflammatory cytokine gene expression in human rheumatoid fibroblast-like synoviocytes. *J Exp Med* 1992;175:613.
236. Tumang J, Ep C, Gietl D, et al. T-helper cell-dependent, microbial superantigen-induced murine B-cell activation: polyclonal and antigen-specific antibody responses. *J Immunol* 1991;147:432.
237. Lindstrom J. Immunobiology of myasthenia gravis, experimental autoimmune myasthenia gravis and Eaton–Lambert syndrome. *Annu Rev Immunol* 1985;3:109.
238. Oosterhuis H. Observations of the natural history of myasthenia gravis and effect of thymectomy. *Ann NY Acad Sci* 1981;377:678.
239. Engel W, Trotter J, McFarlin D, Al E. Thymic epithelial cell contains acetylcholine receptor. *Lancet* 1977;1:1310.
240. Wraith D, Smilek D, Mitchell D, Steinman L, McDevitt H. Antigen recognition in autoimmune encephalomyelitis and the potential for peptide-mediated immunotherapy. *Cell* 1989;59:247–55.
241. Moudgil K, Sercarz E. Dominant determinants in hen egg-white lysozyme correspond to the cryptic determinants within its self-homolog, mouse lysozyme: implications in the shaping of the T cell repertoire and autoimmunity. *J Exp Med* 1993;178:2131–2138.
242. Mamula M. The inability to process a self peptide allows T cells to escape tolerance. *J Exp Med* 1993;177:567–71.
243. Mamula M, Croft J. The expression of self antigenic determinants: implications for tolerance and autoimmunity. *Curr Opin Immunol* 1994;6:882–6.
244. Kelly A, Powis S, Blynne R, Radley E, Beck S, Trowsdale J. Second proteasome-related gene in the human MHC class II region. *Nature* 1991;353:667–8.
245. Ortiz-Navarrete V, Seelig A, Gernold M, Frentzel S, Kloetzel P, Hammerling G. Subunit of the "20S" proteasome encoded by the major histocompatibility complex. *Nature* 1991;353:662–4.
246. Rossman M, Maida B, Douglas S. Monocyte-derived macrophage and alveolar macrophage fibronectin production and cathepsin D activity. *Cell Immunol* 1990;126:268–77.
247. Moreno J, Vignali D, Nadimi F, Fuchs S, Adorini L, Hammerling G. Processing of an endogenous protein can generate MHC class II-restricted T cell determinants distinct from those derived from exogenous antigen. *J Immunol* 1991;147:3306–13.
248. Fatenejad S, Brooks W, Schwartz A, Craft J. Pattern of anti-small nuclear ribonucleoprotein antibodies in MRL/lpr/lpr mice suggests that the intact U1snRNP particle is their autoimmunogenic target. *J Immunol* 1994;152:5523–31.
249. Lou Y, Tung K. T cell peptide of a self protein elicits autoantibody to the protein antigen: implications for specificity and pathogenetic role of antibody in autoimmunity. *J Immunol* 1993;151:5790–9.
250. Stein M, Stadecker M. Characterization and antigen-presenting function of a murine-thyroid derived epithelial cell line. *J Immunol* 1987; 139:1786–91.
251. Betazzo G, Dean B, McNally J, Al E. Role of aberrant HLA-DR expression and antigen presentation in induction of endocrine autoimmunity. *N Engl J Med* 1985;313:353.
252. Gaspari A, Jenkins M, Katz S. Class II MHC-bearing keratinocytes induce antigen-specific unresponsiveness in hapten-specific Th1 clones. *J Immunol* 1988;141:2216–20.
253. Bal V, McIndoe A, Denton G, et al. Antigen presentation by keratinocytes induces tolerance in human T cells. *Eur J Immunol* 1990; 20:1893–7.
254. Bohme J, Haskins K, Stecha P, van Evijk W. Transgenic mice with I-A on islet cells are normoglycemic but immunologically intolerant. *Science* 1989;244:1179.
255. Lo D, Burkly L, Widera G, Cowing C. Diabetes and tolerance in transgenic mice expressing class II MHC molecules in pancreatic b cells. *Cell* 1988;53:159.
256. Guo Y, Mengchao W, Chen H, et al. Effective tumor vaccine generated by fusion of hepatoma cells with activated B cells. *Science* 1994; 263:518–20.
257. Ramarathinam L, Castle M, Wu Y, Liu Y. T cell costimulation by B7/BB1 induces CD8 T cell-dependent tumor rejection: an important role of B7/BB1 in the induction, recruitment, and effector function of antitumor T cells. *J Exp Med* 1994;179:523–32.
258. Governman J, Woods L, Larson L, Weiner H, Hood L, Zaller D. Transgenic mice that express a myelin basic protein-specific T cell receptor develop spontaneous autoimmunity. *Cell* 1993;72:1065–70.
259. Miller J, Heath W. Self-ignorance in the peripheral T-cell pool. *Immunol Rev* 1993;133:131–50.
260. Weston K, Ju S-T, Liu C, Sy M-S. Autoreactive T cells in MRL/MP–lpr/lpr mice. Characterization of the lymphokines produced and

analysis of antigen-presenting cells required. *J Immunol* 1988;141:1941–8.
261. Jabs D, Kuppers R, Saboori A, et al. Effects of early and late treatment with anti-CD4 monoclonal antibody on autoimmune disease in MRL/MP–lpr/lpr mice. *Cell Immunol* 1994;154:66–76.
262. Watanabe-Fukunaga R, Brannan C, Copeland N, Jenkins A, Nagata S. Lymphoproliferative disorder in mice explained by defects in Fas antigen that mediates apoptosis. *Nature* 1992;256:314–7.
263. Herron L, Eisenberg R, Roper E, Kakkanaiah V, Cohen P, Kotzin B. Selection of the T cell receptor repertoire in Lpr mice. *J Immunol* 1993;151:3450–9.
264. Cheng J, Zhou T, Liu C, et al. Protection form Fas-mediated apoptosis by a soluble form of the Fas molecule. *Science* 1994;263:1759–62.
265. Takahashi T, Tanaka M, Brannan C, et al. Generalized lymphoproliferative disease in mice, caused by a point mutation in the Fas ligand. *Cell* 1994;76:969–76.
266. Tsubata T, Murakami M, Honjo T. Antigen-receptor cross-linking induces peritoneal B-cell apoptosis in normal but not autoimmunity-prone mice. *Curr Biol* 1994;4:8–17.
267. Nisitani S, Tsubata T, Murakami M, Okamoto M, Honjo T. The bcl-2 gene product inhibits clonal deletion of self-reactive B lymphocytes in the periphery but not in the bone marrow. *J Exp Med* 1994;178:1247–55.
268. Reininger L, Radaszkiewicz T, Kosco M, Melchers R, Rolink A. Development of autoimmune disease in SCID mice populated with long-term in vitro proliferating (NZB×NZW)F1 pre-B cells. *J Exp Med* 1992;176:1343–53.
269. Bensimon C, Chastagner P, Zouali M. Human lupus anti-DNA autoantibodies undergo essentially primary Vκ gene rearrangements. *EMBO J* 1994;13:2951–62.
270. Wasserman N, Penn A, Freimuth P, et al. Anti-idiotypic route to anti-acetylcholine receptor antibodies and experimental myasthenia gravis. *Proc Natl Acad Sci USA* 1982;79:4810–4.
271. Puccetti A, Koizumi T, Migliorini P, Andre-Schwartz J, Barrett K, Schwartz R. An immunoglobulin light chain from a lupus-prone mouse induces autoantibodies in normal mice. *J Exp Med* 1990;171:1919–30.
272. De Franco M, Gille-Perramant M-F, Mevel J-C, Couderc J. T helper subset involvement in two high antibody responder lines of mice (Biozzi mice): HI (susceptible) and HII (resistant) to collagen-induced arthritis. *Eur J Immunol* 1995;25:132–6.
273. Kennedy M, Torrance D, Picha K, Mohler K. Analysis of cytokine mRNA expression in the central nervous system of mice with experimental autoimmune encephalomyelitis reveals that IL-10 mRNA expression correlates with recovery. *J Immunol* 1992;149:2496–505.
274. Liblau R, Singer S, McDevitt H. Th1 and Th2 CD4+ T cells in the pathogenesis of organ-specific autoimmune disease. *Immunol Today* 1995;16:34–8.
275. Merrill J, Kono D, Clayton J, Ando D, Hinton D, Hoffman F. Inflammatory leukocytes and cytokines in the peptide induced disease of experimental allergic encephalomyelitis in SJL/J and B10.PL mice. *Proc Natl Acad Sci USA* 1992;89:574–8.
276. Racke M, Bonomo A, Scott D, et al. Cytokine-induced immune deviation as a therapy for inflammatory autoimmune disease. *J Exp Med* 1994;180:1961–6.
277. Germann T, Gately M, Schoenhaut D, et al. Interleukin-12/T cell stimulating factor, a cytokine with multiple effects on T helper type 1 (Th1) but not Th2 cells. *Eur J Immunol* 1993;23:1762–70.
278. Leonard J, Waldburger K, Goldman S. Prevention of experimental autoimmune encephalomyelitis by antibodies against interleukin 12. *J Exp Med* 1995;181:381–6.
279. Scott B, Liblau R, Degermann S, Maroni LA, Ogata L, Caton AJ, McDevitt HO, Lo D. A role for non-MHC genetic polymorphism in susceptibility to spontaneous autoimmunity. *Immunity* 1994;1:73–83.
280. Tisch R, Yang X-D, Singer S, Liblau R, Fugger L, McDevitt H. Immune response to glutamic acid decarboxylase correlates with insulitis in non-obese diabetic mice. *Nature* 1993;366:72–6.
281. Lehman D, Wilson C, Dixon F. Interstitial nephritis in rats immunized with heterologous tubular basement membrane. *Kidney Int* 1974;5:187–95.
282. Wilson C. Study of the immunopathogenesis of tubulointerstitial nephritis using model systems. *Kidney Int* 1989;35:938–53.
283. Kelly V, Silvers W, Neilson E. Tolerance to parenchymal self: regulatory role of major histocompatibility complex-restricted, OX8+ suppressor T cells specific for autologous renal tubular antigen in experimental interstitial nephritis. *J Exp Med* 1985;162:1892–903.
284. Kelly C, Roth D, Meyers C. Immune recognition and response to the renal interstitium. *Kidney Int* 1991;31:518–30.
285. Lyon M, Hulse E. An inherited kidney disease of mice resembling human nephronophthisis. *J Med Genet* 1971;8:41–8.
286. Neilson E, McCafferty E, Feldman A, Clayman M, Zakheim B, Korngold R. Spontaneous interstitial nephritis in kdkd mice. I. An experimental model of autoimmune renal disease. *J Immunol* 1984;133:2560–5.
287. Kelly CJ, Neilson EG. Contrasuppression in autoimmunity: abnormal contrasuppression facilitates expression of nephritogenic effector T cells and interstitial nephritis in kdkd mice. *J Exp Med* 1987;165:107–23.
288. Schwartz R. Autoimmunity and autoimmune diseases. In: Paul WE, ed. *Fundamental immunology*. 3rd ed. New York: Raven, 1993:1033–98.
289. Nepom G, Erlich H. MHC-II molecules and autoimmunity. *Annu Rev Immunol* 1991;9:493–526.
290. Campbell R, Milner C. MHC genes in autoimmunity. *Curr Opin Immunol* 1993;5:887–93.
291. Pietromonaco S, Kerjaschki D, Binder S, Ullrich R, Farquhar M. Molecular cloning of a cDNA encoding a major pathogenic domain of the Heymann nephritis antigen gp330. *Proc Natl Acad Sci USA* 1990;87:1811–5.
292. Neilson EG, Sun MJ, Kelly CJ, et al. Molecular characterization of a major nephritogenic domain in the autoantigen of anti-tubular basement membrane disease. *Proc Natl Acad Sci USA* 1991;88:2006–10.
293. Baekkeskov S, Aanstoot H, Christgau S, et al. Identification of the 64K autoantigen in insulin-dependent diabetes as the GABA-synthesizing enzyme glutamic acid decarboxylase. *Nature* 1990;347:151–6.
294. Ota K, Matsui M, Milford E, Mackin G, Weiner H, Hafler D. T-cell recognition of an immunodominant myelin basic protein epitope in multiple sclerosis. *Nature* 1989;346:183–7.
295. Willcox N. Mysathenia gravis. *Curr Opin Immunol* 1993;5:910–7.

Immunologic Renal Diseases,
edited by E. G. Neilson and W. G. Couser.
Lippincott-Raven Publishers, Philadelphia © 1997.

CHAPTER 7

Renal Expression of MHC Antigens

Philip F. Halloran

The genes of the major histocompatibility complex [MHC; in humans the human leukocyte antigen (HLA) complex] encode class I and II products that are crucial to T-cell recognition of antigen. They are necessary for the development of T cells in the thymus and determine the T cell repertoire and thus influence many immune responses. They present antigens to T cells in the initiation and propagation of immune responses and are central to the problem of transplant rejection, serving as the major transplantation antigens, as targets for both T cell and antibody recognition. The MHC genes are expressed in the kidney and were the first genes in the kidney to be shown to undergo increased expression in vivo in inflammatory processes (1,2).

The chapter focuses on the control of the expression of class I and II genes, particularly the role of interferon-gamma (IFN-γ). Other MHC genes [complement proteins, tumor necrosis factors (TNFs), non-classical class I] will not be discussed. Recent reviews of MHC regulation provide additional details (3–7). Many of the mechanisms regulating IFN-γ transcription and production, the mechanisms of IFN signalling, and the key proteins governing MHC transcription have been established. We discuss key points on these topics:

1. The importance of MHC
2. MHC expression in the kidney
3. The principles of gene regulation
4. IFN-t production, the IFN-γ receptor (IFN-γR), and the signalling pathways that link the IFN-γR to MHC transcription
5. The MHC class II regulatory machinery
6. MHC class I regulatory machinery
7. Synthesis: a dynamic view of MHC regulation in the kidney

P. F. Halloran: Department of Medicine, Division of Nephrology and Immunology, University of Alberta, Edmonton, Alberta, Canada.

INTRODUCTION TO MHC EXPRESSION AND REGULATION

What is the MHC?

The MHC is a set of highly polymorphic genes encoding the structures that present antigen to T-cell receptors (TCRs). This complex maps to a region of 3.5 million base pairs (bp) on chromosome 6 (and an analogous region of other mammalian genomes). As shown in Fig. 1, the MHC is divided into the class II region, the class III region, and the class I region. The key MHC genes are the class I genes (e.g., HLA-A and -B) and the class II genes (e.g., *DP, DQ,* and *DR*). The major animal model for understanding MHC in vivo in the kidney is the mouse MHC, H-2.

The MHC Products Present Antigen

The class I and II proteins (Fig. 2A) are type I membrane proteins (i.e., the N terminal points out). The class I protein is a single polypeptide chain with a molecular weight (MW) of 45 kDa, but associated with a smaller 12-kDa protein, β_2 microglobulin (β_2M). The class I molecules present peptide to TCRs of CD8 T cells. The class II protein is a heterodimer of an alpha chain (MW 33 kDa) and a β chain (MW 28 kDa). The class II proteins present peptide to TCRαβ of CD4 T cells. Each MHC molecule contains a groove that presents peptides of eight to 10 amino acids (aa) (class I) or eight to 25 aa (class II) to T cells. The MHC class I and II genes are highly polymorphic in the regions that encode the amino acids lining the groove.

The peptide in the MHC groove is derived from proteins synthesized by the cell or endocytosed by the cell. The class I groove contains peptides derived from endogenously synthesized proteins in the cytosol. The class II groove contains peptides derived from proteins in the

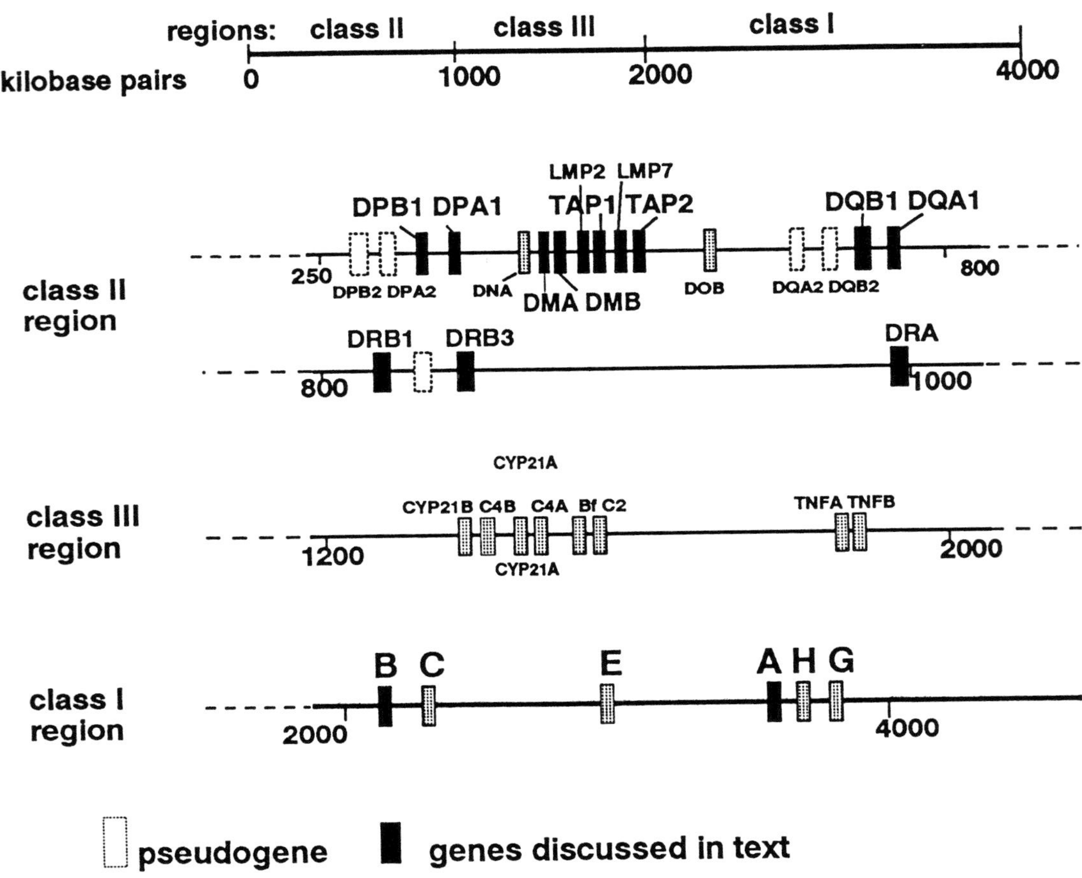

FIG. 1. An overview of the mapping of the HLA genes on chromosome 6. The genes discussed in the text are shown in black. Each class II product requires an A and a B gene; each class I product requires only a single heavy-chain gene because the product associates with β_2M.

endocytic compartment, engulfed by the cell from its environment. The peptide should be regarded as a normal component of the MHC molecule. Usually the peptide engages the MHC molecule grooves shortly after synthesis of the MHC proteins and remains associated for as long as the MHC molecule lasts.

In both class I and II grooves are peptides derived from MHC proteins themselves. In transplantation, peptides derived from donor MHC proteins may be important antigens for triggering host T cell responses. Thus, MHC molecules exist to present antigen to TCRs (Fig. 2B). The MHC–peptide complexes represent a display of peptides derived from the proteins in or near the cell, available to be scrutinized by the T cell for foreign (nonself) peptides. The MHC–peptide complexes may crosslink TCRs and trigger them. The recent solution of the structure of TCRα suggests that MHC molecules may dimerize to cross-link TCRα/β dimers to form an $\alpha_2\beta_2$ tetramer, triggering the TCR-associated signalling apparatus (8). If so, the density of MHC–peptide ligands must be sufficient to permit dimers to form, suggesting a requirement for high MHC expression.

MHC molecules have functions other than peptide presentation to TCRs. They act as the targets for coreceptors CD4 and CD8. CD8 interacts with class I and CD4 interacts with class II. Their ability to interact with both TCRs and CD4 and CD8 coreceptors is important in the role of MHC molecules in the education of T cells in the thymus as well as in triggering TCRs for immune responses. The class I molecules also have a role in regulating natural killer (NK) cells, a complex regulatory function that is still being unravelled (9–12). Candidate NK molecules for the recognition of class I MHC molecules include the murine molecule Ly-49 and the human molecule p58. The principal function of class I molecules in NK recognition may be as a self marker to inhibit random killing

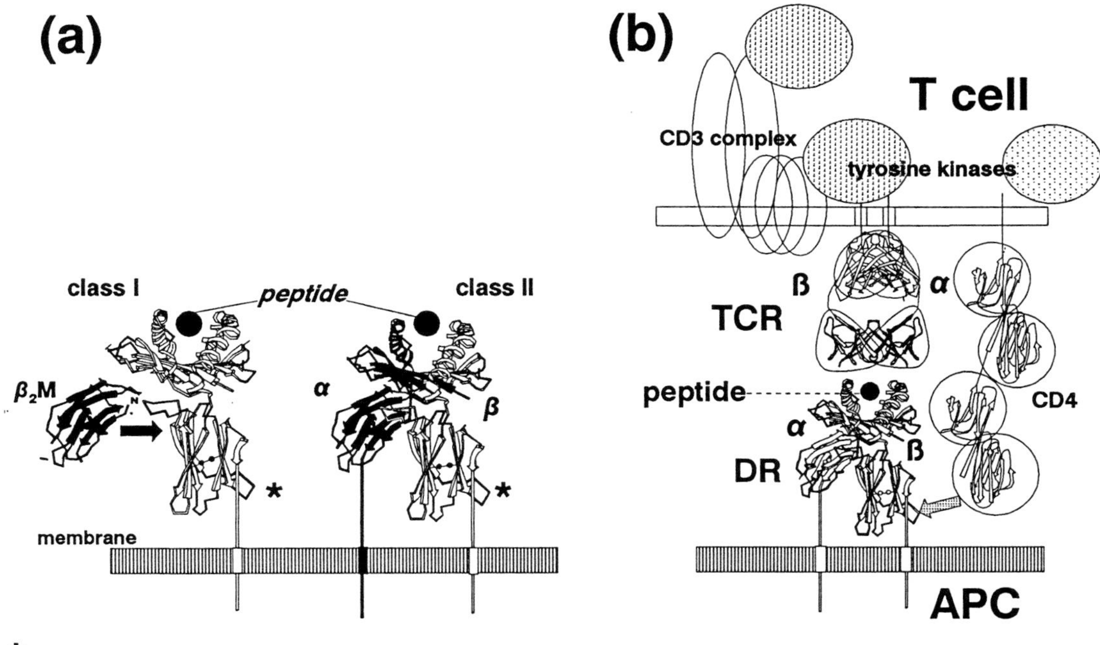

FIG. 2. The structure of MHC class I and II products, and the relationship to T-cell triggering. **A:** A cartoon showing comparison between the class I product, which consists of β_2M, the class I heavy chain, plus peptide; and the class II product, which consists of an alpha chain, the chain, and the peptide. **B:** The class II plus peptide engages the TCR and the CD4 molecule to trigger a T cell. The antigen-presenting cell is below and the T cell is above. Triggering probably involves dimerization of TCRs and of the MHC molecules, triggering the tyrosine kinases. Conformational change in the TCR also may occur.

by NK cells. MHC class II molecules serve to mediate the complex interaction between TCRs and bacterial superantigens, which interact with class II independent of the class II groove.

The components of the antigen presentation system for class I include β_2M, transporters associated with antigen processing (TAP1, TAP2), and large multifunctional protease components (LMP2, LMP7), which contribute to class I antigen presentation. β_2M is associated with class I and stabilizes it: in the absence of β_2M, class I does not fold properly, is not expressed well on the membrane, and is rapidly degraded (13). LMPs are components of the large enzyme complexes called proteasomes, which degrade cytosolic proteins into peptides. The LMPs alter the protease activity of the proteasome (14). The peptide created when proteasomes break down cytosolic proteins are transported by TAP1 and 2 from the cytosol into the endoplasmic reticulum.

Invariant chain (Inv) and DM proteins contribute to class II antigen presentation. Inv stabilizes the newly synthesized class II dimers to prevent them from binding peptide in the endoplasmic reticulum (ER). A region of the invariant chain called CLIP actually blocks access to the groove. Inv then chaperones the class II dimer to the endosomal compartment, where it meets the endocytic vacuoles and binds peptide (15,16). DM proteins are class II–like and help to ensure that class II proteins bind peptide properly by inducing CLIP dissociation from MHC class II and promoting peptide loading (17–19).

MHC Gene and Product Expression

Class I HLA-A and -B products are expressed in most cells, but the amount expressed varies greatly among tissues and cell types. The expression of C products is less than A or B, and the pattern in tissues is not clear; the atypical class I or class Ib proteins are expressed only at specialized tissues or in embryonic life (e.g., HLA-G). The expression of the class II proteins (DR, DQ, DP) is mainly confined to marrow-derived cells, which function as antigen-presenting cells: B cells, some macrophages, and interstitial dendritic cells (IDCs), including skin Langerhans cells. (We use the term IDC to denote class II–positive cells of bone marrow origin and branching morphology seen in tissue sections. The relationship between dendritic cells in different tissues and similar cells isolated in vitro is unclear (20–22). Class II is expressed on many endothelial cells in humans and on some epithelial cells. A variety of other cell types express class II in disease states such as transplant rejection.

Coordinate Regulation

Class I HLA-A and -B genes are coordinately expressed: they are both expressed to about the same degree in the same sites and are "turned on" together by stimuli such as cytokines. Class II genes (*DPA* and *-B, DQA* and *-B, DRA* and *-B*) are also coordinately expressed, but there is more evidence of individuality when comparing class II genes such as *DRB* and *DQB* than there is for class I loci. The important class II genes in transplantation are the DR products; the evidence for a role for *DP* or *DQ* in transplantation is less convincing. Class I and class II are both inducible by stimuli, but with differences in sites and mechanisms, confirming independent control of class I and class II.

Function of MHC and Importance of Regulation of MHC Expression

The limiting factor in T-cell recognition is MHC presentation of antigen. The MHC alleles expressed by an individual are important. Genetic studies of human diseases and murine immune responses established the importance of particular MHC class I and II alleles in determining disease susceptibility and specific immune responses. The ability of particular peptides to engage the class I or II groove reflects the shape of the groove, which in turn reflects the alleles that individual inherits. Thus, MHC polymorphism determines susceptibility to many immunologic diseases (23). However, the quantity of MHC expressed also affects T-cell responses (24). Increased MHC expression increases the probability that a particular antigen will trigger a T-cell response. TCR triggering is limited by MHC–peptide concentration. Thus, the immunogenicity of tissues in transplantation and autoimmunity, as well as the success of an immune response against an infectious agent, is affected by the level of MHC expression (see the section on how this relates to MHC regulation in the kidney).

To maintain a balance between risk of autoimmunity (too much MHC expression) and risk of infection (too little MHC expression), the level of expression of MHC molecules can be adjusted both locally and systemically. Ideally, particularly on parenchymal cells, MHC expression is maintained at a relatively low level, but with the capacity for large increases. MHC product expression is inducible. In inflammatory disease the expression of MHC products can increase by 10-fold or more. This induction is primarily due to an increase in the transcription of the MHC genes. However, if peptides are not available to engage the MHC groove, the survival of the MHC proteins may be reduced. Thus, peptide availability may be another control on MHC product expression, without affecting transcription.

IFN-γ and Other Cytokines Regulate MHC Expression

Many influences from outside the cell can alter MHC expression (Fig. 3), particularly IFNs and cytokines, acting locally or systemically. IFN-γ is the major inducer of MHC expression. IFN-γ is the only cytokine that can induce high levels of MHC class I and II expression when administered systemically and can also induce MHC class I and II locally. IFN-γ also regulates the expression of other components of the antigen-presentation system, including *β_2M, Inv, TAP1, TAP2, LMP2, and LMP7.* This set of genes, along with the cytokines and signal transduction systems, constitutes a sort of unit of the immune or inflammatory response: the cytokine-MHC axis.

IFN-γ production is regulated at the level of transcription, particularly by stimuli that act on the IFN-γ promoter through the calcium–calcineurin pathway that is the target of cyclosporine (CyA). IFN-γ is made by both T cells and NK cells. For example, T cell–deficient nude mice can make abundant IFN-γ when given T cell–independent stimuli (25,26). Other cytokines are also primarily transcriptionally controlled. IFN-γ induces transcription of MHC genes by inducing activation of existing transcription factors and the synthesis of new transcription factors. The newly synthesized MHC proteins must engage other chains (e.g., β_2M for class I, β chain for class II α chain) and bind peptide or they will be degraded. The availability of other chains and of peptide affects MHC expression, although the importance of this control in vivo is not established.

Potential influences on renal MHC expression

infections : bacterial, viral, etc
endotoxin
tissue injury
interferons
cytokines, growth factors
drugs
hormones
malignant transformation, oncogenic viruses
growth, development
interactions with extracellular matrix

FIG. 3. The influences in vivo that could alter MHC expression in the cells of tissues such as kidney.

MHC EXPRESSION IN KIDNEY: WHAT DO WE KNOW?

Class I

Although class I is widely expressed, the level of expression varies greatly between cell types and between tissues. Class I expression is generally highest in marrow-derived cells and endothelial cells, intermediate on epithelial cells, less on parenchymal cells and mesenchymal interstitial cells, little on muscle cells, and least on neurons. There is some soluble class I in body fluids, but its significance and control are not clear (27). Dimeric forms of soluble class I may be able to induce specific unresponsiveness (28).

In the kidney, class I expression is prominent on arterial endothelium and on the endothelial cells of glomeruli, peritubular capillaries, and veins. Expression is weaker on tubule epithelium (29,30). In general, the class I monoclonals stain human kidney tissue sections diffusely, making quantitative differences difficult to assess, but studies in mice can assess quantitative differences. Class I in mouse kidney is expressed on the basolateral membrane of epithelial cells in the induced state (31,32). Class I expression in the rat kidney is similar but is more extensive in tubules in the basal state (33). No significant differences in class I A locus and class I B locus expression have been described in tissues in vivo.

Class II

Class II MHC antigens in the human kidney are expressed prominently on a population of IDCs and the vascular endothelium, with patchy expression in tubule epithelium (29,34). The pattern of expression has been established by studies of indirect immunoperoxidase staining with monoclonal antibodies against DR antigens. The above pattern may not be characteristic of DQ and DP. In general the hierarchy of expression in tissues is DR > DQ > DP.

All mammals express class II abundantly on IDCs, but in the mouse kidney the expression is confined to IDCs, with the A locus product (the DQ equivalent) being more abundant than the E locus product (the DR equivalent). Thus, mice differ from humans in that they rely more on the DQ-like A locus than on the DR-like E locus product. Some mouse strains do not express any E locus product due to errors in the $E\alpha$ gene. Most mouse strains express no class II in kidney epithelial cells in the basal state (1). Class II expression in IDCs does not require IFN-γ because it is normal in mice lacking IFN-γ (35). Rats express class II on IDCs, but some rat strains express class II in renal tubule epithelium (33,36).

MHC Expression Is Inducible in the Kidney and Many Other Tissues

In the mouse and rat kidney, the level of MHC expression can increase three- to 10-fold in response to local injury or inflammatory disease or as part of a systemic response to a remote stimulus. The amount of MHC expressed in the kidney is massively increased by processes that release IFN-γ in vivo (1,37,38), by systemic administration of IFN-γ (39–41), and by local immune responses such as graft rejection (40). Even local nonimmune injury induces MHC expression, such as ischemic acute tubular necrosis (42–45) and aminoglycoside and other toxic injuries (N. Goes and P.F. Halloran, unpublished observations). In general, both class I and class II are induced in these states, although class I is more easily induced by weak stimuli. The class I increase is more generalized, affecting virtually all the cells in the kidney, whereas class II is increased in some sites (proximal tubules) but not others (distal tubules).

DR antigens are strongly induced in the human kidney during transplant rejection (2). In fact, class I is also induced in human kidney rejection, but the methods of studying quantitative changes in class I expression in the human kidney are limited. MHC expression is upregulated in rejection and in inflammatory diseases in all organs (2,46–51).

We now briefly review some principles of transcriptional regulation of gene expression in eukaryotes, focusing on the mechanisms germane to our discussion of MHC regulation.

INTRODUCTION TO THE REGULATION OF GENE TRANSCRIPTION: GENERAL AND SPECIFIC

The main factor determining the expression of a eukaryotic gene is the extent to which it is transcribed by the complex termed RNA polymerase II (pol II). Other factors—posttranscriptional control of the messenger RNA (mRNA) level, translational and posttranslational control, and the rate of turnover and degradation of the protein—are mentioned as appropriate, but these are not the principal sites of in vivo regulation of MHC expression.

Some Factors in the Availability of a Gene for Transcription

Some genes such as IFN-γ are highly cell type and tissue specific; i.e., they are expressed exclusively in certain cell types (T cell and NK cells) (52). Others, such as MHC class I and II, are housekeeping genes that can be expressed in many cells types. These two expression patterns are reflected in the chromatin and nucleosome arrangement and methylation of the regulatory sites in the DNA of that gene, and the specific proteins that interact with those sites.

Chromatin and Nucleosomes

Chromatin is a term denoting DNA packed with proteins, predominantly histones. The DNA of a chromosome is bound up with histone proteins and packed into nucleosomes, which are coils of DNA around histone cores. Nucleosomes are altered in the regulatory regions of a gene that is due for expression, to permit the proteins that mediate transcription to interact with the DNA of a regulatory region (53). The extent to which DNA is sensitive or hypersensitive to digestion by the enzyme DNAse I reflects the extent to which it is packed into chromatin in nucleosomes versus free to interact with proteins. DNAse hypersensitivity is a feature of the regulatory regions of genes in cells that can express those genes, and probably reflects the effect of proteins binding to the DNA. Thus, in many cells the DNA of the regulatory regions of class I and II genes and other housekeeping genes has hypersensitive sites, but regulatory regions of the IFN-γ gene would be unaccessible except in permissive cells such as T cells.

Cytosine Methylation

The degree of methylation of DNA, and specifically of the cytosine residues in DNA, both influences and is influenced by the state of expression or expressibility. Expressed DNA tends to be undermethylated, and undermethylated DNA tends to be expressed. Undermethylation may be an active process that is an early stage in gene expression. The methylation occurs in regions rich in cytosine-guanine dinucleotides, termed CpG islands, which are undermethylated if a gene is expressed or expressible in a cell. Thus, CpG islands represent regions where methylation changes with the expressibility of the gene.

Regulatory Proteins or Transcription Factors

Transcription is controlled by proteins termed transcription factors (TFs) and is controlled by protein–protein and protein–DNA interactions. The proteins can be classified as the general transcription factors (which can act in the transcription of many genes, by recruiting RNA pol II) and the specific transcription factors or transcriptional activators that regulate the transcription of specific genes by influencing the recruitment of the general factors.

General Transcription Factors

The RNA pol II is recruited to the 5′ end of each gene, the transcription initiation site (Fig. 4). But how does transcriptional machinery know where to start and what direction to take? The pol II apparatus requires an assembly of general factors called the preinitiation complex (PIC), just 5′ to and overlapping the start site. The PIC recruits the pol II apparatus to proceed down the gene to make the mRNA copy.

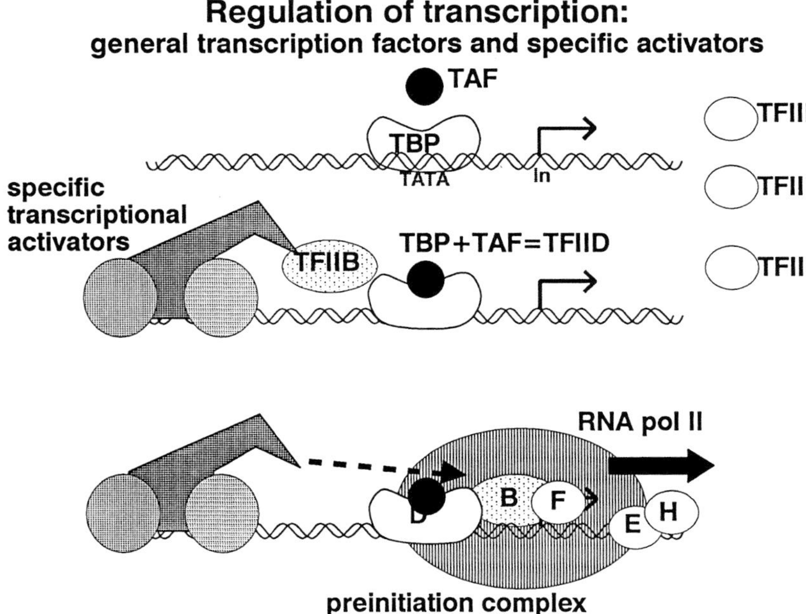

FIG. 4. A cartoon showing a general scheme for the assembly of the general transcription factors and the role of transcriptional activators. Factor TFIIB consists of the TATA box binding protein (TBP) and TBP-associated factors or TAFs. These assemble at the TATA box. Specific transcriptional activators help to assemble the rest of the preinitiation complex, playing a role in the recruitment of TFIIB. However, they play a second role at later stages of activating the factors in the preinitiation complex. The purpose is to control the rate of transcription by polymerase II (POL II).

The PIC is positioned and given direction in many genes by the DNA sequences such as the TATA sequence (often TATAAA) about 25 bp 5′ to the transcription initiation site. A protein termed TATA binding protein (TBP) binds to the TATA box. TATA box binding protein (TBP) is a saddle-shaped protein (54,55) that rests saddlelike on the DNA of the TATA box and assembles other proteins called TBP-associated factors (TAFs). The complex of TBP plus TAFs is termed TFIID. TFIID and TFIIA bind to the promoter and recruit TFIIB and other factors, which recruit RNA pol II (56,57). Thus, TFIID binds to DNA, and TFIIB binds to TBP, which is bound to TATA DNA (58). In genes that lack a TATA box, the PIC assembles in much the same fashion, with TBP and TAFs, etc. The transcription factor SP1 is more important for TATA-less promoters.) The full complex involves factors A, B, D, E, F, and H.

One model for initiation of transcription is that the assembly of general transcription factors causes torsion of the double helix, or "the essential twist" (59). The general factor TFIIH has a component that locally unwinds DNA in an ATP-dependent fashion (59,60). Thus, the PIC recruits pol II, receives signals from the specific TFs, and changes the local DNA structure and possibly the nucleosome arrangement.

Specific Transcription Factors and Transcriptional Activators

The specific transcription factors are the brains of transcriptional regulation. They alter transcription by changing local nucleosome arrangement to a permissive form and contact, recruit, and activate the general transcription factors such as TBP, TAFs, or TFIIB, ultimately influencing pol II. To activate or repress transcription, a transcriptional regulator must be in its active form (often requiring key phosphorylations or dephosphorylations of serines, threonines, or tyrosines, and/or dissociation from inhibitors), located in the nucleus, bound to the DNA of a regulatory site or to a specific factor already bound to the sites. Regulation by extracellular signals must ultimately affect one or more of these processes: the activity, the nuclear localization, binding to other proteins, and binding to DNA. Each transcriptional activator interacts directly or indirectly with other specific transcription factors in a three-dimensional array of protein–protein and protein–DNA interactions. This array of proteins bends and deforms the DNA, and one or more domains from the transcriptional activators contact and alter the general transcription factors. The specific transcriptional activators reverse or prevent inhibition; promote assembly of the correct PIC and prevent nonproductive PIC; alter nucleosomes; and receive and integrate signals from the cytoplasm or membrane receptors.

Specific transcription factors are modular, with a DNA-binding and a dimerization domain, as well as a transcriptional activation domain. Some transcriptional activators lack either DNA binding or transcriptional activation but form dimers with proteins that have such features. Transcriptional activation domains may be acidic (61), proline rich, or glutamine rich. Acidic transcriptional activation domains contact general TFs such as TBP, TAFs, and TFIIB (62,63). The DNA-binding and dimerization domains include such motifs as zinc fingers, helix-turn-helix motifs, homeo domains, and leucine zippers (64,65).

Some Widely Used Transcriptional Activators

The TFs featured in our discussion of IFN-γ and MHC regulation are Jun and Fos, which together comprise activator protein 1 or AP-1; the ETS family; NF-κB and its relatives; and cyclic adenosine monophosphate (cAMP)-regulated element (CRE)-binding protein (CREB).

AP-1, Jun, and Fos

Jun and Fos were discovered as oncogene products but are now known as regulators of many genes that are induced by extracellular stimuli. They control elements known as TPA response elements (TREs), the consensus sequence for which is the palindrome TGAnTCA. The complex binding to such elements can have many different components: Jun–Jun and Jun–Fos (but not Fos–Fos). Both Jun and Fos are member of families of genes: the Jun family contains c-*Jun*, *JunB*, *Jun D*. The Fos family contains c-*fos*, *Fos B*, *Fra*, and *Frb* (Fig. 5). These components are regulated as follows:

1. Via phosphorylation of serine residues in existing Jun and Fos proteins by (a) mitogen-activated protein kinases (MAPK) (66), including ERK-1 and -2; and by (b) the stress-activated protein kinases called Jun N terminal kinases (JNK), which alter Jun tran-

The Jun and Fos protein families

Jun	Fos
c-Jun	c-Fos
JunB	FosB
JunD	Fra-1
	Fra-2

FIG. 5. A table showing the Jun family and the Fos family of transcription factors.

scriptional activity through N terminal serine phosphorylation, and FRK-1, which phosphorylates Fos.
2. Via transcription of the *fos* and *jun* genes. Jun transcription is regulated by *jun* itself, as well as by other TFs. The *jun* gene is controlled by a TRE in the promoter. Fos transcription is controlled by transcription factors such as TCF, Elk-1, and serum response factor, regulated by MAP kinases ERK-1 and ERK-2 (see below).
3. Via assembly with other proteins.
4. Via positive and negative interactions with other TFs.

The c-ETS factors (e.g. elk, EBS, elf, ETS) are constitutively expressed TFs that are controlled by phosphorylation regulated by membrane receptors. ETS transcription factors are regulated by the ras/MAPkinase pathway, specifically MAP kinases such as ERK-2 (66–68). This pathway involves the activation of ras guanosine diphosphate (GDP) to the ras guanosine triphosphate (GTP) form associated with the membrane, which attracts and activates the kinase Raf, which activates the serine/threonine and tyrosine kinase MEK, which activates the ERK1 and 2 kinases (MAP kinases) by serine and tyrosine phosphorylation. The MAP kinases activate transcription factors in the ETS family, such as Elk, which regulate transcription of factors such as Fos. ETS-related transcriptional activators are also regulated by Rb, the retinoblastoma protein. Because Rb is inhibited by hyperphosphorylation (69), this would be another route by which ETS activity could be regulated. ETS consensus binding sites, with a core of GGA, are found in many cytokine promoters, and ETS family members are activated when T cells are triggered, sometimes associating with AP-1 (70).

CREB and CREB-Binding Protein (CBP)

CRE is the DNA element regulated by cAMP receptors. The consensus sequence for CRE is a palindrome, TGACGTCA, which is related to the TRE TGAnTCA. Receptors of the seven-pass family control heterotrimeric G proteins (α, β, γ), which bind GTP and activate adenyl cyclase to generate cAMP. cAMP is a second messenger, which activates protein kinase A, which phosphorylates CREB. Phosphorylated CREB activates cAMP-regulated genes.

NF-κB

This family of Tfs, named for its role in regulating the expression of the light chain of immunoglobulin in B cells, regulates many genes activated in immune and inflammatory responses (Fig. 6). The prototype is a dimer of p50 and p65 components, which exists in many cells in the cytoplasm in its inactive form, bound to its inhibitor, IκB. Signals from outside the cell indicating inflamma-

Nomenclature of NF-κB/rel and IκB families

Common name	protein	gene
NF-κB/rel:		
NF-κB	p50	*NFKB-1*
	p65	*relA*
	p105	*NFKB-1*
Lyt-10(p100)	p100	*NFKB-2*
	p52	*NFKB-2*
c-rel	c-Rel	*c-rel*
relB	RelB	*relB*
dorsal	Dorsal	*dorsal*
IκB:		
IκB-α	IκBα	*MAD-3*
IκB-β	IκBβ	?
IκB-γ and CTR	IκBγ	*NFKB-1*
Bcl-3	Bcl-3	*bcl-3*

Liou and Baltimore 1993

FIG. 6. A table showing the members of the Rel/NF-κB and IκB families. The usual factor called NF-κB is the dimer of p50 and p65.

tion such as the cytokine TNF-α cause IκB to be phosphorylated and degraded by a serine protease. These steps activate NF-κB (71), releasing NF-κB to enter the nucleus, possibly with a protein chaperone. There it engages consensus sequences such as the sequence GGGGATTCCCC in the MHC class I gene, often activating transcription of target genes. The active NF-κB dimers also induce transcription of new IκB, which terminates the response. Some dimers such as p50 homodimers may act as repressors.

The many protein products fall into four types (71):

1. The p50 or p52 members dimerize with themselves or with the p65 or Rel members. The p50 is derived from the p105 product NF-κB1, and the p52 is derived from the p100 NF-κB2 product.
2. The p65 proteins, such as RelA and c-Rel. All of these products have Rel homology domains that mediate many important functions, including dimerization, interaction with IκB, nuclear localization, and DNA binding.
3. The p100 and p105 proteins, which are precursors to small proteins but also have the Rel domain.
4. The IκB members interact with and neutralize the p50 and p65 dimers and lack the Rel domain.

Knockout mice with disruptions of the *p50, RelA,* and *RelB* genes have phenotypes indicating that this family plays vital roles in immunity and inflammation:

1. The disruption of the *NF-κB1* gene in the region that encodes the p50 protein leads to defects in the immune response (72). The phenotype suggests that p50 plays a role in rapid initiation of immune and inflammatory responses. (Whether this phenotype includes abnormal class I or II regulation has not yet been studied (72).
2. Disruption of the *RelA* gene, which encodes p65, causes massive hepatic necrosis at days 15–16 of embryonic life (73). Cells with this defect cannot respond to TNF-α. Thus, p65 is essential for some TNF responses. Whether the active dimer of p65 is p65/p65, p50/p65, or p65/Rel is not clear. The widespread expression of RelA in tissues makes it a good candidate to be a class I regulator.
3. Disruption of the *RelB* gene, which encodes the RelB protein, creates developmental defects in the immune system and multiorgan inflammation (74). RelB may play a suppressive role in inflammation.

Corticosteroids induce IκB expression, thereby inhibiting NF-κB activation (75,76), possibly an important basis of their anti-inflammatory effect. High concentrations of salicylates also inhibit NF-κB activation (77). The immunosuppressive agent 15-deoxyspergualin acts on a chaperone protein, Hsc70, and may inhibit the translocation of NF-κB to the nucleus (78).

MOLECULAR BIOLOGY OF IFN-γ PRODUCTION, RECEPTOR TRIGGERING, AND SIGNAL TRANSDUCTION

Regulation of IFN-γ Expression

IFN-γ is synthesized as a polypeptide chain of 17 kDa (146 aa), and a 20-aa signal peptide does not appear in the mature product. Each IFN-γ monomer has six alpha helical regions, designated A–F. The monomer is glycosylated and dimerizes to create the biologically active form, a head-to-tail dimer. The dimer is symmetrical with two globular domains, each composed of the N terminal four helices of one monomer (A, B, C, and D) and the C terminal two helices of the other (E and F).

The main control on IFN-γ production is transcription. IFN-γ gene is transcribed only in T cells and NK cells. IFN-γ is inducible in vivo by antigenic stimulation, bacterial products such as endotoxin and bacterial superantigens, and by tissue injury, and is also expressed at a low level in the normal host. There is basal expression of IFN-γ mRNA in kidney and other tissues. We have shown that IFN-γ knockout (GKO) mice have deficiencies in basal MHC class I expression in the kidney (35). In addition, GKO mice have multiple severe defects in MHC gene induction. To date IFN-γ is the only cytokine with a proven role in the regulation of MHC expression in vivo. IFN-γ expression is sensitive to immunosuppressive agents such as steroids, CyA, and tacrolimus. In fact, a key role of immunosuppressive treatment is to reduce IFN-γ production and thus reduce MHC expression and antigen presentation (79). CyA inhibits IFN-γ transcription by inhibiting the enzyme calcineurin, a serine-threonine phosphatase, which in turn prevents calcineurin from activating key transcription factors.

Ca^{+}-Calcineurin–Inducible Sites in the IFN-γ Promoter

IFN-γ is regulated like interleukin-2 (IL-2), which is the prototype for cytokine regulation in T cells. IL-2 is regulated by many promoter sites and transcription factors, but a key TF is nuclear factor of activated T cells (NFAT), interacting with the NFAT DNA elements in the IL-2 promoter. CyA-sensitive T-cell cytokines probably all have NFAT binding sites, as listed in Fig. 7 (80). NFAT is a complex with a nuclear component and a cytosolic component (81). At least in some cases the nuclear component is AP-1. NFAT cytosolic components are a family of proteins, the prototype for which is NFATp. NFATp has similarities to NF-κB, and has a Rel-like domain. It is held in the cytosol and released by serine desphosphorylation by the phosphatase calcineurin (82). This releases the activated NFAT to enter the nucleus and

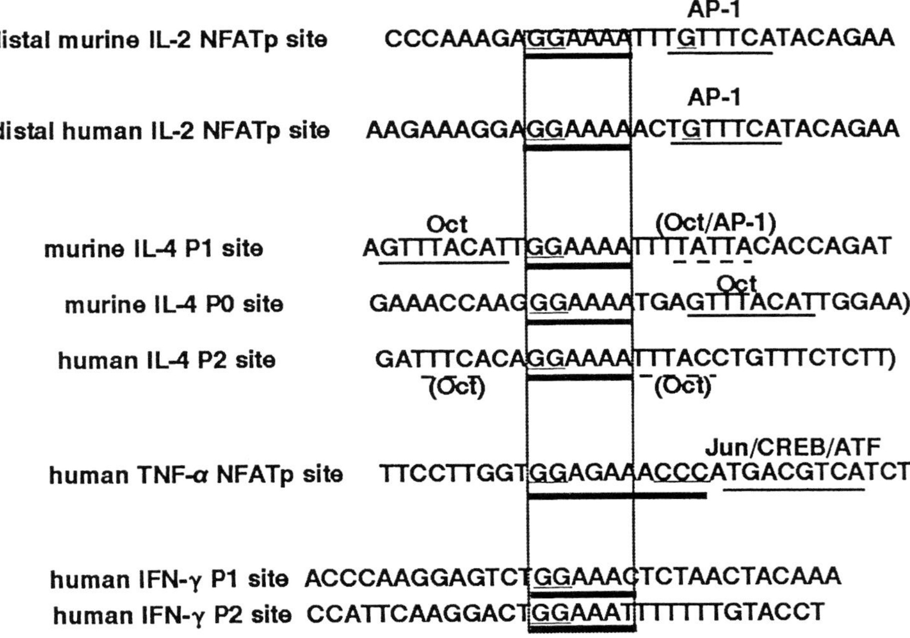

FIG. 7. A map showing sequences in the promoters of various cytokines that are probably regulated by NFAT transcription factors. Thus, each of the cyclosporine-sensitive cytokines expressed in a T cell probably has several NFAT binding sites. The usual NFAT factor is a cytoplasmic component such as NFATp associated with a nuclear component, which in some cases contains Jun/Fos.

engage the NFAT binding site in association with nuclear NFAT components.

The regulatory sites in the IFN-γ gene are outlined in Fig. 8. We have studied the CyA-sensitive sites in detail, seeking homology with NFAT sites in the other cytokine. We found that the IFN-γ promoter has no close homologues of the NFAT sequence in the IL-2 promoter. However, both mouse and human IFN-γ promoters have multiple copies of the consensus sequences ATTTCCnnT, which are homologous to P sequences in the IL-4 promoter that bind NFAT. P oligomers bind a protein that reacts with NFAT antibody, is cytosolic in resting T cells,

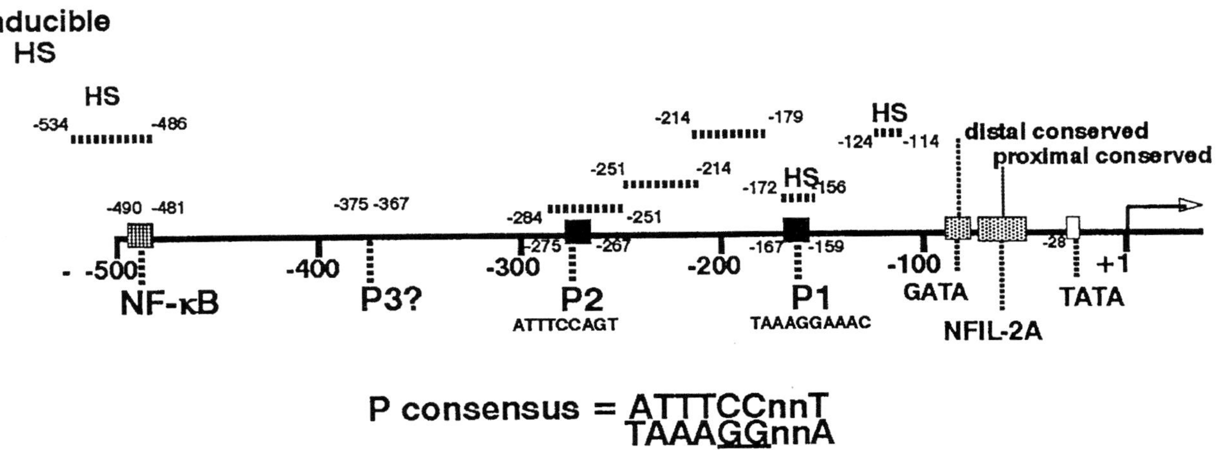

FIG. 8. A map of the human IFN-γ promoter, showing the potential NFAT binding sites (designated P1 and P2). There may be additional NFAT binding sites.

and is nuclear in activated T cells. Tandem repeats of the P sequence conferred calcium ionophore inducibility and CyA sensitivity on a reporter gene. Thus, the P sequences in the IFN-γ promoter are candidate sites of regulation of the IFN-γ gene via NFAT proteins and thus of the IFN-γ–MHC system (83).

It is likely that factors in the NF-κB, ETS, and AP-1 families affect IFN-γ transcription, but the details have not been defined. In our studies of IFN-γ production in mice in vivo, the naturally occurring challenges experienced by the normal host (infections, antigenic stimulation, tissue injury) induce IFN-γ production by CyA-sensitive pathways. Other pathways can induce IFN-γ. For example, basal IFN-γ production is CyA resistant but only involves low levels of expression. Thus, IFN-γ produced by this pathway may induce some basal class I and II expression even in the normal human. Administration of IFN-γ induces IFN-γ mRNA in the kidney, i.e., autoinduction (32): whether this is quantitatively important in the total IFN-t response is dubious.

IFN-α/β

These IFNs are a large and diverse family of 13 different alpha genes and one or two beta genes. They are synthesized by a variety of tissues, not simply lymphocytes. In general they are inducible by virus infections, by mechanisms outside of the immune system. Their in vivo roles have been difficult to assign because of the large number of IFN-α/β genes. IFN-α/β production is CyA and tacrolimus resistant. All act through a single IFN-α/β receptor. Their role in vivo in MHC regulation is less well established than that of IFN-γ, as discussed below.

IFN-γR

The IFN-γR (84) is a multi-unit receptor with at least two subunits, α and β. The a subunit (85) is the high-affinity ligand-binding domain and is a member of the IFN-R family. It is encoded by a gene mapping to chromosome 6q in humans. The IFN-γRα chain (489 aa, 90 kDa) has a 14-aa leader sequence, leaving 475 aa expressed in the mature protein. The amino acids 14–245 form the extracellular domain, 246–266 the transmembrane region, and 267–489 the intracellular portion. In the external portion, there are two immunoglobulinlike domains of about 100 aa each, separated by a linker. Domain 1 has 7 b strands, which fold to form two antiparallel sheets, A, B, E, and G, F, C, and C′, separated by loops. Domain 2 has eight strands, which fold to form two antiparallel sheets, A, B, E, D and G, F, C, and C′, separated by loops. Cysteine residues in each domain hold the sheets together.

Two IFN-γRα chains bind each IFN-γ dimer. The structure of the IFN-γ/2IFN-γRα complex has been solved (86). The V-shaped IFN-γ dimer bends the receptors to form a symmetrical X-shaped mass with the V-shaped IFN-γ dimer in the middle. The principal contact surface in the IFN-γ molecule for the IFN-γRα is formed by the A helix, AB loop, and B helix of one monomer and the F helix and C terminal of the other monomer. The contact site in the IFN-γRα is in the region where the Ig-like domains join: the F and G β strands and the CC′ and EF loops of domain 1, the interdomain linker, and the BC and FG loops of domain 2.

The resulting structure creates sites where the β chain of the receptor can bind, probably with lower affinity, in the N terminal of each member of the IFN-γ dimer and the adjacent Rα chain. The β chain maps to chromosome 21 in humans (87,88). The signalling functions of the a and β chains are distinct. Class I induction requires an accessory factor encoded on chromosome 21 (89,90).

The IFN-γRα chain is constitutively expressed in many tissues. This leaves all or most cells in the kidney and other tissues ready to respond to IFN-γ at all times, with resulting changes in MHC expression. It is important in this respect that IFN-γ is not a growth factor and does not change the function of important cells with life-sustaining roles such as renal epithelium.

Two major features of the intracytoplasmic portion of the a chain are an "LPSX" motif near the membrane, which is critical to binding of Janus kinases (JAKs), and tyrosine (Y) 440 near the C terminal, which is the site that when phosphorylated permits the SH2 domain of p91 signal transducers and activators of transcription (STAT) to dock (91).

JAK–STAT Model for Signalling by IFNs and Other Receptors

In receptors that signal via Y phosphorylation, specific Y phosphorylation occurs in three types of proteins: the tyrosine kinases themselves, the intracytoplasmic components of the receptor, and the target proteins that begin the signal transduction pathways (Figs. 9 and 10). Receptor Y phosphorylation creates docking sites that bind the target proteins via SH2 domains (92) and permits the tyrosine kinases to act on them.

Studies of signalling by the IFN-γR have shown a general pattern for how many receptors selectively induce transcription of target genes via tyrosine kinases, the JAKs acting on members of the STAT family. We call this general model the JAK–STAT mechanism (93–99). JAK–STAT mechanisms are associated with many cytokine, growth factor, and protein hormone receptors in the hematopoietin and IFN receptor family, e.g., IL-4 (100). The JAK–STAT mechanism selectively activates the transcription of a small number of genes, in contrast to the complex serine threonine kinase cascades such as the ras:MAPkinase pathway, that create much more general

IFN-γ triggers JAK1,JAK2 which activate R and p91 STAT1α

- *IFN-γ dimer triggers crosslinks Rα chains*
- *recruits Rβ chain, activates JAK1, JAK2*
- *JAKs tyrosine phosphorylates Rα (Y440)*
- *p91STAT binds R, activated by JAKs*
- *p91 dimerizes, enters nucleus*

FIG. 9. A table showing the probable sequence of events when IFN-τ receptors are triggered.

cell activation. The JAK–STAT mechanism is ideal for selective alteration of gene expression in nonlymphoid cells without changing their other functions.

The elucidation of the JAK–STAT system resulted from genetic experiments. Cell lines were mutated and selected for mutations in which IFN-γ signalling was lost. The deficient cell lines in turn were corrected by transfection with candidate genes. For example, cell line U4A lacks JAK1; U3A lacks p91, etc. (101). These findings were confirmed by over-expression of the candidate genes (JAKs or STATs) in normal cells (95).

JAKs

These studies of mutants lacking IFN-γR and IFN-α/βR signalling showed that JAKs were associated with these receptors: IFN-tR with JAK1 and JAK2, and IFN-a/bR with JAK1 and TYK-2. Studies of other receptors have extended this family. The JAK family of PTKs has four members: JAK1, -2, and -3, plus Tyk-2. Each has a MW of about 130 kDa, with a C terminal kinase domain, a kinaselike domain, and five other domains, but no SH2 and SH3 domains.

JAK Targets: The STAT Family

JAKs activate members of the STAT family, cytosolic precursors of transcription factors (98). STATs are cytosolic proteins that are attracted by their SH2 domains to phosphotyrosine groups on membrane receptors and tyrosine phosphorylated by JAKs. They form multimers and are translocated to the nucleus to interact with specific sequences. This sequence was first identified in the IFN-γ–activated genes and termed the gamma-activated sequence (GAS). The STATs are the only family of transcription factors activated by tyrosine phosphorylation. STATs are distinguished by size, e.g., STAT1a is p91, and STAT1 is p84. STAT2 is p113. p91 and p84 are alternatively spliced variants of the same mRNA, the difference in MW being 38 aa at C terminal. There are now four other STATs described, and more could follow

Hypothesis: how IFN-γ dimers activate the IFN-γ R

IFN-γ dimer crosslinks Rα chains, recruits Rβ chains

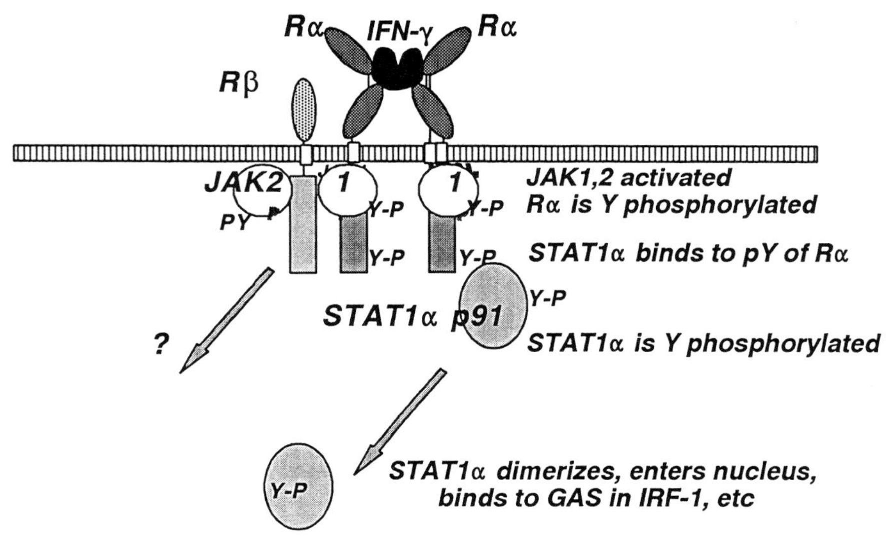

FIG. 10. A cartoon showing how the IFN-γ α chains are crosslinked, recruiting accessory molecules, and triggering the JAK–STAT mechanism. The result is the creation of the active dimer of tyrosine phosphorylated STAT1α. In some cases, STATs may undergo serine phosphorylation by other kinases.

(101). Some of the activities of STAT proteins may require not only tyrosine but also serine phosphorylation, via MAP kinases. This may apply particularly to activated and cycling cells, where MAP kinases are activated (102–104).

Sequence of Events in IFN-γ Signalling

Before ligand binding, IFN-γRα is associated with JAK1 but not JAK2 (101). (IFN-γRβ may associate with JAK2.) The IFN-γR is triggered by dimerization of the IFN-γRα chains, recruiting the IFN-γRβ and JAK2. Receptor aggregation permits the JAKs to activate one another (105–108). The JAKs tyrosine phosphorylate themselves, the α chain of the receptor (on Y 440?), and the STATs (106,109,110). STAT1α p91 dimerizes via SH2-phosphotyrosyl interactions (111) and translocates to the nucleus, where it binds to DNA of GAS. This sequence is found in genes activated directly by IFN-γ, without intermediate protein synthesis, but is not found in the MHC class I or class II promoters. STATs form multimers after IFN-α/βRs are triggered. After triggering of the IFN-γR, STAT1 (p84) is also Y phosphorylated, but its role is uncertain. STAT1α p91 is central to both α and β, but STAT1 p84 and STAT2 p113 are not required for IFN-γ signalling. IFN-γ also induces another STAT related to p91 (112).

Events in IFN-α/βR Triggering

After triggering of the IFN-αR, p84, p91, and p113 are Y phosphorylated and multimerize to form ISGF3α. ISGF3α is not formed after the IFN-γR is triggered. This complexes with a factor called p48 or ISGF3, the principal DNA binding component of the complex, and translocates to the nucleus. p48 ISGF3 is a member of the IRF family [IRF-1, IRF-2, IRF consensus sequence (ICS)BP, and others] and is related to the Myb family of DNA binding proteins (113). It is present in unstimulated cells, but is also IFN-γ induced. There may be two complexes: p48/p84/p113 and p48/p91/p113. p48 ISGF3 has affinity for the DNA sequences known as IFN-stimulated response elements (ISREs).

IFN-Regulated Transcription Factors

There are three types of IFN-regulated transcription factors:

1. First generation or pre-existing cytosolic, the STAT proteins discussed above. These are preformed cytosolic proteins activated by JAKs via Y phosphorylation, multimerization, and translocation, and bind to GAS-like sequences.
2. Second generation, those induced by transcriptional activation and translation via pre-existing transcription factors (the STATs) (and possibly by other pathways). The mRNAs appear without new protein synthesis. The example of these factors is the IRF family. The transcription of the gene for IRF-1 is rapidly induced by STATs after IFN stimulation with no requirement for new protein synthesis. IRF-1 and its relatives often pre-exist in low levels before stimulation, and IRF members may autoregulate and cross-regulate one another, along with STATs. These IRF-related proteins engage DNA at the general IFN-consensus sequences, not the GAS.
3. The third-generation factors [e.g., the class II transactivator (CIITA)] are induced by STATs but also require synthesis of new proteins, probably IRF-1 and perhaps other second generation factors. CIITA is obligatory for class II expression, and is unusual among transcriptional activators in that it does not bind DNA. Thus, in some cases the pre-existing STAT and the induced IRF-like factors work together to induce third-generation factors.

Other transcription factors regulated by IFN-γ are less understood, e.g., NF-X1 factor (114).

IFN-Regulated Consensus Sequences

IFN-regulated genes contain consensus sequences of several types, each of which binds a distinct set of proteins (115). The genes induced by STATs have GAS consensus sequences, and the genes induced by IRF-1 family members have several varieties of related consensus sequences.

Sites Regulated by IFN-γ Alone

The classic GAS (IFN-γ–activated sites) bind dimers of p91 STAT or other STATs. This sequence is found in genes that are immediately activated by IFN-γ. The consensus is TTA/CCnnnAA. For example, the GAS in the IRF-1 gene promoter is TTCCCCGAA. Related GAS-like sequences mediate the action of other STATs.

Sites Regulated by IRF-1 Family Members

The ISRE and the related IFN regulatory factor–binding element (IRF-E) are regulated by IRF family members, at least in part. IRF-1 and IRF-2 (and potentially ISGF3γ) bind to the IRF-E in the IFN-α/β promoters and to the related ISRE in IFN-inducible genes. IRF-2 may be a negative regulator of IRF-1–controlled sites. The IRF-1 knockout (116) has defective antiviral immunity and inducible nitric oxide synthase, and disrupted IFN expression and CD8 development (117). ISREs are regulated by ISGF3 complexes, but at least part of their DNA binding is through p48 ISGF3γ. The ICS in class I MHC genes is related to the ISRE sequence. ICSBP, which is typically found in lymphoid cells and is related to IRF-1 and 2, binds to ISREs and may also be a negative regulator (118,119). ISREs are related to the general IFN consensus sequence, and are repeats of GAAAnn (118), such as GGAAACCGAAACTG (113). The effect of the ISRE is influenced by the flanking DNA sequences (120).

Other Cytokines Potentially Relevant to MHC Expression

The cytokines most frequently implicated in MHC regulation are TNF-α/β, GM-CSF, TGF-β, and IL-10.

TNFs are homotrimers which act on TNF receptors (TNFRs) p55/60 and p75 and trimerize them to activate the sphingomyelin ceramide pathway (121). The members of the NF-κB family are major mediators of the transcriptional effects of TNF-α/β. The immediate agents that transmit the effects to NF-κB are unknown: phospholipase A2, PC-specific phospholipase C, protein kinase C, and possibly PTKs have been incriminated in TNFR signalling. One result is phosphorylation of IκB and release of NF-κB to move to its sites in promoters. Other effects include activation of AP-1, IRF-1, and others (122). In vitro, TNF-α induces MHC class I, particularly in endothelial cells (123). In vivo, TNF-α induces class I weakly but not class II. The principal effect of TNF-α on MHC expression in vivo is its ability to potentiate the effects of IFN-t (124).

GM-CSF induces the differentiation of precursor cells into class II–positive dendritic cells in vitro (125), in cooperation with other cytokines such as TNF-α. However, granulocyte-macrophage colony-stimulating factor (GM-CSF) may not directly induce class II. For example, GM-CSF in mice does not induce class II expression in the kidney in vivo (T. Sims and P. Halloran, unpublished observations). Thus, the in vivo role of GM-CSF in MHC regulation is unknown.

IL-10 acts on an IFN-like receptor (126) and indirectly antagonizes some IFN-γ–induced effects, including antigen presentation (127–129). IL-10 mRNA is found in normal mice and is greatly increased in irradiated mice (130). Administration of IL-10 in vivo to antagonize the effects of IFN-γ has been disappointing, failing to inhibit IFN-γ or MHC induction significantly. IL-10 antagonizes IFN-γ in protracted complex responses such as in parasitic infection, not in short-term assays in vivo. The many contradictions of models involving TH1–TH2 cross-regulation by cytokines have been reviewed recently (131).

TGF-βs are widely expressed cytokine/growth factor proteins subject to complex control at the transcriptional and post-transcriptional levels. TGF-βs are usually considered anti-inflammatory and immunosuppressive and generally suppress cycling cells, although the opposite effects also have been reported. TGF-βs should be considered a family of bifunctional regulators (126) of cell growth. The TGF-β1 knockout mouse develops a fatal multisystem inflammatory disease (55) with increased MHC expression (132). Thus, the usual role for TGF-β1 may be anti-inflammatory, suppressing MHC expression in early life. TGF-β1 suppresses IFN-γ–induced class II induction in vitro in some cell lines (133).

REGULATION OF CLASS II EXPRESSION

In Vivo Regulation of Class II Expression

Class II regulation is a prototype for regulated gene expression in vivo in inflammatory states. Class II expression is a key point at which antigen presentation and thus immune responsiveness is regulated. Class II expression is largely determined by transcription, probably at the level of initiation of transcription rather than elongation, as demonstrated for the mouse *Eβ* gene (134). Hypomethylation of regulating sites in class II is associated with expression (135). There are many class II genes, and, as previously mentioned, all typical class II genes are coordinately regulated, i.e., they tend to be induced as a group, but with some striking features of individuality, more so than in class I genes.

Knowledge Derived from Human Genetic Defects

Transcriptional regulation of class II genes has been studied by a series of steps:

1. Identification of DNAse-hypersensitive sites, CpG islands, and consensus DNA sequences within regulatory regions.
2. Demonstration of protein binding to putative regulatory sequences by electrophoretic mobility shift assays.
3. Transfection of reporter constructs to show whether a particular sequence can indeed respond to regulatory influences in a test cell.
4. Experimentation with mutant and transfected cells and with transgenic and knockout mice.

These approaches proved that some key feature of the behaviour of class II genes is due to the X and Y boxes and proteins that bound to them (5,6). In general, the elements called S, X, and Y are found in the proximal promoter elements of all class II genes, conserved in sequence and position; the element J is conserved in sequence but not position (136). The vital element seems to be the X box.

However, much has been learned from the genetic approach to the rare human inborn errors in which all class II expression is lost (137,138). A number of families have autosomal-recessive defects that manifest as severe combined immunodeficiency with "bare lymphocyte syndrome," a term now used to denote absence of all class II expression, constitutive and induced. Mutant B cell lines that have lost all class II expression have been used in parallel with the studies of cells from patients with bare lymphocyte syndrome (BLS) and represent in vitro counterparts of the same genetic errors. Both sources show that the defects causing deletion of all class II expression are of three types (complementation groups), each corresponding to a defective gene for a molecule that is obligatory for all class II expression but not needed by other genes. These molecules form the core of our knowledge of the unique aspects of class II regulation. However, many other genes and their proteins are involved in class II regulation and can be classified as follows:

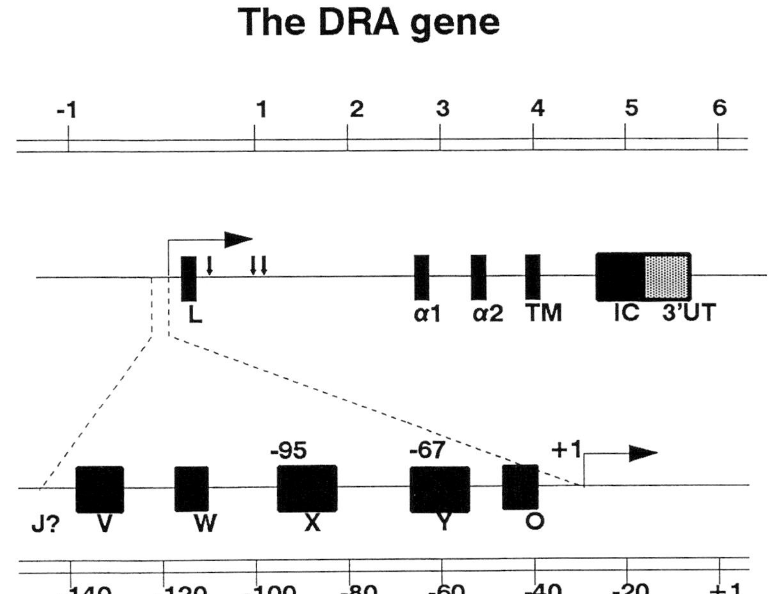

FIG. 11. The class II gene and its promoter. **A:** A class II gene (the DR gene). **B:** The class II promoter, showing the X1, X2, and Y boxes. These boxes each bind proteins and the class II transactivator (CIITA) and engage the bound proteins. Only the genes for CIITA and the RFX5 protein have so far been cloned and shown to be mutated in cases of class II deficiency (BLS).

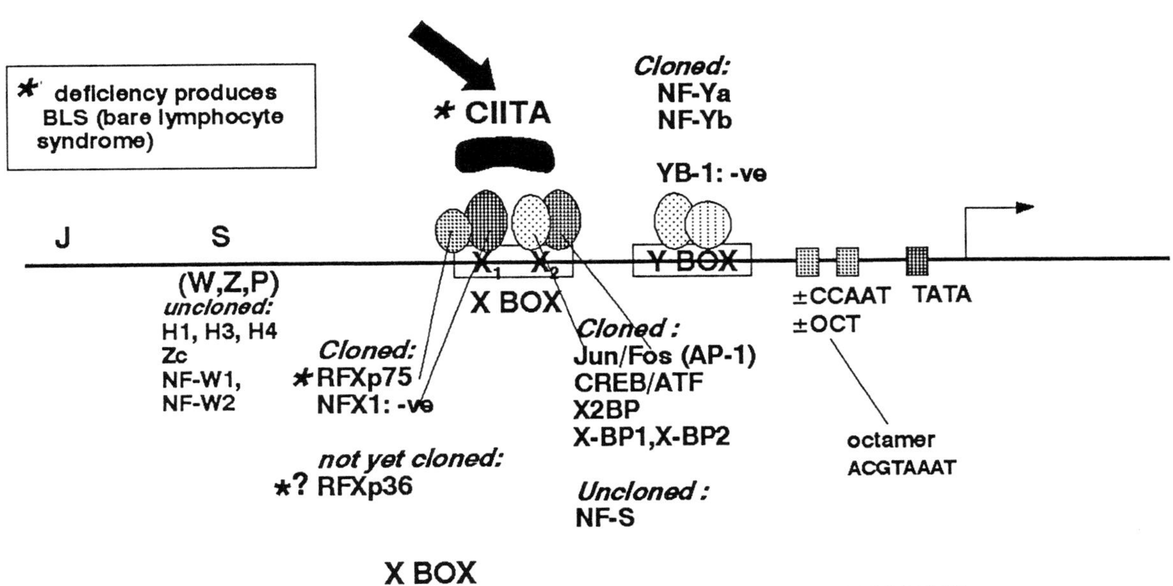

1. Affecting class II expression but also other processes, such that their deletion is nonviable.
2. Affecting class II regulation but redundant; deletion is compensated by proteins with overlapping effects, so that class II expression is not lost.
3. Affecting regulation of one or two class II genes but not all; mutations affect expression of selected class II genes.

We focus here on the general features of all class II gene regulation. Examples of other types of control also are mentioned.

The X and Y Boxes (5,6)

The promoters of class II genes have highly conserved sequences termed the X and Y box, with the X box further subdivided into X1 and X2 (Fig. 11). There are elements 58 to the X-Y region, termed W, H, V, S, or Z. An additional 58 element called J is more variable. The *DRA* gene also has an octamer site 38 to the X and Y elements. Two representative X-Y regions are shown below:

The X, X2, and Y boxes are occupied by proteins in cells expressing or capable of expressing class II, as shown by "footprinting" (139,140). These proteins occupying the promoter give the 5′ region of class II genes a characteristic pattern of DNAse I hypersensitive sites. A variety of sequence-specific DNA binding proteins have been demonstrated to bind to the X1, X2, or Y boxes of various mouse and human genes.

Proteins That Engage the X1 Sequence

The X1 consensus is unique to class II, *Inv,* and *DM* genes. Identification of X1 binding proteins were coupled with genetic studies of BLS families or B cell lines (141), which showed that the X1 binding proteins were class II specific and necessary for all class II expression. A complex designated RFX occupies the X1 box, with at least two components: RFXp36 and RFXp75. The p75 protein has been cloned and designated RFX5 (142). Defects in the RFX1 complex occur in some cases of class II deficiency. In complementation group C (143), the mutations affect the gene for the p75 protein RFX5. In complementation group B, the gene has not been identified but may be the gene that encodes the p36 protein.

Several other proteins bind to X1 in vitro, but their importance in vivo is not clear, and they may not be relevant to class II regulation in vivo. These are RFX1 to RFX4, and NF-X1. These RFX factors are not affected by mutations in the BLS or in mutant class II–negative B cell lines. RFX factors 1 to 4 may not be involved in class II regulation. One potentially significant factor binding to the X1 box is NF-X1, a transcriptional repressor regulated by IFN-γ. It potentially turns off transcription, but its role in vivo is unknown (114).

X2

The X2 box in at least some class II genes is an analog of the CRE consensus sequence (the cAMP-regulated element) consensus, and the related TRE (the TPA regulated site). The X2 box engages proteins related to Jun, Fos, and the cAMP-regulated proteins CREB/ATF. Factors that engage the human X2 box include the X2BP complex, Jun/Fos, and CREB/ATF. Protein hXBP1 is needed for a subset of class II genes and forms a heterodimer with c-Fos (144). In mice, mXBP/CRE-BP2 forms a complex with c-Jun and engages the CRE/ATF sequence in the X2 box in the *Aα* gene (145,146). The nuclear protein CBP interacts with and coactivates the phosphorylated form of CREB (147) and thus could play a role in the regulation of the class II X2 box.

Not surprisingly, no X2-binding proteins are affected by mutations producing BLS. The CRE motif and the proteins engaging it are found in many genes, making isolated class II deficiency an unlikely phenotype for such a mutation. The CRE might be expected to mediate some effects in class II regulation, but this has not been shown in vivo.

The Y Box

The Y box is an inverted CCAAT sequence. CCAAT is a common proximal promoter element found in many eukaryotic genes and binds many proteins. In humans, NF-Y, YB-1, and C/EBP have been described as binding to the Y box. Monocytes express a protein NF-M which could influence the behavior of class II genes in monocytes (148). NF-Y has been shown to play a role in regulating the albumen gene as well as the class II genes (149). The Y box binding protein YB-1 represses IFN-γ activation of class II (150). Thus, the control at the Y box

The human DRA X-Y box:

GGACCCT——CCTAGCAACAGATGCGTCA–(15)——CTGATTGGCCAAAG–(8)—ATTTGCAT—(44)—+1
WBOX____ X1BOX____ X2BOX___ ___YBOX______ OCTAMER

The mouse Aα X-Y box:

AGGCCTC–17–**GCTGGCAACTGTG**ACGTCA–15—CTGATTGGTT
S/H BOX____X1 BOX____ X2 BOX(CRE/ATF)__Y BOX_______

is important but not class II specific. For example, C/EBP knockout mice have defective energy metabolism and die at birth, showing that some non–class II genes regulated by CCAAT boxes are essential for life (151).

CIITA

The human CIITA (152–155) was discovered via a genetic approach, based on complementation cloning of the mutated gene for a missing factor in a subgroup of families with class II deficiency (152–154). CIITA does not bind to DNA but to the proteins bound to the X1, X2, and possibly the Y box in the class II promoters and stabilizes their binding. A functioning CIITA gene is obligatory for all class II expression, constitutive or induced, and silencing of the CIITA gene extinguishes class II expression (153). Developmental extinction of CIITA expression shuts off class II expression in B cells as they differentiate into plasma cells (152). The carboxyl terminus of CIITA may contain the principal transcription activation domain for class II expression (156).

We have found that CIITA mRNA is widely distributed (155) in vivo in mouse tissues, and the expression of CIITA mRNA correlates well with the expression of class II, both basal and induced. In mouse kidney, there is basal CIITA expression, probably in IDC. IFN-γ induces CIITA expression in mouse kidney, probably in epithelial cells. In addition, CIITA is inducible by renal ischemic injury, both via IFN and by non–IFN-γ mechanisms. CIITA is induced by STAT1α but also requires IRF-1; we have shown that CIITA induction is severely impaired in IRF-1 knockout mice (unpublished observations). This explains why CIITA mRNA induction is partially dependent on protein synthesis.

CIITA may either be an on–off switch that permits typical class II genes to express themselves according to gene-specific and cell-specific factors (156) or a quantitative regulator of overall class II expression like a thermostat.

Effect of IFN-γ on Class II Promoters

When IFN-γ induces class II expression, the X1 site in the DRA promoter complex shows no new protein binding. There is increased binding at sites already occupied. This probably reflects IFN-γ stabilizing the binding to the X1, X2, and Y boxes (157) by inducing CIITA. Thus, our current view of the effect of IFN-γ on class II expression is that IFN-γ induces STAT1α and IRF-1, which induce CIITA transcription, and that all effects of IFN-γ on class II transcription are due to CIITA induction (Fig. 12).

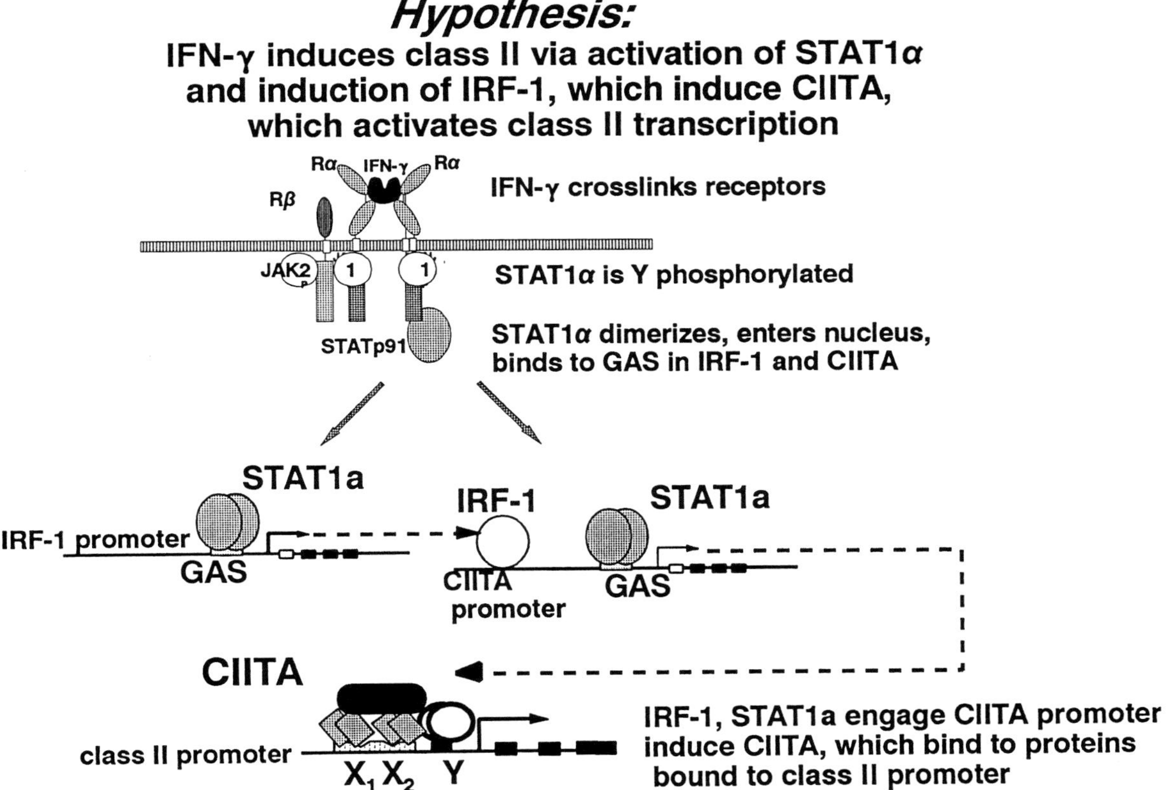

FIG. 12. A cartoon showing our current concept of how interferon-γ can trigger class II expression, acting through STAT1α and IRF-1 on the CIITA promoter.

Effect of TNF on Class II Expression

As mentioned earlier, TNF-α in culture does not consistently induce class II in cells or cell lines but consistently potentiates class II induction by IFN-γ. For some cell types in vitro, TNF-α alone induces class II expression, e.g., endothelial cells (158,159). In murine macrophage cell lines there is induction of class II by TNF-α (160), but the relevance of this for macrophages is unclear. In astrocytes TNF-α does not induce but synergizes with IFN-γ (161). TNF-α actually suppressed transcription of class II in mouse peritoneal macrophages (162). In our in vivo experiments, we demonstrated potentiation of class II induction in mouse kidney by IFN-γ but no induction of class II by TNF-α alone (124). The mechanism by which IFN-γ is potentiated by TNF-α is not known.

Sites for binding of NF-κB and Rel proteins are found in some class II genes but not in others. A TNF-α response element has been described in the DRA promoter (163). A TNF response element (NF-κB) called a T box has been described in some class II genes.

Negative Control of Class II Expression

Two negative transcriptional regulators of human class II are described. NF-X1, isolated from human Raji cells (114), is induced late by IFN-γ and may repress class II transcription and terminate the response by binding to the X box. A Y box binding protein, YB-1, represses IFN-γ–induced transcription of class II (150) but may not be IFN-γ inducible. YB-1 may repress class II by inducing single-stranded regions in the DNA of the promoter (164). Most T cells may be class II negative because the X-Y boxes are suppressed (165). The factor that prevents transcription is not identified. Some pseudogenes in the class II region (e.g., DQA2, DQB2, DOB) have mutations in their promoters that make them silent and noninducible (166).

Other Features of Class II Regulation

The retinoblastoma protein Rb has a general role in the cell cycle. In its hypophosphorylated form it is active, and in its fully phosphorylated form it is inactive. An effect of Rb protein on IFN-γ–induced class II has been described, but whether this is important in noncycling cells is not clear (167).

Class II *Aβ* genes are expressed poorly in kidney epithelium due to a silencer in class II *Aβ* genes (168). This may explain why DR products can be potently induced in epithelial cells but DQ products cannot. In humans, the high inducible expression of DR and the poor inducible expression of other class II genes may be relevant in transplants.

A protein termed high-mobility group protein I/Y (HMG I/Y) has been shown to be important for class II regulation, including IFN-γ induction (169). The protein Oct-2A may activate the DRA octamer region (169).

The *Inv* is coordinately expressed as part of the class II genes and is regulated like a class II gene, with at least some of the W-X1/X2-Y sites in common with the class II α and class II β genes. However, *Inv* also has unique features, such as a κB site, and is induced in some cells by TNF-α (170–172). Thus, *Inv* may be subject to regulation by members of the NF-κB/Rel family (173).

The DM products are important for class II peptide binding (18,19,174,175). *DMA* and *DMB* genes may be crucial to peptide loading in all tisues. They have an X and Y box, as well as several other elements suggesting regulation like other class II genes (174). The *DMA* and *DMB* genes, like the *Inv* gene, have NF-κB sites (174).

Summary of Class II Regulation

The class II genes are coordinately regulated to achieve the typical pattern of basal expression in B cells, antigen-presenting cells, and some endothelial cells, and the pattern of induced expression in many cells such as renal epithelial cells. CIITA integrates the signalling from external signals such as cytokines and injury to class II genes, and probably provides a vital transcriptional activation domain needed for class II expression. The X1 box binding RFX complex (RFX factors p36 and p75) is obligatory and unique for the class II promoter. In addition, in order to be expressed, the class II promoter must be occupied at the X2 box, the Y box, and perhaps other sites, such as the J and S upstream site. Only when this three-dimensional array of proteins is present can CIITA bind to the proteins and activate transcription. Additional controls for specific class II genes confer features on the products of different loci, such as poor inducibility by IFN-γ in some sites. Other genes are needed for class II folding, peptide loading, and product expression, such as the *Inv* and *DMA* and *DMB* genes.

REGULATION OF CLASS I EXPRESSION

The regulation of the class I genes is centered around an element in the promoter of each class I gene called the class I regulatory sequence (CRS) and the ICS. (The CRS is often referred to as CRE, but we use the CRS abbreviation to avoid confusion with the cAMP-regulated element.) In mutations of the CRS, the typical pattern of class I expression is lost. The constitutive and IFN-γ–induced expression of class I are separately controlled, but IFN inducibility is dependent on the program for basal expression with complex interactions. We have recently found that basal class I expression in the endothelium and kidney is reduced in mice lacking IFN-γ (GKO mice) and

IRF-1, indicating that full basal expression requires the participation of IRF-1 binding at the ICS. We also showed that induced expression in mouse kidney requires IRF-1 and is lost in mice lacking IRF-1 (unpublished observations).

Role of the CRS and ICS in Constitutive and Induced Expression

The CRS contains a perfect dyad sequence, GGGGATTCCCC, about 160 bp from the transcription start site. This is also a kB binding site (Fig. 13). Some class I genes have additional repeats and inverted repeats of the same sequence. This CRS is flanked by an ICS homologous to the sequences that bind IRF-1 family proteins. The CRS is divided into three regions (see below):

The transcriptional control of class I has been demonstrated in vivo by nuclear run-on (176). Mutations in the CRS causes loss of typical class I tissue-specific and -inducible expression. Occupancy of class I upstream promoter sites in vivo corresponds with class I expression in mouse tissues (177). However, depending on the proteins that occupy them, the regions of the CRS may have negative effects on class I transcription.

Genetics of Class I Expression

We have seen how genetic experiments have contributed to the analysis of IFN-γ signalling and to the analysis of class II expression. In each case the key factors were identifiable by mutations that deleted the essential functions. In contrast, there are no defined mutations that silence all class I transcription in cell lines or create class I–deficient humans, comparable with the BLS types of class II–deficient humans. However, there are several instructive genetic observations that tell us about class I regulation.

Some class II–deficient humans have low class I expression (178), but this may reflect a lack of cytokines such as IFN-γ rather than a primary event. Similarly, mice lacking IFN-γ or IRF-1 have reduced class I expression in kidney and on arterial endothelium.

Humans with class I deficiency due to TAP mutation have been described (179), indicating that TAP function (and thus peptide availability) is essential for normal class I protein expression in vivo. This is probably a posttranslational mechanism, not a transcriptional effect. The β_2M knockout mice have low class I expression due to rapid degradation of the class I molecule, not decreased transcription.

Many tumors with a general reduction in class I expression have been found. In some of these a correlation with transcription factors in the Rel/NF-κB family has been shown. In melanoma, the oncogene c-*Myc* is overexpressed and suppresses class I transcription through effects on the CCAAT and TATA elements (180,181). (n-Myc may have other effects.) But cell lines that have lost all class I transcription due to a single mutation (analogous to the mutations in the *RFX5* or *CIITA* genes) have not been identified. This may indicate redundancy or that the proteins have other functions essential for cell viability. The one knockout mouse strain that has significantly reduced basal class I expression in vivo is the IRF-1 knockout mouse (Halloran et al., unpublished data).

Transcriptional Activators that Regulate Class I via CRS

The basal level of class I expression in tissues of normal mice (and possibly of humans) reflects the binding of proteins to the CRS (177). Members of the Rel/NF-κB family, including the classical p50/p65 dimers and other proteins (including viral proteins) bind to the CRS in vitro or are implicated in MHC regulation in vivo: members of the Rel/κB family may be the principal proteins regulating the CRS. The p50 homodimers (sometimes called KBF1) may inhibit transcription, whereas the p50/p65 dimers may be the positive regulators. H2TF1 [product of the *NF-κB* gene (182)], and potentially many combinations of Rel, Dorsal, and other family members could also participate. The significance of these proteins in class I regulation will probably be established in knockout mice. Viral products related to the Rel/κB family also affect MHC regulation in virally infected cells: the product of the avian v-*rel* gene promotes class I and II expression in spleen tumors (183). Endogenous c-rel correlates with MHC expression during graft-versus-host disease (GVHD). Whether all of the effects are direct or whether some are indirect (e.g., through cytokines) is unknown. N-myc suppresses class I expression by downregulating p50 subunit of NF-κB (184), as does adenovirus type 12 through a viral protein called E1A (185,186).

The murine K^b CRS

Region II

GGTGAGGTCAGGGGTGGGGAAGCCCAGGGCTGGGGATTCCCCA-161

Region III — Region I (dyad or palindrome)

The murine K^b ICS

167 TTCCCCATCTCCTCAGTTTCACTTCTGCA-139

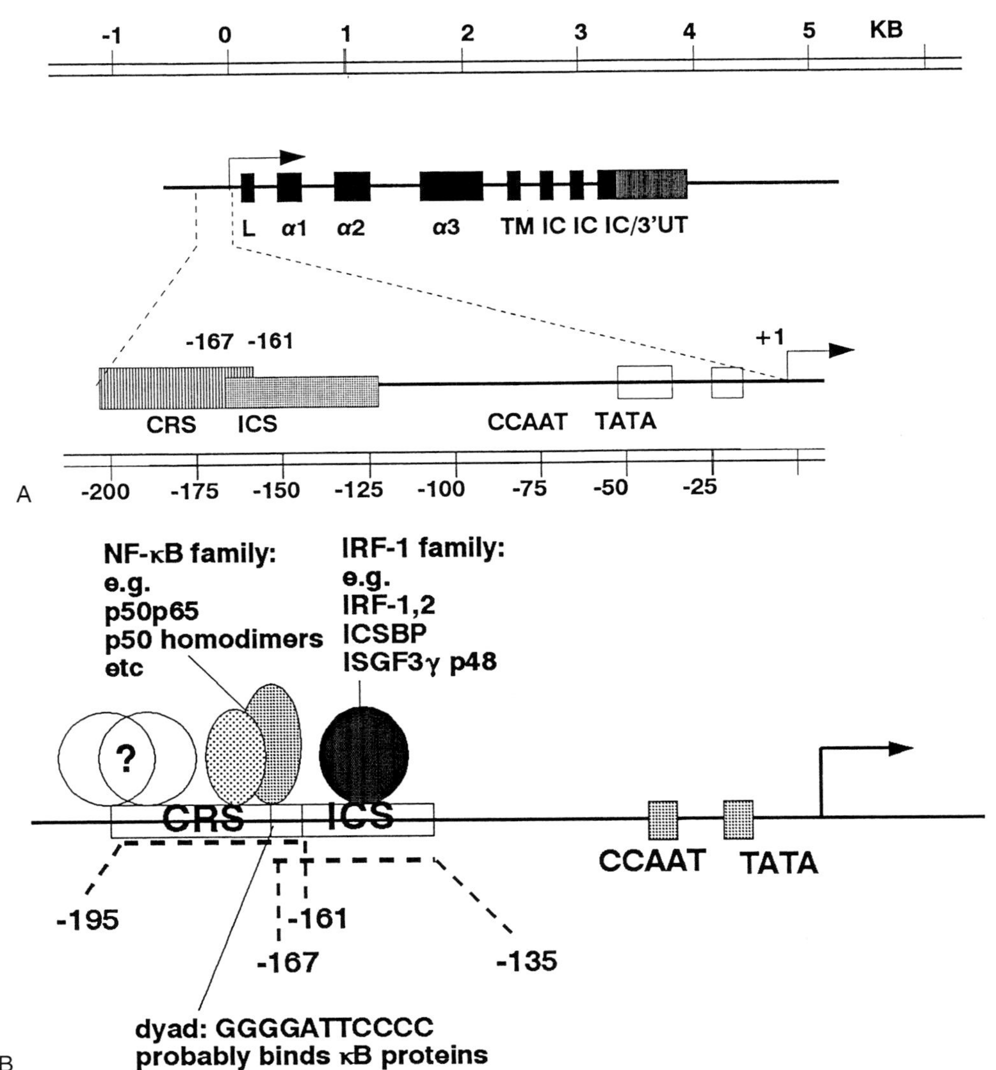

FIG. 13. The class I gene and the class I promoter. **A:** A typical class I gene, the mouse K^b gene. **B:** The class I promoter showing the CRS and the ICS.

To date no single knockout of the gene for a Rel/NF-κB family member has eliminated class I expression, but class I expression in the existing knockouts has not been extensively studied.

Zinc Finger Proteins

MBP-1 and MBP-2 belong to a family of zinc finger proteins that bind to the CRS, specifically to the region I or II sequences. A peptide of MBP-1 protein bound to the GGA trinucleotide of the dyad sequence (187,188). The relationship of MBP-1 and MBP-2 to class I expression in various tissues in vivo is not known.

H-2RIIBP (PXRβ) (189–191) binds to region II of the CRS. H-2RIIBP is a DNA binding protein expressed in many tissues but not correlated with MHC expression. It resembles members of the steroid hormone receptor family, but its ligand is unknown. It is conceivable that by heterodimerization with other proteins, H-2RIIBP participates in hormonal regulation of class I genes (retinoic acid, thyroid hormones, estrogen). Retinoic acid induction of class I involves the NF-kB p50–p65 dimers and retinoic acid receptors (192).

The ICS and the Molecular Basis of Cytokine-Induced Expression (Fig. 14)

Changes in class I genes in response to cytokines occur only after a delay, probably due to a requirement for an intermediate protein such as the members of the IRF family: IRF-1, IRF-2, ICSBP, p48 ISGF3, and possibly others. The possible candidates for IFN-γ–induced positive regulation of class I include IRF-1 (193) and ISGF3 (p48), perhaps in the STAT complex, such as ISGF3 (α

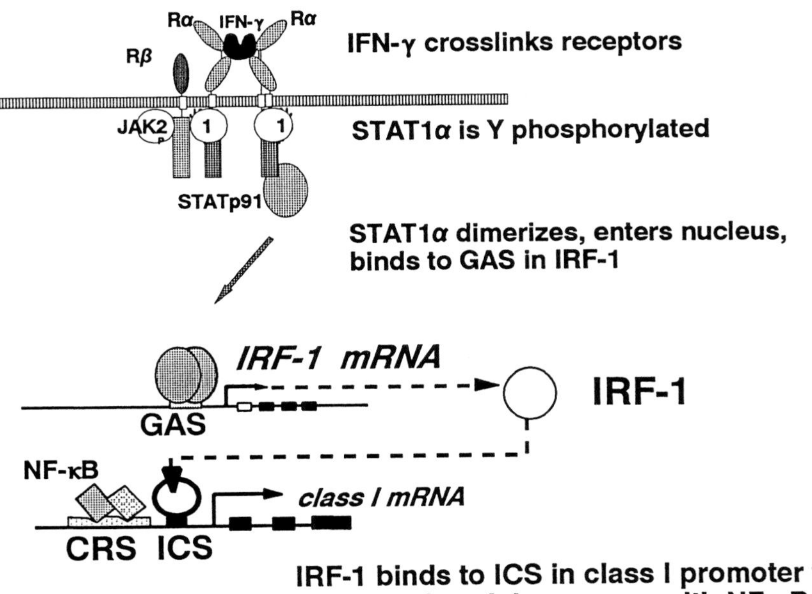

FIG. 14. A hypothesis for how IFN-γ activates class I transcription. In this model, IFN-γ activates STAT1α, which activates IRF-1. IRF-1 then synergizes with preexisting NF-κB and other proteins associated with the CRS to activate transcription.

plus γ). We recently found that IRF-1 knockout mice have defects in both basal and particularly in IFN-γ–induced expression of class I in kidney. Thus, at least IRF-1 has an obligatory role in class I regulation, probably by engaging the ICS and synergizing with κB family members bound to the CRS (194). On the other hand, IRF-1 also may act indirectly, perhaps through other IRF family members or by increasing cytokine production.

TNF-α induces class I relatively well in culture but is a weak inducer in vivo when administered systemically. However, TNF-α potentiates the class I induction by IFN-γ. TNF-α probably acts by altering the Rel/κB proteins, which act on the CRS, but may also induce IRF-1.

Negative Control of MHC Class I Expression

The κB p50 homodimers may act as a repressor at the CRS (195), possibly by preventing the p50–p65 from engaging the CRS. Both IRF-2 and ICSBP could be negative regulators of induced expression at the ICS. IRF-2 in its usual role is a negative regulator (196,197) and has a role in cell cycle regulation by affecting the expression of histone genes (198). ICSBP is principally expressed in lymphoid cells and is a negative regulator of the ICS in lymphoid cells (118,119). Perhaps ICSBP explains why class I expression in lymphoid cells is much less inducible than nonlymphoid cells such as renal tubular epithelium. Class I expression may be negatively regulated by c-jun (199) and human immunodeficiency virus proteins (200).

Some cells can express a molecule that prevents IFN-γ activation of class I genes. This may operate in some tumor cells. A phenomenon called transcriptional knockout has been demonstrated in some tumor cells, i.e., mutations that cause negative regulators to displace positive regulators from the class I promoter.

Other Sites of Class I Regulation

There is little evidence in normal cells for individuality in class I A or B expression. Much work has been done on the effect of polymorphisms in the promoters of class I or II MHC genes, but whether these variations significantly affect MHC expression in kidney or elsewhere is simply not known, and correlations with diseases or graft rejection have not been established.

Summary of Class I Expression

The characteristic patterns of basal and induced class I expression reflect regulatory proteins interacting with the CRS and ICS. The key regulators are Rel/NF-κB members binding to the CRS sites, and IRF-1 binding to the

ICS site. The synergy between TNF and IFN-γ reflects interaction between Rel/NF-κB members at the CRS and IRF-1 at the ICS. The lack of inborn errors, cell lines, or knockout mice that have no class I expression suggest that class I has no unique proteins corresponding to the RFX and CIITA factors for class II. These may reflect considerable redundancy in the proteins that occupy the CRS. More probably, the proteins vital to class I regulation may be vital to other genes, compatible with the ubiquitous nature of class I expression. On the other hand, the ICS is principally positively regulated by IRF-1.

HOW THE MHC PRODUCTS ARE REGULATED IN INFLAMMATORY RESPONSES IN VIVO: A WORKING MODEL OF MHC REGULATION IN KIDNEY

Our laboratory has studied the regulation of MHC expression in vivo in mice (3,201) in normals, in disease and injury states, and in the response to administration of drugs and recombinant cytokines. We present here a hypothesis to explain MHC regulation in the mouse kidney, including observations not yet published. We then extrapolate these findings to the human kidney.

There are three naturally occurring states of MHC expression: basal, systemically induced by IFN-γ, and locally induced by the injury response. (There may be a fourth state, in which only class I expression is induced due to IFN-α/β expression.) We have used GKO mice, IFN-γRα knockout mice (GRKO), and IRF-1 knockout mice to characterize these states. The comparison of normal BALB/c mice to mice treated with anti–IFN-γ and to GKO mice is shown in Fig. 15. All spontaneously occurring MHC expression in kidney corresponds to the following three states.

Basal expression is represented in the kidney of the healthy young adult mouse, free of pathogens. Class I is predominantly expressed on arterial endothelium, with weak expression in the glomerular and peritubular capillary endothelium and virtually none in the tubule epithelium. Class I is part constitutive but part induced by basal IFN-γ production, probably through transcription factor IRF-1: arterial class I staining, and about half of the total class I in the kidney, is lost in mice lacking either IFN-γ, IFN-γRα, or IRF-1. Basal class I expression is resistant to whole-body irradiation and CyA treatment and is normal in germ-free mice. Class II is seen only in IDC. Class II expression declines rapidly after lethal irradiation but is normal in germ-free mice and is resistant to CyA. Class II in renal IDC does not require IFN-γ, IFN-γRα, or IRF-1. Basal class II expression in IDC in the kidney is probably induced, but not by IFN-γ. Stimuli from the extracellular matrix components may be involved, possibly through integrin receptors. Collagen and GM-CSF induces the differentiation of IDC-like cells in culture (202), but their role in vivo is unknown.

Systemically induced expression is represented in the individual releasing IFN-γ and other cytokines systemically due to immune responses, severe local inflammation, or infectious agents, or in mice given IFN-γ. Several in vivo responses induce systemic MHC expression: acute T-cell responses to antigen (oxazalone skin painting), GVHD, allograft rejection, and low-dose streptozotocin. All induce IFN-γ production and massive MHC class I and II expression in the kidney that is abolished by

MHC expression in mouse kidney: anti IFN-γ Mab R46A2 versus GKO

stimulus	*class*	*pattern of expression* *control*	*anti IFN-γ*	*GKO*
basal	**class I**	**+(endo)**	**+(endo)**	**↓↓(endo)**
	class II	**+(IDC)**	**+(IDC)**	**+(IDC)**
allogeneic stimulus	**class I**	**++++**	**+(endo)**	**↓↓(endo)**
	class II	**++++**	**+(IDC)**	**+(IDC)**
LPS	**class I**	**++++**	**+(endo)**	**↓↓(endo)**
	class II	**++++**	**+(IDC)**	**+(IDC)**
Poly IC	**class I**	**+++**	**+++**	**ND**
	class II	**+(IDC)**	**+(IDC)**	**ND**
ischemic injury	**class I**	**++(ep)**	**++(ep)**	**++(ep)**
	class II	**++(ep/IDC)**	**++(ep/DC)**	**++(ep/IDC)**

IDC = interstitial dendritic cells; endo = arterial endothelial cells
ep = epithelium LPS = lipopolysaccaride ND = not yet done

FIG. 15. Experimental results obtained when mouse kidney is examined after a variety of stimuli, in control mice and GKO mice (IFN-γ knockout). In control mice, the stimuli induce MHC expression. Ischemic injury still induces class I and II in anti-IFN-γ–treated mice. In GKO mice, class I is never expressed on arterial endothelium, and there is no induction of class I or II with the stimuli used, except for induction in ischemic injury. Allogeneic stimulus and LPS induce IFN-γ, which induces class I and II; poly IC induces IFN-α/β, which induces only class I. Ischemic injury induces class I and II at least partially through IFN-γ–independent mechanisms.

anti–IFN-γ or CyA and is absent in nude mice. The acute response to bacterial lipopolysaccharide increases IFN-γ production and MHC expression. MHC expression is abolished by anti–IFN-γ or CyA but is normal or increased in T cell–deficient nude mice. Class I is induced in all cells; class II is induced largely in proximal tubules and weakly in arterial endothelium.

The systemic increase of class I and II in inflammatory diseases is lost or greatly reduced in knockout mice lacking IFN-γ, IFN-γRα, or transcription factor IRF-1. Inflammation induces a small increase (10% of normal) in class I expression in such mice, indicating that another pathway is operating, e.g., TNF-α or IFN-α/β on class I expression. Thus, in vivo in models of inflammatory disease and infectious states, systemic MHC induction is an exclusive property of IFN-γ, produced via signals from the CyA sensitive Ca^{2+}–calcineurin pathway and operating via IFN-γ, IFN-γRα, and IRF-1. Thus, systemic MHC induction is uniquely dependent on calcineurin/IFN-γ/IFN-γRα/IRF-1.

Other cytokines probably play a role in synergy or antagonism, e.g., TNF-α, IFN-α/β. Although all of the above systemic responses are accompanied by production of many cytokines, we have found no evidence that IFN-α/β, GM-CSF, or TNF-α plays a significant role in systemic MHC induction in our model responses in vivo when IFN-γ is eliminated, and no cytokine but IFN-γ reproduces the systemic MHC class I and II induction when injected in vivo. Administration of rIFN-α or poly I/C, an artificial inducer of IFN-α/β, induces class I in kidney (203). Perhaps IFN-α/β proteins have a synergistic role, especially in class I expression. TNF-α induces class I weakly, but not class II; GM-CSF injections and IL-10 injections did nothing to MHC expression in our experiments to date.

In the local injury response, MHC expression is increased in models of renal injury (Fig. 16). In renal ischemic injury, IFN-γ and other cytokines, as well as MHC class I and II, are induced, and class II–positive interstitial cells increase, probably reflecting a complex program that we call the injury response (42,44,204,205). Many types of injury attract inflammatory cells, and the class II–positive interstitial cells that accumulate after day 5 in the injured kidney are not unexpected; the dendritic cell is a sentinel for injury (22). However, the induction of class I and II expression in the epithelium was surprising. After describing these events in renal ischemia, we have since found that it is a general characteristic of the injured kidney; a similar pattern of events follows toxins gentamycin and mercuric chloride (206,207). The MHC response to injury is not immune but is partially inhibited by CyA and anti–IFN-γ. The presence of this response in the GKO mice indicates that some injury response is independent of the calcineurin/IFN-γ/IFN-γRα system and probably is T cell independent. It is not clear how IRF-1 is involved in the injury response.

Thus, injury triggers a relatively stereotyped response in the kidney, causing increased MHC expression. The response is confined to the injured kidney and is mainly in sites of epithelial injury, and thus is not a systemic effect of IFN-γ. The injury response reflects both local IFN-γ production and a non–IFN-γ factor. We hypothesize that the non–IFN-γ factor may be local proteins associated with the repair process, signalling through membrane receptors, possibly integrin-like, in the injured cells

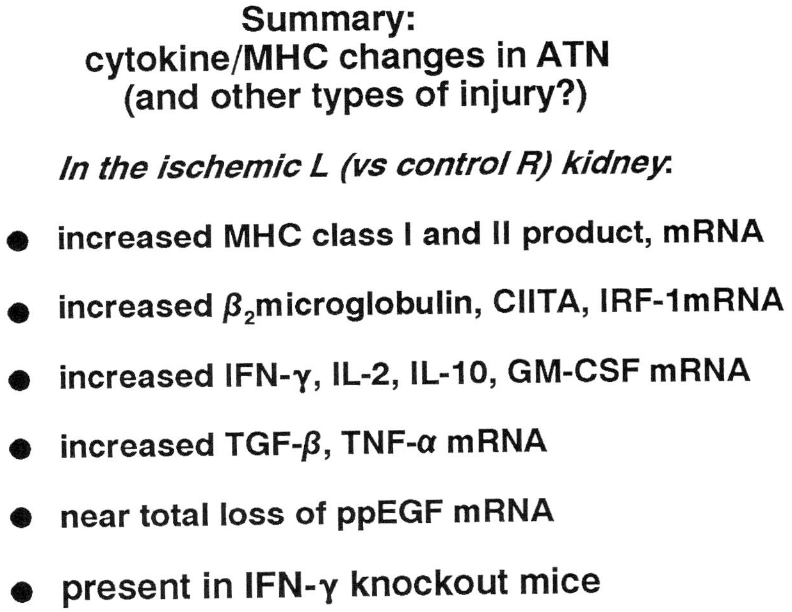

Summary:
cytokine/MHC changes in ATN
(and other types of injury?)

In the ischemic L (vs control R) kidney:

- **increased MHC class I and II product, mRNA**
- **increased $\beta_2$microglobulin, CIITA, IRF-1mRNA**
- **increased IFN-γ, IL-2, IL-10, GM-CSF mRNA**
- **increased TGF-β, TNF-α mRNA**
- **near total loss of ppEGF mRNA**
- **present in IFN-γ knockout mice**

FIG. 16. Summary of the inflammatory changes that occur in mice with unilateral ATN, compared with the contralateral control kidney. In general, these changes occur between days 3 and 5 and decay over the next several weeks. Prepro epidermal growth factor mRNA (ppEGF) is a valuable marker for epithelial integrity and is lost after ischemic ATN.

to induce both class I and class II expression. One or more other cytokine(s) may affect class I or II expression in injury (although no cytokine in vivo has been shown to induce class II except IFN-γ.

In studying renal IDC, we found that some renal interstitial cells express a truncated mRNA of TCRα, which is probably a transcript from an unrearranged TCRα gene from an occult promoter that is activated in the renal interstitium. This mRNA is not expressed in marrow, lymphoid tissues, or other organs (except to some extent in the brain). This unique observation indicates that some marrow-derived IDCs can express mRNAs when resident in kidney that they do not express elsewhere (208,209). It is unlikely that this unusual transcript results in an expressed protein.

Extrapolation to Human Renal MHC Expression

Humans differ from mice in having higher basal class I and II expression in the kidney, as assessed by immunostaining. Unlike mice, humans have class II on their endothelial cells; some humans have class II in their epithelial cells, and human renal epithelial cells are generally class I positive. We have extrapolated our results to humans as follows (Figs. 17 and 18).

Basal class I and II expression in endothelial cells is induced by IFN-γ and reflects the calcineurin/IFN-γ/IFN-γRα/IRF-1 pathway. All expression of MHC in normal endothelial cells may be IFN-γ/IFN-γRα/IRF-1 dependent. (It is possible that an endothelial injury response can induce class I and II in injured endothelium via non–IFN-γ mechanisms.)

Systemic induction of MHC class I and class II is completely dependent on IFN-γ, whether in the response to allogeneic stimulation, LPS, or severe local inflammation or immune responses. The calcineurin/IFN-γ/IFN-γRα/IRF-1 pathway mediates this response. TNF-α and possibly other cytokines potentiate but do not replace IFN-γ. Systemic MHC induction represents a system for activating antigen presentation in the face of the threat of systemic spread of infection. The kidney is very sensitive to systemic class I and II induction.

Local renal injury of many kinds induces MHC class I and II and cytokine expression and a class II–positive interstitial cell infiltrate. These events are partly IFN-γ dependent and partly independent and reflect an attempt to control infection through increased antigen presentation during periods of renal injury.

The increased class I and class II expression in renal transplants or inflammatory disease reflects a combination of basal, systemic IFN-γ induction and local injury response. The local injury response after cadaver renal transplantation may account for the association between poor initial renal function, subsequent acute rejection, and graft loss (210). Furthermore, an acute rejection episode is an episode of renal injury, in turn inducing an injury response that increases the probability of continuing immune activity. The injury response may represent a mechanism perpetuating renal inflammation and injury and thus a mechanism of chronicity and progression in renal disease. In renal transplants this may translate into chronic rejection. In primary renal disease it may represent a disordered repair process that can itself induce injury or interfere with the normal resolution of injury. The progression in the remnant kidney models thus could be based on inflammatory mechanisms as well as abnormal hemodynamics and abnormal growth and repair.

Biologic Significance of Quantitative Variation in MHC Expression

The quantity of MHC expressed is potentially relevant to all functions of the MHC: presentation of peptides for TCR recognition, superantigen presentation by class II to TCRs, CD4 and CD8 coreceptor functions, and class I recognition by NK receptors. In a qualitative sense, MHC expression is necessary for immune recognition of cells, and transfection of MHC genes into nonimmunogenic cells can induce immunogenicity (211). If T-cell triggering reflects the product of the amount of antigen added (peptide) and the amount of MHC expressed to present the antigen, then high MHC expression may be a necessary condition (but is not sufficient) for T-cell recognition of limiting amounts of peptide.

Several observations support the view that in vitro and in vivo MHC expression has an influence on T-cell recognition. It is likely that a threshold level of MHC expression is needed for T-cell recognition. Thus, the quantity of MHC proteins must exceed the threshold. It is also possible that the quantity of MHC proteins expressed above the threshold continues to influence the probability of triggering TCRs, NK receptors, CD4, and CD8 over a considerable range. For example, MHC expression quantitatively affects TCR triggering over a range of concentrations (24,212–214), possibly indicating that the number of surface–TCR–ligand complex interactions is limiting for TCR triggering (215,216). Signalling through the TCR is regulated by the number of ligand–receptor complexes (215). Cells expressing MHC class I molecules with only a single type of peptide in high concentrations (i.e., with high concentrations of a single ligand) are highly immunogenic. In TCR transgenic mice, the efficiency of selection of the transgenic receptor is enhanced in mice that express higher levels of the relevant MHC molecule (217). Low class I expression in neurons correlates with the reduced ability to clear viral infections in neurons, especially in vivo (218). The limiting amount of MHC–peptide to trigger TCRs may explain the need for CD4 and CD8 coreceptors. The requirement for CD8 in T-cell recognition of class I is related to determinant den-

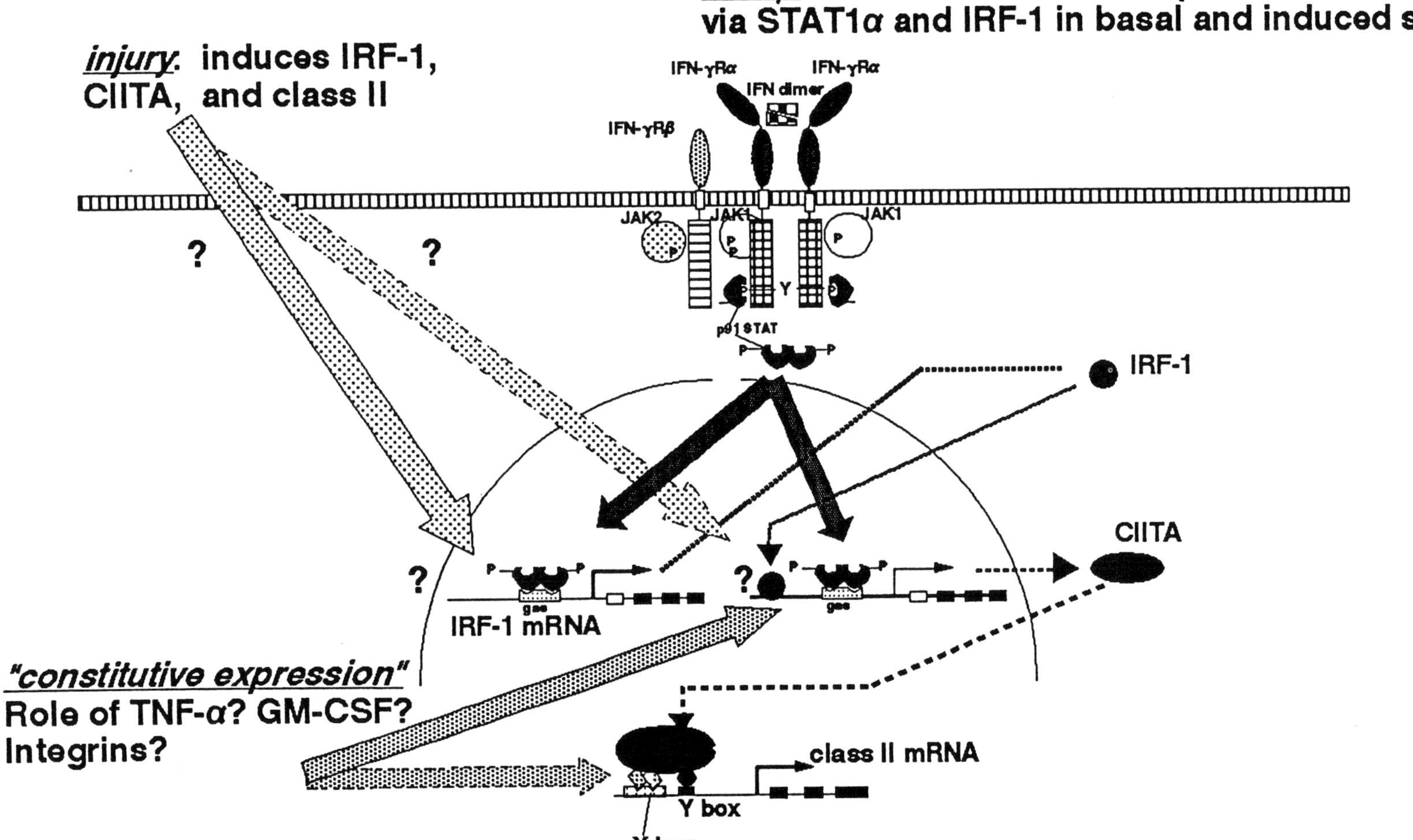

FIG. 17. A model for the three main influences on class II expression: IFN-τ induction, tissue injury, and the mechanisms regulating basal or "constitutive" class II expression, particularly in B cells and IDCs. Which stimuli act exclusively through CIITA, and which stimuli act directly on the promoter, is not yet clear. The role of IRF-1 in renal MHC expression in injury is also not clear.

Three influences on class I expression

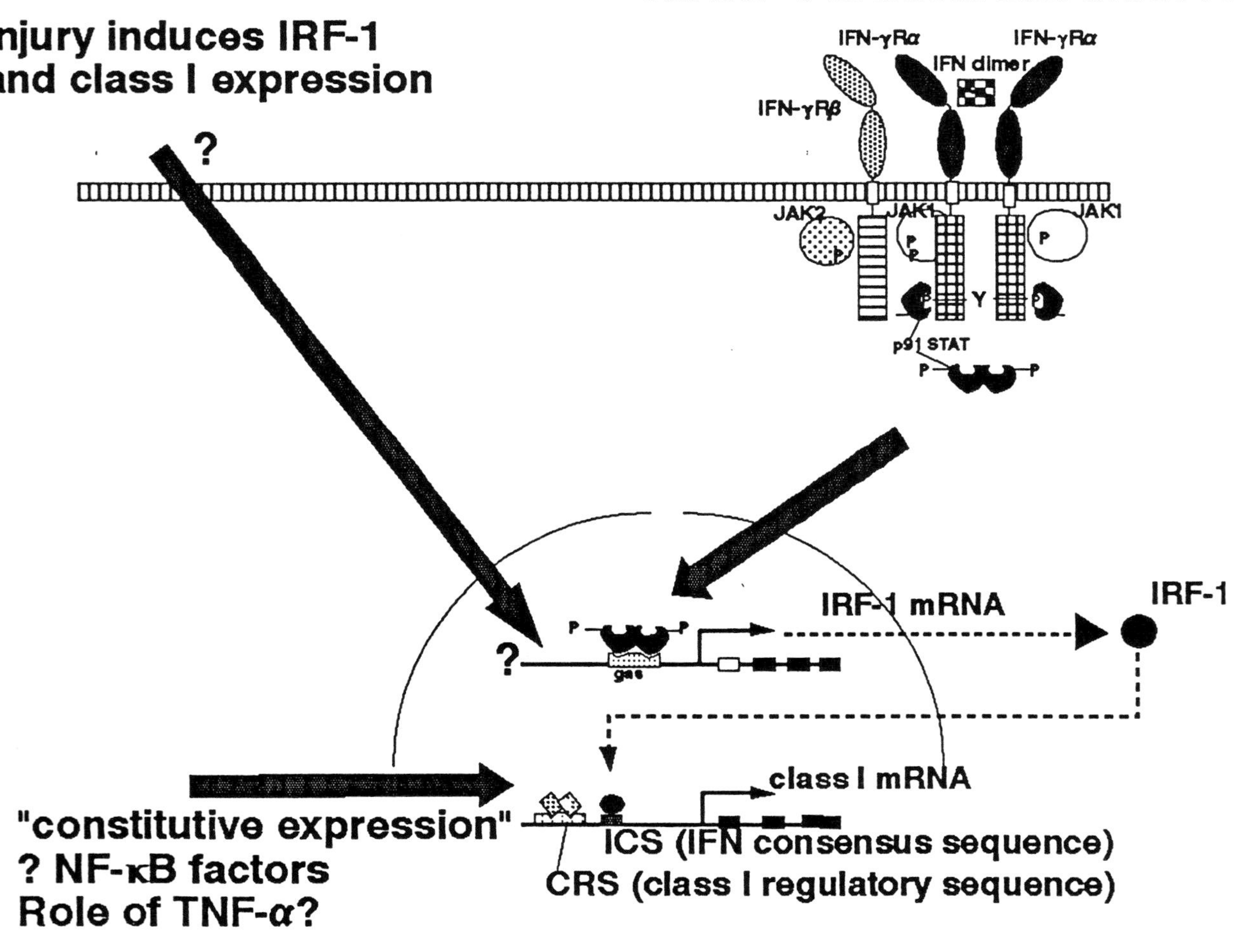

FIG. 18. A hypothesis for the three mechanisms changing class I expression: IFN-τ, and presumably IFN-α/β, act in a parallel fashion (not shown); tissue injury; and the factors regulating basal, IFN-τ–independent expression.

sity: high determinant density reduces the dependency on CD8. Thus, under physiologic conditions where determinant density is limiting, most cytotoxic T-lymphocytes require CD8 (219). But increased signal strength may at some point produce tolerance or anergy: the addition of CD8 recognition to TCR recognition may convert positive to negative selection. Increased signalling of many types of receptors eventually has a negative effect rather than positive, and MHC effects should be expected to have this characteristic (220).

In transplant models, the quantity of MHC expression affects the probability of rejection. The interactions with TCR, CD4/CD8, and NK receptors are potentially affected by the quantity of MHC expressed, and the donor MHC proteins synthesized can be degraded and presented in host MHC molecules on antigen-presenting cells. Both a threshold effect for MHC expression and an additional effect of increased MHC expression above this basal amount may operate. In skin grafting from MHC class I transgenic mice, the level of class I transgene expression correlates with the rate of rejection (221). The reduced level of MHC expression in tissues from immature mice may explain the reduced immunogenicity of tissues from fetal mice (222). The fact that IFN-α can induce acute rejection of renal transplants may be attributable to class I MHC antigen induction (223), and the immunosuppressive effect of anti IFN-γ antibodies in transplantation suggests that IFN-γ–induced activation of the MHC and antigen presentation system contributes to the process of rejection. The quantity of donor and host MHC proteins expressed could affect both the direct and indirect presentation mechanisms (224). Some implications of MHC regulation are listed in Fig. 19.

Observations in tumors suggest that MHC expression affects tumor immunogenicity. Many tumors have reduced MHC expression (225), and oncogenic viruses often suppress MHC expression, e.g., oncogenic adenoviruses. Thus, MHC suppression may permit oncogenic agents to avoid or manipulate immune surveillance. Tumors with low levels of class I alloantigen have a reduced ability to engender immune responses despite remaining susceptible to CTLs (226), conforming to the general rule that triggering the primary response is more demanding than triggering of previously primed cells. Responses to immunotherapy in tumors may correlate with inducibility of MHC antigens: renal cell carcinomas that express high concentrations of MHC class I and II in response to IFNs are more susceptible to growth inhibition by IFNs in nude mice (222).

High MHC expression may predispose toward autoimmunity in some circumstances. Class II induction may be a primary event triggering some forms of autoimmunity. Thyroid autoimmunity has been extensively studied in this regard. The class II genes in thyroid epithelial cells from patients with Grave's disease are hyperinducible by IFN-γ (227). Renal tubule epithelial cells expressing class II can present antigen (228), but class II expression does not automatically trigger autoimmunity (229). Class II induction frequently accompanies autoimmunity (230), and IFN-γ accelerates autoimmune systemic lupus erythematosis (SLE), whereas anti–IFN-γ and CyA inhibit SLE development in mice. Deletion of class II prevents autoimmune SLE in the MRL/1pr mice (231). In rats bearing human B27 class I transgenes, the quantitative level of B27 expression in the transgenics correlates with the development of a spontaneous inflammatory disease (232). Both autoimmune diabetes and autoimmune hepatitis can be induced by expressing IFN-γ in the β cell or the hepatocyte, respectively (233,234). The strong evidence that IFN-γ expression can trigger autoimmunity is suggestive that this effect is mediated through MHC expression, but other mechanisms also could be operating.

However, MHC expression is only one factor in immunogenicity. High levels of renal MHC expression in mice frequently are seen in the absence of pathology in the kidneys and reflect systemic release of IFN-γ (32). In states of perceived threat of systemic infection, induction of MHC expression represents a general but transient activation of antigen presentation for immunologic surveillance and is essentially a benign event, like putting on lights to detect possible intruders. In some transplant models, MHC induction occurs but rejection does not (235,236). Thyroid allografts cultured to reduce antigen-presenting cells and then treated with IFN-γ to induce high levels of MHC expression were not rendered more immunogenic, indicating that loss of antigen-presenting cells cannot be overcome by IFN-γ alone (237). In renal epithelial cells, costimulator B7 expression, not class II expression, correlates with tubule cells stimulating T cells. Thus, class II by itself does not engender T-cell recognition without costimulation (238), perhaps as a safeguard against autoimmunity. MHC expression in the kidney may influence the outcomes of infections, the risk of autoimmunity, and the rejection of transplants. Class I and II overexpression generally favors immunogenicity but does not invariably lead to immune responses. High MHC expression may be either immunogenic or tolerogenic, dependent on other influences: high doses of any ligand will sometimes lead to receptor paralysis. Perhaps the current interpretation of the significance of MHC regulation is that upregulated

Implications of MHC class I and II regulation for transplantation

- ***antigen presentation:***
  direct:
  ✓ ***level of intact donor MHC available***
  ✓ ***level of donor MHC peptide available***
  indirect:
  ✓ ***level of host MHC available to bind donor peptide***
  ✓ ***donor MHC antigen for B cell antibody response***
- ***correlation with induction of other proteins in adhesion and antigen presentation***
- ***susceptibility as targets of CTL and antibody***

FIG. 19. A table showing the potential implications of MHC regulation in renal transplantation.

MHC expression is necessary but not sufficient for T-cell activation. Whether activation, tolerance, or other outcomes follow depends on the other influences operating on the immune system, such as costimulation. Local injury and infiltration by professional antigen-presenting cells such as IDCs may greatly increase the chances that an immune response will follow.

Acknowledgment

This research is supported by grants from the Alberta Heritage Foundation for Medical Research, the Kidney Foundation of Canada, the Medical Research Council of Canada (Operating Grant MT5739), the Muttart Foundation Endowment, the Royal Canadian Legion Kidney Endowment, and Sandoz Canada. I thank P. Publicover for secretarial assistance.

REFERENCES

1. Wadgymar A, Urmson J, Baumal R, Halloran PF. Changes in Ia expression in mouse kidney during acute graft-vs-host disease. *J Immunol* 1984;132:1826–1832.
2. Hall BM, Bishop GA, Duggin GG, Horvath JS, Philips J, Tiller DJ. Increased expression of HLA-DR antigens on renal tubular cells in renal transplants: relevance to the rejection response. *Lancet* 1984;2: 247–251.
3. Halloran PF, Madrenas J. Regulation of MHC transcription. Transplantation overview. *Transplantation* 1990;50:725–738.
4. Guardiola J, Maffei A. Control of MHC class II gene expression in autoimmune, infectious, and neoplastic diseases. *Crit Rev Immunol* 1993;13:247–268.
5. Benoist C, Mathis D. Regulation of major histocompatibility complex class II genes: X, Y and other letters of the alphabet. *Annu Rev Immunol* 1990;8:681–715.
6. Glimcher LH, Kara CJ. Sequences and factors: a guide to MHC class-II transcription. *Annu Rev Immunol* 1992;10:13–49.
7. Ting JPY, Baldwin AS Jr. Regulation of MHC gene expression. *Curr Opin Immunol* 1993;5:8–16.
8. Fields BA, Ober B, Malchiodi EL, et al. Crystal structure of the Vα domain of a T cell antigen receptor. *Science* 1995;270:1821–1824.
9. Held W, Roland J, Raulet DH. Allelic exclusion of Ly49-family genes encoding class I MHC-specific receptors on NK cells. *Nature* 1995;376:355
10. Kane KP. Ly-49 mediates EL4 lymphoma adhesion to isolated class I major histocompatibility complex molecules. *J Exp Med* 1994;179: 1011–1015.
11. Leibson PJ. MHC-recognizing receptors: they're not just for T cells anymore. *Immunity* 1995;3:5–8.
12. Raulet DH, Held W. Natural killer cell receptors: the offs and ons of NK cell recognition. *Cell* 1995;82:697–700.
13. Zijlstra M, Bix M, Simister NE, Loring JM, Raulet DH, Jaenisch R. 2-Microglobulin deficient mice lack CD4-8+ cytolytic T cells. *Nature* 1990;344:742–746.
14. Driscoll J, Brown MG, Finley D, Monaco JJ. MHC-linked LMP gene products specifically alter peptidase activities of the proteasome. *Nature* 1993;365:262–264.
15. Germain RN. MHC-dependent antigen processing and peptide presentation: providing ligands for T lymphocyte activation. *Cell* 76: 287–299.
16. Romagnoli P, Germain RN. The CLIP region of invariant chain plays a critical role in regulating major histocompatibility complex class II folding, transport, and peptide occupancy. *J Exp Med* 1994;180: 1107–1113.
17. Morris P, Shaman J, Attaya M, et al. An essential role for HLA-DM in antigen presentation by class II major histocompatibility molecules. *Nature* 1994;368:551–554.
18. Denzin LK, Cresswell P. HLA-DM induces CLIP dissociation from MHC class II alpha/beta dimers and facilitates peptide loading. *Cell* 1995;82:155–
19. Roche PA. HLA-DM: an in vivo facilitator of MHC class II peptide loading. *Immunity* 1995;3:259–262.
20. Stingl G, Bergstresser PR. Dendritic cells: a major story unfolds. *Immunol Today* 1995;16:330–333.
21. Steinman RM, Swanson J. The endocytic activity of dendritic cells. *J Exp Med* 1995;182:283–288.
22. Ibrahim MAA, Chain BM, Katz DR. The injured cell: the role of the dendritic cell system as a sentinel receptor pathway. *Immunol Today* 1995;16:181.
23. Wucherpfennig KW, Strominger JL. Selective binding of self peptides to disease-associated major histocompatibility complex (MHC) molecules: a mechanism for MHC-linked susceptibility to human autoimmune diseases. *J Exp Med* 1995;181:1597–1601.
24. Matis LA, Glimcher LH, Paul WE, Schwartz RH. Magnitude of response of histocompatibility-restricted T-cell clones is a function of the product of the concentrations of antigen and Ia molecules. *Proc Natl Acad Sci U S A* 1983;80:6019–6023.
25. Jephthah-Ochola J, Urmson J, Farkas S, Halloran PF. Regulation of MHC in vivo. Bacterial lipopolysaccharide induces class I and II MHC products in mouse tissues by a T cell independent, cyclosporine sensitive mechanism. *J Immunol* 1988;141:792–800.
26. Halloran PF, Urmson J, Farkas S, et al. Effects of cyclosporine on systemic MHC expression. Evidence that non T cells produce gamma interferon in vivo and are inhibitable by cyclosporine A. *Transplantation* 1988;46:68S–72S.
27. Priestley CA, Dalchau R, Sawyer GJ, Fabre JW. A detailed analysis of the potential of water-soluble classical class I MHC molecules for the suppression of kidney allograft rejection and in vitro cytotoxic T cell responses. *Transplantation* 1989;48:1031–1038.
28. Abastado J-P, Lone Y-C, Casrouge A, Boulot G, Kourilsky P. Dimerization of soluble major histocompatibility complex–peptide complexes is sufficient for activation of T cell hybridoma and induction of unresponsiveness. *J Exp Med* 1995;182:439–447.
29. Hart DNJ, Fuggle SV, Williams KA, Fabre JW, Ting A, Morris PJ. Localization of HLA-ABC and DR antigens in human kidney. *Transplantation* 1981;31:428–433.
30. Daar AS, Fuggle SV, Fabre JW, Ting A, Morris PJ. The detailed distribution of HLA-A,B,C antigens in normal human kidney. *Transplantation* 1984;38:287–292.
31. Halloran PF, Jephthah-Ochola J, Urmson J, Farkas S. Sytemic immunologic stimuli increase class I and II antigen expression in mouse kidney. *J Immunol* 1985;135:1053–1060.
32. Halloran PF, Autenried P, Ramassar V, Urmson J, Cockfield S. Local T cell responses induce widespread MHC expression. Evidence that IFN-γ induces its own expression in remote sites. *J Immunol* 1992; 148:3837–3846.
33. Hart DN, Fabre JW. Endogenously produced Ia antigens within cells of convoluted tubules of rat kidney. *J Immunol* 1981;126:2109–2113.
34. Daar AS, Fuggle SV, Fabre JW, Ting A, Morris PJ. The detailed distribution of MHC class II antigens in normal human kidney. *Transplantation* 1984;38:293–298.
35. Goes N, Sims T, Urmson J, Vincent D, Ramassar V, Halloran PF. Disturbed MHC regulation in the interferon-γ knockout mouse. *J Immunol* 1995;155:4559–4566.
36. Hart DNJ, Fabre JW. Demonstration and characterization of Ia-positive dendritic cells in the interstitial connective tissues of rat heart and other tissues, but not brain. *J Exp Med* 1981;154:347.
37. Cockfield SM, Ramassar V, Noujaim J, van der Meide PH, Halloran PF. Regulation of IFN-γ expression in vivo. IFN-γ up-regulates expression of its mRNA in normal and lipopolysaccharide-stimulated mice. *J Immunol* 1993;150:717–725.
38. Collins T, Korman AJ, Wake CT, et al. Immune interferon activates multiple class II histocompatibility complex genes and the associated invariant chain gene in human endothelial cells and dermal fibroblasts. *Proc Natl Acad Sci U S A* 1984;81:4917–4921.
39. Skoskiewicz MJ, Colvin RB, Schneeberger EE, Russell PS. Widespread and selective induction of major histocompatibility complex-determined antigens in vivo by interferon. *J Exp Med* 1985;162: 1646–1664.
40. Benson EM, Colvin RB, Russell PS. Induction of Ia antigens in murine renal transplants. *J Immunol* 1985;135:7–9.

41. Skoskiewicz M, Colvin RB, Schneeberger EE, Russell PS. Widespread and selective induction of major histocompatibility complex–determined antigens in vivo by interferon. *J Exp Med* 1985;162:1645–1664.
42. Shoskes D, Parfrey NA, Halloran PF. Increased major histocompatibility complex antigen expression in unilateral ischemic acute tubular necrosis in the mouse. *Transplantation* 1990;49:201–207.
43. Goes N, Urmson J, Vincent D, Halloran PF. Acute renal injury in the interferon-γ knockout mouse: effect on cytokine gene expression. *Transplantation* 1996;60:1560–1564.
44. Goes N, Urmson J, Ramassar V, Halloran PF. Ischemic acute tubular necrosis induces an extensive local cytokine response: evidence for induction of interferon-γ, transforming growth factor-1, granulocyte-macrophage colony-stimulating factor, interleukin-2 and interleukin-10. *Transplantation* 1995;59:565–572.
45. Shackleton CR, Ettinger SL, McLoughlin MG, Scudamore CH, Miller RR, Keown PA. Effect of recovery from ischemic injury on class I and class II MHC antigen expression. *Transplantation* 1990; 49:641–644.
46. Barrett M, Milton AD, Barrett J, et al. Needle biopsy evaluation of class II major histocompatibility complex antigen expression for the differential diagnosis of cyclosporine nephrotoxicity from kidney graft rejection. *Transplantation* 1987;44:223–227.
47. Milton AD, Spencer SC, Fabre JW. Detailed analysis and demonstration of differences in the kinetics of class I and class II major histocompatibility complex antigens in rejecting cardiac and kidney allografts in the rat. *Transplantation* 1986;41:499–508.
48. Milton AD, Spencer SC, Fabre JW. The effects of cyclosporine on the induction of donor class I and class II MHC antigens in heart and kidney allografts in the rat. *Transplantation* 1986;42:337–347.
49. Milton AD, Fabre JW. Massive induction of donor type class I and class II major histocompatibility complex antigens in rejecting cardiac allografts in the rat. *J Exp Med* 1985;161:98–112.
50. Fuggle SV, McWhinnie DL, Morris PJ. Precise specificity of induced tubular HLA-class II antigens in renal allografts. *Transplantation* 1987;44:214–220.
51. Fuggle SV, McWhinnie DL, Chapman JR, Taylor HM, Morris PJ. Sequential analysis of HLA-class II antigen expression in human renal allografts. *Transplantation* 1986;42:144–150.
52. Ernst P, Smale ST. Combinatorial regulation of transcription I: general aspects of transcriptional control. *Immunity* 1995;2:311–319.
53. Adams CC, Workman JL. Nucleosome displacement in transcription. *Cell* 1993;72:305–308.
54. Greenblatt J. Transcription: riding high on the TATA box. *Nature* 1992;360:16–17.
55. Shull MM, Ormsby I, Kier AB, et al. Targeted disruption of the mouse transforming growth factor-1 gene results in multifocal inflammatory disease. *Nature* 1992;359:693–699.
56. Yamashita S, Hisatake K, Kokubo T, et al. Transcription factor TFIIB sites important for interaction with promoter-bound TFIID. *Science* 1993;261:463–466.
57. Hisatake K, Roeder RG, Horikoshi M. Functional dissection of TFIIB domains required for TFIIB–TFIID–promoter complex formation and basal transcription activity. *Nature* 1993;363:744–747.
58. Nikolov DB, Chen H, Halay ED, et al. Crystal structure of a TFIIB–TBP–TATA–element ternary complex. *Nature* 1995;377:119–128.
59. Drapkin R, Reinberg D. The essential twist. *Nature* 1994;369:523–524.
60. Guzder SN, Sung P, Bailly V, Prakash L, Prakash S. RAD25 is a DNA helicase required for DNA repair and RNA polymerase II transcription. *Nature* 1994;369:578–581.
61. Hahn S. Structure(?) and function of acidic transcription activators. *Cell* 1993;72:481–483.
62. Hahn S. Efficiency in activation. *Nature* 1993;363:672–673.
63. Roberts SGE, Ha I, Maldonado E, Reinberg D, Green MR. Interaction between an acidic activator and transcription factor TFIIB is required for transcriptional activation. *Nature* 1993;363:741–744.
64. Tjian R, Maniatis T. Transcriptional activation: a complex puzzle with few easy pieces. *Cell* 1994;77:5–8.
65. Travers AA. The reprogramming of transcriptional competence. *Cell* 1992;69:573–575.
66. Seger R, Krebs EG. The MAPK signaling cascade. *FASEB J* 1995;9: 726–735.
67. Whitmarsh AJ, Shore P, Sharrocks AD, Davis RJ. Integration of MAP kinase signal transduction pathways at the serum response element. *Science* 1995;269:403–407.
68. O'Neill EM, Rebay I, Tijan R, Rubin GM. The activities of two Ets-related transcription factors required for *Drosophila* eye development are modulated by the Ras/MAPK pathway. *Cell* 1994;78:137–147.
69. Weinberg RA. The retinoblastoma protein and cell cycle control. *Cell* 1995;81:323–330.
70. Bassuk AG, Leiden JM. A direct physical association between ETS and AP-1 transcription factors in normal human T cells. *Immunity* 1995;3:223–237.
71. Finco TS, Baldwin AS. Mechanistic aspects of NF-κB regulation: the emerging role of phosphorylation and proteolysis. *Immunity* 1995;3: 263–272.
72. Sha WC, Liou H-C, Tuomanen EI, Baltimore D. Targeted disruption of the p50 subunit of NF-κB leads to mutlifocal defects in immune responses. *Cell* 1995;80:321–330.
73. Beg AA, Sha WC, Bronson RT, Ghosh S, Baltimore D. Embryonic lethality and liver degeneration in mice lacking the RelA component of NF-κB. *Nature* 1995;376:167
74. Weih F, Carrasco D, Durham SK, et al. Multiorgan inflammation and hematopoietic abnormalities in mice with a targeted disruption of RelB, a member of the NF-κB/Rel family. *Cell* 1995;80:331–340.
75. Scheinman RI, Cogswell PC, Lofquist AK, Baldwin AS Jr. Role of transcriptional activation of IκBα in mediation of immunosuppression by glucocorticoids. *Science* 1995;270:283–286.
76. Auphan N, Didonato JA, Rosette C, Helmberg A, Karin M. Immunosuppression by glucocorticoids: inhibition of NF-κB activity through induction of IκB synthesis. *Science* 1995;270:286–290.
77. Kopp E, Ghosh S. Inhibition of NF-κB by sodium salicylate and aspirin. *Science* 1994;265:956–959.
78. Tepper MA, Nadler SG, Esselstyn JM, Sterbenz KG. Deoxyspergualin inhibits κ light chain expression in 7OZ/3 pre-B cells by blocking lipopolysaccharide-induced NF-κB activation. *J Immunol* 1995;155: 2427–2436.
79. Halloran PF, Wadgymar A, Autenried P. Inhibition of MHC product induction may contribute to the immunosuppressive action of ciclosporin. *Prog Allergy* 1986;38:258–268.
80. Rao A. NF-ATp: a transcription factor required for the co-ordinate induction of several cytokine genes. *Immunol Today* 1994;15:274–280.
81. Northrop JP, Ullman KS, Crabtree GR. Characterization of the nuclear and cytoplasmic components of the lymphoid-specific nuclear factor of activated T cells (NF–AT) complex. *J Biol Chem* 1993;268: 2917–2923.
82. Rao A. NFATp, a cyclosplorin-sensitive transcription factor implicated in cytokine gene induction. *J Leukoc Biol* 1995;57:536–542.
83. Campbell PM, Pimm J, Ramassar V, Halloran PF. Identification of a calcium inducible, cyclosporine-sensitive element in the IFN-γ promoter that is a potential NFAT binding site. *Transplantation* 1996;61:933–939.
84. Schreiber RD, Farrar MA. The biology and biochemistry of IFN-γ and its receptor. *Gastroenterol Jpn* 1993;4:88–96.
85. Aguet M, Dembic Z, Merlin G. Molecular cloning and expression of the human interferon-γ receptor. *Cell* 1988;55:273–280.
86. Walter MR, Windsor WT, Nagabhushan TL, et al. Crystal structure of a complex between interferon-γ and its soluble high affinity receptor. *Nature* 1995;376:230–235.
87. Hemmi S, Böhni R, Stark G, Di Marco F, Aguet M. A novel member of the interferon receptor family complements functionality of the murine interferon receptor in human cells. *Cell* 1994;76:803–810.
88. Soh J, Donnelly RJ, Kotenko S, et al. Identification and sequence of an accessory factor required for activation of the human interferon receptor. *Cell* 1994;76:793–802.
89. Kalina U, Ozmen L, Di Padova K, Gentz R, Garotta G. The human gamma interferon receptor accessory factor encoded by chromosome 21 transduces the signal for the induction of 28,58-oligoadenylate-synthetase, resistance to virus cytopathic effect, and major histocompatibility complex class I antigens. *J Virol* 1993;67:1702–1706.
90. Colamonici OR, Domanski P. Identification of a novel subunit of the type I interferon receptor localized to human chromosome 21. *J Biol Chem* 1993;268:10895–10899.
91. Farrar MA, Schreiber RC. A point mutational analysis of the intracellular domain of the IFN receptor. *FASEB J* 1992;6:4519.
92. Pawson T. Protein modules and signalling networks. *Nature* 1995; 373:573–580.

93. Levin D, Constant S, Pasqualini T, Flavell R, Bottomly K. Role of dendritic cells in the priming of $CD4^+$ T lymphocytes to peptide antigen in vivo. *J Immunol* 1993;151:6742–6750.
94. Watling D, Guschin D, Müller M, et al. Complementation by the protein tyrosine kinase JAK2 of a mutant cell line defective in the interferon-γ signal transduction pathway. *Nature* 1993;366:166–170.
95. Silvennoinen O, Ihle JN, Schlessinger J, Levy DE. Interferon-induced nuclear signalling by Jak protein tyrosine kinases. *Nature* 1993;366: 583–585.
96. Sadowski HB, Shuai K, Darnell JE Jr, Gilman MZ. A common nuclear signal transduction pathway activated by growth factor and cytokine receptors. *Science* 1993;261:1739–1744.
97. Shuai K, Ziemiecki A, Wilks AF, et al. Polypeptide signalling to the nucleus through tyrosine phosphorylation of Jak and Stat proteins. *Nature* 1993;366:580–583.
98. Ihle JN, Witthuhn BA, Quelle FW, et al. Signaling by the cytokine receptor superfamily: JAKs and STATs. *TIBS* 1994;19:222–227.
99. Ivashkiv LB. Cytokines and STATs: how can signals achieve specificity? *Immunity* 1995;3:1–4.
100. Hou J, Schindler U, Henzel WJ, Ho TC, Brasseur M, McKnight SL. An interleukin-4–induced transcription factor: IL-4 Stat. *Science* 1994;265:1701–1706.
101. Darnell JE Jr, Kerr IM, Stark GR. Jak–STAT pathways and transcriptional activation in response to IFNs and other extracellular signaling proteins. *Science* 1994;264:1415–1421.
102. Barinaga M. Two major signaling pathways meet at MAP-kinase. *Science* 1995;269:1673.
103. David M, Petricoin E III, Benjamin C, Pine R, Weber MJ, Larner AC. Requirement for MAP Kinase (ERK2) activity in interferon-α– and interferon-γ–stimulated gene expression through STAT proteins. *Science* 1995;269:1721.
104. Wen Z, Zhong Z, Darnell JE Jr. Maximal activation of transcription by Stat1 and Stat3 requires both tyrosine and serine phosphorylation. *Cell* 1995;82:241–250.
105. Greenlund AC, Farrar MA, Viviano BL, Schrieber RD. Ligand-induced IFN receptor tyrosine phosphorylation couples the receptor to its signal transduction system (p91). *EMBO J* 1994;13:1591–1600.
106. Igarashi K, Garotta G, Ozmen L, et al. interferon-γ induces tyrosine phosphorylation of interferon-receptor and regulated association of protein tyrosine kinases, Jak1 and Jak2, with its receptor. *J Biol Chem* 1994;20:14333–14336.
107. Greenlund AC, Schreiber RD, Goeddel DV, Pennica D. IFN-γ induces IFN-γ receptor dimerization under physiologic conditions. *J* 1993;150:205A.
108. Greenlund AC, Schreiber RD, Goeddel DV, Pennica D. Interferon-γ induces receptor dimerization in solution and on cells. *J Biol Chem* 1993;268:18103–18110.
109. Decker T, Lew DJ, Mirkovitch J, Darnell JE Jr. Cytoplasmic activation of GAF, an IFN-γ–regulated DNA-binding factor. *EMBO J* 1991; 10:927–932.
110. Shuai K, Stark GR, Kerr IM, Darnell JE Jr. A single phosphotyrosine residue of Stat91 required for gene activation by interferon-γ. *Science* 1993;261:1744–1746.
111. Shuai K, Horvath CM, Tsai Huang LH, Qureshi SA, Cowburn D, Darnell JE Jr. Interferon activation of the transcription factor Stat91 involves dimerization through SH2–phosphotyrosyl peptide interactions. *Cell* 1994;76:821–828.
112. Guyer NB, Severns CW, Wong P, Feghali CA, Wright TM. IFN-γ induces a p91/Stat1α–related transcription factor with distinct activation and binding properties. *J Immunol* 1995;155:3472–3480.
113. Veals SA, Schindler C, Leonard D, et al. Subunit of an alpha-interferon–responsive transcription factor is related to interferon regulatory factor and Myb families of DNA-binding proteins. *Mol Cell Biol* 1992;12:3315–3324.
114. Song Z, Krishna S, Thanos D, Strominger JL, Ono SJ. A novel cysteine-rich sequence-specific DNA-binding protein interacts with the conserved X-box motif of the human major histocompatibility complex class II genes via a repeated Cys-His domain and functions as a transcriptional repressor. *J Exp Med* 1994;180:1763–1774.
115. Friedman RL, Stark GR. α-interferon–induced transcription of HLA and metallothionein genes containing homologous upstream sequences. *Nature* 1985;314:637–639.
116. Kimura T, Nakayama K, Penninger J, et al. Involvement of the IRF-1 transcription factor in antiviral responses to interferons. *Science* 1994;264:1921–1923.
117. Matsuyama T, Kimura T, Kitagawa M, et al. Targeted disruption of IRF-1 or IRF-2 results in abnormal type I IFN gene induction and aberrant lymphocyte development. *Cell* 1993;75:83–97.
118. Nelson N, Marks MS, Driggers PH, Ozato K. Interferon consensus sequence–binding protein, a member of the interferon regulatory factor family, suppresses interferon-induced gene transcription. *Mol Cell Biol* 1993;13:588–599.
119. Weisz A, Marx P, Sharf R, et al. Human interferon consensus sequence binding protein is a negative regulator of enhancer elements common to interferon-inducible genes. *J Biol Chem* 1992;267: 25589–25596.
120. Strehlow I, Decker T. Transcriptional induction of IFN-γ responsive genes is modulated by DNA surrounding the interferon stimulation response element. *Nucleic Acids Res* 1992;20:3865–3872.
121. Kolesnick R, Golde DW. The sphingomyelin pathway in tumor necrosis factor and interleukin-1 signaling. *Cell* 1994;77:325–328.
122. Schutze S, Machleidt T, Kronke M. Mechanisms of tumor necrosis factor action. *Semin Oncol* 1992;19(Suppl 4):16–24.
123. Collins T, Lapierre LA, Fiers W, Strominger JL, Pober JS. Recombinant human tumor necrosis factor increases mRNA levels and surface expression of HLA-A,B antigens in vascular endothelial cells and dermal fibroblasts in vitro. *Proc Natl Acad Sci U S A* 1986;83:446–450.
124. Halloran PF. Interferon-γ, prototype of the proinflammatory cytokines—importance in activation, suppression, and maintenance of the immune response. *Transplant Proc* 1993;25:10–15.
125. Woo J, Lemster B, Tamura K, Starzl TE, Thomson AW. The antilymphocytic activity of brequinar sodium and its potentiation by cytidine. Effects on lymphocyte proliferation and cytokine production. *Transplantation* 1993;56:374–381.
126. Liu Y, Wei SHY, Ho ASY, de Waal Malefyt R, Moore KW. Expression cloning and characterization of a human IL-10 receptor. *J Immunol* 1994;152:1821–1829.
127. Enk AH, Angeloni VL, Udey MC, Katz SI. Inhibition of Langerhans cell antigen-presenting function by IL-10. A role for IL-10 in induction of tolerance. *J Immunol* 1993;151:2390–2398.
128. de Waal Malefyt R, Haanen J, Spits H, et al. Interleukin 10 (IL-10) and viral IL-10 strongly reduce antigen-specific human T cell proliferation by diminishing the antigen-presenting capacity of monocytes via downregulation of class II major histocompatibility complex expression. *J Exp Med* 1991;174:915–924.
129. Moore KW, O'Garra A, de Waal Malefyt R, Vieira P, Mosmann TR. Interleukin-10. *Annu Rev Immunol* 1993;11:165–190.
130. Broski AP, Halloran PF. Tissue distribution of IL-10 mRNA in normal mice: expression in T and B cells independent and increased by irradiation. *Transplantation* 1994;57:582–592.
131. Kelso A. Th1 and Th2 subsets: paradigms lost? *Immunol Today* 1995; 16:374–379.
132. Geiser AG, Letterio JJ, Kulkarni AB, Karlsson S, Roberts AB, Sporn MB. Transforming growth factor 1 (TGF-1) controls expression of major histocompatibility genes in the postnatal mouse: aberrant histocompatibility antigen expression in the pathogenesis of the TGF-1 null mouse phenotype. *Proc Natl Acad Sci U S A* 1993;90:9944–9948.
133. Devajyothi C, Kalvakolanu I, Babcock GT, Vasavada HA, Howe PH, Ransohoff RM. Inhibition of interferon-γ–induced major histocompatibility complex class II gene transcription by interferon-γ and type 1 transforming growth factor in human astrocytoma cells. Definition of cis-element. *J Biol Chem* 1993;268:18794–18800.
134. Egan RM, Brockman JA, Omer KW, Woodward JG. Transcription of the murine class II Eb gene is regulated primarily at the level of transcriptional initiation. *Cell Immunol* 1994;156:537–543.
135. Scholl T, Pitcock A, Jones B. Hypomethylation of MHC class II Eb gene is associated with expression. *Immunogenetics* 1992;36:255–263.
136. Sugawara M, Scholl T, Mahanta SK, Ponath PD, Strominger JL. Cooperativity between the J and S elements of class II major histocompatibility complex genes as enhancers in normal and class II–negative patient and mutant B cell lines. *J Exp Med* 1995;182:175–184.
137. Mach B, Steimle V, Reith W. MHC class II–deficient combined immunodeficiency: a disease of gene regulation. *Immunol Rev* 1994; 138:207–221.
138. Gronhoj Larsen C, Thomsen MK, Gesser B, et al. The delayed-type hypersensitivity reaction is dependent on IL-8. Inhibition of a tuberculin skin reaction by an anti–IL-8 monoclonal antibody. *J Immunol* 1995;155:2151–2157.
139. Kara CJ, Glimcher LH. Developmental and cytokine-mediated regu-

lation of MHC class II gene promoter occupancy in vivo. *J Immunol* 1993;150:4934–4942.
140. Jennette JC, Falk RJ. Acute renal failure secondary to leukocyte-mediated acute glomerular injury. *Renal Failure* 1992;14:395–399.
141. Reith W, Satola S, Sanchez CH, et al. Congenital immunodeficiency with a regulatory defect in MHC class II gene expression lacks a specific HLA-DR promoter binding protein, RF-X. *Cell* 1988;53:897–906.
142. Steimle V, Durand B, Barras E, Zufferey M, Hadam MR, Mach B, Reith W. A novel DNA-binding regulatory factor is mutated in primary MHC class II deficiency (bare lymphocyte syndrome). *Genes Dev* 1995;9:1021–1032.
143. Sanchez CH, Reith W, Silacci P, Mach B. The DNA-binding defect observed in major histocompatibility complex class II regulatory mutants concerns only one member of a family of complex binding to the X boxes of class II promoters. *Mol Cell Biol* 1992;12:4076–4083.
144. Ono SJ, Liou HC, Davidon R, Strominger JL, Glimcher LH. Human X-box–binding protein 1 is required for the transcription of a subset of human class II major histocompatibility genes and forms a heterodimer with c-*fos*. *Proc Natl Acad Sci U S A* 1991;88:4309–4312.
145. Ivashkiv LB, Liou HC, Kara CJ, Lamph WW, Verma IM, Glimcher LH. *mXBP/CRE-BP2* and c-*Jun* form a complex which binds to the cyclic AMP, but not to the 12-O-tetradecanoylphorbol-13-acetate, response element. *Mol Cell Biol* 1990;10:1609–1621.
146. Whitley MZ, Sisk R, Ivashkiv LB, Finn PW, Glimcher LH, Boothby MR. Non-consensus DNA sequences function in a cell-type–specific enhancer of the mouse class II MHC gene Aα. *Int Immunol* 1991;3: 877–888.
147. Kwok RPS, Lundlad JR, Chrivia JC, et al. Nuclear protein CBP is a coactivator for the transcription factor CREB. *Nature* 1994;370: 223–226.
148. Haas JG, Ströbel M, Leutz A, et al. Constitutive monocyte-restricted activity of NF-M, a nuclear factor that binds to a C/EBP motif. *J Immunol* 1992;149:237–243.
149. Mantovani R, Pessara U, Tonche F, et al. Monoclonal antibodies to NF-Y define its function in MHC class II and albumin gene transcription. *EMBO J* 1992;11:3315–3322.
150. Ting JPY, Painter A, Zeleznik-Le NJ, et al. YB-1 DNA-binding protein represses interferon activation of class II major histocompatibility complex genes. *J Exp Med* 1994;179:1605–1611.
151. Wang N, Finegold MJ, Bradley A, et al. Impaired energy homeostasis in C/EBPα knockout mice. *Science* 1995;269:1108–1112.
152. Silacci P, Mottet A, Steimle V, Reith W, Mach B. Developmental extinction of major histocompatibility complex class II gene expression in plasmocytes is mediated by silencing of the transactivator gene CIITA. *J Exp Med* 1994;180:1329–1336.
153. Steimle V, Siegrist CA, Mottet A, Lisowska-Grospierre B, Mach B. Regulation of MHC class II expression by interferon-γ mediated by the transactivator gene CIITA. *Science* 1994;265:106–109.
154. Steimle V, Otten LA, Zufferey M, Mach B. Complementation cloning of an MHC class II transactivator mutated in hereditary MHC class II deficiency (or bare lymphocyte syndrome). *Cell* 1993;75:135–146.
155. Chang CH, Fontes JD, Peterlin M, Flavell RA. Class II transactivator (CIITA) is sufficient for the inducible expression of major histocompatibility complex class II genes. *J Exp Med* 1994;180:1367–1374.
156. Zhou H, Glimcher LH. Human MHC class II gene transcription directed by the carboxyl terminus of CIITA, one of the defective genes in type II MHC combined immune deficiency. *Immunity* 1995; 2:545–553.
157. Wright KL, Ting JPY. In vivo footprint analysis of the HLA-DRA gene promoter: cell-specific interaction at the octamer site and up-regulation of X box binding by interferon-γ. *Proc Natl Acad Sci U S A* 1992;89:7601–7605.
158. Pober JS, Gimbrone MA Jr, Lapierre LA, et al. Overlapping patterns of activation of human endothelial cells by interleukin 1, tumor necrosis factor, and immune interferon. *J Immunol* 1986;137:1893–1896.
159. Ritchie AJ, Johnson DR, Ewenstein BM, Pober JS. Tumor necrosis factor induction of endothelial cell surface antigens is independent of protein kinase C activation or inactivation. Studies with phorbol myristate acetate and staurosporine. *J Immunol* 1991;146:3056–3062.
160. Freund YR, Dedrick RL, Jones PP. *cis*–acting sequences required for class II gene regulation by interferon gamma and tumor necrosis factor alpha in a murine macrophage cell line. *J Exp Med* 1990;171: 1283–1299.
161. Vidovic M, Sparacio SM, Elovitz M, Benveniste EN. Induction and regulation of class II major histocompatibility complex mRNA expression in astrocytes by interferon-gamma and tumor necrosis factor-alpha. *J Neuroimmunol* 1990;30:189–200.
162. Melhus O, Koerner TJ, Adams DO. Effects of TNF alpha on the expression of class II MHC molecules in macrophages induced by IFN gamma: evidence for suppression at the level of transcription. *J Leukoc Biol* 1991;49:21–28.
163. Panek RB, Moses H, Ting JPY, Benveniste EN. Tumor necrosis factor α response elements in the HLA-DRA promoter: identification of a tumor necrosis factor α–induced DNA–protein complex in astrocytes. *Proc Natl Acad Sci U S A* 1992;89:11518–11522.
164. MacDonald GH, Itoh-Lindstrom Y, Ting JP-Y. The transcriptional regulatory protein, YB-1, promotes single-stranded regions in the DRA promoter. *J Biol Chem* 1995;270:3527–3533.
165. Matsushima GK, Itoh-Lindstrom Y, Ting JPY. Activation of the HLA-DRA gene in primary human T lymphocytes: novel usage of TATA and the X and Y promoter elements. *Mol Cell Biol* 1992;12: 5610–5619.
166. Voliva CF, Tsang S, Peterlin BM. Mapping *cis*-acting defects in promoters of transcriptionally silent DQA2, DQB2, and DOB genes. *Proc Natl Acad Sci U S A* 1993;90:3408–3412.
167. Lu Y, Ussery GD, Muncaster MM, Gallie BL, Blanck G. Evidence for retinoblastoma protein (RB) dependent and independent IFN-γ responses: RB coordinately rescues IFN-γ induction of MHC class II gene transcription in noninducible breast carcinoma cells. *Oncogene* 1994;9:1015–1019.
168. Albert SE, Strutz F, Shelton K, et al. Characterization of a *cis*-acting regulatory element which silences expression of the class II—a gene in epithelium. *J Exp Med* 1994;180:233–240.
169. Abdulkadir SA, Krishna S, Thanos D, Maniatis T, Strominger JL, Ono SJ. Functional roles of the transcription factor Oct-2A and the high mobility group protein I/Y in HLA-DRA gene expression. *J Exp Med* 1995;182:487–500.
170. Kolk DP, Floyd-Smith G. Induction of the murine class-II antigen–associated invariant chain by TNF-α is controlled by an NF-κB–like element. *Gene* 1993;126:179–185.
171. Pessara U, Koch N. Tumor necrosis factor α regulates expression of the major histocompatibility complex class II–associated invariant chain by binding of an NF-κB–like factor to a promoter element. *Mol Cell Biol* 1990;10:4146–4154.
172. Doyle C, Ford PJ, Ponath PD, Spies T, Strominger JL. Regulation of the class II–associated invariant chain gene in normal and mutant B lymphocytes. *Proc Natl Acad Sci U S A* 1990;87:4590–4594.
173. Brown AM, Linhoff MW, Stein B, et al. Function of NF-κB/Rel binding sites in the major histocompatibility complex class II invariant chain promoter is dependent on cell-specific binding of different NF-κB/Rel subunits. *Mol Cell Biol* 1994;14:2926–2935.
174. Radley E, Alderton RP, Kelly A, Trowsdale J, Beck S. Genomic organization of HLA-DMA and HLA-DMB. *J Biol Chem* 1994;269: 18834–18838.
175. Sloan VS, Cameron P, Porter G, et al. Mediation by HLA-DM of dissociation of peptides from HLA-DR. *Nature* 1995;375:802.
176. Drezen JM, Babinet C, Morello D. Transcriptional control of MHC class I and β_2-microglobulin genes in vivo. *J Immunol* 1993;150: 2805–2813.
177. Dey A, Thornton AM, Lonergan M, Weissman SM, Chamberlain JW, Ozato K. Occupancy of upstream regulatory sites in vivo coincides with major histocompatibility complex class I gene expression in mouse tissues. *Mol Cell Biol* 1992;12:3590–3599.
178. Rosen FS, Cooper MD, Wedgwood RJP. The primary immunodeficiencies. *N Engl J Med* 1995;333:431.
179. de la Salle H, Hanau D, Fricker D, et al. Homozygous human TAP peptide transporter mutation in HLA class I deficiency. *Science* 1994; 265:237–241.
180. Versteeg R, Noordermeer IA, Kruse-Wolters M, Ruiter DJ, Schrier PI. c-*myc* down-regulates class I HLA expression in human melanomas. *EMBO J* 1988;7:1023–1029.
181. Peltenburg LTC, Schrier PI. Transcriptional suppression of HLA-B expression by c-Myc is mediated through the core promoter elements. *Immunogenetics* 1994;40:54–61.
182. Potter DA, Larson CJ, Eckes P, et al. Purification of the major histocompatibility complex class I transcription factor H2TF1. The full-length product of the NF-κB2 gene. *J Biol Chem* 1993;268: 18882–18890.

183. Hrdlicková R, Nehyba J, Humphries EH. v-*rel* induces expression of three avian immunoregulatory surface receptors more efficiently than c-*rel*. *J Virol* 1994;68:308–319.
184. van't Veer LJ, Beijersbergen RL, Bernards R. N-*myc* suppresses major histocompatibility complex class I gene expression through down-regulation of the p50 subunit of NF-κB. *EMBO J* 1993;12:195–200.
185. Meijer I, Boot AJM, Mahabir G, Zantema A, Van der Eb AJ. Reduced binding activity of transcription factor NF-κB accounts for MHC class I repression in adenovirus type 12 E1-transformed cells. *Cell Immunol* 1992;145:56–65.
186. Schouten GJ, Van der Eb AJ, Zantema A. Downregulation of MHC class I expression due to interference with p105–NF-κB1 processing by Ad12E1A. *EMBO J* 1995;14:1498–1507.
187. Sakaguchi K, Appella E, Omichinski JG, Clore GM, Gronenborn AM. Specific DNA binding to a major histocompatibility complex enhancer sequence by a synthetic 57-residue double zinc finger peptide from a human enhancer binding protein. *J Biol Chem* 1991;266:7306–7311.
188. Singh H, Le Bowitz JH, Baldwin AS Jr, Sharp PA. Molecular cloning of an enhancer binding protein: isolation by screening of an expression library with a recognition site DNA. *Cell* 1988;52:415–423.
189. Hamada K, Gleason SL, Levy BZ, Hirschfeld S, Appella E, Ozato K. H-2RIIBP, a member of a nuclear hormone receptor superfamily that binds to both the regulatory element of major histocompatibility complex class I genes and the estrogen response element. *Proc Natl Acad Sci U S A* 1989;86:8289–8293.
190. Nagata T, Segars JH, Levi BZ, Ozato K. Retinoic acid–dependent transactivation of major histocompatibility complex class I promoters by the nuclear hormone receptor H-2RIIBP in undifferentiated embryonal carcinoma cells. *Proc Natl Acad Sci U S A* 1992;89:937–941.
191. Marks MS, Hallenbeck PL, Nagata T, et al. H-2RIIBP (RXRβ) heterodimerization provides a mechanism for combinatorial diversity in the regulation of retinoic acid and thyroid hormone responsive genes. *EMBO J* 1992;11:1419–1435.
192. Králová J, Jansa P, Forejt J. A novel downstream regulatory element of the mouse *H-2K^b* class I major histocompatibility gene. *EMBO J* 1992;11:4591–4600.
193. Chang CH, Hammer J, Loh JE, Fodor WL, Flavell RA. The activation of major histocompatibility complex class I genes by interferon regulatory factor-1 (IRF-1). *Immunogenetics* 1992;35:378–384.
194. Johnson DR, Pober JS. HLA class I heavy-chain gene promoter elements mediating synergy between tumor necrosis factor and interferons. *Mol Cell Biol* 1994;14:1322–1332.
195. Plaksin D, Baeuerle PA, Eisenbach L. KBF1 p50 NF-κB homodimer acts as a repressor of H-2K^b gene expression in metastatic tumor cells. *J Exp Med* 1993;177:1651–1662.
196. Harada H, Willison K, Sakakibara J, Miyamoto M, Fujita T, Taniguchi T. Absence of the type I IFN system in EC cells: transcriptional activator (IRF-1) and repressor (IRF-2) genes are developmentally regulated. *Cell* 1990;63:303–312.
197. Harada H, Fujita T, Miyamoto M, et al. Structurally similar but functionally distinct factors, IRF-1 and IRF-2, bind to the same regulatory elements of IFN and IFN-inducible genes. *Cell* 1989;58:729–739.
198. Vaughan PS, Aziz F, van Wijnen AJ, et al. Activation of a cell-cycle–regulated histone gene by the oncogenic transcription factor IRF-2. *Nature* 1995;377:362.
199. Howcroft TK, Richardson JC, Singer DS. MHC class I gene expression is negatively regulated by the proto-oncogene, c-*jun*. *EMBO J* 1993;12:3163–3169.
200. Howcroft TK, Strebel K, Martin MA, Singer DS. Repression of MHC class I gene promoter activity by two-exon TAT of HIV. *Science* 1993;260:1320–1322.
201. Halloran PF, Wadgymar A, Autenried P. The regulation of expression of major histocompatibility complex products. *Transplantation* 1986; 41:413–420.
202. Lu L, Woo J, Rao AS, et al. Propagation of dendritic cell progenitors from normal mouse liver using granulocyte/macrophage colony–stimulating factor and their maturational development in the presence of type-1 collagen. *J Exp Med* 1994;179:1823–1834.
203. Halloran PF, Urmson J, Farkas S, van der Meide P, Autenried P. Regulation of MHC expression in vivo. IFN-α/β inducers and recombinant IFN-α modulate MHC antigen expression in mouse tissues. *J Immunol* 1989;142:4241–4247.
204. Goes N, Urmson J, Vincent D, Ramassar R, Halloran PF. Effect of rh insulin–like growth factor-1 on the inflammatory response to acute renal injury. *JASN* 1996;7:710–720
205. Shoskes DA, Halloran PF. Ischemic injury induces altered MHC gene expression in kidney by an interferon-γ–dependent pathway. *Transplant Proc* 1991;23:599–601.
206. Madrenas J, Parfrey NA, Halloran PF. Interferon γ–mediated renal MHC expression in mercuric chloride-induced glomerulonephritis. *Kidney Int* 1991;39:273–281.
207. Goes N, Urmson J, Ramassar V, Halloran PF. Acute toxic renal injury induces MHC and cytokine gene expression [Abstract]. *J Am Soc Nephrol* 1995;6:979.
208. Madrenas J, Pazderka F, Parfrey NA, Halloran PF. Thymus-independent expression of a truncated T cell receptor-α mRNA in murine kidney. *J Immunol* 1992;148:612–619.
209. Madrenas J, Vincent DH, Kriangkum J, Elliott JF, Halloran PF. Alternatively spliced, germline Jα11-2-Cα mRNAs are the predominant T cell receptor a transcripts in mouse kidney. *Mol Immunol* 1994;31: 993–1004.
210. Halloran PF, Aprile MA, Farewell V, et al. Early function as the principal correlate of graft survival: a multivariate analysis of 200 cadaveric renal transplants treated with a protocol incorporating antilymphocyte globulin and cyclosporine. *Transplantation* 1988;46:223–228.
211. Ostrand-Rosenberg S, Thakur A, Clements V. Rejection of mouse sarcoma cells after transfection of MHC class II genes. *J Immunol* 1990;144:4068–4071.
212. Lechler RI, Norcross MA, Germain RN. Qualitative and quantitative studies of antigen-presenting cell function by using I-A–expressing L cells. *J Immunol* 1985;135:2914–2922.
213. Matis LA, Jones PP, Murphy DB, et al. Immune response gene function correlates with the expression of an Ia antigen II. A quantitative deficiency in Ae:Ea complex expression causes a corresponding defect in antigen presentation. *J Exp Med* 1982;155:508–523.
214. McNicholas JM, Murphy DB, Matis LA, et al. Immune response gene function correlates with the expression of an Ia antigen. I. Preferential association of certain Ae and Ea chains results in a quantitative deficiency in expression of an Ae:Ea complex. *J Exp Med* 1982;155: 490–507.
215. Graber M, Bockenstedt LK, Weiss A. Signaling via the inositol phospholipid pathway by T cell antigen receptor is limited by receptor number. *J Immunol* 1991;146:2935–2943.
216. Karjalainen K. High sensitivity, low affinity—paradox of T-cell receptor recognition. *Curr Opin Immunol* 1994;6:9–12.
217. Berg LJ, Frank GD, Davis MM. The effects of MHC gene dosage and allelic variation on T cell receptor selection. *Cell* 1990;60: 1043–1053.
218. Dhib-Jalbut SS, Xia Q, Drew PD, Swoveland PT. Differential up-regulation of HLA class I molecules on neuronal and glial cell lines by virus infection correlates with differential induction of IFN-γ. *J Immunol* 1995;155:2096–2108.
219. Alexander MA, Damico CA, Wieties KM, Hansen TH, Connolly JM. Correlation between CD8 dependency and determinant density using peptide-induced, Ld-restricted cytotoxic T lymphocytes. *J Exp Med* 1991;173:849–858.
220. Robey EA, Ramsdell F, Kioussis D, Sha W, Loh D, Axel R, Fowikes BJ. The level of CD8 expression can determine the outcome of thymic selection. *Cell* 1992;69:1089–1096.
221. Frels WI, Bordallo C, Golding H, Rosenberg A, Rudikoff S, Singer DS. Expression of a class I MHC transgene: regulation by a tissue-specific negative regulatory DNA sequence element. *New Biol* 1990; 2:1024–1033.
222. Statter MB, Fahrner KJ, Barksdale EM Jr, Parks DE, Flavell RA, Donahoe PK. Correlation of fetal kidney and testis congenic graft survival with reduced major histocompatibility complex burden. *Transplantation* 1989;47:651–660.
223. Magnone M, Holley JL, Shapiro R, et al. Interferon-α–induced acute renal allograft rejection. *Transplantation* 1995;59:1068.
224. Benham AM, Sawyer GJ, Fabre JW. Indirect T cell allorecognition of donor antigens contributes to the rejection of vascularized kidney allografts. *Transplantation* 1995;59:1028–1032.
225. Elliott BC, Carlow DA, Rodricks AM, Wade A. Perspectives on the role of MHC antigens in normal and malignant cell development. *Adv Cancer Res* 1989;53:181–245.
226. Koeppen H, Acena M, Drolet A, Rowley DA, Schreiber H. Tumors with reduced expression of a cytotoxic T lymphocyte recognized antigen lack immunogenicity but retain sensitivity to lysis by cytotoxic T lymphocytes. *Eur J Immunol* 1993;23:2770–2776.
227. Sospedra M, Obiols G, Santamaria Babi LF, et al. Hyperinducibility

of HLA class II expression of thyroid follicular cells from Graves' disease. *J Immunol* 1995;154:4213–4222.

228. Wuthrich RP, Glimcher LH, Yui MA, Jevnikar AM, Dumas SE, Kelley VE. MHC class II, antigen presentation and tumor necrosis factor in renal tubular epithelial cells. *Kidney Int* 1990;37:783–792.
229. Jevnikar AM, Singer GG, Coffman T, Glimcher LH, Rubin-Kelley VE. Transgenic tubular cell expression of class II is sufficient to initiate immune renal injury. *J Am Soc Nephrol* 1993;3:1972–1977.
230. Haverty TP, Watanabe M, Neilson EG, Kelly CJ. Protective modulation of class II MHC gene expression in tubular epithelium by target antigen–specific antibodies. Cell-surface directed down–regulation of transcription can influence susceptibility to murine tubulointerstitial nephritis. *J Immunol* 1989;143:1133–1141.
231. Jevnikar AM, Grusby MJ, Glimcher LH. Prevention of nephritis in major histocompatibility complex class II–deficient MRL-1pr mice. *J Exp Med* 1994;179:1137–1143.
232. Taurog JD, Maika SD, Simmons WA, Breban M, Hammer RE. Susceptibility to inflammatory disease in HLA-B27 transgenic rat lines correlates with the level of B27 expression. *J Immunol* 1993;150:4168–4178.
233. Lee M-S, von Herrath M, Reiser H, Oldstone MBA, Sarvetnick N. Sensitization to self (virus) antigen by in situ expression of murine interferon-γ. *J Clin Invest* 1995;95:486–492.
234. Toyonaga T, Hino O, Sugai S, et al. Chronic active hepatitis in transgenic mice expressing interferon-γ in the liver. *Proc Natl Acad Sci U S A* 1994;91:614–618.
235. Dallman MJ, Wood KJ, Morris PJ. Specific cytotoxic T cells are found in the nonrejected kidneys of blood-transfused rats. *J Exp Med* 1988;165:566–571.
236. Wood KJ, Hopley A, Dallman MJ, Morris PJ. Lack of correlation between the induction of donor class I and class II major histocompatibility complex antigens and graft rejection. *Transplantation* 1988;45:759–767.
237. La Rosa FG, Talmage DW. Major histocompatibility complex antigen expression on parenchymal cells of thyroid allografts is not by itself sufficient to induce rejection. *Transplantation* 1990;49:605–609.
238. Hagerty DT, Evavold BD, Allen PM. Regulation of the costimulator B7, not class II major histocompatibility complex, restricts the ability of murine kidney tubule cells to stimulate CD4+ T cells. *J Clin Invest* 1994;93:1208–1215.

Immunologic Renal Diseases,
edited by E. G. Neilson and W. G. Couser.
Lippincott-Raven Publishers, Philadelphia © 1997

CHAPTER 8

Antigen Presentation by Renal Parenchyma

Rudolf P. Wüthrich, Gary G. Singer, and Vicki Rubin Kelley

INTRODUCTION

Antigen presentation is a complex process whereby foreign peptide antigens are endocytosed, digested, and expressed on the cell surface bound to major histocompatibility complex (MHC) class II molecules. Antigens that have been processed by antigen-presenting cells (APCs) elicit a T-cell response after engagement of the T-cell receptor (TCR) with peptides that are presented by MHC class II molecules. In a broader sense, antigen presentation can also occur with self- (auto-) or alloantigens. MHC class II molecules are constitutively expressed on certain hematopoietically derived cells such as macrophages, B cells, and dendritic cells. These "professional" APCs have the ability to ingest, digest, and present protein antigens efficiently to helper T lymphocytes (Th). CD4+ helper T lymphocytes that have engaged the MHC class II–antigen complex through their TCR then usually respond by antigen-specific proliferation. In the absence of appropriate costimulatory signals, however, the T cell will not proliferate but will become unresponsive (anergic).

Other cells of nonhematopoietic lineage are capable of antigen presentation and include cells located in the gut (1,2), thyroid (3–7), pancreas (8–10), cartilage (11), muscle (12), and kidney (13,14). In general, these "nonprofessional" APCs do not constitutively express MHC class II molecules but can be induced to express these cell surface proteins in response to interferon-gamma (IFN-γ). Important collaborative interaction can thus occur between cells of the immune system and parenchymal cells. Such concerted interaction has been reported in many different organs and is exemplified by studies of T-cell interaction with epithelial cells in the kidney (13–17).

In the following sections, we will discuss the general mechanisms of antigen presentation and highlight differences between hematopoietic and nonhematopoietic APCs. We will then discuss the evidence for antigen presentation processes in the kidney, focusing on the antigen-presenting capacity of tubular epithelial cells, since these cells have been studied in great detail (13,14). Although it is clear that tubular epithelial cells can present antigen to T cells in the context of MHC class II molecules, the usual T-cell response is not proliferation but rather antigen-specific unresponsiveness (17). Antigen processing and presentation by tubular epithelial cells may be responsible for protecting the kidney from autoimmune injury by promoting peripheral T-cell tolerance.

MECHANISM OF ANTIGEN PRESENTATION

Major Histocompatibility Complex and Accessory Cells

It is well known that humoral and cellular immunity are mediated by B and T cells, respectively. T cells recognize a different spectrum of foreign antigens than do B cells. T cells recognize protein antigens, whereas B cells recognize proteins, nucleic acids, lipids, and small chemicals. The induction of T-cell-mediated immune responses to foreign antigens requires the recognition of specific foreign molecular structures by CD4+ helper T cells. Helper T cells—unlike antibodies—are not easily engaged by a foreign antigen. Foreign proteins must be processed by an APC—also termed accessory cell—before they can be displayed to helper T cells in the context of MHC class II molecules.

Helper (CD4+) and cytotoxic (CD8+) T cells recognize foreign protein antigens only when they are properly digested into small peptide fragments of appropriate size

R. P. Wüthrich: Division of Nephrology, University Hospital, 8091 Zürich, Switzerland.

G. G. Singer: Renal Division, Washington University School of Medicine, St. Louis, Missouri 63110.

V. Rubin Kelley: Renal Division, Molecular Autoimmunity Section, Brigham and Women's Hospital, Boston, Massachusetts 02115.

(18). Furthermore, these peptide fragments must be bound to MHC molecules on the surface of APCs to induce a T-cell response (19). The recognition by T cells of this bimolecular complex on the surface of APCs leads to an ordered sequence of events resulting in T-cell activation. Recognition of MHC class II molecules by CD4+ helper T cells induces proliferation or anergy; in comparison, CD8+ cytotoxic T cells induce target cell death upon encountering antigen–MHC class I complex-bearing cells. This selective interaction is determined by the CD4 and CD8 accessory molecules which recognize specific nonpolymorphic regions on MHC class II or class I molecules, respectively. MHC class I molecules are essential in efferent pathways of target recognition. In this review, we focus exclusively on afferent immune interactions mediated by APCs expressing MHC class II molecules.

MHC class II molecules are integral transmembrane proteins encoded by polymorphic genes that lie within the MHC and are members of the immunoglobulin (Ig) gene superfamily. They consist of two polypeptide chains, α (34 kD) and β (28 kD), each of which contains extracellular, transmembrane, and cytoplasmic domains. Associated with the α- and β-chains is a nonpolymorphic (invariant) γ-chain (Ii). The γ-chain is 30 kD in size and is also a member of the Ig gene superfamily. The invariant chain separates from the mature MHC class II αβ heterodimer before it reaches the cell surface. The association of the γ-chain with the αβ complex prior to endosomal transport may prevent the premature binding of endogenously synthesized peptides; the MHC class II binding sites thus remain available for peptides derived from foreign proteins (20).

The conversion of native proteins to MHC class-II-associated peptide fragments is called antigen processing. Foreign proteins enter a cell by endocytosis. Internalized antigens localize to intracellular membrane-bound vesicles (endosomes). APCs then degrade these endocytosed proteins in acidified endosomes or lysosomes. Fusion of these compartments with vesicles containing MHC class II molecules subsequently results in the noncovalent binding of immunodominant peptides (21,22). Intracellular trafficking and fusion of the endosome with the plasma membrane results in presentation of the MHC class II–peptide complex to CD4+ T cells.

The extracellular domain of each chain of the heterodimeric MHC class II molecules can be subdivided into two segments of ~90 amino acids each, termed α_1/α_2 and β_1/β_2, respectively. Our understanding of the interaction between peptide fragments and MHC molecules has been greatly advanced by x-ray crystallographic studies (23–25). The peptide-binding region is formed by the interaction of both chains and involves the α_1 and the β_1 segments of the class II molecule. These segments form a peptide-binding cleft that is composed of two α-helices (sides) and an eight-stranded β-pleated sheet (floor).

The genetic polymorphism of MHC class II molecules determines the physicochemical surface properties of the groove. Based on x-ray crystallographic measurements of HLA molecules, the cleft may accommodate a peptide of 10–20 amino acids. This size is consistent with the size of immunogenic peptides (26), is too small to bind an intact globular protein, and differs from the more planar binding site of antibody molecules.

MHC class-II-restricted antigen presentation is mediated primarily by macrophages, B cells, and dendritic cells. These "professional" APCs not only express class II molecules abundantly, but display costimulatory molecules (membrane glycoproteins and cytokines) that are required to induce a T-cell response. Initial studies suggested that antigen presentation was restricted to the lymphoid organs, which contain large numbers of "professional" APCs. Later studies demonstrated that APCs (macrophages and dendritic cells) were scattered throughout nonlymphoid tissues and that antigen presentation could also occur in these organs. Furthermore, it is now understood that many nonhematopoietic cells, including endocrine tissues, gut epithelium, and various renal parenchymal cells, are capable of expressing MHC class II antigens in response to IFN-γ. The critical property that enables a particular cell to function as an APC appears to be the expression of MHC class II antigens. Therefore, we and others have hypothesized that these parenchymal cells might have antigen-presenting functions.

T-Cell Activation and Accessory Cells

The T-cell response to antigen depends on the expression of specific T-cell surface receptors capable of engaging MHC molecules complexed to antigen. In the majority of T cells, this receptor is composed of two disulfide-linked proteins (α and β). The TCR is noncovalently associated with a complex of invariant chains collectively termed CD3. CD3 is a cluster of at least five cell surface proteins (γ, δ, ε, ζ, and η) closely associated with the TCR. Following TCR engagement, a complex sequence of intracellular signals is generated—mediated in part by CD3—leading to T-cell activation (27).

An initial intracellular signal is generated by the engagement of the TCR with the MHC–peptide complex and is manifested by a rapid increase in intracellular calcium. A host of additional signaling pathways is involved. Activation of phospholipase C causes increased phosphatidylinositol 4,5-bisphosphate breakdown, generating cytosolic diacylglycerol and inositol 1,4,5-trisphosphate. This leads to the translocation of protein kinase C and subsequent protein phosphorylation. The activation of various tyrosine kinases also results in the phosphorylation of numerous intracellular proteins. This complex cascade of intracellular signaling events induces interleukin-2 (IL-2) transcription and ultimately T-cell proliferation.

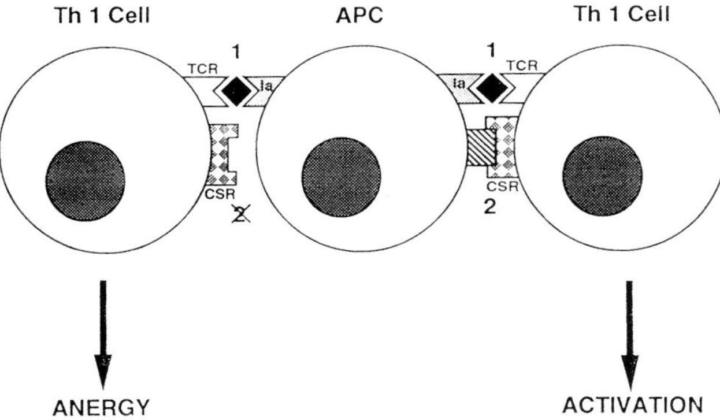

FIG. 1. The two-signal model of T-cell activation. T cells can respond to antigen presented in the context of MHC class II by antigen-presenting cells either by activation if signal 1 (T-cell receptor engagement) plus signal 2 (costimulation) are provided or by anergy if only signal 1 is delivered. From Rubin Kelley and Singer (15).

Occupancy of the TCR alone is insufficient to activate T cells (28). To become activated, a helper T cell must receive two signals from an APC (Fig. 1): engagement of the TCR (signal 1), and a costimulatory signal provided by accessory cells (signal 2). No single molecule has been shown to be a costimulatory signal for all T lymphocytes. In some situations, soluble ligands such as cytokines (IL-1, IL-6, and perhaps IL-12) appear to provide essential costimulatory signals while, in others, costimulation is mediated by membrane proteins (B7 family of cell surface molecules) and requires cell–cell contact (29). Regardless of the second signal, following the influx of calcium that occurs with TCR engagement, the T cell anticipates a second closely timed signal. In the absence of this signal, IL-2 gene activation and T-cell proliferation do not occur, leaving the T cell unable to respond to further stimulation by the same antigen.

The Costimulatory Signal

A costimulatory signal can be regarded as a signal in whose absence TCR occupancy results in anergy. This concept originated from studies exploring B-cell activation and was subsequently applied to T cells (30,31). Various experimental studies have shown that antigen-stimulated T cells can only be induced to proliferate if they also receive a second or costimulatory signal. TCR engagement alone causes anergy, whereas TCR occupancy plus a second signal delivered by the APC leads to T-cell activation (32,33).

Upon antigenic stimulation, CD4+ T helper cells may differentiate into two distinct subpopulations, each producing its own panel of cytokines and mediating separate effector functions. Based on their cytokine secretion profile, Th cells are functionally subdivided into Th1 and Th2 cells (34–36) (Table 1). Th1 cells secrete IL-2, IFN-γ, and TNF-β (lymphotoxin), thereby activating macrophages and inducing delayed-type hypersensitivity responses. In contrast, Th2 cells produce IL-4, IL-5, IL-6, IL-10, and IL-13, thus providing B-cell help and suppressing cell-mediated immunity. Both types of CD4+ cells secrete IL-3, granulocyte-macrophage colony-stimulating factor, and TNF-α. It is well accepted that IL-1 is the costimulatory signal required by Th2 clones. The proliferation of these cells is strictly dependent on IL-1 expression by APCs (37,38). For Th1 cells, the costimulatory signal is more complex. At least four ligands on APCs have been shown to provide proliferative signals for Th1 cells: B7, ICAM-1, VCAM-1, and LFA-3 (39) (Table 2). These accessory molecules provide interaction with the cognate T-cell ligands CD28 (CTLA-4), LFA-1, VLA-4, and CD2, respectively. An additional signal is provided by the direct interaction of CD4 with MHC class II molecules.

TABLE 1. *Cytokine profile of Th1 and Th2 CD4+ helper T cells*

Cell	Cytokines
Th1	IL-2, IFN-γ, TNF-α, TNF-β, IL-3, GM-CSF
Th2	IL-3, IL-4, IL-5, IL-6, IL-10, IL-13, TNF-α, GM-CSF

GM-CSF, granulocyte-macrophage colony-stimulating factor; IL, interleukin; Th, thymocyte; TNF, tumor necrosis factor.

The most potent costimulatory pathway involves the B7 molecule (also termed BB1). B7 represents at least three molecules—B7-1 (CD80), B7-2 (CD86), and B7-3—that interact with the counterreceptors CD28 and CTLA-4 on T cells (40). The extracellular region of the B7-1 and B7-2 molecules is homologous to the Ig supergene family, consisting of two Ig domains (41–44). B7-2 has a longer cytoplasmic tail than B7-1, containing three potential phosphorylation sites. The two ligands for B7—CD28 and CTLA-4—are functionally and structurally related members of the Ig gene superfamily (40,45,46). They are both present on T lymphocytes, CD28 being

TABLE 2. *Costimulatory and accessory molecules*

Molecule	CD	Ligands
B7-1	CD80	CD28, CTLA-4
B7-2	CD86	CD28, CTLA-4
ICAM-1	CD54	LFA-1 (CD11a/CD18) MAC-1 (CD11b/CD18)
VCAM-1	CD106	VLA-4 (CD49d/CD29)
LFA-3	CD58	CD2

ICAM, intracellular adhesion molecule; LFA, lymphocyte-function-associated antigen; MAC, membrane-attack complex; VCAM, vascular cell adhesion molecule.

expressed more abundantly than CTLA-4. They also differ in their binding to B7, CTLA-4 having a much higher affinity than CD28.

The interaction of B7 on APCs with CD28 present on T cells leads to the induction and enhancement of lymphokine gene expression. This process is mediated by intracellular signals distinct from those transduced through the TCR/CD3 complex and is resistant to cyclosporine, which only blocks lymphokine production mediated by signal 1. Thus, the B7–CD28 pathway provides a unique costimulatory signal that leads to T-cell proliferation. On the other hand, absence of this pathway (for example, on tubular epithelial cells) and lack of signal 2 result in anergy.

Another important accessory pathway involves ICAM-1 and LFA-1. ICAM-1, a prototype of a cell adhesion molecule, contains five extracellular Ig-like domains and is expressed by a variety of hematopoietic cells (47,48). Importantly, ICAM-1 is also expressed on many nonhematopoietic cells, for example, kidney mesangial cells (49) and tubular epithelial cells (50). ICAM-1 expression can be upregulated by cytokines, including IFN-γ, TNF-α, and IL-1. LFA-1, the specific counterreceptor of ICAM-1, -2, and -3 is a β_2-integrin whose expression is restricted to leukocytes. The ICAM-1–LFA-1 interaction promotes adhesion between T cells and APCs. Considerable controversy exists as to whether LFA-1 transduces a costimulatory signal. LFA-1-mediated T-cell signal transduction is qualitatively identical to the signals provided by the TCR/CD3 complex. Although augmented T-cell proliferation can be demonstrated by engagement of ICAM-1 with LFA-1, ICAM-1–LFA-1 engagement does not prevent the induction of anergy. In a strict sense, the LFA-1–ICAM-1 pathway is therefore not truly costimulatory.

VCAM-1 is yet another adhesion molecule capable of facilitating interaction between parenchymal cells and T cells (51). Unlike ICAM-1, VCAM-1 has several isoforms generated by alternative splicing (52–54). VCAM-1 interacts with the β_1-integrin ligand VLA-4 (55) and is expressed by endothelial cells (52), bone marrow stromal cells (56), tubular epithelial cells, and mesangial cells (57). VCAM-1 expression is regulated by the same cytokines as ICAM-1. As is the case for ICAM-1–LFA-1 interaction, VCAM-1–VLA-4 interaction augments T-cell proliferation (51). The T-cell signal transduced by VLA-4 is probably similar to the TCR/CD3 signal and does not represent true costimulation (that is, prevention of anergy).

Proliferative Response Versus Anergy

In the absence of a second signal—such as the one provided by the B7–CD28 interaction—the T cell develops a state of antigen-specific unresponsiveness (32,33). Fixed splenocytes, for example, that have processed an antigen can be used as APCs in vitro to render Th1 cells anergic (58,59). The anergic cells are unresponsive to restimulation with untreated splenocytes and antigen, but they remain viable as demonstrated by their proliferation in response to exogenous IL-2. As with T-cell activation, this event is antigen specific and MHC restricted (60).

Anergy is a regulatory process inducing peripheral tolerance. Normally, autoreactive T-cell clones are eliminated in the thymus through the process of negative selection (61,62). However, since not all self-antigens are expressed intrathymically, potentially autoreactive T cells escape clonal deletion and reach the periphery. Failure to differentiate self-antigens from foreign antigens may result in autoimmune disease. Fortunately, additional barriers in peripheral tissues maintain tolerance.

Several mechanisms may explain peripheral tolerance, including attenuation of cell surface TCR (63), reduced visibility of MHC determinants on APCs (64), downregulation of costimulatory molecules, immune suppression, clonal deletion (64a), and antigen-specific unresponsiveness or clonal anergy (32,59). Given that parenchymal cells can express MHC class II molecules and are capable of processing and presenting antigen, and nonproliferative and proliferative responses can be elicited, antigen presentation could generate mechanisms that either thwart or alternatively foster immune and autoimmune processes.

ANTIGEN-PRESENTING FUNCTION OF TUBULAR EPITHELIAL CELLS

Renal tubular epithelial cells possess all of the necessary features to function as APCs (Table 3). Tubular epithelial cells have the ability to express MHC class II molecules (13,65,66) and a variety of costimulatory cell surface proteins and cytokines, including ICAM-1, VCAM-1, and LFA-3. However, the potent costimula-

TABLE 3. *Accessory molecules and cytokines expressed by renal thymic epithelial cells*

Membrane-associated molecules	Secreted molecules
MHC class II	TNF-α
ICAM-1	IL-6
VCAM-1	IL-8
LFA-3	TGF-β
TNF-α	GM-CSF
C3 complement component	MCP-1 and Rantes
	PDGF

GM-CSF, granulocyte-macrophage colony-stimulating factor; ICAM, intracellular adhesion molecule; IL, interleukin; LFA, lymphocyte-function-associated antigen; MHC, major histocompatibility complex; MCP, monocyte chemoattractant factor; PDGF, platelet-derived growth factor; TGF, transforming growth factor; TNF, tumor necrosis factor; VCAM, vascular cell adhesion molecule.

tory molecule B7 is absent on tubular epithelial cells and cannot be induced with IFN-γ stimulation (17).

To study the mechanisms by which tubular epithelial cells interact with T cells in vitro, it is essential to isolate pure tubular epithelial cells devoid of contaminating macrophages and dendritic cells. One approach has been to use freshly isolated tubular epithelial cells (67) or to use tubular epithelial cells that have been grown in primary culture (68). However, the presence of only a few contaminating macrophages could be sufficient to generate a T-cell response. Thus, caution is required in interpreting experimental results from studies using freshly isolated cells. Therefore, we and others have generated homogeneous clonal tubular epithelial cells relying on a strategy of immortalizing tubular epithelial cells with origin-defective SV40 DNA (13) or nonreplicating, non-capsid-forming SV40 virus (14). These cell lines are readily maintained, remain well differentiated, and are thus ideal to investigate T-cell activation and anergy (69).

Major Histocompatibility Complex Class II Expression by Tubular Epithelial Cells

Tubular epithelial cells express few (13) or no MHC class II molecules (14,67). Tubular epithelial cells can be readily induced to express Ia with the addition of IFN-γ. Kinetic studies indicate that surface expression occurs within 24–48 h and reaches maximal levels after 72–96 h in culture (13,66). Removal of IFN-γ results in gradual loss of class II expression over several days. The expression of class II is primarily regulated at the level of gene transcription (13,70,71). Studies on the regulation of MHC class II gene transcription in tubular epithelial cells have not disclosed marked divergence from other cells with antigen-presenting capacity. Concurrent incubation of tubular epithelial cells with IFN-γ and cycloheximide, a potent inhibitor of protein synthesis, results in a loss of MHC class II mRNA induction, suggesting that tubular epithelial cells require de novo protein synthesis for class II transcription (13). This finding is consistent with results in other cell types where induction of MHC class II by IFN-γ requires the synthesis of transacting proteins that specifically bind to 58 upstream sequences (72–74).

Antigen Presentation by Tubular Epithelial Cells in Vitro

Antigen Presentation of Foreign Antigens

Following stimulation with IFN-γ, freshly isolated or cultured tubular epithelial cells can process and present nominal antigen, for example, hen-egg lysozyme (HEL), to MHC-restricted, antigen-specific T-cell hybridomas (13,67). T-cell hybridomas release IL-2 upon engagement of the TCR with processed HEL peptides that are presented by tubular epithelial cell class II molecules. The capacity of T-cell hybridomas to release IL-2 is clearly MHC class II dependent, as specific anti-class-II antibodies completely abrogate the response (13,75).

The release of IL-2 by T-cell hybridomas after exposure to MHC class-II-positive tubular epithelial cells plus antigen is substantially smaller when B cells or macrophages are used in control cocultures (13,67). This could be due to fewer MHC class II antigens on tubular epithelial cells, as it is known that class II density is important in determining the level of a T-cell proliferative response (76). On the other hand, a T-cell response may be elicited by as few as 200–300 MHC–peptide complexes, which may even be below the level of detection by standard immunofluoresence techniques (77). Furthermore, in comparison with classic APCs (macrophages and dendritic cells), tubular epithelial cells are very abundant in the kidney and may thus provide broad interaction with CD4+ T cells. This may account for antigen presentation by tubular epithelial cells even in situations of minimal expression of class II molecules.

Paraformaldehyde fixation of MHC class-II-bearing tubular epithelial cells does not abrogate antigen presentation if cells were previously exposed to native antigen, indicating antigen processing prior to presentation. However, tubular epithelial cells treated with paraformaldehyde prior to exposure to native antigen cannot stimulate T-cell hybridomas, indicating that a critical period is required for tubular epithelial cells to digest protein into immunogenic peptides (13). The level of stimulation by fixed cells is generally less than that of unfixed MHC class-II-bearing cells, which may reflect altered antigenic epitopes or damage to MHC molecules. Alternatively, it may be due to the reduced ability of tubular epithelial cells to provide a costimulatory signal.

Experiments using T-cell hybridomas are useful to assess whether a given cell has the capacity to process and present a foreign antigen. However, T-cell hybridomas are much less stringent in their requirement for costimulatory signals than are T-cell clones. Thus, while the presentation of antigen by tubular epithelial cells is sufficient to stimulate lymphokine production by T-cell hybridomas, additional costimulatory molecules are required to stimulate Th clones.

CD4+ T-cell clones do not proliferate in response to tubular epithelial cells presenting a foreign antigen but rather become anergic (78,79). This may be related to the absence of the costimulatory molecule B7 on tubular epithelial cells (17,78). T-cell clones exposed to MHC class-II-positive tubular epithelial cells and antigen will display some signs of activation, expressing IL-2 receptors, for example. This suggests that engagement by the TCR of MHC class II and antigen has occurred in this situation. The T cells will also remain viable and able to proliferate in response to exogenous IL-2. Overall, cumulative evidence suggests that processing and presentation of foreign antigen by tubular epithelial cells does not elicit a proliferative T-cell response in vivo but rather antigen-specific nonproliferation.

Self-Antigen Presentation by Tubular Epithelial Cells

In addition to foreign antigen presentation, tubular epithelial cells can present autoantigens to T cells. This has led to the speculation that tubular epithelial cells could initiate or participate in autoimmune nephritogenic responses (80,81). In vitro experiments have shown that tubular epithelial cells expressing 3M-1, a target antigen of autoimmune interstitial nephritis, can specifically process and present this self-antigen to nephritogenic 3M-1-reactive helper T cells in the context of MHC class II (14). Similarly, self-antigen can be presented to T-cell hybridomas by freshly isolated tubular epithelial cells (67). Tubular epithelial cells obtained from mice transgenic for the human α_1-antitrypsin can present antigen to an α_1-antitrypsin-specific T-cell hybridoma without the addition of exogenous α_1-antitrypsin to the culture system. Introduction of the α_1-antitrypsin transgene results in tolerance to α_1-antitrypsin. Thus, α_1-antitrypsin can be considered a self-antigen and T-cell hybridomas are capable of recognizing this antigen in the context of self-MHC.

We established that autoreactive T-cell clones from the kidney of MRL-*lpr* mice exclusively proliferate to renal cells. These T cells could have autoreactive potential in murine lupus nephritis (82,83). Interestingly, IFN-γ stimulation of tubular epithelial cells downregulates proliferation of these autoreactive clones, suggesting that in certain situations complex self-regulating mechanisms are elicited to limit autoreactive T-cell expansion (84).

T-Cell Recognition of Allogeneic Tubular Epithelial Cell Antigens

T-cell recognition of allogeneic MHC molecules as foreign peptides is enigmatic. Since tubular epithelial cells can express abundant surface MHC class II molecules, the question arises whether these molecules are capable of eliciting an allogeneic response in mixed-lymphocyte-type reactions. Results in human and canine systems have generated conflicting data. In some studies, tubular epithelial cells were moderately good stimulators in mixed-lymphocyte–kidney-cell cultures, and T cells proliferated to tubular epithelial cells from rejected allografts (85–87). In other studies, not only were poor allogeneic responses observed despite treatment of kidney cells with IFN-γ and surface expression of class II molecules, but, in some instances, these kidney cells became inhibitory to mixed-lymphocyte reactions (66). As with foreign antigens, T-cell activation and proliferation requires appropriate costimulatory signals in addition to the presentation of tubular epithelial cell alloantigens to activate a T cell fully.

Importance of Costimulatory Molecules in T-Cell Activation by Tubular Epithelial Cells

The T-cell response depends not only on the intensity of the TCR/CD3 signal (signal 1) but also on the nature and strength of the costimulatory signal provided by APCs (signal 2). The presence or absence of tubular epithelial cell costimulatory and accessory molecules is a crucial feature whereby the type of T-cell response will be influenced. Experiments have documented that the tubular epithelial cell molecule ICAM-1 is required to induce and maintain a proliferative T-cell hybridoma response (75). It is probable that additional tubular epithelial cell molecules such as LFA-3 (88) and VCAM-1 (51,89) also influence T-cell responses.

Interestingly, the important costimulatory molecule B7 is absent from tubular epithelial cells and cannot be induced (78,79). It appears that the crucial B7–CD28 costimulatory pathway operates only in professional APCs such as macrophages and B cells. Thus, interaction of tubular epithelial cells with T cells through B7–CD28 or CTLA-4 does not occur in vitro and in vivo, thereby depriving tubular epithelial cells of an essential costimulatory pathway.

To elucidate the importance of the B7–CD28 interaction, we transfected B7 into tubular epithelial cells and tested foreign antigen presentation to T-cell hybridomas and to T-cell clones (17). T-cell hybridomas could easily be induced to proliferate to antigen and MHC class-II-positive, B7-positive tubular epithelial cells, whereas T-cell clones did not proliferate to class-II-positive tubular epithelial cells plus antigen even in the presence of B7. By contrast, T-cell clones exposed to B7-positive tubular epithelial cells were not anergic since they could be stimulated to proliferate to antigen-pulsed spleen cells. Thus, T-cell clones became immunologically "ignorant." Interestingly, cocultivation of IFN-γ-stimulated (class-II-positive), antigen-pulsed, B7+ tubular epithelial cells with Th1 cells that had been stimulated through the TCR by using anti-CD3 monoclonal antibody (mAb) caused these Th1 cells to proliferate, a response that was blocked by anti-CD28 and anti-B7 mAb. In another system, transfection of B7 into tubular epithelial cells was sufficient to confer proliferative responses to Th1 helper clones (78). When cultured human tubular epithelial cells are examined for alloantigen presentation in mixed cultures of IFN-γ-stimulated allogeneic tubular epithelial cells and lymphocytes, T-cell stimulation occurs only in the presence of costimulation with anti-CD28 mAb ligation (68). Together, these results suggest that the spectrum of T helper cell (Th1) activation after encountering antigen presented by tubular epithelial cells is broad and is dictated by elements controlling the strength of the TCR/CD3 signal (signal 1) and by the presence or absence of costimulatory signals through the B7–CD28 pathway (signal 2).

Tubular epithelial cells express a number of cytokines that could influence T-cell activation, including TNF-α, IL-6, and TGF-β. IL-1, the second signal for Th2 cell activation, is not produced by tubular epithelial cells. TNF-α production in tubular epithelial cells has been a well-documented response to IL-1 and lipopolysaccharide (65,90), in MRL-*lpr* and NZB/W lupus nephritis (91, 92), and in allograft rejection (93). TNF-α has been shown to enhance T-cell proliferative responses to IL-2 secondary to enhanced expression of IL-2R and to increase T-cell-mediated immune responses to antigen challenge (94–96). IL-6 and TGF-β are additional cytokines that could augment or modify the T-cell response to tubular epithelial cells presenting antigen. However, studies examining the impact of soluble or membrane-bound cytokines in antigen presentation by tubular epithelial cells have not been performed.

The absence in vivo of the B7 antigen on tubular epithelial cells may represent a mechanism whereby T-cell anergy is induced in vivo and may lead to peripheral tolerance. Anergy could be preferred over proliferation and could be biologically protective following random T-cell contact with renal parenchymal cells (97). Then how does autoimmune renal disease or allograft rejection ever occur? It is conceivable that the initiation and maintenance of anergy is a regulated process and that an imbalance of anergic and activating signals might result in autoimmune injury or graft rejection (98).

ANTIGEN PRESENTATION BY OTHER RESIDENT AND NONRESIDENT RENAL CELLS

Few studies have examined antigen presentation by other resident renal cells. Mesangial cells and glomerular visceral epithelial cells are among the resident cells that have been examined for antigen presentation abilities and were indeed found capable of such a mechanism (49,99). However, it is likely that other renal cells are also capable of altering T-cell responses.

Mesangial cells are readily accessible to many cellular and noncellular challenges by virtue of their strategic location in the glomerulus. It is not surprising that mesangial cells have a broad range of functions sharing several properties characteristic of macrophages and endothelial and smooth muscle cells. Mesangial cells secrete cytokines (IL-1, IL-6, IL-10, and TNF-α), phagocytose immune complexes, synthesize prostaglandins, and release reactive oxygen species and nitric oxide. Since mesangial cells are capable of expressing MHC class II products, it has been suggested that mesangial cells may also function as APCs (100). We have established SV4-transformed clonal lines of mesangial cells and have examined these cells for class II expression and accessory functions (49). Clonal lines of mesangial cells do not constitutively express MHC class II but express ICAM-1. Induction with IFN-γ readily induces class II in these cells. IFN-γ and other cytokines such as TNF-α and IL-1 upregulate the accessory molecules ICAM-1 and VCAM-1 in murine mesangial cells (49,57). Mesangial cells are capable of presenting the foreign antigen HEL to T-cell hybridomas in vitro. The T-cell activation induced by mesangial APCs can be blocked with monoclonal antibodies targeting MHC class II antigens and ICAM-1. This accessory molecule not only promotes adherence of T-cell hybridomas, but augments T-cell proliferation. Whether VCAM-1 also functions as an accessory molecule in mesangial cells has not been investigated to date.

Rat glomerular visceral epithelial cells have been examined for antigen presentation (99). Upon stimulation with IFN-γ, they express MHC class II antigens. Processing and presentation of foreign proteins such as HEL occurs in a dose-dependent manner. Interestingly, molecular charge seems to influence antigen presentation by these cells.

Although endothelium can present antigen (101), studies using renal endothelial cells have not been performed. Thus, it remains to be established whether kidney endothelium may also participate in immune responses through antigen processing and presentation to T cells.

In addition to these resident cells, the kidney contains a number of interstitial cells capable of antigen presentation. Interstitial cells are heterogeneous, comprising resident fibroblasts and nonresident dendritic cells and macrophages ("passenger leukocytes") (102). Since these cells express MHC class II molecules, it is likely that they can process and present antigen to T cells. A role for passenger leukocytes is suggested by studies in rats fed a diet deficient in essential fatty acids. This diet causes depletion of passenger leukocytes and prevents renal allograft rejection (103). Additional studies are required to examine the role of resident renal cells and passenger leukocytes in T-cell responses and to establish a causal relationship between antigen presentation and immune renal injury.

ANTIGEN PRESENTATION AND RENAL DISEASES

The renal antigens instrumental in promoting or preventing injury are largely unknown. In kdkd mice, spontaneous interstitial nephritis occurs with an influx of T lymphocytes that bear specificity for a 56-kD glycoprotein component of tubular basement membrane (104). In an induced model of tubulointerstitial nephritis, a unique 30- to 48-kD tubular basement membrane glycoprotein

(3M-1) can be presented to specific T-cell clones and appears to be the target for the disease (14).

Proximal tubular epithelial cell MHC class II expression has been reported in allograft rejection, graft-versus-host disease, and autoimmune and ischemic renal injury. It has been speculated that the expression of MHC class II molecules on tubular epithelial cells initiates organ-specific autoimmune disease by facilitating the presentation of tissue-specific self-antigens to autoreactive CD4+ T cells. Recent experiments have been designed to determine whether MHC class II molecules on tubular epithelial cells are capable of inducing a proliferative T-cell response. Jevnikar et al. have transplanted murine kidneys from transgenic mice expressing the MHC class II molecule I-E abundantly on proximal tubular epithelial cells into bilaterally nephrectomized F_1 hybrids. The transplant recipients maintained stable weights and serum creatinines, and did not become proteinuric. When transplanted mice were killed 5–9 months later, the proximal tubular epithelial cell expression of I-E was maintained, and the kidney was histologically normal without evidence of inflammatory cell infiltrates (105). Thus, MHC class II alone on tubular epithelial cells does not initiate an immune renal injury, but may on the contrary protect the kidney by inducing anergy. On the other hand, MHC class-II-deficient MRL-*lpr* mice develop the characteristic lymphadenopathy but are protected from autoimmune renal disease and do not form autoantibodies (106). In this model, renal and systemic MHC class II expression appears critical for the development of autoaggressive CD4+ T cells, which have been implicated in autoimmune nephritis. These findings clearly dissociate the expansion of the characteristic double-negative T cells (CD4- and CD8-) and the autoimmune renal disease. The definitive importance of MHC class II antigens in autoimmune renal injury remains to be defined. Additional factors, including costimulatory pathways, cytokines, and differential development of Th1- or Th2-type responses, will most probably be implicated.

CONCLUDING REMARKS

Resident renal cells are capable of antigen presentation. An important concept has emerged recently from experimental studies, suggesting that MHC class-II-positive tubular epithelial cells do not necessarily induce a proliferative CD4+ helper T-cell response. In fact, tubular epithelial cells can induce antigen-specific, MHC class-II-restricted unresponsiveness or anergy. Because most individuals do not develop renal parenchymal disease, more signals must be delivered by renal cells to T cells that prevent activation and even induce tolerance than signals that promote T-cell activation. Thus, studies focusing on the interaction of renal parenchymal cells and T cells should not only identify the mechanisms for promoting renal disease, but will uncover crucial events responsible for the maintenance of immunologic tolerance and protection from autoimmune or allogeneic injury.

REFERENCES

1. Mayer L, Shlien R. Evidence for function of Ia molecules on gut epithelial cells in man. *J Exp Med* 1987;166:1471–83.
2. Santos LM, Lider O, Audette J, Khoury SJ, Weiner HL. Characterization of immunomodulatory properties and accessory cell function of small intestine epithelial cells. *Cell Immunol* 1990;127:26–34.
3. Czirjak L, Danko K, Gaulton GN, Stadecker MJ. Thyroid-derived epithelial cells acquire alloantigen-presenting capacities following X-irradiation and class II induction. *Eur J Immunol* 1990;20:2597–601.
4. Grubeck-Loebenstein B, Buchan G, Chantry D, et al. Analysis of intrathyroidal cytokine production in thyroid autoimmune disease: thyroid follicular cells produce interleukin-1 alpha and interleukin-6. *Clin Exp Immunol* 1989;77:324–30.
5. Kimura H, Davies TF. Thyroid specific T cells in the normal Wistar rat. I. Characterization of lymph node T cell reactivity to syngeneic thyroid cells and thyroglobulin. *Clin Immunol Immunopathol* 1991; 58:181–94.
6. Kimura H, Davies TF. Thyroid specific T cells in the normal Wistar rat. II. T cell clones interact with cloned Wistar rat thyroid cells and provide direct evidence of autoantigen presentation by thyroid epithelial cells. *Clin Immunol Immunopathol* 1991;58:195–206.
7. Stein ME, Stadecker MJ. Characterization and antigen-presenting function of a murine thyroid-derived epithelial cell line. *J Immunol* 1987;139:1786–91.
8. Campbell IL, Harrison LC. A new view of the beta cell as an antigen-presenting cell and immunogenic target. *J Autoimmun* 1990;3(Suppl): 53–62.
9. Lo D, Burkly LC, Widera G, et al. Diabetes and tolerance in transgenic mice expressing class II MHC molecules in pancreatic beta cells. *Cell* 1988;53:159–68.
10. Markmann J, Lo D, Naji A, Palmiter RD, Brinster RL, Heber-Katz E. Antigen presenting function of class II MHC expressing pancreatic beta cells. *Nature* 1988;336:476–9.
11. Tiku ML, Liu S, Weaver CW, Teodorescu M, Skosey JL. Class II histocompatibility antigen-mediated immunologic function of normal articular chondrocytes. *J Immunol* 1985;135:2923–7.
12. Rosenberg NL, Kotzin BL. Aberrant expression of class II MHC antigens by skeletal muscle endothelial cells in experimental autoimmune myositis. *J Immunol* 1989;142:4289–94.
13. Wüthrich RP, Glimcher LH, Yui MA, Jevnikar AM, Dumas SE, Kelley VE. Generation of highly differentiated murine renal tubular epithelial cell lines: MHC class II regulation, antigen presentation and tumor necrosis factor production. *Kidney Int* 1990;37:783–92.
14. Haverty TP, Kelly CJ, Hines WH, et al. Characterization of a renal tubular epithelial cell line which secretes the autologous target antigen of autoimmune experimental interstitial nephritis. *J Cell Biol* 1988;107:1359–68.
15. Rubin Kelley VE, Singer GG. The antigen presentation function of renal tubular epithelial cells. *Exp Nephrol* 1993;1:102–11.
16. Heeger PS, Neilson EG. Overcoming tolerance in autoimmune renal disease. *Curr Opinion Nephrol Hypertension* 1994;3:123–32.
17. Yokoyama H, Zheng X, Strom TB, Rubin Kelley VE. B7+-transfectant tubular epithelial cells induce T cell anergy, ignorance or proliferation. *Kidney Int* 1994;45:1105–12.
18. Allen PM. Antigen processing at the molecular level. *Immunol Today* 1987;8:270–3.
19. Hamilos DL. Antigen presenting cells. *Cell Immunol* 1989;8:98–117.
20. Elliott WL, Stille CJ, Thomas LJ, Humphreys RE. A hypothesis on the binding of an amphipathic α helical sequence in Ii to the desetope of class II antigens. *J Immunol* 1987;138:2949–52.
21. Neefjes JJ, Ploegh HL. Intracellular transport of MHC class II molecules. *Immunol Today* 1992;13:179–84.
22. Peters PJ, Neefjes JJ, Oorschot V, Ploegh H, Geuze HJ. Segregation of MHC class II molecules in the Golgi complex for transport to lysosomal compartments. *Nature* 1991;349:669–76.

23. Bjorkman PJ, Saper MA, Samraoui B, Bennett WS, Strominger JL, Wiley DC. Structure of the human class I histocompatibility antigen, HLA-A2. *Nature* 1987;329:506–12.
24. Bjorkman PJ, Saper MA, Samraoui B, Bennett WS, Strominger JL, Wiley DC. The foreign antigen binding site and T cell recognition regions of class I histocompatibility antigens. *Nature* 1987;329: 512–8.
25. Jardetzky TS, Brown JH, Gorga JC, et al. Three-dimensional structure of a human class II histocompatibility molecule complexed with superantigen. *Nature* 1994;368:711–8.
26. Allen PM, Strydon DJ, Unanue ER. Processing of lysozyme by macrophages: identification of the determinant recognized by two T cell hybridomas. *Proc Natl Acad Sci USA* 1984;81:2489–93.
27. Weiss A. Structure and function of the T cell antigen receptor. *J Clin Invest* 1990;86:1015–22.
28. Janeway CA, Bottomly K. Signals and signs for lymphocyte responses. *Cell* 1994;76:275–85.
29. Schwartz RH. Costimulation of T lymphocytes: the role of CD28, CTLA-4, and B7/BB1 in IL-2 production and immunotherapy. *Cell* 1992;71:1065–8.
30. Bretscher P, Cohn M. A theory of self–nonself discrimination: paralysis and induction involve the recognition of one and two determinants on an antigen, respectively. *Science* 1970;169:1042–9.
31. Bretscher P. The two-signal model of lymphocyte activation 21 years later. *Immunol Today* 1992;13:74–76.
32. Mueller DL, Jenkins MK, Schwartz RH. Clonal expansion versus functional clonal inactivation: a costimulatory signalling pathway determines the outcome of T cell antigen receptor occupancy. *Annu Rev Immunol* 1989;7:445–80.
33. Jenkins MK. Models of lymphocyte activation: the role of cell division in the induction of clonal anergy. *Immunol Today* 1992;13:69–73.
34. Mosmann TR, Cherwinski H, Bond MW, Giedlin MA, Coffman RL. Two types of murine helper T cell clone. 1. Definition according to profiles of lymphokine activities and secreted proteins. *J Immunol* 1986;136:2348–57.
35. Mosmann TR, Schumacher JH, Street NF, et al. Diversity of cytokine synthesis and function of mouse CD4+ T cells. *Immunol Rev* 1991; 123:209–29.
36. Seder RA, Paul WE. Acquisition of lymphokine-producing phenotype by CD4+ T cells. *Annu Rev Immunol* 1994;12:635–73.
37. Weaver CT, Hawrylowicz CM, Unanue ER. T helper cell subsets require expression of distinct costimulatory signals by antigen presenting cells. *Proc Natl Acad Sci USA* 1988;85:8181–5.
38. Weaver CT, Unanue ER. The costimulatory function of antigen presenting cells. *Immunol Today* 1990;11:49–55.
39. Springer TA. Adhesion receptors of the immune system. *Nature* 1990;346:425–34.
40. June CH, Bluestone JA, Nadler LM, Thompson CB. The B7 and CD28 receptor families. *Immunol Today* 1994;15:321–31.
41. Freeman GJ, Freedman AS, Segil JM, Lee G, Whitman JF, Nadler LM. B7, a new member of the Ig superfamily with unique expression on activated and neoplastic B cells. *J Immunol* 1989;143:2714–22.
42. Freeman GJ, Gray GS, Gimmi CD, et al. Structure, expression, and T cell costimulatory activity of the murine homologue of the human B lymphocyte activation antigen B7. *J Exp Med* 1991;174:625–31.
43. Azuma M, Ito D, Yagita H, et al. B70 antigen is a second ligand for CTLA-4 and CD28. *Nature* 1993;366:76–9.
44. Freeman GJ, Gribben JG, Boussiotis VA, et al. Cloning of B7-2: a CTLA-4 counterreceptor that costimulates human T cell proliferation. *Science* 1993;262:909–11.
45. June CH, Ledbetter JA, Linsley PS, Thompson CB. Role of the CD28 receptor in T-cell activation. *Immunol Today* 1990;11:211–6.
46. Linsley PS, Brady W, Urnes M, Grosmaire LS, Damle NK, Ledbetter JA. CTLA-4 is a second receptor for the B cell activation antigen B7. *J Exp Med* 1991;174:561–9.
47. Rothlein R, Dustin ML, Springer TA. A human intercellular adhesion molecule (ICAM-1) distinct from LFA-1. *J Immunol* 1986;137: 1270–4.
48. Staunton DE, Marlin SD, Stratowa C, Dustin ML, Springer TA. Primary structure of ICAM-1 demonstrates interaction between members of the immunoglobulin and integrin supergene family. *Cell* 1988; 52:925–33.
49. Brennan DC, Jevnikar AM, Takei F, Rubin-Kelley VE. Mesangial cell accessory functions: mediation by intercellular adhesion molecule-1. *Kidney Int* 1990;38:1039–46.
50. Wüthrich RP, Jevnikar AM, Takei F, Glimcher LH, Kelley VE. Intercellular adhesion molecule-1 (ICAM-1) is upregulated in autoimmune lupus nephritis. *Am J Pathol* 1990;136:441–50.
51. Damle NK, Aruffo A. Vascular cell adhesion molecule-1 induces T cell antigen receptor-dependent activation of CD4+ T lymphocytes. *Proc Natl Acad Sci* USA 1991;88:6403–7.
52. Osborn L, Hession C, Tizard R, et al. Direct expression cloning of vascular cell adhesion molecule-1, a cytokine-induced endothelial protein that binds to lymphocytes. *Cell* 1989;59:1203–11.
53. Hession C, Tizard R, Vassallo C, et al. Cloning of an alternate form of vascular cell adhesion molecule-1 (VCAM-1). *J Biol Chem* 1991; 266:6682–5.
54. Moy P, Lobb R, Tizard R, Olson D, Hession C. Cloning of an inflammation-specific phosphatidylinositol-linked form of murine vascular cell adhesion molecule-1. *J Biol Chem* 1993;268:8835–41.
55. Elices MJ, Osborn L, Takada Y, Hemler ME, Loo R. VCAM-1 on activated endothelium interacts with the leukocyte integrin VLA-4 at a site distinct from the VLA-4/fibronectin binding site. *Cell* 1990;60: 577–84.
56. Miyake K, Weissman IL, Greenberger JS, Kincade PW. Evidence for a role of the integrin VLA-4 in lympho-hemopoiesis. *J Exp Med* 1991;173:599–607.
57. Wüthrich RP. Vascular cell adhesion molecule-1 (VCAM-1) expression in murine lupus nephritis. *Kidney Int* 1992;42:903–14.
58. Jenkins MK, Schwartz RH. Antigen presentation by chemically modified splenocytes induces antigen-specific T cell unresponsiveness in vitro and in vivo. *J Exp Med* 1987;165:302–19.
59. Schwartz RH. A cell culture model for T lymphocyte clonal anergy. *Science* 1990;248:1349–56.
60. Jenkins MK, Ashwell JD, Schwartz RH. Allogeneic non-T spleen cells restore the responsiveness of normal T cell clones stimulated with antigen and chemically modified antigen-presenting cells. *J Immunol* 1988;140:3324–30.
61. Schwartz RH. Acquisition of immunologic self-tolerance. *Cell* 1989; 57:1073–81.
62. Von Boehmer H, Kisielow P. Self–nonself discrimination by T cells. *Science* 1990;248:1369–73.
63. Schonrich G, Kalinke U, Momburg F, et al. Downregulation of T cell receptors on self-reactive T cells as a novel mechanism for extrathymic tolerance induction. *Cell* 1991;65:293–304.
64. Haverty TP, Watanabe M, Neilson EG, Kelly J. Protective modulation of class II MHC gene expression in tubular epithelium by target antigen-specific antibodies: cell surface directed down-regulation of transcription can influence susceptibility to murine tubulointerstitial nephritis. *J Immunol* 1989;143:1133–41.
64a. Sprent J, Webb S. Can self/nonself discrimination be explained entirely by clonal deletion? *Res Immunol* 1992;143:285–7.
65. Wüthrich RP, Yui MA, Mazoujian G, Nabavi N, Glimcher LH, Kelley VE. Enhanced MHC class II expression in renal proximal tubules precedes loss of renal function in MRL/lpr mice with lupus nephritis. *Am J Pathol* 1989;134:45–51.
66. Bishop GA, Waugh JA, Hall BM. Expression of HLA antigens on renal tubular cells in culture. II. Effect of increased HLA antigen expression on tubular cell stimulation of lymphocyte activation and on their vulnerability to cell-mediated lysis. *Transplantation* 1988;46: 303–10.
67. Hagerty DT, Allen PM. Processing and presentation of self and foreign antigens by the renal proximal tubule. *J Immunol* 1992;148:2324–30.
68. Wilson JL, Proud G, Forsythe JLR, Taylor RMR, Kirby JA. Renal allograft rejection: tubular epithelial cells present alloantigen in the presence of costimulatory CD28 antibody. *Transplantation* 1995;59: 91–7.
69. Rubin Kelley VE, Jevnikar AM. Antigen presentation by renal tubular epithelial cells. *J Am Soc Nephrol* 1991;2:13–26.
70. Halloran PF, Autenried P, Wadgymar A. Regulation of HLA antigen expression in human kidney. *Clin Immunol Allergy* 1986;6:411–35.
71. Halloran PF, Madrenas J. Regulation of MHC transcription. *Transplantation* 1990;50:725–38.
72. Basta PV, Sherman PA, Ting JPY. Detailed delineation of an interferon-γ-responsive element important in human HLA-DRα gene expression in a glioblastoma multiform line. *Proc Natl Acad Sci USA* 1988;85:8618–22.

73. Amaldi I, Reith W, Berte C, Mach B. Induction of HLA class II genes by IFN-γ is transcriptional and requires a trans-acting protein. *J Immunol* 1989;142:999–1004.
74. Böttger EC, Blanar MA, Flavell RA. Cycloheximide, an inhibitor of protein synthesis, prevents γ-interferon-induced expression of class II mRNA in a macrophage cell line. *Immunogenetics* 1988;28:215–20.
75. Jevnikar AM, Wüthrich RP, Takei F, et al. Differing regulation and function of ICAM-1 and class II antigens on renal tubular cells. *Kidney Int* 1990;38:417–25.
76. Janeway CA, Bottomly K, Babich J, et al. Quantitative variation in Ia expression plays a central role in immune regulation. *Immunol Today* 1984;5:99–105.
77. Harding CV, Unanue ER. Quantitation of antigen presenting cell MHC class II/peptide complexes necessary for T cell stimulation. *Nature* 1990;346:574–6.
78. Hagerty DT, Evavold BD, Allen PM. Regulation of the costimulator B7, not class II major histocompatibility complex, restricts the ability of murine kidney tubule cells to stimulate CD4+ T cells. *J Clin Invest* 1994;93:1208–15.
79. Singer GG, Yokoyama H, Bloom RD, Jevnikar M, Nabavi N, Rubin Kelley VE. Stimulated renal tubular epithelial cells induce anergy in CD4+ T cells. *Kidney Int* 1993;44:1030–5.
80. Bloom RD, Weiss R, Madaio MP. The nephritogenic immune response. *Curr Opin Nephrol Hypertension* 1993;2:441–8.
81. Meyers CM. T cell regulation of renal immune responses. *Curr Opin Nephrol Hypertension* 1995;4:270–6.
82. Diaz-Gallo C, Jevnikar AM, Brennan DC, Florquin S, Pacheo-Silva A, Rubin Kelley VE. Autoreactive kidney-infiltrating T cell clones in murine lupus nephritis. *Kidney Int* 1992;42:851–9.
83. Kelley VR, Diaz-Gallo C, Jevnikar AM, Singer GG. Renal tubular epithelial and T cell interactions in autoimmune renal disease. *Kidney Int* 1993;43(Suppl 39):S108–15.
84. Diaz-Gallo C, Kelley VR. Self-regulation of autoreactive kidney-infiltrating T cells in MRL-*lpr* nephritis. *Kidney Int* 1993;44:692–9.
85. Roth D, Fuller L, Esquenazi V, Kyriakides GK, Pardo V, Miller J. The biologic significance of the mixed lymphocyte kidney culture in humans. *Transplantation* 1985;40:376–83.
86. Esquenazi V, Fuller L, Pardo V, Roth D, Milgrom M, Miller J. In vivo and in vitro induction of class II molecules on canine renal cells and their effect on the mixed lymphocyte kidney cell culture. *Transplantation* 1987;44:680–92.
87. Ranjan D, Roth D, Esquenazi V, et al. The effects of tissue-associated and MHC class II antigen presentation on in vitro lymphoproliferative responses against canine liver and kidney cell subpopulations. *Transplantation* 1991;51:475–80.
88. Moingeon P, Chang HC, Wallner BP, Stebbins C, Frey AZ, Reinherz EL. CD2-mediated adhesion facilitates T lymphocyte antigen recognition function. *Nature* 1989;339:312–4.
89. Van Seventer GA, Newman W, Shimizu Y, et al. Analysis of T cell stimulation by superantigen plus MHC class II molecules or by CD3 monoclonal antibody: costimulation by purified adhesion ligands VCAM-1, ICAM-1, but not ELAM-1. *J Exp Med* 1991;174:901–13.
90. Jevnikar AM, Brennan DC, Singer GG, et al. Stimulated kidney tubular epithelial cells express membrane associated and secreted TNF-α. *Kidney Int* 1991;40:203–11.
91. Boswell JM, Yui MA, Burt DW, Kelley VE. Increased tumor necrosis factor and interleukin-1 gene expression in the kidneys of mice with lupus nephritis. *J Immunol* 1988;141:3050–4.
92. Brennan DC, Yui MA, Wüthrich RP, Kelley VE. Tumor necrosis factor and IL-1 in New Zealand black/white mice: enhanced gene expression and acceleration of renal injury. *J Immunol* 1989;143:3470–5.
93. Yard BA, Daha MR, Kooymans-Couthino M, et al. IL-1α-stimulated TNF-α production by cultured human proximal tubular epithelial cells. *Kidney Int* 1992;42:383–9.
94. Lee JC, Truneh A, Smith MF, Tsang KY. Induction of interleukin 2 receptor (Tac) by tumor necrosis factor in YT cells. *J Immunol* 1987;139:1935–8.
95. Hurme M. Both interleukin 1 and tumor necrosis factor enhance thymocyte proliferation. *Eur J Immunol* 1988;18:1303–6.
96. Ranges GE, Bombara MP, Aiyer RA, Rice GG, Palladino MA. Tumor necrosis factor-α as a proliferative signal for an IL-2 dependent T cell line: strict species specificity of action. *J Immunol* 1989;142:1203–8.
97. Neilson EG. Is immunologic tolerance self modulated through antigen presentation by parenchymal epithelium? *Kidney Int* 1993;44:927–31.
98. Nickerson P, Steurer W, Steiger J, Zheng X, Steele AW, Strom TB. Cytokines and the Th1/Th2 paradigm in transplantation. *Curr Opin Immunol* 1994;6:757–64.
99. Mendrick DL, Kelly DM, Rennke HG. Antigen processing and presentation by glomerular visceral epithelium in vitro. *Kidney Int* 1991;39:71–8.
100. Martin M, Schewinzer R, Schellekens H, Resch K. Glomerular mesangial cells in local inflammation: induction of the expression of MHC class II antigens by IFN-γ. *J Immunol* 1989;142:1887–94.
101. Cotran RS, Pober JS. Effects of cytokines on vascular endothelium: their role in vascular and immune injury. *Kidney Int* 1989;35:969–75.
102. Kaissling B, Le Hir M. Characterization and distribution of interstitial cell types in the renal cortex of rats. *Kidney Int* 1994;45:709–20.
103. Schreiner GF, Flye W, Brunt E, Korber K, Lefkowith JB. Essential fatty acid depletion of renal allografts and prevention of rejection. *Science* 1988;240:1032–3.
104. Kelly CJ, Korngold R, Mann R, Clayman MD, Haverty TP, Neilson EG. Spontaneous nephritis in kdkd mice. II. Characterization of a tubular antigen specific, H-2k restricted Lyt-2+ effector T cell that mediates destructive tubulointerstitial injury. *J Immunol* 1986;136:526–31.
105. Jevnikar AM, Singer GG, Coffman T, Glimcher LH, Rubin Kelley VE. Transgenic tubular cell expression of class II is insufficient to initiate immune renal injury. *J Am Soc Nephrol* 1992;3:1972–7.
106. Jevnikar AM, Grusby MJ, Glimcher LH. Prevention of nephritis in MHC class II-deficient MRL-*lpr* mice. *J Exp Med* 1994;179:1137–43.

Immunologic Renal Diseases,
edited by E. G. Neilson and W. G. Couser.
Lippincott-Raven Publishers, Philadelphia © 1997.

CHAPTER 9

Membrane Protein Antigens and Other Molecules on Glomerular Cells

Dontscho Kerjaschki

INTRODUCTION

Although much of what is known about immunologically mediated renal injury has been derived from studies of models induced by antibodies to various extracellular matrix components (see Chapter 34), there is increasing evidence, much of it experimental, that antigen-specific immune reactions directed against molecules expressed on the membranes of renal cells (Fig. 1) are important in the pathogenesis of some types of renal disease. Other molecules, such as integrins and podocalyxin, play significant roles in modulating the glomerular response to injury, and still others may be expressed *de novo* in disease as a consequence of injury. In the glomerulus, the classic example is membranous nephropathy induced in rats by antibodies to both protein and glycolipid antigens on the membrane of the glomerular epithelial cell, such as the Heymann nephritis antigenic complex (HNAC). This system is reviewed in detail elsewhere in this book (see Chapters 34 and 37). Whereas antibodies to the HNAC induce injury through activation of the complement system, a variety of monoclonal antibodies directed at other glomerular epithelial cell membrane antigens can trigger a marked alteration in glomerular permeability through a direct effect independent of complement—probably an effect on glomerular epithelial cell activation, adhesion, or both. These studies are also reviewed elsewhere in this book (see Chapters 16 and 30).

The discovery of the Thy-1.1 antigen on glomerular mesangial cells led to the development of the most extensively studied model of immune mesangial injury (antithymocyte-serum model), a model that has provided a wealth of data on the mesangial response to injury, including the roles of platelet growth factors, cytokines, oxidants, proteases, and other mediators in this process (see Chapters 28, 34, and 42). Other mesangial cell membrane proteins have been less well characterized but will likely be elucidated in the near future. To date, there is only one well-defined model of glomerular injury induced by antibodies to antigens expressed on the glomerular endothelial cell (1), although studies of lung injury induced by anti-angiotensin-converting enzyme antibody has taught us much about the kinetics and consequences of immune deposit formation on microvascular endothelium (2). Chapters 29 and 53 review endothelial cell-specific proteins in more detail.

In humans, the study of the role of anti-cell membrane antibodies and cellular reactivity in immune renal disease is still in its infancy. Some antibodies to human glomerular epithelial cells have been reported in selected patients with membranous nephropathy (3), but the principal antibody in the idiopathic form of membranous nephropathy remains elusive (see Chapter 47). Anti-mesangial cell antibodies have been reported by several groups in diseases based in the mesangium, such as IgA nephropathy and Henoch-Schönlein purpura (4,5), and these may contribute to clinical disease. Similarly, there is a growing literature on the presence of anti-endothelial antibodies in a variety of human renal diseases, including lupus nephritis, IgA nephropathy, hemolytic uremic syndrome, ANCA-positive vasculitis, and others (6–8).

Because it is likely that future studies in humans will establish important roles for these proteins, this chapter reviews the technical aspects of the method for isolating and characterizing such proteins and also summarizes some of the results obtained thus far, including identification of a heterogeneous group of amphophilic glomerular proteins, such as β_1-integrin in podocytes (9) and a novel endothelial antigen related to anti-neutrophil antibody

D. Kerjaschki: Institute of Clinical Pathology, University of Vienna, A-1090 Vienna, Austria

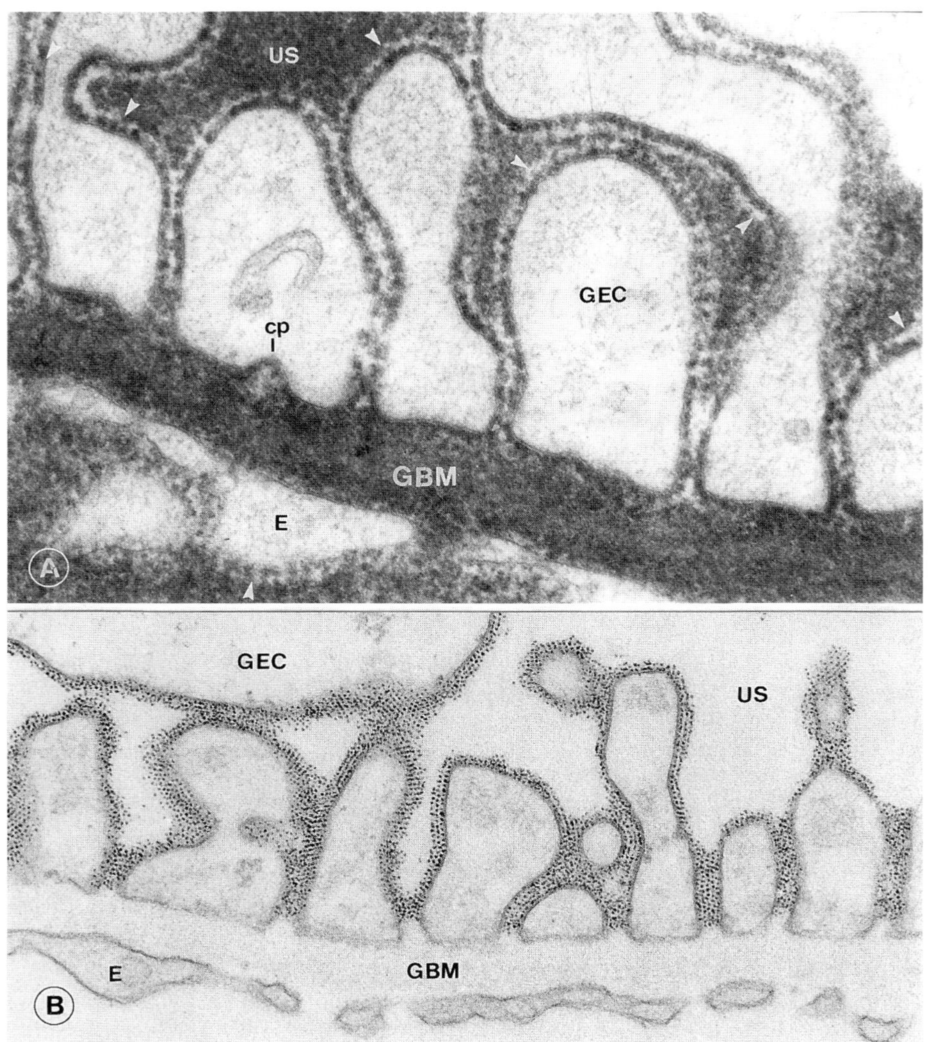

FIG. 1. A: Demonstration of the glycocalyx of the foot processes of rat glomerular epithelial cells. To obtain a "negative staining effect" of the cell surfaces in vivo, horseradish peroxidase was injected intravenously, and after 3 minutes renal cortex was fixed by intraparenchymal injection of hypertonic aldehyde solution, thus trapping the tracer while passing the glomerular filter. This was followed by standard histochemical detection of the enzyme tracer by the diaminobenzidine, yielding an electron-dense reaction product. The surface of podocytes is studded with repetitive units of globular units (*arrowheads*), which are aligned at a fairly constant distance of 200 Å to the cell membrane. A less regular surface coat is also present on the endothelial cell membrane (*E*). **B:** The anionic charges on the surface of podocytes are intensely labeled by polycationic ferritin, which was applied by incubation of unfixed isolated glomeruli. *cp,* coated pit; *US,* urinary space; *GBM,* glomerular basement membrane. × 45,000.

(ANCA) in human glomeruli (8). The major glomerular sialoglycoprotein podocalyxin (10) and proteins synthesized and integrated into glomerular cell membranes as a consequence of immune attack (11) have been enriched by this method.

GLOMERULAR MEMBRANE PROTEIN FRACTIONS

Purification of membrane proteins from intact isolated glomeruli is complicated by the fact that several different types of glomerular cells (epithelial, endothelial, and mesangial) are firmly attached to the glomerular basement membrane and the mesangial matrix. Therefore, conventional membrane fractionation techniques were not practical for isolated glomeruli, but they were successfully employed for cultured glomerular cells (12).

Ideally, a purification protocol for membrane proteins from isolated intact glomeruli should provide efficient detachment of cell membranes from their connections with the extracellular matrix, should remove extrinsic membrane proteins, and positively select for amphophilic proteins that contain membrane-spanning domains. A two-step protocol has been devised that fulfills to some extent these requirements (9). This protocol is described here in some detail, because it could also be useful for analysis of other glomerular membrane proteins.

A Two-Step Protocol for Enrichment of Amphophilic Proteins from Isolated Glomeruli

In a *first step*, freshly isolated rat or human glomeruli were prepared by standard sieving protocols to yield glomerular fractions more than 90% pure. When isolated glomeruli were incubated with 200 mM sodium carbonate (Na_2CO_3) (pH ≈11.5), they disintegrated into fractions consisting of glomerular basement membrane/mesangial matrix, soluble proteins, and small membrane vesicles (Fig. 2). Treatment at high pH was shown to solubilize peripheral, non-transmembrane membrane proteins efficiently while intrinsic transmembrane membrane proteins were retained within membranes of cellular organelles (13). The glomerular basement membrane fractions were collected by low-speed centrifugation, and the membrane vesicles were pelleted by ultracentrifugation (Fig. 2). The vesicular fraction, apparently derived from intercellular and surface membranes of glomerular cells (and presumably also from tubular contaminants), contained cytoplasmic proteins as observed by electron microscopy. To remove these undesired contaminants, it was necessary to introduce a *second step* based on detergent-phase partition (14), in which amphophilic transmembrane proteins with hydrophobic sequences were separated from hydrophilic content proteins. Glomerular membrane vesicles were solubilized in Triton X-114 at 4°C to form small, soluble

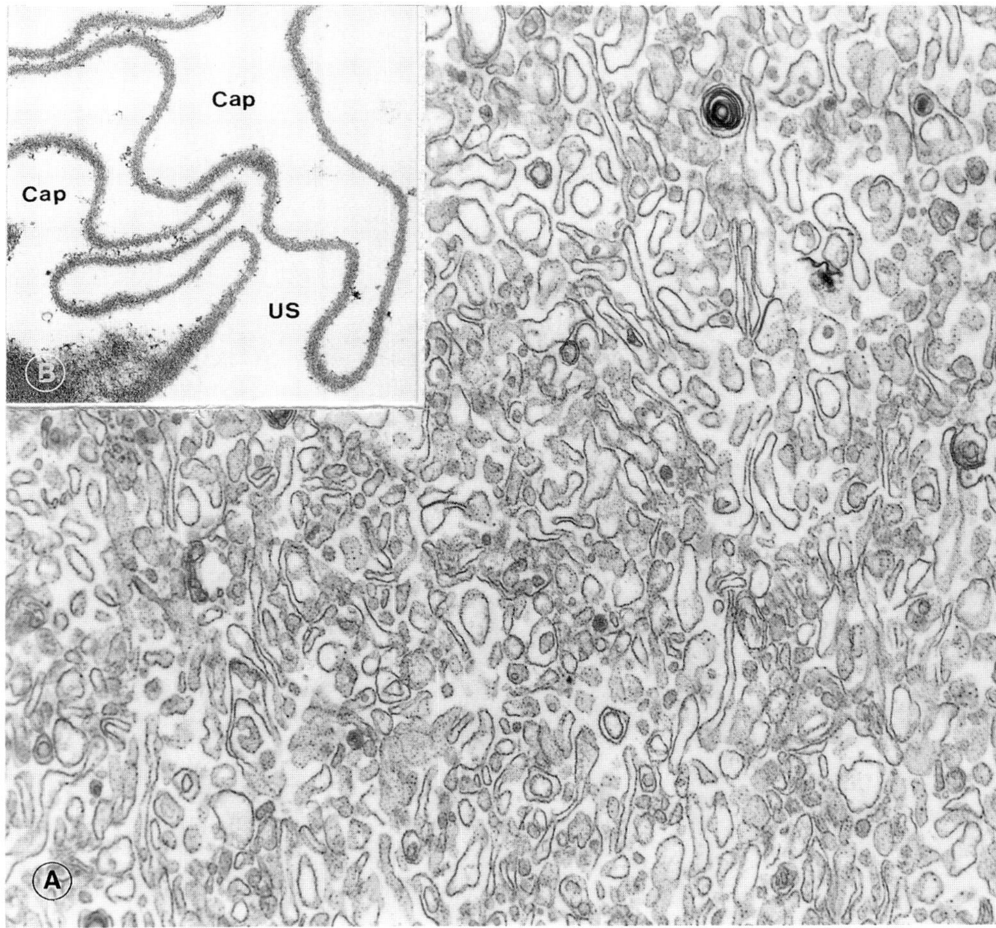

FIG. 2. A: Membrane vesicles are released from isolated glomeruli at high pH. Representative view of a fraction of membrane vesicles obtained from isolated human glomeruli in the first step of the purification procedure by incubation in 200 mM Na2CO3 (pH ≈11.5). Many vesicles contained amorphous and fibrillar material, which was eliminated in a second step of the purification protocol by detergent-phase partitition with Triton X-114, resulting in a concentration of amphophilic membrane proteins. **B:** The glomerular basement membrane is stripped of all cellular material by the high-pH incubation. *US,* urinary space; *cap,* glomerular capillary lumen. A, × 120,000; B, × 25,000.

micellae. Warming to 37°C caused formation and precipitation of large micellae that carried membrane proteins with substantial hydrophobic amino acid sequences. The enrichment of rat glomerular proteins prepared by a one-step Triton X-114 extraction was used previously to raise monoclonal antibodies (15,16).

In summary, this two-step fractionation procedure selects for intrinsic transmembrane proteins, because extrinsic membrane-attached proteins are released because of the high-pH environment. The second step enriches by Triton X-114-phase partition for amphophilic proteins with hydrophobic sequences that concentrate in the detergent-rich phase.

Fractionation of Glomeruli Radiolabeled *In Situ*

Combination of this fractionation technique with *in situ* radiolabeling of glomeruli is useful to determine the localization of membrane proteins. A simple example is given in Figure 3, in which selective radio-iodination of membrane proteins facing the glomerular basement membrane (17) was combined with membrane protein isolation. Briefly, isolated rat kidneys were perfused with the cationic enzyme myeloperoxidase, which was arrested by anionically charged proteoglycans within the glomerular basement membrane. Perfusion was continued with glucose/glucose oxidase and ^{125}I to label tyrosine residues of proteins by myeloperoxidase-mediated halogenation. This resulted in almost selective labeling of basement membrane matrix (Fig. 3), and presumably also of proteins of adjacent membranes of podocytes and endothelial and mesangial cells. Glomeruli were subsequently isolated and subjected to the two-step membrane protein fractionation process, resulting in a greatly simplified pattern of radiolabeled membrane proteins obtained by autoradiography (Fig. 4). These proteins comprise β_1-integrin and several other undefined proteins that presumably face the glomerular basement membrane. The picture obtained may be incomplete, because some membrane proteins may be inaccessible to radioiodination reagents or lack available tyrosine residues. Nevertheless, this protocol permits a first approximation for a molecular analysis of topographically defined glomerular membrane proteins.

The techniques outlined potentially offer the means to establish systematic inventories of human and animal glomerular proteins, especially when combined with N-terminal amino acid sequence analysis and antibody production for precise localization. Obviously, such a "glomerular membrane protein project" is beyond the reach of individual laboratories and calls for a concerted action.

EXAMPLES OF GLOMERULAR MEMBRANE PROTEINS ENRICHED BY THE TWO-STEP FRACTIONATION PROCEDURE

In this section, a heterogenous group of glomerular membrane proteins are discussed that were enriched by the two-step purification protocol. The list comprises several already-defined proteins, such as β_1-integrin, podocalyxin, and cytochrome β_{558} in proteinuric rats with Heymann nephritis, as well as a novel human endothelial antigenic target of ANCA.

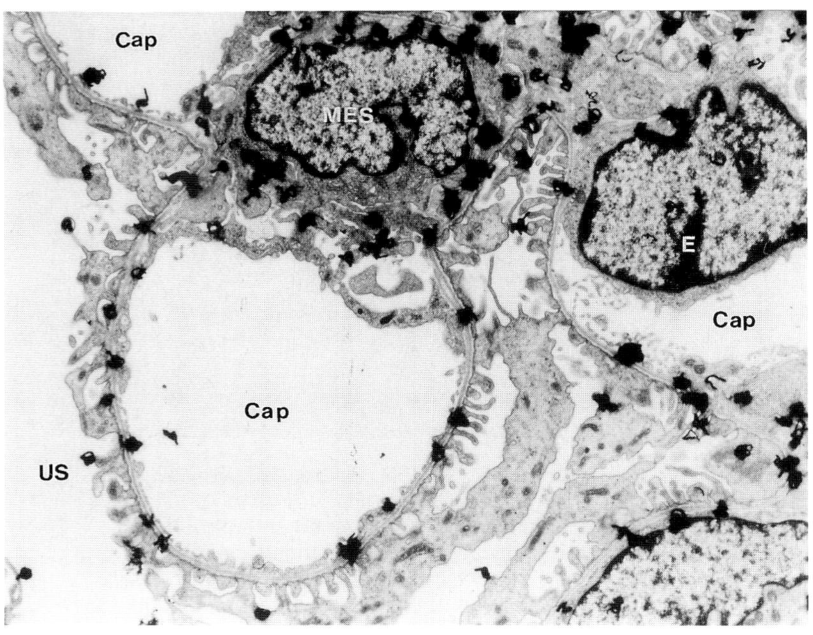

FIG. 3. *In situ* radiolabeling of the glomerular basement membrane and adjacent cell membranes. Proteins labeled with ^{125}I were localized to the glomerular basement membrane and the mesangial matrix by autoradiography. Isolated rat kidneys were perfused in vitro with myeloperoxidase (which adheres to the basement membranes by virtue of its cationic charge), followed by glucose/glucose oxidase as H_2O_2 donor, and ^{125}I. Presumably, the proteins of epithelial, endothelial, and mesangial cell membranes are also radiolabeled. (Specimen prepared by R. Jonson and W. G. Couser). *Cap*, capillary lumen; *Mes*, mesangium; *US*, urinary space; *E*, endothlium. × 12,000

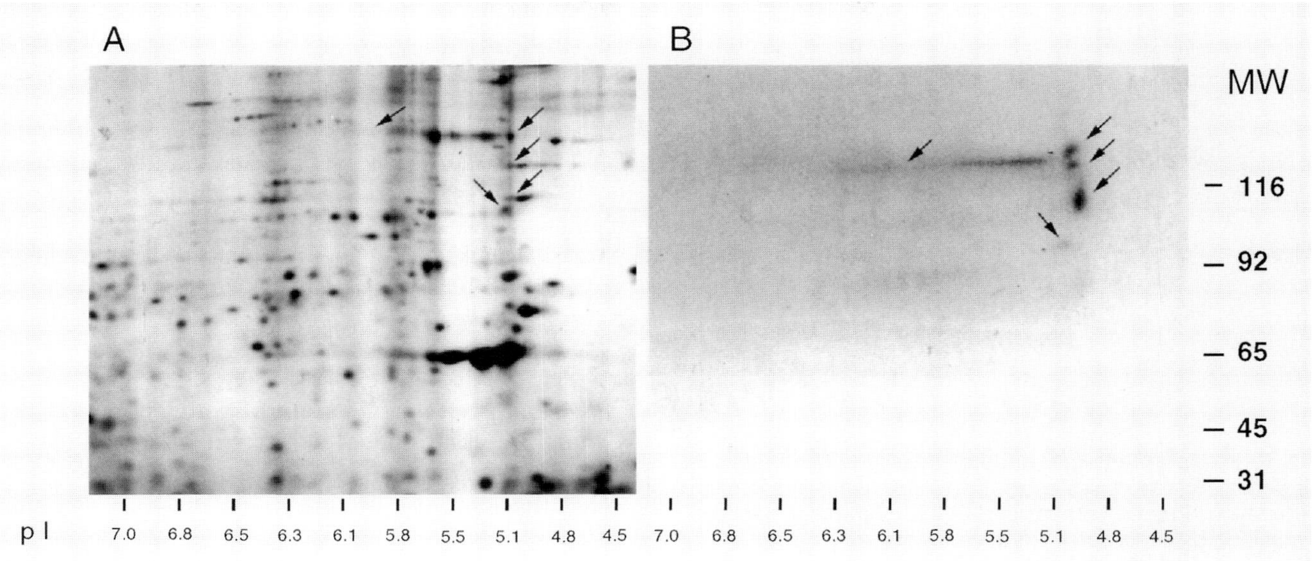

FIG. 4. A: Analysis of glomerular proteins dissolved by SDS from isolated glomeruli from rat kidneys, radio-iodinated by in vitro perfusion as described in Figure 3, by two-dimensional gel electrophoresis and silver staining. A "starry sky" of proteins is resolved. **B:** Autoradiograph of the two-dimensional gel depicted in A. Note that only few proteins are radiolabeled (arrows); these are presumably in contact with the glomerular basement membrane or mesangial matrix. The two proteins with a pI of approximately 5.1 and molecular weights of 120 and 135 kD correspond to b1-integrin. The other proteins are as yet unidentified.

Glomerular β_1-Integrin

The two-step protocol for enrichment of amphophilic proteins was originallly developed to identify and isolate integrins of glomeruli (9). Integrins are transmembrane protein complexes that bind to specific sites on proteins of the extracellular matrix and that transmit intracellular signals, for example, by interaction with elements of the cytoskeleton (18,19). Because the complex architecture of podocytes apparently requires a strict control of adhesion sites on the glomerular basement membrane, it was of interest to identify and precisely localize integrins within glomeruli (9) (see Chapter 30).

We observed that β_1-integrin partitioned quantitatively into the detergent-rich phase (Fig. 5), and it was also detected among the membrane proteins labeled by *in situ* iodination (Fig. 4), indicating that it was located in cell membranes contacting the glomerular basement membrane matrix. This was confirmed by light- and electron-microscopic immunocytochemistry, using polyclonal anti-β_1-integrin antibody (Fig. 6). In peripheral capillary loops, the integrin was found exclusively on the basal cell membranes of foot processes and on the abluminal aspects of endothelial cells. Immunofluorescence studies revealed that the glomerular β_1-integrin was associated with α_3 chains in peripheral capillary loops (20). It was concluded that $\alpha_3\beta_1$-integrin is the major integrin in adult glomeruli and could provide a stable attachment for podocytes and endothelial cells to the basement membrane.

In search of ligands for the glomerular β_1-integrin, it was observed that it functions *in vitro* as a fibronectin receptor, because it was enriched by affinity chromatography on a fibronectin column and was released specifically by the peptide ArgGlySer ASP, but not by a control peptide (9) (Fig. 5). However, when isolated rat kidneys were perfused with blood-free buffer containing a high concentration of ArgGlySer ASP and EDTA (ethylenediaminetetraacetic acid), to detach the β_1-integrin from its ligands, no changes in the architecture of podocytes were observed (D. Kerjaschki, *unpublished observations*), suggesting that β_1-integrin cell attachment to the glomerular basement membrane is mediated by additional binding motifs, or provides only one of several adhesion mechanisms for podocytes and endothelial cells. As there is apparently little fibronectin in normal peripheral capillary loops (21,22), the precise binding partners of the integrin within the GBM remain to be determined.

Distribution and density of β_1-integrin by immunoelectron microscopy were not significantly changed in several human diseases, such as segmental and focal sclerosis, minimal-change nephrosis, and membranous nephropathy (Fig. 6). By contrast, rearrangement of glomerular integrins by immunofluorescence was reported in cases of focal and segmental sclerosis (23), and it will be of inter-

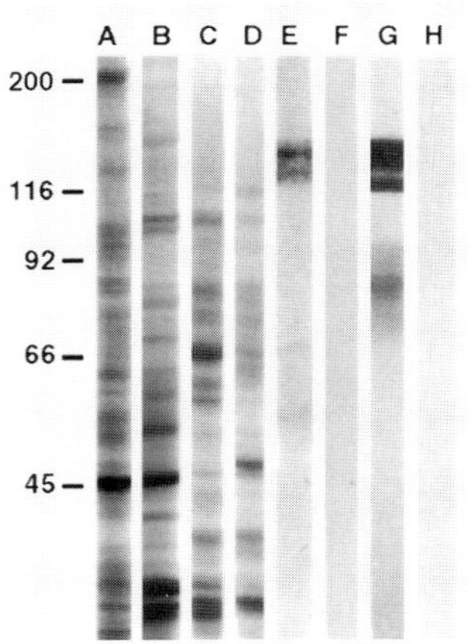

FIG. 5. Human β_1-integrin is quantitatively concentrated in the detergent-rich phase by the two-step membrane protein preparation. Protein composition of the glomerular fractions is obtained by successive extraction with Na_2CO_3 and Triton X-114 (*lanes A–D*) and analyzed in silver-stained 5–10% gradient polyacrylamide SDS gels (performed under reducing conditions), and the β_1-integrin is identified in the membrane protein-enriched fraction (*lane E*). **Lane A:** Protein pattern of isolated glomeruli directly lysed in SDS-sample buffer. Note the prominent bands with apparent molecular weights of 45 kD and 200 kD that migrate at the expected positions of actin and myosin. **Lane B:** Na2CO3-detached membrane vesicles (see Fig. 2). The quantities of actin and myosin are reduced compared with lane A. **Lane C:** Amphophilic molecules that have partitioned into the Triton X-114-rich phase after phase separation. Actin and myosin are almost completely absent, whereas several bands are enriched. **Lane D:** Soluble proteins that do not partition into the Triton X-114 phase but remain in the detergent-poor supernatant after phase separation. **Lane E:** Immune overlay with anti-β_1-integrin antibody of a transfer of amphophilic membrane proteins (compare with the protein pattern in lane C). Two bands with apparent molecular weights of 140 kD and 130 kD are specifically labeled. **Lane F:** Immunoblot with anti-β_1-integrin antibody (prepared against the fibronectin receptor isolated from human placenta) of proteins in the detergent-poor phase after Triton X-114-phase separation (compare with the protein pattern in lane D). The antibody does not bind to any of these proteins. **Lane G:** Immunoblot with anti-β_1-integrin antibody of glomerular proteins that were concentrated by binding to a fibronectin-affinity column and were released specifically by elution with Arg-Gly-Ser-Asp. Note the enrichment of the 130-kD and the 140-kD bands. **Lane H:** Immunoblot with anti-β_1-integrin antibody on glomerular proteins released from a fibronectin-affinity column by elution with the control peptide Gly-Arg-Gly-Glu-Ser-Pro. Collectively, these data indicate that glomerular β_1-integrin is amphophilic and quantitatively partitions into the detergent-rich phase of the two-step membrane protein preparation.

est to explore the possibility that β_1-integrin could be redistributed at sites of podocyte detachment from the glomerular basement membrane that were implicated in the development of proteinuria.

When sera of patients with Goodpasture syndrome and proven anti-glomerular basement membrane activity were immunoblotted on membrane protein preparations enriched for β_1-integrin, no specific binding was observed, suggesting that in this disease antibodies directed against the glomerular β_1-integrin are presumably irrelevant (P. Ojha and D. Kerjaschki, *unpublished observations*). It is, however, possible that antibodies to the β_1-integrin may be involved in experimental anti-glomerular basement membrane disease, because non-complement-fixing nephrotoxic antisera contained antibodies with anti-integrin specificity, which was associated with the rapid development of proteinuria (24) (see Chapter 30).

An H-lamp-2-Related Vasculitis Antigen in Glomerular Endothelial Cells

Identification of membrane proteins on glomerular endothelial cells and in neutrophil granulocytes as antigenic targets for ANCA was based on preparation of membrane proteins of isolated human glomeruli. Anti-neutrophil antibodies are almost regularly found in the blood of patients with various form of vasculitis (25,26) (see Chapter 49). Membrane protein fractions were used to screen ANCA sera by immunoblotting and to raise monoclonal antibodies with properties of natural ANCA (8).

Several forms of vasculitis frequently affect renal glomeruli and cause capillary loop necrosis, capsular crescent formation, and eventually rapid irreversible scarring and functional obsolescence of glomeruli; these correspond to a rapidly progressive glomerulonephritis in clinical terms. As these diseases are associated with the occurrence of ANCA, it was suspected that the auto-antigenic targets of ANCA could be involved in the pathogenesis of vasculitis. This was based on the assumption that neutrophils become activated by ANCA and adhere to endothelial cells of glomerular capillary loops, where they complete their work of destruction by discharge of their granules and extracellular activation of enzymes and free radicals (27–32).

A conceptual problem of this hypothetical explanation of pathogenesis was posed by the fact that auto-antigenic targets of ANCA identified so far were exclusively soluble granular content enzymes, such as myeloperoxidase, protease 3, and elastase (28,33–35) which, however, were not expressed by endothelial cells. For ANCA to cross-link neutrophils to endothelial surfaces directly, a putative "ideal antigen" in this scenario should be exposed both on the endothelial surface and on the neutrophils. Myeloperoxidase electrostatically binds in vitro to the negatively charged surfaces of endothelial cells because of its cationic isoelectric point; however, it is uncertain whether this also occurs in vivo (29). Therefore, the question arose whether genuine transmembrane proteins on surfaces of endothelia and neutrophils could serve as auto-antigenic targets for ANCA.

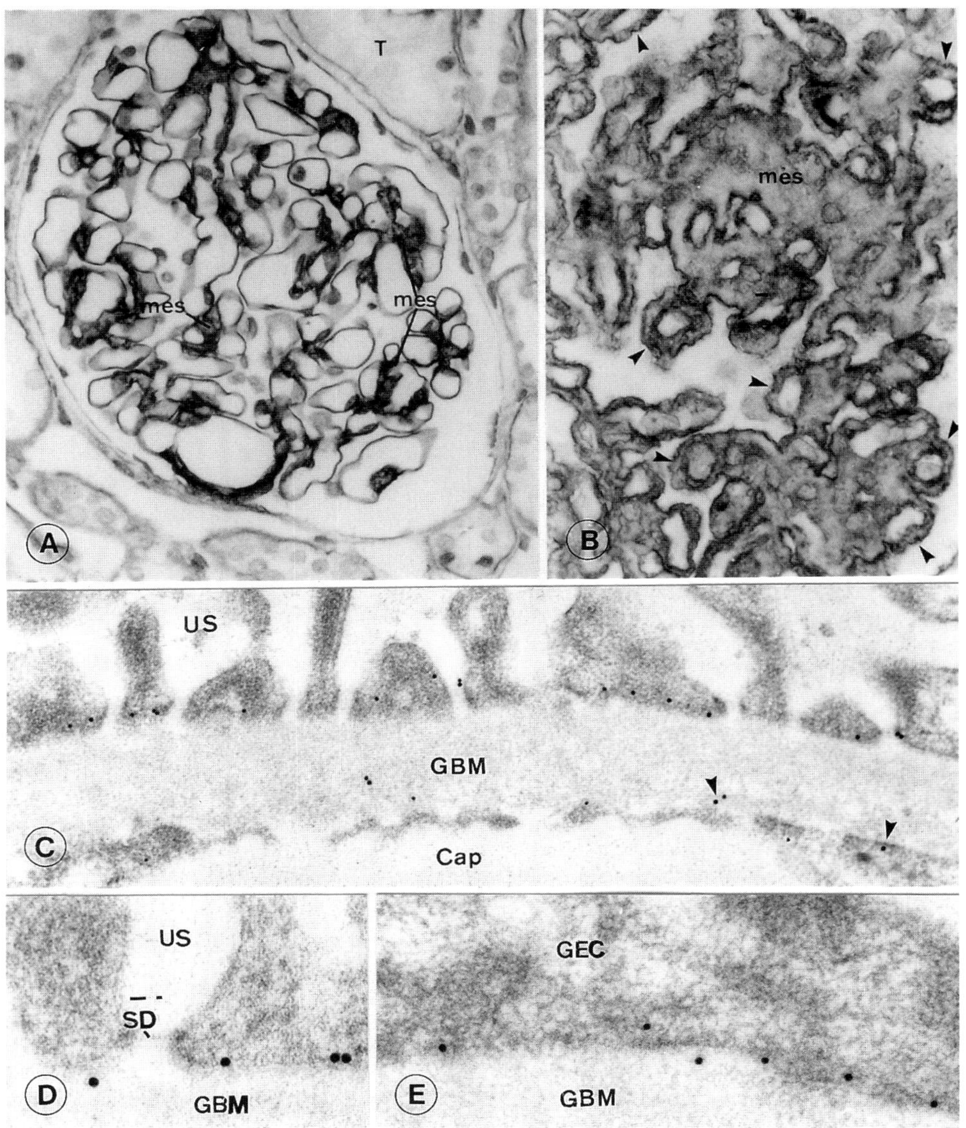

FIG. 6. A,B: Localization of β_1-integrin in human glomeruli of normal individuals and of a patient with membranous glomerulonephritis in paraffin sections using an immunoperoxidase procedure. The β_1-integrin is concentrated in glomeruli in the peripheral capillary loops and also in the mesangium (*mes*). In membranous nephropathy (stage 3), the β_1-integrin is localized in a double contour in the peripheral capillaries because it remains evenly attached to the glomerular epithelial and endothelial cells separated by the thickened basal membrane. **C–E:** Localization of β_1-integrin by immunogold electron microscopy on Lowicryl-K4M-embedded human biopsy specimens of normal kidneys (C,D) and of kidneys from a patient with steroid-sensitive minimal-change nephrosis. The gold grains indicating β_1-integrin are exclusively located at the cell membranes of epithelial and endothelial cells attached to the basement membrane. There is no apparent redistribution of b_1-integrin in minimal-change nephrosis. A,B: × 500; C: × 62,000; D,E: × 80,000.

Membrane protein fractions of isolated human glomeruli were prepared by the two-step protocol outlined previously and used for immunoblotting with the ANCA-containing sera of patients with necrotizing and crescentic glomerulonephritis, and with an international c-ANCA standard derived from the plasmapheresis fluid of a patient with Wegener's granulomatosis (36). More than 50% of the sera specifically bound to a glycoprotein of approximately 138 kD, which was provisionally designated "gp130." When membrane proteins of neutrophil granulocytes were similarly prepared and immunoblotted, two bands with apparent molecular weights of 170 kD and of 80 to 110 kD were specifically immunolabeled (Fig. 7).

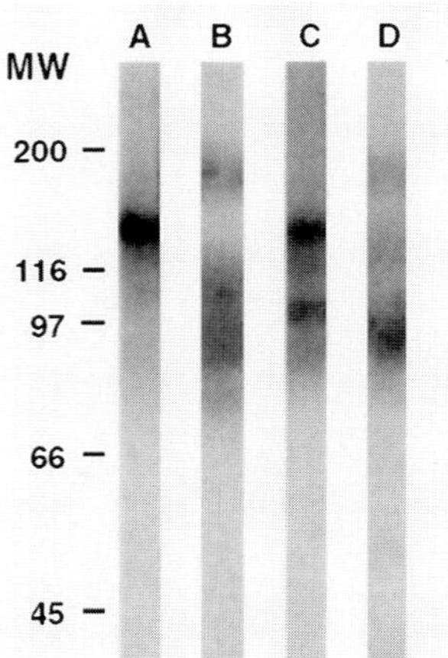

FIG. 7. A,B: Glomerular gp130, a target membrane protein of ANCA, and the lysosomal membrane protein h-lamp-2 are structurally related. Identification of membrane protein antigens with a monoclonal antibody specific for the glomerular endothelial protein gp130 that specifically reacts with ANCA sera of patients with necrotizing and crescentic glomerulonephritis. A membrane protein fraction of human glomeruli (*lane A*) and of isolated human neutrophil granulocytes (*lane B*) were immunoblotted. While the monoclonal antibody specifically labeled a 130-kD membrane protein in glomeruli, it bound a pair of membrane proteins with apparent molecular weights of 170 and 80 to 110 kD in neutrophils. These proteins were found by molecular cloning and sequencing to be identical with the lysosomal membrane glycoprotein h-lamp-2. **C,D:** Immunoblots on membrane proteins of glomeruli (*lane C*), and neutrophils (*lane D*) with a monoclonal antibody specific for h-lamp-2. The same membrane proteins are labeled in both preparations, indicating that ANCA sera of patients, the monoclonal anti-gp130 antibody, and anti-h-lamp-2 IgG all cross-react with these proteins.

Monoclonal antibodies were raised against a human glomerular membrane protein fraction, and a clone producing an anti-130-kD IgG was selected. This monoclonal antibody bound during immunofluorescence to the cytoplasm of neutrophils in a typical c-ANCA pattern (Fig. 8), similar to that of natural ANCA. In sections of normal human kidneys, the antibody specifically labeled endothelial cells of glomeruli and interstitial capillaries (Fig. 9), but no other blood vessels. This monoclonal antibody and a polyclonal anti-gp130 antibody were subsequently used for screening of a γt11 c-DNA library of a human promyelocytic leukemia cell line. A cDNA clone was identified and sequenced, and its predicted amino acid sequence was found to correspond to the human lysosome-associated membrane protein 2 (h-lamp-2 [37,38] or lgp120 [39]) of neutrophils. H-lamp-2 is a member of a family of heavily glycosylated membrane proteins that includes macrosialin, CD56, and others (40,41). Interestingly, there is some evidence that molecules of the lamp family are expressed on cell surfaces (42) and could serve as counter-receptors for selectins (43) that mediate the binding of inflammatory cells to endothelial cell surfaces (see Chapters 24 and 25). Collectively, these data indicated that the ANCA-antigen enriched by the membrane protein protocol from polymorphic neutrophils was h-lamp-2.

The glomerular endothelial membrane protein gp130, which shows apparent cross-reactivity with anti-h-lamp-2 antibodies, is not yet characterized. It is uncertain whether the cross-reactivity depends on shared epitopes in the protein or the carbohydrate moiety, and its molecular identification is currently in progress.

The data obtained so far in this system provide evidence that some natural ANCA sera contain IgG specific for h-lamp-2/gp130 proteins. The fact that these immunologically cross-reactive glycoproteins are constitutively expressed on the surfaces of glomerular endothelial cells and on activated neutrophils suggests that they could assist in ANCA-mediated immobilization of neutrophils in glomerular capillary loops and contribute to glomerular damage in necrotizing and crescentic glomerulonephritis.

Podocalyxin

Podocalyxin is an example of a highly glycosylated membrane protein that is concentrated in the membrane vesicle fraction obtained by the high-pH step of the glomerular membrane protein purification, but then distributes both in the detergent-rich and detergent-poor phases in the Triton X-114 extraction. Podocalyxin belongs apparently to a group of glomerular membrane proteins that contribute to the stability of the complicated structure of glomerular cells by virtue of their anionic charge. It is possible that reduction of negative charges of glomeruli (the "glomerular polyanion" [44]), as visualized by staining with cationic dyes (alcian blue, colloidal iron), could influence the biology of podocytes and glomerular basement membrane permeability. The sialoglycoprotein podocalyxin was originally identified in the rat (Fig. 10), and subsequently similar molecules were found in humans (45) and rabbit glomeruli (46).

Podocalyxin was originally identified in rat glomeruli as a 140-kD protein present in high concentrations in the luminal cell surfaces of podocyte membranes (10) and on endothelial cells (47) (Fig. 11) (see also Chapter 30). The protein was found to be sulfated (48) and heavily sialylated, containing about 20 sialic acid residues per molecule (49). These carriers of negative charge apparently were responsible for binding of the polycationic dyes alcian blue and "stains all." It was proposed that podocalyxin could be involved in the maintenance of podocyte shape, because flattening of foot processes in the course of puromycin nephrosis drastically reduces the content of podocalyxin's sialic acids (44,49). By contrast, other carbohydrate residues and the protein itself appeared unchanged, and the density of podocalyxin on the cell surfaces was not found to be reduced. In addition to the luminal surface of podocytes, podoca-

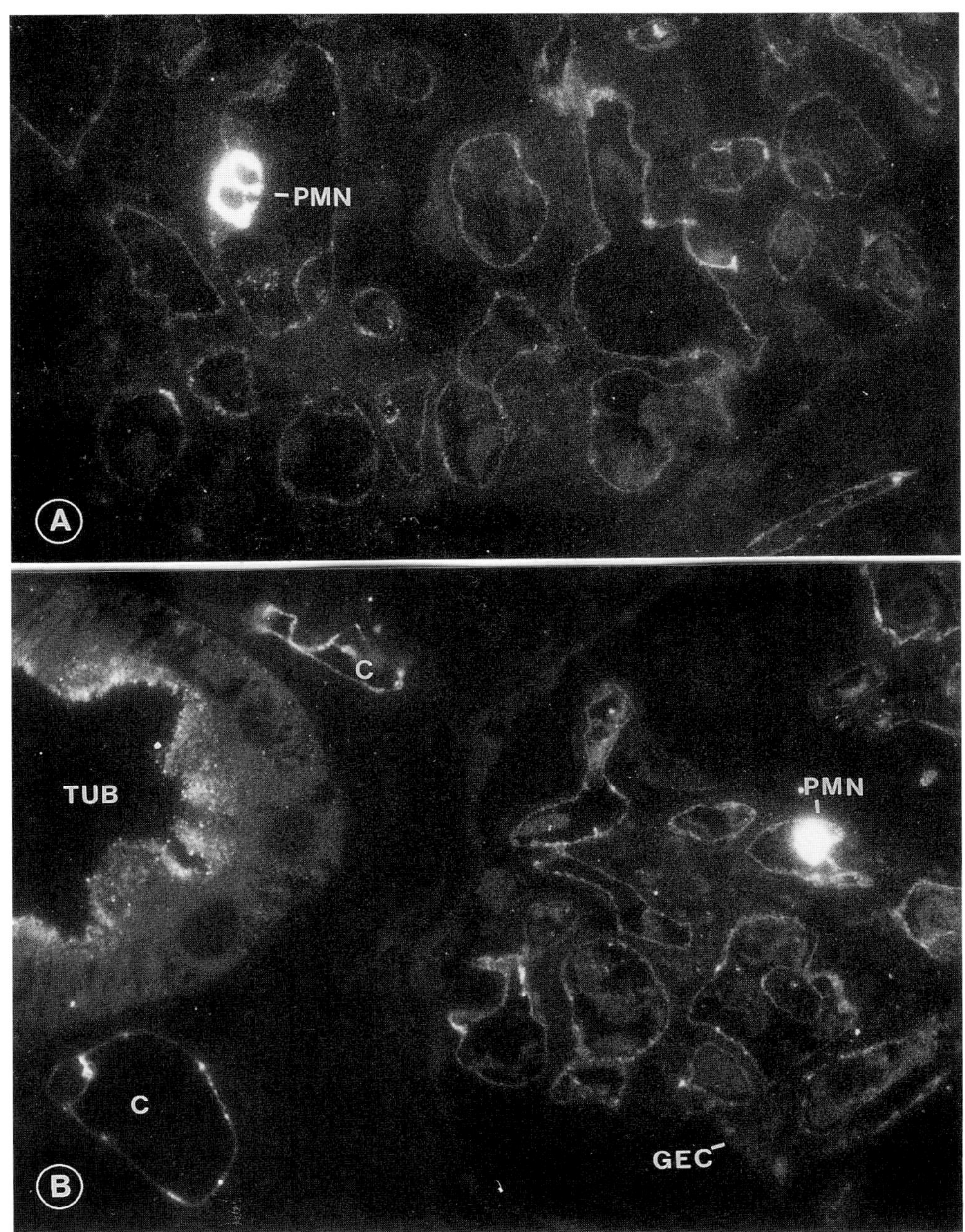

FIG. 8. The ANCA-antigenic target membrane protein gp130 is expressed on endothelial cells and in neutrophil granulocytes. Gp130 was localized by a specific monoclonal antibody in 0.5-μm cryosections of normal human kidney. The glycoprotein is expressed on glomerular endothelial cells and on interstitial capillaries, and is also found in the brush border region of proximal tubules. Neutrophil granulocytes (*PMN*) trapped within capillary loops show intense labeling of their cytoplasm, resembling a c-ANCA pattern frequently found in several forms of vasculitis. ×1200.

lyxin was also observed on endothelial cells and recently on platelets and megakaryocytes (A. Miettinnen, *unpublished observations*).

Glycoproteins similar in charge and distribution to rat podocalyxin were identified in humans (45) and in rabbits (46). In humans, this protein resolved by sodium dodecyl sulfate (SDS) polyacrylamide gel electrophoresis as a doublet with apparent molecular weights of 170 and 160 kD. Recently, molecular cloning of rabbit podocalyxin (designated "podocalyxin-like protein 1") was achieved, revealing a transmembrane protein with a protein backbone of approximately 50 kD (46). Extensive post-translational modifications appear to account for an apparent molecular weight of 140 kD for the complete protein. No homology was found on the amino acid level with other previously described sequences.

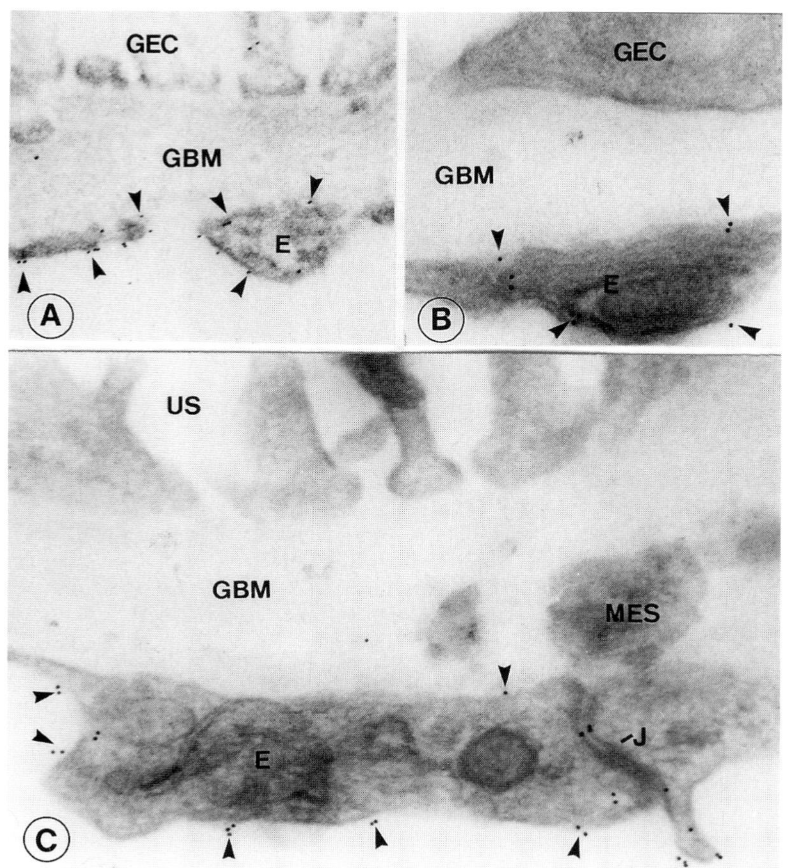

FIG. 9. The ANCA-antigenic target membrane protein gp130 is localized on surfaces of glomerular endothelial cells. Localization of gp130 in human glomerular endothelial cells by immunogold labeling with monoclonal anti-gp130 IgG on ultrathin frozen sections. Gold particles (*arrowheads*) bind exclusively to surfaces of glomerular endothelial cells (*E*), where they are concentrated at the luminal surfaces in a patchy pattern. Occasionally, antigen is also detected at the abluminal side of endothelial cells, and close to intercellular junctions (*J*). There is no specific labeling of glomerular epithelial cells (*GEC*), of the basement membrane (*GBM*), or of extensions of a mesangial cell (*MES*). *US*, urinary space. (Reproduced with permission from ref. 57) × 18,000.

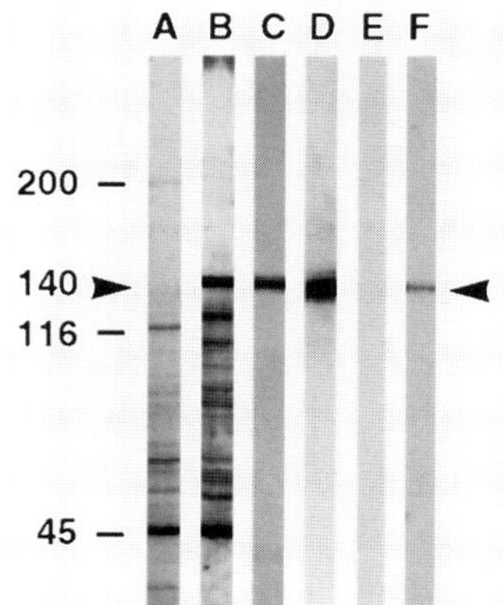

FIG. 10. Identification of the sialoglycoprotein podocalyxin as the major component of the "glomerular polyanion." Extracts of isolated rat glomeruli in SDS-sample buffer were separated on 5–10% gradient SDS gels. **A:** Coomassie blue staining. **B:** Silver staining. **C:** "Stains all," a cationic metachromatic dye, indicative of polyanionic proteins in SDS gels. A prominent, strongly anionic band at approximately 140 kD is visible in B and C, but not in A. **D:** Lectin blot on SDS lysates of rat glomeruli with ^{125}I-labeled wheat germ agglutinin selectively labels the 140-kD band. **E:** Binding of ^{125}I-labeled wheat germ agglutinin is prevented by digestion of the transfer with neuraminidase, indicating that the lectin selectively bound to sialic acid. **F:** Immunoblot with affinity-purified rabbit anti-podocalyxin IgG, which was used for immunolocalization in Fig. 10.

The precise function of podocalyxin remains to be determined. It is possible that it contributes anti-adhesive properties because of its negative charge, but experimental evidence for this speculation has not been provided. Podocalyxin is also expressed on the surface of endothelial cells and could play a role in hemostasis.

MEMBRANE PROTEINS THAT ARE EXPRESSED IN GLOMERULI UNDER PATHOLOGIC CONDITIONS

Podocytes appear to change the profile of membrane proteins synthesized and exposed on their surfaces when they are "activated," for example, by C5b-9 complexes (11,50). In Heymann nephritis in rats, proteins expressed *de novo* comprise receptors that partition into the detergent-rich pellet in the two-step membrane fractionation technique, such as the basic fibroblast growth factor receptor (51).

Cytochrome b_{558} and the NADPH-Oxidoreductase Complex

Whereas some of the proteins expressed *de novo* may protect glomerular cells from extrinsic damaging factors,

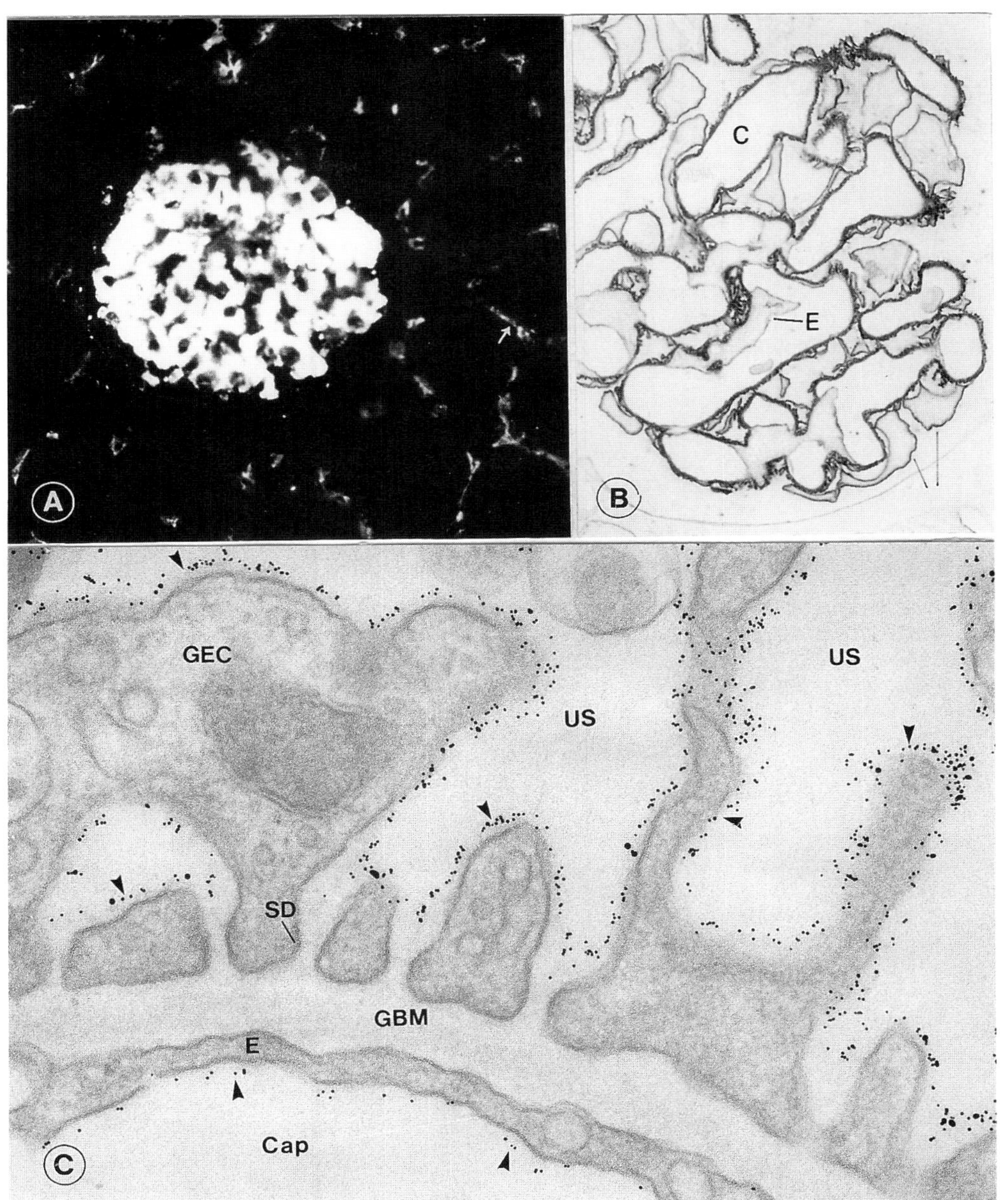

FIG. 11. Podocalyxin is located on surface membranes of glomerular epithelial and endothelial cells. Immunohistochemical localization of podocalyxin in rat kidney, using affinity-purified rabbit antibody. **A:** By indirect immunofluorescence, intense labeling of the glomerulus and of interstitial capillaries is observed. **B:** Localization by immunoperoxidase on a 0.5-µm-thick cryosection of a rat glomerulus. Podocalyxin is observed on the surfaces of epithelial cells, and also more weakly on endothelial cells (*E*). **C:** Localization of podocalyxin on the surfaces of glomerular epithelial and endothelial cells by an indirect immunogold technique. Gold particles are restricted to cell domains facing the urinary (*US*) and capillary (*Cap*) spaces. Whereas the distribution of podocalyxin on epithelial cells is even and dense, it is patchy on the endothelium. A: × 400; B: × 800; C: × 55,000.

others may be harmful. One example is the NADPH-oxidoreductase (reduced nicotinamide adenine dinucleotide phosphate) complex (52), commonly used by granulocytes in the respiratory-burst reaction to produce large amounts of reactive oxygen species (ROS). The NADPH-oxidoreductase enzyme complex consists of several components, one of which is the membrane protein cytochrome b_{558} (53). In granulocytes, the enzyme complex is stored in a dormant, inactivated state in the cell membranes of granules and is inserted into the surface cell membrane by exocytosis of the granules after appropriate stimulation. The sites of ROS production were localized to the cell surfaces of neutrophil granulocytes by ultrastructural cytochemistry using an H_2O_2-cerium precipitation method (54). The NADPH-oxidoreductase complex is apparently widely distributed in low

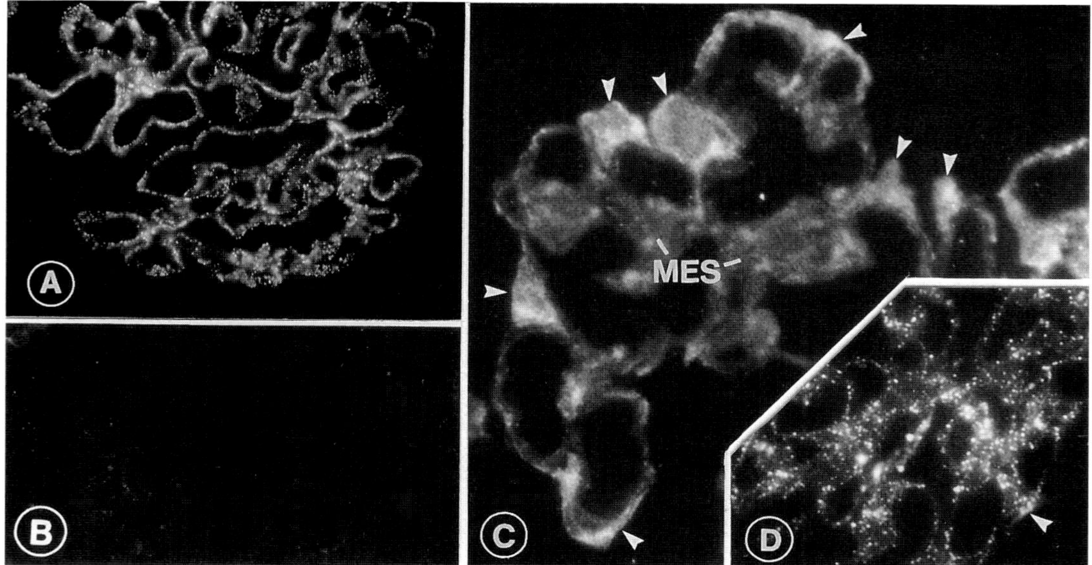

FIG. 12. *De novo* expression of cytochrome b_{558}, a component of the ROS-producing NADPH-oxidoreductase complex, by podocytes in passive Heymann nephritis. Heymann nephritis was induced in rats by injection of sheep antibodies raised against crude renal cortex fractions, resulting in formation of immune deposits and severe proteinuria. Localization of sheep IgG (**A**) and of cytochrome b_{558} (**B–D**) by immunofluorescence on frozen sections. **A:** Localization of sheep IgG in a glomerulus 7 days after injection of nephritogenic IgG, in a fine granular pattern characteristic of passive Heymann nephritis. B: Localization of the B subunit of cytochrome b_{558} in a normal rat glomerulus (1-μm-thick section). At this level of sensitivity of the indirect immunofluorescence technique (the same as used in C and D), the enzyme is visualized only in traces. **C:** Localization of cytochrome b_{558} in a 4-μm cryostat section (to emphasize its overall distribution) of a glomerulus of a proteinuric rat with passive Heymann nephritis. There is intense labeling for cytochrome b_{558} associated with the epithelial cells (*arrowheads*) and a weaker signal also in the mesangial area (*MES*). **D:** In a 1-mm section (to emphasize high resolution) of the same tissue as in C, the cytochrome b_{558} is found in a discrete punctate pattern in glomerular epithelial cells (*arrowhead*), as well as in the mesangium. A,B: × 600; C: × 950; D: × 800. (Reproduced with permission from ref. 57.)

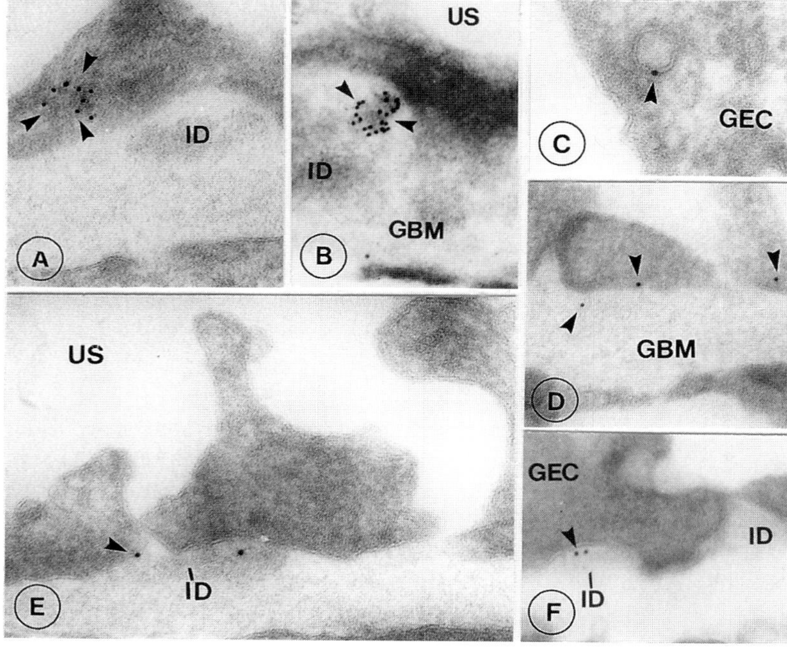

FIG. 13. Cytochrome b_{558} is located on the surface of glomerular cells in passive Heymann nephritis. Localization of cytochrome b_{558} by immunogold electron microscopy on ultrathin frozen sections of glomeruli of proteinuric rats 7 days after injection of IgG prepared against crude renal cortex fractions. **A:** Gold particles outline a vesicle (*arrowheads*) in the glomerular epithelial cellular cytoplasm, corresponding to the granular distribution of this enzyme seen by immunofluorescence. **B:** Extracellularly located cytochrome b_{558} is indicated by a cluster of gold grains adjacent to an immune complex deposit. **C:** Another example of gold particles localized in an intracellular vesicle in a glomerular epithelial cell. **D:** Extracellular localization of cytochrome b_{558} along the cell membrane of a foot process, indicated by gold particles (*arrowheads*). **E,F:** Association of cytochrome b_{558} with the membrane at the "soles" of the glomerular epithelial cells in close proximity to immune complex deposits (*ID*). *US*, urinary space; *GBM*, glomerular basement membrane; *E*, endothelial cell. A,B,D,F: × 32,000; C: × 60,000; E: × 40,000.

concentrations—for example, in fibroblasts (55) and in cultured mesangial cells (56).

The biosynthesis of the NADPH-oxidoreductase complex dramatically increases in passive Heymann nephritis within the glomerulus (57), as detected by immunofluorescence (Fig. 12) and by quantitation of message for cytochrome b_{558} (D. Kerjaschki, *unpublished observations*). At the ultrastructural level, cytochrome b_{558} was exposed on the cell surface of glomerular epithelial cells and also on endothelial cells (Fig. 13). Intriguingly, deprivation of C5b-9 by injection of cobra venom factor in passive Heymann nephritis rats suppressed its *de novo* expression. The functionality of the enzyme complex in podocytes of passive Heymann nephritis rats was demonstrated by perfusion with a Ce^{3+}-containing histochemical medium. An H_2O_2-Ce^{3+} precipitate was found within the glomerular basement membrane in rats with proteinuria, but was absent in non-proteinuric rats (57).

Collectively, these data indicate that the cell membrane-anchored NADPH-oxidoreductase enzyme complex is synthesized *de novo* within glomeruli of rats with passive Heymann nephritis, particularly by glomerular epithelial cells. It further appears that the activation and presumably also the insertion of C5b-9 membrane attack complex into the podocyte membranes (58) could serve as an activator for biosynthesis. The consequence of this expression is flooding of the glomerular basement membrane by toxic ROS, which either directly or indirectly (via lipid peroxidation) cause damage of glomerular basement membrane matrix proteins (59). Preliminary experiments with other experimental models of proteinuria, such as nephrosis induced in rats by puromycin aminonucleoside or doxorubicin, suggests a similar upregulation of the NADPH-oxidoreductase complex and accumulation of ROS within the glomerular basement membranes (T. J. Neale, *unpublished observations*). Thus, it is possible that glomerular cells, in particular the glomerular epithelial cells, could generate ROS by *de novo* induction of oxidoreductase, which causes glomerular damage and proteinuria even in the absence of infiltrating inflammatory cells. It remains to be determined to what extent this concept can be extended to human diseases.

PERSPECTIVE

In this chapter, a simple strategy for enrichment of amphophilic membrane proteins from isolated glomeruli has been outlined. The usefulness of this procedure is illustrated by a few examples. Whereas some of these membrane proteins are expressed constitutively, others are expressed *de novo* after immune complex-mediated C5b-9 attack on the podocyte cell membranes. Some are presumably involved in potentiating agents of glomerular damage, such as the oxygen radical-producing enzymes of the NADPH-oxidoreductase complex, whereas others may serve to protect the integrity of the glomerulus. It will be of interest to define precisely the gene regulatory elements responsible for reprogramming the biosynthetic repertory of glomerular cells. Research on glomerular membrane proteins is still in its beginnings, and the roles of most of these important models in human renal diseases remain to be defined.

ACKNOWLEDGMENT

This work was supported by SFB 5, Project 007.

REFERENCES

1. Matsuo S, Fukatsu A, Taub ML, Caldwell PRB, Brentjens JR, Andres G. Glomerulonephritis induced in the rabbit by antiendothelial antibodies. *J Clin Invest* 1987;79:1798–1811.
2. Barba IM, Caldwell PRB, Downie GH, Camussi G, Brentjens JR, Andres G. Lung injury mediated by antibodies to endothelium. In the rabbit a repeated interaction of heterologous anti-angiotensin-converting enzyme antibodies with alveolar endothelium results in resistance to immune injury through antigenic modulation. *J Exp Med* 1983;158:2141.
3. Douglas M, Rabideau D, Schwartz M, Lewis EJ. Evidence of autologous immune complex nephritis. *N Engl J Med* 1981;305:1326–1329.
4. O'Donoghue DJ, Darvil A, Ballardie FW. Mesangial cell autoantigens in immunoglobulin A nephropathy and Henoch-Schönlein purpura. *J Clin Invest* 1991; 88:1522–1530.
5. Fornasieri A, Pinerolo C, Bernasconi P, Li M, Armelloni S, Gibelli A, D'Amico G. Anti-mesangial and anti-endothelial cell antibodies in IgA mesangial nephropathy. *Clin Nephrol* 1995; 44:71–78.
6. Rosenbaum J, Pottinger BE, Woo P, Black GM, Loizou S, Byron MA, Pearson D. Measurements and characterisation of circulating anti-endothelial cell IgG in connective tissue disease. *Clin Exp Immunol* 1988;72:450.
7. Yap HK, Sakai RS, Bahn L, Rappaport V, Woo KT, Ananthurman V, Lim CH, Chiang GS, Jordan JC. Antivascular endothelial cell antibodies in patients with IgA nephropathy: frequency and clinical significance. *Clin Immunol Immunopathol* 1988;49:450.
8. Kain R, Matsui K, Exner M, Binder S, Schaffner G, Sommer EM, Kerjaschki D. A novel class of autoantigens of anti-neutrophil cytoplasmic antibodies in necrotizing and crescentic glomerulonephritis: the lysosomal membrane glycoprotein h-lamp-2 in neutrophil granulocytes and a related membrane protein in glomerular endothelial cells. *J Exp Med* 1995;181:585–597.
9. Kerjaschki D, Ojha PP, Susani M, Horvat R, Binder S, Hovorka A, Hillemanns P, Pytela R. A beta 1-integrin receptor for fibronectin in human kidney glomeruli. *Am J Pathol* 1989;134:481–489.
10. Kerjaschki D, Sharkey DJ, Farquhar MG. Identification and characterization of podocalyxin—the major sialoglycoprotein of the renal glomerular epithelial cell. *J Cell Biol* 1984;98:1591–1596.
11. Kerjaschki D. Dysfunction of cell biological mechanisms of visceral epithelial cells (podocytes) in glomerular diseases. *Kidney Int* 1994; 45:300–313.
12. Fukatsu A, YY, Olson L, Miller J, Zamlauski-Tucker MJ, J VL, Campagnari A, Niesen N, Patel J, Doi T, Striker L, Striker G, Milgrom F, Brentjens J, Andres GA. Interaction of antibodies with human glomerular epithelial cells. *Lab Invest* 1989;61:389–403.
13. Howell KE, Palade GE. Hepatic Golgi fractions resolved into membrane and content subfractions. *J Cell Biol* 1982;92:822–832.
14. Bordier C. Phase separation of integral membrane proteins in Triton X-114 solution. *J Biol Chem* 1981;256:1604–1607.
15. Miettinen A, Dekan G, Farquhar MG. Monoclonal antibodies against membrane proteins of the rat glomerulus. Immunochemical specificity and immunofluorescence distribution of the antigens. *Am J Pathol* 1990;137:929–944.
16. Dekan G, Miettinen A, Schnabel E, Farquhar MG. Binding of monoclonal antibodies to glomerular endothelium, slit membranes, and

epithelium after in vivo injection. Localization of antigens and bound IgGs by immunoelectron microscopy. *Am J Pathol* 1990;137:913–927.
17. Johnson RJ, Klebanoff SJ, Ochi S, Adler S, Baker P, Sparus L, Couser WG. Participation of the myeloperoxidase-H_2O_2 halide system in immune complex nephritis. *Kidney Int* 1987;32:342–349.
18. Ruoslahti E, Noble NA, Kagami S, Border WA. Integrins. *Kidney Int* 1994;45:S17–S22.
19. Hynes RO. Integrins: versatility, modulation, and signaling in cell adhesion. *Cell* 1992;69:11–25.
20. Korhonen M, Ylanne J, Laitinen L, Virtanen I. The a1-a6 subunits of integrins are characteristically expressed in distinct segments of developing and adult human nephron. *J Cell Biol* 1990;111:1245–1254.
21. Courtoy PJ, Kanwar YS, Hynes RO, Farquhar MG. Fibronectin localization in the rat glomerulus. *J Cell Biol* 1980;87:691–696.
22. Oberley TD, Mosher DF, Mills MD. Localization of fibronectin within the renal glomerulus and its production by cultured glomerular cells. *Am J Pathol* 1979;96:651–667.
23. Kemeny E, Mihatsch JM, Durmüller U, Gudat F. Podocytes loose their adhesive phenotype in focal segmental glomerulosclerosis. *Clin Nephrol* 1995;43:71–83.
24. Adler S, Chen X. Anti-Fx1A antibody recognizes a beta 1-integrin on glomerular epithelial cells and inhibits adhesion and growth. *Am J Physiol* 1992;262:F770–F776.
25. Niles JL. Value of tests for antineutrophil cytoplasmic autoantibodies in the diagnosis and treatment of vasculitis. *Curr Opin Rheumatol* 1993;5:18–24.
26. Jennette JC. Antineutrophil cytoplasmic autoantibody-associated diseases: a pathologist's perspective. *Am J Kidney Dis* 1991;18:164–170.
27. Andrassy K, Koderisch J, Rufer M, Erb A, Waldherr R, Ritz E. Detection and clinical implication of anti-neutrophil cytoplasm antibodies in Wegener's granulomatosis and rapidly progressive glomerulonephritis. *Clin Nephrol* 1989;32:159–167.
28. Falk RJ, Jennette JC. Anti-neutrophil cytoplasmic autoantibodies with specificity for myeloperoxidase in patients with systemic vasculitis and idiopathic necrotizing and crescentic glomerulonephritis. *N Engl J Med* 1988;318:1651–1657.
29. Falk RJ, Terrell RS, Charles LA, Jennette JC. Anti-neutrophil cytoplasmic autoantibodies induce neutrophils to degranulate and produce oxygen radicals in vitro. *Proc Natl Acad Sci U S A* 1990;87:4115–4119.
30. Gaskin G, Savage CO, Ryan JJ, Jones S, Rees AJ, Lockwood CM, Pusey CD. Anti-neutrophil cytoplasmic antibodies and disease activity during long-term follow-up of 70 patients with systemic vasculitis. *Nephrol Dial Transplant* 1991;6:689–694.
31. Kallenberg CG, Brouwer E, Weening JJ, Tervaert JW. Anti-neutrophil cytoplasmic antibodies: current diagnostic and pathophysiological potential. *Kidney Int* 1994;46:1–15.
32. Savage CO, Pottinger BE, Gaskin G, Lockwood CM, Pusey CD, Pearson JD. Vascular damage in Wegener's granulomatosis and microscopic polyarteritis: presence of anti-endothelial cell antibodies and their relation to anti-neutrophil cytoplasm antibodies. *Clin Exp Immunol* 1991;85:14–19.
33. Cameron JS. New horizons in renal vasculitis. *Klin Wochenschr* 1991;69:536–551.
34. Falk RJ. ANCA-associated renal disease [clinical conference]. *Kidney Int* 1990;38:998–1010.
35. Csernok E, Ludemann J, Gross WL, Bainton DF. Ultrastructural localization of proteinase 3, the target antigen of anti-cytoplasmic antibodies circulating in Wegener's granulomatosis. *Am J Pathol* 1990;137:1113–1120.
36. Rasmussen N, Wiik A, Hoier Madsen M, Borregaard N, van der Woude F. Anti-neutrophil cytoplasm antibodies 1988 [Letter]. *Lancet* 1988;1:706–707.
37. Carlsson SR, Fukuda M. Isolation and characterization of leukosialin, a major sialoglycoprotein on human leukocytes. *J Biol Chem* 1986; 261:12779–12786.
38. Carlsson SR, Roth J, Piller F, Fukuda M. Isolation and characterization of human lysosomal membrane glycoproteins, h-lamp-1 and h-lamp-2. Major sialoglycoproteins carrying polylactosaminoglycan. *J Biol Chem* 1988;263:18911–18919.
39. Lewis V, Green SA, Marsh M, Vihko P, Helenius A, Mellman I. Glycoproteins of the lysosomal membrane. *J Cell Biol* 1985;100: 1839–1847.
40. Saitoh O, Piller F, Fox RI, Fukuda M. T-lymphocytic leukemia expresses complex, branched O-linked oligosaccharides on a major sialoglycoprotein, leukosialin. *Blood* 1991;77:1491–1499.
41. Fukuda M. Lysosomal membrane glycoproteins. Structure, biosynthesis, and intracellular trafficking. *J Biol Chem* 1991;266:21327–21330.
42. Holcombe RF, Baethge BA, Stewart RM, Betzing K, Hall VC, Fukuda M, Wolf RE. Cell surface expression of lysosome-associated membrane proteins (LAMPs) in scleroderma: relationship of lamp2 to disease duration, anti-Sc170 antibodies, serum interleukin-8, and soluble interleukin-2 receptor levels. *Clin Immunol Immunopathol* 1993; 67:31–39.
43. Sawada R, Lowe JB, Fukuda M. E-selectin-dependent adhesion efficiency of colonic carcinoma cells is increased by genetic manipulation of their cell surface lysosomal membrane glycoprotein-1 expression levels. *J Biol Chem* 1993;268:12675–12681.
44. Michael AF, Blau E, Vernier RL. Glomerular polyanion: alteration in aminonucleoside nephrosis. *Lab Invest* 1970;23:649–657.
45. Kerjaschki D, Poczewski H, Dekan G, Horvat R, Balzar E, Kraft N, Atkins RC. Identification of a major sialoprotein in the glycocalyx of human visceral epithelial cells. *J Clin Invest* 1986;78:1142–1149.
46. Kershaw DB, Thomas PE, Wharram BL, Goyal M, Wiggins JE, Whiteside CE, C WR. Molecular cloning, expression and characterization of podocalyxin-like protein 1 from rabbits as a transmembrane protein of glomerular podocytes and vascular endothelium. *J Biol Chem* 1995;270:1–8.
47. Horvat R, Hovorka A, Dekan G, Poczewski H, Kerjaschki D. Endothelial cell membranes contain podocalyxin—the major sialoprotein of visceral glomerular epithelial cells. *J Cell Biol* 1986;102: 484–491.
48. Dekan G, Gabel C, Farquhar MG. Sulfate contributes to the negative charge of podocalyxin, the major sialoglycoprotein of the glomerular filtration slits. *Proc Natl Acad Sci U S A* 1991;88:5398–5402.
49. Kerjaschki D, Vernillo AT, Farquhar MG. Reduced sialylation of podocalyxin—the major sialoprotein of the rat kidney glomerulus—in aminonucleoside nephrosis. *Am J Pathol* 1985;118:343–349.
50. Quigg RJ, Cybulsky AV, Salant DJ. Effect of nephritogenic antibody on complement regulation in cultured rat glomerular epithelial cells. *J Immunol* 1991;147:838–845.
51. Floege J, Kriz W, Schulze M, Susani M, Kerjaschki D, Mooney A, Couser WG, Koch KM. Basic fibroblast growth factor augments podocyte injury and induces glomerulosclerosis in rats with experimental membranous nephropathy. *J Clin Invest* 1995;96:2809–2819.
52. Babior BM. Oxygen-dependent microbial killing by phagocytes. *N Engl J Med* 1978;298:659–668.
53. Verhoeven AJ, Bolscher BG, Meerhof LJ, van Zwieten R, Kreijer J, Weening RS, Rood D. Characterization of two monoclonal antibodies against cytochrome b558 of human neutrophils. *Blood* 1989;73: 1686–1694.
54. Briggs RT, Drath DB, Karnovsky ML, Karnovsky MJ. Localization of NADH oxidase on the surface of human polymorphonuclear leukocytes by a new cytochemical technique. *J Cell Biol* 1975;67:566–586.
55. Radeke HH, Cross AR, Hancock JT, Jones JT, Nakamura M, Kraever V, Resch K. Functional expression of NADPH oxidase components (alpha and beta subunits of cytochrome b558 and 45 kD flavoprotein) by intrinsic human glomerular mesangial cells. *J Biol Chem* 1991; 266:21025–21029.
56. Meier B, Radeke HH, Selle S, Younes M, Sies H, Resch K, Habermehl GG. Human fibroblasts release reactive oxygen species in response to interleukin-1 or tumor necrosis factor-alpha. *Biochem J* 1989;263:539–545.
57. Neale TJ, Ullrich R, Ojha P, Poczewski H, Verhoeven AJ, Kerjaschki D. Reactive oxygen species and neutrophil respiratory burst cytochrome b558 are produced by kidney glomerular cells in passive Heymann nephritis. *Proc Natl Acad Sci U S A* 1993;90:3645–3649.
58. Kerjaschki D, Binder S, Kain R, Ojha PP, Susani M, Horvat R, Schulze M, Couser WG. Transcellular transport of the membrane attack complex of complement (MAC) by glomerular epithelial cells in passive Heymann nephritis. *J Immunol* 1989;143:546–552.
59. Neale TJ, Ojha PP, Exner M, Poczewski H, Rüger B, Witztum JL, Davis P, Verjaschki, D. Proteinuria in passive Heymann nephritis is associated with lipid peroxidation and formation of adducts on type IV collagen. *J Clin Invest* 1994;94:1577–1584.

Immunologic Renal Diseases,
edited by E. G. Neilson and W. G. Couser.
Lippincott-Raven Publishers, Philadelphia © 1997

CHAPTER 10

Nephritogenic Antigens in the Glomerular Basement Membrane

Dale R. Abrahamson, Gregory B. Vanden Heuvel, and William L. Clapp

The glomerular basement membrane (GBM), which serves as an adhesive extracellular matrix for both glomerular capillary endothelial cells and epithelial podocytes (1), as well as a charge- and size-selective permeability barrier (2), plays a crucial role in the establishment and maintenance of normal glomerular structure and function (see Chapter 2). However, this basement membrane is a frequent site of deposition of circulating immune complexes (see Chapter 14), and in many individuals, intrinsic GBM molecules are also subject to direct autoimmune attack. Consequently, renal glomeruli can become immunologic battlegrounds, resulting in both acute and chronic loss of kidney function. What we describe here are the principal molecular components of the GBM and mechanisms regulating the synthesis and assembly of these proteins into the matrix. We then discuss which of these constituents become targeted for nephritogenic autoimmune responses.

INTRINSIC BASEMENT MEMBRANE PROTEINS

Numerous thorough reviews on the structure and biochemistry of the several basement membrane proteins recently have appeared (3–10). Here we briefly summarize what we consider to be the most salient points.

Basement membranes are composed of a number of unusually large glycoproteins, and these glycoproteins are only rarely found associated with other extracellular matrices. The most predominant basement membrane components are collagen type IV, the noncollagenous proteins laminin and entactin (also referred to as nidogen), a heparan sulfate proteoglycan (perlecan; HSPG), and to a lesser extent chondroitin sulfate proteoglycans (CSPGs). Undoubtedly there are many more proteins in basement membranes, but only the foregoing have been well characterized in the kidney. Together, these basement membrane molecules form what is characteristically recognized in the electron microscope as a complex meshwork (Fig. 1). In the glomerulus, fenestrated endothelial cells are attached to the inner surface of the GBM, and foot processes of the epithelial podocytes are adherent to the outer surface (Fig. 1). The thickness of the GBM itself measures approximately 0.15 μm in rats and approximately 0.2 μm in humans and has classically been described as having three layers: an inner lamina rara interna, a central lamina densa, and an outer lamina rara externa (Fig. 1). The lamina rara interna contains narrow fibrils that span the approximately 50-nm distance between the adherent endothelial cell layer and the lamina densa. Likewise, similar fibrils extend from the lamina densa and project through the lamina rara externa onto the basal surface of podocyte foot processes (Fig. 1). Although some investigators of electron microscopic studies have concluded that the laminae rarae are artefactual structures (11), certain histochemical evidence (discussed below) nevertheless shows that the molecular organization across the width of the GBM indeed varies.

COLLAGEN TYPE IV

Polymers of type IV collagen are found abundantly in basement membranes. The monomeric subunits are composed of heterotrimers of three α chains with a combined molecular weight (M_r) of approximately 550 to 600 kDa. Each α chain contains (a) a central relatively long collagenous domain, (b) a shorter collagenous domain at the

D. R. Abrahamson: Department of Cell Biology, University of Alabama, Birmingham, Alabama 35294.

G. B. Vanden Heuvel: Section of Nephrology, Department of Medicine, Yale University School of Medicine, New Haven, Connecticut 06510.

W. L. Clapp: Department of Pathology and Laboratory Medicine, University of Florida College of Medicine, Veterans Affairs Medical Center, Gainesville, Florida 32610.

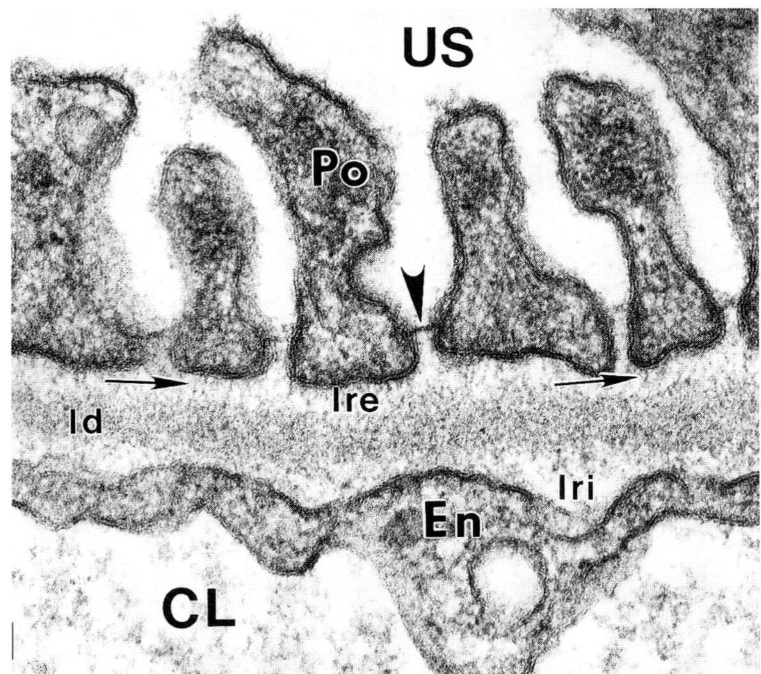

FIG. 1. Electron micrograph of glomerular capillary wall. GBM consists of a mat of extracellular matrix that is more condensed in the central lamina densa (ld). Beneath the endothelium (En) is a looser lamina rara interna (lri). Likewise, a looser lamina rara externa (lre) is beneath the foot processes of epithelial podocytes (Po). Note the fine fibrils *(arrows)* projecting from the lamina densa onto the plasma membranes of the podocytes. CL, capillary lumen; arrowhead, epithelial slit diaphragm, US, urinary space. Original magnification ×75,000.

N-terminus (called the 7S domain), and (c) a C-terminal noncollagenous domain (NC1) (3,5,6,12). Analysis of complementary DNA (cDNA)-derived amino acid sequences from many vertebrate and invertebrate species shows that the 7S and NC1 domains are the most highly conserved regions. Three α chains self-assemble to form monomers consisting of triple helical regions in both the central and N-terminal 7S collagenous domains (3,5,6, 12). Interchain disulfide bonds form between separate monomers at the 7S and NC1 domains and result in a scaffold of polymerized collagen IV (Fig. 2). Specifically, four collagen IV monomers are aligned in an antiparallel fashion at their N-terminal 7S domains, and hydrophobic interactions and disulfide bridges stabilize the alignment to produce a tetramer. Hydrophobic and disulfide bonding also form between the C-terminal NC1 domains on separate monomers. Here, the three α chain C-termini of one monomer crosslink with C-termini of like

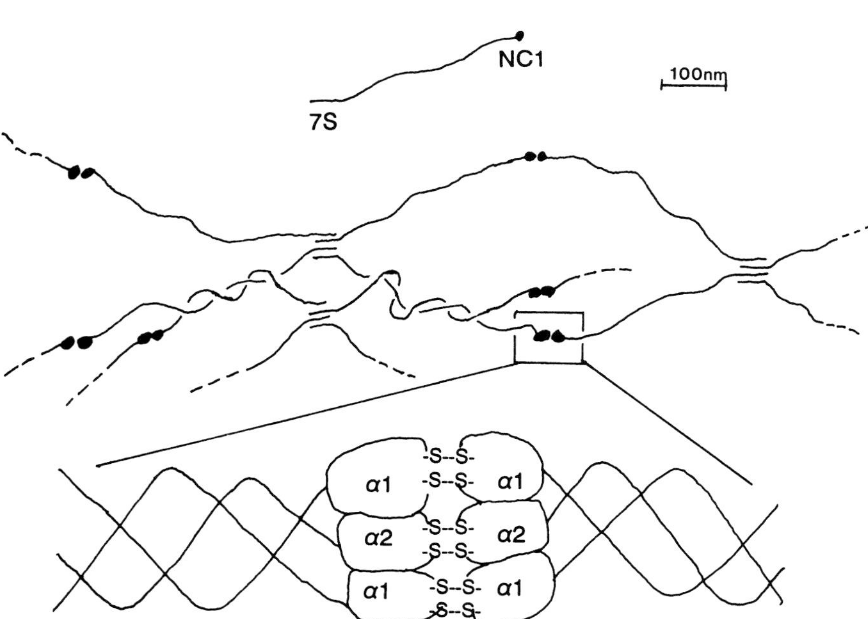

FIG. 2. Diagram showing interactions between separate 7S and NC1 domains of type IV collagen monomers to form an extended meshwork. Lateral interactions between monomers can produce twisted helices. Bottom of figure shows an expanded view of carboxy-terminal globules. The hexamer structure of NC1 domains are stabilized by disulfide crosslinks. [Modified with permission (3,6).]

α chains on the adjacent monomer to produce a fixed hexamer consisting of α chain C-termini (Fig. 2). In addition, noncovalent interactions between monomers probably also take place in the triple helical domains to form twisted helices (Fig. 2). Unlike the fiber-forming collagens (types I, II, and III), type IV chains contain interruptions of the typical Gly-X-Y collagenous repeats in the major collagenous domain. The interruptions are more or less evenly distributed, and, upon alignment of separate α chains, most are in the same position. These breaks in the collagenous sequences allow for much greater flexibility in collagen IV when compared with the relatively rigid collagens I to III and hence may promote the formation of supertwisted collagen IV helices. These interruptions in collagenous sequences are also sites for proteolytic attack and for attachment of collagen IV to other basement membrane molecules (3,5,6,12).

At this writing, six genetically distinct α chains of collagen IV have been completely sequenced and their chromosomal locations identified. Genes encoding the human α1(IV) chain (*COL4A1*) and α2(IV) chain (*COL4A2*) are found on chromosome 13 (13–15); *COL4A3* and *COL4A4* map to chromosome 2q35–37 (16); and *COL4A5* and *COL4A6* are on the X chromosome at q22 (17). The *COL4A1* and *COL4A2* genes are arranged as a head-to-head pair and are coregulated with a bidirectional promoter (13,14). The *COL4A5* and *COL4A6* genes are similarly arranged on the X chromosome (17), and the *COL4A3* and *COLRA4* genes are also thought to be organized in the same way (16).

The most abundant isoform of collagen IV contains two α1(IV) chains and one α2(IV) chain, and this species is believed to occur universally in all basement membranes. Although the α1 and α2(IV) chains are by far the most prevalent, the other chains play important roles in certain basement membrane disorders. As will be discussed in detail below, Goodpasture syndrome is a severe autoimmune disease affecting the GBM (and sometimes lung alveolar basement membranes) in which autoantibodies are directed specifically against a collagenase-resistant epitope found in the NC1 domain of the α3 chain of collagen IV (5,12). Patients with X-linked Alport syndrome, which is not an autoimmune disease but leads to progressive renal failure and is often associated with deafness, have been shown to carry mutations and/or deletions in the α5 and/or α6(IV) chains (12,18). On the other hand, autosomally inherited forms of Alport syndrome seems to be caused by mutations in the α3 and α4(IV) chains.

LAMININ

Laminin is the major noncollagenous basement membrane glycoprotein (3,4,9). The most extensively studied laminin is that isolated from the mouse Englebreth-Holm-Swarm (EHS) tumor and is referred to as laminin-1 (19). This tumor laminin consists of three polypeptides: an α1 chain (formerly called A chain) with an M_r of approximately 400 kDa; a β1 chain (B1 chain, M_r approximately 222 kDa); and a γ1 chain (B2 chain, M_r approximately 210 kDa) (Fig. 3). The cDNAs for the three laminin 1 chains have been cloned and, because all three chains are made up of similar modular domains, the chains exhibit considerable sequence and structural homology (20–22). As is the case for the collagen IV α chains, the separate laminin chains are also found on different chromosomes. In humans the laminin α1 chain gene is located on chromosome 18, the β1 chain gene is found on chromosome 7, and the γ1 is on chromosome 1 (23–25).

The three laminin chains are joined together by intermolecular disulfide bonds to form a cross-shaped molecule with three short and one long arm. Based on the derived amino acid sequences, circular dichroism studies, and electron microscopic analysis of rotary shadowed

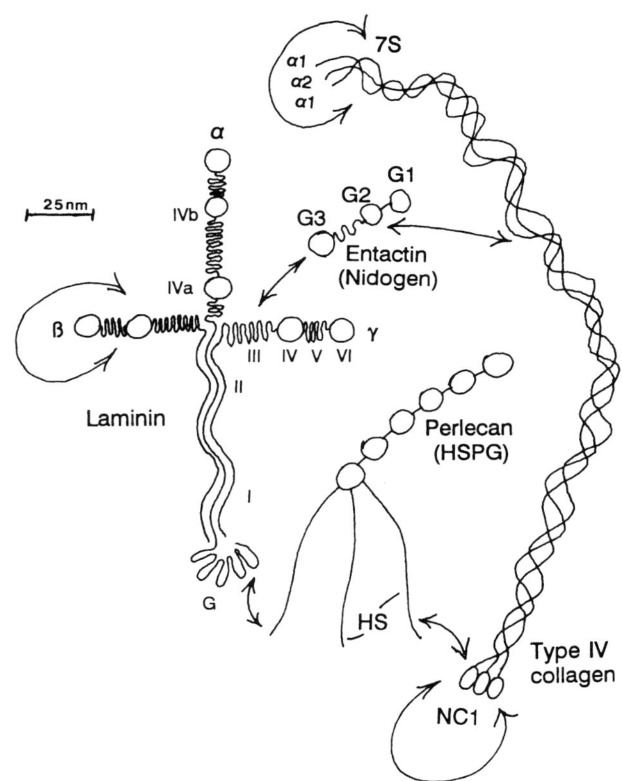

FIG. 3. Diagram showing structures of the laminin α, β, and γ chains, entactin, an α1(IV)2, α2(IV) collagen type IV monomer, and perlecan. Laminin can self-associate through interactions between terminal short-arm domains. The G3 domain of entactin binds to domain III on the laminin chain, and the entactin G2 domain binds to collagen IV. The heparan sulfate (HS) glycosaminoglycan chains of perlecan bind to the terminal globular (G) domain of the laminin α chain and to the NC1 domain of collagen IV. Collagen monomers polymerize through disulfide bonds at the 7S and NC1 domains. [Modified with permission (3,9,10).]

preparations, the α, β, and γ chains interact with one another in domains I and II to form a coiled-coil structure constituting the long arm of laminin (Fig. 3). Analysis of interchain ionic interactions within the coiled-coil domain have demonstrated that three different chains are indeed present and that homodimer and homotrimer formation in this region is unfavorable (26). Domains III and V of the β and γ chains, and domains IIIa, IIIb, and V of the α chain are rich in cysteine residues arranged at regular intervals to form a series of loops that are each stabilized by intrachain disulfide linkages (20–22). These domains show some homology to the cysteine rich region of epidermal growth factor (EGF) and transforming growth factor alpha (TGF-α). Recently, the EGF-like repeat number four in domain III of the γ1 chain has been identified as the binding site for the laminin-associated protein entactin (27) (Fig. 3). Other features of laminin include domains IV and VI, which are found on the N-terminal segments of all three chains and represent the central and terminal globular domains on the short arms. An additional globular domain exists at the end of the long arm, which is contributed solely by the C-terminus of the α chain (21) (Fig. 3).

Numerous biologic activities have been ascribed to laminin, including the mediation or promotion of adhesion, migration, and growth of a variety of cells and induction of neurite outgrowth. Through the use of various proteolytic fragments of the molecule, many of these biologic activities have been assigned to specific domains on laminin. In addition, the cloning of the several chains has provided for the preparation of synthetic or recombinant peptides, which has then led to more precise localization of certain activities to specific peptide sequences (28–31) (Table 1).

Laminin binds to cells through cell surface receptors, including those of the integrin superfamily. Many integrins have been shown to interact with laminin (α1β1, α2β1, α3β1, α6β1, α7β1, αvβ3, $\alpha_{IIb}\beta3$) (32,33), but α6β1 seems to be the primary integrin receptor for laminin. Other nonintegrin laminin-binding proteins probably also exist as well. The sites on the laminin molecule recognized by any of these receptors still are not certain, however. An RGD sequence is present in the N-terminal half of mouse α1 chain, but this site is apparently only active after pepsin digestion of laminin (34). On the other hand, several other studies have shown that a primary cell-binding domain(s) is located on the end of the long arm, on or near the terminal globular domain formed by the C-terminus of the α chain.

In addition to binding to cells, laminin also has been shown to bind specifically to other basement membrane components, including type IV collagen (35,36), HSPG (37), and entactin (38). The binding sites for HSPG also have been identified at the end of the long arm (Fig. 3). Laminin also contains laminin-binding sites, and these are important for the formation of laminin networks (10, 39). Specifically, the laminin-binding sites are located within the short-arm N-terminal globules at each of the three laminin polypeptides (Fig. 3). The most stable laminin polymers seem to occur in a calcium-dependent way in which each short arm of laminin engages short arms from two other laminin molecules (10,39).

In addition to the mouse tumor laminin-1 trimer (α1, β1, γ1), several other distinct laminin-like α, β, and γ chains have been described [α2, α3, α4, α5; β2, β3, β4; γ2 (40,41)], and these can combine with one another to form different laminin isoforms. As is the case for laminin-1, all of the other isoforms of laminin thus far investigated also consist of heterotrimers containing single α, β, and γ chains. These structurally similar but nevertheless unique laminin isoforms presumably impart some specialized functions in the various basement membranes they occupy, but exactly how these functions differ is not known. As discussed below, the laminin-2 isoform appears to replace laminin-1 during GBM development. The presence of many of these laminin isoforms in various tissues have been shown through the use of chain-specific antibodies and/or in situ or Northern hybridization analyses with appropriate probes. Because the homologies among chains are often so similar, however, some falsely

TABLE 1. *Peptide sequences of functional laminin domains*

Sequence	Chain (residues)	Activity
RPVRHAQCRVCDGNSTNPRERH	α (42–63)	Keratinocyte adhesion
KATPMLKMRTSFHGCIK	α (2,615–2,631)	HT1080 cell adhesion
KEGYKVRLDLNITLEFRTTSK	α (2,890–2,910)	Spreading, migration, and outgrowth of neurites
KNLEISRSTFDLLRNSYGVRK	α (2,443–2,463)	Spreading, migration, and outgrowth of neurites
DGKWHTVKTEYIKRKAF	α (2,779–2,795)	Spreading, migration, and outgrowth of neurites
KQNCLSSRASFRGCVRNLRLSR	α (3,011–3,032)	Keratinocyte adhesion
RGD	α (1,118–1,120)	Epithelial and endothelial adhesion, migration, and differentiation
SIKVAV	α (2,099–2,105)	Spreading, migration, and outgrowth of neurites
YIGSR	β (929–933)	Epithelial and endothelial adhesion, migration, and differentiation
RNAIEIIKDA	γ (1,542–1,551)	Cerebellar neurite outgrowth

Data were compiled from refs. 28–31.

positive identifications are probable. Definitive proof of the existence of some isoforms most likely can only be obtained in conjunction with biochemical analysis.

ENTACTIN

Entactin (also referred to as nidogen) is a sulfated glycoprotein (M_r approximately 150 kDa) that has a strong affinity for laminin, and also binds to the NC1 domain of collagen type IV (3,9,42). Mouse entactin consists of a single polypeptide chain of 1,217 amino acids (42,43) and, by rotary shadow electron microscopy, contains three distinct globular domains (G1, G2, G3) connected by rods (44) (Fig. 3). G1 comprises the N-terminal end of the molecule and contains negatively charged residues possessing a calcium-binding, EF hand motif. A second putative calcium-binding domain is located in a short rodlike segment that joins G1 to G2, and binding sites for collagen IV and perlecan are present in G2. Separating G2 and the C-terminal G3 is a second, somewhat longer rodlike domain. G3 is a cysteine-rich domain that bears resemblance to EGF and to the low density lipoprotein (LDL) receptor and is the region that binds entactin to the fourth EGF-like repeat in domain III of the laminin γ1 chain (Fig. 3). Human entactin has been cloned and sequenced and shown to be approximately 84% identical with that of the mouse (45). The gene exists as a single locus on human chromosome 1q43 (46).

Entactin forms ternary complexes between laminin and type IV collagen, as well as between laminin and perlecan (44). Entactin also binds fibronectin and immobilized fibrinogen (47) and is chemotactic for neutrophils (48).

PROTEOGLYCANS

The best characterized HSPG is also that from the EHS tumor. When rotary shadowed and viewed in the electron microscope, the molecule is linear, with six or seven globular domains giving the appearance of beads on a string, hence the name "perlecan" (49) (Fig. 3). The full-length perlecan cDNA has been cloned and sequenced for both mice and humans (49–51), and the derived amino acid sequence shows five different structural domains. The N-terminal domain I is the only region of perlecan that has no significant homology with any other protein. Within a 14–amino acid stretch of domain I are three repeats of the sequence SGD and each of these are the apparent attachment sites for a heparan sulfate glycosaminoglycan side chain. Domain II contains four repeating subunits that are homologous to members of the LDL receptor family. Domain III has homology with the short arms of laminin and contains both cysteine-rich, rodlike regions (correlating to laminin domains III and V) and globular regions (that are similar to domains IV and VI of the laminin α chain). Domain IV of mouse and human perlecan contains a series of fourteen and twenty-one repeats, respectively, and these are similar to the immunoglobulin superfamily and to the neural cell adhesion molecule (N-CAM). Finally, domain V consists of three globular repeats that demonstrate homology with the C-terminal globular domain of the laminin α chain (49–50). The human perlecan gene has been localized to chromosome 1p36 (52).

The heparan sulfate side chains of perlecan (of which there apparently are three) have been shown to contribute to the anionic charge barrier of the GBM (2). As already mentioned, perlecan binds to both laminin and collagen type IV (53) and also may act as a depot for certain growth factors, especially basic FGF (54).

One or more CSPGs are also present within kidney basement membranes (55,56). As of this writing, however, these molecules have not yet been fully cloned or purified in sufficient quantities for biochemical characterization, and their structures therefore remain largely undetermined.

SUPRAMOLECULAR ASSEMBLY OF BASEMENT MEMBRANE PROTEINS

Two separate but convergent approaches have been used to investigate the molecular architecture of basement membranes. First, highly purified preparations of the separate proteins have been incubated together, rotary shadowed with platinum, and then examined by electron microscopy to visualize the intermolecular relationships (10,53). The findings with this technique have indicated that two independent but interwoven polymers probably exist in basement membranes. One polymer consists of a three-dimensional network of collagen type IV stabilized by covalent interactions at N-terminal 7S domains, C-terminal NC1 domains, and noncovalent lateral combinations (3,6,12) (Fig. 2). The second polymer consists of a laminin network established by binding of the terminal globule of each laminin short arm to terminal short arm domains on two other laminin molecules (10). Entactin, through binding of its C-terminus to domain III on the laminin γ1 chain, and of its G2 domain to collagen IV, forms a stabilizing span between the laminin and collagen networks. Likewise, the heparan sulfate glycosaminoglycan side chains of perlecan bind to the C-terminus of the laminin α chain and to the NC1 domain of collagen IV to form what appears to be a fully integrated network (10) (Fig. 3).

The second approach has been to use antibodies against defined epitopes or domains on the various intrinsic proteins and immunomicroscopic techniques to map the distributions of these epitopes in tissue sections. In general, the results from this approach have shown that all of the known basement membrane molecules codistribute throughout the full width of tubular and glomerular basement membranes (57,58), and this is in agreement with the rotary shadowing findings. However, the use of monoclonal antibodies directed specifically against separate polypeptide chains of the various molecules have shown that there can be regional concentrations for certain epitopes (57,59,60). These regional differences emphasize that the matrix is not homogeneous. Many of these regional dissimilarities are particularly evident during basement membrane assembly in development.

BASEMENT MEMBRANE FORMATION DURING NEPHRON DEVELOPMENT

During metanephric kidney development, the ureteric bud invades undifferentiated mesenchyme and, in a temporally and spatially regulated way, the bud epithelium induces the formation of mesenchymal cell condensates (61,62) (see Chapter 2). The induction mechanism is not understood but involves cell–cell contact and the elaboration of specific growth factors as well. Each mesenchymal cell condensate then undergoes a transition to an epithelial phenotype and gives rise to the glomerular and tubular epithelium of a nephron. The first condensates that form go on to develop into juxtamedullary nephrons, whereas the last condensates induced become the most cortical, superficial nephrons. As cells within the condensates convert from a mesenchymal to epithelial phenotype, they stop synthesizing interstitial matrix proteins such as collagen types I and III and begin synthesizing basement membrane proteins (63). These epithelial aggregates are termed vesicles, and they proceed through an orderly sequence of developmental stages described as comma and S-shaped bodies. The lower cleft of the S-shaped body forms the glomerular portion of the nephron, whereas the upper curvature gives rise to the tubular segments. The developing distal tubule soon connects to a branch of the ureteric bud, which functionally matures into the collecting system.

When mouse kidney development is examined by immunofluorescence microscopy, laminin, type IV collagen, and perlecan first appear as discrete spots on aggregating mesenchymal cells, and these then form semicontinuous sheets on the outer surfaces of vesicle, comma- and S-shaped bodies (63). The appearance of these basement membrane molecules early in nephrogenesis suggests roles for these proteins in initial cell aggregation and subsequent epithelial differentiation.

Of the major basement membrane components, the best studied in kidney development is laminin. When kidney mesenchymes are experimentally induced in vitro and examined for the presence of messenger RNA (mRNAs) encoding laminin chains, only the $\beta 1$ and $\gamma 1$ chains are detected 24 hr after induction (64). In contrast, the α chain message does not first appear until 48 hr after induction, and this time frame correlates with the conversion of aggregated mesenchymal cells to an epithelial phenotype. Results of immunolabeling studies with chain-specific antibodies also have shown that the appearance of α chain protein coincides with the formation of basement membranes around the condensing vesicles. This occurs before the appearance of morphologically polarized epithelial cells and therefore places the initial expression of the laminin α chain near the inception of the mesenchyme–epithelial conversion (64). Moreover, application of antibodies against the C-terminal globular domain of the laminin $\alpha 1$ chain, or antisera against an elastase-resistant laminin fragment containing C-termini of all three α, β, and γ chains, effectively blocks epithelial cell polarization in cultured mouse kidneys (64). However, these antisera do not disrupt ureteric bud branching or vesicle formation (65). Hence laminin, especially the C-terminal α chain domain, is crucial for epithelial differentiation in the forming nephron.

GBM ASSEMBLY

As mentioned earlier, the lower, vascular cleft of the S-shaped body is the site from which the glomerulus blossoms. Until recently, glomerular endothelial cells were believed to be derived from angiogenic sprouts growing into the metanephros. However, new evidence has shown that endogenous progenitor endothelial cells (angioblasts) originating from the metanephric mesenchyme establish the renal microvasculature through a vasculogenic, rather than angiogenic, process (66,67). As endothelial (and presumably mesangial) cells migrate into the forming glomerulus, capillary loops rapidly develop, and this process is accompanied by the formation of considerable amounts of basement membrane material (68). Initially, endothelial cells and epithelial podocytes each assemble a separate layer of basement membrane matrix (Fig. 4). With maturation of the glomerular wall, these two layers merge or fuse to produce a common GBM shared on one surface by endothelial cells and on the opposite surface by podocytes. As diameters of the glomerular capillary loops increase, epithelial podocyte foot process interdigitation proceeds, and these cells are still engaged in basement membrane synthesis. This new, podocyte-derived basement membrane is seen as irregular loops of matrix beneath the forming foot processes (Fig. 5). With glomerular maturation, these new basement membrane segments are deposited or spliced into the fused GBM (68).

The mechanisms responsible for basement membrane fusion and splicing are unknown, but they conceivably involve precise spatial and temporal release of matrix proteases to allow for the integration of new material into that already present. There also seem to be temporal

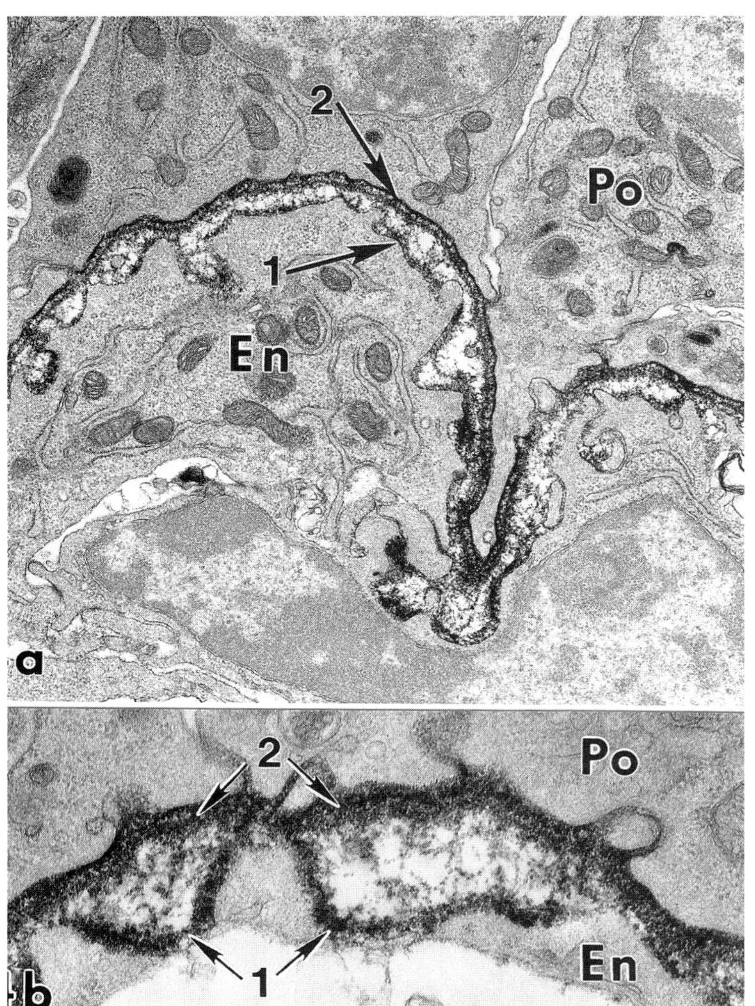

FIG. 4. Immunoelectron micrographs of developing glomerulus in newborn mouse kidney labeled with monoclonal antilaminin IgG conjugated to horseradish peroxidase (HRP). Black, electron-dense HRP reaction product is seen in the subendothelial (1) and subepithelial (2) dual basement membrane. Note that foot processes have not yet formed in the epithelial podocyte layer. En, immature endothelium; Po, immature epithelial podocytes. **a:** Original magnification ×18,000. **b:** Original magnification ×27,500.

changes in patterns of synthesis of certain basement membrane protein isoforms as well. Support for both of these possibilities is provided by immunohistochemical experiments showing changes in GBM structure over time. Certain epitopes on the laminin β1 chain are abundant in immature mouse prefusion GBMs, but these epitopes are undetectable at both the light and electron microscopic level in more mature glomeruli after GBM fusion (69). In addition, the presence of the laminin β2 chain is first observed only after the disappearance of the β1 chain (70). Additional compelling evidence for laminin isoform substitution during glomerular development has come from studies in which homologous recombination was used to generate mice carrying a null mutation in the laminin β2 gene. These animals seem to compensate for a deficiency in the β2 chain by failing to downregulate β1 chain synthesis; hence, considerable β1 chain persists into glomerular maturation (71). Although the GBM in these mice appears morphologically normal, the glomeruli nevertheless contain striking structural and functional abnormalities. Podocyte foot processes fail to form appropriately, and infant mice become massively proteinuric (71). An independent immunofluorescence study of developing human GBM has similarly shown that laminin β1 chain disappears during glomerular maturation, and this correlates with the appearance of the β2 chain (72). The known genetic deficiencies involving other laminin chains, such as mutations in laminin α2 chain in *dy/dy* dystrophic mice (73) and γ2 in human epidermolysis bullosa (74), do not seem to result in structural or functional problems with the GBM or TBM. In situ hybridization studies with riboprobes against rat kidney laminin γ1 chain show that immature rat nephrons synthesize considerable γ1 chains, and mRNAs for this chain are also readily detectable in maturing stage glomeruli, but not in maturing tubules (75). Once again, these findings demonstrate that there are regional differences in basement membrane architecture.

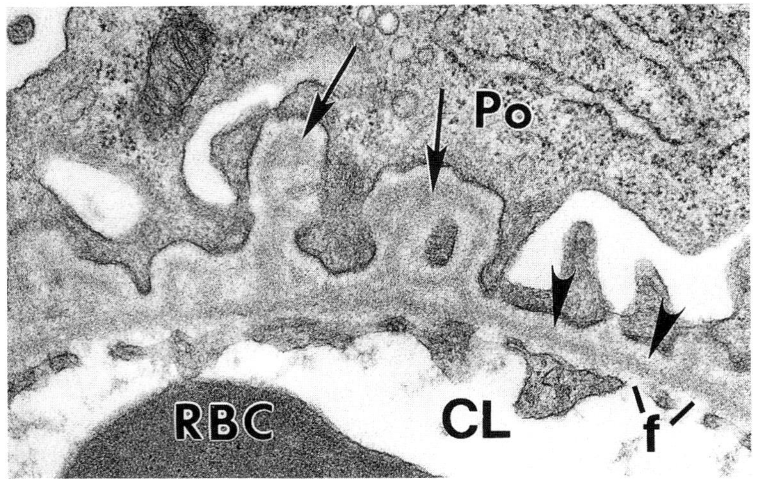

FIG. 5. With continued glomerular maturation, the endothelium flattens and forms fenestrae (f). Areas where the dual basement membrane has fused are seen on the right side of the figure *(arrowheads)*. Newly synthesized segments of basement membrane *(arrows)* derived from podocytes (Po) are located in regions still undergoing foot process development. These segments will somehow be spliced into the fused basement membrane. CL, capillary lumen; RBC, erythrocyte. Original magnification ×36,000.

The time of appearance and distribution of the several collagen type IV α chains during glomerular development has similarly been investigated. Ribonuclease protection assays have shown that kidneys of newborn mice contain abundant collagen IV α1 chain mRNA and little message for α3, 4, or 5 chains (70). Adult mouse kidneys, by contrast, contain abundant mRNAs for all collagen chains. Immunofluorescence labeling with chain-specific antibodies shows that GBM of immature glomeruli in newborn rat kidneys labels intensely for α1 and α2(IV) collagen. In contrast, the GBM of more mature glomeruli was relatively weakly labeled, whereas the mesangium remained positive. Antibodies against the collagen IV α3, 4, and 5 chains labeled maturing glomeruli strongly, but early glomeruli were only weakly labeled. These results therefore show that, like the laminin β2 chain, there is an upregulation of collagen IV α3–5 chains with glomerular maturation (70). Indeed, double-label immunofluorescence microscopy of developing glomeruli has shown that the laminin β1 chain seems to codistribute with collagen IV α1 and α2 chains, and immature GBM is jointly labeled for these polypeptides. Likewise, as GBM assembly progresses, labeling for these molecules diminishes with the appearance of laminin β2 and collagen IV α3–5 chains (70). At the ultrastructural level, monoclonal antibodies have localized the α1(IV) chain mainly to the subendothelial zone (lamina rara interna) of the adult human GBM and throughout mesangial matrices (59). On the other hand, monoclonal antibodies against the α3(IV) chain label the full width of the GBM but not the mesangium (59). Curiously, despite what appears to be the presence of a shared promoter between genes encoding the α5 and α6(IV) collagen chains (discussed further below), only α5 is detectable in the adult human GBM. Anti-α6(IV) antibodies do label Bowman's capsule and distal tubule basement membranes, however (76).

Although entactin (nidogen) appears to play an important stabilizing role in basement membrane networks, only a few studies have examined its synthetic patterns in the kidney. Northern analysis and immunofluorescence microscopy techniques have both shown that entactin is relatively abundant in mouse kidney (77). In addition, antibodies against the entactin binding site on the laminin γ1 chain have been shown to interfere with renal tubule epithelial cell differentiation in vitro (77). However, in situ hybridization studies indicate that entactin actually comes from metanephric mesenchymal cells and not epithelial cells (77). These findings therefore suggest that mesenchymally derived entactin influences renal epithelial development (77).

Beyond immunofluorescence microscopy showing the presence of perlecan in developing kidney basement membranes, there is little information on its synthesis and assembly in the kidney. Immunoelectron microscopy using monoclonal antibodies against the core protein and heparan sulfate side chains showed that both constituents localized primarily to the lamina rara interna of adult human GBM (60). Two recent studies using monoclonal antibodies against domain III of perlecan have indicated that this domain is abundant in the mature GBM (78,79). Northern analysis of mouse kidneys has shown that high levels of perlecan mRNA are detectable in both immature and mature animals (80). In contrast, the same study showed that message levels for collagen IV α1 chain and the laminin α1, β1, and γ1 chain decrease quickly after birth and are almost imperceptible in adult mice (80). There is no information as yet at the molecular level on kidney basement membrane CSPG. An immunohistochemical study showed an unusual transient appearance of the molecule in the GBM of maturing glomeruli of young rats, but in adult rat glomeruli, basement membrane CSPG is present only in the mesangium and the GBM is normally unlabeled (81).

REGULATION OF BASEMENT MEMBRANE GENES

In order for basement membranes to assemble and function properly, the synthesis of the various polypeptide chains of the several basement membrane proteins must somehow be coordinated. Nevertheless, despite considerable progress in understanding the coding sequences, exon/intron structures, and transcription units of the various genes, we still do not understand how, or even if, these genes are centrally regulated. When one examines the regulatory regions of collagen IV genes, some common features appear but the controls for expression of these genes nevertheless seem extremely complex. As mentioned earlier, the genes for the α1 and α2 type IV collagen chains are found to be closely linked on chromosome 13. Genomic sequencing shows that the two genes are oriented head to head in opposite directions and are separated by a 127–base pair region that contains a bidirectional promoter (13). Likewise, the genes for α3 and α4 chains of collagen IV are arranged in a similar manner on chromosome 2, and those for α5 and α6 are found on the X chromosome, except here they are separated by 452 base pairs. The promoter shared by the α1 and α2 chains does not show significant transcriptional activity in either direction; therefore, additional enhancer elements must be necessary to activate transcription. Such elements have been identified in the first exon/intron boundary, and these elements can activate the promoter in either the α1 or α2(IV) direction (13). The promoter itself does not contain a TATA box, which is a sequence present in most eucaryotic promoters transcribed by RNA polymerase II (82). However, the promoter contains a GC box and Sp1 and retinoic acid binding sites. In addition, a somewhat unique CTC box is present, and this motif is also found in certain other extracellular matrix genes, including those encoding the laminin β and γ chains (82,83). Recently, a multimeric CTC box–binding factor has been characterized, and included in this complex is a TATA-binding protein (84). Although the collagen IV promoter lacks the TATA box, other TATA-less promoters are believed to use different promoter-binding factors so that the TATA-binding protein can align RNA polymerase II and initiate transcription. Perhaps the collagen IV α1 and α2 chains are activated in the same way. Nevertheless, how the transcription (or translation) machinery operates to produce collagen IV monomers consisting predominantly of two α1(IV) chains and one α2(IV) chain is not known. Perhaps this chain selection process, like that for the fiber-forming collagens, is mediated in the rough endoplasmic reticulum by the NC1 domains of collagen IV (6).

As mentioned earlier for the α1 and α2 collagen IV genes, the promoter regions for the laminin β and γ chains also share a CTC box . The CTC box is repeated nine times within the mouse γ1 chain promoter and six times in that for the human γ1 chain (85,86). The γ1 promoter also contains many kappa B-like motifs that may be sensitive to interleukin (IL)-1β induction, but whether such elements are important for normal regulation is unknown (87). In the 5′ upstream region of the β1 gene are two CTC boxes, a CCAAT box, and two AP-1 sites (88). Three retinoic acid–responsive elements are also present between –100 and the transcription start site for β1, but these elements are absent in the γ1 gene (88). Based on the regulatory regions of the β1 and γ1 genes, they likely are under different transcriptional controls. Indeed, experiments to quantify laminin message expression have shown that much greater amounts of β chain mRNA are detected than those for α or γ chains, although posttranscriptional regulation events cannot be ruled out (80). The regulatory regions for the other laminin genes have not yet been examined carefully. Nevertheless, these genes are likely to be equally complex.

Unlike *COL4A1* and *COL4A2,* as well as at least some of the laminin genes, TATA boxes are found in human and mouse entactin/nidogen genes (89). Several AP-2 and Sp1 sites are also present (89). Regulatory regions of the human perlecan gene, in contrast, lack TATA motifs, but several GC sites for binding Sp1 transcription factors are also found (90). Due to the diverse promoter control elements and distribution of most of the basement membrane genes to separate chromosomes, considerably more work needs to be conducted before we understand how transcription of these matrix genes is coordinated.

HUMAN ANTI-GBM DISEASE

Human autoimmune disease associated with anti–basement membrane antibodies against GBM and/or alveolar basement membrane has a variety of clinical presentations (see Chapter 4). Broadly, these include Goodpasture syndrome (clinical complex of pulmonary hemorrhage and glomerulonephritis), glomerulonephritis alone without evidence of pulmonary involvement, and pulmonary hemorrhage with little overt evidence of renal disease (91). The underlying pathogenic factors that account for these diverse clinical features remain unknown. Although the following discussion focuses on the glomerulus in anti–basement membrane disease, all three of the above clinical presentations involve the same autoantigen, namely the α3 chain of type IV collagen.

Early in the course of anti-GBM disease the kidney develops striking glomerular lesions characterized by focal segmental proliferation and tuft necrosis, and this evolves into a crescentic glomerulonephritis. Silver stains show GBM destruction by the crescents, which are often circumferential and composed of proliferating parietal epithelial cells and infiltrating monocytes and macrophages. In contrast to other glomerular diseases associated with crescents, endothelial and mesangial cell proliferation is characteristically minimal. With disease progression, the cellular crescents become fibrous, and extensive glomerular obsolescence can result, sometimes within only a few weeks. Discontinuities of the GBM and lucent widening of the subendothelial matrix are observed by electron microscopy. Electron-dense deposits are not present. Immunofluorescence microscopy, which initially elucidated the immunopathogenesis of anti-GBM disease (91), shows a smooth, ribbonlike linear deposition of immunoglobulin (Ig)G along the GBMs of all glomeruli. At the onset of disease, circulating anti-GBM antibody can also be detected with radio- or enzyme-immunoassays in over 95% of patients. Some patients with anti-GBM disease have evidence of vasculitis and accompanying antineutrophil cytoplasmic antibody (92) (see Chapters 43, 49). Conceivably, the severe cell and tissue injury associated with deposition of one autoantibody can lead to the production of a second pathogenic autoantibody that induces a different or overlapping pattern of injury.

From the animal models of human anti-GBM disease, we have gleaned the following general pathologic cascade of glomerular injury (see Chapter 35). The accumulation of autoantibody (IgG) within the GBM activates complement, leading to the generation of chemotactic peptides that attract neutrophils and monocytes, which then accumulate within glomeruli due to enhanced expression of cell adhesion molecules (Fig. 6). The GBM is damaged by proteases and toxic oxygen radicals released from the infiltrating cells. Fibrin leakage through the disrupted glomerular capillary wall into Bowman's space elicits crescent formation. In addition, secondary mediators such as IL-1, transforming growth factor-β, and leukotrienes play a role.

Extensive chemical, immunologic, and molecular studies of type IV collagen extracted from collagenase-digested human GBM have determined that the noncollagenous domain (NC1) at the carboxy-terminus of the α3 chain of type IV collagen contains the autoantigen in anti-GBM disease (12,93). Initial studies with antibodies from patients with anti-GBM disease showed that solubilized GBM contained a reactive 26-kDa polypeptide in the NC1 domain of collagen IV (94,95). In the presence of denaturants, the NC1 hexamer, consisting of six NC1 subunits,

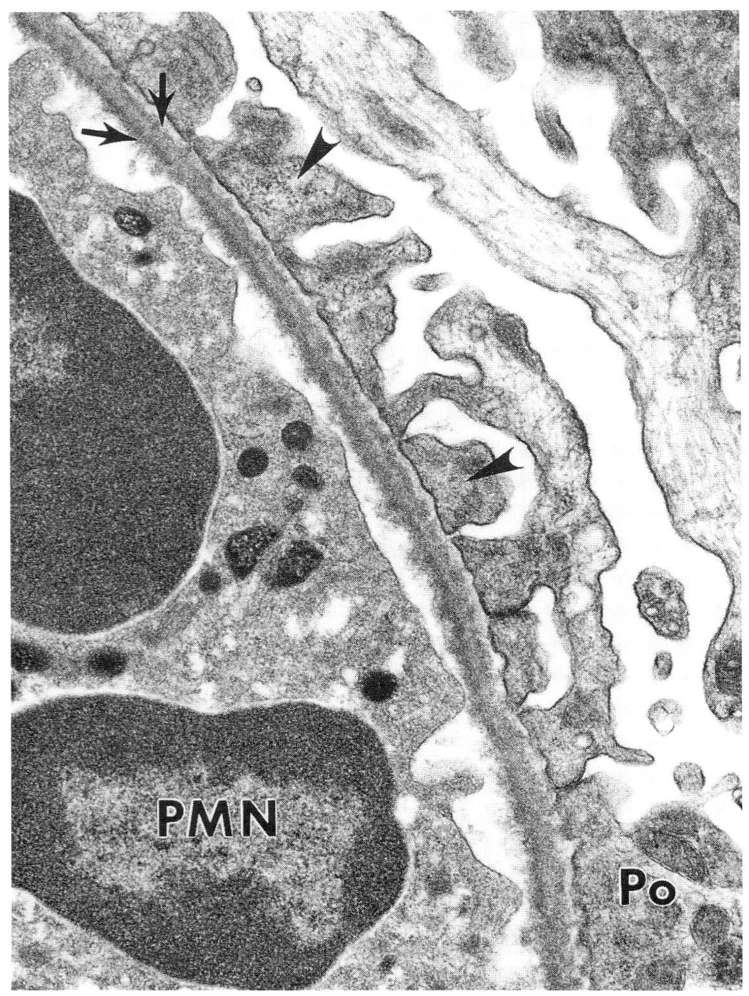

FIG. 6. Glomerular capillary wall from a rat that was immunized against sheep IgG and then received an intravenous injection of sheep antilaminin IgG. A neutrophil (PMN) has completely displaced the endothelium. Note delamination of the normally fused GBM *(arrows)* and foot process broadening *(arrowheads)* by podocytes (Po). Original magnification ×29,000.

dissociated into monomer and dimer forms. Amino-terminal analysis and Western blotting showed the classic α1 and α2 chains of type IV collagen but also identified two novel chains, which were then designated α3 and α4 (96–99). The α3 NC1 domain monomer and dimer bound the anti-GBM antibodies. Subsequently, partial cDNAs encoding the NC1 domain of the α3 chain were obtained, confirming the existence of this chain (100,101).

Complete sequencing of the α3 (IV) chain shows that it contains 1,642 amino acids, including a 232-residue NC1 domain (102). Because it is more homologous to the α1(IV) and α5(IV) chains, the α3 chain is a member of the so-called α1 class. In contrast, the α2, α4, and α6(IV) chains show significant homology and hence are in the α2 class. At both the RNA and protein level, α3 (IV) and α4 (IV) are consistently coexpressed and associate to form $(\alpha3)_2\alpha4$ heterotrimers (102–104). Moreover, the genes *COL4A3* and *COL4A4* encoding α3(IV) and α4(IV), respectively, are located head to head on chromosome 2, likely share a bidirectional promoter, and thus appear to be coregulated (16). Within the adult glomerulus, the α3(IV), α4(IV), and α5(IV) chains are immunolocalized to the lamina densa of the GBM (59,103). In contrast, the α1(IV) and α2(IV) chains are distributed along the subendothelial aspect of the GBM and within the mesangial matrix (59).

Alternative splicing of the mRNA encoding the α3(IV) NC1 domain results in multiple transcripts, the ratio of which appears to be developmentally regulated (105–107). Several of the alternative spliced transcripts lack some of the conserved NC1 domain cysteine residues that are probably required for intermolecular disulfide cross-linking into triple helical monomers (108). What is the biologic significance of this alternative splicing? Whether or not all of the transcripts are translated is not known, but the putative protein isoforms could mediate diverse functions during development and/or maintenance of the GBM. In other words, varying ratios of multiple α3(IV) transcripts may provide a flexible mechanism for controlling the amount of mature α3(IV) that, in turn, is important in regulating the formation and/or maintenance of the polymerized type IV collagen superstructure. Some of the variant α3(IV) transcripts contain truncated forms of the anti-GBM disease autoantigen (Goodpasture syndrome antigen) within the NC1 domain. Thus, varying ratios of α3(IV) isoforms may explain the impaired immunoreactivity of certain human GBM autoantibodies observed on sections of fetal kidney (109,110). Whether a particular ratio of α3(IV) isoforms plays a role in the development of the autoimmune response in anti-GBM disease remains to be determined. Confounding the apparent molecular diversity of the α3(IV) chain is the recent demonstration that a five-residue region (KRGDS) of the Goodpasture syndrome antigen constitutes a serine phosphorylation site (111). Additionally, whether the RGD cell adhesion motif contained within this pentapeptide is modulated by phosphorylation of the adjacent serine is not known.

The location of the Goodpasture syndrome antigen has been verified by strong immunoblot reactivity between anti-GBM antibodies and recombinant α3(IV) NC1 domains (112,113). The ability of recombinant α3(IV) NC1 to inhibit binding of the antibodies to human GBM provides additional evidence that the Goodpasture syndrome antigen indeed resides on α3(IV) NC1 (113). Because these initial findings were based on anti-GBM antibodies from only a few patients, however, a much more comprehensive enzyme-linked immunosorbent assay (ELISA) and two-dimensional immunoblotting analysis was undertaken using sera from 58 patients (114). Anti-GBM antibodies from all of the patients, including 35 with combined glomerulonephritis and pulmonary hemorrhage, 19 with glomerulonephritis alone, and four with pulmonary hemorrhage alone reacted with both bovine and recombinant human α3(IV) NC1 domain (114). Low-level reactivity to the α1(IV) NC1 and α4(IV) NC1 domains was observed in 15% and 3% of the patients, respectively, but the pathologic significance of this finding is unclear. There was no correlation between a particular clinical presentation and antibody reactivity.

Further compelling evidence for the immunopathogenicity of α3(IV) NC1 was provided by the demonstration that autoimmune renal and pulmonary disease similar to human anti-GBM disease can be induced in rabbits by immunization with α3(IV) NC1 but not by analogous NC1 domains of α1(IV), α2(IV), α4(IV), and α5(IV) (115) (see Chapter 35). That the α3(IV) NC1 dimer, but not the α3(IV) NC1 hexamer, induced autoimmune disease suggests that the Goodpasture syndrome epitope is sequestered within the junction of two interacting triple helical monomers. Hence, dissociation of the α3(IV) NC1 hexamer to the dimer form, either experimentally by protein denaturation or possibly by precipitating agents in autoimmune disease, appears to unmask the epitope that then becomes accessible to autoantibody interaction (115,116). Through experiments with modified synthetic α3(IV) NC1 peptides, the Goodpasture syndrome epitope has been sublocalized to the last 36 amino acids of α3 (IV), and its structure is now predicted to be discontinuous (117). Although rats immunized with native, collagenase-solubilized GBM containing α3(IV) NC1 develop an autoimmune glomerulonephritis (118), rats immunized with the above 36-mer peptide alone fail to develop proteinuria or glomerulonephritis despite developing antibodies that are cross-reactive to bovine and human GBM (119). Whether this lack of pathogenicity by the 36–amino acid Goodpasture syndrome epitope is particular to the rat model, or whether the remaining adjacent residues of the α3(IV) NC1 are required to impart a pathogenic conformation to the epitope, is still uncertain. Some progress in this area has recently been obtained in a mouse model (discussed below).

ALPORT SYNDROME

The identification of Alport syndrome as a genetic disorder of type IV collagen has provided new insights into glomerular structure, function, and disease (12,18,120). Although the clinical manifestations vary widely, Alport syndrome is characterized principally by hematuria, distinctive ultrastructural lesions of the GBM, and a positive family history. Over 50% of patients have sensorineural hearing loss as well, and in 15–30% of patients a variety of ocular defects also occur. Rare and poorly understood associated abnormalities include megathrombocytopenia (Epstein syndrome) and megathrombocytopenia with leukocyte inclusions (Fechtner syndrome). More recently, Alport syndrome has been reported in association with esophageal, tracheobronchial, and genital leiomyomatosis.

In the majority of affected families, the syndrome is inherited as an X chromosome–linked dominant trait, and the disorder is therefore more severe in males than in females. Most affected males develop increasing proteinuria and hypertension and slowly progress to end-stage renal disease (ESRD). The rate of disease progression tends to be constant within one family but varies significantly between kindreds. Alport syndrome may be broadly classified as juvenile or adult type depending on the development of ESRD before or after 31 years of age, respectively (121). Most affected females have mild disease and do not develop renal failure. In addition, autosomal forms of Alport syndrome have been well documented. A correlation between clinical phenotype, inheritance pattern, and molecular defect of type IV collagen will continue to be important for diagnosing, understanding, and treating this disease.

The light microscopic findings are nonspecific. Early in the course of the disease, the glomeruli appear normal, may have a fetal appearance, or may demonstrate a mild increase in mesangial cellularity and matrix. With disease progression, segmental and eventual global sclerosis of glomeruli is accompanied by interstitial fibrosis and tubular atrophy. Routine immunofluorescence examination is generally negative or nonspecific. However, the finding that human anti-GBM antibodies do not bind to glomeruli in most male patients with Alport syndrome provided the first solid evidence for a specific molecular defect within the GBM (122,123). Definitive diagnosis of the disease is primarily made by electron microscopy. Characteristic features are irregular thickening, splitting, or lamellation and interspersed thinning of the GBM. On higher magnification, the lamina densa of the GBM is reticulated (basket-weaved) and encloses small granules that likely represent fragments of cell cytoplasm. These lesions are typically diffusely distributed among the glomeruli. Thinning of the GBM may predominate over thickening, especially in children and females. An attractive hypothesis is that the basic ultrastructural lesion of Alport syndrome is the thin GBM. With additional collagen synthesis and matrix accumulation, this abnormally thin GBM then transforms into the split, thick structure seen in more advanced stages. Because some kindreds with Alport syndrome exhibit only thin (or even normal) GBMs (124), molecular methods may be required for a precise diagnosis.

That a defect in collagen type IV is responsible for Alport syndrome has been supported by studies showing that patients with Alport syndrome with posttransplant anti-GBM disease developed antibodies reacting specifically with collagen type IV (125). Subsequently, noncollagenous monomers of type IV collagen reactive with anti-GBM antibodies were shown to be absent in the GBMs from patients with Alport syndrome (126). At the time of these studies, linkage analysis mapped the Alport syndrome defect to the X chromosome (Xq22) (126,127). This finding therefore excluded the *COL4A1* and *COL4A2* genes (encoding the α1 and α2 chains of collagen IV, respectively) as disease loci because these genes localize to chromosome 13 (15). The novel α3 and α4 chains of collagen IV were also being characterized and were later mapped to chromosome 2 (16).

The cDNA encoding the novel α5(IV) chain now has been isolated and this maps to chromosome Xq22, which is the Alport syndrome locus (128,129). Moreover, immunofluorescence microscopy with antiserum against an α5(IV) synthetic peptide shows staining restricted to the GBM (128). Complete sequencing of the α5(IV) chain shows that it is homologous to the α1(IV) chain (130,131). The α5(IV) chain consists of 1,685 amino acids beginning with a 14-residue noncollagenous sequence, long collagenous Gly-X-Y repeat sequences interrupted 22 times by noncollagenous sequence, and a 229-peptide carboxy-terminal NC1 domain that, in turn, contains 12 highly conserved cysteine residues.

The demonstration of mutations in *COL4A5* in three different kindreds firmly established an association between this gene and X-linked Alport syndrome (132). However, more than 70 different mutations of the *COL4A5* gene have now been described in Alport syndrome (18). These mutations include deletions, inversions, insertions and duplications, splicing, and single base mutations dispersed throughout the gene.

Approximately 16% of the *COL4A5* mutations involve variable size deletions that have been primarily detected in males with juvenile Alport syndrome (133). Although uncommon, evidence for the deletion of the entire *COL4A5* gene has been obtained, but the complete absence of α5(IV) chain apparently is no more disruptive to the GBM than abnormal α5 chains arising from more subtle mutations (133,134). Several nonsense and splice site mutations result in a truncated α5(IV) protein (18, 135). Any loss of the carboxy-terminal NC1 domain from α5(IV) could be expected to affect monomer formation and monomer polymerization. Numerous single base mutations have also been identified. Among these, mutations involving glycine substitutions are fairly frequent, and, given the integral structural role played by glycine in the repetitive Gly-X-Y collagenous sequence, these substitutions could interfere with triple-helix formation (136, 137). Strikingly, such glycine mutations may result in a clinical phenotype that does not meet the classifications of Alport syndrome. In approximately 15% of patients, *COL4A5* mutations have been detected in the absence of a family history of Alport syndrome (138).

One curious feature that has emerged from analysis of numerous kindreds with Alport syndrome is that identical or hot spot mutations of *COL4A5* are not present. The clinical phenotype resulting from different mutations also has been difficult to predict or understand. For example, a mutation replacing residue 1563 arginine with glutamine causes juvenile-onset Alport syndrome, whereas when the adjacent residue 1564 cysteine is changed to serine, an adult-type syndrome results (139,140).

As described earlier, the head-to-head arrangement of *COL4A1* and *COL4A2* on chromosome 13, and a similar configuration of *COL4A3* and *COL4A4* on chromosome 2, led investigators to predict and then show that *COL4A5* is also paired with *COL4A6* on the X chromosome (17). The α6(IV) chain consists of 1,691 amino acids, a long collagenous domain containing 25 interruptions in the Gly-x-y tripeptide repeat, and a 228-residue, carboxy-terminal NC1 domain (141). Sequence comparisons show that α6(IV) is most similar to α2(IV) and α4(IV).

Deletions disrupting the 5′ end of both *COL4A5* and *COL4A6* have been found in four independent kindreds with Alport syndrome and associated diffuse leiomyomatosis (17). The delineation of this new contiguous gene deletion syndrome suggests that α5(IV) and/or α6(IV) may play a role in regulating muscle cell growth and differentiation, potentially through cell–matrix interactions. Mutations in *COL4A5* alone or *COL4A6* alone have not yet been reported. However, some patients with Alport syndrome without diffuse leiomyomatosis, known to have 5′ deletions of *COL4A5,* have been shown to have larger deletions of *COL4A6* than in the combined Alport–leiomyomatosis syndrome (142). Taken together, the results suggest that the Alport–leiomyomatosis syndrome may be caused by a dysfunction of the truncated α6(IV) chain.

ANIMAL MODELS OF HUMAN GBM DISEASE

Anti-GBM Disease

Numerous experimental studies have used injections of heterologous antikidney antibodies into experimental animals, most typically rats (143). This system, which was pioneered by Masugi in the 1930s and based on observations originally made by Lindemann at the turn of the century, has in the past been referred to as Masugi or nephrotoxic nephritis. Because of the demonstration that the injected antibodies deposited in linear arrays on glomerular capillary walls and within the GBM, the model is now commonly named anti-GBM nephritis (see also Chapter 35). Historically, the nephrotoxic antibodies have been prepared by immunizing sheep or rabbits with crude homogenates of kidney cortex and/or of GBM preparations purified from isolated glomeruli. When these antisera or purified IgGs are injected into rats, there is a resulting activation of complement and infiltration of neutrophils into glomeruli (Fig. 6), and this is accompanied by significant, acute proteinuria (143).

More recently, several attempts have been made to identify the primary nephritogenic antigen in experimental anti-GBM disease. One approach along these lines has been to intravenously inject into rats or mice antibodies directed against purified basement membrane proteins, as opposed to antibodies against crude cortical homogenates. Although injections of monospecific antibodies against collagen type IV (144), laminin (144,145), or HSPG (146,147) into otherwise normal animals can induce structural and functional renal abnormalities, the spectrum of pathology seen in these cases is generally mild and rarely mirrors that seen after injection of crude anti-GBM antisera (148). Hence, the intrinsic GBM nephritogen that accounts for the dramatic acute changes seen in experimental anti-GBM disease has still not yet been identified, and much of the nephrotoxic IgG may in fact be directed against plasma membrane, not GBM, constituents (149; see also Chapters 9, 17). Nevertheless, that some of the monospecific anti-GBM antibodies have potent nephrotoxic potential has clearly been established. For example, when affinity-isolated sheep antilaminin IgGs are injected into rats preimmunized against sheep IgG, massive glomerular proteinuria is accompanied by neutrophil infiltration, endothelial detachment, GBM delamination, and podocyte foot process derangement (150) (Fig. 6). Among other findings, these results demonstrate that the immunologic status of the animal, including the ability to activate complement (149), is crucial to the outcome of experimental anti-GBM disease. For example, autoimmune anti-DNA antibodies that also bind laminin with high affinity have been isolated from MRL mice, which are a model of human systemic lupus erythematosus (SLE) (151; see also Chapter 13). In addition, autoimmune antilaminin antibodies are generated in Brown-Norway (152) and DZB (153) rats injected with mercuric chloride, which is a model of human membranous glomerulopathy. Although the linkage between GBM laminin antigens and other disorders such as SLE is not clear, the findings nevertheless show that the immunogenetic background, perhaps coupled with some antecedent metabolic or inflammatory event, can result in the formation of autoimmune antibodies that can bind GBM proteins. Preliminary reports from what promises to be a versatile model for human Goodpasture syndrome have recently appeared in which various mice strains are immunized against the NC1 domain of the α3 chain of bovine type IV collagen (154,155). The early findings with this model are that the expression of certain immune response genes and chemokines are necessary for the development of disease.

Hereditary Nephritis

Studies of a family of Samoyed dogs have identified an X-linked hereditary nephritis that in many respects resembles that seen in human Alport syndrome (156). The capillary walls of affected male dogs initially show normal architecture, but beginning several weeks after birth, multilaminar GBM splitting occurs. From birth, there is an absence of the Goodpasture syndrome antigen (156). Nucleotide sequence analysis of collagen α5(IV) cDNAs shows that in affected animals there is a single base mutation that changes a conserved glycine codon (GGA) to a stop codon (TGA). This truncation apparently accounts for the 90% reduction in amount of α5 mRNA in the kidney of affected dogs and may explain the structural GBM defect (157). Although as yet there are no fully developed rodent models for Alport syndrome, kidneys of mice with targeted deficiencies in the gene encoding the α3(IV) collagen chain also resemble those of human Alport patients (J. Miner and J. Sanes, personal communication). Continued experimentation with this new murine model, as well as the mouse Goodpasture syndrome system described earlier, should help unravel the complexities of normal and abnormal GBM biology.

CLOSING COMMENTS

Major strides have been made in the past decade in understanding the normal and abnormal composition of the GBM. A convergence of molecular, biochemical, and immunopathologic analyses have now convincingly demonstrated that human anti-GBM disease may now be more specifically categorized as an anti-α3(IV) NC1 disease. The elucidation of this molecular specificity now provides a foundation for the development of novel molecular therapeutic approaches. In addition, an awareness of the genetic defects responsible for X-linked Alport syndrome has provided some comprehension of the dynamics of GBM collagen IV assembly. Despite recent meaningful progress on basement membranes, numerous questions remain unanswered regarding the complete structure, functions, and pathobiology of these critically important matrices. For example, exactly how is the GBM maintained in health and disease? How is new matrix added and old matrix removed during turnover? What are the central controls for basement membrane gene expression? What kinds of events initiate a humoral autoimmune anti-α3(IV) NC1 response and expose this domain to antibody deposition? We expect that through additional experimentation with animal models, and continued advances in the molecular understanding of human disease, that many of these questions will be answered in the near future.

ACKNOWLEDGMENT

We thank Patricia L. St. John for help with the figures. This work was supported by funds from the American Heart Association and National Institutes of Health (DK 34972).

REFERENCES

1. Kriz W, Elger M, Mundel P, Lemley KV. Structure-stabilizing forces in the glomerular tuft. *J Am Soc Nephrol* 1995;5:1731–9.
2. Farquhar MG. The glomerular basement membrane. A selective macromolecular filter. In: Hay ED, ed. *Cell biology of extracellular matrix.* 2nd ed. New York: Plenum; 1991:365–418.
3. Beck K, Gruber T. Structure and assembly of basement membrane and related extracellular matrix proteins. Richardson PD, Steiner M, eds. *Principles of cell adhesion.* Boca Raton, FL: CRC Press; 1995: 219–52.
4. Engel J. Structure and function of laminin. In: Rohrbach DH, Timpl R, eds. *Molecular and cellular aspects of basement membranes.* San Diego: Academic; 1993:147–76.
5. Hudson BG, Kalluri R, Gunwar S, Noelken ME, Mariyama M, Reeders ST. Molecular characteristics of the Goodpasture autoantigen. *Kidney Int* 1993;43:135–9.
6. Kuhn K. Basement membrane (type IV) collagen. *Matrix Biol* 1994; 14:439–45.
7. Murdoch AD, Iozzo RV. Perlecan: the multidomain heparan sulfate proteoglycan of basement membrane and extracellular matrix. *Virchows Archiv [A]* 1993;423:237–42.
8. Noonan DM, Hassell JR. Proteoglycans of basement membranes. In: Rohrbach DH, Timpl R, eds. *Molecular and cellular aspects of basement membranes.* San Diego: Academic; 1993:189–210.
9. Tryggvason K. The laminin family. *Curr Opin Cell Biol* 1993;5: 877–82.
10. Yurchenco PD, O'Rear JJ. Basal lamina assembly. *Curr Opin Cell Biol* 1994;6:674–81.
11. Chan FL, Inoue S. Lamina lucida of basement membrane: an artifact. *Microsc Res Tech* 1994;28:48–59.
12. Hudson BG, Kalluri R, Tryggvason K. Pathology of glomerular basement membrane nephropathy. *Curr Opin Nephrol Hypertens* 1994;3: 334–9.
13. Poschl E, Pollner R, Kuhn K. The genes for the α1(IV) and α2(IV) chains of human basement membrane collagen type IV are arranged head-to-head separated by a bidirectional promoter of unique structure. *EMBO J* 1988;7:2687–95.
14. Soininene R, Huotari M, Hostikka SL, Prockop DJ, Tryggvasson K. The structural genes for α1 and α2 chains of human type IV collagen are divergently encoded on opposite DNA strands and have an overlapping promoter region. *J Biol Chem* 1988;263:17217–20.
15. Boyd CD, Toth-Fejel S, Gadi IK, et al. The genes coding for human pro α1(IV) and pro α2(IV) collagen are both located at the end of the long arm of chromosome 13. *Am J Human Genet* 1988;42:309–14.
16. Mariyama M, Zheng K, Yang-Feng TL, Reeders ST. Colocalization of the genes for the α3(IV) and α4(IV) chains of type IV collagen to chromosome 2 bands q35–q37. *Genomics* 1992;13:809–13.
17. Zhou J, Mochizuki T, Smeets H, et al. Deletion of the paired α5(IV) and α6(IV) collagen genes in inherited smooth muscle tumors. *Science* 1993;261:1167–9.
18. Tryggvason K, Zhou J, Hostikka SL, Shows TB. Molecular genetics of Alport syndrome. *Kidney Int* 1993;43:38–44.

19. Burgeson RE, Chiquet M, Deutzmann R, et al. A new nomenclature for laminins. *Matrix Biol* 1994;14:209–11.
20. Sasaki M, Kato S, Kohno K, Martin GR, Yamada Y. Sequence of the cDNA encoding the laminin B1 chain reveals a multidomain protein containing cysteine-rich repeats. *Proc Natl Acad Sci U S A* 1987;84: 935–9.
21. Sasaki M, Kleinman HK, Huber H, Deutzmann R, Yamada Y. Laminin, a multidomain protein. The A chain has a unique globular domain and homology with the basement membrane proteoglycan and the laminin B chains. *J Biol Chem* 1988;263:16536–44.
22. Sasaki M, Yamada Y. The laminin B2 chain has a multidomain structure homologous to the B1 chain. *J Biol Chem* 1987;262:17111–7.
23. Pikkarainen T, Eddy R, Fukushima Y, et al. Human laminin B1 chain. A multidomain protein with gene (LAMB1) locus in the q22 region of chromosome 7. *J Biol Chem* 1987;262:10454–62.
24. Vuolteenaho R, Nissinen M, Sainio K, et al. Human laminin M chain (merosin): complete primary structure, chromosomal assignment, and expression of the M and A chain in human fetal tissues. *J Cell Biol* 1994;124:381–94.
25. Pikkarainen T, Kallunki T, Tryggvason K. Human laminin B2 chain. Comparison of the complete amino acid sequence with the B1 chain reveals variability in sequence homology between different structural domains. *J Biol Chem* 1988;262:6751–8.
26. Beck K, Dixon TW, Engel J, Parry DA. Inonic interactions in the coiled-coil domain of laminin determine the specificity of chain assembly. *J Mol Biol* 1993;231:311–23.
27. Mayer V, Nischt R, Poschl E, et al. A single EGF-like motif of laminin is responsible for high affinity nidogen binding. *EMBO J* 1993; 12:1879–85.
28. Daneker GW, Piazza AJ, Steele GD, Mercurio AM. Relationship between extracellular matrix interactions and degree of differentiation of human colon carcinoma cell lines. *Cancer Res* 1989;49:681–6.
29. Graf DS, Iwamoto Y, Sasaki M, et al. Identification of an amino acid sequence in laminin mediating cell attachment, chemotaxis, and receptor binding. *Cell* 1987;48:989–96.
30. Grant DS, Tashiro KI, Segui-Real B, Yamada Y, Martin GR, Kleinman HK. Two different laminin domains mediate the differentiation of human endothelial cells into capillary-like structures in vitro. *Cell* 1989;58:933–43.
31. Skubitz AP, Letourneau PC, Wayner E, Furcht LT. Synthetic peptides from the carboxyl-terminal globular domain of the A chain of laminin: their ability to promote cell adhesion and neurite outgrowth, and interact with heparin and the β1 integrin subunit. *J Cell Biol* 1991; 115:1137–48.
32. Sorokin L, Sonnenberg A, Aumailley M, Timpl R, Ekblom P. Recognition of the laminin E8 cell-binding site by an integrin possessing the α6 subunit is essential for epithelial polarization on developing kidney tubules. *J Cell Biol* 1990;111:1265–73.
33. Weber M. Basement membrane proteins. *Kidney Int* 1992;41:620–8.
34. Aumailley M, Gerl M, Sonnenberg A, Deutzmann R, Timpl R. Identification of the Arg-Gly-Asp sequence in laminin A chain as a latent cell-binding site exposed in fragment P1. *FEBS Lett* 1990;262:82–6.
35. Woodley DT, Rao CN, Hassell JR, Liotta LA, Martin GR, Kleinman HK. Interactions of basement membrane components. *Biochem Biophys Acta* 1983;761:278–83.
36. Aumailley M, Wiedemann H, Mann K, Timpl R. Binding of nidogen and the laminin–nidogen complex to basement membrane collagen type IV. *Eur J Biochem* 1989;184:241–8.
37. Ott U, Odermatt E, Engel J, Furthmayr H, Timpl R. Protease resistance and conformation of laminin. *Eur J Biochem* 1982;123:63–72.
38. Paulsson M, Aumailley M, Deutzmann R, Timpl R, Beck K, Emgel J. Laminin–nidogen complex. Extraction with chelating agents and structural characterization. *Eur J Biochem* 1987;166:11–9.
39. Yurchenco PD, Cheng YS. Self assembly and calcium-binding sites in laminin: a three arm interaction model. *J Biol Chem* 1993;268: 17286–99.
40. Timpl R, Brown JC. The laminins. *Matrix Biol* 1994;14:275–81.
41. Miner JH, Lewis RM, Sanes JR. Molecular cloning of a novel laminin chain, α5, and widespread expression in adult mouse tissues. *J Biol Chem* 1995; 270:28523–6.
42. Durkin ME, Chakravarti S, Bartos BB, Liu S-H, Friedman RL, Chung AE. Amino acid sequence and domain structure of entactin. Homology with epidermal growth factor precursor and low density lipoprotein receptor. *J Cell Biol* 1988;107:2749–56.
43. Mann K, Deutzmann R, Aumailley M, et al. Amino acid sequence of mouse nidogen, a multidomain basement membrane protein with binding activity for laminin, collagen IV, and cells. *EMBO J* 1989;8: 65–72.
44. Aumailley M, Battaglia C, Mayer V, et al. Nidogen mediates the formation of ternary complexes of basement membrane components. *Kidney Int* 1993;43:7–12.
45. Nagayoshi T, Sanborn D, Hickok NJ et al. Human nidogen: complete amino acid sequence and structural domains deduced from cDNAs and evidence for polymorphism of the gene. *DNA* 1989;8:581–94.
46. Olsen DR, Nagayoshi T, Fazio M, et al. Human nidogen: cDNA cloning, cellular expression, and mapping of the gene to chromosome 1q43. *Am J Hum Genet* 1989;44:876–85.
47. Chung AE, Dong L-J, Wu C, Durkin ME. Biological functions of entactin. *Kidney Int* 1993;43:13–9.
48. Senior RM, Gresham HD, Griffin GL, Brown EJ, Chung AE. Entactin stimulates neutrophil adhesion and chemotaxis through interactions between its Arg-Gly-Asp (RGD) domain and the leukocyte response integrin. *J Clin Invest* 1992;90:2251–7.
49. Noonan DM, Fulle A, Valente P, et al. The complete sequence of perlecan, a basement membrane heparan sulfate proteoglycan, reveals extensive similarity with the laminin A chain, low density lipoprotein-receptor, and the neural cell adhesion molecule. *J Biol Chem* 1991; 266:22939–47.
50. Murdoch AD, Dodge GR, Cohen I, Tuan RS, Iozzo RV. Primary structure of the human heparan sulfate proteoglycan from basement membrane (HSPG2/Perlecan). *J Biol Chem* 1992;267:8544–57.
51. Kallunki P, Tryggvason K. Human basement membrane heparan sulfate proteoglycan core protein. *J Cell Biol* 1992;116:559–71.
52. Kallunki P, Eddy RL, Byers MG, Kestila M, Shows TB, Tryggvason K. Cloning of the human heparan sulfate proteoglycan core protein, assignment of the gene (HSPG1) to 1p36.1-p35 and identification of a *Bam*H1 restriction fragment length polymorphism. *Genomics* 1991; 11:389–96.
53. Laurie GW, Bing JT, Kleinman HK, et al. Localization of binding sites for laminin, heparan sulfate proteoglycan and fibronectin on basement membrane (type IV) collagen. *J Mol Biol* 1986;189: 205–16.
54. Folkman J, Klagsburn M, Sasse J, Wadzinski M, Ingber D, Vlodavsky I. A heparin-binding angiogenic protein—basic fibroblast growth factor—is stored within basement membrane. *Am J Pathol* 1988;130:393–400.
55. Kanwar YS, Hascall VC, Farquhar MG. Partial characterization of newly synthesized proteoglycans isolated from the glomerular basement membrane. *J Cell Biol* 1981;90:527–32.
56. McCarthy KJ, Accavitti MA, Couchman JR. Immunological characterization of a basement membrane-specific chondroitin sulfate proteoglycan. *J Cell Biol* 1989;109:3187–98.
57. Abrahamson DR, Irwin MH, St. John PL, et al. Selective immunoreactivities of kidney basement membranes to monoclonal antibodies against laminin: localization of the end of the long arm and the short arms to discrete microdomains. *J Cell Biol* 1989;109:3477–91.
58. Desjardins M, Bendayan M. Heterogeneous distribution of type IV collagen, entactin, heparan sulfate proteoglycan, and laminin among renal basement membranes as revealed by quantitative immunocytochemistry. *J Histochem Cytochem* 1989;37:885–97.
59. Zhu D, Kim Y, Steffes MW, Groppoli TJ, Butkowski RJ, Mauer SM. Application of electron microscopic immunocytochemistry to the human kidney: distribution of type IV and type VI collagen in the normal human kidney. *J Histochem Cytochem* 1994;42:577–84.
60. Van den Born J, Van den Heuvel LPWJ, Bakker MAH, Veerkamp JH, Assmann KJM, Berden JHM. Monoclonal antibodies against the protein core and glycosaminoglyccan side chain of glomerular basement membrane heparan sulfate proteoglycan: characterization and immunohistological application in human tissues. *J Histochem Cytochem* 1994;42:89–102.
61. Saxén L. *Organogenesis of the kidney*. Cambridge, England: Cambridge University Press; 1987.
62. Clapp WL, Abrahamson DR. Development and gross anatomy of the kidney. In: CC Tisher, BM Brenner, eds. *Renal pathology*. 2nd ed. Philadelphia: JB Lippincott; 1994:3–159.
63. Ekblom P. Formation of basement membranes in the embryonic kidney: an immunohistological study. *J Cell Biol* 1981;91:1–10.
64. Ekblom M, Klein G, Mugrauer G, et al. Transient and locally re-

stricted expression of laminin A chain and mRNA by developing epithelial cells during kidney organogenesis. *Cell* 1990;60:337–46.
65. Klein G, Langegger M, Timpl R, Ekblom P. Role of laminin A chain in the development of epithelial cell polarity. *Cell* 1988;55:331–41.
66. Hyink DP, Tucker DC, St. John PL, et al. Endogenous origin of glomerular endothelial and mesangial cells in grafts of embryonic kidneys. *Am J Physiol* 1996;270:F886–899.
67. Robert B, St. John PL, Hyink DP, Abrahamson DR. Evidence that embryonic kidney cells expressing flk-1 are intrinsic, vasculogenic angioblasts. *Am J Physiol* (in press).
68. Abrahamson DR. Glomerulogenesis in the developing kidney. *Semin Nephrol* 1991;11:375–89.
69. Abrahamson DR, St. John PL. Loss of laminin epitopes during glomerular basement membrane assembly in developing mouse kidneys. *J Histochem Cytochem* 1992;40:1943–53.
70. Miner JH, Sanes J. Collagen IV α3, α4, α5 chains in rodent basal laminae: sequence, distribution, association with laminins, and developmental switches. *J Cell Biol* 1994;127:879–91.
71. Noakes PG, Miner JH, Gautam M, Cunningham JM, Sanes JR, Merlie JP. The renal glomerulus of mice lacking s-laminin/laminin β2: nephrosis despite molecular compensation by laminin β1. *Nature Genet* 1995;10:400–6.
72. Virtanen I, Laitinene L, Korhonen M. Differential expression of laminin polypeptides in developing and adult human kidney. *J Histochem Cytochem* 1995;43:621–8.
73. Sunada Y, Bernier SM, Kozak CA, Yamada Y, Campbell KP. Deficiency of merosin in dystrophic dy mice and genetic linkage of laminin M chain gene to dy locus. *J Biol Chem* 1994;269:13729–32.
74. Pulkkinen L, Christiano AM, Airenne T, Haakana H, Tryggvason K, Uitto J. Mutations in the 2 chain gene (LAMC2) of kalinin/laminin 5 in the junctional forms of epidermolysis bullosa. *Nature Genet* 1994; 6:293–7.
75. Vanden Heuvel GB, Leardkamolkarn V, St. John PL, Abrahamson DR. Carboxy-terminal sequence and synthesis of rat kidney laminin γ1 chain. *Kidney Int* 1996;49:752–60.
76. Ninomiya Y, Kagawa M, Iyama K, et al. Differential expression of two basement membrane collagen genes, COL4A6 and COL4A5, demonstrated by immunofluorescence staining using peptide-specific monoclonal antibodies. *J Cell Biol* 1995;130:1219–29.
77. Ekblom P, Ekblom M, Fecker L, et al. Role of mesenchymal nidogen for epithelial morphogenesis in vitro. *Development* 1994;120: 2003–14.
78. Murdoch AD, Liu B, Schwarting R, Tuan RS, Iozzo RV. Widespread expression of perlecan proteoglycan in basement membranes and extracellular matrices of human tissues detected by a novel monoclonal antibody against domain III and by in situ hybridization. *J Histochem Cytochem* 1994;42:239–49.
79. Couchman JR, Ljubimov AV, Sthanam M, Horchar T, Hassell JR. Antibody mapping and tissue localization of globular and cysteine-rich regions of perlecan domain III. *J Histochem Cytochem* 1995;9: 955–63.
80. Vanden Heuvel GB, Abrahamson DR. Quantitation and localization of laminin A, B1 and B2 chain RNA transcripts in developing kidney. *Am J Physiol* 1993;265:F293–9.
81. McCarthy KJ, Bynum K, St John PL, Abrahamson DR, Couchman JR. Basement membrane proteoglycans in glomerular morphogenesis: Chondroitin sulfate proteoglycan is temporally and spatially regulated during development. *J Histochem Cytochem* 1993;41:401–14.
82. Bruggeman LA, Burbelo PD, Yamada Y, Klotman PE. A novel sequence in the type IV collagen promoter binds nuclear proteins from Englebreth-Holm-Swarm tumor. *Oncogene* 1992;7:1497–502.
83. Fischer G, Schmidt C, Opitz J, Cully Z, Kuhn K, Poschl E. Identification of a novel sequence element in the common promoter region of human collagen IV genes involved in the regulation of divergent transcription. *Biochem J* 1993;292:687–95.
84. Genersch E, Eckerskorn C, Lottspeich F, et al. Purification of the sequence-specific transcription factor CTCBF involved in the control of human collagen IV genes: subunits with homology to Ku-antigen. *EMBO J* 1995;14:791–800.
85. Ogawa K, Burbelo PD, Sasaki M, Yamada Y. The laminin B2 chain promoter contains unique repeat sequences and is active in transient transfection. *J Biol Chem* 1988;262:8384–9.
86. Kallunki T, Ikonen J, Chow LT, Kallunki P, Tryggvason K. Structure of the human laminin B2 chain gene reveals extensive divergence from the laminin B1 chain. *J Biol Chem* 1991;266:221–8.
87. Richardson CA, Gordon KL, Couser WG, Bomsztyk K. IL-1 beta increases laminin B2 chain mRNA levels and activates NF-kappa B in rat glomerular epithelial cells. *Am J Physiol* 1995;268:F273–8.
88. Okano R, Mita T, Matsui T. Characterization of a novel promoter structure and its transcriptional regulation of the murine laminin B1 gene. *Biochim Biophys Acta* 1992;1132:49–57.
89. Fazio MJ, O'Leary J, Kahari VM, Chen YQ, Saitta B, Uitto J. Human nidogen gene: structural and functional characterization of the 58 flanking region. *J Invest Dermatol* 1991;97:281–5.
90. Cohen IR, Grassel S, Murdoch AD, Iozzo RV. Structural characterization of the complete human perlecan gene and its promoter. *Proc Natl Acad Sci U S A* 1993;90:10404–8.
91. Lerner RA, Glassock RJ, Dixon J. The role of anti-glomerular basement membrane antibody in the pathogenesis of human glomerulonephritis. *J Exp Med* 1967;126:989–1004.
92. Weber MF, Andrassy K, Pullig O, et al. Anti–neutrophil-cytoplasmic antibodies and antiglomerular basement membrane antibodies in Goodpasture's syndrome and in Wegener's granulomatosis. *J Am Soc Nephrol* 1992;2:1227–34.
93. Hudson BG, Reeders ST, Tryggvason K. Type IV collagen: structure, gene organization, and role in human disease. *J Biol Chem* 1993;268: 26033–6.
94. Wieslander J, Bygren P, Heinegard D. Isolation of the specific glomerular basement membrane antigen involved in Goodpasture syndrome. *Proc Natl Acad Sci U S A* 1984;81:1544–8.
95. Wieslander J, Ban JF, Butkowski RJ, et al. Goodpasture antigen of the glomerular basement membrane: localization to noncollagenous regions of type IV collagen. *Proc Natl Acad Sci U S A* 1984;81: 3838–42.
96. Butkowski RJ, Langeveld JPM, Wieslander J, et al. Localization of the Goodpasture epitope to a novel chain of basement membrane collagen. *J Biol Chem* 1987;262:7874–7.
97. Saus J, Weislander J, Langeveld JPM, et al. Identification of Goodpasture antigen as the α3 (IV) chain of collagen IV. *J Biol Chem* 1988;263:13374–80.
98. Gunwar S, Saus J, Noelken ME, et al. Glomerular basement membrane: identification of a fourth chain, α4, of type IV collagen. *J Biol Chem* 1990;265:5466–9.
99. Gunwar S, Ballester F, Kalluri R, et al. Glomerular basement membrane: identification of the noncollagenous domain (hexamer) of collagen IV and the Goodpasture antigen. *J Biol Chem* 1991;266: 15318–24.
100. Morrison KE, Mariyama M, Yang-Feng TL, et al. Sequence and localization of a partial cDNA encoding the human α3 chain of type IV collagen. *Am J Hum Genet* 1991;49:545–54.
101. Turner N, Mason PJ, Brown R, et al. Molecular cloning of the human Goodpasture antigen demonstrates it to be the α3 chain of type IV chain. *J Clin Invest* 1992;89:592–601.
102. Mariyama M, Leinoven A, Mochizuki T, et al. Complete primary structure of the human α3 (IV) chain. *J Biol Chem* 1994;269: 23013–7.
103. Butkowski RJ, Wieslander J, Kleppel M, et al. Basement membrane collagen in the kidney: regional localization of novel chains related to collagen IV. *Kidney Int* 1989;35:1195–202.
104. Johansson C, Butkowski R, Wieslander J. The structural organization of type IV collagen: identification of three NC1 populations in the glomerular basement membrane. *J Biol Chem* 1992;267:24533–7.
105. Bernal D, Quinones S, Saus J. The human mRNA encoding the Goodpasture antigen is alternatively spliced. *J Biol Chem* 1993;268: 12090–4.
106. Feng L, Xia Y, Wilson CB. Alternative splicing of the NC1 domain of the human α3 (IV) collagen gene. *J Biol Chem* 1994;269;2342–8.
107. Penades JR, Bernal D, Revert F, et al. Characterization and expression of multiple alternatively spliced transcripts of the Goodpasture antigen gene region. *Eur J Biochem* 1995;229:754–60.
108. Siebold B, Deutzmann R, Kuhn K. The arrangement of intra- and intermolecular disulfide bonds in the carboxyterminal, noncollagenous aggregation and cross-linking domain of basement membrane type IV collagen. *Eur J Biochem* 1988;176:617–24.
109. Jeraj J, Fish AJ, Yoshioka K, et al. Development and heterogeneity of antigens in the immature nephron. Reactivity with human antiglomer-

ular basement membrane autoantibodies. *Am J Pathol* 1984;117: 180–3.

110. Yoshioka K, Michael AF, Velosa J, et al. Detection of hidden nephritogenic antigen determinants in human renal and nonrenal basement membranes. *Am J Pathol* 1985;121:156–65.
111. Revert F, Penades JR, Plana M, et al. Phosphorylation of the Goodpasture antigen by type A protein kinases. *J Biol Chem* 1995;270: 13254–61.
112. Neilson EG, Kalluri R, Sun MJ, et al. Specificity of Goodpasture autoantibodies for the recombinant noncollagenous domains of human type IV collagen. *J Biol Chem* 1993;268:8402–5.
113. Turner N, Forstova J, Rees A, et al. Production and characterization of recombinant Goodpasture antigen in insect cells. *J Biol Chem* 1994;269:17141–5.
114. Kalluri R, Wilson CB, Weber M, et al. Identification of the α3 chain of the type IV collagen as the common autoantigen in antibasement membrane disease and Goodpasture syndrome. *J Am Soc Nephrol* 1995;6:1178–85.
115. Kalluri R, Gattone VH, Noelken ME, Hudson BG. The α3 chain of type IV collagen induces autoimmune Goodpasture syndrome. *Proc Natl Acad Sci U S A* 1994;91:6201–5.
116. Wieslander J, Langeveld J, Butkowski R, et al. Physical and immunochemical studies of the globular domain of type collagen: cryptic properties of the Goodpasture antigen. *J Biol Chem* 1985;260:8564–70.
117. Kalluri R, Guwar S, Reeders, ST, et al. Goodpasture syndrome: localization of the epitope for the autoantibodies to the carboxy-terminal region of the α3 (IV) chain of basement membrane collagen. *J Biol Chem* 1991;266:24018–24.
118. Bolton, WK, Luo A-M, Fox PL, et al. Study of EHS type IV collagen lacking Goodpasture's epitope in glomerulonephritis in rats. *Kidney Int* 1995;47:404–10.
119. Bolton WK, Luo A-M, Fox P, et al. Goodpasture's epitope in development of experimental autoimmune glomerulonephritis in rats. *Kidney Int* 1996;49:327–34.
120. Kashtan CE, Sibley RK, Michael AF, Vernier RL. Hereditary nephritis: Alport syndrome and thin glomerular basement membrane disease. In: Tisher CC, Brenner BM, eds. *Renal pathology*. 2nd ed. Philadelphia: JB Lippincott; 1994:1239–66.
121. Atkin CL, Gregory MC. Alport syndrome. In: Schrier RW, Gottscholk CW, eds. *Diseases of the kidney*. 5th ed. Boston: Little, Brown; 1993:571–91.
122. Olson DL, Anand SK, Landing BH, et al. Diagnosis of hereditary nephritis by failure of glomeruli to bind anti-glomerular basement membrane antibodies. *J Pediatr* 1980;96:697–9.
123. McCoy RC, Johnson HK, Stone WJ, Wilson CB. Absence of nephritogenic GBM antigen(s) in some patients with familial nephritis. *Kidney Int* 1982;21:642–52.
124. Rumpelt H-J. Hereditary nephropathy (Alport syndrome): correlation of clinical data with glomerular basement membrane alterations. *Clin Nephrol* 1980;13:203–7.
125. Kashtan CE, Fish AJ, Kleppel MM, et al. Nephritogenic antigen determinants in epidermal and renal basement membranes of kindreds with Alport-type familial nephritis. *J Clin Invest* 1986;78: 1035–44.
126. Kleppel MM, Kashtan CE, Butskowski RJ, et al. Alport-familial nephritis. Absence of 28-kd non-collagenous monomers of type IV collagen in glomerular basement membrane. *J Clin Invest* 1987;80: 263–6.
127. Atkin CL, Hasstedt SJ, Menlov L, et al. Mapping of Alport syndrome to the long arm of the X chromosome. *Am J Hum Genet* 1988;42:249–55.
128. Hostikka SL, Eddy RL, Byers MG, et al. Identification of a distinct type IV collagen alpha chain with restricted kidney distribution and assignment of its gene to the locus of X chromosome-linked Alport syndrome. *Proc Natl Acad Sci U S A* 1990;87:1606–10.
129. Pihlajaniemi T, Pohjalainen E-R, Myers J. Complete primary structure of the triple-helical region and the carboxy-terminal domain of a new type IV collagen chain α5(IV). *J Biol Chem* 1990;265:13758–66.
130. Zhou J, Jerz JM, Leinonen A, Tryggvason K. Complete amino acid sequencing of the human α5 collagen chain and identification of a single base mutation in exon 29 from the 3′ end converting glycine-521 in the collagenous domain to cysteine in an Alport syndrome patient. *J Biol Chem* 1992;267:12475–81.
131. Zhou J, Leinonen A, Tryggvason K. Structure of the human type IV collagen COL4A5 gene. *J Biol Chem* 1994;269:6608–14.
132. Barker DF, Hostikka SL, Zhou J, et al. Identification of mutations in the COL4A5 collagen gene in Alport syndrome. *Science* 1990;248: 1224–7.
133. Antignac C, Knebelmann B, Drouot L, et al. Deletions in the COL4A5 collagen gene in X-linked Alport syndrome. *J Clin Invest* 1994;93:1195–207.
134. Netzer K-O, Renders L, Zhou J, et al. Deletions of the COL4A5 gene in patients with Alport syndrome. *Kidney Int* 1992;42:1336–44.
135. Nomura S, Osawa G, Sai T, et al. A splicing mutation in the α5 (IV) collagen gene of a family with Alport syndrome. *Kidney Int* 1993;43: 1116–24.
136. Boye E, Flinter F, Zhou J, et al. Detection of 12 novel mutations in the collagenous domain of the COL4A5 gene in Alport syndrome patients. *Hum Mutat* 1995;5:197–204.
137. Kawai S, Nomura S, Harano T, et al. The COL4A5 gene in Japanese Alport syndrome patients: spectrum of mutations of all exons. *Kidney Int* 1996;49:814–22.
138. Zhou J, Hertz JM, Tryggvason K. Mutations in the α5(IV) collagen gene in juvenile-onset Alport syndrome without hearing or ocular lesions: detection by denaturing gradient gel electrophoresis of a PCR product. *Am J Hum Genet* 1992;50:1291–300.
139. Zhou J, Gregory MC, Hertz J, et al. Mutations in the codon for a conserved arginine-1563 in the COL4A5 collagen gene in Alport syndrome. *Kidney Int* 1993;43:722–9.
140. Zhou J, Barker D, Gerken SC, et al. Single base mutation in the α5(IV) collagen chain gene converting a conserved cysteine to serine in Alport syndrome. *Genomics* 1991;9:10–8.
141. Zhou J, Ding M, Zhao Z, Reeders ST. Complete primary structure of the sixth chain of human basement membrane collagen, α6(IV). *J Biol Chem* 1994;269:13193–9.
142. Heidet L, Dahan K, Zhou J, et al. Deletions of both alpha-5(IV) and alpha-6(IV) collagen genes in Alport syndrome and in Alport syndrome associated with smooth muscle tumours. *Hum Mol Genet* 1995;4:99–108.
143. Cohen AH, Glassock RJ. Anti-GBM glomerulonephritis including Goodpasture disease. In: CC Tisher, BM Brenner, eds. *Renal pathology*. 2nd ed. Philadelphia: JB Lippincott; 1994:524–52.
144. Yaar M, Foidart JM, Brown KS, Rennard SI, MArtin GR, Liotta L. The Goodpasture-like syndrome in mice induced by intravenous injections of anti–type IV collagen and anti-laminin antibody. *Am J Pathol* 1982;107:79–91.
145. Abrahamson DR, Caulfield JP. Proteinuria and structural alterations in rat glomerular basement membranes induced by intravenously injected anti-laminin immunoglobulin G. *J Exp Med* 1982;156:128–45.
146. Miettinen A, Stow JL, Mentone S, Farquhar MG. Antibodies to basement membrane heparan sulfate proteolgycans bind to the laminae rarae of the glomerular basement membrane (GBM) and induce subepithelial basement membrane thickening. *J Exp Med* 1986;163: 1064–84.
147. van den Born J, van den Heuvel LP, Bakker MA, et al. A monoclonal antibody against GBM heparan sulfate induces an acute selective protein in rats. *Kidney Int* 1992;41:115–23.
148. Eddy AA, Michael AF. Immunopathogenic mechanisms of glomerular injury. In: Tisher CC, Brenner BM, eds. *Renal pathology.* 2nd ed. Philadelphia: JB Lippincott; 1994:162–221.
149. Couser WG. Pathogenesis of glomerulonephritis. *Kidney Int* 1993; 44(suppl):19–26.
150. Feintzeig ID, Abrahamson DR, Cybulsky AV, Dittmer JE, Salant DJ. Nephritogenic potential of sheep antibodies against basement membrane laminin in the rat. *Lab Invest* 1986;54:531–42.
151. Foster MH, Sabbaga J, Line SR, Thompson KS, Barrett KJ, Madaio MP. Molecular analysis of spontaneous nephrotropic anti-laminin antibodies in an autoimmune MRL-lpr/lpr mouse. *J Immunol* 1993; 151:814–24.
152. Druet E, Guery JC, Ayed K, Guilbert B, Avrameas S, Druet P. Characteristics of polyreactive and monospecific IgG anti-laminin autoantibodies in the rat mercury model. *Immunology* 1994;83:489–94.
153. Aten J, Veninga A, Coers W, et al. Autoantibodies to the laminin P1 fragment in $HgCl_2$-induced membranous glomerulopathy. *Am J Pathol* 1995;146:1467–80.
154. Kalluri R, Danoff TM, Neilson EG. Murine anti-α3(IV) collagen dis-

ease: a model of human Goodpasture syndrome and anti-GBM nephritis. *J Am Soc Nephrol* 1995;6:833.

155. Danoff TM, Cook DN, Neilson EG, Kalluri R. Murine anti-α3(IV) collagen disease is abrogated in MIP-1a deficient mice. *J Am Soc Nephrol* 1995;6:827.
156. Thorner P, Jansen B, Baumal R, Valli VE, Goldberger A. Samoyed hereditary glomerulopathy. Immunohistochemical staining of basement membranes of kidney for laminin, collagen type IV, fibronectin, and Goodpasture antigen, and correlation with electron microscopy of glomerular capillary basement membranes. *Lab Invest* 1987;56:435–43.
157. Zheng K, Thorner PS, Marrano P, Baumal R, McInnes RR. Canine X chromosome-linked hereditary nephritis: a genetic model for human X-linked hereditary nephritis resulting from a single base mutation in the gene encoding the α5 chain of collagen type IV. *Proc Natl Acad Sci U S A* 1994;3989–93.

B. Mechanisms of Immune Injury

Immunologic Renal Diseases,
edited by E. G. Neilson and W. G. Couser.
Lippincott-Raven Publishers, Philadelphia © 1997

CHAPTER 11

Pathophysiology of Acute Immune Injury

Roland C. Blantz, Curtis B. Wilson, and Francis B. Gabbai

INTRODUCTION

The expansion of our knowledge of the mechanisms of immune injury to the kidney has been substantial over the past two decades (1–7), and, from an experimental perspective, falls into two broad categories:

1. Understanding of the sequential molecular and cellular events that contribute to glomerular and tubular cell and capillary wall injury.
2. Greater physiologic understanding of the specific mechanisms whereby glomerular filtration rate (GFR) is affected by events occurring within the glomerular capillary, tubulointerstitium and vasculature.

The former investigative area provides the most promise for developing therapies for prevention of renal disease. The latter area of investigation continues to be important because altered GFR is the major consequence of acute immune renal injury often leading to progressive deterioration of renal function and end-stage renal disease. There were pertinent research observations prior to the last two decades both in the clinical setting and in experimental models (8–10). Although these studies recognized the decline in GFR, there was only speculation as to how this deterioration in renal function was achieved, based largely upon pathologic inference from histologic examination of diseased kidneys. It is of interest that this largely intuitive set of conclusions regarding mechanisms proved to be in large part spurious. Understanding of the specific mechanisms whereby GFR decreases has proved to be invaluable to cell and molecular biologists, simply because this information has provided a road map for the reasonable design of appropriate cellular and molecular studies. Physiologic studies have provided clues as to which neurohumoral and/or inflammatory mediator systems are participating.

MECHANISMS OF GLOMERULAR FILTRATION REDUCTION

The mechanisms that determine the GFR and the processes that regulate them are discussed in detail in Chapter 3 of this book. There are only limited mechanisms whereby GFR can decrease with acute immune injury of the kidney (11). For the purposes of evaluating the changes in renal function that occur with immune kidney injury, most studies have been conducted in rats with superficial glomeruli that enable the accurate measurement of all determinants of GFR, including glomerular plasma flow, the glomerular hydrostatic pressure gradient (ΔP), the factors that regulate the permeability of the capillary wall itself to solutes including the total filtering surface area, and the hydraulic permeability characteristics (LpA or Kf).

1. GFR is driven by hydrostatic forces; therefore, the hydrostatic pressure gradient, ΔP, could decrease following injury, either as a consequence of reductions in glomerular capillary hydrostatic pressure or as a result of increases in tubular pressure. Decreases in glomerular pressure could result from afferent arteriolar vasoconstriction or from some impairment of the efferent arteriole leading to reductions in tone or resistance and an inability to sustain normal glomerular capillary pressure. Most renal diseases examined by light microscopy have provided little evidence for damage to either afferent or efferent arteriolar structures, compared with the glomerular capillary. It is certainly quite possible, however, that elevations in tubular pressure might have occurred as a secondary consequence of renal damage. Studies in the

R. C. Blantz: Division of Nephrology, Hypertension and Bioengineering Institute, University of California–San Diego School of Medicine, La Jolla, California 92093.

C. B. Wilson: Department of Immunology, The Scripps Research Institute, La Jolla, California 92037.

F. B. Gabbai: Veterans Affairs Medical Center, San Diego, California 92161.

past certainly implied that the effective filtration pressure should be reduced because of unfavorable changes. When ΔP was directly assessed, this prediction was not verified (1–6,12).

2. Alterations in nephron plasma flow could lead to reductions in GFR. A few early studies measured renal plasma flow with variable results (13,14). These examinations often found a decrease in the filtration fraction, suggesting that plasma flow was reduced to a lesser extent than was GFR. These inferences regarding a role of nephron plasma flow were confounded by the fact that nephron loss could not be distinguished from reductions in plasma flow to each nephron (5). In general, experimental studies in animals have often observed changes in nephron plasma flow, but this finding is a rather inconsistent contribution to reductions in GFR (2,3,12,15).

3. Alterations in colloid osmotic pressure can certainly alter GFR in very special circumstances (11,16). However, significant GFR reductions require substantial increases in plasma colloid osmotic pressure. Such increases are generally not observed in patients with renal disease. Rather the opposite is the case whereby reductions in albumin concentration are observed that favor filtration or at least ameliorate other factors that are causing reductions in GFR.

4. Finally, we are left with alterations in the glomerular ultrafiltration coefficient. This complex determinant of ultrafiltration is derived from other directly measured values whereby GFR = (LpA or Kf) $\times \int(\Delta P - \pi)$ ($\Delta P - \pi$ = effective filtration pressure). LpA or Kf can be reduced either by decreasing the hydraulic conductivity of the glomerular capillary wall (Lp or K) or via significant reductions in the filtering surface area (A or S). Experimental studies in a variety of realistic experimental models of clinical disease have generated the conclusion that acute immune injury causes reductions in GFR most consistently as a consequence of reductions in the glomerular ultrafiltration coefficient (1–6,12,17). However, the specific mechanisms among disease models differ substantially.

The best-studied experimental models of clinical renal disease fall into specific categories. The glomerular diseases include (a) proliferative or endocapillary glomerulonephritis (1–3), (b) membranous nephropathy (1,7,12), (c) mesangiocapillary or membranoproliferative glomerulonephritis (17–19), (d) focal segmental glomerulosclerosis (20), (e) models analogous to minimal change disease in which GFR is usually not reduced (21), (f) tubulointerstitial diseases (22) (see Chapters 35 and 36). All glomerular disease categories that have been studied experimentally demonstrate a strikingly similar pattern with regard to glomerular hemodynamic alterations. Alterations in systemic oncotic pressure do not contribute to the reductions in GFR and, in general, neither do changes in glomerular capillary hydrostatic pressure gradient, ΔP. In most models that have been studied to date, the glomerular capillary hydrostatic pressure gradient is increased, usually due to elevations in glomerular capillary hydrostatic pressure, often from minor reductions in tubular pressure (1–6,12,17). Reductions in nephron plasma flow often occur, but the contributions of vasoconstriction to reductions in GFR are quite variable and are not as consistent as are reductions in the glomerular ultrafiltration coefficient (1–6,12,17). The general pattern observed has been an increase in the hydrostatic pressure gradient and a major reduction in the glomerular ultrafiltration coefficient. Since most experimental animals are at or near filtration pressure equilibrium (11), rather large reductions in the glomerular ultrafiltration coefficient are required to values less than one third of normal before significant reductions in filtration rate have been observed (1–6).

The fact that reductions in the glomerular ultrafiltration coefficient constitute the major pathway for reductions in GFR should come as no surprise to students of glomerular pathology. Glomerulonephritis is often associated with reductions in the number of open capillary lumina as a consequence of scarring and collapse of glomerular capillaries and as a result of obstruction of capillaries with polymorphonuclear or mononuclear inflammatory cells (see Chapters 26 and 28) (3,4). Analysis of the relative contribution of decreases in the hydraulic conductivity of the glomerular capillary wall, however, is somewhat more complex. To a great extent, the separation of hydraulic conductivity from surface area is an artificial or semantic issue. The normal pathway for water and small solute movement across the complex glomerular capillary barrier is undoubtedly via endothelial fenestrae, across the glomerular basement membrane (GBM) and between the epithelial cell foot processes. Slit diaphragms are also present across endothelial fenestrae and between epithelial cell podocytes (21) (see Chapter 31). The specific rate-limiting barrier for water movement in the normal glomerulus has not been specifically defined. It is probably not the same rate-limiting site that restricts albumin and protein movement across the glomerular capillary wall. However, reductions in LpA or Kf and development of proteinuria are events that often go hand in hand with acute immune injury. It is easy to envision by structural correlation that extensive endothelial cell damage, thickening of the basement membrane, or major alterations in the architecture of glomerular epithelial cells could all contribute individually or collectively to reductions in hydraulic conductivity of the capillary wall or, alternatively, the surface area for normal water transit across the capillary wall.

The nearly universal finding of an increase in the glomerular capillary hydrostatic pressure gradient suggests some intrinsic dysregulation of glomerular capillary pressure as a consequence of immune injury (23,24). Whether this finding is a consequence of structural events or the neurohumoral/inflammatory environment remains to be fully defined. Increases in the glomerular capillary hydrostatic pressure gradient may ameliorate the negative effects of other determinants of GFR, but this may be at a significant price. The inability to regulate glomerular capillary hydrostatic pressure normally in response to alterations in blood pressure or the humoral environment may indirectly contribute to further deterioration of glomerular function and progressive damage over time by nonimmune mechanisms. As we will further discuss in this chapter, there is evidence that acute immune injury to the glomerulus impairs, in part, the normal physiologic responses to both blood pressure alterations and neurohumoral modulators of glomerular hemodynamics (24, unpublished observations). We now consider some of the individual experimental animal models of acute immune injury. Although they share similar final common pathways of glomerular hemodynamic alterations, unique aspects characterize each of the individual models.

EXPERIMENTAL MODELS OF GLOMERULONEPHRITIS

Experimental models have been constructed over the past several years that are surprisingly accurate in duplicating the forms of clinical renal disease encountered by clinicians in nephrology practice (see Chapters 35 and 36). These models include (a) proliferative or endocapillary glomerulonephritis (1–4), (b) forms of nephropathy that involve the basement membrane and the external epithelial surface often without evidence of proliferation or inflammatory cells (5,7–9,12), (c) membranoproliferative or mesangiocapillary glomerulonephritis that focuses primarily in the mesangial cell area but with involvement of the GBM (10,17–19,24), and (d) focal segmental glomerulosclerosis (20). These models have sometimes been created by targeting antibodies directed to antigens on the surface of specific glomerular cells.

Proliferative Glomerulonephritis

This experimental model of glomerulonephritis focuses on inflammatory events that are restricted primarily to the endocapillary surface and the capillary lumina, thereby exerting damage to the endothelial surface and the GBM. As these models become more chronic, the glomerular mesangium and other areas of the glomerulus may also become involved (23,25). Administration of anti-GBM antibody produces the classic model of proliferative glomerulonephritis. Within 30 min after administration of anti-GBM antibody, polymorphonuclear leukocytes (PMNs) migrate into the capillary lumina and GFR is reduced almost immediately (3,4) (Fig. 1). The extreme rapidity of inflammatory events is undoubtedly a consequence of the endocapillary location of the antigen on the surface of the GBM (25,26). The fenestrated endothelial cells allow easy access to circulating anti-GBM antibodies. Following antibody deposition, complement is activated locally, promoting the recruitment of PMNs via anaphylatoxins (4). Within 24 h, this cellular response shifts from the PMN to mononuclear inflammatory cells. Endothelial cell swelling and hypertrophy occur, leading to some degree of capillary collapse. The chronic stages are characterized by a diffuse form of sclerosis with GBM thickening and focal scarring with segmental collapse of capillaries (23).

The nephron filtration rate decreases significantly and rapidly, within 30–60 min. Changes in nephron plasma flow contribute somewhat to this reduction in nephron filtration rate, but the contribution of plasma flow is quite variable from antibody to antibody, potent antibodies producing major reductions in nephron filtration rate and significant vasoconstriction (2–4,15,27,28). The universal finding is a major reduction in the glomerular ultrafiltration coefficient and a tendency for the glomerular capillary hydrostatic pressure gradient (ΔP) to increase. This increase in ΔP is usually insufficient to prevent a reduction in the nephron filtration rate, but less potent anti-GBM antibodies produce a reduction in LpA that is effectively neutralized or counteracted by the increase in the hydrostatic pressure gradient, ΔP (15).

The early histologic changes are quite characteristic. There is no histologic correlate to renal vasoconstriction, and the afferent and efferent arterioles appear largely undisturbed within 60–90 min after anti-GBM antibody administration (3,8,25). The endothelial cell is swollen and often detached from the underlying GBM (Fig. 1). PMNs migrate into the capillary, lift the endothelial cells from the underlying GBM, and become firmly adherent to the GBM, thereby partially obstructing glomerular capillary conduits. When one examines the histology in leukocyte-depleted animals, the endothelial cell is usually detached from the GBM, suggesting that antibody deposition per se and complement activation detach the endothelial cell from its normal supports. Detachment of the endothelial cell from the GBM produces a relatively "unstirred layer" that will, in effect, reduce the glomerular ultrafiltration coefficient. Attachment of the PMNs contributes to reductions in the ultrafiltration coefficient, not by reducing capillary surface area directly, but by creating high-resistance pathways that decrease glomerular plasma flow to that capillary conduit, effectively reducing the surface area for filtration by diverting plasma flow away from filtering surfaces (4,26). Studies have also suggested that the PMN may contribute humoral substances such as leukotrienes that may also contribute to the reduction in LpA or Kf (28). Complement anaphylatoxins (C5a), in addition to attracting PMNs, can also produce renal vasoconstriction at the efferent arteriole, contributing to decreases in plasma flow and increases in the glomerular capillary hydrostatic pressure (29). The terminal complement components, C5b-9 (membrane-

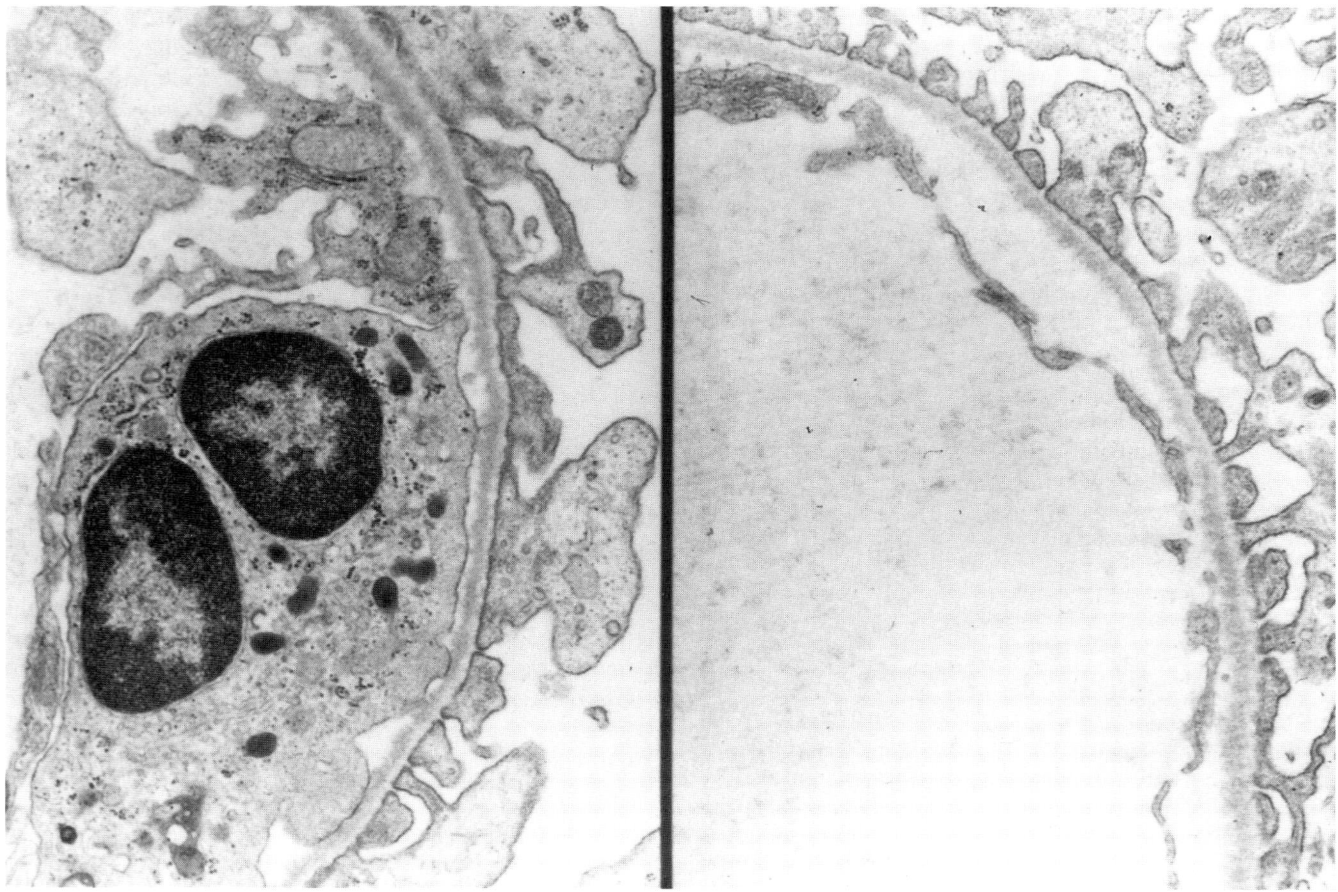

FIG. 1. Electron-microscope studies of a high-dose normal complementemic rat *(left)* and a complement-depleted rat *(right).* The subendothelial aspect of the GBM appeared irregular, presumably representing the fixation of anti-GBM antibody. On the left, a polymorphonuclear leukocyte was found approximated along the GBM displacing the endothelium in the normal complementemic rat. Endothelial separation occurred in the complement-depleted rat seen on the right, but PMN infiltration was almost completely lacking.

attack complex, MAC), produce cell membrane damage and may stimulate release of vasoactive substances from resident glomerular cells as well (see Chapter 18) contribute to the alterations observed in the endothelial cell.

Membranous Nephropathy

Experimental membranous nephropathy is characterized by a relative absence of cellular proliferation and circulating inflammatory cells (7,8,12,30,31). The experimental animal model of membranous nephropathy, known as Heymann nephritis, can be produced either actively or passively, the latter by administration of antibodies directed against Fx1A, which are antigens on the membrane of the glomerular epithelial cell (5,8). Heymann nephritis is discussed in more detail in chapters 35 and 47. This model exhibits characteristics that are remarkably similar to those observed in membranous nephropathy clinically. Antigen–antibody complexes are formed on the subepithelial aspects of the GBM and are associated with considerable distortion or fusion of the epithelial cell foot processes. Several investigators have demonstrated that the antigens of note are located specifically on the surface of the glomerular epithelial cell foot processes and the glomerular epithelial foot-process slit diaphragm (see Chapter 9). Deposition occurs as a result of in situ formation of antigen–antibody complexes rather than as a consequence of trapping circulating immune complexes (7,30–33) (see Chapter 14).

Early in the disease, capillary lumina are entirely patent and free of inflammatory cells (7,12). The endothelial cell surface and the mesangial cells appear quite normal. As a result of the subepithelial location of the antigen–antibody complexes that take several days to develop, the time course for reduction of nephron filtration rate and GFR and the onset of proteinuria is delayed, at least when compared with models such as anti-GBM antibody where antibody

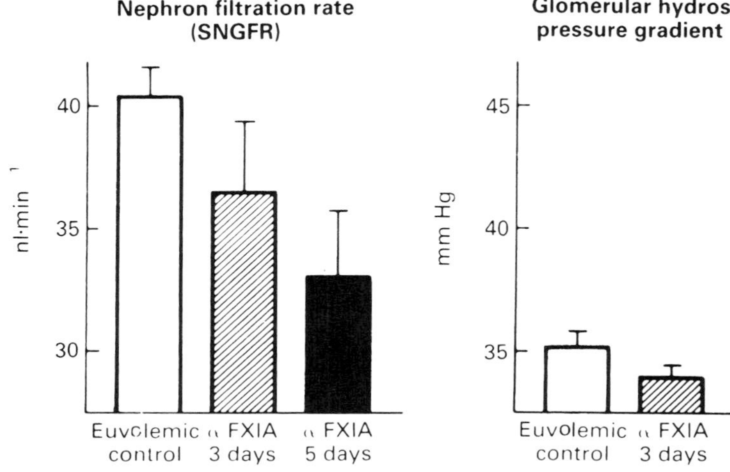

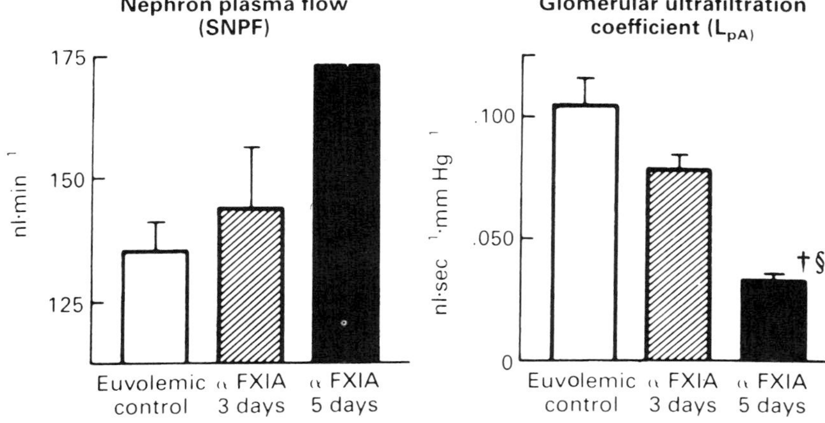

FIG. 2. The alterations in glomerular hemodynamics after anti-Fx1A antibody-induced Heymann nephritis of 3–5 days duration are compared with euvolemic controls + $p < 0.05$ euvolemic control versus 5-day Heymann nephritis. gp < 0.05 3-day Heymann nephritis compared to 5-day Heymann nephritis group.

deposition is maximal within 10 min (3,12). Proteinuria and GFR reductions are first observed in the passive Heymann model 5 days after antibody administration (12). One can, however, observe extensive antibody binding as early as 3 days, prior to the onset of major alterations in epithelial cell foot-process architecture and prior to the onset of proteinuria and GFR alterations. As in models of proliferative nephritis, the reduction in nephron filtration rate and GFR is entirely the consequence of a decrease in the glomerular ultrafiltration coefficient LpA or Kf, which is partially counterbalanced by an increase in the glomerular capillary hydrostatic pressure gradient ΔP (5,12,31,34) (Fig. 2). In the rat model, there is often a modest degree of renal vasoconstriction. The initial reduction in nephron filtration rate is not as severe as observed after the administration of anti-GBM antibody. Structural changes in the glomerular epithelial cell foot processes correlate strongly with the onset of proteinuria and the reduction in nephron filtration rate due to the reduction in LpA. These structural changes are associated with potential elimination of the channels between glomerular epithelial cell foot processes, presumably the normal avenue for water movement. These structural alterations may occur as a result of a "capping and shedding" phenomenon wherein the tertiary architecture of the cell is altered in an attempt to remove the antigen–antibody complexes from the cell surface (12,35). Complement depletion prevents, or at least delays, the onset of proteinuria and the reduction in nephron filtration rate that normally occurs at 5 days after antibody administration (Fig. 3). The complement-dependent attraction of PMNs by anaphylatoxins does not characterize experimental membranous nephropathy. Rather the change in glomerular permeability is mediated primarily by the C5b-9 MAC of complement that inserts into the membrane of the glomerular epithelial cell, resulting in local release of oxidants and proteases (30,36) (see Chapters 18 and 47). In

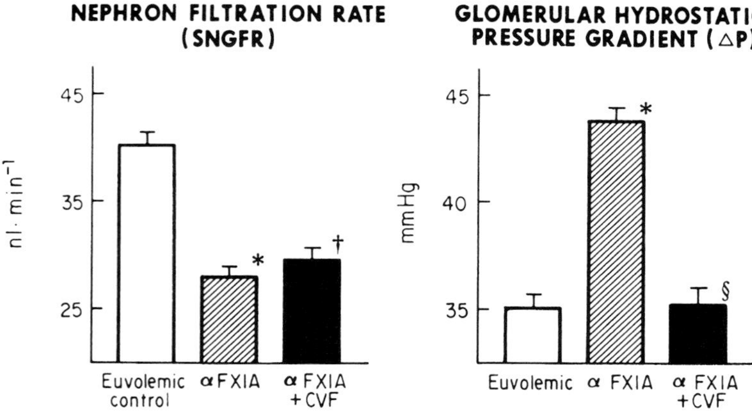

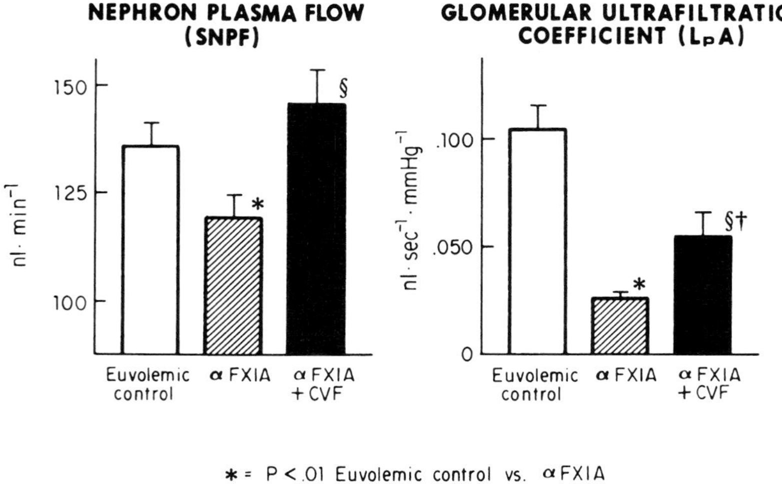

FIG. 3. Glomerular hemodynamics for euvolemic control, passive Heymann nephritis (PHN or αFx1A), rats treated with cobra venom factor (CVF) and rats that received αFx1A antibody. Significance of $p < 0.05$ is reported, using the Bonferroni method to correct the unpaired Student *t* test for multiple groups.

addition, complement depletion delays the events associated with capping and shedding. Quantitative assessments have demonstrated that complement depletion does not prevent antibody binding to the appropriate antigens (12). It only delays the structural alterations in the cell following these events. Capping and shedding requires cytoskeletal rearrangement, and alterations in tertiary architecture may partially depend on complement activation (37). Significantly, administration of angiotensin-converting enzyme inhibitors does not prevent the reduction in LpA following antibody administration and does not prevent alterations in morphology of the glomerular epithelial cells, but increases nephron filtration rate by producing renal vasodilation (34).

Chronic models of glomerulonephritis will develop after the administration of antibodies to Fx1A or with active immunization with the Fx1A antigen (5,8,38). After passive antibody administration, there is an overall homogeneity to changes in nephron filtration rate due to reductions in LpA. After longer periods of time and with active immunization models, some heterogeneity develops in the internephronal responses in experimental membranous nephropathy. In some nephrons, nephron GFR is reduced far more than others and, in certain nephrons, the dominant mechanism appears to be reductions in nephron plasma flow while, in others, reductions in LpA or Kf dominate (5). This disease is only moderately progressive, however, and usually does not produce severe end-stage renal disease in the rat model.

In membranous nephropathy, as in other immune-injury models, the reduction in LpA observed often correlates with the onset of abnormal protein leak across the glomerular capillaries and overt proteinuria. In an effort to examine this apparent association, we have used monoclonal antibodies to specific antigens located on the glomerular epithelial cell slit diaphragm, a thin membrane between glomerular epithelial cell foot processes on the external aspect of the GBM (21). At 2 h after administration of the monoclonal antibody, nephron filtration rate and nephron plasma flow were unchanged, but the glomerular ultrafiltration coefficient was substantially reduced, an effect that was neutralized by an increase in glomerular capillary hydrostatic pressure gradient (Table 1). At this time, there was no significant proteinuria. However, 24 h after the monoclonal antibody was administered, nephron plasma flow and nephron filtration rate increased, the latter also due to restoration of values for the glomerular ultrafiltration coefficient. Administration of cyclooxygenase inhibitors decreased the nephron plasma flow and nephron filtration rate to normal values, suggesting that vasodilatory prostaglandins may have been involved in this process. At 24 h, however, there was a marked increase in urinary protein excretion (21).

There was some aggregation of antigen–antibody complexes by immunocytochemistry between 2 and 24 h, but there were no detectable alterations in the tertiary structure of the glomerular epithelial cell foot processes when using highly quantitative histologic techniques. The GBM was also basically unchanged. These studies suggest that glomerular capillary epithelial slit diaphragm may constitute an important barrier for water movement across the glomerular capillary wall and later may contribute to the albumin leak. These studies do suggest that, after selective administration of antibody to specific glomerular sites, reductions in the glomerular capillary hydraulic conductivity can be effectively separated from increases in macromolecular permeability to albumin (21).

Membranoproliferative or Mesangiocapillary Glomerulonephritis

A reasonable model of membranoproliferative glomerulonephritis can be produced by the administration of antibodies to thymocyte-1 (Thy 1) antigen expressed on the surface of glomerular mesangial cells (see Chapter 35). Acute administration of the antibody results in extensive lysis and damage to glomerular mesangial cells and mesangial detachment from the GBM (17,18,24). The behavior of this model is certainly not static. The injured mesangial cells undergo rapid regeneration and proliferation, and, in fact, when only one dose of antibody is administered—the "single shot" model—recovery of normal architecture is almost complete within 30 days. If antibodies are administered on more than one occasion, however, a model of chronic glomerulosclerosis develops with damage to the mesangium. The glomerular endothelial and epithelial cells remain largely intact and normal in appearance (17,18). The C5b-9 MAC is also important to this model of mesangial cell damage via membrane injury, since complement depletion largely prevents much of the cellular damage after antibody administration and the antibody binds but does not induce injury in the C6-deficient rat (39,39a). Platelets also play a significant role in producing glomerular damage. They play rather specific roles in generating platelet-derived growth factor and other growth factors required for the proliferation phase of this disorder (40). Nephron filtration rate is reduced significantly at the 24-h time period in the lytic phase of the disease, and at 6 days the mesangial cells have proliferated extensively (17). In both cases, nephron filtration is decreased primarily as a consequence of major reductions in the glomerular ultrafiltration coefficient. At 24 h, this reduction in LpA appears the consequence of major disruptions in the normal glomerular architecture as a result of mesangial lysis. Plasma flow transits through the mesangial cell space, and large aneurysmal dilatations of capillaries effectively separate much of the plasma flow from a filtering exchange surface. However, at 6 days, during maximum cellular proliferation the reduction in LpA in all likelihood is a consequence of mesangial cell encroachment upon capillary lumina, possibly reducing capillary surface area. This latter association is less clear cut, and other explanations are possible. Studies performed in the lytic phase of this disease have suggested that the glomer-

TABLE 1. *Glomerular hemodynamics and urine protein excretion 2 and 24 h after monoclonal antibody (mAb) administration*[a]

	SNGFR (nL/min)	SNPF (nL/min)	P_G (mm Hg)	ΔP (mm Hg)	AR (gdyn/s/cm^5)	ER (gdyn/s/cm^5)	LpA (nL/s/mm Hg)	Urine protein excretion (mg/h)
Control	33 ± 2 (n = 29)	111 ± 10 (n = 29)	51 ± 1 (n = 14)	36 ± 1 (n = 14)	22 ± 2 (n = 29)	18 ± 2 (n = 29)	0.063 ± 0.012 (n = 6)	0.26 ± 0.05 (n = 6)
mAb (2 h)	31 ± 3 (n = 27)	100 ± 9 (n = 27)	57 ± 1[b] (n = 11)	41 ± 1[a] (n = 11)	23 ± 2 (n = 27)	20 ± 2 (n = 27)	0.029 ± 0.005[b] (n = 6)	0.10 ± 0.06 (n = 6)
mAb (24 h)	47 ± 2[b,c] (n = 30)	181 ± 8[b,c] (n = 30)	54 ± 1[b,c] (n = 15)	38 ±1[c] (n = 15)	12 ± 1[b,c] (n = 30)	10 ± 1[b,c] (n = 30)	0.043 ± 0.005 (n = 6)	1.78 ± 0.23[b,c] (n = 6)

[a]AR, afferent arteriolar resistance; ER, efferent arteriolar resistance; LpA, ultrafiltration coefficient; ΔP, hydrostatic pressure gradient; PG, glomerular capillary hydrostatic pressure; SNGFR, single nephron glomerular filtration rate; SNPF, single nephron plasma flow.

[b]$p<0.05$ compared with control.

[c]$p<0.05$, 24 compared with 2 h.

ulus is relatively unresponsive to acute volume expansion and the administration of angiotensin II (24). This appears secondary to abnormalities in the regulation of efferent arteriolar resistance associated with mesangial cell damage. Similar studies have not as yet been performed in the mesangial cell proliferation phase of this disorder.

ROLE OF INFLAMMATORY MEDIATORS IN REGULATING GLOMERULAR FILTRATION RATE

Complement

Formation of antigen–antibody complexes activates complement and leads to a significant inflammatory response (see Chapter 18). Localization of these antigen–antibody complexes in the different structures of the glomerular capillary determines the presence or absence and the severity of the inflammatory response. The critical role of complement in immune-mediated injury has been clearly established in the three major models of immune injury: anti-GBM antibody glomerulonephritis, membranous nephropathy, and mesangial cell immune injury. Studies by Blantz et al. have evaluated the role of complement in the anti-GBM antibody glomerular nephritis (4). Intravenous administration of large doses of anti-GBM antibody reduces nephron filtration rate secondary to decreases in nephron plasma flow and major reductions in LpA (3). The role of complement activation in this hemodynamic response to anti-GBM antibody has been analyzed using complement-depleted rats. Administration of cobra venom factor to reduce the systemic concentration of complement factors significantly modifies the hemodynamic response to anti-GBM antibody (4). Complement depletion markedly ameliorates the reduction in nephron filtration rate after anti-GBM antibody by preventing vasoconstriction and by limiting the decrease in the ultrafiltration coefficient. Administration of cobra venom factor not only improves the glomerular hemodynamic response to anti-GBM antibody but also reduces the inflammatory response as indexed by the number of PMNs per glomeruli. The beneficial effects obtained with complement depletion clearly demonstrate the importance of complement activation to both the functional and histologic responses to immune injury, but do not discriminate the mechanism by which complement depletion preserves renal function. Is the beneficial effect mediated by the reduction in PMNs or is there evidence that complement can directly modify glomerular resistances?

Studies by Blantz et al. have analyzed the role of leukocytes in the functional changes associated with anti-GBM antibody (15) (see also Chapter 26). These studies have demonstrated that leukocyte depletion prevents the reduction in LpA, providing important evidence regarding the critical role of PMNs in the reduction of GFR associated with anti-GBM antibody. The vasoactive effect of complement in the absence of immune disease or inflammatory infiltrates has been tested by infusing human C5a in the rat renal artery (29). These studies by Pelayo et al. demonstrated that administration of C5a in normal euvolemic rats increases efferent arteriolar resistance, leading to reductions in nephron plasma flow and nephron filtration rate and increases in ΔP. The aforementioned data establish that, in anti-GBM antibody disease, activation of complement reduces nephron filtration rate by vasoconstricting glomerular arterioles as well as by attracting PMNs that decrease LpA.

Complement activation also plays a critical role in pathogenesis of experimental membranous nephropathy (see Chapters 18 and 47). Studies by Salant et al. using a model of passive Heymann nephritis have demonstrated that development of proteinuria in this experimental model requires the formation of the terminal MAC of complement, C5b-9 (7). In the absence of the C5b-9, administration of anti-Fx1A antibody does not induce proteinuria. Studies by Gabbai et al. have used cobra venom factor to investigate the role of complement activation in the glomerular hemodynamic characteristics of passive Heymann nephritis (31) (Fig. 3). These studies demonstrate that complement depletion resulted in major amelioration of the reduction in LpA observed on day 5 after antibody administration. The improvement in LpA observed with complement depletion, however, did not produce LpA values equal to those of normal rats. Therefore, these micropuncture studies suggest that although complement depletion provides significant improvement in glomerular hemodynamic abnormalities, presumably by modifying the reduction in LpA and preventing the increase in glomerular capillary hydrostatic pressure, there remains a persistent but modest reduction in LpA that may be the result of mechanisms independent of complement activation. Interestingly, the significant amelioration of LpA with complement depletion has no correlate of improved glomerular epithelial cell structure.

Complement also plays a critical role in the anti-Thy-1 antibody model of mesangial cell immune injury (39, 39a). In this experimental model, administration of anti-Thy-1 antibody produces destruction of mesangial cells 24 h after the administration of antibody and proliferation of these cells 3–4 days after antibody administration (41). Studies by Yamamoto and Wilson have elegantly demonstrated that complement depletion prevents mesangial destruction in this immune model (18), and recent studies using a C6-deficient rat model suggest this effect is mediated primarily by C5b-9 (39a). Glomerular hemodynamic studies have established that mesangial cell destruction is associated with significant reductions in nephron filtration rate due to reduction in LpA and variable decreases in nephron plasma flow (17). Functional data regarding the effect of complement depletion in this model are unfortunately not available.

Leukotrienes

Although the previous studies clearly establish the critical role of complement in immune-mediated disease, the presence of an inflammatory infiltrate is associated with generation of multiple mediators that participate in the decrease in GFR associated with the different types of glomerulonephritis. Among the various mediators generated by the presence of PMNs, leukotrienes play a significant role in the glomerular hemodynamic changes associated with immune injury. Studies by Badr et al. in the anti-GBM antibody model have demonstrated that administration of 5-lipoxygenase inhibitor or leukotriene D_4 (LTD_4) receptor antagonist normalize LpA values in this model (28). Interestingly, suppression of leukotriene does not modify the number of white cells per glomerulus, suggesting that the reduction in LpA depends on leukotriene generation from the PMNs and not on the presence of PMNs in the lumen of the glomerular capillaries. The hemodynamic response to leukotriene blockers coupled with increased leukotriene generation in nephritic glomeruli clearly establish the importance of leukotriene generation in the reduction of LpA characteristic of anti-GBM antibody administration.

The importance of leukotrienes in noninflammatory immune-injury models was demonstrated by Katoh et al. Using Heymann nephritis, a model characterized by the lack of inflammatory response, Katoh et al. demonstrated that administration of 5-lipoxygenase inhibitor or LTD_4 receptor blocker normalizes LpA values in this immune-injury model (42). These investigators have also proposed that LTD_4-evoked increases in intraglomerular pressure are, to a large extent, responsible for the presence of proteinuria characteristic of this model. The absence of a PMN infiltrate in passive Heymann nephritis raises questions regarding the source of leukotriene in this experimental model. The studies by Katoh et al. elegantly demonstrate that, in passive Heymann nephritis, leukotriene generation depends on a significant increase in the number of resident macrophages in nephritic glomeruli (42).

Studies by Bresnahan et al. provided important information regarding the role of leukotriene in mesangial cell immune injury. These investigators demonstrated that, in the anti-Thy-1 antibody model, leukotriene blockade partially ameliorates the decrement in the ultrafiltration coefficient (19).

The aforementioned results clearly establish that, in three well-studied experimental models of glomerular immune injury, generation of leukotrienes plays a major role in the reduction of the ultrafiltration coefficient that characterizes these models. Interestingly, studies by Badr suggest that leukotriene generation is antagonized by generation of 15-lipoxygenase products such as lipoxin A_4 (LXA_4) and lipoxin B_4 (LXB_4) that are produced by macrophages (43,44). The glomerular response to immune injury, therefore, depends on the interaction between leukotrienes derived from PMNs and lipoxins generated by macrophages, both types of cells stimulated by the presence of antigen–antibody complexes.

Eicosanoids

The role of cyclooxygenase production in immune renal injury is covered in detail in chapter 22. Thromboxane A_2 (TXA_2) and prostaglandin E_2 (PGE_2) constitute another important group of mediators involved in the glomerular immune response. TXA_2 and PGE_2 are generated by the glomerular cells, including endothelial, mesangial, and epithelial cells (45,46). Multiple studies both in rats and in mice in various experimental models including anti-GBM antibody glomerular nephritis, experimental membranous nephropathy, administration of cationic bovine γ-globulin, immunoglobulin-A nephropathy, and murine lupus have clearly demonstrated that immune injury is associated with increased levels of these eicosanoids (47–53). Generation of TXA_2 is associated with renal vasoconstriction and reduction in the ultrafiltration coefficient. In contrast, increased levels of PGE_2 are associated with renal vasodilation. Most studies in the literature suggest that the presence of vasoconstriction characteristic of the early phases of the immune injury is associated with increased thromboxane generation, whereas normalization of GFR and renal plasma flow at later stages usually depends on the generation of PGE_2. Administration of thromboxane synthesis inhibitors and thromboxane receptor antagonists in the early stages of disease ameliorates the decrease in renal plasma flow and the reduction in LpA. In contrast, administration of cyclooxygenase inhibitors (that is, nonsteroidal anti-inflammatory drugs) during later stages of the disease is frequently associated with reductions in renal plasma flow and GFR (48). In the murine model of lupus, development of renal disease is associated with increased levels of thromboxane (54–56). TXA_2 receptor antagonists and the exogenous administration of prostaglandin provide significant beneficial effects with regard to proteinuria, morphology, and survival in this model (57–60).

Other experimental approaches to evaluate the role of eicosanoids in glomerular immune injury include administration of essential fatty-acid-deficient diet and diets rich in eicosapentaenoic acid (61–64). The rationale for these dietary manipulations is based on the fact that essential fatty-acid-deficient diets decrease the amount of arachidonic acid that is the substrate for the generation of prostanoids. Administration of large quantities of eicosapentaenoic acid leads to the replacement of arachidonic acid by eicosapentaenoic acid and generation of prostaglandin and thromboxane differing in their structure from the arachidonic acid analogue by one additional double bond. Generation of thromboxane A_3 under these conditions leads to significantly less vasoconstriction when compared with thromboxane A_2. Results obtained with these different dietary manipulations are quite promising since improvement in renal function and morphology has been observed in various models of immune injury (63–65). However, some investigators have been unable to establish protection with dietary manipulations (66).

Nitric Oxide

During the past several years, significant interest has developed in the role of nitric oxide (NO) in glomerular immune injury. This subject is covered in more detail in chapter 21. NO is derived from the amino acid L-arginine in the presence of the enzyme nitric oxide synthase (NOS) (67). Two major families of NOS have been characterized: a constitutive form capable of generating nanomolar quantities of NO is responsible for important physiologic functions (neurotransmission and vasoconstriction) and an inducible form, capable of generating micromolar concentrations of NO, is responsible for host defense immune response (68). Both types of enzymes have been demonstrated at the level of the kidneys (69). While constitutive NOS appears to concentrate in the vascular tissue, macula densa, and medullary collecting duct, inducible NOS is present in almost all segments of the kidney. In nephritic glomeruli, NO activity can be generated not only from the normal resident glomerular cells, but also by other cells such as leukocytes, monocytes, macrophages, and platelets (70–73). Mast cells and T lymphocytes also exhibit NOS (74,75). Studies by several investigators have evaluated the role of NO in models of glomerulonephritis (76,77) and have demonstrated both in vivo and in vitro that induction of glomerular nephritis is associated with increased NO activity as indexed by NO_2/NO_3, suggesting the involvement of NO in the mechanism of glomerular injury and the alteration in glomerular hemodynamics under these conditions. Administration of NOS blockers to rats with nephrotoxic glomerulonephritis is associated with significant increases in both glomerular capillary hydrostatic pressure and proteinuria, suggesting that NO generation may act as a vasodilator limiting the effect of other vasoconstrictive mediators (78). Although nephritic glomeruli exhibit increased NO activity, nephritic glomeruli also demonstrate increased arginase activity capable of limiting NO generation (79). L-arginine can be metabolized to NO by NOS or to urea and L-ornithine by arginase. Increased activity of arginase in these nephritic glomeruli constitutes another element that can regulate NO generation in this type of inflammatory process. Recent evidence by two groups of investigators has demonstrated that NO plays a critical role in the lysis of mesangial cells in the anti-Thy-1 antibody model, since NOS blockers prevent the destruction and further proliferation of the mesangial cells in this experimental model (80,81).

ALTERATIONS IN PHYSIOLOGIC RESPONSES BY THE IMMUNE-INJURED KIDNEY

It is becoming increasingly clear that immune injury to the glomerulus and to the tubulointerstitium alters the kidney's capacity to respond physiologically to alterations in blood pressure, volume status, and a variety of neurohumoral control mechanisms. Both clinical and experimental studies have suggested that systemic hypertension coexisting with immune-induced renal disease can accelerate the progressive decline in glomerular function (23,82–85). Several studies in the literature have demonstrated that significant hypertension, when superimposed upon models of glomerular immune injury, results in severe progressive renal dysfunction, observations that are compatible with those derived from human clinical studies. However, even modest hypertension, after application of a renal artery clip, produces significant alterations in glomerular histology over a period of 14–16 weeks (23). Superimposition of modest hypertension upon an anti-GBM antibody disease model resulted in both focal and diffuse glomerulosclerosis and has produced significant reductions in the GFR of glomerulonephritic kidneys (23,83–85, unpublished observations).

More recent studies in an anti-GBM antibody-mediated disease model examined the impact of immune injury upon a variety of parameters. Treatment of hypertension with large doses of an angiotensin-converting enzyme (ACE) inhibitor was much less effective in normalizing blood pressure in nephritic rats (Gabbai, unpublished observations). The extensive focal glomerulosclerosis correlated well with elevations in glomerular capillary pressure and glomerular capillary hydrostatic pressure gradient in nonnephritic rats. In the immune-injury rats, however, glomerulosclerosis correlated only with the absolute level of systolic blood pressure in the awake condition. In addition, there was a loss of correlation between systolic blood pressure and the absolute glomerular capillary pressure in the nephritic rats, a somewhat surprising result suggesting that there are influences affecting the glomerulonephritic kidney other than hemodynamic effects that determine the extent and severity of focal glomerulosclerosis. Plasma angiotensin-II levels were much higher in nephritic rats. In nephritic rats, treatment with an ACE inhibitor was not only less effective in decreasing blood pressure, but ACE inhibitors did not significantly lower plasma angiotensin-II levels. These studies suggest that autoregulation of blood

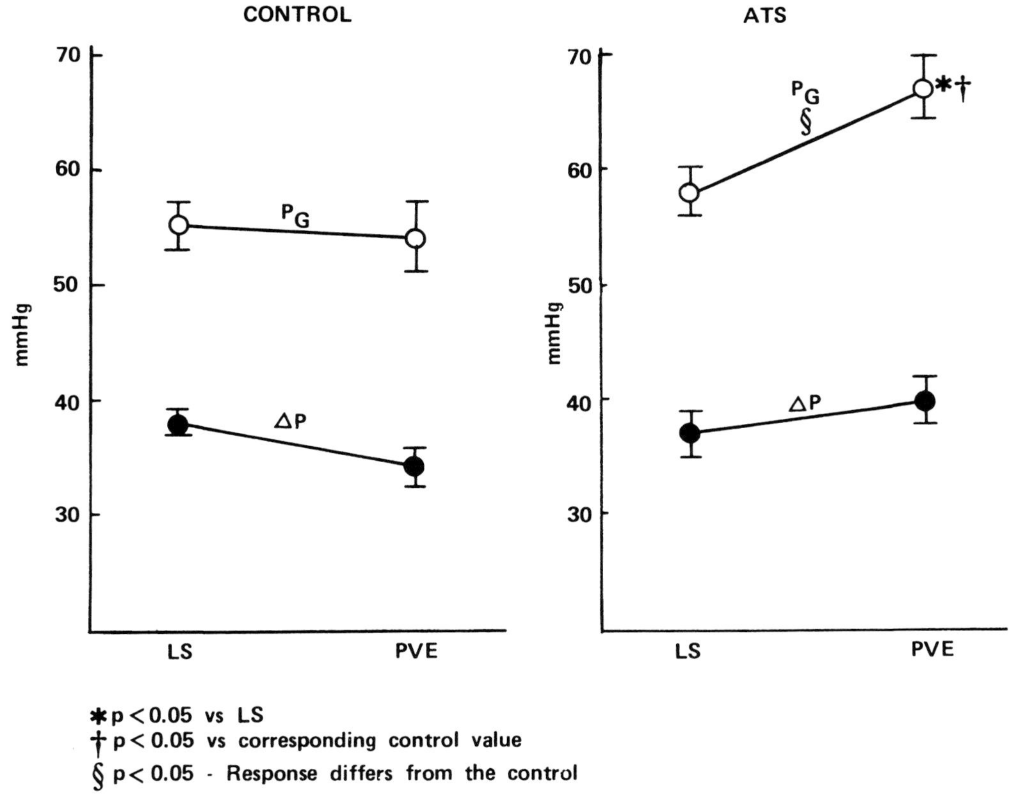

FIG. 4. Response of glomerular capillary hydrostatic pressure (P_G) and glomerular and capillary hydrostatic pressure gradient (ΔP) to plasma volume expansion (PVE) in LS control *(left)* and ATS rats *(right)*. Although pressures remained constant in control animals, PVE caused major increases in P_G in ATS rats. Absolute values for P_G during PVE were significantly higher after ATS than in control group. Mesangial cell lysis and dysfunction result in inability to maintain P_G constant after acute PVE: *$p < 0.05$ versus LS and corresponding control value, and §$p < 0.05$, response differs from control.

flow and glomerular capillary pressure is altered in immune-injury models. However, there is little specific evidence for this conclusion in contrast to models of focal segmental glomerulosclerosis after subtotal nephrectomy (20,86). After subtotal nephrectomy, significant abnormalities of autoregulation of pressure and flow have been observed.

A large component of renal blood flow and presumably pressure autoregulation in the kidney has been attributed to tubuloglomerular feedback activity. Studies in the literature have examined tubuloglomerular feedback activity in models of immune injury and found no major alteration in the capacity for nephron filtration rate to respond appropriately to alterations in delivery of fluid to the distal tubule, macula densa sensing sites (87). Abnormalities might have been predicted because of the fact that LpA or Kf is markedly reduced in these models, leading to a condition of filtration pressure disequilibrium in which normal flow dependence of GFR should be reduced (11). These results suggest that the tubuloglomerular feedback system continued to operate in spite of the fact that there was lesser flow dependency of GFR. However, greater reductions in plasma flow and/or ΔP would be required to achieve a normal feedback SNGFR response. These results are in contrast with those recently observed in a model of tubulointerstitial nephritis, a primarily cellular immune model. Seven days after induction of this disease, tubuloglomerular feedback capacity was essentially eliminated, suggesting abnormalities in either the sensing or effector limb of the system as a result of the tubulointerstitial inflammatory process (Gabbai, unpublished observations).

There are limited studies that address the issue of the neurohumoral status of the kidney with immune injury. Plasma angiotensin-II levels are higher at any given level of blood pressure in both early and later stages of anti-GBM antibody-induced nephritis. Studies have also observed that the number of angiotensin-II receptors in glomeruli are significantly reduced after acute glomerular immune injury (88). It has not been determined whether this is merely a normal response to the elevated plasma angiotensin-II concentrations. Intrarenal angiotensin-II concentrations as determined by radioimmunoassay appear normal early in the disease (unpublished observations). The glomerular hemodynamic response to variations in volume status and to exogenously administered angiotensin II has been evaluated in a model of mesangiocapillary glomerulonephritis after administration of antithymocyte antibody (ATS)(24). In animals with normal NaCl intake, plasma volume expansion increased nephron filtration rate at essentially constant levels of glomerular capillary hydrostatic pressure due to a parallel vasodilator response of the afferent and efferent arterioles. Following plasma volume expansion, nephron filtration rate did not increase in nephritic rats despite increases in single-nephron plasma flow. During the transition from salt depletion (LS) to plasma volume expansion, glomerular capillary hydrostatic pressure increased significantly in nephritic rats as a consequence of afferent arteriolar dilation while efferent resistance remained fixed and elevated (Fig. 4). Angiotensin-II infusion normally decreases nephron filtration rate as a result of reductions in nephron plasma flow and the glomerular ultrafiltration coefficient (89). In rats with mesangial cell injury after anti-Thy-1 antibody administration, angiotensin-II infusion did not change the nephron filtration rate, LpA, or hydrostatic pressure gradient. These in vivo studies suggested that the mesangial cell plays an important role in the regulation of the glomerular ultrafiltration coefficient and contributes to the regulatory behavior of the efferent arteriole, resulting in an absence of normal regulation of glomerular capillary hydrostatic pressure. Responses of the afferent arteriole to both volume expansion and angiotensin-II infusion were basically normal and identical to control animals. Studies during the proliferative phase of this form of mesangiocapillary nephritis have not as yet been conducted. One might predict significant alterations in the normal responses to volume and neurohumoral stimuli.

These studies in the aggregate suggest that there are abnormalities in the regulation of glomerular capillary hydrostatic pressure in various forms of immune-induced glomerular disease. Abnormalities do not appear to be the result of alterations in tubuloglomerular feedback activity, but may result from altered behavior of the efferent arteriolar resistance leading to a disruption of normal relationship between systolic blood pressure, volume status, and the glomerular capillary hydrostatic pressure. Future studies should be performed to determine whether alterations in NO production and/or prostaglandin generation contribute in any way to these alterations in the regulation of glomerular hemodynamics in the immune-injured kidney.

ACKNOWLEDGMENTS

These studies were supported from grants provided by the National Institutes of Health (DK28602, DK40251, DK20043), funds provided by the Research Service of the Department of Veterans Affairs.

REFERENCES

1. Allison M, Wilson CB, Gottschalk CW. Pathophysiology of experimental glomerulonephritis in rats. *J Clin Invest* 1974;53:1402–23.
2. Maddox DA, Bennett CM, Deen WM, et al. Determinants of glomerular filtration in the rat. *J Clin Invest* 1975;55:305–318.
3. Blantz RC, Wilson CB. Acute effects of anti-glomerular basement membrane antibody on the process of glomerular filtration in the rat. *J Clin Invest* 1976;58:899–911.
4. Blantz RC, Tucker BJ, Wilson CB. The acute effects of anti-glomerular basement membrane antibody on the process of glomerular filtration in the rat: the influence of dose and complement depletion. *J Clin Invest* 1978;61:910–21.
5. Ichikawa I, Hoyer JR, Seiler MW, Brenner BM. Mechanism of glomerulotubular balance in the setting of heterogenous glomerular injury. *J Clin Invest* 1982;69:185–98.
6. Blantz RC, Hostetter TM, Brenner BM. Functional adaptations of the kidney to immunological injury. In: Wilson CB, Brenner BM, Stein JH, eds. *Immunologic mechanisms of renal disease*. New York: Churchill Livingston, 1979:122–43.
7. Salant DJ, Belok S, Madiao MP, et al. A new role for complement in experimental membranous nephropathy in rats. *J Clin Invest* 1980;66: 1339–50.
8. Heymann W, Hackel DB, Harwood S, et al. Production of the nephrotic syndrome in rats by Freund's adjuvants and rat kidney suspension. *Proc Soc Exp Med* 1959;100:660–4.
9. Edginton TS, Glassock RJ, Dixon FJ. Autologous immune complex nephritis induced with renal tubular antigen. I. Identification and isolation of the pathogenetic antigen. *J Exp Med* 1968;127:555–72.
10. Mauer SM, Sutherland DER, Howard RJ, et al. The glomerular mesangium. III. Acute immune mesangial injury: a new model of glomerulonephritis. *J Exp Med* 1973;137:553.
11. Tucker BJ, Blantz RC. An analysis of the determinants of nephron filtration rate. *Am J Physiol* 1977;232:F477.
12. Gabbai F, Gushwa L, Wilson CB, et al. An evaluation of the development of experimental membranous nephropathy. *Kidney Int* 1987;31: 1267–78.
13. Bradley SE, Bradley GP, Tyson CJ, Curry J, Blake WD. Renal function in renal diseases. *Am J Med* 1950;9:766.
14. Earle DP, Farber SJ, Alexander JD, Pellegrino ED. Renal function and electrolyte metabolism in acute glomerulonephritis. *J Clin Invest* 1951;30:421.
15. Tucker BJ, Wilson CB, Gushwa LC, et al. Effect of leukocyte depletion on glomerular dynamics during acute glomerular injury. *Kidney Int* 1987;32:652–63.
16. Blantz RC. Effect of mannitol on glomerular ultrafiltration in the hydropenic rat. *J Clin Invest* 1974;54:1135–43.
17. Yamamoto T, Mundy CA, Wilson CB, Blantz RC. Effect of mesangial cell lysis and proliferation on glomerular hemodynamics in the rat. *Kidney Int* 1991;40:705–13.
18. Yamamoto T, Wilson CB. Complement dependence of antibody-induced mesangial cell injury in the rat. *J Immunol* 1987;138:3758–65.
19. Bresnahan BA, Wu S, Fenoy FJ, Roman RJ, Lianos EA. Mesangial cell immune injury: hemodynamic role of leukocyte and platelet derived eicosanoids. *J Clin Invest* 1992;90:2304–12.
20. Brenner BM. Hyperfiltration in remnant nephrons: a potentially adverse response to renal ablation. *Am J Physiol* 1981;241:F85–93.
21. Blantz RC, Gabbai FB, Peterson O. Water and protein permeability is regulated by the glomerular epithelial slit diaphragm. *J Am Soc Nephrol* 1994;4:1957–64.
22. Neilsen EG, Phillips SM. Cell-mediated immunity in interstitial nephritis. II. T lymphocyte effector mechanisms in nephritic guinea pigs: analysis of the renotropic migration and cytotoxic response. *J Immunol* 1979;123:1979.
23. Blantz RC, Gabbai F, Gushwa LC, et al. The influence of concomitant experimental hypertension and glomerulonephritis in the rat. *Kidney Int* 1987;32:652–63.
24. Blantz RC, Gabbai FB, Tucker BJ, Yamamoto T, Wilson CB. Role of mesangial cell in glomerular response to volume and angiotensin II. *Am J Physiol* 1993;264:F158–65.
25. Wilson CB, Blantz RC. Nephroimmunopathology and pathophysiology. *Am J Physiol* 1985;248:F319–31.
26. Blantz RC, Gabbai FB, Wilson CB. Glomerular hemodynamics in experimental glomerulo-nephritis. *Adv Nephrol* 1988;17:3–14.

27. Blantz RC, Tucker BJ, Gushwa L, et al. Glomerular immune injury in the rat: the influence of AII and α-adrenergic inhibitors. *Kidney Int* 1981;20:452–61.
28. Badr KR, Schreiner GF, Wasserman M, et al. Preservation of the glomerular capillary ultrafiltration coefficient during rat nephrotoxic serum nephritis by a specific leukotriene D_4 receptor antagonist. *J Clin Invest* 1988;81:1702–9.
29. Pelayo JC, Chenoweth DE, Hugli TE, Wilson CB, Blantz RC. Effects of anaphylatoxin, C5a, on renal and glomerular hemodynamics in the rat. *Kidney Int* 1986;30:62–7.
30. Groggel GC, Adler S, Rennke HG, et al. Role of the terminal complement pathway in experimental membranous nephropathy in the rabbit. *J Clin Invest* 1983;72:1984.
31. Gabbai FB, Mundy CA, Wilson CB, et al. An evaluation of the role of complement depletion in experimental membranous nephropathy in the rat. *Lab Invest* 1988;58:539–44.
32. Kerjaschki D, Farquhar MG. Immunocytochemical localization of the Heymann nephritis antigen (gp 330) in glomerular epithelial cells of normal Lewis rats. *J Exp Med* 1983;157:667–86.
33. Adler S, Baker JP, Pritzl P, et al. Detection of terminal complement components in experimental glomerular injury. *Kidney Int* 1984;26: 830–7.
34. Gabbai FB, Wilson CB, Blantz RC. Role of angiotensin II in experimental membranous nephropathy. *Am J Physiol* 1988;23:F500–6.
35. Matsuo S, Caldwell PRB, Brentjens JR, et al. In vivo interaction of antibodies with cell surface antigens: a mechanism responsible for in situ formation of immune deposits in the zona pellucida in rabbit oocytes. *J Clin Invest* 1985;75:1369–80.
36. Pruchino CJ, Burns MW, Schulze M, et al. Urinary excretion of C5b-9 reflects disease activity in passive Heymann nephritis. *Kidney Int* 1989;36:65–71.
37. Camussi G, Noble B, Van Liew J, et al. Pathogenesis of passive Heymann nephritis: chlorpromazine inhibits antibody mediated redistribution of cell surface antigens and prevents development of the disease. *Kidney Int* 1986;29:268(abst).
38. Ichikawa I, Rennke HG, Hoyer JR, et al. Role of intrarenal mechanisms in the impaired salt excretion of experimental nephrotic syndrome. *J Clin Invest* 1983;71:91.
39. Yamamoto T, Mundy C, Wilson CB, et al. Antibody induced mesangial cell (MC) lysis and proliferation: glomerular hemodynamic consequences. *Kidney Int* 1988;327(abstr).
39a. Brandt J, Pippin J, Schulze M, et al. Role of the complement membrane attack complex (C5b-9) in mediating experimental mesangioproliferative glomerulonephritis. *Kidney Int* 1995 (in press).
40. Johnson RJ, Garcia RL, Pritzl P, et al. Platelets mediate glomerular cell proliferation in immune complex nephritis induced by antimesangial cell antibodies in the rat. *Am J Pathol* 1990;136:369–74.
41. Yamamoto T, Yamamoto K, Kawaski K, et al. Immunoelectron microscopic demonstration of Thy-1 antigen on the surfaces of mesangial cells in the rat glomerulus. *Nephron* 1987;43:293–8.
42. Katoh T, Lianos EA, Badr KF. Leukotriene D_4 is a mediator of proteinuria and glomerular hemodynamic abnormalities in passive Heymann nephritis. *J Clin Invest* 1993;91:1507–15.
43. Badr KF. 15-Lipoxygenase products as leukotriene antagonists: therapeutic potential in glomerulonephritis. *Kidney Int* 1992;42:S101–8.
44. Badr KF. Five-lipoxygenase products in glomerular immune injury. *J Am Soc Nephrol* 1992;3:907–15.
45. Schlondorff D. Renal prostaglandins synthesis: sites of production and specific actions of prostaglandins. *Am J Med* 1986;81:1–11.
46. Striker GE, Striker LJ. Glomerular cell culture. *Lab Invest* 1985;53: 122–31.
47. Rahman MA, Stork JE, Dunn MJ. The roles of eicosanoids in experimental glomerulonephritis. *Kidney Int* 1987;32:S40–8.
48. Lianos EA, Andres GA, Dunn MJ. Glomerular prostaglandin and thromboxane synthesis in rat nephrotoxic serum nephritis. *J Clin Invest* 1983;72:1429–48.
49. Stork JE, Dunn MJ. Hemodynamic roles of thromboxane A_2 and prostaglandin E_2 in glomerulonephritis. *J Pharmacol Exp Ther* 1985; 233:672–8.
50. Gesualdo L, Emancipator SN, Kesselheim C, Lamm ME. Glomerular hemodynamics and eicosanoid synthesis in a rat model of IgA nephropathy. *Kidney Int* 1992;42:106–14.
51. Thaiss F, Mihatsch MJ, Schoeppe W, Stahl RA. Thromboxane mediates glomerular hemodynamics in a model of chronic glomerular disease. *Eur J Clin Invest* 1992;22:182–9.
52. Stahl RA, Thaiss F, Kahf S, Schoeppe W, Helmohen UM. Immune-mediated mesangial cell injury, biosynthesis and function of prostanoids. *Kidney Int* 1990;38:273–81.
53. Takahashi K, Schreiner GF, Yamashita K, Christman BW, Blair I, Badr KF. Predominant functional roles for thromboxane A_2 and prostaglandin E_2 during late nephrotoxic serum glomerulonephritis in the rat. *J Clin Invest* 1990;85:1974–82.
54. Kelley VE, Sneve S, Musinski S. Increased renal thromboxane production in murine lupus nephritis. *J Clin Invest* 1986;77:252–9.
55. Spurney RF, Onorato JJ, Ruiz P, Pisetsky DS, Coffman TM. Characterization of glomerular thromboxane receptors in murine lupus nephritis. *J Pharmacol Exp Ther* 1993;264:584–90.
56. Spurney RF, Bernstein RJ, Ruiz P, Pisetsky DS, Coffman TM. Physiologic role for enhanced renal thromboxane production in murine lupus nephritis. *Prostaglandins* 1991;42:15–28.
57. Spurney RF, Fan PY, Ruiz P, Sanfilippo F, Pisetsky DS, Coffman TM. Thromboxane receptor blockade reduces renal injury in murine lupus nephritis. *Kidney Int* 1992;41:973–82.
58. Kawakage M, Mizumoto H, Nukui E, Sato S, Karasawa A. Effects of KW-3635, a specific thromboxane A_2-receptor antagonist, on the development of lupus nephritis in NZB × NXW FI mice. *Jpn J Pharmacol* 1993;63:433–8.
59. Zurier RB, Damjanov I, Miller P, Biewer B. Prostaglandin E1 treatment prevents progression of nephritis in murine lupus erythematosus. *J Clin Lab Immunol* 1978;1:95–8.
60. Kelley VE, Winkelstein A, Izui S, Dixon F. Prostaglandin E1 inhibits T-cell proliferation and renal disease in MRL/1 mice. *Clin Immunol Immunopathol* 1981;21:190–203.
61. Clup BR, Titus BG, Lands WE. Inhibition of prostaglandin biosynthesis by eicosapentaenoic acid. *Prostaglandin Med* 1979;3:269.
62. Van Drorp DA. Essential fatty acids and prostaglandins. *Acta Biol Med Ger* 1976;35:1041–9.
63. Prickett JD, Robinson DR, Steinberg AD. Dietary enrichment with the polyunsaturated fatty acid eicosapentaenoic acid prevents proteinuria and prolongs survival in NZA/NZW F1 mice. *J Clin Invest* 1981; 68:556–9.
64. Duboid CH, Foidard JB, Dechenne CA, Mahieu PR. Effects of diet deficient in essential fatty acids on the glomerular hypercellularity occurring in the course of nephrotoxic serum nephritis in rats. *Kidney Int* 1982;21:539–45.
65. Takahashi K, Kato T, Schreiner GF, Ebert J, Badr KF. Essential fatty acid deficiency normalizes function and histology in rat nephrotoxic nephritis. *Kidney Int* 1992;41:1245–53.
66. Thaiss F, Schoeppe W, Germann P, Stahl RAK. Dietary fish oil intake: effects on glomerular prostanoid formation, hemodynamics, and proteinuria in nephrotoxic serum nephritis. *J Lab Clin Med* 1990; 116:172–9.
67. Marletta MA. Nitric oxide synthase structure and mechanism. *J Biol Chem* 1993;268:12,231–4.
68. Moncada S, Palmer RMJ, Higgs EA. Nitric oxide: physiology, pathophysiology and pharmacology. *Pharmacol Rev* 1991;43:109–42.
69. Gabbai FB, Garcia GE, Blantz RC, De Nicola L. Role of nitric oxide in glomerular physiology and pathophysiology. In: Grünfeld JP, Bach JF, Kreis H, Maxwell MH, eds. *Advances in nephrology*. St. Louis: JP Mosby, 1995:3–18.
70. Knowles RG, Salter M, Brooks SL, et al. Anti-inflammatory glucocorticoids inhibit the induction by endotoxin of nitric oxide synthase in the lung, liver, and aorta of the rat. *Biochem Biophys Res Commun* 1990;172:1042–8.
71. McCall TB, Palmer RMJ, Moncada S. Induction of nitric oxide synthase in rat peritoneal neutrophils and its inhibition by dexamethasone. *Eur J Immunol* 1991;21:2523–7.
72. Radomski MW, Palmer RMJ, Moncada S. An L-arginine/nitric oxide pathway present in human platelets regulates aggregation. *Proc Natl Acad Sci USA* 1990;87:5193–7.
73. Wright CD, Mulsch A, Busse R, et al. Generation of nitric oxide by human neutrophils. *Biochem Biophys Res Commun* 1989;160: 813–9.
74. Kirk SJ, Regan MC, Barbul A. Cloned murine T lymphocytes synthesize a molecule with the biological characteristics of nitric oxide. *Biochem Biophys Res Commun* 1990;172:660–5.
75. Salvemini D, Masine E, Anggard E, et al. Synthesis of a nitric oxide-like factor from L-arginine by rat serosal mast cells: stimulation of guanylate cyclase and inhibition of platelet aggregation. *Biochem Biophys Res Commun* 1990;169:596–601.

76. Cattell V, Cook T, Moncada S. Glomeruli synthesize nitrite in experimental nephrotoxic nephritis. *Kidney Int* 1990;38:1056–60.
77. Cook HT, Sullivan R. Glomerular nitrite synthesis in situ immune complex glomerulonephritis in the rat. *Am J Pathol* 1991;139:1047–52.
78. Ferrario R, Takahashi K, Fogo A, Badr KF, Munger KA. Consequences of acute nitric oxide synthesis inhibition in experimental glomerulonephritis. *J Am Soc Nephrol* 1994;4:1847–54.
79. Jansen A, Lewis S, Cattell V, et al. Arginase is a major pathway of L-arginine metabolism in nephritic glomeruli. *Kidney Int* 1992;42:1107–12.
80. Narita I, Border WA, Ketteler M, Nobel NA. Nitric oxide mediates immunologic injury to kidney mesangium in experimental glomerulonephritis. *Lab Invest* 1995;73:17–24.
81. Cattell V, Lianos E, Largen P, Cook T. Glomerular NO synthase activity in mesangial cell immune injury. *Exp Nephrol* 1993;1:36–40.
82. Klahr S. The modification of diet in renal disease study. *N Engl J Med* 1989;320:864–6.
83. Neugarten J, Feiner HD, Schacht RG, Gallo GR, Baldwin DS. Aggravation of experimental glomerulonephritis by superimposed clip hypertension. *Kidney Int* 1982;22:257–63.
84. Raij L, Azar S, Keane W. Mesangial immune injury, hypertension, and progressive glomerular damage in Dahl rats. *Kidney Int* 1984;26:1372–143.
85. Iversen BM, Ofstad J. Effect of hypertension on experimental glomerulonephritis in rats. *Lab Invest* 1984;50:164–73.
86. Pelayo JC, Westcott JY. Impaired autoregulation of glomerular capillary hydrostatic pressure in the rat remnant nephron. *J Clin Invest* 1991;88:101–5.
87. Peterson OW, Gushwa LC, Wilson CB, Blantz RC. Tubuloglomerular feedback activity after glomerular immune injury. *Am J Physiol* 1989;257:F67–71.
88. Timmermans V, Peake PH, Charlesworth JA, McDonald GJ, Pawlak MA. Angiotensin II receptor regulation in anti-glomerular basement membrane nephritis. *Kidney Int* 1990;38:518–24.
89. Blantz RC, Konnen KS, Tucker BJ. Angiotensin II effects upon the glomerular microcirculation and ultrafiltration coefficient of the rat. *J Clin Invest* 1976;57:419–34.

Immunologic Renal Diseases,
edited by E. G. Neilson and W. G. Couser.
Lippincott-Raven Publishers, Philadelphia © 1997.

CHAPTER 12

Development and Expression of Nephritogenic T Cells

Carolyn J. Kelly

INTRODUCTION

Lymphocytes are present within the glomerular or interstitial compartments of the kidney during the natural history of many forms of renal disease. In some settings, the presence of a lymphocytic infiltrate results in the pathologic process being classified as autoimmune or immune mediated. In other situations, T cells within the diseased kidney have been largely dismissed as part of a nonspecific infiltrate whose expression is coincident with progressive tissue destruction. Inflammatory responses injuring the kidney are complex and typically involve both humoral and cellular limbs of the immune system. These immune responses are subject to complex modulation. Current paradigms for understanding the role of T cells in renal injury derive primarily from studies of experimental model systems. This chapter addresses the role of T cells in the expression of different forms of renal disease and outlines how to assess whether T cells are relevant to disease expression. It summarizes studies from human renal disease that implicate T cells in immunopathogenesis and concludes with a summary of information regarding the development and expression of nephritogenic T cells in models of experimental renal disease.

ASSESSING THE RELEVANCE OF T CELLS TO RENAL INJURY

T cells have traditionally been implicated in the pathogenesis of renal disease if such lymphocytes are physically present in the kidney, if their presence is associated with some functional abnormality (for example, proteinuria, abnormalities in tubular reabsorption or secretion, or decrement in glomerular filtration rate), and if they express activation markers [such as the interleukin-2 (IL-2) receptor, transferrin receptor, or class II major histocompatibility complex (MHC)] on the cell surface. The presence of such activation markers is presumptive evidence that the cells are not simply innocent bystanders. Additional supportive evidence for the involvement of T lymphocytes in renal injury would include the correlative finding of disappearance of the cells and functional improvement. The failure to see functional improvement following disappearance of the infiltrate is not typically interpretable, because the replacement of a mononuclear cell infiltrate with areas of extracellular matrix deposition may not result in functional improvement but does not rule out the importance of the initial mononuclear cell infiltrate in the resultant fibrosis. The ability of therapeutics that suppress the activation, proliferation, or effector function of T cells to diminish the severity of the histologic lesion or improve renal function can be taken as supportive evidence for the pathogenicity of the T cells. In experimental models of renal disease, more stringent criteria include the demonstration that T cells are required to transfer the lesion adoptively into a naive host (1,2) or that T cells present in the lesion specifically recognize an antigen expressed in diseased or normal kidney (3–5).

Although these criteria provide useful guidelines, they oversimplify complex processes. To require the presence of lymphocytes in significant numbers in diseased tissue presupposes examination of the tissue at the proper time. A harmful immune response initiated by lymphocytes may be followed by a heavy and numerically more significant nonspecific mononuclear cell infiltrate (for exam-

C. J. Kelly: University of California–San Diego and Veterans Administration Medical Center 111-H, San Diego, California 92161.

ple, natural killer cells and macrophages). Such nonspecific immune cells may dominate the pathologic picture by the time functionally significant organ impairment has occurred. The second problem with this approach is that immunosuppressive therapeutics may not affect the clinical course if added to the therapeutic armamentarium too late. From studies in animal models, it is clear that early intervention is critical in T-cell-initiated pathologies. In experimental models, the requirement that T cells adoptively transfer a lesion is extremely stringent. Although there are models in which this has been accomplished, there are multiple reasons why the adoptive transfer of T-cell subpopulations may not reproduce the same pathologic lesion as seen in the intact animal. For all of these reasons, the potential impact of T cells on various forms of renal injury may be significantly underestimated.

REQUIREMENTS FOR DEVELOPMENT OF NEPHRITOGENIC T CELLS

For priming of the nephritogenic T-cell response to occur, T cells with cell surface antigen receptors capable of recognizing the appropriate processed peptide antigen must be present in the host. An individual of an outbred species or inbred strains may be unresponsive to a self-antigen due to central (thymic) deletion of self-reactive T cells (6,7). Because T cells recognize processed linear peptide sequences in conjunction with polymorphic class I or II MHC molecules (8–10), the MHC antigens expressed by an individual likewise impose important restrictions on the priming of T-cell responses to antigens.

Antigen expression in the kidney has also been seen as a requirement for nephritogenic T-cell function. For those target antigens whose expression is polymorphic [for example, target antigen of antitubular basement membrane (anti-TBM) disease.], a host may develop a nephritogenic immune response in the periphery but not develop renal disease, due to the absence of the target antigen (11–13). In some cases, the antigen expressed within the renal parenchyma may be cross-reactive with a different antigen in the periphery that initially primes the T-cell response: so-called molecular mimicry (14–18). It is also possible, although not yet formally established, that some forms of T-cell-mediated renal injury may not involve infiltration of the glomerular or interstitial compartment with T cells but rather reflect the effects of cytokines released from activated T cells on glomerular/tubular function.

If the antigen, appropriate T-cell receptor (TCR)-bearing T cells, and appropriate MHC are all expressed by the host, priming of such T cells can occur. The outcome of antigen presentation to such T cells may be either to activate or to anergize the T cells, depending on the presence of costimulation (19–21).

PARTICIPATION OF T CELLS IN HUMAN RENAL DISEASE

Interstitial Nephritis

The predominant immune effector mechanism in human interstitial nephritis appears to be cell-mediated immunity. Immune complexes and anti-TBM antibodies are less commonly seen in these settings. Most forms of clinically recognized acute interstitial nephritis occur in association with drug hypersensitivity reactions, infection, or systemic autoimmune diseases (22). In most settings, the majority of the infiltrating mononuclear cells are lymphocytes (>50%) with the remaining cells predominantly monocyte/macrophages, B cells, plasma cells, and natural killer cells (23–27). The CD4/CD8 ratio of the interstitial infiltrate is generally ≥1, although exceptions have been noted (24,28). Both the T cells and tubular epithelial cells can express class II MHC molecules in interstitial nephritis (27,28). The composition of the mononuclear cell infiltrate can be affected by previous immunosuppressive therapy, particularly steroids or cyclosporine, although the latter agent is infrequently used in this setting.

Glomerular Disease

In many lesions classified as primary glomerular diseases, lymphocytes are present within the glomerular and interstitial compartments. This infiltrate is particular striking in primary glomerular diseases accompanied by significant and progressive renal insufficiency. Such entities include crescentic glomerulonephritis (29), progressive immunoglobulin-A nephropathy (30,31), and HIV nephropathy (32). In the latter instance, the glomerular lesion of focal segmental glomerular sclerosis is accompanied by striking infiltration of the interstitium with mononuclear cells. The pathogenesis underlying this infiltrate, frequently seen concomitantly with marked depletion of $CD4^+$ T cells in the periphery, is unclear, but a similar lesion occurs in HIV-1 transgenic mice, in whom *gag* and *pol* gene products are expressed in the absence of active infection (33,34). These mice initially develop focal glomerular sclerosis, which progresses to diffuse glomerular sclerosis. With progressive glomerular sclerosis, the mice develop microcystic changes in the interstitium, with tubular epithelial cell degeneration and interstitial nephritis. It is striking that many of the glomerular lesions that display associated lymphocytic infiltrates within the interstitium are among those that clinically display the most rapid decline in renal function. This observation is consistent with the correlation between severity of interstitial disease and degree of progressive renal failure (35–38).

Occasional lymphocytes are seen within the glomerulus in proliferative forms of glomerulonephritis (29). The number of $CD4^+$ T cells and macrophages in glomeruli and crescents in patients with rapidly progressive glomerulonephritis correlates inversely with responsiveness to methylprednisolone (29). The relative rarity of these cells has made it difficult to evaluate either their function or specificity. Antigen-specific T cells are probably required for the pathogenesis of those forms of glomerular injury classified as antibody mediated: for example, antiglomerular basement membrane (anti-GBM) disease. T cells in this disease may additionally have an effector role distinct from their role to provide B-cell help. Preliminary work has identified a peptide sequence from the $\alpha3$(IV) NC1 domain recognized by a $CD8^+$ T-cell clone from a patient with anti-GBM disease (39).

Minimal-change disease has been hypothesized to be a disorder of activated lymphocytes (40,41), in which lymphocytes and other inflammatory cells are not present within the kidney but a secreted product increases glomerular permeability to protein. Preliminary reports have suggested this protein is a secreted product of activated T cells (42).

STUDIES IN EXPERIMENTAL MODELS OF IMMUNE-MEDIATED RENAL DISEASE

Most of what is known about T cells in renal disease has been derived from model systems of renal injury. Much of the work characterizing T cells in renal disease models has been conducted in models of interstitial nephritis, either spontaneous models (5,43–46) or antigen-in-adjuvant–induced models (2,4,47–80).

Development of T Cells Responsive to Renal Antigens

In the model of antigen-in-adjuvant–induced interstitial nephritis, the priming of antigen-specific T cells occurs in the peripheral lymphoid system. In such model systems, one can study the maturation of the T-cell response from the time that antigen is introduced into the system. T cells isolated from lymph nodes draining the subcutaneous sites of immunization proliferate specifically to antigens in the immunizing regimen and in some cases mediate delayed-type hypersensitivity (DTH) responses or cytotoxicity reactions to these antigens as well (78). Such T cells are either $CD4^+$, $CD8^-$, and class II MHC restricted, or $CD4^-CD8^+$ and class I MHC restricted (4,69). These renal tubular antigen-specific T cells express a repertoire of antigen receptor β chains derived from several different variable regions (55). $CD4^+$ T cells that proliferate to the tubular antigen are also demonstrable in the lymph nodes of immunized mice that, because of their genetic makeup, are not susceptible to anti-TBM disease (4,62). This population differs from the tubular antigen-reactive $CD4^+$ T cells in susceptible mice in that the former are unreactive with a polyclonal antiserum generated against anti-TBM antibodies eluted from nephritic kidneys. Antigen-reactive $CD4^+$ T cells from susceptible mice react with this antiserum (4,78). This differential reactivity may relate to different TCR variable region gene usage by antigen-reactive T cells from susceptible and nonsusceptible mice.

Unlike other organ-specific autoimmune diseases that are primarily mediated by $CD4^+$ T cells, the $CD4^+$ cells primed in susceptible strains do not directly mediate interstitial nephritis. These cells are, however, required for the differentiation of effector T cells that directly initiate interstitial inflammation (57,66,67). Although such antigen-reactive $CD4^+$ T cells do not result in interstitial nephritis following subcapsular transfer in naive mice, antigen-specific $CD8^+$ T cells do result in interstitial infiltrates 5–7 days following adoptive transfer. These cells also express an idiotype cross-reactive with that present on anti-TBM antibodies eluted from nephritic kidneys. These $CD8^+$ effector cells recognize peptide fragments of the target antigen in conjunction with class I MHC molecules (H-$2K^{s,d}$) (69,78). These effector cells are cytotoxic to tubular epithelial cells and additionally mediate DTH responses to the target antigen. This latter property facilitates analysis of the requirements for induction of these effector cells. Effector cells can be induced in vitro by the coculture of naive syngeneic splenocytes, antigen, IL-2, and antigen-specific $CD4^+$ T helper (Th) cells (65,67). Supernatants derived from activated $CD4^+$ Th cells can substitute for the cells themselves (81). The functional activity within Th supernatants does not appear to be a conventional cytokine, and its helper function is antigen specific (57).

Mice susceptible (SJL) and nonsusceptible [B10.S (8R)] to anti-TBM disease also differ in the maturation process of tubular antigen-reactive T cells in the lymph node (4). Following immunization, both $CD8^+$ and $CD4^+$ DTH-reactive T cells are demonstrable in the draining lymph nodes in both strains. The further expansion of these subsets is differentially regulated in SJL and B10.S (8R) mice such that in susceptible mice the $CD8^+$ subset preferentially expands and in the B10.S(8R) the $CD4^+$ subset preferentially expands. Preferential expansion of these two distinct phenotypes of tubular antigen-reactive cells is mediated by regulatory T cells that are differentially expressed in susceptible and nonsusceptible mice (4,62,67). Thus, nonsusceptible mice do not fail to develop a T-cell response to tubular antigen; rather their response results in expansion of tubular antigen-reactive T cells that are not pathogenic under the normal conditions of immunization. The failure of these T cells to be pathogenic may relate in part to the basal low levels of class II

MHC antigen expression on tubular epithelial cells in the kidney. If class II MHC antigen expression is first induced by cytokines such as interferon-γ (IFN-γ), CD4$^+$ DTH-reactive T cells from nonsusceptible mice do mediate interstitial lesions following subcapsular transfer (54). Therefore, these cells have the capacity to cause disease but presumably fail to see their processed antigen along with class II MHC under basal conditions in the kidney. In this regard, it is of interest that the interaction of anti-TBM antibodies with tubular epithelial cells dampens the inducibility of class II MHC molecules by exogenous cytokines (54). Although in the animal model of induced interstitial nephritis, anti-TBM antibody deposition precedes the appearance of a mononuclear cell infiltrate in the interstitium, antigen-specific antibody may play a host-protective role in vivo by inhibiting class II MHC expression and blocking recognition of tubular epithelial cells by CD4$^+$ class-II-restricted effector T cells (54).

In addition to finding renal antigen-specific T cells in lymph nodes draining sites of peripheral immunization, lymph nodes that drain the kidneys are probably also enriched for activated lymphocytes, presumably derived from the renal inflammatory foci. [Macrophages have been demonstrate to traffic to lymph nodes draining the kidney in accelerated anti-GBM disease (82).] Such lymphocytes would be expected to reenter the circulating pool. Antigen-specific proliferative responses may be demonstrable in lymphocytes purified from peripheral blood, probably due to both recirculation and priming of lymphocytes in the periphery. Typically, the magnitude of such responses is not large, given dilution of the antigen-specific population by circulating lymphocytes irrelevant for the specified antigen.

The development of T cells specific for renal antigens in *spontaneous* autoimmune disease is likely a different process than that following immunization. In spontaneous models of autoimmune renal disease, such as the inherited interstitial nephritis of *kdkd* mice, antigen-reactive lymphocytes can be demonstrated in peripheral lymph nodes and spleen (5,46). The disease can be transferred through radiation bone-marrow chimeras but is prevented by thymectomy, demonstrating that thymic education is required for these nephritogenic T cells (46). In *kdkd* mice, the effector T cells that mediate interstitial nephritis following adoptive transfer are CD8$^+$, CD4$^-$, class I MHC-restricted T cells. As in anti-TBM disease, these CD8$^+$ T cells can mediate DTH to collagenase-solubilized TBM antigens (5). The *kdkd* T cells recognize a different target antigen within the TBM preparation. The target antigen for anti-TBM disease is the 3M-1 antigen, a noncollagenous glycoprotein present in the extracellular matrix and synthesized by proximal tubular epithelial cells (50,51,80,83). The *kdkd* T cells recognize a distinct 56-kD protein in collagenase-solubilized TBM (C. Kelly, unpublished observations). Analogous to the situation described above for susceptible and nonsusceptible strains for anti-TBM disease, CBA/Ca mice (the strain from which *kdkd* mice mutated) also have tubular antigen-reactive CD8$^+$ T cells in their peripheral lymphoid organs. The absence of disease in the CBA/Ca is not simply the result of the absence of nephritogenic effector cells but rather the differential regulation of such cells in susceptible and nonsusceptible mice (44). In both models of interstitial nephritis, the development of nephritogenic effector cells maps with the functional expression of T cells reactive with the *Vicia villosa* lectin (44,62). Curiously, ingestion of grasses containing this lectin leads to fulminant interstitial nephritis in cattle, suggesting activation of a nephritogenic population by the lectin (84).

Priming of T Cells by Antigen-Presenting Cells in the Kidney

It is controversial whether renal parenchymal cells, either tissue-based macrophages or tubule epithelial cells, glomerular epithelial cells, endothelial cells, or mesangial cells present antigens to T lymphocytes in a manner that results in T-cell activation (85). Experimental studies using cultured tubular and glomerular epithelial cells support the notion that such cells can present both endogenous (56,86) and foreign antigens to T lymphocytes (86–88). This topic is discussed in detail in Chapter 8. One view is that the ability of parenchymal cells to present antigen to T cells is limited by their relative absence of costimulatory molecules. Antigen presentation to CD4$^+$ helper T cells requires both the expression of class II MHC antigens expressing processed peptide fragments of the target antigen and the presence of costimulatory molecules. Class II MHC molecules are easily induced on renal parenchymal cells with IFN-γ (54,83). Costimulatory molecules such as CD80 and CD86 are not easily induced with either IFN-γ or tumor necrosis factor α (TNF-α) on renal tubular epithelial cells (89). The absence of costimulatory molecules is a potentially important peripheral tolerance mechanism. This applies particularly to tubular epithelial cells that, as highly reabsorptive and endocytic cells, presumably have all of the necessary machinery to process exogenous proteins to peptide fragments and subsequently re-express such peptides with class II MHC molecules on the cell surface. Whether antigen presentation to CD4$^+$ T cells ever occurs in the kidney as an event *initiating* immune injury is uncertain. Presentation by renal epithelial cells may act as an amplifying event leading to further clonal expansion of self-reactive clones should the appropriate costimulatory molecules be expressed. Although recent studies have emphasized the importance of CD80 and CD86 as costimulatory molecules, there are other cell surface molecules that may function in this regard on renal parenchymal cells, including intracellular adhesion molecule 1 (ICAM-1) (90,91), CD40 (92), and vascular cell adhesion molecule (VCAM) (93) and their respective ligands [lymphocyte-function-associated antigen 1 (LFA-1), CD40 ligand (CD40L), and viruslike antigen 4 (VLA-4)] on the T cell.

Diversity of αβ T-Cell Antigen Receptors Expressed on Nephritogenic T Cells

In some organ-specific autoimmune diseases, there are marked biases in the rearranged α- and β-chain receptors expressed on the T cells that cause disease. This tendency toward the usage of a highly restricted set of α and/or β variable (V) regions and hypervariable CDR3 junctional sequences is most obvious in experimental allergic encephalomyelitis (EAE) (94–96). In EAE, the junctional sequences of the antigen receptor β chain display conserved amino acids and are of minimal complexity, suggesting that these autoimmune cells may derive from early in ontogeny, before the full expression of terminal deoxynucleotidyl transferase (97). Other models of autoimmune disease have not demonstrated a V-region repertoire as severely biased as present in EAE (98–100). In immune-mediated renal diseases, the approach to the molecular characterization of T-cell antigen receptors on nephritogenic lymphocytes has been three-pronged: one, by DNA sequencing of α and β antigen receptor chains expressed on cultured T-cell clones relevant to disease expression (55); two, by reverse transcription–polymerase chain reaction (RT-PCR) analysis of cDNA derived from T cells infiltrating diseased kidney (101–103) and, lastly, by performing cytofluorography with Vβ-region-specific antibodies on T cells eluted from diseased kidneys (102). The latter can be performed in conjunction with a marker for activated T cells, to eliminate those cells not involved in the pathologic process. In the murine model of induced interstitial nephritis, evaluation by RT-PCR of cDNA from diseased kidney with a panel of Vβ-region-specific primers demonstrated that a variety of β-chain V regions are expressed on infiltrating T cells (103), without evidence for clonal amplification as assessed by DNA sequencing across the VDJ (variable–diversity–joining) junction. Because most inflammatory foci contain many T cells not specific for the inciting or target antigen, the failure to detect clonal amplification is difficult to interpret. In the rat model of anti-TBM disease, recent studies have detected clonal amplification of discrete Vβ regions by DNA sequence analysis (104). Using cultured T-cell clones responsive to the target antigen of anti-TBM disease, more limited numbers of Vβ regions are detected, but the procedure of long-term in vitro culture may well bias the result (55). In spontaneous models of interstitial nephritis (*kdkd* mice), when only the activated infiltrating T cells are examined, there seems to be selective amplification of Vβ8.2 and Vβ6 sequences, although the junctional sequences of these β chains are not conserved, suggesting perhaps that T cells expressing these Vβ regions are amplified based on stimulation by a superantigen rather than by a processed peptide (101,102).

T-Cell Trafficking to the Kidney

For T cells to come in contact with renal parenchymal cells, they must exit the microcirculation, migrate across both the capillary basement membrane as well as, in the case of tubular epithelial cells, the TBM. The recognition events required for T cells to leave the circulation and enter the interstitial compartment of the kidney have not been thoroughly evaluated. Extrapolating from endothelial cell–lymphocyte interactions in other microvascular compartments, lymphocyte trafficking into the kidney is initiated by slowing of lymphocyte movement in the microvasculature through selectin-dependent rolling along the capillary endothelium (105), followed by a higher-affinity interaction between integrins such as LFA-1 and VLA-4 on the lymphocyte and adhesion molecules, such as ICAM-1 and VCAM, on the endothelial cell (106, 107). This scenario implies activation of the endothelial cell as a required initiating event for the cell transmigration. Interruption of integrin and ICAM interactions by the in vivo administration of monoclonal antibodies can profoundly inhibit various forms of immune-mediated glomerulonephritis (108) and the associated interstitial disease. Antibodies against the α4 integrin (VLA-4, a ligand for VCAM) completely abrogates the interstitial infiltrates seen in mercuric-chloride-induced glomerulonephritis in the Brown Norway rat (109). The continuous endothelium of the microvasculature in the interstitium (as opposed to a microvasculature like the hepatic sinusoid) and the requirement for T cells to additionally traverse the basement membrane (see below) are important barriers to the efflux of autoreactive cells that are capable of inducing renal injury (110). In the setting of inflammatory injury, the expression of both ICAM-1 and VCAM, as well as class II MHC, is typically induced on renal parenchymal cells (54,87,90,91,93). Interruption of T-cell–target-cell interactions may be an additional therapeutic benefit of such monoclonal antibody therapy.

For extravasated T cells to contact a target tubular epithelial cell, they must move across the TBM. Although this process has not been extensively evaluated using renal tubular cells and their elaborated basement membrane in conjunction with nephritogenic T cells, it is clear by both light microscopy and electron microscopy that such movement across TBM occurs in the setting of interstitial inflammation (111). In other systems, T cells have been shown to break down artificial basement membranes through the elaboration of type-IV collagenases (112). The expression of such collagenases by either lymphocytes or nonspecific immune effector cells such as macrophages may be an important marker of pathogenicity that correlates with the ability of T cells to reach the "wrong" side of the basement membrane, both in inflammatory autoimmune renal disease and allograft rejection. At the structural level, this ability to disrupt basement membrane integrity may limit normal regeneration of tubule segments.

T-Cell Effector Functions in the Kidney

Interstitial infiltrates and occasional glomerular localization of T cells have been described in clinical specimens of inflammatory and immune renal injury as well as in experimental model systems. How does the presence of such T cells contribute to structural and functional injury? In general, T-cell effects on organ parenchymal cells can be divided into those that are mediated through cell–cell contact or those that are attributed to the effects of locally high levels of secreted cytokines. It is clear from experimental models of interstitial disease that both $CD4^+$ cells and $CD8^+$ cells can serve as cytotoxic T cells toward renal parenchymal cells, in particular tubular epithelial cells (3,69,70,78). These cytotoxic effects are restricted by class II and class I MHC molecules, respectively, and presumably involve release of cytotoxic mediators following engagement of the TCR antigen receptor by the appropriate MHC–peptide complex on the target cell. Most forms of cell-mediated cytotoxicity are mediated through the actions of granule-associated mediators such as perforin (113) and granzymes (114) or through fas–fas ligand interactions (113). The expression of some of these cytolytic effector proteins, such as perforin, can be downregulated by cytokines such as transforming growth factor β (TGF-β) that also inhibit the ability of T cells to transfer interstitial nephritis (70). Cytotoxicity provides a straightforward explanation for the structural findings of tubular epithelial cell loss in the setting of inflammatory renal disease. Whether cytotoxicity is the dominant mechanism whereby T cells injure epithelial cells in vivo is a difficult question to address. Cytotoxicity in vitro occurs at effector–target-cell ratios that may never be achieved in situ. T cells with or without cytotoxic effector potential in vitro may injure target cells in vivo largely through the release of cytokines that then have adverse effects on target cells. The release of TNF-α might be expected to be associated with cytotoxicity, and TGF-β with the elaboration of augmented amounts of extracellular matrix. The synergistic effects of TNF-α and IFN-γ are probably critical to inducing cellular adhesion molecules and MHC molecules on target epithelial cells (54,87,91). Lastly, granulocyte-macrophage colony-stimulating factor may play an important role in stimulating the expression of costimulatory molecules on renal parenchymal cells, as it does on conventional antigen-presenting cells (115). The elaboration of cytokines may alter renal physiology in the absence of alterations in morphologic structure. For example, IL-1 is known to stimulate Na^+-dependent amino acid and glucose transport by the proximal tubule (116).

Epithelial cells may undergo either lytic death or programmed cell death. This distinction may be an important one in terms of how target cells are destroyed and whether there is resultant amplification or suppression of further inflammatory injury.

In many experimental models, the histologic lesions in the kidney are reminiscent of cutaneous DTH responses (1,117–119). In some model systems, T cells eluted from diseased renal tissue mediate DTH responses to renal target antigens (3–5). These lesions are likely initiated by either $CD4^+$ or $CD8^+$ T cells that express macrophage-activating cytokines (120). Injury to renal parenchymal cells results from cytokines released from both the T cells and activated macrophages as well as from other secreted products of activated macrophages (121), including proteolytic enzymes and oxidants. Some studies have suggested that the development of crescents in the glomerulus is initiated by disruption of the Bowman capsule by activated periglomerular mononuclear cells (122). With DTH-like lesions in either the interstitium or the Bowman space, renal functional effects likely depend on whether the response becomes chronic, fibrotic, and granulomatous, or whether the antigenic stimulation is removed and the DTH reaction subsides.

Although investigative efforts in the area of T-cell–target-cell interactions have regarded target cells as relatively passive participants, it is likely that target cells generate self-protective pathways. One such self-protective pathway was alluded to above and includes the relative inability to induce costimulatory molecules on tubular epithelial cells. Another important mediator system in self-protection is the presence of the cytokine-inducible nitric oxide synthase in multiple tubular segments (123, 124). This molecule is upregulated by cytokines released by infiltrating T cells, including TNF-α and IFN-γ (124, 125), and can be inhibited by steroids, TGF-β, IL-4, or IL-10 (126). The expression of micromolar quantities of NO can induce cytotoxic and/or oxidant related injury to a variety of cell types, and is probably an important mediator of ischemic acute renal failure (127). The generation of nitric oxide could be alternatively a protective event in the setting of lymphocyte initiated and mediated renal injury, as it is in the systemic response generated by staphylococcal enterotoxins (128). Nitric oxide is a potent antiproliferative agent for T lymphocytes (129, 130) and leads to the downregulation of a number of accessory molecules on the surface of both lymphocyte and the target cell, including class II MHC molecules (131), adhesion molecules (132,133), and CD4 (134).

The Th1/Th2 Paradigm in Renal Disease

A common paradigm in understanding pathogenic T-cell responses is based on the notion that the $CD4^+$ T-cell response can be divided into those cells that predominantly secrete IL-2 and IFN-γ (Th1 cells) and those that predominantly secrete IL-4 and IL-10 (Th2 cells) (135). Th1 cells are effector cells for DTH and allow for the differentiation of $CD8^+$ T cells. They also provide help for the induction of IgG2a antibody responses. Th2 cells provide help for the induction of a number of other antibody responses and have been associated with suppressive phenomena mediated by T cells. A strict classification of effector T-cell responses along the lines of the Th1/Th2 paradigm has not been clearly delineated in any model of autoimmune renal disease. In the antigen-in-adjuvant–induced model of murine interstitial nephritis, a panel of $CD4^+$ helper T-cell clones specific for an immunodominant epitope of the target antigen were Th1-like in cytokine profile, in that they expressed IFN-γ and IL-2 but not IL-4 (55). Functional evidence supports the importance of IL-2 in the pathogenesis of lupus nephritis because, antibodies to a subunit of the high-affinity IL-2 receptor protect NZB/NZW F_1 mice from developing renal injury (136). Effector T-cell clones capable of directly mediating interstitial nephritis express a variety of cytokine mRNA species by RT-PCR analysis (71), including IL-2, IL-4, IL-6, TNF-α, and IFN-γ, and therefore do not map as conventional Th1- or Th2-type profiles. The mercuric chloride model of glomerulonephritis in Brown Norway rats displays polyclonal B cell activation, anti-GBM antibodies, and cytokine profiles consistent with a Th2 bias (137).

Antigen-Nonspecific Regulation of Nephritogenic T Cells

The critical role for T cells in both the induction and effector phases of immune responses harmful to the kidney is supported by the ability of a variety suppressive treatments to block the development or progression of autoimmune renal injury in various model systems. Such modalities include immunosuppressive drugs such as cyclophosphamide (47), cyclosporine (138–140), deoxyspergualin (141), and prostaglandin E_1 (81,142) and protein calorie restriction (48,143). In many cases, the utilization of these drugs impairs both the development of antibodies specific for the immunogen as well as the T-cell response. Although the B-cell response is presumably T cell dependent, this is not a surprising outcome when the drugs are administered from the time of admission. In some settings, achieving immunosuppression is highly dependent on the timing of agent administration. For example, administration of exogenous prostaglandin E_1 to mice immunized to produce anti-TBM disease is only efficacious if administered during the first week after immunization. The agent need only be administered during this week to inhibit disease expression 12 weeks later. This treatment has no effect on anti-TBM antibody titers or antibody deposited in the kidney. It inhibits the differentiation of $CD8^+$ antigen-specific effector cells in a reversible manner. The mechanism of this effect appears to be the stimulation of a heat-stable protein that has inhibitor activity. The inhibition can be overcome by recombinant IL-1. Prostaglandin E_1 has also been demonstrated to have beneficial immunosuppressive effects in murine lupus nephritis (144,145). Diets rich in omega-3 fatty acids reduce severity of murine lupus, and this may also be related to alterations in prostaglandin species (146).

In addition to immunosuppressive drugs, antibodies targeting cell surface glycoproteins expressed on T cells, such as CD4, can prevent or ameliorate lupus nephritis in NZB/NZW F_1 mice (147,148). Antibodies to cell surface glycoprotein cells critical for induction of the immune response, such as class II MHC, can similarly serve as effective therapies in autoimmune disease (149,150). Mice in which class II MHC genes have been deleted through targeted gene deletion are not susceptible to develop lupus nephritis (151). Interference with T-cell antigen presentation by blocking class II MHC may occur either in the peripheral lymphoid system or additionally in the target organ, that is, the kidney. Since augmented class II MHC expression has been documented in renal parenchymal cells in many settings of renal inflammatory injury. Interruption of costimulatory signals, such as interactions between CD28 and B7 family molecules, with a CTLA-4 chimeric protein also has profound inhibitory effects on the expression of rat autoimmune anti-GBM glomerulonephritis (152).

An additional antibody that can impair T-cell-mediated autoimmune disease is the antibody to the CD40 ligand. This moiety is expressed transiently on activated T cells and is critical for the induction of B-cell differentiation. Recent studies in two different models of renal disease (membranous nephropathy and murine interstitial nephritis) have demonstrated that administration of an antibody to the CD40 ligand can block the development of disease (153,154). In the case of the membranous nephropathy, the mechanism was presumed to be related to diminished autoantibody responses. In murine interstitial nephritis, however, there was no significant diminution in the nephritogenic antibody response, and the antibody led to a block in T-cell proliferation stimulated by antibodies to CD3. This implies that the CD40–CD40 ligand interaction is additionally important in T–T-cell interactions and T-cell costimulation (155,156).

Antigen-Specific Regulation of Nephritis

A long-standing interest in the inhibition of T-cell-mediated injury has been the development of antigen-specific immunosuppressive modalities. This has been achieved in model systems through immunization with large amounts of tubular antigen in incomplete Freund adjuvant (60), by oral administration of antigen (157), by injection of antigen-reactive T lymphoblasts bearing a cross-reactive idiotype (76), with anti-idiotypic antisera (53), and with induced suppressor T-cell networks (158). This immunosuppressive effect following immunization with tubular antigen and incomplete Freund adjuvant occurs via a $CD8^+$ inhibitory T-cell mechanism (60). In the setting of oral feeding of antigen, the response is concentration dependent and does not map with either inhibition of the antibody response or inhibition of DTH responses to the tubular antigen, although both of those responses are inhibited at defined doses of fed antigen. It may, rather, work via inactivation of the $CD8^+$ effector cell. Inhibitory T cells can also be induced via the injection tubular antigen chemically coupled with 1-ethyl-3-(3-dimethylaminopropyl)carbodiimide (158). This is a technique that has been used in hapten model systems as well and induces two types of inhibitory T cells that are phenotypically and functionally distinct: a $CD4^+$ cell that expresses an idiotype cross-reactive with immunoglobulin eluted from nephritic kidneys and a $CD8^+$ suppressor effector cell that directly inhibits nephritogenic effector T cells. Such suppression is an active event requiring new mRNA and protein synthesis (71). It is critically dependent on the induction of TGF-β in the effector cell, because neutralizing antisera to TGF-β_1 blocks the ability of the suppressor factors to inhibit DTH reactions, the ability to suppress transfer of disease, and the ability to inhibit T-cell-mediated cytotoxicity to tubular epithelial cells (71). TGF-β_1 as a single agent can additionally inhibit the function of nephritogenic effector T cells. As a single exogenous agent, it also inhibits T-cell-mediated cytotoxicity to tubular epithelial cells, where it correlates with diminished expression of cytotoxic mediators, such as perforin, in the effector T cells (70).

TGF-β_1 has emerged as a critical endogenous regulator of T-cell function. The importance of this moiety in the maintenance of peripheral tolerance is supported by the finding that mice that have undergone targeted gene deletion of TGF-β_1 demonstrate multiple-organ mononuclear cell infiltration at several weeks following birth (159). Such inflammation extends to the serosal surface of the kidney. Although TGF-β has been linked to the development of pathologic extracellular matrix production characteristic of progressive renal disease (160–163), in diseases whose expression is dependent on T lymphocytes, TGF-β_1 can be seen more as an immunosuppressive growth factor. Its growth regulatory effect depends on the interaction of TGF-β_1 with its receptors, especially the type-I and type-II receptors. $CD4^+$ nephritogenic T cells that do not exhibit growth inhibition in the presence of TGF-β_1 express mutant type-I receptors on the cell surface. This mutation consists of a leucine-to-glutamine substitution at codon 122, a conserved amino acid in the transmembrane domain of the type-I receptor (49). T cells resistant to TGF-β mediate interstitial lesions that are histologically more severe, presumably because of the loss of the hypoproliferative effects of TGF-β. Other changes in the internal milieu that result in antagonism of TGF-β effects, such as excess IL-2, might similarly be expected to result in a more severe inflammatory lesion. A clinical correlate of this may be the observation that patients receiving recombinant IL-2 and lymphokine-activated killer cells can develop interstitial nephritis (164). A similar lesion is seen in neonatally thymectomized mice after administration of IL-2 (165).

Contribution of T Cells to Immune Amplification Reactions Injuring the Interstitium

It is clear that there is a mononuclear cell infiltrate present in the renal interstitium in the presence of a number of other presumed "primary" insults to the kidney. Such insults include the presence of urinary tract obstruction (166) and multiple forms of proteinuric renal disease (167–169). The mechanisms whereby such diverse insults result in interstitial inflammation are unclear and the focus of an intense research effort. A dominant view has been that the cells within these infiltrates are not antigen specific but rather the result of the stimulated expression of chemoattractants, such as complement (170,171), chemokines (172,173), or lipid chemoattractant mediators (174). An alternate view (not mutually exclusive with the view of chemoattractants as the primary instigators) is that a variety of diverse insults elicit the expression of neoantigens to which the host immune system is not tolerant. One such neoantigen system is inducible heat-shock protein (HSP) (175). Members of the 70-kD family of inducible HSPs are highly immunogenic molecules (176). A number of cellular stresses that are epidemiologically associated with chronic interstitial nephritis and mononuclear cell infiltrates in the interstitium also induce HSP expression (177,178). Such stresses include ionizing radiation, heavy metal toxicity, infection, and antibiotics. HSP-reactive lymphocytes play a role in the pathogenesis of several autoimmune diseases, including adjuvant arthritis (179), autoimmune insulitis in diabetes (180), and encephalomyelitis (181). The chronic administration of cadmium chloride to rodents results in chronic interstitial nephritis, similar to that seen in workers with environmental exposure (182,183). Mice chronically exposed to cadmium chloride demonstrate induced expression of HSP70 in the kidney, particularly within tubular epithelial cells (3). This expression precedes the development of interstitial mononuclear cell infiltrates by at least 4–5 weeks. Cadmium chloride also induces HSP70 expression in cultured tubular epithelial cells. $CD4^+$ TCR αβ-positive T cells specific for an immunodominant HSP70 peptide are cytotoxic to such cadmium-treated renal tubular cells, and these cells mediate an inflammatory interstitial nephritis following adoptive transfer into mice expressing HSP70 in tubular epithelium. T cells isolated from diseased kidneys of mice chronically treated with cadmium chloride are also cytotoxic to heat-shocked or cadmium-chloride-treated tubular cells. These cells can additionally induce interstitial nephritis after passive transfer, indicating their pathogenic significance (3). Therefore, in this model of a heavy metal toxicity, there is clearly a pathogenic immune response mediated by HSP-specific T cells, raising the possibility that similar responses may be in part responsible for pathologic abnormalities in other forms of chronic interstitial nephritis.

Summary of Pathogenetic Information Obtained from Model Systems

The thrust of this chapter has been to summarize what is known (predominantly from model systems) about T-cell-mediated renal injury. Ultimately, this information is valuable if it facilitates a deeper understanding of the pathogenesis of other forms of T-cell-mediated disease and/or enables the development of new therapeutics or prophylactic regimens for the treatment or prevention of renal disease. In addition, endogenous regulatory mechanisms are emerging as important modifiers of the intensity of disease expression. As more becomes known regarding the genetics underlying multiple susceptibility factors in autoimmune diseases, it may be possible to target therapies to populations defined as high risk based on susceptibility genotypes.

REFERENCES

1. Bolton WK, Chandra M, Tyson TM, Kirkpatrick PR, Sadovnic MJ, Sturgill BC. Transfer of experimental glomerulonephritis in chickens by mononuclear cells. *Kidney Int* 1988;45:598–610.
2. Zakheim B, McCafferty E, Mann R, Phillips SM, Clayman M, Neilson EG. Murine interstitial nephritis. II. The adoptive transfer of disease with immune T lymphocytes produces a phenotypically complex interstitial lesion. *J Immunol* 1984;133:234–9.
3. Weiss RA, Madaio MP, Tomaszewski JE, Kelly CJ. T cells reactive to an inducible heat shock protein induce disease in a model of toxin-induced interstitial nephritis. *J Exp Med* 1994;180:2239–50.
4. Neilson EG, McCafferty E, Mann R, Michaud L, Clayman M. Murine interstitial nephritis. III. The selection of phenotypic (Lyt and L3T4) and idiotypic (RE-Id) T cell preferences by genes in IgH-1 and H-2K characterize the cell-mediated potential for disease expression: susceptible mice provide a unique effector T cell repertoire in response to tubular antigen. *J Immunol* 1985;134:2375–82.
5. Kelly CJ, Korngold R, Mann R, Clayman MD, Haverty TP, Neilson EG. Spontaneous nephritis in *kdkd* mice. II. Characterization of a tubular antigen-specific, H-2K restricted Lyt-2^+ effector T cell that mediates destructive tubulointerstitial injury. *J Immunol* 1986;136: 526–31.
6. Kappler J, Wade T, White J, et al. A T cell receptor Vβ segment that imparts reactivity to a class II major histocompatibility complex product. *Cell* 1987;49:263–71.
7. Kappler JW, Roehm N, Marrack N. T cell tolerance by clonal elimination in the thymus. *Cell* 1987;49:273–80.
8. Brown JH, Jardetzsky T, Saper MA, Samraoui B, Bjorkman P, Wiley DC. A hypothetical model of the foreign antigen binding site of class II histocompatibility antigens. *Nature* 1988;332:845–50.
9. Bjorkman PJ, Saper MA, Samraoui B, Bennett WS, Strominger JL, Wiley DC. The foreign antigen binding site and T cell recognition regions of class I histocompatibility antigens. *Nature* 1987;329: 512–8.
10. Bjorkman PJ, Samraoui B, Bennett WS, Strominger JL, Wiley DC. Structure of the human class I histocompatibility antigen, HLA-A2. *Nature* 1987;329:506–11.
11. Lehman DH, Wilson CB, Dixon FJ. Interstitial nephritis in rats immunized with heterologous tubular basement membrane. *Kidney Int* 1974;5:187–95.
12. Sugisaki T, Klassen J, Milgrom F, Andres GA, McCluskey RT. Immunopathologic study of an autoimmune tubular and interstitial renal disease in Brown Norway rats. *Lab Invest* 1973;28:658–71.
13. Wilson CB, Lehman DH, McCoy RC, Gunnells JCJ, Stickel DL. Antitubular basement membrane antibodies after renal transplantation. *Transplantation* 1974;18:447–52.
14. Fasth A, Ahlstedt S, Hanson LA, Jann B, Jann K, Kauser B. Cross-reactions between the Tamm–Horsfall glycoprotein and *Escherichia coli*. *Int Arch Allergy Appl Immunol* 1980;63:303–11.
15. Fitzsimons EJJ, Weber M, Lange CF. The isolation of cross-reactive monoclonal antibodies: hybridomas to streptococcal antigens cross-reactive with mammalian basement membrane. *Hybridoma* 1987;6: 61–9.
16. Kraus W, Beachey EH. Renal autoimmune epitope of a group A streptococci specified by M protein tetrapeptide Lle-Arg-Leu-Arg. *Proc Natl Acad Sci USA* 1988;85:4516–20.
17. Oldstone MB. Molecular mimicry as a mechanism for the cause and a probe uncovering etiologic agent(s) of autoimmune disease. *Curr Top Microbiol Immunol* 1989;145:127–35.
18. Oldstone MBA. Molecular mimicry and autoimmune disease. *Cell* 1987;80:819–20.
19. Hagerty DT, Evavold BD, Allen PM. Regulation of the costimulator B7, not class II major histocompatibility complex, restricts the ability of murine kidney tubule cells to stimulate CD4+ T cells. *J Clin Invest* 1994;93:1208–15.
20. Markmann J, Lo D, Naji A, Palmiter RD, Brinster RL, Heber-Katz E. Antigen presenting function of class II MHC expressing pancreatic beta cells. *Nature* 1988;336:476–9.
21. Schwartz RH. Fugue in T-lymphocyte recognition. *Nature* 1987;326: 738–9.
22. Kelly CJ, Tomaszewski JE, Neilson EG. Immunopathogenesis of tubulointerstitial injury. In: Brenner BM, Tisher CC, eds. *Renal pathology*. Philadelphia: JB Lippincott, 1993:699–722.
23. Husby G, Tung KSK, Williams RC. Characterization of renal tissue lymphocytes in patients with interstitial nephritis. *Am J Med* 1981; 70:31–8.
24. Bender WL, Whelton A, Beschorner WE, Darwish MOP, Hall-Craggs M, Solez K. Interstitial nephritis, proteinuria, and renal failure caused by nonsteroidal anti-inflammatory drugs: immunologic characterization of the inflammatory infiltrate. *Am J Med* 1984;76: 1006–12.
25. Rosenberg ME, Schendel PB, McCurdy FA, Platt JL. Characterization of immune cells in kidneys from patients with Sjögren's syndrome. *Am J Kidney Dis* 1988;11:20–2.
26. Stachura I, Si L, Madan E, Whiteside T. Enumeration in tissue sections with monoclonal antibodies. *Clin Immunol Immunopathol* 1984; 30:362–73.
27. Boucher A, Droz D, Adafer E, Noel LH. Characterization of mononuclear cell subsets in renal cellular interstitial infiltrates. *Kidney Int* 1986;29:1043–9.
28. Cheng H-F, Nolasco F, Cameron JS, Hildreth G, Neild G, Hartlett B. HLA-DR display by renal tubular epithelium and phenotype of infiltrate in interstitial nephritis. *Nephrol Dial Transplant* 1989;4:205–15.
29. Bolton WK, Innes DJ, Sturgill BC, Kaiser DL. T-cells and macrophages in rapidly progressive glomerulonephritis: clinicopathologic correlations. *Kidney Int* 1987;32:869–76.
30. Falk MC, Ng G, Zhang GY, et al. Infiltration of the kidney by alpha beta and gamma delta T cells: effect on progression in IgA nephropathy. *Kidney Int* 1995;47:177–85.
31. Tomino Y, Ohmuro H, Kuramoto T, et al. Expression of intercellular adhesion molecule-1 and infiltration of lymphocytes in glomeruli of patients with IgA nephropathy. *Nephron* 1994;67:302-7.
32. Cohen AH, Nas CC. HIV-associated nephropathy: a unique combined glomerular, tubular, and interstitial lesion. *Mod Pathol* 1988;1:87–97.
33. Kopp JB, Klotman ME, Adler SH, et al. Progressive glomerulosclerosis and enhanced renal accumulation of basement membrane compo-

nents in mice transgenic for human immunodeficiency virus type 1 genes. *Proc Natl Acad Sci USA* 1992;89:1577–81.
34. Dickie P, Felser J, Eckhaus M, et al. HIV-associated nephropathy in transgenic mice expressing HIV-1 genes. *Virology* 1991;185:109–19.
35. Bohle A, Mackensen-Haen S, von Gise H. Significance of tubulointerstitial changes in the renal cortex for excretory function and concentration ability of the kidney: a morphometric contribution. *Am J Nephrol* 1987;7:421–33.
36. Bohle A, Mackensen-Haen S, von Gise H, et al. The consequences of tubulo-interstitial changes for renal function in glomerulopathies. *Pathol Res Pract* 1990;186:135–44.
37. Risdon RA, Sloper JC, de Wardener HE. Relationship between renal function and histological changes found in renal-biopsy specimens from patients with persistent glomerular nephritis. *Lancet* 1968;2: 363–6.
38. Schainuck LI, Striker GE, Cutler RE, Benditt EP. Structural–functional correlations in renal disease. *Hum Pathol* 1970;1:631–41.
39. Merkel F, Kalluri R, Marx M, et al. Autoreactive T-cells in Goodpasture's syndrome recognize the N-terminal NC1 domain on α3 type IV collagen. *Kidney Int* 1996;49:1127–33.
40. Schnaper HW. A regulatory system for soluble immune response suppressor production in steroid-responsive nephrotic syndrome. *Kidney Int* 1990;38:151–159.
41. Shalhoub RJ. Pathogenesis of lipoid nephrosis: a disorder of T cell function. *Lancet* 1974;2:556–557.
42. Koyama A, Fujisaki M, Kobayashi M, Igarashi M, Narita M. A glomerular permeability factor produced by human T cell hybridomas. *Kidney Int* 1991;40:453–60.
43. Harning R, Pelletier J, Van G, Takei F, Merluzzi VJ. Monoclonal antibody to MALA-2 (ICAM-1) reduces acute autoimmune nephritis in *kdkd* mice. *Clin Immunol Immunopathol* 1992;64:129–34.
44. Kelly CJ, Neilson EG. Contrasuppression in autoimmunity: abnormal contrasuppression facilitates expression of nephritogenic effector T cells and interstitial nephritis in *kdkd* mice. *J Exp Med* 1987;165: 107–23.
45. Lyon MF, Hulse EV. An inherited kidney disease of mice resembling human nephronophthisis. *J Med Genet* 1971;8:41–8.
46. Neilson EG, McCafferty E, Feldman A, Clayman MD, Zakheim B, Korngold R. Spontaneous interstitial nephritis in *kdkd* mice. I. An experimental model of autoimmune renal disease. *J Immunol* 1984; 133:2560–5.
47. Agus D, Mann R, Clayman M, et al. The effects of daily cyclophosphamide administration on the development and extent of primary experimental interstitial nephritis in rats. *Kidney Int* 1986;29:635–40.
48. Agus D, Mann R, Cohn D, et al. Inhibitory role of dietary protein restriction on the development and expression of immune-mediated antitubular basement membrane–induced tubulointerstitial nephritis in rats. *J Clin Invest* 1985;76:930–6.
49. Bailey NC, Frishberg Y, Kelly CJ. Loss of high affinity TGF-β_1 binding to a nephritogenic T cell results in absence of growth inhibition by TGF-β_1 and augmented nephritogenicity. *J Immunol* 1996;156: 3009–16.
50. Clayman MD, Martinez-Hernandez A, Michaud L, et al. Isolation and characterization of the nephritogenic antigen producing anti-tubular basement membrane disease. *J Exp Med* 1985;161:290–305.
51. Clayman MD, Michaud L, Brentjens J, Andres GA, Kefalides NA, Neilson EG. Isolation of the target antigen of human anti-tubular basement membrane antibody-associated interstitial nephritis. *J Clin Invest* 1986;77:1143–7.
52. Clayman M, Michaud L, Neilson EG. Murine interstitial nephritis. VI. Characterization of the B cell response in anti-tubular basement membrane disease. *J Immunol* 1987;139:2242–9.
53. Clayman MD, Sun MJ, Michaud L, Brill-Dashoff J, Riblet R, Neilson EG. Clonotypic heterogeneity in experimental interstitial nephritis: restricted specificity of the antitubular basement membrane B cell repertoire is associated with a disease-modifying crossreactive idiotype. *J Exp Med* 1988;167:1296–312.
54. Haverty TP, Watanabe M, Neilson EG, Kelly CJ. Protective modulation of class II MHC gene expression in tubular epithelium by target antigen-specific antibodies: cell-surface directed down-regulation of transcription can influence susceptibility to murine tubulointerstitial nephritis. *J Immunol* 1989;143:1133–47.
55. Heeger PS, Smoyer WE, Saad T, Albert S, Kelly CJ, Neilson EG. Molecular analysis of the helper T cell response in murine interstitial nephritis: T cells recognizing an immunodominant epitope use multiple TCR Vβ genes with similarities across CDR3. *J Clin Invest* 1994; 94:2084–92.
56. Hines WH, Haverty TP, Elias JA, Neilson EG, Kelly CJ. T cell recognition of epithelial self. *Autoimmunity* 1989;5:37–47.
57. Hines WH, Mann RA, Kelly CJ, Neilson EG. Murine interstitial nephritis. IX. Induction of the nephritogenic effector T cell repertoire with an antigen-specific T cell cytokine. *J Immunol* 1990;144:75–83.
58. Kelly CJ, Silvers WK, Neilson EG. Regulatory role of major histocompatibility complex-restricted $OX8^+$ suppressor T cells specific for autologous renal tubular antigen in experimental interstitial nephritis. *J Exp Med* 1985;162:1892–903.
59. Kelly CJ, Silvers W, Neilson EG. Tolerance to parenchymal self: the regulatory role of an RTl-restricted, OX8+ suppressor T cell for autologous renal tubular antigen in experimental interstitial nephritis. *J Exp Med* 1985;162:1892–903.
60. Kelly CJ, Clayman MD, Neilson EG. Immunoregulation in experimental interstitial nephritis: immunization with renal tubular antigen in incomplete Freund's adjuvant induces major histocompatibility complex restricted $OX8^+$ suppressor T cells which are antigen specific and inhibit the expression of disease. *J Immunol* 1986;136:903–7.
61. Kelly CJ, Clayman MD, Hines WH, Neilson EG. Therapeutic immune regulation in experimental interstitial nephritis with suppressor T cells and their soluble factors. *Ciba Found Symp* 1987;129:73–87.
62. Kelly CJ, Mok H, Neilson EG. The selection of effector T cell phenotype by contrasuppression modulates susceptibility to autoimmune injury. *J Immunol* 1988;141:3022–8.
63. Kelly CJ, Roth DA, Meyers CM. Immune recognition and response to the renal interstitium. *Kidney Int* 1991;39:518–31.
64. Mampaso FM, Wilson CB. Characterization of inflammatory cells in autoimmune tubulointerstitial nephritis in rats. *Kidney Int* 1983;23: 448–57.
65. Mann R, Zakheim B, Clayman M, McCafferty E, Michaud L, Neilson EG. Murine interstitial nephritis. IV. Long-term cultured L3T4+ T cell lines transfer delayed expression of disease as I-A-restricted inducers of the effector T cell repertoire. *J Immunol* 1985;135: 286–93.
66. Mann R, Neilson EG. Murine interstitial nephritis. V. The auto-induction of antigen-specific Lyt-2+ suppressor T cells diminishes the expression of interstitial nephritis in mice with antitubular basement membrane disease. *J Immunol* 1986;136:908–12.
67. Mann R, Kelly CJ, Hines WH, et al. Effector T cell differentiation in experimental interstitial nephritis. I. The development and modulation of effector lymphocyte maturation by $I\text{-}J^+$ regulatory T cells. *J Immunol* 1987;136:4200–8.
68. Neilson EG, Kelly CJ, Clayman MD, et al. Murine interstitial nephritis. VII. Suppression of renal injury after treatment with soluble suppressor factor TsF1. *J Immunol* 1987;139:1518–24.
69. Meyers CM, Kelly CJ. Effector mechanisms in organ-specific autoimmunity. I. Characterization of a $CD8^+$ T cell line that mediates murine interstitial nephritis. *J Clin Invest* 1991;88:408–16.
70. Meyers CM, Kelly CJ. Immunoregulation and TGF-β_1: suppression of a nephritogenic murine T cell clone. *Kidney Int* 1994;46:1295–301.
71. Meyers CM, Kelly CJ. Inhibition of murine nephritogenic effector T cells by a clone-specific suppressor factor. *J Clin Invest* 1994;94: 2093–104.
72. Neilson EG, Phillips SM. Cell-mediated immunity in interstitial nephritis. I. T lymphocyte systems in nephritis guinea pigs: the natural history and diversity of the immune response. *J Immunol* 1979; 123:2373–80.
73. Neilson EG, Phillips SM. Cell-mediated immunity in interstitial nephritis. II. T lymphocyte effector mechanisms in nephritis guinea pigs: analysis of the renotropic migration and cytotoxic response. *J Immunol* 1979;123:2381–85.
74. Neilson EG, Jimenez SA, Phillips SM. Cell-mediated immunity in interstitial nephritis. III. T lymphocyte-mediated fibroblast proliferation and collagen synthesis: an immune mechanism of renal fibrogenesis in interstitial nephritis. *J Immunol* 1980;125:1708–14.
75. Neilson EG, Phillips SM. Cell-mediated immunity in interstitial nephritis. IV. Anti-basement membrane antibody functions in antibody dependent cellular cytotoxicity reactions: observations on a nephritogenic effector mechanism acting as an informational bridge between the humoral and cellular immune response. *J Immunol* 1981; 126:1990–3.

76. Neilson EG, Phillips SM. Suppression of interstitial nephritis by auto-anti-idiotypic immunity. *J Exp Med* 1982;155:179–89.
77. Neilson EG, Jimenez SA, Phillips SM. Lymphokine modulation of fibroblast proliferation. *J Immunol* 1982;128:1484–6.
78. Neilson EG, Phillips SM. Murine interstitial nephritis. I. Analysis of disease susceptibility and its relationship to pleiomorphic gene products defining both immune response genes and restrictive requirement for cytotoxic T cells at H-2K. *J Exp Med* 1982;155:1075–85.
79. Neilson EG, Gasser DL, McCafferty E, Zakheim B, Phillips SM. Polymorphism of genes involved in anti-tubular basement membrane disease in rats. *Immunogenetics* 1983;17:555–65.
80. Neilson EG, Sun MJ, Emery J, et al. Molecular characterization of a major nephritogenic domain in the auto-antigen of anti-tubular basement membrane disease. *Proc Natl Acad Sci USA* 1991;88:2006–10.
81. Kelly CJ, Zurier RB, Krakauer KA, Blanchard N, Neilson EG. Prostaglandin E_1 inhibits effector T cell induction and tissue damage in experimental murine interstitial nephritis. *J Clin Invest* 1987;79:782–9.
82. Lan HY, Nikolic-Paterson DJ, Atkins RC. Trafficking of inflammatory macrophages from the kidney to draining lymph nodes during experimental glomerulonephritis. *Clin Exp Immunol* 1993;92:336–41.
83. Haverty TP, Kelly CJ, Hines WH, et al. Characterization of a renal tubular epithelial cell line which secretes the autologous target antigen of autoimmune interstitial nephritis. *J Cell Biol* 1988;107:1358–69.
84. Panciera RJ, Mosier DA, Ritchey JW. Hairy vetch (*Vicia villosa* Roth) poisoning in cattle: update and experimental induction of disease. *J Vet Diagn Invest* 1992;4:318–25.
85. Neilson EG. Is immunologic tolerance of self modulated through antigen presentation by parenchymal epithelium? *Kidney Int* 1993;44:927–31.
86. Hagerty DT, Allen PM. Processing and presentation of self and foreign antigens by the renal proximal tubule. *J Immunol* 1992;148:2324–30.
87. Wuthrich RP, Glimcher LH, Yui MA, Jevnikar AM, Dumas SE, Kelley VE. MHC class II, antigen presentation and tumor necrosis factor in renal tubular epithelial cells. *Kidney Int* 1990;37:783–92.
88. Mendrick DL, Kelly DM, Rennke HG. Antigen processing and presentation by glomerular visceral epithelium in vitro. *Kidney Int* 1991;39:71–8.
89. Yokoyama H, Zheng X, Strom TB, Kelley VR. B7(+)-transfectant tubular epithelial cells induce T cell anergy, ignorance or proliferation. *Kidney Int* 1994;45:1105–12.
90. Wuthrich RP, Jevnikar AM, Takei F, Glimcher LH, Kelley VE. Intercellular adhesion molecule-1 (ICAM-1) expression is upregulated in autoimmune lupus nephritis. *Am J Pathol* 1990;136:441–50.
91. Frishberg Y, Meyers CM, Kelly CJ. Cyclosporine A regulates T cell–epithelial cell adhesion by altering LFA-1 and ICAM-1 expression. *Kidney Int* 1996;50.
92. Yellin MJ, Brett J, Baum D, et al. Functional interactions of T cells with endothelial cells: the role of CD40L–CD40-mediated signals. *J Exp Med* 1995;182:1857–64.
93. Wuthrich RP, Jenkins TA, Snyder TL. Regulation of cytokine-stimulated vascular cell adhesion molecule-1 expression in renal tubular epithelial cells. *Transplantation* 1993;55:172–7.
94. Acha-Orbea H, Steinman L, McDevitt HO. T cell receptors in murine autoimmune diseases. *Annu Rev Immunol* 1989;7:371–405.
95. Kumar V, Kono D, Urban J, Hood L. The T cell receptor repertoire and autoimmune diseases. *Annu Rev Immunol* 1989;7:657–82.
96. Urban JL, Kumar V, Kono DH, et al. Restricted use of T cell receptor V genes in murine autoimmune encephalomyelitis raises possibilities for antibody therapy. *Cell* 1988;54:577–92.
97. Gold D, Offner H, Sun D, Wiley S, Vandenbark A, Wilson D. Analysis of T cell receptor beta chains in Lewis rats with experimental allergic encephalomyelitis: conserved complementarity determining region 3. *J Exp Med* 1991;174:1467–76.
98. Matsuoka M, Bernard N, Concepcion E, Graves P, Ben-Nun A, Davies T. T cell receptor V region beta-chain gene expression in the autoimmune thyroiditis of non-obese diabetic mice. *J Immunol* 1993;151:1691–701.
99. Nakano N, Kikutani H, Nishimoto H, Kishimoto T. T cell receptor V gene usage of islet beta cell-reactive T cells is not restricted in non-obese diabetic mice. *J Exp Med* 1991;173:1091–7.
100. Gold D. TCR V gene usage in autoimmunity. *Curr Opin Immunol* 1994;6:907–12.
101. Smoyer WE, Kelly CJ. Analysis of T cell receptor variable (TCR-V) region gene usage in spontaneous murine interstitial nephritis. *J Am Soc Nephrol* 1991;2:563.
102. Smoyer WE, Madaio MP, Kelly CJ. TCR-Vβ gene usage in murine spontaneous interstitial nephritis. *J Am Soc Nephrol* 1993;4:635.
103. Heeger PS, Smoyer WE, Jones M, Hopfer S, Neilson EG. Heterogeneous T cell receptor Vβ gene repertoire in murine interstitial nephritis. *Kidney Int* 1996;49:1222–30.
104. Deng A, Gold DP, Kelly CJ. Clonal amplification of Vβ19 expressing T cells in Brown Norway rats with autoimmune interstitial nephritis. *J Am Soc Nephrol* 1995;6:827.
105. Ley K, Tedder TF. Leukocyte interactions with vascular endothelium: new insights into selectin-mediated attachment and rolling. *J Immunol* 1995;155:525–8.
106. Picker LJ, Butcher EC. Physiological and molecular mechanisms of lymphocyte homing. *Annu Rev Immunol* 1992;10:561–91.
107. Bevilacqua M. Endothelial–leukocyte adhesion molecules. *Annu Rev Immunol* 1993;11:767–804.
108. Nishikawa K, Guo YJ, Miyasaka M, et al. Antibodies to intercellular adhesion molecule 1/lymphocyte function-associated antigen 1 prevent crescent formation in rat autoimmune glomerulonephritis. *J Exp Med* 1993;177:667–77.
109. Molina A, Sanchez-Madrid F, Bricio T, et al. Prevention of mercuric chloride-induced nephritis in the Brown Norway rat with antibodies against the alpha 4 integrin. *J Immunol* 1994;153:2313–20.
110. Ando K, Guidotti LG, Cerny A, Ishikawa T, Chisari FV. CTL access to tissue antigen is restricted in vivo. *J Immunol* 1994;153:482–8.
111. Olsen TS, Wassef NF, Olsen HS, Hansen HE. Ultrastructure of the kidney in acute interstitial nephritis. *Ultrastruct Pathol* 1986;10:1–16.
112. Romanic AM, Madri JA. The induction of 72-kD gelatinase in T cells upon adhesion to endothelial cells is VCAM-1 dependent. *J Cell Biol* 1994;125:1165–78.
113. Walsh CM, Matloubian M, Liu CC, et al. Immune function in mice lacking the perforin gene. *Proc Natl Acad Sci USA* 1994; 91:10,854–8.
114. Gershenfeld HK, Weissman IL. Cloning of a cDNA for a T cell-specific serine protease from a cytotoxic T lymphocyte. *Science* 1986;232:854–8.
115. Larsen CP, Ritchie SC, Hendrix R, et al. Regulation of immunostimulatory function and costimulatory molecule (B7-1 and B7-2) expression on murine dendritic cells. *J Immunol* 1994;152:5208–19.
116. Kohan DE, Schreiner GF. Interleukin 1 modulation of renal epithelial glucose and amino acid transport. *Am J Physiol* 1988;254(6 Part 2):F879–86.
117. Meyers CM, Kelly CJ. Adoptive transfer of an antigen-specific DTH-reactive T cell clone induces murine interstitial nephritis. *J Am Soc Nephrol* 1991;2:553.
118. Bannister KM, Ulich TR, Wilson CB. Induction, characterization, and cell transfer of autoimmune tubulointerstitial nephritis in the Lewis rat. *Kidney Int* 1987;32:642–51.
119. Lan HY, Nikolic-Paterson DJ, Mu W, Atkins RC. Local macrophage proliferation in multinucleated giant cell and granuloma formation in experimental Goodpasture's syndrome. *Am J Pathol* 1995;147:1214–20.
120. Kennedy TL, Merrow M, Phillips SM, Norman ME, Neilson EG. Macrophage chemotaxis in anti-tubular basement membrane induced interstitial nephritis in guinea pigs. *Clin Immunol Immunopathol* 1985;36:243–8.
121. Nathan C. Secretory products of macrophages. *J Clin Invest* 1987;79:319–26.
122. Lan HY, Nikolic-Paterson DJ, Atkins RC. Involvement of activated periglomerular leukocytes in the rupture of Bowman's capsule and glomerular crescent progression in experimental glomerulonephritis. *Lab Invest* 1992;67:743–51.
123. Ahn KY, Mohaupt MG, Madsen KM, Kone BC. In situ hybridization localization of mRNA encoding inducible nitric oxide synthase in rat kidney. *Am J Physiol* 1994;267(5 Part 2):F748–57.
124. Markewitz BA, Michael JR, Kohan DE. Cytokine-induced expression of a nitric oxide synthase in rat renal tubule cells. *J Clin Invest* 1993;91:2138–43.
125. Deng W, Thiel B, Tannenbaum CS, Hamilton TA, Stuehr DJ. Syner-

gistic cooperation between T cell lymphokines of induction of the nitric oxide synthase gene in murine peritoneal macrophages. *J Immunol* 1993;151:322–9.
126. Oswald IP, Gazzinelli RT, Sher A, James SL. IL-10 synergizes with IL-4 and transforming growth factor-beta to inhibit macrophage cytotoxic activity. *J Immunol* 1992;148:3578–82.
127. Atanasova I, Burke TJ, McMurtry IF, Schrier RW. Nitric oxide synthase inhibition and acute renal ischemia: effect on systemic hemodynamics and mortality. *Ren Fail* 1995;17:389–403.
128. Florquin S, Amraoui Z, Dubois C, Decuyper J, Goldman M. The protective role of endogenously synthesized nitric oxide in staphylococcal enterotoxin B-induced shock in mice. *J Exp Med* 1994;180:1153–8.
129. Fu Y, Blankenhorn EP. Nitric oxide-induced anti-mitogenic effects in high and low responder rat strains. *J Immunol* 1992;148:2217–22.
130. Wei X-Q, Charles IG, Smith A, et al. Altered immune responses in mice lacking inducible nitric oxide synthase. *Nature* 1995;375:408–11.
131. Sicher SC, Chung GW, Vazquez MA, Lu CY. Augmentation or inhibition of IFN-gamma-induced MHC class II expression by lipopolysaccharides: the roles of TNF-alpha and nitric oxide, and the importance of the sequence of signaling. *J Immunol* 1995;155:5826–34.
132. Peng HB, Libby P, Liao JK. Induction and stabilization of I kappa B alpha by nitric oxide mediates inhibition of NF-kappa B. *J Biol Chem* 1995; 270:14,214–9.
133. De Caterina R, Libby P, Peng HB, et al. Nitric oxide decreases cytokine-induced endothelial activation: nitric oxide selectively reduces endothelial expression of adhesion molecule proinflammatory cytokines. *J Clin Invest* 1995;96:60–8.
134. Schwartz I, Frishberg Y, Kelly CJ. Nitric oxide is antiproliferative to nephritogenic T cells and leads to a cell cycle arrest in the G_1 phase. *J Am Soc Nephrol* 1995;6:853.
135. Mosmann TR, Coffman RL. Heterogeneity of cytokine secretion patterns and functions of helper T cells. *Adv Immunol* 1989;46: 111–47.
136. Kelley VE, Gaulton GN, Hattori M, Ikegami H, Eisenbarth G, Strom TB. Anti-interleukin 2 receptor antibody suppresses murine diabetic insulitis and lupus nephritis. *J Immunol* 1988;140:59–61.
137. Prigent P, Saoudi A, Pannetier C, et al. Mercuric chloride, a chemical responsible for T helper cell (Th)2-mediated autoimmunity in brown Norway rats, directly triggers T cells to produce interleukin-4. *J Clin Invest* 1995;96:1484–9.
138. Gimenez A, Leyva-Cobian F, Fierro C, Rio M, Bricio T, Mampaso F. Effect of cyclosporine A on autoimmune tubulointerstitial nephritis in the Brown Norway rat. *Clin Exp Immunol* 1987;69:550–6.
139. Shih W, Hines W, Neilson EG. Effects of cyclosporin A on the development of immune-mediated interstitial nephritis. *Kidney Int* 1987;
140. Thoenes GH, Umscheid T, Sitter T, Langer KH. Cyclosporine A inhibits autoimmune experimental tubulointerstitial nephritis. *Immunol Lett* 1987;15:301–6.
141. Lan HY, Zarama M, Nikolic-Paterson DJ, Kerr PG, Atkins RC. Suppression of experimental crescentic glomerulonephritis by deoxyspergualin. *J Am Soc Nephrol* 1993;3:1765–74.
142. Ulich TR, Ni R-X. Inhibition of experimental autoimmune tubulointerstitial nephritis in Brown–Norway rats by (15S)-15-methyl prostaglandin E_1: analysis of the effect of prostaglandin E_1 on the induction of the humoral immune response and the elicitation of humorally mediated inflammation. *Am J Pathol* 1986;124:286–93.
143. Fernandes G, Yunis EJ, Miranda M, Smith J, Good RA. Nutritional inhibition of genetically determined renal disease and autoimmunity with prolongation of life in *kdkd* mice. *Proc Natl Acad Sci USA* 1978; 75:2888–92.
144. Kelley VE, Winkelstein A, Izui S. Effect of prostaglandin E on immune complex nephritis in NZB/W mice. *Lab Invest* 1979;41:531–7.
145. Zurier RB, Damjanov I, Snyadoff DM, Rothfield NF. Prostaglandin E_1 treatment of NZB/NZW F_1 hybrid mice. *Arthritis Rheum* 1977;20: 1449–56.
146. Alexander NJ, Smythe NL, Jokinen MP. The type of dietary fat affects the severity of autoimmune disease in NZB/NZW mice. *Am J Pathol* 1987;127:106–21.
147. Wofsey D, Seamen WE. Successful treatment of autoimmunity in NZB/NZW F_1 mice with monoclonal antibody to L3T4. *J Exp Med* 1986;161:378–91.
148. Wofsey D, Seaman WE. Reversal of advanced murine lupus in NZB/NZW F_1 mice by treatment with monoclonal antibody to L3T4. *J Immunol* 1987;138:3247–53.
149. McDevitt HO, Perry R, Steinman LA. Monoclonal anti-IA antibody therapy in animal models of autoimmune disease. *Ciba Found Symp* 1987;129:184–93.
150. Adelman NE, Watling DL, McDevitt HO. Treatment of (NZB× NZW)F_1 disease with anti-IA monoclonal antibodies. *J Exp Med* 1987;158:1350–5.
151. Jevnikar AM, Grusby MJ, Glimcher LH. Prevention of nephritis in major histocompatibility complex class II-deficient MRL-*lpr* mice. *J Exp Med* 1994;179:1137–43.
152. Nishikawa K, Linsley PS, Collins AB, Stamenkovic I, McCluskey RT, Andres G. Effect of CTLA-4 chimeric protein in rat autoimmune anti-glomerular basement membrane glomerulonephritis. *Eur J Immunol* 1994;24:1249–54.
153. Biancone L, Andres G, Ahn H, DeMartino C, Stamenkovic I. Inhibition of the CD40–CD40 ligand pathway prevents murine membranous glomerulonephritis. *Kidney Int* 1995;48:458–68.
154. Vance BA, Kelly CJ. Proliferation of a nephritogenic T cell clone is inhibited by an antibody which blocks CD40–CD40L interactions. *J Am Soc Nephrol* 1994;5:772.
155. Van Essen D, Kikutani H, Gray D. CD40 ligand-transduced costimulation of T cells in the development of helper function. *Nature* 1995; 378:620–3.
156. Grewal IS, Xu J, Flavell RA. Impairment of antigen-specific T-cell priming in mice lacking CD40 ligand. *Nature* 1995;378:617–20.
157. Pham K, Archer C, Gabbai F, Kelly CJ. Oral feeding of renal tubular antigen to Brown Norway rats prevents autoimmune interstitial nephritis and progressive renal failure. *J Am Soc Nephrol* 1995;6:848.
158. Neilson EG, McCafferty E, Mann R, Michaud L, Clayman M. Tubular antigen derivatized cells induce a disease protective, antigen-specific, and idiotype-specific suppressor T cell network restricted by IJ and IgH-V in mice with experimental interstitial nephritis. *J Exp Med* 1985;162:215–30.
159. Kulkarni AB, Huh CG, Becker D, et al. Transforming growth factor beta 1 null mutation in mice causes excessive inflammatory response and early death. *Proc Natl Acad Sci USA* 1993;90:770–4.
160. Border WA, Okuda S, Languino LR, Sporn MB, Ruoslahti E. Suppression of experimental glomerulonephritis by antiserum against transforming growth factor beta 1. *Nature* 1990;346:371–4.
161. Border WA, Noble NA, Yamamoto T, et al. Natural inhibitor of transforming growth factor-beta protects against scarring in experimental kidney disease. *Nature* 1992;360:361–4.
162. Yamamoto T, Nakamura T, Noble NA, Ruoslahti E, Border WA. Expression of transforming growth factor beta is elevated in human and experimental diabetic nephropathy. *Proc Natl Acad Sci USA* 1993;90:1814–8.
163. Yamamoto T, Noble NA, Miller DE, Border WA. Sustained expression of TGF-beta 1 underlies development of progressive kidney fibrosis. *Kidney Int* 1994;45:916–27.
164. Feinfeld DA, D'Agati V, Dutcher JP, Werfel SB, Lynn RI, Wiernik PH. Interstitial nephritis in a patient receiving adoptive immunotherapy with recombinant interleukin-2 and lymphokine-activated killer cells. *Am J Nephrol* 1991;11:489–92.
165. Andreu-Sanchez JL, Moreno de Alboran I, Marcos MAR, Sanchez-Morilla A, Martinez C, Kroemer G. Interleukin 2 abrogates the nonresponsive state of T cells expressing a forbidden T cell receptor repertoire and induces autoimmune disease in neonatally thymectomized mice. *J Exp Med* 1991;173:1323–9.
166. Harris KP, Klahr S, Schreiner G. Obstructive nephropathy: from mechanical disturbance to immune activation? *Exp Nephrol* 1993;1: 198–204.
167. Eddy AA. Experimental insights into the tubulointerstitial disease accompanying primary glomerular lesions. *J Am Soc Nephrol* 1994;5: 1273–87.
168. Hooke DH, Gee DC, Atkins RC. Leukocyte analysis using monoclonal antibodies in human glomerulonephritis. *Kidney Int* 1987;31: 964–72.
169. Cameron JS. Tubular and interstitial factors in the progression of glomerulonephritis. *Pediatr Nephrol* 1992;6:292–303.
170. Nath KA, Hostetter MK, Hostetter TH. Pathophysiology of chronic tubulo-interstitial disease in rats: interactions of dietary acid load, ammonia, and complement C3. *J Clin Invest* 1985;76:667–75.
171. Clark EC, Nath KA, Hostetter MK, Hostetter TH. Role of ammonia in tubulointerstitial injury. *Miner Electrolyte Metab* 1990;16:315–21.
172. Gomez-Chiarri M, Ortiz A, Seron D, Gonzalez E, Egido J. The intercrine superfamily and renal disease. *Kidney Int* 1993;43(Suppl 39): S81–5.

173. Heeger P, Wolf G, Sun MJ, Meyers C, Krensky A, Neilson EG. Isolation and characterization of cDNA from renal tubular cells encoding murine Rantes, a small cytokine from the Scy superfamily. *Kidney Int* 1992;41:220–5.
174. Kees-Folts D, Sadow J, Schreiner GF. Tubular catabolism of albumin is associated with the release of an inflammatory lipid. *Kidney Int* 1994;45:1697–709.
175. Lindquist S. The heat shock response. *Annu Rev Biochem* 1986;55: 1151–91.
176. Kaufmann S. Heat shock proteins and the immune response. *Immunol Today* 1991;11:129–36.
177. Emami A, Schwartz J, Borkan S. Transient ischemia or heat stress induces a cytoprotectant protein in rat kidney. *Am J Physiol* 1991; 262:F479–85.
178. Shelton KR, Todd JM, Engle PM. The induction of stress-related proteins by lead. *J Biol Chem* 1986;261:1935–40.
179. Holoshitz J, Naparstek Y, Ben Nun A, Cohen I. Lines of T lymphocytes induce or vaccinate against autoimmune arthritis. *Science* 1983; 219:56–8.
180. Elias D, Markovits D, Reshef T, van der Zee R, Cohen IR. Induction and therapy of autoimmune diabetes in the non-obese diabetic (NOD/Lt) mouse by a 65 kd heat shock protein. *Proc Natl Acad Sci USA* 1990;87:1576–80.
181. Mor F, Cohen IR. T cells in the lesion of experimental autoimmune encephalomyelitis: enrichment of reactivities of myelin basic protein and to heat shock proteins. *J Clin Invest* 1992;90:2447–55.
182. Aughey E, Fell GS, Scott R, Black M. Histopathology of early effects of oral cadmium in the rat kidney. *Environ Health Perspect* 1984;54: 153–61.
183. Goyer RA, Miller CR, Zhu SY. Non-metallothione-bound cadmium in the pathogenesis of cadmium toxicity in the rat. *Toxicol Appl Pharmacol* 1989;101:232–44.

Immunologic Renal Diseases,
edited by E. G. Neilson and W. G. Couser.
Lippincott-Raven Publishers, Philadelphia © 1997.

CHAPTER 13

Molecular Structure and Expression of Nephritogenic Autoantibodies

Mary H. Foster and Michael P. Madaio

Although many forms of nephritis are dependent on B cells and immunoglobulins (Igs), the events leading to B-cell activation, the production of pathogenic autoantibodies, and subsequent immune complex formation are incompletely understood. Recent advances in areas of B-cell development and activation coupled with more precise understanding of Ig structure and function now provide the framework to more precisely decipher both the contribution of these individual components and the sequence of events that lead to the production and deposition of pathogenic Ig. During ontogeny pathogenic B cells are regulated through events involving a diverse group of cell surface receptors, including surface Ig and others. These interactions modulate B-cell activation and differention, Ig secretion and isotype switching, cytokine secretion, and the expression of a variety of cell surface receptors. In this chapter we address these issues with reference to the development and expression of pathogenic Ig. The reader is referred to individual chapters for discussion of specific aspects of B-cell/Ig involvement in particular diseases.

ANTIBODY STRUCTURE AND FUNCTION

Structure and Assembly of Ig

Structure and General Properties

Igs are the soluble form of the B cell's surface antigen receptor, and they are the primary effectors in B cell-mediated immune reactions. All Igs have a similar basic structure (Fig. 1). The prototypic Ig monomer consists of two identical heavy polypeptide chains of 50 to 77 kDa and two identical light chains of approximately 25 kDa covalently linked by disulfide bonds. Each chain has an amino terminal variable (V) region, with a sequence unique to that particular Ig molecule, and a carboxy-terminal constant (C) region common to all Igs of that particular subclass (1–3).

Variable Regions

Three short peptide segments, termed hypervariable or complementarity determining regions (CDRs), within the V region of both the heavy and light chains demonstrate exceptional amino acid variability. These residues are involved in antigen contact and, through tertiary folding of the heavy and light chain V regions, are brought together to create the antigen-binding pocket. The intervening and more conserved peptide segments constitute the framework regions (FRs).

Ig Classes and Subclasses

Five distinct classes of Igs (i.e., isotypes) based on structurally distinct heavy-chain C regions are recognized in most mammals: IgG, IgA, IgM, IgD, and IgE. These heavy chains differ in primary sequence, glycosylation, size, charge, and other physicochemical properties and biologic functions (Table 1) (3,4). IgA1 and IgD are unique in their content of N-acetylgalactosamine in the carbohydrate side chains. IgG has few carbohydrate side chains relative to the other isotypes. Subclasses are recognized within some Ig classes: human IgG (IgG1, IgG2, IgG3, IgG4), human IgA (IgA1, IgA2), and murine IgG (IgG1, IgG2a, IgG2b,

M. H. Foster and M. P. Madaio: Penn Center for Molecular Studies of Kidney Diseases and the Renal-Electrolyte and Hypertension Division, Department of Medicine, University of Pennsylvania School of Medicine, Philadelphia, Pennsylvania 19104.

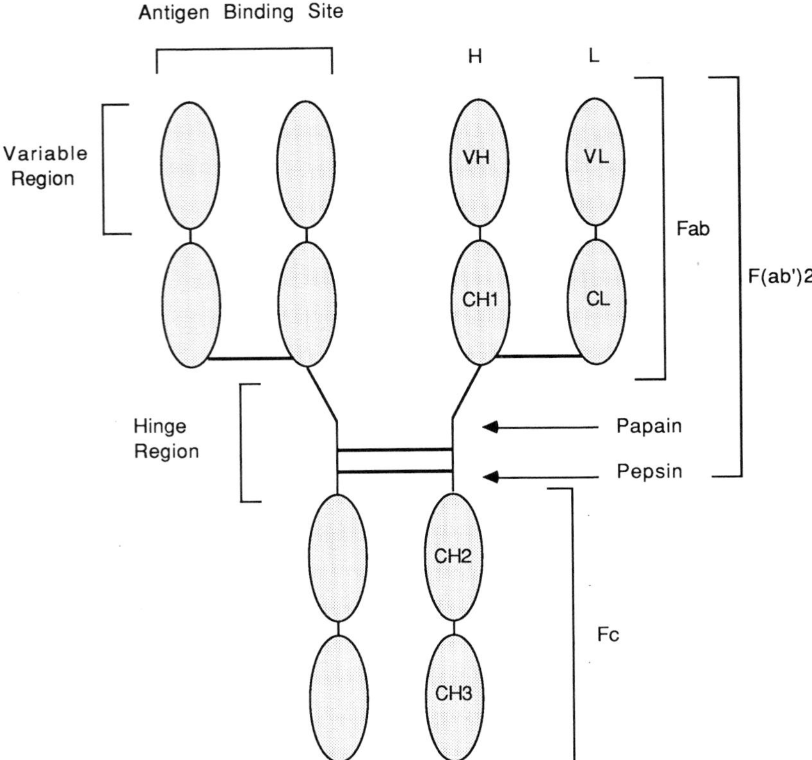

FIG. 1. Basic structure of IgG1. The amino-terminus of the Ig is characterized by marked sequence heterogeneity (hence, variable, or V, region) in both the heavy (V_H) and light (V_L) chains, whereas the carboxy-terminus is a conserved sequence in both chains (constant region, C_H and C_L, respectively) for each class or subclass of Ig. The C_H region includes three discrete structural and functional units (C_H1, C_H2, and C_H3), as well as a hinge segment between C_H1 and C_H2. (The IgM and IgE heavy chains, mu and epsilon, contain an additional C_H unit, C_H4. In these Igs, C_H2 replaces the hinge region). Each C_H unit—C_L, V_H, and V_L—folds into a globular conformation, referred to as a domain, of about 110 amino acid residues stabilized by an intrachain disulphide bond. Each V_H and V_L pair forms an antigen-binding site; thus, IgG is divalent (two antigen-binding sites). Variations of this same basic structure are found in the other Ig classes and subclasses. The fragments generated by enzymatic cleavage with papain (two monovalent Fab fragments and a single Fc region) or pepsin (a single divalent $F(ab')_2$ and smaller Fc portion corresponding to the C_H3 domain) are indicated.

IgG3; unrelated to their human IgG counterparts). Subclasses of IgM, IgD, IgE, and murine IgA are not known. Subclasses are structural variants, encoded by distinct genetic loci, that differ in polypeptide sequence and number and distribution of interchain disulfide bonds. Among the IgG subclasses, IgG3 has a particularly lengthy hinge region with 15 interchain disulfide bonds. Several alleles exist for most of the heavy-chain class and subclass loci, rendering minor variations (termed allotypes) between individuals (i.e., $IgG1^a$ and $IgG1^b$) or strains. These can be identified by antiallotypic reagents.

IgM usually exists as a pentamer consisting of five identical highly glycosylated IgM molecules joined by interchain disulfide bonds and an additional 137–amino acid (15 kDa) polypeptide, the joining chain, that incorporates into the central IgM structure by disulfide bonds. Both IgM and IgA possess an additional C-terminal 18-residue peptide capable of binding the joining chain. This large (970,000-kDa) but highly flexible molecule is the predominant Ig of the primary immune response, and it is largely confined to the intravascular pool. IgD constitutes only a small proportion (<1%) of plasma Ig but is present in large quantities on the membrane of many B cells. IgD executes many of the same functions as IgM, but its unique biologic function remains unknown. The IgG monomer is the major Ig produced in secondary immune responses. IgE, present in only minute quantities in serum, sensitizes the surface membrane of basophils, mast cells, and some mucosal surfaces. It plays a role in immunity to helminthic parasites and mediates many allergic diseases.

IgA is the predominant Ig in external secretions and the major humoral effector mechanism in the lymphoid tissues protecting the body's vast mucosal surfaces (5,6). IgA is also secreted by bone marrow plasma cells and is the second most abundant isotype in serum. IgA circulates either in monomeric or polymeric form; the individual units are joined by joining chains (identical to those present within IgM). In humans the monomer predominates in serum, but in most mammals serum IgA is primarily dimeric. Plasma cells in the lamina propria and epithelium of mucosa-lined organs secrete mainly IgA dimers into the interstitium. Epithelial cells within the mucosa-associated lymphoid tissues (MALTs) express specialized Fc receptors (termed transmembrane polymeric Ig receptors). Secreted IgA binds to these receptors on the basolateral surface of the epithelial cells and is endocytosed via clathrin-coated pits; the IgA/receptor complex is then transcytosed within vesicles to the apical surface (7). Within the transport vesicles, the receptor is cleaved to generate secretory component (a 70-kDa polypeptide). After fusion of the vesicle with the cell membrane, the IgA dimer–secretory component complex is released into the lumen as secretory IgA (sIgA; molecular weight = 380 kDa). sIgA may be of either IgA1 or IgA2

TABLE 1. *Properties and major effector functions of human Ig subclasses*

	Ig type								
	IgG1	IgG2	IgG3	IgG4	IgM	IgA1	IgA2	IgD	IgE
Property									
Heavy chain	γ1	γ2	γ3	γ4	μ	α1	α2	δ	ε
Mean serum concentration (mg/ml)	9	3	1	0.5	1.5	3	0.5	0.03	0.00005
Molecular wt[a] (× 10^{-3})	146	146	170	146	970	160	160	184	188
Half-life (days)	21	20	7	21	10	6	6	3	2
Intravascular distribution (%)	45	45	45	45	80	42	42	75	50
Average carbohydrate (%)	2.5	2.5	2.5	2.5	12	9	9	11.5	12
Effector functions									
Complement fixation[b] (C1q binding)	++	+	+++	−	+++	−[b]	−[b]	−	−
Placental transfer	+	+	+	+	−	−	−	−	−
Binding to *S. aureus* protein A[c]	+++	+++	−[c]	+++	−	−	−	−	−
Binding to streptococcal protein G[d]	+++	+++	+++	+++	−	−	−	−	−
Cell-binding functions[e]									
Mononuclear cells									
FcγRI[f]	+++	−	+++	++	−	−	−	−	−
FcγRIIA	+	−[g]	+	−	−	−	−	−	−
FcγRIIIA[h]									
FcμR	−	−	−	−	+	−	−	−	−
FcεRII	−	−	−	−	−	−	−	−	++
Neutrophils									
FcγRIIA	+	−	+	−	−	−	−	−	−
FcγRIIIB	+	−	+	−	−	−	−	−	−
FcαR	−	−	−	−	−	++	++	−	−
Mast cells/basophils									
FcεRI	−	−	−	−	−	−	−	−	+++
B cells									
FcεRII	−	−	−	−	−	−	−	−	+++

[a] Molecular weight refers to that of the intact Ig monomer (two heavy and two light chains), except for the polymers IgM (pentamer) and sIgA (secretory IgA dimer with secretory component peptide).

[b] Complement fixation via the classic pathway as measured by C1q binding does not necessarily parallel complement cascade activation efficiency. Although IgA does not activate complement via the classic pathway, it efficiently activates the cascade through the alternative pathway (84).

[c] *Staphylococcus aureus* cell wall protein A. Human IgG3 molecules bearing the G3m(st) allotype found in Asian populations do bind Staph protein A. However, allotypes G3m(g) and G3m(b), found in most white populations, do not bind protein A.

[d] Streptococcal cell wall protein G.

[e] Binding functions refer to binding of human Ig to human FcRs. Binding characteristics of only selected (i.e., most studied) human FcR isoforms are shown. The binding functions, structure, and cell distributions of murine FcRs are distinctive (89).

[f] Constitutive FcγRI expression on monocytes is upregulated by IFN-γ, IL-10, and granulocyte colony-stimulating factor, and down-regulated with IL-4; IFN-γ also induces FcγRI expression on neutrophils and eosinophils. FcγRIIA is constitutively expressed on platelets and Langerhans cells. FcγRIIB and –C isoforms are also expressed on B cells. FcγRIIIA is expressed on macrophages and natural killer cells; its expression is upregulated by TNF-β. FcγRIIIB is expressed exclusively on neutrophils. FcμR is expressed by activated B cells but not by T cells or monocytes. Human FcεRI is also expressed on Langerhans cells, eosinophils, and activated monocytes. Human FcεRII is expressed on T cells, eosinophils, platelets, follicular dendritic cells, Langerhans cells, and bone marrow and thymic epithelial cells. Human FcαRI is also expressed on monocytes, macrophages, eosinophils, and mesangial cells. Not shown, the polymeric IgA/IgM receptor expressed on glandular epithelial cells is upregulated by IFN-γ, TNF-α, and IL-4.

[g] The high- and low-responder isoforms of FcγRIIA differ markedly in their binding to human IgG2. The high-responder isoform binds weakly, whereas the low-responder isoform binds strongly.

[h] Binding not known.

subclass. IgA1 is the major subclass in serum, whereas IgA2 predominates in secretions; the latter is due to the sensitivity of IgA1 to cleavage by proteases released by respiratory tract and gastrointestinal microorganisms (8). B cells producing IgA and IgE are concentrated in MALT, although IgM-bearing B cells also are present within these tissues. IgM also can be transported into body secretions via the poly-Ig receptor, thus providing significant mucosal protection for patients with selective IgA deficiency.

The two light-chain types, kappa and lambda, are distinct polypeptides half the length of the heavy chain, encoded independently by genes on different chromosomes. Like heavy chains, light chains consist of two distinct regions: an N-terminal V region with considerable sequence variability between chains and a C-terminal C region. Either light-chain type can combine with any of the heavy-chain types; this contributes to overall antigen-binding diversity.

Genetics of Recombination

Gene Segment Rearrangement

Lymphocytes are uniquely suited to fulfill immununologic functions that require immune receptors with unlimited V region diversity to recognize an enormous range of potential foreign pathogens, yet conserved effector functions. The genetic basis of this paradox was first elucidated in the mouse Vλ system, aided by the small number of *Vλ* genes and the application of recombinant DNA technology in the 1970s. DNA restriction analysis showed that the V and C portions of the heavy and light chains were coded by two separate gene segments that were far apart on the chromosomes of nonlymphoid cells (i.e., germline configuration) but were in close proximity in the DNA of B cells (9), the latter the result of gene segment rearrangement during B-cell development. This form of genetic rearrangement, unique to lymphoid cells, resolved the requirement for both marked sequence heterogeneity (to account for a diverse antigen-binding repertoire) and sequence constancy (to account for similar effector function) in a single Ig chain, as predicted by Dreyer and Bennett (10).

An Ig chain is assembled by a series of rearrangements of germline gene segments. The Ig heavy-chain V region is encoded by three gene segments (*V*, *D*, and *J*); a fourth gene segment encodes the C region (Fig. 2) (11–14). The V_H gene segment encodes the first 294 base pairs of the V region, including CDR1, CDR2, FR1, FR2, and FR3. The short *D* (diversity) gene segment and somatically introduced (non–template-encoded) nucleotides, termed N region nucleotides, encode most of CDR3; the J_H (joining) segment codes for the rest of the V region (FR4). In mice and humans, 100 to 1,000 V_H genes are organized into families based on homology in their framework sequences (15). Ten to 30 *D* gene segments rearrange to four functional J_H segments.

The recombination of *V*, *D*, and *J* gene segments requires base pairing between complementary conserved joining sequences, containing a heptamer–spacer–nonamer motif, within the introns immediately upstream of *D* or *J* genes and downstream of *V* or *D* genes. Intervening intron DNA is subsequently spliced, and the appropriate exons are opposed. Defective recombination prevents generation of functional B or T cells, as in mice with severe combined immune deficiency.

CDR3 is highly variable in both sequence and length (termed joining diversity), due to the multiple mechanisms involved in generating this region (16). Joining of the *D* and *J* genes is imprecise, such that the contribution of 5′ *D* and 3′ *J* gene sequences is variable (i.e., due to deletion of one or more nucleotides at the ends of segments). Furthermore, *D* genes may be joined to J segments either in germline or inverted sequence configuration and in any of three possible reading frames. More than one D segment may join to form a large D region (*D–D* fusion). As noted above, nucleotides can be deleted or added at the D–J_H and V_H–D junctions without the need for a DNA template; this is mediated through the action of exonucleases and the enzyme terminal deoxynucleotidyl transferase (TdT), which randomly adds up to 20 N nucleotides at the *D–J* joint. In mice, such N-region diversity is common in adult cells but rare in neonatal B cells, probably due to low levels of TdT. Nevertheless, the point to be emphasized is that novel sequences, not encoded in germline DNA but not due to mutation, are somatically introduced into CDR3 before antigen contact. Collectively, these mechanisms introduce enormous heterogeneity into the heavy-chain CDR3 and further amplify the diversity of the antibody repertoire.

Light-chain gene rearrangements proceed in a similar fashion, but there are no light-chain *D* genes. One hundred to 350 V_k genes, organized into approximately 16 families (based on 70–80% sequence homology) rearrange directly to join one of four functional J_k genes; there is only one *Ck* gene (in mice, on chromosome 6, and in humans, on chromosome 2). *Vk* encodes residues up to and including codon 95; the precise point at which *Vk* and *Jk* segments join varies, so that codon 96 is encoded by variable contributions from the first three nucleotides in the intron 3′ of *Vk* and those in the first codon of the *Jk* gene. In mice, N region diversity does not occur at this joining site, due to lack of TdT activity at this stage of B-cell development. The genomic organization of the lambda locus (mouse, chromosome 16; human, chromosome 22) is different. The murine lambda locus contains three *V* genes and four *Jλ–Cλ* clusters, and recombination typically occurs within a cluster such that only four combinations are possible. The human lambda locus is more complex, with approximately 100 *Vλ* genes organized similar to the V_H locus; six *Jλ–Cλ* gene pairs are organized 3′ of the *Vλ* genes in sequential fashion, 5′ to 3′ (i.e., *Jλ1–Cλ1*, *Jλ2–Cλ2*, *Jλ3–Cλ3*, etc.).

Early in pre–B-cell development, Ig gene loci rearrangement begins in association with upregulation of the recombination-activating genes, termed *RAG-1* and *RAG-2*, the exact modes of action for which remain incompletely understood (17). The heavy-chain *D* to *J*, followed by *V* to *D-J* gene rearrangement, precedes

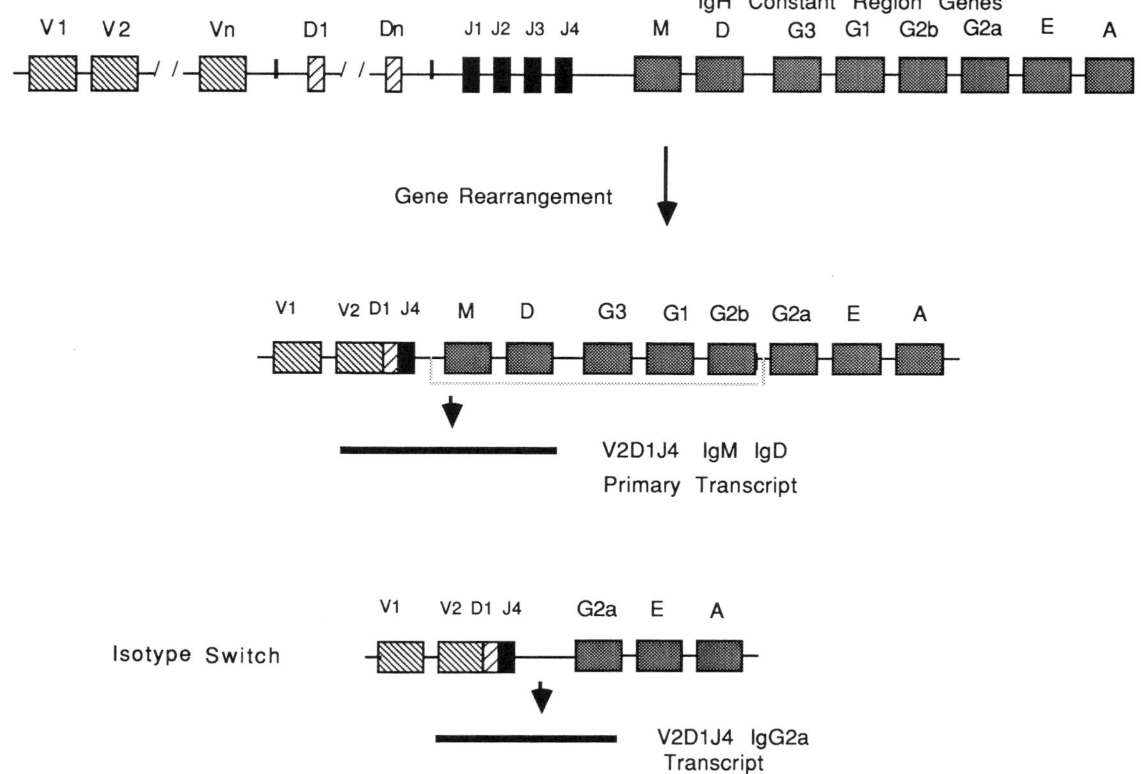

FIG 2. Ig heavy chain gene organization and rearrangement in the mouse. The molecular basis of antibody diversity. During differentiation of the pre-B cell, one of the germline D_H genes becomes apposed to a J_H segment. Subsequently, one of many V_H genes recombines and joins to the *D-J* segment. A variable number of nucleotides may be inserted without a DNA template at the *D–J* and *V–D* junctions, termed N regions. The B cell transcribes a primary RNA transcript that contains this *V-D-J* gene, a long sequence of intervening J segments and introns, and the gene encoding the C region(s) (i.e., IgM and IgD in this figure). RNA processing splices the exons together to form mRNA. Translation begins with the leader or signal sequence, a short hydrophobic peptide encoded by the *V* gene segment that directs transport of the Ig molecule into the endoplasmic reticulum, after which it is cleaved from the mature Ig chain. The heavy-chain C region genes are located approximately 6.5 kb downstream from the J segments (chromosome 12, mouse; chromosome 14, human). Each *C* region gene (except IgD) has a switching sequence in the upstream intron that allows it to recombine with the rearranged *V-D-J* gene. IgD does not have an independent switch sequence. IgM and IgD are transcribed on a single long primary transcript; then either IgM or IgD is generated by differential RNA splicing. Each C region gene contains multiple exons and introns, including one or more exons, encoding the transmembrane domain. Intervening polyadenylation sites determine whether membrane-bound or secreted Ig is formed; the two Igs are identical, with the exception of 20 to 40 amino acid residues in the C terminus.

light-chain *Vk* to *Jk*, followed by *Vλ* to *Jλ* rearrangement. If a rearrangement generates a nonproductive chain (i.e., out-of-frame with stop codons), the cell attempts additional rearrangements. Through poorly understood pathways, functional IgM heavy-chain rearrangement leads to signals that initiate kappa locus rearrangement of *Vk* to *Jk*. If kappa rearrangements are nonfunctional, the lambda locus is signaled to begin rearrangement. Analysis of Ig transgenic models suggests that functional membrane-bound IgM initiates a negative feedback loop that prevents further rearrangements (18). However, recent evidence suggests that *RAG* may remain upregulated, and secondary rearrangements of upstream V_H genes and/or light chains can occur in the presence of functional primary rearrangements (19–21). Although it is unclear whether this phenomenon is limited to primary rearrangements that generate autoreactive Ig, V_H gene replacement (i.e., the insertion of a different upstream V_H gene segment into a previously rearranged *V-D-J* gene) uses a highly conserved switch heptamer found at the 3′ end of the coding region of many V_H genes. This is not unlike gene conversion, a process involving insertion of pseudogenes into the original *V* gene. The latter mechanism is exploited in birds to generate a diverse repertoire from a few functional germline genes.

Somatic Mutation

The mechanisms described above occur during gene rearrangement in the pre–B cell, and this process leads to generation of Ig receptors expressed by naive B cells before antigen contact. The collective population of B cells expressing these diverse but unmutated receptors comprises the preimmune B-cell repertoire, available for subsequent selection and expansion after antigen binding. Potentially unlimited additional diversity can be generated through mutational events. Although poorly understood, mutation appears to be closely (although not exclusively) associated with both B-cell activation via the Ig receptor and Ig class switching (22,23). Most mutations are found in IgG or IgA molecules, whereas the majority of IgM are unmutated (i.e., germline). The *V* gene CDRs (i.e., hypervariable regions) are particularly susceptible to mutation (24–26). It remains unknown whether antigen plays an active role in inducing mutation or merely selects Ig (i.e., engages and activates B-cell surface Ig receptors) in which randomly inserted mutations result in higher affinity. A by-product of the latter mechanism is the generation of many Igs in which point mutations diminish or abolish relevant antigen binding; these B cells may undergo apoptotic death due to lack of stimulation. Alternatively, potentially harmful B cells with autoreactive specificities may be produced, and inability to effectively delete or inactivate these cells may have dire consequences.

Generation of Combining Site Diversity

As evident from the previous discussion, multiple pathways are involved in the generation of *V* region diversity (Table 2) (11,12,16). Somatic recombination allows virtually any *V* gene segment to combine with any *D* or *J* segment; this diversification is amplified by the vagaries of *D* gene contributions and somatic N-nucleotide insertions or deletions at the joining regions. Heavy-chain and light-chain recombinatorial diversity (within conformationally imposed limitations) further expands the potential repertoire exponentially. Finally, additional diversification due to somatic mutation of either or both Ig chains is limitless. Thus, through a combination of germline and somatic events, there is the potential to generate a nearly infinite number of Ig molecules with distinct and diverse antigen-binding functions.

TABLE 2. *Mechanisms for generation of Ig antigen binding diversity*

1. Multiple gene segments[a]:
   50 V_H, 30 D_H, and 6 J_H genes
2. Combinatorial joining of gene segments:
   50 $V_H \times$ 30 $D_H \times$ 6 J_H = 9,000
   80 $V_K \times$ 4 J_K = 320
3. Combinatorial pairing of heavy and light chains:
   9,000 heavy × 320 light = 2,880,000
4. Junctional diversity in CDR3:
   Deletion/insertion of nucleotides at *V–D* and *D–J* junctions
   D gene contributions: multiple reading frames, inversions, *D–D* fusions
   Imprecise joining of V_L and J_L genes
5. Somatic mutations

[a] The number of germline *V* gene segments is only an estimate (i.e., estimates of the number of germline V_H genes range from ~50 to >500). Values are derived from a review of the human Ig *V* gene system (376).

Heavy-Chain Class Switch

Maturation of the immune response involves class switch from a mu heavy chain to another heavy chain class: gamma, epsilon, or alpha. Class switch is largely determined by the presence and nature of T-cell help (Table 3) (27–29); individual cytokines may induce transcription of specific C region genes before switch recombination. Isotype switch (i.e., from IgM to IgG) is often temporally associated with somatic mutation, although the two events can occur independently.

The organization of the murine heavy chain C region genes on chromosome 12 are shown in Fig. 2. In a reaction catalyzed by a switch recombinase, additional DNA rearrangement leads to deletion of intervening DNA such that new downstream C region exons are opposed to the original *V-D-J* gene. Because the new heavy chain retains the original V region, binding specificity is unchanged. At this stage, the B cell produces membrane-bound and secreted Ig of the new isotype (30). Several models have been proposed to explain heavy-chain class switch, including recombination between homologs, unequal sister chromatid exchange, trans-splicing, alternative processing of a long transcript, and looping out and deletion. The latter mechanism is currently favored because recombination by-products of this pathway can been isolated (23, 31,32). An exception to this mechanism occurs with the expression of IgD; there is no switch signal between the mu and delta C region genes. Although immature B cells express membrane-bound IgM (mIgM) exclusively, mature B cells simultaneously express mIgM and mIgD with identical V regions. This is achieved by alternative processing of a single long transcript encoded by the rearranged *V—D-J-*μ*-*δ genes.

Ig Properties and Effector Functions

Igs exist in two forms: as B-cell surface receptors and as soluble secreted Ig. Surface-bound Igs engage, process, and present antigens, and transmit extracellular signals that influence B-cell activation and function. Secreted Igs are also multifunctional molecules; they bind antigens using their Fab regions (Fig. 1), and their Fc regions perform most effector functions, including complement activation and mediation of binding to cell surface Fc receptors (33). These actions are often closely linked physiologically; however, for purposes of discussion, they will be considered separately.

Antigen-Binding (Variable) Region Functions and Properties: Soluble and Membrane-Bound Ig

Antigen Recognition and Specificity

Although B- and T-lymphocytes provide specific recognition for the immune system, the manner in which their surface receptors recognize antigens are quite different. Igs recognize antigens in their native conformation, either in solution or fixed to surfaces, whereas T-cell receptors (TCRs) recognize small polypeptide fragments of antigen presented at the cell surface complexed with major histocompatibility complex (MHC) molecules. The major function of the Ig V region is recognition and binding to a specific antigenic determinant (epitope). This binding occurs in the Ig antigen-binding pocket, formed by Ig heavy and light chain Fab arms (Fig. 1). The hypervariable regions, or CDRs, of the Ig heavy and light chains are brought together during protein folding to form the floor and walls of the antigen-binding cleft, providing the amino acid residues that make contact with the epitope.

Reversible binding occurs through multiple noncovalent bonds formed between particular amino acid residues in the Ig binding site and the epitope. Interaction is dependent on complementary tertiary configurations, and it is often very specific. Small differences in charge, conformation, or amino acid sequence of an epitope may limit the number and strength of intermolecular bonds. Similar constraints apply to antibody interactions. Protein folding may generate multiple smaller binding pockets within some Ig binding clefts so that they are capable of binding more than one antigenic determinant. These binding sites are termed polyfunctional or polyreactive (34). Similar principles apply to consideration of complex antigens and their interactions. Polyreactivity of individual antibodies should be distinguished from multiple antigen-binding specificities typically observed within polyclonal antisera. The specificities of a particular antiserum is the sum of the specificities of individual antibodies; these are typically directed against different epitopes of the same antigen. In some circumstances, however, an epitope may be shared by seemingly divergent antigens (i.e., unrelated by sequence homology). In this case the antibodies (or even a monoclonal antibody) will appear to be cross-reacting with different epitopes, although the interactive region is in fact identical. A classic example of this type of polyreactivity is illustrated by the interaction of monoclonal anti-DNA antibodies with both DNA and cardiolipin. Both antigens share a common phosphodiester backbone that serves as the epitope (35). Another mechanism of polyreactivity occurs when structurally distinct antigens interact with different regions within the Ig binding site [i.e., through different amino acid residues within the site (36)]. The latter may be influenced by the flexibility (adaptability) of the antigen-binding region.

Soluble antigen–antibody interactions (i.e., in blood) are an effective means of either eliminating antigen from the circulation or preventing antigen from localizing at sites where complex formation initiates inflammation. An example of the former is antibody neutralization of bacterial toxin or virus to prevent receptor engagement or cell penetration. Once formed, circulating complexes are eliminated by Fc-bearing phagocytic cells in various organs. This type of interaction is exploited therapeutically with antivenoms, antitoxins, and antibodies directed against drugs (i.e., antidigoxin Ig). With regard to the latter, the role of soluble antigen–antibody complexes during inflammation has been the subject of considerable and ongoing debate over the past three decades. Although earlier work suggested that locally formed immune complexes (i.e., antigen–antibody complexes at the inflammatory site) were necessary to initiate injury, in the 1960s and 1970s the temporal association of circulating immune complexes and inflammation in serum sickness led to the conclusion that complex entrapment initiated the process. However, more recent observations confirm that in situ formation of complexes initiates injury, either by direct binding of antibody to intrinsic tissue-specific antigen or by local antibody interaction with planted antigen. In the latter situation, circulating antigen (either endogenous or exogenous) with an affinity for a particular autoantigen serves as planted antigen for subsequent immune complex formation. For example, cell wall antigens of certain strains of streptococci (exogenous antigen) localize within the kidney, where they serve as a target for circulating antistreptococcal antibodies in post-streptococcal glomerulonephritis, whereas endogenous nuclear antigens or fixed glomerular antigens may serve as targets for lupus autoantibodies. In either case, rheumatoid factors may add to local complex formation to enhance the inflammatory response (see Chapter 14).

In contrast to the pathogenic antigen–antibody interactions just described, antigen engagement by membrane-bound Ig on the surface of B cells typically initiates B-cell activation through one of several signaling pathways. The B-cell response resulting from this interaction depends on multiple factors, including the developmental stage of the B cell, the affinity of interaction, ligation of costimulatory molecules, the presence of T-cell help, cytokines, and other factors outlined elsewhere in this chapter.

Superantigen Recognition

Unconventional antigens that preferentially activate selected populations of B cells through interactions with specific Ig V region framework epitopes (i.e., outside the conventional CDR-framed antigen-binding site) are termed B-cell superantigens. The name is derived from similarity of action with the well-described T-cell superantigens (i.e., murine mammary tumor virus or Mls) that promiscuously bridge the MHC class II molecules on antigen-presenting cells with certain T-cell receptor V_β regions.

Both microbial and endogenous proteins capable of binding particular V_H (or V_L) gene products and acting as B-cell superantigens have been described. The prototype is *Staphylococcus aureus* protein A, a 45-kDa bacterial membrane protein that coincidentally binds to the Fc region of IgG (the basis of its use in IgG purification protocols). *S. aureus* protein A specifically interacts with Fab of selected human Ig (the interaction occurs outside the antigen-binding groove), including most (if not all) Ig-expressing heavy chains derived from the V_H3 family (37). Notably, B cells expressing the V_H3 family appear particularly susceptible to superantigen activation. Other examples include the human immunodeficiency virus type 1 (HIV-1) glycoprotein (gp)120, which binds V_H3 *Fab* and has been implicated in clonal deletion and interference in immune regulation in HIV-1–infected individuals (38); protein Fv, a 175-kDa human hepatic and gut-associated sialoprotein that binds human V_H3 and V_H6 *Fab* (39,40); and peptostreptococcal protein L, which binds human light chain *VκI*, *VκIII*, and *VκIV V* regions (41). B-cell superantigens binding certain murine V_H families also recently have been reported. The in vivo consequences of such interactions remain incompletely understood, but they have been observed to influence Ig production and microbial virulence. They also appear to influence normal immune regulation and tolerance induction among both B and T cells. The role of superantigens and activation of autoreactive B cells is under intense investigation (42).

Valence, Affinity, and Avidity

The noncovalent forces of hydrogen bonding, electrostatic forces, van der Waals forces, and hydrophobic bonds collectively generate considerable binding energy between the antigenic determinant (epitope) and the Ig binding site (paratope). Binding is particularly strong, i.e., high affinity, if the antigen and binding site have complementary surfaces with a high ratio of attractive-to-repulsive forces such that multiple bonds form simultaneously. Antibody affinity, the sum of these forces, is the strength of the bonds between a single epitope and an individual combining site. Amino acid sequence as well as V region glycosylation affect the strength of the interaction (43). Affinity is best measured using a monovalent antigen with a single antigenic determinant, and the Fab fragment of IgG. Interpretation is more difficult with intact, multivalent Ig molecules (i.e., IgG may be bivalent; pentameric IgM may be decavalent) and individual antigens with repeating epitopes. Avidity, the strength of binding between a multivalent Ig and multivalent antigen, is far greater than the sum of the affinities. For this practical reason, avidity is more commonly used to compare antibody–antigen interactions.

Igs with high affinity for specific antigens typically arise by mutation during the process of affinity maturation. However, high-affinity B cells also may arise in the preimmune repertoire from unmutated Ig genes (44). High affinity self-reactive B cells arising in this manner are typically deleted or inactivated by central or peripheral tolerance mechanisms. Ig affinity and avidity also affect the properties of the antibody in biologic interactions. High-affinity Igs are generally more effective in many biologic situations, including virus neutralization, protection against most microbes, immune elimination of antigen, and complement fixation. In some circumstances, high-affinity autoantibodies are more pathogenic; in others, cross-reactive Ig with intermediate affinity appear to be more noxious.

Idiotypes

Because of the unlimited variability of V region sequences, an individual V region domain possesses a unique set of conformational, antigenic determinants unique to that Ig, termed idiotopes (45). By convention, these regions are serologically defined through recognition by other antibodies (anti-idiotopes). Idiotopes may be within or outside the antigen-binding groove. The collective idiotopes of a single Ig variable-region domain—usually defined by either polyclonal antisera derived from an animal immunized with the relevant Ig or a monoclonal antibody produced in a similar manner—constitute the idiotype (Id), and the antibodies that define them are termed anti-idiotypes (anti-Id). An Id may be unique to the individual Ig and B-cell clone (private Id), or it may be shared with other B-cell clones (public, cross-reactive, or recurrent Id). Shared idiotypes among individual Igs imply shared structure; this may be due to similarities in either primary amino acid sequence, tertiary structure, or both.

Natural anti-Id responses are observed during the course of antibody responses (i.e., after antigen exposure), and Id–anti-Id interactions have been implicated in modulating the normal lymphocyte repertoire. It has been suggested that dysregulation of this network may lead to activation of normally suppressed autoreactive B cells and autoantibody production. Both natural and induced anti-Ids (i.e., after intentional immunization of an animal with Ig with known specificity) have been highly useful experimental tools for determining relationships between Ig and investigating regulation (amplification/suppression) of immune network interactions (46–48). In selected circumstances, anti-Ids have been found to share antigen-binding properties with the original antibody, and novel autoantigen-binding specificities among anti-Ids also have been reported (49–51). In the latter situation, anti-Id could amplify autoimmune activity. Attempts at modulation of autoimmune responses after administration of Id or anti-idiotypes have met with variable success: suppression, amplification, and no measurable effect have been observed (52–59). Extrapolation from results of studies in nonautoimmune situations suggest that timing, dosing, and other variables influence the anti-Id effect; therefore, lack of control of these variables during spontaneous autoimmune models probably accounts for some of the observed variability. This unpredictable response in spontaneous autoantibody production has reduced enthusiasm for use of these Igs as solitary immunomodulatory agents. Nevertheless, if used with other immunosuppressive therapies, targeting specific subsets of pathogenic B cells through the Ig receptor may aid in targeted elimination of specific autoantibody responses in selected circumstances.

Size and Charge

Igs within each isotype class demonstrate an extensive charge heterogeneity. Because C regions are identical, charge differences between Igs of the same heavy-chain subtype are largely due to differences in the V regions. Charged residues in these regions appear to influence antigen binding. For example cationic amino acids are commonly found in CDRs of anti-DNA antibodies (60–62). Whether these residues influence the capacity to form immune deposits has not yet been determined, although both anionic and cationic antibodies can be eluted from individuals (mice and humans) with lupus nephritis (63). Of particular relevance, in passive Heymann nephritis, cationic sheep anti-Fx1A antibodies formed subepithelial deposits more rapidly than did their anionic counterparts; however, proteinuria in the heterologous phase of disease is dependent on the complement-fixing properties of the anionic fraction (64). Similar observations have been made in nephrotoxic nephritis (65). Taken together, it appears that in some circumstances positive Ig charge may facilitate immune deposit formation by altering antibody–antigen interactions. Nevertheless, positive Ig charge is not necessarily rate limiting, and in some cases disease appears to be dependent on deposition of relatively anionic antibodies.

Constant Region–Associated Effector Functions

The heavy-chain C region domains (antibody class or subclass) determine the effector functions of Ig by expression of binding sites for complement, bacterial products, and cell surface Fc receptors (FcRs) (4,66–69). Effective engagement of these effectors leads to elimination of immune complexes, initiation of inflammation, and/or necrosis. These effectors also play a major role in autoimmunity. The role of these effectors during nephritis is addressed in forthcoming chapters. In the next few paragraphs, general aspects of Fc and FcR function are discussed.

The CH2 domain of IgG contains the sites responsible for subclass variation as well as the residues responsible for most effector functions. Both peptide and glycosylation residues contribute to the functions of the Fc region, including FcR and C1q binding, C1 activation, and susceptibility to proteolytic degradation; the latter are impaired in aglycosylated IgG (70). Each Ig class and subclass (γ, ε, δ, μ, α, and in some cases allotypes within a subclass) has a unique and distinct profile of interactions with complement components and FcRs expressed on individual cell types. Once engaged, the FcR transmits specific intracellular signals that elicit a variety of cellular responses. These responses are dependent on the FcR class, cell type, state of activation of the cell, costimulatory responses, number of receptors engaged,

TABLE 3. *Cytokine regulation of Ig isotype switching*

Cytokine	Ig isotype[a]	References
IL-4	IgE[b] (mouse and human)	352–355
	IgG1 (mouse)	356
	IgG1, IgG3, IgG4 (human)	357, 358
IL-5	IgA, IgG1 (mouse)	359–361
IL-10	IgG1, IgG3 (human)	362, 363
	IgA[c]	364
IL-12	IgG2a, IgG2b, IgG3 (mouse)	365, 366
IL-13	IgG4, IgE (human)	367, 368
IFN-γ	IgG2a (inhibits IgG1, IgG2b, IgE; variable effect on IgG3)	369–371
TGF-β	IgA[c] (mouse and human)	364, 372
	IgG2b (mouse)	373
Prostaglandin E2	IgE[d], IgG1 (inhibits IgM and IgG3)	374

[a] The isotype response indicated is enhanced by the associated cytokine unless otherwise indicated.

[b] IL-4 is the sole cytokine known to induce IgE synthesis to date; however, multiple cytokines modulate this effect: IFN-α, IFN-γ, TGF-β, and IL-10 are inhibitory, whereas IL-5, IL-6, and TNF-α act synergistically with IL-4 to induce IgE (375).

[c] IL-10 and TGF-β synergize in the induction of IgA isotype switch in humans.

[d] The isotype switch effects of prostaglandin E2 involve synergy with IL-4 and LPS.

receptor cross-linking, and other factors extrinsic to the Fc region of the engaged antibody (66,67,71,72). Novel and recent advances in this area are discussed in the ensuing paragraphs.

Complement Fixation

Complement–Ig interactions are involved in destruction and clearance of immune complexes, opsonization of Ig-coated moieties, activation of phagocytes, and lysis of target cells via formation of the membrane attack complex. Complement activation by the classic pathway depends on the ability of the Ig Fc region to bind the C1q component of the C1 complex. IgG subclasses differ widely in this capacity, with the hierarchy of affinity for C1q by human IgG as follows: IgG3 > IgG1 > IgG2 >> IgG4 (73,74). Site-directed mutagenesis localized the binding site for C1q to the C-terminal half of the CH2 domain of IgG and identified a common sequence motif, Glu-X-Lys-X-Lys at residues 318–322, contributing to C1q–IgG interactions. This motif is contained in all IgG isotypes, with minor but functional differences in some rodent subclasses (75,76). The inability of human IgG4 to activate complement and the poor binding of mouse IgG1 to C1q likely depend on additional amino acid differences in the CH2 domain (33). Additional structural prerequisites for C1 activation include inter–heavy chain disulfide bonds in the CH2 N-terminus, glycosylation of the CH2 domain, intact CH3 domains and multivalent Ig binding to two or more of the six globular domains of intact C1q; the role of Ig hinge region flexibility is unclear (33,77).

Although the efficiency of complement activation roughly parallels the efficiency of C1q binding (human IgG3 and IgG1 are very effective, whereas high concentrations of IgG2 are necessary to activate complement), C1q binding is not the sole determinant of complement activation. IgG subclasses also differ in their relative ability to activate complement component C4 (74,77–79). Human IgG3 binds C1q most efficiently; however, IgG1 is more efficient at mediating cell lysis due to significantly greater efficiency at subsequent C4 activation (74,80,81).

Free circulating pentameric IgM is incapable of activating complement, whereas IgM monomer bound to antigen is a potent complement activator. Alteration of the conformation of pentameric IgM upon binding antigen appears to stabilize the structure and expose cryptic C1q binding sites in the CH3 domain (82,83). IgD and IgE do not significantly activate complement. Although the ability of IgA to activate complement via the classic pathway is unclear, IgA immune complexes effectively activate the alternative pathway (84). Notably, a role for Fc-independent complement activation by antibody also has been proposed (85).

Functions Mediated by Ig Binding to FcRs

Ig interaction with FcRs promotes a variety of functions, as listed in Table 4. Different Ig subclasses interact with different cell types via a complex family of cell surface Fc receptors with differential affinity for Ig, cell distribution, structure, and biologic function (86–89). The binding specificities and cell surface distribution of various FcRs for subclasses of human Igs are provided in Table 1.

Both mouse and human receptors for IgG, FcγR, are members of the Ig superfamily and comprise three distinct groups, including the high-affinity FcγRI (CD64) group, which binds monomeric IgG, and the low-affinity FcγRII (CD32) and FcγRIII (CD16) groups, which interact only with IgG complexes. Multiple genes, allelic variants, and alternative messenger RNA (mRNA) splicing generate multiple FcγR isoforms, which, with the marked differences in transmembrane and cytoplasmic regions, contribute to the functional heterogeneity. This includes the differential capacity for binding of the individual FcγR isoforms to IgG subclasses (particularly human IgG1 and IgG2). Isoform variations have been implicated in susceptibility to certain bacterial infections and differential responses to monoclonal Ig immunosuppression (90–93). Expression of FcγRs varies with the state of cell activation and is regulated by cytokines (Table 1).

There are two distinct IgE Fc receptors (FcεR), including a high-affinity FcεRI (a member of the Ig superfamily) and low-affinity FcεRII (CD23; a member of a serum lectin family). The latter has a diverse hematopoietic cell distribution, including B cells, and it is a counter-receptor for CD21 (complement receptor 2, CR2; involved in modulating B-cell receptor signaling thresholds). The human FcαRIs, members of the Ig superfamily, bind both monomeric and polymeric IgA1 and IgA2 and are widely distributed on different cell types. Differential glycosylation contributes to their heterogeneous phenotype (4,94).

TABLE 4. *Functions of Ig FcRs*

B cell activation[a]
Placental transport of IgG
Coupling of humoral and cellular effector responses
Phagocytosis
Endocytosis
Capping
Enhanced antigen presentation
Release of inflammatory mediators, chemoattractants, and cytokines
Parasite elimination
Antibody-dependent cell-mediated cytotoxicity
Platelet aggregation
Immediate-type hypersensitivity reaction

[a] The reader is referred to other sources for information regarding FcR functions (7,86–88,126,338–351).

The polymeric IgA/IgM receptor was discussed in a previous section of this chapter (95).

Soluble FcRs also have been described, which may derive from either proteolytic cleavage from the cell surface or secretion of alternative mRNA splicing products lacking the transmembrane domain (96–99). They have been implicated in immunoregulation (i.e., inhibition of Ig production in vitro), and they may have therapeutic efficacy in antibody-induced hypersensitivity (99–101).

Bacterial Protein and Rheumatoid Factor Binding

The Fc region of IgG binds fragment B of *S. aureus* protein A via three short peptides in the CH2 and CH3 domains, involving a critical histidine residue at position 435 in CH3. Alternative amino acids at this position in IgG3 molecules bearing the G3m(b) or G3m(g) allotypes renders them incapable of binding protein A. Notably, the majority of rheumatoid factors (RFs) present in the serum of patients with rheumatoid arthritis recognize a common antigen in the IgG Fc region, termed Ga, that overlaps with the *S. aureus* protein A binding site. RFs that do not bind IgG3-G3m(b) or (g) allotypes bind to either the IgG3-G3m(st) allotype or other IgG subclasses (4). Other bacterial cell wall proteins, including streptococcal proteins G and H, bind overlapping sites on IgG (102).

B-CELL ACTIVATION, DIFFERENTIATION, AND DEVELOPMENT

B-Cell Activation and Differentiation

Effective stimulation of resting B cells triggers entry of the cell into G1; this is followed by clonal proliferation and then final differentiation to yield either Ig-secreting plasma cells or memory B cells (103). B cells can be activated either through their antigen receptor (Ig) or by polyclonal stimulators. Antigen-induced B-cell activation may occur either in the absence of helper T cells (for T-independent antigens) or, as is the case for many protein antigens, may require contact with T cells (T-dependent antigens). These different modes of activation induce distinct intracellular signaling and differentiation pathways (104). The expression and activity of these costimulatory molecules and receptors are dependent on numerous factors, including the state of B-cell development and activation, and concomitant stimulation (or lack thereof) through other receptors. These pathways are reviewed in the ensuing paragraphs.

The B-Cell Surface Receptor Complex

The B-cell receptor complex (BCR) is a hetero-oligomer composed of ligand binding and signal transducing subunits (Fig. 3) (103,105–108). mIg monomers form the ligand-binding unit; they are noncovalently associated with a disulfide-bonded transmembrane heterodimer, Igα (CD79a, 34 kDa) and Igβ (CD79b, ~39 kDa, or Igγ, a truncated form of Igβ), encoded by the *mb-1* and *B29* genes, respectively. These members of the Ig superfamily are required for transport, assembly, and signal transduction of mIgM. The membrane forms of the other four Ig classes also associate with the Igα–Igβ heterodimer, but their dependence on these heterodimers for surface transport varies, and they may associate with other surface molecules (109–111). Engagement of accessory molecules and cytokine stimulation modulate the signals initiated by BCR ligation to determine the response of B cells. The fate of B cells is also dependent on their state of maturation and the nature of the stimulus.

B-Cell Receptor Signaling

The intracellular effects of Ig receptor ligation are mediated by tyrosine phosphorylation, involving three major signal transduction pathways: phospholipase Cγ, the *ras* GTPase-activating protein (*ras*GAP), and phosphatidylinositol 3-kinase (PI 3-kinase) (Fig. 3) (103,107,108,112, 113). Strong cross-linking of B-cell surface Ig by multivalent or cell-bound antigen or by anti-Ig triggers phosphorylation of tyrosines within the cytoplasmic tails of the Igα and Igβ molecules. Critical tyrosine residues are located within a common sequence motif, variably termed the antigen receptor homology I (ARH1), antigen recognition activation motif (ARAM), or the immunoreceptor tyrosine-based activation motif (ITAM). This motif also is found in the cytoplasmic domains of other transducing immune recognition receptors, including the TCR complex, FcεRI and FcγRIII, and it is necessary and sufficient to initiate signal transduction through direct interaction with cytoplasmic protein tyrosine kinases (PTK). Several *src* family PTKs, including Blk, Lyn, Fyn, and Lck, associate with the nonphosphorylated ARH1/ITAM of Igα in resting B cells. After receptor-mediated signaling, one or more of these PTKs and Syk may be involved in the phosphorylation of Igα and Igβ, which in turn leads to a cascade of enhanced binding, activation, and further recruitment and phosphorylation of these PTKs. Additional downstream effectors are involved in these different signaling pathways, including phospholipase Cγ1 and Cγ2, SHC, GRB2, Sos, Vav, *ras*GAP, MAP-kinases, and PI 3-kinase (103,107,108, 113). Signaling is downregulated by negative feedback loops, including phosphorylation at negative regulatory sites, dephosphorylation via tyrosine phosphatase activity, and internalization of phosphorylated BCRs. The dominant signaling pathway depends on the stage of B-cell differentiation and the relative activity of individual kinases and cytoplasmic effectors.

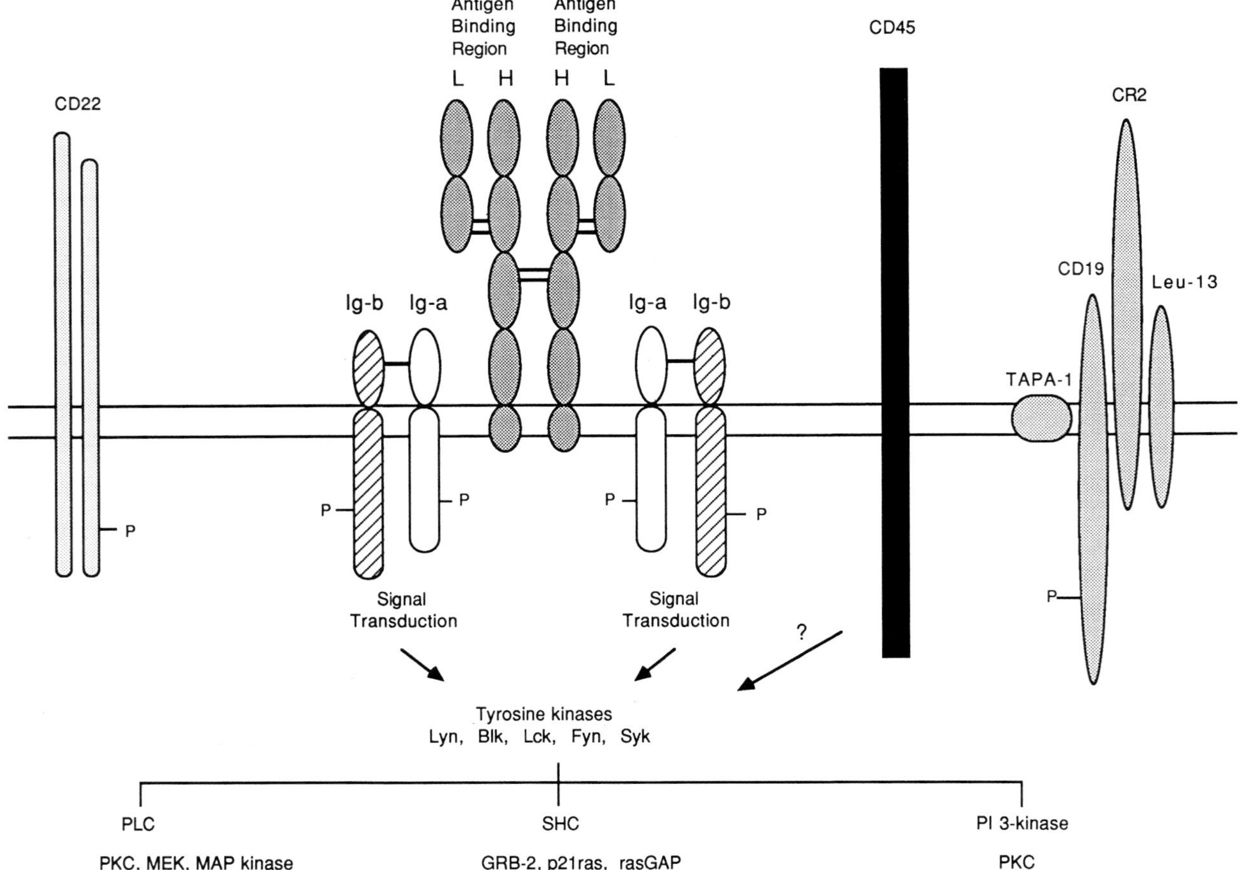

FIG. 3. Structure of the B-cell antigen receptor complex. Membrane-bound Ig is noncovalently associated with a transmembrane signal transducing heterodimer, termed Igα–Igβ. Several transmembrane accessory proteins that function as coreceptors for signal amplification (CD19, CD22) or regulation of B-cell activation (CD45) are indicated. (Adapted from ref. 103.)

Several transmembrane accessory proteins function as coreceptors for signal amplification and are also regulated by reversible tyrosine phosphorylation (Fig. 3) (114). CD19 forms a molecular complex with CD21 (CR2, which binds the complement proteolytic products C3dg and iC3b), TAPA-1, and Leu-13. Cross-linking of this transmembrane complex and the BCR by immune complexes (via complement fragments and antigen, respectively) lowers the threshold for B-cell receptor stimulation (115–119). This pathway may be particularly important for either increasing the sensitivity to low antigen concentration or activation of rare B cells with low-affinity receptors. A similar function for B-cell surface complement receptor 1 (CR1 or CD35) by C3b ligation has been suggested (120). Impaired activation of these pathways in complement-deficient animals may contribute to the observed defects in humoral immunity (121). CD22, a B-cell surface adhesion molecule tyrosine phosphorylated in response to BCR cross-linking, also may modulate signal transduction by the BCR (103).

CD45, a protein tyrosine phosphatase expressed as a 220-kDa isoform on B cells, is required for normal signal transduction through the BCR after antigen ligation. The molecular mechanisms remain poorly understood but may involve the reversible phosphorylation of tyrosine residues via interactions with *src* family PTKs (Fig. 3). CD45 also may regulate the functions of CD19 and CD22 (122). CD23 (low-affinity FcεRII) and CD72 (murine Lyb2), members of the C-type calcium-dependent lectin family, may modulate signal transduction, although their ligands and functions remain controversial (123). CD72 can interact with CD5 (murine Ly-1) on T cells (124). CD5 (Ly-1) is also expressed on a small subset of adult B cells and may transduce costimulatory signals via association with the BCR (125).

B-cell signaling is inhibited by soluble antigen–antibody complexes when FcγRIIB (CD32) and the BCR are brought into close proximity (126,127). This coligation leads to phosphorylation of the cytoplasmic domain of FcγRIIB, with subsequent binding and enhanced activity of the protein tyrosine phosphatase PTP1C (variably termed SH-PTP1, HCP, and SHP). The latter then interferes with phosphorylation and signaling via the mIg–Igα–Igβ complex. Additionally, PTP1C may negatively regulate signaling via the BCR under other conditions. Lack of this function underlies the lymphocyte hyperactivity and autoantibody production seen in *motheaten* mouse strains that exhibit mutations in the gene encoding PTP1C (128–130). The sensitivity of B cells to inhibition via IgG–IC–FcγRIIB signaling can be altered by specific lymphokines [i.e., interleukin (IL)-4 inhibits upregulation of FcγRIIB1 expression], implicating one mechanism through which differential cytokine secretion by TH subsets regulates the humoral response (131).

T-Dependent Responses: T-cell/B-Cell Collaboration and Costimulatory Signals

Activation of B cells by soluble mono- or oligovalent protein antigens (termed T-dependent antigens) typically requires contact with antigen-activated helper T cells, costimulation through CD40, and cytokine stimulation (132,133). The type of B-cell response is highly dependent on the nature of T-cell help and costimulatory signals (134), along with the state of B-cell activation. This cognate interaction is initiated by surface Ig–mediated endocytosis of antigen, followed by processing and presentation of peptides derived from the antigen complexed to class II MHC molecules. The class II–peptide complex is recognized by TCR of a preprimed TH cell. The interaction is stabilized and augmented by the engagement and upregulation of multiple accessory molecules, including adhesion molecules (LFA-1/intercellular adhesion molecule 1, LFA-3/CD2, CD22/CD45 interactions), coreceptors involved in signal amplification (CD19/CD21 in B cells), and additional signal-transducing molecules (Fig. 4) (135).

Two pivotal and interdependent costimulatory signals are transmitted by CD40 ligand (CD40L)/CD40 and B7/CD28 ligand–receptor interactions. Their expression is upregulated during the process. The engagement of these receptors results in reciprocal communication between the T-helper cell and B cell that is crucial to the efficient activation and differentiation of both cell types (29,136–146). Ligation of CD40L, a 39- to 50-kDa membrane protein selectively and transiently expressed on activated T-helper cells, with CD40, a constitutively expressed B-cell surface glycoprotein and member of the nerve growth factor receptor family, triggers B-cell cycling and upregulates B7 expression on the B-cell surface (147–150). Antibodies specific for CD40 induce similar B-cell responses in humans (151). Subsequent ligation of B7.1 (CD80) and B7.2 (CD86) to CD28 and/or CTLA-4 on T

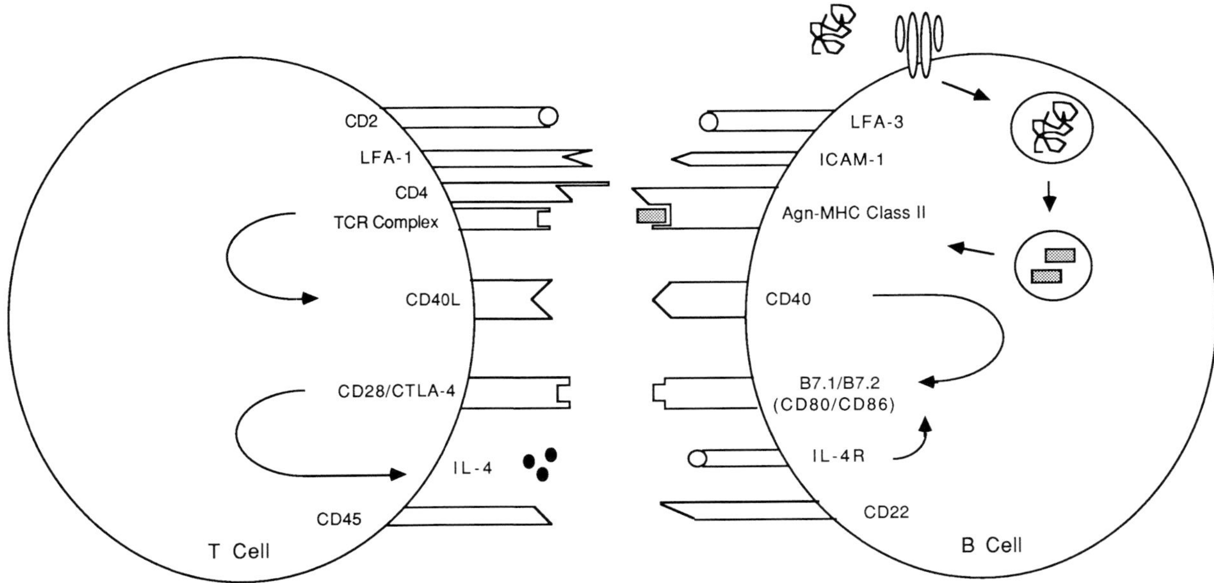

FIG. 4. Costimulatory molecules participating in T-cell/B-cell collaboration. Activation of both the T cell and B cell requires multiple and sequential signals. This cognate (MHC-restricted) interaction is preceded by binding of protein antigen to the B-cell antigen receptor (mIg), leading to cell uptake, intracellular processing, and peptide presentation by a class II MHC molecule and expression of costimulatory molecules (i.e., CD40L, CD28/CTLA4 for T cells; B7, ICAM for B cells). Other less well-characterized transmembrane and soluble molecules (not shown) also participate in lymphocyte activation.

cells fully activates the T cell, inducing production of lymphokines such as IL-4 and IL-5 that regulate subsequent B-cell proliferation and differentiation (133,152–157). Of particular relevance, both ligands and receptors (B7 and CD28/CTLA-4) can be expressed on both T and B cells (depending on the cell activation state), suggesting additional as yet undetermined roles in lymphocyte regulation for this ligand receptor pair (158,159).

CD40/CD40L and B7.2/CD28/CTLA-4 interactions are required for several distinct B-cell functions, including antibody production (for T-dependent antigens), isotype switching, Ig hypermutation, germinal center formation, and induction of memory B cells (28,160–164). Many of these biologic effects appear to be mediated by tyrosine phosphorylation of phosphatidylinositol-3-kinase and phospholipase Cγ2 after activation of the *src* type PTK *lyn* (165,166). Notably, immune regulation by CD40L may lack the redundancy common to many other immune pathways, as demonstrated by the relative lack of compensatory mechanisms and dysregulation observed in CD40L gene knockout studies and human hyper-IgM syndrome (162,167,168). Similarly, blockade of CD40/CD40L or B7/CTLA-4 interactions abrogates or diminishes humoral responses to T-dependent antigens (164,169,170); responses to T-independent antigens are not affected. Nevertheless, once the B-cell response is established (i.e., after immunization), these interventions do not appear to be effective, suggesting that costimulation is not critical in the latter process. As discussed elsewhere, CD40/B7 costimulatory signaling, or lack thereof, also may be crucial to tolerance induction in both T and B cells.

After activation, B cells acquire the ability to respond to cytokines—including IL-1, IL-2, IL-4, IL-5, IL-10, and interferon (IFN)-γ—that synergize with CD40 interactions to promote and modulate B-cell proliferation and differentiation (27,144,171–173). This process involves transient upregulation of MHC class II and B7.2 expression, attachment of the BCR to cytoskeletal microfilaments, upregulation of antigen presentation capabilities, upregulation or de novo synthesis of receptors for growth and differentiation factors, and production of autocrine growth factors (174). TCR–MHC (B-cell) engagement facilitates cytokine–receptor interactions between adherent cells, thus preferentially delivering activation signals to B cells (and vice versa) (175).

Several B-cell functions induced by cognate T-cell/B-cell interactions, including entry into cell cycle and upregulation of adhesion molecules, B7 expression, and antigen presentation (176–178), may be regulated by signals transduced through B-cell surface MHC class II molecules (179). Cross-linking of MHC class II by TCR/CD4 engagement or with monoclonal anti-MHC antibodies induces at least two distinct signaling pathways: one involving protein kinase Cβ, inducing B7 expression, and one involving activation of the PTKs *fgr* and *lyn*, with subsequent activation of phospholipase Cγ1 (179). T-cell superantigens, which stimulate T cells in a TCR-Vβ– or TCR-Vα–restricted fashion, result in similar reciprocal MHC class II–transduced B-cell signals (180–182). Some T-cell superantigens also can stimulate B cells in the absence of T cells, presumably through cross-linking of surface MHC molecules (183). This MHC class II–mediated signaling by T cell superantigens is distinct from Ig V_H- or *Vk*-mediated activation by B-cell superantigens, discussed in a previous section.

Notably, recognition of B-cell surface MHC by T-helper cells is not obligatory for successful T-cell/B-cell collaboration. Certain highly activated and differentiated TH effectors can activate resting B cells regardless of the specificity of the B cell (184–187) or in the absence of class II expression (188). Additionally, some antigens that weakly cross-link the BCR, such as anti-Ig antibodies or SRBC-conjugated haptens, can induce early activation in B cells in the absence of T cells. Further expansion and differentiation of B cells requires T cell–derived lymphokines (189–191). Nevertheless, this "bystander" (non-MHC restricted) help may contribute to nonspecific amplification of humoral responses.

Antigen Processing and Presentation by B Cells

B cells have the unique capacity to selectively and efficiently accumulate and internalize specific protein antigens via their membrane-bound Ig receptors, with subsequent intracellular degradation and processing of antigen into peptides for presentation to MHC class II–restricted TH cells (139,140,172,192–196). B cells also can capture antigens by processes common to professional antigen-presenting cells, and this includes pinocytosis and binding to surface molecules (i.e., MHC or transferrin receptors). This mechanism is considerably less efficient than that involving mIg described above (192,197–200). mIg signaling, lipopolysaccharide (LPS) activation, and class II molecule cross-linking increase the efficiency of Ig-mediated antigen presentation (178,201,202). However efficient antigen internalization and processing can occur under conditions such as low antigen valency or low antigen concentrations, in which mIg cross-linking is insufficient to induce B-cell activation (203–205).

Polyclonal B-Cell Activation and T-Independent Responses

T-independent antigens include polyclonal stimulators (type 1 T-independent antigens, or Ti-1), which activate B cells nonselectively, and type 2 T-independent antigens (Ti-2), which activate B cells through the BCR without T-cell help. Ti-1 antigens include mitogenic lectins (carbohydrate-binding proteins derived from plants and bacteria, i.e., pokeweed mitogen, mitogenic for human B cells), and bacterial LPS (i.e., LPS/lipid A, a major component of the outer membrane of Gram-negative bacteria, mitogenic for mouse B cells). The mechanism by which polyclonal stimulators activate B cells is thought to involve binding to specific receptors on the cell surface (206). At high doses, Ti-1 antigens stimulate clonal expansion and Ig secretion in one-third of all B cells, independent of T-cell help (207). Cytokines, including IL-1 and IL-6, crucial to B-cell activation by LPS may be derived from macrophages, themselves activated by LPS (171,208). At low doses, polyclonal activators may behave as Ti-2 antigens.

Ti-2 antigens activate B cells in the absence of T cells by extensive cross-linking of the BCR (209–211). Typically these antigens are large polymers with repeating polysaccharide or protein determinants [i.e., bacterial dextran, levan, or flagellin (Ficoll)] and are resistant to degradation. They also induce cytokine production by macrophages. B-cell responses (Ig production) to these antigens are more rapid but weaker than to T-dependent antigens, and isotype switch and affinity maturation may not occur. However, T-cell and non-T-cell–derived cytokines can influence the magnitude and quality of the response (104,211–213). At high doses, Ti-2 antigens may behave as polyclonal activators.

B-Cell Superantigens

As discussed earlier, unconventional B-cell antigens, termed B-cell superantigens, can activate selected large populations of B cells through interactions with specific V_H or V_L gene products forming Ig epitopes outside the conventional antigen-binding site. Human Ig expressing a heavy-chain V gene from the V_H3 family appear particularly susceptible to binding by several B-cell superantigens (i.e., protein A).

Regulation of Humoral Immune Responses

The nature of the humoral response depends primarily on the type of TH cell response generated by a particular stimulus or pathogen. In particular, the balance between a TH1 response [characterized by production of IL-2, IFN-γ, and tumor necrosis factor (TNF)-β] and a TH2 response (characterized by IL-10, IL-4, and IL-5) influences the amount, type, and duration of Ig subclass produced (214–222). Several interleukins (IL-2, IL-4, IL-5, IL-10, and IL-13) are potent B-cell growth factors, and IL-6 and IL-10 also markedly enhance B-cell terminal differentiation (29,223–225). IL-6 is a potent growth factor for murine plasmacytomas in vitro (223). Lymphokines are also important in controlling Ig class switch, although the effect of a particular cytokine depends on synergism/antagonism by other cytokines and the differentiative stage of the target B cell (Table 3). T-cell responses dominated by TH2-like cells may be particularly important to mucosal immunity and allergy because IL-4 and IL-5 enhance production of IgE and activate eosinophils and mast cells. Notably, although TH1 cells have been closely linked to immune responses characterized by T-cell activation with low or absent Ig production, TH1-like responses may induce the production of the IgG2a, IgG2b, and IgG3 subclasses, as observed in the response to protein antigens adsorbed to alum. This latter effect may be mediated by synergism of IL-12 and IFN-γ (212,226,227). It has been reported that IgG1 and IgG3 predominate in responses to bacterial protein antigens; IgG4 also increases after chronic stimulation with protein antigens. Bacterial polysaccharides often induce IgG2 responses, although considerable heterogeneity in subclass composition has been observed (67,228).

The cytokines also affect humoral responses indirectly through modulation of T-cell responses (i.e., by shifting the balance between TH1 and TH2 responses) (229–233). The predominant cytokine(s) regulates the development of effector T-helper cell subsets: IL-4 induces a TH2-like response, whereas IL-12 and IFN-γ favor development of a TH1 subset (230,231,233–235).

Control of cell survival is also an important regulatory mechanism in humoral immune responses (236,237). It has been proposed that positive selection of higher affinity B cells during the affinity maturation process and prolonged survival of memory B cells are due to antigen-induced upregulation of the protooncogene *bcl-2*, which promotes cell survival and/or rescues cells from an apoptotic pathway (238). Enhanced cell death also may play a role in terminating antibody responses through downregulation of these responses (236,237). In this regard, expression of a *bcl-2* transgene in murine B-lymphocytes led to an amplified and protracted antibody response and predisposed to a lupuslike autoimmune disease with a high incidence of glomerulonephritis (239).

Removal of antigen from the system by an effective immune response eliminates the stimulus for cell expansion and Ig production. An effective reticuloendothelial system and complement cascade are crucial for this process; the association of systemic autoimmunity with deficiencies of complement components may be due to defective immune complex clearance. Antibody itself participates in a feedback loop, with IgM enhancing and IgG suppressing antibody responses. Although the precise mechanisms responsible for these effects have not been clearly defined, important processes include development of regulatory anti-idiotypes; competitive blocking of antigenic determinants; inhibitory cross-linking of BCR and Fc receptors on B cells; and selective capture of immune complexes by B cells (i.e., by either rheumatoid factors, Fc receptors, or complement receptors on the B-cell surface (120,240,241)). Anti-idiotypes expressed during the neonatal period may have a particularly dramatic and long-lasting effect in modulating specific subsets of B cells. Collectively, these mechanisms also may be responsible for the immunomodulating properties of intravenous Ig (242).

Genetic influences also determine the capacity of individuals to respond to specific antigens. These include influences of both MHC-linked and non-MHC–linked genes. Collectively, they affect both susceptibility and resistance to infection and autoimmune diseases. MHC-linked genes include those encoding MHC molecules and proteins involved in the generation and transport of peptide fragments. Non-MHC–linked genes include those generating the B- and T-cell receptor repertoires (including polymorphisms in *V* genes and endogenous superantigens that induce broad *V* gene deletions) and the genes governing cytokine, enzyme, and adhesion molecule expression.

Analysis of an Antiforeign Immune Response and Affinity Maturation

The immune response evolved to recognize and destroy foreign pathogens. Although the potential B-cell repertoire is enormous, production of high-affinity antibodies with the capacity to eliminate these pathogens requires modulation of the system. B cells that produce Ig with specific antibody activity arise through a process of clonal selection driven by individual antigens, during which B cells expressing the appropriate receptor proliferate rapidly and mature into Ig-producing plasma cells and longer-lived memory cells (243,244). This process will be reviewed below.

Primary antigenic challenge activates virgin B cells expressing mIgM and/or mIgD and alters transcription such that secreted IgM is produced; switch to IgG isotype and greater affinity may occur late in this primary response. Subsequent clonal proliferation and differentiation leads to the production of effector (Ig-producing) cells or long-lived memory B cells. Restimulation of memory cells with the same antigen induces a secondary response, increasing both the effector and memory cell pools. The secondary response differs from the primary response in several respects. The antibody increase appears quicker and persists longer; it reaches a higher titer, and, in a T-dependent response, consists predominantly of IgG with considerably greater affinity (245).

In the early Ig response, T-cell help triggers DNA rearrangement and class switch, typically accompanied or preceded by mutation in the V regions. In the subsequent generations, B cells that bear mutated receptors with higher antigenic affinity preferentially bind antigen (particularly in the presence of low antigen concentration), and this results in expansion of this subset. This process is termed affinity maturation (246,247). During an immune response, a large fraction of antibodies interact with limited regions of the antigen, termed immunodominant epitopes. The factors determining immunodominance are incompletely understood, although physical factors permitting maximization of binding (affinity) and peptide–MHC interactions (promoting specific T-cell help) along with the available TCR and BCR repertoires contribute.

Normal B-Cell Development

B-Cell Lymphopoiesis

Mammalian B cells differentiate from the pluripotent hematopoietic stem cell and common lymphoid progenitor to mature in the fetal omentum and liver and adult bone marrow (248–250). Contact with stromal cells, monocytes/macrophages, and matrix and IL-7 are required for successful lymphopoiesis. Cells committed to the B lineage express different surface differentiation and accessory markers as they mature through developmental stages, from pro-B ($B220^+CD43^+$), pre-B ($B220^+CD43^{+/-}$ HSA^+), immature ($B220^+mIgM^+$), mature ($B220^+mIgM^+$ $mIgD^+$) B cell, and immunoblast ($B220^+mIg^+$), to the terminally differentiated plasmablast and plasmacyte ($B220^+$ mIg^+). In the central (primary) lymphoid organs, B cells express surface Ig receptors (preimmune B-cell repertoire) and undergo positive and negative selection. The murine adult bone marrow produces on average 5×10^7 mature B cells per day. Selected, naive B cells (i.e., not exposed to antigens outside the bone marrow) migrate via the circulation, where they represent 5% to 15% of circulating lymphocytes, into the secondary (peripheral) lymphoid tissues (spleen, lymph nodes, tonsils, Peyer's patches, and other MALTs, as well as adult bone marrow). Other peripheral tissues (i.e., synoviocytes) also have been reported to support the survival and differentiation of B cells (251). Humoral immune responses develop peripherally, where the spleen and lymph nodes filter antigens from the circulation and lymphatics, in close proximity to B-cell follicles. Selected B cells are expanded through antigen contact. During this process, both short-lived effector and long-lived (some surviving over 40 years) memory B cells are generated.

In the microenvironment of the peripheral lymphoid germinal centers, B cells encounter antigen and hypermutate (see previous discussion); selected populations mature into long-lived memory B cells. The latter depends on interaction of maturing B cells with germinal center follicular dendritic cells, which trap, process, and express antigens for extended periods of time, although the events favoring differentiation into memory B cells or shorter-lived plasma cells are incompletely understood (247,252,253). Normally, lymphocytes migrate continuously via blood and lymphatics, with 1% to 2% of the lymphocyte pool (T and B cells) recirculating hourly.

Notably, lymphocytes of the MALT system recirculate primarily back to the mucosal lymphoid system, presumably due to recognition of adhesion molecules selectively expressed on endothelial cells of mucosa venules.

Surrogate Receptors in Pre–B-Cell Development

Two genes, *λ5* and *Vpre-B* (murine), expressed selectively in the pro- and pre–B-cell stages of development, encode surrogate light-chain proteins. These proteins can associate with an Ig gene-derived protein complex, consisting of either truncated D-JH-Cμ (early pre-B) or intact V-D-JH-Cμ (late pre-B) heavy chains, to generate an Ig-like structure expressed on the pre–B-cell surface (254–256). This precedes light-chain rearrangement. These complexes associate with Igβ (and possibly Igα) and are capable of transducing intracellular signals. The requirement for these complexes and Igα expression during B-cell development suggests that their stimulation, via unknown ligand(s), may activate B-cell maturation (257,258) and/or participate in shaping the B-cell repertoire (259).

CD5 B Cells and Natural Autoantibodies

Most B cells during the first few days of life belong to a distinct subset, termed B-1a, which expresses the transmembrane molecule CD5 [previously termed Leu-1 (human) and Ly-1 (mouse)], a counter-receptor of B cell–specific marker CD72 (human), or Lyb-2 (mouse) (260, 261). CD5 also is expressed on normal T cells. Only a small subpopulation (1–2%) of normal adult human spleen or circulating B cells express CD5. In mice, 30% of neonatal splenic B cells express CD5; this high frequency is retained in adult mice among only peritoneal cavity B cells.

CD5 B cells are distinct from conventional (B-2) B cells in that they appear to originate from a unique fetal/neonatal progenitor source, are self-replenishing, use distinct differentiation and signaling pathways, and are associated with a distinct set of B-cell malignancies (262). CD5 B cells may contribute significantly to mucosal immunity and IgA production (263). Ig produced by these cells have a high frequency of autoantibody specificities (i.e., antithymocyte, anti-DNA, and rheumatoid factors), which are predominantly germline encoded (i.e., unmutated) (262,264–266). The repetitive use of certain *V* gene combinations suggests a role for antigen selection in shaping the adult CD5 B-cell repertoire. The CD5 B-cell population is expanded in certain autoimmune strains of mice (NZB and *motheaten* mice) and in certain pathologic conditions in humans (rheumatoid arthritis, Sjogren's syndrome, and primary antiphospholipid syndrome). However, their role in the production of pathogenic autoantibodies in systemic autoimmunity is unclear (125,262,264,267–271). Studies in autoimmune and autoimmune chimeric mice suggest that pathogenic autoantibodies are derived from conventional (bone marrow–derived) B cells (270–272).

CD5 B cells and their sister population, $CD5^-$ $CD45RA^{lo}$ (B-1b) B cells, may be responsible for the production of most of the "natural" autoantibodies generated in the normal (nonautoimmune) preimmune repertoire (250,273–277). IgM derived from both perinatal mice, including germ-free and nude (athymic) mice, and humans exhibit a high frequency of autoreactivity against a variety of self antigens (278–282). These Igs also exhibit a variable degree of polyreactivity and interconnected auto-anti-id activity, bind bacterial antigens, are frequently unmutated, and preferentially express certain *D* gene–proximal V_H gene families (283–286). The cells producing natural autoantibodies are generally believed to have escaped deletion or inactivation due to their low binding affinities for self antigens. Their physiologic role is unclear; however, some have speculated that they participate in regulatory networks, as reservoirs for antiforeign responses, or as APCs in the induction of T-cell tolerance. CD5 cells are capable of hypermutation, suggesting they can provide templates for pathogenic autoantibody production (277,287,288).

Role of Idiotypic Interactions

There is considerable evidence that regulatory idiotypic interactions involved in early stages of B-cell development help shape the adult B-cell repertoire (47,289–291). Studies in normal mice demonstrate that complementary sets of idiotypes and auto-anti-idiotypes emerge spontaneously early in the perinatal period. Moreover, the appearance of anti-id can precede that of Id-positive Ig, and administration of anti-Id either in utero or to newborn mice influences subsequent Id-positive Ig responses in adult animals. These results suggest that auto-anti-Id are important for the functional maturation of some B cell subsets. Negative as well as positive selection have been observed, indicating that the developmental stage of B cells during anti-Id administration determines the response. Notably, there is frequent interconnection of auto-anti-Id activity among perinatal IgM that expresses self reactivity. Such observations have led to the hypothesis that these germline-encoded antibodies regulate pathogenic autoantibody production (250).

Positive Selection of B Cells

Expression of mIg appears to be necessary for positive selection of immature B cells in the bone marrow to protect them from rapid death by apoptosis. The antigens involved in this selection are unknown (258). As noted above, a role for surrogate receptors in positive selection has been postulated (257). The peripheral B-cell repertoire also appears to be positively selected by antigen (292,293).

B-Cell Tolerance and Negative Selection of B Cells

The diversification mechanisms that allow the immune system to protect individual organisms against a vast array of foreign antigens also can readily generate Ig receptors that bind self antigens, with the potential to destroy the host. It is obvious that during various stages of ontogeny (i.e., development, exogenous antigenic stimulation, exposure to hidden autoantigens), the immune system must have effective and efficient mechanisms of either deleting or rendering autoreactive cells unresponsive. This state is generally referred to as immunologic tolerance and is discussed in detail in Chapter 6. In the case of B cells, maintenance of tolerance is complicated by somatic mutation of V genes during exogenous antigenic stimulation. Hypermutation allows potentially high-affinity self-reactive Ig receptors to arise in the periphery at any time (294). Nevertheless, B-cell tolerance is maintained through a variety of ingenious mechanisms (Table 5) (295–308).

Costimulatory molecules involved in lymphocyte activation and cytokines play key roles in the induction and breakdown of tolerance. As previously discussed, both receptor cross-linking and cytokine stimulation are crucial for activation of naive B cells. In most situations, intimate T-cell help is required for this process to proceed, although large polysaccharide antigens also may cross-link Ig receptors. The process is initiated by specific antigen binding mediated by Ig on the surface of B cells. After endocytosis and antigen degradation, peptides derived from the antigen combine with class II molecules in the endoplasmic reticulum. The complex is then transported to the B-cell surface and expressed as a class II peptide complex capable of engaging specific TCR. This process also leads to expression of CD40 on the B-cell surface. T cell receptors engaged by the class II–peptide antigen complexes presented by the B cell become activated, express CD40 ligand (CD40L; formerly termed gp39) and secrete specific cytokines (i.e., IL-4 or IL-2). Along with the receptor-related events just described, B-cell proliferation and differentiation and Ig secretion ensues. Notably, T-cell receptor signaling to a B cell in the absence of a costimulatory signal, via either CD40 ligand or the downstream B7:CD28/CTLA-4 interaction (see Fig. 4), precludes B-cell activation and induces antigen-specific unresponsiveness (tolerance) (145,160,309–312).

TABLE 5. *Major mechanisms regulating the production of autoantibodies*

1. Deletion of self-reactive B cells (clonal deletion)
2. Functional inactivation or downregulation of autoreactive B cells (anergy)
3. Active inhibition of autoreactive B cells (T cell suppression, anti-idiotypic regulation)
4. Receptor editing
5. Competition for lymphoid follicles

Elucidation of the cellular mechanisms involved in self–nonself discrimination in the B-cell compartment has progressed significantly with the development of transgenic models (296,304,305,309,313–321). Mice carrying transgenes encoding high-affinity Ig reactive with self antigens, (i.e., lysozyme, class I antigens, red blood cell membrane antigen, and DNA) under conditions permitting variations in the distribution and timing of self-antigen expression have been particularly useful. It is evident that B-cell unresponsiveness can be mediated by multiple mechanisms (Table 5), that B and T cells may be tolerized independently, and that defects in B-cell tolerance can contribute to, or cause, autoimmunity.

Autoreactive B cells may be eliminated by binding antigen at either immature or mature stages and by encountering self antigen in the bone marrow (central deletion) or in the periphery (peripheral deletion) (309,313–320). Membrane-bound self antigens may be particularly likely to induce clonal deletion. Interestingly, evidence of a stage of arrested development preceding cell death in B cells exposed to deleting autoantigens suggests that central deletion is slow and reversible (322). This may be a stage during which immature B cells are susceptible to a novel mechanism of tolerance, termed receptor editing, which rescues autoreactive B cells from deletion (319, 323–326). After encounter with self antigen, it appears that immature B cells can upregulate the *V(D)J* recombination activator gene (*RAG*) and undergo secondary Ig light-chain gene rearrangements. (This process is facilitated by the particular organization and ordered use of the kappa and lambda loci.) The secondary rearrangement allows self-reactive B cells to alter, or edit, their original autoreactive receptors to generate new receptors with different light chains with nonautoreactive specificities. Editing within the heavy-chain locus, by V_H gene replacement, also has been observed (319). Although the phenomenon of receptor editing was identified and studied primarily in Ig-transgenic B cells, the high frequency of secondary light-chain rearrangements in normal B cells suggests that receptor editing may be operative as a tolerance mechanism during normal B-cell development.

B-cell encounter with soluble self-antigen may be more likely to induce a state of functional inactivation, or anergy, possibly through modulation of surface receptors (327–333). Maintenance of anergy requires persistence of specific signals, and in some conditions, such as removal of antigen, extensive receptor cross-linking. Nevertheless, in the presence of appropriate concentrations of a polyclonal stimulator, anergy can be reversed (334). Notably, 15% to 20% of B cells in normal peripheral lymphoid repositories have the tolerant phenotype. It has been suggested that these anergic B cells may have a physiologic role similar to that postulated for natural autoantibodies (i.e., either as a reservoir of potential anti-foreign B cells or as a source for self antigen–specific APCs to induce unresponsiveness in antiself T-helper cells (305).

Considerable work suggests that tolerance in the B-cell compartment is incomplete, due at least in part to a relatively high binding threshold for tolerance induction. Tolerogenesis may require that receptor occupancy by self antigen exceed a critical threshold, which depends on self antigen concentration and Ig affinity for antigen (294,315). Low-affinity receptor interactions may pose little risk of autoimmune disease, although interaction with a multivalent self antigen that achieves high avidity binding could activate the clone. There may be some parallel with T-cell tolerance induction; although the threshold of tolerization for T cells is much lower than for B cells, a weak interaction of the TCR with self MHC is required for positive selection, and lack thereof leads to T-cell death.

Tolerance in the T-Cell Compartment

B cells depend on T-cell help for activation and differentiation to mount efficient antibody responses to T-dependent antigens. Thus, unresponsiveness of anti-self B cells may be due to tolerance in the anti-self TH cell, rather than or in addition to tolerance in the autoreactive B cell (reviewed in Chapter 6) (335–337).

ACKNOWLEDGMENT

This work was supported by a George M. O'Brien Kidney and Urological Research Center Grant (DK-45191), as well as by individual PHS Awards (DK-33694, DK-47424, and AI-27915) and a Sheryl M. Hirsch Award from the Lupus Foundation of Philadelphia.

REFERENCES

1. Colman PM. Structure of antibody-antigen complexes: implications for immune recognition. *Adv Immunol* 1988;43:99.
2. Kabat EA. Antibody complementarity and antibody structure. *J Immunol* 1988;141(suppl):25.
3. Padlan E. Anatomy of the antibody molecule [Review]. *Mol Immunol* 1994;31:169–217.
4. Jefferis R. Structure–function relationships in human immunoglobulins. *Neth J Med* 1991;39:188–198.
5. Kerr MA. The structure and function of human IgA. *Biochem J* 1990; 271:285–296.
6. Iscaki S, Bouvet J-P. Human secretory immunoglobulin A and its role in mucosal defense. *Bull Inst Pasteur* 1993;91:203.
7. Mostov KE. Transepithelial transport of immunoglobulins. *Annu Rev Immunol* 1994;12:63.
8. Killian M, Mestecky J, Russell MW. Defense mechanisms involving Fc-dependent functions of immunoglobulin A and their subversion by bacterial immunoglobulin A proteases. *Microbiol Rev* 1988;52: 296–310.
9. Hozumi N, Tonegawa S. Evidence for somatic rearrangement of immunoglobulin genes coding for variable and constant regions. *Proc Natl Acad Sci U S A* 1976;73:3628–3632.
10. Dreyer W, Bennett J. The molecular basis of antibody formation: a paradox. *Proc Natl Acad Sci U S A* 1965;54:864–869.
11. Tonegawa S. Somatic generation of antibody diversity. *Nature* 1983; 302:575–581.
12. Rolink A, Melchers F. Molecular and cellular origins of B lymphocyte diversity. *Cell* 1991;66:1081–1094.
13. Schatz DG, Oettinger MA, Schlissel MS. V(D)J recombination: molecular biology and regulation. *Annu Rev Immunol* 1992;10: 359–383.
14. Cook GP, Tomlinson IM. The human immunoglobulin VH repertoire. *Immunol Today* 1995;16:237–42.
15. Rathbun G, Berman J, Yancopoulos C, Alt FW. Organization and expression of the mammalian heavy-chain variable-region locus. In: Honjo T, Alt FW, Rabbits TH, eds. *Immunoglobulin genes*. New York: Academic; 1989:63–90.
16. Sanz I. Multiple mechanisms participate in the generation of diversity of human H chain CDR3 regions. *J Immunol* 1991;147:1720.
17. Oettinger M, Schatz D, Gorka C, Baltimore D. RAG-1 and RAG-2, adjacent genes that synergistically activate V(D)J recombination. *Science* 1990;248:1517–1523.
18. Manz J, Denis K, Witte O, Brinster R, Storb U. Feedback inhibition of immunoglobulin gene rearrangement by membrane mu, but not by secreted mu heavy chains. *J Exp Med* 1988;168:1363–1381.
19. Kleinfield R, Hardy R, Tarlinton D, Dangl J, Herzenberg L, Weigert M. Recombination between an expressed immunoglobulin heavy-chain gene and a germline variable gene segment in a Ly 1+ B-cell lymphoma. *Nature* 1986;322:843–846.
20. Rolink A, Grawunder U, Haasner D, Strasser A, Melchers F. Immature surface Ig+ B cells can continue to rearrange kappa and lambda L chain gene loci. *J Exp Med* 1993;178:1263–1270.
21. Harada K, Yamagishi H. Lack of feedback inhibition of VK gene rearrangement by productively rearranged alleles. *J Exp Med* 1991; 173:409–415.
22. Galibert L, van Dooren J, Durand I, et al. Anti-CD40 plus interleukin-4–activated human naive B cell lines express unmutated immunoglobulin genes with intraclonal heavy chain isotype variability. *Eur J Immunol* 1995;25:733–737.
23. Hengstschlage M, Maizels N, Leung H. Targeting and regulation of immunoglobulin gene somatic hypermutation and isotype switch recombination. *Prog Nucl Acid Res Mol Biol* 1995;50:67–99.
24. Betz AG, Rada C, Pannell R, Milstein C, Neuberger MS. Passenger transgenes reveal intrinsic specificity of the antibody hypermutation mechanism: clustering, polarity, and specific hot spots. *Proc Natl Acad Sci U S A* 1993;90:2385–2388.
25. Betz AG, Milstein C, Gonzalez-Fernandez A, Pannell R, Larson T, Neuberger MS. Elements regulating somatic hypermutation of an immunoglobulin kappa gene: critical role for the intron enhancer/ matrix attachment region. *Cell* 1994;77:239–248.
26. Chang B, Casali P. The CDR1 sequences of a major proportion of human germline Ig VH genes are inherently susceptible to amino acid replacement. *Immunol Today* 1994;15:367–373.
27. Vercelli D, Geha R. Regulation of isotype switching. *Curr Opin Immunol* 1992;4:794–797.
28. Fuleihan R, Ramesh N, Geha R. Role of CD40–CD40-ligand interaction in Ig–isotype switching. *Curr Opin Immunol* 1993;5:963–967.
29. Banchereau J, Briere F, Liu Y, Rousset F. Molecular control of B lymphocyte growth and differentiation. *Stem Cells* 1994;12:278–288.
30. Snapper C, Finkelman F. Rapid loss of IgM expression by normal murine B cells undergoing IgG1 and IgE class switching after in vivo immunization. *J Immunol* 1990;145:3654–3660.
31. Harriman W, Volk H, Defranoux N, Wabl M. Immunoglobulin class switch recombination. *Annu Rev Immunol* 1993;11:361–384.
32. Geha R, Rosen F. The genetic basis of immunoglobulin-class switching [Editorial]. *N Engl J Med* 1994;330:1008–1009.
33. Brekke OH, Michaelsen TE, Sandlie I. The structural requirements for complement activation by IgG:does it hinge on the hinge? *Immunol Today* 1995;16:85–90.

34. Ichiyoshi Y, Casali P. Analysis of the structural correlates for antibody polyreactivity by multiple reassortments of chimeric human immunoglobulin heavy and light chain V segment. *J Exp Med* 1994;180: 885–895.
35. Lafer EM, Rauch J, Andrzejewski C Jr, et al. Polyspecific monoclonal lupus autoantibodies reactive with both polynucleotides and phospholipids. *J Exp Med* 1981;153:897–909.
36. Bentley GA, Boulot G, Chitarra V. Cross-reactivity in antibody–antigen interactions. *Res Immunol* 1994;145:45–48.
37. Hillson JL, Karr NS, Oppliger IR, Mannik M, Sasso EH. The structural basis of germline-encoded VH3 immunoglobulin binding to staphylococcal protein A. *J Exp Med* 1993;178:331.
38. Berberian L, Goodglick L, Kipps TJ, Braun J. Immunoglobulin VH3 gene products: natural ligands for HIV gp120. *Science* 1993;261: 1588–1591.
39. Bouvet JP, Pires R, Lunel-Fabiani F, et al. Protein F. A novel F(ab)-binding factor, present in normal liver, and largely released in the digestive tract during hepatitis. *J Immunol* 1990;145:1176.
40. Silverman GJ, Roben P, Loewer D, Bouvet J-P, Sasano M. Superantigen properties of a human sialoprotein involved in gut-associated immunity. *J Clin Invest* 1995;96:417–426.
41. Nilson BH, Solomon A, Bjorck L, Akerstrom B. Protein L from Peptostreptococcus magnus binds to the kappa light variable domain. *J Biol Chem* 1992;267:2234–2239.
42. Kozlowski L, Kunning S, Zheng Y, Wheatley L, Levinson A. *Staphylococcus aureus* Cowan I–induced human immunoglobulin responses: preferential IgM rheumatoid factor production and VH3 mRNA expression by protein A–binding B cell. *J Clin Immunol* 1995;15:145–151.
43. Wallick SC, Kabat EA, Morrison SL. Glycosylation of a VH residue of a monoclonal antibody against alpha (1–6) dextran increases its affinity for antigen. *J Exp Med* 1988;168:1099–1109.
44. Claflin J, Berry J. Genetics of the phosphocholine-specific antibody response to *Streptococcus pneumoniae.* Germ-line but not mutated T15 antibodies are dominantly selected. *J Immunol* 1988;141:4012–4019.
45. Greenspan N, Bona C. Idiotypes: structure and immunogenicity [Review]. *FASEB J* 1993;7:437–444.
46. Jerne N. Towards a network theory of the immune system. *Ann Immunol (Inst Pasteur)* 1974;125:373.
47. Kearney JF, Vakil M. Idiotype-directed interactions during ontogeny play a major role in the establishment of the adult B cell repertoire. *Immunol Rev* 1986;94:39–50.
48. Shoenfeld Y, Isenberg DA. DNA antibody idiotypes: a review of their genetic, clinical and immunopathologic features. *Semin Arthritis Rheum* 1987;16:215–252.
49. Puccetti A, Madaio MP, Bellese G, Migliorini P. Anti-DNA antibodies bind DNAase 1. *J Exp Med* 1995;181:1797–1804.
50. Pucetti A, Migliorini P, Sabbaga J, Madaio MP. Human and murine anti-DNA antibodies induce the production of anti-idiotypic antibodies with autoantigen binding properties through immune network interactions. *J Immunol* 1990;145:4229–4237.
51. Migliorini P, Ardman B, Kaburaki J, Schwartz RS. Parallel sets of autoantibodies in MRL-lpr/lpr mice. An anti-DNA, anti-SmRNP, anti-gp70 network. *J Exp Med* 1987;165:483–499.
52. Brennan FM, Williams DG, Bovill D, Stocks MR, Maini RN. Administration of monoclonal anti-Sm antibody prolongs the survival and renal function of MRL-lpr/lpr mice. *Clin Exp Immunol* 1986;65:42–50.
53. Hahn BH, Ebling FM. Suppression of NZB/NZW murine nephritis by administration of a syngeneic monoclonal antibody to DNA: possible role of anti-idiotypic antibodies. *J Clin Invest* 1983;71:1728–1736.
54. Hahn BH, Ebling FM. Suppression of murine lupus nephritis by administration of an anti-idiotypic antibody to anti–DNA. *J Immunol* 1984;132:187–190.
55. Ebling FM, Ando DG, Panosian-Sahakian N, Kalunian KC, Hahn BH. Idiotypic spreading promotes the production of pathogenic autoantibodies. *J Autoimmun* 1988;1:47–61.
56. Jacob L, Tron F. Induction of anti-DNA autoanti-idiotypic antibodies in (NZB X NZW)F1 mice: possible role for specific immune suppression. *Clin Exp Immunol* 1984;58:293–299.
57. Mendlovic S, Brocke S, Shoenfeld Y, et al. Induction of a systemic lupus erythematosus-like disease in mice by a common human anti-DNA idiotype. *Proc Natl Acad Sci U S A* 1988;85:2260–2264.
58. Teitelbaum D, Rauch J, Stollar DB, Schwartz RS. In vivo effects of antibodies against a high frequency idiotype of anti-DNA antibodies in MRL mice. *J Immunol* 1984;132:1282–1285.
59. Zanetti M. The idiotype network in autoimmune processes. *Immunol Today* 1985;6:299–302.
60. Seeman NC, Rosenberg JM, Rich A. Sequence-specific recognition of double helical nucleic acids by proteins. *Proc Natl Acad Sci U S A* 1976;73:804.
61. Radic MZ, Mascelli MA, Erikson J, Shan H, Shlomchik M, Weigert M. Structural patterns in anti-DNA antibodies from MRL/lpr mice. *Cold Spring Harb Symp Quant Biol* 1989;54:933–945.
62. Marion T, Bothwell A, Briles D, Janeway J. IgG anti-DNA autoantibodies within an individual autoimmune mouse are the products of clonal selection. *J Immunol* 1989;142:4269.
63. Foster MH, Cizman B, Madaio MP. Nephritogenic autoantibodies in systemic lupus erythematosus: immunochemical properties, mechanisms of immune deposition and genetic origins. *Lab Invest* 1993;69: 494–507.
64. Salant DJ, Belok S, Madaio MP, Couser WG. A new role for complement in experimental membranous nephropathy in rats. *J Clin Invest* 1980;66:1339–1350.
65. Madaio MP, Salant DJ, Adler S, Darby C, Couser WG. Effect of antibody charge and concentration on deposition of antibody to glomerular basement membrane. *Kidney Int* 1984;26:397–403.
66. Morrison SL. In vitro antibodies: strategies for production and application. *Annu Rev Immunol* 1992;10:239–265.
67. Jefferis R, Pound J, Lund J, Goodall M. Effector mechanisms activated by human IgG subclass antibodies: clinical and molecular aspects. *Ann Biol Clin* 1993;52:57–65.
68. Greenspan N, Cooper L. Cooperative binding by mouse IgG3 antibodies: implications for functional affinity, effector function, and isotype restriction. *Springer Semin Immunopathol* 1993;15:275–291.
69. Bredius R, Van de Winkel J, Weening R, Out T. Effector functions of IgG subclass antibodies. *Immunodeficiency* 1993;4:51–53.
70. Tao MH, Morrison SL. Studies of aglycosylated chimeric mouse–human IgG. Role of carbohydrate in the structre and effector functions mediated by the human IgG constant region. *J Immunol* 1989; 143:2595–2601.
71. Horgan C, Brown K, Pincus SH. Alteration in heavy chain V region affects complement activation by chimeric antibodies. *J Immunol* 1990;145:2527.
72. Michaelson TE, Garred P, Aase A. Human IgG subclass pattern of inducing complement-mediated cytolysis depends on antigen concentration and to a lesser extent on epitope patchiness, antibody affinity and complement concentration. *Eur J Immunol* 1991;21:11–16.
73. Schumaker VN, Calcott MA, Spiegelberg HL, Muller-Eberhard. Ultracentrifuge studies of the binding of IgG of different subclasses to the C1q subunit of the first component of complement. *Biochemistry* 1976;15:5175.
74. Bindon CI, Hale G, Bruggemann M, Waldmann H. Human monoclonal IgG isotypes differ in complement activating function at the level of C4 as well as C1q. *J Exp Med* 1988;168:127–142.
75. Burton D, Boyd J, Brampton A, et al. The C1q receptor site on immunoglobulin G. *Nature* 1980;288:338.
76. Duncan AR, Winter G. The binding site for C1q on IgG. *Nature* 1988; 332:738.
77. Michaelson TE, Aase A, Sandlie I. Enhancement of complement activation and cytolysis of human IgG3 by deletion of hinge exons. *Scand J Immunol* 1990;32:517.
78. Bindon CI, Hale G, Waldmann H. Complement activation by immunoglobulin does not depend solely on C1q binding. *Eur J Immunol* 1990;20:277–281.
79. Shaw DR, Khazaeli MB, LoBuglio AF. Mouse/human chimeric antibodies to a tumor-associated antigen: biologic activity of the four human IgG subclasses. *J Natl Cancer Inst* 1988;80:1553–1559.
80. Bruggemann M, Williams GT, Bindon CI, et al. Comparison of the effector functions of human immunoglobulins using a matched set of chimeric antibodies. *J Exp Med* 1987;166:1351.
81. Reichman L, Clark M, Waldmann H, Winter G. Reshaping human antibodies for therapy. *Nature* 1988;332:323.
82. Muraoka S, Shulman MJ. Structural requirements for IgM assembly and cytolytic activity: effects of mutations in the oligosaccharide acceptor site at Asn 402. *J Immunol* 1989;142:695–701.
83. Feinstein A, Richardson NE. Tertiary structure of the constant regions of immunoglobulins in relation to their function. *Monogr Allergy* 1981;17:28–47.
84. Lucisano Valim YM, Lachmann PJ. The effect of antibody isotype

and antigenic epitope density on the complement-fixing activity of immune-complexes: a systematic study using chimeric anti-NIP antibodies with human Fc regions. *Clin Exp Immunol* 1991;84:1–8.
85. Kozlowski L, Lambris JD, Levinson A. B cell superantigen-mediated complement activation in mouse and man. *FASEB J* 1995;9:A518.
86. Ravetch JV, Kinet J-P. Fc receptors. *Annu Rev Immunol* 1991;9:457–492.
87. Capel P, van de Winkel J, van den Herik-Oudijk I, Verbeek J. Heterogeneity of human IgG Fc receptors. *Immunomethods* 1994;4:25–34.
88. Van Den Herik-Oudijk I, Westerdaal N, Henriquez N, Capel P, Van De Winkel J. Functional analysis of human Fc gamma RII (CD32) isoforms expressed in B lymphocytes. *J Immunol* 1994;152:574–585.
89. Hulett MD, Hogarth PM. Molecular basis of Fc receptor function. *Adv Immunol* 1994;57:1–127.
90. Warmerdam P, van de Winkel J, Vlug A, Westerdaal N, Capel P. A single amino acid in the second Ig-like domain of the human Fc gamma receptor II is critical for human IgG2 binding. *J Immunol* 1991;147:1338–1343.
91. Wee S-W, Colvin RB, Phelan JM, et al. Fc receptor for mouse IgG1 (FcRgII) and antibody-mediated cell clearance in patients treated with Leu2a antibody. *Transplantation* 1989;48:1012.
92. Stepleweski Z, Sun LK, Shearman CW, Ghrayeb J, Daddona P, Koprowski H. Biological activity of human–mouse IgG1, IgG2, IgG3 and IgG4 chimeric monoclonal antibodies with anti-tumour activity. *Proc Natl Acad Sci U S A* 1988;85:4852.
93. Rozsnyay Z, Sarmay G, Walker MR, et al. Distinctive role of IgG1 and IgG3 isotypes in FcR-mediated functions. *Immunology* 1989;66:491.
94. Gomez-Guerrerro C, Gonzalez E, Egido J. Evidence for a specific IgA receptor in rat and human mesangial cells. *J Immunol* 1993;151:7172–7181.
95. Mostov K, Friedlander M, Blobel G. The receptor for transepithelial transport of IgA and IgM contains multiple immunoglobulin-like domains. *Nature* 1984;308:37–43.
96. Harrison D, Philips JH, Lanier LL. Involvement of a metalloprotease in spontaneous and phorbol ester–induced release of natural killer cell–associated FcγRIII (CD16–II). *J Immunol* 1991;147:3459–3465.
97. Rappaport EF, Cassel DL, Walterhouse DO, et al. A soluble form of the human Fc receptor FcγRIIA: cloning, transcript analysis and detection. *Exp Hematol* 1993;21:689–696.
98. Fridman WH, Teillaud J-L, Bouchard C, et al. Soluble Fcγ receptors. *J Leukoc Biol* 1993;54:504–512.
99. Astier A, de la Salle H, de la Salle C, et al. Human epidermal Langerhans cells secrete a soluble receptor for IgG (FcγRII/CD32) that inhibits the binding of immune complexes to FcγR+ cells. *J Immunol* 1994;152:201–212.
100. Varin N, Sautes C, Galinha A, Even J, Hogarth PM, Fridman WH. Recombinant soluble receptors for the Fcγ portion inhibit antibody production in vitro. *Eur J Immunol* 1989;19:2263.
101. Ierino FL, Powell MS, McKenzie IFC, Hogarth PM. Recombinant soluble human FcγRII: production, characterization and inhibition of the Arthus reaction. *J Exp Med* 1994;178:1617–1628.
102. Gomi H, Hozumi T, Hattori S, Tagawa C, Kishimoto F, Bjorck L. The gene sequence and some properties of protein H. A novel IgG-binding protein. *J Immunol* 1990;144:4046–4052.
103. Gold MR, DeFranco AL. Biochemistry of B lymphocyte activation. *Adv Immunol* 1994;55:221–295.
104. Pecanha L, Snapper C, Lees A, Mond J. Lymphokine control of type 2 antigen response. IL-10 inhibits IL-5– but not IL-2–induced Ig secretion by T cell–independent antigens. *J Immunol* 1992;148:3427–3432.
105. Reth M. B cell antigen receptors. *Curr Opin Immunol* 1994;6:3–8.
106. Pleiman CM, D'Ambrosio D, Cambier JC. The B-cell antigen receptor complex: structure and signal transduction. *Immunol Today* 1994;15:393–399.
107. Weiss A, Littman DR. Signal transduction by lymphocyte antigen receptors. *Cell* 1994;76:263–274.
108. DeFranco AL. Signalling pathways activated by protein tyrosine phosphorylation in lymphoctyes. *Curr Opin Immunol* 1994;6:364–371.
109. Venkitaraman AR, Williams GT, Dariavach P, Neuberger MS. The B-cell antigen receptor of the five immunoglobulin classes. *Nature* 1991;352:777–781.
110. Kim K, Adachi T, Nielsen P, Terashima M, Lamers M, Kohler G, Reth M. Two new proteins preferentially associated with membrane immunoglobulin D. *EMBO J* 1994;13:3793–3800.
111. Kim K, Reth M. The B cell antigen receptor of class IgD induces a stronger and more prolonged protein tyrosine phosphorylation than that of class IgM. *J Exp Med* 1995;181:1005–1014.
112. Gold M, Law D, DeFranco A. Stimulation of protein tyrosine phosphorylation by the B-lymphocyte antigen receptor. *Nature* 1990;345:810–813.
113. Cambier J, Pleiman CM, Clark MR. Signal transduction by the B cell antigen receptor and its coreceptors. *Ann Rev Immunol* 1994;12:457–486.
114. Clark E, Berberich I, Klaus S, Law C, Sidorenko S. Accessory molecules that influence signaling through B lymphocyte antigen receptors. *Adv Exp Med Biol* 1994;365:35–43.
115. Bradbury L, Kansas G, Levy S, Evans R, Tedder T. The CD19/CD21 signal transducing complex of human B lymphocytes includes the target of antiproliferative antibody-1 and Leu-13 molecule. *J Immunol* 1992;149:2841–2850.
116. Carter RH, Fearon DT. CD19: lowering the threshold for antigen receptor stimulation of B lymphocytes. *Science* 1992;256:105–107.
117. Fearon DT. The CD19–CR2–TAPA-1 complex, CD45 and signaling by the antigen receptor of B lymphocytes. *Curr Opin Immunol* 1993;5:341–348.
118. Tuveson D, Carter R, Soltoff S, Fearon D. CD19 of B cells as a surrogate kinase insert region to bind phosphatidylinositol 3-kinase. *Science* 1993;260:986–989.
119. Fearon DT, Carter RH. The CD19/CR2/TAPA-1 complex of B lymphocytes: linking natural to acquired immunity. *Annu Rev Immunol* 1995;13:127–149.
120. Tuveson D, Ahearn J, Matsumoto A, Fearon D. Molecular interactions of complement receptors on B lymphocytes: a CR1/CR2 complex distinct from the CR2/CD19 complex. *J Exp Med* 1991;173:1083–1089.
121. Van Noesel C, Lankester A, van Lier R. Dual antigen recognition by B cells. *Immunology Today* 1993;14:8–11.
122. Justement LB, Brown VK, Lin J. Regulation of B-cell activation by CD45: a question of mechanism. *Immunol Today* 1994;15:399–406.
123. Gordon J. B-cell signalling via the C-type lectins CD23 and CD72. *Immunol Today* 1994;15:411–417.
124. Van de Velde H, von Hoegen I, Luo W, Parnes J, Thielemans K. The B-cell surface protein CD72/Lyb-2 is the ligand for CD5. *Nature* 1991;351:662–665.
125. Lankester A, van Schijndel G, Cordell J, van Noesel C, van Lier R. CD5 is associated with the human B cell antigen receptor complex. *Eur J Immunol* 1994;24:812–816.
126. Klaus GGB, Bijsterbosch MK, O'Garra A, Harnett MM, Rigley KP. Receptor signalling and crosstalk in B lymphocytes. *Immunol Rev* 1987;99:19.
127. D'Ambrosio D, Hippen KL, Minskoff S, et al. Recruitment and activation of PTP1C in negative regulation of antigen receptor signaling by Fc gamma RIIB1. *Science* 1995;268:293–297.
128. Tsui HW, Siminovitch KA, Souza Ld, Tsui FW. Motheaten and viable motheaten mice have mutations in the haematopoietic cell phosphatase gene. *Nature Genet* 1993;4:124–129.
129. Tsui F, Tsui H. Molecular basis of the motheaten phenotype. *Immunol Rev* 1994;138:185–206.
130. Cyster J, Goodnow C. Protein tyrosine phosphatase 1C negatively regulates antigen receptor signaling in B lymphocytes and determines thresholds for negative selection. *Immunity* 1995;2:13–24.
131. Snapper C, Hooley J, Atasoy U, Finkelman F, Paul W. Differential regulation of murine B cell Fc gamma RII expression by CD4+ T helper subsets. *J Immunol* 1989;143:2133–2141.
132. Noelle R, Snow E. Cognate interactions between helper T cells and B cells. *Immunol Today* 1990;11:361–368.
133. Hodgkin P, Yamashita L, Coffman R, Kehry M. Separation of events mediating B cell proliferation and Ig production by using T cell membranes and lymphokines. *J Immunol* 1990;145:2025–2034.
134. Clark EA, Ledbetter JA. How B and T cells talk to each other. *Nature* 1994;367:425.
135. Dang L, Rock K. Stimulation of B lymphocytes through surface Ig receptors induces LFA-1 and ICAM-1–dependent adhesion. *J Immunol* 1991;146:3273–3279.
136. Rajewsky K, Schirrmacher V, Nase S, Jerne NK. The requirement of more than one antigenic determinant for immunogenicity. *J Exp Med* 1969;129:1131.

137. Mitchison NA. The carrier effect in the secondary response to hapten–protein conjugates. II. Cellular cooperation. *Eur J Immunol* 1971; 1:18.
138. Katz DH, Hamaoka T, Dorf ME, Benacerraf B. Cell interactions between histoincompatible T and B lymphocytes. The H-2 gene complex determines successful physiologic lymphocyte interactions. *Proc Natl Acad Sci U S A* 1973;70:2624.
139. Lanzavecchia A. Antigen-specific interaction between T and B cells. *Nature* 1985;314:537.
140. Lanzavecchia A. Receptor-mediated antigen uptake and its effect on antigen presentation to class II–restricted T lymphocytes. *Annu Rev Immunol* 1990;8:773.
141. Sanders VM, Snyder JM, Uhr JW, Vitetta ES. Characterization of the physical interaction between antigen-specific B and T cells. *J Immunol* 1986;137:2395.
142. Kupfer A, Swain SL, Janeway CA, Singer SJ. The specific direct interaction of helper T cells and antigen presenting B cells. *Proc Natl Acad Sci U S A* 1986;83:6080.
143. Springer T. Adhesion receptors of the immune system. *Nature* 1990; 346:425.
144. Noelle R, Snow EC. T helper cells. *Curr Opin Immunol* 1992;4:333.
145. Banchereau J, Bazan F, Blanchard D, et al. The CD40 antigen and its ligand. *Annu Rev Immunol* 1994;12:881–922.
146. Klaus S, Pinchuk L, Ochs H, et al. Costimulation through CD28 enhances T cell–dependent B cell activation via CD40–CD40L interaction. *J Immunol* 1994;152:5643–5652.
147. Noelle R, Roy M, Shepherd D, Stamenkovic I, Ledbetter J, Aruffo A. A 39-kDa protein on activated helper T cells binds CD40 and transduces the signal for cognate activation of B cells. *Proc Natl Acad Sci U S A* 1992;89:6550–4.
148. Armitage RJ, Fanslow WC, Strockbine L, et al. Molecular and biological characterization of a murine ligand for CD40. *Nature* 1992; 357:80.
149. Freedman A, Freeman G, Horowitz J, Daley J, Nadler L. B7, a B-cell–restricted antigen that identifies preactivated B cells. *J Immunol* 1987;139:3260–3267.
150. Ranheim E, Kipps T. Activated T cells induce expression of B7/BB1 on normal or leukemic B cells through a CD40-dependent signal. *J Exp Med* 1993;177:925–935.
151. Armitage R, Maliszewski C, Alderson M, Grabstein K, Spriggs M, Fanslow W. CD40L: a multi-functional ligand. *Semin Immunol* 1993; 5:401–412.
152. Linsley PS, Clark EA, Ledbetter JA. T-cell antigen CD28 mediates adhesion with B cells by interacting with activation antigen B7/BB-1. *Proc Natl Acad Sci U S A* 1990;87:5031.
153. Gimmi C, Freeman G, Gribben J, et al. B-cell surface antigen B7 provides a costimulatory signal that induces T cells to proliferate and secrete interleukin 2. *Proc Natl Acad Sci U S A* 1991;88:6575–6579.
154. Hathcock KS, Laszlo G, Dickler HB, Bradshaw J, Linsley P, Hodes RJ. Identification of an alternative CTLA-4 ligand costimulatory for T cell activation. *Science* 1993;262:905.
155. Hathcock KS, Laszlo G, Pucillo C, Linsley P, Hodes RJ. Comparative analysis of B7-1 and B7-2 costimulatory ligands: expression and function. *J Exp Med* 1994;180:631.
156. Boussiotis VA, Freeman GJ, Gribben JG, Daley J, Gray GS, Nadler LM. Activated human B lymphocytes express three CTLA-4 counter-receptors that costimulate T cell activation. *Proc Natl Acad Sci* 1993; 90:11059–11063.
157. Lenschow D, Sperling A, Cooke M, et al. Differential up-regulation of the B7-1 and B7-2 costimulatory molecules after Ig receptor engagement by antigen. *J Immunol* 1994;153:1990–1997.
158. Azuma M, Yssel H, Phillips JH, Spits H, Lanier LL. Functional expression of B7/BB1 on activated T lymphocytes. *J Exp Med* 1993; 177:845.
159. Kuiper HM, Brouwer M, Linsley PS, Lier RAWv. Activated T cells can induce high levels of CTLA-4 expression on B cells. *J Immunol* 1995;155:1776–1783.
160. Foy T, Durie F, Noelle R. The expansive role of CD40 and its ligand, gp39, in immunity. *Semin Immunol* 1994;6:259–266.
161. Foy T, Laman J, Ledbetter J, Aruffo A, Claassen E, Noelle R. gp39–CD40 interactions are essential for germinal center formation and the development of B cell memory. *J Exp Med* 1994;180:157–163.
162. Xu J, Foy T, Laman J, et al. Mice deficient for the CD40 ligand. *Immunity* 1994;1:423–431.
163. van den Eertwegh A, Laman J, Noelle R, Boersma W, Claassen E. In vivo T–B cell interactions and cytokine-production in the spleen. *Semin Immunol* 1994;6:327–336.
164. Han S, Hathcock K, Zheng B, Kepler TB, Hodes R, Kelsoe G. Cellular interaction in germinal centers. Roles of CD40 ligand and B7-2 in established germinal centers. *J Immunol* 1995;155:556–567.
165. Ren C, Morio T, Fu S, Geha R. Signal transduction via CD40 involves activation of lyn kinase and phosphatidylinositol-3-kinase, and phosphorylation of phospholipase C gamma 2. *J Exp Med* 1994;179: 673–680.
166. Marshall L, Shepherd D, Ledbetter J, Aruffo A, Noelle R. Signaling events during helper T cell–dependent B cell activation. I. Analysis of the signal transduction pathways triggered by activated helper T cell in resting B cells. *J Immunol* 1994;152:4816–4825.
167. DiSanto J, Bonnefoy J, Gauchat J, Fischer A, de Saint Basile G. CD40 ligand mutations in x-linked immunodeficiency with hyper-IgM. *Nature* 1993;361:541–543.
168. Allen RC, Armitage RJ, Conley ME, et al. CD40 ligand gene defects responsible for X-linked hyper-IgM syndrome. *Science* 1993;259:990.
169. Fanslow W, Anderson D, Grabstein K, Clark E, Cosman D, Armitage R. Soluble forms of CD40 inhibit biologic responses of human B cells. *J Immunol* 1992;149:655–660.
170. Foy T, Shepherd D, Durie F, Aruffo A, Ledbetter J, Noelle R. In vivo CD40–gp39 interactions are essential for thymus-dependent humoral immunity. II. Prolonged suppression of the humoral immune response by an antibody to the ligand for CD40, gp39. *J Exp Med* 1993;178: 1567–1575.
171. Kishimoto T, Hirano T. Molecular regulation of B lymphocyte response. *Annu Rev Immunol* 1988;6:485–512.
172. Vitetta E, Fernandez-Botran R, Myers C, Sanders V. Cellular interactions in the humoral immune response. *Adv Immunol* 1989;45:1–105.
173. Paul W, Seder R. Lymphocyte responses and cytokines. *Cell* 1994; 76:241–251.
174. Boussiotis VA, Nadler LM, Strominger JL, Goldfeld AE. Tumor necrosis factor alpha is an autocrine growth factor for normal human B cells. *Proc Natl Acad Sci U S A* 1994;91:7007–7011.
175. Poo W-J, Conrad L, Janeway CA. Receptor-directed focusing of lymphokine release by helper T cells. *Nature* 1988;332:378.
176. Cambier J, Lehmann K. Ia-mediated signal transduction leads to proliferation of primed B lymphocytes. *J Exp Med* 1989;170:877–886.
177. Nabavi N, Freeman G, Gault A, Godfrey D, Nadler L, Glimcher L. Signalling through the MHC class II cytoplasmic domain is required for antigen presentation and induces B7 expression. *Nature* 1992;360: 266–268.
178. Faassen AE, Pierce SK. Cross-linking cell surface class II molecules stimulates Ig-mediated B cell antigen processing. *J Immunol* 1995; 155:1737–1745.
179. Scholl P, Geha R. MHC class II signaling in B-cell activation [Review]. *Immunol Today* 1994;15:418–422.
180. Mourad W, Scholl P, Diaz A, Geha R, Chatila T. The staphylococcal toxic shock syndrome toxin 1 triggers B cell proliferation and differentiation via major histocompatibility complex–unrestricted cognate T/B cell interaction. *J Exp Med* 1989;170:2011–2022.
181. Fuleihan R, Mourad W, Geha R, Chatila T. Engagement of MHC-class II molecules by staphylococcal exotoxins delivers a comitogenic signal to human B cells. *J Immunol* 1991;146:1661–1666.
182. Tumang J, Posnett D, Cole B, Crow M, Friedman S. Helper T cell–dependent human B cell differentiation mediated by a mycoplasmal superantigen bridge. *J Exp Med* 1990;171:2153–2158.
183. Mourad W, Geha R, Chatila T. Engagement of major histocompatibility complex class II molecules induces sustained, lymphocyte function–associated molecule 1–dependent cell adhesion. *J Exp Med* 1990;172:1513–1516.
184. Tite J, Kaye J, Jones B. The role of B cell surface Ia antigen recognition by T cells in B cell triggering. Analysis of the interaction of cloned helper T cells with normal B cells in differing states of activation and with B cells expressing the xid defect. *Eur J Immunol* 1984; 14:553–561.
185. DeFranco A, Ashwell J, Schwartz R, Paul W. Polyclonal stimulation of resting B lymphocytes by antigen-specific T lymphocytes. *J Exp Med* 1984;159:861–880.
186. Julius M, Rammensee H. T helper cell–dependent induction of resting B cell differentiation need not require cognate cell interactions. *Eur J Immunol* 1988;18:375–379.

187. Croft M, Swain SL. Analysis of CD4+ T cells that provide contact-dependent bystander help to B cells. *J Immunol* 1992;149:3157–3165.
188. Markowitz J, Rogers P, Grusby M, Parker D, Glimcher L. B lymphocyte development and activation independent of MHC class II expression. *J Immunol* 1993;150:1223–1233.
189. Nakanishi K, Howard M, Muraguchi A, Farrar J, Takatsu K, Hamaoka T, Paul W. Soluble factors involved in B cell differentiation: identification of two distinct T cell–replacing factors (TRF). *J Immunol* 1983;130:2219–2224.
190. Leibson H, Gefter M, Zlotnik A, Marrack P, Kappler J. Role of gamma-interferon in antibody-producing responses. *Nature* 1984; 309:799–801.
191. Julius M. A postulated role for the induction of bystander resting B-cell differentiation. *Res Immunol* 1990;141:443–446.
192. Chestnut R, Colon SM, Grey HM. Antigen presentation by normal B cells, B cell tumors and macrophages: functional and biochemical characterization. *J Immunol* 1982;128:1764.
193. Chestnut R, Grey H. Studies on the capacity of B cells to serve as antigen-presenting cells. *J Immunol* 1981;126:1075.
194. Rock K, Benacerraf B, Abbas A. Antigen presentation by hapten-specific B lymphocytes. *J Exp Med* 1984;160:1102.
195. Myers C. Role of B cell antigen processing and presentation in the humoral immune response. *FASEB J* 1991;5:2547–2553.
196. Mitchell RN, Barnes KA, Grupp SA, et al. Intracellular targeting of antigens internalized by membrane immunoglobulin in B lymphocytes. *J Exp Med* 1995;181:1705–1714.
197. Cohen BE, Rosenthal AS, Paul WE. Antigen–macrophage interaction. II. Relative roles of cytophilic antibodies and other membrane sites. *J Immunol* 1973;111:820.
198. Celis E, Chang TW. Antibodies to hepatitis B surface antigen potentiate the response of human T lymphocyte clones to the same antigen. *Science* 1984;224:297.
199. Miettinen HM, Rose JK, Mellman I. Fc receptor isoforms exhibit different capabilities for coated pit localization as a result of cytoplasmic domain heterogeneity. *Cell* 1989;58:317.
200. Snider D, Segal D. Efficiency of antigen presentation after antigen targeting to surface IgD, IgM, MHC, Fc gamma RII, and B220 molecules on murine splenic B cells. *J Immunol* 1989;143:59–65.
201. Mond J, Seghal E, Kung J, Finkelman F. Increased expression of I-region–associated antigen (Ia) on B cells after cross-linking of surface immunoglobulin. *J Immunol* 1981;127:881–888.
202. Casten L, Lakey E, Jelachich M, Margoliash E, Pierce S. Anti-immunoglobulin augments the B-cell antigen-presentation function independently of internalization of receptor–antigen complex. *Proc Natl Acad Sci U S A* 1985;82:5890–5894.
203. Gosselin E, Tony H, Parker D. Characterization of antigen processing and presentation by resting B lymphocytes. *J Immunol* 1988;140: 1408–1413.
204. Tony H, Phillips N. Role of membrane immunoglobulin (Ig) crosslinking in membrane Ig-mediated, major histocompatibility–restricted T cell–B cell cooperation. *J Exp Med* 1985;162:1695–1708.
205. Kakiuchi T. B cells as antigen presenting cells: the requirement for B cell activation. *J Immunol* 1983;131:109.
206. Morrison D, Lei M, Kirikae T, Chen T. Endotoxin receptors on mammalian cells. *Immunobiology* 1993;187:212–226.
207. Andersson J, Coutinho A, Lernhardt W, Melchers F. Clonal growth and maturation to immunoglobulin secretion in vitro of every growth-inducible B lymphocyte. *Cell* 1977;10:27–34.
208. Corbel C, Melchers F. Requirement for macrophages or for macrophage- or T cell–derived factors in the mitogenic stimulation of murine B lymphocytes by lipopolysaccharides. *Eur J Immunol* 1983;13: 528–533.
209. Brunswick M, Finkelman F, Highet P, Inman J, Dintzis H, Mond J. Picogram quantities of anti-Ig antibodies coupled to dextran induce B cell proliferation. *J Immunol* 1988;140:3364–3372.
210. Brunswick M, June C, Finkelman F, Dintzis H, Inman J, Mond J. Surface immunoglobulin-mediated B-cell activation in the absence of detectable elevations in intracellular ionized calcium:a model for T-cell–independent B-cell activation. *Proc Natl Acad Sci U S A* 1989; 86:6724–6728.
211. Mond JJ, Lees A, Snapper CM. T cell–independent antigens type 2. *Annu Rev Immunol* 1995;13:655–692.
212. Snapper C, McIntyre T, Mandler R, et al. Induction of IgG3 secretion by interferon gamma: a model for T cell–independent class switching in response to T cell–independent type 2 antigens. *J Exp Med* 1992; 175:1367–1371.
213. Pecanha L, Snapper C, Finkelman F, Mond J. Dextran-conjugated anti-Ig antibodies as a model for T cell–independent type 2 antigen–mediated stimulation of Ig secretion in vitro. I. Lymphokine dependence. *J Immunol* 1991;146:833–839.
214. Stevens T, Bossie A, Sanders V, et al. Regulation of antibody isotype secretion by subsets of antigen-specific helper T cells. *Nature* 1988; 334:255–258.
215. Croft M, Swain S. B cell response to T helper cell subsets. II. Both the stage of T cell differentiation and the cytokines secreted determine the extent and nature of helper activity. *J Immunol* 1991;147: 3679–3689.
216. Coffman RL. Mechanisms of helper T-cell regulation of B-cell activity. *Ann N Y Acad Sci* 1993;681:25–28.
217. Finkelman F, Holmes J, Katona I, et al. Lymphokine control of in vivo immunoglobulin isotype selection. *Ann Rev Immunol* 1990;8: 303–333.
218. MacLennan ICM. Germinal centers. *Annu Rev Immunol* 1994;12: 117.
219. De Becker G, Sornasse T, Nabavi N, Bazin H, Tielemans F, Urbain J, Leo O, Moser M. Immunoglobulin isotype regulation by antigen-presenting cells in vivo. *Eur J Immunol* 1994;24:1523–1528.
220. O'Garra A, Umland S, De France T, Christiansen J. "B-cell factors" are pleiotropic. *Immunol Today* 1988;9:45–54.
221. Lederman S, Yellin M, Covey L, Cleary A, Callard R, Chess L. Non-antigen signals for B-cell growth and differentiation to antibody secretion. *Curr Opin Immunol* 1993;5:439–444.
222. Bartlett W, Purchio A, Fell H, Noelle R. Cognate interactions between helper T cells and B cells. VI. TGF-beta inhibits B cell activation and antigen-specific, physical interactions between Th and B cells. *Lymphokine Cytokine Res* 1991;10:177–183.
223. Kishimoto T, Akira S, Taga T. Interleukin-6 and its receptor: a paradigm for cytokines. *Science* 1992;258:593–597.
224. Rennick D, Berg D, Holland G. Interleukin 10: an overview. *Prog Growth Factor Res* 1992;4:207–227.
225. Coffman R, Lebman D, Shrader B. Transforming growth factor beta specifically enhances IgA production by lipopolysaccharide-stimulated murine B lymphocytes. *J Exp Med* 1989;170:1039–1044.
226. Germann T, Bongartz M, Dlugonska H, et al. Interleukin-12 profoundly up-regulates the synthesis of antigen-specific complement-fixing IgG2a, IgG2b and IgG3 antibody subclasses in vivo. *Eur J Immunol* 1995;25:823–829.
227. Snapper CM, Paul ES. Interferon-gamma and B cell stimulatory factor-1 reciprocally regulate Ig isotype production. *Science* 1987;236: 944–947.
228. Hammarstrom L, Smith CIE. IgG subclasses in bacterial infections. *Monogr Allergy* 1986;19:122.
229. Mosmann T, Moore K. The role of IL-10 in crossregulation of TH1 and TH2 responses. *Immunol Today* 1991;12:A49–53.
230. Trinchieri G, Scott P. The role of interleukin 12 in the immune response, disease and therapy. *Immunol Today* 1994;15:460–463.
231. Swain S. IL4 dictates T-cell differentiation. *Res Immunol* 1993;144: 616–620.
232. Duncan DD, Swain SL. Role of antigen-presenting cells in the polarized development of helper T cell subsets: evidence for differential cytokine production by Th0 cells in response to antigen presentation by B cells and macrophages. *Eur J Immunol* 1994;24: 2506–2514.
233. Bradley L, Yoshimoto K, Swain SL. The cytokines IL-4, IFN-gamma, and IL-12 regulate the development of subsets of memory effector helper T cells in vitro. *J Immunol* 1995;155:1713–1724.
234. Croft M, Carter L, Swain SL, Dutton RW. Generation of polarized antigen-specific CD8 effector populations: reciprocal action of interleukin (IL)-4 and IL-12 in promoting type 2 versus type 1 cytokine profiles. *J Exp Med* 1994;180:1715–1728.
235. Croft M, Swains SL. Recently activated naive CD4 T cells can help resting B cells, and can produce sufficient autocrine IL-4 to drive differentiation to secretion of T helper 2–type cytokine. *J Immunol* 1995;154:4269–4282.
236. Cohen J, Duke R, Fadok V, Sellins K. Apoptosis and programmed cell death in immunity. *Ann Rev Immunol* 1992;10:267–293.
237. Linette G, Korsmeyer S. Differentiation and cell death: lessons from the immune system. *Curr Opin Cell Biol* 1994;6:809–815.

238. Liu Y, Mason D, Johnson G, et al. Germinal center cells express bcl-2 protein after activation by signals which prevent their entry into apoptosis. *Eur J Immunol* 1991;21:1905–1910.
239. Strasser A, Whittingham S, Vaux D, et al. Enforced BCL2 expression in B-lymphoid cells prolongs antibody responses and elicits autoimmune disease. *Proc Natl Acad Sci U S A* 1991;88:8661–8665.
240. Uhr JW, Moller G. Regulatory effect of the antibody on the immune response. *Adv Immunol* 1968;8:81.
241. Roosnek E, Lanzavecchia A. Efficient and selective presentation of antigen–antibody complexes by rheumatoid factor B cells. *J Exp Med* 1991;173:487–489.
242. Dwyer J. Intravenous therapy with gamma globulin. *Adv Intern Med* 1987;32:111–135.
243. Burnet FM. A modification of Jerne's theory of antibody production using the concept of clonal selection. *Aust J Sci* 1957;20:67.
244. Foote J, Milstein C. Kinetic maturation of an immune response. *Nature* 1991;352:530.
245. Wysocki L, Manser T, Gefter M. Somatic evolution of variable region structures during an immune response. *Proc Natl Acad Sci U S A* 1986;83:1847–1851.
246. Vitetta E, Berton M, Burger C, Kepron M, Lee W, Yin X. Memory B and T cells. *Ann Rev Immunol* 1991;9:193–217.
247. McHeyzer-Williams MG, McLean MJ, Lalor PA, Nossal GJV. Antigen-driven B cell differentiation in vivo. *J Exp Med* 1993;178:295.
248. Rolink A, Melchers F. B lymphopoiesis in the mouse. *Adv Immunol* 1993;53:123–156.
249. Pfeffer K, Mak TW. Lymphocyte ontogeny and activation in gene targeted mutant mice. *Annu Rev Immunol* 1994;12:367.
250. Kearney J, Bartels J, Hamilton A, Lehuen, Solvason N, Vakil M. Development and function of the early B cell repertoire. *Intern Rev Immunol* 1992;8:247–257.
251. Dechanet J, Merville P, Durand I, Banchereau J, Miossec P. The ability of synoviocytes to support terminal differentiation of activated B cells may explain plasma cell accumulation in rheumatoid synovium. *J Clin Invest* 1995;95:456–463.
252. Jacob J, Kelsoe G, Rajewsky K, Weiss U. Intraclonal generation of antibody mutants in germinal centres. *Nature* 1991;354:389.
253. Berek C, Berger A, Apel M. Maturation of the immune response in germinal centers. *Cell* 1991;67:1121.
254. Reth M, Alt FW. Novel immunoglobulin heavy chains are produced from DJH gene segment rearrangements in lymphoid cells. *Nature* 1984;312:418.
255. Sakaguchi N, Melchers F. λ5, a new light chain–related locus selectively expressed in pre-B lymphocytes. *Nature* 1986;324:579–582.
256. Pillai S, Baltimore D. Formation of disulphide-linked μ2ω2 tetramers in pre–B cells by the 18K ω-immunoglobulin light chain. *Nature* 1987;329:172–174.
257. Kitamura D, Kudo A, Schaal S, Muller W, Melchers F, Rajewsky K. A critical role of λ5 protein in B cell development. *Cell* 1992;69:823.
258. Melchers F, Haasner D, Grawunder U, et al. Roles of IgH and L chains and of surrogate H and L chains in the development of cells of the B lymphocyte lineage. *Ann Rev Immunol* 1994;12:209–225.
259. Nishimoto N, Kubagawa H, Ohno T, Gartland G, Stankovic A, Cooper M. Normal pre–B cells express a receptor complex of mu heavy chains and surrogate light-chain proteins. *Proc Natl Acad Sci U S A* 1991;88:6284–6288.
260. Durandy A, Thuillier L, Forveille M, Fischer A. Phenotypic and functional characteristics of human newborns' B lymphocytes. *J Immunol* 1990;144:60.
261. Gadol N, Ault KA. Phenotypic and functional characterization of human Leu 1 (CD5) B cells. *Immunol Rev* 1986;93:23.
262. Hardy RR, Hayakawa K. CD5 B cells, a fetal B cell lineage. *Adv Immunol* 1994;55:297–339.
263. Kroese FG, Butcher EC, Stall AM, Lalor PA, Adams S, Herzenberg LA. Many of the IgA producing plasma cells in murine gut are derived from self-replenishing precursors in the peritoneal cavity. *Int Immunol* 1989;1:75–84.
264. Hayakawa K, Hardy RR, Honda M, Herzenberg LA, Steinberg AD, Herzenberg LA. Ly-1 B cells: functionally distinct lymphocytes that secrete IgM autoantibodies. *Proc Natl Acad Sci U S A* 1984;81: 2494–2498.
265. Herzenberg LA, Stall AM, Lalor PA, et al. The LY-1 B cell lineage. *Immunol Rev* 1986;93:81.
266. Kasturi KN, Mayer R, Bona CA, Scott VE, Sidman CL. Germline V genes encode viable motheaten mouse autoantibodies against thymocytes and red blood cells. *J Immunol* 1990;145:2304–2311.
267. Hayakawa K, Hardy RR, Parks DR, Herzenberg LA. The "Ly-1 B" cell subpopulation in normal, immunodefective, and autoimmune mice. *J Exp Med* 1983;157:202–218.
268. Casali P, Burastero SE, Nakamura M, Inghirami G, Notkins AL. Human lymphocytes making rheumatoid factor and antibody to ssDNA belong to Leu-1+ B-cell subset. *Science* 1987;236:77–81.
269. Kantor A, Herzenberg L. Origin of murine B cell lineages. *Ann Rev Immunol* 1993;11:501–538.
270. Reap EA, Sobel ES, Cohen PL, Eisenberg RA. Conventional B cells, not B-1 cells, are responsible for producing autoantibodies in lpr mice. *J Exp Med* 1993;177:69–78.
271. Reap EA, Sobel ES, Jennette JC, Cohen PL, Eisenberg RA. Conventional B cells, not B1 cells, are the source of autoantibodies in chronic graft-versus-host disease. *J Immunol* 1993;151:7316–7323.
272. Foster MH, MacDonald M, Barrett KJ, Madaio MP. VH gene analysis of spontaneously activated B cells in adult MRL-lpr/lpr mice. The J558 bias is not limited to classic lupus autoantibodies. *J Immunol* 1991;147:1504–1511.
273. Casali P, Notkins AL. Probing the human B cell repertoire with EBV: polyreactive antibodies and CD5+ B lymphocytes. *Annu Rev Immunol* 1989;7:513.
274. Kasaian MT, Casali P. Identification and analysis of a novel human surface CD5– B lymphocyte subset producing natural antibodies. *J Immunol* 1992;148:2690.
275. Kearney J. Formation of autoantibodies, including anti-cytokine antibodies, is a hallmark of the immune response of early B cells. *J Interferon Res* 1994;14:151–152.
276. Ternynck T, Avrameas S. Murine natural monoclonal autoantibodies: a study of their polyspecificities and their affinities. *Immunol Rev* 1986;94:99.
277. Chai SK, Mantovani L, Kasaian MT, Casali P. Natural autoantibodies. *Adv Exp Med Biol* 1994;347:147–159.
278. Pisetsky DS, Caster SA. The B-cell repertoire for autoantibodies: frequency of precursor cells for anti-DNA antibodies. *Cell Immunol* 1982;72:294–305.
279. Dighiero G, Lymberi P, Holmberg D, Lundquist I, Coutinho A, Avrameas S. High frequency of natural autoantibodies in normal newborn mice. *J Immunol* 1985;134:765–771.
280. Underwood JR, Pedersen JS, Chalmers PJ, Toh BH. Hybrids from normal, germ-free, nude and neonatal mice produce monoclonal autoantibodies to eight different intracellular structures. *Clin Exp Immunol* 1985;60:417–426.
281. Streibich CC, Miceli RM, Schulze DH, Kelsoe G, Cerny J. Antigen-binding repertoire and Ig H chain gene usage among B cell hybridomas from normal and autoimmune mice. *J Immunol* 1990;144: 1857–1865.
282. Souroujon M, White-Scharf ME, Andre-Schwartz J, Gefter ML, Schwartz RS. Preferential autoantibody reactivity of the preimmune B cell repertoire in normal mice. *J Immunol* 1988;140:4173–4179.
283. Sanz I, Casali P, Thomas JW, Notkins AL, Capra JD. Nucleotide sequences of eight human natural antibody VH regions reveals apparent restricted use of VH families. *J Immunol* 1989;142:4054.
284. Bellon B, Manheimer-Lory A, Monestier M, et al. High frequency of autoantibodies bearing cross-reactive idiotopes among hybridomas using VH7183 genes prepared from normal and autoimmune murine strains. *J Clin Invest* 1987;79:1044–1053.
285. Holmberg DH. High connectivity, natural antibodies preferentially use 7183 and QUPC 52 VH families. *Eur J Immunol* 1987;17:399–403.
286. Avrameas S. Natural autoantibodies: from "horror autotoxicus" to "gnothi seauton." *Immunol Today* 1991;12:154.
287. Mantovani L, Wilder RL, Casali P. Human rheumatoid B-1a (CD5+ B) cells make somatically hypermutated high affinity IgM rheumatoid factors. *J Immunol* 1993;151:473–488.
288. Ichiyoshi Y, Zhou M, Casali P. A human anti-insulin IgG autoantibody apparently arises through clonal selection from an insulin-specific "germ-line" natural antibody template. *J Immunol* 1995;154: 226–238.
289. Holmberg D, Anderson A, Carlson L, Forsgren S. Establishment and functional implications of B cell connectivity. *Immunol Rev* 1989; 110:889.
290. Elliott M, Kearney J. Idiotypic regulation of development of the B-cell repertoire. *Ann N Y Acad Sci* 1992;651:336–345.

291. Burrows P, Kearney J, Schroede H Jr, Cooper M. Normal B lymphocyte differentiation [Review]. *Baillieres Clin Haematol* 1993;6: 785–806.
292. Gu H, Tarlinton D, Muller W, Rajewsky K, Forster I. Most peripheral B cells in mice are ligand selected. *J Exp Med* 1991;173:1357–1371.
293. Forster I, Rajewsky K. The bulk of the peripheral B cell pool in mice is stable and not rapidly renewed from the bone marrow. *Proc Natl Acad Sci U S A* 1990;87:4781.
294. Goodnow CC, Adelstein S, Basten A. The need for central and peripheral tolerance in the B cell repertoire. *Science* 1990;248: 1373–1379.
295. Klaus G. Irreversible receptor modulation on B lymphocytes and the control of antibody-forming cells by antigen. *Immunol Rev* 1979;43: 96–107.
296. Nemazee D. Mechanisms and meaning of B-lymphocyte tolerance. *Res Immunol* 1992;143:272–275.
297. Nemazee D. Promotion and prevention of autoimmunity by B lymphocytes. *Curr Opin Immunol* 1993;5:866–872.
298. Tsubata T, Murakami M, Nisitani S, Honjo T. Molecular mechanisms for B lymphocyte selection: induction and regulation of antigen-receptor–mediated apoptosis of mature B cells in normal mice and their defect in autoimmunity-prone mice. *Philos Trans R Soc Lond [Biol]* 1994;345:297–301.
299. Nossal GJV. Cellular and molecular mechanisms of B lymphocyte tolerance. *Adv Immunol* 1992;52:283.
300. Nossal GJV. Immunologic tolerance. In: Paul WE, eds. *Fundamental immunology*. 2nd ed. New York: Raven; 1989:571–576.
301. Nossal GJV. Immunologic tolerance: collaboration between antigen and lymphokines. *Science* 1989;245:147–153.
302. Nossal GJ. Tolerance and ways to break it. *Ann N Y Acad Sci* 1993; 690:34–41.
303. Adams TE. Tolerance to self-antigens in transgenic mice. *Mol Biol Med* 1990;7:341–357.
304. Basten A, Brink R, Peake P, et al. Self tolerance in the B-cell repertoire. *Immunol Rev* 1991;122:5–19.
305. Goodnow CC. Transgenic mice and analysis of B-cell tolerance. *Annu Rev Immunol* 1992;10:489–518.
306. Kronenberg M. Self-tolerance and autoimmunity. *Cell* 1991;65: 537–542.
307. Schwartz RH. Acquistion of immunologic self-tolerance. *Cell* 1989; 57:1073–1081.
308. Sinha A, Lopez MT, McDevitt HO. Autoimmune diseases: the failure of self tolerance. *Science* 1990;248:1380–1388.
309. Tsubata T, Wu J, Honjo T. B-cell apoptosis induced by antigen receptor crosslinking is blocked by a T-cell signal through CD40. *Nature* 1993;364:645–648.
310. Durie F, Foy T, Noelle R. The role of CD40 and its ligand (gp39) in peripheral and central tolerance and its contribution to autoimmune disease. *Res Immunol* 1994;145:200–5,244–9.
311. Boussiotis V, Gribben JG, Freeman GJ, Nadler LM. Blockade in the CD28 co-stimulatory pathway: a means to induce tolerance. *Curr Opin Immunol* 1994;6:797–807.
312. Klaus S, Berberich I, Shu G, Clark E. CD40 and its ligand in the regulation of humoral immunity. *Semin Immunol* 1994;6:279–286.
313. Nemazee DA, Burki K. Clonal deletion of B lymphocytes in a transgenic mouse bearing anti-MHC class I antibody genes. *Nature* 1989; 337:562–566.
314. Nemazee D, Buerki K. Clonal deletion of autoreactive B lymphocytes in bone marrow chimeras. *Proc Natl Acad Sci U S A* 1989;86: 8039–8043.
315. Nemazee D, Russell D, Arnold B, Haemmerling G, Allison J, Miller JFAP, Morahan G, Buerki K. Clonal deletion of autospecific B lymphocytes. *Immunol Rev* 1991;122:117–131.
316. Hartley SB, Crosbie J, Brink R, Kantor AB, Basten A, Goodnow CC. Elimination from peripheral lymphoid tissues of self-reactive B lymphocytes recognizing membrane-bound antigens. *Nature* 1991;353: 765–769.
317. Okamoto M, Murakami M, Shimizu A, et al. A transgenic model of autoimmune hemolytic anemia. *J Exp Med* 1992;175:71–79.
318. Murakami M, Tsubata T, Okamoto M, et al. Antigen-induced apoptotic death of Ly-1 B cells responsible for autoimmune disease in transgenic mice. *Nature* 1992;357:77–80.
319. Chen C, Radic MZ, Erikson J, et al. Deletion and editing of B cells that express antibodies to DNA. *J Immunol* 1994;152:1970–1982.
320. Chen C, Nagy Z, Radic MZ, et al. The site and stage of anti-DNA B-cell deletion. *Nature* 1995;373:252–255.
321. Brink R, Goodnow CC, Crosbie J, et al. Immunoglobulin M and D antigen receptors are both capable of mediating B lymphocyte activation, deletion, or anergy after interaction with specific antigen. *J Exp Med* 1992;176:991–1005.
322. Hartley S, Cooke M, Fulcher D, et al. Elimination of self-reactive B lymphocytes proceeds in two stages: arrested development and cell death. *Cell* 1993;72:325–335.
323. Tiegs SL, Russell DM, Nemazee D. Receptor editing in self-reactive bone marrow B cells. *J Exp Med* 1993;177:1009–1020.
324. Gay D, Saunders T, Camper S, Weigert M. Receptor editing: an approach by autoreactive B cells to escape tolerance. *J Exp Med* 1993;177:999–1008.
325. Radic MZ, Erikson J, Litwin S, Weigert M. B lymphocytes may escape tolerance by revising their antigen receptors. *J Exp Med* 1993; 177:1165–1173.
326. Prak EL, Trounstine M, Huszar D, Weigert M. Light chain editing in kappa-deficient animals: a potential mechanism of B cell tolerance. *J Exp Med* 1994;180:1805–1815.
327. Goodnow CC, Crosbie J, Adelstein S, et al. Altered immunoglobulin expression and functional silencing of self-reactive B lymphocytes in transgenic mice. *Nature* 1988;334:676–682.
328. Goodnow CC, Crosbie J, Adelstein S, et al. Clonal silencing of self-reactive B lymphocytes in a transgenic mouse model. *Cold Spring Harb Symp Quant Biol* 1989;54:907–920.
329. Goodnow CC, Crosbie J, Jorgensen H, Brink RA, Basten A. Induction of self-tolerance in mature peripheral B lymphocytes. *Nature* 1989;342:385–391.
330. Tsao BP, Chow A, Cheroutre H, Song YW, McGrath ME, Kronenberg M. B cells are anergic in transgenic mice that express IgM anti-DNA antibodies. *Eur J Immunol* 1993;23:2332–2339.
331. Erikson J, Radic MZ, Camper SA, Hardy RR, Carmack C, Weigert M. Expression of anti-DNA immunoglobulin transgenes in non-autoimmune mice. *Nature* 1991;349:331–334.
332. Erikson J, Radic M, Feld J, Kavaler J, Roark J, Gay D, Weigert M. Tolerance and autoimmunity in anti-DNA transgenic mice [Abstract]. *J Cell Biochem* 1993;17(suppl):248.
333. Bell S, Goodnow C. A selective defect in IgM antigen receptor synthesis and transport causes loss of cell surface IgM expression on tolerant B lymphocytes. *EMBO J* 1994;13:816–826.
334. Cooke MP, Heath AW, Shokat KM, et al. Immunoglobulin signal transduction guides the specificity of B cell–T cell interactions and is blocked in tolerant self-reactive B cells. *J Exp Med* 1994;179:425–438.
335. Adelstein S, Pritchard-Briscoe H, Anderson TA, et al. Induction of self-tolerance in T cells but not B cells of transgenic mice expressing little self antigen. *Science* 1991;251:1223–1225.
336. Kappler J, Roehm N, Marrack P. T cell tolerance by clonal elimination in the thymus. *Cell* 1987;49:273–280.
337. Kappler J, Staerz U, White J, Marrack P. Self-tolerance eliminates T cells specific for Mls-modified products of the major histocompatibility complex. *Nature* 1988;332:35–40.
338. Israel EJ, Simister N, Freiberg E, Caplan A, Walker WA. Immunoglobulin G binding sites on the human foetal intestine: a possible mechanism for the passive transfer of immunity from mother to infant. *Immunology* 1993;79:77–81.
339. Story CM, Mikulska JE, Simister NE. A major histocompatibility complex class I-like Fc receptor cloned from human placenta: possible role in transfer of immunoglobulin G from mother to fetus. *J Exp Med* 1994;180:2377–2381.
340. Salmon JE, Brogle NL, Edberg JC, Kimberly RP. Fcγ receptor III induces actin polymerization in human neutrophils and primes phagocytosis mediated by Fcγ receptor II. *J Immunol* 1991;146:997.
341. Huizinga TWJ, Kemenade Fv, Koenderman L, et al. The 40-kDa Fcγ receptor (FcRII) on human neutrophils is essential for the IgG-induced respiratory burst and IgG-induced phagocytosis. *J Immunol* 1989;142:2365.
342. Miettinen HM, Rose JK, Mellman I. Fc receptor isoforms exhibit different capabilities for coated pit localization as a result of cytoplasmic domain heterogeneity. *Cell* 1989;58:317.
343. Engelhardt W, Gorczytza H, Butterweck A, Monkemann H, Frey J. Structural requirements of cytoplasmic domains of the human macrophage Fcγ receptor IIa and B cell Fcγ receptor IIb2 for the endocytosis of immune complexes. *Eur J Immunol* 1991;21:2227.

344. Miettinen HM, Matter K, Hunziker W, Rose JK, Mellman I. Fc receptor endocytosis is controlled by a cytoplasmic domain determinant that actively prevents coated pit localization. *J Cell Biol* 1992;116: 875–888.
345. Amigorena S, Bonnerot C, Drake JR, et al. Cytoplasmic domain heterogeneity and functions of IgG Fc receptors in B lymphocytes. *Science* 1992;256:1808.
346. Cohen BE, Rosenthal AS, Paul WE. Antigen-macrophage interaction. II. Relative roles of cytophilic antibodies and other membrane sites. *J Immunol* 1973;111:820.
347. Celis E, Chang TW. Antibodies to hepatitis B surface antigen potentiate the response of human T lymphocyte clones to the same antigen. *Science* 1984;224:297.
348. Graziano RF, Fanger MW. FcγRI and FcγRII on monocytes and granulocytes are cytotoxic trigger molecules for tumor cells. *J Immunol* 1987;139:3536.
349. Unkeless JC, Scigliano E, Freedman VH. Structure and function of human and murine receptors for IgG. *Annu Rev Immunol* 1988;6: 251–281.
350. Van de Winkel JGJ, Anderson CL. Biology of human immunoglobulin G Fc receptors. *J Leukoc Biol* 1991;49:511.
351. Hulett MD, Hogarth PM. Molecular basis of Fc receptor function. *Adv Immunol* 1994;57:1–127.
352. Coffman RL, Carty J. A T cell activity that enhances polyclonal IgE production and its inhibition by interferon-γ. *J Immunol* 1986;136: 949.
353. Pene J, Rousset F, Briere F, et al. IgE production by normal human B cells induced by alloreactive T cell clones is mediated by interleukin 4 and suppressed by interferon γ. *J Immunol* 1988;141:1218.
354. Snapper CM, Finkelman FD, Paul WE. Regulation of IgG1 and IgE production by interleukin 4. *Immunol Rev* 1988;102:51.
355. Kuhn R, Rajewsky K, Muller W. Generation and analysis of interleukin-4 deficient mice. *Science* 1991;254:707–710.
356. Isakson P, Pure E, Vitetta ES, Krammer PH. T cell–derived B cell differentiation factor(s). Effect on the isotype switch of murine B cells. *J Exp Med* 1982;155:734–748.
357. Lundgren M, Persson U, Larsson P, et al. Interleukin 4 induces synthesis of IgE and IgG4 in human B cells. *Eur J Immunol* 1989;19: 1311.
358. Fujieda S, Zhang K, Saxon A. IL-4 plus CD40 monoclonal antibody induces human B cells gamma subclass–specific isotype switch: switching to gamma 1, gamma 3, and gamma 4, but not gamma 2. *J Immunol* 1995;155:2318–2328.
359. Coffman RL, Shrader B, Carty J, Mosmann TR, Bond MW. A mouse T cell product that preferentially enhances IgA production. I. Biologic characterization. *J Immunol* 1987;139:3685–3689.
360. Bond MW, Shrader B, Mosmann T, Coffman RL. A mouse T cell product that preferentially enhances IgA production. II. Physicochemical characterization. *J Immunol* 1987;139:3691–3696.
361. Noelle R, Shepherd D, Fell H. Cognate interaction between T helper cells and B cells. VII. Role of contact and lymphokines in the expression of germ-line and mature gamma 1 transcripts. *J Immunol* 1992; 149:1164–1169.
362. Briere F, Servet-Delprat C, Bridon J-M, Saint-Remy J-M, Banchereau J. Human interleukin 10 induces naive surface immunoglobulin D+ (sIgD+) B cells to secrete IgG1 and IgG3. *J Exp Med* 1994;179: 757–762.
363. Mosmann TR. Properties and functions of Interleukin-10. *Adv Immunol* 1994;56:1–26.
364. Defrance T, Vanbervliet B, Briere F, Durand I, Rousset F, Banchereau J. Interleukin 10 and transforming growth factor β cooperate to induce anti–CD40-activated naive human B cells to secrete immunoglobulin A. *J Exp Med* 1992;175:671.
365. Germann T, Bongartz M, Dlugonska H, et al. Interleukin-12 profoundly up-regulates the synthesis of antigen-specific complement-fixing IgG2a, IgG2b and IgG3 antibody subclasses in vivo. *Eur J Immunol* 1995;25:823–829.
366. Trinchieri G, Scott P. The role of interleukin 12 in the immune response, disease and therapy. *Immunol Today* 1994;15:460–463.
367. Punnonen J, Aversa GG, Cocks BG, et al. Interleukin 13 induces interleukin-4–independent IgG4 and IgE synthesis and CD23 expression by human B cells. *Proc Natl Acad Sci U S A* 1993;90:3730.
368. de Vries J, Zurawski G. Immunoregulatory properties of IL-13: its potential role in atopic disease. *Int Arch Allergy Immunol* 1995;106: 175–179.
369. Snapper CM, Paul ES. Interferon-gamma and B cell stimulatory factor-1 reciprocally regulate Ig isotype production. *Science* 1987;236: 944–947.
370. Snapper C, McIntyre T, Mandler R, et al. Induction of IgG3 secretion by interferon gamma: a model for T cell–independent class switching in response to T cell–independent type 2 antigens. *J Exp Med* 1992; 175:1367–1371.
371. Berton M, Uhr JW, Vitetta ES. Synthesis of germline gamma 1 immunoglobulin heavy-chain transcripts in resting B cells: induction by interleukin 4 and inhibition by interferon gamma. *Proc Natl Acad Sci U S A* 1989;86:2829.
372. Coffman R, Lebman D, Shrader B. Transforming growth factor beta specifically enhances IgA production by lipopolysaccharide-stimulated murine B lymphocytes. *J Exp Med* 1989;170:1039–1044.
373. Stavnezer J. Regulation of antibody production and class switching by TGF-β. *J Immunol* 1995;155:1647–1651.
374. Roper R, Brown D, Phipps R. Prostaglandin E2 promotes B lymphocyte Ig isotype switching to IgE. *J Immunol* 1995;154:162–170.
375. Ysse H, Aversa G, Punnonen J, Cocks B, Vries JEd. Regulation of IgE synthesis by T cells and cytokines. *Ann Fr Anesth Reanimation* 1993;12:109–113.
376. Schwartz RS. Jumping genes and the immunoglobulin V gene system. *N Engl J Med* 1995;333:42–44.

Immunologic Renal Diseases,
edited by E. G. Neilson and W. G. Couser.
Lippincott-Raven Publishers, Philadelphia 1997.

CHAPTER 14

Mechanisms of Immune Complex Formation and Deposition in Renal Structures

Christine K. Abrass

The immune system plays a pivotal role in distinguishing self from nonself, a function that is critical to host defense. The immune response to foreign antigens initiates inflammatory reactions that account for clinical manifestations. When appropriately regulated, these reactions are effective in eliminating the foreign invader, usually an infectious agent, and restoring health. When these reactions are ineffective or inappropriately regulated, they lead to perpetual inflammation and/or immunologic response to self-antigens that cause progressive organ damage.

In 1837, the link between the immune response to exogenous antigens and renal disease was reported by Bright in his detailed pathologic descriptions of acute glomerulonephritis (GN) (1). Shortly after von Behring introduced the use of hyperimmune horse serum injections to treat children with diphtheria, reports of toxic reactions known as "serum exanthem" began to appear (2). Recognition that an immune response can initiate inflammation and tissue injury was detailed by Maurice Arthus in 1903 (3) in his classic studies in which intradermal injections of horse serum into sensitized rabbits produced local edema, hemorrhage, and neutrophil infiltration. Shortly thereafter, the systemic form of the reaction typically occurring in recipients of serum therapy was described by von Pirquet and Schick (4). Their monograph described the syndrome of serum sickness that occurs 10 days after serum injection and is typified by fever, skin rash, arthralgia, and lymphadenopathy. By this time, similarities between serum sickness and acute GN were widely appreciated; however, many years passed before a detailed understanding of the pathogenic role of immune complexes (ICs) was achieved.

C. K. Abrass: Department of Medicine, Veterans Affairs Medical Center, Seattle, Washington 98108.

The development of immunofluorescence microscopy in the 1950s was an important advance that allowed the detection of immunoglobulin (Ig) deposits in association with GN. With the use of this tool, human glomerular disease was characterized by the pattern of immune deposits. Virtually all forms of human GN are thought to be immune mediated (Table 1) and approximately 85% have Ig deposits. A number of animal models of GN were developed with histopathologic patterns that mimicked human disease. These models have been invaluable in studies of the immunopathogenesis of GN. The kinetics of IC formation, clearance from the circulation, deposition in tissues, and pathology of glomerular lesions were well described by Germuth, Cochrane, and Dixon (5–11) in studies of rabbits with acute and chronic serum sickness induced by injections of bovine serum albumin. In the ensuing 40 years considerable data have defined the exact nature of the requirements for antigen, antibody, complement components, and IC interactions with cells of the immune system and those intrinsic to the glomerulus. A detailed review of this progress is the subject of this chapter. The reader is also referred to other comprehensive reviews of IC-mediated GN (ICGN) (12–15).

IC FORMATION

Definition

An IC is composed of antigen, primary antibody, and secondarily bound anti-Igs and complement components. Each of the components of the IC takes on new biologic functions as a result of being complexed into this macromolecule. An IC disease is one in which organ dysfunction results from injury caused by formation or deposition of IC in tissues rather than the agent or event that initiates the IC formation. The immune system is tradi-

TABLE 1. *Mechanisms of immune-mediated renal disease*

- I. Antibody-mediated, Ig deposits
  - In situ immune deposit formation
    - Endogenous antigens (e.g., anti-GBM disease, anti-TBM disease)
    - Exogenous antigens (e.g., drug–hapten conjugates and other planted antigens)
  - CIC deposition
    - Endogenous antigens (e.g., SLE)
    - Exogenous antigens (e.g., mixed cryoglobulinemia)
- II. Cell-mediated renal disease, cellular infiltrate without immune deposits
  - e.g., rapidly progressive without immune deposits, Wegeners granulomatosis, most forms of interstitial renal disease
- III. Immune cytokine mediated, no cellular infiltrate or immune deposits
  - e.g., minimal change disease, focal and segmental glomerulosclerosis

tionally divided into the humoral and cellular arms. To some degree this distinction is artificial because the cellular arm is critical to initiation and amplification of antibody production. The resultant IC is critical to activation of the cellular arm, which carries out phagocytosis, cell-mediated cytotoxicity, and other effector responses. Coordinated regulation of these responses is essential to the normal immune response, but when they become dysregulated, ICs accumulate, form, or deposit in tissues and cause disease.

Biochemical Properties of Antigens

Biochemical characteristics of circulating antigen play important roles in determining the biologic activity of ICs (Table 2). The net charge, epitope valence, size, polysaccharide content, blood clearance kinetics, ability to bind to glomerular structures, and similarity of peptide sequences within the antigen to host proteins all influence the properties of the macromolecular IC. Each of these properties of the antigen also has a profound effect on the class, subclass, and affinity of antibody that is produced. In addition to the biochemical characteristics of the antigen, other factors are important (Table 2). Soluble antigens are transported throughout the body by the circulation. These can be endogenous or exogenous, which influences their pathogenic potential. Endogenous antigens are usually continuously present in low concentrations; thus, their persistence leads to perpetual IC formation and chronic progression of disease. Exogenous antigens, particularly viruses, can replicate, leading to a large acute antigen load. If the virus is successfully eliminated from the body, acute nephritis can resolve. When acute inflammation has not been replaced by scar, complete healing can occur. In some cases, similar to endogenous antigens, chronic persistent viral infection (e.g., hepatitis C) leads to chronic ICGN. Tissue-fixed antigens (native or planted) also can participate in IC formation. Their tissue distribution dictates the location and mediation of the inflammatory response. If planted antigens are exogenous in origin, they may cause transient injury. When the fixed antigen is an integral part of the cell or its supporting structure, it is likely that antibody will be continuously deposited, leading to progressive accumulation of glomerular immune deposits.

TABLE 2. *Factors that influence glomerular deposition of ICs*

- Factors related to the kidney
  - Blood flow
  - Intraglomerular pressure
  - Net negative charge of the glomerular capillary wall
  - Kidney receptors (e.g., Fc, C3b)
- Factors related to the IC
  - Quantity
  - Rate of formation
  - Size
  - Antigen
    - Exogenous/endogenous/replicating
    - Size
    - Charge
    - Blood clearance kinetics
    - Sialic acid content
    - Polysaccharide content
    - Valence
    - Ability to bind to glomerular structures
    - Ability to elicit antibody production
  - Antibody
    - Class, subclass
    - Size
    - Charge
    - Affinity, avidity
    - Rheumatoid factors
    - Anti-idiotypic antibodies
    - Blood clearance kinetics
    - Specificity, ability to cross-react with renal structures
    - Precipitability (valence, Fc–Fc interactions)
  - Antigen–antibody ratio
  - Lattice structure
  - Complement content
- Systemic factors
  - Mononuclear phagocyte system function
    - Systemic
    - Local, intrinsic glomerular cells and infiltration by PMNs and monocytes
  - Hemodynamic
    - Blood pressure
    - Turbulence
    - Prostaglandins
    - Angiotensin II
  - Vascular permeability
    - Steroids
    - Vasoactive amines
    - Cytokines (e.g., IL-1)
  - Hormonal status
    - Catecholamines (stress)
    - Diabetes mellitus

Antigen Charge

Molecular charge influences circulating antigen binding to structures within the body (16,17). For instance, the glomerular basement membrane (GBM) is negatively charged as a result of its high content of heparan sulfate proteoglycans; thus, antigens and IC with a net positive charge are more likely to be trapped within the glomerulus. Cationic substances in the body are predominantly intracellular, whereas most cell surfaces and serum proteins are negatively charged. Cationic antigens induce potent immune responses because of charge-facilitated binding to immune cells. DNA, histones, and platelet factor 4 (18) are highly charged, cationic materials. This feature contributes to their immunogenicity and trapping within vascular beds (19). When injected, cationic proteins artificially conjugated to albumin bind to GBM through the cationic moiety (20). Although cationic antigens appear to be more immunogenic and have a propensity for deposition in the glomerular vascular bed, anionic antigens still can participate in ICGN.

Antigen Size and Antigen Valence

Antigen size influences both the valence of the antigen and the final size of the IC. Complex protein antigens usually have several epitopes that serve as binding sites for antibody. This provides the opportunity for several different antibodies to bind to the same antigen and creates the potential for cross-linking between antigens. When ICs are small, they are readily filtered across the glomerular capillary wall and make their way into the mesangium, subendothelial, and sometimes subepithelial spaces. As the glomerular filtrate is formed, solutes and water pass on through, leaving larger proteins and ICs behind. This results in increased local concentration of proteins that are trapped, which facilitates cross-linking of unoccupied antigenic epitopes and unbound antibody leading to lattice formation (21,22). Large lattices are a hallmark of electron-dense deposits, which are frequently identified in glomerular disease by electron microscopy. These larger ICs are resistant to solubilization by complement or excess antigen; therefore, they can persist for long periods of time (23). When an antigen has a limited number of epitopes to which antibody can bind, ICs tend to remain small. These easily penetrate capillary walls and readily deposit in tissues, yet they are also rapidly removed from those sites. Persistence of ICs in tissue with additional cross-linking has been shown to influence their inflammatory potential. These principles are summarized in Figure 1.

Antigen Clearance Kinetics

The structure of the antigen, its size, charge, and polysaccharide side chains all influence clearance kinetics from plasma. The liver contains galactose receptors that remove desialated serum proteins and facilitate clearance of IC containing such modified antigens. In contrast, heavily glycosylated antigens persist in the circulation and may lead to increased glomerular accumulation (24). Antigens that are rapidly cleared by the liver and spleen without need for antibody opsonization influence the rate of IC formation, the amount of IC formed, and, thus, the amount delivered to kidney and other tissues.

Ability to Interact with Glomerular Structures

The glomerular capillary wall is a unique structure in that the endothelial cell is penetrated with fenestrae, the GBM is a dynamic gel with a net negative charge, and a large volume of filtrate transits the capillary wall under high pressure. Furthermore, each of the intrinsic glomerular cells is richly endowed with surface molecules that can interact with antigens or antibodies and may themselves be immunogenic. A multitude of biochemical interactions may favor accumulation of free or complexed antigens in this site. Subsequent binding of antibody can initiate an inflammatory reaction. Specific examples (e.g., apoferritin, cationized albumin or IgG, protamine sulfate, possibly DNA, and streptococcal antigens) are discussed in chapters related to specific diseases.

Antigen Characteristics Influence the Type of Antibody Response

Biochemical characteristics of antigen influence the type and amount of antibody that is produced, as well as the unique peptide sequences that are chosen as epitopes. Antigens are internalized by phagocytes and other antigen-presenting cells where they are enzymatically cleaved to create small peptide fragments. These fragments associate with major histocompatibility complex class II determinants and are expressed on the cell surface. In this context, they are presented to B cells for initiation of antibody synthesis and to T cells for amplification of antibody synthesis and initiation of cell-mediated immune responses. Intracellular enzymes dictate the cleavage products and thus the possible epitopes. Genetic variants in class II antigens determine which proteolytic fragment will become class II bound and thus which epitopes are selected for presentation and antibody recognition (25–27). In turn, the biochemical characteristics of the epitope dictate the class, subclass, charge, and avidity of antibody produced. Thymus-dependent antigens and antigens with repeating polysaccharide polymers are most likely to initiate IgM antibody synthesis. IgG3 is most commonly produced in response to carbohydrate antigens, and IgG1 is usually stimulated by protein antigens. IgA antibodies are produced in response to antigens that enter through the respiratory or gastrointestinal

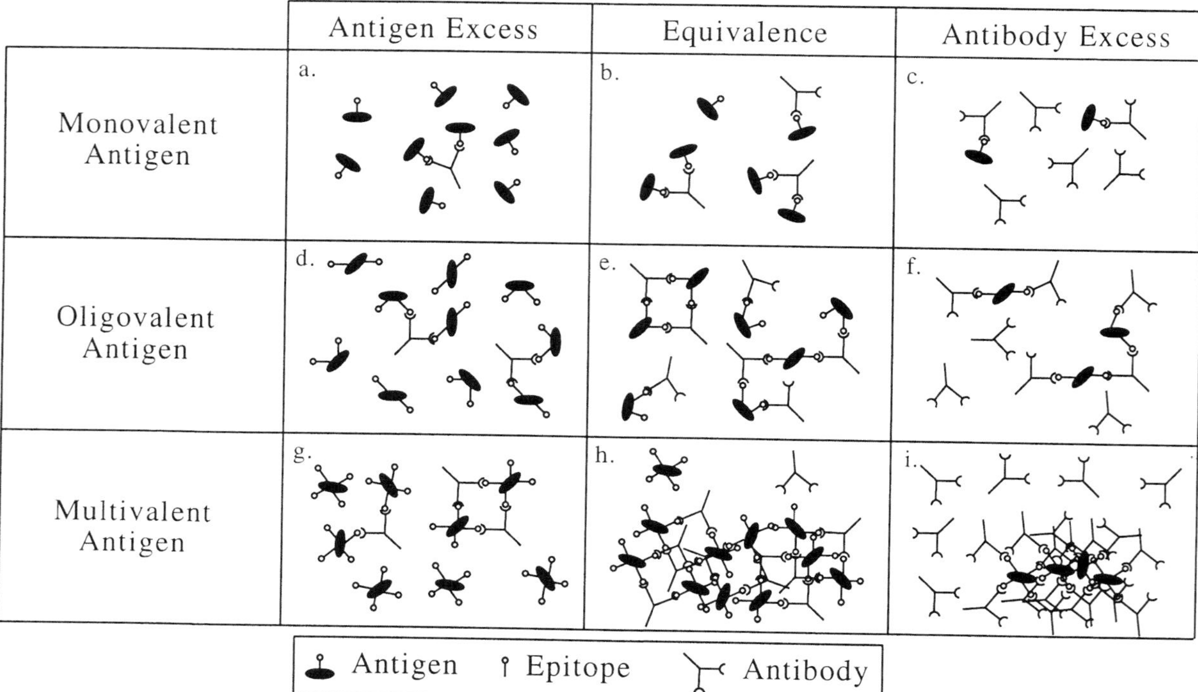

FIG. 1. IC formation is a function of the concentration of antigen and antibody, as well as the number (valence) of epitopes on the antigen. When the antigen is oligovalent (A, B, C), increasing antibody concentration yields higher concentrations of antibodies per antigen molecule, but the size of the lattice is limited. Nonprecipitating ICs result. In the bottom panel a simplified diagram shows what occurs when the antigen has repeating identical epitopes or has multiple different epitopes reactive with different antibodies. Small soluble ICs form when antigen is in excess. These ICs fix complement poorly and evade both Fc- and C3b-receptor–mediated clearance mechanisms. As the antibody to antigen ratio increases, a point of maximum precipitation occurs and is termed equivalence. When adjacent antibodies are in close proximity, hydrogen bonding occurs between Fc regions further compacting the ICs. When these large latticed ICs form in the circulation they are usually rapidly cleared by the MPS. As more antibody is formed and circulates in excess of antigen, multiple antibodies with single occupied antigen combining sites are found. These ICs may be soluble or form precipitates. [Adapted with permission (77).]

tracts, sites of lymphoid tissue rich in IgA-producing B cells. The net charge of antibody formed is usually the opposite of the charge of the antigen. Cationic antigens are also more likely to generate production of rheumatoid factors. The class and subclass of antibody determine complement activation, clearance kinetics, and the ability of ICs to initiate secondary inflammatory reactions (25, 28). In these ways, biochemical characteristics of antigens influence the character of the primary antibody and the biological properties of the ICs that are formed.

Properties of Antibodies

Characteristics of antibodies that influence the biologic properties of the ICs and their ability to deposit in the kidney include class, subclass, idiotype, size, affinity or avidity, charge, cross-reactivities with renal or other endogenous structures, blood clearance kinetics, and complement-fixing ability (Table 2). During the course of an immune response, the spectrum of antibodies generated changes. These changes in turn influence the rate of clearance from the circulation, the ability to deposit in the kidney, and the type and potency of secondary inflammatory reactions. This evolution in character of antibody may account for the commonly observed periods of clinical disease activity and remission such as occurs in lupus and other autoimmune diseases.

Antibody Structure

Antibodies are composed of class-defining heavy chains bound to light chains (Fig. 2). Each chain contains a constant carboxy terminus and a variable amino terminus. The conformational structure created by the variable regions of the combined heavy and light chains determines the antigen-combining site. Antibody affinity is determined by the structure of the antigen-combining site. The likelihood that antibody will stay bound to antigen or avidity is a function of affinity and the number of antigen-combining sites. Each IgG molecule has two and each IgM molecule has ten antigen-binding sites. These features determine the functional activities of the antibody.

Initial stimulation of the entire pool of antigen-reactive B cells leads to a polyclonal response of low-affinity antibodies, predominantly IgM; however, as the antibody response matures, the variable regions that determine antigen specificity are spliced with different constant regions. This generates the final heavy chain class (IgM, IgG, IgA, IgD, IgE) and subclass (IgG1, IgG2, IgG3, IgG4, etc). The population of B cells ultimately responsible for a pathogenic response in GN is a highly selected subset of the original B cells that express surface Ig that recognize a particular antigen. Those cells expressing higher affinity antibody preferentially bind antigen and become amplified by clonal expansion. These antibodies are usually IgG. A small population of B cells gain supremacy to create an oligoclonal response. As these cells are further amplified and driven to secrete antibody, additional somatic mutations alter the fine specificities and cross-reactivities of the antibodies produced. The acquisition of new cross-reactivities may explain the onset of clinical disease in the course of an otherwise benign immune response such as occurs in post-streptococcal GN. Thus, understanding factors that regulate the maturation of this antibody response are critical to understanding disease pathogenesis [generation of antibody diversity has been reviewed elsewhere (25,28,29)]. The application of these principles to GN has been best studied in systemic lupus erythematosis (SLE) and is reviewed in greater detail in Chapter 48.

THE IC AS A MACROMOLECULE

Once antigen has combined with antibody, a new macromolecule exists. By virtue of this reaction, conformational changes occur in both antigen and antibody that expose new regions that through charge or other binding activities may interact with the glomerulus. Whereas individual components of IC may be relatively inert, the IC is not. Conformational changes in bound antibody "activate" complement binding and interaction with Fc receptors (FcRs) of cells of the immune system and intrinsic glomerular cells. When ICs form in situ or passively deposit in glomeruli from the circulation, they can activate infiltrating leukocytes or intrinsic glomerular

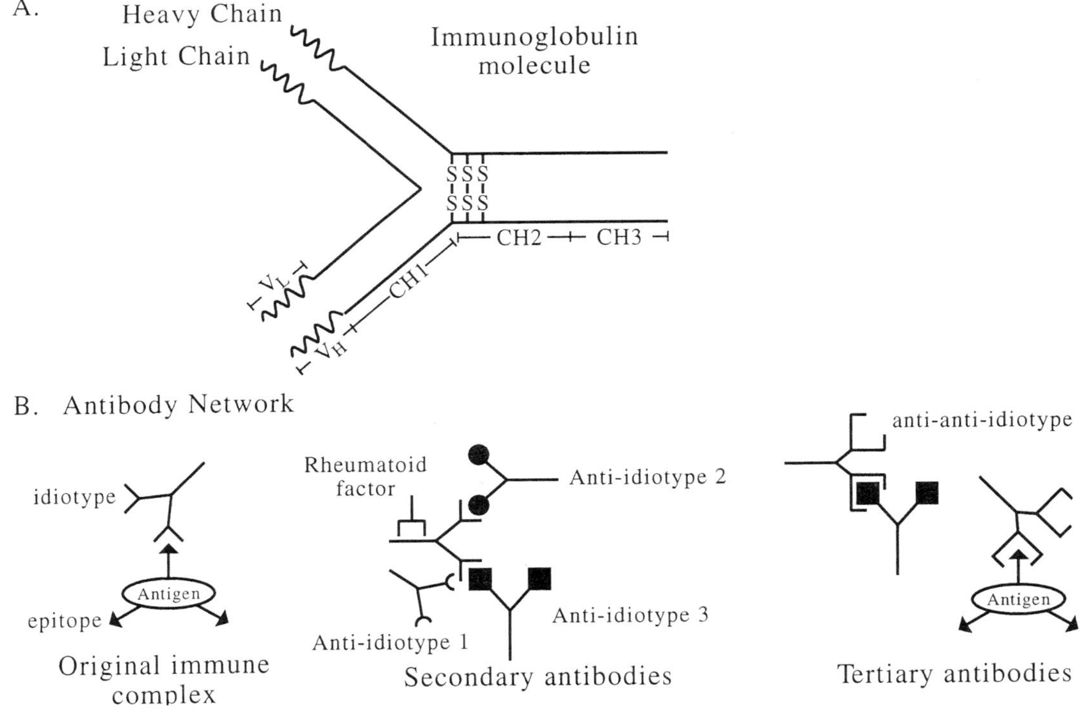

FIG. 2. Antibody structure and anti-idiotypic antibody formation. **A:** The structure of antibody, including the heavy and light chains, the disulfide bridging at the hinge region, the various domains including the CH1 domain, which binds C1q and activates complement, the CH2 domain to which rheumatoid factors bind, and the variable (VH and VL) that determine the antigen combining site. This unique region confers the antigen specificity and presents the immune system with a new antigen. This can give rise to anti-idiotypic antibody formation (**B**). The types of anti-idiotypes that form are schematically represented. [B adapted with permission (77).]

cells to release vasoactive substances, cytokines, and activators of coagulation (30,31). Alternatively, ICs can interact with cells in the circulation or other tissues and initiate the release of inflammatory mediators. These mediators may be delivered to the kidney, where they induce changes in renal blood flow and glomerular filtration rate, proteinuria, and inflammation without local IC accumulation. In this way, ICs may indirectly cause GN. These mechanisms may play a role in minimal change disease and focal and segmental glomerulosclerosis in which Ig deposits are not detected, but other evidence suggests immune system activation (32).

Formation of Macromolecular IC

When an antigen bears few epitopes (oligovalent) or there is excess antigen, ICs tend to be small and soluble. Small ICs are inefficient at complement activation and attachment to FcRs; therefore, they tend to remain in the circulation (Fig. 1). As the antigen:antibody ratio nears equivalence, cross-linking is maximized and large insoluble ICs are formed. Large complexes have a high affinity for binding to FcRs and activate complement. Together with secondary binding to complement receptors, this facilitates phagocytosis. When fewer ICs persist in the circulation, fewer are delivered to vascular beds and fewer are deposited in tissues (33–35). Medium-sized complexes and small complexes that are less well-cleared tend to deposit in tissues and initiate glomerular injury.

IC Size

The size of molecules has been shown to be important in their ability to localize within the glomerulus (30). Large, latticed ICs tend to accumulate in the mesangium and subendothelial space. Small soluble ICs are more likely to penetrate the GBM and collect in the subepithelial space. These ICs are too small to be seen by electron microscopy but can be detected by immunofluorescence (22). Furthermore, as secondary cross-linking reactions develop, they become electron dense (21). In studies of acute and chronic serum sickness in the rabbit (36), it was noted that the entire spectrum of histologic types of GN were observed (7,8). These data indicate that different types of GN can result from the same inciting agent. When low affinity antibody is produced, ICs tend to be smaller and localize in the subepithelial space and membranous nephropathy ensues (37). Alternatively, low-affinity antibodies favor persistence of free antigen, and when antigen or antibody localize alone in the glomerulus, in situ IC formation can subsequently occur. In contrast, when an animal makes high-affinity antibodies and large ICs form, either they are rapidly cleared by phagocytosis and no disease develops or the ICs deposit in the mesangium and subendothelial space, leading to proliferative forms of nephritis. Similarly, when mice are inbred to be either high- or low-affinity antibody producers, animals that produce low-affinity antibody consistently develop membranous nephropathy (38). Thus, the size of the complex influences its ability to deposit and the site of deposition.

IC Diversity

IC formation is a dynamic process that is constantly changing (Fig. 3). It is influenced by the amount and properties of circulating antigen and antibody. No single IC has to be composed of just one antibody class or specificity. Different antibodies may be simultaneously bound to different antigenic epitopes. The proportions of each of the classes and subclasses that arise during an immune response vary with time, nature of the antigen, genetic background of the individual, cytokines that are present, and multiple other variables. Similarly, the character of the IC changes, as does its pathogenicity. Analysis of the composition of ICs in blood and renal eluates has shown that they are heterogeneous, although enrichment for particular subsets may be seen. This observation has confused rather than clarified the immunopathogenesis of GN. Glomerular deposits may contain both nephritic ICs as well as ICs that are passively trapped and have no inflammatory role. Similarly, analysis of the serum may show only the ICs that have been left behind rather than those that are nephritogenic. Moreover, one subset or characteristic of the ICs may influence glomerular localization (nephrotorpic), whereas another characteristic may determine the ability to initiate inflammatory reactions (nephritogenicity) (25). The ongoing task is to understand the biochemical and immunological characteristics that determine these activities.

Secondary Complexing

Once antibody has bound antigen, conformational changes in both molecules occur. This leads to additional changes in the macromolecular complex. Complement-binding sites are exposed, and C1q becomes bound, activating the remainder of the complement cascade. Fc–Fc interactions occur as adjacent antibodies are brought into closer proximity with each other. This compacts the IC and the resultant conformational changes may alter the biologic properties of the new macromolecule. The ICs themselves become immunogenic, and rheumatoid factors (antibodies that bind to the constant region of other antibodies) and anti-idiotypic antibodies (antibodies that bind to the variable regions of other antibodies) are formed. As these antibodies bind to the ICs they also lead to secondary rearrangements and complement activation, thereby changing the pathogenic potential of the ICs.

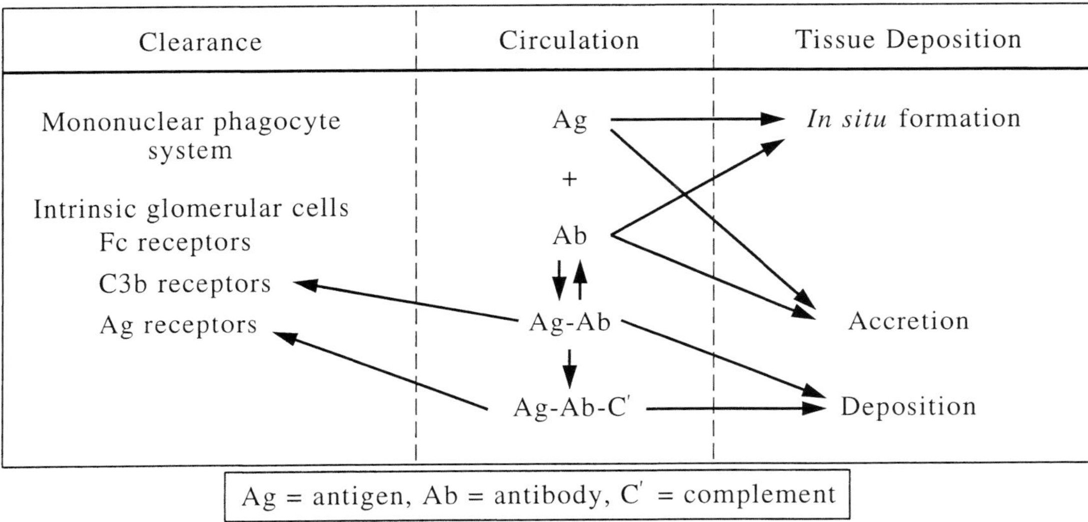

FIG. 3. The dynamic equilibrium. Immune reactants in the circulation are in dynamic equilibrium with each other, with receptors on phagocytes and intrinsic glomerular cells that remove and degrade them, and with the tissues in which they deposit. At one time in this dynamic process, the antigen–antibody ratio and the functional status of the MPS may favor complete clearance of the IC and no tissue deposition will occur. At other times, MPS function may be inadequate or the amounts and biochemical characteristics of antigen, antibody, or ICs will favor tissue deposition. This dynamic equilibrium determines the type of IC, their deposition, and perpetuation within the glomerulus. Ag, antigen; Ab, antibody; C′, complement. [Adapted with permission (77).]

Rheumatoid Factors

Most rheumatoid factors are IgM antibodies that bind to the Fc portion of IgG. They preferentially bind to complexed rather than monomeric IgG, and through these secondary interactions with IC they enhance IC clearance from the circulation and enlarge IC deposits in tissues. The role of rheumatoid factors in GN is poorly understood. GN rarely complicates rheumatoid arthritis, in which these antibodies are common; however, frequently rheumatoid factors are eluted from glomeruli in other forms of ICGN (39). This observation suggests that they may contribute to IC accretion within the glomerulus, but it is likely that other properties unique to the antigen and primary antibody determine the ability to deposit in the kidney.

Anti-idiotypic Antibodies

During maturation of the immune response, clonal expansion of B cells expressing unique variable regions presents the immune system with new structural determinants that are recognized as immunogenic. The unique variable regions are termed idiotypes, and the antibodies to them are anti-idiotypes. Three general types of anti-idiotypic antibodies can form (Fig. 2). Anti-idiotypic antibodies can bind to the variable region of primary antibody adjacent to the antigen-combining site, but not in it. A second type of anti-idiotypic antibody binds to the antigen-combining site and can displace antigen. Both of these antibodies tend to downregulate primary antibody synthesis as antigen is eliminated. A third subset of anti-idiotypic antibodies bind to the antigen-combining site, conformationally represent the internal image of that site, and therefore mimic antigen. These antibodies can act like antigen and stimulate primary antibody synthesis. These antibodies often occur in autoimmune diseases and participate in a positive feedback loop that contributes to chronic disease (40). Anti-idiotypic antibodies have been shown to participate in glomerular IC formation in several models (41). As these antibodies bind to IC containing antigen and primary antibody, the size, complement fixation, and other biological properties of the IC change. The exact role that the addition of anti-idiotypic antibodies to the IC play in growth of tissue-bound IC and initiation of injury is less well defined.

Complement Activation

Once antibody has bound antigen, the conformational change in the CH1 domain of IgG allows C1q to bind, and complement activation is initiated. The incorporation of complement components into the IC changes its biologic properties (12,25,42). The mechanisms and consequences of complement activation are reviewed in detail in Chapter 18. After C1q binds to IgG, a conformational change occurs that exposes a collagenlike region of the C1q molecule. This neoantigen sometimes initiates antibody formation. Anti-C1q–reactive antibodies bind to IC-complexed C1q, but not to free C1q. Anti-C1q antibodies have been described in lupus, idiopathic membranous nephropathy, and hypocomplementemic urticarial vasculitis but are not prominent in other autoimmune diseases (42,43). The prevalence of these antibodies in lupus nephritis and detection of C1q in renal biopsy samples of individuals with lupus nephritis suggests that they play an important pathogenic role, but this remains to be established.

Initiation of Secondary Inflammatory Reactions

ICs are biologically active molecules that play important roles in the regulation of the immune response and initiation of inflammation. ICs bind to B cells and T cells and thereby modify the specificity and amplitude of the antibody response. They similarly modulate cell-mediated reactions. Binding and activation of complement modifies the clearance properties of the ICs and their ability to initiate release of cytokines and other inflammatory mediators. With the exception of ICs binding to FcRs, the interaction of ICs with complement, lymphocytes, macrophages, and intrinsic glomerular cells and the release of cytokines are each described in detail in other chapters of this book; they are thus not reviewed here.

Fc Receptors

Receptors for the Fc region of Ig are heterogenous and expressed on many cells of the immune system and kidney. For additional detail of these receptors and their biologic functions, the reader is referred to several excellent reviews (44–46). Three major classes of receptors for the Fc region of IgG have been described with additional heterogeneity in each class. Some of the heterogeneity is generated by alternative messenger RNA splicing of individual genes and others result from separate gene products. Several FcRs share extracellular domains that confer binding specificity for the same subclass of IgG; however, these proteins differ in their intracellular domains. The variable intracellular domains are responsible for initiating different signal transduction pathways that have different biological consequences. In some cases, this specificity is regulated in individual cell types because they may express only one form of the receptor. In other cases individual cells may express more than one FcR form or may be induced to switch the form of FcR they express. This results in heterogeneity of the consequences of IC binding to the cell. These concepts are shown schematically in Fig. 4.

FcRs initiate a number of well-characterized responses. These include FcR-mediated phagocytosis and antibody-dependent cell-mediated cytotoxicity. The phagocytic function initiated by FcRs is particularly relevant to ICGN. A number of studies have shown that saturation of and/or impairment of FcR-mediated phagocytosis leads to increased tissue delivery and accumulation of ICs (33, 47). Moreover, enhanced FcR-mediated phagocytosis can minimize glomerular accumulation of immune deposits (34). Changes in hormone levels such as insulin in diabetes mellitus (48) and catecholamines during stress (44, 49) can alter FcR function and thereby affect clearance kinetics and tissue deposition of circulating ICs (CICs).

In addition to facilitating IC clearance from the circulation, IC binding to FcRs is crucial to initiation of inflammation. In recent studies, Sylvestre and Ravetch (45) demonstrated that transgenic mice deficient for the γ chain of the FcR complex lack both high- and low-affinity FcRs (Fc RI and Fc RIII). Despite normal inflammatory responses to other stimuli, the response to ICs in these animals is markedly attenuated. A typical Arthus reaction does not follow intradermal formation of ICs in FcR-deficient mice. These data suggest that FcR ligation initiates inflammation, which is amplified by cytokines and activated complement. Thus, FcRs are required for initiation of proinflammatory cytokines. These observations have important implications for therapy because FcR antagonists could be used to treat IC-mediated disease. In this way, interaction with ICs and FcRs on intrinsic glomerular cells is critical to inflammation and activation of scarring.

Recent studies have expanded our knowledge of the mechanisms whereby FcRs induce other effects. FcR ligation stimulates interleukin (IL)-10 release (50). IL-10 in turn has many important consequences (51). IL-10 increases FcR expression, thereby functioning in a positive feedback loop to enhance phagocytosis and other FcR-mediated activities. Enhanced clearance of ICs would ultimately lead to reduction in FcR-mediated activities, and the normal steady state would be reestablished. When the antigen is endogenous, replicating, or ineffectively cleared, chronic IC load would lead to persistent stimulation of FcRs, leading to generation of proinflammatory cytokines as well as those that impair host defense. IL-10 mediates suppression of interferon-γ release, decreases human leukocyte antigen–class II antigen expression, impairs antimicrobial activity, and decreases the generation of Th1 cells and IL-2 release. These consequences of IC binding to FcR contribute to increased susceptibility to infection and reduced tumoricidal responses, common complications of IC diseases. This shows that a delicate balance in immunostimulatory and immunosuppressive reactions exists and is important to host defense and regulation of immune-mediated disease. IC load and their interaction with FcRs are pivotal in this process. Glomerular epithelial cells and mesangial

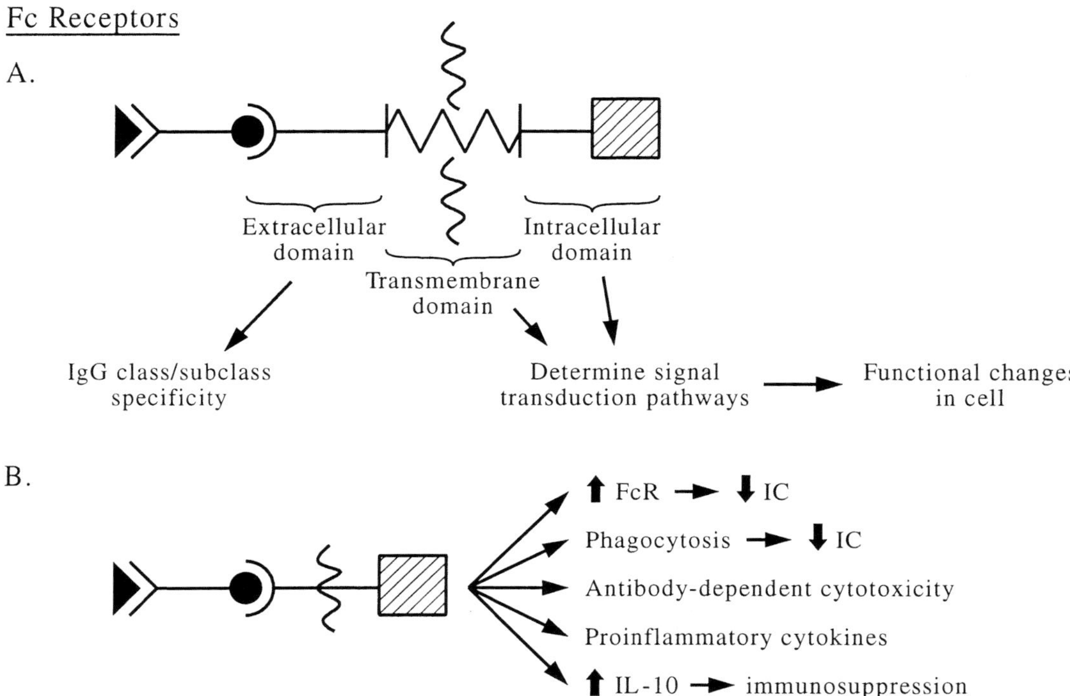

FIG. 4. FcRs. **A:** The schematic structure of an FcR. The extracellular domain determines the class and subclass affinity for the receptor. The transmembrane and intracellular domains determine the signal transduction pathways that are activated and the functional consequences that they initiate. The cell type that expresses the particular FcR form determines the spectrum of effector functions that can be modulated by Ig binding to the FcR. **B:** The variety of consequences of FcR ligation are summarized.

cells express FcRs and phagocytose ICs (52,53); however, the magnitude of the phagocytic response is limited. This suggests that other consequences of FcR ligation on intrinsic glomerular cells may be particularly relevant to mechanisms of IC-mediated glomerular injury. Little is currently known about these activities within the glomerulus.

DEPOSITION IN RENAL STRUCTURES

The kidney is a particularly susceptible target for immune deposit formation. Several characteristics make it different from other capillary beds. Antigens, antibodies, and ICs in the circulation are delivered at a high rate because the kidney receives 25% of the cardiac output. Intraglomerular pressure is higher than in other capillary beds; thus, more protein may be forced across the glomerular capillary wall. The glomerular capillaries provide a large and highly permeable surface through which circulating proteins percolate and can become nonspecifically trapped or directly interact with constituents of the glomerular capillary wall. As the protein-free ultrafiltrate of plasma is formed, serum proteins are prevented from passage into the urinary space by the filtration slits; thus, their local concentration in the glomerular capillary wall increases. As this occurs, interaction between unoccupied antigenic epitopes and antibodies is favored. This facilitates lattice formation, secondary interactions, and the acquisition of properties that activate inflammatory responses.

Immune deposits can form in the glomerular capillary or any other structure by deposition from the circulation, or they can form locally. When antigen and antibody combine to form a macromolecule in the circulation (CICs), they can be cleared by the mononuclear phagocyte system (MPS) or passively deposit in tissues. In situ formation occurs when antibody binds to antigen locally within tissue. Either soluble, uncomplexed, circulating antigen or antibody can bind first to renal structures. When the other member of the pair is subsequently delivered by the circulation, ICs form. In situ IC formation also can occur when the antibody is specifically directed against an intrinsic glomerular antigen. The location of immune deposits that form in situ are determined by the site of expression of the relevant intrinsic glomerular antigen or the site where a nonimmunologic biochemical interaction leads to trapping of antigen or antibody. Once antigen has combined with antibody, free circulating reactants can be delivered to the tissues at a later time, bind to unoccupied sites on antigen or antibody, and lead to progressive IC accretion (Fig. 5).

In the early 1970s, there was considerable debate regarding the relative importance of CIC versus in situ formation of immune deposits. In the intervening 20 years substantial data have accumulated that confirm that ICs can accumulate in the glomerular capillary wall and other sites by both mechanisms. Furthermore, the tissue deposits are in dynamic equilibrium with reactants (antigens, antibodies, and ICs) in the circulation (Fig. 3). Thus, whereas one mechanism may initiate immune deposit formation in tissues, the other mechanism may perpetuate it. Also, the mechanism that predominates may change over the course of the disease. At the present time, debates revolve around the nature of the antigen, because it is important to know whether the antigen is exogenous, endogenous, or intrinsic to the glomerulus and/or renal interstitium. Intrinsic glomerular antigens and other autoantigens cannot be eliminated from the body; thus, therapeutic strategies need to be designed to reduce the autoimmune response to these antigens. In contrast, exogenous antigens need to be eliminated so that the immune response to them will dissipate.

In Situ IC Formation

ICs form in situ when antigen and antibody combine within tissues as opposed to within the circulation. Unbound circulating antibody can combine with antigen that is intrinsic to the glomerulus or has previously been deposited there by virtue of a biochemical interaction between the antigen and a component of the glomerulus (e.g., charge). Once antibody has combined with antigen,

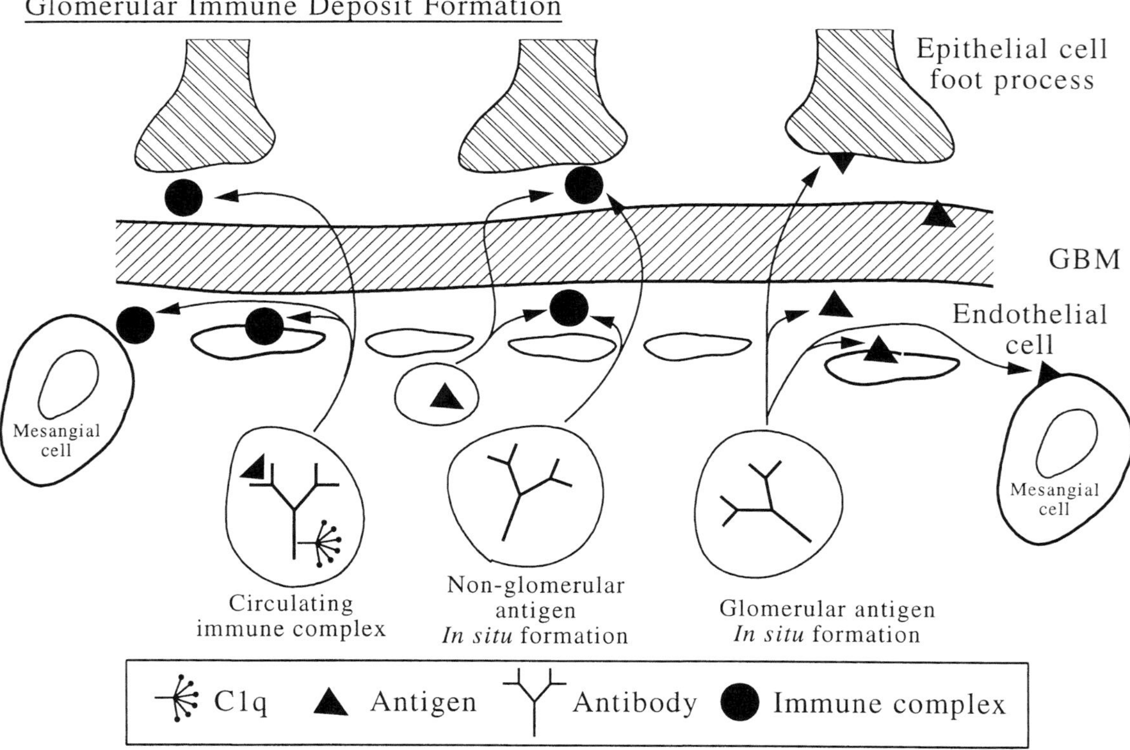

FIG. 5. IC formation in the glomerulus. When antigen and antibody bind in the circulation to form an IC and they are not removed by the MPS they can deposit in the glomerulus. Depending on the size and other biochemical characteristics, deposition in one of three sites—the subdendothelial, subepithelial, or mesangial spaces—is favored. Having deposited, the ICs may undergo further cross-linking with adjacent ICs or subsequently interact with ICs, free antigen, or free antibody that is delivered by the circulation. Alternatively, free antigen or free antibody may have a special biochemical affinity for interaction with a constituent of the glomerulus. Once having been "planted" in this location, it may subsequently bind to the other member of the pair, leading to IC formation within the glomerulus. This IC may then be modified further by any of the mechanisms of IC formation and accumulation. Finally, antibody may specifically bind to an intrinsic glomerular antigen leading to in situ immune deposit formation. In this case the location and rate of IC formation is determined primarily by the location and degree of expression of the relevant antigen within the glomerulus. The concentration, charge, and affinity of antibody also affects the tempo of the IC formation and the injury that ensues.

a conformational change occurs, complement is activated, and secondary inflammatory reactions are initiated as described above. Furthermore, should this occur on the surface of a kidney cell, it may directly change the behavior of that cell. In situ formation of immune deposits was first characterized in the anti-GBM model of GN, where antibody bound directly to GBM, activated complement led to proteinuria and proliferative GN. Because the antigen to which the antibody is bound is continuously distributed in the GBM, immunofluorescence staining of kidney tissue for IgG shows a linear pattern of Ig deposits. In anti-GBM nephritis the antigen is a small peptide region of the noncollagenous domain of the a3 chain of collagen IV (54). This collagen IV chain is expressed predominantly in GBM and alveolar basement membrane, thereby accounting for the clinical pulmonary–renal syndrome known as Goodpasture's disease.

Initially, it was thought that anti-GBM disease was the only form of GN in which ICs formed in situ (55). Subsequently, it was shown that granular immune deposits also could result from in situ formation when the antigens to which antibodies bound were discontinuously distributed within the glomerulus. Such antigens can be components expressed on the surface of glomerular cells or can be structural or secondarily bound components of the extracellular matrix. In the passive Heymann model of membranous nephropathy, heterologous antibody raised to proximal tubular brush border proteins contains antibodies to glycoprotein (gp)330, a member of the LDL-receptor family, which is expressed both on proximal tubular brush border and glomerular epithelial cells (56,57). Although CICs form in this model and can deposit in the glomerulus (58–60), direct perfusion of the kidney with monoclonal antibodies to gp330 shows that antibody can bind directly to gp330 expressed on the surface of glomerular epithelial cell surfaces (56,61). Once antibody binds, complement is activated and the resultant IC is shed from the cell surface and binds to the GBM. Subsequent accretion leads to the subepithelial electron-dense deposits that are typical of membranous nephropathy (61,62). These studies were the first to confirm that granular immune deposits could form by in situ binding of antibody to an intrinsic glomerular antigen (15,55).

In situ formation of ICs in which the antigen is not an intrinsic component of the glomerulus were shown in studies in which concanavalin A was infused (12). Serving as a lectin, concanavalin A binds to glycoproteins rich in mannose and becomes deposited in the glomerulus by this interaction. Having been "planted" in the glomerulus, these antigens are available to bind antibody at a subsequent time. After in situ binding of antibody, an inflammatory reaction ensues. Since completion of these initial studies, many other proteins (e.g., cationized albumin and IgG, various lectins, polycationic molecules such as heparin, laminins, proteoglycans, integrins on the glomerular epithelial cell surface, ACE on endothelial cells, etc.) have been studied that confirm that immune deposits can form locally within tissue when circulating antibody combines with intrinsic tissue antigens or ones that have become "planted" there.

Deposition of CICs

Deposition of CICs is thought to be responsible for the majority of human forms of ICGN (Table 3), although the antigen contained within the glomerular immune deposits is unknown in many cases of human disease. Circulating, soluble antigens are more likely to combine with antibody in the circulation. These antigens can be endogenous or exogenous. Depending on the concentration of each component, CIC size will vary. This is depicted graphically in Fig. 1. Each of the biochemical properties of antigen and antibody discussed above will influence the size and biologic activity of the IC. The factors listed in Table 2 all contribute to tissue deposition of CICs. The role of CICs in initiating tissue inflammation was initially defined in studies of serum sickness in human and animal models. Large quantities of the foreign protein (bovine serum albumin) are administered to rabbits as a single or repeated dose (5–8,36). Shortly after administration of antigen, antibody production begins and CICs form. If the size and biologic properties are favorable, CICs will deposit in tissues and initiate inflammatory reactions.

After formation in the circulation, CICs are delivered to organs containing cells of the MPS (e.g., liver and spleen), which remove them. If the amount of CIC formed does not exceed the clearance capabilities of the MPS, and the biochemical characteristics of the CIC favor high-affinity interactions with Fc, complement, and other receptors on these cells, CICs will be cleared from the circulation and none will remain for deposition in tissues, including the kidney. Should MPS function be impaired, small amounts of CIC may become pathogenic. Alternatively, when the load of CIC exceeds the clearance capacity, tissue deposition is favored. In other cases unique biologic properties of the CIC allow them to escape removal by phagocytes. A number of experimental studies have confirmed these conclusions. Stimulation of phagocyte function with zymosan enhances plasma clearance and reduces glomerular deposition, whereas impairment of the MPS by splenectomy leads to higher levels of CIC and more glomerular deposition (34).

One of the most important lessons from studies of chronic serum sickness in rabbits was the observation that the initiating antigen and the antibody response could be similar; however, different forms of ICGN developed (8). This illustrates the importance of the dynamic equilibrium and the biochemical properties discussed above that determine the degree to which ICs are both nephrotropic and nephritogenic. Large ICs tend to

TABLE 3. *Antigens that are implicated in human IC renal disease*

- Replicating, nonhuman antigens
  - Bacterial
    - Streptococcus
    - Staphylococcus
    - Diplococcus pneumoniae
    - Meningococcus
    - Enterococcus
    - Coliforms
    - Salmonella typhosa
    - Treponema pallidum
    - Mycobacterium
  - Viral
    - Hepatitis B virus
    - Hepatitis C virus
    - Epstein-Barr virus
    - Cytomegalovirus
    - Varicella-zoster virus
    - Measles virus
  - Fungus
    - Coccidioidomycosis
    - Candida albicans
  - Parasitic
    - Malarial organisms
    - Toxoplasma gondii
    - Schistosoma mansoni
    - Filariasis
- Nonreplicating, nonhuman antigens
  - Foreign serum proteins
    - Hepatitis B vaccine
    - Tetanus antitoxin
    - Antisnake venom
    - Antilymphocyte globulin (OKT3)
    - Bovine collagen
  - Drugs and chemicals
    - Penicillin, methicillin
    - Sulfonamides
    - Captopril
    - Penicillamine
  - Food allergens
    - Milk
    - Gluten
- Endogenous antigens
  - Extracellular matrix proteins
    - NC1 domain of a3 chain of collagen IV
    - 3M-1 antigen in tubular basement membrane
    - Laminin
    - Heparan sulfate proteoglycans
    - Collagen I
    - Fibronectin
  - Cellular proteins
    - Proteinase 3
    - Myeloperoxidase
    - gp330
    - Hormone receptors (e.g., for insulin, acetylcholine)
    - Integrins
    - Erythrocyte membrane antigen
  - Nuclear constituents
    - DNA
    - RNA
    - Extractable nuclear antigens (eg, RNP, Sm, Rho, etc)
  - Tumor-specific antigens
    - Carcinoembryonic antigen
    - Melanoma-specific antigen
  - Circulating proteins
    - Thyroglobulin
    - a-1 antitrypsin
    - C1q
    - Insulin
    - Igs (rheumatoid factors, anti-idiotypic antibodies)

deposit in the mesangium, where they may be slowly phagocytosed by mesangial cells. This function of mesangial cells is relatively inefficient; thus, the predominant consequence of IC deposition in the mesangium is interaction with mesangial cells to stimulate the release of cytokines and growth factors. These in turn cause mesangial cell proliferation and changes in the rate of accumulation of mesangial matrix, thereby causing mesangial sclerosis. ICs accumulate in the subendothelial space when the mesangium becomes saturated with ICs, when the unique biochemical characteristics of ICs favor interaction with endothelial cells, when they are too large to penetrate the GBM, or when they begin as small ICs but the load is so high that enhanced local concentration in the subendothelial space favors lattice formation. Usually, ICs trapped in the subendothelial space are large and effective at complement activation. The chemotactic peptides that are released lead to glomerular infiltration with platelets and leukocytes. These typify a proliferative GN. Often proteolytic enzymes are released that digest regions of the GBM leading to leakage of serum proteins into Bowmans space and initiation of crescent formation. Thus, both the immunochemical characteristics of the IC and the location in which they accumulate influence the type of glomerular disease that follows.

In the late 1970s there was controversy regarding the ability of intact IC macromolecules to penetrate the GBM and lead to subepithelial immune deposit formation. A number of studies were performed in an attempt to prove or disprove one of these mechanisms. Considerable new insights were generated. Confirmation that granular subepithelial immune deposits could develop from direct antibody binding to a surface antigen on glomerular epithelial cells was demonstrated using monoclonal antibody to gp330 in the passive model of Heymann nephritis (56). In the active model of Heymann nephritis, glomerular eluates contain antibodies that react with glomerular epithelial cell antigens, as well as nonglomerular antigens and their antibodies (59), thus suggesting that both mechanisms may participate in immune deposit formation in the active model of Heymann nephritis. Injections of small ICs, covalently cross-linked in vitro so that antigen and antibody cannot dissociate, lead to subepithelial localization of the IC, thereby confirming that CICs could give rise to subepithelial immune deposits. Later, Mannik et al. (30,63) showed that small CICs penetrate the fenestra of endothelial cells and become trapped in the subendothelial space. Once there, they dissociate. Each component of the IC then penetrates the GBM, where they again form ICs. As this process is repeated many times, large lattices ultimately form in the subepithelial space, leading to easily identified electron-dense deposits. Thus, these studies demonstrate that ICs can form in the subepithelial space of the glomerulus via a number of mechanisms.

Dynamic Equilibrium

Once antigen has initiated antibody production and ICs have formed, a complex and dynamic system has been put into action (Fig. 3). As discussed above, the biochemical nature of the antigen, its source, and its persistence in the circulation influence the antibody response, the ICs that form, the way in which they are handled, and their biologic properties. These characteristics determine the phlogistic, nephrotropic, and nephritogenic properties of the IC. Over time, additional factors influence the biologic properties, including maturation of the antibody response to include other classes of antibody and antibodies of higher affinity. Complement activation, rheumatoid factors, and anti-idiotypic antibodies further modify the composition and biologic activity of the IC. At each stage, individual components and macromolecules are in dynamic equilibrium with each other in the circulation, MPS, and tissues in which they deposit. Tissue deposits may contain free epitopes and antibodies with unoccupied antigen-combining sites. As additional free antigens and antibodies are delivered to the tissues, solubilization or further cross-linking and accretion may occur. As this happens, the biologic properties of the IC will change again. This feature can be responsible for relapses and remissions of disease activity and is crucial to the progression of glomerular scarring. Further understanding of this dynamic equilibrium is essential to understanding disease progression and the ultimate development of strategies to modify this process.

IC-MEDIATED RENAL DISEASE

An IC disease is one in which the tissue injury that occurs is the consequence of the inflammatory injury initiated by IC rather than the agent or event that stimulated the IC formation. Almost all glomerular diseases are immune mediated, and most glomerular diseases are due to ICs (Tables 1 and 4). ICs can mediate glomerular injury through secondary inflammatory reactions after formation in situ, after deposition from the circulation, or indirectly via interaction with macrophages and lymphocytes that release inflammatory cytokines that affect the kidney. Although IC-mediated interstitial renal disease is an under-studied area, ICs probably account for only a small proportion of all forms of interstitial nephritis. Glomerular diseases are categorized in Table 4 according to the type of IC deposits that form. In many cases, ICs form as a normal consequence of infection or tissue injury from various causes, including myocardial infarction, but they are of no pathogenic significance. It is for this reason that the simple detection of CICs does not always correlate with disease activity or with disease pathogenesis.

TABLE 4. *Human IC-mediated glomerular diseases*

Circulating ICs and nonglomerular antigens
Systemic lupus erythematosus
Poststreptococcal GN
Thyroiditis
Viral infections (e.g., hepatitis B and C)
Membranoproliferative GN type I, with or without mixed cryoglobulinemia and hepatitis C infection
IgA nephropathy
Henoch-Schoenlein purpura
Idiopathic rapidly progressive GN
ICs may be circulating or involve intrinsic renal antigens
Idiopathic membranous nephropathy
IgM mesangial proliferative GN
Systemic lupus erythematosis
ICs involving intrinsic glomerular antigens
Goodpasture's syndrome (anti-GBM disease)

The role of antibody and complement in renal injury was suspected long before the advent of immunofluorescence microscopy, but the development of this technology confirmed their importance. Examination of human biopsy specimens by this technique has shown that antibody deposits can be identified in approximately 85% of all forms of glomerular disease. Although it is possible that nonspecific trapping of serum proteins accounts for the detection of Igs in certain circumstances, in the majority of cases they are thought to play a specific role in the immunopathogenesis of nephritis. Early investigators of GN noted that two distinct patterns of immune deposits were identified: linear and granular. The linear pattern resulted from direct binding of antibody to a component of the GBM that is continuously distributed along the GBM. In contrast, the granular pattern of immune deposits was thought to result solely from deposition of ICs formed in the circulation by antibodies combining with nonrenal antigens and subsequent passive trapping in the glomerular capillary wall. As more biopsies were examined, it was noted that the distribution of the granular deposits varied. Sometimes they were confined to the subepithelial space, looking like a string of beads along the capillary wall. In other cases, they were clustered centrally, corresponding to the mesangium. Finally, they were detected in the mesangium and along the capillary wall with localization to the subendothelial space. Definition of the distribution of ICs, as well as the classes of Igs and complement components that they contain, led to refinements in the classification of glomerular disease. Recent studies have confirmed that intrinsic glomerular antigens that are discontinuously distributed within the glomerulus can participate in in situ immune deposit formation but produce a granular pattern by immunofluorescence. Current diagnostic criteria for glomerular diseases include the light microscopic pattern of inflammatory injury, the findings by immunofluorescence and electron microscopy, associated systemic diseases, serologies, and our present understanding of immunopathogenesis. Improved biochemical techniques have led to specific characterization of the binding specificities of antibodies eluted from diseased glomeruli, and analysis of CICs has led to identification of certain antigens that initiate disease. Each of the clinical forms of ICGN are discussed in greater detail in later chapters. A few specific diseases are described here as examples of mechanisms of immune-mediated renal disease.

One of the best examples of IC disease in which the antigen is an exogenous, replicating antigen is poststreptococcal GN. The clinical course and mechanisms of IC formation in this disease are discussed in detail in Chapter 41. In addition to primary antibody–antigen reaction, IgG rheumatoid factors are easily demonstrated in the circulation of patients with PSGN and in glomerular eluates. Thus, secondary reactions appear to contribute to glomerular injury in this form of ICGN. In most cases, the host response to the acute suppurative infection adequately eliminates the infection. Once the antigen is no longer present, ICs cease to form and antibody titers decrease. When the inflammatory reaction is short-lived, healing can occur without scarring and organ function returns to normal.

Systemic lupus erythematosus (SLE) is an excellent example of an IC disease in which the antigen is endogenous. Because the endogenous antigens are continuously produced in vivo, they provide a chronic stimulus for antibody production and a chronic IC load. CICs are readily detected in patients with lupus and contain a variety of specificities, including antibodies to double-stranded DNA, ribonucleoproteins, gangliosides, C1q, a SPARC-related protein, and laminin. Rheumatoid factors are uncommon in lupus, but anti-idiotypic antibodies appear to play an important role in IC formation and the dysregulation of antibody synthesis that typifies SLE (40). Each of these antibodies can bind to antigens in the circulation, producing CICs, or to tissue antigens, leading to in situ IC formation. Details of the composition of ICs in glomerular deposits and the immune dysregulation leading to autoantibody formation in SLE can be found in Chapter 48.

Considerable progress has been made recently in our understanding of the immunopathogenesis of membranoproliferative GN associated with mixed essential cryoglobulinemia. With the development of a serologic assay for hepatitis C antibody and a polymerase chain reaction (PCR) test for hepatitis C virus RNA, it was quickly recognized that the majority of patients with mixed cryoglobulinemia and membranoproliferative GN had chronic hepatitis C infection (for additional details see Chapter 51). Hepatitis C virus is present in ICs in the circulation and in the kidney. Thus, at the present time this is the best example of a chronic form of glomerular disease that is mediated by deposition of CICs and in which the inciting agent is known. Presumably similar mechanisms will be identified for other histologic forms of glomerular disease as new tests are developed.

The cause of human membranous nephropathy remains unknown. Viral and tumor antigens have been detected in CICs and glomerular immune deposits in humans with membranous nephropathy; thus, both endogenous and exogenous antigens have been implicated in this disorder. At present, it is not known whether these ICs play a pathogenic role or have been secondarily trapped in an injured glomerulus. In the Heymann rat model of membranous nephropathy, ICs form on the subepithelial space by in situ binding of antibody to an antigen expressed on the surface of the glomerular epithelial cell. It is likely that a similar mechanism occurs in human membranous nephropathy, but the antigen has not yet been identified. A detailed discussion of the pathogenesis of membranous nephropathy is included in Chapter 47.

Interstitial Renal Disease

Interstitial renal disease results from both toxic and immunologic mechanisms. The immune mechanisms responsible for tubulointerstitial nephritis (TIN) are identical to those that mediate glomerular disease (and are listed in Table 1); however, the majority of TIN is due to cell-mediated immunologic reactions. In contrast to GN, in which ICs are thought to mediate the majority of human disease, ICs are infrequent in TIN. The potential contributions of intrinsic renal antigens and nonrenal antigens are summarized in Table 5 (64). As in GN, the site of antigen to which antibody binds determines the site of inflammation, and thus the clinical features. For example, in the Heymann model of membranous nephropathy, ICs containing antibodies to brush border antigens localize along the tubular basement membrane (TBM) of proximal tubules. Mild inflammatory reactions are similarly located, and abnormalities in proximal tubular reabsorptive function correlate with the presence of these deposits (65). Immunization with Tamm-Horsfall protein leads to immune deposit formation along the ascending limb of Henle's loop, the site of Tamm-Horsfall protein synthesis. Mild inflammatory reactions develop and are accompanied by defects in urine concentrating ability (66).

TABLE 5. *Antigens involved in human interstitial renal disease*

Intrinsic renal antigens
Heymann nephritis, proximal tubular brush border antigens
Tamm-Horsfall (uromodulin) protein
3M-1 antigen in TBM
Planted antigens
Drug–hapten conjugates
Penicillins
Cephalosporins
Phenytoin
Exogenous antigens that may participate in CIC formation and/or produce cross-reactive antibodies that bind to intrinsic renal antigens because of molecular mimicry
Streptococcus
Coliforms
Viruses
CIC containing nonrenal antigens
Serum sickness
IgA nephropathy
Cryoglobulins
DNA–SLE
Sjogren nephropathy

When antibodies bind to 3M-1, a component of TBM, a prominent cellular infiltrate follows and causes severe interstitial nephritis (67). Although each of these are well-characterized animal models of TIN, their human correlates have not been defined.

A variety of "planted" antigens have been postulated to mediate acute TIN when it accompanies drug exposure. Antibody binding to drug-hapten conjugates in the circulation may produce CICs that passively deposit in the renal interstitium. In situ binding may occur when drug-hapten conjugates biochemically interact with or become concentrated in the renal interstitium as a consequence of glomerular filtration and reabsorption. The penicillins (with methicillin being the most common culprit), cephalosporins, and phenytoin have been implicated in TIN due to this mechanism. These drugs also may incite TIN by purely cell-mediated mechanisms, because often no antibody deposition is detected when these agents are the suspected allergen.

As with GN, a number of bacterial and viral antigens may contribute to CIC formation and deposition in the tubulointerstitium. Additionally, via molecular mimicry cross-reactive antibodies may bind to intrinsic renal interstitial antigens (68). Similar to GN, streptococci, coliforms, and viruses have been implicated in human TIN (69). As discussed above, some antibodies to streptococci cross-react with type IV collagen, a component of TBM. Antibodies to coliforms cross-react with Tamm-Horsfall protein (70). Tubular cells may become infected with cytomegalovirus and express new antigens on their surface, which become targets of antibody or cell-mediated reactions. Although there is experimental evidence that supports the pathogenic role of these mechanisms, none have been proven to be the primary etiology in human disease.

In a number of systemic CIC diseases, CICs also deposit in the renal interstitium and initiate inflammation. Prominent intersitial deposits are not infrequently observed in serum sickness, SLE, IgA nephropathy, Sjogren nephropathy, and cryoglobulinemia. When they accompany severe GN, it is difficult to determine their clinical significance, but experimental data suggest that these deposits can produce interstitial renal injury and contribute to progressive loss of renal function.

ASSAYS FOR CIC

A wide variety of assays to detect ICs in serum have been developed (Table 6). Although the details of each method vary, they all are based on physicochemical properties that are acquired when antibody binds to antigen (71,72). These include an increase in size, increased precipitability in the cold, and complement binding. Most of the assays use a combination of these principles to detect ICs. For example, in the fluid-phase C1q binding assay, serum is mixed with radiolabelled C1q. "Heavy" C1q is precipitated with polyethylene glycol, and the precipitated counts parallel the amount of IC. In the solid-phase C1q binding assay, plastic tubes are coated with C1q and then incubated with serum. Unbound material is washed out, and the bound material is detected by the addition of radiolabelled antibody to Ig. In this manner, molecules containing IgG that bind complement are detected. With the exception of free antibodies that are primarily directed against C1q, only the IgG that has been confor-

TABLE 6. *IC assays*

Conglutinin tests
Conglutinin solid phase assay
Rheumatoid factor tests
Monoclonal RF capillary precipitation test
Monoclonal RF binding inhibition test
Polyclonal RF latex agglutination inhibition assay
Polyclonal RF inhibition radioimmunoassay
C1q tests
Fluid phase C1q binding assay[a]
Solid phase C1q binding assay[a]
C1q deviation test
C1q latex agglutination inhibition test
C1q binding inhibition assay
C3 receptor tests
Raji cell assay[a]
FcR tests
Platelet aggregation assay
Macrophage uptake inhibition assay
Precipitation tests
Enhanced precipitability in polyethylene glycol
Cryoprecipitability[a]

[a]Assays upon which majority of data are based, as well as the assays that are commercially available.

mationally altered as a result of antigen binding will bind C1q; thus, the assay is fairly specific for CICs.

When CIC assays were developed, it was hoped that CIC detection would be of diagnostic utility, would assist in following up patients with diseases such as SLE, and might lead to characterization of antigen, which would presumably define the agent responsible for the disease (71,72). These hopes have been realized only in part. CICs are sometimes detected in association with tissue injury in which they play no direct pathogenic role. In other cases, even those in which ICs mediate tissue injury, the ICs detected in the circulation may represent the subset of CICs that fail to deposit and thus are not pathogenic. Lessons from studies of acute serum sickness have taught us that CICs form, deposit in tissues, and initiate inflammation, and by the time clinical disease is manifested, ICs are no longer present in the circulation. This was confirmed in humans with SLE (73) in whom an increase in the level of CICs 2 months before a clinical flare was predictive of that flare. Levels drawn at the time of presentation of clinical symptoms were less valuable correlates of disease activity. Unless CICs are measured at frequent intervals when patients are clinically quiescent, this predictive utility will not be realized.

Despite these limitations in CIC testing, recent advances have improved their potential utility. Sophisticated technologies in protein biochemistry and molecular biology have improved our ability to analyze the antigenic content of ICs detected by less specific assays. Studies in the active model of Heymann nephritis (58,74) showed that CICs could be isolated and the antigen and antibody specificity determined. In membranoproliferative GN associated with mixed cryoglobulinemia, analysis of the cryoglobulins has shown that they contain antibody reactive with the hepatitic C virus (75). Using PCR techniques, hepatitis C RNA also has been identified in ICs (76). ICs of identical composition have been shown in tissue deposits at sites of IC-mediated injury. It is presumed that similar progress eventually will be made in the analysis of ICs in other diseases.

At the present time CIC analysis can be helpful in the following circumstances: (a) detection of ICs in the circulation may be helpful in circumstances in which the diagnosis is unclear, (b) significant increases in the level of CICs in patients with SLE may be a harbinger of a flare in clinical symptoms, and (c) detection and quantitation of cryoglobulins in patients with hepatitis C infection indicates a significant risk for tissue deposition and injury. Serial measurements can be helpful in monitoring the response to treatment in this disease.

REFERENCES

1. Bright R. *Original papers of Richard Bright on renal diseases.* London: Oxford University Press; 1937.
2. von Behring E, Kitasato O. Ueber das Zustandekommen der Diphtherie-immunitat un der Tetanus-Immunitat bei Thieren. *Deutsch Med Wochenschr* 1890;16:1113.
3. Arthus M. Injections repeté de serum de cheval chez lelapin. *CR Seances Soc Biol Filiales* 1903;55:817.
4. von Pirquet CF, Schick B. *Die serum krankheit.* Vienna, Austria: Franz Deutiche Leipzig; 1905. English translation in: Schick B, ed. *Serum sickness.* Baltimore: Williams & Wilkins; 1951.
5. Germuth FC. Comparative histologic and immunologic study in rabbits of induced hypersensitivity of the serum sickness type. *J Exp Med* 1953;97:257–82.
6. Germuth FC, Pollack AD. The production of lesions of serum sickness in normal rabbits by the passive transfer of antibody in the presence of antigen. *Bull Johns Hopkins Hosp* 1958;104:245–63.
7. Dixon FJ, Vazquez JJ, Weigle WO, Cochrane CG. Pathogenesis of serum sickness. *Arch Pathol* 1958;65:18–28.
8. Dixon FJ, Feldman JD, Vazquez JJ. Experimental glomerulonephritis: the pathogenesis of a laboratory model resembling the spectrum of human glomerulonephritis. *J Exp Med* 1961;113:899–920.
9. Cochrane CG, Koffler D. Immune complex disease in experimental animals and man. *Adv Immunol* 1973;16:185–264.
10. Cochrane CG, Hawkins DJ. Studies on circulating immune complexes: III. Factors governing the ability of circulating immune complexes to localize in blood vessels. *J Exp Med* 1968;127:137–54.
11. Cochrane CG. Mechanisms involved in the deposition of immune complexes in tissues. *J Exp Med* 1971;134(suppl):79–89.
12. Wilson CB. Immunologic aspects of renal diseases. *JAMA* 1992;268: 2904–9.
13. Wilson CB. Immunologic mechanisms of renal disease. In: Brenner BM and Stein JH. *Contemporary Issues in Nephrology.* New York: Churchill-Livingstone, 1979.
14. Mann R, Neilson EG. Pathogenesis and treatment of immune-mediated renal disease. *Med Clin North Am* 1985;69:715–50.
15. Couser WG, Salant DJ. *In situ* immune complex formation and glomerular injury. *Kidney Int* 1980;17:1–13.
16. Kanwar YS. Biophysiology of glomerular filtration and proteinuria. *Lab Invest* 1984;51:7–21.
17. Glass WF, Radnik RA, Garoni J, Kreisberg JI. Urokinase-dependent adhesion loss and shape changes after cyclic adenosine monophosphate elevation in cultured rat mesangial cells. *J Clin Invest* 1988;82: 1992–2000.
18. Barnes JL, Levine SP, Venkatachalam MA. Binding of platelet factor 4 (PF4) to glomerular polyanion. *Kidney Int* 1984;25:759–65.
19. Schmiedeke TM, Stockl FW, Weber R. Histones have high affinity for the glomerular basement membrane. Relevance for immune complex formation in lupus nephritis. *J Exp Med* 1989;169:1879–94.
20. Batsford SR, Mihatsch MJ, Rawiel M. Surface charge distribution is a determinant of antigen deposition in the renal glomerulus: studies employing "charge-hybrid" molecules. *Clin Exp Immunol* 1991;86: 471–7.
21. Mannik M, Agodoa LYC, David KA. Rearrangement of immune complexes in glomeruli leads to persistence and development of electron dense deposits. *J Exp Med* 1983;157:1516–28.
22. Agodoa LYC, Gauthier VJ, Mannik M. Precipitating antigen-antibody systems are required for the formation of subepithelial electron dense immune deposits in rat glomeruli. *J Exp Med* 1983;158: 1259–71.
23. Mannik M, Striker GE. Removal of glomerular deposits of immune complexes in mice by administration of excess antigen. *Lab Invest* 1980;42:483–9.
24. Finbloom DS, Magilavy DB, Harford JB. Influence of antigen on immune complex behavior in mice. *J Clin Invest* 1981;68:214–24.
25. Gauthier VJ, Abrass CK. Circulating immune complexes in renal injury. *Semin Nephrol* 1992;12:379–94.
26. Myers CD. Role of B cell antigen processing and presentation in the humoral immune response. *FASEB J* 1991;5:2547–53.
27. Vitetta ES, Fernandez-Botran R, Myers CD, Sanders VM. Cellular interactions in the humoral immune response. *Adv Immunol* 1989;45: 1–105.
28. Milstein C. From antibody structure to immunological diversification of the immune response. *Science* 1986;231:1261–8.
29. Purkerson J, Isakson P. A two-signal model for regulation of immunoglobulin isotype switching. *FASEB J* 1992;6:3245–52.
30. Wener MH, Mannik M. Mechanisms of immune deposit formation in renal glomeruli. *Springer Semin Immunopathol* 1986;9:219–35.
31. Haakenstad AO, Striker GE, Mannik M. The glomerular deposition

of soluble immune complexes prepared with reduced and alkylated antibodies and with intact antibodies in mice. *Lab Invest* 1976;35: 293–301.
32. Savin VJ. Mechanisms of proteinuria in noninflammatory glomerular disease. *Am J Kidney Dis* 1993;21:347–62.
33. Kijlstra A, Allegonda VDL, Knutson DW, Fleuren GJ, Van Es LA. The influence of phagocyte function on glomerular localization of aggregated IgM in rats. *Clin Exp Immunol* 1978;32:207–17.
34. Abrass CK. Autologous immune complex nephritis in rats. Influence of modification of mononuclear phagocyte system function. *Lab Invest* 1984;51:162–71.
35. Abrass CK, Hori MT. Alterations in plasma clearance and tissue localization of model immune complexes in rats with streptozotocin-induced diabetes. *Immunology* 1987;60:331–6.
36. Fish AJ, Michael AF, Vernier RL, Good RA. Acute serum sickness in the rabbit: an immune deposit disease. *Am J Pathol* 1966;49:997–1022.
37. Iskandar SS, Jennette JC. Influence of antibody avidity on glomerular immune complex localization. *Am J Pathol* 1983;112:155–9.
38. Steward MW. Chronic immune complex disease in mice: the role of antibody affinity. *Clin Exp Immunol* 1979;38:414–23.
39. Ford PM. Interaction of rheumatoid factor with immune complexes in experimental glomerulonephritis—possible role of antiglobulins in chronicity. *J Rheumatol* 1983;10(suppl 11):81–4.
40. Hahn BH, Ebling FM. Idiotypic regulatory networks promote autoantibody formation. *J Rheumatol* 1987;14(suppl 13):143–8.
41. Zanetti M, Wilson CB. A role for antiidiotypic antibodies in immunologically mediated nephritis. *Am J Kidney Dis* 1986;7:445–51.
42. Uwatoko S, Gauthier VJ, Mannik M. Autoantibodies to the collagen-like region of C1q deposit in glomeurli via C1q in immune deposits. *Clin Immunol Immunopathol* 1991;61:268–73.
43. Wener MH, Uwatoko S, Mannik M. Antibodies to the collagen-like region of C1q in patients with autoimmune rheumatic diseases. *Arthritis Rheum* 1989;32:544–51.
44. Abrass CK. Fc receptor-mediated phagocytosis: abnormalities associated with diabetes mellitus. *Clin Immunol Immunopathol* 1991;58: 1–17.
45. Sylvestre DL, Ravetch JV. Fc receptors initiate the arthus reaction: redefining the inflammatory cascade. *Science* 1994;265:1095–8.
46. Ravetch JV, Kinet JP. Fc receptors. *Annu Rev Immunol* 1991;9: 457–92.
47. Mauer SM, Fish AJ, Blau EB, Michael AF. The glomerular mesangium: I. Kinetic studies of macromolecular uptake in normal and nephrotic rats. *J Clin Invest* 1972;51:1092–101.
48. Abrass CK, Hori M. Alterations in Fc receptor function of macrophages from streptozotocin-induced diabetic rats. *J Immunol* 1984;133:1307–12.
49. Abrass CK, O'Connor SW, Scarpace PJ, Abrass IB. Characterization of the β-adrenergic receptor of the rat peritoneal macrophage. *J Immunol* 1985;135:1338–41.
50. Tripp CS, Beckerman KP, Unanue ER. Immune complexes inhibit antimicrobial responses through interleukin-10 production. Effects in severe combined immunodeficiency mice during *Listeria* infection. *J Clin Invest* 1995;95:1628–34.
51. Moore KW, O'Garra A, de Waal Malefyt R, Vieira P, Mosmann TR. Interleukin-10. *Annu Rev Immunol* 1993;11:165–90.
52. Mancilla-Jimenez R, Appay MD, Bellon B, Kuhn J, Bariety J, Druet P. IgG Fc membrane receptor on normal human glomerular visceral epithelial cells. *Virchows Arch* 1984;404:139–58.
53. Neuwirth R, Singhal P, Diamond B, et al. Evidence for immunoglobulin Fc receptor-mediated prostaglandin$_2$ and platelet-activating factor formation by cultured rat mesangial cells. *J Clin Invest* 1988;82: 936–44.
54. Saus J, Wieslander J, Langeveld JP, Quinones S, Hudson BG. Identification of the Goodpasture antigen as the α3(IV) chain of collagen IV. *J Biol Chem* 1988;263:13374–80.
55. Couser WG, Abrass CK. Pathogenesis of membranous nephropathy. *Ann Rev Med* 1988;39:517–30.
56. Kerjaschki D, Farquhar MG. Immunochemical localization of the Heymann nephritis antigen (gp330) in glomerular epithelial cells of normal Lewis rats. *J Exp Med* 1983;157:667–86.
57. Kounnas MZ, Chappell DA, Strickland DK, Argraves WS. Glycoprotein 330, a member of the low density lipoprotein receptor family, binds lipoprotein lipase *in vitro*. *J Biol Chem* 1993;268: 14176–81.
58. Abrass CK, Border WA, Glassock RJ. Circulating immune complexes in rats with autologous immune complex nephritis. *Lab Invest* 1980;43:18–27.
59. Abrass CK. Evaluation of sequential glomerular eluates from rats with Heymann nephritis. *J Immunol* 1986;137:530–6.
60. Abrass CK, Cohen AH. The role of circulating antigen in the formation of immune deposits in experimental membranous nephropathy. *Proc Soc Exp Biol Med* 1986;183:348–57.
61. Kerjaschki D, Miettinen A, Farquhar MG. Initial events in the formation of immune deposits in passive Heymann nephritis. gp330–anti-gp330 immune complexes form in epithelial coated pits and become attached to the glomerular basement membrane. *J Exp Med* 1987;166: 109–28.
62. Couser WG, Steinmuller DR, Stilmant MM, Salant DJ, Lowenstein LM. Experimental glomerulonephritis in the isolated perfused rat kidney. *J Clin Invest* 1978;62:1275–87.
63. Mannik M. Mechanisms of tissue deposition of immune complexes. *J Rheumatol* 1987;14(suppl 13):35–42.
64. Kelly CJ, Tomaszewski JE, Neilson EG. Immunopathogenesis of tubulointerstitial injury. In: Brenner BM, and Tisher CC. *Renal Pathology*. Philadelphia: JB Lippincott; 1993:699–722.
65. Noble B, Andres GA, Brentjens JR. Passively transferred anti-brush border antibodies induce injury of proximal tubules in the absence of complement. *Clin Exp Immunol* 1983;56:281–8.
66. Fasth A, Hoyer JR, Seiler MW. Renal tubular immune complex formation in mice immunized with Tamm-Horsfall protein. *Am J Pathol* 1986;125:555–62.
67. Clayman MD, Michand L, Brentjens J, Andres GA, Kefalides NA, Neilson EG. Isolation of the target antigen of human anti-tubular basement membrane antibody-associated interstitial nephritis. *J Clin Invest* 1986;77:1143–7.
68. Oldstone MBA. Molecular mimicry and autoimmune disease. *Cell* 1987;80:819–20.
69. Lehman DH, Wilson CB, Dixon FJ. Extraglomerular immunoglobulin deposits in human nephritis. *Am J Med* 1975;58:765–86.
70. Wilson CB. Nephritogenic tubulointerstitial antigens. *Kidney Int* 1991;39:501–17.
71. Barnett EV, Knutson DW, Abrass CK, Chia DS, Young LS, Liebling MR. Circulating immune complexes: their immunochemistry, detection, and importance. *Ann Intern Med* 1979;91:430–40.
72. Abrass CK, Hall CL, Border WA, Brown CA, Glassock RJ, Coggins CH, Collaborative Study of the Adult Idiopathic Nephrotic Syndrome. Circulating immune complexes in adults with idiopathic nephroatic syndrome. *Kidney Int* 1980;17:545–53.
73. Abrass CK, Nies KM, Louie JS, Border WA, Glassock RJ. Correlation and predictive accuracy of circulating immune complexes with disease acitivity in patients with systemic lupus erythematosus. *Arthritis Rheum* 1980;23:273–82.
74. Hori MT, Abrass CK. Isolation and characterization of circulating immune complexes from rats with experimental membranous nephropathy. *J Immunol* 1990;144:3849–55.
75. Misiani R, Bellavita P, Fenili D, et al. Hepatitis C virus infection in patients with essential mixed cryoglobulinemia. *Ann Intern Med* 1992;117:573–7.
76. Johnson RJ, Gretch DR, Yamabe H, et al. Membranoproliferative glomerulonephritis associated with hepatitis C virus infection. *N Engl J Med* 1993;328:505–6.
77. Abrass CK. Immune complex diseases. In: Massry SG, and Glassock RJ. *Textbook of Nephrology*. Baltimore: Williams & Wilkins; 1995: 635–43.

Immunologic Renal Diseases,
edited by E. G. Neilson and W. G. Couser.
Lippincott-Raven Publishers, Philadelphia © 1997.

CHAPTER 15

Apoptosis in Acute Renal Inflammation

John S. Savill, Andrew F. Mooney, and Jeremy Hughes

Injury to a cell can lead to cell death. Although there may be many types of cell death, it has proved useful to take an extreme view that regards cell death as proceeding by one of two major mechanisms (1). Necrosis is an "accidental" form of cell death triggered by severely noxious stimuli such as hypoxia, extremes of temperature and high concentrations of toxins. Cells dying by necrosis exhibit diminished adenosine triphosphate (ATP) levels, faulty membrane function, and disruption of organelles, with the result that the dying cell swells and disintegrates. Uncontrolled release of cell contents incites tissue injury and an inflammatory response, particularly because the stimuli initiating necrosis tend to affect fields of cells. Cell death by necrosis is "bad news" for a tissue.

By contrast with necrosis, cell death by apoptosis is frequently a "programmed" and physiological event, often affecting scattered cells within a tissue (2,3). Usually, apoptosis does not incite inflammation because apoptotic cells are swiftly recognized and ingested by phagocytes before the dying cell loses membrane integrity and leaks noxious contents. Furthermore, rather than the apparently passive response to "murderous" stimuli represented by necrosis, apoptosis is an active form of cell "suicide" that can in certain circumstances require macromolecular synthesis. In cells dying by apoptosis, ATP levels are maintained, and the structure and function of the plasma membrane and organelles are retained for many hours. Rather than swelling, cells undergoing apoptosis shrink. Generally speaking, if cells must die, then apoptosis tends to disrupt tissue function less than necrosis. Indeed, the non-inflammatory properties of apoptosis are emphasized by the fact that this is the usual mechanism of cell deletion in physiological tissue turnover, embryogenesis, hormone-dependent tissue atrophy, removal of lymphocytes failing selection in the thymus, and many other processes essential to life.

The purpose of this chapter is to consider the role of apoptosis in acute inflammation of the kidney. There is growing evidence that apoptosis may be "good news" in inflammation, leading to safe and desirable deletion of potentially dangerous leukocytes. Furthermore, apoptosis can promote efficient remodelling of injured tissue by removing excess resident renal cells that have proliferated as part of the normal repair mechanisms associated with the inflammatory response. Persistence of inflammatory tissue injury and/or undesirably increased populations of glomerular cells could result from defects in the normal program of apoptosis. Indeed, renal inflammation may be initiated by defects in lymphocyte homeostasis consequent upon abnormalities of apoptosis in this cell lineage. However, an adverse outcome in renal inflammation also might occur when apoptosis is efficiently but inappropriately engaged. For example, cells exposed to levels of noxious stimuli insufficient to induce necrosis may engage the program of apoptosis: the stricken cell altruistically commits suicide in the manner least likely to disrupt tissue structure and function. Unfortunately, such disruption will be inevitable if too many desirable cells are deleted by apoptosis. Furthermore, loss of precious renal cells may be due to direct induction of apoptosis in target cells of cytotoxic lymphocytes. However, as will become apparent, undesirable renal cell death could result from subtle stimuli that are not obviously noxious.

Because there have been dramatic and exciting advances in understanding of the molecular mechanisms of apoptosis, these will be described in some detail in the first section of the chapter. Next, the role of apoptosis in removal of excess resident renal cells will be addressed, following which we will discuss the role of apoptosis in beneficial leukocyte clearance. Finally we will assess the "dark sides" of apoptosis: the promotion of tissue injury by defects in the program and inappropriate engagement of the program with undesirable loss of cells.

J. S. Savill, A. F. Mooney, and J. Hughes: Division of Renal and Inflammatory Disease, Department of Medicine, University Hospital, Nottingham NG7 2UH, England.

MECHANISMS OF APOPTOSIS

Clues from Morphological Changes

Apoptosis was defined on morphological grounds in 1972 (2). Indeed, in the absence of a definitive molecular marker, the only way to be sure that a cell is dying by apoptosis remains demonstration of the typical, highly stereotyped morphological features. These include cell shrinkage, cytoplasmic condensation (sometimes with vacuolation), and typical condensation of nuclear heterochromatin initially into crescents abutting the nuclear membrane and then later into one or more spheres (Fig. 1). In some cell types there is dramatic "blebbing" of the plasma membrane, which can result in the budding away of membrane-bound "apoptotic bodies," which may contain nuclear fragments. However, in addition to intact apoptotic cells, phagocytes also recognize and ingest these apoptotic bodies.

Morphologists studying apoptosis have long suspected that the process involves enzymatic degradation of key structural proteins and of chromatin itself. Indeed, the internucleosomal cleavage of chromatin to yield oligonucleosomal fragments of DNA, demonstrable upon agarose gel electrophoresis as the classical DNA ladder, was long regarded as the biochemical hallmark of this type of cell death (4). In fact, this may represent a late event in the death program because chromatin condensation can occur without internucleosomal chromatin cleavage, probably because this is usually preceded by higher order cleavage of DNA into 300-kb and 50-kb fragments corresponding to detachment from the nuclear matrix of "rosettes" and "loops" of DNA, respectively (5–8). Nevertheless, as we shall see, morphological predictions of a key role for degradative enzymes in apoptosis have not proved unfounded.

A further morphological entrée to mechanisms has come from comparative biology. Cells dying develop-

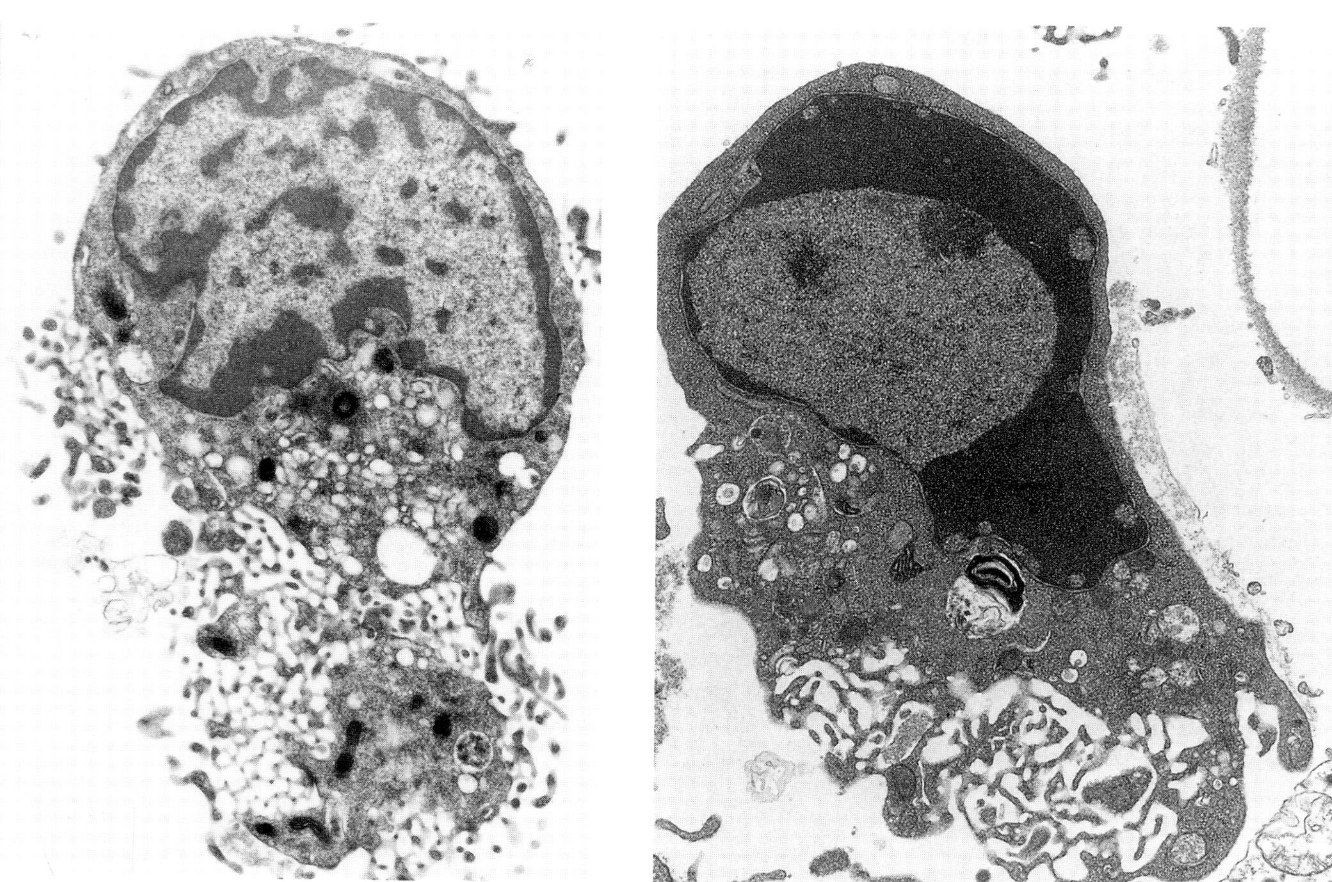

FIG. 1. Ultrastructure of glomerular cell apoptosis. Transmission EM of glomerular cells harvested from enzymatically dissociated glomeruli of rats with nephrotoxic nephritis (original magnification of both images ×13,200). **A:** Normal glomerular endothelial cell. **B:** Cell in early stages of apoptosis. Note nuclear shrinkage with crescent of condensed heterochromatin and prominent nucleolus. Note also cytoplasmic condensation and shrinkage/simplification of cytoplasm and processes.

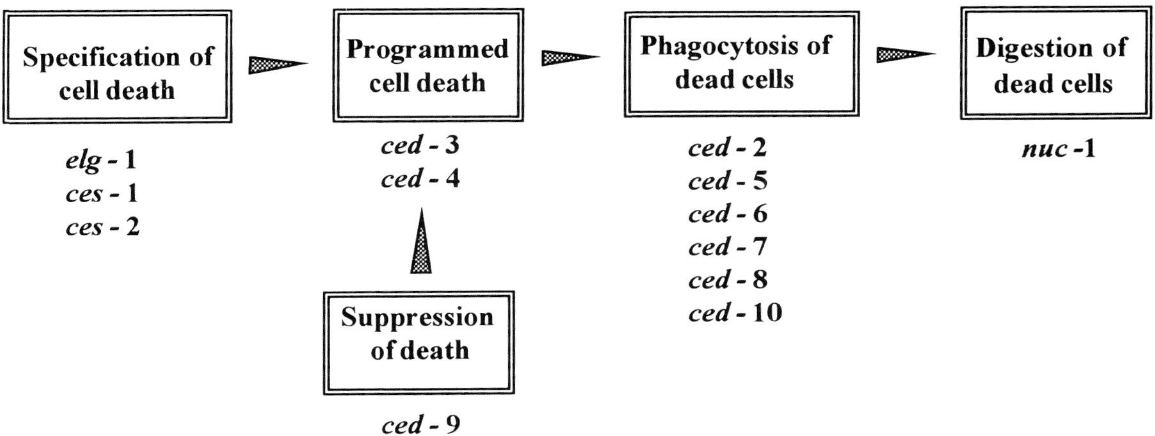

FIG. 2. Cell death program in *C. elegans.* Genes controlling each step are given in italics.

mental deaths during morphogenesis of simple organisms undergo morphological changes very similar to apoptosis. Painstaking vital microscopy of the nematode *Caenorhabditis elegans* has shown that of the 1,090 somatic cells formed during development of an adult hermaphrodite, 131 undergo precisely controlled and predictable programmed cell death (9). However, the number of developmental cell deaths is abnormal in mutant organisms, and analysis of double mutants enables genes controlling the nematode death program to be assigned an order (Fig. 2). Remarkably, a number of these genes have proved to possess structural and functional homology, with mammalian genes controlling apoptosis (see below).

Effector Mechanisms

Many researchers hope that the program of apoptosis could be harnessed to kill undesirable cells, such as those in cancers. For this reason there has been intense activity in attempting to define which proteins drive cell death.

Endogenous Proteases

In the early 1990s, the morphologically based suspicion that proteases could play important roles in apoptosis received indirect support. Cultured monocytes dying by apoptosis, but not necrosis, were found to release mature interleukin (IL)-1, implying proteolytic cleavage of pre-pro–IL-1 (10). Furthermore, studies on apoptosis induced in tumor cell lines by chemotherapeutic agents or in thymocytes by dexamethasone suggested that cleavage of the 116-kDa nuclear protein poly (ADP-ribose) polymerase (PARP) to produce an 85-kDa fragment was a specific marker of apoptosis (11). In addition to this evidence of target protein cleavage, it was found that inhibitors of cysteine and serine proteases could block apoptosis in vitro (12), whereas deliberate introduction of purified proteases could induce apoptosis (13).

However, the most dramatic evidence in support of endogenous proteases driving apoptosis came from cloning of a *C. elegans* gene critically controlling cell death, *ced-3,* which must function for the nematode cell death program to proceed (14). This gene proved to be homologous to the mammalian cysteine protease IL-1–converting enzyme (ICE) (15), already implicated by selective release of processed IL-1 from apoptotic monocytes. Over-expression of ICE in Rat-1 fibroblasts induced typical apoptosis, which could be blocked by point mutations in the region of the molecule with the closest sequence similarity to *ced-3* (16). Indeed, *ICE* proved to be the index member of a gene family including members such as *CPP32* and *Ich-1* (*ICE* and *ced-3* homologue, previously *Nedd-2*), which were found to have effects on cell death (17). For example, alternate transcript splicing yields Ich_L, a protein that when over-expressed can induce apoptosis in mammalian cells, and Ich_S, which can protect fibroblasts against apoptosis induced by serum deprivation.

Nevertheless, growing evidence suggests that rather than ICE itself playing a key role, apoptosis may result from activation of other proteases in the ICE family. Thus, in a cell-free system, purified ICE failed to cleave PARP to yield the putative "apoptotic signature" fragment, although such cleavage could be blocked by protease inhibitors selective for ICE (18). Furthermore, *ICE* –/– "knockout" mice (19) displayed no obvious defects in apoptosis, either in deletion of mammary epithelial cells in postlactation involution of the gland in vivo or in particular models of macrophage and thymocyte apoptosis in vitro. However, when the *ICE* homologue *CPP32β* was expressed as a fusion protein, it was found to cleave PARP and release the "apoptotic" 85-kDa fragment (20). The investigators colorfully suggested that the CPP32β protein should be called "Yama," after the Hindu god of death. Interestingly, Yama is a zymogen requiring proteolytic cleavage for activation and it appears that ICE may cleave Yama, possibly accounting for apoptosis induced by over-expression of ICE. Furthermore, this observation suggests that there may be a cascade of protease activation in apoptosis, which will require careful characterization. Understanding both upstream triggering and downstream targets of "apoptotic" protease activation is now a major goal in the field.

Plasma Membrane Death Receptors

An obvious upstream trigger of apoptotic protease activation could be ligation of cell surface "death receptors." The clearest example of a cell surface receptor that drives programmed death is provided by Fas, a member of the tumor necrosis factor receptor (TNFR) family (21–23). Fas is constitutively expressed (in mice) by cells of the T-lymphocyte line, liver, lung, and ovary. Both in vitro and in vivo (24), binding of Fas with antibody can rapidly trigger apoptosis, a property shared in vitro by the natural Fas ligand, a transmembrane molecule homologous to TNF (25). There is clear evidence for downstream involvement of ICE-like proteases because apoptosis induced by Fas ligation in various cell lines can be blocked by a tetrapeptide inhibitor of ICE and by transfection with an *ICE* antisense complementary DNA (cDNA) construct or the cDNA for the pox virus–derived serine protease inhibitor *crm A,* which is known to block activity of both ICE and Yama (20,26,27). Furthermore, Fas ligation induced ICE-like activity assayed in cells by cleavage of a fluorogenic substrate.

Clearly, therefore, given the central importance of *ced-3* in the nematode cell death program and growing evidence of the importance of ICE-like proteases in many instances of mammalian apoptosis, understanding how Fas engages the lethal protease cascade could have wide importance. There is evidence for involvement in Fas-induced apoptosis of pathways involving the sphingomyelinase/ceramide (28), tyrosine phosphorylation (29), and serine/threonine phosphorylation pathways (30). However, another promising approach has been to employ the yeast two-hybrid system to define proteins binding a cytoplasmic "death" domain shared by Fas and TNFR I (31–33). Three proteins (FADD, TRADD, and the appropriately named RIP) have been identified as binding Fas/TNFR I in a homotypic fashion on the basis of having a homologous domain, but their otherwise unrelated portions are probably those signalling death. Time will tell whether the yeast two-hybrid system will allow investigators to claw their way along signalling pathways impinging on Yama and other ICE-like proteases. An alternative approach could be to exploit the power of *Drosophila* genetics to define death pathways, because the Fas/TNFR I death domain also has homology with reaper (34), a protein upon which most if not all developmental cell death in this organism depends (35).

As implied by the previous paragraph, TNF can induce typical apoptosis in susceptible cells, via both TNFR I and TNFR II (36), which is interesting because the latter does not bear the "death domain," implying still more intracellular pathways capable of signalling death (23). The complexity of receptor-mediated regulation of cell death is further emphasized by the fact that TNF frequently transduces cell activation rather than cell death; indeed, there is even an example of Fas ligation inducing activation rather than cell death (37), which may reflect association of Fas with a protein tyrosine phosphatase (PTP-BAS) that confers resistance to death (38). Furthermore, in certain circumstances apoptosis can be induced by cytokines such as transforming growth factor (TGF-β) (39), or extracellular matrix proteins such as fibronectin (40), each normally involved in active fibrotic responses (41). Finally, while cross-linking of the T-cell receptor induces proliferation in mature T cells, in immature T cells/thymocytes this stimulus causes apoptosis, in which the immediate early gene *nur-77* (which encodes an orphan steroid receptor) plays a key postreceptor role (42). Clearly more investigations are needed before the relationship between exogenous death signals, ligation of cell-surface receptors, and engagement of the death program can be defined.

Nuclear Death Proteins

Elegant experiments suggested that the fundamental effector mechanisms in apoptosis are not nuclear because anucleate cytoplasts could be triggered to undergo morphological changes very similar to apoptosis (43). However, it seems likely that key targets for apoptotic proteases, such as PARP, are nuclear. Indeed, chromatin condensation may depend on proteolytic cleavage of nuclear lamins A-B (5), and there is some evidence (albeit inconsistent, between cell systems) that this event may be regulated by phosphorylation of nuclear lamins by the $p34^{cdc2}$ kinase first implicated in mitosis (44). Lastly, there is compelling evidence that nuclear proteins can drive cell death. When apoptosis occurs as an apparently altruistic response to DNA damage induced by mutagenic/carcinogenic stimuli such as ionizing radiation, elegant studies in knockout mice have confirmed a key effector role for the multifunctional nuclear protein p53 (45). However, precisely how p53 is linked to the apoptotic program remains uncertain (46).

Survival Factors

It should already by apparent that regulation of cell death is likely to involve a complex interplay between factors extrinsic and intrinsic to the cell. So far, we have concentrated on death-promoting effector mechanisms. However, it is becoming ever more apparent that these are normally kept in check by extracellular and intracellular "survival factors."

Extrinsic Survival Factors

During the 1980s, an increasing number of reports indicated that cultured cell lines depended on lineage-specific factors for survival, such as IL-2 for activated lymphocytes (47) or colony-stimulating factors for bone marrow cells (48). Deprivation of such factors resulted in cell death by apoptosis. Because a growing body of evidence, much from neurobiology (49), indicated that cells in vivo also depended on exogenous factors for survival, Raff proposed that all cells (except blastomeres) were dependent on survival factors generated by other cells (50). In the Raff scheme, failure of a given cell to receive a sufficient supply of survival factors results in apoptosis by default. This elegant idea has a number of important ramifications, which include insights into how the size of cell populations may be controlled. For example, gene transfer experiments have shown that although expression of the proto-oncogene *c-myc* drives cells into division, cell number only increases if sufficient survival factors are present in the form of added serum; if not, then apoptosis ensues (51). Indeed, it appears that dividing cells are particularly susceptible to apoptosis triggered by survival factor deprivation. The clear implication is that cell population size will increase if survival factor supply increases. A good example of such "times of plenty" is the enlarged, lactating breast of pregnancy and the puerperium, because when survival factor "famine" ensues as the supply of lactogenic hormones decreases, the breast undergoes involution by apoptosis (52,53). Similarly, interruption of androgen supply by castration results in prostatic atrophy as prostate cells deprived of their key survival factor undergo apoptosis (54). In a healthy tissue with stable populations, such as the kidney, cell birth by mitosis is exactly matched by cell loss by apoptosis. As we shall see, there is evidence that changes in the size of renal cell populations during acute inflammation may reflect imbalance of mitosis and apoptosis consequent upon stimuli selectively signalling mitosis or survival.

If cell population size can be regulated by independent control of cell division and cell survival, then it follows that there may be distinct intracellular pathways signalling "divide" or "survive." Indeed, ligation of the same receptors appears capable of transducing such distinct signals. For example, in serum-deprived fibroblasts transfected with *c-myc*, cytokines such as insulinlike growth factor-1 (IGF-1) can prevent otherwise inevitable apoptosis by mechanisms that are resistant to inhibitors of protein synthesis and other drugs that block intracellular signalling pathways essential for a proliferative response to the same cytokine (55). Recent evidence has implicated both the Ras pathway (56) and phosphatidyl inositol 3-kinase (57) in the signalling of cell survival, but much work remains before we understand how cytokine receptors can selectively regulate cell survival.

A further implication of Raff's ideas is that any cell surface receptor involved in mediating responses such as growth or differentiation also could signal survival. There is abundant evidence that cell contact with extracellular matrix or other cells can direct cell behavior, presumably via cell surface receptors such as integrins and associated cytoplasmic elements including the cytoskeleton (58). For example, establishment of mammary gland alveolar morphology and the coordinated expression of genes related to milk secretion are critically dependent on deposition of a laminin-rich extracellular matrix (58). There is now growing evidence that loss of cell contact may deprive cells of survival signals in addition to those directing differentiation or division, with the result that detaching cells undergo apoptosis (59,60). Frisch and Francis have termed this phenomenon *anoikis,* a word derived from the Greek for "homelessness" (61). In vivo, interruption of survival signals may reflect degradation of extracellular matrix by metalloproteinases, which precedes involution of the lactating breast with associated apoptosis (52). Given that matrix metalloproteinase action may be regulated by local synthesis of both the enzymes and potent tissue inhibitors, and activation of enzymes by proteolysis or reactive oxygen species (ROS), it can be appreciated that regulation of external survival signals from extracellular matrix adds a further level of complexity to the balance between apoptosis and cell survival. Many factors, each subject to regulation, may constitute the "ticket for survival" for any particular cell.

Finally, the Raff hypothesis predicts that there should be close links between survival factor deprivation and the death machinery of the cell. A compelling example is provided by the recent studies of Bissell's group (62). They showed that unlike plastic, laminin-rich extracellular matrix was able to prevent tightly adherent mammary epithelial cells from detaching and undergoing apoptosis. Furthermore, in both cultured mammary cells and in lactating mice, activation of a stromelysin transgene resulted in expression of this matrix metalloproteinase, degradation of matrix, and increased mammary epithelial apoptosis. Survival signals from laminin-rich matrix appeared to be transduced via cell surface integrins, because in mammary epithelial cells cultured on a laminin-rich matrix, apoptosis was induced by function blocking antibody to the $\beta 1$ common chain of the integrins. When apoptosis was induced in vitro and in vivo, increased expression of *ICE* was observed, and a peptide inhibitor of ICE-like proteases and transfected *crm A* blocked apoptosis in cultured cells, demonstrating a close link between lack of survival signals and the effector mechanisms of apoptosis. Similarly, survival pathways seem to interact with the nuclear protein p53 because transfection of dominant-negative inhibitors of wild-type p53 conferred resistance to apoptosis induced by withdrawal of IL-3 from a hematopoietic cell line dependent on this cytokine (63). Clearly, there is a need to understand how failure of sufficient ligation of cell surface receptors for survival signals results in activation of cytoplasmic and nuclear events triggering apoptosis.

CED-9, Bcl-2, and Other Intrinsic Survival Factors

As depicted in Fig. 2, in the *C. elegans* cell death program, the death-promoting CED-3 protease is normally suppressed by an "upstream" gene *ced-9* (9,64). Remarkably, this gene proved to be homologous to the human *bcl-2* protooncogene, originally cloned from the *t*(14:18) chromosomal translocation found in the remarkably long-lived B cells of follicular lymphoma. There is now a mass of evidence from in vitro and in vivo gene transfer experiments to indicate that Bcl-2 is a remarkably ubiquitous "antidote to death," countering apoptosis triggered by multiple stimuli (65–67). Indeed, *bcl-2* may substitute for *ced-9* in preventing developmental cell deaths in *C. elegans.*

Furthermore, there is an ever-expanding family of Bcl-2–related proteins that share homology that is mainly, but not exclusively, sited within the *B*cl-2 *H*omology domains BH-1 and BH-2. These include Bax, Bcl-x_L, Bad, Bak (and Bak-2 and Bak-3), Mcl-1, A-1, and the BHRF-1 and LMW5-HL proteins of the Epstein-Barr and African swine fever viruses (68–74). Most of these proteins have been shown by transfection experiments to regulate cell death. However, although over-expression of family members such as Bcl-x_L mimic Bcl-2 in blocking apoptosis, others, including Bax, Bad, Bak, and Bcl-x_S (the short form of Bcl-x_L), can inhibit the prosurvival properties of Bcl-2 homologues and/or directly promote apoptosis when transfected into various cellular models. Although the in vivo relevance of many of these observations remains to be tested, the *bcl-2* –/– knockout mouse emphasizes the likely central importance of this gene family in regulating cell death (75). For example *bcl-2* –/– mice exhibit progressive loss of their immune system because of postneonatal lymphocyte apoptosis in the thymus and spleen.

A variety of protein–protein interactions seem likely to be critical for the effects of Bcl-2 family members upon cell death. Central among these appears to be the capacity of Bcl-2–related proteins to form hetero- and homodimers via interactions at the BH1 and BH2 domains (76,77). It appears that heterodimerization of Bax by Bcl-2 or Bcl-x_L prevents the formation of Bax homodimers, which promote apoptosis. The protein Bad seems able to displace Bax from Bcl-2 and Bcl-x_L and thereby promote cell death, and binding of Bak to Bcl-x_L may have similar effects (70). A picture is emerging that apoptosis may be regulated by a complex series of competing dimerizations between proteins of the Bcl-2 family. Furthermore, these interactions may in turn be regulated by binding to nonhomologous proteins. These may be endogenous, such as BAG-1 (78), Nip-1, Nip-2, and Nip-3 (79), or may be encoded by viruses such as the E1B 19K adenovirus protein (71). Finally, further levels of regulation are superimposed on such protein–protein interactions. Obviously, there is growing interest in transcriptional controls, and IL-10 has been found to rescue germinal center B-lymphocytes from apoptosis ex vivo by increasing *bcl-2* expression (80). Posttranslational controls on Bcl-2 function such as hyperphosphorylation also may be important in conferring protection against cell death (81).

Interestingly, there are still few insights into how Bcl-2 family proteins regulate cell death. Although some evidence has suggested that Bcl-2 protein might inhibit the generation or action of ROS putatively involved in triggering apoptosis (82), this idea has recently been challenged by data showing that Bcl-2 can prevent apoptosis in a near-anaerobic atmosphere in which the generation of ROS should be much diminished (83,84). Time will test the durability of the equally attractive idea that Bax may be a direct regulator of transcription of the *p53* gene, promoting expression of this nuclear death protein (85).

Research into endogenous survival factors is frenetic to say the least. Many laboratories are seeking new families of survival genes. It should be apparent from the foregoing sections that such genes could fall into many classes. Endogenous survival proteins might include cytokines acting in an autocrine fashion upon survival-promoting receptors; secreted soluble inhibitors preventing ligation of cell surface "death" receptors; cytoplasmic proteins competitively inhibiting binding of signalling molecules to the death domains of receptors such as Fas and TNFR I; protein inhibitors of ICE-like proteases; proteins interfering with dimerizations of the Bcl-2 family; and proteins regulating p53 expression or action. Furthermore, endogenous survival proteins may differ between cell types, as shown by the marked effects of *bcl-2* knockout on lymphoid cells, and at different times, in particular tissues.

BENEFICIAL REMOVAL OF EXCESS RESIDENT CELLS

It should be apparent that apoptosis is the normal means by which excess cells are cleared when physiologically enlarged organs return to normal size; involution of the lactating breast already has been cited as an example (53). Indeed, one of the earliest reports of apoptosis in the kidney highlighted a role for programmed cell death in the regression of tubular hyperplasia (86). Simplistically, an inflamed tissue contains an excess of cells, which are derived from the blood and from proliferation of resident cells. This section describes recent evidence indicating that apoptosis mediates clearance of excess renal cells during resolution of nephritis.

Glomerular Inflammation

Johnson has highlighted the stereotyped response of the glomerulus to injury, which has many similarities to inflammation in other organs (87). First, there is infiltration with leukocytes, which is reversible because these cells can be cleared by mechanisms such as apoptosis. Second, there is an increase in the amount and nature of glomerular extracellular matrix in keeping with wound repair in other organs. Again, this is potentially reversible, and may relate to increased expression of degradative enzymes during resolution of glomerulonephritis. Third, the last component of the triad of glomerular responses to inflammatory injury is proliferation and phenotypic change of resident glomerular cells. Mesangial cells are particularly prone to increase in number, but they also undergo a phenotypic transformation to a myofibroblastlike cell, expressing α smooth muscle actin and interstitial collagens (88,89). Although the mechanisms promoting later loss of this phenotype are unknown, there is now strong evidence that excess mesangial cells are cleared away by undergoing apoptosis, data that will be the focus of this section.

Detection of Apoptosis in Glomerulonephritis

Although apoptosis was first described in 1972, it was not until 1987 that apoptosis was reported in the kidney during the seminal studies of Gobé and Axelsen addressing tubular cell loss after experimentally induced ureteric obstruction (90). Indeed, it was another year before Harrison's careful light microscopical study demonstrated the presence of apoptotic cells in the glomeruli of humans with nephritis (91).

Much of this delay probably reflected the fact that observers familiar with the typical light microscopical features of apoptosis took some time to study glomerulonephritis. Although confirmation by electron microscopy (EM) is always preferable, conventional histological stains do show the typical cell shrinkage, chromatin condensation, and nuclear fragmentation of apoptosis at the light microscopical level (Fig. 3A). A useful technique by which to confirm such findings is to stain appropriately prepared tissue sections with DNA-binding dyes such as propidium iodide, viewing the material by epifluorescence (Fig. 3B). In conventional 4- to 5-micron sections, it is necessary to rack the microscope objective up and down to find apoptotic cells and confirm that nuclear staining is homogenous, but this can be greatly facilitated by using confocal microscopy.

However, a dramatic recent development has been the introduction of a number of related techniques designed to detect DNA cleaved as a consequence of apoptosis, using conventional tissue sections and enzymatic bonding of

A,B

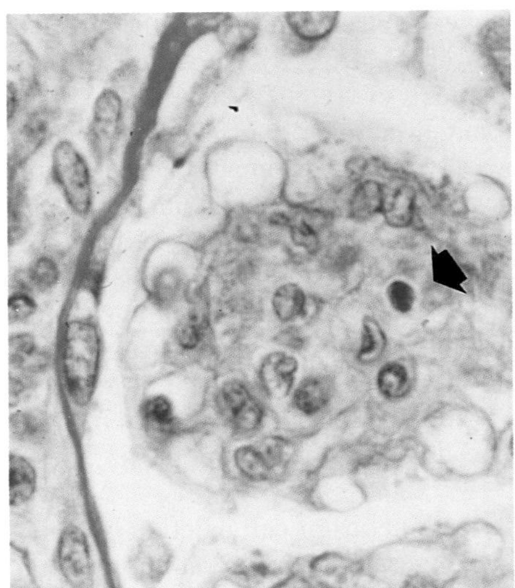

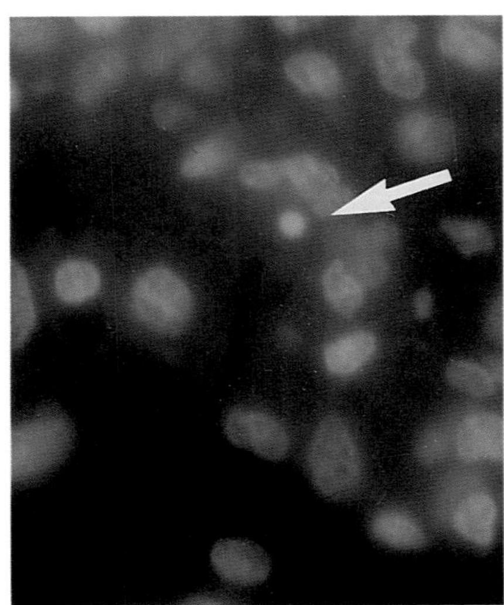

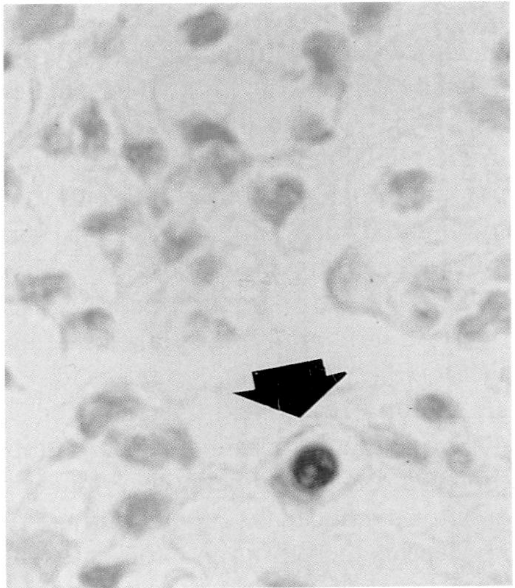

C

FIG. 3. Mesangial cell apoptosis in rat Thyl.1 nephritis. **A:** PAS stain of glomerular tuft at 10 days (*arrow*: apoptotic cell) (original magnification ×900). **B:** Propidium iodide stain of RNase-treated material viewed under epifluorescence (original magnification ×1,200). Note condensed, homogeneous nucleus of apoptotic cell (*arrow*). **C:** TUNEL (TdT-mediated dUTP-biotin nick end labelling) stain for DNA degradation (original magnification ×1,200). Note apoptotic cell within halo (*arrow*). Reproduced from the *Journal of Clinical Investigation* 1994;94:2105–16, by copyright permission of the Society for Clinical Investigation.

labelled nucleotides to the free ends of fragmented DNA (92,93). Great care in interpreting such data are required because these techniques can pick up DNA breaks of any cause and in certain circumstances may erroneously label cells undergoing necrosis. Nevertheless, in our own studies using terminal deoxynucleotidyl transferase-mediated dUTP-biotin nick end-labelling (TUNEL) (Fig. 3C) we found a close agreement with quantitation of apoptosis by light and fluorescence microscopy (94), and others have confirmed these data (95).

Mesangial Cells Can Undergo Apoptosis

Many types of human proliferative glomerulonephritis, in which glomerular mesangial cell numbers increase, are reversible. Examples include immunoglobulin (Ig)A nephropathy, lupus nephritis, and postinfectious glomerulonephritis. Therefore, there must be mechanisms by which excess mesangial cells are cleared. Indeed, this point is emphasized by a well-established rat model of selective and self-limited mesangial proliferation (96,97). Administration of antibody to Thyl.1, which is expressed by mesangial cells in the rat, causes a brisk mesangiolysis. The number of mesangial cells progressively increases from a nadir of approximately one per glomerular cross-section to reach a peak 10–14 days after antibody administration, when mesangial cell number is about double the normal amount. Mesangial cell number then gradually returns to baseline over the next 40–50 days, and normal glomerular structure and function are restored. In this model, as in many types of human glomerulonephritis, mesangial cells express α smooth muscle actin and other features of the myofibroblast (88,98). In skin wounds there were data implying that myofibroblasts could be deleted by apoptosis (99), which suggested that we should determine whether the program of apoptosis is available to mesangial cells. We found that cultured human, rat, or porcine mesangial cells subjected to vigorous deprivation of potential survival factors such as serum and insulin did indeed undergo typical apoptosis, although approximately 90% of human mesangial cells were able to survive for over 8 hours, implying synthesis of endogenous survival factors (94). In keeping with this idea, the protein synthesis inhibitor cycloheximide induced apoptosis in nearly 40% of human mesangial cells within 8 hours. Furthermore, rat mesangial cells were much more susceptible to apoptosis induced by either stimulus.

Clearly, therefore, apoptosis was a candidate mechanism for clearance of excess mesangial cells during resolution of mesangial hyperplasia in Thyl.1 nephritis. We confirmed that apoptosis did indeed occur in Thyl.1 nephritis, using light and electron microscopy (94), data that were confirmed by Shimizu et al. (95). This group sought to confirm the mesangial origin of the apoptotic cells by TUNEL/anti-Thyl.1 double-labelling experiments, but unfortunately this approach is confounded somewhat because in both groups' studies there was clear evidence that apoptotic cells were ingested by healthy mesangial cells. Therefore, Thyl.1-positive cytoplasm around an apoptotic nucleus does not necessarily imply a mesangial cell origin for the apoptotic cell. However, both groups found EM evidence of cells in early stages of apoptosis with cytoplasmic bundles of microfilaments, consistent with a mesangial cell origin. Furthermore, apart from occasional exceptions, apoptotic cells occupied a mesangial position. Lastly, the major clearance task in this model appears to be removal of mesangial cells because the vast majority (>85%) of proliferating nuclear cell antigen (PCNA positive) cells express Thyl.1, and most of the remainder are macrophages, which may leave the glomerulus to meet elsewhere (100). Therefore, in this model of selective changes in mesangial cell number, apoptotic cells appeared very likely to be of mesangial cell origin.

Kinetics of Mesangial Cell Clearance by Apoptosis

In normal rat glomeruli, before administration of Thyl.1 antibody, glomerular cell apoptosis was rare, occurring in only 0.01% of cells (94). Even at its peak, apoptosis was only increased to 0.25% in our studies. How could such apparently small levels of apoptosis achieve large changes in cell number? The answer lies in the speed of cell deletion by apoptosis. Time lapse videomicroscopy has shown that cells adopt apoptotic morphology within minutes. Furthermore, in vitro studies demonstrate that apoptotic cells are ingested and degraded by phagocytes in a series of events that are also measured in minutes (101). Direct observation of cells being deleted by apoptosis in vivo (9), calculations based on known changes in cell number in a given tissue over certain time periods (102), and estimates based on the decrease in numbers of apoptotic cells in vivo after administration of a survival factor (103) all indicate that apoptotic cells are usually degraded beyond histological recognition in 0.5–2.0 h, the so-called clearance time. Thus, in a hypothetical tissue in which there is no cell birth by mitosis and the apoptotic clearance time is 1 h, demonstration of 1% apoptosis implies that in 24 h nearly 24% of cells will be deleted. A little apoptosis goes a long way.

Before dissecting the kinetics of cell deletion by apoptosis in Thyl.1-induced mesangial proliferation in the rat, it appears important and worthwhile to assess whether apoptosis could be an important mode of cell deletion in human glomerulonephritis. Reassuringly, Szabolcs et al. found in renal biopsy samples from normal human kidney glomerular cells that apoptosis was observed with a frequency similar to that of the rat: 0.03 apoptotic cells per ten glomerular cross-sections (104). In acute postinfectious glomerulonephritis, this figure was increased by over 250-fold, which we estimate would imply that roughly 1% of cells are apoptotic at the time of biopsy. In turn, this suggests that perhaps as many as one quarter of the cells identified are destined to be removed in one day if the glomerular apoptotic cell clearance time is 1 h. As we shall demonstrate below, these data are likely to reflect the intense infiltration of glomeruli in this condition, with short-lived neutrophils destined to die by apoptosis. Nevertheless, even in IgA nephropathy or lupus nephritis, proliferative nephritides with less intense leukocyte infiltration, these investigators reported substantial increases in glomerular apoptosis of about 50- to 100-fold. By inference these data imply that in the absence of cell proliferation or recruitment, glomerular cell number might decrease by up to a few percent per day. This figure makes sense because such lesions probably resolve over weeks or months, so that the day-by-day changes in glomerular number required to restore the cell complement to normal would be small. In short, estimates based on observed frequency of apoptosis in human renal biopsy samples are consistent with a potentially major role for this mode of cell death in promoting recovery from glomerulonephritis.

What then of the Thyl.1 model? Is mesangial cell apoptosis the major mechanism for resolution of mesangial hypercellularity? In time course studies (Fig. 4) we found that apoptosis was increased by about fivefold between days 10 and 42, when mean glomerular cell number decreased by about 20% (although mesangial cell number doubles, this cell type only represents a proportion of glomerular cells, so that the total number increases by only about 25–30%). Although this was consistent with apoptosis mediating cell removal, we found that by far the highest frequency of apoptosis (0.25%) was seen at day 5, when mitosis also peaked (94). This was unexpected because in other situations of hyperplasia and regression, a wave of apoptosis is followed by a wave of mitosis (86). Therefore, we undertook a detailed study of the first 14 days of our model of Thyl.1 nephritis. This confirmed that apoptosis did indeed correlate closely with mitosis, but increased apoptosis persisted beyond 10 days, by which time mitosis decreased to baseline and glomerular cell number began to decrease (Fig. 5). From days 3 to 7, during which time glomerular cell number increased, mitosis was about twofold more frequent than apoptosis. However, from days 10 to 14, when cell number was decreasing, apoptosis was about twofold more frequent than mitosis. Therefore, changes in the ratio of apoptosis to mitosis were commensurate with changes in cell number (94).

By making reasonable estimates of the time for which mitosis and apoptosis are histologically detectable, we (105) have been able to take this analysis further (Fig. 5). A large number of diverse studies suggest that mitoses are visible for about 1 h (106,107). By taking an area-under-the-curve approach, we were able to calculate that over the first 10 days the expected increase in glomerular cell number should have been approximately 45, when in fact it was only about 22. By assuming that apoptosis accounted for this shortfall, we calculated that apoptotic cell clearance time was approximately 1.6 h. Indeed, a similar figure was obtained when 10 and 14 days were compared and when any other pair of adjacent time points were assessed. This estimate is in accord with other data on apoptotic cell clearance time and is strong evidence that apoptosis is indeed the major mechanism for mesangial cell clearance in Thyl.1 nephritis.

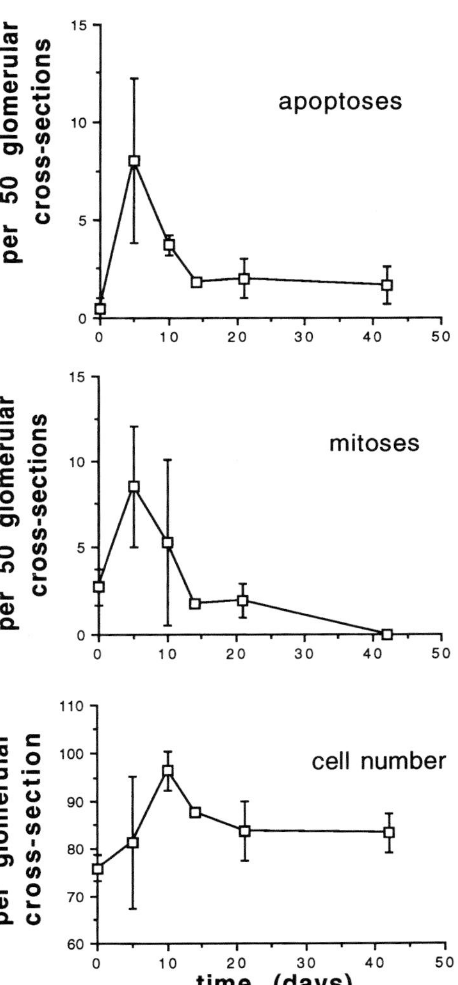

FIG. 4. Histologic time course study of Thyl.1 nephritis. Cell number per glomerular cross-section (bottom) and mitotic figures (middle) and apoptotic cells (top) per 50 glomerular cross-sections. Oil immersion light microscopy of PAS-stained material (mean ± SE). Reproduced from the *Journal of Clinical Investigation* 1994;94:2105–16, by copyright permission of the Society for Clinical Investigation.

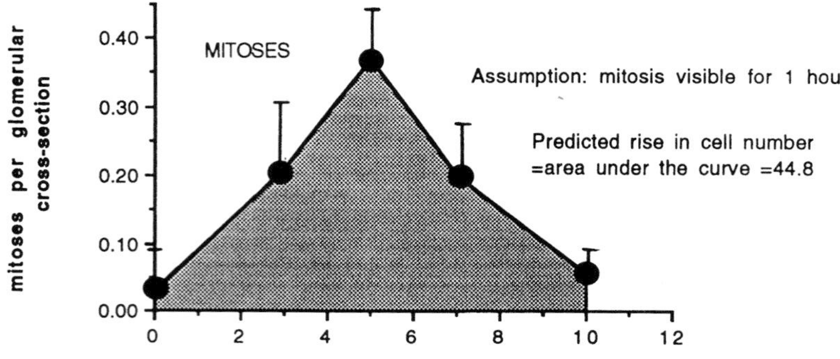

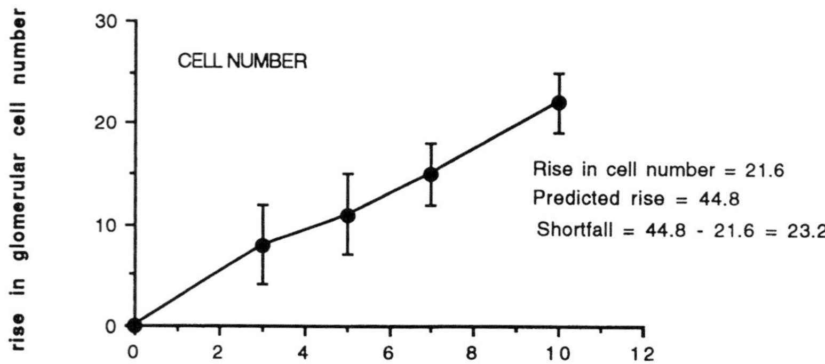

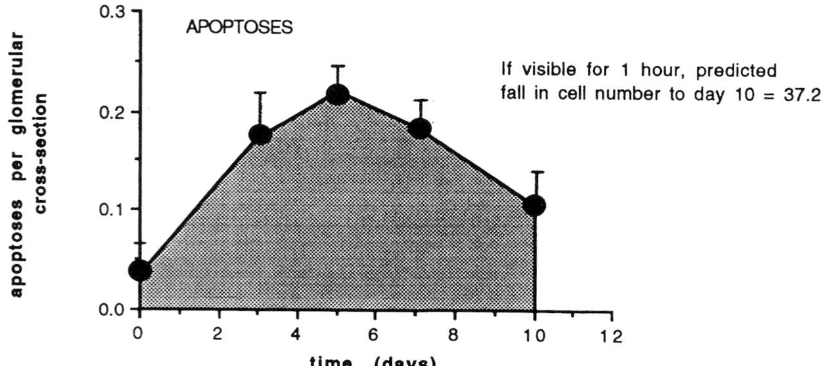

FIG. 5. Kinetic estimates in Thyl.1 nephritis. *Top panel* shows mitoses counted from days 0 to 10. *Shaded area* under the curve corresponds to predicted increase in cell number. If mitoses are visible for 1 h, predicted increase in cell number over 10 days = 44.8. *Middle panel* shows actual increase. Note predicted shortfall of 23.2. *Lower panel* shows apoptosis counts from days 0 to 10. If apoptosis is visible for 1 h, predicted decrease in cell number = 37.2, greater than shortfall. Therefore, assuming all of shortfall due to apoptosis, and mitoses are visible for 1 h, apoptosis clearance time = $1 \times 37.2/23.2$ = 1. 6 h.

Mechanisms Regulating Mesangial Cell Apoptosis

At present little is known of how mesangial cell apoptosis is regulated in the complex microenvironment of the inflamed glomerulus. However, there is evidence that the general principles of a balance between survival and death factors is at play.

First, our observation of an initial correlation between apoptosis and mitosis points to a role for survival factors because (as described above) dividing cells are known to be particularly susceptible to apoptosis if survival factors are in short supply (51). Preliminary data (A. Mooney and J. Savill, unpublished data) indicate that insulinlike growth factor-1, but not platelet-derived growth factor or epidermal growth factor (EGF), is a potent exogenous survival factor for cultured mesangial cells exposed to a range of stimuli likely to promote apoptosis. Furthermore, there is a growing body of in vitro and in vivo data indicating that mesangial cells can express endogenous survival factors such as Bcl-2 and the counter-regulatory element Bax (108–110). Indeed, our finding (discussed above) that a protein synthesis inhibitor promotes apoptosis in cultured mesangial cells is indirect but functional evidence for endogenous synthesis of survival factors

(94). Clearly, therefore, future work will focus on which genes promote mesangial cell survival, particularly because this could be a potentially deleterious event, tending to prevent proper resolution of mesangial hypercellularity and thereby increasing the risk of glomerular scarring should the expanded resident cell population lay down excessive extracellular matrix.

Second, there is evidence that mesangial cell number could be "tailored" by exogenous death factors. Mesangial cells stimulated by lipopolysaccharide (LPS) and proinflammatory cytokines such as TNFα can be induced to express Fas in culture, in which case anti-Fas antibody will trigger apoptosis (111). This is of interest because normal renal tissue can express messenger RNA for Fas ligand (25), which in rats has been localized to the glomerulus (in addition to the proximal tubule) (112). It seems likely that inflamed glomeruli could be infiltrated with activated cytotoxic lymphocytes expressing this membrane-bound homologue of TNF. However, in the only immunofluorescence study available at this writing, preliminary data on human IgA nephropathy and lupus nephritis indicate that although up to about 10 Fas-positive cells may be seen in each glomerular cross-section, these cells are probably not mesangial because they do not stain for a smooth muscle actin (113). Therefore, the in vivo relevance of mesangial cell expression of Fas in vitro remains conjectural. However, there are other mechanisms by which infiltrating cells such as macrophages, which are prominent in the first few days of Thyl.1 nephritis, could direct mesangial cells to die and limit an otherwise potentially over-exuberant reparative response. Both ROS and nitric oxide derivatives generated by myeloid cells can trigger apoptosis in other cell types (82,114). Furthermore, preliminary studies indicate that ROS may induce apoptosis in mesangial cells (115), implying that myeloid cells could induce mesangial cell apoptosis, especially as glomerular nitric oxide production occurs in Thyl.1 nephritis (116). Indeed, a report of *ICE* expression in rat glomeruli suggests that protease cascades capable of driving apoptosis will be found in mesangial cells. Finally, the potential importance of control of mesangial cell number by exogenous death influences is illustrated by the studies of Polunovsky et al. (117), which showed that resolving fibroblastic granulation tissue in the human lung secreted apparently homeostatic death factors that could induce apoptosis in cultured vascular and mesenchymal cells. It may prove possible to adapt this approach to investigate the possible existence of such factors in Thyl.1 nephritis.

Apoptosis in Other Glomerular Cell Types

At present there has been little study of apoptosis in glomerular endothelial or epithelial cells. Although the general principles of control of cell number by balanced mitosis and apoptosis may apply, the visceral epithelial cell appears to be particularly resistant to proliferative stimuli (87,118). One might therefore expect that loss of such cells would be highly undesirable and that they might prove to be resistant to apoptosis. In this regard it is interesting that in normal human kidney the most intense staining for the endogenous survival factor Bcl-2 is indeed found in glomerular epithelial cells (119), but a little disappointing that this is most prominent in parietal epithelial cells. Nevertheless, we have found intense Bcl-2 staining in glomerular crescents (E.M. Thompson, J. Hughes, J. Savill, unpublished data). Clearly, therefore, although there is clinical evidence that epithelial cell proliferation can resolve, the scene is set for glomerular epithelial cells representing "special cases", in which both mitosis and apoptosis are kept firmly in check, although the genes responsible are unknown.

Glomerular endothelial cells appear to represent a cell type with considerably more plasticity than the epithelial cell. Proliferation of endothelial cells is a classical feature of reversible lesions such as postinfectious glomerulonephritis. Furthermore, there is increasing evidence that endothelial cell proliferation and new vessel formation (angiogenesis) may be important features of resolving glomerular inflammation in models such as Thyl.1 nephritis (R.J. Johnson, personal communication). The susceptibility of cultured umbilical and microvascular endothelial cells to apoptosis induced by deprivation of survival factors (120), or by exposure to death factors (117) including TNF (121), implies that the program of apoptosis is readily available to glomerular endothelial cells. In a study of nephrotoxic nephritis in rats (C. Sarraf, J. Savill, unpublished), we have found evidence of glomerular endothelial cell apoptosis (Fig. 1). Furthermore, on reviewing his earlier studies of self-limited glomerular endothelial cell accumulation induced in rats by perfusion of the renal artery with myeloperoxidase and hydrogen peroxide (122), Johnson found evidence of glomerular endothelial cell apoptosis in the resolution phase (123). This opens up a rich vista of future studies on the control of glomerular endothelial cell number.

Tubulointerstitial Inflammation

There is a growing awareness that the outcome of glomerular inflammation may depend crucially on tubulointerstitial changes. Many readers are familiar with the histologic evidence of glomerulonephritis being accompanied by expansion of the interstitium and its infiltration by mononuclear leukocytes. Furthermore, in situations such as chronic pyelonephritis/reflux nephropathy, the tubulointerstitial compartment may represent the main target of injury. Certainly there is evidence that tubulointerstitial injury is reversible, but this short section will emphasize that regarding any role for apoptosis, there are more questions than answers.

Interstitial Myofibroblasts

In keeping with the appearance of myofibroblasts in wounded skin or injured glomeruli, injury of the renal interstitium is associated with accumulation of α smooth muscle actin positive cells of the myofibroblast type. Given recent evidence that apoptosis mediates clearance of excess myofibroblastlike mesangial cells from the injured glomerulus or wounded skin (124), one may speculate that apoptosis of interstitial myofibroblasts may occur, and that it could be an important factor in regulating the outcome of interstitial injury. However, there are no data available to support or refute this idea.

Tubular Cells

By contrast with the paucity of data on interstitial cells of the adult kidney, there is a large and growing body of evidence available indicating that tubular cells can undergo apoptosis induced by ischemia, toxins, or ureteric obstruction in vivo (90,125–128). Furthermore, in health or disease these cells can express many of the key proteins regulating apoptosis, including Fas, Fas ligand, ICE, and Bcl-2, whereas tubular cell number is also likely to be under exogenous control by survival factors such as EGF (129). Indeed, there is evidence that apoptosis may play an important role in remodelling tubular hyperplasia induced by earlier injury (127). However, the extent to which apoptosis is implicated in the tubular response to inflammatory injury is unknown.

LEUKOCYTE CLEARANCE BY APOPTOSIS

Given the lack of data on tubulointerstitial involvement in glomerulonephritis, this section will address briefly the general principles of leukocyte clearance from inflamed sites and will focus on glomerular inflammation.

Leukocyte Fate in Inflammation

Although leukocyte infiltration is a key feature of the inflammatory response, until recently there has been little interest in the fate of leukocytes reaching an inflamed site.

Granulocyte Fate

The archetypal inflammatory leukocyte, the neutrophil, is loaded with toxic contents capable of causing tissue injury. Once neutrophils have emigrated from the circulating pool, there is general agreement that they meet their fate in situ because there is no evidence that they can return to the blood and no data support the possibility of large-scale emigration via the lymphatics (130,131). It has been assumed that the inevitable fate of the inflammatory neutrophil is necrosis and disintegration, but it appears that this is only true if inflammation fails to resolve completely, as in abscess formation. In fact, it has been known since Metchnikoff's seminal work that during resolution of inflammation senescent neutrophils can be recognized while still intact and ingested by macrophages (132). Indeed, in the experimentally inflamed peritoneum, where one can sample the cellular infiltrate at frequent intervals, there is clear evidence that phagocytosis of intact neutrophils is the major clearance mechanism (133). Although less well studied, similar principles appear to apply to eosinophil clearance (134).

However, glomerular inflammation occurs within special structural constraints. Although leukocytes do have direct access to the mesangium and can cross the basement membrane to reach the urinary space, in many types of glomerulonephritis leukocytes appear to accumulate within the lumen of injured glomerular capillaries. In order to examine the fate of neutrophils accumulating in glomerular capillary injury, we have studied a model of this condition induced in rats by perfusion via the renal artery of concanavalin A (ConA) followed by anti-ConA antibody. In situ immune complexes are formed, injuring the glomerular endothelium and triggering marked neutrophil infiltration (135; and J. Hughes, R. Johnson, D. Lombardi, J. Savill, manuscript in preparation). Purified rat neutrophils radiolabelled ex vivo were infused into rats soon after initiation of unilateral glomerular capillary injury, and specific accumulation was observed, peaking at 4 hours. By 24 h, a time at which histologic examination showed that only about 14% of the neutrophils present at 4 h were still detectable, approximately 26% of radiolabel remained in the glomerulus. There was evidence that this reflected macrophage ingestion of neutrophils. Apart from occasional labelled cells on autoradiographs of draining lymph nodes, counts showed no evidence of neutrophil emigration via the lymphatics. Consequently, the data suggest that in glomerular capillary injury, during which most neutrophils remain in the lumen, the majority of recruited cells leave the glomerulus, presumably detaching from injured endothelium and returning to the blood. However, even in this special circumstance roughly one quarter may meet a phagocytic fate in the glomerulus.

Fate of Other Leukocyte Types

Whereas neutrophils have no business in normal tissues, other leukocyte types enter tissues in health. Monocytes leave the blood in order to differentiate and maintain normal tissue levels of resident macrophages (136).

Since the seminal work of Gowans, Ford, and others (137), it has been appreciated that lymphocytes recirculate through normal tissues. Therefore, when increased numbers of monocytes and lymphocytes are summoned to inflamed sites it might be predicted that their fate would differ from the neutrophil. Although the data are limited, it seems highly likely that monocytes/macrophages (and presumably lymphocytes) leave the inflamed kidney to meet their fate in draining lymph nodes (100). Clearly, future work will need to define the mechanisms promoting emigration of leukocytes, but these are beyond the scope of this contribution.

Neutrophil Apoptosis and Phagocytic Clearance

In 1982, Newman et al. (138) discovered that senescent neutrophils, prepared by "aging" blood neutrophils overnight in culture, became recognizable to macrophages and were ingested, just as suggested by Metchnikoff's in vivo work. We showed that both blood and inflammatory neutrophils aging in culture are constitutively programmed to undergo apoptosis and that this change determined recognition by macrophages (101). Subsequently, we have obtained clear histological evidence that neutrophil apoptosis leading to phagocytosis by macrophages occurs at a number of inflamed sites in vivo (139–141). It seems likely that this is an injury-limiting neutrophil clearance mechanism. First, neutrophils undergoing apoptosis lose the capacity to make injurious responses such as degranulation when stimulated by chemotactic factors (142). Second, apoptotic neutrophils retain membrane integrity and are cleared without leakage of toxic granule contents (101). Last, macrophages ingesting apoptotic neutrophils do not make a potentially injurious secretary response, by contrast with uptake of other particles (143). Thus, apoptosis appears to be the desirable and physiologic fate of the inflammatory neutrophil.

Regulation of Neutrophil Apoptosis and Clearance

As emphasized above, apoptosis is subject to internal and external regulation. The neutrophil is no exception. Although we know little of endogenous genes regulating neutrophil death, the fact that inhibitors of protein synthesis accelerate apoptosis in cultured neutrophils is strong evidence in favor of control by endogenously synthesized survival factors (130). Furthermore, proinflammatory mediators, which include the candidate lineage-specific survival factor granulocyte-monocyte colony-stimulating factor (GMCSF), can slow neutrophil apoptosis and prolong functional life-span (144). Teleologically, this could be viewed as a mechanism ensuring that neutrophils recruited early in an inflammatory response retain their microbicidal capacity. However, slowing of neutrophil apoptosis by inflammatory mediators could also be viewed as a matching mechanism, delaying neutrophil apoptosis until phagocytes are ready to clear such cells. Such a delay could be necessary because monocytes must mature into inflammatory macrophages before they acquire the capacity to take up apoptotic cells, a differentiation process that takes 2–3 days in vitro (138).

Proinflammatory cytokines such as IL-1 and TNFα also increase macrophage capacity for phagocytosis of apoptotic neutrophils, in a manner strongly suggestive of a newly recognized negative feedback loop in inflammation. Mediators responsible for recruitment of neutrophils to an inflamed site also ready macrophages to clear granulocytes once they have served their function and undergone apoptosis (145). Intriguingly, the most potent cytokine was GMCSF, which in only 6 h could treble the capacity of human monocyte-derived macrophages to take up apoptotic neutrophils. Perhaps GMCSF is a model for a disposal-matching cytokine, simultaneously slowing neutrophil apoptosis and accelerating the development of capacity for phagocytic clearance.

Neutrophil Apoptosis in Glomerulonephritis

In addition to clear histological evidence of neutrophil apoptosis in human glomerulonephritis (146), we also have obtained definitive confirmation that neutrophil apoptosis leading to phagocytosis by inflammatory macrophages occurs in rat glomeruli injured with nephrotoxic globulin (140). Furthermore, in our recent unpublished studies of experimental glomerular capillary injury there was clear evidence that neutrophils underwent apoptosis and phagocytosis by inflammatory macrophages in the lumen of the capillaries.

However, we also have unequivocal evidence from in vitro and in vivo studies that glomerular mesangial cells can act as "semiprofessional" phagocytes ingesting various cell types undergoing apoptosis, including neutrophils (94,140). Phagocytosis by mesangial cells may represent an important back-up to macrophage clearance of apoptotic cells. This could be particularly important early in an inflammatory response, when recently recruited monocytes have yet to mature into phagocytically competent macrophages.

Nevertheless, it should be pointed out that much work remains. First, the contribution of apoptosis toward removal of neutrophils meeting their fate in the glomerulus needs to be defined. Interestingly, in our studies of ConA–anti-ConA glomerular capillary injury, the observed frequency of neutrophil apoptosis at the peak of infiltration (2.4% at 4 h), taken together with an assumption that clearance time is 1 h, generates an estimate that approximately 25% of recruited neutrophils will be cleared by apoptosis over the next 20 h, a figure close to the proportion of neutrophils believed to die in the glomerulus on the basis of retention of radiolabelled cells. Although this suggests that most, if not all, neutrophils remaining in the glomerulus do indeed undergo apoptosis, it is obvious that many more detailed studies of neutrophil fate will be required. Such studies need to define the relative contributions of "professional" and "semi-professional" phagocytes in the clearance of apoptotic neutrophils. Finally, the consequences of ingestion of apoptotic cells by glomerular phagocytes will need to be investigated.

Phagocyte Recognition of Apoptotic Leukocytes

This is a key feature of the program of cell death by apoptosis, and in inflammation probably serves an important function in injury-limiting clearance of leukocytes undergoing apoptosis (130,147). Indeed, preliminary experiments in our laboratory (Y. Ren, S. Kar, C. Haslett, J. Savill, manuscript in preparation) demonstrate that when apoptotic neutrophils are cocultured with macrophages, all the neutrophils are phagocytosed without release of toxic contents such as elastase. However, when phagocytosis is inhibited by colchicine, apoptotic neutrophils are not taken up, lose their membrane integrity, and leak elastase and other toxic contents. These observations re-emphasise the tissue-protective potential of the phagocytosis of apoptotic cells. Furthermore, because there is a clear inference that defects in this process may be a hitherto unrecognized factor promoting persistence of inflammation, there is a clear need to understand the cell surface mechanisms by which phagocytes recognize and ingest apoptotic cells. These have been extensively renewed elsewhere (147) and will only be outlined here.

Almost all of the data available reflect in vitro studies of phagocytic mechanisms. Only in the case of *C. elegans* mutants with defective phagocytosis of dying cells (Fig. 2) is there in vivo evidence pointing to a role for particular gene products in this process (9). Furthermore, to date the sequence of these genes has yet to be published. Nevertheless, the relevance of these molecules to the human inflammatory response may be limited, because this nematode does not have professional phagocytes, dying cells are eaten by neighbors. Therefore, at present we are forced to identify candidate recognition mechanisms in vitro that need to be checked out with in vivo studies.

Currently, it appears that particular populations of phagocytes use a particular recognition mechanism in the uptake of apoptotic cells irrespective of the lineage of the ingested cell. The best available model of the human inflammatory macrophage, the monocyte-derived macrophage (Mφ; obtained by culture of monocytes adherent to plastic in the presence of serum) uses two cell surface receptors, the $\alpha_v\beta_3$ vitronectin receptor and CD36 to bind the soluble adhesive glycoprotein thrombospondin (TSP), which bridges the phagocyte to unknown sites on the apoptotic cell (141,148–150). Indeed, in the presence of TSP, CD36 gene transfer to cells bearing $\alpha_v\beta_3$ confers capacity for phagocytosis of cells of various lineages undergoing apoptosis (151). The $\alpha_v\beta_3$/CD36/TSP recognition mechanism has been implicated in uptake of apoptotic neutrophils, lymphocytes (152), fibroblasts (151), and eosinophils (M. Stern, J. Savill, C. Haslett, manuscript in preparation). Furthermore, similar mechanisms appear to mediate uptake of apoptotic cells by mouse bone marrow–derived macrophages (153), human glomerular mesangial cells (154), and human fibroblasts (155), although the latter also uses a mannose-inhibitable C-type lectin in phagocytosis.

However, the thioglycollate-elicited murine peritoneal macrophage, a true inflammatory macrophage, does not use the $\alpha_v\beta_3$/CD36/TSP phagocytic mechanism (153,156). Instead, as yet uncharacterized but stereospecific receptors are deployed to recognize the anionic phospholipid phosphatidylserine (PS), which is exposed on apoptotic neutrophils and lymphocytes by reason of loss of the membrane asymmetry that normally dictates that PS is predominantly sited in the inner membrane leaflet. Interestingly, mouse bone marrow–derived macrophages (which use an $\alpha_v\beta_3$/CD36/TSP-like mechanism) can be switched to a PS-dependent mechanism by ingestion of digestible β-glucan particles via an effect dependent on autocrine action of TGF-β (157). However, TGF-β and other cytokines do not switch human Mφ, instead enhancing recognition via the $\alpha_v\beta_3$/CD36/TSP mechanism (145).

Ultimately, if we are to understand phagocyte clearance of apoptotic cells in vivo, we will need to design strategies to assess these and other recognition mechanisms in animal models of glomerulonephritis.

RENAL INFLAMMATION AND DEFECTS IN APOPTOSIS

Defective apoptosis could result in renal inflammation by at least two general mechanisms (146,158). First, defects in cell clearance could exacerbate tissue injury and inflammation, promote accumulation of unwanted cells, and fuel further inflammation by triggering autoimmunity (summarized in Fig. 6). Second, renal inflammation could be initiated or exacerbated by defects in the normal roles of apoptosis in maintaining lymphocyte homeostasis.

Defective Cell Clearance

It should be emphasized that there is no direct evidence that any of the events depicted in Fig. 6 are important in determining the outcome of renal inflammation. However, it is reasonable to propose that failure to clear

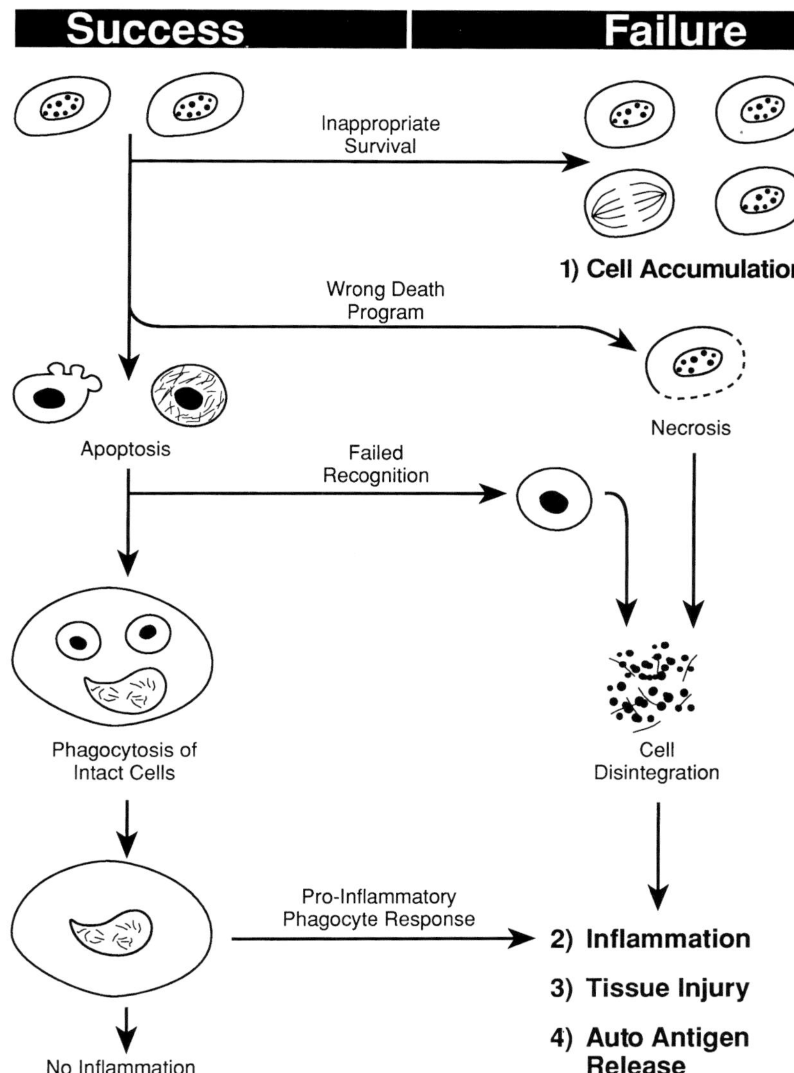

FIG. 6. Potential mechanisms and consequences of failure of safe cell clearance by apoptosis. Reproduced with permission from *European Journal of Clinical Investigation* 1994;24:715–23.

excess glomerular cells because apoptosis is inhibited by exogenous or endogenous survival factors might be an important factor in cases of glomerulonephritis where undesirably expanded mesangial cell populations persist. Although there are no unequivocal supporting data, such an event could favor glomerular scarring.

There is more direct evidence to suggest that defective phagocytosis of apoptotic cells could trigger tissue injury in vivo. For example, when anti-Fas antibody was administered to mice, rapid and widespread hepatocyte apoptosis was induced (24). However, presumably because of insufficient local capacity to clear an unphysiologically massive load of apoptotic cells, hepatocytes disintegrated, releasing cell contents, which led to coagulative necrosis of the liver and death. Furthermore, our own coculture experiments emphasize the potentially dire consequences of defective phagocytosis of apoptotic cells, which eventually undergo postapoptotic or secondary necrosis/disintegration. Indeed, this could be doubly deleterious because preliminary data (M. Stern, J. Savill, C. Haslett, manuscript in preparation) indicate that macrophage ingestion of postapoptotic granulocyte fragments triggers potentially deleterious secretory responses, by contrast with uptake of intact apoptotic cells. Whether there are states in which macrophages or other phagocytes make a proinflammatory response to ingestion of apoptotic cells will also require investigation. Nevertheless, in vitro data suggest that a number of known perturbations of the inflammatory microenvironment, such as low pH (148), accumulation of highly charged molecules (148), and release from extracellular matrix of arg-gly-asp–bearing peptides (149), can all block phagocytosis of apoptotic cells. Therefore, future studies also should seek such conditions in examples of renal inflammation that fail to resolve.

Lastly, there are intriguing links between defective phagocytosis of apoptotic cells and autoimmunity. Keratinocytes exposed to ultraviolet light undergo apoptosis and have been shown to compartmentalize potential autoantigens into the plasma membrane blebs that are so typical of many cell types undergoing apoptosis (159). Ribosomes, SS-A/Ro riboproteins, and fragmented endoplasmic reticulum are directed into a population of small blebs, whereas larger blebs bear nucleosomal DNA. It is possible that such blebs could be found on other cell types undergoing apoptosis, particularly because there is evidence that proteolytic processing may underlie this compartmentalization (160). Once these blebs have budded off from the dying cell as apoptotic bodies, then (differential) failure to ingest these bodies might result in release of cellular constituents to which autoantibodies are so often found in autoimmune diseases such as SLE. Certainly, the detection of circulating free nucleosomes in this condition may point to failed phagocytosis of apoptotic cells (161,162). Indeed, whether there is a specific defect of this process in SLE deserves further investigation, particularly because antiphospholipid autoantibodies may bind apoptotic cells (163) and could block their phagocytosis. In short, defective phagocytosis of apoptotic cells with leakage of potentially immunogenic contents may stoke the fire of autoimmunity, setting up further rounds of inflammatory tissue injury.

Defective Lymphocyte Homeostasis and Autoimmunity

A detailed description of this exciting and active field is beyond the scope of this chapter (164). However, the key concepts need to be outlined. Most important is that there is growing evidence that during generation of the immune repertoire, apoptosis is involved in deletion of lymphocytes recognising self components, probably both in the thymus and in the periphery. Furthermore, apoptosis plays crucial roles in returning expanded lymphocyte populations to their normal size at the end of an immune response.

MLR-*lpr/lpr* mice have defective expression of Fas (165) due to disruption of the *Fas/lpr* gene by integration of an endogenous retrovirus (166), and their cells are resistant to apoptosis induced by Fas ligation. Such mice fail to delete T cells in the periphery, and they accumulate lymphocytes of immature phenotype (CD3 positive, CD4 negative, CD8 negative) and exhibit gross enlargement of lymphoid organs. Furthermore, they develop an autoimmune disease with glomerulonephritis and other similarities to SLE. This engendered great excitement in the possibility that Fas might be defective in human SLE, particularly because lymphocytes isolated from patients with this disorder exhibit increased susceptibility to apoptosis similar to that observed in lymphocytes isolated from MLR-*lpr/lpr* mice (167). However, no consistent defect in Fas protein expression or function was found in human SLE (168). Nevertheless, a recent report (169) has described human Fas mutations in five children with a rare autoimmune lymphoproliferative syndrome characterized by massive nonmalignant lymphadenopathy, expanded populations of CD3-positive, CD4-negative, CD8-negative lymphocytes, and autoimmune phenomena (but only one case of nephritis). It seems likely that other cases could have defects in the Fas ligand, because a point mutation in this structure causes generalized lymphoproliferative disease in mice (170), which has a virtually identical presentation. Given the lack of this phenotype, it therefore seems unlikely that most cases of SLE reflect mutations in Fas or Fas ligand. Nevertheless, these observations establish the principle that autoimmunity triggering renal inflammation can arise from defects in lymphocyte population control by apoptosis. Indeed, this is underscored by the prolonged antibody responses, lymphocyte accumulation, and autoimmune disease with nephritis that are manifest by transgenic mice over-expressing *bcl-2* in the B-cell line (171).

DELETERIOUS ENGAGEMENT OF APOPTOSIS

So far, we have painted a flattering picture of apoptosis, emphasizing the physiological nature of this type of cell death and proposing that apoptosis is critical in the beneficial clearance of unwanted cells from inflamed glomeruli. However, in the penultimate section of this chapter we will emphasize the "dark sides" of apoptosis. First, apoptotic cells detected in renal inflammation could represent previously healthy cells injured by toxic stimuli or cytotoxic lymphocytes. Second, preliminary but tantalizing data from Shimizu et al. imply that loss of glomerular cells by apoptosis could be part of the scarring process (172).

Renal Cell Injury Leading to Apoptosis

We have already discussed data suggesting that ROS and nitric oxide can induce apoptosis in renal cells. Although there is no direct evidence that this is the case in renal inflammation, it seems likely to be a consequence of infiltration of the organ by activated myeloid cells. Furthermore, a probable consequence of autoimmunity to renal cell components may be infiltration of the organ with CD8-positive cytotoxic lymphocytes (CTLs) specific for renal peptides presented by self major histocompatibility complex molecules. It has long been known that although CTLs can induce rapid lysis of target cells, the "lethal hit" is frequently constituted by induction of apoptosis in the target cell (173). In some target cell types this undoubtedly reflects secretion by the CTL of perforin, a pore-forming molecule that allows the CTL to insert proteolytic enzymes A and B (174) into the target cell, an event that probably triggers the protease cascade of apoptosis. However, experiments with CTL from perforin knock-out mice demonstrate that when target cells express Fas, ligation by Fas ligand expressed on the CTL also can trigger apoptosis (175). Whether such mechanisms are involved in renal inflammation induced by autoimmunity is unknown, but it can be appreciated that expression of Fas, driven in some cases by infective or inflammatory stimuli (111), may render renal cells particularly susceptible to the CTL's double "kiss of death."

Cell Loss by Apoptosis During Glomerular Scarring

The first report of apoptosis in the kidney emphasises that this is a mechanism by which desirable cells may be lost; ureteric obstruction induced rapid renal atrophy by initiating widespread tubular cell apoptosis (90). Whether this is important in progressive tubular atrophy in kidneys afflicted by persistent glomerulonephritis will need examination in the future. However, cell loss by apoptosis also may contribute directly to postinflammatory scarring of the glomerulus. It has been emphasized above that a typical early glomerular response to inflammatory injury is proliferation of resident cells, and it is widely believed that an increased complement of resident cells constitutes a risk factor for excessive matrix deposition and later scarring. However, clinical experience indicates that as glomerular scarring progresses, cell number decreases, ultimately leading to disappearance of viable cells from the glomerular remnant. Shimizu et al. have recently presented an interesting study of experimental crescentic glomerulonephritis induced in WKY rats by nephrotoxic globulin (172). Initially, there was infiltration with leukocytes and proliferation of glomerular cells, which was rapidly followed by increased glomerular apoptosis. However, by contrast with Thyl.1 nephritis, where it appears that apoptosis returns to normal levels as glomerular cell number returns to normal, in the model under study the investigators found a progressive increase in apoptosis, such that glomerular cell number progressively decreased as scarring ensued.

The mechanism of glomerular cell loss by apoptosis during scarring is unknown but will be important to define because it might be possible to retard established scarring by inhibiting glomerular cell apoptosis. We think particular attention should be directed to the possibility that disruption of the normal glomerular extracellular matrix results in a failure to provide survival signals. The consequences of interruption of survival signals from extracellular matrix have recently been demonstrated in a study showing that antibodies to endothelial cell surface integrins could trigger apoptosis in the new vessels of tumors (176).

CONCLUSIONS AND FURTHER PROSPECTS

We believe that apoptosis is a fundamental part of renal inflammation. Much evidence suggests that this type of cell death may mediate beneficial deletion of infiltrating leukocytes and excess resident renal cells. We speculate that future studies will show that defects in cell clearance by apoptosis occur in examples of renal inflammation that fail to resolve. If this is the case, then current knowledge already suggests approaches toward therapy. Should inflammatory injury be fuelled by failure of phagocytic clearance of apoptotic leukocytes, then approaches such as CD36 gene transfer may facilitate beneficial increases in local phagocytic capacity (151). Where glomerular hypercellularity fails to resolve, it can be speculated that cell number could be reduced by antagonizing exogenous or endogenous survival factors, for example by administering agents blocking glomerular cell receptors for survival cytokines or by delivering antisense oligonucleotides against genes such as *bcl-2*. However, the consequences of inducing apoptosis in too many glomerular cells would be dire, and we regard such potential therapies as being a long way beyond current horizons.

There is also growing evidence that apoptosis may mediate undesirable loss of renal cells in inflammation of the kidney. In this case the prime therapeutic objective would be to interrupt the mechanisms that promote cell death, but it also might prove useful to inhibit the program of apoptosis. Approaches could include administration of survival factors because EGF can retard tubular cell apoptosis in ureteric obstruction (129). Alternatively, administration of small molecular inhibitors of ICE-like proteases, or *bcl-2* gene transfers, also might be of benefit.

Five years ago many of these proposals would have been impossible to make. However, in that time, knowledge of the basic mechanisms of cell death has grown rapidly. Furthermore, targeted gene therapy of the glomerulus seems to be a realistic prospect. The next 5 years could see the development of candidate therapies for renal inflammation based on genetic manipulation of cell survival and death.

ACKNOWLEDGMENTS

We thank Dr. Catherine Sarraf for the electron micrographs. J.S. has been supported by the Wellcome Trust (013158, 035283, 039737) and the National Kidney Research Fund. J.H. was, and A.M. is, a Medical Research Council Training Fellow. Judith Hayes typed the manuscript.

REFERENCES

1. Duvall E, Wyllie AH. Death and the cell. *Immunol Today* 1986;7: 115–9.
2. *Kerr JFR, Wyllie AH, Currie AR. Apoptosis: a basic biological phenomenon with widespread implications in tissue kinetics.* Br J Cancer 1972;26:239–57.
3. Wyllie AH, Kerr JFR, Currie AR. Cell death: the significance of apoptosis. *Int Rev Cytol* 1980;68:251–306.
4. Wyllie AH. Glucocorticoid-induced thymocyte apoptosis is associated with endogenous endonuclease activation. *Nature* 1980;284: 555–6.
5. Oberhammer FA, Hochegger K, Fröschl G, Tiefenbacher R, Pavelka M. Chromatin condensation during apoptosis is accompanied by degradation of lamin A-B, without enhanced activation of cdc2 kinase. *J Cell Biol* 1994;126:827–37.
6. Oberhammer FA, Wilson JW, Dive C, et al. Apoptotic cell death in epithelial cells: cleavage of DNA to 300 and/or 50 kilobase fragments prior to or in the absence of internucleosomal fragmentation. *EMBO* 1993;12:3679–84.
7. Cohen GM, Sun X-M, Fearnhead H, et al. Formation of large molecular weight fragments of DNA is a key committed step of apoptosis in thymocytes. *J Immunol* 1994;153:507–16.
8. Ucker DS, Obermiller PS, Eckhart W, Apgar JR, Berger NA, Myers J. Genome digestion is a dispensible consequence of physiological cell death mediated by cytotoxic T lymphocytes. *Mol Cell Biol* 1992;12:3060–9.
9. Ellis RE, Yuan J, Horvitz HR. Mechanisms and functions of cell death. *Annu Rev Cell Biol* 1991;7:663–98.
10. Hogquist KA, Nett MA, Unanue ER, Chaplin DD. Interleukin-1 is processed and released during apoptosis. *Proc Natl Acad Sci USA* 1991;88:8485–9.
11. Kaufmann SH, Desnoyers S, Ottaviano Y, Davidson NE, Poirier GG. Specific proteolytic cleavage of poly(ADP-ribose) polymerase: an early marker of chemotherapy-induced apoptosis. *Cancer Res* 1993; 53:3976–85.
12. Sarin A, Adams DH, Henkart PA. Protease inhibitors selectively block T cell receptor-triggered programmed cell death in a murine T cell hybridoma and activated peripheral T cells. *J Exp Med* 1993;178: 1693–700.
13. Williams MS, Henkart PA. Apoptotic cell death induced by intracellular proteolysis. *J Immunol* 1994;153:4247–56.
14. Yuan J, Shaham S, Ledoux S, Ellis HM, Horvitz HR. The C-elegans death gene ced-3 encodes a protein similar to mammalian interleukin 1–converting enzyme. *Cell* 1993;75:641–52.
15. Wilson KP, Black J-AF, Thomson JA, et al. Structure and mechanism of interleukin-1 converting enzyme. *Nature* 1994;370:270–5.
16. Miura M, Zhu H, Rotello R, Hartwig EA, Yuan J. Induction of apoptosis in fibroblasts by IL-1–converting enzyme, a mammalian homolog of the *C. elegans* cell death gene ced-3. *Cell* 1993;75: 653–60.
17. Wang L, Miura M, Bergeron L, Zhu H, Yuan L. Ich-1, an Ice/ced-3–related gene, encodes both positive and negative regulators of programmed cell death. *Cell* 1994;78:739–50.
18. Lazebnik YA, Kaufmann SH, Desnoyers S, Poirer GG, Earnshaw WC. Cleavage of poly(ADP-ribose) polymerase by a proteinase with properties like ICE. *Nature* 1994;371:346–7.
19. Li P, Allen H, Banerjee S, et al. Mice deficient in IL-1–converting enzyme are defective in production of mature IL-1 and resistant to endotoxic shock. *Cell* 1995;80:401–11.
20. Tewari M, Quan LT, O'Rourke K, et al. Yama/CPP32, a mammalian homolog of CED-3, is a CrmA-inhibitable protease that cleaves the death substrate poly(ADP-ribose) polymerase. *Cell* 1995;81:801–9.
21. Itoh N, Yonehara S, Ishii A, et al. The polypeptide encoded by the cDNA for human cell surface antigen Fas can mediate apoptosis. *Cell* 1991;66:233–43.
22. Nagata S, Golstein P. The Fas death factor. *Science* 1995;267: 1449–56.
23. Smith CA, Farrah T, Goodwin RG. The TNF receptor superfamily of cellular and viral proteins: activation, costimulation and death. *Cell* 1994;76:959–62.
24. Ogasawara J, Watanabe-Fukunaga R, Adachi M, et al. Lethal effect of the anti-Fas antibody in mice. *Nature* 1993;364:806–9.
25. Suda T, Takahashi T, Golstein P, Nagata S. Molecular cloning and expression of the Fas ligand. *Cell* 1993;75:1169–78.
26. Enari M, Hug H, Nagata S. Involvement of an ICE-like protease in Fas-mediated apoptosis. *Nature* 1995;375:78–81.
27. Los M, Van de Craen M, Penning LC, et al. Requirement of an ICE/CED-3 protease for Fas/APO-1–mediated apoptosis. *Nature* 1995;375:81–3.
28. Cifone MG, De Maria R, Roncaioli P, et al. Apoptotic signaling through CD95 (Fas/Apo-1) activates an acidic sphingomyelinase. *J Exp Med* 1993;177:1547–52.
29. Eischen CM, Dick CJ, Leibson PJ. Tyrosine kinase activation provides an early and requisite signal for Fas-induced apoptosis. *J Immunol* 1994;153:1947–55.
30. Darnay BG, Reddy SAG, Aggarwal BB. Physical and functional association of a serine-threonine protein kinase to the cytoplasmic domain of the p80 form of the human tumor necrosis factor receptor in human histiocytic lymphoma U-937 cells. *J Biol Chem* 1994;269:19687–90.
31. Hsu H-M, O'Rourke K, Boguski MS, Dixit VM. A novel RING finger protein interacts with the cytoplasmic domain of CD40. *J Biol Chem* 1994;269:30069–72.
32. Chinnaiyan AM, O'Rourke K, Tewari M, Dixit VM. FADD, a novel death domain-containing protein, interacts with the death domain of Fas and initiates apoptosis. *Cell* 1995;81:505–12.
33. Stanger BZ, Leder P, Lee T-H, Kim E, Seed B. RIP: A novel protein containing a death domain that interacts with Fas/APO-1 (CD95) in yeast and causes cell death. *Cell* 1995;81:513–23.
34. Golstein P, Marguet D, Depraetere V. Homology between reaper and the cell death domains of Fas and TNFR1. *Cell* 1995;81:185–6.
35. White K, Grether ME, Abrams JM, Young L, Farrell K, Steller H. Genetic control of programmed cell death in drosophila. *Science* 1994;264:677–83.
36. Grell M, Zimmermann G, Hülser D, Pfizermaier K, Scheurich P. TNF receptors TR60 and TR80 can mediate apoptosis via induction of distinct signal pathways. *J Immunol* 1994;153:1963–71.
37. Alderson MR, Armitage RJ, Maraskovsky E, et al. Fas transduces activation signals in normal human T lymphocytes. *J Exp Med* 1993; 178:2231–5.
38. Sato T, Irie S, Kitada S, Reed JC. FAP-1: A protein tyrosine phosphatase that associates with Fas. *Science* 1995;268:411–5.
39. Oberhammer FA, Pavelka M, Sharma S, et al. Induction of apoptosis in cultured hepatocytes and in regressing liver by transforming growth factor-1. *Proc Natl Acad Sci USA* 1992;89:5408–12.
40. Sugahara H, Kanakura Y, Furitsu T, et al. Induction of programmed cell death in human hematopoietic cell lines by fibronectin via its interaction with very late antigen 5. *J Exp Med* 1994;179:1757–66.
41. Border WA, Ruoslahti E. Transforming growth factor-β in disease: the dark side of tissue repair. *J Clin Invest* 1992;90:1–7.
42. Liu Z-G, Smith SW, McLaughlin KA, Schwartz LM, Osborne BA. Apoptotic signals delivered through the T-cell receptor of a T-cell hybrid require the immediate-early gene nur77. *Nature* 1994;367: 281–4.
43. Jacobson MD, Burne JF, Raff MC. Programmed cell death and Bcl-2 protection in the absence of a nucleus. *EMBO J* 1994;13:1899–910.
44. Shi LS, Nishioka WK, Thíng J, Bradbury EM, Litchfield DW, Greenberg AH. Premature p34cdc2 activation required for apoptosis. *Science* 1994;263:1143–5.
45. Clarke AR, Purdie CA, Harrison DJ, et al. Thymocyte apoptosis induced by p53-dependent and independent pathways. *Nature* 1993;362:849–52.
46. Strasser A, Harris AW, Jacks T, Cory S. DNA damage can induce apoptosis in proliferating lymphoid cells via p53-independent mechanisms inhibitable by Bcl-2. *Cell* 1994;79:329–39.
47. Duke RC, Cohen JJ. IL-2 addiction: withdrawal of growth factor activates a suicide program in dependent T cells. *Lymphokine Res* 1986;5:289–94.
48. Williams GT, Smith CA, Spooncer E, Dexter TM, Taylor DR. Haemopoietic colony stimulating factors promote cell survival by suppressing apoptosis. *Nature* 1990;343:76–8.
49. Barres BA, Hart IK, Coles HSR, et al. Cell death and control of cell survival in the oligodendrocyte lineage. *Cell* 1992;70:31–46.
50. Raff MC. Social controls on cell survival and cell death. *Nature* 1992;356:397–400.
51. Evan GI, Wyllie AH, Gilbert GS, et al. Induction of apoptosis in fibroblasts by c-myc protein. *Cell* 1992;69:119–28.

52. Talhouk RS, Bissell MJ, Werb Z. Co-ordinated expression of extracellular matrix–degrading proteinases and their inhibitors regular mammary epithelial function during involution. *J Cell Biol* 1992;118: 1271–82.
53. Walker NI, Bennett RE, Kerr JFR. Cell death by apoptosis during involution of the lactating breast in mice and rats. *Am J Anat* 1989; 185:19–24.
54. English HF, Kyprianou N, Isaacs JT. Relationship between DNA fragmentation and apoptosis in the programmed cell death of the rat ventral prostate. *Prostate* 1989;15:233–50.
55. Harrington EA, Bennett MR, Fanidi A, Evan GI. Control of c-Myc–induced apoptosis in fibroblasts by cytokines. *EMBO J* 1994; 13:3286–94.
56. Kinoshita T, Yokota T, Arai K, Miyajima A. Suppression of apoptotic death in hematopoietic cells by signalling through the IL-3/GM-CSF receptors. *EMBO J* 1995;14:266–75.
57. Yao R, Cooper GM. Requirement for phosphatidylinositol-3 kinase in the prevention of apoptosis by nerve growth factor. *Science* 1995; 267:2003–6.
58. Lin C, Bissell MJ. Regulation of cell differentiation by extracellular matrix. *FASEB J* 1993;4:737.
59. Bates RC, Buret A, Van Helden DF, Horton MA, Burns GF. Apoptosis induced by inhibition of intercellular contact. *J Cell Biol* 1994; 125:403–15.
60. Ruoslahti E, Reed JC. Anchorage dependence, integrins, and apoptosis. *Cell* 1994;77:477–8.
61. Frisch SM, Francis H. Disruption of epithelial cell-matrix interactions induces apoptosis. *J Cell Biol* 1994;124:619–26.
62. Boudreau N, Sympson CJ, Werb Z, Bissell MJ. Suppression of ICE and apoptosis in mammary epithelial cells by extracellular matrix. *Science* 1995;267:891–2.
63. Gottlieb E, Haffner R, von R‚den T, Wagner EF, Oren M. Down-regulation of wild-type p53 activity interferes with apoptosis of IL-3–dependent hematopoietic cells following IL-3 withdrawal. *EMBO J* 1994;13:1368–74.
64. Hengartner MO, Horvitz HR. *C. elegans* cell survival gene ced-9 encodes a functional homolog of the mammalian proto-oncogene bcl-2. *Cell* 1994;76:665–76.
65. Korsmeyer SJ. Bcl-2: an antidote to programmed cell death. *Cancer Surv* 1992;15:150–68.
66. Reed JC. Bcl-2 and the regulation of programmed cell death. *J Cell Biol* 1994;124:1–6.
67. Vaux DL, Haecker G, Strasser A. An evolutionary perspective on apoptosis. *Cell* 1994;76:777–9.
68. Oltvai ZN, Milliman CL, Korsmeyer SJ. Bcl-2 heterodimerizes in vitro with a conserved homolog, Bax, that accelerates programmed cell death. *Cell* 1993;74:609–19.
69. Boise LH, Garcia MG, Postema CE, et al. bcl-x, a bcl-2–related gene that functions as a dominant regulator of apoptotic cell death. *Cell* 1993;74:597–608.
70. Yang E, Zha J, Jockel J, Boise LH, Thompson CB, Korsmeyer SJ. Bad, a heterodimeric partner for bcl-x_L and bcl-2, displaces bax and promotes cell death. *Cell* 1995;80:285–91.
71. Farrow SN, White JHM, Martinou I, et al. Cloning of a bcl-2 homologue by interaction with adenovirus E1B 19K. *Nature* 1995;374: 731–2.
72. Chittenden T, Harrington EA, OíConnor R, Flemington C, Lutz RJ, Evan GI. Induction of apoptosis by the Bcl-2 homologue Bak. *Nature* 1995;374:733–6.
73. Kiefer MC, Brauer MJ, Powers VC, et al. Modulation of apoptosis by the widely distributed Bcl-2 homologue Bak. *Nature* 1995;374:736–9.
74. Henderson S, Huen D, Rowe M, Dawson C, Johnson G, Rickinson A. Epstein-Barr virus–coded BHRF1 protein, a viral homologue of Bcl-2, protects human B cells from programmed cell death. *Proc Natl Acad Sci USA* 1993;90:8479–83.
75. Veis DJ, Sorenson CM, Shutter JR, Korsmeyer SJ. Bcl-2–deficient mice demonstrate fulminant lymphoid apoptosis, polycystic kidneys, and hypopigmented hair. *Cell* 1993;75:229–40.
76. Yin X-M, Oltvai ZN, Korsmeyer SJ. BH1 and BH2 domains of Bcl-2 are required for inhibition of apoptosis and heterodimerization with Bax. *Nature* 1994;369:321–3.
77. Borner C, Martinou I, Mattmann C, et al. The protein bcl-2a does not require membrane attachment, but two conserved domains to suppress apoptosis. *J Cell Biol* 1994;126:1059–68.
78. Takayama S, Sato T, Krajewski S, et al. Cloning and functional analysis of BAG-1: a novel Bcl-2 binding protein with anti-cell death activity. *Cell* 1995;80:279–84.
79. Boyd JM, Malstrom S, Subramanian T, et al. Adenovirus E1B 19 kDa and Bcl-2 proteins interact with a common set of cellular proteins. *Cell* 1994;79:341–51.
80. Levy Y, Brouet J-C. Interleukin-10 prevents spontaneous death of germinal center B cells by induction of the bcl-2 protein. *J Clin Invest* 1994;93:424–8.
81. May WS, Tyler PG, Ito T, Armstrong DK, Qatsha KA, Davidson NE. Interleukin-3 and bryostatin-1 mediate hyperphosphorylation of BCL2a in association with suppression of apoptosis. *J Biol Chem* 1994;269:26865–70.
82. Hockenberry DM, Oltvai ZN, Yin XM, Milliman CL, Korsmeyer SL. Bcl-2 functions in an antioxidant pathway to prevent apoptosis. *Cell* 1993;75:241–51.
83. Jacobson MD, Raff MC. Programmed cell death and Bcl-2 protection in very low oxygen. *Nature* 1995;374:814–6.
84. Shimizu S, Eguchi Y, Kosaka H, Kamiike W, Matsuda H, Tsujimoto Y. Prevention of hypoxia-induced cell death by Bcl-2 and Bcl-xL. *Nature* 1995;374:811–3.
85. Miyashita T, Reed JC. Tumor suppressor p53 is a direct transcriptional activator of the human bax gene. *Cell* 1995;80:293–9.
86. Ledda-Columbano GM, Columbano A, Coni P, Faa G, Pani P. Cell deletion by apoptosis during regression of renal hyperplasia. *Am J Pathol* 1989;135:657–62.
87. Johnson R. The glomerular response to injury: progression or resolution? *Kidney Int* 1994;45:1769–82.
88. Johnson RJ, Iida H, Alpers CE, et al. Expression of smooth muscle cell phenotype by rat mesangial cells in immune complex nephritis. *J Clin Invest* 1991;87:847–58.
89. Floege J, Johnson RJ, Gordon K, et al. Increased synthesis of extracellular matrix in mesangial proliferative nephritis. *Kidney Int* 1991;40:477–88.
90. Gobé GC, Axelsen RA. Genesis of renal tubular atrophy in experimental hydronephrosis in the rat. Role of apoptosis. *Lab Invest* 1987; 56:273–82.
91. Harrison DJ. Cell death in the diseased glomerulus. *Histopathology* 1988;12:679–83.
92. Gavrieli Y, Sherman Y, Ben-Sasson SA. Identification of programmed cell death in situ via specific labelling of nuclear DNA fragmentation. *J Cell Biol* 1992;119:493–501.
93. Wijsman JH, Jonker RR, Keijzer R, Van de Velde CJH, Cornelisse CJ, Van Direndonck JH. A new method to detect apoptosis in paraffin sections: in situ end-labeling of fragmented DNA. *J Histochem & Cytochem* 1993;41:7–12.
94. Baker AJ, Mooney A, Hughes J, Lombardi D, Johnson RJ, Savill J. Mesangial cell apoptosis: the major mechanism for resolution of glomerular hypercellularity in experimental mesangial proliferative nephritis. *J Clin Invest* 1994;94:2105–16.
95. Shimizu A, Kitamura H, Masuda Y, Ishizaki M, Sugisaki Y, Yamanaka N. Apoptosis in the repair process of experimental proliferative glomerulonephritis. *Kid Int* 1995;47:114–21.
96. Bagchus WM, Hoedemaeker PJ, Rozing J, Bakker WW. Glomerulonephritis induced by monoclonal anti-Thyl. 1 antibodies. A sequential histological and ultrastructural study in the rat. *Lab Invest* 1986;55: 680–7.
97. Johnson RJ, Garcia RL, Pritzl P, Alpers CE. Platelets mediate glomerular cell proliferation induced by anti-mesangial cell antibodies in the rat. *Am J Pathol* 1990;136:369–74.
98. Johnson RJ, Floege J, Yoshimura A, Iida H, Couser WG, Alpers CE. The activated mesangial cell: a glomerular "myofibroblast?" *J Am Soc Nephrol* 1992;2(suppl):190–7.
99. Darby I, Skalli O, Gabbiani G. Alpha-smooth muscle actin is transiently expressed by myofibroblasts during wound healing. *Lab Invest* 1990;63:21–9.
100. Lan HY, Nikolic-Paterson DJ, Atkins RC. Trafficking of inflammatory macrophages from the kidney to draining lymph nodes during experimental glomerulonephritis. *Clin Exp Immunol* 1993;92: 336–41.
101. Savill JS, Wyllie AH, Henson JE, Walport MJ, Henson PM, Haslett C. Macrophage phagocytosis of aging neutrophils in inflammation. Programmed cell death in the neutrophil leads to its recognition by macrophages. *J Clin Invest* 1989;83:865–7.

102. Perry VH, Henderson Z, Linden R. Postnatal changes in retinal ganglion cell and optic axon populations in pigmented rat. *J Comp Neurol* 1983;219:356–68.
103. Coles HSR, Burne JF, Raff MC. Large-scale normal cell death in the developing rat kidney and its reduction by epidermal growth factor. *Dev* 1993;118:777–84.
104. Szabolcs MJ, Ward L, Buttyan R, DíAgati V. Apoptosis in human renal biopsies. *J Am Soc Nephrol* 1994;5:844.
105. Mooney A, Hughes J, Lombardi D, Johnson RJ, Savill J. Kinetic analysis of apoptosis in resolution of the rat thy 1.1 model of mesangial proliferative glomerulonephritis. *J Am Soc Nephrol* 1994;5:797.
106. Pabst R, Sterzel RB. Cell renewal of glomerular cell types in normal rats. An autoradiographic analysis. *Kidney Int* 1983;24:626–31.
107. Avers CJ. In: Avers CJ, ed. *Mitosis and meiosis*. New York: D. Van Nostrand; 1976:449–503.
108. Ortiz A, Karp SL, Danoff TM, Neilson EG. Expression of survival promoting Bcl-2 oncogene by renal cells and whole kidney [Abstract]. *J Am Soc Nephrol* 1993;4:742.
109. Ortiz A, Neilson EG. Expression of bax and bcl-x, members of the bcl-2 gene family, in murine tubular cells and acute renal failure. *J Am Soc Nephrol* 1994;5:906.
110. Uda S, Yoshimura A, Inui K, et al. Glomerular expression of apoptosis-related molecules in rats with mesangial proliferative nephritis. *J Am Soc Nephrol* 1994;5:797.
111. Gonzalez-Cuadrado S, Ortiz A, Karp S, et al. The Fas ligand (FasL)-Fas (CD95) system in the kidney. *J Am Soc Nephrol* 1994;5:748.
112. Terada Y, Tomita K, Yamada T, Nonoguchi H, Marumo F. Apoptosis-related genes IL-1-beta coverting enzyme (ICE). Bcl-2, Fas, Fas-ligand (Fas-L) are expressed in microdissected rat nephron segments and changed in renal damage. *J Am Soc Nephrol* 1994;5:911.
113. Sugenoya Y, Yoshimura Y, Uda S, Inui K, Taira T, Ideura T. Apoptosis-inducible antigen (Fas) is expressed in glomeruli with human proliferative glomerulonephritis. *J Am Nephrol* 1994;5:342.
114. Sarih M, Souvannavong V, Adam A. Nitric oxide synthase induces macrophage death by apoptosis. *Biochem Biophys Res Commun* 1993;191:503–8.
115. Sugiyama H, Kashihara N, Yamasaki Y, et al. Le y is a member predictive of apoptosis and its increased expression is associated with progression of glomerulosclerosis. *J Am Soc Nephrol* 1993;4:783.
116. Cattell V, Lianos E, Largen P, Cook T. Glomerular NO synthase activity in mesangial cell immune injury. *Exp Nephrol* 1993;1:36–40.
117. Polunovsky VA, Chen B, Henke C, et al. Role of mesenchymal cell death in lung remodelling after injury. *J Clin Invest* 1993;92:388–97.
118. Floege J, Kriz W, Schulze M, Kerjcischki D, Couser WG, Koch KM. bFGF augments podocyte injury and glomerulosclerosis in rats with membranous nephropathy but not in normal rats. *J Am Soc Nephrol* 1994;5:778.
119. Chandler D, El-Naggar AK, Brisbay S, Redline RW, McDonnell TJ. Apoptosis and expression of the bcl-2 proto-oncogene in the fetal and adult human kidney. *Hum Pathol* 1994;8:789–96.
120. Araki S, Shimada Y, Kaji K, Hayashi H. Apoptosis of endothelial cells induced by fibroblast growth factor deprivation. *Biochem Biophys Res Commun* 1990;168:1194–9.
121. Robaye B, Mosselmans R, Fiers W, Dumont JE, Galand P. Tumour necrosis factor induces apoptosis (programmed cell death) in normal endothelial cells in vitro. *Am J Pathol* 1991;138:447–53.
122. Johnson RJ, Guggenheim SJ, Klebanoff SJ, et al. Morphologic correlates of glomerular oxidant injury induced by the myeloperoxidase-hydrogen peroxide-halide system of the neutrophil. *Lab Invest* 1988;58:294–301.
123. Savill J, Johnson RJ. Glomerular remodelling after inflammatory injury. *Exp Nephrol* 1995;3:149–58.
124. Desmoulière A, Redard M, Darby I, Gabbiani G. Apoptosis mediates the decrease in cellularity during the transition between granulation tissue and scar. *Am J Pathol* 1995;146:56–66.
125. Schumer M, Sawczuk IS, Colombel MC, et al. Morphologic, biochemical and molecular evidence of apoptosis during the reperfusion phase after brief periods of renal ischemia. *Am J Pathol* 1992;140:831–8.
126. Ortiz A, Neilson EG. Apoptosis related Fas RNA is expressed by renal cells and increased in renal damage. *J Am Soc Nephrol* 1993; 4:496.
127. Nouwen EJ, Verstrepen WA, Buyssens N, Zhu MQ, De Broe ME. Hyperplasia, hypertrophy and phenotypic alterations in the distal nephron after acute proximal tubular injury in the rat. *Lab Invest* 1994;70:479–93.
128. Kennedy WA, Stenberg A, Lackgren G, Hensle TW, Sawczuk IS. Renal tubular apoptosis after partial ureteral obstruction. *J Urol* 1994; 152:658–64.
129. Kennedy WA, Buttyan R, Sawczuk IS. Epidermal growth factor suppresses renal tubular apoptosis following ureteral obstruction. *Am Soc Nephrol* 1993;4:738.
130. Haslett C. Resolution of acute inflammation and the role of apoptosis in the tissue fate of granulocytes. *Clin Sci* 1992;83:639–48.
131. Savill J, Haslett C. Fate of neutrophils. In: Helliwell PG, Williams TJ, eds. *Immunopharmacology of neutrophils*. London: Academic, 1994: 295–314.
132. Metchnikoff E. *Lectures on the comparative pathology of inflammation*. In: Starling FA, Starling EH, eds. (Translated from the French by London: Kegan, Paul, Trench and Trubner, 1893.)
133. Sanui H, Yoshida S-I, Nomoto K, Ohhara R, Adachi Y. Peritoneal macrophages which phagocytose autologous polymorphonuclear leucocytes in guinea-pigs. *Br J Exp Pathol* 1982;63:278–85.
134. Kawabori S, Soda K, Perdue MH, Bienenstock J. The dynamics of intestinal eosinophil depletion in rats treated with dexamethasone. *Lab Invest* 1991;64:224–33.
135. Johnson RJ, Alpers CE, Pruchno C, et al. Mechanisms and kinetics for platelet and neutrophil localisation in immune complex nephritis. *Kidney Int* 1989;36:780–9.
136. Cattell V. Macrophages in acute glomerular inflammation. *Kidney Int* 1994;45:945–52.
137. Harris JE, Ford CE. Cellular traffic of the thymus: experiments with chromosome markers. Evidence that the thymus plays an instructional part. *Nature* 1964;201:884–6.
138. Newman SL, Henson JE, Henson PM. Phagocytosis of senescent neutrophils by human monocyte-derived macrophages and rabbit inflammatory macrophages. *J Exp Med* 1982;156:430–42.
139. Grigg J, Savill J, Sarraf C, Haslett C, Silverman M. Neutrophil apoptosis and clearance from neonatal lungs. *Lancet* 1991;338:720–2.
140. Savill JS, Smith J, Ren Y, Sarraf C, Abbott F, Rees AJ. Glomerular mesangial cells and inflammatory macrophages ingest neutrophils undergoing apoptosis. *Kidney Int* 1992;42:924–36.
141. Savill J. Macrophage recognition of senescent neutrophils. *Clin Sci* 1992;83:649–55.
142. Whyte MKB, Meagher LC, MacDermot J, Haslett C. Impairment of function in aging neutrophils is associated with apoptosis. *J Immunol* 1993;150:5124–34.
143. Meagher LC, Savill JS, Baker A, Haslett C. Phagocytosis of apoptotic neutrophils does not induce macrophage release of thromboxane B2. *J Leukoc Biol* 1992;52:269–73.
144. Lee A, Whyte MKB, Haslett C. Inhibition of apoptosis and prolongation of neutrophil functional longevity by inflammatory mediators. *J Leukoc Biol* 1993;54:283–8.
145. Ren Y, Savill J. Pro-inflammatory cytokines potentiate thrombospondin-mediated phagocytosis of neutrophils undergoing apoptosis. *J Immunol* 1995;154:2366–74.
146. Savill J. Apoptosis in disease. *Eur J Clin Invest* 1994;24:715–23.
147. Savill J, Fadok VA, Henson PM, Haslett C. Phagocyte recognition of cells undergoing apoptosis. *Immunology* 1993;14:131–6.
148. Savill JS, Henson PM, Haslett C. Phagocytosis of aged human neutrophils by macrophages is medicated by a novel "charge sensitive" recognition mechanism. *J Clin Invest* 1989;84:1518–27.
149. Savill J, Dransfield I, Hogg N, Haslett C. Vitronectin receptor mediated phagocytosis of cell undergoing apoptosis. *Nature* 1990;343: 170–3.
150. Savill JS, Hogg H, Ren Y, Haslett C. Thrombospondin cooperates with CD36 an the vitronectin receptor in macrophage recognition of neutrophils undergoing apoptosis. *J Clin Invest* 1992;90:1513–22.
151. Ren Y, Silverstein RL, Allen J, Savill J. CD36 gene transfer confers capacity for phagocytosis of cells undergoing apoptosis. *J Exp Med* 1995;181:1857–62.
152. Akbar AN, Savill J, Gombert W, et al. The specific recognition by macrophages of CD8+, CD45RO+ T cells undergoing apoptosis: a mechanism for T cell clearance during resolution of viral infections. *J Exp Med* 1994;180:1943–7.
153. Fadok V, Savill JS, Haslett C, et al. Different populations of macrophages use either the vitronectin receptor or the phosphatidylserine

receptor to recognise and remove apoptotic cells. *J Immunol* 1992; 149:4029–35.

154. Hughes J, Savill J. The human mesangial cell vitronectin receptor mediates phagocytosis of senescent neutrophils undergoing apoptosis. *J Am Soc Nephrol* 1992;3:566.
155. Hall S, Savill J, Henson P, Haslett C. Apoptotic neutrophils are phagocytosed by fibroblasts with participation of the fibroblast vitronectin receptor and involvement of a mannose/fucose-specific lectin. *J Immunol* 1994;153:3218–27.
156. Fadok VA, Voelker DR, Campbell PA, Cohen JJ, Bratton DL, Henson PM. Exposure of phosphatidylserine on the surface of apoptotic lymphocytes triggers specific recognition and removal by macrophages. *J Immunol* 1992;148:2207–16.
157. Fadok VA, Laszlo DJ, Noble PW, Weinstein L, Riches DWH, Henson PM. Particle digestibility is required for induction of the phosphatidylserine recognition mechanism used by murine macrophages to phagocytose apoptotic cells. *J Immunol* 1992;151:4274.
158. Savill J. Apoptosis and the kidney. *J Am Soc Nephrol* 1994;5:12–21.
159. Casciola-Rosen LA, Anhalt G, Rosen A. Autoantigens targeted in systemic lupus erythematosus are clustered in two populations of surface structures on apoptotic keratinocytes. *J Exp Med* 1994;179: 1317–30.
160. Casciola-Rosen LA, Miller DK, Anhalt GJ, Rosen A. Specific cleavage of the 70-kDa protein component of small nuclear ribonucleoprotein is a characteristic biochemical feature of apoptotic cell death. *J Biol Chem* 1994;269:30757–60.
161. Batsford SR. Cationic antigens as mediators of inflammation. *APMIS* 1991;99:1–9.
162. Bell DA, Morrison B. The spotaneous apoptotic death of normal human lymphocytes in vitro: the release of and immunoproliferative response to nucleosomes in vitro. *Clin Immunol Immunopathol* 1991; 60:13–26.
163. Price B, Lieberthal W, Triaca V, Fitzpatrick J, Koh J, Levine J. The lupus anticoagulant recognises an epitope on the membranes of apoptotic cells. *J Am Soc Nephrol* 1994;5:763.
164. Cohen JJ, Duke RC, Fadok VA, Sellins KS. Apoptosis and programmed cell death in immunity. *Annu Rev Immunol* 1992;10: 267–93.
165. Watanabe-Fukunaga R, Brannon CI, Copeland NG, Jenkins NA, Nagata S. Lymphoproliferation disorder in mice explained by defects in Fas antigen that mediates apoptosis. *Nature* 1992;356:314–7.
166. Wu J, Zhou T, He J, Mountz JD. Autoimmune disease in mice due to integration of an endogenous retrovirus in an apoptosis gene. *J Exp Med* 1993;178:461–8.
167. Emlen W, Niebur J, Kadera R. Accelerated in vitro apoptosis of lymphocytes from patients with systemic lupus erythematosus. *J Immunol* 1994;152:3685–92.
168. Mysler E, Bini P, Drappa J, et al. The apoptosis-1/Fas protein in human systemic lupus erythematosus. *J Clin Invest* 1994;93:1029–34.
169. Fisher GH, Rosenberg FJ, Straus SE, et al. Dominant interfering Fas gene mutations impair apoptosis in a human autoimmune lymphoproliferative syndrome. *Cell* 1995;81:935–46.
170. Takahashi T, Tanaka M, Brannan CI, et al. Generalized lymphoproliferative disease in mice, caused by a point mutation in the Fas ligand. *Cell* 1994;76:969–76.
171. Strasser A, Whittingham S, Vaux DL, et al. Enforced Bcl2 expression in B-lymphoid cells prolongs antibody responses and elicits autoimmune disease. *Proc Natl Acad Sci USA* 1991;88:8661–5.
172. Shimizu A, Nakao N, Muroga K, et al. Apoptosis in progression process of experimental crescentic glomerulonephritis. *J Am Soc Nephrol* 1994;5:769.
173. Berke G. The CTLís kiss of death. *Cell* 1995;81:9–12.
174. Heusel JW, Wesselschmidt RL, Shresta S, Russell JH, Ley TJ. Cytotoxic lymphocytes require granzyme B for the rapid induction of DNA fragmentation and apoptosis in allogeneic target cells. *Cell* 1994;76:977–87.
175. Lowin B, Hahne M, Mattmann C, Tschopp J. Cytolytic T-cell cytotoxicity is mediated through perforin and Fas lytic pathways. *Nature* 1994;370:650–2.
176. Brooks P, Montgomery AMP, Rosenfield M, et al. Integrin a_vb_3 antagonists promote tumor regression by inducing apoptosis of angiogenic blood vessels. *Cell* 1994;79:1157–64.

Immunologic Renal Diseases,
edited by E. G. Neilson and W. G. Couser.
Lippincott-Raven Publishers, Philadelphia © 1997.

CHAPTER 16

Mechanisms of Allograft Rejection

James M. Pattison, Richard K. Sibley, and Alan M. Krensky

INTRODUCTION

Clinical transplantation has been a great success as a result of refinements in immunosuppressive regimens, better treatment of infections, and improvements in tissue typing. Nevertheless, major problems still plague transplantation, especially rejection (both acute and chronic), and the increased incidence of infections and malignancies (1). The immunologic nature of allograft rejection was first demonstrated over 50 years ago by Medawar, who found that skin grafts between genetically disparate rabbits were accepted but rapidly became necrotic (2). The rejection was specific for the donor. Second grafts were rejected rapidly, but third party grafts were rejected more slowly. Much is now known about the molecular and cellular mechanisms of allograft rejection, and this information should lead to the development of more specific immunosuppressants (3–7).

The basic cellular mechanism of allograft rejection is as follows (Fig. 1). Recipient donor T-lymphocytes recognize foreign human leukocyte antigen (HLA) class II molecules in the allograft and are activated to proliferate, differentiate, and secrete a variety of cytokines. Cytokines upregulate expression of HLA class II antigens on engrafted tissues such as vascular endothelium, stimulate B-lymphocytes to produce high-affinity and high-titer antibodies against the allograft, and help cytotoxic T cells (CTLs), macrophages, and natural killer (NK) cells to develop cytotoxicity against the graft.

An understanding of allograft rejection thus requires a knowledge of mechanisms of antigen presentation by major histocompatibility complex (MHC) molecules, T-cell activation and cytotoxicity, leukocyte–endothelial interactions, and the role of various cytokines in mediating inflammatory processes.

J. M. Pattison: Guy's Hospital, London SE1 9RT, England.

R. K. Sibley: Department of Pathology, Stanford University, Stanford, California 94305.

A. M. Krensky: Division of Immunology and Transplantation Biology, Department of Pediatrics, Stanford University, Stanford, California 94305.

Allorecognition

The alloresponse involves recognition of nonself antigens on donor cells by recipient lymphocytes where both donor and recipient are of the same species. At least two distinct pathways are involved (8). In the "direct" pathway, T cells recognize intact nonself MHC molecules on the surface of the donor cells with an array of peptides derived from endogenous proteins present in the peptide-binding groove. In the "indirect" pathway, T cells recognize processed alloantigen as protein fragments (peptides) in the context of self MHC molecules on antigen-presenting cells (9,10). Although the relative contribution of these two pathways remains controversial, the direct pathway dominates. However, evidence also suggests involvement of the indirect pathway, especially in chronic rejection (11,12).

The alloresponse is characterized by its strength in vivo, which is reflected in vitro by the high precursor frequency of T cells responding to any particular MHC type. The strength of the response may be due to the high density of allogeneic MHC molecules on the graft (13), the multitude of different peptides that can be presented (14), and/or the additional involvement of the indirect pathway of antigen presentation (11,12). Another level of complexity is added by the potential variety of T-cell specificities that may be involved in allorecognition (15). Although some T cells are strictly peptide specific (similar to nominal antigen recognition), others recognize different peptides bound by the same MHC molecule (promiscuous) and some are capable of recognizing allogeneic MHC molecules in the absence of bound peptide (empty). In some cases, T-cell recognition may be cross-reactive; e.g., a single T-cell receptor (TCR) can recog-

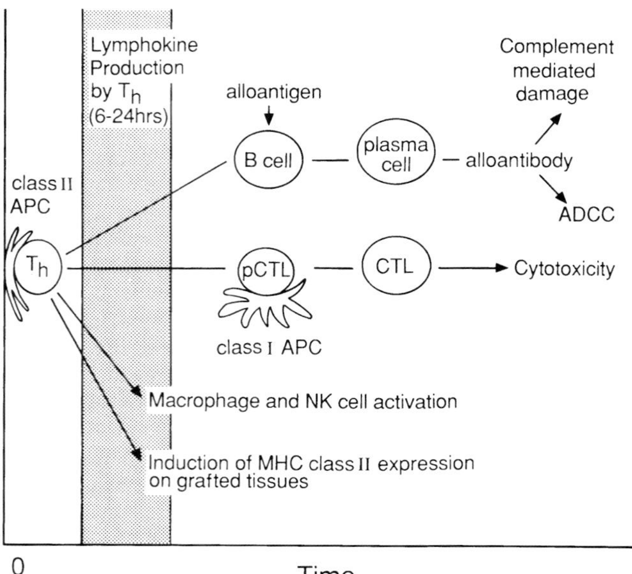

FIG. 1. The activation of a T-helper (Th) cell by an APC expressing MHC class II to produce cytokines. Lymphokines promote the activation, proliferation, and differentiation of numerous effector cells thought to contribute to transplant rejection. pCTL, precursor CTL. Reprinted with permission (4).

nize both self MHC + X and allogeneic MHC. In other cases, a single T cell can express more than one functional TCR gene (16). This may provide an additional explanation for the ability of some T cells to recognize both nominal and allogeneic antigen.

Major Histocompatibility Complex

The genes of the MHC encode for molecules that are the primary antigens responsible for the induction of the immune response to an allograft (17,18). HLAs are encoded on the short arm of chromosome 6 in a 3.5 million base pair region of DNA (19). The MHC locus encodes two major classes of proteins—HLA class I (HLA-A, -B, and -C) and HLA class II (HLA-DP, -DQ, and -DR), as well as other proteins essential for the processing of antigens, including low molecular weight proteins (LMP2 and LMP7), transporter proteins associated with antigen presentation (TAP1 and TAP2), and HLA-DM molecules. Between the class I and class II loci are genes for the complement components C2, Bf, and C4, sometimes referred to as class III genes (Fig. 2). The class I and class II genes probably evolved from a common ancestral gene, and both are members of the immunoglobulin supergene family (20).

Class I Molecules

MHC class I molecules are the major target antigens recognized by CTLs. They are composed of two polypeptide chains: the polymorphic 45-kDa heavy chain, an integral membrane glycoprotein encoded within the MHC, and the 12-kDa light chain, β_2-microglobulin, which is encoded on chromosome 15. Class I antigens are constitutively expressed on the cell surface of all nucleated cells, allowing CTLs to recognize and destroy any cell if an appropriate foreign peptide antigen is bound.

The x-ray crystallographic structure of the human class I molecule shows two immunoglobulin-like domains, corresponding to the membrane proximal portion of the class I heavy chain and to β_2-microglobulin, which support a peptide-binding site composed of a floor of eight beta strands flanked by helical walls, all encoded by the heavy chain (21). Zinkernagel and Doherty showed in 1974 that CTLs are specific for both foreign antigen and self MHC class I molecules (22). This phenomenon of MHC restriction is explained by the fact that CTLs recognize proteolyzed forms of the antigen (peptides) bound to the MHC class I molecule. The crystal structure of HLA-A2 demonstrates discontinuous radiodense material within the groove, which was subsequently shown to be peptide. Peptides bind in an extended beta structure with the amino and carboxy terminal ends fixed tightly into opposite ends of the binding groove (Fig. 3). Most peptides binding to class I are 8 to 10 amino acids in length (23), although longer peptides have been found (up to 12 amino acids) that bulge out of the groove (24). The peptides are characterized by anchor residues, which are present at defined positions and fit into corresponding pockets within the HLA class I binding site (25). The pockets are formed by polymorphic amino acids that lead to different specificities among different class I allelic products.

Most peptides presented by class I molecules are generated in the cytosol (26). The major pathway for protein turnover in the cytoplasm involves proteasomes, which cleave endogenous proteins into peptide fragments capable of binding to the grooves of HLA molecules (27) (Fig. 4). A subset of proteasomes contains two components (large multifunctional protease [LMP]-2 and LMP-7) that are encoded by genes in the MHC. The LMP subunits alter the proteolytic activity of the proteasome such that the peptides are more suitable for binding to the MHC class I molecule. Other proteasome subunits, MB1 and delta, also may be important for improving specificity for antigen processing (28).

Transporter proteins associated with antigen presentation (TAPs) are responsible for the adenosine triphosphate–dependent transport of short peptides (suitable for binding to class I molecules) from the cytoplasm to the endoplasmic reticulum (ER) lumen. The functional trans-

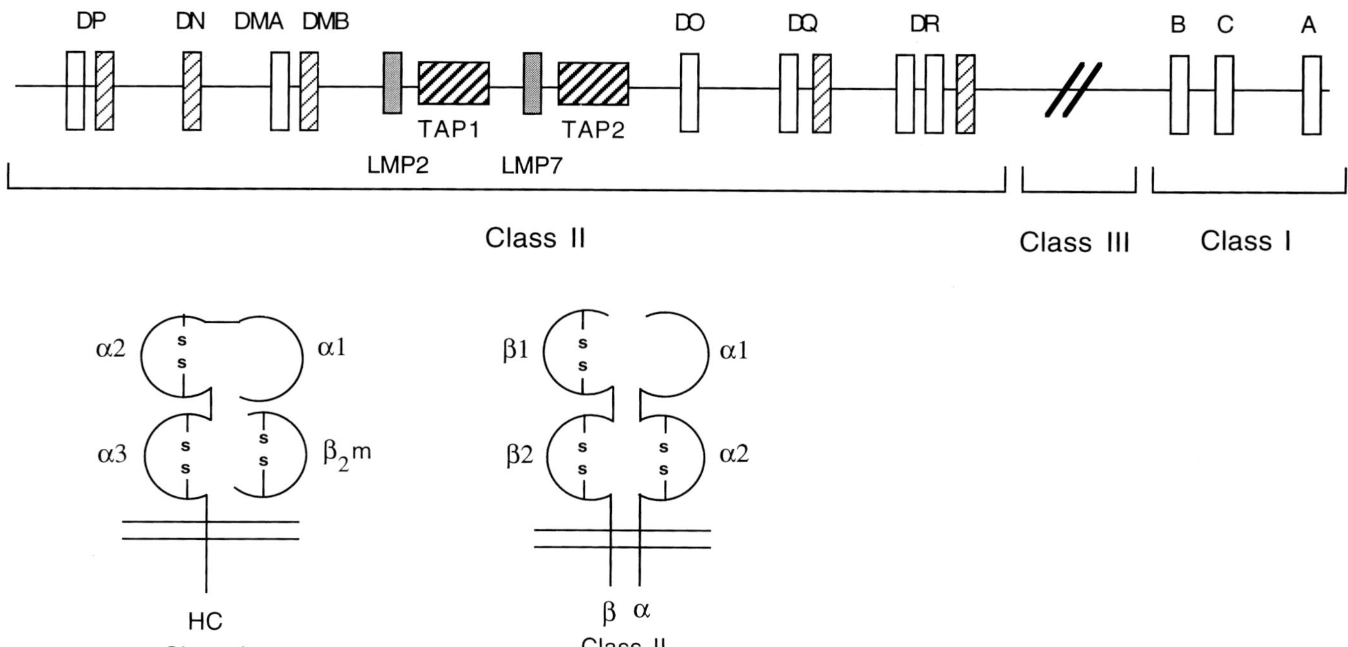

FIG. 2. Genomic organization of the human MHC complex (top) and schematic representation of the HLA class I and II domain organization (bottom). Reprinted with permission (20).

porter complex is a heterodimer composed of TAP1 and TAP2 polypeptide chains. TAPs show size and sequence specificity (29). Peptides matching the optimum size of the class I binding sites are transported most efficiently. The TAP-mediated pathway provides most of the class I binding peptides, although alternative pathways may exist (30).

Assembly of the functional MHC class I complex (consisting of the class I heavy chain, β_2-microglobulin, and a bound peptide) occurs in the ER. Class I heavy chains and β_2-microglobulin are cotranslationally translocated into the lumen of the ER, and peptides derived from the protein degradation in the cytosol are transported into the ER by the TAPs. Peptides are required to stabilize the class I structure. All three components are needed to stabilize the complex and ensure efficient intracellular transport from the ER to the plasma membrane. The resident ER protein calnexin (p68, lp90) binds transiently to peptide-free class I heavy chains. Release from calnexin is necessary for protein movement out of the ER into the Golgi complex. Calnexin thus prevents transport of empty class I chains to the cell surface, providing a quality control mechanism (31). This reduces the likelihood of exogenous peptide acquisition and presentation and ensures that CTLs focus on actively infected cells.

Class II Molecules

MHC class II antigens—HLA-DR, -DQ, and -DP—are encoded upstream of the HLA class I molecules (Fig. 2). Class II proteins present peptides processed from exogenous antigens present in extracellular fluid, and are recognized by $CD4^+$ T helper lymphocytes. Activated T-helper cells produce cytokines that enhance T-cell activity and also lead to secretion of antibodies by B cells, which thus eliminate extracellular antigens.

Class II is a heterodimer of two transmembrane subunits, alpha (33 kDa) and beta (29 kDa), encoded in the MHC. Each of these chains has two extracellular domains and the polymorphic regions are mostly in the outer amino terminal domains (α_1 and β_1). Class II is expressed primarily by B cells, macrophages, monocytes, and dendritic cells, although γ-interferon can upregulate its expression in a variety of other cell types, including endothelium, epithelium, and T-lymphocytes. Class II differs mainly from class I in the separation of the peptide-binding domain into two noncovalently associated halves, with one alpha helix and four beta strands (90 amino acids) contributed by each subunit. Class II binding peptides are longer (12–28 amino acids) and more

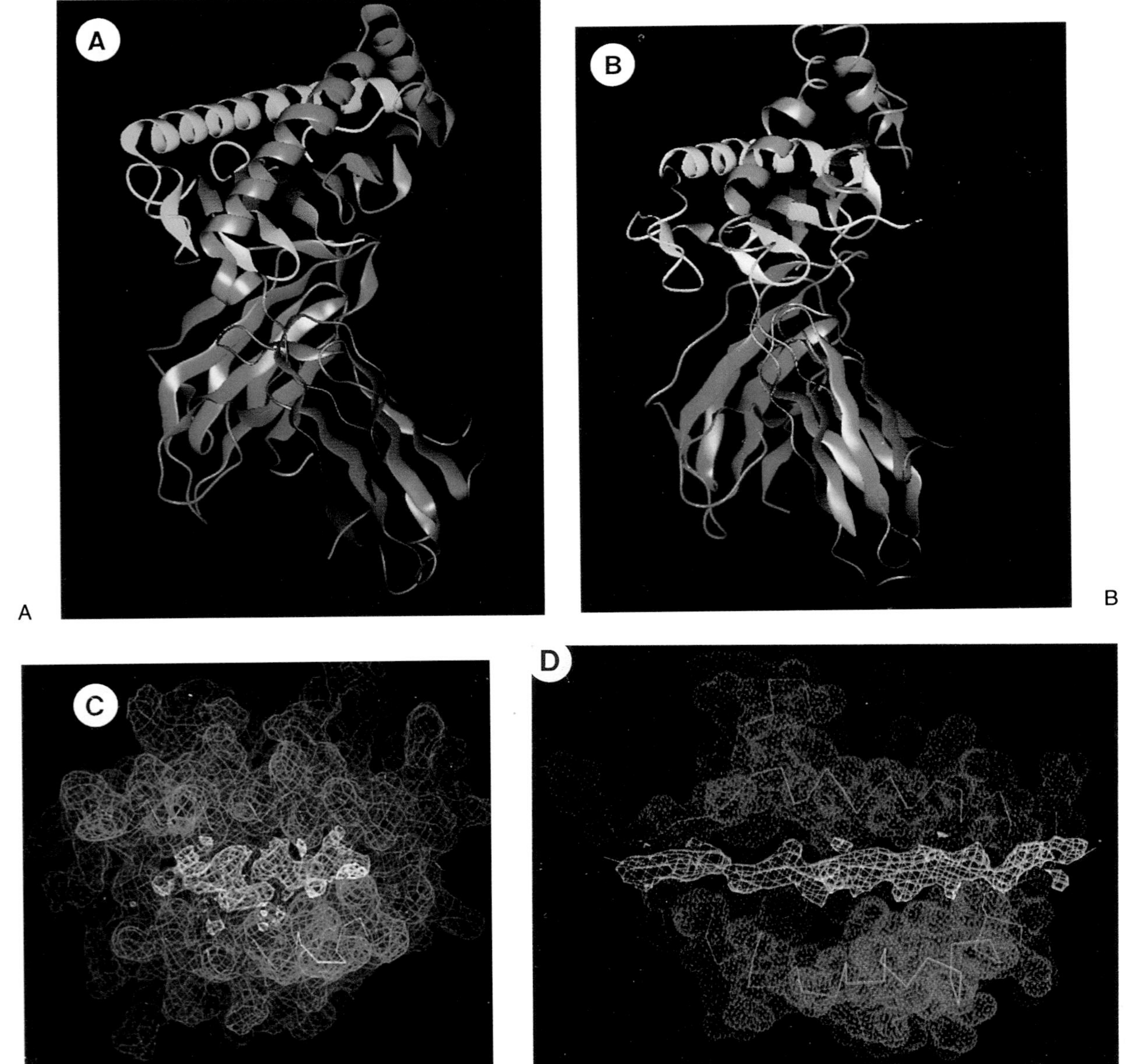

FIG. 3. A: Computer image of the human class I molecule, HLA-B27. The $\alpha1$ domain is shown in yellow, $\alpha2$ in blue, and $\alpha3$ in green. β_2-microglobulin is shown in red. **B:** Computer image of the human class II molecules, HLA-DR1. The $\alpha1$ domain is shown in yellow, $\alpha2$ domain in red, $\beta1$ domain in blue, and $\beta2$ domain in green. For both images, the peptide-binding region is at the top and includes the two α-helices supported by a floor of beta strands. The colors are the same for homologous domains in the two proteins. Van der Waal's surface representation of the top of an MHC class I molecule (HLA-A2) (**C**) and MHC class II molecule (HLA-DR1) (**D**), probably as seen by T cells. Shown in blue are the two α-helices forming the rim of the peptide binding site. Shown in red is the electron density corresponding to bound peptides. **A** and **B:** Reprinted with permission (26). **C:** Reprinted with permission (21). **D:** Reprinted with permission (33).

variable in size than those presented by class I (32). The class II binding site is open at both ends, allowing peptides to bulge out, and the ends of the groove are not involved in anchoring the peptide to the class II molecule (Fig. 3). Class II–associated peptides appear to rest on top of the groove rather than being tightly embedded and have less well-defined anchor residues. Brown observed dimers of the class II alpha and beta heterodimers in crystallographic studies (33). It is possible that such "dimers of dimers" may occur physiologically. Although such

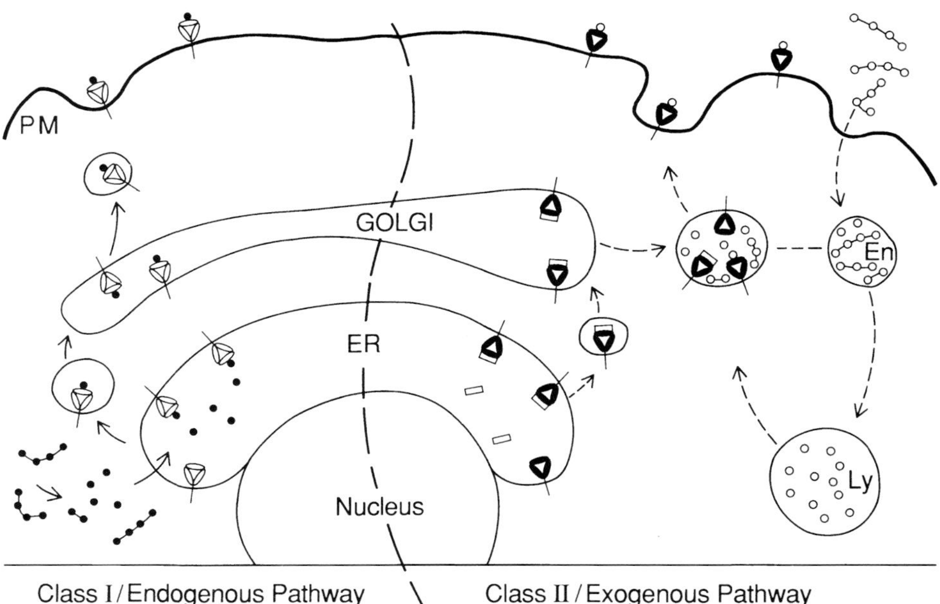

FIG. 4. Antigen processing and presentation. Peptides derived from endogenous proteins bind to HLA class I molecules in the ER and are transported through the Golgi to the plasma membrane (PM). Peptides from exogenous antigens enter the cell by endocytosis and are degraded in endosomes (En) and lysosomes (Ly). Peptides bind to class II molecules in a specialized compartment before transport to the plasma membrane. Reprinted with permission (7).

dimerization might potentiate cytoplasmic signaling events in T-cell activation, the physiologic relevance of this observation remains uncertain.

Class II alpha and beta chains are cotranslationally inserted into the membrane of the ER (Fig. 4). Within the ER, both MHC class II chains associate with a third chain, the invariant chain (Ii). As nonamers $[(\alpha/\beta/Ii)_3]$, the class II complexes leave the ER and travel through the Golgi to early endosomes and the peptide-loading compartment (34). Ii promotes the assembly of class II alpha and beta chain heterodimers. In the absence of Ii, the class II chains form homodimers and are retained in the ER in association with BiP, grp 94, and p72. Ii prevents premature peptide loading in the ER by peptides required by class I molecules. The invariant chain possesses a short internal segment [the class II-associated invariant chain peptide (CLIP) region] that occludes the class II site so that such binding cannot occur. Thus, the Ii plays a key role in differentiating the antigen presentation pathways of both MHC classes. Ii knockout mice show reduced transport of class II from the ER to the Golgi, and they have greatly reduced surface expression of class II (35).

Binding of peptides to class II occurs in a post-Golgi, acidic, proteolytic, intracellular compartment before long-lived surface expression. The compartment of peptide loading (CPL) morphologically resembles spherical multivesicular bodies. The high concentration of proteases and acidic pH make it an ideal compartment to generate a diverse range of peptides. The antigens that will be presented by class II molecules enter the cells by pinocytosis or via receptor-mediated internalization after binding to surface immunoglobulin or the binding of antigen–antibody complexes to Fc receptors. Antigens arrive in the early endosome and are transported to the CPL, where they are processed by such enzymes as cathepsin B, D, and E. In the CPL, the Ii is degraded, and the class II molecules bind processed peptide to stabilize their structure. A further MHC-encoded heterodimer (HLA-DM), which is structurally similar to class II itself, is found within the CPL and appears to be essential for efficient class II–restricted antigen presentation (36,37). The role of HLA-DM is unclear, although it may be involved in the late transport of class II molecules from the CPL to the plasma membrane, the facilitation of the dissociation of Ii, or binding antigenic peptides to prevent them from complete degradation.

Antigen-Presenting Cells

Dendritic cells, macrophages, and B cells are the "professional" antigen-presenting cells, with donor dendritic cells probably the most potent stimulators of rejection (38). Antigen recognition by T cells may occur either peripherally within the graft itself or centrally as a result of the migration of antigen-presenting cells into the recipient lymphoid tissue (39,40). Dendritic cells and macrophages express low levels of class I and class II molecules in the resting state, but upon cytokine stimulation, especially with γ-interferon, the expression of class I, class II, and TAP genes is increased. Peptides are loaded onto these molecules, creating a high-density peptide display. MHC molecule synthesis then decreases, thus fixing an image of antigen previously acquired on the cell surface. The mature dendritic cells, with the stable display of distantly acquired antigens, then migrates into lymphoid tissue where their surface membranes are efficiently scanned by receptors on recirculating T cells. Dendritic cells thus increase the likelihood of an antigen-specific T cell recognizing its antigen. In rodent transplantation models, depletion of dendritic cells from an allograft before transplantation leads to prolonged survival of the allograft after transplantation (41). The role of the dendritic cell in humans may not be so crucial, where in contrast to the rodents, class II MHC is also expressed on the endothelial cells (42). B cells and macrophages express cell surface molecules, which enhance their efficiency for acquiring antigen. Macrophages use their Fc receptors to bind antigen–antibody complexes, and B cells express surface immunoglobulin, which binds antigen. This allows T cells to focus effector function on the specific B cell as a result of processing this particular antigen, providing selective stimulation of antibody production (26). Additional cell types, including tubular epithelial cells and pancreatic islets, can be induced to express MHC class II antigens by γ-interferon and can function in antigen presentation (4).

HLA Typing

The HLA system was initially defined serologically using antibodies derived from large-scale screening of thousands of serum samples from multiparous females. Classical class I HLA proteins, HLA-A, -B, and -C molecules, show high levels of polymorphism. Based on serologic reactivities, 27 distinct antigenic specificities have been defined for the HLA-A locus, 57 for the HLA-B locus, and 10 for the HLA-C locus. However, additional polymorphisms have been defined by nucleotide sequencing. Forty-one alleles have been identified for the HLA-A locus, 61 for the HLA-B locus, and 18 for the HLA-C locus (43). The polymorphism resides within the membrane distal α_1 and α_2 domains of the class I heavy chain in contrast to the α_3 chain, which is highly conserved.

Class II molecules are also highly polymorphic, with most of the polymorphism located in the membrane distal α_1 and β_1 domains. Additional polymorphisms have been detected by RFLP techniques or by class II hybridization with sequence-specific oligonucleotide probes (SSOPs). Due to the difficulty in obtaining and characterizing serologic and cellular reagents, SSOPs are increasingly used for class II typing. All of the polymorphism among HLA-DR molecules is in the beta chain; the alpha chain is almost invariant. Sixty DRB1 allelic products have been identified to date (43). Both HLA-DQα and -β chains are polymorphic. Fourteen DQA1 and 19 DQB1 alleles have been identified. Six HLA-DP specificities have been defined cellularly, although at least eight DPα1 and 40 DPβ1 allele products have been identified by sequencing.

The biologic significance of such polymorphism of MHC molecules is that it provides a mechanism for increasing the number of peptides that can be presented. This is an advantage both at the level of the individual and the species. With increasing polymorphism, the chance of encountering a pathogen against which all members of a population have a poor response and to which they may succumb decreases. Therefore, species that can generate or maintain greater MHC polymorphism have greater collective immunity and are more likely to survive. The phenomenon of allograft rejection is a direct result of the advantage to the species of having more HLA types.

Clinically, the influence of matching for HLA in living related renal transplantation is clear. HLA-identical sibling transplants have a better survival rate than do one-haplotype matches (e.g., parent to child), and these in turn have a better survival rate than do two-haplotype mismatches (e.g., living related sibling). These differences are particularly marked with increasing time after transplantation, even in the cyclosporine era (44). The role of matching in cadaveric transplantation is more controversial. Matching for HLA-A and -B antigens has a modest effect on graft survival, although matching for HLA-DR leads to a more marked improvement (45). Although these correlations were more obvious in the precyclosporine era, they are still present. In the Collaborative Transplant Study of Opelz of around 10,000 patients treated with cyclosporine, there was a 17% better 1-year graft survival rate in recipients matched for HLA-B and -DR antigens compared with those mismatched for all four -B and -DR antigens (46).

Serologic determination of HLA-A and -B antigens has reached a high level of reliability because of international standardization. Typing errors for HLA-A and -B antigens are likely to exert only a small influence on cadaveric transplant matching. This is not the case for HLA-DR antigens. Serologic typing for HLA-DR is technically more demanding and less reliable than typing for HLA-A or -B. Opelz demonstrated that 25% of serologic HLA-DR typings may be incorrect when compared with the DNA-RFLP method (47). The 1-year graft survival for DNA-matched HLA-A, -B, and -DR grafts was 87% compared with 69% for -DR mismatched grafts. The routine use of SSOPs and polymerase chain reaction (PCR)-

based methods are expected to improve matching and, therefore, cadaveric graft survival.

Minor Histocompatibility Antigens

Minor histocompatibility (miH) antigens are less well defined (48). Over 30 minor systems, all with limited polymorphism, have been identified in mice and can result in vigorous rejection in MHC-identical mice. Because minor histocompatibility antigens are recognized as peptides in association with an MHC molecule, rather than as intact antigen, it is extremely difficult to raise antibodies against them. Rather, these antigens are identified by generating T-cell clones in vitro and by skin graft transplant models in vivo. Minor histocompatibility antigens are peptides derived from self proteins, which vary between different members of the species (e.g., mitochondrial proteins) and between the sexes (e.g., H-Y antigen) (49).

T-CELL RECOGNITION

T-Cell Receptor

Antigen specificity in allograft rejection by T cells is provided by clonally restricted TCRs (50). The TCR consists of two chains, alpha and beta, linked by disulfide bridges. Each chain is 40 to 50 kDa in size and contains both constant and variable regions (Fig. 5). (A small proportion of T cells express an alternate, γ/δ, TCR, but the role of these receptors in transplant rejection is unclear, and they are not addressed here.) The variable regions are involved in contacting antigenic peptide in the HLA binding groove, and the HLA molecule. The alpha and beta chains of the TCRs undergo genetic rearrangements of germline sequences similar to those of the immunoglobulin genes in order to generate the diversity of combining sites needed to recognize specifically many different antigens. However, unlike immunoglobulin, the TCR chains are designed to recognize peptide fragments in the context of MHC rather than as isolated specific epitopes of whole proteins.

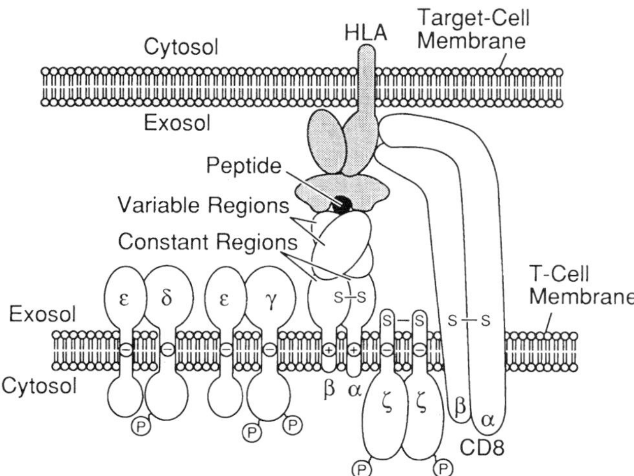

FIG. 5. The TCR complex. The TCR heterodimer (α/β) recognizes a peptide–HLA complex in an antigen-specific manner. The CD3 polypeptides transduce signals from the TCR into the cell. The CD8 molecule transiently associates with the TCR complex, recognizes invariant sequences in the α3 domain of the HLA molecule, and serves as a coreceptor in antigen recognition and signal transduction. Reprinted with permission (7).

The TCR is noncovalently associated with the CD3δ, CD3ε and CD3γ chains and a zeta chain–containing dimer. It is thought that each alpha and beta chain is associated with a CD3εδ and a CD3εγ dimer, although the precise stoichiometry of the chains within the receptor is still not known and may vary in different T-cell clones. The cytoplasmic domains of the invariant chains are much longer (40–113 residues) than are those of the alpha and beta chains (5 residues) and are responsible for coupling the TCR to the intracellular signaling machinery. The cytoplasmic domains of the invariant chains contain a common domain that couples these proteins to intracellular protein kinases (51). This antigen recognition activation motif (ARAM) consists of paired tyrosines and leucines in the consensus sequence (D/E) XXYXXL$(X)_{6-8}$YXXL. This ARAM motif is also found in the cytoplasmic domain of the B-cell receptor (immunoglobulin) and FcεR1. The presence of multiple ARAM sequences within a single oligomeric receptor may provide a means for signal amplification. TCR ligation or cross-linking also could induce aggregation of the ARAMs, making them better substrates for protein kinases. The Src family members, lck and fyn, are two protein kinases that interact with these ARAMs (52,53). They each have a myristylated glycine at position 2, which is responsible for membrane association. In contrast, ZAP-70, a 70-kDa protein tyrosine kinase expressed exclusively in T cells and NK cells (54), is not constitutively located at the plasma membrane, but is rapidly recruited to the zeta and CD3 chains after TCR stimulation. ZAP-70 has two amino-terminal SH_2 domains and a catalytic carboxyl terminal domain. It is likely that the SH_2 domains are responsible for recruiting ZAP-70 to the tyrosine phosphorylated ARAMs. The sequence of events is probably as follows: lck or fyn first phosphorylates the ARAM, resulting in recruitment of ZAP-70 via its SH_2 domains to the membrane receptor complex. Additional interactions between the Src and ZAP-70 families of protein tyrosine kinases modulate the increased catalytic activity observed after receptor stimulation. Recently, two families with autosomal-recessive severe combined immune deficiency were described with a defect in ZAP-70 protein expression and failure of TCR signal transduction (55).

Coreceptors (CD4 and CD8)

Coreceptor molecules act synergistically with the antigen receptors to induce signal transduction events at low levels of receptor occupancy. Cells that express the CD4 coreceptor have TCRs specific for class II and have primarily helper functions, whereas $CD8^+$ cells recognize class I molecules and are mainly cytotoxic (4).

CD4 binds to the β_2 segment of MHC class II (56), whereas CD8 interacts with the α_3 segment of class I (57). Both CD4 and CD8 bind to the cytoplasmic protein tyrosine kinase lck through a cysteine-containing motif shared by their cytoplasmic domains (52). The coreceptor brings lck into proximity with the TCR complex, where it acts early in the signal transduction pathway to phosphorylate tyrosines within the ARAMs of the CD3 and zeta chains. Later the SH_2 domain of CD4-associated lck is engaged by other tyrosine-phosphorylated residues in the TCR complex, thus anchoring CD4/lck to the stimulated TCR complex. This increases the avidity of the TCR–MHC interaction and increases the efficiency of signaling.

The various isoforms of the CD45 protein tyrosine phosphatase are plasma membrane proteins expressed on all cells of the hematopoietic lineage except mature erythrocytes (58). Physiologic ligands have not been established, although CD45 interacts with the B-cell antigen CD22 (59). CD45 is critical to TCR signaling, perhaps by dephosphorylating the negative regulatory site of critical Src family members (60).

T-CELL ACTIVATION

Stimulation of the TCR induces the tyrosine phosphorylation of many cytoplasmic and membrane proteins (61) (Fig. 6). Phosphorylation of phospholipase C-γ1 (PLCγ1) increases its activity and causes the cleavage of phosphatidyl inositol bisphosphate, resulting in the generation of the second messengers, inositol 1,4,5-trisphosphate (IP_3) and diacylglycerol (DG). IP_3 induces a sustained increase in intracellular calcium, and DG activates protein kinase C (PKC). These two signals synergize to induce and activate DNA-binding factors needed for interleukin (IL)-2 gene transcription. The increase in intracellular calcium activates the calcium-dependent serine/threonine phosphatase calcineurin (62), which in some way modi-

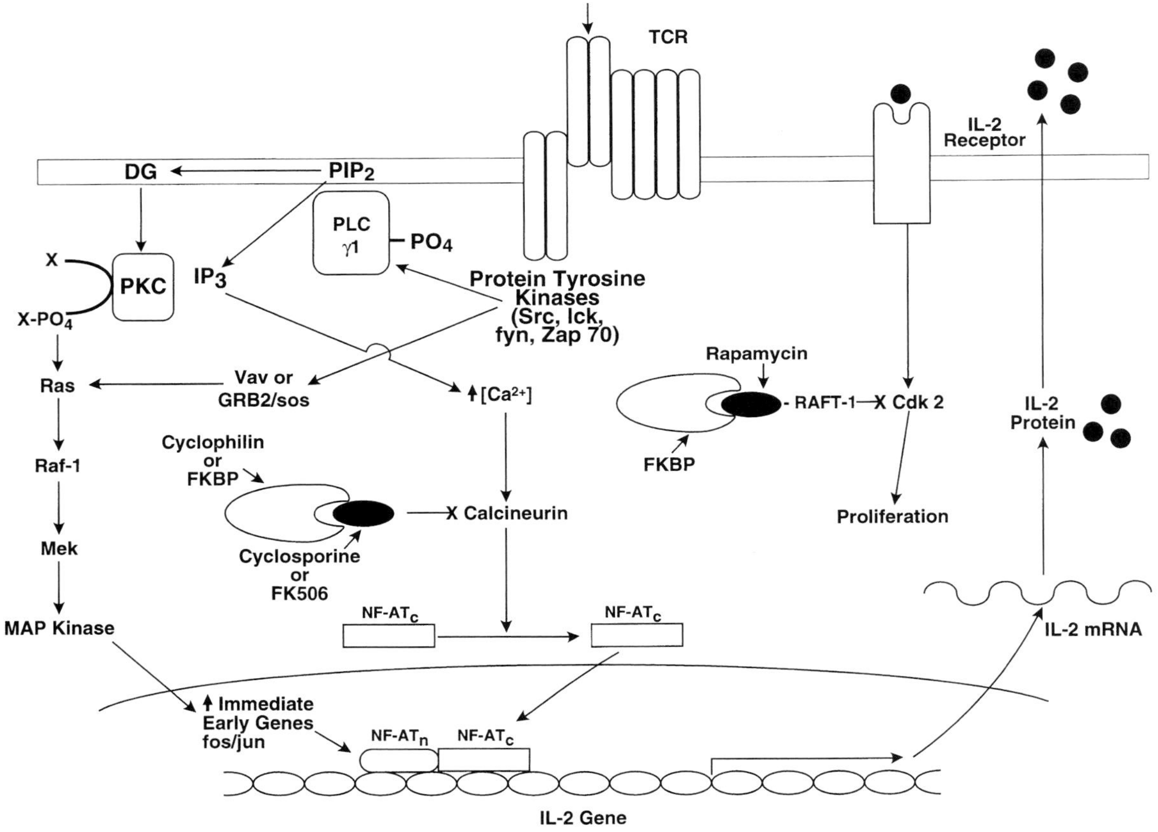

FIG. 6. Downstream signaling pathways induced after TCR stimulation, with sites of action of cyclosporine, FK506, and rapamycin. PIP_2, phosphatidylinositol 4,5-bisphosphate; DG, diacylglycerol; IP_3, inositol 1,4,5-trisphosphate; FKBP, FK506 binding protein; NF-AT, nuclear factor of activated T cells; RAFT-1, rapamycin and FKBP12 target.

fies the constitutively expressed cytoplasmic component of the nuclear factor of activated T cells (NF-AT), allowing it to translocate to the nucleus (63,64). There it combines with newly formed Fra-1 (a member of the fos family) and JunB proteins, induced by the PKC pathway, to form a functional NF-AT complex, which acts as a positively acting transcription factor on the IL-2 enhancer. Cyclosporine and FK506 bind to cytoplasmic proteins called immunophilins, or cyclophilins and FKBPs (FK506 binding proteins), respectively (65). These complexes then bind to calcineurin and inhibit its function, thus preventing NF-AT formation and IL-2 gene transcription. T cells are exquisitely sensitive to cyclosporine and FK506, possibly because they express low levels of calcineurin. Alternatively, T cell–specific proteins yet to be identified are responsible for the specific immunosuppressive effects of these potent drugs.

Tyrosine phosphorylation of vav activates the ras signal transduction pathway (66) (Fig. 6). Ras, a 21-kDa GTP-binding protein with GTPase activity, then interacts directly with the serine-threonine kinase Raf-1, which regulates the activity of a kinase cascade that includes Mek and MAP kinase and leads to nuclear events involved in cell proliferation and differentiation, probably by inducing the c-fos and c-jun transcription factors. Expression of an activated form of ras potentiates IL-2 promoter activity, whereas a dominant negative form of ras greatly inhibits IL-2 promoter activity (67).

TCR stimulation also causes the NFκB transcription factor to translocate to the nucleus (68) and also regulates the stability of several lymphokine messenger RNAs (mRNAs) by the induction of RNA-binding factors (69).

Costimulation

To induce maximal IL-2 production by T cells, antigen-presenting cells (APCs) also must provide antigen nonspecific costimulatory signals. These signals determine if lymphokine production, apoptotic cell death, or anergy is induced by TCR engagement (70). There are several costimulatory molecules on APCs (Table 1). Intracellular adhesion molecule (ICAM)-1 (CD54), ICAM-2 (CD102), and ICAM-3 (CD50) on the APC interact with lymphocyte function-associated antigen (LFA)-1 (CD11a/CD18) on the T cell, and LFA-3 on the APC binds to LFA-2 on the T-lymphocyte. LFA-2 binding LFA-3 promotes cellular adhesion, whereas the LFA-1–ICAM interaction costimulates T-cell proliferation (71). These two interactions probably both increase the total pool of TCR-derived second messengers, thus mimicking a second level of TCR occupancy. IL-1 and IL-6 also may function in costimulation.

TABLE 1. *Ligand–receptor interactions between a T cell and an APC*

T cell	APC
TCR	MHC + peptide
CD4/CD8	MHC
CD28	B7.1, 2, and 3
CTLA-4	B7.1, 2, and 3
LFA-1	ICAM-1, -2, and -3
LFA-2 (CD2)	LFA-3 (CD58)
CD5	CD72

However, the major costimulatory activity required for IL-2–driven proliferation of T cells is mediated by the interaction of the CD28 molecule on the T-cell surface with its ligands, members of the B7 family on the APCs (72). Engagement of the TCR in the absence of this costimulatory signal not only fails to induce an immune response but actually results in anergy. This is because the CD28 signal transduction pathway differs from the TCR pathway.

The CD28 receptor is a homodimeric glycoprotein composed of two disulfide-linked 44-kDa subunits and is a member of the immunoglobulin supergene family. In humans, CD28 is constitutively expressed on 95% of resting $CD4^+$ cells and 50% of resting $CD8^+$ peripheral blood T cells, and its expression increases after activation (73). CD28 is structurally similar to CTLA-4 (31% homology), with the greatest identity found in the cytoplasmic domain (74). This domain contains the sequence MYPPPY, which is perfectly conserved between CD28 and CTLA-4 molecules from all species, suggesting that this sequence may play a fundamental role in signaling. CTLA-4 expression is restricted to activated T cells.

CD28 and CTLA-4 bind to structurally related proteins called B7-1, -2, and -3, which can be induced on a variety of APCs and are members of the immunoglobulin supergene family with a variable and constant domain (75–77). B7-1 and B7-3 are induced slowly (48–72 h) after activation of B cells, whereas B7-2 is induced more rapidly (within 24 h). B7-2 is also constitutively expressed by monocytes and is the major form present on dendritic cells. B7-2 is probably the critical costimulator used by B cells to initiate IL-2 production, and B7-1 and B7-3 may provide later signals. Both B7-1 and -2 are low-affinity receptors for CD28 and high-affinity receptors for CTLA-4.

Polyvalent anti-CD28 antibodies induce the production of IL-2 and the proliferation of human T cell lines stimulated with inactive antigen-pulsed APCs (78). CD28 knockout mice do not produce IL-2 in response to a T-cell mitogen (79). Anti-B7 antibodies or CTLA-4Ig block T-cell proliferation and IL-2 production in response to nominal antigens, alloantigens, or anti-CD3 antibodies (80).

CD28 signals through different pathways than the TCR, explaining the functional synergy observed. CD28 binding leads to tyrosine phosphorylation of a variety of cellular proteins, including the cytoplasmic tail of CD28, and induces the activity of phosphoinositol 3-kinase (PI

3-kinase) (81). Signaling through CD28 induces transcriptional and posttranscriptional effects. There is a CD28 response element in the IL-2 promoter that probably binds a NFκB-like factor (82). CD28 signaling also enhances the mRNA stability of a number of critical lymphokines (83).

T-CELL DIFFERENTIATION

After the complex series of biochemical changes described above, there is a regulated cascade of sequential gene activation leading to the development of differentiated effector T cells (84) (Fig. 7). Two proto-oncogenes, c-*myc* and c-*fos*, are transcribed within minutes of T-cell activation. The products of such immediate early activation genes, together with the effects of ongoing signal transduction, are likely to initiate the next wave of gene activation, which involves transcription of the IL-2 gene and the IL-2 receptor. IL-2 is key to inducing T-cell proliferation, acting via the IL-2 receptor via either an autocrine (acting on the same cell that produces it) or a paracrine (acting on other nearby cells) effect. Subsequently, other cytokines, such as IL-3, -4, -5, and -6 and γ-interferon, are secreted. Once this initial burst of lymphokine secretion has occurred, the T cells divide under the influence of IL-2 and IL-4 and take on differentiated functions such as cytotoxicity. The genes coding for granzymes (serine esterases involved in cytotoxicity) and the chemoattractant cytokine RANTES are transcribed after 3 to 5 days. Finally, a group of very late activation (VLA) molecules of the integrin supergene family are produced after 7 to 14 days.

CD4 T Cells

Activated $CD4^+$ T cells secrete cytokines that modulate and amplify the immune response. They can be subclassified according to their phenotypic pattern of cytokine production: T_{h1} cells secrete mainly IL-2, γ-interferon, and lymphotoxin, and T_{h2} cells produce IL-4, -5, -6, and -10 (85). T_{h1} and T_{h2} cells develop from a common precursor and can cross-regulate each other. Thus, γ-interferon inhibits expression of the T_{h2} program, whereas IL-4 and IL-10 inhibit the T_{h1} program. Rejecting allografts contain $CD4^+$ cells, which are mainly of the T_{h1} phenotype. IL-2 stimulates proliferation of $CD4^+$ cells in an autocrine manner and the activation of $CD8^+$ CTLs. γ-Interferon recruits and activates macrophages, activates endothelial cells, and increases MHC and TAP expression. IL-2 knockout mice are able to reject allografts (86). Other T-cell growth factors—IL-4, -7, -10, -12, and -15—cause IL-2–independent T-cell proliferation. IL-15 binds to the IL-2 receptor beta chain, whereas IL-4 and IL-7 interact with the gamma chain of the IL-2 receptor. Interestingly, a form of human X-linked severe combined immune deficiency is caused by a defect in the IL-2 receptor gamma chain (87).

Although it is useful to think of the coordinate regulation of cytokine gene groups and their mutual inhibitory feedback, it is important to understand that human T cells, both in vitro and in vivo, may not strictly conform to the T_{h1} and T_{h2} phenotypes.

CD8 T Cells

Activated CTLs accumulate within the graft and recognize the MHC class I–peptide complex on the allograft. Once the TCR for antigen is engaged, the target cells are lysed while the CTLs remain viable. There are at least two mechanisms of lymphocyte-mediated cytotoxicity: (a) secretion of cytolytic granules (the "perforin/granzyme" pathway) and (b) induction of apoptosis in the target cells (the "Fas" pathway).

The cytolytic granules contain a variety of cytolytic proteins including the 65-kDa, calcium-dependent lytic protein perforin (88), and a family of serine proteases,

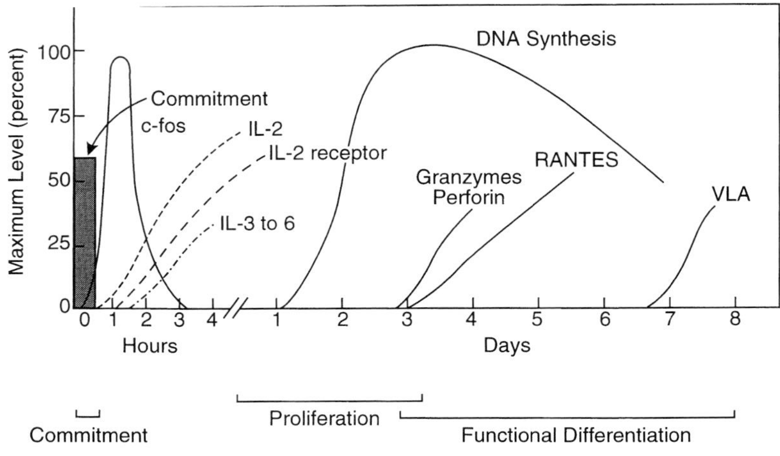

FIG. 7. Sequence of events in T-lymphocyte activation after antigen–MHC triggering. Commitment refers to the time after which the removal of the primary signal no longer limits progression. The time courses represent the activation of transcription as indicated by levels of mRNA. Adapted with permission (4).

called granzymes (89). Perforins are structurally related to the ninth component of complement (C9), which upon activation, polymerize in the target cell membrane to form large pores and thus cause osmotic lysis of the cells. The CD8$^+$ T cells of perforin knockout mice are unable to lyse specific virus-infected cells in vitro, or to clear viral infections in vivo (90). Granzymes are serine proteases. They are somehow involved in the triggering of the DNA fragmentation characteristic of apoptotic cell death by deregulating normal cell-cycle control processes. CTLs from granzyme B knockout mice cause abnormally slow lysis and damage to target cell DNA (91). Granzyme B and perforin transcripts as measured by reverse transcriptase–PCR are highly expressed in acute cellular rejection (92).

A calcium-independent lysis pathway is mediated by the binding of the Fas ligand on activated CD8$^+$ cells to the Fas antigen on target cells, leading to apoptotic cell death (93). These two pathways are complementary. One pathway requires cell–cell contact using a regulated ligand able to lyse only Fas receptor–bearing cells; the second pathway uses a perforin-granzyme–based activity that kills target cells by osmotic lysis. Of particular interest, CTLs are themselves resistant to perforin-granzyme–mediated cytolysis. The mechanism of this resistance is unknown.

Role of Other Cell Types

The primary cell types involved in rejection are T-lymphocytes and macrophages. T lymphocytes are important regulators and effectors in rejection, whereas macrophages and dendritic cells are important in antigen presentation. Cells that are of second-order importance include B cells, NK cells, neutrophils, eosinophils, and platelets. Soluble factors important in rejection include components of the complement system, coagulation factors, leukotrienes, bradykinins, and inflammatory cytokines.

B-Lymphocytes

B cells produce antibodies that then bind to target cells and effector cells (NK cells, macrophages, and T cells), which will bind the Fc region of the antibody, mediating antibody-dependent cellular cytotoxicity (ADCC). Effector cells can be directed against epithelial and endothelial cells. ADCC provides a second-order mechanism for allograft rejection, possibly important in arteritis and chronic rejection (94).

NK Cells

Natural killing is not MHC restricted but does use perforin. The nature of target cell recognition by NK cells is controversial (95), but recognition of MHC class I molecules on target cells inhibits NK-mediated lysis (96). Although phenotypic analysis of cells invading a rejecting allograft shows many NK cells, depletion of NK cells from recipients has no effect on skin, heart, or kidney allograft survival. Furthermore, high levels of NK cell activity can be detected within stably functioning grafts, raising questions about their in vivo significance in transplant rejection (97).

Renal Tubular Epithelial Cells

Recent evidence indicates that epithelial cells are not merely passive targets of the alloresponse but also can modulate the response. Renal tubular cells can process and present exogenous antigen, and γ-interferon upregulates class II expression on these cells (98). The importance of this effect is controversial. The fate of rat islets or cardiac allografts is unaltered by pretreatment with lymphokines to induce MHC class II expression (99). Proximal tubular cells also release cytokines such as tumor necrosis factor (TNF)-α in response to lipopolysaccharide (LPS) and IL-1, and chemoattractant cytokines such as IL-8, MCP-1 and RANTES (100). Finally, IL-1, TNF-α and γ-interferon induce adhesion molecules such as ICAM-1 and vascular cell adhesion molecule (VCAM)-1 in vitro on cultured tubular cells, and expression of ICAM-1 increases on tubular cells during rejection (101).

Endothelium

Inflammatory cytokines such as IL-1, TNF, and γ-interferon induce changes in the endothelium (endothelial cell activation), which include increased expression of class II antigens and of adhesion molecules, which are pivotal to leukocyte migration. In vitro peak expression of E-selectin occurs rapidly after stimulation and is transient, whereas ICAM-1 and VCAM-1 demonstrate sustained expression (102). In human renal allograft biopsies, E-selectin and ICAM-1 expression increases before clinical and pathologic rejection. The expression of ICAM-1 and VCAM-1 is concurrent with active rejection, but E-selectin expression is shut off. The expression of all three adhesion molecules decreases after successful treatment of rejection (103).

The migration of leukocytes across the endothelium has been divided into four sequential steps: tethering, triggering, tight adhesion, and transendothelial migration (104,105) (Fig. 8). First, the flowing leukocyte is tethered and brought into contact with the endothelial wall by selectin-mediated interactions. Tethering allows cytokines on the vessel wall to activate leukocyte adhesion molecules, such as integrins, which result in strong adhesion to the vessel wall. Subsequent migration into the tissue is directed by chemoattractant cytokines that are

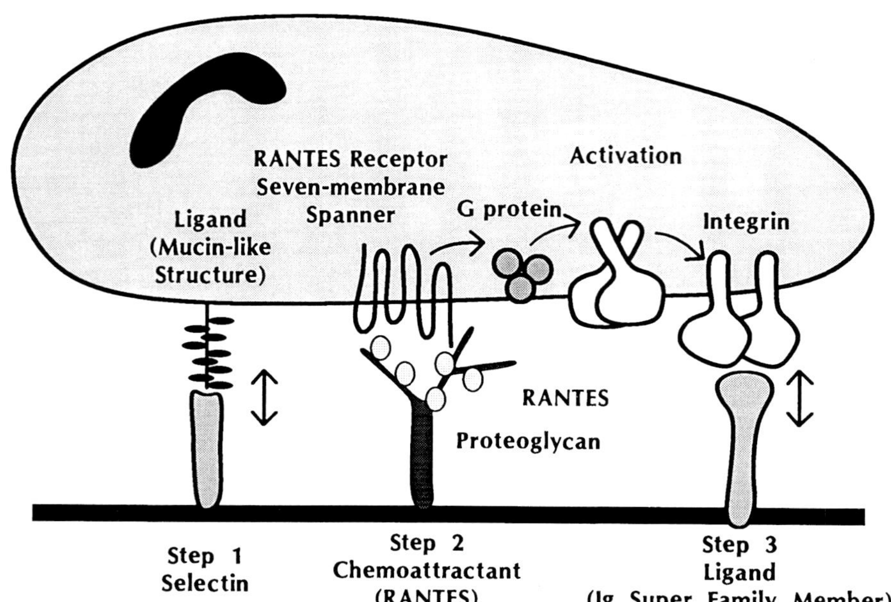

Fig. 8. Three-step model of leukocyte—endothelial interactions. The first step involves tethering of a flowing leukocyte to the vessel wall via selectins. The second step involves chemoattractants, such as RANTES, which are displayed by the endothelium binding to receptors that span the membrane seven times on the surface of leukocytes. These couple to G proteins, which transduce signals that activate integrin adhesiveness, thus resulting in arrest of the rolling leukocyte in the third step.

secreted by graft interstitial cells, inflammatory cells, degranulating platelets, or endothelial cells. The diversity of signals at each step along this pathway explains the selective recruitment of leukocytes in different inflammatory diseases.

Tethering

The initial tethering of leukocytes to the endothelium is mediated by the selectin family. L-selectin is constitutively expressed on most leukocytes, whereas E-selectin is synthesized and expressed on endothelium in response to IL-1 and TNF-α. P-selectin is stored preformed in the Weibel-Palade bodies of endothelial cells and the alpha granules of platelets. In response to activation, P-selectin is rapidly mobilized to the plasma membrane to bind neutrophils and monocytes. The selectin ligands are carbohydrate structures related to sialyl Lewis^x. The fast on and off rates of selectin binding, the flexible structure of the selectins, and the expression of L-selectin on the tips of the leukocyte microvilli are ideal for this tethering role. The transient nature of the interaction allows leukocytes to sample the endothelium for triggering factors that can activate leukocyte integrins and cause adhesion. Without such signals, leukocytes disengage and move on.

Triggering

Strong adhesion of leukocytes to endothelium is mediated by heterodimeric adhesion molecules called integrins (105). Integrins on circulating leukocytes do not bind well unless they are activated. The chemokines (chemoattractant cytokines) are pivotal mediators of this increased adhesion. The chemokines are structurally related 70- to 80-amino acid peptides (8–10 kDa), which are secreted by a variety of immune and nonimmune cells (106). They are potent, resistant to degradation, and act on selective leukocyte subtypes. At least 30 distinct chemokines have been identified, and they can be divided into at least three families based on sequence (around the first two cysteine residues) and function (Table 2). The

TABLE 2. *The chemokine superfamily*

C-X-C	C-C	C
IL-8	MCP-1	Lymphotactin
ENA-78	MCP-2	
SDF-1α/1β	MCP-3	
GCP-2	MIP-1α	
MGSA/*gro* α/β/γ	MIP-1β	
PBP (βTG, CTAP-III, NAP-2)	I309/TCA3	
PF4	RANTES	
IP-10	C10	
mig	Eotaxin	

The name used for each of the chemokines is that of the human protein. Certain chemokines are listed for which no known human homolog has yet been identified (e.g., guinea pig eotaxin). Three proteins with distinct functional activities are proteolytically derived from PBP (TG, CTAP-III, and NAP-2).

PF-4, platelet factor 4; PBP, platelet basic protein; TG, thromboglobulin; CTAP-III, connective tissue activating protein-III; NAP-2, neutrophil activating protein-2; MGSA, melanocyte growth stimulatory activity; mig, monokine induced by IFN-γ; ENA-78, epithelium-derived neutrophil attractant-78; GCP-2, granulocyte chemotactic protein-2; SDF-1, stromal cell derived factors; TCA3, T-cell activation gene 3.

C-X-C chemokines are predominantly chemoattractant for neutrophils, C-C chemokines act mainly on lymphocytes and monocytes, and the C chemokine, lymphotactin, acts only on lymphocytes. The C-C chemokines induce chemoattraction and adhesion of different subsets of T cells. For example, MIP-1α acts on $CD8^+$ T cells, MIP-1β attracts $CD4^+$ T cells, and RANTES preferentially attracts memory T-lymphocytes (107). They are also differentially expressed and presented. Chemokines bind to proteoglycans on the endothelium. The chemokines are thus concentrated at the inflammatory site rather than swept downstream by the flow of blood. RANTES is highly expressed in acute cellular rejection with abundant expression along the vascular endothelium (108). Other mechanisms also exist to preserve a localized endothelial chemokine gradient, including a red blood cell clearance receptor (first identified as the Duffy antigen) and antichemokine antibodies. Chemokines mediate their effects on target cells through interactions with various seven-transmembrane G protein linked receptors (Fig. 8) (109).

Strong Adhesion

Strong adhesion is mediated by leukocyte integrins that bind to counter-receptors on the endothelium. Integrins consist of alpha and beta subunits and are subclassified according to their beta subunits. The β_1 integrins (or VLA proteins) have a common beta chain (CD29), which pairs with different alpha subunits (CD49a-CD49f). The β_2 integrins (or leukocyte cell adhesion molecules) share a beta chain (CD18) paired with CD11a (LFA-1), CD11b (Mac-1), or CD11c (p150, 95). At least five integrins are important in lymphocyte–endothelial interactions, the most important being LFA-1, which binds ICAM-1 and -2 on the endothelium, and VLA-4, which binds VCAM-1.

Transendothelial Migration

After integrin-mediated firm attachment is established, leukocytes can migrate through the endothelial cell layer and basement membrane to enter the tissue. This transmigration is dependent on integrins and the chemokines. T cells also secrete metalloproteinases, which dissolve the basement membrane and allow them to enter the tissue (110).

TYPES OF REJECTION

Hyperacute Rejection

Pre-existing donor-specific antibodies can cause almost immediate rejection of vascularized allografts. The preformed antibodies that cause this hyperacute rejection include anti-ABO antibodies or anti-MHC IgG cytotoxic antibody to donor T-lymphocytes (111). These antibodies cause hyperacute rejection by binding to antigens on the vascular endothelium. The binding of antibody triggers complement activation, coagulation, and the production of chemotactic factors. Histologic features within the first 12 h posttransplantation demonstrate fibrin and platelet thrombi within glomerular and peritubular capillaries associated with a prominent neutrophilic exudate. The thrombotic process also may be evident in the arterioles, but the arteries are usually unaffected at this stage. During the next 12–18 h, as the thrombotic process becomes more widespread, ischemic tubular injury with interstitial edema followed by cortical infarction develops. A similar thrombotic/neutrophil exudative process occurs in the capillary beds of other organ transplants involved by hyperacute rejection. Kidney and heart are more susceptible than liver allografts to hyperacute rejection. Hyperacute rejection has been largely eliminated from clinical practice by routine cross-matching before transplantation.

Acute Vascular Rejection (Accelerated Rejection)

The grafts show glomerular and vascular lesions reminiscent of those seen in hyperacute rejection (112). However, the lesions seem to predominate in the arterial bed rather than in the arteriolar and capillary beds. Lesions are characterized by fibrinoid necrosis of the media, and fibrin/platelet thrombosis of the lumens. Prominent interstitial edema and hemorrhage, tubular necrosis, and foci of cortical infarction are characteristic features. Tubular and interstitial mononuclear cell infiltrates may be found in some cases, varying from minimal to moderate in intensity. Accelerated rejection occurs within 30–90 days after transplantation and usually progresses to loss of the graft within 1 to 6 months. Vascular rejection is probably due to pre-existing donor-specific antibodies present at levels below the limit of detection by standard T-lymphocyte cross-matching but identifiable by flow cytometry.

Acute Cellular, Tubulointerstitial, and Vascular Rejection

The earliest stages of acute cellular rejection in the renal allograft is characterized by a perivenular and periglomerular infiltrate of transformed lymphocytes and macrophages (113). An increased number of mononuclear cells also may be identified in peritubular and glomerular capillaries. This is followed by infiltration of the interstitium and tubular epithelium, predominantly by lymphocytes, although the interstitial infiltrates are pleomorphic, consisting of variably sized lymphocytes, macrophages, eosinophils, plasma cells, and neutrophils. The interstitial infiltrates are often associated with edema, and there also may be extravasation of erythrocytes. Tubular lumens become dilated, brush borders disappear, and, with cellular death, cells are found within the tubular lumens and the basement membranes become denuded.

With vascular involvement, the arteries, and sometimes the arterioles, demonstrate subendothelial infiltrates of lymphocytes and macrophages. The endothelium often is lifted from its basement membrane. In some cases, small deposits of fibrin and platelets are found in relation to the endothelial injury. Uncommonly, the mononuclear cell infiltrates transmurally involve the blood vessel wall, resulting in inflammatory necrotizing arteritis. Similar vascular lesions are found in pancreatic, cardiac, pulmonary, and hepatic transplantation but are only rarely found in cardiac and liver biopsy samples because arteries are rarely encountered.

Cellular rejection of the pancreas is characterized by pleomorphic infiltrates of inflammatory cells involving the acinar and islet parenchyma. Perivenular and bronchiolar infiltrates are characteristic of acute pulmonary rejection, whereas more severe forms demonstrate an interstitial pneumonitis with airway injury. Acute rejection of the cardiac allograft is characterized by interstitial mononuclear infiltrates, with variable distribution throughout the myocardium. Acute liver allograft rejection is characterized by pleomorphic infiltrates, predominantly limited to the portal tracts. Lymphocytes infiltrate bile duct epithelium and are found in the subendothelial aspect of portal venules.

Chronic Rejection

Despite major improvements in 1 year graft survival, the long-term graft survival rate has not improved. The half-life of cadaveric renal allografts remains constant at approximately 7 years (114). The major reason for graft loss is now chronic rejection. Its etiology is not clearly defined, although it probably consists of a combination of immunologic, hemodynamic, and social (compliance) factors.

Several potential risk factors have been implicated in chronic rejection (115) (Table 3). Immunologic factors such as poor HLA matching (116) and more frequent acute rejection episodes are correlated with chronic rejection (117). There is a lower rate of chronic rejection in grafts from living related donors than in cadaveric grafts, and this difference increases over time. HLA-DR mismatching especially influences graft survival. Cytomegalovirus (CMV) infection of the recipient may increase the likelihood of chronic rejection. Experimentally, intimal and smooth muscle hypertrophy increases significantly in rats infected with CMV. ADCC using antibodies directed against endothelial cells may be an effector mechanism in chronic rejection.

Early injury to the graft endothelial cells caused by alloantigen-independent factors such as ischemia and reperfusion also may be important, given the improved graft survival of living unrelated transplants compared with cadaveric transplants. The effect of early ischemia on late function has been reproduced in experimental animal models (118). Ischemia reduces the number of functioning nephrons and induces class II expression on tubular cells. The initial amount of functioning renal mass and the nephron number also determine late graft outcome (119). Kidney allografts most at risk for failure are those with a low ratio of renal weight to recipient body weight. For example, pediatric kidneys transplanted into adults, females into large males, and older donors or blacks with fewer nephrons into whites, all give lower than average graft survival (120).

Chronic rejection is characterized histologically by organ destruction, usually in association with fibro-obliterative vascular lesions (121). The latter predominantly involve the arterial system of the organ and are characterized by cellular myofibroproliferation in the subintimal space, leading to narrowing of the vascular lumen. The media in most cases is of normal architecture and thickness. The fibroproliferative lesions often contain variable numbers of small lymphocytes and macrophages, not only within the fibrous tissue but also in the subendothelial space. In some cases, the subendothelial spaces contain foamy macrophages and a paucity of myofibroblastic cells. In the kidney, these vascular lesions can be associated with tubular atrophy, interstitial fibrosis, and glomerular capillary collapse. In the liver, they are associated with centrilobular cholestasis, ballooning degeneration and cell dropout; in the heart, with myocardial infarction; and in the pancreas, a chronic atrophic pancreatitis with infarction. Chronic rejection of these organs may reflect in part direct immunologic injury of epithelial structures, resulting in tubular atrophy in the kidney, paucity of bile ducts in the liver, destruction of islets and acinar tissue in the pancreas, and obliterative bronchiolitis in the lung. These processes may be "inactive" or "active" in that there may be an associated mononuclear cell infiltrate

TABLE 3. *Risk factors for chronic rejection*

Hypertension
Proteinuria
Duration
Acute rejection episodes
Ischemia time
Cadaver graft
HLA mismatches
Hyperlipidemia
Extremes of age of donor
Smoking history

among the epithelial cells. The glomeruli, in addition to showing collapsing ischemic changes, may show double and multicontoured capillary walls, so-called chronic transplant glomerulopathy. The multicontouring, on ultrastructural study, is found to be secondary to mesangial interposition and endothelial cell basal lamina replication. Increased numbers of mononuclear cells are often present within the glomerular capillaries. Immunofluoresence examination in the latter cases often demonstrates linear and granular deposits of immunoglobulin and complement, along not only capillary walls but also peritubular capillaries.

The periglomerular and perivascular macrophages secrete cytokines that are profibrogenic, including platelet-derived growth factor (PDGF) and transforming growth factor (TGF)-β. In experimental chronic allograft rejection, mRNA transcripts coding for PDGF and the PDGFβ receptor increase. Increased expression of IL-1, TNF, and IL-6 occurs in long-term rat renal allografts (122). Increased ICAM-1 expression is found on the glomeruli of rat renal allografts undergoing chronic rejection, which may then recruit more cells (123).

The gradual functional deterioration caused by the development of glomerulosclerosis and arterial obliteration also may cause systemic hypertension. This causes the remaining functioning glomeruli to hyperfilter before they eventually fibrose, thus establishing a vicious cycle of progressive renal damage (124).

In preliminary studies, both RS61443 (mycophenolate mofetil) and rapamycin diminish the lesions of chronic rejection in heart and kidney grafts (125). Angiotensin-converting enzyme inhibitors, protein restriction, and control of systemic hypertension may attenuate the rate of decline in renal function, as in other progressive renal diseases.

IMMUNOSUPPRESSIVE DRUGS

The use of azathioprine and corticosteroids in the early 1960s was the breakthrough that made clinical transplantation a reality. The introduction of cyclosporine in the 1980s improved 1-year cadaveric renal allograft survival by 15% to 20%, allowing the reduction of corticosteroid dosages, and permitted successful heart, heart-lung, and lung transplant programs to be developed.

Corticosteroids

Corticosteroids are used at low doses to prevent rejection and at higher doses to reverse rejection. Corticosteroids have a variety of immunosuppressive effects (126). They inhibit gene transcription by binding to glucocorticoid receptors, which then bind to the response elements in the promoters of certain key cytokine genes. Glucocorticoids block transcription of the IL-1, TNF, and IL-6 genes in accessory cells (127,128) and the IL-2 gene in T cells (129). In addition, glucocorticoids block the transcription of chemokine genes such as IL-8, *gro*, and MCP-1, thus interfering with recruitment of inflammatory cells into the graft (130). In antirejection doses, corticosteroids cause lysis of lymphocytes. The use of these potent drugs is limited by side effects that include decreased inflammatory and phagocytic capacity resulting in increased susceptibility to infection, glucose intolerance, growth retardation, delayed wound healing, hypertension, avascular necrosis, and psychologic disturbances.

Azathioprine

Azathioprine is a thioether derivative of 6-mercaptopurine. The active mercaptopurine moiety is liberated after absorption and blocks the synthesis of adenine and guanine nucleotides, disrupting DNA and RNA synthesis and blocking cell proliferation. Azathioprine is a powerful inhibitor of primary immune responses and is used to prevent rejection. It does not block secondary responses and is not used to treat rejection (131). It decreases circulating neutrophils and mononuclear cells. The major side effects of azathioprine are neutropenia and thrombocytopenia, megaloblastic anemia, idiosyncratic interstitial pneumonitis, hepatotoxicity (including hepatic veno-occlusive disease), and an increased prevalence of malignancies.

Cyclosporine/FK506

Cyclosporine is a small, fungal, 11–amino acid, cyclic peptide that is potent in preventing acute rejection but is of little use in treating established rejection. Cyclosporine and FK506 (tacrolimus), a macrolide, block T-cell activation by similar mechanisms (Fig. 9). Cyclosporine and FK506 bind to their respective cytoplasmic receptor proteins called immunophilins (cyclophilin and FKBP). Both of these complexes bind calcineurin and inhibit its phosphatase activity, thus inhibiting expression of T-cell activation genes, including IL-2, c-*myc*, and the IL-2 receptor (IL-2R) (132). Cyclosporine may additionally increase the secretion of proimmunosuppressive cytokines such as TGF-β (133) and IL-10 (134). Nephrotoxicity, both acute and chronic, is the major side effect of cyclosporine. Other side effects of cyclosporine include hepatotoxicity, hyperkalemia, hypertension, gingival hypertrophy, neurotoxicity, and hirsutism. FK506 is possibly a more potent immunosuppressant than cyclosporine, allowing it to be used as monotherapy (135), and for the reversal of acute rejection (136). However, it has a more narrow therapeutic index with neurotoxicity, with impaired glucose tolerance, hypertension, and nephrotoxicity being the main side effects (137).

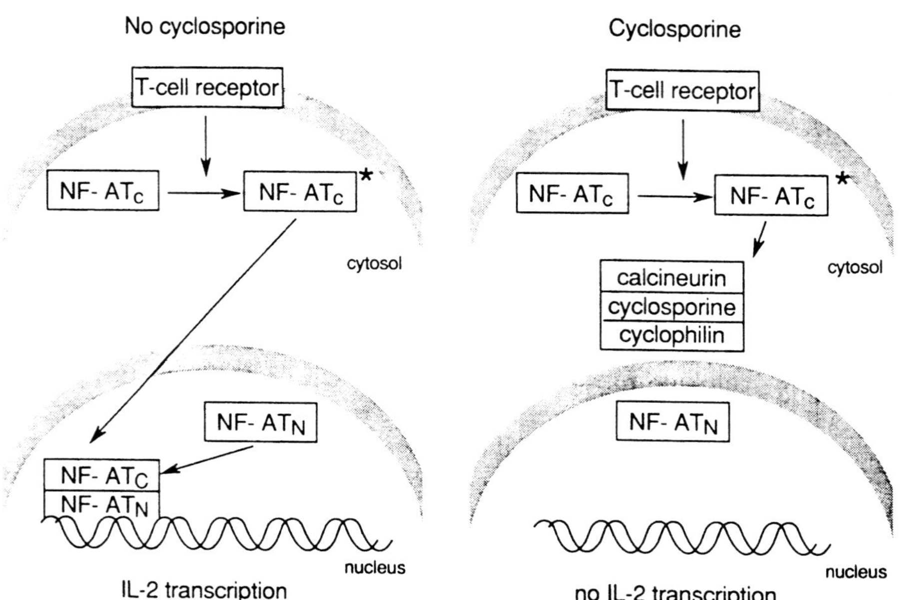

FIG. 9. Mechanism of action of cyclosporine. Normally upon T-cell activation, a cytoplasmic component of the nuclear factor of activated T cells (NF-ATc) enters the nucleus, binds to a nuclear component (NF-ATn), and induces IL-2 transcription. In the presence of cyclosporine, NF-ATc fails to enter the nucleus, and there is no IL-2 gene transcription. Reprinted with permission (5).

Rapamycin

Rapamycin is a macrolide, like FK506, that binds to FKBP but does not block the transcription of cytokine genes. Rather it inhibits signal transduction mediated by IL-2 and other growth factors (Fig. 6). Two cellular proteins of 245 and 34 kDa (rapamycin and FKBP12 targets 1 and 2 = RAFT1 and RAFT2, respectively), with sequence homology to the catalytic domain of the p110 subunit of PI-3 kinase, are potential targets for the rapamycin–FKBP complex (138). Rapamycin also blocks the calcium-independent CD28/CTLA-4–induced costimulatory pathway. Rapamycin and FK506 are pharmacologic antagonists, whereas cyclosporine and rapamycin act synergistically. In animal models, rapamycin is effective at inhibiting vascular disease associated with allograft rejection (139). Rapamycin causes diabetes in rats but not in primates and is reportedly less nephrotoxic than cyclosporine.

Inhibitors of DNA Synthesis

Mycophenolate mofetil, mizoribine, and brequinar inhibit nucleotide biosynthesis, thus halting T- and B-cell proliferation by blocking DNA synthesis. Mycophenolate mofetil and mizoribine inhibit only the de novo (and not the salvage pathway) of purine synthesis. Brequinar is a noncompetitive inhibitor of dihydro-orotate dehydrogenase and blocks the de novo pathway of pyrimidine synthesis. They all are reported to be more selective antiproliferative agents than is azathioprine. Mycophenolate mofetil and mizoribine diminish proliferation of T- and B-lymphocytes, decrease generation of CTLs, suppress antibody formation, and inhibit allograft rejection in rodents (140). Indeed, in rodent models, mycophenolate mofetil can prolong allograft and xenograft survival, reverse advanced rejection, prevent graft vascular disease, and induce unresponsiveness to alloantigen (125). Brequinar is a potent immunosuppressant, effective in advanced mouse heart allograft rejection (141). The combination of cyclosporine and brequinar is synergistic. Although all of these agents have the potential to be myelotoxic, they probably will be used as replacements for azathioprine. Unlike azathioprine, they also may reverse advanced rejection.

Deoxyspergualin

Deoxyspergualin (DSG) appears to act in a very late stage in the response of T- and B-lymphocytes to activation. DSG binds to intracellular heat shock protein 70 family members (142). In preclinical models, DSG appears to exert potent immunosuppressive properties and is claimed to be effective both as maintenance and rescue therapy (143).

Leflunomide (HWA 486)

Leflunomide is a small molecular weight isoxazole derivative that reverses experimental arthritis and is currently being evaluated in clinical trials for rheumatoid arthritis. In vitro, leflunomide blocks T- and B-cell proliferation and blocks the generation of allospecific antibodies. In vivo, leflunomide can prevent or reverse rejection of allografts in rats and synergizes with cyclosporine. Leflunomide may act by blocking the activity of tyrosine kinases associated with certain growth factor receptors and by inhibition of pyrimidine biosynthesis (144).

Antilymphocyte Preparations: Polyclonal Antisera

Polyclonal antilymphocyte globulins or antithymocyte globulins have been used since the 1960s to prevent or reverse allograft rejection (145,146). Such polyclonal immune globulins are generated by injecting animals with human lymphoid cells (e.g., B-cell lymphoblasts, peripheral T-cell lymphocytes, or thymic lymphocytes) and then purifying the resulting immune sera to obtain isolated gamma-globulin fractions. They contain a heterogeneous group of antibodies, only a minority of which are specific to T cells. Such antisera cause clearance of lymphocytes due to reticuloendothelial cell uptake, complement-mediated lysis of lymphocytes, blockade of function of lymphocytes, and possibly expansion of suppressor cell populations. Because each preparation varies in its constituent antibodies, efficacy and side effects are variable. Side effects include thrombocytopenia, neutropenia, serum sickness, and antigen-antibody–induced glomerulonephritis. Anaphylactoid reactions are common due to host antibodies to polyclonal immune globulin. There is an increased risk of infection and malignancies.

Monoclonal Antibodies

OKT3 is the only U.S. Food and Drug Administration (FDA)-approved monoclonal antibody in current use for treatment of transplant rejection. OKT3 is a mouse IgG2a directed against the 20-kDa ε chain of the CD3 complex. OKT3 blocks TCR function, clears TCRs from the cell surface (internalization, shedding), and removes T cells from the circulation (T-cell depletion). Peripheral blood lymphocyte counts fall transiently, and reappearing T-lymphocytes fail to express the TCR/CD3 complex, until OKT3 is stopped. OKT3 is effective as induction therapy (146,147) and for the reversal of rejection (148,149).

The main side effect of OKT3 therapy is related to the massive, transient release of cytokines seen after the first two or three doses, causing a flulike syndrome (fever, chills, rigors), aseptic meningitis, an increase in serum creatinine, and pulmonary edema due to capillary leak (149,150). Viral infections (151) and lymphoproliferative disease occur at increased frequency with prolonged use of OKT3 (152,153). Human antimouse OKT3 antibodies are produced, which neutralize the antibody's efficacy (154). The incidence of anti-OKT3 antibodies decreases with the use of concurrent immunosuppressive treatments (149,155). Construction of human–mouse chimeric antibodies and "humanized" antibodies may decrease or eliminate this anti-antibody response (156).

Antibodies directed against IL-2R are theoretically attractive agents, because IL-2R is only transiently expressed after activation. Therefore, anti–IL-2R monoclonal antibodies should specifically inhibit T cells that have been activated by foreign antigens, but spare the remaining T-cell repertoire. In a mouse model, treatment for only 10 days produces indefinite graft survival in more than 50% of recipients and also can reverse ongoing rejection (157). In clinical trials, anti–IL-2R has been more effective as induction therapy than as antirejection therapy (158). Another approach, which does not require a monoclonal antibody, is to use an IL-2 toxin construct directly to bind to the IL-2R in order to kill activated T cells (159).

The CD4 antigen is an attractive target for antibody therapy because it is implicated in antigen recognition as a coreceptor, in signal transduction, and in tolerance induction. Anti-CD4 monoclonal antibodies transiently deplete $CD4^+$ cells and modulate CD4 at the cell surface. Postgraft treatment with OKT4 in rhesus monkeys prolongs graft survival (160). Clinical trials are in progress with a variety of anti-CD4 antibodies. In experimental animals, donor-specific suppression occurs only several months after anti-CD4 administration (161).

Antibodies against T-cell adhesion molecules, LFA-1 on the T cells and ICAM-1 on the target cell, may interfere with T-cell activation and leukocyte-endothelial interaction. Animal studies (162) and clinical trials (163) suggest that anti–ICAM-1 or anti–LFA-1 antibodies can prolong graft survival.

Other monoclonal antibodies against T-cell surface molecules that have been evaluated for use in transplantation include Campath-1 (anti-CD52), anti-CD2, -CD5, -CD7, -CD8, and -CD45 (157). Campath-1 antibodies bind human complement and lyse all T cells. In a clinical trial, the incidence of rejection was decreased, but major infectious episodes were increased (164). Anti-CD45 antibodies have been used ex vivo to deplete grafts of passenger leukocytes and significantly decreased the incidence of subsequent rejection (165).

Finally, antibodies to various cytokines, including TNF-α and γ-interferon, have been evaluated, but so far none have been successful in animal models of transplantation (166). In contrast, anti–TNF-α antibodies have proven useful for the therapy of rheumatoid arthritis (167). Perhaps a more fruitful approach will involve the use of cytokine receptor antagonists, such as have been described for the IL-1 and IL-4 receptors.

TOLERANCE

The ultimate goal of transplantation is tolerance, the active state of antigen-specific nonresponsiveness, thus abrogating the need for chronic immunosuppression. Burnet reasoned that the introduction of allogeneic cells or tissues early in development would result in them being recognized as self. Billingham demonstrated that the neonatal injection of allogeneic cells prevented subsequent rejection of a skin transplant expressing the same MHC molecules (168). For rodents, this critical early

Two Signals for T-cell Activation

Antigen Responsiveness
- IL-2 secretion
- T-cell proliferation
- normal immune responsiveness

Antigen Unresponsiveness
- no IL-2 secretion
- no T-cell proliferation
- anergy

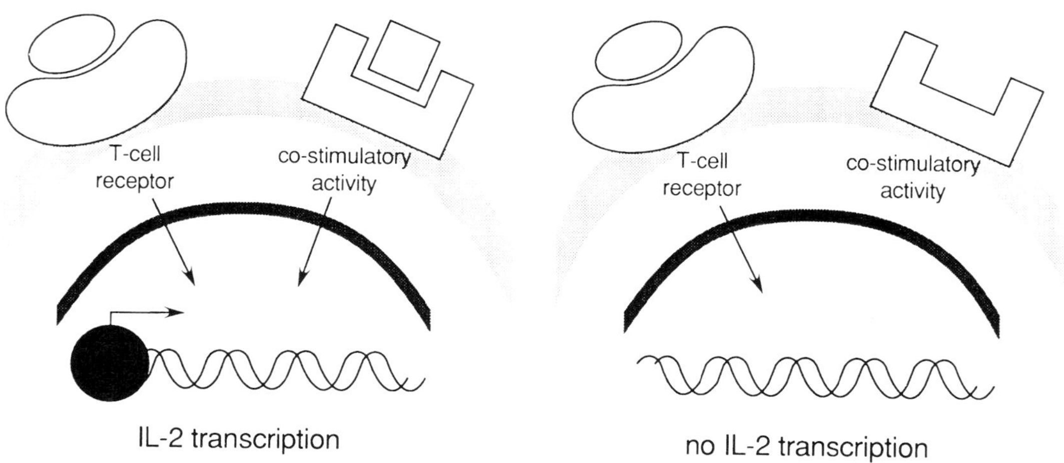

FIG. 10. The two-signal hypothesis for T-cell activation. In order to activate T cells, both the TCR and a second signal must be triggered. If the TCR is triggered without a second signal, anergy results. Reprinted with permission (5).

period lasts until shortly after birth, but for humans this period ends before birth. This obviously limits the application of neonatal tolerance in humans, although protocols involving fetal manipulation are under investigation. Such neonatal tolerance is largely due to clonal deletion by negative selection in the thymus (169).

Adult or peripheral T-cell tolerance may be due to a combination of anergy and suppression, although the molecular mechanisms underlying these processes are just starting to be understood. In order for tolerance to develop, it may be that the immune system must continuously be exposed to alloantigen.

Anergy applies to a state where antigen-specific T cells are present but fail to respond. Schwartz attributes anergy to the failure of two signals to activate the T cell (170). According to the two-signal hypothesis, T-cell activation depends on the simultaneous application of two signals to the T cell: one through the TCR and the other through other receptors on the cell surface (Fig. 10). Engagement of the TCR in the absence of this costimulation leads to anergy. The B7-CD28 costimulation pathway is critical in preventing the induction of anergy. Blocking the costimulatory signals mediated through binding of B7 to CD28/CTLA-4 with anti-B7 monoclonal antibodies or anti-CD28 Fab′ leads to anergy in vitro (171). Treatment in vivo with CTLA-4Ig (a chimeric molecule consisting of the CTLA-4 binding domain attached to the Ig constant region) leads to donor-specific tolerance to xenogeneic human islet cell transplants in mice (172) and prolongs graft survival in a fully mismatched rat cardiac allograft model (173). Anergized T cells can still proliferate in response to exogenous IL-2 (174). Interestingly, allograft rejection is often preceded by viral infections that induce nonspecific inflammation and cytokine release. Anergy may require the continuous presentation of the specific antigen to the T cells. When anergic T cells are removed from a self antigen by adoptive transfer to a mouse strain lacking the specific antigen, the previously anergic cells can regain their normal function (175). Anergy is associated with the absence or decreased expression of some cytokine genes (i.e., IL-2/γ-interferon) (176) and a response defect for others (i.e., IL-4/IL-12) (177).

Suppression is another major mechanism to explain tolerance. Gershon et al. showed that T cells from a tolerant animal could adoptively transfer unresponsiveness to a naive animal (178). Nevertheless, it has been difficult to isolate and characterize these suppressor cells and/or the soluble factors they are thought to produce. Two current models exist. One model suggests that the effects are due to the suppressive effects of T cell–derived cytokines such as IL-4, IL-10, or TGF-β, which inhibit the activation of IL-2–producing cells (179). The other model proposes that antigen-specific T cells that have been rendered nonresponsive suppress other T cells that have the same specificity in a passive manner through competition for ligand and for cytokines such as IL-2 (180).

In vivo studies in tolerant grafts have shown a dramatic decrease in the expression of the proinflammatory IL-2 and γ-interferon cytokines, whereas increased levels of IL-4 and IL-10 are found (181). Thus, the expression of the T_{h2} phenotype is correlated with the induction of tolerance. High levels of IL-4 may skew T_{h0} cells toward a T_{h2} response. IL-10 has a variety of anti-inflammatory effects, including blockade of γ-interferon release, inhibition of proliferation of T_{h1} cells stimulated by macrophages, decreased class II expression on monocytes, and downregulation of B7 expression on macrophages (182). However, IL-10 also can have proinflammatory activities, such as stimulating proliferation and cytotoxicity by CTLs (183). Oral tolerance in an experimental allergic encephalitis model is associated with the appearance of antigen-specific $CD8^+$ cells, which secrete the immunosuppressive cytokine TGF-β in the central nervous system (184).

Other mechanisms invoked to explain peripheral tolerance include microchimerism and veto cells. Starzl reported a high correlation between the presence of small numbers of circulating donor cells and tolerance in liver allografts (185), but further studies in both kidney and heart transplants found microchimerism to be an infrequent event (186), thus raising questions as to its clinical significance. Veto cells may inhibit or eliminate precursor cells, usually cytotoxic precursors, although the molecular mechanisms involved are unclear (187).

Novel Approaches to Tolerance

Given the redundancy of the cytokines, it may be difficult to block or modulate the production of all their proinflammatory effects. However, IL-2R, which binds a number of T-cell growth factors, is an attractive target for inducing tolerance. Numerous other approaches have been proposed to block cytokine release and/or receptor-mediated signaling (158).

Intrathymic injection of rodents with pancreatic islets induces donor-specific unresponsiveness (188). Indeed, intrathymic injection of donor peripheral blood mononuclear cells into the thymus induced indefinite survival of the subsequent renal allografts, as did injection of isolated glomeruli, indicating that acquired thymic tolerance may not be tissue specific (189). Similar observations were seen for cardiac, liver, small bowel, and skin allografts in rodent models (190). Intrathymic injection of 100 μg of a mixture of eight synthetic class II MHC 25–amino acid allopeptides is sufficient to induce systemic unresponsiveness to a subsequent MHC-incompatible renal allograft (191). The induction phase of tolerance appears to be mediated by a state of T-cell anergy, whereas the maintenance phase may involve clonal deletion of the previously anergized T cells. Studies in large animals are needed to confirm the feasibility of the intrathymic approach for tolerance induction. The human thymus involutes in adult life, so the thymic approach might only be applicable in children and young adults. It also is essential to define the role of immunosuppressive drugs on the unresponsive state induced by intrathymic injection of antigen. Current drugs may actually block the active processes of tolerance induction and/or maintenance.

Pretreatment with soluble or membrane-bound donor MHC can induce immune unresponsiveness to a subsequent graft. This may be the basis of the blood transfusion effect in transplantation (192). Recent novel strategies based on treatment with synthetic peptides corresponding to linear sequences of class I and II molecules reproducibly induce tolerance to alloantigens (193). Peptides corresponding to the sequences of the CD8-binding loop of HLA class I molecules block the generation of CTLs but are unable to inhibit pre-existing CTLs, whereas peptides corresponding to the α1 domain of certain class I molecules can block both the generation of CTLs and cytolysis by preexisting CTLs (194). In vivo studies also have demonstrated the efficacy of peptide therapy. Heart allografts were transplanted into recipients undergoing treatment with a synthetic peptide corresponding to residues 75–84 of HLA-B7, combined with two to five doses of cyclosporine. Eighty percent of the allografts survived greater than 200 days. This tolerance was donor specific and mediated by anergic T cells. Oral and intravenous injection of peptides were equally efficacious (195). Similar results have been shown for class II–derived peptides. Early preclinical studies indicate that such synthetic peptides are nontoxic (196). They may prove effective for the induction of tolerance in clinical transplantation.

XENOTRANSPLANTATION

Interest in xenotransplantation has increased with the growing shortage of organs and an increasing knowledge of the mechanisms underlying xenograft rejection (197). Most interest is focused on pigs as potential donors for humans. Their organs are of the appropriate size, and blood group O animals exist. Pig organs undergo hyperacute rejection due to preformed "natural" human antibodies that bind to the pig endothelium and activate the xenogeneic endothelium itself. Preformed naturally occurring antipig antibodies react with the bacterial galα1–3gal epitope (198). IgM antipig antibodies appear more important than IgG isotypes (199). It may be possible to remove antipig antibodies by immunoabsorption of human serum over columns containing carbohydrates with the galα1–3gal linkage. Alternatively, intravenous infusions of specific carbohydrates block antibody binding to the epitopes on the endothelium. Inhibitors of complement activation such as C1 inhibitor and soluble complement receptor 1 are also being investigated. The other approach has been to express human membrane-bound complement regulatory proteins such as CD46 (membrane cofactor protein), CD55 (decay accelerating factor), and CD59 on cultured xenogeneic cells and thus protect these cells from lysis by human serum (200). Transgenic pigs expressing these human proteins on their endothelium are being developed. The rationale for using organs from these animals is that by only inhibiting complement activation locally, the risk of infection associated with systemic anticomplement therapy is avoided.

If hyperacute rejection is prevented by the depletion of xenoreactive antibody and/or the inhibition of complement, delayed acute vascular rejection may be seen in the next few days with vascular thrombosis and an inflammatory cell infiltrate. In some cases this does not occur, but a process termed accommodation allows the xenograft to survive despite the return of xenoreactive antibodies and complement (201). If the humoral barriers to xenografting can be overcome, the cellular immune response must be blocked. Although the cellular immune response to xenoantigens may be similar to alloantigens (202) and may be inhibited by conventional immunosuppression, further investigation is required. Thus, if the humoral and cellular xenoresponses can be overcome, clinical xenotransplantation may become a reality, although other issues, such as the transmission of viruses across species barriers and animal rights concerns, will have to be addressed.

CONCLUSIONS

There has been an explosive increase in our knowledge of the molecular and cellular mechanisms that underlie allorecognition, although much remains to be discovered, especially in the areas of chronic rejection and tolerance. Tolerance induction would allow the ultimate cure for patients with end-stage renal disease. Patients will be maintained without the need for chronic immunosuppressive therapy and the concomitant risks of opportunistic infections and malignancies. The advent of xenotransplantation will overcome the second major obstacle, the lack of sufficient numbers of suitable organs. In light of the progress in the basic science of allograft rejection over the past decade, major advances in clinical transplantation should continue to improve outcome and may soon result in actual cures for patients with renal failure.

Acknowledgments

This work was supported by grants from the National Institutes of Health (DK35008 and AI35125). J.M.P. was a Fellow of the National Kidney Foundation. A.M.K. is a Burroughs Wellcome Scholar in Experimental Therapeutics and the Shelagh Galligan Professor of Pediatrics.

REFERENCES

1. Suthanthiran M, Strom TB. Renal transplantation. *N Engl J Med* 1994;331:365–376.
2. Medawar PB. The behaviour and fate of skin autografts and skin homografts in rabbits. (A report to the War Wounds Committee of the Medical Research Council.) *J Anat* 1944;78:176–185.
3. Hutchinson IV. Cellular mechanisms of allograft rejection. *Curr Opin Immunol* 1991;3:722–728.
4. Krensky AM, Weiss A, Crabtree G, Davis MM, Parham P. T-lymphocyte–antigen interactions in transplant rejection. *N Engl J Med* 1990;322:510–517.
5. Krensky AM. Transplant immunobiology. In: Holliday M, Barrett M, Avner E, eds. *Pediatric nephrology*. 3rd ed. Baltimore: Williams & Wilkins; 1993:1373–1389.
6. Wood KJ. Mechanisms of rejection. *Baillieres Clin Gastroenterol* 1994;8:431–437.
7. Krensky AM. The immunobiology of transplantation. In: Jamison RL, Wilkinson RH, eds. *Nephrology*. London: Chapman Hall; 1996 (in press).
8. Shoskes DA, Wood KJ. Indirect presentation of MHC antigens in transplantation. *Immunol Today* 1994;15:32–38.
9. Benichou G, Takizawa PA, Olson CA, McMillan M, Sercarz EE. Donor major histocompatibility complex (MHC) peptides are presented by recipient MHC molecules during graft rejection. *J Exp Med* 1992;175:305–308.
10. Fangmann J, Dalchau R, Fabre JW. Rejection of skin allografts by indirect allorecognition of donor class I major histocompatibility complex peptides. *J Exp Med* 1992;175:1521–1529.
11. Bradley JA, Mowat AM, Bolton EM. Processed MHC class I alloantigen as the stimulus for $CD4^+$ T-cell dependent antibody-mediated graft rejection. *Immunol Today* 1992;13:434–438.
12. Auchincloss HJ, Lee R, Shea S, et al. The role of "indirect" recognition in initiating rejection of skin grafts from major histocompatibility complex class II-deficient mice. *Proc Natl Acad Sci U S A* 1993;90: 3373–3378.
13. Bevan MJ. High determinant density may explain the phenomenon of alloreactivity. *Immunol Today* 1984;5:128–130.
14. Matzinger P, Bevan MJ. Hypothesis—why do so many lymphocytes respond to major histocompatibility antigens? *Cell Immunol* 1977; 29:1–5.
15. Rotzschke O, Falk K, Faath S, Rammensee H-G. On the nature of peptides involved in T cell allorecognition. *J Exp Med* 1991;174: 1059–1071.
16. Padovan E, Casorati G, Dellabona P, et al. Expression of two T cell receptor α chains: dual receptor T cells. *Science* 1993;262:422–424.
17. Counce S, Smith P, Barth R, Snell GD. Strong and weak histocompatibility gene differences in mice and their role in the rejection of homografts of tumor and skin. *Ann Surg* 1956;144:198–204.
18. Benacerraf B, McDevitt HO. Histocompatibility-linked immune response genes. *Science* 1972;175:273–279.
19. Trowsdale J, Ragoussis J, Campbell RD. Map of the human MHC. *Immunol Today* 1991;12:443–446.
20. Noessner E, Krensky AM. HLA and antigen presentation. In: Tilney NL, Strom TB, Paul LC, eds. *Transplantation biology*. New York: Raven; 1996;31.1–31.13.
21. Bjorkman PJ, Saper MA, Samraoui B, Bennett WS, Strominger JL, Wiley DC. Structure of the human class I histocompatibility antigen, HLA-A2. *Nature* 1987;329:506–512.
22. Zinkernagel RM, Doherty PC. Restriction of in vitro T cell-mediated cytotoxicity in lymphocytic choriomeningitis within a syngeneic or semiallogeneic system. *Nature* 1974;248:701–702.
23. Rotzschke O, Falk K, Deres K, et al. Isolation and analysis of naturally processed viral peptides as recognized by cytotoxic T cells. *Nature* 1990;348:252–254.
24. Guo H-C, Jardetzky TS, Garrett TPJ, Lane WS, Strominger JL, Wiley DC. Different length peptides bind to HLA-Aw68 similarly at their ends but bulge out in the middle. *Nature* 1992;360:364–366.
25. Falk K, Rotzschke O, Stevanovic S, Jung G, Rammensee H-G.

Allele-specific motifs revealed by sequencing of self-peptides eluted from MHC molecules. *Nature* 1991;351:290–296.
26. Germain RN. MHC-dependent antigen processing and peptide presentation. Providing ligands for T cell activation. *Cell* 1994;76:288–299.
27. Goldberg AL, Rock KL. Proteolysis, proteasomes and antigen presentation. *Nature* 1992;357:375–379.
28. Belich MP, Glynne RL, Senger G, Sheer D, Trowsdale J. Proteasome components with reciprocal expression to that of the MHC-encoded LMP proteins. *Curr Biol* 1994;4:769–776.
29. Momburg F, Neefjes JJ, Hammerling GJ. Peptide selection by the MHC-encoded TAP transporter. *Curr Opin Immunol* 1994;6:32–37.
30. Heemels M-T, Ploegh HL. Untapped peptides. *Curr Biol* 1993;3: 380–383.
31. Ou W-J, Cameron PH, Thomas DY, Bergeron JJM. Association of folding intermediates of glycoproteins with calnexin during protein maturation. *Nature* 1993;364:771–776.
32. Chicz RM, Urban RG, Gorga JC, Stern LJ, Lane WS, Strominger JL. Specificity and promiscuity among naturally processed peptides bound to HLA-DR alleles. *J Exp Med* 1993;178:27–47.
33. Brown JH, Jardetzky TS, Gorga JC, et al. The three-dimensional structure of the human class II histocompatibility antigen HLA-DR1. *Nature* 1993;364:33–39.
34. Roche PA, Marks MS, Cresswell P. Formation of a nine-subunit complex by HLA class II glycoproteins and the invariant chain. *Nature* 1991;354:392–394.
35. Viville S, Neefjes JJ, Lotteau V, et al. Mice lacking the MHC class II-associated invariant chain. *Cell* 1993;72:635–648.
36. Fling SP, Arp B, Pious D, et al. HLA-DMA and -DMB genes are both required for MHC class II/peptide complex formation in antigen-presenting cells. *Nature* 1994;368:554–558.
37. Sanderson F, Kleijmeer N, Kelly A, et al. Accumulation of HLA-DM, a regulator of antigen presentation, in MHC class II compartments. *Science* 1994;266:1566–1569.
38. Setum CM, Hegre OD, Serie JR, Moore WV. The potency of splenic dendritic cells as alloantigen presenters in vivo. Quantitation of the number of cells required to achieve graft rejection. *Transplantation* 1990;49:1175–1177.
39. Pederson N, Morris B. The role of the lymphatic system in the rejection of homografts: a study of lymph from renal transplants. *J Exp Med* 1970;131:936–969.
40. Larsen C, Morris P, Austyn J. Migration of dendritic leukocytes from cardiac allografts into host spleens: a novel pathway for initiation of rejection. *J Exp Med* 1990;171:307–314.
41. Lechler R, Batchelor J. Restoration of immunogenicity to passenger cell depleted kidney allografts by the addition of donor strain dendritic cells. *J Exp Med* 1982;155:31–41.
42. Pober J, Cotran R. Immunologic interactions of T lymphocytes with vascular endothelium. *Adv Immunol* 1991;50:261–302.
43. Hansen TH, Carreno BM, Sachs DH. The major histocompatibility complex. In: Paul WE, ed. *Fundamental immunology*. New York: Raven; 1993:577–628.
44. Terasaki PI, ed. *Clinical transplants 1988*. Los Angeles: UCLA Tissue Typing Laboratory; 1988.
45. Morris PJ, Ting A. Studies of HLA-DR with relevance to renal transplantation. *Immunol Rev* 1982;66:103–113.
46. Opelz G. HLA matching should be utilized for improving kidney transplant success rates. *Transplant Proc* 1991;23:46–50.
47. Opelz G. Survival of DNA HLA-DR typed and matched cadaver kidney transplants. *Lancet* 1991;338:461–463.
48. Lindahl KF. Minor histocompatibility antigens. *Trends Genet* 1991;7: 219–224.
49. Simpson E, Chandler P, Goulmy E. Separation of the genetic loci for the H-Y antigen and testis determination on the Y chromosome. *Nature* 1987;326:876–878.
50. Weiss A, Littman DR. Signal transduction by lymphocyte antigen receptors. *Cell* 1994;76:263–274.
51. Irving BA, Weiss A. The cytoplasmic domain of the T cell receptor ζ chain is sufficient to couple to receptor-associated signal transduction pathways. *Cell* 1991;64:891–901.
52. Veillette A, Abraham N, Caron L, Davidson D. The lymphocyte-specific tyrosine kinase p56lck. *Semin Immunol* 1991;3:143–152.
53. Tsygankov AY, Broker BM, Fargnoli J, Ledbetter JA, Bolen JB. Activation of tyrosine kinase p60fyn following T cell antigen receptor cross-linking. *J Biol Chem* 1991;267:18259–18262.
54. Chan AC, Iwashima M, Turck CW, Weiss A. ZAP-70: A 70kd protein kinase that associates with the TCR ζ chain. *Cell* 1992;71:649–662.
55. Chan AC, Kadlacek TA, Elder ME, et al. ZAP-70 deficiency in an autosomal recessive form of severe combined immunodeficiency. *Science* 1994;264:1599–1602.
56. Konig R, Huang L-Y, Germain RN. MHC class II interaction with CD4 mediated by a region analagous to the MHC class I binding site for CD8. *Nature* 1992;356:796–798.
57. Salter RD, Benjamin RJ, Wesley PK, et al. A binding site for the T cell co-receptor, CD8, on the alpha3 domain of HLA-A2. *Nature* 1990;345:41–46.
58. Trowbridge IS. CD45: a prototype for transmembrane protein tyrosine phosphatases. *J Biol Chem* 1991;266:23517–23520.
59. Stamenkovic I, Sgroi D, Aruffo A, Sy M, Anderson T. The B lymphocyte adhesion molecule CD22 interacts with leukocyte common antigen CD45RO on T cells and α2–6 sialytransferase, CD75, on B cells. *Cell* 1991;66:1133–1144.
60. Cooper JA, Gould KA, Cartwright CA, Hunter T. Tyr 527 is phosphorylated in pp60c-src: implication for regulation. *Science* 1986; 231:1431–1434.
61. Secrist JP, Karnitz L, Abraham RT. T-cell antigen receptor ligation induces tyrosine phosphorylation of phospholipase C-τ1. *J Biol Chem* 1991;266:12135–12139.
62. Liu J, Farmer JD, Lane WS, Friedman J, Weissman I, Schreiber S. Calcineurin is a common target of cyclophilin-cyclosporin A and FKBP-FK506 complexes. *Cell* 1991;66:807–815.
63. Northrop JP, Ho SN, Thomas DJ, et al. NF-AT components define a family of transcription factors targeted in T cell activation. *Nature* 1994;369:497–502.
64. Rao A. NF-ATp: a transcription factor required for the coordinate induction of several cytokine genes. *Immunol Today* 1994;15:274–281.
65. Flanagan WM, Corthesy B, Bram RJ, Crabtree GR. Nuclear association of a T-cell transcription factor blocked by FK506 and cyclosporin A. *Nature* 1991;352:803–807.
66. Downward J, Graves J, Cantrell D. The regulation and function of p21/ras in T cells. *Immunol Today* 1992;13:89–92.
67. Rayter SI, Woodrow M, Lucas SC, Cantrell DA, Downward J. p21ras mediates control of IL-2 gene promoter function in T cell activation. *EMBO J* 1992;11:4549–4556.
68. Kang S-M, Tran A-C, Grilli M, Lenardo MJ. NF-kappa B subunit regulation in non-transformed CD4$^+$ T lymphocytes. *Science* 1992; 256:1452–1456.
69. Bohjanen PR, Petryniak B, June CH, Thompson CB, Lindsten T. An inducible cytoplasmic (AU-B) binds selectively to AUUUA multimers in the 38 untranslated region of lymphokine mRNA. *Mol Cell Biol* 1991;11:3288–3295.
70. Jenkins MK, Johnson JG. Molecules involved in T-cell co-stimulation. *Curr Opin Immunol* 1993;5:361–367.
71. Van Seventer GA, Shimuzu Y, Shaw S. Roles of multiple accessory molecules in T cell activation: bilateral interplay of adhesion and costimulation. *Curr Opin Immunol* 1991;3:294–303.
72. Linsley PS, Ledbetter JA. The role of CD28 receptor during T cell responses to antigen. *Annu Rev Immunol* 1993;11:191–212.
73. June CH, Bluestone JA, Nadler LM, Thompson CB. The B7 and CD28 receptor families. *Immunol Today* 1994;15:321–331.
74. Brunet JF, Denizot F, Luciani MF, et al. A new member of the immunoglobulin superfamily—CTLA-4. *Nature* 1987;328:267–270.
75. Freeman GJ, Freedman AS, Segil JM, Lee G, Whitman JF, Nadler LM. B7, a new member of the Ig superfamily with unique expression on activated and neoplastic B cells. *J Immunol* 1989;143:2714–2722.
76. Freeman GJ, Gribben JG, Boussiotis VA, et al. Cloning of B7-2: a CTLA-4 counter-receptor that co-stimulates human T-cell proliferation. *Science* 1993;262:909–911.
77. Boussiotis VA, Freeman GJ, Gribben JG, et al. Activated human B lymphocytes express three CTLA4 binding counter-receptors which co-stimulate T-cell activation. *Proc Natl Acad Sci U S A* 1993;90: 11059–11063.
78. Harding FA, McArthur JG, Gross JA, Raulet DH, Allison JP. CD28-mediated signalling co-stimulates murine T cells and prevents induction of anergy in T-cell clones. *Nature* 1992;356:607–609.
79. Shahinian A, Pfeffer K, Lee KP, et al. Differential T-cell costimulatory requirements in CD28-deficient mice. *Science* 1993;261:609–612.
80. Tan P, Anasetti C, Hansen JA, et al. Induction of alloantigen-specific hypo-responsiveness in human T lymphocytes by blocking interac-

tion of CD28 with its natural ligand B7/BB1. *J Exp Med* 1993;177: 165–173.
81. Truitt KE, Hicks CM, Imboden JB. Stimulation of CD28 triggers an association between CD28 and phosphatidylinositol 3-kinase in Jurkat T cells. *J Exp Med* 1994;179:1071–1076.
82. Fraser JD, Irving BA, Crabtree GR, Weiss A. Regulation of IL-2 gene enhancer by the T cell accessory molecule CD28. *Science* 1991;251: 313–316.
83. Lindsten T, June CH, Ledbetter JA, Stella G, Thompson CB. Regulation of lymphokine messenger RNA stability by a surface-mediated T cell activation pathway. *Science* 1989;144:339–343.
84. Crabtree GR. Contingent genetic regulatory events in T lymphocyte activation. *Science* 1989;243:355–361.
85. Mossman TR, Cherwinski H, Bond MW, Giedlin MA, Coffman RL. Two types of murine helper T cell clone. Definition according to profiles of lymphokine activities and secreted proteins. *J Immunol* 1986; 136:2348–2357.
86. Nickerson P, Steurer W, Steiger J, Zheng X, Steele AW, Strom TB. Cytokines and the Th1/Th2 paradigm in transplantation. *Curr Opin Immunol* 1994;6:757–764.
87. Noguchi M, Yi H, Rosenblatt H, et al. Interleukin-2 receptor τ chain mutation results in X-linked severe combined immunodeficiency in humans. *Cell* 1994;73:147–157.
88. Liu CC, Walsh CM, Young J. Perforin: structure and function. *Immunol Today* 1995;16:194–201.
89. Smyth MJ, Trapiani JA. Granzymes: exogenous proteinases that induce target cell apoptosis. *Immunol Today* 1995;16:202–206.
90. Kagi D, Ledermann B, Burki K, et al. Cytotoxicity mediated by T cells and natural killer cells is greatly impaired in perforin-deficient mice. *Nature* 1994;369:31–37.
91. Heusel JW, Wesselschmidt RL, Shresta S, Russell JH, Ley TJ. Cytotoxic lymphocytes require granzyme B for the rapid induction of DNA fragmentation and apoptosis in allogeneic target cells. *Cell* 1994;76:977–987.
92. Lipman ML, Stevens AC, Strom TB. Heightened intragraft CTL gene expression in acutely rejecting renal allografts. *J Immunol* 1994;152: 5120–5127.
93. Kagi D, Vignaux F, Ledermann B, et al. Fas and perforin pathways as major mechanisms of T cell-mediated cytotoxicity. *Science* 1994; 265:528–531.
94. Kirby JA, Morgan JC, Shenton BK, et al. Renal allograft rejection. Possible involvement of antibody-dependent cell-mediated cytotoxicity. *Transplantation* 1990;50:255–259.
95. Colonna M, Brooks E, Falco M. Generation of allospecific natural killer cells by stimulation across a polymorphism of HLA-C. *Science* 1993;260:1121–1124.
96. Malnati MS, Peruzzi M, Parker KC. Peptide specificity in the recognition of MHC class I by natural killer cell clones. *Science* 1995;267: 1016–1018.
97. Bradley JA, Mason DW, Morris PJ. Evidence that rat renal allografts are rejected by cytotoxic T cells and not by non-specific effectors. *Transplantation* 1985;39:169–175.
98. Kelley VR, Diaz-Gallo C, Jevnikar A, Singer GG. Renal tubular epithelial and T cell interactions in autoimmune renal disease. *Kidney Int* 1993;45(suppl 39);108–115.
99. Ijzermans JNM, Bouwman E, Van der Meide PH, Marquet R. Increase of major histocompatibility complex class II–positive cells in cardiac allografts by interferon-gamma has no impact on graft survival. *Transplantation* 1989;48:1039–1041.
100. Heeger P, Wolf G, Meyers C, et al. Isolation and characterization of cDNA from renal tubular epithelium encoding murine RANTES. *Kidney Int* 1992;41:220–225.
101. Briscoe DM, Cotran RS. Role of leukocyte-endothelial cell adhesion molecules in renal inflammation: in vitro and in vivo studies. *Kidney Int* 1993;44(suppl 42):27–34.
102. Doukas J, Pober JS. IFN-τ enhances endothelial activation induced by tumor necrosis factor but not IL-1. *J Immunol* 1990;145: 1727–1733.
103. Briscoe DM, Yeung A, Schoen EL, et al. Predictive value of inducible endothelial cell adhesion molecule expression for acute rejection of human cardiac allografts. *Transplantation* 1995;59: 204–211.
104. Springer TA. Traffic signals for lymphocyte recirculation and leukocyte emigration: the mutistep paradigm. *Cell* 1994;76:301–314.
105. Adams DH, Shaw S. Leukocyte-endothelial interactions and regulation of leukocyte migration. *Lancet* 1994;343:831–834.
106. Schall TJ. The chemokines. In: Thomson A, ed. *The cytokine handbook.* New York: Academic; 1994:419–460.
107. Taub DD, Conlon K, Lloyd AR, Oppenheim JJ, Kelvin DJ. Preferential migration of activated CD4+ and CD8+ T cells in response to MIP-1α and MIP-1β. *Science* 1993;260:355–358.
108. Pattison J, Nelson P, Huie P, et al. RANTES chemokine expression in cell-mediated transplant rejection of the kidney. *Lancet* 1994;343: 209–211.
109. Kelvin DJ, Michiel DF, Johnston JA, et al. Chemokines and serpentines: the molecular biology of chemokine receptors. *J Leukoc Biol* 1993;54;604–612.
110. Leppert D, Waubant E, Galardy R, Bunnet N, Hauser SL. T cell gelatinases mediate basement membrane transmigration in vitro. *J Immunol* 1995;154:4379–4389.
111. Kissmeyer-Nielsen F, Olsen S, Petersen V, Fjeldborg O. Hyperacute rejection of kidney allografts, associated with pre-existing humoral antibodies against donor cells. *Lancet* 1966;2:662–665.
112. Talseth T, Westre B, Bondevik H, et al. Prognostic information in biopsies of transplanted kidneys with unsatisfactory response to antirejection therapy. *Transplant Proc* 1987;19:1623–1624.
113. Porter KA, Joseph NH, Randall JM, Stolinski C, Hoehn RJ, Calne RY. The role of lymphocytes in the rejection of canine renal homotransplants. *Lab Invest* 1964;18:1080–1085.
114. Paul LC, Benediktsson H. Chronic transplant rejection: magnitude of the problem and pathogenetic mechanisms. *Transplant Rev* 1993;7: 96–113.
115. Azuma H, Tilney NL. Chronic graft rejection. *Curr Opin Immunol* 1994;6:770–776.
116. Kobayashi T, Yokoyama I, Uchida K, Takagi H. HLA-DRB1 matching as a recipient selection criterion in cadaveric renal transplantation. *Transplantation* 1993;55:1294–1297.
117. Almond PS, Matas A, Gillingham KJ, et al. Early versus late acute renal allograft rejection: impact on chronic rejection. *Transplantation* 1993;55:752–757.
118. Yilmaz S, Hayry P. The impact of acute episodes of rejection on the generation of chronic rejection in rat renal allografts. *Transplantation* 1993;56:1153–1156.
119. Brenner BM, Milford EL. Nephron underdosing: a programmed cause of chronic renal allograft failure. *Am J Kidney Dis* 1993;21:66–72.
120. Almond PS, Matas A, Gillingham K, et al. Risk factors for chronic rejection in renal allograft recipients. *Transplantation* 1993;25: 901–903.
121. Solez K, Axelsen RA, Benediktsson H, et al. International standardization of criteria for the histologic diagnosis of renal allograft rejection: the Banff working classification of kidney transplant pathology. *Kidney Int* 1993;44:411–422.
122. Hancock WH, Whitley WD, Tullius SG, et al. Cytokines, adhesion molecules and the pathogenesis of chronic rejection of rat renal allografts. *Transplantation* 1993;56:643–650.
123. Azuma H, Heeman UW, Tullius SG, Tilney NL. Cytokines and adhesion molecules in chronic rejection. *Clin Transplant* 1994;8:168–175.
124. Neuringer JR, Brenner BM. Glomerular hypertension: cause and consequence of renal injury. *J Hypertens* 1992;10:91–97.
125. Allison CA, Eugui EM, Sollinger HW. Mycophenolate mofetil (RS61443): mechanisms of action and effects in transplantation. *Transplant Rev* 1993;7:129–139.
126. Rugstad HE. Antiinflammatory and immunoregulatory effects of glucocorticoids: mode of action. *Scand J Rheumatol* 1988;76:257–264.
127. Han J, Thompson P, Beutler B. Dexamethasone and pentaoxyifylline inhibit endotoxin-induced cachectin/tumor necrosis factor synthesis at separate points in the signaling pathway. *J Exp Med* 1990;172: 391–394.
128. Lee SW, Tsou AP, Chan H, et al. Glucocorticoids selectively inhibit the transcription of the interleukin 1β gene and decrease the stability of interleukin 1β mRNA. *Proc Nat Acad Sci U S A* 1988;85: 1204–1208.
129. Northrop JP, Crabtree GR, Mattila PS. Negative regulation of interleukin 2 transcription by the glucocorticoid receptor. *J Exp Med* 1992;175:1235–1245.
130. Mukaida N, Morita M, Ishikawa Y, et al. Novel mechanism of glucocorticoid-mediated gene repression. *J Biol Chem* 1994;269: 13289–13295.

131. Strom TB. Immunosuppressive agents in renal transplantation. *Kidney Int* 1984;26:353–365.
132. Schreiber SL, Crabtree GR. The mechanism of action of cyclosporin A and FK506. *Immunol Today* 1992;13:136–142.
133. Khanna A, Li B, Stenzel K, Suthanthiran M. Regulation of new DNA synthesis in mammalian cells by cyclosporine: demonstration of a transforming growth factor β–dependent mechanism of inhibition of cell growth. *Transplantation* 1994;57:577–582.
134. Durez P, Abramowicz D, Gerard C, et al. In vivo induction of interleukin 10 by anti-cd3 monoclonal antibody or bacterial lipopolysaccharide: differential modulation by cyclosporin A. *J Exp Med* 1993; 177:551–555.
135. Armitage JM, Fricker FJ, Nido PD, et al. The clinical trial of FK 506 as primary and rescue immunosuppression in pediatric cardiac transplantation. *Transplant Proc* 1991;23:3058–3060.
136. The U.S. Multicenter FK506 Liver Study Group. A comparison of tacrolimus (FK506) and cyclosporine for immunosuppression in transplantation. *N Engl J Med* 1994;331:1110–1115.
137. Fung JJ, Alessiani M, Abu-Elmagd K, et al. Adverse effects associated with the use of FK506. *Transplant Proc* 1991;23:3195–3196.
138. Sabatini DM, Erdjument-Bromage H, Lui M, Tempst P, Snyder S. RAFT-1: a mammalian protein that binds to FKBP12 in a rapamycin-dependent fashion and is homologous to yeast TORs. *Cell* 1994;78: 35–43.
139. Meiser BM, Billingham ME, Morris RE. Effects of cyclosporine, FK506, and rapamycin on graft vessel disease. *Lancet* 1991;338: 1297–1298.
140. Turka LA, Dayton J, Sinclair G, Thompson CB, Mitchell BS. Guanine ribonucleotide depletion inhibits T cell activation: mechanism of action of the immunosuppressive drug mizoribine. *J Clin Invest* 1991; 87:940–948.
141. Murphy MP, Morris RE. Brequinar sodium effectively and potently suppresses allograft rejection in a heterotopic mouse heart transplant model. *Transplant Proc* 1993;25:75–76.
142. Nadler SG, Tepper MA, Schacter B, Mazzucco CE. Interaction of the immunosuppressant deoxyspergualin with a member of the Hsp70 family of heat shock proteins. *Science* 1992;258:484–485.
143. Jiang H, Takahara S, Takano Y, et al. Experience with the administration of 15-deoxyspergualin in rejection in kidney transplant recipients. *Transplant Proc* 1992;24:1726–1729.
144. Morris RE, Huang X, Cao W, Zheng B, Shorthouse RA. Leflunomide (HWA 486) and its analog suppress T- and B-cell proliferation in vitro, acute rejection, ongoing rejection, and antidonor antibody, synthesis in mouse, rat, and cynomolgus monkey transplant recipients as well as arterial thickening after balloon catheter injury. *Transplant Proc* 1995;27:445–447.
145. Hoitsma AJ, Van Lier HJJ, Reekers P, Koene RAP. Improved patient and graft survival after treatment of acute rejections of cadaveric renal allograft with rabbit antithymocyte globulin. *Transplantation* 1985;39:274–280.
146. Hoitsma AJ, Van Lier HJJ, Reekers P, Koene RAP. Improved patient and graft survival after treatment of acute rejections of cadaveric renal allograft with rabbit antithymocyte globulin. *Transplantation* 1985;39:274–280.
147. Vigeral P, Chkoff N, Chatenoud L, et al. Prophylactic use of OKT3 monoclonal antibody in cadaver kidney recipients. *Transplantation* 1986;41:730–737.
148. Cosimi AB, Burton RC, Colvin B, et al. Treatment of acute renal allograft rejection with OKT3 monoclonal antibody. *Transplantation* 1981;32:535–541.
149. Ortho Multicenter Transplant Study Group. A randomized clinical trial of OKT3 monoclonal antibody for acute rejection of cadaveric renal transplants. *N Engl J Med* 1985;313:337–342.
150. Chatenoud L, Ferran C, Legendre C, et al. In vivo cell activation following OKT3 administration: systemic cytokine release and modulation by corticosteroids. *Transplantation* 1990;49:697–703.
151. Oh CS, Stratta RJ, Fox BC, Sollinger HW, Belzer FO, Maki DG. Increased infections associated with the use of OKT3 for treatment of steroid-resistant rejection in renal transplantation. *Transplantation* 1988;45:68–75.
152. Swinnen LJ, Costanzo-Nordin MR, Fisher SG, et al. Increased incidence of lymphoproliferative disorder after immunosuppression with the monoclonal antibody OKT3 in cardiac transplant recipients. *N Engl J Med* 1990;323:1723–1727.
153. Emery RW, Lake KD. Post transplantation lymphoproliferative disorder and OKT3. *N Engl J Med* 1990;324:1437–1442.
154. Chatenoud L, Jonker M, Villemain F, Goldstein G, Bach JF. The human immune response to the OKT3 monoclonal antibody is oligoclonal. *Science* 1986;232:1406–1409.
155. Hricik DE, Zarconi J, Schulak JA. Influence of low-dose cyclosporine on the outcome of treatment with OKT3 for acute renal allograft rejection. *Transplantation* 1989;47:272–279.
156. Winter G, Milstein C. Man-made antibodies. *Nature* 1991;349: 293–299.
157. Kirkman RL, Barrett LV, Gaulton GN, Kelley VE, Ythier A, Strom TB. Administration of an anti-interleukin-2 receptor monoclonal antibody prolongs cardiac allograft survival in mice. *J Exp Med* 1985; 162:358–364.
158. Soulillou JP. Relevant targets for therapy with monoclonal antibodies in allograft transplantation. *Kidney Int* 1994;46:540–553.
159. Pankewycz O, Mackie J, Hassarjian R, Murphy JR, Strom TB, Kelley VE. Interleukin-2-diptheria toxin fusion protein prolongs murine islet cell engraftment. *Transplantation* 1989;47:318–322.
160. Jonker M, Neuhaus P, Zurcher C, Fucello A, Goldstein G. OKT4 and OKT4A antibody treatment as immunosuppression for kidney transplantation in rhesus monkeys. *Transplantation* 1985;39:247–254.
161. Wood KJ, Pearson TS, Darby C, Morris PJ. CD4: a potential target molecule for immunosuppressive therapy and tolerance induction. *Transplant Rev* 1991;5:150–165.
162. Isobe M, Yagita H, Okumura K, Ihara A. Specific acceptance of cardiac allografts after treatment with antibodies to ICAM-1 and LFA-1. *Science* 1992;255:1125–1128.
163. Haug CE, Colvin RB, Delmonico FL, et al. A phase 1 trial of immunosuppression with anti-ICAM-1 (CD54) mAb in renal allograft recipients. *Transplantation* 1993;55:412–419.
164. Friend PJ, Hale G, Waldman H, et al. Campath-1M—prophylactic use after kidney transplantation. A randomized controlled clinical trial. *Transplantation* 1989;48:248–256.
165. Brewer Y, Taube D, Bewick M, et al. Effect of graft perfusion with two CD45 monoclonal antibodies on incidence of kidney allograft rejection. *Lancet* 1989;2:935–937.
166. Dallman MJ, Clark GJ. Cytokines and their receptors in transplantation. *Curr Opin Immunol* 1991;3:729–734.
167. Elliott MJ, Maini RN, Feldmann M, et al. Randomised double-blind comparison of chimeric monoclonal antibody to tumor necrosis factor alpha (cA2) versus placebo in rheumatoid arthritis. *Lancet* 1994;344: 1105–1110.
168. Billingham R, Brent L, Medawar P. Actively acquired tolerance of foreign cells. *Nature* 1953;172:603–606.
169. Kappler JW, Roehm N, Marrack PC. T cell tolerance by clonal elimination in the thymus. *Cell* 1987;49:273–280.
170. Schwartz RH, Mueller DL, Jenkins MK, Quill H. T-cell clonal anergy. *Cold Spring Harb Symp Quant Biol* 1989;2:605–610.
171. Boussiotis VA, Gribben JG, Freeman GJ, Nadler LM. Blockade of the CD28 co-stimulatory pathway: a means to induce tolerance. *Curr Opin Immunol* 1994;6:797–807.
172. Lenschow DJ, Zeng Y, Thistlethwaite JR, et al. Long term survival of xenogeneic pancreatic islet grafts induced by CTLA4lg. *Science* 1992;257:789–792.
173. Linsley PS, Wallace PM, Johnson J, et al. Immunosuppression in vivo by a soluble form of the CTLA-4 T-cell activation molecule. *Science* 1992;257:792–795.
174. Beverly B, Kang K, Lenardo MJ, Schwartz RH. Reversal of in vitro T cell clonal anergy by IL-2 stimulation. *Int Immunol* 1992;4: 661–671.
175. Ramsdell F, Fowlkes BJ. Maintenance of in vivo tolerance by persistence of antigen. *Science* 1994;264:1130–1134.
176. Mueller DL, Chiodetti L, Bacon PA, Schwartz RH. Clonal anergy blocks the response to IL-4, as well as the production of IL-2, in dual-producing T helper cell clones. *J Immunol* 1991;147:4118–4125.
177. Quill H, Bhandoola A, Trinchieri G, Haluskey J, Peritt D. Induction of interleukin 12 responsiveness is impaired in anergic T lymphocytes. *J Exp Med* 1994;179:1065–1070.
178. Gershon RK, Kondo K. Infectious immunological tolerance. *Immunology* 1971;21:903–914.
179. Ding L, Linsley PS, Huang L, Germain RN, Shevach EM. IL-10 inhibits macrophage costimulation activity by selectively inhibiting the upregulation of B7 expression. *J Immunol* 1993;151:1224–1232.

180. Lombardi G, Sidhu S, Batchelor R, Lechler R. Anergic T cells as suppressor cells in vitro. *Science* 1994;264:1587–1589.
181. Begeon L, Cuturi M-C, Hallet M-M, Paineau J, Chabannes D, Soulillou J-P. Peripheral tolerance of an allograft in adult rats—characterization by low interleukin-2 and interferon-τ mRNA levels and by strong accumulation of major histocompatibility complex transcripts in the graft. *Transplantation* 1992;54:219–225.
182. Macatonia SE, Doherty TM, Knight SC, O'Garra A. Differential effect of IL-10 on dendritic cell–induced T cell proliferation and IFNτ production. *J Immunol* 1993;150:3755–3765.
183. Chen W-E, Zlotnik A. IL-10: a novel cytotoxic T cell differentiation factor. *J Immunol* 1991;147:528–534.
184. Miller A, Lider O, Roberts AB, Sporn MB, Weiner HL. Suppressor T cells generated by oral tolerization to myelin basic protein suppress both in vitro and in vivo immune responses by the release of TGF-β following antigenic specific triggering. *Proc Natl Acad Sci U S A* 1992;89:421–425.
185. Starzl TE, Demetris AJ, Murase N, Ilstad S, Ricordi C, Trucco M. Cell migration, chimerism, and graft acceptance. *Lancet* 1992;339: 1579–1582.
186. Suberbielle C, Caillat-Zucman S, Legendre C, et al. Peripheral microchimerism in long-term cadaveric kidney allograft recipients. *Lancet* 1994;343:1468–1469.
187. Thomas JM, Carver FM, Kasten-Jolly J, et al. Further studies of veto activity in rhesus monkey bone marrow in relation to allograft tolerance and chimerism. *Transplantation* 1994;57:101–115.
188. Posselt AM, Barker CF, Tomaszewski JE, Markmann JF, Choti MA, Naji A. Induction of donor-specific unresponsiveness by intrathymic islet transplantation. *Science* 1990;249:1293–1295.
189. Remuzzi G, Rossini M, Imberti O, Perico N. Kidney graft survival in rats without immunosuppressants after intrathymic glomerular transplantation. *Lancet* 1991;337:750–752.
190. Remuzzi G, Perico N, Carpenter CB, Sayegh MH. The thymic way to transplantation tolerance. *J Am Soc Nephrol* 1995;5:1639–1646.
191. Remuzzi G, Noris M, Benigni A, Imberti O, Sayegh MH, Perico N. Thromboxane A2 receptor blocking abrogates donor-specific unresponsiveness to renal allografts triggered by thymic recognition of histocompatibility allopeptides. *J Exp Med* 1994;180:1967–1972.
192. Opelz G, Terasaki PI. Improvements of kidney graft survival with increased munbers of blood transfusions. *N Engl J Med* 1978;299: 799–803.
193. Krensky AM, Clayberger C. The induction of tolerance to alloantigens using HLA-based synthetic allopeptides. *Curr Opin Immunol* 1994;6:791–796.
194. Clayberger C, Parham P, Rothbard J, Ludwig DS, Schoolnik GK, Krensky AM. Inhibition of alloreactive cytotoxic T lymphocytes by peptides from the α2 domain of HLA-A2. *Nature* 1987;325: 625–628.
195. Nisco S, Vriens P, Hoyt G, et al. Induction of allograft tolerance in rats by an HLA class-I–derived peptide and cyclosporine A. *J Immunol* 1994;152:3786–3792.
196. Sayegh MH, Zhang ZJ, Hancock WW, Kwok CA, Carpenter CA, Weiner HL. Down-regulation of the immune response to histocompatibility antigens and prevention of sensitization by skin allografts by orally administered alloantigen. *Transplantation* 1992;53:63–66.
197. Dorling A, Lechler RI. Prospects for xenografting. *Curr Opin Immunol* 1994;6:765–769.
198. Galili U. Interaction of the natural anti-Gal antibody with α-galactosyl epitopes: a major obstacle for xenotransplantation in humans. *Immunol Today* 1993;14:480–482.
199. Platt JL, Fischel RJ, Matas AJ, Reif SA, Bolman RM, Bach FH. Immunopathology of hyperacute xenograft rejection in a swine-to-primate model. *Transplantation* 1991;52:214–220.
200. Rooney IA, Liszewski MK, Atkinson JP. Using membrane-bound complement regulatory proteins to inhibit rejection. *Xenotransplantation* 1993;1:29–35.
201. Magee JC, Platt JL. Xenograft rejection—molecular mechanisms and therapeutic implications. *Ther Immunol* 1994;1:45–58.
202. Murray AG, Khodadoust MM, Pober JS, Bothwell ALM. Porcine aortic endothelial cells activate human T cells: direct presentation of MHC antigens and costimulation by ligands for human CD2 and CD28. *Immunity* 1994;1:57–63.

PART III

Mediation of Immune Renal Injury

A. Humoral Mediators of Immune Injury

Immunologic Renal Diseases,
edited by E. G. Neilson and W. G. Couser.
Lippincott-Raven Publishers, Philadelphia © 1997.

CHAPTER 17

Glomerular Injury Due to Antibody Alone

David J. Salant, Yasuhiro Natori, and Fujio Shimizu

Glomerular injury induced by antibodies in the absence of any known secondary mediator is a well-documented but as yet ill understood phenomenon (1,2). Although it was first described as a noninflammatory form of nephrotoxic serum nephritis, several other models of "antibody-dependent" injury are now recognized, in some of which the nephritogenic antigen has been identified (Table 1). In general, these complement- and leukocyte-independent lesions exhibit substantial, but sometimes transient, albuminuria and normal histology at the light microscopic level. The major histologic features are ultrastructural alterations in podocyte morphology, sometimes accompanied by endothelial swelling and/or detachment.

The ability of antibodies to cause glomerular injury without involving complement and/or leukocytes has been recognized since the early 1960s, when it was found that high doses of duck nephrotoxic serum (NTS) produce proteinuria without fixing complement (3). Before that time, investigators believed that avian antisera, by virtue of their inability to activate mammalian complement, are incapable of directly inducing proteinuria in mammals but require a host immune response to the "planted" glomerular-bound avian immunoglobulin G (IgG) (4). Indeed, the need for complement appeared to derive further support from studies showing that peptic digestion of rabbit antirat NTS, which removes the Fc part of IgG and abolishes its ability to fix complement, substantially reduced its potential to cause proteinuria (5,6). On the other hand, the NTS $F(ab')_2$ fragments derived by peptic digestion did cause some proteinuria, albeit transient and less than that caused by the intact IgG. As with avian NTS (3,7,8), the nephrotoxic effect of rabbit NTS $F(ab')_2$ fragments was seen, especially at high doses, and was accompanied by normal glomerular histology with no visible leukocytes on light microscopy (5,6,9). Subsequently it was found that the non–complement-fixing subclasses of sheep and guinea pig NTS, as well as their $F(ab')_2$ fragments, induce marked proteinuria in the absence of glomerular complement deposits or leukocytes (10–13). In retrospect, it was already evident from the studies of Hammer and Dixon with the globulin fraction of rabbit antirat NTS that proteinuria is reduced but not necessarily abolished in animals depleted of complement as long as sufficient antibody is injected (3). Similarly, it was well documented that nephrotoxic nephritis in both rabbits (1,7,14) and rats (7) has a substantial component of neutrophil-independent proteinuria.

The phenomenon of complement-independent glomerular injury was further established by several studies in guinea pigs. Thus, guinea pigs immunized with glomeruli develop an autoimmune nephritis characterized by heavy proteinuria and linear deposits of IgG on the glomerular capillary wall without complement fixation (15,16). In addition, guinea pigs injected with sheep NTS (containing both complement-fixing and non–complement-fixing antibodies) or the $F(ab')_2$ fragments of sheep NTS develop massive proteinuria in the absence of glomerular complement deposits (17,18). These studies also served to exclude a role for several known systemic inflammatory mediators, including vasoactive amines, kinins, prostanoids, and the coagulation system (18), and suggested a direct nephritogenic effect of the antibody.

Perhaps the most convincing evidence of a direct action of antibody on the glomerulus itself derived from studies in the isolated perfused rat kidney model (19). Thus, isolated rat kidneys, perfused in vitro with sheep NTS in a serum- and leukocyte-free medium, rapidly developed severe albuminuria. This observation strongly supported the idea that complement- and leukocyte-independent glomerular injury is due to a direct interaction of

D. J. Salant: Department of Medicine, Boston University Medical Center, Boston, Massachusetts 02118, U.S.A.

Y. Natori: Research Institute, International Medical Center of Japan, Tokyo, Japan.

F. Shimizu: Institute of Nephrology, Niigata University School of Medicine, Niigata, Japan.

TABLE 1. *Key studies in which complement- and neutrophil-independent, antibody-mediated proteinuria was documented*

Model: Species and manipulation	Source and nature of antibody or immunogen[a]	Reference[b]
Nephrotoxic nephritis		
Complement independence		
Rat	Duck NTS (high dose)	3
Rat: complement-depleted	Rabbit NTS (high dose)	3
Rat	Guinea pig γ1 NTS	10,11
Rat	Rabbit F(ab′)$_2$ NTS	5,6
Rat	Guinea pig γ1 F(ab′)$_2$ NTS	12
Rat: complement-deficient	Rabbit NTS	34
Rat: complement-depleted and isolated perfused kidney	Sheep NTS	19
Rat	Sheep γ2 NTS	40
Rabbit	Sheep γ2 NTS	13
Guinea pig: complement-depleted and C4-deficient	Sheep NTS	17,18
Guinea pig	Sheep F(ab′)$_2$ NTS	17
Neutrophil independence		
Rat: neutrophil-depleted	Rabbit NTS (high dose)	7
Rat: isolated perfused kidney	Sheep NTS	19
Rabbit: neutrophil-depleted	Sheep NTS (high dose)	7
Guinea pig: neutrophil-depleted	Sheep NTS	18
Autoimmune (Steblay) nephritis		
Guinea pig	Human glomerular antigens	15
Other complement- and leukocyte-independent models		
Rat	Sheep F(ab′)$_2$ and Fab′ anti-Fx1A	20
Rat: C6-deficient	Heymann nephritis	58
Rat	Cationized bovine γ globulin	59
Rat	Rabbit anti-DPPIV	21
Rat	Mouse mAb 5-1-6	25

[a] Guinea pig γ1 IgG, sheep γ2 IgG, and avian IgY do not activate mammalian complement.
[b] Only the first publication of a particular model from each laboratory is cited here.

antibody with some critical component of the glomerular capillary wall and served to further exclude a role for systemic inflammatory mediators.

Evidence that this form of glomerular damage is not confined to nephrotoxic nephritis first became apparent when it was found that F(ab′)$_2$ and F(ab′) fragments of sheep IgG antibodies to the rat proximal tubular brush border fraction, Fx1A, cause early-onset proteinuria when injected into rats (20). Later it was noted that monospecific antibodies to a component of proximal tubular brush border, dipeptidyl peptidase IV (DPPIV), also produce complement-independent proteinuria (21, 22). However, it was the application of hybridoma technology that provided a clearer insight into the probable mechanisms underlying this form of injury and the interrelatedness of the various models (23). Until then, nephrotoxic nephritis was considered to be an experimental model of anti–glomerular basement membrane (GBM) nephritis because of the linear staining pattern resembling human Goodpasture syndrome. When subjected to monoclonal dissection, however, NTS was found to contain antibodies to several cell surface antigens in addition to those reactive with extracellular matrix proteins (23,24). Included among the antibodies identified in this way are monoclonal antibodies (mAbs) to DPPIV, glycoprotein (gp)330 (the Heymann nephritis antigen), and p51 (the target of mAb 5-1-6), as well as several non-nephritogenic antigens (23–28).

It is worth emphasizing that although antibody-dependent glomerular injury necessarily involves reactivity to structural components of the glomerular capillary wall, binding of antibodies to extracellular matrix components of the GBM or cell surface antigens in vivo does not always cause glomerular injury. Thus, antibodies to various extracellular matrix (29–31) and cell membrane proteins, including podocalyxin (32), podoendin (33), GLEPP1 (26), and other less well-defined antigens (27, 28), do not produce changes in glomerular structure or function despite substantial deposition in vivo. This implies that the antigens involved in antibody-induced glomerular injury normally serve an important role in maintaining the structural and/or functional integrity of the glomerular capillary wall.

In the rest of this chapter, we describe in more detail some of the models exhibiting this form of injury, discuss possible mechanisms, and speculate on their potential role in human glomerular disease. For convenience, we refer to the phenomenon as antibody-dependent or antibody-mediated injury, recognizing that other factors may also be involved.

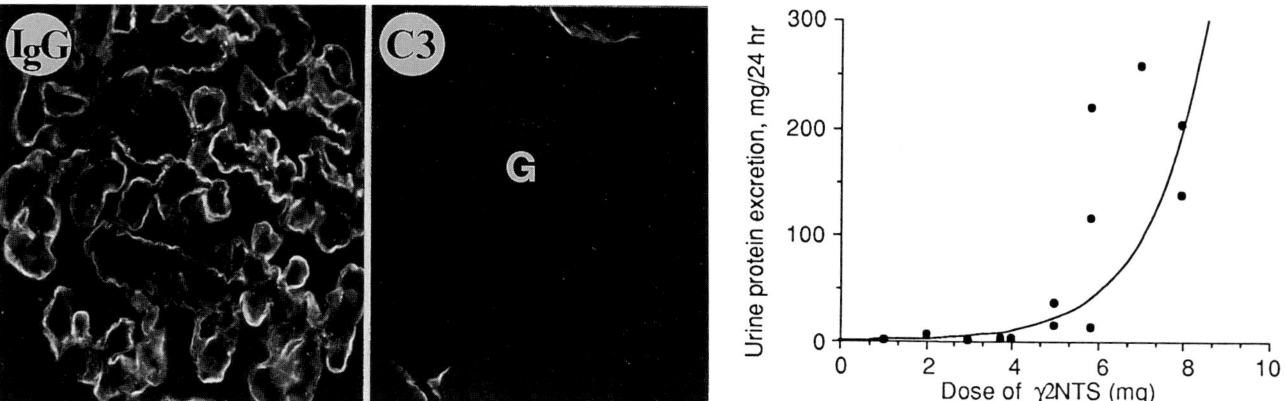

FIG. 1. Proteinuria and glomerular immunofluorescence induced by injection of the γ2 non–complement-fixing subclass of sheep NTS into adult rats. Rats that received ≥5 mg developed proteinuria in the first 24 h, and all rats had pronounced linear staining for sheep IgG but no glomerular (G) staining for C3. The focal extraglomerular C3 staining is typical of that seen in normal kidneys. Original magnification ×400.

NEPHROTOXIC SERUM NEPHRITIS

Features of Complement-Independent Nephrotoxic Nephritis

The features of complement- and leukocyte-independent nephrotoxic nephritis are similar among different species (Table 1) and are well exemplified by our findings with sheep NTS in rats. Proteinuria develops within minutes of antibody injection coincident with the rapid deposition of IgG on the glomerular capillary wall in a linear pattern. Small amounts of rat complement are present in a similar distribution when unfractionated antiserum is used; however, complement depletion has little or no effect on proteinuria (19). When the γ2 non–complement-fixing subclass of NTS IgG is injected, severe proteinuria develops rapidly without complement deposition (Fig. 1). Proteinuria generally subsides over several days, but as in classical complement-dependent nephrotoxic nephritis, it may recur during the autologous phase and persist for life. The mediation of injury in the autologous phase is likely similar to that observed in classical nephrotoxic nephritis (see Chapter 32). Heterologous phase proteinuria may be massive, often in excess of 200 mg/day in rats and guinea pigs, and is mostly composed of albumin. However, formal macromolecular sieving studies have not been performed to define the disturbance in permselectivity. Routine light microscopy shows normal histology with no increase in glomerular cellularity. At the ultrastructural level, the podocytes exhibit variable degrees of damage (Fig. 2). Alterations that have been reported include effacement of foot processes, displace-

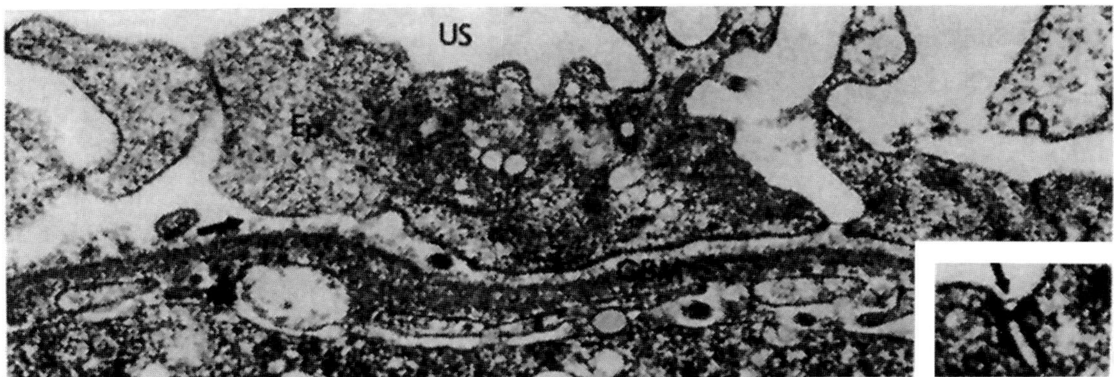

FIG. 2. Representative podocyte alterations in complement-independent nephrotoxic nephritis. Note the effacement and partial detachment *(arrow)* of foot processes, as well as vacuolization of the cytoplasm and condensation of the cytoskeleton. Some slit diaphragms are disrupted or displaced, or replaced with occluding junctions *(inset arrow)*. The endothelial cell is also vacuolated and swollen. US, urinary space; Ep, visceral epithelial cell (podocyte); GBM, glomerular basement membrane En, endothelial cell. Original magnification, ×33,600; inset, ×72,300. Reprinted with permission (34).

ment of the slit-diaphragm and formation of occluding junctions, condensation of the cytoskeleton, microvillous transformation of the apical plasma membrane, vacuolization of the cytoplasm, and focal detachment of foot processes from the basement membrane (10,18,34). In some cases there is also endothelial swelling and detachment. No electron-dense immune deposits are seen in the heterologous phase, but small confluent densities along the GBM interface with epithelial and endothelial cells were noted after passive augmentation of the autologous phase with anti-IgG (35). This may provide a clue that the major nephritogenic antigens are located at these sites.

Characteristics of NTS

Although nephrotoxic nephritis has long been considered an experimental model of anti-GBM nephritis (1), there is still scant evidence that the complement-independent form of injury, induced by heterologous polyclonal NTS, is the result of antibodies reacting with the Goodpasture antigen. In fact, existing data suggest that this form of injury may be due to reactivity with glomerular cell surface antigens.

NTS is usually produced by immunizing sheep, rabbits, or other animals with a crude preparation of glomeruli from an experimental animal (typically rat, rabbit, or guinea pig) (36). The resulting antiserum produces linear staining of the glomerular capillary wall in vitro on normal kidney, and the deposits that form in vivo after injection into experimental animals closely resemble the linear staining pattern seen in human anti-GBM nephritis. The donor animals (particularly sheep and guinea pigs) often develop a severe and sometimes fatal autoimmune nephritis with similar deposits (15,37). Although antibodies to the sheep equivalent of the Goodpasture antigen can be eluted from the kidneys of sheep immunized with purified GBM (38), when NTS is produced with a crude glomerular preparation, the resulting antiserum is polyspecific. Reactivity to the NC1 domain of the $\alpha3$ chain of type IV collagen, the site of the Goodpasture antigen in humans (39), is detectable in such antisera (Kalluri and Salant, unpublished data, 1994), but it is only one of several antibody specificities, and not necessarily the predominant one that causes disease in recipients of the antiserum.

Our own experience with antirat NTS obtained from different sheep over several years exemplifies several of these features. These antisera resemble closely those described by Cochrane and Henson, who found that the non–complement-fixing $\gamma2$ subclass of sheep NTS was capable of inducing severe proteinuria in rabbits (1,13). Although this complement-independent injury requires higher doses of antiserum than does the complement-dependent lesion (1), we have found that as little as 5 mg of $\gamma2$ sheep NTS induces significant proteinuria without complement deposits in adult rats (Fig. 1) (40). This dose is equivalent to about 35 μg of glomerular bound antibody per kidney (35). In complement-depleted rats, 20 mg of the unfractionated IgG produced 140 ± 45 mg urine protein/24 h (19), which is similar to the dose of 289 μg "kidney-fixing antibody" found to cause proteinuria in neutrophil-depleted rats, and somewhat higher than the dose in complement- and neutrophil-replete rats (7). In this regard, guinea pigs are much more sensitive to complement-independent injury and develop severe proteinuria with only 15 μg of antibody in each kidney (17).

Potential Nephritogenic Antigens

GBM Components

The primary nephritogenic target of NTS has not yet been definitively established. The sheep $\gamma2$ NTS produced in our laboratory has detectable reactivity with the GBM matrix components laminin and type IV collagen by enzyme-linked immunosorbent assay (ELISA), although the titer is low. It has 400-fold less reactivity to purified laminin than sheep antilaminin antiserum, an antiserum that does not, in itself, cause heterologous phase proteinuria (29,40,41). Reactivity to the NC1 domain of the $\alpha3$ chain of type IV collagen is present (mean 0.6 ELISA units) at an NTS dilution of 1:50 (Kalluri and Salant, unpublished observations). Although this is significantly higher than the reactivity to the NC1 of other alpha chains of type IV collagen (mean 0.2–0.35 ELISA units; baseline 0.2 ELISA units), it is relatively low by comparison with the titer of this antiserum as measured by indirect immunofluorescence on normal rat kidney (1:1,000) and on cultured glomerular epithelial cells (1:1,000) (40).

Integrins

In seeking alternative glomerular target antigens for NTS, we found immunostaining of basal plasma membrane antigens of glomerular epithelial cells in culture and evidence of strong neutralizing reactivity against a $\beta1$ integrin that is functionally and immunochemically similar to the fibronectin receptor (FnR) and is most likely the $\alpha3\beta1$ integrin (40,42). Thus, sheep $\gamma2$ NTS identifies two glomerular cell membrane antigens of 118 and 135 to 140 kDa on Western blot analysis (Fig. 3). These proteins also are expressed on rat epithelial cells in culture, and antibodies to them can be eluted from glomerular deposits formed in vivo by injecting rats with NTS (Fig. 4) (40). Identity with the $\beta1$ integrin was established by coprecipitation studies with a monospecific anti-FnR antibody and by the profile of adhesion inhibition to collagen, laminin, and fibronectin (40,42). It has not yet been established if this reactivity is responsi-

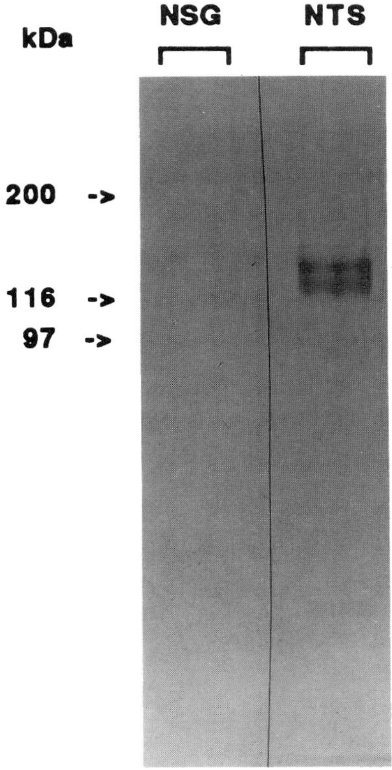

FIG. 3. Western blot analysis of rat glomerular cell membrane proteins with sheep antirat NTS. A cell membrane fraction was prepared from isolated rat glomeruli and equal amounts of solubilized protein per lane (25 μg) were resolved by SDS-PAGE (7.5%) under reducing conditions. Western blotting was performed with 15 μg/ml of the same fraction of NTS as that used to induce proteinuria in Fig. 1. An equal concentration of normal sheep globulin (NSG) served as a negative control. The symbols on the left represent molecular size markers. Note the pair of protein bands specifically identified by NTS at about 118 and 140 kDa. Reprinted with permission (40).

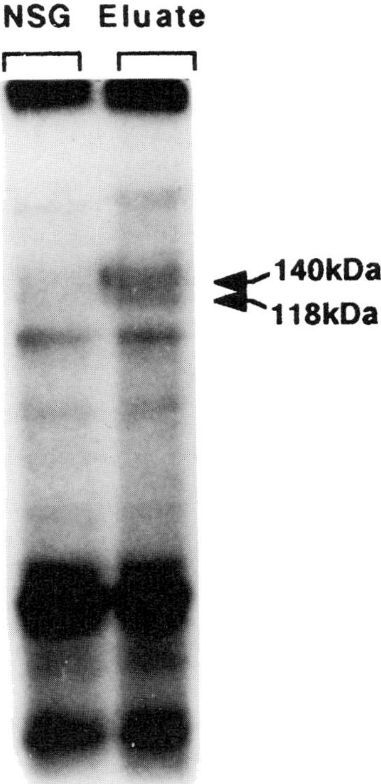

FIG. 4. Autoradiograph of ^{125}I-labeled glomerular epithelial cell membrane proteins immunoprecipitated with IgG eluted from the glomeruli of rats injected with sheep antirat NTS. Cultured rat glomerular epithelial cells were surface labeled with ^{125}I, solubilized, and subjected to immunoprecipitation with pooled IgG (55 μg) that had been acid eluted from the glomeruli of rats injected with a nephritogenic dose of NTS or normal sheep globulin (NSG). A pair of proteins (118 and 140 kDa) was specifically precipitated by the NTS eluate. Modified and reprinted with permission (40).

ble for the nephritogenic effects of NTS; however, preliminary studies suggest that absorption of NTS with GBM and attached basolateral cell membranes reduces both anti-integrin reactivity and proteinuria, whereas absorption with GBM alone reduces neither (O'Meara and Salant, unpublished observations).

These findings are not at all surprising when one considers that NTS is produced by immunization with a mixed preparation of matrix and cell membrane proteins. Indeed, monoclonal dissection of the immune response of mice immunized in this fashion has uncovered a wide array of antibody specificities, including many that react with known and novel cell surface antigens, as well as the predicted reactivity to various extracellular matrix proteins (23,25). Two of the cellular targets identified in this way, namely DPPIV and the antigen recognized by mAb 5-1-6, cause substantial complement-independent proteinuria and are discussed in more detail below. Interestingly, our sheep NTS does not appear to have significant reactivity to either DPPIV or the 51-kDa antigen identified by mAb 5-1-6 (40).

Mediation of Injury in Complement-Independent Nephrotoxic Nephritis

It is still unknown how injury in complement-independent nephrotoxic nephritis is mediated. Classical vasoactive inflammatory mediators, such as kinins, histamine and serotonin, prostanoids, and the coagulation system, were excluded from consideration with pharmacologic blockers (17,18). Furthermore, studies in the isolated perfused kidney model established that local rather than systemic factors are operative (19). Thus, rat kidneys perfused in vitro with a dose of sheep NTS that causes complement-independent proteinuria in vivo developed severe albuminuria in the complete absence of leukocytes, complement, or other known inflammatory mediators (Fig. 5).

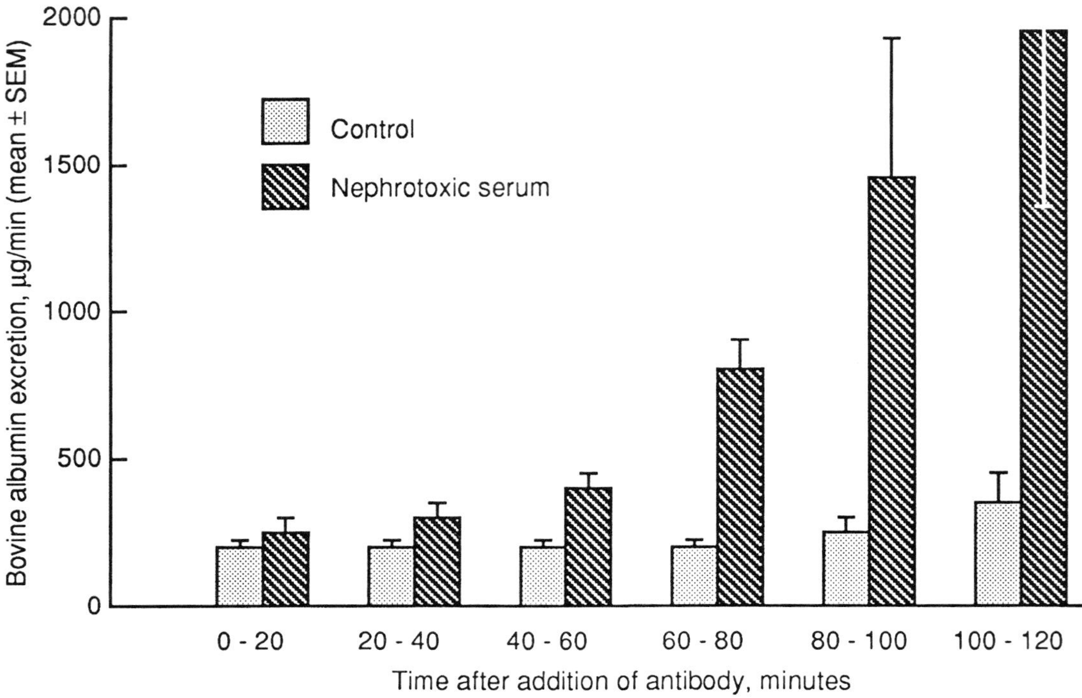

FIG. 5. Urinary excretion of bovine serum albumin by isolated rat kidneys perfused in vitro with physiologic buffer containing BSA and either sheep antirat NTS IgG or nonantibody IgG (control). Experimental values are significantly greater than controls after 60 min. Redrawn and reprinted with permission (19).

To date, the only agents known to play a role in antibody-mediated proteinuria are the cysteine proteinases cathepsins B and L (43) (see Chapter 19 for discussion of proteases). Purified cathepsins B and L have been found capable of degrading GBM in vitro (44,45), and isolated rat glomeruli contain cysteine proteinases with similar activity (46). More significantly, Baricos et al. showed that specific inhibitors of cysteine proteinases, E-64 and Ep-475, significantly reduced the level of proteinuria by about 45% in a complement- and neutrophil-independent model of nephrotoxic nephritis in rats (47). This effect was accompanied by a marked decline in the glomerular activity of cathepsins B and L (47). Moreover, a specific cathepsin L inhibitor, Z-Phe-Tyr(O-t-butyl)CHN_2, reduced proteinuria by 56% and cortical cathepsin L activity by 86% without any change in cathepsin B activity (43).

It is informative to review certain earlier studies of nephrotoxic nephritis in light of these findings and what is now known about GBM composition. Thus, Hawkins and Cochrane showed that neutrophil-dependent injury in rabbits caused nonselective proteinuria with the appearance of GBM fragments and neutrophil cathepsins in the urine, whereas neutrophil-independent injury induced a more selective proteinuria without GBM fragments or proteases in the urine (14). Furthermore, Gang and Kalant noted a loss of "lipid phosphorous from the GBM" in the heterologous phase of rat nephrotoxic nephritis without any change in hexosamine or hydroxyproline content (48). They further noted that the initial change in glomerular permeability and loss of lipid phosphorous occurred before neutrophil infiltration (49). Considering the method used to prepare the GBM for analysis in the latter studies (48,49) and the fact that the GBM does not normally contain phospholipids, it is likely that hydrolysis of phospholipids in adherent cell membranes explains the loss of lipid phosphorous. Furthermore, the absence of change in hexosamine and hydroxyproline content suggests that the proteoglycan and collagenous components of the GBM remained relatively intact, although these techniques are relatively insensitive to small changes. Nonetheless, when taken together these studies suggest that neutrophil-dependent injury causes substantial GBM degradation (likely from neutrophil-derived proteinases), but neutrophil-independent proteinuria may be due to cell membrane damage.

It is presently not understood how acid (cysteine) proteinases operate in nephrotoxic nephritis. If GBM degradation is the mechanism of action, it is conceivable that they act in a relatively acidic microenvironment at the GBM–cell interface. Alternatively, the mechanism could be an indirect one through activation of latent GBM-degrading neutral metalloproteinases in an acidic intracellular compartment. Whatever the mechanism and site of action, the stimulus for cysteine proteinase activity seems most likely to be the result of antibody reacting with a cell surface constituent rather than an extracellular matrix component. For example, cross-linking of integrins or other as yet undefined antigens on the podocyte basal membranes by antibodies in NTS might evoke a signal for the release of proteinases (50,51). This could lead to limited digestion of the matrix components to which the integrins are anchored, which might then disrupt the normal cell–matrix relationship and cause foot process effacement or even detachment without there being substantial degradation of the GBM (52).

NEPHROPATHY INDUCED BY F(AB′)$_2$ AND FAB′ FRAGMENTS OF ANTI-FX1A

Characteristics of the Model

Rats injected with F(ab′)$_2$ or Fab′ fragments of sheep anti-Fx1A develop immediate and transient proteinuria without complement fixation or leukocyte influx in glomeruli (20). This contrasts with the delayed onset of complement C5b-9–mediated proteinuria in passive Heymann nephritis induced by anti-Fx1A IgG (Fig. 6) (53–56). Immunofluorescence microscopy shows a finely granular glomerular capillary wall distribution of heterologous IgG and absent complement deposits. Glomerular histology is normal on light microscopy, and small subepithelial immune deposits are seen on electron microscopy (Fig. 7) (20). Colloidal gold staining for glomerular polyanion is normal, suggesting that the glomerular charge barrier is not grossly disrupted.

Proteinuria in passive Heymann nephritis occurs 4 to 5 days after the injection of complement-fixing anti-Fx1A IgG once sufficient antibody has been deposited in glomeruli to activate complement (approximately 45 μg IgG per kidney), to assemble the membrane attack complex, and to injure the glomerular epithelial cells on whose surface the nephritogenic antigens reside (53,54,57) (see Chapters 9, 18 and 35). Anti-Fx1A F(ab′)$_2$ and Fab′ fragments, on the other hand, deposit rapidly in glomeruli and induce proteinuria when a substantially lower level of antibody has accumulated. Antibody binding, measured after 24 h in glomeruli isolated from individual rats injected with equimolar nephritogenic doses of labeled anti-Fx1A IgG, F(ab′)$_2$, and Fab′ was defined as follows: IgG, 0.17%; F(ab′)$_2$, 0.11%; and Fab′, 0.03% of the administered dose (20).

With regard to the mechanism of proteinuria induced by anti-Fx1A antibody fragments, it is interesting to note that recent studies in C6-deficient PVG/c$^-$ rats suggest that active Heymann nephritis, induced by immunization with Fx1A, also may be mediated by antibody alone in some rat strains (58). This observation is similar to that of complement- and leukocyte-independent proteinuria in another rat model of immune complex nephritis induced with a cationized exogenous antigen (59).

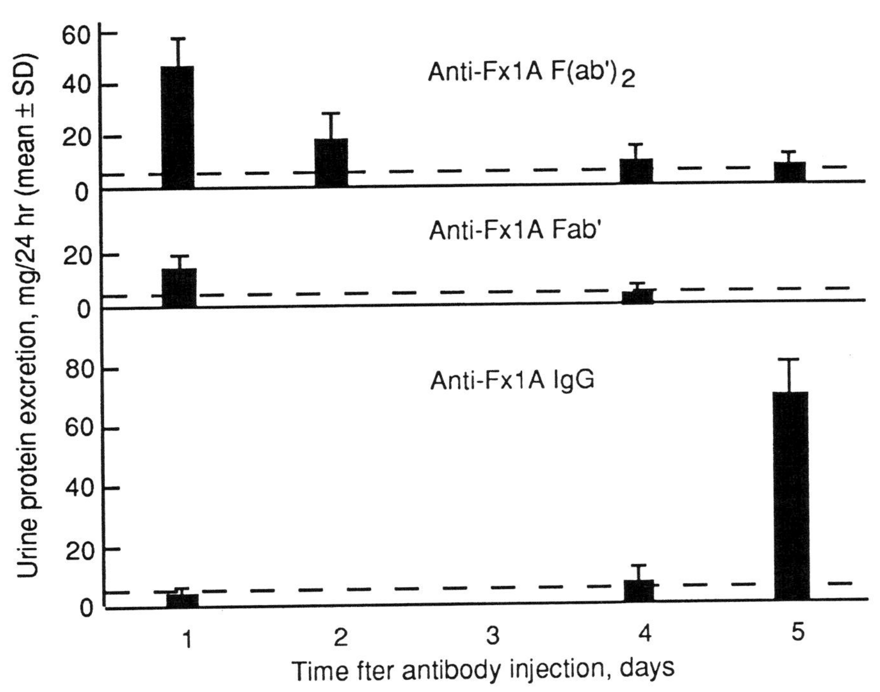

FIG. 6. Proteinuria induced in rats by injecting anti-Fx1A F(ab′)$_2$ and Fab′ fragments, compared with that caused by intact anti-Fx1A IgG (n = 5–16 per time point). The dashed horizontal line indicates the upper 99% confidence interval of 20 normal age-matched rats. Redrawn with permission (20).

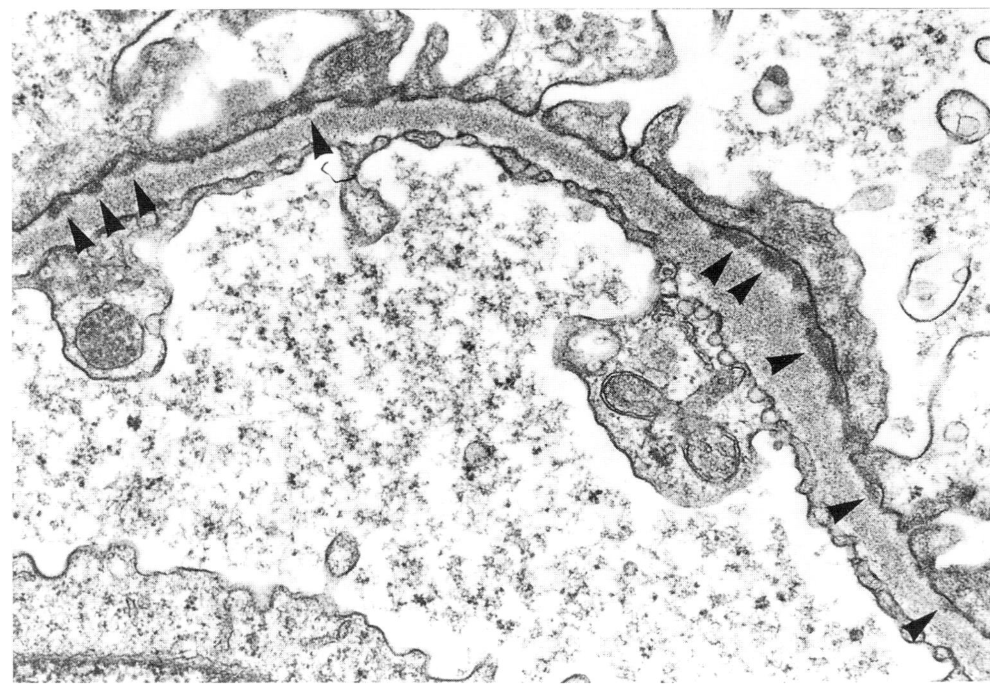

FIG. 7. Electron micrograph obtained 24 h after an injection of anti-Fx1A F(ab′)$_2$. Several small subepithelial electron-dense deposits are present *(arrowheads)* underlying focal areas of podocyte foot process effacement. Original magnification ×31,500. Reprinted with permission (20).

Potential Nephritogenic Antigens

The mechanism of proteinuria induced by anti-Fx1A antibody fragments and the nephritogenic antigens responsible for injury are unknown, but several possibilities merit consideration. Heterologous anti-Fx1A is produced by immunization with a rat renal tubular fraction enriched in proximal tubular brush borders (Fx1A). Fx1A contains several antigens that are also expressed on rat glomerular cell membranes, particularly those of podocytes. The best defined is gp330/megalin, the so-called Heymann nephritis antigen (60,61) (see Chapter 9 for detailed discussion). Antibodies to gp330 and possibly its 39- to 44-kDa receptor-associated protein (62) appear to be most important for antigen redistribution on the podocyte cell surface, shedding of antigen-antibody complexes, and formation of subepithelial immune deposits in passive Heymann nephritis (63). Glycoprotein 330 also may serve as a nonintegrin matrix receptor (64). However, anti-gp330 antibodies do not appear capable of causing proteinuria alone, even when immunopurified from a known nephritogenic preparation of anti-Fx1A (65). Antibodies specific for other antigens contained within Fx1A are necessary to induce substantial proteinuria. This happens when anti-gp330 is accompanied by antibodies to membrane glycolipids present in the brush border fraction. These antiglycolipid antibodies are not capable of depositing in vivo when given alone, but appear to codeposit with anti-gp330, activate complement, and thereby induce proteinuria (65). Thus, it seems that proteinuria in anti-Fx1A F(ab′)$_2$ nephropathy is not readily explained by reactivity to the Heymann nephritis complex and/or reactivity to glycolipid.

Anti-Fx1A also contains significant reactivity to DPPIV, an established target of complement-independent proteinuria. The major difference between the glomerular lesions induced by anti-Fx1A antibody fragments and anti-DPPIV is that electron-dense subepithelial immune deposits are found with the former (Fig. 7) but are not seen when pure anti-DPPIV antibodies are injected (Figs. 8,9) (21,22). It is possible, if not likely, that the subepithelial immune deposits seen with anti-Fx1A antibody fragments are due to reactivity with the Heymann nephritis antigen complex but that the immediate complement-independent proteinuria is due to anti-DPPIV.

Adler also has demonstrated considerable anti-integrin activity in anti-Fx1A (66). The reactivity is directed at the extracellular domain of $\alpha3\beta1$ integrin and is capable of inhibiting glomerular epithelial cell adhesion to extracellular matrix components in vitro (66), similar to that found in NTS (40). Although anti-integrin antibodies have not yet been shown to induce proteinuria in vivo, disruption of the normal relationship between podocytes and the GBM is another potential mechanism whereby anti-Fx1A antibody fragments

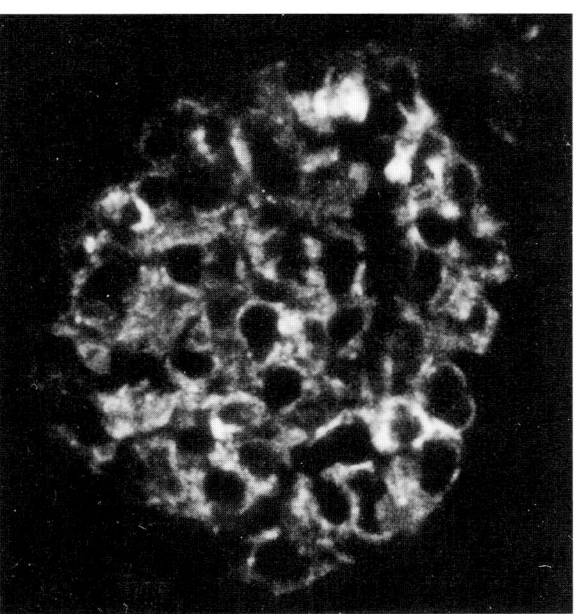

FIG. 8. Representative immunofluorescent micrograph of a rat glomerulus stained for rabbit IgG 24 h after the injection of rabbit anti-DPPIV. Note the diffuse glomerular capillary wall staining. Original magnification ×400. Reprinted with permission (77).

might alter glomerular permeability (67). The possibility that large subepithelial immune deposits cause mechanical distortion of podocyte morphology and displacement of the slit diaphram also has been proposed as a mechanism to account for proteinuria in C6-deficient Heymann nephritic rats (58). Although podocyte stimulation by IgG–Fc receptor interactions and consequent lipid mediator release has been offered as an explanation of complement-independent proteinuria induced by cationized antigen (59), this cannot account for the injury induced by anti-Fx1A Fab′ and $F(ab)'_2$ fragments. Finally, Quigg has shown that sheep antirat Fx1A contains activity that neutralizes glomerular epithelial cell surface regulatory activity of the alternate complement pathway (68). Although this could potentially promote spontaneous activation of the alternate pathway of complement in the vicinity of the glomerular epithelial cell, there is no concrete evidence that this mechanism is at work in anti-Fx1A $F(ab')_2$ nephropathy because of the complete absence of C3 in glomeruli.

Thus, the most promising candidate antigen in anti-Fx1A $F(ab')_2$ nephropathy appears to be DPPIV, although a role for integrins has not been excluded. The definitive experiments—to determine if proteinuria is abolished by depleting anti-Fx1A $F(ab')_2$ fragments of anti-DPP IV or anti-integrin reactivity, or to establish if monospecific anti-β1 integrin antibodies induce proteinuria—have not been reported to date.

PROTEINURIA INDUCED BY ANTI-DPPIV ANTIBODY

DPPIV

DPPIV, also known as gp90 (69,70), gp108 (21), SGP115/107 (24), and CD26 (71), is a cell membrane–bound enzyme that cleaves N-terminal dipeptides from polypeptides primarily when the second residue is proline or alanine (72). Most of its protein mass, including the catalytic moiety, protrudes on the extracellular side (73,74). It is predominantly expressed on the brush border membranes of both renal proximal tubules and intestinal microvilli, but is widely distributed in various tissues and cells in mammals. In glomeruli of rats and mice, DPPIV is detected on the plasma membranes of glomerular endothelial and epithelial cells (75).

DPPIV has been known as one of the major antigens in Fx1A, a renal tubular membrane fraction responsible for the induction of Heymann nephritis (see Chapters 9 and 35). Anti-DPPIV antibody is contained in antirat Fx1A antiserum (21), the administration of which induces passive Heymann nephritis (36). Because anti-DPPIV antibody shows proteinuria-inducing activity as described below, it was once considered a possibility that anti-DPPIV antibody is necessary to fully induce passive Heymann nephritis. However, subsequent studies demonstrated that passive Heymann nephritis can be induced in DPPIV-deficient rats (22), indicating that DPPIV is not essential for induction of the disease.

Characteristics of the Model

Administration of polyclonal antibody raised against DPPIV induces acute and transient proteinuria in rats (21, 76,77). The injected antibody is immediately deposited along glomerular capillary walls, peaking at 4 to 8 h (Fig. 8). It first binds to plasma membranes of glomerular endothelial cells and then to those of glomerular epithelial cells (76; Natori, unpublished observation). In parallel with its early deposition in glomeruli, abnormal urinary protein appears within 8 h. At 24 h or later, when massive proteinuria is observed, the deposition of the antibody also is seen on brush border membranes of proximal tubules. At no time is there any deposition of complement in glomeruli, increase in glomerular cellularity, or interstitial inflammation. Within 4 to 8 h of antibody injection, ultrastructural analysis demonstrates endothelial swelling, wrinkling of the GBM, and focal effacement of epithelial foot processes. After 24 h, at the height of proteinuria, diffuse damage of glomerular epithelial cells is evident, including more extensive effacement of foot processes, formation of numerous apical microvilli and vesicles, vacuolation of the cytoplasm, and appearance of occluding junctions (Fig. 9). No electron-

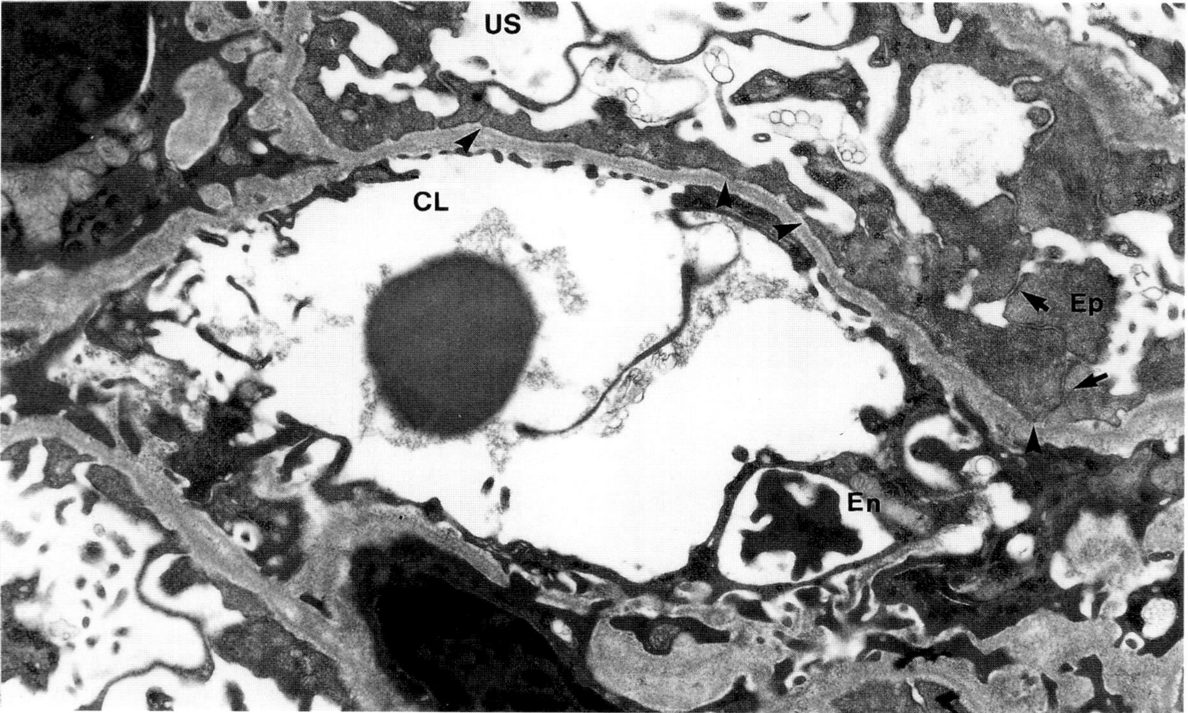

FIG. 9. Representative electron micrograph of a rat glomerulus 24 h after the injection of rabbit anti-DPPIV. Note the diffuse damage of glomerular epithelial cells and swelling of endothelial cells. Extensive effacement of foot processes is present *(between arrowheads),* and there are numerous epithelial apical microvilli and vesicles, cytoplasmic vacuoles, and newly formed occluding junctions *(arrows).* No electron dense deposits are seen either in glomerular capillary walls or mesangial areas. US, urinary space; Ep, visceral epithelial cell; En, endothelial cell; CL, capillary lumen. Original magnification × 17,000.

dense deposits are seen either in glomerular capillary walls or mesangial areas.

Mendrick et al. have demonstrated that a monoclonal anti-DPPIV antibody (K9/9) induces proteinuria in rats given Freund's complete adjuvant (24). As in rats injected with the polyclonal antibody, structural changes of glomerular epithelial cells are prominent, but no deposition of complement or increase of glomerular cellularity is seen. Interestingly, other anti-DPPIV mAbs (K35/4 and K35/64) similarly bind to glomeruli but do not induce proteinuria (78). This indicates the presence of a nephritogenic epitope within the DPPIV molecule that is recognized by K9/9 but not the other mAbs.

DPPIV in Murine Graft-Versus-Host Disease

It also has been suggested that anti-DPPIV antibodies are involved in the pathogenesis of the glomerular lesion of murine chronic graft-versus-host (GvH) disease, a model for human systemic lupus erythematosus (79). GvH is induced by injection of lymphocytes of DBA/2 strain into (C57BL10×DBA/2)F1 hybrid mice. This results in the production and glomerular deposition of autoantibodies accompanied by severe immune complex glomerulonephritis. Autoantibodies eluted from the glomeruli were found to be directed to several antigens, among which were laminin and DPPIV (80). In addition, serum-derived antibodies that had been affinity purified with Fx1A induced subepithelial immune complex formation and proteinuria in naive mice (80). These investigators also showed that a decrease and redistribution of glomerular DPPIV occurs simultaneously with the development of albuminuria in GvH nephritis, whereas other enzymes such as 5′ nucleotidase and adenosine triphosphatase remain stable (81). Although these results suggest that DPPIV may play an important role in the induction of proteinuria in this model, other autoantibodies also may contribute. Furthermore, it has not been determined if the glomerular injury is purely antibody dependent or if other mediators are involved.

Potential Mechanisms of Injury

DPPIV is not only a hydrolase of polypeptides but a nonintegrin receptor for extracellular matrix. It binds to extracellular matrix components such as collagen and fibronectin in vitro (82–85), and anti-DPPIV antibody and an inhibitor of DPPIV enzyme activity interfere with the spreading of fibroblasts and hepatocytes in culture (86). Although the adhesive activity of DPPIV has not yet been demonstrated in glomerular cells, it is conceivable that the mechanism of anti-DPPIV–induced proteinuria involves altered podocyte attachment to GBM by competitive inhibition of DPPIV binding to collagen or other extracellular matrix components. Consistent with this hypothesis are the observations that foot process effacement is pronounced after anti-DPPIV injection (Fig. 9) and that rats injected with anti-DPPIV mAb, K9/9, exhibit podocyte detachment (24).

DPPIV also is located on the cell surface of subpopulations of T- and B-lymphocytes and is known to be involved in the activation and proliferation of T-lymphocytes (87). Some anti-DPPIV mAbs stimulate T-lymphocyte proliferation in humans (71), mice (88), and rats (89), whereas specific DPPIV inhibitors and polyclonal anti-DPPIV antibody inhibit the proliferation of human T-lymphocytes (90). There is presently no direct evidence linking the lymphoproliferative and nephritogenic properties of anti-DPPIV, but it is noteworthy that Freund's complete adjuvant is essential for the induction of proteinuria by monoclonal anti-DPPIV, K9/9 (24). This raises the possibility that the activation of macrophages and/or lymphocytes may play some indirect role in the glomerular injury. It also has been suggested that reactivity of anti-DPPIV autoantibodies with DPPIV expressed on lymphocytes may be involved in the pathogenesis of murine GvH disease (81).

Nephropathy Due to Aminopeptidase A

Another hydrolase, aminopeptidase A (APA), has nephritogenic effects similar to those of DPPIV and a similarly wide distribution. Assmann et al. have shown that monoclonal anti-APA induces proteinuria when injected into mice (91). At least in the early phase, this proteinuria is also complement and leukocyte independent (91). APA is localized on the plasma membranes of glomerular epithelial cells as well as on tubular brush border membranes. It is also present in B-lymphocyte progenitors and is reported to be similar to DPPIV in structure, localization, and function (87). There is no information on the matrix adhesive activity of APA.

DPPIV in Human Kidney Diseases

DPPIV is not detected in normal human glomeruli by immunohistology, but it has been found along glomerular capillary walls in a proportion of patients with various types of primary and secondary glomerular diseases (92). The significance of this finding has not been established. In addition, increased urinary excretion of DPPIV has been reported in glomerular and tubulointerstitial diseases, perhaps as a result of tubular injury (93). In culture, DPPIV is found in human glomerular epithelial cells, and the expression is enhanced by treatment with interferon-γ (94). Thus, there is presently no evidence that DPPIV or APA are directly involved as antigenic targets in human glomerular diseases. On the other hand, the animal models indicate that these molecules are involved in the normal permselective function of the glomerular capillary wall. In addition, the data on DPPIV from humans suggests that its expression may be upregulated in proteinuric diseases or that it may be incorporated during the formation of immune deposits.

NEPHROPATHY INDUCED BY MONOCLONAL ANTIBODY 5-1-6

Characteristics of mAb 5-1-6 and Its Target Antigen

A remarkable model of antibody-dependent proteinuria is that induced by mAb 5-1-6, a murine mAb that identifies a plasma membrane protein on rat glomerular epithelial cells. The mAb was produced by immunizing BALB/C mice with collagenase-digested glomeruli from Wistar rats, and it is an IgG1 kappa antibody with a pI of 5.7 (25). Immunoprecipitation of Nonidet P40-solubilized, ^{125}I surface-labeled rat glomeruli followed by sodium dodecyl sulfate polyacrylamide gel electrophoresis (SDS-PAGE) shows that the molecular weight of the target antigen is about 51 kDa, hence the designation p51. The epitope of p51 identified by mAb 5-1-6 is highly organ and species specific in that reactivity is found only in rat glomeruli. Metabolic labeling studies have shown that p51 is predominantly synthesized during glomerular development (Fig. 10) and is expressed exclusively on the basolateral plasma membrane of developing podocytes from the time they first become distinguishable in the S-shaped body (Fig. 11) (95). As the podocytes mature, mAb 5-1-6 is seen on immunoelectron microscopy to decorate the slit diaphragm and adjacent foot process plasma membrane (Fig. 12). Staining of adult rat kidney sections with mAb 5-1-6 shows immunoperoxidase reaction product on the surface of foot processes, and immunogold particles appear to be concentrated on the slit diaphragm (25). This suggests that p51 is a component of the slit diaphragm or its connections to the podocyte plasma membrane, an observation that may have important bearing on its role as a target of antibody-induced glomerular injury.

Features of mAb 5-1-6–Induced Renal Injury

As illustrated in Fig. 13, a single intravenous injection of mAb 5-1-6 causes severe proteinuria in susceptible rats. No histologic abnormalities are evident on light microscopy, and partial retraction of glomerular epithelial foot processes is the only abnormality observed at the ultrastructural level. Rat immunoglobulins and C3 are not detected in glomeruli during the proteinuric phase (25). There is

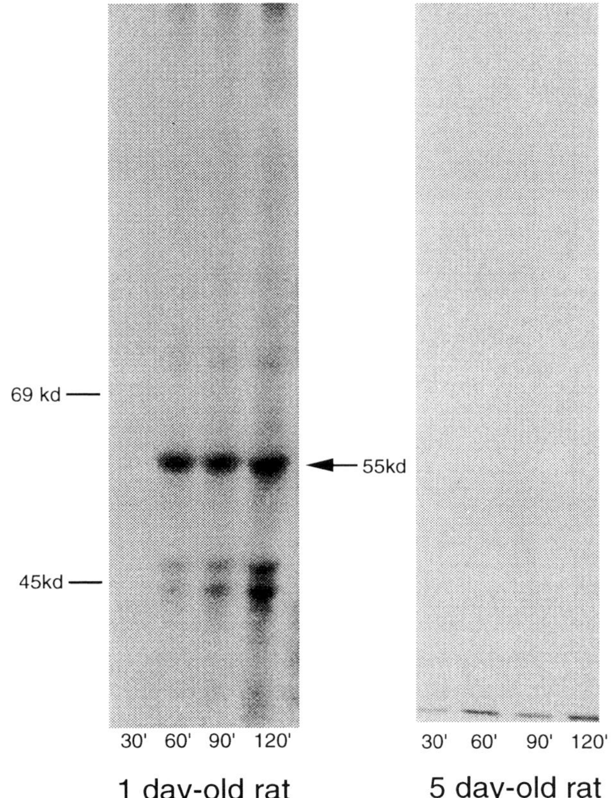

FIG. 10. Immunoprecipitation of glomerular proteins with mAb 5-1-6. Isolated glomeruli from 1-day-old and 5-day-old rats were pulse labeled with [^{35}S]-methionine for 30, 60, 90, 120 min and immunoprecipitated with mAb 5-1-6. A clear band of 55 kDa and two weaker bands of 43 and 46 kDa were detected in 1-day-old rat glomeruli. No bands were detected in 5-day-old rat glomeruli. Reprinted with permission (95).

reduced ruthenium red staining of anionic sites and increased permeation of endogenous globulin, as shown by in situ immunogold labeling of rat albumin and globulin in the glomeruli of drip-fixed kidneys of Munich-Wistar rats (96). Although this suggests that both the charge barrier in the outer zone of the GBM and the size barrier may be disturbed by mAb 5-1-6, this has not been examined functionally by macromolecular clearance studies.

In addition to altering glomerular permselectivity, mAb 5-1-6 induces marked changes in hydraulic conductivity and glomerular hemodynamics. Thus, within 2 h of antibody injection, there is a 50% decrease in the glomerular ultrafiltration coefficient followed by a return to almost control levels after 24 h (97). Interestingly, single-nephron glomerular filtration and plasma flow rates are unchanged after 2 h and increase after 24 h to values that are higher than normal. As yet, the structural and/or functional basis for these changes has not been defined.

Kinetics of Glomerular Antibody and p51 after mAb 5-1-6 Injection

Concomitant with the appearance and resolution of proteinuria, there are notable changes in the in vivo localization of injected mAb 5-1-6 and in the amount, and perhaps distribution, of p51. The immunofluorescence binding pattern of injected mAb 5-1-6 2 h after injection is linear to finely granular (Fig. 14), similar to what is seen in tissue sections incubated with the antibody in vitro (25). Within several days of antibody injection, the staining shifts to a more coarsely granular pattern (Fig. 14) followed by a decrease in the size and intensity of the fluorescent granules by about 2 weeks. On immunoelectron microscopy, the localization of reaction product 2 h after antibody injection is similar to that seen in vitro, but after 48 h, labeling is seen on the urinary surface of the foot processes (98). Over the course of several days, there is progressive uptake of antibody into multivesicular bodies in glomerular epithelial cells and a decrease in staining of the surface of the foot processes, which corresponds to the change in immunofluorescent staining pattern and intensity. Similarly, immunolocalization of p51 with biotinylated mAb 5-1-6 followed by avidin-FITC demonstrates progressively

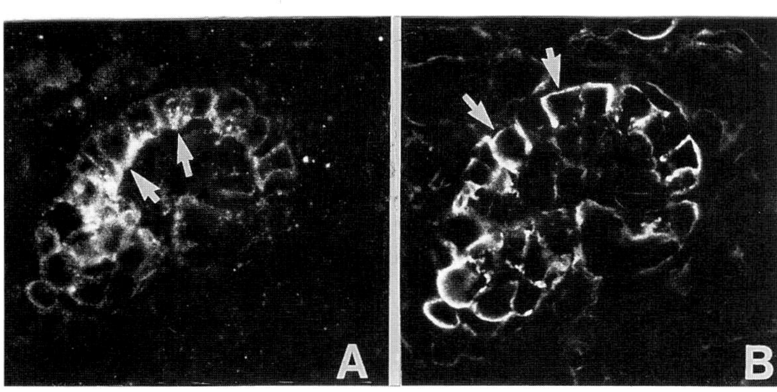

FIG. 11. Localization of p51 and podocalyxin in a developing glomerulus at the early capillary loop stage. A cortical slice of periodate-lysine-paraformaldehyde–fixed 1-day-old rat kidney was sectioned at 5 μm and the same section was stained with mAb 5-1-6 (**A**) and rabbit antipodocalyxin (**B**), and donkey antimouse–CY3 and goat antirabbit–FITC secondary antibodies. In regions where the glomeruli were cut in cross-section, p51 and podocalyxin were detected on opposite surfaces of the epithelial cells. In (**A**) the *arrows* indicate basolateral staining of p51, and in (**B**) they point to apical and lateral staining for podocalyxin in the same developing podocytes. Original magnification ×400. (Data from Salant DJ, Kawachi H, Shimizu F, Brown D, unpublished observation 1995; see also ref. 95.)

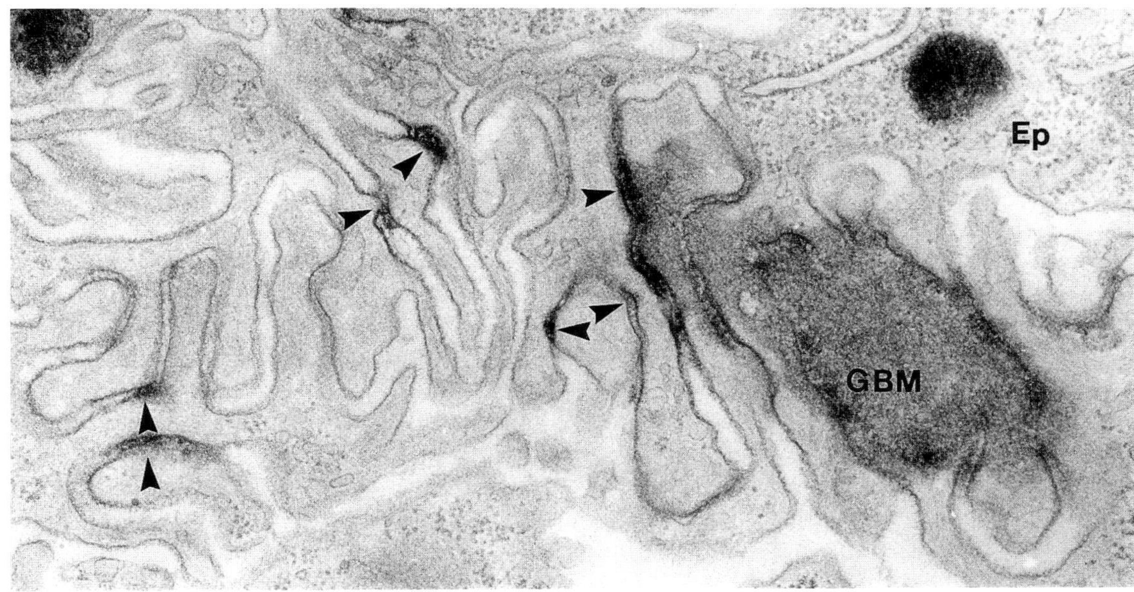

FIG. 12. Immunoperoxidase localization of p51 in the maturing glomerulus in a neonatal rat kidney as determined by sequential injections of mAb 5-1-6 and peroxidase-labeled antimouse IgG. This tangential section of a relatively mature glomerulus shows the formation of interdigitating foot processes with p51 restricted to the podocyte plasma membrane lining the slit pores and the intervening slit diaphragms *(arrows)*. (Original magnification ×34,500.) (Data from Kawachi H, Shimizu F, Abrahamson DR, St. John PL, Salant DJ, unpublished observation, 1995; see also ref. 95.)

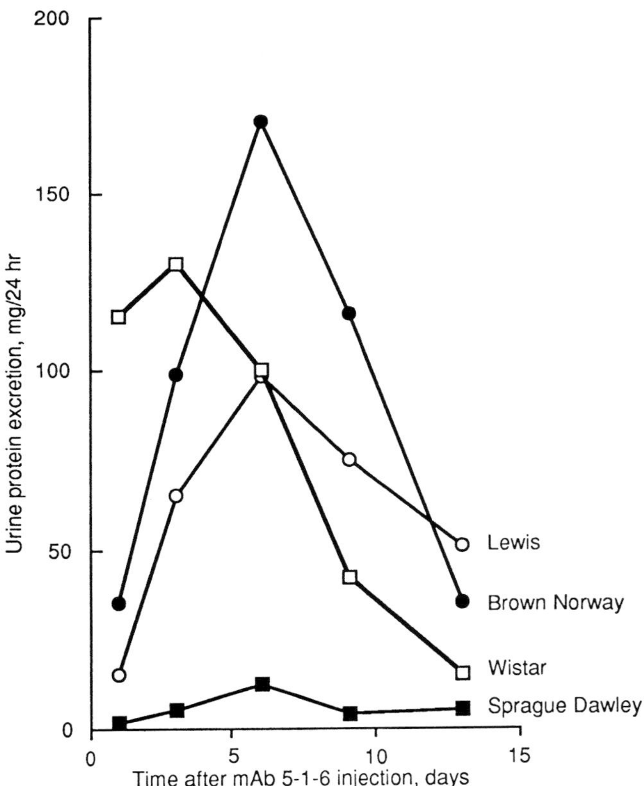

FIG. 13. Susceptibility of different rat strains to the proteinuric effect of mAb 5-1-6. The mean value of 24-h urine protein induced by injecting 5 mg of the mAb is shown. Lewis, Brown Norway, and Wistar rats developed severe proteinuria while Sprague-Dawley rats were resistant to this relatively large dose. Redrawn with permission (102).

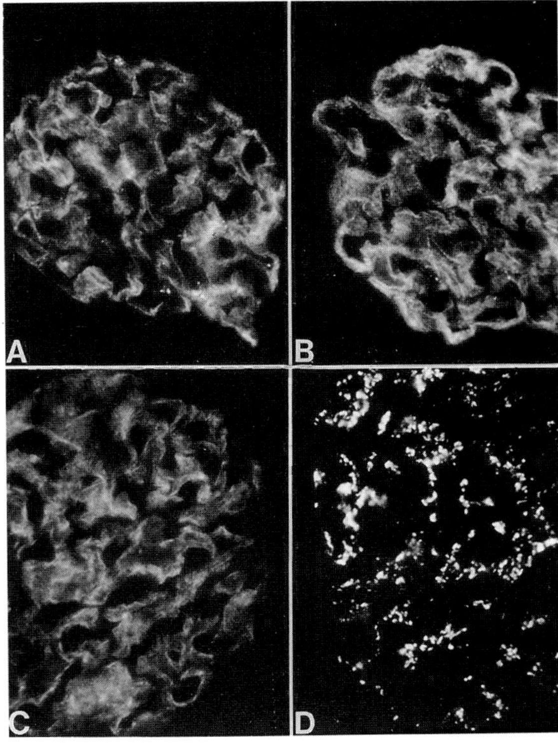

FIG. 14. Direct immunofluorescence with antimouse IgG-FITC of representative glomeruli from Sprague-Dawley (**A and C**) and Lewis (**B and D**) rats injected with mAb 5-1-6. After 2 h (**A and B**), both strains exhibit an interrupted linear staining pattern. After 6 days (**C and D**), this shifted to a more clustered pattern in Lewis (**D**) but remain unchanged in Sprague-Dawley (**C**) rats. Original magnification ×400. Reproduced with permission (102).

reduced immunoreactive antigen with time after injection of antibody. Recovery of p51 immunoreactivity is observed about 30 days later (99).

In vivo kinetics of the injected mAb 5-1-6 and p51 also have been examined quantitatively with ^{125}I-labeled antibody (100). The amount of total kidney-binding antibody (TKAb) determined 1 h after administration of 2 mg of mAb 5-1-6 was 50.8 ± 10.4 μg/2 kidneys and declined to 1.9 ± 0.4 μg/2 kidneys at day 15. In addition, the amount of immunoreactive p51, as determined by the total amount of mAb 5-1-6 bound to glomeruli in vivo and in vitro using radiolabelled antimouse IgG, was found to be less in glomeruli from rats injected with the mAb than in normal rats and was less after 5 days than after 1 h. The minimum injected dose of mAb 5-1-6 required to induce proteinuria is 125 μg, which corresponds to 12.8 μg of TKAb measured at 1 h. This small nephritogenic dose, together with the disappearance of p51 from the cell surface at the peak of proteinuria, further suggests that the antigen occupies a critical position for regulating glomerular capillary permeability.

As described above, corresponding to the peak of proteinuria, there is a shift in immunofluorescence from a pseudo-linear to a finely granular pattern. In general, the extent of this shift in pattern is proportional to the magnitude of proteinuria, and its importance (perhaps reflecting antibody-mediated antigen redistribution) in the pathogenesis of proteinuria is further suggested by two observations. First, intact and $F(ab')_2$ mAb 5-1-6 cause granular deposits and proteinuria in vivo, whereas Fab′ fragments of mAb 5-1-6 produce a persistent linear pattern and no proteinuria despite there being as much antibody deposited (101). Second, it has recently been noted that strain susceptibility to the proteinuric effect of mAb 5-1-6 (Fig. 13) is correlated with a shift in immunofluorescence pattern (102). In all strains examined, a linear-like immunofluorescent staining pattern was observed at 2 h. Although this shifted to a granular pattern 6 days after antibody injection in proteinuric Wistar, Brown Norway, and Lewis rats, it remained linearlike in nonproteinuric Sprague-Dawley rats (Fig. 14). In a related study it was found that the calmodulin-cytoskeleton inhibitor, chlorpromazine, which inhibits both antigen:antibody capping and proteinuria in passive Heymann nephritis (103,104), has no effect on either immune deposit distribution or proteinuria in rats injected with mAb 5-1-6 (98). Thus, there appears to be a chlopromazine-resistant redistribution of antigen in response to mAb cross-linking (as opposed to merely engagement) that is closely coupled to the emergence of proteinuria.

Additional insight into the role of this protein in maintaining normal glomerular permeability may emerge from studies of its behavior in other proteinuric states. Alterations in the amount and/or distribution of p51 have been noted in puromycin aminonucleoside and adriamycin nephroses (105), and in passive Heymann nephritis (PHN) and Masugi (nephrotoxic) nephritis (106). Sequential studies have shown that the distribution of p51 normalizes when proteinuria subsides (99). The observation that immunostaining of glomeruli with mAb 5-1-6 is altered during the proteinuric phase of purine aminonucleoside and is restored with recovery of proteinuria (105) is noteworthy. Puromycin is especially cytotoxic to visceral glomerular epithelial cells, causing podocyte effacement and detachment, apical dislocation, and disruption of the slit diaphragm and reappearance of the ladderlike structures and interepithelial occluding junctions seen during glomerulogenesis (107,108).

These observations lead to the intriguing possibility that the antigen (p51) recognized by mAb 5-1-6 is an integral transmembrane protein of the slit diaphragm and that binding of antibody to its extracellular domain alters the molecular arrangement that constitutes a normally functioning slit diaphragm. An alternative, although no less interesting possibility, is that divalent antibody binding causes p51 to shift from the basolateral surface of the podocyte to the slit diaphragm, where the complex might interfere with the normal molecular arrangement between proteins on the cytoplasmic face, such as ZO-1 (109) and one or more as yet unidentified transmembrane proteins. There are, of course, several other rational mechanisms whereby an mAb directed at a basolateral membrane protein of the podocyte may cause proteinuria. For example, cell activation by antibody acting as a false ligand for a receptorlike protein might stimulate cytoskeleton-mediated cell shape change and slit-pore distortion. Alternatively, cell activation might induce the production of lipid or peptide inflammatory mediators or the release of matrix-degrading proteases into the microenvironment between the GBM and basal surface of the foot processes, thus destroying the constitutive ligands to which podocyte integrins are normally anchored. All of these possibilities merit further study.

RELEVANCE OF ANTIBODY-MEDIATED INJURY IN HUMAN GLOMERULAR DISEASES

As yet, none of the target antigens identified in experimental antibody-dependent proteinuria has been shown to be involved in any human glomerular disease. However, these models are important, not so much because they resemble specific human diseases, but because they provide a means of defining the molecular composition of the normal glomerular capillary wall. It is through a complete understanding of the target antigens that we will gain insight into the structural and functional properties of the glomerular permeability barrier and determine what goes awry in those proteinuric diseases in which components of the glomerular filter, especially the podocyte, are the primary site of injury, for example, minimal change disease, congenital nephrotic syndrome, membranous nephropathy, various forms of focal glomerulosclerosis such as collapsing and human immunodeficiency virus nephropathy, and, arguably, early diabetic glomerulosclerosis.

ACKNOWLEDGMENT

Work reported in this publication was supported in part by research grants DK30932 and DK48236 from the United States Public Health Services (to D.J.S.); a Grant-in-Aid for Scientific Research from the Ministry of Education, Science and Culture of Japan (04670401) and a research grant from the Japan Health Sciences Foundation (2-2-4) (to Y.N.); and a research grant from the Ministry of Education, Science and Culture, Japan (03454188) and a Program project grant from the Ministry of Health and Welfare of Japan (1994) (to F.S.). We thank Drs. Dale Abrahamson and Dennis Brown for their helpful collaboration.

REFERENCES

1. Cochrane CG. Mediation systems in neutrophil-independent immunologic injury of the glomerulus. *Contemp Issues Nephrol* 1979;3:106–121.
2. Couser WG, Salant DJ. Immunopathogenesis of glomerular capillary wall injury in nephrotic states. *Contemp Issues Nephrol* 1982;9:47–83.
3. Hammer DK, Dixon FJ. Experimental glomerulonephritis: II. Immunologic events in the pathogenesis of nephrotoxic serum nephritis in the rat. *J Exp Med* 1963;117:1019–1035.
4. Lange K, Wenk EJ, Wachstein M, Noble J. The mechanism of experimental glomerulonephritis produced in rabbits by avian antikidney sera. *Am J Med Sci* 1958;236:767– 778.
5. Taranta A, Badalamenti G, Cooper NS. Role of complement in nephrotoxic nephritis. *Nature* 1963;200:373–375.
6. Baxter JH, Small PA. Antibody to rat kidney: in vivo effects of univalent and divalent fragments. *Science* 1963;140:1406–1407.
7. Cochrane CG, Unanue ER, Dixon FJ. A role of polymorphonuclear leukocytes and complement in nephrotoxic nephritis. *J Exp Med* 1965;122:99–119.
8. Unanue ER, Dixon F. Experimental glomerulonephritis: V. Studies on the interaction of nephrotoxic antibodies with tissues of the rat. *J Exp Med* 1965;121:697–714.
9. Small PA, Baxter JH. Digestion of anti-kidney antibody: effects on its nephrotoxicity and ability to fix complement. *J Immunol* 1965;95:282–287.
10. Kobayashi Y, Shigematsu H, Tada T. Nephritogenic properties of nephrotoxic guinea pig antibodies: II. Glomerular lesions induced by $F(ab')_2$ fragments of nephrotoxic IgG antibody in rats. *Virchows Arch* 1973;15:35–44.
11. Passos HC, Siqueira M, Martinez OC, Bier OG. Studies on the nephrotoxic activity of guinea-pig gamma-1 and gamma-2 antibodies. *Immunology* 1974;6:407–416.
12. Kobayashi Y, Shigematsu H, Tada T. Nephritogenic properties of nephrotoxic guinea pig antibodies: I. Glomerulonephritis induced by guinea pig IgG antibody in rats. *Virchows Arch* 1973;14:259–271.
13. Henson PM. Release of biologically active constituents from blood cells and its role in antibody-mediated tissue injury. In: Amos B, ed. *Progress in immunology*. New York: Acadamic; 1971:155–171.
14. Hawkins D, Cochrane CG. Glomerular basement membrane damage in immunological glomerulonephritis. *Immunology* 1968;14:665–681.
15. Couser WG, Stilmant MM, Lewis EJ. Experimental glomerulonephritis in the guinea pig: I. Glomerular lesions associated with anti-glomerular basement membrane antibody deposits. *J Immunol* 1973;29:236–243.
16. Couser WG, Spargo BH, Stilmant MM, Lewis EJ. Experimental glomerulonephritis in the guinea pig: II. Ultrastructual lesions of the basement membrane associated with proteinuria. *Lab Invest* 1975;32:46–55.
17. Simpson IJ, Amos N, Evans DJ, Thompson NM, Peters DK. Guinea pig nephrotoxic nephritis: I. The role of complement and polymorphonuclear leukocytes and the effect of antibody subclass and fragments in the heterologous phase. *Clin Exp Immunol* 1975;19:499–511.
18. Couser WG, Stilmant MM, Jermanovich NB. Complement-independent nephrotoxic nephritis in the guinea pig. *Kidney Int* 1977;11:170–180.
19. Couser WG, Darby C, Salant DJ, Adler S, Stilmant MM, Lowenstein LM. Anti-GBM antibody–induced proteinuria in isolated perfused rat kidney. *Am J Physiol* 1985;249:F241–F250.
20. Salant DJ, Madaio MP, Adler S, Stilmant MM. Altered glomerular permeability induced by $F(ab')_2$ and Fab′ antibodies to rat renal tubular epithelial antigen. *Kidney Int* 1982;21:36–43.
21. Natori Y, Hayakawa I, Shibata S. Passive Heymann nephritis with acute and severe proteinuria induced by heterologous antibody against renal tubular brush border glycoprotein gp108. *Lab Invest* 1986;55:63–70.
22. Natori Y, Hayakawa I, Shibata S. Role of dipeptidyl peptidase IV (gp108) in passive Heymann nephritis. Use of dipeptidyl peptidase IV–deficient rats. *Am J Pathol* 1989;134:405–410.
23. Mendrick DL, Rennke HG, Cotran RS, Springer TA, Abbas AK. Monoclonal antibodies against rat glomerular antigens: production and specificity. *Lab Invest* 1983;49:107–117.
24. Mendrick DL, Rennke HG. I. Induction of proteinuria in the rat by a monoclonal antibody against SGP–115/107. *Kidney Int* 1988;33:818–830.
25. Orikasa M, Matsui K, Oite T, Shimizu F. Massive proteinuria induced in rats by a single intravenous injection of a monoclonal antibody. *J Immunol* 1988;141:807–814.
26. Thomas PE, Wharram BL, Goyal M, Wiggins JE, Holzman LB, Wiggins RC. GLEPP1, a renal glomerular epithelial cell (podocyte) membrane protein–tyrosinesphatase. Identification, molecular cloning, and characerization in rabbit. *J Biol Chem* 1994;269:19953–19962.
27. Dekan G, Miettinen A, Schnabel E, Farquhar MG. Binding of monoclonal antibodies to glomerular endothelium, slit membranes, and epithelium after in vivo injection. *Am J Pathol* 1990;137:913–927.
28. Miettinen A, Dekan G, Farquhar MG. Monoclonal antibodies against membrane proteins of the rat glomerulus. *Am J Pathol* 1990;137:929–943.
29. Abrahamson DR, Caulfield JP. Proteinuria and structural alterations in rat glomerular basement membranes induced by intravenously injected anti-laminin immunoglobulin. *J Exp Med* 1982;156:128–145.
30. Wick G, Muller PU, Timpl R. In vivo localization and pathological effects of passively transferred antibodies to type IV collagen and laminin in mice. *Clin Immunol Immunopathol* 1982;23:656–665.
31. Makino H, Gibons JT, Reddy MK, Kanwar YS. Nephritogenicity of antibodies to proteoglycans of the glomerular basement membrane-1. *J Clin Invest* 1986;77:142–156.
32. Kerjaschki D, Sharkey DJ, Farquhar MG. Identification and characterization of podocalyxin—the major sialoprotein of the renal glomerular epithelial cell. *J Cell Biol* 1984;98:1591–1596.
33. Huang TW, Langlois JC. Podoendin: a new cell surface protein of the podocyte and endothelial cell. *J Exp Med* 1985;162:245–267.
34. Pilia PA, Boackle RJ, Swain RP, Ainsworth SK. Complement-independent nephrotoxic serum nephritis in Munich Wistar rats: immunologic and ultrastructural studies. *Lab Invest* 1983;48:585–597.
35. Salant DJ, Adler S, Darby C, et al. Influence of antigen distribution on the mediation of immunological glomerular injury. *Kidney Int* 1985;27:938–950.
36. Salant DJ, Cybulsky AV. Experimental glomerulonephritis. *Methods Enzymol* 1988;162:421–461.
37. Steblay RW. Glomerulonephrits induced in sheep by injection of heterologous glomerular basement membrane and complete Freund's adjuvant. *J Exp Med* 1962;116:253–277.
38. Bygren P, Wieslander J, Heinegärd D. Glomerulonephritis induced in sheep by immunization with human glomerular basement membrane. *Kidney Int* 1987;31:25–31.
39. Hudson BG, Kalluri R, Gunwar S, Noelken ME, Mariyama M, Reeders ST. Molecular characteristics of the Goodpasture autoantigen. *Kidney Int* 1993;43:135–139.
40. O'Meara YM, Natori Y, Minto AW, Goldstein DJ, Manning EJ, Salant DJ. Nephrotoxic antiserum identifies a β1-integrin on rat glomerular epithelial cells. *Am J Physiol* 1992;262:F1083– F1091.
41. Feintzeig ID, Dittmer JE, Cybulsky AV, Salant DJ. Antibody, antigen

and glomerular capillary wall charge interactions: influence of antigen location on in situ immune complex formation. *Kidney Int* 1986; 29:649–657.
42. Bernardi P, Patel VP, Lodish HF. Lymphoid precursor cells adhere to two different sites on fibronectin. *J Cell Biol* 1987;105:489–498.
43. Baricos WH, Shah SV. Glomerular injury and proteolytic enzymes. *Semin Nephrol* 1991;11:327–331.
44. Baricos WH, O'Connor SE, Cortez SL, Wu LT, Shah SV. The cysteine proteinase inhibitor E-64, reduces proteinuria in an experimental model of glomerulonephritis. *Biochem Biophys Res Commun* 1988;155:1318–1323.
45. Thomas GJ, Davies M. The potential role of human kidney cortex cysteine proteinases in glomerular basement membrane degradation. *Biochem Biophys Acta* 1989;990:246–253.
46. Baricos WH, Cortez SL, Le QC, et al. Glomerular basement membrane degradation by endogenous cysteine proteinases present in isolated rat glomeruli. *Kidney Int* 1990;38:395–401.
47. Baricos WH, Zhou Y, Mason RW, Barrett AJ. Human kidney cathepsins B and L. Characterization and potential role in degradation of glomerular basement membrane. *Biochem J* 1988;252:301–304.
48. Gang NF, Kalant N. Nephrotoxic serum nephritis: I. Chemical, morphologic, and functional changes in the glomerular basement membrane during the evolution of nephritis. *Lab Invest* 1970;22:531–540.
49. Gang NF, Mautner W, Kalant N. Nephrotoxic serum nephritis: II. Chemical, morphologic, and functional correlates of glomerular basement membrane at the onset of proteinuria. *Lab Invest* 1970;23: 150–157.
50. Werb Z, Tremble PM, Behrendtsen O, Crowley E, Damsky CH. Signal transduction though the fibronectin receptor induces collagenase and stromelysin gene expression. *J Cell Biol* 1989;109:877–889.
51. Clark EA, Brugge JS. Integrins and signal transduction pathways: the road taken. *Science* 1995;268:233–239.
52. Salant DJ. The structural biology of glomerular epithelial cells in proteinuric diseases. *Curr Opin Nephrol Hypertens* 1994;3:569–574.
53. Salant DJ, Darby C, Couser WG. Experimental membranous glomerulonephritis in rats. *J Clin Invest* 1980;66:71–81.
54. Salant DJ, Belok S, Madaio MP, Couser WG. A new role for complement in experimental membranous nephropathy in rats. *J Clin Invest* 1980;66:1339–1350.
55. Cybulsky AV, Rennke HG, Feintzeig ID, Salant DJ. Complement-induced glomerular epithelial cell injury: the role of the membrane attack complex in rat membranous nephropathy. *J Clin Invest* 1986; 77:1096–1107.
56. Baker PJ, Ochi RF, Schulze M, Johnson RJ, Campbell C, Couser WG. Depletion of C6 prevents development of proteinuria in experimental membranous nephropathy in rats. *Am J Pathol* 1989;135: 185–194.
57. Kerjaschki D, Schulze M, Binder S, et al. Transcellular transport and membrane insertion of the C5b-9 membrane attack complex of complement by glomerular epithelial cells in experimental membranous nephropathy. *J Immunol* 1989;143:546–552.
58. Leenaerts PL, Hall BM, van Damme BJ, Daha MR, Vanrenterghem YF. Active Heymann nephritis in complement component C6 deficient rats. *Kidney Int* 1995;47:106–1614.
59. Rahman MA, Liu CN, Dunn MJ, Emancipator SN. Complement and leukocyte independent proteinuria and eicosanoid synthesis in rat membranous nephropathy. *Lab Invest* 1988; 59:477–483.
60. Kerjaschki D, Farquhar MG. The pathogenic antigen of Heymann nephritis is a membrane glycoprotein of the renal proximal tubule brush border. *Proc Natl Acad Sci U S A* 1982;79:5557–5561.
61. Saito A, Pietromonaco S, Loo AK, Farquhar MG. Complete cloning and sequencing of rat gp330/"megalin," a distinctive member of the low density lipoprotein receptor gene family. *Proc Natl Acad Sci U S A* 1994;91:9725–9729.
62. Orlando RA, Kerjaschki D, Kurihara H, Biemesderfer D, Farquhar MG. gp330 Associates with a 44-kDa protein in the rat kidney to form the Heymann nephritis antigenic complex. *Proc Natl Acad Sci U S A* 1992;89:6698–6702.
63. Kerjaschki D, Miettinen A, Farquhar MG. Initial events in the formation of immune deposits in passive Heymann nephritis. *J Exp Med* 1987;166:109–128.
64. Mendrick DL, Chung DC, Rennke HG. Heymann antigen GP330 demonstrates affinity for fibronectin, laminin, and type 1 collagen and mediates rat proximal tubule epithelial cell adherence to such matrices in vitro. *Exp Cell Res* 1990;188:23–35.
65. Susani M, Schulze M, Exner M, Kerjaschki D. Antibodies to glycolipids activate complement and promote proteinuria in passive Heymann nephritis. *Am J Pathol* 1994;144:807–819.
66. Adler S, Chen X. Anti-Fx1A antibody recognizes a β_1-integrin on glomerular epithelial cells and inhibits adhesion and growth. *Am J Physiol* 1992;262:F770–F776.
67. Adler S. Integrin receptors in the glomerulus: potential role in glomerular injury. *Am J Physiol* 1992;262:F697–F704.
68. Quigg R, Cybulsky AV, Salant DJ. Effect of nephritogenic antibody on complement regulation in cultured rat glomerular epithelial cells. *J Immunol* 1991;147:838–845.
69. Ronco P, Allegri L, Melcion C, et al. A monoclonal antibody to brush border and passive Heymann nephritis. *Clin Exp Immunol* 1984;55: 319–332.
70. Assmann KJM, Ronco P, Tangelder MM, Lange WPH, Verroust P, Koene RAP. Comparison of antigenic targets involved in antibody-mediated membranous glomerulonephritis in the mouse and rat. *Am J Pathol* 1985;121:112–122.
71. Hegen M, Niedobitek G, Klein CE, Stein H, Fleischer B. The T cell triggering molecule Tp103 is associated with dipeptidyl aminopeptidase IV activity. *J Immunol* 1990;144:2908–2914.
72. Hopsu-Havu VK, Glenner GG. A new dipeptide naphthylamidase hydrolyzing glycyl-prolyl-beta-naphthylamide. *Histochemie* 1966;7: 197–201.
73. Kenny AJ, Booth AG, George SG, et al. Dipeptidyl peptidase IV, a kidney brush-border serine peptidase. *Biochem J* 1976;157:169–182.
74. Ogata S, Misumi Y, Ikehara Y. Primary structure of rat liver dipeptidyl peptidase IV deduced from its cDNA and identification of the NH2-terminal signal sequence as the membrane-anchoring domain. *J Biol Chem* 1989;264:3596–3601.
75. Verroust P, Ronco P, Chatelet F. Antigenic targets in membranous glomerulonephritis. *Springer Semin Immunopathol* 1987;9:341–358.
76. Van Leer ECG, De Roo GM, Bruijn JA, Hoedemaeker PJ, De Heer E. Synergistic effects of anti-gp330 and anti-dipeptidyl peptidase type IV antibodies in the induction of glomerular damage. *Exp Nephrol* 1993;1:292–300.
77. Natori Y, Shindo N. Proteinuria induced by anti-dipeptidyl peptidase IV (gp108); role of circulating and glomerular antigen. *Clin Exp Immunol* 1994;95:327–332.
78. Mendrick DL, Rennke HG. II. Epitope specific induction of proteinuria by monoclonal antibodies. *Kidney Int* 1988;33:831–842.
79. Bruijn JA, Bergijk EC, Deheer E, Fleuren GJ, Hoedemaeker PJ. Induction and progression of experimental lupus nephritis: exploration of a pathogenetic pathway. *Kidney Int* 1992;41:5–13.
80. Bruijn JA, Van Leer EHG, Baelde HJJ, Corver WE, Hogendoorn PCW, Fleuren GJ. Characterization and in vivo transfer of nephritogenic autoantibodies directed against dipeptidyl peptidase-IV and laminin in experimental lupus nephritis. *Lab Invest* 1990;63:350–359.
81. Van Leer EHG, Bruijn JA, Prins FA, Hoedemaeker PJ, De Heer E. Redistribution of glomerular dipeptidyl peptidase type IV in experimental lupus nephritis. Demonstration of decreased enzyme activity at the ultrastructural level. *Lab Invest* 1993;68:550–556.
82. Hixson DC, Ponce MD, Allison JP, Walborg EFJ. Cell surface expression by adult rat hepatocytes of a non-collagen glycoprotein present in rat liver biomatrix. *Exp Cell Res* 1984;152:402–414.
83. Walborg EFJ, Tsuchida S, Weeden DS, et al. Identification of dipeptidyl peptidase IV as a protein shared by the plasma membrane of hepatocytes and liver biomatrix. *Exp Cell Res* 1985;158:509–518.
84. Bauvois B. A collagen-binding glycoprotein on the surface of mouse fibroblasts is identified as dipeptidyl peptidase IV. *Biochem J* 1988; 252:723–731.
85. Hanski C, Huhle T, Gossrau R, Reutter W. Direct evidence for the binding of rat liver DPP IV to collagen in vitro. *Exp Cell Res* 1988; 78:64–72.
86. Hanski C, Huhle T, Reutter W. Involvement of plasma membrane dipeptidyl peptidase IV in fibronectin-mediated adhesion of cells on collagen. *Biol Chem Hoppe-Seyler* 1985;366:1169–1176.
87. Shipp MA, Look AT. Hematopoietic differentiation antigens that are membrane-associated enzymes: cutting is the key. *Blood* 1993;82: 1052–1070.
88. Vivier L, Marguet D, Naquet P, et al. Evidence that thymocyte-acti-

vating molecule is mouse CD26 (dipeptidyl peptidase-IV). *J Immunol* 1991;147:447–454.

89. Bristol LA, Sakaguchi E, Apella E, Doyle D, Takacs L. Thymocyte costimulating antigen is CD26 (dipeptidyl-peptidase IV). Costimulating of granulocyte, macrophage, and T lineage cell proliferation via CD26. *J Immunol* 1992;149:367–372.
90. Schön E, Jahn S, Kiessig S, et al. The role of dipeptidyl peptidase IV in human T lymphocyte activation. Inhibitors and antibodies against dipeptidyl peptidase IV suppress lymphocyte proliferation and immunoglobulin synthesis in vitro. *Eur J Immunol* 1987;17: 1821–1826.
91. Assmann KJM, Van Son JPHF, Dijkman HBPM, Koene RAP. A nephritogenic rat monoclonal antibody to mouse aminopeptidase-A. Induction of massive albuminuria after a single intravenous injection. *J Exp Med* 1992;175:623–635.
92. Stiller D, Bahn H, August C. Demonstration of glomerular DPP IV activity in kidney diseases. *Acta Histochem* 1991;91:105–109.
93. Wolf G, Sherberich JE, Nowack A, Stein O, Schoeppe W. Urinary excretion of dipeptidyl aminopeptidase IV in patients with renal diseases. *Clin Nephrol* 1990;33:136–142.
94. Stefanovic V, Ardaillou N, Vlahovic P, Placier S, Ronco P, Ardaillou R. Interferon-gamma induces dipeptidylpeptidase-IV expression in human glomerular epithelial cells. *Immunology* 1993;80:465–470.
95. Kawachi H, Abrahamson DR, St. John PL, et al. Developmental expression of the nephritogenic antigen of monoclonal antibody 5-1-6. *Am J Pathol* 1995;147:823–833.
96. Oka M, Hidaka S, Nagase M, et al. Study on the glomerular alterations in the proteinuric rats induced by a monoclonal antibody 5-1-6. *J Clin Microscopy* 1991;24:5–6.
97. Blantz RC, Gabbai FB, Peterson O, et al. Water and protein permeability is regulated by the glomerular epithelial slit diaphgragm. *J Am Soc Nephrol* 1994;4:1957–1994.
98. Takashima N, Kawachi H, Oite T, Nishi S, Arakawa M, Shimizu F. Effect of chlorpromazine on kinetics of injected monoclonal antibody in MoAb-induced glomerular injury. *Clin Exp Immunol* 1993;91: 135–140.
99. Shimizu F. New concepts of glomerular injury: role of an epitope specific interaction. In: Oite T, ed. *Structural basis for glomerular dysfunction*. Niigata, Japan: Nishimura; 1991:35–51.
100. Kawachi H, Matsui K, Orikasa M, Morioka T, Oite T, Shimizu F. Quantitative studies of monoclonal antibody 5-1-6–induced proteinuric state in rats. *Clin Exp Immunol* 1992;87:215–219.
101. Narisawa M, Kawachi H, Oite T, Shimizu F. Divalency of the monoclonal antibody 5-1-6 is required for induction of proteinuria in rats. *Clin Exp Immunol* 1993;92:522–526.
102. Gollner D, Kawachi H, Oite T, Oka M, Nagase M, Shimizu F. Strain variation in susceptibility to the development of monoclonal antibody 5-1-6 induced proteinuria in rats. *Clin Exp Immunol* 1995;101:341–345.
103. Camussi G, Brentjens JR, Noble B, et al. Antibody-induced redistribution of Heymann antigen on the surface of cultured glomerular visceral epithelial cells: possible role in the pathogenesis of Heymann glomerulonephritis. *J Immunol* 1985;135:2409–2416.
104. Camussi G, Noble B, Van Liew J, Brentjens JR, Andres G. Pathogenesis of passive Heymann glomerulonephritis: chlorpromazine inhibits antibody-mediated redistribution of cell surface antigens and prevents development of the disease. *J Immunol* 1986;136:2127–2135.
105. Okasora T, Nagase M, Kawachi H, et al. Altered localization of antigen recognized by proteinuria-inducing monoclonal antibody in experimental nephrosis. *Virchows Arch [B]* 1991;60:41–46.
106. Shimizu F. Glomerular epithelial cell surface molecule recognized by proteinuria-inducing monoclonal antibody 5-1-6. In: Shimizu F, Oite T, Yamamoto T, Kihara I, eds. *Pathophysiology of glomerular epithelial cell*. Niigata, Japan: Koko-Do; 1993:12–18.
107. Ryan GB, Karnovsky MG. An ultrastructural study of the mechanisms of proteinuria in aminonucleoside nephrosis. *Kidney Int* 1975; 8:219–232.
108. Kurihara H, Anderson JM, Farquhar MG. Diversity among tight junctions in rat kidney: glomerular slit diaphragms and endothelial junctions express only one isoform of the tight junction protein ZO-1. *Proc Natl Acad Sci U S A* 1992;89:7075–7079.
109. Schnabel E, Anderson JM, Farquhar MG. The tight junction protein ZO-1 is concentrated along slit diaphragms of the glomerular epithelium. *J Cell Biol* 1990;111:1255–1263.

Immunologic Renal Diseases,
edited by E. G. Neilson and W. G. Couser.
Lippincott-Raven Publishers, Philadelphia © 1997

CHAPTER 18

Complement and Complement Regulatory Proteins in Renal Disease

Lee A. Hebert, Fernando G. Cosio, and Daniel J. Birmingham

INTRODUCTION

In many experimental models of renal disease, severe renal injury occurs only if the animal's complement system is allowed to function normally. Observations such as these suggest that our kidneys might be better off if there were no complement system. However, such a narrow focus regarding the role of the complement system is not appropriate, even with respect to the kidney. Indeed, when viewed in a larger perspective, it is clear that the overarching role of the complement system with respect to the kidney is to *prevent* renal injury (1). This is particularly true for renal diseases that are caused directly or indirectly by infection (the complement system is a key defense against infection) and for renal diseases that are caused by deposition of antibody in the kidney (the complement system protects against antibody and immune-complex-mediated renal disease by a variety of mechanisms). Only under rare circumstances does the kidney becomes a victim of the "friendly fire" that emanates from activation of the complement system. This chapter examines the mechanisms that activate the complement system and, in that context, shows how the complement system plays either its renoprotective or renoinjurious role. Also discussed is the clinical diagnostic significance of serum complement measurement.

ACTIVATION OF THE COMPLEMENT SYSTEM

The complement system involves 14 plasma proteins: C1q (the q subunit of the first complement protein), C1r, C1s, C2 through C9, factor B, factor D, and properdin. The early steps of activation occur as two distinct pathways. Both pathways converge at a common terminal pathway. Figure 1 provides a general overview of these pathways. Figure 2 details each step in these pathways, as described below.

The Classical Pathway

C1, which initiates classical pathway activation, is composed of an 18-chain C1q molecule, arranged in six triple-helix subunits, and a $C1r_2C1s_2$ tetramer (2,3). The association between C1q and $C1r_2C1s_2$ depends on divalent cations such as Ca^{2-} (4). Activation of the classical pathway occurs when at least two of the six binding sites (globular heads) of C1q become bound (5) (Fig. 2, panel 1) to the Fc regions of two or more closely arranged immunoglobulin (Ig)-G molecules or a single IgM molecule (IgM is a pentamer of the basic Ig structure). C1q cannot bind to IgA (6). Non-IgG-containing substances can also fix the C1 complex. These include viruses, bacterial products, damaged tissue, and mannan-binding protein bound to bacteria (7,8).

Binding of C1q to IgG molecules causes conformational changes in C1q and C1r. These changes in C1r expose proteolytic sites causing cleavage of both C1r molecules. Cleaved C1r activates serine esterase domains in C1r. C1r then cleaves C1s-activating serine esterases within C1s (9).

Activated C1s cleaves C4 into C4a and C4b, and destabilizes an internal thioester group on C4b (panel 2) (10). This reactive thioester enables C4b to bind to nearby structures. There are two allotypic forms of C4: C4A and C4B. C4A preferentially binds to amino groups, whereas C4B preferentially binds to hydroxyl groups (11).

Fluid phase C2 binds to C4b in the presence of Mg^{2-}. If this occurs in proximity to the activated C1 complex, C1s cleaves C2 into C2b and C2a (panel 3) (12). The term

L. A. Hebert, F. G. Cosio, and D. J. Birmingham: Department of Internal Medicine, Ohio State University, Columbus, Ohio 43210.

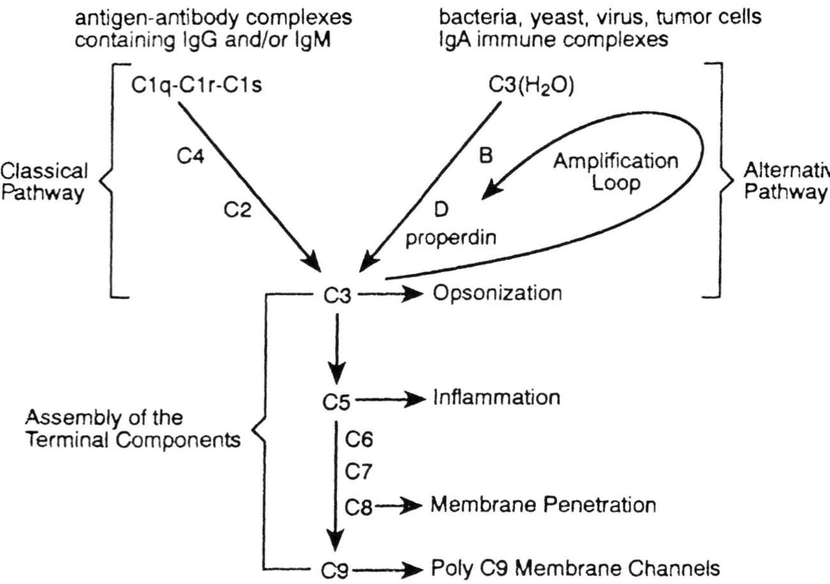

FIG. 1. General overview of the classical, alternative, and terminal pathways of complement activation: *Ig,* immunoglobulin.

"C2b" is used for consistency to designate the larger fragment because the larger fragments of cleaved C3 and C4 are termed C3b and C4b, respectively. However, historically, the larger fragment has been termed C2a.

C4b2b is the classical pathway C3 convertase. The C2b portion contains a serine esterase that cleaves C3 into C3a, an anaphylatoxin and chemokine for eosinophils (13), and C3b (panel 4). The destabilized internal thioester bond on C3b enables it to bind covalently to adjacent structures (14).

C5 binds reversibly to C3b. When this binding occurs close to C4b2b, C5 is cleaved by the serine esterase within C2b (panel 5). Because the cleavage of C5 requires the presence of C3b in close association with C4b2b, this convertase (the classical pathway C5 convertase) is termed C4b2b3b. The cleavage of C5 causes C5a, a potent anaphylatoxin, to be released into the microenvironment.

The Alternative Pathway

The first step in the activation of the alternative pathway requires C3b or a C3b-like molecule. This is provided by the interaction of C3 with water, causing hydrolysis of its internal thioester bond and other changes in structure (panel a) (15,16). This C3b-like molecule, $C3(H_2O)$, binds to factor B in the presence of Mg^{2-}. Factor B, bound to $C3(H_2O)$, is cleaved by factor D (17), causing release of Ba into the microenvironment. Thus, $C3(H_2O)Bb$, the fluid-phase alternative pathway C3 convertase, is formed. Properdin stabilizes this complex (18).

The Bb component of $C3(H_2O)Bb$ contains a serine esterase site that cleaves fluid-phase C3 into C3a and C3b (panel b) (19). This process occurs constantly at a low rate in plasma. Most C3b formed in this manner is rapidly hydrolyzed, inactivating the internal thioester bond, and is degraded by factor I and its cofactors (see below). However, some C3b may bind to a nearby surface if the surface is encountered within microseconds. If the surface inhibits inactivation of bound C3b (for example, by factors H and I), the surface is considered an activator surface because it permits further activation of the alternative pathway (panels c and d).

If C5 binds to C3b adjacent to a C3bBb, the Bb serine esterase cleaves C5 into C5a and C5b (panel e) (20,21). Thus, the complex, C3bBbC3b, is referred to as the alternative pathway C5 convertase.

The Common Terminal Pathway

This pathway is initiated by the formation of C5b by the classical or alternative pathway. C5b binds C6 and then C7, forming a trimolecular complex that produces a labile hydrophobic binding domain (panel I) (22). This complex is released from C3b, inserts into adjacent membranes (panel II), and provides a binding site for C8 and then C9 (23). This initiates a lytic lesion that is completed by polymerization of C9 to form a pore (panel III) (24). These pores can lead to cell activation or lysis.

Control of Complement Activation and Self-Protection

Just discussed were the processes involved in activation of the complement system. Equally important are the processes that inhibit complement activation. This serves (a) to limit the consumption of complement by a given

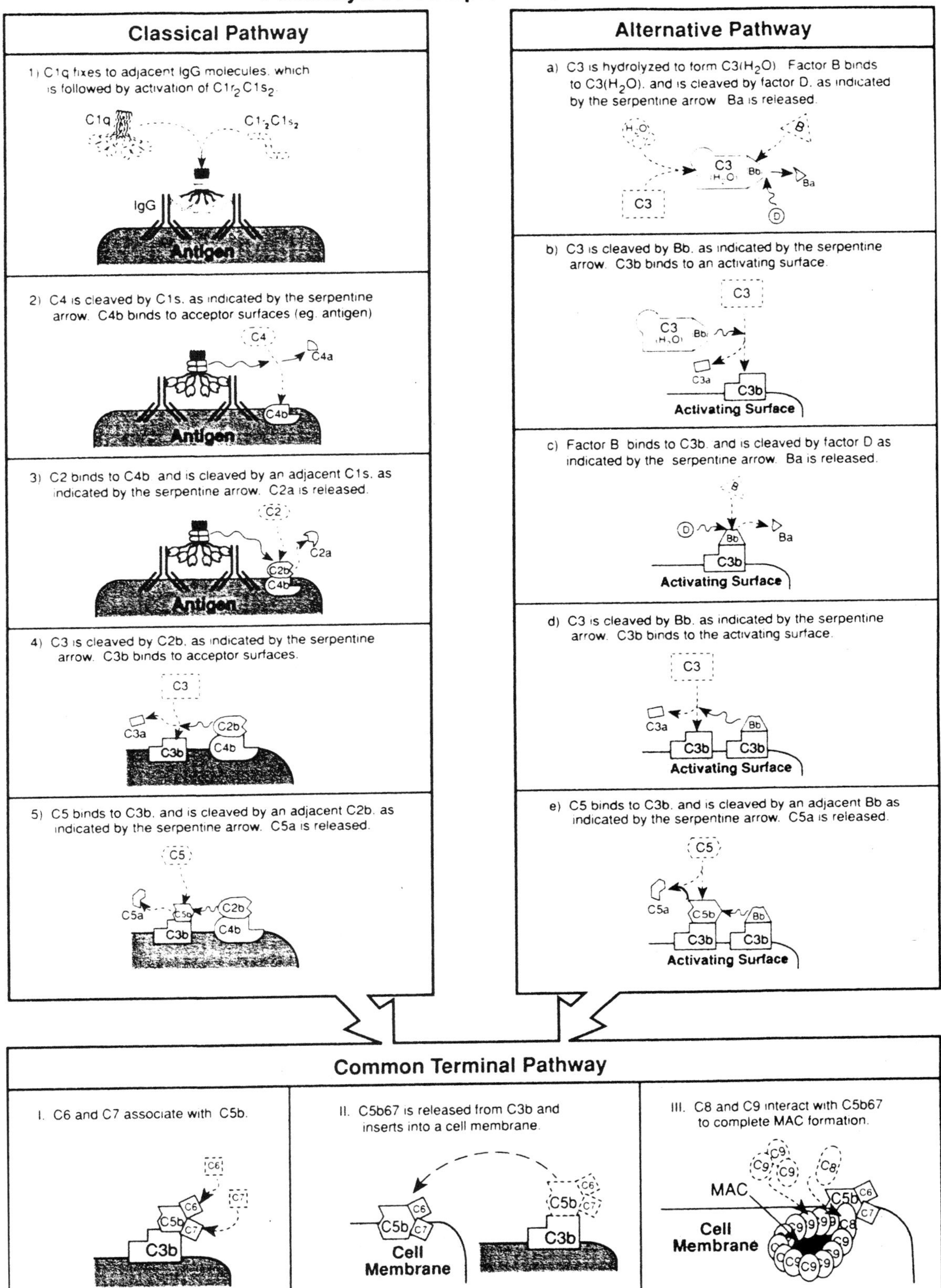

FIG. 2. A detailed analysis of the pathways of complement activation. *MAC*, membrane attack complex.

stimulus, (b) to protect "innocent" bystander cells while allowing sufficient complement activation to damage the intended targets of complement activation (for example, bacteria and abnormal cells), and (c) to control the generation of biologically active complement fragments that can modify both inflammatory and immunologic responses. Complement activation is controlled by plasma proteins and by cell membrane proteins.

Plasma Proteins That Regulate Complement Activation (Table 1)

C1 inhibitor is a serine protease that binds to the activated form of C1 (C1q-2C1r-2C1s) and causes dissociation of C1q from C1r and C1s. C1 inhibitor is extremely efficient. Within 55 s of activation, 90% of activated C1 is bound by C1 inhibitor. As a result, a single C1 complex activates only four C2 molecules and 35 C4 molecules (25).

Factor I, a serine protease, degrades C3 and C4 in the presence of the plasma cofactors C4-binding protein (C4bp) or factor H, or the cell membrane-associated cofactors membrane cofactor protein (MCP) or complement receptor type 1 (CR1). Factor 1 cleaves C4b to C4bi, C4c and C4d, and cleaves C3b to C3bi, C3c, and C3dg. The cleavage of C4 and C3 has at least two effects: (a) inhibition of further C3 and C5 activation by both the classical and alternative pathway, and (b) generation of biologically active products of C3 that remain bound to the activating surface. Cell-bound C3bi and C3dg bind to complement receptor type 3 (CR3) and complement receptor type 2 (CR2), respectively. These events can mediate phagocytosis (26) and modify the immune response (27). C4bp and factor H are incorporated into immune complexes (28), apparently bound to C4b and C3b, and are found in glomeruli in immune-complex diseases (29,30).

Vitronectin (protein S) binds to C5b-7 released into fluid phase, rendering the complex hydrophilic, thereby inhibiting its insertion into the cell membrane lipid bilayer (31). Glomerular vitronectin deposits are present in glomerulonephritis involving complement activation (32). The large plasma glycoprotein clusterin may have functions similar to that of vitronectin (33). Depletion of clusterin increases proteinuria in an in vitro model of Heymann nephritis (34). Clusterin may also play a role in cell remodeling, apoptosis, and renal tubular injury in renal transplant rejection (35).

Cell-Associated Complement Regulatory Proteins (Table 2)

Generation of C3b can result in the following: binding of C3b to innocent bystander cells, activation of more C3b via the alternative pathway, activation of C5 and other terminal complement components and, finally, innocent bystander cell lysis (32,36). However, cells are notoriously resistant to complement-mediated lysis, particularly lysis by homologous complement (37,38). This self-protection is provided by the cell glycocalix (39) and cell-associated complement regulatory proteins (decay-accelerating factor, DAF) (40), MCP (41,42), and CR1 (43,44). These proteins inhibit C3 activation, and thus C5 activation, but by different mechanisms (see Table 2). C8-binding protein (C8bp) (homologous restriction factor) and CD59 (HRF20, MIRL, or gp18) protect the cell from complement-mediated injury by binding to C8 and preventing assembly of the membrane-attack complex (45–48). Human CD59 has higher affinity for human C8 than for nonhuman primate C8. Human CD59 does not bind C8 from nonprimate species (49).

Although DAF, MCP, and CR1 inhibit C3 and C5 deposition in cell membranes, absence or inhibition of

TABLE 1. *Plasma proteins that are regulators of complement activation*

Plasma protein	Mechanism of action	Biologic effects
C1 inhibitor	Binds to activated C1 and dissociates C1q from C1r + C1s	Inhibits activated C1 Inhibits classical pathway activation
C4-binding protein	Binds to C4b and C3b Cofactor for factor I Accelerates C4b2b dissociation	Inhibits classical pathway C4, C3, and C5 activation
Factor H	Cofactor for factor I Binds to C3b Accelerates C3bBb dissociation Inhibits binding of C5 to C3b	Inhibits classical and alternative pathway activation of C3 and C5
Factor I	Serine protease that degrades C4 and C3 in the presence of cofactors	Inhibits classical and alternative pathway activation of C3 and C5 Generates biologically active C3 fragments
Protein S (vitronectin)	Binds to C5b-7 and inhibits its insertion into cell membranes	Inhibits generation of membrane-attack complex on cell membranes
Clusterin	Binds C3, C8, and C9 and inhibits insertion into cell membranes	Same effects as vitronectin

TABLE 2. *Cell membrane proteins that are regulators of complement activation*

Membrane protein	Mechanism of action	Biologic effects
DAF	Prevents formation of C4bC2b and C3bBb Accelerates decay of C3 and C5 convertases	Inhibits classical and alternative pathway activation of C3 and C5 Inhibits complement-mediated cell lysis
MCP	Binds C3b and C4b Cofactor for factor I	Inhibits activation of C3 and C5 With factor I, generates biologically active C3 fragments Inhibits complement-mediated cell lysis
CR1	Binds C3b and C4b Cofactor for factor I Accelerates decay of C3 convertases Inhibits binding of C5 to C3b	Inhibits activation of C3 and C5 With factor I, generates biologically active C3 fragments Mediates binding of C3b-coated particles to cells Inhibits complement-mediated cell lysis
C8bp	Binds to C8	Inhibits binding of C8 to C5b-7 and thus formation of membrane-attack complex Inhibits complement-mediated cell lysis
CD59	Binds homologous C8	Inhibits binding of C8 to C5b-7 and thus formation of membrane-attack complex Inhibits complement-mediated cell lysis

DAF, decay-accelerating factor; MCP, membrane cofactor protein; CR1, complement receptor type 1; C8bp, C8-binding protein.

these proteins does not necessarily result in cell lysis. For example, those with blood group Inab lack DAF on their cells. Nevertheless an acid environment, which activates the alternative pathway, results in marked deposition of C3b but no cell lysis (50). Similarly, patients with paroxysmal nocturnal hemoglobinuria lack DAF, but only those who lack both DAF and CD59 suffer from severe hemolytic episodes (51). Thus, self-protection is conferred by the combined effects of the regulatory proteins shown in Table 2 and perhaps others (52).

Nucleated cells are more resistant to complement-mediated lysis than nonnucleated cells (erythrocytes) in part because self-protection is in part protein synthesis dependent (53). Nucleated cells and nonnucleated cells undergo vesiculation when exposed to terminal complement components (54,55), thereby eliminating those segments of the cell membrane damaged by complement activation (56). However, if the cell cannot synthesize new membrane (for example, erythrocytes), the cell is permanently damaged.

Cell-associated complement regulatory proteins may play a role in the pathogenesis of renal disease (57). We have shown that DAF is present only at low levels in the normal human glomerular mesangium. However, significant mesangial DAF is seen in glomerular diseases with complement activation (58). Also, deposition of terminal complement components on cultured human mesangial cells results in increased synthesis, surface expression, and secretion of soluble DAF (59–61). We demonstrated MCP in the normal human glomerulus and, at much higher concentrations, in the renal tubules. However, glomerular MCP expression was not increased in glomerulonephritis (62). Similarly, complement activation in vitro does not increase MCP synthesis by human mesangial cells (62). Complement activation increases the synthesis of CD59 by human mesangial cells (63). Inhibition of CD59 increases complement-mediated damage in an experimental model of glomerular disease (64). CD59 is present in the normal glomerulus, and its level is increased in patients with glomerulonephritis (65). In human kidney, CR1 is present only in glomerular epithelial cells (GECs) (66). Decreased glomerular CR1 is seen in patients with glomerulonephritis (67). The role of glomerular CR1 is unclear. CR1 is excreted in urine and may reflect the degree of GEC (podocyte) injury (68). In rats, Crry (a DAF and MCP analogue), CD59, and CR1 are present in GECs and confer protection against complement-mediated immune injury (69) and nonimmune injury (70). Crry also appears to confer protection from spontaneous complement attack on the normal kidney (70a).

THE RENOPROTECTIVE ROLE OF THE COMPLEMENT SYSTEM

The ability of the complement system to protect against renal disease has been discussed in detail (1). The following is a summary of that work.

The Complement System Protects Against Renal Disease Caused by Infection

The complement system is particularly important in controlling infections with pyogenic organisms such as *Staphylococcus*, *Streptococcus*, and *Neisseria*. C3, which plays a key role, is normally present in plasma in concentrations of 100–200 mg/dL. Among plasma proteins, only albumin is present in higher concentrations (71).

Bacterial infections can directly damage the kidney or give rise to immune-complex glomerulonephritis (72). Also, certain bacterial infections can precipitate the hemolytic–uremic syndrome (73). The presence of factor-H deficiency may promote infection-related hemolytic–uremic syndrome (74).

The complement system protects against bacterial infection when specific binding of IgG to microorganisms activates the classical pathway, resulting in bacterial lysis. Also, the C3b and C4b deposited on microorganisms facilitates their phagocytosis (75). The alternative pathway protects against infection because bacterial cell walls, particularly those of Gram-negative organisms, activate the alternative pathway (76).

TABLE 3. *Relationship between an inherited deficiency of an individual complement component or complement control protein and the development of systemic lupus erythematosus (SLE) or other immune-complex disease*

Deficient complement	Frequency of SLE or other immune-complex disease[a]	
Complement/ regulator	Complete deficiency	Partial deficiency
C1q, C1r, or C1s	+++	?
C1 inhibitor	+	None reported
C4 (A or B)	++++ (for A and B)	+ (for A only)
C2	+++	+
C3	++++	?
Factor H or I	+	?
C5, 6, 7, 8, or 9	±	?

[a]Frequency of SLE/immune-complex disease: ++++, ~90% or more; +++, ~50–90%; +, above levels in the general population but <25%; ±, probably above levels in the general population; ?, data insufficient for analysis. Estimates of frequency are based on the literature reviewed (see the text).

The Complement System Protects Against Renal Disease Caused by Immune Complexes

The clearest evidence that the complement system protects against immune-complex-mediated diseases[1] is provided by examining the clinical course of patients with genetic deficiency of specific complement components or the regulators of complement activation that can lead to complement deficiency (Table 3). This analysis shows that deficiency of complement components required for classical pathway activation or deficiency of the control proteins that inhibit activation of C3 strongly predisposes one to the development of immune-complex disease, including glomerulonephritis (1,77–80). Predisposition to immune-complex disease in complement deficiency occurs even though C3 deficiency suppresses antibody response and impairs IgM to IgG switching (71). The mechanisms by which specific complement deficiencies predispose one to immune-complex diseases include the following:

1. *Complement deficiencies predispose one to development of infections.* The types of infections seen most commonly in patients with deficiency of a classical pathway component or regulator, or deficiency of an alternative pathway regulator, are infections with "pyogenic" organisms such as *Staphylococcus* and *Streptococcus* (77–80). Patients with deficiency of a terminal pathway component (except for C9) are particularly susceptible to *Neisseria* infections (77–80). Acute infection with certain pyogenic organisms, most notably nephritogenic strains of *Streptococcus* group A can give rise to an acute, postinfectious immune-complex glomerulonephritis (see chapter 41) (72). Chronic bacterial infections can give rise to a chronic immune-complex glomerulonephritis (72). Nevertheless, in many of the patients with deficiency of a classical pathway component or regulator, chronic or recurring infections are not a problem, yet immune-complex disease is nearly universal, particularly in those with a total deficiency of the relevant complement component or regulator (77–80).

2. *Complement deficiency affects the formation, clearance, and solubilization of immune complex.* These mechanisms include inhibition of immune precipitation by complement, and complement-mediated solubilization of precipitated immune complexes. These mechanisms are discussed in chapter 14.

Complement deficiency also impairs the clearance of immune complexes from the circulation. Immune complexes forming in the circulation rapidly become opsonized with C3b and C4b, if the antibodies of the immune complex activate the classical pathway. IgG1, IgG3, and IgM antibodies are especially effective in activating the classical pathway. IgA antibodies activate the alternative pathway. C4b and/or C3b on immune complexes enable the complex to bind to CR1, which are expressed on erythrocytes of only humans and other primates (81). The CR1 on erythrocytes are arranged in fixed clusters that permit firm multipoint binding of C3b/C4b-opsonized immune complexes to the clustered CR1. Neutrophils and monocytes also express CR1; however, the total number of CR1 on circulating leukocytes compared with circulating erythrocytes is relatively small (10–15% versus 85–90%). In addition, the CR1 on resting leukocytes tend not to be arranged in clusters. Thus, almost all of the immune complexes that bind to circulating cells bind to erythrocytes (82–84).

[1]*Immune-complex-mediated disease* refers to disorders in which there is tissue injury associated with substantial accumulation of deposits, which are identified by electron microscopy as *electron dense*, regardless of how these deposits form. These deposits contain immunoglobulin and are associated with complement components, indicating activation of the alternative and/or classic pathways. Hereafter, these disorders are referred to as *immune-complex diseases*.

Immune complexes bound to erythrocyte CR1 are prevented from depositing in vulnerable organs such as the kidney. Instead, the immune complexes remain bound to erythrocytes until the erythrocytes traverse liver or spleen, where the immune complexes are stripped from the erythrocytes and taken up by the macrophages of liver and spleen. The transfer of immune complex from the erythrocyte to the macrophage involves the binding of the Fc regions of the immune complex to macrophage Fc receptors. After transfer of the immune complex from the erythrocyte to the macrophage, which occurs quickly, the erythrocyte then returns to the circulation able once again to participate in what we have termed the *erythrocyte–immune-complex-clearing mechanism* (Fig. 3). If immune complexes in the circulation are unable to bind to erythrocyte CR1, the immune complexes will be trapped in increased amounts in vulnerable organs such as the kidney. Thus, complement-mediated binding of circulating immune complexes to erythrocytes may protect against immune-complex-mediated renal disease (82–84). Erythrocyte CR1 levels are decreased in active immune-complex disease, apparently as a result of damage to the CR1 system from immune-complex–erythrocyte-CR1 interactions in the circulation (83,84). Catabolism of erythrocyte CR1 may also be related to CR1 phenotype (85), age of the erythrocyte (86), or the age of individual (87).

Studies in patients with decreased erythrocyte CR1 levels [systemic lupus erythematosus (SLE) and AIDS] and/or hypocomplementemia have shown decreased binding to erythrocyte CR1 when immune complexes composed of aggregated IgG (88), tetanus-toxoid–anti-tetanus-toxoid (89), or hepatitis B–anti-hepatitis-B (90) are infused intravenously. The decreased binding of immune complex to erythrocyte CR1 was associated with increased rates of immune-complex clearance from the circulation (88–90). Studies in nonhuman primates have shown that decreased binding of immune complexes to erythrocyte CR1 results in decreased uptake of the immune complexes by liver and spleen but increased deposition of immune complexes in kidney (91,92). Thus, the hypocomplementemia and decreased erythrocyte CR1 levels seen in SLE could impair the protective function of the erythrocyte–immune-complex-clearing mechanism. Also, decreased immune-complex binding by erythrocytes increases interaction of immune complexes with neutrophils, resulting in increased interleukin-1 release by neutrophils and increased endothelial permeability (93). This is another mechanism of tissue injury that could result from impaired erythrocyte CR1 function.

Recently we have shown that erythrocyte CR1 expression can be upregulated by stimulating erythropoiesis

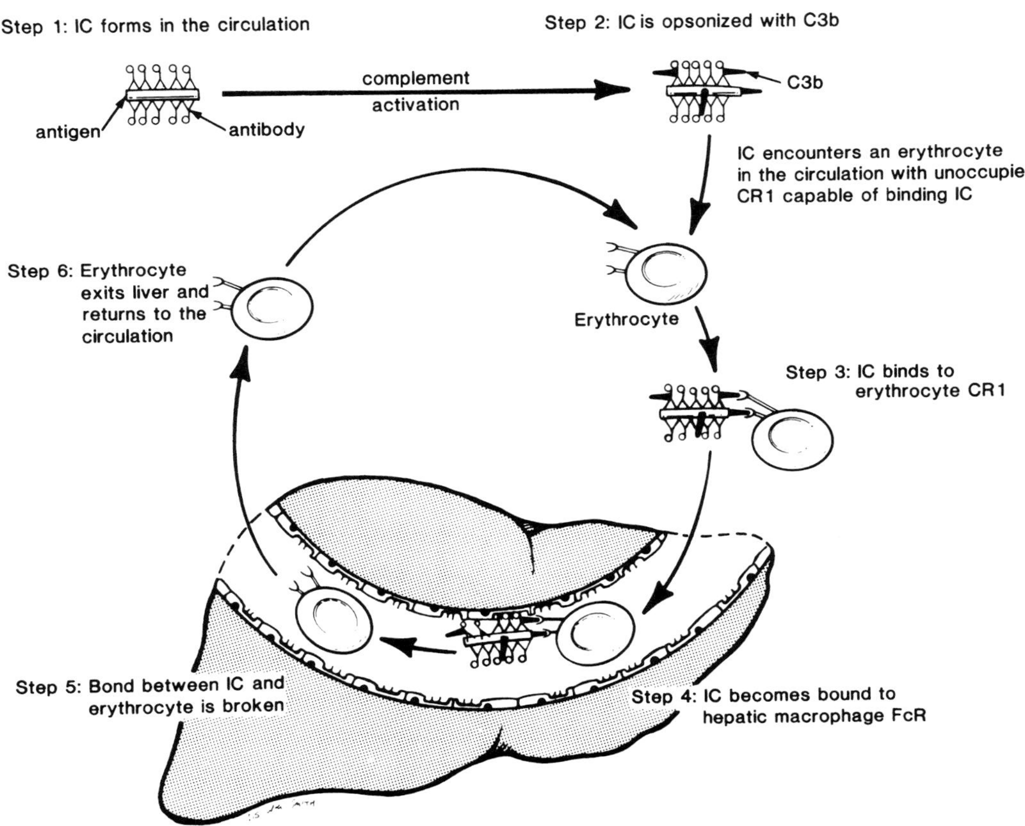

FIG. 3. Schematic representation of the operation of the erythrocyte–immune-complex-clearing mechanism: *CR1*, complement receptor type 1; *IC*, immune complex.

(94,95). Increased erythrocyte CR1 expression could protect against immune-complex-mediated renal diseases. This hypothesis was tested in a model of immune-complex-mediated glomerulonephritis in nonhuman primates (cynomolgus monkeys) (96). We found that monkeys with chronically increased erythrocyte CR1 levels tended to have fewer glomerular immune deposits and less proteinuria than did monkeys without increased erythrocyte CR1 levels; however, these differences did not achieve statistical significance (97). A major caveat in interpreting these studies is that the model of glomerulonephritis used was the traditional model in which antigen was administered as a daily bolus. This method of administering antigen may overwhelm the erythrocyte immune-complex clearance mechanism (98). Also, it is unlikely that antigen enters the circulation as large intermittent boluses in naturally occurring glomerulonephritis (98). Thus, a valid and clinically relevant test of the protective role of the erythrocyte CR1 system would involve a model of glomerulonephritis in which antigen enters the circulation over prolonged periods of time, rather than as large intermittent boluses.

The erythrocyte CR1 system and complement may also participate in the pathogenesis of immune-complex-mediated diseases by playing a role in the regulation of antibody production. Immune complexes bound to erythrocyte CR1 via C3b are rapidly cleaved by factor I with degradation of the C3b sites to C3dg and then to C3d. Immune complexes expressing C3d are then able to bind to the CR2/CD19 complex of B cells. Depending upon the circumstances of ligation, the B cells may either be activated or suppressed (83,84,99).

Nonprimates do not express CR1 on erythrocytes but do express CR1 on platelets. In nonprimates, the platelet CR1 system may be involved in immune-complex clearance in a manner analogous to that of the erythrocyte CR1 mechanism (83,84). However, the biologic value of the platelet immune-complex-clearing mechanism of the nonprimate is not clear. In vitro studies have shown that complement-mediated binding of immune complexes to platelets causes platelets to aggregate irreversibly, thereby releasing inflammatory molecules and activating coagulation (83,84). These events are in contrast to that of the primate erythrocyte immune-complex-clearing mechanism, in which the erythrocyte appears to act as an inert shuttle for the transfer of immune complexes from the circulation to the liver and spleen for safe disposal.

A small number of humans have been identified who express <10% of normal CR1 levels (100). These patients were reported to be healthy. Thus, an intact erythrocyte CR1 system may not be essential to good health. However, these patients might have never been challenged by the formation of a large immune-complex load in the circulation, as could happen during a chronic infection or during a chronic autoimmune state. Under those circumstances, patients who have an inefficient erythrocyte immune-complex-clearing mechanism might be more vulnerable to the development of immune-complex disease.

THE RENOINJURIOUS ROLE OF THE COMPLEMENT SYSTEM

Under certain circumstances, activation of the complement system is detrimental to the kidney. These are discussed next.

Immune Disorders

Excessive Formation of Circulating Immune Complexes

When pathogenic immune complexes form in the circulation at a rate that exceeds the body's capacity to clear the immune complexes safely, the complexes will deposit in vulnerable locations such as the glomerulus. Immune complexes initiate complement activation as they form in the circulation (96). After deposition of the immune complexes, complement activation continues as shown by the C5b-9 that is formed at sites of immune-complex deposition (101–104).

Relatively large amounts of immune complex must be formed in the circulation before net accumulation of immune complex will occur in glomeruli. For example, in an experimental model of immune-complex glomerulonephritis in nonhuman primates, antigen in amounts sufficient to consume all of the circulating precipitating antibody to that antigen must be infused daily for about 3–4 weeks before glomerular immune complexes are readily detectable by electron microscopy (96). This amount of immune-complex formation must be considered "large" because it is virtually all of the insoluble immune complex that the animal is capable of forming to that antigen over a 3- to 4-week period.

If the bulk of the antibody in the circulating immune complexes is IgA, rather than IgG, an "excessive" amount of immune complex might form at a relatively low total amount of circulating immune complex. This is suggested by the fact that IgA immune complexes, which do not activate the classical pathway, will not be influenced by classical pathway inhibition of immune precipitation (105). In addition, compared with IgG immune complexes, IgA immune complexes bind poorly to the erythrocyte CR1, perhaps because IgA fixes C3 poorly (92). Poor binding of IgA immune complexes to erythrocyte CR1 could increase the pathogenicity of IgA immune complexes by decreasing the ability of the erythrocyte–immune-complex-clearing mechanism to clear IgA immune complexes efficiently from the circulation (92,106).

Production or Infusion of Antibodies Directed at Endogenous Glomerular Antigens (See Also Chapter 35)

The classical example of this disorder in man is Goodpasture syndrome, in which the antibodies, almost always IgG, are directed at the noncollagenous domain of the type-IV collagen of glomerular basement membrane (GBM) (72). Also, some forms of idiopathic membranous nephropathy in humans may result from antibodies directed at endogenous antigens expressed on GECs (107) (see chapters 43 and 47).

Examples of experimental glomerulonephritis that are the result of antibodies directed at endogenous glomerular antigens include (a) *Heymann nephritis*. In this model, heterologous or autologous antibodies are directed at glycoproteins expressed on the GECs of Sprague–Dawley rats. This model closely resembles the membranous nephropathy that is seen in humans and is mediated primarily by C5b-9 (107–110). (b) *Thymocyte-1 (Thy-1) glomerulonephritis*. This model uses monoclonal or polyclonal Thy-1 antibodies directed at antigens expressed on rat glomerular mesangial cells (111,111a). The lesion is complement dependent and is mediated primarily by C5b-9 (111,112). (c) *Nephrotoxic serum nephritis*. This model is induced by immunizing the experimental animal to GBM antigens or by infusing the animal with heterologous antibody against GBM (113,114). These models are reviewed in chapter 35.

The glomerular injury in Heymann nephritis and Thy-1 nephritis is primarily mediated by C5b-9 deposition. In nephrotoxic serum nephritis, the glomerular injury is primarily mediated by C5a, which recruits neutrophils to the glomerulus (107,108). This lesion illustrated the role of complement chemotactic products including C5a in the development of glomerulonephritis, although C5b-9 may be involved as well.

Production or Infusion of Antibodies Against Antigens That Are "Planted" in the Glomerulus

In humans, the membranous nephropathy associated with therapy with gold salts or captopril may be examples of glomerulonephritis in which a drug is the planted antigen (107). In experimental animals, the following are examples of glomerulonephritis induced by a planted antigen: (a) *Cationic bovine serum albumin (BSA)*. Cationic BSA infused intravenously binds electrostatically to the GBM, which normally is anionic. If antibodies to BSA are then infused or allowed to develop naturally, glomerulonephritis is induced (115). (b) *Concanavalin A (ConA)*. When this lectin is infused into the renal artery, it binds to renal endothelial cells. When complement-activating antibodies to ConA are infused, a severe glomerulonephritis can be induced (107).

Nonimmune Complement Activation Superimposed on an Immune Renal Disease

Infection with bacterial or viral agents or tissue injury alone can activate the complement system. Intercurrent infections seem to exacerbate immune disorders such as Goodpasture syndrome or Wegener granulomatosis. To test the hypothesis that nonimmune complement activation superimposed on immune renal disease could worsen the renal disease, cobra venom factor (CVF) was infused early or late in the course of experimental nephritis (anti-GBM or $HgCl_2$ nephritis). Infusion of CVF exacerbated proteinuria in both models. The worsening of renal function was neutrophil dependent and probably involves recruitment of complement-activated neutrophils to sites of tissue injury (116).

Experimental Renal Transplant Rejection, Either Xenografts or Allografts

At least part of the injurious aspect of the rejection process in these models is mediated by antibody and complement (117,118).

Production of Autoantibody Nephritic Factors (C3 NeF and C4 NeF)

Autoantibodies that stabilize the alternative or classical pathway C3 convertases (C3 NeF and C4 NeF, respectively) are associated with membranoproliferative glomerulonephritis (MPGN) types I and III. Nephritic factors have generally been regarded as epiphenomena in MPGN types I and III, which are immune complex mediated. Continuous complement activation, however, induced by C3 NeF or C4 NeF might induce renal injury (119,120). The mechanism of injury could involve deposition of C3b at sites of injury and/or activation of neutrophils, which then adhere to sites of tissue injury. Impaired immune complex clearance because of low C3/C4 could also play a role.

Nonimmune Disorders

Nonselective Proteinuria

In glomerular disorders in which large amounts of protein are lost in the urine nonselectively (that is, both large and small molecules are filtered at the glomerulus), all of the components necessary for activation of the alternative complement pathway can be present in the glomerular filtrate (121). In such patients, C5b-9 is present on proximal tubular brush border, and complement split products are present in urine (121). Proteinuria itself leads to tubular injury and interstitial nephritis (122). Thus, the injurious effect of proteinuria may be related, at least in part, to complement activation on proximal tubular brush border (123). Urinary excretion of complement components or fragments may also reflect activity of the glomerular immune injury (124,125).

Ischemic Renal Injury

Exposure of ischemically injured kidneys to the products of complement activation produced by either infusing zymosan intravenously or exposing the animal's blood to cuprophane, delays recovery of the kidneys from the ischemic injury (126). Zymosan and cuprophane are both potent activators of the alternative complement pathway. Patients with acute renal failure show delayed recovery of renal function if hemodialysis is undertaken with bioincompatible dialysis membranes rather than biocompatible membranes (127,128). The mechanism of this adverse effect of bioincompatible membranes may be that these membranes activate complement which activates neutrophils that accumulate at sites of tissue injury in the kidney, particularly the glomerulus (128). Renal infarction also results in complement activation in the affected areas (129).

Atheroembolic Disease

Atheromata activate the classical and alternative complement pathways in vitro (130). Rats infused with atheromatous material or humans experiencing spontaneous or catheter-induced atheromatous embolization can develop hypocomplementemia (decreases in C4 and/or C3 levels). C5b-9 is seen in areas of atheromata formation (131).

Renal Ammonia Production by Diseased Kidneys

In rats with reduced numbers of functioning nephrons, the amount of ammonia produced per nephron is increased. Because ammonia can cause a nucleophilic attack on C3, thereby activating C3, some of the damage in renal insufficiency might be the result of alternative complement pathway activation by excessive renal ammonia production. Oral alkali treatment of animals with ablative nephropathy reduces renal ammonia production, decreases C5b-9 deposits in renal tissue, and preserves kidney function (109,110).

Hypertension-Induced Renal Injury

C5b-9 deposits are present in renal arterioles in patients with hypertensive nephrosclerosis (104). Hypertensive mice that are C5 deficient show less glomerular injury than hypertensive congenic mice that are C5 sufficient (132).

Intravenous Infusion of Both Tumor Necrosis Factor and Lipopolysaccharide

Simultaneous infusion of tumor necrosis factor and lipopolysaccharide mimics the effects of bacterial sepsis. The ability of bacterial sepsis to promote shock and tissue injury in mice is related to activation of the terminal complement pathway because C5-deficient mice infused with tumor necrosis factor and lipopolysaccharide are protected against shock and tissue injury whereas C5-sufficient mice are not (133,134).

Aging of Tissue

Natural aging and aging accelerated by long-standing diabetes mellitus are associated with C5b-9 deposits in glomerulus and renal arterioles and interstitium (104). Complement activation is increased (increased plasma C5b-9) in patients with long-standing type-1 diabetes (104).

MECHANISMS BY WHICH COMPLEMENT ACTIVATION PROMOTES RENAL INJURY

The studies that have provided the most detail regarding the mechanisms of complement-mediated renal injury have involved various models of immune-mediated glomerulonephritis (see also chapters 35 and 36). To assess the role of complement, most studies used intravenous infusion of CVF to induce acute (up to 3 days) complement depletion. More recently, mice with genetic C3, C4, or C5 deficiency, and rabbits or rats with genetic C6 deficiency, have also been studied. The discussion that follows is based on an analysis of these models of complement depletion.

From the studies of complement depletion in the various models of immune-mediated glomerulonephritis, a reasonably clear picture has emerged suggesting that

1. In the heterologous (acute) phase of nephrotoxic serum or anti-GBM nephritis (113,114), the Thy-1 model (111,111a), or the ConA model (107), complement activation has been regarded as the cause of the proteinuria and glomerular hypercellularity. However, recent studies using genetically altered mice ("knockout" of C3 or C4) show that C3 activation via the classical pathway determined glomerular neutrophil accumulation but only partially determined proteinuria (135).
2. In the autologous phase of nephrotoxic serum or anti-GBM nephritis (that is, after the host animal has mounted an immune response to the heterologous antibodies deposited in the glomerulus), complement activation does not play a major role in the pathogenesis of the glomerulonephritis. Instead, monocyte infiltration of the kidney appears to be more important (136).

3. In Heymann nephritis, complement activation apparently mediates the proteinuria in the acute (passive) model (107,108) but not the chronic (active) model of this disorder. The latter is suggested by studies of active Heymann nephritis in the C6-deficient rat that developed proteinuria despite evidence of inability to form C5b-9 (137).

4. In the immune-complex-mediated glomerulonephritis of acute serum sickness in rabbits (138,139), terminal pathway complement activation is not needed to induce glomerular injury but does play a role in mediating proteinuria (139). In models of acute serum sickness in mice (140,141), complement activation appears to be essential to the development of proteinuria. Models of glomerulonephritis involving acute deposition of negatively charged antigens in rodents also requires C5b-9 deposition in glomeruli to express proteinuria fully (142). The mechanisms by which complement activation exerts its effects in glomerulonephritis are discussed next.

Site of Immune-Complex Localization in the Glomerulus as a Determinant of Complement Effects

A key aspect of how complement activation affects the evolution of the glomerulonephritis is whether the complement activation is occurring primarily in the subepithelial space (Heymann nephritis, some models of chronic infusion of heterologous proteins, or acute localization of negatively charged antigens) or whether the complement activation is occurring primarily in or near the glomerular capillary lumen (nephrotoxic serum nephritis, ConA model, or Thy-1 model) (107). Immune complexes that form in the glomerular subepithelial space appear to be less able to induce infiltration of the glomerulus by circulating leukocytes, compared with models in which the immune complexes form in the subendothelial or mesangial space or in the GBM (107). Apparently, C5a generated by complement activation acts more effectively as a chemoattractant for neutrophils and monocytes when the complement activation occurs within the glomerular subendothelial space or the mesangium (107). However, this distinction appears not to be absolute. Complement-mediated localization of monocytes to the kidney may contribute to the pathogenesis of the proteinuria in Heymann nephritis, even though the immune complexes form in the subepithelial space (143).

Effects of Glomerular Subepithelial Immune-Complex Formation

When immune complexes form in the glomerular subepithelial space, the classical pathway is activated because the antibodies are virtually always IgG (107). Complement activation results in deposition of C5b-9 on the GEC membrane. The amount of C5b-9 deposited may be greater if the antibodies bind to epitopes expressed on the GECs rather than to planted antigens in the glomerular subepithelial space (107). If the amount of C5b-9 deposited on the GEC membrane is sublytic (does not result in lysis of the GECs), the cell can become activated to produce collagen (144,145) and products of arachidonic acid metabolism (increased thromboxane, prostaglandin-$F_{2\alpha}$, and prostaglandin-E production) (107). The products of arachidonic acid metabolism could play a protective role as suggested by worsening of nephrotoxic serum nephritis with cyclooxygenase inhibition (146).

Sublytic doses of C5b-9 can also stimulate the production of oxidants and proteinases by GECs (147,148). This could promote proteinuria and impaired kidney function by the following mechanisms: (a) damage to the GECs results in separation of the GECs from GBM. This leads to increased ultrafiltration at that site and increased proteinuria, apparently by bulk flow through the site of increased hydraulic conductivity; (b) loss of GBM anionic charge, which promotes albuminuria; and (c) damage to GBM with the development of shunt pathways that permit nonselective proteinuria (107).

A key role for glomerular C5b-9 deposition in causing proteinuria in membranous nephropathy is indicated by recent studies of C6 depletion in Sprague–Dawley rats with glomerular subepithelial deposits induced by infusion of cationized human IgG (142), and in studies involving complement depletion in the media of isolated glomeruli of Sprague–Dawley rats treated with anti-Fx1A antibody (149). Nevertheless, heavy proteinuria can occur in active Heymann nephritis in the absence of C5b-9 formation, as shown in studies in genetically C6-deficient rats, which are unable to form C5b-9 (137). In those studies, the size of the glomerular subepithelial electron-dense deposits correlated with the magnitude of the proteinuria. Taken together, these studies suggest that the proteinuria induced by glomerular subepithelial immune-complex formation is influenced both by the ability to generate C5b-9 and the mechanical effects of the subepithelial deposits.

Effect of Glomerular Subendothelial or Mesangial Immune-Complex Formation

When immune complexes form in the subendothelial space or when the complement activation is a result of antibodies binding to GBM, the resulting C3b deposition on GBM can itself alter glomerular function and induce proteinuria (150,151). In addition, C3b on glomerular structures permits immune adherence of neutrophils and monocytes via CR1 expressed on those cells (107). Complement activation also promotes adherence of neutrophils and monocytes by inducing upregulation of adhesion molecules on endothelial cells (152,153). Moreover, activated neutrophils can initiate complement activation by release of H_2O_2 (154), creating a "vicious cycle." Infiltrating neutrophils and monocytes release proteases that may be important causes of glomerular injury (155) (see also chapter 26). Neutrophils also release oxidants, which have been shown to induce glomerular injury and proteinuria (107), and eicosanoids, which may be protective (146). The accumulation of neutrophils and monocytes in glomeruli is chiefly the result of the chemotactic effects of C5a (107). C5a can also directly cause renal vasoconstriction and decrease glomerular filtration rate (156) (see chapter 11).

Studies in genetically C6-deficient rats have shown that C5b-9 generation in the glomerulus is necessary to express the lesions of the antithymocyte model of nephritis: mesangial necrosis, glomerular platelet accumulation, mesangial cell proliferation, and proteinuria (157). Nitric oxide, induced by complement activation in antithymocyte nephritis, may play an important role in the glomerular injury of this model (158).

Interaction of complement with complexed antibody and antigen in the vicinity of endothelial cells increases endothelial cell permeability, perhaps as a direct result of C5b67 causing endothelial cells to form gaps but without causing endothelial cell death (159). This complement-mediated increase in capillary permeability would contribute to the inflammatory process.

Complement and Platelets in Glomerulonephritis (see also Chapter 27)

In nonprimates (for example, rodents) platelets may aggregate at sites of glomerular injury via adherence of the platelet CR1 receptors to deposited C3b. Primate platelets, including those of humans, lack CR1 receptors and may be less likely to localize at sites of complement-mediated injury than nonprimate platelets (160). This could be an important difference between the responses of the primate kidney and the nonprimate kidney to complement-induced injury. Indeed, there is impressive evidence that, in nonprimates, complement-dependent platelet accumulation mediates many of the adverse effects of glomerular immune-complex formation, including impaired glomerular filtration rate, proteinuria, and proliferation of resident cells of the glomerulus (161,162). It remains to be determined whether the platelets in humans and other primates can play a similar role.

Production of Complement Components Within the Kidney

Production of complement components C2, C3, C4 and factor B by resident kidney cells (glomerular and tubular) has been demonstrated under various in vivo and in vitro circumstances (163–167). The role of local synthesis of complement components is not clear. However, they could participate in the inflammatory process or serve paracrine or autocrine roles. Of note is that C3 may act as a growth factor (71). Thus, local C3 generation might be part of normal defense/repair/growth processes, which are intensified under conditions of biologic stress.

Other events that promote glomerular injury in immune nephritis, but are not directly the result of complement activation, include the adherence of neutrophils and monocytes via their Fc receptors to the glomerular immune deposits, the adherence of neutrophils and monocytes via adhesion molecules expressed on their surfaces and monocytes (this process can be influenced by complement activation) (152,153), and the recruitment of sensitized T cells to the glomerulus [reviewed by Couser (107)] (see chapters 25–28).

PHARMACOLOGIC APPROACHES TO CONTROL COMPLEMENT-MEDIATED RENAL DISEASE

If immune complexes accumulate within the glomerulus or if complement-activating antibodies bind to endogenous or planted glomerular antigens, the complement system becomes the enemy. Under such conditions, it seems likely that patients would benefit if complement activation could be attenuated, at least temporarily.

There are four basic approaches to diminish the biologic effects of the complement system: (a) activate the complement system to deplete key component(s); (b) administer an inhibitor of complement activation; (c) administer substances that can absorb activated complement components, thereby sparing normal tissue; or (d) remove complement components from the circulation.

Approach a has been used extensively in experimental models when CVF is administered to induce C3 depletion. Animals with experimental complement-mediated diseases usually benefit from CVF treatment. Unfortunately, tissue injury may worsen initially as C3 is depleted by activation of the complement system (116, 152,168). As just discussed, the mechanism involves neutrophil activation by complement causing these inflammatory cells to adhere to sites of tissue injury (116,127,128).

In light of these concerns, approach b (inhibition of complement activation) may be more desirable than approach a (depletion of complement by first activating complement). Presently, heparin is the only inhibitor of complement activation that is available clinically. Unfortunately, use of heparin for this purpose is not clinically feasible because heparin must be administered in amounts much greater than that needed to achieve anticoagulation (91).

Recently, the experimental complement inhibitor soluble recombinant CR1 (sCR1) has been shown to be effective in reducing the acute complement-mediated injury of experimental myocardial ischemia (169,170), xenografts (171–173), gut ischemia (174), thermal and other forms of skin and lung injury (175), experimental allergic encephalomyelitis (176), and experimental nephritis (ConA and antithymocyte serum) (177). sCR1 can also inhibit complement activation by bioincompatible dialysis membranes (178).

The results of sCR1 in experimental models of complement injury are encouraging. However, the clinical utility of sCR1 remains to be established. Of interest is that CR1 is normally shed into the plasma (179), mainly by cleavage of CR1 from neutrophils (180). Thus, plasma CR1 might be a natural mechanism for control of complement activation.

Other inhibitors of complement activation, soluble recombinant MCP (sMCP) and DAF (sDAF) have been developed (181,182). sMCP inhibits complement activation in human and primate systems, but not rodents.

sCR1, sMCP, and sDAF are large proteins that are immunogenic. Thus, if these inhibitors are found to be clinically useful, it will probably be for the acute, not chronic, treatment of complement-mediated disorders.

Approach c (control of complement activation by infusion of a substance that absorbs activated complement components before they can bind to tissue and initiate further complement activation) is currently being used when high doses of intravenous immunoglobulins (IVIgs) are administered. The Fc portion of Ig absorbs C3b and C4b (183), and dimers of IgG (up to 10% of total IgG in IVIg) bind C1 (184). These effects of IVIg could explain some of the benefits attributed to IVIg in the treatment of certain acute immune disorders (183).

Approach d (removal of complement) occurs during plasmapheresis, which also removes other plasma components, including antibodies and coagulation factors. Plasmapheresis is reported to be of value in the management of a number of immune-mediated disorders (185). However, the portion of the benefit of plasmapheresis that is attributable to complement removal is not clear. In SLE patients with severe glomerulonephritis, an 8-week course of plasmapheresis, which had little effect on C3 and C4 levels, did not improve patient outcomes (186).

In summary, there is considerable evidence that the ability to acutely attenuate the effects of complement activation would be beneficial to patients with certain immune-mediated disorders. At present, there is no entirely satisfactory means to achieve this goal. However, the development of specific inhibitors of complement activation offers hope that this goal may be achieved in the not-too-distant future.

DIAGNOSTIC SIGNIFICANCE OF SERUM COMPLEMENT LEVELS

Table 4 shows the principal immune-complex diseases that are associated with hypocomplementemia (187) (see chapter 37). For patients whose complement status is being evaluated for the first time, we recommend the measurement of serum C3 and C4 levels, and CH50 levels from EDTA-treated plasma. The CH50 assay assesses the overall function of the classical and terminal complement pathway components C1 to C8 (C9 is not required for hemolysis in the CH50 assay). Thus, the measurement of CH50 is useful as a screening test for hypocomplementemic states that would be missed if only C3 and C4 levels were measured. The CH50 assay is less useful as a monitor of serial changes in serum complement levels because, for example, C3 and C4 levels may be abnormally low, yet the capacity of the patient's serum to hemolyze the sensitized sheep erythrocytes, the basis for the CH50 assay, may remain within the normal range. In addition, results of the CH50 assay may be more variable because it is more difficult to standardize than nephelometry methods of C3 and C4 measurement (187).

In patients with classical complement pathway activation, C3 and C4 levels change proportionately (Fig. 4) (187). In patients with primarily alternative pathway activation, C4 levels are preserved but C3 levels are decreased. Some reports suggest that in certain immune-complex disorders (for example, type-II cryoglobuline-

TABLE 4. *Immune-complex diseases associated with hypocomplementemia*

Disease[a]	Patterns of hypocomplementemia
SLE	C3 and C4 decreased proportionately
MPGN type 1	C3 decreased more than C4 (effect of C3 NeF)
Cryoglobulinemia	
Types I and III	C3 and C4 decreased proportionately
Type II	C4 may be decreased more than C3
GN of chronic) infection (e.g., endocarditis	C3 and C4 decreased proportionately
Postinfectious (e.g., post-streptococcal) GN	C3 decreased much more than C4
Other conditions[b]	Generally, C3 and C4 decreased proportionately

[a]GN, glomerulonephritis; MPGN, membranoproliferative GN; NeF, nephritic factor; SLE, systemic lupus erythematosus.

[b]Rheumatoid vasculitis, idiopathic vasculitis, repeated injection of foreign proteins, drug-induced SLE, hypersensitivity to drugs, chemotherapy for malignancy with immune-complex formation, thyroid disease and GN, jejunoileal bypass with vasculitis, B-cell lymphoproliferative disorder with immune-complex formation.

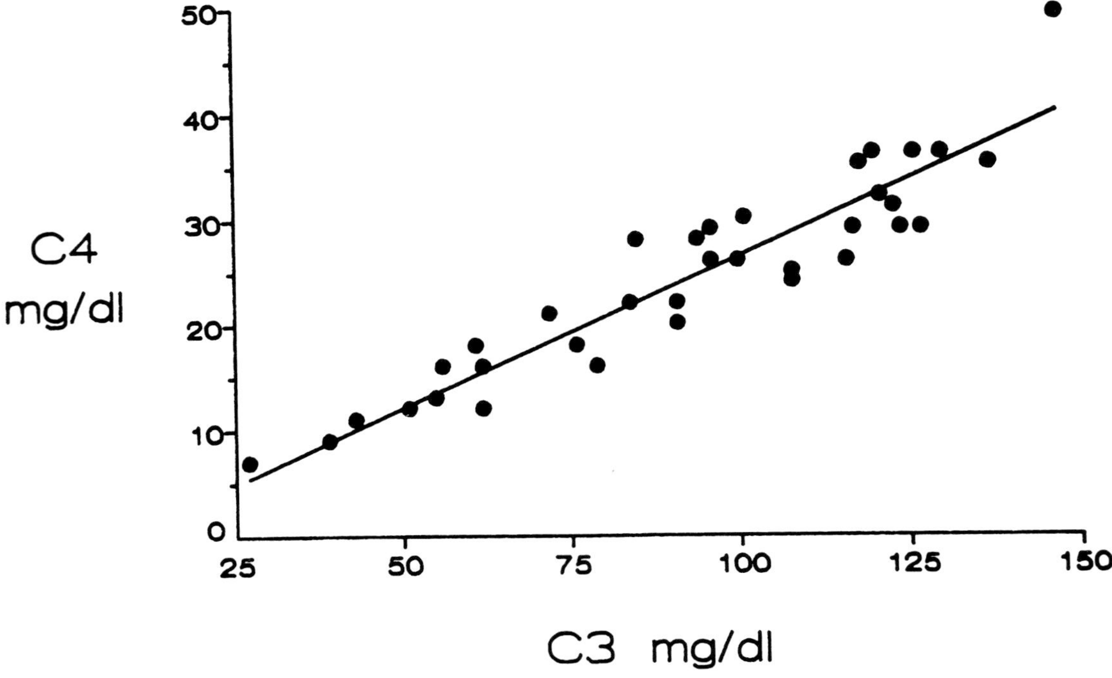

FIG. 4. Relationship between serum C3 and C4 levels in a typical patient with systemic lupus erythematosus and glomerulonephritis. The correlation coefficient of this relationship is 0.93 ($p < 0.001$). The complement levels in this patient were measured by nephelometry.

mia or SLE), C4 levels are disproportionately low compared with C3 levels (188). This has led to the suggestion that in these disorders there may be increased consumption of C4 as compared with C3. It is more likely, however, that the low C4 levels relative to C3 levels in these disorders represent the presence of C4 null genes in the affected individuals. C4 null genes occur commonly in the general population and with increased frequency in immune-complex diseases, such as SLE (187).

Genetic C4 deficiency is a significant risk factor for SLE, particularly in whites (189,190). C4B and total C4 levels tend to be about one-third higher in blacks than whites (190). This should be taken into account when interpreting C4 levels in blacks. Although C4A binds to immune complexes better than does C4B, these isoforms change in parallel during changes in SLE activity (190).

When serum complement levels are measured serially to assess activity of SLE, it is sufficient to measure only C3 levels (191) (see also chapters 37 and 48). Although changes in serum C3 and C4 levels are highly correlated in SLE (Fig. 4), because the normal range for C4 is relatively much greater than that of C3 (an effect of the presence of C4 null genes in the general population), serum C3 levels are more likely to change from normal to abnormal during SLE activity than are serum C4 levels (191).

The role of measurement of products of complement activation (such as C3a des Arg, C3bi, C3dg, Bb, and C5b-9) in assessing clinical activity of immune-complex disease has not been established, but several reports suggest that such measurements can be useful (192,193).

Although hypocomplementemia often predicts or is evidence of active immune-complex-mediated disease, numerous nonimmunologic conditions also can cause hypocomplementemia. It is important to be aware of these conditions because some can induce a systemic disorder that can be easily confused with an immune-complex vasculitis. These conditions are presented in Table 5. In addition, a nonimmunologic condition that causes hypocomplementemia can develop in a patient with an immune-complex disorder that is inactive. If the physician does not recognize that the hypocomplementemia is the result of the nonimmunologic condition, this could lead to incorrect treatment of the patient. The nonimmunologic conditions that could spuriously suggest activity of an immune-complex-mediated disorder, when the nonimmunologic condition develops in a patient with a known immune-complex-mediated disorder, are listed in Table 6.

Not all immune-complex-mediated disorders, or disorders mediated by specific binding of antibody to tissues, are associated with hypocomplementemia. The absence of hypocomplementemia in these disorders is probably related to a lesser mass of antibodies involved in these processes. The immune-complex renal diseases that are rarely or never associated with hypocomplementemia are idiopathic membranous nephropathy, Henoch–Schonlein purpura, IgA nephropathy, Goodpasture syndrome, immunotactoid and fibrillary glomerulonephritis, and C1q glomerulopathy (187).

Certain conditions can raise serum complement levels and, therefore, could offset the effect of an immune-complex disease to lower serum complement levels. Of particular relevance are pregnancy, systemic infections, and noninfectious chronic inflammatory states such as rheumatoid arthritis and idiopathic vasculitis. If these conditions coexist with an active immune-complex disorder, hypocomplementemia might not develop, even though the immune-complex-mediated disease is active. The interaction between a condition that can raise complement levels and a condition that can lower serum complement levels has been particularly well described in SLE patients who become pregnant. In normal pregnancy, serum complement levels often increase to above normal values. Thus, a normal complement level in a pregnant SLE patient could indicate activity of her SLE.

As indicated in Table 6, uncomplicated nephrotic syndrome does not cause hypocomplementemia. Indeed, C3 levels can be increased. When this occurs in patients with idiopathic focal glomerulosclerosis, the prognosis is more favorable than in focal glomerulosclerosis patients with low normal C3 levels (194).

TABLE 5. *Common nonimmunologic diseases that can mimic an immune-complex-mediated vasculitis because they cause multisystem disorders and hypocomplementemia*

Disease	Complement levels[b]	Comment
Atheroembolism	↓C3, ±↓C4	Hypocomplementemia is usually transient, occurring mainly during active embolization[c]
Severe sepsis	↓C3, ↓C4	Development of shock increases likelihood of sepsis causing hypocomplementemia
HUS/TTP[a]	↓C3, ±↓C4	Hypocomplementemia occurs in ~1/2 of cases
Acute pancreatitis	↓C3, ↓C4	Hypocomplementemia clears in a few days[c]

[a]Hemolytic–uremic syndrome/thrombotic thrombocytopenia purpura.
[b]↓, Decreased.
[c]By contrast, the hypocomplementemia of active systemic lupus erythematosus usually requires weeks to return to normal, with successful therapy.

TABLE 6. *Common nonimmunologic conditions that can cause hypocomplementemia and, should they be present in patients with active immune-complex disease, could spuriously suggest activity of the immune-complex disease*

Disease	Complement levels[b]	Comment
The conditions listed in Table 5	See Table 5	See Table 5
Severe malnutrition[a]	↓C3, ±N C4	C1q is also low
Severe liver disease	↓C3, ↓C4	C1q levels are normal
Inherited C4 deficiency	N C3, ±↓C4	20–40% of normals have one or two C4 null genes; SLE patients have a higher incidence of this genetic defect

[a]The protein depletion of uncomplicated nephrotic syndrome does not cause low C3 or C4 levels.
[b]N, normal; ↓, decreased.

REFERENCES

1. Hebert LA, Cosio FG, Birmingham DJ. The role of the complement system in renal injury. *Semin Nephrol* 1992;12:408–27.
2. Reid KBM, Porter KK. Subunit composition and structure of subcomponent C1q of the first component of human complement. *Biochem J* 1976;155:19–23.
3. Sim RB. The human complement system in serine proteases C1r and C1s and their proenzymes. *Methods Enzymol* 1981;80:26–42.
4. Ziccardi RJ. Nature of the metal ion requirement for assembly and function of the first component of complement. *J Biol Chem* 1983; 258:6187–92.
5. Golan MD, Hitschold T, Loos M. The reconstitution of human C1, the first complement component: binding of C1r and C1s to C1q influences the C1q conformation. *FEBS Lett* 1981;128:281–85.
6. Buckman KJ, Moore SK, Ebbin AJ, Cox MB, Dubois EL. Familial systemic lupus erythematosus. *Arch Intern Med* 1978;138:1674–6.
7. Sim RB, Reid KB. C1: molecular interactions with activating systems. *Immunol Today* 1991;12:307–11.
8. Rossen RD, Michael LH, Hawkins HK, et al. Cardiolipin–protein complexes and initiation of complement activation after coronary artery occlusion. *Circ Res* 1994;75:546–55.
9. Porter R, Reid K. Activation of the complement system by antibody–antigen complexes: the classical pathway. *Adv Protein Chem* 1979;33:1–71.
10. Isenman D, Kells DIC. Conformational and functional changes in the fourth component of human complement produced by nucleophilic modification and by proteolysis with C1s. *Biochemistry* 1982;21: 1109–17.
11. Law SKA, Dodds AW, Porter RR. A comparison of the properties of two classes, C4A and C4B, of the human complement component C4. *EMBO J* 1984;3:1819–23.
12. Nagasawa S, Stroud RM. Cleavage of C2 by C1s into the antigenically distinct fragments C2a and C2b: demonstration of binding of C2b to C4b. *Proc Natl Acad Sci USA* 1977;74:2998–3001.
13. Daffern PJ, Pfeifer PH, Ember JA, Hugli TE. C3a is a chemotaxin for human eosinophils but not for neutrophils. I. C3a stimulation of neutrophils is secondary to eosinophil activation. *J Exp Med* 1995;181: 2119–27.
14. Tack BF, Harrison RA, Janatova J, Thomas ML, Prahl JW. Evidence for presence of an internal thiolester bond in third component of human complement. *Proc Natl Acad Sci USA* 1980;77:5764–8.
15. Isenman DE, Kells DI, Cooper NR, Muller-Eberhard HJ, Pangburn MK. Nucleophilic modification of human complement protein C3: correlation of conformational changes with acquisition of C3b-like functional properties. *Biochemistry* 1981;20:4458–67.

16. Pangburn MK, Schreiber RD, Muller-Eberhard HJ. Formation of the initial C3 convertase of the alternative complement pathway: acquisition of C3b-like activities by spontaneous hydrolysis of the putative thioester in native C3. *J Exp Med* 1981;154:856–67.
17. Muller-Eberhard HJ, Gotze O. C3 proactivator convertase and its mode of action. *J Exp Med* 1972;135:1003–8.
18. Fearon DT, Austen KF. Properdin: binding to C3b and the stabilization of the C3b-dependent C3 convertase. *J Exp Med* 1975;142: 856–63.
19. Lachmann PJ, Hughes-Jones NC. Initiation of complement activation. *Springer Semin Immunopathol* 1984;7:143–62.
20. Daha MR, Fearon DT, Austen KF. C3 requirements for formation of alternative pathway C5 convertase. *J Immunol* 1976;117:630–4.
21. Discipio RG. The binding of human complement proteins C5, factor B, β1H and properdin to complement fragment C3b on zymosan. *Biochem J* 1981;199:485–96.
22. Davies KA, Saville J, Walport MJ. In vitro transfer of immune complexes from erythrocytes to monocytes and macrophages. *Complement Inflamm* 1989;6:328.
23. Monahan JB, Sodetz JM. Role of the β-subunit in the interaction of the eighth component of human complement with the membrane-bound cytolytic complex. *J Biol Chem* 1981;256:3258–62.
24. Podack ER. Molecular composition of the tubular structure of the membrane attack complex of complement. *J Biol Chem* 1984;259: 8641–7.
25. Ziccardi RJ. Activation of the early components of the classical complement pathway under physiologic condtions. *J Immunol* 1981;126: 1769–73.
26. Myones BL, Dalzell JG, Hogg N, et al. Neutrophil and monocyte cell surface p150,95 has iC3b-receptor (CR4) activity resembling CR3. *J Clin Invest* 1988;82:640–51.
27. Matsumoto AK, Kopicky-Burd J, Carter RH, Tuveson DA, Tedder TF, Fearon DT. Intersection of the complement and immune systems: a signal transduction complex of the B lymphocyte-containing complement receptor type 2 and CD 19. *J Exp Med* 1991;173:55–64.
28. Sscharstein J, Correa EB, Gallo GR. Human C4-binding protein: association with immune complexes in vitro and in vivo. *J Clin Invest* 1979;63:437–42.
29. Wyatt RJ, McAdams AJ, Forristal J, Snyder J, West CD. Glomerular deposition of complement-control proteins in acute and chronic glomerulonephritis. *Kidney Int* 1979;16:505.
30. Bhaki S, Tranum JJ. Terminal membrane C5b-9 complex of human complement: transition from an amphiphilic to a hydophilic state through binding of the S protein from serum. *J Cell Biol* 1982;94: 755–9.
31. Bariety J, Hinglais N, Bhakdi S, Mandet C, Rouchon M, Kazatchkine MD. Immunohistochemical study of complement S protein (vitronectin) in normal and diseases human kidneys: relationship to neoantigens of the C5b-9 terminal complex. *Clin Exp Immunol* 1989; 75:76–81.
32. Law SK, Levine RP. Interaction between the third complement protein and cell surface macromolecules. *Proc Natl Acad Sci USA* 1977; 74:2701–5.
33. Tschopp J, Chonn A, Hertig S, French LE. Clusterin, the human apolipoprotein and complement inhibitor, binds to complement C7, C8B and the b domain of C9. *J Immunol* 1993;151:2159–65.
34. Saunders JR, Aminian A, McRae JL, O'Farrell KA, Adam WR, Murphy BF. Clusterin depletion enhances immune glomerular injury in the isolated perfused kidney. *Kidney Int* 1994;45:817–27.
35. Dvergsten J, Manivel C, Correa-Rotter R, Rosenberg ME. Expression of clusterin in human renal diseases. *Kidney Int* 1994;45:828–35.
36. Law SK, Lichtenberg NA, Levine RP. Evidence for an ester linkage between the labile binding site of C3b and receptive surfaces. *J Immunol* 1979;123:1388–94.
37. Platts-Mills TAE, Ishizaka K. Activation of the alternate pathway of human complement by rabbit cells. *J Immunol* 1974;113:348.
38. Fearon DT, Austen KF. Activation of the alternative complement pathway with rabbit erythrocytes by circumvention of the regulatory action of endogenous control proteins. *J Exp Med* 1977;146:22–33.
39. Fearon DT. Regulation by membrane sialic acid of B1H-dependent decay–dissociation of amplification C3 convertase of the alternative complement pathway. *Proc Natl Acad Sci USA* 1978;75:1971–5.
40. Lublin DM, Atkinson JP. Decay-accelerating factor: biochemistry, molecular biology and function. *Annu Rev Immunol* 1989;7:35–8.
41. Cole JL, Housley GA, Dykman TR, et al. Identification of an additional class of C3-binding membrane proteins of human peripheral blood leukocytes and cell lines. *Proc Natl Acad Sci USA* 1985;82: 859–63.
42. Liszewski MK, Post TW, Atkinson JP. Membrane cofactor protein (MCP or CD46): newest member of the regulators of complement activation gene cluster. *Annu Rev Immunol* 1991;9:431–55.
43. Holers VM, Cole JL, Lublin DM, Seya T, Atkinson JP. Human C3b and C4b regulatory proteins: a new multi-gene family. *Immunol Today* 1989;6:188–92.
44. Fearon DT. The human C3b receptor. *Springer Semin Immunopathol* 1983;6:159–72.
45. Hansch GM, Hammer CH, Vanguri P, et al. Homologous species restriction in lysis of erythrocytes by terminal complement proteins. *Proc Natl Acad Sci USA* 1981;78:5118–21.
46. Davies A, Simmons DL, Hale G, et al. CD59, and LY-6-like protein expressed in human lymphoid cells, regulates the action of the complement membrane attack complex on homologous cells. *J Exp Med* 1989;170:637–54.
47. Holguin MH, Fredrick LR, Bernshaw NJ, Wilcox LA, Parker CJ. Isolation and characterization of a membrane protein from normal human erythrocytes that inhibit reactive lysis of the erythrocyte of paroxysmal nocturnal hemoglobinuria. *J Clin Invest* 1989;84:7–17.
48. Yamashina M, Ueda E, Kinoshita T, et al. Inherited complete deficiency of 20-kilodalton homologous restriction factor (CD59) as a cause of paroxysmal nocturnal. *N Engl J Med* 1990;323:1184–8.
49. Rollins SA, Zhao J, Ninomiya H, Sims PJ. Inhibition of homologous complement by CD59 is mediated by a species-selective recognition conferred through binding to C8 within C5b-8 or C9 within C5b-9. *J Immunol* 1991;146:2345–51.
50. Holguin MH, Martin CB, Bernshaw N, Parker C. Analysis of the effects of activation of the alternative pathway of complement on erythrocytes with an isolated deficiency of decay accelerating factor. *J Immunol* 1992;148:498–502.
51. Holguin MH, Wilcox LA, Bernshaw NJ, et al. Relationship between the membrane inhibitor of reactive lysis and the erythrocyte phenotypes of paroxysmal nocturnal hemoglobinuria. *J Clin Invest* 1989; 84:1387–94.
52. Quigg RJ, Cybulsky AV, Salant DJ. Effect of nephritogenic antibody on complement regulation in cultured rat glomerular epithelial cells. *J Immunol* 1991;147:838–45.
53. Ramm LE, Whitlow MB, Mayer MM. Complement lysis of nucleated cells: effect of temperature and puromycin on the number of channels required for cytolysis. *Mol Immunol* 1984;21:1015–21.
54. Hamilton KK, Hattori R, Esmon CT, Sims P. Complement proteins C5b-9 induce vesiculation of the endothelial plasma membrane and expose catalytic surface for assembly of the prothrombinase enzyme complex. *J Biol Chem* 1990;265:3809–14.
55. Iida K, Whitlow MB, Nussenzweig V. Membrane vesiculation protects erythrocytes from destruction by complement. *J Immunol* 1991; 147:2638–42.
56. Morgan BP, Dankert JR, Esser AF. Recovery of human neutrophils from complement attack: removal of the membrane attack complex by endocytosis and exocytosis. *J Immunol* 1987;168:246–53.
57. Ichida S, Yuzawa Y, Okada H, Yoshioka K, Matsuo S. Localization of the complement regulatory proteins in the normal human kidney. *Kidney Int* 1994;46:59–96.
58. Cosio FG, Sedmak DD, Mahan JD, Nahman NS Jr. Localization of decay-accelerating factor in normal and diseased kidneys. *Kidney Int* 1989;36:100–7.
59. Shibata T, Cosio FG, Birmingham DJ. Complement activation induces the expression of decay accelerating factor on human mesangial cells. *J Immunol* 1991;147:3901–8.
60. Shibata T, Cosio FG. Complement (C8) stimulates synthesis of a unique form of decay accelerating factor (DAF) by human mesangial cells (MC). *J Am Soc Nephrol* 1991;2:562.
61. Cosio FG, Shibata T, Rovin BH, Birmingham DJ. Effects of complement activation products on the synthesis of decay accelerating factor and membrane cofactor protein by human mesangial cells. *Kidney Int* 1994;46:986–92.
62. Shibata T, Cosio FG. Expression of cell-associated C3 regulatory proteins (CCRP) on human glomerular cells. *J Am Soc Nephrol* 1990;1: 538.
63. Shibata T, Kohsaka T. Effects of complement activation on the

expression of CD59 by human mesangial cells. *J Immunol* 1995;155: 403–9.

64. Matsuo S, Nishikage H, Yoshida F, Nomura A, Piddlesden SJ, Morgan BP. Role of CD59 in experimental glomerulonephritis in rats. *Kidney Int* 1994;46:191–200.
65. Tamai H, Matsuo S, Fukatsu A, et al. Localization of 20-kD homologous restriction factor (HRF20) in diseased human glomeruli: an immunofluorescence study. *Clin Exp Immunol* 1991;84:256–62.
66. Appay M-D, Kazatchkine MD, Levi-Strauss M, Hinglais N, Bariety J. Expression of CR1 (CD35) mRNA in podocytes from adult and fetal human kidneys. *Kidney Int* 1990;38:289–93.
67. Kazatchkine MD, Fearon DT, Appay MD, et al. Immunohistochemical study of the human glomerular C3b receptor in normal kidney and in seventy five cases of renal diseases. *J Clin Invest* 1982;69:900–12.
68. Pascual M, Steiger G, Sadallah S, et al. Identification of membrane-bound CR1 (CD35) in human urine: evidence for its release by glomerular podocytes. *J Exp Med* 1994;179:889–99.
69. Quigg RJ, Sneed AE III. Molecular characterization of rat glomerular epithelial cell complement receptors. *J Am Soc Nephrol* 1994;4: 1912–9.
70. Quigg RJ, Holers VM, Morgan BP, Sneed AE III. Crry and CD59 regulate complement in rat glomerular epithelial cells and are inhibited by the nephritogenic antibody of passive Heymann nephritis. *J Immunol* 1995;154:3437–43.
70a. Nomura A, Nishikawa K, Yuzawa Y, et al. Tubulo-interstitial injury induced in rats by a monoclonal antibody that inhibits function of a membrane inhibitor of complement. *J Clin Invest* 1995;96:2348–56.
71. Hostetter MK. The third component of complement: new functions for an old friend. *J Lab Clin Med* 1993;122:491–6.
72. Glassock RJ, Adler SG, Ward HJ, Cohen AH. Primary glomerular diseases. *Kidney* 1991;1:1182–279.
73. Ives HE, Daniel TO. Vascular diseases of the kidney. *Kidney* 1991;2: 2497–550.
74. Pichette V, Querin S, Schurch W, Brun G, Lehner-Netsch G, Delage J-M. Familial hemolytic–uremic syndrome and homozygous factor H deficiency. *Am J Kidney Dis* 1994;24:936–41.
75. Ross GD. Opsonization and membrane complement receptors. In: Ross GD, ed. Immunobiology of the complement system. Orlando, Florida: Academic Press; 1986;87–114.
76. Pangburn MK. The alternative pathway: immunobiology of the complement system. 1986;45–62.
77. Bach J-F, Crosnier J, Funck-Brentano J-L, eds. *Advances in nephrology;* vol 13. Chicago: Year Book Medical, 1984.
78. Colten HR. Biology of disease: molecular basis of complement deficiency syndromes. *Lab Invest* 1985;52:468–74.
79. Rother K. Hereditary deficiencies in man: summary of reported deficiencies. *Prog Allergy* 39:202–11.
80. Morgan BP, Walport MJ. 1991; Complement deficiency and disease. *Immunol Today* 1986;12:301–6.
81. Nickells MW, Subramanian VB, Clemenza L, Atkinson JP. Identification of complement receptor type 1-related proteins on primate erythrocytes. *J Immunol* 1995;154:2829–37.
82. Hebert LA. The erythrocyte–immune complex–glomerulonephritis connection in man. *Kidney Int* 1987;31:877–85.
83. Hebert LA. Clearance of immune complexes from the circulation of man and other primates. *Am J Kidney Dis* 1991;17:352–61.
84. Hebert LA, Cosio FG, Birmingham DJ, Mahan JD. Biologic significance of the erythrocyte complement receptor: a primate prerequisite. *J Lab Clin Med* 1991;118:301–8.
85. Cohen JHM, Lutz HU, Pennaforte JL, Bouchard A, Kazatchkine MD. Peripheral catabolism of CR1 (the C3b receptor, CD35) on erythrocytes from healthy individuals and patients with systemic lupus erythematosus (SLE). *Clin Exp Immunol* 1992;87:422–8.
86. Pascual M, Lutz HU, Steiger G, Stammler P, Schifferli JA. Release of vesicles enriched in complement receptor 1 from human erythrocytes. *J Immunol* 1993;151:397–404.
87. Shapiro S, Kohn D, Miller B, Gershon H. Erythrocytes from young but not elderly donors can bind and degrade immune complex- and antibody-bound C3 in vitro. *Clin Exp Immunol* 1994;95:181–90.
88. Lobatto S, Daha MR, Breedveld FC, et al. Abnormal clearance of soluble aggregates of human immunoglobulin G in patients with systemic lupus erythematosus. *Clin Exp Immunol* 1988;72:55–9.
89. Schifferli JA, Ng YC, Estreicher J, Walport MJ. The clearance of tetanus toxoid/anti-tetanus toxoid immune complexes from the circulation of humans: complement and erythrocyte complement receptor 1-dependent mechanism. *J Immunol* 1988;140:899–904.
90. Madi N, Pacaud JP, Steiger G, Schifferli JA. Immune adherence of nascent hepatitis B surface antigen–antibody complexes in vivo in humans. *Clin Exp Immunol* 1989;78:201–6.
91. Waxman FJ, Hebert LA, Cornacoff JB, et al. Complement depletion accelerates the clearance of immune complexes from the circulation of primates. *J Clin Invest* 1984;74:1329–40.
92. Waxman FJ, Hebert LA, Cosio FG, et al. Differential binding of immunoglobulin A and immunoglobulin G1 immune complexes to primate erythrocytes in vivo. *J Clin Invest* 1986;77:82–9.
93. Beynon HLC, Davies KA, Haskard DO, Walport MJ. Erythrocyte complement receptor type 1 and interactions between immune complexes, neutrophils, and endothelium. *J Immunol* 1994;153:3160.
94. Hebert LA, Birmingham DJ, Shen X-P, Cosio FG. Stimulating erythropoiesis increases complement receptor expression on primate erythrocytes. *Clin Immunol Immunopathol* 1992;62:301–6.
95. Hebert LA, Birmingham DJ, Cosio FG, Shen X-P, Hebert MM. Erythropoietin therapy in humans increases expression of erythrocyte complement receptor type 1 (CD35). *J Am Soc Nephrol* 1994;4: 1786–91.
96. Hebert LA, Cosio FG, Birmingham DJ, et al. Experimental immune complex-mediated glomerulonephritis in the nonhuman primate. *Kidney Int* 1991;39:44–56.
97. Hebert LA, Birmingham DJ, Mahan JD, et al. Effect of chronically increased erythrocyte complement receptors on immune complex nephritis. *Kidney Int* 1994;45:493–9.
98. Hebert LA, Birmingham DJ, Shen X-P, Cosio FG, Fryczkowski A. Rate of antigen entry into the circulation in experimental versus naturally occurring immune complex glomerulonephritis. *J Am Soc Nephrol* 1994;5(Suppl 1):S70.
99. Molina H, Perkins SJ, Guthridge J, Gorka J, Kinoshita T, Holers VM. Characterization of a complement receptor 2 (CR1, CD21) ligand binding site for C3: an initial model of ligand interaction with two linked short consensus repeat modules. *J Immunol* 1995;154: 5426–35.
100. Moulds JM, Nickells MW, Moulds JJ, Brown MC, Atkinson JP. The C3b/C4b receptor is recognized by the Knops, McCoy, Swain–Langley, and York blood group antisera. *J Exp Med* 1991;173:1159–63.
101. Falk RJ, Dalmasso AP, Kim Y, et al. Neoantigen of the polymerized ninth component of complement: characterization of a monoclonal antibody and immunohistochemical localization in renal disease. *J Clin Invest* 1983;72:560–73.
102. Couser WG, Baker PJ, Adler S. Complement and direct mediation of immune glomerular injury: a new perspective. *Kidney Int* 1985;28: 879–90.
103. Hinglais N, Kazatchkine MD, Bhakdi S, et al. Immunohistochemical study of the C5b-9 complex of complement in human kidneys. *Kidney Int* 1986;30:399–410.
104. Falk RJ, Sisson SP, Dalmasso AP, Kim Y, Michael AF, Vernier RL. Ultrastructural localization of the membrane attack complex of complement in human renal tissues. *Am J Kidney Dis* 1987;9:121–8.
105. Schifferli JA. The classical pathway of complement prevents the formation of insoluble antigen–antibody complexes: biological implications. *Immunol Lett* 1986/1987;14:225–8.
106. Hebert LA. Disposition of IgA-containing circulating immune complexes. *Am J Kidney Dis* 1988;12:388–92.
107. Couser WG. Mediation of immune glomerular injury. *J Am Soc Nephrol* 1990;1:13–29.
108. Cybulsky AV, Quigg RJ, Salant DJ. Role of the complement membrane attack complex in glomerular injury. *Contemp Issues Nephrol* 1988;18:57–86.
109. Nath KA, Hostetter MK, Hostetter TH. Pathophysiology of chronic tubulo-interstitial disease in rats: interactions of dietary acid load, ammonia, and complement component C3. *J Clin Invest* 1985;76: 667–75.
110. Nath KA, Hostetter MK, Hostetter TH. Increased ammoniagenesis as a determinant of progressive renal injury. *Am J Kidney Dis* 1991;17: 654–7.
111. Yamamoto T, Wilson CB. Complement dependence of antibody-induced mesangial cell injury in the rat. *J Immunol* 1987;138:3758–65.
111a. Johnson RJ, Pritzl P, Hiroyuki I, Iida H, Alpers CE. Platelet–complement interactions in mesangial proliferative nephritis in the rat. *Am J Pathol* 1990;138:313–21.

112. Brandt J, Pippin J, Schulze M, et al. Role of the complement membrane attack complex (C5b-9) in mediating experimental mesangioproliferative glomerulonephritis. *Kidney Int* 1996;49:335–43.
113. Holdsworth SR, Neale TJ, Wilson CB. Abrogation of macrophage-dependent injury in experimental glomerulonephritis in the rabbit. *J Clin Invest* 1981;68:686–97.
114. Schreiner GF, Cotran RS, Unanue ER. Modulation of Ia and leukocyte common antigen expression in rat glomeruli during the course of glomerulonephritis and aminonucleoside nephrosis. *Lab Invest* 1984; 51:524–33.
115. Wener MH, Mannik M. Mechanisms of immune deposit formation in renal glomeruli. *Semin Immunopathol* 1986;9:219–35.
116. Savige JA, Dash AC, Rees AJ. Exaggerated glomerular albuminuria after cobra venom factor in anti-glomerular basement membrane disease. *Nephron* 1989;52:29–35.
117. Brauer RB, Baldwin WM III, Ibrahim S, Sanfilippo F. The contribution of terminal complement components to acute and hyperacute allograft rejection in the rat. *Transplantation* 1995;59:288–93.
118. Baldwin WM III, Pruitt SK, Brauer RB, Daha MR, Sanfilippo F. Complement in organ transplantation: contributions to inflammation, injury, and rejection. *Transplantation* 1995;59:797–808.
119. West CD. Nephritic factors predispose to chronic glomerulonephritis. *Am J Kidney Dis* 1994;24:956–63.
120. Mathieson PW, Peters K. Are nephritic factors nephritogenic? *Am J Kidney Dis* 1994;24:964–6.
121. Ogrodowski JL, Hebert LA, Sedmak D, Cosio FG, Tamerius J, Kolb W. Measurement of SC5b-9 in urine in patients with the nephrotic syndrome. *Kidney Int* 1991;40:1141–7.
122. Eddy AA, McCulloch L, Liu E, Adams J. A relationship between proteinuria and acute tubulointerstitial disease in rats with experimental nephrotic syndrome. *Am J Pathol* 1991;138:1111–21.
123. Biancone L, David S, Della Pietra V, Montrucchio G, Cambi V, Camussi G. Alternative pathway activation of complement by cultured human proximal tubular epithelial cells. *Kidney Int* 1994;45:451–60.
124. Brenchley PE, Coupes B, Short CD, O'Donoghue DJ, Ballardie FW, Mallick NP. Urinary C3dg and C5b-9 indicate active immune disease in human membranous nephropathy. *Kidney Int* 1992;41:933–7.
125. Lehto T, Honkanen E, Teppo A-M, Meri S. Urinary excretion of protectin (CD59), complement SC5b-9 and cytokines in membranous glomerulonephritis. *Kidney Int* 1995;47:1403–11.
126. Schulman G, Fogo A, Gung A, Badr K, Hakim R. Complement activation retards resolution of acute ischemic renal failure in the rat. *Kidney Int* 1991;40:1069–74.
127. Hakim RM, Wingard RL, Parker RA. Effect of the dialysis membrane in the treatment of patients with acute renal failure. *N Engl J Med* 1994;331:1338–42.
128. Schulman G, Hakim R. Hemodialysis membrane biocompatibility in acute renal failure. *Adv Renal Replac Ther* 1994;1:75–82.
129. Vakeva A, Meri S, Lehto T, Laurila P. Activation of the terminal complement cascade in renal infarction. *Kidney Int* 1995;47:918–26.
130. Cosio FG, Zager RA, Sharma HM. Atheroembolic renal disease causes hypocomplementaemia. *Lancet* 1985;2:118–21.
131. Seifert PS, Hugo F, Tranum-Jensen J, Zahringer U, Muhly M, Bhakdi S. Isolation and characterization of a complement-activating lipid extracted from human atherosclerotic lesions. *J Exp Med* 1990;172: 547–57.
132. Raij L, Dalmasso AP, Staley NA, Fish AJ. Renal injury in DOCA-salt hypertensive C5-sufficient and C5-deficient mice. *Kidney Int* 1989;36: 582–92.
133. Hsueh W, Sun X, Rioja LN, Gonzalez-Crussi F. The role of the complement system in shock and tissue injury induced by tumour necrosis factor and endotoxin. *Immunology* 1990;70:309–14.
134. Sun X, Hsueh W. Platelet-activating factor produces shock, in vivo complement activation, and tissue injury in mice. *J Immunol* 1991;147: 509–14.
135. Brady HR, Hebert M-J, Takano T, et al. Acute nephrotoxic serum nephritis in complement "knockout" mice: relative roles of the classical and alternate pathways in neutrophil recruitment and proteinuria. *J Am Soc Nephrol* 1995;6:862(abst).
136. Boyce NW, Holdsworth SR. Macrophage–Fc-receptor affinity: role in cellular mediation of antibody initiated glomerulonephritis. *Kidney Int* 1989;36:537–44.
137. Leenaerts PL, Hall BM, Van Damme BJ, Daha MR, Vanrenterghem YF. Active Heymann nephritis in complement component C6 deficient rats. *Kidney Int* 1995;47:1604–14.
138. Wilson CB. The renal response to immunologic injury. *Kidney* 1991; 1:1062–181.
139. Groggel GC, Adler S, Rennke HG, Couser WG, Salant DJ. Role of the terminal complement pathway in experimental membranous nephropathy in the rabbit. *J Clin Invest* 1983;72:1948–57.
140. Sawtell NM, Hartman AL, Weiss MA, Pesce AJ, Michael JG. C3 dependent, C5 independent immune complex glomerulopathy in the mouse. *Lab Invest* 1988;58:287–93.
141. Falk RJ, Jennette JC. Immune complex induced glomerular lesions in C5 sufficient and deficient mice. *Kidney Int* 1986;30:678–86.
142. Couser WG, Ochi RF, Baker PJ, Schulze M, Campbell C, Johnson RJ. C6 depletion reduces proteinuria in experimental nephropathy induced by a nonglomerular antigen. *J Am Soc Nephrol* 2:894–901.
143. Hara M, Batsford SR, Mihatsch MJ, Bitter-Suermann D, Vogt A. 1991; Complement and monocytes are essential for provoking glomerular injury in passive Heymann nephritis in rats: terminal complement components are not the sole mediators of proteinuria. *Lab Invest* 1991;65:168–79.
144. Torbohm I, Schonermark M, Wingen A-M, Berger B, Rother K, Hansch GM. C5b-8 and C5b-9 modulate the collagen release of human glomerular epithelial cells. *Kidney Int* 1990;37:1098–104.
145. Floege J, Johnson RJ, Gordon K, et al. Increased synthesis of extracellular matrix in mesangial proliferative nephritis. *Kidney Int* 1991; 40:477–88.
146. Nagamatsu T, Pippin J, Schreiner GF, Lefkowith JB. Paradoxical exacerbation of leukocyte-mediated glomerulonephritis with cyclooxygenase inhibition. *Am J Physiol* 1992;263:F228–36.
147. Neale TJ, Ullrich R, Ojha P, Poczewski H, Verhoeven AJ, Kerjaschki D. Reactive oxygen species and neutrophil respiratory burst cytochrome b558 are produced by kidney glomerular cells in passive Heymann nephritis. *Proc Natl Acad Sci USA* 1993;50:3645–9.
148. Neale TJ, Ojha PP, Exner M, et al. Proteinuria in passive Heymann nephritis is associated with lipid peroxidation and formation of adducts on type IV collagen. *J Clin Invest* 1994;94:1577–84.
149. Savin VJ, Johnson RJ, Couser WG. C5b-9 increases albumin permeability of isolated glomeruli in vitro. *Kidney Int* 1994;46:382–7.
150. Rehan A, Wiggins RC, Kunkel RG, Till GO, Johnson KJ. Glomerular injury and proteinuria in rats after intrarenal injection of cobra venom factor. Am J Pathol 1986;123:57–66.
151. Boyce NW, Holdsworth SR. Evidence for direct renal injury as a consequence of glomerular complement activation. *J Immunol* 1986;136: 2421.
152. Mulligan MS, Polley MJ, Bayer RJ, Nunn MF, Paulson JC, Ward PA. Neutrophil-dependent acute lung injury. *J Clin Invest* 1992;90:1600–7.
153. Belmont HM, Buyon J, Giorno R, Abramson S. Up-regulation of endothelial cell adhesion molecules characterizes disease activity in systemic lupus erythematosus. *Arthritis Rheum* 1994;37:376–83.
154. Shingu M, Nonaka S, Nishimukai H, Nobunaga M, Kitamura H, Tomo-Oka K. Activation of complement in normal serum by hydrogen peroxide and hydrogen peroxide-related oxygen radicals produced by activated neutrophils. *Clin Exp Immunol* 1992;90:72–8.
155. Baricos WH, Shah SV. Proteolytic enzymes as mediators of glomerular injury. *Kidney Int* 1991;40:161–73.
156. Pelayo JC, Chenoweth DE, Hugli TE, Wilson CB, Blantz RC. Effects of the anaphylatoxin, C5a, on renal and glomerular hemodynamics in the rat. *Kidney Int* 1986;30:62–7.
157. Brandt J, Pippin J, Schulze M, et al. Role of the complement membrane attack complex (C5b-9) in mediating experimental mesangioproliferative glomerulonephritis. *Kidney Int* 1996;49:335–43.
158. Narita I, Border WA, Ketteler M, Noble NA. Nitric oxide mediates immunologic injury to kidney mesangium in experimental glomerulonephritis. *Lab Invest* 1995;72:17.
159. Saadi S, Platt JL. Transient perturbation of endothelial integrity induced by natural antibodies and complement. *J Exp Med* 1995;181: 21–31.
160. Mahan JD, Hebert LA, McAllister C, Birmingham DJ, Shen X-P, Cosio FG. Platelet involvement in experimental immune complex-mediated glomerulonephritis of primates. *Kidney Int* 1993;44:716–25.
161. Couser WG, Johnson RJ. Mechanisms of progressive renal disease in glomerulonephritis. *Am J Kidney Dis* 1994;23:193–8.
162. Johnson RJ. The glomerular response to injury: progression or resolution? *Kidney Int* 1994;45:2769–782.
163. Passwell J, Schreiner GF, Nonaka M, Beuscher HU, Colten HR. Local extrahepatic expression of complement genes C3, factor B, C2, and C4 is increased in murine lupus nephritis. *J Clin Invest* 1988;82:1676–84.

164. Sacks S, Zhou W, Campbell RD, Martin J. C3 and C4 gene expression and interferon-gamma-mediated regulation in human glomerular mesangial cells. *Clin Exp Immunol* 1993;93:411–7.
165. Seelen MAJ, Brooimans RA, Van der Woude FJ, Van Es LA, Daha MR. IFN-gamma mediates stimulation of complement C4 biosynthesis in human proximal tubular epithelial cells (PTEC). *Kidney Int* 1993;44:50–7.
166. Welch TR, Witte DP, Beischel LS. Differential expression and cellular localization of messenger RNA for C3 and C4 in the human kidney. *J Clin Invest* 1993;92:1451–8.
167. Montinaro V, Serra L, Perissutti S, Ranieri E, Tedesco F, Schena FP. Biosynthesis of C3 by human mesangial cells: modulation by proinflammatory cytokines. *Kidney Int* 1995;47:829–36.
168. Regal JF, Fraser DG, Anderson DE, Solem LE. Enhancement of antigen-induced bronchoconstriction after intravascular complement activation with cobra venom factor: reversal by granulocyte depletion. *J Immunol* 1993;150:3496–505.
169. Weisman HF, Bartow T, Leppo MK, et al. Soluble human complement receptor type 1: in vivo inhibitor of complement suppressing post-ischemic myocardial inflammation and necrosis. *Science* 1990; 149:146–51.
170. Homeister JW, Satoh PS, Kilgore KS, Lucchesi BR. Soluble complement receptor type 1 prevents human complement-mediated damage of the rabbit isolated heart. *J Immunol* 1993;150:1055–64.
171. Xia W, Fearon DT, Moore FD Jr, Schoen FJ, Ortiz F, Kirkman RL. Prolongation of guinea pig cardiac xenograft survival in rats by soluble human complement receptor type 1. *Transplant Proc* 1992;24:479–80.
172. Pruitt SK, Kirk AD, Bollinger R, et al. The effect of soluble complement receptor type 1 on hyperacute rejection of porcine xenografts. *Transplantation* 1994;57:363–70.
173. Mieny CJ, Karusseit VOL, Van den Bogaerde JB, Hasa RIR, White DJG. Prolongation of survival of heterotopic heart xenografts by antibody and complement suppression in primates. *Transplant Proc* 1994; 26:1073.
174. Hill J, Lindsay TF, Ortiz F, Yeh CG. Soluble complement receptor type 1 ameliorates the local and remote organ injury after intestinal ischemia–reperfusion in the rat. *J Immunol* 1992;149:1723–8.
175. Mulligan MS, Yeh CG, Rudolph AR, Ward PA. Protective effects of soluble CR1 in complement- and neutrophil-mediated tissue injury. *J Immunol* 1992;148:1479–85.
176. Piddlesden SJ, Storch MK, Hibbs M, Freeman AM, Lassmann H, Morgan BP. Soluble recombinant complement receptor 1 inhibits inflammation and demyelination in antibody-mediated demyelinating experimental allergic encephalomyelitis. *J Immunol* 1994;152:5477–84.
177. Couser WG, Johnson RJ, Young BA, Yeh CG, Toth CA, Rudolph AR. The effects of soluble recombinant complement receptor 1 on complement-mediated experimental glomerulonephritis. *J Am Soc Nephrol* 1995;5:1888–94.
178. Cheung AK, Parker CJ, Hohnholt M. Soluble complement receptor type 1 inhibits complement activation by hemodialysis membranes in vitro. *Kidney Int* 1994;46:1680–87.
179. Pascual M, Duchosal MA, Steiger G, et al. Circulating soluble CR1 (CD35). *J Immunol* 1993;151:1702–11.
180. Danielsson C, Pascual M, French L, Steiger G, Schifferli JA. Soluble complement receptor type 1 (CD35) is released from leukocytes by surface cleavage. *Eur J Immunol* 1994;24:2725–31.
181. Yeh CG, Wu Y-J, Brown M, et al. Recombinant soluble human membrane cofactor protein (MCP) inhibits complement activation in vitro and in vivo. *Int Assoc Inflamm Soc* 1993;73.
182. Moran P, Beasley H, Gorrell A, et al. Human recombinant soluble decay accelerating factor inhibits complement activation in vitro and in vivo. *J Immunol* 1992;149:1736–43.
183. Ruiz de Souza V, Kaveri SV, Kazatchkine MD. Intravenous immunoglobulin (IVIg) in the treatment of autoimmune and inflammatory diseases. *Clin Exp Rheumatol* 1993;11:S33–6.
184. Qi M. Inhibition of complement activation by intravenous immunoglobulins. *Arthritis Rheum* 1995;38:146.
185. Shumak KH, Rock GA. Therapeutic plasma exchange. *N Engl J Med* 1984;310:762–71.
186. Lewis EJ, Hunsicker LG, Lan S-P, Rohde RD, Lachin JM, and the f.t.l.N.C.S.Group. A controlled trial of plasmapheresis therapy in severe lupus nephritis. *N Engl J Med* 1992;326:1373–9.
187. Hebert LA, Cosio FG, Neff JC. Diagnostic significance of hypocomplementemia. *Kidney Int* 1991;39:811–21.
188. Tarantino A, De Vecchi A, Montagnino G, et al. Renal disease in essential mixed cryoglobulinaemia. *Q J Med [New Ser]* 1981;50:1–30.
189. Wilson WA, Perez MC, Armatis PE. Partial C4A deficiency is associated with susceptibility to systemic lupus erythematosus in black Americans. *Arthritis Rheum* 1988;31:1171–5.
190. Moulds JM, Warner NB, Arnett FC. Complement component C4A and C4b levels in systemic lupus erythematosus: quantitation in relation to C4 null status and disease activity. *J Rheumatol* 1993;20:443–7.
191. Ricker DM, Hebert LA, Rohde R, Sedmak DD, Lewis EJ, Clough JD, and the Lupus Nephritis Collaborative Study Group. Serum C3 levels are diagnostically more sensitive and specific for systemic lupus erythematosus activity than are serum C4 levels. *Am J Kidney Dis* 1991;18:678–85.
192. Buyon JP, Tamerius J, Belmont HM, Abramson SB. Assessment of disease activity and impending flare in patients with systemic lupus erythematosus. *Arthritis Rheum* 1992;35:1028–37.
193. Porcel JM, Ordi J, Castro-Salomo A, et al. The value of complement activation products in the assessment of systemic lupus erythematosus flares. *Clin Immunol Immunopathol* 1995;74:283–8.
194. Cosio FG, Hernandez RA. The prognostic value of serum C3 concentration in patients with idiopathic focal glomerulosclerosis. *J Clin Nephrol* (in press).

Immunologic Renal Diseases,
edited by E. G. Neilson and W. G. Couser.
Lippincott-Raven Publishers, Philadelphia © 1997

CHAPTER 19

Proteases and Oxidants in Glomerular Injury

Gur P. Kaushal and Sudhir V. Shah

INTRODUCTION

Numerous mediators have been implicated in glomerular injury (1–3), many of which have been detailed in other chapters in the book. In this chapter, we review the evidence for the role(s) of proteases and reactive oxygen metabolites (ROMs) in both leukocyte-dependent and leukocyte-independent models of glomerular injury. There are several reasons why it is appropriate to consider these two mediators together. Many of the same stimuli that cause generation of ROMs also lead to the release of proteolytic enzymes. Thus, a stimulated neutrophil, for example, generates ROMs and releases proteolytic enzymes. Perhaps equally relevant are the potential interactions between these two mediators. For example, ROMs can convert latent metalloproteinase(s) to their active forms that are capable of glomerular basement membrane (GBM) degradation.

It is well documented that infiltrating leukocytes are present in glomeruli in many proliferative and exudative human and experimental glomerulonephritides. (See also Chapter 26). Several studies have shown that depletion of neutrophils by antineutrophil antibody prevents proteinuria during the heterologous phase of anti-GBM-induced glomerulonephritis (4,5) and in anti-concanavalin-A (ConA)-induced glomerulonephritis (6); and depletion of monocytes by antimonocyte antibody prevents proteinuria during the autologous phase of anti-GBM-induced glomerulonephritis (7). Thus, these studies strongly support the view that leukocytes mediate glomerular injury that results in proteinuria. It is well recognized that leukocytes synthesize and release ROMs and proteases in response to an appropriate stimulus (8–10). We review the evidence that suggests that leukocyte-mediated glomerular injury in experimental models is mediated by the release of ROMs and proteases. In addition, recent studies have documented that resident glomerular cells produce GBM-degrading proteases and are capable of generating ROMs in response to a number of stimuli, indicating that the proteases and oxidants may play a role in leukocyte-independent glomerular disease.

In this chapter, we first describe the proteases and ROMs generated by leukocytes and by resident glomerular cells that may participate in glomerular injury. We include in this section new information related to enzymes involved in the reduction of oxygen to ROMs as well as the identification of new proteolytic enzymes that may be important in extracellular matrix degradation. In recent years, significant advances have been made in understanding the in vitro mechanism of action of proteases and ROMs in mediating GBM damage. We review this aspect in detail, including the important interactions between proteases and oxidants. We also briefly review the other biological effects of proteases and ROMs relevant to glomerular pathophysiology. Finally, we consider in vivo effects of proteases and ROMs and examine their potential role in animal models of glomerular disease.

OXIDANTS AND PROTEASES RELEVANT TO GLOMERULAR INJURY

Leukocyte-Derived Proteases (see also Chapter 26)

Neutrophils contain proteinases belonging to each of the four classes (Table 1) that are capable of degrading GBM under appropriate conditions (9). However, most studies suggest that serine proteinases and metalloproteinases are the neutrophil proteinases physiologically more relevant to GBM degradation because of their neutral pH optima, their ability to degrade extracellular matrix (ECM) components, and their close accessibility to the appropriate site for degradation (Table 2).

G. P. Kaushal and S. V. Shah: Division of Nephrology, University of Arkansas for Medical Sciences, Little Rock, Arkansas 72205.

TABLE 1. *Classes and some general properties of endopeptidases*[a]

Property	Serine	Cysteine	Aspartic	Metallo
Old Name	Serine	Thiol	Carboxyl	Metallo
Enzyme commission #	3.4.21	3.4.22	3.4.23	3.4.24
Active site component	Serine	Cysteine	Aspartic acid	Zn^{2+}
pH range[b]	7–9	3–7	2–6	5–9
Inhibitors (in vitro)	PMSF,SBTI,DIFP	E-64, iodoacetate, organomercurials	Pepstatin	EDTA, o-phenanthroline
Inhibitors (in vivo)	Plasma proteinase inhibitors[c]	Cystatins, α_1-cysteine	Unknown	TIMP-1,TIMP-2, TIMP-3
Location	Intra- and extracellular	Lysosomes[d]	Lysosomes	Intra- and extracellular
Latent forms	Yes	Yes	No	Yes
Examples	Elastase, plasmin Cathepsin G	Cathepsins B and L Calpain, Interleukin-1ß-converting enzyme	Cathepsins D and E	Gelatinase, type IV collagenase Meprin

[a] Used with permission from Kidney International 40:161, 1991 (10).
[b] Varies with substrate and assay conditions
[c] α_1-Proteinase inhibitor, α_2-antiplasmin, α_2-macroglobulin, etc. (99)
[d] Except calpain, the cystolic and membrane-bound $Ca2^+$-dependent cysteine proteinase

Leukocyte-Derived Metalloproteinases

Metalloproteinases are a closely related family of enzymes (which includes collagenases, gelatinases, and stromelysins) capable of degrading one or more of the ECM components (11). Neutrophils synthesize and secrete two metalloproteinases: collagenase (MMP-8) and 92-kD gelatinase (type-IV collagenase, or MMP-9) (Table 2). Neutrophil collagenase is stored in a latent proenzyme form in specific granules (12,13) whereas gelatinase is stored in a latent proenzyme form in distinct secretory granules (14). The proenzymes are released from specific granules in response to stimulation by various growth factors, cytokines, and chemoattractants (15–17). Collagenase activity in neutrophils, first detected in 1968 by Lazarus and co-workers (18), has since been extensively studied. Although initial attempts to purify the enzyme were hindered because of the relatively unstable nature of the enzyme, the purification was recently accomplished using modern techniques (19–22). The enzyme has now been cloned, sequenced, expressed in *Escherichia coli* (23–25) and cocrystallized with the substrate analogue inhibitor Pro-Leu-Gly-NHOH (26). The purified active enzyme is unique in its ability to cleave a chains of type I, II, and III at single site producing one-quarter and three-quarter fragments with preference to type-I collagen (27,28). In addition, the enzyme is capable of degrading fibronectin (29) and proteoglycans (30). Since type-I, II, and III collagens are not present in significant amounts in the GBM, a role for this enzyme in GBM degradation appears limited to the degradation of fibronectin and proteoglycans.

Another member of the metalloproteinase family present in neutrophils is 92-kD gelatinase (MMP-9) (Table 2). The enzyme was originally identified by Sopata and Dancewicz (31) as a gelatinolytic metalloendopeptidase and has been well characterized (32–34). Several independent studies have established that the deduced amino

TABLE 2. *Extracellular matrix degradation by proteolytic enzymes*

Proteinases	Class	Source	Specificity	GBM degradation
Gelatinase B (MMP-9)	Metalloproteinase	Neutrophil	Collagen type IV, V, XI denatured type I collagen	Yes
Collagenase (MMP-8)	Metalloproteinase	Neutrophil	Collagen type I, II, III proteoglycans, fibronectin	–
Elastase and cathepsin G	Serine-proteinase	Neutrophil	Collagen type IV, elastin, laminin, fibronectin	Yes
Proteinase-3	Serine-proteinase	Neutrophil	Collagen type IV, laminin	–
Plasmin	Serine-proteinase	Blood and glomerular cells	Collagen type IV, laminin, gelatin, fibronectin, proteoglycans	Yes
Gelatinase A (MMP-2)	Metalloproteinase	Glomerular mesangial and epithelial cells	Collagen type IV, gelatin, elastin	Yes
Gelatinase B (MMP-9)	Metalloproteinase	Glomerular mesangial and epithelial cells	Collagen type IV, gelatin	Yes
Glomerular metalloproteinase	Metalloproteinase	Glomeruli	Gelatin, collagen type IV, laminin, fibronectin	Yes

acid sequence and various other properties of the enzyme (34–38) are similar to 92- to 95-kD gelatinase secreted by monocyte-macrophages and a number of transformed cells. The purified active enzyme cleaves gelatin and type-IV, V, and XI collagens but not native type-I collagen (33–35). Polymorphonuclear leukocyte (PMN) gelatinase can also degrade intact GBM at neutral pH as shown by studies from our laboratory (39). Of particular interest, neutrophils do not produce tissue inhibitors of metalloproteinase (TIMP) and thus secrete TIMP-free proenzymes. In contrast, other inflammatory cells secrete proenzymes in association with TIMP (40).

Leukocyte-Derived Serine Proteinases

Elastase and cathepsin G are well characterized serine proteinases present in large quantities in primary or azurophil granules of neutrophils (41–47) (Table 2). It is now well established that stimulated intact neutrophils, neutrophil extracts as well as purified PMN elastase and cathepsin G, are capable of degrading GBM at neutral pH in vitro (48–52). In addition, the purified elastase and/or cathepsin G have been shown to degrade key components of the GBM, including type-IV collagen (53), laminin (54,55), fibronectin (56), and proteoglycans (57,58). Proteinases with properties similar to elastase and cathepsin G have also been reported in several tissues and cell types, including macrophages, monocytes, and platelets (41,42,47), raising the possibility that the enzymes from these cells may also contribute to GBM damage.

A third serine proteinase with antibacterial properties, referred to as proteinase 3, has been identified and characterized in PMNs (59,60) (Table 2). Proteinase 3 is capable of degrading several ECM components, including type-IV collagen and laminin (61). In addition, it degrades elastin and causes emphysema when administered to hamsters by tracheal insufflation (60). Ultrastructural immunocytochemical staining revealed that proteinase 3 is localized in the myeloperoxidase (MPO) positive primary granules and on the plasma membrane of the PMNs (62). Proteinase 3 has received considerable attention as it has been recognized as the target antigen for the specific antineutrophil cytoplasmic antibody (ANCA), cANCA, circulating in Wegener granulomatosis (63–65) (see Chapter 49).

Proteases of Resident Glomerular Cells

Recent studies have documented the presence of GBM-degrading proteinases in the freshly isolated glomeruli as well as in cultured glomerular mesangial and epithelial cells, raising the possibility that endogenous glomerular proteinases may contribute to GBM damage in glomerular diseases. Although glomeruli contain proteases from each of the four classes of the proteinases, most likely the physiologically relevant proteases as mediators of GBM damage are endogenous metalloproteinases and serine proteinases.

Metalloproteinases and Their Inhibitors

The major metalloproteinase synthesized and secreted by the glomerular mesangial cells is gelatinase A (72-kD type-IV collagenase), which degrades intact GBM, soluble type-IV collagen, and gelatin, and is the most well-studied metalloproteinase in cultured glomerular cells (see also Chaper 29). The enzyme from rat mesangial cells has been purified, characterized, cloned, and sequenced (66–68). The coding sequence of the enzyme showed 91% sequence homology to 72-kD type-IV collagenase previously cloned and sequenced from human ras-transformed tracheal bronchial epithelial cells. The enzyme shares several structural and functional characteristics with other members of the matrix metalloproteinase family, including synthesis and secretion as an inactive zymogen, maximal activity at neutral pH, activation by 4-aminophenyl mercuric acetate and limited proteolysis, inhibition by endogenous TIMPs, and highly conserved sequences within prodomain, catalytic domain, and zinc-binding domain. The activation of the proenzyme is essential for GBM degradation and thus regulation of activation of the proenzyme is critical in both normal as well as disease conditions (vide infra).

Recent studies show that the process of transcriptional regulation of the gelatinase-A expression by cytokines, phorbol myristate acetate (PMA), and growth factors may be different in human and rat cultured mesangial cells (69,70). In response to interleukin (IL) 1α, tumor-promoting agent, PMA, or transforming growth factor (TGF-β), rat mesangial cells increased the synthesis of gelatinase A, without the induction of gelatinase B (66,69). On the other hand, exposure of human mesangial cells to IL-1α and to PMA induced the synthesis of gelatinase B (92-kD type-IV collagenase) with no effect on the constitutive expression of gelatinase A (70). The constitutive expression of gelatinase A has been previously observed for most connective tissue cells studied. Recent studies on the promoter sequences of the MMP genes have provided some insight for the selective induction of the metalloproteinases by growth factors, cytokines, oncogenes, and tumor promoters. The promoter sequence of the gelatinase-A gene from human cells does not contain an IL-1α or PMA response element (AP1 site) (71,72) but instead possesses an AP2 site that is responsive to TGF-β. In contrast, the promoter site of gelatinase B (collagenase as well as stromelysin 1) contains an AP1 response element, indicating different regulation of the two gelatinases. Since rat but not human mesangial cell gelatinase A responds to IL-1 and PMA, it would be of interest to know whether the gelatinase-A gene from rat mesangial cells possesses an AP1 response element or other elements involved in responses to IL-1 or tumor necrosis factor (TNF) α. The mesangial cells also secrete a metalloproteinase inhibitor, TIMP (67), which may directly regulate the activity of gelatinase A.

Glomeruli isolated from normal rats also contain one or more GBM-degrading activities at neutral pH (73). GBM degradation was markedly inhibited by the metalloproteinase inhibitors, EDTA and 1,10-phenanthroline, but was unaffected by inhibitors of serine [PMSF, leupeptin, alpha-1-proteinase inhibitor (α_1-PI, and soybean trypsin inhibitor I) or cysteine proteinases (E-64 and leupeptin), documenting that metalloproteinase activity was responsible for the GBM degradation. In a separate study, the major gelatin-degrading activity with a molecular mass of 116–125 kD was identified from freshly isolated rat glomeruli (74). This activity was found to be membrane associated, was not inhibited by TIMP, and was not activated by organomercurials, indicating that the glomerular metalloproteinase is distinct from the known members of the metalloproteinase family as well as the mesangial cell gelatinase (75). Further characterization of this distinct enzyme will reveal its molecular and structural features as well as the role of this enzyme in the turnover of the GBM.

Glomerular epithelial cells also synthesize and secrete metalloproteinases that are not inhibited by TIMP and not activated by the organomercurials (see also Chapter 31). Cultured rat glomerular epithelial cells were shown to secrete a major gelatin-degrading activity with a molecular mass of 150 kD and three other activities with molecular masses of 220, 86–93, and 52–54 kD on the gelatin substrate zymogram (76). The gelatinolytic activities were capable of degrading soluble type-IV collagen as well as intact GBM. Like the glomerular metalloproteinase, these activities were not secreted in latent form and were not inhibited by TIMPs, indicating that they are distinct from the known members of the metalloproteinase family. In an another study, gelatinolytic activity with a molecular mass of 68 and 98 kD and 238 kD on gelatin zymograms was reported from the cultures of rat glomerular epithelial cells (77). However, it is not known whether these activities are inhibited by TIMP. Cultured glomerular epithelial cells were recently reported to secrete TIMP-inhibitable gelatin-degrading activity (78). Human glomerular epithelial cells were shown to secrete gelatinase activities with a molecular mass of 72 kD and 92 kD that were inhibited by TIMP-1 and TIMP-2 (78). However, further characterization of these activities is needed in order to identify them among the members of the matrix metalloproteinase family.

Plasmin, Plasminogen Activators, and Their Inhibitors

Plasmin, a serine protease, is produced from its inactive precursor, plasminogen, on activation by plasminogen activators (PAs) that are synthesized and secreted by a variety of cell types (79,80), including the cultured glomerular cells (81–84). Plasmin, best known to degrade fibrin (fibrinolysis), has a broad substrate specificity with the ability to degrade several ECM components (including laminin, fibronectin, proteoglycans, and gelatin) (10,79,85). In addition, plasmin activates latent metalloproteinases, procollagenases, and prostromelysins (86); the latent form of elastase (87); and the latent forms of certain growth factors (88). In view of these properties, plasmin may be an important mediator of glomerular injury.

The formation of plasmin from plasminogen is regulated by the interaction of PAs and their specific inhibitors. Two closely related PAs have been well characterized in mammalian cells and are designated as uPA (urokinase type) and tPA (tissue type) (79,89). The expression of both uPA and tPA has been demonstrated in glomeruli (90–93) as well as in cultured glomerular mesangial cells (84,94–96) and epithelial cells (81,82, 97). However, biochemical analysis shows that human glomerular mesangial cells produce more tPA than uPA (94), whereas glomerular epithelial cells produce more uPA than tPA (98). The two PAs are encoded by two related but distinct genes, and antibodies prepared from purified PAs do not cross-react (79). Both PAs are secreted as single-chain (sc) proenzymes that are processed by limited proteolysis to active two-chain forms. While the sc-uPA form is essentially inactive, the sc-tPA form is active, but much less so than the two-chain form (79). The in vivo activator of pro-uPA is unknown. In vitro, however, partial proteolytic cleavage of pro-uPA by plasmin, kallikrein, factor XIIa, or cathepsin B converts inactive, sc pro-uPA to a two-chain, active enzyme (79,80). Thus, the activation of the PAs provides one of the mechanisms whereby these enzymes are regulated in vivo.

In addition, the activity of the PAs is regulated in vivo by specific inhibitors known as plasminogen activator inhibitors (PAIs). Although four distinct PAIs such as PAI-1, PAI-2, PAI-3, and protease–nexin have been described, PAI-1 is the major physiologic inhibitor of both PAs (99). Thus, the activity of plasmin is controlled by the net effect of PAs and their specific inhibitors, as well as by plasma protease inhibitor, α_2-antiplasmin (100). PAI-1 is produced by a variety of cell types, including glomerular epithelial cells (81–83,98) and mesangial cells (84,94,95,101,102).

Several independent investigations have documented that plasminogen activation involves cell surface attachment of both uPA and plasminogen by specific receptors (103,104). Three receptors such as plasminogen/plasmin receptor, uPA receptor (uPAR), and tPA receptor (tPAR) are expressed by a variety of cells (103,105) and are thought to participate in focalizing plasminogen activation at the cell surface. Plasminogen activation is more efficient by receptor-bound PAs. It is interesting that plasmin associated in the uPA–uPAR complex is protected from its principle inhibitor, α_2-antiplasmin (79, 106). Although uPAR was identified in human glomerular mesangial cells (94,95), its role in ECM degradation could not be observed (94). Plasminogen/plasmin receptors have also been identified in human glomerular epithelial cells (83), but complete characterization of these receptors in kidney cells remains to be determined.

Leukocyte-Derived Oxidants (see also Chapter 26)

In neutrophil-dependent glomerulonephritis, the circulating PMNs are recruited at the site of immune deposits at subendothelial and mesangial areas by a series of events that involve initial adherence and subsequent migration across the endothelium (107–109) (see Chapters 24 and 25). After adherence to the immune site, a wide variety of soluble and particulate stimuli can activate PMNs, resulting in the release of oxidants. Of particular interest is the demonstration that the several immune reactants, such as, serum-treated zymosan (a C_3b receptor stimulus), heat-aggregated immunoglobulin (Ig) G (an Fc receptor stimulus), immune complexes, and complement components have all been shown to trigger the oxidative burst (110,111) (Table 3)

It is now well established that both neutrophils and monocytes exhibit enormous increase in oxygen uptake with the generation of ROMs in response to plasma membrane perturbation by a variety of soluble and particulate stimuli (8,112). The metabolic process of oxygen consumption is often referred to as the respiratory burst. It is catalyzed by the multicomponent enzyme complex known as respiratory-burst oxidase or NADPH oxidase. When neutrophils or monocytes are exposed to appropriate stimuli, the respiratory-burst oxidase is rapidly activated as a result of interaction of specific proteins in the cytoplasm and membrane compartments. The active oxidase then uses its cofactor, NADPH, to reduce molecular oxygen to the superoxide anion (113,114) (Fig. 1)

Superoxide anion then becomes the precursor for the generation of H_2O_2 by rapid dismutation of superoxide anion either spontaneously or by the enzyme, superoxide dismutase (45,115) (Fig. 1). Superoxide and hydrogen peroxide appear to be the primary species generated; these may then play a role in the generation of additional and more reactive oxidants, including the highly reactive hydroxyl radical (or a related highly oxidizing species) in which iron salts play a catalytic role in a reaction, commonly referred to as the metal-catalyzed Haber–Weiss reaction.

There is some controversy whether neutrophils generate hydroxyl radical in vivo (116) because of limited availability of free iron. In other systems, however, results with metal chelators and hydroxyl-radical scavengers indicate an important role of hydroxyl radical or similar oxidants in biological systems vide infra.

Another enzyme, MPO, secreted by neutrophils in large amounts, uses H_2O_2 to oxidize chlorides or other halides to their corresponding hypochlorous or hypohalous acids (112,117) (Fig. 1). The highly toxic hypohalous acids produced by MPO–H_2O_2–halide system are extremely powerful oxidants that rapidly react with biomolecules and are capable of damaging microorganisms

TABLE 3. *Sources of ROMs potentially involved in glomerular injury*

Leukocytes

In vitro studies
- Activation of respiratory burst oxidase by a wide variety of soluble and particulate stimuli, including immune complexes, complement components, and ANCAs (110,112,119)
- Superoxide production by activated respiratory burst oxidase (110,112,119)
- Generation of H_2O_2 from superoxide anion and production of HOCl by the myeloperoxidase–H_2O_2–halide system (6,45)

In vivo studies
- Cytochemical detection of the presence of superoxide- and hydrogen-peroxide-generating leukocytes in anti-thymocyte-1- and anti-GBM-induced glomerulonephritis (120)
- Enhanced superoxide and hydroxyl radical generated by macrophages isolated from glomeruli of rabbits with anti-GBM antibody disease (121)
- Enhanced superoxide generation by macrophages isolated from nephritic glomeruli (antithymocyte serum) (122)

Resident glomerular cells as sources of ROMs for glomerular injury

In vitro studies

Sources	Agents responsible for ROM production
Isolated glomeruli	Phorbol myristate acetate, zymosan, trypsin, chymotrypsin (127,232); adriamycin (125); puromycin aminonucleoside (126)
Mesangial cells	PAF, immune complexes, MAC, TNF-α, IL-1 (127,129,207)
Glomerular epithelial cells	Puromycin aminonucleoside (131)

In vivo studies
- Production of hydrogen peroxide by normal rat kidney glomeruli (124)
- Increased generation of hydrogen peroxide in passive Heymann nephritis (132)

ANCA, antineutrophil cytoplasmic antibody; GBM, glomerular basement membrane; IL-1, interleukin 1; MAC, membrane-attack complex; PAF, platelet-activating factor; ROM, reactive oxygen metabolite; TNF, tumor necrosis factor.

Reproduced with permission from the *Annual Review of Physiology,* volume 57, 1995, by Annual Reviews, Inc.

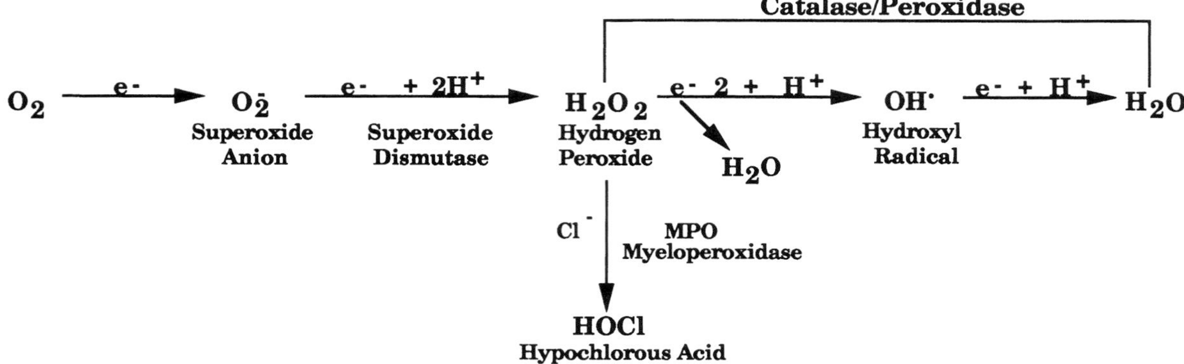

FIG. 1. Formation of reactive oxygen metabolites.

and mammalian cells (112). The hypochlorous acid (HOCl) is also capable of generating long-lived oxidants known as chloramines (118). There is now good evidence in experimental models of neutrophil-mediated glomerular injury that the MPO-H_2O_2 halide system is responsible for much of the tissue damage (6).

ANCAs present in the circulation of patients with pauci-immune necrotizing vasculitis and pauci-immune crescentic glomerulonephritis have been shown to increase significantly the generation of superoxide by neutrophils (119) (see Chapter 49). Thus, stimulated neutrophils or monocytes are potential sources of ROMs in leukocyte-dependent glomerular injury.

In recent years, there has been more direct evidence supporting this concept. Using cytochemical techniques, Poelstra and associates demonstrated the presence of superoxide anion and hydrogen peroxide (H_2O_2)-generating leukocytes in anti-Thy-1- and anti-GBM-induced glomerulonephritis (120). Similarly, enhanced ROM generation by macrophages isolated from glomeruli of rabbits with anti-GBM antibody disease and by macrophages isolated from nephritic glomeruli in the antithymocyte serum model has been demonstrated (121,122). Thus, stimulated neutrophils or monocytes may serve as sources of ROMs in proliferative and exudative glomerulonephritides (Table 3).

Oxidants of Resident Glomerular Cells

There is now ample evidence to support the concept that resident glomerular cells may serve as sources of ROMs in the noninflammatory forms of glomerular disease (Table 3). Because of the presence of phagocytelike cells in the glomerulus (particularly mesangial cells), it was postulated that glomerular cells, like other phagocytic cells, would also generate ROMs in response to a plasma membrane pertubation. Thus, rat glomeruli produced a marked chemiluminescence response (a sensitive measure of ROM generation) when treated with phorbol myristate acetate, a plasma-membrane-perturbing agent (123). In a subsequent study, chymotrypsin or trypsin was shown to increase light emission from isolated glomeruli markedly. Neutral proteases from infiltrating leukocytes and/or renal tissue have been shown to be released in glomerular diseases, suggesting a potential mechanism for the production of ROMs in glomerular diseases. Using aminotriazole-induced inactivation of catalase as a measure of intracellular generation of H_2O_2, the in vivo generation of H_2O_2 by normal glomeruli has been demonstrated (124). Adriamycin, an agent that induces nephrotic syndrome, has been shown to enhance the intracellular generation of ROMs by freshly isolated glomeruli in vitro (125). Puromycin aminonucleoside, which induces a model of minimal change disease, has been shown to enhance the generation of superoxide anion, H_2O_2, and hydroxyl radical when added to freshly isolated glomeruli (126).

These studies with isolated glomeruli have been amply supported by studies using cultured glomerular cells. Mesangial cells have enhanced generation of superoxide and H_2O_2 in response to a variety of stimuli, including opsonized zymosan, immune complexes, membrane-attack complex, and platelet-activating factor (127–129) (see also Chapter 29). Radeke and associates have shown that the human glomerular mesangial cells express all of the three essential components of a plasma-membrane-associated NADPH oxidase system similar to what has been described in neutrophils (130). Thus, the presence of low-potential cytochrome b_{558} α- and β-subunits, a 45-kD or 66-kD flavoprotein, and a 47-kD phosphoprotein have all been shown to be present in mesangial cells. Finally, glomerular epithelial cells have been shown to be the target of injury in many of the noninflammatory forms of glomerular disease, including the nephrotic syndrome induced by the injection of puromycin aminonucleoside (see Chapter 31). In response to puromycin aminonucleoside, cultured glomerular epithelial cells increase the generation of H_2O_2 (131). The ability of glomerular cells to generate ROMs appears to be well established (Table 3). Thus, either leukocytes in inflammatory glomerular diseases or resident glomerular cells in noninflammatory diseases may serve as sources for ROMs.

Recently, in passive Heymann nephritis, it has been shown that cytochrome b_{558}, a major component of the oxidoreductase complex of the respiratory burst, is localized within the visceral glomerular cells. Using an ultrastructural cerium–H_2O_2 histochemical technique, H_2O_2 was detected within the GBM. These data provide evidence that, in rats with passive Heymann nephritis and proteinuria, the glomerular epithelial cells express an externalized respiratory-burst enzyme that generates reactive oxygen species in a manner similar to neutrophils (132) (see also Chapter 47).

EFFECTS OF OXIDANTS AND PROTEASES RELEVANT TO GLOMERULAR INJURY

The major manifestations of glomerular disease are proteinuria, altered glomerular filtration rate (GFR) and, depending on the type of glomerular disease, some morphologic changes. The oxidants and proteases released from stimulated leukocytes or resident glomerular cells may cause proteinuria by damaging the GBM or affecting other factors important in maintaining the glomerular permeability barrier to proteins. The ROMs and proteases may also affect the production of prostaglandins, thromboxanes, and cyclic nucleotides that may affect glomerular hemodynamics. In addition, ROMs at low concentrations may serve as intracellular signals for gene activation involving specific transcriptional factors.

GBM Degradation by Proteases and Oxidants

Studies indicate that proteases and oxidants may work in concert to effect extracellular matrix degradation. Several in vitro studies have documented that superoxide anion as well as H_2O_2 have direct effects on ECM components (133–135). These direct effects of ROMs have been shown to contribute to GBM damage by increasing its susceptibility to proteolytic enzymes (135–137). In addition, both oxidants and proteases can activate latent proteinases and inactivate their inhibitors to potentiate degradation of the GBM and its components further (Fig. 2). Therefore, both oxidant and proteases may work together to have synergistic effects on GBM degradation.

Activation of metalloproteinases is a crucial event for ECM degradation as well as for the regulation of the enzyme activity. Activation of all members of the metalloproteinase family can be achieved in vitro by various agents, including organomercurials, as well as limited proteolysis by trypsin and other proteases that disrupt the cysteine–zinc interaction between the prodomain and the catalytic domain followed by the removal of about a 10-kD fragment from the N-terminus (138). However, the mechanisms of activation in vivo are not completely understood. Of particular interest relevant to glomerular injury is the activation of latent neutrophil gelatinase by endogenous serine proteinases, elastase (139) and cathepsin G (140), and activation of latent neutrophil collagenase by cathepsin G (141,142) and by recombinant stromelysin (143). Although elastase and cathepsin G are demonstrated to be the activators in vitro, they may be involved in activation in vivo under the conditions of PMN-dependent glomerular diseases. A plasma-membrane-dependent activation of the progelatinase A has been described (144–146) that possibly involves a newly discovered "membrane-type" metalloproteinase (MT-MMP) for the activation process (147). A similar plasma-membrane-associated metalloproteinase may be involved in the activation of the mesangial cell gelatinase.

Several independent lines of evidence suggest that ROMs are involved in the activation of latent neutrophil gelatinase and/or collagenase. The degradation of GBM by stimulated neutrophils was shown to be due to the activation of a latent metalloproteinase (most likely gelatinase) by HOCl or a similar oxidant generated by the MPO–H_2O_2–halide system (50). Peppin and Weiss reported that activity of gelatinase in supernatants recovered from triggered neutrophils was considerably inhibited in the presence of catalase, azide, or methionine, indicating that H_2O_2 or its further metabolite such as HOCl generated by the MPO–H_2O_2–halide system was involved in the activation (148). In fact, the addition of HOCl to cell-free supernatants or to purified gelatinase activated the enzyme (148). Similar activation by HOCl has been demonstrated for neutrophil collagenase (149). In addition, the role for this oxidative activation was also studied in neutrophils isolated from human subjects with chronic granulomatous disease (CGD). The CGD neutrophils that are defective in NADPH oxidase failed to activate the neutrophil collagenase, indicating that the generation of ROMs is essential for the activation (149). In an another study, the activation of collagenase was also shown by other ROMs, including hydroxyl radicals generated by hypoxanthine/xanthine oxidase (142). The precise mechanism for ROM activation of latent metalloproteinases is not yet completely known, but it is presumed that this activation by ROMs follows a mechanism similar to that of organomercurial dependent activation. Nevertheless, these observations strongly indicate that interactions between oxidants and metalloproteinases may result in glomerular injury.

Baricos and associates have recently reported the role of PA–plasmin–MMP-2 cascade in ECM degradation by cultured mesangial cells. This cascade initiated by single-chain tPA (sc-tPA) and single chain uPA (sc-uPA) results in the production of plasmin (from the exogenously added plasminogen in the mesangial cell culture) as well as activation of MMP-2, which can act together to degrade ECM (94). Although the details of the pathway are yet established, it was proposed that plasmin initially produced by the less active form of sc-tPA can convert these sc-tPA and sc-uPA forms to the more active two-chain forms, tc-tPA and tc-uPA (80,150), which can generate more plasmin from plasminogen. Furthermore, the tc-uPA form can convert latent MMP-2 to active MMP-2 (151). Thus, both plasmin and active MMP-2 can act together in a cascade to degrade the ECM (94).

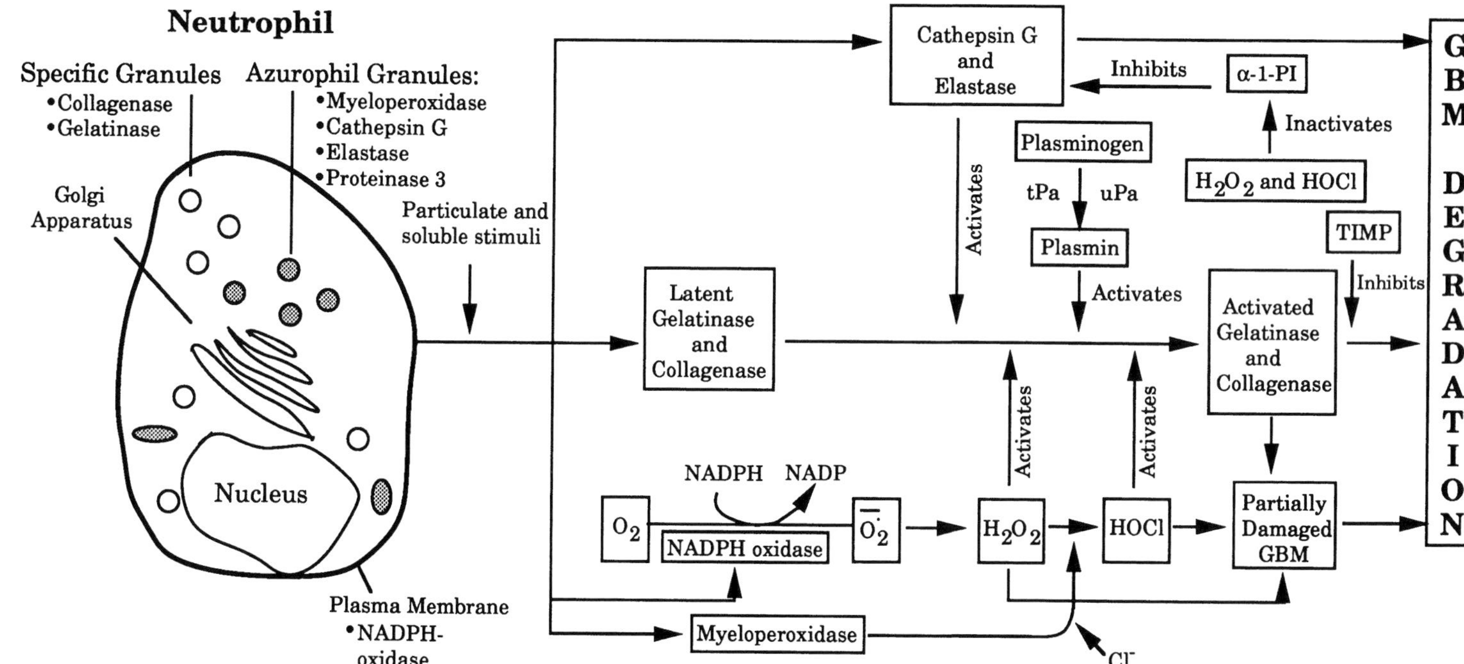

FIG. 2. Scheme of interactions of proteases and oxidants in glomerular injury.

The ability of the proteinase inhibitors to inhibit specific proteolytic activity is an important event in the regulation of proteases. Although several endogenous protease inhibitors have been well identified and characterized (100,152,153), the serine and metalloproteinase inhibitors (α_1-PI, α_2-antiplasmin, PAI-1, and TIMP, respectively] are more relevant to glomerular injury, based on their effects on elastase, gelatinase, and plasmin on GBM and its components (as discussed above). Proteolytic inactivation of elastase inhibitor, α_1-PI in vitro by cathepsin L (154), macrophage elastase (155), and a metalloproteinase secreted by PMA-stimulated human neutrophils (156,157) has been reported. The inactivation of α_1-PI by the neutrophil metalloproteinase is prevented by inhibitors of MPO system and reactivated by the metalloproteinase activator, 4-aminophenylmercuric acetate (156). This indicated that the inactivation of α_1-PI is MPO-dependent autoactivation of the latent metalloproteinase in PMNs. Several other studies have shown that ROMs inactivate α_1-PI (the primary regulator of neutrophil elastase) (158–163) by oxidation of a methionine residue in its active site (162–164). Thus, the inactivation of α_1-PI will allow the released elastase to inflict damage to the extracellular matrix more readily (165). Another study reported the inactivation of PAI-1 by oxidants. PAI-1 has a methionine in its active center that is unusually sensitive to inactivation by oxidants, including H_2O_2 (99).

Okada and co-workers (166) have reported that human neutrophil elastase, trypsin, and chymotrypsin, but not cathepsin G, pancreatic elastase, or plasmin, effectively inactivate TIMP-1, the physiologic inhibitor of matrix metalloproteinases. Neutrophil elastase has been reported to inactivate α_2-antiplasmin (167,168), an inhibitor of plasmin. In addition to these in vitro reactions, in vivo evidence for inactivation of protease inhibitors is indicated by the observation that inactivated α_1-PI can be detected from fluids recovered from the site of inflammation. Although the pathophysiologic significance of these observations to glomerular injury remains to be established, the presence of several of these proteinases in glomeruli (either intrinsically or via infiltrating leukocytes or other cells) raises the possibility that inactivation of one or more proteinase inhibitors could result in increased activity of the corresponding proteinases with subsequent deleterious effects on glomerular structure and function. In keeping with this idea, it is interesting to note that several cases of glomerulonephritis associated with severe genetic deficiency of α_1-PI have been reported (169–172).

Effects of Oxidants on Eicosanoid Metabolism

Increased production of prostaglandins and thromboxane A_2 and B_2 has been demonstrated in various human and experimental glomerulopathies, and they have been implicated as important mediators causing proteinuria and/or a fall in GFR in various experimental models of glomerular disease, including anti-GBM antibody disease, adriamycin-induced nephrotic syndrome in rats, and complement-mediated glomerular injury (173–175). It has been clearly demonstrated that ROMs generated either enzymatically or by stimulated neutrophils increase the synthesis of prostaglandin E_2, $PGF_{2\alpha}$, $6_{keto}PGF_{1\alpha}$, the stable metabolite of prostacyclin, and thromboxane B_2 (Table 4) (176–178). Thus, some of the observed effects

TABLE 4. *Effects of ROMs relevant in glomerular pathophysiology*

Effects of ROMs relevant to the occurrence of proteinuria
- ROMs participate in GBM degradation (50,136)
- Lipid peroxide induces enhanced generation of gelatinase by mesangial cells (235)
- ROMs decrease de novo synthesis of glomerular proteoglycans (225)
- ROMs increase albumin permeability in freshly isolated glomeruli in vitro (224)
- Infusion of phorbol myristate acetate, an activator of neutrophils, results in proteinuria (220) and a fall in GFR (222); these effects are prevented by catalase
- Hydrogen peroxide infused directly into the renal artery causes massive transient proteinuria by inducing a molecular size selectivity defect (223)
- Infusion of MPO–hydrogen peroxide induces proteinuria (117)

Effect of ROMs relevant to altered GFR

ROMs generated enzymatically or by stimulated neutrophils
- Increase glomerular eicosanoid synthesis (176–178)
- ncrease glomerular cyclic AMP content (186,187)
- Induce a reduction in glomerular and mesangial cell planar surface and myosin light-chain phosphorylation; these effects appear to be mediated by PAF (199)
- ROMs have an effect on release and inactivation of TNF-α (128,207)
- Infusion of 8-epi-$PGF_{2\alpha}$, a novel prostanoid produced by noncyclooxygenase mechanism involving lipid peroxidation (179), results in a marked fall in GFR and RPF (180)

Role of ROMs in the morphologic changes
- Infusion of MPO–hydrogen peroxide causes significant proteinuria, marked influx of platelets, endothelial cell swelling, and epithelial cell foot-process effacement; 4–10 days later, a marked proliferative glomerular lesion develops (117,196)
- Scavengers of ROMs prevent the reduction in glomerular ADPase activity and increase in platelet aggregation in anti-thymocyte-1 and anti-GBM antibody disease models (120)
- Rats immunized with MPO and perfused with lysosomal enzyme extract and hydrogen peroxide developed a proliferative glomerulonephritis (197)

GBM, glomerular basement membrane; GRF, glomerular filtration rate; MPO, myeloperoxidase; PAF, platelet-activating factor; PGF, prostaglandin F; ROM, reactive oxygen metabolite; RPF, renal plasma flow; TNF, tumor necrosis factor.

Reproduced with permission from the *Annual Review of Physiology,* volume 57, 1995, by Annual Reviews, Inc.

of ROMs may be mediated through their effect on prostaglandin and thromboxane synthesis.

Roberts and associates identified a series of PGF_2-like compounds that are produced in vivo in humans by a noncyclooxygenase mechanism involving free-radical catalyzed peroxidation of arachidonic acid (179). Intrarenal arterial infusion of small amounts, 0.5 mg/kg/min of one of these compounds, 8-epi-$PGF_{2\alpha}$ resulted in a dose-dependent reduction in GFR and renal plasma flow (180). These changes were completely reversed by thromboxane-A_2 receptor antagonist. Thus, these studies reveal that 8-epi-$PGF_{2\alpha}$ is a potent preglomerular vasoconstrictor acting principally through the thromboxane-A_2 receptor activation. This finding suggests that in those glomerular injuries where free radical mechanisms, including lipid peroxidation, have been implicated, the formation of these novel prostanoids may play an important role in the fall in the GFR and the alterations in renal plasma flow that have been described (Table 4).

Effects of Oxidants and Proteases on Cyclic Nucleotides

Several studies have suggested an important role for cyclic nucleotides in glomerular pathophysiology (181, 182). Infusion of dibutryl cAMP and several hormones that increase the cAMP content of glomeruli cause a fall in the glomerular ultrafiltration coefficient (182). In addition, the cAMP content in glomeruli is altered most strikingly by several local mediators of inflammation, such as serotonin, histamine, and prostaglandins, suggesting that as in other systems (183,184) cAMP may modulate inflammatory and/or immune response in glomerular disease (181,185). It has been shown that xanthine/xanthine oxidase increases cAMP content in freshly isolated glomeruli and the responsible metabolite appears to be H_2O_2 (186). Similarly cell-free supernatants from stimulated neutrophils increase cAMP content in freshly isolated glomeruli and this effect appears to be mediated by H_2O_2 and the product of the MPO–H_2O_2–halide system, HOCl (Table 4) (187).

The ability of proteolytic enzymes including trypsin, elastase, chymotrypsin, and acrosin to alter in vitro the activity of enzymes associated with the metabolism of cAMP and cGMP is well documented (188–192). In addition, trypsin and thrombin have been reported to increase the cAMP content of intact fibroblasts (193) and lymphocytes (191); and thrombin increases the cGMP content of cultured neuroblastoma cells (194). These changes in cyclic nucleotide metabolism require active proteinases, are irreversible, and do not appear to result from inactivation of phosphodiesterases. Although the precise mechanism of action is presently unclear, cleavage of an inhibitory G protein has been postulated in at least one case (192). Similar effects have been observed in freshly isolated glomeruli. Shah has reported that thrombin and trypsin caused a marked increase in the cAMP content of isolated glomeruli (195). Thrombin had no effect on the cGMP content of glomeruli and no effect on either cAMP or cGMP content of tubules. Thrombin did not affect the cAMP phosphodiesterase activity of the glomeruli. The glomerular response to diisopropylfluorophosphate-treated thrombin was markedly reduced, suggesting that proteolytic activity of thrombin is required for the response.

Effects of Oxidants Relevant to Morphologic Changes in Glomerular Disease

Work by several investigators has implicated platelets in glomerular injury. As mentioned above, infusion of MPO and H_2O_2 causes a marked influx of platelets, endothelial cell swelling, and epithelial cell foot-process effacement followed later by a marked proliferative glomerular lesion (196). In addition, low doses of H_2O_2 stimulate the proliferation of cultured rat mesangial cells (197). These findings indicate that ROMs are capable of inducing morphologic changes that are similar to those seen in models of immune-complex glomerulonephritis and anti-GBM antibody disease.

It has been suggested that glomerular ADPase is of major importance in preventing intraglomerular thrombus formation in experimental glomerulonephritis (120). Membrane-associated enzymes are apparently highly susceptible to ROMs (198). There is a marked decrease in the activity of these enzymes in two models of glomerulonephritis (anti-GBM and anti-Thy 1) that are characterized by influx of PMNs (120). Scavengers of ROMs prevented the decrease in glomerular ADPase, suggesting a role of ROMs in the reduction in the glomerular ADPase activity (Table 4) (120).

Necrotizing crescentic glomerulonephritis associated with anti-MPO antibodies is part of the ANCA-associated glomerulonephritis and is characterized by segmental fibrinoid necrosis of the GBM and marked infiltration of neutrophils and mononuclear cells. The close association of pauci-immune necrotizing glomerulonephritis and anti-MPO antibodies suggests a pathogenetic role for anti-MPO-directed immune response. Rats immunized with MPO and perfused with lysosomal enzyme extract and H_2O_2 developed glomerular intracapillary thromboses followed by a proliferative glomerulonephritis characterized by glomerular capillary wall necrosis, extracapillary cell proliferation, infiltration of neutrophils and monocytes, and vasculitis (197). These in vitro and in vivo studies indicate that the ROMs are capable of inducing many of the functional and morphologic changes that are observed in glomerular diseases.

Other Biological Effects of Oxidants Relevant to Glomerular Pathophysiology

The xanthine/xanthine oxidase system has been shown to induce a reduction in the glomerular and mesangial cell planar surface and an increase in the myosin light-chain phosphorylation, a biochemical marker of contraction (199). Interestingly, these effects were completely blocked by platelet-activating factor antagonist, suggesting that the effects of ROMs were mediated by platelet-activating factor. The authors suggested that ROMs, particularly H_2O_2, could modulate the surface area mesangial cells modifying ultrafiltration coefficient and thus explaining the decrease in the GFR in those pathologic conditions characterized by a fall in GFR.

ROMs have usually been regarded as toxic metabolites with cytotoxic properties. At low concentrations, however, they seem to play a significant regulatory role without inducing cell death. The effects of ROMs in altering the cAMP levels have been described above. In addition, regulated generation of low concentrations of ROMs may serve as intracellular signals for gene activation involving specific transcription factors such as NF-kB (200–202) and may represent a second messenger system for generation of cytokines involved in tissue injury and repair. Recently a number of monocyte specific cytokines have been described,including monocyte colony-stimulating factor (CSF-1) and monocyte chemoattractant protein (MCP-1). MCP-1 has been identified as a product of a gene belonging to the small, inducible cytokine family, known in the murine system as the JE gene. CSF-1 is a cytokine required for proliferation, maturation, and activation. Expression of the JE/MCP-1 and CSF-1 genes can be rapidly induced by a number of agents, including TNF. Satriano et al. have shown that scavengers of free radicals attenuated the increase in the mRNA level in response to TNF-α and aggregated IgG (203). Generation of superoxide anion by xanthine oxidase and hypoxanthine increased the mRNA levels of these genes. The authors concluded that the generation of reactive oxygen species possibly by NADPH-dependent oxidase is involved in the induction of the JE/MCP-1 and the CSF-1 genes by TNF-α and IgG complexes (203). Satriano and Schlondorff have provided additional support for the role of ROMs for activation of NF-kB in mesangial cells (204,205). Local generation of ROMs could represent a factor responsible for the expression of JE/MCP-1 in immune-mediated increased expression of monocyte chemoattractant protein in glomeruli from rats with anti-Thy-1 glomerulonephritis (206).

TNF is able to stimulate the generation of ROMs, superoxide anion, and H_2O_2 in glomerular mesangial cells. There is also in vitro evidence of effects of ROMs on the release of TNF-α from lipopolysaccharide-activated mesangial cells (128,207). Although the role of these cytokines in glomerular diseases has not be adequately defined, these results indicate important interactions between ROMs and other mediators. Studies also indicate the regulation of ROM generation by specific cAMP phosphodiesterases (208). For additional examples of such interactions, the reader is referred to a review by Ardaillou and Baud (209).

IN VIVO STUDIES SUPPORTING THE ROLE OF PROTEASES AND OXIDANTS IN GLOMERULAR INJURY

In Vivo Studies Supporting the Role of Proteases in Glomerular Injury

Johnson and co-workers (210) have reported that infusion of microgram quantities of purified PMN elastase or cathepsin G into the renal artery of rats resulted in marked proteinuria in the 24-h period following the infusion. Inactivated elastase or cathepsin G did not cause proteinuria, but both active and inactivated elastase localized equally to the glomerular capillary wall. Rats perfused with cationized IgG failed to develop proteinuria, establishing that neutralization of the anionic charge did not account for the proteinuria. Of particular interest, glomeruli from kidneys perfused with active elastase were histologically normal with no foot-process fusion and no evidence of inflammatory cell involvement or endothelial cell damage (Table 5) (see also Chapter 26). Based on these studies, it was postulated that the proteinuria arises as a result of degradation of the GBM by the infused proteinases. These studies were supported in an experimental

TABLE 5. *In vivo studies suggest a role of proteases in glomerular injury*

- Infusion of purified PMN elastase or cathepsin G into the renal artery of rats results in marked proteinuria (210)
- Injection with anti-GBM antibody results in dose-dependent proteinuria in control mice but not in beige mice with PMN deficient in elastase and cathepsin G (211)
- Acute anti-thymocyte-1.1 glomerulonephritis results in increased number of gelatinase-A-secreting mesangial cells and the localization of the gelatinase along the GBM (75)
- Decreased PA activity along with increased PAI-1 activity in glomeruli isolated from animal models with anti-GBM antibody-induced glomerulonephritis in rats (214) and in rabbits (215), and antithymocyte antibody-induced glomerulonephritis in rats (216)
- Overexpression of PAI-1 in glomeruli from mice with lupus nephritis (217) and in glomeruli from patients with vascular nephropathy and crescentic glomerulonephritis (218)

GBM, glomerular basement membrane; PA, plasminogen activator; PAI, plasminogen activator inhibitor; PMN, polymorphonuclear leukocyte.

model of glomerulonephritis using beige mice with PMNs deficient in elastase and cathepsin G (211). Schrijver and co-workers compared glomerular injury and proteinuria resulting from experimentally induced anti-GBM antibody disease in control and beige mice. Injection of anti-GBM antibody into control mice resulted in a dose-dependent proteinuria during the 24-h period following the injection. In contrast, beige mice injected with identical doses of antibody did not develop proteinuria except at the very high doses of the antibody. Immunofluorescence microscopy showed similar deposits of injected antibody in glomeruli from both groups of mice. In addition, both control and beige mice showed similar degrees of PMN attachment to the GBM, as well as endothelial swelling and necrosis (Table 5). Catalase and deferoxamine had no effect on the proteinuria in control mice, indicating that ROMs are not involved in this model. Thus, these in vivo studies give additional support for proteinase-mediated GBM damage.

Lubec has demonstrated increased collagenase activity in kidneys obtained from rats with anti-GBM antibody disease (212) and immune-complex glomerulonephritis (213). Lovett and colleagues have investigated the expression of gelatinase A and TIMP-1 by immunohistochemistry in glomeruli of normal rats as well as in a model of anti-Thy-1.1 immune-complex-mediated glomerulonephritis. The immunohistochemical studies of the normal glomerulus show the localization of gelatinase A to the mesangial cell area (~10% of the mesangial cell population) exclusively at sites immediately adjacent to the GBM (75) (Table 5). It is suggested that this directional secretion of the enzyme as observed by immunostaining provides an important mechanism for the normal turnover of the basement membrane (75). In addition, the immunoelectron microscopy using anti-TIMP-1 antibody revealed localization of TIMP-1 within the mesangial matrix area as well as within the glomerular capillary endothelial cells. After induction of acute anti-Thy-1.1 glomerulonephritis, there was a significant increase in the number of gelatinase-A-secreting mesangial cells, and the localization of the gelatinase was also detected along the GBM. However, no change was detected in the rates or pattern of TIMP-1 expression. Thus, increased expression of the gelatinase A may cause glomerular injury in a model of immune-complex-mediated glomerulonephritis.

The glomerular production of PA and its inhibitor, PAI-1, has been examined in several experimental and human models of glomerulonephritis. Decreased PA activity along with increased PAI-1 activity was demonstrated in glomeruli isolated from animal models with anti-GBM antibody-induced glomerulonephritis in rats (214) and in rabbits (215), antithymocyte antibody-induced glomerulonephritis in rats (216) (Table 5). In another study, overexpression of PAI-1 was observed in glomeruli from mice with lupus nephritis (217) and in glomeruli from patients with vascular nephropathy and crescentic glomerulonephritis (218) (Table 5). These studies indicate that the plasminogen/plasmin system plays a potential role in the accumulation of ECM components in proliferative glomerulonephritis. Border and co-workers have demonstrated that, in anti-Thy-1.1-induced model of glomerulonephritis, the glomeruli markedly increased the expression of TGF-β and PAI-1. Administration of anti-TGF-β antibody suppressed the overproduction of ECM proteins and decreased the deposition of PAI-1 in nephritic glomeruli (216,219). These studies strongly suggest that TGF-β is an important mediator in regulating the plasminogen/plasmin system and turnover of the ECM components in the glomeruli.

In Vivo Studies Supporting the Role of Oxidants in Glomerular Injury

The direct in vivo effects of ROMs on glomerular function have been examined in several studies (Table 4). Infusion of phorbol myristate acetate (a well-known potent activator of leukocytes) or infusion of cobra venom factor in the renal artery caused significant proteinuria that was prevented by catalase (which destroys H_2O_2) or neutrophil depletion (220–222). In a more recent study, it was shown that H_2O_2 infused directly into the renal artery caused massive transient proteinuria with no effect on GFR and renal plasma flow (223). Fractional clearances of graded sized neutral dextrans of larger molecular radii, an index of glomerular size selectivity, were significantly and substantially elevated after H_2O_2 infusion. More recently, it was demonstrated that infusion of xanthine/xanthine oxidase into freshly isolated glomeruli increases albumin permeability. Similar effects were obtained by incubating glomeruli with activated macrophages. These effects were inhibited by superoxide dismutase, a scavenger of superoxide anion. These results demonstrate that superoxide and/or H_2O_2 can impair the albumin filtration barrier in vitro (Table 4) (224).

These studies indicate that H_2O_2 and/or its metabolites generated by neutrophils can cause proteinuria. Johnson et al. reasoned that H_2O_2-mediated injury may involve the MPO–H_2O_2–halide system. The postulate is particularly attractive in view of the high cationic nature of MPO (isoelectric point >10) and the negative charge of the GBM. They demonstrated that infusion of MPO followed by H_2O_2 in a chloride-containing solution into the renal artery in rats results in significant proteinuria (117) and, 4–10 days later, development of a marked proliferative glomerular lesion (Table 4) (196). In addition, halogenation (as measured by the incorporation of [^{125}I]) of glomeruli and GBM was demonstrated in an in situ model of neutrophil-mediated immune-complex glomerulonephritis (6). These studies indicate the activation of the MPO–H_2O_2–halide system in a model of neutrophil-mediated immune-complex glomerulonephritis and that the MPO–H_2O_2–halide system is capable of inducing glomerular injury that results in proteinuria (see also Chapter 26).

In contrast to the in vitro studies described above demonstrating a role of oxidants in GBM degradation, Kanwar and associates have suggested that synthesis of glomerular heparan sulfate proteoglycans (HSPG) is highly susceptible to oxidant injury (Table 4) (225). Using an isolated perfused kidney model, a marked dose-dependent decrease in the de novo synthesis of proteoglycans in response to xanthine/xanthine oxidase (a system that generates ROMs) was demonstrated. The synthesis of type-IV collagen and laminin was decreased only slightly (~15%). Morphologic studies revealed a 14-fold decrease in the [^{35}S]sulfate-associated autoradiographic grains overlying the GBM. Thus, the nascent core peptide appears to be highly susceptible to "selective" direct damage from ROS during de novo synthesis of HSPG molecules necessary to maintain integrity of the GBM and normal glomerular ultrafiltration.

Studies Suggesting a Role of Reactive Oxygen Metabolites in Animal Models of Glomerular Disease

One of the best-characterized models of complement and neutrophil-dependent glomerular injury is the heterologous phase of anti-GBM antibody disease. In this model of neutrophil-dependent glomerular injury, treatment with catalase markedly reduced the proteinuria, whereas superoxide dismutase had no protective effect (Table 6) (4). In another study, dimethylthiourea, a potent hydroxyl-radical scavenger, or an iron chelator, deferoxamine, significantly attenuated proteinuria in the complement- and neutrophil-dependent heterologous phase of anti-GBM antibody disease in rabbits (226). Although the role of iron is not completely understood, the protective effect of iron chelators has been generally taken as evidence for the participation of hydroxyl radical in tissue injury because iron is critical in the generation of hydroxyl radical (via the Haber–Weiss reaction).

TABLE 6. *Evidence for the role of reactive oxygen metabolites in animal models of glomerular injury*

Scavengers of reactive oxygen metabolites reduce proteinuria in
- Complement- and neutrophil-dependent heterologous phase of anti-GBM antibody disease (4,226)
- Puromycin aminonucleoside model of minimal change disease (227–229,236)
- Adriamycin model of minimal change disease (230)
- Passive Heymann nephritis model of membranous nephropathy (232,234)
- Cationized γ-globulin-induced immune-complex glomerulonephritis (233)

Reproduced with permission from the *Annual Review of Physiology,* volume 57, 1995, by Annual Reviews, Inc.

The ability of glomerular cells to generate ROMs suggests that ROMs may be important mediators of glomerular injury in glomerular diseases that lack infiltrating leukocytes (Table 6). A single intravenous injection of puromycin aminonucleoside results in marked proteinuria and glomerular morphologic changes that are similar to minimal change disease in humans. Diamond et al. reported that allopurinol (an inhibitor of xanthine oxidase) and superoxide dismutase were protective in PAN-induced nephrotic syndrome, suggesting a role for xanthine-oxidase-generated superoxide anion in this model of minimal change disease (227). Beaman and co-workers confirmed the protective effect of superoxide dismutase and, in addition, reported that proteinuria was significantly reduced in rats receiving polyethylene glycol coupled catalase, suggesting a role for both H_2O_2 and superoxide anion in this model of glomerular disease (228). Superoxide anion and H_2O_2 may interact (with iron as a catalyst) to generate the hydroxyl radical. Several studies have, in fact, shown that enhanced generation of H_2O_2 and superoxide anion is accompanied by enhanced generation of hydroxyl radical (or a similar highly oxidizing species). Thakur et al. reported the protective effects of two hydroxyl-radical scavengers and an iron chelator implicating hydroxyl radical in puromycin aminonucleoside-induced nephrotic syndrome (229). Recently, coadministration of α-tocopherol/ascorbic acid resulted in marked reduction in proteinuria, accompanied by reduced foot-process effacement, in this model of minimal change disease (126).

A single intravenous injection of adriamycin (an anthracycline antibiotic used in cancer chemotherapy) causes nephrotic syndrome in rats (127) with morphologic and functional changes similar to those seen in minimal change disease in humans. Adriamycin undergoes a one-electron reduction to a free-radical, semiquinone species catalyzed by microsomes, sarcosomes, mitochondria, nuclei, and cytoplasm (127). Thus, adriamycin-induced nephrotic syndrome appears to be a good model to demonstrate the concept that ROMs generated intracellularly by glomerular cells can cause glomerular injury resulting in proteinuria. However, the evidence from scavenger studies is somewhat controversial. One study showed a protective effect of superoxide dismutase (Table 6) (230), whereas another study did not find any protective effects of scavengers of ROMs (231).

Passive Heymann nephritis, induced by a single intravenous injection of anti-FX1A, is a complement-dependent and neutrophil-independent model of glomerular disease that resembles membranous nephropathy in humans. Shah reported that superoxide dismutase or catalase (native or polyethylene glycol coupled) did not affect the anti-FX1A-induced proteinuria. In contrast, scavengers of hydroxyl radical, and an iron chelator, deferoxamine, markedly reduced the proteinuria (232). The protective effects of both the hydroxyl-radical scavengers and an iron chelator suggest a role for the hydroxyl radical in passive Heymann nephritis. Similarly, Rahman et al. have reported that two hydroxyl-radical scavengers significantly reduced the proteinuria in cationized γ-globulin-induced immune-complex glomerulonephritis, a complement- and neutrophil-independent model of membranous nephropathy (233). Taken together, these studies suggest an important role for hydroxyl radical in animal models of membranous nephropathy. Neale et al. have demonstrated a role for lipid peroxidation in the proteinuria in passive Heymann nephritis (234). They have shown the presence of malondialdehyde adducts localized to GBM. Type-IV collagen was specifically identified as being modified by malondialdehyde adducts. The antioxidant, probucol, inhibited proteinuria, supporting a role for lipid peroxidation in the alteration of glomerular permselectivity that results in proteinuria (234) (see also Chapter 47).

Thus, it appears that leukocytes or resident glomerular cells may serve as sources for ROMs. In vitro and in vivo studies indicate that ROMs have many effects that are relevant to the functional and morphologic changes observed in glomerular injury, and data with scavengers of ROMs document an important role for ROMs in glomerular injury. While most of the studies have emphasized enhanced generation of ROMs, antioxidant defenses are likely to be equally important as determinants of injury.

CONCLUSION

In recent years, some progress has been made in understanding the potential role of proteases and oxidants in glomerulonephritides. However, the complex molecular and cellular mechanisms by which they become activated and released in response to external stimuli have not been fully delineated. Similarly, far less is known on the mechanisms whereby latent proforms of metalloproteinases and latent serine proteinases are activated in vivo. In addition, much of the evidence presented is from experimental models of glomerular disease, and there is negligible information on the importance of oxidants and proteases in human disease. Equally important, it is not certain that proteases and oxidants will be significant once the injury has already been initiated or is ongoing, as is the case in human glomerulonephritides. Nevertheless, better understanding of the role of proteases, oxidants, and other mediators may provide therapeutic tools for the future in an area where treatment is at best empirical.

ACKNOWLEDGMENTS

The authors thank William Baricos, Ph.D., for his critical review of the chapter, and Ellen Satter for secretarial assistance.

REFERENCES

1. Couser WG. Mediation of immune glomerular injury. *J Am Soc Nephrol* 1990;1:13–29.
2. Shah SV. *Mechanisms of glomerular injury*. Philadelphia: WB Saunders, 1991.
3. Johnson RJ, Lovett D, Lehrer RI, Couser WG, Klebanoff SJ. Role of oxidants and proteases in glomerular injury. *Kidney Int* 1994;45: 352–9.
4. Rehan A, Johnson KJ, Wiggins RC, Kunkel RG, Ward PA. Evidence for the role of oxygen radicals in acute nephrotoxic nephritis. *Lab Invest* 1984;51:396–403.
5. Cochrane CG, Unanue ER, Dixon FJ. A role of polymorphonuclear leukocytes and complement in nephrotoxic nephritis. *J Exp Med* 1965;122:95–110.
6. Johnson RJ, Klebanoff SJ, Ochi RF, et al. Participation of the myeloperoxidase–H_2O_2–halide system in immune complex nephritis. *Kidney Int* 1987;32:342–9.
7. Holdsworth SR, Neale TJ, Wilson CB. Abrogation of macrophage-dependent injury in experimental glomerulonephritis in the rabbit. *J Clin Invest* 1981;68:686–98.
8. Shah SV. The role of reactive oxygen metabolites in glomerular disease. *Annu Rev Physiol* 1995;57:245–62.
9. Henson PM, Henson JE, Fittschen C, Bratton DL, Riches DWH. Degranulation and secretion by phagocytic cells. In: Gallin JI, Goldstein IM, Snyderman R, eds. *Inflammation: basic principles and clinical correlates*. New York: Raven, 1992:511–39.
10. Baricos WH, Shah SV. Proteolytic enzymes as mediators of glomerular injury. *Kidney Int* 1991;40:161–73.
11. Matrisian LM. The matrix-degrading metalloproteinases. *BioEssays* 1992;14:455–63.
12. Macartney HW, Tschesche H. Latent and active human polymorphonuclear leukocyte collagenases: isolation, purification and characterisation. *Eur J Biochem* 1983;130:71–8.
13. Murphy G, Reynolds JJ, Bretz U, Baggiolini M. Partial purification of collagenase and gelatinase from human polymorphonuclear leucocytes. *Biochem J* 1982;203:209–21.
14. Dewald B, Bretz U, Baggiolini M. Release of gelatinase from a novel secretory compartment of human neutrophils. *J Clin Invest* 1982;70: 518–25.
15. Hibbs MS, Hasty KA, Kang AH, Mainardi CL. Secretion of collagenolytic enzymes by human polymorphonuclear leukocytes. *Collagen Related Res* 1984;4:467–77.
16. Weissmann G, Smolen JE, Korchak HM. Release of inflammatory mediators from stimulated neutrophils. *N Engl J Med* 1980;303:27–34.
17. Masure S, Proost P, Van Damme J, Opdenakker G. Purification and identification of 91-kDa neutrophil gelatinase: release by the activating peptide interleukin-8. *Eur J Biochem* 1991;198:391–8.
18. Lazarus GS, Daniels JR, Brown RS, Bladen HA, Fullmer HM. Degradation of collagen by a human granulocyte collagenolytic system. *J Clin Invest* 1968;47:2622–9.
19. Hasty KA, Hibbs MS, Kang AH, Mainardi CL. Secreted forms of human neutrophil collagenase. *J Biol Chem* 1986;261:5645–50.
20. Callaway JE, Garcia JA, Hersh CL, Yeh RK, Gilmore-Hebert M. Use of lectin affinity chromatography for the purification of collagenase from human polymorphonuclear leukocytes. *Biochemistry* 1986;25: 4757–62.
21. Mookhtiar KA, Van Wart HE. Purification to homogeneity of latent and active 58-kilodalton forms of human neutrophil collagenase. *Biochemistry* 1990;29:10,620–7.
22. Moloney DB, O'Connor CM, Fitzgerald MX. Human neutrophil collagenase: its isolation and purification. *Biochem Soc Trans* 1991;19: 62S.
23. Hasty KA, Pourmotabbed TF, Goldberg GI, et al. Human neutrophil collagenase: a distinct gene product with homology to other matrix metalloproteinases. *J Biol Chem* 1990;265:11,421–4.
24. Ho TF, Qoronfleh MW, Wahl RC, et al. Gene expression, purification and characterization of recombinant human neutrophil collagenase. *Gene* 1994;146:297–301.
25. Schnierer S, Kleine T, Gote T, Hillemann A, Knauper V, Tschesche H. The recombinant catalytic domain of human neutrophil collagenase lacks type I collagen substrate specificity. *Biochem Biophys Res Commun* 1993;191:319–26.

26. Bode W, Reinemer P, Huber R, Kleine T, Schnierer S, Tschesche H. The X-ray crystal structure of the catalytic domain of human neutrophil collagenase inhibited by a substrate analogue reveals the essentials for catalysis and specificity. *EMBO J* 1994;13:1263–9.
27. Hasty KA, Jeffrey JJ, Hibbs MS, Welgus HG. The collagen substrate specificity of human neutrophil collagenase. *J Biol Chem* 1987;262: 10,048–52.
28. Mallya SK, Mookhtiar KA, Gao Y, et al. Characterization of 58-kilodalton human neutrophil collagenase: comparison with human fibroblast collagenase. *Biochemistry* 1990;29:10,628–34.
29. Tschesche H, Knaufer V, Kramer S, Michaelis J, Oberhoff R, Reinke H. Matrix metalloproteinases and inhibitors. In: Birkedal-Hanson H, Werk Z, Welgus H, Van Wart H, eds. *Matrix supplement no. 1.* Berlin: Gustav Fischer, 1992.
30. Fosang AJ, Last K, Knauper V, et al. Fibroblast and neutrophil collagenases cleave at two sites in the cartilage aggrecan interglobular domain. *Biochem J* 1993;295:273–6.
31. Sopata I, Dancewicz AM. Presence of a gelatin-specific proteinase and its latent form in human leucocytes. *Biochim Biophys Acta* 1974; 370:510–23.
32. Weiss SJ, Peppin GJ. Collagenolytic metalloenzymes of the human neutrophil. *Biochem Pharmacol* 1986;35:3189–97.
33. Hibbs MS, Hasty KA, Seyer JM, Kang AH, Mainard CL. Biochemical and immunological characterization of the secreted forms of human neutrophil gelatinase. *J Biol Chem* 1985;260:2493–500.
34. Murphy G, Ward R, Hembry RM, Reynolds JJ, Kuhn K, Tryggvason K. Characterization of gelatinase from pig polymorphonuclear leucocytes: a metalloproteinase resembling tumour type IV collagenase. *Biochem J* 1989;258:463–72.
35. Pourmotabbed T, Solomon TL, Hasty KA, Mainardi CL. Characteristics of 92 kDa type IV collagenase/gelatinase produced by granulocytic leukemia cells: structure, expression of cDNA in *E. coli* and enzymic properties. *Biochim Biophys Acta* 1994;1204:97–107.
36. Devarajan P, Johnston JJ, Ginsberg SS, Van Wart HE, Berliner N. Structure and expression of neutrophil gelatinase cDNA: identity with type IV collagenase from HT1080 cells. *J Biol Chem* 1992;267: 25,228–32.
37. Graubert T, Johnston J, Berliner N. Cloning and expression of the cDNA encoding mouse neutrophil gelatinase: demonstration of coordinate secondary granule protein gene expression during terminal neutrophil maturation. *Blood* 1993;82:3192–7.
38. Kjeldsen L, Bjerrum O, Hovgaard D, Johnsen A, Sehested M, Borregaard N. Human neutrophil gelatinase: a marker for circulating blood neutrophils—purification and quantitation by enzyme linked immunosorbent assay. *Eur J Haematol* 1992;49:180–91.
39. Baricos WH, Murphy G, Zhou Y, Nguyen HH, Shah SV. Degradation of glomerular basement membrane by purified mammalian metalloproteinases. *Biochem J* 1988;254:609–12.
40. Shapiro SD, Fliszar CJ, Broekelmann TJ, Mecham RP, Senior RM, Welgus HG. Activation of the 92-kDa gelatinase by stromelysin and 4-aminophenylmercuric acetate: differential processing and stabilization of the carboxyl-terminal domain by tissue inhibitor of metalloproteinases (TIMP). *J Biol Chem* 1995;270:6351–6.
41. Havemann K, Gramse M. Physiology and pathophysiology of neutral proteinases of human granulocytes. *Adv Exp Med Biol* 1984;167:1–20.
42. Janoff A. Elastase in tissue injury. *Annu Rev Med* 1985;36:207-16.
43. Sinha S, Watorek W, Karr S, Giles J, Bode W, Travis J. Primary structure of human neutrophil elastase. *Proc Natl Acad Sci USA* 1987; 84:2228–32.
44. Travis J. Structure, function, and control of neutrophil proteinases. *Am J Med* 1988;84:37–42.
45. Weiss SJ. Tissue destruction by neutrophils. *N Engl J Med* 1989;320: 365–76.
46. Salvesen G, Farley D, Shuman J, Przybyla A, Reilly C, Travis J. Molecular cloning of human cathepsin G: structural similarity to mast cell and cytotoxic T lymphocyte proteinases. *Biochemistry* 1987;26: 2289–93.
47. Starkey PM. Elastase and cathepsin G, the serine proteinases of human neutrophil leukocytes and spleen. In: Barret AJ, ed. *Proteinases in mammalian cells and tissues.* Amsterdam: North-Holland, 1977:57.
48. Vissers MCM, Winterbourn CC, Hunt JS. Degradation of glomerular basement membrane by human neutrophils in vitro. *Biochim Biophys Acta* 1984;804:154–60.
49. Bray J, Hume DA, Robinson GB. Degradation of rat or sheep glomerular basement membrane by rabbit neutrophils in vitro: the roles of proteinases, complement and oxygen-derived radicals. *Mol Biol Med* 1983;1:253–69.
50. Shah SV, Baricos WH, Basci A. Degradation of human glomerular basement membrane by stimulated neutrophils: activation of a metalloproteinase/s by reactive oxygen metabolites. *J Clin Invest* 1987;79: 25–31.
51. Davies M, Coles G, Hughes K. Glomerular basement membrane injury by neutrophil and monocyte neutral proteinases. *Renal Physiol* 1980;3:106–11.
52. Baricos WH, Murphy G, Zhou Y, Nguyen HH, Shah SV. Degradation of glomerular basement membrane by purified mammalian metalloproteinases. *Biochem J* 1988;254:609–12.
53. Pipoly DJ, Crouch EC. Degradation of native type IV procollagen by human neutrophil elastase: implications for leukocyte-mediated degradation of basement membranes. *Biochem* 1987;26:5748–54.
54. Heck LW, Blackburn WD, Irwin MH, Abrahamson DR. Degradation of basement membrane laminin by human neutrophil elastase and cathepsin G. *Am J Pathol* 1990;136:1267–74.
55. Bruch M, Landwehr R, Engel J. Dissection of laminin by cathepsin G into its long-arm and short-arm structures and localization of regions involved in calcium dependent stabilization and self-association. *Eur J Biochem* 1989;185:271–9.
56. McDonald J, Kelley D. Degradation of fibronectin by human leukocyte elastase. *J Biol Chem* 1980;255:8848–55.
57. Janusz MJ, Doherty NS. Degradation of cartilage matrix proteoglycan by human neutrophils involves both elastase and cathepsin G. *J Immunol* 1991;146:3922–8.
58. Klebanoff SJ, Kinsella MG, Wight TN. Degradation of endothelial cell matrix heparan sulfate proteoglycan by elastase and the myeloperoxidase–H_2O_2–chloride system. *Am J Pathol* 1993;143:907–17.
59. Campanelli D, Melchior M, Fu Y, et al. Cloning of cDNA for proteinase 3: a serine protease, antibiotic, and autoantigen from human neutrophils. *J Exp Med* 1990;172:1709–15.
60. Kao RC, Wehner NG, Skubitz KM, Gray BH, Hoidal JR. Proteinase 3: a distinct human polymorphonuclear leukocyte proteinase that produces emphysema in hamsters. *J Clin Invest* 1988;82:1963–73.
61. Rao NV, Wehner NG, Marshall BC, Gray WR, Gray BH, Hoidal JR. Characterization of proteinase-3 (PR-3), a neutrophil serine proteinase. *J Biol Chem* 1991;296:9540–8.
62. Csernok E, Ludemann J, Gross WL, Bainton DF. Ultrastructural localization of proteinase 3, the target antigen of anti-cytoplasmic antibodies circulating in Wegener's granulomatosis. *Am J Pathol* 1990;137:1113–20.
63. Goldschmeding R, van der Schoot CE, ten Bokkel Huinink D, et al. Wegener's granulomatosis autoantibodies identify a novel diisopropylfluorophosphate-binding protein in the lysosomes of normal human neutrophils. *J Clin Invest* 1989;84:1577–87.
64. Ludemann J, Utecht B, Gross WL. Anti-neutrophil cytoplasm antibodies in Wegener's granulomatosis recognize an elastinolytic enzyme. *J Exp Med* 1990;171:357–62.
65. Niles JL, McCluskey RT, Ahmad MF, Arnaout MA. Wegener's granulomatosis autoantigen is a novel neutrophil serine proteinase. *Blood* 1989;74:1888–93.
66. Marti H-P, McNeil L, Davies M, Martin J, Lovett DH. Homology cloning of rat 72 kDa type IV collagenase: cytokine and second-messenger inducibility in glomerular mesangial cells. *Biochem J* 1993; 291:441–6.
67. Martin J, Davies M, Thomas G, Lovett DH. Human mesangial cells secrete a GBM-degrading neutral proteinase and a specific inhibitor. *Kidney Int* 1989;36:790–801.
68. Davies M, Thomas GJ, Martin J, Lovett DH. The purification and characterization of a glomerular-basement-membrane-degrading neutral proteinase from rat mesangial cells. *Biochem J* 1988;251:419–25.
69. Marti HP, Lee L, Kashgarian M, Lovett DH. Transforming growth factor-β1 stimulates glomerular mesangial cell synthesis of the 72-kd type IV collagenase. *Am J Pathol* 1994;144:82–94.
70. Martin J, Knowlden J, Davies M, Williams JD. Identification and independent regulation of human mesangial cell metalloproteinases. *Kidney Int* 1994;46:877–85.
71. Tryggvason K, Huhtala P, Tuuttila A, Chow L, Keski-Oja J, Lohi J. Structure and expression of type IV collagen genes. *Differ Dev* 1990; 32:307–12.

72. Frisch SM, Morisaki JH. Positive and negative transcriptional elements of the human type IV collagenase gene. *Mol Cell Biol* 1990;10: 6524–32.
73. Nguyen HH, Baricos WH, Shah SV. Degradation of glomerular basement membrane by a neutral metalloproteinase(s) present in glomeruli isolated from normal rat kidney. *Biochem Biophys Res Commun* 1986;141:898–903.
74. Le Q, Shah S, Nguyen H, Cortez S, Baricos W. A novel metalloproteinase present in freshly isolated rat glomeruli. *Am J Physiol* 1991; 260:F555–61.
75. Lovett DH, Johnson RJ, Marti H-P, Martin J, Davies M, Couser WG. Structural characterization of the mesangial cell type IV collagenase and enhanced expression in a model of immune complex-mediated glomerulonephritis. *Am J Pathol* 1992;141:85–98.
76. Johnson R, Yamabe H, Chen YP, et al. Glomerular epithelial cells secrete a glomerular basement membrane-degrading metalloproteinase. *J Am Soc Nephrol* 1992;2:1388–97.
77. Watanabe K, Kinoshita S, Nakagawa H. Gelatinase secretion by glomerular epithelial cells. *Nephron* 1990;56:405–9.
78. Knowlden J, Martin J, Davies M, Williams JD. Metalloproteinase generation by human glomerular epithelial cells. *Kidney Int* 1995;47: 1682–9.
79. Vassalli J-D, Sappino A-P, Belin D. The plasminogen activator/plasmin system. *J Clin Invest* 1991;88:1067–72.
80. Saksela O, Rifkin DB. Cell-associated plasminogen activation: regulation and physiological functions. *Annu Rev Cell Biol* 1988;4:93–126.
81. Rondeau E, Ochi S, Lacave R, et al. Urokinase synthesis and binding by glomerular epithelial cells in culture. *Kidney Int* 1989;36:593–600.
82. Iwamoto T, Nakashima Y, Sueishi K. Secretion of plasminogen activator and its inhibitor by glomerular epithelial cells. *Kidney Int* 1990; 37:1466–76.
83. Becquemont L, Nguyen G, Peraldi MN, He CJ, Sraer JD, Rondeau E. Expression of plasminogen/plasmin receptors on human glomerular epithelial cells. *Am J Physiol* 1994;267:F303–10.
84. Lacave R, Rondeau E, Ochi S, Delarue F, Schleuning WD, Sraer JD. Characterization of a plasminogen activator and its inhibitor in human mesangial cells. *Kidney Int* 1989;35:806–11.
85. Mackay AR, Corbitt RH, Hartzler JL, Thorgeirsson UP. Basement membrane type IV collagen degradation: evidence for the involvement of a proteolytic cascade independent of metalloproteinases. *Cancer Res* 1990;50:5997–6001.
86. He C, Wilhelm SM, Pentland AP, et al. Tissue cooperation in a proteolytic cascade activating human interstitial collagenase. *Proc Natl Acad Sci USA* 1989;86:2632–6.
87. Chapman HA, Stone OL. Cooperation between plasmin and elastase in elastin degradation by intact murine macrophages. *Biochem J* 1984;222:721–8.
88. Rifkin DB, Moscatelli D, Bizik J, Quarto N, Blei F, Dennis P. Growth factor control of extracellular proteolysis. *Cell Differ Dev* 1990;32: 313–8.
89. Dano K, Andreasen PA, Grondahl-Hansen J, Kristensen P, Nielsen LS, Skriver L. Plasminogen activators, tissue degradation, and cancer. *Adv Cancer Res* 1985;44:139–266.
90. Angles-Cano E, Rondeau E, Delarue F, Hagege J, Sultan Y, Sraer J. Identification and cellular localization of plasminogen activators from human glomeruli. *Thromb Haemost* 1985;54:688–92.
91. Muellbacher W, Maier M, Binder BR. Regulation of plasminogen activation in isolated perfused rat kidney. *Am J Physiol* 1989;256: F787–93.
92. Aya N, Yoshioka K, Murakami K, et al. Tissue-type plasminogen activator and its inhibitor in human glomerulonephritis. *J Pathol* 1992;166:289–95.
93. Sappino A-P, Huarte J, Vassalli J-D, Belin D. Sites of synthesis of urokinase and tissue-type plasminogen activators in the murine kidney. *J Clin Invest* 1991;87:962–70.
94. Baricos WH, Cortez SL, El-Dahr SS, Schnaper HW. ECM degradation by cultured human mesangial cells is mediated by a PA/plasmin/ MMP-2 cascade. *Kidney Int* 1995;47:1039–47.
95. Glass WF, Kreisberg JI, Troyer DA. Two-chain urokinase, receptor, and type 1 inhibitor in cultured human mesangial cells. *Am J Physiol* 1993;264:F532–9.
96. Hagege J, Delarue F, Peraldi M, Sraer J, Rondeau E. Heparin selectively inhibits synthesis of tissue type plasminogen activator and matrix deposition of plasminogen activator inhibitor 1 by human mesangial cells. *Lab Invest* 1994;71:828–37.
97. Brown PAJ, Wilson HM, Reid FJ, et al. Urokinase-plasminogen activator is synthesized in vitro by human glomerular epithelial cells but not by mesangial cells. *Kidney Int* 1994;45:43–7.
98. Kanalas JJ. Analysis of the plasminogen system on rat glomerular epithelial cells. *Exp Cell Res* 1995;218:561–6.
99. Loskutoff DJ, Sawdey M, Mimuro J. Type 1 plasminogen activator inhibitor. *Prog Hemost Thromb* 1989;9:87–115.
100. Travis J, Salvesen GS. Human plasma proteinase inhibitors. *Annu Rev Biochem* 1983;52:655–709.
101. Peraldi M-N, Rondeau E, Medcalf RL, et al. Cell-specific regulation of plasminogen activator inhibitor 1 and tissue type plasminogen activator release by human kidney mesangial cells. *Biochim Biophys Acta* 1992;1134:189–96.
102. Hagege J, Peraldi MN, Rondeau E, et al. Plasminogen activator inhibitor-1 deposition in the extracellular matrix of cultured human mesangial cells. *Am J Pathol* 1992;141:117–28.
103. Bu G, Warshawsky I, Schwartz AL. Cellular receptors for the plasminogen activators. *Blood* 1994;83:3427–36.
104. Miles LA, Levin EG, Plescia J, Collen D, Plow EF. Plasminogen receptors, urokinase receptors, and their modulation on human endothelial cells. *Blood* 1988;72:628–35.
105. Plow E, Felez J, Miles L. Cellular regulation of fibrinolysis. *Thromb Haemost* 1991;66:32–6.
106. Ellis V, Behrendt N, Dano K. Plasminogen activation by receptor-bound urokinase: a kinetic study with both cell-associated and isolated receptor. *J Biol Chem* 1991;266:12,752–8.
107. Eddy AA, Michael AF. Immunopathogenic mechanisms of glomerular injury. In: Tisher CC, Brenner BM, eds. *Renal pathology with clinical and functional correlations.* Philadelphia: JB Lippincott, 1994:162–221.
108. Brady HR, Papayianni A, Serhan CN. Leukocyte adhesion promotes biosynthesis of lipoxygenase products by transcellular routes. *Kidney Int* 1994;45:S90–7.
109. Briscoe D, Cotran R. Role of leukocyte-endothelial cell adhesion molecules in renal inflammation: in vitro and in vivo studies. *Kidney Int* 1993;44:S27–34.
110. Fantone JC, Ward PA. Role of oxygen-derived free radicals and metabolites in leukocyte-dependent inflammatory reactions. *Am J Pathol* 1982;107:397–418.
111. Ward P, Duque R, Sulavik M, Johnson KJ. In vitro and in vivo stimulation of rat neutrophils and alveolar macrophages by immune complexes. *Am J Pathol* 1983;110:297–309.
112. Klebanoff SJ. Oxygen metabolites from phagocytes. In: Gallin JI, Goldstein IM, Snyderman R, eds. *Inflammation: basic principles and clinical correlates.* New York: Raven, 1992:541–88.
113. Chanock SJ, El Benna J, Smith RM, Babior BM. The respiratory burst oxidase. *J Biol Chem* 1994;269:24,519–22.
114. Rotrosen D. The respiratory burst oxidase. In: Gallin JI, Goldstein IM, Snyderman R, eds. *Inflammation: basic principles and clinical correlates.* New York: Raven, 1992:589–601.
115. Weening RS, Wever R, Roos D. Quantitative aspects of the production of superoxide radicals by phagocytizing human granulocytes. *J Lab Clin Med* 1975;85:245–52.
116. Britigan BE, Cohen MS, Rosen GM. Hydroxyl radical formation in neutrophils. *N Engl J Med* 1988;318:858–9.
117. Johnson RJ, Couser WG, Chi EY, Adler S, Klebanoff SJ. New mechanism for glomerular injury. *J Clin Invest* 1987;79:1379–87.
118. Weiss SJ, Lampert MB, Test ST. Long-lived oxidants generated by human neutrophils: characterization and bioactivity. *Science* 1983; 222:625–8.
119. Falk RJ, Terrell RS, Charles LA, Jennette JC. Anti-neutrophil cytoplasmic autoantibodies induce neutrophils to degranulate and produce oxygen radicals in vitro. *Proc Natl Acad Sci USA* 1990;87:4115–9.
120. Poelstra K, Hardonk MJ, Koudstaal J, Bakker WW. Intraglomerular platelet aggregation and experimental glomerulonephritis. *Kidney Int* 1990;37:1500–8.
121. Boyce NW, Tipping PG, Holdsworth SR. Glomerular macrophages produce reactive oxygen species in experimental glomerulonephritis. *Kidney Int* 1989;35:778–82.
122. Oberle GP, Niemeyer J, Thaiss F, Schoeppe W, Stahl RAK. Increased oxygen radical and eicosanoid formation in immune-mediated mesangial cell injury. *Kidney Int* 1992;42:69–74.

123. Shah SV. Light emission by isolated rat glomeruli in response to phorbol myristate acetate. *J Lab Clin Med* 1981;98:46–57.
124. Guidet BR, Shah SV. In vivo generation of hydrogen peroxide by rat kidney cortex and glomeruli. *Am J Physiol* 1989;256:F158–64.
125. Ueda N, Guidet B, Shah SV. Measurement of intracellular generation of hydrogen peroxide by rat glomeruli in vitro. *Kidney Int* 1994;45: 788–93.
126. Ricardo SD, Bertram JF, Ryan GB. Reactive oxygen species in puromycin aminonucleoside nephrosis: in vitro studies. *Kidney Int* 1994;45:1057–69.
127. Shah SV. Role of reactive oxygen metabolites in experimental glomerular disease. *Kidney Int* 1989;35:1093–106.
128. Baud L, Fouqueray B, Philippe C, Amrani A. Tumor necrosis factor alpha and mesangial cells. *Kidney Int* 1992;41:600–3.
129. Radeke HH, Meier B, Topley N, Floge J, Habermehl GG, Resch K. Interleukin 1-α and tumor necrosis factor-α induce oxygen radical production in mesangial cells. *Kidney Int* 1990;37:767–75.
130. Radeke HH, Cross AR, Hancock JT, et al. Functional expression of NADPH oxidase components (α- and β-subunits of cytochrome b_{558} and 45-kDa flavoprotein) by intrinsic human glomerular mesangial cells. *J Biol Chem* 1991;266:21,025–9.
131. Kawaguchi M, Yamada M, Wada H, Okigaki T. Role of active oxygen species in glomerular epithelial cell injury in vitro caused by puromycin aminonucleoside. *Toxicology* 1992;72:329–40.
132. Neale TJ, Ullrich R, Ojha P, Poczewski H, Verhoeven AJ, Kerjaschki D. Reactive oxygen species and neutrophil respiratory burst cytochrome b558 are produced by kidney glomerular cells in passive Heymann nephritis. *Proc Natl Acad Sci USA* 1993;90:3645–9.
133. Greenwald RA, Moy W. Inhibition of collagen gelation by action of the superoxide radical. *Arthritis Rheum* 1979;22:251–9.
134. Curran SF, Amoruso MA, Goldstein BD, Berg RA. Degradation of soluble collagen by ozone or hydroxyl radicals. *FEBS Lett* 1984;176: 155–60.
135. Johnson K, Rehan A, Ward P. The role of oxygen radicals in kidney disease. In: Halliwell B, ed. *Oxygen radicals and tissue injury symposium.* Bethesda: FASEB, 1988:115–22.
136. Vissers MCM, Winterbourn CC. The effect of oxidants on neutrophil-mediated degradation of glomerular basement membrane collagen. *Biochim Biophys Acta* 1986;889:277–86.
137. Wolff SP. Fragmentation of proteins by free radicals and its effect on their susceptibility to enzymic hydrolysis. *Biochem J* 1986;234:399–403.
138. Van Wart HE, Birkedal-Hansen H. The cysteine switch: a principle of regulation of metalloproteinase activity with potential applicability to the entire matrix metalloproteinase gene family. *Proc Natl Acad Sci USA* 1990;87:5578–82.
139. Vissers MCM, Winterbourn CC. Activation of human neutrophil gelatinase by endogenous serine proteinases. *Biochem J* 1988;249: 327–31.
140. Murphy G, Bretz U, Baggiolini M, Reynolds JJ. The latent collagenase and gelatinase of human polymorphonuclear neutrophil leucocytes. *Biochem J* 1980;192:517–25.
141. Capodici C, Muthukumaran G, Amoruso MA, Berg RA. Activation of neutrophil collagenase by cathepsin G. *Inflammation* 1989;13: 245–58.
142. Saari H, Suomalainen K, Lindy O, Konttinen YT, Sorsa T. Activation of latent human neutrophil collagenase by reactive oxygen species and serine proteases. *Biochem Biophys Res Commun* 1990;171:979–87.
143. Knauper V, Wilhelm SM, Seperack PK, et al. Direct activation of human neutrophil procollagenase by recombinant stromelysin. *Biochem J* 1993;295:581–6.
144. Ward RV, Atkinson SJ, Slocombe PM, Docherty AJP, Reynolds JJ, Murphy G. Tissue inhibitor of metalloproteinases-2 inhibits the activation of 72 kDa progelatinase by fibroblast membranes. *Biochim Biophys Acta* 1991;1079:242–6.
145. Brown PD, Kleiner DE, Unsworth EJ, Stetler-Stevenson WG. Cellular activation of the 72 kDa type IV procollagenase/TIMP-2 complex. *Kidney Int* 1993;43:163–70.
146. Strongin AY, Marmer BL, Grant GA, Goldberg GI. Plasma membrane-dependent activation of the 72-kDa type IV collagenase is prevented by complex formation with TIMP-2. *J Biol Chem* 1993;268: 14,033–9.
147. Sato H, Takino T, Okada Y, et al. A matrix metalloproteinase expressed on the surface of invasive tumor cells. *Nature* 1994;370: 61–5.
148. Peppin GJ, Weiss SJ. Activation of the endogenous metalloproteinase, gelatinase, by triggered human neutrophils. *Proc Natl Acad Sci USA* 1986;83:4322–6.
149. Weiss SJ, Peppin G, Ortiz X, Ragsdale C, Test ST. Oxidative autoactivation of latent collagenase by human neutrophils. *Science* 1985; 227:747–9.
150. Ichinose A, Kisiel W, Fujikawa K. Proteolytic activation of tissue plasminogen activator by plasma and tissue enzyme. *FEBS Lett* 1984; 175:412–8.
151. Keski-Oja J, Lohi J, Tuuttila A, Tryggvason K, Varitio T. Proteolytic processing of the 72 kDa type IV collagenase by urokinase plasminogen activator. *Exp Cell Res* 1992;202:471–6.
152. Barrett A, Rawlings N, Davies M, Machleidt W, Salvesen G, Turk V. Cysteine proteinase inhibitors of the cystatin superfamily. In: Barrett AJ, Salvesen G, eds. *Proteinase inhibitors.* Amsterdam: Elsevier, 1986;515.
153. Cawston T. Protein inhibitors of metalloproteinases. In: Barrett AJ, Salvesen G, eds. *Proteinase inhibitors.* Amsterdam: Elsevier, 1986; 589.
154. Johnson DA, Barrett AJ, Mason RW. Cathepsin L inactivates alpha 1-proteinase inhibitor by cleavage in the reactive site region. *J Biol Chem* 1986;261:14,748–51.
155. Banda MJ, Clark EJ, Sinha S, Travis J. Interaction of mouse macrophage elastase with native and oxidized human alpha 1-proteinase inhibitor. *J Clin Invest* 1987;79:1314–7.
156. Ottonello L, Dapino P, Dallegri F. Inactivation of alpha-1-proteinase inhibitor by neutrophil metalloproteinases: crucial role of the myeloperoxidase system and effects of the anti-inflammatory drug, nimesulide. *Respiration* 1993;60:32–7.
157. Desrochers PE, Weiss SJ. Proteolytic inactivation of alpha-1-proteinase inhibitor by a neutrophil metalloproteinase. *J Clin Invest* 1988;81:1646–50.
158. Carp H, Janoff A. In vitro suppression of serum elastase-inhibitory capacity by reactive oxygen species generated by phagocytosing polymorphonuclear leukocytes. *J Clin Invest* 1979;63:793–7.
159. Weiss SJ, Regiani S. Neutrophils degrade subendothelial matrices in the presence of alpha-1-proteinase inhibitor: cooperative use of lysosomal proteinases and oxygen metabolites. *J Clin Invest* 1984;73: 1297–303.
160. Carp H, Janoff A. Phagocyte-derived oxidants suppress the elastase-inhibitory capacity of alpha1-proteinase inhibitor in vitro. *J Clin Invest* 1980;66:987–95.
161. Clark RA, Stone PJ, El Hag A, Calore JD, Franzblau C. Myeloperoxidase-catalyzed inactivation of alpha1-protease inhibitor by human neutrophils. *J Biol Chem* 1981;256:3348–53.
162. Maier K, Matejkova E, Hinze H, Leuschel L, Weber H. Different selectivities of oxidants during oxidation of methionine residues in the alpha-1-proteinase inhibitor. *FEBS Lett* 1989;250:221–6.
163. Matheson N, Wong P, Schuyler M, Travis J. Interaction of human alpha-a-proteinase inhibitor with neutrophil myeloperoxidase. *Biochemistry* 1981;20:331–6.
164. Johnson D, Travis J. The oxidative inactivation of human alpha-1-proteinase inhibitor: further evidence for methionine at the reactive center. *J Biol Chem* 1979;254:4022–6.
165. Donovan KL, Davies M, Coles GA, Williams JD. Relative roles of elastase and reactive oxygen species in the degradation of human glomerular basement membrane by intact human neutrophils. *Kidney Int* 1994;45:1555–61.
166. Okada Y, Watanabe S, Nakanishi I, et al. Inactivation of tissue inhibitor of metalloproteinases by neutrophil elastase and other serine proteinases. *FEBS Lett* 1988;229:157–60.
167. Shieh B-H, Travis J. The reactive site of human α_2-antiplasmin. *J Biol Chem* 1987;262:6055–9.
168. Brower M, Harpel P. Proteolytic cleavage and inactivation of alpha-2-plasmin inhibitor and Ci inactivator by human polymorphonuclear leukocyte elastase. *J Biol Chem* 1982;257:9849–54.
169. Lewis M, Kallenbach J, Zaltzman M, et al. Severe deficiency of alpha 1-antitrypsin associated with cutaneous vasculitis, rapidly progressive glomerulonephritis, and colitis. *Am J Med* 1989;79:489–94.
170. Miller F, Kuschner M. Alpha-1-antitrypsin deficiency, emphysema, necrotizing angitis and glomerulonephritis. *Am J Med* 1969;46: 615–23.

171. Moroz S, Cutz E, Balfe J, Sass-Kortsak A. Membranoproliferative glomerulonephritis in childhood cirrhosis associated with alpha-1-antitrypsin deficiency. *Pediatrics* 1976;57:232–8.
172. Rodriguez-Soriano J, Fidalgo I, Camarero C, Vallo A, Oliveros R. Juvenile cirrhosis and membranous glomerulonephritis in a child with alpha-1-antitrypsin deficiency. *Acta Pediatr Scand* 1978;67:793–6.
173. Cybulsky AV, Lieberthal W, Quigg RJ, Rennke HG, Salant DJ. A role for thromboxane in complement-mediated glomerular injury. *Am J Pathol* 1987;128:45–51.
174. Remuzzi G, Imberti L, Rossini M, et al. Increased glomerular thromboxane synthesis as a possible cause of proteinuria in experimental nephrosis. *J Clin Invest* 1985;75:94–101.
175. Lianos EA, Andres GA, Dunn MJ. Glomerular prostaglandin and thromboxane synthesis in rat nephrotoxic serum nephritis. *J Clin Invest* 1983;72:1439–48.
176. Adler S, Stahl RAK, Baker PJ, Chen YP, Pritzl PM, Couser WG. Biphasic effect of oxygen radicals on prostaglandin production by rat mesangial cells. *Am J Physiol* 1987;252:F743–9.
177. Baud L, Nivez M-P, Chansel D, Ardaillou R. Stimulation by oxygen radicals of prostaglandin production by rat renal glomeruli. *Kidney Int* 1981;20:332–9.
178. Sedor JR, Abboud HE. Hydrogen peroxide stimulates PGE_2 synthesis by cultured rat mesangial cells. *Kidney Int* 1986;29:291.
179. Morrow JD, Hill KE, Burk RF, Nammour TM, Badr KF, Roberts LJ. A series of prostaglandin F_2-like compounds are produced in vivo in humans by a non-cyclooxygenase, free radical-catalyzed mechanism. *Proc Natl Acad Sci USA* 1990;87:9383–7.
180. Takahashi K, Nammour TM, Fukunaga M, et al. Glomerular actions of a free radical-generated novel prostaglandin, 8-epi-prostaglandin F_{2a}, in the rat. *J Clin Invest* 1992;90:136–41.
181. Dousa TP, Shah SV, Abboud HE. Potential role of cyclic nucleotides in glomerular pathophysiology. In: Hamet P, Sands H, eds. *Advances in cyclic nucleotide research.* New York: Raven, 1980:285–99.
182. Dworkin LD, Ichikawa I, Brenner BM. Hormonal modulation of glomerular function. *Am J Physiol* 1983;244:F95–104.
183. Ignarro L. Hormonal control of lysosomal enzyme release from human neutrophils by cyclic nucleotides and autonomic neurohormones. In: Weiss B, ed. *Cyclic nucleotides in diseases.* Baltimore: University Park, 1975:187–210.
184. Lichtenstein L. Hormone receptor modulation of cAMP in the control of allergic and inflammatory responses. In: Beers RF, Bassett EG, eds. *The role of infections, allergic, antiimune processes.* New York: Raven, 1976:339–54.
185. Dousa TP. Cyclic nucleotides in renal pathophysiology. In: Brenner BM, Stein JH, eds. *Contemporary issues in nephrology.* New York: Churchill Livingstone, 1979:251–85.
186. Shah SV. Effect of enzymatically generated reactive oxygen metabolites on the cyclic nucleotide content in isolated rat glomeruli. *J Clin Invest* 1984;74:393–401.
187. Basci A, Wallin JD, Shah SV. Effect of stimulated neutrophils on cyclic nucleotide content in isolated rat glomeruli. *Am J Physiol* 1987;252:F429–36.
188. Anderson WB, Jaworski CJ, Vlahakis G. Proteolytic activation of adenylate cyclase from cultured fibroblasts. *J Biol Chem* 1978;253:2921–6.
189. Wallach D, Anderson W, Pastan I. Activation of adenylate cyclase in cultured fibroblasts by trypsin. *J Biol Chem* 1978;253:24–6.
190. Richert ND, Ryan RJ. Proteolytic enzyme activation of rat ovarian adenylate cyclase. *Proc Natl Acad Sci USA* 1977;74:4857–61.
191. Shneyour A, Patt Y, Trainin N. Trypsin-induced increase in intracellular cyclic AMP of lymphocytes. *J Immunol* 1976;117:2143–9.
192. Johnson RA, Jakobs KH, Schultz G. Extraction of the adenylate cyclase-activating factor of bovine sperm and its identification as a trypsin-like protease. *J Biol Chem* 1985;260:114–21.
193. Gordon EA, Fenton JW, Carney DH. Thrombin-receptor occupancy initiates a transient increase in cAMP levels in mitogenically responsive hamster (NIL) fibroblasts. *Ann NY Acad Sci USA* 1986;485:249–63.
194. Snider R, Richelson E. Thrombin stimulation of guanosine 3′, 5′-monophosphate formation in murine neuroblastoma cells (clone NIE-115). *Science* 1983;221:566–8.
195. Shah SV. Effect of thrombin on cyclic AMP content in glomeruli isolated from rat kidney. *Kidney Int* 1989;35:824–9.
196. Johnson RJ, Guggenheim SJ, Klebanoff SJ, et al. Morphologic correlates of glomerular oxidant injury induced by the myeloperoxidase–hydrogen peroxide–halide system of the neutrophil. *Lab Invest* 1988;5:294–301.
197. Duque I, Puyol MR, Ruiz P, Gonzalez-Rubio M, Marques MLD, Puyol DR. Calcium channel blockers inhibit hydrogen peroxide-induced proliferation of cultured rat mesangial cells. *J Pharmacol Exp Ther* 1993;267:612–6.
198. Bakker WW, Baller JFW, Hardonk MJ. Decrease of glomerular ATPase activity induced by adriamycin is mediated by oxygen free radical species. *Kidney Int* 1987;31:1045–6.
199. Duque I, Garcia-Escribano C, Rodriguez-Puyol M, et al. Effects of reactive oxygen species on cultured rat mesangial cells and isolated rat glomeruli. *Am J Physiol* 1992;263:F466–73.
200. Schreck R, Rieber P, Baeuerle PA. Reactive oxygen intermediates as apparently widely used messengers in the activation of the NF-KB transcription factor and HIV-1. *EMBO J* 1991;10:2247–58.
201. Toledano MB, Leonard WJ. Modulation of transcription factor NF-kB binding activity by oxidation-reduction in vitro. *Proc Natl Acad Sci USA* 1991;88:4328–32.
202. Schreck R, Baeuerle PA. A role for oxygen radicals as second messengers. *Trends Cell Biol* 1991;1:39–42.
203. Satriano JA, Shuldiner M, Hora K, Xing Y, Shan Z, Schlondorff D. Oxygen radicals as second messengers for expression of the monocyte chemoattractant protein, JE/MCP-1, and the monocyte colony-stimulating factor, CSF-1, in response to tumor necrosis factor-α and immunoglobulin G: evidence for involvement of reduced nicotinamide adenine dinucleotide phosphate (NADPH)-dependent oxidase. *J Clin Invest* 1993;92:1564–71.
204. Satriano J, Schlondorff D. Activation and attenuation of transcription factor NF-kB in mouse glomerular mesangial cells in response to tumor necrosis factor-α, immunoglobulin G, and adenosine 3′:5′-cyclic monophosphate. *J Clin Invest* 1994;94:1629–36.
205. Schlondorff D. Cellular mechanism of glomerular injury: metabolic factors in progressive renal injury. *Kidney Int* 1994;45:S54–5.
206. Stahl R, Disser M, Hora K, Schlondorff D. Increased expression of monocyte chemoattractant protein in glomeruli from rats with anti Thy-1 glomerulonephritis. *J Am Soc Nephrol* 1992;3:616.
207. Baud L, Fouqueray B, Philippe C, Ardaillou R. Reactive oxygen species as glomerular autocoids. *J Am Soc Nephrol* 1992;2:S132–8.
208. Chini CCS, Chini EN, Williams JM, Matousovic K, Dousa TP. Formation of reactive oxygen metabolites in glomeruli is suppressed by inhibition of cAMP phosphodiesterase isozyme type IV. *Kidney Int* 1994;46:28–36.
209. Ardaillou R, Baud L. Interactions between glomerular autocoids. *Semin Nephrol* 1991;11:340–5.
210. Johnson RJ, Couser WG, Alpers CE, Vissers M, Schulze M, Klebanoff SJ. The human neutrophil serine proteinases, elastase and cathepsin G, can mediate glomerular injury in vivo. *J Exp Med* 1988;168:1169–74.
211. Schrijver G, Schalkwijk J, Robben JCM, Assmann KJM, Koene RAP. Antiglomerular basement membrane nephritis in beige mice: deficiency of leukocytic neutral proteinases prevents the induction of albuminuria in the heterologous phase. *J Exp Med* 1989;169:1435–48.
212. Lubec G. Collagenase activity of rat kidney with glomerulonephritis during the heterologous phase. *Clin Chim Acta* 1977;76:89–94.
213. Lubec G, Ratzenhofer E. Collagenase activity of rat kidney with immune complex glomerulonephritis. *Clin Chim Acta* 1978;82:205–7.
214. Feng L, Tang WW, Loskutoff DJ, Wilson CB. Dysfunction of glomerular fibrinolysis in experimental antiglomerular basement membrane antibody glomerulonephritis. *J Am Soc Nephrol* 1993;3:1753–64.
215. Malliaros J, Holdsworth SR, Wojta J, Erlich J, Tipping PG. Glomerular fibrinolytic activity in anti-GBM glomerulonephritis in rabbits. *Kidney Int* 1993;44:557–64.
216. Tomooka S, Border WA, Marshall BC, Noble NA. Glomerular matrix accumulation is linked to inhibition of the plasmin protease system. *Kidney Int* 1992;42:1462–9.
217. Loskutoff D, Sawdey M, Keeton M, Schneiderman J. Regulation of PAI-1 gene expression in vivo. *Thromb Haemost* 1993;70:135–7.
218. Rondeau E, Mougenot B, Lacave R, Peraldi MN, Kruithof EK, Sraer JD. Plasminogen activator inhibitor 1 in renal fibrin deposits of human nephropathies. *Clin Nephrol* 1990;33:55–60.

219. Border WA, Okuda S, Languino LR, Sporn MB, Ruoslahti E. Suppression of experimental glomerulonephritis by antiserum against transforming growth factor B1. *Nature* 1990;346:371–4.
220. Rehan A, Johnson KJ, Kunkel RG, Wiggins RC. Role of oxygen radicals in phorbol myristate acetate-induced glomerular injury. *Kidney Int* 1985;27:503–11.
221. Rehan A, Wiggins RC, Kunkel RG, Till GO, Johnson KJ. Glomerular injury and proteinuria in rats after intrarenal injection of cobra venom factor. *Am J Pathol* 1986;123:57–66.
222. Yoshioka T, Ichikawa I. Glomerular dysfunction induced by polymorphonuclear leukocyte-derived reactive oxygen species. *Am J Physiol* 1989;257:F53–9.
223. Yoshioka T, Ichikawa I, Fogo A. Reactive oxygen metabolites cause massive, reversible proteinuria and glomerular sieving defect without apparent ultrastructural abnormality. *J Am Soc Nephrol* 1991;2:902–12.
224. Dileepan KN, Sharma R, Stechschulte DJ, Savin VJ. Effect of superoxide exposure on albumin permeability of isolated rat glomeruli. *J Lab Clin Med* 1993;121:797–804.
225. Kashihara N, Watanabe Y, Makino H, Wallner EI, Kanwar YS. Selective decreased de novo synthesis of glomerular proteoglycans under the influence of reactive oxygen species. *Proc Natl Acad Sci USA* 1992;89:6309–13.
226. Boyce NW, Holdsworth SR. Hydroxyl radical mediation of immune renal injury by desferrioxamine. *Kidney Int* 1986;30:813–7.
227. Diamond JR, Bonventre JV, Karnovsky MJ. A role for oxygen free radicals in aminonucleoside nephrosis. *Kidney Int* 1986;29:478–83.
228. Beaman M, Birtwistle R, Howie AJ, Michael J, Adu D. The role of superoxide anion and hydrogen peroxide in glomerular injury induced by puromycin aminonucleoside in rats. *Clin Sci* 1987;73:329–32.
229. Thakur V, Walker PD, Shah SV. Evidence suggesting a role for hydroxyl radical in puromycin aminonucleoside-induced proteinuria. *Kidney Int* 1988;34:494–9.
230. Okasora T, Takikawa T, Utsunomiya Y, et al. Suppressive effect of superoxide dismutase on adriamycin nephropathy. *Nephron* 1992;60:199–203.
231. Bertolatus JA, Klinzman D, Bronsema DA, Ridnour L, Oberley LW. Evaluation of the role of reactive oxygen species in doxorubicin hydrochloride nephrosis. *J Lab Clin Med* 1991;118:435–45.
232. Shah SV. Evidence suggesting a role for hydroxyl radical in passive Heymann nephritis in rats. *Am J Physiol* 1988;254:F337–44.
233. Rahman MA, Emancipator SS, Sedor JR. Hydroxyl radical scavengers ameliorate proteinuria in rat immune complex glomerulonephritis. *J Lab Clin Med* 1988;112:619–26.
234. Neale TJ, Ojha PP, Exner M, et al. Proteinuria in passive Heymann nephritis is associated with lipid peroxidation and formation of adducts on type IV collagen. *J Clin Invest* 1994;94:1577–84.
235. Kakita N, Sasaguri Y, Kato S, Morimatsu M. Induction of gelatinolytic neutral proteinase secretion by lipid peroxide in cultured mesangial cells. *Nephron* 1993;63:94–9.
236. Ricardo SD, Bertram JF, Ryan GB. Antioxidants protect podocyte foot processes in puromycin aminonucleoside-treated rats. *J Am Soc Nephrol* 1994;4:1974–86.

Immunologic Renal Diseases,
edited by E. G. Neilson and W. G. Couser.
Lippincott-Raven Publishers, Philadelphia © 1997.

CHAPTER 20

Growth Factors and Cytokines

Jürgen Floege and Andrew J. Rees

Cytokines and growth factors comprise a large and rapidly growing class of low molecular weight (Mr) (glyco-)proteins, which act as communicators between cells. Most are secreted, but they also may be expressed in a cell membrane–bound form or may be stored in the extracellular matrix. With few exceptions they can be synthesized by many different types of cells upon adequate stimulation but are not produced constitutively. All cytokines and growth factors exert a wide range of actions. Most actions occur within the close vicinity of the cell of origin, i.e., in an autocrine or paracrine fashion, whereas endocrine actions are prevented by circulating binding molecules, such as α2-macroglobulin. However, some of the cytokines discussed in the following sections (e.g., colony stimulating factors or hepatocyte growth factor) also can exert endocrine actions. Consequently, our attempt is somewhat arbitrary to limit this chapter to locally acting cytokines and growth factors as opposed to growth factors with a primarily endocrine function such as insulin, insulin-like growth factor, growth hormone, angiotensin, endothelin, atrial natriuretic peptide, and so forth. Also, we limit our review to those actions and sources of cytokines and growth factors that are pertinent to nephrology, recognizing that this will cover only a small aspect of the various mediators. Finally, an important family of cytokines, namely the chemokines, are not covered in this chapter but are instead covered in Chapter 24.

Many cytokines and growth factors have been named based on the original cell type from which they were first isolated or the defining bioassay. This practice has frequently created confusion in that it overemphasizes a certain origin or biologic activity, which may in fact be of comparatively low relevance in vivo [e.g., tumor necrosis factor (TNF), transforming growth factor-b (TGF-β)].

For reasons of practicability, we have separated this chapter into reviews of individual factors. However, these factors are all part of a highly complex network of interactions. Such interactions occur in five basic ways:

1. Cascades, i.e., one cytokine/growth factor inducing or activating a second, etc.
2. Amplification loops, i.e., factors inducing their own synthesis.
3. Cytokine/growth factor-induced modulation of receptor expression, affinity, or function.
4. Additive or synergistic biologic effects of individual cytokines and growth factors.
5. Inhibitory effects of one factor on the actions of another, either directly or indirectly via the induction of biologically inactive receptor antagonists, soluble receptors or binding molecules.

To further complicate the situation, cytokines and growth factors are usually produced in characteristic patterns or combinations rather than released individually during disease. Finally, many cytokines and growth factors exhibit a complex regulation of their bioactivity. For example, the bioactivity of TGF-β is regulated at the level of messenger RNA (mRNA) transcription rate, mRNA stability, translation, secretion of the precursor molecule, activation of the biologically inactive precursor, and finally inactivation of bioactive, mature TGF-β by reassociation with parts of the precursor molecule, extracellular matrix proteins, and others. All these factors render the prediction of in vivo biologic effects induced by a single factor difficult. They also imply that great caution is necessary when extrapolating from cell culture data to the in vivo situation.

In view of the above considerations, it is apparent that a biologic effect can only be ascribed to the action of an individual cytokine or growth factor, if several requirements have been fulfilled:

J. Floege: Division of Nephrology, Medical School, Hannover D-30623, Germany.

A. J. Rees: Department of Medicine and Therapeutics, University of Aberdeen, Aberdeen AB9 2ZD, Scotland.

1. The factor exerts the effect in vitro.
2. The effect in vivo is associated with overproduction or release of the factor.
3. The effect is reproduced in vivo by administration or overexpression of the factor.
4. The effect can be abolished or diminished in vivo by specific antagonism of the factor.

The following sections start with a short delineation of general features of the cytokine or growth factor, followed by a brief description of molecular characteristics of the protein, its gene, receptor, and signaling pathways. "Sources" then describes the potential cellular origins of the factor within the kidney and its expression in normal kidney and during renal disease. "Biologic Activity" incorporates in vitro data, data on the association of specific in vivo events with overexpression or release of the factor, and insights gained from the administration of the factor. Finally, "Intervention Studies" describes available data on the effects of specific or nonspecific antagonism of the factor under discussion.

COLONY-STIMULATING FACTORS

Synonyms

Macrophage colony-stimulating factor (M-CSF): CSF-1, macrophage growth factor. Granulocyte-macrophage CSF (GM-CSF): CSF-2, CSF-α, pluripoietin-α. Granulocyte CSF (G-CSF): CSF-3, CSF-β.

Introductory Remarks

CSFs act as differentiation factors initiating irreversible terminal cell differentiation and as survival factors for mature cells. GM-CSF physiologically acts more in a paracrine fashion, whereas G-CSF and M-CSF also exhibit features of hormones (1–3).

Protein Characteristics and Gene Structure

All CSFs are synthesized as precursor molecules. They are not related to each other based on the protein sequence. Both GM-CSF (127-kDa monomer) and M-CSF (224- to 522-kDa homodimers) can be expressed as membrane-bound forms or as secreted proteins. GM-CSF also can complex with heparan sulfate proteoglycans in the extracellular matrix (1–3).

Receptor(s) and Signaling

Characteristics of the various CSF receptors and the signaling pathways involved are given in Table 1 (1–3).

Sources

Normal kidney

CSFs can be produced by T cells, monocytes/macrophages, fibroblasts, and endothelial cells, among others (1–3). Production of GM-CSF, M-CSF, and M-CSF receptor has been demonstrated in cultured mesangial cells and/or glomeruli (4–8). GM-CSF mRNA also has been detected in tubular epithelial cells (9).

Renal Disease

In cultured mesangial cells, expression of M-CSF can be stimulated by immunoglobulin G (IgG) complexes, interleukin (IL)-1, TNF-α, and interferon (IFN)-γ and attenuated by induction of cyclic adenosine monophosphate (cAMP) (5,6,8,10,11). However, during experimental mesangioproliferative glomerulonephritis, glomerular M-CSF mRNA levels did not change (4).

M-CSF expression has been investigated in lupus-prone mice because they exhibit high numbers of mono-

TABLE 1. *Characteristics of receptors for human colony stimulating factors*

Receptor for:	G-CSF	GM-CSF	M-CSF
Active form	Homodimer	Low affinity: α-chain monomer (CDw116) High affinity: α- and β-chain heterodime	Homodimer
Mr	90 kDa	α-chain 45 kDa, β-chain 95 kDa	165 kDa
Signaling involves	Tyrosine and/or serine phosphorylation of intracellular proteins	Tyrosine phosphorylation of intracellular proteins	Autophosphorylation, activation of G protein, *fyn* and *yes* protein kinases
Other characteristics	Soluble form Splice variants	Soluble form Splice variants	Identical to c-*fms* (CD 115)

cytes/macrophages early during the disease. These studies showed that some strains (e.g., MRL-lpr mice), but not all lupus-prone strains, exhibit high M-CSF serum concentrations at young ages, possibly derived from increased renal, particularly glomerular, synthesis (12, 13). Again, the contribution of mesangial cells to this phenomenon remained speculative (5,14).

Increased renal production of GM-CSF has been detected in fibrotic human kidneys (9).

Biologic Activities

CSFs in the kidney may contribute to the recruitment, proliferation, and survival of macrophages. The addition of GM-CSF to cocultures of mesangial cells and monocytes enhanced adherence of monocytes to the mesangial cells via a CD11/CD18-dependent mechanism (15). GM-CSF–primed monocytes also exhibited a higher cytotoxic activity on mesangial cells (15).

M-CSF appears to play a critical role in the regulation of renal macrophage numbers because they are markedly reduced in the kidneys of op/op mice, which have a mutated M-CSF gene (16). In lupus-prone MRL-lpr mice, glomerular macrophages from early stages of disease evolution, presumed to be more immature cells, in contrast to macrophages from later stages of the disease, were found to require M-CSF for proliferation and survival (12). In other renal diseases, a pathogenetic role of M-CSF remains unproven. Thus, in M-CSF–deficient mice with minimal glomerular macrophage numbers, anti–glomerular basement membrane (GBM) nephritis was as severe as in M-CSF–competent control mice (16).

Apart from modulating renal monocytes/macrophages, CSFs also may affect mesangial cells directly, for example, by upregulating mesangial cell expression of Fc receptors for IgG immune complexes (17).

EPIDERMAL GROWTH FACTOR AND TRANSFORMING GROWTH FACTOR-α

Introductory Remarks

Epidermal growth factor (EGF) and transforming growth factor-α (TGF-α) share 40% sequence homology, bind to the same receptor, and are largely indistinguishable in their vitro and in vivo effects in the kidney. Both factors are mitogens for various epithelial and mesenchymal cells and are important in renal development and cell differentiation as well as, possibly, the development of renal cystic disease (18–21).

Protein Characteristics and Gene Structure

Human EGF (6.4 kDa) is synthesized as a 1,207–amino acid precursor (prepro EGF). The EGF precursor, which retains EGF-like biologic activity, is anchored in the plasma membrane (18,20,22). Mature EGF is proteolytically released from its membrane-bound precursor in the kidney. Noncleaved, membrane-bound prepro EGF may itself act as a receptor for as yet unknown ligands or may be involved in juxtacrine growth control mechanisms (18,20). The prepro EGF gene encodes several protein domains, which are homologous to those of other proteins (EGF-like repeats).

TGF-α is a 6-kDa protein that, similar to EGF, is initially translated as an internal part of a 160–amino acid precursor and is then released by proteolysis (18).

Receptor(s) and Signaling

The EGF receptor is a 170-kDa transmembrane glycoprotein with tyrosine kinase activity (22). Two conformational states with low and high EGF binding affinity exist. Parts of the receptor are related to the oncogene products *erb*B and *neu* (22). Soluble forms of the receptor have been described. EGF binding to its receptor results in autophosphorylation, oligomerization, internalization of the receptor, and finally dephosphorylation by phosphotyrosine phosphatases (23). EGF binding, internalization, and dephosphorylation can be modulated by extracellular matrix molecules (23). Subsequent to receptor phosphorylation and phosphorylation of other intracellular proteins, signaling involves MAP kinase, ribosomal S6 kinase, GAP, PI-3 kinase, *raf* kinase, phospholipase-γ1, activation of members of the JAK-STAT signaling pathway, breakdown of inositol lipids, and mobilization of intracellular calcium (20,22,24,25).

Sources

Normal Kidney

High levels of prepro EGF mRNA and EGF protein have been detected in kidneys (20). Little EGF storage is present in the kidney (20). Normally, urine contains about 50 μg/day of mainly intact and/or partially degraded prepro EGF (18,26). Ninety percent of the urinary EGF is believed to be derived from the kidney (20).

EGF is expressed in the thick ascending limb of the loop of Henle and the early distal convoluted tubule, but not in the cells of the macula densa (27–29). In connecting and collecting ducts, some intercalated cells express EGF in their cytoplasm and in long lateral cell projections, which extend between adjacent light cells (27). Other renal localizations of EGF in normal kidney, such as in glomerular endothelial cells, arterioles, and proximal tubules, have not been observed in all studies (27,28,30). TGF-α has been detected in the distal convoluted tubules, connecting ducts, and collecting ducts of normal kidneys (20,27).

In addition to intrinsic renal cells, platelets and macrophages contain EGF and/or TGF–α (19). EGF receptors and/or binding sites are expressed at the basolateral side of proximal and distal tubules, in thin limbs of the loop of Henle, as well as in collecting ducts (31–34). In vitro, mesangial cells (35), glomerular epithelial cells (23,36), proximal tubular cells (33,37,38), inner medullary collecting duct cells (39), and renal interstitial fibroblasts (40) exhibit high- and/or low-affinity EGF receptors.

Renal Disease

Increased distal tubular EGF expression as well as a redistribution of the cellular EGF staining pattern from luminal to diffuse cytoplasmic plus antiluminal staining have been noted after uninephrectomy in rats (41). Renal EGF synthesis, immunostaining, and receptor expression, as well as urinary EGF excretion, decreased in instances of acute or chronic renal injury (42–45). However, transient de novo EGF expression in proximal tubules also has been described after toxic renal injury by some but not all investigators (46,47). EGF receptor expression was enhanced in renal biopsy samples from patients with various glomerulonephritides and transplant rejection in parietal glomerular epithelial cells (particularly adjacent to adhesions), as well as in fibrocellular crescents, distal tubules, and collecting ducts (31,48).

Biologic Activities

A central biologic activity of EGF and/or TGF-α is the induction of cell proliferation. Indeed, mice transgenic for TGF-α are characterized by glomerular hypertrophy and mesangial matrix expansion (49). An EGF and IGF-1 axis also has been suggested to contribute to compensatory renal growth after the loss of renal tissue (50). Indeed, in acute renal injury, elevated intrarenal levels of non–membrane-bound EGF preceded the peak in tubular regeneration (51).

In cell culture, EGF and/or TGF-α are mitogenic for mesangial cells (52), glomerular epithelial cells (23,36), proximal tubular cells (38,53–55), inner medullary collecting duct cells (39), and renal interstitial fibroblasts (40). EGF also may synergize with vasoactive substances, e.g., angiotensin-II, or other factors to stimulate renal cell growth (38,54,56,57). Further pathways of EGF-induced growth may involve stimulation of EGF and/or EGF receptor production by thyroid hormones and others (58,59) or the induction of other mitogens such as platelet-derived growth factor (PDGF) by EGF (60).

Administration of EGF accelerated functional and structural recovery from severe but not mild toxic and ischemic acute renal failure (42,61). In mild acute renal failure, a self-protection mechanism may exist whereby injured renal tissue releases sufficient endogenous EGF to stimulate tissue repair (61). EGF can exert hemodynamic actions by stimulating prostaglandin release in several renal cell types (18,39) and by inducing contraction in mesangial cells (18) as well as in pre- and post-glomerular arterioles (35).

Intervention Studies

After unilateral nephrectomy in mice, injections of a neutralizing antibody against EGF inhibited compensatory tubular cell proliferation but not renal hypertrophy (62).

FIBROBLAST GROWTH FACTORS

Synonyms

Fibroblast growth factor (FGF)-1: acidic FGF, FGF-α, heparin binding growth factor (HBGF)-1, endothelial cell growth factor. FGF-2: basic FGF (bFGF), FGF-β, HBGF class II, endothelial growth factor.

Introductory Remarks

The FGFs represent a group of currently nine proteins. Few findings on FGF-1 and the kidney have been reported. They show that FGF-1 is expressed in glomerular endothelial and mesangial cells, vessel walls, and proximal tubular cells (63–65). FGF-1 may play a role in renal development and in the regulation of glomerular, endothelial, and proximal tubular epithelial cell proliferation (64,66,67). Little or no information relating to the kidney is available for FGF-3 to FGF-9. Therefore, the remainder of this section addresses FGF-2.

FGF-2 is a pleiotropic growth factor with a wide distribution throughout the body. Among other actions, it may play important roles in embryogenesis, vascular homeostasis, atherosclerosis, wound healing, angiogenesis, and cancer (68–71).

Protein Characteristics and Gene Structure

FGF-2 is a basic protein (pI 9.6). Multiple isoforms (Mr 16–24 kDa) arise from alternative mRNA splicing, which determines whether the intracellular isoforms localize to the cytoplasm or nucleus (72). Effects of FGF-2 within the nucleus (i.e., intracrine effects) have been observed, and some isoforms may represent transcriptional regulators (72,73).

Generally, little to no FGF-2 mRNA is detectable under normal circumstances despite widespread expression of the protein, suggesting that most FGF-2 is present in storage form. FGF-2 lacks a signal peptide and is therefore mainly released after lethal or sublethal cell injury (72,74). However, release from noninjured cells via yet unknown pathways also has been described (75). After cellular release, FGF-2 may be sequestered by heparan sulfate proteoglycans. The latter as well as heparin protect FGF-2 from proteolytic inactivation and can modulate bioactivity of FGF-2 (71,72). Matrix-bound FGF-2 can be released in active form by heparin or heparitinase (71).

Receptor(s) and Signaling

Four distinct high-affinity FGF receptors (FGFR1 to FGFR4) have been identified (76). Alternative mRNA splicing also yields multiple forms of FGFR1 (also termed *flg*, CEK-1) and FGFR2 (also termed *bek*, CEK-3). All FGF receptors exhibit intracellular tyrosine kinase activity. FGF-2 binds to FGFR1 to FGFR3 (76). The differential function of the various receptor isoforms is unknown. Binding of FGF-2 to cells usually also requires the presence of low-affinity binding to cell surface heparan sulfate proteoglycans, particularly syndecan (71). Upon binding to the high-affinity receptors, these homo- or heterodimerize, followed by receptor autophosphorylation and phosphorylation of phospholipase C-γ and other, yet unknown intracellular proteins (76). Secondary events include an increase in intracellular calcium, hydrolysis of polyphosphoinositides, and increased transcription of c-*myc* and c-*fos* (76). Receptor binding and FGF-2–induced biologic effects can be inhibited by heparin-derived oligosaccharides, FGF-2–derived oligopeptides, oligodeoxynucleotides, and soluble FGF receptors (77–80).

Sources

Normal Kidney

In the normal kidney or glomeruli, mRNA for FGF-2 is usually not detectable (64,81,82). Immunohistochemical data on the expression of FGF-2 in the kidney are highly variable. This appears to relate to the recognition of different FGF-2 epitopes/isoforms by the various antibodies as well as to fixation conditions (65,83). Thus, in normal glomeruli, FGF-2 has been described as absent (65) or as confined to the mesangium (81) or to podocytes (84,85). FGF-2 expression in tubular epithelium and/or the tubular basement membrane also has been variable (65,83,86). The above data are complemented by in vitro findings, demonstrating various FGF-2 isoforms in mesangial cells (81,87) and glomerular epithelial cells (84). Similar to findings in endothelial cells, FGF-2 release occurred after antibody and complement-mediated mesangial cell injury in vitro (81). Of potential relevance for the kidney, FGF-2 also can be produced by microvascular endothelial cells, fibroblasts, vascular smooth muscle cells, macrophages, and T-lymphocytes (69–71,88). Constitutive excretion of bFGF in the urine can be detected and may derive from both circulating and locally produced bFGF (89).

FGFR1 and FGFR2 mRNA transcripts have been demonstrated in the kidney (82), and by immunohistochemistry, some constitutive tubular FGFR1 expression has been described (90). Other studies have failed to detect FGFR1 expression in normal human or rat kidney (65,91). Low-affinity bFGF binding sites are widespread throughout the kidney (92,93).

Renal Disease

In line with constitutive storage of FGF-2, glomerular FGF-2 expression decreased rapidly after antibody-mediated mesangial cell injury (81). Subsequently, FGF-2 synthesis and FGF receptor mRNA expression increased during the development of mesangioproliferative nephritis (81,91). Importantly, in this case the loss rather than the subsequent overproduction of glomerular FGF-2 was considered to be indicative of an FGF-2–mediated effect (81). Therefore, the biologic relevance of increased renal FGF-2 mRNA levels in lupus-prone NZB/W F1 mice and in rats with puromycin aminonucleoside nephrosis remains unknown (94,95). Mesangial immunostaining for FGF-2 but not mRNA expression also was augmented in early streptozotocin-induced diabetes (96,97). In the renal tubulointerstitium, increased FGF-2 expression has been described in damaged tubular epithelial cells of human immunodeficiency virus (HIV)-transgenic mice (92). Expression of low-affinity FGF-2 binding sites also increased in HIV-transgenic mice as well as in human kidneys with interstitial fibrosis, whereas they decreased in sclerotic glomeruli (93).

Biologic Activities

Biologic FGF-2 activities with relevance for the kidney include its mitogenicity, chemotactic, and angiogenic effects.

Mitogenicity

In vitro, FGF-2 induces cell proliferation in mesangial cells (87,98–100), glomerular endothelial and epithelial cells (67,84), renal tubular epithelial cells (64,92), and vascular smooth muscle cells (71). In some of these cell types, FGF-2 mediates the mitogenic effect of other agonists, such as angiotensin-II (101). Alternatively, it may itself induce other mitogens, such as PDGF (100). In cultured endothelial and mesangial cells FGF-2 governs the basal cell proliferation rate and allows survival via antiapoptotic effects (74,87,102). Consistently, TGF-β1 has been identified as a negative regulator of FGF-2–induced cell proliferation (98,101). Indeed, TGF-β1 may be involved in controlling unrestained FGF-2–induced cell growth because in endothelial cells FGF-2 can activate latent TGF-β1 via inducing plasminogen activator (103). Unexpectedly, in contrast to a strong mitogenic effect on skin fibroblasts, FGF-2 had no proliferative effect on renal fibroblast lines derived from normal or fibrotic kidneys (104). However, these latter findings have not yet been confirmed in nontransformed cells.

Several studies have addressed the in vivo mitogenicity of FGF-2. Normal rats infused with low concentrations of FGF-2 failed to exhibit renal abnormalities (81,105). However, when administered after prior subnephritogenic mesangial cell injury, FGF-2 exerted mitogenic effects on these cells in vivo (81,105). Similarly, after prior immunologic injury to podocytes (i.e., the induction of passive Heymann nephritis) the podocytes became FGF-2 responsive, possibly due to increased FGFR1 expression (90). In damaged podocytes, FGF-2 induced nuclear division but apparently not cell division. In the long term, this was associated with increased glomerulosclerosis, and we have suggested that release of FGF-2 from damaged cells may be an intrinsic mechanism whereby damage of neighboring cells is amplified (90). If markedly higher doses of exogenous bFGF were chronically administered to rats, podocyte damage and progressive glomerulosclerosis could be inflicted even without prior injury to these cells (85,106), whereas in monkeys prominent parietal epithelial cell proliferation prevailed (106). Finally FGF-2–driven autocrine or paracrine tubular cell proliferation has been invoked in the occurrence of microcystic proliferative lesions in HIV-transgenic mice (92).

Chemotaxis and Angiogenesis

FGF-2 is chemotactic for cultured endothelial and vascular smooth muscle cells (71) and may mediate the smooth muscle cell chemotaxis of other substances such as PDGF (107). The proliferative and chemotactic effects of FGF-2 are intricately linked to its angiogenic activity. The latter activity also includes FGF-2 effects on endothelial and smooth muscle cell matrix synthesis (e.g., downregulation of interstitial collagen synthesis, upregulation of proteoglycan synthesis) as well as the induction of collagenase and/or components of the plasminogen proteolytic system in these cells (69–71). FGF-2 effects on the matrix production in renal cells are largely unknown.

Other Biologic Activities of FGF-2

Potentially relevant for the kidney, FGF-2 bolus injections into rats induced a transient NO-mediated vasodilatation (108). FGF-2 also regulates low-density lipoprotein (LDL) receptor expression and LDL uptake in vascular smooth muscle cells (109) as well as the synthesis of the proatherogenic protein osteopontin in smooth muscle cells (110).

Intervention Studies

Inhibition of FGF-2 with a neutralizing antibody before inducing mesangioproliferative nephritis in rats ameliorated mesangial and endothelial cell proliferation (111), suggesting that release of constitutively expressed FGF-2 may indeed be an early trigger of glomerular cell proliferation in response to injury. Heparin, which among other activities modulates FGF-2 bioactivity, also was able to suppress mesangial cell proliferation in vivo and to decrease the glomerular overexpression of FGF-2 during mesangioproliferative nephritis (112).

HEPATOCYTE GROWTH FACTOR

Synonyms

Hepatocyte growth factor is now frequently referred to as HGF/SF (for scatter factor).

Introductory Remarks

Apart from its actions on epithelial cells, HGF may be important in the development of the kidney (113), renal cyst formation (114), as well as in the recruitment of T-lymphocytes to sites of injury (115).

Protein Characteristics and Gene Structure

HGF is produced as an inactive 90-kDa prepro protein (116,117). The precursor is secreted and stored in a matrix-associated form. Afte tissue injury, an HGF-converting enzyme and/or urokinase are activated, which converts the pro-HGF into the active heterodimeric form (118) composed of a 60-kDa alpha subunit and a 30-kDa beta subunit (117). In addition to acting locally, HGF is also a circulating (i.e., endocrine) molecule. Endocrine synthesis of HGF can be stimulated in organs distant from the injured site via a molecule called injurin (119). HGF antagonists, one of which occurs naturally, have been described. These antagonists (HGF/NK1 and HGF/NK2) are no longer mitogenic but still induce some cell scattering.

The HGF gene is composed of 18 exons and spans about 70 kb. HGF/NK2 is encoded by the same gene and is derived from an alternative HGF transcript.

Receptor(s) and Signaling

The high-affinity HGF receptor is a 190-kDa glycoprotein, encoded by the *met* oncogene (120,121). The receptor is a heterodimer of an alpha subunit light chain and a beta subunit heavy chain. The beta subunit bears an intracytoplasmic tyrosine kinase domain. Various isoforms of the receptor, derived from alternative mRNA splicing, have been described. One form is soluble and is released from the cells. Upon ligand binding, receptor homodimerization and cross-phosphorylation occurs. The secondary events, which ultimately lead to mitogenesis or motogenesis (i.e., chemotaxis and scattering), appear to be largely similar to those described for other tyrosine kinase receptors such as the PDGF receptor (121).

Sources

Normal Kidney

In vitro, HGF is produced by fibroblasts (116,117), microvascular endothelial cells (116,117), and mesangial cells (122,123), among others, but not by proximal tubular cells (122). In vivo, one study reported on the immunohistochemical localization of HGF in distal tubules and collecting ducts of normal human and rat kidney (124). However, other studies have detected HGF expression only in peritubular endothelial cells and/or macrophages of the renal interstitium (125).

Expression of the HGF receptor c-*met* as well as HGF-binding has been demonstrated in normal kidney (122,126). In culture it was detected in proximal tubular cells (122) and an inner medullary collecting duct cell line (127). In cultured mesangial cells, HGF and c-*met* are usually nondetectable, but both can be induced by stimulation of the cells with IL-6 (122,128).

Renal Disease

Upregulation of HGF synthesis and/or c-*met* RNA in the kidney (and liver) occurred in various situations, such as uninephrectomy, acute toxic renal injury, and ischemia, and in some studies even after a sham kidney operation (118,125,129–131). Renal injury also led to an increase in plasma HGF levels, possibly related to injurin release, which induces pulmonary HGF production (119).

Biologic Activities

Depending on cell density, HGF can induce proliferation in glomerular and proximal tubular epithelial cells (122,132,133). EGF and acidic FGF were additive to the mitogenic HGF effect, whereas TGF-β inhibited it (122,132,133). Other experiments have shown that HGF can induce scattering, branching tubule formation, and invasiveness into collagen gels in Madin-Darby canine kidney cells and an inner medullary collecting duct cell line (116,117,134). Finally, HGF exhibits angiogenic activity (135,136).

Systemic administration of HGF stimulated renal tubular regeneration, accelerated recovery of renal function, and reduced mortality in experimental acute renal failure (129,137).

INTERFERON-α AND -β

Synonyms include type I IFN (α and β), leukocyte IFN (α), fibroblast IFN (β), and acid-stable IFN (α and β). IFN-α constitutes a group of at least 23 isoforms (including IFN-ω) with Mr ranging from 19 to 26 kDa. IFN-β, which occurs in a single 20-kDa isoform only, is 30% homologous to IFN-α and binds to the same receptor. Production of IFN-α can be induced in many cells, including lymphocytes, monocytes/macrophages, and fibroblasts, whereas IFN-β is produced by fibroblasts and epithelial cells, among others (138,139).

Biologic activities of IFN-α and -β include the inhibition of cell growth in many cell types as well as antiangiogenic, antifibrotic, and anti-inflammatory actions (140). The latter result from a suppression of the production of chemotactic proteins and several proinflammatory cytokines, such as IL-1 or TNF, while at the same time inducing immunosuppressive cytokines such as TGF-β and IL-1 receptor antagonist (140). Furthermore, lymphocytes are driven toward a T-helper (Th)1 phenotype, and natural killer (NK) cells, as well as T-suppressor cells, are activated (138-140).

Relatively little is known about the renal actions of IFN-α and -β. Similar to observations in other cell types and organs, treatment of mice with a mixture of both IFNs results in upregulation of glomerular, tubular, and vascular major histocompatibility complex (MHC) class I antigen expression, while reducing MHC class II antigen expression in renal interstitial cells (141). In newborn, but not in adult, rodents, high-dose IFN-α and -β treatment also induces glomerulosclerosis via yet unknown mechanisms (142). Glomerular injury in patients treated with IFN-α, if present, is usually mild and manifests with proteinuria, although IFN-α and -β also may induce exacerbations of preexisting autoimmune diseases such as lupus erythematodes (138,140,143). On the other hand, IFN-α is used therapeutically to treat the glomerulonephritis types associated with hepatitis virus B and C infections and cryoglobulinemia (144,145).

INTERFERON-γ

Synonyms

Immune IFN, pH2-labile IFN.

Introductory Remarks

IFN-γ is a pleiotropic cytokine involved in nearly all phases of immune and inflammatory responses, including the regulation of growth, activation, differentiation, and apoptosis in T-lymphocytes, B-lymphocytes, macrophages, NK cells, and others (146).

Protein Characteristics and Gene Structure

IFN-γ exists in a single isoform, composed of two 143–amino acid subunits. It is derived from a 166–amino acid precursor and is secreted after cleavage of a signal sequence (146,147). IFN-γ can exist in a form associated with the extracellular matrix.

Receptor(s) and Signaling

The IFN-γ receptor (also known as type II IFN receptor or CDw119) is widely expressed and composed of a high-affinity binding chain and one or more secondary accessory proteins (IFN-γ receptor b-chain) (147). After ligand binding, dimerization and serine-threonine phosphorylation of the receptor occur. Signaling pathways include protein kinase C (PKC), double-stranded RNA-dependent protein kinase, phospholipase A2, arachidonic acid, and members of the JAK-Stat pathway (146–148). Immediate and delayed gene transcription is induced via a consensus IFN-γ activation site (148). Soluble forms of the receptor exist.

Sources

IFN-γ is produced exclusively by lymphocytes (CD4- and CD8-positive T-cells, NK cells, and, to a lesser degree, B cells). The synthesis of IFN-γ is increased by antigens to which the cells are sensitized, nonspecific T-cell mitogens (concanavalin A, phythemagglutinin), or IL-2 in NK cells (146,147). Exogenous TGF-β was found to downregulate the IFN-γ production of a nephritogenic T-cell clone (149).

Increased renal contents of IFN-γ have been noted in the renal cortex of lupus-prone mice and in autoreactive kidney-infiltrating T cells from these latter mice (150). Serum levels of IFN-γ also increase in systemic lupus erythematodes and during (presumably virus-induced) exacerbations of IgA nephropathy (151,152).

Constitutive high-level expression of the IFN-γ receptor has been documented, among others, in tubular epithelial cells and hematopoietic cells (153).

Biologic Activities

Through its multiple activities on immune cells (146, 147) and renal cells (Table 2), IFN-γ is presumed to play an important role in the pathogenesis of immune-mediated glomerular and renal interstitial disease (150).

In addition to its actions on intrinsic renal cells, IFN-γ can induce monocyte proliferation and macrophage activation/differentiation, resulting in increased production of oxygen radicals, nitric oxide (NO), and multiple cytokines, as well as increased MHC class I and II antigen expression, high- and low-affinity Fc receptor expression, and cytotoxicity (163,174,175).

TABLE 2. *Renal actions of IFN-γ in vitro and in vivo*

Activity	Renal target	Reference
MHC class I upregulation	Mesangial cells	154
	Glomerular epithelial cells	154
	Endothelial cells	154
	Tubular cells	154,155
MHC class II upregulation	Mesangial cells	154,156–159
	Endothelial cells	154,160
	Glomerular epithelial cells	154
	Tubular cells	150,154,155
	Smooth muscle cells	161
Upregulation of adhesion molecule expression	Mesangial cells	159,162
	Tubular cells	150,162
Induction of the ability to act as antigen presenting cells	Mesangial cells	159
	Proximal tubular cells	150
	Endothelial cells	160
Inhibition of cell proliferation	Mesangial cells	157,163–165
	Endothelial cells	160
	Smooth muscle cells	161
Induction of inflammatory mediator synthesis	Mesangial cells (MCP-1; NO; IP-10; IL-1; IL-6 only in some studies)	156,166–169
Increased expression of low-affinity Fc receptors	Mesangial cells	165,168
Increased synthesis of complement proteins	Mesangial cells (factor H)	170
	Glomerular epithelial cells (C4)	171
	Tubular epithelial cells (C4)	172
Increased synthesis of matrix proteins	Nephritic glomeruli	163
	Interstitial cells	173

In line with a proinflammatory action of IFN-γ, administration of IFN-γ to lupus-prone mice led to an exacerbation of nephritis (175–177). Similarly, the induction of a systemic lupus erythematodes–like syndrome or exacerbation of a pre-existing lupus have been described in patients treated with IFN-γ (178,179).

Intervention Studies

Experimental studies have demonstrated a beneficial effect of treatment with anti–IFN-γ antibody or soluble IFN-γ receptor in immune-mediated renal disease: (a) prevention of glomerulonephritis and increased survival in lupus-prone mice in some (176,177) but not all studies (180) and (b) reduction of renal MHC class I and II expression in models of immune renal injury (176,177,179).

Nonspecific immunosuppressive therapy, such as corticosteroids or cyclosporine A, reduces the lymphocyte production of IFN-γ, which may in part account for its efficacy in the treatment of systemic lupus erythematodes (151).

In an opposite approach, IFN-γ has been tested as an antifibrotic drug because the cutaneous collagen synthesis in mice has been reported to decrease after treatment with IFN-γ (181). However, neither in models of mesangioproliferative glomerulonephritis nor models of progressive glomerulosclerosis and interstitial fibrosis did IFN-γ therapy exert detectable beneficial effects on matrix accumulation or fibrotic changes (163,182,183). Rather, treatment with IFN-γ promoted the development of glomerulosclerosis, particularly when combined with other proinflammatory cytokines such as IL-1 (183).

INTERLEUKINS

The name interleukin was introduced to describe mediators that were synthesized by leukocytes whose function was to regulate growth and differentiation of other leukocytes. Since then, it is apparent that interleukins are produced by many other cell types and that they have a much broader range of activities than originally suspected. Currently, 17 such molecules have been designed as interleukins, or more if one includes different isoforms (Table 3). Most interleukins are involved in the growth and differentiation of cells. Here we have excluded discussion of those cytokines primarily

TABLE 3. *Interleukins and their receptors*

Cytokine	Family	Sources	Functions	Receptors
IL-1	Trefoil	Mø, PMN, most other cells	See Table 3	Two receptors, Rt1 active, Rt2 (decoy)
IL-2	Hematopoietin	T cells	Growth and differentiation of T cells, Mø activation	Single receptor, α, β,and γ chains
IL-3	Hematopoietin	T cells, mast cells, Eos	Stimulates hematopoietic stem cells, activetes Mø	IL-3Rt (CD123) associates with β-unit common to IL-5 and GM-CSF
IL-4	Hematopoietin	T cells, mast cells, BM stroma	Induces Th2 cells, promotes IgG1 and -4, deactivates Mø	IL-4Rα chain (CD124) associates with IL-2Rγ chain
IL-5	Hematopoietin	T cells, mast cells, Eos	Eosinophil growth and differentiation	IL-5Rα chain (CD125) associates with IL-3β chain
IL-6	Hematopoietin	Mø, most other cells	T- and B-cell growth deactivates Mø	IL-6Rα chain (CD126) associates with β chain (CD130)
IL-7	Hematopoietin	BM and thymic stroma	B- and T-cell development	IL-7Rα chain (CD127) binds IL-2Rγ chain
IL-8	Chemokine	Mø, PMN, most other cells	PMN chemotaxin/activator	Two receptors: high affinity (CD128), low affinity
IL-9	Hematopoietin	T cells (Th2)	Erythroid, mast cell, megakaryocyte growth, T-cell proliferation	IL-9Rα possibly binds IL-2Rγ chain
IL-10	Hematopoietin	Mø, T cells (THO,Th2)	Inhibits Th1 cells, deactivates Mø	Single receptor homologous to IFN receptors
IL-11	Hematopoietin	BM, stroma, fibroblasts	Hematopoietic growth factor	Single receptor possibly associated with IL-6Rβ chain
IL-12	Hematopoietin	Mø, B cells	Induces IFN-γ synthesis by NK and T cells	Single receptor dimerizes on binding IL-12
IL-13	Hematopoietin	Mø, T cells	Similar to IL-4 except promotes IFN-γ by NK cells	Single receptor, possible shares component of IL-4R
IL-14	Hematopoietin	T cells, B cells	Proliferation of activated B cells, inhibits Ig synthesis	Not yet identified
IL-15	Hematopoietin	Mø, epithelial cells, others	Broadly similar to IL-2	Unique α chain associates with IL-2Rβ and γ chains
IL-16	Unknown	CD8 cells, tracheal epithelial	Chemotaxis and proliferation of CD4 cells	Unknown; binds to CD4
IL-17	Unknown	Activated T cells especially CD4)	Proliferation of T cells, IL-6 and -8 secretion by fibroblasts	Type I transmembrane protein; no homologies

Mø, macrophages; PMN, neutrophils; Eos, eosinophils; BM, bone marrow.

involved in hematopoiesis and immune regulation. We have restricted discussion principally to those involved in the control of inflammation. Discussion of cytokines primarily involved in the control of immune responses and chemokines are reviewed in other chapters.

Interleukin-1

Synonyms

Previous names include lymphocyte-activating factor, endogenous pyrogen, leukocyte endogenous mediator, mononuclear cell factor, and catabolin.

Introductory Remarks

IL-1 is one of the most extensively studied cytokines, and probably one of the most important with effects on proliferation and differentiation of many different cell types (184). Its primary function is probably to coordinate the acute inflammatory response, a role it shares with TNF, a cytokine with similar properties. The enormous biologic importance of these molecules is reflected by the degree to which their activities are regulated. Thus, the IL-1 system consists of two active forms of IL-1 (alpha and beta), and a structurally related IL-1 receptor antagonist (IL-1ra); two IL-1 receptors, one of which is a decoy that binds IL-1 but does not transduce a signal; circulating binding proteins in the form of soluble receptors; and finally, intracellular signaling pathways, which are highly complex and can be modulated at many stages (Fig. 1). An exhaustive review of the biology of IL-1 is beyond the scope of this chapter, and the reader is referred to an excellent series of reviews by Dinarello (184–186).

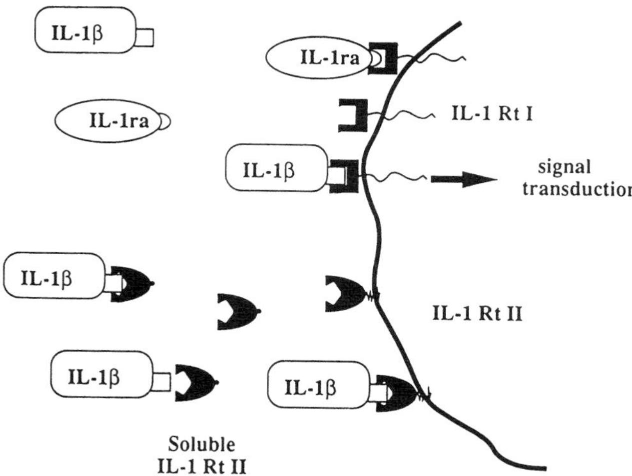

FIG. 1. Diagram to show the relationships between the different components of the IL-1 system.

Protein Characteristics and Gene Structure

IL-1α and IL-1β are products of adjacent genes located on chromosome 2 in both humans (187) and mice (188). They are synthesized as 31-kDa precursor proteins (pro–-IL-1α and β, respectively), which are cleaved to 17-kDa mature forms. The precursor and mature forms of IL-1α have similar biologic activities, whereas pro–IL-1β has little activity. Neither form of IL-1 has a recognizable leader sequence; nevertheless, most IL-1β is released into the fluid phase by a poorly understood mechanism (186). IL-1α, on the other hand, remains cell associated. The gene for IL-1ra is also on chromosome 2 (189), whereas in mice it is on chromosome 1 (190). Three different isoforms of IL-1ra can be produced from a single gene by alternative splicing under the control of different promoters (191). Secretory IL-1ra (sIL-1ra) has a classical 25–amino acid secretory tail and is released by activated neutrophils and monocytes (192,193); the two intracellular forms of IL-1ra (icIL-1ra I and icIL-1ra II) do not have a leader sequence (194,195). All three forms compete with IL-1 for binding to the IL-1 receptor and can inhibit its activity.

There is 18% to 26% amino acid sequence homology between IL-1α, IL-1β, and IL-1ra. X-ray crystallography and nuclear magnetic resonance spectroscopy show that they have a similar beta-trefoil fold topology (196–199). Mutational studies have identified two IL-1 receptor binding sites, one of which is absent in IL-1ra (200,201). Notably, a point mutation in this region converts IL-1ra into a partial IL-1 agonist (202,203).

IL-1 synthesis is controlled in a cell type–specific manner by transcription, translation, and the processing of the precursor peptide (204,205). IL-1 expression is rapidly upregulated when cells are injured or stimulated. The promoter regions contain sequences that bind the ubiquitous transcription factors NF-IL6 and CREB and possibly NF-κB. It also contains tissue-specific binding site Spi-1 (Spi 1), which is responsible for enhanced expression in myeloid cells (205). Both IL-1α and IL-1β genes also have regulatory elements within their first introns, and sequence responsible for message stability is commonly found in endotoxin-inducible cytokines (206).

There is a rapid increase in steady-state IL-1α mRNA without concomitant increase in protein when monocytes are stimulated by adherence, C5a, or thrombin. Addition of low concentrations of IL-1 or LPS stabilizes the message and rapidly removes the translational block (207). About 15% of pro–IL-1α is transported to the cell surface where it remains as active membrane bound IL-1. By contrast, pro–IL-1β is retained in the cytoplasm and is biologically inactive and has to be cleaved by a cysteine protease, IL-1–converting enzyme (ICE), before gaining full activity. The gene *ICE* has been cloned (208,209) and its three-dimentional structure resolved (210). ICE is present in inactive form in most cells and is a member of a family of enzymes that control apoptosis. ICE-defficient knock-out mice make no IL-1β and are susceptible to infection but resistant to LPS (211,212).

Receptor(s) and Signaling

There are two IL-1 receptors, IL-1 receptor type 1 (Rt1 or CD121a) and IL-1 receptor type 2 (Rt2 or CD121b). Both are members of the Ig supergene family and have three Ig domains. IL-1 Rt1 is an 80-kDa transmembrane glycoprotein with a 213–amino acid cytoplasmic tail. IL-1 Rt2 is 60-kDa and has a similar extracellular domain but a much shorter cytoplasmic tail (29 amino acids). Almost all cells express small numbers (about 100) of Rt1 receptors constituitively, whereas Rt2 expression is restricted to B cells and myeloid cells. Rt2 receptor is further induced by anti-inflammatory cytokines such as IL-4, IL-6, and IL-13 (213). The two receptors have entirely different functions: IL-1 signaling occurs exclusively through Rt1 (214), and inhibition of the Rt2 increases the sensitivity of monocytes to IL-1 (213). This suggests that Rt2 acts as a decoy that binds IL-1 and neutralizes it and limits the effect of ambient IL-1 of cells. IL-1α and β bind Rt1 and Rt2 with equal affinity, but, not surprisingly IL-1ra binds poorly to Rt2. Type 2 receptors are released from the cell surface and inhibit IL-1 activity in the fluid phase (215).

Signal transduction through IL-1 Rt1 must be highly efficient because responses are evoked by ligating as few as five receptors. Considerable effort has gone into understanding the signaling, not least because the receptor does not have protein kinase activity and is not homologous to the catalytic subunits of known protein kinases. At least three different sets of pathways have important roles in IL-1 receptor signaling (216,217): (a) multiple MAP kinase cascades that are not unique to IL-1 signaling; (b) a poorly characterized casein kinase activated uniquely by IL-1 and TNF; and (c) a ceramide signaling pathway probably dependent on neutral and acidic sphingomyelinases that may subserve different functions. Four distinct MAP kinase pathways already have been described in mammalian cells (218), and three have been implicated in IL-1 signaling: namely, the ERK (p42/p44 MAPK) cascade; the JNK (SAPK or P54 MAPK) cascade, and the HOG-1 (p40 MAPK) cascade. ERK phosphorylates other signaling molecules in the cytoplasm (including cytoplasmic phospholipase A2, protein kinases, and a variety of the MAP kinases) and translocates to the nucleus. There it activates transcription factors, including c-myc, c-fos/c-jun, NF-IL6, and ATF2, and initiates protein synthesis and proliferation. IL-1 also activates the JNK/SAPK MAP kinase pathway (219, 220), which may inhibit cell proliferation by activating the phosphatases that deactivate MAP kinases (221) and the HOG-1 MAP kinase, which phosphorylates the chaperonin hsp 27.

Much less is known about the casein kinase pathway, which is activated by IL-1–stimulated fibroblasts and endothelial cells. This pathway is highly specific for IL-1 and TNF and is not inhibited by phosphatases. Its natural substrate is unknown, and so is its function. Finally, IL-1 activates sphyngomylases to generate ceramide (222,223) and activates a membrane-bound protein kinase capable of phosphorylating the EGF receptor (224). The ceramide pathway also modulates phosphatase activity (225) and is probably important for generating NO.

Sources

Most cells synthesise IL-1 when injured or activated with proinflammatory cytokines or bacterial products (185). Macrophages and neutrophils are the most abundant producers and synthesize copious IL-1 after phagocytosing particles, or, when exposed to LPS, aggregated IgG or proinflammatory cytokines, including IL-1 itself, IL-2, IL-12, TNF, IFN-α, macrophage inhibitory factor (MIF), and growth factors such as M-CSF and GM-CSF. However, it is much more relevant to consider IL-1 activity in terms of the ratio of IL-1 to IL-1ra. This depends on the mix of cytokines in the cellular environment and differs in monocytes and macrophages. Thus, IL-1, IL-2, and TNF substantially increase the relative concentrations of IL-1, whereas IL-4, IL-6, IL-10, IL-13, TGF, and IFN-α and β decrease it in macrophages (203,226). Non-myeloid cells produce icIL-1ra but little if any of the secreted form (203,227).

Neither IL-1α nor IL-1β are detectable in normal human (228) or rodent kidneys (229,230) assessed by immunohistology, in situ hybridization, or Northern analysis. In culture, rat mesangial cells and visceral epithelial cells can be readily induced to express IL-1α and β (231,232), but the data on human cells is much less certain. Abbott et al. (233) could not detect IL-1 or IL-ra in human mesangial cells stimulated with IL-1α itself or TNF, but small amounts of IL-1α were detected in IL-1β–stimulated cells. Zoja et al. (234) reported that IL-1α stimulated synthesis of IL-1 after binding to IL-1 Rt1 receptors. It is possible that the contradictory results reflect different proportions of cytoplasmic to released IL-1β and IL-1ra in the two studies, analagous to that seen in vascular smooth muscle (227).

Cell damage and numerous specific stimuli have been reported to increase IL-1 synthesis by mesangial cells. Such stimuli include LPS, IL-1, TNF, IFN-α, complement binding, and IgG and IgA containing immune complexes (235). Anti-inflammatory cytokines (and other factors) that diminish mesangial cell IL-1 synthesis have not been examined systematically for their effects on mesangial cells. However, both IL-10 (236) and TGF-β reduce LPS-stimulated expression of IL-1. The effects of IL-4, IL-13, and IFN-α and β on cytokine synthesis by mesangial cells have not been reported, although they decrease IL-1 release from stimulated neutrophils, monocytes, and macrophages.

IL-1 and the Kidney

IL-1 is released from glomeruli purified from the kidneys of rats (237) and patients (238) with crescentic glomerulonephritis. More recently, IL-1α and β have been detected by immunohistology and in situ hybridization in kidneys from patients with severe glomerulonephritis (228). IL-1 is found in glomeruli, tubular epithelium, and interstitial cells in patients with antineutrophil cytoplasmic antibody (ANCA)-associated crescentic glomerulonephritis (239,240). IL-1 is also present in mesangiocapillary glomerulonephritis and severe lupus nephritis (241) but cannot be detected in mesangial IgA disease, Schönlein-Henoch purpura and minimal-change nephropathy (228,241). Presumably these results depend on the degree of inflamation in the kidney, because clinical studies are critically dependent on the timing of the renal biopsy.

Glomerular concentrations of IL-1β in RNA increase in glomeruli of rats during the heterologous phase of nephrotoxic nephritis (NTN) (242,243), especially when injury is amplified by pretreatment with LPS (243–245). The cells responsible have not been identified but probably include intrinsic glomerular cells as well as infiltrating leukocytes. Glomerular IL-1 expression also increases in the autologous phase of NTN (230,246,247); during the acute phase of in situ immune complex glomerulonephritis (248), autoimmune experimental glomerulonephritis (EAG) (249), and lupus nephritis in MRL/lpr mice (250,251); and in autoimmune tubulointerstitial nephritis is Brown Norway rats (252). Thus, IL-1 is readily detectable in acute models of renal injury, but expression is relatively transient. For example, IL-1β mRNA peaks 4 to 6 h after induction of the telescoped model of NTN and is barely detectable 48 to 96 h later (230,246); although some have reported more prolonged synthesis (230,247). Tam et al. (230) analyzed the ratio of IL-1 to IL-1ra, which is probably biologically more important. They showed that initially the IL-1β response dominated in glomerular mRNA but that the opposite was true in the spleen, whereas the IL-1ra was dominant at later time points because expression of IL-1ra was much more persistent. They also showed by in situ hybridization that cells expressing IL-1ra were probably different from those expressing IL-1β. These results are consistent with those obtained in studies of other types of immunologically mediated inflammation (203) and support the idea that the IL-1 system has an important role in control of glomerular inflammation.

Biologic Activities

IL-1 has diverse activities that include roles in differentiation and proliferation of lymphocytes and hematopoietic cells. These have been reviewed extensively elsewhere, so we concentrate here on its effects on inflammation (Table 4). IL-1 amplifies injury of inflammation in the early stages but later modulates the intensity by expressing inhibitors and contains its effects to the site of injury. This is achieved (a) through effects on circulating leukocytes that favor their localization in the tissues (254); (b) by activating endothelium and other fixed cells

TABLE 4. *Actions of IL-1 in the inflammatory response*

Site	Target	Response
Systemic	Hypothalamus	Fever, anorexia
	Liver	Acute phase response (via IL-6)
	Muscle	Catabolism
	Immune system	Stimulates T-cell and B-cell proliferation (via other cytokines)
	Bone marrow	Promotes neutrophil release
Local	Leukocytes	Promotes adhesion, stimulates secretion of other mediators [e.g., chemokines, proinflammatory cytokines (TNFα,IL-1), anti-inflammatory cytokines (IL-1ra, IL-6, IL-4), growth factors (GM-CSF, M-CSF, G-CSF), cyclooxygenase and lipoxygenase products of arachidonic acid]
	Microvasculature	Stimulates adhesion molecule expression, procoagulant effect, promotes transendothelial passage of leukocytes, stimulates secretion of other mediators
	Interstitial cells	Stimulates adhesion of molecule expression, stimulates secretion of other mediators, increases synthesis of collagens and collagenases, promotes proliferation of fibroblasts and mesangial cells

See text for references (reviewed in reference 184).

to release chemotactic factors, express adhesion molecules and procoagulant activity, and secrete cytokines able to activate leukocytes (254); (c) by inducing changes that limit the intensity of inflamation locally (203); and (d) by releasing cytokines that stimulate hepatic synthesis of acute-phase reactants that inhibit the phlogistic effects of inflammatory mediators that leach out of inflammatory foci into the circulation (255). Clearly, local administration of IL-1 causes inflammation and can cause severe tissue injury, but the importance of IL-1 for host defense cannot be understated. For example, ICE knockout mice, which lack detectable IL-1β are resistant to LPS but respond poorly to infection (211,212), and inhibition of IL-1 with pharmacologic doses of IL-1ra exacerbates *Listeria* infection in mice (256) and increases the mortality of *Klebsiella pneumoniae* in rats (257). Aspects of the IL-1 system have been reviewed elsewhere (184,203,258).

Glomerular and tubular cells serve as examples of the effects of IL-1 on fixed cells. The effects of IL-1 on mesangial cells have been studied extensively (reviewed in reference 235). IL-1 promotes DNA synthesis and cell proliferation in rat mesangial cells, but possibly not in humans. This highlights the possible species differences, which also have been suggested by experiments on IL-1–stimulated mesangial cell generation of NO and synthesis of IL-1. Nevertheless, mesangial cells express IL-1 Rt1 (234) and are stimulated by IL-1 to synthesize eicosanoids, principally prostaglandin E2 (PgE2) and thromboxane; cytokines, including IL-6 leukemia inhibitory factor (LIF) (259); chemokines, including IL-8 (260), CINC, MCP-1 (261), and RANTES; enzymes, including type IV collagenases (262) and PUMP-1 (263); and reactive intermediates such as NO (264) and oxygen radicals (264a). There are also reports that IL-1 stimulates rat mesangial cells to make more IL-1 and TNF (265).

Over the past 5 years there has been considerable interest in delineating the biochemical and signaling pathways responsible for these effects. This has been examined extensively for two specific IL-1–driven functions: the synthesis of prostaglandins and the generation of NO. IL-1–treated rat mesangial cells rapidly upregulate group-2 phospholipase A2 (Gp2PLA2) via a mechanism dependent on an MAP kinase (266) and NFκB activation (267). This releases arachidonic acid from the cell membrane (268–271), and the effect is inhibited by dexamethasone, PDGF, and TGF-β (271), as well as by IL-4 (272). IL-1 also augments expression of the inducible cyclo-oxygenase (COX-2), which converts released arachidonic acid into prostaglandins (264,273–275); expression of the constitutive cycloxygenase COX-1 is unaffected (274). This pathway involves activation of the MAP kinase ERK2 and is dependent on tyrosine kinase (273,274) and NADPH oxidase (274). Interestingly, IL-1 also induces expression of three components of NADPH oxidase, namely p22 phox, p47 phox, and p72 phox (264a).

IL-1 increases expression of the inducible form of NO synthase (iNOS) by a tyrosine kinase, NFκB-dependent pathway (273,276). These events are probably initiated by the ceramide signaling pathway using a neutral sphyngomylase located in the plasma membrane (261). NO generation is inhibited by PgE2, although not by prostacyclin (264).

Intervention Studies

Evidence of the role of IL-1 in glomerular inflammation comes from two types of intervention studies. Tomosugi et al. (277) showed that pretreatment with LPS increased injury in rats during the heterologous phase of NTN and that the same effect could be achieved by administration of doses of IL-1β or TNF sufficient to increase the circulatory concentrations into the pathophysiological range. Furthermore, injury in the LPS-enhanced model of NTN could be attenuated by passive immunization against IL-1β or TNF, but not against IL-1α (229). Administration of IL-1ra or soluble TNF or IL-1 receptors was even more effective at abrogating injury (245), and similar results were obtained by administration of IL-6, which decreased circulatory and glomerular concentrations of the cytokines (243). These findings were extended to the conventional heterologous phase model by Tang et al. (242), who showed that glomerular neutrophil infiltration and injury were both diminished by high-dose IL-1ra.

The power of IL-1ra to modulate glomerular injury has been demonstrated even more compellingly in a series of studies of autologous phase injury by the Atkins group, in which groups of rats with telescoped NTN have been treated for 14 days with IL-1ra. They demonstrated marked attenuation of glomerular and tubulointerstitial inflammation, reduced crescent scores, and a significantly lower serum creatinine in the treated rats (278). Macrophage proliferation within crescents was prominent in untreated rats and substantially reduced by IL-1ra (279). Pharmacologic treatment with IL-1ra has not yet been used to treat glomerulonephritis clinically but has been used to treat severe sepsis, rheumatoid arthritis, and graft-versus-host disease after bone marrow transplantation (203).

IL-4 and IL-13

Synonyms

IL-4 was formerly known as B-cell stimulating factor-1 (BSF-1). Murine IL-13 was originally designated P600.

Introductory Remarks

IL-4 and IL-13 are both members of the hematopoietin family of cytokines and have similar properties, gene structure, and location. Both are produced by activated

Th2 cells and have similar (but not identical) anti-inflammatory effects, monocyte and macrophage function, and B-cell differentiation. However, the effects on T cells are different: IL-4 promotes development and proliferation of Th2 lymphocytes, whereas T cells do not express IL-13 receptors (280). They are considered together here because of the similarity of their properties.

Protein Characteristics and Gene Structure

Human and mouse IL-4 are both glycoproteins of 15 to 19 kDa composed of 153 and 140 amino acids, respectively. Resolution of the three-dimensional structure of IL-4 shows a compact globular structure with a hydrophobic core (281). In humans, the gene encoding IL-4 is located on chromosome 5q31 in a cluster that also contains the genes for IL-3, IL-13, GM-CSF, and IL-5. The same genes are encoded in a syntenic region on chromosome 11 in mice. IL-13 is approximately 10 kDa and its primary amino acid sequence has about 30% homology IL-4, which is roughly the same as that between IL-1α and IL-1β.

Receptors and signaling

The IL-4 and IL-13 receptors are both members of the lymphoid group of cytokine receptors and consist of individual primary binding chains (IL-4α and IL-13R, respectively) and a γ chain (γc) common to the receptors for IL-2, IL-7, IL-9, and IL-15 (282). The IL-4 receptor is a heterodimer of IL-4α and γc. A soluble form of the IL-4 receptor is made by alternative splicing (283). It is a strong inhibitor of IL-4 and can be detected in the circulation (284). The IL-13 receptor is more complicated and uses IL-4α as well as IL-13R and γc (280,285), which could explain why IL-13 elicits a subset of the functions of IL-4. Intracellular signaling pathways are complex and involve tryosine kinases (286,287).

Sources

IL-4 is produced by Th0 and Th2 $CD4^+$ T cells and a subset of $CD8^+$ T cells that have a Th2-like cytokine profile. It is also made by mast cells and some B cells. IL-13 also is made by activated T cells. Glomerular and renal tubular cells have not been reported to synthesize IL-4 or IL-13, nor can they be detected in normal kidneys (288,289). However, IL-4–positive cells have been found in the mesangium of patients with IgA nephropathy and proliferative lupus nephritis (289). The IL-4–positive cells were identified as $CD4^+$ T cells and their number correlated with the degree of mesangial proliferation. IL-4 is over-expressed in mercuric chloride–induced autoimmune nephritis in Brown-Norway rats (290,291), but IL-4–producing cells have not been identified in the renal lesions (290). Similarly, abnormalities in IL-4 synthesis have been reported in MRL/lpr mice (292). IL-13 message can be detected in glomerular RNA from rats in the heterologous phase of NTN 2 h after induction of nephritis (293).

Biologic Activities

IL-4 together with IL-12 controls the balance between Th1 and Th2 immune responses and thus has a critical influence on susceptibility to infection and to autoimmune disease. These functions are discussed extensively in Chapter 4, and therefore are not considered further here. IL-13 does not activate T cells but shares most other properties of IL-4 (294). Both cytokines have powerful anti-inflamatory effects on myeloid cells, including human monocytes and polymorphs and murine macrophages (295,296) (Table 3). Briefly, they downregulate the IL-1 system by decreasing IL-1 expression while increasing that of IL-1ra in LPS or cytokine-stimulated monocytes and macrophages. Human neutrophils are similarly inhibited and have been shown to express and release more IL-1 Rt2 (297). Synthesis of TNF, IL-2, IL-6, IL-8, G-CSF, GM-CSF and MCP-1 is also reduced when cells are incubated with IL-4 and IL-13. They also reduce phagocytosis, oxygen radical generation, and production of reactive nitrogen intermediates. Both cytokines selectively increase VCAM-1 and IL-6 expression by endothelium (298), and antagonize the procoagulant effects of TNF and IL-1 on it (299).

IL-4 downregulates proliferation of rat mesangial cells and inhibits prostaglandin synthesis by them (300).

Intervention Studies

There are many reports in the literature on the use of intervention studies to manipulate the balance of Th1 and Th2 responses (301). These show that IL-4 has powerful effects on susceptibility to intracellular infections and that passive immunization against IL-4 increases resistance to *Leishmania* and other intracellular parasites (302). Systemic administration of IL-4 also has been used to decrease injury in diabetes in NOD mice, but it is not clear whether these interventions act principally on the autoimmune response in these models or on effector cells such as macrophages and neutrophils. However, Tam et al. (303) focused on effector systems in their studies of the influence of IL-4 on autologous phase injury in rats with NTN. They observed that IL-4 substantially attenuated injury over the first few days after induction of nephritis. This was associated with a small reduction in macrophage infiltration and evidence of less macrophage activation within the inflamed glomerulus. No intervention studies have been reported using IL-13 to treat inflammatory disease, but in theory its lack of activating T cells might be an advantage.

IL-6

Synonyms

IFN-2, BSF-2, hybridoma/plasmacytoma growth factor, hepatocyte stimulatory factor.

Introductory Remarks

IL-6 is a member of a group of homologous cytokines that includes LIF, oncostatin M, ciliary neurotrophic factor, and IL-11. They are all members of the hematopoietin family of cytokines and their receptors have a common signaling chain (gp130). IL-6 is secreted by most (if not all cells) in response to injury or activation with IL-1 or TNF. It was originally thought to be a proinflammatory cytokine because of the many activities in common with IL-1 and TNF, but it is now clear that IL-6 inhibits inflammation (Table 5). Unlike IL-1 and TNF, it does not activate endothelium but stimulates the pituitary–adrenal axis, inhibits synthesis of proinflammatory cytokines by neutrophils and macrophages, and induces the hepatic acute phase response (304,305).

Protein Characteristics and Gene Structure

IL-6 is a 21- to 28-kDa protein with a 28–amino acid signal sequence. The gene that encodes it is on chromosome 7 (p21-14) in humans and on chromosome 5 in mice. The promoter region of the IL-6 gene contains binding sites for the activating factors NF-IL6 and NF-KB. There is 42% homology between mouse and human proteins, and 58% homology between mouse and rat. The IL-6 receptor consists of an 80-kDa IL-6α chain (CD126 or IL-6R), which binds IL-6 with moderate affinity (K_d 10^{-9} mol/L) but does not transduce a signal (306). IL-6R interacts with gp130 chain (CD 130), and together they have much higher affinity for IL-6 (κ_d 10^{-10} mol/L). In humans the gene for IL-6R is located on chromosome 1, and gp130 has two loci, which are on chromosome 5 and 17, respectively. Gp130 is universally expressed, whereas IL-6R has slightly more restricted distribution: it is expressed by activated but not resting B cells, T cells, neutrophils, monocytes and macrophages, epithelial cells, fibroblasts, vascular smooth muscle cells, and mesangial cells. IL-6 binds to IL-6R either on the cell surface or in the fluid phase, and but unlike IL-1, complexes of IL-6 and its receptor are biologically active and can interact with gp130 on the cell surface. Ligand binding results in the formation of a disulphide-linked gp130 homodimer that activates the tyrosine kinase JAK2 (307). Signal transduction probably involves the Ras-dependent MAP kinase cascade, which results in phosphorylation (and activation) of the transcription factor NF-IL6 (308).

TABLE 5. *Activities of IL-1, TNF, and IL-6*

Biologic property	IL-1	TNF	IL-6
Hepatic acute-phase proteins	+	+	+
Nonspecific resistance to infection	+	+	+
T-cell activation	+	±	+
B-cell activation	+	±	+
B-cell Ig synthesis	±	−	+
Fibroblast proliferation	+	+	−
Endothelial cell activation	+	+	−
Induction of IL-1 and TNF	+	+	−
Induction of IL-6	+	+	−

Sources

Normal Kidney

IL-6 is produced universally by cells exposed to stress and injury or when they are activated by LPS or proinflammatory cytokines such as IL-1 and TNF (304,305). Human (309) and rat (310,311) mesangial cells in culture release small amounts of IL-6 whether proliferating or quiescent, and the amount released is enhanced in dose-dependent fashion by LPS, IL-1, and TNF. Since these original studies, many other stimuli have been reported to enhance IL-6 synthesis. These include ligation of the low-affinity IgG receptor (CD16) (312), aggregated IgG (312,313) and IgA (313,314), IL-6 and IL-4 (315), angiotension-II (316), and lectins. Interestingly the effect of IL-1 and TNF appear to be influenced by the substrate on which mesangial cells grow. Ruef et al. (317) reported that mesangial IL-6 synthesis was augmented in cells grown on collagen type IV and decreased when grown on type I. The closely related cytokine LIF is also expressed by mesangial cells stimulated with IL-1β, TNF-α, PDGF, and LPS (318). IL-6 is also expressed by glomerular epithelial cells in culture (319) and by proximal tubular epithelial cells.

IL-6 is not usually detected in urine, but low levels of expression have been reported in normal human and rodent kidneys. Stimulation of the renal sympathetic nerves has been reported to increase IL-6 mRNA synthesis in Wistar rats, but not in spontaneously hypertensive rats (320). However, it is not clear whether ischemia played a role in these results.

Increased IL-6 expression has been reported repeatedly in proliferative glomerulonephritis, including crescentic nephritis associated with ANCA (321) or anti-GBM antibodies (322), and focal proliferative nephritis caused by mesangial IgA disease (323) or systemic lupus (324,325). IL-6 is expressed in renal tubules and glomeruli from patients with diabetic nephropathy (326). IL-6 excretion in urine is commonly increased in proliferative glomerular disease (310,327,328), and the degree of proliferation and prognosis has been reported to correlate with the magnitude of IL-6 excretion (310,327,328). However, this is not a universal finding (327,330), and urinary IL-6 does not simply reflect renal synthesis but is influenced by tubular function (331). In summary, it is clear that there is widespread overexpression of IL-6 in many pathogenetically different renal diseases: the critical question is whether IL-6 promotes injury or is a response to it.

Biologic Activities

IL-6 has important roles in proliferation and differentiation of many different cell types, both in normal physiology and in response to injury and infection (304,305). IL-6 supports proliferation of T- and B-lymphocytes and stimulates normal B cells to differentiate into plasma cells. It has an obligate role in Ig synthesis irrespective of the isotype. Some plasmacytoma cell lines are IL-6 dependent, and transgenic mice overexpressing IL-6 develop enormous Ig concentrations, which may be pathogenic. IL-6 is also important in hematopoiesis and thrombopoiesis by synergizing with more specific growth factors. IL-6 promotes proliferation of cells that do not originate in the bone morrow, and there is still considerable controversy whether this applies to mesangial cells. IL-6 has been reported to increase proliferation of rat (310,332) and bovine (333) mesangial cells. These results could not be reproduced using human mesangial cells (334,260), and IL-6 was even reported to decrease proliferation of rat mesangial cells (335).

IL-6 also acts as a hormone with wide-ranging anti-inflamatory properties. It directly stimulates the pituitary–adrenal axis and increases circulating adrenocorticotrophic hormone, as well as other anterior pituitary hormones (336). It increases expression of a broader range of hepatic acute-phase proteins than either IL-1 or TNF: these include C-reactive protein, serum amyloid protein, α2-macroglobulin, fibrinogen, and the complement components (337). It also has important anti-inflammatory effects on neutrophils, monocytes, and macrophages. It decreases IL-1 and TNF synthesis by macrophages stimulated with LPS (338) and promotes expression of IL-1ra and soluble IL-1 and TNF receptors in mice (339). In vivo, it decreases the local (340,341) and systemic effects of LPS (340). IL-6 decreases expression of proinflammatory cytokines, including IL-1, IL-8, TNF, and MCP-1 (342), and increases expression of IL-1ra (343) and the IL-1 type 2 (decoy) receptor (344). Oxygen radical generation is also decreased (342).

Intervention Studies

Prolonged exposure to high concentrations of IL-6 is undoubtedly associated with focal proliferative or sclerosing nephritis as demonstrated by mice transgenic for human IL-6 gene (345,346), mice transgenic for the closely related cytokine LIF (347), and mice with bone marrow transplants of stem cells expressing IL-6 (348). This provided strong evidence that prolonged exposure to high concentrations of IL-6 causes renal disease, but they beg the question whether glomerular disease is a direct effect of IL-6 on the mesangium or whether it is an indirect effect of the many other abnormalities present in these mice, for example, polyclonal cell activation with high circulatory IgG concentrations. Certainly IL-6 is not essential for normal development of the mesangium because the kidneys of IL-6 knockout mice are normal (349).

IL-6 is associated with the development of renal injury in other settings. It aggravates glomerulonephritis in NZB/NZW lupus-prone mice, but the effect could have been dependent on the underlying immune response because it was abrogated by cyclosporine (350). This idea is supported by studies demonstrating that administration of a monoclonal antibody to the IL-6 receptor improves the decreased autoantibody concentrations and partially abrogates nephritis (352).

The ability of IL-6 to promote mesangial cell proliferation has been investigated further by Eitner et al. (349), who found that IL-6 knockout mice were not protected from proliferative nephritis induced by Habu snake venom, and that infusions of human recombinant IL-6 did not increase mesangial proliferation when subnephritogenic or nephritogenic doses of anti-Thy 1.1 antibodies were administered to rats.

Karkar et al. (243) assessed the ability of IL-6 to reduce injury in NTN. IL-6 decreased injury in the LPS-enhanced model of NTN and decreased glomerular neutrophil infiltration and expression of IL-1β and the chemokine MIP-2. Studies in the autologous phase of NTN showed that administration of IL-6 was similarly protective and that it did not increase mesangial cell proliferation (353).

IL-10

Synonym

Cytokine synthesis inhibitory factor.

Protein Characteristics and Gene Structure

IL-10 is a homodimeric cytokine with an apparent Mr of 35 to 40 kDa in humans and 17 to 21 kDa in mice. The three-dimensional structure of the molecule is unknown, but it is unusually acid labile. The gene encoding IL-10 is on chromosome 1 in mice and on the syntenic region of chromosome 1 in humans (354).

Receptor(s) and Signaling

The IL-10 receptor is a member of the type II (IFN) receptor family (355). It is expressed in most cells, macrophages, and other hematopoietic cells and cell lines. It is encoded by a gene on chromosome 11. Signaling pathways are uncertain but likely to involve the JAK family of kinases.

Sources

IL-10 is synthesized by human and murine Th0 and Th1 $CD4^+$ T cells and B cells (355). Macrophages also secrete copious amounts of IL-10 when stimulated with LPS, IL-1, or TNF (356), and mast cells and keratinocytes secrete lesser quantities. IL-10 synthesized by glomerular or renal tubular cells has not yet been reported, nor is it expressed in normal human or rodent kidneys or in inflamed kidneys (357). Reduced IL-10 synthesis has been reported in minimal-change nephrotic syndrome (358).

Biologic Effects

IL-10 inhibits synthesis of IL-2 and IFN-γ by Th1 cells and cytotoxic T cells. It has similar effects on NK cells and mast cells and induces differentiation of B cells. IL-10 profoundly influences macrophage function by reducing cytokine synthesis by LPS, IL-1, and TNF stimulated cells (359,360). It increases expression of IL-1ra and IL-1 Rt2 and the release of TNF p55 receptors (361). MHC class II expression is decreased, as is NO synthesis and macrophage-mediated cytotoxicity; the effects are synergistic with those of TGF-β. They are also similar to those of IL-4 and IL-13, but there are striking differences. IL-10 inhibits IL-1 synthesis by rat mesangial cells stimulated with LPS (362).

Intervention Studies

IL-10 is a good candidate for modulating the immune response, and a small number of such studies have been reported. Recombinant IL-10 inhibits LPS-induced TNF synthesis in vivo in mice and protects them from death (363), whereas passive immunization against IL-10 increases mortality from LPS (364). As discussed earlier, IL-10 aggravates injury in MRL/lpr lupus-prone mice, possibly because it inhibits TNF synthesis (365). However, IL-10 decreases delayed-type hypersensitivity in vivo (354) and prevents the development of experimental autoimmune encephalomyelitis in mice (366): this makes it an obvious candidate for further studies in nephritis.

NERVE GROWTH FACTOR

In addition to its neutrotropic actions, nerve growth factor (NGF) also modulates inflammatory and immune reactions and plays a critical role in renal development (367,368). NGF is a 130- to 140-kDa complex of three proteins (α-, β-, γ-NGF). Receptors include a high-affinity receptor ($gp140^{trk}$) and a low-affinity NGF p75 receptor. This latter receptor is expressed in non-neuronal cells that do not respond to neurotrophins. It may facilitate NGF binding to the high-affinity receptor. Cultured mesangial cells and isolated glomeruli produce NGF (369). Immunoreactivity for NGF also has been demonstrated in connecting tubule cells (370). NGF binding sites have been found on lymphocytes and monocytes (368). Expression of the low-affinity NGF receptor has been detected in normal adult kidneys in mesangial areas, peripheral nerves, cortical and medullary interstitial fibroblasts, and periarterial connective tissue (371,372). Upregulation of the low-affinity NGF receptor expression in mesangial and/or interstitial locations was shown to occur in a wide variety of glomerular diseases and in explanted renal allografts (371,373). Renal actions of NGF are largely undefined.

PLATELET-DERIVED GROWTH FACTOR

Synonyms

Fibroblast-derived growth factor, monocyte-derived growth factor.

Introductory Remarks

PDGF is a mitogen and chemoattractant for mesenchymal cells. It is important, for example, in wound healing, atherosclerosis, organ fibrosis, and malignancy (374,375).

Protein Characteristics and Gene Structure

PDGF is composed of a 16-kDa A-chain (also termed PDGF-I) and a 14-kDa B-chain (PDGF-II) (374–376), which exhibit 60% homology. Both chains are released from precursor molecules after cleavage of a signal peptide. The B-chain is encoded by the c-*sis* proto-oncogene. The A- and B-chain combine to three possible isoforms (i.e., AA, AB, BB). PDGF variants arise from differential splicing of the mRNA.

Receptor(s) and Signaling

PDGF receptors consist of an alpha and beta subunit (also termed PDGFRA and PDGFRB), which dimerize upon binding of PDGF. The α-receptor subunit binds all

PDGF isoforms with high affinity, whereas the β-receptor subunit only binds PDGF-BB with high affinity and PDGF-AB with lower affinity (376–378) (Fig. 2). The PDGF receptor possesses tyrosine kinase activity and is autophosphorylated upon ligand binding (375,376). The receptor then interacts with several other cytoplasmic proteins, including phospholipase C (PLC-γ), *ras* GTPase activating protein, phosphatidyl-inositol 3-kinase, and members of the pp60^{src} family of protein tyrosine kinase (376,379). Second messengers include inositol-triphophate and diacylglycerol (374,377,378), intracellular calcium release, and PKC activation (376,379). In the nucleus, PDGF signaling induces various proto-oncogenes and immediate early response genes, including c-*fos*, c-*myc*, and *egr*-1 (380). PDGF antagonists include secreted, truncated receptor forms and PDGF-derived peptides.

Sources

Normal Kidney

Normally expression of PDGF A-chain is confined to podocytes (381). Weak or no glomerular expression of PDGF B-chain can be detected in glomeruli (382–385). In culture, mesangial cells as well as visceral glomerular epithelial cells express PDGF A- and/or B-chain (381, 386–388). Microvascular and glomerular endothelial cells in culture also synthesize PDGF (389), although this has not yet been confirmed in vivo. In the tubulointerstitium, PDGF A- and/or B-chain production has been identified in renal tubular cells (390), cultured inner medullary collecting duct epithelial cells (391), and renal fibroblasts (392). Apart from intrinsic renal cells, PDGF is released upon activation of platelets, monocytes, and macrophages (374–376).

Receptor alpha subunit cannot be detected in normal rat glomeruli (383) but at a low level in human glomeruli and renal interstitium (393). The beta subunit is constitutively expressed on mesangial and parietal glomerular epithelial cells as well as in renal interstitial cells (383, 385,393–395).

Renal Disease

Increased expression of PDGF in glomerular and/or interstitial locations has been documented in a large variety of renal diseases (Table 6). In addition, increased expression of PDGF receptors occurs in experimental and human renal diseases (383,393,394,396). Finally, an increased monocyte content of PDGF B-chain mRNA has been demonstrated in circulating monocytes of patients with IgA nephropathy (397).

Biologic Activities

Glomerular Cell Proliferation

PDGF is an autocrine growth factor for cultured mesangial cells (386). However, normally most of the PDGF released by mesangial cells is PDGF-AA (377), a weak mesangial mitogen as compared with PDGF-BB (409,410). Furthermore, the level of PDGF receptor expression is controlled by the level of endogenous PDGF production, the composition of the extracellular matrix, and other cytokines, such as TGF-β (409,411).

PDGF synthesis is induced in cultured mesangial cells by various mediators, including PDGF itself, EGF, bFGF, TNF-α, TGF-β, angiotensin-II, endothelin, thrombin, lipoproteins, and phospholipids (377,388,411–413). Many of the aforementioned substances may in fact exert

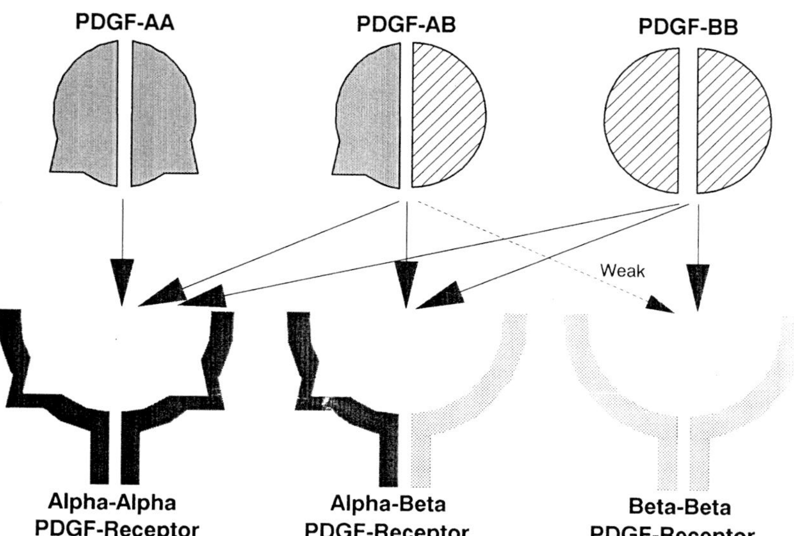

FIG 2. Schematic outline of the binding of the various PDGF isoforms to the various PDGF receptors.

TABLE 6. *Studies showing increased expression of PDGF in experimental or human renal diseases*

Species	Disease	Reference
Mouse	IgA nephropathy	382,398
	Lupus nephritis (NZB/W F1 mice)	398
	Bovine serum albumin nephritis	399
Rat	Mesangial proliferative nephritis	383,384,400
	Remnant kidney model	396
	Puromycin aminonucleoside nephrosis	401
	Anti-GBM nephritis	402
	Passive Heymann nephritis	387
	Streptozotocin-induced diabetes	403
Human	Diffuse proliferative lupus nephritis	404
	Mesangial proliferative nephritis	382,393,394,405–407
	ANCA-positive crescentic nephritis	406
	Crescentic nephritis of other origin	408

their mitogenic effect on mesangial cells through the induction of PDGF (388), although a dissociation of the induction of PDGF B-chain mRNA and mitogenicity also can be observed (411). IL-1, TNF-α, and IL-6 can delay the mitogenic response of PDGF in mesangial cells or inhibit it (410), whereas it is increased by prostaglandin $F_{2\alpha}$ and LDL (414,415).

Functional in vivo studies demonstrated that infusion of recombinant PDGF-BB into rats or transfection of glomeruli in vivo with PDGF B-chain complementary DNA (cDNA) leads to a selective increase of glomerular mesangial cell proliferation (416–418). PDGF-induced mesangial cell proliferation was markedly augmented, if the mesangial cells had suffered a minor (subclinical) injury before the PDGF infusion (416). Finally, in view of the similarity of events occurring during ontogenesis and renal pathology, the observation is of importance that PDGF B-chain plays a critical role in mesangial development (419,420).

Other Biologic Actions of PDGF in the Glomerulus

Some evidence supports a role of PDGF in the regulation of extracellular matrix accumulation. In vitro advanced glycosylation end products (AGEs) can enhance the production of various matrix proteins in mesangial cells via the induction of PDGF (421,422). Type III collagen production in mesangial cells was increased upon direct stimulation with PDGF (422). Accumulation of some, but not all, extracellular matrix proteins also has been noted in PDGF-BB–infused rats or rat kidneys transfected in vivo with a PDGF B-chain cDNA (416,417). Whether these effects are mediated via an induction of TGF-β by PDGF in the mesangial cells remains unknown because divergent observations have been made in vitro and in vivo (417,423). PDGF also acts as a chemoattractant on mesangial cells (424) and leukocytes (376–378). A role of PDGF in the regulation of glomerular hemodynamics is suggested by observations showing that infusion of PDGF into the isolated microperfused glomerulus results in marked increase in intraglomerular pressure, decreased flow rate and a marked increase in the vascular resistance (377). These effects may be due to PDGF-induced contraction of mesangial cells (377,378) and/or synergistic effects of PDGF and inflammatory cytokines, such as IL-1 and IL-6, on mesangial cell prostaglandin production (425).

Finally, PDGF stimulates LDL uptake in human mesangial cells (412).

Renal Interstitial Actions of PDGF

In contrast to proximal tubular epithelial cells (426), renal fibroblasts may proliferate in response to PDGF-BB both in vitro and in vivo (391,418). On the other hand, PDGF A-chain but not B-chain mRNA has been demonstrated in fibroblasts derived from normal or fibrotic human kidneys (392). In those from fibrotic kidneys a higher spontaneous proliferation rate was noted, which similar to observations in skin fibroblasts, appeared to depend on the sequential autocrine production of IL-1 and PDGF-AA (392).

Actions of PDGF on the Immune System

Effects of PDGF on the immune system are only just beginning to be revealed. PDGF has been shown to modulate the biosynthesis of various lymphokines, such as IL-2, IL-4, IL-5, and IFN-γ by activated T-lymphocytes (427).

Intervention Studies

Experiments with a neutralizing antibody against PDGF demonstrated that it can decrease mesangial cell proliferation and matrix accumulation in the anti-Thy 1.1 mesangioproliferative nephritis in rats (428).

Trapidil, an anti-platelet agent, has been shown to inhibit the binding of PDGF to its receptor and to reduce PDGF-induced mesangial cell proliferation (429). This latter finding has been confirmed in the anti-Thy 1.1 model, in which trapidil treatment resulted in a reduction of glomerular cell proliferation (430). Conventional heparin is also effective in inhibiting mesangial cell proliferation (431). This latter effect of heparin was associated with a downregulation of glomerular PDGF receptor beta subunit and PDGF B-chain expression (431). Finally, a low-protein diet in rats using the aminonucleoside nephrosis model has been found to not only attenuate the prevalence of glomerulosclerosis but also to reduce the abnormally high glomerular expression of PDGF A- and B-chain mRNA (401).

TRANSFORMING GROWTH FACTOR BETA

Synonyms

Platelet-derived (endothelial cell) growth inhibitor, polyergin, tumor-inducing factor.

Introductory Remarks

The TGF-βs belong to a superfamily of about 25 peptides involved in development. TGF-β is important in many processes, including wound healing, inflammation, atherosclerosis, organ fibrosis, and malignancy (432–434). Five isoforms of TGF-β have been described, three of which, TGF-β1 to TGF-β3, are expressed in mammals.

Protein Characteristics and Gene Structure

TGF-β1 to -β3 share 70% to 80% amino acid sequence identity, bind to the same receptors, induce similar responses, and for the most part are interchangeable (434, 435). Active, mature TGF–β is a 25-kDa homodimer. All three isoforms are secreted as latent complexes of the homodimer bound noncovalently to the processed mature N-terminal domain of the precursor, an 80-kDa glycoprotein (latency-associated peptide; LAP) (Fig. 3). Although some cells secrete this so-called small latent TGF-β, most others secrete a large latent TGF-β, in which latent TGF binding protein (LTBP-1 = 125–140 kDa; LTBP-2 = 240 kDa) is covalently bound to the LAP (Fig. 3) (435). Small and large latent TGF-β complexes are biologically inactive. They can be activated in vitro by treatment with acid, alkali, heat, urea, or sodium dodecyl sulfate, and in vivo via the action of plasmin, cathepsin D, glycosidases, or thrombospondin (435,436). Active TGF-β may be inactivated by reassociating with LAP, binding to circulating α_2-macroglobulin in serum or to the proteoglycan decorin, which neutralizes some but not all biologic actions of TGF-β (435,437,438). Other binding molecules, including biglycan, type IV collagen, fibronectin, and osteonectin/SPARC may act as scavengers or reservoirs for TGF-β (435).

TGF-β1 to TGF-β3 are encoded by different genes. The individual promoters contain distinct elements, which

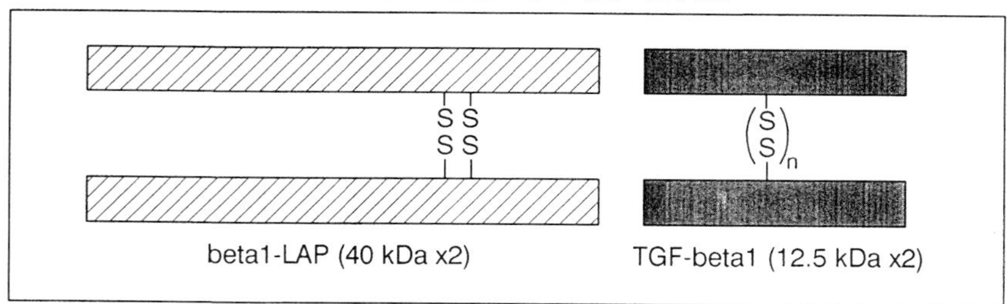

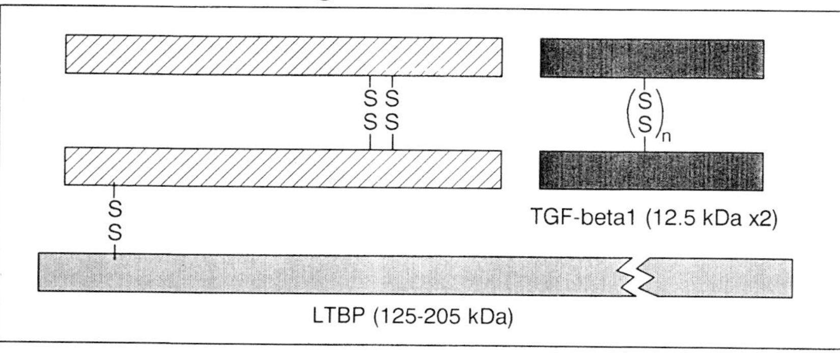

FIG. 3. Structure of small and large latent TGF-β molecule. TGF-β homodimers are bound noncovalently to the processed mature N-terminal domain of the precursor, latency-associated peptide (LAP) (small latent TGF-β) and in other cases also to latent TGF-binding protein (LTBP) (large latent TGF-β).

may confer tissue-specific expression of the TGF-β isoforms. Further regulation of TGF-β expression involves message stability, processing, and secretion.

Receptor(s) and Signaling

Type I (53–65 kDa) and type II (73–95 kDa) TGF-β receptors are transmembrane serine-threonine kinases, which are almost universally expressed (435). After binding of TGF-β to the constitutively autophosphorylated TGF-β receptor II, type I receptor is phosphorylated by the type II receptor chain, and signaling is initiated (439). Subsequent events involve a p42 MAP kinase as well as MAP kinase kinase, G-protein–dependent and –independent pathways, adenylate cyclase, effects on the retinoblastoma susceptibility gene products and the AP-1 complex, and suppression of c-*myc* transcription (434).

In addition to the TGF-β receptors I and II, other TGF-β binding molecules have been described on the cell surface, including betaglycan, heparins, and endoglin (435,440). Betaglycan, also termed TGF-β type III receptor, may enhance the affinity of TGF-βs to the signaling receptors I and II and may release bound TGF-β in an active form after specific cleavage by plasmin (435,440).

Sources

Normal Kidney

In normal glomeruli, absent to abundant amounts of TGF-β1 have been described (441–445). TGF-β1, mostly the small latent form, is also expressed in normal tubules (441). At least in the murine kidney, TGF-β3 follows a similar pattern of expression. TGF-β2 has been detected in glomeruli, mainly in the juxtaglomerular apparatus (444,446).

In cultured renal cells, TGF-β production as well as autoinduction of TGF-β has been described in mesangial cells (447–451) and proximal tubular cells (452,453). Of potential relevance for the kidney, TGF-β also can be detected in cultured vascular smooth muscle cells, endothelial cells, monocytes, macrophages, neutrophils, T- and B-lymphocytes, and platelets (434,454–456).

Renal Disease

Renal overexpression of TGF-β occurs in a multitude of experimental diseases as well as in human pathology (Table 7). Increased renal TGF-β bioactivity and increased urinary excretion of TGF-β in experimental or human renal scarring has been described (457,458). However, given the complexity of TGF-β activation and regulation, in other instances caution is necessary when interpreting data on the renal overexpression of TGF-β.

TABLE 7. *Experimental and human renal diseases associated with overexpression of TGF-β*

Disease	References
Mesangioproliferative nephritis (rat)	461–463
Purine aminonucleoside nephrosis (rat)	465,466
Adriamycin nephropathy (rat)	467
Diabetic nephropathy (mouse, rat)	447,468–470
Unilateral ureteral ligation (rat)	471
Anti-GBM nephritis (rabbit, rat)	458,472
DOCA-salt hypertension (rat)	473
Lupus-prone NZB/I WF1 mice	474
Subtotal nephrectomy (rat)	475
Diabetic nephropathy (human)	442,469
Mesangioproliferative nephritis (human)	442,443,459
Lupus nephritis (human)	442
ANCA-positive glomerulonephritis (human)	476
Focal glomerular sclerosis (human)	443
Membranous nephropathy (human, rat)	442,443,464

Indeed, one study on human renal biopsies has described widespread expression of TGF-β1 LAP, which markedly exceeded that of TGF-β1 (459). Also, instances have been documented in which TGF-β1 mRNA overexpression could be dissociated from TGF-β–induced effects, i.e., stimulation of matrix synthesis (460).

Biologic Activity

Apart from the potential role of TGF-β in renal development (434), two functions of TGF-β are particularly relevant to immunologic renal disease: (a) the modulation of inflammation and (b) the mediation of tissue repair and/or fibrosis.

Modulation of Inflammation

The actions of TGF-β are confusing in that it can exert potent proinflammatory actions but also can act as a potent immunosuppressive agent. This apparent contradictory influence of TGF-β is accounted for in part by the differential effects of TGF-β on resting and activating cells. As a general, but by no means exclusive, rule, resting, immature cells are stimulated by TGF-β, whereas the same cells, once activated, may be inhibited by TGF-β (433).

Early proinflammatory effects of TGF-β as long as its production remains locally confined, include leukocyte chemotaxis, increased expression of adhesion molecules, and autoinduction of TGF-β, as well as induction of other cytokines in leukocytes and weak effects on angiogenesis (432,433). However, when TGF-β was overexpressed in normal rat glomeruli by in vivo transfection, some mesangial cell proliferation but no inflammatory changes ensued (477). Thus, the question of whether TGF-β may be proinflammatory in the kidney is unresolved. Systemic administration or overproduction of TGF-β with increased serum levels mainly results in immunosuppression, which may relate to multiple anti-inflammatory actions, including those listed as follows (433,434,456):

Deactivation of macrophages
Inhibition of IL-2–dependent T-cell proliferation and activation
Suppression of differentiation and proliferation of natural killer cells
Inhibition of Ig secretion by stimulated B cells, as well as a switch of B cells from IgG to IgA production [indeed, in peripheral blood mononuclear cells of patients with IgA nephropathy, increased TGF-β content has been detected (478)]
Inhibition of the IL-1 action by downregulation of IL-1 receptor expression
Inhibition of MHC expression
Suppression of NO generation in macrophages

In vivo evidence for an immunosuppressive role of TGF-β, among other findings, is supported by the following observations:

Suppression of a nephritogenic murine T-cell clone in vivo by TGF-β (479)
Depletion of lymphoid tissue after administration of TGF-β1 to rats (480)
Prolongation of allograft survival after TGF-β administration (456)
Accumulation of TGF-β in the circulation predisposes MRL lupus-prone mice to serious bacterial infections (481)
Genetically TGF-β1 deficient mice die of a multifocal, inflammatory wasting syndrome (482)

Immunosuppressive effects of cyclosporine also may be partially mediated via TGF-β (434). Indeed renal transplant patients treated with cyclosporine exhibit increased TGF-β serum levels (483).

Tissue Repair/Fibrosis

TGF-β is an important regulator of two processes involved in tissue repair and/or scar formation: cell turnover and matrix metabolism.

Proliferation of epithelial and endothelial cells is usually inhibited by TGF-β, which thereby has been suggested to prevent malignant cell transformation (484). TGF-β also has been linked to the induction of programmed cell death (485). A growth inhibitory effect of TGF-β has been confirmed in glomerular epithelial and endothelial cells (486–488). The effects on the growth of mesangial cells or renal interstitial fibroblasts, can be either stimulatory or inhibitory, depending on cell density, the concentration of TGF-β, costimulatory signals, and length of cytokine exposure (450,451,487,489–493). Similar to its action on tubular epithelial cells, TGF-β induces hypertrophy in mesangial cells (450,494). Few data are available on the effects of TGF-β on renal cell turnover in vivo. TGF-β transfection of normal rat glomeruli in vivo resulted in mild, presumably mesangial, cell proliferation (477).

With respect to matrix synthesis, TGF-β regulates the production of some small proteoglycans, namely decorin and biglycan, as well as of fibronectin in cultured glomerular mesangial, epithelial, and endothelial cells as well as tubular cells (448,488,491,495). The effects of TGF-β on the production of the various collagens and laminin are less consistent (448,491,498,499) (Table 8). In vitro data suggest that induction of TGF-β may underlie the increased matrix production induced in renal cells by high glucose or angiotensin II (448,449,468,493). The best evidence for a profibrotic role of TGF-β derives from in vivo data, showing that transfection of normal rat glomeruli in vivo with a TGF-β cDNA resulted in marked expansion of the extracellular matrix, which contained increased amounts of collagen types I and III and, to a lesser degree, collagen type IV (477). Glomerulosclerosis occurred after administration of TGF-β1 to rats (480). TGF-β1 transgenic mice were characterized by accumula-

TABLE 8. *TGF-β effects on the production of matrix proteins by cultured renal cells*

Matrix protein	Glomerular mesangial cells	Glomerular epithelial cells	Glomerular endothelial cells	Proximal tubular cells	Renal interstitial fibroblasts
Collagen I	↑ (448,449)	No change (488)			↑ (500)
Collagen III	↑ (493)	No change (488)			↓ (500)
Collagen IV	No change (491), ↑ (449)	↑ (488)			↑ (500)
Collagen[a]	↑ (450,499)				
Laminin	No change (491)	(↑) (488)			
Fibronectin	(↑) (491) to ↑ (448,495,499)	↑ (488)			
Proteoglycans	↑ (448,491)	↑ (488)	↑ (496)	↑ (497)	

References are cited in parentheses.
(↑), minor increase versus medium control; ↑, increase versus medium control; ↓, decrease versus medium control.
[a] Only the production of collagenase-sensitive protein, but not that of individual collagen types, was assessed in these studies.

tion of glomerular extracellular matrix, thickening of the GBM, crescent formation, and inflammatory arteritis (485). Most studies of TGF effects in vivo have implicated TGF-β1 derived from mesangial cells in mediating mesangial matrix expansion (437,461,462,467). In contrast, in C5b-9 induced disease of the glomerular epithelial cell (passive Heymann nephritis), there is an increase in expression of TGF-β2 and TGF-β3 isoforms (464). Glomerular epithelial cell injury is also associated with upregulation of both TGF-β receptor isotypes, suggesting that the capillary wall thickening and spikes seen in membranous nephropathy may reflect in part effects of TGF-β on the GEC (464) (see also Chapter 47).

TGF-β also can contribute to matrix accumulation by inhibiting matrix-degrading enzymes such as plasmin. In fact, incubation of glomeruli or glomerular cells with TGF-β led to reduced plasmin activity via downregulation of plasminogen activator and upregulation of plasminogen activator inhibitor synthesis (501). The role of increased mRNA expression for mesangial cell collagenase after stimulation with TGF-β remains speculative at present (502). Finally, TGF-β may modulate cell–matrix interactions, for example, by upregulation of integrin expression in nephritic glomeruli (503).

Intervention Studies

Two studies investigated the effects of either a neutralizing antibody against TGF-β or decorin on the transient matrix accumulation in mesangioproliferative nephritis in the rat (437,504). Therapy with antibody to TGF-β at the time of disease induction was shown to markedly reduce the overproduction of proteoglycans and the amount of periodic acid-Schiff (PAS)-positive extracellular matrix. Similarly, repeated injections of decorin led to a marked reduction of glomerular fibronectin EDA+ and tenascin accumulation, as well as of the PAS-positive glomerular matrix. Other studies have shown that a low-protein diet reduces the renal expression of TGF-β (505,506) and that L-arginine may play a central role in this process (507).

TUMOR NECROSIS FACTOR

Synonyms

TNF and lymphotoxin are closely related cytokines sometimes known as TNF-α and TNF-β, respectively. TNF was previously called cachexin, macrophage cytotoxin, and macrophage cytotoxin factor.

Introductory Remarks

TNF and IL-1 are the two really abundant proinflammatory cytokines and are highly synergistic (508).

Protein Characteristics and Gene Structure

TNF-α is synthesized as a prohormone of 26 kDa that is expressed in the plasma membrane, anchored by a single transmembrane domain (509). Mature TNF is a 17.5-kDa polypeptide cleaved from the cell surface by a metalloproteinase (510). Three TNF monomers associate noncovalently to form a trimer, which is the biologically active form. X-ray crystalography shows that it has a "jelly roll" configuration (511,512). In humans, the genes for TNF–α and -β lie adjacent to each other on chromosome 6p21.3 situated among the HLA class III genes. Polymorphisms of the TNF and lymphotoxin genes that affect synthesis have been described (513). Murine TNF is also linked to the MHC on chromosome 17.

Receptor(s) and Signaling

TNF binds to two receptors with similar affinities. The TNF type I receptor (CD 120a) has an Mr of 55 kDa, and the type II receptor (CD 120b) has an Mr of 75 kDa (514). Both are members of the nerve growth factor group of receptors and bind TNF in a complex fashion. One TNF trimer probably engages three receptors, but it is unclear whether signaling results from lattice formation or more conventional change in conformation (515). The cytoplasmic tails of the two TNF receptors are unrelated and presumably engage different signaling pathways, and have different functions. Type I receptors have been reported to initiate the inflammatory effects of TNF (516,517), and the type II receptor may mediate the proliferative activity (518) or cooperate with the type I receptor (519). Studies with knockout mice deficient in type 1 receptors have confirmed their importance in inflammation (520,521), but studies with knockout mice with intact type 2 receptors also showed inflammation inhibition (522).

Intracellular signaling pathways initiated by TNF receptors have not been clearly defined but appear to involve the same cascades described in detail in the section on IL-1. Thus, TNF receptor binding results in engagement of cytoplasmic mediators and initiation of ERK, JNK (SAPK), and HOG-1 MAP kinase cascades; caseinase; and the sphyngomyelase/ceramide pathway (523); the newly expressed proteins are the same as those induced by IL-1. Soluble form type I and II receptors are released from the cell surface by proteolytic cleavage and are able to bind free TNF. They are found in high concentrations in the serum of patients with acute or chronic inflammation (524,525) and can attenuate the effects of TNF; it is possible that they also provide a slow-release preparation of active cytokine. Nevertheless, the balance between TNF-α and the soluble receptors has prognostic significance in meningococcemia and falciparum malaria (526).

Sources

Stimulated monocytes and activated macrophages are the principal sources of TNF, but it is also secreted by neutrophils, lymphocytes, and fibroblasts. It cannot be detected in normal kidneys by immunohistology, in situ hybridization, or Northern analysis. However, injection of large doses of LPS results in the widespread expression of TNF, including in the kidney (527). Both glomerular and proximal tubular cells express TNF, but it is especially prominent in the latter. Unstimulated human and rodent mesangial cells do not release detectable amounts of TNF, but both murine and rat mesangial cells release TNF when stimulated or injured (528,529). Factors that can induce TNF in mesangial cells include aggregated IgGs, LPS, IL-1, TNF, advanced glycosylation end products, and the membrane attack complex (C5-C9) of complement.

TNF is synthesized within the kidney in acute inflammatory renal disease. In clinical studies, TNF has been identified in patients with ANCA-associated crescentic nephritis in glomeruli, tubules, and interstitium (530), as well as in some (531) but not all studies of patients with IgA nephropathy (532). TNF also has been identified in mesangial cells in lupus nephritis (533). Neale et al. (534) identified TNF in podocytes of patients with membranous nephropathy.

Specific TNF messages can be demonstrated in RNA harvested from kidneys and glomeruli of rats injected with a bolus of LPS; message levels are maximal between 4 and 6 h but are sustained for at least 24 h (535,536). TNF is expressed transiently in the heterologous phase of NTN, especially in rats pretreated with LPS (535). It also has been detected early in the course of the autologous phase of NTN (529,537,538) and is expressed in acutely inflamed kidneys of mice with experimental pyelonephritis (539). TNF is expressed in glomerular epithelial cells from rats with adriamycin nephrosis (540), and treatment with cyclosporine decreases both TNF release and proteinuria (541). Mononuclear cells from patients with most acute and chronic inflammatory diseases release increased amounts of TNF (542), so attempts to assess activity of glomerular disease indirectly by assaying TNF released from patients' mononuclear cells is unlikely to be specific. Urinary TNF is increased in some patients with proliferative nephritis (531,543), but excretion does not correlate with TNF expression in renal biopsies (531). Nevertheless, there is a report that patients with progressive of membranous nephropathy have greater urinary TNF excretion than those with stable disease (545).

Biologic Activities

TNF and IL-1 are highly synthesized (508). Their activities are similar, as already described in the section on IL-1 and elsewhere (546–548). Both cytokines activate endothelium and fixed tissue cells and upregulate the proinflamatory properties of neutrophils, monocytes, and macrophages. However, there are some striking differences, and TNF has at least three important properties not shared with IL-1. These are (a) priming neutrophils to increase secretory responses and oxygen radical generation when exposed to chemoattractants; (b) triggering cell death by apoptosis or necrosis (548); and (c) IFN-α–induced macrophage differentiation into cytotoxic cells and macrophage differentiation into inflammatory cells after phagocytosis (549) are both TNF but not IL-1 dependent.

The effect of TNF on mesangial cells is essentially the same as that of IL-1. It stimulates the production of cytokines including IL-6 and the chemokines MCP-1 and CINC; increases surface expression of ICAM-1 and VCAM as well as HLA class I molecules; and promotes synthesis of complement components C4 and factor B and the generation of NO (see section on IL-1 and (528). TNF stimulates glomerular epithelial cells to proliferate (550) and synthesize the third component of complement (C3) (551). In higher concentrations, TNF is toxic for rat mesangial cells (410,540).

Intervention Studies

Administration of large doses of TNF cause circulatory shock and mimic the other effects of LPS (547,548). Small doses of TNF cause glomerular injury in rabbits (552), and smaller doses still cause glomerular neutrophil influx without morphologic or functional evidence of injury in rats (553). Administration of recombinant TNF to achieve serum concentrations in the pathophysiologic range markedly aggravates heterologous-phase injury in NTN, and there is strong synergism with IL-1 when it was administered concurrently (277). These results demonstrate that circulating TNF concentrations have a powerful influence on acute glomerular inflammation, possibly by priming leukocytes and endothelium. However, it has been much more difficult to demonstrate that administered TNF influences autologous-phase injury in NTN (Rees AJ, unpublished observations), maybe because sufficient TNF is generated locally.

Chronic administration of TNF inhibits the development of autoimmune nephritis in NZB/NZW mice injected with 10 mg TNF thrice weekly from 4 months of age. The treated mice survived significantly longer, and this was interpreted in the context of deficient TNF synthesis, which they also found in this strain (554). However, repeated low-dose TNF can cause tolerance to the effect of further TNF (548), so it is possible that the repeated administration paradoxically diminished TNF bioactivity. The recent observation that IL-10 (which reduces TNF synthesis) worsens the prognosis in lupus-prone MRL/lpr mice (365) and that anti-IL10 antibodies improve the prognosis is consistent with a direct effect of TNF, especially because the effect of passive immunization against IL-10 was abrogated by coadministration of antibodies of TNF. However, it is unclear whether these treatments influence prognosis through effects on the autoimmune response or the inflammation it provokes.

TNF can be inhibited specifically by administration of TNF binding proteins, such as anti-TNF antibodies and soluble TNF receptors. Administration of recombinant soluble type I receptor diminishes leukocyte infiltration and injury in the heterologous phase of NTN (555–557). Karkar et al. have reported similar findings in the LPS-enhanced model of heterologous phase injury (556). They showed that pretreatment with either soluble type 1 TNF receptors (556) or anti-TNF antibodies (535) decreased proteinuria and the incidence of glomerular capillary thrombi in this model. The same group also reported that glomerular expression of IL-1 and the neutrophil chemokine, MIP-2, were decreased by the administration of soluble TNF receptors. The autologous phase of NTN is attenuated by passive immunization against TNF, albeit to a surprisingly small degree (558), so it is important to confirm these results using soluble TNF receptors. These data provide compelling evidence that TNF influences acute glomerular injury and provides the basis for studies in humans, especially because administration of soluble TNF receptors has been shown to be highly effective in patients with rheumatoid arthritis (559).

VASCULAR ENDOTHELIAL GROWTH FACTOR/VASCULAR PERMEABILITY FACTOR

Introductory Remarks

Vascular endothelial growth factor (VEGF), also known as vascular permeability factor (VPF), is a relatively unique cytokine because almost all of its biologic activities known to date are related to endothelial cells (560). Important roles of VEGF in angiogenesis, tumor growth, development, and atherosclerosis have been suggested (560–563). VEGF/VPF is probably distinct from the "vascular permeability factor," which has been detected in the circulation of proteinuric patients. Unlike VEGF/VPF, this latter factor is a T-lymphocyte product with a relatively low Mr of about 12 kDa (564).

Protein Characteristics and Gene Structure

VEGF is a dimeric, heavily glycosylated 34- to 45-kDa protein. Four molecular variants of the subunits exist, composed of 121, 165, 189, and 206 amino acids (565). While $VEGF_{121}$ and $VEGF_{165}$ are soluble secreted forms, $VEGF_{189}$ and $VEGF_{206}$ are mostly bound to heparin-containing proteoglycans on the cell surface or in the extracellular matrix (565). Bound forms can be released by proteolysis after plasminogen activation. Four different VEGF RNA species arise from differential splicing (565). The gene contains two regulatory hypoxia-sensing elements (566).

Receptor(s) and Signaling

Two VEGF receptors, both of which belong to the tyrosine kinase family, have been identified: the fms-like tyrosine kinase flt-1 and KDR/flk-1 (567). Recent data suggest that flt-1 may predominantly mediate some of the nonmitogenic effects of VEGF. A truncated receptor form may act as a naturally occurring antagonist of VEGF (568). VEGF binding to its receptors is potentiated by heparin and heparan sulphate proteoglycans (569) and inhibited by suramine and protamine (570). Ligand binding to the receptors induces dimerization; autophosphorylation; phosphorylation of PLC-γ, phosphatidyl-inositol 3-kinase, Ras-GTPase–activating protein, and others and increases intracellular calcium and inositol phosphates (560,571).

Sources

Normal Kidney

High levels of VEGF mRNA have been detected in the kidney, particularly in podocytes (562,572–574). In cell culture, various isoforms of VEGF were found in glomerular epithelial cells (573,574), macrophages, and/or mononuclear cells (572,575), as well as in vascular smooth muscle cells (576,577). Additional studies have described the production of VEGF by cultured human mesangial cells (578), bovine glomerular endothelial cells (579), and SV-40 transformed rat proximal tubular epithelial cells (572). These latter data have not yet been confirmed in vivo and could relate to the pronounced effect of hypoxia on VEGF production. Under normal conditions, the in vivo localization of VEGF in the human and rat kidney is confined to visceral glomerular epithelial cells as well as distal and collecting duct epithelia (562,574,580–582).

Expression for KDR and flt-1 mRNA in normal human kidney has been localized to glomerular and peritubular capillaries as well as to pre- and postglomerular vessels (562,580,582). These studies are corroborated by the demonstration of $^{125}I\text{-}VEGF_{165}$ binding to renal microvessels in glomeruli, the cortical labyrinth, medullar vascular rays, and the papilla (583), as well as to cultured endothelial cells (569,570).

Renal Disease

In acute renal diseases such as florid vascular transplant rejection or necrotizing vasculitis, increased VEGF expression occurred in damaged proximal and distal tubular epithelia plus vascular smooth muscle cells (582), although in more chronic processes such as nephrosclerosis, diabetic nephropathy, and chronic transplant rejection, VEGF synthesis was mostly increased in renal interstitial cells (582). In culture, induction of VEGF synthesis can be stimulated in smooth muscle or mesangial cells by various cytokines, such as IL-1, PDGF, or TGF-β, or by exposure to hypoxia (560,561,575,578).

Messenger RNA expression for KDR in diseased human kidneys was not altered as compared with normal kidneys (582).

Biologic Activities

VEGF is a potent mitogen for endothelial cells, including glomerular endothelial cells, both in vitro and in vivo (579,584). Thus, a paracrine pathway may exist by which endothelial cells can respond to VEGF produced by neighboring cells such as smooth muscle cells or macrophages. In glomerular endothelial cells, an autocrine activity of VEGF has been proposed (579) that so far has not been confirmed in endothelial cells of other origins. Endocrine VEGF actions are largely prevented by rapid inactivation of its biologic activity by circulating α_2-macroglobulin (585).

In addition to its mitogenic activity, VEGF is also chemotactic for endothelial cells as well as for macrophages (560). Both of the mitogenic and chemotactic action on endothelial cells are presumed to contribute to maintaining the endothelial integrity of vessels (560, 577,583). In addition, they constitute an essential part of VEGF's angiogenic activity (560,565). With respect to angiogenesis, the ability of VEGF to modulate the matrix degrading capacity of endothelial cells is also of central importance (560). VEGF also can promote angiogenesis by increasing the permeability of postcapillary venules and small veins for macromolecules, thereby altering the composition of the normal extracellular matrix in a way to promote vessel formation (560). Although angiogenesis has been proposed to occur in the glomerulus (586), the role of VEGF in this process is presently unknown. It is also currently unknown whether VEGF, particularly that produced by glomerular podocytes, is involved in the regulation of glomerular protein permeability (587).

A last biologic activity of VEGF is the induction of an NO-dependent relaxation of small arteries, including the renal vascular bed (587,588).

REFERENCES

1. Demetri GD, Griffin JD. Granulocyte colony-stimulating factor and its receptor. *Blood* 1991;78:2791–2808.
2. Gasson JC. Molecular physiology of granulocyte-macrophage colony-stimulating factor. *Blood* 1991;77:1131–1145.
3. Kawasaki ES, Ladner MB. Molecular biology of macrophage colony-stimulating factor. *Immunol Ser* 1990;49:155–176.
4. Stahl RAK, Thaiss F, Disser M, Helmchen U, Hora K, Schlöndorff D. Increased expression of monocyte chemoattractant protein-1 in anti-thymocyte antibody–induced glomerulonephritis. *Kidney Int* 1993; 44:1036–1047.
5. Brennan DC, Jevnikar AM, Bloom RD, Brissette WH, Singer GG, Kelley VR. Cultured mesangial cells from autoimmune MRL-lpr mice have decreased secreted and surface M-CSF. *Kidney Int* 1992; 42:279–284.
6. Mori T, Bartocci A, Satriano J, et al. Mouse mesangial cells produce colony-stimulating factor-1 (CSF-1) and express the CSF-1 receptor. *J Immunol* 1990;144:4697–4702.
7. Budde K, Coleman DL, Lacy J, Sterzel RB. Rat mesangial cells produce granulocyte-macrophage colony-stimulating factor. *Kidney Int* 1989;257:1065–1078.
8. Zoja C, Wang JM, Bettoni S, et al. Interleukin-1 beta and tumor necrosis factor-alpha induce gene expression and production of leukocyte chemotactic factors, colony-stimulating factors, and interleukin-6 in human mesangial cells. *Am J Pathol* 1991;138:991–1003.
9. Frank J, Engler-Blum G, Rodemann HP, Müller GA. Human renal tubular cells as a cytokine source: PDGF-B, GM-CSF and IL-6 mRNA expression in vitro. *Exp Nephrol* 1993;1:26–35.
10. Hora K, Satriano JA, Santiago A, et al. Receptors for IgG complexes activate synthesis of monocyte chemoattractant peptide 1 and colony-stimulating factor 1. *Proc Natl Acad Sci U S A* 1992;89:1745–1749.
11. Satriano JA, Hora K, Shan Z, Stanley ER, Mori T, Schlöndorff D. Regulation of monocyte chemoattractant protein-1 and macrophage colony-stimulating factor-1 by IFN-gamma, tumor necrosis factor-alpha, IgG aggregates, and cAMP in mouse mesangial cells. *J Immunol* 1993;150:1971–1978.
12. Bloom RD, Florquin S, Singer GG, Brennan DC, Kelley VR. Colony stimulating factor-1 in the induction of lupus nephritis. *Kidney Int* 1993;43:1000–1009.
13. Müller M, Emmendorffer A, Lohmann-Matthes ML. Expansion and high proliferative potential of the macrophage system throughout life time of lupus-prone NZB/w and MRL lpr/lpr mice. *Eur J Immunol* 1991;21:2211–2217.
14. Mishra L, Ooi BS. Biosynthesis of colony-stimulating factor-1 (CSF-1) by mesangial cells of autoimmune mice. *Immunol Invest* 1993; 22:249–255.
15. Brady HR, Denton MD, Jimenez W, Takata S, Palliser D, Brenner BM. Chemoattractants provoke monocyte adhesion to human mesangial cells and mesangial cell injury. *Kidney Int* 1992;42:480–487.
16. Neugarten J, Feith GW, Assmann KJM, Shan Z, Stanley ER, Schlöndorff D. Role of macrophages and colony-stimulating factor-1 in murine antiglomerular basement membrane glomerulonephritis. *J Am Soc Nephrol* 1995;5:1903–1909.
17. Santiago A, Mori T, Satriano J, Schlöndorff D. Regulation of Fc receptors for IgG on cultured rat mesangial cells. *Kidney Int* 1991; 39:87–94.
18. Mendley SR, Toback FG. Autocrine and paracrine regulation of kidney epithelial cell growth. *Annu Rev Physiol* 1989;51:33–50.
19. Harris RC. Potential physiologic roles for epidermal growth factor in the kidney. *Am J Kidney Dis* 1991;17:627–630.
20. Fisher DA, Salido EC, Barajas L. Epidermal growth factor and the kidney. *Annu Rev Physiol* 1989;51:67–80.
21. Wilson PD, Du J, Norman JT. Autocrine, endocrine and paracrine regulation of growth abnormalities in autosomal dominant polycystic kidney disease. *Eur J Cell Biol* 1993;61:131–138.
22. Carpenter G, Cohen S. Epidermal growth factor. *J Biol Chem* 1990; 265:7709–7712.
23. Cybulsky AV, McTavish AJ, Cyr MD. Extracellular matrix modulates epidermal growth factor receptor activation in rat glomerular epithelial cells. *J Clin Invest* 1994;94:68–78.
24. Force T, Kyriakis JM, Avruch J, Bonventre JV. Endothelin, vasopressin, and angiotensin II enhance tyrosine phosphorylation by protein kinase C–dependent and –independent pathways in glomerular mesangial cells. *J Biol Chem* 1991;266:6650–6656.
25. Briscoe J, Guschin D, Müller M. Just another signalling pathway. *Curr Biol* 1994;4:1033–1035.
26. Lakshmanan J, Salido EC, Lam R, Fisher DA. Epidermal growth factor prohormone is secreted in human urine. *Am J Physiol* 1992;263: E142–150.

27. Nouwen EJ, De Broe ME. EGF and TGF-alpha in the human kidney: identification of octopal cells in the collecting duct. *Kidney Int* 1994; 45:1510–1521.
28. Yoshioka K, Takemura T, Murakami K, et al. Identification and localization of epidermal growth factor and its receptor in the human glomerulus. *Lab Invest* 1990;63:189–196.
29. Salido EC, Lakshmanan J, Fisher DA, Shapiro LJ, Barajas L. Expression of epidermal growth factor in the rat kidney. An immunocytochemical and in situ hybridization study. *Histochemistry* 1991;96: 65–72.
30. Lau JLT, Fowler JE, Ghosh L. Epidermal growth factor in the normal and neoplastic kidney and bladder. *J Urol* 1988;139:170–175.
31. Nakopoulou L, Stefanaki K, Boletis J, et al. Immunohistochemical study of epidermal growth factor receptor (EFGR) in various types of renal injury. *Nephrol Dial Transplant* 1994;9:764–769.
32. Nielsen S, Nexo E, Christensen EI. Absorption of epidermal growth factor and insulin in rabbit renal proximal tubules. *Am J Physiol* 1989; 256:E55–E63.
33. Goodyer PR, Kachra Z, Bell C, Rozen R. Renal tubular cells are potential targets for epidermal growth factor. *Am J Physiol* 1988;255: F1191–F1196.
34. Breyer MD, Redha R, Breyer JA. Segmental distribution of epidermal growth factor binding sites in rabbit nephron. *Am J Physiol* 1990;259: F553–558.
35. Harris RC, Hoover RL, Jacobson HR, Badr KF. Evidence for glomerular actions of epidermal growth factor in the rat. *J Clin Invest* 1988;82:1028–1039.
36. Adler S, Chen X, Eng B. Control of rat glomerular epithelial cell growth in vitro. *Kidney Int* 1990;37:1048–1054.
37. Harris RC, Daniel TO. Epidermal growth factor binding, stimulation of phosphorylation, and inhibition of gluconeogenesis in rat proximal tubule. *J Cell Physiol* 1989;139:383–391.
38. Norman J, Badie Dezfooly B, Nord EP, et al. EGF-induced mitogenesis in proximal tubular cells: potentiation by angiotensin II. *Am J Physiol* 1987;253:F299–F309.
39. Harris RC. Response of rat inner medullary collecting duct to epidermal growth factor. *Am J Physiol* 1989;256:F1117–F1124.
40. Alvarez RJ, Sun MJ, Haverty TP, Iozzo RV, Myers JC, Neilson EG. Biosynthetic and proliferative characteristics of tubulointerstitial fibroblasts probed with paracrine cytokines. *Kidney Int* 1992;41:14–23.
41. Miller SB, Rogers SA, Estes CE, Hammerman MR. Increased distal nephron EGF content and altered distribution of peptide in compensatory renal hypertrophy. *Am J Physiol* 1992;262:F1032–1038.
42. Humes HD, Lake EW, Liu S. Renal tubule cell repair following acute renal injury. *Miner Electrolyte Metab* 1995;21:353–365.
43. Storch S, Saggi S, Megyesi J, Price PM, Safirstein R. Ureteral obstruction decreases renal prepro-epidermal growth factor and Tamm-Horsfall expression. *Kidney Int* 1992;42:89–94.
44. Ter Meulen CG, Bilo HJG, Van Kamp GJ, Gans ROB, Donker AJM. Urinary epidermal growth factor excretion is correlated to renal function loss per se and not to the degree of diabetic renal failure. *Neth J Med* 1994;44:12–17.
45. Lev Ran A, Hwang DL, Ahmad B, Bixby H. Immunoreactive epidermal growth factor in serum, plasma, platelets, and urine in patients on chronic dialysis. *Nephron* 1991;57:164–166.
46. Toubeau G, Nonclercq D, Zanen J, et al. Distribution of epidermal growth factor in the kidneys of rats exposed to amikacin. *Kidney Int* 1991;40:691–699.
47. Verstrepen WA, Nouwen EJ, Yue XS, De Broe ME. Altered growth factor expression during toxic proximal tubular necrosis and regeneration. *Kidney Int* 1993;43:1267–1279.
48. Roy Chaudhury P, Jones MC, MacLeod AM, Haites NE, Simpson JG, Power DA. An immunohistological study of epidermal growth factor receptor and neu receptor expression in proliferative glomerulonephritis. *Pathology* 1993;25:327–332.
49. Lowden DA, Lindemann GW, Merlino G, Barash BD, Calvet JP, Gattone VH. Renal cysts in transgenic mice expressing transforming growth factor-alpha. *J Lab Clin Med* 1994;124:386–394.
50. Hammerman MR, Miller SB. The growth hormone insulin-like growth factor axis in kidney revisited. *Am J Physiol* 1993;265: F1–F14.
51. Schaudies RP, Nonclercq D, Nelson L, et al. Endogenous EGF as a potential renotrophic factor in ischemia-induced acute renal failure. *Am J Physiol* 1993;265:F425–434.
52. Ganz MB, Perfetto MC, Boron WF. Effects of mitogens and other agents on rat mesangial cell proliferation, pH, and Ca(2+). *Am J Physiol* 1990;259:F269–278.
53. Zhang G, Ichimura T, Wallin A, Kan M, Stevens JL. Regulation of rat proximal tubule epithelial cell growth by fibroblast growth factors, insulin-like growth factor-1 and transforming growth factor-beta, and analysis of fibroblast growth factors in rat kidney. *J Cell Physiol* 1991;148:295–305.
54. Wolf G, Neilson EG. Angiotensin II induces cellular hypertrophy in cultured murine proximal tubular cells. *Am J Physiol* 1990;259: F768–777.
55. Humes HD, Beals TF, Cieslinski DA, Sanchez IO, Page TP. Effects of transforming growth factor-beta, transforming growth factor-alpha, and other growth factors on renal proximal tubule cells. *Lab Invest* 1991;64:538–545.
56. Marinides GN, Suchard SJ, Mookerjee BK. Role of thrombospondin in mesangial cell growth: possible existence of an autocrine feedback growth circuit. *Kidney Int* 1994;46:350–357.
57. Takuwa N, Ganz M, Takuwa Y, Sterzel RB, Rasmussen H. Studies of the mitogenic effect of serotonin in rat renal mesangial cells. *Am J Physiol* 1989;257:F431–F439.
58. Humes HD, Cieslinski DA, Johnson LB, Sanchez IO. Triiodothyronine enhances renal tubule cell replication by stimulating EGF receptor gene expression. *Am J Physiol* 1992;262:F540–545.
59. Salido EC, Lakshmanan J, Koy S, Barajas L, Fisher DA. Effect of thyroxine administration on the expression of epidermal growth factor in the kidney and submandibular gland of neonatal mice. An immunocytochemical and in situ hybridization study. *Endocrinology* 1990;127:2263–2269.
60. Silver BJ, Jaffer FE, Abboud HE. Platelet-derived growth factor synthesis in mesangial cells: induction by multiple peptide mitogens. *Proc Natl Acad Sci U S A* 1989;86:1056–1060.
61. Seiken G, Grillo FG, Schaudies RP, Johnson JP. Modulation of renal EGF in dichromate-induced acute renal failure treated with thyroid hormone. *Kidney Int* 1994;45:1622–1627.
62. Kanda S, Igawa T, Sakai H, Nomata K, Kanetake H, Saito Y. Anti-epidermal growth factor antibody inhibits compensatory renal hyperplasia but not hypertrophy after unilateral nephrectomy in mice. *Biochem Biophys Res Commun* 1992;187:1015–1021.
63. Zhang G, Ichimura T, Maier JAM, Maciag T, Stevens JL. A role for fibroblast growth factor type-1 in nephrogenic repair. *J Biol Chem* 1993;268:11542–11547.
64. Zhang G, Ichimura T, Wallin A, Kan M, Stevens JL. Regulation of rat proximal tubule epithelial cell growth by fibroblast growth factors, insulin-like growth factor-1 and transforming growth factor-β, and analysis of fibroblast growth factors in rat kidney. *J Cell Physiol* 1991;148:295–305.
65. Hughes SE, Hall PA. Immunolocalization of fibroblast growth factor receptor 1 and its ligands in human tissues. *Lab Invest* 1993;69: 173–182.
66. Witte DP, Nagasaki T, Stambrook P, Lieberman MA. Identification of an acidic fibroblast growth factor-like activity in a mesoblastic nephroma. *Lab Invest* 1989;60:353–359.
67. Ballermann BJ. Regulation of bovine glomerular endothelial cell growth in vitro. *Am J Physiol* 1989;256:C182–C189.
68. Mendley SR, Toback FG. Autocrine and paracrine regulation of kidney epithelial cell growth. *Annu Rev Physiol* 1989;51:33–50.
69. Gospodarowicz D. Biological activities of fibroblast growth factors. *Ann NY Acad Sci* 1991;638:1–8.
70. Baird A. Potential mechanisms regulating the extracellular activities of basic fibroblast growth factor. *Mol Reprod Dev* 1994;39:43–48.
71. Klagsbrun M. Mediators of angiogenesis: the biological significance of basic fibroblast growth factor–heparin and heparan sulfate interactions. *Semin Cancer Biol* 1992;3:81–87.
72. Maciag T, Zhan X, Garfinkel S, et al. Novel mechanisms of fibroblast growth factor 1 function. *Recent Prog Horm Res* 1994;49:105–123.
73. Logan A. Intracrine regulation at the nucleus—a further mechanism of growth factor activity? *J Endocrinol* 1990;125:339–343.
74. D'Amore PA. Modes of FGF release in vivo and in vitro. *Cancer Metastasis Rev* 1990;9:227–238.
75. Mignatti P, Morimoto T, Rifkin DB. Basic fibroblast growth factor, a protein devoid of secretory signal sequence, is released by cells via a pathway independent of the endoplasmic reticulum–golgi complex. *J Cell Physiol* 1992;151:81–93.

76. Johnson DE, Williams LT. Structural and functional diversity in the FGF receptor multigene family. *Adv Cancer Res* 1993;60:1–41.
77. Guvakova MA, Yakubov LA, Vlodavsky I, Tonkinson JL, Stein CA. Phosphorothioate oligodeoxynucleotides bind to basic fibroblast growth factor, inhibit its binding to cell surface receptors, and remove it from low affinity binding sites on extracellular matrix. *J Biol Chem* 1995;270:2620–2627.
78. Tyrrell DJ, Ishihara M, Rao N, et al. Structure and biological activities of a heparin-derived hexasaccharide with high affinity for basic fibroblast growth factor. *J Biol Chem* 1993;268:4684–4689.
79. Baird A, Schubert D, Ling N, Guillemin R. Receptor- and heparin-binding domains of basic fibroblast growth factor. *Proc Natl Acad Sci U S A* 1988;85:2324–2328.
80. Hanneken A, Ying W, Ling N, Baird A. Identification of soluble forms of the fibroblast growth factor receptor in blood. *Proc Natl Acad Sci U S A* 1994;91:9170–9174.
81. Floege J, Eng E, Lindner V, et al. Rat glomerular mesangial cells synthesize basic fibroblast growth factor. Release, upregulated synthesis, and mitogenicity in mesangial proliferative glomerulonephritis. *J Clin Invest* 1992;90:2362–2369.
82. Luqmani YA, Graham M, Coombes RC. Expression of basic fibroblast growth factor, FGFR1 and FGFR2 in normal and malignant human breast, and comparison with other normal tissues. *Br J Cancer* 1992;66:273–280.
83. Kardami E, Murphy LJ, Liu L, Padua RR, Fandrich RR. Characterization of two preparations of antibodies to basic fibroblast growth factor which exhibit distinct patterns of immunolocalization. *Growth Factors* 1990;4:69–80.
84. Takeuchi A, Yoshizawa N, Yamamoto M, et al. Basic fibroblast growth factor promotes proliferation of rat glomerular visceral epithelial cells in vitro. *Am J Pathol* 1992;141:107–116.
85. Kriz W, Hähnel B, Rösner S, Elger M. Long-term treatment of rats with FGF-2 results in focal segmental glomerulosclerosis. *Kidney Int* 1995;48:1435–1450.
86. Cordon-Cardo C, Vlodavsky I, Haimovitz-Friedman A, Hicklin D, Fuks Z. Expression of basic fibroblast growth factor in normal human tissues. *Lab Invest* 1990;63:832–840.
87. Francki A, Uciechowski P, Floege J, Von der Ohe J, Resch K, Radeke HH. Autocrine growth regulation of human glomerular mesangial cells is primarily mediated by basic fibroblast growth factor. *Am J Pathol* 1995;147:1372–1382.
88. Blotnick S, Peoples GE, Freeman MR, Eberlein TJ, Klagsbrun M. T lymphocytes synthesize and export heparin-binding epidermal growth factor–like growth factor and basic fibroblast growth factor, mitogens for vascular cells and fibroblasts: differential production and release by $CD4^+$ and $CD8^+$ T cells. *Proc Natl Acad Sci U S A* 1994;91:2890–2894.
89. Nguyen M, Watanabe H, Budson AE, Richie JP, Hayes DF, Folkman J. Elevated levels of an angiogenic peptide, basic fibroblast growth factor, in the urine of patients with a wide spectrum of cancers. *J Natl Cancer Inst* 1994;86:356–361.
90. Floege J, Kriz W, Schulze M, et al. Basic FGF (FGF-2) augments podocyte injury and induces glomerulosclerosis in rats with experimental membranous nephropathy. *J Clin Invest* 1995;96:2809–2819.
91. Jyo Y, Sasaki T, Tamai H, Nohno T, Itoh N, Osawa G. Demonstration of fibroblast growth factor receptor mRNA in glomeruli in mesangial proliferative nephritis by in situ hybridization. *J Am Soc Nephrol* 1994;5:784.
92. Ray PE, Bruggeman LA, Weeks BS, et al. bFGF and its low affinity receptors in the pathogenesis of HIV-associated nephropathy in transgenic mice. *Kidney Int* 1994;46:759–772.
93. Morita H, Shinzato T, David G, et al. Basic fibroblast growth factor–binding domain of heparan sulfate in the human glomerulosclerosis and renal tubulointerstitial fibrosis. *Lab Invest* 1994;71:528–535.
94. Nakamura T, Ebihara I, Nagaoka I, Osada S, Tomino Y, Koide H. Effect of methylprednisolone on transforming growth factor-beta, insulin-like growth factor-I, and basic fibroblast growth factor gene expression in the kidneys of NZB/W F1 mice. *Renal Physiol Biochem* 1993;16:105–116.
95. Nakamura T, Ebihara I, Fukui M, et al. Messenger RNA expression for growth factors in glomeruli from focal glomerular sclerosis. *Clin Immunol Immunopathol* 1993;66:33–42.
96. Young BA, Johnson RJ, Alpers CE, et al. Cellular events in the evolution of experimental diabetic nephropathy. *Kidney Int* 1995;47:935–944.
97. Karpen CW, Spanheimer RG, Randolph AL, Lowe WL. Tissue-specific regulation of basic fibroblast growth factor mRNA levels by diabetes. *Diabetes* 1992;41:222–226.
98. Jaffer F, Saunders C, Shultz P, Throckmorton D, Weinshell E, Abboud HE. Regulation of mesangial cell growth by polypeptide mitogens. Inhibitory role of transforming growth factor beta. *Am J Pathol* 1989;135:261–269.
99. Mene P, Abboud HE, Dunn MJ. Regulation of human mesangial cell growth in culture by thromboxane A2 and prostacyclin. *Kidney Int* 1990;38:232–239.
100. Silver BJ, Jaffer FE, Abboud HE. Platelet-derived growth factor synthesis in mesangial cells: induction by multiple peptide mitogens. *Proc Natl Acad Sci U S A* 1989;86:1056–1060.
101. Dzau VJ. Cell biology and genetics of angiotensin in cardiovascular disease. *J Hypertens Suppl* 1994;12:3–10.
102. Kondo S, Yin D, Aoki T, Takahashi JA, Morimura T, Takeuchi J. *Bcl-2* gene prevents apoptosis of basic fibroblast growth factor–deprived murine aortic endothelial cells. *Exp Cell Res* 1994;213:428–432.
103. Flaumenhaft R, Abe M, Mignatti P, Rifkin DB. Basic fibroblast growth factor–induced activation of latent transforming growth factor beta in endothelial cells: regulation of plasminogen activator activity. *J Cell Biol* 1992;118:901–909.
104. Lonnemann G, Shapiro L, Engler Blum G, Muller GA, Koch KM, Dinarello CA. Cytokines in human renal interstitial fibrosis. I. Interleukin-1 is a paracrine growth factor for cultured fibrosis–derived kidney fibroblasts. *Kidney Int* 1995;47:837–844.
105. Floege J, Eng E, Young BA, et al. Infusion of platelet-derived growth factor or basic fibroblast growth factor induces selective glomerular mesangial cell proliferation and matrix accumulation in rats. *J Clin Invest* 1993;92:2952–2962.
106. Mazue G, Newman AJ, Scampini G, et al. The histopathology of kidney changes in rats and monkeys following intravenous administration of massive doses of human basic fibroblast growth factor. *Toxicol Pathol* 1993;21:490–501.
107. Sato Y, Hamanaka R, Ono J, Kuwano M, Rifkin DB, Takaki R. The stimulatory effect of PDGF on vascular smooth muscle cell migration is mediated by the induction of endogenous bFGF. *Biochem Biophys Res Commun* 1991;174:1260–1266.
108. Cuevas P, Carceller F, Ortega S, Zazo M, Nieto I, Gimenez-Gallego G. Hypotensive activity of fibroblast growth factor. *Science* 1991;254:1208–1210.
109. Hsu HY, Nicholson AC, Hajjar DP. Basic fibroblast growth factor–induced low density lipoprotein receptor transcription and surface expression. *J Biol Chem* 1994;269:9213–9220.
110. Giachelli CM, Bae N, Almeida M, Denhardt DT, Alpers CE, Schwartz SM. Osteopontin is elevated during neointima formation in rat arteries and is a novel component of human atherosclerotic plaques. *J Clin Invest* 1993;92:1686–1696.
111. Floege J, Hugo C, Gordon K, et al. Basic fibroblast growth factor mediates glomerular mesangial cell and endothelial cell proliferation in experimental mesangioproliferative nephritis. *J Am Soc Nephrol* 1995;6:865.
112. Floege J, Eng E, Young BA, Couser WG, Johnson RJ. Heparin suppresses mesangial cell proliferation and matrix expansion in experimental mesangioproliferative glomerulonephritis. *Kidney Int* 1993;43:369–380.
113. Santos OF, Barros EJ, Yang XM, et al. Involvement of hepatocyte growth factor in kidney development. *Dev Biol* 1994;163:525–529.
114. Horie S, Higashihara E, Nutahara K, et al. Mediation of renal cyst formation by hepatocyte growth factor. *Lancet* 1994;344:789–791.
115. Adams DH, Harvath L, Bottaro DP, et al. Hepatocyte growth factor and macrophage inflammatory protein 1 beta: structurally distinct cytokines that induce rapid cytoskeletal changes and subset-preferential migration in T cells. *Proc Natl Acad Sci U S A* 1994;91:7144–7148.
116. Rubin JS, Bottaro DP, Aaronson SA. Hepatocyte growth factor/scatter factor and its receptor, the *c-met* proto-oncogene product. *Biochim Biophys Acta* 1993;1155:357–371.
117. Mizuno K, Nakamura T. Molecular characteristics of HGF and the gene, and its biochemical aspects. *EXS* 1993;65:1–29.
118. Miyazawa K, Shimomura T, Naka D, Kitamura N. Proteolytic activation of hepatocyte growth factor in response to tissue injury. *J Biol Chem* 1994;269:8966–8970.

119. Matsumoto K, Tajima H, Hamanoue M, Kohno S, Kinoshita T, Nakamura T. Identification and characterization of "injurin," an inducer of expression of the gene for hepatocyte growth factor. *Proc Natl Acad Sci U S A* 1992;89:3800–3804.
120. Comoglio PM. Structure, biosynthesis and biochemical properties of the HGF receptor in normal and malignant cells. *EXS* 1993;65: 131–165.
121. Cantley LG, Cantley LC. Signal transduction by the hepatocyte growth factor receptor, c-met. *J Am Soc Nephrol* 1995;5:1872–1881.
122. Harris RC, Burns KD, Alattar M, Homma T, Nakamura T. Hepatocyte growth factor stimulates phosphoinositide hydrolysis and mitogenesis in cultured renal epithelial cells. *Life Sci* 1993;52:1091–1100.
123. Couper JJ, Littleford KD, Couper RTL, Nakamura T, Ferrante A. High glucose and hyperosmolality stimulate hepatocyte growth factor secretion from cultured human mesangial cells. *Diabetologia* 1994; 37:533–535.
124. Wolf HK, Zarnegar R, Michalopoulos GK. Localization of hepatocyte growth factor in human and rat tissues: an immunohistochemical study. *Hepatology* 1991;14:488–494.
125. Nagaike M, Hirao S, Tajima H, et al. Renotropic functions of hepatocyte growth factor in renal regeneration after unilateral nephrectomy. *J Biol Chem* 1991;266:22781–22784.
126. Tajima H, Higuchi O, Mizuno K, Nakamura T. Tissue distribution of hepatocyte growth factor receptor and its exclusive down-regulation in a regenerating organ after injury. *J Biochem* 1992;111:401–406.
127. Cantley LG, Barros EJ, Gandhi M, Rauchman M, Nigam SK. Regulation of mitogenesis, motogenesis, and tubulogenesis by hepatocyte growth factor in renal collecting duct cells. *Am J Physiol* 1994;267: F271–280.
128. Liu Y, Dworkin LD. Simultaneous induction of HGF and its receptor c-met expression by IL-6 in rat glomerular mesangial cells. *J Am Soc Nephrol* 1995;6:771.
129. Joannidis M, Spokes K, Nakamura T, Faletto D, Cantley LG. Regional expression of hepatocyte growth factor/c-met in experimental renal hypertrophy and hyperplasia. *Am J Physiol* 1994;267: F231–236.
130. Igawa T, Matsumoto K, Kanda S, Saito Y, Nakamura T. Hepatocyte growth factor may function as a renotropic factor for regeneration in rats with acute renal injury. *Am J Physiol* 1993;265:F61–69.
131. Ishibashi K, Sasaki S, Sakamoto H, Hoshino Y, Nakamura T, Marumo F. Expressions of receptor gene for hepatocyte growth factor in kidney after unilateral nephrectomy and renal injury. *Biochem Biophys Res Commun* 1992;187:1454–1459.
132. Igawa T, Kanda S, Kanetake H, et al. Hepatocyte growth factor is a potent mitogen for cultured rabbit renal tubular epithelial cells. *Biochem Biophys Res Commun* 1991;174:831–838.
133. Kawaguchi M, Kawashima F, Ohshima K, Kawaguchi S, Wada H. Hepatocyte growth factor is a potent promoter of mitogenesis in cultured rat visceral glomerular epithelial cells. *Cell Mol Biol* 1994;40: 1103–1111.
134. Weidner KM, Behrens J, Vandekerckhove J, Birchmeier W. Scatter factor: molecular characteristics and effect on the invasiveness of epithelial cells. *J Cell Biol* 1990;111:2097–2108.
135. Grant DS, Kleinman HK, Goldberg ID, et al. Scatter factor induces blood vessel formation in vivo. *Proc Natl Acad Sci U S A* 1993;90: 1937–1941.
136. Bussolino F, Di Renzo MF, Ziche M, et al. Hepatocyte growth factor is a potent angiogenic factor which stimulates endothelial cell motility and growth. *J Cell Biol* 1992;119:629–641.
137. Miller SB, Martin DR, Kissane J, Hammerman MR. Hepatocyte growth factor accelerates recovery from acute ischemic renal injury in rats. *Am J Physiol* 1994;266:F129–134.
138. Dorr RT. Interferon-alpha in malignant and viral diseases. *Drugs* 1993;45:177–211.
139. Sen GC, Lengyel P. The interferon system. *J Biol Chem* 1992;267: 5017–5020.
140. Gutterman JU. Cytokine therapeutics: lessons from interferon alpha. *Proc Natl Acad Sci U S A* 1994;91:1198–1205.
141. Maguire JE, Gresser I, Williams AH, Kielpinski GL, Colvin RB. Modulation of expression of MHC antigens in the kidneys of mice by murine interferon-alpha/beta. *Transplantation* 1990;49:130–134.
142. Gresser I, Maury C, Tovey M, Morel-Maroger L, Pontillon F. Progressive glomerulonephritis in mice treated with interferon preparations at birth. *Nature* 1976;263:420–422.
143. Heremans H, Billiau A, Colombatti A, Hilgers J, De Somer P. Interferon treatment of NZB mice: accelerated progression of autoimmune disease. *Infect Immun* 1978;21:925–930.
144. Johnson RJ, Gretch DR, Couser WG, et al. Hepatitis C virus–associated glomerulonephritis. Effect of alpha-interferon therapy. *Kidney Int* 1994;46:1700–1704.
145. Misiani R, Bellavita P, Fenili D, et al. Interferon alfa-2a therapy in cryoglobulinemia associated with hepatitis C virus. *N Engl J Med* 1994;330:751–756.
146. Sen GC, Lengyel P. The interferon system. *J Biol Chem* 1992;267: 5017–5020.
147. Farrar MA, Schreiber RD. The molecular cell biology of interferon-gamma and its receptor. *Annu Rev Immunol* 1993;11:571–611.
148. Darnell JE, Kerr IM, Stark GR. JAK-STAT pathways and transcriptional activation in response to IFNs and other extracellular signaling proteins. *Science* 1994;264:1415–1421.
149. Meyers CM, Kelly CJ. Immunoregulation and TGF-β1. Suppression of a nephritogenic murine T cell clone. *Kidney Int* 1994;46: 1295–1301.
150. Kelley VR, Diaz Gallo C, Jevnikar AM, Singer GG. Renal tubular epithelial and T cell interactions in autoimmune renal disease. *Kidney Int* 1993;39(suppl):108–115.
151. Yokoyama H, Takabatake T, Takaeda M, et al. Up-regulated MHC-class II expression and gamma-IFN and soluble IL-2R in lupus nephritis. *Kidney Int* 1992;42:755–763.
152. Yokoyama H, Takaeda M, Wada T, et al. Intraglomerular expression of MHC class II and Ki-67 antigens and serum gamma-interferon levels in IgA nephropathy. *Nephron* 1992;62:169–175.
153. Valente G, Ozmen L, Novelli F, et al. Distribution of interferon-gamma receptor in human tissues. *Eur J Immunol* 1992;22: 2403–2412.
154. Mattila PM, Nietosvaara YA, Ustinov JK, Renkonen RL, Häyry PJ. Antigen expression in different parenchymal cell types of rat kidney and heart. *Kidney Int* 1989;36:228–233.
155. Bishop GA, Hall BM, Suranyi MG, Tiller DJ, Horvath JS, Duggin GG. Expression of HLA antigens on renal tubular cells in culture: I. MLC supernatants and gamma interferon increase both class I and class II HLA antigens. *Transplantation* 1986;42:671–678.
156. Kakizaki Y, Kraft N, Atkins RC. Interferon-gamma stimulates the secretion of IL-1, but not of IL-6, by glomerular mesangial cells. *Clin Exp Immunol* 1993;91:521–525.
157. Martin M, Schwinzer R, Schellekens H, Resch K. Glomerular mesangial cells in local inflammation. Induction of the expression of MHC class II antigens by IFN-gamma. *J Immunol* 1989;142:1887–1894.
158. Radeke HH, Emmendorffer A, Uciechowski P, Von der Ohe J, Schwinzer B, Resch K. Activation of autoreactive T-lymphocytes by cultured syngeneic glomerular mesangial cells. *Kidney Int* 1994;45: 763–774.
159. Brennan DC, Jevnikar AM, Takei F, Rubin Kelly VE. Mesangial cell accessory functions: mediation by intercellular adhesion molecule-1. *Kidney Int* 1990;38:1039–1046.
160. Remuzzi G, Zoja C, Perico N. Proinflammatory mediators of glomerular injury and mechanisms of activation of autoreactive T cells. *Kidney Int* 1994;44(suppl):8–16.
161. Hansson GK, Hellstrand M, Rymo L, Rubbia L, Gabbiani G. Interferon gamma inhibits both proliferation and expression of differentiation-specific alpha-smooth muscle actin in arterial smooth muscle cells. *J Exp Med* 1989;170:1595–1608.
162. Wuthrich RP. Vascular cell adhesion molecule-1 expression in murine lupus nephritis. *Kidney Int* 1992;42:903–914.
163. Johnson RJ, Lombardi D, Eng E, et al. Modulation of experimental mesangial proliferative nephritis by interferon-gamma. *Kidney Int* 1995;47:62–69.
164. Kakizaki Y, Kraft N, Atkins RC. Differential control of mesangial cell proliferation by interferon-gamma. *Clin Exp Immunol* 1991;85: 157–163.
165. Santiago A, Mori T, Satriano J, Schlondorff D. Regulation of Fc receptors for IgG on cultured rat mesangial cells. *Kidney Int* 1991;39: 87–94.
166. Grandaliano G, Valente AJ, Rozek MM, Abboud HE. Gamma interferon stimulates monocyte chemotactic protein in human mesangial cells. *J Lab Clin Med* 1994;123:282–289.
167. Gomez-Chiarri M, Hamilton TA, Egido J, Emancipator SN. Expression of IP-10, a lipopolysaccharide- and interferon-gamma–inducible

protein, in murine mesangial cells in culture. *Am J Pathol* 1993;142: 433–439.
168. Radeke HH, Gessner JE, Uciechowski P, Magert HJ, Schmidt RE, Resch K. Intrinsic human glomerular mesangial cells can express receptors for IgG complexes (hFc gamma RIII-A) and the associated Fc epsilon RI gamma-chain. *J Immunol* 1994;153:1281–1292.
169. Shultz PJ, Tayeh MA, Marletta MA, Raij L. Synthesis and action of nitric oxide in rat glomerular mesangial cells. *Am J Physiol* 1991; 261:F600–606.
170. Van den Dobbelsteen MEA, Verhasselt V, Kaashoek JGJ, et al. Regulation of C3 and factor H synthesis of human glomerular mesangial cells by IL-1 and interferon-gamma. *Clin Exp Immunol* 1994;95: 173–180.
171. Zhou W, Campbell RD, Martin J, Sacks SH. Interferon-gamma regulation of C4 gene expression in cultured human glomerular epithelial cells. *Eur J Immunol* 1993;23:2477–2481.
172. Seelen MAJ, Brooimans RA, Van der Woude FJ, Van Es LA, Daha MR. IFN-gamma mediates stimulation of complement C4 biosynthesis in human proximal tubular epithelial cells. *Kidney Int* 1993;44: 50–57.
173. Alvarez RJ, Sun MJ, Haverty TP, Iozzo RV, Myers JC, Neilson EG. Biosynthetic and proliferative characteristics of tubulointerstitial fibroblasts probed with paracrine cytokines. *Kidney Int* 1992;41: 14–23.
174. Nathan CF, Prendergast TJ, Wiebe ME, et al. Activation of human macrophages. Comparison of other cytokines with interferon-gamma. *J Exp Med* 1984;160:600–605.
175. Adam C, Thoua Y, Ronco P, Verroust P, Tovey M, Morel-Maroger L. The effect of exogenous interferon: acceleration of autoimmune and renal diseases in (NZB/W)F1 mice. *Clin Exp Immunol* 1980;40: 373–382.
176. Jacob CO, Van der Meide PH, McDevitt HO. In vivo treatment of (NZB × NZW)F-1 lupus-like nephritis with monoclonal antibody to gamma interferon. *J Exp Med* 1987;166:798–803.
177. Ozmen L, Roman D, Fountoulakis M, Schmid G, Ryffel B, Garotta G. Experimental therapy of systemic lupus erythematosus: the treatment of NZB/W mice with mouse soluble interferon-gamma receptor inhibits the onset of glomerulonephritis. *Eur J Immunol* 1995;25: 6–12.
178. Tolaymat A, Leventhal B, Sakarcan A, Kashima H, Monteiro C. Systemic lupus erythematosus in a child receiving long-term interferon therapy. *J Pediatr* 1992;120:429–432.
179. Graninger WB, Hassfeld W, Pesau BB, Machold KP, Zielinski CC, Smolen JS. Induction of systemic lupus erythematosus by interferon-gamma in a patient with rheumatoid arthritis. *J Rheumatol* 1991;18: 1621–1622.
180. Nicoletti F, Meroni P, Di Marco R, et al. In vivo treatment with a monoclonal antibody to interferon-gamma neither affects the survival nor the incidence of lupus-nephritis in the MRL/lpr-lpr mouse. *Immunopharmacology* 1992;24:11–16.
181. Granstein RD, Murphy GF, Margolis RJ, Byrne MH, Amento EP. Gamma-interferon inhibits collagen synthesis in vivo in the mouse. *J Clin Invest* 1987;79:1254–1258.
182. Ginevri F, Bergamaschi E, Mutti A, et al. Protracted high-dose interferon gamma therapy for chronic experimental nephropathy. *Life Sci* 1994;54:PL-45–PL-50.
183. Montinaro V, Hevey K, Aventaggiato L, et al. Extrarenal cytokines modulate the glomerular response to IgA immune complexes. *Kidney Int* 1992;42:341–353.
184. Dinarello CA. Interleukin-1 and its biologically related cytokines. *Adv Immunol* 1989;44:153–205.
185. Dinarello CA. Interleukin-1. *Rev Infect Dis* 1984;6:51–95.
186. Dinarello CA. The interleukin-1 family: 10 years of discovery. *FASEB J* 1994;8:1314–1325.
187. Webb AC, Collins KL, Auron PE, et al. Interleukin-1 gene (IL1) assigned to long arm of human chromosome 2. *Lymphokine Res* 1986;5:77–85.
188. Silver AJ, Masson WK, George AM, Adam J, Cox R. The IL-1α and genes are closely linked (<70 kbp) on mouse chromosome 2. *Somatic Cell Mol Genet* 1990;16:549–556.
189. Nicklin MJ, Weith A, Duff GW. A physical map of the region encompassing the human interleukin-1 alpha, interleukin-1 beta and interleukin-1 receptor antagonist genes. *Genomics* 1994;19:382–384.
190. Zahedi K, Seldin MF, Rits M, Ezekowitz RAB, Whitehead AS. Mouse IL-1 receptor antagonist. Molecular characterization, gene mapping and expression of mRNA in vitro and in vivo. *J Immunol* 1991;146:4228–4233.
191. Butcher C, Steinkasserer A, Tejura S, Lennard AC. Comparison of two promoters controlling expression of secreted or intracellular IL-1 receptor antagonist. *J Immunol* 1994;53:701–711.
192. Carter DB, Deibel MR Jr, Dunn CJ, et al. Purification, cloning, expression and biological characterization of an interleukin-1 receptor antagonist protein. *Nature* 1990;344:633–638.
193. Eisenberg SP, Evans RJ, Arend WP, et al. Primary structure and funcional expression from complementary DNA of a human interleukin-1 receptor antagonist. *Nature* 1990;343:341–346.
194. Haskill S, Martin G, van Le L, et al. cDNA cloning of an intracellular form of the human interleukin 1 receptor antagonist associated with epithelium. *Proc Natl Acad Sci U S A* 1991;88:3681–3685.
195. Muzio M, Re F, Sironi M, et al. Interleukin-13 induces the production of interleukin-1 receptor antagonist (IL-1ra) and the expression of the mRNA for the intracellular (keratinocyte) form of IL-1ra in human myelomonocytic cells. *Blood* 1994;83:1738–1743.
196. Preistle JP, Schar HP, Grutter MG. Crystallographic refinement of interleukin 1 beta at 2.0 A resolution. *Proc Natl Acad Sci U S A* 1989; 86:9667–9671.
197. Graves BJ, Hatada MH, Hendrickson WA, Miller JK, Madison VS, Satow Y. Structure of interleukin-1α at 2.7 A resolution. *Biochemistry* 1990;29:2679–2684.
198. Vigers GP, Caffes P, Evans RJ, Thompson RC, Eisenberg SP, Brandhuber BJ. X-ray structure of interleukin-1 receptor antagonist at 2.0-A resolution. *J Biol Chem* 1994;269:12874–12879.
199. Stockman BJ, Scahill TA, Strakalatis NA, Brunner DP, Yem AW, Deibel MR Jr. Solution structure of human interleukin-1 receptor antagonist protein. *FEBS Lett* 1994;349:79–83.
200. Grutter MG, van Oostrum J, Priestle JP, et al. A mutational analysis of receptor binding sites of interleukin-1: differences in binding of human interleukin-1 mutants to human and mouse receptors. *Protein Eng* 1994;7:663–671.
201. Evans RJ, Bray J, Childs JD, et al. Mapping receptor binding sites in the IL-1 receptor antagonist and IL-1 by site-directed mutagenesis: identification of a single site in IL-1ra and two sites in IL-1. *J Biol Chem* 1995;270:11477–11483.
202. Ju G, Labriola-Tomkins E, Campen CA, et al. Conversion of the interleukin 1 receptor antagonist into an agonist by site-specific mutagenesis. *Proc Natl Acad Sci U S A* 1991;88:2658–2662.
203. Lennard AC. Interleukin-1 receptor antagonist. *Crit Rev Immunol* 1995;15:77–105.
204. Fenton MJ. Transcriptional and post-transcriptional regulation of interleukin 1 gene expression. *Int J Immunopharmacol* 1992;14: 401–411.
205. Auron PE, Webb AC. Interleukin-1: a gene expression system regulated at multiple levels. *Eur Cytokine Network* 1994;5:573–592.
206. Caput D, Beutler B, Hartog K, Thayer R, Brown-Shimer S, Cerami A. Identification of a common nucleotide sequence in the 38-untranslated region of the mRNA molecules specifying inflammatory mediators. *Proc Natl Acad Sci U S A* 1986;83:1670–1674.
207. Schindler R, Clark BD, Dinarello CA. Dissociation between interleukin-1 mRNA and protein synthesis in human peripheral blood mononuclear cells. *J Biol Chem* 1990;265:10232–10237.
208. Thornberry NA, Bull HG, Calacay JR, et al. A novel heterodimeric cysteine protease is required for interleukin-1 beta processing in monocytes. *Nature* 1992;356:768–774.
209. Cerretti DP, Kozlosky CJ, Mosley B, et al. Molecular cloning of the IL-1 processing enzme. *Science* 1992;256:97–100.
210. Wilson KP, Black JPA, Thomson JA, et al. Structure and mechanism of interleukin-1 converting enzyme. *Nature* 1994;370:270.
211. Li P, Allen H, Banerjee S, et al. Mice deficient in IL-1–converting enzyme are defective in production of mature IL-1 and resistant to endotoxic shock. *Cell* 1995;80:401–411.
212. Kuida K, Lippke JA, Ku G, Harding MW, Livingston DJ, Su MSS, Flavell RA. Altered cytokine export and apoptosis in mice deficient in interleukin-1 converting enzyme. *Science* 1995;267:167–200.
213. Colotta F, Dower SK, Sims JE, Mantovani A. The type II decoy receptor: a novel regulatory pathway for interleukin 1. *Immunol Today* 1994;15:562–566.
214. Kuno K, Matsushima K. The IL-1 receptor signaling pathway. *J Leukoc Biol* 1994;56:542–547.

215. Symons JA, Young PR, Duff GW. Soluble type II interleukin-1 (IL-1) receptor binds and blocks processing of IL-1 beta precursor and loses affinitiy for IL-1 receptor antagonist. *Proc Natl Acad Sci U S A* 1995;92:1714–1718.
216. O'Neill LA. Toward an understanding of the signal transduction pathways for interleukin-1. *Biochim Biophys Acta* 1995;1266:31–44.
217. Saklatvala J. Intracellular signalling mechanisms of interleukin-1 and tumour necrosis factor: possible targets for therapy. *Br Med Bull* 1995;51:401–418.
218. Bokemeyer D, Sorokin A, Yan M, Ahn NG, Templeton DJ, Dunn MJ. Induction of the mitogen-activated protein phosphatase by the stress activated protein kinase signalling pathway but not by extracellular-regulated kinase in fibroblasts. *J Biol Chem* 1996;271:639–642.
219. Kracht M, Shiroo M, Marshall CJ, Hsuan JJ, Saklatvala J. Interleukin 1 activates a novel protein kinase that phosphorylates the EGF receptor peptide T669. *Biochem J* 1994;302:897–905.
220. Kracht M, Truong O, Totty NF, Shiroo M, Saklatvala J. Interleukin 1 activates two forms of p54a MAP kinase in rabbit liver. *J Exp Med* 1994;180:2017–2025.
221. Freshney NW, Rawlinson L, Guesdon F, et al. Interleukin-1 activates a novel protein kinase cascade that results in phosphorylation of Hsp 27. *Cell* 1994;78:1039–1049.
222. Kolesnick R, Golde DW. The sphingomyelin pathway in tumour necrosis factor and interleukin-1 signalling. *Cell* 1994;77:325–328.
223. Hannun YA. The sphingomyelin cycle and the second messenger function of ceramide. *J Biol Chem* 1994;269:3125–3128.
224. Liu J, Mathias T, Yang Z, Kolesnick RN. Renaturation and tumour necrosis factor α stimulation of a 97 kDa ceramide-activated protein kinase. *J Biol Chem* 1994;269:3047–3052.
225. Dobrowsky RT, Kamibayashi C, Mimby MC, Hannun Y. Ceramide activates heterotrimeric protein phosphatase 2A. *J Biol Chem* 1993; 268:15523–15530.
226. Bogdan C, Nathan C. Modulation of macrophage functions by transforming growth factor-β, interleukin-4 and interleukin-10. *Ann NY Acad Sci* 1993;685:713–739.
227. Beasley D, McGuiggin ME, Dinarello CA. Human vascular smooth muscle cells produce an intracellular form of interleukin-1 receptor antagonist. *Am J Physiol* 1995;269:961–968.
228. Waldherr R, Noronha IL, Niemir Z, Kruger C, Stein H, Stumm G. Expression of cytokines and growth factors in human glomerulonephritis. *Pediatr Nephrol* 1993;7:471–478.
229. Karkar AM, Cashman SJ, Dash AC, Bonnfroy J-Y, Rees AJ. Direct evidence that interleukin-1β modulate antibody mediated glomerular injury in rats. *Clin Exp Immunol* 1992;90:312–318.
230. Tam FW, Smith J, Cashman SJ, Wang Y, Thompson EM, Rees AJ. Glomerular expression of interleukin-1 receptor antagonist and interleukin-1 beta genes in antibody-mediated glomerulonephritis. *Am J Pathol* 1994;145:126–136.
231. Lovett DH, Sterzel RB, Ryan JL, Atkins E. Production of an endogenous pyrogen by glomerular mesangial cells. *J Immunol* 1985;134: 670–672.
232. Werber HI, Emancipator SN, Tykocinski ML, Sedor JR. The interleukin-1 gene is expressed by rat glomerular mesangial cells and is augmented in immune complex glomerulonephritis. *J Immunol* 1987; 138:3207–3212.
233. Abbott F, Ryan JJ, Ceska M, Matsushima K, Sarraff CE, Rees AJ. Interleukin-1 beta stimulates human mesangial cells to synthesise and release interleukins-6 and -8. *Kidney Int* 1991;40:597–605.
234. Zoja C, Bettoni S, Morigi M, Remuzzi G, Rambaldi A. Interleukin-1 regulates cytokine gene expression in human mesangial cells through the interleukin-1 receptor type 1. *J Am Soc Nephrol* 1992;2: 1709–1715.
235. Sedor JR, Konieczkowski M, Huang S, et al. Cytokines, mesangial cell activation and glomerular injury. *Kidney Int* 1993;39:S65–70.
236. Fouqueray B, Boutard V, Phillipe C, et al. Mesangial cell–derived interleukin-10 modulates mesangial cell response to lipopolysaccharide. *Am J Pathol* 1995;147:176–182.
237. Matsumoto K. Production of interleukin-1 in glomerular cell cultures from rats with nephrotoxic serum nephritis. *Clin Exp Immunol* 1989; 75:123–128.
238. Matsumoto K, Dowling J, Atkins RC. Production of interleukin-1 in glomerular cell cultures from patients with rapidly progressive crescentic glomerulonephritis. *Am J Nephrol* 1988;8:463–470.
239. Noronha IL, Kruger C, Andrassy K, Ritz E, Waldherr R. In situ production of TNF-alpha, IL-1 beta and IL-2R in ANCA-positive glomerulonephritis. *Kidney Int* 1993;43:682–692.
240. Jenkins DA, Wojtacha DR, Swan P, Fleming S, Cumming AD. Intrarenal localization of interleukin-1 beta mRNA in crescentic glomerulonephritis. *Nephrol Dial Transplant* 1994;9:1228–1233.
241. Takemura T, Yoshioka K, Murakami K, et al. Cellular localization of inflammatory cytokines in human glomerulonephritis. *Virchows Arch* 1994;424:459–464.
242. Tang WW, Feng L, Mathison JC, Wilson CB. Cytokine expression, upregulation of intercellular adhesion molecule-1 and leukocyte infiltration in experimental tubulointerstitial nephritis. *Lab Invest* 1994; 70:631–638.
243. Karkar AM, Tam FW, Proudfoot AE, Meager A, Rees AJ. Modulation of antibody-mediated glomerular injury in vivo by interleukin-6. *Kidney Int* 1993;44:967–973.
244. Karkar AM, Rees AJ. Influence of subclinical infection on glomerular injury in heterologous nephrotoxic nephritis. *Clin Exp Immunol* 1994;98:295–299.
245. Karkar AM, Tam FWK, Steinkasserer A, et al. Modulation of antibody-mediated glomerular injury in vivo by IL-1ra, soluble IL-1 receptor and soluble TNF receptor. *Kidney Int* 1995;48:1738–1746.
246. Feng L, Tang WW, Loskutoff DJ, Wilson CB. Dysfunction of glomerular fibrinolysis in experimental antiglomerular basement membrane antibody glomerulonephritis. *J Am Soc Nephrol* 1993;3: 1753–1764.
247. Onbe T, Kashihara N, Yamasaki Y, Makino H, Ota Z. Expression of mRNA's of cytokines and growth factors in experimental glomerulonephritis. *Res Commun Mol Pathol Pharmacol* 1994;86:131–138.
248. Cook HT, Avey C, Taylor GM. Interleukin-1 beta gene expression in experimental glomerulonephritis in the rat: an in-situ hybridization study. *Int J Exp Pathol* 1994;75:157–163.
249. Nickeleit V, Zagachin L, Nishikawa K, Peters JH, Hynes RO, Colvin RB. Embryonic fibronectin isoforms are synthesised in crescents in experimental autoimmune glomerulonephritis. *Am J Pathol* 1995; 147:965–978.
250. Kiberd BA, Young ID. Modulation of glomerular structure and function in murine lupus nephritis by methylprednisolone and cyclophosphamide. *J Lab Clin Med* 1994;124:496–506.
251. Fan PY, Ruiz P, Pisetsky DS, Spurney RF. The effects of short-term treatment with the prostaglandin E1 (PGE1) analog misoprostol on inflammatory mediator production in murine lupus nephritis. *Clin Immunol Immunopathol* 1995;75:125–130.
252. Tang WW, Feng L, Vannice JL, Wilson CB. Interleukin-1 receptor antagonist ameliorates experimental anti-glomerular basement membrane antibody-associated glomerulonephritis. *J Clin Invest* 1994;93: 273–279.
253. Movat HZ, Cybulsky MI, Colditz IG, Chan MKW, Dinarello CA. Acute inflammation in gram-negative infection: endotoxin, interleukin-1, tumour necrosis factor and neutrophils. *Fed Proc* 1987;46: 97–104.
254. Pober JS, Cotran RS. Effects of cytokines on vascular endothelium: their role in vascular and immune injury. *Kidney Int* 1989;35: 969–975.
255. Baumann H, Prowse KR, Marinkovic S, Won KA, Jahreis GP. Stimulation of hepatic acute phase response by cytokines and glucocorticoids. *Ann NY Acad Sci* 1989;557:280–295.
256. Havell EA, Moldawer LL, Helfgott D, Killian PL, Sehgal PB. Type I IL-1 receptor blockade exacerbates murine listeriosis. *J Immunol* 1992;148:1486–1492.
257. Mancilla J, Garcia P, Dinarello CA. IL-1 receptor antagonist can either protect or enhance the lethality of *Klebsiella pneumoniae* sepsis in newborn rats. *Infect Immun* 1993;61:926–932.
258. Le J, Vilcek J. Interleukin 6: a multifunctional cytokine regulating immune reactions and the acute phase protein response. *Lab Invest* 1989;61:588–600.
259. Hartner A, Sterzel RB, Reindl N, Hocke GM, Fey GH, Goppelt-Struebe M. Cytokine-induced expression of leukemia inhibitory factor in renal mesangial cells. *Kidney Int* 1994;45:1562–1571.
260. Abbott F, Tam FWK, Ryan JJ, Rees AJ. Human mesangial cells synthesise interleukin-1α but not interleukin 1β, interleukin receptor antagonist or tumour necrosis factor. *Nephrol Dial Transplant* 1992; 7:997–1001.
261. Coroneos E, Martinez M, McKenna S, Kester M. Differential regulation of sphingomyelinase and ceramidase activities by growth factors

and cytokines. Implications for cellular proliferation and differentiation. *J Biol Chem* 1995;270:23305–23309.

262. Marti HP, McNeil L, Davies M, Martin J, Lovett DH. Homology cloning of rat 72 kDa type IV collagenase: cytokine and second messenger inducibility in glomerular mesangial cells. *Biochem J* 1993; 291:441–446.
263. Marti HP, McNeil L, Thomas G, Davies M, Lovett DH. Molecular characterisation of a low-molecular-mass matrix metalloproteinase secreted by glomerular mesangial cells as PUMP-1. *Biochem J* 1992; 285:899–905.
264. Kunz D, Walker G, Pfeilschifter J. Dexamethasone differentially affects interleukin-1 and cyclic AMP–induced nitric oxide synthase mRNA expression in renal mesangial cells. *Biochem J* 1994;304: 337–340.
264a. Jones SA, Hancock JT, Jones OT, Neubauer A, Topley N. The expression of NADPH oxidase components in human glomerular mesangial cells: detection of protein and mRNA for p47phox, p67phox, and p22phox. *J Am Soc Nephrol* 1995;5:1483–1491.
265. Baud L, Ardaillou R. Tumour necrosis factor in renal injury. *Miner Electrolyte Metab* 1995;21:336–341.
266. Tetsuka T, Daphna-Iken D, Srivastava SK, Morrison AR. Regulation of heme oxygenase mRNA in mesangial cells: prostaglandin E2 negatively modulates interleukin-1 induced heme oxygenase mRNA. *Biochem Biophys Res Commun* 1995;212:617–623.
267. Walker G, Kunz D, Pignat W, van den Bosch H, Pfeilschifter J. Pyrrolidine dithiocarbamate differentially effects cytokine and cAMP-induced expression of group II phospholipase A2 in rat renal mesangial cells. *FEBS Lett* 1995;364:218–222.
268. Vervoordeldonk MJ, Schalkwijk CG, Vishwanath BS, Aarsman AJ, van den Bosch H. Levels and localization of group II phospholipase A2 and annexin I in interleukin and dexamethasone treated rat mesangial cells: evidence against annexin mediation of the dexamethasone induced inhibition of group II phospholipase A2. *Biochim Biophys Acta* 1994;1224:541–550.
269. Coyne DW, Nickols M, Bertrand W, Morrison AR. Regulation of mesangial cell cyclooxygenase synthesis by cytokines and glucocorticoids. *Am J Physiol* 1992;263:97–102.
270. Schalkwijk CG, de Vet E, Pfeilschifter J, van den Bosch H. Interleukin-1 and transforming growth factor-beta 2 enhance cytosolic high-molecular mass phospholipase A2 activity and induce prostaglandin E2 formation in rat mesangial cells. *Eur J Biochem* 1992;210:169–176.
271. Schalkwijk GG, Veroordeldonk M, Pfeilschifter J, van den Bosch H. Interleukin-1–induced cytosolic phospholipase A2 activity and protein synthesis is blocked by dexamethasone in rat mesangial cells. *FEBS Lett* 1993;333:339–343.
272. Nakazato Y, Okada H, Sato A, et al. Interleukin-4 downregulates cell growth and prostaglandin release of human mesangial cells. *Biochem Biophys Res Commun* 1993;197:486–493.
273. Teksuka T, Morrison AR. Tyrosine kinase activation is necessary for inducible nitric oxide synthase expression by interleukin-1. *Am J Physiol* 1995;269:55–59.
274. Rzymkiewicz DM, DuMaine J, Morrison AR. IL-1 regulates rat mesangial cyclooxygenase II gene expression by tyrosine phosphorylation. *Kidney Int* 1995;47:1354–1363.
275. Srivastava SK, Tetsuka T, Daphna-Iken D, Morrison AR. IL-1 stabilizes COX II mRNA in renal mesangial cells: role of 3′-untranslated region. *Am J Physiol* 1994;267:504–508.
276. Tetsuka T, Daphna-Iken D, Srivastava SK, Baier LD, DuMaine J, Morrison AR. Cross-talk between cyclooxygenase and nitric oxide pathways: prostaglandin E2 negatively modulates induction of nitric oxide synthase by interleukin-1. *Proc Natl Acad Sci U S A* 1994;91: 12168–12172.
277. Tomosugi NI, Cashman SJ, Hay H. Modulation of antibody mediated glomerular injury in vivo by bacterial lipopolysaccharide tumour necrosis factor and IL-1. *J Immunol* 1989;142:3083–3090.
278. Lan HY, Nikolic-Paterson DJ, Zarama M, Vannice JL, Atkins RC. Suppression of experimental crescentic glomerulonephritis by the interleukin-1 receptor antagonist. *Kidney Int* 1993;43:479–485.
279. Lan HY, Nikolic-Paterson DJ, Mu W, Vannice JL, Atkins RC. Interleukin-1 receptor antagonist halts the progression of established crescentic glomerulonephritis in the rat. *Kidney Int* 1995;47:1303–1309.
280. Zurawski SM, Chomarat P, Djossou O, et al. The primary binding subunit of the human interleukin-4 receptor is also a component of the interleukin-13 receptor. *J Biol Chem* 1995;270:13869–13878.
281. Walter MR, Cook WJ, Zhao BG, et al. Crystal structure of recombinant human interleukin-4. *J Biol Chem* 1992;267:20371–20376
282. Ihle N. Cytokine receptor signalling. *Nature* 1995;377:591–594.
283. Mosley B, Beckmann MP, March CJ, et al. The murine interleukin-4 receptor: molecular cloning and characterization of secreted and membrane bound forms. *Cell* 1989;59:335–348.
284. Garrone P, Djossou O, Galizzi JP, Banchereau J. A recombinant extracellular domain of the human interleukin-4 receptor inhibits the biological effects of interleukin-4 on T and B lymphocytes. *Eur J Immunol* 1991;21:1365–1369.
285. Obiri NI, Debinski W, Leondard WJ, Puri RK. Receptor for interleukin 13. Interaction with interleukin 4 by a mechanism that does not involve the common gamma chain shared by receptors for interleukins 2, 4, 7, 9 and 15. *J Biol Chem* 1995;270:8797–8804.
286. Kishimoto T, Taga T, Akira S. Cytokine signal transduction. *Cell* 1994;76:253–262.
287. Wang LM, Keegan A, Frankel M, Paul WE, Pierce JH. Signal transduction through the IL-4 and insulin receptor families. *Stem Cells* 1995;13:360–368
288. Merville P, Pouteil-Noble C, Wijdenes J, Potaux L, Touraine JL, Banchereau J. Detection of single cells secreting IFN-gamma, IL-6 and IL-10 in irreversibly rejected human kidney allografts, and their modulation by IL-2 and IL-4. *Transplantation* 1993;55:639–646.
289. Okada H, Konishi K, Nakazato Y, et al. Interleukin-4 expression in mesangial proliferative glomerulonephritis. *Am J Kidney Dis* 1994;23:242–246.
290. Coers W, Vos JT, Van der Meide PH, Van der Horst ML, Huitema S, Weening JJ. Interferon-gamma (IFN-gamma) and IL-4 expressed during mercury-induced membranous nephropathy are toxic for cultured podocytes. *Clin Exp Immunol* 1995;102:297–307.
291. Gillespie KM, Qasim FJ, Tibbatts LM, Thiru S, Oliveira DB, Mathieson PW. Interleukin-4 gene expression in mercury-induced autoimmunity. *Scand J Immunol* 1995;41:268–272.
292. Tsai CY, Wu TH, Huang SF, et al. Abnormal splenic and thymic IL-4 and TNF-alpha expression in MRL-1pr/1pr mice. *Scand J Immunol* 1995;41:157–163.
293. Lakkis FG, Cruet EN. Cloning of rat interleukin-13 (IL-13) cDNA and analysis of IL-13 gene expression in experimental glomerulonephritis. *Biochem Biophys Res Commun* 1993;197:612–618.
294. Zurawski G, de Vries JE. Interleukin-13, an interleukin-4–like cytokine that acts on monocytes and B cells, but not on T cells. *Immunol Today* 1994;15:19–26.
295. Bogdan C, Nathan C. Modulation of macrophage functions by transforming growth factor-β, interleukin-4 and interleukin-10. *Ann NY Acad Sci* 1994;685:713–739.
296. de Waal Malefyt R, Figdor CG, de Vries JE. Effects of interleukin 4 on monocyte functions: comparison to interleukin 13. *Res Immunol* 1993;144:629–633.
297. Colotta F, Re F, Muzio M, et al. Interleukin-13 (IL-13) induces expression and release of the interleukin-1 (IL-1) decoy receptor in human polymorphonuclear cells. *J Biol Chem* 1994;269:12403–12406.
298. Sironi M, Sciacca FL, Matteucci C, et al. Regulation of endothelial and mesothelial cell function by interleukin-13: selective induction of vascular cell adhesion molecule-1 and amplification of interleukin-6 production. *Blood* 1994;84:1913–1921.
299. Herbert JM, Savi P, Laplace MC, et al. IL-4 and IL-13 exhibit comparable abilities to reduce pyrogen-induced expression of procoagulant activity in endothelial cells and monocytes. *FEBS Lett* 1993;328: 268–270.
300. Nakazato Y, Okada H, Sato A, et al. Interleukin-4 downregulates cell growth and prostaglandin release of human mesangial cells. *Biochem Biophys Res Commun* 1993;197:486–493.
301. Seder RA, Paul WE. Aquisition of lymphokine producing phenotype by $CD4^+$ cells. *Annu Rev Immunol* 1994;12:635–673.
302. Pearce EJ, Reiner SL. Induction of Th2 responses in infectious diseases. *Curr Opin Immunol* 1995;7:497–504.
303. Tam FWK, Smith J, Karkar AM, Pusey CD. Interleukin (IL-4) upregulates decoy receptor for IL-1 and ameliorates nephrotoxic nephritis. *J Am Soc Nephrol* 1995;6:1767.
304. Le J, Vilcek J. Interleukin-6: a multifunctional cytokine regulating immune reactions and the acute phase protein response. *Lab Invest* 1989;61:588–602.
305. Hirano T. Interleukin-6 and its relation to inflammation and disease. *Clin Immunol Immunopathol* 1992;62:60–65.

306. Ihle N. Cytokine receptor signalling. *Nature* 1995;377:591–594.
307. Murakami M, Hibi M, Nakagawa T, et al. IL-6 induced homodimerization of gp 130 and associated activiation of a tyrosine kinase. *Science* 1993;260:1808–1810.
308. Nakajima M, Kinoshita S, Sasagawa T, et al. Phosphorylation at threonine-235 by a ras-dependent mitogen-activated protein kinase cascade is essential for transcription factor NF-IL6. *Proc Natl Acad Sci U S A* 1993;90:2207–2211.
309. Abbott F, Ryan JJ, Ceska M, Matsushima K, Sarraff CE, Rees AJ. Interleukin-1 beta stimulates human mesangial cells to synthesise and release interleukins-6 and -8. *Kidney Int* 1991;40:597–605.
310. Horii Y, Muraguchi A, Iwano M, et al. Involvement of IL-6 in mesangial proliferative glomerulonephritis. *J Immunol* 1989;143: 3949–3955.
311. Ruef C, Budde K, Lacy J, et al. Interleukin-6 is an autocrine growth factor for mesangial cells. *Kidney Int* 1990;38:249–257.
312. Morcos M , Hansch GM, Schonermark M, Ellwanger S, Harle M, Heckl-Ostreicher B. Human glomerular mesangial cells express CD16 and may be stimulated via this receptor. *Kidney Int* 1994;46: 1627–1634.
313. van den Dobbelsteen ME, van der Woude FJ, Schroeijers WE, van den Wall Bake AW, van Es LA, Daha MR. Binding of dimeric and polymeric IgA to rat renal mesangial cells enhances the release of interleukin-6. *Kidney Int* 1994;46:512–519.
314. van den Dobbelsteen MEA, van der Woude FJ, Schroejers WE, van Es LA, Daha MR. Soluble aggregates of IgG and immune complexes enhance IL-6 production by renal mesangial cells. *Kidney Int* 1993; 43:544–553.
315. Sedor JR. Cytokines and growth factors in renal injury. *Seminars in Nephrology* 1992;12:428–440.
316. Moriyama T, Fujibayashi M, Fujiwara Y, et al. Antiotensin II stimulates interleukin-6 release from cultured mouse mesangial cells. *J Am Soc Nephrol* 1995;6:95–101.
317. Ruef C, Kashgarian M, Coleman DL. Mesangial cell-matrix interactions: effects on mesangial cell growth and cytokine secretion. *Am J Pathol* 1992;141:429–439.
318. Hartner A, Sterzel RB, Reindl N, Hocke GM, Fey GH, Goppelt-Struebe M. Cytokine-induced expression of leukemia inhibitory factor in renal mesangial cells. *Kidney Int* 1994;45:1562–1571.
319. Moutabarrik A, Nakanishi I, Ishibashi M. Interleukin-6 and interleukin-6 receptor are expressed by cultured glomerular epithelial cells. *Scand J Immunol* 1994;40:181–186.
320. Nakamura A, Kohsaka T, John EJ. Differential regulation of interleukin-6 production in the kidney by the renal sympathetic nerves in normal and spontaneously hypertensive rats. *J Hypertens* 1993;11: 491–497.
321. Waldherr R, Noronha IL, Niemir Z, Kruger C, Stein H, Stumm G. Expression of cytokines and growth factors in human glomerulonephritis. *Pediatr Nephrol* 1993;7:471–478.
322. Ito Y, Fukatsu A, Baba M, Mizuno M, Ichida S, Sado Y, Matsuo S. Pathogenic significance of interleukin-6 in a patient with anti-glomerular basement membrane antibody-induced glomerulonephritis with multinucleated giant cells. *Am J Kidney Dis* 1995;26: 72–79.
323. Chen WP, Lin CY. Augmented expression of interleukin-6 and interleukin-1 genes in the mesangium of IgM mesangial nephropathy. *Nephron* 1994;68:10–19.
324. Hori Y, Iwano M, Hirata E, et al. Role of interleukin-6 in the progression of mesangial proliferative glomerulonephritis. *Kidney Int* 1993;43(suppl 39):71–75.
325. Malide D, Russo P, Bendayan M. Presence of tumor necrosis factor alpha and interleukin-6 in renal mesangial cells of lupus nephritis patients. *Hum Pathol* 1995;26:558–564.
326. Suzuki D, Miyazaki M, Naka R, et al. In situ hybridization of interleukin 6 in diabetic nephropathy. *Diabetes* 1995;44:233–238.
327. Ohta K, Takano N, Seno A, et al. Detection of clinical usefulness of urinary interleukin-6 in the diseases of the kidney and the urinary tract. *Clin Nephrol* 1992;38:185–189.
328. Hirata E, Iwano M, Hirayama T, et al. Rapid measurement of urinary IL-6 by ELISA: urinary IL-6 as a marker of mesangial proliferation. *Nippon Jinzo Gakkai Shi* 1994;36:33–37.
329. Dohi K, Iwano M, Muraguchi A, et al. The prognostic significance of urinary interleukin-6 in IgA nephropathy. *Clin Nephrol* 1991;35:1–5.
330. Gordon C, Richards N, Howie AJ, et al. Urinary IL-6: a marker for mesangial proliferative glomerulonephritis? *Clin Exp Immunol* 1991; 86:145–149.
331. Nakamura A, Suzuki T, Kohsaka T. Renal tubular function modulates urinary levels of interleukin-6. *Nephron* 1995;70:416–420.
332. Ruef C, Budde K, Lacy J, et al. Interleukin-6 is an autocrine growth factor for mesangial cells. *Kidney Int* 1991;38:249–257.
333. Zoja C, Benigni A, Piccinini G, Figliuzzi M, Longaretti L, Remuzzi G. Interleukin-6 stimulates gene expression matrix components in bovine mesangial cells in culture. *Mediators Inflamm* 1993;2:429–433.
334. Floege J, Topley N, Hoppe J, Barrett TB, Resch K. Mitogenic effect of platelet-derived growth factor in human glomerular mesangial cells: modulation and/or suppression by inflammatory cytokines. *Clin Exp Immunol* 1991;86:334–341.
335. Ikeda M, Ikeda U, Ohara T, Kusano E, Kano S. Recombinant interleukin-6 inhibits the growth of rat mesangial cells in culture. *Am J Pathol* 1992;141:327–334.
336. Naitoh Y, Fukata J, Tominaga T, et al. Interleukin-6 stimulates the secretion of adrenocorticotropic hormone in conscious freely moving rats. *Biochem Biophys Res Commun* 1988;155:1459–1463.
337. Baumann H, Prowse KR, Marinkovic S, Won KA, Jahreis GP. Stimulation of hepatic acute phase response by cytokines and glucocorticoids. *Ann NY Acad Sci* 1989;557:280–295
338. Schindler R, Clark BD, Dinarello CA. Dissociation between interleukin-1 mRNA and protein synthesis in human peripheral blood mononuclear cells. *J Biol Chem* 1990;265:10232–10237.
339. Tilg H, Trehu E, Atkins MB, Dinarello CA, Mier JW. Interleukin-6 (IL-6) as an anti-flammatory cytokine: induction of circulating IL-1 receptor antagonist and soluble tumour necrosis factor receptor p55. *Blood* 1994;83:113–118.
340. Ulich TR, Yin S, Guo K, Yi ES, Remick D, Castillo J. Intratracheal injection of endotoxin and cytokines. II. Interleukin-6 and transforming growth factor beta inhibit acute inflammation. *Am J Pathol* 1991; 138:1097–1101.
341. Denis M. Interleukin-6 in mouse hypersensitivity pneumonitis: changes in lung free cells following depletion of endogenous IL-6 or direct administration of IL-6. *J Leukoc Biol* 1992;52:197–201.
342. Bogdan C, Nathan C. Modulation of macrophage functions by transforming growth factor-β, interleukin-4 and interleukin-10. *Ann NY Acad Sci* 1993;685:713–739.
343. Lennard AC. Interleukin-1 receptor antagonist. *Crit Rev Immunol* 1995;15:77–105
344. Colotta F, Dower SK, Sims JE, Mantovani A. The type II decoy receptor: a novel regulatory pathway for interleukin 1. *Immunol Today* 1994;15:562–566.
345. Suematsu S, Matsuda T, Aozasa K, et al. IgG_1 plasmacytosis in interleukin-6 transgenic mice. *Proc Natl Acad Sci U S A* 1989;86:7547.
346. Fattori E, Della Rocca C, Costa P, et al. Development of progressive kidney damage and myeloma kidney in interleukin-6 transgenic mice. *Blood* 1994;83:2570–2579.
347. Shen MM, Skoda RC, Cardiff RD, Campos-Torres J, Leder P, Ornitz DM. Expression of LIF transgenic mice results in altered thymic epithelium and apparent interconversion of thymic and lymph node morphologies. *EMBO J* 1994;13:1375–1385.
348. Hawley RG, Fong AZ, Burns BF, Hawley TS. Transplantable myeloproliferative disease induced in mice by an interleukin 6 retrovirus. *J Exp Med* 1992;176:1149–1163
349. Eitner F, Westerhuis R, Burg M, et al. On the role of interleukin-6 in mediating mesangial cell proliferation and matirix production in vivo. *Kidney Int* (in press).
350. Ryffel B, Car BD, Gunn H, Roman D, Hiestand P, Mihatsch MJ. Interleukin-6 exacerbates glomerulonephritis in (NZB × NZw) F1 mice. *Am J Pathol* 1994;144:927–937.
351. Finck BK, Chan B, Wofsy D. Interleukin 6 promotes murine lupus in NZB/NZW F1 mice. *J Clin Invest* 1994;94:585–591.
352. Kiberd BA. Interleukin-6 receptor blockage ameliorates murine lupus nephritis. *J Am Soc Nephrol* 1993;4:58–61.
353. Karkar AM, Smith J, Proudfoot A, Rees AJ. Anti-inflammatory effect of IL-6 in experimental nephritis. *Cytokine* 1995;27:619 (abstract).
354. Mosmann TR. Properties and functions of interleukin-10. *Adv Immunol* 1994;56:1–26.
355. Bazan JF. Shared architecture of hormone binding domains in type I and II interferon receptors. *Cell* 1990;61:753–754
356. de Waal Malefyt R, Adrams J, Bennett B, Figdor CG, de Vries JE. Interleukin-10 (IL-10) inhibits cytokine synthesis by human mono-

cytes: an autoregulatory role of IL-10 produced by monocytes. *J Exp Med* 1991:174:1209–1220.
357. Broski AP, Halloran PF. Tissue distribution of IL-10 mRNA in normal mice. Evidence that a component of IL-10 expression is T and B cell–independent and increased by irradiation. *Transplantation* 1994; 57:582–592.
358. Matsumoto K. Decreased release of IL-10 by monocytes from patients with lipoid nephrosis. *Clin Exp Immunol* 1995;102:603–607.
359. Bogdan C, Nathan C. Modulation of macrophage functions by transforming growth factor–β, interleukin-4 and interleukin-10. *Ann NY Acad Sci* 1993;685:713–739.
360. D'Andrea A, Aste-Amezaga M, Valiante NM, Ma X, Kubin M, Trinchieri G. Interleukin-10 (IL-10) inhibits human lymphocyte interferon production by suppressing natural killer cell stimulatory factor IL-12 synthesis in accessory cells. *J Exp Med* 1993;178:1041–1048.
361. Joyce DA, Gibbons DP, Green P, Steer JH, Feldmann M, Brennan FM. Two inhibitors of pro-inflammatory cytokine release, interleukin-10 and interleukin-4, have contrasting effects on the release of soluble p75 tumour necrosis factor receptor by cultured monocytes. *Eur J Immunol* 1994;24:2699.
362. Fouqueray B, Boutard V, Phillipe C, et al. Mesangial cell–derived interleukin-10 modulates mesangial cell response to lipopolysaccharide. *Am J Pathol* 1995;147:176–182.
363. Gerard C, Bruyns C, Marchant A, et al. Interleukin-10 reduces the release of tumour necrosis factor and prevents lethality in experimental endotoxemia. *J Exp Med* 1993;177:547.
364. Marchant A, Bruyns C, Vandenabeele P, et al. IL-10 controls IFN-γ and TNF production during experimental endotoxemia. *Eur J Immunol* 1994;24:1167.
365. Ishida H, Muchamuel T, Sakaguchi S, Andrade S, Menon S, Howard M. Continuous administration of anti–interleukin-10 antibodies delays onset of autoimminuty in NZB/W F1 mice. *J Exp Med* 1994; 179:305–310.
366. Rott O, Fleischer R, Cash E. Interleukin-10 prevents experimental allergic encephalomyelitis in rats. *Eur J Immunol* 1994;24: 1434–1440.
367. Sariola H, Saarma M, Sainio K, et al. Dependence of kidney morphogenesis on the expression of nerve growth factor receptor. *Science* 1991;254:571–573.
368. Otten U, Ehrhard P, Peck R. Nerve growth factor induces growth and differentiation of human B lymphocytes. *Proc Natl Acad Sci U S A* 1989;86:10059–10063.
369. Steiner P, Pfeilschifter J, Boeckh C, Radeke H, Otten U. Interleukin-1 beta and tumor necrosis factor-alpha synergistically stimulate nerve growth factor synthesis in rat mesangial cells. *Am J Physiol* 1991; 261:F792–798.
370. Barajas L, Salido EC, Laborde NP, Fisher DA. Nerve growth factor immunoreactivity in mouse kidney: an immunoelectron microscopic study. *J Neurosci Res* 1987;18:418–424.
371. Alpers CE, Hudkins KL, Ferguson M, Johnson RJ, Schatteman GC, Bothwell M. Nerve growth factor receptor expression in fetal, mature, and diseased human kidneys. *Lab Invest* 1993;69:703–713.
372. Salido EC, Barajas L, Lechago J, Laborde NP, Fisher DA. Immunocytochemical localization of nerve growth factor in mouse kidney. *J Neurosci Res* 1986;16:457–465.
373. Alpers CE, Hudkins KL, Davis CL, et al. Expression of vascular cell adhesion molecule-1 in kidney allograft rejection. *Kidney Int* 1993; 44:805–816.
374. Heldin CH, Ostman A, Westermark B. Structure of platelet-derived growth factor: implications for functional properties. *Growth Factors* 1993;8:245–252.
375. Ross R. Platelet-derived growth factor. *Lancet* 1989;1:1179–1182.
376. Heldin CH, Ostman A, Eriksson A, Siegbahn A, Claesson-Welsh L, Westermark B. Platelet-derived growth factor: isoform-specific signalling via heterodimeric or homodimeric receptor complexes. *Kidney Int* 1992;41:571–574.
377. Abboud HE. Platelet-derived growth factor and mesangial cells. *Kidney Int* 1992;41:581–583.
378. Floege J, Johnson RJ. Multiple roles for platelet-derived growth factor in renal disease. *Miner Electrolyte Metab* 1995;21:271–282.
379. Daniel TO, Kumjian DA. Platelet-derived growth factor receptors and phospholipase C activation. *Kidney Int* 1992;41:575–580.
380. Rupprecht HD, Sukhatme VP, Lacy J, Sterzel RB, Coleman DL. PDGF-induced egr-1 expression in rat mesangial cells is mediated through upstream serum response elements. *Am J Physiol* 1993;265: F351–360.
381. Alpers CE, Hudkins KL, Ferguson M, Johnson RJ, Rutledge JC. Platelet-derived growth factor A-chain expression in developing and mature human kidneys and in Wilms tumor. *Kidney Int* 1995;48: 146–154.
382. Gesualdo L, Pinzani M, Floriano JJ, et al. Platelet-derived growth factor expression in mesangial proliferative glomerulonephritis. *Lab Invest* 1991;65:160–167.
383. Iida H, Seifert R, Alpers CE, et al. Platelet-derived growth factor (PDGF) and PDGF receptor are induced in mesangial proliferative nephritis in the rat. *Proc Natl Acad Sci U S A* 1991;88:6560–6564.
384. Yoshimura A, Gordon K, Alpers CE, et al. Demonstration of PDGF B-chain mRNA in glomeruli in mesangial proliferative nephritis by in situ hybridization. *Kidney Int* 1991;40:470–476.
385. Alpers CE, Seifert RA, Hudkins KL, Johnson RJ, Bowen-Pope DF. Developmental patterns of PDGF B-chain, PDGF-receptor and alpha-actin expression in human glomerulogenesis. *Kidney Int* 1992;42: 390–399.
386. Shultz PJ, DiCorleto PE, Silver BJ, Abboud HE. Mesangial cells express PDGF mRNAs and proliferate in response to PDGF. *Am J Physiol* 1988;255:F674–F684.
387. Floege J, Johnson RJ, Alpers CE, et al. Visceral glomerular epithelial cells can proliferate in vivo and synthesize platelet-derived growth factor B-chain. *Am J Pathol* 1993;142:637–650.
388. Silver BJ, Jaffer FE, Abboud HE. Platelet-derived growth factor synthesis in mesangial cells: induction by multiple peptide mitogens. *Proc Natl Acad Sci U S A* 1989;86:1056–1060.
389. Daniel TO, Gibbs VC, Milfay DF, Garovoy MR, Williams LT. Thrombin stimulates *c-sis* gene expression in microvascular endothelial cells. *J Biol Chem* 1986;261:9579–9582.
390. Frank J, Engler-Blum G, Rodemann HP, Müller GA. Human renal tubular cells as a cytokine source: PDGF-B, GM-CSF and IL-6 mRNA expression in vitro. *Exp Nephrol* 1993;1:26–35.
391. Knecht A, Fine LG, Kleinman KS, et al. Fibroblasts of rabbit kidney in culture. II. Paracrine stimulation of papillary fibroblasts by PDGF. *Am J Physiol* 1991;261:F292–299.
392. Lonnemann G, Müller GA, Koch KM. Regulation of PDGF expression in human renal fibroblasts by interleukin-1 receptor antagonist. *J Am Soc Nephrol* 1994;5:756.
393. Gesualdo L, Di Paolo S, Milani S, et al. Expression of platelet-derived growth factor receptors in normal and diseased human kidney. *J Clin Invest* 1994;94:50–58.
394. Fellström B, Klareskog L, Heldin CH, et al. Platelet-derived growth factor receptors in the kidney—upregulated expression in inflammation. *Kidney Int* 1989;36:1099–1102.
395. Alpers CE, Seifert RA, Hudkins KL, Johnson RJ, Bowen Pope DF. PDGF-receptor localizes to mesangial, parietal epithelial, and interstitial cells in human and primate kidneys. *Kidney Int* 1993;43:286–294.
396. Floege J, Burns MW, Alpers CE, et al. Glomerular cell proliferation and PDGF expression precede glomerulosclerosis in the remnant kidney model. *Kidney Int* 1992;41:297–309.
397. Nakamura T, Ebihara I, Nagaoka I, Tomino Y, Koide H. Activated peripheral blood mononuclear cells in IgA nephropathy express platelet-derived growth factor B-chain messenger RNA. *J Lab Clin Med* 1992;120:212–221.
398. Nakamura T, Ebihara I, Nagaoka I, Tomino Y, Koide H. Renal platelet-derived growth factor gene expression in NZB/W F1 mice with lupus and ddY mice with IgA nephropathy. *Clin Immunol Immunopathol* 1992;63:173–181.
399. Akai Y, Iwano M, Kitamura Y, et al. Intraglomerular expressions of IL-1 alpha and platelet-derived growth factor (PDGF-B) mRNA in experimental immune complex-mediated glomerulonephritis. *Clin Exp Immunol* 1994;95:29–34.
400. Barnes JL, Abboud HE. Temporal expression of autocrine growth factors corresponds to morphological features of mesangial proliferation in Habu snake venom–induced glomerulonephritis. *Am J Pathol* 1993;143:1366–1376.
401. Fukui M, Nakamura T, Ebihara I, Nagaoka I, Tomino Y, Koide H. Low-protein diet attenuates increased gene expression of platelet-derived growth factor and transforming growth factor-beta in experimental glomerular sclerosis. *J Lab Clin Med* 1993;121:224–234.
402. Feng L, Tang WW, Xia Y, Wilson CB. Growth factor, extracellular matrix and protease inhibitor mRNA expression in anti-GBM anti-

body associated glomerulonephritis. *J Am Soc Nephrol* 1992;3:468.
403. Young BA, Johnson RJ, Alpers CE, et al. Cellular events in the evolution of experimental diabetic nephropathy. *Kidney Int* 1995;47:935–944.
404. Frampton G, Hildreth G, Hartley B, Cameron JS, Heldin CH, Wasteson A. Could platelet-derived growth factor have a role in the pathogenesis of lupus nephritis? [Letter]. *Lancet* 1988;2:343
405. Nakajima M, Hewitson TD, Mathews DC, Kincaid Smith P. Platelet-derived growth factor mesangial deposits in mesangial IgA glomerulonephritis. *Nephrol Dial Transplant* 1991;6:11–16.
406. Waldherr R, Noronha IL, Niemir Z, Kruger C, Stein H, Stumm G. Expression of cytokines and growth factors in human glomerulonephritides. *Pediatr Nephrol* 1993;7:471–478.
407. Niemir ZI, Stein H, Noronha IL, et al. PDGF and TGF-beta contribute to the natural course of human IgA glomerulonephritis. *Kidney Int* 1995;48:1530–1541.
408. Yoshimura A, Inui K, Suzuki T, et al. Demonstration of PDGF B-chain mRNA in the cellular crescent in human glomerular diseases. *J Am Soc Nephrol* 1993;4:692
409. Marx M, Daniel TO, Kashgarian M, Madri JA. Spatial organization of the extracellular matrix modulates the expression of PDGF-receptor subunits in mesangial cells. *Kidney Int* 1993;43:1027–1041.
410. Floege J, Topley N, Hoppe J, Barrett TB, Resch K. Mitogenic effect of platelet-derived growth factor in human glomerular mesangial cells: modulation and/or suppression by inflammatory cytokines. *Clin Exp Immunol* 1991;86:334–341.
411. Haberstroh U, Zahner G, Disser M, Thaiss F, Wolf G, Stahl RA. TGF-β stimulates rat mesangial cell proliferation in culture: role of PDGF β-receptor expression. *Am J Physiol* 1993;264:F199–205.
412. Grone EF, Abboud HE, Hohne M, et al. Actions of lipoproteins in cultured human mesangial cells: modulation by mitogenic vasoconstrictors. *Am J Physiol* 1992;263:F686–696.
413. Jaffer FE, Knauss TC, Poptic E, Abboud HE. Endothelin stimulates PDGF secretion in cultured human mesangial cells. *Kidney Int* 1990;38:1193–1198.
414. Grandaliano G, Biswas P, Choudhury GG, Abboud HE. Simvastatin inhibits PDGF-induced DNA synthesis in human glomerular mesangial cells. *Kidney Int* 1993;44:503–508.
415. Mene P, Dunn MJ. Prostaglandins and rat glomerular mesangial cell proliferation. *Kidney Int* 1990;37:1256–1262.
416. Floege J, Eng E, Young BA, et al. Infusion of platelet-derived growth factor or basic fibroblast growth factor induces selective glomerular mesangial cell proliferation and matrix accumulation in rats. *J Clin Invest* 1993;92:2952–2962.
417. Isaka Y, Fujiwara Y, Ueda N, Kaneda Y, Kamada T, Imai E. Glomerulosclerosis induced by in vivo transfection of transforming growth factor-beta or platelet-derived growth factor gene into the rat kidney. *J Clin Invest* 1993;92:2597–2601.
418. Tang WW, Ulich TR, Lacey DL, et al. PDGF-BB induces renal tubulointerstitial myofibroblast formation and tubulointerstitial fibrosis. *Am J Pathol* 1996;148:1169–1180.
419. Soriano P. Abnormal kidney development and hematological disorders in PDGF beta-receptor mutant mice. *Genes Dev* 1994;8:1887–1896.
420. Leveen P, Pekny M, Gebre-Medhin S, Swollin B, Larsson E, Betsholtz C. Mice deficient for PDGF B show renal, cardiovascular, and hematological abnormalities. *Genes Dev* 1994;8:1875–1887.
421. Doi T, Vlassara H, Kirstein M, Yamada Y, Striker GE, Striker LJ. Receptor-specific increase in extracellular matrix production in mouse mesangial cells by advanced glycosylation end products is mediated via platelet-derived growth factor. *Proc Natl Acad Sci U S A* 1992;89:2873–2877.
422. Throckmorton DC, Brogden AP, Min B, Rasmussen H, Kashgarian M. PDGF and TGF-beta mediate collagen production by mesangial cells exposed to advanced glycosylation end products. *Kidney Int* 1995;48:111–117.
423. Abboud HE, Woodruff KA, Synder SP, Bonewald LF. Polypeptide growth factors regulate the production of latent transforming growth factor-1 in human mesangial cells. *J Am Soc Nephrol* 1991;2:434.
424. Barnes JL, Hevey KA. Glomerular mesangial cell migration in response to platelet-derived growth factor. *Lab Invest* 1990;62:379–382.
425. Floege J, Topley N, Wessel K, et al. Monokines and platelet-derived growth factor modulate prostanoid production in growth arrested, human mesangial cells. *Kidney Int* 1990;37:859–869.
426. Humes HD, Beals TF, Cieslinski DA, Sanchez IO, Page TP. Effects of transforming growth factor-beta, transforming growth factor-alpha, and other growth factors on renal proximal tubule cells. *Lab Invest* 1991;64:538–545.
427. Wiedmeier SE, Mu HH, Araneo BA, Daynes RA. Age- and microenvironment-associated influences by platelet-derived growth factor on T cell function. *J Immunol* 1994;152:3417–3426.
428. Johnson RJ, Raines EW, Floege J, et al. Inhibition of mesangial cell proliferation and matrix expansion in glomerulonephritis in the rat by antibody to platelet-derived growth factor. *J Exp Med* 1992;175:1413–1416.
429. Gesualdo L, DiPaolo S, Ranieri E, Schena FP. Trapidil inhibits human mesangial cells proliferation: effect on PDGF beta-receptor binding and expression. *Kidney Int* 1994;46:1002–1009.
430. Futamura A, Iida H, Izumino K, Entani C, Takata M. Effect of the platelet-derived growth factor antagonist trapidil on rat mesangial cell proliferation. *J Am Soc Nephrol* 1992;3:588.
431. Floege J, Eng E, Young BA, Couser WG, Johnson RJ. Heparin suppresses mesangial cell proliferation and matrix expansion in experimental mesangioproliferative glomerulonephritis. *Kidney Int* 1993;43:369–380.
432. Border WA, Noble NA. Transforming growth factor beta in tissue fibrosis. *N Engl J Med* 1994;331:1286–1292.
433. Wahl SM. Transforming growth factor beta: the good, the bad, and the ugly. *J Exp Med* 1994;180:1587–1590.
434. Sharma K, Ziyadeh FN. The emerging role of transforming growth factor-beta in kidney diseases. *Am J Physiol* 1994;266:F829–842.
435. Miyazono K, Ichijo H, Heldin CH. Transforming growth factor-beta: latent forms, binding proteins and receptors. *Growth Factors* 1993;8:11–22.
436. Schultz-Cherry S, Murphy-Ullrich JE. Thrombospondin causes activation of latent transforming growth factor-beta secreted by endothelial cells by a novel mechanism. *J Cell Biol* 1993;122:923–932.
437. Border WA, Noble NA, Yamamoto T, et al. Natural inhibitor of transforming growth factor-beta protects against scarring in experimental kidney disease. *Nature* 1992;360:361–364.
438. Hausser H, Groning A, Hasilik A, Schonherr E, Kresse H. Selective inactivity of TGF-beta/decorin complexes. *FEBS Lett* 1994;353:243–245.
439. Wrana JL, Attisano L, Wieser R, Ventura F, Massague J. Mechanism of activation of the TGF-beta receptor. *Nature* 1994;370:341–347.
440. Massague J. Receptors for the TGF-beta family. *Cell* 1992;69:1067–1070.
441. Ando T, Okuda S, Tamaki K, Yoshitomi K, Fujishima M. Localization of transforming growth factor-beta and latent transforming growth factor-beta binding protein in rat kidney. *Kidney Int* 1995;47:733–739.
442. Iwano M, Akai Y, Fujii Y, Dohi Y, Matsumura N, Dohi K. Intraglomerular expression of transforming growth factor-beta 1 (TGF-beta 1) mRNA in patients with glomerulonephritis. *Clin Exp Immunol* 1994;97:309–314.
443. Yoshioka K, Takemura T, Murakami K, et al. Transforming growth factor-beta protein and mRNA in glomeruli in normal and diseased human kidneys. *Lab Invest* 1993;68:154–163.
444. Mac Kay K, Kondaiah P, Danielpour D, Austin HA, Brown PD. Expression of transforming growth factor-beta 1 and beta 2 in rat glomeruli. *Kidney Int* 1990;38:1095–1100.
445. Flanders KC, Thompson NL, Cissel DS, et al. Transforming growth factor-beta 1: histochemical localization with antibodies to different epitopes. *J Cell Biol* 1989;108:653–660.
446. Ray PE, McCune BK, Gomez RA, Horikoshi S, Kopp JB, Klotman PE. Renal vascular induction of TGF-beta 2 and renin by potassium depletion. *Kidney Int* 1993;44:1006–1013.
447. Pankewycz OG, Guan JX, Bolton WK, Gomez A, Benedict JF. Renal TGF-beta regulation in spontaneously diabetic NOD mice with correlations in mesangial cells. *Kidney Int* 1994;46:748–758.
448. Kagami S, Border WA, Miller DE, Noble NA. Angiotensin II stimulates extracellular matrix protein synthesis through induction of transforming growth factor-beta expression in rat glomerular mesangial cells. *J Clin Invest* 1994;93:2431–2437.
449. Ziyadeh FN, Sharma K, Ericksen M, Wolf G. Stimulation of collagen gene expression and protein synthesis in murine mesangial cells by high glucose is mediated by autocrine activation of transforming growth factor-beta. *J Clin Invest* 1994;93:536–542.

450. Choi ME, Kim EG, Huang Q, Ballermann BJ. Rat mesangial cell hypertrophy in response to transforming growth factor-beta 1. *Kidney Int* 1993;44:948–958.
451. Kaname S, Uchida S, Ogata E, Kurokawa K. Autocrine secretion of transforming growth factor-beta in cultured rat mesangial cells. *Kidney Int* 1992;42:1319–1327.
452. Phillips A, Steadman R, Topley N, Williams J. Elevated D-glucose concentrations modulate TGF-beta1 synthesis by human cultured renal proximal tubular cells: the permissive role of platelet derived growth factor. *Am J Pathol* (in press).
453. Rocco MV, Chen Y, Goldfarb S, Ziyadeh FN. Elevated glucose stimulates TGF-beta gene expression and bioactivity in proximal tubule. *Kidney Int* 1992;41:107–114.
454. Agrotis A, Saltis J, Bobik A. Transforming growth factor-beta 1 gene activation and growth of smooth muscle from hypertensive rats. *Hypertension* 1994;23:593–599.
455. Flaumenhaft R, Abe M, Mignatti P, Rifkin DB. Basic fibroblast growth factor-induced activation of latent transforming growth factor beta in endothelial cells: regulation of plasminogen activator activity. *J Cell Biol* 1992;118:901–909.
456. Waltenberger J, Miyazono K, Funa K, Wanders A, Fellstrom B, Heldin CH. Transforming growth factor-beta and organ transplantation. *Transplant Proc* 1993;25:2038–2040.
457. Kanai H, Mitsuhashi H, Ono K, Yano S, Naruse T. Increased excretion of urinary transforming growth factor beta in patients with focal glomerular sclerosis. *Nephron* 1994;66:391–395.
458. Coimbra T, Wiggins R, Noh JW, Merritt S, Phan SH. Transforming growth factor-beta production in anti-glomerular basement membrane disease in the rabbit. *Am J Pathol* 1991;138:223–234.
459. Niemir ZI, Stein H, Noronha IL, et al. PDGF and TGF-beta contribute to the natural course of human IgA glomerulonephritis. *Kidney Int* 1995;48:1530–1541.
460. Liu ZH, Striker LJ, Pillips C, et al. Mice transgenic for a growth hormone antagonist are protected from diabetic glomerulosclerosis [Abstract]. *J Am Soc Nephrol* 1995;6:1044.
461. Okuda S, Languino LR, Ruoslahti E, Border WA. Elevated expression of transforming growth factor-beta and proteoglycan production in experimental glomerulonephritis. Possible role in expansion of the mesangial extracellular matrix. *J Clin Invest* 1990;86:453–462.
462. Yamamoto T, Noble NA, Miller DE, Border WA. Sustained expression of TGF-beta 1 underlies development of progressive kidney fibrosis. *Kidney Int* 1994;45:916–927.
463. Barnes JL, Abboud HE. Temporal expression of autocrine growth factors corresponds to morphological features of mesangial proliferation in Habu snake venom–induced glomerulonephritis. *Am J Pathol* 1993;143:1366–1376.
464. Shankland SJ, Pippin J, Pichler RH, Gold LI, Gordon KL, Friedman S, Johnson RJ, Couser WG. Differential expression of transforming growth factor (TGF-β) isoforms and receptors in experimental membranous nephropathy. *Kidney Int* 1996;50:116–124.
465. Ding G, Pesek-Diamond I, Diamond JR. Cholesterol, macrophages, and gene expression of TGF-beta 1 and fibronectin during nephrosis. *Am J Physiol* 1993;264:F577–584.
466. Jones CL, Buch S, Post M, McCulloch L, Liu E, Eddy AA. Pathogenesis of interstitial fibrosis in chronic purine aminonucleoside nephrosis. *Kidney Int* 1991;40:1020–1031.
467. Tamaki K, Okuda S, Ando T, Iwamoto T, Nakayama M, Fujishima M. TGF-beta 1 in glomerulosclerosis and interstitial fibrosis of adriamycin nephropathy. *Kidney Int* 1994;45:525–536.
468. Bollineni JS, Reddi AS. Transforming growth factor-beta 1 enhances glomerular collagen synthesis in diabetic rats. *Diabetes* 1993;42:1673–1677.
469. Yamamoto T, Nakamura T, Noble NA, Ruoslahti E, Border WA. Expression of transforming growth factor beta is elevated in human and experimental diabetic nephropathy. *Proc Natl Acad Sci U S A* 1993;90:1814–1818.
470. Shankland SJ, Scholey JW, Ly H, Thai K. Expression of transforming growth factor-beta 1 during diabetic renal hypertrophy. *Kidney Int* 1994;46:430–442.
471. Kaneto H, Morrissey J, Klahr S. Increased expression of TGF-beta 1 mRNA in the obstructed kidney of rats with unilateral ureteral ligation. *Kidney Int* 1993;44:313–321.
472. Lianos EA, Orphanos V, Cattell V, Cook T, Anagnou N. Glomerular expression and cell origin of transforming growth factor-beta 1 in anti-glomerular basement membrane disease. *Am J Med Sci* 1994;307:1–5.
473. Kim S, Ohta K, Hamaguchi A, et al. Role of angiotensin II in renal injury of deoxycorticosterone acetate-salt hypertensive rats. *Hypertension* 1994;24:195–204.
474. Nakamura T, Ebihara I, Fukui M, et al. Renal expression of mRNAs for endothelin-1, endothelin-3 and endothelin receptors in NZB/I WF1 mice. *Renal Physiol Biochem* 1993;16:233–243.
475. Muchaneta-Kubara EC, Sayed-Ahmed N, El Nahas AM. Subtotal nephrectomy: a mosaic of growth factors. *Nephrol Dial Transplant* 1995;10:320–327.
476. Waldherr R, Noronha IL, Niemir Z, Kruger C, Stein H, Stumm G. Expression of cytokines and growth factors in human glomerulonephritides. *Pediatr Nephrol* 1993;7:471–478.
477. Isaka Y, Fujiwara Y, Ueda N, Kaneda Y, Kamada T, Imai E. Glomerulosclerosis induced by in vivo transfection of transforming growth factor-beta or platelet-derived growth factor gene into the rat kidney. *J Clin Invest* 1993;92:2597–2601.
478. Lai KN, Ho RT, Leung JC, Lai FM, Li PK. Increased mRNA encoding for transforming growth factor-beta in CD4+ cells from patients with IgA nephropathy. *Kidney Int* 1994;46:862–868.
479. Meyers CM, Kelly CJ. Immunoregulation and TGF-beta1. Suppression of a nephritogenic murine T cell clone. *Kidney Int* 1994;46:1295–1301.
480. Terrell TG, Working PK, Chow CP, Green JD. Pathology of recombinant human transforming growth factor-beta 1 in rats and rabbits. *Int Rev Exp Pathol* 1993;34:43–67.
481. Lowrance JH, O'Sullivan FX, Caver TE, Waegell W, Gresham HD. Spontaneous elaboration of transforming growth factor beta suppresses host defense against bacterial infection in autoimmune mrl/lpr mice. *J Exp Med* 1994;180:1693–1703.
482. Shull MM, Ormsby I, Kier AB, et al. Targeted disruption of the mouse transforming growth factor-beta 1 gene results in multifocal inflammatory disease. *Nature* 1992;359:693–699.
483. Coupes BM, Newstead CG, Short CD, Brenchley PE. Transforming growth factor beta 1 in renal allograft recipients. *Transplantation* 1994;57:1727–1731.
484. Filmus J, Kerbel RS. Development of resistance mechanisms to the growth-inhibitory effects of transforming growth factor-beta during tumor progression. *Curr Opin Oncol* 1993;5:123–129.
485. Sanderson N, Factor V, Nagy P, et al. Hepatic expression of mature transforming growth factor beta1 in transgenic mice results in multiple tissue lesions. *Proc Natl Acad Sci U S A* 1995;92:2572–2576.
486. Zhang GH, Ichimura T, Wallin A, Kan M, Stevens JL. Regulation of rat proximal tubule epithelial cell growth by fibroblast growth factors, insulin-like growth factor-1 and transforming growth factor-beta, and analysis of fibroblast growth factors in rat kidney. *J Cell Physiol* 1991;148:295–305.
487. Mac Kay K, Striker LJ, Stauffer JW, Doi T, Agodoa LY, Striker GE. Transforming growth factor-beta. Murine glomerular receptors and responses of isolated glomerular cells. *J Clin Invest* 1989;83:1160–1167.
488. Nakamura T, Miller D, Ruoslahti E, Border WA. Production of extracellular matrix by glomerular epithelial cells is regulated by transforming growth factor-beta 1. *Kidney Int* 1992;41:1213–1221.
489. Haberstroh U, Zahner G, Disser M, Thaiss F, Wolf G, Stahl RA. TGF-beta stimulates rat mesangial cell proliferation in culture: role of PDGF beta-receptor expression. *Am J Physiol* 1993;264:F199–205.
490. Wolf G, Sharma K, Chen Y, Ericksen M, Ziyadeh FN. High glucose-induced proliferation in mesangial cells is reversed by autocrine TGF-beta. *Kidney Int* 1992;42:647–656.
491. Border WA, Okuda S, Languino LR, Ruoslahti E. Transforming growth factor-beta regulates production of proteoglycans by mesangial cells. *Kidney Int* 1990;37:689–695.
492. Jaffer F, Saunders C, Shultz P, Throckmorton D, Weinshell E, Abboud HE. Regulation of mesangial cell growth by polypeptide mitogens. Inhibitory role of transforming growth factor beta. *Am J Pathol* 1989;135:261–269.
493. Throckmorton DC, Brogden AP, Min B, Rasmussen H, Kashgarian M. PDGF and TGF-beta mediate collagen production by mesangial cells exposed to advanced glycosylation end products. *Kidney Int* 1995;48:111–117.
494. Fine LG, Holley RW, Nasri H, Badie-Dezfooly B. BSC-1 growth inhibitor transforms a mitogenic stimulus into a hypertrophic stimulus

for renal proximal tubular cells: relationship to Na^+/H^+ antiport activity. *Proc Natl Acad Sci U S A* 1985;82:6163–6166.
495. McKay NG, Khong TF, Haites NE, Power DA. The effect of transforming growth factor beta 1 on mesangial cell fibronectin synthesis: increased incorporation into the extracellular matrix and reduced pI but no effect on alternative splicing. *Exp Mol Pathol* 1993;59: 211–224.
496. Kasinath BS. Glomerular endothelial cell proteoglycans—regulation by TGF-beta 1. *Arch Biochem Biophys* 1993;305:370–377.
497. Humes HD, Nakamura T, Cieslinski DA, Miller D, Emmons RV, Border WA. Role of proteoglycans and cytoskeleton in the effects of TGF-beta 1 on renal proximal tubule cells. *Kidney Int* 1993;43: 575–584.
498. Creely JJ, Di Mari SJ, Howe AM, Haralson MA. Effects of transforming growth factor-beta on collagen synthesis by normal rat kidney epithelial cells. *Am J Pathol* 1992;140:45–55.
499. MacKay K, Striker LJ, Stauffer JW, Doi TA, LY, Striker GE. Transforming growth factor-beta. Murine glomerular receptors and responses of isolated glomerular cells. *J Clin Invest* 1989;83: 1160–1167.
500. Alvarez RJ, Sun MJ, Haverty TP, Iozzo RV, Myers JC, Neilson EG. Biosynthetic and proliferative characteristics of tubulointerstitial fibroblasts probed with paracrine cytokines. *Kidney Int* 1992;41: 14–23.
501. Tomooka S, Border WA, Marshall BC, Noble NA. Glomerular matrix accumulation is linked to inhibition of the plasmin protease system. *Kidney Int* 1992;42:1462–1469.
502. Marti HP, Lee L, Kashgarian M, Lovett DH. Transforming growth factor-beta 1 stimulates glomerular mesangial cell synthesis of the 72-kd type IV collagenase. *Am J Pathol* 1994;144:82–94.
503. Kagami S, Border WA, Ruoslahti E, Noble NA. Coordinated expression of beta 1 integrins and transforming growth factor-beta–induced matrix proteins in glomerulonephritis. *Lab Invest* 1993;69:68–76.
504. Border WA, Okuda S, Languino LR, Sporn MB, Ruoslahti E. Suppression of experimental glomerulonephritis by antiserum against transforming growth factor beta 1. *Nature* 1990;346:371–374.
505. Eddy AA. Protein restriction reduces transforming growth factor-beta and interstitial fibrosis in nephrotic syndrome. *Am J Physiol* 1994; 266:F884–893.
506. Okuda S, Nakamura T, Yamamoto T, Ruoslahti E, Border WA. Dietary protein restriction rapidly reduces transforming growth factor beta 1 expression in experimental glomerulonephritis. *Proc Natl Acad Sci U S A* 1991;88:9765–9769.
507. Narita I, Border WA, Ketteler M, Ruoslahti E, Noble NA. L-Arginine may mediate the therapeutic effects of low protein diets. *Proc Natl Acad Sci U S A* 1995;92:4552–4556.
508. Movat HZ, Cybulsky MI, Colditz IG, Chan MKW, Dinarello CA. Acute inflammation in gram-negative infection: endotoxin, interleukin-1, tumour necrosis factor and neutrophils. *Fed Proc* 1987;46: 97–104.
509. Kriegler M, Perez C, DeFay K. A novel form of TNF/cachectin is a cell surface cytotoxic transmembrane protein: ramifications for the complex physiology of TNF. *Cell* 1988;53:45–53.
510. Gearing AJ, Beckett P, Christodoulou M, et al. Processing of tumour necrosis factor alpha by metalloproteinases. *Nature* 1994;370: 555–557.
511. Smith RA, Baglioni C. The active form of tumour necrosis factor is a trimer. *J Biol Chem* 1987;262:6951–6954.
512. Jones EY, Stuart DI, Walker NP. Structure of tumour necrosis factor. *Nature* 1989;338:225–228.
513. Wilson KP, Black JPA, Thomson JA, et al. Structure and mechanism of interleukin-1 converting enzyme. *Nature* 1994;370:270.
514. Smith CA, Davis T, Anderson D. A receptor for tumour necrosis factor defines an unusual family of cellular and viral proteins. *Science* 1990;248:1019–1023.
515. Bazzoni F, Beutler B. How do tumour necrosis factor receptors work? *J Inflamm* 1995;45:221–238.
516. Engelmann H, Holtmann H, Brakebusch C. Antibodies to a soluble form of a tumour necrosis factor (TNF) receptor have TNF-like activity. *J Biol Chem* 1990;265:14497–14504.
517. Loetscher H, Stueber D, Banner D, MacKay F, Lesslauer W. Human tumour necrosis factor α mutants with exclusive specificity for the 55 kDA or 75 kDa receptors. *J Biol Chem* 1993;268:26350–26357.
518. Tartaglia LA, Goeddel DV, Reynolds C. Stimulation of human T-cell proliferation by specific activation of the 75kDa tumour necrosis factor receptor. *J Immunol* 1993;151:4637–4641.
519. Bigda J, Beletsky I, Brakebusch C. Dual role of the p75 tumour necrosis factor (TNF) receptor in TNF cytotoxicity. *J Exp Med* 1994; 180:445–460.
520. Mackay F, Loetscher H, Stueber D, Gehr G, Lesslauer W. Tumour necrosis factor α (TNF-α) induced cell adhesion to human endothelial cells is under dominant control of one TNf receptor type, TNF-R55. *J Exp Med* 1993;177:1277–1286.
521. Neumann B, Machleidt T, Lifka A, et al. Crucial role of 55-kilodalton TNF receptor in TNF-induced adhesion molecule expression and leukocyte organ infiltration. *J Immunol* 1996;156:1587–1593.
522. Mackay F, Rothe J, Bluethmann H, Loetscher H, Lesslauer W. Differential responses of fibroblasts from wild-type and TNF-R55 deficient mice to mouse and human TNF-α activation. *J Immunol* 1994;153:5274–5284.
523. Bazzoni F, Beutler E. The tumor necrosis factor ligand and receptor families. *New Eng J Med* 1996;334:1717–1725.
524. van Zee KJ, Kohno T, Fischer E. Tumour necrosis factor soluble receptors circulate during experimental and clinical inflammation and can protect against excessive tumour necrosis factor-α in vitro and in vivo. *Proc Natl Acad Sci U S A* 1992;89:4845–4849.
525. Olsson I, Gatanaga T, Gullberg U, Lantz M, Grangers GA. Tumour necrosis factor (TNF) binding proteins (soluble TNF receptor forms) with possible roles in inflammation and malignancy. *Eur Cytokine Network* 1993;4:169–180.
526. Dayer JM, Burger B. Interleukin-1, tumour necrosis factor and their specific inhibitors. *Eur Cytokine Network* 1994;5:563–571.
527. Noiri E, Kuwata S, Nosaka T, et al. Tumour necrosis factor-alpha mRNA expression in lipopolysaccharide-stimulated rat kidney. Chronological analysis of localization. *Am J Pathol* 1994;144: 1159–1166.
528. Baud L, Ardaillou R. Tumour necrosis factor in renal injury. *Miner Electrolyte Metab* 1995;21:336–341.
529. Ortiz A, Alonso J, Gomez-Chiarri M, et al. Fibronectin (FN) decreases glomerular lesions and synthesis of tumour necrosis factor-alpha (TNF-alpha), platelet-activating factor (PAF) and FN in proliferative glomerulonephritis. *Clin Exp Immunol* 1995;101:334–340.
530. Noronha IL, Kruger C, Andrassy K, Ritz E, Waldherr R. In situ production of TNF-alpha, IL-1 beta and IL-2R in ANCA-positive glomerulonephritis. *Kidney Int* 1993;43:682–692.
531. Yoshioka 1K, Takemura T, Murakami K, et al. In situ expression of cytokines in IgA nephritis. *Kidney Int* 1993;44:825–833.
532. Waldherr R, Noronha IL, Niemir Z, Kruger C, Stein H, Stumm G. Expression of cytokines and growth factors in human glomerulonephritis. *Pediatr Nephrol* 1993;7:471–478.
533. Malide D, Russo P, Bendayan M. Presence of tumor necrosis facts alpha and interleukin-6 in renal mesangial cells of lupus nephritis patients. *Hum Pathol* 1995;26:558–564.
534. Neale TJ, Ruger BM, Macaulay H, et al. Tumuor necrosis factor-alpha is expressed by glomerular visceral epithelial cells in human membranous nephropathy. *Am J Pathol* 1995;146:1444–1454.
535. Karkar AM. Passive immunization against tumour necrosis factor-alpha (TNF-α) and IL-1 protects from LPS enhancing glomerular injury in nephrotoxic nephritis in rats. *Clin Exp Immunol* 1992; 90:312–318.
536. Karkar AM, Rees AJ. Influence of subclinical infection on glomerular injury in heterologous nephrotoxic nephritis. *Clin Exp Immunol* 1994; 98:295–299.
537. Tam FW, Smith J, Cashman SJ, Wang Y, Thompson EM, Rees AJ. Glomerular expression of interleukin-1 receptor antagonist and interleukin-1 beta genes in antibody-mediated glomerulonephritis. *Am J Pathol* 1994;145:126–136.
538. Onbe T, Kashihara N, Yamasaki Y, Makino H, Ota Z. Expression of mRNA's of cytokines and growth factors in experimental glomerulonephritis. *Res Commun Mol Pathol Pharmacol* 1994;86:131–138.
539. Rugo HS, O'Hanley R, Bishop AG, et al. Local cytokine production in a murine model of *Escherichia coli* pyelonephritis. *J Clin Invest* 1992;89:1032–1039.
540. Gomez-Chiarri M, Ortiz A, Lerma JL, Mampaso F, Gonzalez E, Egido E. Involvement of tumour necrosis factor and platelet activating factor in the pathogenesis of experimental nephrosis in rats. *Lab Invest* 1994;70:449–459.
541. Bustos C, Gonzales-Cuadrado S, Ruiz-Ortega M, et al. Cyclyosporin

A (CsA) modulates the glomerular production of inflammatory mediators and proteoglycans in experimental nephrosis. *Clin Exp Immunol* 1995;102:608–613.
542. Dinarello CA. Inflammatory cytokines: interleukin-1 and tumour necrosis factor as effector molecules in autoimmune diseases. *Curr Opin Immunol* 1991;3:941–948.
543. Ozen S, Saatci U, Tinaztepe K, Bakkaloglu A, Barut A. Urinary tumour necrosis factor levels in primary glomerulopathies. *Nephron* 1994;66:291–294.
544. Yoshioka K, Hino S, Takemura T, et al. Type IV collagen alpha 5 chain. Normal distribution and abnormalities in X-linked Alport syndrome revealed by monoclonal antibody. *Am J Pathol* 1994;144: 986–996.
545. Honkanen E, Teppo AM, Meri S, Lehto T, Gronhagen-Riska C. Urinary excretion of cytokines and complement SC5b-9 in idiopathic membranous glomerulonephritis. *Nephrol Dial Transplant* 1994;9: 1533–1539.
546. Le J, Vilcek J. Tumour necrosis factor and interleukin-1: cytokines with multiple overlapping biological activities. *Lab Invest* 1987;56: 234–248.
547. Vassalli P. The pathophysiuology of tumour necrosis factors. *Ann Rev Immunol* 1992;10:411–452.
548. Tracy KJ, Cerami A. Tumour necrosis factor: a pleiotropic cytokine and therapeutic target. *Annu Rev Med* 1994;45:491–501.
549. Riches DWH. Signalling heterogeneity as a contributing factor in macrophage functional diversity. *Cell Biol* 1995;6:1–8.
550. Yanagisawa M, Imai H, Fukishima Y, Yasuda T, Miura AB. Effects of tumour necrosis factor alpha and interleukin-1 beta on the proliferation of cultured glomerular epithelial cells. *Virchows Arch* 1994; 424:581–586.
551. Sacks Sh, Zhou, Pani A, Campbell RD, Martin J. Complement C3 gene expression and regulation in human glomerular epithelial cells. *Immunology* 1993;79:348–354.
552. Bertani T, Abbate M, Zoja C. Tumour necrosis factor-α induces glomerular damage in the rabbit. *Am J Pathol* 1989;134:419–430.
553. Tomosugi NI, Cashman SJ, Hay H. Modulation of antibody mediated glomerular injury in vivo by bacterial lipopolysaccharide tumour necrosis factor and IL-1. *J Immunol* 1989;142:3083–3090.
554. Jacob CO, McDevitt HO. Tumour necrosis factor-α in murine autoimmune lupus' nephritis. *Nature* 1988;331:256–258.
555. Mulligan MS, Johnson KJ, Todd RF. Requirements for leucocyte adhesion molecules in nephrotoxic nephritis. *J Clin Invest* 1993;91: 577–587.
556. Karkar AM. Modulation of antibody-mediated glomerular injury in vivo by IL-1ra, soluble IL-1 receptor, and soluble TNF receptor. *Kidney Int* 1995;48:1738–1746.
557. Karkar AM, Tam FW, Proudfoot AE, Meager A, Rees AJ. Modulation of antibody-mediated glomerular injury in vivo by interleukin-6. *Kidney Int* 1993;44:967–973.
558. Hruby ZW, Shirota K, Jothy S, Lowry RP. Antiserum against tumour necrosis factor-alpha and a protease inhibitor reduce immune glomerular injury. *Kidney Int* 1991;40:43–51.
559. Feldmann M, Brennan FM, Elliot M, Katsikis P, Maini RN. TNFα as a therapeutic target in rheumatoid arthritis. *Circ Shock* 1994;43:179–184.
560. Dvorak HF, Brown LF, Detmar M, Dvorak AM. Vascular permeability factor/vascular endothelial growth factor, microvascular hyperpermeability, and angiogenesis. *Am J Pathol* 1995;146:1029–1039.
561. Connolly DT. Vascular permeability factor: a unique regulator of blood vessel function. *J Cell Biochem* 1991;47:219–223.
562. Simon M, Gröne HJ, Johren O, et al. Expression of vascular endothelial growth factor and its receptors in human renal ontogenesis and in adult kidney. *Am J Physiol* 1995;268:F240–250.
563. Gibbons GH, Dzau VJ. The emerging concept of vascular remodeling. *N Engl J Med* 1994;330:1431–1438.
564. Heslan J, MJ, Branellec AI, Pilatte Y, Lang P, Lagrue G. Differentiation between vascular permeability factor and IL-2 in lymphocyte supernatants from patients with minimal-change nephrotic syndrome. *Clin Exp Immunol* 1991;86:157–162.
565. Ferrara N, Houck KA, Jakeman LB, Winer J, Leung DW. The vascular endothelial growth factor family of polypeptides. *J Cell Biochem* 1991;47:211–218.
566. Minchenko A, Salceda S, Bauer T, Caro J. Hypoxia regulatory elements of the human vascular endothelial growth factor gene. *Cell Mol Biol Res* 1994;40:35–39.
567. Neufeld G, Tessler S, Gitay-Goren H, Cohen T, Levi BZ. Vascular endothelial growth factor and its receptors. *Prog Growth Factor Res* 1994;5:89–97.
568. Kendall RL, Thomas KA. Inhibition of vascular endothelial cell growth factor activity by an endogenously encoded soluble receptor. *Proc Natl Acad Sci U S A* 1993;90:10705–10709.
569. Gitay-Goren H, Soker S, Vlodavsky I, Neufeld G. The binding of vascular endothelial growth factor to its receptors is dependent on cell surface–associated heparin-like molecules. *J Biol Chem* 1992;267: 6093–6098.
570. Vaisman N, Gospodarowicz D, Neufeld G. Characterization of the receptors for vascular endothelial growth factor. *J Biol Chem* 1990; 265:19461–19466.
571. Guo D, Jia Q, Song HY, Warren RS, Donner DB. Vascular endothelial cell growth factor promotes tyrosine phosphorylation of mediators of signal transduction that contain SH2 domains. *J Biol Chem* 1995;270:6729–6733.
572. Berse B, Brown LF, Van De Water L, Dvorak HF, Senger DR. Vascular permeability factor (vascular endothelial growth factor) gene is expressed differentially in normal tissues, macrophages, and tumors. *Mol Biol Cell* 1992;3:211–220.
573. Breier G, Albrecht U, Sterrer S, Risau W. Expression of vascular endothelial growth factor during embryonic angiogenesis and endothelial cell differentiation. *Development* 1992;114:521–532.
574. Monacci WT, Merrill MJ, Oldfield EH. Expression of vascular permeability factor/vascular endothelial growth factor in normal rat tissues. *Am J Physiol* 1993;264:C995–1002.
575. Heldin CH, Hellman U, Ishikawa F, Miyazono K. Purification, cloning, and expression of platelet-derived endothelial cell growth factor. *Methods Enzymol* 1991;198:383–391.
576. Tischer E, Mitchell R, Hartman T, et al. The human gene for vascular endothelial growth factor. Multiple protein forms are encoded through alternative exon splicing. *J Biol Chem* 1991;266:11947–11954.
577. Ferrara N, Winer J, Burton T. Aortic smooth muscle cells express and secrete vascular endothelial growth factor. *Growth Factors* 1991;5: 141–148.
578. Iijima K, Yoshikawa N, Connolly DT, Nakamura H. Human mesangial cells and peripheral blood mononuclear cells produce vascular permeability factor. *Kidney Int* 1993;44:959–966.
579. Uchida K, Uchida S, Nitta K, Yumura W, Marumo F, Nihei H. Glomerular endothelial cells in culture express and secrete vascular endothelial growth factor. *Am J Physiol* 1994;266:F81–88.
580. Brown LF, Berse B, Jackman RW, et al. Increased expression of vascular permeability factor (vascular endothelial growth factor) and its receptors in kidney and bladder carcinomas. *Am J Pathol* 1993;143: 1255–1262.
581. Brown LF, Berse B, Tognazzi K, et al. Vascular permeability factor mRNA and protein expression in human kidney. *Kidney Int* 1992; 42:1457–1461.
582. Gröne HJ, Simon M, Gröne EF. Expression of vascular endothelial growth factor in renal vascular disease and renal allografts. *J Pathol* 1995;176:24–31.
583. Jakeman LB, Winer J, Bennett GL, Altar CA, Ferrara N. Binding sites for vascular endothelial growth factor are localized on endothelial cells in adult rat tissues. *J Clin Invest* 1992;89:244–253.
584. Callow AD, Choi ET, Trachtenberg JD, et al. Vascular permeability factor accelerates endothelial regrowth following balloon angioplasty. *Growth Factors* 1994;10:223–228.
585. Soker S, Svahn CM, Neufeld G. Vascular endothelial growth factor is inactivated by binding to alpha 2-macroglobulin and the binding is inhibited by heparin. *J Biol Chem* 1993;268:7685–7691.
586. Iruela-Arispe L, Gordon K, Hugo C, et al. Participation of glomerular endothelial cells in the capillary repair of glomerulonephritis. *Am J Pathol* 1995;147:1715–1727.
587. Klanke B, Gröne HJ, Gros H, Simon M, Stolte H, Weich HA. Effects of vascular endothelial growth factor on hemodynamics and permselectivity of the isolated perfused rat kidney. *J Am Soc Nephrol* 1994;4:582.
588. Ku DD, Zaleski JK, Liu S, Brock TA. Vascular endothelial growth factor induces EDRF-dependent relaxation in coronary arteries. *Am J Physiol* 1993;265:H586–592.

Immunologic Renal Diseases,
edited by E. G. Neilson and W. G. Couser.
Lippincott-Raven Publishers, Philadelphia © 1997.

CHAPTER 21

Endothelin and Nitric Oxide

Tobias A. Marsen and Michael J. Dunn

In most immunologic glomerular diseases, the lesions arise through cell-mediated and humoral mechanisms. Although several possible candidates have been extensively studied, not all aspects of the underlying mechanisms in immunologic renal diseases are clarified. With recent advances in the field of vasoconstrictors and vasodilators, the search for the pathophysiologic mechanism that contributes to this process continues.

Endothelins (ETs), potent endothelium-derived vasoconstrictor peptides (1), contribute to the regulation of glomerular function and may be involved in glomerular disease, both through changes in hemodynamics, in glomerular configuration, and in mesangial proliferation. Nitric oxide (NO), a gaseous molecule with vasodilatory properties (2), plays an important role in control of blood pressure and vascular tone, neurotransmission, mediation of macrophage cytotoxicity, and inhibition of platelet aggregation and is involved in vascular regulation, tissue damage, and immune response.

Changes in the release of either ET or NO may cause marked changes in renal hemodynamics and renal cell function. Thus, they may act as secondary mediators of injurious stimuli to the kidney. It remains questionable if proliferative stimuli or if presently unknown mechanisms directed against the glomerular endothelium and epithelium are crucial for their release. Similar to the action of collagenases, elastases, growth factors, arachidonic acids, and prostaglandins, ET and NO may be dysregulated and may therefore contribute to renal immunologic diseases.

T. A. Marsen: Klinik IV für Innere Medizin, University of Cologne, 50924 Cologne, Germany.

M. J. Dunn: Medical College of Wisconsin, Milwaukee, Wisconsin 53226.

ENDOTHELIN

Structure

Three structurally and pharmacologically distinct ET isoforms are known, they show resemblance to a snake venom, are highly homologous, and share a common structure (3). ETs form a typical hairpin loop configuration, which results from two disulfide bonds at the amino terminal end. They also display a hydrophobic COOH-terminus that contains an aromatic indol side chain at Trp^{21}. Biologic activity requires the COOH-terminus, deletion of Trp^{21} decreases ED_{50} by a factor of 10^3 to 10^4, and deletion of amino acids 17–21 (Leu-Asp-Ile-Ile-Trp) causes complete loss of activity. The two disulfide bonds also are important for bioactivity; their reduction and alkylation reduces ET bioactivity by a factor of 1,000 (4). Differences in the amino acid sequence among the isopeptides are minor but lead to typical pharmacologic characteristics (Table 1).

Synthesis and Secretion

ETs are synthesized via posttranslational proteolytic cleavage of specific prohormones (Fig. 1). Dibasic pair-specific processing endopeptidases, which recognize Arg-Arg or Lys-Arg paired amino acids, cleave prepro ETs and reduce their size from approximately 203 to 39 amino acids. These pro ETs are subsequently proteolytically cleaved at the Trp^{21}-Val^{22} bond by ET-converting enzymes yielding mature ETs. The converting enzymes appear to be metalloproteases and exert different specificities for the ETs; they are localized in the soluble and particulate cell fraction (5,6).

ET secretion depends on polarity because polarized endothelial cells secrete the majority of the peptide into

TABLE 1. *Pharmacologic characteristics of ET isoforms*

	ET-1	ET-2	ET-3
Constrictor activity	+++	++	+
Dilatory activity	+	+	++

their basolateral compartment (7). Secretion occurs at a constant level, suggesting constitutive pathways; however, a variety of stimuli trigger ET synthesis via transcriptional regulation (Table 2).

ET stimulation is endothelium dependent and requires de novo protein synthesis because cycloheximide, a protein synthesis inhibitor, prevents release of the mature peptide. ET is not exclusively released by endothelium but also by nonvascular tissues, albeit at lower levels than endothelial cells. Besides macrovasculature of various tissues, ET synthesis has been detected in breast epithelial cells (8), macrophages (9), vascular smooth muscle cells (10), and brain glial cells (11). Numerous cells in the kidney also produce ET, including microvascular glomerular endothelial cells (12), tubular epithelial cells (13), and glomerular mesangial cells (14).

TABLE 2. *In vivo and in vitro stimuli that alter ET synthesis via transcriptional regulation*

Hormones	Peptides	Physical forces
Insulin	Cytokines	Hypoxia
Adrenalin	Thrombin	Shear stress
Vasopressin	Endotoxins	Osmolarity
Angiotensin	TGF-β	

Renal ET Localization

Various techniques have been used to analyze ET synthesis in the kidney, ranging from radioimmunoassay for ET peptide to immunohistochemistry, Northern analysis, ribonuclease protection assay, and reverse-transcriptase polymerase chain reaction (RT-PCR). The kidney synthesizes ET-1 as well as ET-3 (15). In microdissected rat kidney nephron segments, ET-1 messenger RNA (mRNA) can be found in glomeruli and in inner medullary collecting ducts; however, it is negligible in the cortical collecting duct and undetectable in other nephron segments (Fig. 2) (16,17). These findings correlate with immunoreactive ET-1 production in isolated cell culture as well as neph-

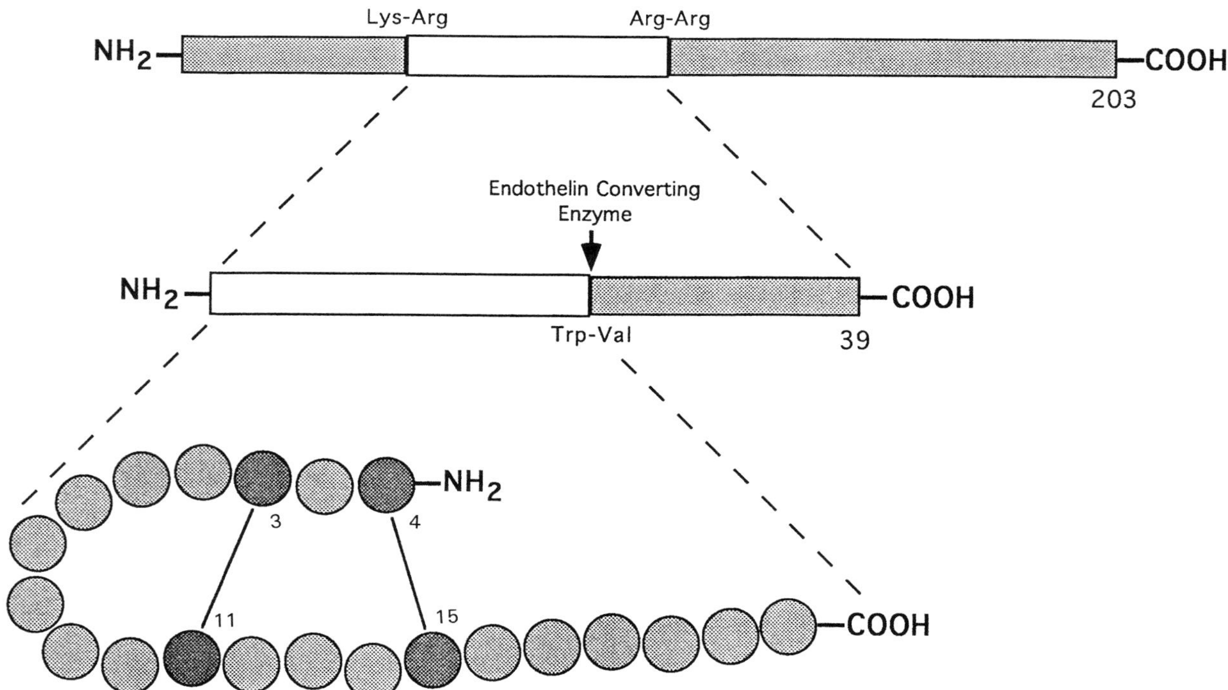

FIG. 1. Proposed pathway of ET synthesis. The prepro ET is cleaved by pair-specific processing endopeptidases at Lys^{51}-Arg^{52} and Arg^{92}-Arg^{93}, to reduce prepro ET from 203 amino acids to 39 and form pro ET. Pro ET is then proteolytically cleaved at Trp^{21}-Val^{22} by ET-converting enzymes, to form the mature ET peptide, which forms a typical hairpin loop-like structure through disulfide bond among Cys^{1}-Cys^{15} and Cys^{3}-Cys^{11}.

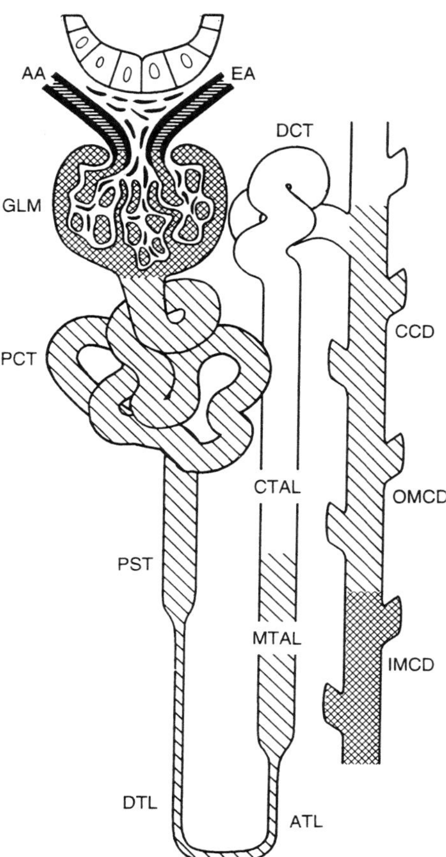

FIG. 2. Proposed ET isoform mRNA distribution pattern in the glomerulus. Distribution of ET-1 and ET-3 synthesis according to their mRNA synthesis in microdissected rat nephrons. Symbols are (▤) ET-1, (▨) ET-3, and (▩) ET-1 and ET-3. AA, afferent arteriole; EA, efferent arteriole; GLM, glomerulus; PCT, proximal convoluted tubule; PST, proximal straight tubule; DTL, descending thin limb of Henle's loop; ATL, ascending thin limb of Henle's loop; MTAL, medullary thick ascending limb; CTAL, cortical thick ascending limb; DCT, distal convoluted tubule; CCD, cortical collecting duct; OMCD, outer medullary collecting duct; IMCD, inner medullary collecting duct. Reprinted with permission (19).

ron segment suspensions. Synthesis of ET-2 in the kidney has not been clarified in detail. ET-2 is expressed in human renal medulla, and renal adenocarcinomas produce exceptionally high levels of ET-2 (18). Immunoreactive ET-1 and ET-3 mRNA are abundantly expressed in distal nephrons (15). In microdissected rat nephrons, using quantitative RT-PCR techniques, the following pattern for ET-3 can be found: outer medullary collecting duct > proximal convoluted tubule > cortical collecting duct > proximal straight tubule > glomerulus > vasa recta bundle. Weak signals are shown in inner medullary collecting duct > terminal inner medullary collecting duct < medullary thick ascending limb > inner medullary limb and arcuate artery (Fig. 2) (19).

ET Renal Binding Sites

ETs bind to two G protein–coupled receptors of approximately 43 to 73 kDa molecular weight, consisting of approximately 415 to 427 amino acids, that have seven transmembrane domains (20,21). ET receptors bind the peptides with selective affinity (20–23). In early studies, using ^{125}I-ET-1 radioligand assays, specific binding sites for ET were mapped in the following order: glomerular cortex and inner medulla region > the inner stripe of the outer medulla > proximal tubule (24,25). In vitro cultured mesangial cells showed heterogeneity for ET-1 and ET-3 receptors (22). Although the existence of two distinct ET receptor subtypes in the kidney was confirmed by Northern analysis (20), specific distribution patterns were determined only recently via RT-PCR (Fig. 3) (26).

ET Gene Regulation

The mechanisms underlying ET isopeptide stimulation are assumed to be transcriptional regulation (27–29). Via gene regulatory domains that are situated upstream of the transcriptional start site, prepro ET-1 gene transcription is upregulated (29–33). Within the 5′ flanking region, binding sites for nuclear factor 1 (NF-1), activator protein-1 (AP-1), and acute-phase reactant (APR) are found. Thus, transforming growth factor (TGF)-β, protein kinase C, as well as acute physical stress are able to exert their actions at the ET gene. Downregulation of ET synthesis is assumed to occur via suppression of protein kinase C–mediated mechanisms (34), through a guanylate cyclase-dependent process and release of cyclic guanosine monophosphate (cGMP) (35,36), or through adenylate cyclase activation (37). Subsequent studies have shown that ET-3 stimulates soluble guanylate cyclase activity and thereby may downregulate its own synthesis. ET-3 stimulates NO formation through receptor-mediated phosphoinositide breakdown and Ca^{2+} mobilization via G protein (38).

PHYSIOLOGIC ACTIONS OF ET ON THE KIDNEY

ET is assumed to exert its hemodynamic effects in nearly all vessels, but the sensitivity of different vasculature varies considerably. The renal together with the mesenteric vasculature has the greatest susceptibility to the peptides (39–41). In the kidney ET-1 increases renal vascular resistance via contraction of glomerular arterioles and arcuate and interlobular arteries and markedly decreases renal blood flow (40,42). Long-lasting vasoconstriction, which is mediated by the ET_A receptor, is temporarily preceded by transient vasodilation (38,41, 43). It is striking that this vasodepressor effect is only present after bolus injection rather than after continuous

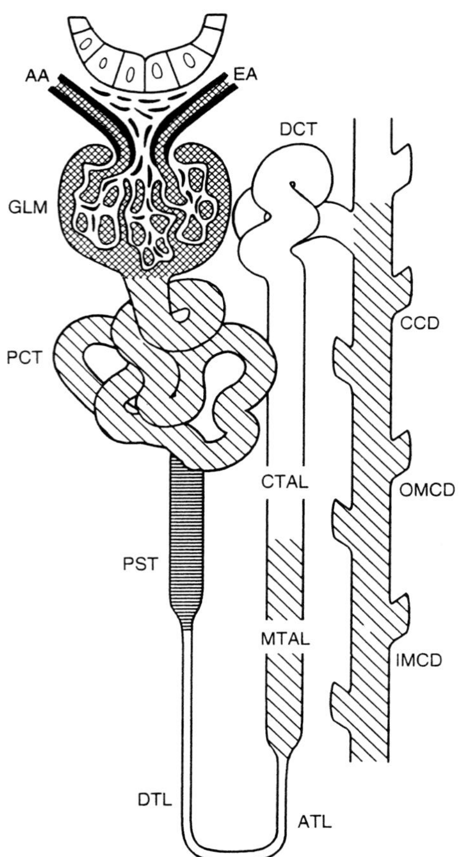

FIG. 3. Proposed ET receptor isoform mRNA distribution pattern in the glomerulus. Distribution of ET_A and ET_B receptor mRNA synthesis in microdissected rat nephrons. Symbols are (▤) ET_A, (▨) ET_B, and (▩) ET_A and ET_B. Reprinted with permission (19).

infusion (43,44). Vasodilation results from ET_B receptor–mediated release of NO (45,46). Coculture experiments of glomerular endothelial and mesangial cells also demonstrate potentiated prostaglandin E_2 synthesis and cyclic adenosine monophosphate (cAMP) release in mesangial cells, which also may exert vasodilatory effects, presumably via an ET-1–dependent paracrine mechanism (47). When assessed by micropuncture techniques, ET-1 generally causes a decline in net filtration pressure and a reduction in the glomerular ultrafiltration coefficient, which results from the extensive constriction of preglomerular afferent and also postglomerular efferent arterioles, regulation of renal blood flow, and the possible mesangial contraction (48,49). Besides alteration of glomerular filtration rate, ETs also influence tubular reabsorption and secretion (Fig. 4) (48).

ROLE OF ET ON GLOMERULAR CELL TYPES

In the glomerular tuft mesangial cells are important targets for ET. ET-1 induces mesangial cell contraction and mitogenesis (50–52). Mesangial cells have several functions, including regulation of glomerular capillary shape, as well as hydraulic properties of the mesangium, control of glomerular hemodynamics, endocytosis of plasma macromolecules, and synthesis and assembly of the glomerular matrix (53). Via release from mesangial and endothelial cells, ET may stimulate contraction of the afferent and efferent arteriole, thus reducing perfusion pressure as well as ultrafiltration rate. Alternately, preglomerular constriction and contraction of the renal mesangium by ET possibly regulates glomerular ultrafiltration in vivo, which is a common finding in postischemic renal failure (49). The most likely underlying mechanism is release of ET by endothelial cells, acting on mesangial cells in a paracrine fashion. Mesangial cells, which express an abundant number of ET receptors, seem especially susceptible to the peptide's actions. The levels of ET released from mesangial cells are by a factor of 100 well below those released from endothelial cells (54). It may therefore not reach biologically active concentrations. However, when ET is secreted in an autocrine fashion by mesangial cells, even low ET concentrations may then exert actions over prolonged periods.

The fact that ET synthesis in endothelial and mesangial cells is stimulated after exposure to proinflammatory agents supports the assumption that ET serves as a biologic signal in glomerular injury and inflammation (55). A large number of proinflammatory substances, such as TGF-β, thromboxane A_2, thrombin, hypoxia, and shear stress, are triggered in response to vascular injury but also stimulate ET gene expression and ET peptide release (14,54) (Table 2).

In glomerular injury, macrophages, neutrophils, and mast cells, which have invaded the capillary narrowing and extracellular space, may be an important source of ET secretion in addition to intrinsic glomerular cell types (14,54). Because ET does not exert chemoattractant properties, it must act itself at these target cells, presumably via coupling to its specific receptors. Such receptor/activator complexes enable initiation of numerous effects that contribute to glomerular inflammation and stimulate contraction, proliferation, and matrix synthesis (56) (Fig. 4). In response to injury, stimulation of ET isopeptide synthesis may cause complex rearrangement of actin microfilament bundles and transforms mesangial cells from a quiescent to an activated status (50). The resulting long-term changes in glomerular cell phenotype would then contribute to immunologic renal disease and glomerulosclerosis.

ET AND IMMUNOLOGIC RENAL DISEASE

Stimulated ET mRNA Expression and Peptide Synthesis

Compared with healthy conditions, during experimental mesangial glomerulonephritis renal hemodynamics

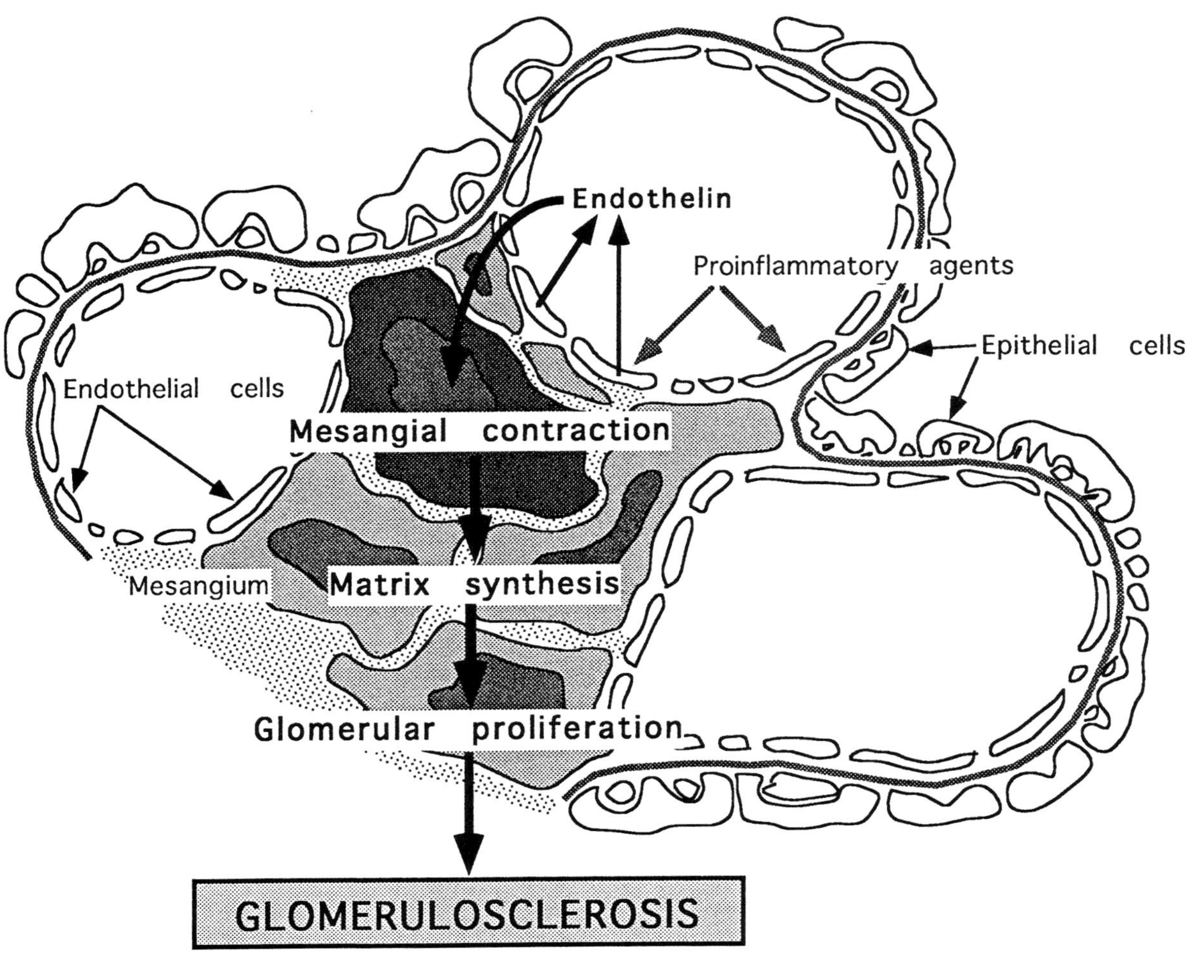

FIG. 4. Proposed pathophysiologic role of ET in immunologic renal disease. Proinflammatory agents, such as various cytokines, hormones, and physical forces, stimulate vascular endothelial cell synthesis of ET. ET is predominantly secreted abluminally and exerts its actions in adjacent tissue. In mesangial cells it is suspected to induce cell contraction, thereby promoting matrix synthesis and glomerular proliferation and ultimately inducing glomerular scarring and renal disease.

become more sensitive to ET, and impaired pressure response has been suggested to contribute to disease progression (57) (Fig. 4). In studies on experimental nephritis in NZB/W F1 mice, ET-1 transcripts but not those for ET-3 increase strongly and ET receptor mRNA expression increases gradually over time during disease progression (58). ET isopeptides also may contribute to renal glomerular disease development and to its progression after renal mass ablation, a model of focal or segmental glomerulosclerosis (55,59,60). In this model, urinary ET secretion significantly correlates with urinary protein excretion as a parameter of disease progression (61) and with the extent of glomerulosclerosis (62). Glomerular injury, histologic changes, and abnormal permeability to proteins can be prevented by ET_A-selective receptor antagonist FR139317, confirming ET_A receptor-mediated pathways in renal disease progression (63,64).

In comparison with experimental investigations, clinical studies are few and primarily assess urinary ET excretion, which increases in several renal diseases and correlates with deterioration of glomerular function and with albumin excretion in glomerulonephritis (59,65,66). The relevance of the clinical studies remains questionable, although growing evidence exists for the role of ET in renal pathophysiologic conditions, and progress will only be achieved by the availability in clinical conditions of ET receptor blockers and ET synthesis inhibitors. During the course of immunologic renal disease, plasma ET levels are elevated in acute poststreptococcal glomerulonephritis (67), and in IgA nephropathy it has been speculated that ET-1 mRNA-expressing peripheral blood monocytes may contribute to the disease progression (68). However, to what extent ET-1 mRNA-expressing activated monocytes may contribute to disease progression and directly affect intrinsic glomerular cells is unclear. Agents that are released from infiltrating macrophages or intrinsic cells contribute to the development and progression of renal glomerular disease, among which ET may act through activation of mesangial cells directly. The putative underlying mechanism of ET is its mitogenic effect on mesangial cells and its stimulatory effect on synthesis of extracellular matrix components such as type I, III, and IV collagen and laminin (62). ET may thereby maintain proliferation and precede glomerulosclerosis (69).

ET Receptor-Mediated Effects

Only limited experimental and clinical data exist on ET receptor-mediated effects in immunologic renal disease. In the remnant kidney model, the renoprotective effect of an ET_A-selective receptor antagonist was demonstrated: segmental glomerulosclerosis, histologic changes, and abnormal permeability to proteins were prevented (63). Similar effects also were demonstrated with an orally active ET_A/ET_B nonselective receptor antagonist, and survival rates were significantly prolonged (64).

In nonimmunologic renal disease, protective effects of ET receptor antagonists on renal function, especially in acute renal failure, have been reported. An unselective ET receptor antagonist, given before experimentally induced acute ischemic renal failure, only leads to partial restitution of morphologic changes in the kidney as well as of renal function itself (70). Selective ET_A receptor antagonist treatment, on the other hand, given before the onset of ischemia, improved clearance and net tubular reabsorption, whereas when applied during the reperfusion period, it was not effective to prevent deterioration of renal function (71). When administered up to 3 h after induction of experimental acute ischemic renal failure, selective ET_A receptor antagonist treatment was able to attenuate loss of renal tubular function and glomerular filtration rate and improved long-term outcome of renal function (72). Neither the number nor the affinity of glomerular ET receptors in the clamped kidney is affected (73).

Contrary to ischemic acute renal failure, in experimental acute renal failure induced by hypertonic glycerol injection into the renal artery, ET receptor mRNA and ET receptor density are upregulated in the renal medulla and cortex. The upregulation is particularly pronounced with the ET_B receptor rather than with the ET_A receptor and may account for renal functional impairment (74,75).

In summary, the response to receptor antagonists appears to be complex. In immunologic renal disease, although only limited data exist, evidence suggests renoprotective effects via ET_A receptor blockade. The possible benefits via the ET_B receptor need further clarification. In nonimmunologic renal disease, ET receptors seem to be refractory to antagonists or "unavailable" after internalization, an effect that also has been reported for ET receptor expression in rat kidneys during pulmonary hypoxia (76) and for ET receptors in hypertension (77), which makes it especially difficult to investigate receptor antagonist effects. However, response to receptor antagonists also may be masked due to inhibition by ET of cAMP response to agonist stimulation. In rat papillary tubules, ET-1 as well as ET-3, and in inner medullary collecting duct, ET-1 exert such effects in a dose-dependent fashion via the ET_B receptor (78,79).

NITRIC OXIDE

Arginine-Citrulline Pathway

NO is a highly reactive and toxic gaseous molecule with a molecular weight of 30 Daltons that is synthesized via enzymatic conversion of L-arginine to L-citrulline by NO synthases (NOS) in a variety of cell types and tissues (Fig. 5). In biologic systems the molecule is labile, with a half-life of a few seconds, and is rapidly oxidized to stable NO_2 and NO_3 (80). Via diffusion, NO reaches its target cell, where it couples to the iron of the heme group of guanylate cyclase and stimulates synthesis of cGMP, which subsequently exerts its local actions (Fig. 6). Although the synthetic pathway is the same in all cell systems, its regulation differs because there are several distinct forms of NOS.

Nitric Oxide Synthases

Three isoforms of NOS have been identified. A calcium-independent, cytokine-inducible form (iNOS) (81, 82) with a molecular weight of 130 kDa is expressed in many ciel types, the list of which is growing, including macrophages, neutrophils, neurons, keratinocytes, astrocytes, hepatocytes, pancreatic islet cells, renal tubular epithelial cells, retinal pigment epithelial cells, respiratory epithelial cells, cardiac myocytes, mesangial cells, endothelial cells, fibroblasts, chondrocytes, osteoclasts, and vascular smooth muscle cells (81,83,84). Two calcium-dependent, apparently constitutive, forms with approximately 60% homology among each other (86–88) and a molecular weight of 150 to 160 kDa are expressed in neuronal tissue (nNOS) (89) and in vascular endothelium (eNOS) (90). NOS are encoded by specific genes, which have been cloned and were used to analyze expression in various tissues (86–88,91–94). The iNOS gene spans 37 kb, eNOS 21 kb, and nNOS 100 kb.

NOS enzymes display recognition sites for cofactors, such as calmodulin, NADPH, flavin adenine dinucleotide, and flavin mononucleotide. After Ca^{2+} has been made available through stimulation by various agents, formation of a Ca^{2+}/calmodulin complex together with oxidative cofactors regulates constitutive eNOS or nNOS enzyme activity and NO formation (89). Synthesis of constitutive NOS peptides is independent of transcriptional regulation, but they can be upregulated and downregulated via hemodynamic changes (95) and shear

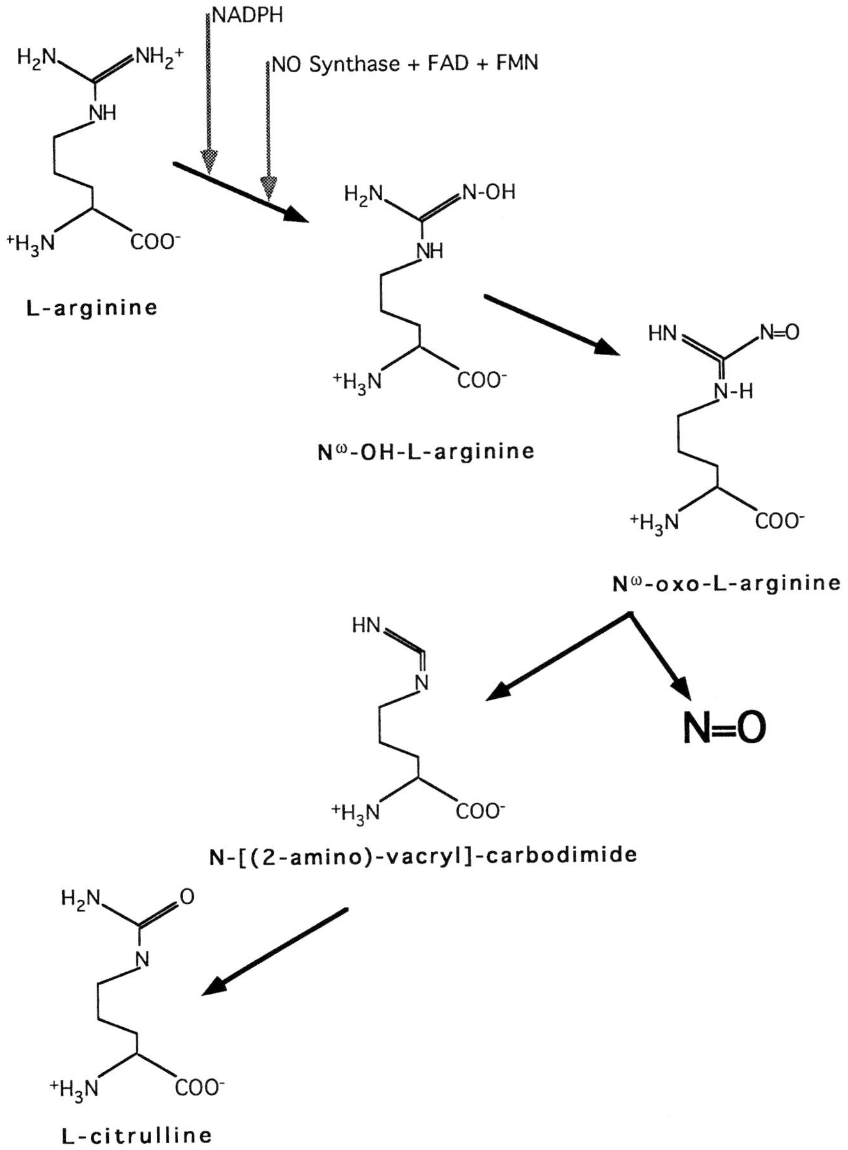

FIG. 5. Biosynthesis of NO. L-arginine is oxidized by catalysis of the flavin adenine dinucleotide (FAD) and flavin mononucleotide (FMN) containing enzyme NOS via several intermediates to yield the gaseous radical NO.

forces (96). iNOS does not require exogenous calcium or calmodulin but challenge with immunologic or inflammatory stimuli and resulting transcriptional regulation to be induced (97). Low basal levels are thereby stimulated many times.

The role of phosphorylation on enzymatic NOS activity is unclear. nNOS is effectively phosphorylated by protein kinase C, cAMP-dependent kinase, and calcium/calmodulin-dependent kinase, but phosphorylation has no effect on its catalytic activity (98,99). Another report states that calmodulin-dependent protein kinase II suppresses nNOS activity, whereas protein kinase C increases its activity (100). iNOS can be phosphorylated by protein kinase C, cAMP-dependent kinase, and calmodulin-dependent kinase II, but the resulting phosphopeptides are different from agonist-stimulated phosphopeptide (T. Michel, personal communication), so that in summary evidence is missing on the role of phosphorylation on direct enzymatic NOS activity.

NOS Gene Regulation

Although regulatory influences on the NOS enzyme activity are extensively evaluated, little is known about the regulation of NOS genes and possible signaling pathways involved. So far it is known that the induction of the iNOS gene by interleukin-1β is regulated by a protein kinase C–independent and Ca^{2+}/calmodulin-independent mechanism (101). Gamma-interferon synergizes with LPS to induce transcription but also stabilizes iNOS mRNA. On the other hand, transforming growth factor-β (TGFβ)destabilizes the transcript and decreases translation, but also accelerates degradation of iNOS protein (102).

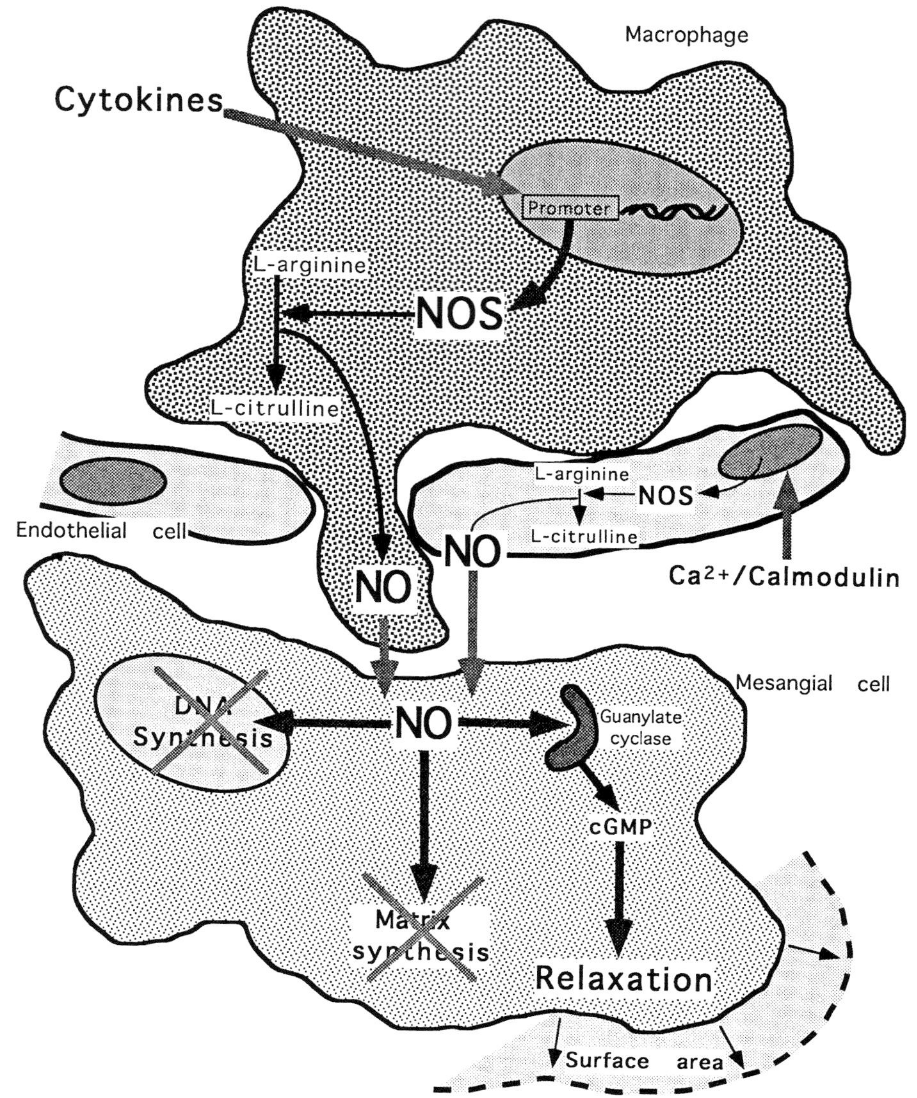

FIG. 6. Postulated NO signaling pathway. Postulated NO signaling pathway leading to inhibition of DNA synthesis, inhibition of matrix synthesis, and cell relaxation.

The eNOS gene is stably expressed, a regulatory mechanism has not been established. However, a preliminary report demonstrated modulation of the eNOS gene by TGF-β, presumably through coupling to an upstream response element (103). Tumor necrosis factor (TNF)-α as well has been reported to decrease steady-state eNOS mRNA levels via destabilization of the transcript (87,96). eNOS mRNA presumably is controlled through induction of a yet unknown protein (104). eNOS plays an important role in vascular tone regulation, prevention of thrombus formation, and modulation of mitogenesis and expresses antiproliferative activity (105). Due to its apparent lack of regulation, eNOS may contribute to a variety of diseases through the relative predominance of bioactive counterparts, for example, vasoconstrictors. Possible mechanisms include inappropriate cGMP synthesis, changes of intracellular ion concentrations, and altered upstream gene regulatory elements (103,106).

Renal NOS Localization

Early, indirect evidence for NO biosynthesis in the kidney was obtained by measurements of the NO end products NO_x and cGMP. NO_2 was detected in isolated glomeruli and cultured mesangial cells (107–111) and cGMP in cultured glomerular endothelial and mesangial cells (112,113). Urinary NO_x excretion was interpreted as an indicator for glomerular NO production (114).

Recently, direct activation of the NO pathway in the glomerulus was demonstrated in Northern analysis and by immunolocalization. However, no reports exist on direct measurement of NO in the glomerulus. eNOS transcripts have been demonstrated in cultured glomerular endothelial cells, as well as in endothelium of renal arterioles (87). nNOS mRNA is localized in the inner medullary collecting duct and, to a lesser extent, in the glomerulus, inner medullary thin limb of Henle's loop, cortical and outer medullary collecting duct, and renal vasculature (115). These findings partially correlate with immunoreactive nNOS protein synthesis, which was detected in the glomerulus, especially the macula densa, juxtraglomerular apparatus, and glomerular capsule in rat and human kidneys (95). iNOS mRNA has been demonstrated in mesangial cells (116), the proximal collecting duct, and inner medullary collecting duct (117), and iNOS protein has been localized to the preglomerular portion of the afferent arteriole (118) and cultured rat mesangial cells (116).

PHYSIOLOGIC ROLE OF NO IN THE GLOMERULUS

The major roles of NO are in the control of blood pressure and vascular tone, neurotransmission, mediation of macrophage cytotoxicity, and inhibition of platelet aggregation. The constitutive enzymes are involved in vascular regulation, whereas the inducible isoform produces high NO concentrations implicated in tissue damage and immune response.

In the kidney, physiologic effects of NO have been evaluated by indirect means. Structural L-arginine analogs, N^G-nitro-L-arginine methyl ester (L-NAME) and N^G-monomethyl-L-arginine (L-NMMA), were used to pharmacologically inhibit the conversion of L-arginine to L-citrulline and NO (119). Acutely, inhibition of NO synthesis increases afferent and efferent arteriolar resistance and causes reduction of cortical blood flow (120) and renal plasma flow (121). Although the glomerular filtration rate is unchanged, the filtration fraction is elevated (122,123), and urine flow and sodium excretion are reduced (121). Chronically, L-NAME inhibition of NO synthesis induces arterial hypertension (124), associated with a large increase in renal vascular resistance, a decrease in renal plasma flow, and marked natriuresis (125). If inhibition of the L-arginine/NO pathway is sustained, proteinuria, glomerulosclerosis and uremia will follow (126,127). Acute as well as chronic effects of NO inhibition can be ameliorated and eventually reversed by the administration of L-arginine. L-arginine positively influences a variety of immunologic renal disease models, such as renal mass reduction (128), diabetic nephropathy (129), and puromycin amino-nucleoside nephrosis (130).

These observations highlight the importance of endogenous NO in control of vascular tone, glomerular filtration, renal perfusion, and renal electrolyte balance. The exact mechanism involved, whether mass balance is modulated and shifted toward vasoconstrictor actions or whether mechanisms such as supersensitization of the renal cortex to vasoconstrictors play a role, is unknown. However, autoregulation of the renal blood flow during L-NAME administration remains intact (131), and endogenous vasoconstrictors only marginally contributes to physiologic effects during NO blockade in the kidney (132).

PHYSIOLOGIC ROLE OF NO ON GLOMERULAR CELL TYPES

Mesangial cells are affected by NO to increase capillary surface area and the glomerular ultrafiltration coefficient (123). In cultured mesangial cells, evidence exists for an inducible NOS and for the activation of guanylate cyclase and synthesis of cGMP (133). As yet, no concrete evidence exists on the presence of either nNOS or eNOS in mesangial cells (115). Mesangial cells, which contain actin and myosin, actively contract to modulate glomerular blood flow through the mesangium (54). NO can inhibit angiotensin II–induced cellular contraction and mesangial cell growth induced by serum-derived and platelet-derived growth factors (134,135). NO donors, such as S-nitroso-N-acetyl-penicillamine (SNAP), isosorbide dinitrate, and sodium nitroprusside (SNP), prevent agonist-induced [^{3}H] thymidine incorporation, a measure of new DNA synthesis. This antiproliferative effect is blocked by NO antagonists, such as hemoglobin and methylene blue, as well as by L-MMA (136). Loss of NO with prevalence of growth factors may therefore stimulate mesangial cell proliferation (137). These data emphasize the important role of NO in glomerular function via changes of mesangial surface area and via attenuation of mesangial cell–mediated matrix production.

Glomerular endothelial cells have not been directly assayed for NO production. The central position of the glomerular mesangium within the glomerulus and the direct juxtaposition of endothelial cells and mesangial cells permits cross-communication. Coculture experiments demonstrated that bovine glomerular endothelial cells induced release of cGMP in mesangial cells. The release could be inhibited by hemoglobin and methylene blue and was calcium dependent, suggesting the physiologic importance of constitutive eNOS (113). 8-bromo-cGMP, a synthetic analog to cGMP, inhibited mesangial cell proliferation in rats only, which demonstrates species-specific antimitogenic effects of NO and of intrinsic cGMP production (134). In human mesangial cells, NO does not require cGMP production to exert its antiproliferative effects. Likewise BALB/3t3 fibroblasts do not require cGMP to be inhibited in their proliferation (138).

NO AND IMMUNOLOGIC RENAL DISEASE

According to current knowledge, NO may contribute to immunologic renal disease through deleterious as well as cytoprotective glomerular cell-dependent processes (Fig. 7).

Cytotoxic Effects

Cytokines that are produced during glomerular injury are responsible for the induction of NOS in infiltrating macrophages and intrinsic glomerular cells such as endothelial and mesangial cells (Fig. 7) Evidence for an active role of NO in glomerular disease has been demonstrated in vitro and in vivo via detection of NO_x excretion, via Northern analysis, and by immunohistochemistry.

NO_x production as an indication for the contribution of the NO pathway in glomerular disease was reported in accelerated nephrotoxic nephritis, which occurs due to macrophage-dependent glomerular injury (140). In immune complex nephritis, too, isolated glomeruli and infiltrating macrophages produce high amounts of NO_x (111). Cellular NO_x secretion and urinary NO_x excretion is augmented, and kidney iNOS mRNA expression is stimulated (110,139,140). L-NMMA in this model is able to prevent onset of glomerulonephritis, thus confirming accelerated glomerular injury by NO (141). There is also evidence for infiltrating macrophages as a major source of NO in active Heymann glomerulonephritis (107). This experimental glomerulonephritis shows induction of NOS, demonstrated by NO_x production, which depends on a complex network of cytokine activation such as IL-1, TNF-α, and TGF-β (142–144). These inflammatory products also attract macrophages. In cultured human mesangial cells, too, NO production depends not only on the rate of macrophage infiltration, but also on the stimulation with multiple cytokines (135). Although proliferative mesangial cells do not spontaneously produce NO_x, together with the anti–Thy 1.1 mesangial proliferative glomerulonephritis model, strong evidence exists for the activation of NOS protein in native or diseased mesangial cells by endotoxins and cytokines (110,111). Mesangial cells are affected by NO to increase capillary surface area and the glomerular ultrafiltration coefficient (123), with consecutive hyperfiltration and possible glomerular scarring (Fig. 7). Not only induction but also long-term outcome of immunologic renal disease is correlated with NO synthesis. Mesangial cell lysis is prevented in experimental glomerulonephritis after NO inhibition with structural analogs (145).

These experiments indicate that a resident population of macrophages in the normal glomerulus can be activated to produce NO under certain conditions. Alternately, elevated NO levels in the nephritic glomerulus may result from intrinsic glomerular mesangial cells directly. However, it cannot be decided what mechanism is involved in neutrophil-mediated glomerular inflammation, with increased neutrophil adherence and expression of leukocyte adhesion molecules (146,147). Through attraction of leukocytes, however, NO may contribute to mesangial cell-dependent matrix production.

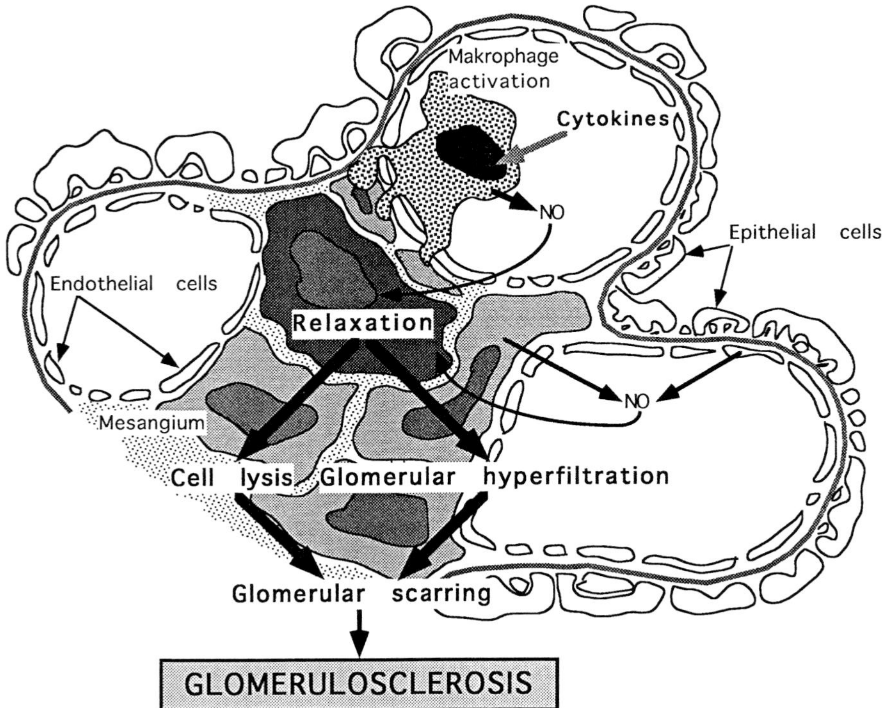

FIG. 7. Proposed pathophysiologic role of NO in immunologic renal disease. Cytokine release during glomerular injury induces NO synthesis in activated infiltrating macrophages and in intrinsic glomerular cells. NO affects mesangial cells to increase capillary surface area by relaxation, thus inducing glomerular hyperfiltration, cell lysis, and matrix synthesis, ultimately leading to glomerular scarring and renal disease.

Cytoprotective Effects

Focal or segmental glomerulosclerosis occurs after reduction of renal mass due to the resulting hyperfiltration and to increased intraglomerular hydraulic pressure (55,59,60,148). Inhibition of NO by structural analogs L-NAME or L-NMMA leads to increased intraglomerular hydraulic pressure, accompanied by renal vasoconstriction, proteinuria, and glomerular sclerosis (129). Glomerular scarring can be prevented and renal vascular resistance is ameliorated in renal mass–ablated animals that have been fed with L-arginine (130). This effect demonstrates the important protective role of NO in glomerular sclerotic lesions.

Another morphologic finding in glomerular injury, thrombosis, is suspected to occur due to NO inhibition, suggesting antithrombotic as well as platelet inhibitory properties for NO (149). These changes presumably involve the endothelial cell rather than other glomerular cell systems, and require activation of the endothelium.

In summary, elevated NO levels in the nephritic glomerulus affect vascular tone, mesangial relaxation, and tissue perfusion via direct endothelium-dependent pathways. The resulting glomerular hyperfiltration is suspected to directly affect glomerular mesangium integrity and ultimately lead to glomerulosclerosis (Fig. 7).

REFERENCES

1. Yanagisawa M, Kurihara H, Kimura S, et al. A novel potent vasoconsrictor peptide produced by vascular endothelial cells. *Nature* 1988; 332:411–415.
2. Furchgott RF, Zawadzki JV. The obligatory role of endothelial cells in the relaxation of arterial smooth muscle by acetylcholine. *Nature* 1980;288:373–376.
3. Inoue A, Yanagisawa M, Kurihara S, et al. The human endothelin family: three structurally and pharmacologically distinct isopeptides predicted by three separate genes. *Proc Natl Acad Sci U S A* 1989;86: 2863–2867.
4. Kimura S, Kasuya Y, Sawamura T, et al. Structure-activity relationships of endothelin: importance of the C-terminal moiety. *Biochem Biophys Res Commun* 1988;156:1182–1186.
5. Ahn K, Beningo K, Olds G, Hupe D. The endothelin-converting enzyme from human umbilical vein is a membrane-bound metalloprotease similar to that from bovine aortic endothelial cells. *Proc Natl Acad Sci U S A* 1992;89:8606–8610.
6. Ohnaka K, Nishikawa M, Takayanagi R, Haji M, Nawata H. Partial purification of phosporamidon-sensitive endothelin converting enzyme in porcine aortic endothelial cells: high affinity for Ricicnus communis agglutinin. *Biochem Biophys Res Commun* 1992;185: 611–616.
7. Wagner OF, Nowotny P, Vierhapper H, Waldhausl W. Plasma concentrations of endothelin in man: arterio-venous differences and release during venous stasis. *Eur J Clin Invest* 1990;20:502–505.
8. Baley PA, Resink TJ, Eppenberger U, Hahn A. Endothelin messenger RNA and receptors are differentially expressed in cultured human breast epithelial and stromal cells. *J Clin Invest* 1990;85:1320–1323.
9. Ehrenreich H, Anderson RW, Ogino Y, et al. Endothelins, peptides with potent vasoactive properties, are produced by human macrophages. *J Exp Med* 1990;172:1741–1748.
10. Resink TJ, Hahn AWA, Scott-Burden T, Powell J, Weber E, Bühler FR. Inducible endothelin mRNA expression and peptide secretion in cultured human vascular smooth muscle cells. *Biochem Biophys Res Commun* 1990;168:1303–1310.
11. MacCumber MW, Ross CA, Snyder SH. Endothelin in brain: receptors, mitogenesis and biosynthesis in glial cells. *Proc Natl Acad Sci U S A* 1990;87:2359–2363.
12. Marsden PA, Dorfman DM, Collins T, Brenner BM, Orkin S, Ballermann BJ. Regulated expression of endothelin 1 in glomerular capillary endothelial cells. *Am J Physiol* 1991;261:F117–F125.
13. Ohta K, Hirata Y, Imai T, et al. Cytokine-induced release of endothelin-1 from porcine renal epithelial cell line. *Biochem Biophys Res Commun* 1990;169:578–584.
14. Sakamoto H, Sasaki S, Hirata Y, et al. Production of endothelin-1 by rat cultured mesangial cells. *Biochem Biophys Res Commun* 1990; 169:462–468.
15. Kohan DE. Endothelin synthesis by rat renal tubule cells. *Am J Physiol* 1991;261:F221–F226.
16. Uchida S, Takemoto F, Ogata E, Kurokawa K. Detection of endothelin-1 mRNA by RT-PCR in isolated rat renal tissues. *Biochem Biophys Commun* 1992;188:108–113.
17. Ujiie K, Terada Y, Nonogushi H, Shunohara M, Tomita K, Marumo F. Messenger RNA expression and synthesis of endothelin-1 along rat nephron segments. *J Clin Invest* 1992;90:1043–1048.
18. Ohkubo S, Ogi K, Hosoya M, et al. Specific expression of human endothelin-2 (ET-2) gene in a renal adenocarcinoma cell line. Molecular cloning of cDNA encoding the precursor of ET-2 and its characterization. *FEBS Lett* 1990;274:136–140.
19. Marsen TA, Simonson MS, Dunn MJ. Renal actions of endothelin: linking cellular signaling pathways to kidney disease. *Kidney Int* 1994;45:336–344.
20. Sakurai T, Yanagisawa M, Tokuwa Y, et al. Cloning of a cDNA encoding a non-isopeptide selective subtype of the endothelin receptor. *Nature* 1990;348:732–735.
21. Arai H, Seiji H, Aramori I, Ohkubo H, Nakanishi S. Cloning and expression of a cDNA encoding an endothelin receptor. *Nature* 1990; 348:730–732.
22. Martin ER, Brenner BM, Ballermann BJ. Heterogeneity of cell surface endothelin receptors. *J Biol Chem* 1990;265:14044–14049.
23. Lin H-Y, Kaji EH, Winkel GK, Ives HE, Lodish HF. Cloning and functional expression of a vascular smooth muscle endothelin-receptor. *Proc Natl Acad Sci U S A* 1990;88:3185–3189.
24. Kohzuki M, Johnston CI, Chai SY, Casley DJ, Mendelsohn FAO. Localization of endothelin-receptors in rat kidney. *Eur J Pharmacol* 1989;160:193–194.
25. Jones CR, Hiley CR, Pelton JT, Miller RC. Autoradiographic localization of endothelin binding sites in the kidney. *Eur J Pharmacol* 1989;163:379–382.
26. Terada Y, Tomita K, Nonagushi H, Marumo F. Different localization of two types of endothelin receptor mRNA in microdissected rat nephron segments using reverse transcriptase and polymerase chain assay. *J Clin Invest* 1992;90:107–112.
27. Horie M, Uchida S, Yanagisawa M, Matsushita Y, Kurokawa K, Ogata E. Mechanisms of endothelin-1 mRNA and peptide induction by TGF-β and TPA in MDCK cells. *J Cardiovasc Pharmacol* 1991; 17(suppl):222–225.
28. Kurihara H, Yoshizumi M, Suguyama T, et al. Transforming growth factor-β stimulates the expression of endothelin mRNA by vascular endothelial cells. *Biochem Biophys Res Commun* 1989;159:1435–1440.
29. Marsden PA, Brenner BM. Transcriptional regulation of the endothelin-1 gene by TNF-α. *Am J Physiol* 1992;262:C854–C861.
30. Inoue A, Yanagisawa M, Takuwa Y, Mitsui Y, Kobayashi M, Masaki T. The human preproendothelin gene. *J Biol Chem* 1989;264: 14954–14959.
31. Wilson D, Dorfman DM, Orkin SH. A nonerythroid GATA-binding protein is required for function of the human preproendothelin-1 promotor in endothelial cells. *Mol Cell Biol* 1990;10:4856–4862.
32. Lee ME, Temizier DH, Clifford JA, Quertermous T. Cloning of GATA-binding protein that regulates endothelin-1 gene expression in endothelial cells. *J Biol Chem* 1991;266:16188–16192.
33. Dorfman DM, Wilson DB, Bruns G, Orkin SH. Human transcription factor GATA-2. *J Biol Chem* 1992;267:1279–1285.
34. Yokokawa K, Mandal AK, Kohno M, et al. Heparin suppresses endothelin-1 action and production in spontaneously hypertensive rats. *Am J Physiol* 1992;32:R1035–R1041.
35. Kohno M, Yasunari K, Yokokawa K, Murakawa K, Horio T, Takeda T. Inhibition by atrial and brain natriuretic peptides on endothelin-1 secretion after stimulation with angiotensin II and thrombin of cultured human endothelial cells. *J Clin Invest* 1991;87:1999–2004.

36. Saijonmaa O, Ristimäki A, Fyhrquist F. Atrial natriuretic peptide, nitroglycerine, and nitroprusside reduce basal and stimulated endothelin production from cultured endothelial cells. *Biochem Biophys Res Commun* 1990;173:514–520.
37. Hu RM, Levin ER, Pedram A, Frank HJL. Atrial natriuretic peptide inhibits the production and secretion of endothelin from cultured endothelial cells. *J Biol Chem* 1992;24:17384–1389.
38. Hirata Y, Emori T, Eguchi S, Kanno K, Imai T, Ohta K, Marumo F. Endothelin receptor subtype B mediates synthesis of nitric oxide by cultured bovine endothelial cells. *J Clin Invest* 1993;91:1367–1373.
39. Miller WL, Redfield MM, Burnett JC Jr. Integrated cardiac, renal, and endocrine actions of endothelin. *J Clin Invest* 1989;83:317–320.
40. Badr KF, Murray JJ, Breyer MD, Takahashi K, Inagami T, Harris RC. Mesangial cell, glomerular, and renal vascular responses to endothelin in the kidney. *J Clin Invest* 1989;83:336–342.
41. Lippton H, Goff J, Hyman A. Effects of endothelin in the systemic and renal vascular beds in vivo. *Eur J Pharmacol* 1988;155:197–199.
42. Hirata Y, Matsuoka H, Kimura K, et al. Renal vasoconstriction by the endothelial cell-derived peptide endothelin in spontaneously hypertensive rats. *Circ Res* 1989;65:1370–1379.
43. Wright CE, Fozard JR. Regional vasodilation is a prominent feature of the hemodynamic response to endothelin in aenesthetized, spontaneously hypertensive rats. *Eur J Pharmacol* 1988;155:201–203.
44. Katoh T, Chang H, Uchida S, Okuda T, Kurokawa K. Direct effects of endothelin in the rat kidney. *Am J Physiol* 1990;258:F397–F402.
45. Namiki A, Hirata Y, Ishikawa M, Moroi M, Aikawa J, Machii K. Endothelin-1 and endothelin-3–induced vasorelaxation via common generation of endothelium-derived nitric oxide. *Life Sci* 1992;50: 677–682.
46. Owada A, Tomita K, Terada Y, Sakamoto H, Nonoguchi H, Marumo F. Endothelin (ET)-3 stimulates cyclic guanosin 3′,5′-monophosphate production via ET_B receptor by producing nitric oxide in isolated rat glomerulus, and in cultured rat mesangial cell. *J Clin Invest* 1994; 93:556–563.
47. Uchida K, Ballermann BJ. Sustained activation of PGE_2 synthesis in mesangial cells cocultured with glomerular endothelial cells. *Am J Physiol* 1992;263:C200–C209.
48. Edwards RM, Trizna WT, Ohlstein EH. Renal microvascular effects of endothelin. *Am J Physiol* 1990;259:F217–F221.
49. Firth JD, Raine AE, Ratcliffe PJ, Ledingham JG. Endothelin: an important factor in acute renal failure. *Lancet* 1988;19:1179–1181.
50. Simonson MS, Dunn MJ. Endothelin-1 stimulates contraction of rat glomerular mesangial cells and potentiates β-adrenergic–mediated cyclic adenosine monophosphate accumulation. *J Clin Invest* 1990; 85:790–797.
51. Simonson MS, Wann S, Mené P, et al. Endothelin stimulates phospholipase C, Na^+/H^+ exchange, *c-fos* expression, and mitogenesis in rat mesangial cells. *J Clin Invest* 1989;83:708–712.
52. Baldi E, Dunn MJ. Endothelin binding and receptor down-regulation in rat glomerular mesangial cells. *J Pharmacol Exp Ther* 1991;256: 581–586.
53. Mené P, Simonson MS, Dunn MJ. Physiology of the mesangial cell. *Physiol Rev* 1989;69:1347–1424.
54. Zoja C, Orisio S, Perico N, et al. Constitutive expression of endothelin gene in cultured human mesangial cells and its modulation by transforming growth factor β, thrombin, and thromboxane A_2 analogue. *Lab Invest* 1991;64:16–25.
55. Simonson MS, Dunn MJ. Endothelin peptides: a possible role in glomerular infammation. *Lab Invest* 1991;64:1–4.
56. Simonson MS, Jones JM, Dunn MJ. Differential regulation of *fos* and *jun* gene expression and AP-1 *cis* element activity by endothelin isopeptides: possible implications for mitogenic signaling by endothelin. *J Biol Chem* 1992;267:8643–8649.
57. Kanai H, Okuda S, Kiyama S, Tomooka S, Hiarakata H, Fujishima M. Effects of endothelin and angiotensin II on renal hemodynamics in experimental mesangial proliferative nephritis. *Nephron* 1993;64: 609–614.
58. Nakamura T, Ebihara I, Fukui M, et al. Renal expression of mRNAs for endothelin-1, endothelin-3 and endothelin receptors in NZB/W F1 mice. *Renal Physiol Biochem* 1993;16:233–243.
59. Orisio S, Benigni A, Bruzzi I, et al. Renal endothelin gene expression is increased in remnant kidney and correlates with disease progression. *Kidney Int* 1993;43:354–358.
60. Benigni A, Perico N, Gaspari F, et al. Increased renal endothelin production in rats with reduced renal mass. *Am J Physiol* 1991;260: F331–F339.
61. Brooks DP, Contino LC, Storer B, Ohlstein EH. Increased endothelin excretion in rats with renal failure induced by partial nephrectomy. *Br J Pharmacol* 1991;104:987–989.
62. Orisio S, Zoja C, Remuzzi G. The role of endothelin in the progression of the renal disease in an experimental model of chronic kidney failure. *Ann Ital Med Int* 1993;8:213–217.
63. Benigni A, Zoja C, Corna D, et al. A specific endothelin subtype A receptor antagonist protects against injury in renal disease progression. *Kidney Int* 1993;44:440–444.
64. Benigni A, Corna D, Zoja C, Remuzzi G. Effect of ET_A/ET_B receptor antagonist in remnant kidney rats [Abstract]. Fourth international Conference on Endothelin, 1995:P129.
65. Abassi ZA, Klein H, Golomb E, Keiser HR. Urinary endothelin: a possible biological marker of renal damage. *Am J Hypertens* 1993;6: 1046–1054.
66. Ohta K, Hirata Y, Shichiri M, et al. Urinary excretion of endothelin in normal subjects and patients with renal disease. *Kidney Int* 1991;39: 307–311.
67. Ozdemir S, Saatci U, Besbas N, Bakkaloglu A, Ozen S, Koray Z. Plasma atrial natriuretic peptide and endothelin levels in acute poststreptococcal glomerulonephritis. *Pediatr Nephrol* 1992;6:519–522.
68. Nakamura T, Ebihara T, Shirato I, Fukui M, Tomino Y, Koide H. Endothelin-1 mRNA expression by peripheral blood monocytes in IgA nephropathy. *Lancet* 1993;342:1147–1148.
69. Klahr S, Schreiner G, Ichikawa I. The progression of renal disease. *N Engl J Med* 1988;318:1657–1666.
70. Kusomoto K, Kubo K, Kandori H, et al. Effects of a new endothelin antagonist, TAK-044, on post-ischemic acute renal failure in rats. *Life Sci* 1994;55:301–310.
71. Chan L, Chittinandana A, Shapiro JI, Shanley PF, Schrier RW. Effect of an endothelin-receptor antagonist on ischemic renal failure. *Am J Physiol* 1994;266:F135–F138.
72. Gellai M, Jugus M, Fletcher T, DeWolf R, Nambi P. Reversal of postischemic acute renal failure with a selective endothelin A receptor antagonist in the rat. *J Clin Invest* 1994;93:900–906.
73. Wilkes BM, Pearl AR, Mento PF, Maita ME, Macica CM, Girardi EP. Glomerular endothelin receptors during initiation and maintenance of ischemic acute renal failure in rats. *Am J Physiol* 1991;260: F110–F118.
74. Roubert P, Gillard-Roubert V, Pourmarin L, et al. Endothelin receptor subtypes A and B are up-regulated in an experimental model of acute renal failure. *Mol Pharmacol* 1994;45:182–188.
75. Roubert P, Cornet S, Plas P, et al. Upregulation of renal endothelin receptors in glycerol-induced acute renal failure in the rat. *J Cardiovasc Pharmacol* 1993;22(suppl):303–305.
76. Li H, Elton TS, Chen YF, Oparil S. Increased endothelin receptor gene expression in hypoxic rat lung. *Am J Physiol* 1994;266: L553–L560.
77. Hayzer DJ, Cicila G, Cockerham C, et al. Endothelin A and B receptors are down-regulated in the hearts of hypertensive rats. *Am J Med Sci* 1994;307:222–227.
78. Woodcock EA, Land SL. Functional endothelin ET_B receptor on renal papillary tubules. *Eur J Pharmacol* 1993;247:93–95.
79. Kohan DE, Padilla E, Hughes AK. Endothelin B receptor mediates ET-1 effects on cAMP and PGE_2 accumulation in rat IMCD. *Am J Physiol* 1993;265:F670–F676.
80. Marletta MA, Yoon PS, Iyengar R, Leaf CD, Wishnok JS. Macrophage oxidation of L-arginine to nitrite and nitrate: nitric oxide is an intermediate. *Biochemistry* 1988;27:8706–8711.
81. Stuehr DJ, Marletta MA. Mammalian nitrate biosynthesis: mouse macrophages produce nitrite and nitrate in response to *Escherichia coli* lipopolysaccharide. *Proc Natl Acad Sci U S A* 1985;82: 7738–7742.
82. Ding A, Nathan CF, Stuehr DJ. Release of reactive nitrogen intermediates and reactive oxygen intermediates from mouse peritoneal macrophages: comparison of activating cytokines and evidence for independent production. *J Immunol* 1988;141:2407–2412.
83. Busse R, Mülsch A. Induction of nitric oxide synthase by cytokines in vascular smooth muscle cells. *FEBS Lett* 1990;275:87–90.
84. Knowles RG, Merrett M, Salter M, Moncada S. Differential induction of brain, lung and liver nitric oxide synthase by endotoxin in the rat. *Biochem J* 1990;270:833–836.

85. Knowles RG, Salter M, Brooks SL, Moncada S. Anti-inflammatory glucocorticoids inhibit the induction by endotoxin of nitric oxide synthase in the lung, liver and aorta of the rat. *Biochem Biophys Res Commun* 1990;172:1042–1048.
86. Sessa WC, Harrison JK, Barber CM, et al. Molecular cloning and expression of a cDNA encoding endothelial cell nitric oxide synthase. *J Biol Chem* 1992;267:15274–15276.
87. Lamas S, Marsden PA, Li GK, Tempst P, Thomas M. Endothelial nitric oxide synthase: molecular cloning and characterization of a distinct constitutive isoform. *Proc Natl Acad Sci U S A* 1992;89: 6348–6352.
88. Janssens SP, Shimoushi A, Quertermous T, Bloch DB, Bloch KD. Cloning and expression of a cDNA encoding human endothelium-derived relaxing factor/nitric oxide synthase. *J Biol Chem* 1992;267: 14517–14522.
89. Bredt DS, Snyder SH. Isolation of nitric oxide synthase, a calmodulin-requiring enzyme. *Proc Natl Acad Sci U S A* 1990;265:133–136.
90. Mayer B, Schmidt K, Humbert P, Böhme E. Biosynthesis of endothelium-derived relaxing factor: a cytosolic enzyme in porcine aortic endothelial cells Ca^{2+}-dependently converts L-arginine into an activator of soluble guanylyl cyclase. *Biochem Biophys Res Commun* 1989; 164:678–685.
91. Bredt DS, Hwang PH, Glatt C, Lowenstein C, Reed RR, Snyder SH. Cloned and expressed nitric oxide synthase structurally resembles cytochrome P-450 reductase. *Nature* 1991;351:714–718.
92. Xie Q-W, Cho HJ, Calaycay J, et al. Cloning and characterization of inducible nitric oxide synthase from mouse macrophages. *Science* 1992;256:225–228.
93. Lowenstein CJ, Glatt CS, Bredt DS, Snyder SH. Cloned and expressed macrophage nitric oxide synthase contrasts with brain enzyme. *Proc Natl Acad Sci U S A* 1992;89:6711–6715.
94. Lyons CR, Orloff GJ, Cunningham JM. Molecular cloning and functional expression of an inducible nitric oxide synthase from a murine macrophage cell line. *J Biol Chem* 1992;267:6370–6374.
95. Bachmann S, Mundel P, Kriz W. Distribution of nitric oxide synthase (NOS) in the kidney. *J Am Soc Nephrol* 1992;3:540–568.
96. Nishida K, Harrison DG, Navas JP, et al. Molecular cloning and characterization of the constitutive bovine aortic endothelial cell nitric oxide synthase. *J Clin Invest* 1992;90:2092–2096.
97. Nathan C. Nitric oxide as a seretory product of mammalian cells. *FASEB J* 1992;6:3051–3064.
98. Brune B, Lapetina EG. Phosphorylation of nitric oxide synthase by protein kinase A. *Biochem Biophys Res Commun* 1991;181:921–926.
99. Bredt DS, Ferris CD, Snyder SH. Nitric oxide synthase regulatory sites: phosphorylation by cyclic AMP dependent protein kinase, protein kinase C, and calcium/calmodulin protein kinase: identification of flavin and calmodulin binding sites. *J Biol Chem* 1992;267: 10976–10981.
100. Nakane M, Mitchell J, Förstermann U, Murad F. Phosphorylation by calcium calmodulin-dependent protein kinase II and protein kinase C modulates the activity of nitric oxide synthase. *Biochem Biophys Res Commun* 1991;180:1396–1402.
101. Kanno K, Hirata Y, Imai T, Marumo F. Induction of nitric oxide synthase gene by interleukin in vascular smooth muscle cells. *Hypertension* 1993;22:34–39.
102. Vodovotz Y, Bogdan C, Paik J, Xie Q-W, Nathan C. Mechanisms of suppression of macrophage nitric oxide release by transforming growth factor beta. *J Exp Med* 1993;178:605–613.
103. Inoue N, Venema RC, Nickenig G, et al. Modulation of constitutive nitric oxide synthase expression by $TGF_{\beta 1}$ in bovine aortic endothelial cells [Abstract]. *Clin Res* 1994;42:181.
104. Yoshizumi M, Perrela MA, Burnett JC Jr, Lee ME. Tumor necrosis factor downregulates an endothelial nitric oxide synthase mRNA by shortening its half-life. *Circ Res* 1993;73:205–209.
105. Garg UC, Hassid A. Nitric oxide-generating vasodilators and 8-bromo-cyclic guanosine monophosphate inhibit mitogenesis and proliferation of cultured rat vascular smooth muscle cells. *J Clin Invest* 1989;83:1774–1777.
106. Boulanger CM, Lüscher TF. Differential effect of cyclic GMP on the release of endothelin-1 from cultured endothelial cells and intact porcine aorta. *J Clin Pharmacol* 1991;17(suppl 7):264–266.
107. Cattell V, Largen P, DeHeer E, Cook T. Glomeruli synthezise nitrite in active Heymann nephritis: the source is infiltrating macrophages. *Kidney Int* 1991;40:847–851.
108. Cattell V, Cook T, Moncada S. Glomeruli synthezise nitrite in experimental nephrotoxic nephritis. *Kidney Int* 1990;38:1056–1060.
109. Cook HT, Sullivan R. Glomerular nitrit synthesis in in situ immune complex glomerulonephritis in the rat. *Am J Pathol* 1991;139: 1047–1052.
110. Cattell V, Lianos E, Largen P, Cook T. Glomerular NO synthase activity in mesangial cell immune injury. *Exp Nephrol* 1993;1:36–40.
111. Pfeilschifter J, Rob P, Multsch A, Fandrey J, Vosbeck K, Busse R. Interleukin 1-β and tumor necrosis factor α induce a macrophage type of nitric oxide synthase in rat mesangial cells. *Eur J Biochem* 1992; 203:251–255.
112. Pfeilschifter J, Schwarzenbach H. Interleukin 1 and tumor necrosis factor stimulate cGMP formation in rat mesangial cells. *FEBS Lett* 1990;273:185–187.
113. Marsden PA, Brock TA, Ballerman BJ. Glomerular endothelial cells respond to calcium-mobilizing agonists with release of EDRF. *Am J Physiol* 1990;258:F1295–F1303.
114. Sever R, Cook T, Cattell V. Urinary excretion of nitrite and nitrate in experimental glomerulonephritis reflects systemic immune activation and not glomerular synthesis. *Clin Exp Immunol* 1992;90:326–329.
115. Terada Y, Tomita K, Nonoguchi H, Marumo F. Polymerase chain reaction localization of constitutive nitric oxide synthase and soluble guanylate cyclase messenger RNAs in microdissected rat nephron segments. *J Clin Invest* 1992;90:659–665.
116. Shultz PJ, Archer SL, Rosenberg ME. Inducible nitric oxide (NO) synthase mRNA and NO production by rat mesangial cells (MC) [Abstract]. *J Am Soc Nephrol* 1992;3:552.
117. Markewitz BA, Michael JR, Kohan DE. Cytokine-induced expression of nitric oxide synthase in rat renal tubule cells. *J Clin Invest* 1993;91: 2138–2143.
118. Tojo A, Gross SS, Zhang L, et al. Immunohistochemical localization of distinct isoforms of nitric oxide synthase in the juxtaglomerular apparatus of the normal kidney. *J Am Soc Nephrol* 1994;4: 1438–1447.
119. Furchgott RF, Vanhoutte PM. Endothelium-derived relaxing and contracting factors. *FASEB J* 1989;3:2007–2018.
120. Walder CE, Thiemermann C, Vane JR. The involvement of endothelium-derived relaxing factor in the regulation of renal cortical blood flow in the rat. *Br J Pharmacol* 1992;102:967–973.
121. Tolins JP, Palmer RMJ, Moncada S, Raji L. Role of endothelium-derived relaxing factor in regulation of renal hemodynamic responses. *Am J Physiol* 1990;258:H655–H672.
124. Lahera V, Salom MG, Fiksen-Olsen MJ, Raij L, Romero JC. Effects of N^G-monomethyl-L-arginine and L-arginine on acetylcholine renal responses. *Hypertension* 1990;15:659–663.
123. Zatz R, DeNucci G. Effects of acute nitric oxide inhibition on rat glomerular microcirculation. *Am J Physiol* 1991;261:F360–F363.
124. Ribeiro MO, Antunes E, deNucci G, Lovisolo SM, Zatz R. Chronic inhibition of nitric oxide synthesis. A new model of arterial hypertension. *Hypertension* 1992;20:298–303.
125. Baylis C, Harton P, Engels K. Endothelial derived relaxing factor controls renal hemodynamics in the normal rat kidney. *J Am Soc Nephrol* 1990;1:875–880.
126. Reyes AA, Karl IE, Klahr S. Role of arginine in health and in renal disease. *Am J Physiol* 1994;267:F331–F346.
127. Baylis C, Mitruka B, Deng A. Chronic blockade of nitric oxide synthesis in the rat produces systemic hypertension and glomerular damage. *J Clin Invest* 1992;90:278–281.
128. Reyes AA, Purkerson ML, Karl I, Klahr S. Dietary supplementation with L-arginine ameliorates the progression of renal disease in rats with subtotal nephrectomy. *Am J Kidney Dis* 1992;20:168–176.
129. Reyes AA, Karl IE, Kissane J, Klahr S. L-arginine administration prevents glomerular hyperfiltration and decreases proteinuria in diabetic rats. *J Am Soc Nephrol* 1993;4:1639–1645.
130. Reyes AA, Porras BH, Chasalow FI, Klahr S. Administration of L-arginine decreases the infiltration of the kidney by macrophages in obstructive nephropathy and puromycin-induced nephrosis. *Kidney Int* 1994;45:1346–1354.
131. Baumann JE, Persson PB, Ehmke H, Nafz B, Kirchheim HR. Role of endothelium-derived relaxing factor in renal autoregulation in conscious dogs. *Am J Physiol* 1992;32:F208–F213.
132. Kohan DE, Padilla E. Endothelin-1 production by rat inner medullary collecting duct: effect of nitric oxide, cGMP, and immune cytokines. *Am J Physiol* 1994;266:F291–F297.

133. Nicolson AG, Haites NE, McKay NG, Wilson HM, MacLeod AM, Benjamin N. Induction of nitric oxide synthase in human mesangial cells. *Biochem Biophys Res Commun* 1993;193:1269–1274.
134. Garg UC, Hassid A. Inhibition of rat mesangial cell mitogenesis by nitric oxide-generating vasodilators. *Am J Physiol* 1989;257:F60–F66.
135. Shultz PJ, Raji L. The glomerular mesangium: role in initiation and progression of renal injury. *Am J Kidney Dis* 1991;17(suppl 1):8–14.
136. Marsden PA, Ballermann BJ. Tumor necrosis factor α activates soluble guanylate cyclase in bovine glomerular mesangial cells via an L-arginine–dependent mechanism. *J Exp Med* 1990;172:1842–1852.
137. Pfeilschifter J. Platelet-derived growth factor inhibits cytokine induction of nitric oxide synthase in rat renal mesangial cells. *Eur J Pharmacol* 1991;208:339–340.
138. Garg UC, Hassid A. Nitric oxide-generating vasodilators inhibit mitogenesis and proliferation of BALB/3t3 fibroblasts by a cyclic GMP-independent mechanism. *Biochem Biophys Res Commun* 1990;171: 474–479.
139. Cook HT, Ebrahim H, Jansen AS, Foster GR, Largen P, Cattell V. Expression of the gene for inducible nitric oxide synthase in experimental glomerulonephritis in the rat. *Clin Exp Immunol* 1994;97: 315–320.
140. Jansen A, Cook T, Taylor GM, et al. Induction of nitric oxide in rat immune complex glomerulonephritis. *Kidney Int* 1994;45:115–1219.
141. Weinberg JB, Granger DL, Pisetsky DS, et al. The role of nitric oxide in the pathogenesis of spontaneous murine autoimmune disease: increased nitric oxide production and nitric oxide synthase expression in MRL-lpr/lpr mice, and reduction of spontaneous glomerulonephritis and arthritis by orally administered N^G-monomethyl-L-arginine. *J Exp Med* 1994;179:651–660.
142. Matsumoto K, Hatano M. Production of interleukin 1 in glomerular cell cultures from rats with nephrotoxic serum nephritis. *Clin Exp Immunol* 1989;75:123–128.
143. Tipping PG, Leong TW, Holdsworth SR. Tumor necrosis factor production by glomerular macrophages in anti-glomerular basement membrane glomerulonephritis in rabbits. *Lab Invest* 1991;65:272–279.
144. Hruby ZW, Shirota K, Jothy S, Lowry RP. Antiserum against tumor necrosis factor-alpha and a protease inhibitor reduce immune glomerular injury. *Kidney Int* 1991;40:43–51.
145. Ketteler M, Narita I, Border WA, Noble NA. Nitric oxide inhibition prevents mesangial cell lysis in experimental glomerulonephrits. *J Am Soc Nephrol* 1993;4:610.
146. McCall TB, Boughton-Smith NK, Palmer RMJ, Whittle BJR, Moncada S. Synthesis of nitric oxide from L-arginine by neutrophils. Release and interaction with superoxide anion. *Biochem J* 1989;261:293–296.
147. Kubes P, Suzuki M, Granger DN. Nitric oxide: an endogenous modulator of leukocyte adhesion. *Proc Natl Acad Sci U S A* 1991;88: 4651–4655.
148. Anderson S, Rennke HG, Brenner BM. Therapeutic advantage of converting enzyme inhibitors in arresting progressive renal disease associated with systemic hypertension in the rat. *J Clin Invest* 1986; 77:1993–2000.
149. Shultz P, Raji L. Endogenously synthezised nitric oxide prevents endotoxin-induced glomerular thrombosis. *J Clin Invest* 1992;90: 1718–1725.

Immunologic Renal Diseases,
edited by E. G. Neilson and W. G. Couser.
Lippincott-Raven Publishers, Philadelphia © 1997.

CHAPTER 22

Prostaglandins and Leukotrienes

Rolf A. K. Stahl

HISTORICAL BACKGROUND

Prostaglandins (PGs) and leukotrienes are metabolites of a family of oxydized 20-carbon fatty acids that exert biologic functions in almost all tissues of the body. The biolog activity of the PGs was independently described by Kurzrock and Lieb (1), Goldblatt (2), and van Euler (3). They observed that extracts of sheep seminal vesicals or human semen had pharmacologic activity and exerted vasodepressor and nonvascular smooth muscle stimulating effects. In the early 1960s, Bergström and Sjövall (4) isolated PGs from sheep prostate gland and elucidated their structures in a series of brilliant studies (5,6). In the mid-1960s Lee et al. (7,8) found that homogenates of rabbit renal medulla exert nonvascular, smooth muscle–stimulating, and vasodepressor activity. Consecutively, Lee et al. (8) described that this bioactivity was at least partially attributed to PGs and they demonstrated that prostaglandin E2 (PGE2) is synthesized in the renal medulla. Since the discovery that PGs are produced in the kidney and that the enzyme cyclooxygenase has a central key role in the production of PGs, their role in renal physiology and pathophysiology has been extensively studied.

The biologic activity of leukotrienes was originally described as a slow-reacting substance of anaphylaxis and has been known for over 50 years (9). They were functionally characterized by the potent bronchoconstricting activity and the increase in the permeabilty of postcapillary venules. Their biosynthesis was first demonstrated in leukocytes, and it has become clear that lipoxygenases are responsible for their formation (10).

Experimental and clinical studies conducted over the past 30 years have elucidated that both PGs and leukotrienes are involved in a multitude of dysfunctions in renal disease. This chapter summarizes the biochemical and pathophysiologic mechanisms of PGs and leukotrienes, with a particular focus on their role in immunologically mediated lesions.

R. A. K. Stahl: Division of Nephrology and Osteology, Department of Medicine, Universitätskrankenhaus Eppendorf, University of Hamburg, 20246 Hamburg, Germany.

BIOSYNTHESIS OF EICOSANOIDS

Biochemistry

Eicosanoids are a family of oxygenated fatty acids that include the prostanoids (PGs and thromboxane), which are formed by the cyclooxygenases; the leukotrienes and the mono-, di-, and trihydroxy acids, which are produced by the lipoxygenase pathway; and the epoxides, which are synthesized by a cytochrome P-450 epoxygenase pathway (Figs. 1–3) (11). The substrates are C20 polyunsaturated fatty acids (12–15), which contain three to five double bonds. The most abundant fatty acid is arachidonic acid (AA) (5,8,11,14-eicosatetraenoic acid; C20:4), which includes 5,8,11,14,17-eicosapentaenoic acid (C20:5), a major compound of fish oil, and the C18 and C22 fatty acids linoleic acid (C18:2) and docosahexaenoic acid (C22:6) (11). AA is an essential fatty acid and gives rise to PGs and thromboxane of the dienoic series, which are indicated by the subscript 2 in their abbreviation. The production of eicosanoids appears in three stages (11):

1. Release of AA from precursors (glycophospholipids, triglycerides, and cholesterol esters) (16).
2. Oxygenation of AA by cyclooxygenases, lipoxygenases, or epoxygenases.
3. Metabolism to end products.

The intracellular concentration of AA is very low, as is the concentration of PGs and leukotrienes. They are produced in response to hormonal stimuli or cell injury by the activation of phopholipases.

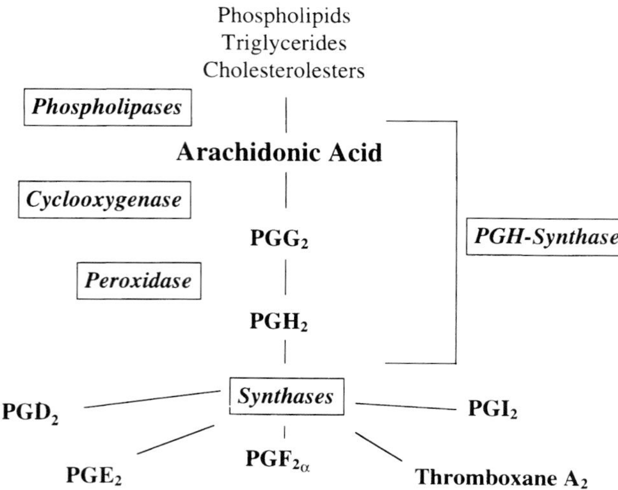

FIG. 1. Phospholipids, triglycerides, and cholesterol esters serve as substrates of the phospholipases, which generate free intracellular AA that is metabolized to PG-endoperoxides (PGH_2) by the PGH-synthase, consisting of a cyclooxygenase and a peroxidase. The biologically active prostanoids are synthesized by PG and thromboxane synthases.

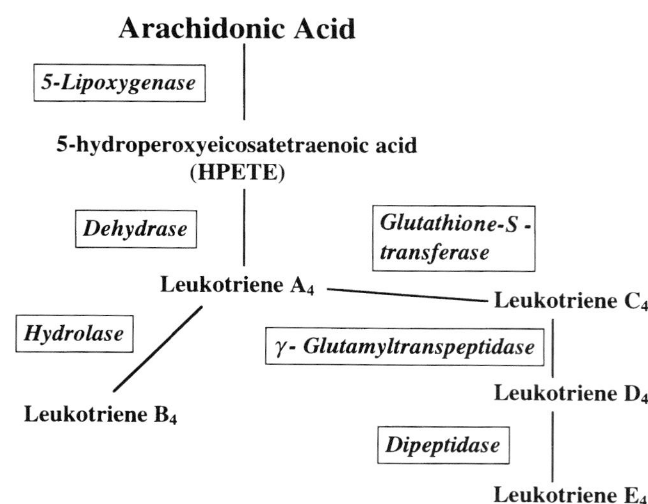

FIG. 2. The 5-lipoxygenase, which plays a central role in the biosynthesis of leukotrienes converts AA to 5-HPETE, but also forms leukotriene A_4. Leukotriene A_4 can be converted by a hydrolase to leukotriene B_4 or by a gluthathione-S-transferase to leukotriene C_4, which serves as a substrate for leukotrienes D_4 and E_4.

Phopholipases

Phospholipases are enzymes that hydrolize phospholipids, and they can be divided into two classes: acylhydrolases (phospholipases A and B) and phophodiesterases (phospholipases C and D). The most important phospholipases for the generation of free cellular AA in the cyclooxygenase pathway is phospholipase A2 (PLA2) (17,18), whereas lipoxygenase and epoxygenase products require the activation of other enzymes (19). PLA2 is a family of enzymes that are classified according to their mass, and they can be divided into secretory and intracellular forms (18,20). PLA2 hydrolizes the 2-acyl-ester and generates AA. PLA2 activation is regulated by a variety of signals, including [Ca^{2+}] (21,22), alkalanic pH (23), protein kinase C (21), and hormonal stimulants (20). After activation, PLA2 is translocated from the cytosol to the membrane and can now release AA from its membrane-bound substrates (24). This mechanism represents the most important component in the acute changes of eicosanoid formation.

Prostaglandin and Thromboxane Formation

In renal cells AA is mainly converted to PGs and thromboxane. AA is metabolized to prostaglandin endoperoxide (PGH2), which includes two reactions that are catalyzed by the same enzyme (PGH synthase) and which includes the cyclooxygenase and the peroxidase activities (25). The cyclooxygenase, but not the peroxidase activity, can specifically be inhibited by aspirin and other nonsteroidal anti-inflammatory drugs (NSAIDs) (26). Whereas aspirin, indomethacin, and meclofenamate lead to an irreversible cyclooxygenase inhibition (27,28), most other NSAIDs are competitive inhibitors of cyclooxygenase (28). There are two PGH synthases: a PGH synthase 1 (also called cyclooxygenase-1 or COX-1) and a PGH synthase 2 (also called cyclooxygenase-2 or COX-2), which have been cloned from several species (29–31). PGH2 was originally isolated from chicken fibroblasts (32) and murine 3T3 cells (33) as an immediate early gene product. Immunohistologic localization studies in the kidney show the abundance of PGH synthetase in a variety of cells in the medulla and cortex, including tubules, vascular endothelial cells, tubular interstitial cells, and glomer-

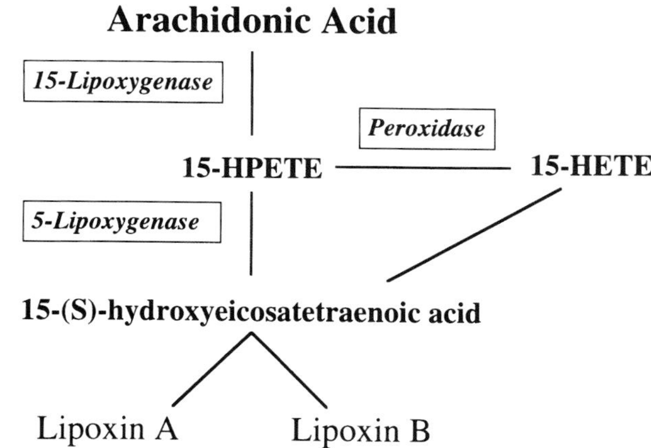

FIG. 3. The lipoxins (A and B) can be formed by nonenzymatic hydrolysis of 15-(S)-HETE, which is the 5-lipoxygenase product of 15-HPETE or also can be formed from 15-HETE.

uli (34,35). PGH2 (COX-2) synthase is drastically upregulated in pathophysiologic conditions under the influence of hormones and inflammatory mediators (36–41), data that suggest that COX-2 may play a major role in renal disease, wheras COX-1 seems to be particularly important for PG formation under physiologic conditions (42–45) (Fig. 2).

The active prostanoids (PGE2, PGD2, PGF2α, PGI2, TxA2, and PGH2) are synthesized in a cell-specific manner, i.e. each cell type produces one of these products as a major metabolite (34,46). Glomerular mesangial cells primarily produce PGE2, the endothelial cells PGI2, and the collecting ducts PGE2, whereas platelets and monocytes synthesize large amounts of thromboxane. Little information is available about enzymes that catalyze the metabolites of PGH2. Thromboxane synthase and prostacyclin synthetase are purified (47,48). PGE2 synthesis requires glutathione and is produced by several isomerases (49).

Lipoxygenase Products

Leukotrienes and mono-, di-, and trihydroxy fatty acids are formed by the lipoxygenase pathway (50). There are three major lipoxygenase pathways. The 5-, 12-, and 15-lipoxygenases include stereospecifically one oxygen molecule at the 5, 12, and 15 positions of the fatty acids. AA is also the major substrate of the lipoxygenases. The initial products are the 5-, 12-, or 15-hydroperoxyeicosatetraenoic acids (5-, 12-, 15-HPETE), which can then be reduced to the hydroxyeicosatetraenoic acids (5-, 12-, 15-HETE). 15-HETE can be transformed in a series of trihdroxy-conjugated tetraens that are called lipoxins (51) (lipoxins A and B).

The 5-lipoxygenase system produces the most potent AA metabolites, which mediate inflammation (52). In competition with its formation to 5-HETE, 5-HPETE can be converted into leukotriene A4 (LTA4), an unstable product that is then converted to LTB4 or LTC4 (Fig. 3). The formation of LTB4 requires the enzyme LTA4 hydrolase, and the formation of the peptide leukotrienes (LTC4, LTD4, and LTE4) requires a specific glutathione-S-transferase. The enzymes of the lipoxygenase pathway are predominantly present in leukocytes; however, the formation of lipoxygenase products has been demonstrated in the kidney in glomeruli (53,54) and cultured glomerular cells (55–58). The formation of lipoxin A4 has been reported in kidney cells in culture; however, the route of the biosynthetic pathway has not been entirely clear (59).

Cytochrome P-450–Dependent Monooxygenase Products

In addition to the metabolism induced by by lipoxygenase and cyclooxygenase, AA can be oxydized in the kidney by microsomal cytochrome P-450 monooxygenases (60–67). This pathway requires the presence of NAPDH and molecular oxygen to form 5,6, 8,9, 11,12, and 14,15 epoxyeicosatrienoic acids (EETs) and their corresponding dihydroyeicosatrienoic acids (DHTs), HETEs, and ω- and 1-hydroxylated metabolites (61,68). There is little information about their mechanisms in the kidney. Vasodilator (69) as well as vasoconstrictor effects (65,70) have been demonstrated in rats. In addition, some monoxygenase products induce natriuresis (8,64) but also inhibit vasopressin actions in the rabbit cortical collecting duct (71).

RENAL RECEPTORS AND INTRACELLULAR SIGNALS OF PROSTAGLANDINS AND LEUKOTRIENES

The presence of PG receptors in the kidney was first reported by Limas (72), who found that PGE2 binds to outer and inner medulla and cortex. In the meantime, several PGE subtype receptors have been cloned and characterized along the nephron. The messenger RNA (mRNA) for the EP1 subtype is expressed in the collecting ducts from the cortex to the papilla (73). Its activation is coupled to intracellular (Ca^{2+}) mobilization. The EP2 subtype, which is linked to stimulation of adenylate cyclase (74,75) is localized in the glomerulus (73). The EP3 receptor is divided into two isoforms (76), which are coupled to the inhibition of adenylate cyclase (EP3A) or an increase in (Ca^{2+}) (EP3B) (77), and they are expressed in tubules of the outer medulla, distal tubules, the thick ascending limb of Henle's loop, and inner medullary collecting ducts of the cortex (73,78,79). All EP receptor subtypes bind PGE2 and PGE1 with a similarly high affinity, whereas other PGs and thromboxane B2 (TxB2) have much lower affinities for these receptors. In glomerular mesangial cells in culture, a thromboxane A2 (TxA2) receptor was partially characterized with the use of a TxA receptor blockers and thromboxane mimetics (80). The receptor binding of the agonist activates phospholipase C, increases cytosolic [Ca^{2+}], and induces the accumulation of inositol triphosphate (81–83). Cellular receptors for leukotrienes were identified in glomeruli (84) and on mesangial cells in culture (85,86). After LTD4 binding, an increase in intracellular (Ca^{2+}) concentration and phosphoinositide hydrolysis appears (85,86).

REGIONAL FORMATION OF PROSTAGLANDINS AND LEUKOTRIENES IN THE KIDNEY

Isolated Glomeruli

After Smith and Bell described in 1978 (35) the antigenicity of cyclooxygenase in glomerular resident cells, several groups described the formation of PGs and thromboxane in isolated glomeruli of animals (87–89) and humans (90,91). The relative abundance of glomerular PGs is different between humans and rat. Whereas prostacyclin is the major product in human glomeruli (90,91), PGE2 and PGF2α are the most abundant prostanoids in rat glomeruli (87). The glomerular PG formation is regulated by several hormones, including vasoactive peptides such as angiotensin II (91–95), norepinephrine (93), arginine vasopressin (AVP) (96), electrolytes (97), (Ca^{2+})-ionophores (98), oxygen radicals (99), or drugs such as the ACE inhibitor captopril (100). Glomeruli also express lipoxygenase activity and produce 12- and 15-HETE (101–103).

Glomerular Mesangial, Endothelial, and Epithelial Cells

Mesangial cells in culture derived from different species produce large amounts of PGs (see also Chapter 29). Whereas in the rat PGE2 is the major product, human cells primarily synthesize PGI2. PG formation is stimulated by a variety of hormonal and inflammatory mediators of disease, including vasoconstrictor peptides, norepinephrine, inflammatory cytokines and growth factors (Table 1). Most of the stimulatory signals are mediated through activation of PLA2 (128–130,141,144) and PLC (128,131–133). The peptide- and cytokine-induced PLC and PLA2 stimulation involves guanosine triphosphate–binding proteins (133–137) and an increase in cytosolic (Ca^{2+}) (131,134,135,138,139). Certain stimulants increase protein kinase C (139,140) and a tyrosine kinase (142); however, cytokine-induced prostanoid formation also depends on the increased formation of cyclooxygenase 2 mass (143,144). Repressors of PG formation in mesangial cells are dexamethasone, transforming growth factor-β, interleukin (IL)-4, and certain antibodies (145–149). Endogenously formed prostanoids exert a variety of effects on mesangial cells. PGE2 and PGI2 are considered to be vasorelaxants, whereas TxB2 and leukotrienes exert vasoconstrictive effects. Several studies show that angiotensin II, AVP, and isoproterenol induce contraction of mesangial cells in culture (150–152), when PG formation is inhibited (153–155), an effect that can be reversed in the presence of PGE2 and PGI2 (155,156). In contrast, TxA2, PGF2α, and leukotrienes C4 and D4 induce mesangial cell contraction (155,157–159).

PGs and leukotrienes also are involved in the regulation of mesangial cell growth, matrix formation, and cell–cell interaction (see also Chapter 29). In rat mesangial cells in culture, the inhibition of cyclooxygenase is associated with an increase in IL-1β– and IL-6–induced cell growth (160–162), effects that are reversed by PGE2 and PGI2 (163). The PGE2-mediated effects are not fully characterized. The inhibition of mitogen-activated kinases due to an increase in cyclic adenosine monophosphate (cAMP) seems to play an important role in PGE1-mediated growth inhibition (164). Whereas PGE2 and PGI2 inhibit mesangial cell growth in culture, thromboxane A2 (163) and epoxyeicosatrienoic acids (165) stimulate mesangial cell proliferation. TxA2 also enhances the formation of extracellular matrix proteins, such as fibronectin and collagen type IV (166,167), whereas PGE2 reduces gene expression, synthesis, and secretion (168, 169) of several collagen types (Fig. 4). PGE2 and thromboxane are also involved in the mesangial cell uptake of immunglobulin complexes and low-density lipoprotein (LDL) particles. Whereas PGE2 inhibits phagocytosis, TxA2 analogs induce IgG complex and LDL uptake by mesangial cells (170,171). TxB2 furthermore stimulates the expression of endothelin and might thereby enhance mesangial cell contraction (172,173).

TABLE 1. *Stimulants of PG formation in mesangial cells*

Stimulant	Product	Species	Reference
Platelet-activating factor (PAF)	PGE_2	Rat, human	104
Angiotensin II	$PGI_2 > PGE_2$	Human	105,107
Angiotensin II	PGE_2	Rat	106,128
Ca^{2+}-ionophore	PGE_2	Rat	106,121
AVP	$PGI_2 > PGE_2$	Human, rat	105,107, 111
Complement components (C5a, MAC)	PGE_2, PGI_2, TxB_2	Rat	108,109, 126
Interleukin 1β	PGE_2	Human	110,120, 121
Tumor necrosis factor α	PGE_2	Human	110,121
Bradykinin	PGE_2, $PGF_{2}\alpha$, PGI_2	Rat	111
Thrombin	PGE_2	Rat	112
Serotonin	PGE_2	Rat	113
Oxygen radicals	PGE_2	Rat	114
Hypoxia	PGE_2, PGI_2, $PGF_{2}\alpha$	Rat	115
Endothelin	PGE_2, PGI_2, TxB_2	Bovine	116,127
Polycations	PGE_2, PGI_2, $PGF_{2}\alpha$, TxB_2	Rat	117
Lipopolysaccharides	PGE_2	Rat	118
Mercuric chloride	PGE_2	Rat	119
Interleukin 6	PGE_2	Rat	122
Poly-L-lysine	PGE_2	Rat	123
LDL	PGE_2	Rat	124
Physical stretching	PGE_2	Rat	125

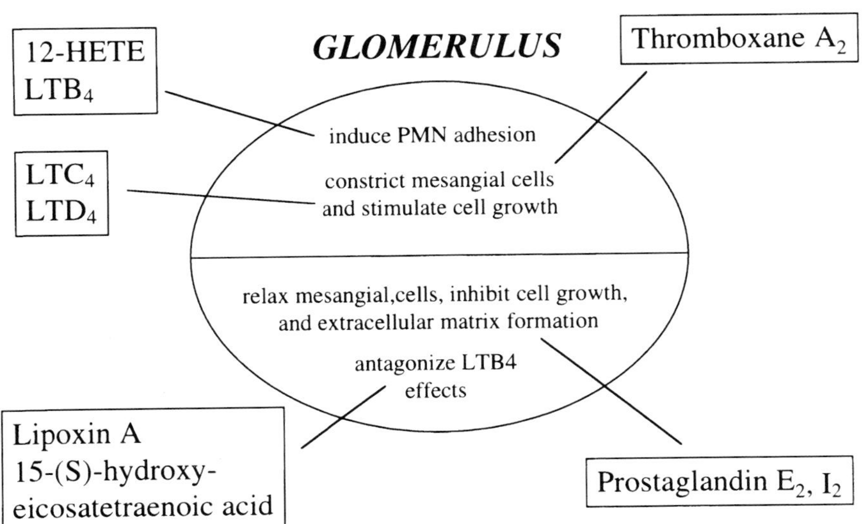

FIG. 4. Lipoxygenase and cyclooxgenase metabolites exert pro- and anti-inflammatory effects in glomerulonephritis. 12-HETE, the leukotrienes (B_4, C_4, D_4) and thromboxane A_2 induce adhesion of PMNs, constrict mesangial cells, and induce glomerular resident cell growth. In contrast, lipoxin A, 15-(S)-HETE and prostaglandins inhibit inflammatory cell recruitment and proliferation, relax mesangial cells, and reduce the formation of extracellular matrix components. The pathophysiologic consequence of altered eicosanoid formation in glomerular immune injury may therefore depend on the predominance of either pro- or anti-inflammatory components or the stage of the disease.

Rat and human epithelial cells in culture also produce PGs and thromboxane (174–177) (see also Chapter 31). The formation is stimulated by angiotensin II, AVP (174, 177), and complement components (178–180). The functional role of eicosanoids in epithelial cells is not completely clear. LTC4 and LTD4 bind to glomerular epithelial cells in culture and induce proliferation (181,182), which would suggest that leukotrienes are mitogenic. Lipoxygenase products induce the adherence of monocytes (LTD4) and neutrophils (LTB4) to glomeruli or mesangial cells in culture, an effect that is modulated by lipoxins and suggests a role of lipoxygenase products in the events of chemoattraction (175,176,183–185). Little information is available about the formation of eicosanoids in glomerular endothelial cells in culture. Bovine cultured endothelial cells primarily produce PGE2 with smaller amounts of PGF2a, TxA2, and PGI2 (186). The synthesis is regulated by PLA2, and the stimulation of prostanoids can be induced by endothelin (187).

PROSTAGLANDINS, LEUKOTRIENES, AND RENAL FUNCTION

Renal Blood Flow and Glomerular Filtration Rate (see also Chapters 2 and 11)

Intra-arterial infusion of PGE2 and PGI2 in dogs and humans produces an increase in renal blood flow (RBF) without affecting the glomerular filtration rate (GFR) (188). In the rat the response is different because PGE1 and PGE2 cause vasoconstriction (189). PGs also affect intrarenal blood flow distribution and induce an increase in outer cortical blood flow (190). Other studies, have shown that PGE2 increases flows to all zones of the kidney, preferentially to the juxtamedullary region (191). The effects of PGs appear to be due to the vasorelaxant action on vascular smooth muscle cells of afferent arterioles, interlobular arteries, and vasa recta (192,193). The normal renal hemodynamic function is not dependent on an intact PG system because the inhibition of PG synthesis in normal animals and humans does not affect renal function (194). Under situations of renal stress, particularly under the influence of vasoconstrictor hormones, which stimulate PG formation (AVP, catecholamines, angiotensin II, cytokines, or inflammatory mediators), renal hemodynamics become PG dependent and the inhibition of cyclooxygenase with NSAIDs increases the vasoconstrictor influences and leads to an impairment of renal function (195–200). This effect is due to the capacity of locally formed PGs to antagonize vasoconstricter influences of peptide hormones, catecholamines, and other lipid mediators. PGs also are involved in tubuloglomerular feedback control and can thereby regulate GFR (201–204). The importance of the intact PG system becomes particularly evident under pathophysiologic conditions, where increased formation of vasoconstrictors is associated with reduced renal perfusion, such as liver cirrhosis, heart failure, nephrotic syndrome, or loss of intact renal tissue (205–208).

Because TxA2 is an unstable cyclooxygenase metabolite, the classical studies of infusion in the kidneys have not been performed. Because endoperoxides bind to a TxA2 receptor (209,210), studies have been performed with PG endoperoxide analogs (211,212). These experiments demonstrate that the PGH2/TxA2 analogs, such as U-46,619 raise afferent and efferent arteriolar resistance in association with a reduction of glomerular capillary flow, single-nephron GFR, and RBF (213). TxA2 analogs can generate TxA2 and PGI2 (28) or eventually leukotrienes, such as LTC4, which might be partially responsible for the changes seen with the application of the analogs (213). TxA2-mediated hemodynamic changes also might derive from effects on the renin-angiotensin system because ACE inhibitors have been demonstrated to improve vasoconstrictor effects induced by TxA2 (214–216).

The lipoxygenase metabolites have vasoconstrictor as well as vasodilator effects. Systemic administration of LTC4 to rats results in a reduction of RBF and GFR (217–219). In micropuncture studies in rats, LTD4 reduced GFR and RBF due to postglomerular vasoconstriction and a reduction in the glomerular capillary ultrafiltration coefficient (Kf). In the dog, leukotrienes particularly increase efferent arteriolar resistance (220). LTB4 is without acute effects on glomerular hemodynamic function (221). In contrast to the vasoconstrictor effects of LTD4 and LTC4, the trihydroxy AA derivates exert vasodilatory effects on arterioles and increase GFR (222). They act probably by competing for the LTD4 receptor on smooth muscle cells (223). It is suggested that lipoxin A4 may act as an antagonist to the 5-lipoxygenase products and may vasodilate afferent and efferent arterioles and relax mesangial cells (222).

Less information is available on the hemodynamic functions of the cytochrome P-450 epoxygenase products. In one study in the rat kidney (224), intrarenal administration led to reduction in GFR, primarily due to afferent arteriolar constriction. It is unknown whether endogenously formed cytochrome P-450 epoxygenase products have functional consequences similar to the noncyclooxygenase prostanoid compound 8-epi-PGF2a, which also reduces afferent, arteriolar resistance, probably by interaction with the TxA2 receptor (225).

Tubulur Functions

The highest biosynthetic cyclooxygenase capacity in the kidney is found in the renal papilla (226). PGE2 is the major product. Vascular, tubular and interstitial cells all are responsible for this prostanoid formation (227–231). The tubular site that demonstrates low PG production is the proximal tubule with the higher biosynthetic capacity in the thin limbs of the loop of Henle and the highest concentrations in the medullary collecting duct (230,232–235). The formation of tubular and interstitial cell prostanoid production is regulated by sodium chloride, potassium, molarity, and bradykinin (230,231,236–239). In contrast to PGE2, the other cyclooxygenase products are only synthesized in small amounts in the medulla. The possible role of PGs on tubular functions has been studied in several ways, including cultured epithelial cells, isolated perfused tubules, and in vivo in animals and humans. In earlier experiments in the isolated perfused cortical collecting duct, PGE2 and PGF2α have been demonstrated to decrease reabsorption of sodium (240–242). Others were unable to confirm these effects (243). However, later studies confirmed the initial findings with different techniques and suggested that PGs may inhibit sodium, water, and potassium reabsorption in the distal tubule and chloride transport in the thick ascending limbs of Henle or the collecting tubule (244,245). There also seem to be species differences between rats and rabbits; for example, PGE1 is an effective inhibitor of salt and water transport in the rabbit cortical collecting duct, whereas it appears to have no significant action in the rat (246). Studies in animals and humans have shown that PGE2 and PGI2 are natriuretic (247,248) without affecting GFR (249). In humans and animals, cyclooxygenase inhibitors decrease salt excretion, which also suggests that PGs are natriuretic (250,251).

In contrast to the still unsettled effects of PGs on sodium chloride transport, there is sufficient evidence that PGE2 is an antagonist of antidiuretic-mediated water reabsorption. Grantham and Orloff (252) found that PGE1 reduced vasopressin-induced water reabsorption by 50% and suggested that PGE1 interferes with the generation of cAMP. In dissected cortical collecting ducts, a dose-dependent effect of PGE2 was demonstrated. Low PGE2 concentrations inhibited AVP-stimulated cAMP, whereas at higher concentrations a stimulatory effect was detected (253). In addition to the possible cAMP inhibitory effect, recent experiments demonstrate that PGE2 can inhibit AVP-mediated water flow due to the stimulation of protein kinase C and intracellular calcium (254,255). In turn, a series of studies have demonstrated that AVP stimulates renal PGE2 formation in humans and animals (256–258). However, it is not entirely clear whether the PGs are derived from collecting tubule cells (259–261) because high concentrations of AVP are necessary to induce PG formation. Therefore, experimental and clinical evidence suggests that PGE2 antagonizes AVP-induced water reabsorption. However, the ultimate mechanisms of action are not entirely clear.

Renin Release

The control of renin release is a multifactorial process and the stimulants and inhibitors act through vascular baroreceptors in the afferent arterioles, renal beta-adrenergic receptors and a group of humoral agents (262). PGs (PGI2 and PGE2) can stimulate renin secretion after infusion or endogenous formation (263–266). PGs seem to stimulate through the increase of intracellular cAMP (267). However, PGs are not essential mediators of renin release because renin can be stimulated despite cyclooxygenase inhibition, when the stimulation is induced by stretch receptors or beta-adrenergic mechanisms (268,269).

PROSTAGLANDINS AND LEUKOTRIENES IN RENAL DISEASE

As already outlined in the preceding paragraph, PGs and leukotrienes are synthesized by glomerular and several tubular cell types. Their production under normal physiologic conditions is low. However, the profile of glomerular and tubular eicosanoid formation dramatically changes when the kidney is under stress. The consequences of the diverse disturbances of kidney integrity on PG and leukotriene formation are not specific but rather depend on the localization of the injury. The resulting response of the kidney tissue with regard to the compartmentalized capacity to produce diverse products also depends on the immediately resulting effects of bone marrow–derived adhesive or infiltrating inflammatory cells. Because PGs and leukotrienes exert their effects at the site of synthesis, the experimental approaches to define their mechanisms of action in renal injury have mainly focused on studies that evaluate biosynthetic capacities of renal tissues after experimental lesions. These approaches have remarkably enhanced the understanding of how diverse renal lesions affect eicosanoid synthesis in the kidney and the role PGs and leukotrienes play. Furthermore, the availability of synthesis inhibitors of the cyclooxygenases and lipoxygenases as well as receptor blockers for some of the cyclooxygenase and lipoxygenase products made it possible to delineate their role in renal pathophysiology.

Immune-Mediated Experimental Glomerular Injuries

In defining the role of PGs and leukotrienes in the mediation of inflammatory glomerular injuries, a variety of animal models have been used to study nephrotoxic serum nephritis (NTN), passive Heymann nephritis (PHN), the lupuslike disease, antithymocyte antibody–induced injury, IgA nephropathy, and other forms of immune complex nephritis.

Nephrotoxic Serum Nephritis (see also Chapter 35)

In the rat model of NTN, Lianos et al. (270) were the first to describe an enhanced glomerular synthesis of the cyclooxygenase products TxB2, PGE2, and PGFa, which appeared within 2 to 3 hr after the induction of the immune injury. The effect on TxB2 formation was more prominent than on PGE2, and thromboxane formation levels remained elevated up to 2 weeks after the induction of the lesion, whereas the glomerular PGE2 formation returned to control levels within a few days. To characterize the biochemical changes in the glomerulus with respect to a hemodynamic role, the authors pretreated the nephritic rats with a thromboxane synthesis inhibitor, a procedure that resulted in an almost complete inhibition of TxB2 formation and prevented the reduction of GFR. In contrast to the thromboxane blockade, a cyclooxygenase inhibitor that reduced PGs further decreased the already compromised renal hemodynamic function. These studies illustrate that in NTN thromboxane is an early mediator of impaired renal hemodynamic function, whereas the elevated production of vasodilatory PGs mediates recovery of renal hemodynamics. Additionally, increased PG formation also prevents the injured kidney from a further decrease in GFR (271,272).

Although several other studies show that TxB2 plays an important role in early hemodynamic changes, the role of thromboxane in the autologous phase of NTN is not entirely clear. One group (273) could not define a role for TxB2 in the impairment of renal hemodynamics; however, others (274) found that 2 weeks after induction of the injury TxB2 was still responsible for the compromised hemodynamic function (274). Cyclooxygenase inhibitors in the autologous phase of NTN have been shown to induce both a decrease (273) and an increase (274) in GFR. Therefore, it seems likely that the role of cyclooxygenase products in the autologous phase of NTN depends on the relative balance of vasodilatory and vasoconstrictive prostanoids at the time of study.

The induction of NTN not only leads to an increase in TxA2 and PGs but also stimulates lipoxygenase products (275). Within hours after the induction of NTN in rats the glomerular formation of 12-HETE (275), as well as the formation of 5-HETE and LTB4 (276–278), is increased. A functional role of 12- and 5-lipoxygenase products in NTN was defined with the LTD4 receptor antagonist SK + F 104353, which maintained GFR by the preservation of the glomerular capillary ultrafiltration coefficient (279). Similarly, other studies describe that LTC4 and 12-HETE also mediate impairment of GFR and RBF (280–282). These studies convincingly demonstrate that in the NTN model, TxB2 and lipoxygenase products are important mediators of impaired renal hemodynamic function, effects that obviously are mediated by afferent and efferent arteriolar constriction and a reduction in Kf, whereas the increased formation of prostanoids seems to protect RBF and GFR.

In NTN, antibody binding is often followed by complement activation with consecutive infiltration of polymorphonuclear granulocytes (PMNs), platelets, monocytes/macrophages, and in a later stage proliferation of resident glomerular cells.

Because infiltrating leukocytes produce eicosanoids, the ensuing questions are which cells in the glomerulus are responsible for the increased eicosanoid formation and which are the endogenous mediators of eicosanoid formation. Several studies have shown that the amount of antibody and the intraglomerular activation of complement are the important mediators of increased formation of lipoxygenase and cyclooxygenase products (276,283).

Furthermore, neutrophils are defined as the major source of lipoxygenase products in NTN. Thus, antibody and complement are the stimulants of glomerular eicosanoid formation, and glomerular resident cells, as well as neutrophils, contribute to the increased glomerular formation of the products (284,285).

Several studies have addressed whether increased glomerular eicosanoids might mediate proteinuria. Although a positive correlation between glomerular TxB2 formation and proteinuria was reported (270,285), the use of a TxB receptor blocker provided little evidence that thromboxane mediates proteinuria in NTN (274,286,287). Another important question concerns the possible role of endogenously formed eicosanoids on glomerular histology. Takahashi et al. (274) could not detect significant changes on glomerular damage or infiltration of ED-1 (+) cells when cyclooxygenase synthesis inhibitors or a thromboxane receptor blocker were applied. However, others observed an increase in glomerular inflammatoy cells in NTN in the presence of an NSAID (288). There is some evidence that 5- and 12-lipoxygenase products mediate glomerular cell growth in NTN (289) because the arachidonate 5-lipoxygenase inhibitor MK886 reduced glomerular cell proliferation. This is consistent with the observation that the 5-lipoxygenase product LTB4 increases PMN infiltration in kidneys that had received nephrotoxic serum (278).

Endogenously formed lipoxygenase metabolites might also exert antiinflammatory actions. The early burst of 5-lipoxygenase products, particularly LTB4, is followed by a reduction in the formation of the AA metabolite. This decrease of LTB4 is paralleled by an increase of 15-(S)-HETE, a 15-lipoxygenase derivative of AA, and a precursor lipoxin A, whose production also increases. Because 15-S-HETE and lipoxin A (290–292) antagonize the proinflammatory action of leukotriene B4 (290,293–295) and reduce its chemotactic actions on PMNs, it might be possible that lipoxin A4 and 15-S-HETE serve as endogenous antagonists of the proinflammatory lipoxygenase product LTB4 (296,297). Lipoxin A4 furthermore antagonizes vasoconstrictive actions of LTD4- and LTC4-induced PMN adhesion to mesangial cells (297,298). Thus, in addition to the cyclooxygenase products, pro- and anti-inflammatory activities also exist in the lipoxygenase pathway.

Passive Heymann Nephritis (see also Chapters 35 and 47)

PHN is a rat model of membranous nephropathy in which the glomerular immune injury is mediated by complement activation that occurs as a consequence of in situ immune complex formation but is independent of infiltrating inflammatory cells (299). In this animal model, antibody binding to glomerular epithelial cells and the consecutive intraglomerular activation of the complement system leads to an increase of TxB2, PGE2, and LTB4 formation (300,301). The increase in leukotriene B4 is also present in the autologous phase of PHN and has been attributed to glomerular infiltrating monocytes and macrophages (302).

The pathophysiologic role of the increased prostanoid and LTB4 synthesis in PHNs is not entirely clear. In one experiment TxB2 formation was almost completely inhibited with a synthesis inhibitor and was without effect on proteinuria (300), whereas others found in the isolated perfused kidney that thromboxane mediates proteinuria (303). There is no information on the possible effect that thromboxane might have on renal hemodynamics in PHN. The role of increased leukotriene formation has been assessed in the autologous form of PHN, and the study shows that an LTD4 receptor blocker normalized impaired glomerular hemodynamic abnormalities by an increase of pre- and postglomeruluar resistances (302). Additionally, the LTD4 receptor antagonist markedly reduced proteinuria, which suggests a role for LTD4 in the mediation of the autologous phase of PHN.

Lupus Nephritis

The models of autoimmune lupus in mice are uniquely valuable to study progressive renal injury and the mediators that might participate in the development of the nephritis. In NZB*NZWF1 hybrid mice the intrarenal synthesis of TxB2 significantly increases as the renal function deteriorates and renal pathologic events progress (304,305). The increased renal TxB2 formation also correlates with a progressive decrease in GFR and with the progressive increase in proteinuria. Treatment of lupus mice with a thromboxane receptor blocker ameliorates the loss of GFR and improves renal histomorphology by reducing crescent formation, interstitial inflammation, and proteinuria (306,307). The mechanisms of the beneficial effects of thromboxane receptor blockade on proteinuria have not been studied in detail. However, effects on glomerular perfusion pressure and direct effects on the filtration barrier may be possible.

LTB4 and LTC4 formation is also increased in kidneys of MRL-lpr mice. Similarly, as with TxB2, LTC4 formation is correlated with histomorphologic abnormalities and the loss of hemodynamic function, and the administration of a specific peptide leukotriene receptor antagonist improved GFR and PAH clearance (308).

Evidence of a hemodynamic role for TxA2 in human lupus nephritis is derived from studies of patients that showed that the infusion of a thromboxane receptor blocker improves impaired GFR (309).

Antithymocyte Antibody–Induced Mesangial Cell Injury

The induction of antithymocyte antibody–mediated mesangioproliferative glomerulonephritis injury leads to a significant increase in glomerular TxB2 formation with no effect on PGE2 and 6-keto PGF1α (310). This increase in TxB2 is dependent on an intact complement system and the infiltration of monocytes (310,311). The increased glomerular TxB2 formation contributes to the reduction in GFR. The formation of LTB4 and 12-HETE is also stimulated in this animal model. 12-HETE synthesis is derived from infiltrating platelets, whereas LTB4 derives from monocytes/macrophages (312). A role for TxB2 in the mediation of histopathologic changes in this disease derives from studies in a chronic model of this lesion which is produced by the repetitive injection of the antithymocyte serum (313). Treatment with a thromboxane synthesis inhibitor and a thromboxane receptor blocker improves proteinuria and glomerular damage in this disease, demonstrating that TxA also mediates extracellular matrix formation (314).

IgA Nephropathy (see Chapter 42)

The development of IgA nephropathy is associated with stimulated glomerular TxB2 formation, which is accompanied by a reduction of GFR and RBF (315). The application of antithromboxane therapy reduced hematuria and normalized RBF, but not GFR, which suggests a role for TxB in IgA nephropathy. In patients with IgA nephropathy and mesangial proliferative glomerulonephritis, increased urinary excretion of 5-lipoxygenase products was detected (316), which suggests that thromboxane and leukotrienes could be involved in the pathogenesis of human IgA nephropathy (316).

Other Models of Immune Complex Glomerulonephritis

In a rat model of immune complex mediated glomerular injury that was induced by daily injection of cationic bovine globuline, elevated formation of TxB2 and PGE2 has been reported. This increase was paralleled by the onset of proteinuria. However, thromboxane synthesis inhibition did not affect proteinuria, whereas cyclooxygenase inhibition reduced GFR and RBF by 40% (317). In the same model, an increase in LTB4 synthesis was described (318). In another model of immune complex injury, which is induced by the intrarenal injection of a cationized human IgG and followed by the intravenous (IV) injection of rabbit human antibody, glomerular TxB2, but not PGE2, formation was stimulated within 24 hr after administration of the antibody. The increased TxB2 formation was associated with a decrease in GFR, an effect that was blunted by treatment with a thromboxane synthesis inhibitor. Proteinuria, which developed in these animals within 48 hr, was unaffected by the thromboxane synthesis inhibitor (319).

These studies in diverse animal models of experimental glomerulonephritis convincingly demonstrate that cyclooxygenase and lipoxygenase products are important mediators of several inflammatory lesions. In the early phases of most injuries, antibody and complement lead to increased formation of TxB2 and LTB4, which are derived from both glomerular resident cells and infiltrating leucocytes. TxB2 and LTD4 seem to be responsible for the reduction in GFR and the impairment of renal plasma flow, whereas LTB4 enhances inflammatory cell recruitment. After the initial lesion, in most injuries an increase in PGE2 and PGI2 can be detected, which serve as counter-regulatory signals to maintain hemodynamic functions, inhibit inflammatory cell recruitment, impair cell proliferation, and ameliorate extracellular matrix formation. Similarly, 15-S-HETE and lipoxin A, which are increased in the later stages of NTN, have anti-inflammatory roles and antagonize LTB4 effects. Thus, the pathophysiologic consequences of PG and leukotriene formation seem to depend on the relative abundance of the pro- or anti-inflammatory mediators of the arachidonic cascade in different stages of disease.

Renal Transplant Rejection (see also Chapter 16)

The process of acute vascular or cellular renal transplant rejection is associated with a marked reduction in RBF and GFR. It is assumed that these hemodynamic impairments are partially mediated by local vasoactive substances, among which thromboxane and leukotrienes play a role. In fact, increased urinary TxB2 excretion is present in patients with renal allograft rejection, and this cyclooxygenase product was used as an indicator of transplant malfunction (320–324). Similarly, increased leukotriene formation also is evident in transplant rejection (325,326). Acute allograft rejection is also characterized by the interstitial infiltration of lymphocytes, PMNs, and monocytes/macrophages, and these cells produce eicosanoids, which induce hemodynamic changes. In experimental studies in which TxB2 receptor blockers, leukotriene receptor antagonists, and lipoxygenase synthesis inhibitors were applied, it was demonstrated that both thromboxane and leukotrienes are involved in hemodynamic and structural changes (327,328). Although TxA2 and leukotrienes seem to mediate the disturbance in renal function in transplant rejection, a protective hemodynamic effect could be shown for PGs, which might improve primary graft function (329). PGs not only mediate the hemodynamic alterations in allografts but also are involved in the immune response due to the immunosuppressive effects of prostaglandins (330). In a placebo-controlled prospective trial, human subjects received misoprostol (PGE1) for the first 12 weeks after transplantation (331). This treatment resulted in an improvement in GFR and a significant reduction of renal transplant rejections, which implies the clinical importance of the prostanoids in renal transplantation.

EICOSANOIDS AS THERAPEUTIC AGENTS IN RENAL IMMUNE INJURY

Treatment of NZB/NZW mice with PGE1 prolongs survival of these animals due to the improvement of renal function. The effect of PGE1 on renal function was characterized by the impairment of renal histologic alterations (332,333). Specifically PGE1 prevents glomerular deposition of immunoglobulins and complement in glomeruli but is without effect on antibody formation (334). Thus, one beneficial effect of PGE1 is due to a reduced immune complex formation in the glomerulus with consequent reduction in local cell proliferation and tissue damage (335–337).

In studies in immune complex glomerulonephritis in mice, McLeish et al. (338) observed that PGE1 reduced immune complex deposition in the glomerulus, improved glomerular histology, and prevented proteinuria. In this model PGE1 and PGE2 significantly reduced antibody levels. However, in contrast to the studies in lupus mice, they could not describe an alteration in the number of antibody-producing cells (339). In additional experiments, lower doses of PGs, which did not inhibit formation of autoantibodies, were ineffective in preventing the disease. This led to the conclusion that the beneficial effect of PGs was due to inhibition of antibody formation (340), which could be attributed to observed changes in T and B cells (341). Similar conclusions were drawn from a long-term study in mercury-induced glomerulonephritis in which PG administration improved glomerular injury due to a reduction of autoantibody binding to the glomerular basement membrane (342).

However, PGE1 also may have local beneficial effects at the site of injury in the glomerulus. In studies in animals with immune complex vasculitis (343) and NTN (344) induced by heterologous antibodies, PGE1 improved the glomerular inflammatory response and inhibited leukocyte infiltration and proteinuria independent of an effect on glomerular antibody binding (345–347).

In a more recent study, the effect of PGE1 on the expression and deposition of extracellular matrix collagens as well as on resident cell growth was evaluated in the antithymocyte antibody–induced model of glomerulonephritis. When animals were treated with PGE1, mRNA expression and extracellular deposition of collagens were markedly reduced. Additionally, PGE1 inhibited the proliferation of mesangial cells and partially prevented the influx of monocytes into the injured glomeruli (348). The therapeutic effects of PGs in glomerular injury thus include the inhibition of autoantibody formation, the secretion of proinflammatory cytokines, such as IL-1β, tumor necrosis factor a, chemokines, and the reduction of extracellular matrix formation (349–351).

Beneficial effects of PGs also have been observed in human renal disease. In a patient with rapidly progressive glomerulonephritis, who was treated with IV PGE1, proteinuria and renal function improved following PG-application. Similarly, in patients with lupus nephritis, PGE1 which was given IV daily for 4 weeks with favorable effects on proteinuria and immunologic parameters (352–356).

DIETARY LIPID INTAKE AND RENAL INJURY

Because cyclooxygenases and lipoxygenases metabolize not only AA, but also other unsaturated fatty acids, changes in the substrate pools have direct effects on these products and can alter the profile of eicosanoids. Because these metabolites have biologic capabilities different from those of the metabolites of AA, changes in the substrates can dramatically alter the biologic functions of PGs and leukotrienes. One of the approaches intensively studied is the effect that dietary fish oil intake may have on renal disease. The renal effects of dietary fish oil intake have been studied in animals and humans, and the clinical outcome varies with respect to the relative role of eicosanoids in the different disease entities (357,358).

Animal Studies

The effect of eicosapentaenoic acid on survival and glomerular injury was studied in the lupus model of NZB x NZWF1 mice. In contrast to control animals that were fed a beef tallow diet, animals that received menhaden oil showed marked impairment in renal disease, less proteinuria, and prolonged survival (359,360). The beneficial effects of fish oils were attributed to a reduction of autoantibody formation, reduction of circulating immune complexes, and impairment of surface antigen expression in macrophages (361–366). Fish oil intake also reduces the formation of dienoic PGs and leukotrienes, such as PGE2 and PGI2 as well as TxB2 and LTB4 (364, 367). Therefore, the reduction of the proinflammatory LTB4 and the vasoconstrictive TxB2 may exert beneficial effects on renal diseases (365,366,368,369). Dietary fish oil also has been shown to have deleterious effects on renal function in the model of subtotal renal nephrectomy (370). Fish oil induces a reduction in PGE2 formation. Because PGE2 is responsible for the maintenance of renal function in this model, fish oil impaired hemodynamic and morphologic integrity.

Human Renal Disease

In 1984 Hamazaki et al. (371) reported that patients with IgA nephropathy who took dietary fish oil had stabilized serum creatinine levels compared with untreated controls, who displayed deterioration of renal function. These data were recently confirmed by Doniado et al. (372), who found that only 6% of patients who received 12 g of fish oil per day had an increase of 50% or more in their serum creatinine, whereas in a group of patients who received olive oil, 33% of the patients had more than a 50% increase in the serum creatinine level. However, others have been unable to demonstrate the beneficial effects of fish oil on proteinuria or creatinine clearance in patients with IgA nephropathy (373,374). Similarly, fish oil in patients with stable lupus erythematosis has no beneficial effects on renal function or lupus-associated disease activity (375–377).

These results in patients with chronic renal injury of different causes who were treated with increased fish oil intake are rather inconclusive. Generally, a tendency toward an improvement of filtration function or a reduction in proteinuria have been observed (378). A recent study in patients with membranous glomerulonephritis and focal segmental sclerosis showed a beneficial effect on proteinuria, when patients received 7 g of eicosapentaenoic acid and docosohexaenoic acid (379).

REFERENCES

1. Kurzrok R, Lieb CC. Biochemical studies on human semen. II. Action of semen on human uterus. *Proc Soc Exper Biol and Med* 1930; 28:268–272.
2. Goldblatt MW. Depressor substance in seminal fluid. *Chem Ind* 1933;52:1056–1057.
3. van Euler US. Über die spezifische blutdrucksenkende Substanz der menschlichen Prostata und des Samenblasensekretes. *Klin Wochenschr* 1935;14:1182–1183.
4. Bergström S, Sjövall J. The isolation of prostaglandin F from sheep prostate glands. *Acta Chem Scand* 1960;14:1693–1719.
5. Bergström S, Sjövall J. The isolation of prostaglandin E from sheep prostate glands. *Acta Chem Scand* 1960b;14:1701–1705.
6. Bergström S, Dressler F, Ryhage R, Samuelsson B, Sjövall J. The isolation of two further prostaglandins from sheep prostate glands. *Arkiv Kemi* 1962;19: 563–567.
7. Lee JB, Hickler RB, Saravis CA, Thorn GW. Sustained depressor effect of renal medullary extract in the normotensive rat. *Circ Res* 1962;26:747.
8. Lee JB, Crowshaw K, Takman BH. Attrep KA Gougoutas JZ. The identification of prostaglandins E2, F2 a and A2 from rabbit kidney medulla. *Biochem J* 1967;105:1251–1260.
9. Kellaway CH, Trethenie QJ. Liberation of slow-reacting smooth muscle–stimulating substance in anaphylaxis. *Exp Physiol Cogn Med Sci* 1940;30:121–145.
10. Samuelsson B. Leukotrienes: mediators of immediate hypersensitivity reactions and inflammation. *Science* 1983;20:568–575.
11. Smith WL. The eicosanoids and their biochemical mechanisms of action. *Biochem J* 1989;259:315–324.
12. Lands WE, Samuelsson B. Phospholipid precursors of prostaglandins. *Biochim Biophys Acta* 1968;164:426–429.
13. Willis AL. Prostaglandins and related lipids. *Handbook of eicosanoids*. Boca Raton, FL: CRC Press; 1987:3–46.
14. Bergström S, Danielsson H, Samuelsson B. The enzymatic formation of prostaglandin E2 from arachidonic acid prostaglandins and related factors. *Biochim Biophys Acta* 1964;90:207–210.
15. van Dorp DA, Beerthuis RK, Nugteren DH, Vonkeman H. The biosynthesis of prostaglandins. *Biochim Biophys Acta* 1964;90: 204–207.
16. Habenicht AJR, Salbach P, Goerig M, et al. The LDL receptor pathway delivers arachidonic acid for eicosanoid formation in cells stimulated by platelet derived growth factor. *Nature* 1990;345:634–636.
17. Flower RG, Blackwell GJ. The importance of phospholipase A2 in prostaglandin synthesis. *Biochem Pharmacol* 1976;25:285–291.
18. Bonventre JV. Phospholipase A2 and signal transduction. *J Am Soc Nephrol* 1992;3:128–150.
19. Rouzer CA. Regulation and structure of human leukocyte 5-lipoxygenase. In: Crooke ST, Wong A. eds. *Lipooxygenases and their products*. San Diego: Academic; 1991:51–65.
20. Waite M. The phospholipases. In: *Handbook of lipid research*. New York: Plenum Press; 1987:5–27.
21. Bonventre JV, Skorecki KL, Kreisberg JI, Cheung JY. Vasopressin increases cytosolic free calcium concentration in glomerular mesangial cells. *Am J Physiol* 1986;251:F94–F102.
22. Bonventre JV, Weber PC, Gronich JH. PAF and PDGF increase cytosolic (Ca2+) and phospholipase activity in mesangial cells. *Am J Physiol* 1988;254:F87–F94.
23. Rordorf G, Uemura Y, Bonventre JV. Characterization of phospholipase A2 (PLA2) activity in gerbil brain. Enhanced activities of cytosolic, mitochondrial and microsomal forms after ischemia and reperfusion. *J Neurosci* 1991;11:1829–1836.
24. Pfeilschifter J. Mesangial cells orchestrate inflammation in the renal glomerulus. *News Physiol Sciences* 1994;9:271–276.
25. Kujubu DA, Herschman HR. Dexamethasone inhibits mitogen induction of the TIS10 prostaglandin synthase/cyclooxygenase gene. *J Biol Chem* 1992;267:7991–7994.
26. Flower RJ, Vane JR. In: Robinson HJ, Vane JR, eds. Prostaglandin synthetase inhibitors. New York: Raven; 1973:9–18.
27. Smith WL, Lands WEM. Stimulation and blockade of prostaglandin biosynthesis. *J Biol Chem* 1971;246:6700–6702.
28. Rome LH, Lands WE. Structural requirements for time-dependent inhibition of prostaglandin biosynthesis by anti-inflammatory drugs. *Proc Natl Acad Sci U S A* 1975;72:486.
29. DeWitt DL, El-Harith EA, Kraemer SA, et al. The aspirin and heme-binding sites of ovine and murine prostaglandin endoperoxide synthases. *J Biol Chem* 1990;265:5192–5198.
30. DeWitt DL, Smith WL. Primary structure of prostaglandin G/H synthase from sheep vesicular gland determined from the complementary DNA sequence. *Proc Natl Acad Sci U S A* 1988;85:1412–1416.
31. Funk CD, Funk LB, Kennedy ME, Pong AS, FitzGerald GA. Human platelet/erythroleukemia cell prostaglandin G/H synthase: cDNA cloning, expression, and gene chromosomal assignment. *FASEB J* 1991;5:2304–2312.
32. Xie W, Chipman JG, Robertson DL, Erikson RL, Simmons DL. Expression of a mitogen-responsive gene encoding prostaglandin synthase is regulated by mRNA splicing. *Proc Natl Acad Sci U S A* 1991; 88:2692–2696.
33. Kujubu DA, Fletcher BS, Varnum BC, Lim RW, Herschman HR. TIS10, a phorbol ester tumor promoter–inducible mRNA from Swiss 3T3 cells, encodes a novel prostaglandin synthase/cyclooxygenase homologue. *J Biol Chem* 1991;266:12866–12872.
34. Smith WL, Bell TG. Immunohistochemical localization of the prostaglandin-forming cyclooxygenase in renal cortex. *Am J Physiol* 1978; 235:F451–F457.
35. Smith WL. Prostaglandin biosynthesis and its compartmentation in vascular smooth muscle and endothelial cells. *Annu Rev Physiol* 1986;48:251–262.
36. Seibert K, Zhang Y, Leahy K, et al. Pharmacological and biochemical demonstration of the role of cyclooxygenase 2 in inflammation and pain. *Proc Natl Acad Sci U S A* 1994;91:12013–12017.
37. Harris RC, McKanna JA, Akai Y, Jacobson HR, Dubois RN, Breyer MD. Cyclooxygenase-2 is associated with the macula densa of rat kidney and increases with salt restriction. *J Clin Invest* 1994;94: 2504–2510.
38. DuBois RN, Tsujii M, Bishop P, Awad JA, Makita K, Lanahan A. Cloning and characterization of a growth factor inducible cyclooxygenase gene from rat intestinal epithelial cells. *Am J Physiol* 1994; 266:G822–G827.

39. O Neil GP, Ford-Hutchinson AW. Expression of mRNA for cyclooxygenase-1 and cyclooxygenase-2 in human tissues. *FEBS Lett* 1993;330:156–160.
40. Salvemini D, Seibert K, Masferrer JL, Misko TP, Currie MG, Needleman P. Endogenous nitric oxide enhances prostaglandin production in a model of renal inflammation. *J Clin Invest* 1994;93:1940–1947.
41. Feng L, Sun W, Xia Y, et al. Cloning two isoforms of rat cyclooxygenase: differential regulation of their expression. *Arch Biochem Biophys* 1993;307:361–368.
42. Akai Y, Homma T, Burns KD, Yasuda Y, Badr KF, Harris RC. Induction of protooncogenes and cyclooxygenase by mechanical stretch/relaxation in cultured rat mesangial cells. *Am J Physiol* 1994; 267:C482–C490.
43. Kester M, Coroneos E, Thomas PJ, Dunn MJ. Endothelin stimulates prostaglandin endoperoxide synthase-2 mRNA expression and protein synthesis through a tyrosine kinase–signaling pathway in rat mesangial cells. *J Biol Chem* 1994;269:22574–22580.
44. Hughes AK, Padilla E, Kutchera WA, Michael JR, Kohan DE. Endothelin-1 induction of cyclooxygenase-2 expression in rat mesangial cells. *Kidney Int* 1995;47:53–61.
45. Rzymkiewicz DM, DuMaine J, Morrisson AR. IL-1β regulates rat mesangial cyclooxygenase II gene expression by tyrosine phosphorylation. *Kidney Int* 1995;47:1354–1363.
46. Smith WL. Prostaglandins and related compounds. In: *Handbook of eicosanoids*. 1987:175–184.
47. DeWitt DL, Smith WL. Purification of prostacyclin synthase from bovine aorta by immunoaffinity chromatography: evidence that the enzyme is a hemoprotein. *J Biol Chem* 1983;258:3285–3293.
48. Ullrich V, Haurand M. Thromboxane synthase as a cytochrome P450 enzyme. *Adv Prostaglandin Thromboxane Leukotrienes Res* 1983;11: 105–110.
49. Tanaka Y, Ward SL, Smith WL. Immunochemical and kinetic evidence for two different prostaglandin H–prostaglandin E isomerases in sheep vesicular gland microsomes. *J Biol Chem* 1987;262: 1374–1381.
50. Samuelsson B, Dahlen SE, Lindgren JA, Rouzer CA, Serhan CH. Leukotrienes and lipoxins: structures, biosynthesis, and biological effects. *Science* 1987;237:1171–1176.
51. Fitzsimmons BJ, Adams J, Evans JF, Leblanc Y, Rokach J. The lipoxins–stereochemical indentification and determination of their biosynthesis. *J Biol Chem* 1985;260:13008–13012.
52. Lewis RA, Austen KF. The biologically active leukotrienes: biosynthesis, metabolism, receptors, functions, and pharmacology. *J Clin Invest* 1984;73:889–897.
53. Sraer J, Rigaud M, Bens M, Rabinovitch H, Ardaillou R. Metabolism of arachidonic acid via the lipoxygenase pathway in human and murine glomeruli. *J Biol Chem* 1983;258:4325–4330.
54. Jim K, Hassid A, Sun F, Dunn MJ. Lipoxygenase activity in rat kidney glomeruli, glomerular epithelial cells and cortical tubules. *J Biol Chem* 1982;257:10294–10299.
55. Baud L, Hagege J, Sraer J, Rondeau E, Perez J, Ardaillou R. Reactive oxygen production by cultured rat glomerular mesangial cells during phagocytosis is associated with stimulation of lipoxygenase activity. *J Exp Med* 1983;158:1836–1852.
56. Sraer J, Bens M, Ardaillou R, Sraer JD. Sulfidopeptide leukotriene biosynthesis and metabolism by rat glomeruli and papilla. *Kidney Int* 1986;29:346.
57. Cattell V, Smith J, Cook HT, Moncada S, Salmon JA. Leukotriene B4 synthesis in normal rat glomeruli. *Kidney Int* 1985;27:254.
58. Lianos EA. Glomerular leukotriene biosynthesis and degradation in the rat: effects of immune injury. *Kidney Int* 1986;29:339.
59. Garrick R, Wong PYK. Enzymatic formation and regulatory function of lipoxins and leukotriene B4 in rat kidney mesangial cells. *Biochem Biophys Res Commun* 1989;162:626–633.
60. Capdevila J, Parkhill L Chacos N, Okita R, Masters BSS, Estabrook RW. The oxidative metabolism of arachidonic acid by purified cytochromes P-450. *Biochem Biophys Res Commun* 1981;101: 1357–1363.
61. Morrison AR, Pascoe N, Metabolism of arachidonic acid through NADPH-dependent oxygenase of renal cortex. *Proc Natl Acad Sci U S A* 1981;78:7375–7378.
62. Oliw EH, Lawson JA, Brash AR, Oates JA. Arachidonic acid metabolism in rabbit renal cortex. *J Biol Chem* 1981;256:9924–9931.
63. Lapuerta L, Chacos N, Falck JR, Jacobson H, Capdevila JH. Renal microsomal cytochrome P-450 and the oxidative metabolism of arachidonic acid. *Am J Med Sci* 1988;295:275–279.
64. Takahashi K, Capdevila J, Karara A, Falck JR, Jacobson HR, Badr KF. Cytochrome P-450 arachidonite metabolites in rat kidney: characterization and hemodynamic responses. *Am J Physiol* 1990;258: F781–F789.
65. Katoh T, Takahashi K, Capdevila J, et al. Glomerular stereospecific synthesis and hemodynamic actions of 8,9-epoxyeicosatrienoic acid in rat kidney. *Am J Physiol* 1991;261:F578–F586.
66. Toto R, Siddhanta A, Manna S, Pramanik B, Falck JR, Capdevila J. Arachidonic acid epoxygenase: detection of epoxyeicosatrienoic acids in human urine. *Biochim Biophys Acta*, 1987;919:132–139.
67. Falck JR, Schueler VJ, Jacobson HR, Siddhanta AK, Pramanik B, Capdevila J. Arachidonate epoxygenase: identification of epoxyeicosatrienoic acids in rabbit kidney. *J Lipid Res* 1987;28:840–846.
68. Carroll MA, Quilley CP, McGiff JC. Novel arachidonate metabolites generated by cytochrome P450-dependent mono-oxygenases. *Pharmacol Res* 1991;23:309–318.
69. Oyekan AO, McGiff JC, Quilley J. Cytochrome P-450–dependent vasodilator responses to arachidonic acid in the isolated, perfused kidney of the rat. *Circ Res* 1991;68:958–965.
70. Carroll MA, Carcia MP, Falck JR, McGiff JC. Cyclooxygenase dependency of the renovascular actions of cytochrome P450-derived arachidonate metabolites. *J Pharmacol Exp Ther* 1992;260: 104–109.
71. Hirt DL, Capdevila J, Falck JR, Breyer MD, Jacobson HR. Cytochrome P450 metabolites of arachidonic acid are potent inhibitors of vasopressin action on rabbit cortcal collecting duct. *J Clin Invest* 1989;84:1805–1812.
72. Limas C, Limas CJ. Prostaglandin receptors in rat kidney. *Arch Biochem Biophys* 1984;233:32–41.
73. Sugimoto Y, Namba T, Shigemoto R, Negischi M, Ichikawa A, Narumiya S. Distinct cellular localization of mRNAs for three subtypes of prostaglandin E receptor in kid. *Am J Physiol* 1994;266:F823–F828.
74. An S, Yang J, Xia M, Goetzl EJ. Cloning and expression of the EP2 subtype of human receptors for prostaglandin E2. *Biochem Biophys Res Commun* 1993;197:263–270.
75. Honda A, Sugimoto Y, Namba T, et al. Cloning and expression of a cDNA for mouse prostaglandin E receptor EP2 subtype. *Biol Chem* 1993;268:7759–7762.
76. Yang J, Xia M, Goetzl EJ, An S. Cloning and expression of the EP3-subtype of human receptors for prostaglandin E2. *Biochem Biophys Res Commun* 1994;198:999–1006.
77. Takeuchi K, Takahashi N, Abe T, et al. Functional difference between two isoforms of rat kidney prostaglandin receptor EP3 subtype. *Biochem Biophys Res Commun* 1994;203:1897–1903.
78. Taniguchi S, Watanabe T, Nakao A, Seki G, Uwatoko S, Kurokawa K. Detection and quantitation of EP3 prostaglandin E2 receptor mRNA along mouse nephron segments by RT-PCR. *Am J Physiol* 1994;266:C1453–C1458.
79. Takeuchi K, Abe T, Takahashi N, Abe K. Molecular cloning and intrarenal localization of rat prostaglandin E2 receptor EP3 subtype. *Biochem Biophys Res Commun* 1993;194:885–891.
80. Spurney RF, Middleton JP, Raymond JR, Coffman TM. Modulation of thromboxane receptor activation in rat glomerular mesangial cells. *Am J Physiol* 1994;267:F467–F478.
81. Mené P, Dubyak GR, Abboud HE, Scarpa A, Dunn MJ. Phospholipase C ativation by prostaglandins and thromboxane A2 in cultured mesangial cells. *Am J Physiol* 1988;255:F1059–F1069.
82. Mené P, Simonson MS, Dunn MJ. Phospholipids in signal transduction of mesangial cells. *Am J Physiol* 1989;256:F375–F386.
83. Mené P, Dubyak GR, Scarpa A, Dunn MJ. Stimulation of cytosolic free calcium and inositol phosphates by prostaglandins in cultured rat mesangial cells. *Biochem Biophys Res Commun* 1987;142:579–586.
84. Ballermann BJ, Lewis RA, Corey EJ, Austen KF, Brenner BM. Identification and characterization of leukotriene C4 receptors in isolated rat renal glomeruli. *Circ Res* 1985;56:324–330.
85. Simonson MS, Mené P, Dubyak GR, Dunn MJ. Identification and transmembrane signaling of leukotriene D4 receptors in human mesangial cells. *Am J Physiol* 1988;255:C771–C780.
86. Badr KF, Mong S, Hoover RL, et al. Leukotriene D4 binding and signal transduction in rat glomerular mesangial cells. *Am J Physiol* 1989; 257:F280–F287.
87. Sraer J, Sraer JD, Chansel D, Russo-Marie F, Kouznetzova B, Ardail-

lou R. Prostaglandin synthesis by isolated rat renal glomeruli. *Mol Cell Endocrin* 1979;16:29–37.

88. Hassid A, Konieczkowski M, Dunn MJ. Prostaglandin synthesis in isolated rat kidney glomeruli. *Proc Natl Acad Sci U S A* 1979;76: 1155–1159.
89. Folkert VW, Schlöndorff D. Prostaglandin synthesis in isolated glomeruli. *Prostaglandins* 1979;17:79–86.
90. Sraer J, Ardaillou N, Sraer JD, Ardaillou R. In vitro prostaglandin synthesis by human glomeruli and papillae. *Prostaglandins* 1982;23: 855–864.
91. Stahl RAK, Paravicini M, Schollmeyer P. Angiotensin II stimulation of prostaglandin E2 and 6-keto-F1a formation by isolated human glomeruli. *Kidney Int* 1984;26:30–34.
92. Schlondorff D, Roczniak S, Satriano JA, Folkert VW. Prostaglandin synthesis by isolated rat glomeruli: effect of angiotensin II. *Am J Physiol* 1980;238:F486–F495.
93. Matsumura Y, Ozawa Y, Suzuki H, Saruta T. Synergistic action of angiotensin II on norepinephrine-induced prostaglandin release from rat glomeruli. *Am J Physiol* 1986;250:F811–F816.
94. Podjarny E, Shapira J, Rathaus M, Kariv N, Bernheim J. Effect of angiotensin II on prostanoid synthesis in isolated rat glomeruli. *Clin Sci* 1986;70:527–530.
95. Scharschmidt LA, Douglas JG, Dunn MJ. Angiotensin II and eicosanoids in the control of glomerular size in the rat and human. *Am J Physiol* 1986;250: F348–F356.
96. Bankir L, Trinh Trang Tan MM, Nivez MP, Sraer J, Ardaillou R. Altered PGE2 production by glomeruli and papilla of rats with hereditary diabetes insipidus. *Prostaglandins* 1980;20:349–365.
97. Rathaus M, Podjarny E, Pomeranz A, Bernheim J. NaC1 modulates captopril effects on glomerular prostaglandin synthesis and glomerular filtration. *Am J Physiol* 1990;258:F382–387.
98. Folkert VW, Yunis M, Schlondorff D. Prostaglandin synthesis linked to phosphatidylinositol turnover in isolated rat glomeruli. *Biochim Biophys Acta* 1984;794:206–217.
99. Baud L, Nivez MP, Chansel D, Ardaillou R. Stimulation by oxygen radicals of prostaglandin production by rat renal glomeruli. *Kidney Int* 1981;20:332–339.
100. Galler M, Backenroth R, Folkert VW, Schlondorff D. Effect of converting enzyme inhibitors on prostaglandin synthesis by isolated glomeruli and aortic strips from rats. *Pharmacol Exp Ther* 1981;220: 23–28.
101. Sraer J, Bens M, Oudinet JP, Ardaillou R. Bioconversion of leukotriene C4 by rat glomeruli and papilla. *Prostaglandins* 1986;31: 909–921.
102. Jim K, Hassid A, Sun F, Dunn MJ. Lipoxygenase activity in rat kidney glomeruli, glomerular epithelial cells, and cortical tubules. *Biol Chem* 1982;257:10294–10299.
103. Sraer J, Rigaud M, Bens M, Rabinovitch H, Ardaillou R. Metabolism of arachidonic acid via the lipoxygenase pathway in human and murine glomeruli. *Biol Chem* 1983;258:4325–4330.
104. Schlondorff D, Satriano JA. Effect of platelet-activating factor and serum-treated zymosan on prostaglandin E2 synthesis, arachidonic acid release, and contraction of cultured rat mesangial cells. *J Clin Invest* 1984;73:1227–1231.
105. Ardaillou N, Hagege J, Nivez MP, Ardaillou R, Schlondorff D. Vasoconstrictor-evoked prostaglandin synthesis in cultured human mesangial cells. *Am J Physiol* 1985;248:F240–F24.
106. Schlondorff D, Perez J, Satriano JA. Differential stimulation of PGE2 synthesis in mesangial cells by angiotensin and A23187. *Am J Physiol* 1985;248:C119–C126.
107. Scharschmidt LA, Dunn MJ. Prostaglandin synthesis by rat glomerular mesangial cells in culture: effects of angiotensin II and arginine vasopressin. *J Clin Invest* 1983;71:1756–1764.
108. Lianos EA, Zanglis A. Effects of complement activation on platelet-activating factor and eicosanoid synthesis in rat mesangial cells. *J Lab Clin Med* 1992;120:459–464.
109. Lovett DH, Haensch GM, Goppelt M, Resch K, Gemsa D. Activation of glomerular mesangial cells by the terminal membrane attack complex of complement. *J Immunol* 1987;138:2473–2480.
110. Topley N, Floege J, Wessel K, et al. Prostaglandin E2 production is synergistically increased In cultured human glomerular mesangial cells by combination of IL-1 and tumor necrosis factor–1a. *J Immunol* 1989;143:1989–1995.
111. Uglesity A, Kreisberg JI, Levine L. Stimulation of arachidonic acid metabolism in rat kidney mesangial cells by bradykinin, antidiuretic hormone, and their analogues. *Prostaglandin Leukot Essent Fatty Acids* 1983;10:83–93.
112. Albrightson CR, Nambi P, Zabko-Potapovich B, Dytko G, Groom T. Effect of thrombin on proliferation, contraction and prostaglandin production of rat glomerular mesangial cells in culture. *J Pharmacol Exp Ther* 1992;263:404–412.
113. Knauss T, Abboud HE. Effect of serotonin on prostaglandin synthesis in rat cultured mesangial cells. *Am J Physiol* 1986;251:F844–F850.
114. Adler S, Stahl RAK, Baker PJ, Chen YP, Pritzl PM, Couser WG. Biphasic effect of oxygen radicals on prostaglandin production by rat mesangial cells. *Am J Physiol* 1987;252:F743–F749.
115. Jelkmann W, Kurtz A, Förstermann U, Pfeilschifter J, Bauer C. Hypoxia enhances prostaglandin synthesis in renal mesangial cell cultures. *Prostaglandins* 1985;30:109–119.
116. Zoja C, Benigni A, Renzi D, Piccinelli A, Perico N, Remuzzi G. Endothelin and eicosanoid synthesis in cultured mesangial cells. *Kidney Int* 1990;37:927–933.
117. Alavi N. Effect of polycations on prostaglandin synthesis in cultured glomerular mesangial cells. *Biochem Biophys Acta* 1990;1042: 221–226.
118. Lovett DH, Bursten SL, Gemsa D, Bessler W, Resch K, Ryan JL. Activation of glomerular mesangial cells by gram-negative bacterial cell wall components. *Am J Pathol* 1988;133:472–484.
119. Sraer JD, Baud L, Sraer J, Delarue F, Ardaillou R. Stimulation of PGE2 synthesis by mercuric chloride in rat glomeruli and glomerular cells in vitro. *Int Soc Nephrol* 1982;(suppl):63–68.
120. Nakazato Y, Simonson MS, Herman WH, Konieczkowski M, Sedor JR. Interleukin-1 alpha stimulates prostaglandin biosynthesis in serum-activated mesangial cells by induction of a non-pancreatic (type II) phospholipase A2. *J Biol Chem* 1991;266:14119–14127.
121. Pfeilschifter J, Muehl H. Interleukin 1 and tumor necrosis factor potentiate angiotensin II– and calcium ionophore–stimulated prostaglandin E2 synthesis in rat renal mesangial cells. *Biochem Biophys Res Commun* 1990;169:585–595.
122. Fukunaga M, Fujiwara Y, Fujibayashi M, et al. Signal transduction mechanism of interleukin 6 in cultured rat mesangial cells. *FEBS Lett* 1991;285:265–267.
123. Pugliese F, Mene P, Anania MC, Cinotti GA. Neutralization of the anionic sites of cultured rat mesangial cells by poly-L-lysine. *Kidney Int* 1989;35:817–823.
124. Wasserman J, Santiago A, Rifici V, et al. Interactions of low density lipoprotein with rat mesangial cells. *Kidney Int* 1989;35:1168–1174.
125. Harris RC, Haralson MA, Badr KF. Continuous stretch–relaxation in culture alters rat mesangial cell morphology, growth characteristics, and metabolic activity. *Lab Invest* 1992;66:548–554.
126. Schoenermark M, Deppisch R, Riedasch G, Rother K, Haensch GM. Induction of mediator release from human glomerular mesangial cells by the terminal complement components C5b-9. *Intern Arch Allergy Appl Immunol* 1991;96:331–337.
127. Fukunaga M, Ochi S, Takama T, et al. Endothelin-1 stimulates prostaglandin E2 production in an extracellular calcium–independent manner in cultured rat mesangial cells. *Am J Hypertens* 1991;4:137–143.
128. Schlondorff D, DeCandido S, Satriano JA. Angiotensin II stimulates phospholipases C and A2 in cultured rat mesangial cells. *Am J Physiol* 1987;253:C113–C120.
129. Maxwell AP, Goldberg HJ, Tay AHN, Li ZG, Arbus GS, Skorecki KL. Epidermal growth factor and phorbol myristate increase expression of cytosolic PL A2 in glomerular mesangial cell. *Biochem J* 1993;295:763–766.
130. Schramek H, Wang Y, Konieczkowski M, Simonson MS, Dunn MJ. Endothelin-1 stimulates cytosolic phospholipase A2 activity and gene expression in rat glomerular mesangial cells. *Kidney Int* 1994;46: 1644–1652.
131. Pfeilschifter J, Kurtz A, Bauer C. Role of phospholipase C and protein kinase C in vasoconstrictor-induced prostaglandin synthesis in cultured rat renal mesangial cells. *Biochem J* 1986;234:125–130.
132. Craven PA, Patterson MC, DeRubertis FR. Role for protein kinase C in the modulation of glomerular PGE2 production by angiotensin II. *Biochem Biophys Res Commun* 1988;152:1481–1489.
133. Schlondorff D, Singhal P, Hassid A, Satriano JA, DeCandido S. Relationship of GTP-binding proteins, phospholipase C, and PGE2 synthesis in rat glomerular mesangial cells. *Am J Physiol* 1989;256: F171–F178.

134. Portilla D, Mordhorst M, Bertrand W, Irwin C, Morrison AR. Different guanosine triphosphate–binding proteins couple vasopressin receptor to phosholipase C and phospholipase A2 in glomerular mesangial cells. *J Lab Clin Med* 1992;120:752–761.
135. Hack N, Clayman P, Skorecki K. A role for G-proteins in the epidermal growth factor stimulation of phospholipase A2 in rat kidney mesangial cells. *Biosci Rep* 1990;10:353–362.
136. Wang J, Kester M, Dunn MJ. Involvement of a pertussis toxin–sensitive G-protein–coupled phospholipase A2 in lipopolysaccharide-stimulated prostaglandin E2 synthesis in cultured rat mesangial cells. *Biochim Biophys Acta* 1988;963:429–435.
137. Pfeilschifter J, Bauer C. Pertussis toxin abolishes angiotensin II–induced phosphoinositide hydrolysis and prostaglandin synthesis in rat renal mesangial Cells. *Biochemistry* 1986;236:289–294.
138. Pfeilschifter J, Fandrey J, Ochsner M, Whitebread S, de Gasparo M. Potentiation of angiotensin II–stimulated phosphoinositide hydrolysis, calcium mobilization and contraction of renal mesangial cells upon down-regulation of protein kinase C. *FEBS Lett* 1990;261:307–311.
139. Bonventre JV, Swidler M. Calcium dependency of prostaglandin E2 production in rat glomerular mesangial cells. Evidence that protein kinase C modulates the Ca2+-dependent activation of phospholipase A2. *J Clin Invest* 1988;82:168–176.
140. Simonson MS, Wolfe JA, Konieczkowski M, Sedor JR, Dunn MJ. Regulation of prostaglandin endoperoxide synthase gene expression in cultured rat mesangial cells: Induction by serum via a protein kinase-C–dependent mechanism. *Mol Endocrinol* 1991;5:441–451.
141. Konieczkowski M, Sedor JR. Cell-specific regulation of type II phospholipase A2 expression in rat mesangial cells. *J Clin Invest* 1993;92:2524–2532.
142. Coyne DW, Morrison AR. Effect of the tyrosine kinase inhibitor, genistein, on interleukin-1 stimulated PGE2 production in mesangial cells. *Biochem Biophys Res Commun* 1990;173:718–724.
143. Coyne DW, Nickols M, Bertrand W, Morrison AR. Regulation of mesangial cell cyclooxygenase synthesis by cytokines and glucocorticoids. *Am J Physiol* 1992;263:F97–F102.
144. Martin M, Neumann D, Hoff T, Resch K, DeWitt DL, Goppelt-Struebe M. Interleukin-1–induced cyclooxygenase 2 expression is suppressed by cyclosporin A in rat mesangial cells. *Kidney Int* 1994;45:150–158.
145. Gronich J, Konieczkowski M, Gelb MH, Nemenoff RA, Sedor JR. Interleukin 1 alpha causes rapid activation of cytosolic phospholipase A2 by phosphorylation in rat mesangial cells. *J Clin Invest* 1994;93:1224–1233.
146. Nakazato Y, Okada H, Sato A, et al. Interleukin 4 downregulates cell growth and prostaglandin release of human mesangial cells. *Biochem Biophys Res Commun* 1993;197:486–493.
147. Tsai CY, Wu TH, Sun KH, Yu CL. Effect of antibodies to double stranded DNA, purified from serum samples of patients with active systemic lupus erythematosus, on the glomerular mesangial cells. *Ann Rheum Dis* 1992;51:162–167.
148. Schalkwijk C, Pfeilschifter J, Maerki F, van den Bosch H. Interleukin-1 beta– and forskolin-induced synthesis and secretion of group II phospholipase A2 and prostaglandin E2 in rat mesangial cells is prevented by transforming growth factor-beta 2. *J Biol Chem* 1992;267:8846–8851.
149. Schalkwijk C, Vervoordeldonk M, Pfeilschifter J, Maerki F, van den Bosch H. Cytokine- and forskolin-induced synthesis of group II phospholipase A2 and prostaglandin E2 in rat mesangial cells is prevented by dexamenthasone. *Biochem Biophys Res Commun* 1991;180:46–52.
150. Ausiello DA, Kreisberg JI, Roy C, Karnovsky MJ. Contraction of cultured rat glomerular cells of apparent mesangial origin after stimulation with angiotensin II and arginine vasopressin. *J Clin Invest* 1980;65:754–760.
151. Kreisberg JI, Venkatachalam M, Troyer D. Contractile properties of cultured glomerular mesangial cells. *Am J Physiol* 1985;249:F457–F463.
152. Foidart J, Sraer J, Delarue F, Mahieu P, Ardaillou R. Evidence for mesangial glomerular receptors for angiotensin II linked to mesangial cell contractility. *FEBS Lett* 1980;121:333–339.
153. Scharschmidt LA, Douglas JG, Dunn MJ. Angiotensin II and eicosanoids in the control of glomerular size in the rat and human. *Am J Physiol* 1986;250:F348.
154. Fandrey J, Jelkmann W. Prostaglandin E2 and atriopeptin III oppose the contractile effect of angiotensin II in rat kidney mesangial cell cultures. *Prostaglandins* 1988;36:249–257.
155. Mené P, Dunn MJ. Eicosanoids and control of mesangial cell contraction. *Circ Res* 1988;62:916–925.
156. Kreisberg JI, Venkatachalam MA, Patel PY. Cyclic AMP–associated shape change in mesangial cells and its reversal by prostaglandin E2. *Kidney Int* 1984;25:874–879.
157. Mené P, Dunn MJ. Contractile effects of TxA2 and endoperoxide analogues on cultured rat glomerular mesangial cells. *Am J Physiol* 1986;251:F1029–F1035.
158. Barnett R, Goldwasser P, Scharschmidt LA, Schlondorff D. Effects of leukotrienes on isolated rat glomeruli and cultured mesangial cells. *Am J Physiol* 1986;250:F838–F844.
159. Simonson MS, Dunn MJ. Leukotriene C4 and D4 contract rat glomerular mesangial cells. *Kidney Int* 1986;30:524–531.
160. Stahl RAK, Thaiss F, Haberstroh U, Kahf S, Shaw A, Schoeppe W. Cyclooxygenase inhibition enhances rat interleukin 1β–induced growth of rat messangial cells in culture. *Am J Physiol* 1990;259:F419–F424.
161. Matsell DG, Gaber LW, Malik KU. Cytokine stimulation of prostaglandin production inhibits the proliferation of serum-stimulated mesangial cells. *Kidney Int* 1994;45:159–165.
162. Nakahama K, Morita I, Murota S. Effects of endogenously produced arachidonic acid metabolites on rat mesangial cell proliferation. *Prostaglandins Leukot Essent Fatty Acids* 1994;51:177–182.
163. Mené P, Abboud HE, Dunn MJ. Regulation of human mesangial cell growth in culture by thromboxane A2 and prostacyclin. *Kidney Int* 1990;38:232–239.
164. Li XM, Schrier RW, Nemenoff RA. Growth factor stimulation of MAP kinase is inhibited by prostaglandin E2 and forskolin in rat renal mesangial cells. *J Am Soc Nephrol* 1994;5:696.
165. Harris RC, Homma T, Jacobson HR, Capdevila J. Epoxyeicosatrienoic acids activate Na+/H+ exchange and are mitogenic in cultured rat glomerular mesangial cells. *J Cell Physiol* 1990;144:429–437.
166. Bruggeman LA, Horigen EA, Horikoshi S, Ray PE, Klotman PE. Thromboxane stimulates synthesis of extracellular matrix proteins in vitro. *Am J Physiol* 1991;261:F488–F494.
167. Mené P, Taranta A, Pugliese F, Cinotti GA, D'Agostino A. Thromboxane A2 regulates protein synthesis of cultured human mesangial cells. *J Lab Clin Med* 1992;120:48–56.
168. Ardaillou N, Nivez MP, Bellon G, Combe C, Ardaillou R. Effect of prostaglandin E2 on proline uptake and protein synthesis by cultured human mesangial cells. *Kidney Int* 1990;38:1151–1158.
169. Zahner G, Disser M, Thaiss F, Wolf G, Schoeppe W, Stahl RAK. The effect of prostaglandin E2 on mRNA expression and secretion of collagens I, III, and IV and fibronectin in cultured rat mesangial cells. *J Am Soc Nephrol* 1994;4:1778–1785.
170. Singhal PC, Gupta S, Shen Z, Schlondorff D. Effects of PGE2 and a thromboxane A2 analogue on uptake of IgG complexes and LDL by mesangial cells. *Am J Physiol* 1991;261:F537–F544.
171. Singhal PC, Ding G, DeCandido S, Franki N, Hays RM, Schlondorff D. Endocytosis by cultured mesangial cells and associated changes in prostaglandin E2 synthesis. *Am J Physiol* 1987;252:F627–F634.
172. Simonson MS, Dunn MJ. Endothelin-1 stimulates contraction of rat glomerular mesangial cells and potentiates β-adrenergic–mediated cyclic adenosine monophosphate accumulation. *J Clin Invest* 1990;85:790–797.
173. Zoja G, Orisio S, Perico N, et al. Constitutive expression of endothelin gene in cultured human mesangial cells and its modulation by transforming growth factor-beta, thrombin, and a thromboxane A2 analogue. *Lab Invest* 1991;64:16–20.
174. Sraer J, Foridart D, Chansel P, Mahiew P, Kouznezova B, Ardaillou R. Prostaglandin synthesis by mesangial and epithelial glomerular cultured cells. *FEBS Lett* 1979;104:420–424.
175. Kreisberg JI, Karnovsky MJ, Levine L. Prostaglandin production by homogeneous cultures of rat glomerular epithelial and mesangial cells. *Kidney Int* 1982;22:355–359.
176. Stollenwerk Petrulis A, Aikawa M, Dunn MJ. Prostaglandin and thromboxane synthesis by rat glomerular epithelial cells. *Kidney Int* 1981;20:469–474.
177. Lieberthal W, Levine L. Stimulation of prostaglandin production in rat glomerular epithelial cells by antidiuretic hormone. *Kidney Int* 1984;25:766–770.

178. Haensch GM, Betz M, Guenther J, Rother KO, Sterzel B. The complement membrane attack complex stimulates the prostanoid production of cultured glomerular eptihelial cells. *Int Arch Allergy Appl Immunol* 1988;85:87–93.
179. Cybulsky AV, Salant DJ, Quigg RJ, Badalamenti J, Bonventre JV. Complement C5b-9 complex activates phospholipases in glomerular epithelial cells. *Am J Physiol* 1989;257:F826–F836.
180. Cybulsky AV. Release of arachidonic acid by complement C5b-9 complex in glomerular epithelial cells. *Am J Physiol* 1991;261: F427–F436.
181. Baud L, Sraer J, Perez J, Nivez MP, Ardaillou R. Leukotriene C4 binds to human glomerular epithelial cells and promotes their proliferation in vitro. *J Clin Invest* 1985;76:374–377.
182. Baud L, Perez J, Cherqui G, Cragoe EJ, Ardaillou R. Leukotriene D4-induced proliferation of glomerular epithelial cells: PKC- and Na+–H+ exchanger-mediated response. *Am Physiol* 1989;257:C232–C239.
183. Baud L, Sraer J, DeLarue F, et al. Lipoxygenase products mediate the attachment of rat macrophages to glomeruli in vitro. *Kidney Int* 1985; 27:855–863.
184. Brady HR, Persson U, Ballermann BJ, Brenner BM. Serhan CN. Leukotrienes stimulate neutrophil adhesion to mesangial cells: modulation with lipoxins. *Am J Physiol* 1990;259:F809–F815.
185. Brady HR, Denton MD, Jimenez W, Takata S, Palliser D, Brenner BM. Chemoattractants provoke monocyte adhesion to human mesangial cells and mesangial cell injury. *Kidney Int* 1992;42:480–487.
186. Nitta K, Simonson MS, Dunn MJ. The regulation and role of prostaglandin biosynthesis in cultured bovine glomerular endothelial cells. *J Am Soc Nephrol* 1991;2:156–163.
187. Uchida K, Ballermann BJ. Sustained activation of PGE2 synthesis in mesangial cells cocultured with glomerular endothelial cells. *Am J Physiol* 1992;263:C200–C209.
188. Johnston HH, Herzog JP, Lauler DP. Effect of prostaglandin E1 on renal hemodynamics, sodium and water excretion. *Am J Physiol* 1967;213:939–946.
189. Malik KU, McGiff JC. Modulation by prostaglandins of adrenergic transmission in the isolated perfused rabbit and rat kidney. *Circ Res* 1975;36:599–609.
190. Chang LCT, Splawinsky JA, Oates JA. Enhanced renal prostaglandin production in the dog. II. Effects on intrarenal hemodynamics. *Circ Res* 1975;36:204–207.
191. Gerber JG, Data JL, Nies AS. Enhanced renal prostaglandin production in the dog. The effect of sodium arachidonate in nonfiltering kidney. *Circ Res* 1978;42:43–45.
192. Arima S, Ren Y, Juncos LA, Carretero OA, Ito S. Glomerular prostaglandins modulate vascular reactivity of the downstream efferent aterioles. *Kidney Int* 1994;45:650–658.
193. Pallone TL. Vasoconstriction of outer medullary vasa recta by angiotensin II is modulated by prostaglandin E2. *Am J Physiol* 1994;266: F850–F857.
194. Dunn MJ. The clinical significance of inhibition of renal prostaglandin synthesis. *Kidney Int* 1987;32:1–12.
195. McGiff JC, Crowshaw K, Terragno NA, Lonigro AJ. Release of a prostaglandin-like substance into renal venous blood in response to angiotensin II. *Circ Res* 1970;26–27:I121–I130.
196. McGiff JC, Crowshaw K, Terragno NA, Malik KU, Lonigro AJ. Differential effect of noradrenaline and renal nerve stimulation on vascular resistance in the dog kidney and the release of a prostaglandin E–like substance. *Clin Sci* 1972;42:223–233.
197. Needleman P, Douglas JR, Jakschik B. Stoecklein PB, Johnson EM. Release of renal prostaglandin by catecholamines: relationship to renal endocrine function. *J Pharmacol Exp Ther* 1974;188:453–460.
198. Finn WF, Arendshorst WJ. Effect of prostaglandin synthetase inhibitors on renal blood flow in the rat. *Am J Physiol* 1976;231: 1541–1545.
199. Satoh S, Zimmerman BG. Influence of the renin–angiotensin system on the effect of prostaglandin synthesis inhibitors in the renal vasculature. *Circ Res* 1975;36—-37:I89–I96.
200. Blackshear JL, Davidman M, Stillman MT. Identification of risk for renal insufficiency from nonsteroidal antiinflammatory drugs. *Arch Intern Med* 1983;143:1130–1134.
201. Ciabattoni G, Cinotti GA, Pierucci A, et al. Effects of sulindac and ibuprofen in patients with chronic glomerular disease. Evidence for the dependence of renal function on prostacyclin. *N Engl J Med* 1984; 310:279–283.
202. Schor N, Ichikawa I, Brenner BM. Mechanisms of action of various hormones and vasoactive substances on glomerular ultrafiltration in the rat. *Kidney Int* 1981;20:442–451.
203. Schnermann J, Briggs JP, Weber PC. Tubuloglomerular feedback, prostaglandins, and angiotensin in the autoregulation of glomerular filtration rate. *Kidney Int* 1984;25:53–64.
204. Chevalier RL, Carey RM, Kaiser DL. Endogenous prostaglandin modulate autoregulation of renal blood flow in young rats. *Am J Physiol* 1987;253:F66–F75.
205. Laffi G, Daskalopoulos G, Kronborg I, Hsueh W, Gentilini P, Zipser RD. Effects of sulindac and ibuprofen in patients with cirrhosis and ascites. An explanation for the renal-sparing effect of sulindac. *Gastroenterology* 1986;90:182–187.
206. Vriesendorp R, DeZeeuw D, DeJong PE, Donker AJM, Pratt JJ, Van Der Hem GK. Reduction of urinary protein and prostaglandin E2 excretion in the nephrotic syndrome by nonsteroidal anti-inflammatory drugs. *Clin Nephrol* 1986;25:105–110.
207. Kimberly RP, Bowden RE, Keiser HR, Plotz PH. Reduction of renal function by newer nonsteroidal antiinflammatory drugs. *Am J Med* 1978;64:804–807.
208. Berg KJ, Talseth T. Acute renal effects of sulindac and indomethacin in chronic renal failure. *Clin Pharmacol Ther* 1985;37:447–452.
209. Wilkes BM, Solomon J, Maita M, Mento PF. Characterization of glomerular thromboxane receptor sites in the rat. *Am J Physiol* 1989;256: F1111–F1116.
210. Folger WH, Halushka PV, Wilcox CS, Guzman NJ. Characterization of rat glomerular thromboxane A2 receptors. Comparison to rat platelets. *Eur J Pharmacol* 1992;2:277–280.
211. Gerber JG, Ellis E, Hollifield J, Nies AS. Effect of prostaglandin endoperoxide analogue on canine renal function. Hemodynamics and renin release. *Eur J Pharmcol* 1979;53:239–246.
212. Feigen LP, Chapnick BM, Flemming JE, Flemming JM, Kadowitz PJ. Renal vascular effects of endoperoxide analogs, prostaglandins, and arachidonic acid. *Am J Physiol* 1977;233:H573–H579.
213. Wilcox CS, Folger WH, Welch WJ. Renal vasoconstriction with U-46,619; role of arachidonate metabolites. *J Am Soc Nephrol* 1994;5: 1120–1124.
214. Welch WJ, Wilcox CS. Modulating role for thromboxane in the tubuloglomerular feedback response in the rat. *J Clin Invest* 1988;81: 1843–1849.
215. Welch WL, Wilcox CS. Feedback response during sequential inhibition of angiotensin and thromboxane. *Am J Physiol* 1990;258: F457–F466.
216. Welch WL, Wilcox CS, Dunbar KR. Modulation of renin by thromboxane: studies with thromboxane synthase inhibitor, receptor antagonists, and mimetic. *Am J Physiol* 1989;257:F554–F560.
217. Badr KF, Baylis C, Pfeffer JM, et al. Renal and systemic hemodynamics response to intravenous infusion of leukotriene C4 in the rat. *Circ Res* 1984;54:492–499.
218. Filep J, Rigter B, Frölich JC. Vascular and renal effects of leukotriene C4 in conscious rats. *Am J Physiol* 1985;249:F739–F744.
219. Badr KF, Brenner BM, Ichikawa I. Effects of leukotriene D4 on glomerular dynamics in the rat. *Am J Physiol* 1987;253:F239–F243.
220. Heller J, Horácek V, Kamarádová S. A possible role for leukotrienes in the regulation of glomerular haemodynamics in the dog. *Pflugers Arch* 1988;412:155–163.
221. Yared A, Albrightson-Winslow C, Griswold D, Takahashi K, Fogo A, Badr KF. Functional significance of leukotriene B4 in normal and glomerulonephritic kidneys. *J Am Soc Nephrol* 1991;2:45–56.
222. Badr KF, Serhan CN, Nicolau KC, Samuelsson B. The action of lipoxin A on glomerular microcirculatory dynamics in the rat. *Biochem Biophys Res Commun* 1987;145:408–414.
223. Badr KF, DeBoer D, Schwartzberg M, Serhan CN. Lipoxin A4 antagonizes cellular and in vivo actions of leukotriene D4 in rat glomerular mesangial cells. Evidence for competition at a common receptor. *Proc Natl Acad Sci U S A* 1989;86:3438–3442.
224. Katoh T, Takahashi K, Capdevila J, et al. Glomerular stereospecific synthesis and hemodynamic actions of 8,9-epoxyeicosatrienoic acid in rat kidney. *Am J Physiol* 1991;261:F578–F586.
225. Takahashi K, Nammour TM, Fukunaga M, et al. Glomerular Actions of a free radical–generated novel prostaglandin, 8-epi-prostaglandin F2α, in the rat. *J Clin Invest* 1992;90:136–141.
226. Van Dorp DA. Aspects of the biosynthesis of prostaglandins. *Prog Biochem Pharmacol* 1967;3:71–82.

227. Bohman SO. Demonstration of prostaglandin synthesis in colecting duct cells and other cell types of the rabbit renal medulla. *Prostaglandins* 1977;14:729–744.
228. Janszen FHA, Nugteren DH. Histochemical localization of prostaglandin synthetase. *Histochemie* 1971;27:159–164.
229. Grenier FC, Smith WL, Formation of 6-keto PGF1a by collecting tubule cells isolated from rabbit renal papillae. *Prostaglandins* 1978; 16:759–772.
230. Schlondorff D, Zanger R, Satriano JA, Folkert VW, Eveloff J. Prostaglandin synthesis by isolated cells from the outer medulla and from the thick ascending loop of Henle of rabbit kidney. *J Pharmacol Exp Ther* 1982;223:120–124.
231. Zusman RM, Keiser HR. Prostaglandin biosynthesis by rabbit renomedullary interstitial cells in tissue culture. Stimulation by angiotensin II, bradykinin, and arginine vasopressin. *J Clin Invest* 1977;60: 215–223.
232. Farman N, Pradelles P, Bonvalet JP. Determination of prostaglandin E2 synthesis along the rabbit nephron by enzyme immunoassay. *Am J Physiol* 1986;251:F238–F244.
233. Farman N, Pradelles P, Bonvalet JP. PGE2, PGF2a, 6-keto-PGF1α, and TxB2 synthesis along the rabbit nephron. *Am J Physiol* 1987;252: F53–F59.
234. Imbert-Teboul M, Siaume S, Morel F. Sites of prostaglandin E2 (PGE2) synthesis along the rabbit nephron. *Mol Cell Endocrinol* 1986;45:1–10.
235. Kirschenbaum MA, Lowe AG, Trizna W, Fine LG. Regulation of vasopressin action by prostaglandins. Evidence for prostaglandin synthesis in the rabbit cortical collecting tubule. *J Clin Invest* 1982;70: 1193–1204.
236. Zusman RM, Keiser HR. Regulation of prostaglandin E2 synthesis by angiotensin II, potassium, osmolality, and dexamethasone. *Kidney Int* 1980;17:277–283.
237. Attallah AA, Stahl RAK, Bloch DL, Ambrus JL, Lee JB. Inhibition of rabbit renal prostaglandin E2 biosynthesis by chronic potassium deficiency. *J Lab Clin Med* 1981;97:205–212.
238. Stahl RAK, Attallah AA, Bloch DL, Lee JB. Stimulation of rabbit renal PGE2 biosynthesis by dietary sodium restriction. *Am J Physiol* 1979;237:F344–F349.
239. Wuthrich RP, Valloton M. Prostaglandin E2 and cyclic AMP response to vasopressin in renal medullary tubular cells. *Am J Physiol* 1986;251:F499–F505.
240. Iino Y, Imai M. Effects of prostaglandins on Na transport in isolated collecting tubules. *Pflugers Arch* 1978;373:125–132.
241. Stokes JB, Kokko JP. Inhibition of sodium transport by prostaglandin E2 across the isolated perfused rabbit collecting tubule. *J Clin Invest* 1977;59:1099–1104.
242. Stokes JB. Effect of prostaglandin E2 on chloride transport across the rabbit thick ascending limb of Henle. Selective inhibition of the medullary portion. *J Clin Invest* 1979;64:495–502.
243. Fine LG, Kirschenbaum MA. Absence of direct effects of prostaglandins on sodium chloride transport in the mammalian nephron. *Kidney Int* 1981;19:797–801.
244. Higashihara E, Stokes JB, Kokko JP, Campbell WB, DuBose TD. Cortical and papillary micropuncture examination of chloride transport in segments of the rat kidney during inhibition of prostaglandin production. Possible role for prostaglandins in the chloruresis of acute volume expansion. *J Clin Invest* 1979;64:1277–1287.
245. Roman RJ, Kauker ML. Renal effect of prostaglandin synthetase inhibition in rats: micropuncture studies. *Am J Physiol* 1978;235: F111–F118.
246. Schafer JA. Salt and water homeostasis—is it just a matter of good bookkeeping. *J Am Soc Nephrol* 1994;4:1933–1950.
247. Johnston HH, Herzog JP, Wauler DP. Effect of prostaglandin E1 on renal hemodynamics, sodium, and water excretion. *Am J Physiol* 1967;213:939–946.
248. Bolger PM, Eisner GM, Ramwell PW, et al. Renal actions of prostacyclin. *Nature* 1978;271:467–469.
249. Strandhoy JW, Ott CE, Schneider EG, et al. Effects of prostaglandins E1 and E2 on renal sodium reabsorption and starling force. *Am J Physiol* 1974;226:1015–1021.
250. Altsheler P, Klahr S, Rosenbaum R, et al. Effects of inhibitors of prostaglandin synthesis on renal sodium excretion in normal dogs and dogs with decreased renal mass. *Am J Physiol* 1978;235: F338–F344.
251. Brater DC. Effect of indomethacin on salt and water homeostasis. *Clin Pharmacol Ther* 1979;25:322–330.
252. Grantham JJ, Orloff J. Effect of prostaglandin E1 on the permeability response of the isolated collecting tubule to vasopressin, adenosine 3, 5-monophosphate, and theophylline. *J Clin Invest* 1968;47: 1154–1161.
253. Sonnenburg WK, Smith WL. Regulation of cyclic AMP metabolism in rabbit cortical collecting tubule cells by prostaglandin. *J Biol Chem* 1988;263:6155.
254. Hébert RL, Jacobsen HR, Breyer MD. PGE2 inhibits AVP-induced water flow in cortical collecting ducts by protein kinase C activation. *Am J Physiol* 1990;259:F318–F325.
255. Chen L, Reif MC, Schafer JA. Clonidine and PGE2 have different effects on Na+ and water transport in the rat and rabbit CCD. *Am J Physiol* 1991;261:F126–F136.
256. Dunn MJ, Greely HP. Renal excretion of prostaglandin E2 and F2α in diabetes insipidus rat. *Am J Physiol* 1978;235:E624–627.
257. Edwards RM. Effects of prostaglandins on vasoconstrictor action in isolated renal arterioles. *Am J Physiol* 1985;248:F779–F784.
258. Walker RM, Brown RM, Stoff JS. Role of renal prostaglandin during antidiuresis and water diuresis in man. *Kidney Int* 1981;21:365.
259. Garcia-Perez A, Smith WL. Apical–basolateral membrane asymmetry in canine cortical collecting tubule cells. *J Clin Invest* 1984;74:63.
260. Garcia-Perez A, Smith WL. Use of monoclonal antibodies to isolate cortical collecting tubule cells. AVP induces PGE release. *Am J Physiol* 1983;244:C211–C220.
261. Kirschenbaum MA, Lowe AG, Trizna W. Regulation of vasopressin action by prostaglandins: evidence for prostaglandin synthesis in the rabbit cortical collecting tubule. *J Clin Invest*, 1982;70:1193.
262. Davis JO, Freeman RH. Mechanisms regulating renin release. *Physiol Rev* 1976;56:1–56.

262. Davis JO, Freeman RH. Mechanisms regulating renin release. *Physiol Rev* 1976;56:1–56.

263. Weber P, Holzgreve H, Stephan R, Herbst R. Plasma renin activity and renal sodium and water excretion following infusion of arachidonic acid in rats. *Eur J Pharmacol* 1975;34:299–304.
264. Weber PC, Larsson C, Anggard E, et al. Stimulation of renin release from rabbit renal cortex by arachidonic acid and prostaglandin endoperoxides. *Circ Res* 1976;39:868–874.
265. Bolger PM, Eisner GM, Ramwell PW, Slotkoff LM. Effect of prostaglandin synthesis on renal function and renin in the dog. *Nature* 1976; 259:244–245.
266. Larsson C, Weber P, Anggard E. Arachidonic acid increases and indomethacin decreases plasma renin activity in the rabbit. *Eur J Pharmacol* 1974;28:391–394.
267. Franco-Saenz R, Suzuki S, Tan SY, Mulrow PJ. Prostaglandin stimulation of renin release: independence of β-adrenergic receptor activity and possible mechanism of action. *Endocrinology* 1980;106: 1400–1404.
268. Seymour AA, Davis JO, Echtenkamp SF, Dietz JR, Freeman RH. Adrenergically induced renin release in conscious indomethacin-treated dogs and rats. *Am J Physiol* 1981;240:F515–F521.
269. Suzuki S, Franco-Saenz R, Tan SY, Mulrow PJ. Effects of indomethacin on plasma renin activity in the conscious rat. *Am J Physiol* 1981;240: E286–E289.
270. Lianos EA, Andres GA, Dunn MJ. Glomerular prostaglandin and thromboxane synthesis in rat nephrotoxic serum nephritis. *J Clin Invest* 1983;72:1439–1448.
271. Kaizu K, Marsh D, Zipser R, Glassock RJ. Role of prostaglandins and angiotensin II in experimental glomerulonephritis. *Kidney Int* 1985; 28:629–635.
272. Macconi D, Benigni A, Morigi M, et al. Enhanced glomerular thromboxane A2 mediates some pathophysiologic effect of platelet-activating factor in rabbit nephrotoxic nephritis: evidence from biochemical measurements and inhibitor trials. *J Lab Clin Med* 1989;113: 549–560.
273. Stork JE, Dunn MJ. Hemodynamic roles of thromboxane A2 and prostaglandin E2 in glomerulonephritis. *J Pharmacol Exp Ther* 1985; 233:672–678.
274. Takahashi K, Schreiner GF, Yamashita K, Christmann BW, Blair I, Badr KF. Predominant functional roles for thromboxane A2 and prostaglandin E2 during late nephrotoxic serum glomerulonephritis in the rat. *J Clin Invest* 1990;85:1974–1982.
275. Lianos EA, Rahman MA, Dunn MJ. Glomerular arachidonate lipoxy-

genation in rat nephrotoxic serum nephritis. *J Clin Invest* 1985;76: 1355–1359.
276. Lianos EA. Synthesis of hydroxyeicosatetraenoic acids and leukotrienes in rat nephrotoxic serum glomerulonephritis: role of anti-glomerular basement membrane antibody dose, complement, and neutrophiles. *J Clin Invest* 1988;82:427–435.
277. Fauler J, Wiemeyer A, Marx KH, Kühn K, Koch KM, Fröhlich JC. LTB4 in nephrotoxic serum nephritis in rats. *Kidney Int* 1989;36: 46–50.
278. Yared A, Albrightson-Winslow C, Griswold D, Takahashi K, Fogo A, Badr KF. Functional significance of leukotriene B4 in normal and glomerulonephritic kidneys. *J Am Soc Nephrol* 1991;2:45–56.
279. Badr KF, Schreiner GF, Wassermann M, Ichikawa I. Preservation of the glomerular capillary ultrafiltration coefficient during rat nephrotoxic serum nephritis by a specific leukotriene D4 receptor antagonist. *J Clin Invest* 1988;81:1702–1709.
280. Wu SH, Bresnahan A, Lianos EA. Hemodynamic role of arachidonate 12- and 5-lipoxygenases in nephrotoxic serum nephritis. *Kidney Int* 1993;43:1280–1285.
281. Albrightson CR, Short B, Dytko G, et al. Selective inhibition of 5-lipoxygenase attenuates glomerulonephritis in the rat. *Kidney Int* 1994;45:1301–1310.
282. Petric R, Ford-Hutchinson AW. Elevated cysteinyl leukotriene excretion in experimental glomerulonephritis. *Kidney Int* 1994;46: 1322–1329.
283. Garcia-Estan J, Roman RJ, Lianos EA, Garancis J. Effects of complement depletion on glomerular eicosanoid production and renal hemodynamics in rat nephrotoxic serum nephritis. *J Lab Clin Med* 1989; 114:389–393.
284. Wu X, Pippin J, Lefkowith JB. Platelets and neutrophils are critical to the enhanced glomerular arachidonate metabolism in acute nephrotoxic nephritis in rats. *J Clin Invest* 1993;91:766–773.
285. Lefkowith JB, Nagamatsu T, Pippin J, Schreiner GF. Role of leukocytes in metabolic and functional derangements of experimental glomerulonephritis. *Am J Physiol* 1991;261:F213–F220.
286. Shinkai Y, Cameron JS. Rabbit nephrotoxic nephritis: effect of a thromboxane synthetase inhibitor on evolution and prostaglandin excretion. *Nephron* 1987;47:211–219.
287. Saito H, Ideura T, Takeuchi J. Effects of a selective thromboxane A2 synthetase inhibitor on immune complex glomerulonephritis. *Nephron* 1984;36:38–45.
288. Nagamatsu T, Pippin J, Schreiner GF, Lefkowith JB. Paradoxical exacerbation of leukocyte-mediated glomerulonephritis with cyclooxygenase inhibition. *Am J Physiol* 1992;F228–F236.
289. Wu SH, Lianos EA. Modulatory effect of arachidonate 5-lipoxygenation on glomerular cell proliferation in nephrotoxic serum nephritis. *J Lab Clin Med* 1993;122:703–710.
290. Fischer DB, Christman JW, Badr KF. Fifteen-S-hydroxyeicosatetraenoic acid (15-S-HETE) specifically antagonizes the chemotactic action and glomerular synthesis of leukotriene B4 in the rat. *Kidney Int* 1992;41:1155–1160.
291. Badr KF. 15-lipoxygenase products as leukotriene antagonist. Therapeutic potential in glomerulonephritis. *Kidney Int* 1992;442(suppl): 101–108.
292. Papayianni A, Serhan CN, Phillips ML, Rennke HG, Brady HR. Transcellular biosynthesis of lipoxin A4 during adhesion of platelets and neutrophils in experimental immune complex glomerulonephritis. *Kidney Int* 1995;47:1295–1302.
293. Badr KF, DeBoer DK, Schwartzberg M, Serhan CN. Lipoxin A4 antagonize cellular and in vivo actions of leukotriene D4 in rat glomerular mesangial cells: evidence for competition at a common receptor. *Proc Natl Acad Sci U S A* 1989;86:3438–3442.
294. Brady HR, Lamas S, Papayianni A, Takata S, Matsubara M Marsden PA. Lipoxygenase product formation and cell adhesion during neutrophil–glomerular endothelial cell interaction. *Am J Physiol* 1995; 268:F1–F12.
295. Takata S, Matsubara M, Allen PG, Janmey PA, Serhan CN, Brady HR. Remodeling of neutrophil phospholipids with 15 (S)-hydroxyeicosatetraenoic acid inhibits leukotriene B4-induced neutrophil migration across endothelium. *J Clin Invest* 1994;93:499–508.
296. Katoh T, Lakkis FG, Makita N, Badr KF. Co-regulated expression of glomerular 12/15-lipoxygenase and interleukin-4 mRNAs in rat nephrotoxic nephritis. *Kidney Int* 1994;46:341–349.
297. Badr KF, DeBoer DK, Schwartzberg M, Serhan CN. Lipoxin A4 antagonizes cellular and in vivo actions of leukotriene D4 in rat glomerular mesangial cells: evidence for competition at a common receptor. *Proc Natl Acad Sci U S A* 1989;86:3438–3442.
298. Brady HR, Persson U, Ballermann BJ, Brenner BM, Serhan CN. Leukotrienes stimulate neutrophil adhesion to mesangial cells: modulation with lipoxins. *Am J Physiol* 1990;259:F809–F815.
299. Couser WG, Steinmuller DR, Stilmant MM, Salant DJ, Lowenstein LM. Experimental glomerulonephritis in the isolated perfused rat Kidney. *J Clin Invest* 1978;62:1275–1287.
300. Stahl RAK, Adler S, Baker PJ, Chen YP, Pritzl PM, Couser WG. Enhanced glomerular prostaglandin formation in experimental membranous nephropathy. *Kidney Int* 1987;31:1126–1131.
301. Lianos EA, Noble B, Hucke B. Glomerular leukotriene synthesis in Heymann nephritis. *Kidney Int* 1989;36:998–1002.
302. Katoh T, Lianos EA, Fukunaga M, Takahashi K, Badr KF. Leukotriene D4 is a mediator of proteinuria and glomerular hemodynamic abnormalities in passive Heymann nephritis. *J Clin Invest* 1993;91: 1507–1515.
303. Cybulsky AV, Lieberthal W, Quigg RJ, Rennke HG, Salant DJ. A role for thromboxane in complement-mediated glomerular injury. *Am J Pathol* 1987;128:45–51.
304. Kelley VE, Sneve S, Musinski S. Increased renal thromboxane production in murine lupus nephritis. *J Clin Invest* 1986;77:252–259.
305. Spurney RF, Bernstein RJ, Ruiz P, Pisetsky DS, Coffman TM. Physiologic role for enhanced renal thromboxane production in murine lupus nephritis. *Prostaglandins* 1991;42:15–28.
306. Spurney RF, Fan PY, Ruiz P, Sanfilippo F, Pisetsky DS, Coffman TM. Thromboxane receptor blockade reduces renal injury in murine lupus nephritis. *Kidney Int* 1992;41:973–982.
307. Salvati P, Lamberti E, Ferrario R, et al. Long–term thromboxane-synthesis inhibition prolongs survival in murine lupus nephritis. *Kidney Int* 1995;47:1168–1175.
308. Spurney RF, Ruiz P, Pisetsky DS, Coffman TM. Enhanced renal leukotriene production in murine lupus: role of lipoxygenase metabolites. *Kidney Int* 1991;39:95–102.
309. Pierucci A, Simonetti BM, Pecci G, et al. Improvement of renal function with selective thromboxane antagonism in lupus nephritis. *N Engl J Med* 1989;320:421–425.
310. Stahl RAK, Thaiss F, Kahf S, Schoeppe W, Helmchen UM. Immune-mediated mesangial cell injury—biosynthesis and function of prostanoids. *Kidney Int* 1990;38:273–281.
311. Oberle GP, Niemeyer J, Thaiss F, Schoeppe W, Stahl RAK. Increased oxygen radical and eicosanoid formation in immune-mediated mesangial cell injury. *Kidney Int* 1992;42:69–74.
312. Lianos EA, Bresnahan BA, Pan C. Mesangial cell immune injury. *J Clin Invest* 1991;88:623–631.
313. Stahl RAK, Thaiss F, Wenzel U, Helmchen UM. Morphologic and functional consequences of immune mediated mesangiolysis: development of chronic glomerular sclerosis. *J Am Soc Nephrol* 1992;2 (suppl):144–148.
314. Stahl RAK, Thais F, Wenzel U Schoeppe W, Helmchen U. A rat model of progressive chronic glomerular sclerosis: the role of thromboxane inhibition. *J Am Soc Nephrol* 1992;2:1568–1577.
315. Gesualdo L, Emancipator SN, Kesselheim C, Lamm ME. Glomerular hemodynamics and eicosanoid synthesis in a rat model of IgA nephropathy. *Kidney Int* 1992;42:106–114.
316. Rifai A, Sakai H, Yagame M. Expression of 5-lipoxygenase and 5-lipoxygenase activation protein in glomerulonephritis. *Kidney Int* 1993;43:95–99.
317. Rahman MA, Emancipator SN, Dunn MJ. Immune complex effects on glomerular eicosanoid production and renal hemodynamics. *Kidney Int* 1987;31:1317–1326.
318. Rahman MA, Nakazawa M, Emancipator SN, Dunn MJ. Increased leukotriene B4 synthesis in immune injured rat glomeruli. *J Clin Invest* 1988;81:1945–1952.
319. Thaiss F, Germann PJ, Kahf S, Schoeppe W, Helmchen U, Stahl RAK. Effect of thromboxane synthesis inhibition in a model of membranous nephropathy. *Kidney Int* 1989;35:76–83.
320. Foegh ML, Zmudka M, Cooley C, Winchester JF, Helfrich GB, Ramwell PW. Urine i-TXB2 in renal allograft rejection. *Lancet* 1981; 2:431–434.
321. Foegh ML, Alijani M, Helfrich GB, Schreiner GE, Ramwell PW. Urine thromboxane as an immunologic monitor in kidney transplant patients. *Transplant Proc* 1984;16:1603–1605.

322. Steinhauer HB, Wilms H, Rüther M, Schollmeyer P. Clinical experience with urine TXB2 in acute renal allograft rejection. *Transplant Proc* 1986;18:98–103.
323. Foegh ML, Khirabadi BS, Shapiro R, et al. Monitoring of rat heart allograft rejection by urinary thromboxane. *Transplant Proc* 1984;16: 1606–1608.
324. Mangino MJ, Anderson CB, DeSchryver K, Tyler JD, Sicard GA, Turk J. Eicosanoid synthesis associated with renal allograft rejection. *Transplant Proc* 1986;18:63–70.
325. Spurney RF, Ibrahim S, Butterly D, Klotman PE, Sanfilippo F, Coffman TM. Leukotrienes in renal transplant rejection in rats. *J Immunol* 1994;152:867–876.
326. Foegh ML, Alijani MR, Helfrich GB, Khirabadi BS, Lim K, Ramwell PW. Lipid mediators in organ transplantation. *Transplant Proc* 1986; 18:20–24.
327. Coffman TM, Yarger WE, Klotman PE. Functional role of thromboxane production by acutely rejecting renal allografts in rats. *J Clin Invest* 1985;75:1242–1248.
328. Mangino MJ, Brunt EM, von Doersten P, Anderson CB. Effects of the thromboxane synthesis inhibitor CGS-12970 on experimental acute renal allograft rejection. *J Pharmacol Exp Ther* 1989;248: 23–28.
329. Neumayer HH, Schreiber M, Wagner K. Prevention of delayed graft function by diltiazem and Iloprost. *Transplant Proc* 1989;21: 1221–1224.
330. Goodwin JS, Ceuppens JL, Gualde N. Control of the immune response in humans by prostaglandins. *Adv Inflamm Res* 1984;7: 79–91.
331. Moran M, Mozes MF, Maddux MS, et al. Prevention of acute graft rejection by the prostaglandin E1 analogue misoprostol in renal-transplant recipients treated with cyclosporine and prednisone. *N Engl J Med* 1990;322:1183–1188.
332. Kunkel SL, Thrall RS, Kunkel RG, McCormick JR, Ward PA, Zurier RB. Suppression of immune complex vasculitis in rats by prostaglandin. *J Clin Invest* 1979;64:1525–1529.
333. Zurier RB, Damjanov I, Miller PL, Biewer BF. Prostaglandin E1 treatment prevents progression of nephritis in murine lupus erythematosus. *J Clin Labor Immunol* 1978;1–2:95–98.
334. Zurier RB, Damjanov I, Sayadoff DM, Rothfield NF. Prostaglandin E1 treatment of NZB/NZW F1 hybrid mice. *Arthritis Rheumatism* 1977;20:1449–1456.
335. Kelley VE, Winkelstein A, Izui S. Effect of prostaglandin E on immune complex nephritis in NZB/W mice. *Lab Invest* 1979;41: 531–537.
336. Izui S, Kelley VE, McConahey PJ, Dixon FJ. Selective suppression of retroviral gp70–anti-gp70 immune complex formation by prostaglandin E1 in murine systemic lupus erythematosus. *J Exp Med* 1980;152: 1645–1658.
337. Winkelstein A, Kelley VE. Effects of PGE1 in murine models of SLE: changes in circulating immune complexes. *Clin Immunol Immunopathol* 1981;20:188–192.
338. McLeish KR, Gohara AF, Gunning WT, Senitzer D. Prostaglandin E1 therapy of murine chronic serum sickness. *Am Fed Clin Res* 1979;96: 470–479.
339. McLeish KR, Gohara AF, Gunning WT. Suppression of antibody synthesis by prostaglandin E as a mechanism for preventing murine immune complex glomerulonephritis. *Lab Invest* 1982;47:147–152.
340. McLeish KR, Gohara AF, Stelzer GT, Wallace JH. Treatment of murine immune complex glomerulonephritis with prostaglandin E2: dose-response of immune complex deposition, antibody synthesis, and glomerular damage. *Clin Immunol Immunopathol* 1983;26: 18–23.
341. McLeish KR, Stelzer GT, Eades DS, Cohen R, Wallace JH. Serial changes in humoral and cellular immunity induced by prostaglandin E2 treatment of murine immune complex glomerulonephritis. *J Lab Clin Med* 1985;106:517–523.
342. Hirszel P, Michaelson JH, Dodge K, Yamase H, Bigazzi PE. Mercury-induced autoimmune glomerulonephritis in inbred rats. II. Immunohistopathology, histopathology and effects of prostaglandin administration. *Surv Synthesis Pathol Res* 1985;4:412–422.
343. Kunkel SL, Thrall RS, Kunkel RG, McCormick JR, Ward PA, Zurier RB. Suppression of immune complex vasculitis in rats by prostaglandin. *J Clin Invest* 1979;64:1525–1529.
344. Kunkel SL, Zanetti M, Sapin C. Suppression of nephrotoxic serum nephritis in rats by prostaglandin E1. *Am J Pathol* 1982;108: 240–245.
345. Nagamatsu T, Suzuki Y. Antinephritic effect of prostaglandin E1 on serum sickness nephritis in rats. *Jpn J Pharmacol* 1986;42:109–116.
346. Nagamatsu T, Kojima J, Ito M, Kondo N, Suzuki Y. Antinephritic effects of PGE1 and thiaprostaglandin E1, TEI-5178 and TEI-6122, on crescentic-type anti-GBM nephritis in rats. *Jpn J Pharmacol* 1989; 51:521–530.
347. Cattell V, Smith J, Cook HT. Prostaglandin E1 suppresses macrophage infiltration and ameliorates injury in an experimental model of macrophage-dependent glomerulonephritis. *Clin Exp Immunol* 1990; 79:260–265.
348. Schneider A, Thaiss F, Rau HP, et al. Prostaglandin E1 inhibits collagen expression in anti-thymocyte antibody induced glomerulonephritis: possible role of TGF-β. *Kidney Int* 1996;50:190–199.
349. Kunkel SL, Wiggins RC, Chensue SW, Larrick J. Regulation of macrophage tumor necrosis factor production by prostaglandin E2. *Biochem Biophys Res Commun* 1986;137:404–410.
350. Haynes DR, Whitehouse MW, Vernon-Roberts B. The prostaglandin E1 analogue, misoprostol, regulates inflammatory cytokines and immune functions in vitro like the natural prostaglandins E1, E2 and E3. *Immunology* 1992;76:251–257.
351. Kunkel SL. The importance of arachidonate metabolism by immune and nonimmune cells [Editorial]. *Lab Invest* 1988;58:119–121.
352. Niwa T, Maeda K, Naotsuka Y, et al. Improvement of renal function with prostaglandin E1 infusion in patients with chronic renal disease. *Lancet* 1982;1:687.
353. Nagayama Y, Namura Y, Tamura T, Muso R. Benefical effect of prostaglandin E1 in three cases of lupus nephritis with nephrotic syndrome. *Ann Allergy* 1988;61:289–295.
354. Niwa T, Asada H, Yamada K. Prostaglandin E1 infusion therapy in chronic glomerulonephritis—a double-blind, crossover trial. *Prostaglandins Leukot Essent Fatty Acids* 1985;19:227–233.
355. Shibasaki T, Kodama K, Ohno I, et al. Adjunctive therapy of lipoprostaglandin E sub(1) in patients with nephrotic syndrome. *Curr Ther Res Clin Exp* 1991;50:356–362.
356. Lin CY. Improvement in steroid and immunosuppressive drug resistant lupus nephritis by intravenous prostaglandin E1 therapy. *Nephron* 1990;55:258–264.
357. Lands WE. *Fish and human health.* Orlando, FL: Academic; 1986.
358. De Caterina R, Endres S, Kristensen SD, Berg Schmidt E. In-depth review. n-3 fatty acids and renal diseases. *Am J Kidney Dis* 1994;24: 397–415.
359. Zurier RB, Damjanov I, Sayadoff DM, Rothfield NF. Prostaglandin E1 treatment of NZB/NZW F1 hybrid mice II. Prevention of glomerulonephritis. *Arthritis Rheum* 1977;20:1449–1456.
360. Prickett JD, Robinson DR, Steinberg AD. Dietary enrichment with the polyunsaturated fatty acid eicosapentaenoic acid prevents proteinuria and prolongs survival in NZB + NZW F1 mice. *J Clin Invest* 1981;68:556–559.
361. Kelley VE, Ferretti A, Izui S, Strom TB. A fish oil diet rich in eicosapentaenoic acid reduces cyclooxygenase metabolites, and suppresses lupus in MRL-1pr mice. *J Immunol* 1985;134:1914–1919.
362. Robinson DR, Prickett JD, Makoul GT, Steinberg AD, Colvin RB. Dietary fish oil reduces progression of established renal disease in (NZB + NZW)F1 mice and delays renal disease in BXSB and MRL/1 strains. *Arthritis Rheumatism* 1986;29:539–546.
363. Westberg G, Tarkowski A, Svalander C. Effect of eicosapentaenoic acid–rich Menhaden oil and MaxEPA on the autoimmune disease of MRL/lpr mice. *Int Arch Allergy Appl Immunol* 1989;88:454–461.
364. Thaiss F, Schoeppe W, Germann P, Stahl RAK. Dietary fish oil intake: effects on glomerular prostanoid formation, hemodynamics, and proteinuria in nephrotoxic serum nephritis. *J Lab Clin Med* 1990; 116:172–179.
365. Kher V, Barcelli U, Weiss M, Pollak VE. Effects of dietary linoleic acid enrichment on induction of immune complex nephritis in mice. *Nephron* 1985;39:261–266.
366. Kher V, Barcelli U, Weiss M, et al. Protective effect of polyunsaturated fatty acid supplementation in apoferritin induced murine glomerulonephritis. *Prostaglandins Leukot Essent Fatty Acids* 1986;22: 323–334.
367. Scharschmidt L, Miller M, Holthofer H, et al. A fish oil preserves renal function in nephrotoxic serum nephritis. *J Lab Clin Med* 1990; 115:405–414.

368. Weise WJ, Natori Y, Levine JS, et al. Fish oil has protective and therapeutic effects on proteinuria in passive Heymann nephritis. *Kidney Int* 1993;43:359–368.
369. Rahman MA, Sauter DC, Young MR. Effects of dietary fish oil on the induction of experimental membranous nephropathy in the rat. *Lab Invest* 1991;64:371–376.
370. Scharschmidt LA, Gibbons NB, McGarry L, et al. Effects of dietary fish oil on renal insufficiency in rats with subtotal nephrectomy. *Kidney Int* 1987;32:700–709.
371. Hamazaki T, Tateno S, Shishido H. Eicosapentanoic acid and IgA nephropathy. *Lancet* 1984;1:1017–1018.
372. Donadio JV, Bergstralh EJ, Offord KP, Spencer DC, Holley KE. A controlled trial of fish oil in IgA nephropathy. *N Engl J Med* 1994; 331:1194–1199.
373. Bennett WM, Walker RG, Kincaid-Smith P. Treatment of IgA nephropathy with eicosapentanoic acid (EPA): a two-year prospective trial. *Clin Nephrol* 1989;31:128–131.
373. Pettersson EE, Rekola S, Berglund L, et al. Treatment of IgA nephropathy with omega-3-polyunsaturated fatty acids: a prospective, double-blind, randomized study. *Clin Nephrol* 1994;41:183–190.
375. Clark WF, Parbtani A, Huff MW, Reid B, Holub BJ, Falardeau P. Omega-3 fatty acid dietary supplementation in systemic lupus erythematosus. *Kidney Int* 1989;36:653–660.
376. Clark WF, Parbtani A, Naylor CD, et al. Fish oil in lupus nephritis: clinical findings and methodological implications. *Kidney Int* 1993; 44:75–86.
377. Westberg G, Tarkowski A. Effect of Maxepa in patients with SLE. A double-blind crossover study. *Scand J Rheumatol* 1990;19:137–143.
378. Bilo HJG, Homan van der Heide JJ, Gans ROB, Donker AJM. Omega-3 polyunsaturated fatty acids in chronic renal insufficiency. *Nephron* 1991;57:385–393.
379. De Caterina R, Caprioli R, Giannessi D, et al. n-3 fatty acids reduce proteinuria in patients with chronic glomerular disease. *Kidney Int* 1993;44:843–850.

Immunologic Renal Diseases,
edited by E. G. Neilson and W. G. Couser.
Lippincott-Raven Publishers, Philadelphia © 1997

CHAPTER 23

Coagulation and Thrombosis in Immunologic Renal Diseases

Carla Zoja and Giuseppe Remuzzi

INTRODUCTION

For many years, activation of the coagulation system has been regarded as a crucial step in starting and amplifying glomerular damage in immunologic renal disease. In several forms of immune-mediated glomerular disease, including human proliferative crescentic glomerulonephritis (GN), fibrin deposits within the glomerular tuft are a prominent finding (1–3), which reflects an abnormal balance between coagulation and fibrinolytic systems. In experimental GN, induced by either chronic immune-complex disease or antiglomerular basement membrane (anti-GBM) antibodies, glomerular injury is similarly associated with fibrin deposition, crescent formation, and renal failure (4–8) (see also Chapter 32).

In 1964, Vassalli and McCluskey (9) were the first to describe fibrin deposits in experimental crescentic anti-GBM GN. The autologous phase of this model either in rabbits or in rats greatly helped the understanding of the mechanisms of glomerular fibrin deposition in GN in the following years. The accumulation of fibrin appears to involve activation of the intrinsic pathway (Fig. 1), as evidenced by the presence in the deposits of factor VIII and factor XII (Hageman factor) (10,11). Activation of the extrinsic pathway of coagulation through the tissue factor procoagulant (factor III, thromboplastin) may also contribute to deposition of fibrin. Studies have suggested an important role for macrophages as initiators of glomerular fibrin deposition in GN by their enhanced expression of tissue factor procoagulant activity (PCA). Thus, in rabbit anti-GBM nephritis, glomerular infiltration by macrophages and increased glomerular synthesis of tissue-factor-like PCA have been shown to coincide with fibrin deposition and crescent formation (12,13). Moreover, fibrin deposition was prevented by depletion of macrophages and could be partially restored by infusion of peritoneal macrophages (12). Similarly, in human crescentic GN, glomerular injury is closely associated with fibrin deposits, macrophage accumulation, and increased tissue factor expression (14) (see also Chapter 32). Macrophages, besides being a source of intraglomerular PCA, release cytokines—interleukin 1 (IL-1) or tumor necrosis factor (TNF)—which in turn stimulate tissue factor synthesis by endothelial cells (15–17). Endothelial cells normally limit the activation of coagulation by a number of functions, which include thrombomodulin-dependent activation of protein C and protein S, the presence of heparinlike proteoglycans on the surface, and the synthesis and secretion of plasminogen activator (PA) and prostacyclin (18,19). Cytokines alter normal endothelial cell function by down-regulating a number of antithrombotic molecules while triggering cell procoagulant activity (20). Thus, IL-1 and/or TNF increase tissue-factor-like activity, PA inhibitor, and von Willebrand factor (vWF) (15–17,21,22). Together these effects act in concert to favor deposition of fibrin and promote intravascular coagulation.

Glomerular endothelial, epithelial, and mesangial cells all have the potential to interact in the coagulation process. Data are available showing that in vitro mesangial cells produce PCA following TNF stimulation (23). PA and its inhibitor, PA inhibitor 1 (PAI-1), are secreted by all the types of glomerular cells. A noteworthy decreased expression of tissue-type PA (tPA) together with upregulation of PAI-1 have been documented in glomeruli from rats and rabbits with anti-GBM GN in association with fibrin accumulation (24–26). In severe forms of human crescentic GN, extracapillary fibrin deposits were associ-

C. Zoja: Mario Negri Institute for Pharmacological Research, 24125 Bergamo, Italy.
G. Remuzzi: Division of Nephrology and Dialysis, Riuniti di Bergamo Ospedali, 24128 Bergamo, Italy.

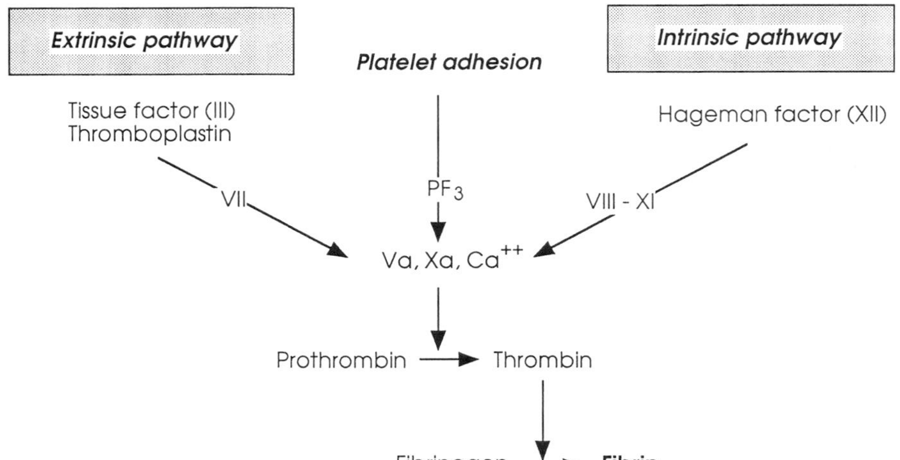

FIG. 1. Intrinsic and extrinsic pathways of coagulation are both involved in the formation of fibrin deposits within glomeruli in immune-mediated glomerulonephritis. Platelet factor 3 (PF_3) released by platelets also participates in the coagulation cascade.

ated with PAI-1, explaining, at least in part, the resistance to fibrinolysis and the persistence of these deposits (27). Thus, changes in PA and PAIs may act synergistically with the augmentation of procoagulant activity to enhance deposition of fibrin in glomeruli and subsequent injury in GN.

ENDOTHELIAL CELLS MODULATE INTRAVASCULAR THROMBUS FORMATION

Vascular endothelial cells are an active nonthrombogenic surface producing substances that maintain the hemostatic balance (18,20) (see also Chapter 30). When perturbed by vascular injury or inflammation, endothelial cells respond with increased expression of procoagulant activity and enhanced platelet adhesion and activation. The adhesion of platelets to the site of injury involves the interaction of glycoprotein (GP) receptors on inactivated platelets with constituents of subendothelial matrix adhesive proteins (28). vWF is essential for initial platelet adhesion by binding to GPIb constitutively expressed on platelet membranes (29). This is a shear-dependent mechanism. While, in the absence of shear forces, no affinity exists between GPIb and vWF, in the presence of shear forces as in the arterial circulation, conformational changes occur in the GPIb molecule with exposure of vWF receptor, which allows subsequent GPIb–vWF binding (28). With fibrinogen, vWF is also able to interlink activated platelets into aggregates by serving as ligand of GPIIb–IIIa on activated platelets (30). Other elements of the subendothelium also may mediate adhesion including fibronectin, lamin, vitronectin, and thrombospondin.

Adherent platelets become a target for other platelets and by a series of platelet–platelet interactions—aggregation events—a platelet mass accumulates, forming the thrombus. Concomitant deposition of fibrin, arising from plasma coagulation, strengthens the developing platelet aggregate by providing additional fibrous links between individual platelets.

The major products of the coagulation cascade are thrombin and fibrinogen. Thrombin, a multifunctional serine protease generated at sites of vascular injury, proteolytically converts fibrinogen to insoluble fibrin (31). Together with collagen, thrombin is the most potent activator of platelets that mediates thrombus formation at sites of vascular injury. Moreover, it has a number of procoagulant effects on endothelial cells, including release of platelet-activating factor, vWF, and tissue factor. Thrombin affects fibrinolytic system by inducing endothelial production of PAI-1. Noteworthy, a cDNA encoding a functional thrombin receptor has been isolated (32). The receptor appears to mediate thrombin-induced platelet activation and a variety of thrombin responses in cultured endothelial cells. The thrombin receptor is expressed in vivo in platelets and in human arteries (normal and atherosclerotic) (33). Abnormal thrombin formation is prevented by a natural anticoagulant system consisting of antithrombin III, heparin cofactor II, protein C, and protein S. Endothelial cells actively participate in the dissolution of fibrin by virtue of their synthesis and secretion of PAs—tPA) or urokinase-type PA (uPA)—which convert the inactive proenzyme plasminogen to plasmin, a serine protease that degrades the fibrin network associated with blood clots (34). The bioactivity of tPA is largely localized to the vasculature due to its high affinity for fibrin, which facilitates its physiologic activity on clot lysis, while uPA predominantly functions within the extravascular compartments (35). Inhibition of the fibrinolytic system may occur at the level of PAs via PAI types 1 and 2 (PAI-1 and PAI-2) or at the level of plasmin, mainly via α_2-antiplasmin. Impairment of this system, caused by an increase in PAI levels or by a reduced release of PAs from endothelial cells, may result in the development of thrombosis. In this context, there are data showing that mice transgenic for PAI-1 form venous thrombi (36). The control of plasminogen activation is also a crucial event in a number of physiologic and pathologic processes, since plasmin, besides having a wide range of activities in fibrinolysis, is also involved in the activation of metalloproteinase and latent transforming growth factor β1, in extracellular matrix degradation, tissue remodeling, and neovascularization (34).

Recent studies have suggested that activated polymorphonuclear leukocytes (PMNs) may impair fibrinolytic potential of the endothelium. Actually cathepsin G, a chymotrypsinlike serine protease released by activated PMNs and known to induce platelet aggregation and endothelial injury, enhanced PAI-1 levels and abolished tPA activity in cultured human endothelial cells (37). Cathepsin G was also able to increase the circulating levels of PAI-1 by promoting its release from activated blood platelets. Thus, a complex system of coordinate interplays between the different blood elements and vascular endothelium operates for the maintenance of normal hemostasis.

CYTOKINES EXERT PROCOAGULANT EFFECTS ON ENDOTHELIAL CELLS

There is now substantial evidence that cytokines affect endothelial cell coagulant properties. In 1984, Bevilacqua et al. (15) (see also Chapter 20) first demonstrated that interleukin-1 (IL-1) markedly increased tissue-factor-like procoagulant activity (PCA) in cultured endothelial cells. IL-1-stimulated endothelial cells acquired the capacity to bind factor VII/VIIa and trigger the extrinsic pathway of the coagulation cascade. IL-1-induced PCA was inhibited by cycloheximide and actinomycin D, which indicated a requirement for RNA and protein synthesis. The increased PCA activity was transient, peaked at 4–8 h after IL-1 treatment, and returned to normal within 24 h even in the presence of the cytokine in the culture medium. TNF had the same effects (16,17). Other studies showed that in vivo infusion of IL-1 into rabbits resulted in an increase of tissue factor activity expressed on the surface of aortic endothelium, with a concomitant blocking of the protein-C anticoagulant activity (38). Thus, both thrombin-mediated protein-C activation and formation of functional activated protein-C–protein-S complex on the endothelial cell surface were considerably decreased. The relevance of these observations to the prothrombotic changes induced by IL-1 in endothelial cells resides in the visualization by scanning electron microscopy of fibrin strands closely associated with the luminal endothelial cell surface of major arteries in rabbits infused with IL-1 (38).

A recently published study has provided important insights on the regulation of the tissue factor gene in porcine endothelial cells (39). It has been documented that the tissue factor promoter region contains potential binding sites for the NFkB element as well as AP-1- and SP-1-like transcription factors whose concerted action appears crucial for tissue factor gene transcription in endothelial cells. Electrophoretic mobility-shift assay experiments have shown that nuclear extracts prepared from cultured porcine endothelial cells stimulated with endotoxin, IL-1, or TNF contained a strongly induced tissue factor NFkB-binding activity, which was absent in unstimulated cells. Constitutive AP-1 and SP-1 binding was revealed.

Besides inducing tissue factor PCA and suppressing the protein-C pathway, cytokines shift the fibrinolytic properties of endothelial cells by decreasing tPA and enhancing PAI-1 secretion over a period of hours, requiring new mRNA and protein synthesis (21). This process occurs both in vitro and in vivo (40).

GLOMERULAR PROCOAGULANT ACTIVITY IN IMMUNE-MEDIATED GLOMERULONEPHRITIS

In 1985, De Prost and Kanfer (41) documented that isolated rat glomeruli contained a procoagulant activity that exhibited the well-established characteristics of thromboplastin/tissue factor. The activity was dependent of the presence of factors VII and X and was suppressed by phospholipase C, an inhibitor of the phospholipid component of tissue factor. The same year, Wiggins et al. (13) measured augmented procoagulant activity in glomeruli and urine of rabbits with nephrotoxic nephritis induced by injection of guinea pig anti-GBM immunoglobulin (Ig) G (see also Chapter 32). The time course for appearance of procoagulant activity corresponded with the appearance of proteinaceous material containing fibrin in the Bowman space. The forms of glomerular and urine procoagulant activity were complex since they seemed to be primarily driven by thromboplastin but also appeared to require the presence of intrinsic coagulation pathway for full expression of PCA. Other studies in rabbit anti-GBM GN documented the presence of fibrin deposition in association with glomerular macrophage accumulation and increased glomerular procoagulant activity (12) (see also Chapters 28, 32). When macrophages were depleted by mustine hydrochloride treatment, fibrin deposition was abrogated and glomerular procoagulant activity reduced. It was speculated that macrophages (by expressing procoagulant activity) were directly involved in glomerular fibrin deposition. Similar conclusions were reached when glomerular procoagulant activity was studied in two patients with rapidly progressive crescentic GN (14). Isolated glomeruli from these patients contained markedly augmented levels of procoagulant activity compared with the levels found in normal glomeruli. This activity had functional and immunologic characteristics of macrophage tissue factor given its dependence on factors VII and V, independence of factors VIII and XII, inhibition by phospholipase C, and association with cell membrane. Moreover, it was inhibited by a specific monoclonal anti-human tissue factor antibody. Activated monocytes, which were present in large numbers within glomeruli from these patients, were suspected as the most likely source of this form of tissue factor. Experimental studies have shown that glomerular PCA synthesis could increase even under circumstances where few monocytes were present in glomeruli. This is the case of mercuric-chloride-induced autoimmune GN in rats where no correlation was found between glomerular procoagulant activity and the number of monocytes/macrophages infiltrating the glomerulus (42). In this setting, glomerular procoagulant activity was maximal at the onset of fibrin formation in the glomeruli. That monocytes/macrophages are not essential for glomerular procoagulant activity expression is consistent with recent data showing that intrinsic glomerular cells synthesize tissue factor and release it locally. Thus, rat glomerular mesangial cells in culture produced tissue factor in small amounts under resting conditions, but following stimulation with TNF or endotoxin, mesangial procoagulant activity significantly increased (23). The above findings support the possibility of a direct participation of mesangial cells in fibrin formation during inflammatory glomerular injury (see also Chapter 29).

GLOMERULAR CELLS MODULATE LOCAL FIBRINOLYSIS POTENTIAL IN IMMUNE-MEDIATED GLOMERULONEPHRITIS

Studies during the last 10 years have established that the kidney is an important source of PAs (43) and that isolated human glomeruli have profibrinolytic activity (44). Specifically, mesangial cells play an active part in regulating fibrinolysis by synthesizing tPA and its inhibitor PAI-1 (see also Chapter 29). Unstimulated human mesangial cells in culture already synthesize tPA and PAI-1 (45), but gene expression and synthetic rate for these components are remarkably upregulated by thrombin, PAI-1 being formed in excess as compared with tPA (46). Thus, thrombin, besides promoting fibrin formation in glomeruli by virtue of its procoagulant potential, also inhibits fibrin degradation by increasing PAI-1 release from mesangial cells. Other in vitro studies have shown that mesangial cell synthesis of PAI-1, but not of tPA, increased in a time- and dose-dependent manner upon stimulation with TNF (47).

It has been consistently documented that glomerular epithelial cells in culture synthesize PA (48–50) and its inhibitor (49) and that cytokines as well as thrombin modulate such a release (see also Chapter 31). In particular, it has been shown by Western immunoblotting analysis that human glomerular epithelial cells secrete both tPA and uPA although uPA, namely, single-chain uPA, is predominant (49). Recent in situ hybridization experiments have demonstrated the cytoplasmic localization of uPA mRNA in epithelial but not mesangial cells (50). Accordingly, uPA antigen was measured only in the supernatants of pure cultures of glomerular epithelial cells. Incubation of human glomerular epithelial cells in culture with increasing concentrations of thrombin significantly increased uPA, tPA, and PAI-1. On the other hand, IL-1 enhanced synthesis and release of tPA and PAI-1, while TNF induced the synthesis of uPA and tPA (49). These findings would suggest that glomerular epithelial cells actively participate in the regulation of extracapillary fibrinolysis in glomeruli and that local inflammatory and immune processes could affect their fibrinolytic activity. Human glomerular epithelial cells express uPA and plasminogen/plasmin receptors on cell membrane surfaces (48,51). The binding of the two proenzymes (pro-uPA and plasminogen) on their receptors allows the generation of bound plasmin, which is protected from its principal inhibitor, α_2-antiplasmin (51). Thrombin decreases uPA receptor number on human glomerular epithelial cells (52) and down-regulates the expression of plasminogen/plasmin receptors (51), thus showing a potent inhibitory effect on cell-surface-associated fibrinolytic activity.

Activation of fibrinolysis probably has a crucial role in immune-mediated GN. Early in vivo studies performed by Giroux et al. in 1979 (53) documented an increase in glomerular fibrinolytic activity, which was related to fibrin deposition and crescent formation, in rats with anti-GBM GN. Glomerular fibrinolytic activity was measured on preparations of isolated glomeruli by using a radioassay based on lysis of ^{125}I fibrin adsorbed on a solid phase. Later, Tomosugi et al. (24) demonstrated increased PAI activity in glomerular culture supernatants from 4 till 24 h after anti-GBM antibody injection in rats with nephrotoxic serum nephritis. Plasma PAI activity peaked at 2 h but decreased rapidly thereafter, returning to normal levels at 24 h. Concomitant administration of TNF resulted in a fivefold increase in PAI activity, with a corresponding increase in glomerular fibrin formation. In agreement with these data are recent experiments by Feng et al. (25) showing that glomerular PAI-1 steady-state mRNA was increased after the induction of an accelerated anti-GBM GN in rats with an antibody that produced large amounts of glomerular capillary fibrin deposition. PAI-1 mRNA expression was noted at 6 h, peaked at 1 day and, although falling thereafter, remained higher than that of the control group through day 17. PAI-1 mRNA correlated with increased PAI-1 bioactivity (as determined by a functional tPA-binding assay) that occurred locally within the glomerulus and was associated with fibrin deposits. uPA and tPA mRNA either remained unchanged or decreased. The latter observation is consistent with studies showing low fibrinolytic activity in immune-mediated GN (26,54,55) but is in contrast with data of Giroux et al. (53) showing increased fibrinolytic activity in anti-GBM GN. Inconsistencies in the above studies have been attributed to differences in the type of anti-GBM antibodies administered. Feng et al. (25), by examining in a rat model the relationship between PAI, uPA, tPA, and cytokines by sequential glomerular mRNA expression determinations, found a maximally upregulated IL-1β mRNA at 6 h that preceded PAI-1 peak and declined by day 3 (see also Chapter 35). TGF-β mRNA began to increase at day 1 in correspondence with the maximal expression of PAI, reached a peak at day 6, and fell only slightly by day 17. It can be derived from these findings that increase in PAI-1 mRNA and bioactivity could be an early function of IL-1β and later on of TGF-β. Of interest, persisting increases in TGF-β and PAI-1 mRNA levels on day 17 were associated with fibrin deposits and thickened GBM, the latter suggestive of the early stages of diffuse glomerulosclerosis. It is likely that inhibition of plasmin generation as a consequence of increased PAI-1 activity may have contributed to the observed thickened GBM.

It is well established that degradation of matrix and basement membrane is mediated by plasmin and cell-surface-associated proteinases (34) and, because PAI inhibits PA activity, increased expression of glomerular PAI would result in decreased proteolytic activity with consequent matrix accumulation.

Recent studies provide compelling evidence that TGF-β plays a pivotal role in the pathologic accumulation of extracellular matrix in several experimental glomerular diseases including anti-thymocyte (Thy)-induced mesangial proliferative GN (56) and adriamycin-induced nephropathy (57) in rats, as well as in experimental and human diabetic nephropathy (58) (see also Chapter 20). Moreover, in vivo transfection of TGF-β gene into rat kidney induced glomerular sclerotic changes with extracellular matrix expansion and increased expression of type-I and-III collagen (59). Evidence is available that TGF-β leads to large increases in renal PAI-1 mRNA (60) and that TGF-β regulates the PAI-1 promoter through at least three different regions (61).These data are in keeping with the observation that incubation of normal glomeruli with TGF-β led to a dramatically increased PAI-1 production with a net decrease in PA activity (62). In the same study, glomeruli from rats with anti-Thy GN showed decreased PA activity and increased PAI-1 synthesis that preceded the glomerular accumulation of extracellular matrix; the administration of anti-TGF-β serum to these animals blocked the increase in glomerular PAI-1 deposition. Thus, TGF-β may indeed decrease matrix turnover in GN by enhancing local generation of PAI-1, which in turn inhibits PA activity.

Overexpression of PAI-1 has been recently described in murine lupus autoimmune disease (63). Expression of PAI-1 mRNA was detectable by in situ hybridization experiments in glomeruli from old (NZB × NZW)F_1 (B/W) lupus-prone mice in which the syndrome was fully expressed, whereas it could not be found in normal glomeruli. Northern and Western blotting of RNA and protein extracted from kidney cortex both confirmed that PAI-1 protein and RNA increased in lupus-prone mice as they aged and developed nephritis. When mice were fed a 40% calorie-restricted diet, the accumulation of PAI-1 protein and the expression of PAI-1 mRNA diminished and the histologic alterations were less severe than in lupus mice fed ad libitum. The authors of this elegant study concluded that PAI-1 might play an active role in the inflammation and accumulation of matrix that is so prominent in this model of lupus and also hypothesized a possible role for TGF-β in the observed upregulation of glomerular PAI-1 gene.

ANTICOAGULANT AND FIBRINOLYTIC THERAPY IN IMMUNE-MEDIATED GLOMERULONEPHRITIS

In 1964, Vassalli and McCluskey (9) suggested that intraglomerular coagulation could play a critical role in the pathogenesis of GN. They demonstrated by immunofluorescence fibrin-related material in glomeruli from rabbits with Masugi nephritis produced by the injection of nephrotoxic sheep serum. Deposits of fibrin were also frequently observed in the Bowman space and associated with the formation of crescents.

Studies performed over the last several decades in experimental GN have provided evidence that accumulation of fibrin in the Bowman space is essential for the formation of crescents, which consist predominantly of mononuclear phagocyte infiltrates and proliferating cells from the parietal epithelium of Bowman capsule (8,64) (see also Chapter 32). The mechanisms triggering the recruitment of inflammatory cells into the glomerulus are only partially understood. Chemotactic factors in the fibrin deposits, such as thrombin or fibronectin fragments, may attract monocytes into the Bowman space (64), a process that is possibly favored by breaks in the glomerular capillary wall or the Bowman capsule. Ig Fc has also been recognized as an important stimulus for macrophage accumulation in some forms of GN (11). Monocytes and macrophages may in turn contribute to crescent formation through increasing fibrin deposition by the release of tissue factor and other procoagulants such as IL-1 and TNF (11) (Fig. 2). Moreover, they can also increase the mass of cells that comprise crescents by stimulating fibroblast and epithelial cell proliferation through the release of growth factors (11,65) (see also Chapter 32).

In the last 20 years, efforts have been devoted to identify drugs with anticoagulant and/or fibrinolytic properties

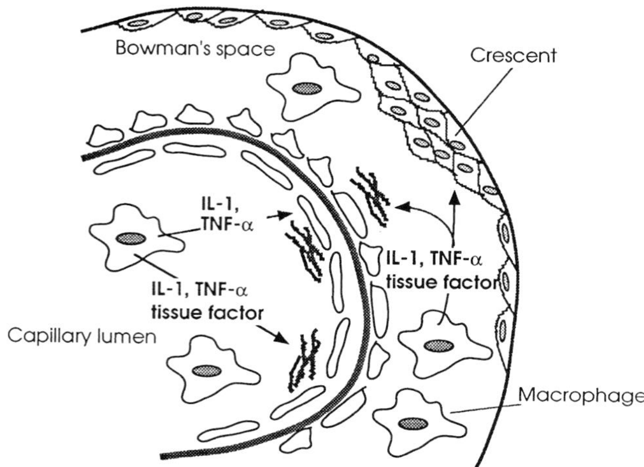

FIG. 2. Potential mechanisms involved in fibrin and crescent formation in immune-mediated glomerulonephritis. Macrophages contribute to crescent formation through increasing fibrin deposits by the release of tissue factor and procoagulant cytokines. Cytokines in turn stimulate proliferation of fibroblasts and epithelial cells that consolidate the crescent structure (see also Chapter 32).

with the aim of limiting the deposition of fibrin and the consequent glomerular obsolescence and progression of the disease. Some investigators reported that heparin prevented fibrin deposition and reduced glomerular hypercellularity, thus limiting crescent formation and glomerular sclerosis in rabbits with anti-GBM GN (4,5,66). This occurred despite persistent proteinuria due to immunologic injury. However, the doses of heparin employed were so large that many animals died from hemorrhage. Other studies were unable to demonstrate an effect of heparin in preventing glomerular fibrin deposition or altering the progression of experimental immune-complex GN or anti-GBM GN in rabbits (67). Heparin was equally ineffective in preventing renal damage in nephrotoxic serum nephritis in rats (68). Reasons for these conflicting results are not obvious and could be attributed to the different severity of the models and differences in second mediators of injury, apart from the difficulty in standardizing anti-GBM antibodies. Another anticoagulant, warfarin, entirely prevented crescent formation and markedly reduced intracapillary damage and hypercellularity in rabbits with nephrotoxic nephritis when given in very high doses before and after an injection of potent anti-GBM antiserum (9). However, fatal hemorrhage often occurred.

Additional evidence for the prominent role of coagulation in immune-mediated GN includes data from Naish et al. (6) and Thomson et al. (7), who showed that treatment with ancrod, a defibrinating agent, reduced glomerular fibrin deposition and crescent formation and protected rabbits with nephrotoxic nephritis from renal function impairment, without causing hemorrhagic complications. In addition, Thomson et al. (7) found that ancrod was effective in preventing crescent formation in rabbits with chronic serum sickness. Taking into account all of these data, McCluskey and Andres (65) concluded that, even with different underlying immunologic mechanisms, crescent formation depends on coagulation and may follow a final common pathway (see also Chapter 32).

Wu et al. (69) recently reported that defibrination by ancrod in rats with immune-complex GN decreased proteinuria as well as the influx of platelets and PMNs into the glomerulus. Fibrinogen has been considered responsible for promoting interactions between platelets and neutrophils, which contributed to neutrophil activation and proteinuria in this model. A marked increase in glomerular fibrinogen receptor (β3-integrin) expression was detected early in the course of the disease in these animals and was predominantly associated with platelets. Fibrinogen receptor blockade with a RGD analog protected against proteinuria almost completely, suggesting a major functional role for receptor upregulation in this model.

We investigated the efficacy of recombinant tPA therapy to prevent deteriorating renal function in rabbit extracapillary GN (70). tPA, a naturally occurring serine protease, isolated in 1981 by Rijken and Collen (71) from a human melanoma cell line, is now produced on a large scale by recombinant DNA technology (72) and employed in the treatment of thromboembolic diseases (73). The property of tPA that distinguishes it from other PAs such as streptokinase and urokinase is that its enzymatic activity is much more greatly increased in the presence of fibrin than that of either streptokinase or urokinase (74). The enhancement of the enzymatic activity of tPA by fibrin results from a conformational change either in tPA or plasminogen, brought about by the binding to fibrin, that promotes the interaction between tPA and plasminogen on the fibrin surface with the subsequent conversion of plasminogen to plasmin (75). Human recombinant tPA given to already proteinuric nephrotoxic nephritis rabbits significantly reduced glomerular fibrin deposition and crescent formation and ameliorated renal function impairment (70). Although treated rabbits had prolonged bleeding times, there were no hemorrhagic complications. These observations could be potentially important for future perspectives of using tPA in humans with crescentic GN and fibrin depositions. As highlighted by McCluskey and Andres (65), there are, however, serious difficulties in evaluating effectiveness of agents that prevent or dissolve glomerular fibrin deposits in human rapidly progressive glomerular diseases as noted from the previous experiences with heparin, warfarin, and antithrombotic agents combined with steroids and immunosuppressive agents or ancrod (76–81). This is essentially due to the fact that crescentic GN is not a homogeneous entity. This group of diseases include forms with many different underlying causes and possibly different mechanisms of renal injury and widely differ in severity and rate of progression. Actually, forms such as anti-GBM nephritis, Wegener granulomatosis, and idiopathic necrotizing and crescentic GN are quite uncommon, and performing controlled trials with a homogeneous group of patients is almost impossible.

As a possible alternative to the anticoagulant and fibrinolytic therapies so far available, a recent study has reported that FK506 significantly reduced thrombus formation and proteinuria and improved renal function in experimental immune-mediated GN (82). Early infiltration of PMNs into the glomeruli was significantly suppressed in the FK506 as compared with the placebo group. Another finding of that study was that the immunosuppressant markedly reduced the increases in serum TNF measured after nephrotoxic serum. The antithrombotic effects of FK506 in these animals (rats) appeared related to inhibition of the synthesis and release of cytokines and possibly other inflammatory mediators rather than to the immunosuppressive actions of FK506.

ACKNOWLEDGMENTS

The authors thank Dr. Simon Oldroyd and Dr. Miriam Galbusera for invaluable help in preparing this manuscript.

REFERENCES

1. Glassock RJ. The pathogenesis of crescentic glomerulonephritis in man. In: Bertani T, Remuzzi G, eds. *Glomerular injury 300 years after Morgagni.* Milan: Wichtig, 1983:195–204.
2. Nield GH, Cameron JS. Primary glomerulonephritis. In: Remuzzi G, Rossi EC, eds. *Haemostasis and the kidney.* London: Butterworths, 1989:56–79.
3. Glassock RJ, Adler SG, Ward HJ, Cohen AH. Primary glomerular diseases. In: Brenner BM, Rector FC, eds. *The kidney.* Philadelphia: Saunders, 1991:1182–279.
4. Kleinerman J. Effects of heparin in experimental nephritis in rabbits. *Lab Invest* 1954;3:495–508.
5. Halpern B, Milliez P, Lagrue G, Fray A, Morard JC. Protective action of heparin in experimental immune nephritis. *Nature* 1965;205:257–9.
6. Naish P, Penn GB, Evans DJ, Peters DK. The effect of defibrination on nephrotoxic serum nephritis in rabbits. *Clin Sci* 1972;42:643–6.
7. Thomson NM, Moran J, Simpson IJ, Peters DK. Defibrination with ancrod in nephrotoxic nephritis in rabbits. *Kidney Int* 1976;10:343–7.
8. Cattel V, Jamieson SW. The origin of glomerular crescents in experimental nephrotoxic serum nephritis in the rabbit. *Lab Invest* 1978;35:584–90.
9. Vassalli P, McCluskey RT. The pathogenic role of the coagulation process in rabbit Masugi nephritis. *Am J Pathol* 1964;45:653–77.
10. Wiggins RC. Hageman factor in experimental nephrotoxic nephritis in the rabbit. *Lab Invest* 1985;53:335–48.
11. Holdsworth SR, Tipping PG. Mechanisms of glomerular fibrin deposition in glomerulonephritis. In: Hatano M, ed. *Nephrology.* Tokyo: Springer-Verlag, 1991:209–21.
12. Holdsworth SR, Tipping PG. Macrophage-induced glomerular fibrin deposition in experimental glomerulonephritis in the rabbit. *J Clin Invest* 1985;76:1367–74.
13. Wiggins RC, Glatfelter A, Brukman J. Procoagulant activity in glomeruli and urine of rabbits with nephrotoxic nephritis. *Lab Invest* 1985;53:156–65.
14. Tipping PG, Dowling JP, Holdsworth SR. Glomerular procoagulant activity in human proliferative glomerulonephritis. *J Clin Invest* 1988;81:119–25.
15. Bevilacqua MP, Pober JS, Majeau GR, Cotran RS, Gimbrone MA Jr. Interleukin (IL-1) induces biosynthesis and cell surface expression of procoagulant activity in human vascular endothelial cells. *J Exp Med* 1984;160:618–23.
16. Bevilacqua MP, Pober JS, Majeau GR, Fiers W, Cotran RS, Gimbrone MA Jr. Recombinant tumor necrosis factor induces procoagulant activity in cultured human vascular endothelium: characterization and comparison with the actions of interleukin-1. *Proc Natl Acad Sci USA* 1986;83:4533–7.
17. Nawroth PP, Stern DM. Modulation of endothelial cell hemostatic properties by tumor necrosis factor. *J Exp Med* 1986;163:740–5.
18. Cotran RS. New roles for the endothelium in inflammation and immunity. *Am J Pathol* 1987;129:407–13.
19. Esmon CT. The regulation of natural anticoagulant pathways. *Science* 1987;235:1348–52.
20. Key NS. Scratching the surface: endothelium as a regulator of thrombosis, fibrinolysis, and inflammation. *J Lab Clin Med* 1992;120:184–6.
21. Bevilacqua MP, Schleef RR, Gimbrone MA Jr, Loskutoff DJ. Regulation of fibrinolytic system of cultured human vascular endothelium by interleukin 1. *J Clin Invest* 1986;78:587–91.
22. Schleef RR, Bevilacqua MP, Sawdey M, Gimbrone MA, Loskutoff DJ. Cytokine activation of vascular endothelium: effects on tissue-type plasminogen activator and type I plasminogen activator inhibitor. *J Biol Chem* 1988;263:5797–803.
23. Wiggins RC, Njoku N, Sedor JR. Tissue factor production by cultured rat mesangial cells: stimulation by TNFα and lipopolysaccharide. *Kidney Int* 1990;37:1281–5.
24. Tomosugi N, Wada T, Naito T, Takasawa K, Yokoyama H, Kida H, Kobayashi K. Role of plasminogen activator inhibitor on nephrotoxic nephritis and its modulation by tumor necrosis factor. *Nephron* 1992;62:213–9.
25. Feng L, Tang WW, Loskutoff DJ, Wilson CB. Dysfunction of glomerular fibrinolysis in experimental antiglomerular basement membrane antibody glomerulonephritis. *J Am Soc Nephrol* 1993;3:1753–64.
26. Malliaros J, Holdsworth SR, Wojta J, Erlich J, Tipping PG. Glomerular fibrinolytic activity in anti-GBM glomerulonephritis in rabbits. *Kidney Int* 1993;44:557–64.
27. Rondeau E, Mougenot B, Lacave R, Peraldi M-N, Kruithof EKO, Sraer J-D. Plasminogen activator inhibitor 1 in renal fibrin deposits of human nephropathies. *Clin Nephrol* 1990;33:55–60.
28. Roth GJ. Platelets and blood vessels: the adhesion event. *Immunol Today* 1992;13:100–5.
29. Stel HV, Sakariassen KS, De Groot PHG, van Mourik JA, Sixma JJ. The von Willebrand factor in the vessel wall mediates platelet adherence. *Blood* 1985;65:823–31.
30. Ruggeri ZM, De Marco L, Gatti L, Bader R, Montgomery RR. Platelets have more than one binding site for von Willebrand factor. *J Clin Invest* 1983;72:1–12.
31. Fenton JW II. Thrombin specificity. *Ann NY Acad Sci* 1981;370:468–95.
32. Vu T-KH, Hung DT, Wheaton VI, Coughlin SR. Molecular cloning of a functional thrombin receptor reveals a novel proteolytic mechanism of receptor activation. *Cell* 1991;64:1057–68.
33. Nelken NA, Soifer SJ, O'Keefe J, Vu T-KH, Charo IF, Coughlin SR. Thrombin receptor expression in normal and atherosclerotic human arteries. *J Clin Invest* 1992;90:1614–21.
34. Vassalli J-D, Sappino A-P, Belin D. The plasminogen activator/plasmin system. *J Clin Invest* 1991;88:1067–72.
35. Bu G, Warshawsky I, Schwartz AL. Cellular receptors for the plasminogen activators. *Blood* 1994;83:3427–36.
36. Erickson LA, Fici GJ, Lund JE, Boyle TP, Polites HG, Marotti KR. Development of venous occlusions in mice transgenic for the plasminogen activator inhibitor-1 gene. *Nature* 1990;346:74–6.
37. Pintucci G, Iacoviello L, Castelli MP, et al. Cathepsin G-induced release of PAI-1 in the culture medium of endothelial cells: a new thrombogenic role for polymorphonuclear leukocytes? *J Lab Clin Med* 1995;122:69–79.
38. Nawroth PP, Handley DA, Esmon CT, Stern DM. Interleukin 1 induces endothelial cell procoagulant while suppressing cell-surface anticoagulant activity. *Proc Natl Acad Sci USA* 1986;83:3460–4.
39. Moll T, Czyz M, Holzmuller H, et al. Regulation of the tissue factor promoter in endothelial cells. *J Biol Chem* 1995;270:3849–57.
40. van Hinsbergh VWM, Kooistra T, Vanderberg EA, Princer HMG, Fiers W, Emeis JJL. Tumor necrosis factor increases the production of plasminogen activator inhibitor in human endothelial cells in vitro and in rats in vivo. *Blood* 1988;72:1467–73.

41. De Prost D, Kanfer A. Quantitative assessment of procoagulant activity in isolated rat glomeruli. *Kidney Int* 1985;28:566–8.
42. Kanfer A, De Prost D, Guettier C, et al. Enhanced glomerular procoagulant activity and fibrin deposition in rats with mercuric chloride-induced autoimmune nephritis. *Lab Invest* 1987;57:138–43.
43. Angles-Cano E, Rondeau E, Delarue F, Hagege J, Sultan Y, Sraer J-D. Identification and cellular localization of plasminogen activators from human glomeruli. *Thromb Haemost* 1985;54:688–92.
44. Bergstein JM, Riley M, Bang NU. Analysis of the plasminogen activator activity of the human glomerulus. *Kidney Int* 1988;33:868–74.
45. Lacave R, Rondeau E, Ochi S, Delarue F, Schleuning WD, Sraer J-D. Characterization of a plasminogen activator and its inhibitor in human mesangial cells. *Kidney Int* 1989;35:806–11.
46. Villamediana LM, Rondeau E, He C-J, et al. Thrombin regulates components of the fibrinolytic system in human mesangial cells. *Kidney Int* 1990;38:956–61.
47. Meulders Q, He C-J, Adida C, et al. Tumor necrosis factor α increases antifibrinolytic activity of cultured human mesangial cells. *Kidney Int* 1992;42:327–34.
48. Rondeau E, Ochi S, Lacave R, et al. Urokinase synthesis and binding by glomerular epithelial cells in culture. *Kidney Int* 1989;36:593–600.
49. Iwamoto T, Nakashima Y, Sueishi K. Secretion of plasminogen activator and its inhibitor by glomerular epithelial cells. *Kidney Int* 1990; 37:1466–76.
50. Brown PAJ, Wilson HM, Reid FJ, et al. Urokinase-plasminogen activator is synthesized in vitro by human glomerular epithelial cells but not by mesangial cells. *Kidney Int* 1994;45:43–7.
51. Becquemont L, Nguyen G, Peraldi M-N, He C-J, Sraer J-D, Rondeau E. Expression of plasminogen/plasmin receptors on human glomerular epithelial cells. *Am J Physiol* 1994;267:F-303–10.
52. He CJ, Rondeau E, Lacave R, Delarue F, Sraer JD. Thrombin stimulates proliferation and decreases fibrinolytic activity of human glomerular epithelial cells. *J Cell Physiol* 1991;146:131–40.
53. Giroux L, Verroust P, Morel-Maroger L, Delarue F, Delauche M, Sraer JD. Glomerular fibrinolytic activity during nephrotoxic nephritis. *Lab Invest* 1979;40:415–22.
54. Stark H, Miller K, Michael AF. Renal cortical fibrinolytic activity in rabbits with chronic immune complex nephritis. *Isr J Med Sci* 1979; 15:610–20.
55. Hara M, Kihara I, Morita T, Oite T, Yamamoto T. The fibrinolytic activity of isolated rat glomerulus by fibrin slide technique: its application to rat Masugi nephritis. *Acta Pathol Jpn* 1981;31:249–55.
56. Okuda S, Languino LR, Ruoslahti E, Border WA. Elevated expression of transforming growth factor-β and proteoglycan production in experimental glomerulonephritis: possible role in expansion of the mesangial extracellular matrix. *J Clin Invest* 1990;86:453–62.
57. Tamaki K, Okuda S, Ando T, Iwamoto T, Nakayama M, Fujishima M. TGF-β1 in glomerulosclerosis and interstitial fibrosis of adriamycin nephropathy. *Kidney Int* 1994;45:525–36.
58. Yamamoto T, Nakamura T, Noble NA, Ruoslahti E, Border WA. Expression of transforming growth factor β is elevated in human and experimental diabetic nephropathy. *Proc Natl Acad Sci USA* 1993;90: 1814–8.
59. Isaka Y, Fujiwara Y, Ueda N, Kaneda Y, Kamada T, Imai E. Glomerulosclerosis induced by in vivo transfection of transforming growth factor-β or platelet-derived growth factor gene into the rat kidney. *J Clin Invest* 1993;92:2597–601.
60. Sawdey M, Loskutoff DJ. Regulation of murine type 1 plasminogen activator inhibitor gene expression in vivo: tissue specificity and induction by lipopolysaccharide, tumor necrosis factor-α, and transforming growth factor-β. *J Clin Invest* 1991;88:1346–53.
61. Keeton M, Eguchi Y, Sawdey M, Ahn C, Loskutoff DJ. Cellular localization of type 1 plasminogen activator inhibitor mRNA and protein in murine renal tissue. *Am J Pathol* 1993;142:59–70.
62. Tomooka S, Border WA, Marshall BC, Noble NA. Glomerular matrix accumulation is linked to inhibition of the plasmin protease system. *Kidney Int* 1992;42:1462–9.
63. Troyer DA, Chandrasekar B, Thinnes T, Stone A, Loskutoff DJ, Fernandes G. Effects of energy intake on type 1 plasminogen activator inhibitor levels in glomeruli of lupus-prone B/W mice. *Am J Pathol* 1995;146:111–20.
64. Silva FG, Hoyer JR, Pirani CL. Sequential studies of glomerular crescent formation in rats with antiglomerular basement membrane-induced glomerulonephritis and the role of coagulation factors. *Lab Invest* 1984;51:404–15.
65. McCluskey RT, Andres GA. Does t-PA have a role in the treatment of crescentic glomerulonephritis? *Lab Invest* 1990;62:1–4.
66. Thomson NM, Simpson IJ, Peters DK. A quantitative evaluation of anticoagulants in experimental nephrotoxic nephritis. *Clin Exp Immunol* 1975;19:301–8.
67. Border WA, Wilson CB, Dixon FJ. Failure of heparin to affect two types of experimental glomerulonephritis in rabbits. *Kidney Int* 1975; 8:140–8.
68. Bone JM, Valdes AJ, Germuth FG Jr, Lubowitz H. Heparin therapy in anti-basement membrane nephritis. *Kidney Int* 1975;8:72–9.
69. Wu X, Helfrich MH, Horton MA, Feigen LP, Lefkowith JB. Fibrinogen mediates platelet–polymorphonuclear leukocyte cooperation during immune-complex glomerulonephritis in rats. *J Clin Invest* 1994; 94:928–36.
70. Zoja C, Corna D, Macconi D, Zilio P, Bertani T, Remuzzi G. Tissue plasminogen activator therapy of rabbit nephrotoxic nephritis. *Lab Invest* 1990;62:34–40.
71. Rijken DC, Collen D. Purification and characterization of the plasminogen activator secreted by human melanoma cells in culture. *J Biol Chem* 1981;256:7035–41.
72. Pennica D, Holmes WE, Kohr WJ, et al. Cloning and expression of human tissue-type plasminogen activator cDNA in *E. coli*. *Nature* 1983;301:214–21.
73. Collen D. Tissue-type plasminogen activator: therapeutic potential in thrombotic disease states. *Drugs* 1986;31:1–5.
74. Ranby M. Studies on the kinetics of plasminogen activation by tissue plasminogen activator. *Biochim Biophys Acta* 1982;704:461–9.
75. Loscalzo J, Braunwald E. Tissue plasminogen activator. *N Engl J Med* 1988;319:925–31.
76. Arieff AI, Pinggera WF. Rapidly progressive glomerulonephritis treated with anticoagulants. *Arch Intern Med* 1972;129:77–84.
77. Brown CB, Wilson D, Turner D, et al. Combined immunosuppression and anticoagulation in rapidly progressive glomerulonephritis. *Lancet* 1974;2:1166–72.
78. Kincaid-Smith P. The kidney: a clinicopathological study. Oxford: Blackwell, 1975:259.
79. Suc JM, Conte J, Mignon-Conte M, Orfila C, Durant D, Ton That H. Short term heparin trial in idiopathic rapidly progressive glomerulonephritis. *Kidney Int* 1975;8:275(abstr).
80. Pollak VE, Glueck HI, Weiss MA, Lebron-Berges A, Miller MA. Defibrination with ancrod in glomerulonephritis: effects on clinical and histologic findings and on blood coagulation. *Am J Nephrol* 1982;2:195–207.
81. Kim S, Wadhwa NK, Kant KS, et al. Fibrinolysis in glomerulonephritis treated with ancrod: renal functional, immunologic and histopathologic effects. *Q J Med* 1988;69:879–905.
82. Hiromura K, Hayashi J, Tsukada Y, et al. FK506 inhibits renal glomerular thrombosis induced in rats by nephrotoxic serum and lipopolysaccharide. *Kidney Int* 1994;45:1572–9.

B. Cellular Mediators of Immune Injury

Immunologic Renal Diseases,
edited by E. G. Neilson and W. G. Couser.
Lippincott-Raven Publishers, Philadelphia © 1997.

CHAPTER 24

The Role of Chemoattractants in Renal Disease

Theodore M. Danoff and Eric G. Neilson

INTRODUCTION

The migration of leukocytes from the circulation into tissue was first described over a century ago (1). This process of leukocyte movement is integral to immune surveillance, to directing immune response to antigen-challenged tissue, and to the accumulation of leukocytes at sites of injury. Both the stage of the immune response and the type of tissue response determine which of the functionally distinct subsets of leukocytes will comprise the immune cell infiltrate. Which subsets of leukocytes make up the infiltrate is in large part determined by the action of multiple interacting molecules. These molecules include cell surface proteins, which mediate adhesion of the leukocytes to the vasculature in areas of inflammation, and diffusible molecules, which direct the movement of these leukocytes through the parenchyma of the inflamed tissue. This latter group of proteins are chemoattractants.

The directed migration of the leukocytes toward the site of immune injury is a result of chemotaxis. Chemotaxis is defined as the unidirectional movement of cells which follow the soluble gradient of a chemical substance, the chemoattractant. A large, diverse group of molecules, including peptides, proteins, and lipids, have been described to possess chemoattractant activity for leukocytes (2). Recent evidence indicates that the role of chemoattractants is more than just directing the flow of cells through the interstitium; chemoattractants are also involved in the process by which the leukocytes exit the circulation and pass through the endothelium. Finally, distinct from their role in eliciting the inflammatory infiltrate, many chemoattractants activate inflammatory cells to release molecules like proteases, free oxygen radicals, and peptide mediators. This chapter reviews the role that chemoattractants play in the renal inflammatory process. The process of cell adhesion is discussed in more detail in Chapter 25.

Focusing only on leukocyte chemoattractants and their role in the inflammatory process places two constraints on the following discussion. First, many of the chemoattractants that are discussed are also intimately involved in other biologic processes. For instance, the chemoattractant C5a is produced when the complement cascade is activated. Obviously, other components of the complement cascade have important effects on the kidney independent of the chemoattractant ability of C5a. For this reason, it is often hard to dissociate completely the role of the chemoattractant from the other effects produced concurrent with the production of the chemoattractant. Second, in addition to leukocyte chemoattractants, a number of molecules have been described that are chemoattractants for nonlymphoid cells like fibroblasts and mesangial cells (3). From the renal perspective, the best studied of these nonleukocyte chemoattractants is platelet-derived growth factor (PDGF). Although PDGF is a mesangial cell chemoattractant (4), its function as a mitogen (4,5) has been most extensively characterized (reviewed in chapter 20). These molecules are not discussed in this chapter.

The classic way that chemoattractants have been studied is with the Boyden-chamber assay (6). A Boyden chamber is basically two reservoirs separated by a porous membrane. The pores in the membrane are large enough to allow the leukocytes to pass through. The cells to be studied are placed in one of the reservoirs and the presumed chemoattractant in the other. If the chemoattractant is chemotactic to the cells, then the cells will migrate across the porous membrane toward the reservoir containing the chemoattractant and hence up the chemoattractant concentration gradient. Potency of the chemoattractant is assessed based upon the concentration of the agent that caused the cell movement and the number of cells that moved.

At one time, it was postulated that chemotaxis to the chemoattractants expressed at sites of immune injury could

T. M. Danoff and E. G. Neilson: Penn Center for the Molecular Studies of Kidney Diseases, Renal-Electrolyte and Hypertension Division, Department of Medicine, University of Pennsylvania, Philadelphia, Pennsylvania 19104.

explain the formation and composition of inflammatory infiltrates. By this theory, chemoattractants produced at sites of inflammation were solely responsible for drawing in the leukocytes, much like cells migrate across the membrane in the Boyden chamber in response to the chemoattractant. Using this analogy, the reservoir containing the cells is the vascular system, the porous membrane is the endothelium, and the reservoir containing the chemoattractant is the underlying tissue.

There are several problems with this simple theory. One is that this theory does not explain how the chemoattractants maintain their gradient localized to the specific site of inflammation. Unlike in the Boyden chamber, blood is constantly flowing. If diffusible chemoattractants were responsible for the formation of the inflammatory infiltrates, then the chemoattractant's gradient should rapidly be washed away by the blood flow. Another significant shortcoming of this theory is that it does not account for the role that the endothelium plays in the inflammatory response. Unlike the porous membrane in the Boyden chamber, the endothelium plays a significant role in regulating the inflammatory response. Because of these and other problems with this model, other models have been developed. It is now clear that although chemoattractants do not completely control the site and composition of the inflammatory response, they still play a central role.

A model for leukocyte trafficking must satisfy several important criteria in order to explain the numerous observations about the regulation of the inflammatory response. The model must help explain how the infiltrate is directed to the site of inflammation and what determines the cellular composition of the inflammatory infiltrate. A current working model for leukocyte trafficking uses a three-step paradigm (7). Each step involves the interaction of specific classes of molecules. Because each of these classes are composed of multiple distinct molecules, whose functions are analogous but unique, great combinatorial diversity of potential interaction is generated. This diversity is what is presumed to regulate the cellular profile of the inflammatory infiltrate.

The three-step model for the recruitment of leukocytes to sites of inflammation (depicted in Fig. 1) incorporates

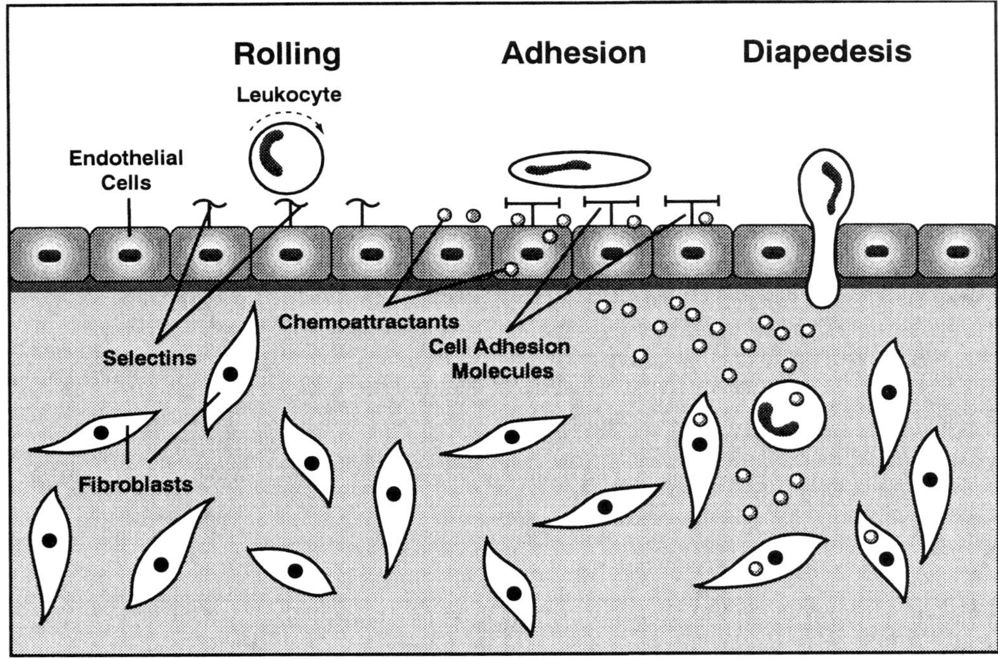

FIG. 1. Schematic of the three-step model for the recruitment of leukocytes to areas of inflammation. In areas of inflammation, the endothelium is stimulated to express selectins. When leukocytes bump into the endothelial cells that express these selectins, they loosely stick to the endothelium as a result of a weak interaction between the selectins on the endothelium and selectin ligands that are constitutively expressed on the leukocytes. This weak interaction is not strong enough to resist the shear force of the blood flow but does keep the leukocyte tethered to the vessel wall; hence, the leukocyte rolls along the endothelial cells. If the leukocyte encounters chemokines, which also adhere to the endothelial wall, then the integrins expressed by the leukocyte become active and can tightly bind to cell adhesion molecules. The expression of these cell adhesion molecules can be induced on endothelial cells by inflammatory cytokines. The interaction of the integrins with the cell adhesion molecules is strong and allows tight adhesion of the leukocyte to the vessel wall. The leukocyte can then move through the vessel wall into the underlying parenchymal tissue. The direction of movement could be directed by chemoattractants released by parenchymal cells.

the important role that cytokines and the endothelium plays in the accumulation of the circulating leukocytes by way of the expression of adhesion molecules, and the important role that the chemoattractants play in initiating the tight adhesion of the leukocytes to the endothelium (7). The formation of the inflammatory infiltrate is initiated when leukocytes flowing through the capillary beds randomly bump up against the capillary walls. In areas of inflammation, the capillary endothelium is activated by inflammatory mediators like thrombin, histamine, tumor necrosis factor (TNF-α) and interleukin 1 (IL-1). These activated endothelial cells express adhesion molecules of the selectin family that include L-selectin and P-selectin (8,9) (for details see chapter 25). When the leukocytes bump up against the activated endothelium, carbohydrate-containing selectin ligands on the leukocyte, such as sialyl-Lewis X, bind to the selectins on the endothelium. These selectin ligands are constitutively expressed by the leukocytes. This interaction between the endothelium's selectins and leukocyte's selectin ligands mediates a loose binding of the leukocytes to the endothelium and enables the leukocyte to roll slowly along the endothelial surface in the direction of flow. This rolling of the leukocyte along the endothelium is ~100 times slower than the rate of blood flow prior to this loose adherence (10). The nature of the inflammatory mediator determines which member of the selectin family gets expressed on the endothelium, and thereby acts as the first step in determining the composition of the inflammatory infiltrate.

Once the selectin-mediated rolling begins, an integrin–integrin-receptor interaction can mediate tight adhesion of the leukocytes to the endothelium. This tight interaction enables the leukocyte to stop rolling and firmly attach to the endothelium. The integrin receptors include the intercellular and vascular cell adhesion molecules (ICAMS, VCAM) as well as fibronectin and iC3b. Like the selectin step, the expression of the integrin receptors on the endothelium is determined in part by inflammatory mediators. In contrast to the constitutive expression of functional selectin ligands by the leukocytes, the integrins expressed on the circulating leukocytes are inactive. In order for the integrins to become activated and initiate the tight interaction between leukocyte and endothelium, the leukocytes must also receive a specific signal. A number of chemoattractants have been shown to deliver this signal (11). In addition to activating the integrins, chemoattractants can also upregulate the number of integrins on the leukocyte cell surface (12).

Once a tight interaction between leukocyte and endothelium has developed, the leukocytes flatten and spread on the endothelium in a process of adhesion strengthening. Tightly bound leukocytes then migrate to intercellular junctions and move between the endothelial cells. Once through the endothelial layer, they enter the extravascular space and migrate to an area of the inflammatory or immune response. The migration through the extravascular space is presumably mediated by a concentration gradient of the chemoattractants.

Although initially it was thought that the only role that chemoattractants played in the formation of the inflammatory infiltrate was in directing movement of the inflammatory cells, it has become clear that chemoattractants serve more than this attractant function. Their initial role in the formation of the inflammatory infiltrate is to act as the signal that converts the inactive integrin to the active integrin, thereby allowing tight adhesion of the rolling leukocyte to the endothelium. Once the leukocytes have stopped rolling, the chemoattractants give direction to their movement. Obviously, the composition of inflammatory infiltrates varies with the nature of the injury and the time after injury. Diversity in the activity of the chemoattractants helps explain this spectrum of inflammatory response. Table 1 lists the major chemoattractants that are thought to be involved in the renal inflammatory process. The "classic" chemoattractants are the complement split product C5a, the chemokines, platelet-activating factor and leukotriene B_4. In addition, among its many biologic activities, transforming growth factor β is a leukocyte chemoattractant, although the physiologic significance of this biologic activity is unknown.

The molecular machinery by which eukaryotic cells respond to a chemoattractant is only now starting to be unraveled (13). As the initial step in monitoring their environment, inflammatory cells detect the presence of chemoattractants through specific cell surface receptors. For the classic chemoattractants, these receptors are composed of seven-transmembrane-spanning domains with an extracellular amino terminus and an intracellular carboxy terminus. These receptors belong to a large superfamily of receptors that detect/transduce signals from a wide range of external stimuli, including neurotransmitters, cytokines, and sensory stimuli such as photons or odorants. The prototypic member of this family is the rhodopsin receptor. Within the seven-transmembrane-spanning receptor superfamily (STRs), five consensus features identify the chemoattractant receptors as a distinct family (11) (Fig. 2). (a) Their sequences are similar in length, ~350 amino acids. They are among the smallest members of the STRs, primarily due to an average-length amino-terminal segment, a very short third intracellular loop, and a relatively short carboxy-terminal segment. (b)

TABLE 1. *Major chemoattractants thought to be involved in the renal inflammatory process*

Proteins
Complement C5a
Chemokines
Osteopontin
Transforming growth factor β_1
Lipids
Leukotrienes
Platelet-activating factor

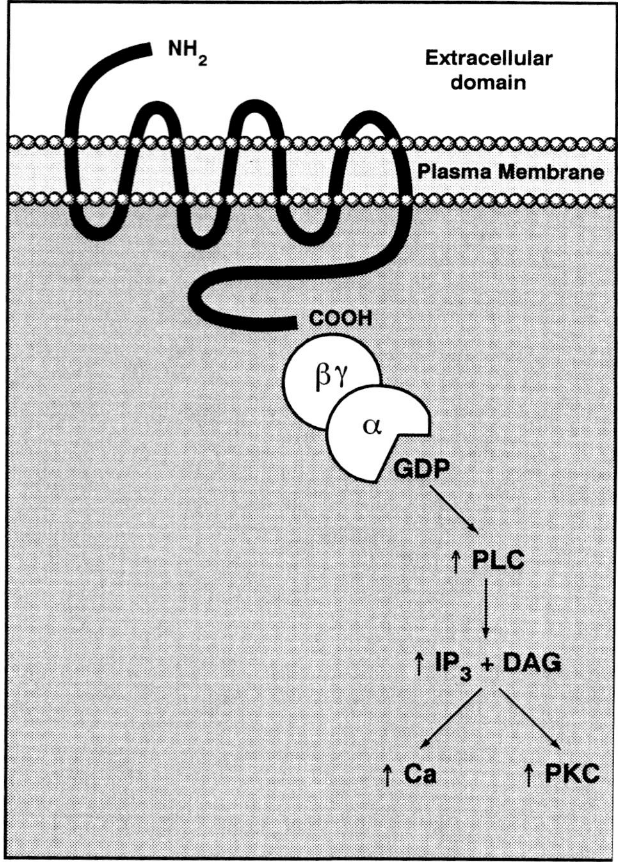

FIG. 2. Schematic diagram of a typical classic chemoattractant receptor and its signaling cascade. The receptor contains seven-transmembrane-spanning segments. When a ligand binds to the receptor, a G protein is activated, which results in the dissociation of the a subunit from the βγ subunits. These activated subunits in turn activate phospholipase C (*PLC*). This activation, in turn, induces the production of two secondary messengers, inositol (1,4,5)-triphosphate (*IP_3*) and diacylglycerol (*DAG*). The IP_3 mobilizes intracellular calcium, while DAG activates protein kinase C (*PKC*). PKC activation and increased intracellular calcium induce cellular responses.

They have >20% amino acid identity overall to each other (>28% excluding the platelet-activating factor receptor). (c) The short third intracellular loop is enriched in basic amino acids and in most cases can be modeled to form a cationic amphipathic α-helix, a motif nested within the much longer corresponding loop of many other members of the STRs. (d) The amino-terminal segments are in most cases unusually acidic (11). (e) Their RNAs are expressed in leukocytes.

These classic chemoattractant receptors share a common intracellular signaling system: namely, they couple to cytosolic G proteins through their carboxy-terminal cytosolic domains (11,14). These G proteins are composed of three subunits, α, β, and γ, of which the α subunit binds guanosine diphosphate in the basal state. However when the specific ligand binds to its cognate receptor, the receptor undergoes a conformational change that induces an exchange of guanosine triphosphate for the guanosine diphosphate. This results in the dissociation of α from βγ subunits. In turn, βγ activates a phosphoinositide-specific phospholipase C, leading to the accumulation of inositol triphosphate and diacylglycerol in the cytoplasm. These products induce mobilization of calcium and activation of protein kinase C, respectively, and they may be involved in the delayed activation of phospholipase D. Early phospholipase-C-mediated and late phospholipase-D-mediated biochemical events have been temporally correlated with the highly sensitive migratory response of phagocytes to chemoattractants (11).

The ability of a cell to identify the directionality of the chemoattractant gradient depends on the difference in the fraction of occupied receptors at the ends of the cell. The cell's accuracy in following the gradient is maximal when the gradient is steep and when the midpoint of the gradient is near the dissociation constant of the chemoattractant for its cell surface receptor. Cells are exquisitely sensitive to chemoattractants with a 10-mm cell able to detect a concentration gradient of ~1% across its length, which corresponds to a difference of only 250 occupied chemoattractant receptors between its ends (13). The cells sense relative rather than absolute levels of chemoattractants, thereby allowing them to move up (toward) areas of increasing concentration. The extension of pseudopodia allows the cell to test the gradient of chemoattractant continuously across the cell diameter in order to identify accurately the direction of increasing chemoattractant concentration. By sensing differences in concentration of the chemoattractant across its diameter and continuously probing out into its environment, motile cells are able to track toward sites of chemoattractant production.

The following sections discuss the major leukocyte chemoattractants that have been studied in the kidney. Most of the functional studies have been performed using animal models; therefore, strict application to human disease is inferential.

C5a

The complement system is a cascade of proteins whose interactions generate a number of biologically relevant products. The cascade is composed of at least 13 effector proteins and at least eight regulatory proteins. A number of products generated by the complement cascade mediate the inflammatory process, including the chemoattractant C5a. It should be noted that only one aspect of the complement system's role in renal pathology is through chemotaxis. For a comprehensive discussion of the role of complement in renal injury, see chapter 18.

Progression down the complement cascade typically involves the proteolytic cleavage of complement components. The result of this proteolytic cleavage is the activation of the complement component. The activated complement components function either independently or through their aggregation with other complement components. In several cases, the proteolytic cleavage yields two fragments, both of which have biologic significance. This is the case for the generation of the complement chemoattractant product C5a. When the fifth component of complement (C5) is cleaved, it generates two fragments: C5a and C5b. C5b is involved with the activation of downstream complement components, while C5a is a potent chemoattractant for neutrophils and monocytes (15–17). This cascade of interacting proteins is depicted in Fig. 3.

The complement cascade can be activated through either the classical or the alternative pathway. The classical pathway is involved in several forms of complement-mediated renal injury such as antiglomerular basement membrane (anti-GBM) disease. The classical pathway is activated when immunoglobulin M (IgM) or IgG (subclasses 1, 2, and 3) class antibodies complex with antigen. The binding of the antibody to its specific antigen induces a conformational change in the Fc region of the antibody. This conformational change allows the sequential binding and proteolytic activation of C1, C4, and C2, leading to the formation of the classic pathway C3 convertase (C4b2a). The alternative pathway also forms a C3 convertase composed of fragments of C3 and factor B (C3bBb). The alternative pathway is activated by basement membrane fragments or bacterial wall components. Some renal diseases, like anti-GBM disease, activate complement through the classical complement pathway while others, like membranoproliferative glomerulonephritis type-II or post-streptococcal glomerulonephritis, activate complement through the alternative pathway. The activity of these two independent pathways converges upon the third component of complement (C3) by their respective formation of a C3 convertase.

When plasma C3 interacts with the C3 convertase, it is cleaved to generate two fragments: C3a and C3b. C3a is a small diffusible peptide that can induce the release of agents such as histamine from basophils and mast cells. These mediators produce biologic effects such as increased vascular permeability, increased expression of adhesion molecules, and contraction of smooth muscle. These effects, although not chemotactic as defined by Boyden-chamber analysis, are obviously important in the formation of inflammatory infiltrates at sites of complement activation by their altering of the circulating leukocytes' adhesion to the endothelium. In terms of chemotaxis, the C3b molecule is more important because it serves as the first step in the activation of the terminal complement complex. Some of the C3b that is generated by the C3 convertase becomes covalently bound to cell membrane via a thioester bond. This membrane-bound C3b can associate with either the classical or alternative C3 convertase to generate a C5 convertase.

The C5 convertase initiates the activation of the terminal components of the complement system. The process begins with the proteolytic cleavage of C5 to generate C5a and C5b. C5b binds to the C5 convertase and anchors the formation of the membrane-attack complex, which is composed of C6, C7, C8, and C9. C5a is a soluble 11-kD amino-terminal fragment of C5. In terms of

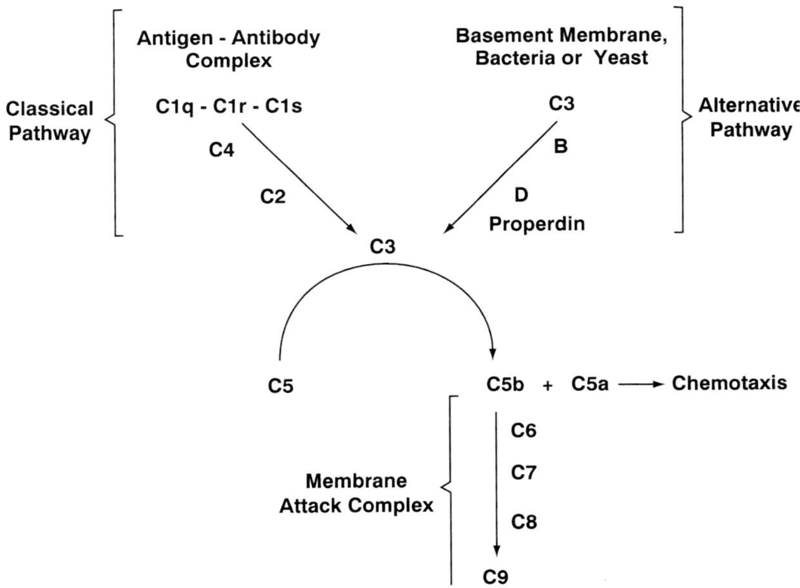

FIG. 3. The classical, alternative and terminal pathways of complement activation. The chemoattractant C5a is generated from the cleavage of C5 by C3.

chemotaxis, C5a is one of the most potent neutrophil and monocyte chemoattractants as yet described and, like C3a, induces increased vascular permeability, increased expression of adhesion molecules, and contraction of smooth muscle (18). All of these biologic activities contribute to C5a's potent effects on the formation of inflammatory infiltrates.

The C5a receptor is a seven-transmembrane-segment receptor that is homologous to the other "classic" chemoattractant receptors. The cloning and sequencing of the receptor (19) have revealed that, among the seven-transmembrane-segment receptors, it is most homologous to the formyl-methionine bacterial chemotactic receptors. It binds C5a with a 1 nM Kd. The extracellular amino-terminal segment is acidic and contains seven negatively charged residues. Because C5a is cationic with multiple arginine and lysine residues in the proposed "recognition domain," the amino terminus of the C5a receptor has been proposed as a potential ligand binding site (19). However, both experiments in which the receptor was mutagenized and experiments in which peptides corresponding to the amino-terminal sequence were used to compete for binding to C5a indicate that the C5a recognition domain of the receptor also includes the third extracellular loop (18).

As can be appreciated even from this brief description of the complement cascade, a large number of biologically active molecules are generated during the activation of the complement system. Although complement can have a profound effect on renal function in the absence of inflammatory cells, the complement cascade is also intimately involved in the formation of inflammatory renal lesions. A number of the molecules generated by the complement cascade are important in the formation of inflammatory infiltrates either by directly or indirectly inducing the production of other chemoattractants or adhesion promoting molecules (20,21), but only C5a is directly chemotactic. Because of the numerous overlapping functions, it is sometimes difficult to be certain which are the direct effects of complement and which are the secondary effects in the formation of the inflammatory infiltrates. Nonetheless, based on complement depletion studies, complement-mediated chemotaxis has been shown to be important in at least one form of immune-mediated renal injury: the heterologous phase of nephrotoxic serum nephritis (NSN) (22).

In NSN, antiserum against glomerular antigen preparations is raised in one species, such as rabbit. This antiserum is then injected into a heterologous species, such as rat. The heterologous antibody rapidly binds to the glomerular basement membrane (GBM) in a linear pattern, with much of it bound in the first pass through the kidney (23,24). Glomerular injury is proportional to the amount of antibody deposited, which is related to both the avidity (25) and charge of the antibody (26). Complement activation, as judged by C3 deposition, occurs essentially immediately after the antibody binding to the GBM (24). Within 15–30 min, glomeruli show a cellular infiltrate that is composed of neutrophils and monocytes (27,28). The neutrophilic infiltrate resolves in <12 h (22), although the mononuclear infiltrate persists. If prior to injection of the nephrotoxic serum, complement is depleted using heat-aggregated human immunoglobulin, then the neutrophilic glomerular infiltrate is abolished (22). This indicates that complement-mediated chemotaxis is important in the formation of this inflammatory infiltrate. This is in contrast to other models of glomerular injury such as passive in situ immune-complex glomerulonephritis (29) in which complement depletion does not abolish the neutrophilic infiltrates.

The characteristics of the heterologous phase of NSN, where complement-mediated chemotaxis is felt to be important, which differentiate it from other renal disease models in which complement-mediated chemotaxis does not seem to be involved is the presence of neutrophils in the infiltrates and the site of the complement activation. The prominence of neutrophils in the infiltrate is intuitively obvious because C5a is one of the most potent neutrophil chemoattractants; therefore, if complement-mediated chemotaxis is involved, neutrophils should be present. NSN has an exuberant neutrophilic infiltrate in the glomerulus, which is greatly reduced by complement depletion (22,30) or if the nephrotoxic serum does not fix complement (22,31). Of course, the formation of neutrophilic infiltrates in the glomerulus is not always C5a dependent, such as in the case of in situ immune-complex formation (29).

The location of the complement activation is the other key feature that determines whether C5a's chemotactic activities will be important in the evolution of the inflammatory response. In glomerulonephritis, if complement activation is in or near the glomerular capillary lumen (as in NSN), then complement-mediated chemotaxis plays a role in the accumulation of neutrophils (32,33). If the complement activation is primarily in the subepithelial space (as in Heymann nephritis or passive immune-complex deposition), then it tends not to induce a complement-mediated chemotactic response. This may be related to the accessibility of the C5a to the circulating neutrophils. In subendothelial or mesangial activation of complement, the C5a is directly accessible to circulating cells and results in their accumulation, whereas C5a production at a subepithelial site is separated from the circulating neutrophils by the overlying GBM and therefore can not attract them (32). However, the distinction between the complement activation occurring in the glomerular subepithelial space versus the capillary lumen/mesangial space appears not to be absolute. Complement has been shown to mediate the localization of monocytes to the kidney in Heymann nephritis, even though the immune complex forms in the subepithelial space (34).

Complement activation and complement-mediated chemotaxis also play an important role in hyperacute rejections of transplants. In nonrodent models of transplant rejection, the classical complement pathway is activated by the binding of circulating natural anti-xenoantibodies to the endothelium of the transplanted organ (35). These naturally occurring antibodies react with multiple antigens on the endothelium of the transplanted organ. The acute rejection is characterized by rapid infiltration of peritubular capillaries by neutrophils, interstitial edema and hemorrhage, and vascular thrombi. Immunohistochemistry reveals the deposition of complement along the endothelial aspect of the vasculature. There is also depletion of circulating complement components. In animal models, this rapid inflammatory response can be abrogated by interventions that inhibit this early activation of complement. Experimental interventions such as depletion of the circulating anti-xenoantibodies or complement depletion (36) have been shown to prolong xenograft survival. In an attempt to make xenotransplants more immunologically compatible, transgenic pigs have been developed that express human complement regulatory proteins on their endothelial cell surfaces. By modulating the complement activation in these xenotransplants, kidneys from these animals do not experience hyperacute rejection when transplanted into primates (37,38).

CHEMOKINE FAMILY OF CHEMOATTRACTANTS

The chemokines are a superfamily of molecules that are both chemoattractants and cytokines; hence, the derivation of the name *chemo-kine* (39). The superfamily is composed of over a dozen members that are all small, secreted proteins that mediate inflammation by inducing chemotaxis and/or activation of a variety of inflammatory cells, including neutrophils, monocytes, eosinophils, and $CD4^+$ as well as $CD8^+$ T cells. Chemokines are synthesized and secreted both by resident renal cells, such as mesangial cells, endothelial cells, and tubular cells, as well as by cell populations that can migrate into the renal parenchyma, such as monocytes/macrophages and T cells. A number of mediators released either by injured renal cells or infiltrating inflammatory cells, such as TNF-α, IL-1, interferon-γ (IFN-γ), and free oxygen radicals, stimulate the production of the chemokines. This diverse superfamily of molecules is involved both in the initial inflammatory response to acute renal injury as well as in the chronic inflammatory response, which is equally important in the progression of renal dysfunction.

Members of the chemokine superfamily have molecular weights in the 6- to 25-kD range, demonstrate 20–45% homology on the amino acid level, are basic heparin-binding proteins, and have a conserved arrangement of cysteines in their sequence. The superfamily is tripartite, with the branches being classified according to the conserved motif of cysteines. The *C-X-C* branch, which includes such molecules as IL-8, platelet factor 4 (PF4), macrophage inflammatory protein 2 (MIP-2), and interferon-inducible protein 10 (γIP-10), is characterized by the separation of the first two of their four cysteines in the primary structure by an intervening amino acid. The C-X-C chemokines can be further divided into ELR containing or lacking proteins. The ELR motif represents the three amino acids Glu-Leu-Arg that immediately precede the first cysteine amino acid residue of the proteins. In the *C-C* branch, which includes RANTES (Regulated upon Activation Normal T cell Expressed presumed Secreted), MIP-1α, MIP-1β, and monocyte chemotactic protein 1 (MCP-1), these first two cysteines are directly adjacent. Recently, a third branch of the chemokine superfamily has been identified that contains only a single cysteine pair (40). This branch has been provisionally designated the *C* branch and contains only one member: lymphotactin. In addition to these physical characteristics that imply an evolutionary relation, each branch of the chemokine family has mapped to the same chromosomal location with the C-X-C clustered on human chromosome 4q12-21 (41), the C-C clustered on chromosome 17q11-21 (42), and the C chemokine on chromosome 1 (40).

The role that the chemokines play in both the acute and chronic inflammatory responses in the kidney stems both from their chemotactic specificity and from their sites of production (43). As a general rule, the specificity of the chemotactic activity of the chemokines can divided along the branches of the chemokine family. Although not exclusive or absolute, the ELR containing C-X-C chemokines, like IL-8 and MIP-2, are potent chemoattractants for neutrophils, while the ELR-negative C-X-C chemokines, like PF4 and IP-10, are only weak chemoattractants for neutrophils. This ELR motif is important in receptor–ligand interactions on neutrophils, and the insertion of the ELR motif into the amino terminus of PF4 converts it to a potent neutrophil activator and attractant that binds to the IL-8 receptor (44). The C-C chemokines are chemoattractants for mononuclear cells, especially monocytes and T cells, and the C chemokine appears to be T cell specific. Table 2 lists the major chemokines that have been identified and their in vitro chemotactic activities. As can be seen from the table, there is a great deal of overlap in the in vitro chemotactic specificity of the various members of the family.

Based on the highly redundant chemotactic activities of the chemokines listed in Table 2, one might postulate that wherever chemokines are expressed the inflammatory infiltrates would be composed of essentially every type of inflammatory cell. In fact, this is not the case. For instance, IL-8 is a very potent neutrophil chemoattractant that can be detected in both proximal and distal epithelial cells in renal biopsy specimens from patients with acute allograft rejection (45). However, neutrophils are not a

TABLE 2. *Major chemokines and their in vitro chemotactic activities*

Name	Target cells in vitro	Site of production in kidney	Stimuli for production
C-X-C chemokines			
IL-8	Neutrophils T cells Monocytes Basophils NK cells	Mesangial cells Renal tubular cells Fibroblasts	TNF-α IL-1 LPS
MIP-2/MGSA	Neutrophils	Mesangial cells	IFN-γ TNF Immune complexes
γIP-10	T cells NK cells	Mesangial cells Glomerular epithelial cells Fibroblasts	IFN-γ
Platelet factor 4	Neutrophils	Platelets	Factors that activate platelets
C-C chemokines			
RANTES	T cells (CD4 > CD8) Monocytes Eosinophils NK cells	Mesangial cells Proximal tubular cells Fibroblasts Platelets Macrophages	TNF-α IL-1 IFN-γ
MIP-1α	T cells (CD8+) Monocytes B cells NK cells	NA	NA
MIP-1β	T cells (CD4+) Monocytes NK cells	NA	NA
MCP-1	Monocytes	Mesangial cells Fibroblasts	TNF-α IL-1 Superoxide Immune complexes

IFN, interferon; IL, interleukin; IP, interferon-inducible protein; LPS, lipopolysaccharide; MCP, monocyte chemotactic protein; MGSA, melanoma growth-stimulating activity; MIP, macrophage inflammatory protein; NA, not available; NK, natural killer; TNF, tumor necrosis factor.

prominent component of acute allograft rejection (46). This disparity between the in vitro chemotactic activity of a chemokine and the composition of the in vivo infiltrate probably stems from two major factors. First, it reflects the complex interactions involved in the formation of inflammatory infiltrates. The composition of the infiltrates represents not only the chemotactic specificity of the chemokine but also the activation state of the endothelium and possibly also the activation state of circulating inflammatory cells. Each of these interactions also poses a challenge in determining the role of the chemokines in specific inflammatory responses. Second, the in vitro chemotactic assays may overrepresent the sensitivity of a cell to a chemoattractant.

The regulation of production of a large number of the chemokines has been investigated and shows certain themes in their mode of regulation. Many of the chemokines are early-response genes, whose rates of synthesis are regulated based on the level of their messenger RNA. The transcript levels of many of the chemokines can be superinduced in the presence of cycloheximide, indicating that their induction occurs in the absence of new protein synthesis and may be under the control of labile repressor proteins. Due to the clustering of the C-C and C-X-C branches of the chemokines on the their respective chromosomes, it has been suggested that there may be regulation at both the individual as well as the regional levels. Regulation of clusters of related genes is well described for other gene families, including β-globin (47) and chicken lysozyme (48).

The regulation of production of the chemokines appears to be predominantly regulated at the level of messenger RNA, with increases in message reflected as an increase in protein production and release. The regulation of a number of the chemokines, including IL-8 (45,49–52), γIP-10 (53–55), MCP-1 (56–63), and RANTES (64,65), by renal cells has been studied in some detail. The message level of each of these genes is regulated at the transcriptional level, and several of them are also regulated at the message-stability level. Upregulation of their messages is induced by free oxygen radicals (60) and by immune complexes (60) and inflammatory cytokines like TNF-α, IFN-γ, and IL-1 (49,50,52,54,56–62,64,65).

An understanding of the transcriptional regulation of these genes has in part been achieved by cloning and sequencing the genes and their 5′ flanking regions. The 5′ flanking region of a gene often contains the transcriptional regulatory elements for the gene. Sequence analysis of the chemokine's 5′ flanking regions reveals a number of transcription factor binding motifs. These motifs are 6–10 base-pair segments of DNA that are recognized by specific transcription factors. When the appropriate transcription factor engages the motif, RNA transcription is upregulated, which leads to elevated levels of message. Among the motifs found in each of the chemokine's 5′ flanking regions studied to date is the DNA sequence to which the transcription factor nuclear factor kappa b (NF-κb) (66) binds. This DNA motif and its cognate transcription factor mediate the transcriptional upregulation of many genes whose message is induced by inflammatory cytokines or cellular stress. At the basal state, NF-κb is maintained in the cytoplasm in an inactive state bound to a labile repressor molecule, I-κB (67). When NF-κb is activated (for example, in response to TNF-α, cellular stress, or reactive oxygen intermediates), I-κB becomes phosphorylated and undergoes proteolysis, thereby releasing the NF-κb. The free NF-κb migrates into the nucleus and upregulates the transcription of those genes with NF-kb motifs in their transcriptional regulatory regions (67). The important role that the NF-κb site plays in the transcriptional regulation of a number of the chemokines, including IL-8 (68), RANTES (69), and MCP-1 (70), has been confirmed by such molecular biologic techniques as gel shift analysis and reporter gene constructs. In addition to TNF-α, Northern blot analysis indicates that IFN-γ plays an important role in the regulation of a number of the chemokines. Message levels of some of the chemokines, such as IP-10, are directly control by IFN-γ while, for others, IFN-γ is synergistic with TNF-α or IL-1 in upregulating the chemokine message level. Consistent with this observation is the presence of the interferon-stimulus response element (ISRE) in the 5′ flanking region of many of the chemokine genes. Unique transcription factors, including interferon-stimulated gene factor (71) and interferon-regulated factors 1 and 2 (72,73), engage ISRE sites and induce or facilitate transcription of the downstream genes.

In addition to regulation of the message level of the chemokine genes at a transcriptional level, many chemokine genes also have a post-transcriptional level of regulation. Several of the chemokines mRNAs, including those of IL-8 and MIP-2 (74,75), contain AUUUA-rich sequences in their 3′ untranslated regions. This sequence has been associated with instability of mRNA (76) and may account for the rapid disappearance of these chemokines' message after the initial induction.

It would seem that essentially every cell population in the kidney is capable of synthesizing any of the chemokines. The resident renal cell populations that have been studied most extensively as to their ability to produce chemokines are the mesangial cells and fibroblasts. Both populations express a message for essentially every one of the chemokines studied to date when the cells are appropriately stimulated. Table 2 provides a more detailed list of which renal cell populations have been shown to produce chemokines and which stimuli upregulate their production. In addition to the resident renal cell populations, infiltrating cells such as monocytes and T cells produce chemokines when appropriately stimulated. Platelets are also a rich source of the chemokines RANTES and PF4. These chemokines are stored preformed in the platelet's granules and are released when the platelets degranulate.

The molecular mechanism by which the chemokines induce chemotaxis is starting to be elucidated. As described in the introductory section, the chemokine receptors are all seven-transmembrane-spanning receptors and belong to a superfamily of seven-transmembrane-spanning receptors. The cloning and characterization of the receptors for the chemokines are still incomplete. To date, five receptors have been cloned, but, based on Scatchard analysis and functional data, there are probably more that have not been characterized. Consistent with the overlap in chemoattractant specificity among the chemokine subfamilies, more than one chemokine can bind to each receptor. For instance, for the C-X-C chemokines, two high-affinity IL-8 receptors have been cloned (77) that are 77% identical at the amino acid level. In addition to each of these receptors binding IL-8 with a dissociation constant (K_d) of 1 nM, one also binds GROα with a comparable K_d. Either IL-8 or GROα can desensitize calcium transients elicited by the other chemokine (11). In addition to the two C-X-C chemokine receptors, there are at least five C-C chemokine receptors that have partially overlapping specificity.

The intracellular signaling pathway for the IL-8 receptor has been best characterized. When IL-8 engages its receptor, there is a rapid rise in intracellular calcium that presumably serves as the intracellular secondary messenger. This calcium flux initiates at least two distinct steps in the recruitment of leukocytes to sites of inflammation. First, it induces the adherence of neutrophils to both endothelial cells and subendothelial matrix (78), which provides a mechanism by which neutrophils can begin accumulating along the endothelium in areas overlying sites of inflammation. This enhanced adhesion is mediated through the activation of integrins on the neutrophil. Second, by acting as a chemotactic factor, IL-8 can induce the migration of the neutrophils from the endothelium into the area of inflammation. In addition, once the neutrophils have accumulated in the area of inflammation, IL-8 can activate the neutrophils to release various molecules, including gelatinases and free oxygen radicals (79), that have been implicated in the tissue injury associated with the inflammatory process. This latter step, although not related to chemotaxis, indicates that the chemokines can mediate tissue injury by means other than attracting inflammatory cells.

In addition to the functional chemokine receptors that engage a limited spectrum of chemokines, a promiscuous chemokine receptor also engages essentially all chemokines yet does not initiate an intracellular signal when it engages its ligand (80,81). This receptor is the protein that is recognized by the antibody that defines the Duffy blood-group antigen and hence has been termed the *Duffy antigen–erythrocyte chemokine receptor* (DFA-ECKR). Although DFA-ECKR was first found on red blood cells, its has subsequently been shown to be expressed on endothelium activated by inflammatory mediators, including the postcapillary venules in the kidney (82). Its recent cloning reveals that it is also a seven-transmembrane-spanning protein that is homologous to the classic chemokine receptors and the C5a receptor (83).

Although the DFA-ECKR can not function as a chemotactic receptor because of its inability to mediate a calcium flux, it probably serves an important ancillary function in the chemotactic process. As can be appreciated from the model for leukocyte migration (Fig. 1), the chemokines that trigger the activation of the integrins thereby initiating the tight binding of the leukocytes to the endothelium must be lining the endothelium in order to allow contact with the leukocytes as they go rolling along. Since the chemokines are heparin-binding proteins, they could bind to the proteoglycans expressed on endothelial cells. In fact, it has been shown that when IL-8 binds to heparin sulfate the chemotactic activity of the IL-8 is enhanced several fold (84). In addition, the DFA-ECKR that is expressed on postcapillary venules could present the chemokines to the rolling leukocytes. Binding sites for RANTES along the endothelium have been shown to be present in renal allografts undergoing cellular rejection (85), although it is not certain whether these binding sites were proteoglycans, DFA-ECKR, or other uncharacterized chemokine-binding sites.

Maybe as important to the control of the inflammatory process as presenting chemokines on the endothelium overlying areas of inflammation is the removal of those chemokines. Removal of the chemokines is theoretically important as a negative feedback step in the inflammatory process as well as for the maintenance of effective chemokine gradients. As a part of the negative feedback system for inflammation, removal of chemokines from the endothelium should block further inflammatory cell accumulation. DFA-ECKR on the circulating red blood cells could act as a sponge to wipe the chemokines from the endothelium. Chemokines share receptors, and the nature of the receptor that the chemokines use is that, once stimulated, the receptor goes through a period of unresponsiveness. Therefore, if excess chemokines started entering the circulation by diffusing out from areas of active inflammation, this could inactivate the chemokine receptors on the inflammatory cells in the circulation. These circulating inflammatory cells would then be unable to respond to appropriate endothelial-bound inflammatory stimuli. DFA-ECKR on red blood cells can act to remove these free, circulating chemokines and in so doing protect circulating inflammatory cells from inappropriate chemokine desensitization.

The exact role of the chemokines in the renal inflammatory response is just starting to be defined. A number of animal models of immune-mediated renal injury indicate that chemokines are involved in the cellular immune response in the glomerulus. The chemokines may also play an important role in the interstitial inflammatory response both in primary interstitial nephritis or following glomerular injury.

In the glomerular inflammatory response, the induction of chemokine synthesis by glomerular cells could be a direct effect of the perturbation of the glomerular cells or may be a response to mediators released by the injured glomeruli. TNF-α and IL-1 can both induce chemokine expression, the production of both of these inflammatory mediators is upregulated in the glomerulus during glomerulonephritis (86–88), exogenous addition of these cytokines increases the glomerular neutrophil infiltrate during experimental glomerulonephritis (89), and blockade of IL-1 function can ameliorate the inflammatory infiltrate (90). Obviously, these cytokines have a multitude of effects on the immune response other than chemokine production, but in the absence of experimental evidence it is tempting to speculate that the modulation of chemokine production may alter the course of glomerular injury.

The role of IL-8 has been examined in both human glomerular disease and experimental acute immune-complex-induced glomerulonephritis. Wada et al. (91) found that urinary levels of IL-8 were elevated in several glomerular diseases, including IgA nephropathy, acute glomerulonephritis, lupus nephritis, purpura nephritis, membranoproliferative glomerulonephritis, and cryoglobulinemia, compared with the IL-8 levels in healthy controls (see Fig. 4). Among the patients with glomerular disease, the urinary IL-8 levels were higher in patients with glomerular leukocyte infiltration than in those without infiltration. For instance, in the patients with IgA nephropathy, the urinary IL-8 levels in patients with acute exacerbation were 203 ± 117 pg/mL • Cr compared with 15 ± 12 pg/mL • Cr in those without acute exacerbation or onset. These elevated urinary IL-8 levels seen during the acute phase or exacerbation of the glomerular disease were found to decrease during spontaneous remission or steroid pulse-therapy-induced convalescence in all patients examined. To identify the source of the urinary IL-8, immunohistochemical examination of biopsy specimens from the patients was performed using an anti-IL-8 monoclonal antibody. In patients without elevated urinary IL-8 levels, no IL-8 was detectable by immunohistochemistry, but in patients with elevated urinary IL-8, IL-8-positive cells were present in glomerular capillaries. The cellular source of the IL-8 could be mesangial cells that secrete IL-8 when stimulated (49,50,52,62), or the IL-8 may be produced by glomerular macrophages (92).

Production of a chemokine during an inflammatory response is supportive evidence that the chemokine is

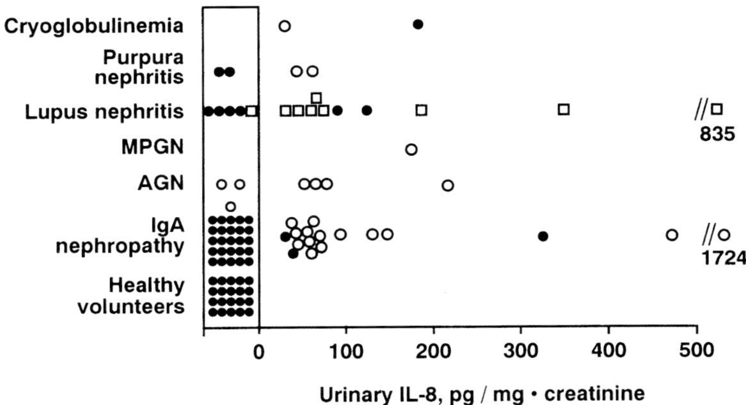

FIG. 4. Urinary interleukin-8 levels in patients with various renal diseases. The *open symbols* indicate patients with acute exacerbation or onset, whereas the *closed symbols* indicate patients without acute exacerbation or onset. For lupus nephritis patients, the *open symbol* indicates patients with an activity index of ≥6. Modified from Wada et al. (91)

involved in the inflammatory process. To satisfy Koch's postulate, however, it is necessary to show that the removal of the chemokine abrogates the inflammatory response. Such work has been done with two animal models of acute glomerulonephritis. The acute phase of glomerulonephritis is characterized by glomerular infiltration with inflammatory cells, particularly neutrophils. The roles of two of the chemokines that are potent neutrophil chemoattractants have been investigated. These two chemokines are IL-8 and MIP-2. In each case, neutralizing antibodies against the chemokines were developed and then injected into experimental animals at the time of induction of the glomerulonephritis. Wada et al. (93) examined the role of IL-8 in a rabbit model of glomerulonephritis induced by the repeated injection of bovine serum albumin into rabbits, causing the deposition of immune complexes consisting of bovine serum albumin and rabbit IgG in glomeruli. Their histologic analysis revealed a small but significant number of neutrophils in the glomeruli from rabbits in which glomerulonephritis was induced (62.7 ± 7.6 neutrophils/50 glomeruli, which was significantly greater than neutrophils in glomeruli from the control rabbits, $p < 0.01$). Treatment with anti-IL-8 reduced the number of neutrophils per glomeruli by >40% (with treatment, 37.7 ± 3.7 neutrophils/50 glomeruli, $p < 0.05$ versus untreated). Although IL-8 is also a monocyte chemoattractant, there was no effect on the mononuclear cell infiltrate with anti-IL-8 treatment. Aside from the histologic changes, there was a statistically significant decrease in urinary levels of protein. These experiments indicate that in this animal model of glomerulonephritis IL-8 participates in the recruitment of neutrophils to the glomerulus and in the impairment of renal function. IL-8's role in the renal function impairment could be due to the recruitment of the neutrophils as well as the activation of the neutrophils (79). The incomplete blockade of the neutrophil infiltrate in the glomerulus by the anti-IL-8 is not surprising given the functional overlap of other chemokines and non-chemokine chemoattractants.

Feng et al. (94) examined the effect of blocking MIP-2 in the accumulation of neutrophils in the glomerulus of rats with NSN. In this model, MIP-2 message was upregulated within 30 min of treatment with anti-GBM antibody, and MIP-2 protein was detectable within 4 h, with both disappearing by 24 h. This expression correlates with the glomerular neutrophil influx. Similar to Wada et al. (93), pretreatment with a neutralizing anti-MIP-2 antibody decreased the number of glomerular neutrophils by 40% at 4 h (glomerulonephritis, 608 ± 26 neutrophils/35 glomeruli; versus glomerulonephritis + anti-MIP-2, 362 ± 6 neutrophils/35 glomeruli, $p < 0.01$) and reduced proteinuria. Presumably, some of the residual neutrophil infiltrate seen in the rats treated with the anti-MIP-2 antibody was due to complement activation and the action of other chemokines. These experiments show that in two separate models of acute glomerulonephritis, characterized by early neutrophil infiltrates, blocking potent neutrophil chemotactic chemokines reduces the neutrophil infiltrate and ameliorates renal injury. Although the long-term use of neutralizing antibodies is not currently practical for human therapy, other chemokine blockers may offer therapeutic efficacy in glomerulonephritis.

Monocytes also play an important role in glomerulonephritis, especially in those forms of glomerulonephritis that do not have significant neutrophilic infiltrates (95). The role of MCP-1 in the recruitment of monocytes to the glomerulus has been examined in both human material and animal models. Renal biopsy specimens from patients with idiopathic crescentic or proliferative glomerulonephritis, Wegener granulomatosis, and systemic lupus erythematosus were found to be positive for MCP-1 by immunohistochemistry (96). When Rovin et al. (96) examined the expression of MCP-1 in a rat model of anti-GBM nephritis, they found that glomerular expression of MCP-1 mRNA and immunoreactive protein was transiently upregulated during the early stages of the glomerulonephritis. The appearance of MCP-1 preceded the influx of monocytes into the glomerulus. The source of the MCP-1 could have been mesangial cells

(56–58,60,62), although they showed that total body irradiation, which depleted circulating monocytes, also resulted in a 73% reduction of MCP-1 message in the glomerulus during the glomerulonephritis. This implies that, like IL-8 (92), infiltrating monocytes are an important source of chemokine production.

Another model in which MCP-1 expression has been examined is antithymocyte antibody-induced glomerulonephritis. In this model, heterologous antithymocyte serum (ATS), directed against the thymocyte-1 (Thy-1) antigen localized on mesangial cells, induces a complement-dependent but C5a-independent influx of monocytes into the glomerulus. The increase in glomerular macrophages is first detectable 30 min after injection of the ATS, reaches a peak by 24 h, and remains elevated for >3 weeks. Stahl et al. (97) examined the MCP-1 expression in rats in which ATS glomerulonephritis was induced. They demonstrated that glomerular expression of MCP-1 message is biphasic, with the first peak at 30 min after ATS injection and a return to baseline by 24 h, but MCP-1 message was again elevated by 5 days and remained elevated for >3 weeks. This pattern of expression of MCP-1 message was also reflected in immunostaining of MCP-1 in glomeruli. These experiments suggest that MCP-1 is involved in the formation of the monocytic glomerular infiltrates.

Finally, there is evidence that γIP-10 expression is also elevated in rat glomeruli in which glomerulonephritis is induced by immunization with ovalbumin (55). Much like the work with MCP-1, the time course of expression of IP-10 in this model precedes the formation of the monocytic and T-cell infiltrates (55).

The role of chemokines in primary interstitial inflammatory responses is less well defined. There is some evidence that chemokines are involved in the interstitial inflammatory response seen during bacterial pyelonephritis. During acute bacterial pyelonephritis, there is an initial interstitial infiltrate of polymorphonuclear leukocytes temporally followed by a mononuclear infiltrate composed of T cells and monocytes (98). It has also been found that there is a marked increase in urinary IL-8 excretion during pyelonephritis (99,100). Direct immunohistologic studies are needed to see if interstitial cells are producing the IL-8. Using a murine model of bacterial pyelonephritis, Rugo et al. (101) showed that message for MIP-1β is upregulated during pyelonephritis. This temporal pattern of chemokine production is consistent with its role in this interstitial inflammatory process.

MCP-1 expression has also been detected in two models of non-immune-initiated renal injury. These models, unilateral ureteral obstruction and ischemic acute renal failure, are characterized by the appearance of interstitial macrophages that have pathologic significance. In unilateral ureteral obstruction, the appearance of interstitial macrophages 4–12 h after obstruction follows the same time course and histologic distribution as MCP-1 expression (102). A similar association between MCP-1 expression and macrophage infiltration has been noted during the recovery phase of acute renal ischemia (103).

Another primary interstitial disease in which chemokines may be involved is acute cell-mediated transplant rejection. Acute cellular rejection of solid organs is characterized by an interstitial infiltrate consisting of T cells, macrophages, and eosinophils. RANTES mRNA was detected by in situ hybridization and RANTES protein was detected by immunohistochemistry in infiltrating mononuclear cells and renal tubular epithelial cells in the rejecting renal transplants (85). RANTES transcript is also increased in rat models of chronic renal allograft rejection at a time suggesting that it plays a key role in mediating the events of the chronic process (104).

In the case of interstitial inflammation after initial glomerular injury, the cellular infiltrate is relatively distant from the immune injury and the infiltrate is relatively devoid of polymorphonuclear leukocytes. Given these criteria, chemoattractants like C5a that are produced at the site of injury and attract neutrophils are likely not involved in the formation of these infiltrates. Chemokines can be released at a site distant from the initial immune injury, since their production can be regulated by diffusible agents like TNF-α or IL-1. Both IL-1 and TNF-α production by glomerular cells is upregulated during glomerular injury and could conceivably reach the interstitial cells. The TNF-α/IL-1-stimulated interstitial cells could then release chemokines and thereby establish a chemoattractant gradient into the interstitium. Direct experimental evidence for this is limited although our laboratory has demonstrated RANTES expression by tubular cells in mice with anti-GBM disease (T. Danoff, unpublished observations).

OSTEOPONTIN

Osteopontin is a highly acidic glycosylated phosphoprotein. It was originally isolated as a matrix molecule in bone (105) but subsequently has been shown to mediate a number of functions. Some of these functions are of immunologic importance, such as chemotaxis and regulation of nitric oxide production (106), while others are not, such as regulation of formation and remodeling of mineralized tissue and inhibiting the growth of calcium oxalate crystals (106,107). Although Boyden-chamber analysis of osteopontin's chemotactic activity toward monocytes has not been reported, osteopontin has been shown to bind to macrophages in vitro, and osteopontin elicits macrophage accumulation when injected subcutaneously (108). The chemotactic signal of osteopontin is transduced not through a classic STRs receptor but rather through CD44 (109), a transmembrane glycoprotein that is involved in a diverse range of functions, including cell–cell and cell–matrix interactions, which are involved in lymphocyte recirculation, homing, and activation (110).

Osteopontin mRNA is abundant in the kidney, and the protein is found in the urine. Under normal conditions, the distribution of osteopontin in the kidney is restricted to the thick ascending limbs of the loop of Henle and to the distal convoluted tubule (111). Osteopontin expression has been shown to be upregulated in a number of interstitial inflammatory models initiated either by immune or nonimmune injury. The immune-mediated models were anti-Thy-1 glomerulonephritis (112) or anti-FX1A glomerulonephritis (Heymann nephritis) (112), and the nonimmune models were puromycin-induced glomerulonephritis (112) or angiotensin-II-induced tubulointerstitial inflammation (113). Each of these models is characterized by the appearance of the accumulation of macrophages in the tubulointerstitium. These infiltrates are typically patchy in nature. In each case, osteopontin message and protein are upregulated in the kidney in a time course consistent with osteopontin playing a role in the formation of the macrophage infiltrate. Because the infiltrate is often patchy, it is possible to see that the site of increased osteopontin expression correlates with the site of inflammatory cell accumulation and tubular injury. Although these studies are very suggestive that osteopontin is involved in the formation of the interstitial infiltrate, appropriate inhibitors are still needed to prove the relative role of osteopontin versus other chemoattractants to the formation of the infiltrate. Also, formal chemotaxis experiments are needed to confirm that osteopontin's role in the formation of the inflammatory infiltrate is due chemotaxis rather than enhanced adhesion of the monocytes.

LEUKOTRIENE B_4

In addition to chemoattractant proteins, lipid compounds play an important proinflammatory role. The proinflammatory lipids can be divided into two basic classes. The first class is referred to as eicosanoids and consists of metabolites of arachidonic acid. The other class is the alkyl-ether glycerophospholipids of which platelet-activating factor has been the most studied (see below).

The metabolism of arachidonic acid (AA) occurs via a number of metabolic pathways to yield a large number of biologically active end products. Some of these end products affect the kidney through their action on glomerular hemodynamics or immune modulation (see chapter 22 for details). One of the pathways for AA metabolism is through oxidation by the enzyme 5-lipoxygenase (5-LO; see Fig. 5) to yield 5-hydroperoxyeicosatrienoic acid (5-HPETE), which is further metabolized to leukotriene A_4 (LTA_4). LTA_4 is then metabolized by either LTA_4 hydrolase or LTC_4 synthase to yield leukotriene B_4 (LTB_4) or the peptidoleukotrienes (114) (LTC_4, LTD_4, and LTE_4),

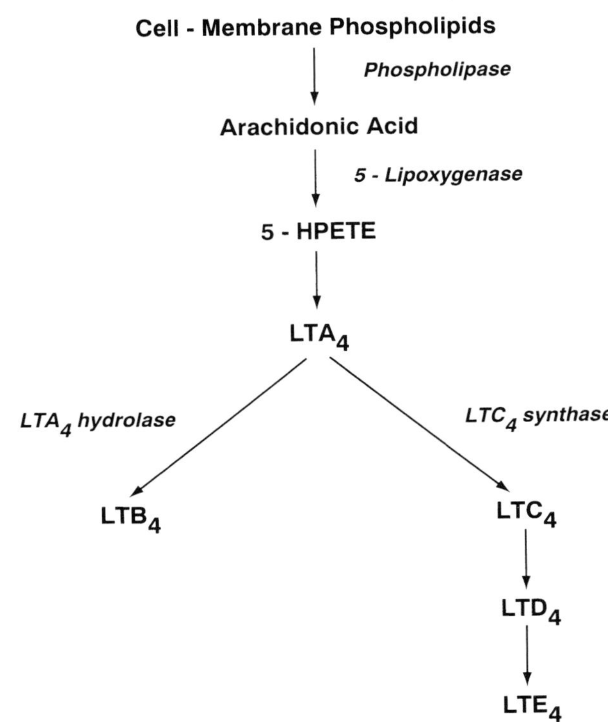

FIG. 5. 5-lipoxygenase pathway for the formation of LTB_4.

respectively. Leukotriene B_4 [(5S,12R)-dihyroxy-6,14-*cis*-8,10-*trans*-eicosatetraenoicacid] is the only AA metabolite with significant chemoattractant activity, being 100- to 1,000-fold more active than AA or its main metabolites (115,116).

LTB_4's primary target appears to be neutrophils, which express high- and low-affinity receptors for LTB_4. Through the high-affinity receptor, LTB_4 functions as a potent chemoattractant as well as an agent that induces neutrophil aggregation and adhesion to the endothelium. Through the low-affinity receptor, LTB_4 acts as a calcium ionophore, leading to neutrophil activation, release of lysosomal enzymes, and an increase in oxidative metabolism. LTB_4's function is partially autocrine in nature, since activated neutrophils are one of the richest sources of LTB_4. The LTB_4 receptor has not been cloned but is thought to belong to the seven-transmembrane-spanning receptor family (11,117).

Studies in rats have demonstrated that normal glomeruli can produce small amounts of LTB_4 (118), but with immunologic injury there is a marked increase in its synthesis. Both proliferative and nonproliferative models of glomerular immune injury show enhanced LTB_4 synthesis. These models include anti-Thy-1 nephritis (119), Heymann nephritis (120), NSN (121–124), and cationic bovine-γ-globulin-induced glomerulonephritis (CBGG glomerulonephritis) (125). LTB_4 production is also enhanced in rat renal allografts undergoing rejection (126) and in a murine model of lupus (127).

The source of LTB_4 production has been examined. The production of LTB_4 in normal glomeruli is predominantly from the resident glomerular macrophages. Although it is clear that LTB_4 production is upregulated during immune injury, the cellular source of the LTB_4 is not absolutely clear. At first glance, it would appear that only neutrophils and monocytes could make LTB_4, since they are the only cell types that contain 5-LO, the enzyme that commits AA metabolism toward LTB_4. It has been shown, though, that LTA_4 can diffuse out of these cells and be converted into LTB_4 by mesangial, endothelial, and epithelial cells (128) that possess LTA_4-hydrolase activity. Regardless of the source, it is clear that, in proliferative glomerulonephritis, invading neutrophils and monocytes are either directly or indirectly responsible for the upregulation of LTB_4 production.

In noninflammatory models of glomerular injury like CBGG glomerulonephritis or anti-Thy-1, the resident glomerular macrophages seem to be the major source of LTB_4 production (119,125).

In inflammatory models of glomerular injury like NSN, there is conflicting data as to the source of LTB_4 synthesis. All of the studies on NSN show that LTB_4 production rises rapidly after induction of disease and peaks at ~1–3 h. This peak represents an increase in LTB_4 production of >5-fold over baseline (121–123). Several studies suggest that the increased LTB_4 production is a result of the invading polymorphonuclear leukocytes. Yared et al. (129) showed a strong correlation between the percent increase of LTB_4 production and glomerular myeloperoxidase activity, a marker for neutrophils. Also, Schreiner et al. (123) showed that temporally the peak of LTB_4 production corresponded to the peak in neutrophil number in the glomerulus, and Lefkowith et al. (124) showed that there is a strong correlation between the amount of urinary LTB_4 and the number of neutrophils per glomeruli. The findings in these studies are in contrast to the results reported by Lianos (121), who showed that the peak of neutrophil infiltration precedes the peak in LTB_4 production and that neutrophil depletion does not significantly reduce LTB_4 production. In addition to the neutrophils, invading monocytes appear to contribute to LTB_4 production. Schreiner et al. (123) showed that by depleting the rats of essential fatty acids, they depleted resident glomerular macrophages as well as the monocytic infiltrate seen 24–72 h after induction of NSN without changing the neutrophil infiltration. These studies indicate that the early peak in LTB_4 production is present but reduced in magnitude, but the later (24–72 h) LTB_4 production is abolished, which suggests that the monocytes also play a critical role in the LTB_4 production.

Although a number of studies have examined the kinetics of LTB_4 production after immunologic injury, there is still no compelling proof that LTB_4 plays a major role an the formation of inflammatory infiltrates in the kidney. This is not to say that there is not abundant evidence that AA metabolites, including LTB_4, do not play an important role in renal pathology (see chapter 22) by mechanisms other than chemotaxis. This lack of proof stems from the fact that essentially all of the studies have been done in rats, and neutrophils in rats are not chemotactic to LTB_4 (130). Since LTB_4 is a very potent chemoattractant for human neutrophils, LTB_4 may play a role in the human glomerular inflammatory response.

PLATELET-ACTIVATING FACTOR

Platelet-activating factor (PAF) is a potent autocoid that participates in the renal inflammatory process as well as in other renal pathophysiologic processes (131,132). It was originally isolated from IgE-stimulated basophils as a potent inducer of platelet aggregation (133). Subsequently, it has been shown to have an important role in the inflammatory process based on its activity as a neutrophil chemoattractant (134); its ability to activate neutrophils, monocytes, and macrophages; and its ability to promote leukocyte adhesion to endothelium (135). In addition to its proinflammatory role, PAF plays a role in a number of pathologic processes in the kidney, including increasing vascular permeability (136), thereby promoting proteinuria (137).

PAF's chemical structure is 1-*O*-alkyl-2-acetyl-*sn*-glycero-3-phosphocholine. The biologic activity of PAF depends on two structural features: an ether linkage at the *sn*-1 position and an acetate group at the *sn*-2 position (135). PAF is not stored in cellular organelles but rather is enzymatically synthesized in response to a variety of stimuli. PAF is generated in one of two ways. In one known as the "remodeling" pathway, PAF is generated from preformed phospholipids through the action of phospholipase A_2 and acetyltransferase. The phospholipase A_2 also generates the precursor for AA metabolism. The other pathway for PAF production is through de novo synthesis. PAF is inactivated through degradation by the enzyme PAF acetylhydrolase, which catalyzes the cleavage of the acetyl group from the PAF molecule.

The PAF receptor has been cloned (138) and, like the classic chemoattractants, belongs to the seven-transmembrane-spanning receptor family. The PAF receptor is somewhat unusual among the classic chemoattractant seven-transmembrane-spanning receptor family in that it is least homologous with the other chemoattractant seven-transmembrane-spanning receptor family, that the calcium mobilization that is elicited by PAF is not blocked by pertusis toxin, and that the sequence contains an unusually large number of cysteines (11). There only appears to be one PAF receptor.

PAF can be produced by a variety of cells. The production of PAF was initially detected in antigen-stimulated IgE-sensitized basophils (133). Subsequently, PAF has been shown to be produced by neutrophils, macrophages/

monocytes, platelets, eosinophils, and endothelial cells (132). However, the amount of PAF secreted varies considerably from cell to cell (139). Moreover, isolated kidneys, isolated glomeruli, and mesangial cells are capable of producing PAF (132).

There are several lines of experimental evidence that PAF participates in renal immune injury. First, PAF can be detected during immune injury. Increased intraglomerular formation of PAF has been detected in several experimental models of renal immune injury, including hyperacute kidney allograft rejection (140), acute serum sickness (141), and nephrotoxic nephritis (142). Direct evidence supporting the role of PAF in the accumulation of neutrophils in the glomerulus comes from two groups of studies. In one, PAF was perfused in the renal circulation, which resulted in a number of physiologic changes, including the accumulation of neutrophils in the capillary lumen (137). In the other, PAF receptor antagonists have been shown to abrogate the accumulation of neutrophils in the glomerulus in NSN (132,142), in an acute, in situ form of immune-complex glomerulonephritis (143), and in a murine model of systemic lupus erythematosus (144). Collectively, this evidence strongly supports a role for PAF in the accumulation of inflammatory infiltrates in various animal models of immune-mediated renal injury.

Given the important role that PAF appears to play in renal immune injury, interruption of the PAF signaling system may prove to have important clinical benefits. Two strategies for blocking PAF activity have been described. One of these strategies is the conventional receptor antagonist, whereas the other is the production of a natural PAF-metabolizing enzyme. A number of receptor antagonists have been produced and shown to be effective in ameliorating various animal models of renal disease (132,142–145). The other strategy uses the enzyme PAF acetylhydrolase, which normally metabolizes PAF to its inactive metabolite lysoplatelet-activating factor. This enzyme has been cloned (146) and the recombinant protein shown to ameliorate several nonrenal models of severe acute inflammation (146). Hopefully, one of these therapeutic modalities will prove to be useful for renal inflammatory processes.

TRANSFORMING GROWTH FACTOR β

Transforming growth factors β (TGF-βs) are multifunctional cytokines that play an important role in renal disease (for a complete discussion, see chapter 20). Among its numerous functions, which have been well studied, are effects on matrix accumulation and on renal parenchymal cell growth and proliferation (147–149). There are five distinct TGF-β isoforms, of which TGF-β_1 has been shown to be an exquisitely potent chemoattractant for monocytes (150), neutrophils (151), and fibroblasts (3). Its in vitro chemotactic activity occurs at concentrations of 50–500 f*M* (10^{-15}M) (150,151), which is >1,000-fold more potent than the other chemoattractants described previously. TGF-β has also been shown to cause the accumulation of mononuclear leukocytes in vivo (152).

TGF-β_1's biologically active form is as a homodimeric polypeptide. Of the TGF-β isoforms expressed in the kidney, it is the most highly expressed. TGF-β_1 is present both in tubular epithelial cells and in the glomerulus. Unlike the "classic chemoattractant" receptors that are linked to G proteins and induce intracellular calcium fluxes, the action of TGF-β is mediated through a distinct receptor system (153). The TGF-β signaling receptors have serine–threonine kinase activity in their cytoplasmic domain, which presumably is involved in the signal transduction pathway for chemotaxis (151).

Although many aspects of TGF-β's role in renal diseases have been carefully examined, its role as a chemoattractant has not been examined. Arguing against a significant role for TGF-β_1's chemotactic activity in renal disease is that it is upregulated in a number of disease models such as acute anti-Thy-1 glomerulonephritis and chronic diabetic models that are associated with matrix accumulation but not with significant inflammatory cell infiltrates. However, in progressive anti-Thy-1 glomerulonephritis, the increased expression of TGF-β is associated with the accumulation of monocytes in the interstitium (154). As discussed previously, there are other monocyte chemoattractants that are upregulated in this model and the relative role of TGF-β_1 has not been assessed.

An ideal means for evaluating the role of the chemotactic activity of TGF-β on the accumulation of inflammatory cells in the kidney would be through the use of mice that have been genetically modified to prevent the production of TGF-β (the so-called knockout mice). Theoretically, one could compare the inflammatory infiltrates in TGF-β_1-deficient mice with those in TGF-β_1-sufficient mice, and the difference would represent the role that the TGF-β played. Such TGF-β_1 knockout mice have been made (155,156), but in contrast to the lack of inflammatory infiltrates that would be expected if TGF-β's primary role were as a chemoattractant, these mice develop a spontaneous inflammatory process that results in wasting and death (157). This suggests that TGF-β plays a crucial role in the homeostatic regulation of the immune system, although maybe not through its chemotactic activity.

CONCLUSIONS

Chemoattractants are important in the formation of inflammatory renal lesions by virtue of their activity as regulators of leukocyte movement and adhesion. Because the regulation of renal inflammation is complex, it is exceedingly hard to dissect the relative role of each chemoattractant in the renal inflammatory process, especially since many chemoattractants and their receptors are seemingly redundant and their generation pathways themselves have physiologic significance.

REFERENCES

1. Harris H. The role of chemotaxis in inflammation. *Physiol Rev* 1954; 34:529.
2. Rot A. The role of leukocyte chemotaxis in inflammation. In: Whicher JT, Evans SW, eds. *Biochemistry of inflammation;* vol. Dordrecht, The Netherlands: Kluwer, 1992;18:271.
3. Postlethwaite AE, Kang AH. Fibroblast chemoattractants. *Methods Enzymol* 1988;163:694.
4. Abboud HE. Role of platelet-derived growth factor in renal injury [Review]. *Annu Rev Physiol* 1995;57:297.
5. Floege J, Eng E, Young BA, Johnson RJ. Factors involved in the regulation of mesangial cell proliferation in vitro and in vivo [Review]. *Kidney Int Suppl* 1993;39:S47.
6. Boyden SE. The chemotactic effect of mixtures of antibody and antigen on polymorphonuclear leukocytes. *J Exp Med* 1962;115:453.
7. Springer TA. Traffic signals for lymphocyte recirculation and leukocyte emigration: the multistep paradigm. *Cell* 76:301.
8. Rabb HAA. Cell adhesion molecules and the kidney. *Am J Kidney Dis* 1994;23:155.
9. Brady HR. Leukocyte adhesion molecules and kidney disease. *Kidney Int* 1994;45:1285.
10. Ley K, Gaehtgens P, Fennie C, Singer MS, Lasky LA, Rosen SD. Lectin-like cell adhesion molecule 1 mediates leukocyte rolling in mesenteric venules in vivo. *Blood* 1991;77:2553.
11. Murphy PM. The molecular biology of leukocyte chemoattractant receptors [Review]. *Annu Rev Immunol* 1994;12:593.
12. Vaddi K, Newton RC. Regulation of monocyte integrin expression by beta-family chemokines. *J Immunol* 1994;153:4721.
13. Caterina MJ, Devreotes PN. Molecular insights into eukaryotic chemotaxis [Review]. *FASEB J* 1991;5:3078.
14. Sozzani S, Locati M, Zhou D, et al. Receptors, signal transduction, and spectrum of action of monocyte chemotactic protein-1 and related chemokines [Review]. *J Leukoc Biol* 1995;57:788.
15. Cochrane CG, Muller-Eberhard HJ. The derivation of two distinct anaphylatoxin activities from the third and fifth components of human complement. *J Exp Med* 1968;127:371.
16. Jensen J. Anaphylatoxin in its relation to the complement system. *Science* 1967;155:1122.
17. Muller-Eberhard HJ. The complement system and nephritis [Review]. *Adv Nephrol Necker Hosp* 1974;4:3.
18. Gerard C, Gerard N. C5a anaphylatoxin and its seven transmembrane-segment receptor. *Annu Rev Immunol* 1994;12:775.
19. Gerard NP, Gerard C. The chemotactic receptor for human C5a anaphylatoxin. *Nature* 1991;349:614.
20. Yamamoto T, Hara M, Yamamoto K, Kihara I. A role of complement receptors on polymorphonuclear leukocytes in the adherence to immune deposits. *Tohoku J Exp Med* 1984;143:149.
21. Tonnesen MG, Smedley LA, Henson PM. Neutrophil–endothelial cell interaction: modulations of neutrophil adhesiveness induced by complement fragments C5a and C5a des arg and formyl-methionyl-leucyl-phenyl-alanine in vitro. *J Clin Invest* 1984;74:1581.
22. Cochrane CG, Unanue ER, Dixon FJ. A role of polymorphonuclear leukocytes and complement in nephrotoxic nephritis. *J Exp Med* 1965;122:99.
23. Stein JH, Boonjarern S, Wilson CB, Ferris TF. Alterations in intrarenal blood flow distribution: methods of measurement and relationship to sodium balance [Review]. *Circ Res* 1973;1:61.
24. Unanue ER, Dixon FJ. Experimental glomerulonephritis: immunological events and pathogenetic mechanisms. *Adv Immunol* 1967;6:56.
25. Shimizu F, Mossmann H, Takamiya H, Vogt A. Effect of antibody avidity on the induction of renal injury in anti-glomerular basement membrane nephritis. *Br J Exp Pathol* 1978;59:624.
26. Madaio MP, Salant DJ, Adler S, Darby C, Couser WG. Effect of antibody charge and concentration on deposition of antibody to glomerular basement membrane. *Kidney Int* 1984;26:397.
27. Morita T, Kihara I, Oite T, Yamamoto T. Participation of blood borne cells in rat Masugi nephritis. *Acta Pathol Jpn* 1976;26:409.
28. Schreiner GF, Cotran RS, Pardo V, Unanue ER. A mononuclear cell component in experimental immunological glomerulonephritis. *J Exp Med* 1978;147:369.
29. Thaiss F, Batsford S, Mihatsch MJ, Heitz PU, Bitter-Suermann D, Vogt A. Mediator systems in a passive model of in situ immune complex glomerulonephritis: role for complement, polymorphonuclear granulocytes and monocytes. *Lab Invest* 1986;54:624.
30. Cochrane CG, Muller-Eberhard HJ, Aiken BS. Depletion of plasma complement in vivo by a protein of cobra venom: its effects on various immunological reactions. *J Immunol* 1970;105:55.
31. Hammer DK, Dixon FJ. Experimental glomerulonephritis. II. Immunologic events in the pathogenesis of nephrotoxic serum nephritis in rats. *J Exp Med* 1963;117:1019.
32. Couser WG. Mediation of immune glomerular injury. *J Am Soc Nephrol* 1990;1:13.
33. Hebert LA, Cosio FG, Birmingham DJ. The role of the complement system in renal injury [Review]. *Semin Nephrol* 1992;12:408.
34. Hara M, Batsford SR, Mihatsch MJ, et al. Complement and monocytes are essential for provoking glomerular injury in passive Heymann nephritis in rats: terminal complement components are not the sole mediators of proteinuria. *Lab Invest* 1991;65:168.
35. Platt J, Vercellotti G, Dalmasso A, et al. Transplantation of discordant xenografts: a review of progress. *Immunol Today* 1990;11:450.
36. Dalmasso AP, Vercellotti GM, Fischel RJ, Bolman RM, Bach FH, Platt JL. Mechanism of complement activation in the hyperacute rejection of porcine organs transplanted into primate recipients. *Am J Pathol* 1992;140:1157.
37. Kaufman CL, Gaines BA, Ildstad ST. Xenotransplantation [Review]. *Annu Rev Immunol* 1995;13:339.
38. Morgan BP. Complement regulatory molecules: application to therapy and transplantation [Review]. *Immunol Today* 1995;16:257.
39. Lindley I, Westwick J, Kunkel S. Nomenclature announcement: the chemokines. *Immunol Today* 1993;14:24.
40. Kelner GS, Kennedy J, Bacon KB, et al. Lymphotactin: a cytokine that represents a new lass of chemokine. *Science* 1994;266:1395.
41. Oppenheim JJ, Zachariae COC, Mukaida N, Matsushima K. Properties of the novel proinflammatory supergene "intercrine" cytokine family. *Annu Rev Immunol* 1991;9:617.
42. Irving SG, Zipfel PF, Balke J, et al. Two inflammatory mediator cytokine genes are closely linked and variably amplified on chromosome 17q. *Nucleic Acids Res* 1990;18:3261.
43. Wenzel UO, Abboud HE. Chemokines and the kidney. *Am J Kidney Dis* 1995;26:982.
44. Clark-Lewis I, Dewald B, Geiser T, Moser B, Baggiolini M. Platelet factor 4 binds to interleukin 8 receptors and activates neutrophils when its N terminus is modified with Glu-Leu-Arg. *Proc Natl Acad Sci USA* 1993;90:3574.
45. Schmouder RL, Strieter RM, Wiggins RC, Chensue SW, Kunkel SL. In vitro and in vivo interleukin-8 production in human renal cortical epithelia. *Kidney Int* 1992;41:191.
46. Lindquist RR, Gutmann RD, Merrill JP, Damimin GJ. Human renal allografts: interpretation of morphology and immunohistochemical observations. *Am J Pathol* 1968;53:851.
47. Crossley M, Orkin SH. Regulation of the beta-globin locus [Review]. *Curr Opin Genet Dev* 1993;3:232.
48. Bonifer C, Hecht A, Saueressig H, Winter DM, Sippel AE. Dynamic chromatin: the regulatory organization of eukaryotic gene loci. *J Cell Biochem* 1991;47:99.
49. Kusner DJ, Luebbers EL, Nowinski RJ, Konieczkowski M, King CH, Sedor JR. Cytokine- and LPS-induced synthesis of interleukin-8 from human mesangial cells. *Kidney Int* 1991;39:1240.
50. Abbott F, Ryan JJ, Ceska M, Matsushima K, Sarraf CE, Rees A. Interleukin-1 beta stimulates human mesangial cells to synthesize and release interleukins-6 and -8. *Kidney Int* 1991;40:597.
51. Brown Z, Fairbanks L, Strieter RM, Neild GH, Kunkel SL, Westwick J. Human mesangial cell-derived interleukin 8 and interleukin 6: modulation by an interleukin 1 receptor antagonist. *Adv Exp Med Biol* 1991;305:137.
52. Brown Z, Strieter RM, Chensue SW, et al. Cytokine-activated human

mesangial cells generate the neutrophil chemoattractant, interleukin 8. *Kidney Int* 1991;40:86.

53. Narumi S, Wyner LM, Stoler MH, Tannenbaum CS, Hamilton TA. Tissue-specific expression of murine IP-10 mRNA following systemic treatment with interferon gamma. *J Leukoc Biol* 1992;52:27.
54. Gomez-Chiarri M, Hamilton TA, Egido J, Emancipator SN. Expression of IP-10, a lipopolysaccharide- and interferon-gamma-inducible protein, in murine mesangial cells in culture. *Am J Pathol* 1993;142:433.
55. Gomez-Chiarri M, Ortiz A, Seron D, Gonzalez E, Egido J. The intercrine superfamily and renal disease [Review]. *Kidney Int Suppl* 1993; 39:581.
56. Largen PJ, Tam FW, Rees AJ, Cattell V. Rat mesangial cells have a selective role in macrophage recruitment and activation. *Exp Nephrol* 1995;3:34.
57. Grandaliano G, Valente AJ, Rozek MM, Abboud HE. Gamma interferon stimulates monocyte chemotactic protein (MCP-1) in human mesangial cells. *J Lab Clin Med* 1994;123:282.
58. Rovin BH, Yoshiumura T, Tan L. Cytokine-induced production of monocyte chemoattractant protein-1 by cultured human mesangial cells. *J Immunol* 1992;148:2148.
59. Rovin BH, Tan LC. Role of protein kinase pathways in IL-1-induced chemoattractant expression by human mesangial cells. *Kidney Int* 1994;46:1059.
60. Satriano JA, Hora K, Shan Z, Stanley ER, Mori T, Schlondorff D. Regulation of monocyte chemoattractant protein-1 and macrophage colony-stimulating factor-1 by IFN-gamma, tumor necrosis factor-alpha, IgG aggregates, and cAMP in mouse mesangial cells. *J Immunol* 1993;150:1971.
61. Satriano JA, Shuldiner M, Hora K, Xing Y, Shan Z, Schlondorff D. Oxygen radicals as second messengers for expression of the monocyte chemoattractant protein, JE/MCP-1, and the monocyte colony-stimulating factor, CSF-1, in response to tumor necrosis factor-alpha and immunoglobulin G: evidence for involvement of reduced nicotinamide adenine dinucleotide phosphate (NADPH)-dependent oxidase. *J Clin Invest* 1993;92:1564.
62. Zoja C, Wang JM, Bettoni S, et al. Interleukin-1 beta and tumor necrosis factor-alpha induce gene expression and production of leukocyte chemotactic factors, colony-stimulating factors, and interleukin-6 in human mesangial cells. *Am J Pathol* 1991;138:991.
63. Hora K, Satriano JA, Santiago A, et al. Receptors for IgG complexes activate synthesis of monocyte chemoattractant peptide 1 and colony-stimulating factor 1. *Proc Natl Acad Sci USA* 1992;89:1745.
64. Heeger P, Wolf G, Meyers C, et al. Isolation and characterization of cDNA from renal tubular epithelium encoding murine RANTES. *Kidney Int* 1992;41:220.
65. Wolf G, Aberle S, Thaiss F, et al. TNF alpha induces expression of the chemoattractant cytokine RANTES in cultured mouse mesangial cells. *Kidney Int* 1993;44:795.
66. Baeuerle PA. The inducible transcription activator NF-κb: regulation by distinct protein subunits. *Biochim Biophys Acta* 1991;1072:63.
67. Grilli M, Chiu JJ, Lenardo MJ. NF-kappa B and Rel: participants in a multiform transcriptional regulatory system [Review]. *Int Rev Cytol* 1993;143:1.
68. Yasumoto K, Okamoto S, Mukaida N, Murakami S, Mai M, Matsushima K. Tumor necrosis factor alpha and interferon gamma synergistically induce interleukin 8 production in a human gastric cancer cell line through acting concurrently on AP-1 and NF-κb-like binding sites of the interleukin 8 gene. *J Biol Chem* 1992;267:22,506.
69. Ortiz B, Krensky A, Nelson P. Kinetics of transcription factors regulating the RANTES chemokine gene reveals a developmental switch in nuclear events during T-lymphocyte maturation. *Mol Cell Biol* 1996;16:202.
70. Ueda A, Okuda K, Ohno S, et al. NF-kappa B and Sp1 regulate transcription of the human monocyte chemoattractant protein-1 gene. *J Immunol* 1994;153:2052.
71. Kessler DS, Veals SA, Fu XY, Levy DE. Interferon-alpha regulates nuclear translocation and DNA-binding affinity of ISGF3, a multimeric transcriptional activator. *Genes Dev* 1990;4:1753.
72. Miyamoto M, Fujita T, Kimura Y, et al. Regulated expression of a gene encoding a nuclear factor, IRF-1, that specifically binds to IFN-beta gene regulatory elements. *Cell* 1988;54:903.
73. Harada H, Fujita T, Miyamoto M, et al. Structurally similar but functionally distinct factors, IRF-1 and IRF-2, bind to the same regulatory elements of IFN and IFN-inducible genes. *Cell* 1989;58:729.
74. Mukaida NM, Shiroo M, Matsushima K. Genomic structure of the human monocyte-derived neutrophil chemotactic factor IL-8. *J Immunol* 1989;143:1366.
75. Tekamp-Olson P, Gallegos C, Bauer D, et al. Cloning and characterization of cDNAs for murine macrophage inflammatory protein 2 and its human homologues. *J Exp Med* 1990;172:911.
76. Sachs AB. Messenger RNA degradation in eukaryotes. *Cell* 1993; 74:413.
77. Horuk R. The interleukin-8-receptor family: from chemokines to malaria [Review]. *Immunol Today* 1994;15:169.
78. Detmer PA, Lo SK, Olesen-Egbert E, Walz A, Baggiolini M, Cohn ZA. Neutrophil-activating protein 1/interleukin-8 stimulates the binding activity of the leukocyte adhesion receptor CD11b/CD18 on human neutrophils. *J Exp Med* 1990;171:1155.
79. Baggiolini M, Watz A, Kunkel SL. Neutrophil activating peptide-1/interleukin 8, a novel cytokine that activates neutrophils. *J Clin Invest* 1989;84:1045.
80. Neote K, Darbonne W, Ogez J, Horuk R, Schall TJ. Identification of a promiscuous inflammatory peptide receptor on the surface or red blood cells. *J Biol Chem* 1993;268:12247.
81. Neote K, Mak JY, Kolakowski LF Jr, Schall TJ. Functional and biochemical analysis of the cloned Duffy antigen: identity with the red blood cell chemokine receptor. *Blood* 1994;84:44.
82. Hadley TJ, Lu ZH, Wasniowska K, et al. Postcapillary venule endothelial cells in kidney express a multispecific chemokine receptor that is structurally and functionally identical to the erythroid isoform, which is the Duffy blood group antigen. *J Clin Invest* 1994; 94:985.
83. Chaudhuri A, Polyakova J, Zbrzezna V, Williams K, Gulati S, Pogo AO. Cloning of glycoprotein D cDNA, which encodes the major subunit of the Duffy blood group system and the receptor for the *Plasmodium vivax* malaria parasite. *Proc Natl Acad Sci USA* 1993;90: 10,793.
84. Webb LMC, Ehrengruber MU, Clark-Lewis I, Baggiolini M, Rot A. Binding to heparin sulfate or heparin enhances neutrophil responses to interleukin 8. *Proc Natl Acad Sci USA* 1993;90:7158.
85. Pattison JM, Nelson PJ, Huie P, Krensky A. RANTES chemokine in cell-mediated transplant rejection of the kidney. *Lancet* 1994;343: 209.
86. Tipping PG, Lowe MG, Holdsworth SR. Glomerular interleukin 1 production is dependent on macrophage infiltration in anti-GBM glomerulonephritis. *Kidney Int* 1991;39:103.
87. Brennan DC, Yui MA, Wuthrich RP, Kelley VE. Tumor necrosis factor and IL-1 in New Zealand Black/White mice: enhanced gene expression and acceleration of renal injury. *J Immunol* 1989;143:3470.
88. Camussi G, Tetta C, Bussolino F, et al. Effect of leukocyte stimulation on rabbit immune complex glomerulonephritis. *Kidney Int* 1990; 38:1047.
89. Tomosugi NI, Cashman SJ, Hay H, et al. Modulation of antibody-mediated glomerular injury in vivo by bacterial lipopolysaccharide, tumor necrosis factor, and IL-1. *J Immunol* 1989;142:3083.
90. Tang WW, Feng L, Vannice JL, Wilson CB. Interleukin-1 receptor antagonist ameliorates experimental anti-glomerular basement membrane antibody-associated glomerulonephritis. *J Clin Invest* 1994; 93:273.
91. Wada T, Yokoyama H, Tomosugi N, et al. Detection of urinary interleukin-8 in glomerular diseases. *Kidney Int* 1994;46:455.
92. Matsumoto K. Spontaneous release of interleukin-8 by glomerular macrophages from patients with rapidly progressive crescentic glomerulonephritis [Letter]. *Nephrol Dial Transplant* 1994;9:1693.
93. Wada T, Tomosugi N, Naito T, et al. Prevention of proteinuria by the administration of anti-interleukin 8 antibody in experimental acute immune complex-induced glomerulonephritis. *J Exp Med* 1994;180: 1135.
94. Feng L, Xia Y, Yoshimura T, Wilson CB. Modulation of neutrophil influx in glomerulonephritis in the rat with anti-macrophage inflammatory protein-2 (MIP-2) antibody. *J Clin Invest* 1995;95:1009.
95. Rovin BH, Schreiner GF. Cell-mediated immunity in glomerular disease. *Annu Rev Med* 1991;42:25.
96. Rovin BH, Rumancik M, Tan L, Dickerson J. Glomerular expression of monocyte chemoattractant protein-1 in experimental and human glomerulonephritis. *Lab Invest* 1994;71:536.
97. Stahl RA, Thaiss F, Disser M, Helmchen U, Hora K, Schlondorff D. Increased expression of monocyte chemoattractant protein-1 in anti-

thymocyte antibody-induced glomerulonephritis. *Kidney Int* 1993; 44:1036.
98. Heptinstall RH. *Pathology of the kidney.* Boston: Little, Brown, 1983:1324.
99. Tullus K, Fituri O, Burman LG, Wretlind B, Brauner A. Interleukin-6 and interleukin-8 in the urine of children with acute pyelonephritis. *Pediatr Nephrol* 1994;8:280.
100. Jacobson SH, Hylander B, Wretlind B, Brauner A. Interleukin-6 and interleukin-8 in serum and urine in patients with acute pyelonephritis in relation to bacterial-virulence-associated traits and renal function. *Nephron* 1994;67:172.
101. Rugo HS, O'Hanley P, Bishop AG, et al. Local cytokine production in a murine model of *Escherichia coli* pyelonephritis. *J Clin Invest* 1992;89:1032.
102. Diamond JR, Kees-Folts D, Ding G, Frye JE, Restrepo NC. Macrophages, monocyte chemoattractant peptide-1, and TGF-beta 1 in experimental hydronephrosis. *Am J Physiol* 1994;266:F926.
103. Safirstein R, Megyesi J, Saggi SJ, et al. Expression of cytokine-like genes JE and KC is increased during renal ischemia. *Am J Physiol* 1991;261:F1095.
104. Nadeau KC, Azuma H, Tilney NL. Sequential cytokine dynamics in chronic rejection of rat renal allografts: roles for cytokines RANTES and MCP-1. *Proc Natl Acad Sci USA* 1995;92:8729.
105. Butler WT. The nature and significance of osteopontin. *Connect Tissue Res* 1989;23:123.
106. Denhardt DT, Guo X. Osteopontin: a protein with diverse functions [Review]. *FASEB J* 1993;7:1475.
107. Hoyer JR, Otvos L Jr, Urge L. Osteopontin in urinary stone formation [Review]. *Ann NY Acad Sci* 1995;760:257.
108. Singh RP, Patarca R, Schwartz J, Singh P, Cantor H. Definition of a specific interaction between the early T lymphocyte activation 1 (Eta-1) protein and murine macrophages in vitro and its effect upon macrophages in vivo. *J Exp Med* 1990;171:1931.
109. Weber GF, Ashkar S, Glimcher MJ, Cantor H. Receptor–ligand interaction between CD44 and osteopontin (Eta-1). *Science* 1996;271:509.
110. Gunthert U. CD44: a multitude of isoforms with diverse functions [Review]. *Curr Top Microbiol Immunol* 1993;184:47.
111. Lopez CA, Hoyer JR, Wilson PD, Waterhouse P, Denhardt DT. Heterogeneity of osteopontin expression among nephrons in mouse kidneys and enhanced expression in sclerotic glomeruli. *Lab Invest* 1993;69:355.
112. Pichler R, Giachelli CM, Lombardi D, et al. Tubulointerstitial disease in glomerulonephritis: potential role of osteopontin (uropontin). *Am J Pathol* 1994;144:915.
113. Giachelli CM, Pichler R, Lombardi D, et al. Osteopontin expression in angiotensin II-induced tubulointerstitial nephritis. *Kidney Int* 1994; 45:515.
114. Lewis RA, Austen KF. The biologically active leukotrienes: biosynthesis, metabolism, receptors, functions, and pharmacology [Review]. *J Clin Invest* 1984;73:889.
115. Goetzl EJ, Sun FF. Generation of unique mono-hydroxy-eicosatetraenoic acids from arachidonic acid by human neutrophils. *J Exp Med* 1979;150:406.
116. Turner SR, Campell JA, Lynn WS. Polymorphonuclear leukocyte chemotaxis toward oxidized lipid components of cell membranes. *J Exp Med* 1975;141:1437.
117. Goetzl EJ, Sherman JW, Ratnoff WD, et al. Receptor-specific mechanisms for the responses of human leukocytes to leukotrienes [Review]. *Ann NY Acad Sci* 1988;524:345.
118. Cattell V, Cook HT, Smith J, Salmon JA, Moncada S. Leukotriene B_4 production in normal rat glomeruli. *Neprol Dial Transplant* 1987; 2:154.
119. Bresnahan BA, Wu S, Fenoy FJ, Roman RJ, Lianos EA. Mesangial cell immune injury: hemodynamic role of leukocyte- and platelet-derived eicosanoids. *J Clin Invest* 1992;90:2304.
120. Lianos EA, Noble B. Glomerular leukotriene synthesis in Heymann nephritis. *Kidney Int* 1989;36:998.
121. Lianos EA. Synthesis of hydroxyeicosatetraenoic acids and leukotrienes in rat nephrotoxic serum glomerulonephritis: role of anti-glomerular basement membrane antibody dose, complement, and neutrophils. *J Clin Invest* 1988;82:427.
122. Fauler J, Wiemeyer A, Marx KH, Kuhn K, Koch KM, Frolich JC. LTB_4 in nephrotoxic serum nephritis in rats. *Kidney Int* 1989;36:46.
123. Schreiner GF, Rovin B, Lefkowith JB. The antiinflammatory effects of essential fatty acid deficiency in experimental glomerulonephritis: the modulation of macrophage migration and eicosanoid metabolism. *J Immunol* 1989;143:3192.
124. Lefkowith JB, Pippin J, Nagamatsu T, Lee V. Urinary eicosanoids and the assessment of glomerular inflammation. *J Am Soc Nephrol* 1992;2:1560.
125. Rahman MA, Nakazawa M, Emancipator SN, Dunn MJ. 1988. Increased leukotriene B_4 synthesis in immune injured rat glomeruli. *J Clin Invest* 81:1945.
126. Spurney RF, Ibrahim S, Butterly D, Klotman PE, Sanfilippo F, Coffman TM. Leukotrienes in renal transplant rejection in rats: distinct roles for leukotriene B_4 and peptidoleukotrienes in the pathogenesis of allograft injury. *J Immunol* 1994;152:867.
127. Spurney RF, Ruiz P, Pisetsky DS, Coffman M. Enhanced renal leukotriene production in murine lupus: role of lipoxygenase metabolites. *Kidney Int* 1991;39:95.
128. Makita N, Funk CD, Imai E, Hoover RL, Badr KF. Molecular cloning and functional expression of rat leukotriene A_4 hydrolase using the polymerase chain reaction. *FEBS Lett* 1992;299:273.
129. Yared A, Albrightson-Winslow C, Griswold D, Takahashi K, Fogo A, Badr KF. Functional significance of leukotriene B_4 in normal and glomerulonephritic kidneys. *J Am Soc Nephrol* 1991;2:45.
130. Kreisle RA, Parker CW, Griffin GL, Senior RM, Stenson WF. Studies of leukotriene B_4-specific binding and function in rat polymorphonuclear leukocytes: absence of a chemotactic response. *J Immunol* 1985;134:3356.
131. Ortiz A, Gomez-Chiarri M, Lerma JL, Gonzalez E, Egido J. The role of platelet-activating factor (PAF) in experimental glomerular injury [Review]. *Lipids* 1991;26:1310.
132. Perico N, Remuzzi G. Role of platelet-activating factor in renal immune injury and proteinuria [Review]. *Am J Nephrol* 1990;1:98.
133. Benveniste J, Henson PM, Cochrane CG. Leukocyte-dependent histamine release from rabbit platelets: the role of IgE, basophils, and a platelet-activating factor. *J Exp Med* 1972;136:1356.
134. Goetzl EJ, Pickett WC. The human PMN leukocyte chemotactic activity of complex hydroxy-eicosatetraenoic acids (HETEs). *J Immunol* 1980;125:1789.
135. Yue TL, Rabinovici R, Feuerstein G. Platelet-activating factor (PAF): a putative mediator in inflammatory tissue injury [Review]. *Adv Exp Med Biol* 1991;314:223.
136. Humphrey DM, McManus LM, Hanahan DJ, Pinckard RN. Morphologic basis of increased vascular permeability induced by acetyl glyceryl ether phosphorylcholine. *Lab Invest* 1984;50:16.
137. Camussi G, Tetta C, Coda R, Segoloni GP, Vercellone A. Platelet-activating factor-induced loss of glomerular anionic charges. *Kidney Int* 1984;25:73.
138. Honda Z, Nakamura M, Miki I, et al. Cloning by functional expression of platelet-activating factor receptor from guinea-pig lung. *Nature* 1991;349:342.
139. Cluzel M, Undem BJ, Chilton FH. Release of platelet-activating factor and the metabolism of leukotriene B_4 by the human neutrophil when studied in a cell superfusion model. *J Immunol* 1989;143:3659.
140. Ito S, Camussi G, Tetta C, Milgrom F, Andres G. Hyperacute renal allograft rejection in the rabbit: the role of platelet-activating factor and of cationic proteins derived from polymorphonuclear leukocytes and from platelets [Review]. *Lab Invest* 1984;51:148.
141. Camussi G, Tetta C, Deregibus MC, Bussolino F, Segoloni G, Vercellone A. Platelet-activating factor (PAF) in experimentally-induced rabbit acute serum sickness: role of basophil-derived PAF in immune complex deposition. *J Immunol* 1982;128:86.
142. Bertani T, Livio M, Macconi D, et al. Platelet activating factor (PAF) as a mediator of injury in nephrotoxic nephritis. *Kidney Int* 1987;31: 1248.
143. Camussi G, Pawlowski I, Saunders R, Brentjens J, Andres G. Receptor antagonist of platelet activating factor inhibits inflammatory injury induced by in situ formation of immune complexes in renal glomeruli and in the skin. *J Lab Clin Med* 1987;110:196.
144. Baldi E, Emancipator SN, Hassan MO, Dunn MJ. Platelet activating factor receptor blockade ameliorates murine systemic lupus erythematosus. *Kidney Int* 1990;38:1030.
145. Gomez-Chiarri M, Ortiz A, Lerma JL, et al. Involvement of tumor necrosis factor and platelet-activating factor in the pathogenesis of experimental nephrosis in rats [see comments]: comment in *Lab Invest* 1994 Apr;70(4):435–6. *Lab Invest* 1994;70:449.

146. Tjoelker LW, Wilder C, Eberhardt C, et al. Anti-inflammatory properties of a platelet-activating factor acetylhydrolase. *Nature* 1995; 374:549.
147. Sharma K, Ziyadeh FN. The emerging role of transforming growth factor-beta in kidney diseases [Editorial review]. *Am J Physiol* 1994;266:F829.
148. Border WA, Ruoslahti E. Transforming growth factor-beta in disease: the dark side of tissue repair [Review]. *J Clin Invest* 1992;90:1.
149. Wahl SM. Transforming growth factor beta: the good, the bad, and the ugly [Review]. *J Exp Med* 1994;180:1587.
150. Wahl SM, Hunt DA, Wakefield LM, et al. Transforming growth factor type beta induces monocyte chemotaxis and growth factor production. *Proc Natl Acad Sci USA* 1987;84:5788.
151. Reibman J, Meixler S, Lee TC, et al. Transforming growth factor beta 1, a potent chemoattractant for human neutrophils, bypasses classic signal-transduction pathways. *Proc the Natl Acad Sci USA* 1991;88:6805.
152. Allen JB, Manthey CL, Hand AR, Ohura K, Ellingsworth L, Wahl SM. Rapid onset synovial inflammation and hyperplasia induced by transforming growth factor beta. *J Exp Med* 1990;171:231.
153. Massague J. Receptors for the TGF-beta family. *Cell* 1992;69:1067.
154. Yamamoto T, Noble NA, Miller DE, Border WA. Sustained expression of TGF-beta 1 underlies development of progressive kidney fibrosis. *Kidney Int* 1994;45:916.
155. Kulkarni AB, Huh CG, Becker D, et al. Transforming growth factor beta 1 null mutation in mice causes excessive inflammatory response and early death. *Proc Natl Acad Sci USA* 1993;90:770.
156. Shull MM, Ormsby I, Kier AB, et al. Targeted disruption of the mouse transforming growth factor-beta 1 gene results in multifocal inflammatory disease. *Nature* 1992;359:693.
157. Kulkarni AB, Karlsson S. Transforming growth factor-beta 1 knockout mice: a mutation in one cytokine gene causes a dramatic inflammatory disease [Review]. *Am J Pathol* 1993;143:3.

Immunologic Renal Diseases,
edited by E. G. Neilson and W. G. Couser.
Lippincott-Raven Publishers, Philadelphia © 1997.

CHAPTER 25

Leukocyte Adhesion

Marie-Josée Hébert and Hugh R. Brady

Migration of leukocytes from circulating blood to the extravascular space was first noted over 150 years ago when Dutrochet made the following observation: "Observing the movement of blood, I have often seen a cell escape laterally from the blood vessel and move in the transparent tissue . . . with a slowness which contrasted strongly with the rapidity of the circulation" (1). More than 50 years later, Metschnikoff recognized the crucial role of this process in host defense in his seminal work on the function of phagocytes: "After bacterial propagation in the subcutaneous tissue, an inflammatory reaction supervenes which attracts many inflammatory cells to the site of battle. The phagocytes then incorporate the parasites and destroy them" (2). Since then, leukocyte trafficking to sites of inflammation has been defined as an orchestrated multistep process that includes directed locomotion up gradients of chemoattractants (chemotaxis), rolling and immobilization of leukocytes on endothelium (margination, adhesion), diapedesis of leukocytes between endothelial cells, and migration through the extracellular matrix to the inflammatory focus. Upon arrival, leukocytes ingest invading micro-organisms (phagocytosis) and destroy them by release of reactive oxygen species, proteases, and other toxic molecules into phagolysosomes. Recruited phagocytes, in turn, release an array of mediators that attract subsequent waves of leukocytes and thereby amplify the inflammatory response. This "appropriate" inflammatory reaction allows efficient destruction of microbes with relative preservation of host tissue. In "inappropriate" inflammatory reactions, such as occur in autoimmune diseases, transplant rejection, and ischemia–reperfusion, the target of leukocyte aggression is usually an antigen that is either adherent to (e.g., "planted" antigen) or an intrinsic component of the host tissue (autoantigen) or an allograft. Under these circumstances, similar mechanisms of leukocyte recruitment are used; however, phagocytosis may be less efficient and incomplete (frustrated phagocytosis) and result in release of cytotoxic species into extravascular tissue (3,4).

Recent advances have identified leukocyte adhesion to endothelial cells as a pivotal event in leukocyte trafficking and have defined the cell surface molecules (leukocyte adhesion molecules) that support these interactions (5–14). Leukocyte adhesion and emigration are mediated through at least four major families of adhesion molecules: (a) selectins, (b) mucins and other selectin ligands, (c) integrins, and (d) immunoglobulin-like (Ig-like) adhesion molecules and other integrin ligands. Complementary *in vitro* and *in vivo* approaches in human and experimental systems suggest that initial loose adhesion of leukocytes and endothelial cells is supported by engagement of leukocyte or endothelial selectins with their molecular partners (Fig. 1). This tethering process supports rolling of leukocytes on the vessel wall where they are exposed to soluble and cell-associated mediators generated by activated endothelium and other cells within the inflammatory milieu. These signals provoke activation of leukocyte integrins and immobilization of leukocytes through binding of integrins to endothelial ligands such as Ig-like proteins. Immobilized leukocytes undergo rapid shape change and diapedesis; the latter process also uses members of the Ig-like adhesion molecule family (Fig. 1).

The biological activity of adhesion molecules far exceeds their role in leukocyte trafficking and encompasses key roles in maturation of hematopoietic cells, lymphocyte homing to peripheral lymph nodes and organs of the reticuloendothelial system, antigen presentation, T-cell activation, cytotoxicity, and transcellular biosynthesis of eicosanoids. In this chapter we summarize the classification, structural characteristics, and cellular distribution of the leukocyte adhesion molecules, discuss the regulation of adhesion by inflammatory mediators, review the

M-J. Hébert and H.R. Brady: Renal Division, Brigham & Women's Hospital, Harvard Medical School, Boston, Massachusetts 02115 and the Department of Medicine and Therapeutics Maler Miseracordiae Hospital, University College Dublin, Ireland.

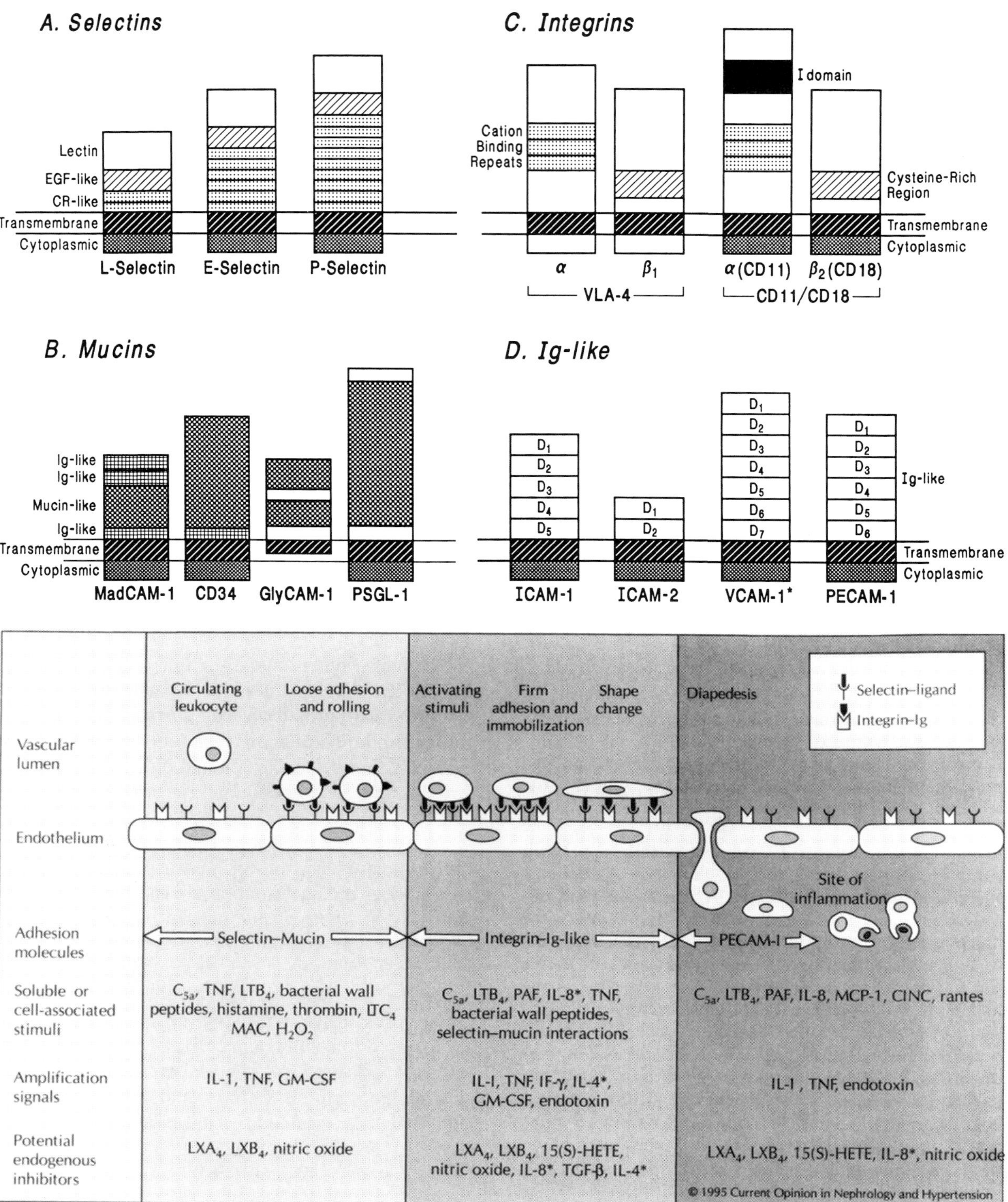

FIG. 1. Overview of leukocyte trafficking to site of extravascular inflammation. Role of selectins, mucins, integrins and Ig-like adhesion molecules. **Upper panel:** Some structural features of the four major families of leukocyte adhesion molecules. CR-like, complement regulatory protein–like domain; D, domain (Modified from Brady HR. Kidney Int. 1994;45:1285–1300; with permission). **Lower panel:** Leukocytes migrate toward the site of inflammation up concentration gradients of chemoattractants (chemotaxis), adhere to endothelial cells (margination/adhesion), and disrupt tight junctions and migrate between endothelial cells (diapedesis). Initial adhesion of leukocytes and endothelial cells is supported by interaction of leukocyte or endothelial cell selectins with carbohydrate-containing ligands, many of which are mucins. Selectin-mediated adhesion supports leukocyte rolling on endothelium, where they are subject to soluble and cell-associated activation signals from endothelium and extravascular tissue. Upon activation, leukocytes are immobilized by interaction of leukocyte integrins with endothelial cell ligands such as ICAM-1 and VCAM-1, members of the Ig-like superfamily. The molecular basis for diapedesis has not been established fully but appears to involve PECAM-1, an Ig-like molecule localized at intercellular junctions. (Modified from Takano T, Brady HR. Current Opinion in Nephrology and Hypertension 1995,4:277–286.)

evidence implicating adhesion as a key event in leukocyte recruitment, highlight the importance of adhesion in other pathophysiologic cell–cell interactions during inflammation, discuss the contribution of adhesion to the pathophysiology of kidney diseases, and summarize current approaches and possible future therapeutic strategies for inhibition of leukocyte adhesion in inflammation.

STRUCTURAL CHARACTERISTICS OF THE MAJOR LEUKOCYTE ADHESION MOLECULES

The classification, structural features, cellular distribution, and ligands of the four major families of leukocyte adhesion molecules are summarized in Fig. 1 and Table 1.

TABLE 1. *Summary of classification, distribution, and ligands of major adhesion molecules*

Family	Members	Distribution	Ligands	Target cells	Renal diseases where implicated
Selectins	L-selectin	Leukocytes	MadCAM-1, GlyCAM-1, ? other mucins, glycoproteins and glycolipids	Endothelial cells	Dialysis (first use syndrome)
	P-selectin	Platelets and endothelium	PSGL-1 and ?other mucins, glycoproteins, and glycolipids	Granulocytes, monocytes, T-cell subsets, some cancer cells	Glomerulonephritis, ischemia–reperfusion
	E-selectin	Endothelium	ESL-1 and ?other mucins, glycoproteins or glycolipids	Neutrophils, monocytes, lymphocyte subsets, some cancer cells	Glomerulonephritis, vasculitis, allograft rejection
Carbohydrate ligands for selectins	PSGL-1	Myeloid cells	P-selectin	Platelets, endothelium	Not reported
	ESL-1	Myeloid cells	E-selectin	Activated endothelium	Not reported
	MadCAM-1	Endothelium of mucosal lymphoid tissue	L-selectin and $\alpha4\beta7$ integrins	Leukocytes, lymphocytes	Not reported
	GlyCAM-1	Lymph node endothelium	L-selectin	Leukocytes	Not reported
Integrins	$\alpha4\beta1$ VLA-4 (β_1)	Monocytes, lymphocytes, eosinophils	VCAM-1, fibronectin	Endothelial, epithelial, mesangial, vascular, smooth muscle	Glomerulonephritis, allograft rejection
	CD11a/ CD18 (β_2)	Leukocytes	ICAM-1, ICAM-2	Endothelial, epithelial, mesangial vascular, smooth muscle	Glomerulonephritis, allograft rejection, ischemia–reperfusion
	CD11b/ CD18 (β_2)	Granulocytes, monocytes	ICAM-1, C3bi, fibrinogen, factor x, other	Endothelial, epithelial, mesangial, vascular, smooth muscle, other	Glomerulonephritis, allograft rejection, ischemia–reperfusion, dialysis (first use)
	CD11c/ CD18 (β_2)	Granulocytes, monocytes	Not characterized	Endothelial, mesangial	Not reported
Ig-like	ICAM-1	Endothelial, epithelial, smooth muscle, mesangial cell	CD11a/CD18	Most leukocytes	Glomerulonephritis, allograft rejection, interstitial nephritis, ischemia–reperfusion
	ICAM-2	Endothelial	CD11a/CD18	Most leukocytes	Not reported
	VCAM-1	Endothelial, epithelial, mesangial, smooth muscle	VLA-4	Monocytes, lymphocytes	Glomerulonephritis, vasculitis, allograft rejection
	PECAM-1	Endothelium, platelets, some leukocytes	? PECAM-1, ? other	Some leukocytes, endothelial	Not reported

Modified from Brady HR. *Kidney Int* 1994;45:1285–1300; with permission.

Selectins

Selectins support both initial rolling of leukocytes on endothelium and leukocyte–platelet interactions within the vascular lumen (5–12). Three selectins have been characterized: leukocyte selectin (L-selectin, CD62L), platelet selectin (P-selectin, CD62P), and endothelial cell selectin (E-selectin, CD62E). Selectins each possess a 120–amino acid NH2 terminal C-type (calcium-dependent) lectin-binding domain, a conserved epidermal growth factor (EGF)-like domain of ~30 amino acids, several 60–amino acid repeat sequences that are homologous to complement regulatory proteins, a single membrane-spanning domain, and a short intracellular COOH-terminal domain (Fig. 1). The genes encoding P-, E-, and L-selectins are present in a cluster on the long arm of chromosome 1 (7,10,11). Selectins are 40% to 60% homologous at the nucleotide and amino acid level and 60% to 70% homologous in their lectin-binding domain.

L-selectin is only expressed on leukocytes (Table 1). It was originally described as a homing receptor involved in the binding of lymphocytes to high endothelial venules of peripheral lymph nodes, a central step in normal lymphocyte migration from the systemic circulation into secondary lymphoid tissue (5–12). Subsequent studies demonstrated that leukocyte adhesion to cytokine-activated endothelium, including cultured glomerular endothelial cells, is attenuated by anti–L-selectin monoclonal antibodies (mAbs) (15,16), suggesting that L-selectin also regulates leukocyte trafficking in nonlymphoid tissue. P-selectin was first described in platelets but also is expressed by endothelial cells (Table 1). In both cell types, P-selectin is stored in cytoplasmic granules (alpha granules for platelets, Weibel-Palade bodies for endothelial cells) and mobilized to the plasma membrane upon cell activation (5–12). P-selectin supports platelet adhesion to neutrophils and monocytes, as well as endothelial cell adhesion to granulocytes, monocytes, and some lymphocytes subsets. P-selectin also supports adhesion of several tumor cell lines, implicating a role for P-selectin in tumor cell migration and metastasis formation. Expression of E-selectin is restricted to endothelial cells and requires induction of de novo synthesis by cytokines (Table 1). E-selectin supports adhesion of granulocytes, monocytes, some memory T-lymphocytes, natural killer (NK) cells, and some carcinoma cells (Table 1).

Mucins and Other Selectin Ligands

The ligands for the selectins are still being defined and are the subject of heated debate. A detailed discussion of this complex area is beyond the scope of this chapter, and interested readers are referred to recent extensive reviews (7,10,11,17,18). The lectin-binding domains of the selectins bear their principal adhesion epitopes, and most selectin ligands are heavily glycosylated structures. Many are sialomucins, typified by regions rich in O-linked sugars that extend beyond the cell glycocalyx and present polyvalent carbohydrates to selectins (Fig. 1) (18). Candidate carbohydrate moieties include sialyl Lewis X (CD15s), a fucosylated tetrasaccharide that decorates many cell surface proteins, and the related molecules Lewis X and sialyl Lewis A (7,10,11,17,18).

Three mucins bind L-selectin: MadCAM-1 (mucosal addressin cellular adhesion molecule), CD34, and GlyCAM-1 (glycosylation-dependent cell adhesion molecule) (Fig. 1, Table 1) (7,17–21). MadCAM-1 is preferentially localized to mucosal lymphoid tissue and supports L-selectin–dependent rolling on endothelium of Peyer's patches (22). Cloning of the gene for MadCAM-1 has demonstrated Ig-like domains similar to those found on Ig-like ligands for integrins, in addition to characteristic mucin motifs. Compatible with this finding, MadCAM-1 is a ligand for the $\alpha4\beta7$ integrin and supports lymphocyte adhesion to endothelium of Peyer's patches (13,17,18). This intriguing molecule may regulate the physiologic trafficking of lymphocytes within mucosal lymphoid tissue. CD34 is expressed on lymphoid and nonlymphoid endothelium and, like MadCAM-1, bears an Ig-like motif. Its role in leukocyte trafficking is unclear. GlyCAM-1 is a sulphated, fucosylated, and sialylated 50-kDa O-glycosylated mucin expressed by HEV of peripheral lymph nodes. Glycosylation-dependent cell adhesion molecule 1 (GlyCAM-1) was originally proposed to be the L-selectin ligand at this location (20,21); however, GlyCAM-1 lacks a cellular anchoring transmembrane–spanning domain and may function as a soluble modulator of L-selectin binding to HEV. Which, if any, of these mucins supports L-selectin mediation of leukocytes to nonlymphoid endothelium remains to be defined.

The ligands for P- and E-selectin are less well defined (7,17,18). In several in vitro systems, P- and E-selectin–dependent adhesion is blocked by mAbs against sialyl Lewis X and the related molecules Lewis X and sialyl Lewis A. P-selectin glycoprotein ligand (PSGL-1), a novel sialomucin, has been cloned and identified as a potential presenter of these and other carbohydrates to P-selectin (23,24). E-selectin binds several sialyl Lewis X-bearing membrane structures in vitro, including L-selectin, CD66, and β_2 integrins; however, the evidence that these interactions are physiologically important is, as yet, far from compelling. ESL-1, a 150-kDa glycoprotein, has been identified recently as a high-efficiency ligand for mouse E-selectin (25). In contrast to PSGL-1, ESL-1 is not a mucin. The predicted amino acid sequence of ESL-1 is 94% identical to the recently identified chicken cysteine-rich fibroblast growth-factor receptor, except for a unique 70–amino acid amino-terminal domain of mature ESL-1. Fucosylation of ESL-1 appears to be imperative for binding of E-selectin (25), a property shared by many selectin ligands (7,17,18). The further identification of ligands for the selectins will undoubtedly be a major focus of adhesion research in the near future.

Integrins

As discussed above, activation of rolling leukocytes triggers binding of leukocyte integrins to Ig-like and other endothelial cell adhesion molecules and causes immobilization of leukocytes on endothelium (Fig. 1). Integrins are heterodimeric glycoproteins composed of noncovalently associated alpha and beta subunits (5–9, 13,14,26) (Fig. 1). The major integrins involved in leukocyte-endothelial cell adhesion are the very late activation antigen-4 β_1 integrin [synonyms: VLA-4 ($\alpha4\beta1$); CD49d/CD29], the CD11/CD18 family of β_2 integrins, and the $\alpha4\beta7$ integrin (ligand for MadCAM-1).

VLA-4 is constitutively expressed by all leukocytes, except neutrophils, and binds to the Ig-like vascular cell adhesion molecule-1 (VCAM-1), thrombospondin, fibronectin and CS-1, an alternatively spliced fragment of fibronectin (5–9,13,27) (Table 1). VLA-4 supports adhesion of lymphocytes, monocytes, NK cells, eosinophils, and basophils to cytokine-activated endothelium. Three β_2 integrins have been characterized: CD11a/CD18, CD11b/CD18, and CD11c/CD18 (CD11 and CD18 referring to their alpha and beta subunits, respectively; Fig. 1) (5–9, 14,26). The CD18 beta subunit, common to all β_2 integrins, is a 678–amino acid protein encoded on chromosome 21. It possesses a short highly conserved cytoplasmic tail of 46 amino acids with several potential phosphorylation sites, a conserved membrane-spanning domain, and a longer extracellular region that contains a conserved cysteine-rich region that is necessary for surface expression. Point mutations in the latter region cause severe immunodeficiency in humans (26). CD11a, CD11b, and CD11c are proteins of 1,063, 1,136, and 1,144 amino acids, respectively, and are encoded by a cluster of genes on chromosome 16. CD11a is constitutively expressed by granulocytes, monocytes, and lymphocytes, whereas CD11b and CD11c are expressed by granulocytes and monocytes, but not lymphocytes (Table 1). CD11b is also expressed on subpopulations of B- and T-lymphocytes and NK cells (28). The major ligands for CD11a/CD18 are the Ig-like intercellular adhesion molecules-1 and -2 (ICAM-1 and ICAM-2) (5–9,14,26). CD11b/CD18 also binds ICAM-1. In addition, CD11b/CD18 supports leukocyte adhesion to cellular and acellular substrates by mechanisms that are independent of ICAM-1 (Table 1). In keeping with these ligand specificities, mAbs against CD11a and CD11b attenuate leukocyte adhesion to ICAM-1 and other ligands on cultured glomerular endothelial and mesangial cells in vitro (Fig. 2) (29). The endothelial counter-receptors for CD11c/CD18 have not been defined, and the role of this molecule in leukocyte trafficking is unclear. As detailed above, $\alpha4\beta7$ integrin is expressed by lymphocytes and may be a key modulator of lymphocyte homing to mucosal lymphoid tissue through its interaction with MadCAM-1, a sialomucin expressed preferentially in Peyer's patches (13).

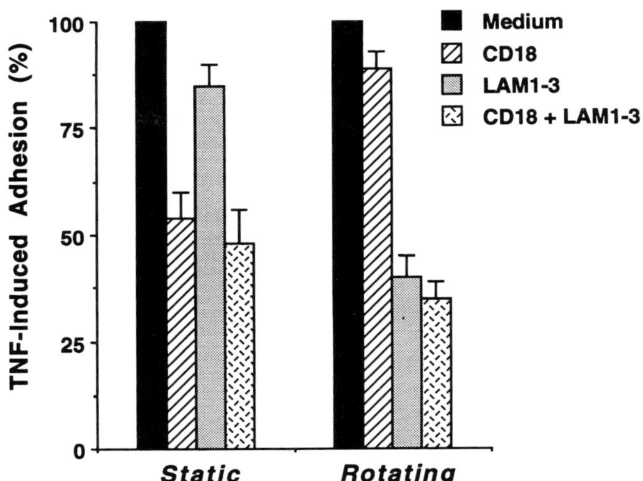

FIG. 2. Neutrophil adhesion to cytokine-activated glomerular endothelial cell (GEN) monolayers in vitro. A model of leukocyte–endothelial cell interactions during the amplification phase of glomerular inflammation. This representative study demonstrates the relative contributions of L-selectin and CD11/CD18 integrins to neutrophil–GEN adhesion under static and simulated flow (rotation) conditions. Neutrophils were incubated for 15 min with saturating concentrations of mAb to either L-selectin (LAM1–3) or CD18 before coincubation with TNF-activated (100 ng/ml for 24 hr) monolayers of GEN for 10 min at 37°C. Anti–L-selectin mAb did not influence neutrophil adhesion to GEN under basal conditions. These data and several other lines of evidence not shown here indicated that TNF induces de novo synthesis of a GEN ligand for leukocyte L-selectin. These observations support the contention that selectin-mediated adhesion is the initial tethering event in leukocyte recruitment that facilitates activation and engagement of leukocyte integrins, immobilization, and diapedesis. (Reprinted from Brady HR et al. *J Immunol* 1992;149:2437–2444; with permission.)

Ig-like Molecules and Other Integrin Ligands

The Ig superfamily of cell surface proteins is subcategorized into the C1-type cell surface proteins, which function in antigen recognition (e.g., CD4, CD8, T-cell receptor), and the C2-type molecules, which mediate complement binding and cell adhesion. Five C2-type Ig-like molecules support leukocyte–endothelial cell interactions: ICAM-1, ICAM-2, VCAM-1, platelet endothelial cell adhesion molecule-1 (PECAM-1), and MadCAM-1 (5–9). Each contains one or more disulphide-bridged loops containing antiparallel beta-pleated strands arranged into two sheets that are homologous to Ig, a transmembrane domain, and a short cytoplasmic tail (5–9) (Fig. 1). ICAM-1 (CD54) is encoded by chromosome 19 and contains five tandem Ig domains (D1–5) (5–9,30). ICAM-1 is a ligand for CD11a/CD18 and CD11b/CD18 but not CD11c/CD18. Single amino acid substitutions in the amino terminal D1 and, to a lesser extent, D2 domains reduce the avidity of ICAM-1 for CD11a/CD18. The third Ig-like domain is a binding site for CD11b/CD18. ICAM-1 is constitutively expressed at low levels by endothelial cells, and its expression is further enhanced on endothelium, and induced de novo on other cell types, after exposure to cytokines (5–9,29) (Table 1). ICAM-1 is also found on lymphocytes, where it mediates important homotypic and heterotypic interactions that subserve lymphocyte costimulation, cytotoxicity, and possibly induction of tolerance.

ICAM-2 (CD102) is a noninducible Ig-like adhesion molecule, encoded by chromosome 17, that is constitutively expressed by endothelial cells. It bears two Ig-like domains and is a ligand for CD11a/CD18, but not other β_2 integrins (Fig. 1, Table 1). Low levels of ICAM-2 are also detected on mononuclear cells, including lymphocytes and NK cells (5–9). Because resting T-lymphocytes express ICAM-2, but little ICAM-1, ICAM-2 may regulate the initial interaction of lymphocytes with antigen-presenting cells (see secion on Antigen Presentation).

VCAM-1 (CD106; INCAM-110) is a 110-kDa glycoprotein that contains seven Ig-like domains, a 22–amino acid transmembrane domain, and a short 19–amino acid cytoplasmic tail (Fig. 1). A second form of VCAM-1, consisting of six Ig-like domains, is generated in some tissues by alternate splicing (31,32). VCAM-1 is constitutively expressed by occasional endothelial cells of most large blood vessels and by parietal epithelial cells of Bowman's capsule (5–9) (Table 1). The functional role of VCAM-1 in the latter location is unclear but fascinating given emerging evidence that VCAM-1 also plays a role in tissue architecture and development (see section on Adhesion Molecule "Knockout" Mice). As with ICAM-1, cytokines induce de novo expression of VCAM-1 by endothelial, mesangial cells, tubular epithelial cells and vascular smooth muscle cells (5–9,33). VCAM-1 supports adhesion of eosinophils, basophils, monocytes, and lymphocytes, but not neutrophils, through interaction with VLA-4 on leukocytes (5–9,13).

PECAM-1 (CD31) is a 130-kDa integral membrane protein expressed by platelets, some leukocytes, and endothelial cells (Fig. 1, Table 1). This Ig-like molecule is constitutively expressed at tight junctions of endothelial cells and appears to regulate leukocyte diapedesis through a homotypic adhesion mechanism (5–9,34,35).

Soluble Adhesion Receptors

Soluble isoforms of the selectins and Ig-like adhesion molecules circulate in blood at levels that inhibit leukocyte-endothelial cell adhesion in vitro (36). Soluble L-selectin (sL-selectin), of which there are at least two isoforms, is 3–5 kDa smaller than its cell surface homologue and is released from leukocytes within minutes of cell activation. Its blood levels are increased in sepsis, human immunodeficiency virus infection, certain leukemias (36) and, interestingly, after leukocyte activation on hemodialysis membranes (126). Soluble P-selectin (sP-selectin) is approximately 3 kDa smaller than cell-associated P-selectin and represents an alternatively spliced form of the latter that lacks a transmembrane domain. It circulates in normal plasma and has been detected in increased concentration in patients with hemolytic uremic syndrome and thrombotic thrombocytopenic purpura, diseases characterized by endothelial and platelet activation. Soluble E-selectin (sE-selectin) is released by endothelial cells in vitro after activation by cytokines. Elevated levels of sE-selectin have been reported in patients with sepsis, polyarteritis nodosa, giant cell arteritis, scleroderma, systemic lupus erythematosus, renal failure, and diabetes mellitus but does not correlate well with disease activity (36). Soluble ICAM-1 (sICAM-1) contains most of the extracellular region of its cell-associated homologue, binds LFA-1 (lymphocyte function associated), and is released by melanoma and ovarian carcinoma cells, peripheral blood mononuclear cells, and endothelial cells in vitro. Elevated sICAM-1 levels have been reported in inflammatory diseases, infection, and cancers. In renal allograft patients, sICAM-1 levels increase during episodes of allograft rejection, and it has been proposed as a means of distinguishing rejection from cyclosporine toxicity (37–41). Several isoforms of soluble VCAM-1 (sVCAM-1) also circulate in healthy individuals, and their levels are increased in patients with inflammatory diseases, cancer, allograft rejection, cytomegalovirus infection and preeclampsia (36,41,42). Indeed, sVCAM-1 correlates closely with disease activity in patients with systemic lupus erythematosus. It will be intriguing to determine if the release of soluble adhesion receptors into the circulation or other body fluids serves as a negative feedback loop to limit leukocyte inflammation and tissue destruction during inflammation, and whether these systems can be modulated pharamacologically for therapeutic gain (see section on Future Strategies for Inhibition of Leukocyte Adhesion).

REGULATION OF LEUKOCYTE ADHESION BY INFLAMMATORY MEDIATORS

To avoid autodestruction of host tissue, it is essential that leukocytes and endothelial cells are maintained in a resting antiadhesive phenotype during health. It is also crucial that these cell types are exquisitely sensitive to the adhesion-promoting actions of inflammatory mediators

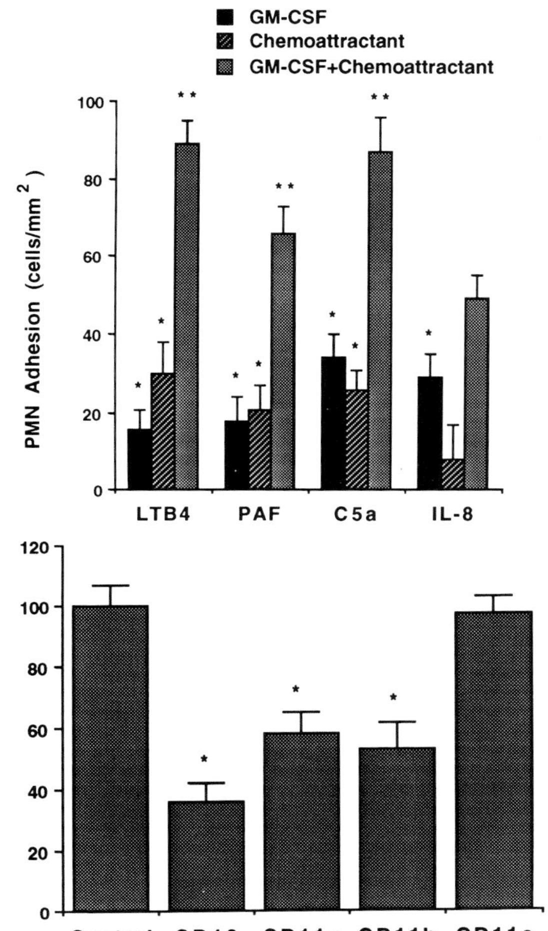

FIG. 3. Rapid regulation of neutrophil adhesion to cultured GEN by lipid-derived and peptide mediators in vitro. A model of leukocyte recruitment during glomerular inflammation. **Upper panel:** The addition of either the lipid-derived mediators LTB_4 or PAF, or peptide mediators C5a or IL-8 to the coincubations of neutrophils and GEN provoked rapid neutrophil–GEN adhesion. Prior exposure of neutrophils to GM-CSF, a cytokine whose levels are frequently increased in acute glomerulonephritis, enhanced their adhesiveness for GEN and primed PMN to the actions of lipid and peptide mediators. **Lower panel:** In this static adhesion assay, neutrophil–GEN adhesion was inhibited, in part, by mAb against either neutrophil CD18, CD11a, or CD11b. Thus, chemoattractants and cytokines can act in a coordinated manner to enhance leukocyte recruitment during the evolution of inflammatory responses by modulation of adhesion molecule biosynthesis, surface expression, and avidity. (Reproduced from Brady HR et al. *Am J Physiol* 1995;268:F1–F12; with permission.)

for efficient host defense. Model in vitro systems provide compelling evidence that leukocyte–endothelial cell adhesion is subject to two general levels of regulation (Fig. 3, Table 2). Initial recruitment of leukocytes is achieved by rapid modulation of the expression and avidity of preformed molecules by inflammatory mediators (seconds to minutes). The inflammatory response is sustained and amplified by cytokine-stimulated de novo synthesis of adhesion molecules (5–9,43–45).

Rapid Modulation of the Expression and Avidity of Preformed Molecules

Many structurally diverse inflammatory mediators rapidly enhance leukocyte adhesiveness for endothelium. These include bacterial cell wall products such as lipopolysaccharide and formyl peptides, the complement component C5a, lipid-derived mediators such as leukotriene B_4 (LTB_4) and platelet-activating-factor (PAF), and cytokines such as monocyte-chemotactic peptide-1 (MCP-1), interleukin-8 (IL-8), granulocyte-macrophage colony-stimulating factor (GM-CSF), and tumor necrosis factor (TNF) (5–9,43–47). The ability of certain mediators to selectively recruit different types of leukocytes (e.g., MCP-1 and monocytes; IL-8 and neutrophils) is probably determined by the differential expression of specific cell surface receptors on subpopulations of leukocytes. Engagement of these receptors triggers a cascade of signal transduction events that induce mobilization of preformed molecules (e.g., CD11b/CD18, CD11c/CD18) from intracellular stores to the cell surface and/or increased the avidity of constitutively expressed molecules for their molecular partners (Fig. 3) (5–9,43–45). In this regard, qualitative changes in avidity appear more important than quantitative changes in surface expression.

The signaling events that transduce engagement of cell surface receptors to alterations in adhesion molecule function are still being defined (5–9,48). Modulation of adhesion by classic chemoattractants such as C5a, LTB_4, and PAF is associated with activation of guanine nucleotide binding proteins and phospholipases C and/or D, hydrolysis of phosphatidylinositol bisphosphate and generation of inositol trisphosphate and diacylglycerol, and elevation of intracellular calcium and stimulation of protein kinases (48,49). These events occur within the same temporal framework as adhesion and pharmacologic inhibitors, many of these processes attenuate chemoattractant-stimulated adhesion. The more distal signaling events that ultimately enhance the avidity of adhesion molecules probably include phosphorylation of adhesion proteins and/or associated cytoskeletal components (9,26). The cytoplasmic domain of the CD18 chain of β_2 integrins possesses multiple serine/threonine residues that are targets for phosphorylation. Many compounds that trigger adhesion (e.g., N-formyl-met-leu-phe [fMLP], phorbol-12-mynistate 13-acetate [PMA]) also cause phosphorylation of these residues, whereas deletion of the cytoplasmic domain of CD18 results in loss of responsiveness. These findings suggest that the avidity of the CD11 ligand-binding chain of β_2 integrins is modulated by the phosphorylation status of the CD18 component.

Endothelial cells are also excitable and are subject to rapid changes in their adhesiveness for leukocytes and other blood components (5–9). Thrombin, histamine, hydrogen peroxide, membrane attack complex of complement, and the lipoxygenase-derived leukotrienes C_4

TABLE 2. *Regulation of leukocyte adhesion by chemoattractants, cytokines, chemokines, and other inflammatory mediators*

Response	Sites of action	Mechanisms	Molecules	Some stimuli
Seconds to minutes	Leukocytes	Increase in avidity and/or expression of preformed adhesion molecules	CD11/CD18,VLA-4, L-selectin	C5a, LTB_4, PAF, IL-8, MCP-1, TNF-α, bacterial wall peptides, E-selectin, ANCA
	Platelets	Increased expression of pre-formed adhesion molecules	P-selectin	ADP, thrombin, histamine
	Endothelium	Increased expression of pre-formed adhesion molecules	P-selectin	Histamine, thrombin, H_2O_2, MAC, LTC_4, LTD_4
	Mesangium	Increase in cell adhesiveness	? Ligand(s)	LTD_4
Hours to days	Leukocytes	De novo synthesis of adhesion molecules	CD11/CD18, L-selectin	GM-CSF
	Endothelium	De novo synthesis of adhesion molecules	ICAM-1, VCAM-1, E-selectin, ligands for L-selectin, ? P-selectin	TNF-α, IL-1β, IFN-τ, IL-4, endotoxin
	Mesangial, smooth muscle, epithelial	De novo synthesis of adhesion molecules	ICAM-1, VCAM-1	TNF-α, IL-1β, IFN-τ, IL-4, endotoxin

ADP, adenosine diphosphate; MAC, membrane attack complex of complement.
Reprinted from Brady HR. *Kidney Int* 1994;45:1285–1300; with permission.

and D_4 (LTC_4 and LTD_4) mobilize P-selectin from Weibel-Palade bodies to the cell surface within minutes, thereby increasing endothelial cell adhesiveness for leukocytes (5,7,8). The mechanism(s) by which these mediators modulate P-selectin expression is being defined. The time course of mobilization of P-selectin by histamine and thrombin (peak 1–2 min) differs markedly from that of LTC_4 and LTD_4 (peak 15–30 min), suggesting the presence of multiple regulatory signaling pathways. L-selectin and P-selectin are rapidly shed and reinternalized, respectively, after cell activation, a process that may limit adhesion and facilitate diapedesis in vivo (9–11).

Induction of De Novo Gene Transcription and Adhesion Molecule Biosynthesis

Cytokines are important amplifiers of leukocyte-mediated inflammation, in part because of their ability to induce de novo biosynthesis of adhesion molecules (Fig. 2, Table 2) (5–9,43–45). The profile of adhesion molecules expressed by cytokine-activated cells can differ dramatically depending on the cell type, time of exposure, and cytokine. With regard to differential expression by different cell types, glomerular endothelial and mesangial cells, tubular epithelial cells, and vascular smooth muscle cells express ICAM-1 and VCAM-1 in abundance after cytokine activation (5–9,43–45), whereas expression of E-selectin is restricted to endothelial cells (5–9,43–45). The importance of time of exposure is best illustrated by comparing the patterns of induction of endothelial ICAM-1, VCAM-1, and E-selectin in vitro. ICAM-1 and VCAM-1 expression is usually sustained for at least 24 to 48 hr in the presence of stimulatory cytokines in vitro (5–9, 43–45), whereas E-selectin expression is typically transient. Finally, certain cytokines are more potent inducers of individual adhesion molecules. For example, TNF-α and -β, IL-1α and -1β, and lipopolysaccharide are each potent inducers of mesangial cell VCAM-1 and ICAM-1 biosynthesis. In contrast, interferon-γ (IFN-γ) typically induces a more marked increase in mesangial cell ICAM-1 than VCAM-1 levels, whereas IL-4 is a relatively selective inducer of VCAM-1 expression and a weak stimulus for ICAM-1 synthesis (50). Interestingly, IFN-γ appears to be a more potent stimulus for adhesion molecule biosynthesis by epithelial cells, including tubular epithelial cells, than either TNF or IL-1 and has been implicated as a central player in renal tubulointerstitial injury. Thus, it is likely that the profile of adhesion molecules expressed by endothelial cells and other cell types within an inflammatory milieu is governed by the relative concentrations of different cytokines and the duration of disease.

The induction of ICAM-1, VCAM-1, and E-selectin is associated with increased messenger RNA (mRNA) expression and can be attenuated by inhibitors of protein and mRNA synthesis. These observations suggest that cytokines enhance adhesion molecule biosynthesis by stimulating gene transcription and have been confirmed by nuclear run-off studies. The mechanism(s) by which cytokines trigger gene transcription is still being defined and appears to involve activation of members of the protein kinase C (PKC) family and triggering of binding of the transcription regulatory protein AP-1, the ICAM-1 promoter (5–9,43–45,48,49).

VCAM-1 and E-selectin transcription is regulated by the pleiotropic transcription regulatory factor NFκB (Nuclear factor kappa B) (Fig. 4) (51–53). The signaling

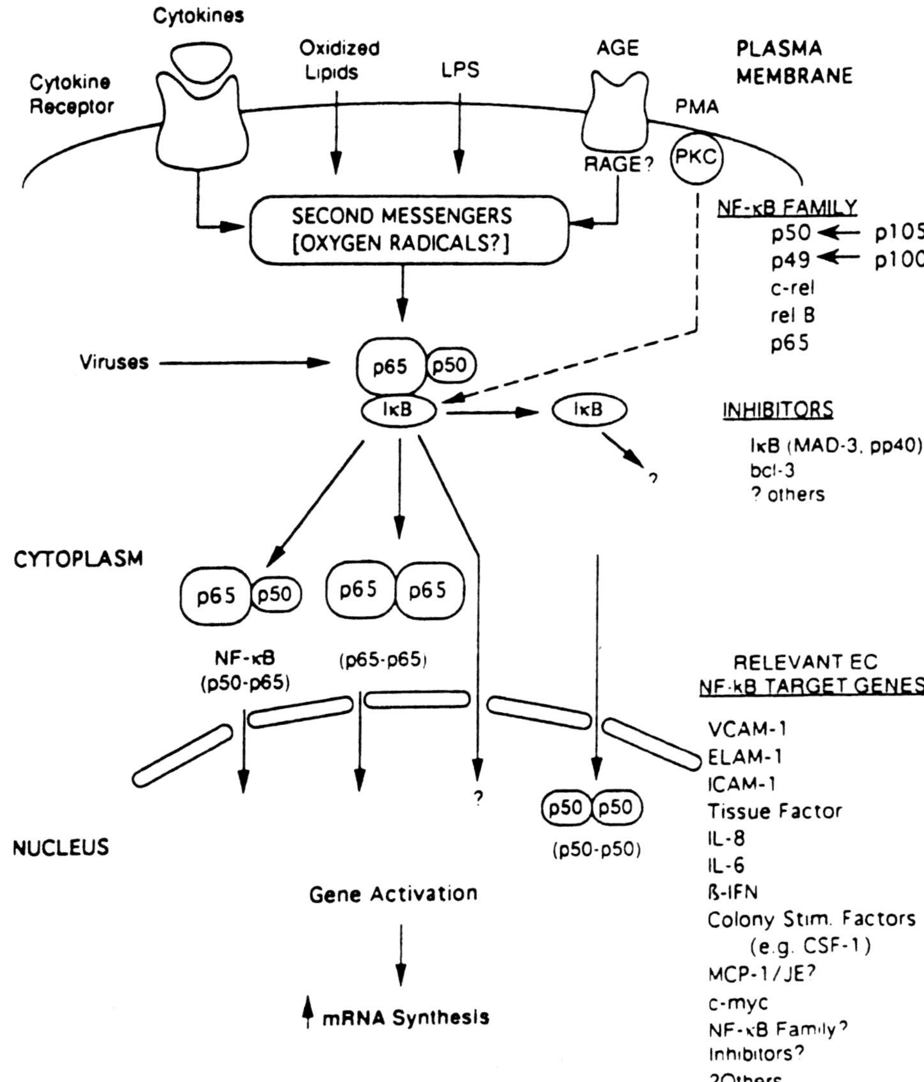

FIG. 4. Cytokines regulate VCAM-1 and E-selectin gene transcription through the pleiotropic regulator factor NFκB. The 5′-flanking regions of the VCAM-1 and E-selectin genes bear multiple NFκB binding sites and many cytokines (e.g., TNF-α, IL-1β, and LPS) that induce the expression of VCAM-1 and E-selectin also induce NFκB binding activity. Purified p50 and p65 subunits of NFκB stimulate transcription of reporter genes linked to the E-selectin or VCAM-1 promoter. Furthermore, site-directed mutagenesis of the NFκB binding sites on the VCAM-1 and E-selectin promoters indicates that the NFκB binding sites are required for cytokine-induced adhesion molecule expression. The 5′-flanking regions of both genes also bear other motifs that are required for induction of transcription by NFκB, namely an ATF-2 binding site, four positive regulatory domains (PRD I–IV), and an HMG-1 site that may facilitate binding of ATF-2 and NFκB to the promoter. (Reprinted from Collins T. *Lab Invest* 1993;68:499–508; with permission.)

events that link cytokine receptors to activation of NFκB are still being defined and may involve free radicals, fatty acids, and/or changes in the cellular redox state. In contrast to ICAM-1, PKC does not appear to be an important modulator of VCAM-1 or E-selectin gene transcription because most cytokines do not activate PKC at concentrations that induce either NFκB activity or expression of VCAM-1 or E-selectin. The mechanism of postinduction transcriptional repression that accounts for the transience of E-selectin expression has yet to be determined. Similarly, the molecular basis for the restriction of E-selectin expression to endothelial cells is under investigation. The further elucidation of the signaling events that modulate adhesion molecule expression and function may suggest novel strategies for inhibition of leukocyte recruitment during inflammation.

ROLE OF ADHESION IN LEUKOCYTE TRAFFICKING IN HOST DEFENSE AND INFLAMMATION

The consensus model for the coordinated interactions of selectin- and integrin-mediated adhesion in leukocyte trafficking (Fig. 1) was initially derived from studies using mAbs in models of the microcirculation (5–9). For example, mAbs against selectins inhibit rolling but not immobilization of leukocytes on endothelium in venules of the hamster cheek pouch, mesentery, and skin. These mAbs also block adhesion of leukocytes to cultured endothelial cells under simulated flow conditions in vitro (Fig. 2) and to purified selectins immobilized on artificial substrates. In contrast, mAbs against integrins or Ig-like molecules have little effect on rolling, but prevent immobilization of activated leukocytes. mAbs can potentially inhibit leukocyte–endothelial cell adhesive interactions in vivo and/or in vitro through indirect mechanisms, such as lysis or sequestration of subpopulations of leukocytes, and activation of leukocytes or endothelial cells with desensitization of adhesion responses. Therefore, it is essential that the functions of different adhesion molecules are confirmed by other techniques. Studies of patients with leukocyte adhesion deficiency (LAD) syndromes and of mice rendered deficient in adhesion molecules by homologous recombination in embryonic stem cells have proved invaluable in this regard.

LAD Syndromes

Two immunodeficiency syndromes graphically illustrate the importance of selectin-mediated leukocyte rolling and β_2 integrin–mediated leukocyte adhesion in normal host defense. LAD syndrome type 1 (LAD-1) is a rare autosomal-recessive inherited disorder in which there is absence of β_2 integrins on the cell surface of all leukocytes as a consequence of mutations in their CD18 beta chain that prevent association with CD11 alpha chains (14,26). Afflicted individuals experience recurrent life-threatening bacterial infections during the first years of life, characterized by persistent systemic neutrophilia and absence of pus formation due to impaired neutrophil migration from blood to extravascular tissue. Neutrophils isolated from patients with LAD-1 roll, but do not immobilize, on endothelium in response to activating signals. In addition, their neutrophils display markedly impaired degranulation and superoxide generation in response to serum opsonized zymosan particles, but not soluble stimuli. Importantly, monocyte and lymphocyte trafficking is relatively preserved, confirming that these cell types can use other adhesion ligands to extravasate from blood.

LAD-2 patients have a systemic congenital abnormality in fucose metabolism, one of the manifestations of which is impaired expression and function of Sialyl-Lewis X, a ligand for selectins (54). Afflicted individuals also experience recurrent bacterial infections, albeit less severe than in LAD-1. Compatible with a role for selectins in initial tethering of leukocytes to endothelium, leukocytes from these children display impaired rolling on endothelium in the microcirculation in vivo but adhere normally to endothelium through β_2 integrins upon cell activation in static adhesion assays in vitro.

Adhesion Molecule "Knockout" Mice

Generation of mice that are deficient in adhesion molecules, by homologous recombination in embryonic stem cells, has helped to further clarify the roles of selectins and Ig-like adhesion molecules in host defense and inflammation. The phenotypes of P-selectin (55), L-selectin (56), E-selectin (57), ICAM-1 (58), and VCAM-1 (59) single mutants have recently been described. Mice that are deficient in either L-selectin, P-selectin, E-selectin, or ICAM-1 are viable and fertile and do not express major physical abnormalities, suggesting that none of these molecules is absolutely necessary for survival. In contrast, deletion of VCAM-1 is lethal, but for unexpected reasons. Initial studies of glomerulonephritis in adhesion molecule "knockout" mice have yielded intriguing insights into the complex cell–cell interactions that occur within the vascular lumen in renal diseases (60).

L-Selectin–Deficient Mice

L-selectin–deficient animals typically have normal circulating white cell counts but small inguinal, axillary, periaortic, and cervical lymph nodes that contain reduced numbers of lymphocytes (56). In keeping with the hypothesis that L-selectin regulates lymphocyte homing, lymphocytes from null mice do not bind high endothelial venules of peripheral lymph nodes. Leukocytic rolling in mesenteric venules is also severely compromised, confirming a role for this ligand in leukocyte–endothelial cell interactions in the general circulation. L-selectin–deficient animals are protected against a number of inflammatory diseases, including thioglycollate-induced peritonitis and allergic contact dermatitis (56,61). The influence of L-selectin deficiency on the course of renal diseases has not been reported to date but clearly warrants study given that cytokine-activated glomerular endothelial cells express a ligand(s) for L-selectin and support L-selectin–dependent adhesion of neutrophils, monocytes, and lymphocytes in vitro (Fig. 2) (16).

P-Selectin–Deficient Mice

In contrast to L-selectin–deficient animals, basal blood neutrophil counts are increased by ~2.4-fold in P-selectin–deficient mice. Leukocyte rolling in the mesenteric venules is notably absent under basal conditions and after exposure of endothelium to stimuli that induce rapid mobilization of P-selectin from Weibel-Palade bodies in normal animals (55). These observations confirm that P-selectin modulates physiologic leukocyte margination in health and initial tethering of leukocytes to endothelial cells during inflammation. In keeping with the latter hypothesis, neutrophil recruitment to the peritoneal cavity in null mice is attenuated early in the course of thioglycollate-induced peritonitis (55,62). Accumulation of neutrophils, monocytes, and $CD4^+$ T-lymphocytes is also significantly blunted in null mice with contact hypersensitivity, indicating a role for P-selectin in leukocyte recruitment in both acute and subacute inflammatory reactions.

P-selectin is expressed by both activated endothelial cells and platelets. Initial studies of glomerulonephritis in P-selectin–deficient mice suggest complex roles for P-selectin in glomerular inflammation that probably also apply to other diseases in which there are prominent platelet–neutrophil interactions. P-selectin–deficient mice are not protected against neutrophil recruitment or proteinuria in a complement-independent model of nephrotoxic serum nephritis (60). Indeed, P-selectin deficient mice experience significantly greater morphologic and functional injury than do wild-type controls. This exaggerated inflammatory response occurs in the context of less efficient transcellular generation of lipoxin A_4 during P-selectin–mediated platelet–polymorphonuclear neutrophils (PMN) interactions within the glomerular capillary lumen (see section on Transcellular Generation of Eicosanoids). These data are intriguing given accumulating evidence that lipoxin A_4 may be an endogenous inhibitor of neutrophil recruitment that limits or reverses acute neutrophil-mediated inflammation in vivo (see section on Endogenous "Stop Signals" of Leukocyte Recruitment).

E-Selectin–Deficient Mice

The phenotype of E-selectin knockout mice is less dramatic than for other selectins. Basal leukocyte counts do not differ significantly from normal mice, and neutrophil migration is not impaired in either thioglycollate-induced peritonitis or delayed-type hypersensitivity reactions (57). However, anti–P-selectin mAbs blunt neutrophil recruitment in these models to a greater extent in E-selectin–deficient mice than in wild-type mice (57). These results suggest that there is overlap of function between P- and E-selectin in acute and subacute inflammation and may explain in part the variable protection afforded by anti–P- and anti–E-selectin mAbs in some experimental renal diseases.

ICAM-1–Deficient Mice

Deletion of ICAM-1 is associated with elevation of peripheral leukocyte counts due to an increased number of circulating neutrophils (two- to sixfold) and lymphocytes (two- to threefold) (58). ICAM-1–deficient mice are somewhat protected from delayed-type hypersensitivity and are also resistant to the lethal effect of high-dose endotoxin. In mixed lymphocyte reactions, lymphocytes from ICAM-1–deficient animals proliferate normally but cannot stimulate maximally an allogeneic response (58). The latter finding supports the hypothesis that ICAM-1 is important for maximal T-cell activation (see section on Antigen Presentation). In aggregate, those experiments highlight the importance of ICAM-1 in T-cell activation, as well as in acute and subacute inflammatory responses.

VCAM-1–Deficient Mice

Fewer than 3% of genetically engineered homozygous VCAM-1–deficient embryos survive embryonic development (59). In most VCAM-1–deficient embryos, there is complete absence of chorioallantoic fusion and demise of the embryo within 10–12 days. Epicardial abnormalities were also common. These unexpected findings indicate a major role for VCAM-1 in placentation and organ development. The few surviving homozygous VCAM-1–deficient animals reported to date appear phenotypically normal but have an increased number of circulating mononuclear leukocytes (59). These data are compatible with those derived from other experimental models that suggest a pivotal role for VCAM-1 in mononuclear cell trafficking.

ROLE OF ADHESION IN OTHER PATHOPHYSIOLOGIC CELL–CELL INTERACTIONS DURING INFLAMMATION

Adhesion, in addition to modulating leukocyte trafficking, promotes several other key events in the inflammatory cascade, including antigen presentation, T-cell activation, free-radical generation, degranulation, cytotoxicity, and transcellular biosynthesis of eicosanoids (Table 3). P-selectin also has been implicated as a modulator of vascular thrombosis. Agents that block leukocyte–endothelial cell adhesion attenuate these pathophysiological events, and it is likely that inhibition of these responses contributes to the anti-inflammatory efficacy of antiadhesion therapies in vivo.

TABLE 3. *Some inflammatory and immunologic events that are dependent on or facilitated by leukocyte adhesion in renal inflammation*

Leukocyte recruitment
Antigen presentation
Free radical generation
Degranulation
Phagocytosis
Cytotoxicity
Transcellular eicosanoid generation
Thrombosis

Antigen Presentation and T-Cell Activation

T-cell activation upon exposure to antigen involves three major steps (63) (Fig. 5). First, T cells adhere to "professional" (e.g., dendritic cells, activated B cells, monocytes/macrophages, and Langerhans cells) or "nonprofessional" [e.g., endothelial cells (64), mesangial cells (65), renal tubular cells (66)] antigen-presenting cells (APCs). This adhesion step can be supported by several molecular interactions: LFA-1–ICAM-1, LFA-3–CD2, CD43–ICAM-1, or VLA-4–VCAM-1. The second major step is recognition of antigen, presented by APCs in the groove of MHC molecules, by the lymphocyte T-cell receptor (TCR)–CD3 complex. This process is facilitated by binding of major histocompatibility complex (MHC) class I on APCs to CD8 on lymphocytes and MHC class II on APCs to CD4 on lymphocytes. After TCR ligation, T cells become receptive to additional costimulatory signals that initiate and enhance clonal expansion and T-cell functional responses. Here again, C-1 type and C-2 type members of the Ig superfamily are central players: signals being transduced through interactions of classic leukocyte adhesion molecules (e.g., LFA-3 with CD2, ICAM-1 with LFA-1) or through more specialized costimulatory interactions involving C-1 type Ig molecules and other receptors (e.g., B7-1 with CD 28, B7-2 with CD 28, B7-1 with CTLA-4, B7-2 with CTLA-4). Blocking of the early adhesion or recognition steps with mAbs against leukocyte adhesion molecules markedly attenuates T-cell activation, clonal expansion, lymphokine release, and cytotoxicity. Disruption of later costimulatory events can induce T-cell anergy (63).

Free-Radical Generation, Degranulation, and Cytotoxicity

Seminal studies of phagocyte function in patients with LAD-1 showed decreased phagocyte binding to the complement opsonin iC3b and reduced phagocytosis and particle-induced oxidative burst and degranulation (26). These findings underscore the complex interdependence of leukocyte adhesion and cytotoxicity responses in host defense. mAbs against CD11/CD18 integrins and ICAM-

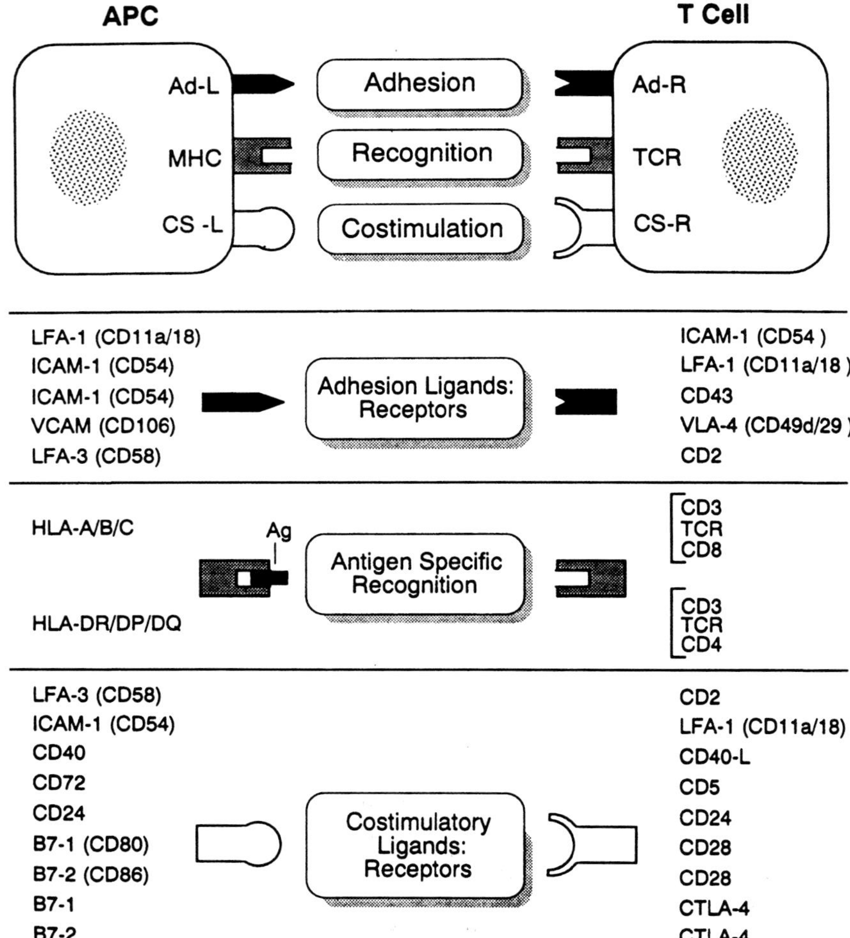

FIG. 5. Role of adhesion molecules in antigen presentation. See text for details. (Reprinted from Guinan EC et al. *Blood* 1994;84:3261–3282; with permission.)

1 attenuate phagocyte toxicity to mesangial cells and killing of tubular epithelial cells by cytotoxic T-lymphocytes in vitro (Fig. 6), suggesting that leukocyte adhesion also promotes renal injury by recruited leukocytes during inflammation (67). Adhesion probably promotes cytotoxicity by at least two mechanisms. First, adhesion primes leukocyte respiratory bursts, degranulation, and other "killing" responses to the actions of inflammatory mediators (9,68–70). Second, adhesion facilitates release of reactive oxygen products, proteases, and other toxic species in close proximity to renal cells, thereby reducing the effectiveness of free-radical scavengers and protease

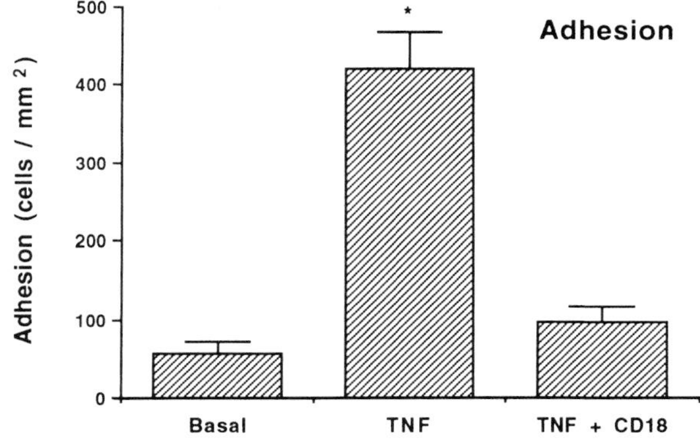

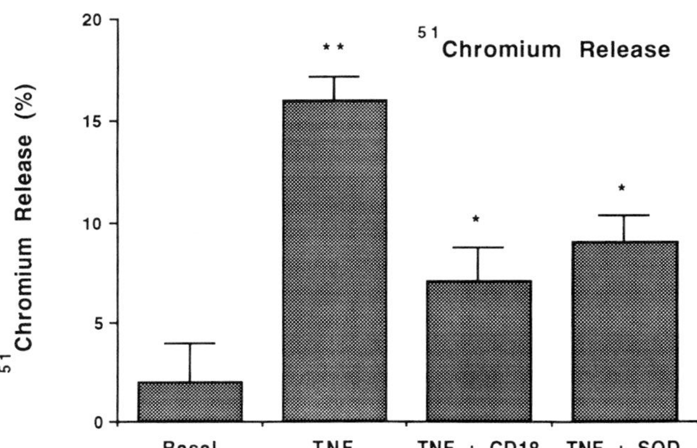

FIG. 6. Leukocyte adhesion promotes leukocyte-mediated injury to renal glomerular mesangial cells in culture. **Upper panel:** Upper graph shows phagocyte adhesion to cultured mesangial cells in vitro that had been exposed to TNF for 24 hr before coincubations. Most phagocyte adhesion was inhibited in the presence of an mAb (CD18) against phagocyte CD11/CD18 integrins. In parallel experiments shown in the lower graph, phagocyte adhesion was associated with cytotoxicity to mesangial cells that was reduced in the presence of anti-CD18 mAb, suggesting that adhesion promotes cell injury. Mesangial cell injury also was reduced in the presence of the free radical scavenger superoxide dismutase (SOD), implicating a role for reactive oxygen species. In experiments not shown, superoxide anion generation by phagocytes was significantly enhanced when phagocytes were adherent to mesangial cells and was attenuated in the presence of anti-CD18 mAb (reprinted from Denton MD et al. *Am J Physiol* 1991;261:F1071–F1079; with permission). **Lower panel:** Some potential mechanisms by which leukocyte adhesion could promote cytotoxicity during glomerular inflammation. Adherent leukocytes, as compared with leukocytes in suspension, release increased quantities of toxic oxygen radicals (O) and lysosomal enzymes (E) upon activation. In addition, adhesion facilitates release of these toxic mediators in close proximity to resident glomerular cells with relative exclusion of endogenous inhibitors (I) present in extracellular fluid. By inference, mAb or other agents that inhibit adhesion may not only confer protection by blocking leukocyte recruitment to sites of inflammation but also inhibit leukocyte-mediated cytotoxicity within a local inflammatory milieu. (Reprinted from Brady HR. *Kidney Int* 1994;45:1285–1300; with permission.)

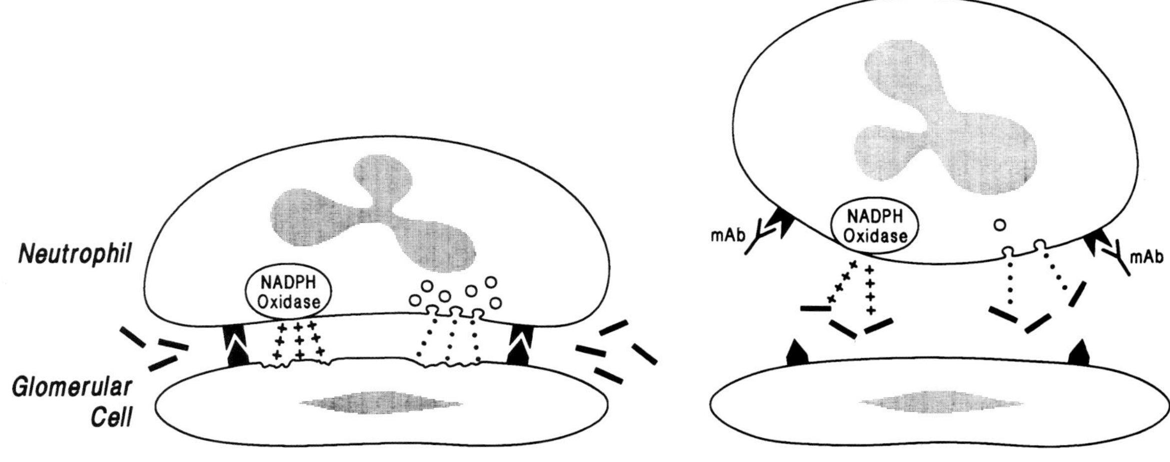

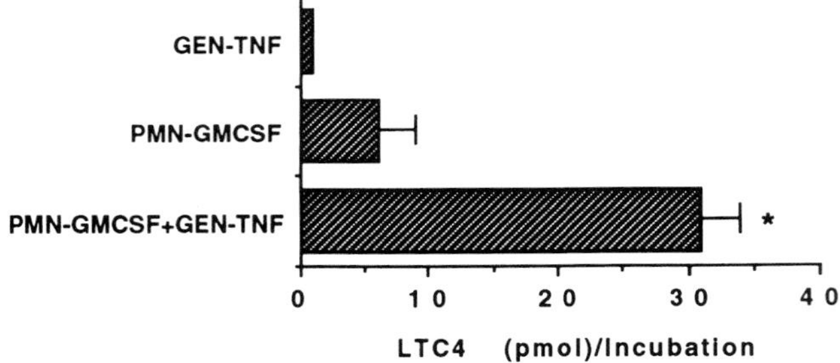

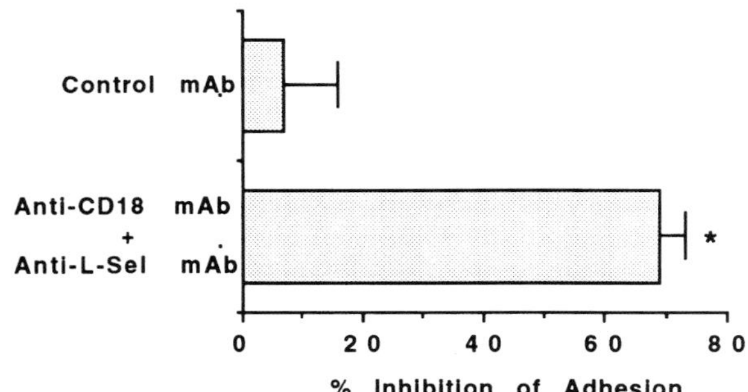

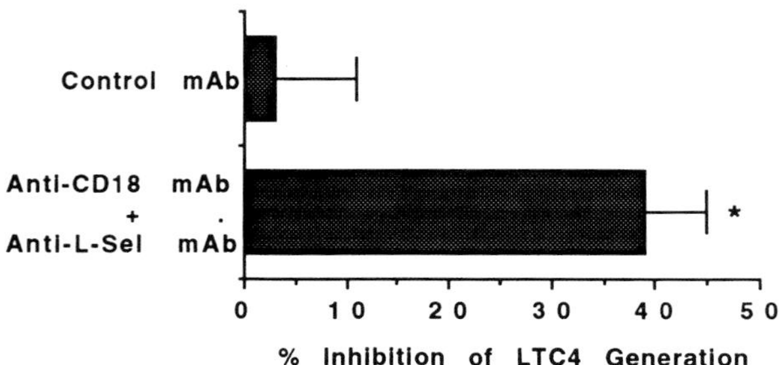

FIG. 7. Leukocyte adhesion promotes the generation of lipoxygenase products by transcellular routes during leukocyte–endothelial cell interactions. **Upper panel:** Upper graph depicts LTC_4 generation triggered by the peptide chemoattractant fMLP in incubations of cytokine-activated (TNF) GEN alone, cytokine-primed (GM-CSF) neutrophils (PMN) alone, and PMN–GEN coincubations under simulated flow conditions. The middle graph demonstrates that most PMN–GEN adhesion is inhibited by mAb against CD18 and L-selectin. The lower graph shows parallel experiments in which these mAbs also attenuated LTC_4 generation during coincubations, suggesting that leukocyte adhesion can promote transcellular eicosanoid generation during multicellular inflammatory responses. (Reprinted from Brady HR, Serhan CN. *Biochem Biophys Res Commun* 1992;186:1307–1314; with permission.) **Lower panel:** GEN lacks 5-lipoxygenase (5-LO) activity but can transform neutrophil-derived LTA_4 to bioactive products. GEN conjugates LTA_4 with glutathione (GSH) to form the vasoconstrictive eicosanoid LTC_4, a reaction catalyzed by LTC_4 synthase (glutathione-S-transferase). mAbs that block leukocyte adhesion to glomerular endothelial cells also block transcellular LTC_4 formation during coincubations in vitro. These observations suggest that adhesion facilitates transfer of LTA_4, an unstable lipophilic and hydrophobic intermediate, from leukocytes to adherent cells. Adhesion could also potentially prime leukocyte lipoxygenase pathways through "outside-in" signaling and enhance LTA_4 biosynthesis. These observations suggest alternate mechanisms by which adhesion blocking agents may confer protection during inflammation and other multicellular vascular events. (Reprinted from Brady HR et al. *Kidney Int* 1994; 45(suppl):90–97; with permission.)

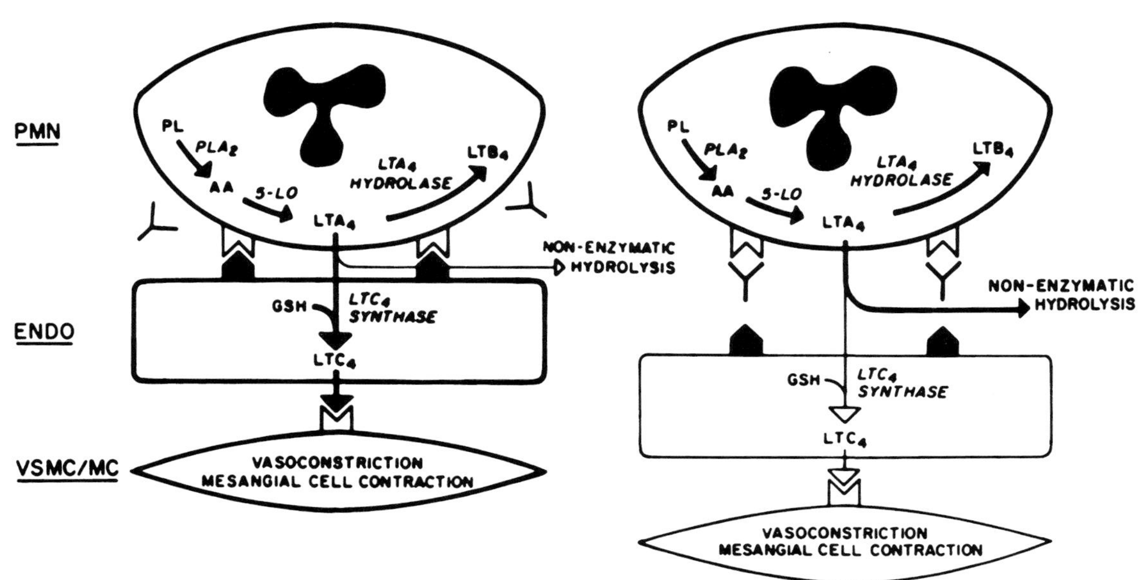

inhibitors in extracellular fluid (9). The molecular basis for this priming of leukocytes through engagement of adhesion molecules (outside-inside signaling) is incompletely understood.

Transcellular Eicosanoid Biosynthesis

Adhesion of leukocytes to other blood cells and resident tissue cells can amplify the levels and diversity of lipid mediators within a local inflammatory milieu by promoting the generation of eicosanoids by transcellular routes (Fig. 7) (71–73). With regard to the kidney, transcellular biosynthesis of leukotrienes has been demonstrated during interactions of neutrophils with both glomerular endothelial cells and mesangial cells in vitro. In these settings, renal parenchymal cells convert the neutrophil-derived arachidonate intermediate LTA_4 to the final bioactive lipoxygenase product. Thus, recruited blood cells and resident tissue cells can effectively pool their enzymatic machinery during cell–cell interactions to form bioactive lipids that neither cell type generates efficiently in isolation.

Compelling evidence for transcellular generation of lipoxins, a relatively recent addition to the families of bioactive eicosanoids, has recently been presented in the concanavalin A (Con A)–ferritin model of immune complex glomerulonephritis in vivo (Fig. 8) (74). Lipoxins (LX) are generated via biosynthetic pathways that initially involve the dual lipoxygenation of arachidonic acid by either 15- and 5-lipoxygenases or 5- and 12-lipoxygenases (*lipox*ygenase *in*teraction product*s*) (75). For example, platelets generate LXA_4 from the neutrophil-derived 5-lipoxygenase product LTA_4 through the action of platelet 12 lipoxygenase/lipoxin synthase during cell–cell interactions in vitro. Platelet–neutrophil transcellular pathways appear to be a rich source of LXA_4 in inflammed kidneys in Con A–ferritin glomerulonephritis because LXA_4 generation is blunted by prior depletion of animals of either neutrophils or platelets. Intriguingly, transcellular LXA_4 biosynthesis occurs in the context of platelet–neutrophil adhesion within the vascular lumen in this model and is blunted by mAbs against P-selectin, a major ligand for platelet–neutrophil adhesion (74). Additional evidence supporting a role for platelet–neutrophil interaction in transcellular LXA_4 generation has been gleaned from studies of LXA_4 generation after induction of nephrotoxic serum nephritis in P-selectin–deficient mice. In this model, abundant LXA_4 generation is again demonstrable in wild-type animals in the presence of morphologic evidence of platelet–neutrophil interactions within the glomerular capillary lumen. LXA_4 generation is blunted in P-selectin–deficient animals (60), an intriguing observation given that these null mice experience more glomerular injury than do wild-type mice and that LXA_4 has been implicated as an endogenous inhibitor of neutrophil trafficking during inflammation (see section on Endogenous "Stop Signals" for Leukocyte Recruitment).

LEUKOCYTE ADHESION MOLECULES AND KIDNEY DISEASES

Adhesion Molecule Expression in Normal Kidneys

E-selectin and P-selectin do not appear to be constitutively expressed in normal kidneys (76–78). There is little or no published information on the distribution of ligands for L-selectin in healthy renal tissue. ICAM-1 is expressed at low levels on the luminal surface of endothelial cells of large vessels, glomeruli, and peritubular capillaries; by some cells in the mesangium; on the luminal surface of some parietal epithelial cells of Bowman's capsule; on the brush border of proximal tubule cells; and by fibroblast-like interstitial cells (Table 1) (79–96). Constitutive expression of VCAM-1 is usually detected only on parietal epithelial cells of Bowman's capsule and occasional endothelial cells of large vessels or peritubular capillaries (93,97–104). Based on a limited number of reports, expression of ICAM-2 and PECAM-1 appears to be restricted to microvascular endothelial cells in normal kidneys.

Glomerulonephritis and Tubulointerstitial Nephritis

The mechanisms by which adhesion molecule expression and function is modulated in glomerulonephritis is complex and involves multiple mediator systems, some of which are illustrated in Fig. 9. Antibody-induced complement activation triggers local generation of C5a, a potent stimulus for β_2 integrin–mediated adhesion, and C5b-9, a stimulus for endothelial P-selectin expression. Immune complexes stimulate the release of an array of proadhesive chemoattractants and cytokines from resident glomerular cells through engagement of Fc receptors and potentially through specific reactivity with cell surface antigens. Secondary mediator systems may further modulate these adhesion responses (3–5). Superoxide anion has been reported to enhance β_2 integrin function, whereas hydrogen peroxide is a stimulus for P-selectin mobilization. Intriguingly, antineutrophil cytoplasmic antibodies (ANCAs) provoke adhesion of cytokine-primed neutrophils to endothelium in vitro (105), suggesting a mechanism by which ANCAs may contribute to the pathophysiology of pauci-immune glomerulonephritis. Against this background, a series of studies have documented the patterns of expression of adhesion molecules in human and experimental glomerular and tubulointerstitial disease (76–104) and evaluated the efficacy of antiadhesion therapy in these settings (106–117).

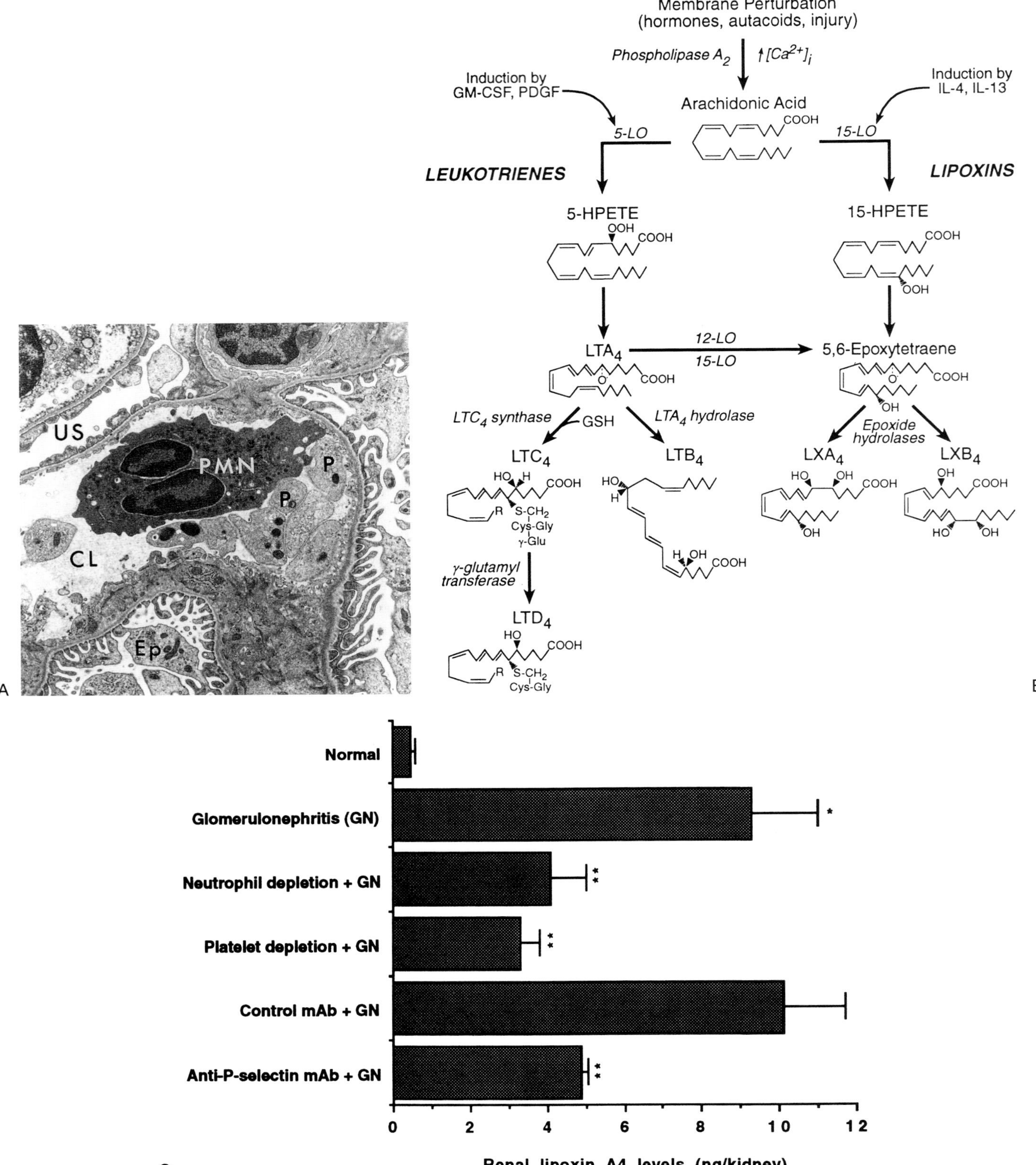
US
PMN
P
P
CL
Ep
A
Membrane Perturbation
(hormones, autacoids, injury)
Phospholipase A_2
$\uparrow[Ca^{2+}]_i$
Induction by
GM-CSF, PDGF
Arachidonic Acid
Induction by
IL-4, IL-13
5-LO
15-LO
LEUKOTRIENES
LIPOXINS
5-HPETE
15-HPETE
LTA_4
12-LO
15-LO
5,6-Epoxytetraene
LTC_4 synthase
GSH
LTA_4 hydrolase
Epoxide hydrolases
LTC_4
LTB_4
LXA_4
LXB_4
γ-glutamyl transferase
LTD_4
B
Normal
Glomerulonephritis (GN)
Neutrophil depletion + GN
Platelet depletion + GN
Control mAb + GN
Anti-P-selectin mAb + GN
0
2
4
6
8
10
12
Renal lipoxin A4 levels (ng/kidney)
C

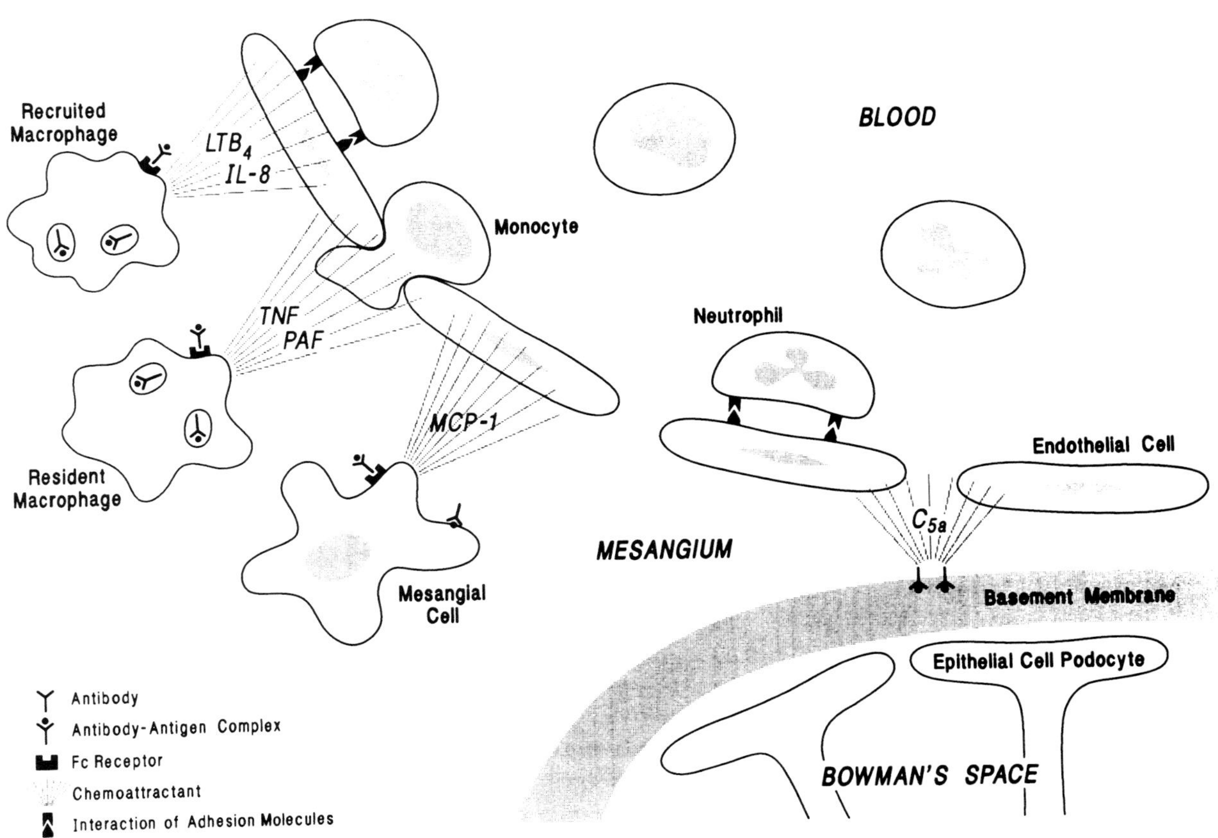

FIG. 9. Some mechanisms by which Ig deposition within the glomerulus can trigger the generation of chemoattractants, cytokines, and chemokines that provoke leukocyte recruitment. Some Ig subclasses activate complement, and the complement component C5a is a stimulus for neutrophil chemotaxis, CD11/CD18–mediated neutrophil adhesion to endothelial cells, and diapedesis. The membrane attack complex of complement also can increase adhesion but via an endothelial cell–directed action, namely mobilization of endothelial cell P-selectin from Weibel-Palade bodies to the cell surface. In addition, Ig can activate resident glomerular macrophages and mesangial cells and induce elaboration of proadhesive mediators through interaction with Fc receptors on their cell surfaces or perhaps through specific interactions with antigenic determinants. It should be noted that adhesion molecules are not absolutely required for leukocyte recruitment because leukocytes also can be recruited through engagement of their own Fc receptors with Ig in a mediator- and adhesion molecule–independent manner (not shown). (Reprinted from Brady HR. *Kidney Int* 1994;45:1285–1300; with permission.)

FIG. 8. P-selectin promotes transcellular LXA_4 generation during adhesion of platelets and neutrophils in the Con A–ferritin model of immune-complex–mediated glomerulonephritis. **Panel A:** Electron microscopic examination of the Con A–ferritin model of acute immune complex–mediated glomerulonephritis. Micrograph shows a glomerular capillary loop with an infiltrating neutrophil (PMN) adherent to a glomerular endothelial cell. A more striking and novel finding was the presence of platelets (P) in close contact with PMN and partially occluding the lumen. (Reprinted from Papayianni A et al. *Kidney Int* 1995;47:1295–1302; with permission.) **Panel B:** Overview of pathways for leukotriene and lipoxin formation by human cells. LT, leukotriene; LX, lipoxin; LO, lipoxygenase; $[Ca]_i$, intracellular calcium concentration; GSH, glutathione; PDGF, platelet-derived growth factor. (Reproduced from Brady HR. *Trends Cardiovasc Med* 1995;5:186–192.) **Panel C:** Role of platelet–neutrophil adhesion in transcellular LXA_4 formation in the Con A–ferritin model of glomerulonephritis. In this model, LXA_4 generation was blunted by prior depletion of either neutrophils or platelets in the animals, suggesting that most LXA_4 was formed by transcellular routes. LXA_4 formation also was inhibited in vivo and in vitro (not shown) by mAbs against P-selectin, an important ligand for platelet–neutrophil adhesion. (Reprinted from Papayianni A et al. *Kidney Int* 1995;47:1295–1302; with permission.)

Patterns of Expression

The pattern of expression of E-selectin and P-selectin in glomerulonephritis and tubulointerstitial inflammation has not been comprehensively studied. Induction of P-selectin expression has been described in some, but not all, models of immune complex glomerulonephritis and has not been studied extensively in human disease. Cytokine-activated renal microvascular endothelial cells express E-selectin in vitro (76–78), and induction of E-selectin has been reported in glomeruli and/or interstitial venules of some patients with acute glomerulonephritis, lupus nephritis, IgA nephropathy, and experimental septic shock, but not in patients with focal segmental glomerulosclerosis or membranous nephropathy (5,45,76–78,106,107). There are no published data on the expression of mucins or other putative ligands for selectins in renal disease.

In contrast to the selectins and their ligands, the pattern of expression of the Ig-like molecules ICAM-1 and VCAM-1 is well documented. Induction of endothelial ICAM-1 is a common finding in human and/or experimental crescentic glomerulonephritis, mesangioproliferative glomerulonephritis, IgA nephropathy, Henoch-Schonlein purpura, proliferative lupus nephritis, and tubulointerstitial nephritis (80–86). In addition, there is usually striking induction of ICAM-1 expression on the luminal surface of proximal tubules, distal convoluted tubules, collecting duct cells, and fibroblast-like interstitial cells (80–84). The level of expression tends to correlate with activity of disease and the number of CD11/CD18-bearing leukocytes in the local environment. Glomerular ICAM-1 levels may revert toward baseline in patients with advanced sclerotic disease. ICAM-1 levels are usually unchanged or reduced in minimal change disease, although induction of ICAM-1 expression has been noted in some patients (80–84). Different patterns of expression of ICAM-1 also have been reported in human focal segmental glomerulosclerosis and membranous nephropathy; some investigators have reported increased mesangial and/or tubulointerstitial staining, and others have noted a focal and segmental decrease in glomerular

TABLE 4. *Efficacy of some adhesion-blocking mAbs in kidney diseases*

Renal disease	Species (strain)	Molecule	Protection	Reference
Nephrotoxic serum nephritis	Rat (Long-Evans)	CD18	Yes	107
		CD11a	No	
		CD11b	Yes	
		VLA-4	Yes	
		ICAM-1	Yes	
		E-selectin	No	
Nephrotoxic serum nephritis	Rat (Lewis)	CD11b	Yes	108
Nephrotoxic serum nephritis	Rat (Wistar)	ICAM-1	Yes	109
Nephrotoxic serum nephritis	Mouse (C57/Bl10)	P-selectin	Yes	106
Nephrotoxic serum nephritis	Rabbit (New Zealand white)	CD18	No	[a]
		ICAM-1	No	
Nephrotoxic serum nephritis	Rabbit (New Zealand white)	CD18	No	[b]
Con A–ferritin nephritis	Rat (Sprague-Dawley)	P-selectin	No	74
Crescentic glomerulonephritis	Rat (Wistar-Kyoto)	CD11a	Yes	110
		ICAM-1	Yes	
		CD11a + ICAM-1	Yes	
Crescentic glomerulonephritis	Rat (Wistar-Kyoto)	CD11a + ICAM-1	Yes	111
Tubulointerstitial nephritis	Mouse (CBA/Ca, kdkd)	ICAM-1	Yes	112
Acute allograft rejection	Monkey (cynomolgus)	ICAM-1	Yes	113
Acute allograft rejection	Human	ICAM-1	Yes	114
Ischemia–reperfusion	Rabbit (New Zealand white)	CD18	No	120
Ischemia–reperfusion	Rabbit (New Zealand white)	CD18	No	[c]
		ICAM-1	No	
Ischemia–reperfusion	Rat (Sprague-Dawley)	Anti–ICAM-1	Yes	115
		Anti–ICAM-1 + anti–LFA-1	Yes	
Ischemia–reperfusion	Rat (Sprague-Dawley)	Anti–ICAM-1	Yes	116
		Anti–P-selectin	Yes	
Ischemia–reperfusion	Rat (Sprague-Dawley)	Anti–ICAM-1	Yes	117

Modified from Brady HR. *Kidney Int* 1994;45:1285–1300; with permission.

[a] O'Meara YM, Salant DJ, Brady HR. XIIth International Congress of Nephrology, Jerusalem, Israel, June 1993.

[b] Tipping PG, Cornthwaite LJ, Holdsworth SR. XIIth International Congress of Nephrology, Jerusalem, Israel, June 1993.

[c] Neuringer J, Brady HR, unpublished observations.

expression (80–84). These differences may reflect sampling at different stages in the disease.

Induction of VCAM-1 is almost always observed on proximal tubule cells of patients with vasculitis and crescentic nephritis, lupus nephritis, IgA nephropathy, and tubulointerstitial nephritis (5,45,50,97,98,100). For unclear reasons, VCAM-1 is not markedly induced on vascular endothelial cells in any of these diseases. Again, VCAM-1 expression is usually most prominent in patients with active inflammation, and there is generally a positive correlation between the level of expression and the magnitude of the surrounding leukocytic infiltrate. Indeed, adhesion of T-cell and macrophage cell lines to kidney sections from mice with lupus nephritis can be inhibited with mAbs against VCAM-1 (86). Striking VCAM-1 expression is also common in proximal tubules of patients with diabetic nephropathy, amyloid, gouty nephropathy, minimal change disease, and membranous nephropathy, diseases that usually are not considered to be inflammatory and leukocyte mediated (5,45,50,97,98, 100). These findings are compatible with the notion that both expression of adhesion molecules and a rich local source of chemoattractants are required for significant leukocyte recruitment.

It is worth noting that the pattern of expression of adhesion molecules does not appear, per se, to dictate the cellular composition of leukocyte infiltrates at sites of inflammation. Most renal cells, either in their basal state or after cytokine activation, express ligands that support granulocyte, monocyte, and lymphocyte adhesion. However, regional differences in the composition of leukocyte infiltrates are frequent in renal diseases, and enhanced expression of adhesion molecules may be observed in the absence of leukocyte infiltration. These observations suggest that leukocyte recruitment is not regulated solely by the profile of adhesion molecules on invading and resident cells, but also by the complex interplay of chemoattractants and other soluble and cell-associated activation signals within a local inflammatory milieu.

Efficacy of Antiadhesion Therapy

The efficacy of antiadhesion mAbs has been assessed in experimental models of glomerulonephritis and tubulointerstitial disease (Table 4) (106–112). Although the results are generally encouraging, it is clear that different ligands that support adhesion depend on the experimental model, species, and time of study. Two studies evaluated the influence of P-selectin mAbs on leukocyte infiltration in experimental immune complex glomerulonephritis with different results. Tipping et al. observed inhibition of neutrophil infiltration and renal injury in a complement-independent model of murine nephrotoxic serum nephritis (106). In contrast, Papayianni et al. did not find a protective effect of anti–P-selectin mAbs in a Con A–ferritin model of glomerulonephritis in rats (74). Only one study has evaluated mAbs against E-selectin in experimental glomerulonephritis and did not observe protection (Fig. 10) (107). The efficacy of inhibition of L-selectin has not been evaluated.

Infusion of anti-CD11b mAbs 16 hr before induction of nephrotoxic serum nephritis in Lewis rats caused a striking decrease in proteinuria and neutrophil infiltration, whereas administration of mAbs 30 min before induction also afforded protection without affecting glo-

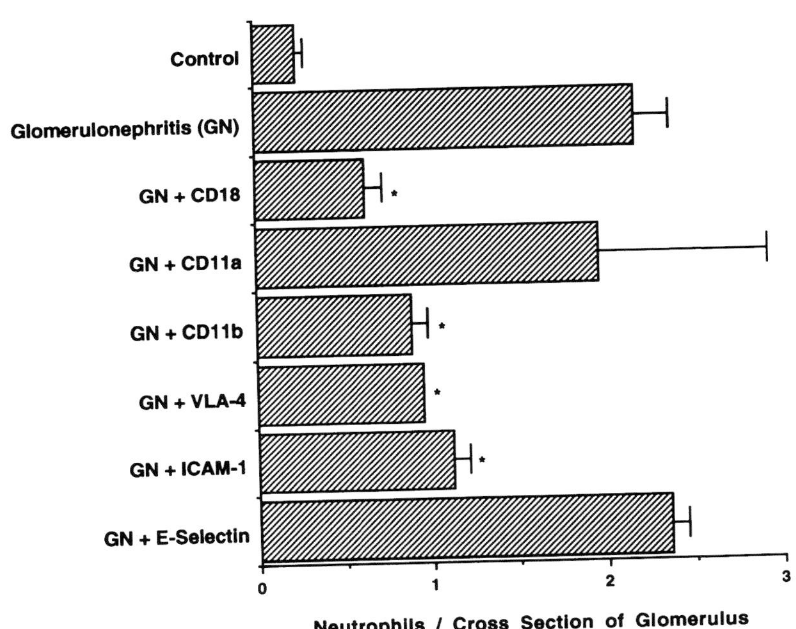

FIG. 10. Influence of mAbs against some selectins, integrins and Ig-like adhesion molecules on neutrophil recruitment in rat nephrotoxic serum nephritis, a model of acute glomerulonephritis. (Reproduced from Mulligan MS et al. *J Clin Invest* 1993;91:577–587; with permission.)

TABLE 5. *Treatment with anti–ICAM-1 mAb reduces clinical disease in the kdkd murine model of autoimmune tubulointerstitial nephritis*

Treatment	n	Mean histologic score (mean ± SD)[a]
Control	3	0.0
Saline	8	3.66 ± 0.23
Rat IgG	7	3.53 ± 0.22
ICAM-1	11	2.09 ± 0.23[b]

Reproduced from Harning R et al. *Clin Immunol Immunopathol* 1992;64:129–134; with permission.

[a] Clinical pathology was measured in a blinded fashion, where 0 = normal kidney and 4 = extensive tubular damage involving greater than 75% of the cortex.

[b] $p < 0.001$ when compared with either saline or rat IgG-treated mice.

merular neutrophil counts (108). These findings underscore the fact that mAbs against leukocyte adhesion molecules may reduce inflammation via mechanisms other than through inhibition of leukocyte–endothelial cell interaction. MAbs against CD11a and ICAM-1 abrogated proteinuria and inhibited crescent formation in two studies of crescentic glomerulonephritis in Wistar-Kyoto rats (110,111), a model characterized by linear deposition of IgG in the glomerular basement membrane, upregulation of ICAM-1 on glomerular endothelium, early infiltration of glomeruli by T-lymphocytes and monocytes/macrophages, crescent formation, and glomerulosclerosis. Importantly, progression of disease was retarded significantly even when treatment was instituted after disease was established (111), an important consideration if such agents are to be useful therapeutically in humans. In contrast to these studies in rats, two different anti-CD18 mAbs failed to protect rabbits against nephrotoxic serum nephritis in rabbits even when administered in doses that saturate CD18 on circulating and glomerular neutrophils, inhibit neutrophil migration to other vascular beds, and attenuate neutrophil-dependent tissue injury in other organs in this species (Table 4).

Administration of anti–ICAM-1 mAbs attenuated leukocyte infiltration, tubular injury, and proteinuria, although not survival, in hereditary autoimmune tubulointerstitial nephritis in the kdkd variant of the CBA/Ca mice (Table 5) (112). These animals have normal kidneys at birth but develop progressive and ultimately lethal tubulointerstitial nephritis beginning after approximately 4 weeks. The disease process is associated with upregulation of ICAM-1 expression in the renal interstitium, on infiltrating leukocytes, and on the basolateral surface of renal tubule epithelium.

Allograft Rejection

In allograft rejection, the initial stimuli for the release of proadhesion inflammatory mediators appear to be reactivity of circulating host antibodies with antigens on allograft endothelium (humoral rejection) and activation of host T cells triggered by interactions with allogeneic MHC molecules. These immune recognition events trigger the release of an array of chemoattractants, cytokines, and chemokines, many of which share stimulation of adhesion as a common bioaction. There is already compelling evidence from studies in experimental models and humans that homotypic and heterotypic leukocyte adhesive interactions are key events in antigen recognition and leukocyte recruitment during allograft rejection (87–95,99–104) and that these interactions are attractive targets for therapeutic intervention (113,114).

Patterns of Expression

The patterns of expression of selectin and Ig-like adhesion molecules in allograft rejection differ from those observed in glomerulonephritis and tubulointerstitial nephritis. The expression of P-selectin or ligands for L-selectin in that setting has not been reported. Variable induction of E-selectin on endothelium has been reported in acute rejection, although this is not a constant finding (93,94). The absence of staining in some patients does not preclude a role for this molecule in leukocyte recruitment because it may reflect the transience of E-selectin expression or extensive endothelial injury. Indeed, focal

TABLE 6. *Influence of prophylactic anti–ICAM-1 mAb on leukocyte infiltration of allografts in nonhuman primates*[a]

Infiltrating cells/10^4 mm^2	Days posttransplant	Mononuclear cells	$CD2^+$ cells	$CD8^+$ cells	$CD4^+$ cells
Controls[b]	7 ± 1	55.6 ± 14.2	27.4 ± 5.3	15.6 ± 4.2	14.0 ± 10.0
(n)		(4)	(4)	(4)	(4)
Anti–ICAM-1	7 ± 1	38.1 ± 16.6	5.3 ± 3.0	3.9 ± 2.8	2.5 ± 2.2
(n)		(8)	(6)	(6)	(6)
p versus control		<0.05	<0.001	<0.001	<0.03

Adapted from Cosimi AB et al. *J Immunol* 1990;144:4604–4612; with permission.

[a] Similar efficacy reported in a phase 1 trial in human renal allograft recipients (Haug CE et al., Transplantation 55: 766–773, 1993).

[b] Treated with nonreactive mAb or no antibody.

absence of PECAM-1, which is constitutively expressed by healthy renal endothelium, has been reported in acute allograft rejection, supporting the latter contention (94).

Glomerular levels of ICAM-1 and VCAM-1 are typically unchanged in acute cellular rejection. In contrast, there is often a striking induction of ICAM-1 on the luminal surface of proximal tubule cells, on some distal tubule and collecting duct cells, and on infiltrating leukocytes (87–95,100). Although ICAM-1 is also induced on vascular endothelium, it is usually more difficult to detect due to the constitutive expression of ICAM-1 at this site or perhaps due to extensive vascular injury and destruction of endothelium. De novo expression of VCAM-1 is usually observed in a focal distribution (30–50% of tubules) toward the basolateral surface of proximal tubule cells and on occasional distal tubules in renal allograft rejection in humans (99–104). In addition, striking induction of VCAM-1 has been reported on the endothelium of peritubular capillaries, venules, and arterioles (104). In a study of 34 renal allograft biopsies, Alpers et al. also noted VCAM-1 expression by some arterial smooth muscle cells and mesangial cells in acute cellular rejection (102). In addition, they reported a small but distinct population of interstitial cells with dendritic morphology that showed focally prominent expression of VCAM-1, nerve growth factor receptor, and CD35. They proposed that VCAM-1–bearing dendritic cells could migrate into host kidney and participate in antigen presentation and cellular rejection process (102). As in the studies of acute glomerulonephritis discussed above, ICAM-1, VCAM-1, and E-selectin expression is usually greatest in areas of leukocyte infiltration, again suggesting that these molecules contribute to the recruitment process.

Efficacy of Antiadhesion Therapy

Several studies have assessed the immunosuppresive and tolerogenic potential of mAbs against different adhesion molecules in vivo. Cosimi et al. observed a marked delay in the onset of renal allograft rejection and increased recipient survival in cynomolgus monkeys when anti–ICAM-1 mAb was used as the sole immunosuppressive agent after transplantation (113). This protective effect of anti–ICAM-1 mAb was associated with partial inhibition of T-lymphocyte (CD2, CD4, and CD8) and monocyte recruitment into the renal interstitium and arterial endothelium, respectively. Anti–ICAM-1 mAbs also reversed established rejection in allograft recipients maintained on subtherapeutic doses of cyclosporine, on this occasion without causing a major change in the intensity of the leukocyte infiltrate. The results of a phase 1 clinical trial of anti–ICAM-1 in high-risk allograft recipients suggests that this mAb also may prevent rejection in humans (114) (Table 6).

Ischemia–Reperfusion

Neutrophils contribute to experimental ischemia–reperfusion injury in many vascular beds, including the pulmonary, coronary, cerebral, and splanchnic circulations. Anti-CD18 mAbs confer protection in many of these models (9). The role of neutrophils and adhesion in renal ischemic–reperfusion injury is less clear (115–121). Several groups have evaluated the role of selectins, integrins, and Ig-like adhesion in ischemic acute renal failure (115–117,120,121). Anti-CD18 alone or CD18 and anti–ICAM-1 did not confer any protection in two studies of renal ischemia–reperfusion in rabbits (Table 4) (120; and Neuringer J, Brady HR, unpublished observations). However, recent reports indicate that anti-CD11/CD18, anti–ICAM-1 and anti–P-selectin antibodies are potent inhibitors of leukocyte recruitment, renal dysfunction, and morphologic injury after renal ischemia in some rat models (Fig. 11) (115–117). Furthermore, ICAM-1 knockout mice are also protected against renal ischemia (121) as exemplified by reduced mortality, better preservation of renal function, and reduced kidney myeloperoxidase activity. The reasons for these varying experiences are unclear, but likely include differences in experimental protocols (e.g., duration and severity of ischemia), species, and spectrum of bioactivities of the mAb. Indeed, neutrophil depletion does not consistently protect the kidney against ischemic injury in many of the commonly used models. ICAM-1 is expressed on the luminal aspect of proximal tubular and some other renal epithelial cells, raising the intriguing possibility that it may serve complex roles in the kidney and regulate processes other than leukocyte recruitment.

Dialysis Membrane Incompatibility

Exposure of circulating blood to new cellulosic hemodialysis membranes frequently results in dramatic changes in CD11/CD18 and L-selectin surface expression on neutrophils and monocytes in association with increased leukocyte adhesiveness. It also may contribute to sequestration of leukocytes in the pulmonary vasculature and systemic granulocytopenia that characterize the dialysis "first-use" syndrome (122–126). In keeping with this hypothesis, granulocytes from normal subjects undergo dramatic degranulation when exposed to cellulosic membranes in vitro, whereas degranulation is markedly attenuated with granulocytes from individuals with LAD-1 disease (125). Initial results suggest that leukocytes are activated by both complement-dependent and -independent pathways in this setting and that leukocyte activation is minimized by using newer biocompatible dialysis membranes.

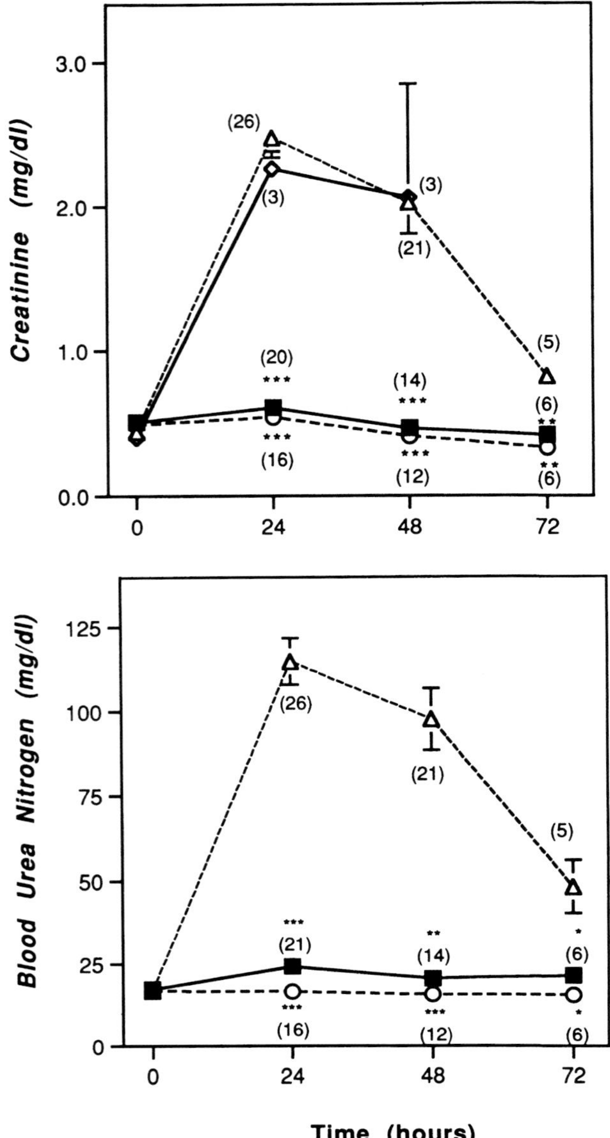

FIG. 11. Influence of anti–ICAM-1 mAb on the course of ischemic acute renal failure in rats. Animals were subjected to sham surgery (open circles), administered vehicle (open triangle), control antibody (open diamonds), or full-strength anti–ICAM-1 mAbs (shaded squares). Plasma creatinine (upper) and BUN (lower) were measured 0, 24, 48, and 72 hr after 30 min of bilateral renal ischemia or sham surgery. *$p < 0.05$; **$p < 0.01$; ***$p < 0.0001$ compared with the vehicle-treated group. Data are means ± SEM. Values in parentheses represent the number of animals studied. (Reproduced from Kelly KJ et al. *Proc Natl Acad Sci U S A* 1994;91:812–816; with permission.)

FUTURE STRATEGIES FOR INHIBITION OF LEUKOCYTE ADHESION IN INFLAMMATORY DISEASES

Soluble Adhesion Receptors

mAbs are of limited use in clinical practice because of their potential immunogenicity and the need for parenteral administration. As discussed above, soluble forms of most selectin and Ig-like adhesion molecules circulate in concentrations that modulate leukocyte–endothelial cell interactions in vitro (36–42,126). There are already encouraging data suggesting that these systems can be manipulated pharmacologically in the treatment of inflammatory disease. Mulligan et al. recently reported dramatic inhibition of neutrophil influx and tissue injury in rats with P-selectin–dependent lung injury who had been treated with soluble SLe^x (127). The efficacy of several other soluble adhesion molecules is presently being assessed.

Antisense Oligonucleotides

Antisense oligonucleotides that hybridize to specific mRNAs for leukocyte adhesion molecules, thereby preventing translation and expression, also hold promise as potential antiadhesion immunotherapy (128–130). Long-lived phosphorothioate antisense oligodeoxynucleotides, in which the phosphodiester backbone has been modified to resist degradation by nucleases, appear particularly attractive in this regard (128). Such nucleotides are potent inhibitors of cytokine-induced endothelial expression of ICAM-1, VCAM-1, and E-selectin expression in vitro and have been demonstrated to block ICAM-1 expression after intravenous injection in vivo (129,130). Interestingly, many phosphorothioate oligonucleotides are concentrated in the kidney and liver, raising the intriguing possibility that they may be particularly suited to treat inflammation in these organs (128). The efficacy and safety of these novel drugs in renal disease will undoubtedly be the focus of intensive investigation in the near future.

Endogenous "Stop Signals" for Leukocyte Recruitment

Most inflammatory responses are self-limiting, raising the possibility that endogenous inhibitors of leukocyte–endothelial cell interactions are generated that act as "stop signals" in inflammatory cascades. Potential candidates in this regard include soluble adhesion receptors, prostacyclin (131), nitric oxide (132,133), IL-4, IL-8, 15-hydroxyeicosatetraenoic acid (15-HETE) (134–138), and lipoxins (72–75,139–143). In the field of nephrology, most attention has focused on the bioactivity of 15-HETE and LXA_4 (139,140)

15-HETE is a lipid-derived eicosanoid, formed via the actions of 15-lipoxygenase, cycooxygenases, and epoxygenases on arachidonic acid, whose levels are frequently elevated in inflammatory tissues or exudates. 15(*S*)-HETE is rapidly esterified into inositol-containing lipids of neutrophil membranes from where it can undergo agonist-induced deacylation and transformation into bioactive products such as lipoxins (137) (Fig. 12). 15(*S*)-HETE–remodeled neutrophils display impaired LTB_4

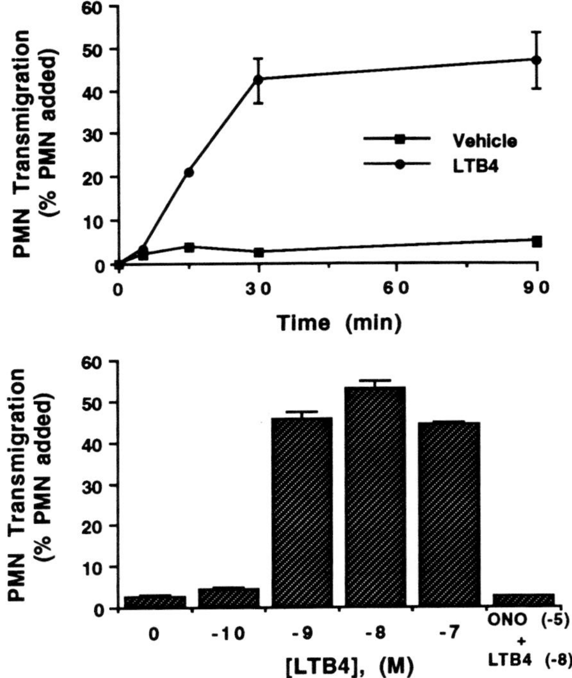

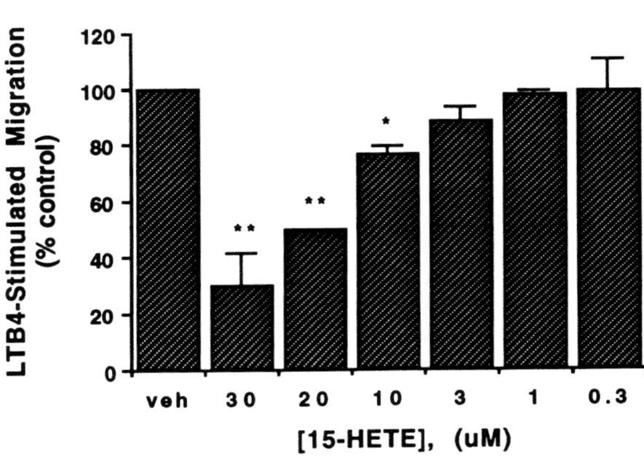

A

FIG. 12. 15(S)-HETE: a potential inhibitor of neutrophil trafficking during inflammation. **Left panel:** Inhibition of LTB_4-induced PMN migration across endothelial monolayers after remodeling of PMN phospholipids with 15(*S*)-HETE. LTB4 provoked rapid (upper graph) and dose-dependent (middle graph) neutrophil transmigration that was almost completely blocked in the presence of a synthetic LTB_4 receptor antagonist (ONO 4057; middle graph) or anti-CD18 mAb (not shown). Esterified 15(*S*)-HETE attenuates neutrophil trafficking by causing a striking reduction in the affinity of LTB_4 cell surface receptors for their ligand and inhibition of LTB_4-triggered stimulus–response coupling. As a result of these actions, esterified 15(*S*)-HETE attenuated the cytoskeletal rearrangements and CD11/CD18–mediated adhesive events (not shown) that subserve directed locomotion of neutrophils across endothelium (lower graph). (Reprinted from Takata S et al. *J Clin Invest* 1994;93: 499–508; with permission.) **Lower panel:** Potential mechanisms by which 15(*S*)-HETE modulates neutrophil responsiveness to receptor-triggered inflammatory stimuli. 15(*S*)-HETE is rapidly esterified into neutrophil cell membrane phospholipids, where it can directly influence receptor function or coupling. In addition, 15(*S*)-HETE may influence cell function after release from esterified stores or after subsequent transformation of deacylated 15(*S*)-HETE to other bioactive lipoxygenase products such as lipoxins. (Reprinted from Takano T, Brady HR. *Curr Opin Nephrol Hypertens* 1995;4: 277–286; with permission.)

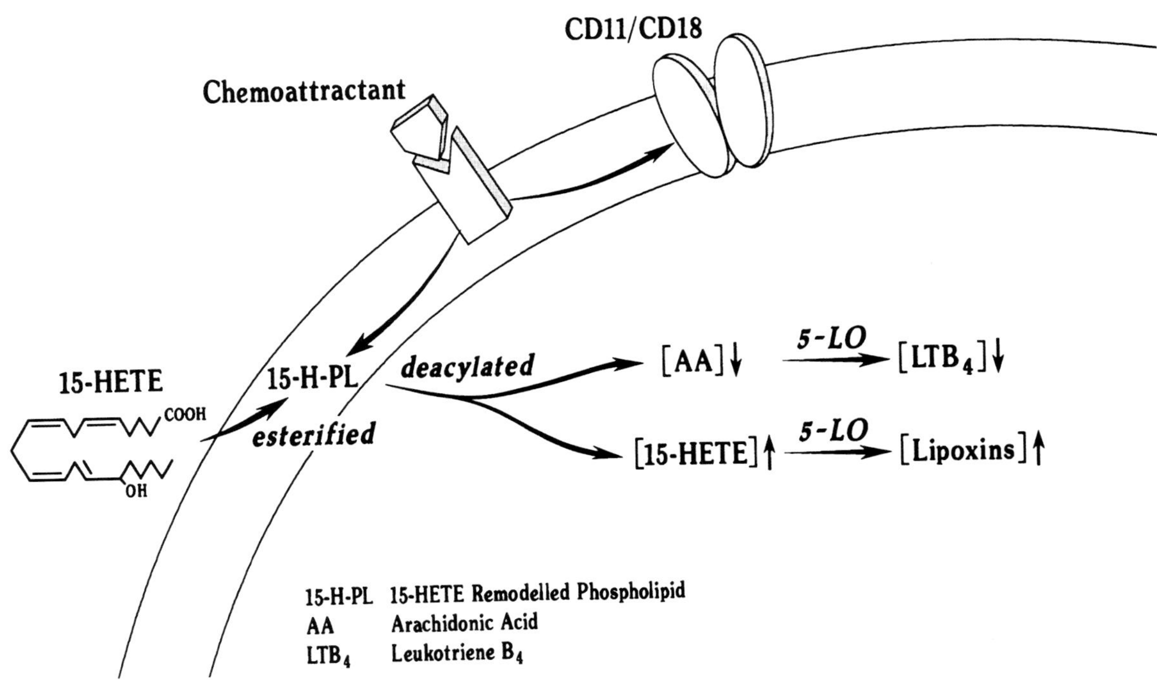

B

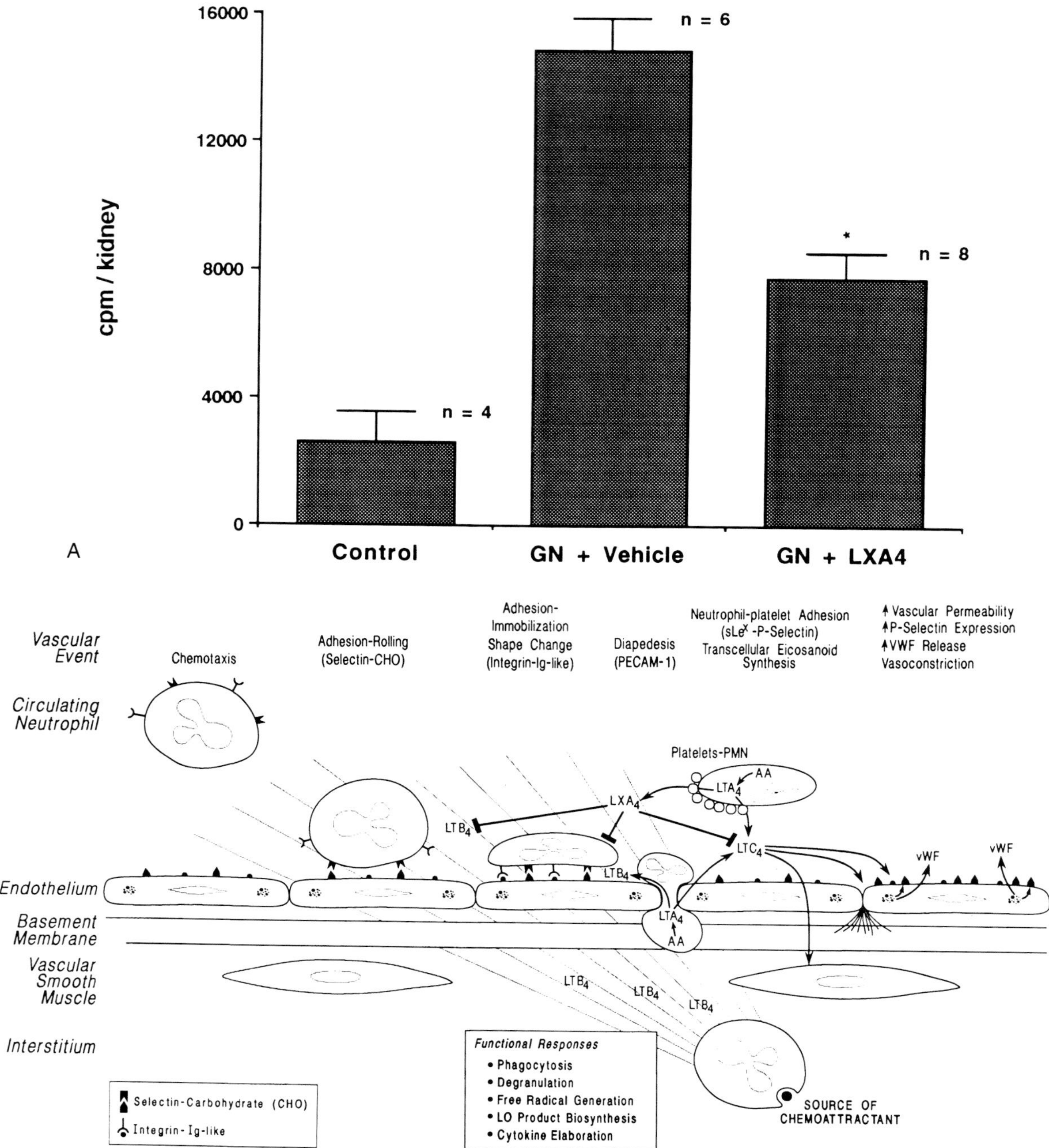

FIG. 13. Modulation of neutrophil recruitment in experimental glomerulonephritis by LXA_4. **Upper panel:** Prior exposure of radiolabeled neutrophils to LXA_4 ex vivo significantly blunted their recruitment to inflammed glomeruli in the Con A–ferritin model of immune complex glomerulonephritis. This outcome supports the contention that lipoxins may represent an endogenous "stop signal" that may contribute to the suppression of neutrophil-mediated tissue injury. (Reprinted from Papayianni A et al. *Kidney Int* 1995;47:1295–1302; with permission.) **Lower panel:** Theoretical scheme depicting some sites at which leukotrienes and lipoxins regulate neutrophil trafficking. LTB_4 is a potent stimulus for neutrophil (PMN) chemotaxis, β_2 integrin–mediated PMN adhesion, and diapedesis, whereas the peptidoleukotrienes LTC_4 and LTD_4 promote increased plasma exudation, endothelial P-selectin expression, adhesiveness for PMN, and vasoconstriction. Lipoxins antagonize the adhesion-promoting actions of LTB_4 and peptidoleukotrienes in vitro via distinct actions with neutrophils and endothelial cells, respectively. In addition, LXA_4 and LXB_4 are potent vasodilators and antagonize the vasoconstrictive actions of peptidoleukotrienes. [Reprinted from Brady HR et al. *Trends Cardiovasc Med* 1995 (in press); with permission.]

formation upon activation and blunted neutrophil chemotaxis, adhesion, and transmigration responses in response to C5a, fMLP, PAF, and/or LTB_4 (134–136). This inhibitory action of 15(*S*)-HETE is stereoselective and mediated in part through attenuation of signal transduction responses within neutrophil cell membranes (134,135). Treatment of glomeruli, isolated from rats with nephrotoxic serum nephritis, with 15(*S*)-HETE also results in impaired LTB_4 production, and neutrophils exposed to 15(*S*)-HETE ex vivo display impaired migration to inflamed glomeruli in vivo (136).

Several lines of evidence suggest that lipoxins and leukotrienes evoke opposing actions on leukocyte-endothelial cell interactions in a manner akin to the regulation of platelet aggregation and vascular tone by thromboxane and prostacyclin. LXA_4 and LXB_4 are potent inhibitors of leukotriene-induced neutrophil chemotaxis and of neutrophil adhesion to endothelial cells supported by neutrophil β_2 integrins and endothelial P-selectin in vitro. In addition, LXA_4 attenuates leukotriene-stimulated neutrophil margination and diapedesis in the hamster cheek pouch in vivo (143). As discussed above, LXA_4 is generated in abundance during P-selectin–dependent adhesive interactions in experimental Con A–ferritin glomerulonephritis in vivo (Fig. 8) (74). Prior exposure of radiolabeled neutrophils to nanomolar concentrations of LXA_4 ex vivo retards their recruitment to inflamed glomeruli in this model (Fig. 13), supporting a potential role for these lipoxins as endogenous inhibitors of neutrophil recruitment. Along these lines, neutrophil recruitment and renal injury is exaggerated in P-selectin–deficient mice, compared with wild-type mice, during nephrotoxic serum nephritis in association with reduced LXA_4 generation (60). Transfusion of null mice with wild-type platelets that express P-selectin rescues LXA_4 generation in this setting and approximates glomerular neutrophil infiltration in P-selectin–deficient and wild-type animals. Thus, the interaction of platelets and neutrophils, which are well-defined proinflammatory cells early in the course of glomerular injury (144), can also initiate formation of lipid-derived mediators that potentially limit neutrophil-mediated renal injury as inflammation progresses (74).

If lipoxins are confirmed to be important inhibitors of neutrophil recruitment, it will be intriguing to define the molecular switches that convert an inflammatory milieu from a proadhesive to an antiadhesive phenotype. Several regulatory mechanisms have been defined that may amplify lipoxin biosynthesis. Transcellular lipoxin biosynthesis through platelet–neutrophil circuits is augmented by some cytokines (GM-CSF, PDGF) (145), disruption of platelet cell membrane, and changes in cell redox potential that depletes glutathione levels, as occurs during oxidant stress due to local ischemia or leukocyte-derived radicals (75). In addition, two T cell–derived cytokines, IL-4 and IL-13, that are upregulated in glomerulonephritic kidneys induce 15-lipoxygenase gene expression and enzyme activity and may promote differential augmentation of lipoxin production as inflammation evolves (146–149). Definitive proof that lipoxins play a pivotal role in the stop programs of host defense and inflammation will require the development of specific approaches for inhibition of lipoxin biosynthesis and/or bioactivity. Pharmacologic manipulation of these negative feedback loops may lead to the development of novel anti-inflammatory agents that are more specific and less toxic than those currently available.

ACKNOWLEDGEMENT

Dr. Hébert is the recipient of a Postdoctoral Fellowship from the Medical Research Council of Canada. Dr. Brady is supported by National Institutes of Health Grant DK44380 and an award from the Research Advisory Group of the Department of Veterans Affairs.

REFERENCES

1. Dutrochet MH. *Recherches anatomiques et physiologiques sur la structure intime des animaux et des végétaux, et sur leur motilité.* Paris: Baillière et Fils; 1824.
2. Metschnikoff E. Sur la lutte des cellules de l'organisme contre l'invasion des microbes. *Ann Institut Pasteur* 1887;1:321–336.
3. Eddy AA, Michael AF. Immunopathogenetic mechanisms of glomerular injury. In: Tisher CC, Brenner BM, eds. *Renal pathology.* Philadelphia: JB Lippincott; 1989:111–155.
4. Couser WG. Mediation of glomerular immune injury. *J Am Soc Nephrol* 1990;1:13–29.
5. Brady HR. Leukocyte adhesion molecules and kidney diseases. *Kidney Int* 1994;45:1285–1300.
6. Springer TA. Adhesion receptors of the immune system. *Cell* 1994; 76:301–314.
7. Carlos TM, Harlan JM. Leukocyte-endothelial adhesion molecules. *Blood* 1994;84:2068–2101.
8. Brady HR. Leukocyte adhesion molecules: potential targets for therapeutic intervention in kidney diseases. *Curr Opin Nephrol Hypertens* 1993;2:171–182.
9. Harlan JM, Liu DY, eds. *Adhesion: its role in inflammatory disease.* New York: Freeman; 1992.
10. Bevilacqua MP, Nelson RM. Selectins. *J Clin Invest* 1993;91:379–387.
11. Lasky LA. Selectins: interpreters of cell-specific carbohydrate information during inflammation. *Science* 1992;258:964–969.
12. Bevilacqua M, Butcher E, Furie B, et al. Selectins: a family of adhesion receptors. *Cell* 1991;67:233.
13. Lobb RR, Hemler ME. The pathophysiologic role of $\alpha4$ integrins in vivo. *J Clin Invest* 1994;94:1722–1728.
14. Arnaout MA. Structure and function of leukocyte adhesion molecules CD11/CD18. *Blood* 1990;75:1037–1050.
15. Spertini O, Luscinskas FW, Gimbrone MA, Tedder TF. Monocyte attachment to activated human vascular endothelium in vitro is mediated by leukocyte adhesion molecule-1 (L-selectin) under nonstatic conditions. *J Exp Med* 1992;175:1789–1792.
16. Brady HR, Spertini O, Jimenez W, Brenner BM, Marsden PA, Tedder TF. Neutrophils, monocytes, and lymphocytes bind to cytokine-activated kidney glomerular endothelial cells through L-selectin (LAM-1) in vitro. *J Immunol* 1992;149:2437–2444.
17. Varki A. Selectin ligands. *Proc Natl Acad Sci U S A* 1994;91:7390–7397.
18. Shimizu Y, Shaw S. Mucins in the mainstream. *Nature* 1993;366: 630–631.
19. Briskin MJ, McEvoy LM, Butcher EC. MadCAM-1 has homology to immunoglobulin and mucin-like adhesion receptors and to IgA1. *Nature* 1993;363:461–466.

20. Lasky LA, Singer MS, Dowbenko D, et al. An endothelial ligand for L-selectin is a novel mucin-like molecule. *Cell* 1992;69:927–938.
21. Imai Y, Lasky LA, Rosen SD. Sulphation requirement for GlyCAM-1, an endothelial ligand for L-selectin. *Nature* 1993;361:555–557.
22. Berg EL, McEvoy LM, Berlin C, Bargatze RF, Butcher EC. L-selectin–mediated lymphocyte rolling on MadCAM-1. *Nature* 1993; 366:695–698.
23. Sako D, Chang XJ, Barone KM, et al. Expression cloning of a functional glycoprotein ligand for P-selectin. *Cell* 1993;75:1179–1186.
24. Barone KM, Pittman D, Shaw G. Structure/function studies of P-selectin glycoprotein ligand (PSGL-1) [Abstract]. *J Cell Biochem* 1994;18(suppl):290.
25. Steegmaler M, Levinovitz A, Isenmann S, et al. The E-selectin-ligand ESL-1 is a variant of a receptor for fibroblast growth factor. *Nature* 1995;373:615–620.
26. Arnaout MA. Leukocyte adhesion molecules deficiency: its structural basis, pathophysiology and implications for modulating the inflammatory response. *Immunol Rev* 1990;114:145–180.
27. Rabb H, Rosen R, Ramirez G. VLA-4 and its ligands: relevance to kidney diseases. *Springer Semin Immunopathol* 1995;16:417–425.
28. Andrew DP, Butcher EC. Subpopulations of B and T lymphocytes express CD11b/CD18 and are capable of CD11b/CD18 mediated adhesion [Abstract]. *J Cell Biochem* 1994;18(suppl):294.
29. Brady HR, Lamas S, Papayianni A, Takata S, Matsubara M, Marsden PA. Lipoxygenase product formation and cell adhesion during neutrophil-glomerular endothelial cell interaction. *Am J Physiol* 1995; 268:F1–F12.
30. Stade BG, Messer G, Riethmuller G, Johnson JP. Structural characteristics of the 58 region of the human ICAM-1 gene. *Immunobiology* 1990;182:79–87.
31. Cybulsky MI, Fries JW, William AJ, et al. Alternate splicing of human VCAM-1 in activated vascular endothelium. *Am J Pathol* 1991;138:815–820.
32. Cybulski MI, Fries JW, Williams AJ, et al. Gene structure, chromosomal location and basis for alternative splicing of the human VCAM-1 gene. *Proc Natl Acad Sci U S A* 1991;88:7859–7863.
33. Osborn L, Hession C, Tizard R, et al. Direct expression cloning of vascular cell adhesion molecule-1, a cytokine-induced endothelial protein that binds to lymphocytes. *Cell* 1989;59:1203–1211.
34. Muller WA, Weigl SA, Deng X, Phillips DM. PECAM-1 is required for transendothelial migration of leukocytes. *J Exp Med* 1993;178: 449–460.
35. Vaporciyan AA, DeLisser HM, Yan H-C, et al. Involvement of platelet–endothelial cell adhesion molecule-1 in neutrophil recruitment in vivo. *Science* 1993;262:1580–1582.
36. Gearing AJH, Newman W. Circulating adhesion molecules in disease. *Immunol Today* 1993;14:506–512.
37. Seth R, Raymond FD, Makgoba MW. Circulating ICAM-1 isoforms; diagnostic prospects for inflammatory and immune disorders. *Lancet* 1991;338:83–84.
38. Rothlein R, Mainolfi EA, Czajkowski M, Marlin SD. A form of circulating ICAM-1 in human serum. *J Immunol* 1991;147:3788–3793.
39. Yokoyama H, Tomosugi N, Takaeda M, et al. Glomerular expression of cellular adhesion molecules and serum TNF alpha and soluble ICAM-1 levels in human glomerulonephritis [Abstract]. *J Am Soc Nephrol* 1992;3:669.
40. Stockenhuber F, Kramer G, Schenn G, et al. Circulating ICAM-1: novel parameter of renal graft rejection. *Transplant Proc* 1993;25: 919–920.
41. Bechtel U, Scheuer R, Landgraf R, Konig A, Feucht HE. Assessment of soluble adhesion molecules (sICAM-1, sVCAM-1, sELAM-1) and complement cleavage products (sC4d, sC5b-9) in urine. Clinical monitoring of renal allograft recipients. *Transplantation* 1994;58: 905–911.
42. Higgins JR, Papayianni A, Brady HR, Darling M, Walshe JJ. Circulating adhesion molecules in toxemia, gestational hypertension and normal pregnancy: evidence for selective dysregulation of VCAM-1 homeostasis in pre-eclampsia [Abstract]. *J Am Soc Nephrol* 195;67: 660.
43. Takano T, Brady HR. The endothelium in glomerular inflammation. *Curr Opin Nephrol Hypertens* 1995;4:277–286.
44. Pober JS, Cotran RS. Cytokines and endothelial cell biology. *Physiol Rev* 1990;70:427–451.
45. Briscoe DM, Cotran RS. Role of leukocyte-endothelial cell adhesion molecules in renal inflammation: in vitro and in vivo studies. *Kidney Int* 1993;44(suppl):27–36.
46. Brady HR, Persson U, Ballermann BJ, Brenner BM, Serhan CN. Leukotrienes stimulate neutrophil adhesion to mesangial cells: modulation with lipoxins. *Am J Physiol* 1990;259:F809–F815.
47. Brady HR, Denton MD, Brenner BM, Serhan CN. Neutrophil adhesion to glomerular mesangial cells: regulation by lipoxygenase-derived eicosanoids. In: Wong PK-Y, Serhan CN, eds. *Cell–cell interaction in the release of inflammatory mediators.* New York: Plenum; 1992:347–359.
48. Weissman G. The role of neutrophils in vascular injury: a summary of signal transduction mechanisms in cell/cell interactions. *Springer Semin Immunopathol* 1989;11:235–258.
49. Myers CL, Desai SN, Schembri-King J, Letts GL, Wallace RW. Discriminatory effects of protein kinase inhibitors and calcium ionophore on endothelial ICAM-1 induction. *Am J Physiol* 1992;262:C365–C373.
50. Marsden PA, Cybulsky Mi, Brenner BM, Brady HR. Regulated expression of vascular cell adhesion molecule (VCAM-1) in human glomerular mesangial cells [Abstract]. *J Am Soc Nephrol* 1991;2:553.
51. Neish AS, Williams AJ, Palmer HJ, Whitley MA, Collins T. Functional analysis of the human vascular cell adhesion molecule-1 (VCAM-1) promoter. *J Exp Med* 1992;176:1583–1593.
52. Shu HB, Agranoff AB, Nabel EG, et al. Differential regulation of VCAM-1 gene expression by specific NFkB subunits in endothelial and epithelial cells. *Mol Cell Biol* 1993;13:6283–6289.
53. Collins T. Endothelial nuclear factor-kappa B and the initiation of the atherosclerotic lesion. *Lab Invest* 1993;68:499–508.
54. Etzioni A, Frydman M, Pollack S, et al. Recurrent severe infections caused by a novel leukocyte adhesion deficiency. *N Engl J Med* 1992; 327:1789–1792.
55. Mayadas TN, Johnson RC, Rayburn H, Hynes RO, Wagner DD. Leukocyte rolling and extravasation are severely compromised in P selectin–deficient mice. *Cell* 1993;74:541–554.
56. Arbones ML, Ord DC, Ley K, et al. Lymphocyte homing and leukocyte rolling and migration are impaired in L-selectin–deficient mice. *Immunity* 1994;1:247–260.
57. Labow MA, Norton CR, Rumberger JM, et al. Characterization of E-selectin–deficient mice: demonstration of overlapping function of the endothelial selectins. *Immunity* 1994;1:709–720.
58. Xu H, Gonzalo JA, St. Pierre Y, et al. Leukocytosis and resistance to septic shock in intercellular adhesion molecule 1–deficient mice. *J Exp Med* 1994;180:95–109.
59. Gurtner GC, Davis V, Li H, McCoy MJ, Sharpe A, Cybulsky MI. Targeted disruption of the murine VCAM1 gene: essential role of VCAM-1 in chorioallantoic fusion and placentation. *Genes Dev* 1995;9:1–14.
60. Mayadas TN, Mendrick DL, Brady HR et al. Acute passive anti-glomerular basement membrane nephritis in P-selectin-deficient-mice. *Kidney Int.* 1996;49:1342–1349.
61. Tedder TF, Steeber DA, Pizcueta P. L-selectin–deficient mice have impaired leukocyte recruitment into inflammatory sites. *J Exp Med* 1995;181:2259–2264.
62. Subramaniam M, Saffaripour S, Watson SR, Mayadas TN, Hynes RO, Wagner DD. Reduced recruitment of inflammatory cells in a contact hypersensitivity response in P-selectin–deficient mice. *J Exp Med* 1995:181;2277–2282.
63. Guinan EC, Gribben JG, Boussiotis VA, Freeman GJ, Nadler LM. Pivotal role of the B7:CD28 pathway in transplantation tolerance and tumor immunity. *Blood* 1994;84:3261–3282.
64. Epperson DE, Pober JS. Antigen-presenting function of human endothelial cells; direct activation of resting CD8 T cells. *J Immunol* 1994; 153:5402–5412.
65. Brennan DC, Jevnikar AM, Takei F, Reubin-Kelley V. Mesangial cell accessory functions: mediation by intercellular adhesion molecule-1. *Kidney Int* 1990;38:1039–1046.
66. Kelley VE, Jevnikar AM. Antigen presentation by renal tubular epithelial cells. *J Am Soc Nephrol* 1991;2:13–26.
67. Suranyi MG, Bishop GA, Clayberger C, et al. Lymphocyte adhesion molecules in T-cell mediated lysis of human kidney cells. *Kidney Int* 1991;39:312–319.
68. Nathan C, Srimal S, Farber C, et al. Cytokine-induced respiratory burst of human neutrophils: dependence on extracellular matrix proteins and CD11/CD18 integrins. *J Cell Biol* 1989;109:1341–1349.
69. Denton MD, Marsden PA, Luscinskas FW, Brenner BM, Brady HR. Cytokine-induced phagocyte adhesion to human mesangial cells: role

of CD11/CD18 integrins and ICAM-1. *Am J Physiol* 1991;261: F1071–F1079.
70. Brady HR, Denton MD, Jimenez W, Takata S, Palliser D, Brenner BM. Chemoattractants provoke monocyte adhesion to human mesangial cells and mesangial cell injury via CD11/CD18–ICAM-1 dependent and independent mechanisms. *Kidney Int* 1992;42:480–487.
71. Brady HR, Serhan CN. Adhesion promotes transcellular leukotriene biosynthesis during neutrophil–glomerular endothelial cell interactions: inhibition by anti-CD18 and L-selectin monoclonal antibodies. *Biochem Biophys Res Commun* 1992;186:1307–1314.
72. Brady HR, Papayianni A, Serhan CN. Leukocyte adhesion promotes lipoxygenase product biosynthesis by transcellular routes. *Kidney Int* 1994;45:590–597.
73. Brady HR, Papayianni A, Serhan CN. Transcellular pathways and cell adhesion as potential contributors to leukotriene and lipoxin biosynthesis in acute glomerulonephritis. *Adv Exp Med Biol* (in press).
74. Papayianni A, Serhan CN, Phillips ML, Rennke HG, Brady HR. Transcellular biosynthesis of lipoxin A_4 during adhesion of platelets and neutrophils in experimental immune complex glomerulonephritis. *Kidney Int* 1995;47:1295–1302.
75. Serhan CN. Lipoxin biosynthesis and its impact in inflammatory and vascular events. *Biochim Biophys Acta* 1994;1212:1–25.
76. Redl H, Dinges HP, Buurman WA, et al. Expression of endothelial leukocyte adhesion molecule-1 in septic but not traumatic/hypovolemic shock in the baboon. *Am J Pathol* 1991;139:461–466.
77. Laszik Z, Nadasdy T, Johnson D, Lerner M, Smith W, Brackett D. Transient expression of ELAM-1 in endotoxin and *E. coli*–induced septic shock in rat kidney [Abstract]. *J Am Soc Nephrol* 1992;3:601.
78. Nikolic-Paterson DJ, Yu Y, Atkins RC. Regulation of glomerular VCAM-1 and ELAM-1 gene expression by inflammatory stimuli [Abstract]. *J Am Soc Nephrol* 1992;3:639–688
79. Bishop GA, Hall BM. Expression of leukocyte and lymphocyte adhesion molecules in the human kidney. *Kidney Int* 1989;36:1078–1085.
80. Muller GA, Markovic-Lipkovski J, Muller CA. Intercellular adhesion molecule-1 expression in human kidneys with glomerulonephritis. *Clin Nephrol* 1991;36:203–208.
81. Lhotta K, Neumayer HP, Joannidis M, Geissler D, Konig P. Renal expression of intercellular adhesion molecule-1 in different forms of glomerulonephritis. *Clin Sci* 1991;81:477–481.
82. Markovic-Lipkovski J, Muller CA, Risler T, Bohle A, Muller GA. Mononuclear leukocytes, expression of HLA class II antigens and intercellular adhesion molecule-1 in focal segmental glomerulosclerosis. *Nephron* 1991;58:286–293.
83. Dal Canton A, Fuiano G, Sepe V, Caglioti A, Ferrone S. Mesangial expression of intercellular adhesion molecule-1 in primary glomerulosclerosis. *Kidney Int* 1992;41:951–955.
84. Waldherr R, Eberlein-Gonska M, Noronha IL, Andrassy K, Ritz E. TNFα and ICAM-1 expression in renal disease. *Transplantation* 1993;56(4):1026–9.
85. Fuiano G, Sepe V, Ferrone S, et al. Expression of intercellular adhesion molecule-1 in necrotizing glomerulonephritis [Abstract]. *J Am Soc Nephrol* 1990;1:560.
86. Wuthrich RP, Jevnikar AM, Takei F, Glimcher LH, Kelley VE. Intercellular adhesion molecule-1 expression is upregulated in autoimmune murine lupus nephritis. *Am J Pathol* 1990;136:441–450.
87. Faull RJ, Russ GR. Tubular expression of intercellular adhesion molecule-1 during renal allograft rejection. *Transplantation* 1989;48: 226–230.
88. Kanagawa K, Ishikura H, Takahashi C, et al. Identification of ICAM-1 positive cells in the nongrafted and transplanted rat kidney: an immunohistochemical and ultrastructural study. *Transplantation* 1991; 52:1057–1062.
89. Matsuno T, Sakagami K, Saito S, et al. Expression of intercellular adhesion molecule-1 and perforin on kidney allograft rejection. *Transplant Proc* 1992;34:1306–1307.
90. Yoshizawa N, Oda T, Nakamura H. Expression of intercellular adhesion molecule-1 and HLA-DR by tubular cells and immune cell infiltration in human renal allografts. *Transplant Proc* 1992;24: 1308–1309.
91. Moolenaar W, Bruijn JA, Schrama E, et al. T-cell receptors and ICAM-1 expression in renal allografts during rejection. *Transplant Int* 1991;4:140–145.
92. Andersen CB, Blaehr H, Ladenfoged S, Larsen S. Expression of intercellular adhesion molecule-1 in human renal allografts and cultured human tubular cells. *Nephrol Dial Transplant* 1992;7:147–154.
93. Brockmeyer C, Ulbrecht M, Schendel DJ, et al. Distribution of cell adhesion molecules (ICAM-1, VCAM-1, ELAM-1) in renal tissue during allograft rejection. *Transplantation* 1993;55:610–615.
94. Fuggle SV, Sanderson JB, Gray DWR, Richardson A, Morris PJ. Variation in expression of endothelial adhesion molecules in pretransplant and transplanted kidneys—correlation with intragraft events. *Transplantation* 1993;55:117–123.
95. von Willebrand E, Loginov R, Salmela K, Isoniemi H, Hayry P. Relationship between intercellular adhesion molecule-1 and HLA class II expression in acute cellular rejection of human kidney allografts. *Transplant Proc* 1993;25:870–871.
96. Hill PA, Lan HY, Nikolic-Paterson DJ, Atkins RC. ICAM-1 directs migration and localization of interstitial leukocytes in experimental glomerulonephritis. *Kidney Int* 1994;45:32–42.
97. Seron D, Cameron JS, Haskard DO: Expression of VCAM-1 in the normal and diseased kidney. *Nephrol Dial Transplant* 1991;6: 917–922.
98. Wuthrich RP, Snyder TL. Vascular cell adhesion molecule-1 (VCAM-1) expression in murine lupus nephritis. *Kidney Int* 1992;42: 903–914.
99. Briscoe DM, Pober JS, Harmon HE, Cotran RS. Expression of vascular cell adhesion molecule-1 in human renal allografts. *J Am Soc Nephrol* 1992;3:1180–1185.
100. Wuthrich RP. Intercellular adhesion molecules and vascular cell adhesion molecule-1 and the kidney. *J Am Soc Nephrol* 1992;3: 1201–1211.
101. Lin Y, Kirby JA, Clark K, et al. Renal allograft rejection: induction and function of adhesion molecules on cultured epithelial cells. *Clin Exp Immunol* 1992;90:111–116.
102. Alpers CE, Hudkins KL, Davis CL, et al. Expression of vascular cell adhesion molecule-1 in kidney allograft rejection. *Kidney Int* 1993; 44:805–816.
103. Lin Y, Kirby JA, Browell DA, Morley AR, Stenton BK, Proud G, Taylor RM. Renal allograft rejection: expression and function of VCAM-1 on tubular epithelial cells. *Clin Exp Immunol* 1993;92: 145–151.
104. Hill PA, Main IW, Atkins RC. ICAM-1 and VCAM-1 in human renal allograft rejection. *Kidney Int* 1995;47:1383–1391.
105. Ewert BW, Becker M, Jennette JC, Falk RJ. Anti-myeloperoxidase antibodies stimulate neutrophils to adhere to cultured human endothelial cells utilizing the beta-2 integrin CD11/CD18 [Abstract]. *J Am Soc Nephrol* 1992;3:585.
106. Tipping PG, Huang XR, Berndt MC, Holdsworth SR. A role for P-selectin in complement-independent neutrophil-mediated glomerular injury. *Kidney Int* 1994;46:79–88.
107. Mulligan MS, Johnson KJ, Todd RF III, et al. Requirements for leukocyte adhesion molecules in nephrotoxic serum nephritis. *J Clin Invest* 1993;91:577–587.
108. Wu X, Pippin J, Lefkowith JB. Attenuation of immune-mediated glomerulonephritis with an anti-CD11b monoclonal antibody. *Am J Physiol* 1993;264:F715–F721.
109. Wada J, Makino H, Shikata K, et al. Role of intercellular adhesion molecule-1 in nephrotoxic serum nephritis [Abstract]. *J Am Soc Nephrol* 1992;3:647.
110. Kawasaki K, Yaoita E, Yamamoto T, Tamatani T, Miyasaki M, Kihara I. Antibodies against intercellular adhesion molecule-1 and lymphocyte function–associated antigen-1 prevent glomerular injury in rat experimental crescentic glomerulonephritis. *J Immunol* 1993; 150:1074–1083.
111. Nishikawa K, Guo Y-J, Miyasaki M, et al. Antibodies to ICAM-1/LFA-1 prevent crescent formation in rat autoimmune glomerulonephritis. *J Exp Med* 1993;177:667–677.
112. Harning R, Pelletier J, Van G, Takei F, Merluzzi VJ. Monoclonal antibody to ICAM-1 reduces acute autoimmune nephritis in kdkd mice. *Clin Immunol Immunopathol* 1992;64:129–134.
113. Cosimi AR, Conti D, Delmonico FL, et al. In vivo effects of monoclonal antibody to ICAM-1 (CD54) in nonhuman primates with renal allografts. *J Immunol* 1990;144:4604–4612.
114. Tolkoff-Rubin N, Rothlein R, Scharschmidt L, et al. A phase I trial of immunosuppression with anti–ICAM-1 (CD54) mAb in renal allograft recipients. *Transplantation* 1993;55:766–773.
115. Kelly KI, Williams WW, Colvin RB, Bonventre JV. Antibody to

intercellular adhesion molecule-1 protects the kidney against ischemia. *Proc Natl Acad Sci U S A* 1994;91:812–816.
116. Rabb H, Mendiola C, Saba SR, et al. Antibodies to P-selectin and ICAM-1 protect kidneys from ischemic-reperfusion injury. *J Am Soc Nephrol* 1994;5:907.
117. Rabb H, Mendiola CC, Saba SR, et al. Antibodies to ICAM-1 protect kidneys in severe ischemic reperfusion injury. *Biochem Biophys Res Commun* 1995;211:67–73.
118. Linas SL, Shanley PF, Whittenburg D, Berger R, Repine JE. Neutrophils accentuate ischemia–reperfusion injury in isolated perfused rat kidneys. *Am J Physiol* 1988;255:F728–F735.
119. Hellberg PO, Kallskog TO. Neutrophil-mediated post-ischemic tubular leakage in the rat kidney. *Kidney Int* 1989;36:555–561.
120. Thornton MN, Winn R, Alpers CE, Zager R. An evaluation of the neutrophil as a mediator of in vivo renal ischemic-reperfusion injury. *Am J Pathol* 1989;135:509–515.
121. Kelly KJ, Williams WW, Colvin RB, et al. Intercellular adhesion molecules-1 (ICAM-1) knock-out mice are protected against renal ischemia. *J Am Soc Nephrol* 1994;5:900.
122. Arnaout MA, Hakim RM, Todd RF III, Dana N, Colten HR. Increased expression of an adhesion-promoting surface glycoprotein in the granulocytopenia of hemodialysis. *N Engl J Med* 1985;312:458–462.
123. Cheung AK, Hohnholt M, Gilson J. Adherence of neutrophils to hemodialysis membranes: role of complement receptors. *Kidney Int* 1991;40:1123–1133.
124. Himmelfarb J, Zaoui P, Hakim R. Modulation of granulocyte LAM-1 and Mac-1 during dialysis—a prospective randomized control trial. *Kidney Int* 1992;41:388–395.
125. Cheung AK, Parker CJ, Hohnholt M. β2 integrins are required for neutrophil degranulation induced by hemodialysis membranes. *Kidney Int* 1993;43:649–660.
126. Rabb H, Agosti SJ, Bittle PA, Fernandez M, Ramirez G, Tedder T. Alterations in soluble and leukocyte surface L-selectin (CD 62L) in hemodialysis patients. *American Journal of Kidney Disease* 1996;27 (2):239–243.
127. Mulligan MS, Paulson JC, Frees SD, Zheng Z-L, Lowe JB, Ward PA. Protective effects of oligosaccharides in P-selectin–dependent lung injury. *Nature* 1993;364:149–151.
128. Rappaport J, Hanss B, Kopp JB, et al. Transport of phosphorathioate oligonucleotides in kidney: implications for molecular therapy. *Kidney Int* 1995;47:1462–1469.
129. Bennett CF, Condon TP, Grimm S, Chan H, Chiang M-Y. Inhibition of endothelial cell adhesion molecules expression with antisense oligonucleotides. *J Immunol* 1994;152:3530–3540.
130. Chiang M-Y, Chan H, Zounes MA, Freier SM, Lima WF, Bennett CF. Antisense oligonucleotides inhibit intercellular adhesion molecule 1 expression by two distinct mechanisms. *J Biol Chem* 1991;266: 18162–18171.
131. Boxer LA, Allen JM, Schmidt M, Yoder M, Baehner RL. Inhibition of polymorphonuclear leukocyte adherence by prostacyclin. *J Lab Clin Med* 1980;95:672–678.
132. Kubes P, Suzuki M, Granger DN. Nitric oxide: an endogenous modulator of leukocyte adhesion. *Proc Natl Acad Sci U S A* 1991;88: 4651–4655.
133. Matsubara M, Takata S, Jimenez W, Marsden PA, Brenner BM, Brady HR. Endothelial cell–derived nitric oxide limits neutrophil migration across TNF-activated endothelial cell monolayers [Abstract]. *J Am Soc Nephrol* 1992;3:547.
134. Takata S, Papayianni A, Matsubara M, Jimenez W, Pronovost PH, Brady H. 15-Hydroxyeicosatetraenoic acid inhibits neutrophil migration across cytokine-activated endothelium. *Am J Physiol* 1994;145: 541–549.
135. Takata S, Matsubara M, Allen PG, Janmey PA, Serhan CN, Brady HR. Remodeling of neutrophil phospholipids with 15(S)-hydroxyeicosatetraenoic acid inhibits leukotriene B4-induced neutrophil migration across endothelium. *J Clin Invest* 1994;93:499–508.
136. Fischer DB, Chiristman JW, Badr K. Fifteen-S-hydroxyeicosatetraenoic acid (15-S-HETE) specifically antagonizes the chemotactic action and glomerular systhesis of leukotriene B_4 in the rat. *Kidney Int* 1992;41:1155–1160.
137. Brezinski ME, Serhan CN. Selective incorporation of (15S)-hydroxyeicosatetraenoic acid in phosphatidylinositol of human neutrophils: agonist-induced deacylation and transformation of stored hydroxyeicosanoids. *Proc Natl Acad Sci U S A* 1990;87:6248–6252.
138. Spector AA, Gordon JA, Moore SA. Hydroxyeicosatetraenoic acids. *Prog Lipid Res* 1988;27:271–323.
139. Brady HR, Papayianni A, Serhan CN. Potential vascular roles for lipoxins in the "stop program" of host defense and inflammation. *Trends Cardiovasc Med* 1995;5:186–192.
140. Badr KF. 15-Lipoxygenase products as leukotriene antagonists: therapeutic potential in glomerulonephritis. *Kidney Int* 1992;38(suppl): 101–108.
141. Lee TH, Crae AE, Gant V, et al. Identification of lipoxin A_4 and its relationship to the sulfidopeptide leukotrienes C_4, D_4 and E_4 in bronchoalveolar lavage fluids from patients with selected pulmonary diseases. *Am Rev Respir Dis* 1990;141:1453–1458.
142. Lee TH, Horton CE, Kyan-Aung U, Haskard D, Crea AEG, Spur W. Lipoxin A_4 and lipoxin B_4 inhibit chemotactic responses of human neutrophils stimulated by LTB_4 and N-formyl-L-methionyl-L-leucyl-L-phenylalanine. *Clin Sci Lond* 1989;77:195–203.
143. Hedqvist P, Raud J, Palmertz J, Haeggstrom J, Nicolau KC, Dahlen S-E. Lipoxin A_4 inhibits leukotriene B_4–induced inflammation in the hamster cheek pouch. *Acta Physiol Scand* 1989;137:571–581.
144. Johnson RJ, Alpers CE, Pruchno C, et al. Mechanisms and kinetics for platelet and neutrophil localization in immune complex nephritis. *Kidney Int* 1989;36:780–789.
145. Fiore S, Serhan CN. Formation of lipoxins and leukotrienes during receptor-mediated interactions of human platelets and recombinant human granulocyte/macrophage colony stimulating factor-primed neutrophils. *J Exp Med* 1990;172:1451–1457.
146. Nassar GM, Morrow JD, Robert J II, Lakkis FG, Badr KF. Induction of 15-lipoxygenase by interleukin-13 in human blood monocyte. *J Biol Chem* 1994;269:27631–27634.
147. Katoh T, Lakkis FG, Makita N, Badr KF. Co-regulated expression of glomerular12/15-lipoxygenase and interleukin-4 mRNAs in rat nephrotoxic nephritis. *Kidney Int* 1994;46:341–349.
148. Lakkins FG, Cruet EN. Cloning of rat interleukin-13 (IL-13) cDNA and analysis of IL-13 gene expression in experimental glomerulonephritis. *Biochem Biophys Res Commun* 1993;197:612–618.
149. Okada H, Konishi K, Nakazato Y, et al. Interleukin-4 expression in mesangial proliferative glomerulonephritis. *Am J Kidney Dis* 1994; 23:242–246.

Immunologic Renal Diseases,
edited by E. G. Neilson and W. G. Couser.
Lippincott-Raven Publishers, Philadelphia © 1997

CHAPTER 26

Neutrophils

Richard J. Johnson, Seymour J. Klebanoff, and William G. Couser

INTRODUCTION

The neutrophil (polymorphonuclear leukocyte, PMN) has been recognized as an important cell in host defense since the sentinel studies by Ehrlich (1) and Metchnikov (2) in the late 1800s. Constituting 50–60% of the total circulating leukocyte population, the neutrophil patrols the circulation, exiting it to do battle with invading microorganisms. Equipped with an arsenal of proteolytic enzymes, cationic proteins, lipid mediators, and reactive oxygen and nitrogen species, the neutrophil is particularly effective at eliminating bacterial and fungal organisms (reviewed in references 3–7). Most of the killing is done by phagocytosis, with the organisms trapped in phagolysosomes where the highly toxic products can be unleashed with impunity (4–7). Immune complexes can also be phagocytosed and degraded in this manner (4–7). However, if phagocytosis is not possible (that is, frustrated phagocytosis), the neutrophil may inadvertently attack the organism or immune complex via the extracellular release of oxidants and proteinases. Moreover, an untoward consequence may be local injury to innocent bystander cells and surrounding extracellular matrix, particularly if local antioxidant and antiprotease mechanisms are overwhelmed. It is in this latter setting that the neutrophil has been implicated as a mediator of inflammatory injury. In this chapter, we review the evidence supporting a role for this important effector cell in mediating capillary wall damage and proteinuria in immune glomerular disease.

NEUTROPHIL BIOLOGY

Neutrophils are produced in the bone marrow under the influence of granulocyte and granulocyte-macrophage colony-stimulating factors. The normal production of neutrophils by the marrow is 10^{11} cells per day, but this can increase over tenfold with infection or inflammation. After maturation in the marrow, neutrophils enter the circulation for only 4–10 h, after which they either marginate or migrate into tissue (4). The migration of neutrophils into tissue is mediated by specific ligand–receptor interactions between adhesion proteins on neutrophils and vascular endothelium (see Chapter 25). Once in tissue, they may survive for 1 or 2 more days, but eventually will succumb to apoptosis and then be phagocytosed by local macrophages or other resident cells (see Chapter 15).

Neutrophil Granules: An Arsenal of Mobilizable Inflammatory Mediators

Neutrophils contain four types of granules: the primary (azurophil) granule, the secondary (specific) granule, the tertiary (C type) granules, and secretory vesicles (5–7). Each of these granules contains various inflammatory mediators that are mobilized to the cell membrane and/or released into the extracellular space following PMN activation (5–7). The primary granule contains myeloperoxidase (MPO), an enzyme important in the generation of powerful oxidants (3). The primary granule also contains the serine proteinases [proteinase 3 (Pr-3), elastase, and cathepsin G] and cationic proteins, such as the defensins, bacterial permeability-increasing protein, and lysozyme (5–7). Interest in the primary granule components has been sparked recently by the observation that antibodies to primary granule components, especially Pr-3 and MPO, are common in patients with vasculitis and rapidly progressive glomerulonephritis (discussed below; see also Chapter 49). The secondary granule contains a variety of proteins, including lactoferrin, lysozyme, thrombospondin, fibronectin, and vitamin B12-binding protein. The tertiary granule contains several proteins, of which the most important is the matrix metalloproteinase 9

R. J. Johnson, S. J. Klebanoff, and W. G. Couser: Department of Medicine, University of Washington, Seattle, Washington 98195.

TABLE 1. *Major inflammatory mediators of the neutrophil*[a]

Category	Specific mediators
Reactive oxygen species	O_2^-, H_2O_2, ·OH, HOCl, $^1O_2$
Proteinases	Proteinase 3, elastase, cathepsin G, MMP-9
Cationic proteins	Defensins, azurocidin, bactericidal permeability increasing, lysozyme
Lipid mediators	Thromboxane A_2, platelet-activating factor, leukotriene B_4, 5-HETE products
Cytokines	Interleukin 1 (IL-1), tumor necrosis factor, IL-6
Reactive nitrogen species:	Nitric oxide, peroxynitrite

[a]For a more complete list, the reader is referred to references 3–7. [b]Recent data suggest that human polymorphonuclear leukocytes (PMNs), unlike PMNs from rodents, do not generate detectable nitric oxide (14). MMP, matrix metalloproteinase 9.

(MMP-9, also referred to as type-IV collagenase or gelatinase), which is a 92-kD protease that is active at neutral pH. Secretory vesicles are particularly involved in the mobilization of various proteins to the PMN cell membrane, such as complement regulatory proteins (CR1 and decay-accelerating factor), phagocyte oxidase components (cytochrome b_{558}), and cell adhesion proteins, Mac-1 or CD11b) (5–7).

Although the neutrophil granules contain a cache of mediators that can be released with activation, neutrophils can also generate other inflammatory mediators from the cytoplasm or cell membrane. A summary of the major types of mediators is provided below and in Table 1.

Reactive Oxygen Species (Fig. 1)

When neutrophils are stimulated, such as by immune complexes, phagocytosis, or complement activation products (C5a), they undergo a respiratory burst characterized by an increased oxygen consumption, increased utilization of glucose by the hexose monophosphate shunt, and the formation of reduced or excited products of oxygen that can function as oxidants (3). Initially, oxygen is univalently reduced to form superoxide anion (O_2^-) by a cell membrane-bound oxidase that utilizes nicotinamide adenine dinucleotide phosphate (NADPH) as a substrate:

$$O_2 + NADPH \xrightarrow{\text{oxidase}} O_2^- + H^+ + NADP$$

Superoxide anion can then dismutate spontaneously (such as in an acidic PMN phagolysosome) or by catalysis by the enzyme superoxide dismutase (SOD) to form hydrogen peroxide (H_2O_2):

$$2O_2^- + 2H^+ \xrightarrow{\text{SOD}} O_2 + H_2O_2$$

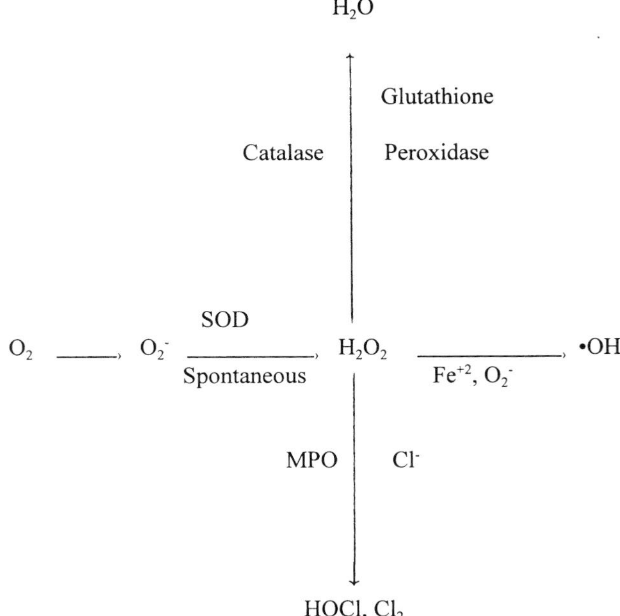

FIG. 1. Pathway for reactive oxygen species generation by neutrophils. MPO, myeloperoxidase; SOD, superoxide dismutase.

Although H_2O_2 is an oxidant, it is relatively weak, and more powerful oxidants can be generated from H_2O_2 by two major mechanisms. The first involves reaction of H_2O_2 with the PMN enzyme MPO to oxidize chloride to generate hypochlorous acid/hypochlorite (bleach). Hypochlorous acid can further react with chloride at acid pH to form chlorine:

$$H_2O_2 + Cl^- + H^+ \xrightarrow{\text{MPO}} H_2O + HOCl$$

$$HOCl + Cl^- \longrightarrow Cl_2 + OH^-$$

Another strong oxidant generated in small amounts by neutrophils is the hydroxyl radical (·OH) that can be formed either by the iron-catalyzed interaction between O_2^- and H_2O_2 (Haber–Weiss reaction) (3)

$$\begin{array}{l} Fe^{+2} + H_2O_2 \longrightarrow Fe^{+3} + \cdot OH + OH^- \\ O_2^- + Fe^{+3} \longrightarrow O_2 + Fe^{+2} \\ \hline O_2^- + H_2O_2 \longrightarrow O_2 + \cdot OH + OH^- \end{array}$$

or by the reaction of HOCl formed by the MPO system with O_2^- (8):

$$H_2O_2 + Cl^- + H^+ \xrightarrow{\text{MPO}} H_2O + HOCl$$

$$HOCl + O_2^- \longrightarrow \cdot OH + O_2 + Cl^-$$

The role of the Haber–Weiss reaction in the generation of ·OH in vivo has been questioned due to the limited availability of free iron (in part because of the presence of lactoferrin) (9). An excited form of oxygen (singlet oxygen, $^1O_2$), in which one of the valence electrons of oxygen is raised to an orbital of higher energy with an inversion of spin, also has been proposed as a product of the respiratory burst of neutrophils. Although earlier studies had questioned the formation of $^1O_2$ in appreciable amounts [reviewed by Klebanoff (3)], the recent detection of $^1O_2$ formation by the Haber–Weiss reaction (10) and by the interaction of hypochlorite formed by the MPO system with H_2O_2 (11)

$$H_2O_2 + Cl^- \longrightarrow H_2O + OCl^-$$

$$OCl^- + H_2O_2 \longrightarrow {}^1O_2 + H_2O + Cl^-$$

has renewed interest in the formation of $^1O_2$ by neutrophils. The participation of oxidants in immune renal damage is covered in Chapter 19.

Proteinases

Activated neutrophils also release proteinases with extracellular matrix-degrading activity. The most important group are the serine proteinases, consisting of Pr-3, elastase, and cathepsin G (4–7). These proteinases are small (<30 kD), cationic, and have maximal activity at neutral pH (4–7). Neutrophils also express a 92-kD neutral metalloproteinase (MMP-9), which is released in a latent form from C-granules and specific granules following cell activation (4–7). Studies have demonstrated that both the MPO–H_2O_2 system (12) and elastase (13) can generate active MMP-9 from its latent form. Finally, neutrophils also can secrete various acid hydrolases, phospholipases, polysaccharidases, and sulfatases (4–7), most of which have not been studied in any detail. The role of proteases in immune renal injury is covered in Chapter 19.

Reactive Nitrogen Species

Neutrophils from many species can also generate nitric oxide (NO) from L-arginine (14). However, very little NO is produced by human PMNs, because they have no detectable levels of the constitutive NO synthase (14). NO has multiple hemodynamic and nonhemodynamic effects. For example, it inhibits contraction and cell proliferation in vascular smooth muscle cells and mesangial cells (15). However, NO also is cytotoxic for various cell types and is a major mechanism by which murine macrophages induce injury (16). NO is discussed at more length in Chapter 21.

Cationic Proteins

Many proteins released from the granules are strongly cationic, including MPO, the serine proteinases, the defensins, lysozyme, bactericidal permeability-increasing protein and azurocidin (5–7). Of particular importance are the defensins, which are a family of four low molecular weight (<3.5 kD) proteins that represent as much as 50% of the protein in the primary (azurophil) granules (17). The defensins have been shown to have significant antimicrobial and cytotoxic activity, and human defensin 1 is also chemotactic for macrophages (17,18).

Lipid Mediators

The neutrophil can also generate various eicosanoids, particularly thromboxane A_2 (19) and various 5-lipoxygenase products, such as leukotriene B_4 (LTB_4) and 5-hydroxyeicosatetraenoic acid (5-HETE) (20). Neutrophils also produce platelet-activating factor (PAF) (21). Neutrophils may also interact with platelets to generate other eicosanoids, including the lipoxins (22,23). The role of eicosanoids in immune renal injury is covered in Chapter 22.

Cytokines

Although neutrophils are classically considered to be terminally differentiated, they do contain small amounts of messenger RNA and are capable of synthesizing several inflammatory cytokines with activation (24). Some of the more important cytokines produced by the neutrophil include interleukin 1β (IL-1β), IL-6, IL-8, interferon-γ, and tumor necrosis factor α (TNF-α) (24).

THE NEUTROPHIL IS AN IMPORTANT MEDIATOR OF GLOMERULAR DISEASE

Strong evidence supports a role for the PMN in mediating glomerular disease (Table 2). This includes evidence that (a) PMNs can injure glomerular cells and degrade GBM in vitro; (b) PMNs are present in many experimental and human glomerular diseases; (c) PMN depletion by irradiation, cytotoxic drugs, or specific antibodies can reduce glomerular injury in experimental models; and (d) administration of neutrophils to PMN-depleted rats with nephritis can reconstitute injury. These criteria are simi-

TABLE 2. *Neutrophils are important mediators of glomerular disease*

1. PMNs can injure glomeruli and degrade GBM in vitro
2. PMNs are present in glomerular disease
3. PMN depletion reduces glomerular injury in experimental models
4. PMN repletion reconstitutes injury in PMN-depleted rats with nephritis

GBM, glomerular basement membrane; PMN, polymorphonuclear leukocyte.

lar to that used by Koch to establish the pathogenesis of the mycobacteria in tuberculosis (25).

Neutrophils may also have a beneficial role in immune-mediated renal disease due to the ability of the PMN to phagocytose and remove immune complexes. Thus, PMN depletion studies have shown that neutrophils have an important role in the clearance of immune complexes from peritubular capillaries in a model of experimental immune-complex nephritis (26).

PMNs Mediate Glomerular Injury and GBM Damage in Vitro

In vitro studies have demonstrated that activated neutrophils can degrade basement membranes and injure glomerular cells. For example, PMNs activated by immune complexes or by phorbol myristate acetate (PMA) will degrade GBM due to the release of proteases, including serine proteases (elastase and cathepsin G) (27,28) and metalloproteinases (MMP-9) (29). The MMP-9-mediated GBM degradation depends on activation of the MMP-9 by oxidants generated by the MPO–H_2O_2–halide system (30). Activated neutrophils can also kill cultured mesangial cells via the release of oxidants (31).

PMNs Are Present in Many Experimental and Human Glomerular Diseases

Human Glomerular Diseases

Many types of glomerular disease are associated with neutrophil infiltration. The classic example is the marked exudative glomerular lesion that accompanies post-streptococcal glomerulonephritis (32–34) (see Chapter 41). In this disease, large numbers of neutrophils, monocytes, and occasionally eosinophils are present in glomeruli (35). Electron microscopy often demonstrates neutrophils abutting basement membrane, occasionally at sites where the subepithelial immune deposits ("humps") are present (33–35). Neutrophils are also frequent in other types of postinfectious nephritis, cryoglobulinemic and idiopathic membranoproliferative nephritis, diffuse proliferative lupus nephritis, Henoch–Schönlein purpura, immunoglobulin (Ig)-A nephropathy, Wegener vasculitis, anti–glomerular basement membrane (anti-GBM) disease, and other types of crescentic nephritis (32–42) (Fig. 2).

Neutrophil cationic proteins have also been localized in glomeruli in a variety of renal diseases, including lupus nephritis (43) and rapidly progressive glomerulonephritis (40–42). MPO, in particular, has been localized to glomerular capillary walls in crescentic nephritis (40), whereas Pr-3 and elastase remain more cell associated in these diseases (41,42).

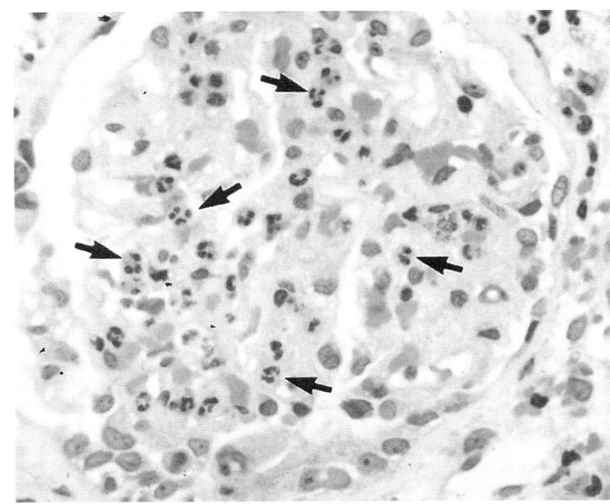

FIG. 2. Exudative glomerulonephritis in a patient with Henoch–Schönlein purpura. Numerous neutrophils are present throughout the glomerulus *(arrows)*. Periodic acid–Schiff reagent, ×400. Courtesy of Dr. Charles E. Alpers, University of Washington, Seattle, WA.

The degree of neutrophil infiltration appears to be greatest in diseases associated with subendothelial immune deposits and/or anti-GBM antibodies, whereas mesangial lesions are associated with fewer neutrophils. Diseases such as membranous nephropathy and minimal change disease are not associated with a PMN infiltrate, presumably because any chemotactic factors generated have relative inaccessibility to the blood due to the opposing filtration pressure and intervening basement membrane. The fact that neutrophils are commonly present in postinfectious glomerulonephritis, which has characteristic subepithelial immune deposits, probably is due to the frequent coexistence of mesangial and subendothelial deposits (33).

Experimental Models of Glomerular Disease

The characteristics of various animal models of immune renal disease are reviewed in Chapters 35 and 36. This section focuses exclusively on the role defined for neutrophils in these lesions. Neutrophils have been recognized as important mediators of glomerular injury since the 1960s (44). The classic model of neutrophil-associated glomerular disease is anti-GBM disease (nephrotoxic nephritis) (45). Rats or rabbits injected with heterologous antibody to either whole glomeruli or isolated GBM develop renal dysfunction with proteinuria and with deposition of the antibody and complement on the GBM (45,46). Early in the course of the disease, a prominent infiltration of neutrophils can be demonstrated, often in association with endothelial cell swelling (44,47). The peak neutrophil infiltration occurs ~2–6 h after anti-GBM antibody injection and then slowly subsides over several days (44). Neutrophils also localize to the lung, where the anti-GBM antibody cross-reacts with alveolar basement membrane (48). Whereas neutrophils represent the major infiltrating cell during the initial course, a mild lymphocyte infiltration has also been noted (49). The increase in glomerular permeability corresponds with the initial PMN influx (46), and the degree of proteinuria correlates with the degree of PMN infiltration (45). By 24 h, monocyte/macrophages are present, and macrophages also represent the principal leukocyte in the later (autologous) phase of the disease (that is, when the rat is making its own antibody to the foreign IgG) (50).

Two models of subendothelial immune-complex disease resembling lupus nephritis have been developed using lectins in which neutrophil infiltration can be massive (51–53). The models are induced in rats by the renal artery perfusion of the lectin, concanavalin A (ConA), or

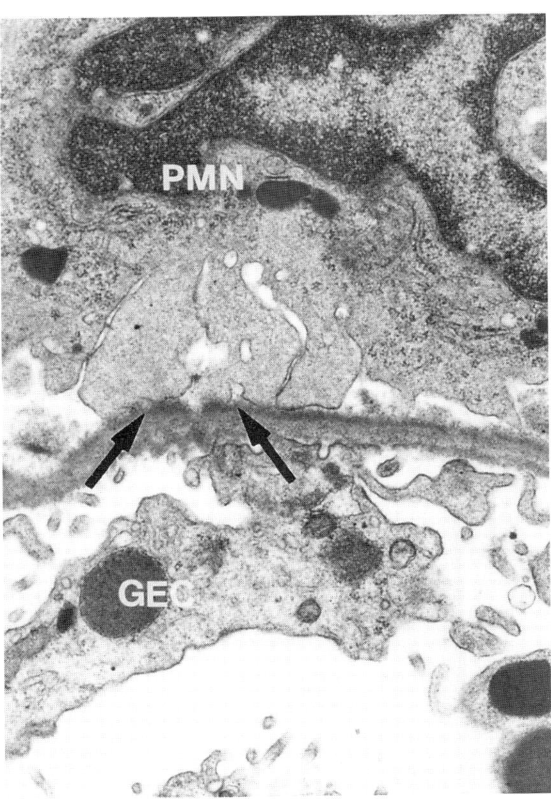

FIG. 3. Electron micrograph of an activated polymorphonuclear leukocyte (PMN) adherent to bare basement membrane in experimental glomerulonephritis. An activated PMN is adherent to the glomerular basement membrane of a rat with concanavalin-A nephritis. Large pseudopodia extend from the PMN to the immune deposits *(arrows)* and GBM. The endothelium is denuded, and severe damage of the glomerular epithelial cell with frank detachment is evident. PMN, neutrophil; GEC, glomerular epithelial cell. ×12,000. Courtesy of Dr. Charles E. Alpers, University of Washington, Seattle, WA.

with Lens culinaris hemagglutinin, both of which bind sugar residues on the glomerular endothelial cell (51–53). Subsequent perfusion with a polyclonal anti-ConA (or anti–Lens culinaris hemagglutinin) antibody results in in situ immune-complex formation, complement activation, and injury to the endothelium and basement membrane (51–53). Immune deposits are rapidly shed from the endothelium into the subendothelial space and later can also be detected in some subepithelial areas (51–54). A dramatic platelet and neutrophil infiltration can be documented, with the platelets peaking at 10 min and the neutrophils between 1 and 4 h (54) (Fig. 3).

PMN Depletion Reduces Injury in Experimental Glomerular Disease

To examine directly the role of the PMN in mediating glomerular injury, several studies have examined the effect of depletion of the PMN population by irradiation, cytotoxic drugs, or anti-PMN antibody (45,54–59). In general, neutrophils appear to be important in models associated with subendothelial or GBM injury, whereas disease models affecting the glomerular epithelial cell are PMN independent (60). Proteinuria, which is a reflection of glomerular injury, can be significantly inhibited by PMN depletion in both the heterologous (45,55) and autologous (56,57) phases of anti-GBM nephritis and in the ConA model (52,54). Neutrophil depletion will also prevent the reduction in the glomerular filtration rate (GFR) and ultrafiltration coefficient (LpA) (58) and ameliorate the lung injury associated with anti-GBM disease (59).

Both the anti-GBM model (45) and the ConA model (54) are also complement dependent, since complement depletion with cobra venom factor (*Naja naja*, CVF) will abolish the PMN influx and prevent proteinuria. The mechanism by which complement mediates the injury in this model is presumably by generating the PMN chemotactic peptide, C5a, but in anti-GBM nephritis part of the proteinuria also depends on the terminal C5b-9 MAC (61,62) (see Chapter 18). High doses of anti-GBM antibody may also result in a complement- and PMN-independent proteinuria (44,63). This may be due to antibodies present in the preparation that bind to integrins involved in the attachment of the glomerular epithelial cell to the GBM (64) (see Chapter 17).

PMN Repletion Reconstitutes Injury in Experimental Glomerular Disease

Studies have also been performed in which PMNs have been infused into rabbits with anti-GBM nephritis that had been previously depleted of their endogenous neutrophils with nitrogen mustard (65). In the absence of neutrophils, proteinuria in these rabbits was prevented; but, following infusion of 7–7.5 × 10^8 neutrophils, mild proteinuria was reconstituted (65).

MECHANISMS FOR PMN-MEDIATED GLOMERULAR INJURY: THE ROLE OF OXIDANTS AND PROTEASES

Most evidence suggests that the mechanisms by which PMNs mediate glomerular damage are primarily due to the release of oxidants and proteases (for review, see references 66–74; also see Chapter 19). Evidence suggests that oxidants may be responsible for much of the cellular injury and some of the increase in glomerular permeability in glomerulonephritis, whereas proteases act primarily to increase glomerular permeability (74). A brief summary of the evidence is provided as follows:

Role of Oxidants in PMN-Mediated Glomerular Injury

The role of neutrophil-derived oxidants in mediating glomerular injury has been shown by (a) examining the effects of oxidants on glomerular cells in culture, (b) documenting oxidant production and oxidative injury in models of nephritis, (c) infusing oxidants directly into the kidney, and (d) administering inhibitors or scavengers of oxidants to animals with glomerular disease. Whereas most studies have focused on the role of neutrophils in mediating glomerular injury, evidence has also been provided that neutrophil-derived oxidants may also have a role in ischemia-reperfusion injury in the kidney (75). Furthermore, oxidants produced by other inflammatory cells (for example, monocytes and macrophages) as well as endogenous glomerular cells are also involved in the pathogenesis of some models of glomerular injury; these are described in detail in Chapter 19.

In Vitro Studies

Neutrophils release oxidants (as measured by chemiluminescence) in response to immune complexes containing GBM and anti-GBM IgG (76,77). PMNs from patients with IgA nephropathy also secrete more H_2O_2 in response to heat-aggregated IgG or opsonized zymosan as compared with PMNs from normal controls (78). PMNs stimulated by PMA are cytotoxic for rat mesangial cells by a H_2O_2 and Fe-dependent mechanism (31). Indeed, the isolated components of the MPO–H_2O_2–halide system are particularly cytotoxic for rat mesangial cells, and inhibition or removal of any component eliminates the toxicity (74). The MPO–H_2O_2–halide system has also been shown to increase albumin permeability in the isolated glomerulus, an effect that was not seen with H_2O_2 alone (79).

PMN-derived oxidants, and especially those derived from the MPO–H_2O_2–halide system, have also been shown to facilitate PMN protease activity by several mechanisms, including the inactivation of antiproteases (such as the α_1-proteinase inhibitor) (80), the activation of the PMN-derived 92-kD type-IV collagenase (MMP-9) (12), and by rendering GBM more susceptible to proteolytic action (81,82). Oxidants can also inactivate proteases, but the balance is in favor of enhanced protease action (82). Shah et al. have shown that activated PMNs degrade GBM partially as a consequence of MPO–H_2O_2-mediated activation of MMP-9 (30).

PMN-Derived Oxidants Are Released in Glomerular Disease

Several studies have demonstrated that PMNs are activated in glomerular disease and release oxidants. For example, in the anti-Thy 1 model of mesangial proliferative nephritis in rats, O_2^-- and H_2O_2-secreting PMNs can be identified within glomeruli (83,84). Evidence for participation of the MPO–H_2O_2–halide system has also been provided in the ConA model of proliferative nephritis (52). Specifically, iodination (halogenation) of the GBM, a consequence of MPO action (85), was demonstrated in rats with ConA nephritis, but was abolished in diseased rats by depletion of PMNs with an anti-PMN antibody (52).

Infusion of Oxidants into the Kidney Induces Glomerular Injury

Johnson et al. infused the PMN cationic enzyme, MPO, into the renal artery, followed by H_2O_2 and a halide (chloride) (86). The MPO localized on the basis of charge to the sites rich in anions on the GBM (principally heparan sulfate proteoglycan) and on the surface of the glomerular epithelial cells (primarily sialoproteins) (86). This allowed the MPO-catalyzed reaction to generate hypohalous acids on the capillary wall. Whereas the infusion of H_2O_2 alone or MPO alone induced no discernible injury, the combination of MPO and H_2O_2 resulted in severe endothelial and mesangial cell loss, marked intraglomerular platelet accumulation, and proteinuria. By including ^{125}I in the perfusate, it was possible to demonstrate iodination (halogenation) of the GBM by autoradiography (86). Several days after the infusion, a dramatic proliferative response of the glomerular cells was documented (87).

Others have also demonstrated the ability of oxidants to induce glomerular injury. Thus, in rabbits, infusion of xanthine/xanthine oxidase (which generates several different oxidants) or H_2O_2 directly into the renal artery results in mesangiolysis with microaneurysm formation (88,89). In rats, infusion of lower concentrations of H_2O_2 for longer periods than in the MPO study will also lead to proteinuria, interestingly with little associated cellular injury documented by electron microscopy (90). The renal artery infusion of the pigment, pheophorbide, followed by exposure to light, which is thought to generate $^1O_2$, also results in severe endothelial and mesangial injury (91).

Effect of Oxidant Scavengers and Inhibitors on Glomerulonephritis

Inhibitors or scavengers of oxidants have also been administered to animals with experimental renal disease, including superoxide dismutase (SOD) (which converts O_2^- to H_2O_2) and catalase (which degrades H_2O_2 to water) (see also Chapter 19). Other agents that have been reported to scavenge ·OH [such as dimethylthiourea (DMTU) and dimethylsulfoxide (DMSO)] or limit ·OH formation by iron chelation [such as with desferrioxamine (DFO)]. However, DFO is not specific, for it will also inhibit oxidant production by the MPO–H_2O_2–halide system (92,93).

Some of the most compelling evidence for oxidants in PMN-mediated glomerular injury was provided by the sentinel studies by Rehan et al. (55,94,95). In addition to studying the anti-GBM models, these investigators established two new models of renal disease, which were produced in rats by the renal artery perfusion of PMA (which stimulates oxidant production in PMNs) or CVF (which, by activating complement, leads to PMN activation) (94, 95). In both of the latter models, a mild proteinuria was induced in association with a PMN infiltrate in glomeruli (94,95). In the PMA model, a decrease in the GFR was also documented (96). Confirmation that these models were PMN dependent was provided by depleting the rats of PMNs by using an anti-PMN antibody that abolished the proteinuria and improved the GFR (55,94–96). Importantly, the injury in these models could also be abolished by catalase but not by SOD, suggesting a critical role for H_2O_2 in mediating the injury (55,94–96).

Oxidant inhibitors have also been administered to animals with anti-GBM nephritis (55,97–99). For example, Adachi et al. reported that daily administration of SOD reduced the proteinuria and histologic injury in the autologous phase of anti-GBM nephritis (97), which is a phase that is thought to be both PMN dependent (56,57) and monocyte dependent (50). Others have not noted any beneficial effect of SOD in an accelerated version of this model (98). Rehan et al. reported that catalase, but not SOD or DMSO, reduced proteinuria in the initial PMN-dependent heterologous phase of anti-GBM nephritis in rats, again suggesting a role for H_2O_2 (55). Others have reported that high-dose SOD or polyethylene-glycol-conjugated catalase both reduce proteinuria in the heterologous phase of a similar model (99). In contrast, in the PMN-dependent heterologous phase of anti-GBM nephritis in rabbits, the proteinuria was found to be ·OH dependent, based on the ability of DFO or DMTU to reduce proteinuria without affecting antibody binding, renal function, complement activity, or PMN counts (100).

One problem with administering antioxidants is that these agents may not reach the site of oxidative injury, due to the fact that PMNs, when adherent to a nonphagocytosable site, release their oxidants into the zones of contact at the cell-substrate interface (101), which is impenetrable to many circulating proteins (80,102). An alternative approach is to induce local antioxidant mechanisms. For example, endogenous glomerular antioxidants have been stimulated in rats by administering steroids (103). Pretreatment of rats with steroids increased their endogenous SOD and glutathione peroxidase levels and protects them from glomerular injury induced by the renal artery perfusion of H_2O_2 (103).

Neutrophil Proteases Mediate Glomerular Injury GBM Damage

Neutrophil proteases also have an important role in mediating glomerular injury (see also Chapter 19). Both the serine proteases (elastase, cathepsin G, and Pr-3) and the 92-kD metalloproteinase (MMP-9) of the neutrophil can degrade GBM in vitro (104–110). Elastase also degrades laminin (111), fibronectin (80), and proteoglycan (112). Neutrophils release their lysosomal granules in response to GBM and anti-GBM antibody (77), and activated PMNs will digest the type-IV collagen in GBM by both serine- and metalloproteinase-dependent pathways (27–30). Neutrophil proteases can also be localized in glomeruli (41,42) and detected in urine (46,113) of experimental and human glomerulonephritis in which PMN infiltration is prominent.

The most direct evidence that PMN proteases injure the GBM is provided by in vivo studies in which the infusion of elastase or cathepsin G into the renal artery of rats resulted in massive proteinuria (114). The mechanism may relate to degradation of heparan sulfate proteoglycan in the capillary wall (115). Pr-3 can also induce proteinuria but requires higher amounts than those used to achieve proteinuria with elastase or cathepsin G (74).

An interesting aspect of these latter studies was that very little cellular injury was observed ultrastructurally (114), suggesting that proteases primarily act to increase glomerular permeability possibly by direct action on the GBM. This was indirectly addressed by studying mice with an inherited defect in their PMNs in which the PMNs released only low amounts of proteases (beige mice) (116). These mice developed cellular injury but not proteinuria after injection of anti-GBM antibody (116). However, the defect in these mice also resulted in less MPO release and oxidant production (117), so this study did not clearly differentiate between the relative importance of oxidants versus proteases in mediating capillary wall damage and proteinuria.

Other Mechanisms for PMN-Mediated Glomerular Injury

It is possible that PMNs may inflict glomerular injury through mechanisms that do not involve proteases or oxidants. For example, cationic proteins, and particularly the low molecular weight defensins, have been demonstrated to be bactericidal and cytotoxic agents in vitro (17,18). Neutrophil cationic proteins have also been localized in glomeruli in experimental and human glomerulonephritis (43). Theoretically, these agents could induce proteinuria either by direct cytotoxic effects (17,18) or by neutralization of the charge barrier in the GBM. However, infusion of a mixture of defensins into the renal artery of rats did not induce proteinuria despite localizing to the mesangium and capillary walls (74).

MECHANISMS FOR PMN RECRUITMENT

The mechanisms for PMN accumulation in glomerulonephritis have been of intense interest, as recent studies suggest that blocking PMN recruitment and adherence may provide a new way to treat glomerular disease. A brief discussion of the chemotactic and adhesive factors involved in PMN recruitment is provided, but a more complete review can be found elsewhere (see Chapters 24 and 25).

Chemotactic Factors

The initial deposition or formation of an immune complex in the glomerulus is usually associated with activation of the complement system with the release of potent chemotactic factors, particularly C5a. A role for complement in mediating PMN recruitment is supported by the observation that complement-depletion prevents the PMN influx that occurs in several models of nephritis (44,54).

An important family of chemotactic factors are the chemokines, which are proteins characterized by four conserved cysteine residues that form two disulfide bonds. Two subfamilies exist, depending on whether there is an intervening amino acid (CXC or α and CC or β subfamily) [reviewed by Gomez-Chiarri et al. (118)]. Members of the CC family are primarily chemotactic for mononuclear cells (monocytes and T cells), whereas members of the CXC family are mainly chemotactic for PMNs. Members of the CXC family include IL-8, cytokine-induced neutrophil chemoattractant (CINC), platelet factor 4, macrophage inflammation protein 2 (MIP-2), and 10-kD interferon-inducible protein (118).

A role for CINC and MIP-2 has been demonstrated in experimental anti-GBM nephritis. CINC and MIP-2 are upregulated in glomeruli by 30 min after anti-GBM antibody injection, and the degree of expression correlates with the PMN infiltrate (119). The PMN infiltration and proteinuria can be reduced by anti-CINC or anti-MIP-2 antibody (120–122), whereas anti-IL-8 antibodies are without effect (120). However, IL-8 is important in acute serum sickness in rabbits, as anti-IL-8 antibody prevents the leukocyte influx, histologic injury, and proteinuria in this model (122). This model is probably mediated by macrophages as opposed to PMNs (123). Anti-IL-8 antibodies also reduce proteinuria in other models of immune-complex-mediated glomerular injury (124). IL-8 is also increased in the urine of patients with IgA nephropathy, lupus, and postinfectious nephritis, and the urinary level correlates with the degree of glomerular PMN infiltration in the renal biopsies (125).

Other chemotactic factors may also be produced by resident or infiltrating cells, including PAF (126), LTB_4 and other lipoxygenase products (127), and various growth factors and cytokines such as IL-1, TNF-α, and platelet-derived growth factor [reviewed by Johnson (128)]. For example, rats with anti-GBM nephritis have elevated urinary (129) and glomerular (130) levels of LTB_4 that correlate with the degree of PMN infiltration in glomeruli. LTB_4 infusion into the renal artery also amplifies injury in anti-GBM nephritis, whereas inhibition of LTB_4 formation with 5-lipoxygenase inhibitors reduces the PMN infiltration and proteinuria (131). Pretreatment of rats with anti-GBM nephritis with endotoxin, IL-1, or TNF-α increases the PMN influx and proteinuria (132). Furthermore, antibodies to TNF-α or to IL-1β also reduce the PMN infiltration and proteinuria in endotoxin-primed rats with anti-GBM nephritis (133). Anti-TNF-α antibody also prevents PMN-mediated glomerular injury in unmodified anti-GBM nephritis (134).

Adherence

Once attracted to the site of injury, the neutrophil will adhere to the immune complexes or to endothelium by specific receptors. Some of the important receptors involved in PMN adherence include the Fc receptor, the C3b (CR1) receptor, and members of the LFA-1, Mac-1 glycoprotein family (CD11/CD18), including the receptor for C3bi (CR3) [reviewed by Carlos and Harlan (135)]. Increased expression of many of these receptors can be documented on activated PMNs. Indeed, the mechanism by which LTB_4 acts to increase PMN adherence to mesangial cells involves upregulation of CD11/CD18 (136). In contrast, the mechanism by which PMNs bind to TNF-α-primed glomerular endothelial cells involves L-selectin expression by the PMN (137).

In addition, endothelium may also express leukocyte adherence proteins, including the selectins (E- and P-selectin), which are involved in mediating the initial rolling of the PMN on the endothelial surface, and intercellular adhesion molecule 1 (ICAM-1) and vascular cell adhesion molecule 1 (VCAM-1), which are members of the Ig superfamily that are involved in PMN adherence. The expression of leukocyte adherence protein on PMNs and endothelium is regulated by numerous substances, including damaged fibronectin, PAF, thromboxane, IL-1, C5a, LTB_4, and TNF-α (135).

The importance of leukocyte adherence proteins in PMN-mediated injury has been documented by blocking studies. Antibodies to Mac-1 (CD11b/CD18) reduce proteinuria in anti-GBM nephritis (134,138), and anti-LFA-1α antibodies reduce the leukocyte infiltration and proteinuria in active and passive anti-GBM nephritis in WKY rats in which crescents develop (139,140). Antibodies to P-selectin and ICAM-1 are also protective in models of anti-GBM disease (134,139–141).

Finally, other factors may also be important in PMN adherence in glomeruli. Several studies suggest that PMN localization is both Fc dependent and complement dependent. In the complement-independent passive autologous model of anti-GBM nephritis in rabbits, the administration of $F(ab')_2$ fragments of antibody to GBM, which lack the Fc portion, resulted in significantly less PMN accumulation (142). Others have shown a role for complement in mediating the PMN accumulation in the acute heterologous phase of anti-GBM nephritis (44), but it is not known whether this is due to the generation of C5a or due to C3b-mediated PMN adherence. The renal artery perfusion of neuraminidase, which is produced by streptococci and other bacteria, also results in a mild PMN infiltrate in glomeruli, which is thought to be due to the liberation of sialic acid from cell surface glycoproteins within the glomerulus (143). Interstitial collagens, which are induced in various glomerular diseases, can also activate PMNs (144).

PMN INTERACTIONS WITH PLATELETS AND OTHER CELLS

There is also evidence that activation of the neutrophil is regulated by infiltrating cells, particularly platelets (145,146) and T lymphocytes (147). In the ConA model of immune-complex nephritis, neutrophils and platelets accumulate rapidly in glomeruli in the first 24 h after induction of disease, and by electron microscopy may occasionally appear to have sites of contact (adhesion) (54). Depletion of platelets reduces the proteinuria in this PMN-dependent model (148). The mechanism by which platelets may mediate injury in this model could relate to the ability of the platelet to release substances that can increase neutrophil chemotaxis, adhesion, aggregation, phagocytosis, or oxidant release (145,146,149,150). Platelet involvement in immune renal disease is covered in Chapter 27.

Neutrophils and platelets also appear to act synergistically to produce eicosanoids. In anti-GBM nephritis in rats, neutrophil generation of LTB_4 is reduced by platelet depletion (151). The mechanism may be mediated by platelet-derived 12-hydroperoxy-icosatetraenoic acid (152). Platelets and neutrophils also interact in this ConA model to generate lipoxin A_4 (153).

MECHANISMS FOR PMN REMOVAL (APOPTOSIS)

The ultimate fate of the neutrophil, after it has discharged its contents in a glomerular lesion, remains open. It is likely that some neutrophils detach from immune deposits and/or endothelium and return to the circulation. Other neutrophils may undergo apoptosis (programmed cell death). Apoptotic neutrophils have been documented in anti-GBM nephritis in rats (154) and likely represent the hematoxylin bodies found in diffuse proliferative lupus nephritis in humans (155). Once apoptotic, the PMN is rapidly phagocytosed by macrophages or by resident mesangial cells (154). Apoptosis is reviewed in Chapter 15.

ANTINEUTROPHIL CYTOPLASMIC ANTIBODY (ANCA)-ASSOCIATED SYNDROMES

Several types of vasculitis may be associated with circulatory antibodies to neutrophil cytoplasmic antigens (156–158) (see Chapter 49). In particular, antibodies to Pr-3 (C-ANCA pattern) are common in Wegener granulomatosis, whereas antibodies to MPO (P-ANCA pattern) are frequent in idiopathic rapidly progressive glomerulonephritis (156–158). Although the ANCA may simply be produced in response to sequestered antigens that are released in vasculitis (159), there is also evidence indicating that they may be pathogenic. For example, IL-1 or TNF-α-primed PMNs release oxidants that mediate endothelial cell killing in the presence of ANCA (160, 161). Infusion of PMN contents into the renal artery of MPO-immunized rats also results in a severe proliferative glomerulonephritis (162), which, in part, may be due to T-cell reactivity to the ANCA antigens (163).

REFERENCES

1. Ehrlich P. Leukocytose. In: *13th congress of internal medicine*. Paris, 1900.
2. Metchnikov E. *Immunity in infectious diseases*. New York: Johnson Reprint, 1905.
3. Klebanoff SJ. Oxygen metabolites from phagocytes. In: Gallin JI, Goldstein IM, Snyderman R, eds. *Inflammation: basic principles and clinical correlates*. 2nd ed. New York: Raven Press, 1992:541–88.

4. Smith JA. Neutrophils, host defense, and inflammation: a double-edged sword. *J Leukoc Biol* 1994;56:672–86.
5. Borregaard N, Lollike K, Kjeldsen L, et al. Human neutrophil granules and secretory vesicles. *Eur J Haematol* 1993;51:187–98.
6. Henson PM, Johnston RB Jr. Tissue injury in inflammation. *J Clin Invest* 1987;79:669–74.
7. Bainton DF. Neutrophilic leukocyte granules: from structure to function. *Adv Exp Med Biol* 1993;336:17–33.
8. Ramos CL, Pou S, Britigan BE, Cohen MS, Rosen GM. Spin trapping evidence for myeloperoxidase-dependent hydroxyl radical information by human neutrophils and monocytes. *J Biol Chem* 1992;267: 8307–12.
9. Cohen MS, Britigan BE, Hassett DJ, Rosen GM. Do human neutrophils form hydroxyl radical? Evaluation of an unresolved controversy. *Free Radic Biol Med* 1988;5:81–8.
10. Khan AU, Kasha M. Singlet molecular oxygen in the Haber–Weiss reaction. *Proc Natl Acad Sci USA* 1994;91:12,365–7.
11. Steinbeck MJ, Khan AU, Karnovsky MJ. Intracellular singlet oxygen generation by phagocytosing neutrophils in response to particles coated with a chemical trap. *J Biol Chem* 1992;267:13,425–33.
12. Peppin GJ, Weiss SJ. Activation of the endogenous metalloproteinase, gelatinase, by triggered human neutrophils. *Proc Natl Acad Sci USA* 1986;83:4322–6.
13. Vissers MCM, Winterbourn CC. Activation of human neutrophil gelatinase by endogenous serine proteinases. *Biochem J* 1988;249: 327–31.
14. Yan L, Vandivier W, Suffredini AF, Danner RL. Human polymorphonuclear leukocytes lack detectable nitric oxide synthase activity. *J Immunol* 1994;153:1825–34.
15. Raij L, Shultz PJ. Endothelium-derived relaxing factor, nitric oxide: effects on and production by mesangial cells and the glomerulus. *J Am Soc Nephrol* 1993;3:1435–41.
16. Hibbs JB Jr, Taintor RR, Vavrin Z, Rachlin EM. Nitric oxide: a cytotoxic activated macrophage effector molecule. *Biochem Biophys Res Commun* 1988;157:87–94.
17. Selested ME, Harwig SSL, Ganz T, Schilling JW, Lehrer RI. Primary structures of three human neutrophil defensins. *J Clin Invest* 1985;76: 1436–9.
18. Ganz T, Selested ME, Szlarek D, et al. Defensins: natural peptide antibiotics of human neutrophils. *J Clin Invest* 1985;76:1427–35.
19. Goldstein IM, Malmsten CM, Kindahl H, et al. Thromboxane generation by human peripheral blood polymorphonuclear leukocytes. *J Exp Med* 1978;48:787–92.
20. Henderson WR Jr. The role of leukotrienes in inflammation. *Ann Intern Med* 1994;121:684–97.
21. Jouvin-Marche JE, Ninio E, Beaurain G, Tencé M, Niaudet P, Benveniste J. Biosynthesis of paf-acether (platelet-activating factor). VII. Precursors of paf-acether and acetyltransferase activity in human leukocytes. *J Immunol* 1984;133:892.
22. Marcus AJ, Safier LB, Ullman HL, et al. Platelet–neutrophil interactions. *J Biol Chem* 1988;263:2223–9.
23. Serhan CN, Sheppard KA. Lipoxin formation during human neutrophil–platelet interactions. *J Clin Invest* 1990;85:772–80.
24. Lloyd AR, Oppenheim JJ. Poly's lament: the neglected role of the polymorphonuclear neutrophil in the afferent limb of the immune response. *Immunol Today* 1992;12:169–71.
25. Koch R. Die Actiologie der Tuberculose. *Berl Klin Wochenschr* 1882;19:221. Trans Dr and Mrs M Pinner. *The actiology of tuberculosis.* Baltimore: Wavery [National Tuberculosis Association], 1932:1–48.
26. Alpers CE, Hudkins KL, Pritzl P, Johnson RJ. Mechanisms of clearance of immune complexes from peritubular capillaries in the rat. *Am J Pathol* 1991;139:855–67.
27. Vissers MCM, Winterbourn CC, Hunt JS. Degradation of glomerular basement membrane by human neutrophils in vitro. *Biochim Biophys Acta* 1984;804:154–60.
28. Donovan KL, Davies M, Coles GA, Williams JD. Relative roles of elastase and reactive oxygen species in the degradation of human glomerular basement membrane by intact human neutrophils. *Kidney Int* 1994;45:1555–61.
29. Vissers MCM, Winterbourn CC. Gelatinase contributes to the degradation of glomerular basement membrane collagen by human neutrophils. *Collagen Related Res* 1988;8:113–22.
30. Shah SV, Baricos WH, Basci A. Degradation of human glomerular basement membrane by stimulated neutrophils: activation of a metalloproteinase(s) by reactive oxygen metabolites. *J Clin Invest* 1987;79: 25–31.
31. Varani J, Taylor CG, Riser B, et al. Mesangial cell killing by leukocytes: role of leukocyte oxidants and proteolytic enzymes. *Kidney Int* 1992;42:1169–77.
32. Hooke DH, Gee DC, Atkins RC. Leukocyte analysis using monoclonal antibodies in human glomerulonephritis. *Kidney Int* 1987;31: 964–72.
33. Sorger K, Gessler U, Hübner FK, et al. Subtypes of acute postinfectious glomerulonephritis: synopsis of clinical and pathological features. *Clin Nephrol* 1987;17:114–28.
34. Camussi G, Caligaris Cappio F, et al. The polymorphonuclear neutrophil (PMN) immunohistological technique: detection of immune complexes bound to the PMN membrane in acute poststreptococcal and lupus nephritis. *Clin Nephrol* 1980;14:280–7.
35. Lewy JE, Salinas-Madrigal L, Herdson PB, Pirani CL, Metcoff J. Clinicopathologic correlations in acute poststreptococcal glomerulonephritis. *Medicine (Baltimore)* 1971;50:453–501.
36. Appel GB, Silva FG, Pirani CL, Meltzer JI, Estes D. Renal involvement in systemic lupus erythematosus (SLE): a study of 56 patients emphasizing histologic classification. *Medicine (Baltimore)* 1978;57: 371–409.
37. Min KW, Györkey F, Györkey P, Yium JJ, Eknoyan G. The morphogenesis of glomerular crescents in rapidly progressive glomerulonephritis. *Kidney Int* 1974;5:47–56.
38. Tarantino A, DeVecchi A, Montagnino G, et al. Renal disease in essential mixed cryoglobulinemia. *Q J Med* 1981;197:1–30.
39. Kincaid-Smith P, Nicholls K, Birchall I. Polymorphs infiltrate glomeruli in mesangial IgA glomerulonephritis. *Kidney Int* 1989;36: 1108–11.
40. Saeki T, Kuroda T, Morita T, Suzuki K, Arakawa M, Kawaski K. Significance of myeloperoxidase (MPO) in rapidly progressive glomerulonephritis (RPGN). *Am J Kidney Dis* 1995;26:13–21.
41. Brouwer E, Huitema MG, Leontine Mulder AH, et al. Neutrophil activation in vitro and in vivo in Wegener's granulomatosis. *Kidney Int* 1994;45:1120–31.
42. Mrowka C, Csernok E, Gross WL, Feucht HE, Bechtel U, Thoenes GH. Distribution of the granulocyte serine proteinases proteinase 3 and elastase in human glomerulonephritis. *Am J Kidney Dis* 1995;25: 253–61.
43. Camussi G, Tetta C, Segoloni G, Coda R, Vercellone A. Localization of neutrophil cationic proteins and loss of anionic charges in glomeruli of patients with systemic lupus erythematosus glomerulonephritis. *Clin Immunol Immunopathol* 1982;24:299–314.
44. Cochrane CG. Immunologic tissue injury mediated by neutrophilic leukocytes. *Adv Immunol* 1968;9:99–162.
45. Cochrane CG, Unanue ER, Dixon FJ. A role of polymorphonuclear leukocytes and complement in nephrotoxic nephritis. *J Exp Med* 1965;122:99–122.
46. Hawkins D, Cochrane CG. Glomerular basement membrane damage in immunological glomerulonephritis. *Immunology* 1968;14:665–80.
47. Kühn K, Ryan GB, Hein SJ, Galaske RG, Karnovsky MJ. An ultrastructural study of the mechanisms of proteinuria in rat nephrotoxic nephritis. *Lab Invest* 1977;36:375–87.
48. Lan HY, Paterson DJ, Hutchinson P, Atkins RC. Leukocyte involvement in the pathogenesis of pulmonary injury in experimental Goodpasture's syndrome. *Lab Invest* 1991;64:330–8.
49. Tipping PG, Neale TJ, Holdsworth SR. T-lymphocyte participation in antibody-induced experimental glomerulonephritis. *Kidney Int* 1985; 27:530.
50. Schreiner GF, Cotran RS, Pardo V, Unanue ER. A mononuclear cell component in experimental immunological glomerulonephritis. *J Exp Med* 1978;147:369–84.
51. Golbus SM, Wilson CB. Experimental glomerulonephritis induced by in situ formation of immune complexes in glomerular capillary wall. *Kidney Int* 1979;16:148–57.
52. Johnson RJ, Klebanoff SJ, Ochi RF, et al. Participation of the myeloperoxidase–H_2O_2–halide system in immune complex nephritis. *Kidney Int* 1987;32:342–9.
53. Sekiyama S, Yoshida F, Yuzawa Y, et al. Mesangial proliferative glomerulonephritis induced in rats by a lentil lectin and its antibodies. *J Lab Clin Med* 1993;121:71–82.
54. Johnson RJ, Alpers CE, Pruchno C, et al. Mechanisms and kinetics

for platelet and neutrophil localization in immune complex nephritis. *Kidney Int* 1989;36:780–9.
55. Rehan A, Johnson KJ, Wiggins RC, Kunkel RG, Ward PA. Evidence for the role of oxygen radicals in acute nephrotoxic nephritis. *Lab Invest* 1984;51:396–403.
56. Naish PF, Thomson NM, Simpson IJ, Peters DK. The role of polymorphonuclear leukocytes in the autologous phase of nephrotoxic nephritis. *Clin Exp Immunol* 1975;22:102–11.
57. Thomson NM, Naish PF, Simpson IJ, Peters DK. The role of C3 in the autologous phase of nephrotoxic nephritis. *Clin Exp Immunol* 1976;24:464–73.
58. Tucker BJ, Gushwa LC, Wilson CB, Blantz RC. Effect of leukocyte depletion on glomerular dynamics during acute glomerular immune injury. *Kidney Int* 1985;28:28–35.
59. Boyce NW, Fernando NS, Neale TJ, Holdsworth SR. Acute pulmonary and renal injury after administration of heterologous anti-lung antibodies in the rat: characterization of ultrastructural binding sites, basement membrane epitopes, and inflammatory mediation systems. *Lab Invest* 1991;64:272–8.
60. Salant DJ, Adler S, Darby C, et al. Influence of antigen distribution on the mediation of immunological glomerular injury. *Kidney Int* 1985;27:938–50.
61. Tipping PG, Boyce NW, Holdsworth SR. Relative contributions of chemo-attractant and terminal components of complement to anti-glomerular basement membrane (GBM) glomerulonephritis. *Clin Exp Immunol* 1989;78:444–8.
62. Groggel GC, Salant DJ, Darby C, Rennke HG, Couser WG. Role of the terminal complement pathway in the heterologous phase of anti-glomerular basement membrane nephritis in the rabbit. *Kidney Int* 1985;27:643–51.
63. Boyce NW, Holdsworth SR. Anti-glomerular basement membrane antibody-induced experimental glomerulonephritis: evidence for dose-dependent, direct antibody and complement-induced, cell-independent injury. *J Immunol* 1985;135:3918–21.
64. O'Meara YM, Natori Y, Minto AWM, Goldstein DJ, Manning EC, Salant DJ. Nephrotoxic antiserum identifies β_1-integrin on rat glomerular epithelial cells. *Am J Physiol* 1992;262(6 Part 2):F1083–91.
65. Henson PM. Pathologic mechanisms in neutrophil-mediated injury. *Am J Pathol* 1972;68:593–604.
66. Baud L, Ardaillou R. Reactive oxygen species: production and role in the kidney. *Am J Physiol* 1986;251:765–76.
67. Shah SV. Role of reactive oxygen metabolites in experimental glomerular disease. *Kidney Int* 1989;35:1093–106.
68. Johnson RJ, Klebanoff SJ, Couser WG. Oxidants in glomerular injury. In: Wilson CW, Brenner BM, Stein J, eds. *Contemporary issues in nephrology*. New York: Churchill-Livingston, 1988:87–110.
69. Shah SV. Oxidant mechanisms in glomerulonephritis. *Semin Nephrol* 1991;11:320–6.
70. Diamond JR. The role of reactive oxygen species in animal models of glomerular disease. *Am J Kidney Dis* 1992;19:292–300.
71. Andreoli SP. Reactive oxygen molecules, oxidant injury and renal disease. *Pediatr Nephrol* 1991;5:733–42.
72. Davies M, Coles GA, Thomas GJ, Martin J, Lovett DH. Proteinases and the glomerulus: their role in glomerular diseases. *Klin Wochenschr* 1990;68:1145–9.
73. Baricos WH, Shah SV. Proteolytic enzymes as mediators of glomerular injury. *Kidney Int* 1991;40:161–73.
74. Johnson RJ, Lovett D, Lehrer RI, Couser WG, Klebanoff J. Role of oxidants and proteases in glomerular injury. *Kidney Int* 1994;45:352–9.
75. Linas SL, Shanley PF, Whittenburg D, Berger E, Repine JE. Neutrophils accentuate ischemia-reperfusion injury in isolated perfused rat kidneys. *Am J Physiol* 1988;255:F728–35.
76. Mossmann H, Hoyer B, Walz W, Himmelspach K, Hammer DK. Antibody-dependent cellular cytotoxicity and chemiluminesence as a tool for studying the mechanism of anti-glomerular basement membrane nephritis: the role of the cytotoxic potential of polymorphonuclear granulocytes and monocytes. *Immunology* 1984;53:545–52.
77. Davies M, Coles GA, Harber MJ. Effect of glomerular basement membrane on the initiation of chemiluminescence and lysosomal enzyme release in human polymorphonuclear leucocytes: an in vitro model of glomerular disease. *Immunology* 1984;52:151–9.
78. Chen H-C, Tomino Y, Yaguchi Y, et al. Oxidative metabolism of polymorphonuclear leukocytes (PMN) in patients with IgA nephropathy. *J Clin Lab Anal* 1992;6:35–9.
79. Li JZ, Sharma R, Dileepan KN, Savin VJ. Polymorphonuclear leukocytes increase glomerular albumin permeability via hypohalous acid. *Kidney Int* 1994;46:1025–30.
80. Campbell EJ, Senior RM, McDonald JA, Cox DL. Proteolysis by neutrophils: relative importance of cell-substrate contact and oxidative inactivation of proteinase inhibitors in vitro. *J Clin Invest* 1982; 70:845–52.
81. McGowan SE, Murray JJ. Direct effects of neutrophil oxidants on elastase-induced extracellular matrix proteolysis. *Am Rev Respir Dis* 1987;135:1286–93.
82. Vissers MCM, Winterbourn CC. The effect of oxidants on neutrophil-mediated degradation of glomerular basement membrane collagen. *Biochim Biophys Acta* 1986;889:277–86.
83. Poelstra K, Hardonk MJ, Koudstall J, Bakker WW. Intraglomerular platelet aggregation and experimental glomerulonephritis. *Kidney Int* 1990;37:1500–8.
84. Poelstra K, Brouwer E, Baller JFW, Hardonk MJ, Bakker WW. Attenuation of anti-Thy 1 glomerulonephritis in the rat by anti-inflammatory platelet-inhibiting agents. *Am J Pathol* 1993;142:441–50.
85. Klebanoff SJ, Clark RA. Iodination by human polymorphonuclear leukocytes: a re-evaluation. *J Lab Clin Med* 1977;89:675–86.
86. Johnson RJ, Couser WG, Chi EY, Adler S, Klebanoff SJ. New mechanism for glomerular injury: myeloperoxidase–hydrogen peroxide–halide system. *J Clin Invest* 1987;79:1379–87.
87. Johnson RJ, Guggenheim S, Klebanoff SJ, et al. Morphologic correlates of glomerular oxidant injury induced by the myeloperoxidase–hydrogen peroxide–halide system of neutrophils. *Lab Invest* 1988;58: 294–301.
88. Stratta P, Canavese C, Mazzucco G, et al. Mesangiolysis and endothelial lesions due to peroxidative damage in rabbits. *Nephron* 1989; 51:250–6.
89. Stratta P, Canavese C, Dogliani M, et al. Experimental evidence for mesangiolysis due to hydrogen peroxide. *J Nephrol* 1989;1:37–41.
90. Yoshioka T, Ichikawa I, Fogo A. Reactive oxygen metabolites cause massive, reversible proteinuria and glomerular sieving defect without apparent ultrastructural abnormality. *J Am Soc Nephrol* 191;2: 902–12.
91. Ito S, Ueda Y, Sugisaki T, Iidaka K. Induction of glomerular injury by singlet oxygen. *Nephron* 1992;60:204–9.
92. Klebanoff SJ, Waltersdorph AM. Inhibition of peroxidase-catalyzed reactions by deferoxamine. *Arch Biochem Biophys* 1988;264:600–6.
93. Vissers MCM, Fantone JC. Inhibition of hypochlorous acid-mediated reactions by desferrioxamine: implications for the mechanism of cellular injury by neutrophils. *Free Radic Biol Med* 1990;8:331–7.
94. Rehan A, Johnson KJ, Kunkel RG, Wiggins RC. Role of oxygen radicals in phorbol myristate acetate-induced glomerular injury. *Kidney Int* 1985;27:503–11.
95. Rehan A, Wiggins RC, Kunkel RG, Till Go, Johnson KJ. Glomerular injury and proteinuria in rats after intrarenal injection of cobra venom factor: evidence for the role of neutrophil-derived oxygen free radicals. *Am J Pathol* 1986;123:57–66.
96. Yoshioka T, Ichikawa I. Glomerular dysfunction induced by polymorphonuclear leukocyte-derived reactive oxygen species. *Am J Physiol* 1989;257:F53–9.
97. Adachi T, Fukuta M, Ito Y, Hirano K, Sugiura M, Sugiura K. Effect of superoxide dismutase on glomerular nephritis. *Biochem Pharmacol* 1986;35:341–5.
98. Webb DB, MacKenzie R. Evidence against a role for superoxide ions in the injury of nephrotoxic nephritis in rats. *Clin Sci* 1985;69:687–9.
99. Birtwistle RJ, Michael J, Howie AJ, Adu D. Reactive oxygen products in heterologous anti-glomerular basement membrane nephritis in rats. *Br J Exp Pathol* 1989;70:207–13.
100. Boyce NW, Holdsworth SR. Hydroxyl radical mediation of immune renal injury by desferrioxamine. *Kidney Int* 1986;30:813–7.
101. Vissers MCM, Day WA, Winterbourn CC. Neutrophils adherent to a nonphagocytosable surface (glomerular basement membrane) produce oxidants only at the site of attachment. *Blood* 1985;66:161–6.
102. Wright SD, Silverstein SC. Phagocytosing macrophages exclude proteins from the zones of contact with opsonized targets. *Nature* 1984; 309:359–61.
103. Kawamura T, Yoshioka T, Bills T, Fogo A, Ichikawa I. Glucocorticoid activates glomerular antioxidant enzymes and protects glomeruli from oxidant injuries. *Kidney Int* 1991;40:291–301.

104. Davies M, Barrett AJ, Travis J, Sanders E, Coles GA. The degradation of human glomerular basement membrane with purified lysosomal proteinases: evidence for the pathogenic role of the polymorphonuclear leucocyte in glomerulonephritis. *Clin Sci Mol Med* 1978; 54:233–40.
105. Davies M, Coles GA, Hughes KT. Glomerular basement membrane injury by neutrophil and monocyte neutral proteinases. *Renal Physiol* 1980;3:106–11.
106. Baricos WH, Murphy G, Zhou Y, Nguyen HH, Shah SV. Degradation of glomerular basement membrane by purified mammalian metalloproteinases. *Biochem J* 1988;254:609–12.
107. Murphy G, Reynolds JJ, Bretz U, Baggiolini M. Partial purification of collagenase and gelatinase from human polymorphonuclear leucocytes. *Biochem J* 1982;203:209–21.
108. Uitto V-J, Schwartz D, Veis A. Degradation of basement-membrane collagen by neutral proteases from human leukocytes. *Eur J Biochem* 1980;105:409–17.
109. Hughes KT, Davies M, Sanders E, Coles GA. A kinetic study of the degradation of human glomerular basement membrane by human polymorphonuclear leucocyte azurophil granules: supportive evidence for the involvement of leucocytes in glomerulonephritis. *Biochem Soc Trans* 1979;7:941–3.
110. Stuffers-Heiman M, Tjoeng-Mutsaerts N, Ferwerda W, Van Es LA. Immunological properties of glomerular basement membrane antigens solubilized by elastase digestion. *J Immunol Methods* 1980;32: 93–102.
111. Heck LW, Blackburn WD, Irwin MH, Abrahamson DR. Degradation of basement membrane laminin by human neutrophil elastase and cathespin G. *Am J Pathol* 1990;136:1267–74.
112. Roughley PJ. The degradation of proteoglycan by leucocyte elastase. *Biochem Soc Trans* 1977;5:443–5.
113. Sanders E, Davies M, Coles GA. On the pathogenesis of glomerulonephritis: a clinico-pathological study indicating that neutrophils attach and degrade glomerular basement membrane. *Renal Physiol* 1980;3:355–9.
114. Johnson RJ, Couser WG, Alpers CE, Vissers M, Schulze M, Klebanoff S. The human neutrophil serine proteinases, elastase and cathepsin G, can mediate glomerular injury in vivo. *J Exp Med* 1988; 168:1169–74.
115. Heeringa P, Brouwer E, Klok PA, et al. Elastase but not proteinase 3 induces proteinuria after in vivo renal perfusion. *J Am Soc Nephrol* 1994;5:781(abst).
116. Schrijver G, Schalkwijk J, Robben JCM, Assmann KJM, Koene RAP. Antiglomerular basement membrane nephritis in beige mice. *J Exp Med* 1989;168:1435–48.
117. Kubo A, Sasada M, Nishimura T, et al. Oxygen radical generation by polymorphonuclear leucocytes of beige mice. *Clin Exp Immunol* 1987;73:658–63.
118. Gomez-Chiarri M, Ortiz A, Seron D, Gonzalez E, Egido J. The intercrine superfamily and renal disease. *Kidney Int* 1993;39:S81–5.
119. Tang WW, Yin S, Wittwer AJ, Qi M. Chemokine gene expression in anti-glomerular basement membrane antibody glomerulonephritis. *Am J Physiol* 1995;269:F323–F330.
120. Wu X, Wittwer AJ, Carr LS, Crippes BA, DeLarco JE, Lefkowith JB. Cytokine-induced neutrophil chemoattractant mediates neutrophil influx in immune complex glomerulonephritis in rats. *J Clin Invest* 1994;94:337–44.
121. Feng L, Xia Y, Yoshimura T, Wilson CB. Prevention of neutrophil influx in glomerulonephritis in the rat with anti-macrophage inflammatory protein-2 (MIP-2) antibody. *J Clin Invest* 1995;95:1009.
122. Wada T, Tomosugi N, Naito T, et al. Prevention of proteinuria by the administration of anti-interleukin 8 antibody in experimental acute immune complex-induced glomerulonephritis. *J Exp Med* 1994;180: 1135–40.
123. Holdsworth SR, Neale TJ, Wilson CB. Abrogation of macrophage-dependent injury in experimental glomerulonephritis in the rabbit. *J Clin Invest* 1981;68:686–98.
124. Harada A, Sekido N, Akahoshi T, Wada T, Mukaida N, Matsushima K. Essential involvement of interleukin-8 (IL-8) in acute inflammation. *J Leukoc Biol* 1994;56:559–64.
125. Wada T, Yokoyama H, Tomosugi N, et al. Detection of urinary interleukin-8 in glomerular diseases. *Kidney Int* 1994;46:455–60.
126. Perico N, Remuzzi G. Role of platelet-activating factor in renal immune injury and proteinuria. *Am J Nephrol* 1990;10(Suppl 1):98–104.
127. Bresnahan BA, Wu S, Fenoy FJ, Roman RJ, Lianos EA. Mesangial cell immune injury: hemodynamic role of leukocyte- and platelet-derived eicosanoids. *J Clin Invest* 1992;90:2304–12.
128. Johnson RJ. The glomerular response to injury: progression or resolution? *Kidney Int* 1994;45:1769–82.
129. Lefkowith JB, Pippin J, Nagamatsu T, Lee V. Urinary eicosanoids and the assessment of glomerular inflammation. *J Am Soc Nephrol* 1992;2:1560–7.
130. Lefkowith JB, Nagamatsu T, Pippin J, Schreiner GF. Role of leukocytes in metabolic and functional derangements of experimental glomerulonephritis. *Am J Physiol* 1991;261:F213–20.
131. Yared A, Albrightson-Winslow C, Griswold D, Takahashi K, Fogo A, Badr KF. Functional significance of leukotriene B_4 in normal and glomerulonephritic kidneys. *J Am Soc Nephrol* 1991;2:45–56.
132. Tomosugi NI, Cashman SJ, Hay H, et al. Modulation of antibody-mediated glomerular injury in vivo by bacterial lipopolysaccharide, tumor necrosis factor, and IL-1. *J Immunol* 1989;142:3083–90.
133. Karkar AM, Koshino Y, Cashman SJ, et al. Passive immunization against tumour necrosis factor-alpha (TNF-alpha) and IL-1 beta protects from LPS enhancing glomerular injury in nephrotoxic nephritis in rats. *Clin Exp Immunol* 1992;90:312–8.
134. Mulligan MS, Johnson KJ, Todd RF III, et al. Requirements for leukocyte adhesion molecules in nephrotoxic nephritis. *J Clin Invest* 1993;91:577–87.
135. Carlos T, Harlan JM. Leukocyte-endothelial adhesion molecules. *Blood* 1994;84:2068–101.
136. Brady HR, Denton MD, Brenner BM, Serhan CN. Neutrophil adhesion to glomerular mesangial cells: regulation by lipoxygenase-derived eicosanoids. *Adv Exp Med Biol* 1991;314:347–59.
137. Brady HR, Spertini O, Jimenez W, Brenner BM, Marsden PA, Tedder TF. Neutrophils, monocytes, and lymphocytes bind to cytokine-activated kidney glomerular endothelial cells through L-selectin (LAM-1) in vitro. *J Immunol* 1992;149:2437–44.
138. Wu X, Pippin J, Lefkowith JB. Attenuation of immune-mediated glomerulonephritis with an anti-CD11b monoclonal antibody. *Am J Physiol* 1993;264:715–21.
139. Kawasaki K, Yaoita E, Yamamoto T, Tamatani T, Miyasaka M, Kihara I. Antibodies against intercellular adhesion molecule-1 lymphocyte function-associated antigen-1 prevent glomerular injury in rat experimental crescentic glomerulonephritis. *J Immunol* 1993;150: 1074–83.
140. Nishikawa K, Guo Y-J, Miyasaka M, et al. Antibodies to intercellular adhesion molecule 1/lymphocyte function-associated antigen 1 prevent crescent formation in rat autoimmune glomerulonephritis. *J Exp Med* 1993;177:667–77.
141. Tipping PG, Huang XR, Berndt MC, Holdsworth SR. A role for P selectin in complement-independent neutrophil-mediated glomerular injury. *Kidney Int* 1994;46:79–88.
142. Sindrey M, Naish P. The mediation of the localization of polymorphonuclear leucocytes in glomeruli during the autologous phase of nephrotoxic nephritis. *Clin Exp Immunol* 1979;35:350–5.
143. Marín C, Mosquera J, Rodríguez-Iturbe B. Neuraminidase promotes neutrophil, lymphocyte and macrophage infiltration in the normal rat kidney. *Kidney Int* 1995;47:88–95.
144. Borel JP, Bellon G, Garnotel R, Monboisse JC. Adhesion and activation of human neutrophils on basement membrane molecules. *Kidney Int* 1992;43:26–9.
145. Weksler BB. Roles for human platelets in inflammation. *Prog Clin Biol Res* 1988;283:611–38.
146. Henson PM. Editorial: interactions between neutrophils and platelets. Lab Invest 1990;62:391.
147. Campbell PA. Editorial review: the neutrophil, a professional killer of bacteria, may be controlled by T cells. *Clin Exp Immunol* 1990;79: 141–3.
148. Johnson RJ, Alpers CE, Pritzl P, et al. Platelets mediate neutrophil-dependent immune complex nephritis in the rat. *J Clin Invest* 1988; 82:1225–35.
149. Del Maschio A, Corvazier E, Maillet F, Kazatchkine MD, Maclouf J. Platelet-dependent induction and amplification of polymorphonuclear leucocyte lysosomal enzyme release. *Br J Haematol* 1989;72:329–35.
150. Coëffier E, Delautier D, Le Couedic J-P, Chignard M, Denizot Y, Benvenist J. Cooperation between platelets and neutrophils for paf-acether (platelet-activating factor) formation. *J Leukoc Biol* 1990;47: 234–43.

151. Wu X, Pippin J, Lefkowith JB. Platelets and neutrophils are critical to the enhanced glomerular arachidonate metabolism in acute nephrotoxic nephritis in rats. *J Clin Invest* 1993;91:766–73.
152. Maclouf J, Fruteau de Laclos B, Borgeat P. Stimulation of leukotriene biosynthesis in human blood leukocytes by platelet-derived 12-hydroperoxy-icosatetraenoic acid. *Proc Natl Acad Sci USA* 1982;79: 6042–6.
153. Papayianni A, Serhan CN, Phillips ML, Rennke HG, Brady HR. Transcellular biosynthesis of lipoxin A_4 during adhesion of platelets and neutrophils in experimental immune complex glomerulonephritis. *Kidney Int* 1995;47:1295–302.
154. Savill J, Smith J, Sarraf C, Ren Y, Abbott F, Rees A. Glomerular mesangial cells and inflammatory macrophages ingest neutrophils undergoing apoptosis. *Kidney Int* 1992;42:924–36.
155. Ordonez NG, Gomez LA. The ultrastructure of glomerular haematoxylin bodies. *J Pathol* 1981;135:259–65.
156. Van der Woude FJ, Rasmussen N, Lobatto S, et al. Autoantibodies to neutrophils and monocytes: a new tool for diagnosis and a marker of disease activity in Wegener's granulomatosis. *Lancet* 1985;2:425–9.
157. Falk RJ, Jennette JC. Anti-neutrophil cytoplasmic autoantibodies with specificity for myeloperoxidase in patients with systemic vasculitis and idiopathic necrotizing and crescentic glomerulonephritis. *N Engl J Med* 1988;318:1651–7.
158. Kallenberg CGM, Brouwer E, Weening JJ, Cohen Tervaert JW. Anti-neutrophil cytoplasmic antibodies: current diagnostic and pathophysiological potential. *Kidney Int* 1994;46:1–15.
159. Johnson RJ. The mystery of the antineutrophil cytoplasmic antibodies. *Am J Kidney Dis* 1995;26:57–61.
160. Falk RJ, Terrell RS, Charles LA, Jennette JC. Anti-neutrophil cytoplasmic autoantibodies include neutrophils to degranulate and produce oxygen radicals in vitro. *Proc Natl Acad Sci USA* 1990;87:4115–9.
161. Savage COS, Pottinger BE, Gaskin G, Pusey CD, Pearson JD. Autoantibodies developing to myeloperoxidase and proteinase in systemic vasculitis stimulate neutrophil cytotoxicity toward cultured endothelial cells. *Am J Pathol* 1992;141:335–42.
162. Brouwer E, Huitema MG, Klok PA, et al. Antimyeloperoxidase-associated proliferative glomerulonephritis: an animal model. *J Exp Med* 1993;177:905–14.
163. Brouwer E, Stegeman CA, Huitema MG, Limburg PC, Kallenberg CGM. T cell reactivity to proteinase 3 and myeloperoxidase in patients with Wegener's granulomatosis (WG). *Clin Exp Immunol* 1994;98:448–53.

Immunologic Renal Diseases,
edited by E. G. Neilson and W. G. Couser.
Lippincott-Raven Publishers, Philadelphia © 1997

CHAPTER 27

Platelets

Jeffrey L. Barnes

INTRODUCTION

Platelets serve as a reservoir for a variety of secretory products required for coagulation and thrombosis during hemostasis. Many of these products are biologically active and have enzymatic, chemotactic, or mitogenic properties that can have multiple effects on target cells during episodes of acute or subacute injury. In an inflammatory setting, a number of these secretory products have the potential to interact with the glomerulus and induce permeability changes favoring immune-complex deposition and/or to elicit cellular proliferation and regulate extracellular matrix synthesis, leading to the deterioration of renal function. A role for platelet activation in renal vascular diseases has been suggested and has been the focus of a several recent reviews (1–3). This chapter discusses the function of the platelet as an inflammatory cell, reexamines the evidence that platelets are involved in clinical renal vascular disease, and discusses experimental data supporting mechanisms of how platelet secretory products might facilitate glomerular deposition of immune complexes, and stimulate cellular behaviors during remodeling that can lead to a distortion of normal glomerular architecture.

THE PLATELET AS AN INFLAMMATORY CELL

Platelets secrete many biologically active products from α-granules, lysosomes, and dense granules and generate lipid mediators from membranes within the canalicular system (Table 1). Several of these products function in coagulation and thrombosis, whereas other platelet products have the potential to interact locally within the microvasculature and mediate cellular events associated with injury or resolution of inflammation (including cell adhesion, migration, proliferation, and extracellular matrix assembly).

Adhesive Proteins and Platelet–Vessel Wall Interactions

Platelets contain a variety of adhesive proteins (including fibronectin, vitronectin, thrombospondin, von Willebrand factor, osteonectin, and fibrinogen) that function in platelet–platelet aggregation and platelet–cell or matrix adhesion and are important in platelet–vessel interactions (1,4). Platelets also have several integrin receptors ($\alpha_{IIb}\beta_3$, $\alpha_v\beta_1$, $\alpha_5\beta_1$, and $\alpha_6\beta$) on their surface that bind these and other adhesive proteins through specific domains within the ligand structure. Such interactions are believed to be instrumental in platelet–platelet interactions in developing platelet thrombi. A variety of cells also display integrin receptors for the adhesive proteins that might be involved in platelet–cell interactions. Moreover, several of the adhesive proteins just mentioned are normal constituents of the cell substratum; thus, integrin receptors on platelet surfaces can be expected to interact with extracellular matrix in situations of cell injury and loss of structural integrity of the microvasculature. Platelet-released adhesive proteins might also have direct biologic effects on target cells and play an instrumental role in cellular reparative processes through mediation of cellular migration and proliferation or by provision of matrix for subsequent accumulation of other matrix proteins (see sections below).

Mediators of Inflammation and Repair

Growth Factors

Platelets contain a variety of mitogens that stimulate a diversity of cell types in culture. Of these, the peptide

J. L. Barnes: Department of Medicine, Division of Nephrology, University of Texas Health Science Center, San Antonio, Texas 78284; and Audie L. Murphy Memorial Veterans Medical Center, San Antonio, Texas 78229.

TABLE 1. *Platelet secretory products*

α-Granule constituents	
Growth factors	**Adhesive proteins**
Platelet-derived growth factor (+,H,C)	Fibronectin (H,C)
Transforming growth factor α (C)	Thrombospondin (H,C)
Transforming growth factor β (H,C)	Vitronectin (H,C)
Epidermal growth factor (C)	Osteonectin (SPARC) (C)
Platelet-derived endothelial growth factor (C)	von Willebrand factor
Hepatocyte growth factor (scatter factor) (+,H,C)	
Insulinlike growth factor 1 (C)	
Basic fibroblast growth factor (+,H,C)	
Interleukin 1γ	
Platelet factor 4 (+,H,C)	
β-Thromboglobulin (+,H,C)	

Lysosomal constituents (enzymes)	
Proteinases	**Acid hydrolases**
Cathepsins (+)	Aryl sulfatase
Collagenase (+)	β-Glucuronidase
Neutral protease	β-Galactosidase
Elastase (+)	N-Acetylglucose-aminidase
	Endoglycosidase (heparitinase) (+,H)

Biologically active lipids and eicosanoids constituents	
Dense	**granule**
Thromboxane A_2 (C)	Serotonin (C)
12-HETE (C)	Histamine (C)
Leukotrienes (C)	Norepinephrine (C)
Malondialdehyde	ADP
Platelet-activating factor (AGEPC) (C)	

AGEPC, 1-O-hexadecyl/octadecyl-2-acetyl-*sn*-glyceryl-3-phosphorylcholine; C, chemotactin; H, heparin-binding protein; 12-HETE, 12-L-hydroxy-5,8,10,14-eicosatetraenoic acid; +, cationic protein or inferred to be cationic by gel chromatography.

growth factors platelet-derived growth factor (PDGF), transforming factor (TGF) α, TGF-β, basic fibroblast growth factor (bFGF), platelet factor (PF) 4, and interleukin (IL) 1 have been implicated as mediators of vascular disease and wound healing and are important mediators in the progression of renal disease (1,3,5,6) (see also chapter 20). Other platelet-associated mitogenic substances include serotonin, thromboxane A_2 (TXA_2), and lipoxygenase products (3). In all, there are over 20 known platelet secretory products that potentiate cell proliferation and may play several roles during tissue remodeling in disease states (Table 1).

Conversely, some factors such as TGF-β and PF4 inhibit proliferation and may have regulatory functions in tissue repair and disease (5–7). Several platelet growth factors, particularly TGF-β, can potentiate extracellular matrix synthesis and may participate in tissue fibrosis (5,6,8,9).

Chemotactins

Nearly all platelet growth factors have been reported to be chemoattractants for a variety of inflammatory and noninflammatory cell types (Table 1) (chapter 24) (1). Several of these products may contribute to repair processes by direct recruitment of blood-borne leukocytes or by mediating migration of intrinsic cells to sites of injury during tissue remodeling. Also, platelet secretory constituents can promote migration of one cell type, yet inhibit another, as demonstrated for vascular smooth muscle cell and endothelial cell migration in response to PDGF, TGF-β, serotonin, histamine, and norepinephrine (10). Thus, cell migration at sites of injury can depend on cell type, the initiating stimulus, and the presence of modulating factors.

Enzymes

Platelets secrete several lysosomal proteases and hydrolases (Table 1). The role of these enzymes is not entirely clear, but they may function in clot resolution, degradation of extracellular matrix at sites of tissue injury, or enhancement of cellular responses to secreted biologically active proteins. Collectively, these enzymes have the potential to digest the majority of extracellular matrix components contained within the glomerular basement membrane (GBM) and mesangial matrix. Thus, these enzymes may have roles in altering glomerular permeability and mediating tissue remodeling (see below).

Lipid Mediators and Eicosanoids

Platelets generate several lipid mediators (Table 1) through conversion of arachidonic acid to bioactive intermediate and end products via lipoxygenase and cyclooxygenase pathways (11,12). For example, TXA_2 is a potent platelet activator and has mitogenic, chemotactic, and hemodynamic properties. 12-HETE (12-hydroxyeicosatetraenoic acid) is a mild chemotactin produced in large quantities by platelets and can be converted by activated neutrophils into a powerful proinflammatory lipid, leukotriene B_4 (LTB_4). Platelets also use lipoxygenase and cyclooxygenase pathways to form oxidants that are cytotoxic to parasites and endothelial cells (3,13) and may have a direct role in tissue damage in inflammatory settings (see Chapter 22) (3). Moreover, an end product of the cyclooxygenase pathway, monodialdehyde, is potentially cytotoxic through its ability to cross-link proteins. Platelets also generate 1-*O*-hexadecyl/octadecyl-2-acetyl-*sn*-glyceryl-3-phosphorylcholine (AGEPC), more commonly referred to as platelet-activating factor (PAF). PAF is a highly potent lipid autacoid that has diverse biologic effects, including induction of platelet aggregation, neutrophil chemotaxis, vasoconstriction, and enhancement of vascular permeability. In short, PAF can evoke nearly all of the well-known cardinal signs of acute inflammation and has been implicated as a primary mediator of immune renal injury (1,14).

Platelet–Inflammatory Cell Interactions

Platelets interact with and adhere to leukocytes, and cross talk between these cells may condition the course of thrombotic and inflammatory diseases (3,15). Platelet-released products such as adenine nucleotides, PF4, PAF, and arachidonate metabolites are chemotactic for leukocytes and can potentiate neutrophil function (3,15–20). Also, direct cell–cell attachment between platelets and neutrophils can occur through selectins expressed on activated platelet surfaces (21) (see also chapters 25 and 26). Products released from platelets can also be converted into more potent biologic substances through transcellular metabolic pathways, as has been previously described for neutrophil conversion of 12-HETE into LTB_4 and several other lipoxygenase metabolites (12). Conversely, platelet–neutrophil adhesion may be instrumental in formation of lipoxins that inhibit neutrophil adhesion, chemotaxis, and diapedesis. Thus, products generated from neutrophil–platelet interactions may be important in suppression of neutrophil-mediated tissue injury (22).

Multiple cell interactions may also occur such as that described in monocyte–platelet coculture [for example, cleavage of platelet basic protein with consequent formation of neutrophil-activating peptide 2, a powerful chemotactin (23)]. Conversely, leukocyte-released factors can modify platelet function. Thus, a reciprocity of stimulatory function between platelets and inflammatory cells may be postulated in cellular injury or hypercellularity in glomerular disease (16–20,22) (see Chapter 26).

EVIDENCE OF PLATELET INVOLVEMENT IN CLINICAL RENAL DISEASE

As just discussed, a myriad of biologically active platelet products can be released at sites of localized cell injury or inflammation and participate in the progression of renal vascular disease. Clinical observations have implicated platelets as mediators of renal disease by reporting platelet destruction, increases in circulating platelet secretory products, and glomerular localization of platelets and/or their related antigens in various forms of glomerular disease.

Platelet Activation in Glomerular Disease

Platelet activation in renal disease has been documented by observations of shortened platelet survival or intrarenal platelet sequestration in patients with membranoproliferative, membranous, lupus glomerulonephritis, focal segmental glomerulosclerosis, and diabetic nephropathy (24–26). Also, thrombocytopenia and glomerular thrombosis are prevalent observations in patients with lupus nephritis and have been implied to represent important factors in determining the subsequent development of glomerulosclerosis (27,28). Accelerated platelet destruction has been found to be most notable in human diffuse proliferative glomerulonephritis in which statistically significant correlations between platelet destruction and intraglomerular cellular proliferation were reported (25,26,28). Platelet and fibrin thrombi in lumens of small arteries and glomerular capillaries are also common renal pathologic features in hemolytic uremic syndrome (29), thrombotic thrombocytopenic purpura, systemic sclerosis (30), acute and chronic transplant rejection (31), and nephropathy associated with essential hypertension (32). In addition, glomeruli in these diseases frequently show mild endothelial and mesangial hypercellularity and, in limited cases, crescents.

Elevated Blood and Urine Levels of Platelet Products

Platelet activation in patients with progressive forms of glomerular disease has been documented by release into the circulation and elevation of plasma levels of platelet secretory products such as PF4, β-TG (thromboglobulin), and serotonin (33–37). Moreover, decreased platelet counts and decreased platelet serotonin levels have been reported in post-streptococcal nephritis (38). Further evidence of platelet activation in glomerular disease is indicated by the observations of platelets or their α-granule constituents (β-TG, PF4, or GMP-140) in the urine of patients with diabetic (39) and immunoglobulin-A (IgA) nephropathies (40,41). Thus, renal structures are exposed to platelet products either through filtration of circulating platelet products or by activation of platelets within the glomerular microvasculature.

Renal Localization of Platelet Secretory Products

Platelets in glomeruli of renal biopsy specimens are infrequently identified in routine histologic preparations. Several explanations for the paucity of morphologically intact platelets in diseased glomeruli have been postulated. The first and most obvious is because platelets in human immune glomerular disease may have little tendency for localization within glomerular structures (42). Conversely, a loss or destruction of structural features of platelets or a "hit and run" phenomenon whereby stimulated platelets are to release their secretory granule contents and then exit the glomerular microcirculation may resolve the absence of visible platelet localization. Because of the complex interplay among inflammatory cells, resident glomerular cells, and platelets, it appears highly likely that platelets are activated during glomerular injury.

Indeed, platelet aggregates have been documented by light and electron microscopy in glomeruli from patients with mesangiocapillary glomerulonephritis, focal and segmental glomerulosclerosis, and IgA nephropathy (43–47). Evidence for platelet activation and release is also supported by the identification of platelet antigens and secretory products within the renal vasculature or diseased glomeruli by immunohistochemistry. For example, intraglomerular localization of undefined platelet antigens has been described in membranoproliferative, diabetic nephropathy and in hemolytic uremic syndrome and accelerated hypertension (47–49). Moreover, Camussi has provided data on the localization of platelet cationic proteins in glomerular capillary walls of lupus patients (Fig. 1), an observation that bears implications for charge interactions of these proteins with glomerular permselectivity and immune-complex deposition (as discussed below). More specifically, PF4, β-TG (47,50), platelet membrane antigen (GPIIb-IIIa) (51), or PDGF (45,52) have been identified in glomerular structures in renal biopsy specimens from patients with post-streptococcal nephritis, lupus nephritis, and mesangioproliferative, membranous, and IgA nephropathy. PF4, GPIIb-IIIa, and β-TG are specific platelet products; but others, including PDGF, TGF-β, and IL-1, can be synthesized by inflammatory cells or resident glomerular cells. Therefore, localization of these products could also be attributed to nonplatelet sources or to localized de novo cellular synthesis.

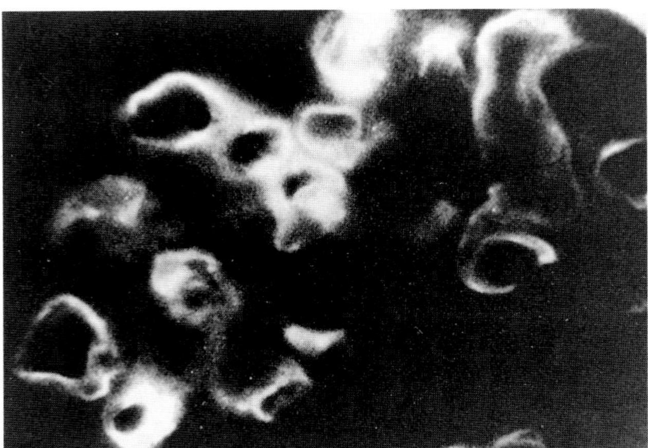

FIG. 1. Capillary walls of a glomerulus from a patient with lupus nephritis showing binding of platelet cationic proteins. From Camussi et al. (49), reproduced by permission of Blackwell Science, Inc.

A precise role for platelets in the pathogenesis of glomerular disease is unclear. However, studies on the normal physicochemical structure of the glomerular capillary wall and the knowledge of the diverse molecular properties and biologic activities of platelet secretory products have fostered the development of a variety to hypotheses to explain increased vascular permeability and development of glomerular hypercellularity, both of which are common features of glomerular disease.

Role for Platelets in Other Renal Vascular Diseases

As just mentioned, platelet activation and glomerular changes are observed in hemolytic uremic syndrome, thrombotic thrombocytopenic purpura, systemic sclerosis, acute and chronic transplant rejection, and essential hypertension (29–32). However, the major pathologic features of these diseases are myointimal proliferation and matrix accumulation within small arteries and arterioles. Such changes have been postulated to be associated with the release of platelet-derived mitogenic factors that could stimulate cell migration and proliferation similar to those described during the pathogenesis of atherosclerotic lesions (29–32). Consistent with this hypothesis are the experimental observations of aggregation of platelets and neutrophils and local release of PAF in the renal vasculature, and localization of platelet and neutrophil cationic proteins within the walls of glomerular capillaries in a rabbit model of hyperacute renal allograft rejection (53).

PLATELETS IN EXPERIMENTAL RENAL DISEASE

The investigations just outlined have established the presence of platelet activation, release, and localization of secretory products in vascular structures during clinical renal disease. These studies, however, do not shed light on whether localization of platelet secretory products in renal structures is an epiphenomenon or whether these products have biologic relevance either in the initiation or progression of renal disease. Answers to these questions have required the examination of several models of experimental renal disease that have platelet aggregation and secretion as morphologic features. Studies of the mechanisms of how platelets and their secretory products can mediate immune-complex localization and alter glomerular cell behavior have been the focus of numerous studies over the last 30 years.

Facilitation of Glomerular Immune-Complex Deposition

Platelet sequestration within glomerular capillaries is a common denominator in several immune-mediated models of glomerulonephritis. These include intrarenal administration of concanavalin-A–anti-concanavalin-A antibody (16,17) or antigen in preimmunized rabbits (54), acute serum sickness (55), and nephrotoxic serum nephritis (56,57). In these models, glomerular immune-complex localization has been associated with alterations in glomerular permeability and/or proteinuria. Early studies examining immune-complex localization in vascular beds described an increased permeability to molecular markers such as colloidal carbon (58,59). The etiologies of these permeability defects have not been resolved, but have been associated with platelets and release of secretory products that have been postulated to have direct effects on glomerular capillary barrier function. PAF-induced release of vasoactive amines from basophils and platelets and subsequent alterations in glomerular permeability to immune complexes have been implicated in immune glomerular diseases (1,14,60). However, contemporary thought suggests that direct charge–barrier interactions between products released from platelets and inflammatory cells and the glomerular capillary wall are causative (see below).

The glomerular capillary wall forms a restrictive barrier to circulating macromolecules through molecule–filter interactions, dependent on pore size, charge, physical integrity of the capillary wall, and hemodynamic forces (61) (see Chapter 3). The GBM is richly endowed with negatively charged moieties derived from the N-sulfated glycosaminoglycan, heparan sulfate; the sialic-acid-containing glycoproteins, laminin and fibronectin; the sulfated glycoprotein, entactin; and carboxyl groups located within various aspects of the basement membrane (61) (see Chapter 10). Surfaces of epithelial and endothelial cells also display polyanions that further contribute to the total negative charge of the capillary wall. Collectively, these negatively charged structures repel circulating negatively charged macromolecules. Positively charged molecules have an affinity for glomerular polyanion; therefore, cationic macromolecules including antibodies, antigens, or their complexes are attracted to and localize within glomerular structures, whereas anionic immune reactants do not (1,18).

Endogenous polycationic macromolecules derived from platelets (49,54,55,62,63) or other inflammatory cell sources (55) also possess an affinity for glomerular polyanion and may effect local alterations in glomerular permeability via charge interactions. Additionally, a variety of platelet secretory products are enzymes and may degrade structural components of the GBM, producing an increase in porosity and/or a loss of repulsive forces of the negatively charged membranes to circulating macromolecules. Platelet products could also alter glomerular hemodynamics fostering enhanced localization of immune complexes. The mechanisms of how platelet secretory products might facilitate glomerular permeability to circulating macromolecules and immune complexes are discussed in detail in the following sections (see also Chaper 14).

Loss of Glomerular Polyanion

A loss of glomerular polyanion preceding increased glomerular permeability or proteinuria has been shown to occur in most models of immune-complex glomerulonephritis. For example, reductions in glomerular polyanion have been reported in disorders marked by glomerular permeability defects, including nephrotoxic serum nephritis (64), acute serum sickness (55), intrarenal Arthus reaction (54), and lupus nephritis (64,65). Because platelet accumulation is common in these models, loss of glomerular polyanions could be related to products released from platelets that may contribute to increased glomerular permeability, proteinuria, and enhancement of immune-complex deposition within glomerular structures.

Loss of glomerular polyanion as effected by platelet products can occur by three mechanisms: (a) polycation-induced neutralization of fixed negative charge, (b) enzymatic degradation of anionic molecules, and (c) a reduction in glomerular cell synthesis of basement membrane constituents. In terms of acute platelet–basement membrane interactions, the first two events represent the most likely candidates for altering membrane permeability.

Neutralization of Fixed Negative Charge of the Glomerular Basement Membrane by Polycations

Synthetic Polycations

Injection or infusion of synthetic polycations, including hexadimethrine bromide, polyethyleneimine, and protamine sulfate, results in binding of these to glomerular polyanion with consequent neutralization of the electrostatic barrier and increased permeability to circulating macromolecules (1,61,67,68). Similarly, high-ionic-strength buffers perfused through rat kidneys can neutralize glomerular polyanion and progressively abolish GBM charge barrier properties, leading to clogging of the membrane by tracer molecules (69). Polycations can also alter size-restrictive barriers (67,68) presumably by binding with polyanion and reducing gel hydration, leading to structural distortion and alterations in porosity (70).

Synthetic polycations such as polyethyleneimine also increase glomerular permeability to passively administered antigen and antibody (71) or preformed immune complexes (72) (Fig. 2), leading to enhanced deposition and altered distribution of immune deposits in glomerular structures. Moreover, neutralization of glomerular poly-

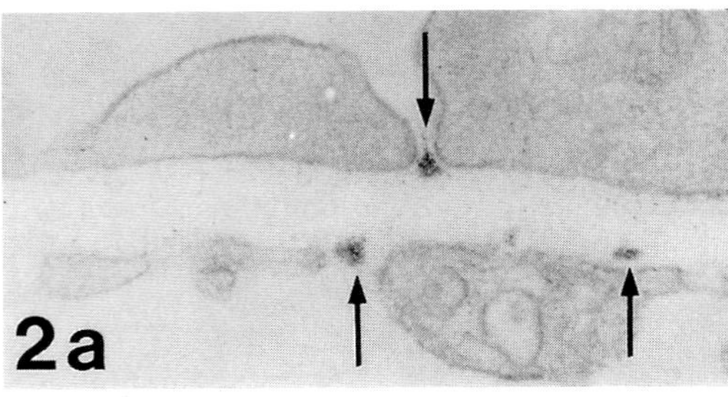

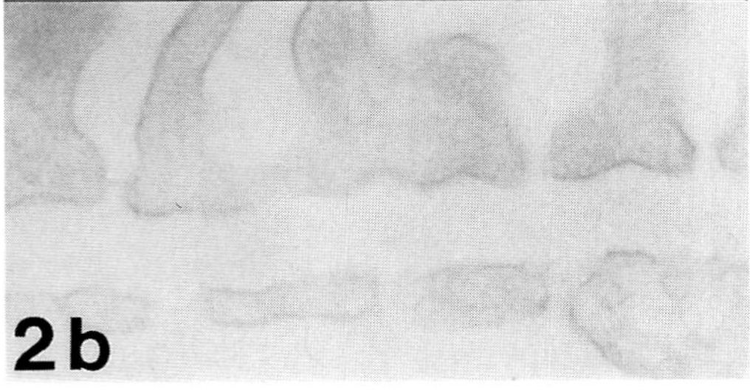

FIG. 2. Enhanced localization of BSA (bovine serum albumin)–anti-BSA immune complexes in a rat treated with polyethyleneimine (a) compared with a diluent control (b). Immunoperoxidase localization of immunoglobulin G is illustrated by electron microscopy in subendothelial and subepithelial *(arrows)* aspects of the glomerular basement membrane in polyethyleneimine-treated rats and absent in the same locations in diluent controls. From Barnes and Venkatachalam (72), reproduced by permission of the Rockefeller University Press.

anion by polyethyleneimine leads to enhancement of anti–renal tubular epithelial antigen IgG fixation to GBM in situ, presumably by a greater accessibility of the antibody to intrinsic fixed antigenic sites (73).

Endogenous Platelet Cationic Proteins

Platelet-released polycationic macromolecules, like synthetic polycations, have the potential to bind to glomerular polyanion and alter the electrostatic and size barriers to circulating macromolecules, thereby facilitating the deposition of immune complexes. Many platelet secretory products are cationic [pI 7.0–10.5 (Table 1)] and have the potential to bind to glomerular polyanion and alter permselectivity. Several of these proteins bind to heparin (Table 1) (and presumably heparan sulfate), and this interaction may explain, in part, the localization of PDGF, PF4, and β-TG in glomerular structures in several disorders (45–47,50,52). Additional platelet secretory products are not cationic, but have heparin binding domains (Table 1). Because heparan sulfate is believed to be the polyanion primarily responsible for maintaining the glomerular charge barrier (61), a role for platelet secretory products in altering glomerular permeability is tenable.

We have shown a strong ionic affinity of PF4 to GBMs in vitro and to subendothelial and subepithelial sites following intravenous injection (62). Binding of PF4 to these structures could be reversed by high-ionic-strength buffers or heparin and by blocking PF4 binding to glomerular polyanion in vivo by prior administration of polyethyleneimine. Similarly, platelet cationic proteins bind to GBM when applied to tissue sections of normal human or rat renal cortex or in glomerular capillary walls of renal biopsy sections from patients with lupus nephritis (49,63). Polyanion staining in both experimental and human tissue could be restored by exposure of sections to high-ionic-strength buffer or heparin. Platelet cationic proteins have been associated with loss of polyanion and increased glomerular permeability in acute serum nephritis (55) and by localized Arthus reaction after infusion of bovine serum albumin into the renal artery of preimmunized rabbits (54). More directly, undefined platelet cationic proteins, when infused intravenously into rats, bind to and neutralize glomerular polyanion and enhance glomerular permeability to ferritin (Fig. 3) (63). These observations are consistent with the interpretation that platelet secretory products can alter glomerular polyanion and enhance permeability in glomerular immune disease. However, the modes by which polycations induce polyanion loss in these experiments remain enigmatic. To date, direct effects of specific platelet cationic proteins on glomerular permeability have not been tested.

Enzymatic Degradation of Glomerular Basement Membrane

Platelets release elastase, collagenase, cathepsins, and endoglyosidase (heparitinase), all of which can digest structural components of the GBM and mesangial matrix (Table 1). Thus, degradation of type-IV collagen, fibronectin, entactin, nidogen, and heparan sulfate, which collectively contribute to polyanion and offer structural framework to the GBM, would conceivably lead to structural defects in porosity and/or charge barriers.

A role for secretory enzymes in glomerular injury and altered permeability has been suggested by the observation of GBM breakdown products in the urine during severe glomerulonephritis, concomitant with increased excretion of cationic cathepsins (74) that could be derived from leukocytes and platelets (see also Chapters 19 and 26). This hypothesis is supported by experiments during which infusion of collagenase (75), heparitinase (76), and neutrophil-derived elastase and cathepsin G (77) into the renal vasculature led to either enhanced glomerular permeability to tracer molecules or proteinuria. In addition, most platelet-derived enzymes are cationic and may promote dual effects of neutralization and degradation of glomerular polyanionic moieties (as outlined above). A role for platelet-derived enzymes as mediators of altered glomerular permselectivity during immune-complex glo-

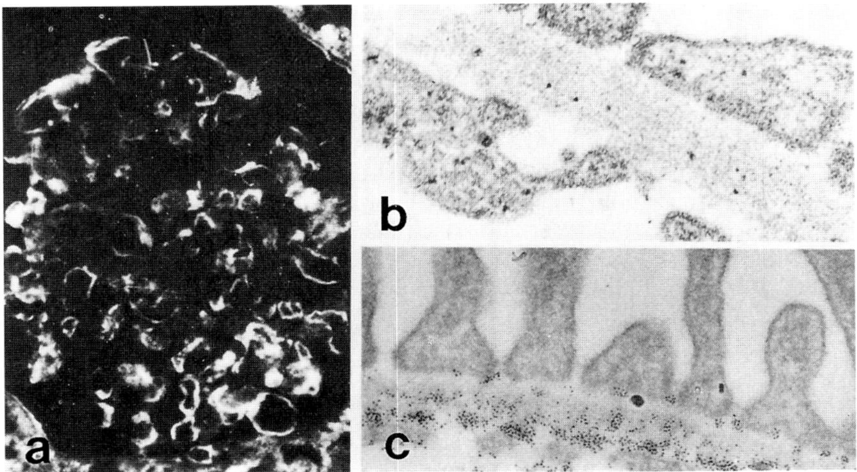

FIG. 3. Glomerular capillary walls after intravenous injection of human platelet cationic proteins into a rat illustrating (a) immunofluorescence localization of cationic proteins and enhanced basement membrane localization of ferritin particles after injection with cationic proteins (c) compared with control receiving ferritin and saline (b). From Tetta et al. (63), reproduced by permission of Birkhäuser Verlag AG.

merulonephritis appears likely, but direct observations have not been documented.

Alterations in Glomerular Hemodynamics

Glomerular hemodynamic influences on glomerular permeability have been examined extensively (78). Vasoactive agents that increase net intraglomerular hydraulic transcapillary pressure often tend to be associated with reductions in flow or glomerular filtration rate and an increase fractional clearance of marker molecules. A variety of platelet secretory products, including PAF (14), TXA_2 (79), histamine (80), PDGF (81), and epidermal growth factor (EGF) (82), can induce mesangial cell contraction in vitro. Moreover, several secretory products have been associated with reductions in glomerular filtration rate or increases in hydraulic capillary pressure when administered in vivo (78,82,83). Glomerular diseases are frequently associated with hemodynamic changes that can include reductions in renal blood flow and glomerular filtration rate. Whether these or other platelet products alter permeability or filtration properties of the glomerular capillary wall through hemodynamic alterations remains to be assessed.

Role for Platelets During Remodeling in Proliferative Glomerular Disease

Not only might platelet secretory products interact with glomerular structures by physicochemical interactions, but nearly all platelet secretory products are biologically active (that is, they are enzymes, chemotactins, or mitogens). Binding of these substances to glomerular polyanion could allow for nonspecific "targeting" to local glomerular structures where they could subsequently exert their specific biologic activities. Platelets secrete a variety of biologically active proteins that might influence glomerular hypercellularity on a local level by a combination of several potential pathways. Many secretory proteins are chemotactins and might influence the infiltration of inflammatory cells into glomerular structures or might directly affect proliferation of resident glomerular cells with a consequent increase in extracellular matrix, distorting normal glomerular structure and function (discussed below).

Experimental Models of Proliferative Glomerulonephritis

Platelets have been implicated as mediators in several experimental models of proliferative glomerular diseases. Methods that lead to platelet aggregation in the renal microvasculature—such as intraarterial infusion of

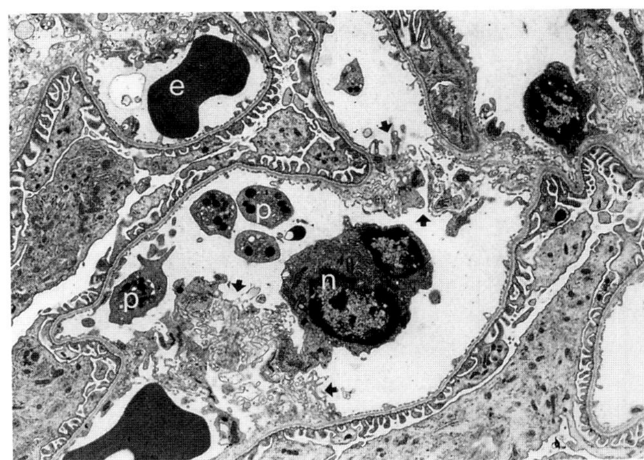

FIG. 4. Electron micrograph showing activated platelets *(p)* and a neutrophil *(n)* in a glomerular capillary loop 4 h after injection of thymocyte-1.1 antibody. From Johnson et al. (157), reproduced with permission by the American Society for Investigative Pathology.

ADP (84), antigen in preimmunized rabbits (85,86), polymeric IgA–concanavalin-A complexes (87), or mesangial lytic models of proliferative glomerulonephritis induced by habu snake venom (88–90) or anti-thymocyte (Thy)-1 antibody (Fig. 4) (91)—lead to proliferation of resident glomerular cells. Moreover, intraglomerular platelet aggregation is present in the early phase of nephrotoxic serum nephritis (56,57) following glomerular injury in rats with reduced renal mass (92,93) and in experimental diabetic glomerulopathy induced by streptozotocin (94). In all of these models, platelet accumulation or glomerular localization of platelet secretory products has been shown to occur before mesangial cell proliferation, further implicating platelets and their secretory products as initiators of glomerular disease. Increase in extracellular matrix synthesis is also common to several of these models; thus, a role for platelets in advanced glomerular disease should also be considered.

Mechanisms of Cell Remodeling

Studies on the mechanisms of how platelet-associated factors might mediate remodeling during glomerular disease have gained considerable attention within the last few years. Clues as to how platelet products might influence glomerular hypercellularity can be extrapolated from studies examining remodeling during embryogenesis, angiogenesis, atherosclerosis, and wound healing. The process of remodeling involves four sequential cellular events: (a) enzymatic degradation of cell substrata, (b) cell migration, (c) cell proliferation, and (d) organization or formation of extracellular matrix (95–98). Platelets contain secretory products that have the potential to mediate all four of these events and may play a role in remodeling during glomerular disease.

Enzymatic Degradation of Glomerular Matrix

Remodeling during embryogenesis, tissue regeneration, and wound healing involves complex interactions between cells and components of the extracellular matrix (99–102). For example, degradation of extracellular matrix precedes cell migration and proliferation in angiogenesis followed by resynthesis of matrix components and a return of the cells to a quiescent state and may be related to facilitation of movement and cell division (97). Similarly, matrix dissolution might be required as the earliest step for glomerular cell response to various growth factors. Glomerular epithelial cells (103) and mesangial cells (104) can synthesize plasminogen activators that may serve autoregulatory functions of cell attachment. A urokinase-dependent adhesion loss and shape change has been observed in stimulated mesangial cells, further implicating a role for plasminogen activators in disruption of adhesion plaques. Plasminogen activators are serine proteases and have been implicated in extracellular matrix turnover during cell migration and tissue remodeling (101). Mesangial cells also produce neutral proteases and protease inhibitors, which have been hypothesized to play a role in mesangial remodeling (105) (see also Chapters 19 and 29).

A variety of platelet-associated products can potentially induce glomerular cell proteolysis. For example, TGF-β, IL-1, PDGF, and EGF stimulate the synthesis and secretion of neutral proteases from cultured mesenchymal cells (105) and TGF-β and IL-1 stimulate protease secretion from mesangial cells (106). Moreover, thrombospondin can bind plasminogen and plasminogen activators (107,108), potentially providing a focus for protease generation (109). We have shown localization of platelet-released thrombospondin associated with mesangial cell migration and expression of plasminogen activator inhibitor 1 during habu snake venom–induced glomerulonephritis, suggesting a similar interaction between thrombospondin and the plasminogen system in vivo (see below). Proteases or their breakdown products can also directly induce cell proliferation (102) suggesting that platelet released enzymes could have the same effects on renal cells during disease.

Migration and Redistribution of Resident Glomerular Cells

Cell migration is an important event in embryogenesis and remodeling during wound repair or pathologic situations such as atherosclerosis and tumor invasion (95–98). A variety of platelet products have been implicated in monocyte or smooth muscle cell migration during atherosclerosis or vascular repair (96–98). Similarly, glomerular mesangial cells, which are analogous to vascular smooth muscle cells, may migrate in response to chemoattractant stimuli during the pathogenesis of glomerular disease (see Chapter 29). Mesangial cells have been shown to migrate after denudation injury to a confluent monolayer in cells in culture (110). Also, studies in our laboratory confirm that mesangial cells can migrate through porous membranes in blind-well chemotaxis chambers toward concentration gradients of platelet releasate, and specifically to PDGF and platelet fibronectin, but not to EGF, TGF-α, TGF-β, or PF4 (111,112). Thus, it seems plausible that platelet secretory products can influence endothelial, mesangial, and/or epithelial cell migration, redistribution, and proliferation in glomerular disease. Migration and redistribution of cells indigenous to the glomerulus may also be operative prior to cell division in other proliferative glomerular diseases characterized by distortion of the normal glomerular architecture.

A role for glomerular cell migration in vivo in proliferative disease has been examined in our laboratory in the habu snake venom model of glomerulonephritis (113).

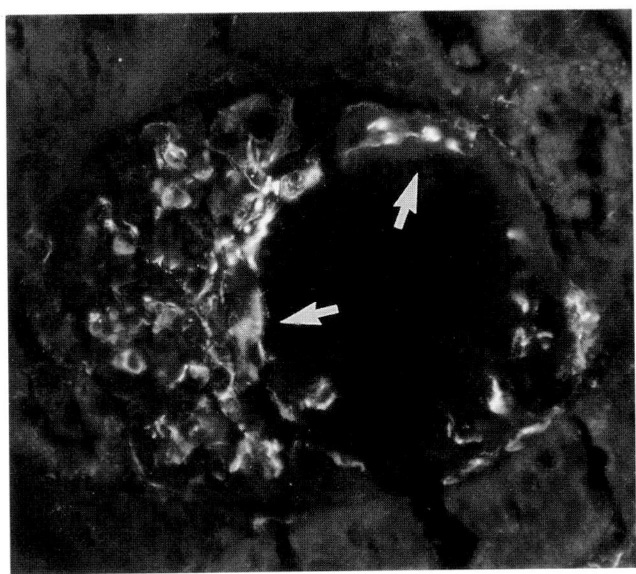

FIG. 5. Immunofluorescence localization of desmin *(arrows)*, an intermediate filament marker for mesangial cells, at the interface between intact glomerular capillary tufts and a microaneurysm 24 h after administration of habu snake venom.

This model is characterized by early mesangiolysis, capillary ballooning, and formation of microaneurysms that quickly fill with platelet aggregates, leukocytes, and blood proteins. Within 3 days after injection of habu snake venom, the lesions develop into proliferative micronodules comprised almost exclusively of mesangial cells. Sequential analysis of the position of mesangial cells over the course of the disease indicated that mesangial cells marginate along the interface between the intact capillary tuft and lesion (Fig. 5) prior to increases in DNA synthesis, suggesting that mesangial cells migrate before cell proliferation during repopulation of glomerular lesions. Both mesangial cell migration and proliferation could be retarded by prior platelet depletion, suggesting that platelet-released products are prerequisites for cell remodeling in this model.

Subsequent studies have shown a temporal course of fibronectin expression first by platelets and macrophages followed by mesangial cells over the course of the disease (114). Early events involving cell migration were associated with localization of an alternatively spliced fibronectin isoform (Fn-EIIIA) (114–116) and thrombospondin (116) derived from platelets and macrophages. Both Fn-EIIIA and thrombospondin have been associated with cell migration and proliferation during embryogenesis and during wound healing (109,117). Thus, the presence of these adhesive proteins in glomerular lesions suggests similar roles during remodeling. Also, mesangial cell expression of PAI-1 mRNA and protein is enhanced at the margins of early habu snake venom–induced glomerular lesions associated with cell migration (118). Components of the plasminogen/plasmin system are expressed in cells and tissues associated with a high rate of cell migration (101), suggesting that mesangial cells respond to platelet-released products over the course of glomerular disease.

A role for platelet secretory products in cell migration during clinical glomerular disease has not been defined. However, platelets have a strong association with membranoproliferative glomerulonephritis, a glomerular disease in which mesangial cells are observed in interpositional areas within capillary walls away from their normal intracapillary position (see Chapter 51). The mechanisms of this transposition are undefined. Similarly, cell migration is probably an early event in the formation of crescents that are comprised of macrophages, fibroblasts, and resident glomerular epithelial cells (see Chapter 32). Preliminary studies in our laboratory, in collaboration with B. S. Kasinath (UTHSCSA), have indicated that glomerular epithelial cells can migrate in response to platelet releasate. Studies are under way to examine specific platelet products that might influence glomerular epithelial cell migration.

Stimulation of Cell Proliferation by Platelet Secretory Products

Platelet-associated growth factors have the potential to stimulate renal cells in culture and during disease settings (1,3,5,6) (see Chapter 20). For example, mesangial cells proliferate in response to PDGF, bFGF, EGF, TGF-α, IL-1, insulinlike growth factor (IGF), TXA_2, serotonin, and fibronectin (see Chapter 29). Glomerular epithelial cells are stimulated by EGF and IL-1, but do not respond to PDGF or IGF-1 (see Chapter 31). TGF-β inhibits cell proliferation by both cell types. Similarly, PF4 inhibits serum- and PDGF-induced mesangial cell proliferation (unpublished data) (119). To date, information on platelet-associated growth factors and glomerular endothelial cell proliferation is limited (see Chapter 30). It appears that glomerular cells are targets of many of the mitogenic products previously identified in platelets and that the cellular responses to specific mitogens depend on the relative concentrations of the growth factors and the target cell population.

Further evidence that platelet secretory products might influence glomerular cell behavior has been provided by Floege et al. (120) in which intravenous infusion of bFGF and PDGF in normal or Thy-1-treated rats specifically stimulated mesangial cell proliferation. Conversely, administration of antibody to PDGF inhibited mesangial cell proliferation in this model (121), supporting a role, in part, for these platelet-released factors in the progression of glomerular disease.

Platelet secretory proteins can also stimulate synthesis of growth factors by a variety of cell types themselves and activate autocrine control of cell growth. For example, mesangial cell secretion of PDGF can be stimulated by PDGF, EGF, TGF-α, and TGF-β (122) (see Chapters 20 and 29). Also, PDGF and EGF stimulate mesangial cell secretion of IL-1 (123). Thus, platelet factors might initiate the early events in glomerular disease, but perpetuation of these events may be directed by autoregulation of intrinsic cells themselves. Such a phenomenon in glomerular disease is supported by the observations that platelet activation precedes increased mesangial expression of PDGF and/or PDGF-β receptor as well as their respective mRNAs in glomeruli in rats with proliferative glomerulonephritis induced by anti-Thy-1 antibody (124), renal ablation (93) and streptozotocin-induced diabetes (94). Cell proliferation is inhibited by prior platelet depletion in several of the above models (see below).

Evidence for autocrine pathways involving peptide growth factors has also been reported in human glomerular disease (see Chapter 20). For example, increased expression of PDGF and PDGF-b receptor has been demonstrated in vascular structures and glomeruli in diverse proliferative diseases, including IgA nephropathy, crescentic glomerulonephritis, focal segmental glomerulosclerosis, chronic transplant rejection, and lupus nephritis (125–128) (see Chapter 20). All of these glomerular diseases are associated with platelet activation. Thus, platelets may initiate early events in glomerular disease, but perpetuation of proliferation of intrinsic cells may involve autocrine pathways.

Platelet Secretory Products and Matrix Accumulation

Progressive glomerular diseases are commonly associated with extracellular matrix accumulation and sclerosis. Glomerulosclerosis has been associated with proliferation in the early phases of these diseases and is believed to be a result of abnormalities in the turnover of matrix by resident glomerular cells (129,130). The mechanisms that lead to increased synthesis of extracellular matrix are unclear, but stimulation by growth factors released from platelets and inflammatory cells (131,132) or through autocrine pathways particularly involving TGF-β have been postulated (6,8,9,130,132) (see Chapters 33, 34). TGF-β inhibits mesangial cell proliferation, but stimulates synthesis of collagen, fibronectin, and proteoglycans by mesangial cells (8,9,133), glomerular epithelial (134), and endothelial cells (135). An elevated expression of TGF-β mRNA has been associated with increased proteoglycan production in anti-Thy-1 experimental glomerulosclerosis (9) and collagen synthesis in nephrotoxic nephritis (136) and habu snake venom–induced proliferative glomerulonephritis (90). Also, infusion of PDGF into anti-Thy-1.1-treated rats induces glomerular matrix expansion with increased expression of type-IV collagen, laminin, and fibronectin mRNAs and their translated proteins (120). Moreover, antibodies to TGF-β (137) and PDGF (121) ameliorate progressive glomerular disease in this model. Whether platelets participate exclusively as initiators of cell proliferation followed by autocrine stimulation of matrix synthesis or whether platelets play a more protracted role over the entire course of these diseases remains to be elucidated.

ANTIPLATELET INTERVENTIONS IN GLOMERULAR DISEASE

Platelet Depletion

The most convincing evidence of a role for platelets in experimental renal diseases is found in studies in which platelets have been depleted from the circulation prior to initiation of the disease. Use of antiplatelet serum to remove circulating platelets has been highly effective in preventing immune-complex deposition and proteinuria in immune nephritis (16,17,57,138–140) and inhibiting cell proliferation in several models of glomerulonephritis (88,91,113) and diabetic nephropathy (94).

Antiplatelet Therapy in Experimental Renal Disease

A role for platelets in the pathogenesis of glomerular and renal vascular disease is further substantiated by the efficacy of an extensive list of antiplatelet drugs that are used to improve renal function and/or histopathology in experimental and clinical settings. This topic has been thoroughly reviewed in previous publications (1–3) and is beyond the scope of this review. The list includes drugs that act on platelet function by diverse mechanisms, including (a) membrane receptor interactions involving PAF and TXA_2; (b) compounds and dietary manipulations that increase platelet cytosolic cAMP, such as dipyridamole or dietary linoleic acid or administration of prostaglandin (PG) E_1, PGE_2, and PGI_2; (c) compounds that interfere with prostaglandin pathways, including inhibitors of cyclooxygenase and thromboxane synthetase or diets rich in fish oil that reduce TXA_2 synthesis; and (d) drugs such as heparin that alter platelet coagulation. Heparin might have multiple roles beyond anticoagulant properties, in that it may directly affect the cell cycle and/or bind to and neutralize many platelet-released growth factors, chemotactic proteins, and enzymes (see Table 1).

Several of the these drugs or dietary manipulations have been associated with an improvement in platelet stability and renal function and proteinuria in clinical glomerular diseases, including membranoproliferative glomerulonephritis, IgA nephropathy, focal sclerosis, and diabetic nephropathy (141–153). However, the efficacy of these therapeutic approaches has been challenged (154–156). Moreover, the these drugs are not specific for platelets and can affect similar pathways in other inflammatory cells. Thus, the interpretation of the efficacy of antiplatelet therapies, even when successful in ameliorating various aspects of glomerular disease, is confounded by the nonspecific nature of their target pathways.

CONCLUSIONS AND FUTURE DIRECTIONS

This chapter presents compelling evidence supporting specific mechanisms through which platelets are involved in the progression of renal vascular disease. Platelets and their secretory products promote a wide range of biologic activities with the potential to facilitate glomerular immune-complex deposition, stimulate inflammatory cell recruitment, and modulate tissue remodeling through resident cell migration, proliferation, and extracellular matrix synthesis. Platelets are but one element of a complex interplay of cell types, including leukocytes and cells intrinsic to the renal parenchyma, that can release biologically active substances involved in paracrine or autocrine pathways during progression of renal disease. Future directions of research will need to define precisely the temporal sequence of events in experimental and human disease by identifying the cellular sources of specific factors that mediate cellular behaviors that result in structural alterations and loss of renal function. Antiplatelet therapies that have targeted platelet function have been unfortunately nonspecific. Future therapeutic approaches may require interventions directed toward specific secretory products and cellular pathways at precise times during the course of disease processes.

REFERENCES

1. Barnes JL. Platelets in renal disease. In: Tetta C, ed. *Immunopharmacology of the renal system: handbook of immunopharmacology.* London: Academic Press, 1993:88–118.
2. Cameron JS. Platelets and renal disease. In: Page C, ed. *Platelets in health and disease.* London: Blackwell Scientific, 1991:228–60.
3. Johnson RJ. Platelets in inflammatory glomerular injury. *Semin Nephrol* 1991;11:276–84.
4. Charo IF, Keiffer N, Phillips DR. Platelet membrane glycoproteins. In: Colman RW, Hirsh J, Marder VJ, Salzman EW, eds. *Hemostasis and thrombosis: basic principles and clinical practice.* Philadelphia: JB Lippincott, 1994:489–507.
5. Kujubu DA, Fine LG. Physiology and cell biology update: polypeptide growth factors and their relations to renal disease. *Am J Kidney Dis* 1989;14:61–73.
6. Abboud HE. Growth factors in glomerulonephritis. *Kidney Int* 1993; 43:252–67.
7. Maione TE, Gray GS, Petro J, et al. Inhibition of angiogenesis by recombinant human platelet factor-4 and related peptides. *Science* 1990;247:77–9.
8. Border WA, Noble NA. Transforming growth factor β in tissue fibrosis. *N Engl J Med* 1994;331:1286–92.
9. Okuda S, Languino LR, Ruoslahti E, Border WA. Elevated expression of transforming growth factor-β and proteoglycan production in experimental glomerulonephritis: possible role in expansion of the mesangial extracellular matrix. *J Clin Invest* 1990;86:453–62.
10. Bell L, Madri JA. Effect of platelet factors on migration of cultured bovine aortic endothelial and smooth muscle cells. *Circ Res* 1989;65: 1057–65.
11. Pinckard RN. The "new" chemical mediators of inflammation. In: Majno G, Cotran RS, Kaufman N, eds. *Current topics in inflammation and infection.* Baltimore: Williams and Wilkins, 1982:38–53.
12. Marcus AJ. Multicellular eicosanoid and other metabolic interactions of platelets and other cells. In: Colman RW, Hirsh J, Marder VJ, Salzman EW, eds. *Hemostasis and thrombosis: basic principles and clinical practice.* Philadelphia: JB Lippincott, 1994:590–602.
13. Slezak S, Symer DE, Shin HS. Platelet-mediated cytotoxicity. *J Exp Med* 1987;166:489–505.
14. Schlondorff D, Neuwirth R. Platelet-activating factor and the kidney. *Am J Physiol* 1986;251:F1–11.
15. Bazzoni G, Dejana E, Del Maschio A. Platelet-dependent modulation of neutrophil function. *Pharmacol Res* 1992;26:269–72.
16. Johnson RJ, Alpers CE, Pritzl P, et al. Platelets mediate neutrophil-dependent immune complex nephritis in the rat. *J Clin Invest* 1988; 82:1225–35.
17. Johnson RJ, Alpers CE, Pruchno C, et al. Mechanisms and kinetics for platelet and neutrophil localization in immune complex nephritis. *Kidney Int* 1989;36:780–9.
18. Couser WG. Pathogenesis of glomerulonephritis. *Kidney Int* 1993;42: s19–26.
19. Wu X, Helfrich MH, Horton MA, Feigen LP, Lefkowith JB. Fibrinogen mediates platelet–polymorphonuclear leukocyte cooperation during immune-complex glomerulonephritis in rats. *J Clin Invest* 1994; 94:928–36.
20. Wu X, Pippin J, Lefkowith JB. Platelets and neutrophils are critical to the enhanced glomerular arachidonate metabolism in acute nephrotoxic nephritis in rats. *J Clin Invest* 1993;91:766–73.
21. McEver RP. Selectins: novel receptors that mediate leukocyte adhesion during inflammation. *Thromb Haemost* 1991;65:223–8.
22. Papayianni A, Serhan CN, Phillips ML, Rennke HG, Brady HR. Transcellular biosynthesis of lipoxin A_4 during adhesion of platelets and neutrophils in experimental immune complex glomerulonephritis. *Kidney Int* 1995;47:1295–302.
23. Walz A, Delwald B, von Tscharner V, Baggiolini M. Effects of the neutrophil-activating peptide NAP-2, platelet basic protein, connective tissue-activating peptide III, and platelet factor 4 on human neutrophils. *J Exp Med* 1989;170:1745–50.
24. Carruthers JA, Ralfs I, Gimlette TMD, Finn R. Platelet survival in acute proliferative glomerulonephritis. *Clin Sci Mol Med* 1974;47: 507–13.
25. Clark WF, Lewis ML, Cameron JS, Parsons V. Intrarenal platelet consumption in the diffuse proliferative nephritis of systemic lupus erythematosus. *Clin Sci Mol Med* 1975;49:247–52.
26. George CRP, Slichter SJ, Quadracci LJ, Striker GE, Harker LA. A kinetic evaluation of hemostasis in renal disease. *N Engl J Med* 1974; 291:1111–5.
27. Kant KS, Pollak VE, Weiss MA, Glueck HI, Miller MA, Hess EV. Glomerular thrombosis in systemic lupus erythematosus: prevalence and significance. *Medicine (Baltimore)* 1981;60:71–86.
28. Parbtani A, Clark WF, Cameron JS. Pathogenic significance of platelet activation in lupus nephritis. *Transplant Proc* 1986;18:657–8.
29. Heptinstall RH. Hemolytic uremic syndrome, thrombotic, thrombocytopenic purpura, and systemic sclerosis (systemic scleroderma). In: Heptinstall RH, ed. *Pathology of the kidney.* Boston: Little, Brown, 1992:1163–233.
30. Amenta PS, Katz SM. Platelets in renal scleroderma. *Arch Pathol Lab Med* 1983;107:439–4.
31. Porter KA. Renal transplantation. In: Heptinstall RH, ed. *Pathology of the kidney.* Boston: Little, Brown, 1992:1799–933.
32. Heptinstall RH. Hypertension I:essential hypertension. In: Heptinstall RH, ed. *Pathology of the kidney.* Boston: Little, Brown, 1992:951–1028.
33. Parbtani A, Cameron JS. Platelet and plasma serotonin concentrations in glomerulonephritis. I. *Thromb Res* 1979;15:109–25.
34. Parbtani A, Frampton G, Cameron JS. Platelet and plasma serotonin concentrations in glomerulonephritis. II. *Clin Nephrol* 1980;14:112–23.
35. Parbtani A, Frampton G, Cameron JS. Measurement of platelet release substances in glomerulonephritis: a comparison of beta-thromboglobulin (β-TG), platelet factor 4 (PF4) and serotonin assays. *Thromb Res* 1980;19:177–89.
36. Parbtani A, Frampton G, Yewdall V, Kasai N, Cameron JS. Platelet and plasma serotonin in glomerulonephritis. III. The nephritis of systemic lupus erythematosus. *Clin Nephrol* 1980;14:164–72.
37. Tomura S, Ida T, Kuriyama R, et al. Activation of platelets in patients with chronic proliferative glomerulonephritis and the nephrotic syndrome. *Clin Nephrol* 1982;17:24–30.

38. Mezzano S, Kunick M, Olivarria F, Ardiles L, Aranda E, Mezzano D. Decreased platelet counts and decreased platelet serotonin in post-streptococcal nephritis. *Nephron* 1995;69:135–9.
39. Hopper AH, Tindall H, Davies JA. Urinary beta-thromboglobulin correlates with impairment of renal function in patients with diabetic nephropathy. *Thromb Haemost* 1986;56:229–31.
40. Taira K, Hewitson TD, Kincaid-Smith P. Urinary platelet factor four (PF4) levels in mesangial IgA glomerulonephritis and thin basement membrane disease. *Clin Nephrol* 1992;37:8–13.
41. Tomino Y, Tsushima Y, Ohmuro H, et al. Detection of activated platelets in urinary sediments by immunofluorescence using monoclonal antibody to human platelet GMP-140 in patients with IgA nephropathy. *J Clin Lab Anal* 1993;7:329–33.
42. Mahan JD, Hebert LA, McAllister C, et al. Platelet involvement in experimental immune complex-mediated glomerulonephritis in the nonhuman primate. *Kidney Int* 1993;44:716–25.
43. Duffy JL, Cinque T, Grishman E, Churg J. Intraglomerular fibrin, platelet aggregation, and subendothelial deposits in lipoid nephrosis. *J Clin Invest* 1970;49:251–8.
44. Kincaid-Smith P, Laver MC, Fairley KF, Mathews DC. Dipyridamole and anticoagulants in renal disease due to glomerular and vascular lesions: a new approach to therapy. *Med J Aust* 1970;1:145–51.
45. Nakajima M, Hewitson TD, Mathews DC, Kincaid-Smith P. Platelet-derived growth factor mesangial deposits in mesangial IgA glomerulonephritis. *Nephrol Dial Transplant* 1991;6:11–6.
46. Woo KT, Junor BJR, Salem H, d'Apice AJF, Whitworth JA, Kincaid-Smith P. Beta-thromboglobulin and platelet aggregates in glomerulonephritis. *Clin Nephrol* 1980;14:92–5.
47. Duffus P, Parbtani A, Frampton G, Cameron JS. Intraglomerular localization of platelet related antigens, platelet factor 4 and β-thromboglobulin in glomerulonephritis. *Clin Nephrol* 1982;17:288–97.
48. Miller K, Dresner IG, Michael AF. Localization of platelet antigens in human kidney disease. *Kidney Int* 1980;18:472–9.
49. Camussi G, Tetta C, Mazzucco G, et al. Platelet cationic proteins are present in glomeruli of lupus nephritis patients. *Kidney Int* 1986;30:555–65.
50. Mezzano S, Burgos ME, Ardiles L, et al. Glomerular localization of platelet factor 4 in streptococcal nephritis. *Nephron* 1992;61:58–63.
51. Deguchi F, Tomura S, Yoshiyama N, Takeuchi J. Intraglomerular deposition of coagulation–fibrinolysis factors and a platelet membrane antigen in various glomerular diseases. *Nephron* 1989;51:377–83.
52. Frampton G, Hildreth G, Hartley B, Cameron JS, Heldin C-H, Westeson A. Could platelet-derived growth factor have a role in the pathogenesis of lupus nephritis? *Lancet* 1988;2:343.
53. Ito S, Camussi G, Tetta C, Milgrom F, Andres G. Hyperacute renal allograft rejection in the rabbit: the role of platelet-activating factor and of cationic proteins derived from polymorphonuclear leukocytes and from platelets. *Lab Invest* 1984;51:148–61.
54. Barnes JL, Camussi G, Tetta C, Venkatachalam MA. Glomerular localization of platelet cationic proteins after immune complex-induced platelet activation. *Lab Invest* 1990;63:755–61.
55. Camussi G, Tetta C, Meroni M, et al. Localization of cationic proteins derived from platelets and polymorphonuclear neutrophils and local loss of anionic sites in glomeruli of rabbits with experimentally-induced acute serum sickness. *Lab Invest* 1986;55:56–62.
56. Poelstra K, Hardonk MJ, Koudstaal J, Bakker WW. Intraglomerular platelet aggregation and experimental glomerulonephritis. *Kidney Int* 1990;37:1500–8.
57. Lianos EA, Zanglis A. Glomerular platelet-activating factor levels and origin in experimental glomerulonephritis. *Kidney Int* 1990;37:736–40.
58. Benacerraf B, McCluskey BT, Patras D. Localization of colloidal substances in vascular endothelium: a mechanism of tissue damage. I. Factors causing the pathologic deposition of colloidal carbon. *Am J Pathol* 1959;35:75–83.
59. Cochrane CG, Hawkins DJ. Studies on circulating immune complexes. III. Factors governing the ability of circulating complexes to localize in blood vessels. *J Exp Med* 1968;127:137–254.
60. Camussi G. Potential role of platelet-activating factor in renal pathophysiology. *Kidney Int* 1986;29:469–77.
61. Kanwar YS, Venkatachalam MA. Ultrastructure of glomerulus and juxtaglomerular apparatus. In: Windhager EE, ed. *Handbook of physiology. Section 8: Renal physiology.* New York: Oxford University, 1992:3–40.
62. Barnes JL, Levine SP, Venkatachalam MA. Binding of platelet factor four (PF4) to glomerular polyanion. *Kidney Int* 1984;25:759–65.
63. Tetta C, Coda R, Camussi G. Human platelet cationic proteins bind to rat glomeruli, induce loss of anionic charges and increase glomerular permeability. *Agents Actions* 1985;16:24–6.
64. Kreisberg JI, Wayne DB, Karnovsky MJ. Rapid and focal loss of negative charge associated with mononuclear cell infiltration early in nephrotoxic serum nephritis. *Kidney Int* 1979;16:290–300.
65. Kelley VE, Cavallo T. Glomerular permeability: focal loss of anionic sites in glomeruli of proteinuric mice with lupus nephritis. *Lab Invest* 1980;42:59–64.
66. Melnick GF, Ladoulis CT, Cavallo T. Decreased anionic groups and increased permeability precedes deposition of immune complexes in the glomerular capillary wall. *Am J Pathol* 1981;105:114–20.
67. Hunsicker LG, Shearer TP, Shaffer SJ. Acute reversible proteinuria induced by infusion of the polycation hexadimethrine. *Kidney Int* 1981;20:7–17.
68. Barnes JL, Radnik RA, Gilchrist EP, Venkatachalam MA. Size and charge selective permeability defects induced in glomerular basement membrane by a polycation. *Kidney Int* 1984;25:11–9.
69. Kanwar YS, Rosenzweig LJ. Clogging of the glomerular basement membrane. *J Cell Biol* 1982;93:489–94.
70. Tanaka T. Gels. *Sci Am* 1981;244:124–38.
71. Barnes JL, Venkatachalam MA. Glomerular interactions of exogenous and endogenous polycations. In: Lambert PP, Bergmann P, Beauwens R, eds. *The pathogenicity of cationic proteins.* New York: Raven, 1983:218–94.
72. Barnes JL, Venkatachalam MA. Enhancement of glomerular immune complex deposition by a circulating polycation. *J Exp Med* 1984;160:286–93.
73. Hogendoorn PCW, De Heer E, Weening JJ, Daha MR, Hoedemaeker PJ, Fleuren GJ. Glomerular capillary wall charge and antibody binding in passive Heymann nephritis. *J Lab Clin Med* 1988;111:150–7.
74. Cochrane CG. Mediation systems in neutrophil-independent immunologic injury of the glomerulus. In: Wilson CB, Brenner BM, Stein JH, eds. *Immunologic mechanisms of renal disease* New York: Churchill Livingstone, 1979:106–21.
75. Schaeverbeke J, Moreau LaLande H, et al. Enhancement of glomerular permeability to anionic ferritin induced by kidney perfusion with collagenase. *Biol Cell* 1985;53:179–85.
76. Kanwar YS, Linker A, Farquhar MG. Increased permeability of the glomerular basement membrane to ferritin after removal of glycosaminoglycans (heparan sulfate) by enzyme digestion. *J Cell Biol* 1980;86:688–93.
77. Johnson RJ, Couser WG, Alpers CE, Vissers M, Schulze M, Klebanoff SJ. The human neutrophil serine proteinases, elastase and cathepsin G, can mediate glomerular injury in vivo. *J Exp Med* 1988;168:1169–74.
78. Anderson S, Garcia DL, Brenner BM. Renal and systemic manifestations of glomerular diseases. In: Brenner BM, Rector FC, eds. *The kidney* Philadelphia: WB Saunders, 1991:831–1870.
79. Mené P, Dunn MJ. Contractile effects of TxA_2 and endoperoxide analogues on cultured rat glomerular mesangial cells. *Am J Physiol* 1986;251:F1029–35.
80. Sedor JR, Abboud HE. Histamine modulates contraction and cyclic nucleotides in cultured rat mesangial cells. *J Clin Invest* 1985;75:1679–89.
81. Mené P, Abboud HE, Dubyak GR, Searpa A, Dunn MJ. Effects of PDGF on inositol phosphates, Ca^{2+}, and contraction of mesangial cells. *Am J Physiol* 1987;253:F458–63.
82. Harris RC, Hoover RL, Jacobson HR, Badr KF. Evidence for glomerular actions of epidermal growth factor in the rat. *J Clin Invest* 1988;82:1028–39.
83. Yoo J, Schlondorff D, Neugarten J. Thromboxane mediates the renal hemodynamic effects of platelet activating factor. *J Pharmacol Exp Ther* 1990;253:743–8.
84. Jørgensen L, Glynn MF, Hovig T, Murphy EA, Buchanan MR, Mustard JF. Renal lesions and rise in blood pressure caused by adenosine diphosphate-induced platelet aggregation in rabbits. *Lab Invest* 1970;23:347–57.
85. Gabbiani G, Badonnel M-C, Vassalli P. Experimental focal glomerular lesions elicited by insoluble immune complexes: ultrastructural and immunofluorescent studies. *Lab Invest* 1975;32:33–45.
86. Shigematsu H, Niwa Y, Takizawa J, Akikusa B. Arthus-type nephri-

tis. I. Characterization of glomerular lesions induced by insoluble and poorly soluble immune complexes. *Lab Invest* 1979;40:492–502.
87. Davin JC, Dechenne C, Lombet J, Rentier B, Foidart JB, Mahieu PR. Acute experimental glomerulonephritis induced by the glomerular deposition of circulating polymeric IgA–concanavalin A complexes. *Virchows Arch [A]* 1989;415:7–20.
88. Cattell V. Focal mesangial proliferative glomerulonephritis in the rat caused by habu snake venom: the role of platelets. *Br J Exp Pathol* 1979;60:201–8.
89. Barnes JL. Glomerular localization of platelet secretory proteins in mesangial proliferative lesions induced by habu snake venom. *J Histochem Cytochem* 1989;37:1075–82.
90. Barnes JL, Abboud HE. Temporal expression of autocrine growth factors corresponds to morphologic features of mesangial proliferation in habu snake venom–induced glomerulonephritis. *Am J Pathol* 1993;143:1366–76.
91. Johnson RJ, Garcia RL, Pritzl P, Alpers CE. Platelets mediate glomerular cell proliferation in immune complex nephritis induced by anti-mesangial cell antibodies in the rat. *Am J Pathol* 1990;136:369–74.
92. Purkerson ML, Hoffsten PE, Klahr S. Pathogenesis of the glomerulopathy associated with renal infarction in rats. *Kidney Int* 1976;9:407–17.
93. Floege J, Burns MW, Alpers CE, et al. Glomerular cell proliferation and PDGF expression precede glomerulosclerosis in the remnant kidney model. *Kidney Int* 1992;41:297–309.
94. Young BA, Johnson RJ, Alpers CE, et al. Cellular events in the evolution of experimental diabetic nephropathy. *Kidney Int* 1995;47:935–44.
95. Folkman J. Angiogenesis: initiation and control. *Ann NY Acad Sci* 1987;401:212–5.
96. Rosen EM, Goldberg ID. Protein factors which regulate cell motility. *In Vitro Cell Dev Biol* 1989;25:1079–87.
97. Madri JA, Bell L, Marx M, Merwin JR, Basson C, Prinz C. Effects of soluble factors and extracellular matrix components on vascular cell behavior in vitro and in vivo: models of de-endothelialization and repair. *J Cell Biochem* 1991;45:123–30.
98. Munro JM, Cotran RS. Biology of disease: the pathogenesis of atherosclerosis—atherogenesis and inflammation. *Lab Invest* 1988;58:249–61.
99. von der Mark K, von der Mark H, Goodman S. Cellular responses to extracellular matrix. *Kidney Int* 1992;41:632–40.
100. Matrisian LM. Metalloproteinases and their inhibitors in matrix remodeling. *Trends Genet* 1990;6:121–5.
101. Vassalli J-D, Sappino A-P, Belin D. The plasminogen activator/plasmin system. *J Clin Invest* 1991;88:1067–72.
102. Scher W. The role of extracellular proteases in cell proliferation and differentiation. *Lab Invest* 1987;57:607–33.
103. Angles-Cano E, Rondeau E, Delarue F, Hagege J, Sultan Y, Sraer JD. Identification and cellular localization of plasminogen activators from human glomeruli. *Thromb Haemost* 1985;54:688–92.
104. Glass WF, Radnik RA, Garoni JA, Kreisberg JI. Urokinase-dependent adhesion loss and shape change after cyclic adenosine monophosphate elevation in cultured rat mesangial cells. *J Clin Invest* 1988;82:1992–2000.
105. Davies M, Martin J, Thomas GJ, Lovett DH. Proteinases and glomerular matrix turnover. *Kidney Int* 1992;41:671–8.
106. Kashgarian M, Sterzel RB. The pathobiology of the mesangium. *Kidney Int* 1992;41:524–9.
107. Silverstein RL, Nachman RL. Thrombospondin–plasminogen interactions: modulation of plasmin generation. *Semin Thromb Hemost* 1987;13:335–42.
108. Harpel PC, Silverstein RL, Pannell R, Gurewich V, Nachman RL. Thrombospondin forms complexes with single-chain and two-chain forms of urokinase. *J Biol Chem* 1990;265:11,289–94.
109. Dixit VM. Thrombospondin and tumor necrosis factor. *Kidney Int* 1992;41:679–82.
110. Person JM, Lovett DH, Raugi GJ. Modulation of mesangial cell migration by extracellular matrix components: inhibition by heparinlike glycosaminoglycans. *Am J Pathol* 1988;133:609–14.
111. Barnes JL, Hevey KA. Glomerular mesangial cell migration in response to platelet-derived growth factor. *Lab Invest* 1990;62:379–82.
112. Barnes JL, Hevey KA. Glomerular mesangial cell migration: response to platelet secretory products. *Am J Pathol* 1991;138:859–66.
113. Barnes JL, Hevey KA, Hastings RR, Bocanegra RA. Mesangial cell migration precedes proliferation in habu snake venom–induced glomerular injury. *Lab Invest* 1994;70:460–7.
114. Barnes JL, Hastings RR, De La Garza MA. Sequential expression of cellular fibronectin by platelets, macrophages, and mesangial cells in proliferative glomerular disease. *Am J Pathol* 1994;145:585–97.
115. Barnes JL, Torres ES, Mitchell RJ, Peters JH. Expression of alternatively spliced fibronectin variants during remodeling in proliferative glomerulonephritis. *Am J Pathol* 1995 (in press).
116. Barnes JL, Mitchell RJ, Torres ES. Expression of cellular fibronectin (Fn-EIIIA) and thrombospondin (TSP) during remodeling in habu snake venom–induced glomerulonephritis. *J Am Assoc Nephrol* 1995 (abst).
117. Hynes RO. *Fibronectin.* New York, Springer-Verlag, 1990.
118. Barnes JL, Mitchell RJ, Torres ES. Expression of plasminogen activator-inhibitor-1 (PAI-1) during cellular remodeling in proliferative glomerulonephritis. *J Histochem Cytochem* 1995;43:895–905.
119. Barnes JL, Abboud HE, Levine SP. Inhibition of mesangial cell proliferation by platelet factor 4 (PF4). *J Am Soc Nephrol* 1992;3:462.
120. Floege J, Eng E, Young BA, et al. Infusion of platelet-derived growth factor or basic fibroblast growth factor induces selective glomerular mesangial cell proliferation and matrix accumulation in rats. *J Clin Invest* 1993;92:2952–62.
121. Johnson RJ, Raines EW, Floege J, et al. Inhibition of mesangial cell proliferation and matrix expansion in glomerulonephritis in the rat by antibody to platelet-derived growth factor. *J Exp Med* 1992;175:1413–6.
122. Silver BJ, Jaffer FE, Abboud HE. Platelet-derived growth factor synthesis in mesangial cells: induction by multiple peptide mitogens. *Proc Natl Acad Sci USA* 1989;86:1056–60.
123. Lovett DH, Larsen A. Cell cycle-dependent interleukin 1 gene expression by cultured glomerular mesangial cells. *J Clin Invest* 1988;82:115–22.
124. Iida H, Seifert R, Alpers CE, et al. Platelet-derived growth factor (PDGF) and PDGF receptor are induced in mesangial proliferative nephritis in the rat. *Proc Natl Acad Sci USA* 1991;88:6560–4.
125. Gesualdo L, Pinzani M, Floriano JJ, et al. Platelet-derived growth factor expression in mesangial proliferative glomerulonephritis. *Lab Invest* 1991;65:160–7.
126. Gesualdo L, Di Paolo S, Milani S, et al. Expression of platelet-derived growth factor receptors in normal and diseased human kidney: an immunohistochemistry and in situ hybridization study. *J Clin Invest* 1994;94:50–8.
127. Rubin K, Tingstrom A, Hasson GK, et al. Induction of B-type receptors for platelet-derived growth factor in vascular inflammation: possible implications for development of vascular proliferative lesions. *Lancet* 1988;1:1353–6.
128. Fellström B, Klareskog L, Heldin CH, et al. Platelet-derived growth factor receptors in the kidney: upregulated expressions in inflammation. *Kidney Int* 1989;36:1099–102.
129. Striker LJ, Doi T, Elliot S, Striker GE. The contribution of glomerular mesangial cells to progressive glomerulosclerosis. *Semin Nephrol* 1989;9:318–28.
130. Couser WG, Johnson RJ. Mechanisms of progressive renal disease in glomerulonephritis. *Am J Kidney Dis* 1994;23:193–8.
131. Clark WF, Naylor CD. The role of platelets in progressive glomerulosclerosis: mechanisms for intraglomerular platelet activation and pathogenetic consequences. *Med Hypotheses* 1989;28:51–6.
132. Sterzel RB, Schulze-Lohoff E, Marx M. Cytokines and mesangial cells. *Kidney Int* 1993;39:s26–31.
133. MacKay K, Striker LJ, Stauffer JW, Doi T, Agodoa LY, Striker GE. Transforming growth factor-beta: murine glomerular receptors and responses of isolated glomerular cells. *J Clin Invest* 1989;83:1160–7.
134. Nakamura T, Miller D, Ruoslahti E, Border WA. Production of extracellular matrix by glomerular epithelial cells is regulated by transforming growth factor-β1. *Kidney Int* 1992;41:1213–21.
135. Kasinath BS, Terhune WC, Davalath S. Glomerular endothelial cell proteoglycans: regulation by TGF-β1. 1993;305:370–7.
136. Coimbra T, Wiggins R, Noh JW, Merritt S, Phan SH. Transforming growth factor-β production in anti-glomerular basement membrane disease in the rabbit. *Am J Pathol* 1991;138:223–34.
137. Border WA, Okuda S, Languino LR, Sporn MB, Ruoslahti E. Suppression of experimental glomerulonephritis by antiserum against transforming growth factor β1. *Nature* 1990;346:371–4.

138. Kniker WT, Cochrane CG. The localization of circulating immune complexes in experimental serum sickness: the role of vasoactive amines and hydrodynamic forces. *J Exp Med* 1968;127:119–35.
139. Ideura T, Ogasawara M, Tomura S, et al. Effect of thrombocytopenia on the onset of immune complex glomerulonephritis. *Nephron* 1992; 60:49–55.
140. Sindrey M, Marshall TL, Naish P. Quantitative assessment of the effects of platelet depletion in the autologous phase of nephrotoxic serum nephritis. *Clin Exp Immunol* 1979;36:90–6.
141. Kincaid-Smith P. Anticoagulants are of value in the treatment of renal disease. *Am J Kidney Dis* 1984;3:299–307.
142. Donadio JV Jr, Anderson CF, Mitchell JC III, et al. Membranoproliferative glomerulonephritis: a prospective clinical trial of platelet-inhibitor therapy. *N Engl J Med* 1984;310:1421–6.
143. Donadio JV Jr, Ilstrup DM, Holley KE, Romero JC. Platelet-inhibitor treatment of diabetic nephropathy: a 10-year prospective study. *Mayo Clin Proc* 1988;63:3–15.
144. Donadio JV Jr. Effects of Omega (gw)-3 polyunsaturated fatty acids in renal disease. In: *Renal nutrition: report on the Eleventh Ross Round Table on Medical Issues.* Columbus, OH: Ross Laboratories, 1991:76–82.
145. Zimmerman SW, Moorthy AV, Dreher WH, Friedman A, Varanasi U. Prospective trial of warfarin and dipyridamole in patients with membranoproliferative glomerulonephritis. *Am J Med* 1983;75:920–7.
146. Barnett AH, Wakelin K, Leatherdale BA, et al. Specific thromboxane synthetase inhibition and albumin excretion rate in insulin-dependent diabetes. *Lancet* 1984;1:1322.
147. Ueda N, Kawaguchi S, Niinomi Y, et al. Effect of dipyridamole treatment on proteinuria in pediatric renal disease. *Nephron* 1986;44:174–9.
148. Grekas D, Alivanis P, Kalekou H, Syrganis C, Tourkantonis A. Are antiplatelet agents of value in the treatment of chronic glomerular disease? *Nephrol Dial Transplant* 1987;2:377–9.
149. Tojo S, Hatano M, Honda N, et al. Natural history of IgA nephropathy in Japan. *Semin Nephrol* 1987;7:386–8.
150. Woo KT, Edmondson RPS, Yap HK, et al. Effects of triple therapy on the progression of mesangial proliferative glomerulonephritis. *Clin Nephrol* 1987:27:56–64.
151. Niwa T, Maeda K, Shibata M, Yamada K. Clinical effects of selective thromboxane A_2 synthetase inhibitor in patients with nephrotic syndrome. *Clin Nephrol* 1988;30:276–81.
152. Sakai H, Watanabe S, Inoue I, et al. Effect of urokinase on preservation of renal function in patients with diabetic nephropathy. *J Diabetic Complications* 1991;5:95–7.
153. Camara S, de la Cruz JP, Frutos MA, et al. Effects of dipyridamole on the short-term evolution of glomerulonephritis. *Nephron* 1991;58: 13–6.
154. Border WA. Anticoagulants are of little value in the treatment of renal disease. *Am J Kidney Dis* 1984;3:308–12.
155. Cattran DC, Cardella CJ, Roscoe JM, et al. Results of a controlled drug trial in membranoproliferative glomerulonephritis. *Kidney Int* 1985;27:436–41.
156. Chan MK, Kwan SYL, Chan KW, Yeung CK. Controlled trial of antiplatelet agents in mesangial IgA glomerulonephritis. *Am J Kidney Dis* 1987;9:417–21.

Immunologic Renal Diseases,
edited by E. G. Neilson and W. G. Couser.
Lippincott-Raven Publishers, Philadelphia © 1997.

CHAPTER 28

Macrophages in Immune Renal Injury

David J. Nikolic-Paterson, Hui Y. Lan, and Robert C. Atkins

THE MONONUCLEAR PHAGOCYTE SYSTEM

The mononuclear phagocyte system is composed of blood monocytes and the resident macrophages present throughout connective tissue and around basement membranes in all organs of the body (1). Mononuclear phagocytes play a central role in inflammatory and cell-mediated immune responses, including defense against microbes, wound healing, defense against tumors and tissue destruction. These functions can be induced directly or in concert with other arms of the immune system, such as complement, antibodies, and T-cells.

An ordered process of proliferation and differentiation by hematopoietic stem cells within the bone marrow gives rise to monoblasts, promonocytes, and finally monocytes that then enter the circulation (1). Blood monocytes can enter tissues, where they undergo a process of differentiation to become resident tissue macrophages. Recruitment of blood monocytes is the main mechanism by which most resident tissue macrophage populations are renewed because they have little, if any, proliferative capacity (1,2). It is also thought that blood monocyte recruitment is the primary mechanism of macrophages that accumulate at sites of acute inflammation (1,3). However, high levels of local proliferation of recruited monocytes recently have been described in cases of severe tissue injury (4,5).

CELL-MEDIATED IMMUNITY

T Cell–Mediated Immunity

T-cell immune responses are dependent on recognition of peptide antigens presented by antigen-presenting cells (6) (see Chapter 4). Dendritic cells, and to a lesser extent macrophages, are the professional antigen-presenting cells that endocytose/phagocytose, process, and then combine antigen peptides with molecules of the major histocompatibility complex (MHC). $CD8^+$ T cells recognize antigen in association with MHC class I molecules, which can lead to the development of antigen-specific cytotoxic Tcells (CTLs). $CD4^+$ T cells recognize antigen associated with MHC class II molecules and can develop one of two major types of responses, termed T_h1 and T_h2, which are not necessarily mutually exclusive (7).

In the T_h1 response, uncommitted or naive T-cells (termed T_h0 cells) commit to a T_h1 phenotype, which is characterized by the production of a specific group of cytokines [interleukin (IL)-2, IL-12, and interferon-τ (IFN-τ)] (see Chapter 4). This leads to T-cell expansion and tissue destruction at sites of antigen deposition. Cytokines produced by T_h1 $CD4^+$ T cells induce monocyte accumulation [via macrophage migration inhibitory factor (MIF)] and macrophage activation (via IFN-τ and MIF) at the site of antigen deposition. These inflammatory macrophages then mediate tissue destruction. A good example is that of rat experimental autoimmune encephalomyelitis in which myelin basic protein–specific $CD4^+$ T cells mediate neuronal damage through the recruitment and activation of macrophages (8). In cases in which antigen or antigen–antibody immune complexes persist, chronic cytokine stimulation of macrophages can lead to the development of granulomatous lesions. Granulomas typically consist of a core of epithelioid cells, macrophages, and multinucleated macrophage giant cells, around which are T cells and a variable number of fibroblasts and collagen deposition (9). T_h1 $CD4^+$ T-cells also may cause tissue damage through production of cytokines such as IL-2, which induce lymphokine-activated killer (LAK) cells and activate natural killer (NK) cells; however, there is little in vivo evidence to support this as a major mechanism of T cell–mediated tissue injury.

In the T_h2 response, naive T_h0 cells commit to a T_h2 response, in which production of cytokines IL-4, IL-5,

D. J. Nikolic-Paterson, H. Y. Lan, and R. C. Atkins: Department of Nephrology, Monash Medical Centre, Clayton, Victoria, Australia.

IL-6, IL-10, and IL-13 predominate (7). B-cell antibody production is augmented by these cytokines and also via direct contact between T_h2 $CD4^+$ T cells and B cells (10). In addition, IL-5 production can attract and activate eosinophils to sites of antigen deposition, resulting in tissue destruction (11).

T-cell cytokines also exert a negative feedback on T-cell responses. Cytokines produced by T_h2 T cells (IL-4 and IL-10) have an inhibitory effect on T_h1 responses, whereas T_h1 cytokines (IFN-τ) inhibit T_h2 responses (7).

Memory T-cell responses are often described as delayed-type hypersensitivity (DTH) or type IV hypersensitivity reactions. These reactions to previously encountered antigen involve the T_h1 response, and a major characteristic of chronic DTH reactions is granuloma formation, which can be seen in the Mantoux reaction to tuberculin, viral infections, and fungal and parasitic diseases (9).

T Cell–Independent Cell-Mediated Immunity

Macrophages can mediate tissue damage independent of T-cell activation by interacting with components of the humoral immune response—immunoglobulin and complement (12). Macrophages express cell surface receptors for the Fc-subunit of immunoglobulin. This enables macrophages to phagocytose antibody-coated microbes and immune complexes and to kill antibody-coated cells through the process of antibody-dependent cell-mediated cytotoxicity (ADCC). In addition, uptake of immune complexes or immunoglobulin (Ig)A can induce macrophage production of IL-1 and reactive oxygen species (ROS), causing tissue damage (13–15). Complement activation can induce monocyte chemotaxis through the action of C5a, whereas macrophage expression of the C3bi receptor (CD11b/CD18, Mac-1) facilitates adhesion to complement-coated surfaces and can trigger production of platelet activating factor (PAF) (16,17).

An alternative mechanism of activation of monocyte/macrophages is through the action of bacterial endotoxin or the proinflammatory cytokines IL-1 and tumor necrosis factor-α (TNF-α). IL-1 and TNF-α prime/activate macrophages to produce various mediators of tissue injury, including ROS, metalloproteinases, and PAF (18–21). These cytokines can be produced by both polymorphonuclear cells and by a variety of nonimmune cells (22). For example, monolayers of colon epithelial cells exposed to different bacterial strains secrete a characteristic pattern of cytokines, including TNF-α, IL-8, and monocyte chemoattractant peptide-1 (MCP-1), which has the potential to recruit and activate blood monocytes (23). A parallel to this is seen in renal tubular epithelial cells, which have been shown to synthesis MCP-1 and TNF-α (24,25).

T CELL–MEDIATED IMMUNITY IN RENAL INJURY

T-cells play an important role in the development of antibody responses within lymphoid tissues, which in turn may, under certain circumstances, result in antibody deposition within the glomerulus and the induction of renal injury. However, T cells within the kidney itself also can play a direct role in mediating renal injury. The application of monoclonal antibodies (mAbs) in immunohistochemistry staining of kidney sections has shown that T cells and macrophages are present in various forms of glomerulonephritides (see Chapter 38). This prompted an investigation of the importance of sensitized T cells and cell-mediated immunity in the pathogenesis of glomerulonephritis. Examination of biopsy material found that significant glomerular T-cell infiltration occurs in the more aggressive forms of glomerulonephritis such as proliferative and crescentic disease (26,27), whereas it is only occasionally present in nonproliferative diseases such as focal segmental sclerosis and minimal-change glomerulonephritis (28,29). In most cases $CD4^+$ T cells predominate over $CD8^+$ T cells, and there is a correlation between the number of glomerular T cells and glomerular macrophage accumulation (27). Although most studies have failed to show a correlation between glomerular T-cell infiltration and renal function, patients with active crescentic glomerulonephritis show activated T-cells within glomeruli (30). In such cases of acute injury, the presence of activated T cells correlated with parameters of renal function and the activity of glomerular crescents in IgA glomerulonephritis (31).

In contrast to the small numbers of T-cells seen within glomeruli, substantial interstitial T-cell infiltration is a feature in all forms of glomerulonephritis (26). The intensity of the interstitial mononuclear cell infiltrate, which consists of approximately equal numbers of T cells (predominantly $CD4^+$) and macrophages, correlates with renal function at the time of biopsy and is predictive of disease progression in both primary and secondary glomerulonephritis (26,28,32–35). Thus, interstitial cell-mediated immunity may be a crucial component of disease progression irrespective of the type of glomerulonephritis.

Determining the contribution of cell-mediated immunity to the induction and progression of glomerulonephritis is complicated by the presence of components of both the humoral and cellular responses in most forms of disease. It is therefore necessary to investigate the cellular immune response in the absence of a humoral response. Indeed, it is well recognized that crescentic glomerulonephritis often occurs in the absence of antibody deposition, suggesting that the cellular arm of the immune response plays a major role in this particular disease (36).

In common with human studies, significant interstitial T-cell infiltration is evident in all animal models of renal injury, whether initiated through an immune (37–39) or nonimmune insult (40–42). In order to determine the potential of cell-mediated immunity to mediate renal injury, two main experimental strategies have been used: (a) passive transfer of disease to naive recipients by T cells in the absence of antibody and (b) depletion of T cells in diseased animals.

The transfer of T cells from a diseased bird to a naive recipient induced a glomerular lesion in an avian model of autoimmune glomerulonephritis in the absence of antibody and complement (43). In a different strategy, the infusion of a hapten-carrier into the left kidney of preimmunized rats resulted in marked glomerular histologic damage in concert with a skin-proven DTH response (44,45). Furthermore, glomerular and interstitial lesions caused by the azobenzenaersonate hapten were induced in naive recipients by adoptive transfer of T cells in the absence of antibody (45). Murine interstitial nephritis also can be adoptively transferred to naive recipients by both $CD4^+$ and $CD8^+$ T cells, although it is the latter that is predominantly responsible for mediating tissue injury (46,47). In addition, interstitial nephritis induced in guinea pigs by active immunization with autologous Tamm-Horsfall protein can be adoptively transferred to naive recipients by lymph node cells in the absence of antibody (48).

An alternative to T-cell transfer is to delete T cells from diseased animals without modifying the humoral immune response. WKY rats develop a severe crescentic disease after injection of nephrotoxic serum. The ability of anti-CD8 mAb treatment to inhibit proteinuria in classical anti-glomerular basement membrane (GBM) glomerulonephritis in these rats demonstrates a crucial role for CTLs or NK cells in this disease model (49). In contrast, using accelerated anti-GBM disease in WKY rats, Huang et al. (50) demonstrated that there is a marked DTH response within the kidney featuring $CD4^+$ T-cell infiltration and granuloma formation. Depletion of $CD4^+$ T cells from these animals inhibited proteinuria, granuloma formation, and the skin DTH response (50). In a rat model of Heymann's nephritis, depletion of either $CD4^+$ or $CD8^+$ T cells caused profound inhibition of proteinuria without affecting antibody titers or complement deposition (38). Depletion of $CD4^+$ T cells inhibits autoantibody formation and the development of lupus glomerulonephritis in susceptible mouse strains (51,52). Using a different approach, Nishikawa et al. (53) demonstrated that the interaction between the T cell CD28/CTLA (inducible cytotoxic T-lymphocyte-associated gene transcript-4) antigen and the B7 molecules on the surface of antigen-presenting cells is essential for development of T cell–mediated renal injury in WKY rats immunized with bovine GBM. Importantly, treatment with a soluble form of CTLA when disease was already established suppressed renal injury and interstitial macrophage accumulation.

T cell–dependent renal injury also can be demonstrated in models in which the initial insult is nonimmune in nature. Depletion of $CD5^+$ T-cells in a rat model of protein overload partially abrogated proteinuria and reduced interstitial macrophage infiltration (42). Also, chronic to administration of adriamycin to rats induces a nephropathy with prominent interstitial leukocytic infiltrate consisting almost exclusively of $CD4^+$ T-cells interstitial infiltrate. Treatment with cycophosphamide abrogated the interstitial infiltrate and suppressed renal impairment, tubular atrophy, and interstitial fibrosis (54).

In summary, T-cell transfer and T-cell depletion studies in animal models support the notion that sensitized T cells play an important role in the pathogenesis of glomerulonephritis. It is well recognized that in human diseases in which the antigen has been identified, such as anti-GBM nephritis (see Chapter 43), cellular as well as humoral immunity to GBM is readily demonstrable (54a, 54b). Most studies indicate that it is the $CD4^+$ T-cell subset that is important in the mediation of renal injury. As described in the previous sections, the main mechanism by which sensitized $CD4^+$ T cells induce renal injury is via the DTH response in which T cells direct recruitment of blood monocytes into a tissue (in this case the kidney) and then promote their activation and differentiation in order to clear the deposited antigen, a process that also results in significant tissue injury. Evidence that $CD4^+$ T cells direct monocyte recruitment into the kidney comes from several studies. A correlation between glomerular T-cell and macrophage accumulation has been shown in human glomerulonephritis (27), and a significant accumulation of $CD4^+$ T cells and macrophages is seen within the renal interstitium in most forms of disease (26). In addition, the inhibition of renal injury in rat models of Heymann's nephritis and accelerated anti-GBM glomerulonephritis resulting from depletion of $CD4^+$ T-cells was associated with blocking renal macrophage infiltration and had no effect on the humoral immune response (38,50). The mechanisms by which T cells promote monocyte recruitment to the kidney and induce macrophage activation (with consequent renal injury) are considered in the following sections.

SIGNIFICANCE OF MACROPHAGE ACCUMULATION WITHIN THE KIDNEY

After our original discovery that large numbers of macrophages were present in glomerular cultures from patients with crescentic glomerulonephritis (55), it became clear that glomerular macrophage accumulation occurs in most forms of primary and secondary glomerulonephritis (26–28,33,35,56–66). Some studies have found a correlation between glomerular macrophage infiltration and the degree of proteinuria at the time of biopsy (35,60,66), whereas other studies have been unable to demonstrate a correlation between glomerular macrophage accumulation and renal function or outcome (26,30,61). However, a consistent finding is that glomerular macrophage accumulation correlates with the degree of glomerular hypercellularity (56–58,60,61,63). Examination of urinary sediments found significantly higher numbers of mononuclear cells in the urine of patients with active IgA nephritis compared with those with noncrescentic and inactive IgA nephritis. In addition, there was a significant correlation between the number of urinary $CD14^+$ macrophages and the presence of glomerular crescents in these patients (67).

Although glomerular macrophage infiltration is evident in most forms of human glomerulonephritis, the role of these cells in progressive renal impairment remains unclear. In contrast, interstitial macrophage infiltration is prominent in all types of glomerulonephritis, except minimal-change disease (26,29,32,35,57,64–66). The interstitial infiltrate is different from that seen in the glomerulus because it consists of approximately equal numbers of macrophages and T cells. The density of the interstitial mononuclear cell infiltrate correlates with renal function at the time of biopsy (26,29,32,33,35) and predicts renal outcome in both primary and secondary glomerulonephritis (33,35,68).

Macrophage accumulation in experimental models of renal injury follows a pattern similar to that observed in human disease. Glomerular and particularly interstitial macrophage accumulation is present in a variety of immune-initiated disease models, including autoimmune and passive anti-GBM glomerulonephritis (37,69–72), acute and chronic immune complex glomerulonephritis (73–76), passive serum sickness (77), lupus nephritis (78), anti–Thy-1 nephritis (79,80), autoimmune anti-THP interstitial nephritis (48), anti-TBM interstitial nephritis (81), Heymann's nephritis (38,82), and streptozotocin-induced diabetic nephropathy (83). Significant macrophage infiltration is also evident in nonimmune initiated models of renal injury, such as puromycin aminonucleoside (PAN)-induced nephrosis and focal segmental glomerulosclerosis (41,84,85), lipid-induced nephritis (86,87), renal ablation (88), ureteral obstruction (40), protein overload (42), angiotensin II–mediated nephritis (89), hypertension-induced renal injury (90), and chronic renal ischemia (91).

A temporal association between macrophage accumulation and renal injury has been described in many of these disease models (37,41,75,78,83,85,86,88,89,92–94). For example, interstitial macrophage accumulation during the evolution of rat anti-GBM glomerulonephritis gives a highly significant correlation with proteinuria, declining creatinine clearance and interstitial fibrosis (37). Similarly, interstitial macrophage accumulation in a PAN-induced rat model of focal and segmental glomerulosclerosis correlates with declining creatinine clearance and interstitial fibrosis (41).

MECHANISMS OF MACROPHAGE ACCUMULATION IN THE KIDNEY

Macrophage accumulation within the kidney is a dynamic process that reflects the balance of monocyte recruitment, macrophage proliferation and death within the kidney, and macrophage drainage from the kidney. There are two main components regulating blood monocyte recruitment into the kidney: (a) immune adherence and monocyte chemotactic molecules and (b) expression of leukocyte adhesion molecules.

Immune Adherence and Chemotactic Molecules (see Chapters 24 and 25)

Glomerular macrophage accumulation through immune adherence to deposited immunoglobulin via Fc-receptor binding has been demonstrated in rat anti-GBM glomerulonephritis (95). Renal deposition of immune complexes bearing C3bi also may induce immune adherence of monocytes through their cell-surface C3bi receptors (CD11b/CD18), although glomerular monocyte recruitment can develop in the absence of complement activation (96). Although there are some reports of glomerular macrophage accumulation in association with subendothelial deposits and glomerular C3 localization (59), most studies of human glomerulonephritis have failed to demonstrate a correlation between the presence or location of immune deposits and macrophage accumulation (60,61,64). Indeed, crescentic glomerulonephritis often is seen in the absence of detectable immunoglobulin deposition (97).

A number of monocyte chemotactic proteins have been implicated in glomerular monocyte recruitment. T cells can direct macrophage accumulation at sites of DTH responses via production of MIF (98), and glomerular MIF bioactivity has been implicated in monocyte recruitment in experimental anti-GBM glomerulonephritis (99). Mesangial cells synthesize MCP-1 after stimulation with IL-1 and aggregated IgG (100–102), and glomerular MCP-1 expression is associated with macrophage accumulation in rat anti-GBM glomerulonephritis, rat anti–Thy-1 nephritis and human glomerulonephritis (103,104). Transforming growth factor-β (TGF-β) is another potent monocyte chemoattractant that is released after platelet activation and can be synthesized by many cell types, including glomerular mesangial cells (105,106). Glomerular mesangial cells also can be induced to express macrophage–colony stimulating factor (M-CSF), which is both a chemoattractant and growth factor for monocytes (107). Glomerular M-CSF expression is induced immediately before glomerular macrophage infiltration during the development of murine lupus nephritis (78). In addition, monocytes can migrate in response to products of complement activation such as C5a, which also induce endothelial P-selectin expression (16,108).

Tubular epithelial cells are also a rich source of monocyte chemotactic molecules. Tubular production of MCP-1 is associated with interstitial macrophage infiltration after unilateral ureteral obstruction (109). Lipid-associated albumin induces proximal tubules to synthesize an extremely potent monocyte-specific chemotactic lipid (110). Suppression of the biosynthesis of this chemotactic lipid may explain the ability of an essential fatty acid–deficient (EFAD) diet to prevent macrophage infiltration and renal injury in animal models of kidney disease (111,112). Induction of osteopontin expression, a molecule that is both chemoattractant and adhesive for monocyte/macrophages, is closely associated with the development of macrophage accumulation around proximal and distal tubules in rat models of Heymann's nephritis, PAN-nephrosis, anti–Thy-1 nephritis and angiotensin II–induced tubulointerstitial nephritis (113,114).

Leukocyte Adhesion Molecules (see Chapter 25)

Adhesion molecules play a critical role in facilitating leukocyte attachment to the endothelium and the subsequent migration of leukocytes between adjacent endothelial cells and into the kidney (115). Studies of renal macrophage infiltration have focused primarily upon expression of intracellular adhesion molecule-1 (ICAM-1; CD54) and vascular cell adhesion molecule-1 (VCAM-1) (CD106) molecules. In human glomerulonephritis, ICAM-1 expression is upregulated on most endothelia, mesangial cells, and tubules, particularly damaged tubules. Increased glomerular ICAM-1 expression is associated with macrophage infiltration and glomerular hypercellularity; however, it has yet to be determined whether upregulation of tubular ICAM-1 expression is associated with macrophage accumulation (28,116–120). In contrast, only weak VCAM-1 staining is seen within the mesangial area in human glomerulonephritis, but the upregulation of tubular VCAM-1 expression does correlate with interstitial macrophage accumulation (116,121).

Direct evidence that adhesion molecules are involved in renal macrophage infiltration has come from studies of animal disease models. Endothelial ICAM-1 expression is upregulated within 1.5 h of induction of rat anti-GBM glomerulonephritis with colocalization of lymphocyte function-associated antigen-1 (LFA-1) and ICAM-1 at sites of monocyte adhesion to activated endothelium in the glomerulus (Fig. 1) and interstitium, as demonstrated by

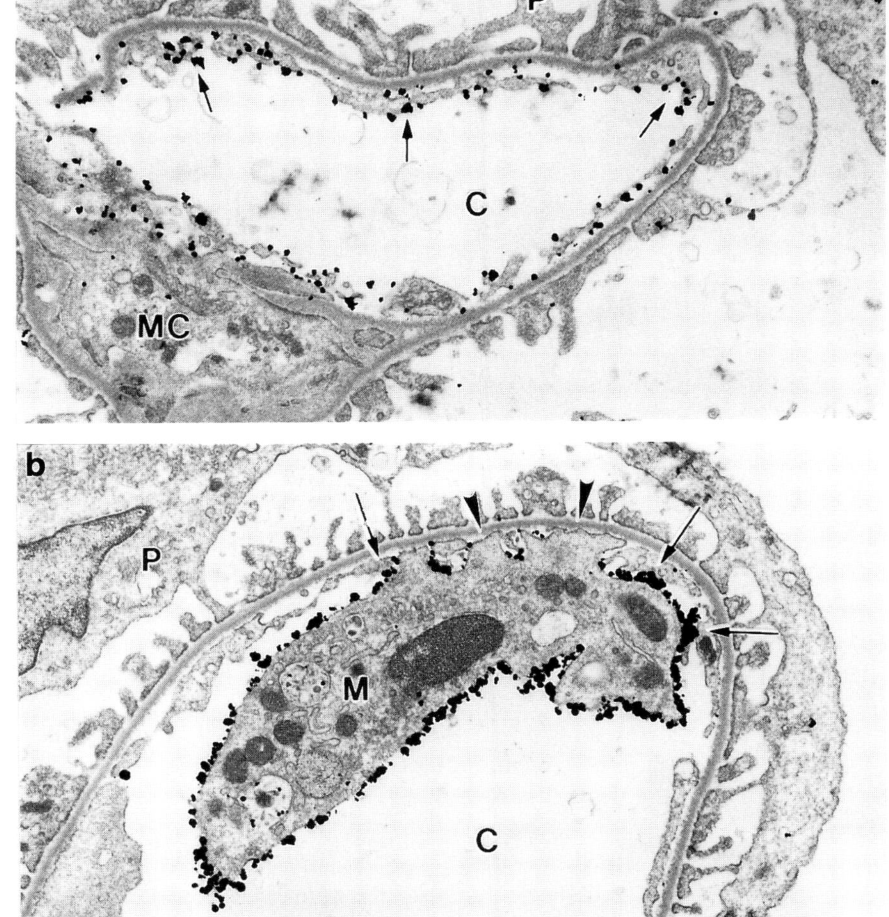

FIG. 1. Immunoelectron microscopy of adhesion molecule expression in rat anti-GBM glomerulonephritis. **A:** ICAM-1 (CD54) is strongly expressed on the glomerular endothelium *(arrows)*. Note the absence of ICAM-1 on mesangial cells (MC) and podocytes (P). **B:** LFA-1 (CD11a) is strongly expressed on the surface of a monocyte/macrophage migrating beneath the glomerular endothelium. LFA-1 is prominent at sites of adhesion of the monocyte to the endothelium *(arrows)* but is absent on the surface attached to the bare GBM. C, capillary lumin; P, podocyte. Reprinted with permission (122).

immunoelectron microscopy (122,123). Upregulation of tubular ICAM-1 expression during development of this disease model is associated with macrophage accumulation and tubular necrosis (123). A temporal association between upregulation of glomerular ICAM-1 expression and the accumulation of LFA-1$^+$ macrophages has been described in lipid-induced glomerular injury in susceptible ExHC rats (124), whereas increased VCAM-1 expression is associated with leukocyte infiltration in the development of murine lupus nephritis (125). The central importance of the ICAM-1/LFA-1 interaction in the recruitment of monocytes and T cells into the kidney is demonstrated by the ability of neutralizing anti–ICAM-1 and/or anti–LFA-1 antibodies to abrogate leukocyte infiltration and proteinuria in rat anti-GBM glomerulonephritis (72).

Macrophage Proliferation Within the Kidney

Resident tissue macrophages have little proliferative capacity and are renewed through constant immigration of blood monocytes (1,2). It is also widely believed that macrophage accumulation at sites of inflammation is the result of recruitment of blood monocytes with little or no

A

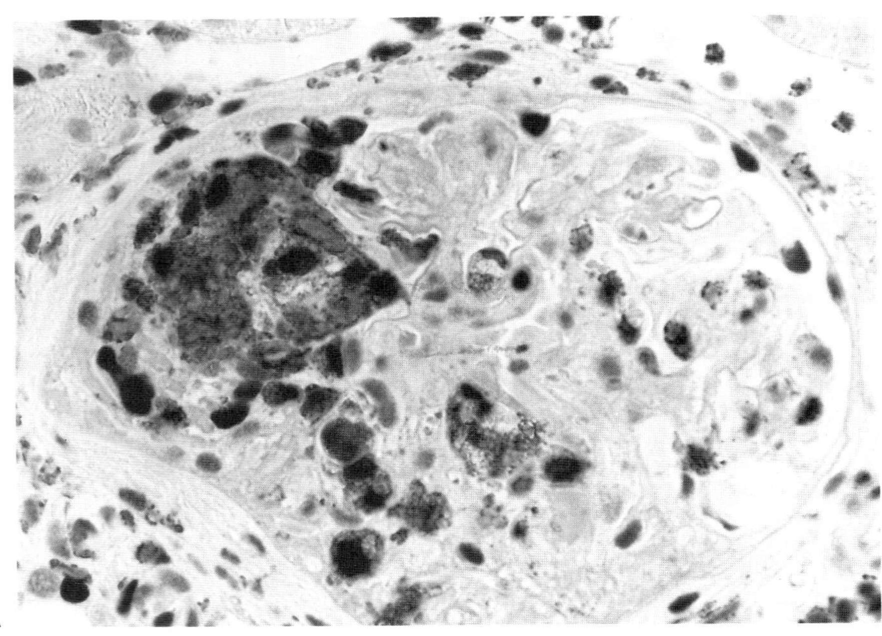

B

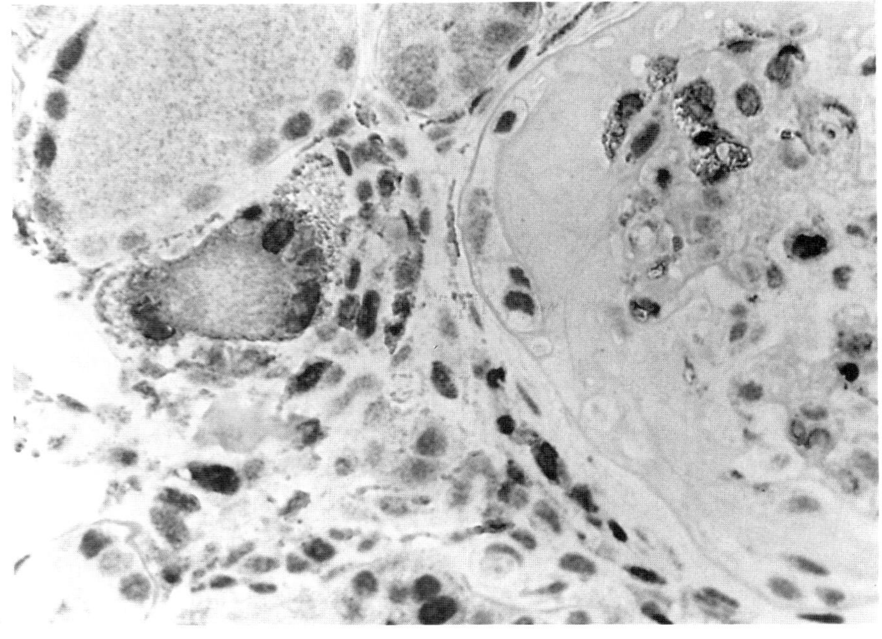

FIG. 2. Macrophage proliferation in renal lesions in rat anti-GBM glomerulonephritis. Cytoplasmic ED1 antibody staining of macrophages and nuclear PCNA staining in paraffin sections counterstain with PAS minus hematoxylin. **A:** Focal area of proliferating macrophages within a glomerular segmental lesion. **B:** Macrophage proliferation within a tubulointerstitial granulomatous lesion in an area of tubular destruction. Note that the multinucleated giant cell is also PCNA-positive.

local proliferation (1,3). However, our recent studies in two rat models of severe renal injury, acute renal allograft rejection, and Goodpasture's syndrome, have challenged this traditional dogma with the demonstration that substantial macrophage proliferation can occur within the inflamed kidney (4,5). Double immunohistochemistry staining found that 42% and 45% to 60% of total $ED1^+$ ($CD68^+$) macrophages in acute allograft rejection and Goodpasture's syndrome, respectively, were proliferating on the basis of expression of the proliferating cell nuclear antigen (PCNA), a marker of G1, S, and G2 phases of the cell cycle (4,5,126). An example of macrophage PCNA expression is shown in Fig. 2. These high levels of macrophage proliferation were confirmed by bromodeoxyuridine (BrdU) incorporation studies and the presence of mitotic figures in $ED1^+$ macrophages (5,127). Macrophage accumulation in the kidney and lung during the first 24 h of this disease model occurred primarily through monocyte recruitment, but high levels of proliferating macrophages were evident thereafter during progressive renal and pulmonary injury (5). The number of $PCNA^+$ macrophages gave an excellent correlation with total macrophage numbers in both the glomerulus and interstitium during disease development ($p < 0.001$), indicating that macrophage proliferation is the primary mechanism of macrophage accumulation after the induction of renal injury in this model (5). These findings raise the questions of whether this proliferation is restricted to the injured tissue and if the proliferating cells are resident tissue macrophages or recruited blood monocytes? The absence of detectable blood monocyte proliferation and unaltered levels of macrophage proliferation in uninvolved tissues suggest that macrophage proliferation in this disease is a localized event (5). In addition, proliferating macrophages within the kidney and lung had a monocyte phenotype, whereas cells with a resident tissue macrophage phenotype exhibited no proliferative activity (5). Proliferating macrophages within the kidney were primarily restricted to focal areas of glomerular and tubulointerstitial lesions (127), as illustrated in Fig. 2. Both total glomerular macrophages and the subset of proliferating macrophages gave a highly significant correlation with glomerular hypercellularity, glomerular segmental lesions, proteinuria, and declining creatinine clearance throughout disease progression (127). In contrast, the subset of nonproliferating glomerular macrophages failed to correlate with these indices of renal injury (127).

An interesting observation was the presence of large numbers of $PCNA^+$ and $BrdU^+$ macrophages within granulomatous lesions, indicating that local proliferation plays an important role in granuloma formation. Furthermore, all nuclei within multinucleated macrophage giant cells were $PCNA^+$ (Fig. 1B) but showed no evidence of BrdU incorporation, suggesting that these giant cells are formed by the fusion of macrophages in the G1 phase of the cell cycle, which then arrest and fail to proceed through the S phase (128).

At present it is not clear what factors drive local macrophage proliferation in severe renal injury. However, studies of murine lupus nephritis suggest that local production of M-CSF within the kidney may play an important role (78).

The degree of local macrophage proliferation within the kidney is related to the severity and progressive nature of the renal injury. The two disease models described above come at the severe end of the spectrum of rapidly progressive renal injury. In contrast, the first demonstration of macrophage proliferation within the kidney was in rat anti–Thy-1 nephritis (a disease featuring mild renal injury), in which only relatively small numbers of glomerular $ED1^+PCNA^+$ macrophages are seen (80,129, 130). Similarly, small numbers of proliferating macrophages have been demonstrated in rat immune complex glomerulonephritis, in which the number of $ED1^+BrdU^+$ glomerular macrophages gives an excellent correlation with the degree of proteinuria (75). A study of a broad cross-section of human glomerulonephritides found little evidence of glomerular leukocyte PCNA expression, although interstitial leukocyte proliferation was not examined (131). Therefore, it would be predicted that the presence of macrophage proliferation in human renal biopsy samples would be indicative of a rapidly progressive disease. As yet, it is unclear whether proliferating macrophages have the capacity to directly cause renal damage through increased production of mediators of injury or if macrophage proliferation is simply a mechanism to regulate the severity of the local inflammatory response.

Macrophage Exit from the Kidney

It has been shown that macrophages in the liver, lung, and gut can migrate to their local lymph nodes (1). However, the fate of infiltrating macrophages at sites of inflammation has received little attention. The finding that substantial local macrophage proliferation can occur at sites of severe tissue injury has brought renewed interest to this question. Total macrophage accumulation within the kidney during rat Goodpasture's syndrome was far less than that predicted by the number of proliferating macrophages, indicating that there was a rapid turnover of macrophages within the kidney (127). There are two possible fates for these cells. First, they may leave the kidney via the lymphatic drainage. Support for this possibility comes from the observation that macrophages account for up to 75% of cells entering the dilated marginal sinus of kidney draining lymph nodes during this disease (132). Second, macrophages may die within the kidney through apoptosis; however, such a mechanism remains to be proven.

MECHANISMS OF MACROPHAGE-MEDIATED RENAL INJURY

Macrophages can produce a wide variety of molecules that can directly or indirectly mediate renal injury (Table 1). Other chapters in this book describe most of these mediators in turn. This section addresses the role of macrophages in the pathogenesis of different renal lesions.

Glomerular Injury

The first direct demonstration that macrophages induce renal injury came from studies in which the monocyte/macrophage population was depleted from experimental animals. Systemic irradiation with kidney shielding prevented glomerular macrophage infiltration and abrogated proteinuria in rat accelerated anti-GBM glomerulonephritis (70). Monocyte depletion using an antimacrophage serum inhibited glomerular macrophage accumulation and proteinuria in anti-GBM glomerulonephritis and acute serum sickness in the rabbit (133). Antimacrophage serum also has proved effective in depleting glomerular macrophages and inhibiting proteinuria in rat accelerated anti-GBM glomerulonephritis and rat Heymann's nephritis (82,134). Furthermore, proliferative lesions and proteinuria were passively transferred by peritoneal mononuclear cells into rabbits made leukopenic by nitrogen mustard treatment during the autologous phase in rabbit anti-GBM glomerulonephritis (135).

Glomerular macrophages can produce ROS in experimental glomerulonephritis and have been shown to damage the GBM and increase protein permeability in vitro (136,137). Macrophages also may cause damage to the GBM through production and activation of metalloproteinases, whereas nitric oxide synthesis may cause direct podocyte toxicity and modulate glomerular hemodynamics. In addition, macrophage-derived cytokines such as IL-1 can stimulate mesangial cell synthesis of ROS, NO, and eicosanoids, as well as endothelial production of PAF (138–141).

TABLE 1. *Mechanisms of macrophage-mediated renal injury*

Macrophage product	Renal damage
Reactive oxygen species	Cell toxicity and basement membrane damage
Nitric oxide	Cell toxicity and possibly hemodynamic alterations
Metalloproteinases	Basement membrane degradation, release of growth factors from matrix, vascular leakage
Procoagulant activity	Fibrin deposition, crescent formation
Thromboxane/ eicosanoids	Alteration of glomerular hemodynamics, mesangial cell proliferation
IL-1	Endothelial activation, adhesion molecule expression, mesangial cell proliferation, fibroblast proliferation and collagen production, and synthesis of cytokines, NO and metalloproteinases
TNFα	Endothelial activation, adhesion molecule expression, cytokine production, cell cytotoxicity, NO synthesis
PAF	Decrease GFR and renal blood flow
IL-6	Mesangial cell proliferation
bFGF	Mesangial cell and fibroblast proliferation
PDGF	Mesangial cell and fibroblast proliferation
TGFβ	Extracellular matrix deposition and macrophage recruitment

Glomerular Hemodynamics (see Chapters 11 and 22)

Transient glomerular neutrophil influx after the induction of renal injury is known to cause an acute decrease in glomerular filtration rate and plasma flow due to large-scale synthesis of five-lipoxygenase products (142) (see Chapter 22). However, there is substantial evidence that macrophage eicosanoid production can mediate glomerular hemodynamic abnormalities. The marked increase in renal thromboxane A2 excretion and the decline in glomerular filtration rate after acute ureteral obstruction in the rat parallels the development of macrophage infiltration (40). Furthermore, macrophage depletion via an EFAD diet prevents macrophage infiltration, blocks eicosanoid production, and inhibits renal injury in this model (143). Glomerular macrophage accumulation is associated with increased leukotriene D4 (LTD4) synthesis during the autologous phase of rat Heymann's nephritis. Treatment of this disease model with a specific LTD4 antagonist inhibited proteinuria and improved glomerular filtration rate, whereas depletion of glomerular macrophages by irradiation blocked LTD4 synthesis, inhibited proteinuria, and improved glomerular filtration rate (144). In addition, treatment of rats with an EFAD diet inhibited glomerular macrophage accumulation, glomerular LTB4, and thromboxane production and proteinuria—but not glomerular neutrophil infiltration—during the heterologous phase of rat anti-GBM glomerulonephritis (145). Indeed, angiotensin II–induced eicosanoid production in normal rat glomeruli is inhibited by depletion of the resident glomerular macrophage population by an EFAD diet (146).

Crescent Formation (see Chapter 32)

The first demonstration that glomerular crescents contain large numbers of macrophages came from glomeru-

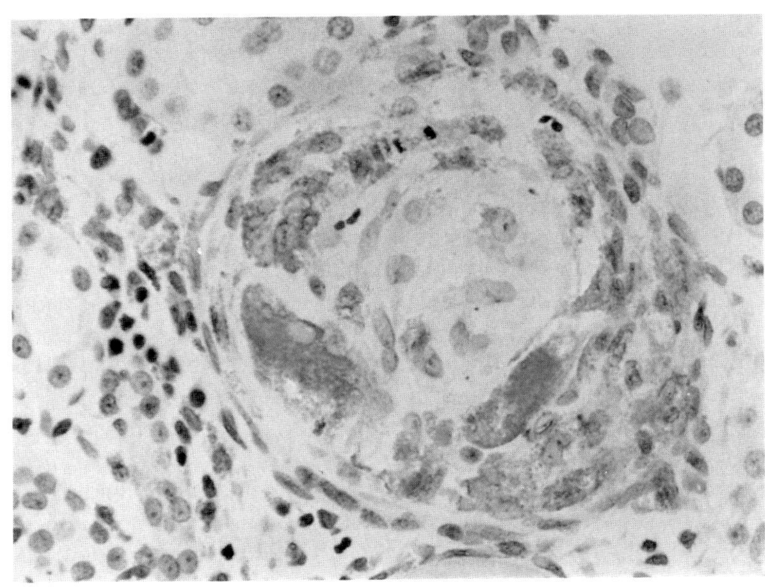

FIG. 3. Macrophages in a glomerular crescent in rat anti-GBM glomerulonephritis. Many ED1$^+$ macrophages (brown cytoplasmic staining) are present within a glomerular crescent. Section was counterstained with hematoxylin.

lar culture studies of patients with rapidly progressive glomerulonephritis (55). Since then a variety of methods have been used to confirm that macrophages are the predominant cell type in most cellular crescents in human and experimental glomerulonephritis (147–149). Figure 3 shows many macrophages within a cellular crescent. Macrophage accumulation within Bowman's space exhibits components of a classical DTH response, being dependent on CD4$^+$ T cells and fibrin deposition. Infiltration of immune activated (IL-2R$^+$) CD4$^+$ T cells and macrophages and fibrin deposition is evident in active IgA crescentic glomerulonephritis (30). Depletion of CD4$^+$ T cells abrogates crescent formation in rat anti-GBM glomerulonephritis, whereas fibrin depletion prevents crescent formation in rat chronic immune complex nephritis (52,150). Infiltrating glomerular macrophages express coagulant tissue factor–like activity in human proliferative glomerulonephritis and experimental anti-GBM disease (151–154). This is thought to promote fibrin deposition within Bowman's space because macrophage depletion abrogates this fibrin deposition without affecting systemic coagulation (154).

Adhesion molecules may play an important role in macrophage accumulation within Bowman's space by facilitating macrophage attachment to parietal epithelial cells or deposited matrix molecules such as hyaluronate (155,156) (see Chapter 25). Parietal epithelial cells constitutively express a number of leukocyte adhesion molecules such as ICAM-1 (CD54) and VCAM-1 (CD106), which are markedly upregulated after the induction of glomerular injury (115,116,119,121,122). Indeed, anti–ICAM-1 antibody treatment inhibits crescent formation in rat autoimmune anti-GBM glomerulonephritis (72). In addition, blocking IL-1 activity in rat anti-GBM glomerulonephritis by treatment with the IL-1 receptor antagonist (IL-1ra) prevents crescent formation even in the presence of significant proteinuria and glomerular macrophage accumulation (157,158). This may be due to the marked reduction in renal ICAM-1 expression seen in IL-1ra–treated animals (159).

A previously unrecognized mechanism of macrophage accumulation within Bowman's space is that of local macrophage proliferation. In rat anti-GBM glomerulonephritis, greater than 50% of glomeruli develop crescent formation by day 21, with ED1$^+$ macrophages accounting for 50% to 80% of total crescent cells (160). A striking finding was that 60% to 75% of macrophages within crescents were PCNA$^+$, indicating a high level of local proliferation within Bowman's space, which was also confirmed by macrophage BrdU incorporation and the presence of macrophage mitotic figures within crescents (161).

An important feature of crescent formation is the process by which cellular crescents become infiltrated by fibroblasts leading to glomerular scarring (see also Chapter 32). It has been shown that rupture of Bowman's capsule is necessary for the entry of interstitial fibroblasts into Bowman's space and fibrotic development (160,162, 163). The integrity of Bowman's capsule also has been shown to determine the composition of glomerular crescents in human and experimental glomerulonephritis (160,164). It generally has been assumed that Bowman's capsule is ruptured by the action of macrophages within Bowman's space. However, this conventional view has been challenged by a study in rat anti-GBM glomerulonephritis in which 25% to 52% of glomerular cross-sections exhibiting Bowman's capsule rupture had no evidence of crescent formation, whereas focal periglomerular accumulation of immune-activated (IL-2R$^+$) CD4$^+$ T cells and macrophages was adjacent to all areas of Bowman's capsule rupture (160). Disruption of Bowman's capsule facilitated the entry of periglomerular fibroblasts and activated (IL-2R$^+$) T cells into Bowman's space and the development of glomerular fibrosis (160). This study suggests that periglomerular leukocytes mediate Bowman's capsule rupture through a DTH-type mechanism, possibly via T-cell activation of macrophage ROS production and the secretion and plasmin activation of metalloproteinases.

The ability of periglomerular leukocytes to mediate rupture of Bowman's capsule is exemplified in a rat model of interstitial nephritis induced by active immunization with autologous Tamm-Horsfall protein. No glomerular changes were evident in this model except for the development of a prominent periglomerular leukocytic infiltrate with immune-activated (IL-2R$^+$) T cells and macrophages, which was associated with Bowman's capsule rupture and the development of mild proteinuria (Q Song, HY Lan, DJ Nikolic-Paterson, RC Atkins, manuscript submitted).

Glomerular Hypercellularity and Glomerulosclerosis (see Chapter 33)

Mesangial hypercellularity is seen in a variety of glomerulonephritides and is thought to contribute to the development of glomerulosclerosis (165). A study of pediatric nephritis found that glomerular hypertrophy in minimal-change disease predicted progression to focal glomerulosclerosis (166). In addition, a repeat biopsy study demonstrated that macrophage infiltration within areas of focal segmental endocapillary proliferation preceded development of focal glomerulosclerosis (167). Animal disease models also have demonstrated a link between mesangial hypercellularity and glomerulosclerosis. Transgenic mice chronically expressing growth hormone or growth hormone–releasing factor develop mesangial proliferation before the appearance of glomerulosclerosis (168). Mesangial cell proliferation precedes the development of glomerulosclerosis in rat models of anti–Thy-1 nephritis, renal ablation, and streptozotocin-induced diabetes (83,94,169,170). Similarly, the peak of mesangial cell proliferation in rat anti-GBM glomerulonephritis is associated with the induction of glomerulosclerosis (158,171).

Glomerular macrophage accumulation frequently is associated with increased mesangial cellularity and indeed contributes in part to this change (56,58,60,61,66, 172). Macrophage depletion prevents mesangial hypercellularity and the consequent mesangial matrix deposition and development of glomerulosclerosis in rat models of renal ablation and PAN-induced nephrosis (173,174). A direct coculture system found that glomerular macrophages in experimental serum sickness are a major stimulus for mesangial cell proliferation (175). Although there is good evidence that glomerular macrophage infiltration plays an important role in progressive mesangial proliferation and the development of glomerulosclerosis, the initial triggering of mesangial proliferation in some models of renal injury is dependent on platelet activation before significant macrophage infiltration (83,94,169,170,176).

There are a number of mechanisms by which glomerular macrophages may stimulate mesangial proliferation and the development of glomerulosclerosis. Infiltrating macrophages are the main source of glomerular IL-1 production in human and experimental glomerulonephritis (93,177–185) (see Chapter 20). IL-1 stimulates mesangial cell proliferation and glomerular epithelial cell collagen synthesis in vitro (186–188), whereas IL-1ra treatment has been reported to inhibit mesangial proliferation in rat anti–Thy-1 nephritis (180). In addition, IL-1ra treatment of rat anti-GBM glomerulonephritis suppressed glomerular cell proliferation, glomerular hypercellularity, and development of glomerulosclerosis in association with a reduction in glomerular macrophage infiltration (157).

Macrophages also can secrete IL-6, basic fibroblast growth factor (bFGF), and platelet-derived growth factor (PDGF), which participate in mesangial cell proliferation in vivo (189–192) (see Chapter 20). However, the relative contribution of infiltrating macrophages compared with that of resident glomerular cells in the synthesis of these growth factors is unclear. Macrophages also may stimulate matrix deposition within the mesangium. Glomerular macrophages synthesize fibronectin in rat proliferative glomerulonephritis and can stimulate fibronectin production by mesangial cells (193,194). Macrophages are also a major source of TGF-β, which plays a central role in the development of glomerulosclerosis (195–197).

Glomerular macrophages also are involved in the development of glomerulosclerosis after lipid accumulation (198). Induction of a high-cholesterol diet in susceptible ExHC rats results in glomerular lipid accumulation, macrophage infiltration, foam cell formation, proteinuria, and the development of glomerulosclerosis (93). Macrophage accumulation and glomerular injury in this model can be inhibited by the use of the antioxidant probucol (199). Macrophage accumulation is also prominent in lipid-induced glomerular injury in Zucker rats (200), and macrophage depletion ameliorates the adverse effects of a high-cholesterol diet in rats with PAN-induced nephrosis (87).

Interstitial Damage and Fibrosis (see Chapter 34)

It is well established that interstitial lesions correlate with declining renal function at the time of biopsy and predict renal outcome (201–208). Tubular necrosis and atrophy, mononuclear cell accumulation, and tubulointerstitial fibrosis are integral components of these interstitial lesions. However, the causal relationship between these components is only now starting to be understood. This is a crucial issue because ongoing interstitial fibrosis is seen as the most important determinant of progression to end-stage renal failure and has become the main focus in developing new therapeutic strategies for the treatment of renal diseases.

Interstitial macrophage and T-cell infiltration occurs in all types of glomerulonephritis and correlates with renal function at the time of biopsy and predicts renal outcome (26,28,29,32,33,35,57,64,65,68). Prominent interstitial macrophage and T-cell infiltration also is seen in animal models of disease, including those induced by nonimmune renal insults (40–42,85,88–91) (see Chapter 36). These findings suggest that irrespective of the nature of the initial insult, progressive interstitial damage and renal impairment is mediated by a common cell-mediated immune mechanism, which may involve a DTH-like response to renal neoantigens (207,209,210).

A number of studies support a causal role for interstitial macrophages in the mediation of tubulointerstitial injury. There is an excellent correlation between interstitial accumulation and activation (IL-2R expression) of $CD4^+$ T cells and macrophages with declining renal function, tubulitis, and tubulointerstitial fibrosis in rat anti-GBM glomerulonephritis (37). The ability of IL-1ra treatment to prevent development of tubulitis and fibrosis in this model is largely attributed to the abrogation of interstitial macrophage infiltration and immune activation of the $CD4^+$ T-cell infiltrate (157,158). In a rat model of focal and segmental glomerulosclerosis induced by PAN and protamine sulphate, prednisolone treatment of established disease markedly suppressed interstitial mononuclear cell infiltration and IL-2R expression in association with improved creatinine clearance and inhibition of interstitial fibrosis, whereas the existing glomerular injury was unaffected in terms of proteinuria, glomerular mononulcear cell infiltration, and glomerulosclerosis (41,211). Macrophage depletion markedly improved renal function in the postobstructive rat kidney and PAN-induced nephrotic syndrome (212,213). Similarly, macrophage depletion of established PAN nephrosis prevented glomerular and interstitial macrophage accumulation and suppressed renal injury (174). In addition, leukocyte depletion prevented the predominant $CD4^+$ T-cell interstitial infiltrate and consequent reduction in renal function, tubular atrophy, and interstitial fibrosis in chronic adriamycin nephropathy in the rat (54).

Although few studies have directly addressed the mechanisms by which macrophages cause tubular injury, there are a number of macrophage products that have the potential to mediate tubular toxicity (Table 1). Infiltrating macrophages have been shown to produce ROS, NO, and TNF-α, which can all directly induce cellular toxicity (136,178,179,181,182,184,214). Macrophages also may damage the tubular basement membrane and increase local vascular permeability through secretion and activation of metalloproteinases (215–218).

Macrophages play an important role in the fibrotic response after tissue injury through production of cytokines and growth factors that promote fibroblast accumulation, proliferation, and matrix synthesis (219) (see also Chapter 34). Infiltrating macrophages are the major source of the proinflammatory cytokine IL-1, which has been implicated in the fibrotic process. IL-1 can stimulate the proliferation of some types of fibroblasts, including fibroblasts isolated from fibrotic human kidney (220, 221). IL-1 also has been reported to stimulate fibroblast collagen synthesis in some, but not all, studies (222,223). Blockade of IL-1 activity inhibits fibrosis during the induction and progression of rat anti-GBM glomerulonephritis and a murine model of pulmonary fibrosis. However, it is not clear whether this is a consequence of inhibiting fibroblast activity or if it reflects inhibition of macrophage infiltration and cytokine production (157, 158,224). Macrophages also can synthesize bFGF and PDGF, two potent fibroblast mitogens that play a major role in the development of active fibrotic lesions (219, 225,226).

TGF-β is the key molecule regulating renal fibrosis (197) (see also Chapter 20). However, the cellular source of TGF-β responsible for progressive tissue fibrosis is not clear. Macrophages can synthesize large amounts of TGF-β, and a number of studies have identified infiltrating macrophages as the major source of TGF-β in human and experimental glomerulonephritis (109,227–232). TGF-β production and the appearance of interstitial myofibroblasts parallels interstitial macrophage accumulation in experimental hydronephrosis, which is abolished by macrophage depletion (109). In addition to being an important source of TGF-β production, macrophages can release extracellular matrix–associated bFGF and TGF-β through local plasminogen activation and also may be involved in the activation of latent TGF-β (233).

FUTURE STRATEGIES TO INHIBIT MACROPHAGE-MEDIATED RENAL INJURY

The beneficial effects of general immunosuppressive drugs such as prednisolone and cyclophosphamide in the treatment of progressive glomerulonephritis have been largely attributed to a reduction in circulating monocyte and T-cell numbers and inhibition of leukocyte accumulation at sites of inflammation (1,35,41,234). However, the doses required to completely suppress cell-mediated immune renal injury cause serious side effects, thus limiting their usefulness in many patients. Therefore, there is great interest in developing better general immunosuppressive drugs that are well tolerated. For example, deoxyspergualin is a new drug that inhibits primary and secondary CTL and antibody responses, as well as macrophage and mesangial cell proliferation, lacks nephrotoxicity, and has only mild side effects, making it an attractive treatment for rapidly progressive glomerulonephritis (4,171,235,236). Apart from its success in suppressing rejection of kidney, liver, and pancreatic islet transplants in humans (237–240), deoxyspergualin has been shown to abrogate renal injury in murine lupus nephritis and rat models of Goodpasture's syndrome, $HgCl_2$-induced glomerulonephritis, and tubulointerstitial nephritis (241–245).

One significant drawback with general immunosuppressive drugs is that the patient is left susceptible to opportunistic infection. Therefore, an alternative approach is to develop new therapeutic agents that target specific mechanisms of macrophage-mediated renal injury. There are three main points at which macrophage-mediated renal injury can be targeted: (a) monocyte entry into the kidney, (b) macrophage activation within the kidney, and (c) the action of macrophage-derived mediators of injury. Table 2 summarizes some possible treatment strategies. Work on these strategies generally has been conducted as individual studies, but there is great potential for targeting multiple aspects of macrophage-mediated renal injury to provide therapeutic strategies tailored to specific disease groups.

Of these new therapeutic strategies, there has been significant progress in blocking the action of IL-1 using recombinant IL-1ra protein. IL-1ra treatment can suppress many different animal models of cell-mediated immune injury (246), even though IL-1 blockade does not inhibit T cell–dependent antibody responses (247). Clinical trials have found no side effects of IL-1ra administration in humans, and phase III trials in rheumatoid arthritis are currently underway. Although IL-1ra treatment does not prevent neutrophil-dependent induction of proteinuria in rat anti-GBM glomerulonephritis (157,248,249),

TABLE 2. *Strategies for inhibiting macrophage-mediated renal injury*

Target	Strategy	Comments
Inhibit monocyte entry to the kidney	Block immune complex deposition via soluble FcG RII.	Depletes circulating immune complexes, inhibits arthus reaction, yet to be proven in renal injury.
	Block monocyte-specific chemotaxis via Ab or sR for MCP-1 or MIF. Block synthesis of monocyte-specific chemotactic lipid or an sR.	Yet to prove that blocking these molecules will inhibit renal injury.
	Block leukocyte adhesion molecules via Ab or sR for molecules such as P-selectin, ICAM-1, LFA-1, VCAM-1.	Ab proven effective in experimental renal injury. Good potential, although targets all leukocyte populations.
	Inhibit M-CSF–driven macrophage proliferation via sR expressed locally within the kidney.	Yet to be proven in renal injury. Requires gene therapy to target kidney without affecting bone marrow monocyte production.
Inhibit macrophage activation	Block macrophage activation through Ab or sR for MIF or IFN-γ, or use cytokines IL-10 or IL-4.	IL-10 and IL-4 suppress models of T cell–dependent macrophage-mediated tissue injury. Potential to inhibit production of many mediators of renal injury such as IL-1, TNFα, NO, ROS and metalloproteinases.
	Block macrophage activation by blocking transcription factors such as NF-ATp.	Unproven in experimental disease models. Good potential if adequately specific in target genes.
Inhibit action of macrophage-derived mediators of injury	Block production of mature IL-1β by inhibiting IL-1β–converting enzyme, block action of IL-1 via IL-1ra, Ab, or sR	IL-1ra suppresses established rat crescentic glomerulonephritis. Good potential therapy.
	Block TNF-α action via Ab or sR.	Anti-TNFα Ab suppresses rat anti-GBM glomerulonephritis. Good potential therapy.
	Block bFGF and PDGF action by Ab or sR.	Anti-PDGF Ab suppresses mesangial proliferation in rat anti–Thy-1 nephritis.
	Block TGF-β action via Ab, sR, or decorin.	Anti-TGFβ Ab and decorin inhibit glomerular sclerosis in rat anti–Thy-1 nephritis. Good therapeutic potential.
	Block macrophage expression or activity of inducible nitric oxide synthase via targeted antisense or antagonist.	Yet to be proven in renal injury. Critical to target macrophage and not endothelial NO production because they play different roles.
	Block ROS production or action via enzyme antagonists or antioxidants such as sodium pyruvate and taurine.	Effective in glycerol-induced acute renal failure and PAN nephrosis.
	Block macrophage procoagulant activity via tissue factor Ab or antagonists.	Anti–tissue factor Ab inhibits endotoxin-induced acute renal injury in baboons.

Ab, antibody; sR, soluble form of cell surface receptor.

IL-1 blockade does prevent the development of glomerular crescent formation, renal function impairment, and tubulointerstitial lesions despite persistent moderate to severe proteinuria (157). Importantly, IL-1ra treatment of established crescentic glomerulonephritis halted a further increase in proteinuria and crescent formation and caused a return to a normal rate of creatinine clearance (158). Thus, a clinical trial of IL-1ra treatment as an adjunct to standard immunosuppressive therapy of rapidly progressive glomerulonephritis is an attractive proposal.

Having identified IL-1 as a good therapeutic target, there is a wide range of possible approaches to blocking IL-1 action reflecting recent advances in biotechnology. Apart from administration of recombinant IL-1ra protein, IL-1 action can be inhibited by neutralizing anti–IL-1 antibodies or by a soluble form of the IL-1 receptor type II. Macrophage production of IL-1β can be suppressed by inhibiting the IL-1β–converting enzyme. As an alternative to injection of recombinant IL-1ra, the protein can be locally administered by gene therapy, which has already proved successful in a rabbit model of arthritis (250).

There has been substantial interest in using gene therapy to introduce therapeutic agents into the kidney, with a number of recent successes in animal models being reported (192,251–254). Gene therapy has many potential benefits such as permitting the local delivery of drugs,which may be toxic/harmful if given systemically, it is substantially cheaper compared with recombinant protein–based drugs, and DNA vectors need only be administered on a monthly basis. In addition, gene therapy can be used to replace a defective gene or to block synthesis of a specific protein within target cells. Although there are a number of outstanding difficulties in the delivery systems, these are likely to be solved during the next few years.

In conclusion, there has been substantial progress during the past 5 years in defining mechanisms of macrophage-mediated immune renal injury. The ability to target specific mechanisms of macrophage-mediated injury together with the explosion in gene therapy technology holds great promise for the development of effective treatment strategies for many different renal diseases.

REFERENCES

1. Van Furth R. Phagocytic cells: development and distribution of mononuclear phagocytes in normal steady state and inflammation. In: Gallin JI, Goldstein IM, Synderman R, eds. *Inflammation: Basic Principles and Clinical Correlates*. New York: Raven; 1988: 281–295.
2. Westermann J, Ronneberg S, Fritz FJ, Pabst R. Proliferation of macrophage subpopulations in the adult rat: comparison of various lymphoid organs. *J Leukoc Biol* 1989;46:263–269.
3. Blussé van Oud Alblas A, van der Linden-Schrever AB, van Furth R. Origin and kinetics of pulmonary macrophages during an inflammatory reaction induced by intravenous administration of heat-killed bacillus Calmette-Guerin. *J Exp Med* 1981;154:235–252.
4. Kerr PG, Nikolic-Paterson DJ, Lan HY, Rainone S, Tesch G, Atkins RC. Deoxyspergualin suppresses local macrophage proliferation in renal allograft rejection. *Transplantation* 1994;58:596–601.
5. Lan HY, Nikolic-Paterson DJ, Atkins RC. Local macrophage proliferation in experimental Goodpasture's syndrome. *Nephrology* 1995; 1:151–156.
6. Swain SL. T cell subsets and the recognition of MHC class. *Immunol Rev* 1983;74:129–142.
7. Powrie F, Coffman RL. Cytokine regulation of T-cell function: potential for therapeutic intervention. *Immunol Today* 1993;14:270–274.
8. Huitinga I, van Rooijen N, de Groot CJ, Uitdehaag BM, Dijkstra CD. Suppression of experimental allergic encephalomyelitis in Lewis rats after elimination of macrophages. *J Exp Med* 1990;172:1025–1033.
9. Williams GT, Williams WJ. Granulomatous inflammation—a review. *J Clin Pathol* 1983;36:723–733.
10. June CH, Bluestone JA, Nadler LM, Thompson CB. The B7 and CD28 receptor families. *Immunol Today* 1994;15:321–331.
11. Terada N, Konno A, Shirotori K et al. Mechanism of eosinophil infiltration in the patient with subcutaneous angioblastic lymphoid hyperplasia with eosinophilia (Kimura's disease). Mechanism of eosinophil chemotaxis mediated by candida antigen and IL-5. *Int Arch Allergy Immunol* 1994;104:18–20.
12. Roitt IM. *Essential Immunology*. 8th ed. Oxford: Blackwell; 1994.
13. Vissers MC, Fantone JC, Wiggins R, Kunkel SL. Glomerular basement membrane–containing immune complexes stimulate tumor necrosis factor and interleukin-1 production by human monocytes. *Am J Pathol* 1989;134:1–6.
14. Matsumoto K. Renal tubular epithelial antigen–containing immune complexes stimulate interleukin-1 production by monocytes from patients with glomerulonephritis. *Int Urol Nephrol* 1992;24:319–326.
15. Padeh S, Jaffe CL, Passwell JH. Activation of human monocytes via their sIgA receptors. *Immunology* 1991;72:188–193.
16. Piquette CA, Robinson-Hill R, Webster RO. Human monocyte chemotaxis to complement-derived chemotaxins is enhanced by Gc-globulin. *J Leukoc Biol* 1994;55:349–354.
17. Elstad MR, Parker CJ, Cowley FS. CD11b/CD18 integrin and a beta-glucan receptor act in concert to induce the synthesis of platelet-activating factor by monocytes. *J Immunol* 1994;152:220–230.
18. Szefler SJ, Norton CE, Ball B, Gross JM, Aida Y, Pabst MJ. IFN-gamma and LPS overcome glucocorticoid inhibition of priming for superoxide release in human monocytes. Evidence that secretion of IL-1 and tumor necrosis factor-alpha is not essential for monocyte priming. *J Immunol* 1989;142:3985–3992.
19. Ward PA, Warren JS, Johnson KJ. Oxygen radicals, inflammation, and tissue injury. *Free Radic Biol Med* 1988;5:403–408.
20. Opdenakker G, Masure S, Grillet B, Van Damme J. Cytokine-mediated regulation of human leukocyte gelatinases and role in arthritis. *Lymphokine Cytokine Res* 1991;10:317–324.
21. Warren JS. Relationship between interleukin-1 beta and platelet-activating factor in the pathogenesis of acute immune complex alveolitis in the rat. *Am J Pathol* 1992;141:551–560.
22. Malyak M, Smith MF Jr, Abel AA, Arend WP. Peripheral blood neutrophil production of interleukin-1 receptor antagonist and interleukin-1 beta. *J Clin Immunol* 1994;14:20–30.
23. Jung HC, Eckmann L, Yang S-K, et al. A distinct array of proinflammatory cytokines is expressed in human colon epithelial cells in response to bacterial invasion. *J Clin Invest* 1995;95:55–65.
24. Schmouder RL, Strieter RM, Kunkel SL. Interferon-τ regulation of human renal cortical epithelial cell–derived monocyte chemotactic peptide-1. *Kidney Int* 1993;44:43–49.
25. Jevnikar AM, Brennan DC, Singer GG. Stimulated kidney tubular epithelial cells express membrane associated and secreted TNF alpha. *Kidney Int* 1991;40:203–211.
26. Hooke DH, Gee DC, Atkins RC. Leukocyte analysis using monoclonal antibodies in human glomerulonephritis. *Kidney Int* 1987;31:964–972.
27. Bolton WK, Innes DJ, Sturgill BC, et al. T-cells and macrophages in rapidly progressive glomerulonephritis: clinicopathologic correlations. *Kidney Int* 1987;32:869–876.
28. Markovic-Lipkovski J, Müller CA, Bohle A, et al. Mononuclear leukocytes, expression of HLA class II antigens and intercellular adhesion molecule 1 in focal segmental glomerulosclerosis. *Nephron* 1991;59:286–293.
29. Markovic-Lipkovski J, Müller CA, Risler T, et al. Association of glomerular and interstitial mononuclear leucocytes with different forms of glomerulonephritis. *Nephrol Dial Transplant* 1990;5:10–17.

30. Li H-L, Hancock WW, Dowling JP, et al. Activated (IL-2R+) intraglomerular mononuclear cells in crescentic glomerulonephritis. *Kidney Int* 1991;39:793–798.
31. Li H, Hancock WW, Hooke DH, et al. Mononuclear cell activation and decreased renal function in IgA nephropathy with crescents. *Kidney Int* 1990;37:1552–1556.
32. Alexopoulos E, Seron D, Hartley RB, et al. Lupus nephritis: correlation of interstitial cells with glomerular function. *Kidney Int* 1990;37:100–109.
33. Alexopoulos E, Seron D, Hartley RB, et al. The role of interstitial infiltrates in IgA nephropathy: a study with monoclonal antibodies. *Nephrol Dial Transplant* 1989;4:187–195.
34. Falk MC, Hg G, Zhang GY, et al. Infiltration of the kidney by αβ and τδ T cells: effect on progression in IgA nephropathy. *Kidney Int* 1995;47:177–185.
35. Ootaka T, Saito T, Yusa A, Munakata T, Soma J, Abe K. Contribution of cellular infiltration to the progression of IgA nephropathy: a longitudinal, immunocytochemical study on repeated renal biopsy specimens. *Nephrology* 1995;1:135–142.
36. Stilmant MM, Bolton WK, Sturgill BC, Schmitt GW, Couser WG. Crescentic glomerulonephritis without immune deposits: clinicopathologic features. *Kidney Int* 1979;15:184–195.
37. Lan HY, Paterson DJ, Atkins RC. Initiation and evolution of interstitial leukocytic infiltration in experimental glomerulonephritis. *Kidney Int* 1991;40:425–433.
38. Quiza CG, Leenaerts PL, Hall BM. The role of T cells in the mediation of glomerular injury in Heymann's nephritis in the rat. *Int Immunol* 1992;4:423–432.
39. Tipping PG, Neale TJ, Holdsworth SR. T lymphocyte participation in antibody-induced experimental glomerulonephritis. *Kidney Int* 1985;27:530–537.
40. Schreiner GF, Harris KPG, Purkerson ML, Klahr S. Immunologic aspects of acute ureteral obstruction: immune cell infiltrate in the kidney. *Kidney Int* 1988;34:487–493.
41. Saito T, Atkins RC. Contribution of mononuclear leucocytes to the progression of experimental focal glomerular sclerosis. *Kidney Int* 1990;37:1076–1083.
42. Eddy AA. Interstitial nephritis induced by protein-overload proteinuria. *Am J Pathol* 1989;135:719–733.
43. Bolton WK, Chandra M, Tyson TM, et al. Transfer of experimental glomerulonephritis in chickens by mononuclear cells. *Kidney Int* 1988;34:598–610.
44. Oite T, Shimizu F, Kagami S, et al. Hapten-specific cellular immune response producing glomerular injury. *Clin Exp Immunol* 1989;76:463–468.
45. Rennke HG, Klein PS, Sandstrom DJ, Mendrick DL. Cell-mediated immune injury in the kidney: acute nephritis induced in the rat by azobenzenearsonate. *Kidney Int* 1994;45:1044–1056.
46. Meyers CM, Kelley CJ. Effector mechanisms in organ-specific autoimmunity. I. Characterisation of a $CD8^+$ T cell line that mediates murine interstitial nephritis. *J Clin Invest* 1991;88:408–416.
47. Mann R, Zakheim B, Clayman M, McCafferty E, Michaud L, Neilson EG. Murine interstitial nephritis. IV. Long-term cultured L3T4+ T cell lines transfer delayed expression of disease as I-A–restricted inducers of the effector T cell repertoire. *J Immunol* 1985;135:286–293.
48. Sato K, Oguchi H, Yoshie T, Koiwai T. Tubulointerstitial nephritis induced by Tamm-Horsfall protein sensitization in guinea pigs. *Virchows Arch [B]* 1990;58:357–363.
49. Kawasaki K, Yaoita E, Yamamoto T, Kihara I. Depletion of CD8 positive cells in nephrotoxic serum nephritis in WKY rats. *Kidney Int* 1992;41:1517–1526.
50. Huang XR, Holdsworth SR, Tipping PG. Evidence for delayed-type hypersensitivity mechanisms in glomerular crescent formation. *Kidney Int* 1994;46:69–78.
51. Carteron NL, Schimenti CL, Wofsy D. Treatment of murine lupus with $F(ab\ )_2$ fragments of monoclonal antibody to L3T4. *J Immunol* 1989;142:1470–1475.
52. Jabs DA, Burek CL, Hu Q, Kuppers RC, Lee B, Prendergast RA. Anti-CD4 monoclonal antibody therapy suppresses autoimmune disease in MRL/Mp–lpr/lpr mice. *Cell Immunol* 1992;141:496–507.
53. Nishikawa K, Linsley PS, Collins AB, Stamenkovic I, McCluskey RT, Andres G. Effect of CTLA-4 chimeric protein on rat autoimmune anti-glomerular basement membrane glomerulonephritis. *Eur J Immunol* 1994;24:1249–1254.
54. Ginevri F, Trivelli A, Mutti A, et al. Progression of chronic adriamycin nephropathy in leukopenic rats. *Nephron* 1993;63:79–88.
54a. Rocklin RE, Lewis EJ, David JR. In vitro evidence for cellular hypersensitivity to glomerular basement membrane antigens in human glomerulonephritis. *N Engl J Med* 1970;283:497–501.
54b. Derry CJ, Ross CN, Lombardi G, et al. Analysis of T cell responses to the autoantigen in Goodpasture's disease. *Clin Exp Immunol* 1995;100:262–268.
55. Atkins RC, Holdsworth SR, Glasgow EF, et al. The macrophage in human rapidly progressive glomerulonephritis. *Lancet* 1976;1:830–832.
56. Hooke DH, Hancock WW, Gee DC, et al. Monoclonal antibody analysis of glomerular hypercellularity in human glomerulonephritis. *Clin Nephrol* 1984;22:163–168.
57. Stachura I, Lusheng SI, Whiteside TL. Mononuclear cell subsets in human idiopathic crescentic glomerulonephritis. *J Clin Immunol* 1984;4:202–208.
58. Monga GM, Mazzucco G, di Belgiojoso GB, et al. Monocyte infiltration and glomerular hypercellularity in human acute and persistent glomerulonephritis. Light and electron microscopic, immunofluorescence, and histochemical investigation on twenty-eight cases. *Lab Invest* 1981;44:381–387.
59. Magil AB, Wadsworth LD, Loewen M. Monocytes and human renal glomerular disease. A quantitative evaluation. *Lab Invest* 1981;44:27–33.
60. Ferrario F, Castiglione A, Colasanti G, et al. The detection of monocytes in human glomerulonephritis. *Kidney Int* 1985;28:513–519.
61. Nolasco FEB, Cameron JS, Hartley B, et al. Intraglomerular T cells and monocytes in nephritis: study with monoclonal antibodies. *Kidney Int* 1987;31:1160–1166.
62. Harry T, Bryant D, Coles GA, et al. The detection of monocytes in human renal biopsies: a prospective study. *Clin Nephrol* 1982;18:29–33.
63. Jothy S, Sawka R. Presence of monocytes in systemic lupus erythematosis-associated glomerulonephritis. *Arch Pathol Lab Med* 1981;105:590–593.
64. Castiglione A, Bucci A, Fellin G, et al. The relationship of infiltrating renal leucocytes to disease activity in lupus and cryoglobulinaemic glomerulonephritis. *Nephron* 1988;50:14–23.
65. D'Agati V, Appel GB, Estes D, et al. Monoclonal antibody identification of infiltrating mononuclear leukocyte in lupus nephritis. *Kidney Int* 1986;30:573–581.
66. Arima S, Nakayama M, Naito M, Sato T, Takahashi K. Significance of mononuclear phagocytes in IgA nephropathy. *Kidney Int* 1991;39:684–692.
67. Hotta O, Taguma Y, Ooyama M, Yusa N, Nagura H. Analysis of CD14+ cells and CD56+ cells in urine using flow cytometry: a useful tool for monitoring disease activity of IgA nephropathy. *Clin Nephrol* 1993;39:289–294.
68. Sabadini E, Castiglione A, Colasanti G, et al. Characterization of interstitial infiltrating cells in Berger's disease. *Am J Kidney Disease* 1988;12:307–315.
69. Bolton WK, May WJ, Sturgill. Proliferative autoimmune glomerulonephritis in rats: a model for autoimmune glomerulonephritis in humans. *Kidney Int* 1993;44:294–306.
70. Schreiner GF, Cotran RS, Pardo V, et al. A mononuclear cell component to experimental immunological glomerulonephritis. *J Exp Med* 1978;147:369–384.
71. Boyce NW, Holdsworth SR, Dijkstra CD, et al. Quantitation of intraglomerular mononuclear phagocytes in experimental glomerulonephritis in the rat using specific monoclonal antibodies. *Pathology* 1987;19:290–293.
72. Nishikawa K, Guo Y-J, Miyasaka M et al. Antibodies to intercellular adhesion molecule 1/lymphocyte function–associated antigen 1 prevent crescent formation in rat autoimmune glomerulonephritis. *J Exp Med* 1993;177:667–677.
73. Hunsicker LG, Shearer TP, Plattner SB, et al. The role of monocytes in serum sickness nephritis. *J Exp Med* 1979;150:413–425.
74. Holdsworth SR, Neale TJ, Wilson CB. The participation of macrophages and monocytes in experimental immune complex glomerulonephritis. *Clin Immunol Immunopathol* 1980;15:510–524.
75. Ren K, Brentjens J, Chen Y, et al. Glomerular macrophage proliferation in experimental immune complex nephritis. *Clin Immunol Immunopathol* 1991;60:384–398.

76. Noble B, Ren K, Taverne J. Mononuclear cells in glomeruli and cytokines in urine reflect the severity of experimental proliferative immune complex glomerulonephritis. *Clin Exp Immunol* 1990;80: 281–287.
77. Striker GE, Mannik M, Tung MY. Role of marrow-derived monocytes and mesangial cells in removal of immune complexes from renal glomeruli. *J Exp Med* 1979;149:127–136.
78. Bloom RD, Florquin S, Singer GG, Brennan DC, Rubin Kelley V. Colony stimulating factor-1 in the induction of lupus nephritis. *Kidney Int* 1993;43:1000–1009.
79. Bagchus WM, Jeunink MF, Elema JD. The mesangium in anti–Thy-1 nephritis. Influx of macrophages, mesangial cell hypercellularity and macromolecular accumulation. *Am J Pathol* 1990;137:215–223.
80. Johnson RJ, Lombardi D, Eng E, et al. Modulation of experimental mesangial proliferative nephritis by interferon-τ. *Kidney Int* 1995;47: 62–69.
81. Bannister KM, Ulich TR, Wilson CB. Induction, characterisation, and cell transfer of an autoimmune tubulointerstitial nephritis in the Lewis rat. *Kidney Int* 1987;32:642–651.
82. Hara M, Batsford SR, Mihatsch MJ, Bitter-Suermann D, Vogt A. Complement and monocytes are essential for provoking glomerular injury in passive Heymann's nephritis in rats. *Lab Invest* 1991;65:168–179.
83. Young BA, Johnson RJ, Alpers CE et al. Cellular events in the evolution of experimental diabetic nephropathy. *Kidney Int* 1995;47: 935–944.
84. Diamond JR, Ding G, Frye J, Diamond IP. Glomerular macrophages and the mesangial proliferative response in the experimental nephrotic syndrome. *Am J Pathol* 1992;141:887–894.
85. Eddy AA, Michael AF. Acute tubulointerstitial nephritis associated with aminonucleoside nephrosis. *Kidney Int* 1988;33:14–23.
86. Hattori M, Yamaguchi Y, Kawaguchi H, Ito K. Characteristic glomerular lesions in the ExHC rat: a unique model for lipid-induced glomerular injury. *Nephron* 1993;63:314–322.
87. Pesek-Diamond I, Ding G, Frye J, Diamond JR. Macrophages mediate adverse effects of cholesterol feeding in experimental nephrosis. *Am J Physiol* 1992;263:F776–F783.
88. van Goor H, Fidler V, Weening JJ, Grond J. Determinants of focal and segmental glomerulosclerosis in the rat after renal ablation. Evidence for involvement of macrophages and lipids. *Lab Invest* 1991; 64:754–765.
89. Giachelli CM, Pichler R, Lombardi D, et al. Osteopontin expression in angiotensin II–induced tubulointerstitial nephritis. *Kidney Int* 1994;45:515–524.
90. Mai M, Geiger H, Hilgers KF. Early interstitial changes in hypertension-induced renal injury. *Hypertension* 1993;22:754–765.
91. Truong LD, Farhood A, Tasby J, Gillum D. Experimental chronic renal ischemia: morphologic and immunologic studies. *Kidney Int* 1992;41:1676–1689.
92. Diamond JR, Ding G, Frye J, Diamond IP. Glomerular macrophages and the mesangial proliferative response in the experimental nephrotic syndrome. *Am J Pathol* 1992;141:887–894.
93. Matsumoto K, Atkins RC. Glomerular cells and macrophages in the progression of experimental focal glomerulosclerosis. *Am J Pathol* 1989;134:933–945.
94. Floege J, Burns MW, Alpers CE, et al. Glomerular cell proliferation and PDGF expression precede glomerulosclerosis in the remnant kidney model. *Kidney Int* 1992;41:297–309.
95. Boyce NW, Holdsworth SR: Macrophage–Fc-receptor affinity: role in cellular mediation of antibody initiated glomerulonephritis. *Kidney Int* 1989;36:537–544.
96. Holdsworth SR, Neale TJ, Wilson CB. Abrogation of macrophage-dependent injury in experimental glomerulonephritis in the rabbit. *J Clin Invest* 1981;68:686–698.
97. David JR. Delayed hypersensitivity in vitro: its mediation by cell-free substances formed by lymphoid cell–antigen interaction. *Proc Natl Acad Sci U S A* 1966;56:72.
98. Cohen S, Pick E, Oppenheim JJ. *Biology of the lymphokines.* New York: Academic; 1979.
99. Boyce NW, Tipping PG, Holdsworth SR. Lymphokine (MIF) production by glomerular T-lymphocytes in experimental glomerulonephritis. *Kidney Int* 1986;30:673–677.
100. Rollins BJ, Pober JS. Interleukin-4 induces the synthesis and secretion of MCP-1/JE by human endothelial cells. *Am J Pathol* 1991;138: 1315–1319.
101. Zoja C, Wang JM, Bettoni S, et al. Interleukin-1 beta and tumor necrosis factor-alpha induce gene expression and production of leukocyte chemotactic factors, colony-stimulating factors, and interleukin-6 in human mesangial cells. *Am J Pathol* 1991;138:991–1003.
102. Satriano JA, Shuldiner M, Hora K, Xing Y, Shan Z, Schlondorff D. Oxygen radicals as second messengers for expression of the monocyte chemoattractant protein, JE/MCP-1, and the monocyte colony-stimulating factor, CSF-1, in response to tumor necrosis factor-alpha and immunoglobulin G. Evidence for involvement of reduced nicotinamide adenine dinucleotide phosphate (NADPH)-dependent oxidase. *J Clin Invest* 1993;92:1564–1571.
103. Rovin BH, Rumancik M, Tan L, Dickerson J. Glomerular expression of monocyte chemoattractant peptide-1 in experimental and human glomerulonephritis. *Lab Invest* 1994;71:536–542.
104. Stahl RAK, Thaiss F, Disser M, Helmchen U, Hora K, Schlondorff D. Increased expression of monocyte chemoattractant peptide-1 in anti-thymocyte antibody–induced glomerulonephritis. *Kidney Int* 1993; 44:1036–1047.
105. Assoian RK, Komoriya A, Meyers CA, Miller DM, Sporn MB. Transforming growth factor-beta in human platelets. Identification of a major storage site, purification, and characterization. *J Biol Chem* 1983;258:7155–7160.
106. Kagami S, Border WA, Miller DE, Noble NA. Angiotensin II stimulates extracellular matrix protein synthesis through induction of transforming growth factor-beta expression in rat glomerular mesangial cells. *J Clin Invest* 1994;93:2431–2437.
107. Baccarini M, Stanley ER. Colony stimulating factor-1. In: Habenicht A, ed. *Growth factors, differentiation factors, and cytokines.* Berlin: Springer-Verlag; 1990:188–199.
108. Foreman KE, Vaporciyan AA, Bonish BK, et al. C5a-induced expression of P-selectin in endothelial cells. *J Clin Invest* 1994;94:1147–1155.
109. Diamond JR, Kees-Folts D, Ding G, Frye JE, Restrepo NC. Macrophages, monocyte chemoattractant peptide-1, and TGF-beta 1 in experimental hydronephrosis. *Am J Physiol* 1994;266:F926–F933.
110. Kees-Folts D, Sadow JL, Schreiner GF. Tubular catabolism of albumin is associated with the release of an inflammatory lipid. *Kidney Int* 1994;45:1697–1709.
111. Rovin BH, Lefkowith JB, Schreiner GF. Mechanisms underlying the antiinflammatory effects of essential fatty acid deficiency in experimental glomerulonephritis: inhibited release of a monocyte chemoattractant by glomeruli. *J Immunol* 1990;145:1238–1245.
112. Diamond JR, Pesek I, Ruggieri S, Karnovsky MJ. Essential fatty acid deficiency during acute puromycin nephrosis ameliorates late renal injury. *Am J Physiol* 1989;257:F798–F807.
113. Pichler R, Giachelli CM, Lombardi D, et al. Tubulointerstitial disease in glomerulonephritis. Potential role of osteopontin (uropontin). *Am J Pathol* 1994;144:915–926.
114. Giachelli CM, Pichler R, Lombardi D. Osteopontin expression in angiotensin II–induced tubulointerstitial nephritis. *Kidney Int* 1994; 45:515–524.
115. Nikolic-Paterson DJ, Main IW, Lan HY, Hill PA, Atkins RC. Adhesion molecules in glomerulonephritis. *Springer Semin Immunopathol* 1994;16:3–22.
116. Bruijn JA, Dinklo NJCM. Distinct patterns of expression of intercellular adhesion molecule-1, vascular adhesion molecule-1, and endothelial-leukocyte adhesion molecule-1 in renal disease. *Lab Invest* 1993;69:329–335.
117. Chow J, Hartley RB, Jagger C, Dilly SA. ICAM-1 expression in renal disease. *J Clin Pathol* 1992;45:880–884.
118. Dal Canton A, Fuiano G, Sepe V, Caglioti A, Ferrone S. Mesangial expression of intercellular adhesion molecule-1 in primary glomerulosclerosis. *Kidney Int* 1992;41:951–995.
119. Lhotta K, Neumayer HP, Joannidis M, Geissler D, Konig P. Renal expression of intercellular adhesion molecule-1 in different forms of glomerulonephritis. *Clin Sci* 1991;81:477–481.
120. Muller GA, Markovski-Lipkovski J, Muller CA. Intercellular adhesion molecule-1 expression in human kidneys with glomerulonephritis. *Clin Nephrol* 1991; 36:203–208.
121. Seron D, Cameron JS, Haskard DO. Expression of VCAM-1 in the normal and diseased kidney. *Nephrol Dial Transplant* 1991;6:917–922.
122. Hill PA, Lan HY, Nikolic-Paterson DJ, Atkins RC. The ICAM-1/LFA-1 interaction in glomerular leukocyte accumulation in anti-GBM glomerulonephritis. *Kidney Int* 1994;45:700–708.

123. Hill PA, Lan HY, Nikolic-Paterson DJ, Atkins RC. ICAM-1 directs migration and localisation of interstitial leukocyte infiltration in experimental glomerulonephritis. *Kidney Int* 1994;45:32–42.
124. Hattori M, Nikolic-Paterson DJ, Lan HY, Kawaguchi H, Ito K, Atkins RC. Up-regulation of ICAM-1 and VCAM-1 expression during macrophage recruitment in lipid-induced glomerular injury in ExHC rats. *Nephrology* 1995;1:221–232.
125. Wuthrich RP. Vascular cell adhesion molecule-1 (VCAM-1) expression in murine lupus nephritis. *Kidney Int* 1992;42:903–914.
126. Morris GF, Mathews, MB. Regulation of proliferating cell nuclear antigen during the cell cycle. *J Biol Chem* 1989;264:13856–13864.
127. Lan HY, Nikolic-Paterson DJ, Mu W, Atkins RC. Local macrophage proliferation in the progression of glomerular and tubulointerstitial injury in rat anti-GBM glomerulonephritis. *Kidney Int* 1995;48:753–760.
128. Lan HY, Nikolic-Paterson DJ, Mu W, Atkins RC. Local macrophage proliferation in multinucleated giant cell and granuloma formation in experimental Goodpasture's syndrome. *Am J Pathol* 1995;147:1214–1220.
129. Johnson RJ, Garcia RL, Pritzl P, Alpers CE. Platelets mediate glomerular cell proliferation in immune complex nephritis induced by anti-mesangial cell antibodies in the rat. *Am J Pathol* 1990;136:369–374.
130. Iida H, Seifert R, Alpers CE, et al. Platelet-derived growth factor (PDGF) and PDGF receptor are induced in mesangial proliferative nephritis in the rat. *Proc Natl Acad Sci U S A* 1991;88:6560–6564.
131. Alpers CE, Hudkins KL, Gown AM, Johnson RJ. Enhanced expression of "muscle-specific" actin in glomerulonephritis. *Kidney Int* 1992;41:1134–1142.
132. Lan HY, Nikolic-Paterson DJ, Atkins RC. Trafficking of inflammatory macrophages to the draining kidney lymph node during experimental glomerulonephritis. *Clin Exp Immunol* 1993;92:336–341.
133. Holdsworth SR, Neale TJ, Wilson CB. Abrogation of macrophage-dependent injury in experimental glomerulonephritis in the rabbit. *J Clin Invest* 1981;68:686–698.
134. Matsumoto K, Hatano M. Effect of antimacrophage serum on the proliferation of glomerular cells in nephrotoxic serum nephritis in the rat. *J Clin Lab Immunol* 1989;28:39–44.
135. Holdsworth SR, Neale TJ. Macrophage induced glomerular injury: cell transfer studies in passive autologous antiglomerular basement membrane antibody–initiated experimental glomerulonephritis. *Lab Invest* 1984;51:172–80.
136. Boyce NW, Tipping PG, Holdsworth SR. Glomerular macrophages produce reactive oxygen species in experimental glomerulonephritis. *Kidney Int* 1989;35:778–782.
137. Dileepan KN, Sharma R, Stechschulte DJ, Savin VJ. Effect of superoxide exposure on albumin permeability of isolated rat glomeruli. *J Lab Clin Invest* 1993;121:797–804.
138. Radeke HH, Meier B, Topley N, Floge J, Habermehl GG, Resch K. Interleukin 1-α and tumor necrosis factor-α induce oxygen radical production in mesangial cells. *Kidney Int* 1990;37:767–775.
139. Pfeilschifter J, Schwarzenbach H. Interleukin 1 and tumor necrosis factor stimulate cGMP formation in rat renal mesangial cells. *FEBS Lett* 1990;273:185–187.
140. Rzymkiewicz DM, DuMaine J, Morrison AR. IL-1β regulates rat mesangial cycooxygenase II gene expression by tyrosine phosphorylation. *Kidney Int* 1995;47:1354–1363.
141. Bussolino F, Arese M, Silvestro L. Camussi G. Involvement of a serine protease in the synthesis of platelet-activating factor by endothelial cells stimulated by tumor necrosis factor-alpha or interleukin-1 alpha. *Eur J Immunol* 1994;24:3131–3139.
142. Badr KF. Five-lipoxygenase products in glomerular immune injury. *J Am Soc Nephrol* 1992;3:907–915.
143. Spaethe SM, Freed MS, De Schryver-Kecskemeti K, Lefkowith JB, Needleman P. Essential fatty acid deficiency reduces the inflammatory cell invasion in rabbit hydronephrosis resulting in suppression of the exaggerated eicosanoid production. *J Pharmacol Exp Ther* 1988;245:1088–1094.
144. Katoh T, Lianos EA, Fukunaga M, Takahasi K, Badr KF. Leukotriene D4 is a mediator of proteinuria and glomerular hemodynamic abnormalities in passive Heymann nephritis. *J Clin Invest* 1993;91:1507–1515.
145. Schreiner GF, Rovin B, Lefkowith JB. The antiinflammatory effects of essential fatty acid deficiency in experimental glomerulonephritis. *J Immunol* 1989;143:3192–3199.
146. Lefkowith JB, Schreiner GF. Essential fatty acid deficiency depletes rat glomeruli of resident macrophages and inhibits antiotensin II–induced eicosanoid synthesis. *J Clin Invest* 1987;80:947–956.
147. Atkins RC, Glasgow EF, Holdsworth SR, et al. Tissue culture of isolated glomeruli from patients with glomerulonephritis. *Kidney Int* 1980;17:515–527.
148. Magil AB, Wadsworth LD. Monocyte involvement in glomerular crescents. A histochemical and ultrastructural study. *Lab Invest* 1982;47:160–166.
149. Hancock WW, Atkins RC. Cellular composition of crescents in human rapidly progressive glomerulonephritis identified using monoclonal antibodies. *Am J Pathol* 1984;4:177–181.
150. Thomson NM, Simpson IJ, Evans DJ, Peters DK. Defibrination with Ancrod in experimental immune complex nephritis. *Clin Exp Immunol* 1975;20:527.
151. Neale TJ, Carson SD, Tipping PG, et al. Participation of cell-mediated immunity in deposition of fibrin in glomerulonephritis. *Lancet* 1988;2:421–424.
152. Hancock W, Atkins RC. Activation of coagulation pathways and fibrin deposition in human glomerulonephritis. *Semin Nephrol* 1985;5:69–77.
153. Tipping PG, Lowe MG, Holdsworth SR. Glomerular macrophages express augmented procoagulant activity in experimental fibrin-related glomerulonephritis in rabbits. *J Clin Invest* 1988;82:1253–1259.
154. Holdsworth SR, Tipping PG. Macrophage-induced glomerular fibrin deposition in the rabbit. *J Clin Invest* 1985;76:1367–1374.
155. Nishikawa K, Andres G, Bhan AK. Hyaluronate is a component of crescents in rat autoimmune glomerulonephritis. *Lab Invest* 1993;68:146–153.
156. Zhao J, Lan HY, Atkins RC, Nikolic-Paterson DJ. CD44 expression in rat anti-GBM glomerulonephritis [Abstract]. *Kidney Int* (in press).
157. Lan HY, Nikolic-Paterson DJ, Zarama M, Vannice JL, Atkins RC. Suppression of experimental glomerulonephritis by the IL-1 receptor antagonist. *Kidney Int* 1993;43:479–485.
158. Lan HY, Nikolic-Paterson DJ, Mu W, Vannice JL, Atkins RC. Interleukin-1 receptor antagonist halts the progression of established rat crescentic glomerulonephritis in the rat. *Kidney Int* 1995;47:1303–1309.
159. Nikolic-Paterson DJ, Lan HY, Hill PA, Vannice JL, Atkins RC. Suppression of experimental glomerulonephritis by the interleukin-1 receptor antagonist: inhibition of intercellular adhesion molecule-1 expression. *J Am Soc Nephrol* 1994;4:1695–1700.
160. Lan HY, Nikolic-Paterson DJ, Atkins RC. Involvement of activated periglomerular leucocytes in the rupture of Bowman's capsule and crescent progression in experimental glomerulonephritis. *Lab Invest* 1992;67:743–751.
161. Lan HY, Nikolic-Paterson DJ, Mu W, Atkins RC. Local macrophage proliferation in progressive renal injury. In: *Proceedings of international symposium on progression of chronic renal diseases.* Basel, Switzerland: Karger AG; 1996;118:100–108.
162. Silva FG, Hoyer JR, Pirani CL. Sequential studies of glomerular crescent formation in rats with antiglomerular basement membrane–induced glomerulonephritis and the role of coagulation factors. *Lab Invest* 1984;51:404–415.
163. Striker LMM, Killen PD, Chi E, Striker GE. The composition of glomerulosclerosis. I. Studies in focal sclerosis, crescentic glomerulonephritis, and membranoproliferative glomerulonephritis. *Lab Invest* 1984;51:181–192.
164. Boucher A, Droz D, Adafer E, Noel LH. Relationship between the integrity of Bowman's capsule and the composition of cellular crescents in human crescentic glomerulonephritis. *Lab Invest* 1987;56:526–533.
165. Eng E, Fleoge J, Young BA, Couser WG, Johnson RJ. Does extracellular matrix expansion in glomerular disease require mesangial cell proliferation? *Kidney Int* 1994;45(Suppl)45:S45–S47.
166. Fogo A, Hawkins EP, Berry P, et al. Glomerular hypertrophy in minimal change disease predicts subsequent progression to focal glomerular sclerosis. *Kidney Int* 1990;38:115–123.
167. Saito T, Ootaka T, Sato H. Participation of macrophages in segmental endocapillary proliferation preceding focal glomerular sclerosis. *J Pathol* 1993;170:179–185.
168. Doi T, Striker LJ, Quaife C, et al. Progressive glomerulosclerosis develops in transgenic mice chronically expressing growth hormone

and growth hormone releasing factor but not in those expressing insulinlike growth factor-1. *Am J Pathol* 1988;131:398–403.
169. Floege J, Alpers CE, Burns MW, et al. Glomerular cells, extracellular matrix accumulation, and the development of glomerulosclerosis in the remnant kidney model. *Lab Invest* 1992;66:485–497.
170. Johnson RJ, Pritzl P, Lida H, Alpers CE. Platelet–complement interactions in mesangial proliferative nephritis in the rat. *Am J Pathol* 1991;138:313–321.
171. Nikolic-Paterson DJ, Tesch GH, Lan HY, Foti R, Atkins RC. Deoxyspergualin inhibits mesangial cell proliferation and MHC class II expression. *J Am Soc Nephrol* 1995;5:1895–1902.
172. Furuta T, Saito T, Ootaka T. The role of macrophages in diabetic glomerulosclerosis. *Am J Kidney Dis* 1993;21:480–485.
173. van Goor H, van der Horst ML, Fidler V, Grond J. Glomerular macrophage modulation affects mesangial expansion in the rat after renal ablation. *Lab Invest* 1992;66:5645–5671.
174. Diamond JR, Pesek-Diamond I. Sublethal X-irradiation during acute puromycin nephrosis prevents late renal injury: role of macrophages. *Am J Physiol* 1991;260:F779–F786.
175. Kasai S. Effects of glomerular macrophages on mesangial cells in rat serum sickness glomerulonephritis: a comparison of histological and co-culture studies. *Pathol Int* 1994;44:107–114.
176. Johnson RJ, Raines EW, Floege J, et al. Inhibition of mesangial cell proliferation and matrix expansion in glomerulosclerosis in the rat by antibody to platelet-derived growth factor. *J Exp Med* 1992;175: 1413–1416.
177. Matsumoto K, Dowling J, Atkins RC. Production of interleukin-1 in glomerular cell cultures from patients with rapidly progressive crescentic glomerulonephritis. *Am J Nephrol* 1988;8:463–470.
178. Noronha IL, Kruger C, Andrassy K, Ritz E, Waldherr R. In situ production of TNF-α, IL-1β and IL-2R in ANCA-positive glomerulonephritis. *Kidney Int* 1993;43:682–692.
179. Yoshioka K, Takemura T, Murakami K. In situ expression of cytokines in IgA nephritis. *Kidney Int* 1993;44:825–833.
180. Tesch G, Nikolic-Paterson DJ, Main IW, Lan HY, Atkins RC. The role of interleukin-1 in mesangial proliferation. *Contrib Nephrol* 1995;111:144–148.
181. Takemura T, Yoshioka K, Murakami K, et al. Cellular localization of inflammatory cytokines in human glomerulonephritis. *Virchows Arch* 1994;424:459–464.
182. Boswell JM, Yui MA, Burt DW, Kelley VE. Increased tumor necrosis factor and IL-1β gene expression in the kidneys of mice with lupus nephritis. *J Immunol* 1988;141:3050–3054.
183. Matsumoto K. Production of interleukin-1 by glomerular macrophages in nephrotoxic serum nephritis. *Am J Nephrol* 1990;10:502–506.
184. Diamond JR, Pesek I. Glomerular tumor necrosis factor and interleukin 1 production during acute aminonucleoside nephrosis. *Lab Invest* 1991;64:21–28.
185. Tipping PG, Lowe MG, Holdsworth SR. Glomerular interleukin-1 production is dependent on macrophage infiltration in anti-GBM glomerulonephritis. *Kidney Int* 1991;39:103–110.
186. Lovett DH, Ryan JL, Sterzel B. Stimulation of rat mesangial cell proliferation by macrophage interleukin-1. *J Immunol* 1983;131: 2830–2836.
187. Kakizaki Y, Kraft N, Atkins RC. Differential control of mesangial cell proliferation by interferon gamma. *Clin Exp Immunol* 1991;85: 157–163.
188. Torbohm I, Berger B, Schonermark M, von Kempis J, Rother K, Hansch GM. Modulation of collagen synthesis in human glomerular epithelial cells by interleukin-1. *Clin Exp Immunol* 1989;75:427–431.
189. Horii Y, Muraguchi A, Iwano M, et al. Involvement of IL-6 in mesangial proliferative glomerulonephritis. *J Immunol* 1989;143: 3949–3955.
190. Gesualdo L, Pinzani M, Floriano JJ, et al. Platelet–derived growth factor expression in mesangial proliferative glomerulonephritis. *Lab Invest* 1991;65:160–167.
191. Floege J, Eng E, Young BA. Infusion of platelet-derived growth factor or basic fibroblast growth factor induces selective glomerular mesangial cell proliferation and matrix accumulation in rats. *J Clin Invest* 1993;92:2952–2962.
192. Isaka Y, Fujiwara Y, Ueda N, Kaneda Y, Kamada T, Imai E. Glomerulosclerosis induced by in vivo transfection of transforming growth factor-α or platelet-derived growth factor gene into the rat kidney. *J Clin Invest* 1993;92:2597–2601.
193. Barnes JL, Hastings RR, De La Garza M. Sequential expression of cellular fibronectin by platelets, macrophages, and mesangial cells in proliferative glomerulonephritis. *Am J Pathol* 1994;145:585–597.
194. Mosquera JA. Increase production of fibronectin by glomerular cultures from rats with nephrotoxic nephritis. *Lab Invest* 1993;68: 406–412.
195. Border WA, Okuda S, Languino LR, et al. Suppression of experimental glomerulonephritis by antiserum against transforming growth factor β1. *Nature* 1990;346:371–374.
196. Yamamoto T, Nakamura T, Noble NA, Ruoslahti E, Border WA. Expression of transforming growth factor beta is elevated in human and experimental diabetic nephropathy. *Proc Natl Acad Sci U S A* 1993;90:1814–1818.
197. Border WA, Noble NA. Transforming growth factor beta in tissue fibrosis. *N Engl J Med* 1994;331:1286–1292.
198. Kees-Folts D, Diamond JR. Relationship between hyperlipidemia, lipid mediators, and progressive glomerulosclerosis in the nephrotic syndrome. *Am J Nephrol* 1993;13:365–375.
199. Hattori M, Ito K, Kawaguchi H, Yamaguchi Y. Probucol reduces renal injury in the ExHC rat. *Nephron* 1994;67:459–468.
200. Magil AB, Frohlich JJ. Monocytes and macrophages in focal glomerulosclerosis in Zucker rats. *Nephron* 1991;59:131–138.
201. Risdon RA, Sloper JC, DeWardner HE. Relationship between renal function and histological changes found in renal biopsy specimens from patients with persistent glomerulonephritis. *Lancet* 1968;2: 363–366.
202. Bohle A, Christ H, Grund KE, Mackensen S. The role of the interstitium of the renal cortex in renal disease. *Contrib Nephrol* 1979;16: 109–114.
203. Mackensen-Haen S, Bader R, Grund KE, Bohle A. Correlations between renal cortical interstitial fibrosis, atrophy of the proximal tubules and impairment of the glomerular filtration rate. *Clin Nephrol* 1981;15:167–171.
204. Abe S, Amagasaki Y, Iyori S, Konishi K, Kato E, Sakaguchi H. Significance of tubulointerstitial lesions in biopsy specimens of glomerulonephritic patients. *Am J Nephrol* 1989;9:30–37.
205. Bogenschutz O, Bohle A, Batz C, et al. IgA nephritis: on the importance of morphological and clinical parameters in the long-term prognosis of 239 patients. *Am J Nephrol* 1990;10:137–147.
206. Wehrmann M, Bohle A, Held H, Schumm G, Kendziorra H, Pressler H. Long-term prognosis of focal sclerosing glomerulonephritis. An analysis of 250 cases with particular regard to tubulointerstitial changes. *Clin Nephrol* 1990;33:115–122.
207. Bohle A, Mackensen-Haen S, von Gise H, et al. The consequences of tubulo-interstitial changes for renal function in glomerulopathies. A morphometric and cytological analysis. *Pathol Res Pract* 1990;186: 135–144.
208. Ong AC, Fine LG. Loss of glomerular function and tubulointerstitial fibrosis: cause or effect? *Kidney Int* 1994;45:345–351.
209. Atkins RC. Pathogenesis of glomerulonephritis 1990. In: Hatano M, ed. *Nephrology*. New York: Springer-Verlag; 1991:4–17.
210. Bohle A, Wehrmann M, Mackensen-Haen S, et al. Pathogenesis of chronic renal failure in primary glomerulopathies. *Nephrol Dial Transplant* 1994;9(Suppl 3):4–12.
211. Saito T, Atkins RC. Interstitial activated (IL–2R+) mononuclear cells and Ia antigens in experimental focal glomerulosclerosis. *Pathology* 1994;26:403–406.
212. Harris KP, Schreiner GF, Klahr S. Effect of leukocyte depletion on the function of the postobstructed kidney in the rat. *Kidney Int* 1989; 36:210–215.
213. Harris KP, Lefkowith JB, Klahr S, Schreiner GF. Essential fatty acid deficiency ameliorates acute renal dysfunction in the rat after the administration of the aminonucleoside of puromycin. *J Clin Invest* 1990;86:1115–1123.
214. Jansen A, Cook T, Taylor GM. Induction of nitric oxide synthase in rat immune complex glomerulonephritis. *Kidney Int* 1994;45: 1215–1219.
215. Shapiro SD, Campbell EJ, Senior RM, Welgus HG. Proteinases secreted by human mononuclear phagocytes. *J Rheumatol* 1991; 27(Suppl):95–98.
216. Welgus HG, Campbell EJ, Cury JD, et al. Neutral metalloproteinases produced by human mononuclear phagocytes. Enzyme profile, regulation, and expression during cellular development. *J Clin Invest* 1990;86:1496–1502.

217. Cohen RL, Xi XP, Crowley CW, Lucas BK, Levinson AD, Shuman MA. Effects of urokinase receptor occupancy on plasmin generation and proteolysis of basement membrane by human tumor cells. *Blood* 1991;78:479–487.
218. Gijbels K, Galardy RE, Steinman L. Reversal of experimental autoimmune encephalomyelitis with a hydroxamate inhibitor of matrix metalloproteinases. *J Exp Med* 1994;94:2177–2182.
219. Kovacs EJ, DiPietro LA. Fibrogenic cytokines and connective tissue production *FASEB J* 1994;8:854–861.
220. Schmidt JA, Mizel AB, Cohen D, Green I. Interleukin-1, a potential regulator of fibroblast proliferation. *J Immunol* 1982;128:2177–2181.
221. Lonnemann G, Shapiro L, Engler-Blum G, Muller GA, Koch KM, Dinarello CD. Cytokines in human renal interstitial fibrosis. I. Interleukin-1 is a paracrine growth factor for cultures fibrosis–derived kidney fibroblasts. *Kidney Int* 1995;47:837–844.
222. Postlethwaite AE, Raghow R, Stricklin GP, Poppleton H, Seyer JM, Kang AH. Modulation of fibroblast functions by interleukin-1: increased steady-state accumulation of type I procollagen messenger RNAs and stimulation of other functions but not chemotaxis by human recombinant interleukin 1α and β. *J Cell Biol* 1988;106:311–318.
223. Bathon JM, Hwang JJ, Shin LH, Precht PA, Towns MC, Horton WE Jr. Type VI collagen–specific messenger RNA is expressed constitutively by cultured human synovial fibroblasts and is suppressed by interleukin-1. *Arthritis Rheum* 1994;37:1350–1356.
224. Piguet PF, Vesin C, Grau GE, Thompson RC. Interleukin 1 receptor antagonist (IL-1ra) prevents or cures pulmonary fibrosis elicited in mice by bleomycin or silica. *Cytokine* 1993;5:57–61.
225. Henke C, Marinelli W, Jessurun J, et al. Macrophage production of basic fibroblast growth factor in the fibroproliferative disorder of alveolar fibrosis after lung injury. *Am J Pathol* 1993;143:1189–1199.
226. Wangoo A, Taylor IK, Haynes AR, Shaw RJ. Up-regulation of alveolar macrophage platelet–derived growth factor-β (PDGF-β) mRNA by interferon-gamma from *Mycobacterium tuberculosis* antigen (PPD)-stimulated lymphocytes. *Clin Exp Immunol* 1993;94:43–50.
227. Sakai H, Naka R, Suzuki D. In situ hybridization analysis of TGFβ in glomeruli from patients with IgA nephropathy. *Contrib Nephrol* 1995;111:107–115.
228. Lianos EA, Orphanos V, Cattell V, Cook T, Anagnou N. Glomerular expression and cell origin of transforming growth factor-beta 1 in anti-glomerular basement membrane disease. *Am J Med Sci* 1994; 307:1–5.
229. Tamaki K, Okuda S, Ando T, Iwamoto T, Nakayama M, Fujishima M. TGF-β1 in glomerulosclerosis and interstitial fibrosis of adriamycin nephropathy. *Kidney Int* 1994;45:525–536.
230. Ding G, Pesek-Diamond I, Diamond JR. Cholesterol, macrophages, and gene expression of TGF-beta 1 and fibronectin during nephrosis. *Am J Physiol* 1993;264:F577–F584.
231. Eddy AA. Protein restriction reduces transforming growth factor-beta and interstitial fibrosis in nephrotic syndrome. *Am J Physiol* 1994; 266:F884–F893.
232. Eddy AA, Giachelli CM. Renal expression of genes that promote interstitial inflammation and fibrosis in rats with protein-overload proteinuria. *Kidney Int* 1995;47:1546–1557.
233. Falcone DJ, McCaffrey TA, Haimovitz-Friedman A, Vergilio JA, Nicholson AC. Macrophage and foam cell release of matrix-bound growth factors. Role of plasminogen activation. *J Biol Chem* 1993; 268:11951–11958.
234. Holdsworth SR, Bellomo R. Differential effects of steroids on leukocyte-mediated glomerulonephritis in the rabbit. *Kidney Int* 1984;26: 162–169.
235. Lan HY, Zarama M, Nikolic-Paterson DJ, Kerr PG, Atkins RC. Suppression of experimental crescentic glomerulonephritis by deoxyspergualin. *J Am Soc Nephrol* 1993;3:1765–1774.
236. Tepper MA. Deoxyspergualin: mechanism of action studies of a novel immunosuppressive drug. *Ann NY Acad Sci* 1993;696:123–132.
237. Okubo M, Tamura K, Kamata K, et al. 15-Deoxyspergualin "rescue therapy" for methylprednisolone-resistant rejection of renal transplants as compared with anti–T cell monoclonal antibody (OKT3). *Transplantation* 1993;55:505–508.
238. Takahashi K, Tanabe K, Ooba S, et al. Prophylactic use of a new immunosuppressive agent, deoxyspergualin, in patients with kidney transplantation from ABO-incompatible or preformed antibody-positive donors. *Transplant Proc* 1991;23:1078–1082.
239. Groth CG, Ohlman S, Ericzon BG, Barkholt L, Reinholt FP. Deoxyspergualin for liver graft rejection. *Lancet* 1990;2:626.
240. Gores PF, Najarian JS, Stephanian E, et al. Insulin independence in type I diabetes after transplantation of unpurified islets from single donor with 15-deoxyspergualin. *Lancet* 1993;341:19–21.
241. Okubo M, Inoue K, Umetani N, et al. Lupus nephropathy in New Zealand F1 hybrid mice treated by (-)15-deoxyspergualin. *Kidney Int* 1988;34:467–473.
242. Okubo M, Umetani N, Inoue K, et al. Reversal of established nephropathy in New Zealand B/W F1 mice by 15-deoxyspergualin. *Nephron* 1991;57:99–105.
243. Lan HY, Nikolic-Paterson DJ, Zarama M, Kerr PG, Atkins RC. Suppression of pulmonary injury in experimental "Goodpasture's syndrome" by deoxyspergualin (DSP). *Clin Exp Immunol* 1994;95: 502–508.
244. Nikolic-Paterson DJ, Kerr PG, Lan HY, Tesch GH, Atkins RC. Deoxyspergualin: a new immunosuppressive drug for the treatment of autoimmune disease. *Nephron* 1995;70:391–396.
245. Schorlemmer HU, Neubauer HP, Czech J, Dickneite G. Immunosuppressive therapy of organ-specific nephritic autoimmune diseases with 15-deoxyspergualin. *Agents Actions* 1993;39:C121–C124.
246. Dinarello CA, Wolff SM. The role of interleukin-1 in disease. *N Engl J Med* 1993;328:106–113.
247. Faherty DA, Claudy V, Plocinski JM, Kaffka K, Kilian P, Thompson RC. Failure of IL-1 receptor antagonism to inhibit antigen-specific immune responses in vivo. *J Immunol* 1992;148:766–771.
248. Mulligan MS, Johnson KJ, Todd RF 3d, et al. Requirements for leukocyte adhesion molecules in nephrotoxic nephritis. *J Clin Invest* 1993;91:577–587.
249. Tang WW, Feng L, Vannice JL, Wilson CB. Interleukin-1 receptor antagonist ameliorates experimental anti-glomerular basement membrane antibody-associated glomerulonephritis. *J Clin Invest* 1994;93: 273–279.
250. Bandara G, Mueller GM, Galea-Lauri J, et al. Intraarticular expression of biologically active interleukin-1-receptor-antagonist protein by ex vivo gene transfer. *Proc Natl Acad Sci U S A* 1993;90:10764–10768.
251. Bosch RJ, Woolf AS, Fine LG. Gene transfer into the mammalian kidney: direct retrovirus-transduction of regenerating tubular epithelial cells. *Exp Nephrol* 1993;1:49–54.
252. Kitamura M, Taylor S, Unwin R, Burton S, Shimizu F, Fine LG. Gene transfer into the rat renal glomerulus via a mesangial cell vector: site-specific delivery, in situ amplification, and sustained expression of an exogenous gene in vivo. *J Clin Invest* 1994;94:497–505.
253. Lien HY, Lai L, Moeckel GW, Xu H, Martin D, Erickson RP. Liposome-mediated gene transfer targeted to the kindey in mice: comparison among intra-renal-arterial (IA), retrograde intrapelvic (IP), and intra-renal-parenchymal (IK) injections [abstract]. *J Am Soc Nephrol* 1994;5:629.
254. Yokoyama H, Naito T, Dranoff G, Mulligan R, Rubin-Kelley V. Gene transfer system establishing constitutive stable, sustained cytokine delivery into the kidney and circulation [Abstract]. *J Am Soc Nephrol* 1994;5:774.

PART IV

Response to Immune Injury

Immunologic Renal Diseases,
edited by E. G. Neilson and W. G. Couser.
Lippincott-Raven Publishers, Philadelphia © 1997.

CHAPTER 29

Glomerular Mesangial Cells

R. Bernd Sterzel and Harald D. Rupprecht

BASIC BIOLOGY OF MESANGIAL CELLS

1. Introduction

History

For long, it was assumed that the capillary tuft of the mammalian glomerulus contained only two cell types, the visceral epithelial and the endothelial cells. In 1929 and 1933, Zimmermann's classic papers were published, demonstrating that the centrolobular or axial space of the glomerulus differed from the endothelial and epithelial cell layers (1,2). This inter- or pericapillary region, harboring a "third cell" type, was termed *mesangium* (2), a structural entity consisting of both cells and extracellular matrix. In 1930, von Möllendorf described this region as the connective tissue of the glomerulus (3). These views were shared by MacCallum, who noticed that, in glomerular diseases, extracellular material was laid down at an intercapillary rather than intracapillary location (4). In 1936, the description by Kimmelstiel and Wilson of nodular alterations of glomerular lobules in diabetic patients further supported the idea of the existence of the intercapillary mesangium (5). In the early 1960s, the ultrastructural aspects of the rat mesangium, including mesangial uptake and trafficking of macromolecular marker substances, were described in beautiful detail by Latta and colleagues (6,7) and Farquhar and Palade (8) and, more recently, by Kriz and coworkers (9,10).

In view of the complex biology and the prominent involvement of the mesangium in the pathogenesis of most glomerular diseases, it is important to understand the mechanisms that control the behavior and function of mesangial cells (MCs) and the composition, turnover, as well as function of the surrounding extracellular matrix (ECM) under both, physiologic and abnormal conditions. Several reviews on the mesangium have been published over the last 15 years (6,11–15).

R. B. Sterzel and H. D. Rupprecht: Medizinische Klinik IV—University of Erlangen-Nürnberg, 91054, Erlangen, Germany.

Ontogeny and Nomenclature of Mesangial Cells

Studies of the embryonic development of the kidney by Yamanaka (16) and by Sorokin and Ekblom (17) have confirmed that, at the initiation of nephrogenesis, the glomerular capillary extends into the S-shaped body from the surrounding vascular system. MCs are thought to be derived from the vascular cell lineage accompanying the endothelial cells and appear to be continuous to the capillary pericyte–smooth muscle cell system during the glomerular development. MCs participate in the subdivision of the capillary network during glomerulogenesis. It has also been reported that glomerular endothelial and mesangial cells could be derived from the nephrogenic mesenchyme (18). The recruitment of MCs to the glomerulus and the development of the mesangium depend on the presence and intact function of the platelet-derived growth factor (PDGF) B/PDGF-β receptor system, as recently shown in studies of glomerulogenesis in mutant mouse embryos deficient for either the ligand (19) or the receptor (20) (see below). These reports also revealed that glomerular capillary tufts fail to develop properly in the absence of MCs. In addition to the ontogenetic findings, location and morphology of MCs in the mature glomerulus are consistent with the concept that they are specialized pericytes. Accordingly, MCs display several characteristics of vascular smooth muscle cells, including the expression of smooth muscle myosin and the intermediate filament protein, desmin (21). In their normal quiescent state, MCs in vivo are negative for smooth muscle α-actin. However, activated MCs express smooth muscle α-actin and acquire additional phenotypic properties of vascular smooth muscle cells (21) (see section 3). Activated MCs can also develop fibroblastlike features, which are manifested by the production of interstitial collagen types I and III in addition to their normal formation of fibronectin, laminin, and collagen type IV (22). The acquisition of properties of smooth muscle cells and fibroblasts in glomerular disease has led some investigators to use the term *glomerular myofibroblasts* for activated MCs (23).

2. Normal Structure and Function of the Glomerular Mesangium and Mesangial Cells

Morphology

The mesangium, containing MCs and matrix, occupies the central region of a glomerular lobule (Fig. 1 and Table 1). The capillary endothelium is in direct contact with the mesangium because the glomerular basement membrane (GBM) is not developed at the endothelium–mesangium interface. The sites where the GBM deviates from the endothelial tube are called mesangial angles. In the juxtacapillary region, processes of MCs branch toward the mesangial angles and frequently extend some distance into the narrowing space between the endothelium and the GBM (9). Of note, in lower species and during embryonic development of mammals as well as in some disease states (for example, mesangiocapillary or membranoproliferative glomerulonephritis), MCs expand into this space, leading to circumferential interposition of the mesangium (see below). In adult rats, MCs represent about one-third of the total 600–750 cells in a glomerulus (24). The turnover rate of MCs in normal adult rats in vivo is low. An autoradiographic study revealed a constant renewal rate of glomerular cells of ~1% per day. The majority of cycling cells noted in glomerular tufts were endothelial. MCs had a lower renewal rate, and podocytes revealed no evidence of cell

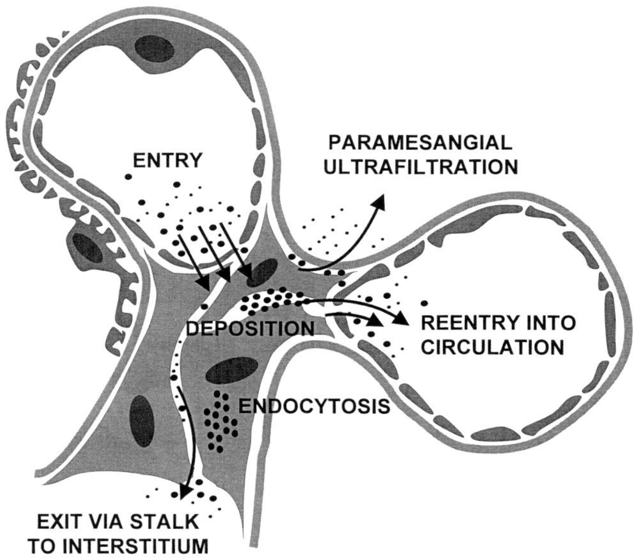

FIG. 1. Trafficking and processing of plasma-derived macromolecules in the mesangium.

TABLE 1. *Functional properties of mesangial cells (MCs)*

1. *Structural support* of glomerular capillary tuft
   - MCs and mesangial matrix as part of the connective tissue tree of the mesangium
   - Production/modeling of mesangial matrix and GBM
2. *Contractility* allowing modulation of glomerular microcirculation and ultrafiltration
   - MCs as target for vasoactive molecules
   - MCs as source of vasoactive molecules
3. *Migration* during embryonic development and reconstitution of damaged glomeruli
4. *Endocytosis/clearing function*
   - Mesangial space provides a coarse filter for plasma constituents
   - Receptor-mediated and fluid-phase uptake of macromolecules from plasma and filtration residues from capillary wall
   - Degradation and removal or trapping and sequestration of filtration residues, antigens, and matrix proteins
5. *Endotheliumlike properties and functions*
   - Subendothelial location on the inner aspect of the GBM
   - Nonthrombogenic surface
   - Nonleukocyte adherent surface
   - Source of vasoactive molecules
6. *Response to local injury*
   - MC proliferation
   - Formation of soluble regulator molecules with autocrine and/or paracrine effects
   - Formation, breakdown, and remodeling of mesangial matrix and GBM
7. *Interaction of activated MCs with immune complexes and immune cells*
   - Binding and uptake of immune complexes via Fc receptors and complement via C3 receptors
   - Upon activation, expression of MHC II molecules
   - Presentation of antigens to T lymphocytes
   - Interaction with leukocytes directly via adhesion molecules (for example, ICAM-1) or indirectly via soluble molecules (for example, cytokines, chemokines, and autacoids)

GBM, glomerular basement membrane; ICAM, intracellular adhesion molecule; MHC, major histocompatibility complex.

replication (25). In glomeruli of normal rats, the mesangium contains two distinct cell types: the vascular smooth muscle cell–like, intrinsic MCs and few bone-marrow-derived, Ia-positive monocyte-macrophages (26). In the mesangium of normal human kidneys, only vascular smooth muscle cell–like, intrinsic MCs but no resident macrophages have been described (27); however, in glomerular disease, inflammatory cells are recruited to the mesangium (see below and section 9).

MCs contain numerous microfilament bundles, predominantly in MC processes. They run mostly transversely from one side of a process to the opposite side. These processes are connected to the GBM, either directly or indirectly through the interposition of extracellular microfibrils, which serve as "microtendons." The GBM, therefore seems to represent the effector structure for MC contractility (see chapter 2).

The mesangial ECM fills spaces between MCs and toward the perimesangial GBM. Small amounts of ECM are also found beneath the endothelium at the endothelium–mesangiium interface. The matrix consists of a dense network of microfibrils that form an extensively interwoven, three-dimensional network. Thus, the mesangial ECM constitutes the centrolobular stroma of the glomerular capillary tuft. In immunocytochemical studies, a variety of ECM components have been localized to the mesangium, including collagen types IV and V, fibronectin, laminin, and nidogen (see also sections 6 and 8). Fibronectin is the most abundant ECM component. It is associated with myofibrils and is thought to link MC surfaces to extracellular structures, including the GBM (28). In addition, MC-derived matrix molecules are thought to be involved in the buildup of the inner layers of the perimesangial GBM, although recent findings in PDGF-deficient mouse embryos, lacking the mesangium but showing normal perimesangial GBM, cast some doubt on this concept (19). Functional aspects of the ECM are addressed in section 8.

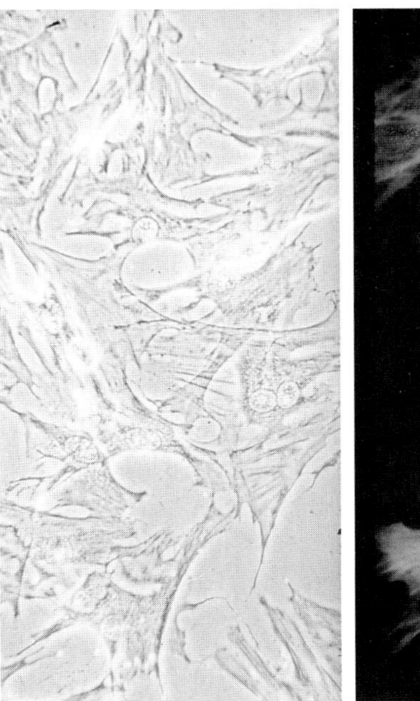
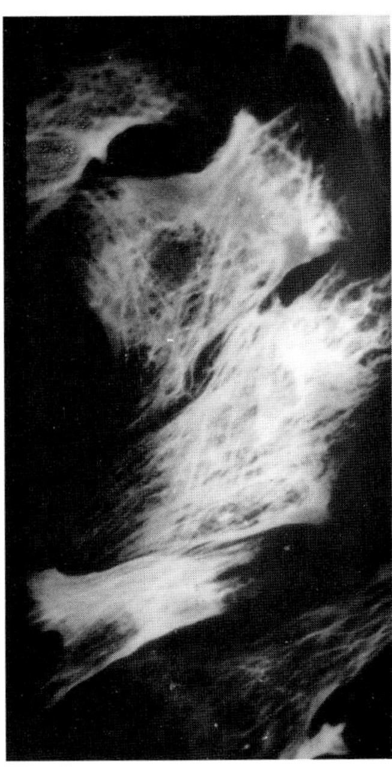

FIG. 2. Human mesangial cells in culture. **Left:** Phase contrast micrograph of subconfluent culture showing large, stellate cells with irregular cytoplasmic projections. Mesangial cells do not form a monolayer. **Right:** Immunofluorescence stain for smooth muscle α-actin showing characteristic fibrillar labeling of all cells. × 280.

Functional Properties of Mesangial Cells

As listed in Table 1, MCs have been shown to possess multiple functional properties. MCs produce ECM components that combine to make up the mesangial matrix. As the connective tissue of the glomerulus, the mesangium provides *structural support* to the glomerular capillary tuft. Similar to vascular smooth muscle cells, MCs in culture stain with antibodies to smooth muscle α-actin and myosin and contain actinomyosin bundles that span their length and insert at the cell membrane (Fig. 2). These "stress fibers" maintain basic cellular tone and are responsible for *contractile responses* of MCs that can be elicited by vasopressors in vitro. Contraction and relaxation of MCs have been observed in response to a variety of agents (see section 6). Growing cells on a flexible silicone rubber substratum has proven useful to study MC contractility. Cell contraction causes increased wrinkling of the supporting silicone film and, at the same time, diminishes the cell surface area, whereas relaxation results in decreased wrinkling, the cell surface remaining unchanged. Results of in vitro studies of MC contraction–relaxation correlate reasonably well with the effects of vasoactive agents observed in vivo (12,13).

A contribution of MCs to the regulation of the *glomerular microcirculation and ultrafiltration* is assumed because of their centrolobular position, contractile smooth muscle cell–like characteristics and their syncytial continuity with cells of the juxtaglomerular apparatus. Moreover, vasoactive agents can decrease the effective glomerular filtration surface by reducing blood flow to selected capillary loops, that is, by intraglomerular shunting of flow away from some capillaries. This may be accomplished by MC contraction. Also, MCs are strategically located at the glomerular hilus, where they surround glomerular capillaries at their branching points and are well suited to regulate the number of perfused glomerular capillaries (13). MC-mediated control of glomerular microcirculation and ultrafiltration depends on a delicate balance between vasoactive substances promoting contraction or relaxation of MCs (see section 6).

In analogy to the known *migratory activities* of smooth muscle cells in vascular walls of arteries and arterioles, it has been proposed that MCs also have the ability to migrate. although migration of the primitive pericytic MCs along with endothelial cells is required during the embryonic development of the glomerular capillary tuft, less convincing data are presently available to show that this also occurs in vivo in the developed normal or diseased kidney. Extension of MC processes into the subendothelial space of the peripheral capillary loop, as seen in some glomerular diseases, appears unlikely to reflect active migration. It is conceivable, however, that reorganization of the mesangium and capillary network following mesangiolytic changes of glomeruli [for example, in rat antithymocyte (anti-Thy)-1.1 nephritis; see below and section 11] involves migratory function of proliferating MCs. The distances in the glomerular tuft are short and might not require extensive migration of MCs. Nevertheless, locomotion of cultured MCs has been described by using a filter assay or a modified Boyden chamber assay (29). In this system, locomotive activity of rat MCs was increased by PDGF (29). No experiments have been reported on potential effects of the composition of the underlying ECM on MC locomotion.

A *clearing function* of MCs for macromolecules and filtration residues has been demonstrated by numerous in vivo experiments (7,8,30–33), showing that intravenously injected macromolecules localize to the glomerular mesangium (Fig. 1). As the mesangium is separated from the bloodstream by only the fenestrated, leaky endothelium without intervening GBM, it is constantly percolated by plasma. Deposition of macromolecules in the mesangium results from the formation of plasma residues due to the ultrafiltration process. Deposit removal is important for the maintenance of mesangial structure and function. In rats, few Ia-positive macrophages are resident in the mesangium and contribute to clear macromolecules and immune complexes. However, there is good evidence that intrinsic MCs also have the potential for nonspecific endocytosis (33) as well as specific, receptor-mediated uptake of opsonized zymosan (34) or immune complex-coated gold particles (35). The removal of immune complexes from the mesangium is of particular relevance for mesangial and glomerular housekeeping. To this account, several investigators have employed immunofluorescence microscopy, immunoblotting, and Northern blot analysis to show the presence of low-affinity Fc receptors on MCs, specifically binding aggregated immunoglobulin (Ig) G or immune complexes (35,36). Fc-dependent uptake of IgG immune complexes led to MC activation, as reflected by formation of eicosanoids, platelet-activating factor (PAT), and various cytokines (35). Uptake of immune complexes was augmented by preincubation of MCs with angiotensin II (37). Infusion of this vasopressor to rats also increased mesangial uptake of ferritin (38). In addition, it was shown that Fc receptors on MCs are regulated, because baseline expression of Fc receptors, as well as IgG binding and uptake, were increased by interferon-γ (IFN-γ) and colony-stimulating factor (CSF)-1 (36). With regard to other phagocytic activities, cultured MCs have been reported to show active uptake and replication of virus (for example, cytomegalovirus and human immunodeficiency virus). The pathobiologic relevance of these observations for in vivo conditions is presently unclear. In addition, MCs are able to ingest cells (for example, neutrophils) undergoing apoptosis (39) (see below and chapter 15).

MCs can express and secrete a large arsenal of substances (see the first two subsections of section 6). Most data on MC *secretory activities* have been obtained in culture or in animal models of glomerulonephritis. Under these conditions, MCs are in an activated state. The biosynthetic profile of quiescent MCs in the healthy glomerulus is less well known, but it can be assumed to serve the maintenance of architecture and function of the mesangium and the glomerular filtration apparatus. MC number, low cell turnover, and maintenance of balanced deposition and degradation of mesangial ECM are regulated by basal secretory activities of MCs. Other functions of MCs include their participation in the local response to glomerular injury as well as MC interactions with immune cells. These issues are addressed in sections 6 and 9.

3. Mesangial Cells in Vivo Versus in Vitro

The technique to isolate and maintain MCs in culture was developed in the 1970s, and MCs from human, bovine, rat, guinea pig, and mouse kidneys can be successfully cultured. Primary MC cultures can be set up by explantation and/or enzymatic isolation. Both methods use isolated glomeruli as the starting material obtained by differential sieving of renal cortex homogenate. In the former, MCs are allowed to grow out from whole glomeruli seeded onto plastic culture flasks and are maintained in supplemented culture medium containing 10–20% fetal calf serum. This method relies on the different growth potentials of the intrinsic glomerular cell types. In the second approach, whole glomeruli are preincubated with proteolytic enzymes that degrade and partly eliminate glomerular matrices to yield glomerular lobules or "cores" that consist predominantly of cells of the mesangium and capillary loops. MCs grow out and can be established in culture as a relatively homogeneous population. Under these conditions, contaminating endothelial cells and podocytes have limited growth potential and are usually lost within 2–3 passages. However, as with the explant method, MCs must undergo many divisions before sufficient numbers are available for meaningful studies (12,40,41). To shift MCs from an actively dividing into a quiescent state, they are incubated in "starvation" medium containing 0.5% fetal calf serum for 3–4 days.

Characterization and definitive proof of purity of MCs in vitro pose certain problems. Unlike endothelial cells, which can be readily identified by the demonstration of factor VIII, no single specific protein marker has as yet been described to enable reliable identification of MCs in culture as well as in tissue sections (42). However, a characteristic pattern of positive and negative markers can be employed to identify rat and human MCs and distinguish them from other cell types in order to exclude contamination (12,40–43) (Table 2).

In culture, MCs grow in an irregular fashion resembling smooth muscle cells or fibroblasts (Fig. 2). They lack close cell–cell contact and the cobblestone appearance typical for endothelial and epithelial cells. Usually, they exhibit two morphologic phenotypes: fusiform, elongated or stellate. In long-term culture, MCs can form nodular protrusions, so-called hillocks, composed of cells embedded in large masses of extracellular matrix (44) (see below). The expression of smooth muscle α-actin, which is readily detected in cultured MCs (10), is not seen in the mesangium of the normal glomerulus in vivo (21). Its de novo expression occurs in vivo only after disruption of the mesangial architecture following, for example, administration of the Thy-1.1 antibody (21), increased glomerular capillary pressure after 5/6 nephrectomy (45), or infusion of angiotensin II (AII) (46). Type IV collagen is the major collagen in the normal glomerulus in vivo while the expression of interstitial type I or III collagens is weak or absent (22,47). In vitro, however, >90% of the collagen synthesized by cultured MCs consists of collagen types I and III, with less type-IV collagen produced (48). Similar to smooth muscle α-actin, interstitial collagens appear in pathologic states in vivo, for example, in patients with focal sclerosis or crescentic or membranoproliferative glomerulonephritis (49) and in rats with experimental anti-Thy-1.1 mesangioproliferative glomerulonephritis (22) or with remnant kidney disease (50).

TABLE 2. *Factors for identification of mesangial cells in vivo and in vitro (12,27,40–42) (immunofluorescence scale: ++, strong; +, moderate; and (+), weak or variable*

	Rat	Human
Staining present		
Thy-1.1 antigen	++	(+)
Cellular ED-fibronectin	++	++
Smooth muscle cell α-actin and myosin	++	+
Desmin	+	+
β_1 integrin	++	+
α_1-chain	++	+
α_2-chain	+	+
α_3-chain	+	(+)
α_5-chain	++	(+)
α_8-chain	++	++
Lectins		
Ricinius communis A	+	+
Wisteria floribunda A	+	+
Staining absent		
Endothelial markers		
Factor VIII		
Glycoprotein 340		
MRC OX-43		
Podocyte markers		
Podocalyxin		
O-acetyl GD3 ganglioside		
Glycoprotein 330		
Tubular cell markers		
Tamm–Horsfall protein		
Brush border proteins		

Main Differences of Mesangial Cells in Phenotypic Characteristics and Behavior

Concerns with Cell Culture

Unlike glomerular epithelial and endothelial cells, MCs in vivo are not polarized but reside within a three-dimensional (3D) ECM. In contrast, in two-dimensional (2D) culture, MCs have their base attached to the plastic surface of a nonflexible culture dish or an ECM substratum whereas the top part of the cell is bathed in medium and its supplements. In the normal adult mammal, MCs have a very low replication rate (25), contrasting with MC proliferation as the sine qua non for cell culture. In culture, MCs undergo a variable number of rounds of replication before being studied. As a result, dedifferentiation and chromosomal aberrations of MCs, particularly in cell lines, can influence cell characteristics and make comparisons with other MCs difficult. Cultured MCs lack contact with other intrinsic or infiltrating glomerular cells. MCs in culture are grown at relatively high concentrations of fetal calf serum to facilitate production of proteins for attachment (for example, fibronectin and laminin) and growth factors (for instance, PDGF) that are necessary for MC replication. Therefore, MCs in culture represent activated cells rather than the quiescent cell type observed in the normal glomerulus in vivo (40–42,51). Moreover, in vivo, MCs are exposed to the glomerular capillary pressure and to the presumably pulsatile flow of plasma, both lacking in conventional culture. To account for this, systems have been developed to culture MCs on flexible surfaces that enable propagation of MCs in a pulsatile environment (52,53).

Phenotypic Differences of Cultured Mesangial Cells

Many similarities as well as some significant differences exist between human and rat MCs (27,40–42). For example, in the rat mesangium, two distinct cell types are found: 98% of cells exhibit features of smooth muscle cell–like, intrinsic MCs and 2% of cells show characteristics of bone-marrow-derived monocyte-macrophages (54). These have receptors for C3b and Fc and bear Ia determinants, allowing antigen presentation to T lymphocytes. In the human mesangium, only intrinsic MCs and no resident macrophages are normally seen. After several passages of culture, neither rat nor human MCs maintain surface proteins of macrophages. However, the synthetic and secretory phenotype of cultured rat versus human MCs differs in many ways, for example, with regard to production of tumor necrosis factor (TNF) α, PDGF, eicosanoids, coagulation factors, and various enzymes [reviewed by Mené et al. (12) and Sraer et al. (27)]. Differences were also found concerning the expression of receptors for TNFα, AII, and Fc/IgG (27). Although both rat and human MCs express the classic receptor for low-density lipoprotein (LDL), only rat MCs possess the scavenger receptor. Also, rat MCs show a four- to five-fold increase in binding of oxidized LDL versus native LDL and preferentially take up oxidized LDL (55,56).

Behavior of MCs in culture is also influenced by the age of the kidney donor. MCs obtained from fetal kidneys or young donors tend to grow faster, requiring lesser amounts of additives, such as fetal calf serum. It has also been observed that a mitogenic response to AII is present in fetal MCs although MCs from adult kidneys only show hypertrophy (57).

Two-Dimensional Versus Three-Dimensional Growth

Marx et al. cultured MCs embedded in a 3D matrix by using native collagen I (58). Although the use of this interstitial collagen type does not represent the complex composition of the mesangial ECM in vivo, it did serve to demonstrate that, in 3D culture, MCs show a low proliferative state. Under these culture conditions, MCs failed to respond to PDGF because of downregulation of its receptor. These observations exemplify the problem with interpreting data obtained in conventional 2D culture (44,58, 59). It is presently unclear whether MCs alter not only their proliferative profile but also their biosynthetic and secretory profiles (for example, ECM synthesis) when grown in 3D instead of 2D culture. Another approach to circumvent the rather artificial 2D culture system is to investigate MC behavior in freshly isolated glomeruli. This multiple cell type system, however, usually does not enable one to ascribe the observed effects to a specific cell type.

In summary, the findings obtained in vitro and in vivo reveal both, consistent and divergent results. Frequently, MC culture data differ from in vivo results obtained in normal glomeruli but are similar to findings obtained in disease states. Under standard cell culture conditions, MCs exhibit the phenotype of an activated cell in vivo. There is no complete dedifferentiation of MCs in culture because most response patterns in vitro have correlates in vivo, either in normal or disease states. In spite of the obvious limitations of analogies between phenotypic responses of MCs in vivo versus in vitro, the available cell culture data have allowed identification of many biologic systems, mechanisms and molecules at the cellular level for in-depth examination in experimental animals and in kidney biopsy tissue from patients with glomerular diseases.

PATHOBIOLOGY OF MESANGIAL CELLS

4. Mesangial Cells in the Context of the Glomerular Capillary Ultrafilter

As detailed above, the mesangium constitutes the highly specialized, branching connective tissue of the glomerular capillary tuft and is normally composed of intrinsic vascular smooth muscle cell–like MCs embedded in the ECM. The mesangium is involved in virtually all types of progressive glomerular disease, be they induced by immunologic or other mechanisms. Based on microscopic examination of such glomerulopathies, histologic abnormalities of the mesangium may include

1. Cell hyperplasia due to intrinsic MC proliferation and/or infiltration of bone-marrow-derived granulocytes or monocyte-macrophages
2. ECM widening due to accumulation of normal or abnormal matrix molecules, which may lead to glomerulosclerosis
3. MC expansion and subendothelial interposition into the circumference of the glomerular capillary wall
4. Mesangiolysis due to necrosis and loss of MCs and ECM
5. Apoptotic cells
6. Mesangial deposits of immune globulins and complement components or other trapped plasma-derived compounds

In glomerular disease, the proliferative and sclerosing abnormalities of the mesangium are the most conspicuous, reflecting major changes of the MC phenotype. Although they are quite nonspecific, hyperplasia and/or increased matrix production of MCs often occur in their response to an immune injury to the glomerular capillary tuft.

Before discussing particular aspects of MC responses to immunologic stimuli, it deserves emphasis that changes in MC phenotype ought to be considered in the context of the biology of the mesangium as a component of the glomerular capillary ultrafilter. Several structural and functional specialities of the mesangium are of particular importance for the pathobiology of MCs, distinguishing their response to injury from that of ordinary vascular smooth muscle cells or pericytes (Fig. 3):

1. Due to the high-flow and high-pressure characteristics of the mammalian glomerular ultrafiltration apparatus, the mesangium is exposed to the physiologic yet relatively high hydrostatic pressure in the glomerular capillary, that is, 45–50 mm Hg. Under conditions of further pressure rise

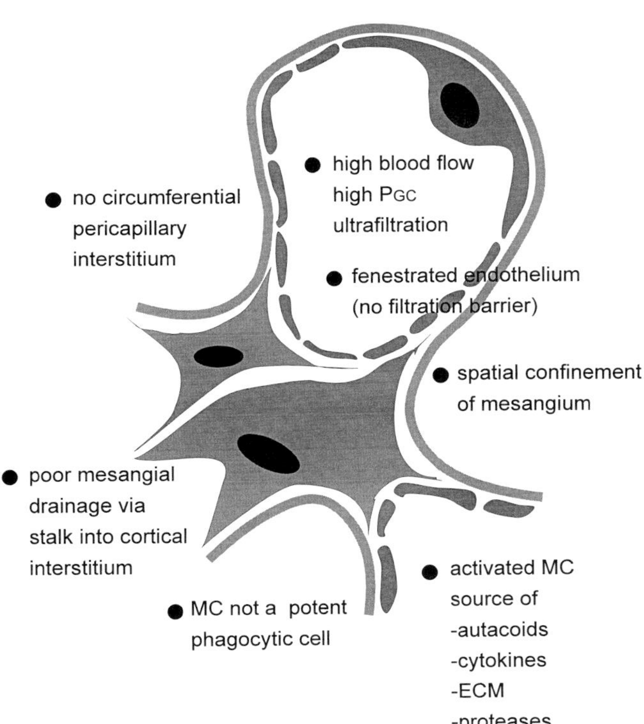

FIG. 3. Structural and functional characteristics of the mesangium as a component of the glomerular capillary ultrafilter in adult mammals ("mesangial handicap"). See the text for details.

(so-called glomerular hypertension), for example, due to loss of renal parenchyma, the increased hydrostatic pressure may cause mechanical injury and activation of MCs.

2. As a result of the ultrafiltration process, the concentration of nonfiltered plasma constituents (for example, macromolecules) increases along the glomerular capillary; thus, their entry into the mesangium near the efferent arteriole can be assumed to be significantly enhanced.

3. MCs are situated under the fenestrated endothelial lining of the capillary lumen, which does not constitute a filtration barrier; thus, they are located at the capillary side of the GBM and are constantly in contact with plasma and all its constituents.

4. MCs and matrix are integral parts of the branching connective tissue tree of the mesangium, joining at the vascular pole with cells of the juxtaglomerular apparatus and the cortical interstitium. Conspicuously, in the kidney of normal adult mammals (in contrast to that of lower species), the mesangium has a centrolobular location and does not extend into the periphery of the capillary loop. Here, the endothelial and epithelial cell layers are separated not by an interstitial space but only by a shared specialized basement membrane so that the GBM ultrafilter is in direct contact with blood and plasma constituents.

5. If one considers the mesangium as the restricted interstitial space of the glomerulus, representing a coarse sieve, the drainage of this area via the narrow glomerular stalk, tightly packed with cells, does not allow easy access to the cortical interstitium. Rather, outflow from the mesangium appears to occur mainly by ultrafiltration via the paramesangial GBM into the urinary space as well as by draining back into the blood, reaching the capillary lumen at a more downstream site toward the efferent arteriole (Figs. 1 and 3). The dynamics and regulation of such transmesangial fluxes, however, have not yet been determined quantitatively.

6. Although MCs have endocytic properties, unlike bone marrow-derived macrophages, they are not "professional" phagocytes. Nonetheless, upon activation, MCs produce a wide spectrum of bioactive mediators.

7. Like the whole glomerulus, the mesangium is confined in space and cannot extend (for example, due to MC proliferation and matrix increase) without reducing the capillary space required for glomerular blood flow and ultrafiltration.

Taken together, these special characteristics of the location, structure, and function of the mesangium (depicted in Fig. 3) render it prone to deposition and trapping of potentially injurious plasma constituents and filtration residues. For example, circulating immune complexes or other macromolecules have constant access to MCs. In case they are not easily removed but instead become trapped and accumulate, they can activate MCs, leading to changes in the proliferative and secretory phenotype. Upon activation, MCs are the source of numerous secretory substances that regulate the inflammatory response to an injury, including changes in the glomerular microcirculation and deposition of ECM, both affecting glomerular function. Thus, it appears as if the mammalian glomerulus has to deal with a "mesangial handicap," introduced to accomplish its main task, which is high-volume ultrafiltration.

5. Mechanisms of Mesangial Injury

General

The glomerular mesangium is the target of different types of injury. Immune-mediated damage can affect MCs by mechanisms of humoral and/or cellular immunity. Many other processes that may accompany or follow and perpetuate the immunologic process can also injure the mesangium. Clearly, the type, extent, and duration of an immune-mediated assault are relevant for the course of the mesangial damage because they determine the inflammatory response that is generated in the glomeruli. The inflammatory response is completed once the injurious agent or mechanism is removed or neutralized and tissue integrity of the mesangium and capillary tuft is restored. Regulation of this process of "wound healing" requires the release of many soluble substances that contribute to the attempt of tissue restoration. This usually includes the recruitment of bone marrow-derived inflammatory cells and requires tissue remodeling, which involves various changes of the proliferative and secretory MC phenotype. An inflammatory response to an acute and transitory injury (for instance, deposition of foreign antigens during acute infections) is usually followed by a phase of resolution. Obviously, if the injury to the mesangium is prolonged (for example, in continuous deposition of immunoglobulins, C3, amyloid, diabetic hyperglycemia, or glomerular hypertension), the inflammatory process becomes chronic, and the ongoing release of mediators and paracrine and autocrine regulators may never lead to a phase of resolution. Complete tissue restoration becomes impossible and the attempted remodeling of the mesangium may cause buildup of ECM, resulting in replacement of the delicate glomerular capillary tuft with inert scar tissue. Partial or complete glomerular sclerosis may initiate additional injury due to hyperfiltration and hypertension in remaining glomerular capillaries and ischemic changes in post-glomerular regions of the renal parenchyma. Conceivably, perpetuation of MC activation may also be due to inadequate downregulation of MC proliferation and secretory activity. Lack of factors that are required to regain and maintain the physiologic MC phenotype with low-rate cell renewal and matrix formation may prevent resolution, causing chronic mesangial and glomerular dysfunction and irreversible damage. Presently, few physiologic downregulators of MC activation are known (see section 10).

Immune-Mediated Mesangial Injury

Humoral Immune Mechanisms

The involvement of humoral immune mechanisms in the pathogenesis of mesangial pathology is well established in vivo and in cell culture, whereas much less is known about specific cellular immune mechanisms affecting MC behavior. Routine application of immunofluorescence microscopy for evaluation of kidney biopsy sections provides nephrologists and pathologists with a reliable tool to demonstrate the deposition of immunoglobulins and complement components in the mesangium and elsewhere in glomeruli and kidney. With few exceptions, the specificity of the deposited antibodies is uncertain. Rarely, the corresponding antigens have been identified as microbial breakdown products (for example, from streptococci, treponema, plasmodium malariae, or viruses) or circulating autoantigens (for instance, DNA, histones, or IgG). They are assumed to enter the mesangium either as part of circulating antigen–antibody immune complexes or separately and form immune complexes within the mesangium. The immunoglobulin class involved most frequently is IgG, but IgM and IgA are also found. IgM may be a component of cryoglobulins that are trapped in the mesangium.

Components of the complement system play a prominent role in immune-mediated mesangial pathology. In many forms of glomerulonephritis, antibodies and complement (C3 cleavage products and the terminal complement complex C5b-9) are deposited in the afflicted areas. Rat and human MCs have been shown to express receptors for C1Q that may facilitate the mesangial deposition of immune complexes in the presence of C1Q, perhaps in cooperation with Fc receptors (60). Complement activation in the mesangium, as it occurs in certain forms of glomerulonephritis, usually does not result in binding of sufficient C5b-9 membrane-attack complex to cause MC necrosis. C5b-9, however, activates MCs and alters their secretory phenotype, thus initiating an inflammatory response (61–63). Recent studies have indicated that complement components, such as C3, can also be synthesized by intrinsic renal cells, including MCs (64,65). Although the mechanisms leading to MC overexpression of complement are presently unclear, it is conceivable that abnormal local synthesis and activation of complement components may contribute to the mesangial deposition of immunoglobulins, thus inducing glomerulonephritis. It remains to be seen whether such a process may be relevant in the pathogenesis of IgA nephropathy, as has been suggested (64).

Cellular Immune Mechanisms

Although T lymphocytes are very rarely found in glomeruli with predominant mesangial pathology, there is evidence that cell-mediated immunity can contribute to mesangial injury and that specific interactions occur between MCs and immune cells. MCs have been shown to be activated by products of T helper cells. Also, MCs secrete costimulatory factors for T lymphocytes such as interleukin 1 (IL-1) and IL-6 (66,67). MCs do not constitutively express major histocompatibility (MHC) class II molecules, but they can be induced in vitro by recombinant T-cell lymphokines, such as IFN-γ. A combination of IFN-γ with IL-1 or TNF-α resulted in enhanced induction (68). IFN-γ, IL-1, and TNF-α also induced MC expression of intercellular adhesion molecule 1 (ICAM-I) (69). MCs, therefore, can function as antigen-presenting cells and substitute for macrophages by meeting the accessory cell requirement in their interaction with T lymphocytes, as has been reported for the small population of Ia-positive cells found in the mesangium of healthy rats (26). The capacity of IFN-γ-treated mouse MCs to process and present exogenous antigen to specific T lymphocytes has been demonstrated (69,70). In these studies, anti-ICAM monoclonal antibodies decreased adhesion and antigen presentation, and anti-MHC class II antibodies abrogated antigen presentation by MCs but did not block adhesion. The functional activity of MHC class II antigen expression on MCs was further demonstrated by coculturing IFN-γ/TNF-α-treated MCs with allogeneic unstimulated lymph node cells. MCs positive for MHC class II were able to stimulate allogeneic lymphocytes (71). It is presently uncertain, however, whether these experimental findings are relevant for mesangial inflammatory changes in patients.

Other Types of Mesangial Cell Injury

Other prominent causes of injury to the mesangium are indicated in Fig. 4. Besides glomerular hypertension, chronic metabolic diseases can disturb structure and function of the mesangium. Of great clinical relevance are chronic and progressive mesangial abnormalities resulting in glomerular hyalinosis and sclerosis, which are associated with long-standing diabetes mellitus. Hyperglycemia has been shown to affect the MC phenotype by multiple mechanisms, many of which induce changes in ECM production and deposition (see below). Amyloidosis can also lead to progressive mesangial widening due to irregular deposition of amyloid fibrils throughout the mesangium. Other causes of MC injury are discussed elsewhere in the book [and reviewed by Mené et al. (12), Lovett and Sterzel (41), and Sterzel and Lovett (72)] and are not discussed here.

Mesangiolysis

Mesangiolytic changes seen in renal tissue sections are characterized by dissolution of mesangial matrix and degeneration and necrosis of MCs, resulting in widening of mesangial areas that stain poorly in tissue sections. The loss of mesangial support structures and attachment points for the GBM causes dilation of the capillary lumina, which become aneurysmatic and resemble "blood cysts." Mesangiolysis is the typical primary lesion in glomerular disease induced in rats by habu snake venom (73) and in anti-Thy-1.1 nephritis (74). In addition to these experimental glomerulopathies, mesangiolysis is occasionally seen in human renal diseases, including various forms of glomerulonephritis, diabetic nephropathy, malignant nephrosclerosis, thrombotic microangiopathic glomerular disease, hemolytic uremic syndrome, renal transplant rejection, and glomerulopathies induced by snake bites (75). Stout et al. found focal mesangiolysis in ~35% of glomerulopathies associated with non-insulin-dependent diabetes (76). Pathogenetic mechanisms leading to mesangiolytic phenomena in human renal disease are likely to be nonspecific. At present, their nature is uncertain.

Secondary Damage to the Mesangium Due to the Inflammatory Responses

The primary immune-mediated insult can activate MCs and lead to synthesis, release, and action of chemotactic and vasoactive mediators (for example, as a consequence of immune-complex deposition and/or complement activation in the mesangium). However, the induction of a local inflammatory response to the initial injury can greatly potentiate the stimulatory effect on the proliferative and secretory phenotype of MCs. Following an acute insult to the mesangium, this amplification is frequently brought about by the recruitment and activation of inflammatory cells (granulocytes, platelets, and monocyte-macrophages), which results in the release of multiple soluble bioactive substances serving to confine the damage, eliminate the injurious agent, and restore tissue integrity (see section 6). In this process, MCs may be induced to proliferate and to produce more paracrine and/or autocrine mediators and matrix constituents that help to control the inflammatory response and reestablish the normal structure and function of the mesangium. Obviously, this concept is quite simplistic; for example, it does not consider the likely interaction or cooperation between glomerular endothelial cells and MCs (see below). Also, presently there is no reliable way to assess the dynamics and control of the extent and temporal sequence of release and action of proinflammatory versus anti-inflammatory mediator substances. In particular, it is unknown whether inadequacy or loss of factors, which function as physiologic downregulators of MC activation [for example, transforming growth factor (TGF) β; heparan sulfate proteoglycan (HSP); and normal amount, composition, and spatial organization of ECM) may contribute to the extent of MC injury. Finally, it is unclear which factors maintain activation of MCs in chronic glomerular disease following an acute immune-mediated insult (for example, progressive glomerulonephritis with MC proliferation and matrix buildup), even though mesangial immune deposits and infiltrating inflammatory cells have diminished or disappeared. It is possible that nonimmune factors, such as glomerular hypertension and inadequately controlled autocrine mechanisms, maintain MC activation, leading to progressive glomerular pathology.

6. Responses of Mesangial Cells to Immune Injury

The most common histopathologic changes of the mesangium in immune-mediated and other inflammatory diseases of glomeruli include MC proliferation with or without circumferential expansion of the mesangium, mesangiolysis, ECM widening, and sclerosis and mesangial immune deposits. Figure 4 depicts a scheme of the causes, phenotypic changes, and consequences of MC activation. The latter will be discussed here briefly because it is covered in detail elsewhere in the book.

Changes in Secretory Phenotype of Mesangial Cells: Soluble Factors

The MC phenotype can be specifically modified by binding of targeted antibodies, immune complexes, com-

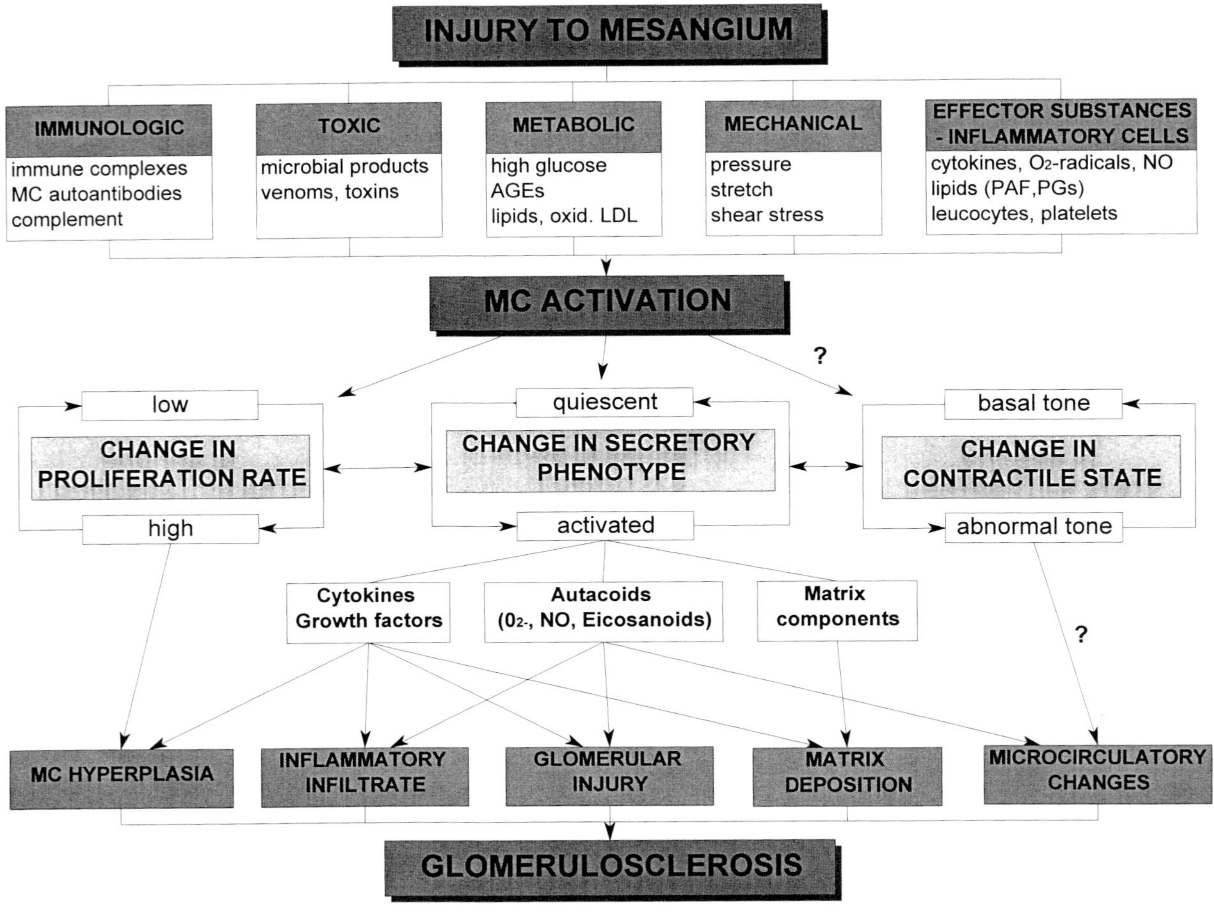

FIG. 4. Diagram of the mesangial response to injury. Pathomechanisms of mesangial injury are related to activation and changes of mesangial cell (MC) phenotype, which may result in glomerulosclerosis. Mechanisms leading to MC deactivation and resolution of inflammatory response (for example, apoptosis) are not indicated.

plement components, and immune cells. Also, it can be nonspecifically influenced by other types of injuries (such as hyperglycemia, abnormal hydrostatic pressure, stretch, and poisons). The precise regulation, however, is achieved in a paracrine manner by soluble mediator molecules derived from inflammatory cells or glomerular endothelial cells. Importantly, many of these soluble regulators are also secreted by activated MCs. They contribute to the inflammatory response by regulating MC behavior in an autocrine fashion or by affecting other cell types, for example, by chemotaxis and activation of monocyte-macrophages. Studies of MCs in culture have revealed a wide array of secretory products with bioactive potential. As listed in Table 3, they include many low molecular weight autacoids, hormones, enzymes, polypeptide cytokines, and growth factors. These MC-derived substances have been shown to exert many specific effects on MC behavior: that is, they can greatly alter the proliferative, synthetic, or contractile MC phenotype. Many secretory products also affect the behavior of other intrinsic or infiltrating cells in the glomerulus (see below). Because the fast-growing amount of information on MC-derived bioactive regulators is covered in detail elsewhere in the book (chapter 20), it is not discussed here further.

Changes in Secretory Phenotype of Mesangial Cells: Insoluble Components of the Extracellular Matrix and Matrix-Degrading Enzymes

The diverse components of the mesangial ECM are listed in Table 4. They can be categorized as microfibril associated, basement membrane associated, and interstitium associated. The fibril-associated components include fibronectin, which mediates binding of microfibrils to MCs and GBM. The basement-membrane-associated components include type IV collagen, laminin, nidogen, HSP, and a specific chondroitin sulfate proteoglycan that is associated with basement membranes other than the GBM (77). The interstitium-associated group includes collagen types I, III, and V and other chondroitin sulfate and dermatan sulfate proteoglycans (77). Depending on their state of activation, MCs can change their synthetic profile and express and secrete the interstitial collagen types I and III, for example, in cell culture and glomerular disease. This switch appears to be critical for the initiation of mesangial sclerosis and scarring. Glomerular ECM deposition is regulated by multiple factors that can affect generation and removal of ECM. MCs produce paracrine and autocrine mediators that enhance ECM production (TGFβ, TNF-α, IL-1, and PDGF) (78,79). This regulation can occur at the level of gene expression, protein synthesis or secretion, and deposition of ECM components.

The expression of mesangial ECM components during glomerular injury has been examined in many experimental glomerular diseases. Border and colleagues have reported that TGFβ plays a central role in ECM accumulation found in prolonged anti-Thy-1.1 nephritis (80). Other models, for example, obese Zucker rats (81) and the multiple-injection purine aminonucleoside nephrosis (PAN) rat model (82), develop progressive glomerular changes. In the PAN rat model, expression of various mesangial ECM components (collagen IV, laminin, and HSP) increased shortly after disease induction and rose with time. In contrast, expression of interstitial collagens (types I and III), not normally found within the glomerulus, was delayed in onset, starting at ~70 days after disease induction (82).

TABLE 3. *Regulators of inflammation secreted by mesangial cells*[a]

Low molecular weight autacoids	
Prostaglandins E_2, D_2, and $F_{2\alpha}$, prostacyclin, and thromboxane A_2	(27)
Hydroeicosatetraenoic acid	(34)
Epoxyeicosatrienoic-acid-like	(103)
Platelet-activating factor	(190)
Reactive oxygen species	(34,192)
Nitric oxide and metabolites	(194)
Hormones	
Endothelin	(197)
Insulin	(187)
Enzymes/proenzymes/inhibitors	
Matrix-degrading enzymes	(Table 5)
Ecto 5′-nucleotidase	(203)
Aminopeptidase N	(203)
Tissue plasminogen activator (tPA)	(208)
Plasminogen activator inhibitor 1 (inhibitor of tPA)	(209)
Tissue factor (thromboplastin)	(210)
Renin	(211)
Complement C3	(65)
Polypeptide mediators[b]	
Platelet-derived growth factor	(185,186)
Basic fibroblast growth factor	(153)
Insulinlike growth factor 1	(187)
Transforming growth factor β	(188,189)
Nerve growth factor	(191)
GM-CSF	(193)
Tumor necrosis factor α	(195)
IL-1	(66)
IL-6	(67,196)
IL-8	(198)
IL-10	(199)
LIF	(200)
RANTES	(201)
Macrophage inflammatory protein 2	(202)
Monocyte chemoattractant factor 1	(204,205)
Colony-stimulating factor 1	(206,207)
Matrix components	(Table 4)

References are in parentheses.

[a]Reviewed by Radeke and Resch (71), Abboud (183), and Sterzel et al. (184).

[b]GM-CSF, granulocyte-macrophage colony-stimulating factor; IL, interleukin; LIF, leukemia inhibitory factor; RANTES, regulated upon activation, normal T-cell expressed and secreted.

Mesangial Matrix-Degrading Proteinases

The turnover and modeling of mesangial ECM requires the secretion and extracellular action of neutral proteinases. MCs have been shown to synthesize and secrete serine proteinases, cysteine proteinases, and metalloproteinases that can cleave and degrade macromolecules of the GBM and mesangial ECM (Table 5). They include a 72-kD matrix metalloproteinase with gelatinase and type-IV collagenase activity (54,83), stromelysin 1 or proteoglycanase, and a stromelysinlike enzyme, termed putative metalloproteinase (PUMP)-1 (84). They are secreted as latent proenzymes and require extracellular activation. The biologic relevance of such matrix proteinases and their inhibitors (for example, tissue inhibitor of metalloproteinase (TIMP)-1) has been examined in experimental glomerular diseases. For example, in rats with anti-Thy-1.1 glomerulonephritis, the abundance of MCs expressing 72-kD type-IV collagenase was markedly augmented (85). MC culture studies have shown that the synthesis of this and other matrix-degrading proteinases can be induced in MCs exposed to IL-1β, TNF-α, or TGFβ (54). In contrast, TGFβ was found to inhibit the MC-derived serine protease, plasminogen activator, while it increased the activity of the inhibitor (86). It is presently unclear whether and in what way these effects might contribute to the fibrogenic potential of TGFβ (see chapter 19).

Changes in Proliferative Phenotype of Mesangial Cells

One of the prominent histopathologic features of many human glomerular diseases is cellular hyperplasia in the mesangium due to MC proliferation. As detailed in Tables 6 and 7, numerous factors of greatly different nature stimulate or inhibit MC proliferation in culture and in vivo. Many of the soluble or insoluble ligands are produced by MCs and, thus, possess autocrine growth-modulating activity. Because the growth rate of MCs in the normal adult mammal is quite low (<1%), quiescent MCs can be assumed to face few mitogens or to be protected due to either downregulation of receptors or presence of growth-inhibitory factors maintaining the low proliferative activity. Regardless of the mechanism, an

TABLE 4. *Extracellular matrix molecules synthesized by mesangial cells in culture and in vivo*

	In vivo/ normal (ref.)	In vivo/diseased (ref.)	In vitro (ref.)
Collagens			
I	Absent (276)	⇑ Thy-1.1 (22), PAN (82,277), renal ablation (50), TGF-β glomerular gene transfer (180)	(145), ⇑ FCS (278); ⇑⇓ HG (279,280)
III		⇑ PAN (82), TGF-β glomerular gene transfer (180)	(145), ⇑ FCS (278)
IV	(77)	⇑ Thy-1.1 (22), PAN (82,277), GH transgenic (281), mGVHD (276), renal ablation (50,282), TGF-β glomerular gene transfer (180), human diabetic nodules (283)	⇑ TGF-β (216), TXA2 (284), HG (93,279); ⇓ PGE2 (285)
V	(77)		
VI	(276)	⇑ mGVHD (276)	⇑ HG (95)
VIII	(137)		(137,286)
Glycoproteins			
Fibronectin	(287)	⇑ Thy-1.1 (80), PAN (277), renal ablation (50), mGVHD (276), human diabetic nodules (283)	⇑ TGF-b (216), HG (93,279), TXA2 (284), AII (222), AVP (288), LDL (289)
Nidogen/entactin	(290)	⇑ Thy-1.1 (22), renal ablation (50)	
Laminin	(77)	⇑ Thy-1.1 (80), PAN (82), GH transgenic (281), renal ablation (50,282), mGVHD (276)	⇑ HG (93,279), FCS (278), TXA2 (284)
Tenascin	(141)	⇑ In most types of human GN, whenever there was expansion of extracellular matrix (141)	(291)
Thrombospondin	(292)		(145)
Proteoglycans			
Heparan sulfate PGs	(293)	⇑ Thy-1.1 (22), PAN (82), GH transgenic (281), renal ablation (50,282), human diabetic nodules (283)	⇑-⇓ HG (294,295)
Chondroitin and dermatan sulfate proteoglycans (versican, decorin, biglycan)	293)	⇑ Thy-1.1 (80), diabetic rats (STZ) (77)	⇑ TGF-β (151), IL-1 (78), TNF-α (78); ⇑-⇓ HG (294,295)

(AII, angiotensin II; AVP, arginine vasopressin; CSS, chronic serum sickness; FCS, fetal calf serum; GH, growth hormone; HG, high-glucose-containing medium; IL-1, interleukin-1; LDL, low-density lipoproteins; mGVHD, murine graft-versus-host disease; PAN, purine aminonucleoside nephrosis; PGE2, prostaglandin E2; TGF-β, transforming growth factor beta; Thy-1.1, anti-thymocyte-1.1 nephritis; TNF-α, tumor necrosis factor alpha; TXA2, thromboxane A2.

imbalance in the control of MC proliferation seems to play an early and perhaps crucial role in the pathogenesis of progressive glomerular injury and glomerular sclerosis. In experimental models of nephritis, MC proliferation frequently precedes and is tightly linked to the development of mesangial ECM expansion and glomerular sclerosis (45,87). Mice transgenic for the SV40 T antigen, which has growth-promoting functions, develop MC proliferation followed by progressive sclerosis (88). Mice transgenic for growth hormone ultimately develop severe progressive mesangial sclerosis and show a fivefold increase in the [^{3}H]thymidine-labeling index of glomerular tuft cells. Interestingly, the labeling index remained high at late time points in densely sclerotic glomeruli (87), indicating that increased MC turnover can be a significant feature associated with sclerosis, both at the onset and in later stages. Moreover, measures that reduce cell proliferation in glomerular disease models, such as treatment with heparin (89), low-protein diet (90), or neutralizing antibodies to PDGF (91), also reduce ECM expansion and sclerotic changes. Further evidence for the role of uncontrolled MC prolif-

TABLE 5. *Matrix-degrading enzymes and their substrates* [a]

Enzyme	Substrates
Serine proteases	
Plasminogen activators	Glycoproteins, protein core of proteoglycans, gelatin, latent metalloproteinases
Matrix metalloproteinases (MMPs)	
Interstitial collagenases MMP-1 (type-I collagenase)	Collagen types I, II, III, VII, X
Type-IV collagenases MMP-2 (72-kD collagenase) MMP-9 (92-kD collagenase)	Gelatin, collagen types IV, V, VII, X, fibronectin
Stromelysins MMP-3 (stromelysin 1, proteoglycanase) MMP-7 (matrilysin, PUMP-1) MMP-10 (stromelysin 2)	Fibronectin, laminin, elastin, collagen types IV, V, VIII, IX, proteoglycans
Cysteine proteinases (cathepsins)	Collagen type I, laminin, proteoglycans
Endo-exoglycosidases	Aminosugar moieties of proteoglycans

[a] Reviewed by Davies et al. (212) and Johnson et al. (213).

TABLE 6. *Regulators of mesangial cell (MC) proliferative phenotype in culture*

Mitogenic	
Platelet-derived growth factor BB	(214)
Platelet-derived growth factor AB	(186)
Basic fibroblast growth factor	(214)
Epidermal growth factor	(214,215)
Insulin	(224)
Insulinlike growth factor 1	(224,227)
Interleukin-1	(66,225)
Interleukin-6	(67,196)
Transforming growth factor β (low conc. 0.01–1 ng/mL)	(215,233)
Arginine vasopressin	(99,100)
Endothelin-1	(235)
Serotonin	(99,220)
Adenosine triphosphate	(237)
Dinucleotides	(239,240)
Prostaglandin $F_{2\alpha}$	(229)
Epoxyeicosatrienoic acid	(103)
Thrombin	(241)
Bradykinin	(220)
Neuropeptide Y	(220)
Oxytocin	(220)
Phorbol myristate acetate	(220)
Low-density lipoprotein, native	(55)
Nephritogenic immunoglobulin-A immune complexes	(242)
Thrombospondin	(147)
Fibronectin	(146)
Stretch	(243)
Antimitogenic	
Transforming growth factor β (high conc. >250 pg/mL)	(215,216)
Interferon-γ	(217)
Interleukin-4	(219)
Interleukin-10	(221)
Prostaglandin E_2	(225)
Prostaglandin I_2 (stable analogue iloprost)	(228,229)
Atrial natiuretic peptide	(232)
Cyclic guonosine monophosphate	(230)
Low-density lipoprotein, oxidized	(55)
Calcium-channel blockers	(234)
Phosphodiesterase-III antagonist	(236)
P450 monooxygenase inhibitors	(103)
Lovastatin	(238)
Simvastatin	(104)
Heparan sulfate proteoglycan	(149)
Heparin	(159)

TABLE 6. *(Continued.)*

Variable	
Tumor necrosis factor a	
⇑	(214)
~/⇓	(218)
Angiotensin II	
~(adult rMCs)	(220)
⇑ (mMCs, fetal hMCs)	(222,223)
Nitric oxide	
~	(226)
⇑	(230,231)
Thromboxane A_2	
⇑ (quiescent)	(228)
⇓ (serum stim.)	(228)
High glucose	
⇑ (after 1–2 days)	(188)
⇓ (after 3–4 days)	(188)
No effect	
Platelet-derived growth factor AA	(186)
Granulocyte colony-stimulating factor	(51)
Macrophage colony-stimulating factor	(51)
Granulocyte-macrophage colony-stimulating factor	(193)
Interleukin-3	(51)
Leukemia inhibitory factor	(200)
Gastrin	(51)
Glucagon	(51)
Secretin	(51)
Somatostatin	(51)
Substance P	(220)
Norepinephrine	(220)
Bombesin	(220)
Endotoxin	(51)

References are in parentheses.

eration in the pathogenesis of sclerosis was provided by work in rats with spontaneous age-related glomerulosclerosis. MCs cultured from these rats showed increased proliferative potential as a function of donor age, whereas in control animals showing no or little glomerular sclerosis the proliferative potential of MCs decreased with age of the donor (92).

However, MC growth and ECM synthesis are not necessarily influenced concordantly. Several groups have demonstrated that cultured MCs, incubated under high glucose conditions, markedly increased synthesis of various ECM components (laminin, fibronectin, and collagens type IV and VI and, inconsistently, type I), whereas proliferation was found to be inhibited (93–95). A recent study showed that the stimulation of fibronectin synthesis by high glucose in cultured MCs closely correlated with the inhibition of MC proliferation. This effect appeared to be mediated via the activation of protein kinase C (96). Its relevance for the in vivo process of diabetic glomerulosclerosis is presently unclear.

Changes in Contractile Phenotype

Combined in vivo and in vitro data indicate that contractile MCs contribute to the regulation of glomerular ultrafiltration. Several vasoactive compounds that contract MCs in culture are capable of reducing the glomerular ultrafiltration coefficient in vivo. Some of these factors, for example, endothelin (ET), thromboxane A_2, and adenosine, are produced by MCs in an autocrine manner. Ligands that cause MC contraction are listed in Table 8. The contractile process is dependent on Ca^{2+} and is accompanied by eicosanoid production. Because vasodilator rather than vasoconstrictor prostaglandins predominate, it is possible that prostaglandin (PG) E_2 (in rat MCs) and PGI_2 (in

TABLE 7. *Regulators of mesangial cell (MC) proliferative phenotype in vivo*

Mitogenic	
Platelet-derived growth factor (PDGF) BB	
⇑ MC proliferation after infusion in normal rats or glomerular gene transfer	(180,244)
⇓ Proliferation after PDGF antibody in anti-Thy-1.1 nephritis	(91)
Basic fibroblast growth factor	
No proliferative response after bolus or 1-week infusion in normal rats, but fivefold increase when given after subnephrotic dose of anti-Thy-1.1	(153,244)
Interleukin-1 (IL-1)	
Constant infusion of IL-1 receptor antagonist reduced proteinuria, hypercellularity and glomerular necrosis in rabbit and rat anti–glomerular basement membrane nephritis	(249–251)
Interleukin-6 (IL-6)	
Mesangioproliferative glomerulonephritis in mice transgenic for human IL-6	(253)
Endothelin-1	
Endothelin-A receptor antagonist in remnant kidney model reduced proteinuria and glomerular injury	(254)
SV40	
Mice transgenic for SV40 T antigen showed MC proliferation and sclerosis after age of 2 months	(256)
Growth hormone (GH)	
Mice transgenic for GH or GH-releasing factor showed MC proliferation followed by progressive sclerosis	(87,257)
Antimitogenic	
Heparin	
Anti-Thy-1.1 nephritis	(89)
Habu snake venom model	(245)
Puromycin aminonucleoside nephrosis	(246)
Remnant kidney model	(247,248)
Interferon-γ	
Reduction of MC proliferation by 44% in anti-Thy-1.1 model, but increase in glomerular macrophages and transforming growth factor β	(171)
Calcium-channel blockers	
Nifedipine reduced MC number and mesangial expansion in anti-Thy-1.1 nephritis	(252)
Angiotensin-converting enzyme inhibitors	
Enalapril had similar effect as nifedipine in anti-Thy-1.1 nephritis	(252)
Phosphodiesterase III or IV antagonists (Lixazinone, Rolipram) reduced proteinuria, α-actin expression, and MC proliferation	(255)

Thy, thymocyte. References are in parentheses.

human MCs) function in a negative-feedback manner to attenuate the contractile action of vasoconstrictors. Importantly, some vasopressors also have indirect and delayed effects on MC behavior with regard to the induction and secretion of growth factors (PDGF, for example) and MC mitogenesis (Table 8). Furthermore, AII was shown to increase macromolecular uptake by MCs in culture. It induced Fc receptor expression and uptake of IgG-coated particles in MCs and increased the uptake of gold particles coated with bovine serum albumin (37). In addition, AII infusion to rats increased mesangial uptake of ferritin (38). It is, therefore, possible that AII excess in vivo facilitates mesangial deposition of filtration residues, which eventually may lead to impairment of mesangial clearing function causing mesangial and glomerular damage. This hypothetical pathomechanism is of interest because several clinical studies have indicated protective effects of angiotensin-converting enzyme inhibitors on the progression of experimental and human glomerular disease that are not entirely explained by alterations in intraglomerular hemodynamics.

7. Postreceptor Signal Transduction Pathways

The phenotype of MCs, similar to that of other anchoring cells, is affected and regulated by multiple soluble, diffusable as well as by solid-phase, nondiffusable signaling molecules. Their ligation to specific MC membrane receptors triggers the activation of various signaling networks. Figure 5 schematically depicts some of the main signal-transducing systems identified in MCs that are affected by soluble agonists. These systems include:

1. Signals originating from G-protein-coupled receptors linked to the activation of phospholipase C (PLC) with consecutive generation of inositol triphosphate (IP_3) and diacylglycerol (DAG). IP_3 induces a rise in intracellular Ca^{2+} concentration, which in turn activates various Ca^{2+}-dependent processes like contraction or activation of phospholipase A_2 (PLA_2) and arachidonic acid (AA) metabolism. DAG leads to activation of protein kinase C (PKC), a key enzyme in a wide variety of intracellular processes. MCs have been reported to express multiple subtypes of PKC, for example, PKC-α (Ca^{2+} dependent) and PKC-δ, PKC-ε, and PKC-ζ (Ca^{2+} independent). No PKC-β or PKC-γ isoforms have as yet been detected (97). Whereas PKC-α, PKC-δ, and PKC-ε immunoreactivity is predominantly present in the particulate fraction of MCs, PKC-ζ is mostly located in the cytosolic fraction (97).
2. Receptor tyrosine-kinase-activated signals that are generated by a multiprotein complex forming at the intracellular domain of these receptors; they are linked to PLC activation and to the cascade of the mitogen-activated protein kinase (MAPK).
3. Signal systems linked to receptors that are coupled to adenylate or guanylate cyclase, causing generation of cAMP or cGMP and activation of the respective cAMP- or cGMP-dependent kinases.

In general, these three main pathways follow a common pattern in that ligand–receptor interaction leads to the acti-

TABLE 8. *Agents influencing contractility and mitogenesis of cultured mesangial cells*[a]

Agonist	Contraction	Relaxation	Proliferation
Peptides			
Angiotensin II	+ (258)		~/⇑ (220,222)
Arginine vasopressin	+ (258)		⇑ (100)
Endothelin 1	+ (259)		⇑ (235)
Serotonin	+ (40)		⇑ (220)
Bradykinin	+ (260)		⇓ (220)
Atriol notrivretic peptide		+ (117)	⇓ (232)
Growth factors			
Platelet-derived growth factor	+ (261)		⇑ (214)
Tumor necrosis factor α	+(262)		~ (214,218)
Autacoids			
Prostaglandin $F_{2\alpha}$	+ (13)		⇑ (229)
Thromboxane A_2	+ (116)		~ (228)
Platelet-activating factor	+ (263)		
Leukotriene C_4/leukotriene D_4	+ (264)		
Prostaglandin E_2		+ (116,265)	⇓ (225)
Prostaglandin I_2 (analogue iloprost)		+ (116)	⇓ (228)
Nitric oxide		+ (231)	~/⇓ (226,230,231)
Others			
Histamine	+ (266)		
Norepinephrine	+ (267)		~ (220)
Dopamine	+ (111)		
Increase in cGMP		+ (117)	⇓ (230)
Increase in cAMP		+ (118)	⇓ (268)
Immune complexes	+ (269)		⇑ (242)
Ca^{2+} ionophore A23187	+ (118)		

[a]See also Mené et al. (12), Schlondorff (13), and Ganz et al. (220). References are in parentheses.

vation of various enzymatic steps that trigger the release of intracellular second messengers. These, in turn, activate a variety of systems, leading to post-translational modification of cellular proteins, the best studied being various kinases. Phosphorylation of multiple substrates by serine/threonine kinases (PKC, PKA, and PKG) or cytoplasmic tyrosine kinases is a final step in extranuclear signaling. These events initiate the intricately regulated modification and activation of nuclear transcription factors that couple short-term events to more prolonged processes involving alteration of gene expression and protein synthesis, ultimately resulting in specific changes of the cellular phenotype. Cross talk between signal transduction pathways, along with the release of eicosanoids and cytokines acting as autocrine or paracrine intercellular mediators, promotes the potential for interactive regulation of glomerular cell functions.

Because some of the most prominent reaction patterns of MCs in glomerular immune injury and inflammation are DNA synthesis, proliferation, and contraction, selected postreceptor signal transduction pathways leading to these phenotypic changes shall be discussed in more detail.

DNA Synthesis and Mesangial Cell Replication

Proliferative stimuli to MCs are generated by binding of mitogens to various receptor superfamilies. Both, serine/threonine and tyrosine kinases are essential elements of the mitogenic signal transduction cascade. Preincubation of MCs with genistein, an inhibitor of protein tyrosine phosphorylation, blocks PDGF-induced MC proliferation (98) and depletion or inhibition of PKC blunts arginine-vasopressin (AVP)-induced mitogenesis (99,100). PKC and nonreceptor protein tyrosine kinase activity (such as pp^{60}c-src) contribute to mitogenic signaling of ET-1 (101). A variety of other intracellular events linked to MC proliferation have been elaborated. ET-1 induces elevation of phosphatidic acid by activation of phospholipase D (PLD), an enzyme linked to mitogenesis in other cell types. PLD activation was shown to be PLC dependent and constitutes an event downstream of PKC activation (102). Sellmayer et al. suggested a role for endogenous arachidonic acid and its metabolites as mediators of MC growth. In particular, products of the P450 monooxygenase system, such as compounds with epoxyeicosatrienoic-acid-like characteristics, could be identified as mediators of the growth response to mitogenic agents (103).

The activation of the MAPK pathway is believed to play a critical role in normal and induced proliferation of MCs. Diverse MC mitogens, such as AVP (104), PDGF, epidermal growth factor (EGF) (105), and ET-1 (106), have all been shown to activate MAPK. Inhibitors of MC growth, like PGE_2 or other cAMP-elevating agents (105) and simvastatin (104) were demonstrated to inhibit

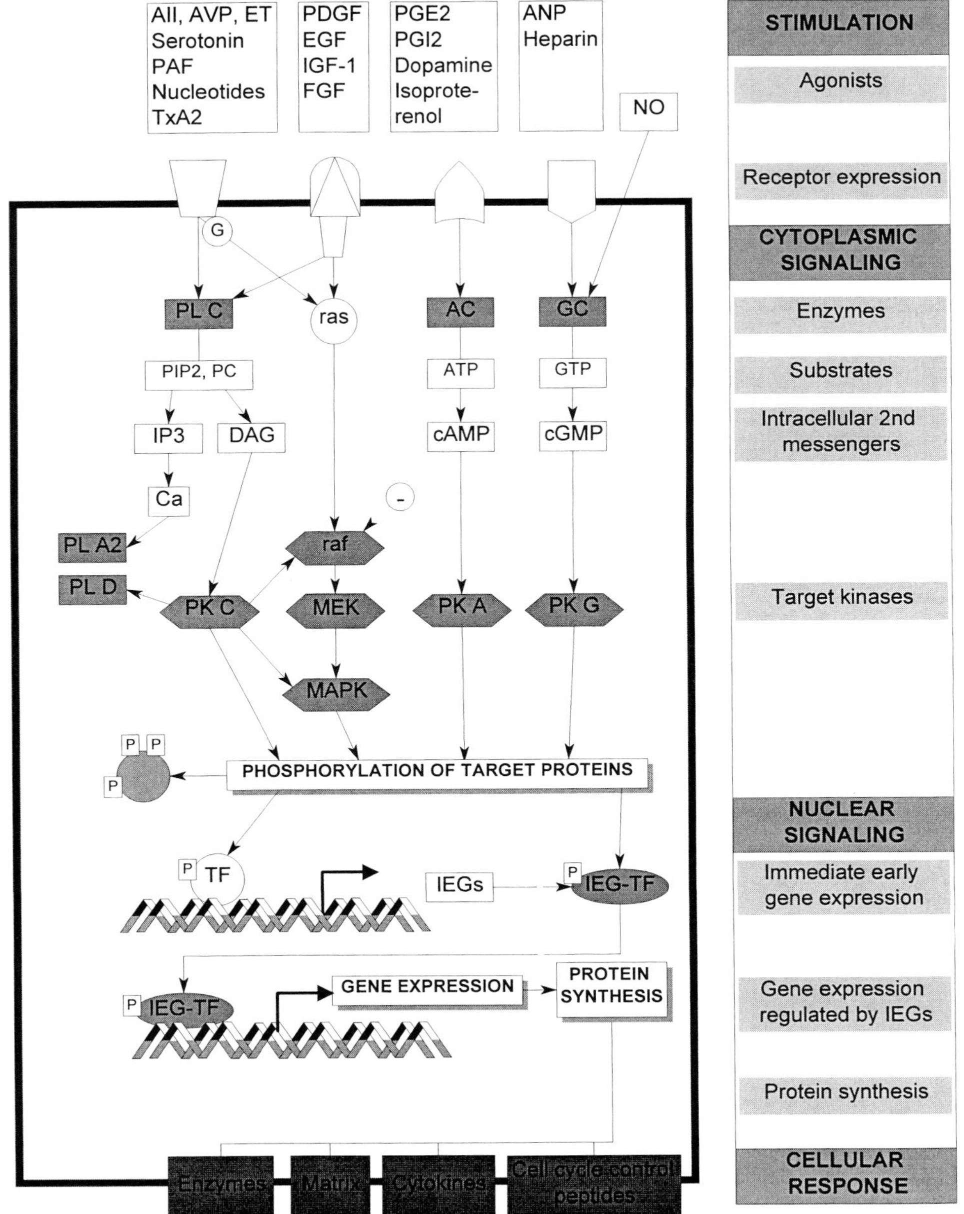

FIG. 5. Scheme of ligand-elicited mechanisms of postreceptor signal transduction resulting in changes of the mesangial cell phenotype: *G,* G protein; *PLC,* phospholipase C, *PLA_2,* phospholipase A_2; *PLD,* phospholipase D; *PIP_2,* phosphatidylinositol-4,5-bisphosphate; *PC,* phosphatidylcholine; *IP_3,* inositol triphosphate; *DAG,* diacylglycerol; *Ca,* intracellular calcium; *AC,* adenylate cyclase; *GC,* guanylate cyclase; *PKA,* protein kinase A; *PKC,* protein kinase C; *PKG,* protein kinase G; *MEK,* mitogen-activated protein kinase kinase; *MAPK,* mitogen-activated protein kinase; *TF,* transcription factor; *IEG,* immediate early gene.

MAPK. Activation of MAPK by ET-1 was shown to occur via at least two pathways, one of which is PKC dependent and one that involves protein tyrosine kinase activity (106), requiring stimulation of ras and the c-Raf-1 kinase (105,107). The activation of the ras/Raf-1/MAPK cascade is one of the major signaling pathways by which growth factors transmit their mitogenic signals from the cell membrane to the nucleus. Here, these signals are translated into early changes of gene expression, the earliest being the induction of the so-called immediate early genes (IEGs). Indeed, transfection of MCs with a plasmid expressing constitutively activated δ Raf-1 activates the serum response element (SRE) in the promoter of the IEG, c-fos. ET-1-induced activation of the c-fos SRE was blocked by transfection of a dominant negative c-Ha ras mutant (107). As shown in a mouse macrophage cell line, MAPK activates SREs not only of the c-fos promoter but also of the promoter of another IEG, the early growth response gene 1 (Egr-1) (108). Rupprecht et al. have shown a very close correlation between the induction of MC growth and the induction of Egr-1 mRNA and protein (98,99,109). By using antisense oligonucleotides to Egr-1, they were able to establish that Egr-1 induction is a necessary step in the mitogenic signal transduction cascade in MCs, because Egr-1 antisense oligonucleotides inhibit PDGF-induced Egr-1 mRNA and protein as well as MC growth. Sense or scrambled control oligonucleotides were without significant effects (110). Importantly, some of the IEGs, like c-fos or Egr-1, encode transcription factors and, as such, initiate the expression of additional genes. Characterization of these downstream genes will be important to elucidate nuclear events following mitogenic MC stimulation.

Mesangial Cell Contraction

Kreisberg et al. suggested a biochemical model of MC contraction in which agonist–receptor binding activates PLC to cleave IP_3 and DAG from membrane phosphoinositides (111). IP_3 releases Ca^{2+} from intracellular stores and, together with extracellular Ca^{2+} influx, leads to an elevation of intracellular Ca^{2+} concentration with consecutive activation of Ca^{2+}-dependent enzymes. One such enzyme is myosin light chain kinase, which phosphorylates myosin, leading to actinomyosin complex formation and development of tension. Ca^{2+} influx into MCs was shown to depend on the extracellular presence of Cl^- ions, which was reflected by a corresponding Cl^- dependence for agonist-induced MC contraction (112). PKC also phosphorylates myosin light chain and other cytoskeletal proteins, and it was suggested that PKC activation results in tonic contraction and a sustained response subsequent to the initial Ca^{2+} signal (113). As expected, phorbol myristate acetate, a PKC agonist, dose-dependently stimulates contraction of MCs. This effect was synergistic with that of the Ca^{2+} ionophore A23187 (114).

A mechanism opposing contraction is the generation of endogenous vasorelaxant autacoids. Because most vasopressors induce PG synthesis in MCs, the release of PGE_2 or PGI_2 is considered to constitute a negative-feedback mechanism. Inhibiting mesangial cyclooxygenase and its major product PGE_2 by nonsteroidal anti-inflammatory drugs augmented MC contraction caused by various stimuli (114,115). The relaxant action of PGE_2 or PGI_2 is considered to be mediated by cAMP accumulation because it was abolished by preincubation of MCs with 2′,5′-dideoxyadenosine, a false substrate for adenylate cyclase (116), and could be mimicked by application of membrane-permeant stable analogues, such as dibutyryl cAMP (117,118). cGMP also has potent inhibitory effects on agonist-induced MC contraction. In keeping with this are new findings which indicate that activation of guanylate cyclase by atrial natriuretic peptide (ANP) or nitric oxide (NO) can inhibit AII-induced MC contraction. This effect was reproduced by 8-bromo cGMP, a stable cGMP analogue (117). [For a more complete overview on signaling cascades in MCs, see the review by Mené et al. (12) and chapter 21.]

8. Mesangial Cell–Matrix Interaction

The phenotype of MCs is affected not only by soluble regulators, such as cytokines and autacoids, but also by signals of the nondiffusible mesangial ECM. These molecules can specifically interact with ECM receptors on the MC surface, inducing and regulating cellular responses, such as adhesion, migration, synthetic, and secretory activities as well as growth. The relevance of cell–matrix interactions was first shown in the process of MC localization, anchoring, and differentiation during embryonic development of the glomerular capillary tuft (16,17). The composition and spatial organization of matrix constitute a 3D context that provides not only structural support for MCs but also specific signals contributing to the regulation of MC behavior. Alterations of the normal "ECM context", as it occurs in glomerular diseases, may then affect the MC phenotype. This could be relevant for diverse processes, such as anchoring and proliferation of MCs and synthesis of cytokines and ECM. During inflammatory responses in the glomerulus, MCs face an altered spectrum of soluble and insoluble regulators, and the "cross talk" between them is likely to be greatly different from normal steady-state conditions. ECM molecules can, through interaction with specific receptors on the MC surface, influence many aspects of cellular behavior.

Molecular Mechanisms

Receptors

The molecular mechanisms of specific cell–ECM interactions have only recently become amenable to thorough investigation. Most cell types express transmembranous surface glycoproteins that specifically interact with ECM components. The widely distributed integrins, a protein superfamily, permit cellular recognition of ECM components. Receptors for ECM molecules also include cell surface proteoglycans. Thus, various types of receptors can specifically mediate attachment of cells to ECM molecules and the effects of ECM on various cellular functions. A summary of ECM receptor expression in the mesangium is presented in Table 9.

Integrins are heterodimeric, noncovalently associated protein complexes consisting of an α-chain and a β-chain. They have been shown to control many cell–matrix interactions, such as adhesion, growth, and differentiation (119). The different distribution patterns of β_1-integrins in the

TABLE 9. *Extracellular matrix receptor expression in the mesangium*[a]

Receptor	Ligands	Human Tissue	Human Cells[b]	Rat Tissue	Rat Cells[b]	References
β_1-Integrins						
α_1	Col IV, Col I, LM	+	++	++	++	(125,128,270)
α_2	Col I, Col IV, LM	+	(+)	(+)	(+)	(125,127,271)
α_3	LM, Col I, FN	+	+	+	+	(125,126,128)
α_4	VCAM I, LM, FN	-	-	-	-	(126,128,270)
α_5	FN, RGD	+	++	+	+	(125,126,128)
α_6	LM (E8 fragment)	-	-	-	-	(125,128)
α_7	FN, multiple	+	+	+	+	
β_3-Integrin						
α_V	VN, FN, RGD, multiple	+	+	+	+	(128,272)
Cell surface proteoglycan						
Syndecan 4	FN, Others?	?	?	?	?	

[a]Detected by immunochemistry.
[b]Results dependent on the extracellular matrix substratum used for mesangial cell culture; see the text for details.
Col, collagen; LM, laminin; FN, fibronectin; RGD, arginine-glycine-aspartic acid; VN, vitronactin; VCAM, vascular cell adhesion molecule.

developing and adult kidney imply their potential role in morphogenesis and maintenance of the normal adult renal architecture [reviewed by Adler (120) and Korhonen et al. (121)]. Cell surface proteoglycans, especially the syndecan family and the cell surface antigen CD44, have also been described to possess ECM receptor qualities. Syndecans constitute a polymorphic family of cell surface proteoglycans with variable glycosylation, bearing heparan sulfate and chondroitin sulfate chains. Woods and Couchman have demonstrated that syndecan 4 is a component of focal adhesions of fibroblasts on ECM substratum (122). Obviously, studies with respect to the potential presence or function of such surface proteoglycans on MCs are of considerable interest.

Signaling by Integrins

Recent cell culture studies have greatly advanced our knowledge of the organization of components involved in specific interactions of an ECM ligand with a cell surface receptor and subsequent cellular transducers [reviewed by Juliano and Haskill (123) and Ruoslahti et al. 124)]. Many cell types, mainly of mesenchymal origin, including fibroblasts, vascular smooth muscle cells, and MCs, when plated on matrix substratum form transmembranous assemblies, which are known as focal contacts or focal adhesions. Focal contacts enable cells to anchor to their ECM environment and may thus facilitate not only cell and tissue organization but also the exertion of tension, for example, in contraction and wound closure. The ECM ligand initiates clustering of adjacent integrins and formation of a focal contact. Indeed, the localization of certain integrin α-chains into focal contacts depends on the specific ECM ligand. For example, use of fibronectin, which is abundant in the mesangial matrix, as the substratum, induces the movement of $\alpha_5\beta_1$ integrin but not of $\alpha_4\beta_1$ or $\alpha_6\beta_1$ into focal contacts of MCs (125–128). Laminin interacts with focal contacts containing $\alpha_1\beta_1$, $\alpha_2\beta_1$, or $\alpha_3\beta_1$ (see Table 9). Thus, on MCs, laminin does not appear to use its specific surface receptor, $\alpha_6\beta_1$, but promiscuous α-chains.

Beside clustered integrins, the cytoplasmic plaque of a focal contact contains a complex of intracellular cytoskeletal proteins, including paxillin, talin, α-actinin, tensin, and vinculin. These and other cytoskeletal components provide linkage to actin microfilament bundles, important for cell shape change, contraction, and motility. Although the cytoplasmic domains of the α- and β_1-integrin chains do not have intrinsic enzymatic activity, the focal contact assembly contains multiple regulator molecules, for example, tyrosine kinases and PKC. It has been reported that the PKC isoform is a focal adhesion component in several cell types (129). Recent studies have shown that a cytoplasmic protein tyrosine kinase, termed focal adhesion kinase (FAK), is involved in the signal transduction pathways initiated by ligand–integrin binding on the cell surface. FAK is rapidly phosphorylated and activated following attachment of fibroblasts to fibronectin-coated surfaces or integrin clustering by antibodies (130). FAK has been localized to focal contacts, consistent with its role in starting the signaling cascade following ligand–integrin interaction (131). However, FAK expression and phosphorylation is also induced in cultured MCs exposed to shear stress, AII (132), or ET (133), indicating its wider relevance in MC signal transduction.

Recent data have demonstrated that fibronectin binding to integrins of fibroblasts promotes SH2 domain-mediated association of the GRB2 adapter protein and the c-src protein tyrosine kinase with FAK in vivo. This results in activation of MAPK (134). Phosphatidylinositol 3-kinase was shown to be a substrate of FAK in vivo and, thus, may serve as an effector of FAK (135). In addition, integrin-mediated attachment of fibroblasts and smooth muscle cells to fibronectin caused an increase in the activity of the transcription factor NF-kB, although a direct involvement of FAK remains to be demonstrated (136). Taken together, these findings indicate that signal transduction events are elicited by interaction of insoluble ECM ligands with integrins and subsequent integrin-mediated FAK phosphorylation. These events are similar to those stimulated by binding of soluble growth factors to receptor tyrosine kinases. The specific relevance of such mechanisms for interactions of MCs with surrounding normal or abnormal ECM and the regulation of MC behavior in vivo needs to be elucidated.

Mesangial Cell Funtions Regulated by Cell–Matrix Interactions

Maintenance of Structural and Functional Integrity of the Glomerular Tuft

The mesangial matrix is characterized by the presence of small bundles of fine fibers. These microfibrils form an extensively interwoven, 3D meshwork that also provides an array of contacts between MCs and the perimesangial GBM (9). Fibronectin, the most abundant molecule in the mesangial matrix has been shown to be associated with microfibrils and could serve to link MC surfaces to these extracellular structures. Therefore, ECM molecules are thought to function as stabilizers of the 3D architecture of the glomerular capillary tuft, counteracting the distending forces (hydraulic pressure gradient across the capillary wall) acting on the GBM by transmitting inwardly directed traction generated by contractile MCs [reviewed by Kriz et al. (9)]. It has been speculated that loss of the ECM linkage of MCs to the GBM is responsible for the development of glomerular capillary microaneurysms (40,77,137) because the GBM is no longer held in a fixed position by its attachment to the mesangium.

Owing to their "intracapillary" location (see above), MCs are subjected to pulsatile stretch and relaxation cycles resulting from changes in intravascular hydraulic pressure. To investigate this effect of mechanical strain on cultured MCs, flexible surfaces have been used that allow cell culture in a pulsatile environment, where stretch–relaxation cycles are regulated by computer-driven devices (53). Cyclic stretching altered cell morphology, stimulated MC proliferation, and increased the production of laminin, fibronectin, and type I, III, and IV collagen (52,138). The extent of stretch-induced MC elongation was found to be directly related to increased type IV collagen expression. Of interest, the expression of type IV collagenase mRNA was unchanged or slightly reduced (52). Based on such findings, it has been proposed that augmented ECM deposition, as seen in states of glomerular hypertension and/or hypertrophy, could be in part due to greater physical forces acting on MCs with consecutive alterations in the ECM synthesis profile. However, the exact mechanisms of how increased glomerular capillary pressure is translated into mesangial ECM accumulation have yet to be clarified.

Dynamic Regulation of Mesangial Cell Adhesion

Anchorage-dependent cells require attachment to ECM to allow growth as well as expression of a differentiated phenotype. Various ECM molecules have been shown to serve as adhesive substrates for MCs in vitro (Table 9) (125,126,128). Initial ECM–integrin interaction and MC attachment are followed by cell spreading and subsequent organization of focal contacts. We assume that the process of specific attachment of MCs to ECM molecules is regulated in a complex and dynamic manner. For example, during proliferation, adhesive forces have to be diminished to allow rounding and division of cells. Although focal contacts of fibroblasts appear to be instrumental in contracting and generating tension to direct wound closure in vivo, it is unclear whether MCs exert tension on the surrounding matrix and capillaries, for example, following a glomerular lesion.

At present, little is known about factors controlling adhesion of MCs to matrix. As discussed above, multiple ECM molecules, notably fibronectin, collagens, and laminin, specifically interact with MC integrins and induce formation of focal adhesion sites. Other ECM glycoproteins, including thrombospondin, SPARC (secreted protein acidic and rich in cysteine, also termed osteonectin), and tenascin, can antagonize the adhesive process. These latter compounds appear to exert antiadhesive functions promoting cell rounding and partial detachment of cells from the substratum (129,139,140). In addition, SPARC has been shown to inhibit progression through the cell cycle in vitro (140). Although these glycoproteins are secreted and retained in the local environment where they can function in an autocrine or paracrine manner, they usually do not function as structural components. A recent immunohistochemical report indicated that tenascin is a component of the mesangial matrix in the normal mature human kidney (141). In biopsies from diseased kidneys, it was noted that expansion of mesangial ECM was associated with increased presence of tenascin. It remains unclear from this descriptive study, however, whether tenascin or other antiadhesive ECM molecules play a protective or detrimental role in the evolution of glomerular diseases. More specifically, it remains to be shown whether and how glycoproteins may influence MC adhesiveness and, possibly, proliferation in glomerular disease.

The formation of focal contacts involving expression of integrin receptors is likely to be also affected by soluble regulators. First studies have shown that TGFβ, EGF, and hepatocycle growth factor (HGF) can affect focal contact formation and/or components of integrin signal transduction pathways in various cell types (142,143). High glucose concentration has also been found to increase expression of β_1-integrin in cultured MCs (144). Clearly, much more information is required to understand better these aspects of cooperative regulation of MC behavior by soluble growth factors and ECM.

Extracellular Matrix Molecules and Growth Regulation

It has been shown in different cell systems that ECM regulates both cell growth and ECM synthesis. For example, MCs plated and cultured on collagen type IV and laminin exhibit increased production and secretion of fibronectin and laminin (145). Freshly seeded MCs do not only plate with much higher efficiency on collagen types I, II, and IV than on plastic but also possess greater replication activity (146). Thrombospondin increases MC proliferation, an effect that might be mediated by upregulation of EGF and PDGF secretion (147). HSP influences cell behavior in a different manner. For example, the rapid attachment of MCs to fibronectin is greatly inhibited by the HSP perlecan (148). Also, several investigators have reported dose-dependent inhibition of MC proliferation by heparan sulfate in culture (149,150). In addition to direct receptor-mediated effects, ECM molecules can indirectly affect the MC phenotype, for example, by binding and sequestering various cytokines. The small proteoglycan decorin, for example, the production of which in MCs is increased by TGFβ (151), can neutralize the action of TGFβ. This effect could reflect an autoregulatory feedback system. Furthermore, the potent MC mitogen basic fibroblast growth factor (bFGF) strongly binds to HSPs (152). Because bFGF has proinflammatory effects in experimental kidney diseases (153), interactions of basement membrane proteoglycans with bFGF may have important regulatory functions. In a recent study, Morita et al. demonstrated that HSPs show enrichment of bFGF-binding domains in fibrotic lesions of the peritubular interstitium (154). Taken together, these reports demonstrate the important function of ECM molecules in binding, sequestering, and neutralizing growth factors. Possibly they could also provide a local "reservoir" of regulatory proteins and present them to adjacent cells in a biologically more active form.

The concept of interdependency of MC growth and ECM synthesis and secretion by MCs was supported by the finding that production of collagens, fibronectin, and laminin paralleled proliferation of cultured MCs (145). Of note, localization of ECM constituents was strictly intracellular until confluency of MCs with cell–cell contacts was reached, when extracellular deposition of collagen IV and laminin appeared, followed by collagen I and fibronectin. On surfaces coated with the GBM components collagen IV and laminin, secretion and deposition of ECM preceded confluency (145). Thus, production and distribution of ECM appears to be affected not only by MC growth but also by cell–cell contact and the composition of deposited ECM.

In summary, there is ample evidence, albeit mostly based on MC culture studies, that mesangial ECM acts not only as a mechanical, inert structural support system of the glomerular capillary tuft. Rather, the ECM affects and regulates cellular events in a specific manner, similar to growth factors and cytokines. ECM molecules can influence many aspects of MC behavior, such as adhesion and growth, migration, differentiation, repair, and possibly apoptosis, as shown for other cells (155).

Extracellular Matrix Organization and Mesangial Cell Differentiation

Based on the evidence provided by studies with MCs, renal epithelial cells, and fibroblasts (notably during embryogenesis and organ development), the ECM-mediated effects on the MC phenotype have to be considered as part of a cooperative control system that also involves the action of soluble regulators and MC interaction with adjacent endothelial and infiltrating cells. The spatial organization and composition of the ECM constitutes a regulated microenvironment of MCs in the glomerulus, thus providing a nonsoluble context that, as such, is likely to affect the regulation of the MC phenotype by soluble factors. As discussed in section 3, it is important to stress that effects of ECM on MCs in vivo or in 3D culture may differ significantly from a situation when MCs are plated onto a 2D ECM substratum covering the culture plate.

In this context, it is of interest that MCs in long-term culture form round protrusions or hillocks, which are nodules of MCs embedded in a supporting 3D meshwork of ECM (44). In the periphery of hillocks, the morphologic MC phenotype is fusiform and elongated while it is stellate and plump in hillock centers. In labeling studies, the central, stellate, and more differentiated MC phenotype was found to be downregulated with regard to DNA replication but showed high secretory activity, producing collagens I and III and fibronectin (J. Grond, R. B. Sterzel, M. Kashgarian, unpublished observations). It is as yet unclear which factors regulate the maintenance of the differentiated, nonproliferating MC phenotype under 3D culture conditions or in vivo. Also, data on differential expression of ECM receptors on MCs grown in 3D as compared with 2D culture are lacking. Thus, the mechanisms of interaction between 3D ECM and MCs in the regulation of the observed cellular phenotypes remain to be clarified.

Extracellular Matrix in Glomerular Repair Processes

Although much work has been published describing abnormal mesangial ECM deposition in glomerular disease, few data exist concerning ECM involvement in repair mechanisms regulating recovery from injury and restoring structural and functional integrity of the glomerulus. In the context of this review, it may be asked whether interactions of glomerular cells with the mesangial ECM play a role in this process. Reversal of abnormal ECM accumulation has to involve modulation of ECM turnover shifting the balance of ECM deposition and proteinase secretion and proteolytic activity toward resolution of the lesion. It is conceivable that inhibitory effects of "abnormal" ECM molecules on this process may be relevant by interfering with recovery.

A novel aspect concerning resolution of glomerular pathology points toward a possible role of MC–matrix interactions in the induction of apoptosis in the recovery phase of glomerulonephritic disease. Baker et al. demonstrated MC apoptosis to be a major cell clearance mechanism counterbalancing MC replication in self-limited anti-Thy-1.1 glomerulonephritis, thereby effecting resolution of glomerular hypercellularity (39). Induction of apoptosis, however, may be dependent on and regulated by the expression of distinct sets of cell adhesion molecules. Recently, Zhang et al. demonstrated in Chinese hamster ovary cells that expression of $\alpha_5\beta_1$-integrin but not of the closely related $\alpha_v\beta_1$-integrin appears to suppress apoptosis using the bcl-2 pathway (155). Thus, one could hypothesize that integrin-mediated signaling regulates induction of apoptosis and, hence, cell survival in vivo and may thereby contribute to glomerular repair processes. Clearly, this field of research requires much work to help elucidate the role of ECM and ECM receptors in resolution and repair after glomerular injury.

9. Mesangial Cell Interaction with Endothelial, Epithelial, and Inflammatory Cells

Little is known about direct and specific interactions between different cell types in the glomerulus, and few coculture studies have addressed this issue in vitro. In vivo, glomerular cell–cell interactions have been examined using depletion studies, an approach applicable only to inflammatory cells infiltrating the glomerulus, that is, granulocytes, macrophages, and platelets.

Interactions with Endothelial and Epithelial Cells

Cultured endothelial cells can release substances that affect the MC phenotype, for example, PDGF, bFGF, IL-1, ETs, NO, and eicosanoids. MCs respond to coculture with endothelial cells with enhanced synthesis of PGE_2, which was dependent on ET-1 release by endothelial cells (156). Coculture also led to a five- to sixfold increase in MC cGMP content, caused by endothelial cell NO production. The local release of the vasoconstrictor ET-1 and the vasodilator NO is likely to participate in the regulation of glomerular hemodynamics through alterations of MC tone. Cross talk between endothelial cells and MCs is also suggested by the finding that a heparin-like molecule extracted from culture medium conditioned by glomerular endothelial cells inhibits MC growth (157). Furthermore, coculture of the two cell types led to an initial inhibition (days 1–3) and a late stimulation (days 3–5) of MC proliferation (158).

Glomerular epithelial cells, like endothelial cells, have also been reported to secrete heparinlike substances into the culture supernatant that inhibit MC growth (159). The in vivo relevance of this finding, however, is unclear. It is presently unknown whether soluble epithelial cell products are able to diffuse across the GBM against a pressure gradient to reach a target cell in a mesangial location.

Interactions with Bone Marrow-Derived Cells

Platelets

Platelets are the source of multiple growth factors for MCs, including PDGF, EGF, insulinlike growth factor 1, IL-1, adenosine triphosphate, serotonin, and thromboxane A_2. Intraglomerular platelet accumulation and aggregation can be observed in several animal models of glomerular disease (73,160) and in human disease (161). Evidence to support a role for platelets in mediating MC proliferation in vivo has been generated by depletion studies. In glomerulopathies caused by habu snake venom or anti-Thy-1.1 IgG in rats rendered thrombocytopenic with antiplatelet serum, mesangiolysis was unaffected, but MC hypercellularity was largely prevented (162,163). Similar effects were seen with the antiplatelet agent dipyridamole (164). Platelets, therefore, do not appear to initiate mesangial injury in these models, but their products are able to stimulate proliferation of activated MCs.

Leukocytes

Complex interactions exist between MCs and immune cells that infiltrate the mesangium during nephritis. On the one hand, MCs produce a variety of immune modulatory cytokines (IL-1, CSF-1, granulocyte-macrophage colony-stimulating factor, TNF-α, and IL-6) and chemokines [RANTES (regulated upon activation normal T cell expressed and secreted), monocyte chemoattractant protein (MCP) 1, macrophage inflammatory protein 2, and IL-8], which may serve in the recruitment of various inflammatory cells to the glomerulus (Table 10).

Indeed, MC expression of MCP-1 and RANTES was associated with macrophage influx to the glomerulus as shown in rat models and human proliferative glomerular diseases (165,166). On the other hand, soluble regulators produced by activated leukocytes [for example, cytokines, chemokines, eicosanoids, NO, reactive oxygen species

TABLE 10. *Mesangial cell release of chemotactic factors for immune cells*

	Chemotactic target cell	Stimulator of release	References
Colony-stimulating factor 1	Monocytes, macrophages	Interferon-γ, immunoglobulin-G complexes, tumor necrosis factor α	(205–207)
RANTES	Monocytes, CD4+ lymphocytes, eosinophilic granulocytes	Lipopolysaccharide, tumor necrosis factor α, immunoglobulin-G complexes	(201)
Monocyte chemoattractant factor 1	Macrophages, monocytes	Interleukin 1β, platelet-derived growth factor, tumor necrosis factor α, interferon-γ, leukemia inhibitory factor, low-density lipoprotein, immunoglobulin-G complexes, thrombin, reactive oxygen species	(200,204, 205,273,274)
Macrophage inflammatory protein 2	Neutrophils	Interleukin 1	(202)
Interleukin 8	Neutrophils and lymphocytes	Interleukin 1, tumor necrosis factor α, lipopolysaccharide	(198,275)

(ROS), proteolytic enzymes, and other pro- and anti-inflammatory substances] can greatly affect the proliferative and synthetic/secretory phenotypes of MCs in a paracrine fashion (Fig. 6). The amount of IL-1 released by macrophages can be 10–100 times greater than that produced by resident MCs. Also, glomerular IL-1 production in a rat anti-GBM nephritis model was shown to be largely dependent on infiltrating macrophages (167). In macrophage depletion studies using the rat model of accelerated anti-GBM nephritis, Matsumoto and Hatano reported a reduction in glomerular and mesangial hypercellularity (168). Furthermore, coculture experiments demonstrated that U937 monocytes can bind to cultured human MCs (169). This process was greatly enhanced by lipopolysaccharide, TNF-α, or phorbol myristate acetate and was inhibitable by prior treatment of MCs with anti-ICAM-1 antibody. Cell adhesion strongly stimulated subsequent MC proliferation, whereas U937-conditioned medium had no effect. These data show that, in addition to secretory products, direct and specific cell–cell interaction can affect glomerular pathobiology. Finally, MCs can also be induced to express MHC class II antigens and

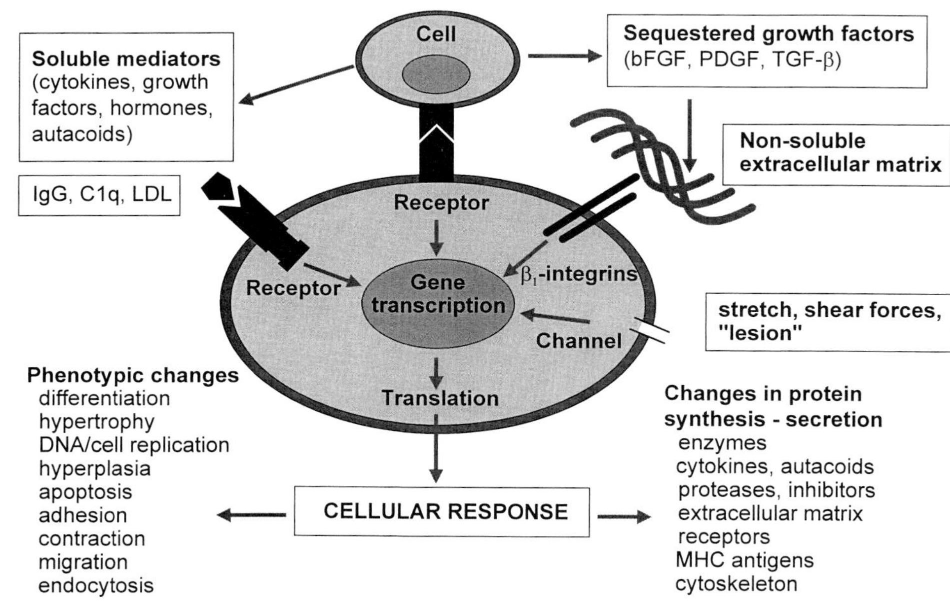

FIG. 6. Control of mesangial cell phenotype by interactions ("cross talk") between cells, soluble ligands, nonsoluble extracellular matrix, and other stimuli.

assume accessory cell functions in the immune response by presenting antigens to T lymphocytes (71).

10. Summary of Mesangial Cell Activation Versus Deactivation

Both in situ and in culture, MCs can assume a differentiated, contractile, nonreplicating phenotype or they can exist as synthetically active, proliferating cells. However, precise markers for differentiation versus dedifferentiation, or activation versus deactivation, or of an MC "phenotype switch" have not been well defined. In the activated state, MCs, like many other cells, express newly produced proteins in response to different needs and stimuli. The highly complex network of MC responses (or "cross talk") to other cells, paracrine or autocrine soluble regulators, nonsoluble ECM components, and physical or toxic stimuli is schematically illustrated in Figs. 6 and 7. In general terms, these responses reflect changes of the synthetic/secretory, proliferative, apoptotic, or contractile MC phenotype (Table 11). Several MC proteins are being used as markers of cell activation, for example, expression of smooth muscle α-actin or formation of interstitial collagens. Expression of these proteins indicates the similarity of activated MCs with vascular smooth muscle cells and fibroblasts, that is, with myofibroblasts (23). Although expression of smooth muscle α-actin and collagens I and III may reflect upregulation of the contractile and/or synthetic phenotype, for example, in response to vasopressor or inflammatory stimuli, it does not necessarily indicate increased DNA synthesis and MC proliferation (23,46, 170,171). Histochemical assessment of these and other phenotypic markers of MCs in renal tissue sections is becoming a very attractive method to gain more information on MC activation in vivo.

Resolution of Mesangial Cell Hyperplasia: Apoptosis

In the normal adult glomerulus, there is a stable balance between cell renewal and cell removal, resulting in maintenance of a constant number of glomerular cells at a low level of proliferation (25). In disease states, this equilibrium is often changed, resulting in hyperplasia of endothelial cells and MCs. The resolution of hypercellularity, therefore, would require reduction of the regeneration rate (even below the very low baseline levels) and/or shortening of cell survival, that is, increased rate of MC death or removal. One way of removing "unwanted" cells is by apoptosis. In the kidney, pathologists first described apoptosis or programmed cell death in renal biopsies from patients with proliferative glomerulonephritis or hemolytic uremic syndrome (172,173). Savill and colleagues showed that MCs are capable of undergoing apoptosis in culture after having been deprived of serum growth factors (39,174). In vivo, the anti-Thy-1.1 model of mesangioproliferative glomerulonephritis is characterized by complete resolution of glomerular hypercellularity. Here, apoptotic cells were seen much more frequently in glomeruli from nephritic rats. Interestingly, mitotic and apoptotic cells often coincided in the same glomerulus (39), suggesting that both processes occur simultaneously. Indeed, apoptosis was upregulated at the beginning of the hypercellular state. Using the same model, Shimizu et al. noted increases of apoptotic cells in glomeruli with a maximum at day 10 to week 2, the majority of apoptotic cells being of MC origin (175). By conventional histology, apoptosis is rather inconspicuous because only a minor part (that is, 1–2 h) of the whole process is apparent. This important phenotypic switch of MCs is difficult to analyze in one-time kidney biopsies of patients. To detect earlier steps of the apoptotic program, current studies are testing for the expression of apoptosis-related proteins in renal tissue sections (see chapter 15). Takemura et al. demonstrated high glomerular expression of Fas antigen in Henoch–Schönlein purpura nephritis and lupus nephritis and high expression of the antiapoptotic molecule Bcl-2 in lupus nephritis and IgA nephritis. Fas antigen and Bcl-2 were expressed by MCs and infiltrating leukocytes (176).

11. Mesangial Cells in Glomerular Disease

Among the available animal models of glomerular immune-mediated disease are several with prominent mesangial pathology. Suitable models include: anti-Thy-1.1 glomerulonephritis, concanavalin-A–anti-concanavalin-A glomerulonephritis, IgA-associated glomerulopathy, and several transgenic mouse models. Because they are described in detail in chapters 11 and 35, they are not covered here.

The great majority of human glomerular diseases show histopathologic changes of MCs and/or the mesangial matrix. The most prevalent causes and types of glomerulopathies with prominent mesangial involvement include most types of proliferative and/or sclerosing glomerulonephritis, diabetic glomerulosclerosis, and glomerulopathies caused by deposits of amyloid and other fibrillar proteins (addressed in detail in chapters 41–48). In addition to conventional diagnostic analysis of renal biopsy sections by light, immunofluorescence, and electron microscopy, recent use of molecular techniques has also addressed the state of MC activation, for example, with regard to the expression of smooth muscle α-actin, DNA and cell replication, hypertrophy, apoptosis, matrix formation, and composition (see section 10). By investigating molecular indicators of the proliferative and/or synthetic phenotype of MCs, it becomes possible to unmask mechanistic and regulatory features of MC behavior by using renal biopsy sections. As in the well-established analysis of neoplastic tumor tissue, the prolif-

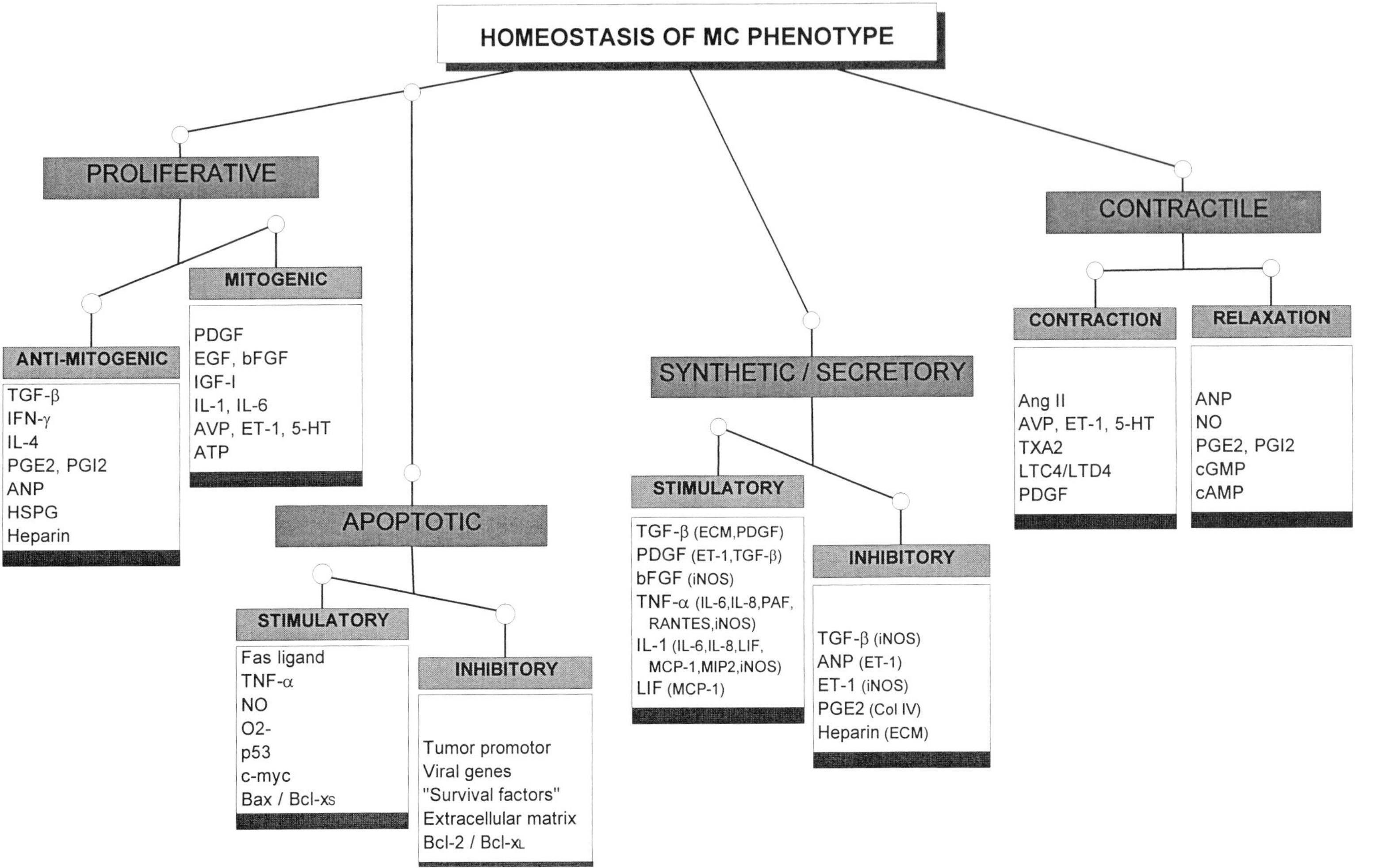

FIG. 7. Homeostasis and selected regulators of the mesangial cell phenotype with respect to cell proliferation, apoptosis, biosynthesis/secretion, and contractility (see the text for details).

TABLE 11. *Phenotypic modulation of mesangial cells (MCs)*

Characteristics expressed	MC activation	MC deactivation
Synthetic/secretory phenotype		
Smooth muscle α-actin	Positive	Negative
Collagen types I and III	Positive	Negative
Proinflammatory mediators (cytokines, autacoids, enzymes)	Increased	Low
Proliferative phenotype		
Proliferation markers (proliferating cell nuclear antigen, Ki67, etc.)	Increased	Low
Uptake of [^{3}H]thymidine, bromodeoxyuridine	Increased	Low
Immediate early genes	Increased	Low
Apoptotic phenotype		
TUNEL (terminal deoxynucleotidyl transferase-mediated dUTP-biotin nick end labeling)	Increased	Low
Bax, bcl2, p53	Increased	Low

erative state of MCs can be assessed by immunohistochemical staining for nuclear protein markers, such as proliferating cell nuclear antigen, Ki67, cyclins, and cyclin-dependent kinases. Enzymes and transcription factors that are relevant in postreceptor transduction of mitogenic signals can be demonstrated on the mRNA and protein levels (for example, PKC isoforms, MAPKs, and immediate early genes). Indicators and regulators of apoptosis (for example, Fas ligand, Bcl-2, and Bax proteins) are also being studied, as are suppressor proteins, for example, retinoblastoma gene product and cyclin-dependent kinase inhibitors. These investigations of the mesangium in renal tissue sections also concern gene expression, synthesis, and release of soluble regulators, such as enzymes, cytokines (notably PDGF, TGFβ, IL-1, and chemokines) and their receptors, matrix components, and β_1-integrins. Most of these analytic procedures on renal tissue are currently being used as research tools. They need further evaluation before being introduced into routine histopathology of small samples of renal tissue obtained by renal biopsy in order to yield reliable and meaningful new information on the pathobiology of MCs and ECM in human glomerular disease.

12. Gene Transfer to Mesangial Cells and Prospects for Gene Therapy

Currently, in the early phase of the gene therapy era, several attempts are being made to achieve kidney-targeted expression of foreign genes. Here, we briefly discuss some of these results as well as future perspectives, with special emphasis on the glomerular mesangium.

There are two main concepts of gene therapy: germline gene therapy aimed at altering reproductive cells, and somatic gene therapy targeted at somatic tissue, for example, the kidney. Because the kidney is an organ with a very low mitotic index, it is not well suited for gene transfer techniques relying on replicating cells, for example, use of retroviral vectors. In recent years, however, several methods for somatic gene transfer have been developed that are applicable to the kidney (177). Delivery of a gene can be achieved either in vivo, where the gene is introduced to the body by a special vehicle (virus, liposomes, or direct injection) or by ex vivo means, where cells are genetically modified outside the body and are then reintroduced into the host. In fact, both routes have been used successfully in the kidney. By in vivo gene transfer, Zhu et al. efficiently transfected virtually all tissues in mice with a single intravenous injection of chloramphenitol acetyl transferase expression plasmid–cationic liposome complexes (178). High expression was found in the kidney but was confined to its vascular compartment. By a modification of the liposome method [liposomes containing DNA were incubated with inactivated hemagglutinating virus of Japan (HVJ) to form HVJ liposomes], Tomita et al. selectively transferred the SV40 T antigen via an aortic catheter into glomerular mesangial and endothelial cells without expressing the gene in other tissues (179). However, expression only lasted for several days. The reason for glomerulus-specific gene expression by this method is not clear, but one possible explanation is that the phagocytic activity of glomerular MCs facilitated uptake of HVJ liposomes. Using this method, Isaka et al. transfected glomeruli in vivo with the TGFβ or PDGF B genes (180). The introduction of either the TGFβ or the PDGF B gene led to glomerulosclerosis. Interestingly, TGFβ affected ECM accumulation rather than glomerular cell proliferation and PDGF affected the latter rather than the former. Finally, Chang et al. showed that MCs, at least in vitro, are susceptible to adenovirus-mediated gene transfer (181). It needs to be established whether this observation holds true in vivo. An ex vivo somatic gene transfer technique to the kidney of rats was developed by Kitamura and colleagues, who used primary cultures of MCs as the vehicle (182). In initial experiments, MCs were stably transfected in vitro with the β-galactosidase gene and injected into the renal artery.

MCs localized to 57% of glomeruli remaining either in glomerular capillaries or repopulating the mesangial area. This led to sustained expression of the β-galactosidase gene in the mesangium for at least 4 weeks. These findings were extended by experiments introducing transfected MCs into kidneys of rats subjected to anti-Thy-1.1 antibodies that elicited mesangiolysis followed by transient MC proliferation and regeneration. Expression of β-galactosidase was amplified up to tenfold and lasted for at least 8 weeks. This approach was used to elucidate the in vivo function of TGFβ (Kitamura et al., 13th International Congress of Nephrology, Madrid, 1995, p. 71). TGFβ cDNA, modified to facilitate the secretion of active TGFβ, was introduced into cultured MCs. When these cells were transferred into rats with anti-Thy-1.1 nephritis, glomerular cell proliferation was significantly reduced.

In the future, further developments and refinements of gene transfer will be needed, with special considerations regarding safety, efficiency, duration, and regulation of gene expression. For certain purposes, low-efficiency gene transfer may suffice whereas, for others, transfer to a high percentage of target cells will be necessary. Short duration of expression may be sufficient or even desirable for some reasons (acute illnesses, for example, rapid progressive glomerulonephritis and acute tubular necrosis) whereas, in other instances, prolonged expression is preferable (for example, chronic glomerulonephritis). Moreover, future studies have to address the issue of regulated and cell-type specific expression, for example, by incorporating cis-acting elements active in the target cell. For MC-directed gene transfer, this will require the identification of MC-specific, transcriptionally regulated genes and characterization of cis-acting elements responsible for MC-specific expression. No such genes are currently known.

At present, one can only speculate about possible applications of gene transfer targeted to the mesangium. Some forms of acute glomerulonephritis are characterized by an initial exudative, inflammatory phase and, in animal models, it was shown that monocyte-macrophages contribute to MC proliferation and subsequent matrix buildup. Because MCs are the source of chemokines, such as RANTES, IL-8, or MCP-1, gene therapy could aim at inhibiting production of these chemoattractants for recruitment of inflammatory cells. Alternatively, because MCs can express cell adhesion molecules (for example, ICAM-1), prevention of the adhesion of inflammatory cells to MCs could be inhibited. By blocking induction of MHC class II antigen expression, the antigen-presenting function of MCs might be abolished. Another approach could be the interference of MC proliferation. This may be achieved by overexpressing growth inhibitory factors (for example, TGFβ) or by eliminating autocrine growth-promoting factors (for instance, PDGF or others), for example, by transfer of antisense oligonucleotides. Additionally, intracellular factors linked to mitogenesis could be targeted. As antisense experiments with cultured MCs have shown, the transcription factor Egr-1 is a necessary component of the mitogenic signaling cascade in MCs and, thus, might be a candidate gene for this approach (see section 7) (110). Alternatively, one could attempt to increase the rate of apoptosis in hypercellular glomeruli by introducing proapoptotic genes. In more chronic stages of glomerular disease, one could envision experiments to interfere at the level of matrix buildup (for example, overexpression of matrix proteases or blocking of their inhibitors).

In addition to these potential therapeutic applications, gene transfer provides nephrologists with a new research tool. It can be employed in studies aimed at overexpressing a single gene or eliminating a gene by transfer of antisense constructs to affect normal glomerular biology or to influence the course of experimental glomerular diseases. Such studies should facilitate determining whether gene transfer to the human kidney is desirable as well as achievable.

REFERENCES

1. Zimmermann KW. Über den Bau des Glomerulus der menschlichen Niere. *Z Mikrosk Anat Forsch* 1929;18:520–52.
2. Zimmermann KW. Über den Bau des Glomerulus der Säugetiere: Weitere Mitteilungen. *Z Mikrosk Anat Forsch* 1933;32:176–277.
3. von Möllendorf W. Der Exkretionsapparat. In: von Möllendorf W, ed. *Handbuch der Mikroskopischen Anatomie des Menschen;* vol 7: *Harn- und Geschlechtsapparat.* Berlin: Springer, 1930:34–64.
4. MacCallum WG. Glomerular changes in nephritis. *Bull Johns Hopkins Hosp* 1934;55:416–32.
5. Kimmelstiel P, Wilson C. Intercapillary lesions in the glomeruli of the kidney. *Am J Pathol* 1936;12:83–105.
6. Latta H. An approach to the structure and function of the glomerular mesangium. *J Am Soc Nephrol* 1992;2:S65–73.
7. Latta H, Maunsbach AB, Madden SC. The centrolobular region of the renal glomerulus studied by electron microscopy. *J Ultrastruct Res* 1960;4:455–72.
8. Farquhar MG, Palade GE. Glomerular permeability. II. Ferritin transfer across the glomerular capillary wall in nephrotic rats. *J Exp Med* 1961;144:699–715.
9. Kriz W, Elger M, Lemley K, Sakai T. Structure of the glomerular mesangium: a biomechanical interpretation. *Kidney Int* 1990;3(Suppl 30):S2–9.
10. Drenckhahn D, Schnittler H, Nobiling R, Kriz W. Ultrastructural organization of contractile proteins in rat glomerular mesangial cells. *Am J Pathol* 1990;137:1343–51.
11. Kashgarian M, Sterzel RB. The pathobiology of the mesangium. *Kidney Int* 1992;41:524–9.
12. Mené P, Simonson MS, Dunn MJ. Physiology of the mesangial cell. *Physiol Rev* 1989;69:1347–424.
13. Schlondorff D. The glomerular mesangial cell: an expanding role for a specialized pericyte. *FASEB J* 1987;1:272–81.
14. Sterzel RB, Lovett DH, Stein HD, Kashgarian M. The mesangium and glomerulonephritis. *Klin Wochenschr* 1982;60:1077–94.
15. Michael AF, Keane WF, Raij L, Vernier RL, Mauer SM. The glomerular mesangium. *Kidney Int* 1980;17:141–54.
16. Yamanaka N. Development of the glomerular mesangium. *Pediatr Nephrol* 1988;2:85–91.
17. Sorokin L, Ekblom P. Development of tubular and glomerular cells of the kidney. *Kidney Int* 1992;41:657–64.
18. Pinson Hyink D, St John PL, Abrahamson DR. Endogenous, not endogenous, origin of glomerular vasculature in fetal kidney grafts. *J Am Soc Nephrol* 1995;6:697.

19. Leveen P, Pekny M, Gebre Medhin S, Swolin B, Larsson E, Betsholtz C. Mice deficient for PDGF B show renal, cardiovascular, and hematological abnormalities. *Genes Dev* 1994;8:1875–87.
20. Soriano P. Abnormal kidney development and hematological disorders in PDGF beta-receptor mutant mice. *Genes Dev* 1994;8:1888-96.
21. Johnson RJ, Iida H, Alpers CE, et al. Expression of smooth muscle cell phenotype by rat mesangial cells in immune complex nephritis: alpha-smooth muscle actin is a marker of mesangial cell proliferation. *J Clin Invest* 1991;87:847–58.
22. Floege J, Johnson RJ, Gordon K, et al. Increased synthesis of extracellular matrix in mesangial proliferative nephritis. *Kidney Int* 1991;40:477–88.
23. Johnson RJ, Floege J, Yoshimura A, Iida H, Couser WG, Alpers CE. The activated mesangial cell: a glomerular "myofibroblast"? *J Am Soc Nephrol* 1992;2:S190–7.
24. Olivetti G, Anversa P, Melissari M, Loud A. Morphometry of the renal corpuscle during postnatal growth and compensatory hypertrophy. *Kidney Int* 1980;17:438–54.
25. Pabst R, Sterzel RB. Cell renewal of glomerular cell types in normal rats: an autoradiographic analysis. *Kidney Int* 1983;24:626–31.
26. Schreiner GF, Kiely J-M, Cotran RS, Unanue ER. Characterization of resident glomerular cells in the rat expressing Ia determinants and manifesting genetically restricted interactions with lymphocytes. *J Clin Invest* 1981;68:920–31.
27. Sraer JD, Adida C, Peraldi MN, Rondeau E, Kanfer A. Species-specific properties of the glomerular mesangium. *J Am Soc Nephrol* 1993;3:1342–50.
28. Courtoy PJ, Kanwar YS, Hynes RO, Farquhar MG. Fibronectin localization in the rat glomerulus. *J Cell Biol* 1980;87:691–6.
29. Barnes JL, Hevey KA. Glomerular mesangial cell migration in response to platelet-derived growth factor. *Lab Invest* 1990;62: 379–82.
30. Lee S, Vernier RL. Immunoelectron microscopy of the glomerular mesangial uptake and transport of aggregated human albumin in the mouse. *Lab Invest* 1980;42:44–58.
31. Leiper JM, Thomson D, MacDonald MK. Uptake and transport of Imposil by the glomerular mesangium in the mouse. *Lab Invest* 1977;37:526–33.
32. Mancilla Jimenez R, Bellon B, Kuhn J, et al. Phagocytosis of heat-aggregated immunoglobulins by mesangial cells: an immunoperoxidase and acid phosphatase study. *Lab Invest* 1982;46:243–53.
33. Sterzel RB, Perfetto M, Biemesderfer D, Kashgarian M. Disposal of ferritin in the glomerular mesangium of rats. *Kidney Int* 1983; 23:480–8.
34. Baud L, Hagege J, Sraer J, Rondeau E, Perez J, Ardaillou R. Reactive oxygen production by cultured rat glomerular mesangial cells during phagocytosis is associated with stimulation of lipoxygenase activity. *J Exp Med* 1983;158:1836–52.
35. Neuwirth R, Singhal P, Diamond B, et al. Evidence for immunoglobulin Fc receptor-mediated prostaglandin 2 and platelet-activating factor formation by cultured rat mesangial cells. *J Clin Invest* 1988;82: 936–44.
36. Santiago A, Mori T, Satriano J, Schlondorff D. Regulation of Fc receptors for IgG on cultured rat mesangial cells. *Kidney Int* 1991; 39:87–94.
37. Singhal PC, Santiago A, Satriano J, Hays RM, Schlondorff D. Effects of vasoactive agents on uptake of immunoglobulin G complexes by mesangial cells. *Am J Physiol* 1990;258:F589–96.
38. Stein HD, Feddergreen W, Kashgarian M, Sterzel RB. Role of angiotensin II-induced renal functional changes in mesangial deposition of exogenous ferritin in rats. *Lab Invest* 1983;49:270–80.
39. Baker AJ, Mooney A, Hughes J, Lombardi D, Johnson RJ, Savill J. Mesangial cell apoptosis: the major mechanism for resolution of glomerular hypercellularity in experimental mesangial proliferative nephritis. *J Clin Invest* 1994;94:2105–16.
40. Davies M. The mesangial cell: a tissue culture view. *Kidney Int* 1994; 45:320–7.
41. Lovett DH, Sterzel RB. Cell culture approaches to the analysis of glomerular inflammation. *Kidney Int* 1986;30:246–54.
42. Holthöfer H, Sainio K, Miettinen A. The glomerular mesangium: studies of its developmental origin and markers in vivo and in vitro. *APMIS* 1995;103:354–66.
43. Kreisberg JI, Karnovsky MJ. Characterization of rat glomerular cells in vitro. In: Cummings NB, Michael AE, Wilson CB, eds. *Immune mechanism in renal disease.* New York: Plenum, 1983:189–200.
44. Sterzel RB, Lovett DH, Foellmer HG, Perfetto M, Biemesderfer D, Kashgarian M. Mesangial cell hillocks: nodular foci of exaggerated growth of cells and matrix in prolonged culture. *Am J Pathol* 1986; 125:130–40.
45. Floege J, Burns MW, Alpers CE, et al. Glomerular cell proliferation and PDGF expression precede glomerulosclerosis in the remnant kidney model. *Kidney Int* 1992;41:297–309.
46. Johnson RJ, Alpers CE, Yoshimura A, et al. Renal injury from angiotensin II-mediated hypertension. *Hypertension* 1992;19:464–74.
47. Abrass CK, Peterson CV, Raugi GJ. Phenotypic expression of collagen types in mesangial matrix of diabetic and nondiabetic rats. *Diabetes* 1988;37:1695–702.
48. Haralson MA, Jacobson HR, Hoover RL. Collagen polymorphism in cultured rat kidney mesangial cells. *Lab Invest* 1987;57:513–23.
49. Striker LJ, Killen PD, Chi E, Striker GE. The composition of glomerulosclerosis. I. Studies in focal sclerosis, crescentic glomerulonephritis, and membranoproliferative glomerulonephritis. *Lab Invest* 1984;51: 181–92.
50. Floege J, Alpers CE, Burns MW, et al. Glomerular cells, extracellular matrix accumulation, and the development of glomerulosclerosis in the remnant kidney model. *Lab Invest* 1992;66:485–97.
51. Floege J, Eng E, Young BA, Johnson RJ. Factors involved in the regulation of mesangial cell proliferation in vitro and in vivo. *Kidney Int Suppl* 1993;39:S47–54.
52. Harris RC, Akai Y, Yasuda T, Homma T. The role of physical forces in alterations of mesangial cell function. *Kidney Int* 1994;45(Suppl 45):S17–21.
53. Banes AJ, Gilbert J, Taylor D, Monabreau O. A new vacuum-operated stress-providing instrument that applies static or variable duration cyclic tension or compression to cells invitro. *J Cell Sci* 1985;75:35–43.
54. Marti HP, Lee L, Kashgarian M, Lovett DH. Transforming growth factor-beta 1 stimulates glomerular mesangial cell synthesis of the 72-kd type IV collagenase. *Am J Pathol* 1994;144:82–94.
55. Coritsidis G, Rifici V, Gupta S, et al. Preferential binding of oxidized LDL to rat glomeruli in vivo and cultured mesangial cells in vitro. *Kidney Int* 1991;39:858–66.
56. Gröne EF, Abboud HE, Hohne M, et al. Actions of lipoproteins in cultured human mesangial cells: modulation by mitogenic vasoconstrictors. *Am J Physiol* 1992;263:F686–96.
57. Ray PE, Aguilera G, Kopp JB, Horikoshi S, Klotman PE. Angiotensin II receptor-mediated proliferation of cultured human fetal mesangial cells. *Kidney Int* 1991;40:764–71.
58. Marx M, Daniel TO, Kashgarian M, Madri JA. Spatial organization of the extracellular matrix modulates the expression of PDGF-receptor subunits in mesangial cells. *Kidney Int* 1993;43:1027–41.
59. Yaoita E. Behavior of rat mesangial cells cultured within extracellular matrix. *Lab Invest* 1989;61:410–8.
60. van den Dobbelsteen ME, van der Woude FJ, Schroeijers WE, Klar Mohamad N, van Es LA, Daha MR. C1Q, a subunit of the first component of complement, enhances the binding of aggregated IgG to rat renal mesangial cells. *J Immunol* 1993;151:4315–24.
61. Lovett DH, Haensch GM, Goppelt M, Resch K, Gemsa D. Activation of glomerular mesangial cells by the terminal membrane attack complex of complement. *J Immunol* 1987;138:2473–80.
62. Hansch GM, Schieren G, Wagner C, Schonermark M. Immune damage to the mesangium: antibody- and complement-mediated stimulation and destruction of mesangial cells. *J Am Soc Nephrol* 1992;2: S139–43.
63. Adler S, Baker PJ, Johnson RJ, Ochi RF, Pritzl P, Couser WG. Complement membrane attack complex stimulates production of reactive oxygen metabolites by cultured rat mesangial cells. *J Clin Invest* 1986;77:762–7.
64. Abe K, Miyazaki M, Furusu A, et al. Intraglomerular C3 synthesis and its activation in IgA nephropathy. *J Am Soc Nephrol* 1995;6:917
65. van den Dobbelsteen ME, Verhasselt V, Kaashoek JG, et al. Regulation of C3 and factor H synthesis of human glomerular mesangial cells by IL-1 and interferon-gamma. *Clin Exp Immunol* 1994;95: 173–80.
66. Lovett DH, Ryan JL, Sterzel RB. Stimulation of rat mesangial cell proliferation by macrophage interleukin 1. *J Immunol* 1983;131:2830–6.
67. Horii Y, Muraguchi A, Iwano M, et al. Involvement of IL-6 in mesangial proliferative glomerulonephritis. *J Immunol* 1989;143:3949–55.
68. Martin M, Schwinzer R, Schellekens H, Resch K. Glomerular mesangial cells in local inflammation: induction of the expression of MHC class II antigens by IFN-gamma. *J Immunol* 1989;142:1887–94.

69. Brennan DC, Jevnikar AM, Takei F, Reubin Kelley VE. Mesangial cell accessory functions: mediation by intercellular adhesion molecule-1. *Kidney Int* 1990;38:1039–46.
70. Brennan DC, Yui MA, Wuthrich RP, Kelley VE. Tumor necrosis factor and IL-1 in New Zealand Black/White mice: enhanced gene expression and acceleration of renal injury. *J Immunol* 1989;143: 3470–5.
71. Radeke HH, Resch K. The inflammatory function of renal glomerular mesangial cells and their interaction with the cellular immune system. *Clin Invest* 1992;70:825–42.
72. Sterzel RB, Lovett DH. Interactions of inflammatory and glomerular cells in the response to glomerular injury. In: Wilson C, ed. *Immunopathology of renal disease.* New York: Churchill Livingstone, 1988:137–73.
73. Cattell V, Bradfield JW. Focal mesangial proliferative glomerulonephritis in the rat caused by habu snake venom: a morphologic study.*Am J Pathol* 1977;87:511–24.
74. Bagchus WM, Hoedemaeker PJ, Rozing J, Bakker WW. Glomerulonephritis induced by monoclonal anti-Thy 1.1 antibodies: a sequential histological and ultrastructural study in the rat. *Lab Invest* 1986;55:680–7.
75. Morita T, Churg J. Mesangiolysis. *Kidney Int* 1983;24:1–9.
76. Stout LC, Kumar S, Whorton EB. Focal mesangiolysis and the pathogenesis of the Kimmelstiel–Wilson nodule. *Hum Pathol* 1993;24: 77–89.
77. Couchman JR, Beavan LA, McCarthy KJ. Glomerular matrix: synthesis, turnover and role in mesangial expansion. *Kidney Int* 1994;45:328–35.
78. Davies M, Thomas GJ, Shewring LD, Mason RM. Mesangial cell proteoglycans: synthesis and metabolism. *J Am Soc Nephrol* 1992;2: S88–94.
79. Sterzel RB, Schulze-Lohoff E, Weber M, Goodman SL. Interactions between glomerular mesangial cells, cytokines, and extracellular matrix. *J Am Soc Nephrol* 1992;2:S126–31.
80. Okuda S, Languino LR, Ruoslahti E, Border WA. Elevated expression of transforming growth factor-beta and proteoglycan production in experimental glomerulonephritis: possible role in expansion of the mesangial extracellular matrix. *J Clin Invest* 1990;86:453–62.
81. Fioretto P, Keane WF, Kasiske BL, O'Donnell MP, Klein DJ. Alterations in glomerular proteoglycan metabolism in experimental non-insulin dependent diabetes mellitus. *J Am Soc Nephrol* 1993;3: 1694–704.
82. Ebihara I, Suzuki S, Nakamura T, et al. Extracellular matrix component mRNA expression in glomeruli in experimental focal glomerulosclerosis. *J Am Soc Nephrol* 1993;3:1387–97.
83. Marti HP, McNeil L, Davies M, Martin J, Lovett DH. Homology cloning of rat 72 kDa type IV collagenase: cytokine and second-messenger inducibility in glomerular mesangial cells. *Biochem J* 1993; 291:441–6.
84. Marti HP, McNeil L, Thomas G, Davies M, Lovett DH. Molecular characterization of a low-molecular-mass matrix metalloproteinase secreted by glomerular mesangial cells as PUMP-1. *Biochem J* 1992;285:899–905.
85. Lovett DH, Johnson RJ, Marti HP, Martin J, Davies M, Couser WG. Structural characterization of the mesangial cell type IV collagenase and enhanced expression in a model of immune complex-mediated glomerulonephritis. *Am J Pathol* 1992;141:85–98.
86. Tomooka S, Border WA, Marshall BC, Noble NA. Glomerular matrix accumulation is linked to inhibition of the plasmin protease system. *Kidney Int* 1992;42:1462–9.
87. Pesce CM, Striker LJ, Peten E, Elliot SJ, Striker GE. Glomerulosclerosis at both early and late stages is associated with increased cell turnover in mice transgenic for growth hormone. *Lab Invest* 1991;65: 601–5.
88. Striker LJ, Peten EP, Elliot SJ, Doi T, Striker GE. Mesangial cell turnover: effect of heparin and peptide growth factors. *Lab Invest* 1991;64:446–56.
89. Floege J, Eng E, Young BA, Couser WG, Johnson RJ. Heparin suppresses mesangial cell proliferation and matrix expansion in experimental mesangioproliferative glomerulonephritis. *Kidney Int* 1993;43:369–80.
90. Fukui M, Nakamura T, Ebihara I, Nagaoka I, Tomino Y, Koide H. Low-protein diet attenuates increased gene expression of platelet-derived growth factor and transforming growth factor-beta in experimental glomerular sclerosis. *J Lab Clin Med* 1993;121:224–34.
91. Johnson RJ, Raines EW, Floege J, et al. Inhibition of mesangial cell proliferation and matrix expansion in glomerulonephritis in the rat by antibody to platelet-derived growth factor. *J Exp Med* 1992;175: 1413–6.
92. Pugliese F, Ferrario RG, Ciavolella A, et al. Growth abnormalities in cultured mesangial cells from rats with spontaneous glomerulosclerosis. *Kidney Int* 1995;47:106–13.
93. Ayo SH, Radnik RA, Glass WF, et al. Increased extracellular matrix synthesis and mRNA in mesangial cells grown in high-glucose medium. *Am J Physiol* 1991;260:F185–91.
94. Nahman NS Jr, Leonhart KL, Cosio FG, Hebert CL. Effects of high glucose on cellular proliferation and fibronectin production by cultured human mesangial cells. *Kidney Int* 1992;41:396–402.
95. Wakisaka M, Spiro MJ, Spiro RG. Synthesis of type VI collagen by cultured glomerular cells and comparison of its regulation by glucose and other factors with that of type IV collagen. *Diabetes* 1994;43: 95–103.
96. Cosio FG. Effects of high glucose concentrations on human mesangial cell proliferation. *J Am Soc Nephrol* 1995;5:1600–9.
97. Huwiler A, Schulze-Lohoff E, Fabbro D, Pfeilschifter J. Immunocharacterization of protein kinase C isoenzymes in rat kidney glomeruli, and cultured glomerular epithelial and mesangial cells. *Exp Nephrol* 1993;1:19–25.
98. Rupprecht HD, Sukhatme VP, Lacy J, Sterzel RB, Coleman DL. PDGF-induced Egr-1 expression in rat mesangial cells is mediated through upstream serum response elements. *Am J Physiol* 1993;265: F351–60.
99. Rupprecht HD, Dann P, Sukhatme VP, Sterzel RB, Coleman DL. Effect of vasoactive agents on induction of Egr-1 in rat mesangial cells: correlation with mitogenicity. *Am J Physiol* 1992;263:F623–36.
100. Ganz MB, Pekar SK, Perfetto MC, Sterzel RB. Arginine vasopressin promotes growth of rat glomerular mesangial cells in culture. *Am J Physiol* 1988;255:F898–906.
101. Simonson MS, Herman WH. Protein kinase C and protein tyrosine kinase activity contribute to mitogenic signaling by endothelin-1: cross-talk between G protein-coupled receptors and pp60c-src. *J Biol Chem* 1993;268:9347–57.
102. Kester M, Simonson MS, McDermott RG, Baldi E, Dunn MJ. Endothelin stimulates phosphatidic acid formation in cultured rat mesangial cells: role of a protein kinase C-regulated phospholipase D. *J Cell Physiol* 1992;150:578–85.
103. Sellmayer A, Uedelhoven WM, Weber PC, Bonventre JV. Endogenous non-cyclooxygenase metabolites of arachidonic acid modulate growth and mRNA levels of immediate-early response genes in rat mesangial cells. *J Biol Chem* 1991;266:3800–7.
104. Ishikawa S, Kawasumi M, Saito T. Simvastatin inhibits the cellular signaling and proliferative action of arginine vasopressin in cultured rat glomerular mesangial cells. *Endocrinology* 1995;136:1954–61.
105. Li X, Schrier RW, Nemenoff RA. Inhibition of growth factor stimulation of mitogen-activated protein kinase by prostaglandin E_2 in rat renal mesangial cells. *Chung Hua I Hsueh Tsa Chih* 1995;75:207–10.
106. Wang Y, Simonson MS, Pouyssegur J, Dunn MJ. Endothelin rapidly stimulates mitogen-activated protein kinase activity in rat mesangial cells. *Biochem J* 1992;287:589–94.
107. Herman WH, Simonson MS. Nuclear signaling by endothelin-1: a Ras pathway for activation of the c-fos serum response element. *J Biol Chem* 1995;270:11,654–61.
108. Hipskind RA, Büscher D, Nordheim A, Baccarini M. Ras/MAP kinase-dependent and -independent signaling pathways target distinct ternary complex factors. *Genes Dev* 1994;8:1803–16.
109. Rupprecht HD, Sukhatme VP, Rupprecht AP, Sterzel RB, Coleman DL. Serum response elements mediate protein kinase C dependent transcriptional induction of early growth response gene-1 by arginine vasopressin in rat mesangial cells. *J Cell Physiol* 1994;159:311–23.
110. Rupprecht HD, Hofer G, Faller G, Sterzel RB, de Heer E, Schöcklmann HO. Expression of the transcriptional regulator Egr-1 in experimental nephritis: correlation with mesangial cell proliferation. *J Am Soc Nephrol* 1995;6:882.
111. Kreisberg JI, Venkatachalam M, Troyer D. Contractile properties of cultured glomerular mesangial cells. *Am J Physiol* 1985;249:F457–63.
112. Kremer SG, Zeng W, Hurst R, Ning T, Whiteside C, Skorecki KL. Chloride is required for receptor-mediated divalent cation entry in mesangial cells. *J Cell Physiol* 1995;162:15–25.
113. Rasmussen H, Takuwa Y, Park S. Protein kinase C in the regulation of smooth muscle contraction. *FASEB J* 1987;1:177–85.

114. Troyer DA, Gonzalez OF, Douglas JG, Kreisberg JI. Phorbol ester inhibits arginine vasopressin activation of phospholipase C and promotes contraction of, and prostaglandin production by, cultured mesangial cells. *Biochem J* 1988;251:907–12.
115. Mene P, Simonson MS, Dunn MJ. Eicosanoids, mesangial contraction, and intracellular signal transduction. *Tohoku J Exp Med* 1992; 166:57–73.
116. Mené P, Dunn MJ. Eicosanoids and control of mesangial cell contraction. *Circ Res* 1988;62:916–25.
117. Appel RG, Wang J, Simonson MS, Dunn MJ. A mechanism by which atrial natriuretic factor mediates its glomerular actions. *Am J Physiol* 1986;251:F1036–42.
118. Singhal PC, Scharschmidt LA, Gibbons N, Hays RM. Contraction and relaxation of cultured mesangial cells on a silicone rubber surface. *Kidney Int* 1986;30:862–73.
119. Albelda SM, Buck CA. Integrins and other cell adhesion molecules. *FASEB J* 1990;4:2868–80.
120. Adler S. Integrin matrix receptors in renal injury. *Kidney Int Suppl* 1994;45:S86–9.
121. Korhonen M, Laitinen L, Ylanne J, Gould VE, Virtanen I. Integrins in developing, normal and malignant human kidney. *Kidney Int* 1992; 41:641–4.
122. Woods A, Couchman JR. Syndecan 4 heparan sulfate proteoglycan is a selectively enriched and widespread focal adhesion component. *Mol Biol Cell* 1994;5:183–92.
123. Juliano RL, Haskill S. Signal transduction from the extracellular matrix. *J Cell Biol* 1993;120:577–85.
124. Ruoslahti E, Noble NA, Kagami S, Border WA. Integrins. *Kidney Int Suppl* 1994;44:S17–22.
125. Petermann A, Fees H, Grenz H, Goodman SL, Sterzel RB. Polymerase chain reaction and focal contact formation indicate integrin expression in mesangial cells. *Kidney Int* 1993;44:997–1005.
126. Cosio FG, Sedmak DD, Nahman NSJ. Cellular receptors for matrix proteins in normal human kidney and human mesangial cells. *Kidney Int* 1990;38:886–95.
127. Adler S. Integrin receptors in the glomerulus: potential role in glomerular injury [Editorial]. *Am J Physiol* 1992;262:F697–704.
128. Grenz H, Carbonetto S, Goodman SL. Alpha 3 beta 1 integrin is moved into focal contacts in kidney mesangial cells. *J Cell Sci* 1993;105:739–51.
129. Couchman JR, Woods A. Transmembrane signaling generated by cell–extracellular matrix interactions. *Kidney Int Suppl* 1995;47: S8–11.
130. Hanks SK, Calalb MB, Harper MC, Patel SK. Focal adhesion protein-tyrosine kinase phosphorylated in response to cell attachment to fibronectin. *Proc Natl Acad Sci USA* 1992;89:8487–91.
131. Parsons JT, Schaller MD, Hildebrand J, Leu TH, Richardson A, Otey C. Focal adhesion kinase: structure and signalling. *J Cell Sci Suppl* 1994;18:109–13.
132. Kondo S, Homma T, Yasuda T, Harris RC. Mechanical stretch augments angiotensin II induced tyrosine phosphorylation of p125FAK and paxillin in rat mesangial cells. *J Am Soc Nephrol* 1995;6:798
133. Josepevitz C, Nord EP. Endothelin stimulates tyrosine phosphorylation of focal adhesion kinase and association with paxillin in mesangial cells. *J Am Soc Nephrol* 1995;6:795.
134. Schlaepfer DD, Hanks SK, Hunter T, van der Geer P. Integrin-mediated signal transduction linked to Ras pathway by GRB2 binding to focal adhesion kinase. *Nature* 1994;372:786–91.
135. Chen HC, Guan JL. Association of focal adhesion kinase with its potential substrate phosphatidylinositol 3-kinase. *Proc Natl Acad Sci USA* 1994;91:10,148–52.
136. Qwarnstrom EE, Ostberg CO, Turk GL, Richardson CA, Bomsztyk K. Fibronectin attachment activates the NF-kappa B p50/p65 heterodimer in fibroblasts and smooth muscle cells. *J Biol Chem* 1994;269:30,765–8.
137. Rosenblum ND. The mesangial matrix in the normal and sclerotic glomerulus. *Kidney Int Suppl* 1994;45:S73–7.
138. Riser BL, Cortes P, Zhao X, Bernstein J, Dumler F, Narins RG. Intraglomerular pressure and mesangial stretching stimulate extracellular matrix formation in the rat. *J Clin Invest* 1992;90:1932–43.
139. Sage EH, Bornstein P. Extracellular proteins that modulate cell–matrix interactions: SPARC, tenascin, and thrombospondin. *J Biol Chem* 1991;266:14,831–4.
140. Lane TF, Sage EH. The biology of SPARC, a protein that modulates cell–matrix interactions. *FASEB J* 1994;8:163–73.
141. Truong LD, Pindur J, Barrios R, et al. Tenascin is an important component of the glomerular extracellular matrix in normal and pathologic conditions. *Kidney Int* 1994;45:201–10.
142. Clark EA, Brugge JS. Integrins and signal transduction pathways: the road taken. *Science* 1995;268:233–9.
143. Bruijn JA, de Heer E. Adhesion molecules in renal diseases. *Lab Invest* 1995;72:387–94.
144. Ihm CG, Park JK, Ahn JH, Lee TW, Cho BS, Kim MJ. Effect of glucose and cytokines on the expression of cell adhesion molecules on mesangial cells. *Kidney Int* 1995;48:S39–42.
145. Ishimura E, Sterzel RB, Budde K, Kashgarian M. Formation of extracellular matrix by cultured rat mesangial cells. *Am J Pathol* 1989;134: 843–55.
146. Simonson MS, Culp LA, Dunn MJ. Rat mesangial cell–matrix interactions in culture. *Exp Cell Res* 1989;184:484–98.
147. Marinides GN, Suchard SJ, Mookerjee BK. Role of thrombospondin in mesangial cell growth: possible existence of an autocrine feedback growth circuit. *Kidney Int* 1994;46:350–7.
148. Gauer S, Schulze-Lohoff E, Schleicher E, Sterzel RB. Glomerular basement membrane derived perlecan inhibits mesangial cell adhesion to fibronectin. *Eur J Cell Biol* 1996;70:233–242.
149. Groggel GC, Marinides GN, Hovingh P, Hammond E, Linker A. Inhibition of rat mesangial cell growth by heparan sulfate. *Am J Physiol* 1990;258:F259–65.
150. Caenazzo C, Garbisa S, Ceol M, et al. Heparin modulates proliferation and proteoglycan biosynthesis in murine mesangial cells: molecular clues for its activity in nephropathy. *Nephrol Dial Transplant* 1995;10:175–84.
151. Border WA, Okuda S, Languino LR, Ruoslahti E. Transforming growth factor-beta regulates production of proteoglycans by mesangial cells. *Kidney Int* 1990;37:689–95.
152. Saksela O, Rifkin DB. Release of basic fibroblast growth factor–heparan sulfate complexes from endothelial cells by plasminogen activator-mediated proteolytic activity. *J Cell Biol* 1990;110: 767–75.
153. Floege J, Eng E, Lindner V, et al. Rat glomerular mesangial cells synthesize basic fibroblast growth factor: release, upregulated synthesis, and mitogenicity in mesangial proliferative glomerulonephritis. *J Clin Invest* 1992;90:2362–9.
154. Morita H, Shinzato T, David G, et al. Basic fibroblast growth factor-binding domain of heparan sulfate in the human glomerulosclerosis and renal tubulointerstitial fibrosis. *Lab Invest* 1994;71:528–35.
155. Zhang Z, Vuori K, Reed JC, Ruoslahti E. The $\alpha_5\beta_1$ integrin supports survival of cells on fibronectin and upregulates bcl-2 expression. *Proc Natl Acad Sci USA* 1995;92:6161–5.
156. Uchida K, Ballermann BJ. Sustained activation of PGE_2 synthesis in mesangial cells cocultured with glomerular endothelial cells. *Am J Physiol* 1992;263:C200–9.
157. Castellot JJ Jr, Hoover RL, Karnovsky MJ. Glomerular endothelial cells secrete a heparinlike inhibitor and a peptide stimulator of mesangial cell proliferation. *Am J Pathol* 1986;125:493–500.
158. Saeki T, Morioka T, Arakawa M, Shimizu F, Oite T. Modulation of mesangial cell proliferation by endothelial cells in coculture. *Am J Pathol* 1991;139:949–57.
159. Castellot JJ Jr, Hoover RL, Harper PA, Karnovsky MJ. Heparin and glomerular epithelial cell-secreted heparin-like species inhibit mesangial-cell proliferation. *Am J Pathol* 1985;120:427–35.
160. Johnson RJ, Alpers CE, Pruchno C, et al. Mechanisms and kinetics for platelet and neutrophil localization in immune complex nephritis. *Kidney Int* 1989;36:780–9.
161. Clark WF, Lewis ML, Cameron JS, Parsons V. Intrarenal platelet consumption in the diffuse proliferative nephritis of systemic lupus erythematosus. *Clin Sci Mol Med* 1975;49:247–52.
162. Cattell V. Focal mesangial proliferative glomerulonephritis in the rat caused by habu snake venom: the role of platelets. *Br J Exp Pathol* 1979;60:201–8.
163. Johnson RJ, Garcia RL, Pritzl P, Alpers CE. Platelets mediate glomerular cell proliferation in immune complex nephritis induced by anti-mesangial cell antibodies in the rat. *Am J Pathol* 1990;136: 369–74.
164. Cattell V, Mehotra A. Focal mesangial proliferative glomerulonephritis in the rat caused by habu venom: the effect of antiplatelet agents. *Br J Exp Pathol* 1980;61:310–4.
165. Stahl RA, Wolf G, Thaiss F. The possible role of chemotactic cytokines in renal disease. *Clin Invest* 1994;72:711–2.

166. Rovin BH, Rumancik M, Tan L, Dickerson J. Glomerular expression of monocyte chemoattractant protein-1 in experimental and human glomerulonephritis. *Lab Invest* 1994;71:536–42.
167. Tipping PG, Lowe MG, Holdsworth SR. Glomerular interleukin 1 production is dependent on macrophage infiltration in anti-GBM glomerulonephritis. *Kidney Int* 1991;39:103–10.
168. Matsumoto K, Hatano M. Effect of antimacrophage serum on the proliferation of glomerular cells in nephrotoxic serum nephritis in the rat. *J Clin Lab Immunol* 1989;28:39–44.
169. Mené P, Fais S, Cinotti GA, Pugliese F, Luttmann W, Thierauch K-H. Regulation of U-937 monocyte adhesion to cultured human mesangial cells by cytokines and vasoactive agents. *Nephrol Dial Transplant* 1995;10:481–9.
170. Alpers CE, Hudkins KL, Gown AM, Johnson RJ. Enhanced expression of "muscle-specific" actin in glomerulonephritis. *Kidney Int* 1992;41:1134–42.
171. Johnson RJ, Lombardi D, Eng E, et al. Modulation of experimental mesangial proliferative nephritis by interferon-gamma. *Kidney Int* 1995;47:62–9.
172. Harrison DJ. Cell death in the diseased glomerulus. *Histopathology* 1988;12:679–83.
173. Arends MJ, Harrison DJ. Novel histopathologic findings in a surviving case of hemolytic uremic syndrome after bone marrow transplantation. *Hum Pathol* 1989;20:89–91.
174. Savill J. Apoptosis and the kidney. *J Am Soc Nephrol* 1994;5:12–21.
175. Shimizu A, Kitamura H, Masuda Y, Ishizaki M, Sugisaki Y, Yamanaka N. Apoptosis in the repair process of experimental proliferative glomerulonephritis. *Kidney Int* 1995;47:114–21.
176. Takemura T, Murakami K, Miyazato H, Yagi K, Yoshioka K. Expression of Fas antigen and Bcl-2 in human glomerulonephritis. *Kidney Int* 1995;48:1886–92.
177. Sukhatme VP. Prospects for gene therapy in the kidney. In: Schlöndorff D, Bonventre JV, eds. *Molecular nephrology.* New York: Marcel Dekker, 1995:913–21.
178. Zhu N, Liggitt D, Liu Y, Debs R. Systemic gene expression after intravenous DNA delivery into adult mice. *Science* 1993;261:209–11.
179. Tomita N, Higaki J, Morishita R, et al. Direct in vivo gene introduction into rat kidney. *Biochem Biophys Res Commun* 1992;186:129–34.
180. Isaka Y, Fujiwara Y, Ueda N, Kaneda Y, Kamada T, Imai E. Glomerulosclerosis induced by in vivo transfection of transforming growth factor-beta or platelet-derived growth factor gene into the rat kidney. *J Clin Invest* 1993;92:2597–601.
181. Chang H, Katoh T, Noda M, et al. Highly efficient adenovirus-mediated gene transfer into renal cells in culture. *Kidney Int* 1995;47:322–6.
182. Kitamura M, Taylor S, Unwin R, Burton S, Shimizu F, Fine LG. Gene transfer into the rat renal glomerulus via a mesangial cell vector: site-specific delivery, in situ amplification, and sustained expression of an exogenous gene in vivo. *J Clin Invest* 1994;94:497–505.
183. Abboud HE. Growth factors and the mesangium. *J Am Soc Nephrol* 1992;2:S185–9.
184. Sterzel RB, Schulze-Lohoff E, Marx M. Cytokines and mesangial cells. *Kidney Int Suppl* 1993;39:S26–31.
185. Abboud HE, Poptic E, DiCorleto P. Production of platelet-derived growth factorlike protein by rat mesangial cells in culture. *J Clin Invest* 1987;80:675–83.
186. Abboud HE, Grandaliano G, Pinzani M, Knauss T, Pierce GF, Jaffer F. Actions of platelet-derived growth factor isoforms in mesangial cells. *J Cell Physiol* 1994;158:140–50.
187. Aron DC, Rosenzweig JL, Abboud HE. Synthesis and binding of insulin-like growth factor I by human glomerular mesangial cells. *J Clin Endocrinol Metab* 1989;68:585–91.
188. Wolf G, Sharma K, Chen Y, Ericksen M, Ziyadeh FN. High glucose-induced proliferation in mesangial cells is reversed by autocrine TGF-beta. *Kidney Int* 1992;42:647–56.
189. Kaname S, Uchida S, Ogata E, Kurokawa K. Autocrine secretion of transforming growth factor-β in cultured rat mesangial cells. *Kidney Int* 1992;42:1319–27.
190. Schlondorff D, Goldwasser P, Neuwirth R, Satriano JA, Clay KL. Production of platelet-activating factor in glomeruli and cultured glomerular mesangial cells. *Am J Physiol* 1986;250:F1123–7.
191. Steiner P, Pfeilschifter J, Boeckh C, Radeke HH, Otten U. Interleukin-1β and tumor necrosis factor-α synergistically stimulate nerve growth factor synthesis in rat mesangial cells. *Am J Physiol* 1991;261:F792–8.
192. Sedor JR, Carey SW, Emancipator SN. Immune complexes bind to cultured rat glomerular mesangial cells to stimulate superoxide release: evidence for an Fc receptor. *J Immunol* 1987;138:3751–7.
193. Budde K, Coleman DL, Lacy J, Sterzel RB. Rat mesangial cells produce granulocyte-macrophage colony-stimulating factor. *Am J Physiol* 1989;257:F1065–78.
194. Beck K-F, Mohaupt MG, Sterzel RB. Endothelin-1 inhibits cytokine-stimulated transcription of inducible nitric oxide synthase in glomerular mesangial cells. *Kidney Int* 1995;48:1893–9.
195. Baud L, Oudinet JP, Bens M, et al. Production of tumor necrosis factor by rat mesangial cells in response to bacterial lipopolysaccharide. *Kidney Int* 1989;35:1111–8.
196. Ruef C, Budde K, Lacy J, et al. Interleukin 6 is an autocrine growth factor for mesangial cells. *Kidney Int* 1990;38:249–57.
197. Zoja C, Orisio S, Perico N, et al. Constitutive expression of endothelin gene in cultured human mesangial cells and its modulation by transforming growth factor-beta, thrombin, and a thromboxane A_2 analogue. *Lab Invest* 1991;64:16–20.
198. Kusner DJ, Luebbers EL, Nowinski RJ, Konieczkowski M, King CH, Sedor JR. Cytokine- and LPS-induced synthesis of interleukin-8 from human mesangial cells. *Kidney Int* 1991;39:1240–8.
199. Fouqueray B, Boutard V, Philippe C, et al. Mesangial cell-derived interleukin-10 modulates mesangial cell response to lipopolysaccharide. *Am J Pathol* 1995;147:176–82.
200. Hartner A, Sterzel RB, Reindl N, Hocke GM, Fey GH, Goppelt-Strübe M. Cytokine-induced expression of leukemia inhibitory factor in renal mesangial cells. *Kidney Int* 1994;45:1562–71.
201. Wolf G, Aberle S, Thaiss F, et al. TNF alpha induces expression of the chemoattractant cytokine RANTES in cultured mouse mesangial cells. *Kidney Int* 1993;44:795–804.
202. Largen PJ, Tam FWK, Rees AJ, Cattell V. Rat mesangial cells have a selective role in macrophage recruitment and activation. *Exp Nephrol* 1995;3:34–9.
203. Ardaillou R, Chansel D, Stefanovic V, Ardaillou N. Cell surface receptors and ectoenzymes in mesangial cells. *J Am Soc Nephrol* 1992;2:S107–15.
204. Rovin BH, Yoshiumura T, Tan L. Cytokine-induced production of monocyte chemoattractant protein-1 by cultured human mesangial cells. *J Immunol* 1992;148:2148–53.
205. Hora K, Satriano JA, Santiago A, et al. Receptors for IgG complexes activate synthesis of monocyte chemoattractant peptide 1 and colony-stimulating factor 1. *Proc Natl Acad Sci USA* 1992;89:1745–9.
206. Schlondorff D, Mori T. Contributions of mesangial cells to glomerular immune functions. *Klin Wochenschr* 1990;68:1138–44.
207. Mori T, Bartocci A, Satriano J, et al. Mouse mesangial cells produce colony-stimulating factor-1 (CSF-1) and express the CSF-1 receptor. *J Immunol* 1990;144:4697–702.
208. Lacave R, Rondeau E, Ochi S, Delarue F, Schleuning WD, Sraer JD. Characterization of a plasminogen activator and its inhibitor in human mesangial cells. *Kidney Int* 1989;35:806–11.
209. Glass WF, Rampt E, Garoni JA, Fenton JW, Kreisberg JI. Regulation of mesangial cell adhesion and shape by thrombin. *Am J Physiol* 1991;261:F336–44.
210. Wiggins RC, Njoku N, Sedor JR. Tissue factor production by rat cultured mesangial cells: stimulation by TNFα and lipopolysaccharide. *Kidney Int* 1990;37:1281–5.
211. Chansel D, Dussaule JC, Ardaillou N, Ardaillou R. Identification and regulation of renin in human cultured mesangial cells. *Am J Physiol* 1987;252:F32–8.
212. Davies M, Martin J, Thomas GJ, Lovett DH. Proteinases and glomerular matrix turnover. *Kidney Int* 1992;41:671–8.
213. Johnson RJ, Lovett D, Lehrer RI, Couser WG, Klebanoff SJ. Role of oxidants and proteases in glomerular injury. *Kidney Int* 1994;45:352–9.
214. Silver BJ, Jaffer FE, Abboud HE. Platelet-derived growth factor synthesis in mesangial cells: induction by multiple peptide mitogens. *Proc Natl Acad Sci USA* 1989;86:1056–60.
215. Jaffer F, Saunders C, Shultz P, Throckmorton D, Weinshell E, Abboud HE. Regulation of mesangial cell growth by polypeptide mitogens: inhibitory role of transforming growth factor beta. *Am J Pathol* 1989;135:261–9.
216. MacKay K, Striker LJ, Stauffer JW, Doi T, Agodoa LY, Striker GE. Transforming growth factor-beta: murine glomerular receptors and responses of isolated glomerular cells. *J Clin Invest* 1989;83:1160–7.
217. Kakizaki Y, Kraft N, Atkins RC. Differential control of mesangial

cell proliferation by interferon-gamma. *Clin Exp Immunol* 1991; 85:157–63.

218. Baud L, Perez J, Friedlander G, Ardaillou R. Tumor necrosis factor stimulates prostaglandin production and cyclic AMP levels in rat cultured mesangial cells. *FEBS Lett* 1988;239:50–4.
219. Nakazato Y, Okada H, Sato A, et al. Interleukin 4 downregulates cell growth and prostaglandin release of human mesangial cells. *Biochem Biophys Res Commun* 1993;197:486–93.
220. Ganz MB, Perfetto MC, Boron WF. Effects of mitogens and other agents on rat mesangial cell proliferation, pH, and Ca^{2+}. *Am J Physiol* 1990;259:F269–78.
221. Osawa H, Yamabe H, Inuma H, et al. Interleukin 10 (IL-10) modulates mesangial cell proliferation and its IL-6 production. *J Am Soc Nephrol* 1995;6:846.
222. Ray PE, Bruggeman LA, Horikoshi S, Aguilera G, Klotman PE. Angiotensin II stimulates human fetal mesangial cell proliferation and fibronectin biosynthesis by binding to AT1 receptors. *Kidney Int* 1994;45:177–84.
223. Wolf G, Haberstroh U, Neilson EG. Angiotensin II stimulates the proliferation and biosynthesis of type I collagen in cultured murine mesangial cells. *Am J Pathol* 1992;140:95–107.
224. Conti FG, Striker LJ, Lesniak MA, MacKay K, Roth J, Striker GE. Studies on binding and mitogenic effect of insulin and insulin-like growth factor I in glomerular mesangial cells. *Endocrinology* 1988; 122:2788–95.
225. Stahl RA, Thaiss F, Haberstroh U, Kahf S, Shaw A, Schoeppe W. Cyclooxygenase inhibition enhances rat interleukin 1 beta-induced growth of rat mesangial cells in culture. *Am J Physiol* 1990;259: F419–24.
226. Mohaupt M, Schoecklmann HO, Schulze-Lohoff E, Sterzel RB. Altered nitric oxide production and exogenous nitric oxide do not affect the proliferation of rat mesangial cells. *J Hypertens* 1994;12:401–8.
227. Doi T, Striker LJ, Elliot SJ, Conti FG, Striker GE. Insulinlike growth factor-1 is a progression factor for human mesangial cells. *Am J Pathol* 1989;134:395–404.
228. Mené P, Abboud HE, Dunn MJ. Regulation of human mesangial cell growth in culture by thromboxane A_2 and prostacyclin. *Kidney Int* 1990;38:232–9.
229. Mené P, Dunn MJ. Prostaglandins and rat glomerular mesangial cell proliferation. *Kidney Int* 1990;37:1256–62.
230. Garg UC, Hassid A. Inhibition of rat mesangial cell mitogenesis by nitric oxide-generating vasodilators. *Am J Physiol* 1989;257:F60–6.
231. Raij L, Shultz PJ. Endothelium-derived relaxing factor, nitric oxide: effects on and production by mesangial cells and the glomerulus [Editorial]. *J Am Soc Nephrol* 1993;3:1435–41.
232. Johnson A, Lermioglu F, Garg UC, Morgan Boyd R, Hassid A. A novel biological effect of atrial natriuretic hormone: inhibition of mesangial cell mitogenesis. *Biochem Biophys Res Commun* 1988;152:893–7.
233. Haberstroh U, Zahner G, Disser M, Thaiss F, Wolf G, Stahl RA. TGF-beta stimulates rat mesangial cell proliferation in culture: role of PDGF beta-receptor expression. *Am J Physiol* 1993;264:F199–205.
234. Shultz PJ, Raij L. Inhibition of human mesangial cell proliferation by calcium channel blockers. *Hypertension* 1990;15:176–80.
235. Simonson MS, Wann S, Mené P, et al. Endothelin stimulates phospholipase C, Na^+/H^+ exchange, c-fos expression, and mitogenesis in rat mesangial cells. *J Clin Invest* 1989;83:708–12.
236. Matousovic K, Grande JP, Chini CC, Chini EN, Dousa TP. Inhibitors of cyclic nucleotide phosphodiesterase isozymes type-III and type-IV suppress mitogenesis of rat mesangial cells. *J Clin Invest* 1995;96:401–10.
237. Schulze-Lohoff E, Zanner S, Ogilvie A, Sterzel RB. Extracellular ATP stimulates proliferation of cultured mesangial cells via P2-purinergic receptors. *Am J Physiol* 1992;263:F374–83.
238. Kasiske BK, O'Donnell MP, Kim Y, Atluru D, Keane WF. Cholesterol synthesis inhibitors inhibit more than cholesterol synthesis. *Kidney Int Suppl* 1994;45:S51–3.
239. Schulze-Lohoff E, Zanner S, Ogilvie A, Sterzel RB. Vasoactive diadenosine polyphosphates promote growth of cultured renal mesangial cells. *Hypertension* 1995;26:899–904.
240. Heidenreich S, Tepel M, Schluter H, Harrach B, Zidek W. Regulation of rat mesangial cell growth by diadenosine phosphates. *J Clin Invest* 1995;95:2862–7.
241. Shultz PJ, Knauss TC, Mené P, Abboud HE. Mitogenic signals for thrombin in mesangial cells: regulation of phospholipase C and PDGF genes. *Am J Physiol* 1989;257:F366–74.
242. Chen A, Chen WP, Sheu LF, Lin CY. Pathogenesis of IgA nephropathy: in vitro activation of human mesangial cells by IgA immune complex leads to cytokine secretion. *J Pathol* 1994;173:119–26.
243. Cortes P, Riser BL, Zhao X, Narins RG. Glomerular volume expansion and mesangial cell mechanical strain: mediators of glomerular pressure injury. *Kidney Int Suppl* 1994;45:S11–6.
244. Floege J, Eng E, Young BA, et al. Infusion of platelet-derived growth factor or basic fibroblast growth factor induces selective glomerular mesangial cell proliferation and matrix accumulation in rats. *J Clin Invest* 1993;92:2952–62.
245. Coffey AK, Karnovsky MJ. Heparin inhibits mesangial cell proliferation in habu-venom-induced glomerular injury. *Am J Pathol* 1985; 120:248–55.
246. Diamond JR, Karnovsky MJ. Nonanticoagulant protective effect of heparin in chronic aminonucleoside nephrosis. *Renal Physiol* 1986;9: 366–74.
247. Purkerson ML, Tollefsen DM, Klahr S. N-desulfated/acetylated heparin ameliorates the progression of renal disease in rats with subtotal renal ablation. *J Clin Invest* 1988;81:69–74.
248. Purkerson ML, Hoffsten PE, Klahr S. Pathogenesis of the glomerulopathy associated with renal infarction in rats. *Kidney Int* 1976;9: 407–17.
249. Lan HY, Nikolic Paterson DJ, Zarama M, Vannice JL, Atkins RC. Suppression of experimental crescentic glomerulonephritis by the interleukin-1 receptor antagonist. *Kidney Int* 1993;43:479–85.
250. Nikolic Paterson DJ, Lan HY, Hill PA, Vannice JL, Atkins RC. Suppression of experimental glomerulonephritis by the interleukin-1 receptor antagonist: inhibition of intercellular adhesion molecule-1 expression. *J Am Soc Nephrol* 1994;4:1695–700.
251. Tang WW, Feng L, Vannice JL, Wilson CB. Interleukin-1 receptor antagonist ameliorates experimental anti-glomerular basement membrane antibody-associated glomerulonephritis. *J Clin Invest* 1994;93: 273–9.
252. Kiyama S, Nanishi F, Tomooka S, Okuda S, Onoyama K, Fujishima M. Inhibitory effects of antihypertensive drugs on mesangial cell proliferation after anti-thymocyte serum (ATS)-induced mesangiolysis in spontaneously hypertensive rats. *Life Sci* 1994;54:1891–900.
253. Suematsu S, Matsuda T, Aozasa K, et al. IgG1 plasmacytosis in interleukin 6 transgenic mice. *Proc Natl Acad Sci USA* 1989;86:7547–51.
254. Benigni A, Zoja C, Corna D, et al. A specific endothelin subtype A receptor antagonist protects against injury in renal disease progression. *Kidney Int* 1993;44:440–4.
255. Tsuboi Y, Shankland S, Grande JP, Walker HJ, Johnson RJ, Dousa TP. Treatment of anti-Thy1.1 mesangioproliferative glomerulonephritis with cyclic-38,58-nucleotide phosphodiesterase (PDE) isozyme antagonists, types PDE-III and PDE-IV. *J Am Soc Nephrol* 1995;6:856.
256. MacKay K, Striker LJ, Pinkert CA, Brinster RL, Striker GE. Glomerulosclerosis and renal cysts in mice transgenic for the early region of SV40. *Kidney Int* 1987;32:827–37.
257. Doi T, Striker LJ, Quaife C, et al. Progressive glomerulosclerosis develops in transgenic mice chronically expressing growth hormone and growth hormone releasing factor but not in those expressing insulinlike growth factor-1. *Am J Pathol* 1988;131:398–403.
258. Ausiello DA, Kreisberg JI, Roy C, Karnovsky MJ. Contraction of cultured rat glomerular cells of apparent mesangial origin after stimulation with angiotensin II and arginine vasopressin. *J Clin Invest* 1980; 65:754–60.
259. Badr KF, Murray JJ, Breyer MD, Takahashi K, Inagami T, Harris RC. Mesangial cell, glomerular and renal vascular responses to endothelin in the rat kidney: elucidation of signal transduction pathways. *J Clin Invest* 1989;83:336–42.
260. Bascands JL, Pecher C, Bompart G, Rakotoarivony J, Tack JL, Girolami JP. Bradykinin-induced in vitro contraction of rat mesangial cells via a B_2 receptor type. *Am J Physiol* 1994;267:F871–8.
261. Mené P, Abboud HE, Dubyak GR, Scarpa A, Dunn MJ. Effects of PDGF on inositol phosphates, Ca^{2+}, and contraction of mesangial cells. *Am J Physiol* 1987;253:F458–63.
262. Camussi G, Turello E, Tetta C, Bussolino F, Baglioni C. Tumor necrosis factor induces contraction of mesangial cells and alters their cytoskeletons. *Kidney Int* 1990;38:795–802.
263. Schlondorff D, Satriano JA, Hagege J, Perez J, Baud L. Effect of platelet-activating factor and serum-treated zymosan on prostaglandin E_2 synthesis, arachidonic acid release, and contraction of cultured rat mesangial cells. *J Clin Invest* 1984;73:1227–31.
264. Simonson MS, Dunn MJ. Leukotriene C_4 and D_4 contract rat glomerular mesangial cells. *Kidney Int* 1986;30:524–31.

265. Dunlop ME, Larkins RG. Insulin-dependent contractility of glomerular mesangial cells in response to angiotensin II, platelet-activating factor and endothelin is attenuated by prostaglandin E_2. *Biochem J* 1990;272:561–8.
266. Sedor JR, Abboud HE. Histamine modulates contraction and cyclic nucleotides in cultured rat mesangial cells: differential effects mediated by histamine H_1 and H_2 receptors. *J Clin Invest* 1985;75:1679–89.
267. Mahieu PR, Foidart JB, Dubois CH, Dechenne CA, Deheneffe J. Tissue culture of normal rat glomeruli: contractile activity of the cultured mesangial cells. *Invest Cell Pathol* 1980;3:121–8.
268. Savic V, Blanchard A, Vlahovic P, Stefanovic V, Ardaillou N, Ardaillou R. Cyclic adenosine monophosphate-stimulating agents induce ecto-58-nucleotidase activity and inhibit DNA synthesis in rat cultured mesangial cells. *Arch Biochem Biophys* 1991;290:202–6.
269. Mené P, Dubyak GR, Emancipator SN, Dunn MJ. Stimulation of cytosolic free calcium and contraction by immune complexes in cultured rat mesangial cells. *Trans Assoc Am Physicians* 1987;100:179–86.
270. Simon EE, McDonald JA. Extracellular matrix receptors in the kidney cortex. *Am J Physiol* 1990;259:F783–92.
271. Baraldi A, Zambruno G, Furci L, Manca V, Vaschieri C, Lusvarghi E. Beta-1 integrins in the normal human glomerular capillary wall: an immunoelectron microscopy study. *Nephron* 1994;66:295–301.
272. Kanahara K, Yorioka N, Arita M, Ohira N, Yamakido M. Immunohistochemical studies of extracellular matrix components and integrins in IgA nephropathy. *Nephron* 1994;66:29–37.
273. Satriano JA, Hora K, Shan Z, Stanley ER, Mori T, Schlondorff D. Regulation of monocyte chemoattractant protein-1 and macrophage colony-stimulating factor-1 by IFN-gamma, tumor necrosis factor-alpha, IgG aggregates, and cAMP in mouse mesangial cells. *J Immunol* 1993;150:1971–8.
274. Goppelt-Strübe M, Ströbel M. Synergistic induction of monocyte chemoattractant protein-1 (MCP-1) by platelet-derived growth factor and interleukin-1. *FEBS Lett* 1995;374:375–8.
275. Brown Z, Strieter RM, Chensue SW, et al. Cytokine-activated human mesangial cells generate the neutrophil chemoattractant, interleukin 8. *Kidney Int* 1991;40:86–90.
276. Bergijk EC, Munaut C, Baelde JJ, et al. A histologic study of the extracellular matrix during the development of glomerulosclerosis in murine chronic graft-versus-host disease. *Am J Pathol* 1992;140: 1147–56.
277. Jones CL, Buch S, Post M, McCulloch L, Liu E, Eddy AA. Renal extracellular matrix accumulation in acute puromycin aminonucleoside nephrosis in rats. *Am J Pathol* 1992;141:1381–96.
278. Ishimura E, Sterzel RB, Morii H, Kashgarian M. Extracellular matrix protein: gene expression and synthesis in cultured rat mesangial cells. *Nippon Jinzo Gakkai Shi* 1992;34:9–17.
279. Pugliese G, Pricci F, Pugliese F, et al. Mechanisms of glucose-enhanced extracellular matrix accumulation in rat glomerular mesangial cells. *Diabetes* 1994;43:478–90.
280. Ziyadeh FN, Sharma K, Ericksen M, Wolf G. Stimulation of collagen gene expression and protein synthesis in murine mesangial cells by high glucose is mediated by autocrine activation of transforming growth factor-beta. *J Clin Invest* 1994;93:536–42.
281. Doi T, Striker LJ, Kimata K, Peten EP, Yamada Y, Striker GE. Glomerulosclerosis in mice transgenic for growth hormone: increased mesangial extracellular matrix is correlated with kidney mRNA levels. *J Exp Med* 1991;173:1287–90.
282. Nakamura T, Ebihara I, Tomino Y, Koide H, Kikuchi K, Koiso K. Gene expression of growth-related proteins and ECM constituents in response to unilateral nephrectomy. *Am J Physiol* 1992;262:F389–96.
283. Tamsma JT, van den Born J, Bruijn JA, et al. Expression of glomerular extracellular matrix components in human diabetic nephropathy: decrease of heparan sulphate in the glomerular basement membrane. *Diabetologia* 1994;37:313–20.
284. Bruggeman LA, Horigan EA, Horikoshi S, Ray PE, Klotman PE. Thromboxane stimulates synthesis of extracellular matrix proteins in vitro. *Am J Physiol* 1991;261:F488–94.
285. Ardaillou N, Nivez MP, Bellon G, Combe C, Ardaillou R. Effect of prostaglandin E_2 on proline uptake and protein synthesis by cultured human mesangial cells. *Kidney Int* 1990;38:1151–8.
286. Rosenblum ND, Karnovsky MJ, Olsen BR. Non-fibrillar collagenous proteins synthesized by rat mesangial cells. *J Am Soc Nephrol* 1990; 1:785–91.
287. Oberley TD, Mosher DF, Mills MD. Localization of fibronectin within the renal glomerulus and its production by cultured glomerular cells. *Am J Pathol* 1979;96:651–62.
288. Wolthuis A, Boes A, Rodemann HP, Grond J. Vasoactive agents affect growth and protein synthesis of cultured rat mesangial cells. *Kidney Int* 1992;41:124–31.
289. Rovin BH, Tan LC. LDL stimulates mesangial fibronectin production and chemoattractant expression. *Kidney Int* 1993;43:218–25.
290. Bender BL, Jaffe R, Carlin B, Chung AE. Immunolocalization of entactin, a sulfated basement membrane component, in rodent tissues, and comparison with GP-2 (laminin). *Am J Pathol* 1981;103:419–26.
291. Truong LD, Majesky MW, Pindur J. Tenascin is synthesized and secreted by rat mesangial cells in culture and is present in extracellular matrix in human glomerular diseases. *J Am Soc Nephrol* 1994;4: 1771–7.
292. Wight TN, Raugi GJ, Mumby SM, Bornstein P. Light microscopic immunolocation of thrombospondin in human tissues. *J Histochem Cytochem* 1985;33:295–302.
293. Kanwar YS, Jakubowski ML, Rosenzweig LJ. Distribution of sulfated glycosaminoglycans in the glomerular basement membrane and mesangial matrix. *Eur J Cell Biol* 1983;31:290–5.
294. Moran A, Brown DM, Kim Y, Klein DJ. Effects of IGF-I and glucose on protein and proteoglycan synthesis by human fetal mesangial cells in culture. *Diabetes* 1991;40:1346–54.
295. Silbiger S, Schlondorff D, Crowley S, et al. The effect of glucose on proteoglycans produced by cultured mesangial cells. *Diabetes* 1993; 42:1815–22.

Immunologic Renal Diseases,
edited by E. G. Neilson and W. G. Couser.
Lippincott-Raven Publishers, Philadelphia © 1997.

CHAPTER 30

Endothelial Responses to Immune Injury

Barbara J. Ballermann

The renal endothelium, like that of all blood vessels, ordinarily serves several physiological functions. It provides an anticoagulant surface; forms a component of the capillary wall barrier to cell, fluid, and macromolecule flux; actively transports molecules to and from the interstitium; and produces mediators that influence the function of adjacent cells. Most prominent among endothelial cell–derived mediators are those that regulate vascular tone and vascular remodeling. During immune-mediated disease, endothelial cells often undergo dramatic phenotypic changes, a process commonly referred to as endothelial cell activation. Cell swelling, vacuolization, or denudation from the basement membrane may be observed. At the molecular level, expression of adhesion molecules and chemokines facilitates leukocyte attachment and transmigration, and endothelial cells may become procoagulant due to reduced anticoagulant and enhanced procoagulant factor expression. Immune injury also results in increased endothelial cell proliferative and apoptotic activity. Endothelial cell activation in response to immune stimuli often is self-limited, but more chronic activation can play an important role in renal injury and remodeling, which leads to glomerular sclerosis and interstitial fibrosis.

Most studies that have examined endothelial cell responses during inflammation represent work with nonglomerular endothelial cells, and many have been performed in vitro. In this review, the presentation of endothelial cell responses to immune injury represents a composite view of what has been learned from such work. Although it is likely that many of the findings also hold for glomerular disease, some responses in the glomerulus may eventually be shown to differ because significant phenotypic variation between endothelial cells in different vascular beds exists (1,2). Wherever possible, work that substantiates a particular finding for the glomerulus in vivo or glomerular endothelial cells in vitro is also cited.

B. J. Ballermann: Department of Medicine, Johns Hopkins University School of Medicine, Baltimore, Maryland 21205.

MORPHOLOGIC FEATURES OF ENDOTHELIAL CELL INJURY

Like all large blood vessels, renal arteries, arterioles, and veins are lined by nonfenestrated endothelium that is separated from medial vascular smooth muscle by an internal elastic lamina. Large vessel endothelium does not normally play a major role in the immune response, except when components of the vessel wall themselves come under immune attack, as is observed during vasculitis. In contrast, capillary and postcapillary venular endothelial cells play a central role during many immune responses because their activation serves to facilitate the recruitment of leukocytes to the locus of inflammation.

Glomerular capillary endothelium forms an extremely thin and highly fenestrated cell layer around the circumference of the glomerular capillary loops (see Chapter 1), where it abuts the trilaminate glomerular basement membrane (GBM). The nuclear region of glomerular endothelial cells usually lies at the hilum of the loop, in close proximity to mesangial cells. Whereas GBM forms the underlying matrix for endothelial cells around the periphery of the loops, GBM is not interposed between mesangial cells and endothelium. In the rat, the diameter of most glomerular capillaries ranges from 5 to 12.5 μm, averaging 7.5 μm, similar to the diameter of normal red blood cells. A few loops with diameters of 15 to 25 μm are also present (3). Glomerular capillary endothelial cells are covered by a negatively charged layer of proteoglycans, composed in part of podocalyxin (4). Fenestral diaphragms are present (5), although these structures are less developed than those of peritubular capillary endothelium (6). Within glomerular endothelial cells, actin microfilaments surround the fenestrae, and it has been proposed that functional adjustments in fenestral size may occur (7). Peritubular blood vessels comprise the cortical peritubular capillaries, and in the medulla vasa rectae with their descending and ascending branches. There are significant regional differences in vasa recta, peritubular capillary and renal venular endothelial cell morphology (6), the endothelia of peritubular capillaries and venules are fenestrated, those of vasa rectae are fenestrated only deep in the inner medulla.

At the ultrastructural level, endothelial cell injury is manifested by cell swelling; loss of fenestrae; vacuolization; widening of the subendothelial cell space due to deposition of immunoglobulins, fibrin, and other proteins; or frank detachment of endothelial cells from the basement membrane. A good example of such changes in glomerular endothelium is shown in Fig. 1. Glomerular endothelial cell swelling is a nonspecific reaction. It can become pronounced in diseases such as pre-eclampsia (8,9) and the hemolytic uremic syndrome (10), in which the endothelium and subendothelial material can obliterate the capillary lumina sufficiently to profoundly reduce capillary perfusion. Furthermore, because wall shear stress is inversely proportional to the third power of the vessel radius, any swelling of glomerular endothelial cells significantly increases the level of shear stress at the vessel wall (3).

Endothelial cell swelling and loss of fenestrae is commonly seen in immune complex–mediated proliferative glomerulonephritis, including systemic lupus erythematosus (SLE), poststreptococcal glomerulonephritis, and Schönlein-Henoch purpura, and in severe cases of immunoglobulin (Ig)A nephropathy. Swelling occurs in areas of subendothelial cell immune complex deposition, and evidence for endothelial cell proliferation with mitotic figures is frequently detected (11,12). Intraendothelial cell inclusions with a characteristic myxoviruslike appearance are seen in SLE (13) and sometimes with IgA nephropathy (14). In cases of anti-GBM–mediated glomerulonephritis, endothelial cell damage is often even more severe. Loss of fenestrae, swelling, adhesion of inflammatory cells, detachment of endothelial cells from the basement membrane, and large rents in the basement membrane can be observed (15,16).

Reactive matrix production and deposition by endothelial cells also occurs. In membranoproliferative glomerulonephritis, electron-dense deposits may take on the appearance of an intramembranous location due to new matrix deposition by endothelial cells around the immune deposits (17). Furthermore, both mesangial and endothelial cells can be found interposed between the layers of old and new basement membrane material, giving the appearance of a duplicated basement membrane (17,18). The ultrastructural findings in membranoproliferative glomerulonephritis suggest that the glomerular endothelial cells can significantly increase their rate of matrix synthesis and that they can migrate.

Vasculitic disorders are characterized, during the initial active phase, by intravascular fibrin deposition, endothelial cell swelling, inflammatory cell infiltration, denudation of the endothelium, and destruction of the underlying elastic lamina (19). During the healing phase, endothelial cells again cover the luminal vessel wall, and significant neointimal hyperplasia and increased matrix deposition are observed. The neointimal thickening is often severe enough to significantly reduce the vessel diameter (20). With microvascular forms of vasculitis, including Wegener's granulomatosus, fibrin deposits are observed early within capillary loops. There also is endothelial cell swelling, denudation, and infiltration of the glomerulus

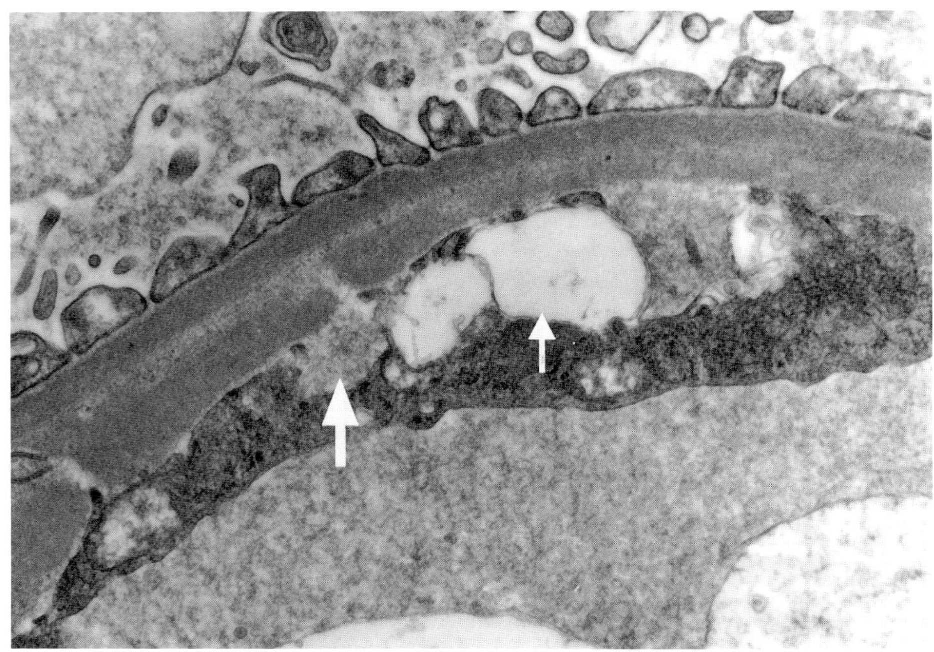

FIG. 1. An example of glomerular capillary endothelial cell swelling, vacuolization *(small arrow)*, loss of fenestrae, and subendothelial deposition of proteinaceous material *(larger arrow)*. The podocyte morphology is normal. The sample was obtained from a patient with HIV-associated thrombotic microangiopathy. (Courtesy of Lorraine Racusen, M.D.)

with inflammatory cells. Destruction of the glomerular capillary tuft, with cell necrosis and overt gaps in the glomerular capillary membrane, is also seen (21,22). During the healing phase, progressive matrix deposition leads to obliteration of glomeruli.

MECHANISMS OF ENDOTHELIAL CELL INJURY AND ACTIVATION

In most cases of immune-mediated injury, endothelial cells are activated by inflammatory cytokines released from tissue monocytes/macrophages, mesangial cells, or other resident cells. In addition, endothelial cells also can come under direct attack themselves. They are subject to infection (e.g., with cytomegalovirus or rickettsia), triggering an immune response. They can be injured by antiendothelial cell antibodies, and they can respond directly to immune complex–mediated complement activation, without requiring paracrine mediators from other cells.

Responses to Viral Infection

Infection of endothelial cells with viruses or other organisms occurs in vivo and in vitro (23–25) and can lead to histologic features in vivo that are indistinguishable from vasculitis (26–28). Endothelial cell infection also may become latent, as is the case with cytomegalovirus and herpes simplex virus type I (29,30). Latent viral infection of the vessel wall may play a role in the chronic vessel wall remodeling that leads to atherosclerosis (29, 30). Like all cells, endothelial cells infected with virus produce interferons. Type I interferons induce expression of major histocompatibility complex (MHC) class I (31). Viral proteins are then presented at the cell surface in the context of MHC class I, which leads to activation of cytotoxic T cells. At the same time, expression of MHC class II molecules is suppressed (32,33). Viral infection also leads to expression of Fas at the cell surface, which promotes binding of Fas ligand on cytotoxic T cells; interaction of these two molecules sets in motion the process of programmed cell death in the cells expressing Fas (34). Fas expression by activated endothelial cells has been documented in human coronary vessels (35).

Cytotoxic T cells (CTLs) interact via their antigen receptor with cells presenting viral proteins on MHC class I. This interaction is highly specific and requires accessory cell adhesion proteins (36). Binding and clustering of the T-cell antigen receptor activates the CTLs to produce a number of soluble cytokines (36), as well as the Fas ligand (34), which remains T cell associated. In addition, T-cell granules move to the cell surface and cluster at the site of endothelial cell contact. Killing of target endothelial cells then proceeds via two distinct and parallel mechanisms. At the site of contact, CTLs exocytose a pore-forming protein (perforin) from their granules, which inserts into the plasma membrane of the target cell and leads to disruption of membrane integrity (37). In addition, the Fas ligand at the CTL surface binds to Fas on the activated endothelial cell, leading to programmed cell death (34). Cells infected by virus also may be destroyed by natural killer (NK) cells, without the degree of specificity with which CTLs act on their target (38).

In addition to the activation of cytotoxic T cells and NK cells, endothelial cells infected by virus also express an array of molecules that are common endothelial cell mediators of the inflammatory response and reflect endothelial cell activation. These include leukocyte adhesion molecules (39,40), procoagulant activity (41), and cytokines (42). Furthermore, viral infection may facilitate formation of antiendothelial cell antibodies (43).

Thus, infection of endothelial cells leads to their removal through the CTL and NK systems. In the case of massive endothelial cell infection, blood vessel wall destruction due to the mobilization of immune effector cells occurs, as is the case in virally induced vasculitis. Because cells infected by virus are also subject to Fas-Fas ligand–mediated apoptosis, virally infected endothelial cells also may lead to formation of autoantibodies specific for proteins mobilized to apoptotic blebs (44).

Direct Antibody-Mediated Endothelial Cell Injury

It is distinctly unusual to visualize antibody or immune complex deposition at the apical surface of vascular endothelial cells in diseased vessels or glomeruli in vivo. The lack of such findings might suggest that direct antibody-mediated endothelial cell injury does not occur. A more likely explanation is that antibody-mediated endothelial cell attack results in cell detachment and/or lysis and that such lethally injured endothelial cells are swept away in the circulation. Evidence for direct antibody-mediated endothelial cell injury in some forms of vasculitis and in xenotransplantation is emerging (45,46). The most prominent and reproducible example is hyperacute xenograft rejection, in which preformed antibodies directed against endothelial cell alpha-galactosyl–bearing glycolipids and glycoproteins mediate the injury (47).

The presence of circulating antiendothelial cell antibodies has been reported in some cases of vasculitis (47–49) and scleroderma (50). In other patients with vasculitis, autoantibodies against vessel wall matrix components play a more important role (51). In SLE, autoantibody formation results from presentation of normally hidden nuclear and inner cell membrane antigens in apoptotic blebs (44). Casciola-Rosen et al. reported that phosphatidylserine, normally confined to the inner surface of the cell membrane, is shifted to the outer leaflet in apoptotic blebs of endothelial cells. Circulating phosphatidylserine-binding proteins such as annexin V then associate with it, and the complex stimulates antiphospholipid autoantibody production (52). Other intracellular and nuclear autoantigens similarly stimulate autoantibody production because of their relocation into membrane blebs of apoptotic cells (53). Thus, autoantibody production in SLE appears to be a specific response to apoptotic cell death. Once autoantibodies have formed, any stimulus that leads to apoptosis of endothelial cells then results in localization of the autoantibodies to the apoptotic blebs of those cells, resulting in complement activation at that site.

Data supporting direct antibody-mediated endothelial cell injury are also emerging from studies in patients with Wegener's granulomatosus and other forms of antineutrophil cytoplasmic antibody (ANCA)-associated vasculitis (54). Whereas endothelial cells themselves do not produce proteinase 3 (55) or myeloperoxidase, the most common ANCA antigens, these enzymes can associate noncovalently with the glycocalyx of endothelial cells (56). It has been postulated that myeloperoxidase and proteinase 3 released from degranulating neutrophils (57) may localize to the endothelial cell glycocalyx, where interaction with ANCA then induces complement-dependent endothelial cell lysis (56). ANCA antigens also appear at the plasma membrane of activated neutrophils and are subject to ANCA binding and stimulation of an oxidative burst (57–59). Neutrophil-derived oxygen-free radicals, proteases, and lipid mediators then lead to endothelial cell injury (58,59).

Endothelial Cell Responses to Complement Components

Interaction of antibodies with endothelial cell antigens leads to complement fixation at the endothelial cell surface and complement-mediated injury (60,61). Deposition of antibody in the subendothelial cell space [e.g., in anti-GBM–mediated glomerulonephritis (62,63)], subendothelial cell immune complex deposition in SLE (64–66), and acute poststreptococcal glomerulonephritis (67) also elicit endothelial cell injury. In this case, endothelial cell injury is mediated, at least in part, through direct effects of complement fixation in close proximity to endothelial cells.

Activation of the classical complement cascade is initiated by the interaction of C1 with antibody–antigen complexes (see Chapter 18). C1 is a multimer composed of one C1q subunit and two each of C1r and C1s (68). Fixation of C1q to the Fc portion of antigen-bound antibody results in the release and activation of C1r and C1s. C1q remains associated with the Fc portion of IgG and IgM, which induces a conformational change allowing it to interact with C1q receptors on cells. Receptors for C1q are expressed by leukocytes, platelets, and mesangial and endothelial cells (69,70). In cells that also express Fc receptors (e.g., mesangial cells), C1q receptors increase immune complex binding and are believed to enhance the efficiency of their phagocytosis (69). In myeloid cells, binding of C1q to C1q receptors similarly enhances immune complex phagocytosis and leads to oxygen metabolite production through a protein kinase C–dependent pathway (71–73). In endothelial cells, which do not express Fc receptors in the quiescent state (74), it recently was shown that antigen-antibody–fixed C1q stimulates endothelial cell expression of the neutrophil adhesion molecules E-selectin, intracellular adhesion molecule-1 (ICAM-1), and vascular cell adhesion molecule-1 (VCAM-1) by activating C1q receptors (75). Thus, the initial response of endothelial cells to immune complex deposition is an increase in leukocyte adhesion molecules stimulated by C1q in the absence of other costimulants. Activation of endothelial cells by viral infection (76) and cytokines (77) stimulates expression of Fc receptors on their surface and may allow endothelial cells to participate in the process of immune complex phagocytosis as well.

Antibody-antigen–mediated activation of the classical complement cascade in turn leads to the release of anapylatoxins C3a, C4a, and C5a, soluble proteins produced by proteolytic cleavage of the inactive C4, C3, and C5 complement components. To date, receptors for C5a, but not C4a or C3a, have been found on endothelial cells (78). In endothelial cells, C5a receptor occupancy activates a pertussis toxin–sensitive G protein to rapidly stimulate the phospholipase C–inositol 1,4,5-triphosphate–calcium–protein kinase C signaling cascade (79). Consequences of C5a receptor activation in endothelial cells include the time- and dose-dependent expression of endothelial P-selectin and secretion of von Willebrand factor (80), enhanced oxygen free radical generation (79), and heparan sulfate proteoglycan release (81) from endothelial cells. The effects of C5a on P-selectin expression and von Willebrand factor release are consistent with C5a-mediated degranulation of endothelial cells because both preformed von Willebrand factor and P-selectin are stored in endothelial cell Weibel-Palade bodies, which can be rapidly mobilized upon appropriate stimulation (82).

C5a also alters neutrophil–endothelial cell interactions through direct but highly concentration-dependent effects on neutrophils (83). At concentrations above 1 nmol/L, C5a promotes neutrophil adhesion to endothelial cells due to expression of endothelial cell adhesion molecules by neutrophils (83,84). In contrast, at concentrations below 1 nmol/L, C5a reduces their adhesion to endothelial cells due to loss of L-selectin on neutrophils (85). Similar to the action of C5a on endothelial cells, neutrophils also generate oxygen free radicals in response to C5a, which in turn participate in endothelial cell injury (86,87). A role of C5a in monocyte/macrophage chemotaxis and endothelial cell transmigration also has been shown. Monocytes produce interleukin (IL)-8 in response to C5a stimulation (88) and respond to C5a with chemotaxis and transendothelial cell migration (89).

The complement membrane attack complex C5b-9, which forms large pores in the plasma membrane, is the ultimate product of complement activation (90). In patients with vasculitis, C5b-9 has been localized to endothelial cells (91), and a functional role for C5b-9 has been observed in endothelial cell destruction after xenotransplantation (92). When present in sufficient quantity in endothelial cell plasma membranes, C5b-9 results in endothelial cell lysis (60,90,93). In patients with glomerulonephritis, C5b-9 has been localized to glomerular capillaries (94), and enhanced excretion of C5b-9 has been documented in some forms of glomerulonephritis (95).

Endothelial cells also produce inhibitors of complement activation. CD59 and homologous restriction factor (HRF) prevent C5b-9 formation at the cell surface. CD59 and HRF are expressed in many cells, but their density appears to be greatest at the apical surface of endothelial cells (96,97), including renal glomerular and peritubular endothelial cells (98,99). These proteins protect cells from complement-mediated endothelial cell damage in a species-specific fashion (100–102). It has been reported that human CD59 protects against xenoantibody-mediated endothelial cell lysis in vivo and in vitro, suggesting that the xenotransplantation barrier might be overcome in part by using organs from animals transgenic for human CD59 (101–103). Endogenous inhibitors of earlier steps in the complement activation cascade, including decay accelerating factor, which inhibits C3 and C5 convertase function, also are expressed by endothelial cells (104–106) and are similarly protective against complement activation (107). Venneker et al. reported markedly reduced expression of complement inhibitors in endothelial cells from dermal lesions of patients with scleroderma (108), raising the possibility that enhanced complement-mediated endothelial injury plays a role in progressive vessel damage in these patients.

Given the prominence of endothelial complement inhibitors, it is not surprising that complement activation does not always lead to endothelial cell death. Indeed, many sublytic effects of C5b-9 are described, most prominent among them the induction of procoagulant activity (109). Formation of sublytic amounts of C5b-9 stimulate the formation of the prothrombinase complex at the endothelial cell surface (110), activate the release of von Willebrand factor and cell-surface expression of P-selectin (111), and markedly enhance endothelial cell tissue factor production (112). Aside from inducing endothelial cell procoagulant activity, the C5b-9 complex also stimulates expression of the leukocyte adhesion molecules E-selectin and ICAM-1 (113). Sublytic C5b-9 furthermore augments synthesis of platelet-derived growth factor and fibroblast growth factor by endothelial cells (114), suggesting that it may participate in the vessel remodeling response to immune injury.

Endothelial Cell Activation by Inflammatory Cytokines

Tumor necrosis factor-α (TNF-α) and IL-1β stimulate endothelial cells to secrete chemokines, to express leukocyte adhesion molecules, and to turn endothelium into a procoagulant surface (115–119). These endothelial cell responses are commonly referred to as endothelial cell activation. TNF-α and IL-1β serve as paracrine signals from tissue macrophages and other resident cells. The most potent stimulus for TNF-α secretion by monocyte/macrophages is bacterial endotoxin [lipopolysaccharide (LPS)], and this response can be markedly augmented in macrophages primed with interferon-γ (120). Macrophages also secrete TNF-α after phagocytosis of opsonized particles, in response to Fc receptor cross-linking (121), upon encountering IgG and IgA immune complexes (122), and in response to C5a (123). Thus, the interaction of immune complexes with resident macrophages is an effective and sufficient stimulus for TNF-α secretion. TNF-α autoinduces its own synthesis (124), providing for a positive amplification loop of secretion. TNF-α also is secreted by T-lymphocytes during the process of T-cell receptor engagement with MHC class II–bound antigens (125,126) and by activated polymorphonuclear neutrophils (127). IL-1β is synthesized by monocytes/macrophages; potent stimuli for its synthesis are LPS and macrophage contact with $CD4^+$ T cells (128, 129). TNF-α strongly stimulates IL-1β synthesis by macrophages and by a number of other cell types, including endothelial cells (119).

Rat mesangial cells in culture also respond to LPS with TNF-α secretion (130), and TNF-α has been found in the mesangium of human renal glomeruli from patients with active lupus nephritis but not in normal individuals (131). In patients with membranous glomerulonephritis, intense TNF-α staining of visceral glomerular epithelial cells and urinary TNF-α excretion suggest that injured podocytes produce TNF-α (132). In IgA nephropathy, TNF-α immunoreactivity was strongest in the mesangial area and colocalized with macrophage markers (133,134). This finding is in keeping with the observation that IgA immune complexes activate TNF-α synthesis by macrophages (122). In acute nephrotoxic serum nephritis in rats, both TNF-α and IL-1β synthesis were induced in renal glomeruli, with TNF-α preceding the appearance of IL-1β (135). In ANCA-associated crescentic glomerulonephritis, Noronha et al. (136) found both TNF-α and IL-1β messenger RNA (mRNA) in the renal interstitium, in glomerular crescents, and in the blood vessel wall at sites of vasculitis. The involvement of TNF-α in glomerulonephritis recently has been reviewed in detail by others (137,138). Finally, Morel et al. (139) found highly significant induction of TNF-α expression by infiltrating inflammatory cells in the interstitium in human renal transplants during rejection. Thus, there is ample evidence for

TNF-α and IL-1β synthesis and action in various immune diseases affecting the kidney. The data suggest that TNF-α and IL-1β are produced primarily by inflammatory cells and other nonendothelial renal cells (139), in keeping with the view that these mediators are paracrine activators of endothelial cells.

Transcriptional Regulation of Endothelial Cell Activation

The response of endothelial cells to inflammatory cytokines is best characterized for TNF-α and IL-1β. The endothelial cell response to TNF-α is elicited by specific cell surface receptors (140), which are members of a family of receptors that includes Fas (34). The mechanism of downstream signaling involves activation of an acidic sphingomyelinase (141) and requires tyrosine kinase activity (142). IL-1β receptors belong to a separate receptor family and share a common extracellular motif with fibroblast growth factor receptors (143).

There now is abundant evidence that both, TNF-α and IL-1β activate the nuclear transcription factor NF-kB/Rel, and thereby trigger the transcription of a number of genes that control the endothelial cell inflammatory response (144). NF-κB/Rel is a dimeric complex consisting of NF-κB and Rel subunits, the former 50 kDa, the latter 65 kDa in size. In nonactivated endothelial cells, the 65-kDa Rel component is either bound to a larger 105-kDa precursor of NF-κB, which requires proteolytic cleavage to the 50-kDa form for activation, or the 50-kDa/65-kDa NF-κB/Rel complex is bound to IκB-α, which masks the NF-κB nuclear targeting sequence. Activation of the NF-κB/Rel complex requires processing of the 105-kDa precursor of NF-κB or degradation of IκB-α via the ubiquitin/proteasome pathway (145–147). It is thought that phosphorylation of IκB-α targets it for degradation (144); indeed, inhibition of IκB-α phosphorylation prevents NF-κB/Rel activation and enhanced expression of leukocyte adhesion molecules by endothelial cells (148). It is furthermore of great interest that nitric oxide (NO), a mediator produced by endothelial cells and activated macrophages, inhibits IκB-α degradation and NF-κB/Rel activation (149). Upon activation, the NF-κB/Rel dimer is rapidly translocated to the endothelial cell nucleus (150) where it interacts with a number of promoters, among them those for leukocyte adhesion molecules E-selectin (144,151), VCAM-1 (152), and ICAM-1 (153,154), procoagulant molecules such as tissue factor (155), and other components of the inflammatory response, for instance the IL-8 promoter (156). However, although binding of NF-κB/Rel is central to the response of endothelial cells to inflammatory stimuli, it is only a component of the transcriptional complex for each of its various targets. Other transcription factors cooperate with NF-κB/Rel to regulate the promoter activity of a number of genes involved in the endothelial cell inflammatory response. For instance, cyclic AMP response element binding protein (CREB) and activating transcription factors (ATFs) interact together with the E-selectin promoter (144), SP1 and interferon regulatory factor-1 (IRF-1) cooperate with NF-κB/Rel to regulate VCAM-1 promoter activity (144,157), and in the tissue factor promotor, AP-1 and SP-1 sites cooperate with NF-κB/Rel sites to increase transcription in response to TNF-α (158,159). Furthermore, cooperativity between two binding sites on the E-selectin promoter is induced by a protein termed high-mobility group (HMG) protein I(Y) and is necessary for transcriptional activation by NF-κB/Rel (160). It is thought that HMG protein I(Y) bends the DNA in the promoter region and thereby facilitates the appropriate three-dimensional conformation of the promoter–transcription factor complex for optimal promoter activation (144). Cooperative binding of transcription factors to promoter elements of genes that are targets for NF-κB/Rel may provide specificity for transcriptional activation of various effector systems in the inflammatory response.

MECHANISMS OF LEUKOCYTE RECRUITMENT

Except for specialized endothelial cells that facilitate continual lymphocyte recirculation through tissues as part of their surveillance function (161), endothelium does not normally support the adhesion and transmigration of inflammatory cells. Recirculation of naive lymphocytes into lymphoid tissues and of tissue-specific memory T cells is mediated by interactions of lymphocytes with postcapillary venule endothelial cells, which allow tissue-specific uptake of appropriate lymphocyte subsets. During the inflammatory response, transmigration of leukocytes occurs locally at sites of infection, antibody-mediated injury, or immune complex deposition. This process requires activation of both endothelial cells and leukocytes and the coordinate expression of matching adhesion molecules on their surfaces.

To activate leukocytes, specific chemokines are secreted by tissue macrophages, other resident cells, and endothelial cells. Chemokines display a significant degree of specificity for leukocyte subsets so that predominantly granulocytes, monocytes, or lymphocytes may be recruited. For instance, in acute immune-complex and anti-GBM antibody-mediated glomerulonephritis, as well as in vasculitic disorders affecting the renal microvasculature, infiltration with neutrophils predominates during the early phase, whereas in more chronic disease, monocyte/macrophage infiltration is more typical (162). Infiltration with T-lymphocytes is much less pronounced in diseased glomeruli, although the presence of T cells has been noted in crescentic glomerulonephritis, minimal-change disease, and focal and segmental glomerulonephritis. In IgA nephritis, and in experimental models of nephrotoxic serum nephritis, the presence of T-lymphocytes, usually $CD4^+$ helper cells, may relate causally to the development of crescents, and T-lymphocyte infiltration is a prominent component of the inflammatory response in the periglomerular and interstitial compartment (162).

Endothelium-Derived Chemokines

Chemokines are a group of mediators that stimulate chemotaxis of leukocytes to areas of inflammation. There are at least 22 proteins in this family, all ranging from 8 to 10 kDa in size and all with heparin-binding activity. The superfamily of chemokines has been divided into two broad groups, alpha and beta, based on chromosomal clustering of their genes and on the structural arrangement of cysteine residues within the molecules (163,164). The alpha family is clustered on human chromosome 4 and is primarily involved in neutrophil chemotaxis. The most studied member of this group is IL-8, formerly known as neutrophil activating protein 1. Genes of the beta family cluster on human chromosome 17 and act principally on monocytes. Monocyte chemotactic proteins 1, 2, and 3 (MCP-1, -2, -3) as well as RANTES are members of this group. A novel chemokine, lymphotactin, which is active toward lymphocytes, recently was identified and is believed to belong to a unique subgroup (164,165). Four different groups of chemokine receptors mediate the cellular actions of these proteins (166,167). There are receptors that display selectivity for specific chemokines, receptors that distinguish only alpha- and beta-chemokines, and a highly promiscuous receptor, the Duffy erythrocyte antigen, which is expressed at high levels in renal postcapillary venules (168) and recognizes a number of alpha and beta chemokines. In addition, herpesvirus homologs of alpha and beta chemokine receptors can bind chemokines on virally infected cells (166,167). This section focuses on IL-8, MCP-1, and RANTES actions because they have been studied most extensively in renal disease (164) and in relationship with endothelial cell activation.

Endothelial activation by TNF-α, IL-1β, and LPS stimulates transcription of the IL-8 and MCP-1 genes and the release of the newly synthesized proteins from the cells (169,170). Recent evidence suggests that these chemokines may remain confined to the endothelial cell surface, where they are presented to leukocytes in characteristic clusters (171). As is the case with other endothelial cell responses to TNF-α, IL-8 transcription is dependent on NF-κB activation (172). Further stimuli for endothelial cell IL-8 synthesis are hypoxia (156), histamine (173), and contact with fibrin (174,175). The latter finding is of interest in view of the procoagulant nature of activated endothelium and because fibrin deposition in glomerular capillaries is commonly observed during glomerulonephritis. Direct interaction of activated monocytes with endothelial cells also induces IL-8 synthesis (176,177), an effect that appears to be mediated by lectin-bound IL-1α at the monocyte surface, which is presented to endothelial cells during cell–cell adhesion (177). In endothelial cells infected with *Rikettsia conorii*, IL-1α synthesis is induced and dramatically stimulates IL-8 synthesis by the same cells in an autocrine fashion (178). A number of mediators modulate cytokine-stimulated IL-8 and MCP-1 synthesis by endothelial cells. For instance, IL-4 and interferon-γ potentiate (170–180), whereas NO (181,182) and transforming growth factor-β (180) significantly inhibit synthesis. Aside from endothelial cells, many other cell types can produce chemokines (164, 183). For example, RANTES is produced by rat glomerular mesangial cells in response to TNF-α (184), monocytes stimulated by C5a synthesize large quantities of IL-8 (185), and neutrophils secrete IL-8 and MCP-1 in response to LPS and cytokines (186,187).

Chemotaxis of polymorphonuclear leukocytes (188–190) and basophils (191) across endothelial cell monolayers is stimulated by IL-8, whereas MCP-1 is chemotactic principally for monocytes (192), and RANTES potently affects eosinophil chemotaxis (193,194). It is also of note that C5a mimics the chemoattractant actions of IL-8 on neutrophils (195,196). The chemotactic action of these molecules is dependent on leukocyte binding to adhesion molecules on endothelial cells (197–201) and does not occur without endothelial cell activation (164). Chemokine-mediated leukocyte activation involves increased expression of adhesion molecules by the leukocyte and the acute alteration in the affinity of the adhesion molecule on the leukocyte for its endothelial cell counter-receptor. For instance, C5a is a powerful chemotactic agent for neutrophils (202), which stimulates increased expression of neutrophil MAC-1 (CD11b/CD18) (200) (Table 1) and increases MAC-1 affinity for endothelial cell receptor ICAM-1 (195,197,203). However, the adhesion response of neutrophils also can be inhibited by the chemotactic mediators IL-8 and C5a. IL-8 directly desensitizes the neutrophil chemotactic response on endothelium (204,205), and both IL-8 and C5a can inhibit and even reverse neutrophil adhesion to endothelium (205,206). This seemingly paradoxical response is partly related to the chemokine concentration encountered by neutrophils; high concentrations of chemokine stimulate adhesion, whereas lower concentrations clearly inhibit adhesion (207–209). Loss of adhesion appears to be mediated by shedding of L-selectin from the neutrophil surface in response to IL-8 and C5a (85). Also, soluble IL-8 presented to neutrophils at the apical surface of endothelial cells inhibits chemotaxis, whereas IL-8 at the basolateral side stimulates chemotaxis of apical neutrophils (210). Taken together, the findings may indicate that the neutrophil chemotactic response depends on a chemokine gradient (85,210). Rot (211) has suggested an alternative possibility, namely that stimulation of leukocytes requires presentation of chemokines in the bound form on the endo-

TABLE 1. *Endothelial–leukocyte adhesion molecules*

Endothelial cell receptor	Activator	Leukocyte counter-receptor	Activator
P-selectin	C5a, C5b-9, thrombin, histamine, platelet-activating factor	PSGL-1 (Mucin)	
E-selectin (ELAM-1)	TNF-α, IL-1β, LPS	ESL-1 (Mucin)	
CD34 (Mucin)	Constitutive	L-selectin	Inhibited by C5a, IL-8
MAd-CAM-1	?		
ICAM-1	TNF-α, IL-1β, LPS	αM/β2 (MAC-1, CD11b/CD18), αL/β2 (LFA-1, CD11a/CD18)	C5a, chemokines
VCAM-1	TNF-α, IL-1β, LPS	α4/β1 (VLA-1, CD49/CD29)	MCP-1, lymphotactin
ICAM-2	Constitutive	αL/β2 (LFA-1, CD11a/CD18)	Chemokines

thelial cell surface, whereas soluble chemokines inhibit leukocyte adhesion. Evidence supporting this view comes from the observation that endothelial cells apparently lack specific high-affinity receptors for IL-8 and are unresponsive to it (212) but that IL-8 nevertheless adheres to endothelial cells via low-affinity binding sites. Endothelial cells in vivo appear to transcytose both IL-8 and RANTES from the interstitium followed by clustering of these chemokines on luminal endothelial cell projections (171). In attached lymphocytes, IL-8 and RANTES stimulate the formation of extensions (uropods) with clustered endothelial cell adhesion molecules at their tip (213). Such findings support the view that the chemokine–leukocyte interaction takes place at the endothelial cell surface, and suggest that chemokines clustered on special extensions are presented by endothelial cells to leukocytes, whereas leukocytes extend uropods with appropriate adhesion molecules toward the endothelial cells. Such feet may do the walking on the endothelium during leukocyte chemotaxis.

At high doses, C5a and IL-8 stimulate neutrophil respiratory burst activity and release of reactive oxygen intermediates, which contribute to endothelial cell injury (196,214–217). Neutrophil-derived superoxide anion appears to be the critical agent (217), whereas generation of hydrogen peroxide during the neutrophil–endothelial cell encounter depends on endothelial cell xanthine oxidase expression (218). In addition, C5a stimulates the translocation of enzymes from neutrophil granules to the cell surface and the release of lysosomal enzymes (219,220). Neutrophil adherence, degranulation, and generation of oxygen metabolites in response to chemokines can induce significant endothelial cell injury.

Endothelial Cell Leukocyte Adhesion Molecules

Activation of endothelial cells by the complement components C1q, C5a, and C5b-9, as well as by inflammatory cytokines, most notably TNF-α and IL1-β, stimulates expression of leukocyte adhesion molecules (144, 221). High levels of adhesion molecule expression are found in tissues during inflammation (221), including glomerular and tubulointerstitial diseases (222,223). It is now held that the leukocyte–endothelial cell interaction occurs in a stepwise fashion (Fig. 2). An initial low-affinity interaction is mediated by selectin–mucin binding, which promotes rolling of leukocytes along the endothelial cells. During selectin-mediated contact, leukocytes encounter IL-8 and other chemokines presented at the endothelial cell surface. These stimulate expression of leukocyte integrins, clustering in uropods, and conformational changes that increase integrin affinity. The integrins expressed at the leukocyte cell surface then bind to endothelial cell adhesion molecules belonging to the immunoglobulin gene family (ICAMs, VCAM-1, and platelet endothelial cell adhesion molecule [PECAM-1]) as well as specific cell matrix binding sites (221,224,225). Integrin-mediated binding to endothelial cells is responsible for arrest and spreading of the leukocytes on the endothelium. Chemokinesis along the endothelial cell surface and migration through the endothelial cell monolayer is dependent on both chemokine stimulation and integrin–CAM interaction (221). Differences in adhesion molecule expression between endothelial cell subtypes and between various stimuli have been described. For instance, selectin expression in the kidney seems to be much greater in peritubular vessels than in glomerular capillary endothelium (223). Differences in the repertoire of adhesion molecules expressed by endothelial cells may play an important role in determining the specific leukocyte subsets to be recruited.

The Selectin Family

There are three known members of the selectin family; L-, P-, and E-selectin. These proteins are structurally related, sharing a calcium-dependent lectin domain at the amino-terminus, and an epidermal growth factor–like domain and several short consensus repeat units homologous to complement-binding proteins in the extracellular portion (226). They are anchored at the cell surface by single transmembrane spanning domains and contain short cytoplasmic tails. Selectins promote cell–cell adhesion by binding carbohydrate moieties on mucinlike glycoproteins and proteoglycans on adjacent cells. Selectin

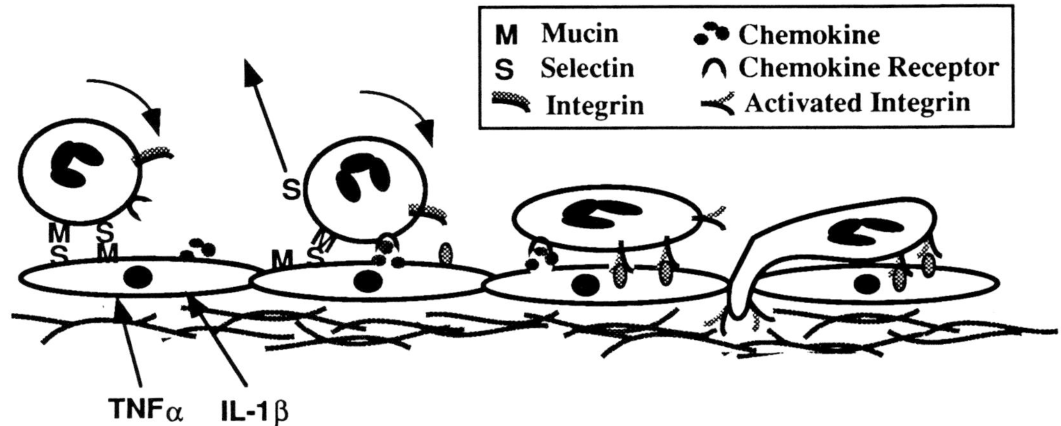

FIG. 2. Schematic representation of leukocyte adhesion and transmigration through the endothelial cell monolayer. Upon activation, endothelial cells express P-selectin and E-selectin (designated S), which interact with specific, highly glycosylated proteins (M, for mucin) on leukocytes. Leukocyte L-selectin also binds to a counter-receptor mucin on endothelial cells. The selectin-mediated low-affinity binding of leukocytes to endothelial cells brings chemokine receptors on leukocytes in contact with chemokines (e.g., IL-8) on the endothelial cell surface, triggering a change in integrin affinity and expression in leukocytes. Leukocyte integrins then bind to the endothelial cell counter-receptors (VCAM, ICAMs), allowing them to spread and transmigrate.

binding affinity is dependent in part on an intact cytoplasmic domain, which may regulate binding affinity (227).

L-selectin is confined to hematopoietic cells and is constitutively expressed by recirculating lymphocyte subsets (161), circulating monocytes, and most circulating neutrophils and eosinophils (226). L-selectin promotes the initial low-affinity interaction of leukocytes with endothelial cells and is cleaved rapidly upon activation of the leukocyte with chemokines, including endothelial cell–derived IL-8 (85). Cleavage is brought about by activation-induced changes in the L-selectin conformation with consequent exposure of epitopes near the membrane-spanning domain that are susceptible to catalysis by an endoprotease (228). Cleaved, soluble L-selectin is shed into the circulation, where it is found in significant concentrations and is believed to function as an inhibitor of leukocyte binding to endothelial cell surfaces (229).

P-selectin is constitutively expressed by endothelial cells and platelets, where it is stored preformed in Weibel-Palade bodies and alpha granules, respectively (230). Activation of endothelial cells with agonists that activate the phospholipase C–inositol phosphate–calcium signaling cascade, including histamine, thrombin, C5a, and C5b-9, result in rapid mobilization of Weibel-Palade bodies to the cell surface, where P-selectin is inserted into the endothelial cell plasma membrane and acts to mediate rapid recruitment of leukocytes (80,111). P-selectin expression also is regulated at the transcriptional level upon stimulation of endothelial cells with LPS and TNF-α (226). Thus, P-selectin is thought to be involved both in early and later phases of endothelial cell activation and consequent leukocyte recruitment.

E-selectin is a highly specific marker for cytokine-activated endothelial cells (115,231,232). E-selectin synthesis and expression at the apical surface of endothelial cells is suppressed under basal conditions and is strongly induced by the inflammatory cytokines TNF-α, IL-1β, and interferon-γ, as well as by LPS. Whereas cytokine-stimulated expression of E-selectin by human umbilical vein endothelial cells in vitro is transient, with a peak at 4 to 6 h after activation and a decline to basal levels by 48 h (231), in vivo E-selectin expression at sites of inflammation persists (226). Upregulation of E-selectin on peritubular capillaries is found in renal allografts during rejection (233), and E- and P-selectin expression has been reported in a case of crescentic glomerulonephritis due to Wegener's granulomatosus (224).

Selectins can bind many carbohydrate molecules in vitro, although binding to most small sialylated and fucosylated oligosaccharides is of low affinity. The tetrasaccharide leukocyte antigen sialyl Lewis^x has been identified as one of the major ligands for E- and P-selectins (226, 234). In addition, several heavily glycosylated, mucinlike proteins have been identified as high-affinity selectin ligands. In mice, MAdCAM-1, GlyCAM-1, and CD34 are L-selectin ligands (226), and high endothelial venules express a 200,000-kDa mucin (235). MAdCAM-1 is preferentially expressed in lymph nodes, and GlyCAM-1 is a circulating L-selectin ligand that may inhibit L-selectin interactions with endothelium. CD34 is expressed both in lymph nodes and constitutively on endothelial cells. Tissue-specific glycosylation of endothelial cell CD34 has been proposed as a mechanism whereby tissue-selective lymphocyte recruitment may be achieved (234,236).

Although activation of endothelial cells (237), including glomerular endothelial cells (238), results in enhanced L-selectin–mediated rolling of leukocytes, findings suggesting that expression of mucins may be induced as part of the endothelial cell activation cascade, evidence for enhanced expression of specific mucins has not been found. E- and P-selectin similarly interact with a number of specific mucins expressed on leukocytes. Among them are P-selectin glycoprotein ligand-1 (PSGL-1) (239) and E-selectin ligand (ESL-1) (240).

Mice deficient in P-, E-, and L-selectin have been generated (241–243); they are developmentally normal and display no enhanced susceptibility to infection. However, challenge with inflammatory stimuli has shown that the rate of leukocyte recruitment in such animals is reduced. Furthermore, monoclonal antibodies directed against selectins reduce tissue inflammation in a number of models (244). It is therefore possible that carbohydrate-based blockers of selectin-mediated leuykocyte–endothelial cell interactions may become therapeutically useful.

Integrin-Based Leukocyte–Endothelial Cell Interactions

Integrins are heterodimeric proteins composed of alpha and beta subunits that interact with their ligands in a calcium-dependent manner (245). The nomenclature for these molecules is based on trivial names, on the alpha and beta subunit configuration, and on their cluster of differentiation antigen (CD) designation (246) (Table 1). Alpha and beta subunits each belong to large families (245). The leukocyte adhesion integrins contain predominantly β1 (CD29) and β2 (CD18) subunits; their specificity is derived predominantly from their diverse alpha subunit partners. The integrin MAC-1 ($a_M\beta_2$; CD11b/CD18) is expressed by granulocytes, monocytes, and NK cells. LFA-1 ($a_L\beta_2$; CD11a/CD18) is expressed by all leukocytes, and VLA-4 ($a_4\beta_1$; CD49/CD29) is expressed by monocytes and T- and B-lymphocytes, but not granulocytes. Leukocyte activation results in both an increase in expression and an increase in affinity of integrins at the leukocyte surface.

The endothelial cell counter-receptors for these molecules are ICAM-1 and -2 and VCAM-1. These proteins display extracellular immunoglobulin–like ligand binding domains and are anchored in the endothelial cell membrane by a single transmembrane-spanning domain (245). They have short cytoplasmic domains that may participate in signaling. ICAM-1 binds both MAC-1 and LFA-1; ICAM-2 interacts with LFA-1; and VCAM-1 interacts with VLA-4 (Table 1). VCAM-1 is not usually expressed by endothelial cells, but the rate of transcription of the VCAM-1 gene is markedly enhanced upon stimulation with cytokines, and the VCAM-1 protein expression at the cell membrane is dramatically induced (144,157,247,248). Similarly, ICAM-1 expression is normally exceedingly low in all endothelia and is dramatically induced upon stimulation of endothelial cells with TNF-α and IL-1β as well as LPS (144,153,154,249–251). In contrast, ICAM-2 is constitutively expressed at the apical surface of endothelial cells and is not altered by endothelial cell activation.

In models of experimental glomerulonephritis, induction of leukocyte adhesion molecules in glomerular endothelial cells in situ has been shown, and infusion of neutralizing ICAM-1 and VCAM-1 antibodies reduced glomerular leukocyte infiltration and crescent formation (252–254). In addition, ICAM-1 was upregulated significantly in endothelial cells of peritubular capillaries in experimental glomerulonephritis (255). In a model of autoimmune lupus nephritis, Wuthrich et al. (256) also found induction of ICAM-1. Similarly, in human lupus glomerulonephritis, crescentic glomerulonephritis, and renal transplant rejection, ICAM-1 and VCAM-1 are expressed and are thought to play a role in promoting leukocyte recruitment (162,223,224,257). It is of further interest that the expression of integrins on circulating leukocytes was increased in patients with active Wegener's granulomatosus (258). These observations lend support to the view that regulation of both leukocyte integrins and their endothelial cell counter-receptors plays an important role in leukocyte recruitment during immune-mediated renal diseases and that interruption of this step in the inflammatory response could become a therapeutic option when pharmacologically active inhibitors of these proteins become available.

ACTIVATION OF ENDOTHELIAL CELL PROCOAGULANT FUNCTIONS

Endothelial cell activation also alters the balance of endothelial cell anticoagulant versus procoagulant activity (115,259,260). Normal endothelium produces a number products that prevent platelet activation and blood coagulation and others that lyse fibrin. These systems are critical for maintaining blood in the fluid state. Nevertheless, endothelial cells also synthesize procoagulant mediators that offset the action of the anticoagulant systems. Injury and cytokine stimulation of endothelial cells has profound effects on the balance between pro- and anticoagulant systems and can turn the endothelium into a frankly procoagulant surface. For instance, highly procoagulant endothelium is observed during disseminated intravascular coagulation (261) and in cases of thrombotic microangiopathy where histologic evidence of platelet and fibrin deposition are readily evident (Fig. 3). In addition, fibrin and platelet deposition are commonly seen in various forms of glomerulonephritis, suggesting that local activation of the coagulation systems and/or reduced fibrinolytic activity are occurring (262–265).

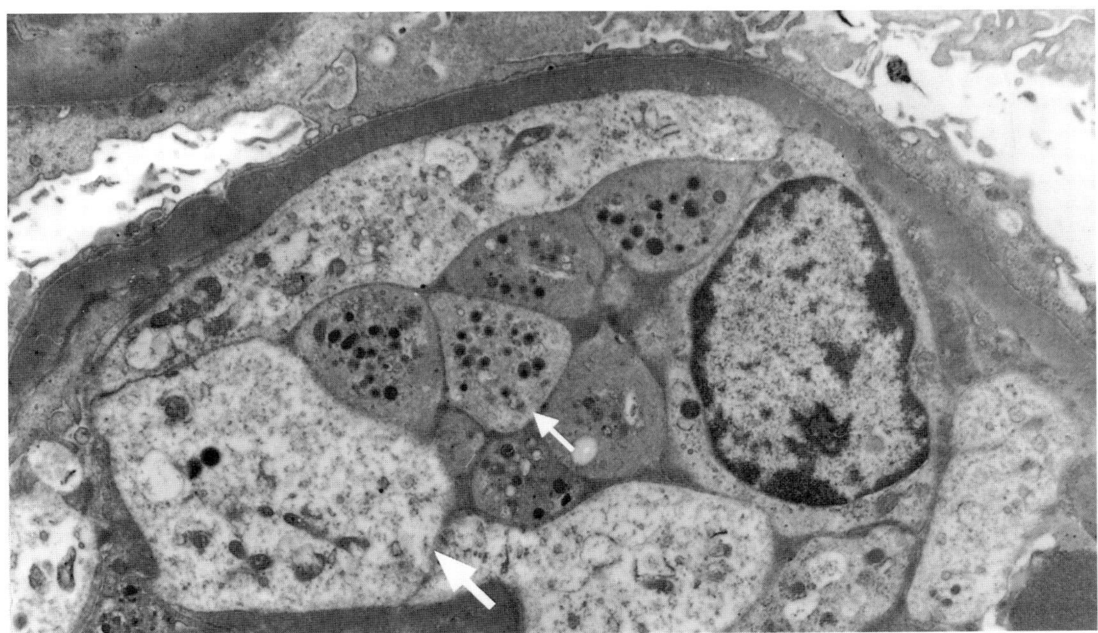

FIG. 3. An example of severe glomerular endothelial cell swelling *(large arrow)* and platelet deposition *(small arrow)* within the glomerular capillary lumen. This sample was obtained from a patient with thrombotic microangiopathy due to FK506 toxicity. (Courtesy of Lorraine Racusen, M.D.)

Endothelial Cell–Derived Mediators Regulating Platelet Aggregation

Von Willebrand Factor

The von Willebrand factor (vWF) is a multimeric glycoprotein produced by endothelial cells and platelets. It is stored in Weibel-Palade bodies within endothelial cells, colocalized with P-selectin (266). Under physiologic conditions, endothelial cells secrete vWF into the subendothelial matrix and into the circulation, where vWF acts as a carrier for factor VIII (266). Binding to vWF protects inactive factor VIII from protein C–mediated cleavage and facilitates its activation by thrombin, thereby enhancing the formation of factor Xa in the coagulation cascade (267) (Fig. 4). The vWF interacts with platelets through the platelet surface glycoprotein receptor GP Ib-IX-V, which in turn results in activation of the platelet integrin αIIbβ3, responsible for platelet adhesion and spreading (268). The platelet activation/adhesion response is amplified by vWF factor release from platelets and by thrombin.

Von Willebrand factor release from endothelial cells is induced by several agonists, including thrombin (269, 270), serotonin (271), platelet-activating factor (272), leukotrienes (273), and C5a (274). The mechanism of release involves activation of the phospolipase C signaling cascade (275), mobilization of intracellular calcium (276), and consequent exocytosis of stored vWF (277). In each case, vWF exocytosis is accompanied by P-selectin expression at the endothelial cell surface (269,273,274, 278). Vasopressin, acting via the adenylate cyclase–coupled V2 receptor, also stimulates endothelial cell vWF release (279,280), although this response appears to be indirect, involving vasopressin-stimulated platelet activating factor release from monocytes (272). The V2 vasopressin receptor selective agonist ddAVP is used clinically to promote hemostasis (280). Viral infection of endothelial cells (281) and exposure to bacterial LPS (282) stimulate vWF release (259). Release in response to bacterial endotoxin is most likely mediated by platelet-activating factor (283). In patients with the hemolytic uremic syndrome, increased vWF release from endothelial cells and platelets takes place (284). In addition to vWF release from endothelium, denudation of endothelial cells from their underlying matrix exposes matrix-associated vWF, thus promoting platelet adhesion and local fibrin deposition (266). Whereas exocytosis of vWF is stimulated by a number of agonists involved in the inflammatory response and endothelial cell lysis due to massive injury results in vWF release, endothelial cell synthesis of vWF appears to be diminished in response to some inflammatory cytokines, including interferon-γ and TNF-α (259).

The vWF circulates as multimers of progressively diminishing size. It has been suggested that the appearance of multiple forms of vWF in the circulation reflects progressive metabolism to smaller isoforms after secre-

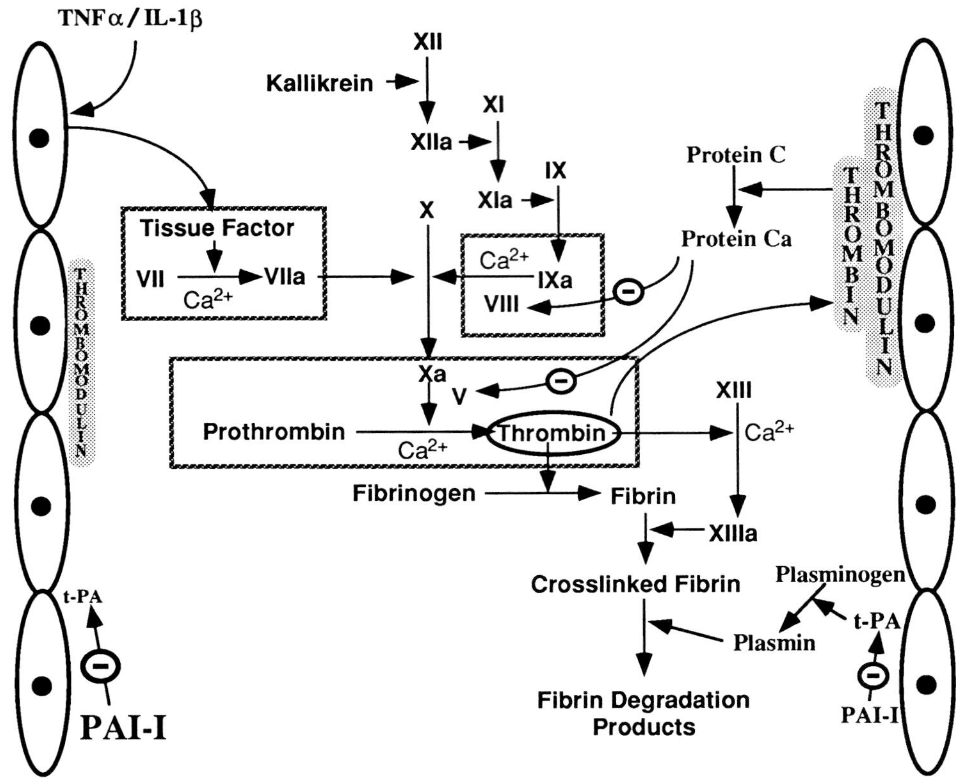

FIG. 4. Schematic representation of the coagulation and fibrinolytic cascades. All of the components interact at the endothelial cell surface. In the nonactivated endothelium (at right), an active thrombomodulin complex interacts with thrombin, causing protein C to be activated, which in turn inactivates clotting factors V and VIII. t-PA generated by nonactivated endothelium promotes plasmin-mediated cleavage of cross-linked fibrin. Endothelium activated by cytokines (at left) produces tissue factor, which can activate the extrinsic coagulation cascade. Thrombomodulin is markedly downregulated on activated endothelium, and plasminogen activator inhibitor (PAI-I) synthesis is markely enhanced. Not shown, von Willebrand factor, which may be secreted acutely from endothelial cells in response C5a and thrombin, and is also present in subendothelial cell matrix, participates in platelet activation and serves as a cofactor for factor VIII. Also, phospholipids derived from activated platelets and from apoptotic or injured endothelial cells facilitate coagulation.

tion of large molecular weight vWF multimer from endothelial cells (269). In the hemolytic uremic syndrome, the accumulation of unusually large vWF multimers in plasma has been reported, and the large molecular weight vWF was proposed to potentiate platelet aggregation in this disorder (285,286). Because multimerization is greatest in endothelial cell Weibel-Palade bodies, an alternative explanation for the greater abundance of large molecular weight vWF multimers in some patients with HUS/TTP may be massive vWF release from injured endothelial cells. Reduced rates of clearance of the multimeric form of vWF also may play a role. Nevertheless, although it is clear that the predominant defect in HUS/TTP is intravascular platelet aggregation and coagulation due to acute endothelial cell injury and vWF release, a direct pathogenic role for unusually large forms of vWF in HUS remains unconfirmed (287).

Prostacyclin

Endothelial cells produce two prominent soluble inhibitors of platelet activation: NO and prostacyclin (288, 289). Both are extremely short lived and function as local inhibitors of platelet activation and smooth muscle cell contraction (290). Prostacyclin synthesis (291) depends on the activation of a series of enzymes, beginning with phospholipase A2, which liberates arachidonic acid from membrane phospholipids, predominantly from phosphadidylcholine. Activation by a number of endothelial cell agonists, including thrombin, bradykinin, and histamine, stimulates cytosolic phospholipase A2. Arachidonic acid is then converted to prostaglandin H2 (PGH2) by two PGH synthase isoenzymes (also known as cyclooxygenases) (292), the rate-limiting step in the reaction (293). PGH2 is the common substrate for prostacyclin, prostaglandins, and thromboxane A2 synthases. In endothelial cells, PGI2 synthase is the most abundant prostaglandin synthase; therefore, mostly PGI2 is produced. All enzymes in the pathway can be regulated transcriptionally in endothelial cells (294), although the most significant inductive stimulus is on PGH synthase-2, which is not expressed at significant levels in quiescent endothelial cells but is impressively upregulated by IL-1α (295), endotoxin, and lysophosphatidylcholine (296,297). PGH synthase-1 autoinactivates during the catalytic step so that endothelial cell prostacyclin production in response to agonists is transient (288), even if continued release of arachidonic acid occurs. Increased expression of cytokine-inducible PGH synthase-2 has been postulated to provide for more sustained prostacyclin release during the endothelial cell response to immune injury/activation (259).

Although data are scarce, it has been postulated that reduced or inadequate prostacyclin synthesis may contribute to intraglomerular fibrin and platelet deposition during immune-mediated (265,298) and microangiopathic glomerular injury (299). Therapeutic infusion of prostacyclin analogs has been attempted in patients with the hemolytic uremic syndrome (299), in NZB/WF1 mice with immune complex–mediated glomerulonephritis (300), and in rats with anti-Thy-1–mediated glomerulonephritis (301). Although the overall inflammatory response appeared diminished (302), convincing effects of prostacyclin analogs on the degree of intraglomerular platelet and fibrin deposition have not been reported.

Nitric Oxide

The second endothelium-derived inhibitor of platelet activation and smooth muscle cell contraction, NO, is produced in endothelial cells by a constitutively expressed NO synthase (eNOS) that converts arginine to citrulline, liberating NO in the process (303–306). NO acts directly on soluble guanylate cyclase to generate the second messenger cyclic guanosine monophosphate. The eNOS is calcium dependent and is activated by a number of agonists that trip the inositol-tris-phosphate-calcium-protein kinase C cascade in endothelial cells, among them thrombin, bradykinin, platelet-activating factor, and histamine (305). Expression of eNOS is increased in anti-Thy-1–mediated glomerulonephritis in rats (307), possibly due to the action of TGF-β1, which is induced in anti–Thy-1 glomerulonephritis (308) and stimulates eNOS transcription in endothelial cells (309).

Although NO production by eNOS may increase during immune-mediated glomerular injury, there also is a profound upregulation of inducible NO synthase in various forms of glomerulonephritis (307,310–312). Inducible NO synthase (iNOS) is expressed in macrophages in response to stimulation by IL-1β and TNF-α, and increased glomerular iNOS expression correlates well with macrophage accumulation. Glomerular mesangial cells (313,314), smooth muscle cells (315,316), and endothelial cells (317,318) also express iNOS when stimulated with IL-1β and TNF-α and interferon-γ. Induction of iNOS in macrophages (319,320), smooth muscle cells (321), and endothelial cells is potentiated by adenylate cyclase–coupled mediators (315,322,323) and inhibited by glucocorticoids and TGF-β (317,324). In vascular smooth muscle cells, induction of iNOS expression also is inhibited by angiotensin II. Mohaupt et al. (325) showed that two isoforms of inducible NOS exist in the kidney: one homologous with the macrophage iNOS was expressed most prominently in glomeruli and tubules, the other in renal vascular smooth muscle cells. Greater induction of the vascular smooth muscle cell than of the macrophage isoform was observed after stimulation by cytokines (325). These findings are consistent with those of Spink et al. (326), who reported that promoter activity of the vascular smooth muscle cell iNOS is regulated by NF-κB in response to cytokines, whereas stimulation of the macrophage isoform by LPS does not involve NF-κB.

In glomerulonephritis, both eNOS and iNOS activity and consequent NO synthesis increase. Because NO is a potent inhibitor of platelet aggregation, blockers of NO synthase in models of glomerulonephritis might be expected to increase platelet deposition. NO also may act to inhibit some immune responses, and it may have direct toxic effects when present at very high concentrations (327,328). In rats with experimental glomerulonephritis, Ferrario et al. (329) found a significant increase in proteinuria, likely related to an increase in glomerular capillary pressure and reduced glomerular neutrophil infiltration in response to NO synthesis inhibition. Waddington et al. (330) observed increased proteinuria when NO synthesis was inhibited in rats with nephrotoxic serum nephritis, but they also found markedly increased intraglomerular platelet deposition and thrombosis. Thus, limited studies so far suggest that overproduction of NO during glomerulonephritis serves to offset other stimuli for platelet deposition and thrombosis.

Activated Endothelium and Coagulation

Thrombin

Thrombin is a multifunctional protease central to the process of coagulation, with additional actions on specific platelet and endothelial cell receptors. Thrombin activates endothelial cell prostacyclin, NO, and vWF release, actions that are mediated via endothelial cell thrombin receptors. Active thrombin is the product of prothromin cleavage by factors Xa and V (Fig. 4). The procoagulant actions of thrombin include induction of platelet aggregation, fibrin formation from fibrinogen, and activation of coagulation factors V, VII, and XIII (259). Healthy endothelial cells strongly inhibit the procoagulant activity of thrombin through thrombomodulin and antithrombin III–mediated effects. During inflammatory disease, there is reduced effectiveness of thrombin interactions with the endothelium; consequently, its procoagulant activity increases.

Thrombomodulin

Thrombomodulin, a potent inhibitor of coagulation, is an integral membrane protein expressed in abundance at the surface of endothelial cells (331). Thrombomodulin binds and induces a conformational change in thrombin, thereby enhancing its affinity for protein C. Protein C, a proenzyme produced by the liver, is then selectively activated by thrombin at the endothelial cell surface, and active protein C cleaves and inactivates clotting factors Va and VIIIa. Endothelial cells produce another component of this system, protein S, a vitamin K–dependent factor that enhances the activity of protein C against factor Va (332,333). Thus, the interaction of thrombin with thrombomodulin serves as a negative feedback inhibitor of the coagulation cascade. The thrombin–thrombomodulin complex is internalized and degraded after thrombin binding, a process that also serves to reduce thrombin action.

When endothelial cells are stimulated with the cytokines TNF-α and IL-1β, thrombomodulin expression at the endothelial cell surface is markedly reduced (334). This effect is mediated through rapid internalization and degradation of cell surface thrombomodulin (335) and reduced thrombomodulin transcription (336,337). Loss of cell surface thrombomodulin, but not the reduced transcription, is mediated by activation of protein kinase C (334,338). Reduced thrombomodulin transcription and cell-surface expression were observed for as long as 24 h after stimulation of endothelial cells with TNF-α. In contrast to the cytokine response, thrombin increases thrombomodulin mRNA expression in endothelial cells and stimulates thrombomodulin internalization and degradation in endothelial cells (339). In keeping with such in vitro findings, Horvat and Palade (340) reported thrombomodulin expression at the apical plasma membrane of endothelial cells in heart, lung, and kidney in vivo. Upon infusion of thrombin, clusters of thrombomodulin and thrombin were found within cells and at the basolateral endothelial cell surface. Such findings suggest that endothelial cells remove active thrombin from the circulation by thrombomodulin-dependent endo- and trans-cytosis (340).

Several investigators have addressed the question of whether altered thrombomodulin expression can be observed in glomerulonephritis and by inference might play a role in increased fibrin and platelet deposition. DeBault (331) found thrombomodulin to be an endothelial cell–specific protein expressed most abundantly in the lung, heart, and intestinal vasculature. Relative to other vessels, renal glomeruli expressed less thrombomodulin. In rats infused with LPS, massive intrarenal platelet aggregation and thrombosis were observed, but glomerular thrombomodulin expression did not differ from control rats (261). Mizutani et al. (341) examined thrombomodulin expression in 100 patients with different forms of glomerulonephritis and found low levels of discernible thrombomodulin under control conditions and no difference from controls in most of the pathologic specimens. However, increased glomerular staining for thrombomodulin was observed in patients with membranoproliferative lupus nephritis. Circulating levels of thrombomodulin were found to be increased in patients with lupus nephritis compared with other patients with a reduced glomerular filtration rate (342). Shiiki et al. (343) examined the expression of thrombomodulin in patients with focal and segmental glomerulosclerosis and found no change in diseased versus normal glomeruli, but a marked upregulation of thrombomodulin protein in glomeruli of patients with focal and segmental glomerulosclerosis (FSGS) in remission. They suggested that thrombomodulin may play a role in the repair process. Thus, although thrombomodulin expression is suppressed in response to stimulation of endothelial cells with inflammatory cytokines in vitro, it is unclear at this time whether changes in this system play a role in glomerular endothelial cell activation in vivo.

Antithrombin III

Heparan sulfate proteoglycans at the endothelial cell surface serve to bind and activate antithrombin III. Antithrombin III is a serine protease inhibitor, which binds thrombin and other serine proteases, including clotting factors Xa, IXa, and XIIa. Binding of thrombin to antithrombin III is markedly accelerated by heparan sulfate (259). The loss of antithrombin III in patients with the nephrotic syndrome is believed to play an important role in the increased susceptibility to intravascular thrombosis (344). In patients with acute renal allograft rejection, depletion of the vascular heparan sulfate proteoglycan-antithrombin III has been reported and was associated with significantly greater intrarenal fibrin deposition (345). Release of heparan sulfate in response to neutrophil-mediated endothelial cell injury is found in vitro (346) and may account for the increase in circulating antithrombin III observed in patients with acute renal allograft rejection (347). In one patient with concomitant antithrombin III deficiency and antiphospholipid antibody syndrome, massive intraglomerular thrombosis has been described (348). However, there is no convincing evidence that glomerular endothelial cell damage in most forms of glomerular immune injury leads to reduced local antithrombin III activity and thrombosis.

Tissue Factor

Tissue factor is an important initiator of coagulation via the extrinsic pathway and is expressed in most tissues (155). It is responsible for the immediate coagulation of blood in case of escape from the vasculature into tissues. Renal glomerular epithelial cells (349) and mesangial cells (350) express tissue factor in vitro, although levels in unstimulated mesangial cells are low. Under normal conditions, endothelial cells produce little if any tissue factor. Nevertheless, because tissue factor expression is under the control of a promoter containing NF-κB response elements (155,159), it is activated in endothelial cells exposed to TNF-α and IL-1β (150,159,351). Thrombin also increases tissue factor abundance at the apical surface of endothelial cells through mechanisms that involve acute mobilization of prestored tissue factor (352) and increased tissue factor gene transcription (339). Endothelial cells infected with measles virus (353) or cytomegalovirus (354) express much greater levels of tissue factor than do noninfected cells. In endothelial cells, activation by TNF-α, thrombin, and other proinflammatory agents results in polarized expression of tissue factor at the apical surface (353,355,356).

Whereas endothelial cells can be stimulated to produce significant amounts of tissue factor in response to proinflammatory cytokines, in glomerular diseases the most abundant source of this factor are activated monocyte/macrophages. Tipping et al. (357) found increased tissue factor expression by resident glomerular cells early in crescentic glomerulonephritis, followed by abundant expression later in the disease when tissue factor mRNA colocalized with macrophages. In rabbits with anti-GBM–mediated glomerulonephritis, the same group reported enhanced tissue factor expression in conjunction with macrophage infiltration and enhanced fibrin deposition (358). In this regard, it is of interest that endothelial cells participate in stimulating monocyte tissue factor expression in a contact-dependent fashion. Lo et al. (359) found that adhesion of monocytes to activated endothelial cells resulted in increased monocyte tissue factor transcription and protein expression. This effect was not observed with unstimulated endothelial cells and was dependent on cell–cell contact. Purified P-selectin mimics this effect of endothelial cells on monocyte tissue factor expression and may represent the critical molecule that triggers the response during monocyte–endothelial cell contact (360).

Studies in human glomerulonephritis (263,361) and animal models (357,358) have suggested that enhanced procoagulant activity participates in the process of fibrin deposition locally, a process that Tipping and Holdsworth (263) suggest is at least partly mediated by increased local tissue factor expression. In hyperacute xenograft rejection, enhanced endothelial cell tissue factor expression, together with other markers of endothelial cell activation, is also observed (362). A tissue factor pathway inhibitor (TFPI) also has been identified (363). This factor is produced in the liver and by endothelial cells, and Wu (259) suggested that endothelium may be a major source. Reduced levels of circulating TFPI were found in patients with active thrombotic thrombocytopenic purpura (364), suggesting that enhanced consumption or deficiency of this factor may promote vascular thrombosis in thrombotic microangiopathy.

Fibrinolytic System and Endothelial Cells

The plasminogen–plasmin system performs two important functions. It is critical for continual surveillance of the vasculature for fibrin strands and their appropriate dissolution, and it acts at cell surfaces to aid in matrix degradation during cell migration (365). Plasminogen is bound by cell surface plasminogen receptors, which are abundant on endothelial cells (366,367). Tissue-type plasminogen activator (t-PA), produced by endothelial cells (368), also binds to cell surface receptors, where it is brought in close apposition to bound plasminogen and cleaves it to produce active plasmin. Small amounts of urokinase-type plasminogen activator (u-PA) also are synthesized by unstimulated endothelial cells (369). t-PA is thought to act primarily in the vascular tree to remove fibrin, whereas u-PA may act predominantly in matrix degradation during cell growth and migration. Active plasmin bound to the cell surface is protected from inactivation, but once released from cells it has a short half-life due to inactivation by α2-antiplasmin (365). Endothelial cells also produce powerful inhibitors of t-PA, plasminogen activator inhibitors I and II (PAI-I, PAI-II) (368, 370). PAI-I associates with endothelial cells by binding to vitronectin at the cell surface (371), and vitronectin is necessary for PAI-I–mediated inactivation of both t-PA and u-PA (372,373). Thus, the process of plasmin activation by t-PA and control over its activation by inhibitors of t-PA is largely confined to the endothelial cell surface by binding to appropriate receptors, vitronectin, and proteoglycans.

During endothelial cell activation by inflammatory cytokines, the balance between t-PA and PAI-I synthesis is profoundly altered. Schleef et al. found that t-PA protein expression by human endothelial cells was reduced to 25% of control values 24 h after TNF-α or IL-1β treatment, whereas PAI activity increased some fivefold (368). The cytokine-induced increase in PAI-I expression is largely due to transcriptional activation (368,374–376). Furthermore, under basal conditions most of the PAI-I immunoreactivity was found in the subendothelial cell compartment, whereas a large amount of PAI-I immunoreactivity appeared at the apical surface of endothelial cells in response to cytokine treatment (377). Although t-PA activity is diminished during endothelial cell activation, u-PA transcription is significantly enhanced by TNF-α treatment (369). Thrombin also induces PAI-I synthesis (378,379) and is involved with neutralizing PAI-I in the context of vitronectin (380). Endothelial cell infection by rickettsia results in profound upregulation of PAI-I expression and reduced t-PA activity at the endothelial cell surface (381). Thus, in conjunction with other mechanisms already discussed, the alteration in the balance between cell surface t-PA and PAI-I activity during endothelial cell activation would tend to enhance endothelial cell procoagulant activity and therefore promote local fibrin deposition.

In immune-mediated glomerular diseases, alterations in the plasminogen/plasmim system have been sought both to understand mechanisms of intraglomerular fibrin deposition and to delineate mechanisms involved in glomerular remodeling. In the normal kidney, t-PA is expressed primarily in glomeruli, whereas u-PA is observed along the tubule epithelium. PAI-I expression is usually low (382,383). Keeton et al. (384) found significant induction of PAI-I mRNA and immunoreactivity in kidneys of MRL/lpr mice with active lupus nephritis. Levels of expression seemed to correlate with disease activity, and much of the PAI-I expression was observed in vessels, including glomeruli, where it seemed to colocalize with endothelial cells (384). In a rabbit model of anti-GBM antibody–mediated glomerulonephritis, diminished t-PA and u-PA activity together with enhanced PAI-I activity were found in glomeruli infiltrated with macrophages during the autologous phase of the disease, when fibrin deposition was also significant. In contrast, these changes were not observed during the heterologous phase, when macrophage infiltration and fibrin deposition were also much less prominent (385). Similar findings were obtained by Feng et al. (386), who reported the greatest alteration in the fibrinolytic profile and fibrin deposits early after induction of anti-GBM disease and postulated that inflammatory cytokines such as IL-1β were at play. In rats injected with TNF-α and in rats with acute nephrotoxic serum nephritis, intraglomerular PAI-I expression also increased rapidly and dissipated after 24 h; however, fibrin deposits were noted early and continued to increase with time (387), suggesting that changes in the fibrinolytic system may operate early, but that other mechanisms must be considered to explain the continued fibrin deposition. In human glomerulonephritis, some evidence favoring an imbalance in the intraglomerular fibrinolytic system has been found (388), and in some patients improvement of glomerular function and a decrease in fibrin deposition was found after treatment with the fibrinolytic agent ancrod (389). Nevertheless, an increase in PAI-I expression does not invariably accompany glomerular fibrin deposition (390). It is more likely that multiple mechanisms cooperate to enhance intraglomerular fibrin deposition in human glomerulonephritis.

The Schwartzman reaction, produced by two consecutive infusions of endotoxin, produces massive intravascular coagulation, glomerular capillary occlusion with fibrin, and, when severe, acute cortical necrosis. Endotoxin infusion in rats was found to markedly reduce t-PA and increase PAI-I expression in renal vessels (383), and infusion of t-PA markedly reduced glomerular fibrin deposits after induction of the Schwartzman reaction in rabbits (391). These findings are consistent with rapid reversal of the normal fibrinolytic capacity of renal endothelium after exposure to endotoxin in vitro. Human renal microvascular endothelial cells express receptors for Shiga toxin and the Shiga-like verotoxin responsible for many cases of childhood hemolytic uremic syndrome (392). In such cells PAI-I expression increased dramatically in response to Shiga toxin, whereas no change in fibrinolytic profile was observed in response to TNF-α. In contrast, the response to Shiga toxin was significantly less in human umbilical vein endothelial cells, whereas PAI-I levels increased and t-PA decreased after cytokine treatment (393). This in vitro finding is consistent with reports of markedly increased circulating PAI-I levels in patients with active hemolytic uremic syndrome (394,395), and together the data are consistent with a significant pathogenic role for excess PAI-I release from endothelial cells in this disease.

CHRONIC RESPONSE TO IMMUNE-MEDIATED GLOMERULAR INJURY

Glomerular endothelial cells participate in the repair response to immune-mediated disease by several mechanisms. First, glomerular injury can be sufficiently severe to cause endothelial cell death via apoptosis or necrosis (19). Proliferation of glomerular endothelial cells to form new capillaries or to cover denuded basement membrane takes place as a component of glomerular repair. Second, immune-mediated glomerular injury is frequently accompanied by enhanced matrix deposition both within the GBM and in the mesangial area. Although mesangial cell matrix synthesis is believed to account for most of the excess matrix, published evidence suggests that endothelial cells also produce matrix as a response to immune injury. Finally, there is a prominent role for growth factors during both the acute and chronic phases of immune-mediated glomerular disease. Endothelial cells produce and activate growth factors that participate in this process.

Endothelial Cell Proliferation and Matrix Synthesis

In normal, mature glomeruli, endothelial cell division is a rare event (396). However, active endothelial cell proliferation is one of the phenomena observed in pathologic specimens from patients with different forms of proliferative glomerulonephritis (11,12). In the experimental model of Habu snake venom–induced glomerulonephritis, prominent endothelial cell proliferation and new capillary formation were observed (397). Also, Iruela-Arispe et al. (398) reported significant endothelial cell proliferation and angiogenesis in the repair phase of anti-Thy-1 antibody–mediated mesangial proliferative glomerulonephritis, a response that was dependent, in part, on basic fibroblast growth factor (bFGF). bFGF is a known angiogenic growth factor released from injured endothelial cells (399) which stimulates glomerular endothelial cell proliferation in vitro (400). In addition to bFGF, upregulation of vascular endothelial cell growth factor and its receptor suggests that vascular endothelial growth factor also participates in stimulating endothelial cell proliferation under these conditions (398). TGF-β also plays a prominent role in the glomerular response to injury in many experimental models of glomerulonephritis, in human glomerulonephritis, and in other human glomerular and interstitial diseases in which excess matrix deposition and fibrosis are important features (401,402). TGF-β1 exerts angiogenic effects in vivo (403) and participates in the process of capillary formation in vitro (404). Thus, it is also possible that angiogenesis during glomerular repair may involve TGF-β1.

Matrix accumulation and GBM thickening are a common feature of glomerular immune injury. In membranous nephropathy, matrix laid down between immune deposits on the epithelial side of the GBM is derived from podocytes. However, enhanced deposition of α3/α4 type IV collagen along the subendothelial surface of the GBM also has been described in membranous glomerulonephritis (405). Because α3/α4 type IV collagen is derived exclusively from glomerular endothelial cells (406), this finding suggests that enhanced endothelial cell type IV collagen synthesis or reduced degradation may participate in GBM thickening. In a rat model of chronic renal transplant rejection, subendothelial cell matrix deposition was similarly observed, suggesting that enhanced endothelial cell matrix synthesis participates in the glomerular remodeling response during chronic transplant rejection (407). Similarly, in patients recovering from pre-eclampsia, increased subendothelial cell matrix components were found (408). It is possible that the increase in subendothelial cell matrix reflects reduced matrix degradation (409). Nevertheless, the findings are consistent with the view that endothelial cells participate in GBM deposition and remodeling as part of the repair response to glomerular injury.

Growth Factors

Endothelial cells produce both growth inhibitory and mitogenic mediators (410). Of note, endothelium-derived vasodilators (NO and prostacyclin) tend to inhibit proliferation of neighboring cells and vasoconstrictors (endothelin-1, angiotensin II, platelet-derived growth factor) tend to promote proliferation of neighboring cells, including vascular smooth muscle cells in arteries and arterioles and mesangial cells in the glomerulus. Evidence for overexpression of several growth factors during glomerular immune injury has been found (135,411–413), and inhibition of some of these growth factors has been reported to reduce cell proliferation and/or matrix deposition (412,414,415). The growth regulators most commonly implicated in glomerular cell proliferation and matrix deposition are PDGF, bFGF, and TGF-β. Prominent sources of PDGF and TGF-β1 are platelets (416), macrophages (412,413,417), and T-lymphocytes (418), although resident mesangial cells also have been shown to produce PDGF, TGF-β1, and bFGF (412,418–421).

Endothelial cells also contribute to the vascular remodeling and repair process by producing PDGF, bFGF, and TGF-β1 (422–424). bFGF is a heparin-binding growth factor that is normally present in the subendothelial cell matrix and is bound to endothelial cell–associated heparan sulfate proteoglycan (425). bFGF is released from subendothelial cell matrix by the endothelial cell–associated plasminogen activator system and is believed to be important for invasion of matrix during angiogenesis and to help re-establish the integrity of the endothelium after denudation (426–429). Furthermore, interaction of endothelial cells with activated platelets and neutrophils also results in release of bFGF from the subendothelial cell matrix and from the cells (430). It recently was shown that bFGF is highly expressed in the repair phase of anti–Thy-1 mesangial proliferative glomerulonephritis in the rat, that endothelial cell proliferation and angiogenesis are observed in this model of immune-mediated glomerular disease, and that bFGF is an important local factor necessary for the repair of the glomerular endothelium (397). Also, because mesangial cell proliferation is in part regulated by bFGF, it is conceivable that glomerular endothelial cell injury and consequent release of bFGF from subendothelial cell matrix exerts paracrine actions on the mesangial cells. Finally, it has been observed that administration of bFGF in rats produces a glomerular lesion similar to that of FSGS, with prominent podocyte hypertrophy (431). It is therefore possible that bFGF release from GBM could be involved in the development of human FSGS.

Endothelial cells also produce PDGF: two homologous growth factors produced from distinct genes, PDGF-A and -B. PDGF-B has potent mitogenic actions on mesangial cells (432,433) and is required during renal morphogenesis for the formation of glomerular mesangial cells (434,435). In renal microvascular endothelial cells, thrombin and TGF-β1 stimulate PDGF synthesis (424, 436–438), whereas bFGF significantly inhibits synthesis and release of PDGF (439). Furthermore, mechanical injury of endothelial cell monolayers in vivo results in enhanced local PDGF-B synthesis (440). Because thrombin and TGF-β1 are likely to act on glomerular endothelial cells during immune injury, endothelium-derived PDGF-B may participate in glomerular remodeling during immune-mediated glomerular injury.

Endothelial cells also may participate in increasing local TGF-β1 concentrations during the response to immune-mediated injury. Like most cells, endothelial cells produce TGF-β1, but during glomerular injury this growth regulator is produced at much higher levels by macrophages and platelets. Nevertheless, TGF-β is released from cells as a latent precursor and must be activated in order to produce biologic effects. Both plasmin (441) and thrombospondin (442,443) activate TGF-β1. Endothelial cell–derived plasmin participates in the release of active TGF-β in pericyte/endothelial cell cocultures through a process that requires immobilization of latent TGF-β at the smooth muscle or pericyte cell membrane (444–446). Whether endothelial cells in the glomerulus play a role in TGF-β activation during immune-mediated injury remains to be determined.

SUMMARY

The renal endothelium participates in every component of the response to immune-mediated injury. It is subject to direct leukocyte- and complement-mediated damage and activation, and it responds with activation to cytokines released by other cells. Endothelial activation is critically important for the process of leukocyte recruitment and promotes local coagulation. It is becoming more and more evident that many of the processes involved in coagulation (249,340,359), leukocyte recruitment (213), and mediator production (171) are restricted to the surface of the endothelium by various binding proteins and receptors and often require cell–cell contact (447). Finally, endothelial cells also participate in the chronic tissue remodeling response observed during repair or ongoing immune injury because it promotes recruitment and adhesion of platelets and leukocytes that release growth factors and because endothelial cells themselves respond to injury with enhanced growth factor synthesis.

It is not yet known to what degree specific responses of renal glomerular and peritubular endothelial cells differ from the generic responses decribed in this chapter. Also, patterns of injury differ signficantly in various diseases; reasons for many such differences remain to be dissected. Further work also is needed to develop pharmaceutical agents that might interrupt deleterious aspects of the endothelial response to immune system activation.

Acknowledgements

Work in the author's laboratory was supported by an American Heart Association Established Investigator Award, by a grant-in-aid from the American Heart Foundation, and by National Institutes of Health Grant DK47023-01. Sidney McGaughey provided expert secretarial assistance.

REFERENCES

1. Risau W. Differentiation of endothelium. *FASEB J* 1995;9:926–933.
2. Bennet HS, Luft JH, Ampton JC. Morphological classification of vertebrate blood capillaries. *Am J Physiol* 1959;196:381–390.
3. Remuzzi A, Brenner BM, Pata V, et al. Three-dimensional reconstructed glomerular capillary network: blood flow distribution and local filtration. *Am J Physiol* 1992;263:F562–F572.
4. Horvat R, Hovoka A, Dekan G, Poczewski H, Kerjaschki D. Endothelial cell membranes contain podocalyxin—the major sialoprotein of visceral glomerular epithelial cells. *J Cell Biol* 1986;102:484–491.
5. Jorgenssen F. *The ultrastructure of the normal human glomerulus*. Copenhagen: Ejnar Munksgaard; 1966.
6. Lemley KV, Kriz W. Structure and function of the renal vasculature. In: Tisher CC, Brenner BM eds. *Renal pathology*. Philadelphia: JB Lippincott; 1994:981–1026.
7. Vasmant D, Maurice M, Feldmann G. Cytoskeleton ultrastructure of podocytes and glomerular endothelial cells in man and in the rat. *Anat Rec* 1984;210:17–24.
8. Faith GC, Trump BF. The glomerular capillary wall in human kidney disease: acute glomerulonephritis, systemic lupus erythematosus, and preeclampsia–eclampsia. Comparative electron microscopic observations and a review. *Lab Invest* 1966;15:1682–1719.
9. Fisher ER, Pardo V, Paul R, Hayashi TT. Ultrastructural studies in hypertension. IV. Toxemia of pregnancy. *Am J Pathol* 1969;55:109–131.
10. Vitsky BH, Suzuki Y, Strauss L, Churg J. The hemolytic–uremic syndrome: a study of renal pathologic alterations. *Am J Pathol* 1969;57:627–647.
11. Fish AJ, Herdman RC, Michael AF, Pickering RJ, Good RA. Epidemic acute glomerulonephritis associated with type 49 streptococcal pyoderma. II. Correlative study of light, immunofluorescent and electron microscopic findings. *Am J Med* 1970;48:28–39.
12. Andres GA, Accinni L, Hsu KC, Zabriskie JB, Seegal BC. Electron microscopic studies of human glomerulonephritis with ferritin-conjugated antibody. Localization of antigen–antibody complexes in glomerular structures of patients with acute glomerulonephritis. *J Exp Med* 1966;123:399–412.
13. Jennette JC, Iskandar SS, Dalldorf FG. Pathologic differentiation between lupus and nonlupus membranous glomerulopathy. *Kidney Int* 1983;24:377–385.
14. Zimmerman SW. Burkholder PM. Immunoglobulin A nephropathy. *Arch Intern Med* 1975;135:1217–1223.
15. Sisson S, Dysart NK Jr, Fish AJ, Vernier RL. Localization of the Goodpasture antigen by immunoelectron microscopy. *Clin Immunol Immunopathol* 1982;23:414–429.
16. Morita T, Suzuki Y, Churg J. Structure and development of the glomerular crescent. *Am J Pathol* 1973;72:349–368.
17. Katz SM. Reduplication of the glomerular basement membrane. A study of 110 cases. *Arch Pathol Lab Med* 1981;105:67–70.
18. Zhang PF, Rao KV, Anderson WR. An ultrastructural study of the membranoproliferative variant of transplant glomerulopathy. *Ultrastruct Pathol* 1988;12:185–194.
19. Serra A, Cameron JS, Turner DR, et al. Vasculitis affecting the kidney: presentation, histopathology and long-term outcome. *Q J Med* 1984;53:181–208.
20. Hotchi M. Pathological studies on Takayasu arteritis. *Heart Vessels* 1992;7(suppl):11–17.
21. Weiss MA, Crissman JD. Renal biopsy findings in Wegener's granulomatosis: segmental necrotizing glomerulonephritis with glomerular thrombosis. *Hum Pathol* 1984;15:943–956.
22. Juncos W, Alexander RW, Marbury TC. Intravascular clotting preceding crescent formation in a patient with Wegener's granulomatosis and rapidly progressive glomerulonephritis. *Nephron* 1979;24:17–20.
23. Grefte A, Giessen MVD, Son WV. The TH. Circulating cytomegaolovirus infected endothelial cells in patients with an active CMV infection. *J Infect Dis* 1993;167:270–277.

24. Waldman, WJ, Knight DA, Huang EH, Sedmak DD. Bidirectional transmission of infectious cytomegalovirus between monocytes and vascular endothelial cells: an in vitro model. *J Infect Dis* 1995;171: 263–272.
25. Moses AV, Bloom FE, Pauza CD, Nelson JA. Human immunodeficiency virus infection of human brain capillary endothelial cells occurs via a CD4/galactosylceramide-independent mechanism. *Proc Natl Acad Sci U S A* 1993;90:10474–10478.
26. Estes PC, Cheville NF. The ultrastructure of vascular lesions in equine viral arteritis. *Am J Pathol* 1970;58:235–253.
27. Phinney PR, Fligiel S, Bryson YJ, Porter DD. Necrotizing vasculitis in a case of disseminated neonatal herpes simplex infection. *Arch Pathol Lab Med* 1982;106:64–67.
28. Golden MP, Hammer SM, Wanke CA, Albrecht MA. Cytomegalovirus vasculitis. Case reports and review of the literature. *Medicine (Baltimore)* 1994;73:246–255.
29. Hendrix MGR, Salimans MM, van Boven CP, Bruggeman CA. High prevalence of latently present cytomegalovirus nucleic acids in arterial walls of patients suffering from grade III atherosclerosis. *Am J Pathol* 1990;136:23–28.
30. Jacob HS, Visser M, Key NS, Goodman JL, Moldow CF, Vercellotti GM. Herpes virus infection of endothelium: new insights into atherosclerosis. *Trans Am Clin Climatol Assoc* 1992;103:95–104.
31. Sen GC, Lengyel P. The interferon system. A bird's eye view of its biochemistry. *J Biol Chem* 1992;267:5017–5020.
32. Sedmak DD, Chaiwiriyakul S, Knight DA, Waldmann WJ. The role of interferon beta in human cytomegalovirus–mediated inhibition of HLA DR induction on endothelial cells. *Arch Virol* 1995;140: 111–126.
33. Sedmak DD, Guglielmo AM, Knight DA, Birmingham DJ, Huang EH, Waldman WJ. Cytomegalovirus inhibits major histocompatibility class II expression on infected endothelial cells *Am J Pathol* 1994; 144:683–692.
34. Nagata S, Golstein P. The Fas death factor. *Science* 1995;267:1449–1455.
35. Dong CM, Wilson JE, Winters GL, Mcmanus BM. Human transplant coronary artery disease—pathological evidence for Fas-mediated apoptotic cytotoxicity in allograft arteriopathy. *Lab Invest* 1996;74: 921–931.
36. Pober JS, Cotran RS. Immunologic interactions of T lymphocytes with vascular endothelium. *Adv Immunol* 1991;50:261–302.
37. Podack ER, Hengartner H, Lichtenheld MG. A central role of perforin in cytolysis? *Ann Rev Immunol* 1991;9:129–157.
38. Trinchieri G. Biology of natural killer cells. *Adv Immunol* 1989;47: 187–376.
39. Brankin B, Hart MN, Cosby SL, Fabry Z, Allen IV. Adhesion molecule expression and lymphocyte adhesion to cerebral endothelium: effects of measles virus and herpes simplex 1 virus. *J Neuroimmunol* 1995;56:1–8.
40. Scholz M, Hamann A, Blaheta RA, Auth MK, Encke A, Markus BH. Cytomegalovirus- and interferon-related effects on human endothelial cells. Cytomegalovirus infection reduces upregulation of HLA class II antigen expression after treatment with interferon-gamma. *Hum Immunol* 1992;35:230–238.
41. Almeida GD, Porada CD, St Jeor S, Ascensao JL. Human cytomegalovirus alters interleukin-6 production by endothelial cells. *Blood* 1994;83:370–376.
42. Bok RA, Jacob HS, Balla J, et al. Herpes simplex virus decreases endothelial cell plasminogen activator inhibitor. *Thromb Haemost* 1993;69:253–258.
43. Delneste Y, Lassalle P, Jeannin P, et al. Production of anti-endothelial cell antibodies by coculture of EBV-infected human B cells with endothelial cells. *Cell Immunol* 1993;150:15–26.
44. Casciola-Rosen LA, Anhalt G, Rosen A. Autoantigens targeted in systemic lupus erythematosus are clustered in two populations of surface structures on apoptotic keratinocytes *J Exp Med* 1994;179: 1317–1330.
45. Cines DB. Disorders associated with antibodies to endothelial cells. *Rev Infect Dis* 1989;11(suppl 4):705–711.
46. Robson SC, Candinas D, Hancock WW, Wrighton C, Winkler H, Bach FH. Role of endothelial cells in transplantation. *Int Arch Allergy Immunol* 1995;106:305–322.
47. LaVecchio JA, Dunne AD, Edge AS. Enzymatic removal of alpha-galactosyl epitopes from porcine endothelial cells diminishes the cytotoxic effect of natural antibodies. *Transplantation* 1995;60: 841–847.
48. Leung DYM, Geha RS, Newberger JW, et al. Two monokines, interleukin-1 and tumor necrosis factor, render cultured vascular endothelial cells susceptible to lysis by antibodies circulating during Kawasaki syndrome. *J Exp Med* 1986;164:1958–1972.
49. Wang CR, Liu MF, Tsai RT, Chuang CY, Chen CY. Circulating intercellular adhesion molecules-1 and autoantibodies including anti–endothelial cell, anti-cardiolipin, and anti-neutrophil cytoplasma antibodies in patients with vasculitis. *Clin Rheumatol* 1993;12:375–380.
50. Holt CM, Lindsey N, Moult J, et al. Antibody-dependent cellular cytotoxicity of vascular endothelium: characterization and pathogenic association in systemic sclerosis. *Clin Exp Immunol* 1989;78: 359–365.
51. Dhingra R, Talwar KK, Chopra P, Kumar R. An enzyme linked immunosorbent assay for detection of anti-aorta antibodies in Takayasu arteritis patients. *Int J Cardiol* 1993;40:237–242.
52. Casciola–Rosen L, Rosen A, Petri M, Schlissel M. Surface blebs on apoptotic cells are sites of enhanced procoagulant activity—implications for coagulation events and antigenic spread in systemic lupus erythematosus. *Proc Natl Acad Sci U S A* 1996;93:1624–1629.
53. Casciola-Rosen LA, Anhalt GJ, Rosen A. DNA-dependent protein kinase is one of a subset of autoantigens specifically cleaved early during apoptosis. *J Exp Med* 1995;182:1625–1634.
54. Chan TM, Frampton G, Jayne DR, Perry GJ, Lockwood CM, Cameron JS. Clinical significance of anti-endothelial cell antibodies in systemic vasculitis: a longitudinal study comparing anti-endothelial cell antibodies and anti-neutrophil cytoplasm antibodies. *Am J Kidney Dis* 1993;22:387–392.
55. King WJ, Adu D, Daha MR, et al. Endothelial cells and renal epithelial cells do not express the Wegeners autoantigen, proteinase 3. *Clin Exp Immunol* 1995;102:98–105.
56. Savage CO, Gaskin G, Pusey CD, Pearson JD. Anti-neutrophil cytoplasm antibodies can recognize vascular endothelial cell–bound anti-neutrophil cytoplasm antibody-associated autoantigens. *Exp Nephrol* 1993;1:190–195.
57. Falk RJ, Terrell RS, Charles LA, Jennette JC. Antineutrophil cytoplasmic autoantibodies induce neutrophils to degranulate and produce oxygen radicals in vitro. *Proc Natl Acad Sci U S A* 1990;87: 4115–4119.
58. Ewert BM, Jennette JC, Falk RJ. Antimyeloperoxidase antibodies stimulate neutrophils to damage human endothelial cells. *Kidney Int* 1992;41:375–383.
59. Savage COS, Pottinger BE, Gaskin G, Pusey CD, Pearson JD. Autoantibodies developing to myeloperoxidase and proteinase 3 in systemic vasculitis stimulate neutrophil cytotoxicity toward cultured endothelial cells. *Am J Pathol* 1992;141:335–342.
60. Camussi G, Biesecker G, Caldwell PR, Biancone L, Andres G, Brentjens JR. Role of the membrane attack complex of complement in lung injury mediated by antibodies to endothelium. *Int Arch Allergy Immunol* 1993;102:216–223.
61. Dalmasso AP, Platt JL, Bach FH. Reaction of complement with endothelial cells in a model of xenotransplantation. *Clin Exp Immunol* 1991;86(suppl 1):31–35.
62. Lerner RA, Glassock RJ, Dixon FJ. The role of antiglomerular basement antibody in the pathogenesis of human glomerulonephritis. *J Exp Med* 1967;126:989–1004.
63. Wilson CB, Dixon FJ. Antiglomerular basement membrane antibody-induced glomerulonephritis. *Kidney Int* 1973;3:74–89.
64. Tateno S, Kobayaski Y, Shigematsu H, Hiki Y. Study of lupus nephritis: its classification and the significance of subendothelial deposits. *Q J Med* 1983;295: 907–918.
65. Frampton G, Hobby P, Morgan A, Taines NA, Cameron JS. A role for DNA in anti-DNA antibodies binding to endothelial cells. *J Autoimmunity* 1991;4:463–478.
66. Chan TM, Frampton G, Staines NA, Hobby P, Perry GJ, Cameron JS. Different mechanisms by which monoclonal anti-DNA antibodies bind to human endothelial cells and glomerular mesangial cells. *Clin Exp Immunol* 1992;88:68–74.
67. Sorger K, Gessler, U, Hubner FK, et al. Subtypes of postinfectious glomerulonephritis: synopsis of clinical and pathological features. *Clin Nephrol* 1982;17:114–128.
68. Schumaker VN, Zavodszky P, Poon PH. Activation of the first component of complement. *Ann Rev Immunol* 1987;5:21–42.

69. van den Dobbelsteen ME, van der Woude FJ, Schroeijers WE, Klar-Mohamad N, van Es LA, Daha MR. C1Q, a subunit of the first component of complement, enhances the binding of aggregated IgG to rat renal mesangial cells. *J Immunol* 1993;151:4315–4324.
70. Peerschke EI, Malhotra R, Ghebrehiwet B, Reid KB, Willis AC, Sim RB. Isolation of a human endothelial cell C1q receptor (C1qR). *J Leukoc Biol* 1993;53:179–184.
71. Goodman EB, Tenner AJ. Signal transduction mechanisms of C1q-mediated superoxide production. Evidence for the involvement of temporally distinct staurosporine-insensitive and sensitive pathways. *J Immunol* 1992;148:3920–3928.
72. Tenner AJ. Functional aspects of the C1q receptors. *Behring Inst Mitt* 1993;93:241–523
73. Sim RB, Reid KBM. C1: molecular interactions with activating systems. *Immunol Today* 1991;12:307–311.
74. Ryan US, Schultz DR, Del Vecchio PJ, Ryan JW. Endothelial cells of bovine pulmonary artery lack receptors for C3b and for the Fc portion of immunoglobulin G. *Science* 1980;208:748–749.
75. Lozada C, Levin RI, Huie M, et al. Identification of C1q as the heat-labile serum cofactor required for immune complexes to stimulate endothelial expression of the adhesion molecules E-selectin and intercellular and vascular cell adhesion molecules 1. *Proc Natl Acad Sci U S A* 1995;92:8378–8382.
76. Cines DB, Lyss AP, Bina M, Corkey R, Kefalides NA, Friedman HM. Fc and C3 receptors induced by herpes simplex virus on cultured human endothelial cells. *J Clin Invest* 1982;69:123–128.
77. Ryan US, Schultz DR, Ryan JW. Fc and C3b receptors on pulmonary endothelial cells: induction by injury. *Science* 1981;214:557–558.
78. Wetsel RA. Expression of the complement C5a anaphylatoxin receptor (C5aR) on non-myeloid cells. *Immunol Lett* 1995;44:183–187.
79. Murphy HS, Shayman JA, Till GO, et al. Superoxide responses of endothelial cells to C5a and TNF-alpha: divergent signal transduction pathways. *Am J Physiol* 1992;263:L51–L59.
80. Foreman KE, Vaporciyan AA, Bonish BK, et al. C5a-induced expression of P-selectin in endothelial cells. *J Clin Invest* 1994;94:1147–1155.
81. Platt JL, Dalmasso AP, Lindman BJ, Ihrcke NS, Bach FH. The role of C5a and antibody in the release of heparan sulfate from endothelial cells. *Eur J Immunol* 1991;21:2887–2890.
82. Wagner DD. The Weibel-Palade body: the storage granule for von Willebrand factor and P-selectin. *Thromb Haemost* 1993;70:105–110.
83. Vogt W. Anaphylatoxins: possible roles in disease. *Complement* 1986;3:177–188.
84. Charo IF, Yuen C, Perez HD, Goldstein IM. Chemotactic peptides modulate adherence of human polymorphonuclear leukocytes to monolayers of cultured endothelial cells. *J Immunol* 1986;136:3412–3419.
85. Moser R, Olgiati L, Patarroyo M, Fehr J. Chemotaxins inhibit neutrophil adherence to and transmigration across cytokine-activated endothelium: correlation to the expression of L-selectin. *Eur J Immunol* 1993;23:1481–1487.
86. Hardy MM, Flickinger AG, Riley DP, Weiss RH, Ryan US. Superoxide dismutase mimetics inhibit neutrophil-mediated human aortic endothelial cell injury in vitro. *J Biol Chem* 1994;269:18535–18540.
87. Jose PJ, Forrest MJ, Williams TJ. Human C5a des Arg increases vascular permeability. *J Immunol* 1981;127:2376–2380.
88. Ember JA, Sanderson SD, Hugli TE, Morgan EL. Induction of interleukin-8 synthesis from monocytes by human C5a anaphylatoxin. *Am J Pathol* 1994;144:393–403.
89. Chuluyan HE, Osborn L, Lobb R, Issekutz AC. Domains 1 and 4 of vascular cell adhesion molecule-1 (CD106) both support very late activation antigen-4 (CD49D/CD29)-dependent monocyte transendothelial migration. *J Immunol* 1995;155:3135–3144.
90. Muller-Eberhard HJ. The membrane attack complex. *Ann Rev Immunol* 1986;4:503–528.
91. Boom BW, Mommaas M, Daha MR, Vermeer BJ. Complement-mediated endothelial cell damage in immune complex vasculitis of the skin: ultrastructural localization of the membrane attack complex. *J Invest Dermatol* 1989;93(suppl):68–72.
92. Rollins SA, Matis LA, Springhorn JP, Setter E, Wolff DW. Monoclonal antibodies directed against human C5 and C8 block complement-mediated damage of xenogeneic cells and organs. *Transplantation* 1995;60:1284–1292.
93. Suttorp N, Bhakdi S. Terminal complement complex and endothelial cells. *Z Kardiol* 1989;78(suppl 6):140–142.
94. Okada M, Yoshioka K, Takemura T, et al. Immunohistochemical localization of C3d fragment of complement and S-protein (vitronectin) in normal and diseased human kidneys: association with the C5b-9 complex and vitronectin receptor. *Virchows Arch [A]* 1993;422:367–373.
95. Lehto T, Honkanen E, Teppo AM, Meri S. Urinary excretion of protectin (CD59), complement SC5b-9 and cytokines in membranous glomerulonephritis. *Kidney Int* 1995;47:1403–1411.
96. Meri S, Mattila P, Renkonen R. Regulation of CD59 expression on the human endothelial cell line EA.hy 926. *Eur J Immunol* 1993;23:2511–2516.
97. Nose M, Katoh M, Okada N, Kyogoku M, Okada H. Tissue distribution of HRF20, a novel factor preventing the membrane attack of homologous complement, and its predominant expression on endothelial cells in vivo. *Immunology* 1990;70:145–149.
98. Brooimans RA, Van der Ark AA, Tomita M, Van Es LA, Daha MR. CD59 expressed by human endothelial cells functions as a protective molecule against complement-mediated lysis. *Eur J Immunol* 1992;22:791–797.
99. Quigg RJ, Morgan BP, Holers VM, Adler S, Sneed AE 3rd, Lo CF. Complement regulation in the rat glomerulus: Crry and CD59 regulate complement in glomerular mesangial and endothelial cells. *Kidney Int* 1995;48:412–421.
100. Hamilton KK, Ji Z, Rollins S, Stewart BH, Sims PJ. Regulatory control of the terminal complement proteins at the surface of human endothelial cells: neutralization of a C5b-9 inhibitor by antibody to CD59. *Blood* 1990;76:2572–2577.
101. McCurry KR, Kooyman DL, Diamond LE, Byrne GW, Logan JS, Platt JL. Transgenic expression of human complement regulatory proteins in mice results in diminished complement deposition during organ xenoperfusion. *Transplantation* 1995;59:1177–1182.
102. Charreau B, Cassard A, Tesson L, et al. Protection of rat endothelial cells from primate complement-mediated lysis by expression of human CD59 and/or decay-accelerating factor. *Transplantation* 1994;58:1222–1229.
103. Charreau B, Cassard A, Tesson L, et al. Permanent expression of human CD59 and/or decay-accelerating factor by rat endothelial cells confers protection from human complement–mediated lysis. *Transplant Proc* 1995;27:336–337.
104. Tsuji S, Kaji K, Nagasawa S. Decay-accelerating factor on human umbilical vein endothelial cells. Its histamine-induced expression and spontaneous rapid shedding from the cell surface. *J Immunol* 1994;152:1404–1410.
105. Moutabarrik A, Nakanishi I, Hara T, et al. Cytokine-mediated regulation of the surface expression of complement regulatory proteins, CD46(MCP), CD55(DAF), and CD59 on human vascular endothelial cells. *Lymphokine Cytokine Res* 1993;12:167–172.
106. Brooimans RA, van Wieringen PA, van Es LA, Daha MR. Relative roles of decay-accelerating factor, membrane cofactor protein, and CD59 in the protection of human endothelial cells against complement-mediated lysis. *Eur J Immunol* 1992;22:3135–3140.
107. Rosengard AM, Cary N, Horsley J, et al. Endothelial expression of human decay accelerating factor in transgenic pig tissue: a potential approach for human complement inactivation in discordant xenografts. *Transplant Proc* 1995;27:326–327.
108. Venneker GT, van den Hoogen FH, Boerbooms AM, Bos JD, Asghar SS. Aberrant expression of membrane cofactor protein and decay-accelerating factor in the endothelium of patients with systemic sclerosis. A possible mechanism of vascular damage. *Lab Invest* 1994;70:830–835.
109. Sims PJ, Wiedmer T. Induction of cellular procoagulant activity by the membrane attack complex of complement. *Semin Cell Biol* 1995;6:275–282.
110. Hamilton KK, Hattori R, Esmon CT, Sims PJ. Complement proteins C5b-9 induce vesiculation of the endothelial plasma membrane and expose catalytic surface for assembly of the prothrombinase enzyme complex. *J Biol Chem* 1990;265:3809–3814.
111. Hattori R, Hamilton KK, McEver RP, Sims PJ. Complement proteins C5b-9 induce secretion of high molecular weight multimers of endothelial von Willebrand factor and translocation of granule membrane protein GMP-140 to the cell surface. *J Biol Chem* 1989;264:9053–9060.

112. Saadi S, Holzknecht RA, Patte CP, Stern DM, Platt JL. Complement-mediated regulation of tissue factor activity in endothelium. *J Exp Med* 1995;182:1807–1814.
113. Kilgore KS, Shen JP, Miller BF, Ward PA, Warren JS. Enhancement by the complement membrane attack complex of tumor necrosis factor-alpha–induced endothelial cell expression of E-selectin and ICAM-1. *J Immunol* 1995;155:1434–1441.
114. Benzaquen LR, Nicholson-Weller A, Halperin JA. Terminal complement proteins C5b-9 release basic fibroblast growth factor and platelet-derived growth factor from endothelial cells. *J Exp Med* 1994;179: 985–992.
115. Pober JS, Cotran R. Cytokines and endothelial cell biology. *Physiol Rev* 1990;70:427–451.
116. Wenzel UO, Abboud HE. Chemokines and renal disease. *Am J Kidney Dis* 1995;26:982–994.
117. Luscinskas FW, Gimbrone MA. Endothelial-dependent mechanisms in chronic inflammatory leukocyte recruitment. *Annu Rev Med* 1996; 47:413–421.
118. Salgado A, Boveda JL, Monasterio J, et al. Inflammatory mediators and their influence on haemostasis. *Haemostasis* 1994;24:132–138.
119. Vassalli P. The pathophysiology of tumor necrosis factors. *Annu Rev Immunol* 1992;10:411–452.
120. Shakhov AN, Collart MA, Vassalli P, Nedospasov SA, Jongeneel VC. Kappa-B–type enhancers are involved in lipopolysaccharide-mediated transcriptional activation of the tumor necrosis factor-alpha gene in primary macrophages. *J Exp Med* 1990;171:35–47.
121. Stein M, Gordon S. Regulation of tumor necrosis factor (TNF) release by murine peritoneal macrophages: role of cell stimulation and specific phagocytic plasma membrane receptors. *Eur J Immunol* 1991; 21:431–437.
122. Laufer J, Boichis H, Farzam N, Passwell JH. IgA and IgG immune complexes increase human macrophage C3 biosynthesis. *Immunology* 1995;84:207–212.
123. Okusawa S, Yancey KB, van der Meer JWM, et al. C5a stimulates secretion of tumor necrosis factor from human mononuclear cells in vitro. Comparison with secretion of interleukin 1ÿE1 and interleukin 1a. *J Exp Med* 1988;168:443–448.
124. Descoteaux A, Matlashewski G. Regulation of tumor necrosis factor gene expression and protein synthesis in murine macrophages treated with recombinant tumor necrosis factor. *J Immunol* 1990;145: 846–853.
125. Trede NS, Heha RS, Chatila T. Transcriptional activation of IL-1β and tumor necrosis factor-α genes by MHC class II ligands. *J Immunol* 1991;146:2310–2315.
126. Steffen M, Ottmann O, Moore M. Simultaneous production of tumor necrosis factor-α and lymphotoxin by normal T cells after induction with IL-2 and anti-T3. *J Immunol* 1988;140:2621–2624.
127. Djeu J, Serbousek D, Banchard DK. Release of tumor necrosis factor by human polymorphonuclear leukocytes. *Blood* 1990;76: 1405–1409.
128. Dinarello CA, Savage N. Interleukin-1 and its receptor. *Crit Rev Immunol* 1989;9:1–20.
129. Dinarello CA. Role of interleukin-1 in infectious diseases. *Immunol Rev* 1992;127:119–146.
130. Baud L, Oudinet JP, Bens M, et al. Production of tumor necrosis factor by rat mesangial cells in response to bacterial lipopolysaccharide. *Kidney Int* 1989;35:1111–1118.
131. Malide D, Russo P, Bendayan M. Presence of tumor necrosis factor alpha and interleukin-6 in renal mesangial cells of lupus nephritis patients. *Hum Pathol* 1995;26:558–564.
132. Neale TJ, Ruger BM, Macaulay H, et al. Tumor necrosis factor-alpha is expressed by glomerular visceral epithelial cells in human membranous nephropathy. *Am J Pathol* 1995;146:1444–1454.
133. Yoshioka K, Takemura T, Murakami K, et al. In situ expression of cytokines in IgA nephritis. *Kidney Int* 1993;44:825–833.
134. Matsumoto K. Increased release of tumor necrosis factor-alpha by monocytes from patients with glomerulonephritis. *Clin Nephrol* 1993;40:148–154.
135. Onbe T, Kashihara N, Yamasaki Y, Makino H, Ota Z. Expression of mRNA's of cytokines and growth factors in experimental glomerulonephritis. *Res Commun Mol Pathol Pharmacol* 1994;86:131–138.
136. Noronha IL, Kruger C, Andrassy K, Ritz E, Waldherr R. In situ production of TNF-alpha, IL-1 beta and IL-2R in ANCA-positive glomerulonephritis. *Kidney Int* 1993;43:682–692.
137. Ortiz A, Bustos C, Alonso J, et al. Involvement of tumor necrosis factor-alpha in the pathogenesis of experimental and human glomerulonephritis. *Adv Nephrol Necker Hosp* 1995;24:53–77.
138. Baud L, Ardaillou R. Tumor necrosis factor in renal injury. *Miner Electrolyte Metab* 1995;21:336–341.
139. Morel D, Normand E, Lemoine C, et al. Tumor necrosis factor alpha in human kidney transplant rejection—analysis by in situ hybridization. *Transplantation* 1993;55:773–777.
140. Paleolog EM, Delasalle SA, Buurman WA, Feldmann M. Functional activities of receptors for tumor necrosis factor-alpha on human vascular endothelial cells. *Blood* 1994;84:2578–2590.
141. Wiegmann K, Schütze S, Machleidt T, Witte D, Krönke M. Functional dichotomy of neutral and acidic sphingomyelinases in tumor necrosis factor signaling. *Cell* 1994;78:1005.
142. Weber C, Negrescu E, Erl W, et al. Inhibitors of protein tyrosine kinase suppress TNF-stimulated induction of endothelial cell adhesion molecules. *J Immunol* 1995;155:445–451.
143. Akeson AL, Mosher LB, Woods CW, Schroeder KK, Bowlin TL. Human aortic endothelial cells express the type I but not the type II receptor for interleukin-1 (IL-1). *J Cell Physiol* 1992;153:583–588.
144. Collins T, Read MA, Neish AS, Whitley MZ, Thanos D, Maniatis T. Transcriptional regulation of endothelial cell adhesion molecules and cytokine-inducible enhancers. *FASEB J* 1995;9:899–909.
145. Palombella VJ, Rando OJ, Goldberg AL, Maniatis T. The ubiquitin–proteasome pathway is required for processing the NF-κB1 precursor protein and the activation of NF-κB. *Cell* 1994;78:773–785.
146. Ciechanover A. The ubiquitin–proteasome proteolytic pathway. *Cell* 1994;79:13–21.
147. Read MA, Neish AS, Luscinskas FW, Palombella VJ, Maniatis T, Collins T. The proteasome pathway is required for cytokine-induced endothelial leukocyte adhesion molecule expression. *Immunity* 1995; 2:493–506.
148. Chen CC, Rosenbloom CL, Anderson DC, Manning AM. Selective inhibition of E-selectin, vascular cell adhesion molecule-1, and intercellular adhesion molecule-1 expression by inhibitors of I kappa B-alpha phosphorylation. *J Immunol* 1995;155:3538–3545.
149. Peng HB, Libby P, Liao JK. Induction and stabilization of I kappa B alpha by nitric oxide mediates inhibition of NF-kappa B. *J Biol Chem* 1995;270:14214–14219.
150. Read MA, Whitley MZ, Williams AJ, Collins T. NF-κB and IκB-α: an inducible regulatory system in endothelial activation. *J Exp Med* 1994;179:503–512.
151. Schindler U, Baichwal VR. Three NF-κB binding sites in the human E-selectin gene required for maximal tumor necrosis factor alpha–induced expression. *Mol Cell Biol* 1994;14:5820–5831.
152. Neish AS, Read MA, Thanos D, Pine R, Maniatis T, Collins T. Endothelial IRF-1 cooperates with NF-κB as a transcriptional activator of vascular cell adhesion molecule-1. *Mol Cell Biol* 1995;15: 2558–2569.
153. Hou J, Baichwal V, Cao Z. Regulatory elements and transcription factors controlling basal and cytokine-induced expression of the gene encoding ICAM-1. *Proc Natl Acad Sci U S A* 1994;91:1641–1645.
154. Jahnke A, Johnson JP. Synergistic activation of intercellular adhesion molecule 1 (ICAM-1) by TNF-α and IFN-τ is mediated by p65/p50 and p65/c-Rel and interferon-responsive factor Stat–1α (p91) that can be activated by both IFN-τ and IFN-α. *FEBS Lett* 1994;354:220–226.
155. Mackman N. Regulation of the tissue factor gene. *FASEB J* 1995;9: 883–889.
156. Karakurum M, Shreeniwas R, Chen J, et al. Hypoxic induction of interleukin-8 gene expression in human endothelial cells. *J Clin Invest* 1994;93:1564–1570.
157. Neish AS, Khachigian LM, Park A, Baichwal VR. Collins T. Sp1 is a component of the cytokine-inducible enhancer in the promoter of vascular cell adhesion molecule-1. *J Biol Chem* 1995;270:28903–28909.
158. Bierhaus A, Zhang Y, Deng Y, et al. Mechanism of the tumor necrosis factor alpha–mediated induction of endothelial tissue factor. *J Biol Chem* 1995;270:26419–26432.
159. Moll T, Czyz M, Holzmuller H, et al. Regulation of the tissue factor promoter in endothelial cells. Binding of NF kappa B–, AP-1–, and Sp1-like transcription factors. *J Biol Chem* 1995;270:3849–3857.
160. Lewis H, Kasuzubska W, DeLamarter JF, Whelan J. Cooperativity between two complexes, mediated by high-mobility–group protein I(Y), is essential for cytokine-induced expression of the E-selectin promoter. *Mol Cell Biol* 1994;14:5701–5709.

161. Butcher EC, Picker LJ. Lymphocyte homing and homeostasis. *Science* 1996;272:60–66.
162. Noris M, Remuzzi G. New insights into circulating cell–endothelium interactions and their significance for glomerular pathophysiology. *Am J Kidney Dis* 1995;26:541–548.
163. Lindley IJD, Westwick J, Kunkel SL. Nomenclature announcement: the chemokines. *Immunol Today* 1993;14:24.
164. Wenzel UO, Abboud HE. Chemokines and renal disease. *Am J Kidney Dis* 1995;26:982–994.
165. Kelner GS, Kennedy J, Bacon KB, et al. Lymphotactin: a cytokine that represents a new class of chemokine. *Science* 1994;266: 1395–1399.
166. Kelvin DJ, Michiel DF, Johnston JA, et al. Chemokines and serpentines: the molecular biology of chemokine receptor. *J Leukoc Biol* 1993;54:604–612.
167. Murphy PM. The molecular biology of leucocyte chemoattractant receptors. *Annu Rev Immunol* 1994;12:593–633.
168. Hadley TJ, Lu ZH, Wasniowsk K, et al. Postcapillary venule endothelial cells in kidney express a multispecific chemokine receptor that is structurally and functionally identical to the erythroid isoform, which is the Duffy blood group antigen. *J Clin Invest* 1994;94:985–991.
169. Strieter RM, Kunkel SL, Showell HJ, et al. Endothelial cell gene expression of a neutrophil chemotactic factor by TNF-α, LPS and IL-1β. *Science* 1989;243:1467–1469.
170. Brown Z, Gerritsen ME, Carley WW, Strieter RM, Kunkel SL, Westwick J. Chemokine gene expression and secretion by cytokine-activated human microvascular endothelial cells. Differential regulation of monocyte chemoattractant protein-1 and interleukin-8 in response to interferon-gamma. *Am J Pathol* 1994;145:913–921.
171. Rot A, Hub E, Middleton J, et al. Some aspects of IL-8 pathophysiology. 3. Chemokine interaction with endothelial cells. *J Leukocyte Biol* 1996;59:39–44.
172. Ferran C, Millan MT, Csizmadia V, et al. Inhibition of NF-kappa B by pyrrolidine dithiocarbamate blocks endothelial activation. *Biochem Biophys Res Commun* 1995;214:212–223.
173. Jeannin P, Delneste Y, Gosset P, et al. Histamine induces interleukin-8 secretion by endothelial cells. *Blood* 1994;84:2229–2233.
174. Qi J, Kreutzer DL. Fibrin activation of vascular endothelial cells. Induction of IL-8 expression. *J Immunol* 1995;155:867–876.
175. Ramsby ML, Kreutzer DL. Fibrin induction of interleukin-8 expression in corneal endothelial cells in vitro. *Invest Ophthalmol Vis Sci* 1994;35:3980–3990.
176. Kaplanski G, Farnarier C, Kaplanski S, et al. Interleukin-1 induces interleukin-8 secretion from endothelial cells by a juxtacrine mechanism. *Blood* 1994;84:4242–4248.
177. Lukas NW, Strieter RM, Elenr V, Evanoff HL, Burdick MD, Kunkel SL. Production of chemokines, interleukin-8 and monocyte chemoattractant protein-1, during monocyte:endothelial cell interactions. *Blood* 1995;86:2767–2773.
178. Kaplanski G, Teysseire N, Farnarier C, et al. IL-6 and IL-8 production from cultured human endothelial cells stimulated by infection with *Rickettsia conorii* via a cell-associated IL-1-alpha–dependent pathway. *J Clin Invest* 1995;96:2839–2844.
179. De Beaux AC, Maingay JP, Ross JA, Fearon KC, Carter DC. Interleukin-4 and interleukin-10 increase endotoxin-stimulated human umbilical vein endothelial cell interleukin-8 release. *J Interferon Cytokine Res* 1995;15:441–445.
180. Chen CC, Manning AM. TGF-beta-1, IL-10 and IL-4 differentially modulate the cytokine-induced expression of IL-6 and IL-8 in human endothelial cells. *Cytokine* 1996;8:58–65.
181. De Caterina R, Libby P, Peng HB, et al. Nitric oxide decreases cytokine-induced endothelial activation. Nitric oxide selectively reduces endothelial expression of adhesion molecules and proinflammatory cytokines. *J Clin Invest* 1995;96:60–68.
182. Villarete LH, Remick DG. Nitric oxide regulation of IL-8 expression in human endothelial cells. *Biochem Biophys Res Commun* 1995;211: 671–676.
183. Kunkel SL, Lukacs N, Strieter RM. Expression and biology of neutrophil and endothelial cell–derived chemokines. *Semin Cell Biol* 1995;6:327–336.
184. Wolf G, Aberle S, Thaiss F, et al. TNF alpha induces expression of the chemoattractant cytokine RANTES in cultured mouse mesangial cells. *Kidney Int* 1993;44:795–804.
185. Ember JA, Sanderson SD, Hugli TE, Morgan EL. Induction of interleukin-8 synthesis from monocytes by human C5a anaphylatoxin. *Am J Pathol* 1994;144:393–403.
186. Kasama T, Strieter RM, Lukacs NW, Lincoln PM, Burdick MD, Kunkel SL. Interferon gamma modulates the expression of neutrophil-derived chemokines. *J Invest Med* 1995;43:58–67.
187. Strieter RM, Kasahara K, Allen RM, et al. Cytokine-induced neutrophil-derived interleukin-8. *Am J Pathol* 1992;141:397–407.
188. Hammond ME, Lapointe GR, Feucht PH, et al. IL-8 induces neutrophil chemotaxis predominantly via type I IL-8 receptors. *J Immunol* 1995;155:1428–1433.
189. Smart SJ, Casale TB. TNF-alpha–induced transendothelial neutrophil migration is IL-8 dependent. *Am J Physiol* 1994;266:L238–L245.
190. Kuijpers TW, Hakkert BC, Hart MH, Roos D. Neutrophil migration across monolayers of cytokine-prestimulated endothelial cells: a role for platelet-activating factor and IL-8. *J Cell Biol* 1992;117:565–572.
191. Krieger M, Brunner T, Bischoff SC, et al. Activation of human basophils through the IL-8 receptor. *J Immunol* 1992;149:2662–2667.
192. Zhang YJ, Rutledgge BJ, Rollins BJ. Structure/activity analysis of human monocyte chemoattractant protein-1 (MCP-1) by mutagenesis. Identification of a mutated protein that inhibits MCP-1 mediated monocyte chemotaxis. *J Biol Chem* 1994;269:15918–15924.
193. Rot A, Krieger M, Brunner T, Bischoff SC, Schall TJ, Dahinden CA. RANTES and macrophage inflammatory protein 1 alpha induce the migration and activation of normal human eosinophil granulocytes. *J Exp Med* 1992;176:1489–1495.
194. Ebisawa M, Yamada T, Bickel C, Klunk D, Schleimer RP. Eosinophil transendothelial migration induced by cytokines. III. Effect of the chemokine RANTES. *J Immunol* 1994;153:2153–2160.
195. Gerard NP, Gerard C. The chemotactic receptor for human C5a anaphylatoxin. *Nature* 1991;349:614–617.
196. Ehrengruber MU, Geiser T, Deranleau DA. Activation of human neutrophils by C3a and C5a. Comparison of the effects on shape changes, chemotaxis, secretion, and respiratory burst. *FEBS Lett* 1994;346: 181–184.
197. Altieri DC. Occupancy of CD11b/CD18 (Mac-1) divalent ion binding site(s) induces leukocyte adhesion. *J Immunol* 1991;147:1891–1898.
198. Chuluyan HE, Osborn L, Lobb R, Issekutz AC. Domains 1 and 4 of vascular cell adhesion molecule-1 (CD106) both support very late activation antigen-4 (CD49d/CD29)–dependent monocyte transendothelial migration. *J Immunol* 1995;155:3135–3134.
199. Chuluyan HE, Schall TJ, Yoshimura T, Issekutz AC. IL-1 activation of endothelium supports VLA-4 (CD49d/CD29)–mediated monocyte transendothelial migration to C5a, MIP-1 alpha, RANTES, and PAF but inhibits migration to MCP-1: a regulatory role for endothelium-derived MCP-1. *J Leukoc Biol* 1995;58:71–79.
200. Issekutz TB. In vivo blood monocyte migration to acute inflammatory reactions, IL-1 alpha, TNF-alpha, IFN-gamma, and C5a utilizes LFA-1, Mac-1, and VLA-4. The relative importance of each integrin. *J Immunol* 1995;154:6533–6540.
201. Monk PN, Barker MD, Partridge LJ. Multiple signalling pathways in the C5a-induced expression of adhesion receptor Mac-1. *Biochim Biophys Acta* 1994;1221:323–329.
202. Mulder K, Colditz IG. Migratory responses of ovine neutrophils to inflammatory mediators in vitro and in vivo. *J Leukoc Biol* 1993;53: 273–278.
203. Lo SK, Detmers PA, Levin SM, Wright SD. Transient adhesion of neutrophils to endothelium. *J Exp Med* 1989;169:1779–1793.
204. Smith WB, Gamble JR, Clark-Lewis I, Vadas MA. Chemotactic desensitization of neutrophils demonstrates interleukin-8 (IL-8)–dependent and IL-8–independent mechanisms of transmigration through cytokine-activated endothelium. *Immunology* 1993;78: 491–497.
205. Luscinskas FW, Kiely JM, Ding H, et al. In vitro inhibitory effect of IL-8 and other chemoattractants on neutrophil-endothelial adhesive interactions. *J Immunol* 1992;149:2163–2171.
206. Westlin WF, Kiely JM, Gimbrone MA Jr. Interleukin-8 induces changes in human neutrophil actin conformation and distribution: relationship to inhibition of adhesion to cytokine-activated endothelium. *J Leukoc Biol* 1992;52:43–51.
207. Jagels MA, Chambers JD, Arfors KE, Hugli TE. C5a- and tumor necrosis factor-alpha–induced leukocytosis occurs independently of beta 2 integrins and L-selectin: differential effects on neutrophil adhesion molecule expression in vivo. *Blood* 1995;85:2900–2909.
208. Molad Y, Haines KA, Anderson DC, Buyon JP, Cronstein BN. Im-

munocomplexes stimulate different signalling events to chemoattractants in the neutrophil and regulate L-selectin and beta 2–integrin expression differently. *Biochem J* 1994;299:881–887.
209. Tonnesen MG, Smedly LA, Henson PM. Neutrophil-endothelial cell interactions. Modulation of neutrophil adhesiveness induced by complement fragments C5a and C5a des arg and formyl-methionyl-leucyl-phenylalanine in vitro. *J Clin Invest* 1984;74:1581–1592.
210. Takahashi M, Masuyama J, Ikeda U, et al. Effects of endogenous endothelial interleukin-8 on neutrophil migration across an endothelial monolayer. *Cardiovasc Res* 1995;29:670–675.
211. Rot A. Endothelial cell binding of NAP-1/IL-8: role in neutrophil emigration. *Immunol Today* 1992;13:291–294.
212. Petzelbauer P, Watson CA, Pfau SE, Pober JS. IL-8 and angiogenesis: evidence that human endothelial cells lack receptors and do not respond to IL-8 in vitro. *Cytokine* 1995;7:267–272.
213. del Pozo MA, Sanchez-Mateos P, Nieto M, Sanchez-Madrid F. Chemokines regulate cellular polarization and adhesion receptor redistribution during lymphocyte interaction with endothelium and extracellular matrix. Involvement of cAMP signaling pathway. *J Cell Biol* 1995;131:495–508.
214. Wozniak A, Betts WH, Murphy GA, Rokicinski M. Interleukin-8 primes human neutrophils for enhanced superoxide anion production. *Immunology* 1993;79:608–615.
215. Baggiolini M, Imboden P, Detmers P. Neutrophil activation and the effects of interleukin-8/neutrophil–activating peptide 1 (IL-8/NAP-1). *Cytokines* 1992;4:1–17.
216. Smith RJ, Sam LM, Leach KL, Justen JM. Postreceptor events associated with human neutrophil activation by interleukin-8. *J Leukoc Biol* 1992;52:17–26.
217. Hardy MM, Flickinger AG, Riley DP, Weiss RH, Ryan US. Superoxide dismutase mimetics inhibit neutrophil-mediated human aortic endothelial cell injury in vitro. *J Biol Chem* 1994;269: 18535–18540.
218. Murphy HS, Shayman JA, Till GO, et al. Superoxide responses of endothelial cells to C5a and TNF-alpha: divergent signal transduction pathways. *Am J Physiol* 1992;263:L51–L59.
219. Nagata S, Kebo DK, Kunkel S, Glovsky MM. Effect of adenylate cyclase activators on C5a-induced human neutrophil aggregation, enzyme release and superoxide production. *Int Arch Allergy Immunol* 1992;97:194–199.
220. Bajaj MS, Kew RR, Webster RO, Hyers TM. Priming of human neutrophil functions by tumor necrosis factor: enhancement of superoxide anion generation, degranulation, and chemotaxis to chemoattractants C5a and F-Met-Leu-Phe. *Inflammation* 1992;16:241–250.
221. Springer TA. Traffic signals for lymphocyte recirculation and leukocyte emigration: the multistep paradigm. *Cell* 1994;76:301–314.
222. Brady H. Leukocyte adhesion molecules. *Kidney Int* 1994;45: 1285–1300.
223. Roy-Chaudhury P, Wu B, King G, et al. Adhesion molecule interactions in human glomerulonephritis: importance of the tubulointerstitium. *Kidney Int* 1996;49:127–134.
224. Muller WA. The role of PECAM-1 (CD31) in leukocyte emigration: studies in vitro and in vivo. *J Leukoc Biol* 1995;57:523–8.
225. Luscinskas FW, Gimbrone MA Jr. Endothelial-dependent mechanisms in chronic inflammatory leukocyte recruitment. *Annu Rev Med* 1996;47:413–421.
226. Tedder TF, Steeber DA, Chen A, Engel P. The selectins: vascular adhesion molecules. *FASEB J* 1995;9:866–873.
227. Tedder TF, Luscinskas W, Kansas GS. Regulation of leukocyte migration by L-selectin: mechanisms, domains and ligands. *Behring Inst Mitt* 1993;92:165–177.
228. Chen A, Engel P, Tedder TF. Structural requirements regulate endoproteolytic release of the L-selectin (CD62L) adhesion receptor from the cell surface of leukocytes. *J Exp Med* 1995;182:519–530.
229. Gearing AJ, Newman W. Circulating adhesion molecules in disease. *Immunol Today* 1994;14:506–512.
230. McEver RP, Beckstead JH, Moore KL, Marshal-Carlson L, Bainton DF. GMP-140, a platelet alpha granule membrane protein, is also synthesized by vascular endothelial cells and is localized in Weibel-Palade bodies. *J Clin Invest* 1989;84:92–99.
231. Bevilaqua MP, Pober JS, Mendrick DL, Cotran RS, Gimbrone MA Jr. Identification of an inducible endothelial-leukocyte adhesion molecule. *Proc Natl Acad Sci U S A* 1987;84:9238–9243.
232. Granger DN, Kubes P. The microcirculation and inflammation: modulation of leukocyte-endothelial cell adhesion. *J Leuk Biol* 1994;55: 662–675.
233. Heemann UW, Tullius SG, Kupiec-Weglinski JW, Tilney NL. Early events in acute allograft rejection: leukocyte/endothelial cell interactions. *Clin Transplant* 1993;7:82–89.
234. Rosen SD, Bertozzi CR. The selectins and their ligands. *Curr Opin Cell Biol* 1994;6:663–673.
235. Hemmerich S, Butcher EC, Rosen SD. Sulfation-dependent recognition of HEV-ligand by L-selectin and MECA 79, an adhesion-blocking mAB. *J Exp Med* 1995;VOL:2219–2226.
236. Shimizu Y, Shaw S. Cell adhesion: mucins in the mainstream. *Nature* 1993;336:630–631.
237. Spertini O, Luscinskas FW, Kansas GS, et al. Leukocyte adhesion molecule-1 (LAM-1, L-selectin) interacts with an inducible endothelial cell ligand to support leukocyte adhesion. *J Immunol* 1991;147: 2565–2573.
238. Brady HR, Spertini O, Jimenez W, Brenner BM, Marsden PA, Tedder TF. Neutrophils, monocytes and lymphocytes bind to cytokine-activated kidney glomerular endothleial cells through L-selectin (LAM-1) in vitro. *J Immunol* 1992;149:2437–2444.
239. Moore KL, Patel KD, Breuhl RE, et al. P-selectin glycoprotein ligand-1 mediates rolling of human neutrophils on P-selectin. *J Cell Biol* 1995;128:661–671.
240. Steegmaler M, Levinovitz A, Isenmann S, et al. The E-selectin ligand ESL-1 is a variant of a receptor for fibroblast growth factor. *Nature* 1995;373:615–620.
241. Labow MA, Norton CR, Rumberger JM, et al. Characterization of E-selectin–deficient mice: demonstration of overlapping function of the endothelial selectins. *Immunity* 1994;1:709–720.
242. Subramaniam M, Saffaripour S, Watson SR, Mayadas TN, Hynes RO, Wagner DD. Reduced recruitment of inflammatory cells in a contact hypersensitivity response in P-selectin–deficient mice. *J Exp Med* 1995;181:2277–2282.
243. Tedder TF, Pizcueta P. L-selectin deficient mice have impaired leukocyte recruitment into inflammatory sites. *J Exp Med* 1995;181: 2259–2264.
244. Albelda SM, Smith CW, Ward PA. Adhesion molecules and inflammatory injury. *FASEB J* 1994;8:504–512.
245. Bevilaqua MP. Endothelial-leukocyte adhesion molecules. *Annu Rev Immunol* 1993;11:767–804.
246. Abbas AK, Lichtman AH, Pober JS. Appendix: principal features of known CD molecules. In: *Cellular and molecular immunology*. Philadelphia: WB Saunders; 1994:431–435.
247. Osborn L, Hession C, Tizard R, et al. Direct expression cloning of vascular cell adhesion molecule 1, a cytokine induced endothelial protein that binds to lymphocytes. *Cell* 1989;59:1203–1211.
248. Elices M, Osborn L, Takada Y, et al. VCAM-1 on activated endothelium interacts with the leukocyte integrin VLA-4 at a site distinct from the VLA-4/fibronectin binding site. *Cell* 1990;60:577–584.
249. Wertheimer SJ, Myers CL, Wallace RW, Parks TP. Intercellular adhesion molecule-1 expression in human endothelial cells. *J Biol Chem* 1992;267:12030–12035.
250. Voraberger G, Schafer R, Stratowa C. Cloning of the human gene for intercellular adhesion molecule 1 and analysis of its 58 regulatory region; induction by cytokines and phorbol ester. *J Immunol* 1991; 147:2777–2786.
251. Ledebur HC, Parks TP. Transcriptional regulation of the intercellular adhesion molecule-1 gene by inflammatory cytokines in human endothelial cells. *J Biol Chem* 1995;270:933–943.
252. Mulligan MS, Johnson KJ, Todd RF III, et al. Requirement for leukocyte adhesion molecules in nephrotoxic nephritis. *J Clin Invest* 1993; 91:577–587.
253. Kawasaki K, Yaoita E, Yamamoto T, Tamatani T, Miyasaka M, Kihara I. Antibodies against intercellular adhesion molecule-1 and lymphocyte function associated antigen-1 prevent glomerular injury in rat experimental glomerulonephritis. *J Immunol* 1991;150: 1074–1083.
254. Nishikawa K, Guo Y-J, Miyasaka M, et al. Antibodies to intercellular adhesion molecule-1/lymphocyte–associated antigen-1 prevent crescent formation in rat autoimmune glomerulonephritis. *J Exp Med* 1993;177:667–677.
255. Hill PA, Lan HY, Nikolic-Paterson DJ, Atkins RC. ICAM-1 directs migration and localization of interstitial leukocytes in experimental glomerulonephritis. *Kidney Int* 1994;43:32–42.

256. Wuthrich RP, Jevnikar AM, Takei F, Limcher LH, Kelley VE. Intercellular adhesion molecule-1 expression is upregulated in autoimmune murine lupus nephritis. *Am J Pathol* 1990;136:441–450.
257. Canton AD. Adhesion molecules in renal disease. *Kidney Int* 1995; 48:1687–1696.
258. Haller, H, Eichhorn J, Pieper K, Gÿ94bel U, Luft FC. Circulating leukocyte integrin expression in Wegener's granulomatosus. *J Am Soc Nephrol* 1996;7:40–48.
259. Wu KK, Thiagarajan P. Role of endothelium in thrombosis and hemostasis. *Annu Rev Med* 1996;47:315–331.
260. Pearson JD. Vessel wall interactions regulating thrombosis. *Br Med Bull* 1994;50:776–788.
261. Laszik Z, Carson CW, Nadasdy T, et al. Lack of suppressed renal thrombomodulin expression in a septic rat model with glomerular thrombotic microangiopathy. *Lab Invest* 1994;70:862–867.
262. Kanfer A. Coagulation factors in nephrotic syndrome. *J Am Soc Nephrol* 1990;10(suppl 1):63–68.
263. Tipping PG, Dowling J,P Holdsworth SR. Glomerular procoagulant activity in human proliferative glomerulonephritis. *J Clin Invest* 1988;81:119–125.
264. Takemura T, Yoshioka K, Akano N, Miyamoto H, Matsumoto K, Maki S. Glomerular deposition of cross-linked fibrin in human kidney diseases. *Kidney Int* 1987;32:102–111.
265. Bergstein JM. Glomerular fibrin deposition and removal. *Pediatr Nephrol* 1990;4:78–87.
266. Ruggeri ZM, Ware J. von Willebrand factor. *FASEB J* 1993;7: 308–316.
267. Koppelman SJ, Koedam JA, van Wijnen M, et al. von Willebrand factor as a regulator of intrinsic factor X activation. *J Lab Clin Med* 1994;123:585–593.
268. Kroll MH, Harris TS, Moake JL, Handin RI, Schafer AI. von Willebrand factor binding to platelet GpIb initiates signals for platelet activation. *J Clin Invest* 1991;88:1568–1573.
269. Collins PW, Macey MG, Cahill MR, Newland AC. von Willebrand factor release and P-selectin expression is stimulated by thrombin and trypsin but not IL-1 in cultured human endothelial cells. *Thromb Haemost* 1993;70:346–350.
270. Storck J, Kusters B, Zimmermann ER. The tethered ligand receptor is the responsible receptor for the thrombin induced release of von Willebrand factor from endothelial cells (HUVEC). *Thromb Res* 1995;77:249–258.
271. Palmer DS, Aye MT, Ganz PR, Halpenny M, Hashemi S. Adenosine nucleotides and serotonin stimulate von Willebrand factor release from cultured human endothelial cells. *Thromb Haemost* 1994;72: 132–139.
272. Hashemi S, Palmer DS, Aye MT, Ganz PR. Platelet-activating factor secreted by DDAVP-treated monocytes mediates von Willebrand factor release from endothelial cells. *J Cell Physiol* 1993;154:496–505.
273. Datta YH, Romano M, Jacobson BC, Golan DE, Serhan CN, Ewenstein BM. Peptido-leukotrienes are potent agonists of von Willebrand factor secretion and P-selectin surface expression in human umbilical vein endothelial cells. *Circulation* 1995;92:3304–3311.
274. Foreman KE, Vaporciyan AA, Bonish BK, et al. C5a-induced expression of P-selectin in endothelial cells. *J Clin Invest* 1994;94: 1147–1155.
275. Carew MA, Paleolog EM, Pearson JD. The roles of protein kinase C and intracellular Ca2+ in the secretion of von Willebrand factor from human vascular endothelial cells. *Biochem J* 1992;286:631–635.
276. Birch KA, Ewenstein BM, Golan DE, Pober JS. Prolonged peak elevations in cytoplasmic free calcium ions, derived from intracellular stores, correlate with the extent of thrombin-stimulated exocytosis in single human umbilical vein endothelial cells. *J Cell Physiol* 1994; 160:545–554.
277. Tranquille N, Emeis JJ. The role of cyclic nucleotides in the release of tissue-type plasminogen activator and von Willebrand factor. *Thromb Haemost* 1993;69:259–261.
278. Kanwar S, Woodman RC, Poon MC, et al. Desmopressin induces endothelial P-selectin expression and leukocyte rolling in postcapillary venules. *Blood* 1995;86:2760–2766.
279. Lethagen S, Nilsson IM. DDAVP-induced enhancement of platelet retention: its dependence on platelet–von Willebrand factor and the platelet receptor GP IIb/IIIa. *Eur J Haematol* 1992;49:7–13.
280. Lusher JM. Response to 1-deamino-8-D-arginine vasopressin in von Willebrand disease. *Haemostasis* 1994;24:276–284.
281. Etingin OR, Silverstein RL, Hajjar DP. von Willebrand factor mediates platelet adhesion to virally infected endothelial cells. *Proc Natl Acad Sci U S A* 1993;90:5153–5156.
282. Schorer AE, Moldow CF, Rick ME. Interleukin 1 or endotoxin increases the release of von Willebrand factor from human endothelial cells. *Br J Haematol* 1987;67:193–197.
283. Koltai M, Hosford D, Braquet PG. Platelet-activating factor in septic shock. *New Horiz* 1993;1:87–95.
284. van de Kar NC, van Hinsbergh VW, Brommer EJ, Monnens LA. The fibrinolytic system in the hemolytic uremic syndrome: in vivo and in vitro studies. *Pediatr Res* 1994;36:257–264.
285. Moake JL, Byrnes JJ, Troll JH, et al. Abnormal VIII: von Willebrand factor patterns in the plasma of patients with the hemolytic-uremic syndrome. *Blood* 1984;64:592–598.
286. Rose PE, Enayat SM, Sunderland R, Short PE, Williams CE, Hill FGH. Abnormalities of factor VIII related protein multimers in the haemolytic uraemic syndrome. *Arch Dis Child* 1984;59:1135–1140.
287. Remuzzi G, Ruggenenti P. The hemolytic uremic syndrome. *Kidney Int* 1995;47:2–19.
288. Sanduja SK, Tsai A-L, Matijevic-Aleksic N, et al. Kinetics of prostacyclin synthesis in PGHS-1 over-expressed endothelial cells. *Am J Physiol* 1994;267:C1459–1466.
289. Walter U, Geiger J, Haffner C, et al. Platelet–vessel wall interactions, focal adhesions, and the mechanism of action of endothelial factors. *Agents Actions* 1995;45(suppl):255–268.
290. Welch GN, Upchurch GR, Loscalzo J. Nitric oxide as a vascular modulator. *Blood Rev* 1995;9:262–269.
291. Vane JR, Botting RM. Formation by the endothelium of prostacyclin, nitric oxide and endothelin. *J Lipid Mediat* 1993;6:395–404.
292. Hla T, Neilson K. Human cyclooxygenase-2 cDNA. *Proc Natl Acad Sci U S A* 1992;89:7384–7388.
293. Xu XM, Ohashi K, Sanduja SK, Ruan KH, Wang LH, Wu KK. Enhanced prostacyclin synthesis in endothelial cells by retrovirus-mediated transfer of prostaglandin H synthase cDNA. *J Clin Invest* 1993;91:1843–1849.
294. Ristimaki A, Viinikka L. Modulation of prostacyclin production by cytokines in vascular endothelial cells. *Prostaglandins Leukot Essent Fatty Acids* 1992;47:93–99.
295. Maier JA, Ragnotti G. An oligomer targeted against protein kinase C alpha prevents interleukin-1 alpha induction of cyclooxygenase expression in human endothelial cells. *Exp Cell Res* 1993;205:52–58.
296. Zembowicz A, Jones SL, Wu KK. Induction of cyclooxygenase-2 in human umbilical vein endothelial cells by lysophosphatidylcholine. *J Clin Invest* 1995;96:1688–1692.
297. Wu KK. Inducible cyclooxygenase and nitric oxide synthase. *Adv Pharmacol* 1995;33:179–207.
298. Tonshoff B, Momper R, Schweer H, Scharer K, Seyberth HW. Increased biosynthesis of vasoactive prostanoids in Schonlein-Henoch purpura. *Pediatr Res* 1992;32:137–140.
299. Bobbio–Pallavicini E, Porta C, Tacconi F, et al. Intravenous prostacyclin (as epoprostenol) infusion in thrombotic thrombocytopenic purpura. Four case reports and review of the literature. *Haematologica* 1994;79:429–437.
300. Utsunomiya Y, Ogura M, Kawamura T, Mitarai T, Maruyama N, Sakai O. Attenuation of immune complex nephritis in NZB/WF1 mice by a prostacyclin analogue. *Clin Exp Immunol* 1995;99: 454–460.
301. Poelstra K, Brouwer E, Baller JF, Hardonk MJ, Bakker WW. Attenuation of anti-Thy1 glomerulonephritis in the rat by anti-inflammatory platelet-inhibiting agents. *Am J Pathol* 1993;142:441–450.
302. Patrono C, Pierucci A. Renal effects of nonsteroidal anti-inflammatory drugs in chronic glomerular disease. *Am J Med* 1986;81:71–83.
303. Busse R, Fleming I. Regulation and functional consequences of endothelial nitric oxide formation. *Ann Med* 1995;27:331–340.
304. Wang Y, Marsden PA. Nitric oxide synthases: biochemical and molecular regulation. *Curr Opin Nephrol Hypertens* 1995;4:12–22.
305. Marsden PA, Brock TA, Ballermann BJ. Glomerular endothelial cells respond to calcium-mobilizing agonists with EDRF release. *Am J Physiol* 1990;258:F1295–F1303.
306. Hattori R, Sase K, Eizawa H, et al. Structure and function of nitric oxide synthases. *Int J Cardiol* 1994;47(suppl 1):71–75.
307. Goto S, Yamamoto T, Feng L0, et al. Expression and localization of inducible nitric oxide synthase in anti–Thy-1 glomerulonephritis. *Am J Pathol* 1995;147:1133–1141.

308. Border WA, Okuda S, Languino LR, Sporn MB, Ruoslahti E. Suppression of experimental glomerulonephritis by antiserum against transforming growth factor beta 1. *Nature* 1990;346:371–374.
309. Inoue N, Venema RC, Sayegh HS, Ohara Y, Murphy TJ, Harrison DG. Molecular regulation of the bovine endothelial cell nitric oxide synthase by transforming growth factor-beta 1. *Arterioscler Thromb Vasc Biol* 1995;15:1255–1261.
310. Jansen A, Cook T, Taylor GM, et al. Induction of nitric oxide synthase in rat immune complex glomerulonephritis. *Kidney Int* 1994;45: 1215–1219.
311. Cattell V, Cook T. The nitric oxide pathway in glomerulonephritis. *Curr Opin Nephrol Hypertens* 1995;4:359–364.
312. Saura M, Lopez S, Rodriguez Puyol M, Rodriguez Puyol D, Lamas S. Regulation of inducible nitric oxide synthase expression in rat mesangial cells and isolated glomeruli. *Kidney Int* 1995;47:500–509.
313. Marsden PA, Ballermann BJ. Tumor necrosis factor activates soluble guanylate cyclase in bovine glomerular mesangial cells via an L-arginine–dependent mechanism. *J Exp Med* 1990;172:1843–1852.
314. Cook HT, Ebrahim H, Jansen AS, Foster GR, Largen P, Cattell V. Expression of the gene for inducible nitric oxide synthase in experimental glomerulonephritis in the rat. *Clin Exp Immunol* 1994;97: 315–320.
315. Koide M, Kawahara Y, Nakayama I, Tsuda T, Yokoyama M. Cyclic AMP-elevating agents induce an inducible type of nitric oxide synthase in cultured vascular smooth muscle cells. Synergism with the induction elicited by inflammatory cytokines. *J Biol Chem* 1993;268: 24959–24966.
316. Koide M, Kawahara Y, Tsuda T, Yokoyama M. Cytokine-induced expression of an inducible type of nitric oxide synthase gene in cultured vascular smooth muscle cells. *FEBS Lett* 1993;318:213–217.
317. Kanno K, Hirata Y, Imai T, Iwashina M, Marumo F. Regulation of inducible nitric oxide synthase gene by interleukin-1 beta in rat vascular endothelial cells. *Am J Physiol* 1994;267:H2318–H2324.
318. Balligand JL, Ungureanu-Longrois D, Simmons WW, et al. Induction of NO synthase in rat cardiac microvascular endothelial cells by IL-1 beta and IFN-gamma. *Am J Physiol* 1995;268:H1293–1303.
319. Vodovotz Y, Bogdan C, Paik J, Xie QW, Nathan C. Mechanisms of suppression of macrophage nitric oxide release by transforming growth factor beta. *J Exp Med* 1993;178:605–613.
320. Hausmann EH, Hao SY, Pace JL, Parmely MJ. Transforming growth factor beta 1 and gamma interferon provide opposing signals to lipopolysaccharide-activated mouse macrophages. *Infect Immunol* 1994; 62:3625–3632.
321. Perrella MA, Yoshizumi M, Fen Z, et al. Transforming growth factor-beta 1, but not dexamethasone, down-regulates nitric-oxide synthase mRNA after its induction by interleukin-1 beta in rat smooth muscle cells. *J Biol Chem* 1994;269:14595–14600.
322. Nakayama I, Kawahara Y, Tsuda T, Okuda M, Yokoyama M. Angiotensin II inhibits cytokine-stimulated inducible nitric oxide synthase expression in vascular smooth muscle cells. *J Biol Chem* 1994;269: 11628–11633.
323. Tetsuka T, Daphna-Iken D, Srivastava SK, Baier LD, DuMaine J, Morrison AR. Cross-talk between cyclooxygenase and nitric oxide pathways: prostaglandin E2 negatively modulates induction of nitric oxide synthase by interleukin 1. *Proc Natl Acad Sci U S A* 1994;91: 12168–12172.
324. Imai T, Hirata Y, Kanno K, Marumo F. Induction of nitric oxide synthase by cyclic AMP in rat vascular smooth muscle cells. *J Clin Invest* 1994;93:543–549.
325. Mohaupt MG, Elzie JL, Ahn KY, Clapp WL, Wilcox CS, Kone BC. Differential expression and induction of mRNAs encoding two inducible nitric oxide synthases in rat kidney. *Kidney Int* 1994;46: 653–665.
326. Spink J, Cohen J, Evans TJ. The cytokine responsive vascular smooth muscle cell enhancer of inducible nitric oxide synthase. Activation by nuclear factor-kappa B. *J Biol Chem* 1995;270:29541–29547.
327. Raij L, Jaimes E, Delcastillo D, Guerra J, Westberg G. Pathophysiology of the vascular wall—the role of nitrix oxide in renal disease. *Prostaglandins Leukotrienes Essent Fatty Acids* 1996;54:53–58.
328. Raij L, Baylis C. Glomerular actions of nitric oxide. *Kidney Int* 1995; 48:20–32.
329. Ferrario R, Takahashi K, Fogo A, Badr KF, Munger KA. Consequences of acute nitric oxide synthesis inhibition in experimental glomerulonephritis. *J Am Soc Nephrol* 1994;4:1847–1854.
330. Waddington S, Cook HT, Reaveley D, Jansen A, Cattell V. L-arginine depletion inhibits glomerular nitric oxide synthesis and exacerbates rat nephrotoxic nephritis. *Kidney Int* 1996;49:1090–1096.
331. DeBault LE, Esmon NL, Olson JR, Esmon CT. Distribution of the thrombomodulin antigen in the rabbit vasculature. *Lab Invest* 1986; 54:172–178.
332. Esmon CT. Thromobmodulin as a model of molecular mechanisms that modulate protease specificity and function at the vessel surface. *FASEB J* 1995;946–955.
333. Walker FJ, Fay P. Regulation of blood coagulation by the protein C system. *FASEB J* 1992;6:2561–2567.
334. Hla T, Hirokawa K, Aoki N. Regulatory mechanisms for thrombomodulin expression in human umbilical vein endothelial cells in vitro. *J Cell Physiol* 1991;147:157–165.
335. Moore KL, Esmon CT, Esmon NL. Tumor necrosis factor leads to the internalization and degradation of thrombomodulin from the surface of bovine aortic endothelial cells in culture. *Blood* 1989;73:159–165.
336. Lenz SR, Tsiang M, Sadler JE. Regulation of thromobmodulin by tumor necrosis factor-a: comparison of transcriptional and posttranscriptional mechanisms. *Blood* 1991;77:542–550.
337. Conway EM, Rosenberg RD. Tumor necrosis factor suppresses transcription of the thrombomodulin gene in endothelial cells. *Mol Cell Biol* 1988;8:5588–5592.
338. Archipoff G, Beretz A, Freyssinet JM, Klein-Soyer C, Brisson C, Cazenave JP. Heterogeneous regulation of constitutive thrombomodulin or inducible tissue-factor activities on the surface of human saphenous-vein endothelial cells in culture following stimulation by interleukin-1, tumour necrosis factor, thrombin or phorbol ester. *Biochem J* 1991;273:679–684.
339. Bartha K, Brisson C, Archipoff G, et al. Thrombin regulates tissue factor and thrombomodulin mRNA levels and activities in human saphenous vein endothelial cells by distinct mechanisms. *J Biol Chem* 1993;268:421–429.
340. Horvat R, Palade GE. Thrombomodulin and thrombin localization on the vascular endothelium; their internalization and transcytosis by plasmalemmal vesicles. *Eur J Cell Biol* 1993;61:299–313.
341. Mizutani M, Yuzawa Y, Maruyama I, Sakamoto N, Matsuo S. Glomerular localization of thrombomodulin in human glomerulonephritis. *Lab Invest* 1993;69:193–202.
342. Tomura S, Deguchi F, Ando R, et al. Plasma thrombomodulin in primary glomerular disease and lupus glomerulonephritis. *Nephron* 1994;67:185–189.
343. Shiiki H, Enomoto Y, Uyama H, et al. Distribution of thrombomodulin in patients with focal and segmental glomerulosclerosis (FSGS). *Nippon Jinzo Gakkai Shi* 1994;36:890–895.
344. Cameron JS. Proteinuria and progression in human glomerular diseases. *J Am Soc Nephrol* 1990;10(suppl 1):81–87.
345. Torry RJ, Labarrere CA, Gargiulo P, Faulk WP. Natural anticoagulant and fibrinolytic pathways in renal allograft failure. *Transplantation* 1994;58:926–931.
346. Key NS, Platt JL, Vercellotti GM. Vascular endothelial cell proteoglycans are susceptible to cleavage by neutrophils. *Arterioscler Thromb* 1992;12:836–842.
347. Schrader J, Gallimore MJ, Eisenhauer T, et al. Parameters of the kallikrein-kinin, coagulation and fibrinolytic systems as early indicators of kidney transplant rejection. *Nephron* 1988;48:183–189.
348. Peddi VR, Kant KS. Catastrophic secondary antiphospholipid syndrome with concomitant antithrombin III deficiency. *J Am Soc Nephrol* 1995;5:1882–1887.
349. Yamabe H, Yoshikawa S, Ohsawa H, et al. Tissue factor production by cultured rat glomerular epithelial cells. *Nephrol Dial Transplant* 1993;8:519–523.
350. Wiggins RC, Njoku N, Sedor JR. Tissue factor production by cultured rat mesangial cells. Stimulation by TNF alpha and lipopolysaccharide. *Kidney Int* 1990;37:1281–1285.
351. Schmid EF, Binder K, Grell M, Scheurich P, Pfizenmaier K. Both tumor necrosis factor receptors, TNFR60 and TNFR80, are involved in signaling endothelial tissue factor expression by juxtacrine tumor necrosis factor alpha. *Blood* 1995;86:1836–1841.
352. Lupu C, Lupu F, Dennehy U, Kakkar VV, Scully MF. Thrombin induces the redistribution and acute release of tissue factor pathway inhibitor from specific granules within human endothelial cells in culture. *Arterioscler Thromb Vasc Biol* 1995;15:2055–2062.
353. Mazure G, Grundy JE, Nygard G, et al. Measles virus induction of

human endothelial cell tissue factor procoagulant activity in vitro. *J Gen Virol* 1994;75:2863–2871.
354. van Dam–Mieras MC, Muller AD, van Hinsbergh VW, Mullers WJ, Bomans PH, Bruggeman CA. The procoagulant response of cytomegalovirus infected endothelial cells. *Thromb Haemost* 1992;68: 364–370.
355. Mulder AB, Hegge-Paping KS, Magielse CP, et al. Tumor necrosis factor alpha–induced endothelial tissue factor is located on the cell surface rather than in the subendothelial matrix. *Blood* 1994;84: 1559–1566.
356. Narahara N, Enden T, Wiiger M, Prydz H. Polar expression of tissue factor in human umbilical vein endothelial cells. *Arterioscler Thromb* 1994;14:1815–1820.
357. Tipping PG, Erlich JH, Apostolopoulos J, Mackman N, Loskutoff D, Holdsworth SR. Glomerular tissue factor expression in crescentic glomerulonephritis. Correlations between antigen, activity, and mRNA. *Am J Pathol* 1995;147:1736–1748.
358. Tipping PG, Lowe MG, Holdsworth SR. Glomerular macrophages express augmented procoagulant activity in experimental fibrin-related glomerulonephritis in rabbits. *J Clin Invest* 1988;82: 1253–1259.
359. Lo SK, Cheung A, Zheng Q, Silverstein RL. Induction of tissue factor on monocytes by adhesion to endothelial cells. *J Immunol* 1995;154: 4768–4777.
360. Celi A, Pellegrini G, Lorenzet R, et al. P-selectin induces the expression of tissue factor on monocytes. *Proc Natl Acad Sci U S A* 1994; 91:8767–8771.
361. Neale TJ, Tipping PG, Carson SD, Holdsworth SR. Participation of cell-mediated immunity in deposition of fibrin in glomerulonephritis. *Lancet* 1988;2:421–424.
362. Blakely ML, Van der Werf WJ, Berndt MC, Dalmasso AP, Bach FH, Hancock WW. Activation of intragraft endothelial and mononuclear cells during discordant xenograft rejection. *Transplantation* 1994;58: 1059–1066.
363. Girard TJ, Broze GJ Jr. Tissue factor pathway inhibitor. *Methods Enzymol* 1993;222:195–209.
364. Kobayashi M, Wada H, Wakita Y, et al. Decreased plasma tissue factor pathway inhibitor levels in patients with thrombotic thrombocytopenic purpura. *Thromb Haemost* 1995;73:10–14.
365. Plow EF, Herren T, Redlitz A, Miles LA, Hoover-Plow JL. The cell biology of the plasminogen system. *FASEB J* 1995;9:939–945.
366. Hajjar KA, Harpel PC, Jaffe EA, Nachmann RL. Binding of plasminogen to cultured human endothelial cells. *J Biol Chem* 1986;261: 11656–11662.
367. Ganz PR, Dupuis D, Dudani AK, Hashemi S. Characterization of plasminogen binding to human capillary and arterial endothelial cells. *Biochem Cell Biol* 1991;69:442–448.
368. Schleef RR, Bevilacqua MP, Sawdey M, Gimbrone MA Jr, Loskutoff DJ. Cytokine activation of vascular endothelium. Effects on tissue-type plasminogen activator and type 1 plasminogen activator inhibitor. *J Biol Chem* 1988;263:5797–5803.
369. van Hinsbergh VW, van den Berg EA, Fiers W, Dooijewaard G. Tumor necrosis factor induces the production of urokinase–type plasminogen activator by human endothelial cells. *Blood* 1990;75: 1991–1998.
370. Ginsburg D, Zeheb R, Yang AY, et al. cDNA cloning of human plasminogen activator–inhibitor from endothelial cells. *J Clin Invest* 1986;78:1673–1680.
371. Preissner KT, Grulich-Henn J, Ehrlich HJ, et al. Structural requirements for the extracellular interaction of plasminogen activator inhibitor 1 with endothelial cell matrix–associated vitronectin. *J Biol Chem* 1990;265:18490–18498.
372. Keijer J, Ehrlich HJ, Linders M, Preissner KT, Pannekoek H. Vitronectin governs the interaction between plasminogen activator inhibitor 1 and tissue-type plasminogen activator. *J Biol Chem* 1991; 266:10700–10707.
373. Kanse SM, Kost C, Wilhelm OG, Andreasen PA, Preissner KT. The urokinase receptor is a major vitronectin-binding protein on endothelial cells. *Exp Cell Res* 1996;224:344–353.
374. van den Berg EA, Sprengers ED, Jaye M, Burgess W, Maciag T, van Hinsbergh VW. Regulation of plasminogen activator inhibitor-1 mRNA in human endothelial cells. *Thromb Haemost* 1988;60:63–67.
375. Bevilacqua MP, Schleef RR, Gimbrone MA Jr, Loskutoff DJ. Regulation of the fibrinolytic system of cultured human vascular endothelium by interleukin 1. *J Clin Invest* 1986;78:587–591.
376. van Hinsbergh VW, Kooistra T, van den Berg EA, Princen HM, Fiers W, Emeis JJ. Tumor necrosis factor increases the production of plasminogen activator inhibitor in human endothelial cells in vitro and in rats in vivo. *Blood* 1988;72:1467–1473.
377. Schleef RR, Loskutoff DJ, Podor TJ. Immunoelectron microscopic localization of type 1 plasminogen activator inhibitor on the surface of activated endothelial cells. *J Cell Biol* 1991;113:1413–1423.
378. Gelehrter TD, Sznycer-Laszuk R. Thrombin induction of plasminogen activator–inhibitor in cultured human endothelial cells. *J Clin Invest* 1986;77:165–169.
379. Heaton JH, Dame MK, Gelehrter TD. Thrombin induction of plasminogen activator inhibitor mRNA in human umbilical vein endothelial cells in culture. *J Lab Clin Med* 1992;120:222–228.
380. Ehrlich HJ, Gebbink RK, Preissner KT, et al. Thrombin neutralizes plasminogen activator inhibitor 1 (PAI-1) that is complexed with vitronectin in the endothelial cell matrix. *J Cell Biol* 1991;115: 1773–1781.
381. Shi RJ, Simpsonhaidaris PJ, Marder VJ, Silverman DJ, Sporn LA. Increased expression of plasminogen activator inhibitor-1 in R-Rickettsii–infected endothelial cells. *Thrombosis Haemostasis* 1996;75: 600–606 .
382. Sappino AP, Huarte J, Vassalli JD, Belin D. Sites of synthesis of urokinase and tissue-type plasminogen activators in the murine kidney. *J Clin Invest* 1991;87:962–970.
383. Keeton M, Eguchi Y, Sawdey M, Ahn C, Loskutoff DJ. Cellular localization of type 1 plasminogen activator inhibitor messenger RNA and protein in murine renal tissue. *Am J Pathol* 1993;142: 59–70.
384. Keeton M, Ahn C, Eguchi Y, Burlingame R, Loskutoff DJ. Expression of type 1 plasminogen activator inhibitor in renal tissue in murine lupus nephritis. *Kidney Int* 1995;47:148–157.
385. Malliaros J, Holdsworth SR, Wojta J, Erlich J, Tipping PG. Glomerular fibrinolytic activity in anti-GBM glomerulonephritis in rabbits. *Kidney Int* 1993;44:557–564.
386. Feng L, Tang WW, Loskutoff DJ, Wilson CB. Dysfunction of glomerular fibrinolysis in experimental antiglomerular basement membrane antibody glomerulonephritis. *J Am Soc Nephrol* 1993;3: 1753–1764.
387. Tomosugi N, Wada T, Naito T, et al. Role of plasminogen activator inhibitor on nephrotoxic nephritis and its modulation by tumor necrosis factor. *Nephron* 1992;62:213–219.
388. Rondeau E, Mougenot B, Lacave R, Peraldi MN, Kruithof EK, Sraer JD. Plasminogen activator inhibitor 1 in renal fibrin deposits of human nephropathies. *Clin Nephrol* 1990;33:55–60.
389. Kim S, Wadhwa NK, Kant KS, et al. Fibrinolysis in glomerulonephritis treated with ancrod: renal functional, immunologic and histopathologic effects. *Q J Med* 1988;69:879–905.
390. Aya N, Yoshioka K, Murakami K, et al. Tissue-type plasminogen activator and its inhibitor in human glomerulonephritis. *J Pathol* 1992;166:289–295.
391. Bergstein JM. Tissue plasminogen activator therapy of glomerular thrombi in the Shwartzman reaction. *Kidney Int* 1989;35:14–18.
392. Obrig TG, Louise CB, Lingwood CA, Boyd B, Barley-Maloney L, Daniel TO. Endothelial heterogeneity in Shiga toxin receptors and responses. *J Biol Chem* 1993;268:15484–15488.
393. Louise CB, Obrig TG. Human renal microvascular endothelial cells as a potential target in the development of the hemolytic uremic syndrome as related to fibrinolysis factor expression, in vitro. *Microvasc Res* 1994;47:377–387.
394. Bergstein JM, Riley M, Bang NU. Role of plasminogen-activator inhibitor type 1 in the pathogenesis and outcome of the hemolytic uremic syndrome. *N Engl J Med* 1992;327:755–759.
395. Menzel D, Levi M, Dooijewaard G, Peters M, ten Cate JW. Impaired fibrinolysis in the hemolytic-uremic syndrome of childhood. *Ann Hematol* 1994;68:43–48.
396. Engerman RL, Phaffenbach D, Davis MD. Cell turnover of capillaries. *Lab Invest* 1967;17:738–743.
397. Kitamura H, Sugisaki Y, Yamanaka N. Endothelial regeneration during the repair process following Habu-snake venom induced glomerular injury. *Virchows Arch* 1995;427:195–204.
398. Iruela-Arispe L, Gordon K, Hugo C, et al. Participation of glomerular

endothelial cells in the capillary repair of glomerulonephritis. *Am J Pathol* 1995;147:1715–1727.

399. Ku PT, D'Amore PA. Regulation of basic fibroblast growth factor (bFGF) gene and protein expression following its release from sublethally injured endothelial cells. *J Cell Biochem* 1995;58:328–343.
400. Ballermann BJ. Regulation of bovine glomerular endothelial cell growth in vitro. *Am J Physiol* 1989;256:C182–C189.
401. Yamamoto T, Noble NA, Miller DE, Border WA. Sustained expression of TGF-beta 1 underlies development of progressive kidney fibrosis. *Kidney Int* 1994;45:916–927.
402. Yamamoto T, Noble NA, Cohen AH, et al. Expression of transforming growth factor-beta isoforms in human glomerular diseases. *Kidney Int* 1996;49:461–469.
403. Roberts AB, Sporn MB, Assoian RK, et al. Transforming growth factor type beta: rapid induction of fibrosis and angiogenesis in vivo and stimulation of collagen formation in vitro. *Proc Natl Acad Sci U S A* 1986;83:4167–4171.
404. Choi ME, Ballermann BJ. Inhibition of capillary morphogenesis and associated apoptosis by dominant negative mutant transforming growth factor-β receptors. *J Biol Chem* 1995;270:21144–21150.
405. Kim Y, Butkowski R, Burke B, et al. Differential expression of basement membrane collagen in membranous nephropathy. *Am J Pathol* 191;139:1381–1388.
406. Lee LK, Pollock AS, Lovett DH. Asymmetric origins of the mature glomerular basement membrane. *J Cell Physiol* 1993;157:169–177.
407. Yilmaz A, Yilmaz S, Kallio E, Rapola J, Hayry P. Evolution of glomerular basement membrane changes in chronic rejection. *Transplantation* 1995;60:1314–1322.
408. Shiiki H, Nishino T, Uyama H, et al. Alterations in extracellular matrix components and integrins in patients with preeclamptic nephropathy. *Virchows Arch* 1996;427:567–573.
409. Tomooka S, Border WA, Marshall BC, Noble NA. Glomerular matrix accumulation is linked to inhibition of the plasmin protease system. *Kidney Int* 1992;42:1462–1469.
410. Luscher TF. Endothelium in the control of vascular tone and growth: role of local mediators and mechanical forces. *Blood Press Suppl* 1994;1:18–22.
411. Couser WG, Johnson RJ. Mechanisms of progressive renal disease in glomerulonephritis. *Am J Kidney Dis* 1994;23:193–198.
412. Border WA. Transforming growth factor-beta and the pathogenesis of glomerular diseases. *Curr Opin Nephrol Hypertens* 1994;3:54–58.
413. Zhang G, el Nahas AM. Platelet-derived growth factor in experimental glomerulonephritis. *Nephrol Dial Transplant* 1995;10:787–795.
414. Johnson RJ, Raines EW, Floege J, et al. Inhibition of mesangial cell proliferation and matrix expansion in glomerulonephritis in the rat by antibody to platelet-derived growth factor. *J Exp Med* 1992;175: 1413–1416.
415. Border WA, Noble NA, Yamamoto T, et al. Natural inhibitor of transforming growth factor-beta protects against scarring in experimental kidney disease. *Nature* 1992;360:361–364.
416. Zoja C, Remuzzi G. Role of platelets in progressive glomerular diseases. *Pediatr Nephrol* 1995;9:495–502.
417. Lan HY, Nikolic-Paterson DJ, Mu W, Atkins RC. Local macrophage proliferation in the progression of glomerular and tubulointerstitial injury in rat anti-GBM glomerulonephritis. *Kidney Int* 1995;48: 753–760.
418. Lai KN, Ho RT, Leung JC, Lai FM, Li PK. Increased mRNA encoding for transforming factor-beta in CD4+ cells from patients with IgA nephropathy. *Kidney Int* 1994;46:862–868.
419. Francki A, Uciechowski P, Floege J, von der Ohe J, Resch K, Radeke HH. Autocrine growth regulation of human glomerular mesangial cells is primarily mediated by basic fibroblast growth factor. *Am J Pathol* 1995;147:1372–1382.
420. Floege J, Eng E, Lindner V, et al. Rat glomerular mesangial cells synthesize basic fibroblast growth factor. Release, upregulated synthesis, and mitogenicity in mesangial proliferative glomerulonephritis. *J Clin Invest* 1992;90:2362–2369.
421. Bhandari B, Woodruff K, Abboud HE. Platelet-derived growth factor B-chain gene expression in mesangial cells: effect of phorbol ester on gene transcription and mRNA stability. *Mol Cell Biochem* 1994;140: 31–36.
422. Schweigerer L, Neufeld G, Friedman J, Abraham JA, Fiddes JC, Gospodarowicz D. Capillary endothelial cells express basic fibroblast growth factor, a mitogen that promotes their own growth. *Nature* 1987;325:257–259.
423. Hannan RL, Kourembanas S, Flanders KC, Rogelj SJ, Faller DV, Klagsbrun M. Endothelial cells synthesize basic fibroblast growth factor and transforming growth factor beta. *Growth Factors* 1988; 1:7–17.
424. Daniel TO, Gibbs VC, Milfay DF, Garovoy MR, Williams LT. Thrombin stimulates c-sis gene expression in microvascular endothelial cells. *J Biol Chem* 1986;261:9579–9582.
425. Bashkin P, Doctrow S, Klagsbrun M, Svahn CM, Folkman J, Vlodavsky I. Basic fibroblast growth factor binds to subendothelial extracellular matrix and is released by heparitinase and heparin-like molecules. *Biochemistry* 1989;28:1737–1743.
426. Gajdusek CM, Carbon S. Injury-induced release of basic fibroblast growth factor from bovine aortic endothelium. *J Cell Physiol* 1989; 139:570–579.
427. Sato Y, Rifkin DB. Autocrine activities of basic fibroblast growth factor: regulation of endothelial cell movement, plasminogen activator synthesis, and DNA synthesis. *J Cell Biol* 1988;107:1199–1205.
428. McNeil PL, Muthukrishnan L, Warder E, D'Amore PA. Growth factors are released by mechanically wounded endothelial cells. *J Cell Biol* 1989;109:811–822.
429. Saksela O, Rifkin DB. Release of basic fibroblast growth factor–heparan sulfate complexes from endothelial cells by plasminogen activator–mediated proteolytic activity. *J Cell Biol* 1990;110: 767–775.
430. Ishai-Michaeli R, Eldor A, Vlodavsky I. Heparanase activity expressed by platelets, neutrophils, and lymphoma cells releases active fibroblast growth factor from extracellular matrix. *Cell Regul* 1990;1: 833–842.
431. Kriz W, Hähnel B, Rösner S, Elger M. Long-term treatment of rats with FGF-2 results in focal and segmental glomerulosclerosis. *Kidney Int* 1995;48:1435–1450.
432. Abboud HE. Role of platelet-derived growth factor in renal injury. *Annu Rev Physiol* 1995;57:297–309.
433. Nitta K, Uchida K, Tsutsui T, Kawashima A, Yumura W, Nihei H. Glomerular endothelial cells promote mesangial cell growth via a PDGF-like substance. *Life Sci* 1994;56:143–150.
434. Leveen P, Pekny M, Gebre-Medhin S, Swolin B, Larsson E, Betsholtz C. Mice deficient for PDGF B show renal, cardiovascular, and hematological abnormalities. *Genes Dev* 1994;8:1875–1887.
435. Soriano P. Abnormal kidney development and hematological disorders in PDGF beta-receptor mutant mice. *Genes Dev* 1994;8: 1888–1896.
436. Starksen NF, Harsh GR 4th, Gibbs VC, Williams LT. Regulated expression of the platelet-derived growth factor A chain gene in microvascular endothelial cells. *J Biol Chem* 1987;262:14381–14384.
437. Daniel TO, Gibbs VC, Milfay DF, Williams LT. Agents that increase cAMP accumulation block endothelial c-sis induction by thrombin and transforming growth factor-beta. *J Biol Chem* 1987; 262:11893–11896.
438. Kavanaugh WM, Harsh GR 4th, Starksen NF, Rocco CM, Williams LT. Transcriptional regulation of the A and B chain genes of platelet-derived growth factor in microvascular endothelial cells. *J Biol Chem* 1988;263:8470–8472.
439. Kourembanas S, Faller DV. Platelet-derived growth factor production by human umbilical vein endothelial cells is regulated by basic fibroblast growth factor. *J Biol Chem* 1989;264:4456–4459.
440. Khachigian LM, Lindner V, Williams AJ, Collins T. EGR-1–induced endothelial gene expression—a common theme in vascular injury. *Science* 1996;271:1427–1431.
441. Flaumenhaft R, Abe M, Mignatti P, Rifkin DB. Basic fibroblast growth factor–induced activation of latent transforming growth factor beta in endothelial cells: regulation of plasminogen activator activity. *J Cell Biol* 1992;118:901–909.
442. Schultz-Cherry S, Lawler J, Murphy-Ullrich JE. The type 1 repeats of thrombospondin 1 activate latent transforming growth factor-beta. *J Biol Chem* 1994;269:26783–26788.
443. Schultz-Cherry S, Murphy-Ullrich JE. Thrombospondin causes activation of latent transforming growth factor-beta secreted by endothelial cells by a novel mechanism. *J Cell Biol* 1993;122:923–932.
444. Antonelli-Orlidge A, Saunders KB, Smith SR, D'Amore PA. An activated form of transforming growth factor beta is produced by co-cul-

tures of endothelial cells and pericytes. *Proc Natl Acad Sci U S A* 1989;86:4544–4548.
445. Sato Y, Okada F, Abe M, et al. The mechanism for the activation of latent TGF-beta during co-culture of endothelial cells and smooth muscle cells: cell-type specific targeting of latent TGF-beta to smooth muscle cells. *J Cell Biol* 1993;123:1249–1254.
446. Dennis PA, Rifkin DB. Cellular activation of latent transforming growth factor beta requires binding to the cation-independent mannose 6-phosphate/insulin-like growth factor type II receptor. *Proc Natl Acad Sci U S A* 1991;88:580–584.
447. Papayianni A, Serhan CN, Phillips ML, Rennke HG, Brady HR. Transcellular biosynthesis of lipoxin A4 during adhesion of platelets and neutrophils in experimental immune complex glomerulonephritis. *Kidney Int* 1995;47:1295–1302.

Immunologic Renal Diseases,
edited by E. G. Neilson and W. G. Couser.
Lippincott-Raven Publishers, Philadelphia © 1997.

CHAPTER 31

Glomerular Epithelial Cells

Stephen Adler

Sitting between the glomerular basement membrane (GBM) and the urinary space, the glomerular epithelial cell (GEC) functions as the last barrier between the forming glomerular ultrafiltrate and the exterior world. As such it is strategically located to perform its functions of regulation of the glomerular filtration of solutes and macromolecules, synthesis and catabolism of the GBM, and structural support to counteract the hydrostatic pressure in the glomerular capillaries. It further appears to play a role in the glomerular response to immune injury and inflammation through its ability to present antigens; catabolize immune deposits; synthesize and degrade cytokines, autacoids, and growth factors; and regulate complement activation. Finally, it acts as the prime target in diseases such as membranous glomerulonephritis and minimal-change disease. Its injury appears to be an important intermediate step on the pathway to glomerulosclerosis, leading to the inexorable decline of renal function, which may be triggered by many different initial glomerular lesions (see Chapter 33).

DEVELOPMENT

The GEC, in contrast to most other epithelial cells, is originally derived from mesenchymal tissues (1) (see Chapter 2). Under the influence of the ureteric buds, the mesenchyme condenses into a comma-shaped and then S-shaped epithelium. At this stage, the cells that give rise to the parietal epithelium of Bowman's capsule and the visceral epithelial cells, or podocytes, can be distinguished (1). The extracellular matrix appears to contribute to the development of tubular epithelial polarity during this stage, with coordinate synthesis of laminin and expression of the $\alpha_6\beta_1$ integrin (a laminin receptor) by the developing tubular epithelium and interference with tubulogenesis by anti-α_6 antibodies in animal studies (1,2). Similar expression of laminin and $\alpha_6\beta_1$ integrins in the developing glomerulus suggest a role there as well (1,3). During further development, as the glomerular cleft deepens and is invaded by the developing glomerular capillaries, there is loss of podocyte expression of $\alpha_6\beta_1$. $\alpha_3\beta_1$ integrin expression, which is first present in the S-shaped body stage, becomes more polarized and distributed along the developing GBM, where it persists into adulthood (3,4). Several cell adhesion molecules (CAMs), which mediate cell–cell adhesion, are expressed in the developing glomerulus on parietal and visceral epithelial cells, including N-CAM, A-CAM and L-CAM (N=neuronal; A=adherens junction associated; L=liver), although their contribution to morphogenesis is unclear (5). In the adult kidney, expression of A-CAM and L-CAM in the glomerulus is restricted to the lateral membranes of parietal epithelial cells (5).

S. Adler: Division of Nephrology, Department of Medicine, New York Medical College, and Renal Center, Westchester Medical Center, Valhalla, New York 10595.

GLOMERULAR EPITHELIAL CELL STRUCTURE

The parietal epithelial cells that line Bowman's capsule are simple, attenuated squamous epithelial cells that end abruptly at the transition to the proximal tubule (6). At the vascular pole, where the transition occurs between the parietal and visceral epithelium, cells resembling visceral epithelial cells (podocytes) (see Chapter 2) may be seen and are referred to as parietal podocytes. They are more common in humans (where they may cover up to 25% of the Bowman's capsule surface) and possess pedicels linked by slit diaphragms, similar to visceral epithelial cells, but have more elongated cell bodies, flatter nuclei, and fewer organelles (7).

The glomerular visceral epithelial cell (podocyte), which overlies the GBM and forms the last layer of the glomerular filtration barrier, is a highly differentiated and structured cell. From the cell body, which sits in the urinary space, arise a series of branching processes (primary, secondary, and tertiary) from each of which sprout a series of interdigitating foot processes that terminate in the outer layer of the GBM (6) (Fig. 1). Located between the foot processes are slits ~25–50 nm wide, the so-called filtration slits, where the actual filtration of water and electrolytes is believed to occur (8). Bridging these slits at their lower ends, ~60 nm from the GBMs, are specialized adaptations of the podocyte membranes referred to as slit diaphragms (6,8). As seen en face, this structure appears to possess a zipperlike arrangement of filaments crossing from the foot processes to a central filament in the slit diaphragm (9,10), although more recently a sheetlike substructure has been suggested along with the possibility of fixation artifact giving rise to the zipper arrangement (11) (see Chapter 2). Tight junctions, which are typical of most epithelia, are not seen in this epithelial cell layer, but the slit diaphragm appears to arise from junctional complexes between epithelial cells during embryogenesis, and ZO-1 protein, which is typically associated with tight junctions, is also present along its cytoplasmic surface (12). The entire surface of the podocyte above the slit diaphragm is covered with a relatively thick glycocalyx, which is rich in negatively charged glycoproteins, mainly owing to sialic acid and sulfate groups, and contains anionic proteins such as podocalyxin, podoendin, and heparan sulfate proteoglycan (6).

On initial examination the visceral epithelial cells covering the glomerular capillaries appear to lack the polarized structure typical of other epithelial cell layers, but on an ultrastructural level it is clear that these cells are indeed polarized with unique differences between the areas of membrane above and below the slit diaphragms. Studies of membrane lipids using the sterol-binding antibiotic filipin demonstrate an abrupt reduction in membrane labeling below the slit diaphragm, suggesting microheterogeneity of the podocyte plasma membrane with respect to protein and/or cholesterol content or mobility within the membrane (13,14). Several podocyte cell surface antigens also display altered distribution above and below the slit diaphragm. For example, podocalyxin, a major sialoglycoprotein of the podocyte, appears on the apical surfaces of future podocytes during the S-shaped body stage and continues to be found above the slit diaphragm in the adult kidney (15,16). β_1 integrins, which mediate podocyte adhesion to the GBM, and 13A antigen are largely restricted to the base of the foot processes, whereas other antigens (ZO-1, 5-1-6) are associated with the slit diaphragm (17–19) (see Chapters 2 and 9).

The highly ordered external structure of the podocyte is reflected in its interior by an extensive network of microtubules, microfilaments, and intermediate filaments. This internal skeleton contains several components of the contractile apparatus of muscle, including actin, myosin, and α-actinin (20), which may function in the regulation of filtration and capillary distention. Microtubules and vimentin containing intermediate filaments tend to be

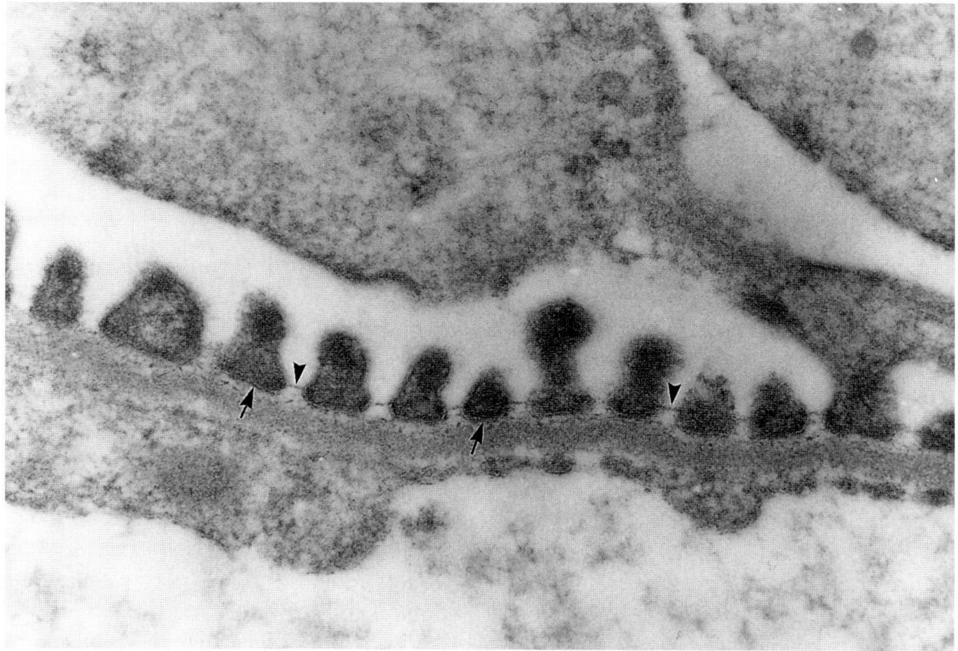

FIG. 1. Electron micrograph of normal glomerular capillary wall showing foot processes *(arrows)* abutting the GBM. Between the foot processes, bridging the lower end of the filtration slits, are slit diaphragms *(arrowheads)*. Original magnification ×20,000.

restricted to the cell body and primary processes (20,21). The foot processes contain longitudinal microfilament bundles that terminate in a dense layer of cytoplasm immediately overlying the sole plate, which is embedded in the outer layer of the GBM (20,21). These bundles contain actin, myosin, and α-actinin and appear to be continuous with a subplasmalemmal network in the primary processes and the cell body (20,22). Expression of desmin in GECs is variable (23). At the sites of termination of these bundles, where the foot process inserts into the GBM, are found talin, vinculin, and paxillin, proteins known to be associated with focal adhesion plaques (20, 24). These proteins, which can interact with actin filaments and integrins, are present in a similar distribution to that of the β_1 integrins, which link the podocyte to the GBM and presumably provide continuity between the extracellular matrix and the cell cytoskeleton (3,4,17). The role of this cytoskeletal, matrix receptor network in maintenance of the normal architecture of the podocyte is supported by experiments with microfilament and microtubule destabilizing agents, which demonstrate alterations in foot process morphology after incubation with intact rat glomeruli (25).

CULTURE OF GLOMERULAR EPITHELIAL CELLS

Understanding of the in vivo function of GECs has been expanded by the study of cultured cells even if certain caveats must be applied to the interpretation of such in vitro studies, including questions about the dedifferentiated state of the cells and their precise origins (26–29). Cultures of these cells have been established from several species, including human, monkey, sheep, dog, rabbit, rat, mouse, and guinea pig kidney (26–33). GEC culture is initiated by the incubation of sterile, isolated glomeruli with relatively enriched medium, usually on plates coated with extracellular matrix components (26,27). Some laboratories have used enzyme treatments to loosen or free individual cells before plating, but in our hands this has tended to decrease the yield of viable epithelial cells. The cloning efficiency of these cells is also low (27; S. Adler, unpublished observations), leading many investigators to attempt to obtain populations of GECs by using media favoring epithelial cell growth and using only the early outgrowth. The nature and purity of such populations of cells is debatable, and every effort should be made to obtain pure populations arising from a single cell.

GECs in culture display a typical polygonal morphology, possess numerous microvilli and one or two cilia, and form domes when plated on a solid substratum (27) (Fig. 2). When allowed to grow in a three-dimensional matrix, such as a type I collagen gel, they form spheroids similar to those reported for tubular epithelial cells (S. Adler, unpublished observations). Characterization of these cells in culture also has relied on their possession of C3 receptors, absence of factor VIII, and phagocytic ability and sensitivity to aminonucleoside of puromycin (26).

The question of whether GECs cultured by conventional techniques originate from the visceral or parietal epithelium has been debated for some time. In vivo, it has been argued that podocytes are terminally differentiated and cannot proliferate (34), although recent work with more sensitive markers suggests that they can duplicate their DNA even if they do not complete cellular mitosis (35). When Norgaard labeled isolated glomeruli in culture with ^{3}H-thymidine, a marker of DNA synthesis, both visceral and parietal epithelial cells incorporated the label and clearly grew out of the glomerulus (36,37). On the basis of morphologic appearance, Norgaard argued that the typical polygonal epithelial cell described in most cultures is of parietal origin. However, morphology may be dependent on the culture substrate, and most investigators culture these cells on collagen-coated plates or collagen gels. Furthermore, when a pure population of rat podocytes is isolated from digested glomeruli using a monoclonal antibody specific for podocytes, the resulting cells can be grown for up to 25 passages and possess the typical small polygonal morphology described by others in GEC cultures (27,38). Thus, it is clear that podocytes can proliferate in vitro, and the appearance of the cells is consistent with that usually described for GECs in culture.

The other arguments concerning the parietal or visceral origin of cultured GECs revolve around the expression, or lack thereof, of cell surface antigens or intermediate filaments characteristic of one or the other cell type in vivo. Some groups have argued that these cells are of parietal origin based on lack of markers normally present on podocytes in vivo, including podocalyxin, GP330, GD3 ganglioside, vimentin, CALLA and C3b receptor, and expression of cytokeratin and thrombospondin, markers of parietal cells in vivo (39,40), although neither of these studies used pure cell populations. On the other hand, several markers specific for podocytes, including complement receptors, Fc receptors, podoendin, CALLA, PHM5, and GSA3, have been reported by others in cultured cells (26,41–45). Although it is true that cytokeratin expression is a marker of parietal epithelium in the normal adult kidney, cytokeratin expression by podocytes in vivo has been reported during glomerulogenesis (46,47). Expression of cytokeratin by cultured GECs may be a marker of dedifferentiation of podocytes rather than evidence of their parietal origin. Although, the question cannot be definitively answered by the above studies, the preponderance of evidence seems to be consistent with a visceral origin of most cultured GECs.

Knowledge of the regulation of proliferation of GECs has been largely derived from in vitro studies. Whether GEC do in fact proliferate in vivo is uncertain. Important mitogenic factors in vitro include epidermal growth factor (EGF), insulin, basic fibroblast growth factor (bFGF),

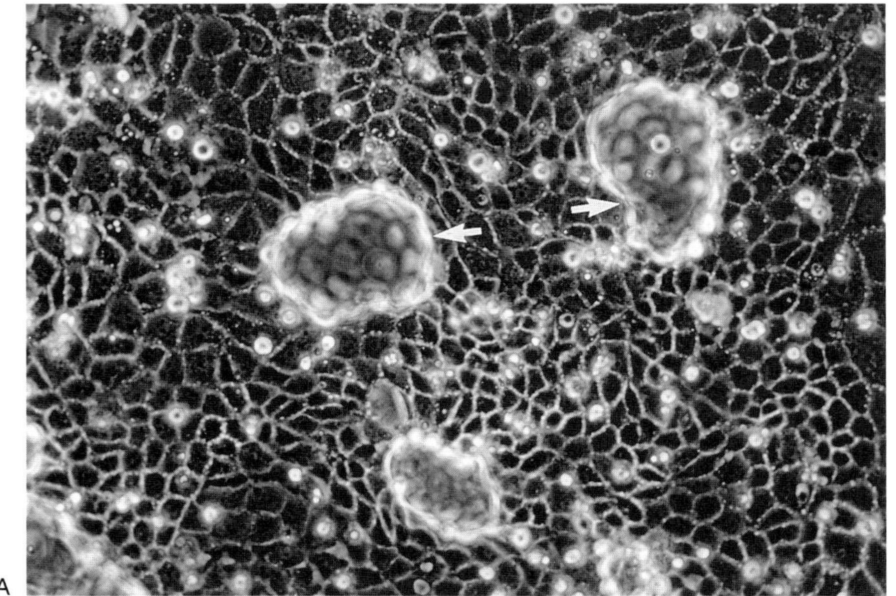

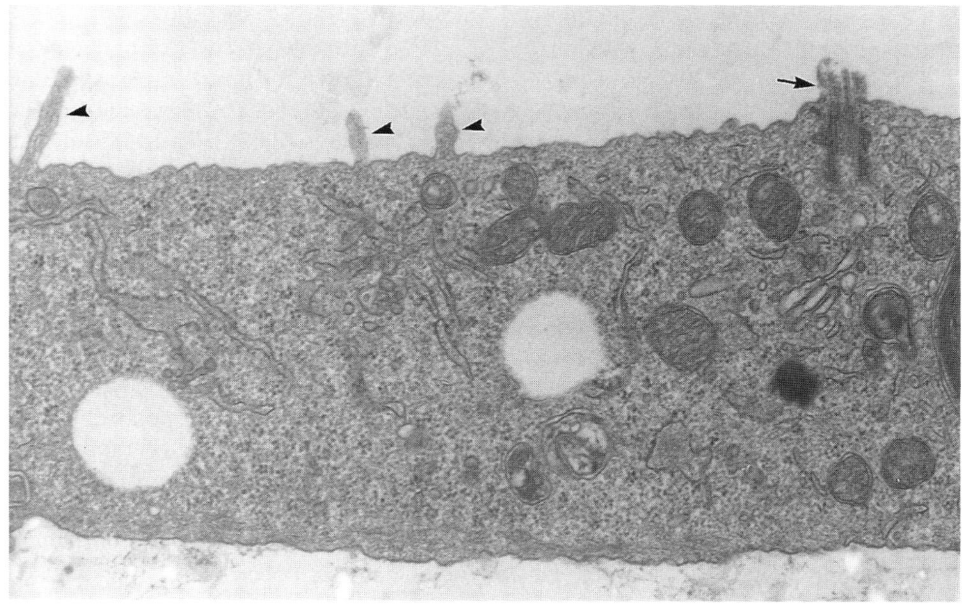

FIG. 2. A: GECs (rat) growing on a solid substrate displaying typical cobblestone morphology and formation of domes *(arrows)*. Original magnification ×100. **B:** Electron micrograph of GEC monolayer showing the base of a cilium *(arrow)* and several microvilli *(arrowheads)*. Original magnification ×10,000.

thrombin, and leukotrienes C_4 and D_4 (48–53). Transforming growth factor-β (TGF-B), heparan sulfate, and heparin inhibit growth (48,54). Fibrin, long blamed as the culprit in initiation of crescent formation, does not stimulate growth in vitro (S. Adler, unpublished observations) and may actually inhibit it (55). Extracellular matrix interactions also play a role in the control of GEC proliferation in vitro. Growth inhibition by heparin (and presumably heparan sulfate) appears to involve stimulation of EGF receptor turnover and EGF degradation, whereas growth stimulation by collagen involves alterations in phospholipid turnover and may be mediated via β_1 integrins (56,57). In vivo, infusions of bFGF increase mitoses and binucleate cells in podocytes in both normal rats and in rats with experimental membranous nephropathy (58,59).

GLOMERULAR EPITHELIAL ANTIGENS AND RECEPTORS

GECs possess numerous antigenic markers and receptors including components of the podocyte glycocalyx (podocalyxin and podoendin), peptidases (aminopeptidase, dipeptidyl peptidase IV and neutral endopeptidase), a tyrosine phosphatase (GLEPP1), receptors for matrix components, complement products, immunoglobulin G (IgG), lipoproteins, vasoactive peptides, plasminogen and growth factors, complement regulatory proteins and various cytoplasmic proteins, glycoproteins (e.g., gp330-megalin, gp108, gp90, SGP115/107) and gangliosides, some of unclear function (19,42,43,60–71) (see Chapter 9). For some of these, their main interest is as targets for antibodies that produce experimental membranous nephropathy (see Chapters 9 and 35). I concentrate here on GEC receptors and antigens that may play a role in normal function and response to injury.

The major extracellular matrix receptors present on the GEC are the β_1 integrins (72,73). Integrins are heterodimeric cell surface proteins that function in cell–cell and cell–matrix interactions (73). In the normal adult human kidney, only $\alpha_3\beta_1$ integrins are present on the podocyte, and their expression is largely restricted to the base of the foot process (17,74–76). This restricted distribution suggests an important role for this integrin in podocyte adhesion to the GBM. In vitro studies with rat GECs demonstrate the presence of $\alpha_3\beta_1$ integrin and document its function as the major receptor for fibronectin, laminin, and collagen on these cells (72). As noted above, this integrin is strategically located to provide a link between the extracellular matrix and the podocyte cytoskeleton and may play a role in regulating glomerular permeability. $\alpha_2\beta_1$ integrin expression also has been shown on these cells in vitro, but its importance is unclear because it is not present in vivo (77,78). Other cell surface proteins expressed by GECs in vivo that demonstrate matrix binding capacity include GP330, dipeptidyl peptidase IV (gp108, sgp115/107), and heparan sulfate proteoglycan (73,79).

The presence of receptors for products of complement activation in the glomerulus was initially recognized by the binding of C3b-coated red blood cells to glomeruli in human kidney sections (80). Further work localized this binding to the cell surface of human podocytes (81–83), and it was subsequently shown to be the CR1 type receptor (84,85). Its presence in rat glomeruli was difficult to demonstrate with rosetting techniques, but it is present in freshly isolated rat glomeruli by Western blotting (86). Cultured rat GECs express both CR1 and CR2 (86,87). Their function on podocytes is unclear but may relate to handling of subepithelial immune complexes. Complement regulatory proteins are also expressed by podocytes in vivo and in culture. Decay accelerating factor (DAF) and membrane cofactor protein, which inhibit formation of C3 and C5 convertases, are present in human glomeruli, and DAF is present on human and rat GECs in culture (88,89). CD59 (protectin) and homologous restriction factor, which inhibit membrane attack complex (C5b-9) formation and insertion, are present on human podocytes and parietal epithelial cells in vivo and in vitro (90). SP-40,40 (clusterin) is present in normal rat but not human glomeruli on podocytes and is synthesized by rat GECs in vitro (91; S. Adler, unpublished observations). The functional activity of DAF and CD59 on cultured cells has been documented by studies in vitro and in vivo in which complement-mediated injury is aggravated by antibodies to the regulatory proteins (88,90,91a,91b,91c). The presence of these regulatory proteins on podocytes may play an important role in diseases where complement activation is occurring on the glomerular capillary wall and products of complement activation, including C5b-9, might be expected to reach the podocytes (see Chapters 18 and 47). This could include both diseases with subepithelial deposits, such as idiopathic membranous and lupus membranous glomerulonephritis, and diseases with subendothelial and GBM deposits such as lupus nephritis, anti-GBM disease, and membranoproliferative glomerulonephritis.

Several other receptors whose presence has been documented on podocytes and may participate in normal function and the response to injury also have been described. Receptors for low-density lipoprotein (LDL) and modified LDL (scavenger receptor) have been demonstrated on human podocytes in vivo and in vitro and are able to mediate LDL uptake by these cells (63,92). They also may be responsible for uptake of lipoproteins into these cells during glomerular injury (63). IgG-F_c receptors are present on human podocytes in vivo and in vitro and appear to be able to mediate uptake of aggregated IgG and immune complexes (44,93) (see Chapter 14). A complete plasminogen activating system is also present on human GECs in culture, including urokinase, plasminogen, and plasmin receptors, which might play a role in responding to fibrin formation in the urinary space (67, 94,95). GLEPP1, a recently described protein tyrosine-phosphatase that is largely restricted to the foot process surface facing the urinary space, has the potential for regulating podocyte function via dephosphorylation of proteins, although its ligand is unknown (68). Specific binding of labeled EGF has been demonstrated in rabbit glomeruli, and specific saturable binding of EGF to a 170-kDa receptor has been found in cultured rat GECs (48,56,96). Receptors for atrial natriuretic peptide, nitric oxide, endothelin, and possibly angiotensin II have been demonstrated on podocytes (21,69,70,97–102). The receptors for atrial natriuretic peptide in the rat are accessible to circulating peptides and mediate increases in cyclic guanosine monophosphate (cGMP) production in podocytes after intra-arterial infusion, raising the possibility that they might contribute to physiologic and pathophysiologic alterations of podocyte function (97,98).

SYNTHETIC PRODUCTS OF PODOCYTES

Much of the work done on the synthetic products of GECs has involved studies of cultured cells. Therefore, questions concerning the origin of these products (i.e., from parietal vs. visceral epithelial cells) remain. The production and secretion of these products in vivo also must remain a question unless it has been directly demonstrated or the product is known to be present in association with GECs in the kidney.

Synthesis and turnover of the GBM is one of the primary functions of the cells lining the GBM, and an important role of podocytes has been demonstrated in this process (see Chapter 10). In the developing kidney, a basement membrane is seen under the future visceral epithelial cells as early as the comma- and S-shaped bodies (103). That this is synthesized by the podocytes is supported by studies with explanted embryonic kidney tissue showing synthesis of type IV collagen, laminin, and heparan sulfate proteoglycans in the developing glomerulus (103–106). In culture, collagen (mainly type IV) is one of the major protein products of rat GECs representing ~0.5% of total protein synthesis (107). These cells also secrete fibronectin into the medium and cell layer (107). Human GECs in culture similarly produce type IV collagen and fibronectin along with variable amounts of type I collagen (108). Analysis of messenger RNA (mRNA) of human and porcine cells demonstrate the presence predominantly of α_1(IV) and α_2(IV) mRNAs and procollagen chains (109). They also express α_2(I) collagen mRNA but do not secrete type I collagen. Although type I collagen is not normally present in the GBM, type I collagen synthesis increases in the glomerulus after injury, and cultured GECs may represent a model of these cells under inflammatory stress. When grown on filters, GEC secretion of type IV collagen and laminin also can be shown to be polarized with most of the protein released at the basal pole of the cells (110). Synthesis of collagen by human and rat GECs is increased by interleukin-1 and the complement–membrane attack complex, respectively (111,112), although another study using antibody-mediated complement activation on GECs did not find an increase in laminin or type IV collagen synthesis (178). TGF-β increased fibronectin but not collagen synthesis by murine GECs, whereas it increased production of type IV collagen, fibronectin, biglycan, and laminin by rat cells (113,114). Thus, thickening of the GBM in states of glomerular injury may be related in part to increased synthesis of some of its components by the podocytes.

Proteoglycans are another important component of the GBM that appear to be synthesized at least in part by podocytes. Rat, murine, and human GECs in culture synthesize and secrete predominantly heparan sulfate proteoglycan with smaller amounts of chondroitin and dermatan sulfate (115–117). Autoradiographic and immunocytochemical evidence further suggest that the podocytes are the source of GBM heparan sulfate proteoglycan in vivo as well (117,118).

Turnover of proteins of the GBM also may be mediated by enzyme systems present on or released by podocytes. Cultured rat GECs secrete metalloproteinases capable of digesting type IV collagen and gelatin that might participate in normal turnover of the GBM as well as contributing to GBM injury (119,120,120a) (see Chapter 19). The major proteinase secreted by cultured rat GECs has been characterized as a 98-kDa enzyme with similarities to human matrix metalloproteinase-9 (gelatinase B) and expression of this protease is increased in experimental membranous nephropathy (119,120a). Interleukin-1β, tumor necrosis factor, and lipopolysaccharide were capable of increasing the secretion of gelatinase by these cells (119). Plasmin is also capable of digesting components of the GBM, including collagens and proteoglycans (121). As noted above, a complete plasminogen activating system is present on the podocyte surface, raising the potential that it also may participate in GBM breakdown.

GECs in vitro produce several autacoids and cytokines that might play a role in normal regulation of glomerular function and in the response to glomerular injury. The relative abundance of prostaglandins produced by these cells has varied from study to study, but they are capable of producing PGE_2, PGI_2 and TxB_2 (122,123) (see Chapter 22). Several factors can increase their prostaglandin release, including neutralization of cell surface charge, angiotensin II, arginine vasopressin, and the complement membrane attack complex (124–127). 12-hydroxyeicosatetraenoic acid, a lipoxygenase metabolite, has been found in early GEC cultures of questionable purity (128). In vivo, expression of mRNA for platelet-derived growth factor, bFGF, and vascular permeability factor, as well as the respective proteins, have been demonstrated in podocytes of rat and human kidneys (53,129,130). Staining for several TGF-β isoforms and receptors is also evident over podocytes and increased in experimental membranous nephropathy, perhaps contributing to basement membrane thickening (131). Other biologically active compounds produced by GECs in vitro include the third and fourth components of complement, platelet-derived growth factor, endothelins 1 and 3, a neutrophil chemotactic factor, plasminogen activators, and plasminogen activator inhibitor (94,95,129,130,132–137). Secretion of some of these components was also shown to be modulated by other inflammatory cytokines (129,133–135). An enzyme system that can produce reactive oxygen species, the NADPH oxido-reductase complex, also has been described in rat podocytes in vivo (137a) (see Chapter 19).

PODOCYTE FUNCTION IN HEALTH AND DISEASE

Several lines of evidence point to the podocyte as an important component of the glomerular filtration barrier (see Chapter 3 for a more detailed discussion of glomerular permeability). In addition to the passive role that was previously assumed, there is an emerging recognition of its potential as an active participant in the regulation of the permeability of the glomerular ultrafilter to solutes and macromolecules. Supporting this possibility are the recognition of a complex contractile cytoskeletal structure within the podocyte, the presence of matrix receptors that provide a link between the cytoskeleton and the GBM, the presence of receptors for vasoactive peptides and ectoenzymes capable of their degradation, and the ability of the podocyte cytoskeleton to respond to those factors.

The contribution of the podocyte to the overall filtration barrier is supported by in vivo observations in human and experimental glomerular disease as well as mathematical modeling of glomerular filtration. The in vivo contribution of the podocytes to restriction of filtration is deduced mainly from observations of abnormalities in proteinuric states. Hypofiltration in nephrotic patients with minimal change disease and membranous nephropathy is largely explained by a decrease in the ultrafiltration coefficient, which in turn correlates well with the reduction in filtration slit frequency seen as a consequence of foot process effacement (138,139). Mathematical modeling further suggests that roughly one half of the total hydraulic resistance of the glomerular capillary wall is due to the filtration slits, with the slit diaphragm being the dominant resistance in the filtration slit (140). Finally, studies of a model of proteinuria in rats induced by a monoclonal antibody to an antigen localized mainly on the slit diaphragm support a role for the slit diaphragm in regulating hydraulic conductivity and protein excretion (141) (see Chapter 17).

The contribution of adhesion of the podocyte to the GBM to limitation of glomerular filtration of macromolecules is similarly supported by studies of proteinuric states (see Chapter 3). Podocyte detachment from the GBM correlates well with the presence and/or onset of proteinuria in several models of injury to GECs, and areas of denuded GBM appear to be sites of protein leakage (142–150). In vitro work comparing filtration through isolated denuded GBM versus intact glomeruli also supports the contribution of the podocyte to restriction of the filtration of proteins (151). Finally, observations of podocytes in human proteinuric states are also consistent with the types of morphologic lesions seen in experimental models (152).

Thus, the simple presence of the podocyte on the exterior aspect of the GBM would seem to contribute significantly to the glomerular filtration barrier. However, a more active role of the podocyte in regulation of ultrafiltration and in the response to injury is also possible. As noted above, the podocyte possesses an extensive cytoskeleton that provides a continuous framework from the cell body, through the primary processes and their branches, into the individual pedicles, and terminating in the sole plate of the foot processes (20–24). Adhesion of the podocyte to the GBM is most likely mediated via β_1 integrins. This is supported by their restricted distribution to the base of the foot process, their colocalization with proteins known to be associated with focal adhesion plaques (i.e., vinculin and talin, which are also known to mediate interactions between the actin cytoskeleton and the cytoplasmic tails of integrins), and the binding properties of the $\alpha_3\beta_1$ integrin, the only β_1 integrin expressed on adult podocytes (3,17,20). In vitro studies using cultured rat GECs have demonstrated the important role played by this integrin in adhesion to fibronectin, laminin, and collagen, components of the GBM (72,77). Other components of the podocyte surface, including dipeptidyl peptidase IV, gp330, and heparan sulfate proteoglycans, also display matrix-binding properties and may participate with the integrins in anchoring the podocytes to the GBM.

The presence of an elaborate contractile system in the podocyte raises questions as to its possible functions. One possibility is the prevention of distention of the glomerular capillaries. Two possible mechanisms involved in preventing capillary distention have been proposed (21,153,154) comparing the podocytes to the flying buttresses of Gothic cathedrals or to nondistensible bands applied to the surface of a balloon, although the longitudinal arrangement of the filaments in the foot processes makes the latter possibility more likely. It is also possible that contraction of the podocytes, by further compressing the GBM, might play a role in regulating GBM permeability as proposed by Kriz et al. (155) (see Chapter 2). The contractile apparatus of the podocyte, influenced by vasoactive peptides and other cytokines acting through receptors outlined above, also might regulate podocyte shape and filtration slit density and might participate in some of the changes in podocyte morphology seen in nephrotic states and after podocyte injury.

Morphologic changes of podocytes seen in response to injury include foot process flattening, spreading, effacement, and retraction, as well as vacuolation, narrowing of filtration slits, formation of occluding junctions between foot processes, microvillous transformation of their apical membranes, and detachment from the GBM (62,152, 156–159) (see Chapter 38). In the past, loss of surface charge of the foot processes was assumed to contribute to these changes, and several studies involving infusion of cations documented reversible proteinuria and associated changes in foot process morphology (143,158). However, other studies suggest that many of these changes involve an active response of the podocyte to injury mediated through autocrine or paracrine pathways.

To postulate a role for a factor in regulating a cell function, the cell should possess receptors for that factor as well as some mechanism for degrading the factor or otherwise turning off its effect. As noted above, podocytes in vivo or in vitro possess receptors for atrial natriuretic peptide (ANP), endothelin, soluble guanylate cyclase, and angiotensin II. They are capable of producing endothelin and autacoids, which might affect the podocytes in an autocrine manner, or they might respond to peptides produced by other glomerular or infiltrating cells in a paracrine manner. The podocytes express several peptidases capable of metabolizing vasoactive factors, giving them the ability to regulate local levels of these factors and thereby their own response to them (61). In vivo, intra-arterial infusion of ANP results in specific increases in cGMP in podocytes (98). Agents such as ANP, nitroprusside, and nitric oxide, which increase glomerular filtration, also increase intracellular cGMP, increase glomerular hydraulic permeability in vitro, and cause disaggregation of the actin cytoskeleton in cultured GECs (71). Conversely, agents such as angiotensin II, which decrease glomerular filtration, also increase cyclic adenosine monophosphate (cAMP) which is associated with decreased hydraulic permeability and actin aggregation in vitro (71). These changes in the actin cytoskeleton could lead to alterations in foot process morphology, which might alter glomerular filtration by changing the size and frequency of filtration slits and slit diaphragms.

Further support for an active role of the podocyte cytoskeleton in regulating foot process morphology comes from in vivo studies. Flattening and spreading of podocytes occurs with dehydration and renal ischemia in experimental animals and humans, and possible effects of vasopressin or angiotensin II have been proposed (156,159). Cytochalasin, which interferes with actin polymerization and inhibits formation of contractile filaments, produces foot processes that appear taller and have narrower bases than normal, leading to wider filtration slits and suggesting that the actin cytoskeleton normally contributes to foot process morphology through its basal tone (25). Increases in cGMP might be expected to produce similar morphologic changes by leading to cytoskeletal disaggregation (see above). Cytochalasin also prevents the broadening and flattening of the foot processes, as well as the loss of foot processes and filtration slits, which occur after prolonged incubation of glomeruli in vitro or after removal of cell surface charge with neuraminidase (25,157,159). Kerjaschki similarly demonstrated that cytochalasin, as well as low temperature and low calcium, attenuated the decrease in podocyte foot processes produced by renal perfusion with protamine sulfate, although the formation of tight junctions was not prevented (160). These studies suggest that foot process alterations after injury may require energy and an intact contractile apparatus. The reorganization of the filtration slits that occurs with protamine infusion is associated with increased phosphorylation of the ZO-1 protein associated with the slit diaphragms, further demonstrating that active signal transduction is occurring in the podocyte during its reorganization in response to injury (24).

RESPONSE OF GLOMERULAR EPITHELIAL CELLS TO INJURY

The podocyte is the target of injury in several models of immunologic and toxic glomerular injury and in human renal disease (see Chapters 9, 32–34, and 41–47). It appears to be the major target in several proteinuric diseases such as membranous nephropathy, where injury is due to subepithelial immune deposits and complement activation, as well as minimal change disease and focal glomerulosclerosis, where the initiators of injury are still unclear. Its responses to injury include morphologic alterations, possibly proliferation, synthesis of autacoids, oxygen radicals, vasoactive peptides, cytokines, and extracellular matrix components. It also modulates the response to injury by endocytosis of immune complexes and complement components by acting as an antigen-presenting cell and by limiting intraglomerular complement activation. These responses, or lack of response, also may be involved in the progression of renal injury eventuating in GBM thickening and/or focal sclerosis (see Chapter 33).

Proliferation of GECs is perhaps most prominent in crescentic glomerulonephritis. It is now generally accepted that crescents are composed predominantly of proliferating parietal epithelial cells and infiltrating macrophages and that the proliferative potential of podocytes is limited or non-existent (see Chapter 32). The experimental basis for this is largely based on studies involving ^{3}H-thymidine labeling, which is very insensitive (161). Morphologic and immunohistochemical studies have suggested a contribution of podocyte proliferation to crescents, especially in focal sclerosis (161–163). Recent studies using more sensitive markers of DNA synthesis (e.g., proliferating cell nuclear antigen [PCNA]) have suggested that DNA synthesis and mitosis do occur in podocytes in response to injury or growth factors (38,58,59). In passive Heymann nephritis, where podocyte injury secondary to the complement membrane attack complex occurs, evidence of DNA synthesis is present in podocytes (38). Further study of the interaction of FGF with podocytes in this model demonstrated upregulation of FGF receptors and the ability of FGF to augment podocyte damage, worsen proteinuria, and accelerate development of glomerulosclerosis (58). Although these studies did not suggest that FGF affected podocytes in normal glomeruli, another group, using an order of magnitude greater dose, documented podocyte mitosis, injury, and development of sclerosis even in normal rats treated for a prolonged period (59). The potential inability of GECs to complete cell division and truly proliferate in states of glomerular hypertrophy has been cited as one factor contributing to progression to focal sclerosis (see Chapter 33).

Interactions between GECs and the GBM or Bowman's capsule basement membrane also may play a role in the cells' proliferative response. Both heparin and heparan sulfate inhibit proliferation of rat GECs in culture, possibly via accelerated catabolism of EGF (54,56). Stimulation of phospholipases in the same cells by interactions with collagen via β_1 integrins also may affect responsiveness to EGF through an effect of eicosanoids on EGF receptor activation (57,164). Synthesis of eicosanoids by GECs has been demonstrated in vitro and is increased in response to neutralization of cell surface charge, angiotensin II, vasopressin, and the complement–membrane attack complex (see above), raising the possibility that eicosanoids produced in the glomerulus during injury, by the epithelial cells or other glomerular cells, might affect the responsiveness of these cells to growth factors (see Chapter 22).

Knowledge of some of the mediators responsible for podocyte injury in vivo have come from the study of models of glomerular injury where the podocyte is the primary target. Study of models of toxic podocyte damage, by compounds such as puromycin aminonucleoside and adriamycin, have implicated oxygen radicals in the podocyte injury that leads to proteinuria (165–167). In passive Heymann nephritis, a model of experimental membranous nephropathy in the rat, amelioration of proteinuria also has been demonstrated using scavengers of oxygen radicals, raising the possibility of oxygen radicals contributing to podocyte damage initiated by immunologic injury as well (168,169) (see Chapter 19). The source of oxygen radicals in passive Heymann nephritis may be the podocytes themselves. During the course of injury in this model, increased levels of cytochrome b_{558}, a component of the oxidoreductase complex that produces the respiratory burst in leukocytes, and H_2O_2 are present in the podocytes (137a). Furthermore, peroxidation products are found in the podocyte membranes and the GBM, including modified type IV collagen in the GBM, suggesting a role of oxygen radical generation by podocytes in podocyte injury and modification of the adjacent GBM (170). Oxygen radicals also increase cAMP levels in glomeruli, which could lead to actin aggregation in podocytes, as outlined above, resulting in altered morphology and proteinuria (171).

Another mediator of podocyte injury is the complement–membrane attack complex (C5b-9) which plays a major role in the production of proteinuria in models of membranous nephropathy (172). In addition to playing a role in the production of proteinuria in vivo, numerous effects of the membrane attack complex that may play a role in glomerular injury have been documented in vitro (see Chapters 18 and 47). Exposure of cultured GECs to the membrane attack complex results in increased synthesis of type IV collagen, increased intracellular calcium, activation of phospholipases, and release of arachidonic acid, diacylglycerol, prostaglandins, and thromboxane (112,173–175). However, in vivo, enhanced production of type IV collagen by podocytes in experimental membranous nephropathy has not been demonstrated, although type I collagen mRNA and possibly protein are transiently increased (176–178). Synthesis of SPARC, a so-called antiadhesive glycoprotein, the GEC 98-kDa matrix metalloproteinase, and TGF-β is increased in podocytes in vivo in complement-mediated podocyte injury, possibly contributing to alterations in GBM structure or function (120a,131,179).

As noted above, podocytes possess several defensive mechanisms against complement-mediated attack, including CR1,2 and DAF (which inhibit C3 and C5 convertases) and CD59, homologous restriction factor, and clusterin, which inhibit membrane attack complex formation and insertion. Membrane attack complex triggered increases in calcium and diacylglycerol, resulting in protein kinase C activation, appear to play a role in protecting the podocyte from complement-induced injury in vitro (180). Perhaps, analogous to human mesangial cells, complement activation might increase production of some of these complement regulatory proteins (181). Finally, the podocyte possesses an active endocytic pathway, involving coated pits, which mediates uptake, transcytosis, and discharge into the urinary space of membrane-inserted membrane attack complexes (182). This endocytic pathway may play a role in clearing other macromolecules, including immune complexes (62,183). Attempts have been made to measure alterations in rates of podocyte endocytosis in vivo in nephrotic states using protamine–heparin complexes with conflicting results (184–186).

Several other features of podocytes described in vivo or in vitro also may contribute to the response of the glomerulus to injury. In vitro, cultured podocytes can process and present antigens, and they may contribute to cell-mediated immune injury in the glomerular capillary wall (38). Altered synthesis of proteoglycans by podocytes after injury may contribute to some of the alterations in charge density described in models of podocyte injury (187–191). Uptake of lipoproteins into human GECs occurs via a receptor-mediated mechanism in vitro, and increased amounts of lipoproteins are present in podocytes in experimental nephrosis, possibly contributing to podocyte damage (192,193). The plasminogen activating system present on GECs (see above) may participate in a glomerular fibrinolytic system as well as in regulation of other glomerular proteases capable of degrading GBM.

SUMMARY

The GEC, especially the visceral epithelial cell, is now recognized as an important participant in both the normal functioning of the glomerulus and the response to injury. It contributes to synthesis of the GBM and major components of the glomerular negative charge barrier and helps to maintain the structural integrity of the GBM. Through its contractile cytoskeleton and receptors for vasoactive substances, it may contribute to regulation of ultrafiltration of solutes and macromolecules. It is a frequent target in glomerular injury and may play a protective role through the uptake of immune complexes and regulation of complement activation. However, it is also a potential source of oxygen radicals, autacoids, and cytokines and may respond to these in an autocrine or paracrine fashion. Dysfunction of the podocyte may contribute to altered GBM turnover, resulting in GBM thickening, and may be an important step along the pathway to glomerulosclerosis.

REFERENCES

1. Sorokin L, Ekblom P. Development of tubular and glomerular cells of the kidney. *Kidney Int* 1992;41:657–664.
2. Ekblom P, Klein G, Ekblom M, Sorokin, L. Aspects of renal growth during fetal and neonatal development. Laminin isoforms and their receptors in the developing kidney. *Am J Kidney Dis* 1991;17:603–605.
3. Korhonen M, Ylanne J, Laitinen L, Virtanen I. The α_1-α_6 subunits of integrins are characteristically expressed in distinct segments of developing and adult human nephron. *J Cell Biol* 1990;111:1245–1254.
4. Korhonen M, Laitinen L, Ylanne J, Gould VE, Virtanen I. Integrins in developing, normal and malignant human kidney. *Kidney Int* 1992;41:641–644.
5. Nouwen EJ, Dauwe S, Van Der Biest I, De Broe ME. Stage- and segment-specific expression of cell-adhesion molecules N-CAM, A-CAM, and L-CAM in the kidney. *Kidney Int* 1993;44:147–158.
6. Tisher CC, Madsen KM. Anatomy of the kidney. In: Brenner BM, Rector FC, eds. The Kidney. Philadelphia: WB Saunders; 1986:3–60.
7. Gibson IW, Downie I, Downie TT, Han SW, More IAR, Lindop GBM. The parietal podocyte: a study of the vascular pole of the human glomerulus. *Kidney Int* 1992;41:211–214.
8. Karnovsky MJ. The ultrastructure of glomerular filtration. *Ann Rev Med* 1979;30:213–224.
9. Rodewald R, Karnovsky MJ. Porous substructure of the glomerular slit diaphragm in the rat and mouse. *J Cell Biol* 1974;60:423–433.
10. Schneeberger EE, Levey RH, McCluskey RT, Karnovsky MJ. The isoporous substructure of the human glomerular slit diaphragm. *Kidney Int* 1975;8:48–52.
11. Ohno S, Hora K, Furukawa T, Oguchi H. Ultrastructural study of the glomerular slit diaphragm in fresh unfixed kidneys by a quick-freezing method. *Virchows Arch [B]* 1992;61:351–358.
12. Schnabel E, Anderson JM, Farquhar MG. The tight junction protein ZO-1 is concentrated along slit diaphragms of the glomerular epithelium. *J Cell Biol* 1990;111:1255–1263.
13. Orci L, Singh A, Amherdt M, Brown D, Perrelet A. Microheterogeneity of protein and sterol content in kidney podocyte membrane. *Nature* 1981;293:646–647.
14. Orci L, Brown D, Amherdt M, Perrelet A. Distribution of intramembrane particles and filipin–sterol complexes in plasma membranes of kidney I. Corpuscle of malpighi. *Lab Invest* 1982;46:545–553.
15. Schnabel E, Dekan G, Miettinen A, Farquhar MG. Biogenesis of podocalyxin—the major glomerular sialoglycoprotein—in the newborn rat kidney. *Eur J Cell Biol* 1989;48:313–326.
16. Sawada H, Stukenbrok H, Kerjaschki D, Farquhar MG. Epithelial polyanion (podocalyxin) is found on the sides but not the soles of the foot processes of the glomerular epithelium. *Am J Pathol* 1986;125:309–318.
17. Kerjaschki D, Ojha PP, Susani M, et al. A β_1–integrin receptor for fibronectin in human kidney glomeruli. *Am J Pathol* 1989;134:481–489.
18. Orikasa M, Matsui K, Oite T, Shimizu F. Massive proteinuria induced in rats by a single intravenous injection of a monoclonal antibody. *J Immunol* 1988;141:807–814.
19. Tissari J, Holthofer H, Miettinen A. Novel 13A antigen is an integral protein of the basolateral membrane of rat glomerular podocytes. *Lab Invest* 1994;71:519–527.
20. Drenckhahn D, Franke RP. Ultrastructural organization of contractile and cytoskeletal proteins in glomerular podocytes of chicken, rat, and man. *Lab Invest* 1988;59:673–682.
21. Kriz W, Mundel P, Elger M. The contractile apparatus of podocytes is arranged to counteract GBM expansion. *Contrib Nephrol* 1994;107:1–9.
22. Andrews PM, Bates SB. Filamentous actin bundles in the kidney. *Anat Rec* 1984;210:1–9.
23. Yaoita E, Kawasaki K, Yamamoto T, Kihara I. Variable expression of desmin in rat glomerular epithelial cells. *Am J Pathol* 1990;136:899–908.
24. Kurihara H, Anderson JM, Farquhar MG. Increased Tyr phosphorylation of ZO-1 during modification of tight junctions between glomerular foot processes. *Am J Physiol* 1995;268:514–524.
25. Andrews PM. Investigations of cytoplasmic contractile and cytoskeletal elements in the kidney glomerulus. *Kidney Int* 1981;20:549–562.
26. Kreisberg JI, Hoover RL, Karnovsky MJ. Isolation and characterization of rat glomerular epithelial cells in vitro. *Kidney Int* 1978;14:21–30.
27. Harper PA, Robinson JM, Hoover RL, Wright TC, Karnovsky MJ. Improved methods for culturing rat glomerular cells. *Kidney Int* 1984;26:875–880.
28. Lovett DH, Sterzel RB. Cell culture approaches to the analysis of glomerular inflammation. *Kidney Int* 1986;30:246–254.
29. Striker GE, Lange MA, MacKay K, Bernstein K, Striker L. Glomerular cells in vitro. *Adv Nephrol* 1987;16:169–186.
30. Holdsworth SR, Glasgow EF, Atkins RC, Thomson NM. Cell characteristics of cultured glomeruli from different animal species. *Nephron* 1978;22:454–459.
31. Striker GE, Killen PD, Farin FM. Human glomerular cells in vitro: isolation and characterization. *Transplant Proc* 1980;12:88–99.
32. Oberley TD, Muth JV, Murphy-Ullrich JE. Growth and maintenance of glomerular cells under defined conditions. *Am J Pathol* 1980;101:195–204.
33. Foidart JB, Dechenne CA, Mahieu P, Creutz CE, De Mey J. Tissue culture of normal rat glomeruli. Isolation and morphological characterization of two homogeneous cell lines. *Invest Cell Pathol* 1979;2:15–26.
34. Fries JW, Sandstrom DJ, Meyer TW, Rennke HG. Glomerular hypertrophy and epithelial cell injury modulate progressive glomerulosclerosis in the rat. *Lab Invest* 1989;60:205–218.
35. Floege J, Johnson RJ, Alpers CE, Richardson CA, Gordon K, Couser WG. Visceral glomerular epithelial cells can proliferate in vivo and synthesize PDGF B-chain. *Am J Pathol* 1993;142:637–650.
36. Norgaard JOR. Cellular outgrowth from isolated glomeruli. Origin and characterization. *Lab Invest* 1983;48:526–542.
37. Norgaard JOR. Rat glomerular epithelial cells in culture. Parietal or visceral epithelial origin? *Lab Invest* 1987;57:277–290.
38. Mendrick DL, Kelly DM, Rennke HG. Antigen processing and presentation by glomerular visceral epithelium in vitro. *Kidney Int* 1991;39:71–78.
39. Holthofer H, Sainio K, Miettinen A. Rat glomerular cells do not express podocytic markers when cultured in vitro. *Lab Invest* 1991;65:548–557.
40. Weinstein T, Cameron R, Katz A, Silverman M. Rat glomerular epithelial cells in culture express characteristics of parietal, not visceral, epithelium. *J Am Soc Nephrol* 1992;3:1279–1287.
41. Delarue F, Virone A, Hagege J, et al. Stable cell line of T-SV40 immortalized human glomerular visceral epithelial cells. *Kidney Int* 1991;40:906–912.
42. Huang TW, Langlois JC. Podoendin. A new cell surface protein of the podocyte and endothelium. *J Exp Med* 1985;162:245–267.
43. Hancock WW, Atkins RC. Monoclonal antibodies to human glomerular cells: a marker for glomerular epithelial cells. *Nephron* 1983;33:83–90.
44. Mancilla-Jimenez R, Appay MD, Bellon B, Kuhn J, Bariety J, Druet P. IgG Fc membrane receptor on normal human glomerular visceral epithelial cells. *Virchows Arch* 1984;404:139–158.
45. Nosaka K, Nishi T, Imaki H, et al. Permeable type I collagen membrane promotes glomerular epithelial cell growth in culture. *Kidney Int* 1993;43:470–478.
46. Fleming S, Symes CE. The distribution of cytokeratin antigens in the kidney and in renal tumours. *Histopathology* 1987;11:157–170.

47. Moll R, Hage C, Thoenes W. Expression of intermediate filament proteins in fetal and adult human kidney: modulations of intermediate filament patterns during development and in damaged tissue. *Lab Invest* 1991;65:74–86.
48. Adler S, Chen X, Eng B. Control of rat glomerular epithelial cell growth in vitro. *Kidney Int* 1990;37:1048–1054.
49. Cybulsky, AV, Bonaventre JV, Quigg RJ, Wolfe, LS, Salant DJ. Extracellular matrix regulates proliferation and phospholipid turnover in glomerular epithelial cells. *Am J Physiol* 1990;259:F326–F337.
50. He CJ, Rondeau E, Medcalf RL, Lacave R, Schleuning WD, Sraer JD. Thrombin increases proliferation and decreases fibrinolytic activity of kidney glomerular epithelial cells. *J Cell Physiol* 1991;146: 131–140.
51. Baud L, Sraer J, Perez J, Nivez, MP, Ardaillou R. Leukotriene C4 binds to human glomerular epithelial cells and promotes their proliferation in vitro. *J Clin Invest* 1985;76:374–377.
52. Baud L, Perez J, Cherqui G, Cragoe EJ, Ardaillou R. Leukotriene D_4-induced proliferation of glomerular epithelial cells: PKC- and Na+-H+ exchanger-mediated response. *Am J Physiol* 1989;257:232–239.
53. Takeuchi A, Yoshizawa N, Yamamoto M, et al. Basic fibroblast growth factor promotes proliferation of rat glomerular visceral epithelial cells in vitro. *Am J Pathol* 1992;141:107–116.
54. Adler S. Inhibition of rat glomerular visceral epithelial cell growth by heparin. *Am J Physiol* 1988;255:781–786.
55. Yang AH, Chang HJ. Effects of fibrin matrix on growth of glomerular cells. *Am J Pathol* 1992;140:569–579.
56. Adler S. Heparin alters epidermal growth factor metabolism in cultured rat glomerular epithelial cells. *Am J Pathol* 1991;139:169–175.
57. Cybulsky AV, Carbonetto S, Cyr MD, McTavish AJ, Huang Q. Extracellular matrix–stimulated phospholipase activation is mediated by β_1-integrin. *Am J Physiol* 1993;264:323–332.
58. Floege J, Kriz W, Schulze M, et al. Basic FGF augments podocyte injury and induces glomerulosclerosis in rats with experimental membranous nephropathy. *J Clin Invest* 1996 (in press).
59. Kriz W, Hähnel B, Rösener S, Elger M. Long-term treatment of rats with FGF-2 results in focal segmental glomerulosclerosis. *Kidney Int* 1995;48:1435–1450.
60. Brentjens JR, Andres G. Interaction of antibodies with renal cell surface antigens. *Kidney Int* 1989;35:954–968.
61. Ronco PM, Ardaillou N, Verroust P, Lelongt B. Pathophysiology of the podocyte: a target and a major player in glomerulonephritis. *Adv Nephrol* 1994;23:91–131.
62. Kerjaschki D. Dysfunction of cell biological mechanisms of visceral epithelial cell (podocytes) in glomerular diseases. *Kidney Int* 1994; 45:300–313.
63. Takemura T, Yoshioka K, Aya N, et al. Apolipoproteins and lipoprotein receptors in glomeruli in human kidney diseases. *Kidney Int* 1993;43:918–927.
64. Mundel P, Gilbert P, Kriz W. Podocytes in glomerulus of rat kidney express a characteristic 44 KD protein. *J Histochem Cytochem* 1991; 39:1047–1056.
65. Kerjaschki D, Sharkey DJ, Farquhar MG. Identification and characterization of podocalyxin—the major sialoprotein of the renal glomerular epithelial cell. *J Cell Biol* 1984;98:1591–1596.
66. Kerjaschki D, Poczewski H, Dekan G, et al. Identification of a major sialoprotein in the glycocalyx of human visceral glomerular epithelial cells. *J Clin Invest* 1986;78:1142–1149.
67. Becquemont L, Nguyen G, Peraldi M, He C, Sraer J, Rondeau E. Expression of plasminogen/plasmin receptors on human glomerular epithelial cells. *Am J Physiol* 1994;267:F303–F310.
68. Thomas PE, Wharram BL, Goyal M, Wiggins JE, Holzman LB, Wiggins RC. GLEPP1, a renal glomerular epithelial cell (podocyte) membrane protein-tyrosine phosphatase. *J Biochem* 1994;269:19953–19962.
69. Hori S, Komatsu Y, Shigemoto R, Mizuno N, Nakanishi S. Distinct tissue distribution and cellular localization of two messenger ribonucleic acids encoding different subtypes of rat endothelin receptors. *Endocrinology* 1992;130:1885–1895.
70. Yamada H, Sexton PM, Chai SY, Adam WR, Mendelsohn FA. Angiotensin II receptors in the kidney. Localization and physiological significance. *Am J Hypertens* 1990;3:250–255.
71. Sharma R, Lovell HB, Wiegmann TB, Savin VJ. Vasoactive substances induce cytoskeletal changes in cultured rat glomerular epithelial cells. *J Am Soc Nephrol* 1992;3:1131–1138.
72. Adler S. Characterization of glomerular epithelial cell matrix receptors. *Am J Pathol* 1992;141:571–578.
73. Adler S. Integrin receptors in the glomerulus: potential role in glomerular injury. *Am J Physiol* 1992;262:697–704.
74. Korhonen M, Ylanne J, Laitinen L, Virtanen I. Distribution of β_1 and β_3 integrins in human fetal and adult kidney. *Lab Invest* 1990;62: 616–625.
75. Cosio FG, Sedmak DD, Nahman NS Jr. Cellular receptors for matrix proteins in normal human kidney and human mesangial cells. *Kidney Int* 1990;38:886–895.
76. Simon EE, McDonald JA. Extracellular matrix receptors in the kidney cortex. *Am J Physiol* 1990;259:783–792.
77. Cybulsky AV, Carbonetto S, Huang Q, McTavish AJ, Cyr MD. Adhesion of rat glomerular epithelial cells to extracellular matrices: role of β_1 integrins. *Kidney Int* 1992;42:1099–1106.
78. Mendrick DL, Kelly DM. Temporal expression of VLA-2 and modulation of its ligand specificity by rat glomerular epithelial cells in vitro. *Lab Invest* 1993;69:690–702.
79. Mendrick DL, Chung DC, Rennke HG. Heymann antigen GP330 demonstrates affinity for fibronectin, laminin, and type I collagen and mediates rat proximal tubule epithelial cell adherence to such matrices in vitro. *Exp Cell Res* 1990;188:23–35.
80. Gelfand MC, Frank MM, Green I. A receptor for the third component of complement in the human renal glomerulus. *J Exp Med* 1975;142: 1029–1034.
81. Shin ML, Gelfand MC, Nagle RB, Carlo JR, Green I, Frank MM. Localization of receptors for activated complement on visceral epithelial cells of the human renal glomerulus. *J Immunol* 1977;118:869–873.
82. Burkholder PM, Oberley TD, Barber TA, Beacom A, Koehler C. Immune adherence in renal glomeruli. *Am J Pathol* 1977;86:635–654.
83. Kazatchkine MD, Fearon DT, Appay MD, Mandet C, Bariety J. Immunohistochemical study of the human glomerular C3b receptor in normal kidney and in seventy-five cases of renal diseases. *J Clin Invest* 1982;69:900–912.
84. Fischer E, Appay MD, Cook J, Kazatchkine MD. Characterization of the human glomerular C3 receptor as the C3b/C4b complement type one (CR1)receptor. *J Immunol* 1986;136:1373–1377.
85. Appay MD, Kazatchkine MD, Levi-Strauss M, Hinglais N, Bariety J. Expression of CR1 (CD35) mRNA in podocytes from adult and fetal human kidneys. *Kidney Int* 1990;38:289–293.
86. Quigg RJ, Galishoff ML, Sneed AE III, Kim D. Isolation and characterization of complement receptor type 1 from rat glomerular epithelial cells. *Kidney Int* 1993;43:730–736.
87. Kasinath BS, Maaba MR, Schwartz MM, Lewis EJ. Demonstration and characterization of C3 receptors on rat glomerular epithelial cells. *Kidney Int* 1986;30:852–861.
88. Quigg RJ, Nicholson-Weller, A, Cybulsky AV, Badalamenti J, Salant DJ. Decay accelerating factor regulates complement activation on glomerular epithelial cells. *J Immunol* 1989;142:877–882.
89. Ichida S, Yuzawa Y, Okada H, Yoshioka K, Matsuo S. Localization of the complement regulatory proteins in the normal human kidney. *Kidney Int* 1994;46:89–96.
90. Rooney IA, Davies A, Griffiths D, et al. The complement-inhibiting protein, protectin (CD59 antigen), is present and functionally active on glomerular epithelial cells. *Clin Exp Immunol* 1991;83:251–256.
91. Eddy AA, Fritz IB. Localization of clusterin in the epimembranous deposits of passive Heymann nephritis. *Kidney Int* 1991;39:247–252.
91a. Quigg RJ, Holers VM, Morgan BP, Sneed AE. Crry and CD59 regulate complement in rat glomerular epithelial cells and are inhibited by the nephritogenic antibody of passive Heymann nephritis. *J Immunol* 1995;154:3437–3443.
91b. Matsuo S, Nishikage H, Yoshida F, Nomura A, Piddlesden SJ, Morgan BP. Role of CD59 in experimental glomerulonephritis in rats. *Kidney Int* 1994;46:191–200.
91c. Quigg RJ, Morgan PB, HolersVM, Adler S, Sneed AE, Lo CF. Complement regulation in the rat glomerulus: Crry and CD 59 regulate complement in glomerular mesangial and endothelial cells. *Kidney Int* 1995;48:412–421.
92. Grone HJ, Walli AK, Grone E, Kramer A, Clemens MR, Seidel D. Receptor mediated uptake of apo B and apo E rich lipoproteins by human glomerular epithelial cells. *Kidney Int* 1990;37:1449–1459.
93. Mizoguchi Y, Horiuchi Y. Localization of IgG-Fc receptors in human glomeruli. *Clin Immunol Immunopathol* 1982;24:320–329.
94. Rondeau E, Ochi S, LaCave R, He C, Medcalf R, Delarue F, Sraer JD.

Urokinase synthesis and binding by glomerular epithelial cells in culture. *Kidney Int* 1989;36:593–600.
95. Brown PAJ, Wilson HM, Reid FJ, et al. Urokinase-plasminogen activator is synthesized in vitro by human glomerular epithelial cells but not by mesangial cells. *Kidney Int* 1994;45:43–47.
96. Breyer MD, Redha R, Breyer JA. Segmental distribution of epidermal growth factor binding sites in rabbit nephron. Am J Physiol 1990;259: 553–558.
97. Koseki C, Kanai Y, Hayashi Y, Ohnuma N, Imai M. Intrarenal localization of receptors for alpha-rat atrial natriuretic polypeptide: an autoradiographic study with [^{125}I]-labeled ligand injected in vivo into the rat aorta. *Jpn J Pharmacol* 1986;42:27–33.
98. Chevalier RL, Fern RJ, Garmey M, El-Dahr SS, Gomez RA, De Vente J. Localization of cGMP after infusion of ANP or nitroprusside in the maturing rat. *Am J Physiol* 1992;262:417–424.
99. Rebibou JM, He CJ, Delarue F, Peraldi MN, Adida C, Rondeau E, Sraer JE. Functional endothelin-1 receptors on human glomerular podocytes and mesangial cells. *Nephrol Dial Transplant* 1992;7:288–292.
100. Chansel D, Pham P, Nivez MP, Ardaillou R. Characterization of atrial natriuretic factor receptors in human glomerular epithelial and mesangial cells. *Am J Physiol* 1990;259:619–627.
101. Mundel P, Gambarayan S, Bachmann S, Koesling D, Kriz W. Immunolocalization of soluble guanylyl cyclase subunits in rat kidney. *Histochemistry* 1995;103:75–79.
102. Ardaillou N, Nivez MP, Ardaillou R. Stimulation of cyclic GMP synthesis in human cultured glomerular cells by atrial natriuretic peptide. *FEBS* 1986;204:177–182.
103. Abrahamson DR. Structure and development of the glomerular capillary wall and basement membrane. *Am J Physiol* 1987;253:783–794.
104. Sariola H, Timpl R, von der Mark K, et al. Dual origin of glomerular basement membrane. *Dev Biol* 1984;101:86–96.
105. Kanwar YS, Jakubowski ML, Rosenzweig LJ, Gibbons JT. De novo cellular synthesis of sulfated proteoglycans of the developing renal glomerulus in vivo. *Proc Natl Acad Sci U S A* 1984;81:7108–7111.
106. Bernstein J, Cheng F, Roszka J. Glomerular differentiation in metanephric organ culture. *Lab Invest* 1981;45:183–190.
107. Foidart JM, Foidart JB, Mahieu PR. Synthesis of collagen and fibronectin by glomerular cells in culture. *Renal Physiol* 1980;3:183–192.
108. Striker GE, Striker LJ. Glomerular cell culture. *Lab Invest* 1985;53: 122–131.
109. Scheinman JI, Tanaka H, Haralson M, Wang SL, Brown O. Specialized collagen mRNA and secreted collagens in human glomerular epithelial, mesangial, and tubular cells. *J Am Soc Nephrol* 1992;2:1475–1483.
110. Natori Y, O'Meara YM, Manning EC, et al. Production and polarized secretion of basement membrane components by glomerular epithelial cells. *Am J Physiol* 1992;262:131–137.
111. Torbohm I, Berger B, Schonermark M, Von Kempis J, Rother K, Hansch GM. Modulation of collagen synthesis in human glomerular epithelial cells by interleukin 1. *Clin Exp Immunol* 1989;75:427–431.
112. Torbohm I, Schonermark M, Wingen AM, Berger B, Rother K, Hansch GM. C5b-8 and C5b-9 modulate the collagen release of human glomerular epithelial cells. *Kidney Int* 1990;37:1098–1104.
113. MacKay K, Striker LJ, Stauffer JW, Doi T, Agodoa LY, Striker GE. Transforming growth factor-β. Murine glomerular receptors and responses of isolated glomerular cells. *J Clin Invest* 1989;83:1160–1167.
114. Nakamura T, Miller D, Ruoslahti E, Border WA. Production of extracellular matrix by glomerular epithelial cells is regulated by transforming growth factor-β1. *Kidney Int* 1992;41:1213–1221.
115. Stow JL, Soroka CJ, MacKay K, Striker L, Striker G, Farquhar MG. Basement membrane heparan sulfate proteoglycan is the main proteoglycan synthesized by glomerular epithelial cells in culture. *Am J Pathol* 1989;135:637–646.
116. Foidart JB, Pirard YS, Winand RJ, Mahieu PR. Tissue culture of normal rat glomeruli. *Renal Physiol* 1980;3:169–173.
117. Klein DJ, Oegema TR Jr, Fredeen TS, van-der-Woude F, Kim Y, Brown DMAD. Partial characterization of proteoglycans synthesized by human glomerular epithelial cells in culture. *Arch Biochem Biophys* 1990;277:389–401.
118. Stow JL, Sawada H, Farquhar MG. Basement membrane heparan sulfate proteoglycans are concentrated in the lamina rarae and in podocytes of the rat renal glomerulus. *Proc Natl Acad Sci U S A* 1985;82: 3296–3300.
119. Watanabe K, Kinoshita S, Nakagawa H. Gelatinase secretion by glomerular epithelial cells. *Nephron* 1990;56:405–409.
120. Johnson R, Yamabe H, Chen YP, et al. Glomerular epithelial cells secreate a glomerular basement membrane-degrading metalloproteinase. *J Am Soc Nephrol* 1992;2:1388–1397.
120a. McMillan JI, Riordan JW, Couser WG, Pollock AS, Lovett DH. Characterization of a glomerular epithelial cell metalloproteinase as matrix metalloproteinase-9 with enhanced expresion in a model of membranous nephropathy. *J Clin Invest* 1996;1094–1101.
121. Davies M, Martin J, Thomas GJ, Lovett DH. Proteinases and glomerular matrix turnover. *Kidney Int* 1992;41:671–678.
122. Petrulis AS, Aikawa M, Dunn MJ. Prostaglandin and thromboxane synthesis by rat glomerular epithelial cells. *Kidney Int* 1981;20: 469–474.
123. Kreisberg JI, Karnovsky MJ, Levine L. Prostaglandin production by homogeneous cultures of rat glomerular epithelial and mesangial cells. *Kidney Int* 1982;22:355–359.
124. Ardaillou R, Sraer J, Chansel D, Ardaillou N, Sraer JD. The effects of angiotension II on isolated glomeruli and cultured glomerular cells. *Kidney Int* 1987;31:74–80.
125. Pugliese F, Singh AK, Kasinath BS, Kreisberg JI, Lewis EJ. Glomerular epithelial cell, polyanion neutralization is associated with enhanced prostanoid production. *Kidney Int* 1987;32:57–61.
126. Hansch GM, Betz M, Gunther J, Rother KO, Sterzel B. The complement membrane attack complex stimulates the prostanoid production of cultured glomerular epithelial cells. *Int Arch Allergy Appl Immunol* 1988;85:87–93.
127. Lieberthal W, Levin L. Stimulation of prostaglandin production in rat glomerular epithelial cells by antidiuretic hormone. *Kidney Int* 1984; 25:766–770.
128. Jim K, Hassid A, Sun F, Dunn MJ. Lipoxygenase activity in rat kidney glomeruli, glomerular epithelial cells and cortical tubules. *J Biol Chem* 1982;257:10294–10299.
129. Floege J, Johnson RJ, Alpers CE, et al. Visceral glomerular epithelial cells can proliferate in vivo and synthesize platelet-derived growth factor B-chain. *Am J Pathol* 1993;142:637–650.
130. Brown LF, Berse B, Tognazzi K, et al. Vascular permeability factor mRNA and protein expression in human kidney. *Kidney Int* 1992;42: 1457–1461.
131. Shankland SJ, Pippin J, Pichler RH, Gold L, Gordon K, Johnson RJ. Differential expression of transforming growth factor isoforms and receptors in experimental membranous nephropathy [Abstract]. *J Am Soc Nephrol* 1995;6:853.
132. Kasinath BS, Fried TA, Davalath S, Marsden PA. Glomerular epithelial cells synthesize endothelin peptides. *Am J Pathol* 1992;141: 279–283.
133. Cybulsky AV, Stewart DJ, Cybulsky MI. Glomerular epithelial cells produce endothelin-1. *J Am Soc Nephrol* 1993;3:1398–1404.
134. Watanabe K, Nakagawa H. Cytokines enhance the production of a chemotactic factor of polymorphonuclear leukocytes by rat renal glomerular epithelioid cells. *Nephron* 1990;54:169–175.
135. Iwamoto T, Nakashima Y, Sueishi K. Secretion of plasminogen activator and its inhibitor by glomerular epithelial cells. *Kidney Int* 1990; 37:1466–1476.
136. Sacks SH, Zhou W, Pani A, Campbell RD, Margin J. Complement C3 gene expression and regulation in human glomerular epithelial cells. *Immunology* 1993;79:348–354.
137. Zhou W, Campbell RD, Martin J, Sacks SH. Interferon–gamma regulation of C4 gene expression in cultured human glomerular epithelial cells. *Eur J Immunol* 1993;23:2477–2481.
137a. Neale TJ, Ullrich R, Ojha P, Poczewski, H, Verhoeven AJ, Kerjaschki D. Reactive oxygen species and neutrophil respiratory burst cytochrome b_{558} are produced by kidney glomerular cells in passive Heymann nephritis. *Proc Natl Acad Sci U S A* 1993;90:3645–3649.
138. Ting RH, Kristal B, MyersBD. The biophysical basis of hypofiltration in nephrotic humans with membranous nephropathy. *Kidney Int* 1994;45:390–397.
139. Guasch A, Myers BD. Determinants of glomerular hypofiltration in nephrotic patients with minimal change nephropathy. *J Am Soc Nephrol* 1994;4:1571–81.
140. Drumond MC, Deen WM. Structural determinants of glomerular hydraulic permeability. *Am J Physiol* 1994;266:F1–F12.
141. Blantz RC, Gabbai FB, Peterson O, Wilson CB, Kihara I, Kawachi H, Shimizu F, Yamamoto T. Water and protein permeability is regulated by the glomerular epithelial slit diaphragm. *J Am Soc Nephrol* 1994; 4:1957–1964.

142. Kanwar YS, Rosenweig LJ. Altered glomerular permeability as a result of focal detachment of the visceral epithelium. *Kidney Int* 1982;21: 565–574.
143. Kanwar YS. Biophysiology of glomerular filtration and proteinuria. *Lab Invest* 1984;51:7–21.
144. Ryan GB, Karnovsky MJ. An ultrastructural study of the mechanisms of proteinuria in aminonucleoside nephrosis. *Kidney Int* 1975; 8:219–232.
145. Whiteside C, Prutis K, Cameron R, Thompson J. Glomerular epithelial detachment, not reduced charge density, correlates with proteinuria in adriamycin and puromycin nephrosis. *Lab Invest* 1989;61:650–660.
146. Hostetter TH, Olson JL, Rennke HG, Venkatachalam MA, Brenner BM. Hyperfiltration in remnant nephrons: a potentially adverse response to renal ablation. *Am J Physiol* 1981;241:F85–F93.
147. Messina A, Davies DJ, Dillane PC, Ryan GB. Glomerular epithelial abnormalities associated with the onset of proteinuria in aminonucleoside nephrosis. *Am J Pathol* 1987;126:220–229.
148. Olson JL, Hostetter TH, Rennke HG, Brenner BM, Venkatachalam MA. Altered glomerular permselectivity and progressive sclerosis following extreme ablation of renal mass. *Kidney Int* 1982;22:112–126.
149. Weening JJ, Rennke HG. Glomerular permeability and polyanion in adriamycin nephrosis in the rat. Kidney Int 1983;24:152–159.
150. Weening JJ, Van Guldener C, Daha MR, Klar N, Van Der Wal A, Prins FA. The pathophysiology of protein-overload proteinuria. *Am J Pathol* 1987;129:64–73.
151. Daniels BS. Increased albumin permeability in vitro following alterations of glomerular charge is mediated by the cells of the filtration barrier. *J Lab Clin Med* 1994;124:224–230.
152. Cohen AH, Mampaso F, Zamboni L. Glomerular podocyte degeneration in human renal disease. An ultrastructural study. *Lab Invest* 1977; 37:30–42.
153. Salant DJ. The structural biology of glomerular epithelial cells in proteinuric diseases. *Curr Opin Nephrol Hypertens* 1994;3:569–574.
154. Kriz W, Hackenthal E, Nobiling R, Sakai T, Elger M. A role for podocytes to counteract capillary wall distension. *Kidney Int* 1994;45: 369–376.
155. Kriz W, Elger M, Mundel P, Lemley KV. Structure-stabilizing forces in the glomerular tuft. *J Am Soc Nephrol* 1995;5:1731–1739.
156. Racusen LC, Prozialeck DH, Solez K. Glomerular epithelial cell changes after ischemia or dehydration. Possible role of angiotension II. *Am J Pathol* 1984;114:157–163.
157. Andrews PM, Coffey AK. Cytoplasmic contractile elements in glomerular cells. *Fed Proc* 1983;42:3046–3052.
158. Seiler MW, Rennke HG, Venkatachalam MV, Cotran RS. Patholgenesis of polycation-induced alterations ("fusion") of glomerular epithelium. *Lab Invest* 1977;36:48–61.
159. Andrews P. Morphological alterations of the glomerular (visceral) epithelium in response to pathological and experimental situations. *J Elect Microsc Tech* 1988;9:115–144.
160. Kerjaschki D. Polycation-induced dislocation of slit diaphragms and formation of cell junctions in rat kidney glomeruli. *Lab Invest* 1978; 39:430–440.
161. Sterzel RB, Pabst R. The temporal relationship between glomerular cell proliferation and monocyte infiltration in experimental glomerulonephritis. *Virchows Arch [B]* 1982;38:337–350.
162. Morita T, Suzuki Y, Churg J. Structure and development of the glomerular crescent. *Am J Pathol* 1973;72:349–368.
163. Hancock WW, Atkins RC. Cellular composition of crescents in human rapidly progressive glomerulonephritis identified using monoclonal antibodies. *Am J Nephrol* 1984;4:177–181.
164. Cybulsky AV, Goodyer PR, Cyr MD, McTavish AJ. Eicosanoids enhance epidermal growth factor receptor activation and proliferation in glomerular epithelial cells. *Am J Physiol* 1992;262:F639–F646.
165. Diamond JR, Bonventre JV, Karnovsky MJ. A role for oxygen free radicals in aminonucleoside nephrosis. *Kidney Int* 1986;29:478–483.
166. Ricardo SD, Bertram JF, Ryan GB. Antioxidants protect podocyte foot processes in puromycin aminonucleoside-treated rats. *J Am Soc Nephrol* 1994;4:1974–1986.
167. Thakur V, Walker PD, Shah SV. Evidence suggesting a role for hydroxyl radical in puromycin aminonucleoside-induced proteinuria. *Kidney Int* 1988;34:494–499.
168. Lotan D, Kaplan BS, Fong JSC, Goodyer PR, De Chadarevian J-P. Reduction of protein excretion by dimethyl sulfoxide in rats with passive Heymann nephritis. *Kidney Int* 1984;25:778–788.
169. Shah SV. Evidence suggesting a role for hydroxyl radical in passive Heymann nephritis in rats. *Am J Physiol* 1988;254:F337–F344.
170. Neale TJ, Ojha PP, Exner M, et al. Proteinuria in passive Heymann nephritis is associated with lipid peroxidation and formation of adducts on type IV collagen. *J Clin Invest* 1994;94:1577–1584.
171. Shah SV. Effect of enzymatically generated reactive oxygen metabolites on the cyclic nucleotide content in isolated rat glomeruli. *J Clin Invest* 1984;74:393–401.
172. Couser WG. Mediation of immune glomerular injury. *J Am Soc Nephrol* 1990;1:13–29.
173. Cybulsky AV, Salant DJ, Quigg RJ, Badalamenti J, Bonventre JV. Complement C5b-9 complex activates phospholipases in glomerular epithelial cells. *Am J Physiol* 1989;257:F826–F836.
174. Cybulsky AV. Release of arachidonic acid by complement C5b-9 complex in glomerular epithelial cells. *Am J Physiol* 1991;261: F427–F436.
175. Cybulsky AV, Cyr MD. Phosphatidylcholine-directed phospholipase C: activation by complement C5b-9. *Am J Physiol* 1993;265: F551–F560.
176. Fogel MA, Boyd CD, Leardkamolkarn V, Abrahamson DR, Minto AWM, Salant DJ. Glomerular basement membrane expansion in passive Heymann nephritis. *Am J Pathol* 1991;138:465–475.
177. Minto AW, Fogel MA, Natori Y, et al. Expression of type I collagen mRNA in glomeruli of rats with passive Heymann nephritis. *Kidney Int* 1993;43:121–127.
178. Floege J, Johnson RJ, Gordon K, et al. Altered glomerular extracellular matrix synthesis in experimental membranous nephropathy. *Kidney Int* 1992;42:573–585.
179. Floege J, Alpers CE, Sage EH, et al. Markers of complement-dependent and complement-independent glomerular visceral epithelial cell injury in vivo. *Lab Invest* 1992;67:486–497.
180. Cybulsky AV, Bonventre JV, Quigg RJ, Lieberthal W, Salant DJ. Cytosolic calcium and protein kinase C reduce complement–mediated glomerular epithelial injury. *Kidney Int* 1990;38:803–811.
181. Cosio FG, Shibata T, Rovin BH, Birmingham DJ. Effects of complement activation products on the synthesis of decay accelerating factor and membrane cofactor protein by human mesangial cells. *Kidney Int* 1994;46:986–992.
182. Kerjaschki D, Schulze M, Binder S, et al. Transcellular transport and membrane insertion of the C5b-9 membrane attack complex of complement by glomerular epithelial cells in experimental membranous nephropathy. *J Immunol* 1989;143:546–552.
183. Singh AK, Rahman MA. Intracellular processing of immune complexes formed on the surface of glomerular epithelial cells. *Am J Physiol* 1994;266:F246–F253.
184. Schwartz MM, Sharon Z, Pauli BU, Lewis EJ. Inhibition of glomerular visceral epithelial cell endocytosis during nephrosis induced by puromycin aminonucleoside. *Lab Invest* 1984;51:690–696.
185. Schwartz MM, Bidani AK, Lewis EJ. Glomerular epithelial cell function and pathology following extreme ablation of renal mass. *Am J Pathol* 1987;126:315–324.
186. Schwartz MM, Bidani AK, Lewis EJ. Glomerular epithelial cell structure and function in chronic proteinuria induced by homologous protein-load. *Lab Invest* 1986;55:673–679.
187. Lelongt B, Makino H, Sanwar YS. Status of glomerular proteoglycans in aminonucleoside nephrosis. *Kidney Int* 1987;31:1299–1310.
188. Klein DJ, Dehnel PJ, Oegema TR, Brown DM. Alterations in proteoglycan metabolism in the nephrotic syndrome induced by the aminonucleoside of puromycin. *Lab Invest* 1984;50:543–551.
189. Groggel GC, Hovingh P, Border WA, Linker A. Changes in glomerular heparan sulfate in puromycin aminonucleoside nephrosis. *Am J Pathol* 1987;128:521–527.
190. Kerjaschki D, Vernillo AT, Farquhar MG. Reduced sialylation of podocalyxin—the major sialoprotein of the rat kidney glomerulus—in aminonucleoside nephrosis. *Am J Pathol* 1985;118:343–349.
191. Kasinath BS, Singh AK, Kanwar YS, Lewis EJ. Effect of puromycin aminonucleoside on HSPG core protein content of glomerular epithelial cells. *Am J Physiol* 1988;255:F590–F596.
192. Kramer A, Nauck M, Pavenstadt H, et al. Receptor-mediated uptake of IDL and LDL from nephrotic patients by glomerular epithelial cells. *Kidney Int* 1993;44:1341–1351.
193. van Goor H, van-der-Horst ML, Atmosoerodjo J, Joles JA, van-Tol A, Grond J. Renal apolipoproteins in nephrotic rats. *Am J Pathol* 1993;142:1804–1812.

Immunologic Renal Diseases,
edited by E. G. Neilson and W. G. Couser.
Lippincott-Raven Publishers, Philadelphia © 1997.

CHAPTER 32

Glomerular Inflammation and Crescent Formation

Roger C. Wiggins, Lawrence B. Holzman, and Daniel J. Legault

Crescent formation is a glomerular response to inflammation. An understanding of the biology of crescent formation requires an understanding of inflammatory and immunologic events and the reaction of glomerular cells and macromolecular structures to these processes and their products. The reader is referred to previous reviews on this topic (1,2).

THE SITE OF IMMUNE COMPLEX ACCUMULATION IN THE GLOMERULUS IN PART DETERMINES THE OUTCOME

Normally, macromolecules that accumulate on the glomerular filter surface are cleared into the mesangial space, where they are catabolized by mesangial cells (3). Immune complexes, with specificity for glomerular structures [e.g., anti–glomerular basement membrane (GBM) antibody], or possessing specific physicochemical characteristics (charge and size), or present in large amounts, tend to accumulate in the glomerulus at one of three major sites. The sites include (a) the mesangial region, (b) the glomerular endothelial cell surface and subendothelial space, and (c) the subepithelial region.

Clinical experience suggests that the site in the glomerulus at which an immune complex accumulates often is directly correlated to the observed clinical syndrome (Fig. 1). Generally, crescent formation is associated with immune complex accumulation along the inner surface of the glomerular capillary wall (on the endothelial cell surface and in the subendothelial space). This includes both antigen–antibody complexes [containing immunoglobulin (Ig)G, complement, IgM, or IgA] and anti-GBM antibody (IgG), which binds to the NC1 domain of the $\alpha3$ chain of type IV collagen located in the GBM (4). At this location, immune complex accumulation is directly accessible to circulating inflammatory mediators. Cell adherence and activation occurs via Fc and C3b expression, C5a release, and production of cytokines that lead to expression of adhesion molecules by both endothelial and inflammatory cells (5–7). The consequent accumulation of activated inflammatory cells producing oxidants and enzymes results in damage to the filter surface, dysfunction of the filter, and leakage of cells and protein into the filtrate (8).

FORCES DRIVING GLOMERULAR INFLAMMATION ARISING OUTSIDE THE GLOMERULUS

For the reasons outlined above, the glomerulus is a major site for immune complex accumulation and a prominent target for inflammatory cell attack whenever systemic immune complex activation occurs (8). Glomerular immune complex deposition does not occur in isolation. It occurs as part of the overall immune activation taking place in the host. Even when the kidney (glomerulus) appears to be the only organ involved (primary glomerular disease), this appearance may be artifact, perhaps because urinalysis provides a simple and sensitive diagnostic window that allows detection of renal involvement before systemic involvement becomes clinically apparent at other sites.

Host immune system activation includes antigen presentation in local lymph nodes, activation of T cells and B cells, antibody production, and macrophage activation throughout the reticuloendothelial system. This is accompanied by increased secretion and circulation of cytokines and other mediators.

Thus, whether detectable inflammation and injury occurs probably depends on both targeting mechanisms as well as the degree of activation of circulating cells. For example, individuals with IgA nephropathy have glomer-

R. C. Wiggins, L. B. Holzman, and D. J. Legault: Nephrology Division, Department of Internal Medicine, University of Michigan, Ann Arbor, Michigan 48109.

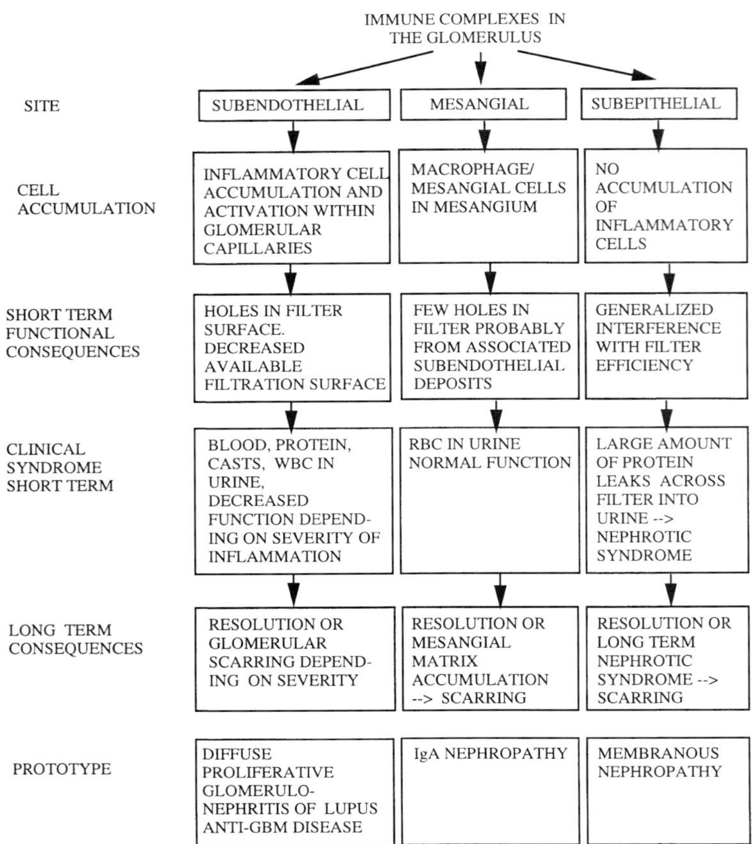

FIG. 1. Simplified illustration of the relationship between the site of immune complex accumulation and the associated pathologic and clinical syndromes.

ular IgA deposits at times when there is no apparent acute inflammatory disease; however, episodes of hematuria are often preceded by upper respiratory tract infection (9,10). In patients with anti-GBM disease, individuals may have circulating anti-GBM antibodies and have little or no glomerular inflammation. It has been observed that an episode of sepsis or upper respiratory tract infection may precede a focused inflammatory response at sites of anti-GBM antibody deposition (11). This phenomenon can be reproduced by injection of cytokines such as interleukin (IL)-1 and tumor necrosis factor-α (TNF-α) into experimental animals with circulating anti-GBM antibodies (12). These observations are compatible with the concept that a nonspecific response to infection or other stimuli may modulate the pre-existing immune homeostasis and thereby either upregulate or downregulate glomerular inflammation.

FACTORS THAT TARGET IMMUNE ATTACK TO THE GLOMERULUS

A range of immune mechanisms result in glomerular inflammation and crescent formation (Fig. 2). They can be conveniently divided into three groups with respect to targeting of immune attack to the glomerulus: (a) those with immune complexes in glomeruli, (b) those with linear anti-GBM antibody, and (c) those with little or no antibody or complement present (pauci-immune) (8). Where immunoglobulins and complement proteins are easily demonstrated in the glomerulus, a reasonable argument can be made for their participation in targeting injury to the glomerulus. However, in the pauci-immune group, which are usually ANCA positive (90%) this is not the case. ANCA-dependent mechanisms of targeting injury are discussed in detail in Chapter 49.

ESSENTIAL BARRIER STRUCTURES OF THE GLOMERULUS

Bowman's space may be conceptualized as bounded by two major barriers that prevent the spread of inflammatory mediators from initiation sites within the glomerular capillary lumen (site of immune complex accumulation) or the interstitial compartment. These two barriers are the glomerular capillary wall (filtration surface) and Bowman's capsule (Fig. 3). During glomerular inflammation, major disruptions in both of these barriers have been observed in the form of holes (Fig. 4) (13,14). Simplisti-

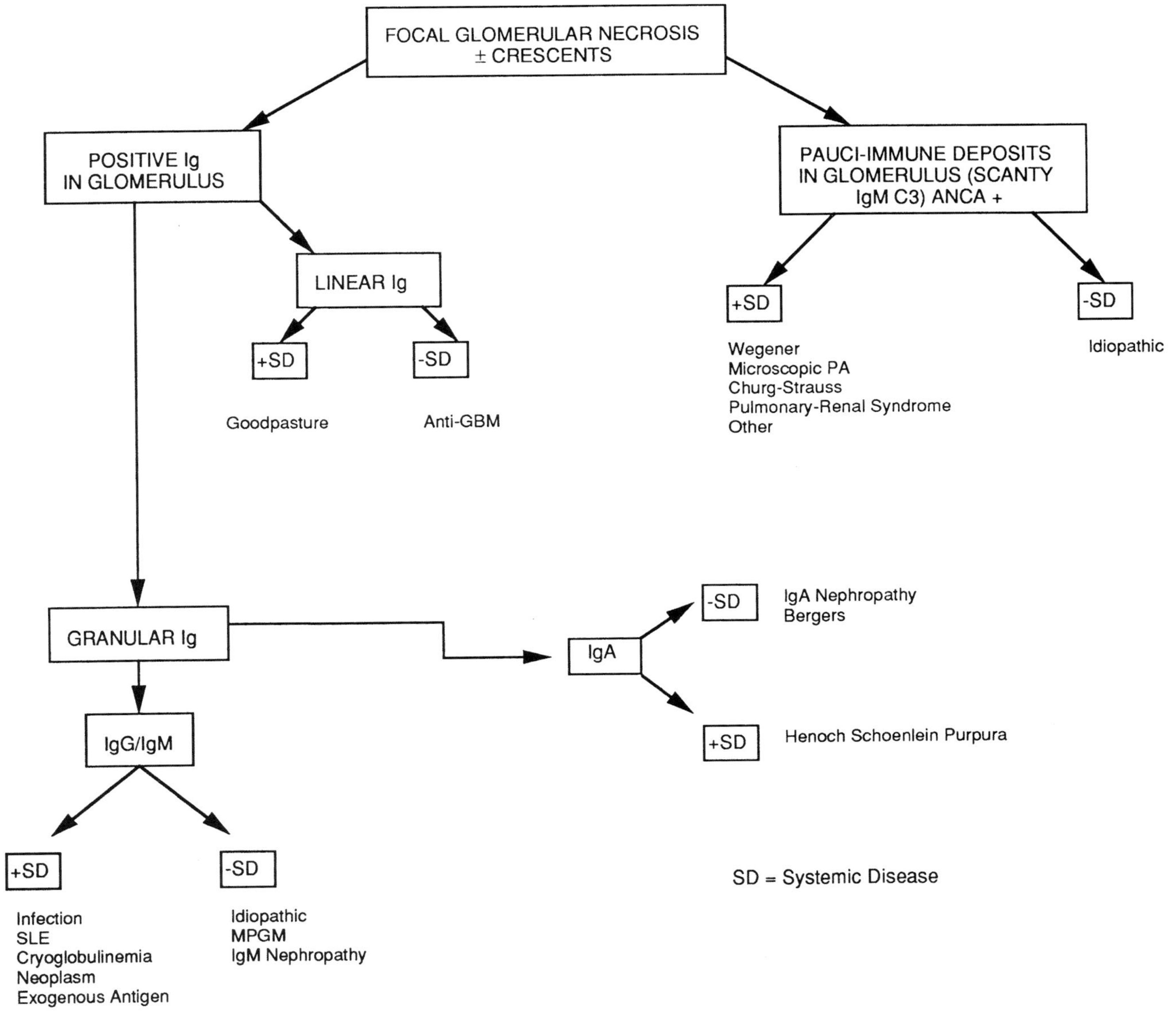

FOCAL GLOMERULAR NECROSIS
± CRESCENTS
POSITIVE Ig
IN GLOMERULUS
PAUCI-IMMUNE DEPOSITS
IN GLOMERULUS (SCANTY
IgM C3) ANCA +
LINEAR Ig
+SD
-SD
Goodpasture
Anti-GBM
+SD
-SD
Wegener
Microscopic PA
Churg-Strauss
Pulmonary-Renal Syndrome
Other
Idiopathic
GRANULAR Ig
IgA
-SD
IgA Nephropathy
Bergers
+SD
Henoch Schoenlein Purpura
IgG/IgM
+SD
-SD
Infection
SLE
Cryoglobulinemia
Neoplasm
Exogenous Antigen
Idiopathic
MPGM
IgM Nephropathy
SD = Systemic Disease

FIG. 2. Diagrammatic illustration of the major underlying mechanisms driving focal necrotizing glomerulitis with crescent formation.

INTERSTITIUM
BARRIER I
(Glomerular
capillary
wall)
BOWMAN'S
SPACE
BLOOD
BARRIER II
(Bowman's
capsule)

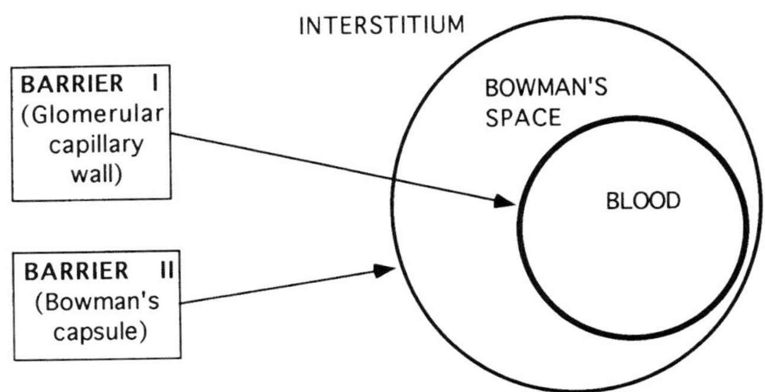

FIG. 3. Diagrammatic illustration of the major barriers of the glomerulus that delineate Bowman's space.

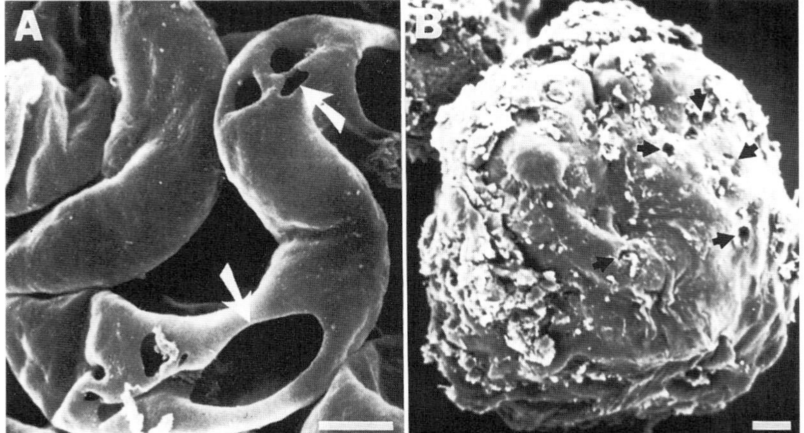

FIG. 4. Scanning electron micrographs showing holes in the GBM (**A**) and Bowman's capsule (**B**). **A:** Glomerular capillary loop with cells removed showing holes *(white arrows)*. The bar represents 10 mm. Adapted with permission (13). **B:** Isolated glomerulus with intact Bowman's capsule from a rabbit with anti-GBM disease showing Bowman's capsule hugging the underlying structures and penetrated by holes *(black arrows)*. The bar represents 10 mm.

cally viewed, damage to these barriers may allow the passage of macromolecules/mediators (small holes) or cells (large holes). Light microscopic illustrations of crescents with and without loss of integrity of Bowman's capsule are shown in Fig. 5. Therefore, the future of an inflamed glomerulus may depend in part on its success in defending, repairing, and maintaining these two major barriers.

IMPORTANCE OF THE TYPE OF INFLAMMATORY CELL THAT ACCUMULATES IN THE GLOMERULUS

The extent of injury and the mediator systems that are activated depend on the cell types that accumulate in the inflamed glomerulus. This point is emphasized in Fig. 6.

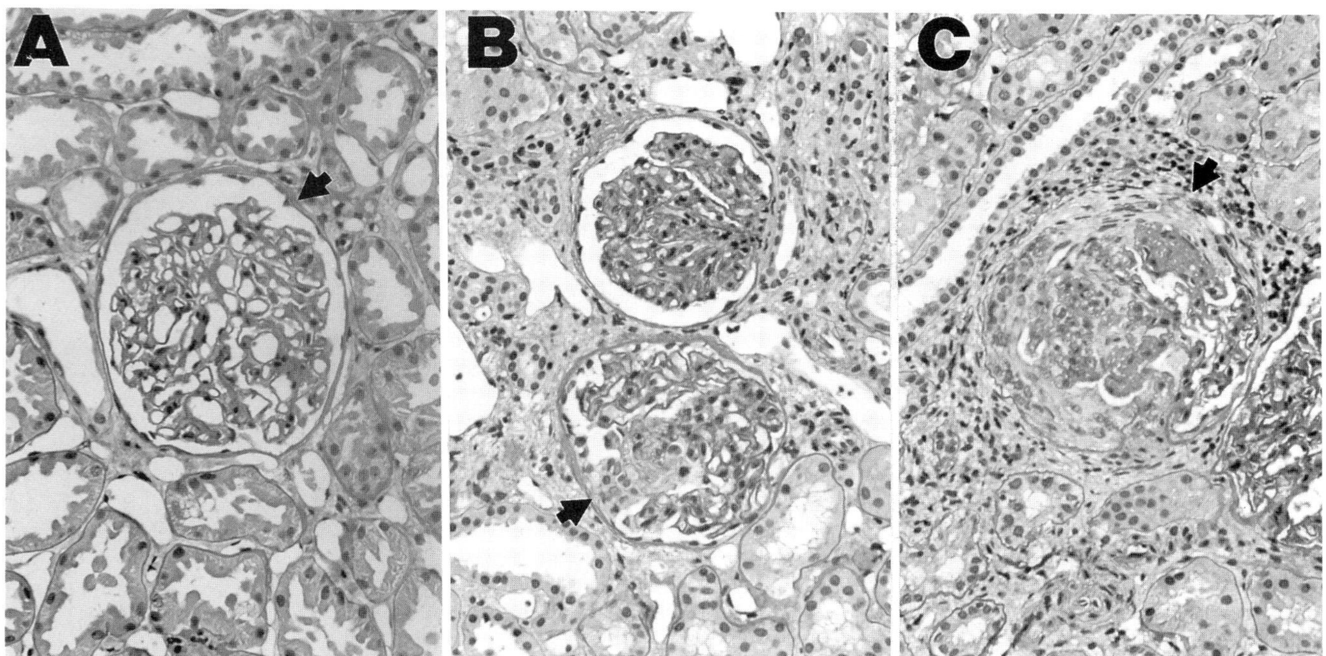

FIG. 5. Photomicrographs stained with periodic acid-Schiff to demonstrate the integrity of Bowman's capsule. **A:** Normal glomerulus with intact Bowman's capsule *(arrow)*. **B:** Lower glomerulus shows a focal necrotizing glomerular lesion with fibrin formation and a small cellular crescent without detectable loss of integrity in Bowman's capsule *(arrow)*. **C:** Major disruption of Bowman's capsule *(arrow)* with extensive cellular crescent and cellular traffic between Bowman's space and the interstitial compartment.

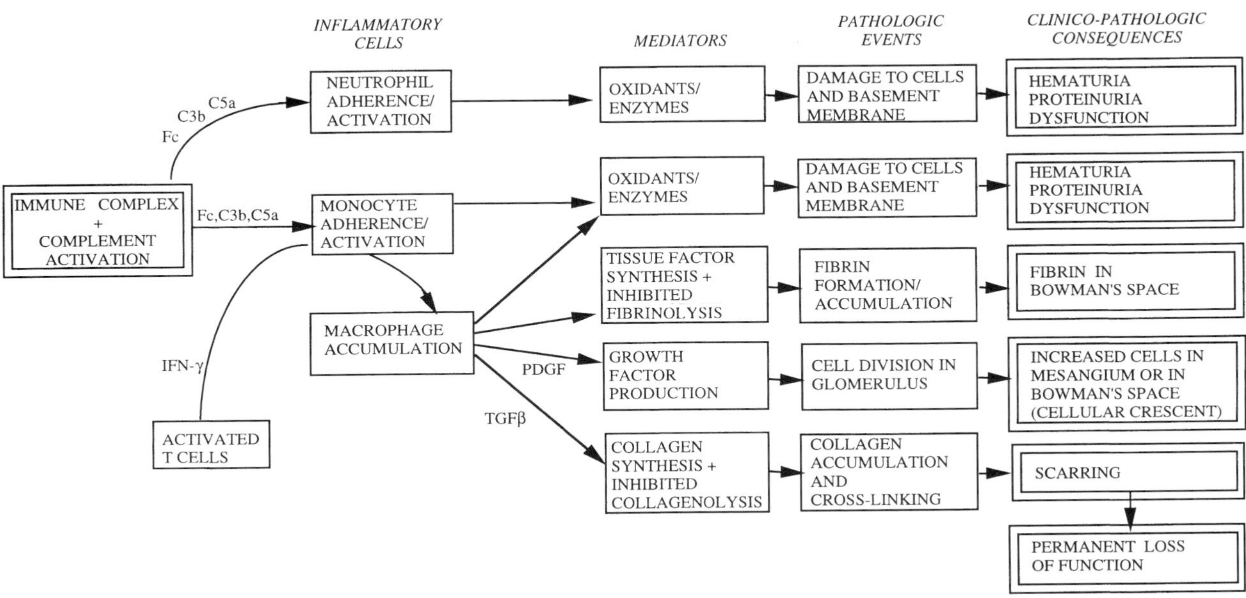

FIG. 6. Tabular representation of the repertoire of mechanisms by which inflammatory cells can participate in progression of crescent formation.

Thus, accumulation of neutrophils alone such as usually occurs in poststreptococcal glomerulonephritis results in acute injury and dysfunction, but usually does not lead to crescent formation. On the other hand, if accumulation of monocytes and activated T cells occurs for any reason, then monocytes may be activated to macrophages. Macrophages migrate into Bowman's space and there produce various factors that drive the glomerulus through a series of stages that can result in damage to the glomerular filter wall, fibrin formation in Bowman's space, cellular crescent formation, collagen synthesis, and obliteration of that glomerulus by scar (2).

STAGES OF GLOMERULAR INFLAMMATION LEADING TO CRESCENT FORMATION

Inflammatory changes in the glomerulus can be considered as a series of stages through which a glomerulus passes en route to irreversible scarring. This sequence is based largely on experimental models of anti-GBM disease (2,15). Five morphologic stages can be recognized and related to particular pathogenetic mechanisms as illustrated in Fig. 7. These stages are inter-related and form a continuum. Events of one stage modify events of another. However, for dissection of pathogenetic processes it is convenient to consider each stage separately.

Stage 0: The Normal Glomerulus

The mechanisms by which circulating inflammatory cells are prevented from being activated on the glomerular endothelial cell surface include those used by endothelial cells at other sites (16). These include the minimal expression of adhesion proteins (17), a highly effective fibrinolytic and anticoagulant system (18), and high levels of adenosine diphosphatase, which hydrolyzes adenosine diphosphate and prevents platelet activation in the glomerulus as well as production of mediators such as prostaglandin (PG)I_2 and PGE_2, which inhibit inflammatory cell activation (19). However, there are several factors that could be postulated to make the glomerular endothelial cell surface especially susceptible to inflammatory cell attack:

1. The glomerular endothelial cell is the inner surface of a blood filter that collectively receives 20% of cardiac output. Because there is a net 20% flux of fluid across the glomerular filter, cell density must increase, leading to probable increased frequency of interaction between circulating cells and the filter surface.
2. Like any filter, the glomerulus tends to collect large unfilterable material on its surface that could attract and activate inflammatory cells and promote their adherence.

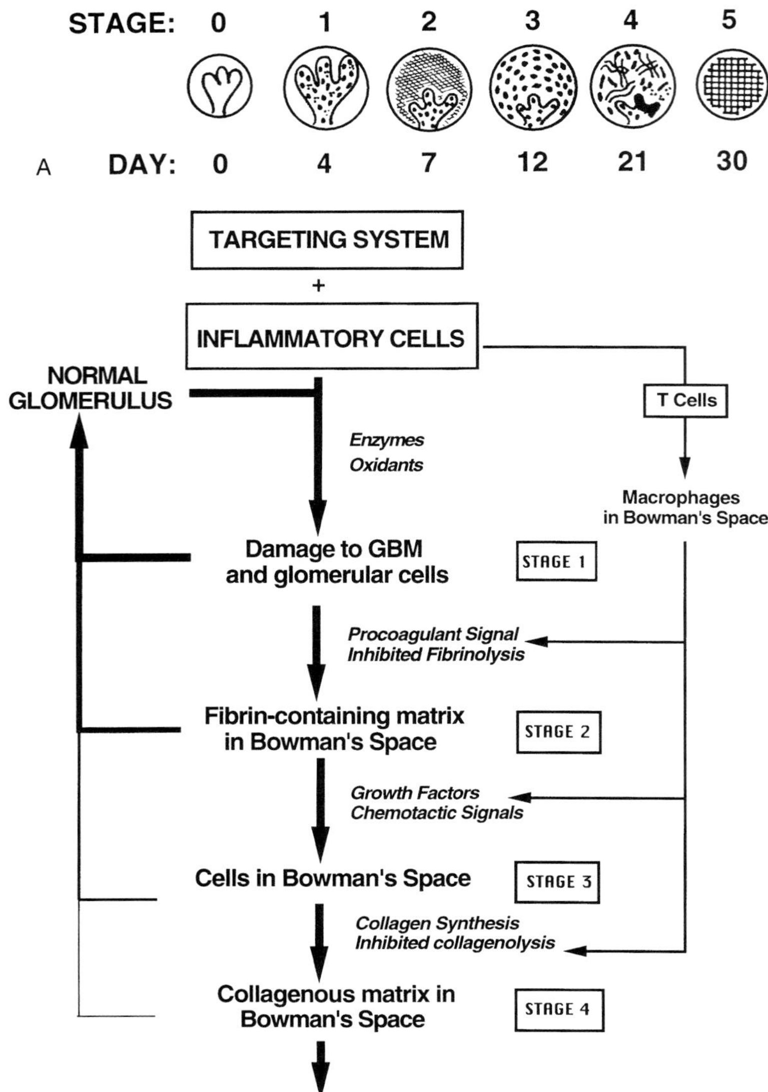

FIG. 7. **A:** Diagrammatic representation of the stages of glomerular crescent formation. **B:** Diagrammatic illustration of the sequential steps through the five stages of crescent formation. The further down the sequence that the glomerulus passes, the less likely it is that the glomerulus will be capable of returning to normal.

3. Glomerular endothelial cell fenestrations tend to allow direct contact of circulating cells with the subendothelial surface and molecules that have collected at that site.

Stage 1: Inflammatory Cell Accumulation Within the Glomerular Capillary Lumen Leading to Damage of the Glomerular Filter and Leakage of Cells and Protein into the Filtrate

The mechanisms of inflammatory cell adherence to the glomerular endothelial cell surface and the roles of inflammatory cells in promoting proteinuria have been extensively studied (8). These topics are examined in detail in Chapter 25. A brief discussion of this process is provided here, focusing particularly on models of anti-GBM disease that develop crescents. Other models in which injury is produced by in situ immune complex accumulation behave in a similar manner.

Complement- and Neutrophil-Dependent Injury

Models of acute glomerular injury secondary to antibodies against GBM show two stages of glomerular inflammation. The first stage occurs within 24 h of antibody injection and is associated with accumulation of complement and neutrophils in the glomerulus (20). Neutrophil accumulation and glomerular injury can be prevented by prior removal of circulating C3 using cobra venom factor. Thus, neutrophil accumulation is complement dependent in this model. Similarly, the amount of protein appearing in urine can be reduced by inhibitors of oxidants and proteolytic enzymes, indicating that these agents are mediators of this type of injury (21–23).

Monocyte- and Macrophage-Dependent Injury

Monocytes and macrophages are present in glomeruli in many forms of glomerular injury, both in humans and in experimental models (24–27). In the anti-GBM model, the second or autologous phase of glomerular injury typically evolves over 5 days after initial injury. During this period the host animal produces antibodies to the experimentally introduced anti-GBM antibodies. In this phase, proteinuria is prevented by macrophage depletion (28, 29), but not by complement or neutrophil depletion. Therefore, glomerular injury in the second phase is monocyte and macrophage dependent.

In the anti-GBM disease model, neutrophils and large numbers of monocytes accumulate such that the glomerular cell number per histologic cross-section more than doubles. However, within 3 days, only a relatively small proportion of monocytes remain in glomeruli. At this time point, activated macrophages are found in Bowman's space (30), where they are thought to promote crescent formation (31). As shown in Fig. 6, macrophages, possibly under the influence of activated T cells, are capable of activating each of the stages of crescent development. Macrophage production of cytokines and other factors likely play an important role in crescent development. For example, the production of IL-1 within the inflamed glomerulus is macrophage dependent (32).

T Cell–Induced Injury

The autologous phase of the anti-GBM disease model requires T-cell activation in order to mount the immune response. The conclusion is supported by the fact that T cells transferred from immunized animals to control animals can cause glomerular injury (33). Activated T cells are present in glomeruli in severe glomerular injury both in models and in humans (34–39). Frequently, T cells are present in a periglomerular distribution in severe glomerular injury and probably contribute to the destruction of Bowman's capsule, fibroblast activation, and the fibrotic process (40). These periglomerular T cells are initially class II negative but subsequently become class II positive (30), suggesting that they accumulate through local chemotactic mechanisms and become activated within the periglomerular region as a result of local activation mechanisms.

Platelets

Platelets have been shown to play an important role in mesangial models of glomerular injury (41,42); they have not yet been shown to play an important role in crescent formation. Frequently, aggregated platelets are seen in inflamed glomeruli (43) and thrombocytopenia may occur in association with crescent formation. Platelets release mediators [e.g., transforming growth factor-β (TGF-β), platelet-derived growth factor (PDGF), fibroblast growth factor (FGF), and other growth factors] (44–46), which likely promote the inflammatory and fibrogenic process.

Role of Adhesion Molecules in Crescent Formation

The recruitment of a leukocytic infiltrate from the vasculature is the basis of any inflammatory process. At the site of inflammation, several classes of cell adhesion molecules act sequentially to promote leukocyte–endothelial cell adherence (6,7). With regard to glomerulonephritis, the spatiotemporal expression of these molecules and their role in inflammation is only now being elucidated (47). The importance of adhesion molecules was confirmed in two animal models of glomerulonephritis. In a murine anti-GBM disease model, pretreatment of mice with anti–P-selectin inhibited glomerular neutrophil accumulation and proteinuria (48). Additionally, in a rat experimental crescentic glomerulonephritis model, pretreatment of rats with antibodies to intercellular adhesion molecule 1 (ICAM-1) and/or antibodies to β1 or β2 integrins markedly reduced accumulation of inflammatory cells, proteinuria, and crescent formation (49–51).

Mediators of Glomerular Structural Injury

Inflammatory injury to the glomerular capillary wall sufficient to increase protein leak into the filtrate occurs by several mechanisms (8). Hematuria that accompanies glomerular inflammation is due to holes punched in the glomerular capillary wall by inflammatory cell products (Fig. 4A) (14). The enzymes that produce these holes may be from inflammatory cells (52) or from intrinsic glomerular cells (53–56). The enzymes involved may include metalloproteinases, cysteine or serine proteinases from macrophages, or intrinsic glomerular cells. Proteolytic digestion of GBM is markedly enhanced by prior treatment with oxidants (57). This suggests one mechanism by which the combination of oxidants and proteolytic enzymes may enhance injury.

Stage 2. Accumulation of a Proteinaceous Cast (Fibrin Formation) in Bowman's Space

The presence of fibrin in Bowman's space is well established to be associated with crescent formation (58). The importance of this process for subsequent formation of the cellular crescent was suggested by experiments that showed that removal of circulating fibrinogen by injection of Malayan pit viper venom (Ancrod) (59) or treatment of animals with tissue plasminogen activator (t-PA) (60) prevented crescent formation in models of anti-GBM disease in the rabbit.

Glomerular Procoagulant Signal

Fibrin formation appears in glomeruli in association with procoagulant activity that is predominantly tissue factor-like (61). The major procoagulant signal expressed during glomerular inflammation is tissue factor produced by macrophages (61–63). Additionally, cytokines produced by macrophages such as IL-1 and TNF-α collaborate to induce tissue factor production by endothelial and other cells (64,65). Other procoagulant molecules such as prothrombinase are also induced by activated T cells (66). In normal glomeruli, tissue factor is expressed by glomerular epithelial cells, so that leakage of blood into Bowman's space would be expected to result in fibrin formation without additional procoagulant activity (67). Therefore, one would expect that cells other than macrophages would significantly contribute to the procoagulant signal. However, the experimental data available suggest that macrophages are key cells for inducing glomerular procoagulant signal (62,63), possibly via production of cytokines that induce tissue factor production by intrinsic glomerular cells (32,68) as well as by macrophages. T cells are required for this response (68).

Inhibited Fibrinolysis in the Glomerulus

Fibrinolysis occurs when plasminogen is activated to plasmin by either of the two plasminogen activators: urokinase (u-PA) or tissue plasminogen activator (t-PA). t-PA is the principle physiologic mediator of thrombolysis, whereas u-PA regulates matrix degradation and tissue remodeling (69,70). PA activity is regulated at several levels. This includes synthesis and secretion by particular cells, binding of PAs to fibrin and matrix molecules, and the specific inhibitor plasminogen activator inhibitor-1 (PAI-1) (71). The normal glomerulus produces large amounts of fibrinolytic activity as u-PA and t-PA (72, 73). During inflammation PAI-1 is produced by macrophages and other cells, which reduces plasminogen activation in glomeruli (74) and serves to tip the balance toward a net procoagulant signal and fibrin formation and accumulation. In experimental anti-GBM disease, glomerular PA activity decreases in association with the appearance of fibrin in Bowman's space (72–74) and can be prevented by treatment of animals with t-PA (75). These changes are probably regulated by macrophages (76). Thus, the fibrinolytic system appears to play an important role in this type of glomerular injury.

Role of the Proteinaceous Cast in Bowman's Space

In the developing crescent, the evolving composition of the extracellular matrix likely participates in signaling progressive changes in cellular composition and function by affecting cellular differentiation, migration, and proliferation, as has been demonstrated in other systems such as wound healing (2). Fibronectin plays an important role in this process (77).

Stage 3: Accumulation of Cells (Cellular Crescent) in Bowman's Space

The cells in Bowman's space that constitute the crescent may include macrophages, epithelial cells, fibroblast-like cells, and T cells. The outcome of crescentic nephritis appears to correlate with the composition of cells that accumulate in Bowman's space. In turn, crescent cellular composition correlates with the integrity of Bowman's capsule.

Macrophages that Have Migrated into Bowman's Space

The first cells to accumulate in Bowman's space during severe glomerular inflammation are macrophages derived from the influx of cells into the glomerular capillary loop (78–81). The potential influence of these cells in this setting has been discussed above.

Epithelial Cells in Bowman's Space that Have Undergone Cell Division Under the Influence of Growth Factors

In most reported studies, the predominant cell in the glomerular crescent is a derivative of an epithelial cell (82–85). It is likely that this cell is derived from parietal epithelial cells, although visceral glomerular epithelial cells also can undergo cell division in vivo in response to injury (86). The particular growth factors responsible for driving epithelial cell division have not yet been identified. Possible candidates include PDGF, FGFs and erythrocyte growth factor/TGF-α. These growth factors could be derived from macrophages or from intrinsic glomerular cells, including mesangial cells, which can secrete a range of growth factors (87). Glomerular epithelial cells probably do not produce interstitial collagens. They may undergo apoptosis and disappear without leaving major permanent injury in the glomerulus.

Fibroblasts in Bowman's Space

The major cell types that accumulate in the periglomerular region during glomerular inflammation are T cells, macrophages, and collagen-producing fibroblastlike cells from interstitium (30,40,88). The destruction of Bowman's capsule correlates with the translocation of these cells from the periglomerular region to the glomerular domain (89–93). The fibroblastlike cells may be of myofibroblast origin (94–96); however, the precise origin of these collagen-producing cells is not well established. As outlined above, the interaction of these cells with the proteinaceous matrix in Bowman's space may have important consequences in determining whether these cells produce matrix materials, which may in turn influence outcome.

Fibronectin

Fibronectin metabolism is an important regulatory protein in wound healing (77). In the crescentic glomerulus, large amounts of fibronectin are present (97–99). Initially, fibronectin originating from the serum is deposited in the glomerulus (99). At this time, fibronectin catabolism is rapid, with more than 80% of fibronectin molecules being fragmented. Later, as the cellular crescent develops, cells that form the crescent synthesize fibronectin. Hence, fibronectin deposition is two phased and its turnover is complex and rapid (99). The generation of fibronectin fragments (the products of fibronectin catabolism) may be critical to crescentic glomerulonephritis because they have been found to be chemoattractants for fibroblasts (100,101).

Stage 4: Scarring in the Glomerulus (Sclerosis), in the Cellular Crescent, and in the Periglomerular Region

The secretion and cross-linking of interstitial collagens plays an important role in determining the fate of the inflamed glomerulus, preventing restoration of normal glomerular structure and function. Under some conditions, basement membrane collagens also may participate in replacing glomerular structure, leading to glomerulosclerosis independent of crescent formation.

Interstitial collagens type I, III, and V are produced by fibroblastlike cells, including myofibroblasts, pericytes, and mesangial cells under the influence of TGF-β and other mediators (102–104). These cells produce metalloproteinases, the collagenolytic enzymes that normally break down and turn over secreted collagen (105). Collagenolytic metalloproteinases are regulated by a group of inhibitors called tissue inhibitors of metalloproteinases (TIMPs) (106,107). Induced by TGF-β, TIMPs are secreted by a variety of cells, including intrinsic glomerular cells (108). At this stage of the injury process, TGF-β coordinates a net collagen synthetic response to injury by stimulating collagen secretion and cross-linking and preventing collagen removal.

In vitro, TGF-β has been shown to be chemoattractant for monocytes (109) and fibroblasts (110); therefore, TGF-β may participate with other cytokines in the recruitment of cells to the developing cellular crescent. TGF-β promotes the differentiation of immature fibroblasts (104,111) and stimulates fibroblasts and mesangial and other cells to synthesize collagen and other matrix proteins (103,112,113), as well as TIMPs (106,107). Thus, the net effect of TGF-β secretion is accumulation and cross-linking of collagen and scar. Normal glomeruli constitutively produce TGF-β in an inactive form (114). In a model of crescentic glomerulonephritis, glomeruli isolated at early stages produce activated TGF-β. In another model of glomerular injury, inhibition of activated TGF-β via a neutralizing antibody resulted in decreased collagen and matrix proteoglycan synthesis (115, 116). Thus, TGF-β is likely to be one important factor driving collagen synthesis in crescent formation, as in other models of glomerular injury.

Stage 5: The Scarred Glomerulus

Complete (global) scarring of the glomerulus and replacement by interstitial collagen signals irreversible loss of that glomerulus. Once extensive accumulation of cross-linked interstitial (type I/III) collagens has occurred, the chances of recovery are small. However, if the glomerular tuft itself remains intact, then remodeling of interstitial collagens may be possible, particularly if collagen cross-linking is limited.

INTERSTITIAL COMPARTMENT IN SEVERE GLOMERULAR INFLAMMATION

Glomerular inflammation severe enough to result in significant crescent formation is accompanied by interstitial inflammation and accumulation of extracellular matrix. As with other forms of glomerular disease, it is probably the degree of interstitial scarring that correlates best with outcome (117–120).

Periglomerular Scarring

Scarring in the periglomerular region is common after glomerular injury of any cause. The cells that cause this scarring are probably mainly the periglomerular myofibroblastlike cells, which can be considered as analagous to the cells that form the normal vascular adventitial compartment.

Inflammatory Cell Accumulation and Activation in the Interstitial Compartment as a Consequence of Glomerular Injury

The mechanisms by which signals from the inflamed glomerulus induce inflammatory cells to accumulate in the interstitial (and particularly the periglomerular) region are poorly understood. In the model of anti-GBM disease, because the glomerular capillary is the initial site of injury, it is likely that inductive signals derived from the glomerulus result in the accumulation of cells in the interstitium. Soon after initial injury, macrophages, T cells, and fibroblastlike cells begin to accumulate in the periglomerular interstitium (30,40). Initially, T cells that accumulate at this site are class II negative but subsequently become class II positive, indicating T-cell activation (30,93). Accumulation of cells in this compartment likely results from complex mechanisms, including recruitment along chemotactic gradients, recruitment due to alterations in tissue adhesion molecule expression, in situ proliferation or phenotypic differentiation under the influence of cytokines, and changes in the composition of the extracellular matrix.

Fibroblast Activation and Recruitment from the Interstitial Compartment

Normally, perivascular adventitial cells are resident in the interstitial collagen cuff surrounding arterioles, arteries, venules, and veins, where they are presumed to synthesize perivascular type I collagen. After initial glomerular injury, these perivascular adventitial cells are induced to express type I collagen messenger RNA (mRNA) (88). A soluble mediator is likely responsible for this induction because the site of injury is distant from the site of response. Here, TGF-β is a candidate mediator because activated TGF-β has been detected in isolated glomeruli derived from the anti-GBM model shortly after initial injury (114). At later time points, numerous type I collagen–producing cells are present in the interstitial compartment. Again, activated TGF-β may play a role in recruiting peri-adventitial fibroblasts or other myofibroblast or fibroblastlike cells in the interstitial compartment to the inflamed glomerulus. An additional chemotactic factor for fibroblasts being produced by these glomeruli at this time are fibronectin fragments generated by the degradation of fibronectin deposited in the glomerulus (101).

TIME COURSE OF GLOMERULAR PROGRESSION TO SCARRING

Correlation of histologic and functional data from a rabbit model of anti-GBM disease emphasizes that after induction of injury, only a short window of opportunity exists for institution of therapy before the accumulation of collagen (2). Figure 8 shows various parameters of collagen metabolism that change over time in this model. Importantly, at day 4, when red cell casts and protein are first present in urine and renal function is only slightly abnormal, renal cortical collagen mRNA content and collagen synthetic rate are already markedly induced. Serum creatinine concentration begins to increase by day 7, when collagen transcription and translation are already maximally switched on. Histology shows no scarring at this time point, and renal cortical hydroxyproline content is not yet significantly elevated. At day 14, hydroxyproline content of the renal cortex has begun to rise, although histologic measurement of scar accumulation by Masson-Trichrome staining remains not significantly abnormal. By day 21, hydroxyproline content is markedly abnormal, and histologic evidence of scarring is obviously present. Widespread scarring is present in both glomerular and interstitial compartments at day 30.

The glomeruli effected in the rabbit model of anti-GBM antibody–induced crescentic glomerulonephritis move synchronously through the stages of glomerular inflammation. In human disease, this is often not the case. Here, glomeruli representing all stages are often simultaneously observed. The degree of synchronicity as well as the extent of inflammation is likely to impact on acuteness of presentation and the likely response to treatment.

REVERSIBILITY OF THE CRESCENT

Not all cellular crescents progress to glomerular sclerosis. Crescent formation is a common response to injury produced by a large group of disease entities (120). Nevertheless, renal survival differs markedly among these diseases. In one study of patients with IgA nephropathy, 100% of individuals had crescents present during an episode of gross hematuria. In contrast, only 21% of individuals demonstrated crescents in renal biopsies obtained at a time point greater than 30 days after an episode of gross hematuria (117). This observation implies that crescents are reversible. In a retrospective study on patients with rapidly progressive glomerulonephritis (RPGN), Hind et al. found that 63% of 27 patients without anti-GBM antibodies (probably representing mainly ANCA-positive RPGN) recovered some renal function. No correlation was found between the degree of crescent formation or other histologic characteristics and eventual recovery (118). In the same study, none of 21 patients with anti-GBM antibody disease recovered function. Glomerular pathology and extraglomerular pathology responsible for renal dysfunction may vary among diseases and be responsible for differences in their natural history and response to therapy.

Evidence from animal models further support the concept that glomerular crescents are not obligated to progress to sclerosis. In a rabbit model of anti-GBM antibody–induced crescentic nephritis, by day 7 after induction of injury, 90% of glomeruli examined demonstrate acute inflammatory changes. However, by day 50, only approximately 50% of glomeruli examined appeared sclerotic, whereas nearly 50% of the remaining glomeruli appeared histologically normal by light microscopy (119,

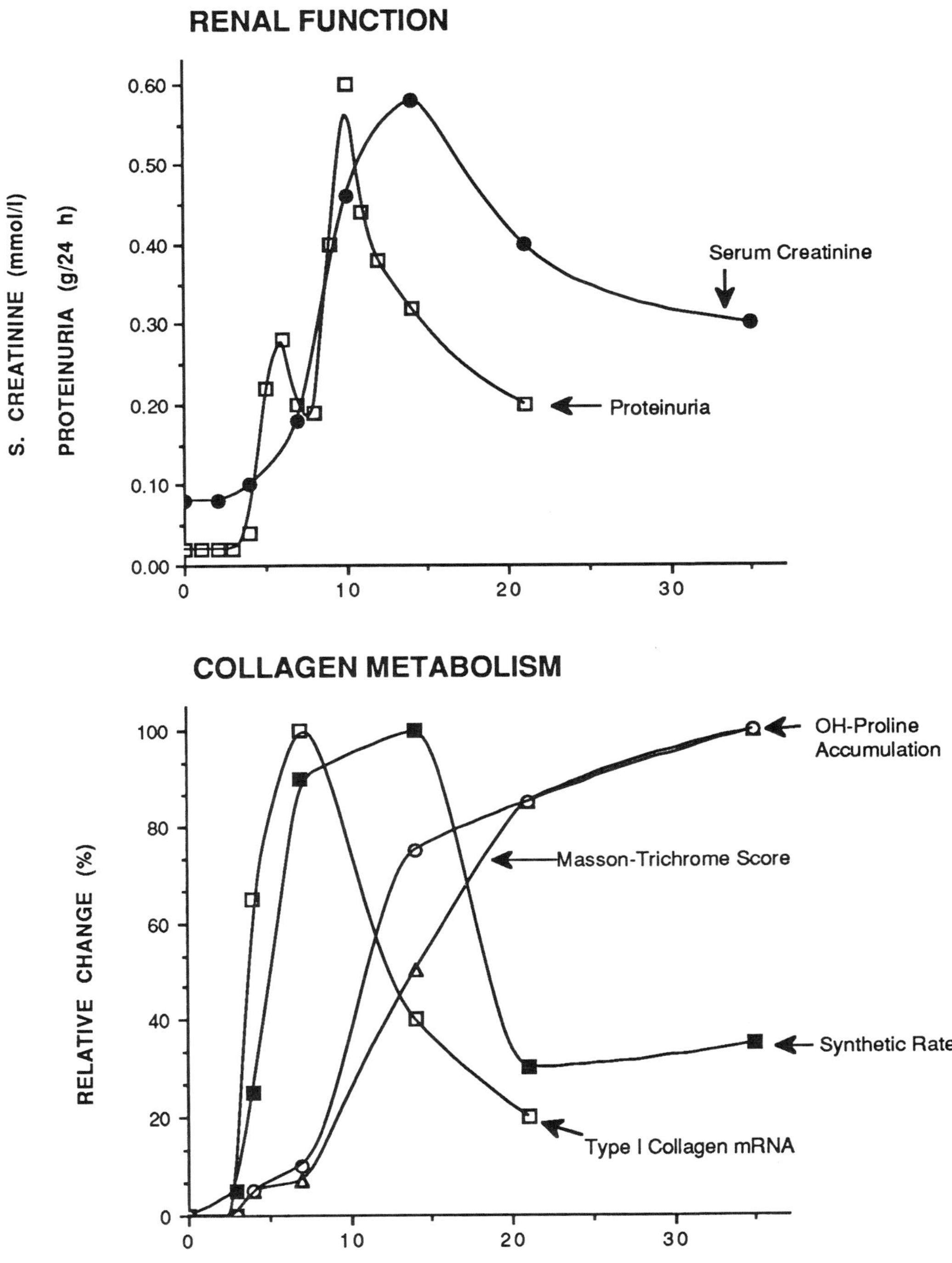

FIG. 8. Time course of fibrosis in a model of crescentic nephritis in relation to commonly measured clinical parameters (serum creatinine and protein excretion). The parameters of collagen synthesis are cortical α1(I) procollagen mRNA relative to 28S recombinant RNA content; cortical collagen synthetic rate; cortical hydroxyproline content per dry weight; and Masson-Trichrome stainable matrix on histologic section. The time course of collagen synthesis is rapid. Collagen synthesis is maximally turned on before serum creatinine has increased significantly. Hydroxyproline accumulates before matrix is recognizably present by histologic staining in renal cortex, probably reflecting a delay in the cross-linking process.

120). This phenomenon is partially anti-GBM antibody dose dependent. Silva et al. made similar observations in a rat model of anti-GBM antibody–induced glomerulonephritis (15).

The factors influencing and the mechanisms responsible for determining the outcome of the glomerular crescent, progression to sclerosis, or resolution have not been experimentally determined.

LESSONS FOR CLINICAL PRACTICE

In crescentic nephritis, treatment strategies must be aimed at preventing collagen synthesis and scarring in both glomerular and interstitial compartments. The job of the physician is to create conditions that favor prevention of scar and replacement of normal structure.

To achieve effective therapy for severe glomerular inflammation, the physician must reverse the inflammatory event driving the process as rapidly as possible without jeopardizing the life of the patient. Corticosteroids with addition of plasma exchange (to remove soluble factors) and cyclophosphamide (to inhibit T-cell, macrophage, and fibroblast cell division) are probably useful. On the other hand, cyclophosphamide tends to delay recovery of normal cells. Newer investigatory agents directed toward specific steps in the inflammatory cascade (49,50,121–123) as well as the rational use of well-tried agents (124) promise alternative opportunities to intervene more effectively.

Pivotal to the therapeutic plan of severe glomerular inflammation is expeditious diagnosis allowing early treatment before the commencement of diffuse glomerular scarring. This requires teaching primary care physicians and general internists to recognize patients with RPGN and urgently refer them for diagnosis and treatment. Nephrologists must be aware that acute nephritis is a medical emergency requiring urgent renal biopsy for diagnosis and development of a rational therapeutic strategy. The biopsy is necessary (a) to confirm the underlying pathologic process (crescent formation), (b) to determine the factor(s) driving the inflammatory process (by immunofluorescent analysis) and thereby assess appropriate treatment strategies, and (c) to assess the potential reversibility of the process (degree of scarring). The urgency of the renal biopsy is governed by the rate of deterioration of renal function, but it should probably be performed and analyzed, including immunofluorescent analysis, within 24 h in most cases to allow for optimal treatment to prevent scar formation.

In summary, crescent formation in the glomerulus is part of the glomerular response to injury. The cellular crescent itself is one step in a series of events that if not stopped often leads to scarring of the glomerulus and irreversible loss of function. The time course to irreversible injury in severe glomerulonephritis is short. We must educate front line physicians and nephrologists to treat severe glomerulonephritis as a medical emergency.

REFERENCES

1. Salant DJ. Immunopathogenesis of crescentic glomerulonephritis and lung purpura. *Kidney Int* 1987;32:408–425.
2. Holzman LB, Wiggins RC. Glomerular crescent formation. *Semin Nephrol* 1991;11:346–353.
3. Michael AF, Nevins TE, Raij L, et al. Macromolecular transport in the glomerulus: studies of the mesangium and epithelium in vivo and in vitro. In: Wilson CB, Brenner BM, Stein JH, eds. *Immunologic mechanisms of renal disease*. New York: Churchill Livingstone; 1978: 167–213.
4. Hudson BG, Reeders ST, Tryggvason K. Type IV collagen structure, gene organization and role in human diseases. Molecular basis of Goodpasture's syndrome and Alport's syndrome and diffuse leiomyomatosis. *J Biol Chem* 1993;268:26033–26036.
5. Ward PA, Marks RM. The acute inflammatory reaction. *Curr Opin Immunol* 1989;2:5–9.
6. Cronstein BN, Weissman G. The adhesion molecules of inflammation. *Arthritis Rheum* 1993;36:147–159.
7. Carlos TM, Harlan JM. Leukocyte-endothelial adhesion molecules. *Blood* 1994;84:2068–2101.
8. Couser WG. Mediation of immune glomerular injury. *Clin Invest* 1993;71:508–811.
9. Rodicio JL. Idiopathic IgA nephropathy. *Kidney Int* 1984;25: 717–729.
10. Kincaid-Smith P, Nicholls K. Mesangial IgA nephropathy. *Am J Kidney Dis* 1983;111:90–102.
11. Rees AJ, Lockwood CM, Peters DK. Nephritis due to antibodies to GBM. In: Kincaid-Smith P, d'Apice AJF, Atkins RC, eds. *Progress in glomerulonephritis*. New York: Wiley Medical; 1979:347–384.
12. Tomosugi NI, Cashman SJ, Hay H, et al. Modulation of antibody-mediated glomerular injury in vivo by bacterial lipopolysaccharide, tumor necrosis factor and IL-1. J *Immunol* 1989;142:3083–3090.
13. Bonsib SM. Glomerular basement membrane necrosis and crescent organization. *Kidney Int* 1988;33:966–974.
14. Wiggins RC. Rapidly progressive glomerulonephritis: resolution and scarring. In: Pusey CD, Rees AJ, eds. *Rapidly progressive glomerulonephritis*. Oxford, England: Oxford University Press; 1993.
15. Silva FG, Hoyer JR, Pirani CL. Sequential studies of glomerular crescent formation in rats with antiglomerular basement membrane–induced glomerulonephritis and the role of coagulation factors. *Lab Invest* 1984;51:404–415.
16. Pober JS, Cotran RS. Cytokines and endothelial cell biology. *Physiol Rev* 1990;70:427–451.
17. Seron D, Cameron JS, Haskard DO. Expression of VCAM-1 in the normal and diseased kidney. *Nephrol Dial Transplant* 1991;6: 917–922.
18. Sueishi K, Yasunaga C, Murata T, Kumamoto M, Nakagawa K, Kono S. Endothelial function in thrombosis and thrombolysis. *Jpn Circ J* 1992;56:192–198.
19. Poelstra K, Baller JF, Hardonk MJ, Bakker W. Intraglomerular thrombotic tendency and glomerular ADPase. Unilateral impairment of ADPase elicits a proaggregatory microenvironment in experimental glomerulonephritis. *Lab Invest* 1991;64:520–526.
20. Cochrane CG. Immunologic tissue injury mediated by neutrophilic leukocytes. *Adv Immunol* 1968;9:97–162.
21. Rehan A, Johnson KJ, Wiggins RC, et al. Evidence for the role of oxygen radicals in acute nephrotoxic nephritis. *Lab Invest* 1984;51: 396–403.
22. Shah SV. Oxidant mechanisms in glomerulonephritis. *Semin Nephrol* 1991;11:320–326
23. Baricos W, Shah SV. Glomerular injury and proteolytic enzymes. *Semin Nephrol* 1991;11:327–331.
24. Schreiner GF, Cotran RS, Pardo V, et al. A mononuclear cell component in experimental immunologic glomerulonephritis. *J Exp Med* 1978;147:369–384.
25. Magil AB, Wadsworth LD, Loewen M. Monocytes and human renal glomerular disease. *Lab Invest* 1981;44:27–33.

26. Sterzel B, Pabst R. The temporal relationship between glomerular cell proliferation and monocyte infiltration in experimental glomerulonephritis. *Virchows Arch* 1982;38:337–350.
27. Schreiner GF. The role of the macrophage in glomerular injury. *Semin Nephrol* 1991;11:268–275.
28. Lavelle KJ, Durland BD, Yum MN. The effect of antimacrophage anti-serum on immune complex glomerulonephritis. *J Lab Clin Med* 1981;98:195–205.
29. Holdsworth SR, Neale TJ, Wilson CB. Abrogation of macrophage-dependent injury in experimental glomerulonephritis in the rabbit. *J Clin Invest* 1981;68:686–698.
30. Eldridge C, Merritt S, Goyal M, et al. Analysis of T cells and MHC class I and class II mRNA and protein content and distribution in anti-GBM disease in the rabbit. *Am J Pathol* 1991;139:1021–1035.
31. Clarke BE, Ham KN, Tange JD, et al. Macrophages and glomerular crescent formation. Studies with rat nephrotoxic nephritis. *Pathology* 1983;15:75–81.
32. Tipping PG, Lowe MG, Holdsworth SR. Glomerular interleukin-1 production is dependent on macrophage infiltration in anti-GBM glomerulonephritis. *Kidney Int* 1991;39:103–110.
33. McCluskey RT, Bhan AK. Cell-mediated immunity in renal disease. *Hum Pathol* 1986;17:146–153.
34. Tipping PG, Neale TJ, Holdsworth SR. T lymphocyte participation in antibody-induced experimental glomerulonephritis. *Kidney Int* 1985; 27:530–537.
35. Bolton WK, Innes DJ Jr, Sturgill BC, et al. T-cells and macrophages in rapidly progressive glomerulonephritis: clinicopathologic correlations. *Kidney Int* 1987;32:869–876.
36. Nolasco FEB, Cameron JS, Hartley B, et al. Intraglomerular T cells and monocytes in nephritis: study with monoclonal antibodies. *Kidney Int* 1987;31:1160–1166.
37. Hooke DH, Gee DC, Atkins RC. Leukocyte analysis using monoclonal antibodies in human glomerulonephritis. *Kidney Int* 1987;31: 964–972.
38. Li HL, Hancock WW, Dowling JP, Atkins RC. Activated (IL-2R+) intraglomerular mononuclear cells in crescentic glomerulonephritis. *Kidney Int* 1991;3:793–798.
39. Main IW, Nikolic-Peterson DJ, Atkins RC. T cells and macrophages and their role in renal injury. *Semin Nephrol* 1992;12:395–407.
40. Lan HY, Nikolic-Paterson DJ, Atkins RC. Involvement of activated periglomerular leukocytes in the rupture of Bowman's capsule and glomerular crescent progression in experimental glomerulonephritis. *Lab Invest* 1992;67:743–751.
41. Johnson RJ. Platelets in inflammatory glomerular injury. *Semin Nephrol* 1991;11:276–284.
42. Johnson RJ. The glomerular response to injury: progression or resolution? *Kidney Int* 1994:1769–1782.
43. Miller K, Dresner IG, Michael AF. Localization of platelet antigens in human kidney disease. *Kidney Int* 1980;18:472–479.
44. Assoian RK, Komoriya A, Meyers CA, et al. Transforming growth factor-β in human platelets. *J Biol Chem* 1983;258:7155–7159.
45. Johnson R, Iida H, Yoshimura A, et al. Platelet-derived growth factor: a potentially important cytokine in glomerular disease. *Kidney Int* 1992;41:590–594.
46. Alpers CE, Seifert RA, Hudkins KL, et al. PDGF-receptor localizes to mesangial, parietal epithelial, and interstitial cells in human and primate kidneys. *Kidney Int* 1993;43:286–294.
47. Briscoe DM, Cotran RS. Role of leukocyte-endothelial cell adhesion molecules in renal inflammation: in vitro and in vivo studies. *Kidney Int* 1993;44(suppl):27–34.
48. Tipping PG, Huang XR, Brendt MC, Holdsworth SR. A role for P-selectin in complement-independent neutrophil-mediated glomerular injury. *Kidney Int* 1994:46;79–88.
49. Kawasaki K, Yaoita E, Yamamoto T, et al. Antibodies against intercellular adhesion molecule-1 and lymphocyte function–associated antigen-1 prevent glomerular injury in rat experimental crescentic glomerulonephritis. *J Immunol* 1993;150:1074–1083.
50. Nishikawa K, Guo Y, Miyasaka M, et al. Antibodies to intercellular adhesion molecule 1/lymphocyte function–associated antigen 1 prevent crescent formation in rat autoimmune glomerulonephritis. *J Exp Med* 1993;177:667–677.
51. Mulligan MS, Johnson KJ, Todd RF, 3rd, et al. Requirements for leukocyte adhesion molecules in nephrotoxic nephritis. *J Clin Invest* 1993;91:577–587.
52. Vissers MCM, Wiggins RC, Fantone JC. Comparative ability of human monocytes and neutrophils to degrade glomerular basement membrane in vitro. *Lab Invest* 1989;60:831–838.
53. Martin J, Davies M, Thomas G, et al. Human mesangial cells secrete a GBM-degrading neutral protease and a specific inhibitor. *Kidney Int* 1989;36:790–801.
54. Baricos WH, Cortex SL, Le QC, et al. Glomerular basement membrane degradation by endogenous cysteine proteinases in isolated rat glomeruli. *Kidney Int* 1990;38:395–401.
55. Le Q, Shah S, Nguyen H, et al. A novel metalloproteinase present in freshly isolated glomeruli. *Am J Physiol* 1991;260:F555–F561.
56. Lovett DH, Johnson RJ, Marti HP, et al. Structural characterization of the mesangial cell type IV collagenase and enhanced expression in a model of immune complex glomerulonephritis. *Am J Pathol* 1992; 141:85–98.
57. Fligiel SE, Lee EC, McCoy J, Johnson KJ, Varani J. Protein degradation following treatment with hydrogen peroxide. *Am J Pathol* 1984; 115:418–25.
58. Srarer J-D, Kanfer A, Rondeau E, et al. Glomerular hemostasis in normal and pathologic conditions. *Adv Nephrol* 1988;17:27–56.
59. Naish P, Penn GB, Evans DJ, et al. The effect of defibrinogenation on nephrotoxic serum nephritis in rabbits. *Clin Sci* 1972;42:643–646.
60. Zoja C, Corna D, Macconi D, et al. Tissue plasminogen activator therapy of rabbit nephrotoxic nephritis. *Lab Invest* 1990;62:34–40.
61. Wiggins RC, Glatfelter A, Brukman J. Procoagulant activity in glomeruli and urine of rabbits with nephrotoxic nephritis. *Lab Invest* 1985;53:156–165.
62. Tipping PG, Holdsworth SR. The participation of macrophages, glomerular procoagulant activity, and factor VIII in glomerular fibrin deposition. Studies on anti-GBM antibody–induced glomerulonephritis in rabbits. *Am J Pathol* 1986;124:10–17.
63. Tipping PG, Lowe MG, Holdsworth SR. Glomerular macrophages express augmented procoagulant activity in experimental fibrin–related glomerulonephritis in rabbits. *J Clin Invest* 1988;82:1253–1259.
64. Bevilacqua MP, Pober JS, Majeau GR, Cotran RS, Gimbrone MAJ. Interleukin 1 (IL-1) induces biosynthesis and cell surface expression of procoagulant activity in human vascular endothelial cells. *J Exp Med* 1984;160:618–623.
65. Prydz H, Pettersen KS. Synthesis of thromboplastin (tissue factor) by endothelial cells. *Haemostasis* 1988;18:215–223.
66. Altieri DC, Edgington TS. Sequential receptor cascade for coagulation proteins on monocytes. Constitutive biosynthesis and functional prothrombinase activity of a membrane form of factor V/Va. *J Biol Chem* 1989;264:2969–2972.
67. Drake TA, Morrissey JH, Edgington T. Selective cellular expression of tissue factor in human tissues. Implications for disorders of hemostasis and thrombosis. *Am J Pathol* 1989;134:1087–1097.
68. Neale TJ, Carson SD, Tipping PG, et al. Participation of cell-mediated immunity in deposition of fibrin in glomerulonephritis. *Lancet* 1988;2:421–424.
69. Dano K, Andreason PA, Grondahl-Hanson J, et al. Plasminogen activator, tissue degradation, and cancer. *Adv Cancer Res* 1985;44: 139–266.
70. Laiho M, Keski-Oja J. Growth factors in the regulation of pericellular proteolysis: a review. *Cancer Res* 1989;49:2533–2553.
71. Loskutoff DJ, Sawdey M, Mimuro J. Type 1 plasminogen activator inhibitor. In: Collier B, ed. *Progress in hemostasis and thrombosis*. Philadelphia: WB Saunders; 1988:87–115.
72. Hara M, Kihara I, Morita T, et al. The fibrinolytic activity of isolated rat glomerulus by fibrin slide technique. Its application to rat Masugi nephritis. *Acta Pathol Jpn* 1981;31:249–255.
73. Tomasugi N, Wada T, Takero N, et al. Role of plasminogen activator inhibitor on nephrotoxic nephritis and its modulation by tumor necrosis factor. *Nephron* 1992;62:213–219.
74. Feng L, Tang WW, Loskutoff DJ, et al. Dysfunction of glomerular fibrinolysis in experimental antiglomerular basement membrane antibody glomerulonephritis. *Am J Soc Nephrol* 1993;3:1753–1764.
75. Zoja C, Corna D, Macconi D, et al. Tissue plasminogen activator therapy of rabbit nephrotoxic nephritis. *Lab Invest* 1990;62:34–40.
76. Vassalli L-D, Dayer J-M, Wohlwend A, et al. Concomitant secretion of prourokinase and of a plasminogen activator inhibitor by cultured human monocyte-macrophages. *J Exp Med* 1984;159:1653–1668.
77. Clark RAF. Potential roles of fibronectin in cutaneous wound repair. *Arch Dermatol* 1988:124:201–206.

78. Cattell V, Jamieson SW. The origin of glomerular crescents in experimental nephrotoxic serum nephritis in the rabbit. *Lab Invest* 1978;39: 584–590.
79. Hancock WW, Atkins RC. Cellular composition of crescents in rapidly progressive glomerulonephritis identified using monoclonal antibodies. *Am J Nephrol* 1984;4:177–181.
80. Hooke DH, Hancock WW, Gee DC, et al. Monoclonal antibody analysis of glomerular hypercellularity in human glomerulonephritis. *Clin Nephrol* 1984;22:163–168.
81. Magil AB. Histogenesis of glomerular crescents: immunohistochemical demonstration of cytokeratin in crescent cells. *Am J Pathol* 1985; 120:222–229.
82. Stachura I, Si L, Madan E, et al. Mononuclear cell subsets in human renal disease enumeration in tissue sections with monoclonal antibodies. *Clin Immunol Immunopathol* 1984;30:362–373.
83. Jennette JC, Hipp CG. The epithelial antigen phenotype of glomerular crescent cells. *Am J Clin Pathol* 1986;86:274–280.
84. Harrison DJ, Macdonald MK. The origin of cells in the glomerular crescent investigated by the use of monoclonal antibodies. *Histopathology* 1986;10:945–952.
85. Floege J, Johnson RJ, Alpers CE, et al. Visceral glomerular epithelial cells can proliferate in vivo and synthesize platelet-derived growth factor B-chain. *Am J Pathol* 1993;142:637–650.
86. Abboud HE. Nephrology forum: growth factors in glomerulonephritis. *Kidney Int* 1993;43:252–267.
87. Wiggins R, Goyal M, Merritt S, et al. Vascular adventitial cell expression of collagen I mRNA in anti-GBM antibody–induced crescentic nephritis in the rabbit. A cellular source for interstitial collagen synthesis in inflammatory renal disease. *Lab Invest* 1993;68:557–565.
88. Striker GE, Cutler RE, Huang TW, et al. Renal failure, glomerulonephritis and glomerular epithelial cell hyperplasia. In: Kincaid-Smith P, Mathew TH, Becker EL, eds. *Perspectives in Nephrology and Hypertension.* Vol 1. New York: John Wiley & Sons; 1973:657–675.
89. Min KW, Gyorkey F, Gyorkey P, et al. The morphogenesis of glomerular crescents in rapidly progressive glomerulonephritis. *Kidney Int* 1974;5:47–56.
90. Silva FG, Hoyer JR, Pirani CL. Sequential studies of glomerular crescent formation in rats with antiglomerular basement membrane–induced glomerulonephritis and the role of coagulation factors. *Lab Invest* 1984;51:404–415.
91. A clinicopathologic study of crescentic nephritis in 50 children. A report of the Southwest Pediatric Nephrology study Group. *Kidney Int* 1985;27:450–458.
92. Boucher A, Droz D, Adafer E, et al. Relationship between the integrity of Bowman's capsule and the composition of cellular crescents in human crescentic glomerulonephritis. *Lab Invest* 1987;56: 526–533.
93. Grinnell F. Fibroblasts, myofibroblasts, and wound contraction. *J Cell Biol* 1994;124:401–404.
94. Estes JM, Vande Berg JS, Adzick NS, MacGillivray TE, Desmouliere A, Gabbiani G. Phenotypic and functional features of myofibroblasts in sheep fetal wounds. *Differentiation* 1994;56:173–181.
95. Zhang K, Rekhter MD, Gordon D, Phan SH. Myofibroblasts and their role in lung collagen gene expression during pulmonary fibrosis. A combined immunohistochemical and in situ hybridization study. *Am J Pathol* 1994;145:114–112.
96. Petterson EA, Colvin RB. Cold-insoluble globulin (fibronectin, LETS protein) in normal and diseased human glomeruli: papain-sensitive attachment to normal glomeruli and deposition in crescents. *Clin Immunol Immunopathol* 1978;11:425–436.
97. Weiss MA, Ooi BS, Ooi YM, Engvall E, Rouslahti E. Immunoflourescent localization of fibronectin in human kidney. *Lab Invest* 1979;41:340–347.
98. Goyal M, Wiggins R. Fibronectin mRNA and protein accumulation, distribution and breakdown in rabbit antiGBM disease. *J Am Soc Neph*rol 1991;1:1334–1342.
99. Postlethwaite AE, Keski-Oja J, Balian G, Kang AH. Induction of fibroblast chemotaxis by fibronectin. Localization of the chemotactic region to a 140,000–molecular weight non–gelatin-binding fragment. *J Exp Med* 1981;15:494–499.
100. Phan SH, Wolber F, Wiggins R. Fibronectin is the major fibroblast chemotactin in crescentic nephritis. *J Am Soc Nephrol* 1992;3:576.
101. Desmouliere A, Geinoz A, Gabbiani F, Gabbiani G. Transforming growth factor-beta 1 induces alpha-smooth muscle actin expression in granulation tissue myofibroblasts and in quiescent and growing cultured fibroblasts. *J Cell Biol* 1993;122:103–111.
102. Glick AD, Jacobson HR, Haralson MA. Mesangial deposition of type I collagen in human glomerulosclerosis. *Hum Pathol* 1992;23: 1373–1379.
103. Raghow R. Role of transforming growth factor-beta in repair and fibrosis. *Chest* 1991;99(suppl):61–65.
104. Murphy G, Willenbrock F, Crabbe T, et al. Regulation of matrix metalloproteinase activity. *Ann NY Acad Sci* 1994;732:31–41.
105. Woessner JF. Matrix metalloproteinases and their inhibitors in connective tissue remodeling. *FASEB J* 1991;5:2145–2154.
106. Denhardt DT, Feng B, Edwards DR, Cocuzzi ET, Malyankar UM. Tissue inhibitor of metalloproteinases (TIMP, aka EPA): structure, control of expression and biological functions. *Pharmacol Ther* 1993; 59:329–341.
107. Carome MA, Striker LJ, Peten EP, et al. Human glomeruli express TIMP-1 mRNA and TIMP-2 protein and mRNA. *Am J Physiol* 1993; 264:F923–F929.
108. Wahl SM, Hunt DA, Wakefield LM, et al. Transforming growth factor type b induces monocyte chemotaxia and growth factor production. *Proc Natl Acad Sci U S A* 1987;84;5788–5792.
109. Postlethwaite AE, Keski-Oja J, Moses HL, et al. Stimulation of the chemotactic migration of human fibroblasts by transforming growth factor β. *J Exp Med* 1987;165:251–256.
110. Roberts AB, Heine UI, Flanders KC, Sporn MB. Transforming growth factor beta. Major role in regulation of extracellular matrix. *Ann NY Acad Sci* 1990;580:225–232.
111. Johnson RJ, Floege J, Yoshimura A, et al. The activated mesangial cell: a glomerular "myofibroblast"? *J Am Soc Nephrol* 1992;2(suppl): 190–197.
112. Haralson MA. Extracellular matrix and growth factors: an integrated interplay controlling tissue repair and progression to disease. *Lab Invest* 1993;69:369–372.
113. Coimbra TM, Wiggins RC, Noh JW, et al. Transforming growth factor-β production in anti-glomerular basement disease in the rabbit. *Am J Pathol* 1990;138:223–234.
114. Border WA, Okuda S, Languino LR, et al. Suppression of experimental glomerulonephritis by antiserum against transforming growth factor β1. *Nature* 1990;346:371–374.
115. Border WA, Noble NA, Yamamoto T, et al. Natural inhibitor of transforming growth factor-β protects against scarring in experimental kidney disease. *Nature* 1992;360:361–364.
116. Couser WG. Rapidly progressive glomerulonephritis: classification, pathogenetic mechanisms and therapy. *Am J Kidney Dis* 1988;11: 449–464.
117. Bennett WM, Kincaid-Smith P. Macroscopic hematuria in mesangial IgA nephropathy. *Kidney Int* 1983;23:393–400.
118. Hind CRK, Lockwood CM, Peters DK, et al. Prognosis after immunosuppression of patients with crescentic nephritis requiring dialysis. *Lancet* 1983;1:263–265.
119. Downer G, Phan S, Wiggins R. Analysis of renal fibrosis in a rabbit model of crescentic nephritis. *J Clin Invest* 1988;82:998–1005.
120. Merritt SE, Killen PD, Phan SH, et al. Analysis of α1 (I) procollagen, α1 (IV) collagen and β-actin mRNA in glomerulus and cortex of rabbits with experimental anti-GBM disease. Evidence for early extraglomerular collagen biosynthesis. *Lab Invest* 1990;63:762–769.
121. Lan HY, Nikolic-Paterson DJ, Zarama M, et al. Suppression of experimental crescentic glomerulonephritis by the interleukin-1 receptor antagonist. *Kidney Int* 1993;43:479–485.
122. Lan HY, Zarama M, Nikolic-Paterson DJ, et al. Suppression of experimental crescentic glomerulonephritis by deoxyspergualin. *J Am Soc Nephrol* 1993;3:1765–1774.
123. McClurkin C Jr, Phan SH, Hsu CH, et al. Moderate protection of renal function and reduction of fibrosis by colchicine in a model of anti-GBM disease in the rabbit. *J Am Soc Nephrol* 1990;1:257–265.
124. Koyayashi Y, Sigematsu H, Masaki Y, et al. Effect of methylprednisolone on progressive Magsugi nephritis in the rabbit. *Virchows Arch [B]* 1980;35:45–61.

Immunologic Renal Diseases,
edited by E. G. Neilson and W. G. Couser.
Lippincott-Raven Publishers, Philadelphia © 1997.

CHAPTER 33

Pathophysiology of Progressive Renal Disease

Agnes B. Fogo and Valentina Kon

Renal scarring, be it glomerular and/or tubulointerstitial, is the pathologic process underlying progressive decline in the glomerular filtration rate (GFR) and occurs with any number of different primary diseases, whether immune, metabolic, or degenerative. The ultimate anatomical feature of glomerular sclerosis is the accumulation of extracellular matrix in the glomerulus and collapse of capillary lumina. Tubulointerstitial scarring is characterized by tubular atrophy and an accumulation of interstitial matrix, which may emanate from fibroblasts or tubular cells themselves. Progression occurs even when the primary disease process has been treated or becomes inactive, indicating that secondary adaptive mechanisms play an important role in ongoing damage. The remarkably similar histologic appearance of chronic renal diseases, regardless of the primary insult, is additional evidence suggesting such a common final pathway. The alterations and adaptations in nephrons remaining after the initial insult are thought to ultimately cause scarring and further nephron loss and, thus, perpetuate a vicious cycle that results in the end-stage kidney (1–3). The downward course is so predictable that serum measurements of GFR, assessing the rate of change in renal function, allow prediction of a time course until dialysis or transplantation will be needed (4). In addition to assessment of GFR, progression can be evaluated clinically by monitoring urinary protein excretion and morphologically by renal biopsy. How we approach each of these parameters and evaluate their inter-relationships has evolved greatly in recent years. Thus, the focus has switched from documentation of the status quo of lesions to assessment of prognostic indices and information that has relevance for therapeutic responsiveness. Tubulointerstitial processes are the focus of Chapters 34 and 36. We focus in this chapter on glomerular events in progression. Recent evidence for heterogeneity regarding incidence of disease, rates of progression, and mechanisms of progression in different animal models and human diseases is reviewed.

A. Fogo and V. Kon: Departments of Pathology and Pediatrics, Vanderbilt University Medical Center, Nashville, Tennessee 37232.

GLOMERULAR DETERMINANTS OF INJURY

Mechanisms of glomerulosclerosis could relate to increased matrix production and/or decreased matrix degradation. Possible sources of increased matrix include all of the glomerular resident cells, as well as tubular epithelial cells and fibroblasts. Dynamic interactions between each of these components occur and are affected by infiltrating cells and release of cytokines with effects on cell proliferation versus cell death (Fig. 1). Even the glomerular filtrate, which contributes factors from circulating and/or glomerular sites, can modulate downstream processes that mediate fibrogenesis in the tubulointerstitium (5).

Endothelial Cell

The position of endothelial cells at the interface between circulating blood and the vascular wall emphasizes their potential importance, both as targets and as effectors of injury. Endothelial cells are heterogeneous, both phenotypically and in their response to a given injury (6). Even within a normal glomerulus, heterogeneous expression of messenger RNAs (mRNAs) for glomerular basement membrane components is seen. Notably, collagen type IV α-1 and α-2 localize to endothelial cells in small-diameter capillary loops (7). The long half-life of the glomerular endothelial cell can result in delay of manifestation of structural injury. Thus, after radiation- or mitomycin-induced injury, endothelial swelling and thrombosis with resultant thrombotic microangiopathy occurs weeks to months after the insult (8) (Fig. 2). Some of the factors upregulated after injury such as plasminogen activators and their inhibitors and collagenases not only affect coagulation and thrombosis but also have been

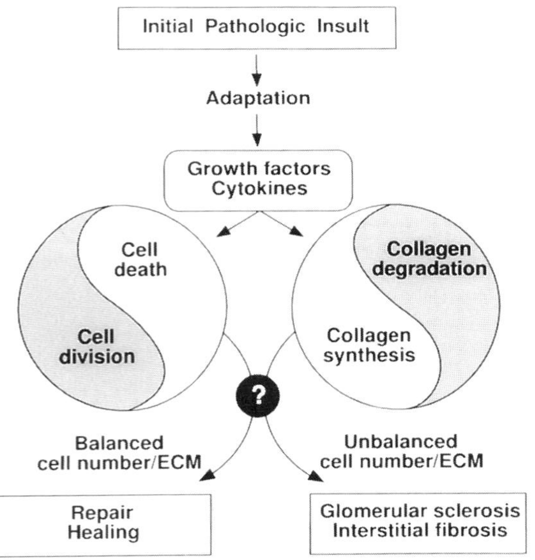

FIG. 1. Glomerulosclerosis is postulated to result from the net effects of growth promoters and inhibitors on cell growth and matrix accumulation. The balance of cell proliferation versus apoptosis and matrix production versus degradation determine whether scarring or healing ensues in response to injury. (ECM; extracellular matrix.)

linked to matrix remodeling. Thus, scarring may be a late sequela of endothelial cell injury. Endothelial cells release cytokines that affect vascular tone and express adhesion molecules for circulating cells (Chapter 30). Normally, endothelial cells inhibit smooth muscle cell migration and proliferation. When injured, they release growth factors that promote proliferation and matrix, lipoproteins, and cholesterol accumulation (9–11).

Epithelial Cell

The glomerular epithelial cell is an integral component of the glomerular capillary wall, contributing to permselectivity, and is also the primary target in many human glomerular diseases (see Chapter 31). Epithelial cells are injured in the experimental models of nephrotic syndrome, adriamycin and puromycin aminonucleoside nephropathies, diseases ultimately characterized by increased mesangial matrix and sclerosis. Glomerular epithelial cells also contain specific antigens, e.g., megalin, that are targets in immune-mediated glomerulonephritis (12,13). Epithelial cells are a source of matrix in both physiologic and pathophysiologic settings. The limited capability of the glomerular epithelial cell to undergo hyperplasia results in epithelial cell detachment when the glomerulus enlarges in response to injury. These denuded areas are associated with areas of hyalinosis and are believed to play a role in progressive scarring due to injury from exudation of plasma proteins (14,15).

Epithelial cells normally produce an endogenous heparinlike substance that inhibits mesangial cell growth. Epithelial cell injury may decrease this growth-inhibitory effect and allow mesangial growth to occur in response to other mediators. Epithelial cells are the main renal source of vascular endothelial growth factor, an endothelial cell–specific mitogen that plays a key role in both physiologic and pathologic angiogenesis (16,17). Epithelial cell integrins are key modulators of cell interactions and cell–matrix binding, and antibodies to β1 integrins or epithelial slit pores caused proteinuria acutely (18,19). In early sclerotic lesions, α-3 and α-5 integrins were segmentally decreased and lost polar distribution. More severe loss of integrins and loss of filamentous actin were associated with advanced sclerotic lesions (20). Together these

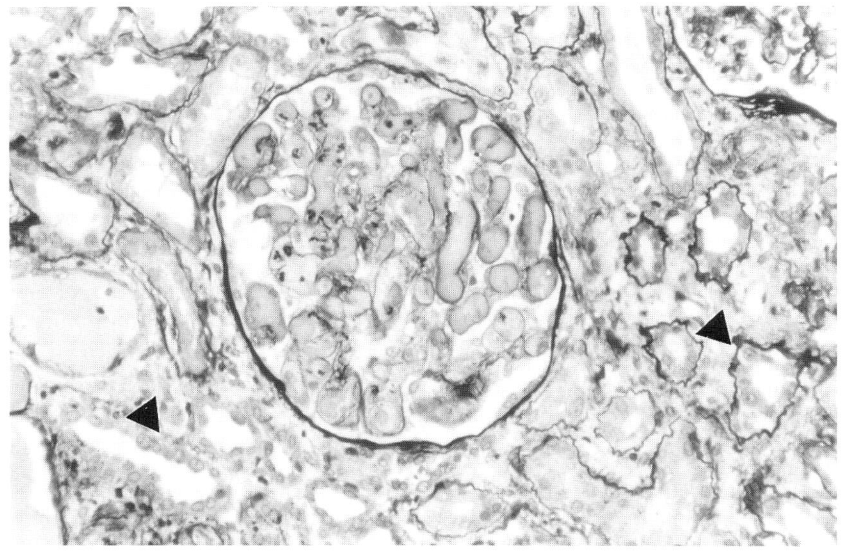

FIG. 2. Glomerular thrombosis with early tubulointerstitial fibrosis 6 months after mitomycin treatment. Thus, glomerular endothelial cell injury manifestation can be delayed and activate fibrotic processes *(arrowheads)* in the interstitium (Jones' silver stain, original magnification ×200). (Case kindly shared by Dr. Robert G. Horn.)

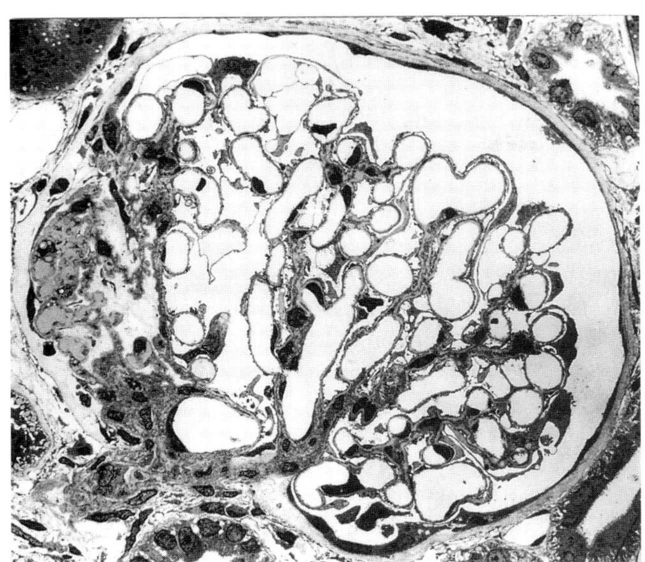

FIG. 3. Preferential localization of visceral epithelial cell injury at the vascular pole in the nephrectomized Fawn-hooded rat. Glomerulosclerosis has developed inside an adherent tuft area at the vascular pole. The capillary loops are either collapsed or filled with hyaline materials. Signs of cellular proliferation are not apparent (transmission electron micrograph, original magnification ×700).(Courtesy of Professor Wilhelm Kriz.)

structural changes may underly the foot process fusion and altered cell–cell and cell–matrix interactions. Of note, glomerular epithelial cells at the vascular pole show the earliest alterations in animal models (21) (Fig. 3). The vascular pole is also the site of the earliest capillary dilatation after uninephrectomy in rats (22). This specific segmental localization suggests the possibility that glomerular epithelial cells may be heterogeneous in susceptibility to injury and/or that injury is initially limited to this site.

Mesangial Cell

The mesangial cell's pivotal position within the glomerulus provides both anatomical support and allows it to modulate several glomerular functions (see Chapter 29). Because sclerosis ultimately is comprised of obliterated capillary loops and excess mesangial matrix, the mesangial cell presumably plays a central role in the process of glomerular sclerosis. The mesangial cells share many characteristics with vascular smooth muscle cells: they contract and proliferate in response to numerous cytokines and vasoactive substances, such as angiotensin II (Ang II) and to altered shear stress (2). Mesangial cell contraction also promotes vasoconstriction through capillary/vascular narrowing or collapse and facilitates trapping of circulating cells that, in turn, are a key source for initiation of many glomerular injuries (23,24).

Cells with the morphologic appearance of mesangial cells are not uniform within the entire glomerulus. Thus, the extraglomerular mesangial cells, as part of the juxtaglomerular apparatus, are uniquely situated to be an active component of the renin angiotensin system because this region shows the highest expression of Ang II type I receptor within the glomerulus (25). This has implications for many injurious processes because sclerosis often starts in the axial component. In human focal segmental glomerular sclerosis there is, indeed, heterogeneity in localization of the sclerotic regions that may impact not only pathogenesis but also response to therapy. In adult renal biopsy samples, a hilar position of sclerotic lesions was much more frequent and prominent than in children whose biopsy samples more frequently had small peripheral lesions (26). Further study of underlying heterogeneity and receptor expression of mesangial cells in these anatomical sites can shed light on the mechanisms underlying heterogeneity of sclerosis.

MECHANISMS OF SCLEROSIS

Glomerulosclerosis is the end result of complex interactions of these resident cells, influenced by both the systemic and local environment. Possible mechanisms include, but are not limited to, hemodynamic factors, shear stress, growth factors, and metabolic factors such as a diabetic milieu and hyperlipidemia. In addition, injury may be initiated or modified via elaboration of reactive oxygen species, activation of platelets and coagulation, complement activation, and/or macrophage recruitment (see Chapters 23, 27 and 28). The interplay of these factors determines the balance of cell growth and proliferation versus cell death by necrosis or apoptosis, and the balance of matrix accumulation versus degradation. The end result after injury is then healing with remodeling and resolution of damage, or ongoing sclerosis (Fig. 1).

Systemic and Glomerular Hypertension

Systemic hypertension often accompanies renal disease. It is both the result of and a contributor to progression of renal damage. Hypertension accelerates progression of chronic renal disease in humans. Systemic blood pressure not only can affect the glomerulus by transmission of pressures but may affect other determinants of progressive injury. In addition, the unique aspects of kidney structure and function are important. The glomerulus has both an afferent and efferent arteriole, which permits modulation of perfusion and pressure within the glomerular capillary bed differentially from systemic blood pressure. Therefore, attention has been focused on the potential impact of local, i.e., glomerular, hemodynamic changes in structural glomerular injury.

Numerous studies in the past decade have examined the remnant kidney, or renal ablation model of progression, in the rat. In this model, removal of a large portion of renal mass (i.e., removal of one entire kidney and two-thirds of the contralateral kidney, resulting in a total of five-sixths nephrectomy), results in progressive hyperperfusion, hyperfiltration, and sclerosis in a heterogeneous pattern, i.e., focal and segmental glomerulosclerosis (1,27,28). Kidney weight increases and tubular and glomerular growth occur. The structural changes after loss of nephrons include hyperplasia and hypertrophy. So-called glomerular hypertrophy represents both cellular hypertrophy (increase in cell size) and hyperplasia (increase in cell number). As noted above, glomerular visceral epithelial cells are limited in their capacity for hyperplasia and respond primarily by hypertrophy, whereas mesangial cells and glomerular endothelial cells and renal tubular cells can undergo both hyperplasia and hypertrophy. Renal ablation causes rats to develop hypertension, azotemia, proteinuria, and progressive glomerular sclerosis. The striking similarity in this animal model to the histologic changes in human renal disease led to extensive investigation of potential pathogenetic mechanisms of the progressive changes that ultimately afflict these initially normal remnant nephrons. The postulated intermediary factors for progressive glomerulosclerosis also have been investigated in other models where nephrons are not removed and the initial injury is more diffuse. Both the puromycin aminonucleoside and adriamycin models of renal disease show initial proteinuria and epithelial cell damage similar to human minimal change disease, followed by progressive focal and segmental glomerulosclerosis.

The initial observations that single-nephron function was increased after renal ablation led to further studies, and the hypothesis was advanced that hyperfiltration was injurious (1,29). It was postulated that this maladaptive change after removal of nephrons results in the ongoing loss of glomeruli, thus perpetuating a cycle of hyperfiltration and glomerulosclerosis (30). Manipulations of hyperfiltration by feeding a low-protein diet or by giving angiotensin I–converting enzyme inhibitors (ACEI), lipid lowering agents, or heparin were effective in ameliorating glomerular sclerosis. However, in some studies glomerular sclerosis was decreased without altering glomerular hyperfiltration (31,32). In addition, experimental maneuvers that actually increased glomerular hyperperfusion, such as thromboxane synthetase inhibitors or exercise training, not only did not accelerate progression, but actually slowed the process. Finally, glomerular sclerosis was noted to occur even in the absence of intervening hyperperfusion (2,3).

Glomerular hypertension is typical in many models of chronic renal failure. Maneuvers that increase glomerular capillary pressure, such as therapy with erythropoietin, glucocorticoids, or a high-protein diet, usually accelerate glomerulosclerosis. Maneuvers that induce systemic and/or glomerular hypertension, such as uninephrectomy, superimposed on other forms of renal disease, including nephrotoxic serum nephritis, immune complex nephritis, or diabetic nephropathy, worsen both functional and structural deterioration (2,3). There appears to be better correlation between increased glomerular pressure and glomerulosclerosis than between hyperfiltration/hyperperfusion and sclerosis. Thus, many of the maneuvers that had been used to ameliorate glomerulosclerosis also affected glomerular pressures. Decreased glomerular pressure, in response to dietary protein restriction (33) or antihypertensive drugs (2,3,34,35), for example, is associated with slower progression. As discussed below, these maneuvers also have other effects. Of special interest are the findings of protection against glomerulosclerosis with inhibition of Ang II by ACEI or a newly developed Ang II receptor antagonist. These agents are not only effective systemic antihypertensive agents, but they also appear to be more efficacious than other, nonspecific antihypertensive agents in protecting against progressive glomerulosclerosis (36,37). This has been postulated to relate to ACEI's unique actions to decrease glomerular capillary pressure by preferential dilatation of the efferent arteriole (3,38). However, inhibition of Ang II can affect parameters other than vasomotor tone, including mesangial and vascular smooth muscle cell growth and matrix production (see below).

Thus, factors other than pressure likely contribute to glomerular damage. One study in rats examined the heterogeneous changes in function in individual nephrons after renal ablation. Glomerular filtration and pressure were assessed repeatedly by micropuncture in the same nephrons over a 6-week period. When the single-nephron GFR and glomerular capillary pressure were correlated with the degree of sclerosis in the same glomerulus, no correlation was found between the level of these hemodynamic parameters and the degree of sclerosis. Thus, the nephrons with the greatest hyperfiltration or highest glomerular capillary pressure did not show the most severe sclerosis at the end of the study, indicating that glomerular hypertension or hyperperfusion per se did not directly account for the glomerular damage (39). Similar conclusions were reached based on experiments in another model, the puromycin aminonucleoside nephropathy, in which ACEIs were effective in slowing glomerulosclerosis, although glomerular capillary pressure was not affected (40).

Also relevant are observations of disorders characterized by glomerular hypertension which do not develop sclerosis. For example, in the diabetic nephropathy model in the rat, although glomerular capillary hypertension is typically seen, only mild mesangial expansion results rather than overt glomerulosclerosis (3,41). In another study, hyperfiltration was induced either by removal of nephrons or by diversion of urine into the peritoneal cavity. Two-thirds ablation of the right kidney was combined with ureteral diversion, total nephrectomy, or sham operation on the left. Similar degrees of glomerular hyperperfusion, hyperfiltration, and hypertension developed in the remaining right kidneys in both ureter-diverted and renal ablation groups. Glomeruli of the ureter-diverted rats did not enlarge, whereas those of the renal ablation rats did. Significant glomerulosclerosis developed only in the renal ablation group (35). Overall, these findings indicate that glomerulosclerosis can develop in settings without glomerular hypertension, and glomerulosclerosis can be ameliorated without altering glomerular hemodynamics. These results suggest that glomerular hyperfiltration, hyperperfusion, or glomerular hypertension alone do not fully explain the development of glomerular growth or sclerosis.

On the other hand, it has been postulated that the interaction of glomerular growth and glomerular pressures heightens injury by increasing wall tension, postulated to be a mechanism for glomerulosclerosis. Increased wall tension is predicted by LaPlace's law when the diameter of the glomerular capillary increases (42–44). However, glomerular enlargement after nephrectomy in rats occurs through lengthening and branching of the capillaries rather than by increased capillary diameter (32). Another pattern of glomerular growth was observed in diabetes and lithium-induced nephropathy, in which new capillary branching without increased diameter, rather than lengthening, was the mechanism for increased glomerular size (45,46). These observations cast doubt on whether increased wall tension actually occurs, at least in such settings of glomerular growth. This reservation is further fueled by the findings in renal biopsies from children with reflux nephropathy. In these patients, glomerular growth resulted from increased capillary branching and not increased capillary diameter (47).

Shear Stress

Increased systemic blood pressure may either directly or indirectly activate other synergistic contributors to progressive damage. Thus, systemic pressures may modulate glomerular sclerosis either by direct transmission of pressures, shear stress, and/or altering the elaboration of vasoactive substances. In vitro studies have investigated mechanisms by which increased pressure promotes sclerosis. Mesangial cells in culture were subjected to pulsatile mechanical stretch/relaxation. The cells changed both the type and amount of collagen production to a wound-healing phenotype, which may be pivotal in the scarring process in vivo (48). Of interest, recent preliminary studies subjecting mesangial cells in culture to increased pressure without stretch showed increased proliferation and altered myosin heavy-chain expression (49). The contribution of shear stress to injury may be particularly relevant in the renal circulation. Thus, capillaries within other systems such as joints are subject to profound changes in pressure and shear stress, which directly reflect the normal systemic pressure variations with change in posture or exertion. However, the unique anatomy of the glomerulus allows independent modulation of local hemodynamic as well as shear pressures. Changes in the efferent arteriolar resistance alter pressure and shear stress within the glomerular capillary bed, which in turn elicits responses in endothelial and mesangial cells that may be pivotal in determining subsequent injury.

The response of glomerular endothelial cells to shear stress is not linear. Depending on the degree and nature of the shear stress imposed, the net response may induce proliferation or inhibition of growth in other glomerular cells (50,51). For example, brief and low fluid shear stress increases endothelin production, whereas sustained and higher shear stress had the opposite effects (52–54). Thus, injury that causes capillary narrowing and collapse induces changes in laminar flow and shear stress that can stimulate mitogenic factors such as endothelin and platelet-derived growth factor (PDGF). The change in shear stress also stimulates other cytokines (e.g., nitric oxide), which dampen this aftermath. Media from glomerular endothelial cells subjected to shear stress induced proliferation in both mesangial and epithelial cells (51). These responses may in turn effect matrix accumulation (see below). Increased shear stress may also affect progression by altered rheology due to changes in laminar flow. Altered rheologic properties of blood may directly affect flow and pressure or alter cytokine production. Blood viscosity may also directly affect proteinuria by modulating glomerular permselectivity to macromolecules. Evidence for this includes amelioration of glomerular sclerosis with anemia, contrasting worsening injury along with increased systemic and glomerular pressures in response to erythropoietin, with consequent increased hematocrit (3,55). Of interest, ACEI, in addition to hemodynamic and matrix effects, has a beneficial effect on rheology in patients with renal disease (56).

Glomerular Growth

After initial loss of nephrons, growth promoters are increased and act on remaining glomeruli. Glomerular growth often is closely associated with glomerular sclerosis in a variety of animal and human diseases (2). Stimuli that induce glomerular growth often accelerate glomerular sclerosis, and this has focused research on possible roles of these growth factors in progression of renal disease (Fig. 1). Uninephrectomy, a stimulus for growth, accelerates glomerular sclerosis (2,3). In oligomeganephronia, a congenital renal disease characterized by a decreased number of nephrons, there is extreme glomerulomegaly and an increase in development of focal segmental glomerulosclerosis (FSGS) (57). Recent studies postulate that once maximal compensatory increase in glomerular size is achieved in several disease settings, focal segmental glomerulosclerosis may ensue (58).

In the remnant kidney in rats, similar to human FSGS, glomerulosclerosis occurs initially in the deep juxtamedullary glomeruli (59,60). Of interest, injury after renal ablation is more severe in young animals in which maturational growth is occurring than in adults (61,62). Detailed analysis of the distribution of this glomerular injury showed more focal and severe glomerulosclerosis in the deep versus superficial glomeruli in the young rats. Hemodynamic factors were not different between young and adult rats. Although glomerular enlargement occurred to a greater degree in the young compared to the adult rat after renal ablation, glomerular enlargement occurred proportionally in both superficial and deep nephron populations. The more severe injury of the deep glomeruli in the young immature rat was therefore postulated to be related to factors unique in the young growing kidney, which is characterized by centripetal growth and differentiation (62). Marked glomerular growth and accelerated glomerulosclerosis also occur in response to excess growth hormone, whether endogenously produced, i.e., in transgenic mice (63), or exogenously produced (64,65). Even in normal young rats, recombinant human growth hormone caused glomerular growth and severe sclerosis (65). Although these normal rats did not develop uremia over the course of observation, these findings raise important issues for the treatment of children with recombinant human growth hormone.

Although growth stimuli accelerate glomerular sclerosis, the converse is also true: decreasing the growth response is associated with less severe glomerular sclerosis. Dwarf rats with a defect in growth hormone or with a specific growth hormone receptor deletion are resistant to the development of glomerulosclerosis after renal ablation (64,66). A rat strain characterized by a larger number of small glomeruli and a minimal growth response to loss of nephrons, the PVGc strain, has proved resistant to the development of glomerulosclerosis after the removal of one kidney (2). Many interventions that ameliorate glomerulosclerosis also dampen glomerular growth. Treatment with low protein diets ameliorates sclerosis; however, it may be effective only when the diet is low enough in calories to inhibit growth (67). Antihypertensive drugs also inhibit both glomerular growth and glomerulosclerosis through their direct or indirect actions on growth factors.

The association of abnormal glomerular growth and sclerosis also is seen in human diseases. In vivo and in vitro experimental evidence point to the capability of many cytokines to promote growth of glomerular cells and to enhance extracellular matrix release, thus promoting sclerosis as well as growth. Stimuli to abnormal growth include hypoxia, as seen in cyanotic heart disease; sickle cell disease; obesity-associated sleep apnea; limited renal mass, as in transplantation; removal of more than one kidney; and unilateral renal agenesis (2). In diabetic nephropathy and idiopathic FSGS, the glomerular enlargement appears to result from primary pathogenic mechanisms and not be secondary to nephron loss or hypoxia. Thus, in diabetic nephropathy, glomeruli enlarge and hyperfunction from the onset of diabetes, well before any sclerosis is present (68,69). In FSGS, glomerular enlargement also was observed even at early stages. Adult patients with existing focal segmental glomerulosclerosis had significantly larger glomerular size than did adult patients with minimal change disease. In patients with glomerular tip lesions, i.e., sclerosis local-

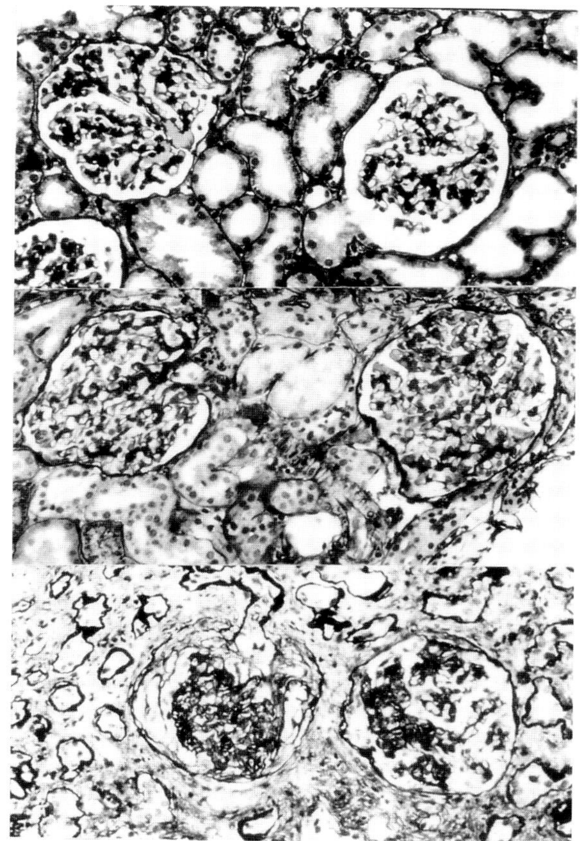

FIG. 4. Glomerular size in FSGS versus MCD. The two top panels show initial biopsy samples from patients with apparent MCD. The 5-year-old girl's initial biopsy sample in the middle panel was indistinguishable from age-matched typical MCD **(top panel)** except for marked glomerular enlargement. Her subsequent biopsy sample **(bottom panel)** 50 months later, showed FSGS. (Jones' silver stain, original magnification ×160). Reproduced with permission (71).

ized to the tubular pole of the glomerulus, prognosis is thought to be similar to that of minimal change disease, and glomerular enlargement was not found (70). In a study of pediatric patients with apparent minimal change disease, patients who subsequently developed overt focal segmental glomerulosclerosis indeed had larger glomeruli than either normal age-matched controls or patients with typical minimal change disease who had benign clinical courses and, on rebiopsy, also had minimal change disease (71) (Fig. 4). These findings were confirmed in a recent study by Mauer and Steffes et al. (72).

Of interest, increased glomerular size also predicted subsequent glomerular sclerosis in the setting of recurrent FSGS in the transplant. Thus, children who received an adult transplant who did not develop FSGS in their transplants did not show increased glomerular size over the initial months after transplantation. In contrast, those children who developed recurrent FSGS had marked, abnormal glomerular growth, preceding overt manifestation of FSGS (73). Glomerular enlargement could therefore be a marker in the early phase of disease, before overt sclerosis is detectable, for aberrant growth factor expression ultimately leading to scarring of the kidney. Molecular detection of these early processes could potentially be an even earlier, more sensitive marker of progression.

Growth factors also appear to play key roles in progression of glomerular and tubulointerstitial scarring. Increased release of growth factors may be triggered by local increase in shear stress, hydraulic pressures, or by insults that include but are not limited to increased glomerular metabolism, heightened reactive oxygen species, altered ammonia or phosphate metabolism, altered lipid metabolism, and intraglomerular hypercoagulability (2,3, 74–76). The particular growth factors and the roles they play may differ at the various stages of injury. The focus of research in this area reflects not only interest in unraveling mechanisms of progression, but identification of therapeutic targets. Altered gene expressions in pathophysiologic settings implicate some factors: PDGF, transforming growth factor-β, (TGF-β), TGF-α, insulin-like growth factor-1 (IGF-1), growth hormone, epidermal growth factor, interleukins 1 and 6, tumor necrosis factor-α, endothelin, and Ang II, among others (2,77–79). The contribution of Ang II is particularly relevant because it can be inhibited by currently clinically available agents. So far, results regarding the relative importance of these specific growth factors in in vivo settings are limited. A recent study showed that inhibition of a specific growth factor, TGF-β or PDGF, could decrease mesangial matrix expansion in the anti-Thy1 model (80,81). However, effects of inhibiting these factors in progressive disease models have not yet been determined. Further study is necessary to determine the specific role each of these factors plays at varying stages of glomerular injury.

Metabolic Factors

Diabetes Mellitus

Only 40% of all patients with diabetes develop diabetic nephropathy. However, predictors of development of diabetic nephropathy have not been identified. Control of glucose has always been advocated to minimize complications of diabetes, and recent data have indicated that tight control of glucose decreases the rate of GFR loss (82). A tight correlation also has been found between degree of glucose control and mesangial matrix expansion in diabetic kidney transplant patients (83). Hyperfiltration has been suggested as another risk factor for development of subsequent diabetic nephropathy (41). However, antihypertensive therapy, initially advocated for its potential effects on such deleterious hemodynamic mechanisms (e.g., hyperfiltration and glomerular hypertension), now is used even in normotensive diabetic patients (84). This has focused research efforts on additional nonhemodynamic modulators of initiation and progression of diabetic nephropathy. These include abnormal growth and hormonal factors, metabolic products consequent to hyperglycemia, and other genetic determinants.

As in focal segmental glomerulosclerosis, abnormal renal growth precedes development of sclerosis. Patients with diabetic nephropathy showed significantly larger mean glomerular size and mesangial volume compared with both normal controls and diabetics without nephropathy (85). In addition, there was a strong correlation between severity of glomerular sclerosis and glomerular size. However, the results of biopsies performed at early stages of microalbuminuria showed variable lesions (86,87). The potential importance of the diabetic milieu in promoting the glomerular growth and mesangial matrix expansion of diabetic nephropathy was evident in a study of diabetic patients with renal and pancreas transplants. Only minimal mesangial expansion was seen in the transplant kidneys from patients with combined transplant who had metabolic cure of their diabetes. The pancreas transplant patients also had smaller mean glomerular volume and mesangial volumes than did control patients (88). In contrast, diabetic patients receiving only kidney transplant without abolishment of their underlying disease showed more severe diabetic lesions. In addition, although the lesions in type I and type II diabetes may be due to a similar pathogenetic mechanism, the glomerular volume remains normal in patients with type II diabetes, contrasting with enlarged glomeruli in type I diabetes mellitus. There are no long-term studies establishing whether the degree and/or presence of glomerular enlargement or mesangial expansion are reliable markers of long-term progression (89).

Development of glomerulosclerosis in patients with diabetes may be affected by several hormonal/cytokine systems. IGF-1 is one key growth factor altered in progressive renal diseases, including diabetes. The circulating level is under the control of growth hormone, although many factors may affect its biological actions. IGF-1 induces renal and glomerular growth in vivo, as demonstrated in transgenic mice, and causes mesangial cell hyperplasia in vitro, but may require synergistic actions of other cytokines to result in a sclerotic lesion (63). Specific receptors for IGF show increased expression in diabetic rat mesangial cells (90,91). Several other growth factors, including basic fibroblastic growth factor (FGF), PDGF, and EGF, may be altered in diabetes and affect glomerular growth and sclerosis (90,91). Although somatostatin analogs protected against injury in diabetic animal models, the specific growth factors of key importance have not yet been defined in diabetes (92).

Hyperglycemia results in accumulation of other metabolic products, which can also modulate glomerulosclerosis. Thus, polyamines and glucose levels both affect mesangial cell growth and matrix accumulation (90,93). Advanced glycosylation end products (AGEs) are formed by effects of increased glucose on proteins. The glycosylated products can form stable adducts (AGEs) via protein cross-linking and polymerization. AGEs are increased in diabetes and also in aging. AGEs have direct effects to upregulate multiple cytokines, which in turn augment matrix production. Furthermore, AGEs also may prevent normal protease digestion of collagens to which they bind. Infusion of AGEs into normal mice lead to glomerular growth and increased expression of matrix genes, whereas inhibition of AGE cross-linking with aminoguanidine significantly blunted these effects (94). Longer time course of administration of AGEs resulted in significant glomerulosclerosis and proteinuria. These abnormalities were decreased by cotreatment with aminoguanidine (93). Aminoguanidine had a similar beneficial effect on mesangial expansion in diabetic animal models without altering glucose levels, strongly implicating AGEs in the progressive lesion (95,96). Similarly, increased circulating AGE levels paralleled the severity of renal dysfunction in patients with diabetic nephropathy (97).

Lipids

Lipids are important in modulating glomerular sclerosis in rats, although studies are incomplete in humans (75, 98). Glomerulosclerosis shares several features with atherosclerosis; both are affected by macrophages, PDGF, and lipids (99). Histologic evidence of abnormal renal lipid accumulation has long been noted. Lipid deposits were described in early studies of kidneys of patients with nephrotic syndrome. Extensive fatty degeneration was observed in patients with end-stage renal disease. Glomerular lipid deposits are seen in diabetic nephropathy. Glomerular disease has been reported in the rare familial disease lecithin cholesterol acyltransferase deficiency, and with excess apolipoprotein E. Gross obesity is associated with the development of focal segmental glomerular sclerosis (100). However, renal disease is not a common finding in the more common forms of primary hyperlipidemias. Patients with minimal change disease or membranous glomerulonephritis, characterized by hyperlipidemia as part of their nephrotic syndrome, usually do not develop glomerular scarring (75).

Evidence of the effects on progression of renal disease of manipulation of lipids currently is limited to animal studies. Hypercholesterolemia modulates vascular tone by reducing vasodilators and increasing vasoconstrictors such as thromboxane A_2 and endothelin. Indirect effects of hypercholesterolemia include altered fatty acid metabolism (see ensuing section on reactive oxygen species). However, glomerular injury was increased in experimental models of kidney disease when excess cholesterol was added to diets of rats with pre-existing glomerular disease, ablation nephropathy, or hypertension (75). The degree of injury was proportional to glomerular size, and the glomerular pressures were not affected. Similar effects of cholesterol were produced in the puromycin aminonucleoside rat model. Conversely, lipid-lowering agents decrease glomerular injury in several models. The glomerular injury in rats with renal ablation was lessened by lovistatin without affecting systemic or glomerular pressures or glomerular growth (101). Probucol, another lipid-lowering agent, was effective in decreasing injury in puromycin nephropathy and in the remnant kidney model (102,103). Zucker rats, which have an autosomal-recessive disorder associated with hyperphagia, hyperlipidemia, and glomerular sclerosis, do not have glomerular hemodynamic abnormalities. Their lean littermates develop neither lipid abnormalities nor glomerular lesions. Lipid-lowering agents lessen both the hyperlipidemia and glomerulosclerosis in the affected rats (104).

Macrophage accumulation resulting from high cholesterol levels has been postulated to be a key early step for glomerulosclerosis, analogous to atherosclerosis (99, 105). These cells are potential sources of numerous cytokines that affect the glomerulus. Increased cholesterol intake in puromycin-treated rats increased macrophage infiltration and concomitantly increased TGF-β mRNA levels (106). Further evidence supporting a role of macrophages in lipid injury is seen with the protective effects of essential fatty acid deficiency, closely associated with decreased macrophage influx (107). Direct effects of lipids include mesangial cell cytotoxicity mediated by oxidized low-density lipoprotein (75). Endothelial cells may be affected directly or by increased adhesion of monocytes (108). Elevated lipids may thus contribute to glomerulosclerosis through effects on different glomerular cell types. Some lipid-lowering therapies have additional effects. Thus, alpha tocopherol decreases lipids and is also an effective antioxidant. Thus, the mechanism of its efficacy in progressive adriamycin nephropathy may result from these dual actions (109). These results further illustrate the interaction of pathogenic mechanisms and multiple actions of therapies to target these processes.

Reactive Oxygen Species

Reactive oxygen species (ROS), in addition to well-described effects in acute tubular injury, are increased in settings in which sclerosis may ensue, including glomerular diseases (110–114), ischemic renal failure (115), and toxic nephropathies (116,117) (see Chapter 19). Conversely, scavengers of oxygen radicals are protective in these settings. Fish oil increases antioxidant genes and also decreases cytokines and eicosanoid production, thus resulting in increased defense against ROS and decreased infiltration of inflammatory cells, a potent source of ROS (118). Fish oil's benefit on renal function in stable renal transplant patients and in immunoglobulin A (IgA) nephropathy may be related in part to these mechanisms (118–120). ROS plays a role in several animal models, including puromycin aminonucleoside or adriamycin nephropathies (121,122). Vitamin E, an antioxidant, decreased ROS, ameliorated proteinuria, and lessened glomerular growth, sclerosis, and tubular interstitial scarring in the adriamycin model (123). Intrarenal infusion of hydrogen peroxide acutely induced marked proteinuria, without changes in glomerular hemodynamics or histologic abnormalities, indicating that ROS can directly induce a transient sieving defect (124–126). The proteinuria could be prevented in this setting by antioxidant pretreatment, which also reduced proteinuria in other models (126). This transient ROS-induced proteinuria without apparent glomerular damage appears particularly relevant to human exercise-induced proteinuria.

Proteinuria

Proteinuria itself has been proposed to be injurious by affecting glomerular mesangial and epithelial cells or by cast formation, causing subsequent tubular epithelial damage and interstitial inflammation (127). In support of such proposals are the observations that glomerular disease accompanied by severe proteinuria has a worse prognosis than when proteinuria is less. Whether proteinuria is merely a marker of injury or a contributor to progressive injury has been debated. Little is known about tubulointerstitial mechanisms in progression; it has been suggested that these may play a role or may be primary in progressive renal disease. Overload proteinuria induces tubulointerstitial scarring associated with macrophage influx (128,129). Filtered neutral lipid in proteinuric states may have additional pathogenic effects on matrix accumulation, and further proteinuria induces inflammatory mediators (130,131). Indeed, the severity of proteinuria correlated with tubulointerstitial nephritis in puromycin nephropathy (132). Although correlation of proteinuria and glomerulosclerosis has been shown in the remnant kidney at the whole kidney level, sclerosis and proteinuria in individual glomeruli do not correlate with each other. Rather, proteinuria originates largely from nonsclerotic glomeruli (133).

Further divergence between sclerosis in glomeruli and proteinuria is illustrated by experiments in analbuminemic rats. These rats when treated with adriamycin developed the same degree of glomerular sclerosis and renal failure despite 70% reduction of proteinuria, compared with Sprague-Dawley counterparts (134). Moreover, amelioration of early proteinuria in rats with puromycin nephropathy did not affect the subsequent severity of glomerulosclerosis, strengthening the postulate that proteinuria is not causal in glomerulosclerosis (135). These observations impact on assessment of therapeutic interventions specifically targeting proteinuria. Thus, therapeutic interventions have been shown in some patients to affect proteinuria, but effects on sclerosis have not been proven. This relates in part to uncertainty as to the nature of factors that cause proteinuria. In this connection, plasmapheresis with a protein A adsorptive column decreased proteinuria and induced remission in several patients with recurrent FSGS (136,137). Infusion of the adsorbed factor obtained from several of these patients into rats induced proteinuria. Although the specific identity of such a circulating factor(s) is not yet known, promising data from an intriguing ex vivo model are emerging and point to a cytokine as a primary effector of increased glomerular permeability (138). Possible sources for the postulated cytokine include activated T cells and/or monocytes. Furthermore, whether the substance(s) effecting the proteinuria also are causal in glomerulosclerosis has not been established.

MECHANISMS OF HETEROGENEITY OF SCLEROSIS

Stage of Injury

Glomerulosclerosis is not a uniform, linear process over time. Rather, the process is affected by different mediators at each stage. Progression after initial injury likely involves numerous acute-phase reactants and proto-oncogenes, many of which are shown to be upregulated at this early stage. It is likely that at each stage of progression, a balance exists between factors that control matrix accumulation versus degradation and cell proliferation/regeneration versus apoptosis. This balance then determines whether healing or scarring results from the injury (Fig. 1).

Early, but after the initial injury phase, PDGF-B mRNA is increased in several animal models (139,140). In addition, investigators of progressive renal diseases also have recently started mapping human renal biopsies for expression of various cytokines. These observations show increased PDGF in proliferative glomerulonephritides, but not in those processes that do not have proliferation, such as minimal change disease (141). Increased PDGF-B receptor expression has been detected in glomerular as well as interstitial areas in proliferative human diseases, providing a mechanism for autocrine activation of proliferation (142). As destructive processes continue, PDGF-B expression wanes and may reflect the downregulation of its receptor, which occurs in response to enhanced matrix accumulation (143). Thus, in the remnant kidney model, glomeruli with early sclerotic lesions had enhanced PDGF-B chain protein, whereas those glomeruli with more advanced sclerosis did not show such expression. This enhanced expression was normalized by treatment with Ang II receptor antagonist, but not with nonspecific antihypertensive treatment (144). The stage of injury with upregulated PDGF may therefore be particularly sensitive to therapies that inhibit Ang II, known to affect PDGF expression.

In the later stages, TGF-β is increased in association with sclerosis. Glomerular TGF-β expression was increased in biopsy samples from patients with overt diabetic nephropathy compared with samples from patients with nonprogressive renal disease (minimal change disease and thin basement membrane disease) (145). Quantity of staining correlated with the severity of glomerular sclerosis. Increased mature and/or latency-associated peptide and mRNA for TGF-β1 also were increased in proliferative human nephritides (146,147). mRNA intensity did not correlate with infiltrating cells, implicating glomerular resident cells as a source of TGF-β at this stage (146). It is important to note that although a time course has been described for maximum activation of several growth factors described above, there is likely to be overlap in this sequence. Thus, the development of glomerulosclerosis likely will unfold as analogous to the activation of the clotting cascade with complex interactions of multiple factors.

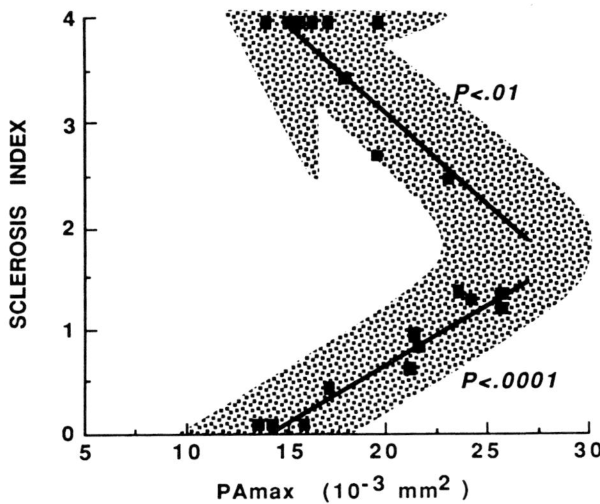

FIG. 5. Relationship of glomerular growth and sclerosis in individual glomeruli within one kidney at 12 weeks after five-sixths nephrectomy. When sclerosis index (scale of 0–4 by serial section) and maximum planar area (PAmax) were evaluated for each of 22 glomeruli in a single remnant rat kidney 12 weeks after subtotal nephrectomy, a significant correlation with a biphasic pattern was found between these parameters. Thus, there was a negative correlation for the glomeruli with advanced sclerosis and a positive correlation for the glomeruli with early-stage sclerosis, pointing to a potential linkage between the pathogenesis of glomerular growth and sclerosis. Reproduced with permission (230).

Glomerular Heterogeneity

Heterogeneity in modulators at each stage of injury is attended by the well-known observation of heterogeneous (i.e., focal/segmental) glomerular injury even at a specific time point. This heterogeneity is observed in both humans and animals with a biphasic correlation of glomerular enlargement and sclerosis. At early stages of sclerosis, glomerular growth and sclerosis are positively correlated, whereas the glomerulus becomes smaller as it approaches end-stage sclerosis (148,149) (Fig. 5). The distribution of severity of glomerular lesions has important implications for pathogenesis and potential response to therapy, in that glomeruli at early stages of injury are still potentially amenable to optimum therapies. However, detection of segmental and focal lesions may not be accurate by assessment on a single slide. Instead, serial section analysis is necessary to precisely examine stage of injury in individual glomeruli. In one recent study, the distribution of sclerosis in adult and pediatric patients with FSGS was indeed focal, sparing some glomeruli. Of interest, only 23% of glomeruli were involved by sclerosis at time of biopsy in children versus 48% in adults. A similar three-dimensional analysis in patients with a solitary kidney who also had undergone partial nephrectomy for renal cell carcinoma showed extensive total sclerosis. Only 8% of glomeruli were intact by serial section analysis. Sclerosis was distributed multifocally, suggesting that pathologic processes occur simultaneously at anatomically discrete locations within the glomerulus (150) (Fig. 6). FSGS tended to show a peripheral pattern of sclerosis in children, whereas multiple areas of the tuft, including a prominent hilar component, tended to be involved in adults (Fig. 7) (26). Although further studies are required, these observations may reflect differences in pathogenesis between children and adults. Of note, different diseases also show varying nature of sclerotic lesions. In diabetic nephropathy, peripheral mesangial nodules of

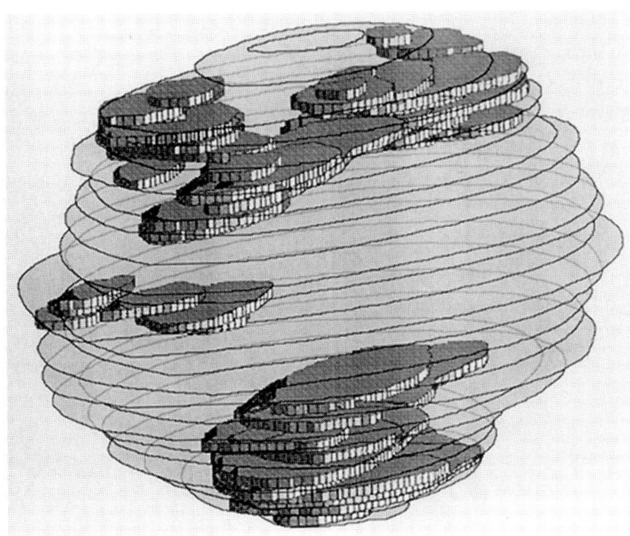

FIG. 6. Multifocal distribution of sclerotic areas in a patient after loss of more than one kidney. The lesions were mapped by three-dimensional computer-assisted analysis. Reproduced with permission (150).

sclerosis predominate in a regular, horseshoe-shaped distribution, in contrast to the hilar location of sclerosis in many cases of adult FSGS, or the random peripheral scarring seen late in vasculitic renal diseases (151).

The heterogeneity of disease processes within the glomerulus also may affect response to therapy. In this regard, response to therapy in children with FSGS appears better than in adults. Heterogeneity of scarring is paralleled by heterogeneity in the distribution of several key growth factors. Ang II type I receptors are particularly highly expressed in the mesangial axial areas (25), and ACEI is particularly effective in progressive renal disease in animal models and in humans. It is possible therefore that benefits of ACEI therapy could be linked to its potential greatest effect on mediators, which are particularly activated in the mesangial axial areas. Inhibition of Ang II actions per se, or indirect effects of Ang II inhibition on other cytokines such as PDGF, may underlie ACEI efficacy on sclerosis (142,144,152). Of further interest, PDGF receptor is localized in both mesangial and parietal epithelial cells in the human kidney (153), and inhibition of PDGF matrix–promoting effects might therefore affect both hilar and peripheral lesions.

Increased TGF-β was especially evident in severely sclerosed glomeruli in human biopsy specimens, a stage that appears refractory to therapeutic impact of ACEI (145,149). These observations impact the findings that tubulointerstitial fibrosis is associated with more chronic stages of glomerulosclerosis and may relate in part to the marked effects of TGF-β on both glomeruli and tubules at this stage of injury. TGF-β effects on the tubulointerstitium may occur in part via increased α1 and β1 integrin expression. These integrins serve as receptors for extracellular matrix components, and their upregulation in turn may affect cell–cell and cell–matrix interaction and increase glomerular and interstitial matrix accumulation. TGF-β circulates in inactive form, bound to the latency-associated peptide (LAP), and disruption of LAP (e.g., by plasmin) activates TGF (154,155). For example, while transfection of TGF-β results in increased matrix deposition (156), it also decreases matrix degradation by inducing protease inhibitors and inhibiting collagenases (155). TGF-β also affects inflammatory cells. TGF-β inhibits T-cell proliferation, and TGF-β1 knock-out mice have T-cell anergy (157,158). Increased TGF-β stimulates decorin, a proteoglycan that is an endogenous inhibitor of TGF activity. Of note, increased TGF-β occurs in response to several other key factors implicated in sclerosis, including PDGF-B and Ang II (155). Ang II also promotes conversion of TGF-β to its active form (159), indicating that maximal TGF activation may follow increased Ang II. Thus, therapies aimed at inhibiting

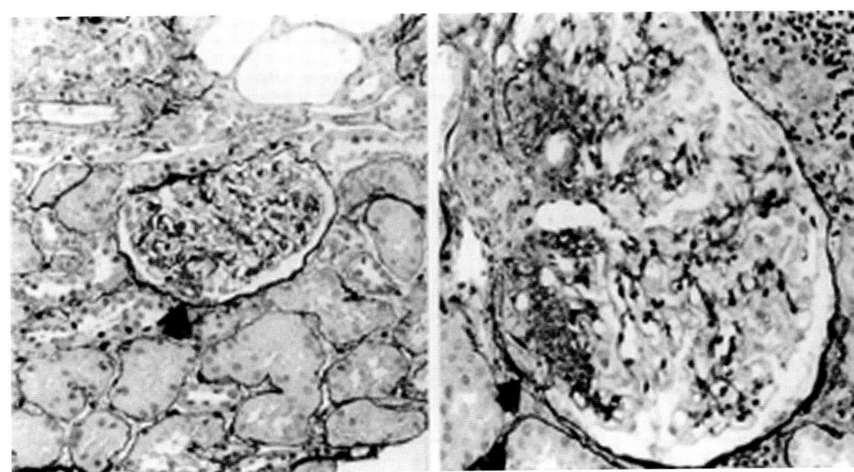

FIG. 7. Hilar distribution of sclerosis in adults (right) versus peripheral distribution in children *(left)* with focal segmental glomerulosclerosis *(arrows)*. Reproduced with permission (26).

TGF-β at established stages of disease may not affect more proximal and/or other matrix-promoting mechanisms that advance the fibrotic process.

Modulation of Matrix

Recent evidence suggests that upregulation of collagen, in addition to its role in the sclerotic process, may offer a sensitive index of progression from one stage of injury to the next. Of note, marked increase in collagen mRNAs by in situ polymerase chain reaction (PCR) from microdissected individual glomeruli was evident in several animal models even at stages of minimal sclerosis (Fig. 8). These findings suggest that this increase in collagen mRNA may not merely mirror existing sclerosis but may have a predictive value early in the disease. A lesser degree of structural damage in another model showed correspondingly lesser elevation of type IV collagen (160,161). In human renal tissue, a correlation also was found between the level of glomerulosclerosis and expression of collagen type IV mRNA (162). Thus, the slope of progression of a given type of glomerulosclerosis was postulated to parallel that of extracellular matrix mRNAs. Preliminary studies of diabetic mice transgenic for a functional antagonist of growth hormone showed upregulated TGF-β but no upregulation of collagen IV mRNA. These diabetic growth hormone antagonist transgenic mice did not develop glomerular lesions or increased matrix, contrasting nontransgenic diabetic controls (163). These studies suggest that collagen IV expression, rather than TGF-β per se, may be a more direct indicator of risk for sclerosis. Furthermore, diverse growth factors likely underlie matrix gene upregulation in various settings. Given that response to therapy is strongly linked to stage of injury, such molecular predictors may soon become widely used.

Matrix degradation also is actively modulated during sclerosis and healing. Tissue inhibitors of metalloproteinases 1 and 2 were expressed in normal human glomeruli and were upregulated in tissue from patients with glomerulosclerosis (164). Thus, degradation of collagen may be impaired in concert with upregulation of matrix-producing genes, both promoting sclerosis.

Competitive PCR on 1/10 Normal Glomerulus for mα_1IV Collagen

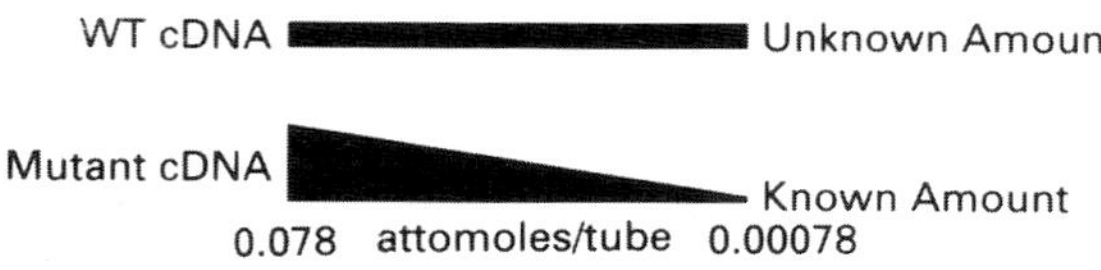

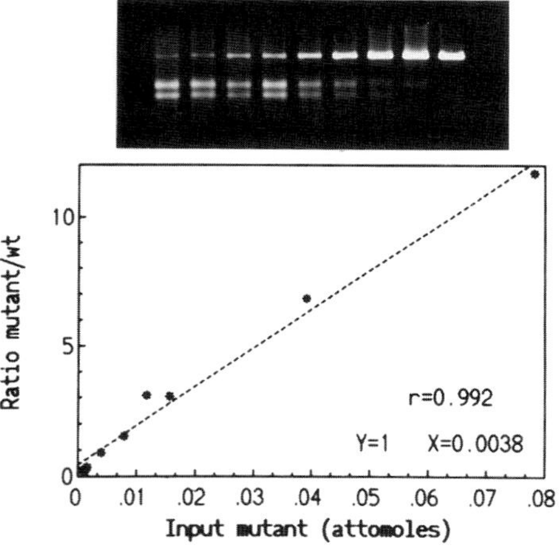

FIG. 8. Competitive PCR for α-1 type IV collagen in one tenth of a normal mouse glomerulus. Each tube has an added unknown amount of wild-type (WT) cDNA and known amounts of mutant cDNA (top panel schema). Mutants were constructed to differ from WT by adding a *Bcl* I restriction enzyme site. The middle panel shows the resulting ethidium bromide–stained gel after PCR amplification. After PCR, the PCR products were exposed to *Bcl* I, and WT and mutant bands were analyzed via densitometry. The bottom panel shows the ratio of mutant to WT density, versus the amount of mutant cDNA per tube. Amount of cDNA in the unknown sample is then calculated from the equivalence point (y = 1). Reproduced with permission (231).

Modulation of Cell Turnover

The rather static appearance of sclerosis in a renal biopsy histological slide belies the fact that sclerosis is an ongoing dynamic process. Even in the late phases of sclerosis, there is increased cell turnover and apoptosis in various animal models and in human FSGS. Even late-stage glomerulosclerosis demonstrates a marked increase in glomerular cell turnover (fourfold) by ^{3}H-thymidine labeling index, predominantly due to cells in the mesangial regions (165). Markers for cell proliferation also are upregulated in tissue repair and remodeling (166). A specific role for apoptosis has not yet been established in progressive renal diseases; however, increased cell growth is accompanied by increased apoptosis and altered regulators of this process both in proliferative and sclerotic glomerular diseases, as well as in acute and chronic tubular injuries (167,168). Increased apoptosis has been reported in human glomerular diseases, especially focal segmental glomerulosclerosis (167). The balance of apoptosis and proliferation (e.g., angiogenesis) is postulated to determine the ultimate phenotype of the glomerulus (140,169,170). Apoptosis may serve as a healing mechanism, minimizing stimulation of immune/inflammatory mechanisms and cytokines that occur in response to necrosis (171). However, apoptosis in disproportionate amounts also may serve to promote scarring, removing cells that may effect healing and matrix reabsorption. Mechanisms of apoptosis appear to vary among cell types and depend on the type of stimulus. Recent intriguing speculations postulate that ongoing subcellular apoptotic mechanisms may be important in regulating protein trafficking, clearing defective or other cellular elements by mechanisms similar to apoptosis (i.e., reabsorption/death by active processes that do not induce inflammation) (172).

INTERVENTION: MECHANISMS OF ACTIONS

Assessment of Interventions

Glomerular Filtration Rate

Regardless of the primary disease, progressive decline of GFR is used as a marker of ongoing structural damage. However, it is important to consider the determinants of GFR in this setting. Whole-kidney GFR reflects not only the number of functioning glomeruli but the sum of filtration in each of the heterogeneously affected glomeruli, which vary not only in degree of sclerosis but also degree of adaptation, including both hyperfiltration and growth. Even at advanced stages of structural injury, these compensatory mechanisms elevate GFR toward or even into the normal range. Injury perturbs glomerular function, proteinuria, and structure; however, the impact on each of these parameters is often divergent. Recently, the mechanisms underlying the divergence between function and structure were examined in a chronic cyclosporine-induced rat model. A combined antagonist against the endothelin A and endothelin B receptors offered a remarkable preservation in renal function but no benefit in the structural damage (173). By contrast, treatment with ACEI was associated with profound hypofiltration but ameliorated structural injury. The ACEI-linked hypoperfusion relates to augmentation of bradykinin and its specific effect to decrease efferent arteriolar tone and therefore decrease glomerular capillary pressure (174–176). These observations are particularly relevant because interruption of the renin angiotensin system by ACEI has become an important therapeutic intervention in lowering of blood pressure, decreasing proteinuria, and forestalling chronic deterioration in renal function. However, although renal vasodilatation and renal sparing are desirable therapeutic end points, a decrease in vascular resistance can also decrease glomerular capillary pressure, thereby removing an important compensatory mechanism to maintain GFR. This may be particularly important under conditions in which glomerular filtration is critically dependent on the heightened renin angiotensin system, which promotes efferent arteriolar maintenance of intraglomerular hydraulic pressure and, thus, GFR. The decrease in GFR in response to ACEI in such settings occurs even in the absence of profound systemic hypotension (176–178). Indeed, ACEI has been found to be the second most common cause of treatment-related decrease in GFR (179).

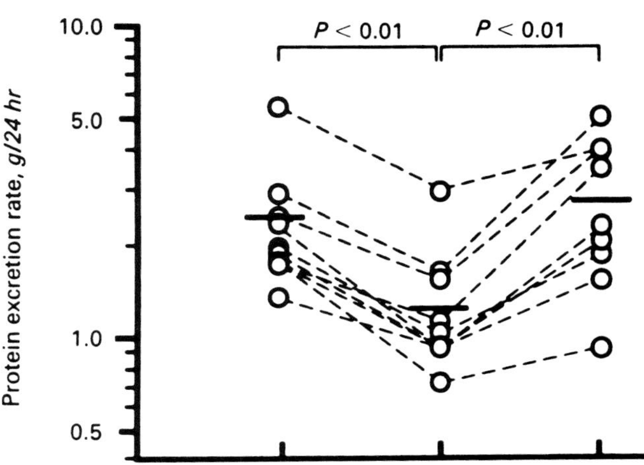

FIG. 9. Acute and reversible decrease of proteinuria in patients with IgA nephropathy with ACEI therapy. Reproduced with permission (180).

Proteinuria

The apparent level of proteinuria that has been widely used as an index of disease activity is also impacted by the hemodynamic effects of ACEI. Thus, changes in the magnitude of proteinuria have been taken to reflect the efficacy of therapeutic intervention, including dietary manipulation or antihypertensive treatment. However, it is now recognized that a given degree of proteinuria encompasses two separate components: one is acutely reversible (functional) proteinuria and the other is acutely nonreversible (fixed) proteinuria. Thus, ACEI acutely decreased not only proteinuria but also GFR in patients with IgA nephropathy, effects that were reversed upon discontinuation of ACEI treatment (180) (Fig. 9). That these functional antiproteinuric effects of ACEI relate to bradykinin was shown in animals because a bradykinin antagonist promptly dampened the antiproteinuric effects of ACEI (135). Thus, separate pathogenic mechanisms influence proteinuria. These observations underscore that efficacy of a given therapeutic intervention cannot be extrapolated from early effects on proteinuria. The beneficial effects of a given therapy on proteinuria may reflect its effects on intraglomerular hemodynamics or may reflect restoration toward normal glomerular capillary permeability.

Impact of Genetics

Heterogeneity in the extent or virulence of a given disease among individuals has long been recognized. Even when patients are stricken with a given disease, the risk of progression varies greatly. Only a portion of patients with, for example, diabetes mellitus, IgA nephropathy, or postinfectious glomerulonephritis develop progressive glomerulosclerosis. Recent efforts have been directed at

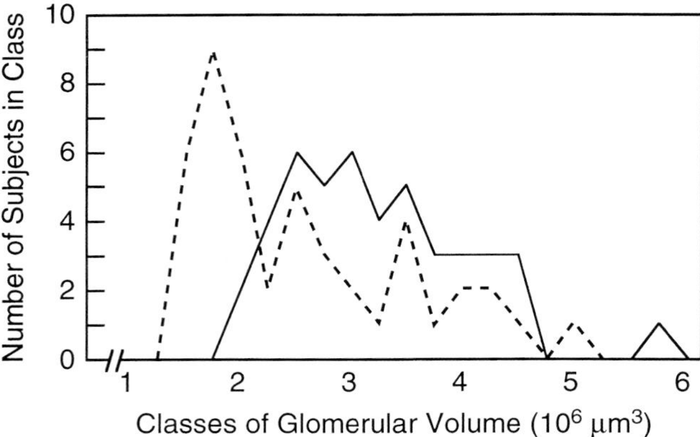

FIG. 10. Distribution of mean glomerular volume values in normal African Americans (n = 45, solid line) and Caucasians (n = 45, dotted line). Values from the total population are shown by the open bars. Each size class is identified by the lowest glomerular volume value. Redrawn with permission (187).

identifying risk for occurrence and progression of disease both by analysis of genetic susceptibilities and by molecular analysis of kidney tissue. A patient's genetic burden thus impacts assessment of progression due to increased variability of this process and influences the choice and efficacy of therapeutic interventions.

Genetic background can affect disease incidence. African Americans have a fourfold higher incidence of end-stage renal disease than do Caucasians. Abnormal glomerular size distribution was assessed as a possible indicator of underlying differences in populations in severity and incidence of risks for progressive renal disease. Kidneys from normal African American and Caucasian adults who died suddenly were assessed morphometrically (181). Average glomerular size in African Americans was significantly greater than in Caucasians. Of note, the distribution, while gaussian in African Americans, showed a biphasic distribution in Caucasians (Fig. 10). The subpopulation of Caucasians with larger glomeruli were postulated to have increased risk for progressive renal disease, comparable to the African American population. Other ethnic groups also have a disproportionately high occurrence of chronic renal failure. Pima Indians are particularly susceptible to non–insulin-dependent diabetes mellitus with nephropathy, and this population also has enlarged glomeruli even at baseline before nephropathy develops (182). The potential link between genotypes, altered matrix/sclerosing mechanisms, and increased glomerular size discussed above has not yet been examined.

Certain genotypes have been identified as potentially contributing to the occurrence of renal diseases (see Chapter 5). In African Americans, human leukocyte antigen (HLA)-DR3 was consistently associated with end-stage renal disease due to hypertension, diabetic nephropathy due to insulin-dependent diabetes mellitus, or membranous glomerulonephritis. In Caucasians, no association of HLA-DR3 with end-stage renal disease due to hypertension, IgA nephropathy, or FSGS was seen. However, excess HLA-D3 was present in Caucasians with end-stage renal disease when end-stage renal disease was caused by insulin-dependent diabetes mellitus, lupus, or membranous glomerulonephritis. The possibility that the HLA class II association is due to linkage disequilibrium with the HLA class III tumor necrosis factor locus is currently being investigated due to the close physical proximity of these two genes on chromosome 6 (183). Based on evidence thus far, differences in genetic makeup among different racial groups appear to influence the occurrence of renal disease.

There is also accumulating evidence that genes modulate the course and rate of progression. Polymorphisms in several genes within the renin angiotensin system, including ACE, angiotensinogen, and the receptor, have been linked with cardiovascular disorders, including hypertension, myocardial infarction, and cardiac hypertrophy (184–188). Polymorphisms of all three genes were recently evaluated in a cohort of Caucasian American patients with IgA nephropathy. The ACE DD genotype frequency was increased in the patients who ultimately experienced progressive decline in renal function during follow-up compared with those whose function remained stable over the same time. Notably, exclusion of patients with known risk factors for progression, such as hypertension and significant proteinuria, strengthened the association of the DD genotype and progression of renal dysfunction in IgA nephropathy (189) (Fig. 11). Two studies of Japanese and British populations observed similar linkage between progressive renal damage and ACE DD genotype in IgA nephropathy (190,191). Although environmental and other genetic factors may contribute, similar ACE polymorphism distributions in progressive IgA nephropathy in genetically distinct and geographically remote populations point to a significant functional role for the deletion allele of the ACE polymorphism.

Scrutiny of the sequence of ACE intron 16 encompassing the I/D segment showed a repeated 14–base pair (bp) sequence, comprising 14 terminal bases of one end of the insert and flanking the opposite end, comprising the next 14 bases that follow. The arrangement of these two repeats suggests a possible origin of the D allele. During meiosis, one of these two repeats could align with the complement of the other, thus producing a loop-out of the intervening 287-bp fragment. This observation suggests that the mutational event may actually occur by a deletion rather than by an insertion (192). Interestingly, in normal Caucasians, those with the II genotype have the lowest serum ACE levels, DD subjects have the highest, and those with the ID genotype have intermediate levels, supporting the notion that the D allele contributes to the activation of ACE (193). This suggests that the insert may contain a silencer element, the absence of which activates the ACE gene. Furthermore, normotensive men with the

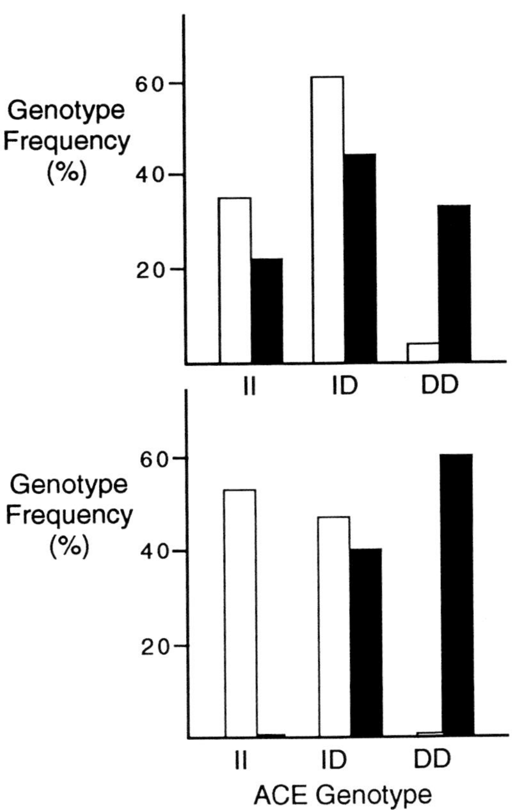

FIG. 11. Top: Frequency of ACE genotypes in patients who maintained stable renal function *(open bars)* and those who developed progressive renal dysfunction *(filled bars)*. **Bottom:** Frequency of ACE genotypes in patients without hypertension or heavy proteinuria who maintained stable renal function *(open bars)* and those who developed progressive renal dysfunction *(filled bars)*. Note, no II patient in this group progressed, whereas no DD patient remained stable. Reproduced with permission (189).

DD genotype had increased systemic pressor responsiveness to infusion of Ang I when compared with II genotypes, strengthening the postulate that the ACE polymorphism has functional relevance (194). The plasma concentrations of Ang II were also higher across the dose range of Ang I infusion, implying increased generation of Ang II in the DD individuals. Nonetheless, it is also possible that the identified polymorphic locus, although affecting ACE levels, may only be a marker for another gene variant that more directly contributes to renal functional deterioration.

Mechanisms of Therapeutic Interventions

Renin Angiotensin System

Morphologic and molecular heterogeneity discussed above affect responsiveness to therapies. Recently, antihypertensives have become the mainstay of warding off progressive renal destruction. Therapies that inhibit the renin angiotensin system appear particularly effective in both human and animal models. However, the efficacy in humans has been assessed only by GFR and not by effects on structural lesions. The mechanisms of actions of antihypertensive therapies rely not only on decreasing blood pressure but include effects on growth. Treatment with ACEI markedly attenuated glomerular growth and ameliorated glomerulosclerosis in the renal ablation model (34,149,195) and decreased glomerulosclerosis even in a nonhypertensive model (135). Furthermore, ACEI attenuated hypertrophy of nonrenal blood vessels independently of its vasodilative effects in animals with hypertension (196). The mechanisms by which Ang II affects growth and matrix include both direct and indirect effects via thrombospondin, fibronectin, tenascin, glucosaminoglycan expression, and induction of other growth factors, including basic FGF, PDGF, and TGF-β (2,155). The effects of angiotensin to induce plasminogen activator inhibitor provides a link of the renin angiotensin system to thrombosis and may be mediated by the Ang IV ligand (197,198). In addition, Ang II affects migration of endothelial cells and vascular smooth muscle cells and induces both hypertrophy and hyperplasia of both smooth muscle cells and mesangial cells (2,199). Ang II is present in monocytes, which may thus serve as yet another source of Ang II in immune-mediated glomerular injuries (200). Recent studies have shown that local transfection to the carotid artery of ACE resulted in increased DNA synthesis and medial hypertrophy, associated with local Ang II generation without systemic changes (201,202). Glomerular transfection in vivo with angiotensinogen or renin similarly induced activation of mesangial cells and increased matrix (203). The net effect of Ang II thus depends on the balance of its induction of proliferative growth factors such as PDGF and basic FGF, versus TGF-β1, which inhibits or promotes cellular proliferation depending on the specific conditions.

Recent observations further complicate predictions regarding consequences of long-term Ang II inhibition. In this regard, knockout mice deficient for angiotensinogen surprisingly developed pronounced vascular lesions and mesangial matrix expansion, despite hypotension (204,205). These lesions were accompanied by upregulated PDGF-B and TGF-β in the cortex and in vascular lesions. Similarly, in transgenic growth hormone mice treated with high-dose ACEI or Ang II receptor antagonist, vascular thickening and juxtaglomerular apparatus hyperplasia occurred (206). These findings point to the interactions of growth factors in maintaining not only normal tone of the vasculature, but also normal structure. Taken together, these observations reiterate that a balance among growth factors is key in both development as well as intervention in disease processes.

The similar effects on preservation of structure with ACEI and Ang II receptor antagonists in several models

(135,196) have been taken as evidence for the key role of Ang II in structural injury. However, recent evidence points to a role of aldosterone in progressive injury. Added benefits were seen with addition of aldosterone antagonism over angiotensin inhibition alone in experimental renal disease (207). In addition to aldosterone's well-defined effects on electrolyte transport, aldosterone is now recognized to modulate cardiovascular collagen accumulation and ventricular hypertrophy (208). These effects appear to not be dependent on sodium and volume status, but may rather be linked to aldosterone effects on potassium, and potassium's tropic effects (209).

There is accumulating evidence that response to therapy depends on the stage of injury. Animal studies with delayed onset of treatment to mimic the clinical setting showed that progressive sclerosis was only attenuated in glomeruli with a mild degree of sclerosis when ACEI therapy was started. In contrast, those glomeruli with more advanced sclerosis (greater than 50% of the tuft sclerosed) showed continued, progressive sclerosis (149). These findings emphasize that early aggressive treatment is important not only in limiting initial injury, but in controlling progression, or even potentially allowing remodeling of early lesions. Of great interest, higher doses of ACEI (having the same hemodynamic effects) showed even greater efficacy (149). In some animals glomerular sclerosis was even reversed after high-dose treatment with ACEI. This potential to decrease established glomerulosclerosis also was demonstrated in a study of rats with puromycin aminonucleoside nephropathy that were treated with a low-protein diet and ACEI (210). Reversal of vascular lesions also was seen in resistance vessels in hypertensive patients treated with ACEI, but not in those treated with beta-blocker (211). It remains uncertain whether ACEI-induced decrease of sclerosis actually reverses the same course that advanced the structural damage, or if ACEI remodels glomerular structure into an altered phenotype. Current evidence supports the notion that ongoing dynamic remodeling of the glomerulus occurs even at stages of established sclerosis. The glomerular size in the above high-dose ACEI studies did not return to normal, but rather remained abnormally enlarged, indicating that ongoing remodeling indeed is a dynamic process, not merely passively returning the glomerulus to a baseline status. Thus, the presence of nonsclerosed glomeruli in human FSGS provides a rationale for aggressive therapy to effectively ameliorate, or even reverse, ongoing sclerogenic mechanisms. The application of these conclusions is currently being investigated in patients with diabetes with normal renal function and absence of overt proteinuria. Further molecular studies may pinpoint key mediators in the microenvironment of the glomerulus. This molecular staging in combination with assessment of the patient's individual risk profile determined by genotype, may provide accurate prediction of risk for progression and form the basis for optimal effective intervention.

Dietary Protein

A high-protein diet accelerates progression of renal disease in rats regardless of the primary injury (30,212). A high-protein diet increases expression of other growth factors, including those of the renin angiotensin system (213). Protection with a low-protein diet has been observed in several rat models (214). Studies have attempted to unravel exactly which component(s) of the low-protein diets are critical for this beneficial effect. However, the altered dietary protein also resulted in changes in other dietary components. Postulated dietary mediators of progressive renal disease include calcium, salt, phosphate, and fat. Reduction in calorie intake per se may be a pivotal factor in the protection against progressive injury (67). A low-protein diet slowed progression in the nonhypertensive puromycin aminonucleoside nephropathy model; when combined with ACEI therapy, sclerosis was even reversed (210). A high-protein diet that accelerated progression augmented gene expression of the renin angiotensin system both in normal rats and in those with renal ablation (215). These findings provide a potential basis for the augmented effects of the combined ACEI and low-protein therapy. Additional mechanisms postulated for the effect of low-protein diets include altered T-cell function, decreases in macrophage influx, decreased TGF-β expression (38), calcium-phosphate precipitation–induced tubular injury, proteinuria, oxygen radicals (216), and decreased plasma IGF-1 (217).

The recently published data of the Modification of Diet in Renal Disease Study did not demonstrate the expected dramatic effects of protein restriction on progression, perhaps not surprising in view of the diverse underlying conditions in the populations studied (218). The resistance to therapy in some diseases, such as polycystic kidney disease, may reflect the heterogeneous mechanisms in different renal diseases. A further caveat in extrapolating from these studies is to consider the differences of the experimental models and human renal disease (216). The renal ablation model in the rat is characterized by marked compensatory growth as well as ongoing maturational growth. Rats continue to have renal and especially glomerular growth during most of their life span, contrasting with humans, in whom glomerular growth is complete when body growth is completed. Therefore, the effects of restricted diets that affect both maturational and pathophysiologic growth processes may be more extreme in rats than it is in humans.

Glucocorticoids

Glucocorticoids have long been used in the treatment of glomerulonephritides having an immunologic/inflammatory component and affect many processes involved in progressive renal damage. They may provide benefit by decreasing chemotaxis, inhibiting antibody production or suppression of infiltrating leukocyte accumulation, inhibition of cytokine secretion, and lessening cell adhesion interactions (219–221). However, glucocorticoids also have been shown to be effective in renal diseases without an apparent immunologic/inflammatory component. Interestingly, animal models, such as puromycin aminonucleoside nephropathy, which closely resembles human minimal change disease but lacks clear evidence for immunologic or inflammatory events, responds to glucocorticoid treatment (222,223). Glucocorticoids may effect nonimmunologic pathways, which include modulation of ROS and modulation of growth or cellular proliferation. Each of these factors may in turn affect progression of renal disease. Glucocorticoids also can modulate apoptosis (224,225), eliminating certain populations of cells and leaving resistant cells, thus decreasing potential cytokine release from cells more susceptible to injury.

Glucocorticoids may be beneficial in ROS-mediated injuries through their capacity to upregulate antioxidant enzymes, particularly manganese superoxide dismutase (MnSOD). Treatment with methylprednisolone significantly increased glomerular levels of antioxidants, especially MnSOD, and induced tolerance to a variety of oxidant stresses (125). Conversely, depletion of MnSOD exacerbated puromycin nephropathy in rats (226). These glucocorticoid-mediated effects showed cell specificity in the regulation of the MnSOD gene that was under transcriptional control (29). Thus, glomerular endothelial cells and mesangial cells, but not glomerular epithelial cells, responded to glucocorticoid treatment. The benefit from glucocorticoid-induced antioxidants in renal disease also may reflect effects on circulating cells, another key source of oxygen radicals. Thus, the elevated superoxide production from neutrophils harvested from patients with antineutrophil cytoplasmic antibody-positive nephritis could be normalized by glucocorticoid treatment (227). Of note, glucocorticoids also have potential adverse effects. These include increased systemic pressure and indirect inhibition of collagenase (2). Of note, glucocorticoid did not protect against glomerulosclerosis in chronic puromycin nephropathy, although proteinuria was mildly decreased (228). Recently, a direct effect of glucocorticoid to induce ACE gene expression was documented in vitro. This induction occurred in both endothelial and vascular smooth muscle cells, but endothelial cells were more sensitive (229). These findings imply that glucocorticoids can affect vascular remodeling, and also impact on therapeutic consequences of long-term glucocorticoid treatment.

SUMMARY

Progression cannot be summarized as a linear culmination of events common to all diseases in which glomeruli scar. Disease- and stage-specific mechanisms are just being studied at a higher resolution, including via molecular profiles. Evidence is emerging that the genetically fixed components (patient's DNA) may significantly influence the dynamic molecular responses (mRNA of matrix promoting factors). The newly available techniques to develop animal models with specific enhancement or deletion of genes at targeted sites, along with sophisticated methods to apply molecular analysis to small tissue samples, herald exciting advances in investigation of these mechanisms of progression. This new era includes consideration not only of stage of injury, mapping heterogeneity of injury, and molecular indices in glomerular and extraglomerular renal tissues, but also the potential impact of the patient's own genetic burden. Information thus analyzed can then predict not only nature and magnitude of injury, but also dictate stage-specific optimal therapy and predict response in individual patients.

ACKNOWLEDGMENT

Agnes Fogo and Valentina Kon are recipients of Established Investigator Awards from the American Heart Association.

REFERENCES

1. Hostetter TH, Olson JL, Rennke HG, Venkatachalam MA, Brenner BM. Hyperfiltration in remnant nephrons: a potentially adverse response to renal ablation. *Am J Physiol* 1981;241:F85–F93.
2. Fogo A, Ichikawa I. Glomerular growth promoter—the common channel to glomerular sclerosis. In: Mitch WE, ed. *Contemporary issues in nephrology: the progressive nature of renal disease.* 2nd ed. New York: Churchill Livingstone; 1992:23–54.
3. Neuringer JR, Anderson S, Brenner BM. The role of systemic and intraglomerular hypertension. In: Mitch WE, ed. *The progressive nature of renal disease.* Vol 26. New York: Churchill Livingstone; 1992:1–21.
4. Mitch WE, Walser M, Buffington GA, Lemann JJ. A simple method of estimating progression of chronic renal failure. *Lancet* 1976;2:1326–1328.
5. Danoff TM, Chiang MY, Ortiz A, Neilson EG. Transcriptional regulation of murine RANTES (MuR) in proximal tubular cells [Abstract]. *J Am Soc Nephrol* 1993;4:599.
6. Ott MJ, Olsen JL, Ballermann BJ. Phenotypic differences between glomerular capillary (GE) and aortic (AE) endothelial cells in vitro [Abstract]. *J Am Soc Nephrol* 1993;4:564.
7. Lee LK, Pollock AS, Lovett DH. Asymmetric origins of the mature glomerular basement membrane. *J Cell Physiol* 1993;157:169–177.
8. Zager RA. Acute renal failure in the setting of bone marrow transplantation. *Kidney Int* 1994;46:1443–1458.
9. Gerritsen ME, Bloor CM. Endothelial cell gene expression in response to injury. *FASEB J* 1993;7:523–532.
10. Haijar DP, Pomerantz KB. Signal transduction in atherosclerosis: integration of cytokines and the eicosanoid network. *FASEB J* 1992;6:2933–2941.
11. Casscells W. Migration of smooth muscle and endothelial cells: critical events in restenosis. *Circulation* 1992;86:723–729.
12. Bruijn JA, de Heer E. Adhesion molecules in renal disease. *Lab Invest* 1995;72:387–394.
13. Farquhar MG, Kerjaschki D, Lundstrom M, Orland RA. gp330 and RAP: the Heyman nephritis antigenic complex. *Ann NY Acad Sci* 1994;737:96–113.
14. Fries JWU, Sandstrom DJ, Meyer TW, Rennke HG. Glomerular hypertrophy and epithelial cell injury modulate progressive glomerulosclerosis in the rat. *Lab Invest* 1989;60:205–218.

15. Rennke HG. How does glomerular epithelial cell injury contribute to progressive glomerular damage? *Kidney Int* 1994;45(suppl 45): 58–63.
16. Aiello LP, Avery RL, Arrigg PG, et al. Vascular endothelial growth factor in ocular fluid of patients with diabetic retinopathy and other retinal disorders. *N Engl J Med* 1994;331:1480–1487.
17. Pe'er J, Shweiki D, Itin A, Hemo I, Gnessin H, Keshet E. Hypoxia-induced expression of vascular endothelial growth factor by retinal cells is a common factor in neovascularizing ocular diseases. *Lab Invest* 1995;72:638–645.
18. Adler S, Chen X. Anti-Fx1A antibody recognizes a β1-integrin on glomerular epithelial cell and inhibits adhesion and cell growth. *Am J Physiol* 1992;31:F770–F776.
19. Salant DJ. The structural biology of glomerular epithelial cells in proteinuric diseases. *Curr Opin Nephrol Hypertens* 1994;3:569–574.
20. Kemeny E, Mihatsch MJ, Durmuller U, Gudat F. Podocytes loose their adhesive phenotype in focal segmental glomerulosclerosis. *Clin Nephrol* 1995;43:71–83.
21. Kriz W, Hosser H, Simons JL, Provoost AP. In Fawn-hooded (FHH) rats focal segmental glomerulosclerosis (FSGS) preferentially develops at the vascular pole [Abstract]. *J Am Soc Nephrol* 1995;6:1019.
22. Nagata M, Schärer K, Kriz W. Glomerular damage after uninephrectomy in young rats. I. Hypertrophy and distortion of capillary architecture. *Kidney Int* 1992;42:136–147.
23. Fogo A, Kawamura T, Ikoma M, Kon V, Ichikawa I. Role for the mesangium in glomerular neutrophil entrapment [Abstract]. *Kidney Int* 1990;37:551.
24. Ichikawa I, Yoshioka T, Fogo A, Kon V. Role of angiotensin II in altered glomerular hemodynamics in congestive heart failure. *Kidney Int* 1990;38(suppl 30):123–126.
25. Kakinuma Y, Fogo A, Inagami T, Ichikawa I. Intrarenal localization of angiotensin II type 1 receptor mRNA in the rat. *Kidney Int* 1993; 43:1229–1235.
26. Fogo A, Glick AD, Horn SL, Horn RG. Is focal segmental glomerulosclerosis really focal? Distribution of lesions in adults and children. *Kidney Int* 1995;47:1690–1696.
27. Morrison AB, Howard RM. The functional capacity of hypertrophied nephrons: effect of partial nephrectomy on the clearance of inulin and PAH in the rat. *J Exp Med* 1966;123:829–844.
28. Shimamura T, Morrison AB. A progressive glomerulosclerosis occurring in partial five-sixths nephrectomized rats. *Am J Pathol* 1975; 79:95–106.
29. Yoshioka T, Kawamura T, Meyrick BO, et al. Induction of manganese superoxide dismutase by glucocorticoids in glomerular cells. *Kidney Int* 1994;45:211–219.
30. Brenner BM, Meyer TW, Hostetter TH. Dietary protein intake and the progressive nature of kidney disease: the role of hemodynamically mediated glomerular injury in the pathogenesis of progressive glomerular sclerosis in aging, renal ablation, and intrinsic renal disease. *N Engl J Med* 1982;307:652–659.
31. Nath KA, Kren SM, Hostetter TH. Dietary protein restriction in established renal injury in the rat. Selective role of glomerular capillary pressure in progressive glomerular dysfunction. *J Clin Invest* 1986;78:1199–1205.
32. Nyengaard JR. Number and dimensions of rat glomerular capillaries in normal development and after nephrectomy. *Kidney Int* 1993;43: 1049–1057.
33. Hostetter TH, Meyer TW, Rennke HG, Brenner BM, Noddin JA, Sandstrom DJ. Chronic effects of dietary protein in the rat with intact and reduced renal mass. *Kidney Int* 1986;30:509–517.
34. Anderson S, Meyer TW, Rennke HG, Brenner BM. Control of glomerular hypertension limits glomerular injury in rats with reduced renal mass. *J Clin Invest* 1985;76:612–619.
35. Yoshida Y, Fogo A, Ichikawa I. Glomerular hemodynamic changes vs. hypertrophy in experimental glomerular sclerosis. *Kidney Int* 1989;35:654–660.
36. Kasiske BL, Kalil RSN, Ma JZ, Liao M, Keane WF. Effect of antihypertensive therapy on the kidney in patients with diabetes: a meta-regression analysis. *Ann Intern Med* 1993;118:129–138.
37. Yoshida H, Nakamura M. Inhibition by angiotensin converting enzyme inhibitors of endothelin secretion from cultured human endothelial cells. *Life Sci* 1992;50:PL195–200.
38. Okuda S, Nakamura T, Yamamoto T, Ruoslahti E, Border WA. Dietary protein restriction rapidly reduces transforming growth factor β1 expression in experimental glomerulonephritis. *Proc Natl Acad Sci U S A* 1991;88:9765–9769.
39. Yoshida Y, Fogo A, Shiraga H, Glick AD, Ichikawa I. Serial micropuncture analysis of single nephron function in the rat model of subtotal renal ablation. *Kidney Int* 1988;33:855–867.
40. Fogo A, Yoshida Y, Glick AD, Homma T, Ichikawa I. Serial micropuncture analysis of glomerular function in two rat models of glomerular sclerosis. *J Clin Invest* 1988;82:322–330.
41. Anderson S, Rennke HG, Brenner BM. Short and long term effects of antihypertensive therapy in the diabetic rat. *Kidney Int* 1989;36: 526–536.
42. Daniels BS, Hostetter TH. Adverse effects of growth in the glomerular microcirculation. *Am J Physiol* 1990;258:F1409–F1416.
43. Dworkin LD, Levin RI, Bernstein JA, et al. Effects of nifedipine and enalapril on glomerular injury in rats with deoxycorticosterone-salt hypertension. *Am J Physiol* 1990;259:F598–F604.
44. Dworkin LD, Feiner HD, Parker M, Tolbert E. Effects of nifedipine and enalapril on glomerular structure and function in uninephrectomized SHR. *Kidney Int* 1991;39:1112–1117.
45. Marcussen N, Nyengaard JR, Christensen S. Compensatory growth of glomeruli is accomplished by an increased number of glomerular capillaries. *Lab Invest* 1994;70:868–874.
46. Nyengaard JR, Rasch R. The impact of experimental diabetes mellitus in rats on glomerular capillary number and sizes. *Diabetologia* 1993;36:189–194.
47. Akaoka K, White RHR, Raafat F. Glomerular morphometry in childhood reflux nephropathy, emphasizng the capillary changes. *Kidney Int* 1995;47:1108–1114.
48. Harris RC, Haralson MA, Badr KF. Continuous stretch-relaxation in culture alters mesangial cell morphology, growth characteristics, and metabolic activity. *Lab Invest* 1992;66:548–554.
49. Kawata Y, Fujii Z, Sakumura T, Umemoto S, Yamakawa K. High pressure promotes the proliferation of rat cultured mesangial cells in vitro [Abstract]. *J Am Soc Nephrol* 1995;6:1017.
50. Morigi M, Zoja C, Figliuzzi M, Remuzzi G, Remuzzi A. Supernatant of endothelial cells exposed to laminar flow inhibits mesangial cell proliferation. *Am J Physiol* 1993;264:C1080–C1083.
51. Ott MJ, Ballermann BJ. Shear stress augments glomerular endothelial cell (GEN) PDGF mRNA expression and mitogen production. *J Am Soc Nephrol* 1992;3:476.
52. Yoshizumi M, Kurihara H, Sugiyama T, et al. Hemodynamic shear stress stimulates endothelin production by cultured endothelial cells. *Biochem Biophys Res Commun* 1989;161:859–864.
53. Kuchan MJ, Frangos JA. Shear stress regulates endothelin-1 release via protein kinase C and cGMP in cultured endothelial cell. *Am J Physiol* 1993;264:H150–H156.
54. Malek AM, Greene AL, Izumo S. Regulation of endothelin 1 gene by fluid shear stress is transcriptionally mediated and independent of protein kinase C and cAMP. *Proc Natl Acad Sci U S A* 1993;90: 5999–6003.
55. Garcia DL, Anderson S, Rennke HG, Brenner BM. Anemia lessens and its prevention with recombinant human erythropoietin worsens glomerular injury and hypertension in rats with reduced renal mass. *Proc Natl Acad Sci U S A* 1988;85:6142–6146.
56. Shand BI, Bailey RR, Lynn KL, Robson RA. Effect on enalapril on hemorheology in hypertensive patients with renal disease. *Clin Exp Hypertens* 1995;17:689–700.
57. Elfenbein IB, Baluarte HJ, Gruskin AB. Renal hypoplasia with oligomeganephronia. *Arch Pathol* 1974;97:143–149.
58. Bhathena DB. Nephronopenic focal segmental glomerulosclerosis (FGS) and glomerular size [Abstract]. *J Am Soc Nephrol* 1995;6:1010.
59. Rich AR. A hitherto undescribed vulnerability of the juxta-medullary glomeruli in lipoid nephrosis. *Bull Johns Hopkins Hosp* 1957;100: 173–186.
60. Aschinberg LC, Koskimies O, Bernstein J, Nash M, Edelmann CM Jr, Spitzer A. The influence of age on the response to renal parencymal loss. *Yale J Biol Med* 1978;51:341–345.
61. O'Donnell MP, Kasiske BL, Raij L, Keane WF. Age is a determinant of the glomerular morphologic and functional responses to chronic nephron loss. *J Lab Clin Med* 1985;106:308–313.
62. Ikoma M, Yoshioka T, Ichikawa I, Fogo A. Mechanism of the unique susceptibility of deep cortical glomeruli of maturing kidneys to severe focal glomerular sclerosis. *Pediatr Res* 1990;28:270–276.

63. Doi T, Striker LJ, Gibson CC, Agodoa LYC, Brinster RL, Striker GE. Glomerular lesions in mice transgenic for growth hormone and insulinlike growth factor-I. I. Relationship between increased glomerular size and mesangial sclerosis. *Am J Pathol* 1990;137:541–552.
64. El Nahas AM, Bassett AH, Cope GH, Le Carpentier JE. Role of growth hormone in the development of experimental renal scarring. *Kidney Int* 1991;40:29–34.
65. Allen DB, Fogo A, El-Hayek R, Langhough R, Friedman AL. Effects of prolonged growth hormone administration in rats with chronic renal insufficiency. *Pediatr Res* 1992;31:406–410.
66. Yoshida H, Mitarai T, Kitamura M, et al. The effect of selective growth hormone defect in the progression of glomerulosclerosis. *Am J Kidney Dis* 1994;23:302–312.
67. Tapp DC, Wortham WG, Addison JF, Hammonds DN, Barnes JL, Venkatachalam MA. Food restriction retards body growth and renal pathology in remnant kidneys regardless of protein intake. *Lab Invest* 1989;60:184–195.
68. Østerby R, Parving HH, Nyberg G, et al. A strong correlation between glomerular filtration rate and filtration surface in diabetic nephropathy. *Diabetologia* 1988;31:265–270.
69. Mauer SM, Steffes MW, Ellis EN, Sutherland DER, Brown DM, Goetz FC. Structural–functional relationships in diabetic nephropathy. *J Clin Invest* 1984;74:1143–1155.
70. Jennette JC, Marquis A, Falk RJ, Bodick N. Glomerulomegaly in focal segmental glomerulosclerosis (FSGS) but not minimal change glomerulopathy (MCG) [Abstract]. *Lab Invest* 1990;62:48.
71. Fogo A, Hawkins EP, Berry PL, et al. Glomerular hypertrophy in minimal change disease predicts subsequent progression to focal glomerular sclerosis. *Kidney Int* 1990;38:115–123.
72. Vats AN, Basgen JM, Steffes MW, Mauer M. Mean glomerular volume (GV) in minimal change nephrotic syndrome (MCNS), focal segmental glomerulosclerosis (FSGS), normal children and adults [Abstract]. *J Am Soc Nephrol* 1994;5:797.
73. Fogo A, Hawkins EP, Verani R, MacDonell RC Jr, Ichikawa I. Focal segmental glomerulosclerosis (FGS) in renal transplants is associated with marked glomerular hypertrophy [Abstract]. *J Am Soc Nephrol* 1991;2:797.
74. Nath KA, Hostetter MK, Hostetter TH. Increased ammoniagenesis as a determinant of progressive renal injury. *Am J Kidney Dis* 1991;17: 654–657.
75. Keane WF, Mulcahy WS, Kasiske BL, Kim Y, O'Donnell MP. Hyperlipidemia and progressive renal disease. *Kidney Int* 1991;39 (suppl 31):41–48.
76. Klahr S, Schreiner G, Ichikawa I. Nonimmunologic mechanisms of glomerular injury. *Lab Invest* 1988;59:564–578.
77. Fine LG, Hammerman MR, Abboud HE. Evolving role of growth factors in the renal response to acute and chronic disease. *J Am Soc Nephrol* 1992;2:1163–1170.
78. Abboud HE. Growth factors and the mesangium. *J Am Soc Nephrol* 1992;2(suppl):185–189.
79. Striker LJ, Peten EP, Elliott SJ, Doi T, Striker GE. Mesangial cell turnover: effect of heparin and peptide growth factors. *Lab Invest* 1991;64:446–456.
80. Johnson RJ, Raines EW, Floege J, et al. Inhibition of mesangial cell proliferation and matrix expansion in glomerulonephritis in the rat by antibody to platelet-derived growth factor. *J Exp Med* 1992;175: 1413–1416.
81. Border WA, Okuda S, Languino LR, Sporn MB, Ruoslahti E. Suppression of experimental glomerulonephritis by antiserum against transforming growth factor β1. *Nature* 1990;346:371–374.
82. The Diabetes Control and Complications Trial Research Group. The effect of intensive treatment of diabetes on the development and progression of long-term complications in insulin-dependent diabetes mellitus. *N Engl J Med* 1993;329:977–986.
83. Barbosa J, Steffes MW, Sutherland DER, Connett JE, Rao KV, Mauer SM. Effect of glycemic control on early diabetic renal lesions: A 5-year randomized controlled clinical trial of insulin-dependent diabetic kidney transplant recipients. *JAMA* 1994;272:600–606.
84. Mathiesen ER, Hommel E, Giese J, Parving HH. Efficacy of captopril in postponing nephropathy in normotensive insulin dependent diabetic patients with microalbumionuria. *Br Med J* 1991;303:81–87.
85. Bilous RW, Mauer SM, Sutherland DER, Steffes MW. Mean glomerular volume and rate of development of diabetic nephropathy. *Diabetes* 1989;38:1142–1147.
86. Bangstad HJ, Østerby R, Dahl-Jørgensen K, et al. Early glomerulopathy is present in young, type 1 (insulin-dependent) diabetic patients with microalbuminuria. *Diabetologia* 1993;36:523–529.
87. Chavers BM, Bilous RW, Ellis EN, Steffes MW, Mauer SM. Glomerular lesions and urinary albumin excretion in type I diabetes without overt proteinuria. *N Engl J Med* 1989;320:966–970.
88. Bilous RW, Mauer SM, Sutherland DER, Najarian JS, Goetz FC, Steffes MW. The effects of pancreas transplantation on the glomerular structure of renal allografts inpatients with insulin-dependent diabetes. *N Engl J Med* 1989;321:80–85.
89. Breyer J. Diabetic nephropathy in insulin-dependent patients. *Am J Kidney Dis* 1992;20:533–547.
90. Ziyadeh FN. The extracellular matrix in diabetic nephropathy. *Am J Kidney Dis* 1993;22:736–744.
91. Kreisberg JI. Hyperglycemia and microangiopathy. Direct regulation by glucose of microvascular cells. *Lab Invest* 1992;67:416–426.
92. Flyvbjerg A, Marshall SM, Frystyk J, Hansen KW, Harris AG, Ørskov H. Octreotide administration in diabetic rats: effects on renal hypertrophy and urinary albumin excretion. *Kidney Int* 1992;41: 805–812.
93. Vlassara H, Striker LJ, Teichberg S, Fuh H, Li YM, Steffes M. Advanced glycation end products induce glomerular sclerosis and albuminuria in normal rats. *Proc Natl Acad Sci U S A* 1994;91: 11704–11708.
94. Yang C-W, Vlassara H, Peten EP, He CJ, Striker GE, Striker LJ. Advanced glycation end products up-regulate expression found in diabetic glomerular disease. *Proc Natl Acad Sci U S A* 1994;91: 9436–9440.
95. Cohen MP, Sharma K, Jin Y, et al. Prevention of diabetic nephropathy in db/db mice with glycated albumin antagonists: a novel treatment strategy. *J Clin Invest* 1995;95:2338–2345.
96. Yang C-W, Vlassara H, Striker GE, Striker LJ. Administration of AGEs in vivo induces genes implicated in diabetic glomerulosclerosis. *Kidney Int* 1995;47(suppl 49):55–58.
97. Makita Z, Radoff S, Rayfield EJ, et al. Advanced glycosylation end products in patients with diabetic nephropathy. *N Engl J Med* 1991; 325:836–842.
98. Moorhead JF. Lipids and progressive kidney disease. *Kidney Int* 1991;39(suppl 31):35–40.
99. Diamond JR. Effect of lipid abnormalities on the progression of renal damage. Analogous pathobiologic mechanisms in glomerulosclerosis and atherosclerosis. *Kidney Int* 1991;39(suppl 31):29–34.
100. Jennette JC, Charles L, Grubb W. Glomerulomegaly and focal segmental glomerulosclerosis associated with obesity and sleep-apnea syndrome. *Am J Kidney Dis* 1987;10:470.
101. Kasiske BL, O'Donnell MP, Garvis WJ, Keane WF. Pharmacologic treatment of hyperlipidemia reduces glomerular injury in rat 5/6 nephrectomy model of chronic renal failure. *Circ Res* 1988;62: 367–374.
102. Hirano T, Morchoshi T. Treatment of hyperlipidaemia with probucol suppresses the development of focal and segmental glomerulosclerosis in chronic aminonucleoside nephrosis. *Nephron* 1992;60:443–447.
103. Modi K, Schreiner GF, Purkerson ML, Klahr S. Effects of probucol on renal function and structure in rats with subtotal kidney ablation. *J Lab Clin Med* 1992;120:310–317.
104. Kasiske BL, O'Donnell MP, Cleary MP, Keane WF. Treatment of hyperlipidemia reduces glomerular injury in obese Zucker rats. *Kidney Int* 1988;33:667–672.
105. van Goor H, Fidler V, Weening JJ, Grond J. Determinants of focal and segmental glomerulosclerosis in the rat after renal ablation. Evidence for involvement of macrophages and lipids. *Lab Invest* 1991;64:754.
106. Ding G, Pesek-Diamond I, Diamond JR. Cholesterol, macrophages, and gene expression of TGF-β1 and fibronectin during nephrosis. *Am J Physiol* 1993;33:F577–F584.
107. Schreiner GF, Rovin BH, Lefkowith JB. The anti-inflammatory effects of essential fatty acid deficiency in experimental glomerulonephritis: the modulation of macrophage migration and eicosanoid metabolism. *J Immunol* 1989;143:3192–3199.
108. Keane WF, Kasiske BL, O'Donnell MP. Hyperlipidemia and the progression of renal disease. *Am J Clin Nutr* 1988;47:157–160.
109. Washio M, Nanishi F, Okuda S, Onoyama K, Fujishima M. Alpha tocopherol improves focal glomerulosclerosis in rats with adriamycin-induced progressive renal failure. *Nephron* 1994;68:347–352.
110. Shah SV. Effect of enzymatically generated reactive oxygen metabo-

lites on the cyclic nucleotide content in isolated rat glomeruli. *J Clin Invest* 1984;74:393–401.
111. Shah SV, Baricos WH, Basci A. Degradation of human glomerular basement membrane by stimulated neutrophils: activation of a metalloproteinase/s by reactive oxygen metabolites. *J Clin Invest* 1987;79: 25–31.
112. Rehan A, Johnson KJ, Wiggins RC, Kunkel RG, Ward PA. Evidence for the role of oxygen radicals in acute nephrotoxic nephritis. *Lab Invest* 1984;51:396–403.
113. Rehan A, Johnson KJ, Kunkel RG, Wiggins RC. Role of oxygen radicals in phorbol myristate acetate-induced glomerular injury. *Kidney Int* 1985;27:503–511.
114. Rehan A, Wiggins RC, Kunkel RG, Till GO, Johnson KJ. Glomerular injury and proteinuria in rats after intrarenal injection of cobra venom factor. *Am J Physiol* 1986;123:57–66.
115. Paller MS, Hoidal JR, Ferris TF. Oxygen free radicals in ischemic acute renal failure in the rat. *J Clin Invest* 1984;74:1156–1164.
116. Walker PD, Shah SV. Evidence suggesting a role for hydroxyl radical in gentamicin-induced acute renal failure in rats. *J Clin Invest* 1988; 81:334–341.
117. Walker PD, Shah SV. Gentamicin enhanced production of hydrogen peroxide by renal cortical mitochondria. *Am J Physiol* 1987;253: 495–499.
118. Chandrrasekar B, Fernandes G. Decreased pro-inflammatory cytokines and increased antioxidant enzyme gene expression by omega-3 lipids in murine lupus nephritis. *Biochem Biophys Res Commun* 1994; 200:893–898.
119. van der Heide JJH, Bilo HJG, Donker JM, Wilmink JM, Tegzess AM. Effect of dietary fish oil on renal function and rejection in cyclosporine-treated recipients of renal transplants. *N Engl J Med* 1993;329: 769–773.
120. Donadio JV, Bergstrahl EJ, Offord KP, Spencer DC, Holley KE. A controlled trial of fish oil in IgA nephropathy. *N Engl J Med* 1994; 331:1194–1199.
121. Ricardo SD, Bertram JF, Ryan GB. Antioxidants protect podocyte foot processes in puromycin aminonucleoside-treated rats. *J Am Soc Nephrol* 1994;4:1974–1986.
122. Ricardo SD, Bertram JF, Ryan GB. Reactive oxygen species in puromycin aminonucleoside nephrosis: in vitro studies. *Kidney Int* 1994; 45:1057–1069.
123. Trachtman H, Schwob N, Maesaka J, Valderrama E. Dietary vitamin E supplementation ameliorates renal injury in chronic puromycin aminonucleoside nephropathy. *J Am Soc Nephrol* 1995;5:1811–1819.
124. Yoshioka T, Bills T, Moore-Jarrett T, Greene HL, Burr IM, Ichikawa I. Role of intrinsic antioxidant enzymes in renal oxidant injury. *Kidney Int* 1990;38:282–288.
125. Kawamura T, Yoshioka T, Bills T, Fogo A, Ichikawa I. Glucocorticoid activates glomerular antioxidant enzymes and protects glomeruli from oxidant injuries. *Kidney Int* 1991;40:291–301.
126. Yoshioka T, Ichikawa I, Fogo A. Reactive oxygen metabolites cause massive, reversible proteinuria and glomerular sieving defect without apparent ultrastructural abnormality. *J Am Soc Nephrol* 1991;2: 902–912.
127. Remuzzi G, Bertani T. Is glomerulosclerosis a consequence of altered glomerular permeability to macromolecules? *Kidney Int* 1990;38: 384–394.
128. Eddy AA, Giachelli CM. Renal expression of genes that promote interstitial inflammation and fibrosis in rats with protein-overload proteinuria. *Kidney Int* 1995;47:1546–1557.
129. Eddy AA. Experimental insights into the tubulointerstitial disease accompanying primary glomerular lesions. *J Am Soc Nephrol* 1994;5: 1273–1287.
130. Thomas ME, Schreiner GF. Contribution of proteinuria to progressive renal injury: consequences of tubular uptake of fatty acid bearing albumin. *Am J Nephrol* 1993;13:385–398.
131. Kees-Folt D, Sadow JL, Schreiner GF. Tubular catabolism of albumin is associated with the release of an inflammatory lipid. *Kidney Int* 1994;45:1697–1709.
132. Eddy AA, McCulloch L, Liu E, Adams J. A relationship between proteinuria and acute tubulointerstitial disease in rats with experimental nephrotic syndrome. *Am J Pathol* 1991;138:1111–1123.
133. Yoshioka T, Shiraga H, Yoshida Y, et al. "Intact nephrons" as the primary origin of proteinuria in chronic renal disease: a study in the rat model of subtotal nephrectomy. *J Clin Invest* 1988;82:1614–1623.
134. Okuda S, Oochi N, Wakisaka M, et al. Albuminuria is not an aggravating factor in experimental focal glomerulosclerosis and hyalinosis. *J Lab Clin Med* 1992;119:245–253.
135. Tanaka R, Kon V, Yoshioka T, Ichikawa I, Fogo A. Angiotensin converting enzyme inhibitor modulates glomerular function and structure by distinct mechanisms. *Kidney Int* 1994;45:537–543.
136. Artero ML, Sharma R, Savin VJ, Vincenti F. Plasmapheresis reduces proteinuria and serum capacity to injure glomeruli in patients with recurrent focal glomerulosclerosis. Am J Kidney Dis 1994;23:574–581.
137. Dantal J, Bigot E, Bogers W, et al. Effect of plasma protein adsorption on protein excretion in kidney-transplant recipients with recurrent nephrotic syndrome. *N Engl J Med* 1994;330:7–14.
138. Savin VJ, Sharma M, McCarthy ET, Swan SK, Ellis E, Lovell H, Warday B, Gunwar S, Chonko AM, Artero M, Vincenti F. Circulating factor associated with increased glomerular permeability to albumin in recurrent focal segmental glomerulosclerosis. *N Engl J Med* 1996;334:878–883.
139. Floege J, Alpers CE, Burns MW, et al. Glomerular cells, extracellular matrix accumulation, and the development of glomerulosclerosis in the remnant kidney model. *Lab Invest* 1992;66:485–497.
140. Johnson RJ. The glomerular response to injury: progression or resolution? *Kidney Int* 1994;45:1769–1782.
141. Nabeshima K, Yoshimura A, Inui K, et al. Relationship of PDGF β-chain mRNA expression identified by in situ hybridization (ISH) and disease severity in various human glomerular diseases [Abstract]. *J Am Soc Nephrol* 1993;4:777.
142. Gesualdo L, DiPaolo S, Milani S, et al. Expression of platelet-derived growth factor receptors in normal and diseased human kidney: an immunohistochemistry and in situ hybridization study. *J Clin Invest* 1994;94:50–58.
143. Marx M, Daniel TO, Kashgarian M, Madri JA. Spatial organization of the extracellular matrix modulates the expression of PDGF-receptor subunits in mesangial cells. *Kidney Int* 1993;43:1027–1041.
144. Tanaka R, Sugihara K, Tatematsu A, Fogo A. Internephron heterogeneity of growth factors and sclerosis—modulation of platelet derived growth factor by angiotensin II. *Kidney Int* 1995;47:131–139.
145. Yamamoto T, Nakamura T, Noble NA, Ruoslahti E, Border WA. Expression of transforming growth factor B is elevated in human and experimental diabetic nephropathy. *Proc Natl Acad Sci U S A* 1993; 90:1814–1818.
146. Yoshioka K, Takemura T, Murakami K, et al. Transforming growth factor-β protein and mRNA in glomeruli in normal and diseased human kidneys. *Lab Invest* 1993;68:154–163.
147. Iwano M, Akai Y, Fujii Y, Horii Y, Dohi Y, Dohi K. Glomerular expression of TGF-β mRNA in human glomerulonephritis [Abstract]. *J Am Soc Nephrol* 1993;4:680.
148. Fogo A, Ikoma M, Burke BA, Nath KA, Glick AD, Ichikawa I. Biphasic morphologic pattern of glomerular hypertrophy in progression of human focal glomerulosclerosis (FGS) [Abstract]. *Lab Invest* 1991;64:977A.
149. Ikoma M, Kawamura T, Fogo A, Ichikawa I. Cause of variable therapeutic efficiency of angiotensin converting enzyme inhibitor on the glomerular mesangial lesions. *Kidney Int* 1991;40:195–202.
150. Remuzzi A, Mazarska M, Gephardt GN, Novick AC, Brenner BM, Remuzzi G. Three-dimensional analysis of glomerular morphology in patients with subtotal nephrectomy. *Kidney Int* 1995;48:155–162.
151. Sandison A, Newbold KM, Howie AJ. Evidence for unique distribution of Kimmelstiel-Wilson nodules in glomeruli. *Diabetes* 1992;41: 952–955.
152. Floege J, Burns MW, Alpers CE, et al. Glomerular cell proliferation and PDGF expression precede glomerulosclerosis in the remnant kidney model. *Kidney Int* 1992;41:297–309.
153. Alpers CE, Seifert RA, Hudkins KL, Johnson RJ, Bowen-Pope DF. PDGF-receptor localizes to mesangial, parietal epithelial, and interstitial cells in human and primate kidneys. *Kidney Int* 1993;43:286–294.
154. Sharma K, Ziyadeh FN. The emerging role of transforming growth factor-β in kidney diseases. *Am J Physiol* 1994;35:F829–F842.
155. Ketteler M, Noble NA, Border WA. Transforming growth factor-β and angiotensin II: the missing link from glomerular hyperfiltration to glomerulosclerosis? *Annu Rev Physiol* 1995;57:279–295.
156. Isaka Y, Fujiwara Y, Ueda N, Kaneda Y, Kamada T, Imai E. Glomerulosclerosis induced by in vivo transfection of transforming growth factor-β or platelet-derived growth factor gene into the rat kidney. *J Clin Invest* 1993;92:2597–2601.

157. Christ M, McCartney-Francis NL, Kulkami AB, et al. Immune dysregulation in TGF-beta 1–deficient mice. *J Immunol* 1994;153:1936–1946.
158. Ahuja SS, Paliogianni F, Yamada H, Balow JE, Boumpas DT. Mechanism of inhibition of T cell proliferation by transforming growth factor-β1 (TGF-β1) [Abstract]. *J Am Soc Nephrol* 1992;3:572.
159. Gibbons GH, Pratt RE, Dzau VJ. Vascular smooth muscle cell hypertrophy vs. hyperplasia. *J Clin Invest* 1992;90:456–461.
160. Yang CW, Striker LJ, Pesce C, et al. Glomerulosclerosis and body growth are mediated by different portions of bovine growth hormone. Studies in transgenic mice. *Lab Invest* 1993;68:62–70.
161. Peten EP, Striker LJ, Garcia-Perez A, Striker GE. Studies by competitive PCR of glomerulosclerosis in growth hormone transgenic mice. *Kidney Int* 1993;43(suppl):55–58.
162. Peten EP, Striker LJ, Carome MA, Elliot SJ, Yang CW, Striker GE. The contribution of increased collagen synthesis to human glomerulosclerosis: a quantitative analysis of α2IV collagen mRNA expression by competitive polymerase chain reaction. *J Exp Med* 1992;176:1571–1576.
163. Liu Z-H, Striker LJ, Phillips C, et al. Mice transgenic for a growth hormone antagonist are protected from diabetic glomerulosclerosis [Abstract]. *J Am Soc Nephrol* 1995;6:1044.
164. Carome MA, Striker LJ, Peten EP, et al. Human glomeruli express tissue inhibitor of metalloproteinase-1 (TIMP-1) mRNA and TIMP-2 protein and mRNA. *Am J Physiol* 1993;264:F923–F929.
165. Pesce CM, Striker LJ, Peten E, Elliot SJ, Striker GE. Glomerulosclerosis at both early and late stages is associated with increased cell turnover in mice transgenic for growth hormone. *Lab Invest* 1991;65:601–605.
166. Nadasdy T, Laszik Z, Blick KE, Johnson LD, Silva FG. Proliferative activity of intrinsic cell populations in the normal human kidney. *J Am Soc Nephrol* 1994;4:2032–2039.
167. Szabolcs MJ, Ward L, Buttyan R, D'Agati V. Apoptosis elucidated by labeling for DNA fragmentation in human renal biopsies [Abstract]. *Lab Invest* 1994;70:160.
168. Oikawa T, Kakuchi J, Fogo A. Interleukin 1β converting enzyme (ICE) is increased in settings of increased apoptosis in vivo [Abstract]. *Lab Invest* 1995;72:160.
169. Baker AJ, Mooney A, Hughes J, Lombardi D, Johnson RJ, Savill J. Mesangial cell apoptosis: the major mechanism for resolution of glomerular hypercellularity in experimental mesangial proliferative nephritis. *J Clin Invest* 1994;94:2105–2116.
170. Kitamura H, Shimizu A, Masuda Y, et al. Capillary regeneration during progression or recovery of glomerulonephritis (GN) [Abstract]. *J Am Soc Nephrol* 1995;6:872.
171. Savill J. Apoptosis in disease. *Eur J Clin Invest* 1994;24:715–723.
172. de Almeida JB, Holtzman EJ, Peters P, Ercolani L, Ausiello DA, Stow JL. Targeting of chimeric G alpha i proteins to specific membrane domains. *J Cell Sci* 1994;107:507–515.
173. Kon V, Hunley TE, Fogo A. Combined antagonism of endothelin A/B receptors links endothelin to vasoconstriction whereas angiotensin II effects fibrosis. *Transplantation* 1995;60:89–95.
174. Burdmann EM, Lindsley J, Elzinga L, Andoh T, Bennett WM. Role of the renin-angiotensin system in experimental chronic cyclosporine (CSA) nephrotoxicity [Abstract]. *J Am Soc Nephrol* 1992;3:721.
175. Kon V, Fogo A, Ichikawa I. Bradykinin causes selective efferent arteriolar dilation during angiotensin I converting enzyme inhibition. *Kidney Int* 1993;44:545–550.
176. Yoshioka T, Yared A, Kon V, Ichikawa I. Impaired preservation of GFR during hypotension in preexistent renal hypoperfusion. *Am J Physiol* 1989;256:F314–F320.
177. Hricik DE, Browning PJ, Kopelman R, Goorno WE, Madias NE, Dzau VJ. Captopril-induced functional renal insufficiency in patients with bilateral renal-artery stenosis in a solitary kidney. *N Engl J Med* 1983;308:373–376.
178. Deedwania PC. Angiotensin-converting enzyme inhibitors in congestive heart failure. *Arch Intern Med* 1990;150:1798–1805.
179. Boiskin M, Marcussen N, Kjellstrand C. ACE inhibitors are now the second most common cause of acute, iatrogenic renal failure [Abstract]. *J Am Soc Nephrol* 1992;3:720.
180. Remuzzi A, Perticucci E, Ruggenenti P, Mosconi L, Limonta M, Remuzzi G. Angiotensin converting enzyme inhibition improves glomerular size-selectivity in IgA nephropathy. *Kidney Int* 1991;39:1267–1273.
181. Pesce C, Schmidt K, Fogo A, et al. Glomerular size and the incidence of renal disease in African Americans and Caucasians. *J Nephrol* 1994;7:355–358.
182. Schmidt K, Pesce C, Liu Q, et al. Large glomerular size in Pima Indians: lack of change with diabetic nephropathy. *J Am Soc Nephrol* 1992;2:229–235.
183. Freedman BI, Bowden DW. The role of genetic factors in the development of end-stage renal disease. *Curr Opin Nephrol Hypertens* 1995;4:230–234.
184. Cambien F, Poirier O, Lecerf L, et al. Deletion polymorphism in the gene for angiotensin-converting enzyme is a potent risk factor for myocardial infarction. *Nature* 1992;359:641–644.
185. Schunkert H, Hense H-W, Holmer SR, et al. Association between a deletion polymorphism of the angiotensin-converting enzyme gene and left ventricular hypertrophy. *N Engl J Med* 1994;330:1634–1638.
186. Bonnardeaux A, Davies E, Jeunemaitre X, et al. Angiotensin II type 1 receptor gene polymorphisms in human essential hypertension. *Hypertension* 1994;24:63–69.
187. Tiret L, Bonnardeaux A, Poirer O, et al. Synergistic effects of angiotensin-converting enzyme and angiotensin-II type I receptor gene polymorphisms on risk of myocardial infarction. *Lancet* 1994;334:910–913.
188. Jeunemaitre X, Soubrier F, Kotelevtsev YV, et al. Molecular basis of human hypertension: role of angiotensinogen. *Cell* 1992;71:169–180.
189. Hunley TE, Julian BA, Phillips JA, Summar ML, Yoshida H, Horn RG, Brown NJ, Fogo A, Ichikawa I, Kon V. Angiotensin converting enzyme gene polymorphism: potential silencer motif and impact on progression in IgA nephropathy. *Kidney Int* 1996;49:571–577.
190. Yoshida H, Mitarai T, Kawamura T, et al. Role of the deletion polymorphism of the angiotensin converting enzyme gene in the progression and therapeutic responsiveness of IgA nephropathy. *J Clin Invest* 1995;96:2100–2102.
191. Harden PN, Geddes C, Rowe PA, et al. Polymorphisms in angiotensin-converting-enzyme gene and progression of IgA nephropathy. *Lancet* 1995;345:1540–1542.
192. Hunley T, Summar ML, Phillips JA, Ichikawa I, Kon V. Mutational loop-out may be the mechanism for the deletion/insertion polymorphism of the angiotensin converting enzyme gene [Abstract]. *J Am Soc Nephrol* 1995;6:722.
193. Rigat B, Hubert C, Alhenc-Gelas F, Cambien F, Corvol P, Soubrier F. An insertion/deletion polymorphism in the angiotensin I-converting enzyme gene accounting for half the variance of serum levels. *J Clin Invest* 1990;86:1343–1346.
194. Ueda S, Elliott HL, Morton JJ, Connell JMC. Enhanced pressor response to angiotensin I in normotensive men with the deletion geneotype (DD) for angiotensin-converting enzyme. *Hypertension* 1995;25:1266–1269.
195. Anderson S, Rennke HG, Brenner BM. Therapeutic advantage of converting enzyme inhibitors in arresting progressive renal disease associated with systemic hypertension in the rat. *J Clin Invest* 1986;77:1993–2000.
196. Kakinuma Y, Kawamura T, Bills T, Yoshioka T, Ichikawa I, Fogo A. Blood-pressure independent effect of angiotensin inhibition on vascular lesions of chronic renal failure. *Kidney Int* 1992;42:46–55.
197. Kerins DM, Hao Q, Vaughan DE. Angiotensin induction of PAI-1 expression in endothelial cells is mediated by the hexapeptide angiotensin IV. *J Clin Invest* 1995;96:2515–2520.
198. Vaughan DE, Lazos SA, Tong K. Angiotensin II regulates the expression of plasminogen activator inhibitor-1 in cultured endothelial cells. *J Clin Invest* 1995;95:995–1001.
199. Orth SR, Weinreich T, Bönisch S, Weih M, Ritz E. Angiotensin II induces hypertrophy and hyperplasia in adult human mesangial cells. *Exp Nephrol* 1995;3:23–33.
200. Kitazono T, Padgett RC, Armstrong ML, Tompkins PK, Heistad DD. Evidence that angiotensin II is present in human monocytes. *Circulation* 1995;91:1129–1134.
201. Morishita R, Gibbons GH, Ellison KE, et al. Evidence for direct local effect of angiotensin in vascular hypertrophy: in vivo gene transfer of angiotensin converting enzyme. *J Clin Invest* 1994;94:978–984.
202. Gibbons GH. Mechanisms of vascular remodeling in hypertension: role of autocrine-paracrine vasoactive factors. *Curr Opin Nephrol Hypertension* 1995;4:189–196.
203. Arai M, Wada A, Isaka Y, et al. In vivo transfection of genes for renin and angiotensinogen into the glomerular cells induced phenotypic

change of the mesangial cells and glomerular sclerosis. *Biochem Biophys Res Commun* 1995;206:525–532.
204. Niimura F, Labosky PA, Kakuchi J, et al. Gene targeting in mice reveals a requirement for angiotensin in the development and maintenance of kidney morphology and growth factor regulation. *J Clin Invest* 1995;96:2947–2954.
205. Tanimoto K, Sugiyama F, Goto Y, et al. Angiotensin-deficient mice with hypotension. *J Biol Chem* 1994;269:31334–31337.
206. Peten EP, Striker LJ, Fogo A, Ichikawa I, Patel A, Striker GE. The molecular basis of increased glomerulosclerosis after blockade of the renin angiotensin system in growth hormone transgenic mice. *Mol Med* 1994;1:104–115.
207. Hostetter TH, Rosenberg ME, Kren S, Greene E. Aldosterone (ALDO) induces glomerular sclerosis in the remnant kidney [Abstract]. *J Am Soc Nephrol* 1995;6:1016.
208. Pitt B. "Escape" of aldosterone production in patients with left ventricular dysfunction treated with an angiotensin converting enzyme inhibitor: implications for therapy. *Cardiovasc Drug Ther* 1995;9: 145–149.
209. Ray PE, McCune BK, Gomez RA, Horikoshi S, Kopp JB, Klotman PE. Renal vascular induction of TGF-β2 and renin by potassium depletion. *Kidney Int* 1993;44:1006–1013.
210. Marinides GN, Groggel GC, Cohen AH, Border WA. Enalapril and low protein reverse chronic puromycin aminonucleoside nephropathy. *Kidney Int* 1990;37:749–757.
211. Schiffrin EL, Deng LY, Larochelle P. Progressive improvement in the structure of resistance arteries of hypertensive patients after two years of treatment with an angiotensin I–converting enzyme inhibitor: comparison with effects of a β-blocker. *Am J Hypertens* 1995;8: 229–236.
212. O'Donnell MP, Kasiske BL, Schmitz PG, Keane WF, Daniels F. High protein intake accelerates glomerulosclerosis independent of effects on glomerular hemodynamics. *Kidney Int* 1990;37:1263–1269.
213. Rosenberg ME, Chmielewski D, Hostetter TH. Effect of dietary protein on rat renin and angiotensinogen gene expression. *J Clin Invest* 1990;85:1144–1149.
214. Mitch WE. Dietary manipulation and progression of chronic renal failure. *Child Nephrol Urol* 1991;11:134–139.
215. Smith LJ, Rosenberg ME, Correa-Rotter R, Hostetter TH. The renin-angiotensin system in chronic renal disease. In: Mitch WE, ed. *The progressive nature of renal disease.* Vol 26. 2nd ed. New York: Churchill Livingstone; 1992:55–76.
216. Abrams JR, Tapp DC, Venkatachalam MA. Dietary influences and pathologic changes. In: Mitch WE, ed. *The progressive nature of renal disease.* Vol 26. New York: Churchill Livingstone; 1992:133–148.
217. Hirschberg R, Kopple JD. Response of insulin-like growth factor I and renal hemodynamics to a high- and low-protein diet in the rat. *J Am Soc Nephrol* 1991;1:1034–1040.
218. Klahr S, Levey AS, Beck GJ, et al. The effects of dietary protein restriction and blood-pressure control on the progression of chronic renal disease. *N Engl J Med* 1994;330:877–884.
219. Holdsworth SR, Bellomo R. Differential effect of steroids on leukocyte-mediated glomerulonephritis in the rabbit. *Kidney Int* 1984;26: 162–169.
220. Schreiber AD, Parson J, McDermott P, Cooper RA. Effects of corticosteroids on human monocyte IgG and complement receptors. *J Clin Invest* 1975;56:1189–1197.
221. Werb Z. Biochemical actions of glucocorticoids on macrophages in culture. Specific inhibition of elastase, collagenase and plasminogen activator secretion and effects on other metabolic functions. *J Exp Med* 1978;147:1685–1712.
222. Lu CY, Sicher SC, Vazquez MA. Prevention and treatment of renal allograft rejection: new therapeutic approaches and new insights into established therapies. *J Am Soc Nephrol* 1993;4:1239–1256.
223. Nakamura T, Ebihara I, Fukui M, Tomino Y, Koide H. Effects of methylprednisolone on glomerular and medullary mRNA levels for extracellular matrices in puromycin aminonucleoside nephrosis. *Kidney Int* 1991;40:874–881.
224. Thompson EB. Apoptosis and steroid hormones. *Mol Endocrinol* 1994;8:665–673.
225. Wyllie AH. Glucocorticoid-induced thymocyte apoptosis is associated with endogenous endonuclease activation. *Nature* 1980;284: 555–556.
226. Hara T, Miyai H, Iida T, Futehnma A, Nakamura S, Kato K. Aggravation of puromycin aminonucleoside nephrosis by the inhibition of endogenous superoxide dismutase [Abstract]. *Proceedings of the XIth International Congress on Nephrology*. 1990:442.
227. Macconi D, Zanoli AF, Orisio S, et al. Methylprednisolone normalizes superoxide anion production by polymorphs from patients with ANCA-positive vasculitides. *Kidney Int* 1993;44:215–220.
228. Trachtman H, Del Pizzo R, Valderrama E, Gauthier B. The renal functional and structural consequences of corticosteroid and angiotensin-converting enzyme inhibitor therapy in chronic puromycin aminonucleoside nephropathy. *Pediatr Nephrol* 1990;4:501–504.
229. Fishel RS, Eisenberg S, Shai S-Y, Redden RA, Bernstein KE, Berk BC. Glucocorticoids induce angiotensin-converting enzyme expression in vascular smooth muscle. *Hypertension* 1995;25:343–349.
230. Fogo A, Ichikawa I. Evidence for the central role of glomerular growth promoters in the development of sclerosis. *Semin Nephrol* 1989;9:329–342.
231. Fogo A, Striker LJ. Advances in diagnostics of the kidney. In: O'Leary, ed. *Advanced diagnostic methods in pathology.* (in press).

Immunologic Renal Diseases,
edited by E. G. Neilson and W. G. Couser.
Lippincott-Raven Publishers, Philadelphia © 1997

CHAPTER 34

Renal Fibrogenesis and Progression

Frank Strutz and Gerhard A. Müller

THE PROGRESSION OF CHRONIC RENAL DISEASE

There are currently >172,000 Americans undergoing dialysis treatment because of end-stage renal disease (ESRD) (1). The most common causes of ESRD include diabetic nephropathy, chronic glomerulopathies, hypertensive nephrosclerosis, chronic pyelonephritis, and polycystic kidney disease (2). In the great majority of cases, progression to end-stage renal failure occurs over a period of several to many years. It is now clear that many factors are involved in the continuous decline in renal function independent of the primary inflammatory process (3). Whereas in a number of cases the initiating disease process remains active throughout progression, in many patients renal failure progresses despite resolution of the initial injury by spontaneous remission or therapy (4). Responsible for progression are so-called progression promoters, which include glomerular hyperfiltration (5), intraglomerular and systemic hypertension (6,7), and glomerular and tubular hypertrophy (8,9), as well as tubulointerstitial disease (10). In fact, all forms of chronic renal disease are accompanied by changes in the tubulointerstitium (11). These changes consist of interstitial inflammation followed by fibrosis, tubular atrophy, and dilatation. Progression of chronic renal failure eventually results in a cirrhotic organ (12). Thus, renal fibrosis (along with glomerulosclerosis) is the final common pathway of a relatively uniform response of the kidney to sustained inflammation independent of its origin. When the point of no return is reached, progression invariably ensues despite the resolution of the inflammatory process. The degree of tubulointerstitial fibrosis correlates well with the decline in renal function (13). Preventing or reversing interstitial fibrosis means prevention of progression of chronic renal failure. This chapter deals with the role of the tubulointerstitial area in chronic renal failure, its pathogenesis, and the possibilities for therapeutic preservation of renal function.

F. Strutz and G. A. Müller: Department of Nephrology and Rheumatology, Georg-August University Medical Center, Göttingen, Germany.

THE ROLE OF THE TUBULOINTERSTITIAL SPACE IN THE PROGRESSION OF RENAL DISEASE

It seems obvious that tubulointerstitial changes are important for progression of primary interstitial disease. However, the significance of these changes for primary glomerular and vascular disease has long been neglected despite evidence that changes in the tubulointerstitial compartment are a strong determinant of renal progression. As early as 1844, Henle and Pfeufer described a 25-year-old girl with Bright disease (as glomerulopathies were called at the time) who died of anasarca (14). They concluded from their histologic examination that tubulointerstitial fibrosis rather than glomerular alterations was responsible for the disease process. A similar view was propagated by Toynbee in England (15). Conversely, in subsequent years, tubulointerstitial changes in glomerulopathies attracted less attention and were finally considered trivial (16). The importance of the tubulointerstitium for renal function was again noted in 1953 by Spühler and Zollinger studying patients with primary interstitial nephritis caused by excessive intake of nonsteroidal anti-inflammatory drugs (17). Regarding glomerular disease, a study by Hutt et al. rerecognized the significance of tubulointerstitial involvement in glomerular disease. This group studied biopsy specimens from 15 patients with acute glomerulonephritis and compared the histologic with the clinical findings (18). To their surprise, they found that the creatinine clearance was lowest in patients with additional tubulointerstitial lesions, whereas the glomerular changes did not correlate with renal function. These findings were subsequently consolidated by Risdon et al. (19) and Schainuck and Striker and colleagues (20,21). The latter group examined 70 patients with various forms of glomerulopathy and compared the histologic changes with glomerular filtration rate and effective renal plasma flow, as well as concentrating and acidifying capacities. To the surprise of the authors, the results indicated a clear relationship between changes in the tubulointerstitial space and impairment of renal function (20). However, the most systematic examination of tubulointerstitial changes in well-defined glomerular diseases was performed by the group of Bohle and co-workers, whose analyses include primary glomerulonephrites such as mesangioproliferative (22), membranous (23), focal sclerosing (24), and membranoproliferative (25) glomerulonephrites as well as secondary forms of glomerular disease including diabetic glomerulosclerosis (26) and glomerular amyloidosis (27). All studies concurred that there was a strong positive correlation between the morphometrically measured interstitial volume and the serum creatinine, whereas there was a negative correlation between the clearances for creatinine, inulin, and para-aminohippurate (PAH) and the relative interstitial volume. In addition, both the extent of interstitial infiltration as well as the degree of interstitial fibrosis were relatively accurate predictors of renal function 5 or more years later (13). Conversely, even severe glomerular changes did not correlate with renal function in membranoproliferative glomerulonephritis, diabetic glomerulosclerosis, and renal amyloidosis as long as the cortical interstitial space was not affected (28). These findings were confirmed and extended by Jepsen and Mortensen (29), Katafuchi et al. (30), Abe et al. (31), Alexopoulos and co-workers (32), and Lane et al. (33). Figure 1 illustrates the importance of the tubulointerstitial area on renal function in several examples. An exception may be immunoglobulin-A nephropathy, where Bennett et al. were unable to find any correlation between the glomerular filtration rate and the interstitial volume in serial biopsies (34). However, an increase in the interstitial volume may be caused solely by infiltrating inflammatory cells and edema without fibrosis being present. Thus, the sole presence of interstitial widening may not always predict renal progression accurately, whereas fibrosis invariably does.

In conclusion, an overwhelming body of evidence points to a very important role of tubulointerstitial disease in the progression of glomerulopathies. Additionally, interstitial changes are of great importance in diabetic nephropathy (35), chronic pyelonephritis (36), so-called benign nephrosclerosis (7), and polycystic kidney disease (37). One histomorphometric study in 105 patients with various degrees of diabetic nephropathy revealed a robust correlation between the renal interstitial volume and the decline in renal function (26). Similar results were published in smaller studies by Thomsen et al. (38) and Mauer et al. (39). In addition, each of the three studies demonstrated a correlation between interstitial and mesangial expansion. A recent study by Lane and co-workers confirmed the relationship between interstitial lesions, mesangial expansion, and global glomerulosclerosis and their correlation to renal function in 84 patients with insulin-dependent diabetes mellitus (33). Regarding chronic pyelonephritis, the presence of infiltrating leukocytes predicted progressive loss of tubules and interstitial fibrosis in one study in mice (40). Mai et al. examined interstitial changes in hypertension-induced renal injury and found that these changes are essential for the progression of hypertensive nephrosclerosis (41).

The strong significance of the tubulointerstitial compartment comes as no surprise, since the interstitial space accompanies ~80 percent of the renal volume (42). The mechanisms of progression of renal disease caused by tubulointerstitial disease are incompletely understood. Nevertheless, a number of theories have emerged and are discussed in the next section.

MECHANISMS OF PROGRESSION

Possible mechanisms of increasing deterioration of renal function include the obliteration of postglomerular capillaries, the generation of atubular glomeruli, and the formation of atrophic tubules.

FIG. 1. Significance of the tubulointerstitial area for renal function. **A and B:** Biopsy sections from two patients with membranoproliferative glomerulonephritis (MPGN) (type I). Periodic acid–Schiff stain, ×4O. **A:** A 51-year-old woman without significant tubulointerstitial involvement. Serum creatinine, 0.6 mg/dL; creatinine clearance, 120 mL/min/1.73 m2. **B:** A 37-year-old man with diffuse interstitial fibrosis and tubular atrophy. Serum creatinine 14.1 mg/dL. **C and D:** Biopsy sections from two patients with renal amyloidosis. Semithin sections, Movat silver stain, ×128. **C:** A 46-year-old woman with normal tubulointerstitium. Creatinine, 0.8 mg/dL; clearance, 119 mL/min/1.73 m2. **D:** A 37-year-old woman with advanced interstitial fibrosis and tubular atrophy. Serum creatinine, 6.9 mg/dL. **E and F**: Biopsy sections from two patients with diabetic nephropathy. Periodic acid–Schiff stain, ×128. **E:** A 48-year-old woman y. Nodular diabetic glomerulosclerosis without tubulointerstitial changes. Serum creatinine, 0.8 mg/dL. **F:** A 65-year-old man with diffuse diabetic glomerulopathy with diffuse interstitial fibrosis and tubular atrophy. Creatinine, 4.5 mg/dL. All biopsies specimens are from Bohle et al. (28), courtesy of A. Bohle, with permission from the publisher.

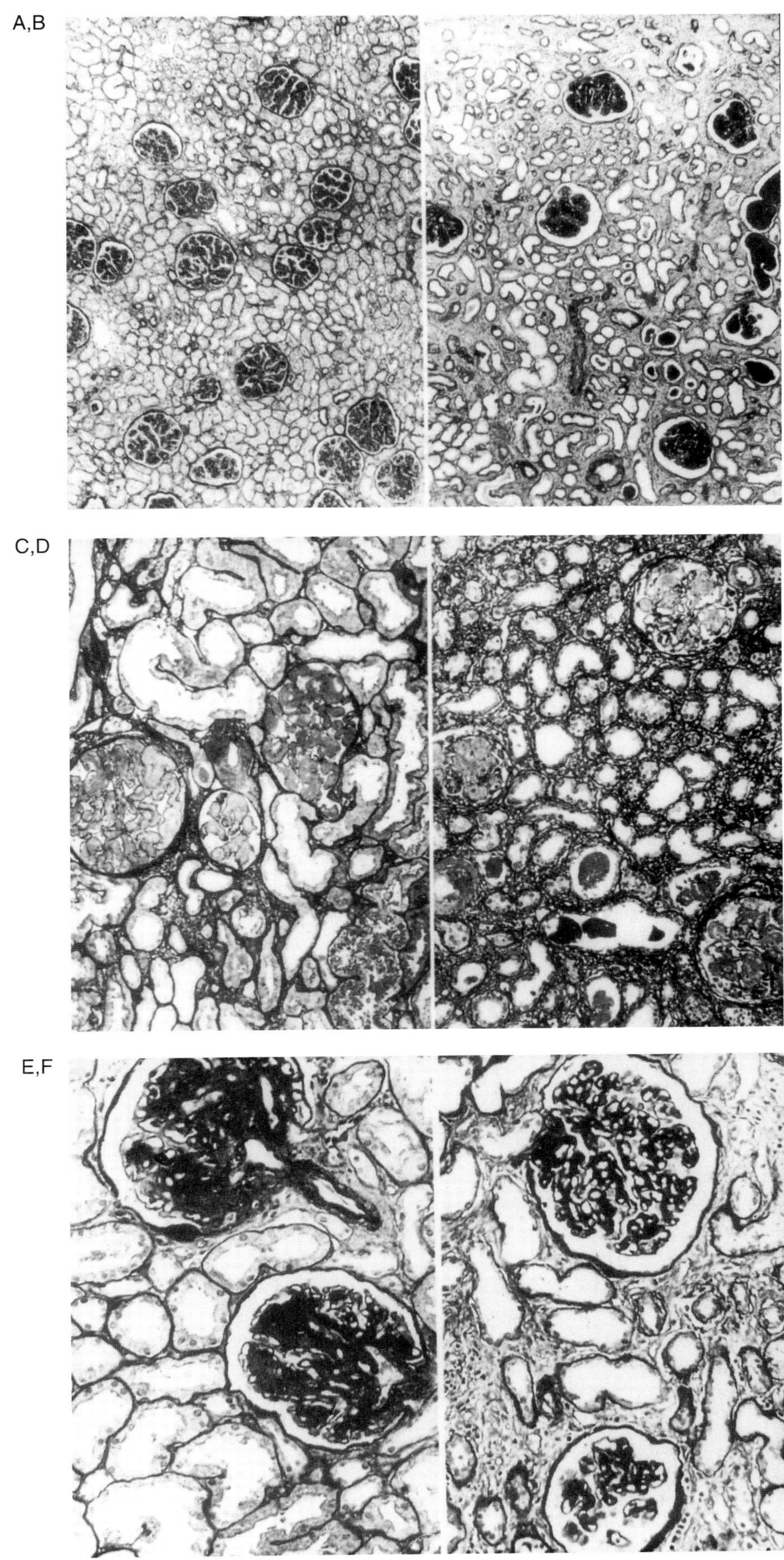
A,B
C,D
E,F

Obliteration of Postglomerular Capillaries

The progressive obliteration of postglomerular capillaries in areas of interstitial inflammation or fibrosis was first described by Ljungquist in 1963 (43). In 1981, Bohle and co-workers examined the number and area of intertubular capillaries in biopsy specimens from patients with primary glomerulopathy in whom the increase of interstitial volume was due to fibrosis (44). The result of their study was a strong correlation between a decrease in renal function (measured by a rise in the serum creatinine) and a reduction in number and area of postglomerular capillaries. Bader et al. observed similar changes in biopsy specimens from patients with diabetic nephropathy (26). The degree of arteriolar hyalinization and occlusion correlated directly with tubulointerstitial fibrosis and glomerular sclerosis. The ensuing ischemia due to capillary obliteration may initially cause an impairment of tubular cell metabolism due to ischemia and increased diffusion length (45). Eventually, the loss of tubular cells due to necrosis, apoptosis, or atrophy may result (46). Conversely, in one morphometric investigation of chronic obstructive nephropathy, the relative volume of interstitial fibrosis had to be increased threefold before any reduction in length or surface area of cortex capillaries could be demonstrated (47). However, peritubular blood flow may be compromised not only by structural changes but also by vasoconstrictory peptides such as platelet-derived growth factor (PDGF), angiotensin II, and endothelin. All three peptides display strong vasoconstrictive activity and are secreted by tubular epithelial cells (48–50). Increased secretion of these mediators may result in vasoconstriction and ensuing tubular damage. Furthermore, tubules may be damaged alternatively by increased filtration of toxic molecules or by direct immune-mediated injury as proposed by Fine and coworkers (51).

Atubular Glomeruli and Atrophic Tubules

Loss of tubular function causes loss of renal function by the formation of atubular glomeruli and the tubuloglomerular feedback mechanism (12). The formation of atubular glomeruli in chronic renal disease was first assumed by Oliver in 1939, who by the use of microdissection noted a heterogeneous population of nephrons (52). Some of the nephrons were hypertrophied and others were aglomerular, whereas in others only the glomerulus remained (atubular glomeruli). Atubular glomeruli cause a decrease in filtration rate because the passing blood can not get filtered (53). Their presence is not easily demonstrated because light microscopy does not reveal whether a glomerulus is atubular (54). However, the existence of atubular glomeruli has been well documented in humans and animals by stereologic and morphometric methods (55,56). Human diseases in which disconnected glomeruli have been detected include renal artery stenosis (57), chronic pyelonephritis (56), and chronic diabetic nephropathy (53). The percentage of atubular glomeruli was lowest in diabetic nephropathy at 8.8% and highest in renal artery stenosis, reaching 52% of all glomeruli (53,57). In the study on patients with chronic pyelonephritis, only 50% of the glomeruli were connected to normal proximal tubules, 35% were without tubular connection, and 15% were joined with atrophic tubules (56). There was a good correlation between the number of atubular glomeruli and the degree of tubulointerstitial fibrosis. Atubular glomeruli are smaller than their normal counterparts and have a reduced number of glomerular capillaries, whereas the number is increased in hypertrophic glomeruli (58). The pathogenesis of the formation of atubular glomeruli is not entirely clear, but it must be due to tubular destruction or atrophy (54). Atubular glomeruli have open capillaries and may provide blood for the intertubular capillary network (54). However, they do not participate in the formation of urine resulting in a loss of nephron function. Thus, the formation of atubular glomeruli results in a continuous decline in renal function. In fact, the percentage of glomeruli deprived of tubular connection correlated in several studies with renal function as measured by plasma creatinine (57,59). However, the correlation with serum creatinine was even more significant with the number of glomeruli with normal proximal tubules. This reflects that some glomeruli are connected to atrophic tubules that may deliver some ultrafiltration but whose contribution to renal function is negligible (54).

What causes tubular atrophy and thus the formation of atubular glomeruli or nonfunctioning tubuli? Tubular atrophy can be a consequence of retrograde tubular breakdown, tubular ischemia, apoptosis, and/or tubulitis. Apoptosis, or programmed cell death, is an especially intriguing mechanism for tubular atrophy. In fact, it was recently demonstrated that apoptosis plays an important role in the loss of functioning renal tissue in polycystic kidney disease (60). In the same study, apoptosis was not detectable in other forms of renal disease. However, the number of cases studied was small, and it was not revealed whether interstitial fibrosis was present. Thus, apoptosis might be an important mechanism for the formation of atrophic tubules.

FIBROBLASTS AND FIBROGENESIS

Tubulointerstitial fibrosis is the hallmark of chronic renal failure independent of the primary disease process. It is characterized by production and secretion of large amounts of extracellular matrix (61). Renal interstitial matrix consists of various types of collagen, fibronectin, and proteoglycans. Interstitial collagens include the fibrillar collagen types I, III, and V, as well as the nonfibrillar collagen type VI (62). In the physiologic state, a bal-

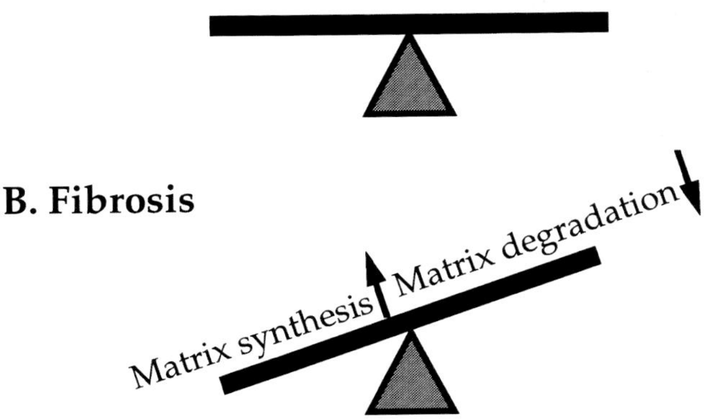

FIG. 2. In physiologic state, a balance exists between matrix deposition and matrix degradation (*A*). This balance is disturbed during fibrogenesis, which is characterized by increased matrix synthesis and decreased matrix degradation.

ance exists between matrix formation and matrix degradation as indicated in Fig. 2 (63). This balance is disrupted in fibrogenesis, which is characterized by an increased matrix production and a decreased matrix degradation.

Phases of Fibrogenesis and Reversibility of Fibrosis

Regular wound healing can be divided into three phases: induction, matrix deposition, and resolution (64). The first phase consists of the promotion of growth, motility, and proliferation of matrix-producing cells. This phase is consists of the influx of inflammatory cells into the tubulointerstitium and subsequent release of cytokines. The phase of matrix production is characterized by increased synthesis and deposition of extracellular matrix. The adhesive protein fibronectin is commonly secreted first, providing a scaffold for the ensuing deposition of collagens. Fibronectin is also a chemotactic factor for fibroblasts, thus resulting in increased fibroblast accumulation (65). In addition, extracellular matrix may have other interactive effects on cells. In fact, the interaction between extracellular matrix and cells is often underappreciated. Wang et al., for example, suggested that matrix proteins may transduce signals through the cell membrane and cytoskeleton into the nucleus (66). Lee and coworkers demonstrated that sudden contraction of a collagen matrix may trigger exocytosis of fibroblast vesicles (67). Moreover, fibroblasts embedded in mechanically relaxed collagen gels displayed a decrease in PDGF-stimulated receptor autophosphorylation, an effect that may play a role in tempering the effects of cytokines in fibrogenesis (68). Cell–matrix interactions also play an important role in the differentiation of epithelial cells. Disruption of cell–matrix contact may induce apoptosis in epithelial cells (69). Similarly, transgenic mice overexpressing stromelysin 1, a matrix-degrading protease, display unscheduled apoptosis during pregnancy and progressive fibrosis, as well as the development of neoplasias after birth (70). Thus, disruption of the basement membrane plays a key role in apoptosis and stromal fibrosis (as well as cancer) of the mammary gland (71). As outlined above, apoptosis may play a role in tubular atrophy, though this effect remains to be demonstrated in the kidney.

Finally, during the phase of resolution, matrix production ceases and matrix degradation increases. These phases are part of the normal wound healing-process (72). In fact, early matrix deposition is fully reversible, as demonstrated by Jones et al. in a model of puromycin aminonucleoside (PAN) nephrosis (73). The initial reversibility is mainly due to an increased activity of matrix-degrading metalloproteinases (MMPs). MMPs are a family of mainly zinc-dependent endopeptidases that have the capability to degrade specific extracellular matrix components at neutral pH (74). The MMP family can be divided by specificity into interstitial collagenases, type-IV collagenases/gelatinases, and stromelysin/transin (75). In addition, members of the MMP family may form complexes resulting in enhanced activity (76). Figure 3 presents an overview of the activation and inactivation of metalloproteinases. A key role in the resolution of the fibrogenic process is played by the tissue inhibitors of matrix metalloproteinases (TIMP), which inhibit all active forms of MMPs by tight binding (77), and by the plasminogen activator–inhibitor (PAI) 1 (78). At least three TIMPs (TIMP-1 to TIMP-3) have been described in humans (79–81). TIMP-1 is upregulated in animal models of PAN nephrosis (82), protein-overload proteinuria (83). and antitubular basement membrane (anti-TBM) disease (84) during active matrix deposition, whereas the matrix proteinases display no or only modest changes in expression. Both TIMP-1 and TIMP-2 are expressed in normal human glomeruli; their level of expression, however, increased by three- to fourfold in one study on human glomerular sclerosis (85). Transgenic mice overexpressing TIMP-1 have delayed matrix degradation and involution process in the mammary gland (71). The main sources of TIMP-1 secretion are endothelial cells and macrophages (84,86). The origin of TIMP-3 is still unknown, but, in one study in mice, the highest levels of TIMP-3 expression were found in kidneys (87). Nonetheless, expression of TIMP-3 did not change in the model of protein-overload proteinuria (83). Conversely, PAI-1 levels were significantly increased in the same model at 2 weeks, when matrix deposition is at its peak (83). PAI-1 inhibits the proteolytic cleavage of plasminogen into the serine protease plasmin. Plasmin, in addition to its function in the coagulation cascade, plays a major role in matrix turnover, since it may activate latent MMPs and has the capability to degrade many matrix proteins directly (78). Inhibition of

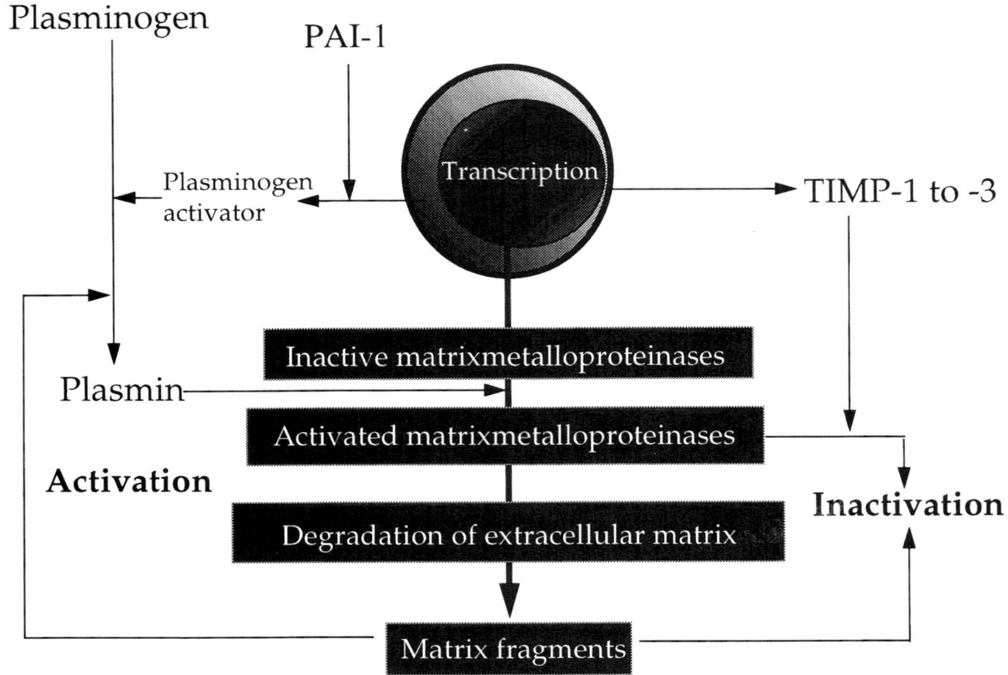

FIG. 3. Schematic illustration of the mechanisms that activate and inactivate metalloproteinases. See the text for explanation.

plasmin activation by increased PAI-1 expression has been described in antithymocyte (anti-Thy)-1.1 glomerulopathy (88). Recently, a discrete increase in PAI-1 mRNA levels was noted in a rat model of bovine serum albumin (BSA)-induced proteinuria (83).

However, resolution does not occur in renal fibrosis. Conversely, fibrosis is characterized by the continued synthesis of extracellular matrix, often despite the resolution of the primary inflammatory process. Thus, we propose a three-step model of fibrogenesis: induction followed by inflammatory matrix synthesis, which in turn precedes postinflammatory matrix synthesis. Table 1 provides an overview. The true difference between regular wound healing and fibrogenesis is the third phase. There is no true resolution in fibrogenesis. It is still unclear what kind of mechanisms are responsible for the perpetuation of matrix synthesis and deposition, but autocrine stimulation of (myo)fibroblasts is likely to play a role. One of these autocrine mechanisms was recently described by Lonnemann et al., who examined the effects of interleukin (IL) 1 on human fibroblasts (89,90). IL-1β had either no influence or even inhibited proliferation in normal fibroblasts, whereas it had a strong mitogenic effect on fibrosis-derived fibroblasts that could be prevented by addition of IL-1 receptor antagonist (IL-1Ra) (89). IL-1Ra expression was reduced in fibrosis-derived fibroblasts (G. Lonnemann, personal communication), whereas there was no difference in IL-1β synthesis (90). Thus, a decrease in IL-1Ra expression may represent one way in which fibroblasts become autonomous from inflammatory stimuli. Additionally, other cytokines, such as transforming growth factor (TGF) α, TGF-β, and fibroblast growth factor (FGF), which are known to play a major role in the self-perpetuation of hepatic myofibroblasts, may play a role as well but are unproven in renal fibrogenesis (91). Besides, continued stimulation by tubular epithelial cells may have an additional effect. Our own studies showed that mRNA expression for PDGF and granulocyte–monocyte colony-stimulating factor (GM-CSF) was increased by 72% and 54%, respectively, in human tubular epithe-

TABLE 1. *Phases of renal fibrogenesis*

I. Induction
Tubulointerstitial infiltration of inflammatory cells
Release of profibrogenic cytokines
Activation and proliferation of resident fibroblasts
Transdifferentiation of tubular epithelial cells (?)
II. Inflammatory matrix synthesis
Continuous release of profibrogenic cytokines by inflammatory cells
Increased matrix synthesis and deposition
Decreased matrix degradation
III. Postinflammatory matrix synthesis
Cessation of the inflammatory stimuli
Autocrine stimulation of (myo)fibroblasts
Continuous matrix synthesis and deposition

lial cells from patients with fibrosis compared with nondiseased kidney-derived tubular cells (92).

Fibroblasts

The origin of matrix-producing cells or fibroblasts in renal fibrogenesis is still controversial. Most authors seem to favor resident interstitial cells, originally classified by Bohman as type-I interstitial cells (93). In 1867, Cohnheim published a classic paper on mechanisms of inflammation, stating that fibroblasts (contractile cellular elements, as they were called at the time) are descendants of migrating leukocytes (94). This theory was widely believed until 1970, when Ross et al., using parabiotic rats, proved that fibroblasts are of local origin (95). In fact, it is assumed that during the process of fibrogenesis resident interstitial fibroblasts convert to so-called myofibroblasts due to the acquisition of smooth-muscle-like features such as α-smooth muscle actin (96,97). The radical change in phenotype is often underappreciated (98). Rodemann and Müller demonstrated the presence of two proteins in human kidney fibrosis-derived fibroblasts not found in normal human fibroblasts by two-dimensional gel electrophoresis (99). One of these proteins proved highly specific for mitotic fibrosis-derived fibroblasts and was subsequently named *fibrosin* (100). Whereas the function of this protein is still unclear, these studies proved that fibroblasts from kidneys with interstitial fibrosis are different from their normal counterparts. Furthermore, our group found that the relative percentage of fibroblasts was markedly increased in cultures from fibrotic kidneys (47% versus 7% in controls) (100). In addition, fibroblasts from fibrotic kidneys had a higher mitotic activity and displayed a higher resistance to the cytostatic drug mitomycin C (101). There was a three- to fivefold increase in the rate of collagen synthesis in fibrosis-derived cells as measured by incorporation of ^{3}H-proline.

However, as is discussed below, it is unclear whether all (activated) myofibroblasts are of resident fibroblast origin. Even resident fibroblasts are a heterogeneous population of cells [reviewed by Müller and Strutz (102)]. Studies on rabbit fibroblasts, for example, revealed significant differences in basal growth, cytokine response (for example, to PDGF), and protein expression (49,103). Renal fibroblasts can be classified according to growth potential and morphology into three mitotic and three postmitotic stages in vitro (101). In vivo studies in human kidneys found that a small subgroup of interstitial fibroblasts constitutively express a-smooth muscle actin and the PDGF receptor β chain (104). In various forms of renal injury, the number of α-smooth muscle positive cells was robustly increased (104,105); however, it remains currently unclear whether this is due to upregulation of the protein in formerly nonexpressing cells or rather a sign of proliferation of these few α-actin-positive cells. Thus, in conclusion, some myofibroblasts are clearly of local origin, probably derived from a subpopulation of resident interstitial cells.

The Role of Transdifferentiation

Other cellular elements besides resident interstitial cells may be involved in renal and nonrenal fibrogenesis (106). In hepatic fibrogenesis, for example, Ito cells (lipocytes, located in the space of Disse) lose their vitamin-A-storing function and transdifferentiate into matrix-synthesizing (myo)fibroblasts (107), whereas resident interstitial fibroblasts do not or only minimally participate in matrix deposition (108). Regarding pulmonary and renal fibrosis, the situation is less clear. The origin of matrix-producing cells remains to be established in pulmonary fibrogenesis (109). Similarly, several cell types besides resident interstitial fibroblasts have been proposed to produce extracellular matrix in the kidney, including tubular epithelial cells (110,111) and perivascular adventitial cells (112). Wiggins and co-workers examined the pathogenesis of interstitial changes in a rabbit model of antiglomerular basement membrane (anti-GBM) nephritis by in situ hybridization with the α_2 chain of collagen type I. Although they were not able to localize any collagen-producing cells under normal conditions, perivascular adventitial cells started collagen type-I synthesis 4 days after disease induction (112). Interstitial cells became positive only at later stages. Our own studies came to similar conclusions, though with one important addition (111). Studies on fibroblasts have long been hindered due to the lack of fibroblast-specific markers. Very few of these markers have been described in the literature (63). A careful analysis of interstitial cells in the rat cortex was recently performed by Kaissling and Le Hir using immunostaining and electron microscopy (113). They found that fibroblasts and dendritic cells constitute the majority of cells in the tubulointerstitial space. Both cell types could be distinguished by specific antigens (ecto-5′-nucleotidase for fibroblasts and MHC class II for dendritic cells) as well as by morphology alone (113). Unfortunately, it remains unclear if all ecto-5′-nucleotidase-positive cells are in fact fibroblasts or rather fibroblastlike cells with different functions, for example, the production of erythropoietin (114). Thus, we used a differential and subtractive hybridization approach to clone a fibroblast-specific marker from a murine fibroblast cDNA library (111,115). One of the cloned cDNAs proved specific for fibroblasts and was named fibroblast-specific protein (FSP) 1. Under physiologic conditions, only few scattered interstitial cells in the kidney (and other organs) expressed FSP-1 as determined by immunohistology (111). Conversely, in mouse models of anti-TBM and anti-GBM disease interstitial staining was robustly increased pointing to resident fibroblast proliferation (111,116). Similar to the findings by Wiggins et al., initial staining was accentuated perivascularly. In addition, however, selected tubular epithelial cells started de novo expression of FSP-1 in both models of chronic renal disease. The acquisition of a fibroblast marker by tubular epithelial cells may indicate that these cells transdifferentiate into matrix-producing (myo)fibroblasts (117). Transdifferentiation is defined as a change of phenotype in a differentiated cell (118). Although unproven in vivo, tubular epithelial cells are capable of producing extracellular matrix in vitro (119). TGF-β, for example, induced collagen production in rat tubular epithelial cells (110) as well as fibronectin and proteoglycan synthesis in rabbit proximal tubule cells (120). Moreover, increased collagen gene transcription has been shown in mouse proximal tubule cells exposed to high-glucose-containing medium (121). Recently, Nadasdy and co-workers performed immunohistologic analyses on human kidneys with tubulointerstitial fibrosis (122). They described mesenchymal-appearing cells in the fibrotic interstitium that expressed three epithelial markers specific for the distal nephron (122). Of course, it is not possible to deduce from that study whether the interstitial cells were transdifferentiated tubular cells or rather fibroblasts that had acquired certain epithelial markers.

Epithelial–mesenchymal transdifferentiation has been demonstrated in a number of cells, including epithelial cells from the thyroid and mammary gland as well as from the embryonic heart and retina (123–126). In fact, as was demonstrated by many groups, differentiated epithelia retain the ability to turn on the mesenchymal genetic program (127). A variety of growth factors such as basic FGF and TGF-β have been shown to be capable of inducing transdifferentiation (124,126). Activation of the epidermal growth factor (EGF) receptor accelerates transdifferentiation in renal tubular epithelia (E. G. Neilson and H. Okada, unpublished observations). In addition, the extracellular matrix plays a key role in transdifferentiation. For example, in a study by Greenburg and Hay, transdifferentiation was induced by type-I collagen, whereas the presence of basement membrane inhibited the process (123). Likewise, collagen type-I matrix induced transdifferentiation in tubular epithelial cells (111). Clearly, further studies are required to establish the exact role of transdifferentiation in renal fibrogenesis.

MEDIATORS OF TUBULOINTERSTITIAL INFLAMMATION AND FIBROSIS

The exact pathogenetic mechanisms leading to tubulointerstitial fibrosis and tubular atrophy in primary glomerular, vascular, or even interstitial disease are still unknown. Almost all forms of primary or secondary interstitial disease are characterized by the formation of inflammatory infiltrates [reviewed by Strutz and Neilson (128)]. Tubulointerstitial infiltrates are the hallmark of any form of primary interstitial nephritis. The hallmark of tubulointerstitial nephritis is tubulitis, which is defined as a situation in which inflammatory cells are localized between tubular epithelial cells and/or between these and the TBM (129). These infiltrates consist in varying degrees of macrophages, neutrophils, T and B lymphocytes, plasma cells, as well as natural killer cells with usually a predominance of monocytes/macrophages and T cells (130,131). The exact nature and significance of primary tubulointerstitial disease is discussed elsewhere in this volume (see Chapter 36). Furthermore, interstitial infiltrates are present in secondary interstitial disease as well. Hooke et al., for example, studied the presence of infiltrating leukocytes in primary glomerulopathies in humans and were able to find them in all forms with the exception of minimal-change disease (132). Interstitial infiltrates are also present in different forms of vasculitis and are particularly common in Wegener granulomatosis (133,134). Tubulitis, as defined by Iványi and Olsen (129), has been described in primary glomerulonephritis, systemic vasculitis, chronic renal ischemia (135), and acute renal allograft rejection (136). The majority of infiltrating lymphocytes in secondary interstitial nephritis are CD2+ lymphocytes (131) with a predominance of CD4+ helper cells (137). Conversely, CD8+ cells predominate in allograft rejection, lupus nephritis, and PAN nephrosis (32,138). Our group has shown that the number of infiltrating CD4+ (and somewhat weaker CD8+) T lymphocytes correlated well with kidney function in humans (139). On the other hand, there was no correlation between kidney function and infiltrating CD14+ monocytes/macrophages. The latter finding has been disputed by others (86). That infiltrating lymphocytes may directly lead to organ fibrosis was demonstrated by Piguet et al. in a model of lung fibrosis (140). This group treated rats after bleomycin induction with anti-CD4+ or anti-CD8+ antibodies and saw a significant decrease in lung fibrosis. Treating animals with both antibodies simultaneously resulted in complete abrogation of fibrosis (140).

A number of factors have been implicated that may mediate secondary interstitial inflammation and fibrosis. These factors are summarized in Table 2 and will be discussed briefly.

TABLE 2. *Factors that mediate secondary tubulointerstitial infiltrates*

Calcium phosphate
MeProteinuria
Immune deposits
Cytokines
Chemokines
Tubular epithelial cells
tabolic acidosis
Lipids

Proteinuria

The degree of proteinuria often correlates well with the progression of various glomerulopathies (141,142), and it has been suggested that proteinuria itself may cause tubulointerstitial infiltrates (143). However, there are clear differences in various proteins in their potential to induce interstitial inflammation. Sanders et al. used a tubular perfusion system to analyze a number of low molecular weight proteins and found a great variability in their potential to induce tubular damage (144). Patients with sole albuminuria, for example, do rarely get interstitial disease (42). In fact, as was recently demonstrated, albumin rather has a protective effect on disease progression. Purified albumin from rats with adriamycin nephropathy caused a downregulation of interstitial collagens in mesangial cells and fibroblasts as determined by SDS–polyacrylamide gel electrophoresis and immunoprecipitation (145).

Few studies in humans have examined interstitial inflammation in patients with proteinuria. Yoshioka and co-workers analyzed cytokine expression in infiltrating interstitial cells in patients with immunoglobulin-A nephropathy and found a good correlation with the number of IL-6-positive cells (146). However, many studies in animals support the concept of proteinuria-induced interstitial inflammation. The degree of proteinuria, for example, paralleled interstitial infiltration in adriamycin-induced rat glomerulosclerosis (147,148). In the PAN nephrosis model, protein-overload proteinuria resulted in marked interstitial inflammation, whereas protein restriction resulted in a decrease in interstitial matrix formation (138,149).

Proteinuria may induce peritubular inflammation by direct tubular toxicity and by indirect effects. Potential direct toxicity may be mediated by enhanced lysosomal activity in tubular cells due to the increased protein reabsorption, as proposed by Maack et al. (150). In fact, Olbricht and co-workers were able to demonstrate that the activity of the two proteases cathepsin B and L was increased in rats with PAN nephrosis (151). Additionally, increased filtration of complement factors such as C5b-9 may play a role, because the urine level of C5b-9 correlated well with the degree of proteinuria (152), albeit there is some controversy about whether C5b-9 is actually filtered or formed by in situ complement activation (152–154). A novel chemotactic factor has recently been described in the model of BSA-induced overload proteinuria (155). The factor was generated in rat proximal tubule cells as a result of metabolism-induced albumin-borne fatty acids and was not detectable when lipid-depleted BSA was used. Another factor that has been implicated in the pathogenesis of proteinuria-induced secondary interstitial inflammation is iron, which may be released from filtered transferrin–iron complexes (156, 157). Iron can lead to the formation of hydroxyl radicals via the Haber–Weiss reaction (157), and iron depletion results in significant less interstitial inflammation compared with animals with normal iron stores in nephrotoxic serum nephritis (156).

Immune Deposits

Immune deposits often induce primary glomerular disease. In addition, they may play a role in tubulointerstitial disease. In experimental animal models, interstitial infiltrates can be observed in areas adjacent to linear TBM deposits of heterologous anti-GBM antibodies in anti-GBM disease (158). Moreover, subepithelial TBM deposits often accompany subepithelial GBM immune complexes in Heymann nephritis (159). In that model, complement depletion did not change the extent of interstitial infiltrates. Thus, the pathogenetic antibody may interact with the Fc receptor of monocytes/macrophages, causing the interstitial infiltrate, as described by Holdsworth and Neale for glomerular injury (160). Descriptions of extraglomerular immune deposits in human disease, though, have been rare. Only one series found extraglomerular immune deposits in up to 30% of studied patients (with type-I membranoproliferative glomerulonephritis) (161). All other descriptions of nonglomerular antibody formation were simple case reports (162–164), making it unlikely that immune deposits play a major role in the induction of tubulointerstitial infiltrates.

Cytokines

Cytokines play a crucial role in the formation of tubulointerstitial infiltrates and subsequent fibrogenesis. The most important cytokines for secondary interstitial disease will be discussed briefly (see Chapter 20 for a thorough discussion of the individual cytokines). Cytokines that may be involved in the accumulation of interstitial infiltrates and the promotion of fibrogenesis include the various interleukins (IL-1 to IL-7); interferon (IFN)-α, IFN-β, IFN-γ; PDGF-A and PDGF-B, tumor necrosis factor (TNF) α and TNF-β; FGF, EGF, insulinlike growth factor (IGF) 1; and TGF-α and TFG-β (165). Lan and co-workers studied the primary localization of interstitial infiltrates in anti-GBM nephritis and concluded that the perivascular sheaths of hilar arterioles were the primary site of infiltration (166). Thus, direct release of cytokines from inflammatory cells within the glomerulus may initiate interstitial inflammation. The two classic proinflammatory cytokines are IL-1 and TNF-α. Both are upregulated early in the disease process and both can cause interstitial infiltration of various leukocytes (167).

Since tubulointerstitial infiltrates precede almost any form of renal fibrosis, the question arises as to how infiltrating cells induce fibrogenesis. Again, cytokines are thought to play a key role. T lymphocytes may induce matrix production directly or indirectly. Direct stimulation is the result of cytokine release, which has a direct influence on matrix-producing cells, while indirect stimulation is mediated via the stimulation of monocytes/macrophages, which in turn secrete fibrogenic cytokines (128). Both T cells and monocytes/macrophages synthesize TGF-β, which is probably the most important cytokine for fibrogenesis (168,169). TGF-β induces the production of fibronectin, collagen, and proteoglycans (170), and inhibits matrix degradation by increased synthesis of PAI-1 (171). In vitro studies on renal fibroblasts revealed that TGF-β enhanced type-I and type-IV collagen production while reducing that of types II and V (115). Increased levels of TGF-β have been detected in models of renal (88), pulmonary (172), and hepatic fibrosis (173). TGF-β expression was elevated in several models of tubulointerstitial fibrosis, including chronic anti-Thy-1.1 glomerulopathy (88), Heymann nephritis (149), anti-GBM disease (174), PAN nephrosis (149), adriamycin-induced nephrosis (175), protein-overload proteinuria (83), and hypertensive (176) and obstructive nephropathy (177). Moreover, the induction of PAI-1 activity was recently demonstrated in a murine model of glomerulonephritis (178). Studies with inhibitors of TGF-β have been performed in models of glomerulosclerosis (179, 180) but not in interstitial renal disease. These inhibition studies were able to prevent glomerulosclerosis. Still, the influence of TGF-β on progression of renal disease was challenged recently, suggesting that it rather has a role in limiting the extent of the injury (181). Clearly, inhibition studies need to be performed in progressive interstitial fibrosis to clarify the role of this cytokine. In addition, TGF-β may have a monocyte chemotactic effect (182) and thus may participate in the generation of interstitial infiltrates. Other cytokines that may induce increased matrix synthesis and deposition include TNF-α and FGF. TNF-α has been shown to play a key role in pulmonary fibrosis (140). The expression of TNF-α was increased in several models of renal disease, though its exact role in interstitial inflammation and fibrosis remains to be determined (183,184).

However, fibrogenesis is not only characterized by increased matrix production per single cell (100) but also by proliferation of matrix-producing cells. Major mitogens for fibroblasts include PDGF, IGF-1, EGF, TGF-α, IL-1, and endothelin. Stimulated macrophages secrete large amounts of PDGF, which is a potent mitogen for fibroblasts but has only marginal effects on extracellular matrix production (185,186). In one study in renal rabbit fibroblasts, PDGF had robust mitogenic effects on papillary but not on cortical fibroblasts (49). Conversely, EGF and IGF-1 stimulated growth in both cell types in the same study. Both cytokines can be detected early in models of interstitial fibrosis, possibly because of their mitogenic effect on tubular epithelial cells (187). In the model of subtotal nephrectomy in rats, however, expression of IGF-1 was also localized in the interstitium and perivascular area coinciding with interstitial fibrosis (187). TGF-α expression has been shown to be upregulated considerably in a model of pulmonary fibrosis (188), but its role in renal fibrosis remains to be established. IL-1 has a number of biologic functions besides the potential effect as an autocrine growth factor for fibroblasts (see above), including the induction of proliferation and collagen production in normal fibroblasts (189). In addition, it has been shown that tubular epithelial cells produce increased amounts of type-IV collagen under the influence of IL-1 (190). Recently, it has been demonstrated that fibroblasts from patients with systemic sclerosis constitutively express IL-1α and IL-1β, whereas normal skin fibroblasts do not (191). Endothelin (ET) 1 is a mitogen and chemoattractant, at least for pulmonary fibroblasts (192). Furthermore, ET-1 and ET-3 stimulated collagen synthesis and inhibited collagenase production in cardiac fibroblasts (193). The effect of endothelins on renal fibroblasts remains to be established.

Chemokines

Chemokines (intercrines) are thought to play an important role in the recruitment of certain leukocyte subtypes during inflammation (194). The expression of chemokines is inducible by various cytokines, lectins, bacterial products, and viruses in a number of renal cells, including tubular epithelial cells and fibroblasts (195). Thus, it has been speculated that the primary inflammatory process in the glomerulus causes a release in cytokines that in turn results in an increased synthesis of chemokines in tubular epithelial cells and subsequently attracts inflammatory cells. However, currently this hypothesis, while intriguing, is still unproven.

According to the spacing of the two cysteine residues, two families may be distinguished (195), but additional families may exist, as was recently demonstrated by Kelner et al. (196) (see also Chapter 24). One of the best-studied members of the chemokine family is IL-8, which belongs to the CXC subfamily. IL-8 is a potent chemoattractant for neutrophils and certain lymphocytes (197). Its production has been described in human tubular epithelial cells in vitro and in vivo (198). In addition, IL-8 has been detected in normal and fibrosis-derived fibroblasts (89). Another member of the CXC subfamily, platelet factor 4, is also a chemoattractant for neutrophils and for monocytes and fibroblasts (199). Members of the CC subfamily, on the other hand, are mainly responsible for the recruitment of mononuclear leukocytes. Thus, they are particularly attractive candidates as mediators of interstitial mononuclear infiltrates. Monocyte chemoattractant protein (MCP) 1 is the prototype of this subfamily. As the name implies, it is chemotactic for monocytes but not for neutrophils (194). In a study of anti-TBM disease in rats, MCP-1 expression preceded the infiltration of mononuclear leukocytes (200). Similarly, increased levels of MCP-1 mRNA and the de novo appearance of MCP-1 protein were detectable in the model of PAN nephrosis (42) and anti-Thy-1.1 glomerulonephritis (201). Moreover, MCP-1 production has been demonstrated in human tubular epithelial cells in various glomerulopathies (202), and its synthesis could be increased by inflammatory cytokines such as IFN-γ, IL-1α, and TNF-α (202,203). Nevertheless, other data do not support the relevance of MCP-1 for interstitial monocyte/macrophage infiltration. MCP-1 expression, for example, was not elevated until week 2 after induction of protein-overload proteinuria in rats, well after the increase in interstitial macrophages (83). Moreover, MCP-1-neutralizing antiserum failed to reduce the number of infiltrating cells in the PAN nephrosis model, indicating that other factors may be implicated in the pathogenesis of interstitial infiltrates (42). RANTES is another member of the CC subfamily. It is expressed in proximal tubular and mesangial cells (204,205). Like MCP-1, RANTES is also a strong chemoattractant for monocytes as well as for eosinophils and basophils (194,206). RANTES expression is increased in interstitial inflammation due to allograft rejection and HIV nephropathy (207). Recently, reactive oxygen intermediates have been implicated in the formation of chemokines such as MCP-1 and RANTES (208), and novel members of the CC subfamily have been described (206). The significance of these findings for renal disease remains to be determined.

Tubular Epithelial Cells

Tubular epithelial cells have a key role in the mediation of secondary interstitial infiltrates. As indicated above, tubular epithelial cells are affected by a variety of cytokines and by proteinuria. In response, they secrete cytokines and chemokines and express certain adhesion molecules. All of these factors may participate in the initiation of interstitial inflammation. Adhesion molecules whose expression is upregulated in interstitial inflammation include intercellular adhesion molecule (ICAM) 1 and vascular adhesion molecule (VCAM) 1. ICAM-1 binds specifically to the CD11a–CD18 complex [formerly known as the lymphocyte-function-associated antigen (LFA) 1], a β_2-integrin that is expressed on a variety of leukocytes (209). Very late antigen (VLA) 4 ($\alpha_4\beta_1$-integrin) binds monocytes to VCAM-1, which is expressed by peritubular capillaries and tubular epithelial cells (210). Under normal conditions, tubular epithelial cells express ICAM-1 not at all or only weakly. Induction is possible by IFN-γ, IL-1, and TNF-α (211,212). A study of anti-TBM disease showed that infiltrating CD18+ leukocytes were present in areas of upregulated ICAM-1 expression (200). Otherwise, ICAM-1 expression has been studied mainly in allograft rejection, where its expression is upregulated. Moreover, a significant role of ICAM-1 in interstitial disease is suggested by the capability of anti-ICAM-1 antibodies to reduce interstitial infiltrates in anti-GBM nephritis (213), renal allograft rejection (214), rapid progressive glomerulonephritis (215) and autoimmune interstitial nephritis (216). Similarly, anti-VLA-4 antibodies are capable of attenuating interstitial disease in rats with mercuric-chloride-induced nephritis (217). Conversely, in a recent study by Eddy and co-workers, ICAM-1 and VCAM-1 expression in tubular epithelial cells was not upregulated in the model of protein-overload proteinuria (83). In that model, however, ICAM-1 and VCAM-1 were upregulated on infiltrating interstitial cells, thus pointing to a role of interactions within the tubulointerstitial infiltrate rather than initiation of interstitial inflammation. In other models, increased expression of ICAM-1 an VCAM-1 on tubular epithelial cells has been demonstrated (129). However, as has been recently demonstrated by immunogold localization technique, ICAM-1 expression is localized to the brush border and VCAM-1 to the basolateral part of the tubular epithelial cell, pointing to a potentially more important pathogenetic role for VCAM-1 (218).

Another molecule that is often implicated in the pathogenesis of tubulointerstitial infiltrates is osteopontin, which is a cell–matrix adhesion molecule, originally described in bone matrix (219), that is synthesized and secreted by tubular epithelial cells (220). Increased osteopontin expression has been described in various glomerulopathies (221), angiotensin-II-induced interstitial fibrosis (222), and glomerulosclerosis (223). A good correlation between the expression of osteopontin (localized mainly in distal tubules and collecting ducts) and monocyte/macrophage accumulation was described in angiotensin-II-induced nephropathy (222). Moreover, de novo osteopontin expression by cortical tubular epithelial cells was noted in the protein-overload model (83) and cyclosporine-induced nephropathy in rats (224). Osteopontin expression was observed in regenerating and non-regenerating cells. Interstitial macrophage infiltration was identified adjacent to osteopontin-positive tubules (83,224). Specific blocking studies are needed to evaluate further the role of osteopontin in the pathogenesis of interstitial infiltrates. Another potentially important chemoattractant for monocytes is vascular endothelial growth factor (VEGF). VEGF is constitutively expressed in podocytes but not in tubular epithelial cells (225). Its expression, however, is inducible by hypoxia (226). The role of VEGF in the formation of interstitial infiltrates awaits further study.

Another important factor in the mediation of tubulointerstitial inflammation may be the expression of major histocompatibility complex (MHC) class II antigens. These antigens are constitutively expressed on tubular epithelial cells, albeit at low level (227). Increased and aberrant MHC class II expression has been demonstrated in a variety of glomerulopathies (228). Initially, it had been proposed that tubular epithelial cells may function as antigen-presenting cells, providing another explanation for secondary interstitial inflammation (229,230). T cells, however, need additional stimuli for activation, such as the expression of cofactors (for example, BB1/B7, which interacts with CD28); otherwise, they become anergic (231). In fact, transplanting kidneys overexpressing MHC class II antigens into syngeneic mice was insufficient to induce tubulointerstitial inflammation (232). Conversely, MHC class I antigens may actually be more important than previously thought. Injection of monoclonal anti-DNA antibody into mice usually results in autoimmune systemic lupus erythematosus. Knockout mice for b_2-microglobulin, however, which are incompetent for MHC class I expression, failed to develop autoimmune disease (233).

Tubular epithelial cells are important mediators for interstitial inflammation. As outlined above, our group was able to show that human tubular epithelial cells from patients with glomerulopathies had a higher level of expression of certain cytokines such as GM-CSF and PDGF compared with tubular cells from kidneys without glomerular disease (92). The expression of both cytokines could be induced by TNF-α and IL-1α. GM-CSF has strong chemoattractive capacities for leukocytes and may induce fibroblast proliferation (234).

Another potential mechanism for tubulitis is the generation of autoreactive oxygen radicals (11). Surviving nephrons in chronic renal disease are characterized by a rise in oxygen consumption that is due to an increase in sodium reabsorption (235). The increased oxygen metabolism may in turn result in a increase in ammoniagenesis and generation of autoreactive oxygen radicals (236). The potential importance of autoreactive oxygen radicals was underlined by a study by Nath and Hudeen (237). Healthy rats were fed a diet deficient in selenium and vitamin E, both scavengers of free oxygen radicals. After 14 days, the rats without selenium and vitamin-E supplements developed acute tubulointerstitial nephritis (237).

Calcium Phosphate

Chronic renal failure is often characterized by a tendency to retain phosphate. Calcium–phosphate precipitations may form even at creatinine values of <1.5 mg/dL (132 mmol/L) (238). These deposits may in turn result in tubulointerstitial inflammation (239). In fact, it has been shown at least experimentally that a normal phosphorus intake is associated with interstitial infiltrates (240), whereas phosphate restriction may reduce tubulointerstitial inflammation (241). Ibels et al. studied rats with $1^3/_4$ nephrectomy and found that dietary phosphorus restriction improved histologic changes and preserved renal function after 24 weeks (242). Likewise, Lumlertgul et al. compared two groups of $^5/_6$ nephrectomized rats that were both fed a normal diet, with one group also receiving a phosphate binder (243). After 12 weeks, the group receiving the phosphate binder had a significantly higher creatinine clearance and less severe histologic scarring than the control group. However, prospective studies in humans on the effects of phosphate binders and low-protein diet on the progression to ESRD are currently not available.

Metabolic Acidosis

Excretion of hydrogen ions is one of the most important functions of the kidney. In chronic renal failure, ammonium secretion is the prominent mechanism for pH stability. Thus, due to the reduced number of functioning nephrons, each remaining nephron has to secrete more ammonium. Ammonium, on the other hand, may cause complement activation, which in turn results in interstitial inflammation. Therapy with alkalizing substances is capable of decreasing interstitial infiltrates in animal models (244). The application of alkaline therapy in humans is unproven.

Lipids

Fatty-acid-depleted rats do not develop interstitial infiltrates in PAN nephrosis (245,246). Thus, it has been proposed that lipid factors may play a role in secondary interstitial inflammation. However, the mechanism is not clear. Houglum and co-workers found that increased lipid peroxidation induced collagen expression in cultured human fibroblasts (247). Administration of D-α-tocopherol prevented this increase. Conversely, the lipid-lowering drugs lovastatin and probucol were able to reduce the severity of tubulointerstitial infiltrates in PAN nephrosis (42). Further studies are necessary to define the role of lipids in interstitial disease.

PREVENTION OF PROGRESSION

This textbook deals with mechanisms of disease rather than therapeutic options. However, preventing the progression to end-stage renal failure is a central goal for any intervention in renal disease. Thus, the following sections discuss briefly the current possibilities for therapeutic intervention in chronic renal failure: the ones that are clinically established and those that are still experimental.

Clinical Treatment

Treatment of the underlying inflammatory process represents the first-line therapy against the progression of renal disease. Corticosteroids are often a mainstay of therapy for renal inflammation. In fact, corticosteroids have been shown to be capable of inhibiting the binding of the proinflammatory cytokine IL-1 to type-I receptors (which are localized on T cells, fibroblasts, and endothelial cells)

(248,249). Moreover, they stop the synthesis of IL-1 and TNF-α, either directly or indirectly via the neuroendocrine axis (249). Besides, corticosteroids have other modes of action, such as the suppression of T lymphocytes and anticomplementary effects. Nevertheless, the success of a corticosteroid therapy is often limited (with the exception of minimal-change nephrosis), and additional therapies are indicated to prevent progression (250).

Hyperglycemia and hypertension are well-established risk factors for the progression of renal disease (7,251). Therapy of hyperglycemia is of particular benefit when initiated before overt diabetic nephropathy (defined by a constantly positive urine dipstick for protein) develops. Intensified antiglycemic therapy can delay the progression of microalbuminuria, at least in type-I diabetics (252). It can not, however, slow the rate of progression once overt nephropathy has developed. Thus, other factors are involved in diabetic nephropathy besides hyperglycemia, including intraglomerular hypertension and glomerular hypertrophy. Antihypertensive therapy is therefore a mainstay to prevent the progression to ESRD in diabetics as well as in nondiabetics. Angiotensin-converting enzyme (ACE) inhibitors are particularly well suited to retard progression because they reverse the angiotensin-II-induced resistance at the efferent arteriole (253). However, ACE inhibitors may have additional modes of action, such as an improvement of size selectivity of the GBM (254). In fact, the therapeutic effect of ACE inhibitors is often independent of its antihypertensive actions since it can be observed in normotensives as well. Angiotensin II is a growth factor for glomerular and tubular cells (255). It may directly stimulate collagen synthesis, an effect that is mediated by TGF-β (256). Thus, in theory, inhibiting angiotensin II should reduce the accumulation of extracellular matrix. In fact, it has been demonstrated that ACE inhibitors may attenuate matrix deposition in models of obstructive nephropathy (257) and PAN nephrosis (258). Nevertheless, the potential of ACE inhibitors to halt progression to ESRD is well documented exclusively in insulin-dependent diabetics (259). Similar effects may be obtained by the use of the new class of angiotensin-II receptor antagonists. These drugs have similar effects on blood pressure as ACE inhibitors (260), with possibly fewer side effects (261). They have been shown to be capable of reducing protein excretion (262) and proved equally effective against progression of renal failure in one smaller study (263). Moreover, an angiotensin-II receptor antagonist ameliorated tubulointerstitial fibrosis in the unilateral ureteral obstruction model comparable to an ACE inhibitor (264). Their long-term effects, though, await further study.

Besides ACE inhibitors and the new angiotensin-II receptor blockers, other antihypertensives have been evaluated in their protential to halt progressive renal failure. Calcium channel blockers have been shown to be effective in smaller studies (265,266), whereas other classes of antihypertensive drugs are much less likely to attenuate progression, because they do not decrease glomerular hypertrophy (267). Finally, protein restriction has been propagated for the prevention of progression because it can reverse glomerular hyperfiltration and hypertrophy (268,269). Additionally, protein-restricted diet may result in decreased expression of selected cytokines such as PDGF and TGF-β (270,271). Large controlled studies in humans, however, yielded conflicting results (272,273). Currently, a modest protein restriction of 0.8–1.0 g/kg is recommended, with the lower value used in patients with proven progression (274).

Experimental Forms of Therapy

As in any form of chronic inflammation, it is critical in glomerular and nonglomerular disease to treat the inflammatory process as early as possible. Unfortunately, there are many forms of chronic renal disease which prove treatable with only little or no success. Thus, therapeutic regimens have been developed to inhibit the prevention of renal fibrosis, the final common pathway of chronic renal disease. Most of these forms of therapy are still at a very experimental stage; few have been tested in animal models of renal disease and even fewer in human patients. Figure 4 provides an overview of currently used experimental strategies for antifibrotic therapy. The most important approaches are discussed below. It should be kept in mind, however, that none of the therapies listed here is kidney specific nor is the effect on matrix synthesis restricted to areas with fibrosis. Obtaining organ- and disease-specific targeting represents one of the major challenges for kidney research. Specific targeting to the kidney is achievable by the use of gene transfer of kidney-specific enzymes or by the use of prodrugs that are activated by kidney-specific enzymes. Finding and characterizing these organ specific genes represents an exciting goal for the next decade.

Inhibition of Fibroblast Activation

Inhibiting interstitial inflammation has been efficient against matrix deposition in models of pulmonary (140,275) and renal fibrosis (276). One experimental approach is to block adhesion molecules that play a role in interstitial inflammation. As outlined above, antibodies to ICAM-1 and LFA-1 prevented crescent formation and tubulointerstitial fibrosis in autoimmune glomerulonephritis when given before disease induction (213). The administration of both antibodies still attenuated interstitial and glomerular changes. Likewise, as indicated above, anti-ICAM-1 antibodies attenuated or prevented interstitial disease in models of primary and secondary interstitial nephritis.

Thus, efforts to inhibit fibroblast activation have concentrated on the inactivation of certain cytokines that are

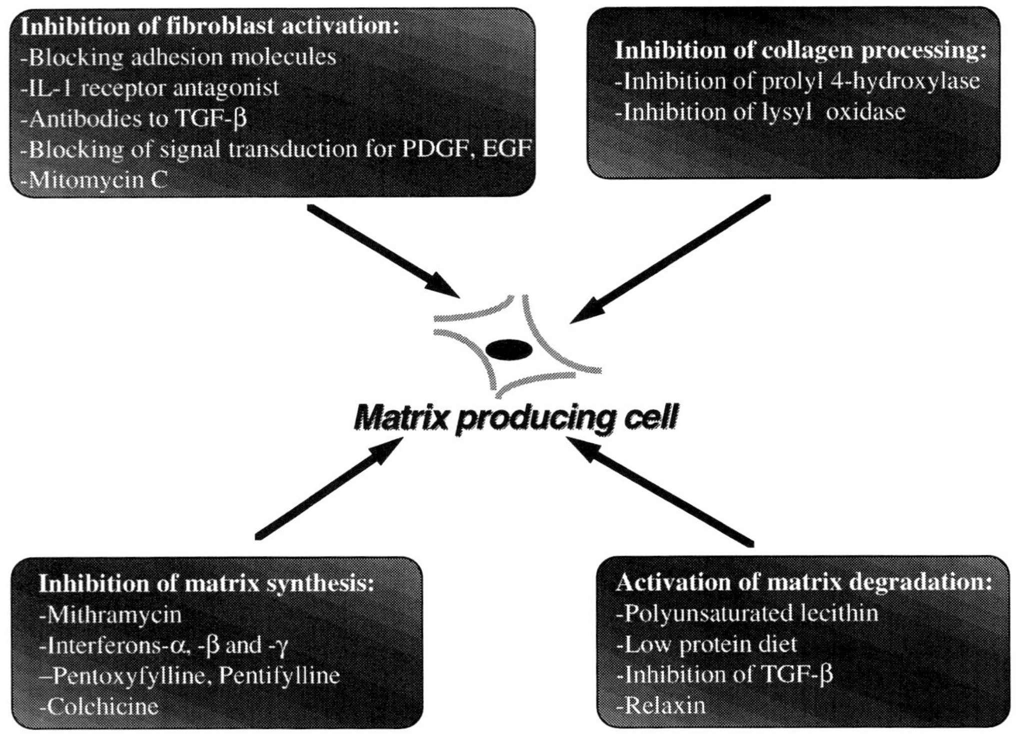

FIG. 4. Experimental strategies for the prevention of chronic renal disease. See the text for explanation.

actively involved in fibrogenesis, including TGF-β, PDGF, IGF-1, EGF, IL-1, and endothelin. Blocking the effects of the proinflammatory cytokine IL-1 has been tried experimentally, especially by use of the IL-1 receptor antagonist. Application of IL-1Ra to rats with anti-GBM disease resulted in a >50% decrease in macrophage accumulation within glomeruli and tubulointerstitium (277). Interestingly, this result could be obtained even when therapy was delayed until day 7 after induction of the disease. Similar results were obtained by Tang and co-workers (278), who found reductions in neutrophil and monocyte/macrophage infiltration by 40% and 30%, respectively, 4 h after the onset of anti-GBM nephritis. However, proteinuria was only reduced from 150 to 75 mg/day. This finding is not surprising, since other falters such as TNF-α production are not checked by IL-1Ra (250). Nevertheless, the use of IL-1Ra represents currently one of the most exciting forms of therapy for the prevention of progressive renal disease. Moreover, application of IL-1Ra has been of benefit in nonrenal fibrosis. Addition of IL-1Ra to rats with hepatic and mice with pulmonary fibrosis attenuated the interstitial matrix deposition (279,280).

As outlined above, TGF-β is one of the most important cytokines in fibrogenesis. Antibodies against TGF-β prevented the accumulation of extracellular matrix in the anti-Thy-1.1 model of mesangioproliferative glomerulonephritis (179). Similarly, decorin, a proteoglycan that is a natural inhibitor of TGF-β, also inhibited glomerular scarring in experimental glomerulonephritis (180). Neutralizing antibodies or decorin have not been used for the prevention of tubulointerstitial fibrosis, but antibodies to TGF-β_1 and TGF-β_2 protected against bleomycin- and immune-induced pulmonary fibrosis, at least partially (281,282). Nevertheless, similar to what has been said about the use of antiadhesion therapies, anti-TGF-β therapy must be initiated relatively early in the disease course. Furthermore, as discussed, TGF-β has prominent anti-inflammatory properties that may limit the use of its inhibitors in vivo (283).

Inhibition of fibroblast proliferation has been tried by substances that block signal transduction via the receptor-specific tyrosine kinase of PDGF receptors and EGF receptors (284). These so-called tyrphostins were successful in attenuating fibroblast proliferation in vitro (284), their effect has not been tested in vivo. Blocking the effects of endothelin by the new endothelin receptor antagonists represents another promising approach to antifibrogenic therapy (285), because endothelins may have profibrogenic effects on fibroblasts (192,193). Endothelin receptor antagonists, though representing an interesting therapeutic option, have not been tested in renal fibroblasts yet. Additionally, inhibition of fibroblast proliferation has been tried experimentally by antiproliferative agents. PDGF-stimulated fibroproliferation, for example, could be significantly attenuated by colchicine, cysteamine, N-actetylcysteine, and by various methyxanthines, including pentoxifylline (286). Furthermore, our group has demonstrated that mitomycin C can be effective in inhibiting fibroblast proliferation (99). However, higher doses were needed for fibroblasts derived from fibrotic kidneys. Moreover, mitomycin induced differentiation in fibroblasts (100), which is often accompanied by an increase in matrix synthesis (287). Thus, the ideal compound would block fibroblast proliferation without influencing differentiation.

Inhibition of Matrix Synthesis

As outlined above, interstitial matrix consists of collagens, various glycoproteins, and proteoglycans. However, the major interstitial matrix protein is collagen type I, which is usually a heterotrimer that is formed by two α_1 and one α_2 chains. Occasionally, homotrimers consisting entirely of α_1 chains are formed. Expression of the α_1 chain is mainly transcriptionally regulated (288). Promoter activity depends on the interaction of transcription factors NF-1 and Sp1 with the relative response elements. Binding of these factors can be blocked. Mithramycin, for example, inhibits binding of Sp1 to the promoter site, resulting in reduced as well as TGF-β-stimulated α_1(I) gene expression in human embryonic lung fibroblasts (289). Conversely, binding of NF-1 to the collagen type-I promoter could be blocked by interferons (IFN)-α, IFN-β, IFN-γ, pentoxifylline, and pentifylline (290). The antifibrotic properties of IFN-γ have long been known (291). In fact, IFN-γ inhibits the increase in collagen production induced by TGF-β in normal human fibroblasts (292). Moreover, IFN-γ may reduce fibroblast proliferation and activation, as shown by Desmoulière et al. (293). IFN-γ has already been tested clinically. Treatment of 14 patients with systemic sclerosis resulted in a significant reduction in pulmonary and skin fibroses (294). Nevertheless, IFN-γ has the potential disadvantage of increasing proteoglycan and glycoprotein synthesis in fibroblasts (295). IFN-α and IFN-β may not have that effect, whereas both compounds suppress collagen type-I synthesis in similar fashion (295). Colchicine has also been proposed in the prevention of fibrosis. It may decrease collagen expression, increase collagenase production, and have additional anti-inflammatory properties (296,297). The compound has been shown to be of benefit in one study in primary biliary cirrhosis (298). Clearly, further studies are needed to establish the role of colchicine in fibrogenesis. Regulation of collagen α_1(I) gene expression is often cell specific (299), providing a potential target for specific therapy. Unfortunately, no kidney-specific inhibition of collagen synthesis is currently known.

Inhibition of Collagen Processing

Post-translational modifications are an essential part of collagen biosynthesis. The classic triple helix of collagen molecules can be formed only if hydroxylation of proline residues occurs by the specific prolyl 4-hydroxylase. Inactivity of this enzyme causes unstable triple helices (300). Recently, two competitive inhibitors of prolyl 4-hydroxylase have been developed (301). Both were found to be effective in reducing liver hydroxyproline content as well as overall mortality in models of liver fibrosis (302). However, while human trials were already under way, one of the compounds (HOE 077) had to be withdrawn because of cataract formation in dogs (303). Moreover, concerns have been raised about the effects on other (collagen containing) tissues because of sustained inhibition of prolyl 4-hydroxylase necessary for a clinically useful reduction in collagen deposition (304). Another enzyme necessary for post-translational collagen stabilization is lysyl oxidase, which catalyzes the oxidative deamination of ε-amino groups of lysyl and hydroxylysyl residues (304). The activity of lysyl oxidase may be increased in fibrogenesis (305); thus, the enzyme represents a potential target for inhibitors, resulting in more unstable collagen molecules (303). In fact, a number of potent lysyl-oxidase inhibitors have been described in the literature and are currently undergoing experimental trials in animal models (304,306).

Activation of Matrix Degradation

All experimental strategies outlined above have the potential disadvantage that therapy has to initiate rather early in the course of the disease to prevent progression. Stimulation of matrix degradation, on the other hand, may initiate at any time, though, in order to preserve as much organ function as possible, an early begin may seem advisable. A stimulation of MMP-1 (type-I collagenase) is possible by the application of polyunsaturated lecithin. In fact, this compound has been shown capable of preventing alcohol-induced liver fibrosis in baboons (307). Inhibiting the effects of TIMPs represents another way of activating matrix degradation. As discussed above, the expression of TIMPs is often upregulated in the phase of active matrix deposition. In the PAN nephrosis model in rats, lower levels in TIMP-1 and TIMP-2 expression were obtained by a restriction of protein intake, an effect possibly mediated by the attenuation of TGF-β expression (270). TIMP expression can also be downregulated by the human hormone relaxin, which has a natural function in cervical softening and uterine involution in and after pregnancy (308). The hormone causes a downregulation of TIMP-1 and an upregulation in MMP-1 expression. Its use in two rodent models of skin fibrosis resulted in a significant reduction in matrix deposition (309). However, it has not been evaluated in nonskin fibrosis.

SUMMARY

Tubulointerstitial inflammation and particularly fibrosis are of great importance for the prognosis of any form

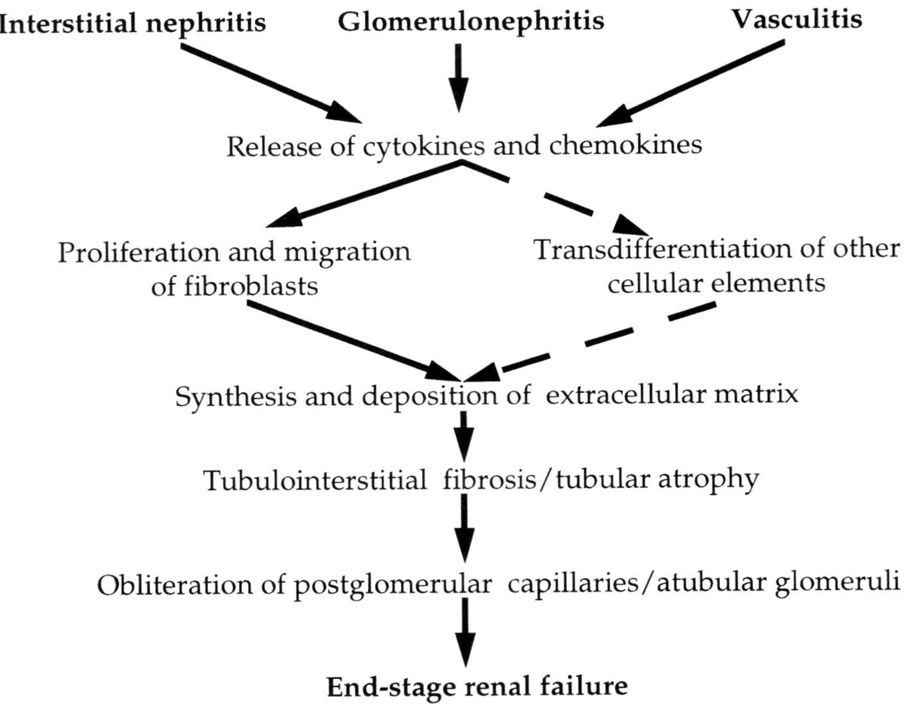

FIG. 5. pathogenesis of progression to end-stage renal failure.

of renal disease. Whereas the exact pathogenesis of secondary tubulointerstitial involvement is still unknown, it has become increasingly clear that interstitial inflammation is mainly a consequence of proteinuria and the release of cytokines and chemokines by tubular epithelial and inflammatory cells. Depositions of immune complexes, calcium phosphate, lipids, and metabolic acidosis play only minor roles. Secondary interstitial infiltrates result in the release of cytokines that in turn stimulate resident fibroblasts and possibly additional resident cells to (trans)differentiate, proliferate, and start extracellular matrix synthesis. Concurrently, matrix degradation is inhibited by upregulation of TIMPs. Experimental models have demonstrated that resolution of the fibrogenic process is possible as in regular wound healing. Otherwise, fibrosis ensues as a consequence of postinflammatory matrix synthesis and deposition due to autocrine and paracrine fibroblast stimulation. Figure 5 summarizes our current view of the pathogenesis of progression to end-stage renal failure. Therapy to prevent the progression of interstitial fibrosis has made much progress in recent years thanks especially to ACE inhibitors. Other forms of therapy are still very much experimental, but some hold great promise for the future.

ACKNOWLEDGMENTS

This work was made possible in part by grants from the Deutsche Forschungsgemeinschaft to F.S. (DFG 388/1-1) and G.A.M. (DFG Mu 523/7-1).

REFERENCES

1. The magnitude of the ESRD problem. *Am J Kidney Dis* 1990;16 (Suppl 2):17–21.
2. *US Renal Data System:* annual data report. Bethesda, MD: National Institute of Diabetes and Digestive and Kidney Diseases, National Institutes of Health, March 1993.
3. Jacobson HR, Klahr S. Chronic renal failure: pathophysiology; management. *Lancet* 1991;338:419–23.
4. Dodd S. The pathogenesis of tubulointerstitial disease and mechanisms of fibrosis. *Curr Top Pathol* 1995;88:51–67.
5. Brenner BM, Meyer TW, Hostetter TH. Dietary protein intake and the progressive nature of kidney disease: the role of hemodynamically mediated glomerular injury in the pathogenesis of progressive glomerular sclerosis in aging, renal ablation, and intrinsic renal disease. *N Engl J Med* 1982;307:652–9.
6. Anderson S, Rennke HG, Brenner BM. Therapeutic advantages of converting enzyme inhibitors in arresting progressive renal disease associated with systemic hypertension in the rat. *J Clin Invest* 1986; 77:1993–2000.
7. Walker WG. Hypertension-related renal injury: a major contributor to end-stage renal disease. *Am J Kidney Dis* 1993;22:164–73.
8. Zatz R, Fujihara CK. Glomerular hypertrophy and progressive glomerulopathy: is there a definite pathogenetic correlation? *Kidney Int* 1994;45:527–9.
9. Wolf G, Neilson EG. Angiotensin II as a renal growth factor. *J Am Soc Nephrol* 1993;3:1531–40.
10. Bohle A, Strutz F, Müller GA. On the pathogenesis of chronic renal failure in primary glomerulopathies. *Exp Nephrol* 1994;2:205–10.
11. Nath KA. Tubulointerstitial changes as a major determinant in the progression of renal damage. *Am J Kidney Dis* 1992;20:1–17.
12. Strutz F, Müller GA. On the progression of chronic renal disease. *Nephron* 1995;69:371–9.
13. Bohle A, Wehrmann M, Bogenschütz O, et al. The long-term prognosis of the primary glomerulonephritides. *Pathol Res Pract* 1992;188: 908–24.
14. Henle J, Pfeufer C. Morbus Bright, klinische Mitteilungen. *Z Rationelle Med Zurich* 1844;1.
15. Toynbee J. On the intimate structure of the human kidney and on the

changes of its several component parts under Bright's disease. *Med Chir Trans* 1846;29:304–24.
16. Allen AC. *The kidney:* medical and surgical diseases. New York: Grune, 1951.
17. Spuhler O, Zollinger HU. Die chronische interstitielle Nephritis. *Z Klin Med* 1953;131:1–50.
18. Hutt MSR, Pinniger JL, de Wardener HE. The relationship between the clinical and the histological features of acute glomerular nephritis. *Q J Med* 1958;106:265–91.
19. Risdon RA, Sloper JAC, de Wardener HE. Relationship between renal function and histological changes found in renal biopsy specimens from patients with persistent glomerular nephritis. *Lancet* 1968; 2:363–6.
20. Schainuck LI, Striker GE, Cutler RE, Benditt EP. Structural–functional correlations in renal disease. II. The correlations. *Hum Pathol* 1970;1:631–41.
21. Striker GE, Schainuck LI, Cutler RE, Benditt EP. Structural–functional correlations in renal disease. I. A method for assaying and classifying histopathologic changes in renal disease. *Hum Pathol* 1970;1: 615–30.
22. Bohle A, Bader R, Grund KE, Mackensen S, Neunhoeffer J. Serum creatinine concentration and renal interstitial volume: analysis of correlations in endocapillary (acute) glomerulonephritis and moderately severe mesangioproliferative glomerulonephritis. *Virchows Arch [A]* 1977;375:87–96.
23. Bohle A, Grund KE, Mackensen S, Tolon M. Correlations between renal interstitium and level of serum creatinine: morphometric investigations of biopsies in perimembranous glomerulonephritis. *Virchows Arch [A]* 1977;373:15–22.
24. Wehrmann M, Bohle A, Helol H, Schumm G, Kendziorra H, Pressler H. Long-term prognosis of focal sclerosing glomerulonephritis: an analysis of 250 cases with particular regard to tubulointerstitial changes. *Clin Nephrol* 1990;33:115–22.
25. Fischbach H, Mackensen S, Grund KE, Kellner A, Bohle A. Relationship between glomerular lesions, serum creatinine and interstitial volume in membranoproliferative glomerulonephritis. *Klin Wochenschr* 1977;55:603–8.
26. Bader R, Bader H, Grund KE, Mackensen-Haen S, Christ H, Bohle A. Structure and function of the kidney in diabetic glomerulosclerosis: correlations between morphological and functional parameters. *Pathol Res Pract* 1980;167:204–16.
27. Mackensen S, Grund KE, Bader R, Bohle A. The influence of glomerular and interstitial factors on the serum creatinine concentration and serum creatinine concentration in renal amyloidosis. *Virchows Arch [A]* 1977;375:159–68.
28. Bohle A, Mackensen-Haen S, Von Gise H. Significance of tubulointerstitial changes in the renal cortex for the excretory function and concentration ability of the kidney: a morphometric contribution. *Am J Nephrol* 1987;7:421–33.
29. Jepsen FL, Mortensen PB. Interstitial fibrosis of the renal cortex in minimal change lesion and its correlation with renal function. *Virchows Arch [A]* 1979;393:265–70.
30. Katafuchi R, Takebayashi S, Taguchi T, Harada T. Structural functional correlations in serial biopsies from patients with glomerulonephritis. *Clin Nephrol* 1987;28:169–73.
31. Abe S, Amagasaki Y, Iyori S, Konishi K, Kato E, Sakaguchi H. Significance of tubulointerstitial lesions in biopsy specimens of glomerulonephritis patients. *Am J Nephrol* 1989;9:30–7.
32. Alexopoulos E, Seron D, Hartley RB, Cameron JS. Lupus nephritis: correlation of interstitial cells with glomerular function. *Kidney Int* 1990;37:100–9.
33. Lane PH, Steffes MW, Fioretto P, Mauer SM. Renal interstitial expansion in insulin-dependent diabetes mellitus. *Kidney Int* 1993;43: 661–7.
34. Bennett WM, Walker RG, Kincaid-Smith P. Renal cortical interstitial volume in mesangial IgA nephropathy. *Lab Invest* 1982;47:330–5.
35. Ziyadeh FN, Goldfarb S. The diabetic renal tubulointerstitium. *Curr Top Pathol* 1995;88:175–202.
36. Roberts JA. Mechanisms of renal damage in chronic pyelonephritis (reflux nephropathy). *Curr Top Pathol* 1995;88:265–87.
37. Wilson PD, Falkenstein D. The pathology of human renal cystic disease. *Curr Top Pathol* 1995;88:1–50.
38. Thomsen OF, Andersen A, Christiansen JS, Deckert T. Renal changes in long-term type I (insulin-dependent) diabetic patients with and without clinical nephropathy: a light microscopic, morphometric study of autopsy material. *Diabetologia* 1984;26:361–5.
39. Mauer SM, Steffes MW, Ellis EN, Sutherland DER, Brown DM, Goetz FC. Structural–functional relationships in diabetic nephropathy. *J Clin Invest* 1984;74:1143–55.
40. Johnson DE, Russell RG, Lockatell CV, Zulty JC, Warren JW. Urethral obstruction of 6 hours or less causes bacteriuria, bacteremia, and pyelonephritis in mice challenged with "nonuropathogenic" *Escherichia coli*. *Infect Immun* 1993;61:3422–8.
41. Mai M, Geiger H, Hilgers KF, et al. Early interstitial changes in hypertension-induced renal injury. *Hypertension* 1993;22:754–65.
42. Eddy AA. Experimental insights into the tubulointerstitial disease accompanying primary glomerular lesions. *J Am Soc Nephrol* 1994;5:1273–87.
43. Ljungquist A. The intrarenal arterial pattern in the normal and diseased human kidney. *Acta Med Scand* 1963;174(Suppl 401):5–34.
44. Bohle A, Von Gise H, Mackensen-Haen S, Stark-Jakob B. The obliteration of the postglomerular capillaries and its influence on the function of both glomeruli and tubuli. *Klin Wochenschr* 1981;59:1043–51.
45. Von Gise H, Von Gise V, Stark B, Bohle A. Nephrotic syndrome and renal insufficiency in association with amyloidosis: a correlation between structure and function. *Klin Wochenschr* 1981;59:75–82.
46. Savill J, Mooney A, Hughes J. Apoptosis and renal scarring. *Kidney Int* 1996(Suppl).
47. Møller JC. Dimensional changes of proximal tubules and cortical capillaries in chronic obstructive renal disease. *Virchows Arch [A]* 1986;410:153–8.
48. Ong ACM, Jowett TP, Firth JD, Burton S, Kitamura M, Fine LG. Human-tubular derived endothelin in the paracrine regulation of renal interstitial fibroblast function. *Exp Nephrol* 1994.
49. Knecht A, Fine LG, Kleinman KS, et al. Fibroblasts of rabbit kidney in culture. II. Paracrine stimulation of papillary fibroblasts by PDGF. *Am J Physiol* 1991;261:F292–9.
50. Wolf G. Regulation of renal tubular growth: effects of angiotensin II. *Exp Nephrol* 1994;2:107–14.
51. Fine LG, Ong AC, Norman JT. Mechanisms of tubulo-interstitial injury in progressive renal diseases. *Eur J Clin Invest* 1993;23:259–65.
52. Oliver J. *Architecture of the kidney in chronic Bright's disease.* New York: Hoeber, 1939.
53. Marcussen N. Biology of disease: atubular glomeruli and the structural basis for chronic renal failure. *Lab Invest* 1992;66:265–84.
54. Marcussen N. Atubular glomeruli in chronic renal disease. *Curr Top Pathol* 1995;88:145–74.
55. Heptinstall RH, Kissane JM, Still WJS. Experimental pyelonephritis: morphology and quantitative histochemistry of glomeruli in pyelonephritic scars in the rat. *Bull Johns Hopkins Hosp* 1963;112:299–311.
56. Marcussen N, Olsen TS. Atubular glomeruli in patients with chronic pyelonephritis. *Lab Invest* 1990;62:467–78.
57. Marcussen N. Atubular glomeruli in renal artery stenosis. *Lab Invest* 1991;65:558–72.
58. Marcussen N, Nyengaard JR, Christensen S. Compensatory growth of glomeruli is accompanied by an increased number of glomerular capillaries. *Lab Invest* 1994;70:868–74.
59. Marcussen N, Ottosen PD, Christensen S, Olsen TS. Atubular glomeruli in lithium-induced chronic nephropathy in rats. *Lab Invest* 1989;61:295–302.
60. Woo D. Apoptosis and loss of renal tissue in polycystic kidney disease. *N Engl J Med* 1995;333:18–25.
61. Müller GA, Markovic-Lipkovski J, Rodemann HP. The progression of renal diseases: on the pathogenesis of renal interstitial fibrosis. *Klin Wochenschr* 1991;69:576–86.
62. Oomura A, Nakamura T, Arakawa M, Ooshima A, Isemura M. Alterations in the extracellular matrix components in human glomerular diseases. *Virchows Arch [A]* 1989;415:151–9.
63. Strutz F. Novel aspects of renal fibrogenesis. *Nephrol Dial Transplant* 1995;10:1526–32.
64. Kuncio GS, Neilson EG, Haverty T. Mechanisms of tubulointerstitial fibrosis. *Kidney Int* 1991;39:550–6.
65. Phan S, Wolber F, Wiggins R. Fibronectin is the major fibroblast chemotactin in crescentic nephritis. *J Am Soc Nephrol* 1992;3:610.
66. Wang N, Butler JP, Ingber DE. Mechanotransduction across the cell surface and through the cytoskeleton. *Science* 1993;260:1124–7.
67. Lee T-L, Lin Y-C, Mochitate K, Grinnell F. Stress–relaxation of fibroblasts in collagen matrices triggers ectocytosis of plasma mem-

brane vesicles containing actin, annexins II and VI, and β_1 integrin receptors. *J Cell Sci* 1993;105:167–77.

68. Lin Y-C, Grinnell F. Decreased level of PDGF-stimulated receptor autophosphorylation by fibroblasts in mechanically relaxed collagen matrices. *J Cell Biol* 1993;122:663–72.
69. Frisch SM, Francis H. Disruption of epithelial cell matrix interactions induces apoptosis. *J Cell Biol* 1994;124:619–26.
70. Sympson CJ, Talhouk RS, Alexander CM, et al. Targeted expression of stromelysin-1 in mammary gland provides evidence for a role of proteinases in branching morphogenesis and the requirement for an intact basement membrane for tissue-specific gene expression. *J Cell Biol* 1994;125:681–93.
71. Werb Z, Sympson CJ, Alexander CM, et al. Extracellular matrix remodeling and the regulation of epithelial–stromal interactions during differentiation and involution. *Kidney Int* 1996 (in press).
72. Gailit J, Clark RAF. Wound repair in the context of extracellular matrix. *Curr Opin Cell Biol* 1994;6:717–25.
73. Jones CL, Buch S, Post M, Culloch LM, Liu E, Eddy AA. Renal extracellular matrix accumulation in acute puromycin aminonucleoside nephrosis in rats. *Am J Pathol* 1992;141:1381–96.
74. Costigan M, Chambers DA, Boot-Handford RP. Collagen turnover in renal disease. *Exp Nephrol* 1995;3:114–21.
75. Matrisian LM. The matrix-degrading metalloproteinases. *BioEssays* 1992;14:455–63.
76. Goldberg GI, Strongin A, Collier IE, Genrich LT, Marmer BL. Interaction of 92-kDa type IV collagenase with the tissue inhibitor of metalloproteinases prevents dimerization, complex formation with interstitial collagenase and activation of the proenzyme with stromelysin. *J Biol Chem* 1992;267:4583–91.
77. Stetler-Stevenson WG, Liotta LA, Kleiner DE. Extracellular matrix 6: Role of matrix metalloproteinases in tumor invasion and metastasis. *FASEB J* 1993;7:1434–41.
78. Vassalli J-D, Sappino A-P, Belin D. The plasminogen activator/plasmin system. *J Clin Invest* 1991;88:1067–72.
79. Docherty AJP, Lyons A, Smith BJ, et al. Sequence of human tissue inhibitor of metalloproteinases and its identity to erythroid-potentiating activity. *Nature* 1985;318:66–9.
80. Stetler-Stevenson WG, Krutzsch HC, Liotta LA. Tissue inhibitor of metalloproteinase (TIMP-2): a new member of the metalloproteinase inhibitor family. *J Biol Chem* 1989;264:17,374–8.
81. Silbiger SM, Jacobsen VL, Cupples RL, Koski RA. Cloning of cDNAs encoding human TIMP-3, a novel member of the tissue inhibitor of metalloproteinase family. *Gene* 1994;141:293–8.
82. Jones CL, Fecondo J, Kelynack K, Forbes J, Walker R, Becker G. Tissue inhibitor of the metalloproteinases and renal extracellular matrix accumulation. *Exp Nephrol* 1995;3:80–6.
83. Eddy AE, Giachelli CM, McCulloch L, Liu E. Renal expression of genes that promote interstitial inflammation and fibrosis in rats with protein-overload proteinuria. *Kidney Int* 1995;47:1546–57.
84. Tang WW, Feng L, Xia Y, Wilson CB. Extracellular matrix accumulation in immune-mediated tubulointerstitial injury. *Kidney Int* 1994;45:1077–84.
85. Carome MA, Striker LJ, Peten EP, et al. Human glomeruli express TIMP-1 mRNA and TIMP-2 protein and mRNA. Am J Physiol 1993;264:F923–9.
86. Eddy AA. Interstitial macrophages as mediators of renal fibrosis. *Exp Nephrol* 1995;3:76–9.
87. Leco KJ, Kohara R, Pavloff N, Hawkes SP, Edwards DR. Tissue inhibitor of metalloproteinases-3 (TIMP-3) is an extracellular matrix associated with a distinctive pattern of expression in mouse cells and tissues. *J Biol Chem* 1994;269:9352–60.
88. Yamamoto T, Noble NA, Miller DE, Border WA. Sustained expression of TGF-β_1 underlies development of progressive kidney fibrosis. *Kidney Int* 1994;45:916–27.
89. Lonnemann G, Shapiro L, Engler-Blum G, Müller GA, Koch KM, Dinarello CA. Cytokines in human renal interstitial fibrosis. I. IL-1 is an autocrine growth factor for cultured fibrosis-derived kidney fibroblasts. *Kidney Int* 1995;47:837–44.
90. Lonnemann G, Engler-Blum G, Müller GA, Koch KM, Dinarello CA. Cytokines in human renal interstitial fibrosis. II. Intrinsic interleukin (IL)-1 synthesis and IL-1-dependent production of IL-6 and IL-8 by cultured kidney fibroblasts. *Kidney Int* 1995;47:845–54.
91. Gressner AM. Transdifferentiation of hepatic stellate cells (Ito cells) to myofibroblasts: a key event in hepatic fibrogenesis. *Kidney Int* 1996(Suppl).
92. Frank J, Engler-Blum G, Rodemann HP, Müller GA. Human renal tubular cells as a cytokine source: PDGF-B, GM-CSF and IL-6 mRNA expression in vitro. *Exp Nephrol* 1993;1:26–35.
93. Bohman SO. The ultrastructure of the rat renal medulla as observed after improved fixation methods. *J Ultrastruct Res* 1974;47:329–60.
94. Cohnheim J. Über Entzündung und Eiterung. *Virchows Arch* 1867;40:1–79.
95. Ross R, Everett NB, Tyler R. Wound healing and collagen formation. VI. The origin of the wound: fibroblast studied in parabiosis. *J Cell Biol* 1970;44:645–54.
96. Darby I, Skalli O, Gabbiani G. α-Smooth muscle actin is transiently expressed by myofibroblasts during experimental wound healing. *Lab Invest* 1990;63:21–30.
97. Gabbiani G. The biology of the myofibroblast. *Kidney Int* 1992;41:530–2.
98. Grinnell F. Fibroblasts, myofibroblasts, and wound contraction. *J Cell Biol* 1994;124:401–4.
99. Rodemann HP, Müller GA. Abnormal growth and clonal proliferation of fibroblasts derived from kidneys with interstitial fibrosis. *J Exp Biol Med* 1990;195:57–63.
100. Müller GA, Rodemann HP. Characterization of human renal fibroblasts in health and disease. I. Immunophenotyping of cultured tubular epithelial cells and fibroblasts derived from kidneys with histologically proven interstitial fibrosis. *Am J Kidney Dis* 1991;17:680–3.
101. Rodemann HP, Müller GA. Characterization of human renal fibroblasts in health and disease. II. In vitro growth, differentiation, and collagen synthesis of fibroblasts from kidneys with interstitial fibrosis. *Am J Kidney Dis* 1991;17:684–6.
102. Müller GA, Strutz FM. Renal fibroblast heterogeneity. *Kidney Int* 1995;48(Suppl 50):S33–6.
103. Rodemann HP, Müller GA, Knecht A, Norman JT, Fine LG. Fibroblasts of rabbit kidney culture. I. Characterization and identification of cell-specific markers. Am J Physiol 1991;261:F283–91.
104. Alpers CE, Hudkins KL, Floege J, Johnson RJ. Human renal cortical interstitial cells with some features of smooth muscle cells participate in tubulointerstitial and crescentic glomerular injury. *J Am Soc Nephrol* 1994;5:201–10.
105. Hewitson TD, Becker GJ. Interstitial myofibroblasts in IgA glomerulonephritis. *Am J Nephrol* 1995;15:111–7.
106. Strutz F, Müller GA, Neilson EG. Transdifferentiation: a new angle on renal fibrosis. *Exp Nephrol* 1996 (in press).
107. Bachem MG, Sell K-M, Melchior R, Kropf J, Eller T, Gressner AM. Tumor necrosis factor alpha (TNFα and transforming growth factor β_1 (TGFβ_1) stimulate fibronectin synthesis and the transdifferentiation of fat-storing cells in the rat liver into myofibroblasts. *Virchows Arch [B]* 1993;63:123–30.
108. Friedman SL. The cellular basis of hepatic fibrosis. *N Engl J Med* 1993;328:1828–35.
109. Zhang K, Rekter MD, Gordon D, Phan SH. Myofibroblasts and their role in lung collagen gene expression during pulmonary fibrosis. *Am J Pathol* 1994;145:114–25.
110. Creely JJ, Di Mari SJ, Howe AM, Haralson MA. Effects of transforming factor-β on collagen synthesis by normal rat kidney epithelial cells. *Am J Pathol* 1992;140:45–55.
111. Strutz F, Okada H, Lo CW, et al. Identification and characterization of fibroblast-specific protein 1 (FSP1). *J Cell Biol* 1995;130:393–405.
112. Wiggins R, Goyal M, Merritt S, Killen PD. Vascular adventitial cell expression of collagen I messenger ribonucleic acid in anti-glomerular basement membrane antibody-induced crescentic nephritis in the rabbit. *Lab Invest* 1993;68:557–65.
113. Kaissling B, Le Hir M. Characterization and distribution of interstitial cell types in the renal cortex of rats. *Kidney Int* 1994;45:709–20.
114. Bachmann S, Le Hir M, Eckardt K-U. Co-localization of erythropoietin mRNA and ecto-5′-nucleotidase immunoreactivity in peritubular cells of rat renal cortex indicates that fibroblasts produce erythropoietin. *J Histochem Cytochem* 1993;41:335–41.
115. Alvarez RJ, Sun MJ, Haverty TP, Iozzo RV, Meyers JC, Neilson EG. Biosynthetic and proliferative characteristics of tubulointerstitial fibroblasts probed with paracrine cytokines. *Kidney Int* 1992;41:14–23.
116. Strutz F, Caron R, Tomaszewski J, Fumo P, Ziyadeh F, Neilson EG. Transdifferentiation: a new concept in renal fibrogenesis. *J Am Soc Nephrol* 1994;5:819(abst).
117. Strutz F, Lo C, Neilson EG. On the origin of fibroblasts: a molecular biological approach. *Kidney Int* 1995;47:1002(abst).

118. Eguchi G, Kodama R. Transdifferentiation. *Curr Opin Cell Biol* 1993;5:1023–8.
119. Haverty TP, Kelly CJ, Hines WH, et al. Characterization of a renal tubular epithelial cell line which secretes the autologous target antigen of autoimmune experimental interstitial nephritis. *J Cell Biol* 1988;107:1359–67.
120. Humes HD, Nakamura T, Cieslinski DA, Miller D, Emmons RV, Border WA. Role of proteoglycans and cytoskeleton in the effects of TGF-β_1 on renal proximal tubule cells. *Kidney Int* 1993;43: 575–84.
121. Ziyadeh F, Snipes ER, Watanabe M, Alvarez RJ, Goldfarb S, Haverty TP. High glucose induces cell hypertrophy and stimulates collagen gene transcription in proximal tubule. Am J Physiol 1990;259: F704–14.
122. Nadasdy T, Laszik Z, Blick KE, Johnson DL, Silva FG. Tubular atrophy in the end-stage kidney: a lectin and immunohistochemical study. *Hum Pathol* 1994;25:22–8.
123. Greenburg G, Hay ED. Cytoskeleton and thyroglobulin expression change during transformation of thyroid epithelium to mesenchyme-like cells. *Development* 1988;102:605–22.
124. Miettinen PJ, Ebner R, Lopez AR, Derynck R. TGF-b induced transdifferentiation of mammary epithelial cells to mesenchymal cells: involvement of type I receptors. *J Cell Biol* 1994;127:2021–36.
125. Potts JD, Runyan RB. Epithelial–mesenchymal cell transformation in the embryonic heart can be mediated, in part, by transforming growth factor β. *Dev Biol* 1989;134:392–401.
126. Opas M, Dziak W. bFGF-induced transdifferentiation of RPE to neuronal progenitors is regulated by the mechanical properties of the substratum. *Dev Biol* 1994;161:440–54.
127. Hay ED. Extracellular matrix alters epithelial differentiation. *Curr Opin Cell Biol* 1993;5:1029–35.
128. Strutz F, Neilson EG. The role of lymphocytes in the progression of interstitial disease. *Kidney Int* 1994;45(Suppl 45):SlO6–lO.
129. Iványi B, Olsen S. Tubulitis in renal disease. *Curr Top Pathol* 1995; 88:117–41.
130. Boucher A, Droz D, Adafer E, Laure-Helene N. Characterization of mononuclear cell subsets in renal cellular interstitial infiltrates. *Kidney Int* 1986;29:1043–9.
131. Markovic-Lipkovski J, Müller CA, Risler T, Bohle A, Müller GA. Association of glomerular and interstitial mononuclear leucocytes with different forms of glomerulonephritis. *Nephrol Dial Transplant* 1990;5:10–7.
132. Hooke DH, Gee DC, Atkins RC. Leukocyte analysis using monoclonal antibodies in human glomerulonephritis. *Kidney Int* 1987;31: 964–72.
133. Cameron JS. New horizons in renal vasculitis. *Klin Wochenschr* 1991;69:536–51.
134. Mignon F, Mery J-P, Morel-Maroger L, Mougenot B, Ronco P, Roland J. Granulomatous tubulointerstitial nephritis. *Adv Nephrol* 1984;13:219–45.
135. Truong LD, Farhood A, Tasby J, Gillum D. Experimental chronic renal ischemia: morphologic and immunologic studies. *Kidney Int* 1992;41:1676–89.
136. Solez K, Axelsen RA, Benediktsson H, et al. International standardization of criteria for the histologic allograft rejection: the Banff working classification of kidney transplant pathology. *Kidney Int* 1993;44:411–22.
137. Müller GA, Markovic-Lipkovski J, Frank J, Rodemann HP. The role of interstitial cells in the progression of renal diseases. *J Am Soc Nephrol* 1992;2:S198–205.
138. Eddy AA, Michael AF. Acute tubulointerstitial nephritis associated with aminonucleoside nephrosis. *Kidney Int* 1988;33:14–23.
139. Müller GA, Rodemann HP, Markovic-Lipkovski J, Müller CA, Mackensen-Haen S, Bohle A. Consequences of tubulointerstitial changes on renal function. In: D'Amico G, Colasantini G, eds. *Issues in nephrosciences:* dialysis strategies, *interstitial infiltrates in glomerulonephritis, diabetic nephropathy.* Milan: Wichtig, 1991: 1062–181.
140. Piguet PF, Collart MA, Grau GE, Kapanci Y, Vassaili P. Tumor necrosis factor/cachectin plays a key role in bleomycin-induced pneumopathy and fibrosis. *J Exp Med* 1989;170:655–63.
141. Cameron JS. Proteinuria and progression in human glomerular diseases. *Am J Nephrol* 1990;10(Suppl 1):81–7.
142. D'Amico G. The clinical role of proteinuria. *Am J Kidney Dis* 1991; 17:48–52.
143. Williams JD, Cole GA. Proteinuria: a direct cause of renal morbidity? *Kidney Int* 1994;45:443–50.
144. Sanders PW, Herrera GA, Chen A, Booker BB, Galla JH. Differential nephrotoxicity of low molecular weight proteins including Bence-Jones proteins in the perfused rat nephron in vivo. *J Clin Invest* 1988; 82:2086–96.
145. Ghiggeri GM, Altieri P, Oleggini R, et al. Intact renal albumin down-regulates the extracellular matrix expression by mesangial cells and renal fibroblasts in vitro. *Nephron* 1994;68:353–9.
146. Yoshioka K, Tohda M, Takemura T, et al. Distribution of type I collagen in human kidney diseases in comparison with type III collagen. *J Pathol* 1990;162:141–8.
147. Bertani T, Cutillo F, Zoja C, Broggini M, Remuzzi G. Tubulo-interstitial lesions mediate renal damage in adriamycin glomerulopathy. *Kidney Int* 1986;30:488–96.
148. Bertani T, Rocchi G, Sacchi G, Mecca G, Remuzzi G. Adriamycin-induced glomerulosclerosis in the rat. *Am J Kidney Dis* 1986;7:12–9.
149. Eddy A. Protein restriction reduces transforming growth factor and interstitial fibrosis in chronic purine aminonucleoside nephrosis. Am J Physiol 1994;266:F884–93.
150. Maack T, Park CH, Camargo MJF. Renal filtration, transport, and metabolism of proteins. In: Seldin GGDW, ed. *The kidney:* physiology and pathophysiology. New York: Raven, 1985:1773–803.
151. Olbricht CJ, Cannon JK, Tisher CC. Cathepsin B and L in nephron segments of rats with puromycin aminonucleoside nephrosis. *Kidney Int* 1987;32:354–61.
152. Ogrodowski JL, Hebert LA, Sedmak D, Cosio FG, Tamerius J, Kolb W. Measurement of SC5b-9 in urine in patients with nephrotic syndrome. *Kidney Int* 1991;40:1141–7.
153. Schulze M, Baker PJ, Perkinson DT. Increased urinary excretion of C5b-9 distinguishes passive Heymann nephritis in the rat. *Kidney Int* 1989;35:60–8.
154. Schulze M, Donadio JV, Pruchno CJ, Baker PJ. Elevated urinary excretion of the C5b-9 complex in membranous nephropathy. *Kidney Int* 1991;40:533–8.
155. Kees-Folts D, Levis Sadow J, Schreiner GF. Tubular catabolism of albumin is associated with the release of an inflammatory lipid. *Kidney Int* 1994;45:1697–709.
156. Alfrey AC, Fromment DH, Hammond WS. Role of iron in tubulointerstitial injury in nephrotoxic serum nephritis. *Kidney Int* 1989;36: 753–9.
157. Howard RL, Buddington B, Alfrey AC. Urinary albumin, transferrin and iron excretion in diabetic patients. *Kidney Int* 1991;40:923–6.
158. Eddy AA. Tubulointerstitial nephritis during the heterologous phase of nephrotoxic serum nephritis. *Nephron* 1991;59:304–13.
159. Eddy AA, Ho GC, Thorner PS. The contribution of antibody-mediated cytotoxicity and immune-complex formation to tubulointerstitial disease in passive Heymann nephritis. *Clin Immunol Immunopathol* 1992;62:42–55.
160. Holdsworth SR, Neale TJ. Macrophage-induced glomerular injury: cell transfer studies in passive autologous antiglomerular basement membrane antibody-initiated experimental glomerulonephritis. *Lab Invest* 1984;51:172–80.
161. Lehman DH, Dixon FJ. Extraglomerular immunoglobulin deposits in human nephritis. *Am J Med* 1975;58:765–96.
162. Campbell-Boswell MV, Linder D, Naylor BR, Brooks RE. Kidney tubule basement membrane alterations in type II membranoproliferative glomerulonephritis. *Virchows Arch [A]* 1979;382:49–61.
163. Levy M, Guesry P, Loirat C, Dommergues JP, Nivet H, Habib R. Immunologically-mediated tubulo-interstitial nephritis in children. *Contrib Nephrol* 1979;16:132–40.
164. Morel-Maroger L. Antitubular basement antibodies in rapidly progressive post-streptococcal glomerulonephritis. *Clin Immunol Immunopathol* 1974;2:185–94.
165. Strutz F, Müller GA. The role of tubulo-interstitial processes in progression of primary renal diseases. *Nephrol Dial Transplant* 1994;9 (Suppl):10–20 [*International yearbook of nephrology dialysis transplantation 1994*].
166. Lan HY, Paterson DJ, Atkins RC. Initiation and evolution of interstitial leukocytic infiltration in experimental glomerulonephritis. *Kidney Int* 1991;40:425–33.
167. Wardle EN. Cytokines: an overview. *Eur J Med* 1993;2:417–23.
168. Wahl SM, Francis-McCartney N, Mergenhagen SEM. Inflammatory and immunomodulatory roles of TGF-β. *Immunol Today* 1989;10: 258–61.

169. Border WA, Noble NA. Mechanisms of disease: transforming growth factor β in tissue fibrosis. *N Engl J Med* 1994;331:1286–92.
170. Roberts AB, McCune BK, Sporn MB. TGF-β: regulation of extracellular matrix. *Kidney Int* 1992;41:557–9.
171. Tomooka S, Border WA, Marshall BC, Noble NA. Glomerular matrix accumulation is linked to inhibition of the plasmin protease system. *Kidney Int* 1992;42:1462–9.
172. Khalil N, Bereznay O, Sporn M, Greenburg AH. Macrophage production of transforming growth factor β and fibroblast collagen synthesis in chronic pulmonary inflammation. *J Exp Med* 1991;170:727–37.
173. Bachem MG, Meyer D, Melchior R, Sell KM, Gressner AM. Activation of rat liver perisinusoidal lipocytes by transforming growth factors derived from myofibroblast-like cells: a potential mechanism of self perpetuation in liver fibrogenesis. *J Clin Invest* 1992;89:19–27.
174. Downer G, Phan SH, Wiggins RC. Analysis of renal fibrosis in a rabbit model of crescentic nephritis. *J Clin Invest* 1988;82:998–1006.
175. Tamaki K, Okuda S, Ando T, Iwamoto T, Nakayama M, Fujishima M. TGF-β_1 in glomerulosclerosis and interstitial fibrosis of adriamycin nephropathy. *Kidney Int* 1994;45:525–36.
176. Hamaguchi A, Kim S, Ohta K, et al. Transforming growth factor-β_1 expression and phenotypic modulation in the kidney of hypertensive rats. *Hypertension* 1995;26:199–207.
177. Kaneto H, Morrissey J, Klahr S. Increased expression of TGF-β_1 mRNA in the obstructed kidney of rats with unilateral ureteral ligation. *Kidney Int* 1993;44:313–21.
178. Moll S, Menoud P-A, Fulpius T, et al. Induction of plasminogen activation inhibitor type 1 in murine lupus-like glomerulonephritis. *Kidney Int* 1995;48:1459–68.
179. Border WA, Okuda S, Languino LR, Sporn MB, Ruoslahti E. Suppression of experimental glomerulonephritis by antiserum against transforming growth factor β_1. *Nature* 1990;346:371–4.
180. Border WA, Noble NA, Yamamoto T, et al. Natural inhibitor of transforming growth factors protects against scarring in experimental kidney disease. *Nature* 1992;360:361–4.
181. Niemir ZI, Stein H, Noronha IL, et al. PDGF and TGF-β contribute to the natural course of human IgA glomerulonephritis. *Kidney Int* 1995; 48:1530–41.
182. Wahl SM, Hunt DA, Wakefield LM, et al. Transforming growth factor type β induces monocyte chemotaxis and growth factor production. *Proc Natl Acad Sci USA* 1987;90:10,759–63.
183. Bertani T, Abbate M, Zoja C. Tumor necrosis factor induces glomerular damage in the rabbit. *Am* J Pathol 1989;134:419–30.
184. Diamond JR, Pesek I. Glomerular tumor necrosis factor and interleukin-1 during acute phase aminonucleoside nephrosis: an immunohistochemical study. *Lab Invest* 1991;64:21–8.
185. Paulsson Y, Hammacher A, Heldin C-H, Westermark B. Possible autocrine feedback in the prereplicative phase of human fibroblasts. *Nature* 1987;328:715–7.
186. Kovacs EJ. Fibrogenic cytokines: the role of immune mediators in the development of scar tissue. *Immunol Today* 1991;12:17–23.
187. Muchaneta-Kubara EC, Sayed-Ahmed N, El-Nahas AM. Subtotal nephrectomy: a mosaic of growth factors. *Nephrol Dial Transplant* 1994;10:320–7.
188. Madtes DK, Busby HK, Strandjord TP, Clark JG. Expression of transforming growth factor-alpha and epidermal growth factor receptor is increased following bleomycin-induced lung injury in rats. *Am J Respir Cell Mol Biol* 1994;11:540–51.
189. Freundlich B, Bomalaski JS, Neilson E, Jiminez SA. Regulation of fibroblast proliferation and collagen synthesis by cytokines. *Immunol Today* 1986;7:303–7.
190. Torbohm I, Berger B, Schönermark M, Van Kempis J, Rother K, Hansch GM. Modulation of collagen synthesis in human glomerular epithelial cells by interleukin-1. *Clin Exp Immunol* 1989;75: 427–31.
191. Kawaguchi Y. IL-1α gene expression and protein production by fibroblasts from patients with systemic sclerosis. *Clin Exp Immunol* 1994;97:445–50.
192. Cambrey AD, Harrison NK, Dawes KE, et al. Increased levels of endothelin-1 in bronchoalveolar lavage fluid from patients with systemic sclerosis contribute to fibroblast mitogenic activity in vitro. *Am J Respir Cell Mol Biol* 1994;11:439–45.
193. Guarda E, Katwa LC, Myers PR, Tyagi SC, Weber KT. Effects of endothelins on collagen turnover in cardiac fibroblasts. *Cardiovasc Res* 1993;27:2130–4.
194. Baggiolini M, Dahinden CA. CC chemokines in allergic inflammation. *Immunol Today* 1994;15:127–33.
195. Gomez-Chiarri M, Ortiz A, Seron D, Gonzalez E, Egido J. The intercrine superfamily and renal disease. *Kidney Int* 1993;43(Suppl 39): S81–5.
196. Keiner GS, Kennedy J, Bacon KB, et al. Lymphotactin: a cytokine that represents a new class of chemokine. *Science* 1994;266:1395–9.
197. Baglioni M, Walz A, Kinkel SL. Neutrophil-activating-peptide-1/interleukin 8, a novel cytokine that activates neutrophils. *J Clin Invest* 1989;84:1045–9.
198. Schmouder RL, Strieter RM, Wiggins RC, Chensue SW, Kunkel SL. In vitro and in vivo interleukin-8 production in human renal cortical epithelia. *Kidney Int* 1992;41:191–8.
199. Maione TE, Grey GS, Petro J, et al. Inhibition of angiogenesis by recombinant platelet factor 4 and related peptides. *Science* 1990;247: 77–9.
200. Tang WW, Feng L, Mathison JC, Wilson CB. Cytokine expression, upregulation of intercellular adhesion molecule-1, and leucocyte infiltration in experimental tubulointerstitial nephritis. *Lab Invest* 1994;70:631–8.
201. Stahl RA, Thaiss F, Disser M, Helmchen U, Hora K, Schlöndorff D. Increased expression of monocyte chemoattractant protein-1 in anti-thymocyte antibody-induced glomerulonephritis. *Kidney Int* 1993;44: 1036–47.
202. Prodjosudjadi W, Gerritsma JSJ, Klar-Mohamed N, et al. Production and cytokine-mediated regulation of monocyte chemoattractant protein-1 by human proximal tubular epithelial cells. *Kidney Int* 1995;48: 1477–86.
203. Schmouder RL, Strieter RM, Kunkel SL. Interferon-γ regulation of human renal cortical epithelial cell-derived monocyte chemotactic peptide-1. *Kidney Int* 1993;44:43–9.
204. Heeger P, Wolf G, Meyers C, Sun MJ, Neilson EG. Isolation and characterization of cDNA from renal tubular epithelium encoding murine Rantes. *Kidney Int* 1992;41:220–5.
205. Wolf G, Aberie S, Thaiss F, Stahl RK. TNFα induces expression of the chemoattractant cytokine RANTES in cultured mouse mesangial cells. *Kidney Int* 1993;44:795–804.
206. Alam R, Forsythe P, Stafford S, et al. Monocyte chemotactic protein-2, monocyte chemotactic protein-3, and fibroblast-induced cytokine: three new chemokines induce chemotaxis and activation of basophils. *J Immunol* 1994;153:3155–9.
207. Pattison J, Nelson PJ, Huie P, et al. RANTES chemokine expression in cell-mediated transplant rejection of the kidney. *Lancet* 1994;343: 209–11.
208. Schlöndorff D. The role of chemokines in the initiation and progression of renal disease. *Kidney Int* 1995;47(Suppl 49):S44–7.
209. Springer TA. Adhesion receptors of the immune system. *Nature* 1990;346:425–34.
210. Lin Y, Kirby JA, Browell DA, et al. Renal allograft rejection: expression and function of VCAM-1 on tubular epithelial cells. *Clin Exp Immunol* 1993;92:145–51.
211. Jevnikar AM, Wüthrich RP, Takei F, et al. Differing regulation and function of ICAM-1 and class II antigens on renal tubular cells. *Kidney Int* 1990;38:417–25.
212. Wüthrich RP, Glimcher LH, Yui MA, Jevnikar AM, Dumas SE, Kelley VE. MHC class II, antigen presentation and tumor necrosis factor in renal tubular epithelial cells. *Kidney Int* 1990;37:783–92.
213. Nishikawa K, Guo Y-J, Miyasaka M, et al. Antibodies to intercellular adhesion molecule 1/lymphocyte function-associated antigen 1 prevent crescent formation in rat autoimmune glomerulonephritis. *J Exp Med* 1993;177:667–77.
214. Cosimi AB, Conti D, Delmonico FL, et al. In vivo effects of monoclonal antibody to ICAM-1 (CD 54) in nonhuman primates with renal allografts. *J Immunol* 1990;144:4604–12.
215. Kawasaki K, Yaoita E, Yamamoto T, Tamatani T, Miyasaki M, Kihara I. Antibodies against intercellular adhesion molecule-1 and lymphocyte function-associated antigen-1 prevent glomerular injury in rat experimental crescentic glomerulonephritis. *J Immunol* 1993;150:1074–83.
216. Harning R, Pelletier J, Van G, Takei F, Merluzzi VJ. Monoclonal antibody to MALA-1 (ICAM-1) reduces acute autoimmune nephritis in *kdkd* mice. *Clin Immunol Immunopathol* 1992;64:129–34.
217. Molina A, Bricio T, Martin A, Mampaso F. Prevention of $HgCl_2$-induced nephritis in the Brown Norway (BN) rat by treatment with antibodies against VLA-4 integrin. *J Am Soc Nephrol* 1993;4:621(abst).

218. Hill PA, Main IW, Atkins RC. ICAM-1 and VCAM-1 in human renal allograft rejection. *Kidney Int* 1995;47:1383–91.
219. Oldberg A, Franzen A, Heinegard D. Cloning and sequence of rat bone sialoprotein (osteopontin) cDNA reveals an Arg-Gly-Asp cell-binding sequence. *Proc Natl Acad Sci USA* 1986;83:8819–23.
220. Nemir M, De Vouge MW, Mukherjee BB. Normal rat kidney cells secrete both phosphorylated and nonphosphorylated forms of osteopontin showing different physiological properties. *J Biol Chem* 1989; 264:18,202–8.
221. Pichler R, Giachelli CM, Lombardi D, Alpers CE, Schwartz SM, Johnson RJ. Tubulointerstitial disease in glomerulonephritis: potential role of osteopontin (uropontin). *Am* J Pathol 1994;144:915–26.
222. Giachelli CM, Pichler R, Lombardi D, et al. Osteopontin expression in angiotensin II-induced tubulointerstitial nephritis. *Kidney Int* 1994; 45:515–24.
223. Lopez CA, Hoyer JR, Wilson PD, Waterhouse P, Denhardt DT. Heterogeneity of osteopontin expression among nephrons in mouse kidneys and enhanced expression in sclerotic glomeruli. *Lab Invest* 1993;69:355–63.
224. Pichler RH, Franceschini N, Young BA, et al. Pathogenesis of cyclosporine nephrotoxicity: roles of angiotensin II and osteopontin. *Am J Soc Nephrol* 1995;6:1186–96.
225. Floege J, Gröne H-J. Progression of renal failure: what is the role of cytokines? *Nephrol Dial Transplant* 1995;10:1575–86.
226. Simon M, Gröne H-J, Jöhren O, Plate KH, Risau W, Fuchs E. Expression of vascular endothelial growth factor and its receptors in human renal ontogenesis and in adult kidney. Am J Physiol 1995;268: F240–50.
227. Havry P, Von Willebrand E, Andersson LC. Expression of HLA-ABC and -DR locus antigens on human kidney, endothelial, tubular and glomerular cells. *Scand J Immunol* 1980;11:303–10.
228. Markovic-Lipkovski J, Müller CA, Risler T, Bohle A, Müller GA. Mononuclear leucocytes, expression of HLA class II antigens and of intercellular adhesion molecule I in focal segmental glomerulosclerosis. *Nephron* 1991;59:286–93.
229. Hagerty DT, Allen PM. Processing and presentation of self and foreign antigens by the renal proximal tubule. *J Immunol* 1992;148:2324–30.
230. Rubin-Kelley V, Diaz-Gallo C, Jevnikar AM, Singer GG. Renal tubular epithelial and T cell interactions in autoimmune renal disease. *Kidney Int* 1993;43(Suppl 39):SlO8–15.
231. Harding FA, McArthur JG, Gross JA, Raulet DH, Allison JP. CD28-mediated signalling co-stimulates murine T-cells and prevents induction of anergy in T-cell clones. *Nature* 1992;356:607–9.
232. Jevnikar AM, Singer GG, Coffman T, Glimcher LH, Rubin-Kelley VE. Transgenic tubular cell expression of class II is insufficient to initiate immune renal injury. *J Am Soc Nephrol* 1993;3:1972–7.
233. Mozes E, Kohn LD, Hakim F, Singer DS. Resistance of MHC class I-deficient mice to experimental systemic lupus erythematosus. *Science* 1993;261:91–4.
234. Rubbia-Brandt L, Sappino AP, Gabbiani G. Locally applied GM-CSF induces the accumulation of α-smooth muscle actin containing myofibroblasts. *Virchows Arch [B]* 1991;60:73–82.
235. Harris DCH, Chan L, Schrier RW. Remnant kidney hypermetabolism and progression of chronic renal failure. Am J Physiol 1988;254: F267–76.
236. Nath KA, Croatt AJ, Hostetter TH. Oxygen consumption and oxidant stress in surviving nephrons. Am J Physiol 1990;258:F1354–62.
237. Nath KA, Hudeen AKS. Induction of renal growth and injury in the intact rat kidney by dietary deficiency of antioxidants. *J Clin Invest* 1990;86:1179–92.
238. Gimenez LF, Solez K, Walker WG. Relation between renal calcium content and renal impairment in 246 human renal biopsies. *Kidney Int* 1987;31:93–9.
239. Loghman-Adham M. Role of phosphate retention in the progression of renal failure. *J Lab Clin Med* 1993;122:16–26.
240. Laouri D, Kleinknecht C, Courmot-Witmer G, Habib R, Mounier F, Broyer M. Beneficial effect of low phosphorus diet in uraemic rats: a reappraisal. *Clin Sci* 1982;1982:539–48.
241. Haut LL, Alfrey AC, Guggenheim S, Buddington B, Schrier N. Renal toxicity of phosphate in rats. *Kidney Int* 1980;17:722–31.
242. Ibels LS, Alfrey AC, Haut L, Huffer WE. Preservation of function in experimental renal disease by dietary restriction of phosphate. *N Engl J Med* 1978;298:122–6.
243. Lumlertgul G, Burke TJ, Gillum DM. Phosphate depletion arrests progression of chronic renal failure independent of protein intake. *Kidney Int* 1986;29:658–66.
244. Nath KA, Hostetter MK, Hostetter TH. Pathophysiology of chronic tubulointerstitial disease in rats: interactions of dietary acid load, ammonia, and complement component C3. *J Clin Invest* 1985;76: 667–75.
245. Diamond JR, Pesek I, Ruggeri S, Karnovsky MJ. Essential fatty acid deficiency during acute puromycin nephrosis ameliorates late renal injury. Am J Physiol 1989;257:F798–807.
246. Harris KPG, Lefkowith JB, Klahr S, Schreiner G. Essential fatty acid deficiency ameliorates acute renal dysfunction in the rat after the administration of the aminonucleoside of puromycin. *J Clin Invest* 1990;86:1115–23.
247. Houglum K, Brenner DA, Chojkier M. D-α-tocopherol inhibits collagen α_1(I) gene expression in cultured human fibroblasts: modulation of constitutive collagen gene expression by lipid peroxidation. *J Clin Invest* 1991;87:2230–5.
248. Chizzonite R, Truitt T, Kilian PL, et al. Two high affinity interleukin 1 receptors represent separate gene products. *Proc Natl Acad Sci USA* 1989;86:8029–33.
249. Barnes PJ, Adcock I. Anti-inflammatory actions of steroids: molecular mechanisms. *Trends Pharmacol Sci* 1993;14:436–40.
250. Wardle EN. Neutralizing inflammatory cytokines in nephritis. *Nephron* 1995;69:223–7.
251. Wardle EN. Cell biology and the functional changes of diabetic nephropathy. *Nephrol Dial Transplant* 1992;7:889–95.
252. Group TDCaCTR. The effects of intensive insulin treatment of diabetes on the development and progression of long-term complications in insulin-dependent diabetes mellitus. *N Engl J Med* 1993;329: 977–86.
253. Anderson S, Jung FF, Ingelfinger JR. Renal renin–angiotensin system in diabetes: functional, immunohistochemical, and molecular biological correlations. *Am J Physiol* 1993;265:F477–86.
254. Remuzzi A, Puntorieri S, Battaglia C, Bertani T, Remuzzi G. Angiotensin converting enzyme inhibition ameliorates glomerular filtration of macromolecules and water and lessens glomerular injury in the rat. *J Clin Invest* 1990;85:541–9.
255. Wolf G, Neilson EG. Cellular biology of tubulointerstitial growth. *Curr Top Pathol* 1995;88:69–97.
256. Kagami S, Border W, Miller DE, Noble NA. Angiotensin II stimulates extracellular matrix synthesis through induction of transforming growth factor-β expression in rat glomerular mesangial cells. *J Clin Invest* 1994;93:2431.
257. Kaneto H, Morrissey J, McCracken R, Reyes A, Klahr S. Enalapril reduces type IV collagen synthesis and expansion of the interstitium in the obstructed kidney. *Kidney Int* 1994;45:1637–47.
258. Diamond JR, Anderson S. Irreversible tubulointerstitial damage associated with chronic aminonucleoside nephrosis: amelioration by angiotensin I converting enzyme inhibition. *Am* J Pathol 1990;137: 1323–32.
259. Lewis EJ, Hunsicker LG, Bain RP, Rohde RD. The effect of angiotensin-converting-enzyme inhibition on diabetic nephropathy. *N Engl J Med* 1993;329:1456–62.
260. Gradman AH, Arcuri KE, Goldberg AI, et al. A randomized, placebo-controlled, double-blind, parallel study of various doses of losartan potassium compared with enalapril maleate in patients with essential hypertension. *Hypertension* 1995;25:1345–50.
261. Goldberg AI, Dunley MC, Sweet CS. Safety and tolerability of losartan potassium, an angiotensin II receptor antagonist, compared with hydrochlorothiazide, atenolol, felodipine ER, and angiotensin-converting enzyme inhibitors for the treatment of systemic hypertension. *Am J Cardiol* 1995;75:793–5.
262. Gansevoort RT, De Zeeuw D, De Jong PE. Is the antiproteinuric effect of ACE inhibition mediated by interference in the renin–angiotensin system? *Kidney Int* 1994;45:861–7.
263. Jover B, Mimran A. Angiotensin II receptor antagonists versus angiotensin converting enzyme inhibitors: effects on renal function. *J Hypertens* 1994;12(Suppl 9):S3–9.
264. Ishidoya S, Morrissey J, McCracken R, Reyes A, Klahr S. Angiotensin II receptor antagonist ameliorates renal tubulointerstitial fibrosis caused by unilateral ureteral obstruction. *Kidney Int* 1995;47:1285–94.
265. Bakris GL. Effects of diltiazem or lisinopril on massive proteinuria associated with diabetic nephropathy. *Ann Intern Med* 1990;112: 707–8.

266. Boehlen L, De Courten M, Weidmann P. Comparative study of the effect of ACE-inhibitors and other antihypertensive agents on proteinuria in diabetic patients. *Am J Hypertens* 1994;7(9 Part 2):84S–92S.
267. Anderson S, Rennke HG, Garcia DL, Brenner BM. Short and long term effects of antihypertensive therapy in the diabetic rat. *Kidney Int* 1989;36:526–36.
268. Meyer TW, Anderson SA, Rennke HG, Brenner BM. Reversing glomerular hypertension stabilizes established glomerular injury. *Kidney Int* 1987;31:752–9.
269. Miller PL, Scholey JW, Rennke HG, Meyer TW. Glomerular hypertrophy aggravates epithelial cell injury in nephrotic rats. *J Clin Invest* 1990;85:1119–26.
270. Nakamura T, Fukui M, Ebihara I, Tomino Y, Koide H. Low protein diet blunts the rise in glomerular gene expression in focal glomerulosclerosis. *Kidney Int* 1994;45:1593–605.
271. Fukui M, Nakamura T, Ebihara I, Nagaoka I, Tomino Y, Koide H. Low-protein diet attenuates increased gene expression of platelet-derived growth factor and transforming growth factor-β in experimental glomerular sclerosis. *J Lab Clin Med* 1993;121:224–34.
272. Locatelli F, Alberti D, Graziani G, Buccianti G, Raedelli B, Giangrande A. Prospective, randomized, multicentre trial of effect of protein restriction on progression of chronic renal insufficiency. *Lancet* 1991;337:1299–304.
273. Klahr S. Low-protein diets and angiotensin-converting enzyme inhibition in progressive renal failure. *Am J Kidney Dis* 1993;22:114–9.
274. Jacobson HR, Striker GE, for the Workshop and Group. Report on a workshop to develop management recommendations for the prevention of progression of chronic renal disease. *Am J Kidney Dis* 1995; 25:103–6.
275. Dennis M, Bisson D. Blockade of leucocyte function-associated antigen (LFA-1) in a murine model of lung inflammation. *Am J Respir Cell Mol Biol* 1994;10:481–6.
276. Saito T, Atkins RC. Contribution of mononuclear leucocytes to the progression of experimental focal glomerular sclerosis. *Kidney Int* 1990;37:1076–83.
277. Lan HY, Nikolic-Paterson DJ, Zarama M, Vannice JL, Atkins RC. Suppression of experimental crescentic glomerulonephritis by the interleukin-1 receptor antagonist. *Kidney Int* 1993;43:479–85.
278. Tang WW, Feng L, Vannice JL, Wilson CB. IL-1 receptor antagonist ameliorates experimental anti-GBM antibody associated glomerulonephritis. *J Clin Invest* 1994;93:273–9.
279. Piquet PF, Vesin C, Grau GE, Thompson RC. IL-1 receptor antagonist prevents or cures pulmonary fibrosis elicited in mice by bleomycin or silica. *Cytokine* 1993;5:57–61.
280. Mancini R, Benedetti A, Jezequel AM. An interleukin-1 receptor antagonist decreases fibrosis induced by dimethylnitrosamine in rat liver. *Virchows Arch* 1994;424:25–31.
281. Giri SN, Hyde DM, Hollinger MA. Effect of antibody to transforming growth factor β on bleomycin induced accumulation of lung collagen in mice. *Thorax* 1993;48:959–66.
282. Denis M. Neutralization of transforming growth factor-beta 1 in a mouse model of immune-induced lung fibrosis. *Immunology* 1994; 82:584–90.
283. Shull MM, Ormsby I, Kier AB, et al. Targeted disruption of the mouse transforming growth factor beta 1 results in multifocal inflammatory disease. *Nature* 1992;359:693-9.
284. Levitzki A. Tyrphostins: tyrosine kinase blockers as novel antiproliferative agents and dissectors of signal transduction. *FASEB J* 1992;6:3275–82.
285. Clozel M, Breu V, Burri K, et al. Pathophysiological role of endothelin revealed by the first orally active endothelin receptor antagonist. *Nature* 1993;365:759–61.
286. Peterson TC, Isbrucker RA, Hooper ML. In vitro effects of platelet-derived growth factor on fibroproliferation and effect of cytokine antagonists. *Immunopharmacology* 1994;28:259–70.
287. Bayreuther K, Rodemann HP, Hommel R, Dittmann K, Albiez M, Francz PI. Human skin fibroblasts in vitro differentiate along a terminal cell lineage. *Proc Natl Acad Sci USA* 1988;85:5112–6.
288. Nehls MC, Rippe R, Veloz L, Brenner DA. Transcription factor nuclear factor 1 and Sp1 interact with the murine collagen α_1(I) promoter. *Mol Cell Biol* 1991;11:4065–73.
289. Nehls MC, Brenner DA, Gruss H-J, Dierbach H, Mertelsmann R, Herrmann F. Mithramycin selectively inhibits collagen-α_1(I) gene expression in human fibroblast. *J Clin Invest* 1993;93:2916–21.
290. Duncan MR, Hasan A, Berman B. Pentoxifylline, pentifylline, and interferons decrease type I and III procollagen mRNA levels in dermal fibroblasts: evidence for mediation by nuclear factor 1 down-regulation. *J Invest Dermatol* 1995;104:282–6.
291. Duncan MR, Berman B. γ Interferon is the lymphokine and β interferon the monokine responsible for inhibition of fibroblast collagen production and late but not early fibroblast proliferation. *J Exp Med* 1985;162:516–27.
292. Varga J, Olsen A, Herhal J, Constantine G, Rosenbloom J, Jiminez SA. Interferon-g reverses the stimulation of collagen but not fibronectin gene expression by transforming growth factor-β in normal human fibroblasts. *Eur J Clin Invest* 1990;20:487–93.
293. Desmoulière A, Rubbia-Brandt L, Abdiu A, Walz T, Macieira-Coelho A, Gabbiani G. a-Smooth muscle actin is expressed in a subpopulation of cultured and cloned fibroblasts and is modulated by γ-interferon. *Exp Cell Res* 1992;201:64–73.
294. Hein R, Behr J, Hündgen M, et al. Treatment of systemic sclerosis with γ-interferon. *Br J Dermatol* 1992;126:496–501.
295. Duncan MR, Berman B, Nseyo UO. Regulation of the proliferation and biosynthetic activities of cultured human Peyronie's disease fibroblasts by interferons-alpha, -beta and -gamma. *Scand J Urol Nephrol* 1991;25:89–94.
296. Kershenobich D, Vargas F, Garcia-Tsao G. Colchicine in the treatment of cirrhosis of the liver. *N Engl J Med* 1988;318:1709–13.
297. Kershenobich D, Rojkind M, Quiroga A. Effect of colchicine for primary biliary cirrhosis. *Hepatology* 1990;11:205–9.
298. Shibata J, Fujuyama S, Honda Y, Sato T. Combination therapy with ursodeoxycholic acid and colchicine for primary biliary cirrhosis. *J Gastroenterol Hepatol* 1992;7:277–82.
299. Houglum K, Buck M, Alcorn J, Contreras S, Bornstein P, Chojkier M. Two different cis-acting regulatory regions direct cell-specific transcription of the collagen α_1(I) gene in hepatic stellate cells and in skin and tendon fibroblasts. *J Clin Invest* 1995;96:2269–76.
300. Pihlajaniemi T, Myllylä R, Kivirikko K. Prolyl 4-hydroxylase and its role in collagen synthesis. *J Hepatol* 1991;13(Suppl 3):S2–7.
301. Wu J, Danielsson A. Inhibition of hepatic fibrogenesis: a review of pharmacologic candidates. *Scand J Gastroenterol* 1994;29:385–91.
302. Bickel M, Baader E, Brocks DG. Beneficial effects of inhibitors of prolyl 4-hydroxylase CCl_4-induced fibrosis of the liver in rats. *J Hepatol* 1991;13(Suppl 3):S26–34.
303. Arthur MJP. Pathogenesis, experimental manipulation and treatment of liver fibrosis. *Exp Nephrol* 1995;3:90–5.
304. Franklin TJ. Opportunities for the discovery of novel therapies for fibrotic diseases. *Exp Nephrol* 1995;3:143–7.
305. Wakasaki H, Ooshima A. Synthesis of lysyl oxidase in experimental fibrosis. *Biochem Biophys Res Commun* 1990;166:1201–4.
306. Tang SS, Simpson DE, Kagan HM. β-Quinone directed irreversible inhibitors of lysysl oxidase. *J Biol Chem* 1984;264:12,963–9.
307. Lieber CS, DeCarli LM, Mak KM. Attenuations of alcohol-induced hepatic fibrosis by polyunsaturated lecithin. *Hepatology* 1990;12: 1390–8.
308. Kakouris H, Eddie LW, Summers RJ. Relaxin: more than just a hormone of pregnancy. *Trends Pharmacol Sci* 1993;14:4–5.
309. Unemori EN, Beck LS, Lee WP, et al. Human relaxin decreases collagen accumulation in vivo in 2 rodent models of fibrosis. *J Invest Dermatol* 1993;101:280–5.

PART V

Animal Models of Immunologic Renal Diseases

Immunologic Renal Diseases,
edited by E. G. Neilson and W. G. Couser.
Lippincott-Raven Publishers, Philadelphia © 1997.

CHAPTER 35

Immune Models of Glomerular Injury

Curtis B. Wilson

The use of models of immune renal injury has been central to our understanding of the basic immune mechanisms that initiate glomerular and tubulointerstitial injury (1–8). In addition, they have served to study the contribution of immune mediator systems in the amplification of the injury induced by the specific immune reaction (8–11). This chapter will deal with the former, other chapters being devoted to the study of the individual mediation pathways that often utilize the model systems described herein.

Immune renal injury in humans is generally categorized relative to the mechanisms identified in model systems. The clinical extrapolation of mechanisms lags considerably behind the level of experimental knowledge, due, in part, to limitations in the ability to study human kidney tissue at appropriate times to understand the events that initiate the injury, as well as those responsible for its recovery or progression. Most clinical assessments rely on a single renal biopsy that is used to determine a morphologic classification (light and electron microscopy) and to characterize the type of immune deposit present, using immunofluorescence or immunohistochemical approaches. Additional study may be done, for example, to identify the phenotype of the inflammatory cells present and/or the presence of mediators or their expression at the protein and mRNA levels. Rarely are etiologic studies undertaken. Subsequent clinical sampling is usually limited to the urine or blood components, which provide only indirect evidence of the activity of the nephritic immune processes.

The information from the biopsy and serum studies is used to suggest a possible immunopathogenic mechanism based on its similarity to one or more of the established experimental models. The best example is perhaps in anti-glomerular basement membrane (GBM) antibody (Ab)-induced glomerulonephritis (GN), in which linear Ig deposits in glomeruli and detection of anti-GBM Abs (glomerular bound or circulating) confirm the immune mechanism. In this particular disease, very convincing clinical evidence was developed nearly seven decades after studies of the animal counterpart were begun. Although most often development of models preceded identification of similar processes in human renal disease, in some instances when no model system is appropriate, efforts are made to establish one. Some examples would be in the case of IgA nephropathy, hemolytic uremic syndrome/thrombotic thrombocytopenic purpura, or the so-called pauci-immune necrotizing and crescentic glomerular lesion that is associated with vasculitis and the presence of antineutrophil cytoplasmic Abs (ANCA).

In this chapter, the models will be discussed in relationship to how the particular immune response appears to lead to initiation of renal injury based on the antigen (Ag) involved (Table 1). The Ags may be part of the structural makeup of the kidney, such as the GBM, the tubular basement membrane (TBM), or renal cell surface Ags. Alternatively, the Ags that are involved in formation of glomerular immune deposits can be nonrenal materials from the circulation that lead to the deposits via immune complex (IC) mechanisms, which include a continuum of glomerular accumulation of circulating IC and trapped or planted Ag mechanisms. The nephritogenic immune response most often is predominately humoral; however, examples in which nephritogenic cellular immune responses predominate are also known.

The models utilize passive or active induction of Ab or cellular nephritogenic immune responses, as well as examination of instances in which immune renal injury is part of a spontaneous disease process, often associated with infection or autoimmune responses. The models offer the user the opportunity to determine the time course and evolution of the lesion, thereby allowing the selection of an appropriate stage of injury to best address the question posed. This may entail selection of the appropriate species, strain, age, and/or sex of the experi-

C. B. Wilson: Department of Immunology, The Scripps Research Institute, La Jolla, California 92037.

TABLE 1. *Models of immune mechanisms of glomerular injury*

Ab reactions with glomerular Ags
Basement membrane Ags and glomerular cell Ags
Ab reactions with circulating Ags
IC mechanisms and planted Ag mechanisms
Cellular immune reactions with glomerular Ags
Immune activation of mediator systems

mental subject. In passive models, the amounts of Abs (or cells) given can be quantitated and used to govern the severity of the lesion, independent from the host's immune response. The passive models are generally more rapid in onset and are well suited for the study of mediator contributions.

In active models, more variation may occur due to different levels of immune response among recipients; however, it is still possible to provide quantitative estimates of Ab binding by elution study (12). Elution, particularly with a mixture of Abs such as is found in systemic lupus erythematosus (SLE), may not provide a truly representative sampling of the glomerular-bound Ab, due to differences in binding strength of the different Abs and denaturation of Ab recovered with harsh elution procedures needed to remove the more tightly bound Abs. The level of the systemic immune response can be assessed for correlation with the severity of the lesion. Studies in which manipulations are done to understand mechanisms or actions of mediators must include monitoring of active and/or passive immune aspects of the lesion to exclude unsuspected effects on the immune parameters that could independently affect outcome. For quantitation, estimates of the amounts of Ab bound within the kidney are needed. The model's cellular immune response component can also be characterized by enumeration of the phenotype of infiltrative leukocytes, as well as by other parameters of the cellular immune response, including changes in expression of major histocompatibility complex (MHC) molecules and T cell receptors (TCR).

Studies of isolated glomeruli can be used to assess immune components or mediators using binding studies, enzymatic assays, or molecular measurements. All three glomerular cells are now available in culture and, in some studies, can be used to address questions not well suited to in vivo study. In addition to whole animal studies, in situ or ex vivo kidney perfusion protocols are available to exclude systemic effects. The isolated erythrocyte perfused kidney system in the rat has been found to maintain essentially normal function for studies of 1–2 hr duration (13). Glomerular hemodynamic studies using micropuncture techniques have been used to assess immune and mediator effects on function and are also applicable in the isolated perfused kidney (see Chapter 11) (14). Genetically altered animals using transgenic or homologous recombination technology and gene transfer are just beginning to open up new avenues of study.

ANTI-GBM AB DISEASE

The Problem in Humans

Anti-GBM Ab disease is the clearest example of Ab-induced glomerular injury with the Ab reacting with GBM (and TBM in about 70% of patients) and causing pulmonary hemorrhage (Goodpasture syndrome) through its reaction with alveolar basement membrane (ABM) in about half of patients (15). The disease, in reality, is an anti-GBM/TBM/ABM disease. A separate anti-TBM Ab not reactive with GBM is associated tubulointerstitial nephritis (TIN) (see Chapter 36). The role of anti-GBM Ab in GN was shown in 1967 when the Ab was identified bound to the GBM in a linear pattern, as had been seen in its experimental counterparts, and the Ab was recovered from the circulation or eluted from the kidney (16). The immunopathogenic significance of the Ab was shown by transfer of GN to nonhuman primates using the recovered anti-GBM Ab. Recurrence of the GN in transplants placed in patients with circulating anti-GBM Ab also confirmed its nephritogenic potential.

The nephritogenic GBM/ABM Ag(s) is now recognized as the globular noncollagenous carboxyl NC1 domain of the α3 chain of type IV collagen [α3(IV)], with possible additional reactivity with NC1 domains of other type IV collagen α-chains (17,18). GN, often rapidly progressive, is found in most patients with anti-GBM Ab. Goodpasture syndrome (GN and pulmonary hemorrhage) occurs in patients in whom the Ab fixes to ABM, probably in association with factors that alter accessibility of the reactive Ags to the circulating Ab. Occasionally, lung involvement without clinically detected glomerular damage (proteinuria, hematuria) is seen.

Fixation to TBM is associated with increased tubulointerstitial leukocyte infiltration (19). The factors responsible for induction of anti-GBM Ab in humans remain obscure; however, evidence exists of clustering with certain MHC loci (20,21).

Models of Anti-GBM Ab Disease

The anti-GBM/TBM/ABM Ab human counterparts have been studied in both passive and active forms and remain as some of the most useful models available for assessing actions of mediators in glomerular inflammation and other facets of immunologically induced glomerular pathophysiology.

Models Using Passive Administration of Anti-GBM Abs

Heterologous Phase Injury

Induction of GN using heterologous antikidney Ab was first reported by Lindeman in 1900. The model was extensively studied by Masugi and co-workers during the 1930s, and the terms *nephrotoxic nephritis* or *Masugi nephritis*, coined during the early studies, are occasionally still used today (22,23). Subsequently, the GBM was found to contain the major nephritogenic Ags, and the model as well as its human counterpart have come to be known as *anti-GBM Ab-induced GN*.

It should be understood that the "GBM" Ag preparations used to induce the heterologous Abs in these models usually are very crude, and although predominately GBM, they do contain variable amounts of TBM and other elements of renal extracellular matrix, cell membrane fragments, and serum proteins. In turn, the anti-GBM Abs raised contain additional reactivity to a variety of proteins trapped in the basement membrane preparations, including cell membranes and serum protein Ags. These extraneous Abs must be absorbed with circulating whole blood cells and serum before administration to prevent or minimize systemic reactions. Ab reactive with non-GBM capillary wall Ags, such as those on glomerular endothelium, may or may not be removed by the usual absorption procedures. Without care in handling, the heterologous anti-GBM antisera may become contaminated with bacterial lipopolysaccharide (LPS), which can result in cytokine activation in the recipient, with worsening of the glomerular lesion (24–26). The heterologous anti-GBM models are generally similar but may have unique features relative to each individual anti-GBM Ab preparation used and the various Ab(s) or contaminants it contains. The ability of the Ab Ig molecules of various species to activate mediator systems also will influence the inflammatory response; avian Ab, for example, activates mammalian complement (C) ineffectively.

The anti-GBM Abs react in a linear pattern predominantly along the GBM when administered intravenously. In contrast, the Abs react with virtually all basement membranes throughout the tissues of the body when studied by indirect immunofluorescent techniques on tissue sections, which indicates that the basement membrane Ags have varying accessibility to Ab in the circulation. The type of GN and its severity induced by heterologous anti-GBM Abs varies among species and presumably relates both to characteristics of the particular anti-GBM Ab used and, more importantly, to the capacity of the recipient to respond to rapid glomerular deposition of Ab with cellular and humoral mediator activation. Among species commonly used or studied, rabbits typically develop more aggressive, neutrophil- and C-mediated crescentic glomerular lesions than do rats, and mice have a less severe and often delayed onset of lesions with more mononuclear inflammatory cell involvement. Nonhuman primates have also been studied (27).

The GN induced with heterologous anti-GBM Abs occurs in both an acute (heterologous) phase, beginning within a few minutes after administration of Ab, and a delayed (autologous) phase, onsetting 7–10 days later when the recipient produces and binds its own Ab reactive with the heterologous immunoglobulin (Ig) previously fixed in its kidneys. The heterologous phase injury can be related in a dose-response fashion to the amount of Ab bound, and the autologous phase can be manipulated by active or passive means to alter the host's immune response to the heterologous immunoglobulin.

For many types of studies, quantitation of the amount of heterologous anti-GBM Ab bound is important. Typically, quantitation is done using radiolabeled Ab fractions, with the paired label radioisotope technique being among the most practical and precise way of making the measurements because it corrects for any nonspecific entrapment in glomeruli, kidney, or other organs of interest (28). Using such a technique, the induction of injury can be related to the micrograms of Ab bound per gram of kidney or in terms of molecules per glomerulus. The species vary in their sensitivity to induction of GN with heterologous anti-GBM Abs, so that rats develop proteinuria after fixation of approximately 75 μg of Ab per gram of kidney (29). In contrast, sheep require only 5 μg of Ab bound per gram of kidney to induce heterologous phase injury; rabbits are intermediate in their sensitivity, requiring 15 μg per gram of kidney (30,31). Years ago, it was calculated that proteinuria could be induced in the rat when approximately 1.2×10^{10} molecules of heterologous anti-GBM Ab were fixed per glomerulus, or approximately 1 Ab molecule for every 26 μm^2 of glomerular capillary filtering surface (29). Morphologic procedures using immunogold electron microscopy have been suggested to provide relative quantitation at the GBM level (32). The amounts of anti-GBM Ab bound to induce injury for non-C-fixing Abs or Ab fractions are generally greater than the C-fixing counterparts.

To be effective, the heterologous anti-GBM Abs are administered intravenously because they will bind to tissue basement membrane components if injected by other routes, reducing the amount of Ab available for kidney fixation. Following intravenous administration, the anti-GBM Abs bind rapidly, with as much as 63–70% bound in a single pass through the kidney (33). Studies have determined that the individual Abs contained in these polyclonal antisera have varying affinity/avidity for the glomerular capillary wall, and considerable dissociation and reassociation of Ab occurs. Temporal factors of binding also influence the nephritogenicity of anti-GBM Ab fixation seen in studies when similar amounts of Ab are delivered as a bolus or after prolonged administration (34). Anti-GBM or antilaminin Ab fixation within the kidney, as would be expected, is related to perfusion and development of glomeruli, as in the newborn rats (35,36).

The accessibility/location of the Ag and characteristics of the particular Ab, including such things as charge as well as ability to initiate inflammation, contribute also to the binding characteristics and quantitation (37–39).

Heterologous anti-GBM Ab-induced GN tends to develop more slowly and with less neutrophil involvement in mice than in rats or rabbits (40) and is little affected by altering the autologous phase immune response; however, crescentic lesions have been described (40–42). Heterologous anti-GBM Ab GN can also be induced in nude (nu/nu) mice deficient in T cells (43,44). Success with heterologous Ab to homologous GBM or TBM is reported, and anti-GBM Ab GN has been used in beige mice, which lack certain neutrophil enzymes, to show the role of these enzymes in disease induction (45,46).

The GBM was shown to be the major antigenic material in induction of "nephrotoxic serum" in studies by Krakower and Greenspon (47,48), who demonstrated that the amount of reactive Ag in various organs could be related to the content of vascular tissue, with kidney, lung, and placenta being the best sources of Ag tested. The GBM is composed of a variety of collagenous and noncollagenous proteins. Studies in the past suggested little reactivity to interstitial collagen and that the nephritogenic reactivity was directed toward noncollagenous proteins in the GBM. In general, Abs reactive with selected GBM components have been less nephritogenic than are Abs produced to cruder intact basement membrane fractions.

Antisera reactive with type IV collagen cause pulmonary injury in mice, with mild histologic changes in glomeruli and lungs (49,50). In these studies, Abs to laminin were less nephritogenic. Comparative binding between antilaminin and anti-type IV collagen Abs support a quantitative difference for these findings (50). An autologous phase injury induced by antilaminin Abs in rats is reported (51). Heterologous antilaminin Ab bound to a renal transplant served as a planted Ag to produce GN in a recipient immunized against heterologous Ig (52). Antiheparan sulfate proteoglycan Abs are reported to produce mild nephritogenicity as well (53,54). The lesion varies among strains and can be enhanced with an augmented autologous phase response (55–57). Studies using the bovine counterpart of the human α3(IV) chain in active immunization protocols produced GN and lung injury (see later) (58).

Heterologous anti-GBM Abs produce injury that is largely confined to the kidney, with the glomeruli the major inflammatory target. Tubulointerstitial infiltration of cells also may be a feature of heterologous anti-GBM Ab-induced injury (59,60) (see Chapter 36). In some instances, pulmonary edema and hemorrhage have been reported after administration of nephrotoxic Ab, and heterologous anti-lung Abs clearly can induce lung lesions, as well as glomerular injury (61,62). Lung involvement is also reported in augmented anti-GBM disease in rats, with an influx of PMNs during the first 12 hours, followed by ED1+ macrophages and, somewhat later, T cells (63). For the most part, reactive lung Ags appear to be sequestered from the circulation and are available for binding of heterologous anti-GBM Abs only after injury to the lung induced by such experimental maneuvers as oxygen toxicity, intratracheal gasoline administration, or administration of proinflammatory cytokines (64–67).

The glomerular injury induced by heterologous anti-GBM Abs and compounded by the autologous phase results from the activation of a number of systems of mediation of immune injury. Proteinuria alone may occur only with Ab fixation or Ab plus C binding, which can be demonstrated in studies using isolated perfused kidneys (68–70). Most mammalian anti-GBM Abs fix C and induce a transient influx of neutrophils within minutes in

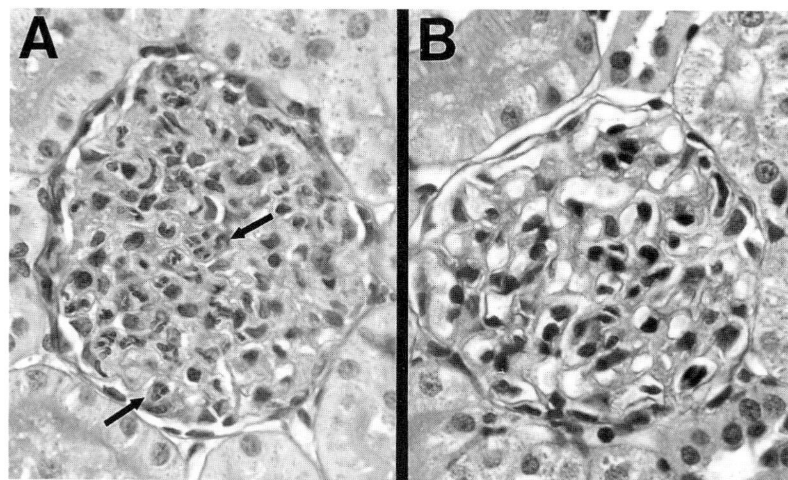

FIG. 1. A: A rat glomerulus is filled with neutrophils *(arrows)* 4 hours after intravenous administration of anti-GBM Ab. **B:** By 24 hours, most of the neutrophils have disappeared, with a modest mononuclear infiltrate and residual damage to the glomerular capillary wall.

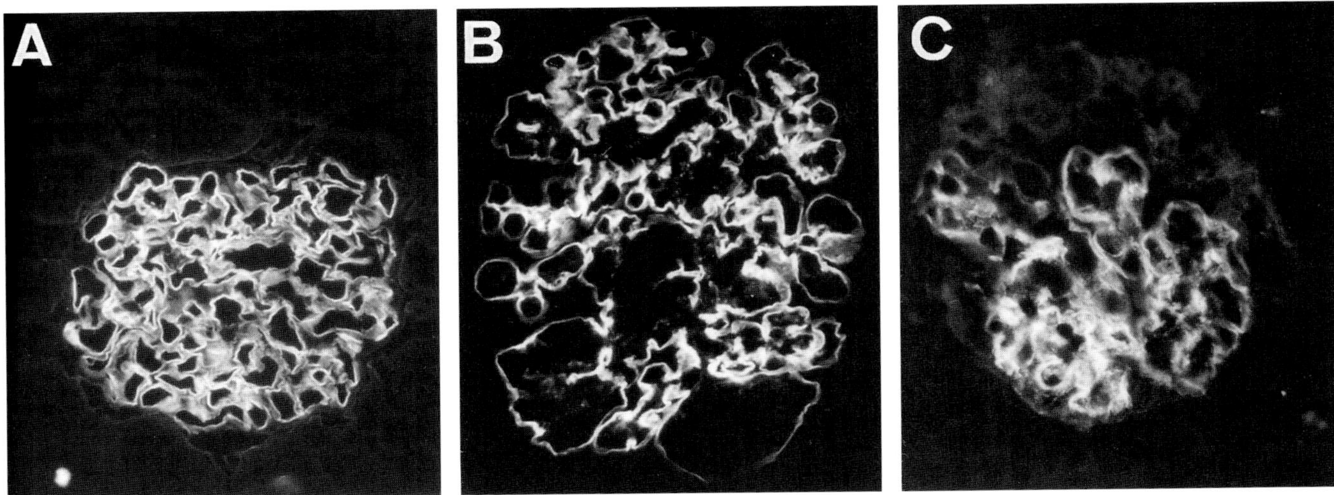

FIG. 2. A: Heterologous IgG deposits are found along the GBM within minutes after injection of anti-GBM Ab. **B:** Several days later, the linear pattern of deposition is less uniform when the architecture of the glomerular capillary wall becomes distorted by the inflammatory response. **C:** After additional time, the glomeruli become even more distorted, with the pattern of IgG (heterologous and autologous) corresponding to the deranged architecture.

rats and rabbits. The neutrophil accumulation peaks within the first 4–6 hours and then resolves, being replaced with varying numbers of mononuclear leukocytes (Fig. 1). Neutrophil as well as monocyte enzymes are capable of disrupting GBM, with fragments appearing in the urine. Hematuria may occur when gaps are produced in the GBM. Varying amounts of crescent formation occur, with rabbits more susceptible than rats. An anti-GBM model developed in the Wistar Kyoto (WKY) rat, either by anti-GBM Ab administration or by immunization to GBM Ags, evolves into a crescentic GN with additional elements of cellular immune responses (see later).

By immunofluorescence, the lesion is typified by continuous linear binding of heterologous anti-GBM Ab Ig along the GBM (Fig. 2A), with minimal focal fixation to segments of TBM (see Chapter 36). During the autologous phase, Abs reactive with host Ig are found in a continuous linear pattern in the GBM. As the GBM becomes progressively injured from the inflammatory response, the Ab deposits may become altered, reflecting inflammation-related distortion of the GBM (Fig. 2B). IgG deposits are accompanied by recipient C deposits, and fibrin deposits are generally striking in areas of crescent formation. The Ig deposits can be visualized at the electron-microscopic level as wispy structures and can be detected by immunohistochemistry. Neutrophils can be observed displacing the endothelium and attaching themselves to the denuded GBM. Local changes in GBM permeability can be demonstrated. Electron dense deposits may occur along the basement membrane in later stages of the disease; however, the composition of these deposits has not been clearly established.

Autologous Phase Injury

The autologous phase of anti-GBM GN induced by heterologous anti-GBM Abs is a natural consequence of the host's immune response to the glomerular-bound heterologous Ig. Studies have shown that small amounts of Ab, clearly sufficient to be visualized by immunofluorescent techniques but insufficient to induce acute injury, can still result in induction of autologous injury 7–10 days later, during the host's immune response to the heterologous Ig bound to the GBM. As little as 5 μg of heterologous anti-GBM Ab bound per gram of kidney is sufficient for autologous phase disease induction in the rat (71).

A number of experimental maneuvers has been employed to enhance or manipulate the autologous phase of injury. A so-called augmented autologous phase model is frequently used in which the host is preimmunized to the Ig of the species producing the heterologous anti-GBM Ab. The immunization is usually given in incomplete Freund's adjuvant to avoid any influence on inflammatory cells produced by complete Freund's adjuvant, and it is given 3–5 days prior to administration of the heterologous anti-GBM Ab to avoid large amounts of circulating Ab, which could induce circulating IC formation and/or anaphylaxis. Alternatively, the autologous phase can be induced by passive transfer of Ab reactive with the heterologous Ig given usually a few hours after fixation of the heterologous anti-GBM Ab. In rabbits, for example, passive autologous phase injury results in the rapid onset of a monocyte/macrophage-induced GN (Fig. 3) (72). The autologous phase can be purposely modulated by immunosuppression. As noted above, quantitation of Ab binding

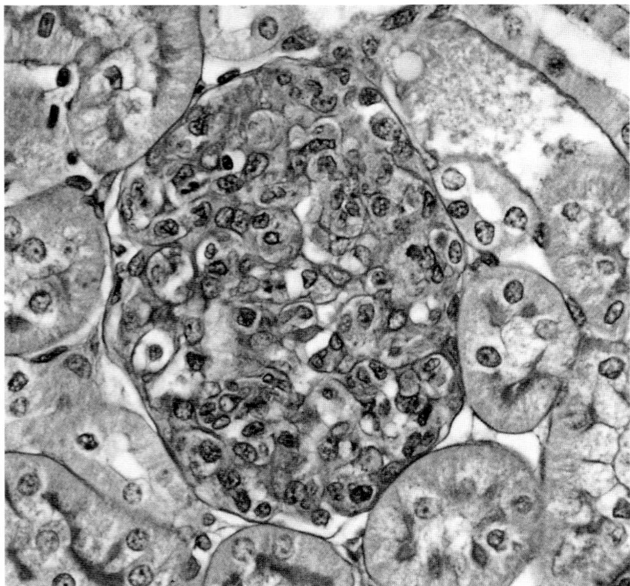

FIG. 3. Passive autologous phase anti-GBM Ab GN in the rabbit is characterized by an initial intense mononuclear cell infiltrate, in contrast to the typical neutrophil, followed by mononuclear cell infiltrates characteristic of the heterologous phase of injury in this species.

should be assessed during any modulatory studies to assure that the immune response to the heterologous Ab is also not being altered. Autologous phase injury has been observed in nude mice that may have an impaired, but not absent, immune Ab response to the heterologous IgG (73).

Models of Active (Autoimmune) Anti-GBM Disease

Immunization with Basement Membrane Ags

Several models of anti-GBM Ab-induced injury have been developed by immunizing animals with basement membrane Ags, usually in complete Freund's adjuvant, with or without additional adjuvants. The classic model developed by Steblay (74) involved repeated immunization of sheep with heterologous or homologous GBM in complete Freund's adjuvant (75). Sheep prove to be particularly susceptible and to develop a rapidly progressive, crescentic form of GN and die within 1 to 3 months. The serum Ab of affected sheep can transfer the GN to normal sheep. The disease can also be caused to recur in renal allografts (76). Studies have indicated that the Ab formed in sheep following immunization with human GBM is directed at the collagen type IV NC1 domain, found to be the major reactive site in human anti-GBM Ab disease (77). Of interest, sheep immunized with heterologous GBM or ABM in adjuvants capable of inducing severe GN do not develop lung lesions or lung Ab fixation (77,78).

Immunization of rats with GBM or other renal basement membrane preparations elicit anti-basement-membrane Ab responses to GBM/TBM/ABM Ag systems, often associated with the development of GN of varying severity; the immunizations sometimes also may induce selective anti-TBM Abs associated with TIN. The rat Abs reactive with the GBM/TBM Ags can be detected in human anti-GBM Ab assays, indicating their similarity to those found naturally in humans. The selective anti-TBM Abs are reactive only with TBM of rat strains (or heterologous species) that express the relevant TBM Ag (TBM Ag+), such as the Brown Norway (BN) strain, and not with TBM Ag- strains, such as the Lewis (LEW) (see Chapter 36). Rat renal basement membrane preparations may be contaminated with renal tubular brush border Ags, which may in turn lead to induction of Heymann nephritis-like lesions after a few weeks, thereby complicating the rat model if studied at later times (see later).

Anti-GBM and anti-TBM Abs are induced in BN rats by immunization with heterologous GBM, with the anti-TBM Ab tubulointerstitial disease preceding the glomerular disease (79). Anti-GBM Ab induction with heterologous GBM was studied in several strains and found most striking in BN rats (80). LEW rats immunized with BN rat renal basement membranes develop Abs to TBM with granulomatous TIN and may, in addition, form Abs reactive with the GBM/TBM Ag system and little or no glomerular or lung disease (see Chapter 36) (81). Immunization of rats with trypsin-solubilized and purified bovine GBM induce Abs reactive with GBM, which induces GN and some pulmonary hemorrhage; however, Ab fixation in the lung has not been detected (82–85). In studies using this Ag, the severity, GBM staining, and histologic picture varied with the strain of the rat used (84). This bovine Ag fraction has been suggested to be similar to the α3 type IV collagen NC1 Ag involved in human anti-GBM disease (86). The lesion is reported to be transferable with Ab from the urine of infected rats (87), as well as with isologous monoclonal Ab from hybridomas derived from the immunized rat spleens.

Active immunization of BN rats with collagenase solubilized homologous (Sprague Dawley) GBM can induce anti-GBM Ab, peaking after 6 weeks with a focal GN (88); T cell transfer results in priming the anti-GBM Ab response (89). Cyclosporine is effective in reducing Ab production and GN (90); Abs to CD4+ T cells also reduced circulating anti-GBM Ab formation and prevented disease in this BN model (91).

WKY rats immunized with GBM Ags or given anti-GBM Abs develop crescentic anti-GBM Ab GN with added cellular immune features (see later) (84,92). Alterations in GBM structure induced by feeding the proline analog 2,3-dehydroproline are reported to induce Ab reactive with altered, but not normal, GBM (93).

In rabbits, a bovine type IV collagen α3 NC1 dimer has been used to induce Abs that react with both GBM and ABM associated with inflammatory changes in glomeruli and pulmonary hemorrhage (58). Minimum pulmonary lesions were also reported in rabbits immunized with choroid plexus, which has a structure and basement membrane not unlike that of the glomerulus (94).

Of interest, the urine of normal subjects contains Ags that are cross-reactive with the GBM and can be used to induce anti-GBM Abs when used to immunize rabbits (95). The nephritogenicity of the anti-GBM Ab in this model was shown by transfer using Ab fractions eluted from kidneys. The excretion of urinary GBM Ags increases in association with glomerular injury (96). GBM Ags can also be detected in the circulation of nephrectomized animals, suggesting that they are derived, at least in part, from systemic basement membrane breakdown and may normally find their way into the urine.

In mice, bovine α3(IV) Ag (as noted earlier in rabbits) has been used to induce a slowly developing anti-GBM Ab-associated glomerular lesion with cellular immune contributions (97). Active anti-GBM models have also been described in nonhuman primates and in other species, including dogs and guinea pigs (98–101). Guinea pigs can also be induced to develop anti-TBM Ab-associated TIN with a nonnephritogenic anti-GBM Ab present directed toward collagenous GBM Ags (102).

We have observed spontaneous formation of anti-GBM Abs in older mice of several strains and have confirmed their presence with elution studies, although their role in the glomerulosclerosis observed in older mice is not defined. Spontaneous development of anti-GBM Ab has also been observed in three horses with linear Ig deposits, with elution confirmation of the anti-GBM Ab in one of the animals.

Anti-GBM Abs Associated with Polyclonal B Cell Activation and Molecular Mimicry

A number of autoimmune GN models have been induced by measures that lead to a polyclonal B cell activation and production of autoantibodies, including Abs reactive with GBM Ags (103,104). Examples also include SLE-associated autoantibodies, anti-myeloperoxidase (MPO) Ab, and vasculitis (see later). Mercuric chloride administration to BN rats induces autoantibodies, including anti-DNA Abs and Abs reacting with GBM Ags (105–110). Monoclonal anti-GBM Abs derived from spleen cells from mercuric chloride-treated rats can produce mild proteinuria in naive BN rats (111). Other strains of rat are also susceptible to induction of anti-GBM reactivity, although the glomerular histologic lesions may be more membranous than acute and proliferative, as seen with heterologous anti-GBM Ab.

The immune responses to basement membrane components in the mercuric chloride model include laminin as a prominent immunoreactant, as well as noncollagenous fractions of type IV collagen and fibronectin (112,113). Because Abs in this model can be detected in our radioimmunoassay for human anti-GBM Abs and do cross-react with other human GBM preparations, reactions with α3 type IV collagen are suggested (114). A granular form of immune deposit GN is observed later in the mercuric chloride model (115). Abs eluted from the mercuric chloride-treated rat kidneys react with laminin and type IV collagen (synthesized by cultured glomerular visceral epithelial cells), which perhaps leads to the formation of the granular immune deposits (116). Disseminated intravascular coagulation has been reported to occur in mercuric chloride-treated rats (117).

Some strains of mice are susceptible to a glomerular lesion after mercuric chloride in which immune deposits are found in the mesangium (118,119). In rabbits, mercuric chloride also induces Abs reactive with GBM, as well as other elements of the extracellular matrix, with eventual development of a membranous immune deposit disease suggested to involve soluble collagen polysaccharides (120). A number of other toxins, including sodium aurothiopropanol sulfonate or D-penicillamine are also noted to induce anti-GBM Abs that share idiotypes similar to those seen in anti-GBM Abs induced by the polyclonal B cell activation associated with graft-versus-host disease (121,122). Cadmium toxicity is also reported to induce GN and B cell activation in rats (123).

In graft-versus-host disease, a transfer of DBA/2 lymphocytes into a C57 BL/10 X DBA/2 F1 hybrid is associated with Abs reactive with both nuclear Ags and laminin, among other GBM components, as well as with glomerular dipeptidyl peptidase IV (124,125). In graft-versus-host disease in BALB/c mice that have received (A/J X BALB/c) F1 hybrid cells, anti-GBM Abs are observed, as are antitubular epithelial Abs (126).

Although lacking any compelling clinical association with anti-GBM disease, a cross-reactivity or molecular mimicry between GBM Ags and streptococcal proteins has been observed and studied in the past. The concept of molecular mimicry is used to define the cross-reactivity of antigenic epitopes shared between two disparate molecules that carry the potential for induction of an "autoimmune" response (127). More recently, monoclonal Abs to glomerular Ags and streptococcal Ags were reported to be cross-reactive (128,129). Antistreptococcal cell membrane monoclonal Abs bind to glomerular and lung Ags in the basement membrane regions of mice, with a granular rather than linear pattern of reactivity and target organ injury noted (130,131). A shared amino acid sequence has been identified in a portion of certain streptococcal M proteins and vimentin (132–134).

AB REACTIONS WITH OTHER GLOMERULAR CELL AGS

The Problem in Humans

The exact mechanism responsible for immune deposit formation in most human GN is unknown. An increasing awareness of experimental models in which Ab reactions with cell surface or other glomerular Ag lead to immune deposits, often irregular in pattern, raises the possibility that human counterparts will be confirmed. To date, no examples have been established with the same certainty of anti-GBM Ab disease. The finding that some Ab identified in murine SLE can bind directly to glomerular sites (see later) suggests that similar findings might be identified in humans. Antiendothelial cell Abs have been reported in human SLE, other connective tissue diseases (135–137), and other forms of vasculitis (see later).

Membranous GN seen in association with tumors and infections or with no obvious clinical associations resembles, morphologically, some forms of experimental serum sickness GN (see later) and, more closely, the model known as *Heymann nephritis* (HN) in rats. In HN, an Ab reactive with Ags on the glomerular epithelial cells (also present on the proximal tubular brush border) has been shown as the mechanism of immune deposit formation (see later). Abs reactive with tubular brush border Ags are occasionally reported in human allografts and urinary tract infections or reflux. The possible association between human membranous GN and HN is the subject of review (138,139).

Antimesangial cell Ab reactivity is sporadically suggested in IgA nephropathy (140,141). Patients with IgA nephropathy have also been reported to have Abs reactive with the collagen region of type IV collagen (142). IgA–fibronectin complexes that can bind to collagen are also reported (143). Ab to nidogen/entactin are suggested to contribute to granular GBM deposits (144,145).

Although lacking well-confirmed examples in human GN, the several model systems to be discussed have provided considerable new insight into possible immune mechanisms of human GN. They suggest new directions to be taken in defining subsets of the large numbers of patients with glomerular immune deposits of uncertain causation.

Models Involving Other Glomerular Ags

Models Using Glomerular Cell Ags

A number of models has been developed in which Ab reactions to glomerular cell surface Ags may result in direct (lytic) cell injury and/or immune deposit formation.

Thy-1 and Mesangial Cell Ags

The anti-Thy-1 Ab model was developed when Thy-1, a phosphatidylinositol-anchored glycoprotein, was recognized to be present on rat mesangial cells. The molecule has a molecular mass of 18 kD, with about one-third being carbohydrate, and its complementary DNA indicates 143 amino acids with a hydrophobic transmembrane domain (146,147). Thy-1 Abs were used for a number of years to identify T cells. Thy-1 is not observed in the renal mesangia of other species, although it has been reported in proximal tubular epithelial cells and in Bowman's capsule in humans.

We were successful in using polyclonal antithymus serum (ATS) reactive with Thy-1-like mesangial cell surface Ag to injure the mesangial cells (148,149); other models using ATS or anti-Thy-1 monoclonal Abs are also reported (150–152). The commercially available anti-Thy-1.1 monoclonal OX7 is also effective. From a quantitative standpoint, the amount of Ab needed to induce glomerular lysis is small, with only 11 μg of Ab bound in the total glomerular mass sufficient for lesion induction (149). This contrasts with the 150–175 μg of Ab bound to both kidneys needed to induce immune injury with anti-GBM Abs or anti-concanavalin A (Con A) Abs in the rat (see other sections).

The lesion induced by ATS is much different than that induced by immune deposit formation and subsequent mediator activation. Instead, the Ab reaction with the mesangial cell, followed by C fixation, results in selective lysis of the mesangial cell itself, which is repaired during a subsequent mesangial-proliferative response. The C dependence of the lysis can be shown in studies using C depletion or with monoclonal Abs of Ig subclasses that do not fix C (150,153,154). Glomerular deposits of C5b-9, the membrane attack complex (MAC), suggest its involvement in the lytic reaction (154). Electron-microscopic evidence of 90 Å doughnut-shaped lesions in cultured mesangial cells treated with ATS were typical of those associated with MAC lesions in other nucleated cells (153). Our observations with studies in the isolated perfused kidney using ATS and C sources deficient in terminal C components also support a role for the MAC in lysis of mesangial cells.

The C-dependent mesangiolytic phase of injury occurring between 1 hour and 2 days is rapidly replaced (days 3–5) by a phase of mesangial proliferation and hypercellularity (Fig. 4). The lesion can be modified by altering the dose of Ab used, in that very large doses with excess lysis will delay the proliferative phase of the lesion, and readministration of the Ab during the hypercellular phase will result in a second lytic episode, although the lysis may not be as effective as the initial administration, perhaps related to alterations in Thy-1 expression on the proliferating mesangial cells. In addition to the proliferating

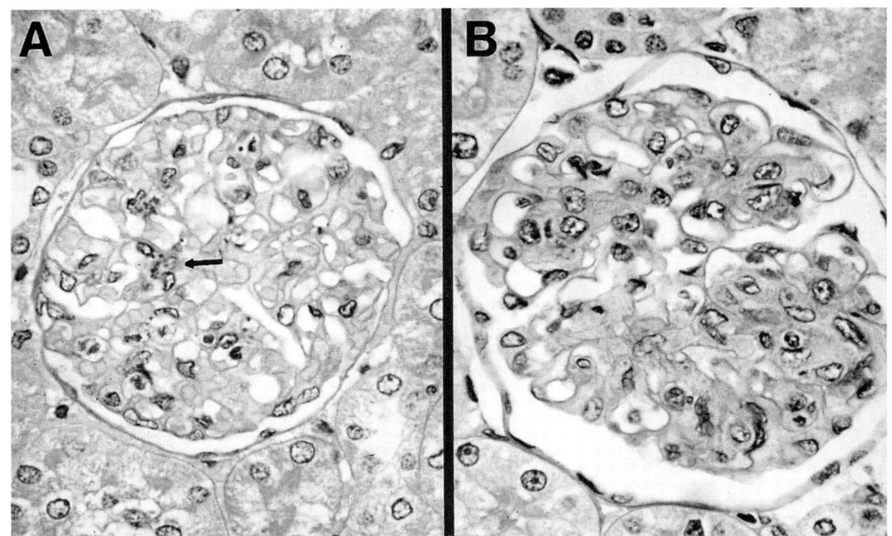

FIG. 4. A: Mesangial cell necrosis *(arrow)* is observed within a few hours of administration of anti-Thy-1 Ab in the rat. **B:** Within 4 days, mesangial proliferation and some mononuclear leukocyte infiltration is apparent.

mesangial cells, monocytes and macrophages are also present (155), with a few neutrophils observed during the acute lytic phase. The chemokine, monocyte chemoattractant protein-1 (MCP-1), is expressed in glomeruli after ATS (156). Depletion of monocytes and macrophages has a modulating effect on the lesion (157,158). The proliferative lesion is prevented if the initial lysis is inhibited by C depletion, but not by maneuvers to deplete neutrophils, such as with irradiation or with antineutrophil Ab (148,154). Platelet depletion is also reported to modulate the lesion (159), as is treatment with nucleotidases that affect adenine nucleotides (160).

Typically, the mesangial-proliferative phase resolves over 3–6 weeks, with minimal to mild focal mesangial sclerosis, depending on the severity of initial insult. Heparin decreases mesangial proliferation, and its administration can reduce the amount of focal mesangial matrix increase (161). Repeated administration of Ab will enhance mesangial sclerosis, which can be augmented by uninephrectomy or modulated by thromboxane inhibition (162–164). Hyperglycemia in streptozoticin-induced diabetes also accentuates mesangial sclerosis in the anti-Thy-1 model (165).

The mesangial cell lesion has found wide use in studying glomerular mesangial cell responses to injury, including the expression of smooth muscle α-actin (166). Both TGFβ and PDGF have been shown to participate in the mesangial cell proliferative response and the accumulation of matrix within the mesangium (167–169). Administration of neutralizing anti-TGFβ or -PDGF Ab decreases the mesangial matrix increase (170–171). A similar effect can be obtained with decorin, a regulator of TGFβ (172).

The anti-Thy-1 lesion has also been used to study mesangial function, such as the uptake of macromolecules (heat-aggregated human IgG or BSA or preformed complexes) (149). Development of proteinuria in the model varies among rat strains. Heavy proteinuria is a feature of the lesion produced in Wistar rats by a new monoclonal anti-Thy-1.1 Ab, which is reported to recognize a different epitope than that seen with OX7 (see later) (173). Glomerular hemodynamic measurements in the model reveal a decrease in glomerular ultrafiltration coefficient related to thromboxane A2 and 5-lipoxygenase products and suggest a role for mesangial cells in glomerular filtration rate (174,175).

Ab attack focused on mesangial cells has also been induced using Abs against materials previously phagocytized by the mesangium (176). A monoclonal Ab that reacts with mesangial matrix in vivo can induce immune deposits (see later) (177). Other models in which mesangial cell damage can be induced have included the use of snake venoms (178–180).

Endothelial Cell Ags

The importance of glomerular endothelial cell/leukocyte interactions in inflammatory infiltrates and vasculitic injury has been emphasized (181–184). Endothelial cell injury is also involved in induction of thrombotic states such as those associated with hemolytic uremic syndrome (see later).

A model of endothelial injury has been reported using the angiotensin converting enzyme (ACE) present on endothelium as an Ag, following ideas used to induce experimental lung injury (185–187). Injections of the anti-ACE Ab into the aorta above the renal artery resulted in binding to the glomerular endothelium as granular aggregates (188). Systemic administration of the Ab produced fine granular deposits on the glomerular endothelium, with C3 on day 2 and a shift to a more linear pattern on days 3–5, at which time the deposit was localized near the base of the epithelial cell foot processes and filtration slits. Endothelial swelling and blebbing was observed. Induction of increased expression of ACE by captopril did not affect the glomerular lesion. The amounts of Ab bound in isolated perfused kidney were in the range of 33 μg. The lesion may have involved shedding of endothelial surface Ag complexes, which were subsequently retained at the level of the podocytes and filtration slits. Von Willebrand's factor (vWF) is present on endothelium, and anti-vWF Abs result in endothelial and mesangial deposits in perfused kidneys, with C fixation, limited leukocyte influx, and scattered electron-dense deposits (189). The interaction of preformed Ab with glomerular endothelial surface Ag is involved in hyperacute rejection or xenograft rejection.

Heymann Nephritis and Epithelial Cell Ags

The HN model in rats, a model for the study of human membranous GN, was first described by Heymann et al. (190) in 1959 as an active model using immunization of rats with fractions of rat kidney in Freund's adjuvant. The active model was refined in the late 1960s, using an Ag termed *Fx1A*, which represented a sediment derived by ultracentrifugation of the supernatant remaining from low-speed centrifugation of rat cortical fractions pressed through stainless steel sieves to remove glomerular and tubular fragments (191). A subfraction of Fx1A, termed *RTEα5*, which could induce active HN after immunization with as little as 3 μg, was reported (192,193). Proteinuria onsets after 4–6 weeks following immunization. Ab fixation to the glomerular capillary wall occurs in a fine granular pattern with C fixation and the development of subepithelial electron dense deposits (Fig. 5). In 1975, Feenstra et al. (194) described a passive version of HN in which heterologous anti-Fx1A Abs were used. When the crude Fx1A is used to immunize animals for production of heterologous Abs for passive HN models, the Abs generated are rather complex, reacting with diverse glomerular and tubular epithelial sites, as well as with glomerular endothelium, GBM components, and T cells (195–198).

Early on, active HN was thought to represent a circulating IC mechanism in which small amounts of RTEα5 in the circulation served as an Ag for IC formation with the induced Ab, and it was sometimes referred to as *autologous immune complex nephritis* (AICN). Circulating ICs were detected in HN in some laboratories but not in others (199–203). The presence or absence of circulating ICs may relate to the particular contents of the Fx1A preparation used for immunization. Fx1A Ag was reported to bind to glomeruli, and other suggestions of IC disease based on changes in mononuclear phagocytic clearance and function were also used to support this idea (204,205).

In two lines of evidence, direct binding of Ab to Fx1A-related Ags in glomeruli was shown to be the major mechanism responsible for this model. Studies employing in vivo or in vitro perfusion of rat kidneys with heterologous anti-Fx1A Ab were used to demonstrate binding to subepithelial sites (206,207). In other studies, concentrated eluates from rats with active HN were found to bind directly to glomerular Ags in tissue sections (201). The Ags were distributed in punctate foci at the junction of epithelial cell foot processes in the GBM (201,208). When Abs eluted from kidneys with active HN were infused into isolated perfused kidneys, direct binding was demonstrated that could be competitively inhibited with heterologous anti-Fx1A Ab (209,210). The demonstration of direct glomerular binding in both active and pas-

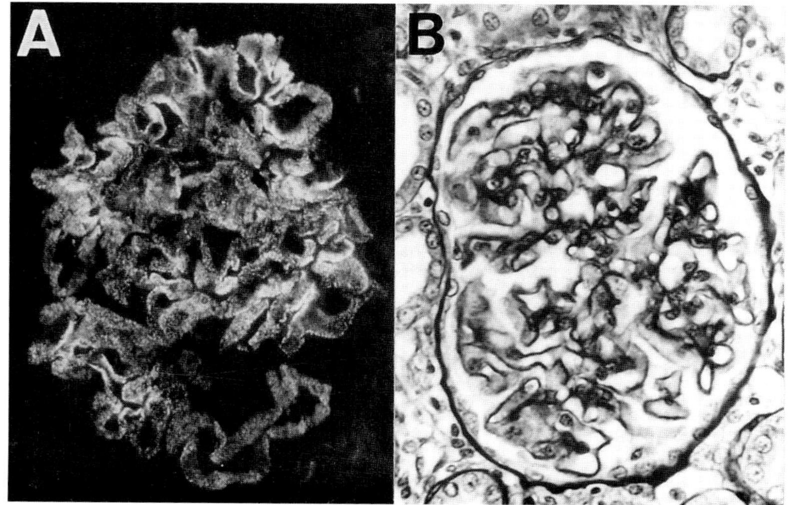

FIG. 5. A: Fine granular deposits of IgG (and C) are found in the glomerular capillary wall of rats developing active HN. **B:** The histologic picture is that of membranous GN. When studied by electron microscopy, subepithelial electron-dense deposits corresponding to those found in human membranous GN are present along the GBM (not shown).

sive HN models indicated that the Abs reacted directly with the glomerular capillary wall, with any additional contribution of circulating ICs unclear.

The exact nature of the nephritogenic HN Ag(s) represented in the Fx1A extracts has been the subject of study over many years. These studies indicate that the major Ag in this model is a molecule originally designated as a glycoprotein of 330 kD or, simply, *gp330* (recently renamed *megalin*) (211-213). Recent cloning studies have shown that gp330 has partial homology with the LDL and α2-macroglobulin receptors (214) and, as such, aid in the uptake of several molecules including plasminogen, protease–protease-inhibitor complexes, apolipoprotein-E-enriched very low-density lipoproteins, and lactoferrin. The gp330 is associated with another protein termed the *receptor-associated protein* (RAP), which, as its name implies, binds to these receptor molecules (215). The exact role of the associated molecules, termed the *HN antigenic complex*, is under study (216–218). Monoclonal Abs or IgG-RAP fusion proteins have been used to detect gp330 in clathrin-coated pits on glomerular epithelial cells, at the bases, and, in some studies, surfaces of microvilli on proximal tubular cells (219–224).

Comparisons between the disease induced by crude Fx1A and gp330 indicates Fx1A is often associated with more severe forms of injury, inducing Abs to gp330 as well as other glomerular Ags (138,225). The epitope specificity of the anti-gp330 Abs also contribute to the development of proteinuria, and the form of the gp330 is reported to vary (226,227). Monoclonal Abs produced against rat brush border Ags can induce glomerular deposits like those of passive HN and can react with tubular sites as well; some monoclonal anti-gp330 Ab can induce proteinuria (228-231). A monoclonal Ab to a 120-kD rat brush border Ag reacted with glomerular deposits induced by gp330 (232).

Tubular and glomerular epithelial cell dipeptidylpeptidase IV (DPP IV) has been suggested to contribute and polyclonal or monoclonal Ab to it may be individually nephrogenic (229,233,234). Other monoclonal Abs may have reactions with similar Ags (235). Expression of DPP IV varies among rat strains, and its expression is upregulated by IFNγ (236). DPP IV is detected on human glomerular epithelial cells, whereas gp330 is not (237).

Quantitative studies on the glomerular uptake of Fx1A Ab indicate that binding occurs slowly, with 12 μg bound to glomeruli at 4 hours and 48 μg bound at 48 hours after 10 μg of immune Ig was administered (238). Binding of 38 μg on day 3 increased to 52 μg per 7.7×10^4 glomeruli at the onset of proteinuria on day 4, which correlated with electron-dense subepithelial deposits in the effacement of foot processes (239). Aminonucleoside of puromycin alters binding of Ab to glomeruli, affecting glomerular accumulation of deposits in active HN as well (240-243). Aminonucleoside treatment was observed to alter binding of active HN eluates to kidneys (201). As with anti-GBM Ab binding, passively administered anti-Fx1a Ab binds in developing glomeruli relative to blood flow (244).

The mechanism by which Abs reactive with components of Fx1A, including gp330, induce HN appears to represent binding of the Abs to the Ags present on the epithelial cell surface with cross-linking of antigenic sites, leading to shedding of the resultant Ag–Ab complexes as an immune deposit in the adjacent subepithelial aspect of the basement membrane (245–249). Ab binding is associated with a change in detergent solubility of the Ag and binding to the cytoskeleton mediated by microfilaments (250). Rapid binding of Ab to the coated pits of the epithelial cell foot processes produces electron deposits that are located under the slit diaphragms at 1 day (251). Serial sections indicate that the deposits that coisolate with GBM maintain contact with the coated pits as well. Studies using monoclonal and polyclonal Abs to human epithelial cell Ags, when administered to human and monkey kidneys, indicate the potential for redistribution of glomerular Ags in these species, as well as in the rat (252). Because the gp330 is a receptor, its alteration via Ab may lead to changes in handling molecules normally taken up by the epithelial cells, molecules which, in turn, might add to the electron-dense subepithelial deposits.

As opposed to the reaction with anti-Thy-1 Ab in the mesangium, epithelial cell loss is not a major feature of HN, although the changes in epithelial cell podocytes leading to effacement are associated with development of proteinuria within 3 to 5 days after administration of heterologous anti-Fx1A Ab. In passive HN, C is a major mediator in the proteinuria, which entails activity of the MAC (253–256). The ability of anti-Fx1A to induce C in MAC-dependent lysis of cultured glomerular epithelial cells (257) does leave open the possibility of direct glomerular epithelial cell damage or even death. Although depletion of C may prevent proteinuria, it does not prevent all effects of passive anti-Fx1A Ab as monitored in glomerular micropuncture studies (258). An anti-glycolipid Ab reactive with glycolipids of the microvilli is suggested to be responsible for the C activation (259).

A model of membranous GN involving glomerular epithelial Ags has been developed in mice using a rabbit Ab to a pronase-treated mouse Fx1A with formation of subepithelial deposits during the autologous immune response (260). Modulation of the autologous immune response via inhibition of the CD40-CD40 ligand pathway prevented the membranous lesion in this model (261).

The rabbits immunized to produce anti-Fx1A Ab may develop glomerular injury; however, deposits are usually more prominent in tubulointerstitial tissues (see Chapter 36) (262). Anti-Fx1A Abs, as well as Abs to other tubular Ags, induce a glomerular lesion in rabbits with somewhat different time courses of induction of proteinuria and epitope reactivity than in the rat (263,264).

Rabbits develop GN spontaneously, which is characterized by segmental irregular IgG and C3 deposits along the GBM (265,266). Deposits are present on the subepithelial aspect of the GBM as multiple irregular accumulations of electron-dense material in a more diffuse, less circumscribed manner than the deposits typical of HN or human membranous nephritis. When Abs are recovered from the glomeruli of the involved rabbit by elution techniques, they can be demonstrated to bind to normal rabbit glomerular cross-sections in an irregular glomerular capillary wall pattern, with some binding to arteriole capillary walls. By immunoelectron microscopy, the binding appears to be confined to the regions where the epithelial cell foot processes abut the GBM (266). It would appear from these studies that the GN that develops spontaneously in these rabbits likely involves an anti-glomerular epithelial cell Ab, which may lead to the formation of deposits in a manner similar to those described above for HN. The eluted rabbit Ab binds to human glomeruli and suggests that an Ag would be present in human glomeruli to which autoantibodies could react and lead to disease similar to that observed spontaneously in the rabbit (266).

Models Using Other Glomerular Ags

Other Glomerular Ags

A number of other potentially nephritogenic Ag/Ab reactions are less well defined but nonetheless of interest. A model has been reported in which antiglomerular Abs are thought to be involved in penicillamine-induced nephrotoxicity (267). The Abs recovered from kidneys with this lesion do react with normal glomeruli in a linear pattern; however, the nature of the Ag has not been completely defined.

Fibronectin is present in the mesangial area, and Abs to fibronectin can react after in vivo administration (268, 269). When rabbits were immunized with human plasma fibronectin, Abs reactive with a 27-kD fragment of rabbit fibronectin developed, and dense deposits were observed in glomeruli (270). Fibronectin also may be involved in trapping Ags for nephritogenic immune reactions (271). Nephritogenic glycopeptides have been recovered from glomeruli, and their relationship to other antibasement membrane Abs remains to be fully defined (272,273). The Ag has been sequenced and is a glycopeptide that can bind Con A (274). Conceivably, Ags present in glomerular cells as a result of an infectious process could serve as targets for nephritogenic Ab reactions.

Other Monoclonal Ab Reactions with Glomerular Ags

Monoclonal Abs reactive with a wide variety of defined and to-be-defined glomerular Ags have a potential for providing many additional models by direct binding with induction of injury or by serving as planted Ags. The use of monoclonal Abs in identifying Ags and mechanisms have been referred to in other sections, including HN with anti-gp330 and anti-DDV-IV Abs (see earlier); OX7, the anti-Thy-1 monoclonal Ab used in mesangial cell injury (see earlier); and a number of glomerular reactive monoclonal Abs in murine SLE (see later). As noted in the section on anti-GBM Abs, isologous monoclonal Abs were found to induce anti-GBM GN in rats (275).

A number of molecules have been identified within the glomerulus that may serve as Ags as monoclonal Abs to some of them bind to glomeruli following injection (276–279). Monoclonal Abs to a glomerular epithelial cell Ag, presumed to be podocalyxin, can bind to neuraminidase-treated rat kidney, raising the question of hidden Ags and factors that might expose them (280). Often, administration of monoclonal Abs may not prove to be particularly nephritogenic and may require additional measures, such as administration of complete Freund's adjuvant (177, 235). One of these latter Abs, K9/9, causes alterations in glomerular epithelial cells in vivo, which is noted to involve an epitope-specific interaction between a cell surface moiety and the monoclonal Ab (281). The formation of subepithelial dense deposits in rats has been reported by monoclonal Ab against glomerular surface Ag (282), and anti-mesangial Ag monoclonal Ab, designated *1G10*, has been reported useful in detecting mesangial hypercellularity in human kidney (283).

A monoclonal Ab 5-1-6 reactive with Ags present in the area of the podocyte and their slit diaphragms is able to induce severe proteinuria when administered to rats (284). About 13 μg of Ab bound are required for induction of the proteinuria (285). Sprague-Dawley rats are less susceptible than are BN, LEW, or Wistar (286) rats. Studies suggest that the Ab must be divalent and the proteinuria is C independent (287). The Ag p51 is synthesized primarily during initial glomerular development and is concentrated in the slit pores of mature podocytes (288). Chlorpromazine, which inhibits movement of the HN Ag, was not able to alter the monoclonal Ab reaction (289). Glomerular hemodynamic studies suggest that in this model, glomerular capillary hydraulic conductivity can be separated from increases in macromolecular permeability (290).

Aminopeptidases are present on glomerular epithelial cells such as aminopeptidase A, also called *angiotensinase A*, which splits an N-terminal aspartic acid from angiotensin II, reducing the activity of the hormone (291). Monoclonal Ab aminopeptidase A can cause GN with proteinuria and can bind to proximal tubular sites, as well (292).

Monoclonal Ab 1-22-3 produced in mice immunized with rat glomeruli appears to react with a different epitope on Thy-1 than that seen by OX7 and, in turn, induces heavy proteinuria (173). Just 2 μg bound is sufficient to initiate proteinuria (293). Progressive glomerulosclerosis occurs when the Ab is given to unilaterally nephrectomized rats (294). A monoclonal Ab JM-403 raised against GBM heparan sulfate can induce a transient and selective proteinuria (295).

NEPHRITOGENIC AB REACTIONS INVOLVING CIRCULATING AGS

The Problem in Humans

Most GN in humans has irregular glomerular immune deposits, sometimes involving particular glomerular locations (mesangium, capillary wall) with specific classes of Ig or mediator molecules and characteristic morphologic responses. The irregular pattern of immune deposit differs from the linear fixation of Ab representative of anti-GBM Ab fixation. Although experimental models characterized by irregular glomerular Ig deposit are known that involve structural glomerular Ags (see earlier), the majority of such deposits have been assumed to represent deposition/formation of immune deposits involving soluble circulating Ags based on similarities to model systems. It is suspected that many soluble Ags may be involved in what has been termed *IC mechanisms*, involving a continuum of concepts from (a) deposition of circulating ICs to (b) in situ IC formation with planted Ags in which glomerular binding of soluble Ags occurs for subsequent Ab interaction.

The types of GN involved include mesangial proliferative, diffuse proliferative, membranoproliferative, membranous, and crescentic—each with its clinical presentation, course, and response to therapy. In diseases such as SLE, multiple histologic forms of GN are found with transition from one form to another (296). In other instances, the disease is defined by the immune deposits as in IgA nephropathy (see later). In most patients, the suspected soluble Ags have not been identified; however, in some instances of GN associated with infection, tumors, therapeutics, or autoimmune diseases, the Ags present in glomerular deposits have been identified. Direct identification of the Ag in the deposit using immunofluorescence/immunohistochemistry or the study of Ab eluted from the kidney represent the two most common approaches. Alternatively, circulating IC can be isolated and studied. A number of assays for circulating ICs have been developed; however, they have been used more for studying disease activity than for identification of etiologic mechanisms. A listing of many of the Ag/Ab systems identified in human GN has been compiled (297).

Models Involving Circulating IC and Planted Ag Mechanisms

A wide variety of nephritogenic immune reactions involve Ab reactions with soluble Ags that reach the kidney from the circulation. The Ags may arrive in the glomeruli before Ab is formed, bind to the glomerular capillary wall, then react with Ab when it is produced by the host, leading to a planted Ag mechanism with in situ IC formation. Alternatively, Ag may first induce an immune response in the host and then become part of a circulating IC that then accumulates in the glomerular filter via "a circulating IC mechanism." These two mechanisms are clearly different at their extremes; however, in many instances they blur into one another when circulating Abs are present and when Ags (or Abs) have a physicochemical propensity to bind to glomerular structures (see later).

One of the clearest examples of an Ag becoming trapped in the glomerulus for a subsequent nephritogenic immune reaction would be the heterologous Ig bound to the glomerulus after administration of anti-GBM Ab. Within 7 to 10 days, the host's immune response to the glomerular bound foreign Ig serves to induce the autologous phase of anti-GBM Ab-induced injury (see earlier). Other early examples include the use of aggregated Ig that is taken up by the mesangium to produce a planted Ag that can be reacted upon by anti-Ig Ab introduced into the circulation (176). Probably the clearest example of a circulating IC mechanism is acute serum sickness in the rabbit using bovine serum albumin (BSA) as the Ag.

Models With Circulating IC Mechanisms

Von Pirquet, in 1911, recognized that serum sickness was related to the host's immune response to foreign serum proteins. In the 1950s, it was determined that circulating ICs could be induced by immunizing animals with serum protein and that these circulating ICs were associated with glomerular and sometimes other vascular deposits. Circulating ICs were then defined as the toxic products of the immune response that had been envisioned by Von Pirquet. It must be understood that an IC is a dynamic interaction of Ag and Ab, rather than a permanent physical structure or unit that can be identified or studied in the circulation or bound in a vascular site. The mechanism can be viewed only in terms of the dynamics of the Ag–Ab reaction and the multiple factors that can influence these dynamics. The composition of the IC can change, either in the circulation or after deposition within tissue, related to the relative concentration of Ag or Ab in the immediate environment. The situation becomes more complicated as multiple Abs of different Ab classes and of different affinities reactive with multiple epitopes on the Ag become involved during the course of the immune response. The overlap between a purely circulating IC disease and one involving a trapped Ag relates to any physicochemical selectivity of fixation on the part of the Ag (or the Ab) for structures within the affected vascular bed, such as the glomerulus. When circulating Ab is present, its Ag, even if capable of binding to the glomerulus, would reach that site in the form of an IC. In all but the simplest systems, it is virtually impossible to quantitate the role of free versus complexed Ag in the accumulation of the glomerular immune deposit. The IC mechanism of immune deposit formation is the subject of review (3,5, 8,298–301).

Acute Serum Sickness

The best example of circulating IC disease is the classic acute serum sickness model in rabbits induced by a single, large bolus of the foreign serum protein BSA. If the BSA is radiolabeled, it is possible to follow its clearance from the vascular compartment, with its half-disappearance time being in the order of 4 days. Ab to the BSA appears beginning on days 4 or 5 and is completely complexed to the excess of circulating Ag. These initial complexes remain small because they cannot cross-link or aggregate in the presence of the initial Ag excess; therefore, they are not easily removed by the body's mononuclear phagocytic system. As Ab production increases, the ratios of Ag and Ab shift, and with increased cross-linking, the ICs reach a size, between days 9 and 10, at which they are rapidly cleared from the circulation by the mononuclear phagocytic system. During this so-called immune elimination stage, but not prior to it, a very small fraction of the complexed BSA accumulates in the glomerulus and other vessels, initiating an acute GN and vasculitis. Variations in the immune deposit and the severity of the lesion relate to IC size, Ab avidity, release of vasoactive substances, rate of IC removal from the circulation by the mononuclear phagocytic system, and other parameters that contribute to the ability of the IC to accumulate in the glomerulus.

In quantitative terms, in rabbits receiving a dose of 250 mg/kg of BSA, only 20 μg of BSA or 4.4×10^8 molecules per glomerulus deposit in the glomerulus during the immune elimination phase, which removes all Ag from the circulation (302,303). The deposited BSA disappears from the glomerulus with a half-disappearance time of approximately 10 days. The glomerular BSA-anti-BSA immune deposits continue to grow in size as free anti-BSA Ab present in the circulation after immune elimination continues to react with unbound epitopes on the BSA in the initial glomerular deposits.

There is little or no evidence that the BSA accumulates in the glomerulus prior to immune elimination, although studies using a perfused kidney have suggested that alternate infusions of BSA and anti-BSA can lead to deposits in what may be a nonphysiologic situation (304). For example, it has been shown that even brief ischemia will allow serum proteins such as albumin and IgG to enter the GBM, a situation that is reversible with reestablishment of the circulation (305).

The difficulty experienced in passively inducing serum sickness-like glomerular injury with preformed ICs has questioned the role of the IC per se in the formation of deposits with circulating Ags. From what has already been said and what will be said later, the reader should

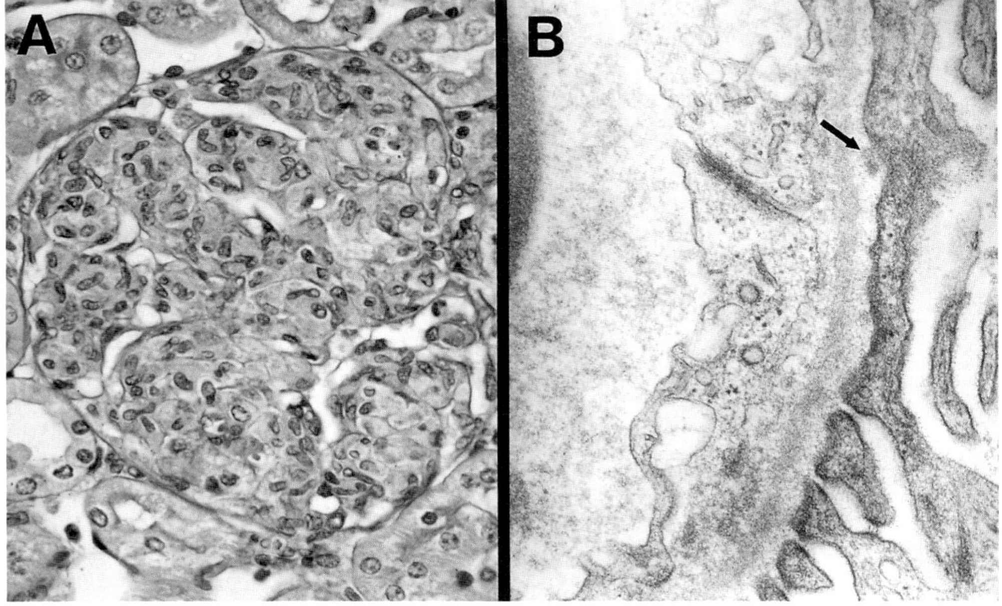

FIG. 6. A: In acute serum sickness, a striking infiltrative GN is seen in a rabbit on the day of immune elimination of a large intravenous dose of BSA given 10 days earlier. The infiltrate is dominated by mononuclear cells and is accompanied by a striking increase in urinary protein excretion. **B:** By electron microscopy, the granular deposits of IgG and BSA that typify this lesion are seen as very small subepithelial electron-dense deposits *(arrow)*.

readily identify that it would be virtually impossible to reproduce the dynamics of the IC formation, growth, and elimination that occur naturally. Although infusion of preformed complexes usually leads to little more than transient mesangial accumulation, some studies have suggested greater glomerular capillary wall localization with the more characteristic lesions of serum sickness (306–308).

The acute serum sickness in the rabbit is heralded by a neutrophil and mononuclear cell infiltrates in glomeruli (Fig. 6) with sudden onset of heavy but transient proteinuria. C and neutrophils, although present, are not essential, whereas antimacrophage serum can inhibit the lesion (72). T cells are also suggested to be involved (309), and migration inhibitory factor, a lymphokine involved in monocyte/macrophage accumulation, is present (310, 311). The lesion is characterized initially by fine granular glomerular capillary wall deposits of Ig, C, and BSA, with increased Ig and less easily detectable BSA during the days following immune elimination, when free Ab is present in the circulation and continues to bind to the BSA epitopes exposed in the initial deposits. During this time, the striking proteinuria resolves.

Maneuvers are often used to heighten the immune response, such as prior administration of anti-BSA Ab to aggregate a portion of the initial BSA for better presentation to the immune system or administration of LPS. This is done to increase the percentage of rabbits that develop GN 10 days later, during the stage of immune elimination in acute serum sickness.

Chronic Serum Sickness

Chronic serum sickness has been studied since the early 1950s (312) and is induced by repeated, often daily injections of foreign serum proteins for periods of several weeks, which results in Ab and IC formation and glomerular immune deposit accumulation containing the foreign serum protein and host Ab. In rabbits, two types of models are used. In one, a fixed dose of the Ag is injected, allowing the rabbits to self-select which will develop nephritogenic IC glomerular deposits, based on the balance between their individual immune response and the fixed amount of Ag administered (313). In the other, the dose of Ag is varied to balance the individual rabbit's immune response, with the daily dose changed weekly as Ab levels increase or decrease (314). A higher yield of nephritic animals is generated by the variable dose approach. Rabbits receiving very high doses of BSA (30–250 mg/day) are particularly susceptible to anaphylactic-like reactions, and the BSA dosage must be divided. Small initial doses complex the bulk of the circulating Abs without forming sufficient insoluble complexes in the lung vasculature that could cause respiratory distress or death prior to administration of the remaining larger amounts of Ag. For example, an initial small BSA dose (10 mg) leads to complexing of most of the circulating anti-BSA Ab as a visible precipitate in the plasma, with loss of circulating leukocytes and platelets trapped in the lung vasculature within the precipitate. The material trapped in the lungs is cleared rather rapidly, and the circulating cells increase over the first hour. The precipitate may actually be dissolved in part as the remainder of the daily dose is given, changing the Ag:Ab environment within the vasculature into one of Ag excess.

Considerable variations in the relative amounts of Ab and Ag occur during any 24-hour period, and the dynamics of the circulating IC formation, as well as interaction of free Ab or Ag (before or after the daily injection), with its counterpart already deposited within glomeruli, renders exact quantitation of direct interaction of Ab/Ag with the glomerular capillary wall deposits, versus interaction with circulating Ag/Ab ICs, virtually impossible. Situations, however, can be set up in which it is possible to quantitate the direct glomerular interactions using transplantation or perfusion situations that eliminate circulating Ab and exclude circulating IC formation (see later).

Rabbits injected daily with BSA have detectable circulating anti-BSA Ab within about 10 days, with levels of Ab varying widely among individual outbred rabbits. Rabbits with poor immune responses or those given inadequate amounts of Ag to balance active Ab production fail to develop GN. A proper situation for development of nephritogenic immune deposits related to the IC formation occurs only in rabbits in which Ag and Ab levels are balanced, irrespective of the absolute amounts of either. Rabbits with high Ab levels receiving large amounts of Ag develop immune deposits more rapidly and have more aggressive glomerular histologic changes and increased proteinuria. Purposeful alteration of Ab responses using immunosuppressants will obviously affect IC deposition, depending on the relative levels of Ag and Ab involved. It is interesting that daily injections of Ag proceed for about 4 weeks before significant glomerular immune deposit formation occurs. Once the immune deposit formation begins, it very rapidly progresses, with attendant histologic change. When examined at this critical transition point, the immune deposits appear to shift from the initial low-level mesangial localization to the glomerular capillary wall, where the deposits are observed by electron microscopy as subepithelial electron dense masses.

If radiolabeled BSA is substituted for a daily dose, the amount of deposition can be quantitated. During the daily injections, prior to the onset of detected GN with proteinuria, only about 50 μg or roughly 0.04% of the daily dose of between 50 and 200 μg of BSA deposits in the kidney daily. When overt GN and proteinuria develop, the deposition increases on average to 600 μg, representing 0.5% of the individual daily dose (303). The half-disappearance rate of the daily BSA deposit is about 5 days and can

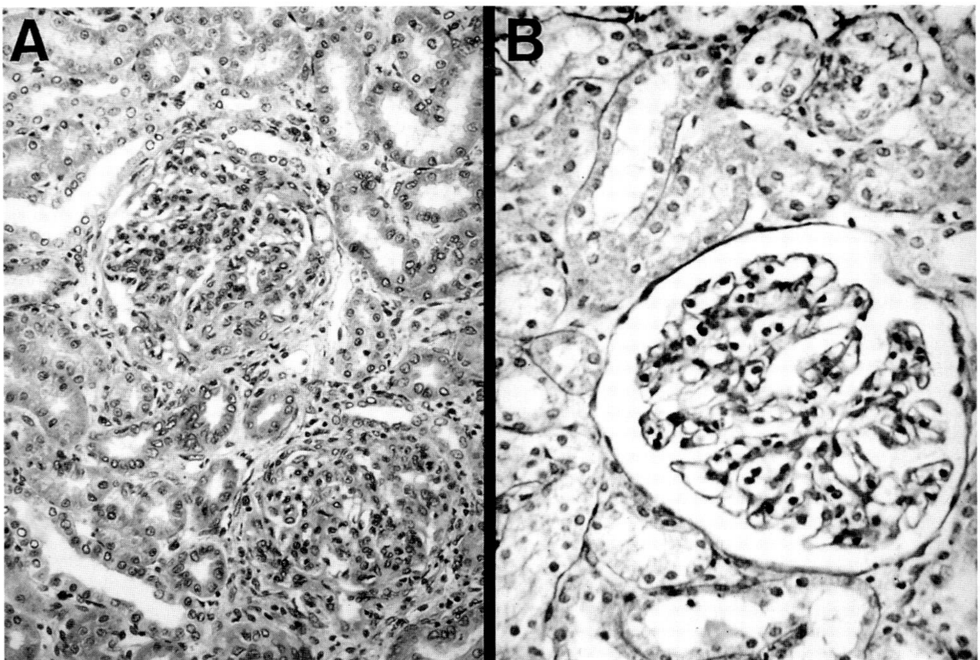

FIG. 7. A: Two glomeruli from a rabbit with chronic serum sickness induced by daily injections of BSA are shown with severe proliferative GN. The rabbit had an active immune response to the BSA and was receiving a moderate daily dose of BSA. **B:** The rabbit shown in this panel had a very poor anti-BSA immune response and was receiving only small amounts of BSA daily over a prolonged period of time. A membranous form of GN was observed, with limited evidence of an active infiltrative element.

be altered by administration of huge Ag excess to dissolve the IC and actually remove the deposits from the glomerular capillary wall (303).

Depending on the immune response and amount of Ag given to balance this response, the histologic lesions of the BSA-induced chronic serum sickness model in rabbits vary and resemble several different forms of human GN (315,316) (Fig. 7). Rabbits with very high anti-BSA immune responses develop fulminant crescentic GN, whereas those having moderate immune responses develop infiltrative/proliferative forms of glomerular injury, marked by large numbers of inflammatory cells, glomerular capillary wall thickening, and severe proteinuria. In the severe forms of GN, renal failure and death occur within 1 to 3 weeks of onset of proteinuria. In rabbits with poor immune responses that receive low doses of BSA, a slow accumulation of glomerular IC deposits leads to a more membranous, less infiltrative form of GN with massive proteinuria, edema, and nephrotic syndrome. Glomerulosclerosis is the sequela if the lesion is not too rapidly fatal.

Each rabbit with chronic serum sickness is somewhat unique, and for comparative study, the rabbits must be grouped by Ab response, dose of BSA used, and histologic response. In the fixed Ag protocols, the rabbits self-select which ones will respond with the correct amount of Ab to cause a nephritogenic IC formation at the dose chosen. The percentage of rabbits that develop GN will be lower than in the variable dose scheme, but the lesions will be more uniform. In contrast, the variable dose models allow comparisons of different levels of severity and forms of histologic response, much like the selection of patients for clinical trials.

Although the predominant localization of the Ag, Ab, and C containing immune deposits is subepithelial (Fig. 8), evidence of deposits among the fibrils of the GBM and in the mesangial matrix, as well as evidence of those deposits being endocytosed by glomerular endothelial cells, has been observed (317–319). In addition, particularly in rabbits with active immune responses having large amounts of circulating ICs, widespread vascular accumulation of Ag, Ab, and C deposits are observed similar to that seen in patients with SLE. The extrarenal immune deposit formation has been quantitated (320).

Several other species are susceptible to induction of chronic serum sickness by often using priming doses to initiate the immune response, followed at a later point by repeated, usually daily, injections of foreign protein. Such models have been described in mice and in rats (321–327), as well as in chickens and in cats (328–330). The chronic serum sickness model has also been duplicated in nonhuman primates (331,332). As with rabbits, chronic sclerosing end-stage glomerular disease is the outcome in rats (333). Uptake of radiolabeled BSA has

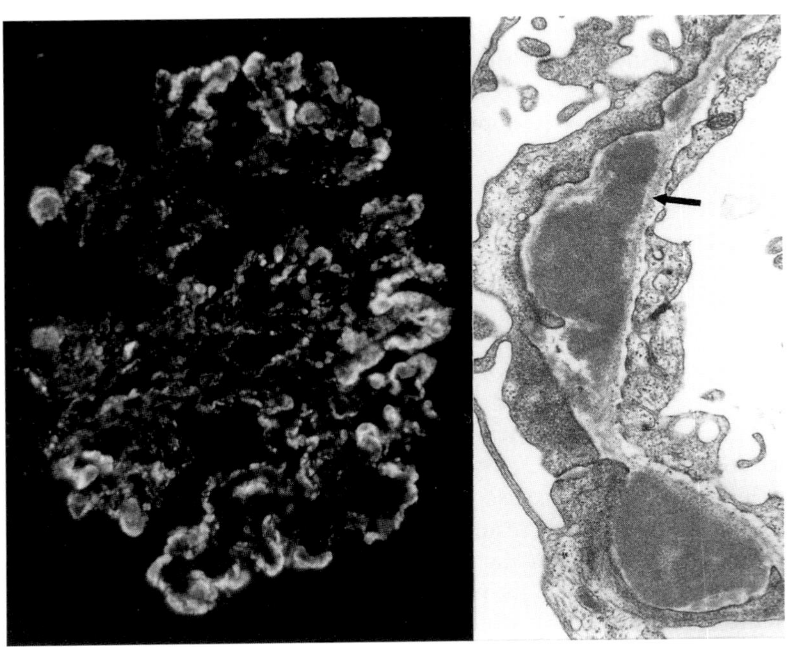

FIG. 8. A: Large amounts of immune deposit form in the chronic serum sickness model in the rabbit. The striking coarse granular BSA deposits shown here are accompanied by IgG and C3 in the same pattern. **B:** The immune deposits are seen as large electron-dense deposits *(arrow)* along the subepithelial aspect of the GBM.

been quantitated in rat serum sickness models, as has distribution in other organs (334,335).

Variations in size of Ag suggest that large Ags, such as thyroglobulin, result in predominant mesangial lesions in rabbits, whereas small Ags, such as ovalbumin, that are easily filtered through the glomerulus, can induce glomerular dysfunction without evidence of localization of immune deposits in the glomerulus (336,337). Ferritin, a large Ag visible by electron microscopy, has been used to produce predominately mesangial IC deposits in mice, and apoferritin induces GN in mice, with a histologic pattern related to dose and immune response of the particular strain used (338,339).

A very large number of studies has been done over the last 20–30 years to determine the factors that relate to the accumulation of immune deposits in the glomerular capillary wall in association with serum sickness models. These studies are too numerous to review here (see earlier); however, factors such as blood flow, efficiency of systemic mononuclear phagocytic clearance versus the rate of IC formation, hydraulic pressure, glomerular permeability, IC size, Ab affinity, preceding glomerular damage, and clearance by the mesangial region of the glomerulus have all been suggested to contribute to varying degrees (reviewed in 8; see also Chapter 14). Among these multiple factors, the clearance of ICs from the circulation has had more recent attention in studies dealing with cell surface receptors for the Fc portion of IgG (Fcγ) and, in addition, receptors for C fragments such as C3b in clearance and metabolism of ICs. The Fc receptors are members of the Ig superfamily, with IgG Fc receptors FCγRI (CD64), FcγRII (CD32), and FcγIII (CD16), their isoforms, and other Ig class receptors defined (340,341). They function in clearance and in cell signaling (342,343). Soluble Fcγ receptors are identified in the circulation, and auto-Abs can form to the receptors (344,345). FcγRII present on platelets that are reported to aid in clearance of IC in serum sickness. Mesangial binding of IC via Fcγ receptors is also noted. C may contribute to dissolution of ICs, and ICs via their bound C3b (and C4b) can interact with C receptor (Cr1) on erythrocytes and leukocytes (346–348).

Glomerular Interaction of IC Components and Overlap with In Situ or Planted Ag Mechanisms of Immune Deposit Formation

A major feature affecting immune deposit formation in chronic serum sickness is the in situ interaction of the individual components of the glomerular immune deposit with their counterparts (free or bound in ICs) from the circulation. This interaction has been shown, using kidneys with BSA containing immune deposits transplanted into animals, to allow free BSA to bind in the absence of circulating Ab, with in situ perfusions to exclude formation of additional complexes, or with ex vivo perfusions in which it was found that, as might be expected, the interchange of Ag or Ab was related to the relative state of Ag or Ab excess of the glomerular deposit (349,350) (C.B. Wilson, *unpublished observations*). Due to this interchange, huge excesses of Ag can dissolve ICs in chronic serum sickness, with a gram of BSA able to cause a five-fold increase in the disappearance rate of glomerular-bound radiolabeled Ag (303). Ag excess has also been successful in removing glomerular immune deposits in models in mice (351,352). The dissolution is Ag-specific in multiple Ag IC models (353). The effect of the interchange also can be shown, using covalent cross-linked ICs that cannot rearrange and do not persist in the glomerular capillary wall in association with their counterparts, which are dissociable (354). When cationized (see later) nondissociating ICs are used, they will bind to the glomerular capillary wall via charge interactions (355). Factors that alter the ability of the complex to dissociate, such as secondary binding of anti-idiotypic Ab or rheumatoid factor, may also contribute (356–360).

We were able to show the presence of autoanti-idiotypic Abs in glomeruli from rabbits given daily BSA immunizations to develop chronic serum sickness (361). Anti-idiotypic Abs were also found in glomerular deposits after polyclonal B cell activation in mice (362, 363). Complexes containing idiotype/anti-idiotype Abs were found in models, using antiphosphorylcholine immune responses, or during polyclonal B cell activation, using African trypanosomes (364,365). Immunization of rabbits with altered homologous IgG of defined allotype were able to induce anti-idiotypic rheumatoid factor-like activity in the glomerular deposits (366). Auto-Abs to C, such as seen in C3 nephritic factor or in other immunoconglutinins, would also be expected to alter the dissociability of the complex.

Cryoglobulins can form through FcFc interactions with Ig, such as those seen with IgG3, rheumatoid factors in lupus mice that react with IgG2a, with induction of glomerular lesions (367–369). The lesion has a characteristic wire loop appearance with subendothelial deposits developing 5–8 days after intraperitoneal injection of hybridoma cells producing IgG3 (370). Infusion of human cryoglobulin in mice can induce glomerular lesions (371).

In addition to the secondary factors affecting dissociation, the dynamic interchange of Ag and Ab within immune deposits in the glomerular capillary walls would be expected to be altered by many factors, such as the affinity of the Ag/Ab interaction, the localization of the complex, and the concomitant inflammatory response with associated morphologic, hemodynamic, and physiologic disturbances within the microenvironment. Infusion of proteolytic enzymes, for example, is reported to alter the disappearance of ICs (372,373).

Perhaps, the most important element that influences dissociation, rearrangement, or local formation would be any physicochemical property of the Ag (or Ab) that allowed it to adhere to the glomerular capillary wall, thereby moving the kinetics of the reaction from a circulating IC mechanism toward that of an in situ or planted Ag mechanism. This means simply that the Ag (or Ab) is no longer free to participate in the fluid dynamics of IC formation but has the added restraints of a fixed Ag that limits its ability to diffuse away from the site. Charge interactions between Ag (or Ab) and the polyanionic glomerular capillary wall are the most studied of these systems.

In the case of BSA, the classic Ag used in developing the models in rabbits, its slightly anionic pI appears to endow the BSA molecule with little or no glomerular binding, as opposed, for example, to purposely cationized IgG or other cationic molecules which bind and, in the absence of circulating Ab, would serve simply as planted Ags for in situ IC formation. In the presence of circulating Ab, any Ag would reach the glomerulus as an IC with a propensity to bind to the polyanionic capillary wall related to the charges present in the resulting IC.

Numerous model systems have employed cationic Ags in serum sickness protocols, in preformed IC protocols, and in planted Ag protocols for glomerular capillary wall in situ immune deposit formation. When native BSA is cationized, it can be shown to bind to the glomerulus, and when it is used in chronic serum sickness protocols in rabbits, it results in much more rapid accumulation of glomerular capillary wall immune deposits (2 weeks) than does its native BSA counterpart (374). Preimmunization models in rabbits with either acute or chronic administration of cationized BSA are also described (375). Highly anionic BSA is also noted to bind to some glomerular sites (376). Alternate perfusions of cationic or natural molecules and Ab indicated the need for a cationic Ag in forming glomerular deposits in the rabbit in this situation (377).

Mice chronically immunized with cationic bovine γ-globulin develop deposits in the glomerular capillary wall, whereas the anionic counterparts of the molecules tend to accumulate in the mesangium (378). Cationic Ags lead to development of glomerular immune deposits in mice with poor immune responses, in contrast to native Ag counterparts (379). Preformed IC containing cationic BSA localize in glomeruli of mice (380–382). Preimmunized mice are also susceptible to rapid development of GN, glomerular capillary thrombosis, and crescent formation after administration of cationic bovine γ-globulin (383).

Cationic Ags are used in models in rats presensitized to the Ag, followed by repeated injections (373,384). This model appears to be C- and neutrophil-independent in terms of its mediation (385). Even a cationic region in a molecule with an overall anionic charge may allow binding to the glomerular capillary wall in the rat (386). Only the initial binding of cationic BSA may be charge-related, with subsequent condensation related to other factors (387).

Cationic Ags can be fixed to the glomerular capillary wall by perfusion and can be reacted with active or passively administered Ab to cause in situ immune deposit formation in rats (388–392). Native cationic avidin can also act as a planted Ag in rats (393). When cationic ferritin is used, it can be visualized, and the initial subendothelial deposits are observed to move to subepithelial locations (394). Anionic sites on the epithelial cells are altered when cationic Ags are administered (395). The binding of cationic protein varies among different rat strains, suggesting some genetic variation in anionic sites (396). Epitope density of substituted cationic carrier molecules may influence the severity of the lesion (397,398). The charge of the Ab may also affect its glomerular localization. Both cationic and anionic Abs have been recovered from glomeruli with HN (399). When cationic and anionic Ab fractions are compared, glomerular binding of cationic Ab has usually been favored, and the location of the Ag also contributes (enhanced binding of cationic Ab to subepithelial Ag), with the charge of the Ag itself an additional factor (400,401). Cationic Abs bind to the glomerular capillary wall and can then interact with Ag to form immune deposits (402). IC with cationic Abs deposit more effectively in glomeruli than do cationic Abs alone (403). A small proportion of cationic Abs in IC is sufficient to cause their deposition in glomeruli (404).

The permeability characteristics of the glomerular capillary wall can be altered by administration of polycationic materials, with alterations in podocyte structure demonstrable (405–407). Heparin is reported to enhance removal of cationic BSA deposits from glomeruli (408). Alteration of heparan sulfate proteoglycan-rich anionic sites through heparitinase treatment also will alter binding of cationic ICs within the glomerular capillary wall (409). Injection of protamine sulfate, a polycation, affects binding of cationized Ag; however, this is less effective in established lesions, with the amount of Ab cross-linking present affecting the amount of protamine to dislodge cationic deposits (410–412).

A number of materials from cells that are potentially phlogogenic are also cationic, and these materials from platelets or leukocytes can bind in glomerular capillary wall (413–416). Naturally occurring charged molecules, such as MPO, may be involved in the so-called pauci-immune GN (see later). Non-Ab-containing complexes of charged proteins, such as cationized BSA-phosphorylcholine conjugated with DNP-BSA, are reported to be nephritogenic by inducing thrombotic microangiopathy and C fixation within glomeruli of mice (417).

Other In Situ IC or Planted Ag Models of Immune Deposit Formation

The ability of cationic molecules to bind to the glomerular capillary wall for subsequent nephritogenic interaction with Ab, leading to immune deposit formation, was discussed in the preceding section and is an important mechanism of in situ IC formation, including that in SLE (see later). Studies with both DNA binding to the glomerular capillary wall (see later) and lectin binding using concanavalin A (Con A) (see later) had set the stage for the cationic Ag studies.

In finding a foreign substance that would bind to the glomerular capillary wall and, in turn, serve as a nephritogenic planted Ag, we used the lectin, Con A, a glucose- and mannose-binding protein that fixes to the glomerular endothelium and subendothelial aspects of the GBM. Unilateral administration of 500 μg of Con A into the renal artery after flushing the vascular compartment with saline resulted in binding of approximately 75 μg of Con A in the glomerulus (418). By immunofluorescence, the fixation was in an irregular linear pattern along the glomerular capillary wall (Fig. 9A). The unperfused kidney had little or no Con A binding and could be used as a control. GN producing histologic changes and proteinuria could be induced by subsequent administration of anti-Con A, so that approximately 70 μg of the Ab bound per gram of kidney, an amount of binding similar to that described above for heterologous anti-GBM Ab. Con A could be infused into the renal artery of a rat that had been immunized previously with Con A, which resulted in binding of the actively formed anti-Con A Ab. Of interest, the Con A could be removed from the glomerulus by administration of a competitive inhibitor, α-methyl mannoside (418).

The Con A lesion is characterized by a striking neutrophil infiltrate (Fig. 9C) and was used to demonstrate the role of MPO present in neutrophils as a system involved in generating reactive oxygen species in glomeruli (419). A Con A model also has been developed in preimmunized beagles (420). Con A coupled to Ig has been used to induce glomerular inflammation with 500 μg of polymeric IgA–Con A complex, inducing a segmental proliferative GN with infiltration of neutrophils, fixation of C3, and production of fibrin (421,422).

Infusion of the lectin *Helix pomatia* agglutinin, which binds to glomerular endothelial cells, was used as a planted Ag for subsequent interaction with Ab (423). A similar model using the lectin *Lens culinaris* hemagglutinin, which binds to glomerular endothelial cells, has also been reported (424). The binding of different lectins to unique glomerular sites suggests that additional models will be described, limited only by accessibility of the bound lectin to circulating Ab. (425,426).

Lectins from infectious agents are thought to utilize a similar mechanism, in that Ags from *Dirofilaria immitis* (canine heartworm) have been reported to bind to GBM, with subsequent linear binding of Ab (427). Experimentally, an infusion of extract from *D. immitis* into the renal artery of hyperimmunized dogs can reproduce the glomerular lesion (428). *D. immitis* Ag has been found in glomeruli and serum of dogs infected with this organism using monoclonal Abs. Schistosoma Ags have been suggested to bind in a model in baboons (429). It is suggested that poststreptococcal GN may involve direct glomerular binding of a streptococcal Ag, with such Ags identified in the glomeruli of humans in the days early after infection (430,431). An Ag, endostreptosin, recovered from nephritogenic group A streptococci will bind to rat GBMs and is associated with rat IgG and C, with circulating Abs to the Ag after 8 days (432).

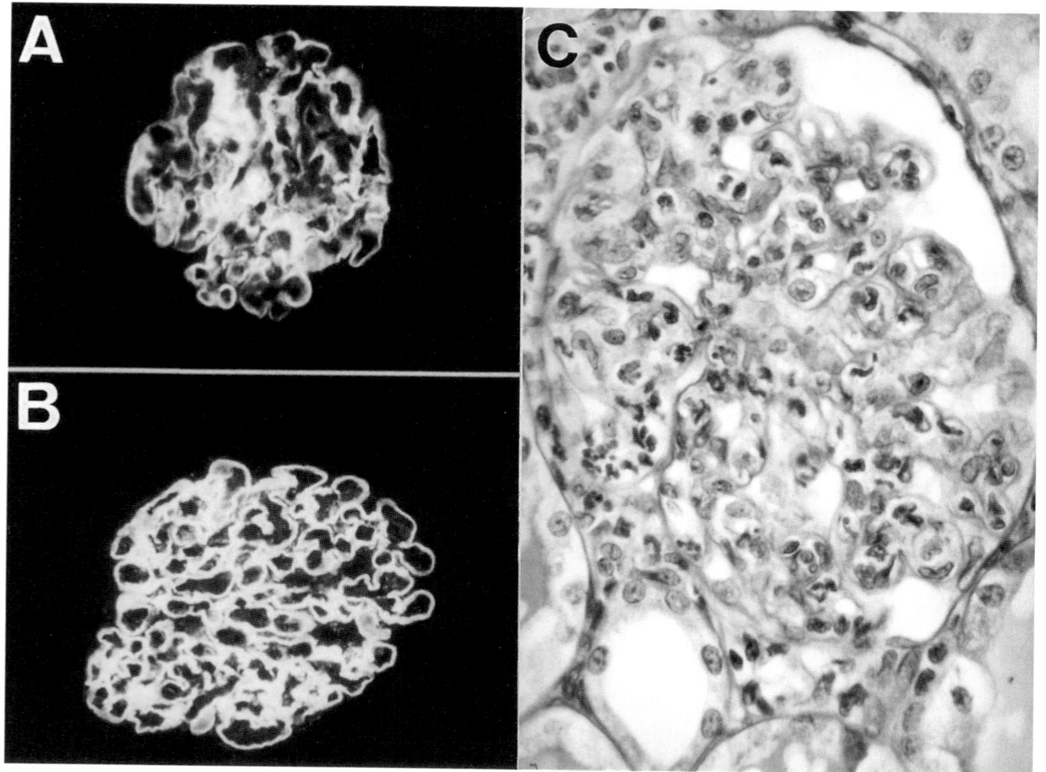

FIG. 9. A: Con A is seen along the glomerular capillary wall in an irregular linear pattern after infusion of Con A into the renal artery of a rat. **B.** When anti-Con A Ab is infused into a rat that has received Con A, the IgG binds to the planted Con A in a linear pattern. The Ab reaction induces a severe GN. **C:** The infiltrative and proliferative GN has a striking neutrophil influx, as seen in a rat that had been immunized to Con A and had been infused with Con A in the renal artery 5 days earlier.

Other Models with IC Mechanisms Involving Exogenous Ags

Granular glomerular deposits of Ig and C are not uncommon in laboratory animals, particularly as the animals age, and this background of deposits must be considered and controlled for. The frequent glomerular immune deposits found in many mice strains are thought most likely to be related to ICs associated with retroviral infections.

A number of models of IC GN, as defined above, in which exogenous Ags contribute to the glomerular IC accumulation has been studied. These models are most frequently associated with infection, and only a few examples will be mentioned here. The chronic lymphocytic choriomeningitis virus (LCMV) infection of mice is perhaps one of the oldest recognized. Mice infected as neonates have lifelong infections with LCMV-anti-LCMV IC detectable in the circulation and in glomerular immune deposits (433,434). Of the approximately 60 μg of Ig that can be eluted from each kidney in this model, about half is anti-LCMV Ab. The Aleutian disease of mink has a viral Ag-associated GN (435).

Attempts at modeling poststreptoccal GN have been inconclusive, with consideration given to planted Ag mechanisms (see earlier), C activation, and cryoglobulin formation. A number of other infections have been associated with IC forms of GN, with varying evidence of Abs/Ags related to the infectious agents in glomerular immune deposits. These include *Plasmodium* infections (436,437), *Schistosoma* infections (438–441), *Trypanosoma* infection (442), and *Leishmania* infection (443–447). Hydatid disease (*Echinococcus granulosus*) in sheep is associated with hydatid Ag in glomerular IC deposits (448). Even trout are reported to have an IC form of GN associated with *Renibacterium salmoninarum* infection.

Other Models with IC Mechanisms Involving Endogenous Ags

Of the models of immune deposit formation, SLE has received the most attention. Models of SLE in mice have had extensive study regarding the mechanisms of immune deposit formation, as well as the immunologic basis for the polyclonal B cell activation and autoimmune responses. In SLE, the mechanisms of immune deposit formation appear to include elements of direct Ab binding, in situ IC formation, and circulating IC accumulations.

The New Zealand black (NZB) mouse was first noted to develop Coombs-positive hemolytic anemia, GN, and positive lupus erythematosus tests in the early 1950s (449,450). The GN developed late in life, with most animals dying of renal failure by 18–24 months. A cross between the NZB and the New Zealand white (NZW) strain (NZBxNZW) F1 led to a more rapid onset of GN, with most mice dying between 8 and 12 months. In both the NZB and (NZBxNZW) F1, the onset of renal disease and death was earlier in females (451). Two additional strains developed in the mid-1970s that had murine SLE were compared with the NZB and (NZBxNZW) F1 (452). In these studies, the MRL/*lpr* mice had much more prominent lymphoid hyperplasia than did the NZB and had an earlier onset of GN and renal failure, with most mice of both sexes dead by 8 months (females slightly sooner than males). In the BXSB strain, GN developed in the males, with most dead by 8 months. The GN in the BXSB was neutrophilic and proliferative; that in the MRL/*lpr* was proliferative with some crescent formation; and that in the (NZB/NZW) F1 and NZB demonstrated more evidence of mesangial proliferation, matrix increase, and other elements of chronicity (Fig. 10). Vasculitis was present in the MRL/*lpr*, as was arthritis, and all strains had evidence of myocardial infarcts in some individuals. Immune deposits were found in the mesangium and peripheral glomerular capillary walls, with greater proportions of capillary wall deposits in the BXSB males and MRL/*lpr* than in the other strains, although there was considerable overlap. Retroviral gp70 deposits were present in glomeruli; however, their contributions to the disease were questioned when anti-gp70 Abs were not concentrated in renal eluates compared to serum, in contrast with specific concentration for anti-DNA Abs. The autoimmune response and diseases of these and other inbred strains of mice have been the subject of extensive reviews (453–455).

Environmental stimuli, such as LPS exposure, enhance the polyclonal B cell activation of these murine SLE strains (456). Immunization to LPS is reported to induce GN in normal mice (457–459). Graft-versus-host disease, with its attendant polyclonal B cell activation, also can create a form of auto-Ab response resembling SLE (460,461).

Numerous studies have focused on the genetic factors, including MHC, responsible for the development of autoimmunity and GN in the murine SLE strains and their human counterparts (462,463). These studies have identified the multigenic NZB and single-locus mutations *lpr* (lymphoproliferation) and *lpr*^{cg}, *gld* (generalized lymphoproliferative disease), and the *Yaa* (Y-chromosome linked autoimmune accelerator) found in the BXSB male (464–467). The *lpr* and *lpr*^{cg} mutations have been recognized in the *Fas* gene, which is involved in apoptosis, including that of T cells, allowing their accumulation (468, 469). The *lpr* represents an insertion in intron 2, which causes premature termination and aberrant splicing. The *lpr*^{cg} is the result of a replacement of isoleucine by asparagine, which affects the *Fas* apoptotic signal (470). When the mutation of *lpr* is corrected with a transgenic *Fas* gene, lymphadenopathy and GN are eliminated (471). The *gld* relates to a point mutation in the *Fas* ligand gene (472,473). Construction of a mouse transgenic for BCL-2, which decreases susceptibility to apoptosis, resulted in greater B cell growth and auto-Ab production with SLE-like renal disease (474). The mutations and the

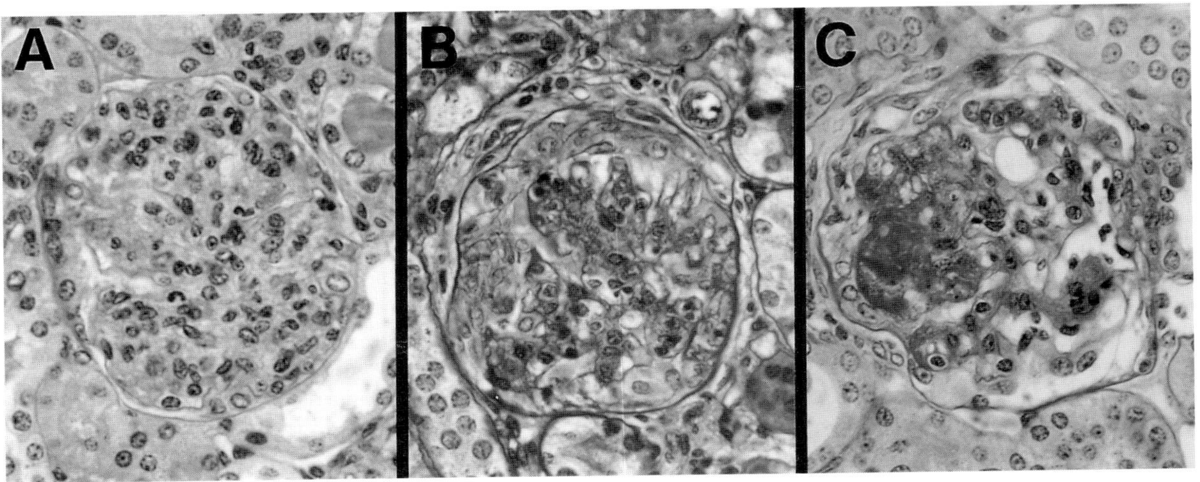

FIG. 10. A: A glomerulus from a male BXSB mouse is shown demonstrating an active infiltrative and proliferative GN. **B:** A glomerulus from a female MRL/*lpr* mouse is shown with an active proliferative GN and evidence of crescent formation. **C:** A glomerulus from a female (NZBxNZW)F1 mouse has a proliferative GN with a striking increase in mesangial matrix and some thickening of the glomerular capillary wall.

role of apoptosis in autoimmunity are the subject of review (475–478), as is the mechanism of the autoimmune response, which includes the contribution of anti-idiotypic Abs (479–483). In addition, apoptosis and removal of intraglomerular inflammatory cells or damaged glomerular cells also play a role in GN (484–486).

Sera of mice with murine SLE, as well as sera from patients with SLE, have large amounts of material detected in various IC assays. Although DNA deposits are found in glomeruli of both mice and humans with SLE, circulating DNA-anti-DNA ICs are less frequently identified, and certain anti-DNA idiotypes may be more pathogenic (487–491). An assay using DNAse-sensitive glomerular binding was used to imply DNA containing IC (492). Extrinsic DNA has also been suggested to be involved in IC and in induction of anti-double-stranded (ds) DNA Ab responses (459,493,494).

Many studies indicate that multiple mechanisms for immune deposit formation are involved in SLE. DNA has been reported to bind to the glomerular capillary wall and, as such, could serve as a site for in situ IC or planted Ag immune deposit formation (457,495). DNA or DNA-anti-DNA ICs are also able to react with fibronectin in a process involving C1q (496).

Attention has now shifted to histones, histone–DNA complexes (nucleosomes), and their Ab ICs as elements from the circulation that could lead to glomerular immune deposits via charge-related binding to heparan sulfate, a component of the GBM/glomerular capillary wall (497–507). Circulating DNA in SLE is reported to be bound to histones (508). Sequential perfusion of histones, DNA, and monoclonal anti-dsDNA resulted in glomerular capillary wall deposits, and perfusion with DNA alone followed by anti-dsDNA Ab resulted in lesser numbers of deposits (500). Monoclonal anti-DNA Abs bound to DNA fix to the glomerulus when complexed with histones (509). Histones have been found in glomerular deposits in (NZBxNZW) F1, and auto-Ab specific for nucleosome core particles have been found in MRL/*lpr* mice (510,511). Ab reactive with heparan sulfate proteoglycan enhances glomerular injury in (NZBxNZW) F1 mice (512). Antiubiquitin Abs are also recognized (513).

Nucleosome-restricted Abs are reported to precede the development of anti-ds DNA Abs, and antihistone Abs in MRL/*lpr* and the antinucleosome Abs are recovered in the kidney eluates (514). Immunization to nuclear Ags in murine SLE and humans may be related to exposure to chromatin released during apoptosis, with anti-dsDNA Abs only a subset of a wide spectrum of antichromatin Abs (515,516).

In addition to the possible circulating and in situ IC mechanisms in SLE, Abs recovered from eluates or produced as monoclonal Ab from SLE lymphoid cells have been found to bind directly to glomerular Ags, with cross-reactivity between DNA and glomerular components, including laminin (499,517–524) (see Chapter 13). In some instances, the binding may result from DNA bound to glomerular structures (525–527). In perfusion studies, mouse and human anti-DNA Abs can induce proteinuria that is blocked when the Abs are absorbed with DNA (528). Some of the anti-DNA monoclonal Abs can penetrate living cells and bind to nuclei (529,530).

The charge of the anti-DNA Ab may also contribute to the binding with cationic Abs found in human SLE serum (531,532). The ability of anti-DNA Abs to bind to strongly charged Ag (histone or heparan sulfate and DNA complexes) has a structural basis (533).

Cryoglobulins can also contribute to the glomerular lesions in murine SLE (see earlier). A concomitant of the SLE disorder is the antiphospholipid syndrome (534, 535). A model is described in male (NZWxBXSB) F1 mice (536). Antiphosphorylcholine Abs deposit in glomeruli and may cause renal dysfunction (537). Glomerular structural functional relationships in the MRL/*lpr* over time have been studied (538).

Transgenes that code anti-DNA Ab can be expressed in mice and lead to GN (539). Human lymphocytes transferred to mice with severe combined immunodeficiency express anti-DNA Abs with some evidence of glomerular deposits (540). Other autoimmune diseases in animals can be associated with GN, such as experimental thyroiditis in rabbits (541,542). The relationship between IC disease and diabetes is unclear; however, insulin containing immune deposits and elutable anti-insulin Abs are reported in inherited diabetes in mice (543).

NEPHRITOGENIC CELLULAR IMMUNE REACTIONS

The Problem in Humans

Most human immune glomerular diseases are defined by the presence of Ig deposits of one type or another. The added role of cellular immune responses in glomerular diseases with and without Ig deposits remains to be quantitated. A cellular immune response is suggested by the variable presence of T cell subsets and monocytes/macrophages in glomerular disease, and the role of cellular immune contributions is the subject of review (544–546). Clearly, interaction of humoral and cellular arms of the immune response are involved in initiation of the nephritogenic immune response. Cellular immune processes appear to be more prominent in tubulointerstitial disease, as outlined in Chapter 36.

In addition, there have been a series of observations that suggest that T cell abnormalities may contribute to the minimal change nephrotic syndrome/focal glomerulosclerosis most often seen in children. T cell-related factors produce glomerular changes and proteinuria when transferred to animals (see later).

Models of Cellular Immune Glomerular Injury

In many experimental situations, humoral immune mechanisms are sufficient for inducing severe glomerular disease. This is probably best exemplified during the rapid onset (minutes) of glomerular inflammation following passive administration of anti-GBM Ab. Even in this situation, lymphocytes are present early on (547), and mononuclear cell involvement increases at later stages. In some strains or species, such as the WKY rat or the SJL mouse, more features suggesting a specific cellular immune effector mechanism are emerging. In augmented autologous anti-GBM models, T cells and lymphokine production may play a role, with the numbers of these cells reduced by cyclosporine treatment (548). In augmented models, the level of Ab production to the heterologous Ab remains a major factor (549). A role for cellular immune mechanisms is usually demonstrated by disease transfer with immune T cells in the absence of Ab production.

Early models of cellular immune injury used transfer of lymphoid cells sensitized to heterologous Ig to induce mononuclear infiltrates in glomeruli containing heterologous Ig planted as anti-GBM Abs or preformed ICs (550, 551). T cells have also been suggested to play a role in glomerular injury induced using cationized conjugates of trinitrophenol and bovine serum albumin planted in the kidneys of rats previously sensitized to these Ags (552). Recently, azobenzenearsonate, a haptenic material that is capable of modifying surface proteins, thereby inducing delayed-type hypersensitivity, has been used to induce cellular immune glomerular injury by infusion in one kidney of BN rats previously sensitized to the Ag (553). The lesion is transferable with immune cells but not with Ab. Phytohemagglutinin administered shortly after transplantation was used to induce an acute cell-mediated glomerular injury in rats receiving renal allografts (554). Phytohemagglutinin also enhances the severity of lymphocyte infiltration in acute serum sickness in rabbits (555).

An interesting model of cellular immune GN has been developed in chickens immunized with GBM, in which a role for humoral immunity can be excluded by cyclophosphamide-induced bursectomy that removes Ab-forming cells (556–558). In these chickens, the nephritic lesion can be transferred with sensitized lymphoid cells given to syngeneic chickens, clearly showing the role of a specific cellular immune process (559).

Passive administration of heterologous anti-GBM Ab to WKY rats induces a mononuclear infiltrative and crescentic form of GN with increased Ab-dependent cellular cytotoxicity (560). Active immunization of this strain with heterologous GBM induces a similar histologic response (84). The lesion is characterized by an early mononuclear cell infiltrate, and the WKY strain is noted for increased natural killer cell activity. It is possible to modulate the crescentic lesion in this strain by depletion of CD8+ cells, which includes the natural killer cell population (561). Treatment with anti-CD5 or anti-CD4 Abs also modulates crescent formation in the WKY model (562). The passive anti-GBM Ab GN of the WKY rat has been modulated using Abs against ICAM-1 and LFA-1 (563). ICAM expression is reported to increase in glomerular endothelial cells after anti-GBM Ab in other strains of rats, an effect modulated by administration of the IL-1 receptor antagonist (564,565). The active anti-GBM model in the WKY rat also has been used to demonstrate the protective effects of Ab reactive with ICAM-1 and LFA-1 (566). CTLA-4, which can interfere with T cell costimulatory factors, modulates the WKY anti-GBM Ab model of GN, as it does in murine SLE (567,568).

Acid-treated, collagenase-digested bovine GBM has been used to induce a severe anti-GBM Ab-associated glomerular lesion in the WKY rat (92). Delayed type hypersensitivity and T cell responses to the acid-treated Ag are demonstrable. Homologous GBM from rats with Masugi nephritis, but not from normal rats, were successful in inducing proteinuria and GN in WKY rats (569).

Activated T cells are reported in the glomeruli of rabbits with anti-GBM Ab-induced GN (570). T cells and migration inhibition factor expression are found early in acute serum sickness (309–311). Activated T cells are also suggested to play a role in development of glomerular crescents associated with rupture in Bowman's capsule in passive augmented anti-GBM Ab disease in rats (571).

A relationship between cellular immunity and minimal change nephrotic syndrome has been suggested in humans. Factors in serum or produced by lymphocytes related to the CD4+ T cell population from patients with this disease are reported to increase permeability of capillaries and to produce alterations in glomerular epithelial cell foot processes and anionic sites following infusion into the renal artery (572–575). The vascular permeability factor found in the serum of patients with active minimal change nephrotic syndrome is also reported to reduce glomerular anionic sites (576,577).

MODELING SPECIFIC NEPHRITOGENIC LESIONS

IgA Nephropathy

The Problem in Humans

IgA nephropathy is one of the most commonly recognized forms of GN characterized by IgA, C3, and often IgG deposits in the mesangium, associated with a mesangial proliferation and frequently heralded by gross hematuria in association with a mild infectious disease process. The etiology is incompletely understood and the subject of numerous reviews (578–586) (see also Chapter 42). Consideration is given to abnormalities in control of IgA production, with increases in polymeric IgA. The IgA appears to be from bone marrow, rather than having a mucosal origin.

The glomerular accumulation of IgA is presumed to represent ICs, with suggestions that Ags from food or mucosal infective agents, as well as, perhaps, glomerular structures, are suspected but not generally confirmed. Other mechanisms of accumulation are suggested as representing macromolecular species of IgA, perhaps rheumatoid factor or other complexes involving proteins such as fibronectin.

Models of IgA Nephropathy

Several models of glomerular IgA deposition have been developed and their relationship to IC mechanisms reviewed (587–593). Both active and passive models are available. DNP-conjugated BSA and IgA MOPC-15 myeloma anti-DNP Ab can produce IgA deposits in glomeruli, using either in vivo or in vivo-formed complexes when the IgA is polymeric (594,595). Interaction of IgA from the circulation with the glomerular deposits is reported (596). In another variation, the anti-DNP and DNP conjugated with IgA antiphosphorylcholine Ab was used to trap phosphorylcholine-conjugated molecules in the glomerulus with phosphorylcholine-conjugated pneumococcal C polysaccharide that was more phlogogenic than either Ficol or BSA (597).

Mesangial IgA deposits are also produced by administration of TECP-15 hybridoma-derived IgA-anti-phosphorylcholine and phosphorylacholine conjugated to a variety of molecules (598). DNP-conjugated anti-Thy-1 Ab has also been used to fix Ag in the glomerulus for interaction with polymeric rat IgA Abs (599). Oral immunization has also been used to induce glomerular IgA deposits. Both systemic and oral administration of dextran can lead to mesangial IgA lesions (600–602). Diethylaminoethyl dextran, which is polycationic, and myeloma-derived murine IgA-antidextran Ab also led to IC localization in the mesangial areas (603). Dextranase treatment reduced mesangial IgA and dextran deposits in passive and active models of dextran sulfate and in monoclonal antidextran IgA or IgM nephropathy (604). Oral immunization with gluten or its lectinlike fraction, gliadin, in addition to ovalbumin or human γ-globulin, was able to induce IgA deposits in mice (605). Glomerular eluates of the immunized mice contained antigliadin IgA; however, this was not specific because renal eluates of control mice also contained these Abs, a finding suggested to relate to glutin in mouse chow. A model using oral immunization of lactalbumin was enhanced by impairing phagocytic function with colloidal carbon.

Studies using aggregated IgA or IgG revealed that, although mesangial uptake is similar, the IgA persists for a greater period of time, suggesting that even though IgA may be the predominant finding, consideration should be given to concomitant IgG deposits (606).

N-nitrosodimethylamine or D-galactosamine have been found to increase serum IgA levels in rats associated with glomerular IgA deposits (607). The fungal contaminant of cereal grains (vomitoxin) is able to increase serum IgA levels with Abs to bacterial and self-antigens, as well as mesangial IgA deposits without C3 in B6C3F1 and other mice (608–610). Hybridomas derived from Peyer's patches of BALB/c mice given oral vomitoxin have been found to react with a variety of self- and non-self-antigens (611). The IgA recovered from the glomeruli of vomitoxin-fed mice following elution react with inulin, DNA, and caseine (612).

The ddY mice develop a spontaneous glomerular deposition of IgA as they age (613). These mice also have mammary or lymphoid neoplasia. Glomerular deposits occur as serum IgA levels increase, and studies using eluates suggest that the more acidic IgA molecules in the polyclonal expansion lead to the mesangial deposits (614). Glomerular complexes of retroviral gp70, as well as histones, have also been reported in other studies in the ddY mice (615,616). The antihistone reaction reminiscent of that reported in murine lupus nephropathy occurs in the absence of anti-DNA Ab. The gp70 deposit varies among substrains of ddY mice and is not essential for the IgA deposition to occur (617). A sheep anti-type-IV collagen antisera is reported to accelerate the deposition of IgA in the ddY mouse by a mechanism suggested to relate to delayed mesangial transport of heterologous IgA (618). An increase in glomerular extracellular matrix components in the ddY mouse is observed (619,620). PDGF A and B chain mRNA expression is increased only slightly with age (621). Rat antimurine CD4 monoclonal Ab is reported to reduce glomerular IgA deposits in the ddY mouse without affecting IgA serum levels (622). Of interest, no change in the rate of ECM accumulation was noted after anti-CD4 Ab treatment in these mice, although glomerular IgA deposits were decreased. Neonatal thymectomy is reported to decrease IgA deposition, again without altering IgA levels (623). A form of spontaneous IgA nephropathy has been reported in dogs (624).

Sendai virus infection is noted to induce a model of IgA nephropathy with characteristics that appear to resemble the IgA nephropathy of humans seen in association with respiratory infection (625). Either a natural infection or purposeful immunization of mucosa with Sendai virus, followed by intravenous administration of virus preparations, induces glomerular deposits with Sendai virus and IgA, and other immunoglobulins (626). The physical form of the viral Ag used in the challenge affects the changes observed.

IgA deposits in the mesangium have also been associated with forms of hepatic damage. IgA deposits are observed in experimental carbon tetrachloride induced liver damage or after bile duct ligation (627–630). This may relate to alterations in normal hepatic clearance of IgA complexes via transport into the bile (631,632). Rats with liver damage induced using a lipotrope-deficient diet and oral alcohol have IgA deposits in their hepatic sinusoid, suggesting impaired transport from blood to bile, and have mesangial IgA deposits (633). Alcohol is also suggested to have direct effects on mesangial cells (634). The particular deposits are characterized by the presence of a secretory component, as are glomerular localizations of IgA associated with bile duct ligation, followed by oral immunization with protein Ags (635,636). These findings are similar to those of the IgA deposits in patients with alcoholic cirrhosis and biliary atresia, in which secretory IgA is present in the mesangium (637).

Pauci-Immune Necrotizing and Crescentic GN

The Problem in Humans

The so-called pauci-immune necrotizing and crescentic GN associated with Wegener's granulomatosis and other forms of microvasculitis is a form of severe GN with scant or no evidence of immune deposits and is associated with circulating Ab reactive with neutrophil cytoplasmic Ags collectively termed *antineutrophil cytoplasmic Ab* (ANCA) (638–640). Two patterns of ANCA are described related to their indirect immunofluorescence staining pattern on ethanol-fixed neutrophils. In one, a diffuse cytoplasmic stain is seen, designated *c-ANCA*, in which the major reactive Ag is proteinase 3 (641,642). In the other, termed *p-ANCA*, MPO assumes a perinuclear localization during fixation (643). Other neutrophil components are also recognized to produce p-ANCA reactions (644). c-ANCA is associated with Wegener's granulomatosis, and p-ANCA is seen in a variety of conditions in patients, including those with anti-GBM Abs. Activated neutrophils are identified in glomeruli of patients with ANCA and Wegener's granulomatosis (645), and cells positive for TNFα, IL-1β, and IL-2 receptors are found in periglomerular sites (646).

ANCA can induce degranulation, as well as an oxidative burst in neutrophils in vitro (647,648). Neutrophils activated in the presence of cytokines/LPS cause injury to endothelial cell cultures (649). The pathogenic potential is the subject of review, as is the contribution of anti-endothelial Ab, leukocyte adhesion molecules, and other aspects of endothelial function (184,650,651).

Models of Pauci-Immune Necrotizing and Crescentic GN

MPO binds to GBM in vivo and can induce oxidative reactions (652). Humoral and cellular immune responses can be induced in rats with human MPO, with cross-reactivity to rat MPO demonstrated (653). Perfusion of MPO into the renal artery of a rat preimmunized with neutrophil extracts and hydrogen peroxide leads to MPO and Ig being found along the GBM accompanied by inflammation (654). The Ig deposits are transient as related to strain, use of hydrogen peroxide, and duration of immunization; granulomatous vasculitis of small vessels also was noted (655). Renal ischemia/reperfusion is found to substitute for the hydrogen peroxide (656). In the model, glomerular epithelial podocytes expressed MHC class I and II molecules and ICAM-1 (657). Additional studies infusing MPO with hydrogen peroxide in rats relate the degree of injury to the intensity of the immune deposit, concluding that an IC, rather than the pauci-immune mechanism, was responsible (658).

Vasculitis can be a striking feature of acute serum sickness in rabbits, with the base of the coronary arteries a particular focus. The spontaneous lupus nephritis strains in mice also have varying frequencies of vasculitis, and ANCA have been detected among the numerous autoantibodies. A recombinant inbred strain derived from BXSB and MRL\l was recently reported to have crescentic GN and small vessel vasculitis with somewhat fewer glomerular deposits than the parent strains (659).

Anti-MPO-ANCA have been found among the auto-Abs, including anti-GBM Abs induced by the polyclonal B cell activation induced in BN rats by mercuric chloride (660,661). The ANCA reaction is associated with necrotizing vasculitis, particularly in the intestine, where it can be modulated by antimicrobial treatment. Serum transfer has been unsuccessful in inducing tissue injury (662). Heterologous antirat MPO Ab is reported to augment glomerular injury induced by heterologous anti-GBM Ab in rats (663).

Hemolytic Uremic Syndrome/Thrombotic Thrombocytopenic Purpura

The Problem in Humans

Hemolytic uremic syndrome (HUS) and thrombotic thrombocytopenic purpura (TTP) are the clinical presentations associated with a number of circumstances that appear to involve injury to the vascular endothelium with generation of a thrombotic microangiopathy. The clinical picture includes hemolytic anemia, thrombocytopenia, renal failure, and microthrombi in arterioles and capillaries of the kidney and elsewhere, with CNS involvement a feature of TTP. The HUS/TTP are associated with infectious (often bloody) diarrhea, drug toxicity, pregnancy, and neoplasia, as well as with familial forms. A number of findings have been suggested to contribute to the genesis of HUS/TTP, including abnormalities in platelet aggregation related to changes in von Willebrand factor and its polymers (664–667) or decreases in prostacyclin (PGI_2) (668–670). Abs to endothelial cell Ags are reported (671,672). Alterations in fibrinolysis related to an increase in plasminogen activator inhibitor-1 (PAI-1) or other factors may play a role in the same manner as suggested for other forms of glomerular coagulopathy (673–675). Elevation of IL-1 and TNF levels occurs in HUS/TTP, and the chemokine IL-8, a neutrophil attractant/activator, is also elevated (676,677). P-selectin is increased in the plasma of patients with HUS/TTP (678). Low C3 and elevated white blood cell counts are associated with more severe episodes (679).

There is great interest in the possible role of bacterial cytotoxins released by certain strains of *E. coli*, such as O157:H7 during its bloody diarrhea-HUS/TTP thrombotic microangiopathy presentation (680–683). The two phage-encoded cytotoxins are termed *Shigalike toxin* (SLT-I, SLT-II) or *verotoxin* (VT-1, VT-2) (with variants) and can cause injury to endothelial cells bearing their glycolipid receptors, with the toxicity produced in a manner similar to that of the toxic plant lectin, ricin. Each toxin has two subunits. The A subunit is about 33,000 molecular weight and is responsible for the cytotoxic activity via inhibition of protein synthesis, having a highly specific N-glycosidase that removes adenine from one particular adenosine residue in the 28S RNA of the 60S ribosomal subunit (684). Each toxin molecule has five B subunits of about 7500 molecular weight that function to bind to receptors on the cell surface. The major receptor is a glycolipid, globotriaosylceramide (Gb3) (685). Studies in human biopsies have shown increased binding of labeled SLT to glomeruli of infants compared with adults, which corresponds to the development of HUS in pediatric patients (686).

Models of HUS/TTP

Parallels have been drawn with glomerular intravascular coagulation seen in sepsis following bacterial lipopolysaccharide (LPS) exposure and cytokine release in which nitric oxide plays a role (687,688). As noted above, endotoxin augments and worsens anti-GBM Ab-induced GN (25). Anti-GBM Ab GN and associated thrombosis are associated with an increase in PAI-1, suggesting impaired fibrinolysis (689). FK506 inhibits glomerular thrombosis in rats induced by anti-GBM Ab and LPS (690). An association of HUS/TTP with drug therapy, including chemotherapeutics and agents such as cyclosporine, has been noted in patients, and a model of mitomycin-induced HUS kidney injury has been reported in the rat (691).

The possible role of the VTs in induction of HUS/TTP is under study. GB3 is 50 times higher in renal endothelial cells than in umbilical endothelial cells. Preexposure of umbilical cells to TNF or LPS increased Gb3 coincident with increases in sensitivity to cytotoxic and protein synthesis inhibitory effects of VT/SLT (692,693). IL-1β incubation with HUVEC induced the Gb3 receptor for VT. LPS enhances the sensitivity of cells to the cytotoxic effects of VT (694,695).

Efforts to induce glomerular thrombotic microangiopathy lesions of HUS/TTP using VT have not been satisfactory to date. VT-1 given to rabbits caused thrombotic microangiopathy in cecum, brain, and spinal cord but failed to replicate the HUS kidney lesion (696). VT producing *E. coli* infection in rabbits caused apoptosis of surface epithelium (697), and SLT induces apoptosis rather than necrosis in rabbit intestine (698). O157:H7 infection in piglets caused vascular damage and small infarcts in the cerebellum (699). VT glycolipid receptors determine the localization of the microangiopathic process in rabbits given SLT (700). VT induced TNF synthesis in the kidney, with tubular damage present in these studies (701). VT-2 is reported to induce acute renal cortical necrosis and death, with damage limited to renal cortical tubule epithelial cells (702). Binding was detected to cortical tubule and medullary duct epithelial cells, and the LD50 dose of VT-II was 400 times lower than VT-I (703).

The baboon has recently been reported to develop an HUS-like disease upon exposure to VT (704). This model revealed elevation in endothelin without a compensatory rise in nitric oxide, with one of six animals developing glomerular thrombotic microangiopathy. Alterations in the endothelin/nitric oxide axis were suggested to contribute to the acute renal failure observed in all animals.

OTHER CONSIDERATIONS

Immune Activation of Mediator Pathways

In some instances, glomerular injury may result from immune activation of mediator molecules, as is postulated to occur in the so-called hypocomplementemic membranoproliferative GN most often seen in children. The patients develop auto-Abs reactive with the alternative C pathway C3/C5 convertase, with the Ab termed *C3 nephritic factor* (C3Nef). The glomerulonephritic lesion of Finnish Landrace lambs has certain similarity to that found in hypocomplementemic membranoproliferative GN in humans (705,706). In studies in rabbits, evidence is found for idiotypic control of the auto-Ab formed to the alternative C pathway C3/C5 convertase (C3Nef) (707). The GN that is found in dogs with C3 deficiency or with levan in rabbits may also have some usefulness in understanding GN with C abnormalities (708-710); a number of deficiencies of C in humans are associated with glomerulonephritic complications. The possibility that ANCA activates neutrophil pathways of injury may represent another example of this type of mechanism (see earlier).

Sequelae of Immune Glomerular Injury

The discussion of the immune models of glomerular injury in this chapter has focused on the initiation of injury, with some mention of cellular immune processes that may contribute to chronicity of injury in some situations. For the most part, in the induced models discussed, the inflammatory responses resolve with varying degrees of glomerular scarring/sclerosis and attendant renal functional impairment, unless continued or repeated episodes of immune injury are used to hasten glomerular destruction. The immune models have had some use in studying factors responsible for glomerulosclerosis, such as that of growth factors (711) (see earlier); however, models utilizing chemical injury, such as the aminonucleoside of puromycin and adriamycin, reduction of renal mass, hypertension, and diabetes, as well as the effects of aging, particularly in rats, have found wider study (712–714). The fawn-hooded rat, for example, develops glomerulosclerosis (715). The FGS/Nga strain of mice has been reported to be a model of focal glomerulosclerosis with immune deposits, including retroviral gp70 (716). These models and progressive renal injury are topics of other chapters. In addition, the contribution of tubulointerstitial inflammation and fibrosis that is associated with most forms of glomerular injury is discussed in Chapter 36.

Here, only a few considerations of the use of immune models in the study of chronic stages of glomerular injury will be mentioned. Because reduction of renal mass is one feature in progressive renal injury, its effects must be considered when serial sampling is used to monitor an immune injury model. Immune glomerular injury may be more severe in an animal with only one kidney, so that sampling by nephrectomy or large biopsies may affect outcome, and appropriate controls are needed. Occasionally, uninephrectomy has been used to "concentrate" the effect of a poorly nephritogenic Ab or immune mechanism on a smaller renal mass; however, the results may not be striking.

Another consideration is that of superimposed hypertension in immune models, which can be done by clipping the renal artery (717–719). In our own studies, clip hypertension added an element of segmental glomerulosclerosis (characteristic of clip hypertension) to the more diffuse glomerulosclerosis associated with progressive augmented anti-GBM Ab GN (718) (Fig. 11). The hypertension-associated glomerular lesions can be prevented by treatment of the hypertension, particularly using ACE inhibitors (719,720). When glomeruli are protected from increased glomerular pressure by preglomerular vasoconstriction, as in the spontaneously hypertensive rat, the hypertensive effects on experimental GN are less evident (721,722). Factors such as nitric oxide serve to counteract the effects of angiotensin and are antiinflammatory. Dietary changes can be used to alter eicosanoid production, lipid metabolism, or the immune response, thereby altering outcome of an immune glomerular lesion.

Another consideration in progressive renal injury with changes in extracellular matrix accumulation in glomeruli would be some unusual contribution of the Ab used

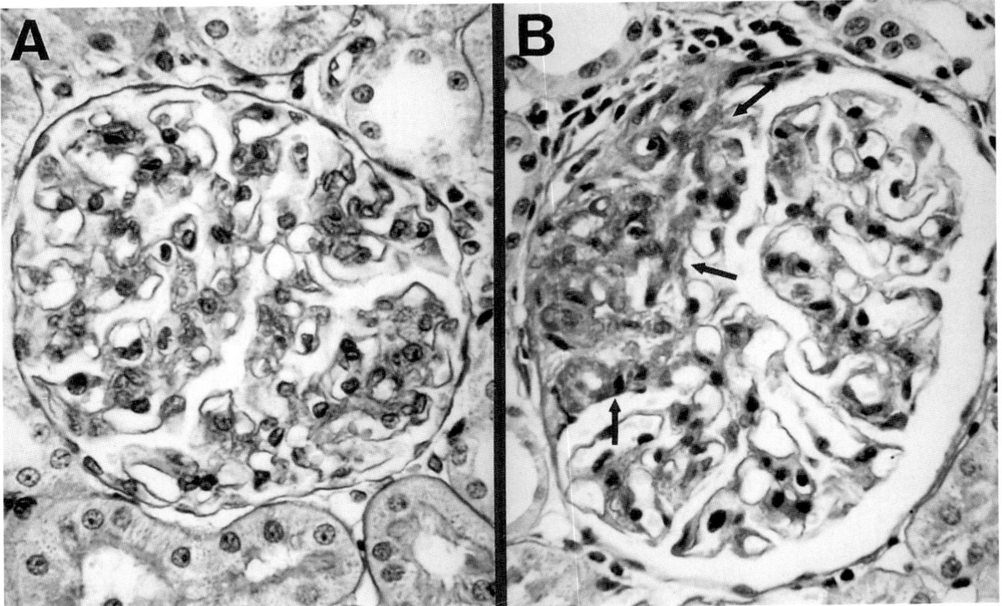

FIG. 11. A: The glomerulus from a rat with long-standing augmented autologous phase anti-GBM Ab GN demonstrates a diffuse glomerulosclerotic process with an increase in thickness of the GBM and some increase in mesangial matrix. **B:** When clip hypertension is superimposed on a rat with this type of anti-GBM Ab GN, a focal/segmental glomerulosclerotic lesion *(arrows)* is superimposed.

for induction of the immune lesion. For example, anti-Fx1A Abs are reported to recognize β1 integrins on glomerular epithelial cells and could, in turn, alter cell adhesion and interaction with the extracellular matrix (723).

Use of Genetically Altered Animals in the Study of Immune Glomerular Injury

Studies in genetically altered animals are gaining increasing usefulness in addressing the effects of over- or underexpression of various gene products on mediation of immune injury, as well as on the more basic aspects of induction of nephritogenic immune reactions. Some of these have been referred to in various situations earlier. A number of very different transgenic mice have been reported to suffer from glomerulosclerosis, including those with interruption of endogenous genes (724), overexpression of growth factors or cytokines (725-729), overexpression of renin (730), and expression of viral genes such as SV40 T Ag, HIV, or other retroviruses (731–735). The roles of TGF-β and PDGF in glomerulosclerosis have been substantiated in mice via in vivo transfection for these growth factors (736). Alterations in TGF-β expression may enhance inflammatory responses, pointing to the multiple roles of this growth factor (737–742).

Additional examples of the use of transgenic animals include ectopic expression of Thy-1 in glomerular epithelial podocytes of transgenic mice, which results in severe proteinuria (743). Glomerular Ig deposits were found in mice with a transgene that altered lymphocyte/granulocyte function (744). Mice transgenic for human IL-8, a neutrophil chemoattractant chemokine, have altered neutrophil involvement in inflammation (745). MIP-1α knockout mice are noted to have somewhat less severe autoimmune GN induced by immunization with bovine α3(IV) collagen (746).

Genetically altered mice also are finding use in studies aimed at better understanding of the autoimmune response (747–749). For example, elimination of B cells blocks SLE in mice of the *lpr/lpr* background (750). Alterations in MHC class II molecule expression is related to induction of autoimmune responses (751). Mice transgenic for pathogenic anti-DNA Abs require a contribution of the MHC (752). TGFb knockout mice can have anti-DNA Abs and a Sjogren's syndrome-like presentation (753). Studies of self-antigen presentation by renal cells (glomerular or tubular), as it may contribute to induction of autoimmune responses, have been considered with interest (754,755). When this was studied in transgenic mice with tubular overexpression of class II molecules, additional factors appeared to be necessary (756).

In vivo transfection and gene therapy are also receiving intense interest as a means of providing selective gene manipulation for short-term study, as well as eventually for correction of genetic defects. Integration of genes into glomerular and other kidney cells has been achieved on at least a short-term basis by several methods. Arterial infusion of DNA-liposome complexes, Sendai virus and liposomes, and the renin promoter and liposomes has been used (757–759). Transfer of retrovirally mediated transfer of transfected metanephrons placed under the renal capsule has also been successful (760). Mesangial trapping of previously transfected cultured mesangial cells (761) and renal artery or retrograde ureteral catheter perfusion with replication-deficient adenoviral vectors offer additional promising methods (762).

Acknowledgments

This work was supported in part by United States Public Health Service Grant DK20043.

REFERENCES

1. Salant DJ, Cybulsky AV. Experimental glomerulonephritis. *Methods Enzymol* 1988;162:421–461.
2. Hoedemaeker PJ, Aten J, Hogendoorn PC, Kawasaki K, van Leer EH, de Heer E, Fleuren GJ. Pathogenesis of glomerulonephritis: experimental models revisited. *Adv Nephrol Neck Hosp* 1991;20:73–90.
3. Wilson CB. Autoimmune renal disease. In: Bona C, Siminovitch K, Zanetti M Theofilopoulos A, eds. *The Molecular Pathology of Autoimmune Diseases*. Langhorne, PA: Harwood Academic Publishers, 1993:673–704.
4. Yee J, Neilson EG. Immune modulation of biologic systems in renal somatic cells. *Kidney Int* 1993;43:128–134.
5. Wilson CB, Tang WW. Immunological renal diseases. In: Frank MM, Austin KF, Claman HN, Unanue ER, eds. *Samter's Immunological Diseases*, 5th ed. Boston: Little Brown and Co, 1994;2:1033–1060.
6. Wilson CB, Tang WW, Feng L, Xia Y, Ward DM. Renal diseases. In: Stites DP, Terr A Parslow TG, eds. *Basic and Clinical Immunology*, 8th ed. Norwalk: Appleton & Lange, 1994:478–491.
7. O'Meara YM, Feehally J, Salant DJ. The nephritogenic immune response. *Curr Opin Nephrol Hyperten* 1994;3:318–328.
8. Wilson CB. Renal response to immunologic glomerular injury. In: Brenner BM, ed. *The Kidney*, 5th ed. Philadelphia: Saunders, 1996; 1253–1391.
9. Makker SP. Mediators of immune glomerular injury. *Am J Nephrol* 1993;13:324–336.
10. Couser WG. Pathogenesis of glomerulonephritis. *Kidney Int* 1993; 44(Suppl 42):S19–S26.
11. Couser WG. New insights into mechanisms of immune glomerular injury. *West J Med* 1994;160:440–446.
12. Woodroffe AJ, Wilson CB. An evaluation of elution techniques in the study of immune complex glomerulonephritis. *J Immunol* 1977;118: 1788–1794.
13. Gabbai FB, Peterson OW, Khang S, Wilson CB, Blantz RC. Glomerular hemodynamics in cell-free and erythrocyte-perfused isolated rat kidney. *Am J Physiol* 1994;267:F423–F427.
14. Gabbai F, Wilson CB, Blantz RC. Glomerular hemodynamic consequences of immune injury. *Semin Nephrol* 1991;11:367–372.
15. Wilson CB. Goodpasture's syndrome and other anti-basement membrane antibody diseases. In: Rich R, ed. *Clinical Immunology: Principles and Practice*. St. Louis: Mosby Year Book, Inc., 1995; 1185–1191.
16. Lerner RA, Glassock RJ, Dixon FJ. The role of anti-glomerular basement membrane antibody in the pathogenesis of human glomerulonephritis. *J Exp Med* 1967;126:989–1004.
17. Hudson BG, Kalluri R, Gunwar S, Noelken ME, Mariyama M, Reeders ST. Molecular characteristics of the Goodpasture autoantigen. *Kidney Int* 1993;43:135–139.

18. Kalluri R, Wilson CB, Weber M, Gunwar S, Chonko AM, Neilson EG, Hudson BG. Identification of the α3 chain of type IV collagen as the common autoantigen in anti-basement membrane disease and Goodpasture syndrome. *J Am Soc Nephrol* 1995;6:1178–1185.
19. Andres G, Brentjens J, Kohli R, Anthone R, Anthone S, Baliah T, Montes M, Mookerjee BK, Prezyna A, Sepulveda M, Venuto R, Elwood C. Histology of human tubulo-interstitial nephritis associated with antibodies to renal basement membranes. *Kidney Int* 1978;13: 480–491.
20. Huey B, McCormick K, Capper J, Ratliff C, Colombe BW, Garovoy MR, Wilson CB. Associations of HLA-DR and HLA-DQ types with anti-GBM nephritis by sequence-specific oligonucleotide probe hybridization. *Kidney Int* 1993;44:307–312.
21. Burns AP, Fisher M, Li P, Pusey CD, Rees AJ. Molecular analysis of HLA class II genes in Goodpasture's disease. *Q J Med* 1995;88: 93–100.
22. Unanue ER, Dixon FJ. Experimental glomerulonephritis: immunologic events and pathogenetic mechanisms. *Adv Immunol* 1967;6: 1–90.
23. Dixon FJ, Wilson CB. The development of immunopathologic investigation of kidney disease. *Am J Kidney Dis* 1990;16:574–578.
24. Tomosugi NI, Cashman SJ, Hay H, Pusey CD, Evans DJ, Shaw A, Rees AJ. Modulation of antibody-mediated glomerular injury in vivo by bacterial lipopolysaccharide, tumor necrosis factor, and IL-1. *J Immunol* 1989;142:3083–3090.
25. Karkar AM, Koshino Y, Cashman SJ, Dash AC, Bonnefoy J, Meager A, Rees AJ. Passive immunization against tumour necrosis factor-alpha (TNF-α) and IL-lβ protects from LPS enhancing glomerular injury in nephrotoxic nephritis in rats. *Clin Exp Immunol* 1992;90:312–318.
26. Karkar AM, Rees AJ. Influence of an established acute phase response on the severity of experimental nephritis. *Clin Exp Immunol* 1994;98:295–299.
27. Battifora HA, Markowitz AS. Nephrotoxic nephritis in monkeys. Sequential light, immunofluorescence, and electron microscopic studies. *Am J Pathol* 1969;55:267–281.
28. Wilson CB, Dixon FJ, Fortner JG, Cerilli GJ. Glomerular basement membrane-reactive antibody in anti-lymphocyte globulin. *J Clin Invest* 1971;50:1525–1535.
29. Unanue ER, Dixon FJ. Experimental glomerulonephritis. V. Studies on the interaction of nephrotoxic antibodies with tissues of the rat. *J Exp Med* 1965;121:697–714.
30. Lerner RA, Dixon FJ. Transfer of ovine experimental allergic glomerulonephritis (ERAG) with serum. *J Exp Med* 1966;124:431.
31. Unanue ER, Dixon FJ, Feldman JD. Experimental allergic glomerulonephritis induced in the rabbit with homologous renal antigens. *J Exp Med* 1967;125:163–176.
32. Weening JJ, Prins FA, Fransen JAM, van der Wal A, Hoedemaeker PJ. Ultrastructural localization and quantitation of nephritogenic antibodies in experimental glomerulonephritis. *Lab Invest* 1986;55:372–376.
33. Stein JH. Boonjarern S, Wilson CB, Ferris TS. Alterations in intrarenal blood flow distribution. Methods of measurement and relationship to sodium balance. *Circ Res* 1973;32:61s–72s.
34. Van Zyl Smit R, Rees AJ, Peters DK. Factors affecting severity of injury during nephrotoxic nephritis in rabbits. *Clin Exp Immunol* 1983;54:366–372.
35. Hammer DK, Vazquez JJ, Dixon FJ. Nephrotoxic serum nephritis in newborn rats. *Lab Invest* 1963;12:8.
36. Abrahamson DR, Caulfield JP. Distribution of laminin within rat and mouse renal, splenic, intestinal, and hepatic basement membranes identified after the intravenous injection of heterologous antilaminin IgG. *Lab Invest* 1985;52:169–181.
37. Madaio MP, Salant DJ, Adler S, Darby C, Couser WG. Effect of antibody charge and concentration on deposition of antibody to glomerular basement membrane. *Kidney Int* 1984;26:397–403.
38. Salant DJ, Adler S, Darby C, Capparell NJ, Groffel GC, Feintzeig ID, Rennke HG, Dittmer JE. Influence of antigen distribution on the mediation of immunological glomerular injury. *Kidney Int* 1985;27: 938–950.
39. Salant DJ, Cybulsky AV, Feintzeig ID. Quantitation of exogenous and endogenous components of glomerular immune deposits. *Kidney Int* 1986;30:255–263
40. Nishihara T, Kusuyama Y, Gen E, Tamaki N, Saito K. Masugi nephritis produced by the antiserum to heterologous glomerular basement membrane. I. Results in mice. *Acta Pathol Jpn* 1981;31:85–92.
41. Kusuyama Y, Nishihara T, Gen E, Saito K. Effect of cyclophosphamide on murine nephrotoxic nephritis. *Nephron* 1983;33:220–223.
42. Wheeler J, Morley AR, Appleton DR. Anti-glomerular basement membrane (GBM) glomerulonephritis in the mouse: Development of disease and cell proliferation. *J Exp Pathol* 1990;71:411–422.
43. Kusuyama Y, Nishihara T, Saito K. Nephrotoxic nephritis in nude mice. *Clin Exp Immunol* 1981;46:20–26.
44. Okada K, Oite T, Kihara I, Morita T, Yamamoto T. Masugi nephritis in the nude mice and their normal littermates. Acta Pathol Jpn 1982; 32:1–11.
45. Assmann KJM, Tangelder MM, Lange WPJ, Schrijver G, Koene RAP. Anti-GBM nephritis in the mouse: Severe proteinuria in the heterologous phase. *Virchows Arch A* 1985;406:285–300.
46. Schrijver G, Schalkwijk J, Robben JCM, Assmann KJM, Koene RAP. Antiglomerular basement membrane nephritis in beige mice. Deficiency of leukocyte neutral proteinases prevents the induction of albuminuria in the heterologous phase. *J Exp Med* 1989;169: 1435–1448.
47. Krakower CA, Greenspon SA. Localization of the nephrotoxic antigen within the isolated renal glomerulus. *Arch Pathol* 1951;51: 629–639.
48. Krakower CA, Greenspon SA. The localization of the "nephrotoxic" antigen(s) in extraglomerular tissues. Observations including a measure of its concentration in certain locales. *Arch Pathol* 1958;66: 364–383.
49. Wick G, Müller PU, Timpl R. In vivo localization and pathological effects of passively transferred antibodies to type IV collagen and laminin in mice. *Clin Immunol Immunopathol* 1982;23:656–665.
50. Yaar M, Foidart JM, Brown KS, Rennard SI, Martin GR, Liotta L. The Goodpasture-like syndrome in mice induced by intravenous injections of anti-type IV collagen and anti-laminin antibody. *Am J Pathol* 1982;107:79–91.
51. Abrahamson DR, Caulfield JP. Proteinuria and structural alterations in rat glomerular basement membranes induced by intravenously injected anti-laminin immunoglobulin G. *J Exp Med* 1982;156: 128–145.
52. Feintzeig ID, Abrahamson DR, Cybulsky AV, Dittmer, JE, Salant DJ. Nephritogenic potential of sheep antibodies against glomerular basement membrane laminin in the rat. *Lab Invest* 1986;54:531–542.
53. Makino H, Gibbons JT, Reddy MK, Kanwar YS. Nephritogenicity of antibodies to proteoglycans of the glomerular basement membrane-I. *J Clin Invest* 1986;77:142–156.
54. Miettinen A, Stow JL, Mentone S, Farquhar MG. Antibodies to basement membrane heparan sulfate proteoglycans bind to the laminae rarae of the glomerular basement membrane (GBM) and induce subepithelial GBM thickening. *J Exp Med* 1986;163:1064–1084.
55. Makino H, Lelongt B, Kanwar YS. Nephritogenicity of proteoglycans. II. A model of immune complex nephritis. *Kidney Int* 1988;34: 195–208.
56. Makino H, Lelongt B, Kanwar YS. Nephritogenicity of proteoglycans. III. Mechanism of immune deposit formation. *Kidney Int* 1988; 34:209–219.
57. Lelongt B, Kashihara N, Makino H, Kanwar YS. Influence of genetics on the nephritogenic potential of proteoglycans. *Am J Pathol* 1992;141:561–569.
58. Kalluri R, Gattone VH II, Noelken ME, Hudson BG. The α3 chain of type IV collagen induces autoimmune Goodpasture syndrome. *Proc Natl Acad Sci U S A* 1994;91:6201–6205.
59. Eddy AA. Tubulointerstitial nephritis during the heterologous phase of nephrotoxic serum nephritis. *Nephron* 1991;59:304–313.
60. Lan HY, Paterson DJ, Atkins RC. Initiation and evolution of interstitial leukocytic infiltration in experimental glomerulonephritis. *Kidney Int* 1991;40:425–433.
61. Willoughby WF, Dixon FJ. Experimental hemorrhagic pneumonitis produced by heterologous anti-lung antibody. *J Immunol* 1970;104: 28–37.
62. Boyce NW, Fernando NS, Neale TJ, Holdsworth SR. Acute pulmonary and renal injury after administration of heterologous anti-lung antibodies in the rat. Characterization of ultrastructural binding sites, basement membrane epitopes, and inflammatory mediation systems. *Lab Invest* 1991;64:272–278.
63. Lan HY, Paterson DJ, Hutchinson P, Atkins RC. Leukocyte involvement in the pathogenesis of pulmonary injury in experimental Goodpasture's syndrome. *Lab Invest* 1991;64:330–338.

64. Jennings L, Roholt OA, Pressman D, Blau M, Andres GA, Brentjens JR. Experimental anti-alveolar basement membrane antibody-mediated pneumonitis. I. The role of increased permeability of the alveolar capillary wall induced by oxygen. *J Immunol* 1981;127:129–134.
65. Downie GH, Roholt OA, Jennings L, Blau M, Brentjens JR, Andres GA. Experimental anti-alveolar basement membrane antibody-mediated pneumonitis. II. Role of endothelial damage and repair, induction of autologous phase, and kinetics of antibody deposition in Lewis rats. *J Immunol* 1982;129:2647–2652.
66. Yamamoto T, Wilson CB. Binding of anti-basement membrane antibody to alveolar basement membrane after intratracheal gasoline instillation in rabbits. *Am J Pathol* 1987;126:497–505.
67. Queluz, TH, Pawlowski I, Brunda MJ, Brentjens JR, Vladutiu AO, Andres G. Pathogenesis of an experimental model of Goodpasture's hemorrhagic pneumonitis. *J Clin Invest* 1990;85:1507–1515.
68. Boyce NW, Holdsworth SR. Anti-glomerular basement membrane antibody-induced experimental glomerulonephritis: Evidence for dose-dependent, direct antibody and complement-induced, cell independent injury. *J Immunol* 1985;135:3918–3921.
69. Couser WG, Darby C, Salant DJ, Adler S, Stilmant MM, Lowenstein LM. Anti-GBM antibody-induced proteinuria in isolated perfused rat kidney. *Am J Physiol* 1985;249:F241–F250.
70. Boyce NW, Holdsworth SR. Direct antiGBM antibody induced alterations in glomerular permselectivity. *Kidney Int* 1986;30:666–672.
71. Unanue ER, Dixon FJ. Experimental glomerulonephritis. VI. The autologous phase of nephrotoxic serum nephritis. *J Exp Med* 1965; 121:715–725.
72. Holdsworth SR, Neale TJ, Wilson CB. Abrogation of macrophage-dependent injury in experimental glomerulonephritis in the rabbit. Use of an antimacrophage serum. *J Clin Invest* 1981;68:686–698.
73. Sato T, Oite T, Nagase M, Shimizu F. Nephrotoxic serum nephritis in nude rats: The roles of host immune reactions. *Clin Exp Immunol* 1991;84:139–144.
74. Steblay RW. Glomerulonephritis induced in sheep by injections of heterologous glomerular basement membrane and Freund's complete adjuvant. *J Exp Med* 1962;116:253–272.
75. Steblay RW, Rudofsky UH. Experimental autoimmune glomerulonephritis induced by anti-glomerular basement membrane antibody. II. Effects of injecting heterologous, homologous, or autologous glomerular basement membranes and complete Freund's adjuvant into sheep. *Am J Pathol* 1983;113:125–133.
76. James MP, Herdson PB, Gavin JB. Recurrence of antiglomerular basement membrane glomerulonephritis in sheep renal allografts. *Pathology* 1981;13:335–344.
77. Bygren P, Wieslander J, Heinegärd D. Glomerulonephritis induced in sheep by immunization with human glomerular basement membrane. *Kidney Int* 1987;31:25–31.
78. Steblay RW, Rudofsky UH. Experimental autoimmune antiglomerular basement membrane antibody-induced glomerulonephritis. I. The effects of injecting sheep with human, homologous or autologous lung basement membranes and complete Freund's adjuvant. *Clin Immunol Immunopathol* 1983;27:65–80.
79. Robertson JL, Hill GS, Rowlands DT Jr. Tubulointerstitial nephritis and glomerulonephritis in Brown-Norway rats immunized with heterologous glomerular basement membrane. *Am J Pathol* 1977;88:53–64.
80. Stuffers-Heiman M, Günther E, Van Es LA. Induction of autoimmunity to antigens of the glomerular basement membrane in inbred Brown-Norway rats. *Immunology* 1979;36:759–767.
81. Bannister KM, Ulich TR, Wilson CB. Induction, characterization, and cell transfer of autoimmune tubulointerstitial nephritis in the Lewis rat. *Kidney Int* 1987;32:642–651.
82. Sado Y, Okigaki T, Takamiya H, Seno S. Experimental autoimmune glomerulonephritis with pulmonary hemorrhage in rats. The dose-effect relationship of the nephritogenic antigen from bovine glomerular basement membrane. *J Clin Lab Immunol* 1984;15:199–204.
83. Sado Y, Watanabe K, Okigaki T, Takamiya H, Seno S. Isolation and characterization of nephritogenic antigen from bovine glomerular basement membrane. *Biochim Biophys Acta* 1984;798:96–102.
84. Sado Y, Naito I, Akita M, Okigaki T. Strain specific responses of inbred rats on the severity of experimental autoimmune glomerulonephritis. *J Clin Lab Immunol* 1986;19:193–199.
85. Naito I, Sado Y. Early changes of rat experimental autoimmune glomerulonephritis induced with the nephritogenic antigen from bovine renal basement membranes. *J Clin Lab Immunol* 1989;28:187–193.
86. Sado Y, Kagawa M, Naito I, Okigaki T. Properties of bovine nephritogenic antigen that induces anti-GBM nephritis in rats and its similarity to the Goodpasture antigen. *Virchows Arch B* 1991;60:345–351.
87. Sado Y, Naito I, Okigaki T. Transfer of anti-glomerular basement membrane antibody-induced glomerulonephritis in inbred rats with isologous antibodies from the urine of nephritic rats. *J Pathol* 1989; 158:325–332.
88. Pusey CD, Holland MJ, Cashman SJ, Sinico RA, Lloveras J-J, Evans DJ, Lockwood, CM. Experimental autoimmune glomerulonephritis induced by homologous and isologous glomerular basement membrane in Brown Norway rat. *Nephrol Dial Transplant* 1991;6:457–465.
89. Reynolds J, Sallie BA, Syrganis C, Pusey CD. The role of T-helper lymphocytes in priming for experimental autoimmune glomerulonephritis in the BN rat. *J Autoimmun* 1993;6:571–585.
90. Reynolds J, Cashman SJ, Evans DJ, Pusey CD. Cyclosporin A in the prevention and treatment of experimental autoimmune glomerulonephritis in the Brown Norway rat. *Clin Exp Immunol* 1991;85:28–32.
91. Reynolds J, Pusey CD. In vivo treatment with a monoclonal antibody to T helper cells in experimental autoimmune glomerulonephritis in the BN rat. *Clin Exp Immunol* 1994;95:122–127.
92. Bolton WK, May WJ, Sturgill BC. Proliferative autoimmune glomerulonephritis in rats: A model for autoimmune glomerulonephritis in humans. *Kidney Int* 1993;44:294–306.
93. Lubec G. A new model for autoimmunity and the kidney. *Nephron* 1991;57:129–130.
94. McIntosh RM, Koss MN, Chernack WB, Griswold WR, Copack PB, Weil R III. Experimental pulmonary disease and autoimmune nephritis in the rabbit produced by homologous and heterologous choroid plexus (experimental Goodpasture's syndrome). *Proc Soc Exp Biol Med* 1974;147:216–223.
95. Lerner RA, Dixon FJ. The induction of acute glomerulonephritis in rabbits with soluble antigens isolated from normal homologous and autologous urine. *J Immunol* 1968;100:1277–1287.
96. Hawkins D, Cochrane CG. Glomerular basement membrane damage in immunological glomerulonephritis. *Immunology* 1968;14:665–681.
97. Kalluri R, Danoff TM, Neilson EG. Murine anti-α3(IV) collagen disease: A model of human Goodpasture Syndrome and anti-GBM nephritis. *J Am Soc Nephrol* 1995;6:833.
98. Steblay RW. Glomerulonephritis induced in monkeys by injections of heterologous glomerular basement membrane and Freund's adjuvant. *Nature* 1963;197:1173–1176.
99. Unanue ER, Dixon FJ. Experimental allergic glomerulonephritis induced in rabbits with heterologous renal antigens. *J Exp Med* 1967; 125:149–162.
100. Steblay RW. Studies on experimental autoimmune glomerulonephritis: Their relevance to human diseases. In: Rose NR, Milgrom F, eds. *International Convocation on Immunology*. Basel: Karger, 1968; 286–299.
101. Couser WG, Stilmant M, Lewis EJ. Experimental glomerulonephritis in the guinea pig. I. Glomerular lesions associated with antiglomerular basement membrane antibody deposits. *Lab Invest* 1973;29:236–243.
102. Lehman DH, Marquardt H, Wilson CB, Dixon FJ. Specificity of autoantibodies to tubular and glomerular basement membranes induced in guinea pigs. *J Immunol* 1974;112:241–248.
103. Hoedemaeker PHJ. Glomerular antigens in experimental glomerulonephritis. *Int Rev Exp Pathol* 1988;30:159–229.
104. Goldman M, Baran D, Druet P. Polyclonal activation and experimental nephropathies. *Kidney Int* 1988;34:141–150.
105. Sapin C, Druet E, Druet P. Induction of anti-glomerular basement membrane antibodies in the Brown-Norway rat by mercuric chloride. *Clin Exp Immunol* 1977;28:173–179.
106. Michaelson JH, McCoy JP Jr, Bigazzi PE. Antibodies to glomerular basement membrane: Detection by an enzyme-linked immunosorbent assay in the sera of Brown Norway rats. *Kidney Int* 1981;20:285–288.
107. Bellon B, Capron M, Druet E, Verroust P, Vial M-C, Sapin C, Girard JF, Foidart JM, Mahieu P, Druet P. Mercuric chloride induced autoimmune disease in Brown-Norway rats: Sequential search for anti-basement membrane antibodies and circulating immune complexes. *Eur J Clin Invest* 1982;12:127–133.
108. Pusey CD, Bowman C, Peters DK, Lockwood CM. Effects of cyclophosphamide on autoantibody synthesis in the Brown Norway rat. *Clin Exp Immunol* 1983;54:697–704.
109. Aten J, Bosman CB, Rozing J, Stijnen T, Hoedemaeker PJ, Weening

JJ. Mercuric chloride-induced autoimmunity in the Brown Norway rat. Cellular kinetics and major histocompatibility complex antigen expression. *Am J Pathol* 1988;133:127–138.

110. Hue J, Pelletier L, Berlin M, Druet P. Autoimmune glomerulonephritis induced by mercury vapour exposure in the Brown Norway rat. *Toxicology* 1993;79:119–129.
111. Hirsch F, Druet E, Vendeville B, Cormont F, Bazin H, Druet P. Production of monoclonal anti-glomerular basement membrane antibodies during autoimmune glomerulonephritis. *Clin Immunol Immunopathol* 1984;33:425–430.
112. Makker SP, Kanalas JJ. Renal antigens in mercuric chloride induced, anti-GBM autoantibody glomerular disease. *Kidney Int* 1990;37:64–71.
113. Guéry J-C, Druet E, Glotz D, Hirsch F, Mandet C, De Heer E, Druet P. Specificity and crossreactive idiotypes of anti-glomerular basement membrane autoantibodies in $HgCl_2$-induced autoimmune glomerulonephritis. Eur *J Immunol* 1990;20:93–100.
114. Michaelson JH, McCoy JP Jr, Hirszel P, Bigazzi PE. Mercury-induced autoimmune glomerulonephritis in inbred rats. I. Kinetics and species specificity of autoimmune responses. *Surv Synth Pathol Res* 1985;4:401-411.
115. Houssin D, Druet E, Hinglais N, Verroust P, Grossetete J, Bariety J, Druet P. Glomerular and vascular IgG deposits in $HgCl_2$ nephritis: Role of circulating antibodies and of immune complexes. *Clin Immunol Immunopathol* 1983:29:167–180.
116. Fukatsu A, Brentjens JR, Killen PD, Kleinman HK, Martin GR, Andres GA. Studies on the formation of glomerular immune deposits in Brown Norway rats injected with mercuric chloride. *Clin Immunol Immunopathol* 1987;45:35–47.
117. Michaud A, Sapin C, Leca G, Aiach M, Druet P. Involvement of hemostasis during an autoimmune glomerulonephritis induced by mercuric chloride in Brown Norway rats. *Thromb Res* 1983;33:77–88.
118. Eneström S, Hultman P. Immune-mediated glomerulonephritis induced by mercuric chloride in mice. *Experientia* 1984;40:1234–1240.
119. Hultman P, Eneström S. The induction of immune complex deposits in mice by peroral and parenteral administration of mercuric chloride: strain dependent susceptibility. *Clin Exp Immunol* 1987;67: 283–292.
120. Roman-Franco AA, Turiello M, Albini B, Ossi E, Milgrom F, Andres GA. Anti-basement membrane antibodies and antigen–antibody complexes in rabbits injected with mercuric chloride. *Clin Immunol Immunopathol* 1978;9:464–481.
121. Guéry J-C, Tournade H, Pelletier L, Druet E, Druet P. Rat anti-glomerular basement membrane antibodies in toxin-induced autoimmunity and in chronic graft-vs-host reaction share recurrent idiotypes. Eur *J Immunol* 1990;20:101–105.
122. Tournade H, Pelletier L, Pasquier R, Vial MC, Mandet C, Druet P. D-penicillamine-induced autoimmunity in Brown-Norway rats. Similarities with $HgCl_2$-induced autoimmunity. *J Immunol* 1990;144: 2985–2991.
123. Joshi BC, Dwivedi C, Powell A, Holschyer M. Immune complex nephritis in rats induced by long-term oral exposure to cadmium. *J Comp Pathol* 1981;91:11–15.
124. Bruijn JA, Hogendoorn PCW, Corver WE, van den Broek LJCM, Hoedemaeker PJ, Fleuren GJ. Pathogenesis of experimental lupus nephritis: A role for anti-basement membrane and anti-tubular brush border antibodies in murine chronic graft-versus-host disease. *Clin Exp Immunol* 1990;79:115–122.
125. Bruijn JA, van Leer EHG, Baelde HJJ, Corver WE, Hogendoorn PCW, Fleuren GJ. Characterization and *in vivo* transfer of nephritogenic autoantibodies directed against dipeptidyl peptidase IV and laminin in experimental lupus nephritis. *Lab Invest* 1990;63:350–359.
126. Florquin S, Abramowicz D, DeHeer E, Bruijn JA, Doutrelepont J-M, Goldman M, Hoedemaeker P. Renal immunopathology in murine host-versus-graft disease. *Kidney Int* 1991;40:852–861.
127. Bona CA. Molecular mimicry of self-antigen. *Immunology Series* 1991;55:239–246.
128. Fitzsimons EJ Jr, Weber M, Lange CF. The isolation of cross-reactive monoclonal antibodies: Hybridomas to streptococcal antigens cross-reactive with mammalian basement membrane. *Hybridoma* 1987;6: 61–69.
129. Goroncy-Bermes P, Dale JB, Beachey EH, Opferkuch W. Monoclonal antibody to human renal glomeruli cross-reacts with streptococcal M protein. *Infect Immun* 1987;55:2416–2419.
130. Fitzsimons EJ, Lange CF. Hybridomas to specific streptococcal antigen induce tissue pathology in vivo; autoimmune mechanisms for post-streptococcal sequelae. *Autoimmunity* 1991;10:115–124.
131. Lange CF. Localization of [^{14}C] labeled anti-streptococcal cell membrane monoclonal antibodies (anti-SCM) mAb) in mice. *Autoimmunity* 1994;19:179–191.
132. Kraus W, Beachey EH. Renal autoimmune epitope of group streptococci specified by M protein tetrapeptide Ile-Arg-Leu-Arg. *Proc Natl Acad Sci U S A* 1988;85:4511–4520.
133. Kraus W, Ohyama K, Snyder DS, Beachey EH. Autoimmune sequence of streptococcal M protein shared with the intermediate filament protein, vimentin. *J Exp Med* 1989;169:481–492.
134. Kraus W, Dale JB, Beachey EH. Identification of an epitope of type 1 streptococcal M protein that is shared with a 43-kDa protein of human myocardium and renal glomeruli. *J Immunol* 1990;145: 4089–4093.
135. Cines DB, Lyss AP, Reeber M, Bina M, DeHoratius RJ. Presence of complement-fixing anti-endothelial cell antibodies in systemic lupus erythematosus. *J Clin Invest* 1984;73:611–625.
136. Rosenbaum J, Pottinger BE, Woo P, Black CM, Loizou S, Byron MA, Pearson JD. Measurement and characterisation of circulating anti-endothelial cell IgG in connective tissue diseases. *Clin Exp Immunol* 1988;72:450–456.
137. D'Cruz DP, Houssiau FA, Ramirez G, Baguley E, McCutcheon J, Vianna J, Haga H-J Swana GT, Khamashta MA, Taylor JC, Davies DR, Hughes GRV. Antibodies to endothelial cells in systemic lupus erythematosus: A potential marker for nephritis and vasculitis. *Clin Exp Immunol* 1991;85:254–261.
138. van Leer EH, Ronco P, Verroust P, de Roo GM, Hoedemaeker PJ, de Heer E. Heymann nephritis: a model of human membranous glomerulopathy. A study of the role of additional antigens. *Nephrol Dial Transplant* 1992;7(Suppl 1):1–8.
139. Cavallo T. Membranous nephropathy. Insights from Heymann nephritis. *Am J Pathol* 1994;144:651–658.
140. Lowance DC, Mullins JD, McPhaul JJ Jr. Immunoglobulin A (IgA)-associated glomerulonephritis. *Kidney Int* 1973;3:167–176.
141. O'Donoghue DJ, Darvill A, Ballardie FW. Mesangial cell autoantigens in immunoglobulin A nephropathy and Henoch-Schönlein purpura. *J Clin Invest* 1991;88:1522–1530.
142. Cederholm B, Wieslander J, Bygren P, Heinegård D. Patients with IgA nephropathy have circulating anti-basement membrane antibodies reacting with structures common to collagen I,II, and IV. *Proc Natl Acad Sci U S A* 1986:83:6151–6155.
143. Cederholm B, Wieslander J, Bygren P, Heinegård D. Circulating complexes containing IgA and fibronectin in patients with primary IgA nephropathy. *Proc Natl Acad Sci U S A* 1988;85:4865–4868.
144. Saxena R, Bygren P, Butkowski R, Wieslander J. Entactin: A possible auto-antigen in the pathogenesis of non-Goodpasture anti-GBM nephritis. *Kidney Int* 1990;38:263–272.
145. Saxena R, Bygren P, Cederholm B, Wieslander J. Circulating anti-entactin antibodies in patients with glomerulonephritis. *Kidney Int* 1991;39:996–1004.
146. Seki T, Chang H-C, Moriuchi T, Denome R, Ploegh H. A hydrophobic transmembrane segment at the carboxyl terminus of Thy-1. *Science* 1985;227:649–651.
147. Seki T, Moriuchi T, Chang H-C, Denome R, Silver J. Structural organization of the rat Thy-1 gene. *Nature* 1985;313:485–487.
148. Yamamoto T, Wilson CB. Antibody-induced mesangial cell damage: The model, functional alterations, and effects of complement. *Kidney Int* 1986;29:296.
149. Yamamoto T, Wilson CB. Quantitative and qualitative studies of antibody-induced mesangial cell damage in the rat. *Kidney Int* 1987;32: 514–525.
150. Bagchus WM, Hoedemaeker PJ, Rozing J, Bakker WW. Acute glomerulonephritis after intravenous injection of monoclonal anti-thymocyte antibodies in the rat. *Immunol Lett* 1986;12:109–113.
151. Bagchus WM, Hoedemaeker PhJ, Rozing J, Bakker WW. Glomerulonephritis induced by monoclonal anti-Thy 1.1 antibodies. A sequential histological and ultrastructural study in the rat. *Lab Invest* 1986; 55:680–687.
152. Ishizaki M, Masuda Y, Fukuda Y, Sugisaki Y, Yamanaka N, Masugi Y. Experimental mesangioproliferative glomerulonephritis in rats induced by intravenous administration of anti-thymocyte serum. *Acta Pathol Jpn* 1986;36:1191–1203.
153. Yamamoto T, Wilson CB. Mesangial cell (MC) injury and prolifera-

tion produced by antibody: A role for the membrane attack complex (MAC). *Kidney Int* 1987;31:333.
154. Yamamoto T, Wilson CB. Complement dependence of antibody-induced mesangial cell injury in the rat. *J Immunol* 1987;138: 3758–3765.
155. Roy-Chaudhury P, Wu B, McDonald S, Haites NE, Simpson JG, Power DA. Phenotypic analysis of the glomerular and periglomerular mononuclear cell infiltrates in the Thy 1.1 model of glomerulonephritis. *Lab Invest* 1995;72:524–531.
156. Stahl RA, Thaiss F, Disser M, Helmchen U, Hora K, Schlondorff D. Increased expression of monocyte chemoattractant protein-1 in anti-thymocyte antibody-induced glomerulonephritis. *Kidney Int* 1993;44: 1036–1047.
157. Bagchus WM, Jeunink MF, Elema JD. The mesangium in anti-Thy-1 nephritis. Influx of macrophages, mesangial cell hypercellularity, and macromolecular accumulation. *Am J Pathol* 1990;137:215–223.
158. van Diemen-Steenvoorde R, Lambers A, van der Wal A, van Rooyen N, Dijkstra C, Hoedemaeker PhJ, de Heer E. Macrophages are responsible for mesangial cell injury and extracellular matrix (ECM) expansion in anti-Thy-1 nephritis in rats. *J Am Soc Nephrol* 1991;2:585.
159. Johnson RJ. Platelets in inflammatory glomerular injury. *Semin Nephrol* 1991;11:276–284.
160. Poelstra K, Heynen ER, Baller JF, Hardonk MJ, Bakker WW. Modulation of anti-Thy 1 nephritis in the rat by adenine nucleotides. Evidence for an anti-inflammatory role for nucleotidases. *Lab Invest* 1992;66:555–563.
161. Tang WW, Wilson CB. Heparin decreases mesangial matrix accumulation following selective antibody-induced mesangial cell injury. *J Am Soc Nephrol* 1992;3:921–929.
162. Stahl RA, Thaiss F, Wenzel U, Helmchen U. Morphologic and functional consequences of immune-mediated mesangiolysis: Development of chronic glomerular sclerosis. *J Am Soc Nephrol* 1992;2(10 Suppl):S144–S148.
163. Stahl RAK, Thaiss F, Wenzel U, Schoeppe W, Helmchen U. A rat model of progressive chronic glomerular sclerosis: The role of thromboxane inhibition. *J Am Soc Nephrol* 1992;2:1568–1577.
164. Morita H, Maeda K, Obayashi M, Shinzato T, Nakayama A, Fujita Y, Takai I, Kobayakawa H, Inoue I, Sugiyama S, Asai J, Nakashima I, Isobe K-I. Induction of irreversible glomerulosclerosis in the rat by repeated injections of a monoclonal anti-Thy-1.1 antibody. *Nephron* 1992;60:92–99.
165. Yoshida F, Isobe K, Matsuo S. In vivo effects of hyperglycemia on the outcome of acute mesangial injury in rats. *J Lab Clin Med* 1995; 125:46–55.
166. Johnson RJ, Iida H, Alpers CE, Majesky MW, Schwartz SM, Pritzl P, Gordon K, Gown AM. Expression of smooth muscle phenotype by rat mesangial cells in immune complex nephritis. α-smooth muscle actin is a marker of mesangial cell proliferation. *J Clin Invest* 1991;87: 847–858.
167. Okuda S, Languino LR, Ruoslahti E, Border WA. Elevated expression of transforming growth factor-β and proteoglycan production in experimental glomerulonephritis. Possible role in expansion of the mesangial extracellular matrix. *J Clin Invest* 1990;86:453–462.
168. Floege J, Johnson RJ, Gordon K, Iida H, Pritzl P, Yoshimura A, Campbell C, Alpers CE, Couser WG. Increased synthesis of extracellular matrix in mesangial proliferative nephritis. *Kidney Int* 1991;40: 477–488.
169. Floege J, Burns MW, Alpers CE, Yoshimura A, Pritzl P, Gordon K, Seifert RA, Bowen-Pope DF, Couser WG, Johnson RJ. Glomerular cell proliferation and PDGF expression precede glomerulosclerosis in the remnant kidney model. *Kidney Int* 1992;41:297–309.
170. Border WA, Okuda S, Languino LR, Sporn MB, Ruoslahti E. Suppression of experimental glomerulonephritis by antiserum against transforming growth factor beta 1. *Nature* 1990;346:371–374.
171. Johnson RJ, Raines EW, Floege J, Yoshimura A, Pritzl P, Alpers C, Ross R. Inhibition of mesangial cell proliferation and matrix expansion in glomerulonephritis in the rat by antibody to platelet-derived growth factor. *J Exp Med* 1992;175:1413–1416.
172. Border WA, Noble NA, Yamamoto T, Harper JR, Yamaguchi Y, Pierschbacher MD, Ruoslahti E. Natural inhibitor of transforming growth factor-β protects against scarring in experimental kidney disease. *Nature* 1992;360:361–363.
173. Kawachi H, Orikasa M, Matsui K, Iwanaga T, Toyabe S, Oite T, Shimizu F. Epitope-specific induction of mesangial lesions with proteinuria by a MoAb against mesangial cell surface antigen. *Clin Exp Immunol* 1992;88:399–404.
174. Yamamoto T, Mundy CA, Wilson CB, Blantz RC. Effect of mesangial cell lysis and proliferation on glomerular hemodynamics in the rat. *Kidney Int* 1991;40:705–713.
175. Bresnahan BA, Wu S, Fenoy FJ, Roman RJ, Lianos EA. Mesangial cell immune injury. Hemodynamic role of leukocyte- and platelet-derived eicosanoids. *J Clin Invest* 1992; 90:2304–2312.
176. Mauer SM, Sutherland DER, Howard RJ, Fish AJ, Najarian JS, Michael AF. The glomerular mesangium. III. Acute immune mesangial injury: A new model of glomerulonephritis. *J Exp Med* 1973;137: 553–570.
177. Mendrick DL, Rennke HG. Immune deposits formed in situ by a monoclonal antibody recognizing a new intrinsic rat mesangial matrix antigen. *J Immunol* 1986;137:1517–1526.
178. Morita T, Kihara I, Oite T, Yamamoto T, Suzuki Y. Mesangiolysis. Sequential ultrastructural study of Habu venom-induced glomerular lesions. *Lab Invest* 1978;38:94–102.
179. Cattell V, Bradfield JWB. Focal mesangial proliferative glomerulonephritis in the rat caused by Habu snake venom: A morphologic study. *Am J Pathol* 1977;87:511–524.
180. Coffey AK, Karnovskey MJ. Heparin inhibits mesangial cell proliferation in Habu-venom-induced glomerular injury. *Am J Pathol* 1985; 120:248–255.
181. Pober JS, Cotran RS. Immunologic interactions of T lymphocytes with vascular endothelium. *Adv Immunol* 1991;50:261–302.
182. Savage COS, Bogle R. Resident glomerular cells in glomerular injury: Endothelial cells. *Semin Nephrol* 1991;11:312–319.
183. Bevilacqua MP. Endothelial-leukocyte adhesion molecules. *Annu Rev Immunol* 1993;11:767–804.
184. Pall AA, Savage CO. Mechanisms of endothelial cell injury in vasculitis. *Springer Semin Immunopathol* 1994;16:23–37.
185. Caldwell PRB, Wigger HJ, Fernandez LT, D'Alisa RM, Tse-Eng D, Butler VP Jr, Gigli I. Lung injury induced by antibody fragments to angiotensin-converting enzyme. *Am J Pathol* 1981;105:54–63.
186. Barba LM, Caldwell PRB, Downie GH, Camussi G, Brentjens JR, Andres G. Lung injury mediated by antibodies to endothelium. 1. In the rabbit a repeated interaction of heterologous anti-angiotensin-converting enzyme antibodies with alveolar endothelium results in resistance to immune injury through antigenic modulation. *J Exp Med* 1983;158:2141–2158.
187. Camussi G, Caldwell PRB, Andres G, Brentjens JR. Lung injury mediated by antibodies to endothelium. II. Study of the effect of repeated antigen-antibody interactions in rabbits tolerant to heterologous antibody. *Am J Pathol* 1987;127:216–228.
188. Matsuo S, Fukatsu A, Taub ML, Caldwell PRB, Brentjens, JR, Andres G. Glomerulonephritis induced in the rabbit by antiendothelial antibodies. *J Clin Invest* 1987;79:1798–1811.
189. Ito S, Hirabayashi K, Nielsen N, Ueda Y, Brentjens JR, Gans RO. Von Willebrand factor in the rat kidney: Its localization and the effects of its in vivo interaction with specific antibodies. *Nephron* 1994;66:200–207.
190. Heymann W, Hackel DB, Harwood S, Wilson SGF, Hunter JLP. Production of nephrotic syndrome in rats by Freund's adjuvants and rat kidney suspensions. *Proc Soc Exp Biol Med* 1959;100:660–664.
191. Edgington TS, Glassock RJ, Dixon FJ. Autologous immune complex nephritis induced with renal tubular antigen. I. Identification and isolation of the pathogenetic antigen. *J Exp Med* 1968;127:555–571.
192. Edgington TS, Glassock RJ, Dixon FJ. Autologous immune complex pathogenesis of experimental allergic glomerulonephritis. *Science* 1967;155:1432–1434.
193. Glassock RJ, Edgington TS, Watson JI, Dixon FJ. Autologous immune complex nephritis induced with renal tubular antigen. II. The pathogenetic mechanism. *J Exp Med* 1968;127:573–587.
194. Feenstra K, Lee Rvd, Greben HA, Arends A, Hoedemaeker PhJ. Experimental glomerulonephritis in the rat induced by antibodies directed against tubular antigens. 1. The natural history: a histologic and immunohistologic study at the light microscopic and the ultrastructural level. *Lab Invest* 1975;235–242.
195. Bakker WW, Bagchus WM, Vos JTWM, Kooistra K, Hoedemaeker PhJ. The specificity of nephritogenic antibodies: I. Evidence on anti-T-cell specificity in nephritogenic antibodies detected by cytotoxicity and MIF assays. *Immunobiology* 1981;159:235–243.

196. Jeraj K, Vernier RL, Sisson SP, Michael AF. A new glomerular antigen in passive Heymann's nephritis. *Br J Exp Pathol* 1984;65: 485–498.
197. Bakker WW. The specificity of nephritogenic antibodies. III. Binding of anti-Fx1A antibodies in glomeruli is dependent on dual specificity. *Clin Exp Immunol* 1986;63:639–647.
198. Hogendoorn PCW, Bruijn JA, vd Broek LJCM, De Heer E, Foidart JM, Hoedemaeker PhJ, Fleuren GJ. Antibodies to purified renal tubular epithelial antigens contain activity against laminin, fibronectin, and type IV collagen. *Lab Invest* 1988;58:278–286.
199. Abrass CK, Border WA, Glassock RJ. Circulating immune complexes in rats with autologous immune complex nephritis. *Lab Invest* 1980;43:18–27.
200. Zanetti M, Bellon B, Verroust P, Druet P. A search for circulating immune complex-like material during the course of autoimmune complex glomerulonephritis in Lewis and Brown Norway rats. *Clin Exp Immunol* 1980;42:86–94.
201. Neale TJ, Wilson CB. Glomerular antigens in Heymann's nephritis: reactivity of eluted and circulating antibody. *J Immunol* 1982;128: 323–330.
202. Cattran DC, Chodirker WB. Experimental membranous glomerulonephritis. The relationship between circulating free antibody and immune complexes to subsequent pathology. *Nephron* 1982;31: 260–265.
203. Hori MT, Abrass CK. Isolation and characterization of circulating immune complexes from rats with experimental membranous nephropathy. *J Immunol* 1990;144:3849–3855.
204. Abrass CK. Autologous immune complex nephritis in rats. Influence of modification of mononuclear phagocyte system function. *Lab Invest* 1984;51:162–171.
205. Abrass CK, Cohen AH. The role of circulating antigen in the formation of immune deposits in experimental membranous nephropathy. *Proc Soc Exp Biol Med* 1986;183:348–357.
206. Van Damme BJC, Fleuren GJ, Bakker WW, Vernier RL, Hoedemaeker PhJ. Experimental glomerulonephritis in the rat induced by antibodies directed against tubular antigens. V. Fixed glomerular antigens in the pathogenesis of heterologous immune complex glomerulonephritis. *Lab Invest* 1978;38:502–510.
207. Couser WG, Steinmuller DF, Stilmant MM, Salant DJ, Lowenstein LM. Experimental glomerulonephritis in the isolated perfused rat kidney. *J Clin Invest* 1978;62:1275–1287.
208. Fleuren GJ, Grond J, Hoedemaeker PhJ. The pathogenetic role of free-circulating antibody in autologous immune complex glomerulonephritis. *Clin Exp Immunol* 1980;41:205–217.
209. Neale TJ, Couser WG, Salant DJ, Lowenstein LM, Wilson CB. Specific uptake of Heymann's nephritic kidney eluate by rat kidney. Studies *in vivo* and in isolated perfused kidneys. *Lab Invest* 1982; 46:450–453.
210. Madaio MP, Salant DJ, Cohen AJ, Adler S, Couser WG. Comparative study of in situ immune deposit formation in active and passive Heymann nephritis. *Kidney Int* 1983;23:498–505.
211. Saito A, Pietromonaco S, Loo AK, Farquhar MG. Complete cloning and sequencing of rat gp330/"megalin," a distinctive member of the low density lipoprotein receptor gene family. *Proc Natl Acad Sci U S A* 1994;91:9725–9729.
212. Farquhar MG. The unfolding story of megalin (gp330): now recognized as a drug receptor. *J Clin Invest* 1995;96:1184.
213. Farquhar MG, Saito A, Kerjaschki D, Orlando RA. The Heymann nephritis antigenic complex: megalin (gp330) and RAP. *J Am Soc Nephrol* 1995;6:35–47.
214. Raychowdhury R, Niles J, McCluskey RT, Smith JA. Autoimmune target in Heymann nephritis is a glycoprotein with homology to the LDL-receptor. *Science* 1989;244:1163–1165.
215. Pietromonaco S, Kerjaschki D, Binder S, Ullrich R, Farquhar MG. Molecular cloning of a cDNA encoding a major pathogenic domain of the Heymann nephritis antigen gp330. *Proc Natl Acad Sci U S A* 1990;87:1811–1815.
216. Strickland DK, Ashcom JD, Williams S, Battey F, Behre E, McTigue K, Battey JF, Argraves WS. Primary structure of α_2-macroglobulin receptor-associated protein. *J Biol Chem* 1991;266:13364–13369.
217. Orlando RA, Kerjaschki D, Kurihara H, Biemesderfer D, Farquhar MG. gp330 associates with a 44-kDa protein in the rat kidney to form the Heymann nephritis antigenic complex. *Proc Natl Acad Sci U S A* 1992;89:6698–6702.
218. Farquhar MG, Kerjaschki D, Lundstrom M, Orlando RA. gp330 and RAP: the Heymann nephritis antigenic complex. *Ann NY Acad Sci* 1994;737:96–113.
219. Kerjaschki D, Noronha-Blob L, Sackktor S, Farquhar MG. Microdomains of distinctive glycoprotein composition in the kidney proximal tubule brush border. *J Cell Biol* 1984;98:1505–1513.
220. Bhan A, Schneeberger E, Baird L, Collins A, Kamata K, Bradford D, Erikson M, McCluskey RT. Studies with monoclonal antibodies against brush border antigens in Heymann nephritis. *Lab Invest* 1985; 53:421–432.
221. Chatelet F, Brianti E, Ronco P, Roland J, Verroust P. Ultrastructural localization by monoclonal antibodies of brush border antigens expressed by glomeruli. I. Renal distribution. *Am J Pathol* 1986;122: 500–511.
222. Chatelet F, Brianti E, Ronco P, Roland J, Verroust P. Ultrastructural localization by monoclonal antibodies of brush border antigens expressed by glomeruli. II. Extrarenal distribution. *Am J Pathol* 1986; 122:512–519.
223. van Leer EH, de Roo GM, Bruijn JA, Hoedemaeker PJ, de Heer E. Synergistic effects of anti-gp330 and anti-dipeptidyl peptidase type IV antibodies in the induction of glomerular damage. *Exp Nephrol* 1993;1:292–300.
224. Abbate M, Bachinsky D, Zheng G, Stamenkovic I, McLaughlin M, Niles JL, McCluskey RT, Brown D. Localization of gp330/α2M receptor-associated protein (α_2-MRAP) and its binding sites in kidney: distribution of endogenous α_2-MRAP is modified by tissue processing. *Eur J Cell Biol* 1993;61:139–149.
225. Kamata K, Baird LG, Erikson ME, Collins AB, McCluskey RT. Characterization of antigens and antibody specificities involved in Heymann nephritis. *J Immunol* 1985;135:2400–2408.
226. Van Leer EHG, Ronco P, Verroust P, van der Wal AM, Hoedemaeker PJ, De Heer E. Epitope specificity of anti-gp330 autoantibodies determines the development of proteinuria in active Heymann nephritis. *Am J Pathol* 1993;142:821–829.
227. Bachinsky DR, Zheng G, Niles JL, McLaughlin M, Abbate M, Andres G, Brown D, McCluskey RT. Detection of two forms of GP330. Their role in Heymnann Nephritis. *Am J Pathol* 1993;143: 598–611.
228. Ronco P, Melcion C, Geniteau M, Ronco E, Reininger L, Galceran M, Verroust P. Production and characterization of monoclonal antibodies against rat brush border antigens of the proximal convoluted tubule. *Immunology* 1984;53:87–95.
229. Ronco P, Allegri L, Melcion C, Pirotsky E, Appay M-D, Bariety J, Pontillon F, Verroust P. A monoclonal antibody to brush border and passive Heymann nephritis. *Clin Exp Immunol* 1984;55:319–332.
230. Ronco P, Neale TJ, Wilson CB, Galceran M, Verroust P. An immunopathologic study of a 330-kD protein defined by monoclonal antibodies and reactive with anti-RTE-alpha-5 antibodies and kidney eluates from active Heymann nephritis. *J Immunol* 1986;136:125–130.
231. Luca ME, Deelder AM, Hogendoorn PC, Daha MR, Galceran M, van Es LA, de Heer E. Glomerulopathy induced by a single monoclonal autoantibody against gp330. *Nephrol Dial Transplant* 1995;10: 490–496.
232. Tsukada Y, Ono K, Maezawa A, Yano S, Naruse T. A major pathogenic antigen of Heymann nephritis is present exclusively in the renal proximal tubule brush border—studies with a monoclonal antibody against pronase-digested tubular antigen. *Clin Exp Immunol* 1994;96: 303–310.
233. Natori Y, Hayakawa I, Shibata S. Identification of gp108, a pathogenic antigen of passive Heymann nephritis, as dipeptidyl peptidase IV. *Clin Exp Immunol* 1987;70:434–439.
234. Natori Y, Hayakawa I, Shibata S. Role of dipeptidyl peptidase IV (gp108) in passive Heymann nephritis. Use of dipeptidyl peptidase IV-deficient rats. *Am J Pathol* 1989;134:405–410.
235. Mendrick DL, Rennke HG. I. Induction of proteinuria in the rat by a monoclonal antibody against SGP-115/107. *Kidney Int* 1988;33: 818–830.
236. Stefanovic V, Ardaillou N, Vlahovic P, Placier S, Ronco P, Ardaillou R. Interferon-γ induced dipeptidylpeptidase IV expression in human glomerular epithelial cells. *Immunology* 1993;80:465–470.
237. Ronco P, Allegri L, Brianti E., Chatelet F., Van Leer EH, Verroust P. Antigenic targets in epimembranous glomerulonephritis. Experimental data and potential applications in human pathology. *Appl Pathol* 1989;7:85–98.

238. Salant DJ, Darby C, Couser WG. Experimental membranous glomerulonephritis in rats. Quantitative studies of glomerular immune deposit formation in isolated glomeruli and whole animals. *J Clin Invest* 1980;66:71–81.
239. Gabbai FB, Gushwa LC, Wilson CB, Blantz RC. An evaluation of the development of experimental membranous nephropathy. *Kidney Int* 1987;31:1267–1278.
240. Bertani T, Nolin L, Foidart J, Vandewalle A, Verroust P. The effect of puromycin on subepithelial deposits induced by antibodies directed against tubular antigens: a quantitative study. *Eur J Clin Invest* 1979; 9:465–472.
241. Couser WG, Salant DJ, Stilmant MM, Arbeit LA, Darby C, Sliogeris VG. The effects of aminonucleoside of puromycin and nephrotoxic serum on subepithelial immune-deposit formation in passive Heymann nephritis. *J Lab Clin Med* 1979;94:917–932.
242. Couser WG, Jermanovich NB, Belok S, Stilmant MM. Effect of aminonucleoside nephrosis on immune complex localization in autologous immune complex nephropathy in rats. *J Clin Invest* 1978;61: 561–572.
243. Salant DJ, Belok S, Stilmant MM, Darby C, Couser WG. Determinants of glomerular localization of subepithelial immune deposits. Effects of altered antigen to antibody ratio, steroids, vasoactive amine antagonists, and aminonucleoside of puromycin on passive Heymann nephritis in rats. *Lab Invest* 1979;41:89–99.
244. Challice J, Barabas AZ, Cornish J, Bruce JW, Lannigan R. Passive Heymann nephritis in pre- and post-natal rats. *Br J Exp Pathol* 1986; 67:915–924.
245. Camussi G, Brentjens JR, Noble B, Kerjaschki D, Malavasi F, Roholt OA, Farquhar MG, Andres G. Antibody-induced redistribution of Heymann antigen on the surface of cultured glomerular visceral epithelial cells: Possible role in the pathogenesis of Heymann glomerulonephritis. *J Immunol* 1985;135:2409–2416.
246. Camussi G, Noble B, Van Liew J, Brentjens JR, Andres G. Pathogenesis of passive Heymann glomerulonephritis: Chlorpromazine inhibits antibody-mediated redistribution of cell surface antigens and prevents development of the disease. *J Immunol* 1986;136: 2127–2135.
247. Allegri L, Brianti E, Chatelet F, Manara GC, Ronco P, Verroust P. Polyvalent antigen-antibody interactions are required for the formation of electron-dense immune deposits in passive Heymann's nephritis. *Am J Pathol* 1986;126:1–6.
248. Brentjens JR, Andres GA. Interaction of antibodies with renal cell surface antigens. *Kidney Int* 1989;35:954–968.
249. Camussi G, Kerjaschki D, Gonda M, Nevins T, Rielle J-C, Brentjens J, Andres G. Expression and modulation of surface antigens in cultured rat glomerular visceral epithelial cells. *J Histochem Cytochem* 1989;37:1675–1687.
250. Cybulsky AV, Quigg RJ, Badalamenti J, Salant DJ. Anti-Fx1A induces association of Heymann nephritis antigens with microfilaments of cultured glomerular visceral epithelial cells. *Am J Pathol* 1987; 129:373–384.
251. Kerjaschki D, Miettinen A, Farquhar MG. Initial events in the formation of immune deposits in passive Heymann nephritis: gp330-anti-gp330 immune complexes form in epithelial coated pits and rapidly become attached to the glomerular basement membrane. *J Exp Med* 1987;166:109–128.
252. Fukatsu A, Yuzawa Y, Olson L, Miller J, Milgrom M, Zamlauski-Tucker MJ, Van Liew JB, Campagnari A, Niesen N, Patel J, Doi T, Striker L, Striker G, Milgrom F, Brentjens J, Andres G. Interaction of antibodies with human glomerular epithelial cells. *Lab Invest* 1989; 61:389–403.
253. Salant DJ, Belok S, Madaio MP, Couser WG. A new role for complement in experimental membranous nephropathy in rats. *J Clin Invest* 1980;66:1339–1350.
254. Cybulsky AV, Quigg RJ, Salant DJ. The membrane attack complex in complement-mediated glomerular epithelial cell injury: Formation and stability of C5b-9 and C5b-7 in rat membranous nephropathy. *J Immunol* 1986;137:1511–1516.
255. Cybulsky Av, Rennke HG, Feintzeig ID, Salant DJ. Complement-induced glomerular epithelial cell injury. Role of the membrane attack complex in rat membranous nephropathy. *J Clin Invest* 1986; 77:1096–1107.
256. Salant DJ, Quigg RJ, Cybulsky AV. Heymann nephritis: Mechanisms of renal injury. *Kidney Int* 1989;35:976–984.
257. Quigg RJ, Cybulsky AV, Jacobs JB, Salant DJ. Anti-Fx1A produces complement-dependent cytotoxicity of glomerular epithelial cells. *Kidney Int* 1988;34:43–52.
258. Gabbai FB, Mundy C, Wilson CB, Blantz RC. An evaluation of the role of complement depletion in experimental membranous nephropathy in the rat. *Lab Invest* 1988;58:539–544.
259. Susani M, Schulze M, Exner M, Kerjaschki D. Antibodies to glycolipids activate complement and promote proteinuria in passive Heymann nephritis. *Am J Pathol* 1994;144:807–819.
260. Assmann KJM, Tangelder MM, Lange WPJ, Tadema TM, Koene RAP. Membranous glomerulonephritis in the mouse. *Kidney Int* 1983;24:303–312.
261. Biancone L, Andres G, Ahn H, DeMartino C, Stamenkovic I. Inhibition of the CD40-CD40 ligand pathway prevents murine membranous glomerulonephritis. *Kidney Int* 1995;48:458–468.
262. Barabas AZ, Lannigan R. Immune-complex nephritis in the rabbit produced by injections of rat renal tubular fraction 3 antigen. *Br J Exp Pathol* 1981;62:94–102.
263. Barabas AZ, Cornish J, Lannigan R. Passive Heymann-like nephritis in the rabbit. *Br J Exp Pathol* 1985;66:357–364.
264. Nicol MJ, Miller JH, Neale TJ. Tubular antigen-associated renal disease in New Zealand white rabbits. *Clin Exp Immunol* 1986;63: 629–638.
265. Neale TJ, Wilson CB. Non-GBM glomerular antigen in spontaneous nephritis in rabbits. *Kidney Int* 1978;14:715.
266. Neale TJ, Woodroffe AJ, Wilson CB. Spontaneous glomerulonephritis in rabbits: Role of a glomerular capillary antigen. *Kidney Int* 1984; 26:701–711.
267. Donker AJ, Venuto RC, Vladutiu AO, Brentjens JR, Andres GA. Effects of prolonged administration of D-penicillamine or captopril in various strains of rats. Brown Norway rats treated with D-penicillamine develop autoantibodies, circulating immune complexes, and disseminated intravascular coagulation. *Clin Immunol Immunopathol* 1984;30:142–155.
268. Murphy-Ullrich JE, Oberley TD, Mosher DF. Glomerular and vascular injury in mice following immunization with heterologous and autologous fibronectin. *Virchows Arch B* 1982;39:305–321.
269. Zanetti M, Takami T. Mesangial immune deposits induced in rats by antibodies to fibronectin. *Clin Immunol Immunopathol* 1984;31: 353–363.
270. Murphy-Ullrich JE, Oberley TD, Mosher DF. Detection of autoantibodies and glomerular injury in rabbits immunized with denatured human fibronectin monomer. *Am J Pathol* 1984;117:1–11.
271. Cosio FG, Mahan JD, Sedmak DD. Experimental glomerulonephritis induced by antigen that binds to glomerular fibronectin. *Am J Kidney Dis* 1990;15:160-168.
272. Shibata S, Miura K. A third glycopeptide (nephritogenoside) isolated from the glomerular basement membrane. *J Biochem* 1981;89: 1737–1749.
273. Natori Y, Shibata S. Enzyme linked immunosorbent assay for Heymann's antigen as a contaminating minor component in nephritogenic glycopeptide, nephritogenoside. *Clin Exp Immunol* 1983;51: 595–599.
274. Shibata S, Takeda T, Natori Y. The structure of nephritogenoside. A nephritogenic glycopeptide with α-N-glycosidic linkage. *J Biol Chem* 1988;263:12483–12485.
275. Sado Y, Kagawa M, Rauf S, Naito I, Moritoh C, Okigaki T. Isologous monoclonal antibodies can induce anti-GBM glomerulonephritis in rats. *J Pathol* 1992;168:221–227.
276. Miettinen A, Dekan G, Farquhar MG. Monoclonal antibodies against membrane proteins of the rat glomerulus. Immunochemical specificity and immunofluorescence distribution of the antigens. *Am J Pathol* 1990;137:929–944.
277. Dekan G, Miettinen A, Schnabel E, Farquhar MG. Binding of monoclonal antibodies to glomerular endothelium, slit membranes, and epithelium after *in vivo* injection. Localization of antigens and bound IgGs by immunoelectron microscopy. *Am J Pathol* 1990;137:913–927.
278. Ronco P, Sahali D, Cittanova ML, van Leer EH, Chatelet F, Verroust P. Monoclonal antibodies to glomerular antigens. *Nephrol Dial Transplant* 1992;7(Suppl 1):9–15.
279. Tissari J, Holthöfer H, Miettinen A. Novel 13A antigen is an integral protein of the basolateral membrane of rat glomerular podocytes. *Lab Invest* 1994;71:519–527.
280. Ozaki I, Ito Y, Fukatsu A, Suzuki N, Yoshida F, Watanabe Y,

Sakamoto N, Matsuo S. A plasma membrane antigen of rat glomerular epithelial cells. Antigenic determinants involving N-linked sugar residues in a 140-kilodalton sialoglycoprotein of the podocytes. *Lab Invest* 1990;63:707–716.
281. Mendrick DL, Rennke HG. II. Epitope specific induction of proteinuria by monoclonal antibodies. *Kidney Int* 1988;33:831–842.
282. Nishikawa K, Fukatsu A, Tamai H, Suzuki N, Ito Y, Sakamoto N, Matsuo S. Formation of subepithelial dense deposits in rats induced by a monoclonal antibody against the glomerular cell surface antigen. *Clin Exp Immunol* 1991;83:143–148.
283. Kagami S, Okada K, Funai M, Matui K, Oite T, Kawachi H, Shimizu F, Kuroda Y. A monoclonal antibody (1G10) recognizes a novel human mesangial antigen. *Kidney Int* 1992;42:700–709.
284. Orikasa M, Matsui K, Oite T, Shimizu F. Massive proteinuria induced in rats by a single intravenous injection of a monoclonal antibody. *J Immunol* 1988;141:807–814.
285. Kawachi H, Matsui K, Orikasa M, Morioka T, Oite T, Shimizu F. Quantitative studies of monoclonal antibody 5-1-6-induced proteinuric state in rats. *Clin Exp Immunol* 1992;87:215–219.
286. Gollner D, Kawachi H, Oite T, Oka M, Nagase M, Shimizu F. Strain variation in susceptibility to the development of monoclonal antibody 5-1-6-induced proteinuria in rats. *Clin Exp Immunol* 1995;101: 341–345.
287. Narisawa M, Kawachi H, Oite T, Shimizu F. Divalency of the monoclonal antibody 5-1-6 is required for induction of proteinuria in rats. *Clin Exp Immunol* 1993;92:522–526.
288. Kawachi H, Abrahamson DR, St John PL, Goldstein DJ, Shia MA, Matsui K, Shimizu F, Salant DJ. Developmental expression of the nephritogenic antigen of monoclonal antibody 5-1-6. *Am J Pathol* 1995;147:823–833.
289. Takashima N, Kawachi H, Oite T, Nishi S, Arakawa M, Shimizu F. Effect of chlorpromazine on kinetics of injected monoclonal antibody in MoAb-induced glomerular injury. *Clin Exp Immunol* 1993;91: 135–140.
290. Blantz RC, Gabbai FB, Peterson O, Wilson CB, Kihara I, Kawachi H, Shimizu F, Yamamoto T. Water and protein permeability is regulated by the glomerular epithelial slit diaphragm. *J Am Soc Nephrol* 1994; 4:1957–1964.
291. Stefanovic V, Vlahovic P, Ardaillou N, Ronco P, Ardaillou R. Cell surface aminopeptidase A and N activities in human glomerular epithelial cells. *Kidney Int* 1992;41:1571–1580.
292. Assmann KJM, van Son JPHF, Dijkman HBPM, Koene RAP. A nephritogenic rat monoclonal antibody to mouse aminopeptidase A. Induction of massive albuminuria after a single intravenous injection. *J Exp Med* 1992;175:623–635.
293. Kawachi H, Oite T, Shimizu F. Quantitative study of mesangial injury with proteinuria induced by monoclonal antibody 1-22-3. *Clin Exp Immunol* 1993;92:342–346.
294. Cheng QL, Orikasa M, Morioka T, Kawachi H, Chen XM, Oite T, Shimizu F. Progressive renal lesions induced by administration of monoclonal antibody 1-22-3 to unilaterally nephrectomized rats. *Clin Exp Immunol* 1995;102:181–185.
295. van den Born J, van den Heuvel LPWJ, Bakker MAH, Veerkamp JH, Assmann KJM, Berden JHM. A monoclonal antibody against GBM heparan sulfate induces an acute selective proteinuria in rats. *Kidney Int* 1992;41:115–123.
296. Kashgarian M. Lupus nephritis: lessons from the path lab. *Kidney Int* 1994;45:928–938.
297. Wilson CB. The renal response to immunologic injury. In: Brenner BM, Rector FC, Jr. eds. *The Kidney*, 4th ed. Philadelphia: Saunders, 1991;1:1062–1181.
298. Mannik M. Experimental models for immune complex-mediated vascular inflammation. *Acta Med Scand [Suppl]* 1987;715:145–155.
299. Mannik M. Mechanisms of tissue deposition of immune complexes. *J Rheumatol* 1987;14(Suppl 13):35–42.
300. Furness PN. The formation and fate of glomerular immune complex deposits. *J Pathol* 1991;164;195–202.
301. Gauthier VJ, Abrass CK. Circulating immune complexes in renal injury. *Semin Nephrol* 1992;12:379–394.
302. Wilson CB, Dixon FJ. Antigen quantitation in experimental immune complex glomerulonephritis. I. Acute serum sickness. *J Immunol* 1970;105:279–290.
303. Wilson CB, Dixon FJ. Quantitation of acute and chronic serum sickness in the rabbit. *J Exp Med* 1971;134:7S–18S.
304. Fleuren G, Grond J, Hoedemaeker PJ. In situ formation of subepithelial glomerular immune complexes in passive serum sickness. *Kidney Int* 1980;17:631–637.
305. Ryan GB, Karnovsky MJ. Distribution of endogenous albumin in the rat glomerulus: Role of hemodynamic factors in glomerular barrier function. *Kidney Int* 1976;9:36–45.
306. Koyama A, Niwa Y, Shigematsu H, Taniguchi M, Tada T. Studies on passive serum sickness. II. Factors determining the localization of antigen-antibody complexes in the murine renal glomerulus. *Lab Invest* 1978;38:253–262.
307. Germuth FC Jr, Rodriguez E, Lorelle CA, Trump EI, Milano L, Wise O. Passive immune complex glomerulonephritis in mice: Models for various lesions found in human disease. I. High avidity complexes and mesangiopathic glomerulonephritis. *Lab Invest* 1979;41:360–365.
308. Germuth FG Jr, Rodriguez E, Lorelle CA, Trump EI, Milano LL, Wise O. Passive immune complex glomerulonephritis in mice: models for various lesions found in human disease. II. Low avidity complexes and diffuse proliferative glomerulonephritis with subepithelial deposits. *Lab Invest* 1979;41:366–371.
309. Lowe MG, Holdsworth SR, Tipping PG. T lymphocyte participation in acute serum sickness glomerulonephritis in rabbits. *Immunol Cell Biol* 1991;69:81–87.
310. Boyce NW, Tipping PG, Holdsworth SR. Lymphokine (MIF) production by glomerular T-lymphocytes in experimental glomerulonephritis. *Kidney Int* 1986;30:673–677.
311. Parra G, Mosquera J, Rodriguez-Iturbe B. Migration inhibition factor in acute serum sickness nephritis. *Kidney Int* 1990;38:1118–1124.
312. McLean CR, Fitzgerald JDL, Younghusband OZ, Hamilton JD. Diffuse glomerulonephritis induced in rabbits by small intravenous injections of horse serum. *AMA Arch Pathol* 1951;51:1–11.
313. Germuth FG Jr, Rodriguez E. *Immunopathology of the Renal Glomerulus: Immune Complex Deposit and Antibasement Membrane Disease*. Boston: Little, Brown, 1973.
314. Dixon FJ, Feldman JD, Vazquez JJ. Experimental glomerulonephritis. The pathogenesis of a laboratory model resembling the spectrum of human glomerulonephritis. *J Exp Med* 1961;113:899–920.
315. Wilson CB, Dixon FJ. The renal response to immunological injury. In: Brenner BM, Rector FC Jr, eds. *The Kidney*. Philadelphia: Saunders, 1976:838–940.
316. Noble B, Van Liew JB, Brentjens JR. A transition from proliferative to membranous glomerulonephritis in chronic serum sickness. *Kidney Int* 1986;29:841–848.
317. Wang YM, al-Nawab MD, Evans B, Das AK, Thomas JH, Davies DR. Glomerular epithelial cell endocytosis of horseradish peroxidase-polylysine conjugate in immune-complex glomerulonephritis. *Nephrol Dial Transplant* 1990;5:771–776.
318. al-Nawab MD, Bass PS, Das AK, Davies DR. Immunoelectron microscopy of cationized bovine serum albumin-induced glomerulonephritis in the rabbit. *J Pathol* 1992;167:33–40.
319. Nakazawa K, Ohno S, Naramoto A, Takami H, Duan H-J, Itoh N, Shigematsu H. Immune deposits in the glomerular extracellular matrix detected by the quick-freezing and deep-etching method. *Nephron* 1992;62:203–212.
320. Neuland C, Albini B, Brentjens J, Grossberg AI, Andres GA. Antigen concentration in tissues of rabbits with systemic chronic serum sickness. *Int Arch Allergy Appl Immunol* 1981;64:385–394.
321. Peress NS, Tompkins DC. Rat CNS in experimental chronic serum sickness. Integrity of the zonulae occludentes of the choroid plexus epithelium and brain endothelium in experimental chronic serum sickness. *Neuropathol Appl Neurobiol* 1979;5:279–288.
322. Noble B, Olson KA, Milgrom M, Albini B. Tissue deposition of immune complexes in mice receiving daily injections of bovine serum albumin. *Clin Exp Immunol* 1980;42:255–262.
323. Noble B, Milgrom M, Van Liew JB, Brentjens JR. Chronic serum sickness in the rat: influence of antigen dose, route of antigen administration and strain of rat on the development of disease. *Clin Exp Immunol* 1981; 46:499–507.
324. Yamamoto T, Kihara I, Hara M, Kawasaki K, Yaoita E. Bovine serum albumin (BSA) nephritis in rats. II. Histological findings and complement activation by immune complex in SHR rats. *Br J Exp Pathol* 1983;64:660–669.
325. Yamamoto K, Oite T, Kihara I, Shimizu F. Experimental glomerulonephritis induced by human IgG in rats. *Clin Exp Immunol* 1984;57: 575–582.

326. McLeish KR, Stelzer GT, Cohara AF, Wallace JH. Variable susceptibility to immune complex glomerulonephritis among mice sharing the same major histocompatibility complex. *Immunol Invest* 1986;15:541–547.
327. Noble B, Brentjens JR. Experimental serum sickness. *Methods Enzymol* 1988;162:484–501.
328. Albini B, Brentjens J, Olson K, et al. Studies on the immune response of rabbits and chickens with chronic serum sickness. In: Milgrom F, Albini B, eds, *Immunopathology*. Sixth International Convocation on Immunology. Basel: S Karger, 1979;207–211.
329. Bishop SA, Stokes CR, Lucke VM. Experimental proliferative glomerulonephritis in the cat. *J Comp Pathol* 1992;106:49–60.
330. Bishop SA, Bailey M, Lucke VM, Stokes CR. Antibody response and antibody affinity maturation in cats with experimental proliferative immune complex glomerulonephritis. *J Comp Pathol* 1992;107: 91–102.
331. Stills HF Jr, Bullock BC, Clarkson TB. Increased atherosclerosis and glomerulonephritis in cynomolgus monkeys (Macaca fascicularis) given injections of BSA over an extended period of time. *Am J Pathol* 1983;113:222–234.
332. Hebert LA, Cosio FG, Birmingham DJ, Mahan JD, Sharma HM, Smead WL, Goel R. Experimental immune complex-mediated glomerulonephritis in the nonhuman primate. *Kidney Int* 1991;39:44–56.
333. Hogendoorn PC, Bruijn JA, Gelok EW, Van den Broek LJ, Fleuren GJ. Development of progressive glomerulosclerosis in experimental chronic serum sickness. *Nephrol Dial Transplant* 1990;5:100–109.
334. Miyazaki S, Kawasaki K, Yaoita E, Yamamoto T, Kihara I. Bovine serum albumin (BSA) nephritis in rats. III. Antigen distribution in various organs. *Clin Exp Immunol* 1985;59:293–299.
335. Miyazaki S, Kawasaki K, Yaoita E, Yamamoto T, Kihara I. Bovine serum albumin nephritis in rats. V. Kinetic studies of antigen localization in various organs and the phagocytic role of polymorphonuclear leukocytes. *Am J Pathol* 1985;119:412–419.
336. Lawler W. Experimental mesangial proliferative glomerulopathy. *J Pathol* 1981;133:107–122.
337. Valdes AJ, Germuth FG, Rodriguez E. Fatal immune complex glomerulonephritis without deposits. *Fed Proc* 1975;34:878.
338. Hagstrom GL, Bloom PM, Yum MN, Lavelle KJ, Luft FC. Ferritin- and apoferritin-induced immune complex glomerulonephritis in mice. *Nephron* 1979;24:127–133.
339. Iskandar SS, Gifford DR, Emancipator SN. Immune complex acute necrotizing glomerulonephritis with progression to diffuse glomerulosclerosis. A murine model. *Lab Invest* 1988;59:772–779.
340. Neville ME, Lischner HW. Activation of Fc receptor-bearing lymphocytes by immune complexes. 1. Stimulation of lymphokine production by nonadherent human peripheral blood lymphocytes. *J Immunol* 1982;128:1063–1069.
341. Fridman WH. Fc receptors and immunoglobulin binding factors. FASEB J 1991;5:2684–2690.
342. Unkeless JC, Boros P, Fein M. Structure, signalling and function of Fc gamma receptors. In: Gallin JI, Goldstein IM, Snyderman R, eds. *Inflammation: Basic Principles and Clinical Correlates*, 2nd ed. New York: Raven Press, 1992:497–510.
343. Lin CT, Shen Z, Boros P, Unkeless JC. Fc receptor-mediated signal transduction. *J Clin Immunol* 1994;14:1–13.
344. Boros P, Muryoi T, Spiera H, Bona C, Unkeless JC. Autoantibodies directed against different classes of FcγR are found in sera of autoimmune patients. *J Immunol* 1993;150:2019–2024.
345. Fridman WH, Teillaud JL, Bouchard C, Teillaud C, Astier A, Tartour E, Galon J, Mathiot C, Sautes C. Soluble Fc gamma receptors. *J Leukoc Biol* 1993;54:504–512.
346. Schifferli JA, Taylor RP. Physiological and pathological aspects of circulating immune complexes. *Kidney Int* 1989;35:993–1003.
347. Hebert LA, Cosio FG, Birmingham DJ, Mahan JD. Biologic significance of the erythrocyte complement receptor: a primate perquisite. *J Lab Clin Med* 1991;118:301–308.
348. Pascual M, Schifferli JA. The binding of immune complexes by the erythrocyte complement receptor 1 (CR1). *Immunopharmacology* 1992;24:101–106.
349. Ward DM, Lee S, Wilson CB. Direct antigen binding to glomerular immune complex deposits. *Kidney Int* 1986;30:706–711.
350. Fornasieri A, Moullier PM, Wilson CB. Dynamic interchange and factors influencing disappearance of antigen (Ag) and/or antibody (Ab) within glomerular (G) immune deposits (ID). *Kidney Int* 1990;37:413.
351. Mannik M, Striker GE. Removal of glomerular deposits of immune complexes in mice by administration of excess antigen. *Lab Invest* 1980;42:483–489.
352. Haakenstad AO, Striker GE, Mannik M. Removal of glomerular immune complex deposits by excess antigen in chronic mouse model of immune complex disease. *Lab Invest* 1983;48:323–331.
353. Haakenstad AO. Removal of glomerular deposits induced by either preformed immune complexes or by a chronic immune complex model in NZB/W mice. *J Immunol* 1987;138:4192–4199.
354. Mannik M, Agodoa LYC, David KA. Rearrangement of immune complexes in glomeruli leads to persistence and development of electron-dense deposits. *J Exp Med* 1983;157:1516–1527.
355. Caulin-Glaser T, Gallo GR, Lamm ME. Nondissociating cationic immune complexes can deposit in glomerular basement membrane. *J Exp Med* 1983;158:1561–1572.
356. Lambert PH, Goldman M, Rose LM, Morel PA. A possible role for idiotypic interactions in the pathogenesis of immune complex glomerulonephritis. *Transplant Proc* 1982;14:543–546.
357. Ford PM. Interaction of rheumatoid factor with immune complexes in experimental glomerulonephritis—possible role of antiglobulins in chronicity. *J Rheumatol* 1983;10(Suppl 11):81–84.
358. Zanetti M, Wilson CB. A role for antiidiotypic antibodies in immunologically mediated nephritis. *Am J Kidney Dis* 1986;7:445–451.
359. Ford PM. Rheumatoid factor and experimental glomerular disease. *Monogr Allergy* 1989;26:240–250.
360. Miyazaki M, Endoh M, Suga T, Yano N, Kuramoto T, Matsumoto Y, Eguchi K, Yagame M, Miura M, Nomoto Y, Sakai H. Rheumatoid factors and glomerulonephritis. *Clin Exp Immunol* 1990;82:250–255.
361. Zanetti M, Wilson CB. Participation of auto-anti-idiotypes in immune complex glomerulonephritis in rabbits. *J Immunol* 1983;2781–2783.
362. Rose LM, Goldman M, Lambert P-H. The production of anti-idiotypic antibodies and of idiotype-anti-idiotype immune complexes after polyclonal activation induced by bacterial LPS. *J Immunol* 1982; 128:2126–2133.
363. Goldman M, Rose LM, Hochmann A, Lambert PH. Deposition of idiotype-anti-idiotype immune complexes in renal glomeruli after polyclonal B cell activation. *J Exp Med* 1982;155:1385–1399.
364. Rose LM, Lambert PH. The natural occurrence of circulating idiotype-anti-idiotype complexes during a secondary immune response to phosphorylcholine. *Clin Immunol Immunopathol* 1980;15:481–492.
365. Rose LM, Goldman M, Lambert P-H. Simultaneous induction of an idiotype, corresponding anti-idiotypic antibodies, and immune complexes during African trypanosomiasis in mice. *J Immunol* 1982;128: 79–85.
366. Cavalot F, Miyata M, Vladutiu A, Terranova V, Dubiski S, Burlingame R, Tan E, Brentjens J, Milgrom F, Andres G. Glomerular lesions induced in the rabbit by physicochemically altered homologous IgG. *Am J Pathol* 1992;140:581–600.
367. Gyotoku Y, Abdelmoula M, Spertini F, Izui S, Lambert P-H. Cryoglobulinemia induced by monoclonal immunoglobulin G rheumatoid factors derived from autoimmune MRL/MpJ-*lpr/lpr* mice. *J Immunol* 1987;138:3785–3792.
368. Abdelmoula M, Spertini F, Shibata T, Gyotoku Y, Luzuy S, Lambert P-H, Izui S. IgG3 is the major source of cryoglobulins in mice. *J Immunol* 1989;143:526–532.
369. Berney T, Shibata T, Izui S. Murine cryoglobulinemia: pathogenic and protective IgG3 self-associating antibodies. *J Immunol* 1991;147: 3331–3335.
370. Lemoine R, Berney T, Shibata T, Fulpius T, Gyotoku Y, Shimada H, Sawada S, Izui S. Induction of "wire-loop" lesions by murine monoclonal IgG3 cryoglobulins. *Kidney Int* 1992;41:65–72.
371. Fornasieri A, Li M, Armelloni S, de Septis CP, Schiaffino E, Sinico RA, Schmid C, D'Amico G. Glomerulonephritis induced by human IgMK-IgG cryoglobulins in mice. *Lab Invest* 1993;69:531–540.
372. Nakazawa M, Emancipator SN, Lamm ME. Removal of glomerular immune complexes in passive serum sickness nephritis by treatment in vivo with proteolytic enzymes. *Lab Invest* 1986;55:551–556.
373. White RB, Lowrie L, Stork JE, Iskandar SS, Lamm ME, Emancipator SN. Targeted enzyme therapy of experimental glomerulonephritis in rats. *J Clin Invest* 1991;87:1819–1827.
374. Border WA, Ward HJ, Kamil ES, Cohen AH. Induction of membranous nephropathy in rabbits by administration of an exogenous cationic antigen. Demonstration of a pathogenic role for electrical charge. *J Clin Invest* 1982;69:451–461.

375. Koyama A, Inage H, Kobayashi M, Narita M, Tojo S. Effect of chemical cationization of antigen on glomerular localization of immune complexes in active models of serum sickness nephritis in rabbits. *Immunology* 1986;58:529–534.
376. Barnes JL, Reznicek MJ, Radnik RA, Venkatachalam MA. Anionization of an antigen promotes glomerular binding and immune complex formation. *Kidney Int* 1988;34:156–163.
377. Ward HJ, Cohen AH, Border WA. In situ formation of subepithelial immune complexes in the rabbit glomerulus: Requirement of a cationic antigen. *Nephron* 1984;36:257–264.
378. Gallo GR, Caulin-Glaser T, Emancipator SN, Lamm ME. Nephritogenicity and differential distribution of glomerular immune complexes related to immunogen charge. *Lab Invest* 1983;48:353–362.
379. Iskandar SS, Zhang J, Rodriguez E. Nephropathy induced in a nephritis-resistant inbred mouse strain with the use of a cationized antigen. *Am J Pathol* 1986;123:67–72.
380. Gallo GR, Caulin-Glaser T, Lamm ME. Charge of circulating immune complexes as a factor in glomerular basement membrane localization in mice. *J Clin Invest* 1981;67:1305–1313.
381. Koyama A, Inage H, Kobayashi M, Nakamura H, Narita M, Tojo S. Effect of chemical modification of antigen on characteristics of immune complexes and their glomerular localization in the murine renal tissues. *Immunology* 1986;58:535–540.
382. Koyama A, Inage H, Kobayashi M, Ohta Y, Narita M, Tojo S, Cameron JS. Role of antigenic charge and antibody avidity on the glomerular immune complex localization in serum sickness of mice. *Clin Exp Immunol* 1986;64:606–614.
383. Sawtell NM, Weiss MA, Pesce AJ, Michael JG. An immune complex glomerulopathy associated with glomerular capillary thrombosis in the laboratory mouse. A highly reproducible accelerated model utilizing cationized antigen. *Lab Invest* 1987;56:256–263.
384. Yamamoto T, Miyazaki S, Kawasaki K, Yaoita E, Kihara I. Rat bovine serum albumin (BSA) nephritis. VI. The influence of chemically altered antigen. *Clin Exp Immunol* 1986;65:51–56.
385. Rahman MA, Liu CN, Dunn MJ, Emancipator SN. Complement and leukocyte independent proteinuria and eicosanoid synthesis in rat membranous nephropathy. *Lab Invest* 1988;59:477–483.
386. Batsford SR, Mihatsch MJ, Rawiel M, Schmiedeke TM, Vogt A. Surface charge distribution is a determinant of antigen deposition in the renal glomerulus: Studies employing 'charge-hybrid' molecules. *Clin Exp Immunol* 1991;86:471–477.
387. Gauthier VJ, Mannik M. Only the initial binding of cationic immune complexes to glomerular anionic sites mediated by charge-charge interactions. *J Immunol* 1986;136:3266–3271
388. Batsford SR, Takamiya H, Vogt A. A model of in situ immune complex glomerulonephritis in the rat employing cationized ferritin. *Clin Nephrol* 1980;14:211–216.
389. Batsford S, Oite T, Takamiya H, Vogt A. Anionic binding sites in the glomerular basement membrane: possible role in the pathogenesis of immune complex glomerulonephritis. *Renal Physiol* 1980;3:336–340.
390. Oite T, Batsford SR, Mihatsch MJ, Takamiya H, Vogt A. Quantitative studies of *in situ* immune complex glomerulonephritis in the rat induced by planted cationized antigen. *J Exp Med* 1982;155:460–474.
391. Vogt A, Rohrbach R, Shimizu F, Takamiya H, Batsford S. Interaction of cationized antigen with rat glomerular basement membrane: *In situ* immune complex formation. *Kidney Int* 1982;22:27–35.
392. Oite T, Shimizu F, Kihara I, Batsford SR, Vogt A. An active model of immune complex glomerulonephritis in the rat employing cationized antigen. *Am J Pathol* 1983;112:185–194.
393. Kaseda N, Uehara Y, Yamamoto Y, Tanaka K. Induction of *in situ* immune complexes in rat glomeruli using avidin, a native cation macromolecule. *Br J Exp Pathol* 1985;66:729–736.
394. Oite T, Shimizu F, Suzuki Y, Vogt A. Ultramicroscopic localization of cationized antigen in the glomerular basement membrane in the course of active, in situ immune complex glomerulonephritis. *Virchows Arch B* 1985;48:107–118.
395. Suzuki Y, Maruyama Y, Arakawa M, Oite T. Preservation of fixed anionic sites in the GBM in the acute proteinuric phase of cationic antigen mediated in-situ immune complex glomerulonephritis in the rat. *Histochemistry* 1984;81:243–246.
396. Boulton Jones JM, Chandrachud L, Mosely H. Inherited variations in glomerular handling of antigen between Lewis and DA rats. *Clin Sci* 1986;71:565–572.
397. Kagami S, Miyao M, Shimizu F, Oite T. Active *in situ* immune complex glomerulonephritis using the hapten-carrier system: role of epitope density in cationic antigens. *Clin Exp Immunol* 1988;74:121–125.
398. Kagami S, Kawakami K, Okada K, Kuroda Y, Morioka T, Shimizu F, Oite T. Mechanism of formation of subepithelial electron-dense deposits in active *in situ* immune complex glomerulonephritis. *Am J Pathol* 1990;136:631–639.
399. Madaio MP, Adler S, Groggel GC, Couser WG, Salant DJ. Charge selective properties of the glomerular capillary wall influence antibody binding in rat membranous nephropathy. *Clin Immunol Immunopathol* 1986;39:131–138.
400. Adler S, Baker P, Pritzl P, Couser WG. Effect of alterations in glomerular charge on deposition of cationic and anionic antibodies to fixed glomerular antigens in the rat. *J Lab Clin Med* 1985;106:1–11.
401. Feintzeig ID, Dittmer JE, Cybulsky AV, Salant DJ. Antibody, antigen, and glomerular capillary wall charge interactions: influence of antigen location on in situ immune complex formation. *Kidney Int* 1986;29:649–657.
402. Agodoa LYC, Gauthier VJ, Mannik M. Antibody localization in the glomerular basement membrane may precede *in situ* immune deposit formation in rat glomeruli. *J Immunol* 1985;134:880–884.
403. Mannik M, Gauthier VJ, Stapleton SA, Agodoa LYC. Immune complexes with cationic antibodies deposit in glomeruli more effectively than cationic antibodies alone. *J Immunol* 1987;38:4209–4217.
404. Gauthier VJ, Mannik M. A small proportion of cationic antibodies in immune complexes is sufficient to mediate their deposition in glomeruli. *J Immunol* 1990;145:3348–3352.
405. Hunsicker LG, Shearer TP, Shaffer SJ. Acute reversible proteinuria induced by infusion of the polycation hexadimethrine. *Kidney Int* 1981;20:7–17.
406. Barnes JL, Radnik RA, Gilchrist EP, Venkatachalam MA. Size and charge selective permeability defects induced in glomerular basement membrane by a polycation. *Kidney Int* 1984;25:11–19.
407. Bertolatus JA, Hunsicker LG. Glomerular sieving of anionic and neutral bovine albumins in proteinuric rats. *Kidney Int* 1985;28:467–476.
408. Furness PN, Drakeley S. Heparin causes partial removal of glomerular antigen deposits by a mechanism independent of its anticoagulant properties. *J Pathol* 1992;168:217–220.
409. Kanwar YS, Caulin-Glaser T, Gallo GR, Lamm ME. Interaction of immune complexes with glomerular heparan sulfate-proteoglycans. *Kidney Int* 1986;30:842–851.
410. Adler SG, Wang H, Ward HJ, Cohen AH, Border WA. Electrical charge. Its role in the pathogenesis and prevention of experimental membranous nephropathy in the rabbit. *J Clin Invest* 1983;71: 487–499.
411. Oite T, Shimizu F, Batsford SR, Vogt A. The effect of protamine sulfate on the course of immune complex glomerulonephritis in the rat. *Clin Exp Immunol* 1986;64:318–322.
412. Raj AS, Tuscan M, Shapiro B, Glatfelter A, Kunkel R, Wiggins RC. Amount of antibody is critical for immune complex displacement by charge competition from both rabbit glomeruli and anionic beads. *Clin Exp Immunol* 1986;64:629–637.
413. Camussi G, Tetta C, Segoloni G, Coda R, Vercellone A. Localization of neutrophil cationic proteins and loss of anionic charges in glomeruli of patients with systemic lupus erythematosus glomerulonephritis. *Clin Immunol Immunopathol* 1982;24:299–314.
414. Barnes JL, Venkatachalam MA. The role of platelets and polycationic mediators in glomerular vascular injury. *Semin Nephrol* 1985;5: 57–68.
415. Camussi G, Tetta C, Meroni M, Torri-Tarelli L, Roffinello C, Alberton A, Deregibus C, Sessa A. Localization of cationic proteins derived from platelets and polymorphonuclear neutrophils and local loss of anionic sites in glomeruli of rabbits with experimentally induced acute serum sickness. *Lab Invest* 1986;55:56–62.
416. Camussi G, Tetta C, Mazzucco G, Monga G, Roffinello C, Alberton M, Dellabona P, Malavasi F, Vercellone A. Platelet cationic proteins are present in glomeruli of lupus nephritis patients. *Kidney Int* 1986; 30:555–565.
417. Chen A, Chou W-Y, Ding S-L, Shaio M-F. Glomerular localization of nephritogenic protein complexes on a nonimmunologic basis. *Lab Invest* 1992;67:175–185.
418. Golbus SM, Wilson CB. Experimental glomerulonephritis induced by in situ formation of immune complexes in glomerular capillary wall. *Kidney Int* 1979;16:148–157.
419. Johnson RJ, Klebanoff SJ, Ochi RF, Adler S, Baker P, Sparks L,

Couser WG. Participation of the myeloperoxidase-H_2O_2-halide system in immune complex nephritis. *Kidney Int* 1987;32:342–349.
420. Longhofer SL, Frisbie DD, Johnson HC, Culham CA, Cooley AJ, Schultz KT, Grauer GF. Effects of thromboxane synthetase inhibition on immune complex glomerulonephritis. *Am J Vet Res* 1991;52: 480–487.
421. Davin J-C, Nagy J, Lombet J, Foidart J-B, Dechenne C, Mahieu PR. Experimental glomerulonephritis induced by the glomerular deposition of IgA-concanavalin A complexes. *Contr Nephrol* 1988;67:111–116.
422. Davin JC, Dechenne C, Lombet J, Rentier B, Foidart JB, Mahieu PR. Acute experimental glomerulonephritis induced by the glomerular deposition of circulating polymeric IgA-concanavalin A complexes. *Virchows Arch A* 1989;415:7–20.
423. Matsuo S, Yoshida F, Yuzawa Y, Hara S, Fukatsu A, Watanabe Y, Sakamoto N. Experimental glomerulonephritis induced in rats by a lectin and its antibodies. *Kidney Int* 1989;36:1011–1021.
424. Sekiyama S, Yoshida F, Yuzawa Y, Fukatsu A, Suzuki N, Sakamoto N, Matsuo S. Mesangial proliferative glomerulonephritis induced in rats by a lentil lectin and its antibodies. *J Lab Clin Med* 1993;121:71–82.
425. Holthöfer H. Lectin binding sites in kidney. A comparative study of 14 animal species. *J Histochem Cytochem* 1983;31:531–537.
426. Kizaki T, Takeda Z, Watanabe M, Hanioka K, Itoh H. Histochemical analysis of changes in lectin binding in murine glomerular lesions. *Acta Pathol Jpn* 1989;39:31–41.
427. Abramowsky CR, Powers KG, Aikawa M, Swinehart G. Dirofilaria immitis. 5. Immunopathology of filarial nephropathy in dogs. *Am J Pathol* 1981;104:1–12.
428. Grauer GF, Culham CA, Dubielzig RR, Longhofer SL, Grieve RB. Experimental *Dirofilaria immitis*-associated glomerulonephritis induced in part by in situ formation of immune complexes in the glomerular capillary wall. *J Parasitol* 1989;75:585–593.
429. Houba V, Sturrock RF, Butterworth AE. Kidney lesions in baboons infected with *Schistosoma mansoni*. *Clin Exp Immunol* 1977;30: 439–449.
430. Lange K, Seligson G, Cronin W. Evidence for the in situ origin of poststreptococcal glomerulonephritis: glomerular localization of endostreptosin and the clinical significance of the subsequent antibody response. *Clin Nephrol* 1983;19:3–10.
431. Vogt A, Batsford S, Rodriguez-Iturbe B, Garcia R. Cationic antigens in poststreptococcal glomerulonephritis. *Clin Nephrol* 1983;20:271–279.
432. Cronin WJ, Lange K. Immunologic evidence for the in situ deposition of a cytoplasmic streptococcal antigen (endostreptosin) on the glomerular basement membrane in rats. *Clin Nephrol* 1990;34:143–146.
433. Oldstone MBA, Dixon FJ. Pathogenesis of chronic disease associated with persistent lymphocytic choriomeningitis viral infection. 1. Relationship of antibody production to disease in neonatally infected mice. *J Exp Med* 1969;129:483–505.
434. Oldstone MBA, Dixon FJ. Immune complex disease in chronic viral infection. *J Exp Med* 1971;134:32s–40s.
435. Portis JL, Coe JE. Deposition of IgA in renal glomeruli of mink affected with Aleutian disease. *Am J Pathol* 1979;96:227–236.
436. Delvinquier B, Goumard P, Dubarry M, Tronchin G, Camus D. Renal deposits of lipoprotein-immunoglobulin complexes in *Plasmodium chabaudi*-infected mice. *J Immunol* 1984;133:2243–2249.
437. Haines H, Farmer JN. Glomerular filtration rate and plasma solutes in BALB/c mice infected with *Plasmodium berghei*. *Parasitol Res* 1991; 77:411–414.
438. Van Marck EAE, Deelder AM, Gigase PLJ. *Schistosoma mansoni:* anodic polysaccharide antigen in glomerular immune deposits of mice with unisexual infection. *Exp Parasitol* 1981;52:62–68.
439. El-Dosoky I, Van Marck EAE, Deelder AM. Presence of *Schistosoma mansoni* antigens in liver, spleen and kidney of infected mice: A sequential study. *Z Parasitenkd* 1984;70:491–497.
440. El-Sherif AK, Befus D. Predominance of IgA deposits in glomeruli of *Schistosoma mansoni* infected mice. *Clin Exp Immunol* 1988;71: 39–44.
441. Sobh M, Moustafa F, Ramzy R, Saad M, Deelder A, Ghoneim M. *Schistosoma mansoni* nephropathy in Syrian golden hamsters: Effect of dose and duration of infection. *Nephron* 1991;59:121–130.
442. Costa RS, Monteiro RC, Lehuen A, Joskowicz M, Noel LH, Droz D. Immune complex-mediated glomerulopathy in experimental Chagas' disease. *Clin Immunol Immunopathol* 1991;58:102–114.
443. Oliveira AV, Rossi MA, Roque-Barreira MC, Sartori A, Campos-Neto A. The potential role of *Leishmania* antigens and immunoglobulins in the pathogenesis of glomerular lesions of hamsters infected with *Leishmania donovani*. *Ann Trop Med Parasitol* 1985;79: 539–543.
444. Oliveira AV, Roque-Barreira MC, Sartori A, Campos-Neto A, Rossi, MA. Mesangial proliferative glomerulonephritis associated with progressive amyloid deposition in hamsters experimentally infected with *Leishmania donovani*. *Am J Pathol* 1985;120:256–262.
445. Sartori A, de Oliveira AV, Roque-Barreira MC, Rossi MA, Campos-Neto A. Immune complex glomerulonephritis in experimental kala-azar. *Parasite Immunol* 1987;9:93–103.
446. Sartori A, Roque-Barreira MC, Coe J, Campos-Neto A. Immune complex glomerulonephritis in experimental kala-azar. II. Detection and characterization of parasite antigens and antibodies eluted from kidneys of *Leishmania donovani*-infected hamsters. *Clin Exp Immunol* 1992;87:386–392.
447. Nieto CG, Navarrete I, Habele MA, Serrano F, Redondo E. Pathological changes in kidneys of dogs with natural *Leishmania* infection. *Vet Parasitol* 1992;45:33–47.
448. Albano Edelweiss MI, Lizardo-Daudt HM. Naturally existing model of glomerulonephritis mediated by immune complexes associated with hydatidosis in sheep. *Nephron* 1991;57:253–254.
449. Bielschowsky M, Bielschowsky F. Reaction of the reticular tissue of mice with autoimmune haemolytic anaemia to 2-aminofluorene. *Nature* 1962;194:692.
450. Helyer BJ, Howie JB. Renal disease associated with positive lupus erythematosus tests in a cross-bred strain of mice. *Nature* 1963;197: 197.
451. Howie JB, Helyer BJ. The immunology and pathology of NZB mice. *Adv Immunol* 1968;9:215–266.
452. Andrews BS, Eisenberg RA, Theofilopoulos AN, Izui S, Wilson CB, McConahey PJ, Murphy ED, Roths JB, Dixon FJ. Spontaneous murine lupus-like syndromes. *J Exp Med* 1978;148:1198–1215.
453. Theofilopoulos AN, Dixon FJ. Murine models of systemic lupus erythematosus. *Adv Immunol* 1985;37:269–358.
454. Jacob L, Viard J-P, Louvard D, Bach JF. Recent advances in the pathogenesis of systemic lupus erythematosus. *Adv Nephrol* 1990;19: 237–256.
455. Morel L, Rudofsky UH, Longmate JA, Schiffenbauer J, Wakeland EK. Polygenic control of susceptibility to murine systemic lupus erythematosus. *Immunity* 1994;1:219–229.
456. Granholm NA, Cavallo T. Bacterial lipopolysaccharide enhances deposition of immune complexes and exacerbates nephritis in BXSB lupus-prone mice. *Clin Exp Immunol* 1991;85:270–277.
457. Izui S, Lambert P-H, Fournie, GJ, Turler H, Miescher PA. Features of systemic lupus erythematosus in mice injected with bacterial lipopolysaccharides. Identification of circulating DNA and renal localization of DNA-Anti-DNA complexes. *J Exp Med* 1977;145:1115–1130.
458. In S, Le Lann AD, Oksman F, Fournie EL, Labarre J-F, Benoist H, Fournie GJ. An *in vivo* model for the experimental selection of drugs able to prevent immune complex glomerulonephritis. *Int J Immunopharmacol* 1992;14:871–876.
459. Gilkeson GS, Ruiz P, Howell D, Lefkowith JB, Pisetsky DS. Induction of immune-mediated glomerulonephritis in normal mice immunized with bacterial DNA. *Clin Immunol Immunopathol* 1993;68: 283–292.
460. Bruijn JA, Bergijk EC, de Heer E, Fleuren GJ, Hoedemaeker PJ. Induction and progression of experimental lupus nephritis: exploration of a pathogenetic pathway. *Kidney Int* 1992;41:5–13.
461. van Leer EH, Bruijn JA, Prins FA, Hoedemaeker PJ, de Heer E. Redistribution of glomerular dipeptidyl peptidase type IV in experimental lupus nephritis. Demonstration of decreased enzyme activity at the ultrastructural level. *Lab Invest* 1993;68:550–556.
462. Drake CG, Kotzin BL. Genetic and immunological mechanisms in the pathogenesis of systemic lupus erythematosus. *Curr Opin Immunol* 1992;4:733–740.
463. Arnett FC, Reveille JD. Genetics of systemic lupus erythematosus. *Rheum Dis Clin North Am* 1992;18:865–892.
464. Cohen PL, Eisenberg RA. *Lpr* and *gld:* single gene models of systemic autoimmunity and lymphoproliferative disease. *Annu Rev Immunol* 1991;9:243–269.
465. Kimura M, Ogata Y, Shimada K, Wakabayashi T, Onoda H, Katagiri T, Matsuzawa A. Nephritogenicity of the lpr^{cg} gene on the MRL background. *Immunology* 1992;76:498–504.
466. Rosenblatt N, Hartmann K-U, Loor F. The Yaa mutation induces the

development of autoimmunity in mice heterozygous for the *gld* (generalized lymphadenopathy disease) mutation. *Cell Immunol* 1994; 156:519–528.

467. Merino R, Iwamoto M, Gershwin ME, Izui S. The Yaa gene abrogates the major histocompatibility complex association of murine lupus in (NZB x BXSB) F[1] hybrid mice. *J Clin Invest* 1994;94:521–525.
468. Watson ML, Rao JK, Gilkeson GS, Ruiz P, Eicher EM, Pisetsky DS, Matsuzawa A, Rochelle JM, Seldin MF. Genetic analysis of MRL-lpr mice: relationship of the *Fas* apoptosis gene to disease manifestations and renal disease-modifying loci. *J Exp Med* 1992;176:1645–1656.
469. Gillette-Ferguson I, Sidman CL. A specific intercellular pathway of apoptotic cell death is defective in the mature peripheral T cells of autoimmune *lpr* and *gld* mice. *Eur J Immunol* 1994;24:1181–1185.
470. Nagata S, Suda T. Fas and Fas ligand: *lpr* and *gld* mutations. *Immunol Today* 1995;16:39–43.
471. Wu J, Zhou T, Zhang J, He J, Gause WC, Mountz JD. Correction of accelerated autoimmune disease by early replacement of the mutated *lpr* gene with the normal *Fas* apoptosis gene in the T cells of transgenic MRL-*lpr* /*lpr* mice. *Proc Natl Acad Sci U S A* 1994; 91:2344–2348.
472. Ramsdell F, Seaman MS, Miller RE, Tough TW, Alderson MR, Lynch DH. *gld/gld* mice are unable to express a functional ligand for Fas. *Eur J Immunol* 1994;24:928–933.
473. Takahashi T, Tanaka M, Brannan CI, Jenkins NA, Copeland NG, Suda T, Nagata S. Generalized lymphoproliferative disease in mice, caused by a point mutation in the Fas ligand. *Cell* 1994;76:969–976.
474. Strasser A, Whittingham S, Vaux DL, Bath ML, Adams JM, Cory S, Harris AW. Enforced *BCL2* expression in B-lymphoid cells prolongs antibody responses and elicits autoimmune disease. *Proc Natl Acad Sci U S A* 1991;88:8661–8665.
475. Steinberg AD. MRL-*lpr/lpr* disease: theories meet Fas. *Semin Immunol* 1994;6:55–69.
476. Tan EM. Autoimmunity and apoptosis. *J Exp Med* 1994;179: 1083–1086.
477. Singer GG, Carrera AC, Marshak-Rothstein A, Martinez-A C, Abbas AK. Apoptosis, Fas and systemic autoimmunity: the MRL-*lpr/lpr* model. *Curr Opin Immunol* 1994;6:913–920.
478. Eisenberg RA, Sobel ES, Reap EA, Halpern MD, Cohen PL. The role of B cell abnormalities in the systemic autoimmune syndromes of lpr and *gld* mice. *Semin Immunol* 1994;6:49–54.
479. Diamond B, Katz JB, Paul E, Aranow C, Lustgarten D, Scharff MD. The role of somatic mutation in the pathogenic anti-DNA response. *Annu Rev Immunol* 1992;10:731–757.
480. Marion TN, Tillman DM, Jou N-T, Hill RJ. Selection of immunoglobulin variable regions in autoimmunity to DNA. *Immunol Rev* 1992;128:123–149.
481. Theofilopoulos AN, Balderas RS, Baccala R, Kono DH. T-cell receptor genes in autoimmunity. *Ann NY Acad Sci* 1993;681:33–46.
482. Stollar BD. Molecular analysis of anti-DNA antibodies. *FASEB J* 1994;8:337–342.
483. Shoenfeld Y. Idiotypic induction of autoimmunity: a new aspect of the idiotypic network. *FASEB J* 1994;8:1296–1301.
484. Savill J, Smith J, Sarraf C, Ren Y, Abbott F, Rees A. Glomerular mesangial cells and inflammatory macrophages ingest neutrophils undergoing apoptosis. *Kidney Int* 1992;42:924–936.
485. Baker AJ, Mooney A, Hughes J, Lombardi D, Johnson RJ, Savill J. Mesangial cell apoptosis: the major mechanism for resolution of glomerular hypercellularity in experimental mesangial proliferative nephritis. *J Clin Invest* 1994;94:2105–2116.
486. Shimizu A, Kitamura H, Masuda Y, Ishizaki M Sugisaki Y, Yamanaka N. Apoptosis in the repair process of experimental proliferative glomerulonephritis. *Kidney Int* 1995;47:114–121.
487. Muryoi T, Sasaki T, Hatakeyama A, Shibata S, Suzuki M, Seino J, Yoshinaga K. Clonotypes of anti-DNA antibodies expressing specific idiotypes in immune complexes of patients with active lupus nephritis. *J Immunol* 1990;144:3856–3861.
488. Suzuki M, Hatakeyama A, Kameoka J, Tamate E, Yusa A, Kurosawa K, Saito T, Sasaki T, Yoshinaga K. Anti-DNA idiotypes deposited in renal glomeruli of patients with lupus nephritis. *Am J Kidney Dis* 1991;18:232–239.
489. Segal R, Globerson A, Zinger H, Mozes E. Induction of experimental systemic lupus erythematosus (SLE) in mice with severe combined immunodeficiency (SCID). *Clin Exp Immunol* 1992;89:239–243.
490. Malide D, Londoño I, Russo P, Bendayan M. Ultrastructural localization of DNA in immune deposits of human lupus nephritis. *Am J Pathol* 1993;143:304–311.
491. Waisman A, Mendlovic S, Ruiz PJ, Zinger H, Meshorer A, Mozes E. The role of the 16/6 idiotype network in the induction and manifestations of systemic lupus erythematosus. *Int Immunol* 1993;5: 1293–1300.
492. Bernstein KA, Bolshoun D, Lefkowith JB. Serum glomerular binding activity is highly correlated with renal disease in MRL/*lpr* mice. *Clin Exp Immunol* 1993;93:418–423.
493. Terada K, Okuhara E, Kawarada Y. Antigen DNA isolated from immune complexes in plasma of patients with systemic lupus erythematosus hybridizes with the *Escherichia coli* lac Z gene. *Clin Exp Immunol* 1991;85:66–69.
494. Gilkeson GS, Pritchard AJ, Pisetsky DS. Specificity of anti-DNA antibodies induced in normal mice by immunization with bacterial DNA. *Clin Immunol Immunopathol* 1991;59:288–300.
495. Izui S, Lambert P-H, Miescher PA. In vitro demonstration of a particular affinity of glomerular basement membrane and collagen for DNA. A possible basis for a local formation of DNA-anti-DNA complexes in systemic lupus erythematosus. *J Exp Med* 1976;144: 428–443.
496. Gupta RC, Simpson WA, Raghow R. Interaction of fibronectin with DNA/Anti-DNA complexes from systemic lupus erythematosus: role of activated complement C1 in modulation of the interactions. *Clin Immunol Immunopathol* 1988;46:368–381.
497. Jacob L, Viard JD, Allenet B, Anin M-F, Slama FBH, Vandekerckhove J, Primo J, Markovits J, Jacob F, Bach J-F, Le Pecq, J-B, Louvard D. A monoclonal anti-double-stranded DNA autoantibody binds to a 94-kDa cell-surface protein on various cell types via nucleosomes or a DNA-histone complex. *Proc Natl Acad Sci U S A* 1989;86: 4669–4673.
498. Schmiedeke TMJ, Stöckl FW, Weber R, Sugisaki Y, Batsford SR, Vogt A. Histones have high affinity for the glomerular basement membrane. *J Exp Med* 1989;169:1879–1894.
499. Termaat RM, Brinkman K, Van Gompel F, Van Den Heuvel LPWJ, Veerkamp J, Smeenk RJT, Berden JHM. Cross-reactivity of monoclonal anti-DNA antibodies with heparan sulfate is mediated via bound DNA/histone complexes. *J Autoimmunity* 1990;3:531–545.
500. Termaat R-M, Assmann KJM, Dijkman HBPM, von Gompel F, Smeenk RJT, Berden JHM. Anti-DNA antibodies can bind to the glomerulus via two distinct mechanisms. *Kidney Int* 1992;42: 1363–1371.
501. Mohan C, Adams S, Stanik V, Datta SK. Nucleosome: A major immunogen for pathogenic autoantibody-inducing T cells of lupus. *J Exp Med* 1993;177:1367–1381.
502. Vogt A, Batsford S, Morioka T. Nephritogenic antibodies in lupus nephritis. *Tohoku J Exp Med* 1994;173:31–41.
503. van Bruggen MC, Kramers C, Hylkema MN, Smeenk RJ, Berden JH. Pathophysiology of lupus nephritis: the role of nucleosomes. *Netherlands J Med* 1994;45:273–279.
504. Mohan C, Datta SK. Lupus: key pathogenic mechanisms and contributing factors. *Clin Immunol Immunopathol* 1995;77:209–220.
505. Bernstein KA, Valerio RD, Lefkowith JB. Glomerular binding activity in MRL lpr serum consists of antibodies that bind to a DNA/histone/type IV collagen complex. *J Immmunol* 1995;154:2424–2433.
506. Di Valerio R, Bernstein KA, Varghese E, Lefkowith JB. Murine lupus glomerulotropic monoclonal antibodies exhibit differing specificities but bind via a common mechanism. *J Immunol* 1995;155: 2258–2268.
507. Tax WJM, Kramers C, van Bruggen MCJ, Berden JHM. Apoptosis, nucleosomes, and nephritis in systemic lupus erythematosus. *Kidney Int* 1995;48:666–673.
508. Rumore PM, Steinman CR. Endogenous circulating DNA in systemic lupus erythematosus. Occurrence as multimeric complexes bound to histone. *J Clin Invest* 1990;86:69–74.
509. Morioka T, Woitas R, Fujigaki Y, Batsford SR, Vogt A. Histone mediates glomerular deposition of small size DNA anti-DNA complex. *Kidney Int* 1994;45:991–997.
510. Schmiedeke T, Stoeckl F, Muller S, Sugisaki Y, Batsford S, Woitas R, Vogt A. Glomerular immune deposits in murine lupus models may contain histones. *Clin Exp Immunol* 1992;90:453–458.
511. Losman JA, Fasy TM, Novick KE, Massa M, Monestier M. Nucleosome-specific antibody from an autoimmune MRL/Mp-*lpr/lpr* mouse. *Arthritis Rheum* 1993;36:552–560.

512. Kashihara N, Makino H, Szekanecz Z, Waltenbaugh CR, Kanwar YS. Nephritogenicity of anti-proteoglycan antibodies in experimental murine lupus nephritis. *Lab Invest* 1992;67:752–760.
513. Elouaai F, Lule J, Benoist H, Appolinaire-Pilipenko S, Atanassov C, Muller S, Fournie GJ. Autoimmunity to histones, ubiquitin, and ubiquitinated histone H2A in NZB x NZW and MRL-lpr/lpr mice. Antihistone antibodies are concentrated in glomerular eluates of lupus mice. *Nephrol Dial Transplant* 1994;9:362–366.
514. Amoura Z, Chabre H, Koutouzov S, Lotton C, Cabrespines A, Bach JF, Jacob L. Nucleosome-restricted antibodies are detected before anti-dsDNA and/or antihistone antibodies in serum of MRL-Mp lpr/lpr and +/+mice, and are present in kidney eluates of lupus mice with proteinuria. *Arthritis Rheum* 1994;37:1684–1688.
515. Burlingame RW, Rubin RL, Balderas RS, Theofilopoulos AN. Genesis and evolution of antichromatin autoantibodies in murine lupus implicates T-dependent immunization with self antigen. *J Clin Invest* 1993;91:1687–1696.
516. Burlingame RW, Boey ML, Starkebaum G, Rubin RL. The central role of chromatin in autoimmune responses to histones and DNA in systemic lupus erythematosus. *J Clin Invest* 1994;94:184–192.
517. Viard J-P, Bach J-F, Jacob L. Splenocytes from MRL/MP-lpr/lpr mice spontaneously produce antibodies against a cell-surface protein cross-reacting with DNA. *Clin Immunol Immunopathol* 1987;45:516–521.
518. Jacob L, Lety M-A, Monteiro RC, Jacob F, Bach J-F, Louvard D. Altered cell-surface protein(s), crossreactive with DNA, on spleen cells of autoimmune lupic mice. *Proc Natl Acad Sci U S A* 1987;84:1361–1363.
519. Madaio MP, Carlson J, Cataldo J, Ucci A, Migliorini P, Pankewycz O. Murine monoclonal anti-DNA antibodies bind directly to glomerular antigens and form immune deposits. *J Immunol* 1987;138:2883–2889.
520. Sabbaga J, Peres Line SR, Potocnjak P, Madaio MP. A murine nephritogenic monoclonal anti-DNA autoantibody binds directly to mouse laminin, the major non-collagenous protein component of the glomerular basement membrane. *Eur J Immunol* 1989;19:137–143.
521. Sabbaga J, Pankewycz OG, Lufft V, Schwartz RS, Madaio MP. Cross-reactivity distinguishes serum and nephritogenic anti-DNA antibodies in human lupus from their natural counterparts in normal serum. *J Autoimmunity* 1990;3:215–235.
522. Vlahakos DV, Foster MH, Adams S, Katz M, Ucci AA, Barrett KJ, Datta SK, Madaio MP. Anti-DNA antibodies form immune deposits at distinct glomerular and vascular sites. *Kidney Int* 1992;41:1690–1700.
523. Foster MH, Cizman B, Madaio MP. Nephritogenic autoantibodies in systemic lupus erythematosus: immunochemical properties, mechanisms of immune deposition, and genetic origins. *Lab Invest* 1993;69:494–507.
524. Termaat R-M, Assmann KJM, van Son JPHF, Dijkman HBPM, Koene RAP, Berden JHM. Antigen-specificity of antibodies bound to glomeruli of mice with systemic lupus erythematosus-like syndromes. *Lab Invest* 1993;68:164–173.
525. Brinkman K, Termaat R, Berden JHM, Smeenk RJT. Anti-DNA antibodies and lupus nephritis: the complexity of crossreactivity. *Immunol Today* 1990;11:232–234.
526. Frampton G, Hobby P, Morgan A, Staines NA, Cameron JS. A role for DNA in anti-DNA antibodies binding to endothelial cells. *J Autoimmunity* 1991;4:463–478.
527. Chan TM, Frampton G, Staines NA, Hobby P, Perry GJ, Cameron JS. Different mechanisms by which anti-DNA MoAbs bind to human endothelial cells and glomerular mesangial cells. *Clin Exp Immunol* 1992;88:68–74.
528. Raz E, Brezis M, Rosenmann E, Eilat D. Anti-DNA antibodies bind directly to renal antigens and induce kidney dysfunction in the isolated perfused rat kidney. *J Immunol* 1989;142:3076–3082.
529. Vlahakos D, Foster MH, Ucci AA, Barrett KJ, Datta SK, Madaio MP. Murine monoclonal anti-DNA antibodies penetrate cells, bind to nuclei, and induce glomerular proliferation and proteinuria in vivo. *J Am Soc Nephrol* 1992;2:1345–1354.
530. Yanase K, Smith RM, Cizman B, Foster MH, Peachey LD, Jarett L, Madaio MP. A subgroup of murine monoclonal anti-deoxyribonucleic acid antibodies traverse the cytoplasm and enter the nucleus in a time- and temperature-dependent manner. *Lab Invest* 1994;71:52–60.
531. Suenaga R, Abdou NI. Cationic and high affinity serum IgG anti-dsDNA antibodies in active lupus nephritis. *Clin Exp Immunol* 1993;94:418–422.
532. Suzuki N, Harada T, Mizushima Y, Sakane T. Possible pathogenic role of cationic anti-DNA autoantibodies in the development of nephritis in patients with systemic lupus erythematosus. *J Immunol* 1993;151:1128–1136.
533. Ohnishi K, Ebling FM, Mitchell B, Singh RR, Hahn BH, Tsao BP. Comparison of pathogenic and non-pathogenic murine antibodies to DNA: antigen binding and structural characteristics. *Int Immunol* 1994;6:817–830.
534. Frampton G, Perry GJ, Chan TM, Cameron JS. Significance of anti-cardiolipin and antiendothelial cell antibodies in the nephritis of lupus. *Contrib Nephrol* 1992;99:7–16.
535. Piette J-C, Cacoub P, Wechsler B. Renal manifestations of the antiphospholipid syndrome. *Semin Arthritis Rheum* 1994;23:357–366.
536. Limpanasithikul W, Ray S, Diamond B. Cross-reactive antibodies have both protective and pathogenic potential. *J Immunol* 1995;155:967–973.
537. Hashimoto Y, Kawamura M, Ichikawa K, Suzuki T, Sumida T, Yoshida S, Matsuura E, Ikehara S, Koike T. Anticardiolipin antibodies in NZW x BXSB F1 mice. A model of antiphospholipid syndrome. *J Immunol* 1992;149:1063–1068.
538. Kiberd BA. The functional and structural changes of the glomerulus throughout the course of murine lupus nephritis. *J Am Soc Nephrol* 1992;3:930–939.
539. Tsao BP, Cheroutre H, Ohnishi K, Teitell M, Ebling FM, Mixter P, Kronenberg M, Hahn BH. Nephritis in normal mice expressing transgenes encoding an antibody to DNA. *Arthritis Rheum* 1990;33:S19 .
540. Duchosal MA, Eming SA, McConahey PJ, Dixon JF. The hu-PBL-SCID mouse model. Long-term human serologic evolution associated with the xenogeneic transfer of human peripheral blood leukocytes into SCID mice. *Cell Immunol* 1992;139:468–477.
541. Weigle WO,Nakamura RM. Perpetuation of autoimmune thryroiditis and production of secondary renal lesions following periodic injections of aqueous preparations of altered thyroglobulins. *Clin Exp Immunol* 1969;4:645–657.
542. Weigle WO, High GJ. The behavior of autologous thyroglobulin in the circulation of rabbits immunized with either heterologous or altered homologous thryroglobulin. *J Immunol* 1967;98:1105–1114.
543. Meade CJ, Brandon DR, Smith W, Simmonds RG, Harris S, Sowter C. The relationship between hyperglycemia and renal immune complex deposition in mice with inherited diabetes. *Clin Exp Immunol* 1981;43:109–120.
544. Atkins RC, Holdsworth SR. Cellular mechanisms of immune glomerular injury. In: Wilson CB, Brenner BM, Stein, eds. *Contemporary Issues in Nephrology*, vol 18. New York: Churchill Livingstone, 1988:111–135.
545. Rovin BH, Schreiner GF. Cell-mediated immunity in glomerular disease. *Annu Rev Med* 1991;42:25–33.
546. Florquin S, Goldman M. T cell subsets in glomerular diseases. *Springer Semin Immunopathol* 1994;16:71–80.
547. Kreisberg JI, Wayne DB, Karnovsky MJ. Rapid and focal loss of negative charge associated with mononuclear cell infiltration early in nephrotoxic serum sickness. *Kidney Int* 1979;16:290–300.
548. Tipping PG, Neale TJ, Holdsworth SR. T lymphocyte participation in antibody-induced experimental glomerulonephritis. *Kidney Int* 1985;27:530–537.
549. Lowry RP, Clarke Forbes RD, Blackburn JH. Immune reactivity and immunosuppressive intervention (TLI) in experimental nephritis. I. Immunopathologic correlates in the accelerated autologous form of nephrotoxic serum nephritis. *J Immunol* 1984;132:1001–1006.
550. Bhan AK, Schneeberger EE, Collins AB, McCluskey RT. Evidence for a pathogenic role of a cell-mediated immune mechanism in experimental glomerulonephritis. *J Exp Med* 1978;148:246–260.
551. Bhan AK, Collins AB, Schneeberger EE, McCluskey RT. A cell-mediated reaction against glomerular-bound immune complexes. *J Exp Med* 1979;150:1410–1420.
552. Oite T, Shimizu F, Kagami S, Morioka T. Hapten-specific cellular immune response producing glomerular injury. *Clin Exp Immunol* 1989;76:463–468.
553. Rennke HG, Klein PS, Sandstrom DJ, Mendrick DL. Cell-mediated immune injury in the kidney: Acute nephritis induced in the rat by azobenzenearsonate. *Kidney Int* 1994;45:1044–1056.
554. Andres GA, Cerra F, Elti G, Casciani C, Cortesini R, Hsu KC. Lym-

phocyte and blast cell glomerulonephritis in renal allografts of rats injected with phytohaemagglutinin. *Cell Immunol* 1974;13:146–163.
555. Camussi G, Tetta C, Bussolino F, Turello E, Brentjens J, Montrucchio G, Andres G. Effect of leukocyte stimulation on rabbit immune complex glomerulonephritis. *Kidney Int* 1990;38:1047–1055.
556. Bolton WK, Tucker FL, Sturgill BC. Experimental autoimmune glomerulonephritis in chickens. *J Clin Lab Immunol* 1980;3:179–184.
557. Bolton WK, Tucker FL, Sturgill BC. New avian model of experimental glomerulonephritis consistent with mediation by cellular immunity. Nonhumorally mediated glomerulonephritis in chickens. *J Clin Invest* 1984;73:1263–1276.
558. Tucker FL, Sturgill BC, Bolton WK. Ultrastructural studies of experimental autoimmune glomerulonephritis in normal and bursectomized chickens. *Lab Invest* 1985;53:563–570.
559. Bolton WK, Chandra M, Tyson TM, Kirkpatrick PR, Sadovnic MJ, Sturgill BC. Transfer of experimental glomerulonephritis in chickens by mononuclear cells. *Kidney Int* 1988;34:598–610.
560. Granados R, Mendrick DL, Rennke HG. Antibody-induced crescent formation in WKY rats: potential role of antibody-dependent cell cytotoxicity (ADCC) in vivo. *Kidney Int* 1990;37:414.
561. Kawasaki K, Yaoita E, Yamamoto T, Kihara I. Depletion of CD8 positive cells in nephrotoxic serum nephritis of WKY rats. *Kidney Int* 1992;41:1517–1526.
562. Huang XR, Holdsworth SR, Tipping PG. Evidence for delayed-type hypersensitivity mechanisms in glomerular crescent formation. *Kidney Int* 1994;46:69–78.
563. Kawasaki K, Yaoita E, Yamamoto T, Tamatani T, Miyasaka M, Kihara I. Antibodies against intercellular adhesion molecule-I and lymphocyte function-associated antigen-1 prevent glomerular injury in rat experimental crescentic glomerulonephritis. *J Immunol* 1993; 150:1074–1083.
564. Hill PA, Lan HY, Nikolic-Paterson DJ, Atkins RC. The ICAM-1/LFA-1 interaction in glomerular leukocytic accumulation in anti-GBM glomerulonephritis. *Kidney Int* 1994;45:700–708.
565. Tang WW, Feng L, Vannice JL, Wilson CB. Interleukin-1 receptor antagonist ameliorates experimental anti-glomerular basement membrane antibody-associated glomerulonephritis. *J Clin Invest* 1994;93: 273–279.
566. Nishikawa K, Guo Y-J, Miyasaka M, Tamatani T, Collins AB, Sy M-S, McCluskey RT, Andres G. Antibodies to intercellular adhesion molecule 1/lymphocyte function-associated antigen 1 prevent crescent formation in rat autoimmune glomerulonephritis. *J Exp Med* 1993;177:667–677.
567. Nishikawa K, Linsley PS, Collins AB, Stamenkovic I, McCluskey RT, Andres G. Effect of CTLA-4 chimeric protein on rat autoimmune anti-glomerular basement membrane glomerulonephritis. *Eur J Immunol* 1994;24:1249–1254.
568. Chu EB, Hobbs MV, Wilson CB, Romball CG, Linsley PS, Weigle WO. Intervention of CD4- cell subset shifts and autoimmunity in the BXSB mouse by murine CTLA4Ig[1]. *J Immunol* 1996;156:1262–1268.
569. Tsuji Y, Okuyama K, Kobayashi K, Shibata T, Saito K, Kitazawa K, Sugisaki T. Studies on cell-mediated immunity (CMI) in the glomeruli. Immunization with GBM antigen from Masugi nephritis in Wistar-Kyoto rats. *Nippon Jinzo Gakkai Shi* 1994;36:95–102.
570. Eldredge C, Merritt S, Goyal M, Kulaga H, Kindt TJ, Wiggins R. Analysis of T cells and major histocompatibility complex class I and class II mRNA and protein content and distribution in antiglomerular basement membrane disease in the rabbit. *Am J Pathol* 1991;139: 1021–1035.
571. Lan HY, Nikolic-Patterson DJ, Atkins RC. Involvement of activated periglomerular leukocytes in the rupture of Bowman's capsule and glomerular crescent progression in experimental glomerulonephritis. *Lab Invest* 1992;67:743–751.
572. Maruyama K, Tomizawa S, Shimabukuro N, Fukuda T, Johshita T, Kuroume T. Effect of supernatants derived from T lymphocyte culture in minimal change nephrotic syndrome on rat kidney capillaries. *Nephron* 1989;51:73–76.
573. Yoshizawa N, Kusumi Y, Matsumoto K, Oshima S, Takeuchi A, Kawamura O, Kubota T, Kondo S, Niwa H. Studies of a glomerular permeability factor in patients with minimal-change nephrotic syndrome. *Nephron* 1989;51:370–376.
574. Tanaka R, Yoshikawa N, Nakamura H, Ito H. Infusion of peripheral blood mononuclear cell products from nephrotic children increases albuminuria in rats. *Nephron* 1992;60:35–41.
575. Dantal J, Bigot E, Bogers W, Testa A, Kriaa F, Jacques Y, Huralt de Ligny B, Niaudet P, Charpentier B, Soulillou JP. Effect of plasma protein adsorption on protein excretion in kidney-transplant recipients with recurrent nephrotic syndrome. *N Engl J Med* 1994;330:7–14.
576. Wilkinson AH, Gillespie C, Hartley B, Williams DG. Increase in proteinuria and reduction in number of anionic sites on the glomerular basement membrane in rabbits by infusion of human nephrotic plasma in vivo. *Clin Sci* 1989;77:43–48.
577. Levin M, Gascoine P, Turner MW, Barratt TM. A highly cationic protein in plasma and urine of children with steroid-responsive nephrotic syndrome. *Kidney Int* 1989;36:867–877.
578. Emancipator SN. Immunoregulatory factors in the pathogenesis of IgA nephropathy. *Kidney Int* 1990;38:1216–1229.
579. Waldo FB. Role of IgA in IgA nephropathy. *J Pediatr* 1990;116: S78–S85.
580. van Es LA. Pathogenesis of IgA nephropathy. *Kidney Int* 1992;41: 1720–1729.
581. Schena FP, Gesualdo L, Montinaro V. Immunopathological aspects of immunoglobulin A nephropathy and other mesangial proliferative glomerulonephritides. *J Am Soc Nephrol* 1992;2:S167–S172.
582. Williams DG. Pathogenesis of idiopathic IgA nephropathy. *Pediatr Nephrol* 1993;7:303–311.
583. Emancipator SN. IgA nephropathy: Morphologic expression and pathogenesis. *Am J Kidney Dis* 1994;23:451–462.
584. Endo Y, Kanbayashi H. Etiology of IgA nephropathy syndrome. *Pathol Int* 1994;44:1–13.
585. Ibels LS, Györy AZ. IgA nephropathy: analysis of the natural history, important factors in the progression of renal disease, and a review of the literature. *Medicine (Baltimore)* 1994;73:79–102.
586. Yoshikawa N, Nakamura H, Ito H. IgA nephropathy in children and adults. *Springer Semin Immunopathol* 1994;16:105–120.
587. Rifai A. Experimental models for IgA-associated nephritis. *Kidney Int* 1987;31:1–7.
588. Hebert LA. Disposition of IgA-containing circulating immune complexes. *Am J Kidney Dis* 1988;12:388–392.
589. Montinaro V, Gesualdo L, Schena FP. Primary IgA nephropathy: The relevance of experimental models in the understanding of human disease. *Nephron* 1992;62:373–381.
590. Emancipator SN, Rao CS, Amore A, Coppo R, Nedrud JG. Macromolecular properties that promote mesangial binding and mesangiopathic nephritis. *J Am Soc Nephrol* 1992;2:S149–S158.
591. Rifai A. Immunopathogenesis of experimental IgA nephropathy. *Springer Semin Immunopathol* 1994;16:81–95.
592. Chen A, Wei C-H, Lee W-H, Lin C-Y. Experimental IgA nephropathy: factors influencing IgA-immune complex deposition in the glomerulus. *Springer Semin Immunopathol* 1994;16:97–103.
593. Fornasieri A, D'Amico G. Experimental IgA mesangial nephropathy: the role of antigen and antibody. *Contrib Nephrol* 1995;111:149–154.
594. Rifai A, Small PA Jr, Teague PO, Ayoub EM. Experimental IgA nephropathy. *J Exp Med* 1979;150:1161–1173.
595. Brenner BM, Meyer TW, Hostetter TH. Dietary protein intake and the progressive nature of kidney disease: the role of hemodynamically mediated glomerular injury in the pathogenesis of progressive glomerular sclerosis in aging, renal ablation, and intrinsic renal disease. *N Engl J Med* 1982;307:652–659.
596. Chen A, Wong SS, Rifai A. Glomerular immune deposits in experimental IgA nephropathy. A continuum of circulating and in situ formed immune complexes. *Am J Pathol* 1988;130:216–222.
597. Montinaro V, Esparza AR, Cavallo T, Rifai A. Antigen as mediator of glomerular injury in experimental IgA nephropathy. *Lab Invest* 1991; 64:508–519.
598. Chen A, Ding S-L, Sheu L-F, Song Y-B, Shieh S-D, Shaio M-F, Chou W-Y, Ho Y-S. Experimental IgA nephropathy. Enhanced deposition of glomerular IgA immune complex in proteinuric states. *Lab Invest* 1994;70:639–647.
599. Stad RK, Bruijn JA, van Gijlswijk-Janssen DJ, van Es LA, Daha MR. An acute model for IgA-mediated glomerular inflammation in rats induced by monoclonal polymeric rat IgA antibodies. *Clin Exp Immunol* 1993;92:514–521.
600. Isaacs K, Miller F, Lane B. Experimental model for IgA nephropathy. *Clin Immunol Immunopathol* 1981;20:419–426.
601. Isaacs K, Miller F. Dextran-induced IgA nephropathy. *Contrib Nephrol* 1984;40:45–50.
602. Hirabayashi A, Hamaguchi N, Shigemoto K, Ochiai M, Okushin S,

Kobayashi M, Wada K, Yorioka N, Yamakido M, Hata J. Experimental IgA nephropathy induced by oral administration of dextran. *Hiroshima J Med Sci* 1986;35:53–58.
603. Isaacs KL, Miller F. Antigen size and charge in immune complex glomerulonephritis. II. Passive induction of immune deposits with dextran–anti-dextran immune complexes. *Am J Pathol* 1983;111:298–306.
604. Gesualdo L, Ricanati S, Hassan MO, Emancipator SN, Lamm ME. Enzymolysis of glomerular immune deposits in vivo with dextranase/protease ameliorates proteinuria, hematuria, and mesangial proliferation in murine experimental IgA nephropathy. *J Clin Invest* 1990;86;715–722.
605. Coppo R, Mazzucco G, Martina G, Roccatello D, Amore A, Novara R, Bargoni A, Piccoli G, Sena LA. Gluten-induced experimental IgA glomerulopathy. *Lab Invest* 1989;60:499–506.
606. Ward DM, Spiegelberg HL, Wilson CB. Persistence of IgA aggregates in the glomerular mesangium in mice. *Kidney Int* 1979;16:801.
607. Stad RK, Bogers WMJM, Muizert Y, Van Es LA, Daha MR. Deposition of IgA is associated with macrophage influx in the kidney of rats. *Scand J Immunol* 1991;34:81–89.
608. Dong W, Sell, JE, Pestka JJ. Quantitative assessment of mesangial immunoglobulin A (IgA) accumulation, elevated circulating IgA immune complexes, and hematuria during vomitoxin-induced IgA nephropathy. *Fund Appl Toxicol* 1991;17:197–207.
609. Rasooly L, Pestka JJ. Vomitoxin-induced dysregulation of serum IgA, IgM and IgG reactive with gut bacterial and self antigens. *Food Chem Toxicol* 1992;30:499–504.
610. Greene DM, Bondy GS, Azcona-Olivera JI, Pestke JJ. Role of gender and strain in vomitoxin-induced dysregulation of IgA production and IgA nephropathy in the mouse. *J Toxicol Environ Health* 1994;43:37–50.
611. Rasooly L, Abouzied MM, Brooks KH, Pestka JJ. Polyspecific and autoreactive IgA secreted by hybridomas derived from Peyer's patches of vomitoxin-fed mice: characterization and possible pathogenic role in IgA nephropathy. *Food Chem Toxicol* 1994;32:337–348.
612. Rasooly L, Pestka JJ. Polyclonal autoreactive IgA increase and mesangial deposition during vomitoxin-induced IgA nephropathy in the BALB/c mouse. *Food Chem Toxicol* 1994;32:329–336.
613. Imai H, Nakamoto Y, Asakura K, Miki K, Yasuda T, Miura AB. Spontaneous glomerular IgA deposition in ddY mice: An animal model of IgA nephritis. *Kidney Int* 1985;27:756–761.
614. Muso E, Yoshida H, Takeuchi E, Shimada T, Yashiro M, Sugiyama T. Pathogenic role of polyclonal and polymeric IgA in a murine model of mesangial proliferative glomerulonephritis with IgA deposition. *Clin Exp Immunol* 1991;84:459–465.
615. Takeuchi E, Doi T, Shimada T, Muso E, Maruyama N, Yoshida H. Retroviral gp70 antigen in spontaneous mesangial glomerulonephritis of ddY mice. *Kidney Int* 1989;35:638–646.
616. Wakui H, Imai H, Nakamoto Y, Kobayashi R, Itoh H, Miura AB. Anti-histone autoantibodies in ddY mice, an animal model for spontaneous IgA nephritis. *Clin Immunol Immunopathol* 1989;52:248–256.
617. Shimizu M, Tomino Y, Abe M, Shirai T, Koide H. Retroviral envelope glycoprotein (gp70) is not a prerequisite for pathogenesis of primary immunoglobulin A nephropathy in ddY mice. *Nephron* 1992;62:328–331.
618. Masuda Y, Ishizaki M, Yamanaka N, Sugisaki Y, Masugi Y. Evidence of delayed mesangial transport of human IgA in glomeruli of ddY mice pretreated with sheep anti-type IV collagen serum. *Acta Pathol Jpn* 1989;39:289–295.
619. Tomino Y, Nakamura T, Ebihara I, Funabiki K, Yaguchi Y, Shimizu M, Shirato I, Koide H. Altered steady-state levels of mRNA coding for extracellular matrices in renal tissues of ddY mice, an animal model of IgA nephropathy. *J Clin Lab Anal* 1991;5:106–113.
620. Duan HJ, Nagata T. Glomerular extracellular matrices and anionic sites in aging ddY mice: a morphometric study. *Histochemistry* 1993;99:241–249.
621. Nakamura T, Ebihara I, Nagaoka I, Tomino Y, Koide H. Renal platelet-derived growth factor gene expression in NZB/W F1 mice with lupus and ddY mice with IgA nephropathy. *Clin Immunol Immunopathol* 1992;63:173–181.
622. Tomino Y, Shimizu M, Koide H, Abe M, Shirai T. Effect of monoclonal antibody CD4 on glomerulonephritis of ddY mice, a spontaneous animal model of IgA nephropathy. *Am J Kidney Dis* 1993;21:427–432.
623. Nagasawa R, Mitarai T, Utsunomiya Y, Yoshida H, Kitamura M, Yamura W, Maruyama N, Isoda K, Sakai O. Neonatal thymectomy diminishes renal IgA deposition in IgA nephropathy-prone ddY mice. *Nephron* 1994;66:326–332.
624. Harris CH, Krawiec DR, Gelberg HB, Shapiro SZ. Canine IgA glomerulonephropathy. *Vet Immunol Immunopathol* 1993;36:1–16.
625. Jessen RH, Nedrud JG, Emancipator SN. A mouse model of IgA nephropathy induced by Sendai virus. *Adv Exp Med Biol* 1987;216B:1609–1618.
626. Jessen RH, Emancipator SN, Jacobs GH, Nedrud JG. Experimental IgA-IgG nephropathy induced by a viral respiratory pathogen. Dependence on antigen form and immune status. *Lab Invest* 1992;67:379–386.
627. Gormly AA, Smith PS, Seymour AE, Clarkson AR, Woodroffe AJ. IgA glomerular deposits in experimental cirrhosis. *Am J Pathol* 1981;104:50–54.
628. Melvin T, Burke B, Michael AF, Kim Y. Experimental IgA nephropathy in bile duct ligated rats. *Clin Immunol Immunopathol* 1983;27:369–377.
629. Woodroffe AJ, Gormly AA, Clarkson AR, Seymour AE, Lomax-Smith JD. Experimental cirrhosis and deposition of glomerular IgA immune complexes. *Contrib Nephrol* 1984;40:51–54.
630. Iida H, Izumino K, Matsumoto M, Takata M, Mizumura Y, Sugimoto T. Glomerular deposition of IgA in experimental hepatic cirrhosis. *Acta Pathol Jpn* 1985;35:561–567.
631. Russell MW, Brown TA, Mestecky J. Role of serum IgA. Hepatobiliary transport of circulating antigen. *J Exp Med* 1981;153:968–976.
632. Brown TA, Russell MW, Mestecky J. Hepatobiliary transport of IgA immune complexes: molecular and cellular aspects. *J Immunol* 1982;128:2183–2186.
633. Amore A, Coppo R, Roccatello D, Piccoli G, Mazzucco G, Gomez-Chiarri M, Lamm, ME. Experimental IgA nephropathy secondary to hepatocellular injury induced by dietary deficiencies and heavy alcohol intake. *Lab Invest* 1994;70:68–77.
634. Smith SM, Leaber R, Lefebre A, Leung MF, Baricos WH. Leung WC. Pathogenesis of IgA nephropathy in ethanol consumption: animal model and cell culture studies. *Alcohol* 1993;10:477–480.
635. Emancipator SN, Gallo GR, Razaboni R, Lamm ME. Experimental cholestasis promotes the deposition of glomerular IgA immune complexes. *Am J Pathol* 1983;113:19–26.
636. Gallo GR, Emancipator SN, Lamm ME. Experimental cholestasis and deposition of glomerular IgA immune complexes. *Contrib Nephrol* 1984;40:55–61.
637. Abramowsky CR, Christiansen DM. Secretory immunoglobulin deposits in renal glomeruli of children with extrahepatic biliary atresia: studies in a human counterpart of experimental ligation of the bile ducts. *Hum Pathol* 1987;18:1126–1131.
638. Jennette JC, Falk RJ. Antineutrophil cytoplasmic autoantibodies and associated disease: a review. *Am J Kidney Dis* 1990;15:517–529.
639. Niles JL, Pan G, Collins AB, Shannon T, Skates S, Fienberg R, Arnaout MA, McCluskey. Antigen-specific radioimmunoassays for anti-neutrophil cytoplasmic antibodies in the diagnosis of rapidly progressive glomerulonephritis. *J Am Soc Nephrol* 1991;2:27–36.
640. Kallenberg CGM, Brouwer E, Weening JJ, Cohen Tervaert JW. Anti-neutrophil cytoplasmic antibodies: current diagnostic and pathophysiological potential. *Kidney Int* 1994;46:1–15.
641. Niles JL, McCluskey RT, Ahmed MF, Arnaout MA. Wegener's granulomatosis autoantigen is a novel neutrophil serine proteinase. *Blood* 1989;74:1888–1893.
642. Goldschmeding R, van der Schoot CE, ten Bokkel Huinink D, Hack CE, van den Ende ME, Kallenberg CGM, von dem Borne AEGKr. Wegener's granulomatosis autoantibodies identify a novel diisopropylfluorophosphate-binding protein in the lysosomes of normal human neutrophils. *J Clin Invest* 1989;84:1577–1587.
643. Falk RJ, Jennette JC. Anti-neutrophil cytoplasmic autoantibodies with specificity for myeloperoxidase in patients with systemic vasculitis and idiopathic necrotizing and crescentic glomerulonephritis. *N Engl J Med* 1988;318:1651–1657.
644. Wiik A, Stummann L, Kjeldsen L, Borregaard N, Ullman S, Jacobsen S, Halberg P. The diversity of perinuclear antineutrophil cytoplasmic antibodies (pANCA) antigens. *Clin Exp Immunol* 1995;101(Suppl 1):15–17.
645. Brouwer E, Huitema MG, Leontine Mulder AH, Herringa P, van Goor H, Cohen Tervaert JW, Weening JJ, Kallenberg CGM: Neutro-

phil activation *in vitro* and *in vivo* in Wegener's granulomatosis. *Kidney Int* 1994;45:1120–1131.
646. Noronha IL, Krüger C, Andrassy K, Ritz E, Waldherr R: *In situ* production of TNF-α, IL-1β and IL-2R in ANCA-positive glomerulonephritis. *Kidney Int* 1993;43:682–692.
647. Falk RJ, Terrell RA, Charles LA, Jennette JC: Anti-neutrophil cytoplasmic autoantibodies induce neutrophils to degranulate and produce oxygen radicals in vitro. *Proc Natl Acad Sci U S A* 1990;87:4115–4119.
648. Charles LA, Caldas MLR, Falk RJ, Terrell RS, Jennette JC: Antibodies against granule proteins activate neutrophils in vitro. *J Leukoc Biol* 1991;50:539–546.
649. Ewert BH, Jennette JC, Falk RJ: Antimyeloperoxidase antibodies stimulate neutrophils to damage human endothelial cells. *Kidney Int* 1992;41:375–383.
650. Jennette JC: Pathogenic potential of anti-neutrophil cytoplasmic autoantibodies. *Lab Invest* 1994;70:135–137.
651. Kain R, Matsui K, Exner M, Binder S, Schaffner G, Sommer EM, Kerjaschki D. A novel class of autoantigens of anti-neutrophil cytoplasmic antibodies in necrotizing and crescentic glomerulonephritis: the lysosomal membrane glycoprotein h-lamp-2 in neutrophil granulocytes and a related membrane protein in glomerular endothelial cells. *J Exp Med* 1995;181:585–597.
652. Johnson RJ, Couser WG, Chi EY, Adler S, Klebanoff SJ. New mechanism for glomerular injury. Myeloperoxidase-hydrogen peroxide-halide system. *J Clin Invest* 1987;79:1379–1387.
653. Brouwer E, Weening JJ, Klok PA, Huitema MG, Cohen Tervaert JW, Kallenberg CGM. Induction of an humoral and cellular (auto) immune response to human and rat myeloperoxidase (MPO) in Brown-Norway (BN), Lewis and Wistar Kyoto (WKY) rat strains. *Adv Exp Med Biol* 1993;336:139–142.
654. Brouwer E, Huitema MG, Klok PA, de Weerd H, Cohen Tervaert, Weening JJ, Kallenberg CGM. Antimyeloperoxidase-associated proliferative glomerulonephritis: an animal model. *J Exp Med* 1993;177:905–914.
655. Kettritz R, Yang JJ, Kinjoh K, Jennette JC, Falk RJ: Animal models in ANCA-vasculitis. *Clin Exp Immunol* 1995;101(Suppl 1):12–15.
656. Brouwer E, Klok PA, Huitema MG, Weening JJ, Kallenberg CG: Renal ischemia/reperfusion injury contributes to renal damage in experimental anti-myeloperoxidase-associated proliferative glomerulonephritis. *Kidney Int* 1995;47:1121–1129.
657. Coers W, Brouwer E, Vos JT, Chand A, Huitema S, Heeringa P, Kallenberg CG, Weening JJ: Podocyte expression of MHC class I and II and intercellular adhesion molecule-1 (ICAM-1) in experimental pauci-immune crescentic glomerulonephritis. *Clin Exp Immunol* 1994;98:279–286.
658. Yang JJ, Jennette JC, Falk RJ: Immune complex glomerulonephritis is induced in rats immunized with heterologous myeloperoxidase. *Clin Exp Immunol* 1994;97:466–473.
659. Kinjoh K, Kyogoku M, Good RA: Genetic selection for crescent formation yields mouse strain with rapidly progressive glomerulonephritis and small vessel vasculitis. *Proc Natl Acad Sci U S A* 1993;90:3413–3417.
660. Mathieson PW, Thiru S, Oliveira DBG: Mercuric chloride-treated Brown Norway rats develop widespread tissue injury including necrotizing vasculitis. *Lab Invest* 1992;67:121–129.
661. Esnault VL, Mathieson PW, Thiru S, Oliveira DBG, Lockwood CM: Autoantibodies to myeloperoxidase in Brown Norway Rats treated with mercuric chloride. *Lab Invest* 1992;67:114–120.
662. Qasim FJ, Mathieson PW, Thiru S, Oliveira DB, Lockwood CM: Further characterization of an animal model of systemic vasculitis. *Adv Exp Med Biol* 1993;336:133–137.
663. Kobayashi K, Shibata T, Sugisaki T: Aggravation of rat Masugi nephritis by heterologous anti-rat myeloperoxidase (MPO) antibody. *Clin Exp Immunol* 1993;93(Suppl 1):20.
664. Moake JL, Rudy CK, Troll JH, Weinstein MJ, Colannino NM, Azocar J, Seder RH, Hong SL, Deykin D. Unusually large plasma factor VIII: von Willebrand factor multimers in chronic relapsing thrombotic thrombocytopenic purpura. *N Engl J Med* 1982;307:1432–1435.
665. Asada Y, Sumiyoshi A, Hayashi T, Suzumiya J, Kaketani K. Immunohistochemistry of vascular lesion in thrombotic thrombocytopenic purpura. *Thromb Res* 1985;38:469–479.
666. Moake JL, McPherson PD. von Willebrand factor in thrombotic thrombocytopenic purpura and the hemolytic-uremic syndrome. *Transfus Med Rev* 1990;4:163–168.
667. Bloom AL. von Willebrand factor: Clinical features of inherited and acquired disorders. *Mayo Clin Proc* 1991;66:743–751.
668. Remuzzi G, Misiani R, Mecca G, de Gaetano G, Donati MB. Thrombotic thrombocytopenic purpura—a deficiency of plasma factor regulating platelet-vessel-wall interaction. *N Engl J Med* 1978;299:311.
669. Defreyn G, Proesmans W, Machin SJ, Lemmens F, Vermylen J. Abnormal prostacyclin metabolism in hemolytic uremic syndrome: Equivocal effect of prostacyclin infusions. *Clin Nephrol* 1982;18:43–49.
670. Walters MD, Levin M, Smith C, Nokes TJ, Hardisty RM, Dillon MJ, Barratt TM. Intravascular platelet activation in the hemolytic uraemic syndrome. *Kidney Int* 1988;33:107–115.
671. Leung DYM, Moake JL, Havens PL, Kim M, Pober JS. Lytic anti-endothelial cell antibodies in haemolytic-uremic syndrome. *Lancet* 1988;2:183–186.
672. Dillon MJ, Tizard EJ. Anti-neutrophil cytoplasmic antibodies and anti-endothelial cell antibodies. *Pediatr Nephrol* 1991;5:256–259.
673. Bergstein JM, Riley M, Bang NU. Role of plasminogen-activator inhibitor type 1 in the pathogenesis and outcome of the hemolytic uremic syndrome. *N Engl J Med* 1992;327:755–759.
674. Louise CB, Obrig TG. Human renal microvascular endothelial cells as a potential target in the development of the hemolytic uremic syndrome as related to fibrinolysis factor expression, *in vitro*. *Microvasc Res* 1994;47:377–387.
675. Menzel D, Levi M, Dooijewaard G, Peters M, ten Cate JW. Impaired fibrinolysis in the hemolytic-uremic syndrome of childhood. *Ann Hematol* 1994;68:43–48.
676. Fitzpatrick MM, Shah V, Trompeter RS, Dillon MJ, Barratt TM. Interleukin-8 and polymorphoneutrophil leucocyte activation in hemolytic uremic syndrome. *Kidney Int* 1992;42:951–956.
677. Wada H, Kaneko T, Ohiwa M, Tanigawa M, Tamaki S, Minami N, Takahashi H, Deguchi K, Nakano T, Shirakawa S. Plasma cytokine levels in thrombotic thrombocytopenic purpura. *Am J Hematol* 1992;40:167–170.
678. Katayama M, Handa M, Araki Y, Ambo H, Kawai Y, Watanabe K, Ikeda Y. Soluble P-selectin is present in normal circulation and its plasma level is elevated in patients with thrombotic thrombocytopenic purpura and haemolytic uremic syndrome. *Brit J Haematol* 1993;84:702–710.
679. Robson WLM, Leung AKC, Fick GH, McKenna AI. Hypocomplementemia and leukocytosis in diarrhea-associated hemolytic uremic syndrome. *Nephron* 1992;62:296–299.
680. Richardson SE, Karmali MA, Becker LE, Smith CR. The histopathology of the hemolytic uremic syndrome associated with verocytotoxin-producing *Escherichia coli* infections. *Human Path* 1988;19:1102–1108.
681. Ashkenazi S. Role of bacterial cytotoxins in hemolytic uremic syndrome and thrombotic thrombocytopenic purpura. *Annu Rev Med* 1993;44:11–18.
682. Pickering LK, Obrig TG, Stapleton FB. Hemolytic-uremic syndrome and enterohemorrhagic *Escherichia coli*. *Pediatr Infect Dis J* 1994;13:459–476.
683. Boyce TG, Swerdlow DL, Griffin PM. *Escherichia coli* O157:H7 and the hemolytic-uremic syndrome. *N Engl J Med* 1995;333:364–368.
684. O'Brien AD, Tesh VL, Donohue-Rolfe A, Jackson MP, Olsnes S, Sandvig K, Lindberg AA, Keusch GT. Shiga toxin: Biochemistry, genetics, mode of action, and role in pathogenesis. *Cur Top Microbiol Immunol* 1992;180:65–94.
685. Lingwood CA. Verotoxins and their glycolipid receptors. Review. *Adv Lipid Res* 1993;25:189–211.
686. Lingwood CA. Verotoxin-binding in human renal sections. *Nephron* 1994;66:21–28.
687. Abbas AK, Lichtman AH, Pober JS. *Cellular and Molecular Immunology*. Philadelphia: WB Saunders, 1991;225–243.
688. Shultz PJ, Raij L. Endogenously synthesized nitric oxide prevents endotoxin-induced glomerular thrombosis. *J Clin Invest* 1992;90:1718–1725.
689. Feng L, Tang WW, Loskutoff DJ, Wilson CB. Dysfunction of glomerular fibrinolysis in experimental antiglomerular basement membrane antibody glomerulonephritis. *J Am Soc Nephrol* 1993;3:1753–1764.
690. Hiromura K, Hayashi J, Tsukada Y, Ono K, Tsuchida A, Yano S, Naruse T. FK506 inhibits renal glomerular thrombosis induced in rats by nephrotoxic serum and lipopolysaccharide. *Kidney Int* 1994;45:1572–1579.

691. Cattell V. Mitomycin-induced hemolytic uremic kidney. An experimental model in the rat. *Am J Pathol* 1985;121:88–95.
692. van de Kar NCAJ, Monnens LAH, Karmali MA, van Hinsbergh VWM. Tumor necrosis factor and interleukin-1 induce expression of the verocytotoxin receptor globotriaosylceramide on human endothelial cells: Implications for the pathogenesis of the hemolytic uremic syndrome. *Blood* 1992;80:2755–2764.
693. Obrig TG, Louise CB, Lingwood CA, Boyd B, Barley-Maloney L, Daniel TO. Endothelial heterogeneity in Shiga toxin receptors and responses. *J Biol Chem* 1993;268:15484–15488.
694. Louis CB, Obrig TG. Shiga toxin-associated hemolytic uremic syndrome: Combined cytotoxic effects of Shiga toxin and lipopolysaccharide. *Infect Immun* 1992;60:1536–1543.
695. Kaye SA, Louise CB, Boyd B, Lingwood CA, Obrig TG. Shiga toxin-associated hemolytic uremic syndrome: interleukin-1β enhancement of Shiga toxin cytotoxicity toward human vascular endothelial cells in vitro. *Infect Immun* 1993;61:3886–3891.
696. Richardson SE, Rotman TA, Jay V, Smith CRD, Becker LE, Petric M, Olivieri NF, Marmali MA. Experimental verocytotoxemia in rabbits. *Infect Immun* 1992;60:4154–4167.
697. Pai CH, Kelly JK, Meyers GL. Experimental infection of infant rabbits with a verotoxin-producing Escherichia coli. *Infect Immun* 1986; 51:16–23.
698. Keenan KP, Sharpnack DD, Collins H, Formal SB, O'Brein AD. Morphologic evaluation of the effects of Shiga toxin and E coli shiga-like toxin on the rabbit intestine. *Am J Pathol* 1986;125:69–80.
699. Tzipori S, Chow CW, Powell HR. Cerebral infection with Escherichia coli o157:H7 in humans and gnotobiotic piglets. *J Clin Pathol* 1988;41:1099–1103.
700. Zoja C, Corna D, Farina C, Sacchi G, Lingwood C, Doyle MP, Padhye VVV, Abbate M, Remuzzi G: Verotoxin glycolipid receptors determine the localization of microangiopathic processes in rabbits given verotoxin-1. *J Lab Clin Med* 1992;120:229–238.
701. Harel Y, Silva M, Giroir B, Weinberg A, Cleary TB, Beutler B. A reporter transgene indicates renal-specific induction of tumor necrosis factor (TNF) by Shiga-like toxin. Possible involvement of TNF in hemolytic uremic syndrome. *J Clin Invest* 1993;92:2110–2116.
702. Wadolkowski EA, Sung LM, Burris JA, Samuel JE, O'Brien AD. Acute renal tubular necrosis and death of mice orally infected with Escherichia coli strains that produce Shiga-like toxin type II. *Infect Immun* 1990;58:3959–3965.
703. Tesh VL, Burris JA, Owens JW, Gordon VM, Wadolkowski EA, O'Brein AD, Samuel JE. Comparison of the relative toxicities of Shiga-like toxins type I and type II in mice. *Infect Immun* 1993;61: 3392–3402.
704. Siegler RL, Taylor FB Jr, Tesh VL, Edwin SS, Cook JB, Dudley DJ. The endothelin-nitric oxide axis in a primate model of shiga-like toxin induced hemolytic uremic syndrome. *J Am Soc Nephrol* 1995;6:989.
705. Angus KW, Gardiner AC, Sykes AR, Davidson AM. A rapidly progressing mesangio-capillary glomerulonephritis in Finnish Landrace lambs. *Vet Rec* 1973;92:337–338.
706. Frelier PF, Pritchard J, Armstrong DL, Nagge WT, Lewis RM. Spontaneous mesangiocapillary glomerulonephritis in Finn cross lambs from Alberta. *Can J Comp Med* 1984;48:215–218.
707. Spitzer RE, Stitzel AE, Tsokos GC. Study of the idiotypic response in autoantibody to the alternative pathway C3/C5 convertase in normal individuals, patients with membranoproliferative glomerulonephritis, and experimental animals. *Clin Immunol Immunopathol* 1992;62: 291–294.
708. Stark H, Alkalay A, Ben-Bassat M, Hazaz B, Joshua H. Levan-induced glomerulitis in rabbits: a possible role for direct complement activation in situ. *Br J Exp Pathol* 1985;66:165–171.
709. Blum JR, Cork LC, Morris JM, Olson JL, Winkelstein JA. The clinical manifestations of a genetically determined deficiency of the third component of complement in the dog. *Clin Immunol Immunopathol* 1985;34:304–315.
710. Cork LC, Morris JM, Olson JL, Krakowka S, Swift AJ, Winkelstein JA. Membranoproliferative glomerulonephritis in dogs with a genetically determined deficiency of the third component of complement. *Clin Immunol Immunopathol* 1991;60:455–470.
711. Johnson RJ. The glomerular response to injury: Progression or resolution? *Kidney Int* 1994;45:1769–1782.
712. Olson JL, Heptinstall RH. Nonimmunologic mechanisms of glomerular injury. *Lab Invest* 1988;59:564–578.
713. Neuringer JR, Brenner BM. Hemodynamic theory of progressive renal disease: A 10-year update in brief review. *Am J Kidney Dis* 1993;22:98–104.
714. Striker GE, Peten EP, Yang CW, Striker LJ. Glomerulosclerosis: Studies of its pathogenesis in humans and animals. *Contrib Nephrol* 1994;107:124–131.
715. Provoost AP. Spontaneous glomerulosclerosis: Insights from the fawn-hooded rat. *Kidney Int* 1994;45(suppl 45):S2–S5.
716. Yoshida F, Matsuo S, Fujishima H, Kim H-K, Tomita T. Renal lesions of the FGS strain of mice: A spontaneous animal model of progressive glomerulosclerosis. *Nephron* 1994;66:317–325.
717. Neugarten J, Feiner HD, Schacht RG, Gallo GR, Baldwin DS. Aggravation of experimental glomerulonephritis by superimposed clip hypertension. *Kidney Int* 1982;22:257–263.
718. Neugarten J, Kaminetsky B, Feiner H, Schacht RG, Liu DT, Baldwin DS. Nephrotoxic serum nephritis with hypertension: Amelioration by antihypertensive therapy. *Kidney Int* 1985;28:135–139.
719. Blantz RC, Gabbai F, Gushwa LC, Wilson CB. The influence of concomitant experimental hypertension and glomerulonephritis. *Kidney Int* 1987;32:652–663.
720. Gabbai FB, De Nicola L, Thomson SC, Peterson OW, Tucker BJ, Keiser JA, Wilson CB, Blantz RC. Effect of chronic converting enzyme inhibitor (CEI) in rats with chronic glomerulonephritis with (GC) and without hypertension (G). *J Am Soc Nephrol* 1991;2:678.
721. Raij L, Azar S, Keane WF. Role of hypertension in progressive glomerular immune injury. *Hypertension* 1985;7:398–404.
722. Stein HD, Sterzel RB, Hunt JD, Pabst R, Kashgarian M. No aggravation of the course of experimental glomerulonephritis in spontaneously hypertensive rats. *Am J Pathol* 1986;122:520–530.
723. Adler S, Chen X. Anti-Fx1A antibody recognizes a β_1-integrin on glomerular epithelial cells and inhibits adhesion and growth. *Am J Physiol* 1992;262:F770–F776.
724. Weiher H, Noda T, Gray DA, Sharpe AH, Jaenisch R. Transgenic mouse model of kidney disease: Insertional inactivation of ubiquitously expressed gene leads to nephrotic syndrome. *Cell* 1990;62: 425–434.
725. Doi T, Striker LJ, Quaife C, Conti FG, Palmiter R, Behringer R, Brinster R, Striker GE. Progressive glomerulosclerosis develops in transgenic mice chronically expressing growth hormone and growth hormone releasing factor but not in those expressing insulinlike growth factor-1. *Am J Pathol* 1988;131:398–403.
726. Quaife CJ, Mathews LS, Pinkert CA, Hammer RE, Brinster RL, Palmiter RD. Histopathology associated with elevated levels of growth hormone and insulin-like growth factor 1 in transgenic mice. *Endocrinology* 1989;124:40–48.
727. Suematsu S, Matsuda T, Aozasa K, Akira S, Nakano N, Ohno S, Miyazaki J-I, Yamamura K-I, Hirano T, Kishimoto T. IgG1 plasmacytosis in interleukin 6 transgenic mice. *Proc Natl Acad Sci U S A* 1989;86:7547–7551.
728. Peten EP, Yang C-W, Striker GE, Striker LJ. Gene activation in glomerulosclerosis: A role for growth promoting hormones. *Kidney Int* 1994;45(suppl 45):S48–S50.
729. Fattori E, Della Rocca C, Costa P, Giorgio M, Dente B, Pozzi L, Ciliberto G. Development of progressive kidney damage and myeloma kidney in interleukin-6 transgenic mice. *Blood* 1994;83: 2570–2579.
730. Springate JE, Feld LG, Ganten D. Renal function in hypertensive rats transgenic for mouse renin gene. *Am J Physiol* 1994;266:F731–F737.
731. MacKay K, Striker LJ, Pinkert CA, Brinster RL, Striker GE. Glomerulosclerosis and renal cysts in mice transgenic for the early region of SV40. *Kidney Int* 1987;32:827–837.
732. Dickie P, Felser J, Eckhaus M, Bryant J, Silver J, Marinos N, Notkins AL. HIV-associated nephropathy in transgenic mice expressing HIV-1 genes. *Virology* 1991;185:109–119.
733. Kopp JB, Klotman ME, Adler SH, Bruggeman LA, Dickie P, Marinos NJ, Eckhaus M, Bryant JL, Notkins AL, Klotman PE. Progressive glomerulosclerosis and enhanced renal accumulation of basement membrane components in mice transgenic for human immunodeficiency virus type 1 genes. *Proc Natl Acad Sci U S A* 1992;89: 1577–1581.
734. Ray PE, Bruggeman LA, Weeks BS, Kopp JB, Bryant JL, Owens JW, Notkins AL, Klotman PE. bFGF and its low affinity receptors in the pathogenesis of HIV-associated nephropathy in transgenic mice. *Kidney Int* 1994;46:759–772.

735. Weiher H. Glomerular sclerosis in transgenic mice: The *Mpv*-17 gene and its human homologue. *Adv Nephrol* 1993;22:37–42.
736. Isaka Y, Fujiwara Y, Ueda N, Kaneda Y, Kamada T, Imai E. Glomerulosclerosis induced by in vivo transfection of transforming growth factor-β or platelet-derived growth factor gene into the rat kidney. *J Clin Invest* 1993;92:2597–2601.
737. Gresham HD, Ray CJ, O'Sullivan FX. Defective neutrophil function in the autoimmune mouse strain MRL/*lpr*. Potential role of transforming growth factor-β_1. *J Immunol* 1991;146:3911–3921.
738. Shull MM, Ormsby I, Kier AB, Pawlowski S, Diebold RJ, Yin M, Allen R, Sidman C, Proetzel G, Calvin D, Annunziata N, Doetschman T. Targeted disruption of the mouse transforming growth factor-β_1 gene results in multifocal inflammatory disease. *Nature* 1992;359:693–699.
739. Kulkarni AB, Huh C-G, Becker D, Geiser A, Lyght M, Flanders KC, Roberts AB, Sporn MB, Ward JM, Karlsson S. Transforming growth factors-β_1 null mutation in mice causes excessive inflammatory response and early death. *Proc Natl Acad Sci U S A* 1993;90:770–774.
740. Kulkarni AB, Karlsson S. Transforming growth factor-β_1 knockout mice. A mutation in one cytokine gene causes a dramatic inflammatory disease. *Am J Pathol* 1993;143:3–9.
741. Wahl SM. Transforming growth factor β: The good, the bad, and the ugly. *J Exp Med* 1994;180:1587–1590.
742. Sanderson N, Factor V, Nagy P, Kopp J, Kondaiah P, Wakefield L, Roberts AB, Sporn MB, Thorgeirsson SS. Hepatic expression of mature transforming growth factor β1 in transgenic mice results in multiple tissue lesions. *Proc Natl Acad Sci U S A* 1995;92:2572–2576.
743. Kollias G, Evans DJ, Ritter M, Beech J, Morris R, Grosveld F. Ectopic expression of Thy-1 in the kidneys of transgenic mice induces functional and proliferative abnormalities. *Cell* 1987;51:21–31.
744. Lo D, Quill H, Burkly L, Scott B, Palmiter RD, Brinster RL. A recessive defect in lymphocyte or granulocyte function caused by an integrated transgene. *Am J Pathol* 1992;141:1237–1246.
745. Simonet WS, Hughes TM, Nguyen HQ,Trebasky LD, Danilenko DM. Long-term impaired neutrophil migration in mice overexpressing human interleukin-8. *J Clin Invest* 1994;94:1310–1319.
746. Danoff TM, Cook DN, Neilson EG, Kalluri R. Murine anti-α3(IV) collagen disease is abrograted in MIP-1α deficient mice. *J Am Soc Nephrol* 1995;6:827.
747. Campbell RD, Milner CM. MHC genes in autoimmunity. *Curr Opin Immunol* 1993;5:887–893.
748. Miller JF, Flavell RA. T-cell tolerance and autoimmunity in transgenic models of central and peripheral tolerance. *Curr Opin Immunol* 1994;6:892–899.
749. Meyers CM. T-cell regulation of renal immune responses. *Curr Opin Nephrol Hyperten* 1995;4:270–276.
750. Shlomchik MJ, Madaio MP, Ni D, Trounstein M, Huszar D. The role of B cells in *lpr/lpr*-induced autoimmunity. *J Exp Med* 1994;180: 1295-1306.
751. Merino R, Iwamoto M, Fossati L, Muniesa P, Araki K, Takahashi S, Huarte J, Yamamura K-I, Vassalli J-D, Izui S. Prevention of systemic lupus erythematosus in autoimmune BXSB mice by a transgene encoding I-E α chain. *J Exp Med* 1993;178:1189–1197.
752. Song YW, Tsao BP, Hahn BH. Contribution of major histocompatibility complex (MHC) to upregulation of anti-DNA antibody in transgenic mice. *J Autoimmun* 1993;1:1–9.
753. Dang H, Geiser AG, Letterio JJ, Nakabayashi T, Kong L, Fernandes G, Talal N. SLE-like autoantibodies and Sjogren's syndrome-like lymphoproliferation in TGF-beta knockout mice. *J Immunol* 1995; 155:3205–3212.
754. Hagerty DT, Allen PM. Processing and presentation of self and foreign antigens by the renal proximal tubule. *J Immunol* 1992;148: 2324–2330.
755. Mendrick DL, Kelly DM, Rennke HG. Antigen processing and presentation by glomerular visceral epithelium in vitro. *Kidney Int* 1991; 39:71–78.
756. Jevnikar AM, Singer GG, Coffman T, Glimcher LH, Kelley VE. Transgenic tubular cell expression of class II is insufficient to initiate immune renal injury. *J Am Soc Nephrol* 1993;3:1972–1977.
757. Nabel EG, Gordon D, Yang ZY, Xu L, San H., Plautz GE, Wu BY, Gao X, Huang L, Nabel GJ. Gene transfer in vivo with DNA-liposome complexes: Lack of autoimmunity and gonadal localization. *Hum Gene Ther* 1992;3:649–656.
758. Tomita N, Higaki J, Morishita R, Kato K, Mikami H, Kaneda Y, Ogihara T. Direct in vivo gene introduction into rat kidney. *Biochem Biophys Res Commun* 1992;186:129–134.
759. Yamada T, Horiuchi M, Morishita R, Zhang L, Pratt RE, Dzau VJ. In vivo identification of a negative regulatory element in the mouse renin gene using direct gene transfer. *J Clin Invest* 1995;96: 1230–1237.
760. Woolf AS, Bosch RJ, Fine LG. Gene transfer into the mammalian kidney: First steps towards renal gene therapy. *Kidney Int* 1993;39: S116–S119.
761. Kitamura M, Taylor S, Unwin R, Burton S, Shimizu F, Fine LG. Gene transfer into the rat renal glomerulus via a mesangial cell vector: Site-specific delivery, in situ amplification, and sustained expression of an exogenous gene in vivo. *J Clin Invest* 1994;94: 497–505.
762. Moullier P, Friedlander G, Calise D, Ronco P, Perridaudet M, Ferry N. Adenoviral-mediated gene transfer to renal tubular cells in vivo. *Kidney Int* 1994;45:1220–1225.

Immunologic Renal Diseases,
edited by E. G. Neilson and W. G. Couser.
Lippincott-Raven Publishers, Philadelphia © 1997.

CHAPTER 36

Immune Models of Tubulointerstitial Injury

Curtis B. Wilson

Tubulointerstitial renal lesions are increasingly recognized as contributors to renal failure, with the relationship between tubulointerstitial fibrosis and the loss of renal function a major focus of study (1,2). The tubular injury and fibrosis may be the sequelae of immune glomerular injury or the result of primary tubular injury, such as the result of an immune tubulointerstitial lesion as well as vascular, metabolic, drug, or toxic insults (3–7). Although a specific immune process has not been defined in many of the latter causes of injury, infiltration of monocytes/macrophages and lymphocytes suggests that the mediation of the progressive injury, if not specifically "immune," may be similar, involving the effects of these inflammatory cells on processes that foster progressive injury and fibrosis. Discussions of the mediator pathways of the injury and tubulointerstitial fibrosis are the subject of review (8–13).

Model systems of immune tubular injury, as with the study of glomerular immune disease, have provided our current level of understanding of the mechanisms of induction and mediation of tubulointerstitial nephritis (TIN) (14–19). In TIN, as in glomerulonephritis (GN), groupings of endogenous structural or cellular Ags as well as exogenous Ags have been identified in induced or spontaneous development of TIN. Humoral and cellular immune processes direct the selectivity of the immune attack, which is magnified by immune mediator systems. The models allow both acute inflammatory and more chronic, progressive, and sclerosing stages of injury to be investigated. Various segments of the nephron and regions of the tubulointerstitial tissue can be the focus of the immune attack. Human examples of some models are known, whereas the relationship to known human disease is less obvious in others. In turn, much of human TIN is not clearly related to a particular model; however, the features of the inflammatory process of human TIN can be mimicked for detailed study, including its functional effects (20).

In a general way, the same types of immune processes that initiate injury to glomeruli have also been identified in TIN (Table 1). The accessibility of tubular cell-associated antigens (Ags) may be less than in the glomerulus, in which both the glomerular basement membrane (GBM) and the mesangium have direct contact with the vascular compartment. In contrast, the basal aspect of the tubular cells is separated from the vascular compartment by the peritubular capillary and the tubular basement membrane (TBM). The peritubular capillary endothelium is fenestrated, and tracers such as catalase (240 kD) and ferritin (500 kD) can penetrate into the interstitium rather freely,

TABLE 1. *Models of immune tubular injury*

Models associated with antibasement membrane Ab
Anti-GBM/TBM models
Anti-TBM models
Drug-associated anti-TBM Abs
Spontaneous anti-TBM Abs
Models of immune deposit formation
Soluble circulating Ags
Arthus reaction
Planted Ags
Other tubular materials, i.e., infectious Ags
Models involving renal tubular cell Ags
Brush-border Ags
Tamm-Horsfall Ags
Other tubular Ags?
Models of predominant cellular immunity
Delayed-type hypersensitivy reaction
Infectious Ags
Tubular Ags
Toxin-induced models
Spontaneous TIN
Models in which immune mediator pathways may induce injury

Department of Immunology, The Scripps Research Institute, La Jolla, California 92037.

including the basal infoldings of tubular cells except those of the proximal tubule (21). Basolateral endocytosis of protein by isolated perfused proximal tubules is reported, however (22).

The luminal aspect of the tubular cell can be reached by molecules that pass through the glomerular filter or are produced by the tubular cells themselves. The glomerular filter normally excludes cells and most immunoglobulin (Ig) molecules from the tubular fluid. In contrast to the makeup of the GBM, the TBM appears to have regional differences in antigenicity, probably related to compositional variations relative to its functional requirements. For example, the TBM Ag of guinea pig or rat anti-TBM antibody (Ab) TIN is confined to the cortical TBM and does not extend into Bowman's capsule. The Heymann nephritis Ag complex is localized to the brush border of proximal tubular cells, whereas the Tamm-Horsfall protein is present normally only in the ascending limb of the loop of Henle and the distal nephron. Models involving these Ags, in turn, focus on the areas in which the Ags are located.

ANTI-GBM/TBM AB- AND ANTI-TBM AB-ASSOCIATED DISEASES

The Problem in Humans

At least two patterns of anti-TBM Ab reactivity, presumably related to two different Ag systems, are found in patients. In one, the anti-TBM Ab is part of a larger anti-GBM, TBM, alveolar basement membrane (ABM), etc., reaction, as seen in antibasement membrane Ab diseases such as Goodpasture's syndrome. The Ag is believed to be in the noncollagenous C-terminal (NC1) region of the $\alpha 3$ chain of type IV collagen and its distribution among basement membranes varies (23–25). In the other pattern, the anti-TBM Ab reactivity is confined largely to the TBM, although in some instances other basement membranes, such as the intestinal basement membrane, may be involved. An example of the first type of anti-TBM Ab is that identified in about 70% of patients with anti-GBM Ab disease (26–28). In these patients, at least two patterns of TBM reactivity are found among the anti-GBM/-TBM Abs. In one, the Abs react with only a portion of tubules in a cross section by indirect immunofluorescence, compared with others that are more diffusely reactive. This varied reactivity suggests that quantitative or qualitative differences in anti-TBM Ab or its Ag may be involved. In those individuals with anti-GBM Ab disease who have added anti-TBM reactivity, increased tubulointerstitial inflammation has been reported, although TIN is overshadowed by the rapidly progressive glomerular lesion, at least early on in the disease (29).

Anti-TBM reactions alone are found infrequently to be primary (linear TBM deposits of Ig and circulating anti-TBM Abs are present without evidence of glomerular disease) (30–34). More commonly, although still infrequently, the anti-TBM Abs are associated with some form of non-anti-GBM Ab-associated glomerular disease, perhaps with tubular dysfunction, such as Fanconi syndrome. Anti-TBM Abs have been seen late in the course of poststreptococcal GN (35), in children with presumed immune complex (IC) forms of glomerular injury (36–39), and occasionally in systemic lupus erythematosus (SLE) (40). In one infant with intractable diarrhea and anti-TBM Abs associated with severe membranous glomerulopathy, antijejunal basement membrane Abs in addition to anti-TBM Abs were identified in renal eluates (Wilson CB, *unpublished observations*). Anti-TBM Abs are reported in a patient with nephrotic syndrome and celiac disease, possibly in villous atrophy of the small intestine, and in a patient with oxalosis and chronic TIN associated with an intestinal bypass (37, 41,42).

Anti-TBM Abs can also infrequently complicate drug-related forms of TIN (43,44), sometimes being associated with methicillin (45,46)-, phenytoin (47)-, and possibly allopurinol (48)-related TIN. Drug breakdown products bind to TBM and may serve as in hapten-carrier mechanisms of Ab formation, leading to Abs reactive with the TBM (46,47). The most frequent occurrence of anti-TBM Abs is in renal transplant recipients, although their nephritogenic contribution to the chronic inflammation often associated with a transplant is unclear (49,50). The anti-TBM Abs can form in response to allogenic differences in TBM Ags between donor and recipient (51). More commonly, no allogenic differences are detected, and the mechanism responsible for induction of an anti-TBM response in the immunosuppressed posttransplant recipient is undefined. Anti-TBM Abs associated with the patient's primary disease can also sometimes be detected after renal transplantation (39,52,53).

Models of Anti-GBM/TBM and Anti-TBM Ab-Associated TIN

The two major categories of anti-TBM Ab identified in humans have been studied experimentally. One is typified by the combined GBM, TBM, and other basement membrane reactivities seen in heterologous anti-GBM Abs. The other is the predominant anti-TBM reactivity seen in autoimmune models of anti-TBM Ab-associated TIN. In the latter, the reactive Ags are confined to segments of the TBM with expression genetically determined, at least in rats and humans. In rats, the GBM/TBM Ag system appears to be shared by all strains; however, the selective TBM Ag is strain-related, and the different strains can be designated *TBM* Ag^{+} and *TBM* Ag^{-}.

Models Involving Autoimmune and Heterologous Anti-GBM/TBM Abs

Autoimmune models of anti-GBM/TBM Ab-associated GN or TIN/GN Abs have been induced by immunization with homologous GBM/TBM (54) or heterologous GBM Ags (55), respectively. The latter model also has evidence of lung lesions. The presence of glomerular injury complicates the study of tubulointerstitial injury, even though a TIN is prominent early in the former model. It is unclear whether both the GBM/TBM and TBM Ag systems are involved in this model. Anti-GBM/TBM Abs can also be induced in rats given mercuric chloride (see Chapter 35), with GN the predominant problem (56). Lewis (LEW) rats immunized with BN renal basement membrane (RBM) to induce a granulomatous interstitial lesion (see later) can develop anti-GBM/TBM Abs in addition to anti-TBM Abs (57).

Anti-TBM Ab reactivity is typically found in heterologous anti-GBM Abs used for induction of experimental models of GN (see Chapter 35). Although these Abs react strongly with GBM, TBM, and ABM in vitro (indirect immunofluorescence, etc.), when given in vivo, they fix poorly to TBM or ABM, usually with only weak, focal TBM fixation at most (Fig. 1). This relative lack of fixation is probably related, in part, to absorption by GBM and to accessibility of the circulating Ab to the TBM or ABM Ags. The in vivo anti-ABM reaction, for example, is favored by local events that alter pulmonary anatomic barriers, such as induced oxygen, hydrocarbon, or cytokine toxicity in the lung (58–61). The focal TBM binding is favored by increasing the amount of Ab administered; it also seems to vary among heterologous anti-GBM Ab preparations. For example, comparison of anti-rabbit "GBM" or "TBM" Abs revealed GBM and TBM reactions in both but greater tubular fixation and involvement in rabbits receiving the "anti-TBM" antiserum, although tubular changes were found after either preparation (32).

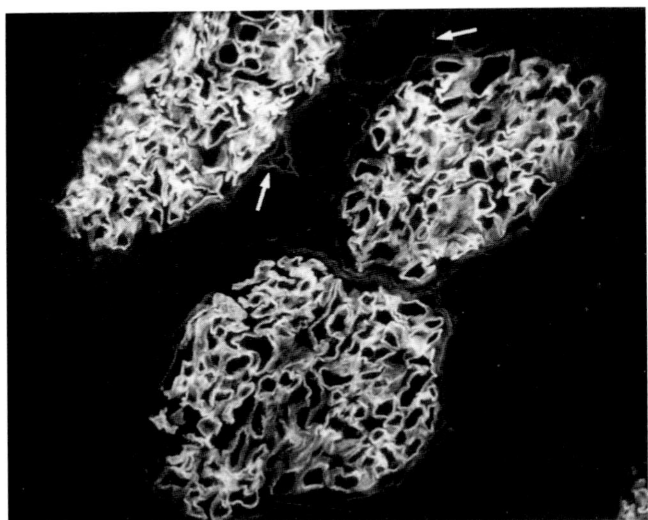

FIG. 1. Intravenous administration of a typical rabbit anti-rat glomerular basement membrane (anti-GBM/TBM) Ab to a rat results in intense Ig fixation to the GBM in a continuous linear distribution along the GBM and faint linear binding to the TBM of some renal tubules, particularly those adjacent to glomeruli (*arrows*). This same Ab would bind strongly to the TBM of sections of normal rat kidney when studied by indirect immunofluorescence, hence its designation as *anti-GBM/TBM* (see text). GBM, glomerular basement membrane; TBM, tubular basement membrane; Ab, antibody.

Tubulointerstitial inflammation observed in models of GN induced by anti-GBM/TBM Abs is associated with focal fixation of anti-TBM Abs (62). The Ab deposit is accompanied by neutrophil and monocyte/macrophage accumulation at 24 hours, which increases between 3 and 7 days as a mononuclear infiltrate with monocytes/macrophages and some cytotoxic lymphocytes. The interstitial lesion is reported to be C-independent, based on C depletion studies using cobra venom, and not part of the autologous phase of injury, in which the recipient forms Abs that are reactive with the renal-bound heterologous Ig.

Models Involving Autoimmune Anti-TBM Abs

Autoimmune models of TIN in guinea pigs, rats, and mice are characterized by the production and tubular fixation of anti-TBM Abs (Fig. 2). These models are induced by immunization with homologous or heterologous TBM, less purified fractions of kidney homogenate (with adjuvants), or, in some instances, with passive transfer of Ab or immune cells from immunized donors. The models form the basis for much of what is known regarding the immunopathogenesis of anti-TBM Ab TIN in humans. In the different species, varying contributions of humoral (Ab) and cellular (effector T cell) immune mechanisms have been identified, which allows relatively selective study of the two immune mechanisms.

Models in Guinea Pigs

Experimentally, anti-TBM Ab-associated TIN was first induced in guinea pigs in 1971 by immunization with rabbit renal cortical basement membrane in adjuvants (63) and subsequently with bovine (Bov) TBM (64). The interstitial lesion was characterized by a striking mononuclear infiltrate, giant cell formation, and tubular dysfunction (glycosuria). The giant cells were reported to contact the TBM, with suggestions of perforation and phagocytosis of TBM fragments (65). Anti-GBM and anti-ABM Abs (63,64,66) were also present, but neither GN nor lung injury was a prominent feature of the model. In guinea pigs immunized with Bov TBM, the

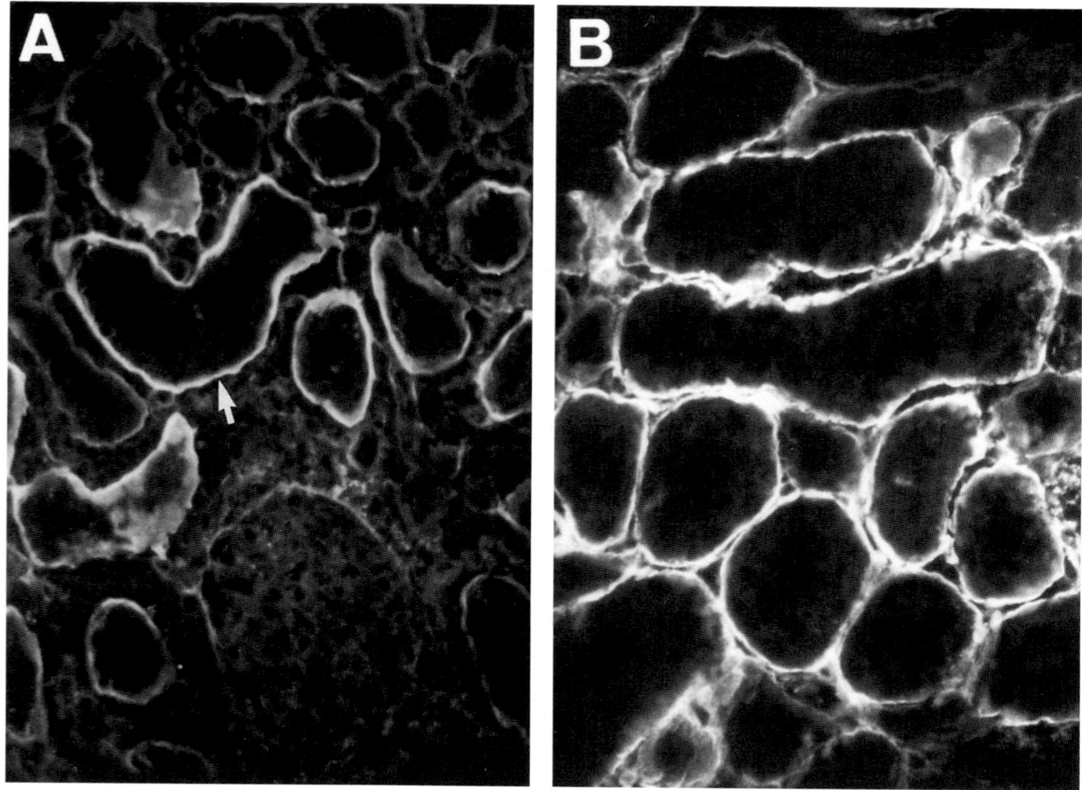

FIG. 2. Circumferential linear deposits of Ig (*arrow*), beginning about 7 days after immunization, are observed along the TBMs of TBM Ag^+ rats immunized with heterologous TBM (*Bov*) in adjuvants (**A**). The tubules are spread apart by the extensive interstitial inflammatory cell infiltration associated with the Ab binding. The anti-TBM Ab reactivity of the Ig can be confirmed by using Ig eluted from an involved kidney [such as that in (**A**)], as shown in the indirect immunofluorescence study using a normal TBM Ag^+ BN kidney section (**B**).

nephritogenic anti-TBM Abs reacted with noncollagenous portions of the TBM, whereas the minimally nephritogenic anti-GBM Abs were reactive with collagenous determinants (64); nephritogenic anti-GBM Abs typically are reactive with noncollagenous GBM components. The guinea pig susceptibility to induction of anti-TBM Ab TIN segregated to the strain XIII major histocompatibility complex (MHC) (67).

Anti-TBM Ab TIN in guinea pigs is easily transferred with Ab, but not with immune cells (68,69) obtained from an involved subject, so that studies in both active or passive models are possible. Both IgG_1 and IgG_2 can transfer the lesion and generate self-production of anti-TBM Ab by the recipient (70). Transplacental transfer of anti-TBM Ab has been detected but apparently is insufficient to induce disease (71). Anti-TBM Ab production and disease development can be modulated with heterologous anti-idiotypic Ab (72). Cyclophosphamide (Cytoxan, NEOSAR) inhibition of Ab production modulates the lesion (73). Ab transfer of disease was inhibited in recipients depleted of complement (C) with cobra venom factor; however, the disease developed in immunized C4-deficient guinea pigs, suggesting a role for alternative C pathway activation (74,75). Radiation-induced leukopenia blocked the transfer lesion, which could be reconstituted with bone marrow but not with lymphoid cells (76,77). Cellular sensitivity to chaotrope-solubilized immunogen was present, with trafficking of such cells to the kidney (78,79). A chemoattractant for macrophages was reported in the renal venous blood coincident with macrophage influx (80).

Models in Rats

When Brown Norway (BN) rats were immunized with Sprague-Dawley rat kidney homogenate in adjuvants, anti-TBM Ab TIN was found (beginning 1–2 weeks after immunization), followed by TIN and, later, a form of Heymann nephritis (5–6 weeks) (81). Anti-TBM Abs were present in the circulation and could be eluted from the kidneys. Large amounts (12 mL) of immune serum were reported to transfer a mild TIN in a portion of recipients. Anti-TBM Abs and a Heymann nephritis-like lesion have also been induced by immunization of Wistar-King-Aptekman rats with the mouse Engelbreth-Holm-Swarm tumor (a source of basement membrane components) (82).

The heterologous Ag, Bov TBM, induced anti-TBM Ab and severe TIN in BN rats without the compounding problem of Heymann nephritis or anti-GBM Ab and, as such, has served as a useful model for the study of autoimmune TIN (83). The Bov TBM is prepared by sonication of cortical renal tissue retained on a 150-mesh sieve after most glomeruli have been pressed through with a spatula. Immunization is given in the tail base with complete Freund's adjuvant, and the rats also receive a separate injection of pertussis vaccine. The temporal development of the interstitial infiltrate, as well as the severity of the lesion, are greatly influenced by the quality of the immunization. The induction of disease can be related to quantitative binding of Ig to the kidney [elution study (83)]. Rabbit TBM, as well as solubilized fractions of various heterologous TBMs, including chaotropic extracts, can induce similar autoimmune disease in rats (84–86).

Initially, the inflammatory cell infiltrate in the BN Bov TBM-TIN is dominated by neutrophils, beginning when anti-TBM Ab and C deposition occurs 7–8 days after immunization (Figs. 2,3). The neutrophils are replaced by a mononuclear infiltrate over the next 1–3 days, with the time course related to the Ag batch and the quality of immunization.

By day 13, cells recovered from the infiltrate are 10% Ig^+ (B cells), 60% $W3/25^+$ (includes T helper cells), 9% $OX8^+$ (includes cytotoxic T cells), and 9% $esterase^+$ (monocytes/macrophages) (87). Augmented natural killer (NK) activity is reported (88). Monocytes/macrophages detected as $esterase^+$ cells increase in number, approaching 40% of the total cells recovered by day 28 at a time when fibrosis and other histologic evidence of chronicity of the lesion are found. Monocytes/macrophages may represent a higher percentage of the early mononuclear infiltrate based on ED-1 identification. Multinucleate giant cell formation is found. These cells may derive from monocytes/macrophages that had evolved into epithelioid cells (89–93). A temporal association is noted between the expression of interleukin-1β (IL-1β), tumor necrosis factor α (TNFα), monocyte chemoattractant protein-1 (MCP-1), IL-6, and upregulation of intracellular adhesion molecule-1 (ICAM-1) with leukocyte infiltration (94). Interstitial extracellular matrix accumulation is associated with an increase in expression of proteinase inhibitors (95).

In rats, the nephritogenic TBM Ag is an alloantigen that is present in BN rats (a TBM Ag^+ strain) and is not accessible in the LEW rat (a TBM Ag^- strain) (81,83). Other TBM Ag^+ strains include Fisher 344, Sprague Dawley, August, ACI, and Buffalo, with Maxx and Wistar-Furth noted to be TBM Ag^-. The TBM Ag^- LEW rats produce high levels of anti-TBM Abs when immunized with Bov TBM Ags, but these Abs do not bind to the LEW TBM in vivo or in vitro (indirect immunofluorescence), although reactive Ag can be recovered after enzymatic dissolution of the LEW TBM (96). In contrast, the LEW GBM/TBM Ag cross-reactive with human anti-GBM Abs is present. The allotypic difference in TBM Ags will induce anti-TBM Abs if a TBM Ag^+ BN or LEW x BN F_1 kidney is transplanted into a TBM Ag^- LEW recipient (97,98). This mimics the situation reported in humans when a TBM Ag^- individual receives a TBM Ag^+ renal transplant (51).

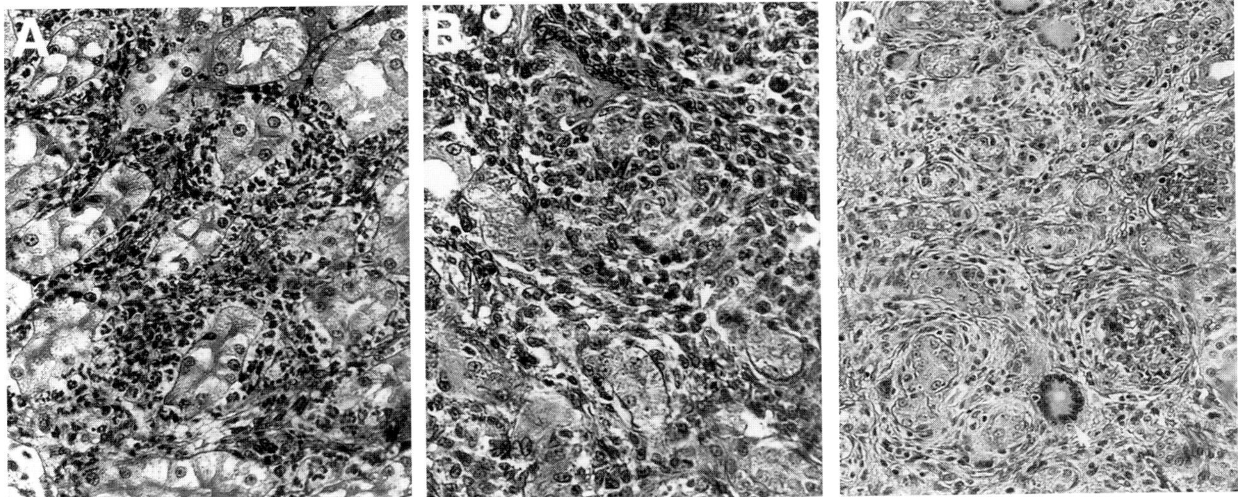

FIG. 3. A diffuse infiltrative TIN is induced in TBM Ag^+ BN rats by immunization with heterologous TBM (*Bov*) in adjuvants. The lesion onsets on days 7–8, with Ab and C fixation along the TBM and an intense peritubular neutrophil infiltration [*arrow, **A*** (day 8)]. Within 1 to 3 days, the neutrophils are replaced by a diffuse mononuclear infiltrate (*arrow*) and the presence of occasional multinucleate giant cells [**B** (day 10)]. Within a few days, the lesion displays less intense infiltrates, evidence of myofibroblasts, interstitial fibrosis, and increased numbers of multinucleate giant cells (*arrow*) [**C** (day 14)]

Several studies exploiting the TBM Ag allogenic differences include the induction of anti-TBM Abs in a TBM Ag^+ F_1 hybrid given parenteral TBM Ag^- lymphocytes (33,99,100). Of interest, female LEW rats with anti-TBM Abs transfer these transplacentally to F_1 TBM Ag^+ hybrids and, in turn, the rat pups may have some tubular atrophy and mild inflammatory changes (101). LEW rats with long-standing Fisher 344 renal allografts develop anti-TBM Ab associated TIN in the transplant and transplant glomerulopathy as well, in which Abs reactive with punctate glomerular Ags were found (102). The TBM alloantigens are inherited as a dominant gene outside the MHC (RT1) (103–105), with expression linked to the genes for pinkeye dilution and albinism (84,106). The spontaneously hypertensive rat background appears to have a strong suppressive effect on anti-TBM Ab (107–109).

The circulating Abs in Bov TBM-immunized rats react with both Bov and BN TBM Ags, whereas the Abs eluted from the kidneys with TIN displayed major reactivity against BN particulate and collagenase-solubilized BN TBM Ags (96). Heterologous anti-idiotypic Abs raised to the eluted anti-TBM Abs were able to suppress development of TIN, with a decrease in anti-BN collagenase-solubilized BN TBM Abs independent of any effect on antiBov particulate or collagenase-solubilized TBM reactivity and an insignificant lowering of anti-BN particulate TBM Ab (110). Anti-idiotypic Abs induced by immunization with T cells from rats with TIN also inhibited disease development (111). An anti-idiotypic Ab (induced by immunization with several monoclonal anti-TBM Abs) was found to react with a cross-reactive epitope; it was protective when given at immunization, and it was modulating when given 2 weeks postimmunization (112). The cross-reactive idiotype localized to the CDR3 region of the heavy chain (113). Rats immunized to produce disease do not exhibit an expected autologous anti-idiotypic Ab response related to a cyclophosphamide-sensitive suppressor cell, which appears to limit the host's ability to regulate the self-destructive anti-TBM Ab response (114).

In contrast to the guinea pig, passive transfer of anti-TBM Ab-associated TIN using immune serum is difficult in the rat (81,85,100). This may relate, in part, to the quantities of nephritogenic Ab available. Relatively small amounts (3–5 mL) of LEW anti-BN RBM Ab are able to transfer the lesion (115) (Fig. 4). The lack of a reactive TBM Ag in the LEW would prevent absorption of the relevant Ab, thereby increasing its concentration in the immune serum. The lesion induced by the LEW anti-BN RBM Ab is similar to that present in the actively immunized BN rat. The transfer makes it possible to study the quantitative parameters of Ab fixation in the TIN model (115). The paired-label isotope technique [which corrects for nonspecific tissue trapping of Abs (116)] demonstrated that Ab fixation increases gradually and reaches its peak 5–6 days after administration before beginning to fall. The onset of the cellular infiltration occurs about 24 hours after Ab administration, when about 170 μg of Ab per gram of kidney has bound. In comparison, about 75 μg of anti-GBM Ab per gram (which binds within a few minutes) is sufficient to induce an acute neutrophil infiltrate in glomeruli of rats (117). The quantitative paired-label studies were confirmed by elution of Ig from pooled kidneys of serum recipients, which showed increasing fixation over 6 days. The elution study also demonstrated that the anti-collagenase-solubilized BN RBM Ab reactivity in the eluate was concentrated, compared with that in serum on day 6. Such assessments of specific concentration of Ab in eluate versus serum relative to Ig content are necessary to exclude nonspecific trapping of circulating Ab during elution studies.

Initially, the transferred anti-RBM Ab bound in a linear pattern to the TBM of foci of tubules. Corresponding

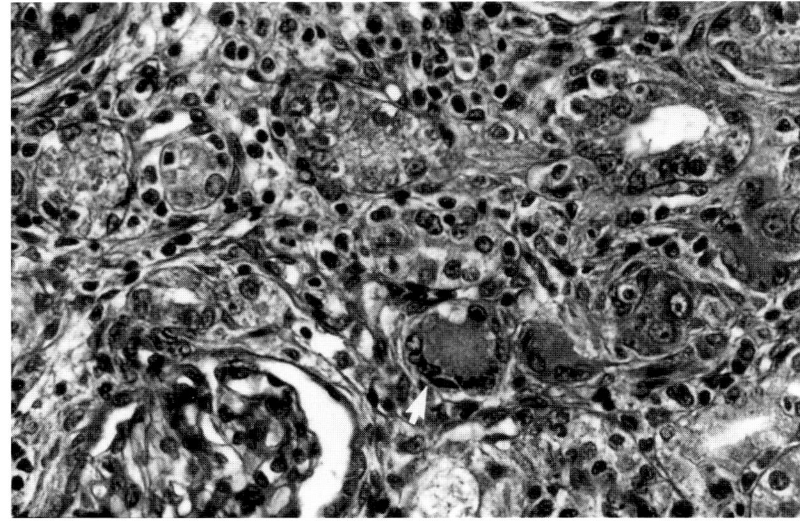

FIG. 4. The anti-TBM Ab-associated TIN of the BN rat can be induced by passive transfer of anti-TBM Ab obtained from a TBM Ag^- LEW rat immunized with TBM Ag^+ BN rat renal basement membrane. The lesion (shown on day 12 after serum transfer) is similar to that induced by active immunization, including the presence of multinucleate giant cells (*arrow*).

to this, the TIN transfer lesion appears as a focal accumulation of inflammatory cells, which are predominately mononuclear, with lesser numbers of neutrophils associated with foci of tubular injury. With time as well as increasing dose, the distribution of the linear Ig deposits becomes more diffuse, with areas of brighter fixation. The histologic lesion also becomes more diffuse and is characterized by mononuclear infiltrates, tubular destruction, and giant cells, much as the active lesion.

Because the TIN induced by the passive transfer contained C3 deposits in areas of cellular infiltration, the role of C was studied. C was depleted by administration of cobra venom factor prior to administering the anti-BN RBN Ab. This treatment diminished the number of destructive lesions without affecting Ab fixation (115). If cobra venom factor is used to decomplement BN rats during the development of active TIN after immunization with Bov TBM Ags, the early neutrophil phase is greatly diminished without evidence that Ab binding is altered (118). Some mononuclear cell infiltration persists, suggesting that a portion of the mononuclear component is not dependent on the initial C-associated neutrophil influx.

In the BN TIN model, the infiltrating T cells were sensitized to Bov TBM, as well as to purified protein derivative (PPD) (from the complete Freund's adjuvant); however, no sensitization to a variety of autologous BN renal Ags was detected (85). Immune cells from rats immunized with Bov TBM placed under the renal capsule did transfer a very mild circumscribed TIN (119). Systemic transfer of immune cells that had been propagated with the immunizing Bov TBM Ag did transfer TIN to normal BN recipients accompanied by the production and tubular fixation of anti-TBM Abs (85).

The development of BN TIN can be altered by preimmunization using Ag with incomplete Freund's adjuvant, which is a means of inducing suppressor cells (120). Although not normally responsive to autologous TBM Ags, BN rats will develop TIN if treated with cyclophosphamide to impair a population of suppressor cells that normally appears to maintain tolerance to self (121). In contrast to low-dose cyclophosphamide, which altered suppressor mechanisms, high-dose cyclophosphamide, when given during established disease (day 12), reduced progression (122). Cyclosporine has also been reported to inhibit induction of the BN TIN lesion (123–125). Dietary protein restriction and the stable analogue of PGE_1 (15S-15-methyl PGE_1) also inhibited the lesion, as did 15-deoxyspergualin (126–129).

Characterization of the TBM Ags of the Autoimmune TIN Models

The selective presence of Ag reactive with anti-TBM Abs in different tubular segments suggests that the antigenic molecule is probably important in the function of the particular nephron segment. Trypsin digests of murine or human TBM contain a 30-kD Ag that can induce anti-TBM Ab and TIN without detected GBM reactions in goats and BALB/c mice (130,131). In the BN TIN induced by immunization with Bov TBM, an Ag (42–45 kD) solubilized from BN TBM by collagenase was shown to account for about 70% of the reactivity of the eluted anti-TBM Ab detected using particulate BN TBM (96). Of interest, small amounts of reactive Ag were found in collagenase digests of the TBM Ag^- LEW TBM, suggesting that sequestered reactive epitopes may be present in this strain. A 45-kD Ag extracted from LEW TBM by trypsin digestion was reported to induce TIN in BALB/c mice; however, the ability of the eluted Ab to react with both BN and LEW rat TBM suggest an additional Ag system (132). A monoclonal Ab reactive with BN, but not LEW, TBM was used to isolate a noncollagenous nephritogenic Ag, termed *3M-1*, of about 48 kD from collagenase-solubilized rabbit TBM fractions (133). This Ag was localized to the most lateral aspects of the TBM bordering the interstitium by immunoelectron microscopy. The cDNA for the 3M-1 framework domain has been isolated (134). The domain has partial homology to mouse and rat intermediate filament-associated proteins related to cell–cell and extracellular matrix interactions. A peptide deduced from the cDNA bound the anti-3M-1 monoclonal Ab, stimulated the growth of 3M-1-reactive T helper cells, and induced nephritogenic T cells. The anti-3M-1 monoclonal Ab noted above (133) was used to recover a 48-kD Ag from collagenase-solubilized human RBM; the Ag reacted with two human anti-TBM Abs but not with anti-GBM Ab containing sera (135). A monoclonal Ab isolated from a BN rat given mercuric chloride identifies the same Ag but a different epitope (136).

An Ag reactive with human anti-TBM Abs has been extracted from rabbit TBM using guanidine and is composed predominately of a 58-kD form with small amounts of other components (137,138). The extraction procedure should not cleave peptide bonds, as do the enzymatic solubilization techniques and, in turn, may better preserve the true size of the reactive molecule. Monoclonal Abs to the isolate recognize minor components up to 300 kD (139). These high molecular weight fractions are reported to be more efficient in inducing TIN in BN rats than is the 58 kD form (140). The 58-kD Ag is present in highest amounts in proximal tubular and ileal basement membrane structures, which support epithelia with large absorptive capacity, suggesting a role in function (139). In other studies, 54- and 48-kD Ags with many of the same properties have been recovered from collagenase-digested Bov TBM and have been shown to be present along the interstitial side of the TBM in association with collagen fibers (141–143). These rabbit and Bov TBM Ags, like 3M-1, have little similarity to known basement membrane components. The 58-kD Ag has been shown to interact with laminin and type IV collagen and to promote cell adhesion (144). In addition, the molecule can interfere with the ability of laminin to self-associate. The ability of chemicals to alter TBM components used in induction of experimental renal cystic disease has been associated with a decrease in TBM Ag (145–150). In nephronophthisis, decreased reactivity of TBM with human anti-TBM Abs, but not monoclonal anti-TBM Abs, has been suggested to correlate with defective TBM structure (151).

Models in Mice

As in rats, mice develop anti-GBM and/or anti-TBM Ab after immunization with heterologous GBM/TBM preparations (152–155) or homologous TBM Ags (86). The TIN in mice induced by immunization with heterologous TBM is relatively slow in onset, with much more evidence of a predominant cellular immune mechanism than that in rats or guinea pigs (156,157). The SJL mouse is most susceptible, with A.CA, A.SW, T.TL, BALB/c, and NZB also responding. Mononuclear cell infiltrates appear in most immunized SJL mice after 5–7 weeks, even though anti-TBM Ab appears much earlier. Linear fixation of IgG to both GBM and TBM was observed. Susceptibility to TIN was not related to C5 status but was linked to MHC phenotypic traits other than autoantibody response (157). Comparison of the anti-TBM Abs among the mouse strains that do or do not develop TIN revealed no difference in amount of Ab, epitopic specificity of the response, or difference in the idiotype of the anti-TBM Ab eluted from the kidney (158). Murine monoclonal IgG_1 anti-TBM Ab that bound to BALB/c mouse TBM did not cause inflammation in BALB/c (159), and a monoclonal IgM rat TBM Ab that bound mouse TBM had only minimal inflammatory potential (160).

A $CD8^+$ T effector cell was shown early on to play a prominent role in the pathogenesis in the SJL TIN model (161). $CD8^+$ T cells taken from SJL mice with TIN could transfer TIN to naive recipients after 4–6 weeks, while transfer of immune serum produced a less striking and more delayed lesion (162). Attempts to reproduce the serum transfer failed (163). The $CD8^+$ effector T cell expressed idiotypes shared with kidney-bound anti-TBM Ab and, if recovered from interstitial infiltrates, could transfer disease in 5 days if placed under the kidney capsule (164). A $CD4^+$ T cell line also could transfer TIN after 12 weeks, and studies suggested that the line induced $CD8^+$ effector cells (165). A $CD8^+$ T cell line termed *M52*, which mediates Ag-specific delayed type hypersensitivity to 3M-1 and is cytotoxic to 3M-1-expressing renal tubular epithelial cells in vitro, can transfer TIN to naive syngeneic recipients (166). Clonal analysis reveals distinct functional phenotypes within the M52 cell line. The ability of the M52.26 clone to transfer TIN is inhibited by TGF-β1 (167). Studies suggest that TGF-β1 may be involved in clone-specific suppression of the M52.26 nephritogenic response (168). The $CD4^+$ Th1 cells that induce the $CD8^+$ effector cells recognize a 14-amino-acid residue in 3M-1 and have a repertoire of Vβ T cell receptors with some preference for Vβ14 (169). The oligoclonality of the T cell receptor response appears to relate to conservation of amino acid sequences in the Vβ/Dβ/Jβ junction.

Both $CD8^+$ effector and $CD4^+$ nephritogenic T cells were developed initially in in vitro studies of mice susceptible and nonsusceptible to murine TIN (170). In the nonsusceptible strains, the $CD8^+$ effector cell was inhibited via a mechanism suggested to involve countersuppression (171). Suppressor cell networks and factors are thought to contribute to control of this nephritogenic immune response, and a protective $CD8^+$ suppressor cell can be induced by injection of tubular Ag-coupled lymphocytes (168,172–174). The detailed discussion of the cellular immune mechanisms identified during studies of the SJL TIN model are the subject of review (17,18) (see Chapter 12)

The proximal tubular cell, which can express MHC class II molecules, may serve as an Ag presenting cell (175,176). The MHC molecules have grooves that allow them to selectively bind peptides and activate T cells via the T cell receptor molecules. MHC class I molecules are configured to present peptides present in the endoplasmic reticulum to C8+ T cells, and MHC class II molecules primarily deal with peptides reaching endocytic pathways, often from exogenous sources, with presentation to CD4+ T cells (177). A murine proximal tubular cell that expressed 3M-1 tubular Ag had both MHC class I and class II molecules on its surface and could stimulate cloned T cells reactive with 3M-1 (178). The MHC class II expression is modulated by anti-3M-1 Ab (179). Proximal tubular cells can present foreign Ag (180), although overexpression of class II molecules does not initiate immune renal injury (181,182). The role of costimulatory molecules necessary to complete the expansion of reactive T cell clones appears to determine the contribution of tubular cell Ag presentation in immune stimulation or anergy (183–187).

Models of Anti-TBM Abs Associated with Drugs

Sodium aurothiomalate (gold)-induced tubular injury was reported to induce anti-TBM Ab in the guinea pig (188). The anti-TBM Ab appeared 20 weeks after administration of gold salt. Ab also was present, reactive with renal tubular Ags (prepared like the Heymann nephritis Ag, Fx1A), and some animals had glomerular mesangial deposits. Ab reactive with the renal tubular Ags also reacted with the glomerular deposits. Antibasement membrane Abs have also been found in other forms of heavy metal-induced nephrotoxicity, e.g., anti-GBM Ab is seen with mercuric chloride toxicity in rats (189). Sodium aurothiomalate was used to aid in induction of murine TIN in the usually resistant C57Bl/6 mouse strain (190). Mice were treated with the gold compound prior to immunization with syngeneic TBM Ag. The mechanism for the effect was suggested to relate to inhibition of a suppressor activity.

Infrequent Spontaneous Appearance of Anti-TBM Abs

Anti-TBM Abs have been found in the lupus-prone New Zealand black/white hybrid mice (156). Anti-TBM Abs were also reported in a Samoyed dog with TIN (191). The Samoyed suffers from an X-linked hereditary nephritis not unlike Alport's syndrome in humans, a condition associated with alterations in GBM structure and Ag content (192). The Samoyed disease differs from the autosomal hereditary nephritis noted in the bull terrier, which has GBM Ags that are missing in the Samoyed (193).

AB REACTIONS THAT INDUCE IMMUNE DEPOSIT FORMATION AND TIN

The Problem in Humans

Irregular granular deposits of Ig and C in the tubulointerstitial tissue are sometimes observed in the kidneys of patients associated with IC forms of GN. Patients with SLE have relatively large quantities of immune reactants (Abs and ICs) in their circulation, and more than 50% of biopsies from such patients have granular Ig, C3, and DNA deposits in TBM, peritubular capillaries, and larger vessels (27,194). The presence of these deposits is so common that it can assist in making a diagnosis of SLE. The contribution of the deposits in producing tubulointerstitial inflammation has not been quantitated (195–197). Mediation systems, including the C5b-9 complex, are suggested to contribute (198), along with cells of which CD4+ T cells are prominent (199). The tubulointerstitial disease with renal tubular acidosis can overshadow the glomerular disease in SLE (200). Granular tubulointerstitial immune deposits are occasionally found in other presumed IC forms of GN, as well as in renal allografts (27,201–203). Exogenous Ags, such as those from a viral infection of tubular cells, can serve as a target for Ab reactions in humans (204). The possible mechanisms of immune deposit formation are largely extrapolated from several models in which IC formation and direct reactions with tubular cell Ags have been identified.

Models of Immune Deposit Formation with Soluble Circulating or Trapped Ags

Models with Circulating Ags, IC Formation, and Renal Accumulation

In the chronic serum sickness models of renal injury, particularly those in rabbits, induced by daily injection of soluble serum protein Ags, such as bovine serum albumin (BSA), extraglomerular immune deposits in the TBM and peritubular capillary areas representing ICs (Ig and Ag) can be prominent (205) (Fig. 5). In our experience, the extraglomerular IC accumulations are most striking in rabbits, in which very large quantities of circulating IC are fostered. This occurs when large amounts of Ab are present and when correspondingly large amounts of Ag are given daily.

As outlined in Chapter 35 in the discussion of IC mechanisms of glomerular disease, there is a dynamic

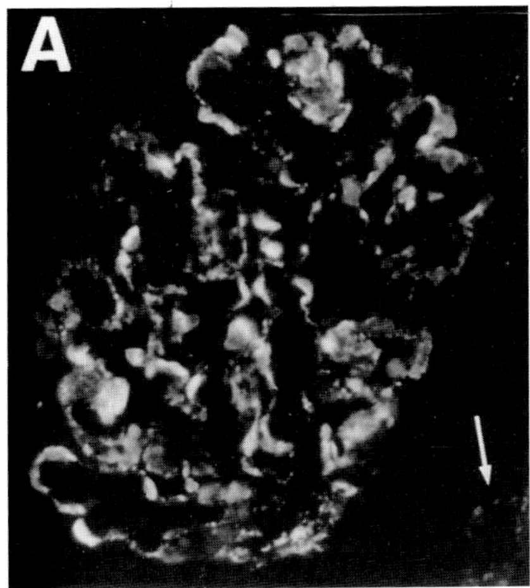

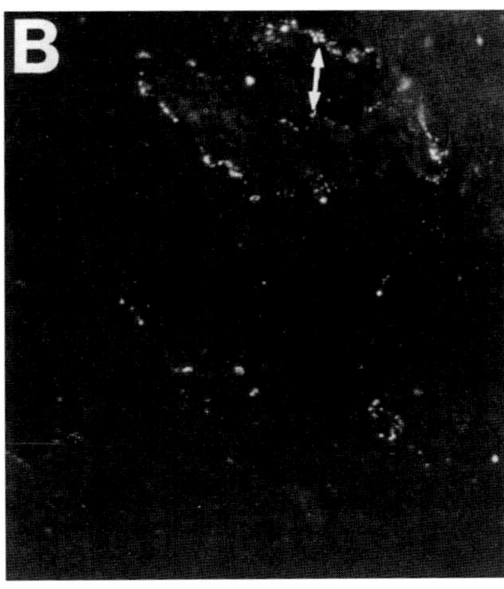

FIG. 5. Rabbits given daily intravenous doses of BSA sufficient to balance their Ab production develop chronic serum sickness GN with coarse granular deposits of BSA, Ig, and C in their glomeruli (**A**). Rabbits with very active immune responses that receive large amounts of BSA and, in turn, form large amounts of circulating ICs develop immune deposits in vessel walls (*arrow*, **A**) and along the TBM (*arrows*, **B**).

interrelationship between the relative amounts of Ag and Ab that are free to interchange and constantly reshape the composition of the renal immune deposit (206). In trying to determine why deposits accumulate and persist, the multiple events that influence the dynamics of this interchange must be considered. These factors include the size of the complex, its clearance from the circulation, any factor that increases its physical attraction to a particular site, such as its charge, and perhaps interactions with tissue receptors, such as tubulointerstitial Fc receptors, which may focus the IC localization (207–209). Secondary events such as anti-idiotypic Abs or rheumatoid Abs, which could cross-link the IC components and change the dynamics of the subsequent Ag and Ab interactions, may favor retention at the site (210).

In addition to the prominent GN, Ig and C3 deposits in the TBM and small vessels of the kidney as well as in extrarenal deposits often are found in the (NZB x NZW) F_1 and other lupus-prone mouse strains (211). The multiple potential mechanisms, including IC formation, that may contribute to immune deposits in glomeruli in lupus remain the subject of study (see Chapter 35) and are no better defined in tubulointerstitial immune deposit formation. These immune deposits in the tubulointerstitial areas may be found in areas with or without evidence of an inflammatory response, suggesting that quantitative and temporal features of the deposition influence the response, much as is found in the glomerulus. Lysozyme treatment of the NZB/W F_1 is reported to displace ICs from the glomerulus into the urine with their subsequent tubular uptake (212). Increased renal cortical expression of IL-1 and TNF is found in lupus mice (213–215). Enhanced expression of ICAM-1 and vascular cell adhesion molecule-1 (VCAM-1) is thought to contribute to cellular infiltration in the mice (216–218). Proximal tubular cell expression of MHC class II molecules precedes loss of renal function (219), and autoreactive T cell clones, which produce IL-4, TNFα, and interferon γ (IFN γ), can be recovered from the cortical interstitium of MRL/lpr mice (220). The IFNγ decreases the ability of tubular epithelial cells to induce proliferation of the T cell clones and may contribute to self-regulatory control of the T cell response (221).

Models Involving Arthus-Type Reactions

The Arthus reaction occurs when soluble Ag and Ab meet at a vessel wall, form IC locally, interact with Fc-receptors, activate mediator systems, and, in turn, incite an inflammatory response (222,223). Active or passive immunization to an Ag followed by injection of the Ag into a tissue site or, alternatively, administration of a soluble Ag and injection of Ab into a tissue site will induce this type of reaction if the amounts of Ab and Ag are properly balanced. The reaction also varies among species and at different sites. As a way to study drug-induced renal interstitial reactions, hapten–protein conjugates were introduced into the renal interstitium of mice actively or passively immunized to the haptens (224). In this study, intrarenal injection of preformed IC using the same Ag and Ab also induced disease.

Models in Which Circulating Ags are Planted or Trapped in the Kidney

The dynamic IC mechanisms of immune deposit formation move easily into the idea of planted Ag mechanisms. In the latter, the soluble antigenic material (endogenous or exogenous) becomes trapped at a renal site, where it is subsequently accessible to Ab. In theory, the trapping could occur as free Ag or as Ag already in an IC, once circulating Ab is present. The general mechanism was defined in immune glomerular disease (see Chapter 35), in which molecules bound to the glomerular capillary wall for immune or other physicochemical reasons (such as lectin binding or charge binding) served as targets for nephritogenic Ab reactions.

In rats given cationized BSA, which normally binds to GBM, treatment with highly cationic polyethyleneimine can displace the BSA to the peritubular capillary (225). Cationized trinitrophenol-conjugated ovalbumin was bound to the TBM, whereas its noncationized counterpart was taken up by the tubular epithelium, suggesting that molecules that are filtered through the glomerulus can be handled differently by the tubular cell, depending on charge. These molecules bound to the TBM potentially could serve as Ags for nephritogenic immune reactions.

The lectin concanavalin A (ConA) binds to glomerular and peritubular capillary endothelial cells and can serve as a planted Ag for subsequent IC formation if anti-ConA Ab is introduced. In the peritubular capillary, C is fixed, and neutrophils and platelets may be attracted to the site (226). Clearance of the complexes from the peritubular capillary is rapid (hours) and is slowed by measures that deplete neutrophils or C. A planted Ag mechanism would be attractive in drug-induced immune tubular injury; however, other than a few drug-regulated products associated with anti-TBM Ab formation (see above), examples are scarce (227).

Models in Which Ags May Originate from Renal Infections

One might speculate that Ag from infections of the renal tubule may provide a source of surface Ag for subsequent interaction with humoral (or cellular) (see later) immune responses leading to cytotoxic damage. Experimental infections, such as leptospirosis, which can damage the tubulointerstitium, have Ags detected early but do not have a clear immune pathogenesis, even though C deposits are reported (228,229).

TIN ASSOCIATED WITH ABS REACTIVE WITH RENAL TUBULAR CELL AGS

The Problem in Humans

Local formation of immune deposits could occur through the reactions of Ab with an Ag located on a tubular cell surface or released from it. The former could lead to direct cell injury in addition to possible immune deposit formation, whereas the latter could cause immune deposits to form adjacent to the cell of origin. Anti-tubular brush border, anti-Tamm-Horsfall, and other anti-tubular cell Abs have been reported after renal transplantation, associated with urinary tract infection, urinary obstruction, and with renal tubular acidosis or Sjogren's syndrome (230–242).

Models Involving Tubular Ags.

Models Induced in Rabbits

Immune deposit formation in the extracellular space between the TBM and the plasma membranes of tubular cells occurs in rabbits immunized with homologous tubular Ag fractions (243,244). The location of the deposit relative to the plasma membrane and basement membrane is similar to that described for thyroglobulin containing immune deposits in experimental thyroiditis, in which Ag leaving the cells meets Ab in the potential space between the plasma membrane and the basement membrane (245). Human tubular brush border Ags prepared like Fx1A (246,247) (*unpublished observations*), as well as repeated renal transplants, can cause similar deposits in rabbits (248). For example, heterologous Ab reactive with rabbit Fx1A bind to glomerular and tubular Ags when administered in vivo (Fig. 6). Ab recovered from active tubular deposits by elution reacted with Ags in the renal tubular brush border and cytoplasm (249). A monoclonal Ab raised to rabbit visceral yolk sac endothelial cells reacts with the apical region of the proximal renal tubule with a distribution similar to Fx1A, although it was not detected in glomeruli (250).

In another rabbit model, heterologous Abs reactive with angiotensin-converting enzyme (ACE), which is expressed on the apical surface of the proximal tubular cells, was used to induce a mild and transient immune deposit in the basolateral compartment (251). In this study, perfusion of isolated rabbit kidney with the Ab also induced deposits in the basal region of the proximal tubular cells. In most rabbits, the deposits were not accompanied by histologic abnormalities, although a few had mild tubular changes and interstitial infiltrates. The authors suggest that Ab passing through the TBM reacted with ACE that may be on the basolateral membranes of the proximal tubular cell. When the Abs were given to rabbits rendered proteinuric by a cationic Ag form of glomerular injury, the anti-ACE Ab was able to bind to the proximal tubular brush border.

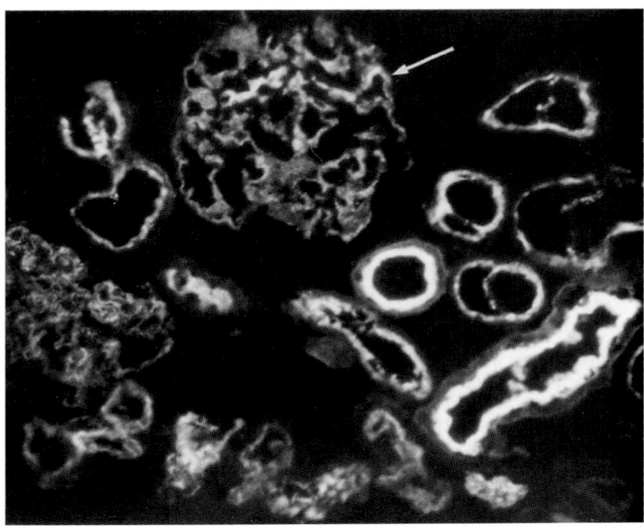

FIG. 6. Intravenous administration of goat anti-rabbit Fx1A Ab to rabbits results in glomerular fixation of Ab (*arrow*) and binding to renal tubular brush border, with some deposits in the basal regions of the renal tubules. The sections were obtained 24 hours after Ab administration.

Models Involving Tubular Ags in Rats, Mice, and Other Species

Brush Border Ags of the Proximal Tubule

Rats immunized with Fx1A develop Heymann nephritis, a model of membranous glomerulopathy (246,247). Because the Ag is present on the proximal tubular brush border, any Ab that reaches the tubular fluid could bind. Indeed, rats with long-standing Heymann nephritis have Ab binding to the brush border, C3 fixation, and tubular abnormalities, including intraluminal rosettes of cells surrounding brush border fragments (252,253). When looked at in detail, the fixation of the Ab to the brush border and cytolytic injury to proximal tubular cells correlates with the onset of proteinuria beginning 5–7 weeks after immunization, when high levels of circulating Ab are present (254). Immune deposit formation also occurs in the basal areas of the cell in the area of the TBM. If rats are made proteinuric by induction of serum sickness, passively administered anti-Fx1A Ab is able to pass into the tubular fluid and bind to the brush border Ags, to fix limited amounts of C as detected by C3 binding, and to produce lysis of proximal tubular cells (255). The tubular cell lesions are C-independent (studies using C depletion with cobra venom factor). The authors felt that Ab-related clumping and shedding of brush border was likely to be the mechanism for the cell damage (256).

Passively administered Ab also causes deposits at the basolateral aspect of the cells associated with focal clusters of interstitial macrophages (257) (Fig. 7). A similar mechanism of immune deposit formation is believed to be responsible for the immune deposit formation in the glomeruli in Heymann nephritis. That is when Ab reacts with Ag present on glomerular epithelial cell podocytes, a capping and shedding of the Ag–Ab complex as an immune deposit occurs along the subepithelial aspect of the GBM, with injury related to a C-dependent mechanism (258–265). The tubular damage associated with Heymann nephritis is accompanied by decreases in three proteins in the apical membranes of proximal tubular cells, namely, clathrin, gp330, and a proton-pumping adenosine triphosphatase (266).

As outlined in the discussion of the glomerular lesion of Heymann nephritis (see Chapter 35), the major antigenic molecule, shared between the brush border and the glomerular epithelial cell, is thought to be gp330 [recently renamed *megalin* (267,268)]. This glycoprotein has been cloned and has homology with the low density lipoprotein (LDL) and α2-macroglobulin receptors (269). An associated protein, the receptor-associated protein (RAP), binds to these receptors and has also been cloned (270). Its relationship to Heymann nephritis as

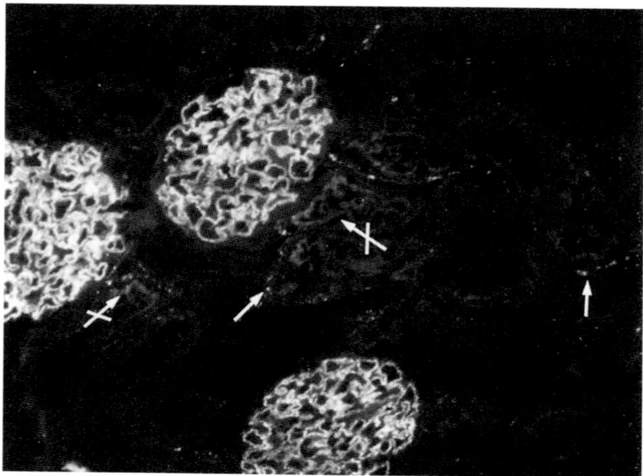

FIG. 7. Granular Ig deposits are found in the brush border (*hatched arrow*) and in the basal regions of the proximal renal tubules in rats with passive Heymann nephritis induced by intravenous administration of goat anti-rat Fx1A Ab. The majority of the Ab fixation is in glomeruli as a fine granular deposit. The sections were obtained 7 days after Ab administration.

part of the Heymann nephritis antigenic complex is under study (271–273). gp330 is present in coated pits on glomerular epithelial cells and at the base of microvilli on cells of the proximal renal tubule, as well as in some studies on the surface of the microvilli using monoclonal Abs or an Ig-RAP fusion protein (274–278).

Monoclonal Abs produced against rat brush border Ags can induce glomerular deposits like those of passive Heymann nephritis and can react with tubular sites as well (279–281). Abs reactive with other tubular brush border Ags, such as aminopeptidase A, can cause GN and bind to proximal tubular sites as well (282). A monoclonal Ab to a 120-kD rat brush border Ag reacted with glomerular deposits induced by gp330 (283).

Tamm-Horsfall Protein of the Distal Nephron

Another renal tubular Ag that can contribute to formation of immune deposits in the tubulointerstitial tissue is the glycosyl-phosphatidylinositol-linked Tamm-Horsfall protein, also known as *uromodulin*, whose gene is found on chromosome 16p13.11 (284–291). The Tamm-Horsfall protein is located on the surface of tubular cells in the ascending limb of the loop of Henle and distal convoluted tubule (292,293), and, although its function remains incompletely understood, it is a major urinary constituent. When rats are immunized with the Tamm-Horsfall protein, the Ab that forms can bind the tubular Ag, which leads to immune deposit formation at the bases of distal tubular cells that contain Tamm-Horsfall protein (294,295). The immune deposits disappear quite rapidly (within 2 weeks) in the affected kidney if it is transplanted into a normal rat to prevent additional exposure to circulating Ab (296). Similar deposits, as well as a mild mononuclear cell infiltrate, can be induced by passive immunization with heterologous anti-Tamm-Horsfall Abs (297). When mice were immunized with Tamm-Horsfall protein, they also developed immune deposits within the basal and lateral intercellular spaces of the ascending limb (298). Rabbits immunized with Tamm-Horsfall protein or homologous urine developed TIN; however, interstitial immune deposits were not seen, in spite of the presence of circulating Ab (299,300). Peripheral lymphocytes sensitized to the Tamm-Horsfall protein were found, and a cellular immune pathogenesis was suggested (299).

If the recipient is first made proteinuric, anti-Tamm-Horsfall Ab will bind to the luminal surface of the ascending limb of the loop of Henle with C3 fixation. Ab deposits are also visible in the basal areas of the cells (301). Increased mitotic activity is found within the cells of the ascending limb of the loop of Henle. This type of reaction allows the study of Ab-induced injury to the luminal aspect of cells in the distal nephron, in a manner similar to that described above for the proximal tubular injury in active or passive Heymann nephritis. Binding of Ab to Tamm-Horsfall protein is also suggested as a monitor of proteinuria in individual nephrons (302).

The Tamm-Horsfall protein may be redistributed retrograde or into interstitial tissue during urinary obstruction or reflux (303,304). Ab to Tamm-Horsfall protein and deposits has been noted in a pig model of reflux nephropathy (305,306). The Tamm-Horsfall protein can bind to the extracellular matrix and can interact with and activate neutrophils and mononuclear phagocytes (307–310). Tamm-Horsfall protein binds IgG (311), and Bence Jones proteins can bind to Tamm-Horsfall protein, causing cast nephropathy or myeloma kidney (312–315); human kappa light chains are toxic to the rat proximal tubular cells (316).

Possible Models Using Tubular Ags Recognized by Monoclonal Abs

Monoclonal antibodies can be used to characterize segments of the renal tubule; however, their ability to produce selective injury to study the effects of localized tubular injury has not been extensively evaluated. Monoclonal Abs have been raised reactive with numerous brush border and other tubular Ags (317–322) or known markers such as specific enzymes, receptors, or transport protein, which help identify specific tubular segments (323–332). Human monoclonal cold agglutinins recognize collecting ducts and other segments of the tubules (333). Monoclonal Abs have been used to isolate selected tubular cells to establish renal tubular cell cultures (334,335). In some instances, these Abs might have a nephritogenic potential, directly or as planted Ags, during an active or passive autologous immune response to the foreign trapped Ig.

CELLULAR IMMUNITY IN TUBULOINTERSTITIAL INJURY AND TIN

The Problem in Humans

The contribution of cellular immunity to the characteristic mononuclear cell infiltration in human TIN is being increasingly appreciated. In the drug-associated TINs, the distal tubule is reported to be the focus of the greatest cellular influx (336). Numerous studies document the presence of large numbers of interstitial T cells of somewhat varying CD4+:CD8+ ratios in TIN, cytomegalovirus-associated TIN, renal allografts, and in various forms of GN, including minimal change nephropathy and SLE (337–340). The interstitial infiltrates in Sjogren's syndrome have prominent CD4+ T cells and nodules of B cells (341,342). TIN related to drug reactions often has prominent T cell infiltrates, with the relationship of $CD4^+$:$CD8^+$ T cells reported to vary among drug classes (343–346). The granulomatous nephritis that is sometimes found in drug reactions, as well as in other conditions, including sarcoidosis, tuberculosis, and Wegener's granulomatosis (347,348), has a striking similarity to a model of cellular immunity produced in LEW rats (see later). Patients, often adolescent girls, are described with TIN with an eosinophilic component, uveitis, and with the variable presence of hypergammaglobulinemia, circulating ICs, granulomas in bone marrow, and generally negative renal immunofluorescence findings (349–355).

Models of TIN in Which Cellular Immunity Plays a Prominent Role

Models Using Interstitial Delayed-Type Hypersensitivity Reactions

It is possible to induce delayed-type hypersensitivity (DTH) reactions in the interstitium, much as in the skin. For example, DTH reactions can be induced in the renal interstitium of rats by injection of aggregated, but not soluble, Bov γ globulin following presensitization to this Ag in adjuvant (356). The aggregated Ag presumably favors the reaction by remaining in the cortical interstitium for greater periods of time than its soluble counterpart. It is possible to transfer induction of lesions with immune cells but not with serum. Other proteins, including purified protein derivative and dodecanoic acid conjugated BSA, have been used to induce similar lesions in guinea pigs (357). It is tempting to suspect that drugs or their breakdown products could be used as an Ag for a DTH-like reaction to mimic drug-related mononuclear leukocyte infiltrates.

Models Related to Infection

Mice infected with lymphocytic choriomeningitis virus have interstitial lesions associated with an IC type of GN (358). The absence of immune deposits associated with the interstitial cellular infiltration led the authors to propose that persistence of viral Ag elicited a cell-mediated immune reaction. A similar sequence is suggested in the renal disease of Aleutian mink, in which an Aleutian disease parvovirus Ag–Ab IC type of GN and a cellular interstitial disease are seen (359). Viral replication is found in renal tubular cells by in situ hybridization with T cells around the infected tubules in the absence of immune deposits.

Models Induced with Kidney Ags or Alloantigens

A mild mononuclear infiltrate was observed in LEW rats after immunization with LEW kidney homogenate (360). It was possible to transfer a mild lesion using immune cells but not serum; no Ab deposition was found. DA rats that had been sensitized to LEW cells via skin grafts reacted with an interstitial infiltrate when LEW lymphocytes were placed in the renal cortex (361). The interstitial infiltrate of renal allograft rejection also has many similarities to the mononuclear infiltrates associated with TIN and, in turn, could serve as a model for some questions.

A nodular granulomatous tubulointerstitial lesion was induced in the TBM Ag$^-$ LEW rat by immunization with TBM Ag$^+$ BN rat RBM (57). RBMs from other TBM Ag$^+$ rat strains also were able to induce the disease, whereas heterologous TBM Ag$^+$ RBMs were less effective. The RBM was obtained as the extensively washed residue of homogenized and repeatedly sonicated whole BN kidneys. Focal macroscopic granuloma-like lesions developed by day 9 after immunization. The focal lesions were composed of epithelioid cells, giant cells, and mononuclear cell infiltrates scattered throughout the cortex and outer medulla, often in a periglomerular location (Fig. 8). The large epithelioid cells in the center of the inflammatory foci were not stained with the pan T cell reagent OX19 or T cell subset reagents W3/25 or OX8. In contrast, 50–60% of the surrounding mononuclear cells were positive for OX19 and W3/25, with only 1–5% being OX8$^+$. The rats developed elevated serum creatinine levels but no proteinuria or glycosuria.

The TBM Ag$^-$ LEW rats immunized with the TBM Ag$^+$ RBM developed circulating anti-TBM Abs, with the Ab capable of transferring TIN to the BN rat (115). Of interest, very occasional segments of TBM within the nodular LEW lesion fixed IgG in a linear pattern, suggesting anti-TBM Ab binding. As noted above, LEW TBM was shown to contain small amounts of Ags reactive with anti-BN TBM Abs after enzymatic digestion, which may have resulted from the inflammatory cell proteinases present in the lesion (96). As the lesion progresses, occasional rats developed Abs reactive with LEW GBM/TBM (also ABM) Ags, much like those discussed above (54,362).

The granulomatous lesion was transferable to naive LEW rats with cells (but not by Ab). Extensive transfer lesions were found by day 7 that were similar to those produced 14–21 days after active immunization (Fig. 8). No Ab deposits were present, and irradiated cells did not transfer the lesion.

Models Induced with Toxins

TIN associated with renal toxin exposure, such as to cadmium, has been reported to be related to the induction of heat shock protein (HSP)-reactive T cells in SJL/J mice (363). The HSPs have multiple effects on the immune response and, in turn, have been associated with autoimmune responses (364,365). Chronic administration of $CdCl_2$ (1–3 mg/kg/day intraperitoneally) induced interstitial infiltration beginning at 8–10 weeks and resulted in expression of HSP70 antedating the infiltrate. Cattle grazing in pastures with the forage source *Vicia villosa* (hairy vetch) are reported to develop TIN, among other toxic manifestations (366).

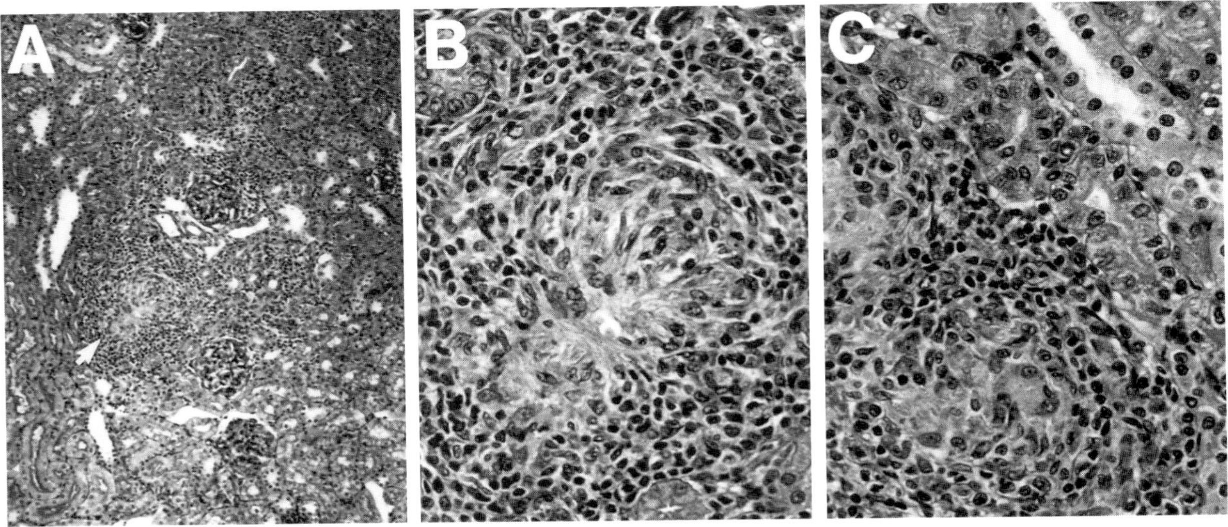

FIG. 8. A focal granulomatous form of TIN can be induced in TBM Ag$^-$ LEW rats by immunization with BN or other TBM Ag$^+$ rat renal basement membrane in adjuvant (**A**). The focal lesion marked by the arrow in (A) is seen at high magnification in (**B**). The lesion can be transferred to naive LEW rats with immune cells obtained from an immunized LEW rat (**C**). Both the active and transferred lesions are at 14 days.

Spontaneous Models of TIN

An autosomal recessive form of TIN develops in the kdkd mouse, a congenic subline derived from the CBA/Ca strain (367). A link to the gene markers, waltzer and grizzled on chromosome 10, was suggested. The mice develop proteinuria by 10 weeks and polyuria later. A peritubular infiltrate develops and tubular dilatation occurs, with distortion of the tubular architecture. The glomeruli are not involved. Death occurs by 24–30 weeks. The development and progression of the disease was decreased or eliminated by restricting daily food intake (368). No immunoglobulin deposits were detected. No antikidney reactivity was present in sera or renal eluates, and the TIN in the kdkd mice was suggested to be cell-mediated (369). The disease can be transferred with kdkd to CBA/Ca bone marrow chimeras and is prevented in CBA/Ca to kdkd chimeras. A DTH reaction is detected in cyclophosphamide-treated recipients using collagenase-solubilized CBA/Ca TBM (370). Cyclophosphamide treatment was used to impair T cells from CBA/Ca mice that could suppress disease development (371). The disease could be transferred using kdkd lymph node cells into CBA/Ca mice that had been thymectomized, irradiated, and given T cell-depleted CBA/Ca bone marrow to eliminate suppressor cells. kdkd lymph node cells administered directly under the renal capsule of cyclophosphamide-treated CBA/Ca mice also could establish a lesion. The effector cells were H-2K restricted and of a $CD8^+$ phenotype. The onset of disease in the kdkd mice was related to a functional inactivation of normally present suppressor T cells in young kdkd and CBA/Ca mice by an Ag-specific set of countersuppressor T cells (371). The regulatory T cell population that is permissive for the interstitial lesion in kdkd mice is suggested to bear a distinct form of CD45 (372). The majority of T cells in the interstitial lesion express either Vβ8 or Vβc T cell receptors (373). Anti-ICAM-1 Ab is reported to decrease leukocyte infiltration in the kdkd mice (374). A parallel has been suggested between the kdkd mouse disease and the possible autoimmune pathogenesis of medullary cystic disease–familial juvenile nephronophthisis complex (375).

POSSIBLE IMMUNE MEDIATOR-RELATED PATHWAYS OF TUBULOINTERSTITIAL INJURY

Immune mediator activation in tubulointerstitial tissue, perhaps unrelated to a specific immune response, could contribute to injury. The brush border area of the proximal tubule and walls of renal vessels can activate the alternative C pathway in vitro (376,377). C localization to brush border without C1q or C4 is said to correlate with urinary C3 excretion in humans (378).

C components, including those associated with the C5b-9 complex, are found in the TBM region in chronic interstitial injury (379). It has been suggested that increasing ammonia found after reduction in renal mass or hypokalemic nephropathy could activate the alternative C pathway, leading to C3 deposition (380–383). The C3 deposition can be reduced by dietary $NaHCO_3$ supplementation of the rats, which reduces tubulointerstitial injury.

A relationship exists between proteinuria, such as that induced in puromycin aminonucleoside nephrosis (PAN), and the development of tubulointerstitial injury associated with T cell infiltrates in the interstitium, although T cell depletion does not affect the outcome (384–386). Proteinuria in PAN lesions is modulated by Abs to IL-1β and/or TNFα (387). Prednisolone decreases the T cell infiltrate, and interstitial fibrosis can be the sequela of this lesion (388–390). Iron-related oxidative toxicity, potentially caused by a glomerular leak of transferrin, among other proteins, has been suggested as one of the possible causes of the proteinuria-associated tubular injury (391). A lipid derived from albumin that is chemotactic for macrophages has been associated with protein-overload proteinuria and interstitial macrophage infiltration (392).

IL-2 is reported to alter the normal unresponsiveness of T cells in neonatally thymectomized CBA/H mice, leading to autoimmune manifestations, including interstitial nephritis (393). Enhanced expression of osteopontin in renal tubules, in association with experimental glomerular injury, is suggested to enhance interstitial monocyte/macrophage accumulation (394).

Mice transgenic for various growth factors or other molecules may suffer from glomerular and tubular changes, including renal cysts (395–400). Tsukuba hypertensive mice have been developed from mice transgenic for the human renin gene or the human angiotensinogen gene (401). Mice transgenic for portions of the HIV genome have glomerulosclerosis and tubulointerstitial injury (402,403).

OTHER FORMS OF TUBULOINTERSTITIAL INJURY WITH MONONUCLEAR INTERSTITIAL INFILTRATES

A number of other models of renal injury result in accumulation of inflammatory cells in renal tubular cell injury, often with accumulation of interstitial inflammatory cells and, subsequently, interstitial fibrosis. Detailed discussion of these nonimmune lesions is beyond the scope of this presentation; however, these models may have value in understanding the overall mechanisms of tubulointerstitial injury, and some will be mentioned in closing.

Hypertension and models such as the remnant kidney are associated with interstitial injury (404,405). Systemic hypertension induced by chronic angiotensin II infusion is associated with tubulointerstitial injury, with the suggestion that overexpression of the RGD containing phosphoprotein, osteopontin, may facilitate monocyte/macrophage accumulation (406).

Renal ischemia induced by unilateral renal artery clamping leads to interstitial inflammatory infiltration (407–409). Ureteral ligation induces interstitial infiltration and interstitial fibrosis (410–412). Models of experimental pyelonephritis (413,414), as well as of polycystic disease (415–418), might also have some usefulness. Spontaneous TIN associated with an increase in interstitial vimentin is found in cattle and dogs (419,420).

Papillary necrosis and chronic tubulointerstitial injury can be induced in rats with 2-bromoethylamine hydrobromide (421,422). Cyclosporine toxicity includes tubulointerstitial injury (423–425), as does drug-induced tubular injury, such as with antibiotics (426–429). Alternatives to in vivo models are also attracting increased interest, including in vitro approaches to study tubular cell responses to injurious agents (430–433).

REFERENCES

1. Bohle A, Mackensen-Haen S, Gise H. Significance of tubulointerstitial changes in the renal cortex for the excretory function and concentration ability of the kidney: a morphometric contribution. *Am J Nephrol* 1987;7:421–433.
2. Nath KA. Tubulointerstitial changes as a major determinant in the progression of renal damage. *Am J Kidney Dis* 1992;20:1–17.
3. Katafuchi R, Takebayashi S, Taguchi T, Harada T. Structural-functional correlations in serial biopsies from patients with glomerulonephritis. *Clin Nephrol* 1987;28:169–173.
4. Abe S, Amagasaki Y, Iyori S, Konishi K, Kato E, Sakaguchi H. Significance of tubulointerstitial lesion in biopsy specimens of glomerulonephritic patients. *Am J Nephrol* 1989;9:30–37.
5. Yee J, Kuncio GS, Neilson EG. Tubulointerstitial injury following glomerulonephritis. *Semin Nephrol* 1991;11:361–366.
6. Singh AB, Mann RA. Chronic interstitial nephritis. In: Jacobson HR, Striker GF, Klahr S, eds. *The Principles and Practice of Nephrology*. Philadelphia: BC Decker, 1991;356–366.
7. Appel GB. Acute interstitial nephritis. In: Jacobson HR, Striker GF, Klahr S, eds. *The Principles and Practice of Nephrology*. Philadelphia: BC Decker, 1991;348–355.
8. Kuncio GS, Neilson EG, Haverty T. Mechanisms of tubulointerstitial fibrosis. *Kidney Int* 1991;39:550–556.
9. Cameron JS. Tubular and interstitial factors in the progression of glomerulonephritis. *Pediatr Nephrol* 1992;6:292–303.
10. Alvarez RJ, Sun MJ, Haverty TP, Iozzo RV, Myers JC, Neilson EG. Biosynthetic and proliferative characteristics of tubulointerstitial fibroblasts probed with paracrine cytokines. *Kidney Int* 1992;41:14–23.
11. Eddy AA. Experimental insights into the tubulointerstitial disease accompanying primary glomerular lesions. *J Am Soc Nephrol* 1994;5:1273–1287.
12. Strutz F, Neilson EG. The role of lymphocytes in the progression of interstitial disease. *Kidney Int* 1994;45(Suppl 45):S106–S110.
13. Couser WG, Johnson RJ. Mechanisms of progressive renal disease in glomerulonephritis. *Am J Kidney Dis* 1994;23:193–198.
14. Wilson CB. Study of the immunopathogenesis of tubulointerstitial nephritis using model systems. *Kidney Int* 1989;35:938–953.
15. Neilson EG. Pathogenesis and therapy of interstitial nephritis. *Kidney Int* 1989;35:1257–1270.
16. Wilson CB. Nephritogenic tubulointerstitial antigens. *Kidney Int* 1991;39:501–517.
17. Kelly CJ, Roth DA, Meyers CM. Immune recognition and response to the renal interstitium. *Kidney Int* 1991;39:518–530.
18. Neilson EG. The nephritogenic T lymphocyte response in interstitial nephritis. *Semin Nephrol* 1993;13:496–502.
19. Meeus F, Rossert J, Druet P. Cellular immunity in interstitial nephropathy. *Ren Fail* 1993;15:325–329.
20. Gabbai FB, Peterson OW, Kelly CJ. Activity of the tubuloglomerular feedback system (TGFS) in rats with autoimmune tubulointerstitial nephritis (TIN). *J Am Soc Nephrol* 1995;6:1013.
21. Venkatachalam MA, Karnovsky MJ. Extravascular protein in the kidney. An ultrastructural study of its relation to renal peritubular capillary permeability using protein tracers. *Lab Invest* 1972;27:435–444.
22. Nielsen JT, Christensen EI. Basolateral endocytosis of protein in isolated perfused proximal tubules. *Kidney Int* 1985;27:39–45.
23. Wieslander J, Barr JF, Butkowski RJ, Edwards SJ, Bygren P, Heinegard D, Hudson BG. Goodpasture antigen of the glomerular basement membrane: localization to noncollagenous regions of type IV collagen. *Proc Natl Acad Sci USA* 1984;81:3838–3842.
24. Weber M, Pullig O. Different immunologic properties of the globular NC1 domain of collagen type IV isolated from various human basement membranes. *Eur J Clin Invest* 1992;22:138–146.
25. Kalluri R, Wilson CB, Weber M, Gunwar S, Chonko AM, Neilson EG, Hudson BG. Identification of the α3 chain of type IV collagen as the common autoantigen in anti-basement membrane disease and Goodpasture syndrome. *J Am Soc Nephrol* 1995; 6:1178–1185.
26. Wilson CB, Dixon FJ. Anti-glomerular basement membrane antibody-induced glomerulonephritis. *Kidney Int* 1973;3:74–89.
27. Lehman DH, Wilson CB, Dixon FJ. Extraglomerular immunoglobulin deposits in human nephritis. *Am J Med* 1975;58:765–786.
28. Graindorge PP, Mahieu PR. Radioimmunologic method for detection of antitubular basement membrane antibodies. *Kidney Int* 1978;14:594–606.
29. Andres G, Brentjens J, Kohli R, Anthone R, Anthone S, Baliah T, Montes M, Mookerjee BK, Presyna A, Sepulveda M, Venuto M, Elwood C. Histology of human tubulo-interstitial nephritis associated with antibodies to renal basement membranes. *Kidney Int* 1978;13:480–491.
30. Bergstein J, Litman N. Interstitial nephritis with anti-tubular-basement-membrane antibody. *N Engl J Med* 1975;292:875–878.
31. Andres GA, McCluskey RT. Tubular and interstitial renal disease due to immunologic mechanisms. *Kidney Int* 1975;7:271–289.
32. Rakotoarivony J, Orfila C, Segonds A, Giraud P, Durand D, DuBois Ch, Mahieu Ph, Suc J-M. Human and experimental nephropathies associated with antibodies to tubular basement membrane. *Adv Nephrol* 1981;10:187–212.
33. Brentjens JR, Matsuo S, Fukatsu A, Min I, Kohli R, Anthone R, Anthone S, Biesecker G, Andres G. Immunologic studies in two patients with antitubular basement membrane nephritis. *Am J Med* 1989;86:603–608.
34. Lindqvist B, Lundberg L, Wieslander J. The prevalence of circulating anti-tubular basement membrane-antibody in renal diseases, and clinical observations. *Clin Nephrol* 1994;41:199–204.
35. Morel-Maroger L, Kourilski O, Mignon F, Richet G. Antitubular basement membrane antibodies in rapidly progressive poststreptococcal glomerulonephritis. Report of a case. *Clin Immunol Immunopathol* 1974;2:185–194.
36. Tung KSK, Black WC. Association of renal glomerular and tubular immune complex disease and antitubular basement membrane antibody. *Lab Invest* 1975;32:696–700.
37. Levy M, Guesry P, Loirat C, Dommergues JP, Nivet H, Habib R. Immunologically mediated tubulo-interstitial nephritis in children. *Contrib Nephrol* 1979;16:132–140.
38. Wood EG, Brouhard BH, Travis LB, Cavallo T, Lynch RE. Membranous glomerulonephropathy with tubular dysfunction and linear tubular basement membrane IgG deposition. *J Pediatr* 1982;101:414–417.
39. Katz A, Fish AJ, Santamaria P, Nevins TE, Kim Y, Butkowski RJ. Role of antibodies to tubulointerstitial nephritis antigen in human anti-tubular basement membrane nephritis associated with membranous nephropathy. *Am J Med* 1992;93:691–698.
40. Makker SP. Tubular basement membrane antibody-induced interstitial nephritis in systemic lupus erythematosus. *Am J Med* 1980;69:949–952.
41. Zawada ET Jr, Johnston WH, Bergstein J. Chronic interstitial nephritis. Its occurrence with oxalosis and anti-tubular basement membrane antibodies after jejunoileal bypass. *Arch Pathol Lab Med* 1981;105:379–383.
42. Ellis D, Fisher SE, Smith WI Jr, Jaffe R. Familial occurrence of renal and intestinal disease associated with tissue autoantibodies. *Am J Dis Child* 1982;136:323–326.

43. Appel GB. A decade of penicillin related acute interstitial nephritis-more questions than answers. *Clin Nephrol* 1980;13:151–154.
44. Kleinknecht D, Vanhille Ph, Morel-Maroger L, Kanfer A, LeMaitre V, Mery JP, Laederich J, Callard P. Acute interstitial nephritis due to drug hypersensitivity. An up-to-date review with a report of 19 cases. *Adv Nephrol* 1983;12:277–308.
45. Baldwin DS, Levine BB, McCluskey RT, Gallo GR. Renal failure and interstitial nephritis due to penicillin and methicillin. *N Engl J Med* 1968;279:1245–1252.
46. Border WA, Lehman DH, Egan JD, Sass HJ, Glode JE, Wilson CB. Antitubular basement-membrane antibodies in methicillin-associated interstitial nephritis. *N Engl J Med* 1974;291:381–384.
47. Hyman LR, Ballow M, Knieser MR. Diphenylhydantoin interstitial nephritis. Roles of cellular and humoral immunologic injury. *J Pediatr* 1978;92:915–920.
48. Grussendorf M, Andrassy K, Waldherr R, Ritz E. Systemic hypersensitivity to allopurinol with acute interstitial nephritis. *Am J Nephrol* 1981;1:105–109.
49. Klassen J, Kano K, Milgrom F, Menno AB, Anthone S, Anthone R, Sepulveda M, Elwood CM, Andres GA. Tubular lesions produced by autoantibodies to tubular basement membrane in human renal allografts. *Int Arch Allergy Appl Immunol* 1973;45:675–689.
50. Rotellar C, Noel LH, Droz D, Kreis H, Berger J. Role of antibodies directed against tubular basement membranes in human renal transplantation. *Am J Kidney Dis* 1986;7:157–161.
51. Wilson CB, Lehman DH, McCoy RC, Gunnells JC Jr, Stickel DL. Antitubular basement membrane antibodies after renal transplantation. *Transplantation* 1974;18:447–452.
52. Cattran DC. Circulating anti-tubular basement membrane antibody in a variety of human renal diseases. *Nephron* 1980;26:13–19.
53. Jordan SC, Barkley SC, Lemire JM, Sakai RS, Cohen A, Fine RN. Spontaneous anti-tubular-basement-membrane antibody production by lymphocytes isolated from a rejected allograft. *Transplantation* 1986;41:173–176.
54. Sado Y, Naito I. Experimental autoimmune glomerulonephritis in rats by soluble isologous or homologous antigens from glomerular and tubular basement membranes. *Br J Exp Path* 1987;68:695–704.
55. Robertson JL, Hill GS, Rowlands DT Jr. Tubulointerstitial nephritis and glomerulonephritis in Brown-Norway rats immunized with heterologous glomerular basement membrane. *Am J Pathol* 1977;88: 53–64.
56. Sapin C, Druet E, Druet P. Induction of anti-glomerular basement membrane antibodies in the Brown-Norway rat by mercuric chloride. *Clin Exp Immunol* 1977;28:173–179.
57. Bannister KM, Ulich TR, Wilson CB. Induction, characterization, and cell transfer of autoimmune tubulointerstitial nephritis in the Lewis rat. *Kidney Int* 1987;32:642–651.
58. Jennings L, Roholt OA, Pressman D, Blau M, Andres GA, Brentjens JR. Experimental anti-alveolar basement membrane antibody-mediated pneumonitis. I. The role of increased permeability of the alveolar capillary wall induced by oxygen. *J Immunol* 1981;127:129–134.
59. Downie GH, Roholt OA, Jennings L, Blau M, Brentjens JR, Andres GA. Experimental anti-alveolar basement membrane antibody-mediated pneumonitis. II. Role of endothelial damage and repair, induction of autologous phase, and kinetics of antibody deposition in Lewis rats. *J Immunol* 1982;129:2647–2652.
60. Yamamoto T, Wilson CB. Binding of anti-basement membrane antibody to alveolar basement membrane after intratracheal gasoline instillation in rabbits. *Am J Pathol* 1987;126:497–505.
61. Queluz TH, Pawlowski I, Brunda MJ, Brentjens JR, Vladutiu AO, Andres G. Pathogenesis of an experimental model of Goodpasture's pneumonitis. *J Clin Invest* 1990;85:1507–1515.
62. Eddy AA. Tubulointerstitial nephritis during the heterologous phase of nephrotoxic serum nephritis. *Nephron* 1991;59:304–313.
63. Steblay RW, Rudofsky U. Renal tubular disease and autoantibodies against tubular basement membrane induced in guinea pigs. *J Immunol* 1971;107:589–594.
64. Lehman DH, Marquardt H, Wilson CB, Dixon FJ. Specificity of autoantibodies to tubular and glomerular basement membranes induced in guinea pigs. *J Immunol* 1974;112:241–248.
65. Andres GA, Szymanski C, Albini B, Brentjens J, Milgrom M, Noble B, Ossi E, Steblay R. Structural observations on epithelioid and giant cells in experimental autoimmune tubulointerstitial nephritis in guinea pigs. *Am J Pathol* 1979;96:21–34.
66. Milgrom M, Albini B, Noble B, O'Connell D, Brentjens J, Andres GA. Antibodies in guinea-pigs immunized with kidney and lung basement membranes. *Clin Exp Immunol* 1979;38:249–258.
67. Hyman LR, Steinberg AD, Colvin RB, Bernard EF. Immunopathogenesis of autoimmune tubulointerstitial nephritis. II. Role of an immune response gene linked to the major histocompatibility complex. *J Immunol* 1976;117:1894–1897.
68. Steblay RW, Rudofsky U. Transfer of experimental autoimmune renal cortical tubular and interstitial disease in guinea pigs by serum. *Science* 1973;180:966–968.
69. Van Zwieten MJ, Bhan AK, McCluskey RT, Collins AB. Studies on the pathogenesis of experimental anti-tubular basement membrane nephritis in the guinea pig. *Am J Pathol* 1976;83:531–546.
70. Hall CL, Colvin RB, Carey K, McCluskey RT. Passive transfer of autoimmune disease with isologous IgG_1 and IgG_2 antibodies to the tubular basement membrane in strain XIII guinea pigs. Loss of self-tolerance induced by autoantibodies. *J Exp Med* 1977;146:1246–1260.
71. Albini B, Milgrom M, Noble B, Albini C, Ossi E, Andres GA. Transplacental transmission of antibodies to tubular basement membrane in guinea-pigs with autoimmune tubulointerstitial nephritis. *Clin Exp Immunol* 1984;56:153–158.
72. Brown CA, Carey K, Colvin RB. Inhibition of autoimmune tubulointerstitial nephritis in guinea pigs by heterologous antisera containing anti-idiotype antibodies. *J Immunol* 1979;123:2102–2107.
73. Idikio H. Experimental autoimmune tubulointerstitial nephritis in guinea-pigs: effects on renal lesions of cyclophosphamide administered before and after tubular basement membrane immunization on renal lesions. *Immunology* 1982;46:833–839.
74. Rudofsky UH, McMaster PRB, Ma W-S, Steblay RW, Pollara B. Experimental autoimmune renal cortical tubulointerstitial disease in guinea pigs lacking the fourth component of complement (C4). *J Immunol* 1974;112:1387–1393.
75. Rudofsky UH, Steblay RW, Pollara B. Inhibition of experimental autoimmune renal tubulointerstitial disease in guinea pigs by depletion of complement with cobra venom factor. *Clin Immunol Immunopathol* 1975;3:396–407.
76. Rudofsky UH, Pollara B. Studies on the pathogenesis of experimental autoimmune renal tubulointerstitial disease in guinea pigs. I. Inhibition of tissue injury in leukocyte-depleted passive transfer recipients. *Clin Immunol Immunopathol* 1975;4:425–439.
77. Rudofsky UH, Pollara B. Studies on the pathogenesis of experimental autoimmune renal tubulointerstitial disease in guinea pigs. II. Passive transfer of renal lesions by anti-tubular basement membrane autoantibody and nonimmune bone marrow cells to leukocyte-depleted recipients. *Clin Immunol Immunopathol* 1976;6:107–114.
78. Neilson EG, Phillips SM. Cell-mediated immunity in interstitial nephritis. I. T lymphocyte systems in nephritic guinea pigs: the natural history and diversity of the immune response. *J Immunol* 1979; 123:2373–2380.
79. Neilson EG, Phillips SM. Cell-mediated immunity in interstitial nephritis. II. T lymphocyte effector mechanisms in nephritic guinea pigs: analysis of the renotropic migration and cytotoxic response. *J Immunol* 1979;123:2381–2385.
80. Kennedy TL, Merrow M, Phillips SM, Norman M, Neilson EG. Macrophage chemotaxis in anti-tubular basement membrane-induced interstitial nephritis in guinea pigs. *Clin Immunol Immunopathol* 1985;36:243–248.
81. Sugisaki T, Klassen J, Milgrom F, Andres GA, McCluskey RT. Immunopathologic study of an autoimmune tubular and interstitial renal disease in Brown Norway rats. *Lab Invest* 1973;28:658–671.
82. Kazama T, Nakamura T, Morioka T, Oite T, Sato Y, Shimizu F. A nephropathy induced by immunization of rats with EHS tumour. *Clin Exp Immunol* 1985;62:104–111.
83. Lehman DH, Wilson CB, Dixon FJ. Interstitial nephritis in rats immunized with heterologous tubular basement membrane. *Kidney Int* 1974;5:187–195.
84. Neilson EG, Gasser DL, McCafferty E, Zakheim B, Phillips SM. Polymorphism of genes involved in anti-tubular basement membrane disease in rats. *Immunogenetics* 1983;17:55–65.
85. Ulich TR, Bannister KM, Wilson CB. Tubulointerstitial nephritis induced in the Brown Norway rat with chaotropically solubilized bovine tubular basement membrane: the model and the humoral and cellular responses. *Clin Immunol Immunopathol* 1985;36:187–200.
86. Ueda S, Wakashin M, Wakashin Y, Yoshida H, Azemoto R, Iesato K,

Mori T, Mori Y, Ogawa M, Okuda K. Autoimmune interstitial nephritis induced in inbred mice. Analysis of mouse tubular basement membrane antigen and genetic control of immune response to it. *Am J Pathol* 1988;132:304–318.
87. Mampaso FM, Wilson CB. Characterization of inflammatory cells in auto-immune tubulointerstitial nephritis in rats. *Kidney Int* 1983;23: 448–457.
88. Bricio T, Mampaso F. Natural killer function in the rat with interstitial nephritis. *Scand J Immunol* 1991;33:639–645.
89. Langer KH, Thoenes W. Characterization of cells involved in the formation of granuloma. An ultrastructural study on macrophages, epithelioid cells, and giant cells in experimental tubulo-interstitial nephritis. *Virchows Arch B* 1981;36:177–194.
90. Thoenes W, Sonntag W, Heine W-D, Langer KH. Cell fusion as a mechanism for the formation of giant cells (Langhans' type). Autoradiographic findings in autoimmune tubulo-interstitial nephritis of the rat. *Virchows Arch A* 1982;41:45–50.
91. Langer KH, Thoenes W. Endocytotic activity in epithelioid and Langhans' giant cells. Tracer studies with ferritin in the tubulointerstitial (anti-TBM) nephritis model. *Virchows Arch B* 1984;47:177–182.
92. Baum H-P, Thoenes W. Differentiation of granuloma cells (epithelioid cells and multinucleated giant cells): a morphometric analysis. Investigations using the model of experimental autoimmune (anti-TBM) tubulo-interstitial nephritis. *Virchows Arch B* 1985;50:181–192.
93. Baum HP, Thoenes W. Freeze-fracture features of epithelioid cells, multinucleated giant cells, and phagocytic macrophages. Investigations using the model of experimental autoimmune (anti-TBM) tubulo-interstitial nephritis. *Virchows Arch B* 1987;53:13–22.
94. Tang WW, Feng L, Mathison JC, Wilson CB. Cytokine expression, upregulation of intercellular adhesion molecule-1, and leukocyte infiltration in experimental tubulointerstitial nephritis. *Lab Invest* 1994;70: 631–638.
95. Tang WW, Feng L, Xia Y, Wilson CB. Extracellular matrix accumulation in immune-mediated tubulointerstitial injury. *Kidney Int* 1994; 45:1077–1084.
96. Zanetti M, Wilson CB. Characterization of anti-tubular basement membrane antibodies in rats. *J Immunol* 1983;130:2173–2179.
97. Lehman DH, Lee S, Wilson CB, Dixon FJ. Induction of antitubular basement membrane antibodies in rats by renal transplantation. *Transplantation* 1974;17:429–431.
98. Ulich TR, Ni RX, Hewitt CW, Black KS, Go C, Martin DC. The development of humoral immunity to tissue-specific tubular basement membrane alloantigens after renal transplantation across the major histocompatibility barrier in rats immunomodulated with blood transfusions and cyclosporin. *Proc Soc Exp Biol Med* 1988;188:328–334.
99. Hart DNJ, Fabre JW. Kidney-specific allo- and autoantibodies in the alloantibody response to rat kidney: the use of kidney homogenate as a target for serological analysis. *Clin Exp Immunol* 1980;40:111–119.
100. Sugisaki T, Kano K, Andres G, Milgrom F. Antibodies to tubular basement membrane elicited by stimulation with allogeneic kidney. *Kidney Int* 1982;21:557–564.
101. Sugisaki T, Kano K, Andres G, Milgrom F. Transplacental transfer of antibodies to tubular basement membrane. *J Clin Lab Immunol* 1982;7:167–171.
102. De Heer E, Davidoff A, van der Wal A, van Geest M, Paul LC. Chronic renal allograft rejection in the rat. Transplantation-induced antibodies against basement membrane antigens. *Lab Invest* 1994; 70:494–502.
103. Hart DNJ, Fabre JW. Kidney-specific alloantigen system in the rat. Characterization and role in transplantation. *J Exp Med* 1980;151: 651–666.
104. Krieger A, Thoenes GH, Gunther E. Genetic control of autoimmune tubulointerstitial nephritis in rats. *Clin Immunol Immunopathol* 1981;21:301–308.
105. Paul LC, Carpenter CB. Antigenic determinants of tubular basement membranes and Bowman's capsule in rats. *Kidney Int* 1982;21: 800–807.
106. Matsumoto K, McCafferty E, Neilson EG, Gasser DL. Mapping of the genes for tubular basement membrane antigen and a submaxillary gland protease in the rat. *Immunogenetics* 1984;20:117–123.
107. Schlegerová D, Panczak A, Stejskal J, Kren V. Anti-Tubular basement membrane rejection nephropathy in rat kidney transplantation across multiple non-major histocompatibility complex alloantigenic differences. *Transplant Proc* 1990;22:2539–2540.
108. Panczak A, Schlegerová D, Stejskal J, Křen V. Complex genetic determination of the antitubular basement membrane disease in the rat. *Transplant Proc* 1990;22:2568–2569.
109. Panczak A, Schlegerová D, Pravenec M, Stejskal J, Kren V. Further study of the anti-TBM response in the spontaneously hypertensive rat using a panel of recombinant inbred strains. *Transplant Proc* 1993; 25:2828.
110. Zanetti M, Mampaso F, Wilson CB. Anti-idiotype as a probe in the analysis of autoimmune tubulointerstitial nephritis in the Brown Norway rat. *J Immunol* 1983;131:1268–1273.
111. Neilson EG, Phillips SM. Suppression of interstitial nephritis by auto-anti-idiotypic immunity. *J Exp Med* 1982;179–189.
112. Clayman MD, Sun MJ, Michaud L, Brill-Dashoff J, Riblet R, Neilson EG. Clonotypic heterogeneity in experimental interstitial nephritis. Restricted specificity of the anti-tubular basement membrane B cell repertoire is associated with a disease-modifying crossreactive idiotype. *J Exp Med* 1988;167:1296–1312.
113. Karp SL, Kieber-Emmons T, Sun MJ, Wolf G, Neilson EG. Molecular structure of a cross-reactive idiotype on autoantibodies recognizing parenchymal self. *J Immunol* 1993;150:867–879.
114. Neilson EG, McCafferty E, Phillips SM, Clayman MD, Kelly CJ. Anti-idiotypic immunity in interstitial nephritis. II. Rats developing anti-tubular basement membrane disease fail to make an antiidiotypic regulatory response: the modulatory role of an RT7.1$^+$, OX8$^-$ suppressor T cell mechanism. *J Exp Med* 1984;159:1009–1026.
115. Bannister KM, Wilson CB. Transfer of tubulointerstitial nephritis in the Brown Norway rat with anti-tubular basement membrane antibody: quantitation and kinetics of binding and effect of decomplementation. *J Immunol* 1985;135:3911–3917.
116. Wilson CB, Dixon FJ, Fortner JG, Cerilli GJ. Glomerular basement membrane-reactive antibody in anti-lymphocyte globulin. *J Clin Invest* 1971;50:1525–1535.
117. Unanue ER, Dixon FJ. Experimental glomerulonephritis. V. Studies on the interaction of nephrotoxic antibodies with tissues of the rat. *J Exp Med* 1965;121:97–714.
118. Ulich TR, Bannister KM, Wilson CB. Inhibition of the neutrophilic infiltrate of experimental tubulointerstitial nephritis in the Brown-Norway rat by decomplementation. *Clin Immunol Immunopathol* 1987;42:288–297.
119. Lehman DH, Wilson CB. Role of sensitized cells in antitubular basement membrane interstitial nephritis. *Int Arch Allergy Appl Immunol* 1976;51:168–174.
120. Kelly CJ, Clayman MD, Neilson EG. Immunoregulation in experimental interstitial nephritis: immunization with renal tubular antigen in incomplete Freund's adjuvant induces major histocompatibility complex-restricted, OX8$^+$ suppressor T cells which are antigen-specific and inhibit the expression of disease. *J Immunol* 1986;136:903–907.
121. Kelly CJ, Silvers WK, Neilson, EG. Tolerance to parenchymal self. Regulatory role of major histocompatibility complex-restricted, OX8$^+$ suppressor T cells specific for autologous renal tubular antigen in experimental interstitial nephritis. *J Exp Med* 1985;162:1892–1903.
122. Agus D, Mann R, Clayman M, Kelly C, Michaud L, Cohn D, Neilson EG. The effects of daily cyclophosphamide administration on the development and extent of primary experimental interstitial nephritis in rats. *Kidney Int* 1986;29:635–640.
123. Shih W, Hines H, Neilson EG. Effects of cyclosporin on the development of immune-mediated interstitial nephritis. *Kidney Int* 1988;33:1113–1118.
124. Thoenes GH, Umscheid T, Sitter T, Langer KH. Cyclosporin A inhibits autoimmune experimental tubulointerstitial nephritis. *Immunol Lett* 1987;15:301–306.
125. Gimenez A, Leyva-Cobian F, Fierro C, Rio M, Bricio T, Mampaso F. Effect of cyclosporin A on autoimmune tubulointerstitial nephritis in the Brown Norway rat. *Clin Exp Immunol* 1987;69:550–556.
126. Agus D, Mann R, Cohn D, Michaud L, Kelly C, Clayman M, Neilson EG. Inhibitory role of dietary protein restriction on the development and expression of immune-mediated anti-tubular basement membrane-induced tubulointerstitial nephritis in rats. *J Clin Invest* 1985; 76:930–936.
127. Ulich TR, Ni R-X. Inhibition of experimental autoimmune tubulointerstitial nephritis in Brown-Norway rats by (15S)-15-methyl prostaglandin E_1. Analysis of the effect of prostaglandin E_1 on the induction of the humoral immune response and the elicitation of humorally mediated inflammation. *Am J Pathol* 1986;124:286–293.

128. Ulich TR, Ni R-X, Gutmam GA, Zhou D. The effects of a stable analogue of PGE_1 on the IgG subclass response to particulate bovine tubular basement membrane in the Brown-Norway rat. *Proc Soc Exp Biol Med* 1987;185:441–447.
129. Schorlemmer HU, Neubauer HP, Czech J, Dickneite G. Immunosuppressive therapy of organ-specific nephritic autoimmune diseases with 15-deoxyspergualin. *Agents Actions* 1993;39:C121–C124.
130. Wakashin M, Wakashin Y, Ueda S, Takei I, Mori Y, Mori T, Iesato K, Okuda K. Murine autoimmune interstitial nephritis and associated antigen: purification of a soluble tubular basement membrane antigen from mice kidneys. *Renal Physiol* 1980;3:360–367.
131. Wakashin Y, Takei I, Ueda S, Mori Y, Iesato K, Wakashin M, Okuda K. Autoimmune interstitial disease of the kidney and associated antigen purification and characterization of a soluble tubular basement membrane antigen. *Clin Immunol Immunopathol* 1981;19:360–371.
132. Yoshida H, Wakashin Y, Ueda S, Azemoto R, Iesato K, Yamamoto S, Mori T, Ogawa M, Mori Y, Wakashin M. Detection of nephritogenic antigen from the Lewis rat renal tubular basement membrane. *Kidney Int* 1990;37:1286–1294.
133. Clayman MD, Martinez-Hernandez A, Michaud L, Alper R, Mann R, Kefalides NA, Neilson EG. Isolation and characterization of the nephritogenic antigen producing anti-tubular basement membrane disease. *J Exp Med* 1985;161:290–305.
134. Neilson EG, Sun MJ, Kelly CJ, Hines WH, Haverty TP, Clayman MD, Cooke NE. Molecular characterization of a major nephritogenic domain in the autoantigen of anti-tubular basement membrane disease. *Proc Natl Acad Sci USA* 1991;88:2006–2010.
135. Clayman MD, Michaud L, Brentjens J, Andres GA, Kefalides NA, Neilson EG. Isolation of the target antigen of human anti-tubular basement membrane antibody-associated interstitial nephritis. *J Clin Invest* 1986;77:1143–1147.
136. Guery J-C, Hedrich HJ, Mercier P, Reetz IC, Mandet C, Mahieu P, Neilson EG, Druet P. Mapping of a gene for the M_r 48 000 tubular basement membrane antigen in the rat. *Immunogenetics* 1989;29:350–354.
137. Fliger FD, Wieslander J, Brentjens JR, Andres GA, Butkowski RJ. Identification of a target antigen in human anti-tubular basement membrane nephritis. *Kidney Int* 1987;31:800–807.
138. Butkowski RJ, Langeveld JPM, Wieslander J, Brentjens JR, Andres GA. Characterization of a tubular basement membrane component reactive with autoantibodies associated with tubulointerstitial nephritis. *J Biol Chem* 1990;265:21091–21098.
139. Butkowski RJ, Kleppel MM, Katz A, Michael AF, Fish AJ. Distribution of tubulointerstitial nephritis antigen and evidence for multiple forms. *Kidney Int* 1991;40:838–846.
140. Crary CS, Katz A, Fish AJ, Michael AF, Butkowski RJ. Role of a basement membrane glycoprotein in anti-tubular basement membrane nephritis. *Kidney Int* 1993;43:140–146.
141. Yoshioka K, Morimoto Y, Iseki T, Maki S. Characterization of tubular basement membrane antigens in human kidney. *J Immunol* 1986;136:1654–1660.
142. Yoshioka K, Hino S, Takemura T, Miyasato H, Honda E, Maki S. Isolation and characterization of the tubular basement membrane antigen associated with human tubulo-interstitial nephritis. *Clin Exp Immunol* 1992;90:319–325.
143. Miyazato H, Yoshioka K, Hino S, Aya N, Matsuo S, Suzuki N, Suzuki Y, Sinohara H, Maki S. The target antigen of anti-tubular basement membrane antibody-mediated interstitial nephritis. *Autoimmunity* 1994;18:259–265.
144. Kalfa TA, Thull JD, Butkowski RJ, Charonis AS. Tubulointerstitial nephritis antigen interacts with laminin and type IV collagen and promotes cell adhesion. *J Biol Chem* 1994;269:1654–1659.
145. Kanwar YS, Carone FA. Reversible changes of tubular cell and basement membrane in drug-induced renal cystic disease. *Kidney Int* 1984;26:35–43.
146. Butkowski RJ, Carone FA, Grantham JJ, Hudson BG. Tubular basement membrane changes in 2-amino-4,5-diphenylthiazole-induced polycystic disease. *Kidney Int* 1985;28:744–751.
147. Carone FA, Hollenberg PF, Nakamura S, Punyarit P, Glogowski W, Flouret G. Tubular basement membrane change occurs pari passu with the development of cyst formation. *Kidney Int* 1989;35:1034–1040.
148. Carone FA, Bacallao R, Kanwar YS. Biology of polycystic kidney disease. *Lab Invest* 1994;70:437–448.
149. Ehara T, Carone FA, McCarthy KJ, Couchman JR. Basement membrane chondroitin sulfate proteoglycan alterations in a rat model of polycystic kidney disease. *Am J Pathol* 1994;144:612–621.
150. Carone FA, Butkowski RJ, Nakamura S, Polenaković M, Kanwar YS. Tubular basement membrane changes during induction and regression of drug-induced polycystic kidney disease. *Kidney Int* 1994;46:1368–1374.
151. Cohen AH, Hoyer JR. Nephronophthisis. A primary tubular basement membrane defect. *Lab Invest* 1986;55:564–572.
152. Avasthi PS, Avasthi P, Tokuda S, Anderson RE, Williams RC Jr. Experimental glomerulonephritis in the mouse. I. The model. *Clin Exp Immunol* 1971;9:667–676.
153. Bolton WK, Benton FR, Sturgill BC. Autoimmune glomerulotubular-nephropathy in mice. *Clin Exp Immunol* 1978;463–473.
154. Erard D, Moulonguet-Doleris D, Auffredou MT, Graindorge P, Mahieu P, Galanaud P, Dormont J. Specificity of antibodies to heterologous glomerular and tubular basement membranes in BALB/c mice. *Clin Exp Immunol* 1979;38:259–264.
155. Moulonguet-Doleris D, Erard D, Auffredou MT, Foidart JM, Mahieu P, Dormont J. Specificity of antibodies to heterologous glomerular and tubular basement membranes in various strains of mice with different H-2 types. *Clin Exp Immunol* 1981;46:35–43.
156. Rudofsky UH. Spontaneous and induced autoantibodies to renal and nonrenal basement membranes in mice. *Clin Immunol Immunopathol* 1980;15:200–212.
157. Rudofsky UH, Dilwith RL, Tung KSK. Susceptibility differences of inbred mice to induction of autoimmune renal tubulointerstitial lesions. *Lab Invest* 1980;43:463–470.
158. Clayman MD, Michaud L, Neilson EG. Murine interstitial nephritis. VI. Characterization of the B cell response in anti-tubular basement membrane disease. *J Immunol* 1987;139:2242–2249.
159. Rudofsky UH, Dilwith RL, Lynes M, Flaherty L. Murine monoclonal antikidney autoantibodies. 1. Anti-renal proximal tubular basement membrane autoantibodies. *Clin Immunol Immunopathol* 1982;25:165–178.
160. Chen XM, Tanaka T, Kobayashi Y, Shigematsu H, Okumura K. Tubulointerstitial nephritis induced by monoclonal anti-proximal tubular basement membrane antibodies in mice. *Clin Immunol Immunopathol* 1990;54:40–52.
161. Neilson EG, Phillips SM. Murine interstitial nephritis. I. Analysis of disease susceptibility and its relationship to pleiomorphic gene products defining both immune-response genes and a restrictive requirement for cytotoxic T cells at H-2K. *J Exp Med* 1982;155:1075–1085.
162. Zakheim B, McCafferty E, Phillips SM, Clayman M, Neilson EG. Murine interstitial nephritis. II. The adoptive transfer of disease with immune T lymphocytes produces a phenotypically complex interstitial lesion. *J Immunol* 1984;133:234–239.
163. Evans BD, Dilwith RL, Balaban SL, Rudofsky UH. Lack of passive transfer of renal tubulointerstitial disease by serum or monoclonal antibody specific for renal tubular antigens in the mouse. *Int Arch Allergy Appl Immun* 1988;86:238–242.
164. Neilson EG, McCafferty E, Mann R, Michaud L, Clayman M. Murine interstitial nephritis. III. The selection of phenotypic (Lyt and L3T4) and idiotypic (RE-Id) T cell preferences by genes in Igh-1 and H-2K characterizes the cell-mediated potential for disease expression: susceptible mice provide a unique effector T cell repertoire in response to tubular antigen. *J Immunol* 1985;134:2375–2382.
165. Mann R, Zakheim B, Clayman M, McCafferty E, Michaud L, Neilson EG. Murine interstitial nephritis. IV. Long-term cultured $L3T4^+$ T cell lines transfer delayed expression of disease as I-A-restricted inducers of the effector T cell repertoire. *J Immunol* 1985;135:286–293.
166. Meyers CM, Kelly CJ. Effector mechanisms in organ-specific autoimmunity. I. Characterization of a $CD8^+$ T cell line that mediates murine interstitial nephritis. *J Clin Invest* 1991;88:408–416.
167. Meyers CM, Kelly CJ. Immunoregulation and TGF-β_1. Suppression of a nephritogenic murine T cell clone. *Kidney Int* 1994;46:1295–1301.
168. Meyers CM, Kelly CJ. Inhibition of murine nephritogenic effector T cells by a clone-specific suppressor factor. *J Clin Invest* 1994;94:2093–2104.
169. Heeger PS, Smoyer, WE, Saad T, Albert S, Kelly CJ, Neilson EG. Molecular analysis of the helper T cell response in murine interstitial nephritis. T cells recognizing an immunodominant epitope use multiple T cell receptor Vβ genes with similarities across CDR3. *J Clin Invest* 1994;94:2084–2092.
170. Mann R, Kelly CJ, Hines WH, Clayman MD, Blanchard N, Sun MJ,

Neilson EG. Effector T cell differentiation in experimental interstitial nephritis. l. The development and modulation of effector lymphocyte maturation by I-J+ regulatory T cells. *J Immunol* 1987;138:4200–4208.
171. Kelly CJ, Mok H, Neilson EG. The selection of effector T cell phenotype by contrasuppression modulates susceptibility to autoimmune injury. *J Immunol* 1988;141:3022–3028.
172. Neilson EG, McCafferty E, Mann R, Michaud L, Clayman M. Tubular antigen-derivatized cells induce a disease-protective, antigen-specific, and idiotype-specific suppressor T cell network restricted by I-J and Igh-V in mice with experimental interstitial nephritis. *J Exp Med* 1985;162:215–230.
173. Mann R, Neilson EG. Murine interstitial nephritis. V. The auto-induction of antigen-specific Lyt-2+ suppressor T cells diminishes the expression of interstitial nephritis in mice with antitubular basement membrane disease. *J Immunol* 1986;136:908–912.
174. Neilson EG, Kelly CJ, Clayman MD, Hines WH, Haverty T, Sun MJ, Blanchard N. Murine interstitial nephritis. VII. Suppression of renal injury after treatment with soluble suppressor factor $TsF_1{}^1$. *J Immunol* 1987;139:1518–1524.
175. Rubin-Kelley VE, Jevnikar AM. Antigen presentation by renal tubular epithelial cells. *J Am Soc Nephrol* 1991;2:13–26.
176. Kelley VR, Singer GG. The antigen presentation function of renal tubular epithelial cells. *Exp Nephrol* 1993;1:102–111.
177. Germain RN. The biochemistry and cell biology of antigen processing and presentation. *Annu Rev Immunol* 1993;11:403–450.
178. Haverty TP, Kelly CJ, Hines WH, Amenta PS, Watanabe M, Harper RA, Kefalides NA, Neilson EG. Characterization of a renal tubular epithelial cell line which secretes the autologous target antigen of autoimmune experimental interstitial nephritis. *J Cell Biol* 1988;107: 1359–1368.
179. Haverty TP, Watanabe M, Neilson EG, Kelly CJ. Protective modulation of class II MHC gene expression in tubular epithelium by target antigen-specific antibodies. Cell-surface directed down-regulation of transcription can influence susceptibility to murine tubulointerstitial nephritis. *J Immunol* 1989;143:1133–1141.
180. Hagerty DT, Allen PM. Processing and presentation of self and foreign antigens by the renal proximal tubule. *J Immunol* 1992;148: 2324–2330.
181. Jevnikar AM, Singer GG, Coffman T, Glimcher LH, Rubin Kelley VE. Renal tubular cell expression of MHC class II (l-E^b) is insufficient to initiate immune injury in a transgenic kidney transplant model. *Transplant Proc* 1993;25:142–143.
182. Jevnikar AM, Singer GG, Coffman T, Glimcher LH, Rubin Kelley VE. Transgenic tubular cell expression of class II is insufficient to initiate immune renal injury. *J Am Soc Nephrol* 1993;3:1972–1977.
183. Neilson EG. Is immunologic tolerance of self modulated through antigen presentation by parenchymal epithelium? *Kidney Int* 1993;44: 927–931.
184. Singer GG, Yokoyama H, Bloom RD, Jevnikar AM, Nabavi N, Rubin Kelley V. Stimulated renal tubular epithelial cells induce anergy in CD4+ T cells. *Kidney Int* 1993;44:1030–1035.
185. Rubin Kelley V, Diaz-Gallo C, Jevnikar AM, Singer GG. Renal tubular epithelial and T cell interactions in autoimmune renal disease. *Kidney Int* 43(Suppl 39);1993:S108–S115.
186. Hagerty DT, Evavold BD, Allen PM. Regulation of the costimulator B7, not class 11 major histocompatibility complex, restricts the ability of murine kidney tubule cells to stimulate CD4+ T cells. *J Clin Invest* 1994;93:1208–1215.
187. Yokoyama H, Zheng X, Strom TB, Rubin Kelley V. B7+—transfectant tubular epithelial cells induce T cell anergy, ignorance or proliferation. *Kidney Int* 1994;45:1105–1112.
188. Ueda S, Wakashin M, Wakashin Y, Yoshida H, Iesato K, Mori T, Mori Y, Akikusa B, Okuda K. Experimental gold nephropathy in guinea pigs: detection of autoantibodies to renal tubular antigens. *Kidney Int* 1986;29:539–548.
189. Druet E, Sapin C, Gunther E, Feingold N, Druet P. Mercuric chloride-induced anti-glomerular basement membrane antibodies in the rat. Genetic control. *Eur J Immunol* 1977;7:348–351.
190. Ueda S, Wakashin M, Wakashin Y, Mori T, Yoshida H, Mori Y, Iesato K, Ogawa M, Azemoto R, Kato I, Okuda K. Suppressor system in murine interstitial nephritis. Analysis of tubular basement membrane (TBM)-specific suppressor T cells and their soluble factor in C57BL/6 mice using a syngeneic system. *Clin Immunol Immunopathol* 1987; 45:78–91.
191. Mezza LE, Seiler RJ, Smith CA, Lewis RM. Antitubular basement membrane autoantibody in a dog with chronic tubulointerstitial nephritis. *Vet Pathol* 1984;21:178–181.
192. Thorner P, Jansen B, Baumal R, Valli VE, Goldgerger A. Samoyed hereditary glomerulopathy. Immunohistochemical staining of basement membranes of kidney for laminin, collagen type IV, fibronectin, and Goodpasture antigen, and correlation with electron microscopy of glomerular capillary basement membranes. *Lab Invest* 1987;56: 435–443.
193. Hood JC, Savige J, Hendtlass A, Kleppel MM, Huxtable CR, Robinson WF. Bull terrier hereditary nephritis: a model for autosomal dominant Alport syndrome. *Kidney Int* 1995;47:758–765.
194. Brentjens JR, Sepulveda M, Baliah T, Bentzel C, Erlanger BF, Elwood C, Montes M, Hsu KC, Andres GA. Interstitial immune complex nephritis in patients with systemic lupus erythematosus. *Kidney Int* 1975;7:342–350.
195. Magil AB, Tyler M. Tubulo-interstitial disease in lupus nephritis. A morphometric study. *Histopathology* 1984;8:81–87.
196. O'Dell JR, Hays RC, Guggenheim SJ, Steigerwald JC. Tubulointerstitial renal disease in systemic lupus erythematosus. *Arch Intern Med* 1985;145:1996–1999.
197. Park MH, Agati VD, Appel GB, Pirani CL. Tubulointerstitial disease in lupus nephritis: relationship to immune deposits, interstitial inflammation, glomerular changes, renal function, and prognosis. *Nephron* 1986;44:309–319.
198. Biesecker G, Katz S, Koffler D. Renal localization of the membrane attack complex in systemic lupus erythematosus nephritis. *J Exp Med* 1981;154:1779–1794.
199. Caligaris-cappio F, Bergui L, Tesio L, Ziano R, Camussi G. HLA-Dr+ T cells of the Leu 3 (helper) type infiltrate the kidneys of patients with systemic lupus erythematosus. *Clin Exp Immunol* 1985; 59:185–189.
200. Gur H, Kopolovic Y, Gross DJ. Chronic predominant interstitial nephritis in a patient with systemic lupus erythematosus: a follow up of three years and review of the literature. *Ann Rheum Dis* 1987;46: 617–623.
201. Burden RP, Cotton RE, Wallington TB, Reeves WG. Immune deposits in extraglomerular vessels: their correlation with circulating immune complexes. *Clin Exp Immunol* 1980;42:483–489.
202. Frasca GM, Vangelista A, Biagini G, Bonomini V. Immunologic tubulo-interstitial deposits in IgA nephropathy. *Kidney Int* 1982;22: 184–191.
203. Nojima Y, Terai C, Takano K, Takehara K, Yamada A, Takaku F. Tubulointerstitial immune complex nephritis in a patient with cutaneous vasculitis. *Clin Nephrol* 1986;25:48–51.
204. Yuzawa Y, Aoi N, Fukatsu A, Ichida S, Yoshida F, Akatsuka Y, Minami S, Kodera Y, Matsuo S. Acute renal failure and degenerative tubular lesions associated with in situ formation of adenovirus immune complexes in a patient with allogeneic bone marrow transplantation. *Transplantation* 1993;55:67–72.
205. Brentjens JR, O'Connell DW, Pawlowski IB, Andres GA. Extraglomerular lesions associated with deposition of circulating antigen-antibody complexes in kidneys of rabbits with chronic serum sickness. *Clin Immunol Immunopathol* 1974;3:112–126.
206. Wilson CB. Renal response to immunologic glomerular injury. In: Brenner BM, ed. *The Kidney*, 5th ed, vol 2. Philadelphia: Saunders, 1996;1253–1391.
207. Gelfand MC, Frank MM, Green I, Shin ML. Binding sites for immune complexes containing IgG in the renal interstitium. *Clin Immunol Immunopathol* 1979;13:19–29.
208. Vogt A, Batsford S. Local immune complex formation and pathogenesis of glomerulonephritis. *Contr Nephrol* 1984;43:51–63.
209. Aarli A, Matre R, Thunold S. IgG Fc receptors on epithelial cells of distal tubuli and on endothelial cells in human kidney. *Int Arch Allergy Appl Immunol* 1991;95:64–69.
210. Zanetti M, Wilson CB. A role for anti-idiotypic antibodies in immunologically mediated nephritis. *Am J Kidney Dis* 1986;6:445–451.
211. Andrews BS, Eisenberg RA, Theofilopoulos AN, Izui S, Wilson CB, McConahey PJ, Murphy ED, Roths JB, Dixon FJ. Spontaneous murine lupus-like syndromes. Clinical and immunopathological manifestations in several strains. *J Exp Med* 1978;148:1198–1215.
212. Yamamoto T, Nagase M, Hishida A, Honda N. Specific increases in urinary excretion of anti-DNA antibodies in lupus mice induced by lysozyme administration: further evidence for DNA–anti-DNA

immune complexes in the pathogenesis of nephritis. *Clin Exp Immunol* 1993;91:115–120.
213. Boswell JM, Yui MA, Endres S, Burt DW, Kelley VE. Novel and enhanced IL-1 gene expression in autoimmune mice with lupus. *J Immunol* 1988;141:118–124.
214. Boswell JM, Yui MA, Burt DW, Kelley VE. Increased tumor necrosis factor and IL-1 β gene expression in the kidneys of mice with lupus nephritis. *J Immunol* 1988;141:3050–3054.
215. Brennan DC, Yui MA, Wuthrich RP, Kelley VE. Tumor necrosis factor and IL-1 in New Zealand black/white mice. Enhanced gene expression and acceleration of renal injury. *J Immunol* 1989;143:3470–3475.
216. Jevnikar AM, Wuthrich RP, Takei F, Xu H-W, Brennan DC, Glimcher LH, Rubin-Kelley VE. Differing regulation and function of ICAM-1 and class II antigens on renal tubular cells. *Kidney Int* 1990;38:417–425.
217. Wuthrich RP, Jevnikar AM, Takei F, Glimcher LH, Kelley VE. Intercellular adhesion molecule-1(ICAM-1) expression is upregulated in autoimmune murine lupus nephritis. *Am J Pathol* 1990;136:441–450.
218. Wuthrich RP. Vascular cell adhesion molecule-1 (VCAM-1) expression in murine lupus nephritis. *Kidney Int* 1992;42:903–914.
219. Wuthrich RP, Yui MA, Mazoujian G, Nabavi N, Glimcher LH, Kelley VE. Enhanced MHC class II expression in renal proximal tubules precedes loss of renal function in MRL/*lpr* mice with lupus nephritis. *Am J Pathol* 1989;134:45–51.
220. Díaz-Gallo C, Jevnikar AM, Brennan DC, Florquin S, Pacheco-Silva A, Rubin Kelley V. Autoreactive kidney infiltrating T-cell clones in murine lupus nephritis. *Kidney Int* 1992;42:851–859.
221. Díaz-Gallo C, Rubin Kelley V. Self-regulation of autoreactive kidney-infiltrating T cells in MRL-*lpr* nephritis. *Kidney Int* 1993;44:692–699.
222. Cochrane CG, Weigle WO. The cutaneous reaction to soluble antigen-antibody complexes. A comparison with the Arthus phenomenon. *J Exp Med* 1958;108:591–604.
223. Colten HR. Drawing a double-edged sword. *Nature* 1994;371:474–475.
224. Joh K, Shibasaki T, Azuma T, Kobayashi A, Miyahara T, Aizawa S, Watanabe N. Experimental drug-induced allergic nephritis mediated by antihapten antibody. *Int Arch Allergy Appl Immunol* 1989;88:337–344.
225. Joh K, Aizawa S, Ohkawa K, Morioka T, Oite T, Shimizu F, Batsford S, Vogt A. Selective planting of cationized, haptenized ovalbumin on the rat tubular basement membrane. *Virchows Arch* 1994;424:587–591.
226. Alpers CE, Hudkins KL, Pritzl P, Johnson RJ. Mechanisms of clearance of immune complexes from peritubular capillaries in the rat. *Am J Pathol* 1991;139:855–867.
227. Kleinknecht D, Vanhille Ph, Morel-Maroger L, Kanfer A, Lemaitre V, Mery JP, Laederich J, Callard P. Acute interstitial nephritis due to drug hypersensitivity. An up-to-date review with a report of 19 cases. *Adv Nephrol* 1983;12:277–308.
228. Sitprija V, Pipatanagul V, Koesoemowardojo M, Boonpucknavig V, Boonpucknavig S. Pathogenesis of renal disease in leptospirosis: clinical and experimental studies. *Kidney Int* 1980;17:827–836.
229. Alves VAF, Gayotto LCC, Yasuda PH, Wakamatsu A, Kanamura CT, DeBrito T. Leptospiral antigens (*L. interrogans* serogroup *icterohaemorrhagiae*) in the kidney of experimentally infected guinea pigs and their relation to the pathogenesis of the renal injury. *Exp Pathol* 1991;42:81–93.
230. Shwayder M, Ozawa T, Boedecker E, Guggenheim S, McIntosh RM. Nephrotic syndrome associated with Fanconi syndrome. Immunopathogenic studies of tubulointerstitial nephritis with autologous immune-complex glomerulonephritis. *Ann Intern Med* 1976;84:433–437.
231. Paul LC, Stuffers-Heiman M, Van Es LA, De Graeff J. Antibodies directed against brush border antigens of proximal tubules in renal allograft recipients. *Clin Immunol Immunopathol* 1979;14:238–243.
232. Fasth A, Ahlstedt S, Hanson LA, Jann B, Jann K, Kaijser B. Cross-reactions between the Tamm-Horsfall glycoprotein and Escherichia coli. *Int Arch Allergy Appl Immunol* 1980;63:303–311.
233. Pascal RR, Sian CS, Brensilver JM, Kahn M, Lefavour GS. Demonstration of an antibody to tubular epithelium in glomerulonephritis associated with obstructive urology. *Am J Med* 1980;69:944–948.
234. Morrison EB, Kozlowski EJ, McPhaul JJ Jr. Primary tubulointerstitial nephritis caused by antibodies to proximal tubular antigens. *Am J Clin Pathol* 1981;75:602–609.
235. Cotran RS. Glomerulosclerosis in reflux nephropathy. *Kidney Int* 1982;21:528–534.
236. Hemstreet GP, Brown AL, Fine PR, Molay MP, Wheat R. *Salmonella minnesota* Re 595 lipid A induced nephritis. *J Urol* 1982;127:374–378.
237. Gaarder PI, Heier HE. A human autoantibody to renal collecting duct cells associated with thyroid and gastric autoimmunity and possibly renal tubular acidosis. *Clin Exp Immunol* 1983;51:29–37.
238. Fasth A, Bjure J, Hjalmas K, Jacobsson B, Jodal U. Serum autoantibodies to Tamm-Horsfall protein and their relation to renal damage and glomerular filtration rate in children with urinary tract malformations. *Contrib Nephrol* 1984;39:285–295.
239. Yamada K, Tamura Y, Tomioka H, Kumagai A, Yoshida S. Possible existence of anti-renal tubular plasma membrane autoantibody which blocked parathyroid hormone-induced phosphaturia in a patient with pseudohypoparathyroidism Type II and Sjogren's syndrome. *J Clin Endocrinol Metab* 1984;58:339–343.
240. Feye GL, Hemstreet GP III, Klingensmith C, Cruse JM, Lewis RE, Anderson IC. Auto-antibody to kidney tubular cells during retrograde chronic pyelonephritis in rats. *Nephron* 1985;39:371–376.
241. Chambers R, Groufsky A, Hunt JS, Lynn KL, McGiven AR. Relationship of abnormal Tamm-Horsfall glycoprotein localization to renal morphology and function. *Clin Nephrol* 1986;26:21–26.
242. Benkovic J, Jelakovic B, Cikes N. Antibodies to Tamm-Horsfall protein in patients with acute pyelonephritis. *Eur J Clin Chem Clin Biochem* 1994;32:337–340.
243. Unanue ER, Dixon FJ, Feldman JD. Experimental allergic glomerulonephritis induced in the rabbit with homologous renal antigens. *J Exp Med* 1967;125:163–175.
244. Klassen J, McCluskey RT, Milgrom F. Nonglomerular renal disease produced in rabbits by immunization with homologous kidney. *Am J Pathol* 1971;63:333–358.
245. Clagett JA, Wilson CB, Weigle WO. Interstitial immune complex thyroiditis in mice. The role of autoantibody to thyroglobulin. *J Exp Med* 1974;140:1439–1456.
246. Edgington TS, Glassock RJ, Watson JI, Dixon FJ. Characterization and isolation of specific renal tubular epithelial antigens. *J Immunol* 1967;99:1199–1210.
247. Edgington TS, Glassock RJ, Dixon FJ. Autologous immune complex nephritis induced with renal tubular antigen. I. Identification and isolation of the pathogenetic antigen. *J Exp Med* 1968;127:555–572.
248. Klassen J, Milgrom F. Autoimmune concomitants of renal allografts. *Transplant Proc* 1969;1:605–608.
249. Klassen J, Milgrom FM, McCluskey RT. Studies of the antigens involved in an immunologic renal tubular lesion in rabbits. *Am J Pathol* 1977;88:135–144.
250. Meads TJ, Wild AE. Apical expression of an antigen common to rabbit yolk sac endoderm and kidney proximal tubule epithelium. *J Reprod Immunol* 1993;23:247–264.
251. Fukatsu A, Yuzawa Y, Niesen N, Matsuo S, Caldwell PRB, Brentjens JR, Andres G. Local formation of immune deposits in rabbit renal proximal tubules. *Kidney Int* 1988;34:611–619.
252. Klassen J, Sugisaki T, Milgrom F, McCluskey RT. Studies on multiple renal lesions in Heymann nephritis. *Lab Invest* 1971;25:577–585.
253. Allison MEM, Wilson CB, Gottschalk CW. Pathophysiology of experimental glomerulonephritis in rats. *J Clin Invest* 1974;53:1402–1423.
254. Mendrick DL, Noble B, Brentjens JR, Andres GA. Antibody-mediated injury to proximal tubules in Heymann nephritis. *Kidney Int* 1980;18:328–343.
255. Noble B, Mendrick DL, Brentjens JR, Andres GA. Antibody-mediated injury to proximal tubules in the rat kidney induced by passive transfer of homologous anti-brush border serum. *Clin Immunol Immunopathol* 1981;19:289–301.
256. Noble B, Andres GA, Brentjens JR. Passively transferred anti-brush border antibodies induce injury of proximal tubules in the absence of complement. *Clin Exp Immunol* 1983;56:281–288.
257. Eddy AA, Ho GC, Thorner PS. The contribution of antibody-mediated cytotoxicity and immune-complex formation to tubulointerstitial disease in passive Heymann nephritis. *Clin Immunol Immunopathol* 1992;62:42–55.
258. Salant DJ, Belok S, Madaio MP, Couser WG. A new role for complement in experimental membranous nephropathy in rats. *J Clin Invest* 1980;66:1339–1350.

259. Camussi G, Brentjens JR, Noble B, Kerjaschki D, Malavasi F, Roholt OA, Farquhar MG, Andres G. Antibody-induced redistribution of Heymann antigen on the surface of cultured glomerular visceral epithelial cells: possible role in the pathogenesis of Heymann glomerulonephritis. *J Immunol* 1985;135:2409–2416.
260. Cybulsky AV, Quigg RJ, Salant DJ. The membrane attack complex in complement-mediated glomerular epithelial cell injury: formation and stability of C5b-9 and C5b-7 in rat membranous nephropathy. *J Immunol* 1986;137:1511–1516.
261. Cybulsky AV, Rennke HG, Feintzeig ID, Salant DJ. Complement-induced glomerular epithelial cell injury: role of the membrane attack complex in rat membranous nephropathy. *J Clin Invest* 1986;77: 1096–1107.
262. Camussi C, Noble B, Van Liew J, Brentjens JR, Andres G. Pathogenesis of passive Heymann glomerulonephritis: chlorpromazine inhibits antibody-mediated redistribution of cell surface antigens and prevents development of the disease. *J Immunol* 1986;136:2127–2135.
263. Camussi G, Salvidio G, Biesecker G, Brentjens J, Andres G. Heymann antibodies induce complement-dependent injury of rat glomerular visceral epithelial cells. *J Immunol* 1987;139:2906–2914.
264. Quigg RJ, Cybulsky AV, Salant DJ. The nephritogenic antibody (AB) of passive Heymann nephritis (PHN) directs complement (C)-mediated cytotoxicity of cultured glomerular visceral epithelial cells (GEC). *Kidney Int* 1987;31:328a.
265. Cybulsky AV, Quigg RJ, Badalamenti J, Salant DJ. Anti-Fx1A induces association of Heymann nephritis antigens with microfilaments of cultured glomerular visceral epithelial cells. *Am J Pathol* 1987;129:373–384.
266. Gutmann EJ, Niles JL, McCluskey RT, Brown D. Loss of antigens associated with the apical endocytotic pathway in proximal tubules from rats with Heymann Nephritis. *Am J Pathol* 1991;138:1243–1255.
267. Saito A, Pietromonaco S, Loo AK, Farquhar MG. Complete cloning and sequencing of rat gp330/"megalin," a distinctive member of the low density lipoprotein receptor gene family. *Proc Natl Acad Sci USA* 1994;91:9725–9729.
268. Farquhar MG. The unfolding story of megalin (gp330): now recognized as a drug receptor. *J Clin Invest* 1995;96:1184.
269. Raychowdhury R, Niles J, McCluskey RT, Smith JA. Autoimmune target in Heymann nephritis is a glycoprotein with homology to the LDL-receptor. *Science* 1989;244:1163–1165.
270. Pietromonaco S, Kerjaschki D, Binder S, Ullrich R, Farquhar MG. Molecular cloning of a cDNA encoding a major pathogenic domain of the Heymann nephritis antigen gp330. *Proc Natl Acad Sci USA* 1990;87:1811–1815.
271. Strickland DK, Ashcom JD, Williams S, Battey F, Behre E, McTigue K, Battey JF, Argraves WS. Primary structure of α_2-macroglobulin receptor-associated protein. *J Biol Chem* 1991;266:13364–13369.
272. Orlando RA, Kerjaschki D, Kurihara H, Biemesderfer D, Farquhar MG. gp330 associates with a 44-kDa protein in the rat kidney to form the Heymann nephritis antigenic complex. *Proc Natl Acad Sci USA* 1992;89:6698–6702.
273. Farquhar MG, Kerjaschki D, Lundstrom M, Orlando RA. gp330 and RAP: the Heymann nephritis antigenic complex. *Ann NY Acad Sci* 1994;737:96–113.
274. Kerjaschki D, Noronha-Blob L, Sackktor S, Farquhar MG. Microdomains of distinctive glycoprotein composition in the kidney proximal tubule brush border. *J Cell Biol* 1984;98:1505–1513.
275. Bhan A, Schneeberger E, Baird L, Collins A, Kamata K, Bradford D, Erikson M, McCluskey RT. Studies with monoclonal antibodies against brush border antigens in Heymann nephritis. *Lab Invest* 1985; 53:421–432.
276. Chatelet F, Brianti E, Ronco P, Roland J, Verroust P. Ultrastructural localization by monoclonal antibodies of brush border antigens expressed by glomeruli. I. Renal distribution. *Am J Pathol* 1986;122: 500–511.
277. Chatelet F, Brianti E, Ronco P, Roland J, Verroust P. Ultrastructural localization by monoclonal antibodies of brush border antigens expressed by glomeruli. II. Extrarenal distribution. *Am J Pathol* 1986; 122:512–519.
278. Abbate M, Bachinsky D, Zheng G, Stamenkovic I, McLaughlin M, Niles JL, McCluskey RT, Brown D. Localization of gp330/α_2M receptor-associated protein (α_2-MRAP) and its binding sites in kidney: distribution of endogenous α_2-MRAP is modified by tissue processing. *Eur J Cell Biol* 1993;61:139–149.
279. Ronco P, Allegri L, Melcion C, Pirotsky E, Appay M-D, Bariety J, Pontillon F, Verroust P. A monoclonal antibody to brush border and passive Heymann nephritis. *Clin Exp Immunol* 1984;55:319–332.
280. Ronco P, Neale TJ, Wilson CB, Galceran M, Verroust P. An immunopathologic study of a 330-kD protein defined by monoclonal antibodies and reactive with anti-RTE-alpha-5 antibodies and kidney eluates from active Heymann nephritis. *J Immunol* 1986;136: 125–130.
281. Ronco P, Melcion C, Geniteau M, Ronco E, Reininger L, Galceran M, Verroust P. Production and characterization of monoclonal antibodies against rat brush border antigens of the proximal convoluted tubule. *Immunology* 1994;53:87–95.
282. Assmann KJM, van Son JPHF, Dijkman HBPM, Koene RAP. A nephritogenic rat monoclonal antibody to mouse aminopeptidase A. Induction of massive albuminuria after a single intravenous injection. *J Exp Med* 1992;175:623–635.
283. Tsukada Y, Ono K, Maezawa A, Yano S, Naruse T. A major pathogenic antigen of Heymann nephritis is present exclusively in the renal proximal tubule brush border—studies with a monoclonal antibody against pronase-digested tubular antigen. *Clin Exp Immunol* 1994;96: 303–310.
284. Tamm I, Horsfall, Jr. FL. A mucoprotein derived from human urine which reacts with influenza, mumps, and Newcastle disease viruses. *J Exp Med* 1952;95:71–97.
285. Pennica D, Kohr WJ, Kuang W-J, Glaister D, Aggarwal BB, Chen EY, Goeddel DV. Identification of human uromodulin as the Tamm-Horsfall urinary glycoprotein. *Science* 1987;236:83–88.
286. Rindler MJ, Naik SS, Li N, Hoops TC, Peraldi M-N. Uromodulin (Tamm-Horsfall glycoprotein/uromucoid) is a phosphatidylinositol-linked membrane protein. *J Biol Chem* 1990;265:20784–20789.
287. Brown D, Waneck GL. Glycosyl-phosphatidylinositol-anchored membrane proteins. *J Am Soc Nephrol* 1992;3:895–906.
288. Jeanpierre C, Whitmore SA, Austruy E, Cohen-Salmon M, Callen DF, Junien C. Chromosomal assignment of the uromodulin gene (UMOD) to 16p13.11. *Cytogenet Cell Genet* 1993;62:185–187.
289. Pook MA, Jeremiah S, Scheinman SJ, Povey S, Thakker RV. Localization of the Tamm-Horsfall glycoprotein (uromodulin) gene to chromosome 16p12.3-16p13.11. *Ann Hum Genet* 1993;57:285–290.
290. Thomas DB, Davies M, Williams JD. Tamm-Horsfall protein: an aetiological agent in tubulointerstitial disease? *Exp Nephrol* 1993;1: 281–284.
291. Yu H, Papa F, Sukhatme VP. Bovine and rodent Tamm-Horsfall protein (THP) genes: cloning, structural analysis, and promoter identification. *Gene Expr* 1994;4:63–75.
292. Hoyer JR, Seiler MW. Pathophysiology of Tamm-Horsfall protein. *Kidney Int* 1979;16:279–289.
293. Sikri KL, Alexander DP, Foster CL. Localization of Tamm-Horsfall glycoprotein in the normal rat kidney and the effect of adrenalectomy on its localization in the hamster and rat kidney. *J Anat* 1982;135: 29–45.
294. Hoyer JR. Tubulointerstitial immune complex nephritis in rats immunized with Tamm-Horsfall protein. *Kidney Int* 1980;17:284–292.
295. Seiler MW, Hoyer JR. Ultrastructural studies of tubulointerstitial immune complex nephritis in rats immunized with Tamm-Horsfall protein. *Lab Invest* 1981;45:321–327.
296. Hoyer JR, Seiler MW. Influence of renal transplantation in rats on glomerular and tubular immune complexes. *Am J Kidney Dis* 1986;7: 69–75.
297. Friedman J, Hoyer JR, Seiler MW. Formation and clearance of tubulointerstitial immune complexes in kidneys of rats immunized with heterologous antisera to Tamm-Horsfall protein. *Kidney Int* 1982;21: 575–582.
298. Fasth A, Hoyer JR, Seiler MW. Renal tubular immune complex formation in mice immunized with Tamm-Horsfall protein. *Am J Pathol* 1986;125:555–562.
299. Mayrer AR, Kashgarian M, Ruddle NH, Marier R, Hodson CJ, Richards EF, Andriole VT. Tubulointerstitial nephritis and immunologic responses to Tamm-Horsfall protein in rabbits challenged with homologous urine or Tamm-Horsfall protein. *J Immunol* 1982;128: 2634–2642.
300. Berke ES, Mayrer AR, Miniter P, Andriole T. Tubulointerstitial nephritis in rabbits challenged with homologous Tamm-Horsfall protein: the role of endotoxin. *Clin Exp Immunol* 1983;53:562–572.
301. Ishidate T, Hoyer JR, Seiler MW. Influence of altered glomerular per-

meability on renal tubular immune complex formation and clearance. *Lab Invest* 1983;49:582–588.
302. Ishidate T, Hebert D, Seiler MW, Hoyer JR. Immunomorphometric studies of proteinuria in individual nephrons of rats. *Lab Invest* 1992;67:369–378.
303. Resnick JS, Sisson S, Vernier RL. Tamm-Horsfall protein: abnormal localization in renal disease. *Lab Invest* 1978;38:550–555.
304. Dziukas LJ, Sterzel RB, Hodson CJ, Hoyer JR. Renal localization of Tamm-Horsfall protein in unilateral obstructive uropathy in rats. *Lab Invest* 1982;47:185–193.
305. Cotran RS, Hodson CJ. Extratubular localization of Tamm-Horsfall in experimental reflux nephropathy in the pig. In: Hodson CJ, Kincaid-Smith P, eds. *Reflux Nephropathy*. New York: Masson Publishing, 1979;213.
306. Mayrer AR, Dziukas L, Hodson CJ, Andriole VT. Antibody to Tamm-Horsfall protein in porcine reflux nephropathy. *Kidney Int* 1980;19:187a.
307. Lambert C, Brealey R, Steele J, Rook GAW. The interaction of Tamm-Horsfall protein with the extracellular matrix. *Immunology* 1993;79:203–210.
308. Thomas DBL, Davies M, Williams JD. Release of gelatinase and superoxide from human mononuclear phagocytes in response to particulate Tamm Horsfall protein. *Am J Pathol* 1993;142:249–260.
309. Yu C-L, Tsai C-Y, Lin W-M, Liao T-S, Chen H-L, Sun K-H, Chen K-H. Tamm-Horsfall urinary glycoprotein enhances monokine release and augments lymphocyte proliferation. *Immunopharmacology* 1993;26:249–258.
310. Toma G, Bates JM Jr, Kumar S. Uromodulin (Tamm-Horsfall protein) is a leukocyte adhesion molecule. *Biochem Biophys Res Commun* 1994;200:275–282.
311. Rhodes DCJ, Hinsman EJ, Rhodes JA. Tamm-Horsfall glycoprotein binds IgG with high affinity. *Kidney Int* 1993;44:1014–1021.
312. Koss MN, Pirani CL, Osserman EF. Experimental Bence Jones cast nephropathy. *Lab Invest* 1976;34:579–591.
313. Sanders PW, Booker BB. Pathobiology of cast nephropathy from human Bence Jones proteins. *J Clin Invest* 1992;89:630–639.
314. Huang Z-Q, Kirk KA, Connelly KG, Sanders PW. Bence Jones proteins bind to a common peptide segment of Tamm-Horsfall glycoprotein to promote heterotypic aggregation. *J Clin Invest* 1993;92: 2975–2983.
315. Sanders PW. Pathogenesis and treatment of myeloma kidney. *J Lab Clin Med* 1994;124:484–488.
316. Sanders PW, Herrera GA, Galla JH. Human Bence Jones protein toxicity in rat proximal tubule epithelium in vivo. *Kidney Int* 1987;32: 851–861.
317. Bander NH, Cordon-Cardo C, Finstad CL, Whitmore WF Jr, Vaughn ED Jr, Oettgen HF, Melamed M, Old LJ. Immunohistologic dissection of the human kidney using monoclonal antibodies. *J Urol* 1985; 133:502–505.
318. Andreesen R, Baier W, Corvol P, Pinet F, Celio MR. Monoclonal antibodies against a human juxtaglomerular epithelioid granular cell tumour. *Acta Anat* 1991;140:130–134.
319. Shimokama T, Watanabe T. Monoclonal antibodies to rat renal tissue: an approach to the immunohistological analysis of the nephron-collecting duct system, and ultra-structural localization of antigens. *Histochem J* 1991;23:13–21.
320. Okot-Opiro P, Baier W, Celio MR. Monoclonal antibodies against rat kidney antigens. *Acta Anat* 1992;144:213–224.
321. Tauc M, Koechlin N, Jamous M, Ouaghi EM, Gastineau M, Le Moal C, Poujeol P. Principal and intercalated cells in primary cultures of rabbit renal collecting tubules revealed by monoclonal antibodies. *Biol Cell* 1992;76:55–65.
322. Birk H-W, Ogiermann M, Altmannsberger M, Schütterle G, Haase W, Koepsell H. Monoclonal antibodies against luminal membranes of renal proximal tubules which are kidney-specific. *Biochim Biophys Acta* 1993;1148:67–76.
323. Davis ID, LeBien TW, Lindman BJ, Platt JL. Biochemical and histochemical characterization of a murine tubular antigen. *J Am Soc Nephrol* 1991;1:1153–1161.
324. Mirshahi M, Razaghi A, Vandewalle A, Cluzeaud F, Tarraf M, Faure J-P. Immunodetection and localization of protein(s) related to retinal S-antigen (arrestin) in kidney. *Biol Cell* 1992;76:175–184.
325. Verpooten GF, Nuyts GD, Hoylaerts MF, Nouwen EJ, Vassanyiova Z, Dlhopolcek P, De Broe ME. Immunoassay in urine of a specific marker for proximal tubular S3 segment. *Clin Chem* 1992;38: 642–647.
326. Nishi N, Kagawa Y, Miyanaka H, Oya H, Wada F. An anti-probasin monoclonal antibody recognizes a novel 40-kDa protein localized in rat liver and a specific region of kidney urinary tubule. *Biochim Biophys Acta* 1992;1117:47–54.
327. Blake PG, Madrenas J, Halloran PF. Ly-6 in kidney is widely expressed on tubular epithelium and vascular endothelium and is up-regulated by interferon gamma. *J Am Soc Nephrol* 1993;4:1140–1150.
328. Barlet-Bas C, Arystarkhova E, Cheval L, Marsy S, Sweadner K, Modyanov N, Doucet A. Are there several isoforms of Na,K-ATPase α subunit in the rabbit kidney? *J Biol Chem* 1993;268:11512–11515.
329. Kloth S, Aigner J, Brandt E, Moll R, Minuth WW. Histochemical markers reveal an unexpected heterogeneous composition of the renal embryonic collecting duct epithelium. *Kidney Int* 1993;44:527–536.
330. Nouwen EJ, De Broe ME. Human intestinal versus tissue-nonspecific alkaline phosphatase as complementary urinary markers for the proximal tubule. *Kidney Int* 1994;46(Suppl 47):S43–S51.
331. Bastani B, Yang L, Steinhardt G. Immunocytochemical localization of vacuolar H-ATPase in the opossum (*Monodelphis domestica*) kidney: comparison with the rat. *J Am Soc Nephrol* 1994;4:1558–1563.
332. Byrne DE, MacPhee M, Mulholland M, McCue P, Callahan HJ, Mulholland SG. Urinary tract glycoprotein: distribution and antigenic specificity. *World J Urol* 1994;12:21–26.
333. Raghunath M, Grupp C, Neumann I, Heidtmann A, Roelcke D. Polylactosamine sugar chains expressed by epithelia of Henle's loop and collecting duct in rat and human kidney are selectively recognized by human cold agglutinins anti-I/i. *Tissue Antigens* 1994;44:159–165.
334. Stanton RC, Mendrick DL, Rennke HG, Seifter JL. Use of monoclonal antibodies to culture rat proximal tubule cells. *Am J Physiol* 1986;251:C780–C786.
335. Poujeol P, Ronco P, Tauc M, Geniteau M, Chatelet F, Sahali D, Vandewalle A, Verroust P. Immunological segmentation of the rabbit distal, connecting, and collecting tubules. *Am J Physiol* 1987;252:F412–F422.
336. Iványi B, Marcussen N, Kemp E, Olsen TS. The distal nephron is preferentially infiltrated by inflammatory cells in acute interstitial nephritis. *Virchows Arch A* 1992;420:37–42.
337. Platt JL, Sibley RK, Michael AF. Interstitial nephritis associated with cytomegalovirus infection. *Kidney Int* 1985;28:550–552.
338. Shorr RI, Longo WL, Oberley TD, Bozdech MJ, Walter DL. Cytomegalovirus-associated tubulointerstitial nephritis in an allogeneic bone marrow transplant recipient. *Ann Intern Med* 1987;107: 351–352.
339. Atkins RC, Holdsworth SR. Cellular mechanisms of immune glomerular injury. In: Brenner BM, Stein JH, Wilson CB, eds. *Contemporary Issues in Nephrology*. New York: Churchill Livingstone, 1988:111–135.
340. Main IW, Nikolic-Paterson DJ, Atkins RC. T cells and macrophages and their role in renal injury. *Semin Nephrol* 1992;12:395–407.
341. Takaya M, Ichikawa Y, Shimizu H, Uchiyama M, Taniguchi R. T lymphocyte subsets of the infiltrating cells in the salivary gland and kidney of a patient with Sjogren's syndrome associated with interstitial nephritis. *Clin Exp Rheumatol* 1985;3:259–263.
342. Rosenberg ME, Schendel PB, McCurdy FA, Platt JL. Characterization of immune cells in kidneys from patients with Sjogren's syndrome. *Am J Kidney Dis* 1988;11:20–22.
343. Finkelstein A, Fraley DS, Stachura I, Feldman HA, Gandy DR, Bourke E. Fenoprofen nephropathy: lipoid nephrosis and interstitial nephritis. A possible T-lymphocyte disorder. *Am J Med* 1982;72: 81–87.
344. Watson AJS, Dalbow MH, Stachura I, Fragola JA, Rubin MF, Watson RM, Bourke E. Immunologic studies in cimetidine-induced nephropathy and polymyositis. *N Engl J Med* 1983;308:142–145.
345. Bender WL, Whelton A, Beschorner WE, Darwish MO, Hall-Craggs M, Solez K. Interstitial nephritis, proteinuria, and renal failure caused by nonsteroidal anti-inflammatory drugs. Immunologic characterization of the inflammatory infiltrate. *Am J Med* 1984;76:1006–1012.
346. Gimenez A, Mampaso F. Characterization of inflammatory cells in drug-induced tubulointerstitial nephritis. *Nephron* 1986;43:239–240.
347. Magil AB. Drug-induced acute interstitial nephritis with granulomas. *Human Pathol* 1983;13:36–41.
348. Mignon F, Mery J-Ph, Mougenot B, Ronco P, Roland J, Morel-Maroger L. Granulomatous interstitial nephritis. *Adv Nephrol* 1984; 13:219–245.

349. Steinman TI, Silva P. Acute interstitial nephritis and iritis. Renal-ocular syndrome. *Am J Med* 1984;77:189–190.
350. Iida H, Terada Y, Nishino A, Takata M, Mizumura Y, Sugimoto T, Kubota S. Acute interstitial nephritis with bone marrow granulomas and uveitis. *Nephron* 1985;40:108–110.
351. Vanhaesebrouck P, Carton D, DeBel C, Praet M, Proesmans W. Acute tubulo-interstitial nephritis and uveitis syndrome (TINU syndrome). *Nephron* 1985;40:418–422.
352. Burnier M, Jaeger P, Campiche M, Wauters J-P. Idiopathic acute interstitial nephritis and uveitis in the adult. *Am J Nephrol* 1986;6:312–315.
353. Gafter U, Ben-Basat M, Zevin D, Komlos L, Savir H, Levi J. Anterior uveitis, a presenting symptom in acute interstitial nephritis. *Nephron* 1986;42:249–251.
354. Gafter U, Kalechman Y, Zevin D, Korzets A, Livni E, Klein T, Sredni B, Levi J. Tubulointerstitial nephritis and uveitis: association with suppressed cellular immunity. *Nephrol Dial Transplant* 1993;8:821–826.
355. Bunchman TE, Bloom JN. A syndrome of acute interstitial nephritis and anterior uveitis. *Pediatr Nephrol* 1993;7:520–522.
356. Van Zwieten MJ, Leber PD, Bahn AK, McCluskey RT. Experimental cell-mediated interstitial nephritis induced with exogenous antigens. *J Immunol* 1977;118:589–593.
357. Vargas Arenas RE, Turner DR. Pathology of interstitial nephritis induced in guinea pigs by exoantigens. *Nephron* 1982;32:170–179.
358. Accinni L, Archetti I, Branca M, Hsu KC, Andres G. Tubulo-interstitial (TI) renal disease associated with chronic lymphocytic choriomeningitis viral infection in mice. *Clin Immunol Immunopathol* 1978;11:395–405.
359. Mori S, Nose M, Miyazawa M, Kyogoku M, Wolfinbarger JB, Bloom ME. Interstitial nephritis in Aleutian mink disease. Possible role of cell-mediated immunity against virus-infected tubular epithelial cells. *Am J Pathol* 1994;144:1326–1333.
360. Sugisaki T, Yoshida T, McCluskey RT, Andres GA, Klassen J. Autoimmune cell-mediated tubulointerstitial nephritis induced in Lewis rats by renal antigens. *Clin Immunol Immunopathol* 1980;15:33–43.
361. Baldamus CA. Immunologically induced tubulo-interstitial nephritis: experimental models in rats. *Contrib Nephrol* 1980;19:104–109.
362. Sado Y, Okigaki T, Takamiya H, Seno S. Experimental autoimmune glomerulonephritis with pulmonary hemorrhage in rats. The dose-effect relationship of the nephritogenic antigen from bovine glomerular basement membrane. *J Clin Lab Immunol* 1984;15:199–204.
363. Weiss RA, Madaio MP, Tomaszewski JE, Kelly CJ. T cells reactive to an inducible heat shock protein induce disease in toxin-induced interstitial nephritis. *J Exp Med* 1994;180:2239–2250.
364. DeNagel DC, Pierce SK. Heat shock proteins in immune responses. *Crit Rev Immunol* 1993;13:71–81.
365. Kaufmann SHE. Heat shock proteins and autoimmunity: a critical appraisal. *Int Arch Allergy Appl Immunol* 1994;103:317–322.
366. Odriozola E, Paloma E, Lopez T, Campero C. An outbreak of Vicia villosa (hairy vetch) poisoning in grazing Aberdeen Angus bulls in Argentina. *Vet Hum Toxicol* 1991;33:278–280.
367. Lyon MF, Hulse EV. An inherited kidney disease of mice resembling human nephronophthisis. *J Med Genetics* 1971;8:41–48.
368. Fernandes G, Yunis EJ, Miranda M, Smith J, Good RA. Nutritional inhibition of genetically determined renal disease and autoimmunity with prolongation of life in kdkd mice. *Proc Natl Acad Sci USA* 1978;75:2888–2892.
369. Neilson EG, McCafferty E, Feldman A, Clayman MD, Zakheim B, Korngold R. Spontaneous interstitial nephritis in kdkd mice. 1. An experimental model of autoimmune renal disease. *J Immunol* 1984;133:2560–2565.
370. Kelly CJ, Korngold R, Mann R, Clayman M, Haverty T, Neilson EG. Spontaneous interstitial nephritis in kdkd mice. II. Characterization of a tubular antigen-specific, H-2K-restricted Lyt-2$^+$ effector T cell that mediates destructive tubulointerstitial injury. *J Immunol* 1986;136:526–531.
371. Kelly CJ, Neilson EG. Contrasuppression in autoimmunity. Abnormal contrasuppression facilitates expression of nephritogenic effector T cells and interstitial nephritis in kdkd mice. *J Exp Med* 1987;165:107–123.
372. Smoyer WE, Kelly CJ. Inherited interstitial nephritis in kdkd mice. *Intern Rev Immunol* 1994;11:245–251.
373. Smoyer W, Madaio MP, Kelly CJ. TCR-Vβ gene usage in murine spontaneous interstitial nephritis. *J Am Soc Nephrol* 1994;4:635.
374. Harning R, Pelletier J, Van G, Takei F, Merluzzi VJ. Monoclonal antibody to MALA-2 (ICAM-1) reduces acute autoimmune nephritis in kdkd mice. *Clin Immunol Immunopathol* 1992;64:129–134.
375. Kelly CJ, Neilson EG. Medullary cystic disease: an inherited form of autoimmune interstitial nephritis? *Am J Kidney Dis* 1987;10:389–395.
376. Camussi G, Rotunno M, Segoloni G, Brentjens JR, Andres GA. In vitro alternative pathway activation of complement by the brush border of proximal tubules of normal rat kidney. *J Immunol* 1982;128:1659–1663.
377. Camussi G, Tetta C, Mazzucco G, Vercellone A. The brush border of proximal tubules of normal human kidney activates the alternative pathway of the complement system in vitro. *Ann NY Acad Sci* 1983;420:321–324.
378. Camussi G, Stratta P, Mazzucco G, Gaido M, Tetta C, Castello R, Rotunno M, Vercellone A. In vivo localization of C3 on the brush border of proximal tubules of kidneys from nephrotic patients. *Clin Nephrol* 1985;23:134–141.
379. Falk RJ, Dalmasso AP, Kim Y, Tsai CH, Scheinman JI, Gewurz H, Michael AF. Neoantigen of the polymerized ninth component of complement. Characterization of a monoclonal antibody and immunohistochemical localization in renal disease. *J Clin Invest* 1983;72:560–573.
380. Nath KA, Hostetter MK, Hostetter TH. Pathophysiology of chronic tubulo-interstitial disease in rats. Interactions of dietary acid load, ammonia, and complement component C3. *J Clin Invest* 1985;76:667–675.
381. Tolins JP, Hostetter MK, Hostetter TH. Hypokalemic nephropathy in the rat. Role of ammonia in chronic tubular injury. *J Clin Invest* 1987;79:1447–1458.
382. Nath KA, Hostetter MK, Hostetter TH. Increased ammoniagenesis as a determinant of progressive renal injury. *Am J Kidney Dis* 1991;17:654–657.
383. Clark EC, Nath KA, Hostetter MR, Hostetter TH. Role of ammonia in progressive interstitial nephritis. *Am J Kidney Dis* 1991;17:15–19.
384. Eddy AA, Michael AF. Acute tubulointerstitial nephritis associated with aminonucleoside nephrosis. *Kidney Int* 1988;33:14–23.
385. Eddy AA, McCulloch L, Liu E, Adams J. A relationship between proteinuria and acute tubulointerstitial disease in rats with experimental nephrotic syndrome. *Am J Pathol* 1991;138:1111–1123.
386. Burton CJ, Walls J. Proximal tubular cell, proteinuria and tubulo-interstitial scarring. *Nephron* 1994;68:287–293.
387. Martin A, Molina A, Bricio T, Mampaso F. Passive dual immunization against tumour necrosis factor-alpha (TNF-alpha) and IL-1 beta maximally ameliorates acute aminonucleoside nephrosis. *Clin Exp Immunol* 1995;99:283–288.
388. Jones CL, Buch S, Post M, McCulloch L, Liu E, Eddy AA. Pathogenesis of interstitial fibrosis in chronic purine aminonucleoside nephrosis. *Kidney Int* 1991;40:1020–1031.
389. Jones CL, Buch S, Post M, McCulloch L, Liu E, Eddy AA. Renal extracellular matrix accumulation in acute puromycin aminonucleoside nephrosis in rats. *Am J Pathol* 1992;141:1381–1396.
390. Saito T, Atkins RC. Interstitial activated (IL-2R$^+$) mononuclear cells and Ia antigens in experimental focal glomerulosclerosis. *Pathology* 1994;26:403–406.
391. Alfrey AC, Froment DH, Hammond WS. Role of iron in the tubulo-interstitial injury in nephrotoxic serum nephritis. *Kidney Int* 1989;36:753–759.
392. Kees-Folts D, Sadow JL, Schreiner GF. Tubular catabolism of albumin is associated with the release of an inflammatory lipid. *Kidney Int* 1994;45:1697–1709.
393. Andreu-Sanchez JL, Moreno de Alboran IM, Marcos MA, Sanchez-Movilla A, Martinez-A C, Kroemer G. Interleukin 2 abrogates the nonresponsive state of T cells expressing a forbidden T cell receptor repertoire and induces autoimmune disease in neonatally thymectomized mice. *J Exp Med* 1991;173:1323–1329.
394. Pichler R, Giachelli CM, Lombardi D, Pippin J, Gordon K, Alpers CE, Schwartz SM, Johnson RJ. Tubulointerstitial disease in glomerulonephritis. Potential role of osteopontin (Uropontin). *Am J Pathol* 1994;144:915–926.
395. Trudel M, D'Agati V, Constantini F. *c-myc* as an inducer of polycystic kidney disease in transgenic mice. *Kidney Int* 1991;39:665–671.
396. Kelley KA, Agarwal N, Reeders S, Herrup K. Renal cyst formation and multifocal neoplasia in transgenic mice carrying the Simian Virus 40 early region. *J Am Soc Nephrol* 1991;2:84–97.

397. Striker LJ, Doi T, Striker GE. Transgenic mice in renal research. *Adv Nephrol* 1991;20:91–108.
398. Schaffner DL, Barrios R, Massey C, Banez EI, Ou CN, Rajagopalan S, Aguilar-Cordova E, Lebovitz RM, Overbeek PA, Lieberman MW. Targeting of the rasT24 oncogene to the proximal convoluted tubules in transgenic mice results in hyperplasia and polycystic kidneys. *Am J Pathol* 1993;142:1051–1060.
399. Lowden DA, Lindemann GW, Merlino G, Barash BD, Calvet JP, Gattone VH II. Renal cysts in transgenic mice expressing transforming growth factor-α. *J Lab Clin Med* 1994;124:386–394.
400. Gattone VH II, Lowden DA, Cowley BD Jr. Epidermal growth factor ameliorates autosomal recessive polycystic kidney disease in mice. *Develop Biol* 1995;169:504–510.
401. Fukamizu A, Watanabe M, Inoue Y, Kon Y, Shimada S, Shiota N, Sugiyama F, Murakami K. Cortical expression of the human angiotensinogen gene in the kidney of transgenic mice. *Kidney Int* 1994;46: 1533–1535.
402. Dickie P, Felser J, Eckhaus M, Bryant J, Silver J, Marinos N, Notkins AL. HIV-associated nephropathy in transgenic mice expressing HIV-1 genes. *Virology* 1991;185:109–119.
403. Ray PE, Bruggeman LA, Weeks BS, Kopp JB, Bryant JL, Owens JW, Notkins AL, Klotman PE. bFGF and its low affinity receptors in the pathogenesis of HIV-associated nephropathy in transgenic mice. *Kidney Int* 1994;46:759–772.
404. Faraj AH, Morley AR. Remnant kidney pathology after five-sixth nephrectomy in rat. 1. A biochemical and morphological study. *APMIS* 1992;100:1097–1105.
405. Mai M, Geiger H, Hilgers KF, Veelken R, Mann JF, Dammrich J, Luft FC. Early interstitial changes in hypertension-induced renal injury. *Hypertension* 1993;22:754–765.
406. Giachelli CM, Pichler R, Lombardi D, Denhardt DT, Alpers CE, Schwartz SM, Johnson RJ. Osteopontin expression in angiotensin II-induced tubulointerstitial nephritis. *Kidney Int* 1994;45:515–524.
407. Truong LD, Farhood A, Tasby J, Gillum D. Experimental chronic renal ischemia: morphologic and immunologic studies. *Kidney Int* 1992;41:1676–1689.
408. Matejka GL, Jennische E. IGF-I binding and IGF-I mRNA expression in the post-ischemic regenerating rat kidney. *Kidney Int* 1992;42: 1113–1123.
409. Shimizu A, Masuda Y, Ishizaki M, Sugisaki Y, Yamanaka N. Tubular dilatation in the repair process of ischaemic tubular necrosis. *Virchows Arch* 1994;425:281–290.
410. González-Avila G, Vadillo-Ortega F, Pérez-Tamayo R. Experimental diffuse interstitial renal fibrosis. A biochemical approach. *Lab Invest* 1988;59:245–252.
411. Sharma AK, Mauer SM, Kim Y, Michael AF. Interstitial fibrosis in obstructive nephropathy. *Kidney Int* 1993;44:774–788.
412. Kaneto H, Morrissey J, McCracken R, Reyes A, Klahr S. Enalapril reduces collagen type IV synthesis and expansion of the interstitium in the obstructed rat kidney. *Kidney Int* 1994;45:1637–1647.
413. Tokunaga S, Ohkawa M, Nakamura S. An experimental model of ascending pyelonephritis due to Candida albicans in rats. *Mycopathologia* 1993;123:149–154.
414. Tsuchimori N, Hayashi R, Shino A, Yamazaki T, Okonogi K. Enterococcus faecalis aggravates pyelonephritis caused by Pseudomonas aeruginosa in experimental ascending mixed urinary tract infection in mice. *Infect Immun* 1994;62:4534–4541.
415. Ozawa Y, Nauta J, Sweeney WE, Avner ED. A new murine model of autosomal recessive polycystic kidney disease. *Nippon Jinzo Gakkai Shi* 1993;35:349–354.
416. Torres VE, Mujwid DK, Wilson DM, Holley KH. Renal cystic disease and ammoniagenesis in Han:SPRD rats. *J Am Soc Nephrol* 1994;5:1193–1200.acute gentamicin nephropathy.
417. Schafer K, Gretz N, Bader M, Oberbaumer I, Eckardt KU, Kriz W, Bachmann S. Characterization of the Han:SPRD rat model for hereditary polycystic kidney disease. *Kidney Int* 1994;46:134–152.
418. Schafer K, Bader M, Gretz N, Oberbaumer I, Bachmann S. Focal overexpression of collagen IV characterizes the initiation of epithelial changes in polycystic kidney disease. *Exp Nephrol* 1994;2:190–195.
419. Scanziani E, Grieco V, Salvi S. Expression of vimentin in the tubular epithelium of bovine kidneys with interstitial nephritis. *Vet Pathol* 1993;30:298–300.
420. Vilafranca M, Domingo M, Ferrer L. Tubular vimentin metaplasia in canine nephropathies. *Res Vet Sci* 1994;57:248–250.
421. Murray G, Wyllie RG, Hill GS, Ramsden PW, Heptinstall RH. Experimental papillary necrosis of the kidney. 1. Morphologic and functional data. *Am J Pathol* 1972;67:285–302.
422. Uemasu J, Fujiwara M, Munemura C, Kawasaki, H. Long-term effects of enalapril in rat with experimental chronic tubulo-interstitial nephropathy. *Am J Nephrol* 1993;13:35–42.
423. Burdmann, EA, Rosen S, Lindsley J, Elzinga L, Andoh T, Bennett WM. Production of less chronic nephrotoxicity by cyclosporine G than cyclosporine A in a low-salt rat model. *Transplantation* 1993;55; 963–966.
424. Ferguson CJ, von Ruhland C, Parry-Jones DJ, Griffiths DF, Salaman JR, Williams JD. Low-dose cyclosporin nephrotoxicity in the rat. *Nephrol Dial Transplant* 1993;8:1259–1263.
425. Lash LH, Tokarz JJ, Woods EB. Renal cell type specificity of cephalosporin-induced cytotoxicity in suspensions of isolated proximal tubular and distal tubular cells. *Toxicology* 1994;94:97–118.
426. Jones DB, Elliott WC. Gentamicin-induced loss of basolateral surface area of rat proximal convoluted tubules. *Lab Invest* 1987;57: 412–420.
427. Güezmes A, Fernández F, Garijo F, Val-Bernal F. Correlation between tubulointerstitial nephropathy and glomerular lesions induced by adriamycin. *Nephron* 1992;62:198–202.
428. Chagnac A, Korzets A, Ben-Bassat M, Zevin D, Hirsh J, Meckler J, Levi J. Uninephrectomy aggravates tubulointerstitial injury in rats with adriamycin nephrosis. *Nephron* 1994;66:176–180.
429. Ohtani H, Wakui H, Komatsuda A, Satoh K, Miura AB, Itoh H, Tashima Y. Induction and intracellular localization of 90-kilodalton heat-shock protein in rat kidneys with acute gentamicin nephropathy. *Lab Invest* 1995;72:161–165.
430. Lash LH, Zalups RK. Mercuric chloride-induced cytotoxicity and compensatory hypertrophy in rat kidney proximal tubular cells. *J Pharmacol Exp Ther* 1992;261:819–829.
431. Racusen LC. Cell shape changes and detachment in cell culture: models of renal injury. *Nephrol Dial Transplant* 1994;9(suppl 4):22–25.
432. Morshed KM, Jain SK, McMartin KE. Acute toxicity of propylene glycol: an assessment using cultured proximal tubule cells of human origin. *Fund Appl Toxicol* 1994;23:38–43.
433. Jalal F, Dehbi M, Berteloot A, Crine P. Biosynthesis and polarized distribution of neutral endopeptidase in primary cultures of kidney proximal tubule cells. *Biochem J* 1994;302:669–674.

PART VI

Clinical Aspects of Immunologic Renal Diseases

A. Patient Evaluation and General Considerations

Immunologic Renal Diseases,
edited by E. G. Neilson and W. G. Couser.
Lippincott-Raven Publishers, Philadelphia © 1997.

CHAPTER 37

Clinical Evaluation and Management of Hematuria and Proteinuria

Karl G. Koenig and W. Kline Bolton

HEMATURIA

Hematuria is the presence of an abnormal number of red blood cells (RBCs) in the urine. It is a common finding in the general population and may herald significant underlying pathology. In screening 6,000 people (5,000 men, 1,000 women) applying for life insurance, Wright found an overall prevalence of hematuria of 3% if more than 3 RBCs per high-power field (HPF) defines hematuria (1). The clinical importance is emphasized by the fact that up to 26% of adults presenting with hematuria are discovered to have a malignancy, depending on the population studied (2). Therefore, in order to expeditiously identify and treat reversible causes of hematuria, including malignancy, a thorough yet tailored cost-effective evaluation is needed. Such an evaluation is problematic, however, given the difficulties in defining, detecting, and localizing hematuria, as well as the potential morbidity and cost of the process. The following discussion addresses these and other issues while developing a complete yet prudent approach to the evaluation of hematuria in the adult patient.

Definition

There is a marked variability in the "normal" number of RBCs in adult urine, owing to the different methods of determination. Quantitatively, an Addis count of less than 500,000 RBCs per 12-h urine collection (3,4) or 1,000–3,000 RBCs/ml (5,6) are the most commonly accepted limits for the normal number of urinary RBCs. These direct quantitative measures, although accurate, are tedious and used only rarely in the clinical situation. Counting RBCs per HPF in a spun urinary sediment is the usual clinical standard, with 2–3 RBCs/HPF as an accepted norm (7–10). Because of difficulties in the technique of urine collection, females are, in general, allowed one more RBC per HPF than males. However, in any given patient the appearance of just 1 RBC/HPF that was not previously present may signify pathology. Unfortunately, quantitative measurements of urinary RBCs such as the Addis count or RBCs per milliliter do not correlate well with counting RBCs per HPF because of fluctuating variables in the preparation of the urinary sediment. Froom et al. clearly demonstrated the wide range of RBCs per milliliter in unspun urine for any given level of RBCs per HPF in urinary sediment. The sensitivity of 1–3 RBCs/HPF or 2–4 RBCs/HPF to detect greater than 2,000 RBCs/ml was only 63% and 54%, respectively (11). However hematuria is defined, one must always account for situations before urine collection that may result in transient hematuria such as vigorous exercise, mild trauma, digital prostate examination, sexual activity, menses, or viral illness.

Detection

Gross hematuria results when there is greater than 5×10^6 RBC/mm^3 of urine, which corresponds to less than 1 ml RBCs/L urine (12). Microscopic hematuria is detected by using cellulose test strips impregnated with orthotolidine and peroxidase buffers. The peroxidase activity of heme inside urinary RBCs, free urinary hemoglobin, or myoglobin catalyzes the oxidation of orthotolidine, resulting in a subjective color change on the reagent strip. This dipstick method is 91% to 100% sensitive and 65% to 99% specific in detecting greater than 2 RBCs/HPF (2,13,14). Causes of false-negative and false-posi-

K. G. Koenig and W. Kline Bolton: Division of Nephrology, University of Virginia Health Sciences Center, Charlottesville, Virginia 22908.

TABLE 1. *Dipstick for hematuria: false positives and false negatives*

False positives (1–35%)	False negatives (0–9%)
Oxidizing contaminants	Interferes with perioxidase reaction
Bacterial oxidases	Vitamin C
Povidone	Preservatives in tetracycline
Hypochlorite	Substantial proteinuria
Copper	Formaldehyde contaminant
Halogens	Urine pH <5.1
Free hemoglobin	Concentrated urine
Myoglobin	

tive dipstick results are listed in Table 1. The urine dipstick is more sensitive to free hemoglobin than hemoglobin within RBCs. Thus, a small number of RBCs in a concentrated urine sample produces little free hemoglobin due to limited RBC lysis and results in a falsely negative test. Vitamin C, ascorbate preservatives in tetracycline, formaldehyde contaminants, heavy proteinuria, and an acid urine interfere with the peroxidase reaction and account for the remainder of the false-negative results. Similarly, oxidizing compounds listed in Table 1 can give false-positive results for urinary RBCs, as can free hemoglobin or myoglobin in the urine.

A simple systematic approach to the patient presenting with red urine is helpful in establishing true hematuria and eliminating pigmenturia, hemoglobinuria, and myoglobinuria as causes before embarking on an extensive and expensive evaluation of hematuria. A thorough history and physical examination is followed by a urinalysis and examination of the urinary sediment. Ten milliliters of urine is spun for 3 to 4 min at 3,000 to 4,000 revolutions per minute. Characteristics of the resultant supernatant and pellet direct further evaluation (Fig. 1):

1. Clear supernatant/red pellet. This represents true hematuria. The supernatant is poured off, and the pellet is resuspended in ≤0.5 ml of residual supernatant and examined under the microscope for more clinical clues such as crystals or dysmorphic RBCs.
2. Red (or brown) supernatant that tests dipstick negative. This represents pigmenturia, which can occur in porphyria (protoporphyrins do not oxidize the orthotolidine reagent of the urinary dipstick), various drugs such as the bladder analgesic phenazopyridine (Pyridium, Parke-Davis, Morris Plains, NJ) or in genetically predisposed individuals who ingest fresh beets or berries (15). See Table 2 for a more extensive list.
3. Red (or brown) supernatant that tests dipstick positive. This represents the presence of free urinary hemoglobin (e.g., from hemolytic anemia) or myoglobin (e.g., from rhabdomyolysis). These can be distinguished by centrifuging a tube of the patient's blood. The plasma supernatant will be red in hemoglobinuria and appear normal color in myoglobinuria.

The majority of plasma hemoglobin released by hemolysis exists as a tetramer (2 alpha, 2 beta chains) and/or is rapidly bound to haptoglobin with a molecular weight (MW) of 68 kilodaltons (kDa). Both free and protein-bound hemoglobin are too large to cross the glomerular basement membrane and therefore do not result in pigmenturia. However, a small portion of released hemoglobin

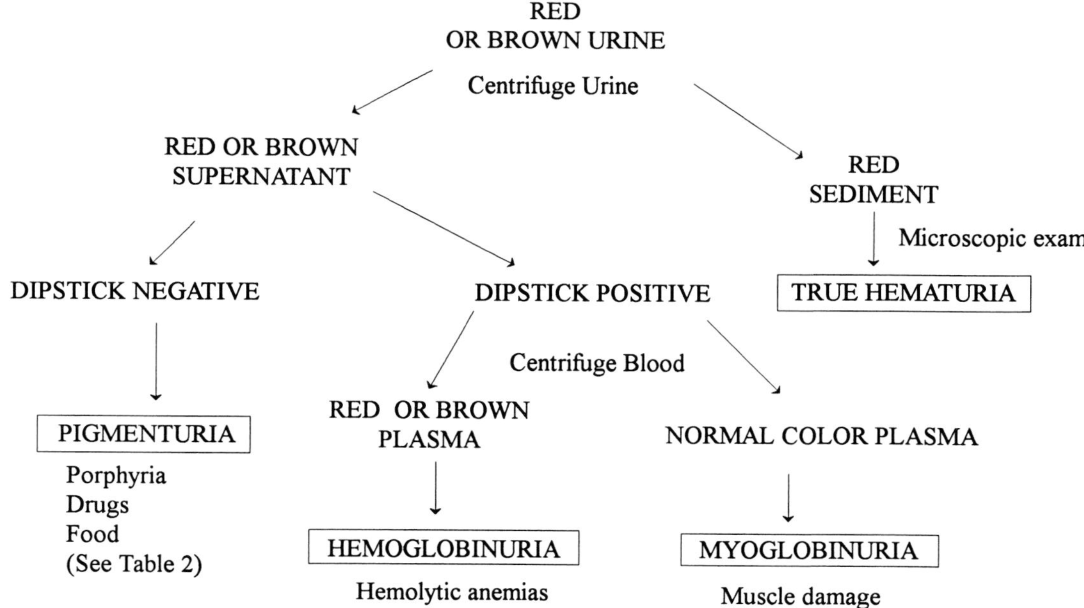

FIG. 1. Initial evaluation of the patient with red or brown urine. Adapted with permission (212).

TABLE 2. *Causes of pigmenturia*

Porphyria, rhabomyolysis, severe hemolytic anemia	
Drugs	
Phenazopyridine (pyridium)	Primaquine, chloroquine
Rifampin	Methocarbamol
Doxorubicin	Phenytoin
Phenothiazines	Deferoxamine
Phenolphthalein	Aminosalicylic acid[a]
Levodopa	Methyldopa[a]
Dimethyl sulfoxide	Cascara-containing laxatives
Foods	
Beets and berries (anthocyanin)	
Rhubarb	
Fava beans	
Food coloring	
Other	
Serratia marcescens urinary tract infection	
Serratia marcescens diaper infection	

[a] Must react with hypochorites (toilet bowl cleaners) to produce a red color.
Adapted with permission (210).

exists as a smaller dimer (MW 34 kDa) that is not protein bound and therefore gets filtered. In massive intravascular hemolysis, the capacity of the proximal tubules to reabsorb the filtered dimer can be overwhelmed, resulting in hemoglobinuria with a positive urine dipstick reaction, and the spun plasma remains red from the large tetrameric protein-bound hemoglobin that cannot be filtered.

In contrast, myoglobin released from damaged muscle is small (MW 17 kDa), is not as highly protein bound, and is therefore rapidly excreted in the urine. Thus, in the absence of renal failure, myoglobin does not accumulate in the plasma. The result is a positive urinary dipstick from myoglobinuria with a normal-appearing plasma.

In the clinical setting, hemoglobinuria and myoglobinuria are rare causes of a positive urinary dipstick. More commonly, hypotonic urine results in the osmotic rupture of RBCs as the urine-specific gravity falls below 1.010 mOsm/kg, releasing free hemoglobin, which is readily detected as demonstrated by Vaughan and Wyker (16). It is important to recognize this phenomenon when evaluating a patient with a positive urinary dipstick for heme with few or no RBCs seen in the urinary sediment.

Localization

Once true hematuria is identified, localizing its origin is helpful in guiding further evaluation. If the patient has gross hematuria primarily in the initial or terminal part of the urinary stream, a urethral or bladder trigone (bladder neck or prostatic lesion) source of the bleeding is implicated, respectively. Hematuria throughout voiding suggests renal, renal pelvis, ureteral, or diffuse bladder bleeding. Likewise, sequential collection of the urinary stream and comparing the number of RBCs in each portion may provide similar localization (three glass test). Identification of ureteral bleeding also can be done at the time of cystoscopy using dipstick sampling of ureteral urine samples (17). A thorough search for a source above the bladder on the affected side should ensue once unilateral bleeding is identified. Retrograde pyelography has classically been used to look for ureteral and calyceal pathology, but recent innovations in endourologic exploration, consisting of rigid or flexible retrograde ureteropyeloscopy and percutaneous pyeloscopy, have proven valuable in elucidating and treating ureteral pathology (18,19).

Distinguishing glomerular from nonglomerular bleeding is crucial to an appropriately focused workup of hematuria. Clinical clues from the urine collection and microscopic examination may implicate glomerular disease. Proteinuria of over 2 g/24 h or finding oval fat bodies (lipid-laden cells) and lipid droplets in the form of Maltese crosses with a polarized microscope (Fig. 2) is highly suggestive of glomerular disease. These are not pathognomonic, however, because tubulointerstial dis-

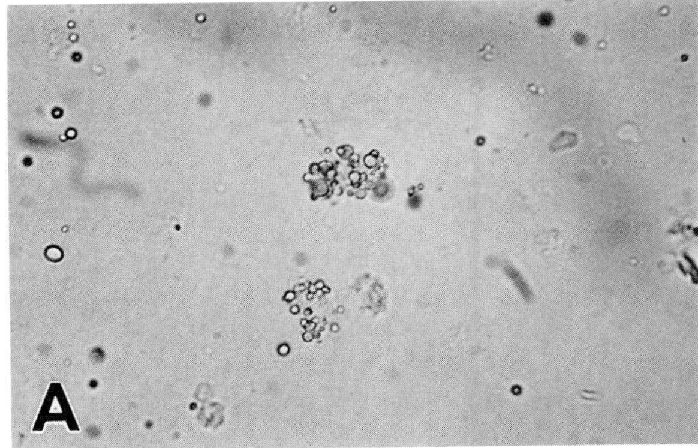

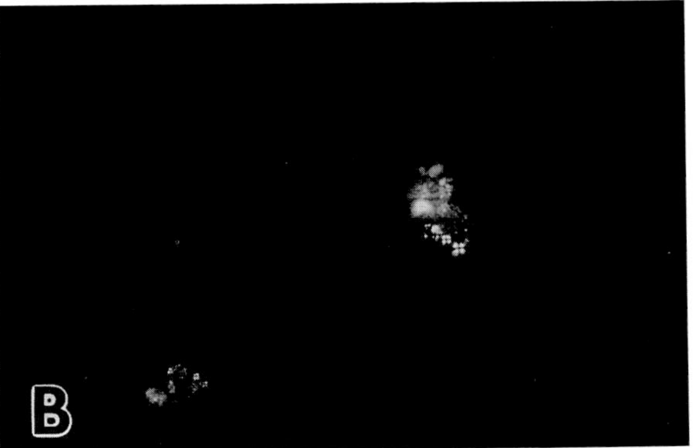

FIG. 2. Oval fat bodies and Maltese crosses under light (**A**) and and polarized (**B**) microscopy. Reprinted with permission (213).

ease can occasionally result in this degree of proteinuria, and polycystic kidney disease, bacterial prostatitis, and strenuous exercise can cause lipiduria (20,21). RBC casts are nearly pathognomonic for glomerular bleeding but false-positive results also can occur.

The concept of dysmorphic RBCs implicating glomerular pathology using phase-contrast microscopy was introduced in 1979 by Birch and Fairley (22). When RBCs squeeze through an abnormal glomerular basement membrane, they become deformed and assume different sizes and shapes (Fig. 3). In addition, exposure to the high osmolality and acid environment while passing through the tubules also may contribute to RBC dysmorphism (23). In contrast, urinary RBCs of uniform size and shape, termed isomorphic, imply a nonglomerular source of bleeding. Phase-contrast microscopy is 90% to 100% sensitive and specific in identifing dysmorphic RBCs (24–26), but a lack of availability and substantial variability in technique and interpretation are associated disadvantages.

Given the above limitations of phase microscopy, a readily available reliable method of identifying glomerular bleeding would be helpful in evaluating hematuria. Sayer and others (27–30) used the Coulter counter to generate urinary RBC size distribution curves to predict glomerular pathology. In general, urinary RBCs of glomerular origin are smaller compared with those of nonglomerular origin. Although readily available, inexpensive, and not affected by overnight storage or centrifugation, this technique is limited by its variable results, especially in urine with fewer than 45 RBCs/HPF. Its accuracy then relies on concentrating multiple urine specimens, which is time intensive and limits its clinical utility. Many other methods also have been reported, but most are unavailable to the clinician and not cost effective (31–38).

Approach to Glomerulonephritis

If a glomerular etiology of hematuria is suspected but not confirmed by a thorough history, physical examination, and analysis of the urinary sediment, appropriate serologic blood tests can be drawn and plans made to perform a percutaneous renal biopsy. At times there may be no clinical clues for a specific glomerular process, and a battery of blood tests are empirically ordered. However, Howard et al. demonstrated that prebiopsy serologies were of no diagnostic value in a series of patients with idiopathic nephrotic syndrome and added several hundred dollars to the cost of their care (39). Therefore, judicious use of serologic tests is recommended, tailored to the clinical presentation.

Unfortunately, the clinical presentation of the glomerulonephritides (Table 3) is often confusing. There may be few if any clues in the history and physical examination, and many of the glomerulonephritides have substantial overlap in their presentations. Formulation of a specific

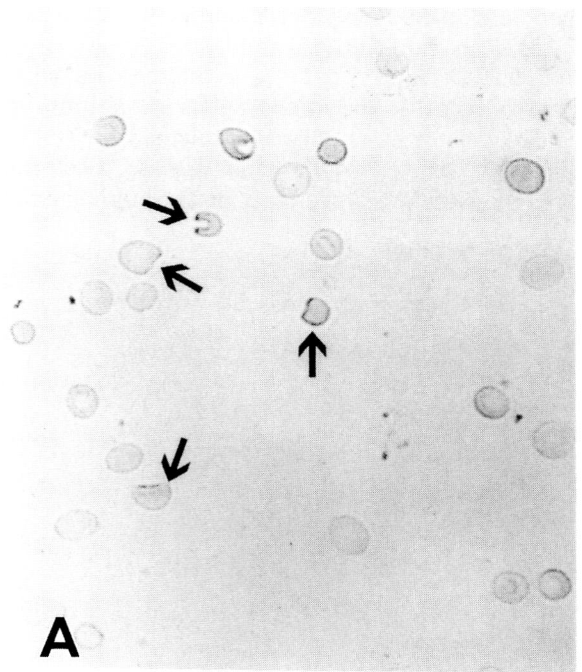

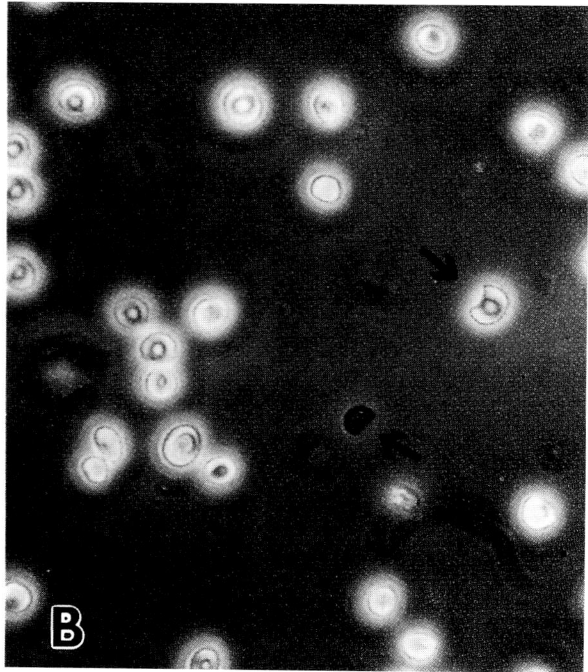

FIG. 3. Isomorphic and dysmorphic *(arrows)* RBCs under light (**A**) and phase contrast (**B**) microscopy. Reprinted with permission (213).

TABLE 3. *Glomerular etiologies of hematuria*

Systemic diseases
Postinfectious glomerulonephritis[a]
Poststreptococcal glomerulonephritis (pharynx, skin, pneumonia) (90%)
Subacute bacterial endocarditis (90%)
Ventricular–peritoneal shunt infections (90%)
Visceral abscess (complement usually normal)
Systemic lupus erythematosus[a] (75%–90%)
Essential mixed cryoglobulinemia[a] (85%)
Alport's syndrome
Diabetes mellitus
Vasculitis
Wegener's granulomatosis
Polyarteritis nodosa (macroscopic or microscopic)
Schönlein-Henoch purpura
Churg-Strauss
Bechet's syndrome
Relapsing polychondritis
Idiopathic
Vasculopathy
Thrombotic thrombocytopenic purpura
Hemolytic uremic syndrome
Diseases intrinsic to the kidney
IgA nephropathy
Thin basement membrane disease
Membranoproliferative glomerulonephritis[a] (60–90%)
Idiopathic rapidly progressive glomerulonephritis
Drug-induced

[a]Hypocomplementemic disorders. Percentages indicate the general incidence of low serum complement levels.

TABLE 4. *Major causes of hematuria in adults*

Infection	Glomerular
Pyelonephritis	Glomeronephritis (e.g., IgA nephropathy[a])
Cystitis	Hereditary nephritis
Prostatitis[a]	Thin basement membrane disease
Epididymitis	Alport's syndrome
Urethritis	Vasculitis/vasculopathies
Renal tuberculosis	Exercise[a]
Malignancy	Interstitial
Renal cell carcinoma	Interstitial nephritis
Transitional cell carcinoma[a]	Polycystic kidney disease
Prostatic carcinoma	Papillary necrosis
Endometrial carcinoma	
Cervical or vaginal cancer	Vascular
	Malignant hypertension
Metabolic/drug/other	Atheroemboli
Calculi[a]	Renal infarct
Hypercalciuria	Renal vein thrombosis
Hyperuricosuria	
Benign prostatic hypertrophy[a]	
Anticoagulants	
Coagulopathy (e.g., hemophilia)	
Menses	
Sickle cell disease	
Cyclophosphamide	
Trauma	

[a]Most common causes.

approach to the evaluation of glomerulonephritis is therefore difficult and of limited clinical utility. However, certain serologic findings such as low complement levels can help narrow a broad differential diagnosis, as indicated in Table 3. Furthermore, serologies such as complement levels and anti-neutrophil cytoplasmic antibody (ANCA) titers may be helpful in following disease activity long term in selected individuals. In general, however, a timely renal biopsy is essential to diagnose the cause of glomerulonephritis and to guide therapy.

Causes of Hematuria

The major causes of hematuria in adults are listed in Table 4. Referring to such a list may be useful if the history, physical examination, and localization procedures are unsuccessful in determining an etiology of the hematuria. However, reviewing the common causes with respect to age and sex (Table 5) is often more helpful in directing further evaluation. Overall, males have a much greater prevalence of hematuria as well as a higher probability of having significant lesions, including urologic malignancies, compared with females. Bard followed 177 women with asymptomatic hematuria over 10 years and found, similar to men, an increased prevalence of hematuria in individuals over 50 years of age. However, only seven women had significant lesions (four calculi, one obstruction, one papillary necrosis, and one benign renal mass), and no malignancies were found (40).

Although a detailed discussion of every major cause of hematuria in adults is beyond the scope of this chapter,

TABLE 5. *Common causes of hematuria by age and sex*

Age 0–20 yr
Glomerulonephritis
Urinary tract infection
Congenital urinary tract anomalies
Age 20–40 yr
Urinary tract infection (females>males)
Calculi
Bladder cancer
Age 40–60 yr
Urinary tract infection (females>males)
Bladder cancer
Calculi
Age ≥60 yr (men)
Benign prostatic hypertrophy
Bladder cancer
Urinary tract infection
Age ≥60 yr (women)
Urinary tract infection
Bladder cancer

Adapted with permission (211).

certain etiologies warrant further discussion, such as exercise-induced hematuria or pigmenturia. March hemoglobinuria results when pounding of feet on hard surfaces causes lysis of RBCs as they pass through the foot capillaries, although Yoshimura postulates a hemolyzing factor produced by the spleen during exercise (41). Rhabdomyolysis and myoglobinuria can occur after intensive, strenuous exercise and may be more common in untrained individuals with pre-existing muscle abnormalities (42). Gross or microscopic hematuria may occur from direct trauma to the kidneys, ureter, or bladder in punishing contact sports such as boxing, hockey, and football. Traumatic bladder contusions in long-distance runners have been cystoscopically documented by Blacklock (43). The likely mechanism is repeated impact of the relatively flaccid posterior wall of an empty bladder against the more rigid fixed base that comprises the trigone, resulting in hematuria of bladder origin (44).

However, not all sports-related hematuria is traumatic in nature. Alyea and Parish demonstrated that hematuria occurred regardless of whether the sport was traumatic or nontraumatic, and in fact was more common in swimmers than in football players (45). This glomerular source of bleeding occurs in proportion to the duration and intensity of the exercise. The purported mechanism is renal vasoconstriction during exercise to redistribute blood flow to skeletal muscle, as well as a relative increase in efferent versus afferent arteriolar constriction mediated by angiotensin. Nephron hypoxia and increased filtration pressure ensue, resulting in increased glomerular permeability with exudation of RBCs into the urinary space (46).

Although exercise-related pigmenturia or hematuria may be common in the right clinical setting, other pathology may coexist. In patients less than 40 years of age, normalization of their urinalysis 24 to 72 h after the sporting event confirms the diagnosis of exercise-related hematuria. Further evaluation may be indicated in individuals over 50 years of age given that hematuria can be intermittent in malignancy and its prevalence rises rapidly in this patient population.

Another relatively common clinical dilemma is how extensively to evaluate an anticoagulated patient with hematuria. In 1986 the American College of Chest Physicians and the Heart, Lung and Blood Institute recommended a decrease in the intensity of anticoagulation (47). Before that, episodes of hematuria were felt to be directly related to the degree of anticoagulation. In a recent prospective evaluation of 243 anticoagulated patients, there was no increased incidence or prevalence of hematuria compared with control subjects and no correlation between the degree of anticoagulation and the frequency of hematuria (48). Therefore, with current standards of anticoagulation, gross or microscopic hematuria may indicate significant underlying pathology and should be appropriately evaluated in anticoagulated patients.

Hypercalciuria is a common cause of macroscopic or microscopic hematuria in children, presumably due to crystalluria, because these children are at increased risk of nephrolithiasis long term (49). It is now well-documented that adults have similar consequences from hypercalciuria and/or hyperuricosuria, with 55% to 67% responding to therapy with hydrochlorothiazide or allopurinol (50,51). In patients less than 40 years of age with hematuria and hypercalciuria (>4 mg/kg/day) and/or hyperuricosuria (>700 mg/day) and no other identifiable cause, the workup of hematuria can stop short of imaging studies. However, hematuria in patients over 50 years of age may merit further evaluation given the rising incidence of malignancy in this age group.

Economic Considerations

Consideration of economic factors is important before proceeding with further discussion on the evaluation and approach to hematuria. First, certain epidemiologic factors and patient characteristics predict a higher prevalence of significant underlying disease and therefore help select those who should undergo extensive evaluation:

1. Patients referred for hematuria. The prevalence of urologic malignancy is greater than 10% in a referral population (52–54), compared with a prevalence of 0–4% in the general population (52,55).
2. Male sex. Life-threatening lesions are more common in men than in women (40,56).
3. Age greater than 50 years. The overwhelming majority of patients with significant pathology, particularly neoplasia, are over 50 years of age (52–54).
4. Gross hematuria. In a recent review of the literature, the chance of finding urologic cancer is much higher with gross hematuria (22.5%) compared with microscopic hematuria (5%) (57).

Therefore, the economic implications based on disease prevalence alone suggest that a 60-year-old man referred for gross hematuria needs an exhaustive evaluation, whereas a 30-year-old woman with asymptomatic microscopic hematuria discovered on an insurance physical requires a more tailored, prudent approach.

Second, the cost-effectiveness of tests and procedures conducted during an evaluation of hematuria depend in part on their ability to exclude significant urologic disease, i.e., a high degree of specificity. In a prospective study of over 1,000 patients using intravenous pyelography (IVP), cystoscopy, renal ultrasound (US), and urine cytology as standards of evaluation, Murikami et al. found that these tests were 99% to 100% specific in excluding moderately significant (urolithiasis, renal parenchymal disease) and highly significant (cancer) lesions (58). This confirms and reassures our suspicions that the standard tests used in the evaluation of hematuria are not only valuable clinical tools but cost effective as well in their ability to exclude disease.

Third, the risk-benefit ratio of undergoing an evaluation has economic impact. Cost containment is an achievable goal if there is little risk of patient morbidity and mortality when undergoing various procedures. Mariani's evaluation of 1,000 patients with microscopic hematuria (IVP, cystoscopy, urine culture and cytology, and other studies as indicated) resulted in only three life-threatening complications (0.3% incidence). Furthermore, the risk of serious adverse consequences during the workup based on procedure complication rates documented in the literature remained low at 1.1% (56). Thus, it appears that a typical evaluation of hematuria carries little risk and therefore adds minimal morbidity-related costs to patient care.

Finally, the actual cost of investigating hematuria must be considered. In the same study, Mariani et al. found the average direct cost of their hematuria evaluation to be $777, which is comparable with a similar evaluation at our institution. He also discovered that the average cost to diagnose and treat three patients with urologic malignancy for 17 months who sought medical care late in the course was $49,000 more per patient compared with three similar patients who presented for evaluation at the first sign of hematuria. They found the overall cost effectiveness of discovering life-threatening lesions on evaluation, including direct medical costs and the risk-benefit of adverse effects, to be favorable in all patients except women less than 40 years of age with microscopic hematuria (56). This group was composed of a small number of patients, which precludes drawing conclusions about the appropriateness or economics of the hematuria evaluation.

In summary, the tests and procedures used in evaluating hematuria have been proven to accurately exclude significant disease with few complications and therefore add little to the cost of investigating hematuria. The key to cost effectiveness, then, rests with identifying those patients at risk for significant disease and embarking on a thorough yet prudent workup.

Hematuria Evaluation

An algorithm outlining a stepwise, thorough, and cost-effective approach to the patient with hematuria is depicted in Fig. 4. A thorough history and physical examination followed by urinalysis and examination of the urinary sediment are always essential first steps in the evaluation of hematuria. This excludes pigmenturia as discussed previously (Fig. 1). Urine culture is an integral part of the early investigation even in asymptomatic patients because it accounts for a significant proportion of hematuria in all age groups. A positive culture necessitates antibiotics, but repeat culture and/or empiric therapy are reasonable if the clinical suspicion for infection is high. If glomerulonephritis is suggested by the history and physical examination and/or analysis of the urinary sediment, appropriate serologic tests should be ordered and renal biopsy performed (see earlier section on Approach to Glomerulonephritis). If the investigation is nonproductive to this point, a complete blood count, coagulation profile, chemistry panel containing calcium and uric acid, and 24-h urine analysis for protein, creatinine, calcium, and uric acid should be obtained. This assesses renal function, identifies a coagulopathy that may be contributing (but does not preclude an anatomic evaluation), and may uncover primary hyperparathyroidism, hypercalciuria, hyperuricosuria, or other etiologies. A sickle cell preparation or hemoglobin electrophoresis should be ordered in African Americans. Men over 50 years of age should proceed with an anatomic workup given their rapidly increasing prevalence of urologic malignancy even if the results of these laboratory tests suggest a cause of their hematuria (e.g., hypercalciuria).

If no information emerges to direct further testing, an anatomic evaluation is next in order, consisting of an IVP, cystoscopy, and possibly retrograde pyelography or uroendoscopic procedures. If the patient has significant renal insufficiency, a renal US can be substituted for the IVP to avoid radiocontrast-induced nephrotoxicity. A renal parenchymal lesion on IVP or US should be imaged in more detail with computed tomography (CT) or magnetic resonance imaging (MRI). MRI may be preferable in patients where it would be advantageous to avoid radiocontrast dye. A cystoscopy should follow a lesion of the renal pelvis or ureters seen on IVP. Retrograde pyelography or urologic endoscopic exploration is indicated for unilateral bleeding discovered on cystoscopy and for any ureteral abnormalities not well defined on IVP. If the results of both IVP and cystoscopy are normal, three first morning urine samples for cytology and CT or MRI should be ordered in all patients over 40 years of age in an effort to identify transitional cell carcinoma in situ and renal cell carcinoma, respectively. Even if renal US were performed, it cannot reliably detect lesions less than 3 cm in diameter (59,60) and may miss renal cell carcinoma that has not disrupted the kidney contour or is isodense to normal renal parenchyma.

An evaluation for urologic tuberculosis should be conducted in patients of any age who have a history of infection or exposure. A chest roentgenogram, skin testing, and analysis of three first morning urine samples for acid-fast bacilli stain and culture are indicated.

At this stage, all patients with a negative hematuria evaluation result need to be followed long term, with a history and physical examination, urinalysis, and examination of the urinary sediment every 6 months. Although controversial, we feel repeated anatomic studies every 2 to 3 years are warranted in patients ≥40 years of age who were referred for hematuria, a group at relatively high risk of malignancy.

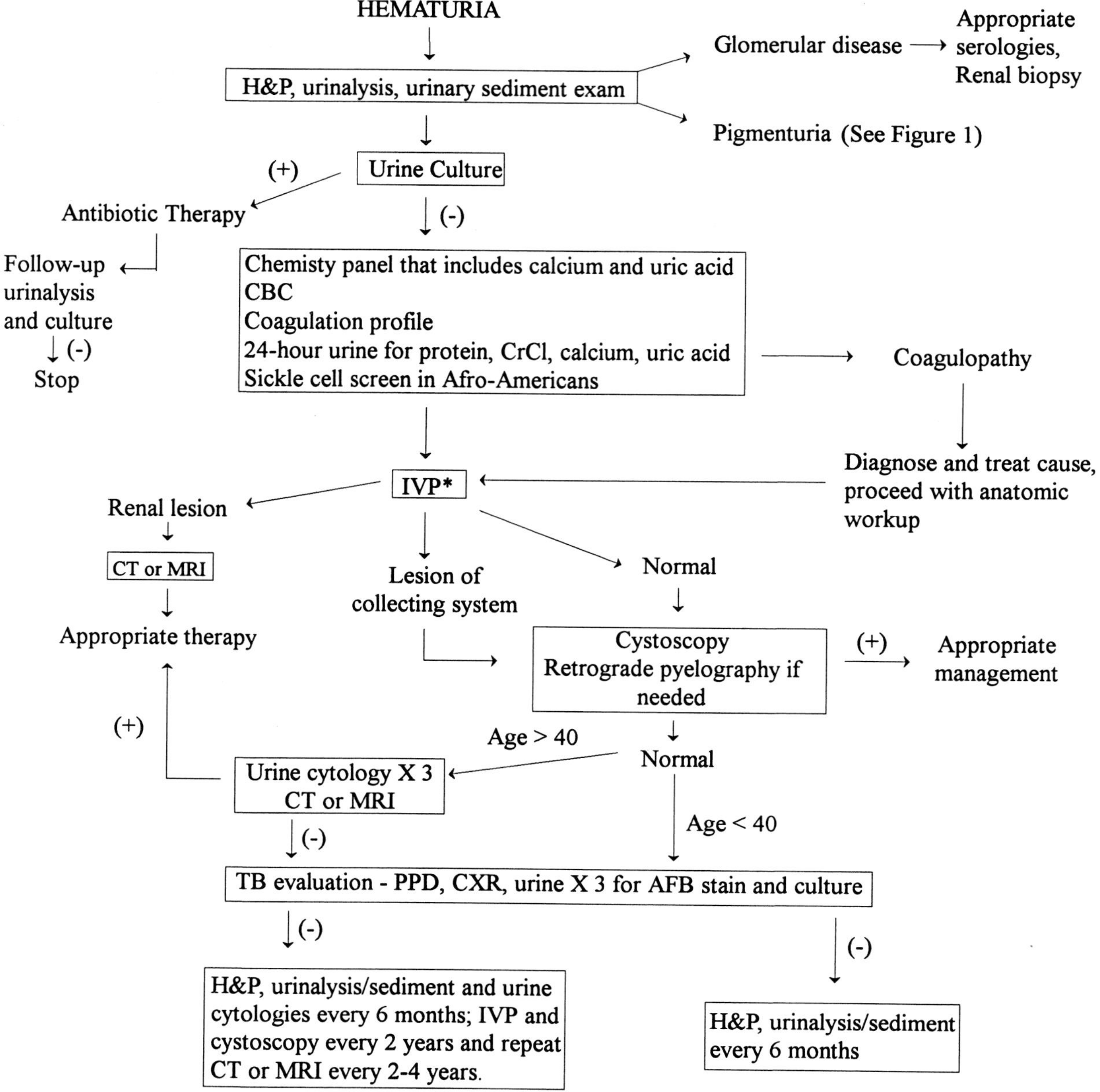

* Substitute renal US in patients at significant risk for contrast-induced nephrotoxicity

(H&P - History and physical, CrCl - Creatinine clearance, TB - Tuberculosis, PPD - Purified protein derivative, CXR - Chest roentogram, AFB - Acid fast bacilli)

FIG. 4. Approach to hematuria.

Of note is that renal arteriography does not appear in the algorithm. CT has a sensitivity, specicticity, positive predictive value, and negative predictive value of 96% to 98% in detecting space-occupying lesions, better than that of US, IVP, or angiography (61). The accuracy of an angiogram cannot compare overall, and the potential complications from arteriotomy, a higher volume of contrast dye, and cholesterol embolization make it a more risky procedure. Arteriography is useful in mapping tumor blood supply preoperatively and is essential for preoperative embolization of tumor vessels to facilitate nephrectomy (62), but its role in the diagnosis and staging of renal mass lesions is currently limited. The fact that angiography is no longer necessary in most patients with renal cell carcinoma also has resulted in considerable cost reduction in evaluating renal lesions (63).

PROTEINURIA

Proteinuria can be transient, orthostatic, or constant in nature, of glomerular and/or tubular origin, and associated with myriad diseases. Some cases are benign and associated with a favorable outcome, such as orthostatic proteinuria, whereas others have a more serious prognosis. In fact, the degree of proteinuria itself has been associated with the progression of renal failure (64–70). An understanding of the pathophysiology, definition, detection, and classification is therefore essential to an organized, complete, and cost-effective approach to the patient with proteinuria.

Normal Physiology and Definition of Proteinuria

Approximately 150 to 180 L of plasma is filtered by our glomeruli each day, some crossing the glomerular capillaries into Bowman's space, moving into the tubules and ultimately forming 1 to 2 L of urine. Each liter of plasma contains 60 to 80 g of protein, creating a potential for 12,000 g of protein that could appear in the urine each day. That only 150 mg of protein is normally excreted per day (71) is explained by two main factors: the glomerulus restricts the filtration of proteins and the tubules reabsorb the majority of proteins that get filtered. The glomerulus allows the passage of only 2 to 4 g of the 12,000 g of protein filtered each day. Factors regulating the transglomerular movement of protein are discussed in detail in Chapter 3. Of the 2–4 g/day of protein that reaches the tubules, 0.5 to 1.0 g is albumin. Yet only 20–40 mg/day of albumin ends up in the urine, the rest reabsorbed and catabolized primarily by the proximal convoluted tubules. Many low molecular weight, freely filtered proteins and peptides [lysozyme, beta-2-microglobulin, light chains of immunoglobulins, insulin, parathyroid hormone (PTH)] are similarly reabsorbed and degraded by the renal tubules, leaving only 10 to 20 mg/day in the final urine. The remaining 40% of our normal protein excretion is composed of the uroepithelial secretory proteins, Tamm-Horsfall glycoprotein, and secretory immunoglobulin A (IgA). Trace amounts of other proteins derived from the lower urinary tract and prostate gland also can be found in normal human urine.

The normal physiology discussed above provides the basis for understanding the pathophysiology of abnormal proteinuria. The mechanisms of excessive protein excretion are listed as follows:

1. Increased glomerular permeability leading to excessive filtration of normal plasma proteins that overwhelms the reabsorptive capacity of the tubules (microalbuminuria, nephrotic syndrome).
2. Tubular defects or disease interfering with the tubules capacity to reabsorb normally filtered plasma proteins or causing a leak of tubular enzymes (e.g., pyelonephritis, Fanconi syndrome).
3. Filtration of abnormal amounts of low molecular weight plasma proteins that exceed the reabsorptive capacity of the tubules (e.g., immunoglobulin light chains).
4. Increased secretion of Tamm-Horsfall mucoprotein and IgA by uroepithelial cells in response to inflammation (e.g., pyelonephritis).
5. Renal hemodynamic factors. In times of stress (physical or emotional), the adrenergic and renin-angiotensin systems can cause afferent and efferent arteriole vasoconstriction. With afferent constriction, glomerular capillary plasma flow is reduced, favoring the movement of albumin and other large molecular weight proteins across the glomerular basement membrane. If efferent arteriolar tone, mediated by angiotensin, exceeds that of the afferent arteriole, glomerular capillary hydrostatic pressure and filtration fraction increase. Plasma proteins can more readily traverse the glomerular basement membrane because of the excessive diffusive forces across the capillary wall.

These effects that lead to increased proteinuria are functional in nature and do not imply a change in glomerular pore size or charge (e.g., exercise-induced proteinuria).

One or more of these pathophysiologic mechanisms can account for abnormal proteinuria in any given patient (e.g., a patient with glomerulonephritis who demonstrates alterations in glomerular permeability and tubulointerstitial inflammation), and they provide a foundation for the classification of proteinuria.

Classification of Proteinuria

Proteinuria can be classified as intermittent or constant, with constant being further subdivided into tubulointerstitial and glomerular categories.

Intermittent Proteinuria

The intermittent proteinurias are probably the most common causes of abnormal protein excretion and are defined as those disorders associated with transient proteinuria that have an inactive urinary sediment and no long-term morbidity such as renal insufficiency or hypertension (71,72).

Functional proteinuria refers to proteinuria that occurs concomitantly with conditions such as fever, strenuous exercise, congestive heart failure, exposure to cold, emotional stress, seizures, and other hyperadrenergic states, and it may be present in as many as 10% of emergency medical admissions (73). It resolves within several days after the acute precipitating event and carries no long-lasting effects. The mechanism of functional proteinuria stems mainly from renal hemodynamic effects on the glomerular capillary bed that favor increased filtration of albumin and other plasma proteins (46), as discussed in the last section. There may also be a tubular component to functional proteinuria, especially in exercise-related proteinuria (74,75).

Idiopathic transient proteinuria is another common category of intermittent proteinuria found in children and young adults (72,76–78). It is defined as proteinuria in an asymptomatic apparently healthy individual found incidentally on routine screening (such as for athletic, pre-employment, or insurance physicals) that disappears on subsequent testing. Again, there are no long-term sequelae of this disorder, although a positive test for urinary protein tends to recur in some people but remains a transient phenomenon (79,80). Wolman showed that if urine samples are tested often enough in healthy young men, proteinuria will be occasionally detected (77), suggesting that idiopathic transient proteinuria is a physiologic and not a pathologic phenomenon. Therefore, when this type of proteinuria is discovered, no further evaluation is necessary. Repeating urinalyses two to three times is necessary to exclude this condition before embarking on an extensive investigation in patients presenting with proteinuria.

Idiopathic intermittent proteinuria is defined as those cases in which approximately 50% of random urine samples show abnormal amounts of protein that is not orthostatic in nature and cannot be attributed to any identifiable etiology. Patients with this pattern of protein excretion are heterogeneous, showing an unpredictable variety of associated disease states and renal histopathology. In the only biopsy study published in these patients, Muth found normal or minimal histologic changes in 39%, chronic glomerulonephritis in 24%, chronic pyelonephritis in 24%, and focal or proliferative glomerulonephritis in 13% (81). The long-term outcome of idiopathic intermittent proteinuria is difficult to relate to any underlying disease because of the variety of conditions, including normal kidneys, that are associated with it. In general, these patients are young (<30 years of age) and asymptomatic with normal blood pressure and renal function, and appear to have a favorable prognosis because proteinuria disappears in most within a few years (82). Hypertension and progressive renal insufficiency are the exception rather than the rule in this age group. Given the small amount of uncertainty, however, patients with idiopathic intermittent proteinuria should be monitored (every 6–12 months) for the development of constant proteinuria, hypertension, renal insufficiency, and the stigmata of systemic disease.

Orthostatic proteinuria is the last type of proteinuria in the intermittent category. First, it is important to recognize that protein excretion increases upon standing in normal subjects (83,84) as well as in those with underlying glomerular disease (85,86). Orthostatic proteinuria is defined as abnormal amounts of protein that are excreted solely in the upright position with a normal amount of protein excreted in the supine position. In other words, this subset of patients excretes protein at the normal rate of less than 150 mg/day when they are recumbent but at higher abnormal rates when they are upright.

In general, orthostatic proteinuria occurs most commonly in adolescents and may account for over 60% of proteinuria seen in this age group (87). It is rarely seen in persons more than 30 years of age. These individuals are usually asymptomatic healthy young men with a normal history and physical examination, normal renal function, and a benign urinary sediment who excrete less than 1 g of protein in 24 h.

Patients with orthostatic proteinuria have an excellent long-term prognosis. Follow-up of such patients over several decades has documented that most (>80%) have resolution of their proteinuria, do not develop renal insufficiency or hypertension, and have normal histology or only minor glomerular lesions (mild mesangial expansion, mild hypercellularity, or focal foot process fusion) on renal biopsy (88–90).

The pathophysiology behind orthostatic proteinuria remains unclear, but renal hemodynamic effects discussed earlier that promote movement of protein across the glomerular basement membrane are felt to play a significant role (91). Of interest are reports that suggest entrapment of the left renal vein by the aorta or superior mesenteric artery may create passive congestion in the left renal vein and therefore promote proteinuria (92).

Despite an overall favorable prognosis for orthostatic proteinuria, approximately 10% of individuals have had definite glomerular pathology documented by biopsy (90), and Burns et al. reported a case of focal glomerulosclerosis in a 15-year-old boy who presented 1 year earlier with orthostatic proteinuria (93). Because these developments are difficult to predict, regular (every 6–12 months) long-term monitoring of these patients for the development of hypertension, renal insufficiency, or an active urinary sediment is indicated.

Constant Proteinuria

Constant proteinuria is defined as abnormal amounts of proteinuria throughout a 24-h period regardless of activity level, position, or functional status. It can be further divided into tubulointerstitial and glomerular categories.

Tubulointerstitial Proteinuria

Many different tubulointerstitial diseases (such as pyelonephritis) and primary tubular disorders (such as Fanconi syndrome) interfere with the tubules' capacity to reabsorb the protein normally filtered by the glomeruli. Thus, the pattern of proteinuria seen in tubulointerstitial disease is composed of small amounts of albumin, enzymes such as lysozyme, and other small, freely filtered plasma proteins that the tubules normally reabsorb. The amount of tubular proteinuria in these disorders rarely exceeds 2 g/day because the glomerular filtration barrier is intact. Significant albuminuria in a patient with known tubulointerstitial disease should stimulate a search for coexistent glomerular pathology.

A second group of disorders classified under tubulointerstitial proteinuria is tubular overload. Overproduction of a filterable plasma protein overloads the tubules' capacity for reabsorption, resulting in the presence of that protein in the final urine. The glomerulus is intact, so albuminuria should be minimal and perhaps undetectable, resulting in a negative urinary dipstick. Multiple myeloma is probably the most common cause of tubular overload in adults, in whom large quantities of immunoglobulin light chains (lambda or kappa) are produced. Because they are neutral or cationic in charge and have a relatively small molecular weight (~25 kDa), light chains are filtered in large amounts, overwhelming the reabsorptive capacity of the tubules, resulting in Bence-Jones proteinuria. The amount of light chains excreted varies but is usually over 500 mg/day and may exceed several grams per day with a heavy tumor burden. Other examples of tubular overload proteinuria include lysozymuria in patients with monocytic or myelomonocytic leukemia (94), hemoglobinuria in severe hemolytic anemia, myoglobinuria in rhabdomyolysis, and urinary amylase in pancreatitis.

Glomerular Proteinuria

Glomerular proteinuria results from a defect in the glomerular filtration barrier with increased glomerular permeability, leading to the excretion of proteins in amounts not found in normal urine.

Isolated proteinuria is defined here as a constant protein excretion of less than 3.5 g/day (non-nephrotic) that is likely glomerular in origin but is not associated with postural changes or any identifiable systemic illness. This type of proteinuria is difficult to categorize because some patients may indeed have chronic tubulointerstitial changes, but our review of the available biopsy literature in adults with persistent isolated proteinuria showed the majority of abnormal biopsies to have glomerular pathology as opposed to tubulointerstitial disease (95–98). Therefore, we classify this type of constant proteinuria as glomerular.

With these stipulations in mind, the principal causes in this category are an as yet unrecognized systemic disease that affects the glomerulus, such as malignancy or amyloidosis, or an early or mild form of disease intrinsic to the glomerulus, such as diabetes or any of the glomerulopathies listed in Table 7 under the Nephrotic Syndrome section.

With variable biopsy results, a paucity of signs or symptoms of a systemic illness at presentation, and confounding factors such as hypertension, diabetes, and peripheral vascular disease, attributing isolated proteinuria to a specific cause is often problematic. Few long-term follow-up studies have been performed, but King followed 92 such patients for an average of 6 years and found that most had developed an abnormal urinary sediment and approximately 50% had developed hypertension (99,100). Therefore, the only way to predict progression of disease in patients with isolated proteinuria is close follow-up. A change in urinary sediment, a substantial increase in proteinuria, the development of hypertension, the onset or worsening of renal insufficiency, or the clinical emergence of a systemic disease should prompt further evaluation with renal biopsy and serologies as indicated.

Microalbuminuria is a second type of proteinuria classified as glomerular in etiology. It is defined as the excretion of 30 to 300 mg of albumin per day, 30 to 300 mg of albumin per gram of urine creatinine in a spot urine sample, or 20 to 200 μg/min on a timed urine collection (101). This small amount of albuminuria is not readily identifiable using the routine urinary dipstick method. The ability to detect and measure microalbuminuria has considerable clinical importance because it predicts the progression of diabetic nephropathy in insulin-dependent diabetes (102,103), is related to patient mortality in non–insulin-dependent diabetes (103–105), and may portend a poor prognosis for renal function in conditions such as essential hypertension and systemic sclerosis (106). We refer the reader to subsequent sections of this chapter for

TABLE 6. *Causes of false-positive and false-negative reactions in qualitative tests for proteinuria*

False positives	False negatives
Urine dipstick	
Highly concentrated urine	Very dilute urine
Gross hematuria	
Overlong immersion	Immunoglobulins
Alkaline urine (pH >8)	Light chains
Urea-splitting bacteria	Mucoproteins (Tamm-Horsfall)
Turbidimetric tests	
Highly concentrated urine	Very dilute urine
Gross hematuria	Alkaline urine (pH >8)
Hematuria plus dilute urine	
Penicillins, cephalosporins	
Sulfonamide metabolites	
Tolbutamide metabolites	
Tolmetin	

specifics on the detection and measurement of microalbuminuria.

The nephrotic syndrome as a class of proteinuria is addressed in detail later in this chapter.

Detection and Measurement of Proteinuria

As discussed in preceding sections, most healthy adults excrete less than 150 mg/day of protein. However, routinely collecting 24-h urine samples for quantitation of protein excretion is cumbersome, prone to collection errors, and costly. Therefore, routine tests for proteinuria are usually conducted on random specimens using qualitative tests, such as the colorimetric dipstick method and/or a turbidimetric method (e.g., sulfosalicylic acid). Attempts also have been made to simplify the quantitation of daily protein excretion using spot urine samples. The qualitative detection and quantification of proteinuria are discussed below.

Qualitative Detection

It must be remembered that qualitative tests of urinary protein can only estimate a range of protein concentration, and interpretation of the results is highly subjective and variable.

Urinary Dipstick

The most common clinically used method to detect protein in the random urine sample is the dipstick method. A plastic strip with a cellulose indicator region for protein (as well as other regions for blood, glucose, etc.) is impregnated with a pH-sensitive indicator, typically tetrabromphenol blue and a citrate buffer, which fixes the pH of the reactive region at 3 so the indicator is not affected by the pH of normal urine. The reaction of the protein indicator region with the amino groups of urinary albumin causes a color change that is qualitatively proportional to the concentration of urinary albumin over a range of 30 mg/dl to 2 g/dl. The reagent is sensitive to albumin at concentrations greater than 10–15 mg/dl but does not approach 100% sensitivity until it reaches 30 mg/dl. Above 2 g/dl, no further color change occurs. Albumin avidly binds the tetrabromphenol blue and therefore causes a change in color far more readily than other proteins such as globulins (107). The dipstick method then, should be regarded as specific for albuminuria. The urine dipstick is so insensitive to other proteins that it may fail to detect Bence-Jones proteinuria even when it exceeds 100 mg/dl.

Turbidimetric Method

Turbidimetric tests for urinary protein overcome some disadvantages of the urinary dipstick method because they readily detect nonalbumin proteins, as well as albumin, down to a level as little as 5–10 mg/dl. This qualitative method works by precipitating proteins at an acid pH by heating then adding glacial acetic acid or, more commonly, by adding an equal volume of 3% sulfosalicylic acid (SSA) to an equal volume of centrifuged urine. Any resulting turbidity is visually graded from trace to 4+ using urine plus water as the standard for a negative test for protein. A trace-positive result is equivalent to approximately 20 mg/dl of urinary protein, whereas a 4+ result corresponds to 1 g/dl or more. The combination of a negative urine dipstick and a positive SSA test may be indicative of the presence of urinary globulins such as Bence-Jones proteins and should prompt further investigation, including a urine protein electrophoresis.

False-Positive and False-Negative Test Results

The false-positive and false-negative reactions for both the dipstick and turbidimetric qualitative methods are shown in Table 6. Because both the urine dipstick method and the turbidimetric tests estimate the concentration of urinary protein, a very concentrated or very dilute urine can yield false-positive or false-negative reactions, respectively. Furthermore, a dilute urine sample containing RBCs with a specific gravity of less than 1.010 lyse most of the RBCs, releasing free hemoglobin that is detected by turbidity tests (16). Thus, urine specimens with specific gravities of less than 1.010 and greater than 1.025 should be submitted to dipstick analysis with caution. Alternatively, the urine protein concentration can be adjusted for the urine specific gravity: the last two digits of the specific gravity represents the upper limit of normal for protein concentration, e.g., 5 mg/dl for a specific gravity of 1.005, and 30 mg/dl for a specific gravity of 1.030 (108). In addition, gross hematuria often results in substantial proteinuria in isotonic, concentrated, or dilute urine (109), rendering both qualitative tests for proteinuria useless under these conditions.

Quantitative Measurement of Proteinuria

Timed Collection

The definitive method for documenting an abnormal amount of protein excretion is a 24-h urine collection. Shorter collection periods are prone to error because they magnify confounding factors such as fever, exercise, and orthostatic variation in protein excretion. The first morning urine specimen should be discarded and all subsequent specimens over the following 24 h collected, including the next morning's void. Ideally, the urine specimen should be kept refrigerated, especially if the ambient temperature is above 75°F or if there will be a delay in submitting the specimen to the laboratory. In the laboratory the volume of urine is measured, as is the concentration of protein and creatinine in a well-mixed aliquot. This allows calculation of the daily protein excretion and creatinine clearance, as well as estimation of the adequacy of the urine collection (14–18 mg creatinine/kg/day in females, 18–26 mg/creatinine/kg/day in males). In adults, a protein excretion of up to 150 mg/24 h is considered normal.

Single-Voided Urine Method

Given that 24-h urine collections are time consuming, cumbersome, and therefore prone to noncompliance, a method of estimating quantitative proteinuria from single-voided urine samples was developed (110,111). This method is particularly valuable in those individuals who have difficulty with the 24-h collection, such as children, the elderly, and incontinent patients. Its accuracy is based on the fact that creatinine excretion, being proportional to lean body mass, is nearly constant throughout the day in any given individual. Therefore, the ratio of protein-to-creatinine excretion should provide a reasonable measurement of daily protein excretion. That is, the protein-to-creatinine ratio (mg/dl protein per mg/dl creatinine) in a single-voided urine numerically approximates the 24-h protein excretion in grams, automatically corrected for body surface area. Thus, normal subjects have a ratio of less than 0.2, corresponding to less than 200 mg/day proteinuria, and nephrotic individuals have a ratio of 3.5 or more, corresponding to ≥3.5 g of protein excretion per day.

Factors that alter the rate of protein but not creatinine excretion, such as upright and recumbent positions, fever, and exercise, decrease the ability of the protein-to-creatinine ratio to accurately quantitate proteinuria. Therefore, it is recommended that single urine samples be obtained during normal daylight activity in the absence of an intercurrent illness. With these caveats in mind, we advocate the use of the protein-to-creatinine ratio to measure daily protein excretion in patients who, for whatever reason, are unable to comply with a 24-h urine collection.

Detection and Measurement of Microalbuminuria

Qualitative tests for the detection of microalbuminuria recently have been developed. Micral (Boehringer-Mannheim) and Microbumitest (Ames) are two of the more convenient, available, and cost-effective methods because they have short assay times and do not require special equipment (112). Micral is a semiquantitative test that ranges from 0 to 100 mg/L, with greater than 20 mg/L producing a positive result. Microbumitest is strictly qualitative: a positive test corresponds to a urine albumin concentration of greater than 40 mg/L. Although sensitive (>90%), their specificities are relatively low at 82% and 87%, respectively, when compared with radioimmunoassay, the standard for measuring microalbuminuria (112).

The above qualitative tests are helpful in initially screening patients, but microalbuminuria is most accurately diagnosed using quantitative radioimmunoassays. A 24-h urine collection yields reliable results but has the same drawbacks as the 24-h collections for overt proteinuria, namely inconvenience and patient noncompliance. A single first morning voided specimen using a radioimmunoassay to measure albumin also reliably quantitates microalbuminuria with a sensitivity of 94% and specifity of 96% when compared with 24-h collections (112). A range of 30 to 300 mg of albumin per gram of urine creatinine defines microalbuminuria using this method (101). However, microalbuminuria can initially be intermittent and can be affected by exercise, ketoacidosis, and urinary tract infections (101). Thus, using single-voided urine samples to estimate 24-h excretion of albumin should be avoided in these circumstances. We advocate 24-h collections to diagnose microalbuminuria whenever feasible and use the albumin-creatinine ratio from the first morning void when necessary, such as in noncompliant or incontinent patients.

Testing for Orthostatic Proteinuria

Confirming or excluding the presence of orthostatic proteinuria can provide important prognostic information regarding the development of hypertension or renal insufficiency as previously discussed. The first morning urine should be discarded, followed by collection of all subsequent specimens in a single container during normal daily activities, including the void just before or 1 h after going to bed. These specimens constitute the upright collection, and the time interval of collection is noted. All urine voided during the night, including the first morning specimen, is collected in a second container, and the time interval of collection is again recorded. This is the recumbent collection. The amount of protein from each sample is measured and then extrapolated to 24 h. Patients with orthostatic proteinuria have increased rates of excretion (>150 mg/24 h) in the upright position and normal rates of excretion (<150 mg/24 h) in the recumbent position. Total protein excretion generally does not exceed 1 g/day. If both specimens contain excessive amounts of protein, even though the upright specimen may have more than the recumbent specimen, the condition cannot be labeled orthostatic.

Alternatively, the diagnosis of orthostatic proteinuria can be made using the protein-to-creatinine ratio. A single-voided specimen just before bed would represent the upright collection, and the first morning void would represent the recumbent collection. A ratio of less than 0.2 in the recumbent urine and greater than 0.2 in the upright urine is diagnostic of orthostatic proteinuria.

Clinical Evaluation of Proteinuria

With the definitions and classification of proteinuria in mind, a rational, stepwise, and cost-effective approach to its evaluation can be developed (Fig. 5). A complete history and physical examination, urinalysis, and careful examination of the urinary sediment should be performed initially. Any evidence of an underlying systemic or renal disease should be pursued with the appropriate workup. (A detailed discussion of specific diseases is covered in detail in subsequent chapters.) Optimally, the urine should be qualitatively tested for protein using both the dipstick method and a turbidimetric method, usually SSA. From this, three possibilities emerge, which form the basis for the subsequent evaluation.

Dipstick-Positive/SSA-Positive

This is usually indicative of true proteinuria, but false-positive results must first be ruled out as previously discussed and shown in Table 6.

If the SSA shows a significantly higher protein concentration (i.e., is more positive) than the dipstick method, substantial amounts of nonalbumin proteins are being excreted. These patients may have both tubulointerstitial and glomerular disease processes and should be evaluated as such. More likely, they have a primarily tubulointerstitial disorder, with the inability of the tubules to reabsorb filtered albumin accounting for the dipstick positivity. An overabundance of filtered plasma proteins plus their decreased tubular reabsorption creates a more positive SSA result. In either case, an evaluation of tubulointerstitial proteinuria should ensue.

Dipstick and SSA tests that are equally positive on repeat testing are indicative of constant albuminuria. Once constant proteinuria is identified, the amount should be quantified and evaluated as in Fig. 5.

Dipstick-Negative/SSA-Positive

This combination of qualitative tests is pathognomonic for tubulointerstitial proteinuria. Bence-Jones proteinuria or lysozymuria are two of the more common causes in adults. Quantifying and identifying the proteins by urine protein electrophoresis (UPEP) and urine immunoelectrophoresis (UIEP) are helpful in guiding further diagnostic tests and subsequent therapy.

Dipstick-Negative/SSA-Negative

Once false-negative reactions common to both qualitative methods (i.e., very dilute urine) are excluded, intermittent proteinurias become the leading diagnostic possibilities. Repeating the dipstick and SSA two to three times over the course of 1 to 2 months determines the extent of the necessary workup.

If follow-up testing is all negative, then the initial proteinuria was likely functional or idiopathic transient proteinuria, and no further evaluation or follow-up is required.

Repeat testing positive for protein one or more times indicates orthostatic or idiopathic intermittent proteinuria as possibilities. Determination of renal function should follow, with an elevated serum creatinine suggesting underlying renal pathology, followed by an evaluation as indicated in Fig. 5.

If renal function is normal and the protein excretion is not orthostatic but remains intermittent in nature, a diagnosis of idiopathic intermittent proteinuria should be considered. To briefly review, this is a class of proteinuria ill defined in the literature with little data on its long-term sequela. The available information suggests that it is a relatively benign process in individuals less than 30 years of age (95). Therefore, we recommend long-term follow-up similar to that for orthostatic proteinuria: a history, physical examination, and urine examination, as well as serum creatinine determination every 12 months. Older patients with idiopathic intermittent proteinuria may be at increased risk for developing hypertension, renal insufficiency, or a systemic disease and should be seen by a physician at least every 6 months.

If follow-up qualitative test results for proteinuria are positive but the serum creatinine is normal, the patient should first undergo evaluation for orthostatic proteinuria. If present, they can then be followed yearly with a history and physical examination, urinalysis, review of urinary sediment, and repeat serum creatinine. If the proteinuria resolves over time, no further follow-up is required. If the patient continues to demonstrate orthostatic proteinuria, follow-up should be continued as above. If constant proteinuria develops, the patient should be followed/evaluated as discussed above.

NEPHROTIC SYNDROME

Definition

The classic definition of nephrotic syndrome is a protein excretion of $\geq$3.5 g/day/1.73 m^2 body surface area (or a protein-to-creatinine ratio of $\geq$3.5) associated with hypoalbuminemia, edema, hyperlipidemia, and lipiduria. However, all these criteria need not be present to confirm the diagnosis because it may be a mild form or early in the disease process. Medical nomenclature commonly reserves the term nephrotic syndrome for $\geq$3.5 g/day proteinuria associated with at least one of the above features, whereas excretion of $\geq$3.5 g/day without any of the above criteria is labeled nephrotic proteinuria or nephrotic-range proteinuria. Clinically,

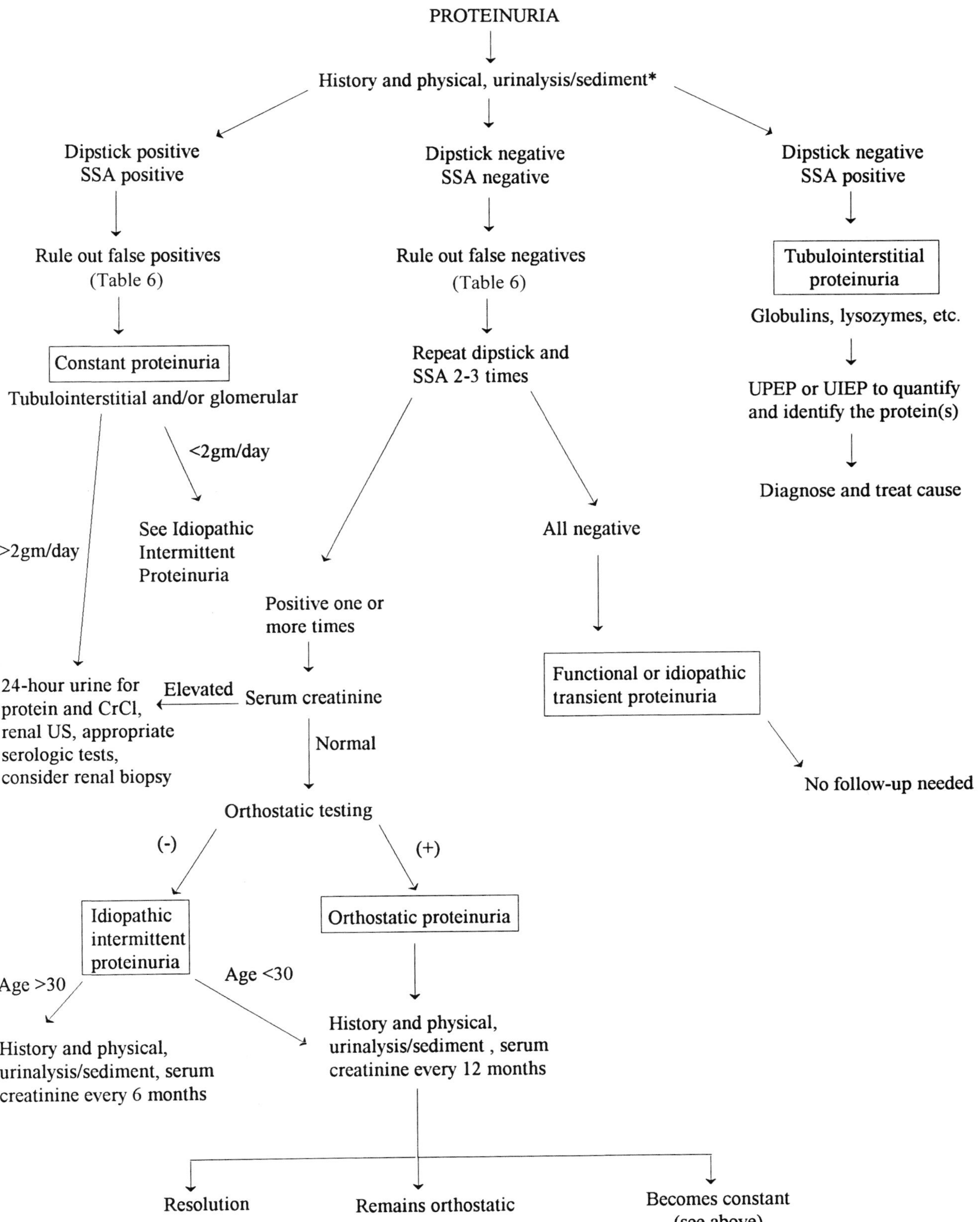

FIG. 5. Evaluation of proteinuria.

this distinction is a matter of semantics because the accompanying features of nephrotic syndrome likely develop in those with sufficient proteinuria over a long enough period of time. Thus, our clinical approach to patients with the nephrotic syndrome or nephrotic proteinuria is identical.

Although 3.5 g proteinuria/day is the hallmark of the nephrotic syndrome, certain caveats apply. Patients with severe disease may have a low serum albumin concentration, causing a marked decrease in the filtration of albumin and excretion of substantially less than 3.5 g/day of protein. A significant impairment of renal function can similarly decrease the filtration of albumin and result in less than nephrotic-range proteinuria. Correcting the amount of proteinuria for these clinical circumstances is an inexact process at best. In such cases, proceeding with a workup for suspected nephrotic syndrome would be a reasonable approach.

Pathophysiology

The nephrotic syndrome results from a defect in the glomerular filtration barrier, covered in detail in Chapter 3.

Etiology and Classification

A wide variety of glomerular lesions may be associated with the nephrotic syndrome in adults. Thus, any list of causes can be nearly endless. It is helpful to separate the adult nephrotic syndrome into primary (idiopathic) and secondary categories. Primary nephrotic syndrome is defined as a disorder with distinct clinicopathologic characteristics and natural history but is not associated with any identifiable cause. Secondary nephrotic syndrome may be pathologically similar to the primary forms but is directly associated with known toxins or systemic disease processes. The classification and major causes of adult nephrotic syndrome are listed in Table 7. As shown, secondary nephrotic syndrome can be further divided into subcategories very similar to those for a fever of unknown origin, an approach we find clinically useful.

TABLE 7. *Classification and major causes of nephrotic syndrome*

- Primary (idiopathic)
  - Minimal change disease (Nil)
  - Focal glomerulosclerosis (FGS)
  - Membranous nephropathy (MN)
  - Membranoproliferative glomerulonephritis (MPGN)
  - Other proliferative glomerulonephritis (OPGN)
- Secondary[a]
  - Infections
    - HIV disease (FGS)
    - Hepatitis B (MN)
    - Hepatitis C (MPGN, cryoglobulinemia)
    - Syphilis (MN)
    - Malaria (MN)
    - Schistosomiasis (MN)
    - Tuberculosis (amyloid)
    - Leprosy (MN)
  - Malignancies
    - Solid adenocarcinomas such as lung, breast, colon (MN)
    - Hodgkins lymphoma (Nil)
    - Multiple myeloma (myeloma kidney and/or Bence Jones proteinuria, amyloid)
    - Renal cell carcinoma (amyloid)
  - Connective tissue diseases
    - Systemic lupus erythematosis (MN, MPGN, OPGN)
    - Rheumatoid arthritis (amyloid, or rarely MN)
    - Mixed connective tissue disease (variable)
  - Drugs and toxins
    - Nonsteroidal anti-inflammatory agents (Nil)
    - Gold (MN)
    - Penicillamine (MN)
    - Probenecid (MN)
    - Mercury (MN)
    - Captopril (MN)
    - Intravenous heroin (FGS), "Skin popping" heroin (amyloid)
  - Other
    - Diabetes mellitus
    - Amyloidosis
    - Pre-eclampsia
    - Chronic allograft rejection
    - Vesicoureteral reflux (FGS)
    - Bee sting

[a]Associated histopathologic lesions are indicated in parentheses.

Clinical Evaluation

With the etiologic classification of the adult nephrotic syndrome in mind, the first and most important step in evaluating such patients is a thorough history and physical examination, urinalysis, and careful examination of the urinary sediment. Serum concentrations of albumin, cholesterol, and triglycerides are also helpful in assessing nephrotic syndrome. Identification of a drug, toxin, or systemic disease implicating a secondary cause should prompt withdrawal of the offending agent or a diagnostic evaluation with subsequent treatment of the underlying disease. In such cases, resolution of proteinuria requires no further evaluation or follow-up provided renal function remains normal. Nonsteroidal anti-inflammatory drug–induced interstitial nephritis and the diagnosis/treatment of secondary syphilis complicated by nephrotic syndrome are examples of this scenario. If the nephrotic syndrome fails to resolve or there is progression of disease, renal US (to document the size, presence, and echotexture of two kidneys), the appropriate serologic blood tests, and a renal biopsy are indicated to diagnose the disorder and potentially guide therapy, as illustrated in Figure 6.

Without any information to guide further evaluation, attention turns to the primary or idiopathic nephrotic syndromes (Table 7). Their clinical presentation often can overlap, but certain clinical and epidemiologic characteristics can help distinguish these syndromes from one another. The age, race, and sex of the patient, urinary sediment, renal function, presence of hypertension, and serum complement levels are key distinguishing factors, as detailed in Table 8. Table 8 is not meant to be diagnostic but can be used as a general guideline in assessing and prioritizing the differential diagnosis of idiopathic nephrotic syndrome. The results of a renal biopsy will provide a diagnosis, prognosticate long-term renal function, and guide treatment in the idiopathic nephrotic syndromes.

Serologic blood tests for glomerular disease are commonly used to diagnose or exclude secondary causes of nephrotic syndrome. However, they can add hundreds of dollars to the evaluation, yet add little diagnostic information in most cases, as demonstrated by Howard et al. (39). Therefore, serologic testing should be selective, not empiric in nature, and limited to those situations for which it will be of diagnostic benefit or assist in monitoring disease activity or therapy.

Recent developments may aid in the follow-up and assessment of disease activity in the nephrotic syndrome. The urinary excretion of terminal complement complexes (C5b-9) in membranous nephropathy may identify a subset of patients with ongoing immunologic damage, providing a marker for initiating, intensifying, or tapering therapy (113–116). Other measures of immunologic activity in the human glomerulus also have been studied, such as the excretion of soluble interleukin 2 receptors in lupus nephritis (117) and the plasma and urine levels of tumor necrosis factor-alpha in focal glomerulosclerosis and membranous nephropathy (118). We refer the reader to Chapters 46–48 for detailed discussion of these topics.

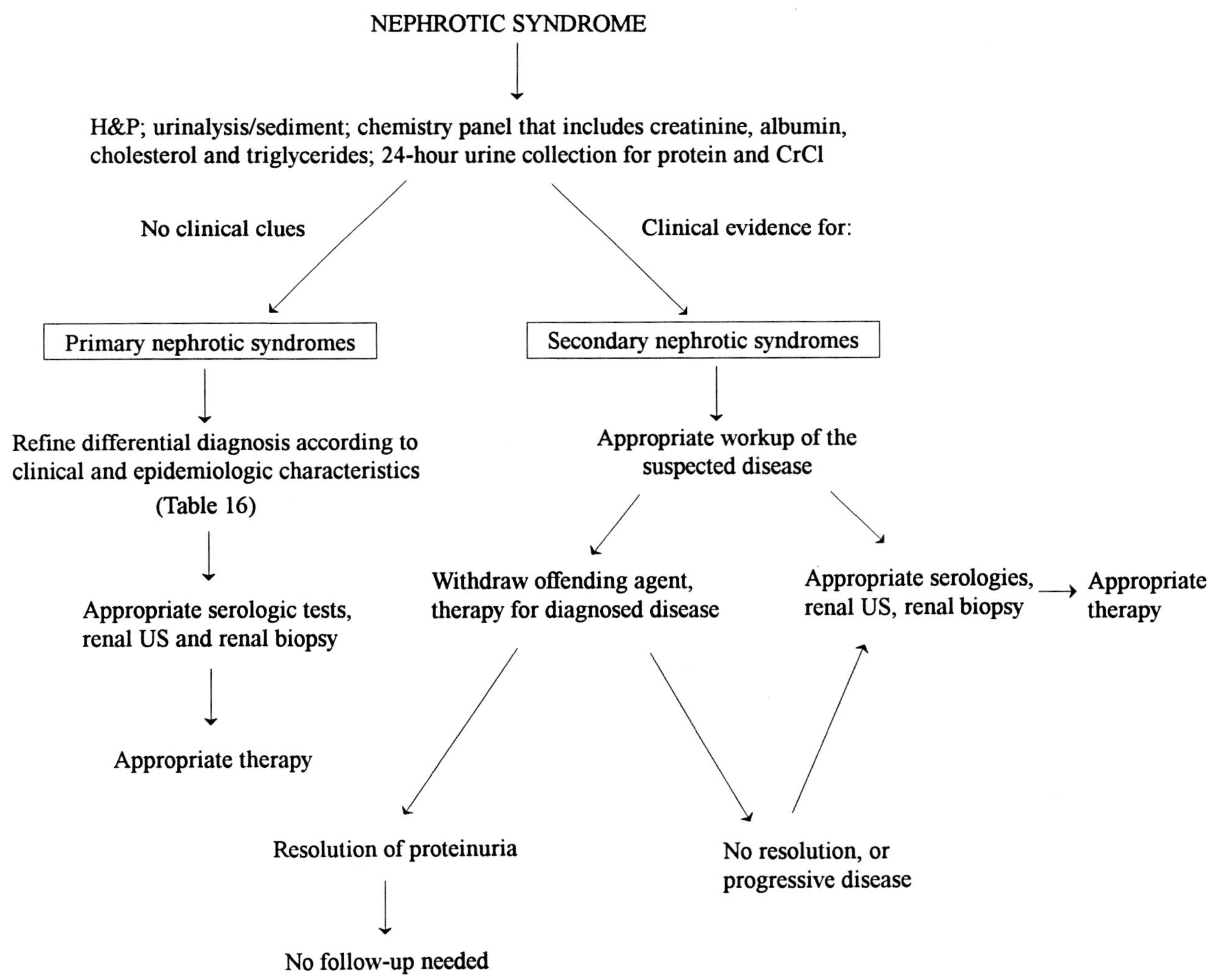

FIG. 6. Approach to the nephrotic syndrome..

TABLE 8. *Clinical and epidemiologic characteristics of the primary or idiopathic nephrotic syndromes in adults*

	Overall prevalence	Age-related prevalence	Hypertension	Urinary sediment	Serum creatinine	Complement
Minimal change disease	~25%	85% of NS <15 yr of age	Frequent in edematous phase; one third of those in remission	Benign; hematuria in <20%	Normal	Normal
Focal glomerulosclerosis	~15%	Over 70% of adult cases occur before age 50 yr	Frequently present	Active; RBCs, granular casts are typical	Elevated (may be normal in mild or early disease)	Normal
Membranous nephropathy	~30%	90% of adult cases occur after age 35 yr; prevalence increases with increasing age	Frequent in edematous phase; <1/3 of those in remission	Usually benign, but up to 50% have hematuria	Normal or elevated	Normal
Membrano-proliferative glomerulo-nephritis	~10%	Most common at 10–30 yr of age	+/–	Active; hematuria, granular and cellular casts not unusual	Elevated (may be normal in mild or early disease)	Depressed ~70% of cases in Type I
Other proliferative glomerulo-nephritis	~20%	Even distribution across all adult age groups	Usually absent, except in crescentic GN	Depends on underlying disease	Depends on underlying disease	Normal

NS, nephrotic syndrome; GN, glomerulonephritis.

Complications of the Nephrotic Syndrome

Hypoalbuminemia

The hypoalbuminemia of the nephrotic syndrome results from the perturbation of albumin's normal homeostatic mechanisms. The plasma albumin concentration can vary in patients with identical urinary protein losses, depending on the balance between dietary protein intake, the rate of hepatic synthesis, urinary losses of albumin, shifts in its body distribution and the rate of catabolism by renal and extrarenal sources.

Synthesis

The liver normally synthesizes 12 to 14 g of albumin daily and can increase production up to threefold if necessary. However, hepatic synthesis increases only slightly in nephrotic patients, which appears to be inadequate to avoid hypoalbuminemia (119). Moreover, in nephrotic patients the synthetic rate of albumin does not correlate with the serum albumin level (120). Thus, hypoalbuminemia itself does not trigger an appropriate response in hepatic albumin synthesis.

Catabolism

The glomerulus filters 2 to 4 g albumin/day, the vast majority of which is reabsorbed and catabolized by the proximal convoluted tubules. With increased glomerular permeability, the proximal tubules encounter large quantities of filtered albumin, potentially exceeding 50 g/day (121), and redistribution of albumin from the extravascular pool to the intravascular space in nephrotic patients (119) only serves to enhance its filtration fraction. Normally the tubules are responsible for only 10% of total body albumin catabolism but may account for as much as 50% in the nephrotic syndrome, i.e., a higher fractional catabolic rate of albumin (122–124). This concept may help explain how some patients excrete only 3.5 g protein/day yet seemingly have disproportionately low serum albumin concentrations.

However, it is well documented that the absolute level of albumin catabolism by the kidney is decreased in adequately fed patients and animals with nephrotic syndrome (119,122–126). This could mask any effects of increased fractional albumin catabolism that may occur. Therefore, the kidney's net albumin catabolism and its contribution to hypoalbuminemia in the nephrotic syndrome remains unclear.

Dietary Protein

High-protein diets fed to nephrotic rats and nephrotic humans increase the hepatic synthesis of albumin (125, 126). However, the filtered load and urinary excretion of albumin also increase, resulting in a decrease in the serum albumin concentration. Therefore, protein-supplemented diets increase albumin production but cannot replenish plasma or body stores of albumin due to increased urinary losses. Modest protein restriction in humans (0.8–1.0 g/kg/day) with the nephrotic syndrome decreased synthesis but also decreased its catabolism and urinary excretion. The net result was an increase in serum albumin concentration (126). Therefore, dietary protein should not be supplemented but mildly restricted in adults with nephrotic syndrome.

Edema

Periorbital and/or extremity edema is the clinical hallmark of an expanded extracellular fluid volume and is usually present in all patients with nephrotic syndrome sometime during the course of disease. Hypoalbuminemia certainly plays a role, as evidenced by the fact that edema usually occurs when serum albumin levels decrease below approximately 2.5 g/dl. However, sodium and water retention by the renal tubules is also essential to maintain the progressive extracellular volume expansion seen in nephrotic syndrome.

The mechanisms by which the above occurs remain controversial. The traditional view is that renal sodium retention is in response to intravascular volume depletion consequent to the hypoalbuminemia: the underfill hypothesis. Although this classic theory is logical, many studies have demonstrated normal circulatory volume in nephrotic patients (127–129) and variable or lack of the expected natriuresis with volume expansion (130,131). Therefore, the natural conclusion is that renal sodium retention is a primary event in volume expansion and edema formation in the nephrotic syndrome: the overflow hypothesis. In all likelihood, both mechanisms are operative in any given patient. Predominance of any one mechanism would largely depend on a multitude of unpredictable factors, such as sodium intake, effects of diuretic or steroid therapy, degree of renal insufficiency, underlying glomerular lesion, and presence of associated cardiac or hepatic disease.

A third pathophysiologic factor in the formation of edema in the nephrotic syndrome involves local factors at the level of the capillary bed that normally defend against edema. The decreased serum oncotic pressure of the nephrotic syndrome would be expected to favor the flux of fluid across the capillaries into the interstitial space. However, fluid tends not to accumulate in the interstitium because of several local buffering mechanisms: an increase in interstitial hydrostatic pressure, a decline in interstitial oncotic pressure, and an increase in lymphatic flow. The result is the movement of fluid back into the intravascular space, either directly or by lymphatic drainage. In the presence of unrelenting sodium and water retention, however, the capillary hydrostatic pressure increases, the above mechanisms are overwhelmed, and edema develops. The factors involved in edema formation in the nephrotic syndrome are illustrated in Figure 7.

Hyperlipidemia and Hyperlipoproteinemia

Although not necessary to make the diagnosis, hyperlipidemia often accompanies the nephrotic syndrome. The typical pattern of blood lipid, lipoprotein, and apolipoprotein (Apo) abnormalities seen in nephrotic syndrome are shown in Table 9. In general, serum cholesterol is usually elevated, whereas triglyceride levels are normal or slightly increased. Low-density lipoprotein (LDL) concentration is nearly always elevated and very low density lipoprotein (VLDL) levels are often increased as well (132–134). Serum high-density lipoprotein (HDL) concentrations are variable and have been reported to be high, low, or normal (132–135). This variability may arise from the unpredictable urinary excretion of HDL in nephrotic individuals (136), different levels of renal function affecting HDL levels, and differences in study design (137). Regardless of changes in total HDL, the LDL:HDL ratio is generally increased (134), subclass HDL_2 levels are decreased, and HDL_3 concentrations are increased (132,138), disturbances that have been associated with an increased risk of atherogenesis (139). Furthermore, lipoprotein (a) levels also may be elevated in proteinuric states, adding to the risk of atherosclerosis (140,141).

Apo abnormalities in the nephrotic syndrome are generally related to the changes of their parent lipoproteins. Thus, elevations in serum levels of Apo B, C, and E are consistent with increases in LDL and VLDL typically seen in nephrotic patients. Apo AI and AII (associated with HDL) are no different in nephrotic patients versus normal subjects (133,142). Although both are elevated, the ratio of CIII to CII is increased in nephrotic syndrome and may have the net effect of suppressing lipoprotein lipase activity, thus reducing lipoprotein catabolism that is seen in the nephrotic syndrome (143).

These abnormalities in plasma lipid, lipoprotein, and Apo concentrations result from a combination of an increased rate of synthesis, a decreased rate of catabolism, and a decreased negative feedback loop. Increased hepatic lipoprotein production may be stimulated by hypoalbuminemia itself, a decrease in plasma oncotic pressure, urinary loss of a substance that regulates lipid metabolism, increased hepatic delivery of the cholesterol precursor mevalonate, and/or faulty negative feedback on lipid synthesis, mediated by the defective hepatic uptake of IDL and LDL (137).

Altered lipoprotein catabolism in the nephrotic syndrome is similarly multifactorial in nature and appears to be primarily mediated by impaired lipoprotein lipase function and reduced lecithin: cholesterol acyltransferase activity, both key enzymes in lipoprotein catabolism

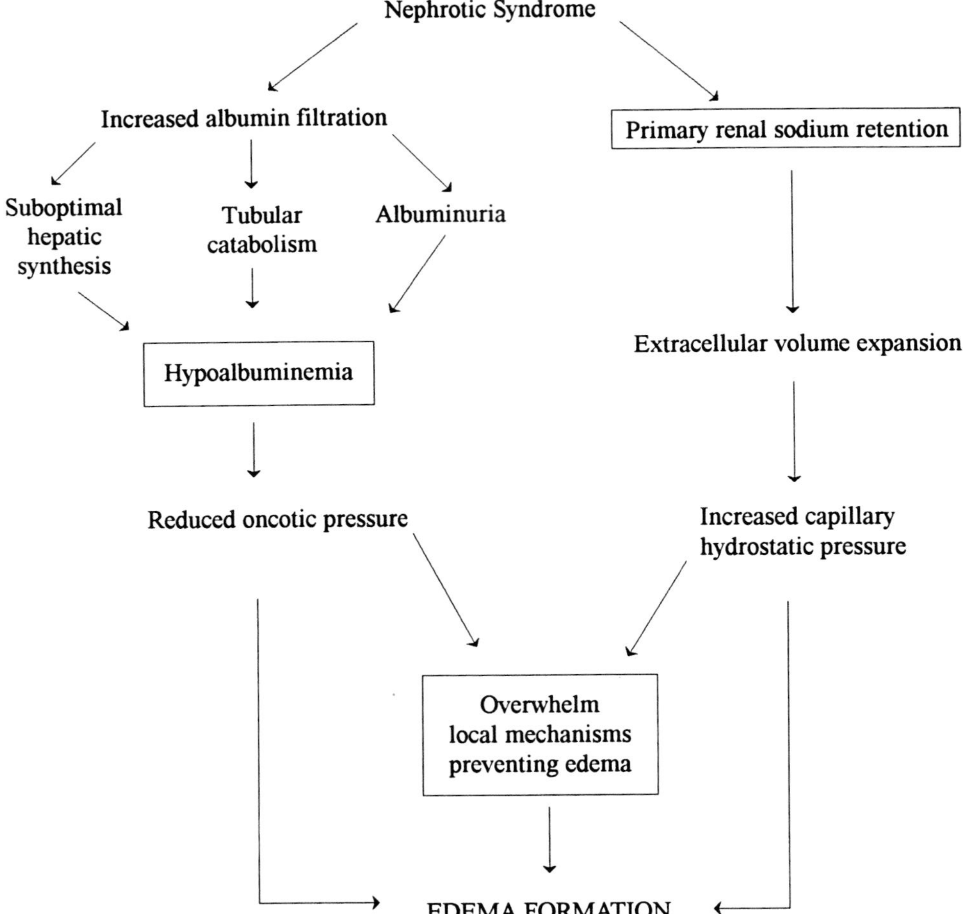

FIG. 7. *Pathophysiology of edema formation in the nephrotic syndrome.*

(137). Specific factors responsible for these defective catabolic pathways have yet to be fully elucidated.

So much attention has been given to lipid abnormalities in the nephrotic syndrome because of the potential for cardiovascular disease (139,144–146). Well-controlled prospective studies are nonexistent (due to inherent difficulties in design) and retrospective studies have shown inconsistent results (147–151). However, an autopsy study in 20 young nephrotic patients with age-matched controls (152) and a recent large retrospective evaluation (153) provide persuasive data supporting an increased incidence of coronary disease in the nephrotic syndrome. Further studies are needed, but with currently available evidence it seems reasonable to conclude that unrelenting nephrotic syndrome engenders a serious risk for atherosclerosis.

A second potential consequence of hyperlipidemia in nephrotic syndrome is progression of renal disease. There is only limited evidence in support of this, but factors potentially contributing to progressive renal injury include the deposition of lipoproteins in the glomerulus and interstitium, setting up a chronic inflammatory reaction with mononuclear cell infiltration and altered cytokine production and release. This causes mesangial and interstitial cell death and the proliferation of matrix, eventually leading to irreversible scarring (154,155). Studies are ongoing, but there is no evidence as of yet that treatment of hyperlipidemia in nephrotic syndrome decreases the risk of renal failure in humans.

Hypercoagulability

Thrombotic events are one of the most feared complications of the nephrotic syndrome. The overall incidence of vascular thrombosis in adults is about 30% to 35% and ranges from 2% to 62% (156). Deep venous thrombosis, renal vein thrombosis, and pulmonary embolism are the most frequent thromboembolic complications. Depending on the series, renal vein thrombosis may be present in as many as 60% of nephrotic adults, particularly those with heavy proteinuria secondary to membranous nephropathy. It usually has a silent or insidious presentation as opposed to the classic triad of acute flank pain, hema-

TABLE 9. *Lipids, lipoproteins, and apolipoproteins in nephrotic syndrome*

	Serum levels
Cholesterol	↑
Triglycerides	→,↑
VLDL	↑
IDL	↑
LDL	↑
HDL	↑,→,↓
LDL:HDL ratio	↑
Chylomicrons	↑
HDL_2	↓
HDL_3	↑
Lipoprotein (a)	↑
Apo AI	→
Apo AII	→
Apo B	↑
Apo CII, CIII	↑
CIII:CII ratio	↑
Apo E	↑

turia, and renal insufficiency (156,157). Although renal vein thrombosis is felt to have a high rate of embolization, there are usually little or no symptoms. This and the fact that 15% to 20% of asymptomatic adult patients with nephrotic syndrome had abnormal ventilation–perfusion scan results suggest that the true incidence of thromboembolism in the nephrotic syndrome may be even higher than reported (157,158). Even though most affected adults have venous events, arterial thrombosis, including coronary, pulmonary, and renal arteries, also has been reported (158,159).

Multiple abnormalities in coagulation factors and cofactors, the fibrinolytic system, and platelet function, as well as individual patient characteristics, can account for the hypercoagulability of the nephrotic syndrome (Table 10). However, inconsistent conflicting data and variable patient and disease characteristics prevent a unifying hypothesis for the predisposition toward thromboembolic events. For example, loss of antithrombin III in the urine of nephrotic individuals is often blamed for hypercoagulability, but alpha-2 macroglobulin increases so that plasma antithrombin activity is actually normal or even elevated (159).

Infection

Before the widespread use of antibiotics, infection was the leading cause of death in the nephrotic syndrome, particularly from encapsulated organisms. Mechanisms predisposing to infection in the nephrotic syndrome include abnormalities in both humoral and cell-mediated immunity, and in the complement system. Loss in the urine and increased catabolism and/or decreased synthesis account for low levels of IgG, IgA, and gamma globulins characteristically found in nephrotic syndrome (160,161). Complement levels themselves are not reduced, but the loss of opsonization factor B in the urine makes destruction of encapsulated bacteria difficult (162). A decrease in the number and function of circulating T cells accounts for the defects in cell-mediated immunity. Urinary losses of transferrin and zinc and the presence of hyperlipidemia play a role in these defects (163–167). Malnutrition, splits in skin integrity secondary to edema, steroids, and other immunosuppressant therapy can further compromise defective host defenses in nephrotic patients.

Endocrine Abnormalities

Calcium and Bone Metabolism

Vitamin D is an important modulator of calcium and bone metabolism in humans. Both 25-hydroxycholecalciferol [25(OH)D] and 1,25-dihydroxycholecalciferol [1,25$(OH)_2$D] circulate in plasma tightly bound (>99%) to vitamin D–binding protein (DBP). Given its molecular weight of approximately 59 kDa, DBP is readily filtered by nephrotic glomeruli, along with its attached 25(OH)D and 1,25$(OH)_2$D moieties. Indeed, ample evidence exists for their excretion in nephrotic urine, resulting in low total serum levels of DBP, 25(OH)D, and 1,25$(OH)_2$D (168–173), although some have found

TABLE 10. *Coagulability in the nephrotic syndrome*

Procoagulant	Anticoagulant
Coagulation factors and cofactors	
Increased factors VII, X	Decreased factors II, IX, XI, XII
Increased cofactors V and VIII	
Increased fibrinogen	
Coagulation inhibitors	
Decreased antithrombin III	Increased alpha-2 macroglobulin
Protein S deficiency,	
Platelet function	
Thrombocytosis	
Increased aggregation	
Increased beta-thromboglobulin	
Fibrinolytic system	
Decreased plasminogen	Decreased antiplasmins
Increased alpha-2 antiplasmin	Alpha-1 antitrypsin alpha-2 antitrypsin
Patient characteristics	
Severe hypoalbuminemia	Mild hypoalbuminemia
Intravascular volume depletion	Volume replete
Diuretics	Renal insufficiency causing platelet dysfunction
Steroids	
Associated adenocarcinoma	
Lupus anticoagulant	

normal levels of 1,25(OH)$_2$D (174). Because 1,25(OH)$_2$D functions to stimulate the gastrointestinal absorption of calcium, suppresses the synthesis of PTH, and helps maintain normal bone turnover, one would expect significant urinary losses to result in hypocalcemia, secondary hyperparathyroidism with eventual osteitis fibrosa cystica, and/or osteomalacia. However, only a minority of adult nephrotic patients demonstrate one or more of these findings.

One reason for the equivocal results may rest with the assay for 1,25(OH)$_2$D, the biologically active form of vitamin D. The standard method measures total 1,25(OH)$_2$D, which includes both the protein-bound and free portions. Because free 1,25(OH)$_2$D is the physiologically active portion, measuring total levels may invalidate any conclusions drawn regarding its effect on calcium homeostasis, PTH, and bone histomorphometry. In the only study to directly measure free 1,25(OH)$_2$D in nephrotic subjects, total 1,25(OH)$_2$D levels were decreased, but the free levels remained normal (175). Thus, 1,25 (OH)$_2$D activity may be maintained even though significant amounts of the protein-bound fraction are lost in the urine.

Therefore, the net effects of the nephrotic syndrome on calcium, vitamin D, PTH, and bone metabolism remain uncertain. Free 1,25 (OH)$_2$D levels, as well as the patient's age, duration and severity of disease, renal function, and steroid therapy, may all play a role. Further studies are needed to clarify these issues.

Other Hormone Abnormalities

In a manner similar to DBP, urinary losses of thyroxin-binding protein, corticosteroid-binding globulin, and sex hormone–binding protein suggest the possibility of hypothyroidism, hypoadrenalism, and hypogonadism in the nephrotic syndrome. However, these patients generally remain clinically euthyroid with normal adrenal and gonadal function, probably as a result of increased synthesis and/or an increased percentage of the physiologically active free hormone (176,177).

Renal Failure

Causes of renal failure in the nephrotic syndrome are listed in Table 11.

Acute Renal Failure

Although intravascular volume may be normal, nephrotic patients are prone to prerenal azotemia from diuretics, surgical procedures, and gastrointestinal losses such as vomiting or diarrhea, all sources of decreased renal perfusion (178,179). Nonsteroidal anti-inflammatory drugs causing afferent arteriole vasoconstriction are included in this category. Because nephrotic patients are more susceptible to infection with encapsulated organisms, acute tubular necrosis from sepsis or aminoglycoside therapy also needs to be considered in the differential diagnosis of acute renal failure, as does allergic interstitial nephritis from penicillin or cephalosporins. Vascular complications, such as bilateral renal vein thrombosis or unilateral renal vein thrombosis with compromised function of the contralateral kidney, are possible given the hypercoagulability of the nephrotic syndrome. Although rare, renal artery thrombosis also has been reported (159).

Acute reversible renal failure also may result from compression of tubules by renal interstitial edema (nephrosarca) in severe cases of nephrotic syndrome, which may respond to diuretic therapy (180). Furthermore, in the six patients in whom renal hemodynamics were measured, afferent vasoconstriction did not appear to play a role (180). Other reports indicate that renal interstitial edema is more likely to cause acute renal failure in older nephrotic patients with anasarca, hypertension, and/or arteriosclerosis (181,182). Although intriguing, nephrosarca as a definitive cause of acute renal failure in the nephrotic syndrome is difficult to prove, other than by exclusion.

Chronic Renal Failure

Proteinuria with resultant hyperfiltration has been linked to progressive glomerular damage and sclerosis (183) and therefore may play a role in the progression of renal failure in patients with persistent nephrotic syndrome. In addition, tubulointerstitial damage has been documented in humans with nephrotic syndrome (184), and evidence exists linking proteinuria to tubulointerstitial injury (185). More recently, hyperlipidemia has been implicated in the pathogenesis of glomerulosclerosis and tubulointerstitial fibrosis (186–188), although its role in

TABLE 11. *Causes of renal failure in nephrotic syndrome*

Acute renal failure
Prerenal azotemia (diuretics, general anesthesia, etc.)
Nonsteroidal anti-inflammatory drugs
Acute tubular necrosis (aminoglycosides, sepsis)
Renal vein thrombosis
Renal artery thrombosis (rare)
Nephrosarca
Chronic renal failure
Glomerulosclerosis from proteinuria/hyperfiltration
Tubulointerstitial damage/fibrosis
Hyperlipidemia
Glomerulosclerosis
Tubulointerstitial damage/fibrosis

the progression of renal disease in human nephrotic syndrome remains undetermined.

Miscellaneous Complications

Protein malnutrition is possible in nephrotic adults with massive loss of protein in the urine, poor oral intake, and a high catabolic rate. Hypoalbuminemia can lead to a decrease in protein binding and an increase in the free unbound fraction of highly protein-bound drugs, resulting in drug toxicity. Clofibrate and warfarin are examples that may require dose reduction and/or close monitoring in the nephrotic syndrome (189,190).

Once considered unusual, hypertension is being increasingly recognized as a complication of minimal-change disease and membranous nephropathy in adults. It seems to be associated with the edematous state but not with renal failure or steroid therapy. Kuster et al. reported that 78% of adults with minimal-change disease and 89% with membranous nephropathy had elevated blood pressures in the edematous phase before therapy, decreasing to 33% and 30%, respectively, with partial or complete remission (191). Altered sodium handling and loss of nitric oxide in the urine of nephrotic individuals are postulated etiologies (192), but the cause of hypertension in these patients remains speculative at this time.

Nonspecific Therapy of the Nephrotic Syndrome

Treatment of specific causes of the nephrotic syndrome is detailed in the following chapters under the specific disease state. Nonspecific therapy targets treating the complications of nephrotic syndrome and is outlined in Table 12.

TABLE 12. *Nonspecific therapy for the nephrotic syndrome*

Complication	Therapy
Edema	Bed rest; sodium and water restriction; support stockings
	Loop diuretics
	If resistance, sequential nephron blockade; add thiazide, metalazone and/or acetazolamide
	Salt-poor albumin (25%) plus furosemide in refractory cases
Hypoalbuminemia	Modest dietary protein restriction 0.8–1.2 g/kg/day (adults only)
	Angiotensin-converting enzyme inhibitor (ACEI)
	Consider nonsteroidal anti-inflamatory agents if renal function is normal
	Medical or surgical nephrectomy when renal function is poor and proteinuria is massive
Hyperlipidemia	Low-cholesterol, low-fat diet
	Regular exercise
	Weight loss if obese
	HMG CoA reductase inhibitors for unremittant cases
Hypercoagulability	Avoid volume depletion and immobility
	High clinical suspicion for thromboembolic events, low threshold for investigation
	Heparin 5,000 U subcutaneously twice daily when immobilized
	Systemic anticoagulation for event
Calcium and bone complications	1,25(OH)$_2$D therapy if hypocalcemia, GFR <50 cm^3/min, osteomalacia or hyperparathyroidism are present
Acute and chronic renal failure	Avoid over-diuresis, nephrotoxins if possible
	Reduction of proteinuria (diet, ACEI)
	Therapy of hyperlipidemia (see above)
Hypertension	Diuresis
	ACEI (drug of choice given effects on proteinuria)
	Calcium channel blocker
Drug toxicity from highly protein-bound drugs	Close clinical monitoring for signs of toxicity
	Drug levels (especially free drug levels), if available

RENAL BIOPSY

Since the 1950s, percutaneous renal biopsy has played an increasing role in the practice of nephrology. As a research tool, it has been instrumental in broadening our understanding of the pathogenesis of many renal diseases, especially with the advent of immunofluorescence and electron microscopy. In the clinical setting, it has proven invaluable in the diagnosis of disease, prognosticating long-term renal survival and guiding therapy. The following summarizes the current indications, contraindications, technique and complications of percutaneous renal biopsy.

Indications

In general, a percutaneous renal biopsy is warranted to obtain a diagnosis, to provide prognostic information, and/or to guide therapy. However, there are varying opinions among nephrologists as to the exact indications for biopsy in specific clinical situations. Few investigators would argue the value of biopsy to identify a renal lesion for which there is accepted beneficial therapy, such as rapidly progressive glomerulonephritis. Circumstances under which renal biopsy and its timing may be based more on individual preference include the assessment of renal failure, isolated hematuria or proteinuria, or even the nephrotic syndrome. Table 13 shows the clinical situations for which percutaneous renal biopsy can assist in the management of kidney disease in adults.

Acute Renal Failure

When the cause of acute renal failure is not evident from the clinical, laboratory, and radiologic evaluation,

TABLE 13. *Indications for renal biopsy in adults*

Acute renal failure
  Unknown cause or atypical for acute tubular necrosis
  Rapidly progressive glomerulonephritis
Chronic renal failure
  Acute on chronic renal failure
  Consider biopsy if cause of renal failure is unknown and patient is a transplant candidate
Microscopic hematuria
  With evidence of glomerular disease
  Consider in isolated hematuria lasting longer than 6 mo where anatomic studies are negative
Non-nephrotic proteinuria
  Greater than 2 g/day and cause is unknown
  Associated with hypertension and progressive renal dysfunction
Nephrotic syndrome
  Nearly all adults
Systemic disease
  Atypical diabetes mellitus
  Systemic lupus erythematosus with renal involvement
  In others to diagnose disease (vasculitis, amyloid, cryoglobulinemia, etc.)
Pregnancy
  Unexplained acute renal failure
  Unexplained severe nephrotic syndrome, if therapy will be affected
Transplant kidney
  Rule out rejection, recurrent or de novo disease, drug-induced disease

a percutaneous renal biopsy can be helpful in the diagnosis. Unsuspected acute tubular necrosis is a common finding, but crescentic glomerulonephritis, vasculitis, or interstitial nephritis also may be found. In addition, renal biopsy is crucial early in the course of rapidly progressive glomerulonephritis to differentiate pauci-immune, immune complex, and antiglomerular basement membrane types and therefore determine optimal therapy.

Chronic Renal Failure

A widely accepted pretense is that patients with small contracted kidneys (<9 cm) are unlikely to harbor reversible disease, and renal biopsy only puts them at risk for complications. Although the risk is increased, the benefits derived may justify biopsy in certain patients. A series of 120 percutaneous biopsies in undiagnosed chronic parenchymal renal diseases identified ten cases of potentially treatable disease (193). Of particular importance were three patients with primary oxalosis, a diagnosis that would potentially prohibit transplantation or certainly change pretransplant management. Several other biopsy series also identified renal histopathology that changed management or therapy in a substantial number of patients with advanced renal failure, even obviating the need for dialysis and altering transplantation plans in some (194–196). Thus, it is our practice to consider renal biopsy in patients with undiagnosed progressive renal failure, particularly those who are transplant candidates.

Microscopic Hematuria

As discussed in the hematuria section, evidence of glomerular disease makes renal biopsy an integral part of the evaluation. Biopsy also should be considered in cases of persistent isolated hematuria with a negative anatomic workup to rule out treatable forms of glomerulonephritis.

Non-Nephrotic Proteinuria

If protein excretion exceeds 2 g/day, then a glomerular etiology is likely and biopsy is indicated. Regardless of the magnitude of the proteinuria, the development of hypertension and renal dysfunction suggests the need for biopsy given the progressive nature of the disease.

Nephrotic Syndrome

Practically all adults with nephrotic syndrome should undergo biopsy for diagnostic, prognostic, and therapeutic reasons, unless the withdrawal of a drug or treatment of an obvious disease results in resolution of the proteinuria.

Systemic Disease

The role of renal biopsy in an undiagnosed systemic disease involving the kidney is clear. Knowledge of the histopathology is essential in lupus erythematosus to classify the nephritis and identify those patients who would benefit from cyclophosphamide therapy. Diabetics, particularly type I, who develop nephrotic proteinuria early in the course of the disease in the absence of retinopathy or neuropathy may have another glomerulopathy besides diabetic nephropathy. Reports of minimal-change disease, membranous glomerulonephritis, and other diseases responsive to therapy in both type I and type II diabetic patients (197–200) make biopsy a reasonable approach under these circumstances.

Pregnancy

Although it can be done safely, percutaneous renal biopsy during pregnancy is rarely indicated unless unexplained acute renal failure and/or severe nephrotic syndrome develops that would significantly alter management. Women with mild to moderate proteinuria and preserved renal function can be followed closely throughout pregnancy and may undergo biopsy several weeks postpartum if necessary.

Transplant Kidney

Percutaneous allograft biopsy is pivotal in diagnosing and characterizing the type and severity of rejection, diagnosing recurrent or de novo glomerulopathy in transplant recipients with proteinuria, and assessing drug-induced disease such cyclosporine toxicity.

Contraindications

Table 14 summarizes the absolute and relative contraindications to percutaneous renal biopsy.

Absolute Contraindications

All nephrologists would avoid performing a renal biopsy until prothrombin time, partial thromboplastin time, and platelet counts are normal. Less clear is the risk of a prolonged bleeding time. Although no study has linked an increased risk of bleeding after biopsy with a prolonged prebiopsy forearm skin bleeding time, our practice is to normalize bleeding time before renal biopsy by withdrawal of an inciting agent (nonsteroidal anti-inflammatory agents or aspirin) or by administration of the vasopressin analog DDAVP.

Because the risk for complications after biopsy is related to the degree of blood pressure elevation (201), control of systolic and diastolic pressures prebiopsy is essential. Although the absolute limits are not well established, we prefer to keep blood pressure persistently less than 160/95 mm Hg if possible. Finally, an uncooperative patient introduces inordinate risks and excludes renal biopsy as a diagnosic option.

TABLE 14. *Contraindications to percutaneous renal biopsy*

Absolute
Bleeding diathesis
Systolic BP > 160 mm Hg
Diastolic BP > 95 mm Hg
Uncooperative patient
Relative
Single functioning kidney
Kidneys <9 cm
Renal infection (pyelonephritis, abscess)
Renal mass or cysts
Hydronephrosis
Massive obesity

Relative Contraindications

Percutaneous biopsy of a single functioning kidney carries an inherent risk of losing the only source of renal function should a serious complication occur. The risk of nephrectomy after percutaneous renal biopsy, approximately one in 2,000, is comparable with the risk of death with general anesthesia in an American Society of Anesthesiology (ASA) status class 2 patient (202). From this aspect, choosing percutaneous biopsy of a solitary kidney in a patient with an ASA class 2 or higher risk for general anesthesia would seem to be a prudent approach. Therefore, we classify a solitary kidney as a relative and not an absolute contraindication to closed renal biopsy.

Perhaps an optimal approach in patients with a single functioning kidney would be a modified open procedure that uses local anesthesia and a small incision. This would also be true for patients at a higher risk of bleeding, such as uremic patients, patients with small kidneys, or those patients who have a coagulopathy.

Another relative contraindication to a percutaneous procedure is biopsy of a renal mass whose vascularity is in doubt or undocumented. These are best managed with a total or partial nephrectomy as indicated. Pyelonephritis, renal abscess, urinary tract infections, and hydronephrosis also preclude percutaneous biopsy unless absolutely necessary.

Technique

Preparation

The prebiopsy evaluation should exclude contraindications discussed previously, and the patient counseled regarding the risks and benefits of the procedure. We prefer to perform percutaneous biopsies in the morning if possible so that any major bleeding complications can be recognized and treated with a full compliment of support personnel during normal working hours. A sedative is given intramuscularly 30 to 60 min before the procedure, and an intravenous catheter is placed in the event that intravenous medications or fluids are needed. The patient is placed in the prone position with a rolled up towel or sheets positioned under the abdomen to fix the kidneys to the posterior abdominal musculature, preventing the kidneys from being pushed away by the biopsy needle.

Localization

The accuracy, efficiency, and manuverability of present-day renal US makes it the mode of choice to localize the lower pole of the kidney. Other advantages of US include its ability to relocalize in the event of an unsuccessful biopsy attempt, the immediate identification of perinephric hematoma formation postbiopsy, and the capability to perform real-time biopsies with continuous monitoring of the needle as it is passed into the kidney.

Biopsy Needles

The Franklin modification of the Vim-Silverman needle and the disposable Tru-Cut needle (Baxter Healthcare, McGraw Park, IL) are manually operated needles available for percutaneous renal biopsy. We prefer the automated spring-loaded devices available in reusable or disposable form because of their ease of use and minimal time the needle is actually within the kidney.

Biopsy Technique

Both kidneys are imaged and the skin marked over the lower pole of the kidney most accessible to biopsy during normal patient respiration. The perpendicular distance from the skin to the lower pole is measured to help approximate the depth of the needle placement. After anesthetizing the skin, a 21- or 22-gauge spinal needle is advanced with the patient holding their breath at end-expiration. A pop through the capsule of the kidney and/or an increase in resistance indicates the needle is in place. Adequate excursion of the spinal needle with respiration and evident arterial pulsations also indicate the appropriate needle placement. The tract is anesthetized as the spinal needle cannula is withdrawn, and the distance to the kidney is noted. After a small stab incision is made in the skin, the biopsy needle is advanced in an identical fashion to the depth of the kidney. The trigger mechanism is then fired and the needle withdrawn, all while the patient holds his or her breath on normal expiration. We routinely visualize the core with a dissecting microscope to ascertain the adequacy of tissue. If a core biopsy of renal tissue is not obtained, a sterile sleeve can be placed over the US transducer, and the biopsy is repeated with constant monitoring of the needle as it approaches and enters the kidney. This real-time method is also helpful when the kidney cannot be located with the finder needle (it may be deep, or the lower pole may be angled away from the approach of the needle), or it can be used as the initial method of biopsy.

End-inspiration (either normal or deep) also can be used for localization with the finder needle if the kidney does not descend below the 12th rib on normal respiration. However, sudden expulsion of air after deep inspiration carries a risk of laceration if the needle lodges against the 12th rib as the kidney moves cephalad during forced expiration. For this reason we prefer end expiration for needle placement, if possible.

Postbiopsy

The kidney examined via biopsy is revisualized via US to assess for developing hematoma. The patient then rests in the supine position for at least 4 to 6 h with appropriate monitoring of vital signs, urine color, urine output, and hematocrit. If performed on an outpatient basis, the patient is followed closely for 4 to 6 h, then discharged home if all parameters remain stable. This is the preferred method in our practice. Otherwise, the patient can be admitted overnight for monitoring.

Other Methods of Renal Biopsy

Transjugular renal biopsy uses a transvenous route to the kidney as opposed to the percutaneous route. This method may be useful in patients with unacceptably high risks for general anesthesia associated with standard open biopsies, such as morbid obesity, severe coronary artery disease, or chronic obstructive pulmonary disease. Mal et al. performed 200 transjugular renal biopsies with an 86% success rate (operator dependent) and a complication rate no higher than that for the percutaneous approach (203).

An open renal biopsy may become necessary if the percutaneous approach carries too many risks. The standard method of open biopsy requires general anesthesia and several days' recuperation in the hospital. Modified, limited open procedures using local anesthesia and a smaller incision make the surgical approach a more attractive option by avoiding the morbidity and mortality of general anesthesia. In a series of 123 patients, Chodak et al. had a 100% yield and a 5% complication rate (no deaths) with their modified approach to open renal biopsy (204).

Complications

Table 15 summarizes the complications of percutaneous renal biopsy. The overall incidence of obtaining adequate renal tissue for pathologic examination using US guidance has been reported to be 90% to 95% (202). Bleeding is the major complication of biopsy, but microscopic and gross hematuria as well as subcapsular bleeding is usually self limited and asymptomatic. Transfusions are required in 0.1% to 3.0% of patients, and surgical or angiographic intervention is necessary in less than 0.2% of percutaneous biopsies (201,205). Arteriovenous fistulas are relatively common if sought but rarely require intervention (206). Significant infections after renal biopsy are rare, except in the presence of pyelonephritis, where bacteremia can develop (207). The risk for nephrectomy after a percutaneous renal biopsy is approximately 0.02% to 0.06% (1/1,600 to 1/5,000] (202–208). The risk of death stems primarily from direct complications of severe bleeding and ranges from less than 0.1% to 0.2% of percutaneous biopsies (205,209).

TABLE 15. *Complications of renal biopsy*

Complication	Incidence (%)
Inadequate tissue	5–10
Bleeding	
Microscopic hematuria	100
Gross hematuria	5–9
Perinephric hematoma	90
Symptomatic	<20
Transfusion required	<3
Surgical/radiologic intervention	<0.2
Adjacent organ trauma	1
Infection	<1
Arteriovenous fistula	15–18
Requiring intervention	1
Nephrectomy	0.02–0.06
Death	<0.1–0.2

Acknowledgment

This work was supported in part by National Institutes of Health Grant DK44107 from the National Institute of Digestive, Diabetic and Kidney Diseases. We thank Terry Herring, Heather Crissman, Peggy Nees and Gail Maffett for their assistance in preparing the manuscript.

REFERENCES

1. Wright WT. Cell counts in urine. *Arch Intern Med* 1959;103:76–78.
2. Woolhandler S, Pels RJ, Bor DH, Himmelstein DU, Lawrence RS. Dipstick urinalysis screening of asymptomatic adults for urinary tract disorders. *JAMA* 1989;262:1215–1219.
3. Addis T. The number of formed elements in the urinary sediment of normal individuals. *J Clin Invest* 1926;2:409–415.
4. Gadeholt H. Quantitative estimation of cells in urine. *Acta Med Scand* 1968;183:369–374.
5. Kesson AM, Talbott JM, Gyory AZ. Microscopic examination of urine. *Lancet* 1978;2:809–812.
6. Gyory AZ, Kesson AM, Talbott JM. Microscopy of urine—now you see it, now you don't. *Am Heart J* 1980;99:537–538.
7. Larcom RC, Carter GH. Erythrocytes in urinary sediment: identification and normal limits. *J Lab Clin Med* 1948;33:875–880.
8. Sanders C. Clinical urine examination and the incidence of microscopic hematuria in apparently normal males. *Practitioner* 1963;191: 192–198.
9. Alwall N, Lohi A. A population study on renal and urinary tract diseases. *Acta Med Scand* 1973;194:529–535.
10. Froom P, Gross M, Froom J, Margaliot S, Benbassat J. The effect of age on the prevalence of asymptomatic hematuria. *Am J Clin Pathol* 1986;86:656–657.
11. Froom P, Gross M, Froom J, Margaliot S, Benbassat J. Sensitivity of the high-power field method in detecting red blood cells in the urinary sediment. *Isr J Med Sci* 1987;23:1118–1120.
12. Boyd PJR. Hematuria. *Br Med J* 1977;2:445–446.
13. Arm JP, Peile EB, Rainford DJ, Strike PW, Tettmor RE. Significance of dipstick hematuria: part 1. *Br Med J* 1986;58:211–217.
14. Messing EM, Young TB, Hunt VB, Emoto SE, Wehbie JM. The significance of asymptomatic microhematuria in men 50 or more years old: findings of a home screening study using urinary dipsticks. *J Urol* 1987;137:919–922.
15. Baran RB, Rowles E. Factors affecting coloration of urine and feces. *J Am Pharm Assoc* 1979;13:139–142.
16. Vaughn ED, Wyker AW. Effect of osmolality on the evaluation of microscopic hematuria. *J Urol* 1971;105:709–713.
17. Jacobellis U, Fabiano A, Tallarigo C. New technique to localize the origin of idiopathic microscopic hematuria. *J Urol* 1982;127: 475–476.
18. Desgrandchamps F, Piergiovanni M, Cussenot O, et al. Exploration and endoscopic treatment of unilateral primary haematuria: is non-specific diffuse pyelitis a real entity? *Eur Urol* 1994;26:109–114.
19. Andersen JR, Kristensen JK. Ureteroscopic management of transitional cell tumors. *Scand J Urol Nephrol* 1994;28:153–157.
20. Duncan KA, Cuppage FE, Grantham JJ. Urinary lipid bodies in polycystic kidney disease. *Am J Kid Dis* 1985;5:49–53.
21. Fairley KF, Birch DF. Microscopic urinalysis in glomerulonephritis. *Kidney Int* 1993;44:509–512.
22. Birch DF, Fairly KF. Hematuria: glomerular or non-glomerular? *Lancet* 1979;2:845–846.
23. Kitamoto Y, Yide C, Tomita M, Sato T. The mechanism of glomerular dysmorphic red cell formation in the kidney. *Tohoku J Exp Med* 1992;167:93–105.
24. Fassett RG, Horgan BA, Mathew TH. Detection of glomerular bleeding by phase contrast microscopy. *Lancet* 1982;1:1432–1434.
25. Roman GV, Peod L, Lee HA, Maskell R. A blind controlled trial of phase microscopy by 2 observers for evaluating the source of hematuria. *Nephron* 1986;44:304–308.
26. Mohammed KS, Bdesha AS, Snell ME, Witherow RO, Coleman DV. Phase contrast microscopic examination of urinary erythrocytes to localize source of bleeding: an overlooked technique? *J Clin Pathol* 1993;46:642–645.
27. Sayer J, McCarthy MP, Schmidt JD. Identification and significance of dysmorphic versus isomorphic hematuria. *J Urol* 1990;143:545–548.
28. Shichiri M, Hosoda k, Nishio Y, et al. Red cell volume distribution curves in the diagnosis of glomerular and non-glomerular hematuria. *Lancet* 1988;1:908–911.
29. Docci D, Delvecchio C, Turci F, Turci A, Baldrati L, Martinelli A. Detection of glomerular bleeding by urinary red cell size distribution. *Nephron* 1988;50:380–382.
30. DeCaestecker MP, Hall CL, Basterfield PT, Smith JG. Localization of hematuria by red cell analyzers and phase microscopy. *Nephron* 1989;52:170–173.
31. Fasset RG, Horgan B, Gove D, Matthew TH. Scanning electron microscopy of glomerular and non-glomerular red blood cells. *Clin Nephrol* 1983;20:11–16.
32. Tanaka M, Kitamoto Y, Sato T, Ishii T. Flow cytometric analysis of hematuria using flourescent antihemoglobin antibody. *Nephron* 1993; 65:354–358.
33. Voghenzi A, Soriani S, Antonio W, Camerini G. Osmotic resistance of urinary red cells in glomerular and nonglomerular haematuria. *Exp Nephrol* 1993;1:196–197.
34. Tomita M, Kitamoto Y, Nakayama M, Sato T. A new morphological classification of urinary erythrocytes for differential diagnosis of glomerular hematuria. *Clin Nephrol* 1992;37:84–89.
35. Verwiebe R, Weber MH, Kallerhoff M, Ruschitzka F, Warneke G, Scheler F. Differentation between renal and postrenal type of hematuria and proteinuria measuring urinary apolipoprotein A1 excretion. *Contrib Nephrol* 1993;101:151–157.
36. DiPaolo N, Garosi G, Capotondo L, diPaolo M. A new method of evaluating urinary erythrocyte dysmorphisms in glomerulonephritis. *Clin Nephrol* 1993;39:50–52.
37. Janssens PM, Kormaat N, Tieleman R, Monnens LA, Willems JL. Localizing the site of hematuria by immunocytochemical staining of erythrocytes in urine. *Clin Chem* 1992;38:216–222.
38. Kitamoto Y, Tomita M, Akamine M, Inoue T, Itoh J, Takamori H, Sato T. Differentiation of hematuria using a uniquely shaped red cell. *Nephron* 1993;64:32–36.
39. Howard AD, Moore J, Gouge SF, et al. Routine serologic tests in the differential diagnosis of the adult nphrotic syndrome. *Am J Kidney Dis* 1990;15:24–30.
40. Bard RH. The significance of asymptomatic microhematuria in women and its economic implications. *Arch Intern Med* 1988;148:2629–2632.
41. Yoshimura H. Anemia during physical training (sports anemia). *Nutr Rev* 1970;28:251–253.
42. Knochel JP, Carter NW. The role of muscle cell injury in the pathogenesis of acute renal failure after exercise. *Kidney Int* 1976;10:58–64.
43. Blacklock NJ. Bladder trauma in the long-distance runner: "10,000 metres haematuria." *Br J Urol* 1977;49:129–132.
44. Abarbenel J, Benet A, Lask D, Kimche D. Sports hematuria. *J Urol* 1990;143:887–890.

45. Alyea EP, Parish HH, Durham NC. Renal response to exercise: urinary findings. *JAMA* 1958;167:807–813.
46. Cianflocco AJ. Renal complications of exercise. *Clin Sports Med* 1992;11:437–451.
47. ACCP-NHLBI National Conference on Antithrombotic Therapy. American College of Chest Physicians and the National Heart, Lung, Blood Institute. *Chest* 1986;89(2 Suppl):1015–1065.
48. Culclasure TF, Brag VJ, Hasbargen JA. The significancy of hematuria in the anticoagulated patient. *Arch Intern Med* 1994;154:649–652.
49. Stapelton FB. Idiopathic hypercalciuria: association with isolated hematuria and risk for urolithiasis in children. *Kidney Int* 1990;37: 807–811.
50. Andres A, Praga M, Bello I, Rolon JAD, Millet VG, Morales JM, Rodicio JL. Hematuria due to hypercalceuria and hyperuricosuria in adult patients. *Kidney Int* 1989;36:96–99.
51. Levy FL, Kemp D, Breyer JA. Macroscopic hematuria secondary to hypercalciuria and hyperuricosuria. *Am J Kid Dis* 1994;24:515–518.
52. Mohr DN, Offord KP, Owen RA, Melton LJ. Asymptomatic microhematuria and urologic disease. *JAMA* 1986;256:224–229.
53. Messing EM, Vaillancourt MA. Hematuria screening for bladder cancer. *J Occup Med* 1990;32:838–845.
54. Carson CC, Segura JW, Greene LF. Clinical importance of microhematuria. *JAMA* 1979;241:149–150.
55. Thompson IM. The evaluation of microscopic hematuria: a population-based study. *J Urol* 1987;138:1189–1190.
56. Mariani AJ, Mariani MC, Machionni C, Stams UK, Hariharan A, Moriera A. The significance of adult hematuria: 1,000 hematuria evaluations including a risk-benefit and cost-effectiveness analysis. *J Urol* 1989;141:350–355.
57. Sutton JM. Evaluation of hematuria in adults. *JAMA* 1900;263: 2475–2480.
58. Murikami S, Igarashi T, Hara S, Shimazaki J. Strategies for asymptomatic microscopic hematuria: a prospective study of 1,034 patients. *J Urol* 1990;144:99–101.
59. Warshauer DM, McCarthy SM, Street L, et al. Detection of renal masses: sensitivities and specifications of excretory urography/linear tomography, US and CT. *Radiology* 1988;169:363–365.
60. Barbario ZL. *Principles of genitourinary radiology.* 2nd ed. New York: Thieme Medical; 1994:165–169.
61. Palko A, Kuhn E, Grexa E, Hertelendy A. Renal cell carcinoma: value of imaging examinations in diagnosis and staging. *Rofo Fortschr Geb Rontgenstr Neyen Bildgeb Verfahr* 1990;153:585–590.
62. Craven WM, Redmond PL, Kumpe DA, Durham JD, Wettlaufer JN. Planned delayed nephrectomy after ethanol embolization of renal carcinoma. *J Urol* 1991;146:704–708.
63. Zimmer WD, Williamson B, Hartman GW, Hattery RR, O'Brien PC. Changing patterns in the evaluation of renal masses. *Am J Roentgenol* 1984;143:285–289.
64. Williams PS, Fass G, Bone JM. Renal pathology and proteinuria determine progression in untreated mild/moderate chronic renal failure. *Q J Med* 1988;252:343–354.
65. Stenvinkel P, Alvestrand A, Bergstrom J. Factors influencing progression in patients with chronic renal failure. *J Intern Med* 1989;226: 183–188.
66. Walser M. Progression of chronic renal failure in man. *Kidney Int* 1990;37:1195–1210.
67. Walser M. Weighted least squares regression analysis of factors contributing to progression of chronic renal failure. *Contrib Nephrol* 1989;75:127–133.
68. Cameron JS. Proteinuria and progression in human glomerular diseases. *Am J Nephrol* 1990;10(suppl 1):81–87.
69. D'Amico G. The clinical role of proteinuria. *Am J Kidney Dis* 1991; 17(suppl 1):48–52.
70. Wight JP, Salzano S, Brown CB, el Nahas AM. Natural history of chronic renal failure: a reappraisal. *Nephrol Dial Transplant* 1992;7: 379–383.
71. Abuelo JG. Proteinuria: diagnostic principles and procedures. *Ann Intern Med* 1983;98:186–191.
72. King SE, Gronbeck C. Benign and pathological albuminuria: a study of 600 hospitalized cases. *Ann Intern Med* 1952;36:765–785.
73. Reuben DB, Watchel TJ, Brown PC, Driscoll JL. Transient proteinuria in emergency medical admissions. *N Engl J Med* 1982;306:1031–1033.
74. Portmans JR, Brauman H, Staroukine M, Verniory A, Deckaestecker C, Leclercq R. Indirect evidence of glomerular/tubular mixed-type postexercise proteinuria in healthy humans. *Am J Physiol* 1988;254: F277–F283.
75. Robertshaw M, Chueng CK, Fairly I, Swaminathan R. Protein excretion after prolonged exercise. *Ann Clin Biochem* 1993;30:34–37.
76. Wagner MD, Smith FG, Tinglof BO, Cornberg E. Epidemiology of proteinuria: a study of 4807 school children. *J Pediatr* 1968;73: 825–832.
77. Wolman IJ. The incidence, causes and intermittency of proteinuria in young men. *Am J Med Sci* 1945;210:86–100.
78. Von Bonsdorff M, Koskenvuo K, Salmi HA, Pasternack A. Prevalence and causes of proteinuria in 20-year-old Finnish men. *Scand J Urol Nephrol* 1981;15:285–290.
79. Randolph MF, Greenfield M. Proteinuria: a six-year study of normal infants, preschool and school-age populations previously screened for urinary tract diseases. *Am J Dis Child* 1967;114:631–638.
80. Larsen SO, Thysell H. Four years' follow up of asymtomatic isolated proteinuria diagnosed in a general health survey. *Acta Med Scand* 1969;186:375–381.
81. Muth RG. Asymptomatic and mild intermittent proteinuria: a percutaneous renal biopsy study. *Arch Intern Med* 1965;115:569–574.
82. Levitt JI. The prognostic significance of proteinuria in young college students. *Ann Intern Med* 1967;66:685–696.
83. Robinson RR, Glenn WG. Fixed and reproducile proteinuria IV, urinary albumin excretion by healthy human subjects in the recumbent and upright postures. *J Lab Clin Med* 1964;64:717–723.
84. Van Acker BA, Stroomer MK, Goose link MA, Koomen GC, Koopman MG, Arisz L. Urinary protein excretion in normal individuals: diurnal changes influence of orthostasis and relationship to the renin–angiotensin system. *Contrib Nephrol* 1993;101:143–150.
85. Devarajan P. Mechanisms of orthostatic proteinuria: lessons from a transplant doctor. *J Am Soc Nephrol* 1993;4:36–39.
86. Cruz HM, Cruz J, Castro MC, Marcondes M. Effect of posture and physical activity on urinary protein excretion by patients with glomerular proteinuria. *Braz J Med Res* 1989;22:1191–1194.
87. Norman ME. An office approach to hematuria and proteinuria. *Pediatr Clin North Am* 1987;34:545–560.
88. Rytand DA, Spreiter S. Prognosis in postural proteinuria. *N Engl J Med* 1981;305:618–621.
89. Glassock RJ. Postural (orthostatic) proteinuria; no cause for concern. *N Engl J Med* 1981;305:639
90. Springberg PD, Garnett LE, Thompson AL, Collins NF, Lordon RE, Robinson RR. Fixed and reproducible proteinuria: results of a 20-year follow-up study. *Ann Intern Med* 1982;97:516–519.
91. Vehaskari N. Mechanism of orthostatic proteinuria. *Pediatr Nephrol* 1990;4:328–330.
92. Shintaku N, Takahasi Y, Akaishi K, Sano A, Kuroda Y. Entrapment of left renal vein in children with orthostatis proteinuria. *Ped Nephrol* 1990;4:324–327.
93. Burns JS, McDonald B, Gaudio KM, Siegel JN. Progression of orthostatic proteinuria to focal and segmental glomerulosclerosis. *Clin Pediatr* 1986;25:165–166.
94. Pruzanski W, Platts ME. Serum and urinary proteins, lysozyme (muramidase), and renal dysfunction in mono- and myelomonocytic leukemia. *J Clin Invest* 1970;49:1694–1708.
95. Phillippi PJ, Reynolds J, Yamauchi H, Beering SC. Persistent proteinuria in asymptomatic individuals: renal biopsy study on 50 patients. *Milit Med* 1966;131:1311–1317.
96. Pollack VE, Pirani CL, Muehreke RC, Kark RM. Asymptomatic persistent proteinuria: studies by renal biopsies. *Guys Hosp Rep* 1958; 353–372.
97. Sinniah R, Law CH, Pwee HS. Glomerular lesions in patients with asymptomatic persistent and orthostatic proteinuria discovered on routine medical examination. *Clin Nephrol* 1977;7:1–14.
98. Phillippi PJ, Robinson RR, Langlier PR. Percutaneous renal biopsy. *Arch Intern Med* 1961;108:739–750.
99. King SE. Diastolic hypertension and chronic protenuria. *Am J Cardiol* 1962;9:669–674.
100. King SE. Albuminuria in renal diseases: II. Preliminary observations on the clinical course of patients with orthostatic proteinuria. *NY State J Med* 1969;59:825–835.
101. American Diabetes Association, National Kidney Foundation. Consensus development conference on the diagonosis and management of nephrology in patients with diabetes mellitus. *Diabetes Care* 1994; 17:1357–1361.

102. Viberti GC. Early functional and morphological changes in diabetic nephropathy. *Clin Nephrol* 1979;12:47–53.
103. Mogensen CE. Microalbuminuria predicts clinical proteinuria and early mortality in maturity-onset diabetics. *N Engl J Med* 1984;310: 356–360.
104. Neil A, Hawkins M, Potok M, Thorogood M, Cohen D, Mann J. A prospective population-based study of microalbuminuria as a predictor of mortality in NIDDM. *Diabetes* 1993;16:996–1003.
105. Mattock MD, Morrish JM, Viberti V, Keen H, Fitzgerald AP, Jackson G. Prospective study of microalbuminuria as predictor of mortality in NIDDM. *Diabetes* 1992;41:736–741.
106. Shihabi ZK, Konen JC, O'Conner ML. Albuminuria vs. total urinary protein for detecting chronic renal disease. *Clin Chem* 1991;37: 621–624.
107. Bowie L, Smith S, Gochman N. Characteristics of binding between reagen strip indicators and urinary proteins. *Clin Chem* 1977;23: 128–130.
108. McCracken BH. Estimations of quantitative proteinuria. *N Engl J Med* 1984;310:1464
109. Tapp DC, Copley JB. Effect of red blood cell lysis on protein quantitation in hematuric states. *Am J Nephrol* 1988;8:190–193.
110. Ginsberg JM, Chang BS, Matarese RA, Garella S. Use of single voided urine samples to estimate quantitative proteinuria. *N Engl J Med* 1983;309:1543–1546.
111. Shaw AB, Risdon P, Lewis-Jackson JD. Protein-creatinine index and albustix in assessment of proteinuria. *Br Med J* 1983;287:929–932.
112. Tiu SC, Lee SS, Chen MW. Comparison of six commercial techniques in the measurement of microalbuminuria in diabetic patients. *Diabetes Care* 1993;16:616–620.
113. Kerjaschki D, Schulze M, Binder S, et al. Transcellular transport and membrane insertion of the C5b-9 membrane attack complex of complement by glomerular epithelial cells in experimental membranous nephropathy. *J Immunol* 1989;143:546–552.
114. Pruchno CJ, Burns MM, Schulze M, et al. Urinary excretion of the C5b-9 membrane attack complex of complement is a marker of immune disease activity in autologous immune disease nephritis. *Am J Pathol* 1991;138:203–211.
115. Schulze M, Donadio JV, Pruchno CJ, et al. Elevated urinary excretion of the C5b-9 complex in membranous nephropathy. *Kidney Int* 1991; 40:533–538.
116. Brenchley PE, Coupes B, Short CD, O'Donoghue DJ, Ballardie FW, Mallick NP. Urinary C3dg and C5b-9 indicate active immune disease in human membranous nephropathy. *Kidney Int* 1992;41:933–937.
117. Tsai CY, Wu TH, Sun KH, Lin WM, Yu CL. Increased excretion of soluble interleukin 2 receptors and free light chain immunoglobulins in the urine of patients with active lupus nephritis. *Ann Rheum Dis* 1992;51:168–172.
118. Suranyi MG, Guasch A, Hall B., Myers BD. Elevated levels of tumor necrosis factor-alpha in the nephrotic syndrome in humans. *Am J Kidney Dis* 1993;21:251–259.
119. Jensen H, Rossing N, Anderson SB. Albumin metabolism in the nephrotic syndrome in adults. *Clin Sci* 1967;33:445–457.
120. Kaysen GA, Martinez CA. The metabolism of serum proteins in nephrosis. *Am Kidney Found Nephrol Letter* 1988;5:31–46.
121. Hardwicke J, Squire JR. The relationship between plasma albumin concentration and protein excretion in patients with proteinuria. *Clin Sci* 1955;14:509–530.
122. Gitlin D, Janeway CA, Farr LE. Studies on the metabolism of plasma proteins in the nephrotic syndrome. I. Albumin, gammaglobulin and iron-binding globulin. *J Clin Invest* 1956;35:44–56.
123. Katz J, Bonorris G, Sellars AL. Albumin metabolism in aminonucleoside nephrotic rats. *J Lab Clin Med* 1963;62:910–934.
124. Katz J, Bonorris G, Sellars AL. Effect of nephrectomy on plasma catabolism in experimental nephrosis. *J Lab Clin Med* 1964;63:680–686.
125. Kaysen GA, Kirkpatrick WG, Couser WG. Albumin homeostasis in nephrotic rats: nutritional considerations. *Am J Physiol* 1984;47: F192–F202.
126. Kaysen GA, Gambertoglio J, Jiminez I, Jones H, Hutchison FN. Effect of dietary protein intake on albumin homeostasis in nephrotic patients. *Kidney Int* 1986;29:572–577.
127. Dorhout Mees EJ, Roos JC, Boer P, Oei HY, Simatupang TA. Observations on edema formation in the nephrotic syndrome in adults with minimal lesions. *Am J Med* 1979;67:378–384.
128. Koomans HA, Braam B, Geers AB, Roos JC, Dorhout Mees EJ. The importance of plasma proteins for blood volume and blood pressure homeostasis. *Kidney Int* 1986;30:730–735.
129. Fadnes HO, Pape JF, Sundsford JA. A study on oedema mechanism in nephrotic syndrome. *Scand J Clin Lab Invest* 1986;46:533–538.
130. Koomans HA, Geers AB, van der Meiracker AH, Roos JC, Boer P, Dorhout Mees EJ. Effects of plasma volume expansion on renal salt handling in patients with the nephrotic syndrome. *Am J Nephrol* 1984;4:234
131. Brown EA, Markandu ND, Sagnella GA, Squires M, Jones BE, MacGregor GA. Evidence that some mechanism other than the renin system causes sodium retention in the nephrotic syndrome. *Lancet* 1982; 2:1237–1240.
132. Muls E, Rosseneu M, Daneels R, Schurgers M, Boelart J. Lipoprotein distribution and compsition in the human nephrotic syndrome. *Atherosclerosis* 1985;54:225–237.
132. Joven J, Villabona C, Villella E, Masana L, Alberti R, Valles M. Abnormalities of lipoprotein metabolism in patients with the nephrotic syndrome. *N Engl J Med* 1990;323:579–584.
134. Warwick GL, Caslake MJ, Boulton-Jones JM, Dagen M, Rackard CJ, Shepherd J. Low-density lipoprotein metabolism in the nephrotic syndrome. *Metabolism* 1990;39:187–192.
135. Joven J, Rubies-Pratt J, Espinel E, Ras MR, Piera L. High-density lipoproteins in untreated idiopathic nephrotic syndrome without renal failure. *Nephrol Dial Transplant* 1987;2:149–153.
136. Lopes-Virella M, Viressa G, DeBeukelaer M, Owens CJ, Colwell JA. Urinary high-density lipoprotein in minimal change glomerular disease and chronic glomerulopathies. *Clin Chim Acta* 1979;94:73–81.
137. Wheeler DC, Bernard DB. Lipid abnormalities in the nephrotic syndrome: causes, consequences and treatment. *Am J Kidney Dis* 1994; 23:331–346.
138. Short CD, Durington PN, Mallick NP, Hunt LP, Tetlow L, Ishola M. Serum and urine high-density lipoproteins in glomerular disease with proteinuria. *Kidney Int* 1986;29:1224–1228.
139. Miller NE, Hammet F, Saltissi S, et al. Relation of angiographically defined coronary artery disease to plasma protein lipoprotein subfractions and apolipoproteins. *Br Med J* 1981;282:1741–1744.
140. Thomas ME, Freestone AL, Persaud JW, Varghese Z, Moorehead JF. Lipoprotein (a) in patients with proteinuria. *Nephrol Dial Transplant* 1992;7:597–601.
141. Karadi I, Romies L, Palos G, et al. Lp (a) lipoprotein concentration in serum of patients with heavy proteinuria of different origin. *Clin Chem* 1989;35:2121–2123.
142. Ohta T, Matsuda I. Lipid and apolipoprotein levels in patients with nephrotic syndrome. *Clin Chim Acta* 1981;117:133–143.
143. Brown WV, Baginski ML. Inhibition of lipoprotein lipase by an apolipoprotein of human very low-density lipoprotein. *Biochem Biophys Res Commun* 1972;46:375–382.
144. Anderson KM, Castelli WP, Levy D. Cholesterol and mortality. Thirty years follow-up from the Framingham study. *JAMA* 1987;257: 2176–2180.
145. Lewis B, Chait A, Wootton IDP, et al. Frequency of risk factors for ischemic heart disease in a healthy british population with particular reference to serum lipoprotein levels. *Lancet* 1974;1:141–146.
146. Rosengren A, Wilhelmsen L, Eriksson E, Risberg B, Wedel H. Lipoprotein (a) and coronary heart disease: a prospective case-control study in a general population sample of middle aged men. *Br Med J* 1990;301:1248–1251.
147. Wass VJ, Jarret RJ, Chilvers C, Cameron JS. Does the nephrotic syndrome increase the risk of cardiovascular disease? *Lancet* 1979;2: 664–667.
148. Alexander JH, Schapel GJ, Edwards KDG. Increased incidence of coronary heart disease associated with combined elevation of serum triglyceride and cholesterol concentrations in the nephrotic syndrome in man. *Med J Aust* 1974;2:119–122.
149. Gilboa N. Incidence of coronary heart disease associated with nephrotic syndrome. *Med J Aust* 1976;1:207–208.
150. Vosnides G, Cameron JS. Hyperlipidemia in renal disease. *Med J Aust* 1974;2:855
151. Wass V, Cameron JS. Cardiovascular disease and the nephrotic syndrome. The other side of the coin. *Nephron* 1981;27:58–61.
152. Curry RC, Roberts WC. Status of the coronary arteries in the nephrotic syndrome. Analysis of 20 necropsy patients aged 15 to 35 years to determine if coronary arterosclerosis is accelerated. *Am J Med* 1977;63:183–192.

153. Ordonez JD, Hiatt RA, Killebrew EJ, Fireman BH. The increased risk of coronary heart disease associated with nephrotic syndrome. *Kidney Int* 1992;44:638–642.
154. Moorhead JF, Wheeler DC, Varghese Z. Glomerular structures and lipids in progressive renal disease. *Am J Med* 1989;87:5N–12N.
155. Neugarten J, Schlondorff D. Lipoprotein interactions with glomerular cells and matrix. *Contemp Issues Nephrol* 1991;24:173–206.
156. Llach F. Hypercoagulability, renal vein thrombosis and other thrombotic complications of nephrotic syndrome. *Kidney Int* 1985;28: 429–439.
157. Llach F, Papper S, Massry SG. The clinical spectrum of renal vein thrombosis: acute and chronic. *Am J Med* 1980;69:819–827.
158. Cameron JS. Coagulation and thromboembolic complications in the nephrotic syndrome. *Adv Nephrol* 1984;13:75–114.
159. Sullivan MJ III, Hough DR, Agodoa LCY. Peripheral arterial thrombosis due to the nephrotic syndrome. The clinical spectrum. *South Med J* 1983;76:1011–1016.
160. Heslan JM, Lautie JP, Intrator L, Blanc C, Lagvue G, Sobel AT. Impaired IgG synthesis in patients with the nephrotic syndrome. *Clin Nephrol* 1982;18:144–147.
161. Aro M, Hardwicke J. Subclass composition of monomeric and polymeric IgG in the serum of patients with nephrotic syndrome. *Clin Nephrol* 1984;22:244–252.
162. McLean RH, Forsgren A, Bjorksten B, Kim Y, Quie PG, Michael AF. Decreased serum factor B concentration associated with decreased opsonization of *Escherichia coli* in the idiopathic nephrotic syndrome. *Pediatr Res* 1977;11:910–916.
163. Fodor P, Saitua MT, Rodriguez E, Gonzales B, Schesinger L. T-cell dysfunction in minimal change nephrotic syndrome of childhood. *Am J Dis Child* 1982;136:713–717.
164. Chapman S, Taube D, Brown Z, Williams D. Impaired lymphocyte transformation in minimal change nephropathy in remission. *Clin Nephrol* 1982;18:34038
165. Warshaw BL, Check IJ, Aymes LC, DiRusso SC. Decreased serum transferrin concentration in children with nephrotic syndrome: effect on lymphocyte proliferation and correlation with serum immunoglobulin levels. *Clin Immunol Immunopathol* 1984;33: 210–219.
166. Dardenne M, Pleau J, Nabarra B, et al. Contribution of zinc and other metals to the biologic activity of the serum thymic factor. *Proc Natl Acad Sci U S A* 1982;79:5370–5373.
167. Lenarsky C, Jordan SC, Ladisch S. Plasma inhibition of lymphocyte proliferation in nephrotic syndrome: correlation with hyperlipidemia. *J Clin Immunol* 1982;2:276–281.
168. Alon U, Chan JCM. Calcium and vitamin D homeostasis in the nephrotic syndrome: current status. *Nephron* 1984;36:1–4.
169. Goldstein DD, Haldimann B, Sherman D, Normal AW, Massry SG. Vitamin D metabolites in calcium metabolism in patients with nephrotic syndrome and normal renal function. *J Clin Endocrinol Metab* 1981;52:116–121.
170. Malluche HH, Goldstein DA, Massry SG. Osteomalacia and hyperparathyroid bone disease in patients with nephrotic syndrome. *J Clin Invest* 1979;63:494–500.
171. Lambert PW, DeGrea PB, Fu IY, et al. Urinary and plasma vitamin D metabolites in the nephrotic syndrome. *Metab Bone Dis Rel Res* 1982;4:7–15.
172. Auwerx J, DeKeyser L, Bouillon R, DeMoor P. Decreased free 1,25-dihydroxy-cholecalciferol index in patients with the nephrotic syndrome. *Nephron* 1986;42:231–235.
173. Tessitore N, Bonucci E, D'Angelo A, et al. Bone histology and calcium metabolism in patients with nephrotic syndrome and normal or reduced renal function. *Nephron* 1984;37:153–159.
174. Korkor A, Schwartz J, Bergfield M, et al. Absence of metabolic bone disease in adult patients with the nephrotic syndrome and normal renal function. *J Clin Endocrinol Metab* 1983;56:496–500.
175. Koenig KG, Lindberg JS, Zerwekh JE, Padalino PK, Cushner HM, Copley JB. Free and total 1,25-dihydroxyvitamin D levels in subjects with renal disease. *Kidney Int* 1992;41:161–165.
176. Harris CR, Ischmail N. Extrarenal complications of the nephrotic syndrome. *Am J Kidney Dis* 1994;23:477–497.
177. Vaziri ND. Endocrinological consequences of the nephrotic syndrome. *Am J Nephrol* 1993;13:360–364.
178. Yamauchi H, Hoopor J, MCCormack K. Blood volume and fainting in nephrosis. *Clin Res* 1960;8:195
179. Chamberlain MJ, Pringle A, Wrang OM. Oliguric renal failure in the nephrotic syndrome. *Q J Med* 1966;35:215–235.
180. Lowenstein J, Schacht RG, Baldwin DS. Renal failure in minimal change nephrotic syndrome. *Am J Med* 1981;70:227–233.
181. Jennette JC, Falk RJ. Adult minimal change glomerulopathy with acute renal failure. *Am J Kidney Dis* 1990;16:532–437.
182. Smith JD, Harplett JP. Reversible renal failure in the nephrotic syndrome. *Am J Kidney Dis* 1992;19:201–213.
183. Brenner BM, Meyer TW, Hostetter TH. Dietary protein intake and the progressive nature of kidney disease: the role of hemodynamically mediated glomerular injury in the pathogenesis of progressive glomerular sclerosis in aging, renal ablation and instrinsic renal disease. *N Engl J Med* 1982;307:652–659.
184. Sticler G, Hayles AB, Power MH, Ulrich JA. Renal tubular dysfunction complicating the nephrotic syndrome. *Pediatrics* 1960;26:75–85.
185. Agarwal A, Nath KA. Effect of proteinuria on renal interstitium. Effect of products of nitrogen metabolism. *Am J Nephrol* 1993;13: 376–384.
186. Moorehead JF, Chan EK, El-Nahas M, Varghese Z. Hypothesis—lipid nephrotoxicity in chronic progressive glomerular and tubulointerstitial disease. *Lancet* 1982;2:1309–1311.
187. Appel G. Lipid abnormalities in renal disease. *Kidney Int* 1991;39: 169–183.
188. Kees-Folts D, Diamond JR. Relationship between hyperlipidemia, lipid mediators, and progressive glomerulosclerosis in the nephrotic syndrome. *Am J Nephrol* 1993;13:365–375.
189. Brodgman JF, Rosen SM, Thorp JM. Complications during clofibrate treatment of nephrotic syndrome hyperlipoproteinaemia. *Lancet* 1972;2:506–509.
190. Ganeval D, Fischer AM, Barre J, et al. Pharmacokinetics of warfarin in the nephrotic syndrome and effect of vitamin K–dependent clotting factors. *Clin Nephrol* 1986;25:75–80.
191. Kuster S, Mehls O, Seidel C, Ritz E. Blood pressure in minimal change and other types of nephrotic syndrome. *Am J Nephrol* 1990; 76:76–80.
192. Stamler JS, Jaraki O, Osborne J, et al. Nitric oxide circulates in mammalian plasma primarily as an S-nitroso adduct of serum albumin. *Proc Natl Acad Sci U S A* 1992;89:7674–7677.
193. Sobh M, Moustafa F, Ghoniem M. Value of renal biospy in chronic renal failure. *Int Urol Nephrol* 1988;20:77–83.
194. Curtis JJ, Rakowski TA, Argy WP, Schreiner GE. Evaluation of percutaneous kidney biopsy in advanced renal failure. *Nephron* 1976;17: 259–269.
195. Bennett WM, Lee T. Tissue diagnosis by closed renal biopsy in severe renal failure. *Dial Transplant* 1976;31–34.
196. Kroop KA, Shapiro RS, Jhunjhunwala JS. Role of renal biopsy in end stage renal failure. *Urology* 1978;13:631–634.
197. Urizar RE, Schwartz A, Top F Jr, Vernier RL. The nephrotic syndrome in children with diabetes mellitus of recent onset: report of five cases. *N Engl J Med* 1969;281:173–181.
198. Brulles A, Caralps A, Vilardell M. Nephrotic syndrome with minimal glomerular lesion in an adult diabetic patient. *Arch Pathol* 1977; 101:270
199. Amoah E, Glickman JL, Malchoff CD, Sturgill BC, Kaiser DLB, Bolton WK. Clinical identification of non-diabetic renal disease in diabetic patients with type I and type II disease presenting with renal dysfunction. *Am J Nephrol* 1988;8:204–211.
200. Richards NT, Greaves I, Lee SJ, Howie AJ, Adu D, Michael J. Increased prevalence of renal biopsy findings other than diabetic glomerulopathy in type II diabetes mellitus. *Nephrol Dial Transplant* 1992;7:397–399.
201. Diaz-Buxo JA, Donadio JV Jr. Complications of percutaneous renal biopsy: an analysis of 1,000 consecutive biopsies. *Clin Nephrol* 1975; 4:223–227.
202. Madaio MP. Nephrology forum: renal biopsy. *Kidney Int* 1990;38: 529–543.
203. Mal F, Meyrier A, Cullard P, Kleinknecht D, Altman JJ, Beaugrand M. The diagnostic yield of transjugular renal biopsy. Experience in 200 cases. *Kidney Int* 1992;41:445–449.
204. Chodak GW, Gill WB, Wald V, Spargo B. Diagnosis of renal parenchymal disease by a modified open kidney biopsy technique. *Kidney Int* 1983;24:804–806.
205. Wickre CG, Gulper TA. Complications of percutaneous needle biopsy of the kidney. *Am J Nephrol* 1982;2:173–178.

206. Bennett AR, Weiner SN. Intrarenal arteriovenous fistula and aneurysm: a complication of percutaneous renal biopsy. *Am J Roentgenol* 1965;95:372–382.
207. Jackson GG, Poirer KP, Grieble HG. Concepts of pyelonephritis: experience with renal biopsies and long-term clinical observations. *Ann Intern Med* 1957;47:1165–1183.
208. Welt L (cited in Kark RM). Renal biopsy. *JAMA* 1968;205:220–226.
209. Parrish AE. Complications of percutaneous renal biopsy: a review of 37 years' experiences. *Clin Nephrol* 1992;38:135–141.
210. Paola AS. Hematuria: Essentials of diagnosis. *Hosp Pract* 1990;25: 144.
211. Wyker AW Jr. Standard diagnostic considerations. In: Gillenwater JY, Grayhack JT, Howards SS, Duckett JW eds. *Adult and pediatric urology.* Chicago: Year Book Medical; 1987:68.
212. Rose BD. *Pathophysiology of renal disease.* New York: McGraw-Hill; 1987:11.
213. Ringsrud, KM, Linne JJ, eds. Urinalysis and body fluids: a colortext and atlas. 1st ed. St. Louis: Mosby Year Book; 1995.

Immunologic Renal Diseases,
edited by E. G. Neilson and W. G. Couser.
Lippincott-Raven Publishers, Philadelphia © 1997.

CHAPTER 38

Morphologic Evaluation of Immune Renal Disease

Michael Kashgarian

INTRODUCTION

The involvement of immunologic mechanisms in the pathogenesis of renal disease was suggested almost 80 years ago by Von Pirquet (1) and was confirmed in the 1950s after immunofluorescence techniques were used to study renal biopsy tissue. By 1968, two major immunofluorescence patterns and potential immune mechanisms in glomerular injury had been defined (2). The first was a smooth linear deposition of immunoglobulin resulting from the binding of antibodies to fixed structural antigens in glomerular basement membrane, and the second was a granular pattern attributed to discrete complexes of antibody bound to antigens unrelated to the kidney.

Advances in our understanding of the immunologic basis of nephritis since that period of time have led to revisions of this classic concept of two different types of humorally mediated renal immunologic injury (3). Important renal antigens have been biochemically and immunologically characterized, and the processes of immune complex deposition have been better elucidated. Information concerning the regulatory mechanisms involved in immunity and auto-immunity and identification of new inflammatory mediators and pathways of tissue injury also have altered our concepts of immune-mediated renal disease. Evidence now supports the involvement of both T-cell-mediated hypersensitivity and polyclonal B-cell activation in specific disease instances, in addition to humoral immune reactions to specific antigens. Furthermore, the role of local glomerular hemodynamic factors and the functional characteristics of specific glomerular structures such as the mesangium in the development of chronic glomerular disease have been highlighted. All this information emphasizes the importance of evaluating renal biopsy specimens not only histologically but also with imaging techniques designed to identify the immunologic mechanisms involved.

M. Kashgarian: Department of Pathology, Yale University School of Medicine, New Haven, Connecticut 06520.

EXAMINATION OF THE RENAL BIOPSY SPECIMEN

The complex anatomy of the kidneys and the small amount of tissue available for study in percutaneous renal biopsy specimens require that tissues be routinely examined by light, immunofluorescence, and electron microscopy in every case. Light microscopic examination is best performed on thin (3 to 4 mm), serial sections using multiple stains, including hematoxylin-eosin, periodic acid–Schiff, Masson trichome, and Jones silver methenamine. This extensive examination is needed for an accurate evaluation of lesions, especially those that may be focal and segmental in distribution or minor in degree.

Terminology is as important as description. The term *focal* is taken to mean disease affecting some but not all glomeruli, in contrast to *diffuse*, which denotes disease affecting all or nearly all glomeruli. *Segmental* refers to a lesion involving only a portion of a glomerulus, whereas *global* describes lesions involving the entire glomerulus. Lesions that can be identified by light microscopy include proliferation of mesangial, endothelial, and epithelial cells, mesangial sclerosis, glomerular hyalinosis, capillary thrombosis, necrosis, and leukocytic infiltration.

Immunofluorescence microscopy should be performed to determine the presence or absence of immunoglobulins in glomerular lesions. Routine staining for IgG, IgM, IgA, C3, C1 or C4, fibrinogen and albumin, and κ and λ chains should be performed. In special instances, other antigens should also be investigated, including IgE, properdin, and specific antigens such as tumor antigens or hepatitis virus antigens. The major patterns that can be described are shown in Table 1. They include continuous

TABLE 1. *Basic patterns of immunofluorescence in the kidney*

Pattern	Distribution	Location	Protein	Example of entity
Glomerular linear	Continuous	GBM	IgG, IgM, IgA	Anti-GBM disease
		Albumin, IgG	Diabetes	
Fine granular	Scattered	Peripheral capillary Subepithelial	IgG, IgM	Acute GN
	Confluent	Peripheral capillary Subepithelial Intramembranous	IgG, C3, IgM	Membranous GN
Coarse granular	Irregular	Peripheral capillary Subendothelial	IgG, IgM, IgA	Mesangiocapillary GN
Focal granular	Arborized	Mesangial	IgG, IgA	Berger's disease
	Nodular	Mesangial Peripheral capillary	C3	Dense-deposit disease
	Segmental	Mesangial	IgM	FSGS
Peritubular				
Linear	Continuous	TBM	IgG, IgM, IgA	Anti-TBM disease
Granular	Scattered	Peritubular	IgG, IgM, IgA	Lupus

GBM, glomerular basement membrane; GN, glomerulonephritis; FSGS, focal segmental glomerulosclerosis; TBM, tubular basement membrane.

linear deposits in glomerular or tubular basement membranes, granular deposits in the peripheral capillary loops, granular deposits in the mesangium, and granular deposits in tubular and vascular structures.

Electron microscopic studies should be performed to assess glomerular architecture more precisely—in particular, epithelial cell morphology, mesangial morphology, and the localization of electron-dense deposits, which correspond to accumulations of immune complexes. The latter can be seen in three major patterns, including mesangial, subendothelial, and subepithelial localizations. By using all three morphologic modalities, an extremely precise diagnostic categorization can be made and information can be gained regarding the nature of the immunologic process that has initiated the injury. Precise diagnosis, classification, and identification of pathogenetic mechanisms enhance the clinical utility of the renal biopsy in the evaluation of patients with renal disease.

Molecular diagnostic examination is still in its infancy. Molecular evaluation of pathology has primarily been applied in the evaluation of genetic alterations occurring in malignant neoplastic conditions, and most fruitfully in the diagnosis of infectious diseases, particularly those of viral origin. The techniques available for use in tissue samples as an adjunct to more routine morphologic techniques include *in situ* hybridization, *in situ* reverse transcription, and polymerase chain reaction amplification (4). In the case of renal biopsy, diagnostic application of these new techniques has largely been restricted to the detection and verification of specific viral diseases (5–9). This has been especially useful in evaluation of allograft biopsy specimens for cytomegalovirus infection and for Epstein-Barr virus in post-transplant lymphoproliferative diseases. Viral identification in glomerular nephritides associated with specific infections has also been applied particularly in the hepatitis B and C infections related to mesangiocapillary glomerulonephritis. Viral etiology in interstitial nephritis is yet another similar application. The potential use of these techniques is undoubtedly greater than the present degree of application suggests. Experimental studies largely done on a variety of experimental models of glomerular and interstitial injury have utilized these techniques to obtain greater insight into pathogenesis. Cytokine and growth factor expression has been studied both in experimental situations and in human renal biopsy material, but findings have not added to the diagnostic categorization of the lesions (10–14). Matrix protein gene expression and metalloprotease gene expression have been investigated to explain mechanisms of glomerular sclerosis and interstitial fibrosis (15–18). Proliferative activity using proliferation-associated nuclear markers such as proliferating cell nuclear antigen and KI-67 have been applied not only to experimental forms of tubular diseases, such as cystic disease and acute renal failure, but also to human biopsy material. Identification of immune cell subsets, idiotypic markers, and auto-antigens has not yet been widely applied in models of renal injury, but it may add significantly to our interpretation of the potential immune responses mediating the various types. Although the application of molecular diagnostic techniques is currently limited, the potential is there, and both application and utility of such techniques are likely to increase.

The importance of the role of the renal biopsy in immune renal disease is further underscored by the fact that a large number of histopathologic entities lead to a limited number of clinical presentations (19–22). The clinical syndromes recognized by nephrologists include the nephrotic syndrome, persistent proteinuria, acute nephritis, persistent or recurrent hematuria, hypertension, urinary tract infections, acute renal failure, and chronic renal failure. The problem is illustrated in Table 2, which correlates the clinical presentations of acute glomerulonephritis, recurrent hematuria, persistent proteinuria, and nephrotic syndrome with the spectrum of histologic appearances seen in each of these presentations. It is obvious that in the majority of instances, the specific histopathologic diagnosis or the pathogenic mechanisms that underlie it cannot be predicted with certainty. Despite this lack of correlation, it is convenient to classify the various histopathologic entities in broad groupings that relate to their more common clinical presentations. Thus, glomerular lesions can be characterized as proliferative lesions (usually associated with acute nephritis or hematuria) or lesions without prominent cellular proliferation (usually associated with the nephrotic syndrome or persistent proteinuria). In addition, tubulointerstitial and vascular lesions can either accompany the primary glomerular lesions or be of importance independent of any glomerular involvement.

GLOMERULAR LESIONS ASSOCIATED WITH A PROLIFERATIVE RESPONSE

Proliferative glomerular lesions are usually associated with the acute nephritic syndrome. Acute nephritis is characterized by hematuria, azotemia, oliguria, and mild to moderate hypertension. Urinalysis reveals an "active" sediment consisting of red blood cells, leukocytes, and red blood cell casts. Proteinuria is generally present but is rarely in the nephritic range. Edema when present is usually mild and frequently is manifested as facial puffiness. A variant of this clinical syndrome is the fulminant form of rapidly progressive glomerulonephritis. Milder forms may be characterized by the presence of microscopic hematuria and non-nephritic proteinuria, occasionally associated with mild hypertension. Gross hematuria or microscopic hematuria alone form another variant. The histopathologic lesions accompanying this clinical presentation vary.

Acute Post-infectious Glomerulonephritis

The natural history of acute post-infectious glomerulonephritis is better studied than that of any other form of renal disease (23,24). Although it has been known for a long time that acute glomerulonephritis follows certain acute infections, studies have established the most common cause to be infection with group A hemolytic streptococci of specific types, including types 12, 3, 1, and 49 (25–29). Less commonly, a variety of other infectious agents, including viruses, protozoa, spirochetes, mycobacteria, and bacteria other than streptococci (staphylococci, salmonellae, and enterococci) have all been implicated as potential antigens (30–32). On the basis of experimental observations in animals with immunologically induced renal disease and studies of human biopsy material, it is generally thought that the immunohistopathologic lesion is an immune complex-mediated inflammatory response within the glomerulus. Pathogenesis has been compared with that of single-shot serum sickness, in which a humorally mediated immune response follows a single antigenic challenge. This type of response results in the formation of immune complexes of different sizes and avidity and a corresponding evolution of glomerular immune complex deposition from subendothelial to subepithelial to mesangial locations.

Post-streptococcal glomerulonephritis is the prototypic form of acute nephritis, and the severity of both the clinical and pathologic findings varies (23–25,33–36). Usually, the onset of renal symptoms occurs after a latent period of 1 to 4 weeks. In most instances, the streptococcal infection affects the upper respiratory system, but skin infections with nephrogenic streptococci are also important. Because the clinical syndrome may be quite

TABLE 2. *Correlation of clinical presentations with histologic appearance*

Histologic appearance	Clinical presentations, % of cases			
	AGN	RH	PP	NS
Minor or absent glomerular proliferation				
Minimal changes	0	6	10	84
Membranous nephropathy	2	0	21	77
Focal (segmental) glomerulosclerosis	1	6	42	51
Obvious glomerular proliferation				
Proliferative and exudative (endocapillary)	76	4	5	15
Mesangial proliferative	30	18	14	38
Predominantly extracapillary proliferative (>80% crescents)	74	1	5	20
Mesangiocapillary glomerulonephritis	2	8	25	45
Focal proliferative and/or necrotizing glomerulonephritis	4	26	40	30
Chronic glomerulonephritis	6	8	41	45

AGN, acute glomerulonephritis; RH, recurrent hematuria; PP, persistent symptomless proteinuria; NS, nephrotic syndrome.

distinctive and the general prognosis is usually excellent, biopsies are not generally performed on patients with this syndrome unless some atypical features complicate the presentation, such as nephrotic syndrome, oliguria, persistent or severe hypertension, or failure to show significant recovery within 4 to 6 weeks.

By light microscopy, the glomeruli show a diffuse hypercellularity, with obliteration of the capillary lumina caused by proliferation and swelling of endothelial cells and leukocytic infiltration (Fig. 1). The severity of the proliferative response varies, but generally all the glomeruli are involved equally. Segmental necrosis and thrombosis associated with crescent formation are usually not seen, although they may rarely occur. A necrotizing arteritis has also been reported in unusual instances.

Immunofluorescence microscopy shows the deposition of IgG and C3 and a peripheral granular and mesangial pattern. C1q or C4 and other immunoglobulins are generally not present. Fibrinogen may be present in a predominantly mesangial pattern.

Electron microscopy of very early biopsy specimens usually demonstrates the presence of small subendothelial deposits. The most characteristic finding, however, is seen in later biopsies—subepithelial, electron-dense deposits called *humps* (Fig. 2). These deposits vary in size and number and are often inhomogeneous in density. There is effacement of foot processes, endothelial cell swelling, and prominent mesangial widening caused by proliferation of mesangial cells, infiltration of mononuclear leukocytes, and some increase in mesangial matrix. Serial studies have shown that a gradual resolution of the histopathologic changes takes place. Cellularity gradually decreases, with a disappearance of immunofluorescence and electron microscopic deposits. Complete restoration to normal histology may be seen as early as 6 months and certainly by 2 to 3 years (37). Only a small percentage of cases appear to have residual changes, which may include persistent mesangial hypercellularity and mesangial deposits seen by electron microscopy and immunofluorescence.

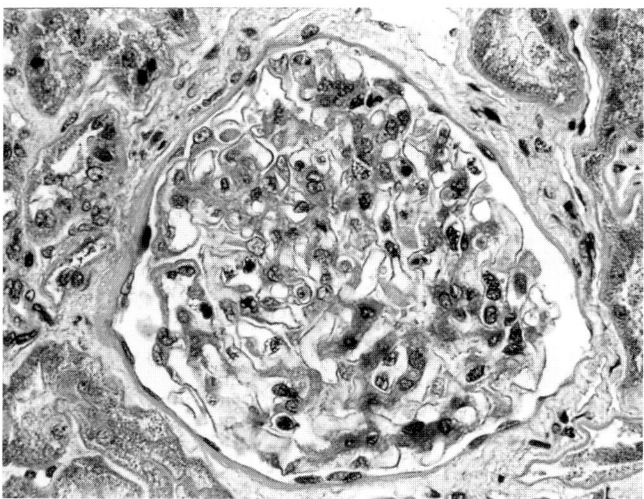

FIG. 1. Acute glomerulonephritis. The glomerulus is hypercellular as a result of proliferation and swelling of mesangial and endothelial cells and infiltration with occasional leukocytes. No necrosis or sclerosis is present. H&E, ×500.

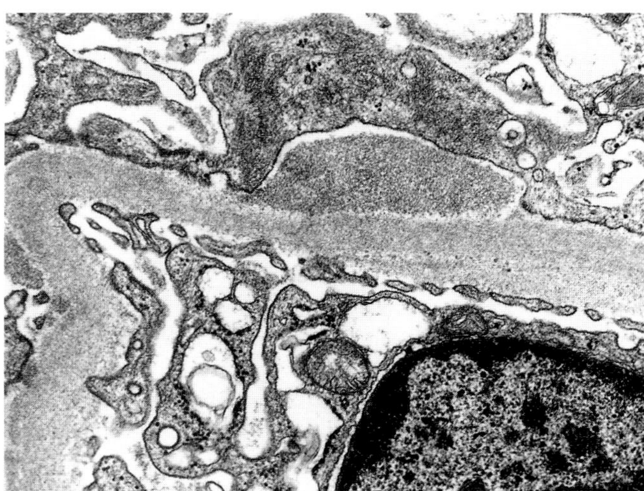

FIG. 2. Acute glomerulonephritis. Electron micrograph demonstrates a typical subepithelial hump as seen in post-infectious glomerulonephritis. The basement membrane shows no significant thickening, and the subepithelial electron-dense deposit is distinctly separated from the basement membrane and pushes the overlying effaced foot processes of the epithelial cell away from the basement membrane. ×24,300.

Diffuse Crescentic Glomerulonephritis

Rapidly progressive glomerulonephritis is a variant of the acute nephritic syndrome in which acute glomerulonephritis is associated with a rapid onset of severe acute renal failure (38). The onset of the disease is characterized by oliguria, advancing azotemia, proteinuria of varying degree, hematuria with cellular casts, and hypertension that is sometimes in the malignant range. The nephrotic syndrome is occasionally present. In a few patients, renal function eventually stabilizes at an impaired level after several weeks, but in most patients, progression to end-stage renal insufficiency occurs. The clinical pathologic entity can be divided into three subgroups (39–41). The first is severe post-infectious glomerulonephritis in which the pathogenic mechanism is immune complex-mediated. In the second, an antibody to glomerular basement membrane can be identified and the immune mechanism is related directly to antibody binding to basement membrane components. In the third, termed *pauci-immune*, antibody deposition is not present and no definite relationship to a particular antigen can be identified, although patients in this group often have an anti-neutrophil cytoplasmic antibody in their serum (42–44).

Light microscopy demonstrates the presence of glomerular crescents. The crescents may be cellular or fibrous, depending the stage of evolution of the glomerular lesion (45,46) (Fig. 3). The crescents consists of accumulations of cells derived from the parietal epithelium and infiltrating monocytes in Bowman's space, and their formation appears to be initiated by deposition of fibrin across gaps or disruptive lesions of the glomerular capillary with extrusion of fibrin into Bowman's space. As the crescents mature, collagen is deposited and fibroepithelial and finally fibrous crescents are formed. Segmental areas of necrosis of the glomerular capillaries are usually present, as well as areas of glomerular capillary collapse and focal increases in mesangial matrix. The light microscopic picture is similar in all three types of pathogenic mechanisms, which are better characterized on the basis of immunofluorescence and electron microscopy.

By immunofluorescence, the findings are variable and fall into the three subgroups (47). In those patients in whom immune complex mediation can be implicated, a granular deposition of IgG and C3 is seen in a pattern similar to that of acute glomerulonephritis. Patients with anti-glomerular basement membrane disease have diffuse linear staining of the glomerular basement membranes, usually revealing IgG but occasionally IgM or IgA antibodies (48) (Fig. 4), and associated granular deposition of complement is present. Fibrinogen is usually seen deposited focally within the capillary loops and in Bowman's space associated with the crescents. Linear staining for immunoglobulins may also be found along tubular basement membranes associated with a tubulointerstitial nephritis. In the third group, no specific immunoglobulin deposition is identified by immunofluorescence microscopy. Complement components in fibrinogen may be present and are usually are seen in association with the crescents. This lack of immunoglobulin deposition has given rise to the term *pauci-immune*.

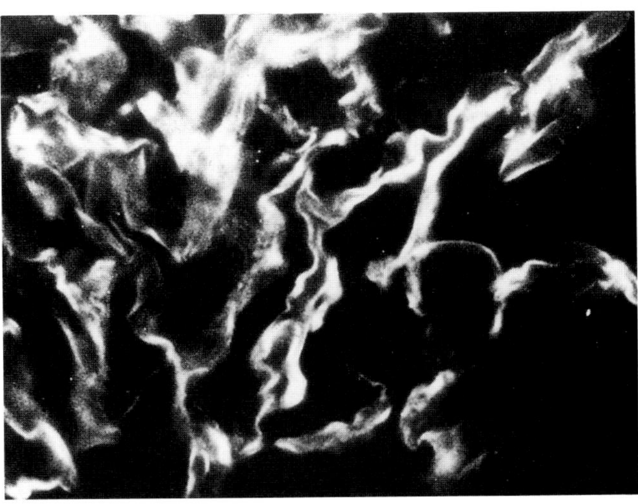

FIG. 4. Immunofluorescence micrograph of a glomerulus of a patient with rapidly progressive glomerulonephritis secondary to anti-glomerular basement disease. There is a smooth linear deposition of immunoglobulin along the entire capillary wall. The mesangial areas are free of immunoglobulin deposition. ×500.

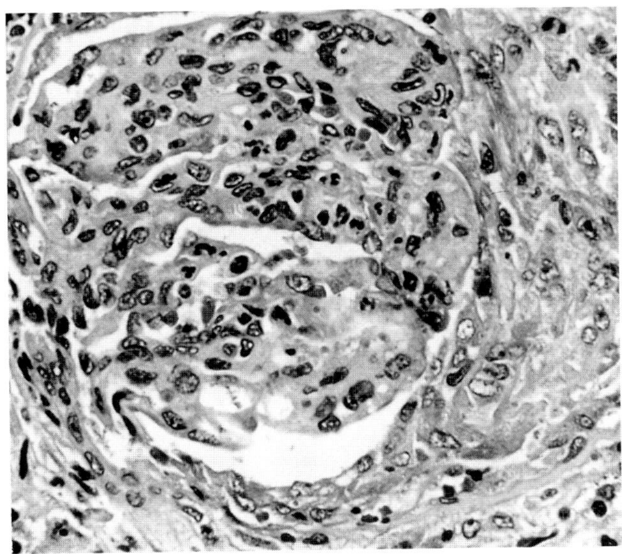

FIG. 3. Rapidly progressive glomerulonephritis. The normal architecture of the glomerulus is obliterated by a striking increase in cellularity, which includes mesangial cells, swollen endothelial cells, and numerous leukocytes. In addition, a marked proliferation of epithelial cells forms an epithelial crescent and fills Bowman's space. Occasional leukocytes can be seen in the crescent. In the glomerulus adjacent to the crescent, there is a focus of necrosis. H&E, ×500.

Findings of electron microscopy are also variable but generally fall into two subgroups. In patients with granular deposition of IgG by immunofluorescence, subepithelial humps, mesangial deposits, and occasionally subendothelial electron-dense deposits are seen. Specimens from patients with anti-glomerular basement membrane disease and those with pauci-immune disease do not demonstrate electron-dense deposits. In most instances, fibrin deposition is prominent and often associated with breaks within the capillary wall and basement membrane.

Diffuse Mesangial Proliferative Glomerulonephritis

Diffuse mesangial proliferation may occur in a variety of conditions, including systemic diseases such as lupus erythematosus and Henoch-Schönlein purpura, or as part of the spectrum of primary nephrotic syndrome. A distinct group of patients without evidence of systemic disease, however, have gross or microscopic hematuria, proteinuria, or combined proteinuria and hematuria, and biopsy reveals a diffuse mild mesangial proliferation (49–51). Some of these patients have mild, resolving or persistent post-infectious glomerulonephritis. The majority of the patients in this group have elevated serum IgA levels and deposition of IgA immune complexes in the mesangium. This condition has been termed *IgA nephropathy* or *Berger's disease*. These patients generally have a favorable prognosis, although most show a slow but progressive course to chronic renal failure (52–56). It is likely that this lesion corresponds to the experimental lesion in which relatively small numbers of stable immune complexes of intermediate size formed with antibodies of high affinity and high avidity accumulate in the mesangium as a result of the mesangial clearing system for removal of macromolecules (84). Because of the relatively small number of complexes characteristic of this lesion, the mesangial system does not become overloaded and the complexes can be sequestered in the mesangium, where they are degraded and removed so that initiation of an inflammatory response is prevented. This explanation of accumulation and restriction of immune complexes to the mesangium assigns no specific characteristics either to the nature of the antigen or to the nature of antibody. Increasing evidence, however, suggests that specific characteristics of both antigen and antibody are involved in localization of complexes to distinct glomerular sites. Fibronectin is an important component of the mesangial matrix, and given its capacity to interact with aggregates of immunoglobulins and immune complexes in the circulation, its presence in the mesangium may play a role in this type of localization. Regardless of the mechanisms involved in mesangial localization, the sequestration of such complexes to this site allows for their isolation from inflammatory mediators and results in a relatively benign, non-inflammatory lesion.

Light microscopy shows expansion of the mesangial areas caused by an increase in mesangial cells and mesangial matrix (Fig. 5). The endothelial cells are not swollen, there is no evidence of proliferation, and the capillary lumina remain patent. The expansion of the mesangium may be mild, with only small clusters of four or more cells per mesangial area, or more diffuse and prominent, with numerous cells and a marked increase in mesangial matrix.

Immunofluorescence microscopy correlates closely with the light microscopic findings (57) (Fig. 6). The presence of IgG and C3 alone is consistent with post-infectious or latent glomerulonephritis. The presence of IgA and C3 in a mesangial pattern is characteristic of IgA nephropathy. It should be noted that marked similarities exist between the morphologic findings in Berger's disease and in Henoch- Schönlein purpura and that the separation of these two categories is predominantly on the basis of the clinical presentation.

Electron microscopy shows mesangial changes that consist of an increase in mesangial cells and matrix and the presence of electron-dense deposits (Fig. 7). Occasionally, electron deposits are also seen in the paramesangial subendothelial region, but there is no evidence of involvement of the peripheral capillary loops. In rare instances, small subepithelial humps may also be found.

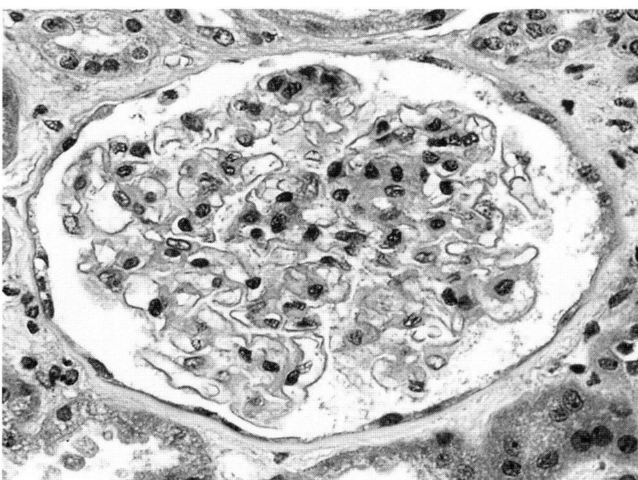

FIG. 5. Diffuse mesangial proliferative glomerulonephritis. There is marked widening of the mesangium and increased cellularity, with more than four nuclei crowded in a mesangial area. The peripheral capillary loops are patent, and no leukocytes are seen. H&E, ×400.

Mesangiocapillary Glomerulonephritis

Mesangiocapillary glomerulonephritis is known by a variety of other names, including *membranoproliferative glomerulonephritis*, *hypocomplementemic glomerulonephritis*, and *lobular glomerulonephritis*. This entity

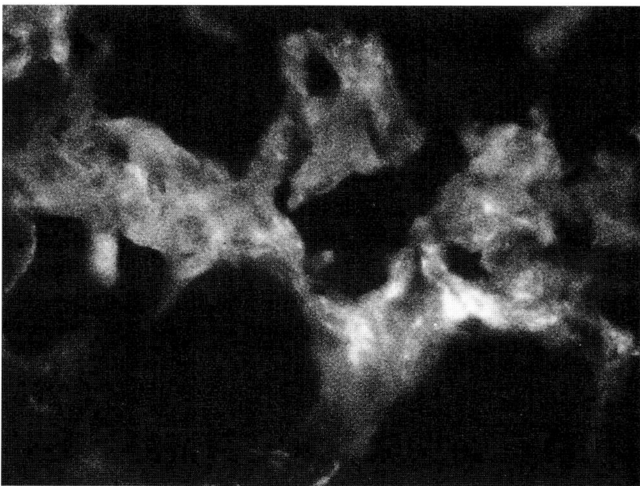

FIG. 6. Immunofluorescence micrograph of a mesangial area of a patient with mesangial proliferative glomerulonephritis with IgA (IgA nephropathy). There is a granular deposition of IgA in the mesangium. The peripheral capillary loops are free of immunoglobulin deposition. ×600.

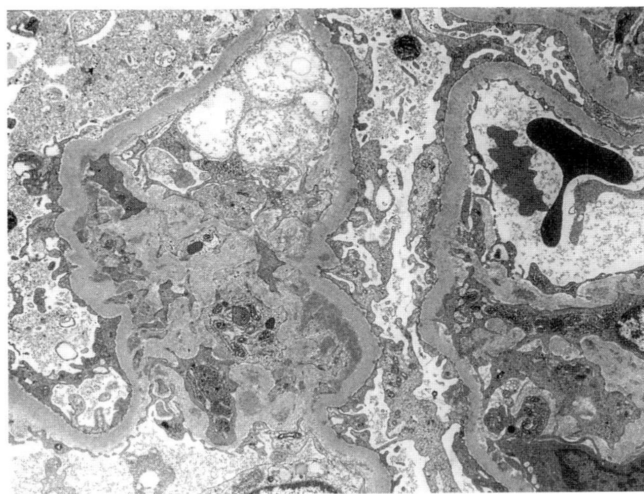

FIG. 7. Mesangial proliferative glomerulonephritis. Electron micrograph of a glomerulus demonstrates marked mesangial widening, with an increase in mesangial matrix and mesangial dense deposits. The mesangial dense deposits extend to the paramesangial subendothelial space. ×2650.

is defined more by its morphology than by a specific clinical presentation or etiology. The classic clinical presentation consists of a combination of acute nephritis, the nephrotic syndrome, and hypertension. A history of infection preceding the onset is not uncommon, but a causal or even temporal relationship has not been confirmed. The clinical course is variable but is generally characterized by a slowly progressive and gradual loss of renal function.

By light microscopy, the most prominent finding is glomerular enlargement and accentuation of the lobular architecture (Fig. 8). Mesangial areas are expanded by increased numbers of mesangial cells and matrix. In some instances, a nodular accumulation of matrix exists within the lobule, giving rise to what has been termed *lobular glomerulonephritis*. The hypercellularity is predominantly mesangial, but infiltration with leukocytes is common and may be extensive. Another characteristic feature is thickening of the peripheral capillary wall. This is the result of the extension of mesangial cells and matrix around the peripheral capillary to produce a double contour or "tram track" appearance with special stains, such as Masson or silver methenamine. Necrosis is uncommon but when present is often accompanied by cellular crescents. Rarely, focal forms in which only a portion of the glomeruli are involved may be found. There are at least two and perhaps three subtypes, which differ in their immunofluorescence and electron microscopic findings and in pathogenesis (21).

The findings of type I mesangiocapillary glomerulonephritis indicate that it is an immune complex-mediated disease (58–60). Immunofluorescence reveals deposition of immunoglobulins, most frequently IgG and IgM but also occasionally IgA. The immunoglobulins are distributed in a granular pattern in the peripheral capillary loops and sometimes in large granules within the mesangial areas. They are accompanied by abundant deposition of C3, and complement components early in the classic pathway—C1q, C4, and C2—are occasionally found, as is properdin of the alternative pathway. Fibrinogen is occasionally present. In some cases, complement components are present but not immunoglobulins.

Findings of electron microscopy correlate with the light microscopic picture. There is extensive mesangial cell proliferation, with mesangialization of the peripheral capillary loops by extension of mesangial cells and mesangial matrix to the periphery of the capillary wall (Fig. 9). The peripheral capillary basement membrane is usually identifiable as a distinct basement membrane, but it is separated from endothelial cells by mesangial cells and matrix continuous with the mesangial area, thus giving rise to the double contour or tram track appearance. In addition, there is a prominent increase in mesangial matrix. Electron-dense deposits are found in the subendothelial and mesangial regions. Occasionally, subepithelial humps are present, and when this is a prominent feature, a distinct subgroup has been suggested (type III of Burkholder) (61). In areas of mesangialization of the peripheral capillary loop, the electron-dense deposits may lie in the reduplicated subendothelial mesangial matrix. The epithelial cells show effacement of foot processes, and inflammatory cells, including polymorphonuclear leukocytes, are seen; monocytes are often present within the capillary lumen and sometimes in a subendothelial site.

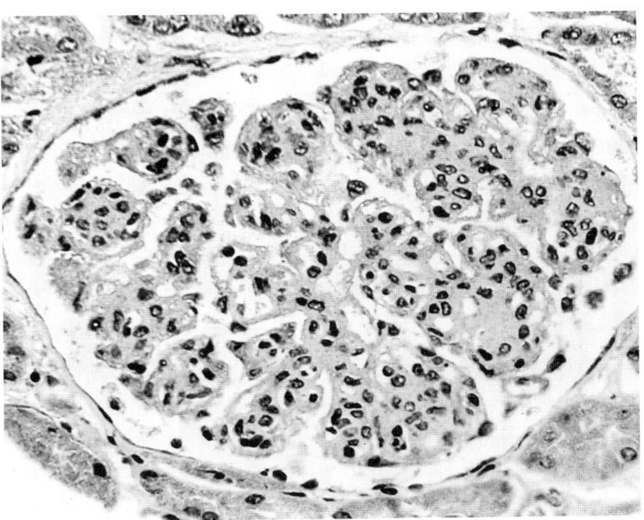

FIG. 8. Mesangiocapillary (membranoproliferative) glomerulonephritis. There is striking lobular accentuation of the glomerular architecture as a result of marked hyperplasia of mesangial cells, with extension of mesangial cells around the peripheral capillary loop. Some of the capillary lumina contain leukocytes. H&E, ×500.

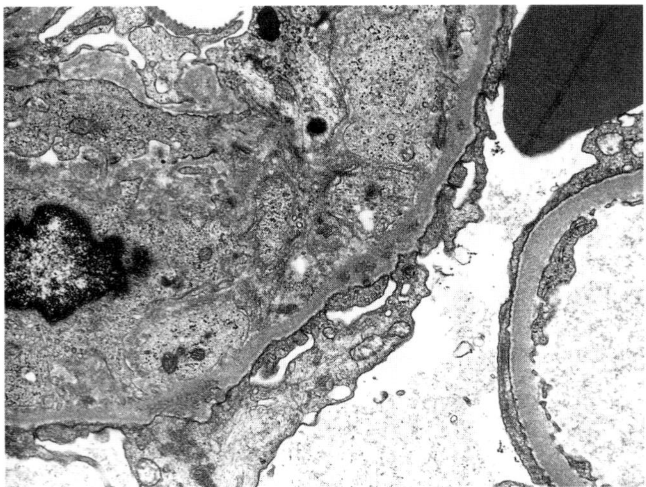

FIG. 9. Mesangiocapillary glomerulonephritis. The electron micrograph demonstrates the mesangialization of a peripheral capillary loop. Mesangial cells have extended between the endothelial cell and the basement membrane, and small submembranous deposits are present. The capillary wall is markedly thickened by layering of epithelial cell, basement membrane, mesangial cell, mesangial matrix, and finally endothelial cell lining the capillary lumen. The mesangial extension results in the lobular accentuation seen by light microscopy. ×10,500.

The localization of immune complexes to the subendothelial region, where they have access to plasma inflammatory mediators, is a critical step in initiating the pattern of mesangiocapillary glomerulonephritis. It is likely that large numbers of intermediate-sized complexes or large complexes formed by high-affinity antibodies overwhelm the mesangial ability to clear macromolecules. As a result, these complexes accumulate in a paramesangial subendothelial location and then ultimately in the peripheral capillary loops. Here, they have access to circulating inflammatory mediators, such as complement and platelets, as well as cellular mediators of inflammation, including monocyte macrophages and cytotoxic lymphocytes, which can secrete cytokines that promote proliferation of the intrinsic glomerular cells, including mesangial cells. Mesangial cells stimulated in this scenario are also sources of secreted cytokines and growth factors that contribute to the proliferative response. The nature of the antigen and antibody may also contribute to the deposition in a subendothelial location in this lesion. Characteristics of certain nephrotropic antibodies, such as cationic charge, could permit binding of complexes that contain such antibodies to negative charges within the glomerular capillary wall. If the complexes are large and highly cationic, they will bind and fix to the closest anionic charges that are encountered at the subendothelial location. Following the initial binding of what might be only a small population of nephrotropic antibodies, activation of inflammatory cytokines could increase the permeability of the capillary wall, thus allowing other complexes to be deposited. Another significant factor is the activation of endothelial adhesion molecules, including I-CAM and V-CAM, which both initiate and modulate the inflammatory response. The immunofluorescence and electron microscopic findings, which strongly suggest that the pathogenesis of this subtype is an immune complex disease, also suggest that the idiopathic forms are perhaps related to an infectious agent. The fact that the exact same histologic picture is seen in the glomerulonephritis associated with infected ventricular-atrial shunts and bacterial endocarditis and hepatitis B and C adds strength to this argument.

Type II mesangiocapillary glomerulonephritis is also known as *dense-deposit disease* (62,63). In addition to the clinical features shared with type I, most cases of type II are characterized by the presence of C3 nephritic factor (NeF) in the serum. There is an apparent familial incidence of this type, which is associated with partial peripheral lipodystrophy. By light microscopy, in addition to the findings of type I, the basement membranes sometimes have a refractile appearance and take up histologic stains more intensely. The immunofluorescence findings in type II mesangiocapillary glomerulonephritis are very distinct. There is extensive deposition of C3 along the peripheral capillary walls (Fig. 10). Depending on the extent of deposition, it can be irregularly linear or discontinuous. Mesangial deposition of complement is also prominent. Immunoglobulins are usually absent, although occasionally IgM may be noted. Fibrin is also occasionally present. The most striking change is detected by electron microscopy. A very electron-dense material is present within the lamina densa of the glo-

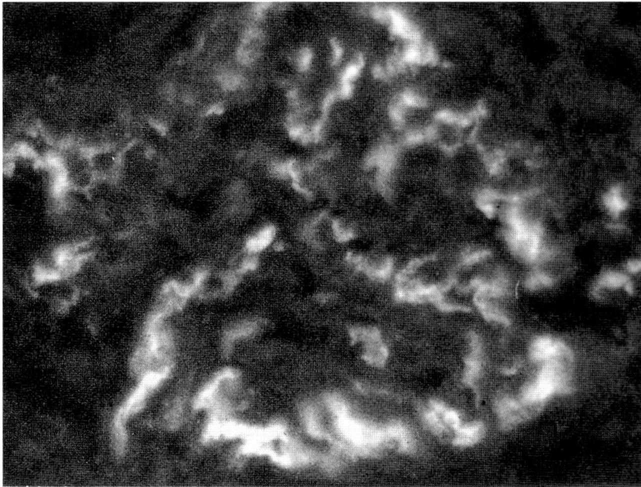

FIG. 10. Immunofluorescence micrograph of type II mesangiocapillary glomerulonephritis (dense-deposit disease). There is peripheral capillary deposition of complement in an interrupted and focally pseudolinear pattern. No associated immunoglobulins are identified. ×400.

merular capillary basement membrane, which is often widened by the presence of the deposit. The deposit forms a long ribbon of hazy, electron-dense material. In some instances, the ribbon is discontinuous and the electron-dense material has a sausagelike appearance (Fig. 11). In some individual cases, subepithelial electron-dense humps similar to deposits observed in post-streptococcal glomerulonephritis are identified. The epithelial foot processes are effaced. The dense deposits are sometimes also identified in the tubular basement membrane as well.

The pathogenesis of this subtype is likely to be a combination of genetic and extrinsic factors. The anatomic characteristics of the deposits suggest that there may be a genetic alteration in the composition of the glycoproteins of the basement membrane. The association in some cases with a familial partial lipodystrophy helps support this concept. The deposition of complement following activation of the complement pathway with formation of C3bB-NeF is likely secondary to an external stimulus, such as an antecedent infection, but could also reflect an intrinsic defect in the complement cascade (64,65).

Burkholder et al. (61,66,67) described a third type (type III) of mesangiocapillary glomerulonephritis. Like type I, it is likely an immune complex-mediated disease. Deposits are located in the subepithelial region, however, and there are gaps in the glomerular basement membrane.

One particular form of mesangiocapillary glomerulonephritis that deserves special note is associated with the presence of cryoglobulins (5,7,68,69). Cryoglobulinemia has been demonstrated in patients with a variety of infectious processes, recently in particular with hepatitis C infection (70,71), and in individuals with primary or essential cryoglobulinemia associated with a dysproteinemia. Up to half of patients with cryoglobulins in their serum may have renal manifestations; a distinct syndrome characterized by the combination of purpura, arthralgias, and glomerulonephritis has been described in such patients. By light microscopy, in addition to the diffuse proliferative glomerulonephritis with lobular accentuation characteristic of mesangiocapillary glomerulonephritis, intraluminal eosinophilic proteinaceous thrombi are present. Immunofluorescence shows characteristic large peripheral capillary deposits containing both immunoglobulins and complement in a granular pattern along the capillary walls. By electron microscopy, subendothelial deposits and mesangial deposits are prominent and are associated with the intracapillary thrombi (Fig. 12). The deposits have a distinct organized appearance and fall into two different pathologic patterns: a random array of fibrils (*fibrillary glomerulonephritis*) or microtubular structures (*immunotactoid glomerulopathy*). Rhomboid, crystalline structures are also often seen, particularly in association with mixed cryoglobulinemias.

Lupus Nephritis

Lupus erythematosus is an autoimmune disease with renal manifestations that cover the entire spectrum of immune-mediated glomerular injury. Both autopsy and

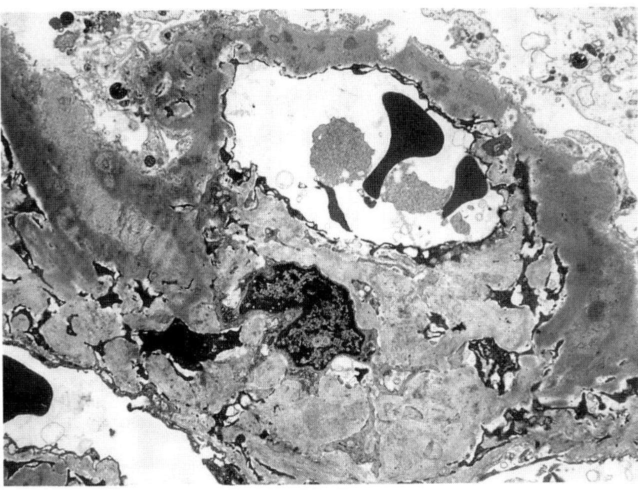

FIG. 11. Electron micrograph of type II mesangiocapillary glomerulonephritis (dense-deposit disease). The peripheral capillary basement is irregularly thickened by the presence of intramembranous dense deposit, which is focally inhomogeneous. The intramembranous dense material corresponds to the deposition of complement seen by immunofluorescence. ×3300.

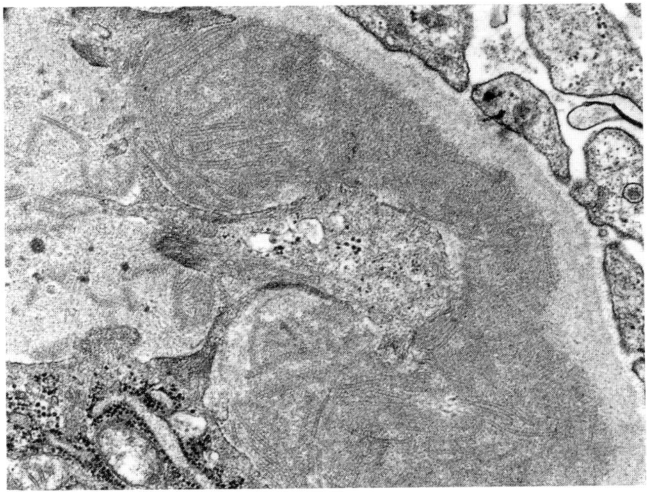

FIG. 12. Electron micrograph of mesangiocapillary glomerulonephritis associated with cryoglobulinemia. Electron-dense deposits seen in a subendothelial location have an organized appearance consisting of a haphazard arrangement of microtubule-like structures. The fibrils are much larger than those seen with amyloidosis and have a distinct crystalline appearance.×2400.

biopsy studies of patients with the clinical diagnosis of systemic lupus erythematosus have documented that renal involvement is a frequent and serious complication of the disease, making the renal biopsy an important part of the clinical management of these patients (72,73). Numerous reports have documented the unpredictable course of lupus nephritis and the role of the renal biopsy in the evaluation of individual patients with isolated unusual clinical features (74–81.) The nature of the lesion on renal biopsy gives direct information relating to the severity of the autoimmune response within the kidney, thereby aiding in selecting the appropriate therapies and predicting both the short-term and long-term outcome in individual patients. Because the histology is varied and the pathogenesis is thought to be similar to that of various forms of experimental immune-complex glomerulonephritis, the various patterns of lupus nephritis are best considered in the context of the potential pathogenetic mechanisms that might be involved in their evolution. A classification scheme for lupus nephritis developed by the World Health Organization (WHO) provides a basis for this type of application (82). It combines all the morphologic modalities of biopsy interpretation, including light, immunofluorescence, and electron microscopic findings. The classification system, along with a semiquantitative assessment of severity, is now in general use and has been accepted by clinical nephrologists and renal pathologists alike.

In class I, the renal biopsy reveals essentially a normal kidney by light, electron, and immunofluorescence microscopy. Minor non-specific changes, such as irregular thickening of the basement membrane, occasionally are observed on electron microscopy, but these changes usually are not associated with a functional abnormality. Because this class is defined in reality by the absence of morphologic evidence of glomerular damage, it denotes a lack of significant renal involvement in systemic lupus erythematosus. Although some reports suggest that all patients with lupus may have renal immune complex deposition even in the absence of clinical evidence, about 25% of affected patients exhibit no significant glomerular findings and thus could be assigned to this group.

Class II is characterized by purely mesangial lesions. It has been subdivided into class IIA and IIB. In the former, lesions have minimal or no significant changes by light microscopy, although immunofluorescence may present evidence of immune deposits confined to the mesangium and electron microscopy reveals corresponding electron-dense deposits in this location. In cases of class IIB, light microscopy shows definite glomerular mesangial hypercellularity confined to the centrilobular areas away from the vascular pole. There is no involvement of the peripheral glomerular capillary walls. Immunofluorescence reveals mesangial immunoglobulin deposition, and electron microscopy discloses dense deposits confined to the mesangial regions. In some cases, deposits are occasionally seen in the paramesangial subendothelial areas. Tubular, interstitial, and vascular changes are usually insignificant. Patients with class II lesions generally have minimal clinical evidence of renal involvement, with mild to moderate proteinuria, hematuria, or both and little or no evidence of renal insufficiency (83). This lesion corresponds to the experimental lesion in which the generation of relatively small numbers of stable immune complexes of intermediate size formed with antibodies of high affinity and high avidity accumulate in the mesangium as a result of the mesangial clearing system for removal of macromolecules as discussed previously (84).

Class III is characterized by light microscopic findings of a focal and segmental glomerulonephritis (Fig. 13). Fewer than 50% of the involved glomeruli show only focal damage occupying less than 50% of the glomerular surface. The segmental changes can be proliferative, necrotizing, sclerosing, or a combination of these alterations. Segmental intracapillary and extracapillary cell proliferation with obliteration of the capillary lumina is sometimes found in addition to generalized mesangial widening. Segmental necrotic lesions may be associated with crescent formation and progress to segmental scars with focal capsular adhesions. These segmental lesions are usually superimposed on a minimal degree of mesangial hypercellularity (85,86).

Immunofluorescence and electron microscopic findings show major differences in comparison with those of class II. Immunofluorescence reveals peripheral granular as well as mesangial deposits of immunoglobulins, and electron microscopy demonstrates subendothelial deposits in addition to the presence of mesangial deposits (Fig. 14). The similarity of the immunofluorescence and electron microscopic findings of class III to those of class IV suggests that these two classes actually may be variations of the same immunopathologic lesion and that the focal nature of

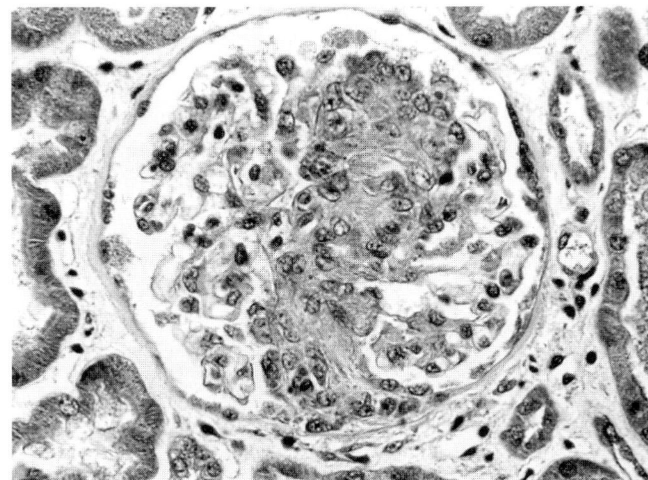

FIG. 13. Focal and segmental necrotizing lupus glomerulonephritis WHO class III. There is a segmental area of necrosis and hypercellularity involving the glomerulus, with adhesion to Bowman's capsule. Nuclear debris is scattered in the necrotic region. The remainder of the glomerulus shows a relatively normal architecture. H&E, ×475.

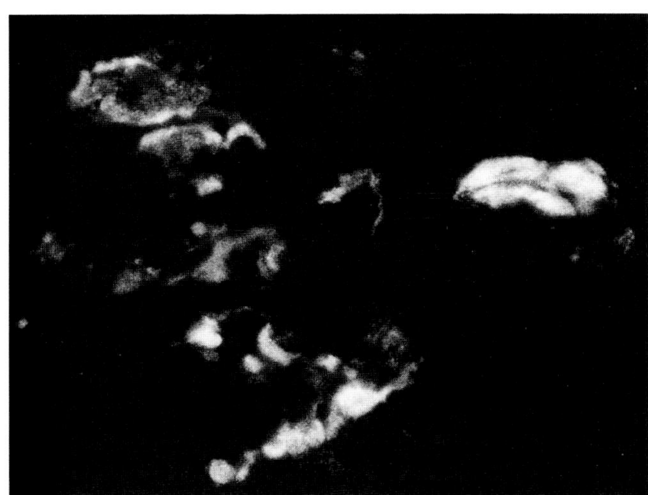

FIG. 14. Immunofluorescence findings in focal segmental lupus glomerulonephritis WHO class III. There is abundant peripheral capillary deposition of immunoglobulins, which is focally more concentrated in areas of necrosis and proliferation. The immunoglobulins are usually accompanied by complement components and fibrinogen. ×300.

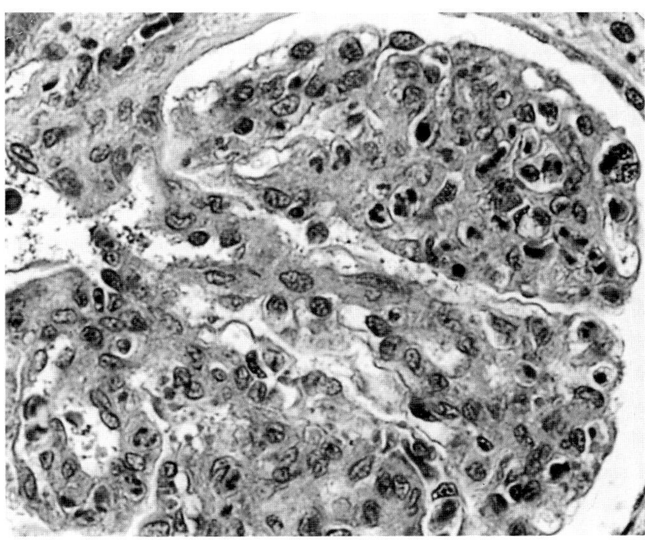

FIG. 15. Diffuse lupus glomerulonephritis WHO class IV. The glomerulus is markedly enlarged; lobular accentuation is associated with marked mesangial hypercellularity, endocapillary proliferation, and leukocyte infiltration. The peripheral capillary walls are focally thickened, and leukocytes can be seen in the capillary lumina. H&E, ×500.

class III lesions represents a quantitative rather than a qualitative difference. Class III has been broken down into three subclasses: active necrotizing lesions, necrotizing and sclerosing lesions, and purely sclerosing lesions. The clinical significance of this subclassification is not clear. The natural history of patients with class III lesions is similar to that of patients having class IV lesions, again suggesting that these two classes represent a continuum of the same lesion (87,88).

Class IV, the most common form of lupus nephritis, is characterized by a diffuse proliferative glomerulonephritis (Fig. 15). The majority or all of the glomeruli are involved, and each glomerulus shows diffuse hypercellularity. As with class III, segmental areas of necrosis can occur, occasionally associated with focal areas of crescent formation. Nuclear debris represented by hemotoxiphil bodies can also be seen. Some segments of peripheral capillary loop can be dramatically thickened to form the so-called wire loop lesion. Segmental areas of sclerosis are an indicator either of previous segmental necrosis or of chronicity. The variety of patterns that can be encountered in this class range from diffuse mesangial hypercellularity without necrosis to a severe necrotizing and crescentic glomerulonephritis with focal and global areas of sclerosis. About a quarter of cases exhibit lobular accentuation with mesangial extension around the peripheral loops, creating a pattern similar to that of other forms of mesangiocapillary glomerulonephritis.

Immunofluorescence microscopy reveals a coarsely granular pattern of immunoglobulin deposition both in the mesangium and the peripheral capillary walls. Multiple immunoglobulins are frequently encountered and are generally accompanied by evidence of activation of inflammatory mediators, such as deposition of complement components, fibrinogen, and properdin. This pattern has been referred to as a "full house" of immunoglobulin deposition.

Electron microscopic findings are similar to those of class III. Abundant subendothelial deposits are accompanied by large mesangial deposits (Fig. 16). These deposits are generally larger and more abundant than

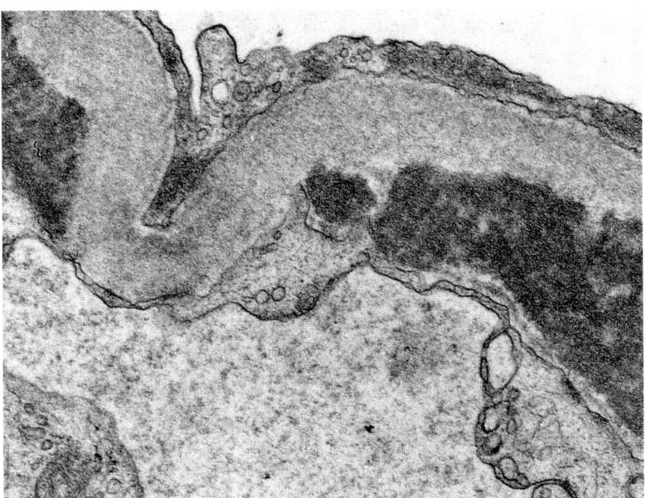

FIG. 16. Electron micrograph of the peripheral capillary loop of a glomerulus from a patient with diffuse lupus glomerulonephritis WHO class IV. A large subendothelial deposit with a somewhat organized appearance that is irregular in electron density separates the endothelial cell from the basement membrane. ×2600.

those in other classes of lupus nephritis. Epimembranous deposits are often present. Mesangial hypercellularity with circumferential mesangial interposition is associated with the light microscopic pattern of a mesangiocapillary glomerulonephritis. Occasionally, the electron-dense deposits show an organized or crystalline pattern, referred to as a "fingerprint" pattern. This organized appearance is most frequently seen in the presence of abundant endothelial deposits but can be present in all classes of lupus nephritis. The crystalline structure is thought by some to represent the presence of cryoglobulins, because similar structures are seen in patients with idiopathic mixed cryoglobulinemia (89). They might also represent a pattern of crystalline DNA (90). Endothelial cell swelling and proliferation are prominent, and occasional mitotic figures of glomerular cellular components suggest active proliferation and regeneration secondary to activation of inflammatory cytokines in growth factors. Intra-endothelial tubular reticular structures resembling myxoviruses have been identified in a majority of all patients with lupus nephropathy (Fig. 17). The significance of these structures is unclear, but some evidence suggests that they are induced by the cytokine interferon-α (91,92). It is likely that this form of lupus nephritis is caused by large numbers of intermediate-sized complexes or large complexes formed by high-affinity antibodies that overcome the mesangial ability to clear these macromolecules (93–95). As a result, these complexes accumulate in a paramesangial subendothelial location and then ultimately in the peripheral capillary loops. Here, they have access to circulating inflammatory mediators, such as complement and platelets, as well as cellular mediators of inflammation, including monocyte macrophages and cytotoxic lymphocytes. The nature of the antigen and antibody may also contribute to the predominance of subendothelial localization in this class (96–98). Some lupus antibodies have been identified to be cationic and therefore nephrotropic, whereas others have been shown to cross-react with native glomerular components. Activation of endothelial adhesion molecules including I-CAM and V-CAM (99,100) is also a prominent feature. A major consequence of severe glomerular inflammation with necrosis is the development of glomerular scarring and sclerosis, resulting in decreased glomerular filtration surface and contributing to progressive renal scarring and loss of function. Class III and class IV lesions represent the most severe form of glomerular involvement in lupus, and patients with class III or class IV pathologic lesions usually have significant clinical renal disease, including proteinuria that is frequently in the nephrotic range, renal insufficiency, and an active urinary sediment.

The class V lesion describes a diffuse membranous glomerulonephropathy. Light microscopy reveals a generalized, diffuse thickening of the peripheral capillary walls that with silver methenamine-Masson staining exhibits a so-called spike-and-dome pattern (Fig. 18). The spikes are outward projections of membranelike material between domes that correspond to the subepithelial and intramembranous deposits seen on immunofluorescence and electron microscopy. A variable degree of mesangial widening may be present, representing both an increase of mesangial cells and mesangial matrix.

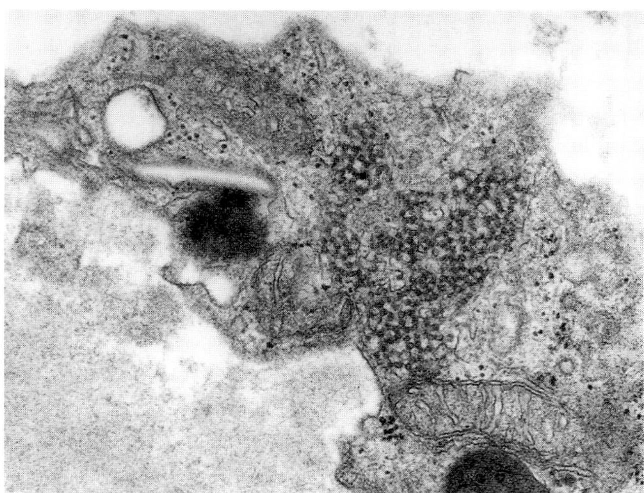

FIG. 17. Electron micrograph of an endothelial cell demonstrating tubular reticular inclusions. These inclusions, seen in almost all patients with lupus glomerulonephritis, are thought to represent activation of the endothelial cells by interferon-α.

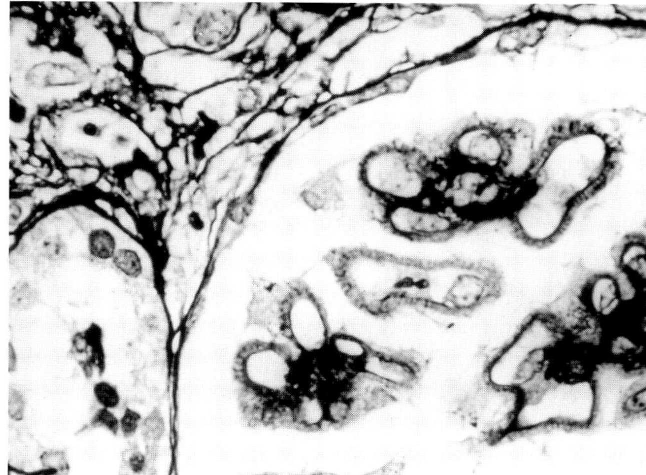

FIG. 18. Membranous lupus glomerulonephropathy WHO class V. There is diffuse thickening of the peripheral capillary wall, and silver staining of the basement membrane demonstrates the typical spike-and-dome pattern produced by the basement membrane spikes that lie between the epimembranous deposits. Jones silver methenamine-Masson stain, ×800.

Immunofluorescence demonstrates a classic confluent peripheral granular deposition of immunoglobulins and occasionally mesangial granular deposits (Fig. 19). Electron microscopy reveals a typical epimembranous nephropathy with subepithelial and intramembranous deposits of varying electron density (Fig. 20). The pattern is essentially identical to that seen in idiopathic membranous glomerulonephropathy (discussed later), except that mesangial deposits are frequently present. The nature of the antigen is likely a major determinant in the pathogenesis of this lesion in lupus. The sera of all patients with lupus contain antibodies directed against a number of auto-antigens, including native and single-stranded DNA, histones, and small ribonuclear proteins of both nuclear and cytoplasmic origin. Of particular importance is the fact that histones are highly cationic and potentially have a high affinity for the anionic sites of the glomerular basement membrane (98). Once bound to the glomerular basement membrane, they can act as a target antigen and a focus for *in situ* complex formation. Such patients would be predicted to have marked proteinuria as the most prominent clinical feature and an indolent course similar to that seen in patients with idiopathic membranous nephropathy (101).

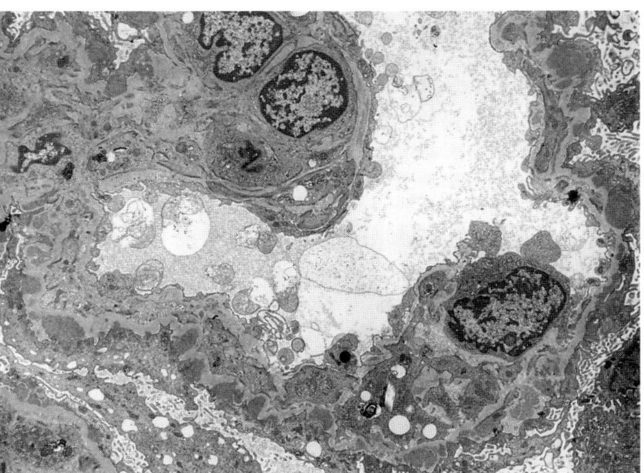

FIG. 20. Electron micrograph of membranous lupus glomerulonephropathy WHO class V. There are abundant subepithelial deposits along the peripheral basement membrane separated by spikes of less electron-dense basement membrane material. Mesangial deposits are also identified. ×3000.

GLOMERULAR LESIONS WITHOUT PROMINENT CELLULAR PROLIFERATION

Lesions that fall into this category are usually associated with the nephrotic syndrome or significant proteinuria in the absence of an "active" sediment indicative of glomerular inflammation. The nephrotic syndrome is characterized clinically by massive proteinuria, hypoproteinemia, edema, and hyperlipidemia. It is the consequence of a major pathophysiologic abnormality of selective glomerular permeability, the mechanism by which serum proteins, in particular albumin, are filtered into the urine and excreted at a rate of more than 3.5 g/24 hours. A spectrum of renal histologic findings has been correlated with this defect, including both immune-mediated and metabolic lesions. Putatively immune-mediated lesions are those of primary nephrotic syndrome with minimal glomerular change and membranous glomerulonephropathy. Metabolic lesions include those associated with diabetes mellitus, amyloidosis, and various forms of hereditary and congenital nephritis.

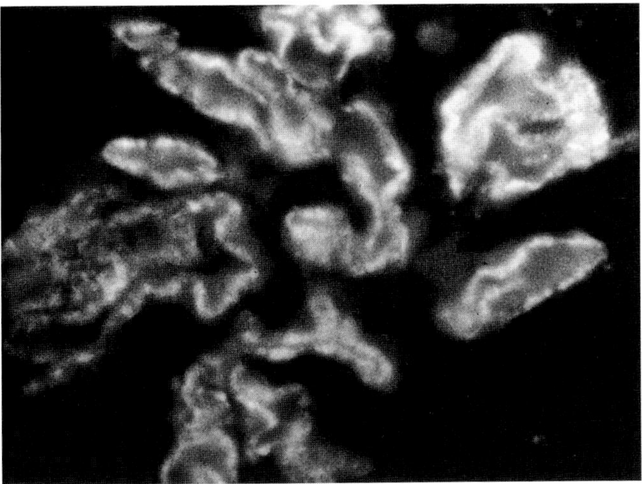

FIG. 19. Immunofluorescence micrograph of membranous lupus glomerulonephropathy WHO class V. In contrast to the findings in class III and class IV (bulky subendothelial deposits), peripheral granular deposition of immunoglobulins in an orderly pseudolinear pattern is seen. ×350.

Minimal-Change Glomerulopathy

Minimal-change disease has been variously called *lipoid nephrosis*, *nil disease*, *minimal-change disease*, *foot process disease*, *visceral epithelial disease*, and *primary nephrotic syndrome*. The term *lipoid nephrosis* was used by pathologists before the advent of electron microscopic examination, as the most prominent feature by light microscopy is vacuolization of the tubular epithelium. Minimal-change disease is 10 to 15 times more common in children than in adults. More than 80% of children with nephrosis have minimal-change disease, whereas only 20–30% of adults with nephrotic syndrome fall into this category (102–104). Among children, boys are affected more often than girls. In the vast majority of pediatric cases, the lesion does not progress to renal insufficiency, although the disease frequently exhibits a relapsing or a cyclical course. Spontaneous remissions can occur, and relapses diminish in frequency after puberty. The onset often follows a viral prodrome, and because the vast majority of children respond to glucocorticoid therapy, the mechanism is thought to be immune-mediated even though antibody deposition is not present. Minimal-change nephrotic syndrome often first appears in adults in their fifth, sixth, and seventh decades at a time when other, unrelated renal abnormalities—such as hypertension, nephrosclerosis, diabetes, or chronic pyelonephritis—may be present (102). A greater percentage of adults appears to be resistant to steroid therapy, and longer periods of therapy are often required to elicit a response. Similarly, whereas the long-term outcome in children is extremely favorable, it is less so in adults, especially when the condition is superimposed on a background of renal vascular disease. Progression to renal insufficiency appears to be more common in adults than in children.

The term *minimal-change disease* comes from the light microscopic histologic picture. Light microscopic examination generally reveals essentially normal-appearing glomeruli ("minimal change") (Fig. 21).Subtle abnormalities can sometimes be identified, including swelling of visceral epithelial cells and a proteinaceous precipitate in Bowman's capsule. In some patients, there may be mild mesangial prominence caused by increases in mesangial cellularity, mesangial matrix, or both. In some instances, the mesangial widening is enough to warrant use of the term *mesangial proliferative glomerulonephritis*. The proximal tubular epithelial cells may be vacuolated or show prominent hyaline droplets or lipid resorption droplets. A loss of staining with colloidal iron and alcian blue in the glomerulus reflects the loss of negatively charged glomerular glycoproteins and therefore of the charge barrier of filtration. Glomerulosclerosis, focal areas of tubular atrophy, and interstitial scarring are generally absent or inconspicuous in children. In adults, the presence of glomerulosclerosis associated with aging or hyaline arteriolosclerosis may make the distinction between minimal-change disease and focal segmental glomerulosclerosis more difficult. In children who have had multiple relapses, subsequent biopsies may show segmental or global sclerosing lesions. The presence of these lesions does not necessarily indicate a change to a more progressive lesion, as it does in focal segmental glomerulosclerosis.

In the majority of cases, results of immunofluorescence examination are usually completely negative. Small amounts of complement and fibrinogen may be found in a commalike pattern in the peripheral capillary walls or in the mesangium. In some patients with mesangial prominence, IgM and complement may be found in a typical mesangial pattern. On very rare occasions, mesangial IgE has been observed. The presence of these proteins does not seem to indicate any adverse clinical effects, such as steroid resistance or potential for progression to renal insufficiency.

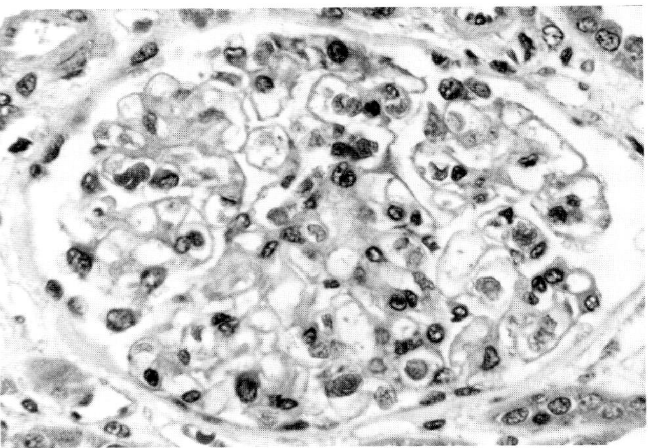

FIG. 21. Minimal-change nephropathy. The architecture is entirely nomal by light microscopy. There is no significant increase in cellularity, and the peripheral capillary loops are thin and delicate with a lacy appearance. The epithelial cells do appear somewhat more prominent. H&E, ×500.

Electron microscopic examination of glomeruli is the gold standard for the diagnosis of this entity. The most prominent changes are found in the visceral epithelial cells. Extensive loss of the normal epithelial cell foot processes occurs on the urinary side of the glomerular basement membrane, so-called foot process fusion with basal condensation of the cytoplasmic microfilaments (Fig. 22). The cell bodies of the visceral epithelial cells in Bowman's space show formation of microvilli and large intracellular pseudocysts. The glomerular basement

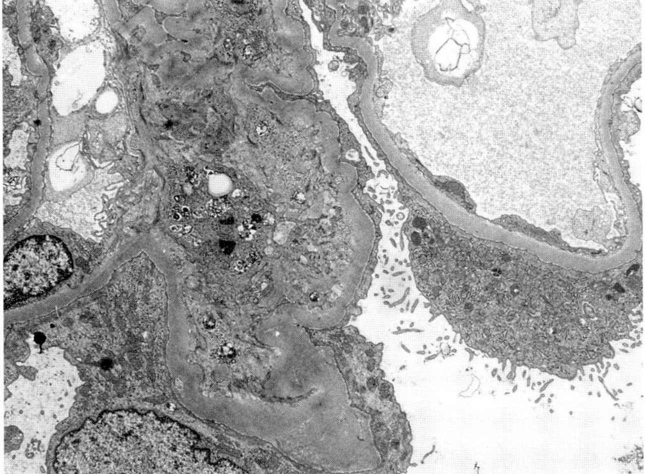

FIG. 22. Minimal-change glomerulonephropathy. Electron micrograph demonstrates a normal peripheral capillary basement membrane with extensive effacement of the epithelial cell foot processes. Microvillus transformation of the epithelial cell is also identified. No deposits are seen, either in the peripheral capillary loops or in the mesangial regions. ×4000.

membrane is of normal thickness and no evidence of immune complex deposition is identified, although focal subendothelial fibrillar material may be found. It should be noted, however, that although the epithelial cell changes are characteristic of this entity, the diagnosis is essentially one of exclusion.

One particular histologic variant of the primary nephrotic syndrome deserves some discussion. In 10–20% of patients within the spectrum of minimal-change disease, there is a more pronounced degree of mesangial hypercellularity and increase in mesangial matrix (105–108). This is often associated with immunofluorescence staining for IgM and C3 and the presence of small mesangial electron-dense deposits by electron microscopy. It is thought that this deposition of IgM is not evidence of immune complex deposition but rather an expression of increased macromolecular transit through the mesangium. Generally, the clinical course of these patients generally is not significantly different from that of patients with very minimal changes, although some may have hematuria and hypertension.

The etiology and pathogenesis of minimal-change disease are unknown, as is the mechanism of the glomerular permeability defect. The association in some cases with a viral prodrome and the occurrence of an identical lesion in a few patients with Hodgkin's disease suggests that a T-cell-mediated immune response may be involved. The recent identification of circulating factors suggests that cytokines may be involved in the permeability defect. The transfer of proteinuria from one animal to others using T-cell transfers is consistent with this proposed mechanism (109). Although many data strongly suggest the involvement of T-cell-mediated immunity, there are insufficient findings to draw any substantive conclusion as to the role of T cells or other immune mechanisms in pathogenesis.

The most important variant in the spectrum of lesions comprising the primary nephrotic syndrome is the presence of focal and segmental glomerulosclerosis (110–113) (Fig. 23). Although the lesion itself is relatively non-specific in that it can be associated with a variety of types of glomerular injury, its presence in patients with the idiopathic nephrotic syndrome makes it a distinct clinical pathologic entity. These patients are initially clinically indistinguishable from individuals with uncomplicated minimal-change disease. A diagnosis of focal segmental sclerosis is considered only after atypical features are noted, such as hypertension, renal insufficiency, hematuria, non-selective proteinuria, or, most commonly, poor or no response to steroid therapy.

By light microscopy, the glomerulosclerosis involves only portions of the glomerular tuft (segmental) of a limited number of glomeruli (focal). Recently, there has been some discussion as to whether the location of the sclerotic lesions has any clinical significance. It has been suggested that the presence of "tip" lesions at the proximal tubular pole of the glomerulus indicates a good prognosis, whereas multiple segmental lesions or hilar lesions are more likely to be steroid-resistant and associated with renal insufficiency (114). Although there may be differences in the pathogenesis of the "tip" versus the "hilar" lesion, at present there is no convincing evidence that the distribution of lesions has any clinical pathologic significance. The sclerotic lesions are generally more common in juxtamedullary glomeruli. Hyaline material is frequently seen in the vascular pole of the glomerulus and in the arterioles. Occasionally, synechiae are present between the segmental sclerotic lesions and Bowman's capsule. Uninvolved portions of the glomerulus may be entirely normal or show mild mesangial hypercellularity and widening (mesangial proliferative glomerulonephritis with focal segmental glomerulosclerosis). Interstitial fibrosis and tubular atrophy are often prominent and may be the only finding in some renal biopsy specimens because of sampling error. Global glomerulosclerosis becomes more prominent as the lesion progresses. Immunofluorescence findings are variable and similar to those of minimal-change glomerulonephropathy but more often reveal the presence of IgM and C3 in a mesangial pattern. By electron microscopy, the sclerotic lesions contain abundant matrix material associated with wrinkled and collapsed glomerular capillary loops . The hyaline deposits observed by light microscopy are electron-dense material that does not have the typical characteristics of immune complexes. The epithelial cells show changes very similar to those of minimal-change disease, with obliteration of the epithelial cell foot processes, but

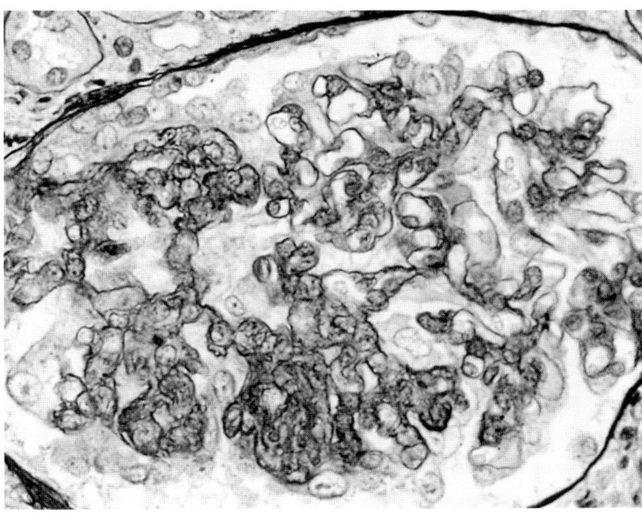

FIG. 23. Focal segmental glomerulosclerosis. Whereas most of the glomerulus has a normal appearance with normal mesangium and lacy peripheral capillary loops, a segmental area of sclerosis is demonstrated by increased amounts of basement membrane-like material stained by silver with obliteration of the normal capillary architecture. Jones silver methenamine-Masson stain, ×500.

occasionally they exhibit more pronounced alterations, including detachment from the basement membrane and denudation of the basement membrane.

Although the pathogenesis of the sclerosis is unclear, several possible mechanisms have been suggested. These include protein overload, hyperfiltration, disordered lipid metabolism, and enhanced intraglomerular coagulation. One interesting explanation offered is that epithelial injury with detachment of visceral epithelial cells from the basement membrane causing focal denudation leads to adhesion to the parietal epithelial cells of Bowman's capsule and formation of a nidus of sclerosis.

Membranous Glomerulonephropathy

Membranous glomerulonephropathy (also termed *membranous nephropathy*, *membranous glomerulonephritis*, *extramembranous glomerulonephritis*, and *epimembranous nephropathy*) is functionally similar to primary nephrotic syndrome with minimal-change nephropathy in that it is characterized by massive proteinuria and the nephrotic syndrome. In contrast to minimal-change nephropathy, however, there is an increased permeability of the glomerular capillaries to serum proteins of high as well as low molecular weight and, in the majority of instances, a gradual but progressive reduction in surface area for ultrafiltration, which leads to some renal insufficiency. In most series of adults with nephrotic syndrome, membranous nephropathy is the most common diagnosis, occurring in approximately 25–30% of all adults with the nephrotic syndrome (115). However, the percentage and incidence of membranous nephropathy in different populations varies. This is likely a consequence of the fact that some cases of so-called idiopathic membranous glomerulonephropathy are associated with a specific identifiable antigen or are secondary to a malignancy, infection, or drug or toxin exposure. Membranous nephropathy is unusual in children. The incidence increases among patients approaching young adulthood (116).

By light microscopy, the glomeruli usually appear moderately enlarged and the mesangium has a mild to moderate degree of prominence. The increase in thickness of the peripheral capillary walls varies from minimal to striking, depending on the stage of the disorder. Where the change is minimal, a stiffness of the glomerular capillary loops is sometimes apparent (Fig. 24). Silver methenamine-Masson stains are particularly useful in evaluating membranous nephropathy, because they reveal a classic spike-and-dome pattern with vacuolization of the thickened peripheral capillary walls. The interstitium may show varying degrees of scarring and tubular atrophy. Some studies suggest that the degree of tubulointerstitial alteration is the best predictor of progression to renal insufficiency. Glomerular capillary thrombosis may occasionally occur and suggests the possibility of large renal vein thrombosis. Margination of the polymorphonuclear leukocytes in the peripheral glomerular capillaries sometimes accompanies renal vein thrombosis.

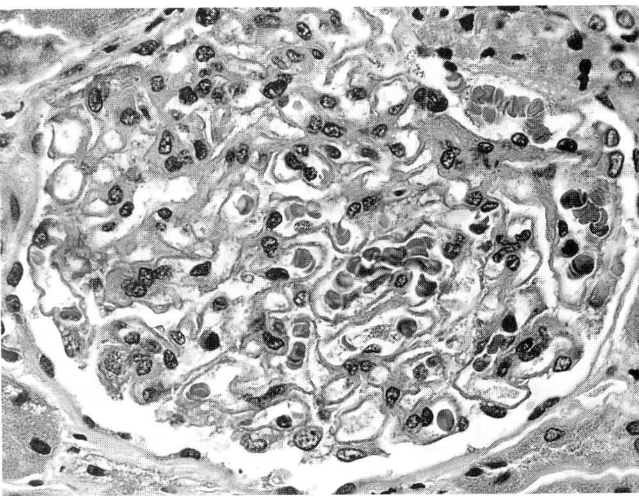

FIG. 24. Membranous glomerulonephropathy. The glomerulus is not strikingly hypercellular. The peripheral capillary loops are thickened and have a rigid appearance. A slight increase in mesangial cellularity is seen focally, with crowding of three to four nuclei. H&E, ×650.

Immunofluorescence staining generally reveals a granular peripheral capillary staining for immunoglobulins (Fig. 25). The extent of the granularity may be so great as to give a pseudolinear appearance. The immunoglobulins most commonly involved in order are IgG, IgM, and IgA. It is of interest that in studies in which IgG subtypes have

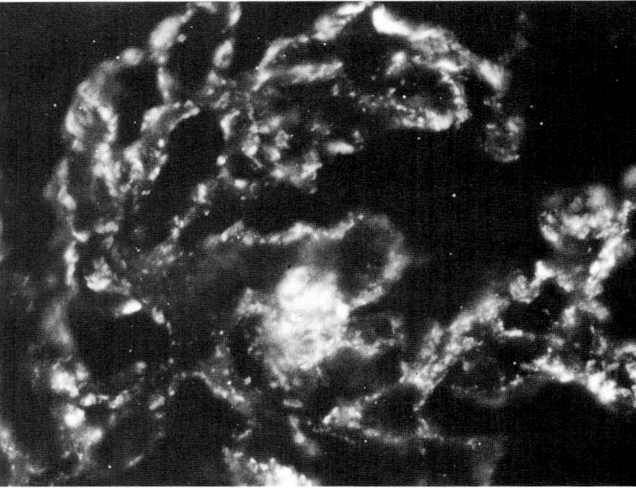

FIG. 25. Membranous glomerulonephropathy. Immunofluorescence demonstrates abundant granular peripheral capillary deposition of immunoglobulin. Complement is frequently found to exist in a similar pattern. The mesangial areas do not show significant immunofluorescence. ×300.

been identified, the IgG in membranous glomerulonephropathy is most commonly IgG4. A granular deposition of C3 is also common; other complement components have not been demonstrated as consistently in a granular pattern. The membrane attack complex C5b-9 has also been found. Mesangial deposits are present in a minority of cases. The finding of mesangial immunoglobulin deposits strongly suggests that an identifiable antigen, such as hepatitis B virus, may be involved.

Electron microscopic studies have described four stages of development of the membranous lesion (117). Although these stages may be useful for descriptive purposes, it is likely that there is a continuum of change from initial immune complex formation to incorporation into the basement membrane and final dissolution. In stage 1 (Fig. 26), scattered electron-dense deposits are noted in an epimembranous pattern, with a relatively normal-appearing glomerular basement membrane. Foot process effacement occurs in relationship to these deposits. The deposits are few and scattered along different portions of the capillary loops. In stage 2 (Fig. 27), subepithelial deposits are more abundant and are separated from each other by the deposition of basement membrane-like material, giving rise to the classic spike-and-dome appearance by light microscopy. In stage 3 (Fig. 28), the apical portions of the spikes form an enclosed basement membrane-like structure so that the deposits are now completely surrounded by basement membrane material and are intramembranous rather than epimembranous. In stage 4 (Fig. 29), there is dissolution of the deposits with rarefaction and evidence of the irregular thickening of glomerular basement membrane repair.

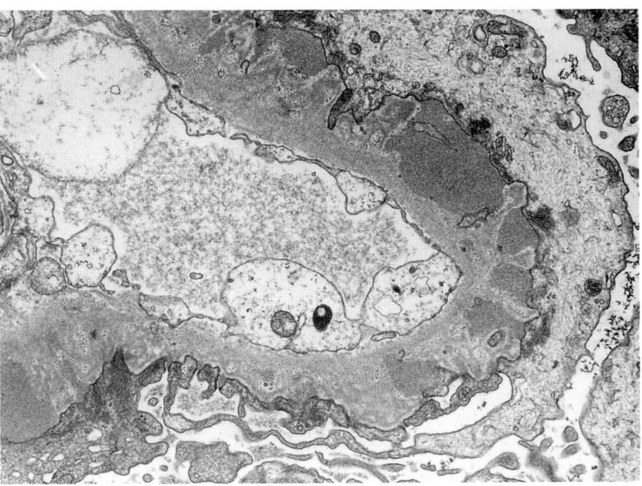

FIG. 27. Membranous glomerulonephropathy stage 2. The subepithelial deposits are more abundant, and basement membranelike material is seen separating the deposits. This gives rise to the spike-and-dome patterns seen with silver methenamine-Masson stains. The result is an irregular thickening of the basement membrane. ×10,500.

Several possible pathogenic mechanisms have been proposed. All suggest that the immune complexes identified by immunofluorescence and electron microscopy are formed at specific sites (3,58). According to one idea, relatively low numbers of circulating immune complexes formed with antibodies of low affinity and avidity

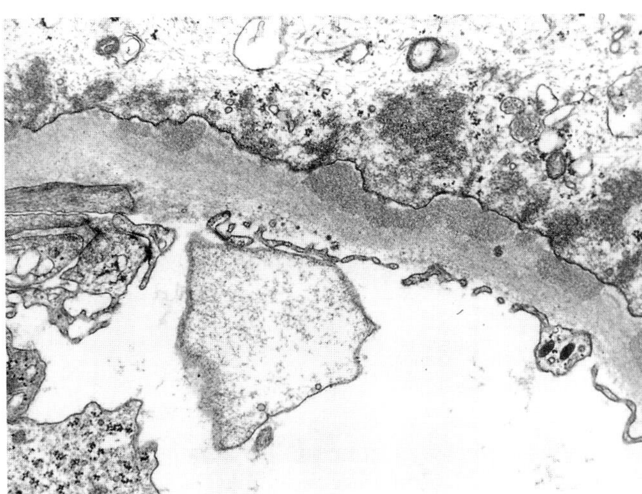

FIG. 26. Membranous glomerulonephropathy stage 1. Electron micrograph demonstrates epimembranous deposits underneath the effaced epithelial cell foot processes. The basement membrane architecture is still preserved; the deposits appear to sit on top of the basement membrane, and only minimal amounts of intervening membrane material are identified. ×15,000.

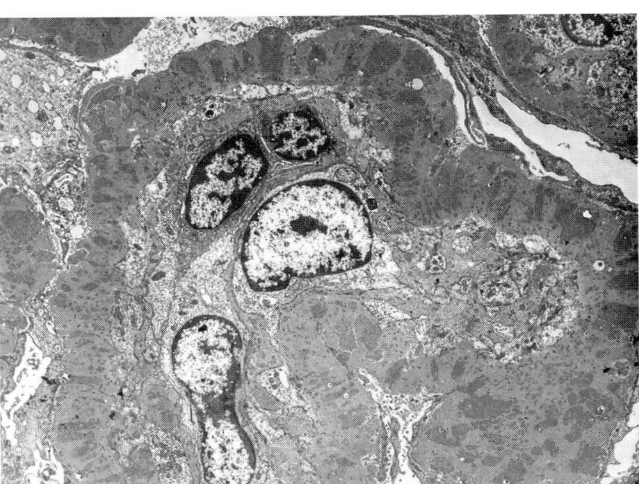

FIG. 28. Membranous glomerulonephropathy stage 3. The basement membrane is irregularly thickened, and electron-dense deposits appear to be incorporated in the basement membrane, with the electron-lucent, basement membrane-like material surrounding the electron-dense deposits. ×2650.

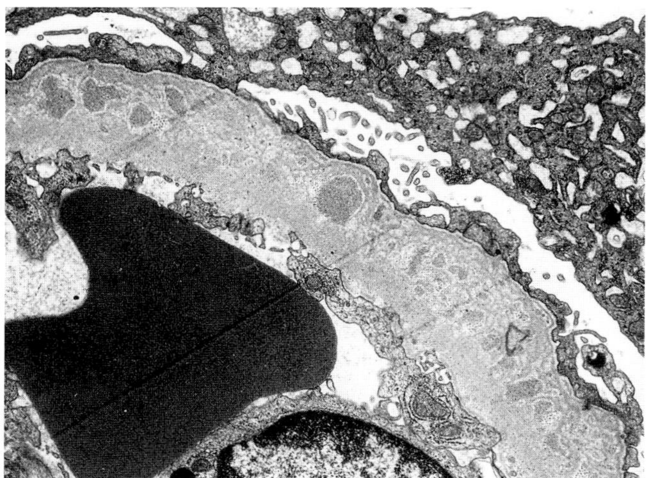

FIG. 29. Membranous glomerulonephropathy stage 4. The basement membrane is irregularly thickened, in some focal areas with electron-dense deposits and in other areas by lucent material; these presumably are regions of basement membrane material that have replaced deposits that have been resorbed. ×8500.

dissociate the antigens localized to the glomerular basement membrane by filtration and form new complexes *in situ* that are stabilized in the basement membrane. A second theory suggests that intrinsic antigens such as specific basement membrane-associated glycoproteins or planted antigens such as bacterial components or lectins serve as the antigenic component of immune complexes formed *in situ*.

AMYLOIDOSIS AND LIGHT CHAIN DISEASE

Although amyloidosis and light chain disease cannot be strictly considered to be immunologically mediated, deposition of these proteins in the kidney is frequently associated with disorders of immune regulation or neoplasia of immunoresponsive cells. Involvement by amyloid and light chains frequently causes heavy proteinuria, with the nephrotic syndrome and renal insufficiency. Although the deposition is often not restricted to the glomerulus, the glomerular manifestations are usually the most prominent. Modulation of glomerular injury is not directed at the glomerulus itself but rather depends on modulation or control of a primary initiating process.

Amyloidosis

Although the single term *amyloidosis* denotes a histopathologic entity characterized by the deposition of a hyaline material, the disease process itself is diverse in terms of clinical manifestations, pathogenesis, and biochemical and immunologic aspects (118,119). The primary fibrillar protein that is seen by electron microscopy and stains with Congo red is amyloid A protein, which forms β-pleated sheets. The amyloid A protein is associated with other proteins, depending on the etiology of the amyloidosis. The most recent classification of amyloidosis is based on the constituent proteins of the fibrils (120). Amyloid AA is formed from a serum precursor called *SAA (serum amyloid-associated) protein* that is synthesized by the liver and circulates together with lipoproteins. AA amyloidosis is usually associated with chronic inflammatory conditions and presumably with chronic immunologic stimulus. A second major type is AL amyloidosis, in which the proteins are composed of immunoglobulin light chains, chiefly of the λ type. AL amyloidosis is associated with multiple myeloma and other monoclonal B-cell proliferations. Less frequently encountered forms of amyloidosis are hereditary types, not all of which are characterized by renal involvement, and several minor forms that are localized to non-renal tissues.

Regardless of the nature of the amyloid protein deposited in the kidney, the histologic findings are essentially identical. Amyloid is an amorphous, homogeneous-appearing substance with a characteristic fibrillar structure by electron microscopy and a β-pleated structure by X-ray defraction. Its structural characteristics make amyloid resistant to proteolysis and are undoubtedly responsible for its accumulation and persistence in tissues. Amyloid deposits usually predominate in the glomeruli and appear as an amorphous eosinophilic material. Congo red stains display an apple green birefringence when examined with polarized light. Amyloid deposits may also involve the tubular basement membranes and vessel walls. Immunofluorescence in amyloid AA may reveal the accumulation of immunoglobulins in the amyloid deposits in a non-specific pattern. AL amyloidosis is characterized by specific deposition of monoclonal λ or κ chains. Electron microscopy reveals regular, non-branching amyloid fibrils ranging from 70 to 120 Å in width and variable in length (Fig. 30). They are generally seen deposited in the mesangium and peripheral capillary basement membrane and may be present as large masses of fibrils that have traversed the glomerular capillary wall to form spikes of basement membrane mixed with amyloid.

Light Chain Disease

In approximately 10% of patients with multiple myeloma, and in an undetermined percentage of patients with other lymphoproliferative disorders, there can be an extracellular deposition of light chains in the blood vessels of many organs, similar to that of amyloidosis (121,122). The glomerulus is a particularly common site of deposition, which causes altered selective permeability and proteinuria (123,124). By light microscopy, the glomeruli show capillary wall thickening and sometimes

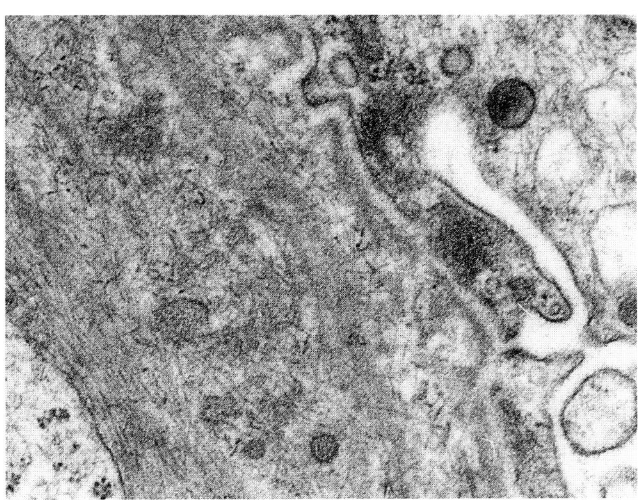

FIG. 30. Glomerular amyloidosis. Electron micrograph demonstrates the deposition of 70- to 100-Å filaments throughout the basement membrane, disrupting the normal basement membrane structure. The fibrils are thin and haphazardly arranged. ×30,000.

a nodular glomerulosclerosis that resembles diabetic glomerulopathy. Immunofluorescence microscopy demonstrates a linear deposition of monoclonal light chains of either κ or λ type. The electron microscopic findings are rather characteristic and show granular electron-dense deposits on the subendothelial side of glomerular basement membranes in a diffuse or sometimes discontinuous linear pattern.

IMMUNE-MEDIATED TUBULOINTERSTITIAL NEPHRITIS

It is now widely recognized that a large variety of drugs—including β-lactam antibiotics, non-steroidal anti-inflammatory drugs, diuretics, anticonvulsants, and an increasingly diverse group of other drugs—can be associated with an allergic, acute tubular interstitial nephritis (125–128). Although the clinical manifestations may be variable, they are usually heralded by fever and hematuria as well as azotemia. Eosinophilia occurs in a majority of cases. Urinalysis reveals hematuria, sterile pyuria, and moderate proteinuria. Eosinophils may be detected in the urinary sediment (129). A skin rash is seen in some patients, lending support to the concept that the renal disease may be a manifestation of a systemic immunologic reaction. The azotemia may be severe, and acute renal failure may develop, prompting the use of renal biopsy as a diagnostic procedure.

Evidence suggests that this form of interstitial nephritis is both immunologically mediated and idiosyncratic. The evidence, which is circumstantial, consists of the frequent presence of a rash and eosinophilia and the fact that the nephritis occurs in only a minority of patients taking normal or subnormal doses of the offending drug (130,131). The nephritis frequently responds to corticosteroid therapy, and there are reports that the disease recurs on re-exposure to the drug. The exact immune mechanisms involved have not been clearly defined, but it is likely that cell-mediated hypersensitivity is involved, as the histologic lesion is very similar to that seen in allograft rejection.

One of the most distinguishing features of acute, drug-induced tubulointerstitial nephritis is the nature of the interstitial infiltrate. The interstitium is edematous, with tubules separated by a pale-staining interstitium (in contrast to the dense staining of fibrosis) and infiltrated with a significant number of eosinophils and mononuclear cells. The infiltrate is characteristically focal and most prominent at the cortical-medullary junction, and it often surrounds individual tubules. The mononuclear portion of the infiltrate is predominantly lymphocytes with some macrophages and plasma cells that sometimes form granulomas. The eosinophils tend to concentrate in small foci and may form eosinophilic microabscesses. Neutrophils can be present but are uncommon. A second distinguishing characteristic is the presence of tubulitis. Particularly with periodic acid–Schiff stains, lymphocytes can be seen invading the tubules beneath the tubular basement membrane. Variable degrees of tubular epithelial cell damage with evidence of regeneration (presence of mitotic figures and pleomorphic nuclei) are almost always found, but extensive necrosis of the epithelium is rare. Additional evidence that the process is immune-mediated has been derived from immunohistochemical analysis of biopsy specimens of such patients. The infiltrate usually has a predominance of T lymphocytes expressing the CD4 antigen, and in most cases there is an enhanced expression of HLA class II antigens on the tubular epithelium (132–135). Immunofluorescence and electron microscopy of such cases have not revealed the presence of immune deposits, further suggesting that the immune process is cell-mediated. The glomeruli are usually not affected, and evidence of vasculitis is generally not seen but does occur in a minority of cases. Although drugs have been implicated in most cases of allergic interstitial nephritis, a similar picture can be found in patients with lupus nephritis (136–139) and rarely in association with anti-tubular basement membrane antibodies. Both the clinical and pathologic findings of lupus interstitial nephritis and anti-tubular basement membrane disease are similar to those seen in allergic, drug-induced tubular interstitial nephritis. Biopsy-proven instances of acute oliguric tubular interstitial nephritis with a similar histologic picture but without any known drug exposure have also been reported (140–142). In one syndrome, occurring mainly in adolescent girls and young women, acute interstitial nephritis is associated with with uveitis and bone marrow and lymph node granulomas (143,144). Granulomas are present in the kidney, and sarcoid involvement must be ruled out.

In considering the differential diagnosis, it must be noted that if the interstitial infiltrate is not prominent, it may be difficult to distinguish acute, drug-induced tubular interstitial nephritis from nephrotoxic tubular injury or ischemic acute tubular necrosis, as a minimal infiltrate with occasional eosinophils has been described in each of these entities. When the interstitial infiltrate is so intense that it forms granulomas, the differential diagnosis must include sarcoidosis. In general, however, sarcoid involvement of the kidney is characterized by the presence of distinct granulomas, with or without areas of central necrosis, that are randomly distributed (145,146). When the granulomas are confluent, involving the glomeruli, or necrosis is prominent, the differential diagnosis must include Wegener's granulomatosis (146–148). Furthermore, whenever an allergic interstitial nephritis with prominent eosinophilic infiltration is identified, the glomeruli and vessels should be carefully examined for the presence of focal and segmental areas of necrosis. The combination of focal and segmental necrotizing glomerulonephritis, even in rare glomeruli, and an acute allergic interstitial nephritis is characteristic of small-vessel vasculitides, including Wegener's granulomatosis (149).

RENAL ALLOGRAFT PATHOLOGY

Evaluation of the renal morphology in allograft patients is used to answer two major questions. Is the failure of the graft caused by rejection or some other, unrelated lesion? If rejection is present, is the lesion potentially reversible with available therapeutic approaches? In the absence of rejection, it should be ascertained whether the graft failure results from acute tubular necrosis, acute infectious pyelonephritis, obstruction of the vasculature or urinary outflow tract, recurrence or onset of glomerular disease, or toxicity associated with the therapeutic agents used to modulate the immune response (150,151). In assessing whether or not rejection lesions are potentially reversible, it is necessary to evaluate not only the intensity but also the nature of the rejection episode.

The Banff schema for the classification of renal allograft pathology is now an internationally accepted, standardized classification of the morphologic changes associated with various types of rejection (152). Interstitial infiltration of activated lymphocytes with tubulitis, characteristic of cellular rejection, and intimal arteritis, characteristic of vascular rejection, are considered the main lesions indicative of acute rejection episodes. A scoring system has been developed to produce an acute or chronic numeric index for purposes of evaluation of severity. The goal of the use of this schema is to give a diagnostic biopsy grade that will provide a prognostic and therapeutic tool. The standardized classification also promotes international uniformity in reporting of renal allograft pathology and is useful to facilitate the performance of multicenter trials of new therapeutic modalities.

Hyperacute Rejection

Hyperacute rejection refers to allograft failure that occurs within minutes or hours after transplantation. It is thought to result from the direction of pre-existing circulating antibodies of the recipient against antigens in the grafted endothelium. Presensitization of the recipient is often related to previous pregnancies, blood transfusions, or other previous antigenic stimuli. However, hyperacute rejections may also be related to endothelial damage that is not immunologic in nature. A separate form of acute graft failure that is not immunologic, termed *acute imminent transplant nephropathy*, has been related to injury occurring in the graft during the preservation phase.

Microscopically, fibrin thrombi are seen in all renal vessels, including the glomerular capillaries and peritubular venules. The vascular thrombosis is associated with infarction and tubular necrosis. Immunofluorescence may show linear staining for immunoglobulins along the capillary walls of the peritubular venules, but this is not a constant finding. Electron microscopy demonstrates platelets, fibrin-sludged red blood cells, and necrosis of glomerular capillaries and other vascular structures.

Acute Rejection

Acute rejection, despite its name, can occur at any time during the course of the life of the allograft. It is most frequently seen during the initial months after grafting but can also occur later in graft life, particularly when disturbances of graft therapy are incurred (153,154). In the Banff classification, the severity is determined by the degree of tubulitis and the presence or absence of intimal arteritis.

Borderline Changes

This category is used to describe acute interstitial cellular rejection of very mild degree. No intimal arteritis is present, and only mild or moderate focal mononuclear cell infiltration in rare foci of mild tubulitis (defined as one to four mononuclear cells per tubular cross-section) is present. This degree of rejection is frequently encountered and probably does not require additional therapy.

Banff Grade I

Grade I or mild acute rejection is characterized by edema and infiltration of the interstitium by immunoblasts, lymphocytes, plasma cells, macrophages, and a scattering of polymorphonuclear leukocytes and eosinophils. The infiltrate is generally diffuse but appears somewhat more concentrated around vessels in glomeruli. More than 25% of the parenchyma is affected, and numerous foci of moderate tubulitis with more than four mononuclear cells per tubular cross-section or group of ten tubular cells are considered characteristic. Analysis of the lymphocytes in the infiltrate demonstrates a large population of T cells (identified by the C3 antigen) and a greater number of cytotoxic T cells (identified by the CD8 antigen) than helper-inducer T cells (identified by the CD4 antigen). The ratio of activation antigens RO and RA is also of use in identifying the activity of the rejection.

Banff Grade II

Grade IIA or moderate acute interstitial cellular rejection is characterized by a significant interstitial infiltrate and foci of severe tubulitis, with more than 10 mononuclear cells per tubular cross-section, but no significant intimal arteritis. Endothelial swelling may be present, but infiltration of the vascular wall by lymphocytes is not. This is essentially a more severe form of grade I allograft rejection that is characterized primarily by the absence of any evidence of significant vascular rejection. This degree of rejection generally has a good response to antirejection therapy.

Grade IIB or moderate acute rejection with a vascular component consists of cases with mild to moderate intimal arteritis in addition to any degree of interstitial cellular rejection. Intimal arteritis is defined as intimal thickening with inflammation of the arterial subendothelial space ranging, from rare intimal inflammatory cells to necrosis of the endothelium with deposition of fibrin, platelets, and inflammatory cells. The cellular infiltrate is composed of lymphocytes and monocytes. Severity is determined by the number of vessels affected as well as the intensity of the individual lesions. Mild degrees of intimal arteritis seen in this category are often focal. Response to therapy is more variable in this group.

Banff Grade III

Grade III is characterized by a severe, acute combination of cellular and vascular rejection. These are cases with severe intimal arteritis or transmural arteritis, defined by injury and inflammation of the whole arterial wall including the media, necrosis of medial smooth muscles, fibrin deposition, and cellular infiltration with mononuclear as well as polymorphonuclear leukocytes. Focal infarction and interstitial hemorrhage without other obvious cause can be assumed to be associated with vascular lesions consistent with this degree of rejection. Rejection episodes of this severity are often associated with graft loss.

Chronic Rejection

Chronic rejection occurs anywhere from several months to several years after transplantation (155–159). Clinically, it is associated with a slow and gradual decrease in renal function, in contrast to the more sudden loss of renal function seen in acute rejection. Microscopically, the picture is similar to that of nephrosclerosis. There is arterial and arteriolar narrowing of the interlobular arcuate and radial arteries by myointimal proliferation and medial hypertrophy. The vascular lesions are associated with a diffuse interstitial fibrosis and tubular atrophy. The glomerular lesions of chronic rejection consist of ischemic glomerular capillary collapse, thickening of the capillary walls, and segmental and global sclerosis. By electron microscopy, the glomeruli show varying degrees of glomerulosclerosis, with an increase in mesangial matrix, mesangial interposition, and irregular thickening of basement membrane (transplant glomerulopathy). Occasionally, there is separation of the endothelial cells from the basement membrane with the accumulation of a granular material in the subendothelial space. Chronic allograft nephropathy has also been graded in the Banff schema: grade I denotes mild interstitial fibrosis and tubular atrophy; grade II, moderate degrees; grade III, severe interstitial tubular atrophy and tubular loss. The mechanisms involved are still unknown, but humoral immunity directed against vascular cellular antigens has been suggested as a likely possibility (155,160–162).

REFERENCES

1. Von Pirquet C. Allergy. *Arch Intern Med* 1911;7:259.
2. Dixon F. The pathogenesis of glomerulonephritis. *Am J Med* 1968;44: 493–495.
3. Couser WG. Pathogenesis of glomerulonephritis. *Kidney Int* 1993;42 [Suppl]:S19–26.
4. Barnes JL, Milani S. *In situ* hybridization in the study of the kidney and renal diseases. *Semin Nephrol* 1995;15:9–28.
5. Alpers CE. Immunotactoid (microtubular) glomerulopathy: an entity distinct from fibrillary glomerulonephritis? [see Comments]. *Am J Kidney Dis* 1992;19:185–191.
6. Kimmel PL, Phillips TM, Ferreira-Centeno A, Farkas-Szallasi T, Abraham AA, Garrett CT. HIV-associated immune-mediated renal disease. *Kidney Int* 1993;44:1327–1340.
7. Lin CY. Hepatitis B virus deoxyribonucleic acid in kidney cells probably leading to viral pathogenesis among hepatitis B virus associated membranous nephropathy patients. *Nephron* 1993;63:58–64.
8. Nadasdy T, Park CS, Peiper SC, Wenzl JE, Oates J, Silva FG. Epstein-Barr virus infection-associated renal disease: diagnostic use of molecular hybridization technology in patients with negative serology. *J Am Soc Nephrol* 1992;2:1734–1742.
9. Nadasdy T, Miller KW, Johnson LD, Hanson-Painton O, DeBault LE, Burns DK, Hawkins E, Silva FG. Is cytomegalovirus associated with renal disease in AIDS patients? *Mod Pathol* 1992;5:277–282.
10. Waldherr R, Noronha IL, Niemir Z, Kruger C, Stein H, Stumm G. Expression of cytokines and growth factors in human glomerulonephritides. *Pediatr Nephrol* 1993;7:471–478.
11. Safirstein R, Megyesi J, Saggi SJ, Price PM, Poon M, Rollins BJ, Taubman MB. Expression of cytokine-like genes JE and KC is increased during renal ischemia. *Am J Physiol* 1991;261:F1095–1101.
12. Johnson RJ, Floege J, Couser WG, Alpers CE. Role of platelet-derived growth factor in glomerular disease [Editorial]. *J Am Soc*

Nephrol 1993;4:119–128 [published erratum appears in *J Am Soc Nephrol* 1993;4:1237].
13. Jenkins DA, Wojtacha DR, Swan P, Fleming S, Cumming AD. Intrarenal localization of interleukin-1 beta mRNA in crescentic glomerulonephritis. *Nephrol Dial Transplant* 1994;9:1228–1233.
14. Alpers CE, Seifert RA, Hudkins KL, Johnson RJ, Bowen-Pope DF. PDGF-receptor localizes to mesangial, parietal epithelial, and interstitial cells in human and primate kidneys. *Kidney Int* 1993;43: 286–294.
15. Bruijn JA, Roos A, de Geus B, de Heer E. Transforming growth factor-beta and the glomerular extracellular matrix in renal pathology. *J Lab Clin Med* 1994;123:34–47.
16. Pichler R, Giachelli C, Young B, Alpers CE, Couser WG, Johnson RJ. The pathogenesis of tubulointerstitial disease associated with glomerulonephritis: the glomerular cytokine theory. *Miner Electrolyte Metab* 1995;21:317–327.
17. Alpers CE, Hudkins KL, Floege J, Johnson RJ. Human renal cortical interstitial cells with some features of smooth muscle cells participate in tubulointerstitial and crescentic glomerular injury. *J Am Soc Nephrol* 1994;5:201–209.
18. Ziyadeh FN. Mediators of hyperglycemia and the pathogenesis of matrix accumulation in diabetic renal disease. *Miner Electrolyte Metab* 1995;21:292–302.
19. Kashgarian M, Hayslett J, Spargo B. Renal disease. *Am J Pathol* 1977;89:187–272.
20. Pirani C, Salinas-Madrigal L, Koss M. Evaluation of percutaneous renal biopsy. In: Sommers S, ed. *Kidney Pathology Decennial, 1966–1975*. New York: Appleton-Century-Crofts; 1975.
21. Churg J, Bernstein J, Glassock R. *Renal Disease*. New York: Igaku-Shoin; 1995 (classification and atlas of glomerular diseases).
22. Zollinger H, Mihatsch N. *Renal Pathology and Biopsy*. Berlin: Springer-Verlag; 1978 (light, electron, and immunofluorescent microscopy and clinical aspects).
23. Whitley K, Keane WF, Vernier RL. Acute glomerulonephritis. A clinical overview. *Med Clin North Am* 1984;68:259–279.
24. Simckes AM, Spitzer A. Poststreptococcal acute glomerulonephritis. *Pediatr Rev* 1995;16:278–279.
25. Earle D. Natural history of acute glomerulonephritis in adults. In: Metcoff J, ed. *Acute Glomerulonephritis*. Boston: Little, Brown; 1967.
26. Reid HF, Bassett DC, Gaworzewska E, Colman G, Poon-King T. Streptococcal serotypes newly associated with epidemic post-streptococcal acute glomerulonephritis. *J Med Microbiol* 1990;32:111–114.
27. Kostrzynska M, Schalen C, Wadstrom T. Specific binding of collagen type IV to *Streptococcus pyogenes*. *FEMS Microbiol Lett* 1989;50: 229–233.
28. Gunzenhauser JD, Longfield JN, Brundage JF, Kaplan EL, Miller RN, Brandt CA. Epidemic streptococcal disease among army trainees, July 1989 through June 1991. *J Infect Dis* 1995;172:124–131.
29. Cronin W, Deol H, Azadegan A, Lange K. Endostreptosin: isolation of the probable immunogen of acute post-streptococcal glomerulonephritis (PSGN). *Clin Exp Immunol* 1989;76:198–203.
30. Jeffrey RF, More IA, Carrington D, Briggs JD, Junor BJ. Acute glomerulonephritis following infection with *Chlamydia psittaci*. *Am J Kidney Dis* 1992;20:94–96.
31. Quigg RJ, Gaines R, Wakely PE Jr, Schoolwerth AC. Acute glomerulonephritis in a patient with Rocky Mountain spotted fever. *Am J Kidney Dis* 1991;17:339–342.
32. Rosenberg HG, Vial SU, Pomeroy J, Figueroa S, Donoso PL, Carranza C. Acute glomerulonephritis in children. An evolutive morphologic and immunologic study of the glomerular inflammation. *Pathol Res Pract* 1985;180:633–643.
33. Dodge W, Spargo B, Bass J, Travis L. The relationship between the clinical and pathologic features of poststreptococcal glomerulonephritis. A study of the early natural history. *Medicine* 1986;47: 227–267.
34. Jennings R, Earle D. Post-streptococcal glomerulonephritis. Histopathologic and clinical studies of the acute, subsiding acute, and early chronic latent phases. *J Clin Invest* 1961;40:1525–1595.
35. Michael A, Drummond K, Good R, Vernier R. Acute post-streptococcal glomerulonephritis. Immune deposit disease. *J Clin Invest* 1966; 45:237–248.
36. Travis L, Dodge W, Bethard G, Spargo B, Lorentz W, Carvajal H, Bergen M. Acute glomerulonephritis in children. A review of the natural history with emphasis on prognosis. *Clin Nephrol* 1973;1:169–181.
37. Tornroth T. The fate of subepithelial deposits in acute poststreptococcal glomerulonephritis. *Lab Invest* 1976;35:461–474.
38. Bancani R, Valasquez F, Kanter A, Pirani C, Pollak V. Rapidly progressive (nonstreptococcal) glomerulonephritis. *Ann Intern Med* 1968;69:463–485.
39. Glassock R. A clinical and immunopathologic dissection of rapidly progressive glomerulonephritis. *Nephron* 1978;2:253–264.
40. Andrassy K, Kuster S, Waldherr R, Ritz E. Rapidly progressive glomerulonephritis: analysis of prevalence and clinical course. *Nephron* 1991;59:206–212.
41. Ferrario F, Tadros MT, Napodano P, Sinico RA, Fellin G, D'Amico G. Critical re-evaluation of 41 cases of "idiopathic" crescentic glomerulonephritis. *Clin Nephrol* 1994;41:1–9.
42. Jennette JC, Falk RJ, Wilkman AS. Anti-neutrophil cytoplasmic autoantibodies—a serologic marker for vasculitides. *Ann Acad Med Singapore* 1995;24:248–253.
43. Mrowka C, Csernok E, Gross WL, Feucht HE, Bechtel U, Thoenes GH. Distribution of the granulocyte serine proteinases proteinase 3 and elastase in human glomerulonephritis. *Am J Kidney Dis* 1995;25: 253–261.
44. Saeki T, Kuroda T, Morita T, Suzuki K, Arakawa M, Kawasaki K. Significance of myeloperoxidase in rapidly progressive glomerulonephritis. *Am J Kidney Dis* 1995;26:13–21.
45. Olsen S. Extracapillary glomerulonephritis. *Acta Pathol Microbiol Scand* 1974;82[Suppl 249]:29–54.
46. Stilmant M, Bolton W, Sturgill B, Schmitt G, Couser W. Crescentic glomerulonephritis without immune deposits. Clinicopathologic features. *Kidney Int* 1979;15:184–195.
47. Lewis E, Cavallo T, Harrington J, Cotran R. An immunopathologic study of rapidly progressive glomerulonephritis in the adult. *Hum Pathol* 1971;2:185–208.
48. Wilson C, Dixon F. Anti-glomerular basement membrane antibody induced glomerulonephritis. *Kidney Int* 1973;3:74–89.
49. Berger J, Hinglais N. Les dépots intercapillaires d'IgA-IgG. *J Urol Nephrol* 1968;74:694–695.
50. D'Amico G, Imbasciati E, Barbiano Di Belgioioso G, Bertoli S, Fogazzi G, Ferrario F, Fellin G, Ragni A, Colosanti G, Minetti L, Ponticelli C. Idiopathic IgA mesangial nephropathy. Clinical and histological study of 374 patients. *Medicine* 1985;64:49–60.
51. West C. Asymptomatic hematuria and proteinuria in children. Causes and appropriate diagnostic studies. *J Pediatr* 1976;89:173–182.
52. D'Amico G. The natural history of IgA disease. *Contrib Nephrol* 1989;70:116–120.
53. D'Amico G, Ragni A, Torpia R. Factors of progression in IgA mesangial nephropathy. *Contrib Nephrol* 1989;75:76–81.
54. Habib R, Murcia I, Beaufils H, Niaudet P. Primary IgA nephropathies in children. *Biomed Pharmacother* 1990;44:159–162.
55. Magil AB, Ballon HS. IgA nephropathy. Evaluation of prognostic factors in patients with moderate disease. *Nephron* 1987;47:246–252.
56. Okada K, Funai M, Kawakami K, Kagami S, Yano I, Kuroda Y. IgA nephropathy in Japanese children and adults: a comparative study of clinicopathological features. *Am J Nephrol* 1990;10:191–197.
57. Jennette JC. The immunohistology of IgA nephropathy. *Am J Kidney Dis* 1988;12:348–352.
58. Couser WG, Salant DJ. *In situ* immune complex formation and glomerular injury. *Kidney Int* 1980;17:1–13.
59. Zamurovic D, Churg J. Idiopathic and secondary mesangiocapillary glomerulonephritis. *Nephron* 1984;38:145–153.
60. D'Amico G, Ferrario F. Mesangiocapillary glomerulonephritis. *J Am Soc Nephrol* 1992;2[10 Suppl]:S159–166.
61. Burkholder PM, Marchand A, Krueger RP. Mixed membranous and proliferative glomerulonephritis. A correlative light, immunofluorescence, and electron microscopic study. *Lab Invest* 1970;23:459–479.
62. Habib R, Gubler MC, Loirat C, Ben Maiz H, Levy M. Dense deposit disease. A variant of membranoproliferative glomerulonephritis. *Kidney Int* 1975;7:204–215.
63. Bennett WM, Fassett RG, Walker RG, Fairley KF, d'Apice AJ, Kincaid-Smith P. Mesangiocapillary glomerulonephritis type II (dense-deposit disease): clinical features of progressive disease. *Am J Kidney Dis* 1989;13:469–476.
64. Strife CF, Leahy AE, West CD. Antibody to a cryptic solid phase C1Q antigen in membranoproliferative nephritis. *Kidney Int* 1989;35: 836–842.
65. Cameron JS, Turner DR, Heaton J, Williams DG, Ogg CS, Chantler

C, Haycock GB, Hicks J. Idiopathic mesangiocapillary glomerulonephritis. Comparison of types I and II in children and adults and long-term prognosis. *Am J Med* 1983;74:175–192.
66. Burkholder PM, Hyman LR, Krueger RP. Characterization of mixed membranous and proliferative glomerulonephritis: recognition of three varieties. *Perspect Nephrol Hypertens* 1973;1:557–589.
67. Burkholder PM. Immunopathology of renal disease. *Clin Lab Med* 1986;6:55–83.
68. Alpers CE. Fibrillary glomerulonephritis and immunotactoid glomerulopathy: two entities, not one [Editorial; Comment]. *Am J Kidney Dis* 1993;22:448–451.
69. D'Amico G, Fornasieri A. Cryoglobulinemic glomerulonephritis: a membranoproliferative glomerulonephritis induced by hepatitis C virus. *Am J Kidney Dis* 1995;25:361–369.
70. Johnson RJ, Gretch DR, Yamabe H, Hart J, Bacchi CE, Hartwell P, Couser WG, Corey L, Wener MH, Alpers CE, et al. Membranoproliferative glomerulonephritis associated with hepatitis C virus infection [see Comments]. *N Engl J Med* 1993;328:465–470.
71. Davda R, Peterson J, Weiner R, Croker B, Lau JY. Membranous glomerulonephritis in association with hepatitis C virus infection. *Am J Kidney Dis* 1993;22:452–455.
72. Muehrcke RC, Kark RM, Pirani CL, Pollak VE. Lupus nephritis: a clinical and pathologic study based on renal biopsies. *Medicine* 1957;36:1–145.
73. Klemperer P, Pollack AD, Baehr G. Pathology of disseminated lupus erythematosus. *Arch Pathol* 1941;32:569–631.
74. Baldwin D, Lowenstein J, Rothfield N, Gallo G, McCluskey R. The clinical causes of the proliferative and membranous form of lupus nephritis. *Ann Intern Med* 1970;73:929.
75. Baldwin DS, Gluck MG, Lowenstein MJ, Gallo GR. Lupus nephritis: Clinical causes as related to morphological forms and their transitions. *Am J Med* 1977;62:12–30.
76. Comerford FR, Cohen AS. The nephropathy of systemic lupus erythematosus: an assessment of clinical, light and electron microscopic criteria. *Medicine* 1967;46:425.
77. Pollak V, Pirani C. Renal histologic findings in systemic lupus erythematosus. *Mayo Clin Proc* 1969;44:63.
78. Estes D, Christian CL. The natural history of systemic lupus erythematosus by prospective analysis. *Medicine* 1971;50:85–95.
79. Ginzler EM, Diamond HS, Weiner M, Schlesinger M, Fries JF, Wasner C, Medsger TA, Zieger G, Klippel JH, Hadler NM, Albert DA, Hess EV, Spencer-Green G, Grayzel A, Worth D, Hahn BH, Barnett EV. A multicenter study of outcome of systemic lupus erythematosus. Entry variables as predictors of progress. *Arthritis Rheum* 1982;25: 601–611.
80. Wallace DJ, Podell T, Weiner J, Klinenberg JR, Forouzesh S, Dubois EL. Systemic lupus erythematosus—survival patterns. Experience with 609 patients. *JAMA* 1981;245:934–938.
81. Wallace DJ, Podell TE, Weiner JM, Cox MB, Klinenberg JR, Forouzesh S, Dubois EL. Lupus nephritis. Experience with 230 patients in a private practice from 1950–1980. *Am J Med* 1982;72: 209–220.
82. McCluskey R. Lupus nephritis. *Kidney Pathology*. New York: Appleton-Century-Crofts; 1975:456–459.
83. Domoto DT, Kashgarian M, Hayslett JP, Adler M, Siegel NJ. The significance of electron dense deposits in mild lupus nephritis. *Yale J Biol Med* 1980;53:314–324.
84. Germuth F, Rodriguez E. *Immunopathology of the Renal Glomerulus*. Boston: Little, Brown; 1973.
85. Monga G, Mazzucco G, di Belgiojoso B, Busnach G. The presence and possible role of monocyte infiltration in human chronic proliferation glomerulonephritis. *Am J Pathol* 1979;94:271–284.
86. Schreiner GF, Cotran RS, Pardo V, Unanue EM. A mononuclear cell component in experimental immunological glomerulonephritis. *J Exp Med* 1978;147:369–384.
87. Appel G, Silva F, Pirani C, Meltzer J, Estes D. Renal involvement in systemic lupus erythematosus. *Medicine* 1978;57:371.
88. Hayslett J, Kashgarian M, Cook CD, BH S. The effect of azathioprine on lupus glomerulonephritis. *Medicine* 1970;49:411.
89. Grishman E, Porush J, Rosen S, Churg J. Lupus nephritis with organized deposits in the kidneys. *Nephron* 1973;10:25.
90. Kim Y, Choi Y, Reiner L. Ultrastructural fingerprint in cryoprecipitate and glomerular deposits. A case report of systemic lupus erythmatosus. *Hum Pathol* 1991;12:86.
91. Riche SA. Human lupus inclusions and interferon. *Science* 1981; 213:772.
92. Schaff Z, Barry DW, Grimley PM. Cytochemistry of tubuloreticular structures in lymphocytes from patients with systemic lupus erythematosus and in cultured human lymphoid cells: comparison to a paramyxovirus. *Lab Invest* 1973;29:557–586.
93. Sakamoto H, Ooshima A. Activation of neutrophil phagocytosis of complement-coated and IgG-coated sheep erythrocytes by platelet release products. *Br J Haematol* 1985;60:173.
94. Johnson R, Couser W, Chi E, Adler S, Klebanott D. New mechanisms for glomerular injury. Myeloperoxidase-hydrogen peroxide-halide system. *J Clin Invest* 1987;79:1379.
95. Johnson R, Alpers C, Pritzi P, Schulze N, Baker P, Oruchno C, Couser W. Platelet-mediated neutrophil-dependent immune complex nephritis in the rat. *J Clin Invest* 1988;82:1225.
96. Vlahakos D, Foster M, Adams S, Katz M, Ucci A, Barrett K, Datta S, Madaio M. Anti-DNA antibodies form immune deposits at distinct glomerular and vascular sites. *Kidney Int* 1992;41:1690–1700.
97. Termaat R, Assmann K, Dijkman H, Van Gompel F, Smeenk R, Berden J. Anti-DNA antibodies can bind to the glomerulus via two distinct mechanisms. *Kidney Int* 1992;42:1363–1371.
98. Schmiedeke T, Stockli FW, Weber R, Sugisaki Y, Batsford SR, Voat A. Histones have high affinity for the glomerular basement mebrane. *J Exp Med* 1989;169:1879–1894.
99. Bruijn J, Dinklo J. Distinct patterns of expression of ICAM-1, VCAM-1 and ELAM-1 in renal disease. *Lab Invest* 1993;69: 329–335.
100. Nishikawa K, Guo Y, Miyasaka M, Tamatani T, Collins A, Sy M, McCluskey R, Andres G. Antibodies to 1CAM-1/CFA-1 prevent crescent formations in rat autoimmune glomerulonephritis. *J Exp Med* 1993;177:667–677.
101. Schwartz MM, Kawala K, Roberts JL, Humes C, Lewis EJ. Clinical and pathological features of membranous glomerulonephritis of systemic lupus erythematosus. *Am J Nephrol* 1984;29:311.
102. Cameron JS, Turner DR, Ogg CS, Sharpstone P, Brown CB. The nephrotic syndrome in adults with "minimal change" glomerular lesions. *Q J Med* 1974;43:461–488.
103. Churg J, Habib R, White RHR. Pathology of the nephrotic syndrome in children. A report for the International Study of Kidney Disease in Children. *Lancet* 1970;1:1299–1302.
104. Anonymous. Report of the International Study of Kidney Disease in Children: nephrotic syndrome in children. Prediction of histopathology from clinical and laboratory characteristics at time of diagnosis. *Kidney Int* 1978;13:159–165.
105. Anonymous. Report of the Southwest Pediatric Nephrology Study Group: childhood nephrotic syndrome associated with diffuse mesangial hypercellularity. *Kidney Int* 1983;23:87–94.
106. Anonymous. Report of the International Study of Kidney Disease in Children: primary nephrotic syndrome in children. Clinical significance of histopathologic variants of minimal change and of diffuse mesangial hypercellularity. *Kidney Int* 1981;20:765–771.
107. Glassock RJ. Natural history and treatment of primary proliferative glomerulonephritis: a review. *Kidney Int Suppl* 1985;17:S136–142.
108. Siegel NJ, Gaudio KM, Krassner LS, McDonald BM, Anderson FP, Kashgarian M. Steroid-dependent nephrotic syndrome in children: histopathology and relapses after cyclophosphamide treatment. *Kidney Int* 1981;19:454–459.
109. Ritz E. Pathogenesis of "idiopathic" nephrotic syndrome [Editorial; Comment]. *N Engl J Med* 1994;330:61–62.
110. Anonymous. Focal segmental glomerulosclerosis in children with idiopathic nephrotic syndrome. A report of the Southwest Pediatric Nephrology Study Group. *Kidney Int* 1985;27:442–449.
111. Cameron JS, Turner DR, Ogg CS, Chantler C, Williams DG. The long-term prognosis of patients with focal segmental glomerulosclerosis. *Clin Nephrol* 1978;10:213–218.
112. Siegel NJ, Kashgarian M, Spargo BH, Hayslett JP. Minimal change and focal sclerotic lesions in lipoid nephrosis. *Nephron* 1974;13:125–137.
113. Kashgarian M. Lipoid nephrosis and focal sclerosis. Distinct entities on spectrum of disease. *Nephron* 1974;13:105–108.
114. Huppes W, Hene RJ, Kooiker CJ. The glomerular tip lesion: a distinct entity or not? *J Pathol* 1988;154:187–190.
115. Cameron JS. Membranous nephropathy and its treatment. *Nephrol Dial Transplant* 1992;7[Suppl 1]:72–79.

116. Habib R, Kleinknecht C. The primary nephrotic syndrome of childhood. Classification and clinicopathologic study of 406 cases. *Pathol Annu* 1971;6:417–474.
117. Ehrenreich T, Churg J. Pathology of membranous nephropathy. *Pathol Annu* 1968;3:145–186.
118. Cohen AS, Jones LA. Amyloid and amyloidosis. *Curr Opin Rheumatol* 1992;4:94–105.
119. Bohle A, Wehrmann M, Eissele R, von Gise H, Mackensen-Haen S, Muller C. The long-term prognosis of AA and AL renal amyloidosis and the pathogenesis of chronic renal failure in renal amyloidosis. *Pathol Res Pract* 1993;189:316–331.
120. Kyle RA. Monoclonal proteins and renal disease. *Annu Rev Med* 1994;45:71–77.
121. Morel-Maroger L, Verroust P. Glomerular lesions in dysproteinemias. *Kidney Int* 1974;5:249–252.
122. Pozzi C, Fogazzi GB, Banfi G, Strom EH, Ponticelli C, Locatelli F. Renal disease and patient survival in light chain deposition disease. *Clin Nephrol* 1995;43:281–287.
123. Picken MM, Shen S. Immunoglobulin light chains and the kidney: an overview. *Ultrastruct Pathol* 1994;18:105–112.
124. Sanders PW, Herrera GA. Monoclonal immunoglobulin light chain-related renal diseases. *Semin Nephrol* 1993;13:324–341.
125. Neelakantappa K, Gallo GR, Lowenstein J. Ranitidine-associated interstitial nephritis and Fanconi syndrome. *Am J Kidney Dis* 1993; 22:333–336.
126. Rashed A, Azadeh B, Abu Romeh SH. Acyclovir-induced acute tubulo-interstitial nephritis. *Nephron* 1990;56:436–438.
127. Smith WR, Neill J, Cushman WC, Butkus DE. Captopril-associated acute interstitial nephritis. *Am J Nephrol* 1989;9:230–235.
128. Vanherweghem JL, Tielemans C, Simon J, Depierreux M. Chinese herbs nephropathy and renal pelvic carcinoma. *Nephrol Dial Transplant* 1995;10:270–273.
129. Corwin H, Korbet SM, Schwartz MM. Clinical correlates of eosinophiluria. *Arch Intern Med* 1985;145:1097–1099.
130. Adler S, Cohen AH, Border WA. Hypersensitivity phenomenon and the kidney: role of drugs and environmental agents. *Am J Kidney Dis* 1985;5:75–96.
131. Houghton DC, English J, Bennett WM. Chronic tubulointerstitial nephritis and renal insufficiency associated with long-term "subtherapeutic" gentamicin. *J Lab Clin Med* 1988;112:694–703.
132. Brentjens J, Noble B AG. Immunologically mediated lesions of kidney tubules and interstitium in laboratory animals and in man. *Semin Immunopathol* 1982;5:357–378.
133. Bender WL, Whelton A, Beschorner WE, Darwish MO, Hall-Craggs M, Solez K. Interstitial nephritis, proteinuria, and renal failure caused by nonsteroidal anti-inflammatory drugs. Immunologic characterization of the inflammatory infiltrate. *Am J Med* 1984;76:1006–1012.
134. Brunati C, Brando B, Confalonieri R, Belli LS, Lavagni MG, Minetti L. Immunophenotyping of mononuclear cell infiltrates associated with renal disease. *Clin Nephrol* 1986;26:15–20.
135. Chow J, Hartley RB, Jagger C, Dilly SA. ICAM-1 expression in renal disease. *J Clin Pathol* 1992;45:880–884.
136. Boucher A, Droz D, Adafer E, Noel LH. Characterization of mononuclear cell subsets in renal cellular interstitial infiltrates. *Kidney Int* 1986;29:1043–1049.
137. Kashgarian M. Lupus nephritis: lessons from the path lab. *Kidney Int* 1994;45:928–938.
138. Magil AB, Tyler M. Tubulo-interstitial disease in lupus nephritis. A morphometric study. *Histopathology* 1984;8:81–87.
139. Park MH, D'Agati V, Appel GB, Pirani CL. Tubulointerstitial disease in lupus nephritis: relationship to immune deposits, interstitial inflammation, glomerular changes, renal function, and prognosis. *Nephron* 1986;44:309–319.
140. Greising J, Trachtman H, Gauthier B, Valderrama E. Acute interstitial nephritis in adolescents and young adults. *Child Nephrol Urol* 1990; 10:189–195.
141. Hawkins EP, Berry PL, Silva FG. Acute tubulointerstitial nephritis in children: clinical, morphologic, and lectin studies. A report of the Southwest Pediatric Nephrology Study Group. *Am J Kidney Dis* 1989;14:466–471.
142. Spoendlin M, Moch H, Brunner F, Brunner W, Burger HR, Kiss D, Wegmann W, Dalquen P, Oberholzer M, Thiel G, et al. Karyomegalic interstitial nephritis: further support for a distinct entity and evidence for a genetic defect. *Am J Kidney Dis* 1995;25:242–252.
143. Vanhaesebrouck P, Carton D, De Bel C, Praet M, Proesmans W. Acute tubulo-interstitial nephritis and uveitis syndrome (TINU syndrome). *Nephron* 1985;40:418–422.
144. Cacoub P, Deray G, Le Hoang P, Baumelou A, Beaufils H, de Groc F, Rousselie F, Jouanneau C, Jacobs C. Idiopathic acute interstitial nephritis associated with anterior uveitis in adults [see Comments]. *Clin Nephrol* 1989;31:307–310.
145. Hannedouche T, Grateau G, Noel LH, Godin M, Fillastre JP, Grunfeld JP, Jungers P. Renal granulomatous sarcoidosis: report of six cases. *Nephrol Dial Transplant* 1990;5:18–24.
146. Mignon F, Mery JP, Mougenot B, Ronco P, Roland J, Morel-Maroger L. Granulomatous interstitial nephritis. *Adv Nephrol Necker Hosp* 1984;13:219–245.
147. Kallenberg CG, Brouwer E, Weening JJ, Tervaert JW. Anti-neutrophil cytoplasmic antibodies: current diagnostic and pathophysiological potential. *Kidney Int* 1994;46:1–15.
148. Savage CO, Gaskin G, Pusey CD, Pearson JD. Anti-neutrophil cytoplasm antibodies can recognize vascular endothelial cell-bound anti-neutrophil cytoplasm antibody-associated autoantigens. *Exp Nephrol* 1993;1:190–195.
149. Singh AB, Mann RA. Tubulointerstitial nephritis and vasculitis. *Curr Opin Nephrol Hypertens* 1993;2:484–490.
150. Diethelm AG, Deierhoi MH, Hudson SL, Laskow DA, Julian BA, Gaston RS, Bynon JS, Curtis JJ. Progress in renal transplantation. A single-center study of 3359 patients over 25 years. *Ann Surg* 1995; 221:446–458.
151. Hume DM MJ, Miller BF. Experiences with renal homotransplantation in the human. *J Clin Invest* 1955;34:327–381.
152. Solez K. International standardization of criteria for histologic diagnosis of chronic rejection in renal allografts. *Clin Transplant* 1994;8: 345–350.
153. Basadonna GP, Matas AJ, Gillingham KJ, Payne WD, Dunn DL, Sutherland DE, Gores PF, Gruessner RW, Najarian JS. Early versus late acute renal allograft rejection: impact on chronic rejection. *Transplantation* 1993;55:993–995.
154. Basadonna GP, Matas AJ, Gillingham KJ, Payne WD, Dunn DL, Sutherland DE, Gores PF, Gruessner RW, Arrazola L, Najarian JS. Relationship between early versus late acute rejection and onset of chronic rejection in kidney transplantation. *Transplant Proc* 1993;25: 910–911.
155. Azuma H, Tullius SG, Heemann UW, Tilney NL. Nonimmune factors may contribute to chronic rejection of kidney transplants. *Transplant Proc* 1994;26:2109–2110.
156. Hayry P, Yilmaz S. Chronic allograft rejection: an update. *Transplant Proc* 1994;26:3159–3160.
157. Isoniemi H, Nurminen M, Tikkanen MJ, von Willebrand E, Krogerus L, Ahonen J, Eklund B, Hockerstedt K, Salmela K, Hayry P. Risk factors predicting chronic rejection of renal allografts. *Transplantation* 1994;57:68–72.
158. Matas A. Chronic rejection in renal transplant recipients—risk factors and correlates. *Clin Transplant* 1994;8:332–335.
159. Paul LC. Functional and histologic characteristics of chronic renal allograft rejection. *Clin Transplant* 1994;8:319–323.
160. Bechtel U, Scheuer R, Landgraf R, Konig A, Feucht HE. Assessment of soluble adhesion molecules (sICAM-1, sVCAM-1, sELAM-1) and complement cleavage products (sC4d, sC5b-9) in urine. Clinical monitoring of renal allograft recipients. *Transplantation* 1994;58: 905–911.
161. de Heer E, Davidoff A, van der Wal A, van Geest M, Paul LC. Chronic renal allograft rejection in the rat. Transplantation-induced antibodies against basement membrane antigens. *Lab Invest* 1994;70: 494–502.
162. Gaciong Z, Koziak K, Religa P, Lisiecka A, Morzycka-Michalik M, Rell K, Kozlowska-Boszko B, Lao M. Increased expression of growth factors during chronic rejection of human kidney allograft. *Transplant Proc* 1995;27:928–929.

Immunologic Renal Diseases,
edited by E. G. Neilson and W. G. Couser.
Lippincott-Raven Publishers, Philadelphia © 1997

CHAPTER 39

Mechanisms and Risks of Immunosuppressive Therapy

Angelo M. de Mattos, Ali J. Olyaei, and William M. Bennett

INTRODUCTION

As understanding of the molecular basis for the immune response has expanded rapidly, so have the possibilities for designing therapeutic interventions that are more effective, more specific, and safer than current treatment options. Nowhere is the understanding of molecular mechanisms, pathophysiology, and targeted therapy more relevant than in the field of renal transplantation, which makes up much of the clinical data base for the use of immunosuppressive therapy for renal disease. Despite the recent advances in basic immunology, clinical validation of new agents and approaches is lacking for most drugs at present. This chapter covers the pharmacology, actions relevant for immunologic renal disease, and toxicities of therapies. Details of individual drug use in specific diseases are covered in depth elsewhere in the book. It should be recognized that clinical pharmacology and experience with newer agents are limited and potential utility is based largely on experimental data.

INHIBITORS OF PURINE AND PYRIMIDINE SYNTHESIS

Since the initial studies 4 decades ago demonstrating the antiproliferative effects of purine and pyrimidine synthesis inhibitors, much knowledge has been accumulated showing additional actions beyond simply inhibition of DNA and RNA synthesis (1). Adenosine triphosphate (ATP) is critical for a multitude of energy-requiring processes. Cyclic adenosine monophosphate (cAMP)is a second messenger molecule. Guanosine triphosphate (GTP) acts in intracellular signaling via the G proteins. Uridine triphosphate and guanosine diphosphate (GDP) are essential for the glycosylation of several proteins, including adhesion molecules (2). Purine and pyrimidine nucleotide biosynthesis is accomplished by two routes: the de novo and the salvage pathways (Fig. 1). Both synthetic pathways are present in all cell types, but some tissues utilize a single pathway more heavily. The importance of the de novo pathway to cells of the immune system is attested to by the profound T and B lymphocyte deficiency seen in individuals with congenital absence of key enzymes involved in this pathway (1,3). On the other hand, the lack of a critical enzyme of the salvage pathway (as observed in Lesch–Nyhan syndrome) leads to significant neurologic abnormalities but intact lymphocyte function (2).

Azathioprine

Azathioprine is an imidazole analogue synthesized in the early 1950s as a prodrug of 6-mercaptopurine (6-MP). The imidazole group of azathioprine prevents the rapid in vivo inactivation of the thiopurine structure of 6-MP. This slow liberation provides azathioprine with a superior therapeutic immunosuppressive index and less toxicity than 6-MP (4).

Absorption

Azathioprine is rapidly absorbed following oral administration. The oral bioavailability, defined as the area-under-the-concentration curves (AUCs) oral divided by intravenous (AUC p.o./AUC i.v.), following a dose is ~20%. However, the bioavailability of its major metabolite, 6-MP is ~40–45%. Therefore, ~60% of drug is absorbed orally before undergoing first-pass metabolism.

A. M. de Mattos, A. J. Olyaei, and W. M. Bennett: Division of Nephrology, Hypertension and Clinical Pharmacology, Oregon Health Sciences University, Portland, Oregon 97201.

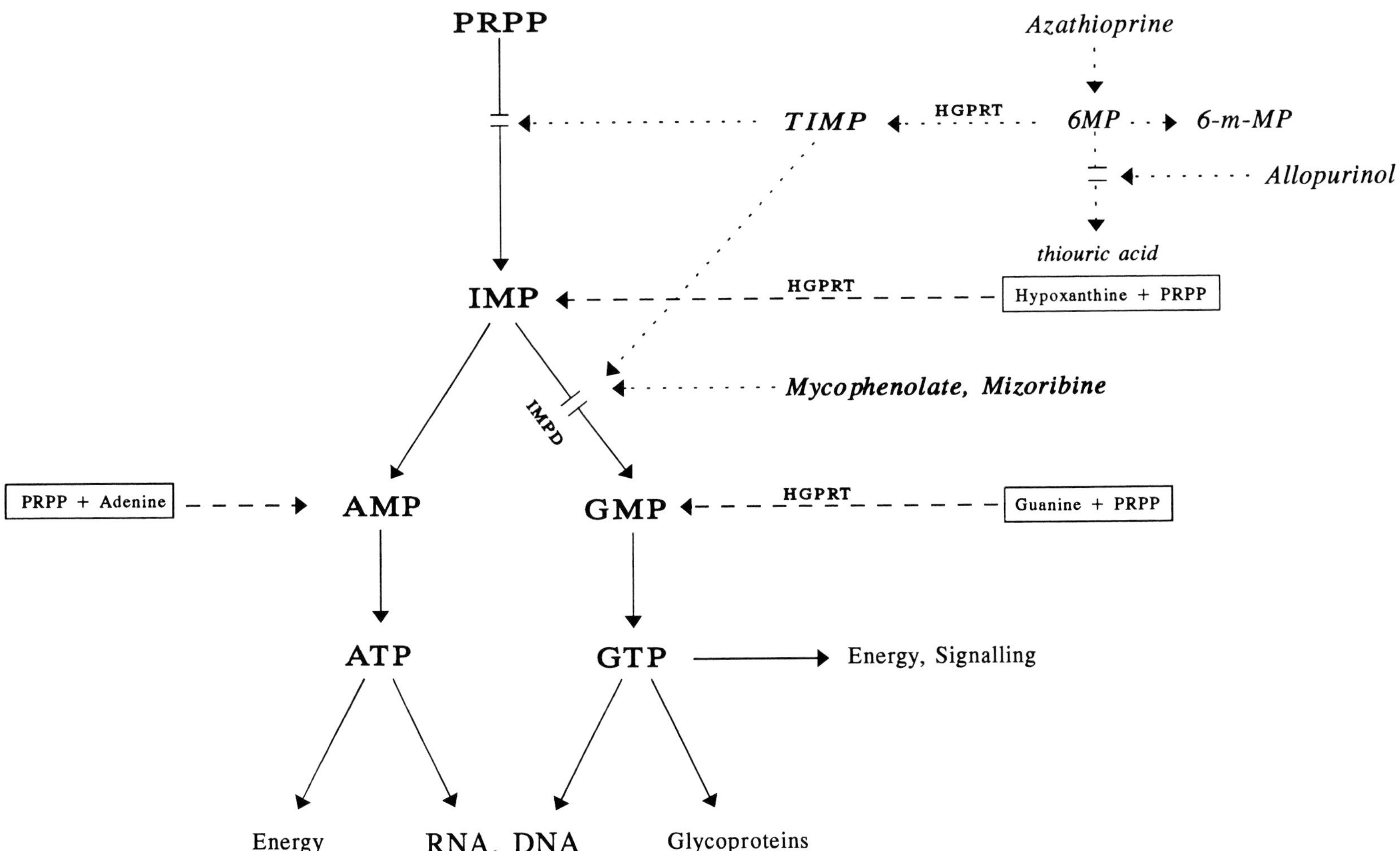

FIG. 1. Purine nucleotide synthesis: *salvage* and *de novo* pathways. Thick solid lines, de novo pathway; dashed lines, salvage pathway; PRPP, phosphororiboysyl pyrophosphate; HGPRT, hypoxanthine-quanine phosphorboysyl transferase; IMP, inosine monophosphate; IMPD, inosine-monophosphate dehydrogenase; 6MP, 6-mercaptopurine; 6-m-MP, 6-methyl-mercaptopurine; TIMP, thioniosine.

TABLE 1. *Summary of agents most commonly used in immunologic renal diseases*

Drug	Dosage	Monitoring	Toxicity	Cost
Cyclosporine Sandimmune, Sandoz Pharmaceutical, NJ	*Starting dose:* 4–5 mg/kg/day. Adjust for therapeutic target level. Cyclosporine dose i.v. is ⅓ of oral dose. Cyclosporine i.v. should be given by continuous infusion over 24 h.	Cyclosporine levels should be measured in whole blood and reported with statement about assay. CSA, CBC, creatinine, glucose, and electrolytes twice per week × 3 months. CSA, creatinine, and glucose weekly after first 3 months.CSA and creatinine monthly thereafter.	Nephrotoxicity, hypertension. Gingival hyperplasia (increased with phenytoin and nifedipine). Hirsutism, hepatotoxicity, neurotoxicity, hypomagnesia, hyperkalemia.	Gelcaps: $1.32/25 mg $2.65/100 mg Liquid: $5.20/100 mg (p.o.) $23.50/250 mg ampule (i.v.)
Azathioprine Imuran, Burroughs-Wellcome, NC	*Starting dose:* 1–3 mg/kg/day. Dose i.v. equals ½ of oral dose. Decrease dose 50% for WBC drop of 50%. Hold dose for WBC < 3,000.	CBC and electrolytes. Reduce dose by 75% with allopurinol administration.	Leukopenia, anemia, thrombocytopenia, aplastic anemia (rare), hepatitis, pancreatitis, alopecia.	$1.17/50-mg tablet $91.96/100-mg vial (i.v.)
Prednisone Geneva Pharmaceuticals, CO Roxane, OH Upjohn, MI	*Starting dose:* 1–2 mg/kg/day of prednisone (higher doses in transplantation). Prednisone taper schedule (variable).	CBC, electrolytes, glucose, and cholesterol.	Fat redistribution, hypertension. Hyperglycemia, increased appetite. Poor healing, sodium retention. Night sweats, insomnia, mood changes. Blurred vision and cataract.	$0.015/5-mg tablet
FK-506 Tacrolimus, Prograf, Fujisawa Pharmaceutical, IL	*Starting dose:* 0.15–0.3 mg/kg/day in 2 divided doses orally, or 0.05–0.1 mg/kg/day as a continuous infusion over 24 h i.v.	FK-506 levels should be measured in whole blood. FK-506, CBC, creatinine, glucose, and electrolytes twice weekly for 3 months. FK-506 and creatinine weekly after first 3 months and monthly thereafter.	Nephrotoxicity, hypertension, hepatotoxicity, pancreatitis, diabetes (rare). Seizures, headache, insomnia, tremor, paresthesia.	$2.18/1-mg capsule $10.92/5-mg capsule $222.00/5-mg ampule
Colchicine Merck, PA Eli Lilly, IN Abbott Laboratories, IL	*Starting dose:* 0.5–2 mg/day orally. (Do not exceed 4 mg/day)	CBC and electrolytes weekly for 1 month. Monthly thereafter.	Nausea, vomiting, diarrhea, abdominal pain, alopecia, dermatitis, peripheral neuropathy, nephrotic syndrome, muscle weakness. Hemolytic anemia (G6PD deficiency), pancytopenia (rare).	$0.19–0.25/500-mg tablet
Cyclophosphamide Cytoxan, Bristol-Myers Squibb, NJ Elkins-Sinn, NJ	*Starting dose:* 1–2 mg/kg/day orally, 0.5–1 g/m^2 BSA i.v. monthly. *Cumulative dose* not to exceed 250 mg/kg.	CBC, BUN, creatinine, and urinalysis weekly. Adjust dose per leukocyte count: half the dose for WBC < 5,000 and hold dose for WBC < 3,000 or hematuria.	Bone marrow depression, hemorrhagic cystitis, gonad toxicity, bladder fibrosis and cancer, other malignancies. Seizures (rare).	$1.50/25-mg tablet $2.75/50-mg tablet
Fish oils Advanced Nutritional, NJ J. R. Carlson Laboratories, IL	*Starting dose:* 1–2 capsules t.i.d. (suggested).	Glucose and lipids profile.	Glucose intolerance, weight gain, unpleasant postdose breath.	$0.09/capsule (EPA-Max)
Interferon-α 2B Intron-A, Schering, NJ	*Starting dose* (HBV): 5 million units/day subcutaneous × 16 weeks or 10 million units t.i.w. × 16 weeks. *Starting dose* (HCV): 3 million units t.i.w. × 6 months.	CBC, electrolytes, ALT, AST, HBeAg, and HBsAg weekly for the first month and monthly thereafter.	Fever, chills, fatigue, headache, myalgia, nausea, vomiting, diarrhea, leukopenia, anemia, thrombocytopenia.	$29.87/3 mIU $49.78/5 mIU
Chlorambucil Leukeran, Burroughs Wellcome, NC	*Starting dose:* 0.15 mg/kg/day orally. Cumulative dose not to exceed 7–10 mg/kg.	CBC, BUN, creatinine, and urinalysis weekly. Adjust dose like cyclophosphamide.	Same as cyclophosphamide.	$1.10/2-mg tablet

ALT, alanine aminotransferase; AST, aspartate aminotransferase; BSA, bovine serum albumin; BUN, blood urea nitrogen; CBC, cell blood count; CSA, cyclosporin A; EPA= eicosapentaneoic acid; G6PD, glucose-6-phosphate dehydrogenase; HBeAG, hepatitis-B e antigen; HBsAG, hepatitis-B surface antigen; HBV, hepatitis-B virus; HCV, hepatitis C virus; SC, subcutaneous; WBC, white blood cells.

After administration of azathioprine orally, peak plasma concentration is achieved within 2 h (4).

Metabolism

The imidazole group of azathioprine protects the sulfhydrate of 6-MP from oxidation. The initial site of metabolism can occur on either side of the S atom. This is mainly achieved by nucleophilic attachment by glutathione, which is abundant in the liver and erythrocytes. Hypoxanthine–guanine phosphorybosyl transferase (HGPRT, an enzyme of the salvage pathway) will then act on the newly formed 6-MP, forming thiopurine ribonucleosides and ribonucleotides. These compounds are thought to be responsible for most of the immunosuppressive activity of azathioprine (see Fig. 1 and *Mechanisms of action* below). There are two primary pathways leading to 6-MP degradation before it reaches HGPRT. The first is the through direct oxidation to 8-hydroxy-6-MP by xanthine oxidase (the enzyme inhibited by allopurinol). The second is via methylation by thiopurine methyltransferase (TPMT) producing 6-methyl-mercaptopurine (6-m-MP). Patients on allopurinol are more susceptible to toxicity when exposed to azathioprine. The level of expression of TPMT varies widely in the general population, making the susceptibility of individuals to myelotoxicity (or under-immunosuppression) also quite variable (5). Azathioprine may also bypass the conversion to 6-MP by being oxidized to 8-hydroxy-azathioprine. Both 8-hydroxy-6-MP, 8-hydroxy-azathioprine, and 6-m-MP are then methylated at the S atom, leading to the final inactive metabolite: 6-thiuric acid (5,6). Monitoring of blood or plasma concentrations has little value in dosing of azathioprine since the efficacy of azathioprine correlates with tissue rather than serum concentration of thiopurine nucleotide.

Elimination

The half-lives of azathioprine and 6-MP are 50 and 75 min, respectively. The final elimination occurs in the kidneys. By 8 h following oral or intravenous administration of azathioprine, neither azathioprine nor its metabolite 6-MP are detectable in the urine. Impaired renal function does not alter the pharmacokinetics of azathioprine or 6-MP. However, hepatic dysfunction may attenuate the pharmacodynamic properties of azathioprine secondary to decreased metabolism and accumulation of active metabolite moieties (4).

Mechanism of Immunosuppressive Action

Azathioprine is nonenzymatically converted inside cells to 6-MP plus a methylnitroimidazole moiety by glutathione and other sulfhydryl-containing molecules. Regarding the azathioprine immunosuppressive action, there is likely a dual mechanism of action involving both compounds. Intracellularly, 6-MP is converted by HGPRT to thio–inosine monophosphate (TIMP) and subsequently to thionucleotides that inhibit phospho-rybosyl-pyrophosphate (PRPP) synthetase, preventing adenosine monophosphate production (Fig. 1). Inosine monophosphate dehydrogenase (IMPD), an enzyme involved in GMP production, is also inhibited by thio-MP. Very small amounts of thio-MP is also incorporated into nucleic acids (RNA and DNA). Addition of adenine and hypoxanthine in vitro can reverse the antiproliferative effect of 6-MP but not azathioprine, suggesting an additional role of the methylnitroimidazole moiety (7). It has been suggested that azathioprine inhibits cell proliferation through a mechanism independent of its effect on the purine metabolic pathways (3,8). The methylnitroimidazole ring interacts with cell membrane molecules rich in sulfhydryl and amino groups interfering with intracellular processes like antigen recognition, adherence and cell-mediated cytotoxicity (1). After prolonged therapy with azathioprine, some lymphocyte clones mutate and become HGPRT-deficient, escaping partially from the drug immunosuppressive actions. Although 6-MP crosses the placenta, fetal tissues are deficient in HGPRT, so the fetus is protected against the effects of this drug (7).

Adverse Reactions to Azathioprine

The major adverse effect of azathioprine is bone marrow suppression. The dosage of the drug is usually monitored by following the peripheral white blood cell count. Although granulocytopenia is the most common hematologic manifestation of excessive azathioprine, all cell lines may be depressed. Reduction of the dosage is usually followed by recovery of white blood cell counts within 5–10 days. Gene polymorphisms of azathioprine metabolic enzyme pathways may identify subgroups of patients who are predisposed to development of extreme leukopenias. However, there are no clinically useful tests that will predict excessive marrow suppression. Persistent leukopenia not only increases the risk of infection, but also reduces graft survival because of the need to reduce azathioprine dose (9,10). Rare cases of pure red cell aplasia and isolated thrombocytopenia have been reported, but complete myelosuppression involving all hemopoietic cell lines is rarely noted (11). Azathioprine has been associated with the development of liver disease, which is fortunately quite rare. A reversible, dose-related acute cholestasis with pruritus occasionally can be due to azathioprine (12). Hepatic venoocclusive disease due to obliteration of the central or sublobular hepatic veins has been associated with azathioprine use (13–15). Progressive portal hypertension develops after an illness characterized by jaundice, hepatomegaly, and ascites. The mortality rate is high even if the azathioprine is discontinued, although some improvement can occur. There is a male predominance in this disorder for unclear reasons. Azathioprine has been associated with reversible interstitial pneumonitis (16) as well as an increased prevalence of malignancy in organ transplant recipients treated with this drug for long periods of time.

Clinical Uses

Azathioprine has been used, in addition to its well-established role in human renal transplantation, in conditions like lupus nephritis (17), steroid-resistant nephrotic syndrome (18,19), and rapidly progressive glomerulonephritis (20).

Alkylating Agents (Cyclophosphamide, Chlorambucil, and Melphalan)

Clinical use of derivatives of nitrogen mustard marked the beginning of the modern era of cancer chemotherapy. Subsequently, their use expanded to the treatment of immune-mediated renal diseases. As cyclophosphamide is the agent of this class used far more frequently, we focus our review on this agent (Table 1).

Pharmacology of Cyclophosphamide

Cyclophosphamide is an alkylating agent with incomplete absorption and variable metabolism. The drug must be metabolized in liver microsomes to be biologically active. Various drug metabolites are excreted in the urine. Its action on B lymphocytes is more pronounced than on T cells, making cyclosphosphamide an important suppressor of the humoral immune response.

Mechanism of Immunosuppressive Action

The mechanism of action of alkylating agents is related to their ability to bind to several target molecules covalently through alkylation. Their cytotoxic effect is mediated mainly through attachment to nucleotides, especially guanosine, inducing alkylation of the DNA leading to miscoding, interruption of transcription, and chromosome breaks. The so-called bifunctional agents can alkylate two molecules at once, forming cross-linking of two nucleic acid chains or the linkage of a nucleic acid and a protein. As expected, those agents are quite mutagenic and carcinogenic, which is the reason why their prolonged use is of major concern. They are quite effective as antiproliferative agents and are cytotoxic to rapid-dividing cells like lymphocytes because the mechanisms of DNA repair are overwhelmed (21). Cyclophosphamide needs activation via the hepatic cytochrome-P450 system. It is converted to 4-hydroxy cyclophosphamide, which is in steady state with its tautomer, aldophosphamide, the active alkylating agent. The liver is protected against these molecules by inactivating oxidizing enzymes. Acrolein, which is a metabolite of aldophosphamide, is the compound implicated in hemorrhagic cystitis and bladder cancer. Chlorambucil has a similar mechanism of action, but some claim it is less myelotoxic than cyclophosphamide (21).

Adverse Reactions to Alkylating Agents

The major side effects of cyclophosphamide are leukopenia, alopecia and, with prolonged use, interstitial cystitis. Hydration and dilution of the urine are effective antidotes toward drug-induced cystitis and neoplasia, both of which are seen with high cumulative doses. These considerations are worrisome in patients treated for long periods for medical renal diseases. In hemorrhagic cystitis due to cyclophosphamide, hemorrhage may be severe, protracted, and even life-threatening. Cyclophosphamide has been implicated as a causative agent in carcinoma of the bladder and renal pelvis (22). Gonadal toxicity is also common with cumulative doses of chlorambucil and cyclophosphamide greater than 7 mg/kg and 200 mg/kg, respectively (18). Excessive immunosuppression leading to malignancies must be considered when weighing the decision whether to use alkylating agents for chronic diseases such as immunologically mediated renal disease. The hazard of malignancy increases with cumulative doses of higher than 82 g for cyclophosphamide and 7 g for chlorambucil (18). Most recently, intermittent high-dose intravenous cyclophosphamide ("pulse" therapy) has been used with fewer side effects, yet with same efficacy, when compared with oral continuous regimens (23–26). This maneuver has allowed a reduction of the cumulative dose of cyclophosphamide. Long-term follow up of these studies should demonstrate a proportional decrease on the incidence of malignancies.

A structural analogue of cyclophosphamide, ifosfamide, has been introduced into chemotherapeutic regimens in recent years. Ifosfamide can also cause hemorrhagic cystitis and, in addition, occasional cases of irreversible renal failure have been reported (27). The frequency of these nephrotoxic reactions may be increased in patients with preexisting renal dysfunction and/or prior therapy with cisplatinum for malignancy. Ifosfamide causes enzymuria, suggesting proximal tubular injury in virtually all patients receiving the drug. Although sodium 2-mercaptoethane sulfonate (mesna) has become available, enabling higher doses of ifosfamide to be used, tubular and glomerular dysfunction has been increasingly reported (28).

Clinical Uses

Alkylating agents have been used extensively in conditions like lupus nephritis (17,26,29,30), Wegener granulomatosis (24,31,32), crescentic glomerulonephritis (23, 25,33,34), minimal change (18), membranous glomerulonephritis (18,35–38), renal amyloidosis (39–41), and steroid-dependent idiopathic nephrotic syndrome (42). Concerns about carcinogenesis have limited the use of those agents for prolonged periods (18). The role of other alkylating agents like melphalan, mechlorethamine, and mitoxine in the treatment of nephropathies is less well established (18). There are no clinical trials using ifosfamide for immunologic renal disease.

GLUCORTICOIDS

Glucocorticoids are members of a class of drugs known as adrenocortical steroids. Naturally occurring glucocorticoids in humans are cortisone and cortisol. Glucocorticoids were first extracted from adrenal glands in 1930 and used for treatment of rheumatoid arthritis in 1949. Since their discovery, glucocorticoids have become mainstays in the treatment and management of asthma, autoimmune disorders, cerebral edema found in patients with brain tumors, and as a basic immunosuppressive agent in solid organ transplantation (Table 1).

Pharmacokinetics of Glucocorticoids

Plasma concentrations of glucocorticoids have not been a critical factor in the dosing of these agents in the clinical setting, since there is a poor correlation between this parameter and the biological activity of glucocorticoids. This has resulted in numerous empiric dosing schedules in the management of renal disorders. To illustrate the dissociation of pharmacokinetics and pharmacodynamics, consider the plasma half-lives of 30 min for cortisone, 1 h for prednisone, and 2–3 h for dexamethasone. The corresponding biological half-lives are 8–12 h, 18–36 h, and 36–54 h, respectively. Thus, individual dosing is done empirically to obtain desirable outcomes and to avoid clinical adverse reactions. Table 2 summarizes the half-lives, equivalent doses, absorption and protein binding of the most frequently used glucocorticoids.

Distribution

Several factors influence the pharmacokinetics of glucocorticoids: circadian rhythm, age, gender, obesity, drug–drug interactions, and underlying disease state. The release of cortisol and its binding to plasma protein and its clearance follow a circadian rhythm (43). The highest activity occurs during the early morning hours, with random bursts during the ensuing 24 h. In spite of these fluctuations, the same total prednisolone AUCs have been reported after morning and evening dosing. The age, obesity, and gender of patients have been shown to be significant interpatient variables in the disposition of glucocorticoids. Children aged 8–12 exhibit a greater clearance compared with that of adults (44). The elderly show a decrease in the amount of unbound prednisolone clearance. Similarly, females also display a 20% decrease in unbound prednisolone clearance. Prednisolone clearance increases with the degree of obesity. Thus, this drug should be dosed according to actual body weight not ideal body weight. In contrast, methylprednisolone should be dosed on the basis of ideal body weight, since total clearance of this drug decreases as the degree of obesity increases. Therefore, less frequent doses should be considered in markedly overweight patients.

Induction of drug metabolizing enzymes by phenytoin, phenobarbital, rifampin, and carbamazepine increases elimination of prednisolone and methylprednisolone. Inhibition of glucocorticoid metabolism by oral contraceptives, conjugated estrogens, erythromycin, ketoconazole, indomethacin, and isoniazid can decrease clearance.

Certain renal disease states affect the disposition of the glucocorticoid. Patients with nephrotic syndrome, particularly those with a serum albumin <2.5 mg/dL, experience more glucocorticoid-related toxicity compared with those with higher albumin levels. Chronic renal failure may increase the free prednisone level as much as 70% in some patients (45). Methylprednisolone exhibited no variability on pharmacokinetic properties when given to patients with renal disease (46) and should be considered as the glucocorticoid of choice for patients with decreased renal function. Concomitant immunosuppressive agents such as cyclosporine and FK-506 as used clinically may alter elimination rate and affect steroid response (47).

Glucocorticoid Receptor

Glucocorticoids in the blood are either bound to serum protein (cortisol-binding globulin) or in a free form,

TABLE 2. *Half-lives, equivalent doses, adsorption, and protein binding of the most frequently used glucocorticoids*

Drug	Biological half-life (h)	Plasma half-life (min)	Absorption	Protein binding	Equivalent dose
Cortisone	8–12	30	100% (i.v.)	90%	25
Hydrocortisone	8–12	80–120	96% (p.o.)	90%	20
Prednisone	18–36	60	92% (p.o.)	70%	5
Methylprednisolone	18–36	100–200	100% (i.v.)	70%	4
Prednisolone	18–36	80–190	84% (p.o.)	95%	5

which is the pharmacologically active fraction (48). The free glucocorticoids, due to their small molecular radius and hydrophobicity, diffuse easily across plasma membranes to interact with their intracellular receptors, which are present in all cell types and are highly conserved among species (48–50). The receptor is conjugated to a dimer of a heat-shock protein of molecular weight of 90 kD (HSP-90), which increases its affinity for the unbound hormone. The dimer is displaced upon the receptor binding of the steroid (50,51). Both the steroid receptor and HSP-90 are phosphorylated in their non-steroid-bound status. A mechanism of phosphorylation and dephosphorylation must operate in receptor recycling (51). The bound receptor is found mainly in the nucleus (that is, the glucocorticoid receptor (GR)–ligand complex translocates) in a dimer configuration essential for glucocorticoid action (49,52). The GR belongs to a family of glycoproteins known as ligand–receptor factors and includes receptors that bind other steroids (progesterone, mineralocorticoids, estrogens, and androgens) and nonsteroid molecules (vitamin D, retinoic acid, and thyroid hormones). The receptor consists basically of three domains, and the presence of all of them is needed for function (50,51): The first domain of the receptor is called "immunogenic" or "modulatory" since it is related to gene activation via its specific interaction with other proteins such as RNA polymerase II. The second domain, located centrally in the molecule, is the DNA-binding domain, which has a highly conserved sequence that interacts with small DNA sequences known as glucocorticoid responsive elements (GREs). This domain is composed of 60–70 amino acids arranged in a "double Zinc finger" configuration. These transcription factors modulate gene transcription (50,52).

The third domain is the least conserved of all three. It is located at the 58 end of the molecule and is called the "ligand" domain since it interacts with the specific hormone (factor) as well the HSP-90 dimer. It is involved in the dimerization and translocation of the GR–steroid complexes into the nucleus (49). Different glucocorticoids may differ in their affinity for this receptor domain as well as influencing interactions with GREs.

Mechanisms of Immunosuppressive Action

Glucocorticoid Induction of Genes

The number of genes that are activated primarily by the glucocorticoid in each target cell type is quite small, particularly if one considers the multitude of hormonal effects that these hormones produce (50). The current model for gene activation assumes that GR–ligand complex interacts with DNA by scanning it and, as it randomly finds GREs, will bind to them using the DNA-binding domain acting as an on–off switch based on variable affinity. Once a GRE is occupied, a series of events leading to a specific gene transcription take place. It has been speculated that genes with multiple GREs are "early responders" by attracting more GR–ligand complexes. Genes with high-affinity GREs may be "superinduced" (50). It has been postulated before that genes with "negative" GREs would bind GR–ligand complexes and prevent "enhancing factors" interaction with the DNA.

Regulation of Gene Expression by Nuclear Transcription Factors

Because few "negative GREs" have been identified so far, an alternative mechanism for steroid transrepression (inhibition of gene transcription) has been proposed (53). Some transcription factors are constitutively expressed or induced in the nucleus upon activation via membrane receptors similar to the mode of action of cytokines. One of these nuclear transcription factors is the so-called AP-1 complex (activating protein). AP-1 is formed by homodimers or heterodimers of the Jun and Fos proteins (coded by the c-Jun and c-Fos protooncogenes, respectively). These complex proteins form a structure named "leucine zipper," which facilitates their interaction with the DNA-binding sites. This particular transcription factor is involved, along with several other cytokines and growth factors, in the interleukin (IL)-2-induced T-cell proliferative response. It is now known that AP-1 and the GR–steroid complex exert mutual antagonism due to ill-defined interaction between the two molecules (49,54–58). The same mechanism has been proposed in the glucocorticoid modulation of the IL-6 gene expression (53).

Mechanisms of Glucocorticoid Inhibition of the Inflammatory Response

Glucocorticoids decrease expression or release of several cytokines and growth factors [for example, IL-1, IL-2, IL-3, IL-4, IL-6, insulinlike growth factor 1, tumor necrosis factor (TNF), interferon (IFN)-γ, IL-8, RANTES, macrophage chemotactic and activating factor (MCAF), and platelet-activating factor (PAF)] (59,60) as well as some of their receptors (for example, IL-2R). Glucocorticoids are also involved in the downregulation gene expression for proteases like elastases, collagenases, and plasminogen activator (54,55,59). Glucocorticoids can inhibit vasodilatation and decrease vascular permeability. Glucocorticoids in vitro can inhibit major histocompatibility complex classII expression (61). The administration of glucocorticoids leads to a decreased number of all leukocytes except neutrophils (59). Glucocorticoids induce expression of neural endopeptidase, which is responsible for degrading several neuropeptides, including substance P and bradykinin, that mediate vasodilatation (59,62). Glucocorticoids have multiple effects on endothelial cells. They affect shape, contractility, and the expression of adhesion molecules (for example, endothelium-leukocyte adhesion molecule and intracellular adhesion molecule 1) and chemoattractants produced by these cells (59,62).

Nontranscriptional Effects

Dexamethasone exerted no inhibition of IL-1β messenger-RNA (mRNA) production after in vitro stimulation of human monocytes with lipopolysaccharide. However, its extracellular release was markedly decreased due to a inhibition of translation of the IL-1β precursor (63). The same can be said about dexamethasone and TNF mRNA translation (64).

Many of the anti-inflammatory actions of glucocorticoid were thought to be mediated by a group of proteins called lipocortins (formerly annexins). They are small proteins that bind intracellular calcium as well as negatively charged phospholipids (65,66). Lipocortins may inhibit chemotaxis and prevent release of reactive oxygen radicals (66). The potential action of lipocortins as inhibitors of cyclooxygenase enzyme expression is debatable. In cell culture experiments (including renal mesangial cells) (60,67,68), most of the anti-inflammatory effects were thought to be mediated via local inhibition of the arachidonic acid production from plasma membrane phospholipids by blockade of phospholipase-A_2 activity. This could lead to a decrease in eicosanoid production and release at sites of inflammation. However, these findings could not be confirmed in other studies (69). Glucocorticoids prevent endothelial activation and vasodilation, and increase neutrophil number, but decrease chemotaxis and inhibit the production of reactive oxygen metabolites. Some studies have shown that glucocorticoids can inhibit mRNA production of a cytokine-dependent inducible cyclooxygenase (70). Glucocorticoids prevent the de novo mRNA synthesis of an inducible, calcium-independent nitric oxide synthetase (71,72). In pathologic processes, nitric oxide promotes vasodilation and increases neutrophil chemotaxis. Besides the aforementioned effects on soluble factors, glucocorticoids in the pharmacologic doses used clinically prevent the IFN-γ induction of HLA classI and classII membrane antigens on activated T cells and endothelial cells while blocking the blastogenesis and proliferative response of T lymphocytes in allogeneic mixed-lymphocyte reaction (61).

Interaction with Other Medications

Many drug interactions with corticosteroids probably affect other immunosuppressive therapy. Inducers of hepatic metabolizing enzymes reduce the immunosuppressive effects of glucocorticoids. Patients who are taking concomitant rifampicin, phenytoin, and phenobarbital reduce the AUC of free nonprotein bound prednisolone. This could lead to lessened immunosuppressive effects for any given dose. These interactions have been confirmed in vitro in renal transplantation (73). Thus, with concomitant enzyme inducers, increases in steroid dosage on a mg/kg basis may be necessary to maintain immunosuppressive action. It is not known whether blockers of hepatic enzyme metabolic pathways influence the immunosuppressive effects and toxicities of usually prescribed doses of corticosteroids, but there are likely acute effects of massive doses of corticosteroids on the pharmacokinetics of other immunosuppressive agents (like cyclosporin A). Azathioprine does not effect prednisolone pharmacokinetics (74).

Adverse Reactions Related to Treatment of Renal Diseases with Glucocorticoids

The adverse effects of corticosteroids are well known to most clinicians. Those of particular relevance to patients with parenchymal renal disease are listed in Table 3. Probably of most concern to renal patients is the increased propensity to infection and the metabolic abnormalities produced by steroids. Hypertension, together with glucose intolerance and hyperlipidemia, probably all contribute to the increased risk of premature death from atherosclerotic heart disease in renal and, in particular, renal transplant patients (75–77).

TABLE 3. *Complications of corticosteroids pertinent for renal patients*

Cardiovascular
Hypertension
Sodium retention
Hypokalemic alkalosis
Central nervous system
Psychosis
Pseudotumor cerebri
Gastrointestinal
Peptic ulcer with or without bleeding
Pancreatitis
Endocrine
Delayed growth
Secondary amenorrhea
Impaired wound healing
Metabolic
Centripetal obesity
Glucose intolerance and type-II diabetes
Hyperlipidemia
Ophthalmologic
Glaucoma
Posterior subcapsular cataracts
Predisposition to infection

Effects of Glucocorticoids on Bones and Cartilage

Osteoporosis has been recognized for more than 40 years as one of the most serious and incapacitating sequelae of chronic glucocorticoid therapy. Despite extensive research, the mechanisms underlying it remain elusive (78–80). Glucocorticoids produce a net negative calcium balance due to decreased intestinal absorption, suppression of renal tubular reabsorption and, increased bone mobilization of calcium and phosphorus. Osteoporosis is partially related to the steroid dosage, occurs early after starting therapy, and seems to be directly related to this class of drugs' mechanism of action. Osteoporosis affects both genders equally and does not seem to be clearly related to the same risk factors described in non-steroid-users. It affects particularly the trabecular bone and portions of bones at high structural risk of collapse and spontaneous fractures (vertebral bodies and head of the femur and humerus) (78,80). Bone effects of glucocorticoids do not seem to be related to stimulation of osteoclastic activity, but rather to a decrease osteoblastic remodeling. Studies on the role of IL-1 and TNF as growth factors for osteoblast precursors in the bone marrow have been published recently (81). Although not clearly mediated by hyperparathyroidism, osteoporosis may be aggravated by increased levels of parathyroid hormone. Steroid-induced osteoporosis is largely independent of vitamin D. Steroid-induced myopathy may contribute to osteoporosis by decreasing mobilization and preventing bone remodeling induced by muscle activity (78).

Besides dose reduction (or even discontinuation) of the steroid involved, there is no other measure that is proven effective. Increased calcium intake, vitamin-D supplementation, and treatment with agents that decrease calcium reabsorption and thus increase deposition in the bones (i.e., calcitonin, biphosphonates, estrogens, or androgens) have not undergone well-controlled larger clinical trials. Recent data suggest that deflazacort, a new oxazoline derivative of prednisolone used in Europe, induces less bone loss while retaining its immunosuppressive effectiveness (82–86).

Deflazacort

Deflazacort is a new glucocorticoid not available yet in the United States. Deflazacort is an oxazoline derivative of prednisolone with a more favorable side-effect profile. Studies done in Europe suggest that this compound is at least as potent as the glucocorticoids commonly used, yet induces less hyperglycemia and less hypercalciuria, preventing bone loss in adults and growth arrest in pediatric patients (82–87). Further larger studies have to be done with this agent to establish its clinical usefulness.

Clinical Uses

Glucocorticoids, besides being considered the drug of choice for nephrotic syndrome, especially that due to minimal-change glomerulonephritis (18,88), have also been used in most of the immunologic renal diseases [i.e., crescentic glomerulonephritis (20,23,25,33,34,88–90), immunoglobulin (Ig)-A nephropathy (20,88,91), idiopathic membranous glomerulonephritis (18,35,37,38), anti–glomerular basement membrane (20,89), renal amyloidosis (40,41), Wegener granulomatosis (31,33), lupus nephritis (17,30), and other systemic vasculitis (92)] and is still a key agent in renal transplantation (93).

CYCLOSPORINES

Cyclosporines belong to a class of immunosuppressive agents that have revolutionized solid organ transplantation. The prototype drug cyclosporin A is a cyclic undecapeptide produced by a fungus isolated from Norwegian soil (*Tolypocladium inflatum*). Even though cyclosporin A was discovered in 1969, it was not until 1972 that it was shown to possess potent immunosuppressive activity (94). The drug has also been used for treatment of primary renal and systemic autoimmune diseases involving the kidney (Table 1).

Absorption

Cyclosporin A is available in oral and intravenous preparations. The oral dosage forms are available as soft gelatin capsules or as active drug dissolved in olive oil solution that is then diluted in water, milk, or orange juice, at room temperature, to make it more palatable. These dosage forms are mainly absorbed from the upper small intestine and depend on the presence of bile. Absorption of cyclosporin A by oral administration is slow, erratic, and incomplete, with a mean bioavailability of ~30% (95). It has been reported that the AUC after oral cyclosporin A administration tends to increase gradually after several weeks of treatment in renal transplantation (96). It has also been reported that the bioavailability increases with continued therapy after 2 weeks of treatment from 10.4% to 56.8%. The absorption of cyclosporin A is inter- and intrapatient variable and can be affected by many different factors. Foods of different fat content are a major factor that accounts for inconsistent absorption. Other factors that can affect the bioavailability of oral cyclosporin A involve the physical condition of individual patients. Impairment of oral cyclosporin-A bioavailability has been demonstrated in liver and bone marrow transplant recipients with diarrhea or external bile drainage and in patients with cholestatic liver disease

(96). Concomitant drugs can also affect the bioavailability of cyclosporin A. Metoclopramide, a drug that increases gastric emptying, increases the oral bioavailability of cyclosporin A. The physical length of the small bowel and the availability of bile acids within the intestinal lumen are also important determinants of the absorption of cyclosporin A (96).

A maximum blood concentration is usually achieved 2–6 h after administration of oral dosage forms of cyclosporin A. The kinetics of cyclosporin A have been described as being complex following zero-order or a series of first-order processes (96). Some investigators have described the occurrence of a second peak concentration 4–6 h after the first peak measured in plasma or whole blood following the administration of the oral dosage forms. The reason for this second peak is unknown, but may be due to enterohepatic recycling, delayed drug absorption, or metabolites converting back to cyclosporin A. This second peak has been noticed when oral cyclosporin A is taken with a meal or with a meal plus bile acid tablets, whereas only one peak was noticed when cyclosporin A was taken under fasting conditions. The second peak concentration can exceed the first peak quantitatively.

Distribution

Cyclosporin A is widely distributed throughout the body tissues. The volume of distribution ranges from an average of 3.5–13 L/kg. Because cyclosporin A is lipophilic and accumulates in body fat, women tend to have higher volumes of distribution than men. In whole blood, approximately 50–70% of cyclosporin A is found bound to cellular elements with 30–40% bound in the plasma fraction. In the cellular fraction, cyclosporin A is primarily bound to erythrocytes (80%), whereas lymphocytes bind to 4–9%. The proportion of cyclosporin A found in the cellular fraction increases as temperature decreases and as hematocrit increases. In the plasma fraction, 90% of cyclosporin A is bound to plasma proteins, particularly low-density lipoproteins (96). The volume of distribution varies with age; this may be due to the age-related difference in lipoprotein concentrations (96). High-fat meals have been reported to increase cyclosporin-A volume of distribution compared with low-fat meals. Because cyclosporine is highly bound to erythrocytes and the its concentration changes depending on the temperature, monitoring of the whole blood is preferred.

Metabolism

Cyclosporin A is extensively metabolized (~99%). At least 25 metabolites have been isolated. Most of the metabolites are hydroxylated, N-demethylated, or both. The major metabolite is a monohydroxylated metabolite, M_1. The trough level of this metabolite may exceed those of parent cyclosporin A (96). Other relatively active metabolites that are present in human blood are M_9, M_{4N}, and M_{19}. The data dealing with the immunosuppressive activity of these metabolites (especially M_1) are controversial as are the data on nephrotoxicity of these compounds. The cytochrome P450 liver microsomal enzyme system is the quantitatively most important metabolic pathway for cyclosporine (96). The human intestinal mucosa also contains a high concentration of cytochrome P450; therefore, cyclosporin A is metabolized in the wall of the gastrointestinal tract as it is absorbed, contributing to its poor oral bioavailability. Biliary excretion is the major route of elimination of cyclosporin A and its metabolites. Enterohepatic recirculation of cyclosporine and/or its metabolites probably occurs in some patients (96). The second peak serum level appears to be due to continued reabsorption of cyclosporine eliminated in the bile.

The clearance of cyclosporin A from the blood is ~5–7 mL/min/kg in adult recipients of liver or kidney transplants, and seems to be age dependent. It has also been suggested that the blood cyclosporine clearance is higher during the night than during the day. The clearance of cyclosporin A is diminished with continued therapy due to cyclosporine's ability to inhibit its own metabolism (96).

Excretion

Only a small amount (that is, ~1% of administered dose) of cyclosporin A is excreted unchanged in the urine. Approximately 3% of the administered dose is excreted into the urine as cyclosporin A plus metabolites. Just as the trough levels of the metabolites may exceed those of cyclosporin A, the urinary concentrations of these metabolites may be higher than parent cyclosporin A. Age also has been reported to influence the renal clearance of cyclosporin A. It has been shown that patients <25 years of age have a twofold increase in renal clearance when compared with older patients (96). The presence of renal dysfunction does not appear to impair cyclosporine clearance or pharmacokinetics.

Mechanisms of Action

Since its discovery as an immunosuppressive agent, the understanding of cyclosporine's mechanism of action has paralleled the development of molecular immunology. There is still controversy and many theories about how cyclosporines act specifically to produce clinical immunosuppression (97,98). Cyclosporines act by disrupting the calcium-dependent cascade of events that normally follows membrane antigen binding to the T-cell receptor leading to activation (transition in the cell cycle from G_0 to G_1 phase) and proliferation of T lymphocytes (transition from G_1 to S phase) (99). This is accomplished by preventing the translocation of cytosolic transcription factors into the nucleus, where they normally interact with genes coding for growth and differentiation factors. Thus, cyclosporine prevents the propagation of extracellular activation signals by interfering with intracellular second messengers. Cyclosporines are involved in the suppression of genes involved in early activation of T lymphocytes like c-myc, as well as genes for cytokines as IL-2, IL-3, IL-4, IL-5, and IFN-γ, as well as cytokine receptors like IL-2 receptor (100). Cyclosporine also affects other cells of the immune system as macrophages (inhibition of TNF synthesis), monocytes, dendritic cells, and B lymphocytes (antigen-presenting cells) (101).

Cyclosporines gain entry into target cells by diffusion through a "facilitated" transport mechanism via an undefined membrane receptor. Cyclosporines may be considered "prodrugs" since they need to bind a ligand inside cells to become active compounds. These ligands are a group of small proteins present in large quantities in all cell types and quite developmentally conserved with a high degree of homology among species: the immunophilins (99,102,103). Among the several proteins included into the "immunophilin family" are those that bind cyclosporines (called cyclophilins) and those that bind to tacrolimus (FK-506) and rapamycin (the FK-binding proteins). These proteins function as PPIases (peptidyl-prolyl *cis-trans* isomerases). The PPIases are involved in "folding" other proteins in the cytosol. Binding to cyclophilin is necessary but not sufficient to explain the immunosuppressive effects of cyclosporine. It has been shown that the antiproliferative effects of cyclosporines are not related to the isomerase function of the cyclophilin since non-immunosuppressive cyclosporine analogues can inhibit the isomerase action (99,102). So far, four cyclosporine-binding proteins have been characterized: Cyp A, Cyp B, Cyp C, and Cyp D (98). The binding of the cyclosporines to the different cyclophilins is governed by their structure (104). Most of the studies so far have focused on the Cyp A.

Role of Calcineurin

Cyclosporine–Cyp complexes bind in the cytosol to a calcium–calmodulin-dependent serine–threonine phosphatase, calcineurin. This highly conserved protein is composed of at least one "regulatory" part and a "catalytic" subunit. The cyclosporine–cyclophilin complex binds to the catalytic unit, rendering the calcineurin complex inactive. Calcineurin is the cyclosporine- and tacrolimus-sensitive component of the T-cell receptor signal transduction pathway (102,105). T-lymphocyte activation is commonly a calcium-dependent event with a sequence of phosphorylation of cytosolic proteins when membrane-bound receptors encounter their ligands. Following phosphorylation, some of these proteins (transcription factors) gain access to the cell nucleus (translocate), where they act upon gene transcription by interacting with small DNA-binding sequences located in the promoter region of a given gene.

Models of Cyclosporine Mechanism of Action

The Interleukin-2 Gene Transcription Model

Cyclosporine inhibits early T-cell signal transaction pathways leading to activation of lymphokine genes (106,107). Most of the current understanding of cyclosporine repression of gene transcription came from the study of the IL-2 gene due to the pivotal role of this cytokine in T-cell activation and proliferation. Following complexing with Cyp A, the cyclosporin–Cyp-A complex binds the calcineurin complex, inhibiting its phosphatase activity (108). This prevents the cytosolic part of the nuclear factor of activated lymphocytes (NF-ATc) from translocating to the nucleus where it binds to the nuclear subunit of the transcription factor (NF-ATn). By preventing ligation of the transcription factor to DNA at the promoter region of the IL-2 gene, cyclosporine inhibits gene transcription (109). It has also been shown that cyclosporine inhibits phosphorylation of other non-T-lymphocyte specific transcription factors like AP-1, AP-3, OAP, Oct-1, and probably NF-kB. The significance of this finding in terms of immunosuppressive effect is still under investigation (98,102,110). These effects have also been observed with tacrolimus (111).

The Transforming Growth Factor-β Hypothesis

An alternative hypothesis for cyclosporine's mechanism of action has been proposed, involving the upregulation of transforming growth factor (TGF)-β mRNA expression by cyclosporines. This multifunctional cytokine has been shown in vitro to inhibit T-lymphocyte growth and activation. TGF-β increases production of extracellular matrix and expression of endothelin 1 in endothelial cells (112). These effects could account for most of the clinically observed actions and adverse effects of cyclosporines (i.e., immunosuppression, renal fibrosis, and hypertension). The mechanism of inhibition involves transcription factors like Oct-1, which binds to upstream regions of the IL-2 promoter or, alternatively, via inhibition of c-myc promoter by a protein coded by the growth-suppressive retinoblastoma gene (110). Interestingly, glucocorticoids have also been shown to increase TGF-β_1 gene expression in normal human T lymphocytes (113).

Cyclosporine Effects on B Cells and Other Cells of the Immune System

Cyclosporine affects B-lymphocyte function not just via the indirect effects due to the decrease in the T-cell-derived cytokines, IL-4 and IL-6. Cyclosporin A can directly inhibit B-cell response to calcium-dependent signals like surface Ig receptor ligation (114). CD40 ligand is a membrane glycoprotein expressed in B lymphocytes and is directly involved in cooperation with T lymphocytes bearing the CD40 surface molecule. CD40-ligand gene expression is inhibited by cyclosporine via a mechanism also involving the blockage of NF-ATc phosphorylation (115). This could imply a disruption in the pathway for antibody production. In vitro blockage of the mast cell and neutrophil and basophil degranulation have been described (116,117). Effects on macrophages and antigen-presenting cells are less evident (114), but inhibition of TNF-α production by monocytes stimulated by superantigen has been observed in vitro (100).

The effects of cyclosporine in bone and connective tissues do not seem to be directly mediated by T lymphocytes. In an experimental model of adjuvant arthritis, cyclosporine protected against bone loss. However, cyclosporine in vitro inhibits bone reabsorption caused by decreased levels of IL-1, parathyroid hormone, 1,25-dihydroxy-vitamin D_3 and prostaglandin E_2 (101,118). Osteoblasts have been shown in vitro to express major histocompatibility complex class II on their surface upon stimulation with IL-1, and may function as antigen-presenting cells. This effect is blocked by cyclosporine (101). The role of cytokines in the proliferation and differentiation of osteoblasts and osteoclasts in the bone marrow has been studied recently (81).

The Nontranscription Effect of Cyclosporines

Inhibition of chemotaxis might involve the inhibition of extracellular release of cyclophilin, which functions there as a chemotactic factor for eosinophils and neutrophils (119,120).

Cyclosporine and Mesangial Cells

It has been shown in rat mesangial cell culture that cyclosporine and some of its metabolites inhibit the expression of an inducible form of cyclooxygenase (COX_2), decreasing the production of vasodilatory prostaglandins (121). Interestingly, in rodents, cyclosporin-induced renal vasoconstriction may only partially be mediated via nitric oxide deficiency. However, the addition of nitric oxide appears to modify vasoconstriction (122).

Cyclosporine Effects on the Renin–Angiotensin System

In an experimental model of chronic cyclosporine administration, there was no intrarenal increase in production of renin mRNA. However, cells along the afferent arterioles contained more renin than did controls, suggesting a post-transcriptional regulation of renin or a downregulation of angiotensin receptor-1 expression in the kidney due to negative feedback by locally produced angiotensin II (123). Studies using bovine endothelial cells demonstrated that cyclosporine induces thromboxane B_2 and prostacyclin breakdown while increasing endothelin release (124).

Cyclosporine and the Vasculature

Cyclosporine has interactions with blood vessels that are implicated in clinical adverse reactions noted with the drug. Local platelet activation, imbalance between vasodilatory and vasoconstrictive mediators (eicosanoids, endothelin, nitric oxide, and renin–angiotensin system), increased responsiveness to catecholamines, and direct effects on endothelial cells are among the mechanisms investigated. Clinically, hypertension, thrombotic episodes, accelerated atherosclerosis, and hemolytic–uremic syndrome have been described. Cyclosporine in vitro induces expression of endothelin 1 by endothelial cells that in turn induces proliferation of cultured smooth muscle cells. This effect was blocked by an antibody against endothelin 1 and by a calcium channel antagonist (125). Cyclosporin A induces platelet hyperaggregability when stimulated by ADP, collagen, and epinephrine (126). Cyclosporine contributes to the hyperlipidemia seen often in renal transplant recipients (127–130). Cyclosporine has a concentration-dependent prooxidant effect on plasma low-density lipoproteins, increasing their affinity to macrophages and contributing to the accelerated atherosclerosis seen in patients receiving this drug (131).

Interaction with Other Drugs (Table 4)

Some groups have suggested that medications like diltiazem (a calcium-channel antagonist) and omega-3 fatty acids might augment the immunosuppressive effects of cyclosporin A while decreasing its nephrotoxicity (132–136). Both compounds inhibit cyclosporine-induced endothelin production (125). Nifedipine has been shown to decrease cyclosporine-induced interstitial fibrosis (137).

Adverse Effects of Cyclosporine

The major adverse effect of cyclosporine is dose-related nephrotoxicity and associated hypertension (138–

140). This is particularly relevant when cyclosporine is used for treatment of immunologic renal disease outside the setting of renal transplantation, where adverse effects on renal structure and function could offset any putative advantages in turning off the primary immunologically mediated disease process. Other cyclosporine-related side effects, such as hepatotoxicity, neurologic disturbances, and hyperuricemia, and epidermal abnormalities, such as hirsutism and gingival hyperplasia, can be managed by therapeutic drug monitoring and adjustment.

Cellular Mechanisms of Nephrotoxicity

The inhibition of calcineurin may be associated with nephrotoxicity as well as immunosuppressive action since non-immunosuppressive analogues of cyclosporine, which bind to and inhibit enzymatic action of calcineurin produce, neither immunosuppression nor nephrotoxicity (141,142). Another mechanism proposed is the cyclosporine-induced inhibition of the multidrug transporter p-glycoprotein (143), which is normally expressed on proximal tubular cells and confers drug resistance on renal tubule cells by facilitating efflux of chemotherapeutic drugs. Cyclosporine can reverse multidrug resistance in human and rodent tumors and can impair secretion of other substrates such as cardiac glycosides (144). The role of p-glycoprotein inhibition and accumulation of an endogenous or exogenous cytotoxic substance has not been explored as a mechanism of cyclosporine nephrotoxicity. Cyclosporine also may generate oxygen-free radicals that induce lipid peroxidation and cellular damage. Renal microsomes show an increased lipid peroxidation when they are associated with decreased glutathione content after exposure to cyclosporine (145,146). Oxygen-free radicals may also react with endogenously generated nitric oxide, producing both reactive chemical species and impairment of vasorelaxation responses.

Clinical Nephrotoxicity

The effects of cyclosporine on the kidneys and systemic vasculature result in a variety of nephrotoxic syndromes (147). However, renal hemodynamics in patients treated with cyclosporin A without discernible renal dysfunction often improve when the drug is withdrawn or the dosage is reduced. This suggests that cyclosporin A may affect the kidney to some extent in most individuals receiving the drug. The most common manifestation of cyclosporine nephrotoxicity is an asymptomatic rise in serum creatinine. Hypertension, fluid retention, hyperkalemia, hyperchloremic metabolic acidosis, and high blood cyclosporine levels are nonspecific and are frequently seen with cyclosporine nephrotoxicity, but can be a manifestation of allograft rejection, in recipients of a kidney transplant. In treatment of primary renal disease with cyclosporine, increases in serum creatinine are most likely due to the drug, although it can be difficult to distinguish this from progression of the primary disease. Other manifestations of cyclosporine nephrotoxicity include hypomagnesemia, hyperuricemia, hypocalcemia, and mild increases in blood urea nitrogen. Declines in renal function are usually reversible within 1 week with appropriate dosage reduction. In the immediate postoperative period following a renal transplant, cyclosporine can be one of the factors responsible for delayed allograft function. The impact of cyclosporine's vasoactive effects on graft function has been minimized at most transplant centers by delaying the onset of drug administration until renal function has been clearly established in the allograft (140). The pathologic changes seen in the renal transplant recipient with cyclosporine therapy are nonspecific. The drug may lead to isometric vacuolization and giant mitochondria within proximal tubular cells; however, these histopathologic changes are not correlated with renal dysfunction and may simply be a marker of therapy. In the renal transplant setting, the most common histopathologic finding in patients with clinically diagnosed cyclosporin-A nephrotoxicity is a biopsy confirming the absence of rejection.

The most serious clinical adverse renal effect of cyclosporin A is a progressive chronic nephropathy that has been reported predominantly in liver or heart transplants and in patients with primary autoimmune diseases treated with cyclosporine (148,149). Some patients have progressed to end-stage renal disease. This chronic nephropathy has been reported in patients who received low-dose cyclosporine for dermatologic disorders such as psoriasis (150,151). Both experimentally and clinically, tubulointerstitial renal disease can progress despite lowering of the cyclosporine dose or even drug withdrawal. There is a characteristic histopathologic lesion of chronic cyclosporine nephropathy consisting of afferent arteriolopathy and a striped pattern of tubulointerstitial atrophy and fibrosis (152). The arteriolar lesions consist of nodular, insudative myointimal protein deposits that may ultimately compromise the vascular lumen. It is difficult to distinguish arteriolar hyalinosis and tubular and interstitial fibrosis caused by cyclosporine from vascular disease caused by acute or chronic rejection. Involvement of arterial-sized vessels with intimal proliferation and atherosclerosis is most characteristic of chronic rejection. The fibrosis and atrophy in cyclosporine chronic nephropathy is usually present in bands or stripes that correspond to the arteriolar lesion. This striped pattern is probably due to lesions beginning in the outer medullary rays. In a small biopsy sample, however, this pattern often is difficult to discern. Unfortunately, cyclosporine blood level monitoring has little correlation with chronic histopathologic changes.

Clinically, cyclosporin-A nephropathy presents as a slowly progressive renal dysfunction associated with hypertension and occasionally mild hyperchloremic metabolic acidosis with hyperkalemia. Urine often shows small amounts of protein and an otherwise bland urinary sediment. Cyclosporine nephrotoxicity can be manifested by the hemolytic uremic syndrome (153). Although this has been most often reported in bone marrow transplant recipients, this rare manifestation of cyclosporine nephrotoxicity has also been observed in renal transplantation (154). Diffuse capillary thrombi are noted in glomerular tufts and small vessels associated with microangiopathic hemolytic anemia and severe hypertension. Treatment with plasmapheresis or plasma infusions has shown a beneficial effect on renal function, although the prognosis of this type of toxicity is guarded.

Arterial hypertension often complicates cyclosporine therapy even in the face of stable kidney function (155, 156). Even when the serum creatinine is normal, a high percentage of successful cardiac recipients and patients with primary renal disease develop high blood pressure. The hypertension is dose related, but can be observed with blood cyclosporine concentrations within the therapeutic range. Although plasma renin activity is usually normal or mildly suppressed, suggesting a volume-dependent mechanism for blood pressure elevation, activation of the intrarenal renin–angiotensin system is suggested by the prominent juxtaglomerular apparatus hyperplasia noted in cyclosporine-treated kidneys (157,158).

Pathogenesis of Cyclosporine Nephrotoxicity

Cyclosporine produces dose-related afferent arteriolar vasoconstriction when given chronically to experimental animals (159). There are marked decreases in glomerular filtration rate and renal blood flow associated with high renal vascular resistance seen with doses from 5–100 mg/kg in various species. At the nadir of renal blood flow, renal tubular function is well maintained and histologic examination shows no evidence of proximal tubular damage. Associated with these hemodynamic changes, fractional excretion of sodium is low and lithium reabsorption by the proximal tubule is maximized, suggesting intact tubular transport function. Impairment in glomerular filtration can also be due to reduction of the glomerular ultrafiltration coefficient due to heightened mesangial cell contractility (157). The timely improvements in renal hemodynamics following drug withdrawal support renal vasoconstriction as a primary pathogenic mechanism in cyclosporine's acute nephrotoxic effects. The Cremophor EL vehicle for intravenous cyclosporine produces vasoconstriction when formulated with cyclosporin A, whereas cyclosporine in other vehicles such as intralipid is less vasoactive (160). In animals, cyclosporine therapy increases renin release, juxtaglomerular cell prorenin, and plasma renin activity (161). Angiotensin-II receptor blockade or converting-enzyme inhibition does not normalize glomerular filtration rate, despite improving renal vascular resistance (162). Cyclosporine increases sympathetic nervous system activity (163), and this correlates with immunosuppressive activity, as assessed by inhibition of the NF-AT phosphorylation (164). However, denervated animals still can develop acute hemodynamic changes produced by cyclosporine. Cyclosporine alters the vasoconstrictor–vasodilator balance between arachidonic acid and cyclooxygenase metabolites (165), favoring vasoconstriction. Cyclosporine augments thromboxane A_2 generation, which increases renal vascular resistance and mesangial cell contraction. Experimentally, thromboxane receptor antagonists and thromboxane synthesis inhibitors improve renal hemodynamics (161). The clinical results of inhibition of thromboxane have been much less impressive. Eicosapentaenoic acid, an inhibitor of renal eicosanoids, reduces cyclosporine nephrotoxicity in experimental and clinical studies (166, 167). Endothelin seems to play a major role in cyclosporine-mediated vasoconstriction (168,169). Thromboxane mimetic agonists also increase endothelin release, whereas endothelin affects glomerular hemodynamics in a similar way to the action of cyclosporin A (168,170). Anti-endothelin antibodies and endothelin receptor antagonists protect against the acute vasoconstriction produced by cyclosporin A. Although inhibition of endothelin improves renal hemodynamics, it does not improve tubulointerstitial fibrosis in an animal model of chronic cyclosporine nephropathy (171). Recently, using a low-salt diet to stimulate the renin–angiotensin system, an animal model for the striped fibrosis of chronic cyclosporine nephropathy in rats, with the characteristic afferent arteriolar lesions, was developed (172). Although salt-repleted animals develop reductions in renal blood flow that are similar to those produced in salt-depleted animals, the former developed no structural changes. Thus, chronic ischemia does not seem to be a satisfactory explanation for the chronic lesions produced by cyclosporine. Cyclosporine also modifies extracellular matrix accumulation (173). Early in the development of the chronic cyclosporine lesion in animals, interstitial macrophage accumulation occurs as well as the upregulation of the proximal tubular chemoattractant molecule, osteopontin. This macrophage chemoattractant interestingly is angiotensin dependent (174). Blockade of angiotensin-II type-1 receptors with specific antagonists blocks fibrosis, despite producing hypotension in this model.

Although the renal transplant recipient with acute and/or chronic rejection modified by concomitant immunosuppressive drugs presents a complex problem in discerning the precise pathophysiologic role of cyclosporine in renal scarring, the drug may alter the renal cytokine profiles of infiltrating cells, favoring fibrosis and increased matrix synthesis (173). Preliminary data support a role of

TGF-β and thromboxane in these processes that may be enhanced by the angiotensin-II stimulation provided by salt depletion (175). The distribution of interstitial fibrosis and arteriolopathy in the transplanted kidney and experimental model of cyclosporine nephrotoxicity corresponds to the distribution of the angiotensin-II type-1 receptor mRNA in the renal parenchyma (176).

In cyclosporine-treated patients, endothelial cells in the kidney develop vacuolar changes. Factor-VIII-related antigen may be increased (177,178). Since the hemolytic uremic syndrome follows vascular endothelial changes, cyclosporine-induced endothelial effects probably cause this unusual type of cyclosporine nephrotoxicity. Increased thromboxane and decreased prostaglandin I_2 promote platelet aggregation at the sites of endothelial damage. Bacterial endotoxemia, which occurs frequently in bone marrow transplant patients, may explain the preponderance of reports of hemolytic uremic syndrome when cyclosporine is used in this setting. Endotoxin and cyclosporine both stimulate endothelin synthesis and are synergistic with respect to many mediators activated by sepsis (179). Cyclosporine-associated hemolytic uremic syndrome can resolve spontaneously with dose reduction or cyclosporine withdrawal with some resolution of glomerular fibrin deposition (180,181). Plasma infusions and plasmapheresis have been used with anecdotal success. Some patients can be switched to tacrolimus, resulting in clinical remission.

The pathogenesis of cyclosporine-induced hypertension is unclear (182). It is probably multifactorial, depending on the type of organ transplant, duration of any preexisting hypertension, dose of concomitant corticosteroids, and concomitant parenchymal disease in the kidney. In every situation where cyclosporine is used clinically, de novo or exacerbated preexisting hypertension is frequent (183). Peripheral vascular resistance progressively increases during the first weeks of therapy. Similar hemodynamics have been noted in conscious sheep that develop increased blood pressure but no renal dysfunction with cyclosporine (184). Although sympathetic nerve traffic is increased by cyclosporine, renal vasoconstriction due to cyclosporine can occur experimentally in functionally denervated renal transplants. Disturbance by cyclosporine of local vasoconstrictor and vasorelaxation factors in resistance vessels subsequent to platelet activation probably contributes to increased vascular resistance. Endothelin is transiently elevated in the urine of kidney recipients after cyclosporin A and in the circulation of liver recipients, which may contribute to increases in renal vascular resistance (183). Nitric oxide inhibition by cyclosporine produces an increase of normal vascular tone. Cyclosporine impairs endothelium-dependent vasodilation in human subcutaneous resistance vessels and in addition reduces the sensitivity to non-endothelium-dependent relaxation in hypertensive rats (185,186). Nitric oxide synthase inhibitors increase blood pressure and produce nephrotoxicity in rodents at doses that are clinically relevant for humans. Endothelin-mediated vasoconstriction is known to be enhanced by nitric oxide inhibition. Locally induced ischemia generates oxygen-free radicals that react with locally produced nitric oxide, reducing nitric oxide vasodilating capacity (187). In normotensive rats receiving large doses of cyclosporine, endothelial relaxation induced by acetylcholine is perturbed after 1 week (186). These experimental and clinical data must be considered in prescribing this drug to people with primary renal disease, since hypertension can lead to disease progression independent of the primary cause of the disease.

Clinical Uses

Cyclosporin A has promoted human renal transplantation to the therapy of choice for most patients with end-stage renal disease. It has also been used in steroid-dependent and steroid-resistant nephrotic syndrome of several etiologies (i.e., membranous, IgA, minimal change, focal segmental, and membranoproliferative) in pediatric (42, 188–190) as well as adult (190–195) patients, as well as in progressive glomerulonephritis (20).

The Neoral Cyclosporin-A Formulation

To reduce the high degree of variability of cyclosporine absorption and provide more consistent pharmacokinetic characteristics, Neoral, a self-emulsifying formulation of cyclosporine, has been developed by Sandoz Pharmaceutical (East Hanover, NJ) (196,197). The Neoral formulation of cyclosporine releases cyclosporin A quickly from the gelatin capsule where it stays in aqueous mixed phase in the gastrointestinal tract. In addition, the physiologic state of gastrointestinal tract, such as presence of bile, food, gastrointestinal motility, and pancreatic juice, does not affect the pharmacokinetics of the Neoral formulation (198). Neoral formulation offers advantages over gelatin capsules or oral solutions of cyclosporine with respect to rate and extent of absorption, greater AUC, higher C_{max}, and faster T_{max}. The increased cyclosporine AUC and C_{max} have not been associated with the increased renal nephrotoxicity or hypertension (199). Overall, Neoral formulation provides more predictable and consistent pharmacokinetics with safety and adverse reaction profiles comparable to other formulations of cyclosporine (199,200).

TACROLIMUS (FK-506)

Tacrolimus is a macrolide antibiotic isolated from *Streptomyces tsukubaensis,* a fungal organism found in Japanese soil. The pharmacokinetics of tacrolimus (FK-506) have been best described in the liver transplant population.

TABLE 4. *Clinically relevant drug interactions with cyclosporine*

Drug	Effect	Mechanism	Management
Diltiazem	↑ CSA blood levels	↓ CSA metabolism	↓ CSA dose 30–40%
Nicardipine	↑ CSA blood levels	↓ CSA metabolism	↓ CSA dose 20%
Verapamil	↑ CSA blood levels	↓ CSA metabolism	↓ CSA dose 20–25%
Erythromycin	↑ CSA blood levels, possible ↑ renal dysfunction	↓ CSA metabolism	↓ CSA dose 50% (p.o.) ↓ CSA dose 25% (i.v.)
Clarithromycin	↑ CSA blood levels, possible ↑ renal dysfunction	↓ CSA metabolism	NA
Ketoconozole	↑ CSA blood levels, possible ↑ renal dysfunction	↓ CSA metabolism	↓ CSA dose 75–80%
Methylprednisolone (high dose only)	↑ CSA blood levels, convulsions	Unknown	Monitor closely
Carbamazepine	↓ CSA blood levels	↑ CSA metabolism	Rapid onset/slow offset, monitor closely
Phenobarbital	↓ CSA blood levels	↑ CSA metabolism	Slow onset/slow offset, monitor closely
Phenytoin	↓ CSA blood levels	↑ CSA metabolism	Rapid onset/rapid offset, monitor closely
Rifampin	↓ CSA blood levels	↑ CSA metabolism	Maximum effect in 3 days to 2 weeks, ↑ CSA dose up to 60%, monitor closely
Aminoglycosides	↑ Renal dysfunction	Additive nephrotoxicity	Avoid if possible, monitor closely
Amphotericin B	↑ Renal dysfunction	Additive nephrotoxicity	Give 250-mL bolus NS before and after Ampho B dose, consider pentoxifylline, 400 mg t.i.d.–q.i.d.
Cimetidine	↑ Serum dysfunction	Competes with creatinine for renal tubular secretion	Consider other H_2 receptor antagonists
SMZ/TMP	↑ Serum dysfunction	TMP competes with creatinine for renal tubular secretion	
Lovastatin	↓ Lovastatin metabolism	Myositis, ↑ CPK, rhabdomyolysis	Avoid doses > 20 mg

Ampho B, amphotericin B; CPK, creatine phosphokinase; CSA, cyclosporin A; NA, not available; NS, normal saline; SMZ/TMP, sulfamethoxazole–trimethoprim.

Tacrolimus has recently been approved by the FDA and has been used in kidney transplantation and other immunologically mediated nephropathies (201) (Table 1).

Absorption

The absorption of tacrolimus from gastrointestinal tract after an oral dose is incomplete and unpredictable. The average bioavailability is ~20% with a range of 15–25%. Similar to cyclosporine, absorption of tacrolimus has inter- and intrapatient variability and can be affected by food and other drugs. Food has been shown to decrease the bioavailability by as much of 25% as compared with taking the drug on an empty stomach. The peak blood concentration occurs usually 0.5–8 h after oral administration. In contrast to cyclosporine, hepatic dysfunction does not alter oral absorption, but instead increases the terminal half-life and the AUC of tacrolimus. Tacrolimus absorption is bile independent (202).

Distribution

The volume of distribution, clearance, and half-life values depend on temperature (203,204). The concentration of tacrolimus is 10–30 times greater in whole blood compared with plasma concentration. Therefore, blood rather than plasma would more accurately describe the pharmacokinetic properties of tacrolimus. Tacrolimus is highly protein bound, ranging from 75% to 95% at any given time. It is mainly bound to albumin and α_1 acid glycoprotein and is also highly bound to erythrocytes (203,204).

Metabolism

Metabolism of tacrolimus occurs primarily in the liver: >98% of a dose is metabolized via the cytochrome-P450–3A4 system. The major mechanism of biotransformation appears to include demethylation and hydroxylation (205,206). There are many potential drug interactions with tacrolimus. Tacrolimus should be used with caution in patients who are concurrently taking P450–3A4 inhibitors and inducers. Drugs that have been reported to increase tacrolimus levels by inhibition of metabolism include ketoconazole, erythromycin, fluconazole, diltiazem, and glucocorticoids. Drugs that may potentially decrease tacrolimus levels include P450–3A4 enzyme inducers such as phenytoin, phenobarbital, carbamazepine, and rifampin. The monitoring parameters for tacrolimus are still unclear. Optimal therapeutic serum levels have not been established. Studies that have assessed therapeutic 12-h trough levels have reported a range from 5–50 ng/mL. Future studies should reveal more helpful data regarding the monitoring of tacrolimus (204).

Mechanism of Action

Even though tacrolimus bears little structural similarity with the cyclosporines, it shares many similar molecular targets and inhibits expression of the same cytokines as cyclosporine (100,111). Like cyclosporine, tacrolimus must bind intracellularly to its receptor, the FK-binding protein (FK-BP) (201,207,208). These highly conserved proteins are members of the immunophilin family and, as such, function as PPIases. No significant sequence homologies have been found between the FK-BPs and the cyclophilins. Tacrolimus inhibits the rotamase activity of FK-BP, but not of cyclophilin, and vice versa (103). The inhibition of the isomerase function of FK-BPs by tacrolimus does not seem to be involved in its immunosuppressive effects (103). The FK-BP–tacrolimus complex binds to the same target as cyclosporine—calcineurin—inhibiting its ability to remove phosphates from transcription factors like NF-AT, AP-3, and Oct-1. This ultimately leads to inhibition of transcription of certain early T-lymphocyte activation genes like IL-2, IL-3, IL-4, TNF-α, and IFN-γ. Tacrolimus appears to exert its effects in vitro in concentrations at least 50 times lower than cyclosporin A (111). Activation of lymphocytes via the CD28 antigen pathway is resistant to inhibition by both tacrolimus and cyclosporine (208). With the discovery of rapamycin, it became clear that T lymphocytes use two distinct signal transmission pathways that can be inhibited by either cyclosporine/tacrolimus (calcium dependent) or rapamycin (calcium independent) (209–211). The immunosuppressive action of tacrolimus is directly related to its inhibition of the phosphatase activity of calcineurin (141,208). In vitro studies have shown that tacrolimus inhibits degranulation of polymorphonuclear leukocytes (116). Some in vitro data suggest that tacrolimus might be less toxic than cyclosporine to endothelial cells (124). Because cyclosporine and tacrolimus share the same mechanism of action and side-effect profile, it is unlikely that these drugs will ever be used in combination.

Adverse Effects of Tacrolimus

Although the exact mechanism of immunosuppression of tacrolimus is similar to that of cyclosporin A, the mechanism of nephrotoxicity remains unclear. The cellular target of the tacrolimus–FK-BP-binding protein is the serine–threonine phosphatase enzyme calcineurin (106). Similar to cyclosporine, tacrolimus also inhibits the multidrug resistance transporter in proximal tubular cells. It is of interest that tacrolimus and cyclosporine exhibit pharmacologic antagonism. The implications of this for nephrotoxicity in clinical immunosuppression remains unclear.

Clinical Manifestations of Nephrotoxicity

Serum creatinines are frequently elevated in liver and heart transplant recipients (201). There is limited use of tacrolimus in autoimmune or primary renal diseases. The incidence of nephrotoxicity is comparable to cyclosporine and, as with cyclosporin A, therapeutic drug monitoring is only loosely correlated with renal function. Asymptomatic elevations of serum creatinine are difficult to distinguish from allograft rejection in renal transplant recipients. Tacrolimus may produce less change in renal hemodynamics than cyclosporine, although this is largely an experimental phenomenon not yet demonstrated clearly in humans. There is limited human histopathologic material, but what is known suggests that tacrolimus causes vacuolar change in myocytes and tubular cells (212). Chronic administration of tacrolimus can produce striped interstitial fibrosis and arteriolar hyalinosis. Renal function may deteriorate rapidly when tacrolimus is used in patients also receiving cyclosporine. Hyperkalemia, hyperuricemia, and hypomagnesemia all occur with tacrolimus similar to that seen with cyclosporine. Blood pressure elevations are less frequent and less severe in liver transplant recipients receiving tacrolimas instead of cyclosporine. In general, patients receiving tacrolimus require less antihypertensive drug therapy perhaps because tacrolimus is relatively steroid sparing.

Pathophysiology of Tacrolimus Nephrotoxicity

Although tacrolimus differs structurally from cyclosporine, the nephrotoxicity is qualitatively similar (213). Very large doses of acutely administered tacrolimus produce little or no increase, however, in renal vascular resistance. This is consistent with the contention that tacrolimus causes less hypertension and increased peripheral vascular resistance than cyclosporine. Tacrolimus also does not increase renal dysfunction in rats with renal ischemia (214). In some animal species such as certain rat strains and dogs, tacrolimus produces medial arterial necrosis and widespread vasculitis. This has not been seen clinically to date. Human endothelial cells showed no expression of endothelin-1 mRNA or endothelin-1 secretion in clinically relevant doses (124,215). This contrasts with cyclosporin A. Given subacutely or chronically to animals, tacrolimus can produce acute renal dysfunction reversed by calcium antagonists and angiotensin-II receptor blockade. Chronic tacrolimus nephrotoxicity can be produced in animals maintained on a low-salt diet. Hypertension is putatively less frequent and severe with tacrolimus than cyclosporin A. This is largely based on clinical observations in liver transplant recipients in whom cyclosporine induces a larger increase in systemic blood pressure and peripheral vascular resistance than tacrolimus, while affecting renal function similarly. In vitro, tacrolimus causes less impairment of endothelin-dependent relaxation than cyclosporin A (216). These comparative studies, however, are difficult to interpret due to the complex pharmacokinetics of these lipophilic immunosuppressive drugs.

Other Adverse Effects

Although cyclosporine produces more nephrotoxicity than neurotoxicity, the converse seems to be true of tacrolimus. Headache, seizures, tremor, and other neurologic manifestations are more common with therapeutic blood levels of tacrolimus than cyclosporine. Hirsutism and gingival hyperplasia are less frequent with tacrolimus. This may be an advantage in female recipients as well as children.

Clinical Uses

Tacrolimus was developed as a immunosuppressive agent for solid organ transplantation. Unlike cyclosporine, tacrolimus, in uncontrolled studies, was able to reverse acute allograft rejection, a quality probably related to its potency (208). Small series have suggested that tacrolimus may be useful in steroid-resistant nephrotic syndrome (217).

OMEGA-3 FATTY ACIDS (FISH OILS)

Polyunsaturated fatty acids represent <2% of the daily fat intake in the United States diet and can be classified into two major categories: the linoleic (LA) (omega-6) and the α-linoleic (α-LA)(omega-3) series of fatty acids. Omega-3 fatty acids (n-3 FAs) belong to a series of polyunsaturated fatty acids characterized by the first double bound at the third position from the methyl end of the molecule (218). n-3 FAs account for <5% of total polyunsaturated fatty acid in the US diet (219). The n-3 FAs are considered essential because mammals cannot synthesize such long fatty-acid chains, although they can desaturate and elongate the aliphatic chain (220). The linoleic acids come from vegetable oils, and their metabolism produces arachidonic acid and its derivatives. On the other hand, metabolism of the α-linoleic acids results in eicosapentaenoic acid (EPA) and docosahexaenoic acid (DHA). Fatty fish and poultry are our main source of EPA and DHA, respectively (219) (Table 1).

Mechanisms of Action

Both the LA and α-LA metabolic pathways utilize the same catabolic enzymes but produce diverse products (Fig. 2) with no interconversion between them. The main purpose behind the use of greater amounts of n-3 FAs would be increased production, by increasing substrates, of metabolites with favorable vasculoprotective and hemodynamic profile (220). n-3 FAs decrease the production of compounds that promote chemotaxis and inflammation (leukotriene 4, LT-4), vasoconstriction (prostaglandin $F_{2\alpha}$), mesangial cell growth (LT-4) and platelet activation (PAF). Renal thromboxane-A_2 production is reduced by n-3 FAs, which correlates with improvement in proteinuria (221) and cyclosporine-induced vasoconstriction (134). In a model of passive Heymann nephritis, n-3 FAs had a protective and therapeutic effect upon proteinuria (222). The beneficial effect of n-3 FAs has been difficult to show in other animal models of renal disease (223,224). In healthy human volunteers, n-3 FAs increased renal plasma flow and glomerular filtration rate, while decreasing intrarenal vascular resistance (225). Theoretically, n-3 FAs would be better agents than nonsteroid anti-inflammatory drugs because they would divert the eicosanoid balance toward the α-LA arm rather than just inhibiting the AA metabolic pathway. Those changes, however, are quite subtle and their clinical significance is still questionable (220). The production of platelet-derived growth factor, IL-1, IL-2, and TNF is

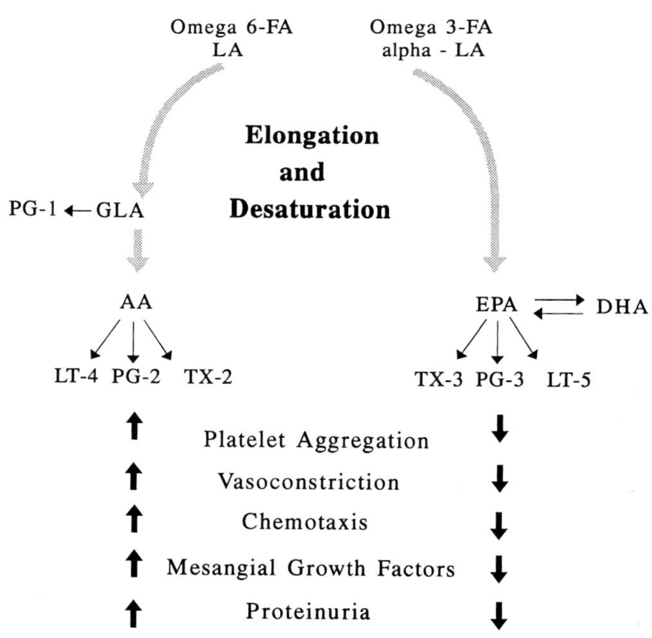

FIG. 2. Metabolic pathways of omega fatty acids.

also affected by fish oils through an undefined none-icosanoid pathway. n-3 FAs have been shown in vitro to inhibit T-lymphocyte proliferation via a noneicosanoid pathway (226). Other potential benefits of n-3 FAs would be ameliorating the dyslipidemia that is commonly found in patients with renal disease, favorable effects on blood viscosity and red blood cell deformability, systemic hypotensive effects, and decreased vascular permeability. The mechanisms underlying these beneficial effects are still unknown (220,227).

Omega-3 Fatty-Acid Adverse Effects

There have been limited clinical applications of n-FAs in the treatment of renal disease and for the purpose of reducing nephrotoxicity of immunosuppressive agents such as cyclosporine (166). To date, the studies in people have used a variety of doses and dose regimens. The effective dose for changing the thromboxane prostaglandin profile is ~1–2 g of active n-FA daily. The lower limits of efficacy are not well established. There seem to be few serious side effects. The caloric effects of these oils could be significant in causing weight gain, and theoretically platelet dysfunction could lead to excessive bleeding. In the clinical trials to date, however, no excessive bleeding has been noted. The most common side effect has been an unpleasant postdose breath, which has limited the acceptance of fish oil by some patients (167).

Clinical Uses

Clinical studies are difficult to compare due to nonstandardization of commercially available fish-oil products regarding proportional concentration and bioavailability of the n-3 FAs (228). Most of the human studies have focused in IgA nephropathy (229,230), cyclosporin-A nephrotoxicity (133,135,136), systemic lupus erythematosus (231), and other chronic glomerular diseases. Some reports showed some improvement in biological markers like proteinuria (221), but clinically significant benefits have been demonstrated only in these few settings (220).

INTERFERONS

IFNs are proteins synthesized by eukaryotic cells with potent antiviral, antiproliferative, and immunomodulatory properties. They have been classified according to the cell of origin and spectrum of action into three groups (α, β, and γ) (232,233). IFN-α is the only agent of this class used clinically in immune-mediated renal disease, and our review will be restricted to it. IFN-α is composed of a group of proteins, with similar amino acid sequences but diverse biological effects in human cells (Table 1).

Absorption

The subcutaneous or intramuscular bioavailability following a single injection of IFN-α is near 80%. A peak plasma concentration is usually achieved 4–8 h after single-dose administration. An exponential increase in plasma concentration of IFN-α after administration of higher doses has been reported (234).

Distribution

A volume of distribution ranging from 30–370 liters has been reported following systemic administration of IFN-α in normal volunteers and patients with leukemia, respectively. IFN-α does not readily distribute throughout the body tissue. Only low levels (<1%) of IFN-α are detectable in cerebrospinal fluid, respiratory secretions, and eye (234,235).

Metabolism

A small fraction of injected IFN-α is metabolized or excreted in bile. Clearance rates reported for IFN-α after intravenous infusion range from 157 to 272 mL/min. IFN-α is totally filtered by glomeruli with minimal tubular reabsorption. Following filtration, IFM-α undergoes rapid degradation that results in no detectable amounts of the drug in the urine (234).

Mechanism of Action

The mechanisms of action of IFNs are multifaceted and driven by the virus studied and is also biased by the cell system used (232). IFN-α binds to its plasma membrane receptor and activates gene transcription of a large number of proteins that interfere with several steps of viral cycle, like cell penetration, synthesis of viral mRNA, and translation of proteins. IFN-α also inhibits viral assembly and cell release of viral particles (236). Type-I IFN receptor binds to either IFN-α or IFN-β. After binding to its ligand, the receptor is phosphorylated in its serine/threonine residues. The mechanism of signal transduction is not fully understood yet, but it involves activation of preformed cytoplasmic transcription factors (named IFN-stimulated gene factors) that would then translocate to the cell nucleus (232). A highly conserved 14 base-pair DNA sequence is found in the promoter region of genes from most IFN-induced proteins. It is called IFN-responsive element and it is the binding site of transcription factors induced by IFN–IFN receptor interaction (237). IFN promotes indirect antiviral effects by means of enhancing nonspecific steps of the immune response as increasing of the major histocompatibility complex antigen expression, increasing Fc expression and adhesion molecule density on the surface of lymphocytes and accessory cells, enhancing the cytolytic properties of natural killers cells and macrophages, increasing production of proinflammatory cytokines and expression of their receptors, and promoting antibody formation and antibody-dependent cellular cytotoxicity (233,236,237). IFN also down regulates the level of expression of a few proteins (232). It is shown that, in the case of hepatitis-B virus, IFN-α interferes with the assembly of the virus core particle (237).

Adverse Effects

Unfortunately, IFN therapy is marked by high dropout rates due to significant adverse reactions to the drug (238). The most commonly reported side effects are fever, chills, myalgia, nausea, vomiting, and headache following the first doses (234,239). Anorexia, weight loss, persistent fatigue, insomnia, thrombocytopenia, leukopenia, elevation of liver enzymes, and alopecia were present during the duration of the treatment. In some series, these side effects were ameliorated by reduction of dosage (240,241). Due to the putative immune activation induced by IFN, the use of these agents after renal transplantation is still controversial (242). Isolated reports implicate IFN-α as a causative agent of glomerulopathies (243,244).

Clinical Uses

IFN-α has been used successfully in the treatment of glomerulopathies related to chronic hepatitis B (245–247 and C (241,248–250). IFN-α has been used in the past decade for treatment of mixed cryoglobulinemia (240, 251,252) and has been effective (at least during short follow-up period) in treating hepatitis-B and -C viremia (253) and may halt histologic liver disease progression, even in dialysis patients (238,254). Studies with longer follow-up periods are needed to exclude late recurrence. Safety and efficacy of IFN-α use after kidney transplantation are still under investigation (239,242).

REFERENCES

1. Elion GB. The pharmacology of azathioprine. *Annals NY Acad Sci* 1993;685:401–7.
2. Cory JG. Purine and pyrimidine nucleotide metabolism. In: Devlin TM, ed. *Textbook of biochemistry:* with clinical correlations. New York: Wiley–Liss, 1992:529–73.
3. St Georgiev V. Enzymes of the purine metabolism: inhibition and therapeutic potential. *Ann NY Acad Sci* 1993;685:207–16.
4. Chan GLC, Canafax DM, Johnson CA. The therapeutic use of azathioprine in renal transplantation. *Pharmacotherapy* 1987;7:165–77.
5. Chocair PR, Duley JA, Simmonds HA, Cameron JS. The importance of thiopurine methyltransferase activity for the use of azathioprine in transplant recipients. *Transplantation* 1992;53:1051–6.
6. Allison AC, Eugui EM. Inhibitors of de novo purine and pyrimidine synthesis as immunosuppressive drugs. *Transplant Proc* 1993;25: 8–18.
7. Lu CY, Sicher SC, Vazquez MA. Prevention and treatment of renal allograft rejection: new therapeutic approaches and new insights into established therapies. *J Am Soc Nephrol* 1993;4:1239–56.
8. Mitchell BS, Dayton JS, Turka LA, Thompson CB. IMP dehydrogenase inhibitors as immunomodulators. *Ann NY Acad Sci* 1993;685: 217–24.
9. Lennard I, Brown CB, Fos M, Maddocks JL. Azathioprine metabolism in kidney transplant recipients. *Br J Clin Pharmacol* 1984;18: 693–700.
10. Pollak R, Nishikawa RA, Mozes M, Johasson O. Azathioprine-induced leukopenia: clinical significance in renal transplantation. *J Surg Res* 1980;29:258–64.
11. DeClerck YA, Ettinger RB, Ortega JA, Pennisi AJ. Macrocytosis and pure RBC anemia caused by azathioprine. *Am J Dis Child* 1980;134: 377–9.
12. Sparburg M, Simon N, DeGreco F. Intrahepatic cholestasis due to azathioprine. *Gastroenterology* 1969;57:439–41.
13. Pettrelli M, Ricanati ES, McCullough AJ. Hepatic veno-occlusive disease associated with renal transplantation and azathioprine therapy. *Ann Intern Med* 1986;104:651–5.
14. Ware AJ, Luby JP, Hollinger B, et al. Etiology of liver diseases in renal transplantation patients. *Ann Intern Med* 1979;91:364–71.
15. Weir M, Kirkman RL, Strom TB, Tilney NL. Liver disease in recipients of long functioning renal allografts. *Kidney Int* 1985;28:839–44.
16. Bedrossian CW, Sussman J, Conklin RH, Kahan BD. Azathioprine associated interstitial pneumonitis. *Am J Clin Pathol* 1984;82: 148–54.
17. Donadio JV Jr, Glassock RJ. Immunosuppressive drug therapy in lupus nephritis. *Am J Kidney Dis* 1993;21:239–50.
18. Ponticelli C, Passerini P. Alkylating agents and purine analogues in primary glomerulonephritis with nephrotic syndrome. *Nephrol Dial Transplant* 1991;6:381–8.
19. Cade R, Mars D, Privette M, et al. Effect of long-term azathioprine administration in adults with minimal-change glomerulonephritis and nephrotic syndrome resistant to corticosteroids. *Arch Intern Med* 1986;146:737–41.
20. Keller F, Oehlenberg B, Kunzendorf U, Schwarz A, Offermann G. Long-term treatment and prognosis of rapidly progressive glomerulonephritis. *Clin Nephrol* 1989;31:190–7.
21. Calabresi P, Chabner BA. Antineoplastic agents. In: Gilman AG, Rall TW, Niew AS, Taylor P, eds. *Goodman and Gilman's The pharmacological basis of therapeutics.* New York: Pergamon, 1990:1209–36.
22. Fraiser LH, Kanekal S, Kehrer JP. Cyclophosphamide toxicity. *Drugs* 1991;42:781–95.
23. Rondeau E, Kourilsky O, Peraldi M-N, Alberti C, Kanfer A, Sraer J-D. Methylprednisolone and cyclophosphamide pulse therapy in crescentic glomerulonephritis: safety and effectiveness. *Ren Fail* 1993; 15:495–501.
24. Hoffman GS, Leavitt RY, Fleisher TA, Minor JR, Fauci AS. Treatment of Wegener's granulomatosis with intermittent high-dose intravenous cyclophosphamide. *Am J Med* 1990;89:403–10.
25. Kunis CL, Kiss B, Williams G, D'Agati V, Appel GB. Intravenous "pulse" cyclophosphamide therapy of crescentic glomerulonephritis. *Clin Nephrol* 1992;37:1–7.
26. Austin HA III, Klippel JH, Balow JE, et al. Therapy of lupus nephritis. *N Engl J Med* 1986;314:614–9.
27. Vogelzang NJ. Nephrotoxicity from chemotherapy: prevention and management. *Oncology* 1991;5:97–110.
28. Patterson WP, Khojasteh A. Ifosfamide induced renal tubular defects. *Cancer* 1989;63:649–51.
29. McCune WJ, Golbus J, Zeldes W, Bohlke P, Dunne R, Fox DA. Clinical and immunologic effects of monthly administration of intravenous cyclophosphamide in severe systemic lupus erythematosus. *N Engl J Med* 1988;318:1423–31.
30. Levey AS, Lan S-P, Corwin HL, et al. The Lupus Nephritis Collaborative Study Group: progression and remission of renal disease in the lupus nephritis collaborative study. *Ann Intern Med* 1992;116: 114–23.
31. Fauci AS, Haynes BF, Katz P, Wolff SM. Wegener's granulomatosis: prospective clinical and therapeutic experience with 85 patients for 21 years. *Ann Intern Med* 1983;98:76–85.
32. Haubitz M, Frei U, Rother U, Brunkhorst R, Koch KM. Cyclophos-

phamide pulse therapy in Wegener's granulomatosis. *Nephrol Dial Transplant* 1991;6:531–5.
33. Palmer A, Cairns T, Dische F, et al. Treatment of rapidly progressive glomerulonephritis by extracorporeal immunoadsorption, prednisolone and cyclophosphamide. *Nephrol Dial Transplant* 1991;6: 536–42.
34. Couser WG. Rapidly progressive glomerulonephritis: classification, pathogenetic mechanisms, and therapy. *Am J Kidney Dis* 1988;11: 449–64.
35. Ponticelli C, Passerini P. The natural history and therapy of idiopathic membranous nephropathy. *Nephrol Dial Transplant Suppl* 1990;1: 37–41.
36. Murphy BF, McDonald I, Fairley KF, Kincaid-Smith PS. Randomized controlled trial of cyclophosphamide, warfarin and dipyridamole in idiopathic membranous glomerulonephritis. *Clin Nephrol* 1992;37: 229–34.
37. Bruns FJ, Adler S, Fraley DS, Segel DP. Sustained remission of membranous glomerulonephritis after cyclophosphamide and prednisone. *Ann Intern Med* 1991;114:725–30.
38. Falk RJ, Hogan SL, Muller KE, Jennette JC, Glomerular Disease Collaborative Network. Treatment of progressive membranous glomerulopathy: a randomized trial comparing cyclophosphamide and corticosteroids with corticosteroids alone. *Ann Intern Med* 1992;116: 438–45.
39. Maezawa A, Hiromura K, Mitsuhashi H, et al. Combined treatment with cyclophosphamide and prednisolone can induce remission of nephrotic syndrome in a patient with renal amyloidosis, associated with rheumatoid arthritis. *Clin Nephrol* 1994;42:30–2.
40. Gertz MA, Kyle RA, Greipp PR. Response rates and survival in primary systemic amyloidosis. *Blood* 1991;77:257–62.
41. Goddard IR, Jackson R, Boulton Jones JM. AL amyloidosis: therapeutic response in two patients with renal involvement. *Nephrol Dial Transplant* 1991;6:592–4.
42. Niaudet P, French Society of Paediatric Nephrology. Comparison of cyclosporin and chlorambucil in the treatment of steroid-dependent idiopathic nephrotic syndrome: a multicentre randomized controlled trial. *Pediatr Nephrol* 1992;6:1–3.
43. English J, Dunne M, Marks V. Diurnal variation in prednisolone kinetics. *Clin Pharmacol Ther* 1983;33:381–5.
44. Rose JQ, Nickelsen JA, Ellis EF, Middleton E, Jusko WJ. Prednisolone disposition in steroid-dependent asthmatic children. *J Allergy Clin Immunol* 1981;67:188–93.
45. Miller PFW, Bowmer CJ, Wheeldon J, Brocklebank JT. Pharmacokinetics of prednisolone in children with nephrosis. *Arch Dis Child* 1990;65:196–200.
46. Jusko WJ, Milad MA, Ludwig EA, Lew KH, Kohli RK. Methylprednisolone pharmacokinetics and pharmacodynamics in chronic renal failure. *Clin Nephrol* 1995;43:S16–9.
47. Gambertoglio JG, Amend WJC, Benet LZ. Pharmacokinetics and bioavailability of prednisone and prednisolone in healthy volunteers and patients: a review. *J Pharmacokinet Biopharm* 1980;8:1–47.
48. Boumpas DT, Chrousos GP, Wilder RL, Cupps TR, Balow JE. Glucocorticoid therapy for immune-mediated diseases: basic and clinical correlates. *Ann Intern Med* 1993;119:1198–208.
49. Karin M, Yang-Yen H-F, Chambard J-C, Deng T, Saatcioglu F. Various modes of gene regulation by nuclear receptors for steroid and thyroid hormones. *Eur J Clin Pharmacol* 1993;45:S9–15.
50. Miesfeld RL. Molecular genetics of corticosteroid action. *Am Rev Respir Dis* 1990;141:S11–7.
51. Munck A, Mendel DB, Smith LI, Orti E. Glucocorticoid receptors and actions. *Am Rev Respir Dis* 1990;141:S2–10.
52. Wright APH, Zilliacus J, McEwan IJ, et al. Structure and function of the glucocorticoid receptor. *J Steroid Biochem Mol Biol* 1993;47: 11–9.
53. Ray A, Sehgal PB. Cytokines and their receptors: molecular mechanism of interleukin-6 gene repression by glucocorticoids. *J Am Soc Nephrol* 1992;2:S214–21.
54. Yang-Yen H-F, Chambard J-C, Sun Y-L, et al. Transcriptional interference between c-Jun and the glucocorticoid receptor: mutual inhibition of DNA binding due to direct protein–protein interaction. *Cell* 1990;62:1205–15.
55. Schule R, Rangarajan P, Kliewer S, et al. Functional antagonism between oncoprotein c-Jun and the glucocorticoid receptor. *Cell* 1990;62:1217–26.
56. Vacca A, Felli MP, Farina AR, et al. Glucocorticoid receptor-mediated suppression of the interleukin 2 gene expression through impairment of the cooperativity between nuclear factor of activated T cells and AP-1 enhancer elements. *J Exp Med* 1992;175:637–46.
57. Krane SM. Some molecular mechanisms of glucocorticoid action. *Br J Rheumatol* 1993;32:3–5.
58. Paliogianni F, Raptis A, Ahuja SS, Najjar SM, Boumpas DT. Negative transcriptional regulation of human interleukin 2 (IL-2) gene by glucocorticoids through interference with nuclear transcription factors AP-1 and NF-AT. *J Clin Invest* 1993;91:1481–9.
59. Schleimer RP. An overview of glucocorticoid anti-inflammatory actions. *Eur J Clin Pharmacol* 1993;45:S3–7.
60. Pfeilschifter J, Mühl H, Pignat W, Märki F, van den Bosch H. Cytokine regulation of group II phospholipase A_2 expression in glomerular mesangial cells. *Eur J Clin Pharmacol* 1993;44:S7–9.
61. Celada A, McKercher S, Maki RA. Repression of major histocompatibility complex IA expression by glucocorticoids: the glucocorticoid receptor inhibits the DNA binding of the X box DNA binding protein. *J Exp Med* 1993;177:691–8.
62. Williams TJ, Yarwood H. Effect of glucocorticosteroids on microvascular permeability. *Am Rev Respir Dis* 1990;141:S39–43.
63. Kern JA, Lamb RJ, Reed JC, Daniele RP, Nowell PC. Dexamethasone inhibition of interleukin 1 beta production by human monocytes. *J Clin Invest* 1988;81:237–44.
64. Han j, Thompson p, Beutler B. Dexamethasone and pentoxifylline inhibit endotoxin-induced cachectin/tumor necrosis factor synthesis at separate points in the signaling pathway. *J Exp Med* 1990;172: 391–4.
65. Peers SH, Flower RJ. The role of lipocortin in corticosteroid actions. *Am Rev Respir Dis* 1990;141:S18–21.
66. Goulding NJ, Guyre PM. Regulation of inflammation by lipocortin 1. *Immunol Today* 1992;13:295–297.
67. Rota S, Rambaldi A, Gaspari F, et al. Methylprednisolone dosage effects on peripheral lymphocyte subpopulations and eicosanoid synthesis. *Kidney Int* 1992;42:981–90.
68. Coyne DW, Nickols M, Bertrand W, Morrison AR. Regulation of mesangial cell cyclooxygenase synthesis by cytokines and glucocorticoids. *Am J Physiol* 1992;263:F97–102.
69. Alwani WY, Hadro ET, Strom TB. Evidence that glucocorticoid-mediated immunosuppressive effects do not involve altering second messenger function. *Transplantation* 1991;52:133–40.
70. O'Banion MK, Winn VD, Young DA. c-DNA cloning and functional activity of a glucocorticoid-related inflammatory cyclooxygenase. *Proc Natl Acad Sci USA* 1992;89:4888–92.
71. Radomski MW, Palmer RMJ, Moncada S. Glucocorticoids inhibit the expression of an inducible, but not the constitutive, nitric oxide synthase in vascular endothelial cells. *Proc Natl Acad Sci USA* 1990;87: 10,043–7.
72. Geller DA, Nussler AK, Di Silvio M, et al. Cytokines, endotoxin, and glucocorticoids regulate the expression of inducible nitric oxide synthase in hepatocytes. *Proc Natl Acad Sci USA* 1993;90:522–6.
73. Gambertoglio T, Frey F, Holford N, et al. Prednisone and prednisolone bioavailability in renal transplant patients. *Kidney Int* 1982;21: 621–6.
74. Gambertoglio JG, Holford NH, Lizak PS, Birnbaum JL, Salvatierra O, Amend WJ. The absence of effect of azathioprine on prednisolone pharmacokinetics following maintenance prednisone doses in kidney transplant patients. *Am J Kidney Dis* 1984;3:425–9.
75. Ong CS, Pollock CA, Caterson RJ, Mahony JF, Waugh DA, Ibels LS. Hyperlipidemia in renal transplant recipients: natural history and response to treatment. *Medicine (Baltimore)* 1994;73:215–23.
76. Sharma AK, Myers TA, Hunninghake DB, Matas AJ, Kashtan CE. Hyperlipidemia in long-term survivors of pediatric renal transplantation. *Clin Transplant* 1994;8:252–7.
77. Ingulli E, Tejani A, Markell M. The beneficial effects of steroid withdrawal on blood pressure and lipid profile in children posttransplantation in the cyclosporine era. *Transplantation* 1993;55:1029–33.
78. Lukert BP, Raisz LG. Glucocorticoid-induced osteoporosis: pathogenesis and management. *Ann Intern Med* 1990;112:352–64.
79. Russell RGG. Cellular regulatory mechanisms that may underlie the effects of corticosteroids on bone. *Br J Rheumatol* 1993;32:6–10.
80. Hodgson SF. Corticosteroid-induced osteoporosis. *Endocrinol Metab Clin North Am* 1990;19:95–111.
81. Manolagas SC, Jilka RL. Bone marrow, cytokines, and bone remodel-

ing: emerging insights into the pathophysiology of osteoporosis. *N Engl J Med* 1995;332:305–11.
82. Avioli LV. Potency ratio: a brief synopsis. *Br J Rheumatol* 1993;32 (Suppl 2):24–6.
83. Olgaard K, Storm T, Wowern NV, et al. Glucocorticoid-induced osteoporosis in the lumbar spine, forearm, and mandible of nephrotic patients: a double-blind study on the high-dose, long-term effects of prednisone versus deflazacort. *Br J Rheumatol* 1993;32(Suppl 2): 15–23.
84. Ferraris JR, Pasqualini T. Therapy with a new glucocorticoid: effects of deflazacort on linear growth and growth hormone secretion in renal transplantation. *J Rheumatol* 1993;20(Suppl 37):43–6.
85. Gennari C. Differential effect of glucocorticoids on calcium absorption and bone mass. *Br J Rheumatol* 1993;32(Suppl 2):11–4.
86. Elli A, Rivolta R, Di Palo FQ, et al. A randomized trial of deflazacort versus 6-methylprednisolone in renal transplantation: immunosuppressive activity and side effects. *Transplantation* 1993;55:209–12.
87. Scudeletti M, Castagnetta L, Imbimbo B, Puppo F, Pierri I, Indiveri F. New glucocorticoids. *Ann NY Acad Sci* 1990;595:368–82.
88. Davison AM. Steroid therapy in primary glomerulonephritis. *Nephrol Dial Transplant Suppl* 1990;1:23–8.
89. Bolton WK, Sturgill BC. Methylprednisolone therapy for acute crescentic rapidly progressive glomerulonephritis. *Am J Nephrol* 1989;9: 368–75.
90. Bruns FJ, Adler S, Fraley DS, Segel DP. Long-term follow-up of aggressively treated idiopathic rapidly progressive glomerulonephritis. *Am J Med* 1989;86:400–6.
91. Schena FP, Montenegro M, Scivittaro V. Meta-analysis of randomised controlled trials in patients with primary IgA nephropathy (Berger's disease). *Nephrol Dial Transplant Suppl* 1990;1:47–52.
92. D'Amico G, Sinico RA. Treatment and monitoring of systemic vasculitis. *Nephrol Dial Transplant Suppl* 1990;1:53–7.
93. Hricik DE, Almawi WY, Strom TB. Trends in the use of glucocorticoids in renal transplantation. *Transplantation* 1994;57:979–89.
94. Yee GC, Mcguire TR. Pharmacokinetic drug interactions with cyclosporine (part II). *Clin Pharmacokinet* 1990;19:400–15.
95. Lake KD. Management of drug interactions with cyclosporine. *Pharmacotherapy* 1991;11:110S–8S.
96. Yee GC, Salomon DR. Cyclosporine. In: Evans WE, Schentag JJ, Jusko WJ, eds. *Applied pharmacokinetics: principles of therapeutic drug monitoring.* Vancouver, WA: Applied Therapeutics, 1992:28: 1–40.
97. Erlanger BF. Do we know the site of action of cyclosporin? *Immunol Today* 1992;13:487–90.
98. Schreiber SL, Crabtree GR. The mechanism of action of cyclosporin A and FK506. *Immunol Today* 1992;13:136–42.
99. Kunz J, Hall MN. Cyclosporin A, FK506 and rapamycin: more than just immunosuppression. *Trends Biochem Sci* 1993;18:334–8.
100. Andersson J, Nagy S, Groth CG, Andersson U. Effects of FK506 and cyclosporine A on cytokine production studied in vitro at a single-cell level. *Immunology* 1992;75:136–42.
101. Russell RGG, Graveley R, Coxon F, et al. Cyclosporin A: mode of action and effects on bone and joint tissues. *Scand J Rheumatol* 1992; 21(Suppl 95):9–18.
102. Wiederrecht G, Lam E, Hung S, Martin M, Sigal N. The mechanism of action of FK-506 and cyclosporin A. *Ann NY Acad Sci* 1993;696: 9–19.
103. Schreiber SL. Chemistry and biology of the immunophilins and their immunosuppressive ligands. *Science* 1991;251:283–7.
104. Fliri H, Baumann G, Enz A, et al. Cyclosporins: structure–activity relationships. *Ann NY Acad Sci* 1993;696:47–53.
105. Clipstone NA, Crabtree GR. Calcineurin is a key signaling enzyme in T lymphocyte activation and the target of the immunosuppressive drugs. *Ann NY Acad Sci* 1993;696:20–30.
106. Bierer BE, Holländer G, Fruman D, Burakoff SJ. Cyclosporin A and FK506: molecular mechanisms of immunosuppression and probes for transplantation biology. *Curr Opin Immunol* 1993;5:763–73.
107. Fischer G, Wittman-Liebold B, Lang K, Kiefhaber T, Schmid FX. Cyclosphilin and peptidyl-prolyl *cis-trans* isomerase are probably identical proteins. *Nature* 1989;337:476–8.
108. Clipstone NA, Crabtree GR. Identification of calcineurin as a key signalling enzyme in T lymphocyte activation. *Nature* 1992;357: 695–7.
109. McCaffrey PG, Perrino BA, Soderling TR, Rao A. NF-ATp: a T lymphocyte DNA-binding protein that is a target for calcineurin and immunosuppressive drugs. *J Biol Chem* 1993;268:3747–52.
110. Brabletz T, Pfeuffer I, Schorr E, Siebelt F, Wirth T, Serfling E. Transforming growth factor β and cyclosporin A inhibit the inducible activity of the interleukin-2 gene in T cells through a noncanonical octamer-binding site. *Mol Cell Biol* 1993;13:1155–62.
111. Henderson DJ, Naya I, Bundick RV. Comparison of the effects of FK-506, cyclosporine-A and rapamycin on IL-2 production. *Immunology* 1991;73:316–21.
112. Khanna A, Li B, Sehajpal PK, Sharma VK, Suthanthiran M. Mechanism of action of cyclosporine: a new hypothesis implicating transforming growth factor-β. *Transplant Rev* 1995;9:41–8.
113. Ayanlar Batuman O, Ferrero AP, Diaz A, Jimenez SA. Regulation of transforming growth factor-β1 gene expression by glucocorticoids in normal human T lymphocytes. *J Clin Invest* 1991;88:1574–80.
114. Thomson AW. The effects of cyclosporin A on non-T cell components of the immune system. *J Autoimmun* 1992;5(A):167–76.
115. Fuleihan R, Ramesh N, Horner A, et al. Cyclosporin A inhibits CD40 ligand expression in T lymphocytes. *J Clin Invest* 1994;93:1315–20.
116. Forrest MJ, Jewell ME, Koo GC, Sigal NH. FK-506 and cyclosporin A: selective inhibition of calcium ionophore-induced polymorphonuclear leukocyte degranulation. *Biochem Pharmacol* 1991;42:1221–8.
117. Hultsch T, Albers MW, Schreiber SL, Hohman RJ. Immunophilin ligands demonstrate common features of signal transduction leading to exocytosis or transcription. *Proc Natl Acad Sci USA* 1991;88: 6229–33.
118. Russell RGG, Graveley R, Skjodt H. The effects of cyclosporin A on bone and cartilage. *Br J Rheumatol* 1993;32:42–6.
119. Xu Q, Leiva MC, Fischkoff SA, Handschumacher RE, Lyttle CR. Leukocyte chemotactic activity of cyclophilin. *J Biol Chem* 1992; 267:11,968–71.
120. Sherry B, Yarlett N, Strupp A, Cerami A. Identification of cyclophilin as a proinflammatory secretory product of lipopolysaccharide-activated macrophages. *Proc Natl Acad Sci USA* 1992;89:3511–5.
121. Martin M, Neumann D, Hoff T, Resch K, Dewitt DL, Goppelt-Struebe M. Interleukin-1-induced cyclooxygenase 2 expression is suppressed by cyclosporin A in rat mesangial cells. *Kidney Int* 1994; 45:150–8.
122. Bobadilla NA, Tapià E, Franco M, et al. Role of nitric oxide in renal hemodynamic abnormalities of cyclosporin nephrotoxicity. *Kidney Int* 1994;46:773–9.
123. Tufro-McReddie A, Gomez A, Norling LL, Omar AA, Moore LC, Kaskel FJ. Effect of CsA on the expression of renin and angiotensin type 1 receptor genes in the rat kidney. *Kidney Int* 1993;43:615–22.
124. Benigni A, Morigi M, Perico N, et al. The acute effect of FK506 and cyclosporine on endothelial cell function and renal vascular resistance. *Transplantation* 1992;54:775–80.
125. Bunchman TE, Brookshire CA. Cyclosporine-induced synthesis of endothelin by cultured human endothelial cells. *J Clin Invest* 1994; 88:310–4.
126. Markell MS, Fernandez J, Naik UP, Ehrlich Y, Kornecki E. Effects of cyclosporine-A and cyclosporine-G on ADP-stimulated aggregation of human platelets. *Ann NY Acad Sci* 1993;696:404–7.
127. Webb AT, Reaveley DA, O'Donnell M, O'Connor B, Seed M, Brown EA. Does cyclosporin increase lipoprotein (a) concentrations in renal transplant recipients? *Lancet* 1993;341:268–70.
128. Webb AT, Brown EA. Letters and comments to editor: author's reply. *Lancet* 1993;341:767.
129. Castelao AM, Barberá MJ, Blanco A, et al. Lipid metabolic abnormalities after renal transplantation under cyclosporine and prednisone immunosuppression. *Transplant Proc* 1992;24:96–8.
130. Kuster GM, Drexel H, Bleisch JA, et al. Relation of cyclosporine blood levels to adverse effects on lipoproteins. *Transplantation* 1994; 57:1479–83.
131. Apanay DC, Neylan JF, Ragab MS, Sgoutas DS. Cyclosporine increases the oxidizability of low-density lipoproteins in renal transplant recipients. *Transplantation* 1994;58:663–9.
132. Kunzendorf U, Walz G, Brockmoeller J, et al. Effects of diltiazem upon metabolism and immunosuppressive action of cyclosporine in kidney graft recipients. *Transplantation* 1991;52:280–4.
133. Homan van der Heide JJ, Bilo HJG, Donker JM, Wilmink JM, Tegzess AM. Effect of dietary fish oil on renal function and rejection in cyclosporine-treated recipients of renal transplants. *N Engl J Med* 1993;329:769–73.

134. Kelley VE, Kirkman RL, Bastos M, Barrett LV, Strom TB. Enhancement of immunosuppression by substitution of fish oil for olive oil as a vehicle for cyclosporine. *Transplantation* 1989;48:98–102.
135. Homan van der Heide JJ, Bilo HJG, Donker AJM, Wilmink JM, Sluiter WJ, Tegzess AM. Dietary supplementation with fish oil modifies renal reserve filtration capacity in postoperative, cyclosporin A-treated renal transplant recipients. *Transpl Int* 1990;3:171–5.
136. Berthoux FC, Guerin C, Burgard G, Berthoux P, Alamartine E. One-year randomized controlled trial with omega-3 fatty acid fish oil in clinical renal transplantation. *Transplant Proc* 1992;24:2578–82.
137. McCulloch TA, Harper SJ, Donnelly PK, et al. Influence of nifedipine on interstitial fibrosis in renal transplant allografts treated with cyclosporin A. *J Clin Pathol* 1994;47:839–42.
138. Myers BD, Ross J, Newton L, Luetscher J, Perlroth M. Cyclosporine-associated chronic nephropathy. *N Engl J Med* 1984;311:699–705.
139. Perico N, Remuzzi G. Cyclosporine-induced renal dysfunction in experimental animals and humans. *Transplant Rev* 1991;5:63–80.
140. Kahan BD. Cyclosporine. *N Engl J Med* 1989;321:1725–38.
141. Dumont FJ, Staruch MJ, Koprak SL, et al. The immunosuppressive and toxic effects of FK-506 are mechanistically related: pharmacology of a novel antagonist of FK-506 and rapamycin. *J Exp Med* 1992; 176:751–60.
142. Sigal NH, Dumont F, Durette P, et al. Is cyclophilin involved in the immunosuppressive and nephrotoxic mechanism of action of cyclosporin-A? *J Exp Med* 1991;172:619–28.
143. Thiebaut F, Tsuruo T, Hamada H, Gottesman MM, Pastan I, Willingham MC. Cellular localization of the multidrug-resistance gene product P-glycoprotein in normal human tissues. *Proc Natl Acad Sci USA* 1987;84:7735–8.
144. Okamura N, Hirai M, Tanigawara Y, et al. Digoxin–cyclosporin A interaction: modulation of the multidrug transporter P-glycoprotein in the kidney. *J Pharmacol Exp Ther* 1993;266:1614–9.
145. Serino F, Grevel J, Napoli KL, Kahan BD, Strobel HW. Generation of oxygen free radicals during the metabolism of cyclosporine A: a cause–effect relationship with metabolism inhibition. *Mol Cell Biochem* 1993;122:101–12.
146. Walker PD, Lazzaro VA, Duggin GG, Horvat JS, Tiller DJ. Evidence that alteration in renal metabolism and lipid peroxidation may contribute to nephrotoxicity. *Transplantation* 1990;50:487–92.
147. Bennett WM. The nephrotoxicity of immunosuppressive drugs. *Clin Nephrol* 1995;43(Suppl 1):53–7.
148. Myers BD, Ross J, Newton L, Luetscher J, Perlroth M. Cyclosporine associated chronic nephropathy. *N Engl J Med* 1984;311:699–705.
149. Myers BD, Newton L, Boshkos C. Chronic injury of human renal microvessels with low-dose cyclosporine therapy. *Transplantation* 1988;46:694–703.
150. Young EW, Ellis CN, Messana JM. A prospective study of renal structure and function in psoriasis patients treated with cyclosporine. *Kidney Int* 1994;46:1216–22.
151. Zachariae H, Hansen HE, Kragballe K, Olsen S. Morphologic renal changes during cyclosporine treatment of psoriasis. *J Am Acad Dermatol* 1992;26:415–9.
152. Mihatsch MJ, Antonovych T, Bohman S-0. Cyclosporin A nephropathy: standardization of the evaluation of kidney biopsies. *Clin Nephrol* 1994;41:23–32.
153. Shulman H, Striker G, Deeg JH, Kennedy M, Storb R, Thomas ED. Nephrotoxicity of cyclosporine A after allogenic marrow transplantation: glomerular thrombosis and tubular injury. *N Engl J Med* 1981; 305:1392–5.
154. Giroux L, Smeesters C, Corman J, et al. Hemolytic uremic syndrome in renal allografted patients treated with cyclosporin. *Can J Physiol Pharmacol* 1987;65:1125–31.
155. Curtiss JJ. Hypertension and kidney transplantation. *Am J Kidney Dis* 1986:181–96.
156. Bennett WM, Burdmann EA, Andoh TF, Houghton DC, Lindsley J, Elzinga LW. Nephrotoxicity of immunosuppressive drugs. *Nephrol Dial Transplant* 1994;9:141–5.
157. Barros EJG, Boim MA, Ajzen H, Ramos OL, Schor N. Glomerular hemodynamics and hormonal participation on cyclosporine nephrotoxicity. *Kidney Int* 1985;32:19–25.
158. Bantle JP, Paller MS, Bourdreau RM, Olivari MT, Ferris TF. Long-term effects of cyclosporine on renal function in organ transplant recipients. *J Lab Clin Med* 1990;115:233–40.
159. English J, Evan A, Houghton DC, Bennett WM. Cyclosporine-induced acute renal dysfunction in rat. *Transplantation* 1987;44: 135–41.
160. Burdmann EA, Andoh TF, Franceschini N, Fugihara C, Zatz R, Bennett WM. Acute renal failure after intravenous cyclosporine administration: role of the vehicle. *J Am Soc Nephrol* 1994;5:918(abst).
161. Perico N, Zoja C, Benigni A, Ghilardi F, Gualandris L, Remuzzi G. Effect of short-term cyclosporine administration in rats on renin–angiotensin and thromboxane A_2: possible relevance to the reduction in glomerular filtration rate. *J Pharmacol Exp Ther* 1986;239: 229–35.
162. McAuley FT, Whiting PH, Thomson AW, Simpson JG. The influence of enalapril or spronolactone on experimental cyclosporin nephrotoxicity. *Biochem Pharmacol* 1987;36:699–703.
163. Moss NG, Powell SL, Falk RJ. Intravenous cyclosporine activates afferent and efferent renal nerves and causes sodium retention in innervated kidneys in rats. *Proc Natl Acad Sci USA* 1985;82:8222–6.
164. Lyson T, Ermel LD, Belshaw PJ, Alberg DG, Schreiber SL, Victor RG. Cyclosporine and FK506-induced sympathetic activation correlates with calcineurin-mediated inhibition of T cell signaling. *Circ Res* 1993;73:596–602.
165. Coffman TM, Carr DR, Yarger WE, Klotman PE. Evidence that renal prostaglandin and thromboxane production is stimulated in chronic cyclosporine nephrotoxicity. *Transplantation* 1987;43:282–5.
166. Van der Heide JJH, Bilo HJG, Donker JM, Wilmink JM, Tegzecs AM. Effects of dietary fish oil on renal function and rejection in cyclosporine-treated recipients of renal transplants. *N Engl J Med* 1993; 329:769–73.
167. Bennett WM, Carpenter CB, Shapiro ME, et al. Delayed omega-3 fatty acid supplements in renal transplantation: a double blind placebo controlled study. *Transplantation* 1995;59:452–6.
168. Kon V, Sugiura M, Inagami T, Harrie BR, Ichikawa I, Hoover RL. Role of endothelin in cyclosporine-induced glomerular dysfunction. *Kidney Int* 1990;37:1487–91.
169. Fogo A, Hellings SE, Inagami T, Kon V. Endothelin receptor antagonism is protective in in vivo acute cyclosporine toxicity. *Kidney Int* 1992;42:770–4.
170. Conger JD, Kim GE, Robinette JB. Effects of ANG II, ETA, and TxA_2 receptor antagonists on cyclosporin A renal vasoconstriction. *Am Physiol Soc* 1994;267:F443–9.
171. Hunley T, Fogo A, Iwasaki S, Kon V. Endothelin A receptor (EtA) mediates functional but not structural damage in chronic cyclosporine nephrotoxicity (Cy). *J Am Soc Nephrol* 1994;5:581.
172. Elzinga L, Rosen S, Bennett WM. Dissociation of glomerular filtration rate from tubulointerstitial fibrosis in experimental chronic cyclosporine nephropathy: role of sodium intake. *J Am Soc Nephrol* 1993;4:214–21.
173. Ghiggeri GM, Altieri P, Oleggini R, Valente F, Perfumo F, Gusmano R. Selective enhancement of collagen expression by cyclosporin with renal cells in vitro. *J Am Soc Nephrol* 1994;4:753.
174. Pichler R, Franceschini N, Young B. Does angiotensin II mediate cyclosporine nephropathy? *J Am Soc Nephrol* 1994;5:929(abst).
175. Shihab FS, Andoh TF, Tanner AM, Noble NA, Franceschini N, Bennett WM. Fibrosis in chronic renal cyclosporine (CsA) toxicity: preferential expression in medulla. *J Am Soc Nephrol* 1995;6:1004.
176. Meister B, Lippoldt A, Bunnemann B, Inagami T, Ganten D, Fuxe K. Cellular expression of angiotensin type-1 receptor mRNA in the kidney. *Kidney Int* 1993;44:331–6.
177. Nield GH, Reuben R, Hartley RB. Glomerular thrombi in renal allografts associated with cyclosporin treatment. *J Clin Pathol* 1983;38: 253–8.
178. Lau DCW, Wong K-L, Hwang WS. Cyclosporine toxicity on cultured rat microvascular endothelial cells. *Kidney Int* 1989;35:604–13.
179. Sugiura M, Inagami T, Kon V. Endotoxin stimulates endothelin-release in vivo and in vitro as determined by radioimmunoassay. *Biochem Biophys Res Commun* 1989;161:1220–7.
180. Van Buren D, Van Buren CT, Flechner SM, Maddox AM, Verani R, Kahan BD. De novo hemolytic uremic syndrome in renal transplant recipients immunosuppressed with cyclosporine. *Surgery* 1985;98: 54–62.
181. McCauley J, Bronsther O, Fung J, Todo S, Starzl TE. Treatment of cyclosporin-induced haemolytic uraemic syndrome with FK506. *Lancet* 1989;23/30:1516.
182. Textor SC, Canzanello VJ, Taler SJ, et al. Cyclosporine-induced hypertension after transplantation. *Mayo Clin Proc* 1994;69:1182–93.

183. Textor SC, Wiesner R, Wilson DJ, et al. Systemic and renal hemodynamic differences between FK506 and cyclosporine in liver transplant recipients. *Transplantation* 1993;55:1332–9.
184. Tresham JJ, Whitworth JA, Scoggins B, Bennett WM. Cyclosporine-induced hypertension in sheep: role of thromboxanes. *Transplantation* 1990;49:144–8.
185. Richards NT, Poston L, Hilston PJ. Cyclosporin A inhibits endothelium-dependent, prostanoid-induced relaxation in human subcutaneous resistance vessels. *J Hypertens* 1990;8:159–63.
186. Roullet JB, Xue H, McCarron DA, Holcomb S, Bennett WM. Vascular mechanisms of cyclosporine-induced hypertension in the rat. *J Clin Invest* 1994;93:2244–50.
187. Diederich D, Yang Z, Lüscher TF. Chronic cyclosporine therapy impairs endothelium-dependent relaxation in the renal artery of the rat. *J Am Soc Nephrol* 1992;2:1291–7.
188. Tanaka R, Yoshikawa N, Kitano Y, Ito H, Nakamura J. Long-term cyclosporin treatment in children with steroid-dependent nephrotic syndrome. *Pediatr Nephrol* 1993;7:249–52.
189. Tejani A, Butt K, Trachtman H, Suthanthiran M, Rosenthal CJ, Khawar MR. Cyclosporine A induced remission of relapsing nephrotic syndrome in children. *Kidney Int* 1988;33:729–34.
190. Niaudet P, Broyer M, Habib R. Treatment of idiopathic nephrotic syndrome with cyclosporin A in children. *Clin Nephrol* 1991;35 (Suppl 1):S31–6.
191. Nyrop M, Olgaard K. Cyclosporin A treatment of severe steroid resistant nephrotic syndrome in adults. *J Intern Med* 1990;227:65–8.
192. Meyrier A, Noel L-H, Auriche P, Callard P. Long-term renal tolerance of cyclosporin A treatment in adult idiopathic nephrotic syndrome. Collaborative Group of the Societe de Nephrologie. *Kidney Int* 1994;45:1446–56.
193. Meyrier A, Condamin MC, Broneer D, Collaborative Group of the French Society of Nephrology. Treatment of adult idiopathic nephrotic syndrome with cyclosporin A: minimal change disease and focal–segmental glomerulosclerosis. *Clin Nephrol* 1991;35(Suppl 1):S37–42.
194. Ponticelli C. Treatment of the nephrotic syndrome with cyclosporin A. *J Autoimmun* 1992;5(Suppl A):315–24.
195. Cattran DC. Current status of cyclosporin A in the treatment of membranous, IgA and membranoproliferative glomerulonephritis. *Clin Nephrol* 1991;35:S43–7.
196. Vonderscher J, Meinzer A. Rationale for the development of Sandimmune Neoral. *Transplant Proc* 1994;26:2925–7.
197. Levy G, Grant D. Potential for CsA—Neoral in organ transplantation. *Transplant Proc* 1994;26:2932–4.
198. Holt DW, Mueller EA, Kovarik JM, van Bree JB, Kutz K. The pharmacokinetics of Sandimmun Neoral: a new oral formulation of cyclosporine. *Transplant Proc* 1994;26:2935–9.
199. Kahan BD, Dunn J, Fitts C, et al. The Neoral formulation: improved correlation between cyclosporine through levels and exposure in stable renal transplant recipients. *Transplant Proc* 1994;26:2940–3.
200. Frei U, Taesch S, Niese D. Use of Sandimmun Neoral in renal transplant patients. *Transplant Proc* 1994;26:2928–31.
201. Peters DH, Fitton A, Plosker GL, Faulds D. Tacrolimus: a review of its pharmacology, and therapeutic potential in hepatic and renal transplantation. *Drugs* 1993;46:746–94.
202. Venkataramanan R, Jain A, Warty VW, et al. Pharmacokinetics of FK 506 following oral administration: a comparison of FK 506 and cyclosporine. *Transplant Proc* 1991;23:931–3.
203. Beysens AJ, Wijnen RMH, Beuman GH, van der Heyden J, Kootstra G, van As H. FK506: monitoring in plasma or in whole blood? *Transplant Proc* 1991;23:2745–7.
204. Jusko WJ, D'Ambrosio R. Monitoring FK 506 concentrations in plasma and whole blood. *Transplant Proc* 1991;23:2732–5.
205. Warty VS, Venkataramanan R, Zendehrouh P, et al. Practical aspects of FK 506 analysis (Pittsburgh experience). *Transplant Proc* 1991; 23:2730–1.
206. Venkataramanan R, Jain A, Warty VS, et al. Pharmacokinetics of FK 506 in transplant patients. *Transplant Proc* 1991;23:2736–40.
207. Harding MW, Galat A, Uehling DE, Schreiber SL. A receptor for the immunosuppressant FK506 is a *cis-trans* peptidyl-prolylisomerase. *Nature* 1989;341:758–60.
208. Morris RE. New small molecule immunosuppressants for transplantation: review of essential concepts. *J Heart Lung Transplant* 1993;12 (6, Part 2):S275–86.
209. Bierer BE, Mattila PS, Standaert RF, et al. Two distinct signal transmission pathways in T lymphocytes are inhibited by complexes formed between an immunophilin and either FK506 or rapamycin. *Proc Natl Acad Sci USA* 1990;87:9231–5.
210. Parsons WH, Sigal NH, Wyvratt MJ. FK-506: a novel immunosuppressant. *Ann NY Acad Sci* 1993;685:22–36.
211. Sigal NH, Dumont FJ. Cyclosporin A, FK-506, and rapamycin: pharmacologic probes of lymphocyte signal transduction. *Annu Rev Immunol* 1992;10:519–60.
212. Thompson AW. FK-506: profile of an important new immunosuppressant. *Transplant Rev* 1990;4:1–13.
213. Randhawa PS, Shapiro R, Jordan ML, Starzl TE, Demetris AJ. The histopathological changes associated with allograft rejection and drug toxicity in renal transplant recipients maintained on FK506. *Am J Surg Pathol* 1993;17:60–8.
214. Nalesnik MA, Lai HS, Murase N, Todo S, Starzl TE. The effect of FK506 and CyA on the Lewis rat renal ischemia model. *Transplant Proc* 1990;22:87–9.
215. Takeda Y, Yoneda T, Ito Y, Miyamori I, Takeda R. Stimulation of endothelin mRNA and secretion in human endothelial cells by FK506. *J Cardiovasc Pharmacol* 1992;22(Suppl 8):S310–2.
216. Roullet JB, Xue H, Andoh TF, et al. Cardiovascular and renal consequences of immunosuppression: adverse effect of FK506 on vascular reactivity. *J Hypertens* 1994;12(Suppl 3):S121.
217. McCauley J, Shapiro R, Scantlebury VP, et al. FK 506 in the management of transplant-related nephrotic syndrome and steroid-resistant nephrotic syndrome. *Transplant Proc* 1991;23:3354–6.
218. Nordøy A. Is there a rational use for omega-3 fatty acids (fish oils) in clinical medicine? *Drugs* 1991;42:331–42.
219. Raper NR, Cronin FJ, Exler J. Omega-3 fatty acid content of the U.S. food supply. *J Am Coll Nutr* 1992;11:304–8.
220. De Caterina R, Endres S, Kristensen SD, Schmidt EB. n-3 fatty acids and renal diseases. *Am J Kidney Dis* 1994;24:397–415.
221. De Caterina R, Caprioli R, Giannessi D, et al. n-3 fatty acids reduce proteinuria in patients with chronic glomerular disease. *Kidney Int* 1993;44:843–50.
222. Weise WJ, Natori Y, Levine JS, et al. Fish oil has protective and therapeutic effects on proteinuria in passive Heymann nephritis. *Kidney Int* 1993;43:359–68.
223. Scharschmidt LA, Gibbons NB, McGarry L, et al. Effects of dietary fish oil on renal insufficiency in rats with subtotal nephrectomy. *Kidney Int* 1987;32:700–9.
224. Clark WF, Parbtani A, Philbrick DJ, Spanner E, Huff MW, Holub BJ. Dietary protein restriction versus fish oil supplementation in the chronic remnant nephron model. *Clin Nephrol* 1993;39:295–304.
225. Düsing R, Struck A, Göbel BO, Weisser B, Vetter H. Effects of n-3 fatty acids on renal function and renal prostaglandin E metabolism. *Kidney Int* 1990;38:315–9.
226. S yland E, Nenseter MS, Braathen L, Drevon CA. Very long chain n-3 and n-6 polyunsaturated fatty acids inhibit proliferation of human T-lymphocytes in vitro. *Eur J Clin Invest* 1993;23:112–21.
227. Connor WE. Omega-3 fatty acids and heart disease. In: Kritchevsky D, Carroll KK, eds. *Nutrition and disease update:* heart disease. Champaign, IL: American Oil Chemists' Society, 1994:7–42.
228. Ackman RG. The absorption of fish oils and concentrates. *Lipids* 1992;27:858–62.
229. Donadio JV Jr, Bergstralh EJ, Offord KP, Spencer DC, Holley KE, Mayo Nephrology Collaborative Group. A controlled trial of fish oil in IgA nephropathy. *N Engl J Med* 1994;331:1194–9.
230. Bennett WM, Walker RG, Kincaid-Smith P. Treatment of IgA nephropathy with eicosapentanoic acid (EPA): a two-year prospective trial. *Clin Nephrol* 1989;31:128–31.
231. Clark WF, Parbtani A, Naylor CD, et al. Fish oil in lupus nephritis: clinical findings and methodological implications. *Kidney Int* 1993; 44:75–86.
232. Sen GC, Ransohoff RM. Interferon-induced antiviral actions and their regulation. *Adv Virus Res* 1993;42:57–102.
233. Samuel CE. Minireview: antiviral actions of interferon—interferon-regulated cellular proteins and their surprisingly selective antiviral activities. *Virology* 1991;183:1–11.
234. Wills RJ. Clinical pharmacokinetics of interferons. *Clin Pharmacokinet* 1990;19:390–9.
235. Smith RA, Norris F, Palmer D, Bernhardt L, Wills RJ. Distribution of alpha interferon in serum and cerebrospinal fluid after systemic administration. *Clin Pharmacol Ther* 1985;37:85–8.

236. Hayden FG. Antiviral agents. In: Mandell GL, Bennett JE, Dolin R, eds. *Mandell, Douglas and Bennett's principles and practice of infectious diseases.* New York: Churchill Livingstone, 1995:411–50.
237. Staeheli P. Interferon-induced proteins and the antiviral state. *Adv Virus Res* 1990;38:147–200.
238. Koenig P, Vogel W, Umlauft F, et al. Interferon treatment for chronic hepatitis C virus infection in uremic patients. *Kidney Int* 1994;45: 1507–9.
239. Rostaing L, Izopet J, Baron E, Duffaut M, Puel J, Durand D. Treatment of chronic hepatitis C with recombinant interferon alpha in kidney transplant recipients. *Transplantation* 1995;59:1426–31.
240. Bonomo L, Casato M, Afeltra A, Caccavo D. Treatment of idiopathic mixed cryoglobulinemia with alpha interferon. *Am J Med* 1987;83: 726–30.
241. Misiani R, Bellavita P, Fenili D, et al. Interferon alfa-2a therapy in cryoglobulinemia associated with hepatitis C virus. *N Engl J Med* 1994;330:751–6.
242. Thervet E, Pol S, Legendre Ch, Gagnadoux M-F, Cavalcanti R, Kreis H. Low-dose recombinant leukocyte interferon-α treatment of hepatitis C viral infection in renal transplant recipients: a pilot study. *Transplantation* 1994;58:625–8.
243. Kimmel PL, Abraham AA, Phillips TM. Membranoproliferative glomerulonephritis in a patient treated with interferon-alpha for human immunodeficiency virus infection. *Am J Kidney Dis* 1994;24: 859–63.
244. Lederer E, Truong L. Unusual glomerular lesion in a patient receiving long term interferon alpha. *Am J Kidney Dis* 1992;20:516–8.
245. Lisker-Melman M, Webb D, Di Bisceglie AM, et al. Glomerulonephritis caused by chronic hepatitis B virus infection: treatment with recombinant human alpha-interferon. *Ann Intern Med* 1989;111: 479–83.
246. Wong S-N, Yu ECL, Lok ASF, Chan K-W, Lau Y-L. Interferon treatment for hepatitis B-associated membranous glomerulonephritis in two Chinese children. *Pediatr Nephrol* 1992;6:417–20.
247. Mizushima N, Kanai K, Matsuda H, et al. Improvement of proteinuria in a case of hepatitis B-associated glomerulonephritis after treatment with interferon. *Gastroenterology* 1987;92:524–6.
248. Yamabe H, Johnson RJ, Gretch DR, et al. Membranoproliferative glomerulonephritis associated with hepatitis C virus infection responsive to interferon-α. *Am J Kidney Dis* 1995;25:67–9.
249. Johnson RJ, Willson R, Yamabe H, et al. Renal manifestations of hepatitis C virus infection. *Kidney Int* 1994;46:1255–63.
250. Johnson RJ, Gretch DR, Yamabe H, et al. Membranoproliferative glomerulonephritis associated with hepatitis C virus infection. *N Engl J Med* 1993;328:465–70.
251. Casato M, Laganà B, Antonelli G, Dianzani F, Bonomo L. Long-term results of therapy with interferon-α for type II essential mixed cryoglobulinemia. *Blood* 1991;78:3142–7.
252. Knox TA, Hillyer CD, Kaplan MM, Berkman EM. Mixed cryoglobulinemia responsive to interferon-α. *Am J Med* 1991;91:554–5.
253. Romeo R, Pol S, Berthelot P, Brechot C. Eradication of hepatitis C virus RNA after alpha-interferon therapy. *Ann Intern Med* 1994;121: 276–7.
254. Duarte R, Huraib S, Said R, et al. Interferon-alpha facilitates renal transplantation in hemodialysis patients with chronic viral hepatitis. *Am J Kidney Dis* 1995;25:40–5.

Immunologic Renal Diseases,
edited by E. G. Neilson and W. G. Couser.
Lippincott-Raven Publishers, Philadelphia © 1997.

CHAPTER 40

Interpretation of Clinical Studies of Renal Disease

Tom Greene, Joseph Lau, and Andrew S. Levey

INTRODUCTION

Recent decades have seen progressively more complex statistical concepts incorporated in the design and analysis in studies of renal diseases. However, incomplete understanding of these concepts is now a serious obstacle to the optimal design and accurate interpretation of clinical studies. In this chapter, we attempt to bridge this gap by describing the main statistical concepts in clinical nephrology research. We first describe the challenges involved in conducting clinical studies of immunologic renal diseases. Then, we provide a brief overview of the types of clinical studies and the principles of randomized trials. In particular, the difficulties in assessing the progression of renal disease are considered in detail. The chapter concludes with a discussion of the principles of meta-analysis and a review of some of the meta-analyses of immunologic renal diseases.

CHALLENGES INVOLVED IN CLINICAL STUDIES OF IMMUNOLOGIC RENAL DISEASES

Table 1 compares features of laboratory and clinical studies in renal disease. In the laboratory, all attempts are made to minimize variability in the experimental model of renal disease and the treatment to be tested. Experimental animals are selected to be of similar age, sex, and strain. The disease is induced in a uniform manner; for example, a uniform dose of nephritogenic antigen is administered at standard intervals. Similarly, the treatment regimen is administered in a uniform dose and at standard intervals. In addition, measurements of renal function and structure are performed using the most sensitive and specific instruments available. By these steps, investigators minimize variability in the clinical response and maximize the ability to detect the response.

In contrast, it is difficult to minimize variability in humans. Investigations are usually undertaken in heterogenous populations, including patients in different stages of the same disease or with different causes of disease. Therefore, patients may vary in their response to the therapeutic intervention being studied. Furthermore, whereas renal biopsy may be performed at the beginning of the study, it is usually performed infrequently or not at all during follow-up, and measurements of renal function are often limited to those that can be performed with the least inconvenience and cost. Thus, it is more difficult to detect the therapeutic response. Consequently, it is usually necessary to enroll a large number of patients to have a high probability of detecting a beneficial effect, if therapy is indeed beneficial. For these reasons, it has been more difficult to determine the effectiveness of therapies of renal disease in humans than in laboratory animals.

These limitations are particularly evident in immunologic renal disease (Table 2). By definition, in idiopathic or primary immunologic renal diseases, the cause is unknown. Instead, these diseases are defined by common morphologic features; for example, the presence of mesangial IgA deposits in IgA nephropathy, or the presence of uniform subepithelial immune complexes in membranous nephropathy. Even in secondary renal diseases, the cause of the systemic disease—for example, systemic lupus erythematosus or vasculitis associated with antineutrophil cytoplasmic antibodies—may be un-

T. Greene: Department of Biostatistics and Epidemiology, Cleveland Clinic Foundation, Cleveland, Ohio 44195.

J. Lau: Division of Clinical Care Research, Department of Medicine, New England Medical Center, Boston, Massachusetts 02111.

A. S. Levey: Department of Medicine, New England Medical Center, Boston, Massachusetts 02111.

TABLE 1. *Differences in design of studies in animals and humans on the progression of renal disease*

	Animal studies	Human studies
Characteristics of population	Uniform	Variable
Characteristics of renal disease	Uniform	Variable
Outcome measurement	Accurate, precise	Convenient
Sample size requirement	Small	Large

known. Possibly, there are multiple causes of these primary and secondary diseases that may respond differently to different therapeutic interventions.

In both primary and secondary renal diseases, the onset of disease may be asymptomatic. Consequently, patients may present themselves for medical care at various phases of illness. Even in patients with renal disease of the same cause, the duration of illness, severity of illness, and prior treatment may affect the prognosis and response to interventions.

The effectiveness of an intervention can be assessed by immunologic, renal, and extrarenal responses. However, assessment of multiple parameters can cause confusion in determining the response to therapy. The different manifestations of disease may not correlate well in individual patients, and therapeutic agents may have varying efficacy for different manifestations. In general, changes in immunologic and extrarenal manifestations are usually not specific enough to assess the progression and remission of renal disease. However, changes in renal function also may lack specificity for this assessment. For example, renal insufficiency may be caused by a variety of pathologic lesions that may respond differently to different therapeutic agents. Inflammation may improve with immunosuppressive therapy while fibrosis does not. Furthermore, assessment of renal function may not be sensitive enough to reveal pathologic evidence of progression. As is discussed later, the glomerular filtration rate (GFR) may remain normal in patients with substantial proteinuria, and progressive glomerular sclerosis may occur despite stable reduction in GFR.

TABLE 2. *Features of immunologic renal disease making it difficult to study*

- Variability among patients
  - Multiple causes of disease
  - Variation in duration, severity, and prior treatment
- Limitations in outcome measurements
  - Poor correlations among immunologic, renal, and extrarenal outcomes
  - Limited specificity and sensitivity of measurements of renal function to assess progression of renal disease
  - Slow rate of progression
  - Complications of immunosuppressive therapy
- Limitations in statistical power
  - Low prevalence in the population

Perhaps the most important and simple outcome to assess is the occurrence of renal failure. For patients undergoing a rapid decline in renal function—for example, cases of rapidly progressive glomerulonephritis—this may be a reasonable strategy. However, in patients with slowly progressive renal diseases, a long duration of follow-up would be necessary to detect the beneficial effect of an intervention on the occurrence of renal failure. Therefore, surrogate outcomes must be selected to assess progression, despite recognized limitations in sensitivity and specificity. In addition, repeated assessment of outcomes during a long follow-up interval requires complicated longitudinal statistical methods.

Whether or not immunosuppressive therapies are effective in causing remission or slowing the progression of renal disease, they can lead to important complications, such as infection or malignancy. These complications must be precisely defined, and sensitive and specific tests must be used to detect them to determine accurately the risks of immunosuppressive therapies. Even when the risk is known, it is difficult to compare the benefit of slowing the progression of renal disease with the harm of a serious infection or malignancy. Many studies use the combined endpoint of the occurrence of death or renal failure. However, as described above, this strategy requires a sufficient duration of follow-up to assess the occurrence of renal failure and late complications of therapy.

Finally, the most difficult aspect of studying immunologic renal diseases is their low prevalence in the population. Clinical trials with adequate statistical power usually require a large sample size, available only through collaboration among a large number of investigators at multiple centers. Appropriate statistical techniques are necessary to address the possibility of differences among populations. Randomized clinical trials have become the standard method to conduct such studies. However, they are expensive, and failure to include sufficient number of patients may result in inconclusive results or apparent inconsistencies among trials. As discussed below, even a well-designed randomized controlled trial usually can answer a limited number of questions. Increasingly, meta-analysis is being used to pool results from multiple studies to resolve apparent inconsistencies or address questions that were not of primary importance in the clinical trial.

STUDY DESIGN AND THE STRENGTH OF EVIDENCE: RANDOMIZED VERSUS NONRANDOMIZED STUDIES

The type of study design determines the strength of the conclusions that can be made from a research study. A

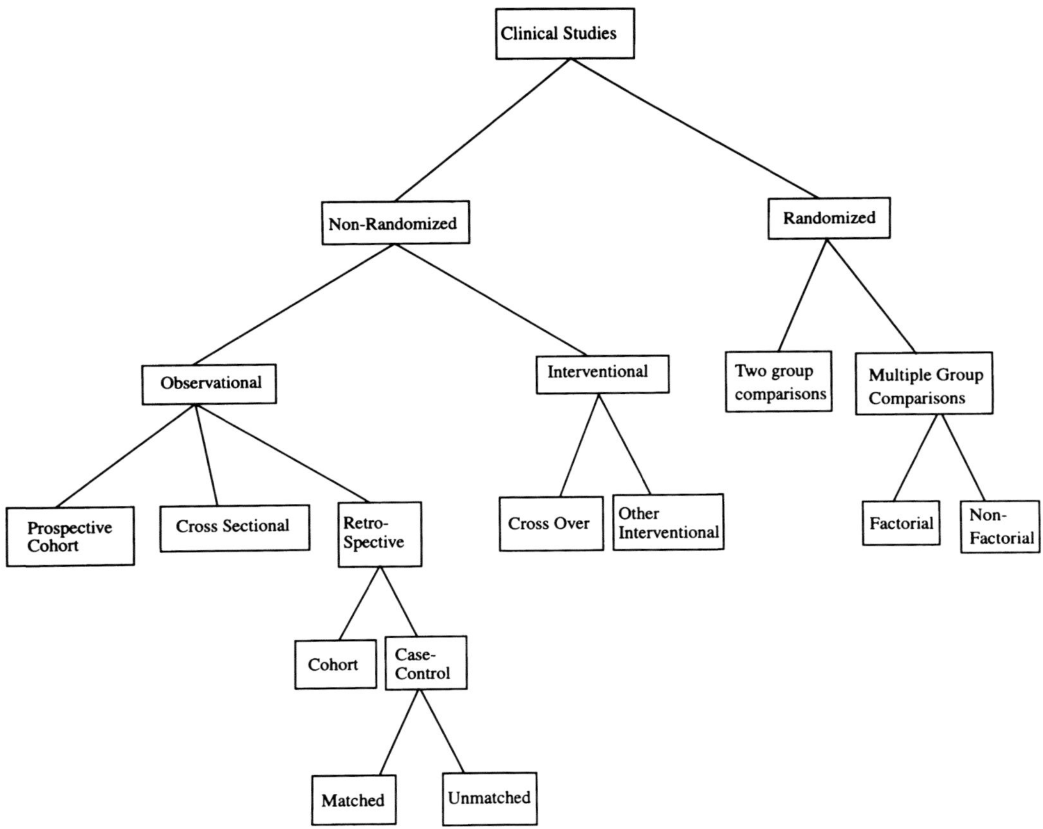

FIG. 1. Types of studies.

classification of common study designs used in nephrology research is given in Figure 1.

The first division in Figure 1 distinguishes between *randomized* and *nonrandomized* studies (1–3). Well-conducted nonrandomized studies give essential information regarding associations between variables in specified patient populations, provide evidence supporting or opposing previously hypothesized causal relationships (4–7), and generate new hypotheses regarding potential interventions. The great majority of published clinical studies are nonrandomized. However, although nonrandomized studies may "suggest" causal relationships, with few exceptions randomized studies are required to *demonstrate firmly* a causal effect of an intervention on patient outcome (1,8).

Consider, for example, the problem of determining whether reducing blood pressure to a lower-than-usual level slows the progression of renal disease in patients with chronic glomerulonephritis. One might investigate this question by assessing the correlation between blood pressure level and the rate of change in a marker for renal function (such as GFR) in a cohort of patients with glomerulonephritis. This is an example of a nonrandomized study, as the blood pressure levels were not controlled based on random assignment. An inverse correlation between observed blood pressure and rate of change in GFR among patients with blood pressure at or below the "usual level" would suggest that lowering blood pressure reduced the rate of loss of renal function. However, a causal effect of lowering blood pressure would not be conclusively demonstrated, as the study design cannot rule out alternative explanations for the association between blood pressure and rate of decline in GFR. One alternative explanation is that *confounding* variables may have jointly affected both blood pressure and loss of renal function so that the latter variables are correlated even though one does not affect the other. For example, patients with higher blood pressure levels may have also had higher levels of risk factors such as proteinuria or auto-antibodies, which are themselves associated with a more rapid loss of renal function. Additionally, it is hard to rule out the possibility of *reverse causality*, that is, the declining renal function caused blood pressure to increase. In this case, the association between blood pressure and the rate of loss of renal function could be a consequence of the effects of declining renal function, rather than conversely.

Alternatively, one might randomly allocate patients to two different levels of blood pressure (say a "low" level and a "usual" level). The randomization assures "approximate equivalence" of the two groups on all other variables, with the exception of the level of blood pressure. This precludes spurious relationships caused by confounding variables, as occurs in nonrandomized studies. Moreover, reverse causality is not possible, because the assignment of blood pressure group has been made randomly by the investigators and thus cannot be influenced by the rate of decline in renal function. Therefore, if a significant difference in the rate of decline in renal function is observed between the randomized blood pressure groups, it will be possible to conclude that the difference was caused by the assigned blood pressure interventions. It is true that the randomization may by chance allocate more rapidly progressing patients to one or the other group. However, as this is completely attributable to the randomization process, such imbalances are generally small, and those that do occur are fully accounted for by measures of probability such as p values and confidence intervals (see below) (2,9).

TYPES OF NONRANDOMIZED STUDIES

Observational Studies

In *observational studies*, measurements are obtained without assignment of patients to treatment interventions. Although numerous specific types of observational studies have been described (2,10), they can be broadly grouped into three classes: prospective cohort studies, in which a cohort of patients is followed up longitudinally over time; cross-sectional studies, in which a defined group of patients is assessed at a single time point; and retrospective studies, in which measurements are obtained by retrospective review of medical records or administrative data. These three classes of studies are described below.

Prospective Cohort (Longitudinal) Studies

Often called *natural history studies*, these studies utilize multiple measurements over time to characterize clinical and physiologic changes associated with disease progression or remission (11). Such studies are particularly well suited to *prediction*; factors measured at the beginning of the study can be correlated with the long-term disease outcomes to determine the risk factors associated with progression or remission of renal disease. The longitudinal measurements in prospective natural history studies are also well suited to identifying early markers for subsequent worsening or improvements in disease status.

Cross-sectional Studies

Cross-sectional studies lack longitudinal assessment, and in this respect are less useful than prospective cohort studies for identifying risk factors for subsequent progression or remission and for suggesting cause-and-effect relationships. However, as discussed below, multivariable statistical analysis may be used to relate prognostic factors to outcomes of interest while controlling for measured confounding variables.

Retrospective Studies

An advantage of prospective cohort and cross-sectional studies is that the measurements are planned in advance, and quality-control procedures can be implemented to monitor the accuracy of these measurements. In retrospective studies, data are obtained from chart review or administrative records, and the investigator must make do with whatever measurements happen to be available, often with little quality control. However, retrospective studies require no measurements beyond those already obtained and thus are a cost-effective way to collect data.

Retrospective studies may compare defined cohorts of patients. One commonly used study design is the *case-control study* (12), in which the investigator compares a group of patients with the disease (cases) with another group without the disease (controls), using defined targets for the numbers of cases and controls. Case-control designs are often used for relatively rare diseases to ensure a sufficient number of cases for comparisons with the controls. A related design is a matched case-control study, in which the investigator compares the cases with controls that are matched to cases based on potential confounding factors. This design efficiently controls for any biases associated with the matching variables by ensuring that these factors are equivalent between cases and controls (13–15). However, only a limited number of matching variables can be used in a single study, and it is difficult to rule out biases caused by confounding factors not included in the matching procedure.

Multiple Regression Analysis in Observational Studies

A chief limitation of all observational studies is the possibility that relationships observed between a predictor variable and an outcome are caused by influences of confounding variables. When confounding variables are known to the investigator and measured as part of the study design, then *multiple regression analysis* may be used to assess the association between the predictor and outcome variables while controlling statistically for the measured confounding factors (16–18). Although classic multiple regression applies to the limited situation in which the outcome variable is normally distributed with independent measurements with the same variability, recent advances have extended multiple regression methodology in numerous directions. Modern multiple regression methods are now available for outcome variables with non-normal distributions (19) whose measurements may be correlated (20) or censored (21), or may have differing levels of variability (22). Techniques have been developed for explanatory variables and covariates that are measured with error (23), and for situations in which the type of relationship between the explanatory variables and the outcome is unknown (24–26). Diagnostic methods for identifying influential observations and violations of assumptions have proliferated (27,28). The appropriate use of multiple regression methods often involves complex statistical issues, so collaboration with a statistician is recommended.

When used appropriately, multiple regression methods can greatly strengthen the inferences that can be made from observational studies. However, it is essential to remember that no statistical technique can control for confounding factors that are unknown to the researchers. Because it is usually impossible to rule out further confounding variables not controlled for in the analysis, it is essential not to lose sight of the principle that whereas multiple regression may reduce confounding effects, it cannot completely remove the limitations associated with nonrandomized studies (29–31).

Prospective Interventional Studies

In this class of studies, patients are treated according to a defined protocol, and the course of their disease is followed longitudinally (over time). However, patients are not randomized to different treatment groups. Changes in parameters can be measured and multivariate analysis can be used to minimize the influence of confounding variables, but inferences regarding cause and effect may not be definitive. In certain areas of medical research (particularly oncology), studies of this type are used in the early stages of investigation of new therapeutic agents to assess safety (phase I clinical trials) (32) and biologic efficacy (phase II clinical trials) (33,34). Final conclusions regarding clinical effectiveness are provided by randomized trials (phase III clinical trials).

Because of the slow rate of progression of many chronic renal diseases, a frequently used study design in nephrology is a variation of the prospective interventional study, the *cross-over design*, in which patients are assigned to two or more treatments in sequence (35–38). For example, the rate of change in GFR may be assessed first in a control period (period A, say) and then in a subsequent period while patients are assigned to a specified treatment (period B, say). The rate of change in GFR is compared between periods A and B in an attempt to assess the effects of the treatment as compared with the control. The cross-over study design has the advantage of controlling for variation between patients by using each patient as his or her own control. The primary drawbacks are that (a) treatments effects in period A may carry over into period B; (b) there may be "period effects" unrelated to the actual interventions—for example, the rate of change in GFR may change in the course of the disease, irrespective of the treatment applied; and (c) the comparisons of mean rates of change may be biased by *regression to the mean*. Regression to the mean is a statistical phenomenon that can lead to artificial changes in a parameter when the distribution of that parameter differs between patients included and patients excluded from a study (39,40). Because of these potential drawbacks, it is usually difficult to be certain that a difference between two treatment periods would not have occurred even if the latter treatment had not be applied.

The above-mentioned shortcomings to cross-over designs can largely be remedied by randomizing patients to sequences such as AB or BA, and by utilizing longer sequences such as ABA or BAB (41). Such designs allow direct comparisons between randomized groups that diminish the likelihood of the types of bias described above.

RANDOMIZED CLINICAL TRIALS

Well-designed randomized clinical trials ensure that potential confounding factors are approximately balanced between the treatment groups. However, randomized trials also have potential drawbacks that may limit the interpretation of results (42–44).

Internal Versus External Validity

To ensure that results accurately reflect the effect of therapeutic interventions, protocols of most randomized trials stipulate provisions intended to maximize the uniformity of extraneous factors with potential effects on outcome. Inclusion and exclusion criteria are defined to limit the study population to a well-defined disease in which an effect of the treatment is expected to be detectable. A baseline or run-in period is often used to assess the likely compliance of potential patients for the study procedures, and patients who demonstrate a high likelihood of noncompliance are excluded from randomization. These provisions are used to assure the *internal validity* of the trial—that is, that the trial accurately answers the research question within the randomized study population under the controlled conditions of the trial.

External validity refers to the degree to which the trial results extend to actual clinical practice in the target patient population. Highly controlled trials are often criticized because the patient selection criteria are so strict that a large percentage of the target patient population is excluded, or because the conditions of the trial are artificial and do not represent the practical alternatives for medical care. Because the patients who are actually randomized in clinical trials are rarely a representative sample from the target patient population, generalization of the results of a clinical trial typically must draw in part from existing biomedical knowledge, basic science laboratory research, animal studies, epidemiologic studies, and related randomized trials (45,46). Such inferences are facilitated by documentation of the comparability of the randomized patients with those patients who were screened but not randomized. A well-known example of the problems that arise when this is not done is the series of studies of lupus nephritis conducted by the National Institutes of Health (NIH), which required that patients have no serious extrarenal disease, have stable renal function for 3 months before entry into the study, and be referred to the NIH for treatment (47). The number of patients excluded by these criteria is not known, nor are the possible differences in patient characteristics that may be related to the effects of therapy.

Frequently, there is a tension between the internal and external validity of a trial (48). Although it is always necessary to strike a balance between internal and external validity, researchers in the methodology of experimental design generally give some level of priority to internal validity. This viewpoint is based on the notion that poor internal validity precludes the possibility of any valid conclusions, even under the controlled conditions of the study. In this situation, external validity becomes irrelevant, as there are no conclusions to generalize.

Validity of Outcome Measures

Clinical trials may include many outcome measures reflecting different dimensions of the therapeutic effects of interventions. As discussed earlier, trials in immunologic renal diseases usually attempt to assess immunologic parameters and extrarenal disease as well as measures of renal function and patient survival. With a large number of different outcomes, there is a high probability that at least one of them would differ significantly between the treatment groups, even in the absence of any true treatment effect. This is known as the problem of *multiple comparisons* (49). To prevent such false-positive results, it is usually advised that a single outcome be designated as the primary outcome, to be used for the main study conclusions. The remaining outcomes are regarded as secondary outcome variables, and they are used to amplify the comparisons of the primary outcome and suggest hypotheses to be tested in future trials (1,2).

The selection of the appropriate primary outcome is of fundamental importance. Considerations include the sensitivity of the outcome to detect the effects of the interventions, the accuracy of measurement or ascertainment of the outcome, the clinical importance of the outcome to the patient, and the connection between the outcome and the research question under investigation. In large-scale clinical trials, the criterion that the outcome be relevant to the patient is of major importance, as this is the main factor determining whether a new therapeutic intervention will be widely used.

Compliance

The evaluation of the efficacy of a treatment therapy requires that patients in each treatment group comply with, or adhere to, the assigned treatment (50). In a trial with poor compliance, it may be impossible to determine whether a negative result is a consequence of lack of efficacy of the treatment or of poor compliance. A related problem in drug or diet trials are "cross-overs," patients in whom clinical conditions develop that require therapies from one or more of the other arms of the study rather than the arm to which the patient was randomized. It is therefore essential that clinical trials monitor adherence to the treatment interventions, and include provisions to improve adherence when poor adherence is identified. Measures of adherence include pill counts in drug trials, frequent blood pressure measurements in trials evaluating efficacy of blood pressure control, and accurate assessments of dietary intake in trials of dietary modification.

Even with high degrees of noncompliance, the principles of experimental design require in most instances that the primary analysis be conducted on an *intent-to-treat* basis, in which patients are analyzed according to the group to which they were originally randomized, regardless of whether the patient actually adhered to the intervention (1,51). Even in the presence of a high rate of noncompliance, the intent-to-treat analysis evaluates the hypothesis that the treatment protocol, as employed in the study, leads to a beneficial effect. Because compliance is unlikely to be better in the general patient population than in the patients participating in the clinical trial, this analysis provides an indication of the maximum impact that treatment interventions can be expected to achieve in practice. However, the main reason for the primacy of the intent-to-treat analysis is that it fully utilizes the randomization to preclude biases caused by confounding variables.

In addition to the primary intent-to-treat analysis, supplemental *as-treated* analyses are often conducted to correlate the treatment the patients actually receive with outcome. Whereas the intent-to-treat analyses assess the impact of an intervention in practice (*effectiveness*), as-treated analyses are intended to address the biological *efficacy* of a therapy. For example, in a drug trial the as-treated analyses would relate the outcome to estimates of the actual drug therapy received by the patient. In a dietary trial, the as-treated analyses would correlate the actual dietary intake during follow-up with the outcome. Such analyses of efficacy can be of interest, but they are subject to the previously noted limitations of nonrandomized studies, as they are not based on comparisons of the randomized groups. Subgroup analyses restricted to compliant patients are subject to *selection biases* of a similar nature (52,53). The major complication is the observation that compliant patients may differ from noncompliant patients in biologic and psychologic characteristics that may correlate with outcome. Without a complete knowledge of these specific characteristics, it is difficult to determine the appropriate comparison for an unbiased estimate of the biologic effect of the therapy. In recent years, some of the limitations of as-treated analyses have been addressed by extending the techniques of *causal modeling* (5) to model the biologic efficacy of a drug while controlling for certain types of noncompliance (54–56).

Subgroup Analyses

Supplemental analyses may also be conducted in which the treatment groups are compared within clinically relevant subgroups (57,58). This is another situation in which false-positive results may occur because of the problem of multiple comparisons, as it is common to perform a large number of subgroup analyses. Hence, it is essential that publications reporting subgroup analyses indicate all the subgroups considered.

One approach to the problem of multiple comparisons in subgroup analyses is to strengthen the criterion for judging a result in any subgroup as statistically significant, so that the probability of false-positive results in all subgroup analyses combined is kept below a prespecified level. Unfortunately, clinical trials are typically designed to have a sample size just large enough to detect a clinically important effect of the intervention in an analysis of all patients. Hence, the power of the study to detect an effect within a subgroup is often marginal at best, and is further worsened if the criterion for statistical significance is made more stringent to account for multiple comparisons. The above problems can be partly controlled by specifying in advance (in the study protocol) a small number of key subgroups in which the main subgroup analyses will be conducted.

Comparisons of More Than Two Groups

In general, the most efficient design with the fewest interpretational difficulties is a two-group design in which equal numbers of patients are randomized to the experimental group receiving the therapeutic intervention and to a control group receiving the current standard of medical care. Given a fixed number of available patients, allocation of patients to more than two groups reduces the number of patients randomized in each individual group and hence reduces the power of the individual comparisons in the trial. Largely for this reason, the two-group design is by far the most common design in randomized clinical trials.

In situations in which it is desired to investigate two or more new therapeutic interventions, a multigroup design will generally require fewer total patients to achieve the same level of power as would be required by multiple two-group trials. Moreover, randomizing patients in a single trial ensures a balance of patient characteristics in each group being compared, which would not be possible in multiple two-group trials. An especially efficient multigroup design is the *factorial design*, in which patients are randomized simultaneously to more than one treatment (factor) (59). For example, the Modification of Diet in Renal Disease (MDRD) study consisted of two 2-by-2 factorial clinical trials in which patients were simultaneously randomized to two levels of dietary protein and two levels of blood pressure (60) (Table 3). Factorial designs are most appropriate when the treatments are

TABLE 3. *Two-by-Two Factorial Design in the MDRD study A[a]*

	Usual MAP group (target MAP ≤107 mm Hg)	Low MAP group (target MAP ≤92 mm Hg	Both MAP groups
Usual-protein diet (target protein intake 1.3 g/kg/d)	Mean Usual MAP, usual protein (n = 145)	Mean Low MAP, usual protein (n = 149)	Overall mean Usual protein (n = 294)
Low-protein diet (target protein intake 0.58 g/kg/d)	Mean Usual MAP, low protein (n = 140)	Mean Low MAP, low protein (n = 151)	Overall mean Low protein (n = 291)
Both diet groups	Overall mean Usual MAP (n = 285)	Overall mean Low MAP (n = 300)	Grand mean (N = 585)

MDRD, modification of diet in renal disease; MAP, mean arterial pressure.

[a]A two-by-two factorial design allows comparison of patient results for two interventions using the same number of patients that would have been needed to make one comparison, assuming the two interventions do not interact in their effect on study outcome. In the MDRD study A, a total of 585 patients provided sample sizes of 294 and 291 for testing the diet intervention, and at the same time provided sample sizes of 285 and 300 for testing the blood pressure intervention. Baseline glomerular filtration rate is 25 to 55 mL/min/1.73 m^2.

known to operate independently of each other, such that the effect of one treatment is the same at both levels of the other treatment. In this situation, the effect of one of the treatments can be tested by comparing all patients assigned to the respective levels of that treatment irrespective of the level of the other treatment. In the MDRD study, the blood pressure intervention was tested by comparing patients assigned to the low blood pressure goal with patients assigned to the usual blood pressure goal, irrespective of their diet group. Similarly, the dietary intervention was tested by comparing patients assigned to the usual protein diet with patients assigned the low-protein diet, irrespective of their blood pressure group. In this way, all patients are used for testing each factor, so in effect, two separate clinical trials have been conducted using the same number of patients required for a single trial.

The chief limitation of factorial designs is that one usually does not know in advance whether the effects of the two treatments are independent. If they are not independent (i.e., if there is an *interaction*), the effects of each treatment must be evaluated separately at each level of the other treatment, thus sacrificing the added efficiency of the factorial design. It is usually difficult to detect an interaction statistically (61,62), so that studies are rarely designed with a sufficient sample size to determine clearly whether a clinically important interaction is present. Hence, in most settings factorial designs should be used only when there is considerable confidence *a priori* that an interaction is not present.

THE LANGUAGE OF STATISTICS

This section provides an overview of the statistical concepts that form the basis of the description of the results of a clinical trial or other research study.

Measuring the Effect: Effect Size

The estimated magnitude of the effect of a predictor variable, such as the therapeutic intervention, on the outcome is known as the *effect size*. We first consider the special case of a two-group randomized clinical trial comparing the treatment group with the control group, and then examine some more general situations.

The expression of the effect size depends on the nature of the outcome variable. For *continuous variables*, the effect size is usually expressed as the difference between the mean of the outcome variable in the treatment and control groups. An effect size of 0 indicates no difference between treatment and control groups. The larger the effect size, the greater the difference. For example, after the first 4 months of follow-up in the MDRD study, the mean rate of change (slope) in GFR was 2.8 mL/min/y in the low-protein diet group, compared with 3.8 mL/min/y in the usual-protein diet group (60). The effect size is the difference in these mean slopes, or 1.0 mL/min/y. That is, on average, the GFR declined 1.0 mL/min/y less rapidly in the low-protein diet group than in the usual-protein diet group.

The effect size can be expressed in several different ways for *dichotomous variables* (Fig. 2). In general, dichotomous variables are summarized as a two-by-two contingency table, which reports the number of patients in the treatment and control groups with and without an event (3,10). The proportion of patients in the treatment or control group who experience the event is termed the *group event rate*. The *risk difference* is the arithmetic difference in the event rate between the treatment and control groups. The risk difference provides an absolute difference between two treatments and is analogous to the difference between means used to express the effect size for continuous variables. A risk difference of 0 indicates no difference between treatment and control groups, and therefore no effect of treatment.

The *risk ratio* is the ratio of the event rates in the treatment group and control group. A risk ratio of 1 indicates no effect of treatment. If a reduction in the event rate is desirable, the standard convention holds that a risk ratio of less than 1 denotes a benefit. The risk ratio provides a relative indication of the treatment benefit, but to determine the degree of absolute benefit, one must also consider the magnitude of the event rate in the control group.

Also commonly used is the *odds ratio*, the ratio of the odds of the event between the treatment and control groups. The odds of an event is the ratio of the proportion of patients with the event to the proportion of patients without the event. For example, an odds of 1 (even odds) indicates that equal numbers of patients in the study group do and do not have the event. An odds ratio of 1 indicates no difference between the treatment and control

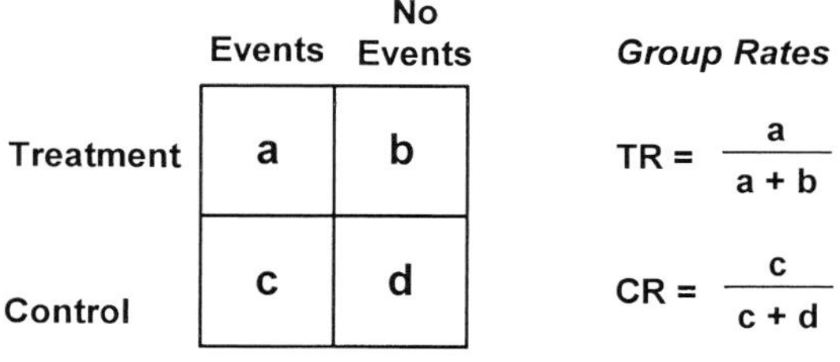

FIG. 2. Definition of treatment effects from a two-by-two contingency table.

group, even if the odds in each group differs from 1. As with the risk ratio, an odds ratio of less than 1 denotes a beneficial effect. The odds ratio is usually used in case-control or other retrospective studies in which the entire study population is not available. If the event rate is low, the odds approaches the event rate, and the odds ratio approaches the risk ratio. However, if the event rate is high, the odds exceeds the event rate, and the odds ratio may differ from the risk ratio.

To illustrate the different methods of expressing the effect size for dichotomous variables, in the Captopril in Diabetic Nephropathy study (63), the event rate for renal failure or death was 23/207 (11.1)% in the treatment group, compared with 42/202 (20.8%) in the control group. The corresponding risk difference, risk ratio, and odds ratio are 11.1 – 20.8% = –10.9%; 11.1%/20.8% = 0.53; and [(23/184)/(42/160)] = 0.48, respectively.

Rather than simply counting whether or not an event occurs, one can perform a *time-to-event analysis*, a potentally more powerful analysis that evaluates the amount of time from randomization until the occurrence of the event (64). In a time-to-event analysis, the simplifying assumption is often made that the ratio of the hazards (instantaneous risks) of the event between the treatment and control groups is constant over time. The effect size in a time-to-event analysis is usually expressed in terms of the hazard ratio, which is analogous to the risk ratio. For example, in the Captopril in Diabetic Nephropathy study, the hazard ratio for renal failure or death was 0.50, indicating that the instantaneous risk for this combined endpoint was reduced by 50% in the group treated with captopril. In general, a hazard ratio of less than 1 partly reflects a delay until the onset of the event rather than prevention of the event. If the risk of the event is constant over time in both treatment groups (a very strong assumption), the hazard ratio is intuitively interpreted as the ratio of the median times until the occurrence of the event between the treatment and control groups.

In more complex settings, regression analysis may be used to relate a quantitative independent variable to the outcome. For example, an important analysis in the MDRD study was a multiple regression relating achieved mean arterial pressure (MAP) to the rate of decline in GFR (65). (Note that this is an example of an as-treated analysis, as described above.) In multiple regression analyses, the effect size is given by the regression coefficient; this indicates the mean difference in the outcome variable that is associated with a specified difference in the independent variable. In the MDRD study A, the regression coefficient relating GFR slope to MAP was –0.17 mL/min/y per mm Hg. This indicates that a 1 mm Hg higher MAP was associated with a 0.17 mL/min/y steeper average GFR slope. Because 1 mm Hg may be too small a difference in MAP to be meaningful, the regression coefficient be expressed in terms of a difference of 10 mm Hg, for example, 1.7 mL/min/y per 10 mm Hg.

Is There Really an Effect? The *p* Value

Under the null hypothesis of no treatment effect, the mean difference or the risk difference, on average, is 0. However, in a particular study, random variations will almost certainly cause the effect size to be different from 0, even if the null hypothesis is true. Similarly, the risk ratio or odds ratio cannot be expected to be exactly equal to 1. This raises the question of whether an observed effect size different from the null hypothesis is the consequence of an effect of treatment or random fluctuations in the outcome variable.

Statistically, this problem is handled by the *p* value. A large *p* value indicates that the observed effect size is compatible with random fluctuations in the outcome variable from the null hypothesis. A small *p* value indicates that the observed effect size is highly unlikely to occur if the null hypothesis is true. Typically, *p* values smaller than a designated threshold, usually 1% or 5% (often referred to as the α level), are regarded as *statistically significant*, in which case one can reasonably conclude that there is in fact a real effect. The α level represents the probability of falsely concluding that an effect is present when in fact it is not. This is often referred to as the probability of committing a *type I error*.

The concepts of statistical and clinical significance are very often confused in the biomedical literature. *Clinical significance* refers to the magnitude of an effect size that is clinically important to the patient—this is a clinical judgement beyond the scope of statistics. *Statistical significance* indicates the degree to which one can be confident that the null hypothesis of no effect is not true. In studies with small sample sizes, the estimated effect may be quite large and clearly significant clinically, but not statistically significant. On the other hand, in large studies even minute effects may be statistically significant but so small as to be of no clinical importance.

Precision of the Estimate: The Confidence Interval

Reporting the effect size of a therapeutic intervention provides only a limited assessment of the results of a study unless the estimate of the effect size is accompanied by an indication of its precision. In small studies, the observed effect size may be very large, but so imprecisely estimated that it provides little indication as to the size of the true effect in the target population. Consequently, it is recommended that estimates of the effect size be accompanied by the *confidence interval*, which indicates the margin of error of the observed effect (66). Alternatively, a confidence interval can be viewed as providing the range of possible values for the effect being estimated in the population that are compatible with the effect actually observed in the study.

For example, in the Captopril in Diabetic Nephropathy study, the 95% confidence interval for the risk ratio in the time-to-event analysis of renal failure or death was 0.18 to 0.70. This means we can be "95% confident" that the actual risk ratio in the population is somewhere within this range. There is a connection between confidence intervals and statistical significance: A 95% confidence interval contains the value of the effect under the null hypothesis if and only if the effect is *not* statistically significant at the 5% level. In this example, the confidence interval for the risk ratio does not contain 1, which indicates that the p value for the risk ratio is smaller than 5%.

Confidence intervals are particularly important for the interpretation of negative studies in which statistical significance is not reached. If the range of the confidence interval is small and includes only minimal-effect sizes that are not regarded as clinically important, then the study has demonstrated a true negative result. One can confidently rule out an effect large enough to be clinically important. On the other hand, if the range of the confidence interval is large and contains effects that are regarded as clinically important, then the study is inconclusive. One does not know if there is truly no effect or if there is a clinically important effect that was undetected by the study.

Precision of a Study: Statistical Power

The *statistical power* of a study is the probability that the study would detect a statistically significant effect if there is a clinically significant effect in the population. The probability of failure to observe a statistically significant effect in the presence of a clinically significant effect in the population is known as the β *error* or the probability of committing a *type II error*. The concept of statistical power is closely connected to the confidence interval. A high statistical power to detect an effect typically means that the confidence interval for the effect size is narrow, indicating a small margin of error. Whereas the confidence interval is best suited to describing the precision of the effect after the study has been completed, computation of statistical power is most useful in the planning stages of a study, during which the sample size and study design are determined.

There is an extensive literature dealing with the computation of statistical power in different circumstances (1, 67). In general, the power of a clinical trial depends on several factors, including the sample size in each treatment group, the variability of the outcome measure, the event rate in the control group (for time-to-event analyses), the magnitude of the minimal clinically important effect, compliance with the study interventions, the rates of drop-out and loss to follow-up, the patterns of enrollment of patients into the study, and the characteristics of the statistical test that is conducted for the primary analysis. We now consider in more detail the first three of these factors.

1. Sample size. In most settings, the margin of error for a confidence interval, or the magnitude of the minimal effect that can be detected with a specified power, is inversely proportional to the square root of the sample size. For example, quadrupling the sample size leads to an approximate halving of the minimal detectable effect.
2. Variability of the outcome measure. The variability of the outcome measure is directly proportional to the minimal detectable effect size. The variability of the outcome depends on the precision by which it is measured, and on the heterogeneity of the outcome among the randomized patients. This is one rationale for conducting clinical trials in relatively focused, well-defined patient populations.
3. Event rate in the control group. In time-to-event analyses, statistical power is directly related to the event rate in the control group. If there are few events in the control group, then it is difficult to establish that the event rate is reduced in the treatment group. An analogous issue in clinical trials of slowing progression in chronic renal disease using quantitative outcomes is that the mean rate of decline in renal function in the control group must be substantially different from 0 to have sufficient power to demonstrate a reduction in the rate of decline in the treatment group.

PROBLEMS IN THE DESIGN OF CLINICAL TRIALS OF THE PROGRESSION OF RENAL DISEASE

This section provides an overview of some of the problems that are particularly relevant to clinical trials of the efficacy of therapeutic interventions to slow the progression of renal disease.

Surrogate Outcomes Versus Clinical Endpoints

Reviewers have often argued that when feasible, the primary outcome variable for a large randomized clinical trial should be a "hard" clinical endpoint rather than a "soft" surrogate outcome (1,68). This assertion is based on the observation that demonstration of a benefit of an intervention on a hard endpoint is necessary to provide unequivocal proof that the intervention benefits the patient, and such proof is necessary if the trial is to set a new standard of clinical practice.

In the context of chronic renal disease, the hard clinical endpoints usually are taken to mean renal failure (defined by initiation of dialysis or renal transplantation) or death. The difficulty with using renal failure or death as the primary endpoint is that the event rate must be high enough to have sufficient statistical power. In clinical trials of chronic renal disease, the number of renal failure events in the control group depends on the following factors: (a) the mean level of renal function at the beginning of the trial (i.e., baseline GFR); (b) the mean rate and distribution of rates of decline in renal function (i.e., follow-up GFR slopes); (c) the duration of follow-up; and (d) the number of randomized patients.

Table 4 demonstrates the interrelationship of these factors by considering scenarios with initial renal function in the moderate (baseline GFR of 30 to 70 mL/min/1.73 m^2) or advanced (baseline GFR of 13 to 30 mL/min/1.73 m^2) range, mean rates of GFR decline of either –2, –4, or –6 mL/min/1.73 m^2/y, and low or high levels of variability of the GFR slopes. The low level of variability of GFR slopes was selected as slightly smaller than the variability seen in patients with polycystic disease in the MDRD study, and thus represents the variability that might be expected in highly focused studies of a single renal disease, whereas the higher level of variability was selected as somewhat larger than that seen in the full population of MDRD patients, who had a wide variety of renal diseases (60). The table provides the expected percentage of patients in the control group reaching renal failure during follow-up under each scenario for different follow-up times. To achieve 80% power to detect a 30% reduction in the event rate in the treatment group, approximately 135 to 147 events in the control group would be necessary. Thus, in a study with two groups, a clinical trial of moderate duration (around 4 years) with 300 to 900 patients can be expected to achieve a sufficient number of events for adequate power for patients who have advanced disease (baseline GFR of $\leq$30 mL/min/1.73 m^2) or who have rapidly progressing disease (i.e., mean GFR slope steeper than –6 mL/min/1.73 m^2/y). However, trials with a longer duration, a larger sample size, or both would be necessary to achieve a comparable event rate for patients with moderate renal disease (mean baseline GFR of >30 mL/min/1.73 m^2) and slower mean decline in GFR (less steep than -6 mL/min/1.73 m^2/y).

Because of relatively short planned durations of follow-up, recent clinical trials in moderate renal disease have used surrogate outcomes based on the rate of change in renal function, such as GFR slope (as in the MDRD study), or the time until doubling of initial serum creatinine (as in the Captopril in Diabetic Nephropathy study). The premise of this approach is that interventions that are effective in slowing the progression of renal disease also should be effective in slowing the decline in renal function, and that these outcome measures should be sensitive enough to detect differences in the rate of decline in renal function. Examinations of surrogate endpoints in a more general setting are provided by the articles of Prentice (69) and Kirby and colleagues (70). We now turn to special problems in assessing the rate of change in renal function.

Measuring Renal Function in Chronic Renal Disease

The GFR is generally accepted as the best overall index of renal function in health and disease (71). In recent years, alternative methods and markers to measure GFR have been developed that are more convenient than the traditional method of measuring renal clearance of inulin during a continuous intravenous infusion (72). In particular, the renal clearance of iothalamate I 125 after subcutaneous bolus injection has been found to be an accurate and precise method for measurement of GFR in multicenter

TABLE 4. *Percentage of patients reaching renal failure in control group of clinical trial of patients with chronic renal disease*

Level of renal disease progression			Patients reaching renal failure during years of follow-up, %					
Mean slope (mL/min/173 m^2/y)	Initial level of renal disease[a]	Slope variability[b]	2 y	3 y	4 y	6 y	8 y	12 y
−2	Moderate	Low	0.0	0.2	1.5	7.1	15.3	31.3
−2	Moderate	High	0.2	1.9	5.4	14.8	24.1	37.4
−4	Moderate	Low	0.0	1.3	5.1	19.0	33.5	54.9
−4	Moderate	High	0.5	4.1	10.4	25.6	38.2	53.0
−6	Moderate	Low	0.1	4.6	13.8	38.1	57.6	78.2
−6	Moderate	High	1.2	8.5	19.6	41.2	56.0	70.7
−2	Advanced	Low	7.0	17.5	27.9	43.9	53.2	62.9
−2	Advanced	High	12.1	24.5	34.3	45.8	52.2	58.5
−4	Advanced	Low	18.3	38.5	55.4	72.5	80.0	86.2
−4	Advanced	High	23.8	41.6	53.4	66.0	71.6	76.8
−6	Advanced	Low	36.6	65.3	80.3	91.2	94.9	97.0
−6	Advanced	High	38.4	60.9	72.7	82.6	86.6	89.8

[a] Baseline glomerular filtration rate: 30–70 mL/min/1.73 m^2 for moderate disease; 13–30 for advanced disease.

[b] Slope standard deviation: 3 (low) or 4.5 (high) mL/min/1.73 m^2 for moderate disease; 2.5 (low) or 3.75 (high) mL/min/1.73 m^2 for advanced disease.

clinical trials (73,74). Nonetheless, technical limitations remain, and to minimize inconvenience and cost, many clinical trials measure creatinine clearance (C_{cr}) or serum (or plasma) creatinine (P_{cr}) as an estimate of GFR. The theoretical relationships among C_{cr}, P_{cr}, and GFR have been described previously (75) and are shown below.

Creatinine is excreted by both glomerular filtration and tubular secretion. The creatinine excretion rate ($U_{cr}V$) can be expressed as follows:

$$U_{cr}V = GFR \cdot P_{cr} + TS_{cr} \qquad \text{(Equation 1)}$$

where TS_{cr} is the rate of creatinine secretion.

Based on the definition of renal clearance,

$$C_{cr} = U_{cr}V/P_{cr} \qquad \text{(Equation 2)}$$

The determinants of C_{cr} are demonstrated by substitution of equation 1 into equation 2:

$$C_{cr} = GFR + C_{TScr} \qquad \text{(Equation 3)}$$

where C_{TScr} is the clearance of creatinine by secretion (TS_{cr}/P_{cr}).

In chronic renal disease, creatinine is eliminated both by renal and extrarenal routes:

$$U_{cr}V = G_{cr} - E_{cr} \qquad \text{(Equation 4)}$$

where G_{cr} is the rate of creatinine generation from endogenous and exogenous sources and E_{cr} is the rate of creatinine elimination by extrarenal routes.

The determinants of P_{cr} are shown by substitution of equation 4 into equation 1 and rearrangement:

$$P_{cr} = (G_{cr} - E_{cr} - TS_{cr})/GFR \qquad \text{(Equation 5)}$$

It is clear, therefore, that C_{cr} and P_{cr} are affected by factors in addition to the GFR. In principal, changes in C_{cr} and P_{cr} can be caused by changes in the generation, extrarenal elimination, or secretion of creatinine in addition to changes in GFR.

It is well-known that changes in generation, extrarenal elimination, and secretion of creatinine occur in chronic renal disease and that these changes can be of sufficient magnitude to cause changes in the rate of decline C_{cr} and $1/P_{cr}$ even if there is no change in the rate of decline in GFR (76). Thus, the rates of decline in C_{cr} or $1/P_{cr}$ may not provide an accurate estimate of the rate of decline in GFR. In the MDRD study, correlations (r) between the rates of change in C_{cr} and GFR and between the rates of change in $1/P_{cr}$ and GFR were significant ($p < 0.001$), but were only 0.64 to 0.79 and 0.79 to 0.85, respectively (77). Thus, less than two thirds of the variability in GFR slopes could be accounted for by variability in C_{cr} or $1/P_{cr}$ slopes. More importantly, the MDRD study also showed that the interventions being investigated to slow the progression of renal disease affected the determinants of creatinine clearance and serum creatinine in addition to affecting the GFR. Dietary protein restriction accelerated the decline in creatinine secretion and reduced creatinine excretion (presumably because of reduced creatinine generation), whereas strict blood pressure control slowed the decline in creatinine secretion (77). As a result of these effects on creatinine excretion and secretion, the effects of the interventions on the rate of decline in C_{cr} and $1/P_{cr}$ differed from the effects on the GFR decline (the primary outcome variable). If changes in C_{cr} or $1/P_{cr}$ had been the primary outcome variable for the clinical trial, these differences would have resulted in different interpretations of the primary results of the clinical trial. Thus, despite the additional inconvenience and cost, it appears that studies assessing the effects of interventions on the progression of renal disease should measure GFR in addition to C_{cr} and P_{cr}.

It would not be appropriate, however, to suggest that the only limitations to assessing the progression of renal disease from changes in GFR are caused by technical difficulties in measuring GFR. First, changes in GFR may not be sufficiently sensitive to the effects of renal disease. For example, the earliest changes in glomerular diseases appear to be associated with alterations in structure and permeability to macromolecules. In diabetic nephropathy, mesangial matrix and urinary excretion of albumin increase before GFR declines (78). In systemic lupus erythematosus, glomerular sclerosis may progress despite stable, although reduced, GFR (79).

Second, a change in GFR is not specific for remission or progression of renal disease. Table 5 lists factors in addition to progressive renal injury that may influence GFR (80). The effects of lowering arterial blood pressure, specific classes of antihypertensive agents, and dietary protein restriction are especially important, because these interventions have been frequently tested and shown to slow the progression of renal disease. The MDRD study showed that these interventions have short-term effects on GFR that are the opposite of their hypothesized long-term beneficial effects (81). Indeed, as discussed below, a critical weakness in the design of the MDRD study was that the short-term reduction in GFR resulting from these interventions was sufficient to obscure their potential benefit in slowing the decline in GFR. In principle, a similar diffi-

TABLE 5. *Factors potentially affecting glomerular filtration rate in clinical trials of progressive renal disease*

Progression or remission of renal disease
Diurnal variation
Relationship to meals
Habitual protein intake
Blood glucose control (in diabetics)
Level of arterial blood pressure
Class of antihypertensive agents
Marked surfeit or deficit of extracellular fluid volume
Pregnancy
Reduction in renal mass

From Levey, ref. 80, with permission.

culty might be encountered in a clinical trial of strict glucose control on the progression of diabetic renal disease.

Despite these limitations, a progressive and large decline in GFR or rise in serum creatinine over a long duration of follow-up in patients with chronic renal disease is a clinically meaningful outcome. Thus, it is necessary to design clinical trials carefully to ensure proper interpretation of changes in parameters of renal function.

Assessing Changes in Renal Function

The simplest design to assess the change in a parameter of renal function would be to measure the parameter in each patient before the intervention (baseline) and once again after the intervention (during follow-up). To allow the greatest change in renal function, the follow-up measurement could be obtained just before the initiation of dialysis or renal transplantation in patients reaching renal failure and at the end of the scheduled follow-up in patients who survive without renal failure. Although straightforward, this approach has serious limitations. First, because only a single measurement of renal function is obtained at baseline and follow-up, this method is susceptible to error in either measurement. Second, it is not feasible to obtain the follow-up measurements in patients who drop out or die before the end of the study. These patients would have to be excluded from the primary analysis, which conflicts with the intent-to-treat principle. Third, the pattern of change in renal function during follow-up might be important, and this could not be determined with only one follow-up measurement.

Because of these drawbacks, it is desirable to measure renal function at baseline and then at regular intervals throughout follow-up. Typically, clinical trials using changes in GFR or creatinine clearance as the primary endpoint have included measurements every 3, 4, or 6 months during follow-up. Trials using changes in serum creatinine as the primary endpoint may contain more frequent measurements, because of the lower cost and greater convenience. When periodic measurements are available, the change in renal function may be assessed as the slope of a regression line fit through the sequence of measurements. The mean slope of GFR, creatinine clearance, or reciprocal of serum creatinine concentration represents the estimate of the mean rate of change in renal function during follow-up. Alternatively, the change in renal function may be assessed as the time required for renal function to decline by a specified amount from the baseline value. The latter approach is exemplified by several clinical trials that have used time to doubling of serum creatinine as the primary outcome.

Special Problems in Slope-Based Analyses

The slope-based approach presents several statistical issues. The most straightforward analysis is to carry out a standard statistical test, such as the two-sample *t* test, which compares the average slopes in the treatment and control groups. The chief drawback of this approach is that some patients will have a short follow-up because of drop-out, rapid progression to renal failure, or death early in the trial, leading to imprecise and highly variable slope estimates in these patients (82). The relationship between duration of follow-up and variability of slope estimates is illustrated by Figure 3, in which the GFR slopes observed in the MDRD study are plotted versus follow-up time. In

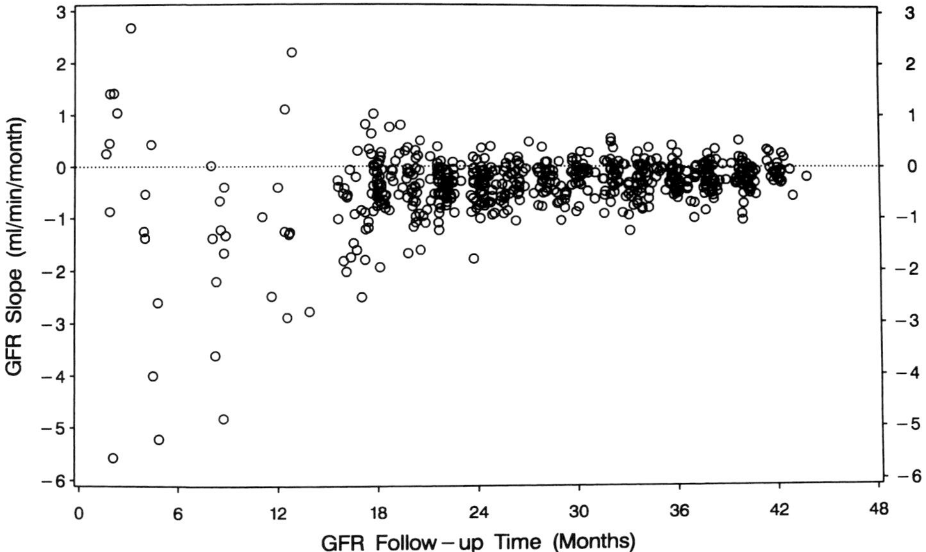

FIG. 3. Relationship between GFR slope and follow-up time in the MDRD study A.

a simple analysis comparing average slopes between the treatment groups, the extreme slopes from patients with short follow-up have a disproportional influence, leading to substantially increased variability in the outcome measure and consequent reduction in statistical power.

To minimize the impact of imprecise slope estimates from patients with short follow-up, slopes from patients with longer follow-up or more measurements of renal function can be assigned more weight in the analysis. A rigorous basis for obtaining optimal analyses of slopes in the presence of differential follow-up between patients has been provided by the mixed-effects modeling framework described by Laird and Ware (83). The Laird-Ware model contains a fixed-effects component, which takes into account the mean effect of the interventions on the rate of change in renal function, and a random-effects component, which models the variability of individual patients' slopes as well as the variability of individual renal function measurements around the individual patient regression lines. The PROC MIXED program in the statistical package SAS and the BMDP5V program can be used to fit these models (84,85).

The Laird-Ware mixed-effects modeling approach is appropriate for quantitative data with an approximately normal distribution. A more general method for categorical and quantitative data that may not be normally distributed has recently been proposed by Liang and Zeger (20). This approach, known as *generalized estimating equations* (*GEE*), provides estimates of the regression coefficients and their standard errors, which are unbiased in large samples under very general assumptions about the correlations among individual patients' measurements.

A limitation of both the Laird-Ware and GEE approaches is that their estimates of mean slope can be biased if the pattern of missing data is *informative*. The pattern of missing data is informative if the likelihood that a measurement is missing is related to the underlying slope in a way that is not fully accounted for by the renal function measurements that are observed (86,87). In studies of chronic renal disease, this type of missing data pattern may arise if patients reach renal failure, which may preclude further measurements of renal function. Bias will arise if the time to renal failure is correlated with the slope of the renal function parameter and this correlation cannot be fully accounted for by the observed renal function measurements before renal failure. Intuitively, in the presence of informative censoring of this type, the Laird-Ware and GEE approaches give too little weight to the patients with rapidly declining renal function, thereby leading to underestimation of the mean decline in renal function.

In the last several years, a number of techniques have been proposed to account for informative censoring in the statistical model (86,88–90). For example, the primary analysis of patients with advanced renal disease in the MDRD study (study B; GFR of 13 to 24 mL/min/1.73 m^2) was conducted using an informative censoring model that assumed a multivariate normal distribution for the GFR slope and intercept, and the logarithm of the time until renal failure or death was reached (89). More generally, these techniques posit models that relate the censoring time to the mean slopes being estimated. If the assumed models are true, these methods produce valid estimates of the mean slopes.

Slope-Based Analysis Versus Time-to-Event Analysis

It can be shown theoretically that the Laird-Ware approach comparing mean slope between treatment and control groups is optimal if the basic assumptions of the model are satisfied. However, recent experience with the MDRD study and other studies (60,77,81) has shown that analyses of mean slope can be seriously limited by two key factors.

First, clinical trials may include some patients whose renal function does not decline during the course of the trial. This is problematic if the therapeutic intervention is hypothesized to benefit only those patients with declining renal function. Inclusion of patients with stable renal function raises the mean slope in the control group toward 0, thereby reducing the statistical power of the study. In essence, the inclusion of patients with stable renal function "dilutes" the beneficial effect of the intervention. The ideal solution to this problem would be to identify and exclude patients with stable renal function from the trial before randomization. However, depending on the renal disease being studied, this may not be feasible.

A second problem with the analysis of mean slope is the observation that several therapeutic interventions hypothesized to slow the progression of renal disease—including dietary protein restriction, strict blood pressure control, and use of specific antihypertensive agents, such as angiotensin-converting-enzyme (ACE) inhibitors—lead to short-term reductions in renal function. As discussed earlier, during a short duration of follow-up, these short-term effects may partially or completely cancel the long-term hypothesized beneficial effect. The follow-up time required for a clinical trial to show that an intervention has preserved renal function depends on the relative magnitudes of the short-term and long-term effects. In general, a longer duration of follow-up is required if the short-term effect is large or if the hypothesized long-term beneficial effect is small.

In certain conditions, a time-to-event approach may be substantially less susceptible than slope-based analysis to the effects of inclusion of patients with stable renal function or of short-term effects of interventions on renal function. For example, consider a clinical trial in which the outcome is the amount of time until (a) GFR declines by at least 25 mL/min/1.73 m^2 from its baseline value, (b) renal failure is reached, or (c) death occurs. Only patients with rapid decline in GFR would be expected to reach any of these events, and it is likely that the first event based on GFR would comprise most events in the analysis. In a time-to-event analysis, patients with stable or slowly declining renal function would not reach events in either the control or experimental groups, and would thus be censored from the analysis. Thus, the time-to-event analysis avoids "diluting" the potential beneficial effect by patients with stable renal function.

Additionally, it may be reasonable to hypothesize that the magnitude of the beneficial effect is proportional to the rate of decline in renal function that would have occurred in the absence of an intervention. Under this "proportional effect" hypothesis, the magnitude of the effect size among patients with more rapid GFR decline will be greater than the mean effect size in the full study population. Therefore, a shorter duration of follow-up would be required to overcome the short-term effect in patients with more rapid GFR decline.

Recent work carried out in conjunction with the design of the African American Study of Kidney Disease has led to the following observations concerning the relative statistical power of slope-based analysis and the time-to-event approach (91): The analysis of mean slopes is favored if (a) short-term effects are not anticipated, (b) a negligible proportion of patients have stable or slowly declining renal function, and (c) the hypothesized beneficial effect is independent of the rate of decline in renal function in the absence of the intervention. In contrast, the time-to-event approach is favored if (a) short-term effects are anticipated, (b) a substantial proportion of patients have stable or slowly declining renal function, and (c) the hypothesized benefit of the intervention is proportional to the rate of decline in renal function in the absence of the intervention.

INTRODUCTION TO META-ANALYSIS

Although the randomized controlled trial is now considered the gold standard for the evaluation of therapeutic interventions, uncertainties may arise when small clinical trials produce statistically insignificant results and controversies occur when trials report discrepant findings. Results of approximately 5000 to 10,000 clinical trials are published each year, so the task of monitoring therapeutic developments is difficult. Traditional journal review articles and textbook chapters, on which most clinicians rely for therapeutic guidance, generally do not include an exhaustive review of the literature, may be biased in their selection of supporting evidence, and usually do not provide a quantitative synthesis of the data (92).

Meta-analysis, also known as *systematic overview* or *quantitative synthesis*, is the discipline of performing critical reviews of existing data using quantitative methods to combine available evidence (93–96). Meta-analysis was first introduced into clinical medicine in the late 1970s, and since then it has been applied to all major clinical disciplines. By pooling results from studies with inadequate sample size, a more precise and statistically significant estimate of the treatment effect may be obtained. By applying regression analysis, heterogeneity of treatment effects and differences across studies may be explained.

The development of meta-analysis parallels the explosion in the number of biomedical publications and the increasing need to provide unbiased and quantitative syntheses in the era of "evidence-based" medicine. Meta-analysis of randomized controlled trials of therapeutic studies, in particular, has experienced rapid growth in the last decade because of the availability of large numbers of randomized controlled trials. In addition to being used to combine the results of therapeutic trials, meta-analysis has also been applied to epidemiologic studies to derive better risk estimates, and to diagnostic test evaluations to obtain more reliable estimates of test performance. In this discussion, we primarily focus on the basic steps of conducting a meta-analysis of therapeutic trials.

Basic Steps of Conducting a Meta-analysis

The goal of a meta-analysis of therapeutic trials is to identify all relevant studies addressing a similar question and combine their results to provide a common estimate of the treatment effect. For the result of a meta-analysis to be reliable and reproducible, the original studies included must be of high quality and the steps must be well delineated.

Establishing the Protocol

Meta-analysis should start with clearly defined questions, and the answers to them should be clinically useful. For example, an appropriate question might be, "Do cytotoxic agents reduce the development of renal failure in idiopathic membranous nephropathy?" (97). Better still would be to address the question to a more specific population of patients and to a more specific stage or severity of disease. However, published data seldom allow one to construct such detailed subgroup analyses.

Items to be specified in the inclusion criteria of studies to be used in a meta-analysis should include study design, patient characteristics, disease characteristics, treatments being compared, study duration, and outcomes considered. Most authorities recommend using only randomized controlled trials in meta-analysis of therapies, because as discussed before, this study design minimizes observer and patient assignment bias.

Another issue with study selection concerns heterogeneity across studies. Studies may vary in their treatment effects, patient populations, and stage or severity of disease. Pooling studies that have similar treatment effects but different patient populations with varying severity of illness is more likely to be accepted and generalizable than pooling studies with different characteristics and different treatment effects. Pooling heterogeneous studies has been criticized as comparing "apples and oranges" (98), although the use of regression analysis may explain heterogeneity among trials (99,100).

Performing the Literature Search

An important principle of meta-analysis is that it should be comprehensive. All relevant studies should be included to avoid selection bias. A thorough search of the literature usually begins with the MEDLINE electronic database maintained by the National Library of Medicine. Because of difficulties in indexing the original studies, use of key words to search for randomized controlled trials typically yields fewer than two thirds of all studies eventually identified. Electronic searches should be supplemented by searches of the bibliographies of retrieved articles and relevant review articles. Sometimes, this can be augmented by inquiries with experts, review of *Current Contents*, and review of journals devoted to the specific domain. Several articles provide details on search strategies (101,102).

Negative studies are more likely to remain unpublished, and their inclusion may affect the results of a meta-analysis (103). Some authors advocate searching for unpublished studies and asking individual investigators for their data. Others have argued that unpublished data have not been evaluated by peer review, are of dubious quality, and should not be trusted. Although a potential source of concern, omission of unpublished studies is not likely to cause a significant problem because such studies tend to be small and would have minimal impact on the overall result.

Selecting Studies and Performing Quality Assessment on the Original Studies

The selection of studies to be included in a meta-analysis is one of the most difficult steps. Studies identified through the literature search should be evaluated according to a prespecified protocol. Failure to adhere to a strict protocol may produce misleading results and invite harsh criticism, especially if the exclusion of a study leads to alteration of statistical significance of the pooled results. Some valid reasons for excluding a study from an analysis are the lack of reported data for an outcome, or extreme differences in the patient or disease characteristics. Another reason, as discussed below, is poor quality of study design. Studies excluded from the analysis should be listed and the reasons stated.

The studies included in a meta-analysis must have high degree of internal validity to produce reliable results. Meta-analyses typically combine clinical trials from different sources, and even though they address a similar question, it is likely they vary in quality. For example, a recent study on the method of randomization found larger reported treatment effects in studies in which the randomization is not well concealed (104). Study protocols should be scrutinized so that only those in which patients were properly randomized are included.

Several investigators have proposed methods to assess the quality of the original studies. Quality assessment forms have been developed to score a variety of items in the methods, conduct, and analysis sections of the original studies. One investigator even regularly performed quality assessments while blinded to authors, source, results, and discussion (105). Resultant quality scores have been used to apply a threshold value to decide whether to include a study, but defining an appropriate quality score for cut-off is arbitrary. Quality scores can also be used to rank studies and as a determinant of the treatment effect. However, in one study (105), there was no consistent relationship of the quality score and treatment effect in seven meta-analyses. On the other hand, others have criticized the use of an aggregate quality score because it may obscure individual trial characteristics that may better explain observed differences in treatment effects (106).

Performing Quantitative Synthesis of Data

The distinguishing feature of a meta-analysis compared with a traditional narrative review is the quantitative synthesis of the data. In a meta-analysis, a weighted average of the outcomes of the individual studies is performed using one of several statistical methods.

Measuring the Treatment Effect

The majority of randomized control trials report dichotomous outcome data, such as survival or death, survival with or without renal failure, or remission or progression of renal disease. As discussed before, the treatment effect is estimated as the effect size using one of three measures: risk difference, risk ratio, and odds ratio (Fig. 2). Most frequently, the pooled risk ratio is used to provide a measure of the relative efficacy of one treatment over another. The pooled odds ratio is often used to approximate the risk ratio. However, as discussed before, this approximation is valid only if the event rate is low. The odds ratio provides no advantage in the evaluation of randomized controlled trials and may overestimate pooled treatment effects when there are large differences in event rates across studies.

Continuous variables, such as differences in renal function, can also be pooled in a meta-analysis. However, difficulty arises if the same outcome variable is not measured in all studies—for example, decline in GFR, creatinine clearance, or reciprocal of serum creatinine concentration. One method to combine treatment effects across studies with different outcome measures is to calculate a dimensionless unit from each study (107). The disadvantage of this method is that it lacks a clinically intuitive scale and is thus difficult to interpret.

Choosing a Statistical Model

It is also necessary to decide whether to use a fixed-effects or random-effects statistical model to pool the data. A fixed-effects model assumes that the true treatment effect is the same across all studies; differences among studies are a consequence only of random variation. In a fixed-effects model, individual studies are weighted by the number of events and the study size in calculating a weighted average. The random-effects model assumes that the treatment effect is not the same across all studies; differences among studies are the consequence of a combination of random variation as well as of true differences in treatment effects across studies with different characteristics.

There has been much discussion concerning the choice of the fixed-effects or the random-effects model to pool data. Some argue that only studies demonstrating statistical homogeneity of treatment effects should be pooled. Others propose the use of a random-effects model when pooling studies with heterogeneous treatment effects. In practice, important differences in the results between these two statistical models occur infrequently. The fixed-effects model produces narrower confidence intervals with the addition of more studies and patients. The random-effects model is more conservative, producing broader confidence intervals for the pooled results. When there is no statistical heterogeneity of treatment effects across studies, the random-effects and the fixed-effects models give similar results. When heterogeneity of treatment effects is suspected, the random-effects model should be used.

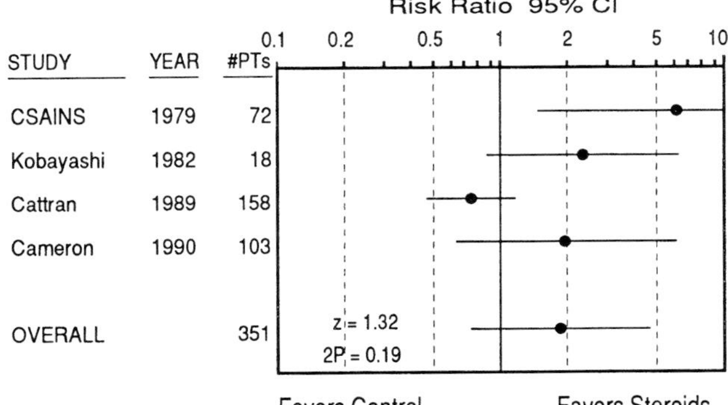

FIG. 4. Displaying the results of a meta-analysis. Point estimate and 95% confidence intervals for individual studies and the pooled result. (Data calculated Hogan et al., ref. 108.)

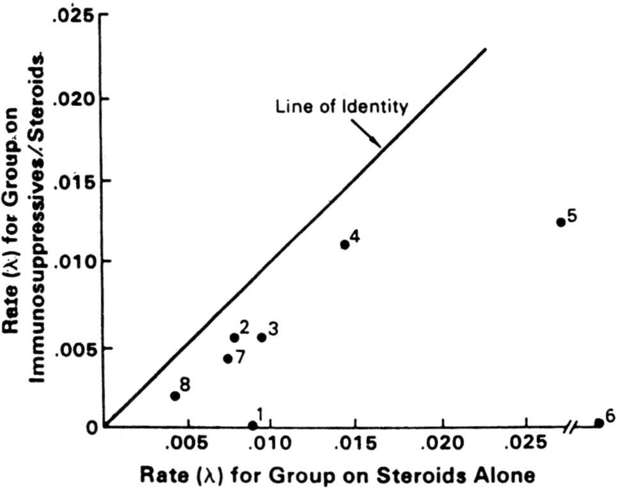

FIG. 5. Displaying the results of a meta-analysis. Rate of renal deterioration in patients treated with steroids alone and in those treated with a combination of immunosuppressive drugs and steroids. Each *point* represents a study. (From Felson and Anderson, ref. 109, with permission.)

Displaying the Results

Pooled results are typically reported as a point estimate and the associated 95% confidence interval. The results are best appreciated by graphically plotting the individual studies, the pooled estimates, and their confidence intervals on an appropriate scale (108) (Fig. 4). A scatter plot of treatment rate against control rate has also been advocated to examine heterogeneity across all the studies pooled (109) (Fig. 5).

Performing a Sensitivity Analysis

A meta-analysis is not complete without testing for the robustness of the pooled results and exploring heterogeneities that may exist among the studies. One form of sensitivity analysis is to delete one study at a time and reassess the impact on the pooled results. Subgroup analyses can be conducted by stratifying studies into clinically meaningful subgroups and pooling them separately. Sex, age, and severity of disease are common variables used. Hypotheses can also be tested by altering the inclusion criteria of the meta-analysis protocol.

Cumulative Meta-Analysis and Meta-Regression

New clinical trials are continuously appearing, and meta-analyses need to be updated to keep the results current. Cumulative meta-analysis is an approach to performing a new pooling with the addition of a new study (Fig. 6). The impact of a new study on the previously pooled results can then be assessed and the cumulative results displayed for the trends that it presents. Performed retrospectively, a cumulative meta-analysis of studies arranged in chronologic order can identify the year when a treatment effect could have been identified. For example, a cumulative meta-analysis on the use of thrombolytic therapy in acute myocardial infarction found that sufficient evidence from randomized controlled trials was available by 1973 to demonstrate a beneficial effect on mortality, but this therapy was not approved by the U.S. Food and Drug Administration until 1988 (110). Performed prospectively, continuous updating of meta-analyses can provide the earliest recognition of treatment efficacy.

Cumulative meta-analysis can also examine relationships between treatment effects and variables of interest (111). For example, a cumulative meta-analysis of studies arranged by increasing or decreasing drug dose could be used to examine a possible dose-response relationship. A trend toward greater treatment effects as studies with increasing doses are pooled would demonstrate that a beneficial dose-response relationship exists.

The use of cumulative meta-analysis to investigate relationships between variables and the treatment effects in clinical trials is similar to the more formal statistical method of meta-regression (99). In a meta-regression, the unit of analysis is the individual study meeting inclusion criteria in the meta-analysis. Variables reported in each of the studies, such as mean dosage, mean age, mean urine protein excretion, mean serum creatinine level, and mean duration of disease, could be extracted from each study and used as the independent variable. The treatment effect, for

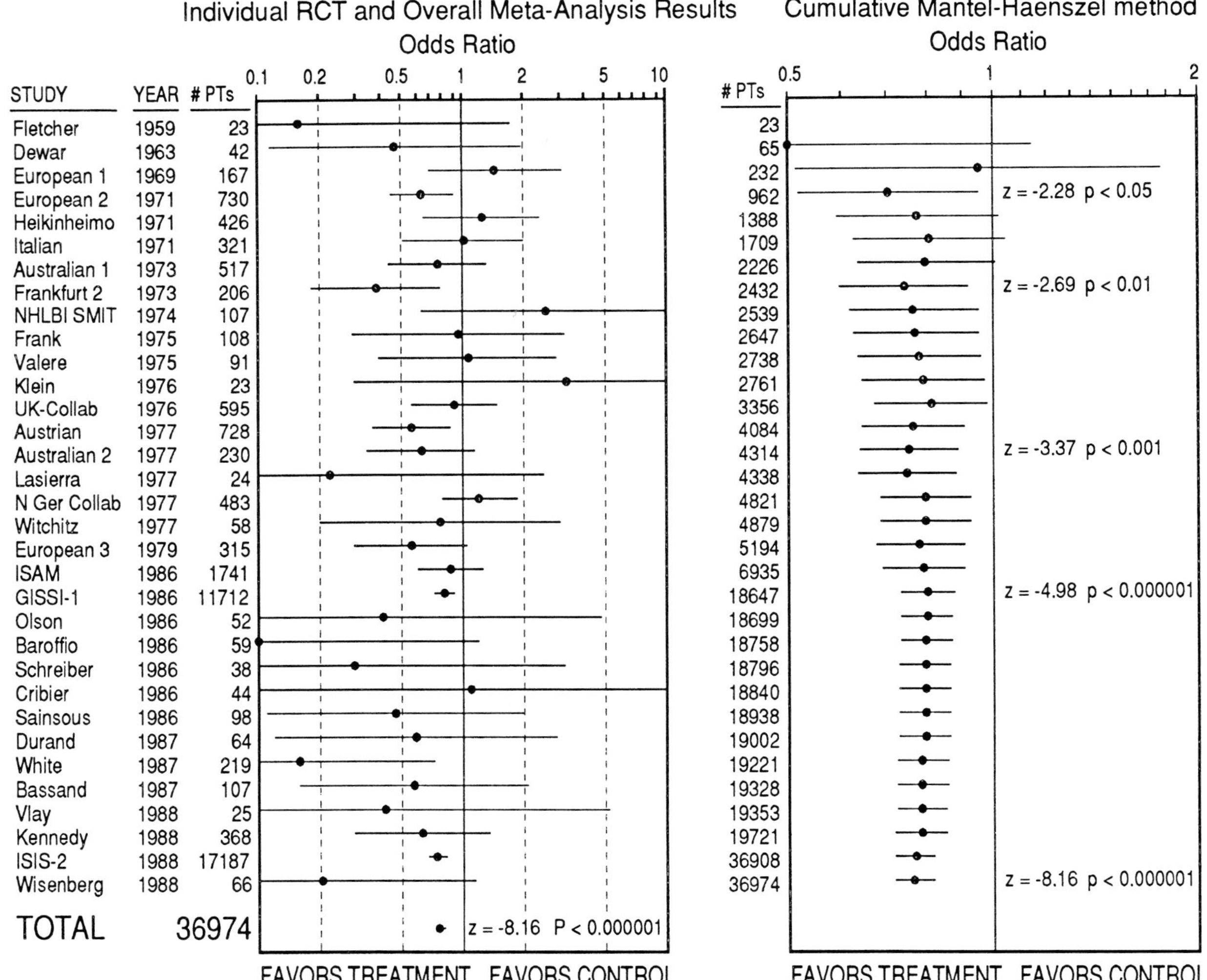

FIG. 6. Displaying the results of a cumulative meta-analysis. (From Lau et al., ref. 110, with permission.)

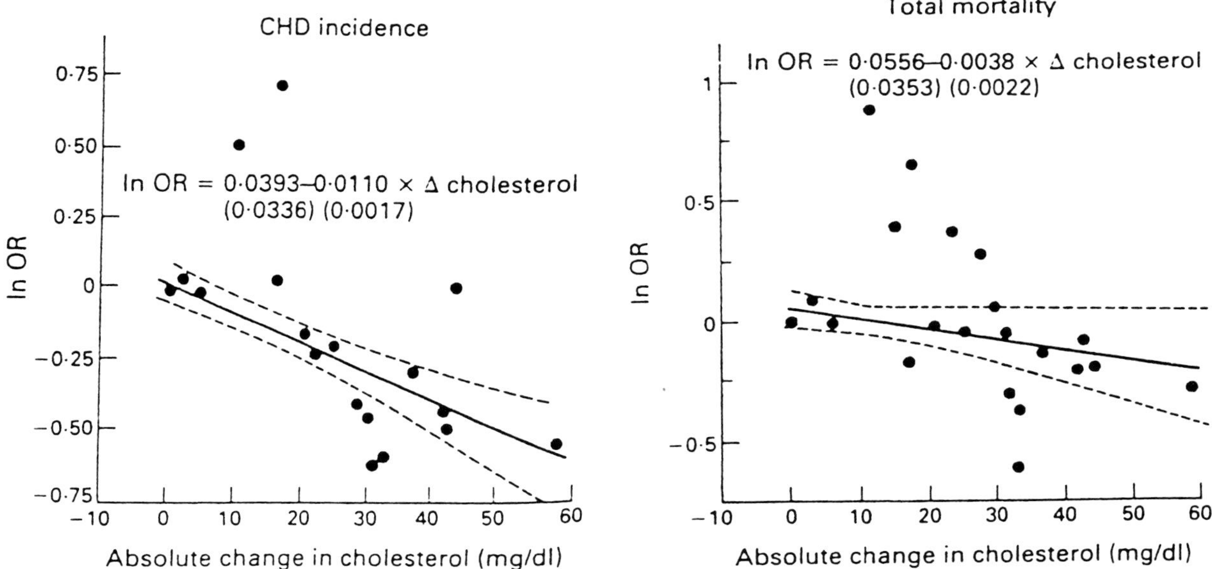

FIG. 7. Displaying the results of a meta-regression analysis. Relation between logarithm of the odds ratio (OR) for coronary heart disease *(CHD; left panel)* or total mortality *(right panel)* and absolute change in plasma cholesterol. (From Holme, ref. 112, with permission.)

example, the risk ratio, is the dependent variable for the analysis. Weighted linear regression on an appropriate scale is typically used. The slope of the regression line provides an estimate of the changes of treatment effect with changing characteristics of interest. Figure 7 shows an example of a meta-regression analysis of the effects of lowering serum cholesterol on the incidence of coronary heart disease and total mortality in randomized trials (112). One of the earliest meta-regression analyses in nephrology was a study by Kasiske et al. (113) that demonstrated greater reduction in urinary protein excretion with ACE inhibitors compared with other classes of antihypertensive agents in patients with diabetes mellitus, controlling for the blood pressure-lowering effects. Recently, a similar effect in nondiabetic patients has also been shown (114).

Reading and Interpreting a Meta-Analysis

Quantitative methods give an aura of credence to any analysis. A meta-analysis, like any clinical study, must be read carefully and its strengths and limitations recognized. The same rules for conducting a meta-analysis should be applied to the interpretation of a meta-analysis. The article should provide the protocol and data from individual studies in sufficient detail to allow the reader to verify the results. Several articles provide a detailed discussion of the assessment of a published meta-analysis (115,116). The basic questions that the clinician and investigator should asked are as follows:

1. Was the meta-analysis performed according to a defined protocol?
2. Were the questions well formulated and would the answers to them be clinically useful?
3. Was a thorough literature search done and the search strategy reported in sufficient detail?
4. Were adequate explanations given for exclusion of studies?
5. Were the studies used in the meta-analysis assessed for their internal validity?
6. Were the treatments well described and similar to what I would plan to use?
7. Were the patients included in the meta-analysis similar to my patients?
8. Were the clinical outcomes well defined and useful?
9. Were the characteristics of the individual studies listed with sufficient detail to allow an assessment of the appropriateness of their inclusion?
10. Were the outcome data provided for the treatment and control groups?
11. Was the definition of the treatment effect meaningful?
12. Were confidence intervals, rather than p values, given for pooled results?
13. Did the meta-analysis provide an estimate of the baseline risk?
14. Were limitations of the meta-analysis discussed?

Review of Selected Meta-Analyses of Therapy for Immunologic Renal Diseases

In this section, several meta-analyses dealing with therapies for immunologic renal disease are briefly reviewed and discussed.

Lupus Nephritis

In one of the earliest published meta-analyses, Felson and Anderson (109) examined evidence for the use of cytotoxic agents in addition to corticosteroids in the management of lupus nephritis. They identified eight randomized controlled trials with 250 patients that compared prednisone alone with prednisone plus cyclophosphamide or azathioprine. All eight trials had 50 patients or less, and no consistent beneficial effect was found on any outcome. Three outcome events were defined for the meta-analysis: decline in renal function, renal failure, or death related to renal disease. An intent-to-treat analysis plan was used, even if a different analysis was reported in the original study. Because of variation in the duration of follow-up in the studies, the mean rate of occurrence of each event was estimated in the two treatment groups in each study and the estimates were pooled. The risk ratio for the pooled estimates of the event rate of each outcome was approximately 0.5 in patients assigned to cytotoxic therapy compared with patients assigned to prednisone alone. Although exact confidence intervals were not reported, the p value for each of the three comparisons was <.05. Subgroup analyses on the efficacy of cytotoxic agents according to biopsy classification revealed a significant benefit in patients with diffuse proliferative glomerulonephritis, but not in patients with a less severe pathologic class. Subgroup analyses of the efficacy of specific agents (cyclophosphamide or azathioprine) showed a similar risk ratio to that of the group as whole, but the results were generally not significant, perhaps because of the small number of patients in the subgroups. The authors concluded that the cytotoxic agents in addition to prednisone were superior to prednisone alone in preventing progression of renal disease in lupus nephritis, and that previously published trials had reached false-negative conclusions because of small sample sizes. This meta-analysis satisfied most of the criteria mentioned above, although quality assessment of the individual studies was not performed and the method of weighing of individual studies in the pooling was not explicitly described. Nonetheless, the superiority of cytotoxic immunosuppressive agents in addition to prednisone alone for diffuse proliferative glomerulonephritis was not generally accepted until the results were replicated in a single large clinical trial (47).

Membranous Nephropathy

Three meta-analyses have been published on the treatment of idiopathic membranous nephropathy. Couchoud et al. (117) reported their results in an editorial containing few details on the methods and results. They reviewed 70 studies and selected eight prospective controlled trials comparing 271 patients treated with prednisone alone or other immunosuppressive agents and 255 patients treated with placebo or no specific therapy. They computed the odds ratio for four endpoints, which were not defined explicitly: "renal death, impairment of renal function, complete remission, and improvement in proteinuria." They reported no beneficial effect on renal death, probably because the duration of follow-up in the trials was too short to allow an adequate number of events. There was also no beneficial effect on complete remissions, again because of the low number of events, but also because of inconsistent definition of this outcome. There was a significant but inconsistent beneficial effect on renal function, and a significant beneficial effect on proteinuria, but the magnitude of the benefits was not reported. This meta-analysis is not convincing because so few details were provided regarding the methods or results, especially the definitions of endpoints. In addition, the authors chose not to make recommendations based on the results and instead recommended a long-term prospective trial.

Hogan et al. (108) reviewed 69 articles and selected seven randomized trials for inclusion in two meta-analyses. One meta-analysis pooled four randomized controlled trials comparing corticosteroids in 176 patients and no specific treatment in 175 patients. The second meta-analysis pooled three randomized trials comparing cytotoxic therapy in 72 patients with no specific treatment in 70 patients. In addition, they also assessed the efficacy of these therapies from a pooled analysis including the seven randomized trials mentioned above, three prospective cohort studies, and 22 retrospective studies. The duration of follow-up in the controlled trials was relatively short, and renal failure developed in few patients. Hence, the main outcome for both meta-analyses was remission of proteinuria. The relative risk (and 95% confidence interval) for remission in patients treated with corticosteroids compared with untreated patients was 1.55 (0.99 to 2.44). The relative risk in patients treated with cytotoxic therapy compared with untreated patients was 4.8 (1.44 to 15.9). The pooled analyses showed overall similar results, but there was no evidence of a beneficial effect in reducing the risk for renal failure. They concluded that cytotoxic agents, but not corticosteroids, are effective in inducing remission of nephrotic syndrome, but that neither treatment improves renal survival in idiopathic nephropathy glomerulopathy. The protocol and the methods of the meta-analysis were well described, but close examination of the data and results raises a number of questions about the validity of the conclusions.

The authors used the χ^2 test to assess heterogeneity of the studies used in the meta-analysis and used only the fixed-effect model to pool the data. The χ^2 test test is acknowledged by most experts to be an insensitive test of treatment effects heterogeneity in a meta-analysis, and the random-effects model is preferred. An examination of the four studies used in the meta-analysis of corticosteroids showed that they may in fact be quite different. Two of the studies had a low rate of spontaneous complete remissions among the control group, 6% and 8%. Two other studies had much higher rates, 33% and 36%. The discrepancies in the event rate in the control group may represent significant clinical differences among the study cohorts or differences in the definition of the clinical outcomes. Pooling of these studies may in fact give erroneous impressions. The meta-analysis on the efficacy of cytotoxic agents excluded one study because there were no remissions in either treatment arm. Thus, the meta-analysis is based on only two studies that used two different treatment regimens—methylprednisolone and chlorambucil in alternating months in one study and cyclophosphamide, warfarin, and dipyridamole in the other study. Overall, the results of the meta-analysis do not appear robust. Although the pooled analyses provide a similar overall result, it is important to remember that nonrandomized studies cannot establish cause and effect. Similar limitations apply to pooled analysis of nonrandomized studies.

Imperiale et al. (97) reviewed 28 studies and selected five prospective controlled trials for inclusion in the meta-analysis. They assumed that there is no benefit of prednisone alone in membranous nephropathy. They compared prednisone and cytotoxic agents (cyclophosphamide in three studies and chlorambucil in two studies) with prednisone alone (in three studies) or no specific therapy (in two studies). Altogether, 228 patients were included. Two endpoints were defined: complete resolution of proteinuria, and partial or complete resolution of proteinuria. Based on the five studies, the risk ratio (and 95% confidence interval) of complete resolution was 4.6 (2.2 to 9.3) and of partial or complete resolution was 2.3 (1.7 to 3.2) in patients treated with prednisone and cytotoxic therapy compared with patients treated with prednisone alone or nonspecific therapy. They concluded there was a significant beneficial effect of prednisone and cytotoxic therapy. In addition to the risk ratio, the number needed to treat (NNT) (118) was also calculated. In this context, the NNT represents the number of patients needed to be treated with a cytotoxic agent to achieve one case of complete or partial remission. The NNTs (and 95% confidence intervals) for complete and for partial or complete remission were 4.7 (3.2 to 8.4) and 2.9 (2.1 to 4.4), respectively. A major finding in this study is that the treatment effects of the studies were found to be homogeneous. Thus, the beneficial effect of cytotoxic therapy did not appear to be a consequence of the inclusion of patients in the control group who did not receive any specific therapy. One limitation of this study is that the outcome data from the individual studies were not reported, and so the results of the meta-analysis could not be verified by the reader. Another limitation is that the conclusions are based on remission of nephrotic syndrome rather than the "hard" endpoint of slowing progression to renal failure.

Overall, it seems clear that cytotoxic agents are more effective than prednisone alone in inducing a remission of proteinuria. Whether prednisone alone is effective in inducing remission remains unclear, and neither therapy has been shown conclusively to slow the progression of renal disease. These meta-analysis highlight the paucity of well-conducted randomized controlled trials of membranous nephropathy and further strengthen the call for higher-quality studies to answer important clinical questions.

IgA Nephropathy

Schena et al. (119) compared a variety of immunosuppressive, anticoagulant, and antiplatelet regimens to nonspecific therapy for primary IgA nephropathy. The analysis combined data from five randomized controlled trials including 80 patients in the treatment group and 68 patients in the control group. The literature search strategy as well as the inclusion and exclusion criteria were not well defined. Patients in all trials had proteinuria, although the magnitude of proteinuria was not reported. Two endpoints were defined: complete or partial remission of proteinuria (data available in only 110 patients) and reduced renal function (data available in all 148 patients). Results were pooled using a fixed-effects model for the odds ratios; the confidence interval was not reported. The pooled odds ratio for remission of proteinuria in the treatment group compared with the control group was 2.6 (p = .02), which corresponded to a risk ratio of 1.7. The test for heterogeneity among studies was significant, and subgroup analysis confirmed a greater effect of therapy on remissions in patients with heavy proteinuria. Despite the beneficial effect on proteinuria, the percentage of patients with renal insufficiency was not different between the treated and control groups—78% and 71%, respectively, after a mean follow-up of 3.2 years. The authors concluded that immunosuppressive medications are beneficial in patients with IgA nephropathy and heavy proteinuria. The major limitations of this study are that no two studies had the same treatment comparisons and the lack of evidence of efficacy on the progression of decline of renal function.

Idiopathic Glomerular Diseases of Various Histopathology

In an earlier meta-analysis, Schena and Cameron (120) reviewed the outcome of immunosuppressive drug treatment for proteinuric idiopathic glomerulonephritis. They selected 35 articles involving 1653 adult patients with urinary protein excretion greater than 1 g/d and the following histopathologies: minimal-change disease, focal segmental glomerulosclerosis, membranous nephropathy, or membranoproliferative glomerulonephritis. Separate analyses of controlled trials and retrospective studies were performed for each of the four histopathologies. They defined outcomes based on proteinuria, serum creatinine, and survival. The event rate for each of the outcomes was calculated from pooling of event counts among studies, rather than pooling the differences between treated and untreated patients among studies. The authors noted a higher incidence of complete remission of proteinuria in patients with minimal-change disease treated with immunosuppressive agents compared with untreated patients. In focal segmental glomerulosclerosis and membranoproliferative glomerulonephritis, there was a low incidence of remission of proteinuria or stable renal function in treated and untreated patients. In membranous nephropathy, they judged the results to be inconclusive because of a higher rate of remissions of proteinuria among untreated patients in controlled trials compared with untreated patients in uncontrolled trials. This study has major limitations. The literature search strategy was not provided. Fewer than half of the studies used in the analysis were randomized controlled trials. The method of pooling event counts is not generally recommended, as it may give rise to the well-known problem of Simpson's paradox (121), in which the rates obtained from pooling of event counts may give a result that is the opposite of the results observed in the individual studies.

Cyclosporine Withdrawal After Renal Transplantation

Kasiske et al. (122) performed a two-part meta-analysis to determine the safety of elective withdrawal of cyclosporine therapy. This study satisfied most of the quality issues listed earlier in this section concerning adequate descriptions of the conduct of the meta-analysis. Randomized and nonrandomized studies were used, and the results were reported together as well as separately. A random-effects model using rate differences was used to pool the data. Sensitivity analyses were performed. Continuation of cyclosporine therapy and elective withdrawal were compared with conventional therapy after renal transplantation. In the first analysis, the authors combined ten randomized and seven nonrandomized trials and compared the outcomes of transplantation in 634 patients in whom cyclosporine was withdrawn with those of 702 patients who continued taking cyclosporine. They found that cyclosporine withdrawal was followed by a higher risk for acute rejection (0.126 more episodes of rejection per patient; 95% confidence interval, 0.085 to 0.167), but there were no differences in graft loss or mortality during a mean follow-up of 27 months. In the second analysis, they combined three randomized and three nonrandomized trials and compared the outcomes of transplantation in 414 patients in whom cyclosporine was withdrawn with those of 400 patients who never received cyclosporine. They found no difference in graft loss, although a separate pooling of only the three randomized studies found a higher rate of graft loss in patients who never received cyclosporine (0.0382 more grafts lost per patient per year; 95% confidence interval, 0.0002 to 0.0762). Based on the results of both analyses, they concluded that elective cyclosporine leads to an increased incidence of acute rejection but does not affect short-term graft or patient survival.

This brief review of published meta-analyses of therapy for immunologic renal disease demonstrates some of the strengths and weaknesses of this discipline. In lupus nephritis, meta-analysis revealed treatment efficacy of cytotoxic agents long before the results of a single large clinical trial. In membranous nephropathy, meta-analysis helped to consolidate the view that cytotoxic agents are efficacious. In renal transplantation, meta-analysis showed convincingly that cyclosporine withdrawal was followed by a higher risk for acute rejection, but not a higher risk for graft loss or patient death. However, there is not yet a standard to which all meta-analyses adhere, and the quality of published meta-analyses is variable. Consequently, not all the analyses reviewed above have had an impact on clinical practice. For example, none of the studies reviewed above used formal quality assessment of individual trials or meta-regression analysis. They used a variety of outcome measures to assess treatment effects. In attempting to combine studies, some meta-analyses had to resort to defining surrogate outcomes that are not universally accepted. Many of the difficulties and inconsistencies may be traced to the weakness of the original publications, such as small sample size, nonuniform definition of outcomes, variable duration of studies, variations in treatment protocols, and nonreporting of data.

Summary of Meta-analysis

Meta-analysis has been applied to clinical medicine for less than two decades, and it is playing an increasingly important role in summarizing evidence for therapeutic decision making. As with any statistical procedure, inappropriate use can lead to misleading results. Meta-analysis has been described as both a tool and a weapon (123). Meta-analysis is an evolving science, and new methods are being developed to provide a more reliable quantitative synthesis of the data. Meta-regression techniques may provide explanations of differences in clinical trials and generate hypotheses for additional studies. Several studies have shown that meta-analyses of small studies yielded similar results when compared with large individual trials (124). Analysis of differences between the results of large trials and of meta-analyses of small trials, rather than demonstrating the unreliability of meta-analysis, has instead provided new insights into the interpretation of clinical trials.

A limitation often faced by those performing meta-analysis is the lack of detailed data reporting in the primary studies. Although little can be done about the quality of the past studies, future trials could be improved by adhering to a higher standard and through the use of structured reporting of clinical trials that is increasingly being advocated (125). It is important to recognize that a single clinical trial is only one data point in a continuum of all other trials. Clinical trials should be planned with the idea that they will be incorporated with other similar studies in a meta-analysis. In addition, meta-analysis of existing trials can be used to identify gaps in the knowledge base, define new research questions, and assist in the planning of future studies. To capitalize on the potentials of this approach, better and more complete reporting of studies must be made.

Meta-analysis is about interpreting the results of a collection of clinical trials addressing a similar problem. The pooling of data from clinical trials to obtain a statistically significant common estimate is useful when treatment effects are homogeneous. More importantly, investigation of heterogeneity between studies can provide insights into why different studies may give different results. When conducted and applied properly, meta-analysis can help us to understand clinical processes and increase the impact of clinical trials on the practice on medicine.

REFERENCES

1. Meinert CL. *Clinical Trials: Design, Conduct, and Analysis*. New York: Oxford University Press; 1986.
2. Friedman LM, Furberg CD, DeMets DL. *Fundamentals of Clinical Trials*. Littleton, MA: John Wright—PSG; 1983.
3. Kelsey JL, Thompson WD, Evans AS. *Methods in Observational Epidemiology*. New York: Oxford University Press; 1986.
4. Cochran WG. *Planning and Analysis of Observational Studies*. New York: John Wiley; 1983.
5. Rubin DB. Estimating causal effects of treatment in randomized and nonrandomized studies. *J Educ Psychol* 1974;66:688–701.
6. Rosenbaum PR. From association to causation in observational studies: the role of tests of strongly ignorable treatment assignment. *JASA* 1984;79:41–48.
7. Lavori PW, Dawson R, Mueller TB. Causal estimation of time-varying treatment effects in observational studies: application to depressive disorder. *Stat Med* 1994;13:1089–1100.
8. Miettinen O. The clinical trial as a paradigm for epidemiologic research. *J Clin Epidemiol* 1989;42:491–496.
9. Byar DP, Simon RM, Friedewald WT. Randomized clinical trials: perspectives on some recent ideas. *N Engl J Med* 1976;295:74–80.
10. Kleinbaum DG, Kupper LL, Morgenstern H. *Epidemiologic Research: Principles and Quantitative Methods*. New York: Van Nostrand Reinhold; 1982.
11. Breslow NE, Day NE. *The Design and Analysis of Cohort Studies*. Lyon: International Agency for Research on Cancer; 1987 (*Statistical Methods in Cancer Research*; vol 2).
12. Schlesselman JJ. *Case-Control Studies*. New York: Oxford University Press; 1982.
13. Karon JM, Kupper LL. In defense of matching. *Am J Epidemiol* 1982; 116:852–866.
14. Kupper LL, Karon JM, Kleinbaum DG, Morgenstern H, Lewis DK. Matching in epidemiological studies: validity and efficiency considerations. *Biometrics* 1991;37:271–291.
15. Friedlander Y, Merom DL, Kark JD. A comparison of different matching designs in case-control studies: an empirical example using continuous exposures, continuous confounders and incidence of myocardial infarction. *Stat Med* 1993:993–1004.
16. Kleinbaum DG, Kupper LL, Muller KE. *Applied Regression Analysis and Other Multivariable Methods*. 2nd ed. Boston: PWS-Kent; 1988.
17. Kaplan RM, Berry CC. Adjusting for confounding variables. In: Sechrest L, Perrin E, Bunker J, eds. *Research Methodology: Strengthening Causal Interpretations of Nonexperimental Data*. Washington, DC: US DHHS publication no 90–3454; 1990:105–114.
18. Greene T, Ernhart CB. Adjustment for cofactors in pediatric research. *J Dev Behav Pediatr* 1991;12:378–385.
19. McCullagh P, Nelder JA. *Generalized Linear Models*. 2nd ed. New York: Chapman and Hall; 1989.
20. Liang KY, Zeger SL. Longitudinal data analysis using generalized linear models. *Biometrika* 1986;73:13–22.
21. Cox DR. Regression models and life tables (with discussion). *J R Stat Soc B* 1972;34:187–220.
22. Carrol RJ, Ruppert D. *Transformation and Weighing in Regression*. New York: Chapman and Hall; 1988.
23. Fuller WA. *Measurement Error Models*. New York: John Wiley; 1987.
24. Hastie T, Tibshirani R. *Generalized Additive Models*. New York: Chapman and Hall; 1990.
25. Hardle W. *Applied Nonparametric Regression*. New York: Cambridge University Press; 1990.
26. Burrleman S, Simon R. Flexible regression models with cubic splines. *Stat Med* 1989;8:551–561.
27. Cook RD, Weisberg S. *Residuals and Influence in Regression*. New York: Chapman and Hall; 1982.
28. Chatterjee S, Hadi AS. *Sensitivity Analysis in Linear Regression*. New York: John Wiley; 1988.
29. Davey SG, Phillips AN. Confounding in epidemiological studies: why "independent" effects may not be all they seem. *Br Med J* 1992; 305:757–759.
30. Davey SG, Phillips AN, Neaton JD. Smoking as an "independent" risk factor for suicide: illustration of an artifact from observational epidemiology? *Lancet* 1992;340:709–712.
31. Cuzick J, Szarewski A. Confounding in epidemiological studies. *Br Med J* 1992;305:1097.
32. Storen BE. Design and analysis of phase I clinical trials. *Biometrics* 1989;45:925–937.
33. Herson J. Statistical aspects in the design and analysis of Phase II clinical trials. In: Buyse ME, Muarice JS, Sylvester RJ, eds. *Cancer Clinical Trials: Methods and Practice*. New York: Oxford University Press; 1984.
34. Moore TD, Korn EJ. Phase II trial design considerations for small-cell lung cancer. *J Natl Cancer Inst* 1992;84:150–154.
35. Mitch WE, Walser M, Steinman TI, Hill S, Zeger S, Tungsarga K. The effect of a keto acid-amino acid supplement to a restricted diet on the progression of chronic renal failure. *N Engl J Med* 1984;311: 623–629.
36. Walser M. Progression of chronic renal failure in man. *Kidney Int* 1990;37:1195–1210.
37. Walker JD, Bendirg JJ, Dodds RA, et al. Restriction of dietary protein and progression of renal failure in diabetic nephropathy. *Lancet* 1989; 2:1411–1415.
38. Parving H-H, Andersen AR, Smidt UM, Svendsen PA. Early antihypertensive treatment reduces rate of decline in kidney function in diabetic nephropathy. *Lancet* 1983;1:1175–1179.
39. Senn SJ, Brown RA. Estimating treatment effects in clinical trials subject to regression to the mean. *Biometrics* 1985;41:555–560.
40. Levey AS, Gassman JJ, Hall PM, Walker WG. Assessing the progression of renal disease in clinical studies: effects of duration of follow-up and regression to the mean. *J Am Soc Nephrol* 1991;1: 1087–1094.
41. Williams GW, Schluchter MD. Statistical considerations for assessing the influence of therapy on progression of chronic renal failure. In: Mitch WE, ed. *The Progressive Nature of Renal Disease*. 2nd ed. New York: Churchill Livingstone.1992:247–276.
42. Pocock SJ, Huges MD, Lee RJ. Statistical problems in reporting of clinical trials. *N Engl J Med* 1987;317:426–432.
43. Cowman CD, Wittes J. Intercept studies, clinical trials, and cluster experiments: to whom can we extrapolate? *Control Clin Trials* 1994; 15:24–29.
44. Howel D, Bhopal R. Assessing cause and effect from trials: a cautionary note. *Control Clin Trials* 1994;15:331–334.
45. Davis C. Generalizing from clinical trials. *Control Clin Trials* 1994; 15:11–14.
46. Bailed K. Generalizing the results of randomized clinical trials. *Control Clin Trials* 1994;15:15–23.

47. Austin HA III, Klippel JH, Balow JE, le Riche NG, Steinberg AD, Plotz PH, et al. Therapy of lupus nephritis: controlled trial of prednisone and cytotoxic drugs. *N Engl J Med* 1986;314:614–619.
48. Yusuf S, Held P, Teo KK, Toretsky ER. Selection of patients for randomized controlled trials: implications of wide or narrow eligibility criteria. *Stat Med* 1990;9:73–86.
49. Miller RG. Simultaneous Statistical Inference. New York: Springer; 1981.
50. Haynes RB, Dantes R. Patient compliance and the conduct and the interpretation of therapeutic trials. *Control Clin Trials* 1987;8:12–19.
51. Last JM. *A Dictionary of Epidemiology*. Oxford: Oxford University Press; 1988.
52. Ellenberg JH. Selection bias in observational and experimental studies. *Stat Med* 1994;13:557–567.
53. Lee YJ, Ellenberg JH, Hirtz DG, Nelson KB. Analysis of clinical trials by treatment actually received: is it really an option? *Stat Med* 1991;10:1595–1605.
54. Efron B, Feldman D. Compliance as an explanatory variable in clinical trials. *JASA* 1991;86:9–26.
55. Albert JM, DeMets DL. On a model-based approach to estimating efficacy in clinical trials. *Stat Med* 1994;13:2323–2335.
56. Mark SD, Robbins JM. A method for the analysis of randomized trials with compliance information: an application to the multiple risk factor intervention trial. *Control Clin Trials* 1993;14:79–97.
57. Yusuf S, Wittes J, Probstfield J, Tyroler A. An analysis and interpretation of treatment effects in subgroups of patients in randomized clinical trials. *JAMA* 1991;266:93–98.
58. Bulpitt CJ. Subgroup analysis. *Lancet* 1988;2:31–34.
59. Byar DP, Piantadosi S. Factorial designs for randomized clinical trials. *Cancer Treat Rep* 1985;69:1055–1062.
60. Klahr S, Levey AS, Beck GJ, Caggiula AW, Hunsicker L, Kusek JW, Striker G, Modification of Diet in Renal Disease Study Group. The effects of dietary protein restriction and blood pressure control on the progression of renal disease. *N Engl J Med* 1994;330:877–884.
61. Brittain E, Wittes J. Factorial designs in clinical trials: the effects of noncompliance and subadditivity. *Stat Med* 1989;8:161–171.
62. Xiang AH, Sather HN, Azen SP. Power considerations for testing an interaction in a 2 × K factorial design with a failure outcome. *Control Clin Trials* 1994;15:489–502.
63. Lewis E, Hunsicker L, Bain R, Rohde R, et al. The effect of angiotensin-converting enzyme inhibition on diabetic nephropathy. *N Engl J Med* 1993;329:1456–1462.
64. Marubini E, Valsecchi MG. *Analyzing Survival Data from Clinical Trials and Observational Studies*. New York: John Wiley; 1995.
65. Peterson JC, Adler S, Burkart JM, Greene T, Hebert LA, Hunsicker LG, King AJ, Klahr S, Massry SG, Seifter JL for the Modification of Diet in Renal Disease Study Group. Blood pressure control, proteinuria, and the progression of renal disease. *Ann Intern Med* 1995;123: 754–762.
66. Bulpitt CJ. Confidence intervals. *Lancet* 1987;1:494–497.
67. Cohen J. *Statistical Power for the Behavioral Sciences*. New York: Academic Press; 1977.
68. Fleming TR. Evaluating therapeutic interventions. some issues and experiences. *Stat Sci* 1992;7:428–456.
69. Prentice RL. Surrogate endpoints in clinical trials: definition and operational criteria. *Stat Med* 1989;8:431–440.
70. Kirby JJ, Gala N, Munoz A. Sample size estimation using repeated measurements on biomarkers as outcomes. *Control Clin Trials* 1994; 15:165–172.
71. Smith HW. Diseases of the kidney and urinary tract. *The Kidney: Structure and Function*. New York: Oxford University Press; 1951: 836–887.
72. Levey AS. Use of glomerular filtration measurements to assess the progression of renal disease. *Semin Nephrol* 1989;9:370–379.
73. Perrone R, Steinman T, Beck GJ, Skibinksi CI, Royal H, Lawlor M, Hunsicker L, Modification of Diet in Renal Disease Study Group. Utility of radioisotopic filtration markers in chronic renal insufficiency: simultaneous comparison of ^{125}I-iothalamate, ^{169}Yb-DTPA, ^{99m}Tc-DTPA to inulin. *Am J Kidney Dis* 1990;16:224–225.
74. Levey AS, Greene T, Schluchter MD, Cleary PA, Teschan PI, Lorenz RA, Molitch ME, Mitch WE, Siebert C, Hall PM, Steffes MW, Modification of Diet in Renal Disease Study Group, Diabetes Control and Complications Trial Research Group. Glomerular filtration rate measurements in clinical trials. *J Am Soc Nephrol* 1993;4:1159–1171.
75. Levey AS, Madaio MP, Perrone RD. Laboratory assessment of renal disease: clearance, urinalysis and renal biopsy. In: Brenner BM, Rector FC Jr, eds. *The Kidney*. 4th ed. Philadelphia: WB Saunders; 1991: 919–968.
76. Levey AS. Nephrology forum: measurement of renal function in chronic renal disease. *Kidney Int* 1990;38:167–184.
77. Modification of Diet in Renal Disease Study Group (prepared by Levey AS, Bosch JP, Coggins CH, Greene T, Mitch WE, Schluchter MD, Schwab SJ). Effects of diet and antihypertensive therapy on creatinine clearance and serum creatinine in the Modification of Diet in Renal Disease Study. *J Am Soc Nephrol* 1996;7:556–566.
78. Mauer SM, Steffes MW, Ellis EN, Sutherland DER, Brown DM, Boetz FC. Structural-functional relationships in diabetic nephropathy. *J Clin Invest* 1984;74:1143–1155.
79. Chagnac A, Kiberd BA, Farinas MC, Strober S, Sibley RK, Hoppe R, Myers BD. Outcome of acute glomerular injury in proliferative lupus nephritis. *J Clin Invest* 1989;84:922–930.
80. Levey AS. Assessing the effectiveness of therapy to prevent the progression of renal disease. *Am J Kidney Dis* 1993;1:207–214.
81. Modification of Diet in Renal Disease Study Group (prepared by Levey AS, Beck GJ, Bosch JP, Caggiula AW, Greene T, Hunsicker LG, Klahr S). Short-term effects of protein intake, blood pressure antihypertensive therapy on glomerular filtration rate in the Modification of Diet in Renal Disease Study. *J Am Soc Nephrol* 1996 (*in press*).
82. Wu MC. Sample size for comparison of changes in the presence of right censoring caused by death, withdrawal, and staggered entry. *Control Clin Trials* 1988;9:32–46.
83. Laird NM, Ware JH. Random-effects models for longitudinal data. *Biometrics* 1982;38:963–974.
84. *SAS/STAT Software: Changes and Enhancements through Release 6.11*. Cary, NC: SAS Institute; 1996.
85. *BMDP Statistical Software Manual*; version 7.0, vol 2. Berkeley, CA: University of California Press; 1992.
86. Wu MC, Carroll RJ. Estimation and comparison of changes in the presence of informative right censoring by modelling the censoring process. *Biometrics* 1988;44:175–188.
87. Little RJA, Rubin DB. *Statistical Analysis with Missing Data*. New York: John Wiley; 1987.
88. Wu MC, Bailey K. Estimation and comparison of changes in the presence of informative right censoring: conditional linear model. *Biometrics* 1989;45:939–955.
89. Schluchter MD. Methods for the analysis of informatively censored longitudinal data. *Stat Med* 1992;11:1861–1870.
90. Gilks WR, Wang CC, Yvonnet B, Coursaget P. Random-effects models for longitudinal data using Gibbs sampling. *Biometrics* 1993;49: 441–452.
91. Greene T, Beck GJ, Gassman JJ, Kutner MH, Paranandi L, Wang S-R, MDRD Study Group, AASK Study Group. Comparison of time-to-event and slope-based analyses in nephrology clinical trials. *Control Clin Trials* 1995;16:65S(abst).
92. Mulrow CD. The medical review article: state of the science. *Ann Intern Med* 1987;106:485–488.
93. Sacks HS, Berrier J, Reitman D, Ancona-Berk VA, Chalmers TC. Meta-analyses of randomized controlled trials. *N Engl J Med* 1987; 316:450–455.
94. L'abbe KA, Detsky AS, O'Rourke K. Meta-analysis in clinical research. *Ann Intern Med* 1987;107:224–233.
95. Thacker SB. Meta-analysis. A quantitative approach to research integration. *JAMA* 1988;259:1685–1689.
96. Dickersin K, Berlin J. Meta-analysis: state-of-the-science. *Epidemiol Rev* 1992;14:154–176.
97. Imperiale TF, Goldfarb S, Berns JS. Are cytotoxic agents beneficial in idiopathic membranous nephropathy? A meta-analysis of the controlled trials. *J Am Soc Nephrol* 1995;5:1553–1558.
98. Goldman L, Feinstein AR. Anticoagulants and myocardial infarction: the problems of pooling, drowning, and floating. *Ann Intern Med* 1979;90:92–94.
99. Greenland S. Quantitative methods in the review of epidemiologic literature. *Epidemiol Rev* 1987;9:1–30.
100. Berlin A, Antman EM. Advantages and limitations of meta-analytic regressions of clinical trials data. *Online J Curr Clin Trials* 1994; document no 134.
101. Jadad AR, McQay HJ. A high-yield strategy to identify randomized

controlled trials for systematic reviews. *Online J Curr Clin Trials* 1993; document no 33.

102. Haynes RB, Wilczynski N, McKibbon A, Walker C, Sinclair JC. Developing optimal search strategies for detecting clinically sound studies in MEDLINE. *J Am Med Inform Assoc* 1994;1:447–458.
103. Easterbrook PJ, Berlin KA, Gopalan R, Matthews DR. Publication bias in clinical research. *Lancet* 1991;337:867–872.
104. Schultz KF, Chalmers I, Hayes RJ, Altman DG. Empirical evidence of bias: dimensions of methodological quality associated with estimates of treatment effects in controlled trials. *JAMA* 1995;273:408–412.
105. Emerson JD, Burdick E, Hoaglin DC, Mosteller F, Chalmers TC. An empirical study of the possible relation of treatment differences to quality scores in controlled randomized clinical trials. *Control Clin Trials* 1990;11:339–352.
106. Greenland S. Invited commentary: a critical look at some popular meta-analytic methods. *Am J Epidemiol* 1994;140:290–296.
107. Hedges LV, Olkin I. *Statistical Methods for Meta-analysis*. San Diego: Academic Press; 1985.
108. Hogan SL, Muller KE, Jennette JC, Falk RJ. A review of therapeutic studies of idiopathic membranous glomerulopathy. *Am J Kidney Dis* 1995;25:862–875.
109. Felson DT, Anderson J. Evidence for the superiority of immunosuppressive drugs and prednisone over prednisone alone in lupus nephritis. *N Engl J Med* 1984;311:1528–1533.
110. Lau J, Antman EM, Jimenez-Silva J, Kupelnick B, Mosteller F, Chalmers TC. Cumulative meta-analysis of therapeutic trials for myocardial infarction. *N Engl J Med* 1992;327:248–254.
111. Lau J, Schmid CH, Chalmers TC. Cumulative meta-analysis of clinical trials builds evidence for exemplary medical care. *J Clin Epidemiol* 1995;48:45–57.
112. Holme I. Relation of coronary heart disease incidence and total mortality to plasma cholesterol reduction in randomized trials: use of meta-analysis. *Br Heart J* 1993;69[Suppl 1]:S42–S47.
113. Kasiske BL, Kalil RSN, Ma JZ, Liao M, Keane WF. Effect of antihypertensive therapy on the kidney in patients with diabetes: a meta-regression analysis. *Ann Intern Med* 1993;118:129–138.
114. Gansevoort RT, Sluiter WJ, Hemmelder MH, de Zeeuw D, de Jong PE. Antiproteinuric effect of blood-pressure-lowering agents: a meta-analysis of comparative trials. *Nephrol Dial Transplant* 1995;10:1963–1974.
115. Henry DA, Wilson A. Meta-analysis: part 1: an assessment of its aims, validity and reliability. *Med J Aust* 1992;156:31–38.
116. Oxman AD, Cook DJ, Guyatt GH. Users' guides to the medical literature. VI. How to use an overview. *JAMA* 1994;272:1367–1371.
117. Couchoud C, Laville M, Boissel JP. Treatment of membranous nephropathy: a meta-analysis. *Nephrol Dial Transplant* 1994;9:469–470.
118. Laupacias A, Scakett DL, Robert RS. An assessment of clinically useful measures of the consequences of treatment. *N Engl J Med* 1988;318:1728–1733.
119. Schena FP, Montenegro M, Scivittaro V. Meta-analysis of randomised controlled trials in patients with primary IgA nephropathy (Berger's disease). *Nephrol Dial Transplant* 1990;5[Suppl 1]:47–53.
120. Schena FP, Cameron JS. Treatment of proteinuric idiopathic glomerulonephritis in adults: a retrospective survey. *Am J Med* 1988;85:315–326.
121. Rothman KJ. *Modern Epidemiology*. Boston: Little, Brown; 1986:89.
122. Kasiske BL, Heim O, Duthoy K, Ma JZ. Elective cyclosporine withdrawal after renal transplantation. A meta-analysis. *JAMA* 1993;269:395–400.
123. Bodin WE. Meta-analysis in clinical trials reporting: has a tool become a weapon? *Am J Cardiol* 1992;69:681–686.
124. Villar J, Carroli G, Belizan JM. Predictive ability of meta-analysis of randomised controlled trials. *Lancet* 1995;345:772–776.
125. The Standards of Reporting Trials Group. A proposal for structured reporting of randomized controlled trials. *JAMA* 1994;272:1926–1931.

B. Primary Glomerular Diseases

Immunologic Renal Diseases,
edited by E. G. Neilson and W. G. Couser.
Lippincott-Raven Publishers, Philadelphia © 1997.

CHAPTER 41

Postinfectious Glomerulonephritis

William G. Couser and Richard J. Johnson

INTRODUCTION

A number of infectious illnesses are accompanied by acute and chronic manifestations of renal disease. These include infections caused by bacteria, viruses, parasites, and several other pathogens (Table 1). Some postinfectious glomerulonephritides, such as post-streptococcal glomerulonephritis (PSGN), were once common causes of renal disease worldwide but are now seen primarily in developing countries. Many postinfectious processes, such as malarial nephropathy, have always been diseases of undeveloped nations. However, the prevalence of others, such as AIDS and hepatitis C nephropathy, is now increasing in developed countries. This chapter reviews the mechanisms and clinical manifestations of the most common postinfectious, immunologically mediated renal diseases. AIDS nephropathy is considered separately in Chapter 54.

GLOMERULONEPHRITIS CAUSED BY BACTERIAL INFECTIONS

Post-streptococcal Glomerulonephritis (Bright's Disease)

Background

The association of hematuria and proteinuria with bacterial infection was noted in the early eighteenth century following epidemics of scarlet fever and was first reported in the early nineteenth century (1,2). Bright (3) linked GN to scarlatina, an observation that resulted in the disease subsequently being called *Bright's disease* (3). Studies in the early 1900s documented the role of group A (β-hemolytic) streptococci (4). In 1953, it was recognized by Rammelkamp and colleagues (5,6) that only certain strains of group A streptococci were nephritogenic, particularly type 12. The classic description of the morphology of PSGN was provided by Jennings and Earle in 1961 (7). Although it is now less common than other types of GN in adults, PSGN is the prototype of acute GN, with all the clinical features of the acute nephritic syndrome (see below). Post-streptococcal glomerulonephritis is also recognized as the prototype of clinical glomerular disease caused by the deposition of immune complexes containing an exogenous antigen; the pathogenetic mechanisms are presumably analogous to those of the acute serum sickness model in rabbits (see Chapter 35), although this hypothesis has not been completely verified in humans.

Etiology and Incidence

The etiologic agent in PSGN is clearly established as a group A streptococcus of nephritogenic M type, which includes primarily type 12 but a number of other types as well (8,9). In GN following pharyngitis, the most common nephritogenic types are 12, 4, 1, 3, 25, and 49 (9–11). Nephritis following a skin infection (pyoderma or impetigo) usually occurs in association with types 49, 55, 2, 57, or 60 (10–19). Because the nephritogenic antigen is probably not an M protein, which confers type specificity on the streptococcus, other strains may sometimes be nephritogenic as well. Occasional cases have been reported following infection with group C streptococci (13–16) or those of group G (17). Post-streptococcal GN contrasts with rheumatic fever, which can be induced by any type of group A streptococcus (18,19). The clinical attack rate is quite variable, even with infections of a single M type, suggesting that other important host factors,

W. G. Couser: Division of Nephrology, Department of Medicine, University of Washington, Seattle, Washington 98195.
R. J. Johnson: Division of Nephrology, Department of Medicine, University of Washington Medical Center, Seattle, Washington 98195.

TABLE 1. *Infectious agents and diseases associated with glomerulonephritis*

Bacterial	Viral
α-Hemolytic streptococci	Arbovirus
β-Hemolytic streptococci	Coxsackievirus
(group A)	Cytomegalovirus
Actinobacillus	Dengue
Actinomyces	Echovirus
Bacillus cereus	Enterovirus
Bacillus subtilis	Epstein-Barr virus
Brucella suis	Guillain-Barré
Campylobacter jejuni	syndrome
Cardiobacterium comitans	Hantaan virus
Cardiobacterium hominis	Hepatitis B, C
Cat scratch disease	Herpes simplex
Chlamydia psittaci	HIV
Corynebacterium bovis	Influenza A and B
Coxiella burnetii	Measles
Diplococcus pneumoniae	Mumps
Diphtheroids	Oncornavirus
Escherichia coli	Ross River virus
Haemophilus aphrophilus	Varicella
Haemophilus	
parainfluenzae	Parasitic
Klebsiella pneumoniae	*Echinococcus*
Legionella	*granulosus*
Leptospira	Filariasis
Moraxella osloensis	*Loa loa*
Mycobacterim gordonae	*Plasmodium falciparum*
Mycobacterim leprae	*Plasmodium malariae*
Mycobacterim tuberculosis	*Schistosoma*
Mycoplasma pneumoniae	*haematobium*
Neisseria meningitidis	*Schistosoma mansoni*
Peptococcus	*Toxoplasma gondii*
Propionibacterium acnes	*Trichinella spiralis*
Proteus mirabilis	*Trypanosoma*
Psittacosis	
Pseudomonas aeruginosa	Rickettsial
Salmonella typhosa	Rocky Mountain spotted
Serratia	fever
Staphylococcus aureus	Scrub typhus
Staphylococcus	
epidermidis	Fungal
Streptococcus mitis	*Aspergillus*
Streptococcus mutans	*Candida albicans*
Streptococcus pneumoniae	Mumps
Streptococcus viridans	*Candida parapsilosis*
Treponema pallidum	*Coccidioides immitis*
Yersinia enterocolitica	*Histoplasma*

most likely immunogenetic ones, are operative (20–25). Clinical attack rates with nephritogenic strains vary from 1% to more than 30% but average 10–12% (20,23,24). However, careful study including urinalysis by nephrologists suggests that the true attack rate including subclinical cases is probably 3 to 4 times this figure (23). Poststreptococcal GN may account for more than 50% of cases of acute GN in children (25–27). In adults, it represents the diagnosis in fewer than 5% of all renal biopsies (28–29). The overall prevalence of PSGN has declined significantly during the past two decades in the United States as well as in many other countries of the world where such data are available (30–32). Presumably, this reflects improved hygiene and public health measures as well as better antibiotic efficacy and perhaps decreased prevalence of the primary nephritogenic M types, such as 4 and 12 (33).

Pathogenesis and Pathophysiology

The immunopathologic features of PSGN suggest that it is an immune complex disease (see below). The mechanisms involved are believed to be analogous to those defined in the acute serum sickness model in rabbits induced by injection of a soluble foreign protein (see Chapters 14 and 35). Thus, the deposits that occur in mesangial and subendothelial sites presumably derive from glomerular trapping of preformed soluble immune complexes from the circulation (see Chapter 14). Circulating immune complex levels are elevated in patients with PSGN, although not more than in patients with rheumatic fever or with impetigo without nephritis (34–36), and they may contain streptococcal antigens (37). The subepithelial "humps" that are so characteristic of PSGN may represent the local re-formation of immune complexes trapped on the inner aspect of the capillary wall that subsequently dissociate and re-form in a subepithelial site, or local formation of complexes containing a low-molecular-weight cationic antigen or cationic antibody (see Chapter 14 and the discussion of how subepithelial deposits form in Chapter 47). However, as subendothelial and mesangial deposits are present but not prominent in PSGN, preformed immune complex trapping is not very nephritogenic, and subepithelial deposits generally do not cause inflammation, there are clearly mechanisms involved in this disease that have not yet been well defined.

The composition of the immune complex deposits in PSGN is also poorly defined. Although circulating immune complexes in PSGN may contain streptococcal antigens (38), the only available studies of antibody eluted from glomeruli in PSGN have not identified any antibody reactivity with known streptococcal antigens; they have documented the presence only of anti-IgG rheumatoid factor activity in relatively high concentration (39,40). Several laboratories have worked for decades to establish the nature of the putative deposited streptococcal antigen in PSGN. Lange et al. have described endostreptosin (ESS), a cytoplasmic protein antigen from groups A, X, and C streptococci (37,41,42). Endostreptosin has a molecular weight of 40,000 to 50,000 kD and is localized in mesangial and subendothelial distributions in early PSGN. Moreover, most patients with PSGN have antibody reactive with ESS (but so do many patients without nephritis and normal controls). Endostreptosin is anionic in charge, so its mechanism of glomerular localization is uncertain. Moreover, it is not localized in subepithelial humps (41,42). Yoshizawa et al. (43) have further studied ESS by purifying a fraction called *pre-absorbing antigen* (*PA-antigen*) and demonstrated antibodies to it in 30 of 31 patients with PSGN, whereas antibody was virtually absent in patients with uncomplicated group A streptococcal infection or normal controls (43). Pre-absorbing antigen, like ESS, was also demonstrated by immunofluorescence in mesangial areas of glomeruli of some patients with early PSGN (43). An interesting feature of this protein is that it functions as a direct activator of the alternative pathway of complement, suggesting that it may localize in glomeruli independently of IgG and generate a local inflammatory reaction, although this phenomenon has not been documented in vivo (43). A protein termed *protein SIC* has also been isolated from several nephritogenic strains of streptococci and has a complement-inhibitory function (44).

Another potential nephritogenic streptococcal antigen is called *nephritis strain-associated protein* (*NSAP*); this protein has been isolated from group 12 streptococci and is probably identical to streptokinase C (45). Nephritis strain-associated protein activates plasminogen and also activates C3 via the alternative complement pathway. Moreover, it has been shown to localize in glomeruli in vivo independently of IgG (46,47). In rabbits and mice given purified NSAP, glomerular lesions develop with some features of PSGN (46,47), and antibody to NSAP is more commonly found in patients with nephritis than in those without (10,28,48,49). However, NSAP has not been convincingly shown to be localized consistently in the immune deposits or subepithelial humps of patients with acute PSGN.

Another recently studied streptococcal antigen is streptococcal pyrogenic exotoxin B (SPEB), an antigen derived from nephritogenic group A streptococci. Antibodies to SPEB are higher in PSGN than in rheumatic fever or scarlet fever, and the antigen has been demonstrated in 4 of 15 biopsy specimens from patients with PSGN (50).

Others have pursued the hypothesis that streptococci induce antibodies that cross-react with native glomerular antigens. Lange and co-workers (51,52) have documented reactivity of antibody to streptococcal cell membrane proteins with glomeruli, sometimes in a granular pattern. Others have demonstrated the presence of antibodies to heparan sulfate proteoglycan, laminin, and type 4 collagen in patients with PSGN, but these observations have not been well correlated with clinical evidence of nephritis, nor is the pattern of immune deposition in PSGN suggestive of anti-glomerular basement membrane (anti-GBM) antibody activity (53).

Other possible mechanisms would involve streptococcal infection as an etiologic mechanism but would not implicate immune complexes containing streptococcal antigens in development of glomerular immune deposits. McIntosh, Rodriguez-Iturbe, and others (54–56) have postulated that the antigen in PSGN is autologous IgG altered by exposure to streptococcal neuraminidase to become antigenic and elicit an anti-IgG rheumatoid factor response, which may lead to formation of cryoglobulins. This is in accord with the observation that IgG eluted from glomeruli in PSGN has rheumatoid factor activity but no detectable antibody to known streptococcal antigens (39,40). However, neuraminidase is produced by non-nephritogenic streptococci as well, and patients with streptococcal infection without nephritis may also have cryoglobulins and rheumatoid factor (57). Moreover, experimental GN induced with cationized IgG results in a primarily membranous type of lesion (58,59).

Another recent observation of potential relevance to the pathogenesis of PSGN is that both streptococcal M proteins and pyrogenic exotoxins can act as superantigens that cause a marked expansion of T cells expressing specific T-cell receptor β-chain variable gene segments (60–62). Super-antigens can induce a selective increase in T-cell receptor β+ cells and massive T-cell activation, with release of T cell-derived lymphokines such as interleukin 1 and interleukin 6 (63–65). Super-antigens also induce polyclonal B-cell activation and production of auto-antibody (66). Elevated levels of the inflammatory cytokines (interleukin 6 and tumor necrosis factor-α) have been reported in PSGN (67). A role for methicillin-resistant *Staphylococcus aureus* (MRSA) in the pathogenesis of a postinfectious immune complex nephritis via a super-antigen mechanism has been suggested (68). Cryoglobulins, rheumatoid factors, and other autoimmune phenomenon do occur in PSGN (see above), and a role for streptococcal super-antigens in the initiation of GN is worthy of further study.

In short, despite more than three decades of rather intensive study of a large number of patients by many investigators, the pathogenesis of PSGN, the prototypic acute immune complex nephritis in humans, remains unclear. Whatever the mechanism by which deposits form in this disease, it is likely that the inflammatory response is complement-mediated, largely through chemotactic factors and recruitment of the neutrophils and monocytes that are prominent in the early lesion (see below).

Pathology

Light Microscopy

The light microscopic appearance of PSGN is that of a diffuse, proliferative GN (13,19,28,29,69–73). Glomerular involvement is generally uniform, and enlarged glomeruli often fill Bowman's space (Fig. 1). There is also a marked and diffuse increase in glomerular cells. The hypercellularity represents both proliferation of endogenous glomerular mesangial and endothelial cells (endocapillary GN) and infiltration by neutrophils, monocytes, and sometimes eosinophils (exudative GN) that are located both within

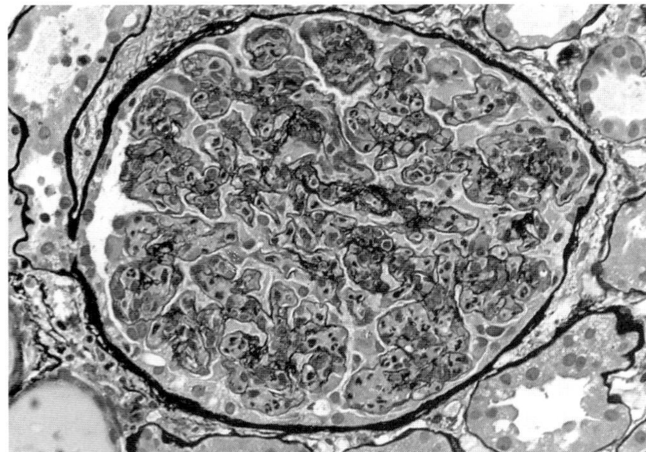

FIG. 1. Light micrograph illustrating diffuse proliferative glomerulonephritis in a patient with acute PSGN. There is a uniform hypercellularity representing a marked inflammatory cell infiltrate of neutrophils and monocytes as well as proliferation of endogenous glomerular cells. Capillary lumina are compromised, and the glomerulus has a somewhat lobular configuration. Original magnification ×400. (Photomicrograph provided by Dr. Charles Alpers.)

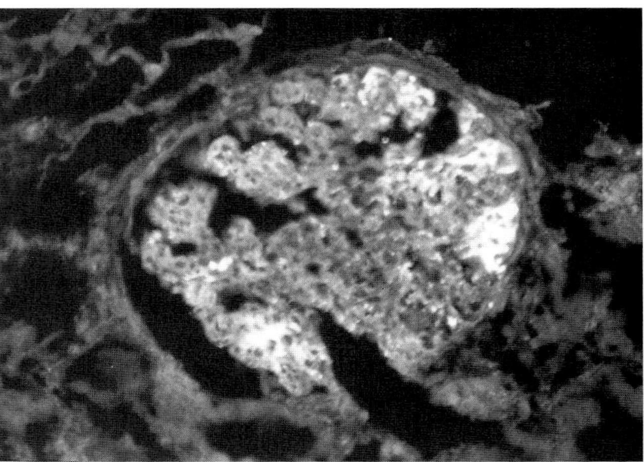

FIG. 2. Immunofluorescent staining for IgG in the biopsy specimen of a patient with PSGN. Large granular deposits of IgG are distributed regularly on capillary walls and on the mesangium. These deposits are presumed to represent passively trapped immune complexes, although the composition of the deposits remains uncertain (see text). Original magnification ×250. (Photomicrograph provided by Dr. Charles Alpers.)

glomerular capillaries and in mesangial areas (Fig. 1). The cellular proliferation and exudation may occlude glomerular capillaries, but basement membranes are grossly intact. Thin sections with trichrome stain may reveal subepithelial humps (see below). Glomeruli with extensive cell proliferation may have a lobular appearance (Fig. 1). Crescent formation may be seen in severe cases, and when present in more than 30% of glomeruli may accompany a clinical picture of rapidly progressive glomerulonephritis (RPGN) (see Chapter 49) (28,29,74–76). The interstitium may exhibit edema and focal cellular infiltrates but is not primarily involved. Some cases of vasculitis associated with PSGN with vascular lesions in the kidney have been reported (77–79). Inflammatory cell infiltrates and glomerular cell proliferation are maximal early in the disease and resolve over a period of several weeks. However, there may be residual mesangial hypercellularity that can last for months or even years.

Immunofluorescence

The first documentation of immunoglobulin and complement deposition as a cause of PSGN was provided by Freedman and colleagues in 1960 (80). Immunofluorescence findings in PSGN are diffuse granular deposition of IgG (Fig. 2), C3 (Fig. 3), or both; this may occur in several patterns. Thirty percent of patients exhibit a "starry sky" pattern of immune deposits consisting of relatively finely granular, diffusely distributed deposits on all capillary walls and in the mesangium (81,82) (Fig. 3). This pattern is seen early and is associated with both cellular proliferation and inflammatory cell infiltration. Forty-five percent of patients exhibit an exclusively mesangial pattern of deposits with accompanying mesangial cell proliferation. This pattern is usually seen early in the disease and is associated with a favorable prognosis, but it can also be seen in resolving stages of PSGN (83). Thirty-five percent of patients exhibit a "garland" pattern of deposits, in which large granular deposits are seen primarily on peripheral capillary walls with relatively few mesangial deposits. This pattern is more common in male patients and is asso-

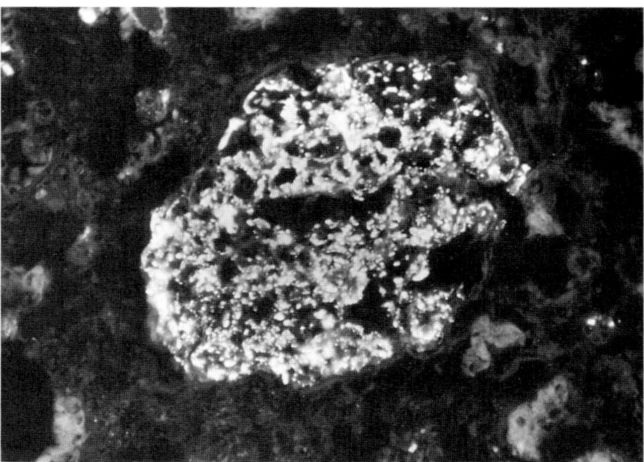

FIG. 3. Immunofluorescent staining for C3 in the glomerulus of a patient with PSGN. Staining for C3 is more intense and more uniform than staining for IgG and may be seen in the absence of IgG, particularly during resolution of disease (see text). Original magnification ×250. (Photomicrograph provided by Dr. Charles Alpers.)

ciated with a greater degree of proteinuria and a less favorable long-term prognosis (14,84). The composition of immune deposits in PSGN is also variable. Usually IgG and C3 are seen, but C3 may be seen in the absence of IgG (28,29). C1q and C4 are generally absent, suggesting complement activation via the alternative rather than the classic pathway, as occurs also in membranoproliferative glomerulonephritis (MPGN) type I (see Chapter 51). Although most deposits resolve within 6 weeks, mesangial immune deposits may persist for months or even years associated with some residual mesangial hypercellularity. When vasculitis is present, immunoglobulin deposits may be seen in vessel walls as well (77–79).

The immune deposits in PSGN are presumed to represent glomerular trapping of preformed immune complexes that contain some nephritogenic streptococcal antigen (see above). Variations in pattern of deposits presumably reflect variations in complex size, charge, and solubility, in turn reflecting different ratios of antigen to antibody and variations in antibody avidity (see Chapter 14).

Electron Microscopy

Post-streptococcal glomerulonephritis is characterized by the unique appearance of multiple large, discrete, dome-shaped deposits that project from the outer surface of the basement membrane beneath effaced epithelial cell foot processes ("humps") (13,28,29,69,85) (Fig. 4). Humps are present early and usually resolve within 6 to 8 weeks (86,87). The GBM is generally normal except for areas of rarefaction beneath the humps. Although the humps are the most striking ultrastructural finding, mesangial and subendothelial immune complex deposits are also often seen in association with "starry sky" and mesangial patterns of immunofluorescence (28,29). Because formation of subepithelial immune complex deposits is not generally associated with an inflammatory reaction (see Chapters 14 and 47), these subepithelial and mesangial deposits are likely important mediators of the cellular reactions seen in PSGN. In other respects, electron microscopy confirms findings by light microscopy of capillary obliteration by infiltrating and proliferating cells.

Clinical Manifestations

Although PSGN is more common in children with a mean age of 6 to 7 years, it has been reported in adults as well (9,28,29,88,89). However, it is rare in children less than 3 years of age and in adults over 50 (9,29). Males

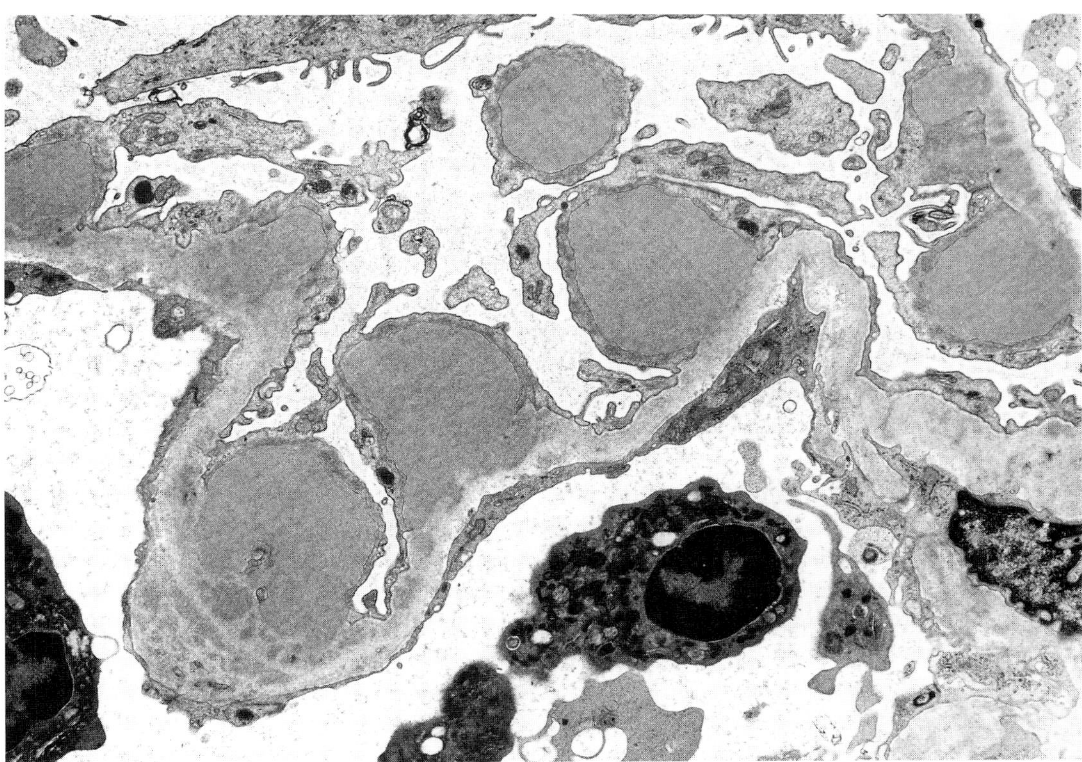

FIG. 4. Electron micrograph of a single glomerular capillary wall in the biopsy specimen of a patient with PSGN. Several large, electron-dense humps, characteristic of PSGN, are present on the subepithelial surface of the capillary wall. A portion of a neutrophil *(dark intraluminal cell)* is also seen. Original magnification ×7700. (Photomicrograph provided by Dr. Charles Alpers.)

are affected about twice as commonly as females (9,28,29). Although some proteinuria and microscopic hematuria may accompany the acute streptococcal infection (24), this usually resolves and is followed by a characteristic "latent period" between the time of infection and the abrupt onset of nephritis. The latent period in PSGN averages about 10 days (range, 6–21) with pharyngitis and 3 weeks with pyoderma (90). Streptococcal infection may also exacerbate another underlying glomerular disease, usually IgA nephropathy, to produce signs of GN in the absence of a latent period (synpharyngitic nephritis) (9,24).

The clinical presentation is usually one of abrupt onset of acute nephritic syndrome, although many asymptomatic cases with mild renal involvement are known to occur (9,29,69,70). A decline in urine output with dark or smoky urine reflecting gross hematuria occurs in about 70% of patients. About 80% of cases display edema and hypertension (9,24,84,70,91). Often edema is more pronounced in the upper body (periorbital region, eyelids, and hands) and worse in the early morning. Hypertension is usually volume-dependent, not severe, and present only during the phase of sodium and fluid retention that may be associated with symptoms of volume overload, including dyspnea, cough, elevated venous pressure, and sometimes frank congestive heart failure (28,29). Circulatory problems are particularly prominent in young children and older adults (9,88,89). In children, additional extrarenal symptomatology may be prominent, including encephalopathy with headaches, confusion, and even seizures (9,69,70). Loin and abdominal pain may be present acutely (9,69,70).

Several laboratory features characterize PSGN and are useful in making a diagnosis. Often urinalysis reveals concentrated urine with low sodium and fractional excretion of sodium (29,91), along with proteinuria, hematuria, and red blood cell casts (9,28,29,91). White cells may predominate in the sediment, particularly in the first few days. Proteinuria is usually not in the nephrotic range, with 50% of patients excreting less than 500 mg/day, but in up to 20% of patients nephrotic syndrome develops during the recovery phase of the disease (69,70, 91). Red cells are generally dysmorphic.

Glomerular filtration rate (GFR) is impaired but usually is greater than 50% of normal, and serum creatinine and blood urea nitrogen levels may not rise out of the normal range (9,28,29). The degree of salt and water retention is not related to the decrease in GFR. In fewer than 5% of patients, acute renal failure develops with a picture of RPGN (see Chapter 49) (75,92,93).

Throat and skin cultures are positive for group A streptococci in only a minority of patients, particularly if antibiotic therapy has already been administered (17,18, 21–29). However, recent infection with streptococci can usually be documented by serologic measurements of antibodies to several different streptococcal antigens. These include anti-streptolysin O (ASO); anti-streptokinase (ASKase); antihyaluronidase (AHase); anti-deoxyribonuclease B (ADNase B); and anti-nicotyladenine dinucleotidase (AN-ADase) (29). Most patients with pharyngitis have an elevated ASO titer in 3 to 5 weeks that persists for several months, but the rise in ASO titer is blunted by antibiotics and may not occur with skin infections. ADNase B and AHase titers are more useful (24,28,29). The Streptozyme test increases sensitivities by combining four different antigens (ASO, ADNase B, AN-ADase, AHase) in a single assay (28,94). However, anti-streptococcal antibody levels do not predict nephritogenicity, do not correlate with disease severity, and may be falsely positive with elevated cholesterol levels and some paraproteins (28,95). Circulating cryoglobulins, rheumatoid factors, and immune complexes are also detectable in most patients early in the disease but are probably not involved in causing nephritis (28,29), although rheumatoid factor has been eluted from glomeruli in PSGN (39). Another useful laboratory test in PSGN is measurement of complement levels. Total serum hemolytic complement (CH_{50}) and C3 levels are reduced in more than 90% of patients for 4 to 6 weeks (28,96–102). Levels of early classic complement pathway components (C1q, C2, and C4) are usually normal or minimally depressed (99–101) and properdin is decreased (99), suggesting predominantly alternate complement pathway activation, which may be induced by nephritogenic antigens directly rather than by immune complexes (see above). Persistent hypocomplementemia should suggest alternative diagnoses, such as MPGN (Chapter 51), endocarditis (see below), and systemic lupus erythematosus (Chapter 48).

Two variants of the typical clinical features of PSGN have been described with sufficient frequency to warrant mention. Several patients with typical PSGN have been reported with histologically documented vasculitis in the arcuate and interlobular arteries of the kidney and sometimes at extrarenal sites as well (77–79). Often these patients have had severe disease with renal failure, hypertension, nephrotic syndrome, and sometimes gastrointestinal or pulmonary manifestations (77–79). However, most have fully recovered with or without steroid therapy. In another group of patients, about 1–2% in most series, a typical RPGN develops with extensive crescents and often acute renal failure (75,92,93). About half of these patients have also recovered normal renal function spontaneously, although a period of dialytic support may be required (92,93,103–105).

Course and Prognosis

More than 95% of patients with acute PSGN recover normal renal function within a period of 3 to 6 weeks (28, 29,69,70). Complement levels usually normalize within 6 weeks (96,99,102). Gross hematuria lasts for 1 to 2 weeks, but microscopic hematuria may persist for a year and proteinuria is sometimes present for up to 2 years (24,78,79,106,107). In general, the disease is less severe in children than in adults (9,28,29) and in patients with epidemic as opposed to sporadic forms of the disease. Acute anuric renal failure requiring dialysis occurs in fewer than 5% of patients in most series (75,92,93,103–105) and may persist for up to a month with full recovery of renal function (92).

Because of the previous frequency of the disease, many studies have addressed the question of long-term prognosis. With complete recovery from the initial episode, long-term prognosis is excellent (24,28,29,106,107–118). Studies of long-term prognosis in patients with epidemic PSGN have revealed few sequelae (116–119). A careful study of 534 patients 11 to 17 years after an epidemic PSGN in Trinidad revealed abnormalities in urinalysis in 3.5%, elevated creatinine in 2.5%, and death from chronic renal failure in 0.3%, but similar figures for a control population are unknown (115). In contrast, other studies containing more endemic cases and a larger percentage of adults by Baldwin and associates (107,116) in New York have suggested that up to 50% of patients may have persistent proteinuria, hypertension, and reduced renal function. However, there is no documentation that a significant number of patients with these abnormalities progress to end-stage renal disease. In the rare elderly patient with PSGN, the prognosis is generally poor (88,89). The presence of persistent proteinuria suggests a worse long-term prognosis (106–108). However, in those patients with acute PSGN who exhibit complete clinical healing with normal GFR and less than 500 mg of protein per day in the urine, the likelihood of later development of progressive renal disease leading to renal failure is very small (119). Because exposure to a nephritogenic subtype of *Streptococcus* confers lifelong immunity, recurrences or second episodes of PSGN are possible but extremely rare (120,121,149,150).

Differential Diagnosis

The differential diagnosis of acute PSGN includes all the other entities that can cause acute GN, including IgA nephropathy, RPGN, vasculitis, systemic lupus erythematosus, and occasionally MPGN. Because other bacteria can induce a similar clinical syndrome, documentation that the lesion is a consequence of streptococcal infection can be established only by bacteriologic and serologic studies. Differentiation from acute IgA nephropathy is usually suggested by the latent period of 10 days to 3 weeks that is not present in IgA nephropathy and confirmed by serologic studies demonstrating antibodies to streptococcal antigens and hypocomplementemia. Because most patients with PSGN have prominent hypocomplementemia, the two entities that most commonly mimic the disease are acute lupus nephritis (see Chapter 48) and MPGN type I (see this chapter and Chapter 51). In addition to the multiorgan involvement and increased antinuclear antibody levels seen in systemic lupus erythematosus, the complement profile is different from that of PSGN, with most patients exhibiting classic pathway activation and depressed levels of C1q and C4, which are usually normal in PSGN (99,100). Type I MPGN may look very similar clinically to PSGN, and in some cases it may actually follow a streptococcal infection (see Chapter 51) (120–122). Membranoproliferative glomerulonephritis is suggested by the presence of nephrotic syndrome or hypocomplementemia that persists beyond 6 weeks.

There is probably no clinical indication for a renal biopsy in classic cases of PSGN with mild renal impairment and typical clinical and serologic findings. However, if renal failure is severe or if the disease does not largely resolve within 6 weeks, a biopsy is indicated to confirm the diagnosis and exclude RPGN or MPGN.

Treatment

There is no evidence that disease-specific therapy is useful in PSGN, and treatment is largely symptomatic. Early antibiotic therapy does not prevent subsequent PSGN as it does acute rheumatic fever, but it may reduce the severity of disease (28,123). For patients with volume expansion and circulatory overload, restrictions of fluid and sodium along with aggressive diuretic therapy are indicated. Potassium-sparing diuretics should be avoided because of the tendency to hyperkalemia (124). Hypertension is usually associated with sodium retention and low renin levels, and if antihypertensive therapy is required, vasodilators are more likely to be effective. In patients with severe renal failure, dialysis may be required. In patients with a severe crescentic GN, treatment with pulse steroids, immunosuppressive agents, or both (see Chapter 49) should be considered (125). However, there are no data to establish the safety or efficacy of such treatment, and spontaneous recovery is quite common.

Infective Endocarditis

Glomerulonephritis secondary to endocarditis has diminished considerably in frequency as rheumatic heart disease has become rare and antibiotic therapy has improved. The most commonly affected valves are now prosthetic ones. However, the increased prevalence of intravenous drug abuse has resulted in some increase in cases reported. About 20% of patients with infective endocarditis have GN (126). *Staphylococcus aureus* is the most common organism, particularly in cases of acute endocarditis and right-sided endocarditis (126). However, a variety of other gram-positive as well as gram-negative organisms can cause a similar lesion (127–131) (Table 1). *Streptococcus viridans* is a common pathogen in patients with subacute or chronic endocarditis. Symptoms of endocarditis usually precede signs of GN. Proteinuria and hematuria, which may be gross, are usual, and nephrotic syndrome is seen or develops in 25% of patients (132). Significant elevations in blood urea nitrogen and creatinine are uncommon unless other nephrotoxic insults have occurred (9,126,132), but RPGN with crescents has been described (126,133). Serologic studies commonly reveal cryoglobulins, rheumatoid factor, and low complement levels with classic pathway activation (126,134). Renal biopsy may reveal focal embolic lesions caused by embolized valvular vegetations (135–137), but the more common lesion is a focal or diffuse proliferative GN with granular deposits of IgG, IgM, and C3 in the mesangium and on both sides of the capillary walls (137–139). Fibrin deposits and focal necrosis are also common. In some cases bacterial antigens have been localized in deposits (140) and antibody to antigens derived from the infecting organisms has been found in the circulation, suggesting an immune complex formation or trapping mechanism as a cause of the glomerular disease (128, 137,140). Treatment consists of appropriate antibiotic therapy of the endocarditis, and the renal lesion gradually resolves with normalization of serologic studies within a few weeks (126). There is no established role for steroid or immunosuppressive therapy in such patients.

Shunt Nephritis

A postinfectious GN occurs in about 4% of children with infected ventriculoatrial shunts for hydrocephalus, but it is much less common with the newer ventriculoperitoneal shunts (141–145). The most common organism is *Staphylococcus albus*, which accounts for 75% of cases, but a wide variety of other organisms has been reported. Usually, the shunt has been in place for several years, but occasionally the lesion develops within weeks (145). Although fever and leukocytosis are common, culturing the organism from blood or spinal fluid is often difficult, and direct culture of the shunt itself may be required. In children, lethargy, weight loss, anorexia, and arthralgias are often seen along with hepatosplenomegaly (145). The usual renal manifestations are hematuria and proteinuria, with nephrotic syndrome developing in about 30% of cases (141–145). As in other postinfectious forms of GN, cryoglobulins, rheumatoid factor, elevated circulating immune complexes, and low complement levels are generally seen (143–147). The glomerular lesion usually resembles type 1 MPGN (see Chapter 51), with a mesangial proliferative lesion, lobulation, and mesangial and subendothelial immune complex deposits that generally contain IgG, IgM, and C3 (144,145). Bacterial antigens may also be present, suggesting an immune complex pathogenesis (143). Therapy requires appropriate antibiotics, but shunt removal is generally required as well (9,28). Complete recovery occurs in about 50% of patients but may require months or even years (132,143, 147). Another 50% will exhibit renal dysfunction, and progression to end-stage renal disease has occasionally been described (145).

Visceral Abscesses

A form of relatively severe postinfectious nephritis has been reported in patients with pulmonary, hepatic, and retroperitoneal abscesses in the absence of positive blood cultures (90,148). The renal lesion may be quite severe, with oliguria and renal failure, but glomerular immune deposits may be scant or absent, complement levels may be normal, and rheumatoid factor is usually negative (148); this is in contrast to what occurs in other forms of postinfectious nephritis. Cryoglobulins are often present and may correlate with disease activity (132). Renal biopsy demonstrates focal segmental proliferation or mesangioproliferative GN, often with C3 deposition revealed by immunofluorescence (90,132,148). The pathogenesis of this lesion is unclear, but it may not involve glomerular immune complex formation. Treatment requires drainage or resection of the abscess, and renal failure may develop if this is unsuccessful.

VIRUS-ASSOCIATED VASCULITIS AND GLOMERULONEPHRITIS

Viral infections may also be associated with GN or vasculitis, particularly if the infection is chronic and associated with persistent viremia or antigenemia. Because most viral infections are eliminated by cell-mediated immunity as opposed to humoral mechanisms, it is not uncommon for chronic viremias to persist despite a strong antibody response, thus setting up the host for chronic immune complex disease. The histolopathologic lesion is usually a proliferative or membranoproliferative glomerulonephritis (MPGN), but membranous nephropathy (MN) has also been reported. It has been postulated that the earlier lesions of virus-associated GN are more likely to show a proliferative histology (possibly with vasculitis), whereas the later lesions are more likely to resemble MPGN (151).

In animals, immune complex GN has been reported with a variety of viral infections, including Aleutian mink disease, hog cholera, and lymphocytic choriomeningitis in mice (reviewed in [152]). Persistent viremia, circulating immune complexes, systemic complement activation, and the localization of viral antigens in the glomerular immune deposits have been documented in these animals (152). In humans, the viral infections most commonly associated with GN include HIV (discussed in Chapter 54), hepatitis B virus (HBV), and hepatitis C virus (HCV). A discussion of the major renal syndromes associated with the latter two viruses follows.

Hepatitis B Virus-Associated Glomerulonephritis

Definition and Historical Perspective

Hepatitis B virus was discovered by Blumberg and associates (153) while screening sera for allo-antigens. The Australia antigen, which is now known to be the hepatitis B surface antigen (HBsAg), was found in the serum of an Australian aborigine and also in patients with leukemia, suggesting to Blumberg that he might have found a marker of leukemia (153). However, it was not until one of the workers in Blumberg's laboratory contracted acute hepatitis after working with the infected sera that it was realized that the Australia antigen represented the long-sought-after marker for "serum" hepatitis, also known as *hepatitis B*.

It soon became apparent that HBV was a major cause of acute hepatitis, chronic active hepatitis, cirrhosis, and even hepatocellular carcinoma. The appreciation that there were extrahepatic manifestations was a little more delayed. However, reports of an association of chronic HBV infection were reported in 1970 for polyarteritis nodosa (PAN) (154,155), in 1971 for MN (156), in 1973 for MPGN (157), in 1977 for cryoglobulinemia (158, 159), and in 1971 for acute HBV infection with a serum sickness-like syndrome (160,161).

Hepatitis B Virus-Associated Polyarteritis Nodosa

(See also Chapter 49.)

Epidemiology

Almost all patients with HBV-associated vasculitis have chronic infection with circulating HBsAg (162). Interestingly, reported cases of HBV-associated PAN are almost always in adults and also in areas of the world where the overall carrier rate in the general population is low (reviewed in [163]). Thus, HBV-PAN has been reported in Europe and the United States, where infection is usually acquired in adulthood by a parenteral route (162). In contrast, HBV-associated PAN has only rarely been reported in children (164). HBV-PAN is also uncommon in regions such as Asia, where infection frequently occurs at birth or during childhood (163).

The percentage of cases of PAN associated with HBV infection also varies depending on the location (165–176) (Table 2). Variations may relate to the underlying prevalence of intravenous drug abuse and the HBV carrier rate at the various centers. Thus, in New York up to 40% of PAN is associated with HBV infection, whereas in less endemic areas of the United States the prevalence of HBV infection in patients with PAN is lower (Table 2).

TABLE 2. *Prevalence of the HBV carrier state in polyarteritis nodosa*

Country	Rate (%)	Reference	Year
United States			
New York	6/16 (38%)	(165)	1971
Ann Arbor	1/16 (6%)	(166)	1975
Ann Arbor	4/17 (24%)	(167)	1987
Rochester (Mayo Clinic)	3/27 (11%)	(168)	1980
Bethesda (NIH)	6/17 (35%)	(169)	1979
Detroit	4/11 (36%)	(154)	1970
England			
Bristol	2/25 (8%)	(170)	1982
London	4/17 (24%)	(171)	1979
Ireland (Dublin)	0/9 (0%)	(172)	1987
France			
Paris	3/17 (18%)	(173)	1983
Lyons	30/55 (54%)	(174)	1974
Paris	21/27 (84%)[a]	(175)	1991
Switzerland	3/10 (30%)	(176)	1986

[a]This study used a more sensitive test for detecting HBsAg (a radioimmunoassay using a monoclonal antibody).

Pathogenesis and Pathophysiology

Most evidence suggests that the HBV vasculitis and serum sickness syndromes result from passive deposition of circulating immune complexes containing HBV antigens in the vasculature and synovia, followed by complement activation and leukocyte infiltration (163). Circulating immune complexes containing HBsAg and anti-HBs have been detected in most patients with HBV serum sickness (177,178) and PAN (174,179,180), and their presence correlates with disease activity (181). Systemic complement activation with depressed C3, C4, and total hemolytic complement levels has been observed in HBV-PAN and serum sickness (160–162). HBsAg, IgG, IgM, and C3 have been identified by immunofluorescence and HBV particles by electron microscopy in blood vessels and glomeruli of patients with vasculitis (165,179,182, 183). Of the various HBV antigens, HBsAg is the most common antigen localized to the lesions (165,179,182, 183). The observation that IgM is more commonly identified in lesions than IgG (154,165,182,183), coupled with the observation that HBV-PAN frequently occurs during the early convalescence phase of acute hepatitis (180, 184–186), suggests that IgM rather than IgG immune complexes may be principally involved. Although IgM immune complexes have generally not been thought to be involved in experimental models of serum sickness or

GN, a precedent for IgM in mediating vascular disease has been shown in Kawasaki disease, in which an IgM auto-antibody is directed against an induced endothelial cell antigen (187). Finally, in the event that HBsAg is cleared from the circulation, either spontaneously (174) or with interferon-α (188), remission of the vasculitis occurs.

It has been suggested that the presence of HBsAg in vessels and glomeruli may simply reflect secondary trapping of immune reactants in injured tissue. The demonstration of HBsAg in glomeruli and capillaries in renal infarcts (189) or focally sclerosed glomeruli (190) would support this concept. However, in some studies HBsAg has been identified only in areas of acute injury as opposed to scar, and the HBsAg is elutable only in the presence of antibody-antigen– dissociating buffers (182). Others have reported that proteins such as albumin or α_2-macroglobulin do not co-localize with HBsAg, further arguing against a nonspecific trapping mechanism (191).

Alternative pathogenic mechanisms have been proposed. Polyarteritis nodosa associated with HBV could result from local immune complex formation, such as initial planting of HBsAg followed by anti-HBs, similar to what has been described in experimental models of glomerular disease (192). The observation that HBV antigens and antibodies are not always present in the vascular lesions may represent rapid clearance and degradation of immune complexes at these sites (193), but would also be consistent with a cell-mediated response. A cellular immune response can be induced in the vessels of mice that have been sensitized to vascular smooth muscle (194). Chronic HBV liver disease may also be associated with the development of auto-antibodies, including anti-neutrophil cytoplasmic antibodies (ANCAs) (195). Theoretically, an auto-antibody against a vessel wall antigen could be present, such as has been shown in Kawasaki disease, or an ANCA-related mechanism could be present. However, ANCAs are uncommon in patients with HBV-associated vasculitis, and currently the favored pathogenic mechanism is the deposition of HBsAg-containing immune complexes.

Pathology

The pathology in HBV-PAN consists of a focal vasculitis involving the small and medium-sized arteries, particularly at bifurcation sites. The lesions are classically panmural, at different stages, and characterized by varying degrees of fibrinoid necrosis with leukocyte infiltration, fibrin deposition, and occasional aneurysm formation (163). Rarely, involvement of the post-capillary venules occurs, in which case the symptoms may include palpable purpura and a lesion suggestive of cryoglobulinemia or Henoch-Schönlein purpura (180).

The renal pathology usually involves the small and medium-sized arteries, often with sparing of the glomeruli ("classic PAN"). In this situation, glomeruli display primarily signs of ischemia, such as wrinkling of the GBM (189). Glomerulonephritis may also accompany HBV-PAN, and diffuse proliferative GN, MPGN, MN, and mesangial proliferative GN have been reported (162, 182). Interestingly, "microscopic PAN," characterized by segmental necrosis of glomerular capillary loops, often with crescent formation, is only rarely seen with HBV-PAN (182).

The liver pathology in patients with HBV-PAN usually shows a chronic active hepatitis or chronic persistent hepatitis (162,196), and occasionally acute hepatitis (162). A normal liver histology is distinctly unusual.

Clinical Manifestations and Laboratory Findings

Polyarteritis nodosa associated with HBV occurs almost exclusively in adults, although rare cases have been reported in children (164). Most commonly, HBV-PAN develops within weeks to months after a clinically mild episode of acute, anicteric hepatitis (184–186,196). Rarely, HBV-PAN may precede the clinical onset of hepatitis, and occasionally HBV-PAN develops in patients with chronic hepatitis (196).

The clinical manifestations of HBV-PAN vary greatly depending on the site of involvement. Often, patients have fever, arthralgias, and purpura, suggestive of a serum sickness-like syndrome. However, unlike the HBV serum sickness-like syndrome, which tends to resolve spontaneously, HBV-PAN progresses (171,196). The vasculitis can affect any organ; it may cause mesenteric ischemia with abdominal pain and occasionally perforation, myocardial ischemia subsequent to coronary involvement, mononeuritis multiplex secondary to vasculitis of the vasa nervorum, and cerebrovascular accidents subsequent to involvement of the cerebral vessels (168, 171,196). Renal involvement is also common and may be associated with renin-dependent hypertension, non-nephrotic or nephrotic proteinuria, microhematuria, and occasionally renal failure (168,171,196).

Liver enzymes (alanine and aspartate aminotransferase levels) are mildly elevated in the majority of patients (165,196). HBsAg and anti-HBc are almost always present in the circulation, and serum is negative for anti-HBs (165,181–183). Rare cases have been reported in which serum is positive for both HBsAg and anti-HBs (197). Complement levels (C3, C4, and CH_{50}) are depressed in only a minority (20%) of patients (165), and ANCA is usually absent. Circulating immune complexes (C1q-binding) are commonly detected (174,180).

Diagnosis of HBV-PAN can be made by skeletal muscle, peripheral nerve, kidney, or even testicular biopsy (170). Angiography may also be useful to look for saccular or fusiform aneurysms or abnormal narrowing of the blood vessels (198). The presence of aneurysms has been correlated with clinically severe disease (167). Angiography of the renal or celiac arteries usually provides the highest diagnostic yield (167).

Differential Diagnosis

Polyarteritis nodosa associated with HBV may mimic other types of vasculitis, including idiopathic PAN, Wegener's granulomatosis, mixed cryoglobulinemia, Henoch-Schönlein purpura, and small-vessel (leukocytoclastic) vasculitis. Unlike HBV-associated PAN, idiopathic PAN is less commonly associated with elevated liver enzymes and more commonly associated with serous otitis (196,199). In addition, although HBV infection is the most common viral infection associated with PAN, PAN (and mixed cryoglobulinemia) have also been reported with HCV infection (200) and HIV infection (201). Polyarteritis nodosa can also develop in humans (202) or animals (203,204) that have been repeatedly injected with foreign proteins, such as horse serum.

Treatment

Treatment of both idiopathic PAN and HBV-PAN has usually consisted of steroids, cytotoxic agents, or both (165,168,184). Although most studies have been uncontrolled, general mortality rates at 5 years have improved from 12% in untreated cases to 50% with steroids and 80% with steroids and cytotoxic agents (169,170,205, 206). A common regimen is the National Institues of Health (NIH) protocol to treat Wegener's disease; it consists of prednisone (1 mg/kg/d) for 2 to 3 months with taper and oral cyclophosphamide (2 mg/kg/d) for 6 to 12 months. Cyclophosphamide is renally excreted, and the dosage should be adjusted for the degree of renal impairment. Intravenous pulse cyclophosphamide has also been administered, but debate continues over whether it is as effective as oral cyclophosphamide in the vasculitis syndromes (207,208). Plasmapheresis has also been used in anecdotal reports (209).

The treatment of aggressive vasculitis usually requires immunosuppressive therapy, but such treatment also impairs the ability of the patient to eliminate the HBV virus. Normally, the HBV virus is eliminated by a cell-mediated response in which cytotoxic T cells and natural killer cells kill infected hepatocytes that express hepatitis B core antigen (HBcAg) on their cell surface (210,211). Indeed, the development of the chronic carrier state is the consequence of a defective cell-mediated response (211–213), and explains why the carrier state is common in disorders such as Down syndrome, uremia, and chronic lymphocytic leukemia. In neonates, the high carrier rate may relate to a relatively insufficient production of interferon-γ (214), or to the maternal transfer of blocking anti-HBc antibodies (211).

Steroids and cytotoxic agents act to suppress cell-mediated immunity further and increase the degree of HBV viremia and the number of infected hepatocytes (215). Some patients who were originally positive for anti-HBs have had a re-emergence of HBsAg following immunosuppressive therapy (216,217). If the cell-mediated immunity is completely suppressed, the liver disease may be clinically silent despite viremia, and results of liver function tests may remain normal. However, cell-mediated immunity is usually only partially suppressed, and the enhanced HBV viral replication may lead to progressive liver disease, such as is frequently observed after organ transplantation (218,219). Furthermore, patients are also at risk following the sudden cessation of immunosuppressive therapy, not only for relapse of the vasculitis but also for sudden worsening of their liver disease (220,221).

Given these considerations, some groups are now initiating treatment with steroids and plasmapheresis, followed by the addition of antiviral agents such as interferon-α or adenosine arabinoside (188,222). Interferon-α has been previously shown to eliminate HBV viremia and convert hepatitis B e antigen (HBeAg) to anti-HBe in as many as 40–50% of patients with chronic hepatitis, although the percentage of patients who become negative for HBsAg is less (in the range of 20%) (223). In one study, prednisone (1 mg/kg/d) was administered for 2 weeks along with plasma exchange (9 to 12 sessions in 3 weeks) and adenosine arabinoside (222). Although 8 of 33 patients died, 76% remained alive at 7 years, with remission in the 36% that became positive for anti-HBe (222). Even more exciting has been the recent report describing a similar regimen with prednisone, plasma exchange, and interferon-α (188). All 6 patients survived and underwent remission, with the development of anti-HBe antibodies in 4 and anti-HBs antibodies in 3 (188).

Prognosis and Outcome

As discussed above, treatment of HBV-PAN has improved survival rates to 80% at 5 years, but the immunosuppressive therapy may have a deleterious consequence on the underlying liver disease. The addition of interferon-α either at the time of initiation of immunosuppresive therapy or shortly after may lead to better long-term survival rates. Unlike remission of idiopathic PAN, remission of HBV-PAN is often extended, and although relapse can occur, it is not inevitable (165). Transplantation is not considered a viable option in HBV-PAN unless the viremia (HBV DNA and HBeAg) clears subsequent to interferon-α therapy.

Membranous Nephropathy Secondary to Infection with Hepatitis B Virus

Association and Epidemiology

The strongest association of chronic HBV infection with GN is with membranous nephropathy (HBV-MN). Idiopathic MN is discussed in Chapter 47. This section discusses only MN associated with HBV. HBV-MN most commonly occurs in children, especially in areas of the world where the endemic carrier rate is high (reviewed in [163]). In these areas, the chronic carrier rate is high because of vertical transmission from mothers to children at the time of birth (224), or horizontal transmission from infected siblings or other children (225). In the United States, HBV-MN appears to be more common in black children (226). HBV-MN can also occur in adults, and the prevalence, although lower, generally mirrors the underlying prevalence of the carrier rate in the general population (163). In adults, the mode of HBV infection is often unknown, although cases have been reported in patients with a history of intravenous drug abuse, blood transfusion, homosexuality, and AIDS (reviewed in [163]).

Other types of GN have also been reported with HBV infection. The most common nephritis associated with chronic HBV infection after HBV-MN is membranoproliferative glomerulonephritis (HBV-MPGN) (157, 227). Cryoglobulinemic MPGN secondary to HBV has also been observed, in which circulating cryoglobulins have been shown to be concentrated with the HBV virus and anti-HBV antibodies (158,159). Less commonly, IgA nephropathy, diffuse proliferative nephritis, and even minimal-change disease have been reported to be associated with HBsAg antigenemia (227,228). The significance of these latter associations has been challenged (229).

Pathogenesis and Pathophysiology

Most evidence suggests that HBV-MN results from the deposition or formation of immune complex deposits containing HBeAg and anti-HBe antibodies in the subepithelial space (230). First, HBeAg is the most commonly detected viral antigen in the immune deposits, although HBsAg and HBcAg have also been identified in the glomerular capillary wall in some cases (231–236). HBeAg and anti-HBe antibody have also been eluted from renal biopsy specimens (237,238). Second, circulating HBeAg is often present in these patients and correlates with disease activity (234). Clearance of HBeAg with the appearance of anti-HBe antibodies often correlates with remission of the disease, even in the presence of continued HBsAg antigenemia (234). When biopsy specimens from patients with HBV-MN are negative for HBeAg, it usually is late in the disease, when the active immunologic mechanisms that initiated the disease may no longer be operative (234).

The mechanism by which immune complexes containing HBeAg localize to the subepithelial space is uncertain. The general mechanisms of subepithelial immune deposit formation are reviewed in more detail in Chapter 47. Most studies suggest that circulating immune complexes rarely if ever penetrate across the GBM to the subepithelial space, unless they are very small and cationic (239). HBeAg is small (3 to 9×10^4 D). Although HBeAg is anionic, anti-HBe antibodies are often cationic (pI, 5.8 to 10.2) (240), and when complexed with HBeAg they shift the isoelectric point to the range of 6.4 to 8.4. Circulating immune complexes containing HBeAg have also been identified in 40% of children with HBV-MN; they are relatively small (2.5×10^5 D) (230,241)) and correlate with disease activity (241). It is therefore possible that a circulating immune complex mechanism is operative.

A more likely mechanism would be the *in situ* formation of immune complexes in the subepithelial space. In experimental animals, it has been shown that immune complexes can be formed locally by the sequential localization of either a cationic antigen or antibody to the highly negatively charged sialoproteins present on the glomerular epithelial cell, followed by the respective antibody or antigen (192). This sequence would be particularly favored in situations in which the immune complexes are easily dissociable, as in an antigen excess state or when the immune complexes are of low avidity, and is consistent with observations in experimental models of MN and in cases of idiopathic MN and lupus MN in humans (242,243) (see also Chapter 13). HBV-MN is also associated with persistent antigenemia. Therefore, one might posit a mechanism involving the sequential localization of cationic anti-HBe antibody followed by HBeAg.

In contrast to HBV-MN, in HBV-MPGN the pathogenic antigen in the mesangial and subendothelial immune deposits appears to be HBsAg (157,227). Anti-HBs has been eluted from the renal tissue in a case of HBV-MPGN, and circulating immune complexes have been shown to contain HBsAg and anti-HBs antibodies (244). Infusion of HBsAg-containing plasma into baboons has also resulted in an MPGN-like lesion (245). Because the infusion of preformed immune complexes in experimental animals does result in their localization to the subendothelial and mesangial spaces (246), one does not need to infer an *in situ* mechanism in the pathogenesis of the disease. However, there is some evidence that HBV may also be able to infect glomerular cells (190,247,248), so that antigen expression on the mesangial surface could lead to the formation of immune complexes locally. Hepatitis B virus has been shown to infect other cells besides hepatocytes, including pancreatic acinar cells and monocytes (247,249,250). HBcAg has been localized in mesangial cell nuclei in two patients with HBV infection and IgA nephropathy (248). In one patient with HBV-MPGN, whole HBV virions were noted by immunoelectron microscopy and appeared to be budding from the mesangial cell membrane (190). Hepatitis B viral DNA has also been identified in glomeruli of patients with HBV-associated GN, although the most frequent site in which HBV DNA is localized are the tubular epithelial cells (251). However, these two findings may reflect the infiltration of infected monocytes into glomeruli and the uptake of HBV particles that have escaped into the urine as a consequence of proteinuria, respectively.

Finally, it is possible that in some cases of HBV-GN the pathogenesis may relate to the induction of auto-antibodies as a consequence of chronic liver disease. Liver disease of diverse etiologies is often accompanied by immune complex deposition in glomeruli (252,253). Some authors have argued that the presence of HBV antigens may simply reflect passive trapping of antigens in damaged tissue, or that the detection system to identify the antigens may be faulty as a consequence of not controlling for the presence of rheumatoid factors or of cross-reactivity with the secondary detecting antibodies (254). In addition, auto-antibodies are not uncommon in patients with chronic HBV hepatitis; these include antinuclear, anti-neutrophil cytoplasmic, and even anti-rat renal tubular brush border antibodies (255,256). The possibility of the generation of auto-antibodies to glomerular antigens remains to be excluded. However, most evidence still favors a mechanism involving HBeAg and HBsAg immune complexes in HBV-MN and HBV-MPGN, respectively.

Pathology

Histologically, HBV-MN is similar to classic idiopathic MN, with thickening of the GBM and the presence of subepithelial spikes by silver methenamine staining (see Chapter 47). Occasionally, mild mesangial hypercellularity is superimposed. Interstitial fibrosis is usually not prominent. Immunofluorescence shows positive capillary wall staining for IgG (100%), C3 (75%), IgM (50%), and IgA (10%) (234,257). HBeAg can also be frequently detected in a distribution similar to that of the IgG and C3 (257,258). By electron microscopy, immune deposits are mainly in the subepithelial space, but unlike the deposits of idiopathic MN they may also be observed to a lesser degree in the mesangium or subendothelial areas (230–235). Immunoelectron microscopy has documented HBeAg and the membrane attack complex of complement in the immune deposits (259). Occasional biopsy specimens also have viruslike particles noted by electron microscopy in mesangial, subendothelial, and subepithelial areas, or even within glomerular endothelial and mesangial cells (260). In many of these studies, the morphology and size of the viral particles are not consistent with the 22- or 42-nm HBV particles, but in at least one study the 42-nm HBV virion could be identified by immunoelectron microscopy within mesangial lysosomes and along the subendothelial and subepithelial aspect of the GBM (261).

In HBV-MPGN, the histologic lesion shows mesangial hypercellularity with lobulation of the glomerular tuft and occasional splitting and "tram tracking" of the GBM (157,262). Immunofluorescence usually shows capillary wall deposition of IgG, IgM, and C3. Electron microscopy usually reveals immune deposits in the subendothelial space, but occasionally small subepithelial and mesangial deposits may also be present, consistent with an MPGN type III lesion (227,262). HBsAg is often localized to the mesangium and capillary wall, and in cases with an MPGN type III pattern, HBeAg may also be detected (263,264).

Clinical Manifestations and Laboratory Findings

Children with HBV-MN usually present with nephrotic syndrome or non-nephrotic proteinuria, microhematuria, and normal or minimally depressed renal function (265). Classically, symptoms appear in children between the ages of 2 and 12 (mean, 6 years) and show a male predominance (230–235). Clinically, liver disease is often silent, but elevated aminotransferase levels are common. Liver biopsy most commonly shows a chronic persistent hepatitis; however, normal histology, chronic active hepatitis, and cirrhosis have all been reported (230–235).

The clinical presentation of adults with HBV-MN is very similar to that of childhood HBV-MN, except that hypertension and renal dysfunction are slightly more common (as is observed in adult idiopathic MN) (232). In addition, adults with HBV-MN are more likely than children to have a history of viral hepatitis several years before the onset of renal disease, and also to have more severe liver histology revealed by biopsy (usually chronic active hepatitis) (reviewed in [163]).

In almost all cases of HBV-MN, circulating HBsAg and anti-HBc are present (233,234). The majority (60–80%) are also positive for HBeAg, especially those with active disease (233,234). Anti-HBe antibodies are present in the remaining 20% of patients. Circulating immune complexes have also been reported in up to 80% of patients with HBV-MN (266). Serum complement levels (C3 and C4) are depressed in 20–50% of cases (231,267).

In HBV-associated MPGN, patients present with nephrotic syndrome and microhematuria, often with hypertension (30–60%) and mild to moderate renal insufficiency (10–30%) (262). As with HBV-MN, circulating HBsAg and anti-HBc are universally present in the early phases of the disease, but rare cases have been described in which clearance of HBsAg from the circulation may occur later despite continued presence of HBsAg deposits in the glomeruli (157).

As in HBV-MN, many patients have no clinical evidence of liver disease on examination nor a history of clinical hepatitis. However, results of liver function tests are mildly abnormal in the majority of cases, and if liver biopsy is performed, a chronic active hepatitis or cirrhosis is often diagnosed.

Differential Diagnosis

HBV-MN may clinically mimic primary or other secondary types of MN, including those caused by drugs (gold, penicillamine), heavy metals (mercury), autoimmune diseases (systemic lupus erythematosus, autoimmune lupoid hepatitis), cancer, or other infections (HCV, leprosy, syphilis). Unlike primary MN, HBV-MN is more likely to be associated with elevated liver enzymes, depressed serum complement, and immune deposits in the mesangium and subendothelial areas in addition to the classic subepithelial location (231).

In the setting of elevated liver enzymes, the major two additional diagnoses to consider would be HCV (diagnosed by testing for anti-HCV and HCV RNA) and autoimmune hepatitis (diagnosed by the presence of antinuclear antibodies, anti-smooth muscle cell antibodies, anti-liver kidney microsomal antibodies, or all of these) (210,268,269). HBV-MPGN may also present clinically as idiopathic MPGN or cryoglobulinemic MPGN. Although HBV is clearly a cause of mixed cryoglobulinemia and MPGN (158,159), most cases of mixed cryoglobulinemia are associated with HCV infection (see below). In addition, HCV infection may present as MPGN in the absence of detectable cryoglobulins (200).

The association of HBV infection with other types of GN has been reported, including IgA nephropathy (with or without coincident membranous changes), focal sclerosis, crescentic nephritis, lupus nephritis, and minimal-change disease (228,270–275). However, the strength and potential pathogenicity of these associations continue to be debated (228,229).

Treatment and Prognosis

HBV-MN has often been thought to have a good prognosis, with the majority of cases not progressing to renal failure. However, in one recent study as many as 20% of untreated adult patients with HBV-MN had progressive renal failure, and 10% required dialysis (232). Children with HBV-MN have a better prognosis, with the majority of cases undergoing spontaneous remission within 5 years (233,267,276). Remission is usually accompanied by clearance of HBeAg and the *de novo* appearance of anti-HBe antibodies in the blood, and less frequently with the clearance of HBsAg (234,277). However, remission does not always correlate with disappearance of HBeAg from the circulation (233). Spontaneous remissions are much less common for patients with HBV-MPGN, but they have been reported (278).

The use of steroids to treat HBV-associated GN does not appear to provide any benefit (265,279), and it may be deleterions due to the ability of immunosuppressive treatment to increase viral replication and potentiate liver disease (279). Indeed, transplantation is generally withheld for patients with chronic HBV infection, because immunosuppressive treatment often results in increasing viremia and progressive worsening of liver disease (218).

In those patients with symptomatic nephrotic syndrome or progressive renal insufficiency, treatment with interferon-α has been tried with limited success (232, 258,280–283). Treatment with interferon-α induces remission in the majority of adults and children with HBV-MN (282,283), although it is less effective if the adults are from endemic areas where they likely acquired the infection in childhood (232). Response is often associated with clearing of HBeAg and, less often, HBsAg from the blood (282,283). HBV-MPGN appears to respond less readily to interferon-α (282). We therefore recommend a trial of interferon-α for those patients who have symptomatic nephrotic syndrome or progressive disease. Other therapies, such as adenine arabinoside monophosphate with or without thymic extract, have also been tried and do appear to reduce proteinuria and suppress or eradicate viremia (284,285), but treatment with adenine arabinoside may be limited because of the occasional induction of painful neuropathies (286).

Glomerulonephritis Secondary to Hepatitis C Virus

Historical Perspective

The hepatitis C virus (HCV) was discovered in 1989 when Choo et al. (287) cloned and expressed an RNA virus from the blood of an infected chimpanzee. Hepatitis C virus is now recognized to be a major cause of sporadic and transfusion-associated non-A–non-B hepatitis, chronic active hepatitis, cirrhosis, and hepatocellular carcinoma (288). Infection with HCV is persistent in as many as 90% of cases (289) and is associated with a prominent humoral response (288), an ideal setting for the development of chronic immune complex-mediated diseases. In chronic HCV infection, circulating immune complexes containing HCV and anti-HCV antibodies are common (290), and hypocomplementemia, cryoglobulinemia, and circulating rheumatoid factors are present in 82% (291), 36–54% (292–294), and 70% (292) of patients, respectively. Whereas many of these patients are asymptomatic, others manifest various extrahepatic syndromes. The major associations are with mixed cryoglobulinemia (with or without nephritis) and MPGN (reviewed in 295–297). Other associations include MN, PAN, acute arthritis, porphyria cutanea tarda, lichen planus, Mooren's corneal ulcer, lymphoproliferative disorders, and a sicca-like syndrome resembling Sjögren's syndrome (reviewed in 295–297).

Definition

Patients with HCV-associated GN may present with renal disease as part of a general presentation of mixed cryoglobulinemia (298–302), or with nephrotic syndrome or nephritis without any other extrarenal symptoms (299). In both settings, the renal biopsy may be consistent with a diagnosis of either MPGN or acute proliferative GN (299,303,304) (see Chapter 51). In the majority of patients whose symptoms are suggestive of primary renal disease, cryoglobulinemia or circulating rheumatoid factors are present, suggesting that they may have an incomplete presentation of essential mixed cryoglobulinemia (EMC) (305,306). Silent cryoglobulinemia has also been observed in a third of patients with idiopathic MPGN type I in France (307). Some patients with HCV-MPGN may never have detectable cryoglobulinemia (299); because these patients clinically resemble other patients with cryoglobulinemic MPGN, we believe that the pathogenesis is still a consequence of circulating immune complexes but that the immune complexes in these cases either form cryoprecipitates below detectable limits or do not form cryoprecipitates at all (305).

Epidemiology

Hepatitis C viral infection is strongly associated with EMC (Table 3), particularly in patients with HCV infection of more than 10 years' duration and chronic active hepatitis or cirrhosis on liver biopsy (293,294,295,297). Both type II (monoclonal IgM and polyclonal IgG) EMC and type III (polyclonal IgM and IgG) EMC are associated with HCV infection. In patients with type II EMC, the monoclonal IgM is usually an IgM κ that is a rheumatoid factor of the WA cross-idiotype (308). As many as 30% of cases of EMC are not caused by HCV; in these patients underlying conditions include HBV infection (309,310), bacterial endocarditis, PSGN, and other autoimmune diseases, such as lupus and rheumatoid arthritis (311). Glomerular disease in dysproteinemias unrelated to HCV are reviewed in Chapter 52.

Hepatitis C viral infection remains a very common cause of cryoglobulinemic MPGN (295–297,303,312–314). It is also a common cause of adult MPGN in general, accounting for 10–20% of cases in the United States and up to 60% in northern Japan (298,315,316) (see also Chapter 52). In contrast, HCV infection does not appear to be a major cause of idiopathic MPGN type I in Hong Kong or France (317,318). Hepatitis C virus is not associated with childhood MPGN, which is discussed in detail in Chapter 52 (319).

Pathogenesis and Pathophysiology

The mechanism for the development of rheumatoid factors and cryoglobulinemia in HCV infection is unknown. Several mechanisms have been proposed. The finding that the WA idiotype is encoded by germ line genes (320) and that B-cell clones expressing WA acquire rheumatoid activity only following somatic diversification (321) suggest that the WA idiotype may initially represent an antibody response to a foreign antigen such as HCV (322). However, one study could not demonstrate any intrinsic binding activity of the IgM rheumatoid factors to several HCV antigens (298).

An alternative hypothesis is that chronic HCV infection may predispose to auto-antibody formation in general, either as a consequence of chronic liver disease or the ability of HCV to infect B lymphocytes (323). Auto-antibodies have been documented in chronic HCV infection,

TABLE 3. *Association of HCV infection with mixed cryoglobulinemia*

		Serum, % (rate)		Cryoprecipitate, % (rate)		
Year	Country	EIA-2	RNA	EIA-2	RNA	Reference
1991	France	70 (21/30)				(383)
1991	Italy	54 (28/52)				(384)
		91 (41/45)	86 (36/42)			(385)
1991	Italy	48 (14/29)				(386)
1992	USA	42 (8/19)	84 (16/19)	25 (1/4)	100 (4/4)	(308)
1992	Italy	80 (129/161)				(387)
1992	Switzerland	87 (13/15)	70 (5/7)			(388)
1992	Italy	98 (50/51)	81 (13/16)	41 (21/51)		(300)
1994	France	80 (12/15)	60 (9/15)	78 (11/14)	93 (14/15)	(389)
1994	France	52 (33/63)	63 (10/16)	75 (12/16)		(390)
	Total	73 (349/480)	77 (89/115)	53 (45/85)	95 (18/19)	

EIA-2, immunoassay enzyme; RNA, ribonucleic acid.

including antinuclear antibodies, anti-smooth muscle cell antibodies, anti-neutrophil cytoplasmic antibodies (P-ANCA), anti-GOR antibodies (directed against a nuclear antigen), and others (292,324–326). Ferri et al. (323,326) have suggested that HCV infection of B cells may lead to a dysregulated immune response with auto-antibody formation, as well as clonal expansion that may favor the development of non-Hodgkin's lymphomas. The observation that chronic liver disease of other etiologies may be associated with auto-antibodies (292,294,325) suggests that the liver injury itself may also contribute to the pathogenesis of the rheumatoid factor formation.

In some cases, the rheumatoid factor in HCV infection may not be a classic rheumatoid factor with Fc binding activity but rather may be an anti-idiotype antibody to anti-HCV IgG. Some evidence has been provided that the rheumatoid factor in patients with cryoglobulinemia has characteristics of an anti-idiotypic antibody (327). In one study, there was indirect evidence that the IgM rheumatoid factor had greater affinity for anti-HCV to the C22 antigen, as opposed to control IgG, in several patients (298). Further studies are needed to clarify which of these various mechanisms is responsible for the induction of rheumatoid factor activity in these patients.

HCV-MPGN is thought to result from the deposition of circulating immune complexes containing HCV antigens, anti-HCV IgG, and IgM rheumatoid factors in the subendothelial and mesangial regions of the glomerulus (295–297). Circulating immune complexes and cryoprecipitates can be shown to contain HCV RNA that is concentrated relative to serum (298,308). Anti-HCV IgG is also present in the cryoprecipitates, especially antibody to the core region (C22) of HCV (298,300). Hepatitis C viral antigens have also been localized in dermal vasculitic lesions (328). Most recently, the HCV C22 antigen and core antigen have been localized to the glomerular capillary wall in patients with HCV-MPGN (329,330). Whereas the circulating immune complexes in most patients contain anti-HCV IgG and IgM rheumatoid factors, in one patient with immune complex-mediated GN the IgM antibody was not a rheumatoid factor and was directed against the C22 antigen (331).

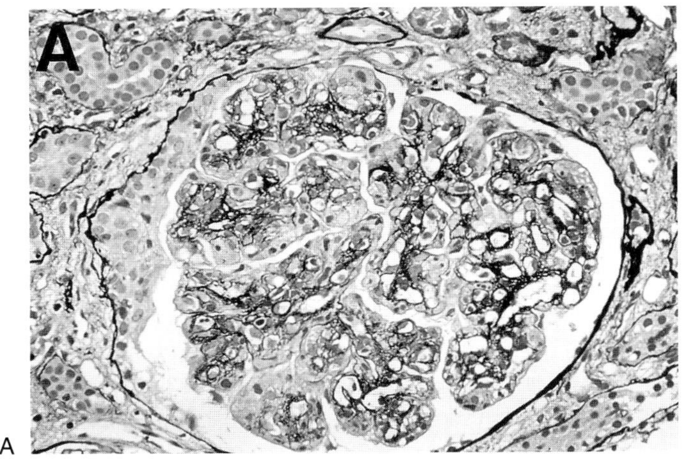

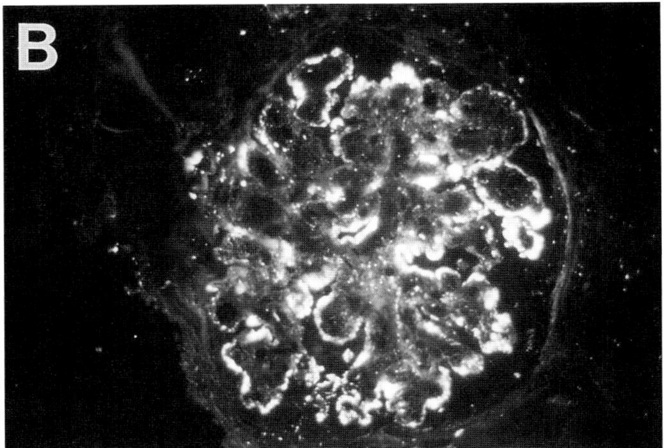

FIG. 5. Membranoproliferative GN caused by HCV. **A:** The glomerulus shows increased cellularity with expansion of the mesangial matrix and various degrees of thickening and splitting of peripheral capillary walls. PAS, ×250. **B:** Capillary wall deposits of IgM are indicated by immunofluorescence. ×250. **C:** Electron microscopy shows subendothelial immune deposits *(arrows)* that are fibrillar in structure and compatible with cryoglobulins. (Photomicrograph provided by Dr. Charles Alpers.)

The deposition of immune complexes is thought to result in complement activation and C5a-mediated accumulation of leukocytes (332). Monocytes and neutrophils, which are common in glomeruli in MPGN (333), then release oxidants and proteases (such as cathepsin D) that cause glomerular injury (334) (see discussion in Chapter 26 regarding neutrophil-mediated glomerular injury).

An experimental model of cryoglobulinemic GN has been induced in mice by injection of cryoprecipitates (335). Glomerulonephritis was induced in mice receiving cryoprecipitates from patients with cryoglobulinemia and nephritis but not from patients with cryoglobulinemia in the absence of nephritis (335). Because no difference in IgG subclass, rheumatoid factor idiotype, or isoelectric point could be identified in nephritogenic and non-nephritogenic cryoprecipitates, the differences in pathogenicity were attributed to differences in intrinsic glomerular binding activity (335). Recently, it has been shown that this glomerular binding activity may involve the binding of the IgM κ to cellular fibronectin (336).

In addition to inducing glomerular injury, it is thought that macrophages and neutrophils participate in the removal of the immune complexes (333,337), which may account for the observation that immune deposits in HCV-MPGN may be scant and that the lesion may resemble acute proliferative GN (299,304).

Whereas the deposition of immune complexes remains the principal hypothesis to explain the pathogenesis of HCV-MPGN, it is also possible that some cases may result from auto-antibodies to glomerular antigens. As discussed above, auto-antibodies are common with chronic HCV infection, including antinuclear antibody (21%), rheumatoid factors (70%), anti-smooth muscle antibody (21%), P-ANCA (37%), and even antibodies to glomerular antigens (292,325,326,338).

Pathology

The renal biopsy in HCV-MPGN shows a proliferative lesion with lobular accentuation and occasional double-contouring of the capillary basement membranes (Fig. 5). Mesangial proliferation or sclerosis may be present (298, 299). By immunofluorescence, IgM, IgG, and C3 are present in the capillary wall in a granular pattern, although the deposits are frequently modest and in a third of cases the IgG may be absent (299) (Fig. 5). Electron microscopy usually shows subendothelial immune deposits, and occasionally mesangial and subepithelial deposits. Granular, finely fibrillar, or immunotactoid structures suggestive of cryoglobulins may also be present (Fig. 5) (298,299). In one patient with a proliferative GN, virus-like particles were identified in paramesangial deposits (304). Tubulointerstitial inflammation with scarring is common, and occasional patients may have a vasculitis of small and medium-sized arteries (298,299).

Clinical Manifestations and Laboratory Findings

The majority of patients with HCV infection and cryoglobulinemia have no symptoms attributable to the cryoglobulinemia (292–294). However, other patients have symptoms and signs of EMC, with weakness, nonpruritic purpura, arthralgias, and neuropathy (300,308,339). A minority of patients with HCV-EMC have renal involvement; in one series, only 8% of patients with HCV-EMC had MPGN (339).

Patients with HCV-MPGN present with nephrotic or, less commonly, non-nephrotic proteinuria, and mild to moderate renal insufficiency (299). Some patients have an aggressive course suggestive of RPGN (299) (*unpublished data,* R. Johnson, 1996). Extrarenal signs or symptoms compatible with EMC are observed in half of the patients; these may manifest as palpable purpura, arthralgias, or peripheral neuropathy (299,300). Some patients have more severe involvement, with myocardial infarction or congestive heart failure, abdominal pain from vasculitis that occasionally leads to intestinal perforation, and pulmonary fibrosis (299). Clinical evidence for liver disease is frequently lacking (299).

The serum is positive for anti-HCV IgG by second- or third-generation enzyme-linked immunosorbent assay (ELISA) and HCV RNA by polymerase chain reaction (PCR) (299,300,340). Genotype analysis has revealed no predilection for any genotype in most studies of HCV-EMC or HCV-MPGN (299,316,341,342). In one study, an increase in genotype 2a (III) was observed in patients with cryoglobulinemia relative to HCV patients without cryoglobulinemia (343).

Liver transaminases are elevated in two thirds of cases, although usually only twofold (299,300). Despite the minimal elevation of liver enzymes and lack of physical findings, liver biopsy usually shows a chronic active hepatitis, with or without cirrhosis (299). Rare cases with normal liver histology have also been described (344).

Other laboratory findings include hypocomplementemia, with depressed CH_{50} in 90%, C4 in 75%, and C3 in 50% (299,300). Rheumatoid factors are present in 70% (299,300). Cryoglobulins are present in 60% at presentation, and are detectable in another 20% during the course of the disease (299). The ANCA test is usually negative (299).

Other Glomerulonephritis Associated with Hepatitis C Virus: Membranous Nephropathy

HCV infection has also been reported in MN (see also Chapter 47) (301,302,345,346). In these patients, the serum is positive for anti-HCV IgG and HCV RNA (301, 345,346). The pathogenesis may relate to the deposition of the core antigen (C22) of HCV in the subepithelial space (because it is cationic; discussed in [346]), followed by the binding of anti-HCV IgG. Recently, C22 has been localized to the capillary wall in two patients with HCV-MN (346). Clinically, these cases mimic idiopathic MN, except that liver enzymes are usually mildly elevated (345,346). The renal biopsy may also show small deposits in the mesangium and subendothelial areas in addition to the classic localization in the subepithelial space (299,300,345,346).

Several cases of IgA nephropathy have also been reported with HCV infection (347). However, most series do not show an increased frequency of HCV infection in patients with IgA nephropathy (316).

Differential Diagnosis

Cases of HCV-MPGN may present as classic EMC, with purpura and arthralgias and sometimes vasculitis of visceral organs (299,300). In this setting, the differential diagnosis would include other causes of cryoglobulinemia, Henoch-Schönlein purpura, and PAN. HCV-MPGN may also present as a primary glomerular disease with either a nephrotic or nephritic picture. Although the clinical course is usually indolent, the disease may also be rapidly progressive, similar to RPGN. HCV-MN clinically resembles idiopathic and other secondary forms of MN (see Chapter 47).

Hepatitis C Viral Glomerulonephritis in Transplantation

HCV-MPGN may be seen in renal transplant patients, either *de novo* or as a recurrence (340,348,349). In some patients, the biopsy specimen may resemble transplant glomerulopathy (349). The frequency of HCV-MPGN may approach 5% in HCV-infected renal transplant patients (348). Peripheral manifestations may include purpura and other manifestations of cryoglobulinemia (340,348,349). However, cryoglobulins and hypocomplementemia occur less frequently than in nontransplant patients with HCV-MPGN (340,348,349).

HCV-MPGN and mesangial proliferative GN have also been reported to develop in liver transplant patients, sometimes within months of transplantation (331,350).

Finally, HCV-MN has been reported in bone marrow transplant (301) and renal transplant (351) patients, and clinically resembles idiopathic MN.

Prognosis and Treatment

The ideal treatment for cryoglobulinemic and noncryoglobulinemic HCV-MPGN has not been determined. Because of evidence that interferon-α is beneficial in chronic HCV hepatitis (352), several groups have treated either HCV-EMC or HCV-MPGN with interferon-α (Table 4). In general, treatment with interferon in HCV-EMC has been associated with a reduction in purpura, improvement in levels of liver enzymes, and reduction in cryocrit in the 50–70% of patients in whom HCV viremia is suppressed (353–356). In patients with HCV-MPGN, treatment with interferon-α (3 mU three times weekly for 6 months) results in suppression of viremia in 60% of patients and is associated with a reduction in proteinuria and an improvement or stabilization of renal function (299). However, response typically takes 1 to 3 months, and relapse of viremia and renal disease is the rule after completion of therapy (299). There is a report of one patient who received higher doses of interferon-α and appears to have been cured of his HCV infection with a complete remission of the MPGN (357). Side effects are common with interferon-α, consisting of influenzalike symptoms and, less commonly, insomnia, psychiatric problems, unmasking of hypothyroidism, leukopenia, thrombocytopenia, and worsening of neuropathies (299, 353–356).

The reason for the lack of efficacy of interferon-α is likely multifactorial. Therapy has been shown to be less effective in the presence of high degrees of viremia and

TABLE 4. *Interferon-α therapy in HCV-associated mixed cryoglobulinemia*

Patients, No.	Year	Treatment regimen	Outcome	Reference
18[a]	1991	3 mU/d × 3 mo, then 3 mU qod	↓LFTs, ↓purpura, ↓creatinine	(353)
26	1993	2 mU qd × 1 mo, qod × 5 mo Methylprednisone 4-8 mg/d	↓LFTs, ↓purpura	(354)
53[b]	1994	3 mU tiw × 6 mo	↓purpura, ↓cryocrit, ↓creatinine	(355)
65	1994	3 mU tiw × 1 y (n=15)	53% remission	(356)
		3 mU tiw + prednisone 16 mg/d (n=17)	53% remission	
		Prednisone 16 mg/d (n=18)	17% remission	
		Placebo (n=15)	7% remission	

LFTs, liver function tests.

[a] These patients had essential mixed cryoglobulinemia but were not tested for HCV.

[b] Clinical response occurred in only 15 of 25 patients randomized to interferon, and correlated with suppression of the HCV viremia by PCR testing.

severe liver disease (358), which are common in patients with HCV-MPGN (299). Genotype 1, also associated with resistance to interferon-α therapy (358), is common in patients with HCV-MPGN and HCV-EMC (299,316, 341,342). However, patients with other genotypes have relapsed as well (299).

Although HCV-MPGN is often chronic with a vacillating course, it can be associated with rapid renal deterioration. In this latter setting, it may be best to treat for RPGN using pulse steroids with or without plasma exchange and cytotoxic agents. Studies of the treatment of cases of cryoglobulinemic MPGN (the majority which are now known to be caused by HCV) with pulse steroids have shown a rapid improvement in renal function (359). In contrast, interferon-α requires 1 to 3 months to show efficacy and therefore would not be suited for treatment in a setting suggestive of RPGN (299).

Whereas immunosuppressive agents appear to control the disease in some patients (359,360), the observation that GN can develop in transplant patients while they are receiving immunosuppressive regimens (340,348,349) emphasizes that response is not universal. Furthermore, in a controlled study, corticosteroids (16 mg prednisone daily) resulted in a remission of 17%, compared with 53% for those treated with natural interferon-α (356). Immunosuppression also results in increased HCV viremia (361,362), with potentially serious consequences for the liver. In liver transplant patients, for example, hepatitis C viral infection recurs universally, and in half of patients it is associated with an accelerated recurrence of chronic liver disease (362).

At this time, we would recommend the following treatment regimen: In patients with symptomatic nephrotic syndrome or renal insufficiency, we would administer long-term interferon-α therapy starting at 3 mU three times weekly and tapering after 6 months to the lowest dose that suppresses viremia (by PCR). We would not give immunosuppressive medicines for chronic HCV-associated MPGN. However, in patients with an aggressive RPGN-like course or with systemic signs of severe vasculitis (such as abdominal pain or myocardial dysfunction), we would initially administer pulse steroids with or without plasmapheresis, followed by rapid tapering of the steroids and institution of interferon therapy.

Glomerulonephritis Associated With Cytomegalovirus Infection

Cytomegalovirus (CMV) was originally postulated to have a significant etiologic role in two major glomerular disease syndromes. In 1981, Richardson et al. (363) reported that in renal transplant patients a distinctive glomerulopathy characterized by endothelial cell swelling and necrosis could develop in association with CMV infection. Subsequently, it was shown that this lesion was not specific for CMV infection and probably represented a type of rejection (364). In 1988, Gregory et al. (365) reported that CMV antigens were present in 31 of 31 renal biopsies from patients with IgA nephropathy versus none of 37 controls. However, it was later shown that the staining was not specific for CMV (366). Furthermore, the presence of CMV DNA in renal biopsy tissue could not be shown to be specifically associated with IgA nephropathy (367).

Nevertheless, a rare case of mesangial proliferative nephritis with immune deposits containing CMV antigens has been described in a patient with CMV pneumonitis (368). Two cases of congenital CMV infection with proliferative and/or necrotizing GN have also been reported (369). In one of these cases, CMV viral particles could be identified in the glomerular endothelial cells (369).

Other Viral Infections

Infection with hepatitis A virus (HAV) has generally not been associated with glomerular disease. However, a single case of nephrotic syndrome with a mesangial proliferative histology has been reported in a patient with acute hepatitis A (370).

PARASITE-ASSOCIATED GLOMERULAR DISEASE

Schistosomal Glomerulopathy

Schistosomiasis may be associated with glomerulopathy (reviewed in [371]). Most cases have been reported in Africa or South America in patients with hepatosplenic disease caused by *Schistosoma mansoni* (371). However, other cases have been described in Asia caused by *S. japonicum* and in Africa caused by *S. haematobium*.

Schistosomiasis affects nearly 200 million people worldwide, but hepatosplenic disease develops in only 4.5%, and renal abnormalities develop in 10% of these. Although most of the time the renal disease is asymptomatic, those patients who do present with clinical disease usually manifest nephrotic syndrome in the second to fourth decade of life. Circulating immune complexes and rheumatoid factors are common, and hypocomplementemia may be present. Some patients may have concomitant urinary tract infection with *Salmonella* (372). Renal biopsy can show a variety of lesions, including mesangial proliferative GN, MPGN, acute proliferative GN, or focal sclerosis (371) (Table 5). Immunofluorescence demonstrates IgM, IgG, and C3 in mesangial or capillary wall patterns. IgA is usually absent. The pathogenesis of the lesion is thought to be related to the deposition of immune complexes containing schistosomal antigens. Schistosomal antigens (373–375) can be identified

TABLE 5. *Principal clinicopathologic features of schistosomal glomerulopathy*

Class	Histopathologic pattern	Glomerular deposits detected by immunofluorescence	Commonly associated infections	Hepatic fibrosis	Features of renal involvement: Asymptomatic proteinuria	Nephrotic syndrome	Hypertension	Progression to ESRD	Response to treatment
I	Mesangioproliferative a. "Minimal lesion" b. Focal antigens c. Diffuse	Mesangial: IgM, C3, schistosomal gut antigens	–	±	+++	+	±	?	±?
II	Exudative	Endocapillary: C3, *Salmonella* antigens	Salmonellosis	+	–	+++	–	?	+++
III	A. Mesangiocapillary	Mesangial: IgG, C3, schistosomal gut antigens (early), IgA (late)	–	+++	+	++	++	++	–
	B. Mesangiocapillary (type III)	Mesangial & subepithelial: IgG, C3, schistosomal gut antigens (early), IgA (late)	Hepatitis B	+++	+	+++	+	++	–
IV	Focal & segmental glomerulosclerosis	Mesangial: IgG, IgM, IgA	–	+++	+	+++	+++	+++	–
V	Amyloidosis	Mesangial: IgG	?Salmonellosis, ?*E. coli* UTI	±	+	+++	±	+++	–

From Barsoum, ref. 371, with permission.
ESRD, end-stage renal disease.

in glomerular lesions, and anti-schistosomal antibody has been eluted from tissue sections (373). In those patients with coexistent *Salmonella* infection, *Salmonella* antigens have also been localized to the glomerular lesion (372). Liver disease is thought to result in decreased hepatic removal of immune complexes, thus resulting in their accumulation in glomeruli.

The prognosis of schistosomal glomerulopathy is variable. The course of patients with an MPGN-type histology progresses at the same rate as the course of patients with idiopathic MPGN (374). Anti-schistosomal therapy does not appear to benefit most patients with schistosomal nephropathy (374,375). However, in those patients with acute proliferative GN from coexistent *Salmonella* and schistosomal infection, there is evidence that antibacterial and antiparasitic therapy may be beneficial (371, 372). Immunosuppressive therapy has not been shown to be of benefit, and schistosomal nephropathy can recur in renal transplant patients (376).

Malaria-Associated Nephropathy

Malaria may be associated with glomerular disease. Whereas acute malaria caused by *Plasmodium vivax* or *P. ovale* typically is not associated with renal disease, acute infection with *P. falciparum* may be associated with acute nephritis, nephrotic syndrome, or acute tubular necrosis from massive hemolysis ("blackwater fever") (reviewed in [377,378]). In patients with *P. falciparum* infection, an acute proliferative GN has been documented, with positive immunofluorescence for IgG, IgM, C3 and *P. falciparum* antigens (377). Renal function typically improves with control of the parasitemia (377).

A more common and serious glomerular disease has been reported in Africa in patients with quartan malaria (*P. malariae*) documented by parasitemia and/or the presence of high titers of anti-*P. malariae* antibodies. (377,378). Clinically, quartan malaria nephropathy typically presents as a steroid-resistant nephrotic syndrome in childhood (ages 5 to 10 years) (379). Microhematuria is frequently observed, but blood pressure is usually normal (379). Renal biopsy shows thickening of the basement membrane, often with double contours, caused by the accumulation of basement membranelike material in the subendothelial regions that stains positively with periodic acid–Schiff (PAS). Small lacunae may also be present in the GBM (379). Histologically, this condition may resemble "tropical nephropathy" (380), but immune deposits containing IgM, IgG, and C3 are often seen in malaria-associated nephropathy, whereas they are generally absent in tropical nephropathy (379,380). Malaria antigens have also been identified in the immune deposits (377,378,381).

Management of quartan malaria nephropathy is supportive, as neither antiparasitic nor immunosuppressive therapy appears to be of benefit (377–379,381). Spontaneous remissions are rare, and the course often slowly progresses to renal failure within 3 to 5 years (377–379,381).

Other Parasitic Diseases

Other parasites may also be associated with glomerular disease. In the tropics, glomerular disease may accompany infection with filariae, such as *Wuchereria bancrofti*, *Onchocerca volvulus*, and *Loa loa* (reviewed in [378]). A nephrotic syndrome with a membranous histology has also been reported in congenital toxoplasmosis (382).

REFERENCES

1. Wells WC. *Transactions of a Society for the Improvement of Medical and Surgical Knowledge*. London: T. Gillet for C. Dilly, The Society; 1812:3,16,194.
2. Blackall J. *Observations on the Nature and Cure of Dropsies*. London: Longman, Hurst, Rees, Orme and Brown; 1818:44.
3. Bright R. *Reports of Medical Cases, Selected with a View of Illustrating the Symptoms and Cure of Disease by Reference to Morbid Anatomy*; vol 1. London: Longman, Rees, Orme, Brown and Green; 1827.
4. Longcope WT. The pathogenesis of glomerular nephritis. *Bull Johns Hopkins Hosp* 1929;45:335–360.
5. Rammelkamp CH Jr, Weaver RS. Acute glomerulonephritis: the significance of variations in the incidence of disease. *J Clin Invest* 1953; 32:345–358.
6. Rammelkamp CH Jr. Acute hemorrhagic glomerulonephritis. In: McCarty M, ed. *Streptococcal Infections*. New York: Columbia University Press; 1954.
7. Jennings RB, Earle DOP. Post-streptococcal glomerulonephritis: histopathologic and clinical studies of the acute, subsiding acute and early chronic latent phases. *J Clin Invest* 1961;40:1525–1595.
8. Jordan SC, Lemire JM. Acute glomerulonephritis. Diagnosis and treatment. *Pediatr Clin North Am* 1982;29:857–873.
9. Cole BR, Salinas-Madrigal L. Acute proliferative glomerulonephritis and crescentic glomerulonephritis. In: Avner, ed. *Glomerular Diseases*. London: Williams & Wilkins; 1994:697–718 (*Pediatric Nephrology*; section 6).
10. Rodriguez-Iturbe B, Gastillo L, Valbuena R, Cuenca L. Acute post-streptococcal glomerulonephritis: a review of recent developments. *Paediatrician* 1979;8:307–324.
11. Holm SE. The pathogenesis of acute post-streptococcal glomerulonephritis in new lights. *APMIS*;1988:189–193.
12. Rodriguez-Iturbe B, Garcia R. Acute glomerulonephritis. In: Holliday MA, Baratt TM, Vernier RI, eds. *Pediatric Nephrology*. 2nd ed. London: Williams and Wilkins; 1987:411–417.
13. Fish AJ, Herdman RC, Michael AF, Pickering RJ, Good RA. Epidemic acute glomerulonephritis associated with type 49 streptococcal pyoderma II: correlative study of light, immunofluorescent and electron microscopic findings. *Am J Med* 1970;48:28–39.
14. Dillon HC Jr, Reeves MS. Streptococcal immune responses in nephritis after skin infections. *Am J Med* 1974;56:333.
15. Svartman M, Finklea JF, Earle DP, Potter EV, Poon-King T. Epidemic scabies and acute glomerulonephritis in Trinidad. *Lancet* 1972;1: 249–251.
16. Barnham M, Thornton TJ, Lange K. Nephritis caused by *Streptococcus zooepidemicus* (Lancefield group C). *Lancet* 1983;101.1:945–948.
17. Read SE, Reid HFM, Bassett DCJ, Poon-King T, Zabriskie JB. The group G streptococcus: its role as a possible pathogen. In: Kimura Y, Kotami S, Shiokawa Y, eds. *Recent Advances in Streptococci and Streptococcal Diseases*. Berks, England: Reedbooks; 1985:70.
18. Dillon HC. Streptococcal infections of the skin and their complications: impetigo and nephritis. In: Wannamaker IW, Matsen JM, eds. *Streptococci and Streptococcal Diseases*. New York: Academic Press; 1972:571.
19. Rodriguez-Iturbe B. Epidemic post-streptococcal glomerulonephritis [Clinical Conference]. *Kidney Int* 1984;25:129–136.
20. Rodriguez-Iturbe B, Rubio L, Garcia R. Attack rate of post-streptococcal nephritis in families: a prospective study. *Lancet* 1981;1: 401–403.
21. Read SE, Reid H, Poon-King T, Fischetti VA, Zabriskie JB, Rapaport FT. HLA and predisposition to the nonsuppurative sequelae of group A streptococcal infections. *Transplant Proc* 1977;9:543–546.
22. Anthony BF, Kaplan EL, Wannamaker LW, Briese FW, Chapman SS. Attack rates of acute nephritis after type 49 streptococcal infection of the skin and of the respiratory tract. *J Clin Invest* 1969;48: 1697–1704.
23. Stetson CA, Rammelkamp CH, Krause RM, et al. Epidemic acute nephritis: studies on etiology, natural history and prevention. *Medicine* 1995;34:431.
24. Nissenson AR, Baraff LJ, Fine RN, Knutson DW. Post-streptococcal acute glomerulonephritis: fact and controversy. *Ann Intern Med* 1979;91:76–86.
25. Treser G, Semar M, Sagel I, et al. Independence of the nephritogenicity of group A streptococci from their M types. *Clin Exp Immunol* 1971;9:57–62.
26. Mota-Hernandez F, Briseno-Mondragon E, Gordillo-Paniagua G. Glomerular lesions and final outcome in children with glomerulonephritis of acute onset. *Nephron* 1976;16:272–281.
27. Habib R, Kleinknecht C, Royer P. Primary nephrotic syndrome in children: classification and anatomoclinical study of 406 cases. *Arch Fr Pediatr* 1971;28:277–319.
28. Glassock RJ, Adler SG, Cohen AH. Primary glomerular diseases. In: Brenner BM, ed. *The Kidney*. 5th ed. Philadelphia: WB Saunders, 1996;2:1392– 1497.
29. Pankewycz OG, Sturgill BC, Bolton WK. Proliferative glomerulonephritis: post-infectious, non-infectious and crescentic forms. In: Tisher CC, Brenner BM, eds. *Renal Pathology*. Philadelphia: JB Lippincott; 1994:222–257.
30. Bodaghi E, Vazirian S, Abtahi MT, Honarmand MT, Madani A, Zia Shamsa AM. Glomerular diseases in children: "the Iranian experience." *Pediatr Nephrol* 1989;3:213–217.
31. Roy S, Stapleton FB. Changing perspectives in children hospitalized with post-streptococcal acute glomerulonephritis. *Pediatr Nephrol* 1990;4:585–588.
32. Alkjaersig NK, Fletcher AP, Lewis ML, Cole BR, Ingelfinger JR, Robson AM. Pathophysiological response of the blood coagulation system in acute glomerulonephritis. *Kidney Int* 1976;10:319–328.
33. Schwartz B, Facklam RR, Breiman RF. Changing epidemiology of group A streptococcal infection in the USA. *Lancet* 1990;336:1167–1171.
34. Rodriguez-Iturbe B, Carr RI, Garcia R, Rabideau D, Rubio L, McIntosh RM. Circulating immune complexes and serum immunoglobulins in acute post-streptococcal glomerulonephritis. *Clin Nephrol* 1980;13:1–4.
35. Yoshizawa N, Treser G, McClung JA, Sagel I, Takahashi K. Circulating immune complexes in patients with uncomplicated group A streptococcal pharyngitis and patients with acute post-streptococcal glomerulonephritis. *Am J Nephrol* 1983;3:23–29.
36. Mezzano S, Olavarria F, Ardiles L, et al. Incidence of circulating immune complexes in patients with acute post-streptococcal glomerulonephritis and in patients with streptococcal impetigo. *Clin Nephrol* 1987;26:61–65.
37. Lange K, Seligson G, Cronin W. Evidence for the *in situ* origin of post-streptococcal glomerulonephritis: glomerular localization of endostreptosin and the clinical significance of the subsequent antibody response. *Clin Nephrol* 1983;19:3–10.
38. Friedman J, van de Rijn I, Ohkuni H, Fischette VA, Zabriskie JB. Immunological studies of post-streptococcal sequelae: evidence for

presence of streptococcal antigens in circulating immune complexes. *J Clin Invest* 1984;74:1027–1034.
39. Rodriguez-Iturbe B, Rabideau D, Garcia R, Rubio L, McIntosh RM. Characterization of the glomerular antibody in acute post-streptococcal glomerulonephritis. *Ann Intern Med* 1980;92:478–481.
40. Mezzano S, Burgos E, Mahabir R, Kemeny E, Zabriskie JB. Failure to detect unique reactivity to streptococcal streptokinase in either the sera or renal biopsy specimens of patients with acute post-streptococcal glomerulonephritis. *Clin Nephrol* 1992;38:305–310.
41. Lange K, Cronin W, Seligson G. Endostreptosin: its characteristics and clinical significance. In: Holm SE, Christensen P, eds. *Basic Concepts of Streptococci and Streptoccal Disease*. Windsor, England: Reedbooks; 1988:260.
42. Cronin WJ, Lange K. Immunologic evidence for the *in situ* deposition of a cytoplasmic streptococcal antigen (endostreptosin) on the glomerular basement membrane in rats. *Clin Nephrol* 1990;34:143–146.
43. Yoshizawa N, Oshima S, Sagel I, Shimizu J, Treser G. Role of a streptococcal antigen in the pathogenesis of acute post-streptococcal glomerulonephritis: characterization of the antigen and a proposed mechanism for the disease. *J Immunol* 1992;148:3110–3116.
44. Akesson P, Sjoholm AG, Bjorck L. Protein SIC, a novel extracellular protein of *Streptococcus pyogenes* interfering with complement function. *J Biol Chem* 1996;271:1081–1088.
45. Johnston KH, Zabriskie JB. Purification and partial characterization of the nephritis strain-associated protein from *Streptococcus pyogenes*, group A. *J Exp Med* 1986;163:697–712.
46. Peake PW, Pussell BA, Karplus TE, Riley EH, Charlesworth JA. Post-streptococcal glomerulonephritis: studies on the interaction between nephritis strain-associated protein (NSAP), complement and the glomerulus. *APMIS* 1991;99:460–466.
47. Holm SE, Bergholm AM, Johnston KH. A streptococcal plasminogen activator in the focus of infection and in the kidneys during the intial phase of experimental streptococcal glomerulonephritis. *APMIS* 1988;96:1097–1108.
48. Ohkuni H, friedman J, van der Rijn I, Fischetti VA, Poon-King T, Zabriskie JB. Immunological studies of post-streptococcal sequelae: serological studies with an extracellular protein associated with nephritogenic streptococci. *Clin Exp Immunol* 1983;54:185–193.
49. Holm SE, Bergholm AM, Johnston KH. A possible role of NSAP in the pathogenesis of the initial phase of experimental APSGN. In: *Abstracts of the 10th Lancefield International Symposium of Streptococci and Streptoccal Disease*. Cologne, 1987:41–43(abst).
50. Cu GA, Zabriskie JB. Streptococcal pyrogenic exotoxin B (SPEB) in acute post-streptococcal glomerulonephritis (APSGN). *J Am Soc Nephrol* 1995;3:416(Abstr).
51. Lange CF, Wever M, Nayyar RP. Age effects on the reactivity of anti-streptococcal cell membrane antisera to murine glomerular basement membrane: in vitro versus in vivo analysis. *Ren Physiol* 1986;9: 148–159.
52. Zelman ME, Lange CF. Immunochemical studies of streptococcal cell membrane antigens immunologically related to glomerular basement membrane. *Hybridoma* 1995;14:6:529–536.
53. Kefalides NA, Pegg MT, Ohno N, Poon-King T, Zabriskie J, Fillit H. Antibodies to basement membrane collagen and to laminin are present in sera from patients with post-streptococcal glomerulonephritis. *J Exp Med* 1986;163:588–602.
54. McIntosh RM, Garcia R, Rubio L, et al. Evidence of an autologous immune complex pathogenic mechanism in acute post-streptococcal glomerulonephritis. *Kidney Int* 1978;14:501–510.
55. Kanwar YS, Farquhar MG. Detachment of endothelium and epithelium from the glomerular basement membrane produced by kidney perfusion with neuraminidase. *Lab Invest* 1980;42:375–384.
56. Rodriguez-Iturbe B, Silva-Beauperthuy V, Parra G, Rubio L, Garcia E. Skin window immune response to normal human IgG in patients with rheumatoid arthritis and acute post-streptococcal glomerulonephritis. *Am J Clin Pathol* 1981;76:270–275.
57. Jacobson HR, Striker GE, Klahr S. *The Principles and Practice of Nephrology*. Philadelphia: BC Becker; 1991:262–265.
58. Oite T, Batsford SR, Mihatsch MJ, Takamiya H, Vogt A. Quantitative studies of *in situ* immune complex glomerulonephritis in the rat induced by planted cationized antigen. *J Exp Med* 1982;155:460–474.
59. Couser WG, Ochi RF, Baker PJ, et al. Depletion of C6 reduces proteinuria in a model of membranous nephropathy induced with a non-glomerular antigen. *J Am Soc Nephrol* 1991;2:894–901.
60. Tomai M, Kotb M, Majumdar G, Beachey EH. Superantigenicity of streptococcal M protein. *J Exp Med* 1990;172:359–362.
61. Abe J, Forrester J, Nakahara T, Lafferty JA, Kotzin BL, Leung DY. Selective stimulation of human T cells with streptococcal erythrogenic toxins A and B. *J Immunol* 1991;146:3747–3750.
62. Kotzin BL, Leung DY, Kappler J, Marrack P. Superantigens and their potential role in human disease. *Adv Immunol* 1993;54:99–166.
63. Mourad W, Mehindate K, Schall TJ, McColl SR. Engagement of major histocompatibility complex class II molecules by superantigen induces inflammatory cytokine gene expression in human rheumatoid fibroblast-like synoviocytes. *J Exp Med* 1992;175:613–616.
64. Gjorloff A, Fischer H, Hedlund G, et al. Induction of interleukin-1 in human monocytes by the superantigen staphylococcal enterotoxin A requires the participation of T cells. *Cell Immunol* 1991;137:61–71.
65. Herman A, Kappler JW, Marrack P, Pullen AM. Superantigens: mechanism of T-cell stimulation and role in immune responses. *Annu Rev Immunol* 1991;9:745–772.
66. Friedman SM, Posnett DN, Tumang JR, Cole BC, Crow MK. A potential role for microbial superantigens in the pathogenesis of systemic autoimmune disease. *Arthritis Rheum* 1991;34:468–480.
67. Parra G, Soto H, Rodriguez-Iturbe B. Circulating levels of cytokines in post-streptococcal glomerulonephritis. *90th International Congress of Nephrology*. Madrid, 1995:301(Abstr).
68. Koyama A, Kobayashi M, Yamaguchi N, et al. Glomerulonephritis associated with MRSA infection: a possible role of bacterial superantigen. *Kidney Int* 1995;47:207–216.
69. Lewy JE, Salinas Madrigal L, Herdson PB, Pirani CL, Metcoff J. Clinicopathologic correlations in acute post-streptococcal glomerulonephritis: a correlation between renal functions, morphologic damage and clinical course of 46 children with acute post-streptococcal glomerulonephritis. *Medicine (Baltimore)* 1971;50:453–501.
70. Dodge WF, Spargo BH, Bass JA, Travis LB. The relationship between the clinical and pathologic features of post-streptococcal glomerulonephritis: a study of the early natural history. *Medicine (Baltimore)* 1968;47:227–267.
71. Burkholder PM, Bradford WD. Proliferative glomerulonephritis in children: a correlation of varied clinical and pathologic patterns utilizing light, immunofluorescence and electron microscopy. *Am J Pathol* 1969;56:423–467.
72. Neustein HB, Davis W. Acute glomerulonephritis: a light and electron microscopy study of eight serial biopsies. *Am J Clin Pathol* 1965; 44:613–626.
73. Churg J, Bernstein J, Glassock R. *Renal Disease: Classification and Atlas of Glomerular Disease*. 2nd ed. New York: Igaku-Shoin; 1994.
74. Parrish AE, Kramer NC, Hatch FE, et al. The relation between glomerular function and histology in acute glomerulonephritis. *J Lab Clin Med* 1961;58:197.
75. Leonard CD, Nagle RB, Striker GE, Cutler RE, Scribner BH. Acute glomerulonephritis with prolonged oliguria: an analysis of 29 cases. *Ann Intern Med* 1970;73:703–711.
76. Hinglais N, Garcia-Torres R, Kleinknecht D. Long-term prognosis in acute glomerulonephritis. *Am J Med* 1974;56:52–60.
77. Bodaghi E, Kheradpir KM, Maddah M. Vasculitis in acute streptococcal glomerulonephritis. *Int J Pediatr Nephrol* 1987;8:69–74.
78. Inglefinger JR, McCluskey RT, Schneeberger EE, Grupe WE. Necrotizing arteritis in acute post-streptococcal glomerulonephritis: report of a recovered case. *J Pediatr* 1977;91:228–232.
79. Fordham CC III, Epstein FH, Hiffines WD, Harrington JT. Polyarteritis and acute post-streptococcal glomerulonephritis. *Ann Int Med* 1964;61:1:89–97.
80. Freedman PJ, Peters JH, Kark RM. Localization of gamma-globlulin in the diseased kidney. *Arch Intern Med* 1960;105:524.
81. Sorger K, Gessler U, Hubner FK, et al. Subtypes of post-infectious glomerulonephritis: synopsis of clinical and pathological features. *Clin Nephrol* 1982;17:114–128.
82. Sorger K, Balun J, Hubner FK, et al. The garland type of acute post-infectious glomerulonephritis: morphological characteristics and follow-up studies. *Clin Nephrol* 1983;20:17–26.
83. Edelstein CL, Bates WD. Subtypes of acute post-infectious glomerulonephritis: a clinicopathological correlation. *Clin Nephrol* 1992;38: 311-317.
84. Nand N, Argent NB, Morley AR, Ward MK. Garland pattern post-streptococcal glomerulonephritis. *Nephrol Dial Transplant* 1992;7: 155–157.

85. Andres GA, Accinni L, Hsu KC, Zabriskie JB, Seegal BC. Electron microscopic studies of human glomerulonephritis with ferritin-conjugated antibody. *J Exp Med* 1966;123:399–412.
86. Richet G, Chevet D, Morel-Maroger L. Serial biopsies in diffuse proliferative glomerulonephritis in adults: an attempt for a better understanding of sporadic acute glomerulonephrits. In: Kincaid-Smith P, Mathew TH, Becker EL, eds. *Glomerulonephritis*: Part 1. New York: John Wiley; 1972:363–381.
87. Tornroth T. The fate of subepithelial deposits in acute post-streptococcal glomerulonephritis. *Lab Invest* 1976;35:461–474.
88. Lee HA, Stirling G, Sharpstone P. Acute glomerulonephritis in middle-aged and elderly patients. *Br Med J* 1966;2:1361–1363.
89. Washio M, Oh Y, Okuda S, et al. Clinicopathological study of post-streptococcal glomerulonephritis in the elderly. *Clin Nephrol* 1994; 41:265–270.
90. Levy M. Infections and glomerular diseases. *J Allergy Clin Immunol* 1986;6:405–435.
91. Madaio MP, Harrington JT. Current concepts: the diagnosis of acute glomerulonephritis. *N Engl J Med* 1983;309:1299–1302.
92. Anand SK, Trygstad CW, Sharma HM, Northway JD. Extracapillary proliferative glomerulonephritis in children. *Pediatrics* 1975;56:434–442.
93. Ferrario F, Kourilsky O, Morel-Maroger L. Acute endocapillary glomerulonephritis in adults: a histologic and clinical comparison between patients with and without initial acute renal failure. *Clin Nephrol* 1983;19:17–23.
94. Bergner-Rabinowitz S, Fleiderman S, Ferne M, et al. The new streptozyme test for streptococcal antibodies. *Clin Pediatr* 1975;14:804–809.
95. Seligmann M, Danon F, Basch A, Bernard J. IgG myeloma cryoglobulin with antistreptosin activity. *Nature* 1968;220:711–712.
96. Hebert LA, Cosio FG, Neff JC. Diagnostic significance of hypocomplementemia (Editorial). *Kidney Int* 1991;39:811–821.
97. Matsell DG, Roy SD, Tamerius JD, Morrow PR, Kolb WP, Wyatt RJ. Plasma terminal complement complexes in acute post-streptococcal glomerulonephritis. *Am J Kidney Dis* 1991;17:311–316.
98. McLean RH, Schrager MA, Rothfield NF, Berman MA. Normal complement in early post-streptococcal glomerulonephritis. *Br Med J* 1977;1:1326.
99. Lewis EJ, Carpenter CB, Schur PH. Serum complement component levels in human glomerulonephritis. *Ann Intern Med* 1971;75:555–560.
100. Cameron JS, Vick RM, Ogg CS, Seymour WM, Chantler C, Turner DR. Plasma C3 and C4 concentrations in management of glomerulonephritis. *Br Med J* 1973;3:668–672.
101. Sjoholm AG. Complement components and complement activation in acute post-streptococcal glomerulonephritis. *Int Arch Allergy Appl Immunol* 1979;58:274–284.
102. Wyatt RJ, Forristal J, West CD, Sugimoto S, Curd JG. Complement profiles in acute post-streptococcal glomerulonephritis. *Pediatr Nephrol* 1988;2:219–223.
103. Gill DG, Turner DR, Chantler C, Cameron JS. The progression of acute proliferative post-streptococcal glomerulonephritis to severe epithelial crescent formation. *Clin Nephrol* 1977;8:449–452.
104. Fairley C, Mathews DC, Becker GJ. Rapid development of diffuse crescents in post-streptococcal glomerulonephritis. *Clin Nephrol* 1987;28:256–260.
105. Modai D, Pik A, Behar M, et al. Biopsy proven evolution of post-streptococcal glomerulonephritis to rapidly progressive glomerulonephritis of a post-infectious type. *Clin Nephrol* 1985;23:198–202.
106. Baldwin DS, Gluck MC, Schacht RG, Gallo G. The long-term course of post-streptococcal glomerulonephritis. *Ann Intern Med* 1974;80: 342–358.
107. Baldwin DS. Post-streptococcal glomerulonephritis: a progressive disease? *Am J Med* 1977;62:1–11.
108. Buzio C, Allegri L, Mutti A, Perazzoli F, Bergamaschi E. Significance of albuminuria in the follow-up of acute post-streptococcal glomerulonephritis. *Clin Nephrol* 1994;41:259–264.
109. Drachman R, Aladjem M, Vardy PA. Natural history of an acute glomerulonephritis epidemic in children: an 11-12 year follow-up. *Isr J Med Sci* 1982;18:603–607.
110. Vogl W, Renke M, Mayer-Eichberger D, Schmitt H, Bohle A. Long-term prognosis for endocapillary glomerulonephritis of post-streptococcal type in children and adults. *Nephron* 1986;44:58–65.
111. Nissenson AR, Mayon-White R, Potter EV, et al. Continued absence of clinical renal disease 7-12 years after post-streptococcal acute glomerulonephritis in Trinidad. *Am J Med* 1979;67:255–262.
112. Travis LB, Dodge WF, Beathard GA, et al. Acute glomerulonephritis in children: a review of the natural history with emphasis on prognosis. *Clin Nephrol* 1973;1:169–181.
113. Kaplan EL, Vernier RL. Progressive nephritis after strep infection questioned [Letter]. *Am J Med* 1978;64:910–911.
114. Potter EV, Abidh S, Sharrett AR, et al. Clinical healing 2-6 years after post-streptococcal glomerulonephritis in Trinidad. *N Engl J Med* 1978;298:767–772.
115. Potter EV, Lipschultz SA, Abidh S, Poon-King T, Earle DP. Twelve to seventeen year follow-up of patients with post-streptococcal acute glomerulonephritis in Trinidad. *N Engl J Med* 1982;307:725–729.
116. Baldwin DS, Schacht RG. Late sequelae of post-streptococcal glomerulonephritis. *Annu Rev Med* 1976;27:49–55.
117. Garcia R, Rubio L, Rodriguez-Iturbe B. Long-term prognosis of epidemic post-streptococcal glomerulonephritis in Maracaibo: follow-up studies 11-12 years after the acute episode. *Clin Nephrol* 1981;15: 291–298.
118. Popovic-Rolovic M, Kostic M, Antic-Peco A, Jovanovic O, Popovic D. Medium- and long-term prognosis of patients with acute post-streptococcal glomerulonephritis. *Nephron* 1991;58:393–399.
119. Williams W. Post-streptococcal glomerulonephritis: how important is it as a cause of chronic renal diseases? *Transplant Proc* 1987;19:2: 97–100.
120. Edelmann CM Jr, Greifer I, Barnett HL. The nature of kidney disease in children who fail to recover form apparent acute glomerulonephritis. *J Pediatr* 1964;64:879–886.
121. Vernier RL, Worthen HG, Wannamaker LW, Good RA. Renal biopsy studies of the acute exacerbation in glomerulonephritis. *Am J Dis Child* 1964;133:653.
122. Habib R, Kleinknecht C, Gubler MC, Levy M. Idiopathic membranoproliferative glomerulonephritis in children: report of 105 cases. *Clin Nephrol* 1973;1:194–214.
123. Weinstein L, Le Frock J. Does antimicrobial therapy of streptococcal pharyngitis of pyoderma alter the risk of glomerulonephritis? *J Infect Dis* 1971;124:229–231.
124. Don BR, Schabelan M. Hyperkalemia in acute glomerulonephritis due to transient hyporeninemic hypoaldosteronism. *Kidney Int* 1990; 38:1159–1163.
125. Couser WG. Rapidly progressive glomerulonephritis: classification, pathogenetic mechanisms and therapy. *Am J Kidney Dis* 1988;11: 449–464.
126. Neugarten J, Baldwin DS. Glomerulonephritis in bacterial endocarditis. *Am J Med* 1984;77:297–304.
127. Moroz, SP, Cutz E, Bulte JW, Sass-Kortsak A. Membranoproliferative glomerulonephritis in childhood cirrhosis associated with alpha$_1$-antitrypsin deficiency. *Pediatrics* 1976;232–238.
128. Levy RL, Hong R. The immune nature of subacute bacterial endocarditis (SBE) nephritis. *Am J Med* 1973;54:645–652.
129. Hurwitz D, Quismorio FOP, Friou GJ. Cryoglobulinaemia in patients with infectious endocarditis. *Clin Exp Immunol* 1975;19:131–141.
130. Hall GH, Hart RJ, Davies SW, George M, Head AC. Glomerulonephritis associated with *Coxiella burnetii* endocarditis [Letter]. *Br Med J* 1975;2:275.
131. Perez-Fontan M, Huarte E, Tellez A, Rodriguez-Carmona A, Picazo ML, Martinez- Ara J. Glomerular nephropathy associated with chronic Q fever. *Am J Kidney Dis* 1988;11:298–306.
132. Adler S, Cohen A, Glassock RJ. Secondary glomerular diseases. *The Kidney*. 5th ed. Philadelphia: WB Saunders; 1996:1547–1589.
133. Rovzar MA, Logan JL, Ogden DA, Graham AR. Immunosuppressive therapy and plasmapheresis in rapidly progressive glomerulonephritis associated with bacterial endocarditis. *Am J Kidney Dis* 1986;7:428–433.
134. Williams RC, Kunkel HG. Rheumatoid factor complement and conglutinin aberrations in patients with subacute bacterial endocarditis. *J Clin Invest* 1962;41:666–675.
135. Baehr G. Glomerular lesions of subacute bacterial endocarditis. *J Exp Med* 1912;15:330.
136. Baehr G, Laude H. Glomerulonephritis as a complication of subacute streptococcus endocarditis. *JAMA* 1920;75:789.
137. Morel-Maroger L, Sraer JD, Herremen G, Godeau P. Kidney in subacute endocarditis: pathological and immunofluorescence findings. *Arch Pathol* 1972;94:205–213.

138. Boulton-Jones JM, Sissons JG, Evans DJ, Peters DK. Renal lesions of subacute infective endocarditis. *Br Med J* 1974;2:11–14.
139. Gutman RA, Striker GE, Gilliland BC, Cutler RE. The immune complex glomerulonephritis of bacterial endocarditis. *Medicine (Baltimore)* 1972;51:1–25.
140. Yum M, Wheat LJ, Maxwell D, Edwards JL. Immunofluorescent localization of *Staphylococcus aureus* antigen in acute bacterial endocarditis nephritis. *Am J Clin Pathol* 1978;70:832–835.
141. Groenveld AB, Nommensen FE, Mullink H, Ooms EC, Bode WA. Shunt nephritis associated with *Propionibacterium acnes* with demonstration of the antigen in the glomeruli. *Nephron* 1982;32:365–369.
142. Schoenbaum SC, Gardner P, Shillito J. Infections of cerebrospinal fluid shunts: epidemiology, clinical manifestations and therapy. *J Infect Dis* 1975;131:543–552.
143. McKenzie SA, Hayden K. Two cases of "shunt nephritis." *Pediatrics* 1974;54:806–808.
144. Black JA, Challacombe DN, Ockenden BG. Nephrotic syndrome associated with bacteremia after shunt operations for hydrocephalus. *Lancet* 1965;2:921.
145. Arze RS, Rashid H, Morley R, Ward MK, Ker DN. Shunt nephritis: report of two cases and review of the literature. *Clin Nephrol* 1983; 19:48–53.
146. Levy M, Gubler MC, Habib R. Pathology and immunopathology of shunt nephritis in children: report of 10 cases. In: *Proceedings of the 8th International Congress of Nephrology*. Basel: Karger; 1981:290.
147. Kaufman DB, McIntosh R. The pathogenesis of the renal lesion in a patient with streptococcal disease, infected ventriculoatrial shunt, cryoglobulinemia and nephritis. *Am J Med* 1971;50:262–268.
148. Beaufils M, Morel-Maroger L, Sraer JD, Kanfer A, Kourilsky O, Lrichet G. Acute renal failure of glomerular origin during visceral abcesses. *N Engl J Med* 1976;295:185–189.
149. Sanjad S, Tolaymat A, Whitworth J, Levin S. Acute glomerulonephritis in children: a review of 153 cases. *South Med J* 1977;70:1202–1206.
150. Roy SD, Wall HP, Etteldorf JN. Second attacks of acute glomerulonephritis. *J Pediatr* 1969;75:758–767.
151. Rennke H. Secondary membranoproliferative glomerulonephritis. *Kidney Int* 1995;47:643–656.
152. Oldstone MB, Dixon FJ. Immune complex disease in chronic viral infections. *J Exp Med* 1971;134(Suppl):32–40.
153. Blumberg B, Alter H, Visnich S. A "new" antigen in leukemia sera. *JAMA* 1965;191:541–546.
154. Gocke DJ, Hsu K, Morgan C, Bombardieri S, Lockshin M, Christian CL. Association between polyarteritis and Australia antigen. *Lancet* 1970;2:1149–1153.
155. Trepo C, Thivolet J. Hepatitis associated antigen and periarteritis nodosa (PAN). *Vox Sang* 1970;19:410–411.
156. Combes B, Shorey J, Barrera A, et al. Glomerulonephritis with deposition of Australia antigen-antibody complexes in glomerular basement membrane. *Lancet* 1971;2:234–237.
157. Myers BD, Griffel B, Naveh D, Jankielowiiz T, Klajman A. Membranoproliferative glomerulonephritis associated with persistent viral hepatitis. *Am J Clin Pathol* 1973;60:222–228.
158. Levo Y, Gorevic PD, Kassab HJ, Zucker Franklin D, Franklin EC. Association between hepatitis B virus and essential mixed cryoglobulinemia. *N Engl J Med* 1977;296:1501–1504.
159. Levo Y, Gorevic PD, Kassab H, Zucker Franklin D, Gigli I, Franklin EC. Mixed cryoglobulinemia—an immune complex disease often associated with hepatitis B virus infection. *Trans Assoc Am Physicians* 1977;90:167–173.
160. Onion DK, Crumpacker CS, Gilliland BC. Arthritis of hepatitis associated with Australia antigen. *Ann Intern Med* 1971;75:29–33.
161. Alpert E, Isselbacher KJ, Schur PH. The pathogenesis of arthritis associated with viral hepatitis. Complement-component studies. *N Engl J Med* 1971;285:185–189.
162. Duffy J, Lidsky MD, Sharp JT, et al. Polyarthritis, polyarteritis and hepatitis B. *Medicine (Baltimore)* 1976;55:19–37.
163. Johnson RJ, Couser WG. Hepatitis B infection and renal disease: clinical, immunopathogenetic and therapeutic considerations. *Kidney Int* 1990;37:663–676.
164. Reznik VM, Mendoza SA, Self TW, Griswold WR. Hepatitis B-associated vasculitis in an infant. *J Pediatr* 1981;98:252–254.
165. Gocke DJ, Hsu K, Morgan C, Bombardieri S, Lockshin M, Christian CL. Vasculitis in association with Australia antigen. *J Exp Med* 1971; 134(Suppl) (3)p:330
166. Sack M, Cassidy JT, Bole GG. Prognostic factors in polyarteritis. *J Rheumatol* 1975;2:411–420.
167. Ewald EA, Griffin D, McCune WJ. Correlation of angiographic abnormalities with disease manifestations and disease severity in polyarteritis nodosa. *J Rheumatol* 1987;14:952–956.
168. Cohen RD, Conn DL, Ilstrup DM. Clinical features, prognosis, and response to treatment in polyarteritis. *Mayo Clin Proc* 1980;55: 146–155.
169. Fauci AS, Katz P, Haynes BF, Wolff SM. Cyclophosphamide therapy of severe systemic necrotizing vasculitis. *N Engl J Med* 1979;301: 235–238.
170. Scott DG, Bacon PA, Elliott PJ, Tribe CR, Wallington TB. Systemic vasculitis in a district general hospital 1972–1980: clinical and laboratory features, classification and prognosis of 80 cases. *Q J Med* 1982;51:292–311.
171. Travers RL, Allison DJ, Brettle RP, Hughes GR. Polyarteritis nodosa: a clinical and angiographic analysis of 17 cases. *Semin Arthritis Rheum* 1979;8:184–199.
172. Reeves A, Bresnihan B. Clinical features, treatment and outcome of polyarteritis nodosa. *Ir J Med Sci* 1987;156:90–92.
173. Ronco P, Verroust P, Mignon F, et al. Immunopathological studies of polyarteritis nodosa and Wegener's granulomatosis: a report of 43 patients with 51 renal biopsies. *Q J Med* 1983;52:212–223.
174. Trepo CG, Zucherman AJ, Bird RC, Prince AM. The role of circulating hepatitis B antigen/antibody immune complexes in the pathogenesis of vascular and hepatic manifestations in polyarteritis nodosa. *J Clin Pathol* 1974;27:863–868.
175. Marcellin P, Calmus Y, Takahashi H, et al. Latent hepatitis B virus (HBV) infection in systemic necrotizing vasculitis. *Clin Exp Rheumatol* 1991;9:23–28.
176. Budmiger H, Turina J, Streuli R, Bollinger A. Diagnosis and clinical course of periarteritis nodosa [in German]. *Schweiz Med Wochenschr* 1986;116:1634–1639.
177. Popp JW Jr, Harrist TJ, Dienstag JL, et al. Cutaneous vasculitis associated with acute and chronic hepatitis. *Arch Intern Med* 1981;141: 623–629.
178. Wands JR, Mann E, Alpert E, Isselbacher KJ. The pathogenesis of arthritis associated with acute hepatitis-B surface antigen-positive hepatitis. Complement activation and characterization of circulating immune complexes. *J Clin Invest* 1975;55:930–936.
179. Drueke T, Barbanel C, Jungers P, et al. Hepatitis B antigen-associated periarteritis nodosa in patients undergoing long-term hemodialysis. *Am J Med* 1980;68:86–90.
180. Gupta RC, Kohler PF. Identification of HBsAg determinants in immune complexes from hepatitis B virus-associated vasculitis. *J Immunol* 1984;132:1223–1228.
181. Fye KH, Becker MJ, Theofilopoulos AN, Moutsopoulos H, Feldman JL, Talal N. Immune complexes in hepatitis B antigen-associated periarteritis nodosa. Detection by antibody-dependent cell-mediated cytotoxicity and the Raji cell assay. *Am J Med* 1977;62:783–791.
182. Michalak T. Immune complexes of hepatitis B surface antigen in the pathogenesis of periarteritis nodosa. A study of seven necropsy cases. *Am J Pathol* 1978;90:619–632.
183. Nowoslawski A, Krawczynski K, Nazarewicz T, Slusarczyk J. Immunopathological aspects of hepatitis type B. *Am J Med Sci* 1975; 270:229–239.
184. Razzak IA, Bauer W, Itzel W. Hepatitis-B-antigenemia with panarteritis, diffuse proliferative glomerulitis and malignant hypertension. *Am J Gastroenterol* 1975;63:476–480.
185. Heathcote EJ, Dudley FJ, Sherlock S. Association of polyarteritis and Australia antigen. *Gut* 1972;13:319.
186. Trepo C, Thivolet J, Lambert R. Four cases of periarteritis nodosa associated with persistent Australia antigen. *Digestion* 1972;5:100–107.
187. Leung DY, Collins T, Lapierre LA, Geha RS, Pober JS. Immunoglobulin M antibodies present in the acute phase of Kawasaki syndrome lyse cultured vascular endothelial cells stimulated by gamma interferon. *J Clin Invest* 1986;77:1428–1435.
188. Guillevin L, Lhote F, Sauvaget F, et al. Treatment of polyarteritis nodosa related to hepatitis B virus with interferon-alpha and plasma exchanges. *Ann Rheum Dis* 1994;53:334–337.
189. Gerber MA, Brodin A, Steinberg D, Vernace S, Yang CP, Paronetto F. Periarteritis nodosa, Australia antigen and lymphatic leukemia. *N Engl J Med* 1972;286:14–17.
190. Knieser MR, Jenis EH, Lowenthal DT, Bancroft WH, Burns W, Shal-

houb R. Pathogenesis of renal disease associated with viral hepatitis. *Arch Pathol* 1974;97:193–200.

191. Nowoslawski A, Krawczy'nski K, Brzosko WJ, Madali'nski K. Tissue localization of Australia antigen immune complexes in acute and chronic hepatitis and liver cirrhosis. *Am J Pathol* 1972;68: 31–56.
192. Couser WG, Salant DJ. *In situ* immune complex formation and glomerular injury. *Kidney Int* 1980;17:1–13.
193. Cream JJ, Bryceson AD, Ryder G. Disappearance of immunoglobulin and complement from the Arthus reaction and its relevance to studies of vasculitis in man. *Br J Dermatol* 1971;84:106–109.
194. Hart MN, Tassell SK, Sadewasser KL, Schelper RL, Moore SA. Autoimmune vasculitis resulting from in vitro immunization of lymphocytes to smooth muscle. *Am J Pathol* 1985;119:448–455.
195. Dalekos G, Tsianos E. Anti-neutrophil antibodies in chronic viral hepatitis. *J Hepatol* 1994;20:561.
196. Sergent JS, Lockshin MD, Christian CL, Gocke DJ. Vasculitis with hepatitis B antigenemia: long-term observation in nine patients. *Medicine (Baltimore)* 1976;55:1–18.
197. Naber AH, De Vlaam AM, Breed WP. Chronic active hepatitis and periarteritis nodosa in a patient with co-occurrence of circulatory hepatitis Bs antigen and anti-HBs. *Neth J Med* 1986;29:189–191.
198. Fisher RG, Graham DY, Granmayeh M, Trabanino JG. Polyarteritis nodosa and hepatitis-B surface antigen: role of angiography in diagnosis. *AJR Am J Roentgenol* 1977;129:77–81.
199. Gocke DJ. Extrahepatic manifestations of viral hepatitis. *Am J Med Sci* 1975;270:49–52.
200. Stehman-Breen C, Willson R, Alpers CE, Gretch D, Johnson RJ. Hepatitis C virus-associated glomerulonephritis. *Curr Opin Nephrol Hypertens* 1995;4:287–294.
201. Gherardi R, Belec L, Mhiri C, et al. The spectrum of vasculitis in human immunodeficiency virus-infected patients. A clinicopathologic evaluation. *Arthritis Rheum* 1993;36:1164–1174.
202. Rich A. The role of hypersensitivity in periarteritis nodosa as indicated by seven cases developing during serum sickness and sulfonamide therapy. *Bull Johns Hopkins Hosp* 1942;71:123–140.
203. Rich A, Gregory J. The experimental demonstration that periarteritis nodosa is a manifestation of hypersensitivity. *Bull Johns Hopkins Hosp* 1943;72:65–88.
204. Germuth FJ. A comparative histologic and immunologic study in rabbits of induced hypersensitivity of the serum sickness type. *J Exp Med* 1953;97:257–282.
205. Frohnert PP, Sheps SG. Long-term follow-up study of periarteritis nodosa. *Am J Med* 1967;43:8–14.
206. Leib ES, Restivo C, Paulus HE. Immunosuppressive and corticosteroid therapy of polyarteritis nodosa. *Am J Med* 1979;67:941–947.
207. Haubitz M, Frei U, Rother Y, Brunkhorst R, Kock K. Cyclophosphamide pulse therapy in Wegener's granulomatosis. *Nephrol Dial Transplant* 1991;6:531–535.
208. Hoffman G, Leavitt R, Fleisher T, Minor J, Fauci A. Treatment of Wegener's granulomatosis with intermittent high-dose intravenous cyclophosphamide. *Am J Med* 1990;89:403–410.
209. Chalopin JM, Rifle G, Turc JM, Cortet P, Severac M. Immunological findings during successful treatment of HBsAg-associated polyarteritis nodosa by plasmapheresis alone. *Br Med J* 1980;280:368.
210. Thomas HC, Lok AS. The immunopathology of autoimmune and hepatitis B virus-induced chronic hepatitis. *Semin Liver Dis* 1984;4: 36–46.
211. Thomas HC, Lever AM. Has immunology become important to hepatologists? *Prog Liver Dis* 1986;8:179–189.
212. Ikeda T, Lever AM, Thomas HC. Evidence for a deficiency of interferon production in patients with chronic hepatitis B virus infection acquired in adult life. *Hepatology* 1986;6:962–965.
213. Tolentino P, Dianzani F, Zucca M, Giacchino R. Decreased interferon response by lymphocytes from children with chronic hepatitis. *J Infect Dis* 1975;132:459–461.
214. Bryson YJ, Winter HS, Gard SE, Fischer TJ, Stiehm ER. Deficiency of immune interferon production by leukocytes of normal newborns. *Cell Immunol* 1980;55:191–200.
215. Scullard GH, Smith CI, Merigan TC, Robinson WS, Gregory PB. Effects of immunosuppressive therapy on viral markers in chronic active hepatitis B. *Gastroenterology* 1981;81:987–991.
216. Wands JR, Chura CM, Roll FJ, Maddrey WC. Serial studies of hepatitis-associated antigen and antibody in patients receiving antitumor chemotherapy for myeloproliferative and lymphoproliferative disorders. *Gastroenterology* 1975;68:105–112.
217. Nagington J. Reactivation of hepatitis B after transplantation operations. *Lancet* 1977;1:558–560.
218. Parfrey PS, Forbes RD, Hutchinson TA, et al. The impact of renal transplantation on the course of hepatitis B liver disease. *Transplantation* 1985;39:610–615.
219. Harnett JD, Zeldis JB, Parfrey PS, et al. Hepatitis B disease in dialysis and transplant patients. Further epidemiologic and serologic studies. *Transplantation* 1987;44:369–376.
220. Flowers MA, Heathcote J, Wanless IR, et al. Fulminant hepatitis as a consequence of reactivation of hepatitis B virus infection after discontinuation of low-dose methotrexate therapy. *Ann Intern Med* 1990;112:381–382.
221. Hanson CA, Sutherland DE, Snover DC. Fulminant hepatic failure in an HBsAg carrier renal transplant patient following cessation of immunosuppressive therapy. *Transplantation* 1985;39:311–312.
222. Guillevin L, Lhote F, Leon A, Fauvelle F, Vivitski L, Trepo C. Treatment of polyarteritis nodosa related to hepatitis B virus with short term steroid therapy associated with antiviral agents and plasma exchanges. A prospective trial in 33 patients. *J Rheumatol* 1993;20: 289–298.
223. Carreno V, Bartolom'e J, Castillo I. Long-term effect of interferon therapy in chronic hepatitis B. *J Hepatol* 1994;20:431–435.
224. Takekoshi Y, Tanaka M, Shida N, Satake Y, Saheki Y, Matsumoto S. Strong association between membranous nephropathy and hepatitis-B surface antigenaemia in Japanese children. *Lancet* 1978;2:1065–1068.
225. Hsu HC, Lin GH, Chang MH, Chen CH. Association of hepatitis B surface (HBs) antigenemia and membranous nephropathy in children in Taiwan. *Clin Nephrol* 1983;20:121–129.
226. Venkataseshan VS, Lieberman K, Kim DU, et al. Hepatitis B surface antigenemia in North American children with membranous glomerulonephropathy. Southwest Pediatric Nephrology Study Group. *J Pediatr* 1985;106:571–578.
227. Iida H, Izumino K, Asaka M, et al. Membranoproliferative glomerulonephritis associated with chronic hepatitis B in adults: pathogenetic role of HBsAg. *Am J Nephrol* 1987;7:319–324.
228. Lai KN, Lai FM, Lo S, Leung A. Is there a pathogenetic role of hepatitis B virus in lupus nephritis? *Arch Pathol Lab Med* 1987;111: 185–188.
229. Iida H, Izumino K, Asaka M, Fujita M, Takata M, Sasayama S. IgA nephropathy and hepatitis B virus. IgA nephropathy unrelated to hepatitis B surface antigenemia. *Nephron* 1990;54:18–20.
230. Takekoshi Y, Tanaka M, Miyakawa Y, Yoshizawa H, Takahashi K, Mayumi M. Free "small" and IgG-associated "large" hepatitis B e antigen in the serum and glomerular capillary walls of two patients with membranous glomerulonephritis. *N Engl J Med* 1979;300: 814–819.
231. Yoshikawa N, Ito H, Yamada Y, et al. Membranous glomerulonephritis associated with hepatitis B antigen in children: a comparison with idiopathic membranous glomerulonephritis. *Clin Nephrol* 1985;23: 28–34.
232. Lai KN, Li PK, Lui SF, et al. Membranous nephropathy related to hepatitis B virus in adults. *N Engl J Med* 1991;324:1457–1463.
233. Hsu HC, Wu CY, Lin CY, Lin GJ, Chen CH, Huang FY. Membranous nephropathy in 52 hepatitis B surface antigen (HBsAg) carrier children in Taiwan. *Kidney Int* 1989;36:1103–1107.
234. Ito H, Hattori S, Matusda I, et al. Hepatitis B e antigen-mediated membranous glomerulonephritis. Correlation of ultrastructural changes with HBeAg in the serum and glomeruli. *Lab Invest* 1981;44:214–220.
235. Slusarczyk J, Michalak T, Nazarewicz de Mezer T, Krawczy'nski K, Nowoslawski A. Membranous glomerulopathy associated with hepatitis B core antigen immune complexes in children. *Am J Pathol* 1980; 98:29–43.
236. Lai KN, Lai FM, Chan KW, Chow CB, Tong KL, Vallance Owen J. The clinicopathologic features of hepatitis B virus-associated glomerulonephritis. *Q J Med* 1987;63:323–333.
237. Hattori S, Furuse A, Matsuda I. Presence of HBe antibody in glomerular deposits in membranous glomerulonephritis is associated with hepatitis B virus infection. *Am J Nephrol* 1988;8:384–387.
238. Venkataseshan VS, Lieberman K, Kim DU, et al. Hepatitis-B-associated glomerulonephritis: pathology, pathogenesis, and clinical course. *Medicine* 1990;69:200–216.

239. Lew AM, Tovey DG, Steward MW. Localization of covalent immune complexes on the epithelial side of the glomerular basement membrane in mice. *Int Arch Allergy Appl Immunol* 1984;75:242–249.
240. Neurath AR, Strick N. Host specificity of a serum marker for hepatitis B: evidence that "e antigen" has the properties of an immunoglobulin. *Proc Natl Acad Sci U S A* 1977;74:1702–1706.
241. Gregorek H, Jung H, Ulanowicz G, Madali'nski K. Immune complexes in sera of children with HBV-mediated glomerulonephritis. *Arch Immunol Ther Exp (Warsz)* 1986;34:73–83.
242. Ooi BS, Ooi YM, Hsu A, Hurtubise PE. Diminished synthesis of immunoglobulin by peripheral lymphocytes of patients with idiopathic membranous glomerulonephropathy. *J Clin Invest* 1980;65: 789–797.
243. Germuth FG Jr, Senterfit LB, Dreesman GR. Immune complex disease. V. The nature of the circulating complexes associated with glomerular alterations in the chronic BSA-rabbit system. *Johns Hopkins Med J* 1972;130:344–357.
244. Ozawa T, Levisohn P, Orsini E, McIntosh RM. Acute immune complex disease associated with hepatitis. Etiopathogenic and immunopathologic studies of the renal lesion. *Arch Pathol Lab Med* 1976; 100:484–486.
245. Gyorkey F, Hollinger FB, Eknoyan G, et al. Immune-complex glomerulonephritis, intranuclear particles in hepatocytes, and in vivo clearance rates in sub-human primates inoculated with HBs Ag-containing plasma. *Exp Mol Pathol* 1975;22:350–365.
246. Gauthier VJ, Striker GE, Mannik M. Glomerular localization of preformed immune complexes prepared with anionic antibodies or with cationic antigens. *Lab Invest* 1984;50:636–644.
247. Dejean A, Lugassy C, Zafrani S, Tiollais P, Brechot C. Detection of hepatitis B virus DNA in pancreas, kidney and skin of two human carriers of the virus. *J Gen Virol* 1984;65(Pt 3):651–655.
248. Lai KN, Lai FM, Tam JS, Vallance Owen J. Strong association between IgA nephropathy and hepatitis B surface antigenemia in endemic areas. *Clin Nephrol* 1988;29:229–234.
249. Shimoda T, Shikata T, Karasawa T, Tsukagoshi S, Yoshimura M, Sakurai I. Light microscopic localization of hepatitis B virus antigens in the human pancreas. Possibility of multiplication of hepatitis B virus in the human pancreas. *Gastroenterology* 1981;81:998–1005.
250. Yoffe B, Noonan CA, Melnick JL, Hollinger FB. Hepatitis B virus DNA in mononuclear cells and analysis of cell subsets for the presence of replicative intermediates of viral DNA. *J Infect Dis* 1986;153: 471–477.
251. Lin CY. Hepatitis B virus deoxyribonucleic acid in kidney cells probably leading to viral pathogenesis among hepatitis B virus associated membranous nephropathy patients. *Nephron* 1993;63:58–64.
252. Crawford DH, Endre ZH, Axelsen RA, et al. Universal occurrence of glomerular abnormalities in patients receiving liver transplants. *Am J Kidney Dis* 1992;19:339–344.
253. Endo Y, Matsushita H, Nozawa Y, Nishikage S, Matsuya S, Hara M. Glomerulonephritis associated with liver cirrhosis. *Acta Pathol Jpn* 1983;33:333–346.
254. Maggiore Q, Bartolomeo F, L'Abbate A, Misefari V. HBsAg glomerular deposits in glomerulonephritis: fact or artifact? *Kidney Int* 1981; 19:579–586.
255. Slusarczyk J, Michalak T. Antibodies reacting with brush borders of rat kidney tubules in sera from children with chronic hepatitis and chronic glomerulonephritis. *Mater Med Pol* 1984;16:15–17.
256. Reed WD, Stern RB, Eddleston AL, et al. Detection of hepatitis-B antigen by radioimmunoassay in chronic liver disease and hepatocellular carcinoma in Great Britain. *Lancet* 1973;2:690–694.
257. Hirose H, Udo K, Kojima M, et al. Deposition of hepatitis B e antigen in membranous glomerulonephritis: identification by F(ab')2 fragments of monoclonal antibody. *Kidney Int* 1984;26:338–341.
258. Lisker Melman M, Webb D, Di Bisceglie AM, et al. Glomerulonephritis caused by chronic hepatitis B virus infection: treatment with recombinant human alpha-interferon. *Ann Intern Med* 1989;111:479–483.
259. Akano N, Yoshioka K, Aya N, et al. Immunoelectron microscopic localization of membrane attack complex and hepatitis B e antigen in membranous nephropathy. *Virchows Arch A Pathol Anat Histopathol* 1989;414:325–330.
260. Ishihara T, Akamatsu A, Takahashi M, et al. Ultrastructure of kidney from three patients with HBeAg-associated nephropathy with special reference to virus-like particles in the glomerular tufts. *Acta Pathol Jpn* 1988;38:339–350.
261. Moriyama M, Fukuda Y, Ishizaki M, Sugisaki Y, Masugi Y. Membranous glomerulonephritis associated with active liver cirrhosis both involved by HBs antigen. *Acta Pathol Jpn* 1976;26:237–250.
262. Lee HS, Choi Y, Yu SH, Koh HI, Kim MJ, Ko KW. A renal biopsy study of hepatitis B virus-associated nephropathy in Korea. *Kidney Int* 1988;34:537–543.
263. Collins AB, Bhan AK, Dienstag JL, et al. Hepatitis B immune complex glomerulonephritis: simultaneous glomerular deposition of hepatitis B surface and e antigens. *Clin Immunol Immunopathol* 1983;26: 137–153.
264. Amemiya S, Ito H, Kato K, Sakaguchi H, Hasegawa O, Hajikano H. A case of membranous proliferative glomerulonephritis type III (Burkholder) with the deposition of both HBeAg and HBsAg. *Int J Pediatr Nephrol* 1983;4:267–273.
265. Wyszy'nska T, Jung H, Madali'nski K, Morzycka M. Hepatitis B mediated glomerulonephritis in children. *Int J Pediatr Nephrol* 1984; 5:147–158.
266. Furuse A, Hattori S, Terashima T, Karashima S, Matsuda I. Circulating immune complex in glomerulonephropathy associated with hepatitis B virus infection. *Nephron* 1982;31:212–218.
267. Wong SN, Yu EC, Chan KW. Hepatitis B virus associated membranous glomerulonephritis in children—experience in Hong Kong. *Clin Nephrol* 1993;40:142–147.
268. Whittingham S, Mackay IR, Irwin J. Autoimmune hepatitis. Immunofluorescence reactions with cytoplasm of smooth muscle and renal glomerular cells. *Lancet* 1966;1:1333–1335.
269. Penner E. Nature of immune complexes in autoimmune chronic active hepatitis. *Gastroenterology* 1987;92:304–308.
270. Lai KN, Lai FM, Tam JS. IgA nephropathy associated with chronic hepatitis B virus infection in adults: the pathogenetic role of HBsAg. *J Pathol* 1989;157:321–327.
271. Looi LM, Prathap K. Hepatitis B virus surface antigen in glomerular immune complex deposits of patients with systemic lupus erythematosus. *Histopathology* 1982;6:141–147.
272. Lai KN, Lai FM, Lo S, Ho CP, Chan KW. IgA nephropathy associated with hepatitis B virus antigenemia. *Nephron* 1987;47:141–143.
273. Nammalwar BR, Sankar VS, Ramesh S, Thiagarajan SP, Subramaniam S. Hepatitis B virus infection and glomerulonephritis. *Indian J Pediatr* 1987;54:7597–7663.
274. Lai KN, Lai FM, Lo ST, Lam CW. IgA nephropathy and membranous nephropathy associated with hepatitis B surface antigenemia. *Hum Pathol* 1987;18:411–414.
275. Brzosko WJ, Krawczy'nski K, Nazarewicz T, Morzycka M, Nowoslawski A. Glomerulonephritis associated with hepatitis-B surface antigen immune complexes in children. *Lancet* 1974;2:477–482.
276. Kleinknecht C, Levy M, Peix A, Broyer M, Courtecuisse V. Membranous glomerulonephritis and hepatitis B surface antigen in children. *J Pediatr* 1979;95:946–952.
277. Cadrobbi P, Bortolotti F, Zacchello G, Rinaldi R, Armigliato M, Realdi G. Hepatitis B virus replication in acute glomerulonephritis with chronic active hepatitis. *Arch Dis Child* 1985;60:583–585.
278. Knecht GL, Chisari FV. Reversibility of hepatitis B virus-induced glomerulonephritis and chronic active hepatitis after spontaneous clearance of serum hepatitis B surface antigen. *Gastroenterology* 1978;75:1152–1156.
279. Lai KN, Tam JS, Lin HJ, Lai FM. The therapeutic dilemma of the usage of corticosteroid in patients with membranous nephropathy and persistent hepatitis B virus surface antigenaemia. *Nephron* 1990;54: 12–17.
280. de Man RA, Schalm SW, van der Heijden AJ, ten Kate FW, Wolff ED, Heijtink RA. Improvement of hepatitis B-associated glomerulonephritis after antiviral combination therapy. *J Hepatol* 1989;8: 367–372.
281. Garcia G, Scullard G, Smith C, et al. Preliminary observation of hepatitis B-associated membranous glomerulonephritis treated with leukocyte interferon. *Hepatology* 1985;5:317–320.
282. Conjeevaram HS, Hoofnagle JH, Austin HA, Park Y, Fried MW, Di Bisceglie AM. Long-term outcome of hepatitis B virus-related glomerulonephritis after therapy with interferon alfa. *Gastroenterology* 1995;109:540–546.
283. Lin C-Y. Treatment of hepatitis B virus-associated membranous nephropathy with recombinant alpha-interferon. *Kidney Int* 1995;47: 225–230.
284. Lin CY, Lo SC. Treatment of hepatitis B virus-associated membra-

nous nephropathy with adenine arabinoside and thymic extract. *Kidney Int* 1991;39:301–306.

285. Esteban R, Buti M, Vall'es M, Allende H, Guardia J. Hepatitis B-associated membranous glomerulonephritis treated with adenine arabinoside monophosphate [Letter]. *Hepatology* 1986;6:762–763.
286. Garcia G, Smith CI, Weissberg JI, et al. Adenine arabinoside monophosphate (vidarabine phosphate) in combination with human leukocyte interferon in the treatment of chronic hepatitis B. A randomized, double-blinded, placebo-controlled trial. *Ann Intern Med* 1987;107:278–285.
287. Choo QL, Kuo G, Weiner AJ, Overby LR, Bradley DW, Houghton M. Isolation of a cDNA clone derived from a blood-borne non-A, non-B viral hepatitis genome. *Science* 1989;244:359–362.
288. Esteban J, Genesca J, Alter H. Hepatitis C: molecular biology, pathogenesis, epidemiology, clinical features, and prevention. In: Boyer J, Ockner R, eds. *Progress in Liver Disease*; vol X. New York: WB Saunders; 1992:235–282.
289. Gretch D, Corey L, Wilson J, et al. Assessment of hepatitis C virus RNA levels by quantitative competitive RNA polymerase chain reaction: high-titer viremia correlates with advanced stage of disease. *J Infect Dis* 1994;169:1219–1225.
290. Hijikata M, Shimizu YK, Kato H, et al. Equilibrium centrifugation studies of hepatitis C virus: evidence for circulating immune complexes. *J Virol* 1993;67:1953–1958.
291. Itoh K, Tanaka H, Shiga J, et al. Hypocomplementemia associated with hepatitis C viremia in sera from voluntary blood donors. *Am J Gastroenterol* 1994;89:2019–2024.
292. Pawlotsky JM, Ben Yahia M, Andre C, et al. Immunological disorders in C virus chronic active hepatitis: a prospective case-control study (see Comments). *Hepatology* 1994;19:841–848.
293. Tanaka K, Aiyama T, Imai J, Morishita Y, Fukatsu T, Kakumu S. Serum cryoglobulin and chronic hepatitis C virus disease among Japanese patients. *Am J Gastroenterol* 1995;90:1847–1852.
294. Lunel F, Musset L, Cacoub P. Cryoglobulinemia in chronic liver diseases: role of hepatitis C virus and liver damage. *Gastroenterology* 1994;106:1291–1300.
295. Gumber SC, Chopra S. Hepatitis C: a multifaceted disease. Review of extrahepatic manifestations. *Ann Intern Med* 1995;123:615–620.
296. D'Amico G, Fornasieri A. Cryoglobulinemic glomerulonephritis: a membranoproliferative glomerulonephritis induced by hepatitis C virus. *Am J Kidney Dis* 1995;25:361–369.
297. Johnson R, Willson R, Yamabe H, et al. Renal manifestations of hepatitis C virus infection. *Kidney Int* 1994;46:1255–1263.
298. Johnson RJ, Gretch DR, Yamabe H, et al. Membranoproliferative glomerulonephritis associated with hepatitis C virus infection (see Comments). *N Engl J Med* 1993;328:465–470.
299. Johnson RJ, Gretch DR, Couser WG, et al. Hepatitis C virus-associated glomerulonephritis. Effect of alpha-interferon therapy. *Kidney Int* 1994;46:1700–1704.
300. Misiani R, Bellavita P, Fenili D, et al. Hepatitis C virus infection in patients with essential mixed cryoglobulinemia. *Ann Intern Med* 1992;117:573–577.
301. Davda R, Peterson J, Weiner R, Croker B, Lau JY. Membranous glomerulonephritis in association with hepatitis C virus infection. *Am J Kidney Dis* 1993;22:452–455.
302. Rollino C, Roccatello D, Giachino O, Basolo B, Piccoli G. Hepatitis C virus infection and membranous glomerulonephritis [Letter]. *Nephron* 1991;59:319–320.
303. Pasquariello A, Ferri C, Moriconi L, et al. Cryoglobulinemic membranoproliferative glomerulonephritis associated with hepatitis C virus [Letter]. *Am J Nephrol* 1993;13:300–304.
304. Horikoshi S, Okada T, Shirato I, et al. Diffuse proliferative glomerulonephritis with hepatitis C virus-like particles in paramesangial dense deposits in a patient with chronic hepatitis C virus hepatitis. *Nephron* 1993;64:462–464.
305. Wener M, Johnson R, Sasso E, Gretch D. Hepatitis C virus and rheumatic disease—an editorial review. *J Rheumatol* 1996;23:953–959.
306. D' Amico G. Is type II mixed cryoglobulinaemia an essential part of hepatitis C virus (HCV)-associated glomerulonephritis? (Editorial). *Nephrol Dial Transplant* 1995;10:1279–1282.
307. Druet P, Letonturier P, Contet A, Mandet C. Cryoglobulinaemia in human renal diseases. A study of seventy-six cases. *Clin Exp Immunol* 1973;15:483–496.
308. Agnello V, Chung RT, Kaplan LM. A role for hepatitis C virus infection in type II cryoglobulinemia (see Comments). *N Engl J Med* 1992; 327:1490–1495.
309. Levo Y, Gorevic PD, Kassab HJ, Zucker Franklin D, Franklin EC. Association between hepatitis B virus and essential mixed cryoglobulinemia. *N Engl J Med* 1977;296:1501–1504.
310. Levo Y, Gorevic PD, Kassab H, Zucker Franklin D, Gigli I, Franklin EC. Mixed cryoglobulinemia—an immune complex disease often associated with hepatitis B virus infection. *Trans Assoc Am Physicians* 1977;90:167–173.
311. Gorevic PD, Kassab HJ, Levo Y, et al. Mixed cryoglobulinemia: clinical aspects and long-term follow-up of 40 patients. *Am J Med* 1980; 69:287–308.
312. Harl'e JR, Disdier P, Dussol B, Bolla G, Casanova P, Weiller PJ. Membranoproliferative glomerulonephritis and hepatitis C infection (Letter; Comment). *Lancet* 1993;341:904.
313. Gonzalo A, Bárcena R, Mampaso F, Zea A, Ortuno J. Membranoproliferative glomerulonephritis and hepatitis C virus infection (Letter) (see Comments). *Nephron* 1993;63:475–476.
314. Ramos A, Vinhas J, Carvalho MF. Mixed cryoglobulinemia in a heroin addict. *Am J Kidney Dis* 1994;23:731–734.
315. Biesemier K, Jethwa VS, Falk R, Folds J, Jennette J. Prevalence of antibodies to hepatitis C in patients with glomerular disease. *Lab Invest* 1994;70:157A.
316. Yamabe H, Johnson RJ, Gretch DR, et al. Hepatitis C virus infection and membranoproliferative glomerulonephritis in Japan. *J Am Soc Nephrol* 1995;6:220–223.
317. Lai FM, Tam JS, Liew CT, Ip M, Lai KN. Low prevalence of hepatitis C virus antibodies with primary membranous nephropathy and membranoproliferative glomerulonephritis in Hong Kong [Letter]. *Nephron* 1995;70:367–368.
318. Rostoker G, Deforges L, Ben Maadi A, et al. Low prevalence of antibodies to hepatitis C virus among adult patients with idiopathic membranoproliferative type I glomerulonephritis in France [Letter]. *Nephron* 1995;69:97.
319. Nowicki MJ, Welch TR, Ahmad N, et al. Absence of hepatitis B and C viruses in pediatric idiopathic membranoproliferative glomerulonephritis. *Pediatr Nephrol* 1995;9:16–18.
320. Gorevic PD, Frangione B. Mixed cryoglobulinemia cross-reactive idiotypes: implications for the relationship of MC to rheumatic and lymphoproliferative diseases. *Semin Hematol* 1991;28:79–94.
321. Knight GB, Agnello V, Bonagura V, Barnes JL, Panka DJ, Zhang QX. Human rheumatoid factor cross-idiotypes. IV. Studies on WA XId-positive IgM without rheumatoid factor activity provide evidence that the WA XId is not unique to rheumatoid factors and is distinct from the 17.109 and G6 XIds. *J Exp Med* 1993;178:1903–1911.
322. Abel G, Zhang QX, Agnello V. Hepatitis C virus infection in type II mixed cryoglobulinemia. *Arthritis Rheum* 1993;36:1341–1349.
323. Ferri C, Monti M, La Civita L, et al. Infection of peripheral blood mononuclear cells by hepatitis C virus in mixed cryoglobulinemia. *Blood* 1993;82:3701–3704.
324. Michel G, Ritter A, Gerken G, Meyer Zum Buschenfelse K-H, Decker R, Manns M. Anti-GOR and hepatitis C virus in autoimmune liver diseases. *Lancet* 1992;339:267–269.
325. Dalekos GN, Tsianos EV. Anti-neutrophil antibodies in chronic viral hepatitis [Letter]. *J Hepatol* 1994;20:561.
326. Ferri C, Longombardo G, La Civita L, et al. Hepatitis C virus chronic infection as a common cause of mixed cryoglobulinaemia and autoimmune liver disease. *J Intern Med* 1994;236:31–36.
327. Geltner D, Franklin E, Frangione B. Anti-idiotypic activity in the IgM fractions of mixed cryoglobulins. *J Immunol* 1980;125:1530–1535.
328. Sansonno D, Cornacchiulo V, Iacobelli AR, Di Stefano R, Lospalluti M, Dammacco F. Localization of hepatitis C virus antigens in liver and skin tissues of chronic hepatitis C virus-infected patients with mixed cryoglobulinemia. *Hepatology* 1995;21:305–312.
329. Yamabe H, Inuma H, Osawa H, et al. Glomerular deposition of hepatitis C virus in membranoproliferative glomerulonephritis. *Nephron* 1996;72–741.
330. Sansonno D, Gesualdo L, Manno C, Schena F, Dammaco F. Localization of HCV antigens (AGS) in renal tissue of HCV-infected patients with cryoglobulinemic mesangiocapillary glomerulonephritis (MCGN): an immunohistochemical study. *J Am Soc Nephrol* 1995; 5:431.
331. Davis C, Gretch D, Perkins J, et al. Hepatitis C-associated glomerular

disease in liver transplant recipients. *Liver Transpl Surg* 1995;1: 166–175.
332. Cochrane CG. Mediation of immunologic glomerular injury. *Transplant Proc* 1969;1:949–958.
333. Roccatello D, Isidoro C, Mazzucco G, et al. Role of monocytes in cryoglobulinemia-associated nephritis. *Kidney Int* 1993;43:1150–1155.
334. Johnson RJ, Lovett D, Lehrer RI, Couser WG, Klebanoff SJ. Role of oxidants and proteases in glomerular injury. *Kidney Int* 1994;45: 352–359.
335. Fornasieri A, Li M, Armelloni S, et al. Glomerulonephritis induced by human IgMK-IgG cryoglobulins in mice. *Lab Invest* 1993;69: 531–540.
336. Fornasieri A, Armelloni S, Bernasconi P, et al. High binding of immunoglobulin M rheumatoid factor from type II cryoglobulins to cellular fibronectin: a mechanism for induction of *in situ* immune complex glomerulonephritis? *Am J Kidney Dis* 1996;27:476–483.
337. Alpers CE, Hudkins KL, Pritzl P, Johnson RJ. Mechanisms of clearance of immune complexes from peritubular capillaries in the rat. *Am J Pathol* 1991;139:855–867.
338. Dolcher MP, Marchini B, Sabbatini A, et al. Autoantibodies from mixed cryoglobulinaemia patients bind glomerular antigens. *Clin Exp Immunol* 1994;96:317–322.
339. Mazzaro C, Tulissi P, Moretti M, et al. Clinical and virological findings in mixed cryoglobulinaemia. *J Intern Med* 1995;238:153–160.
340. Cruzado J, Gil-Vernet S, Ercilla G, et al. Hepatitis C virus associated membranoproliferative glomerulonephritis in renal allografts. *J Am Soc Nephrol* 1996 [*in press*].
341. Willems M, Sheng L, Roskams T, et al. Hepatitis C virus and its genotypes in patients suffering from chronic hepatitis C with or without a cryoglobulinemia-related syndrome. *J Med Virol* 1994; 44:266–271.
342. Pawlotsky JM, Roudot Thoraval F, Simmonds P, et al. Extrahepatic immunologic manifestations in chronic hepatitis C and hepatitis C virus serotypes. *Ann Intern Med* 1995;122:169–173.
343. Zignego AL, Ferri C, Giannini C, et al. Hepatitis C virus genotype analysis in patients with type II mixed cryoglobulinemia. *Ann Intern Med* 1996;124(1 Pt 1):31–34.
344. Sechi LA, Pirisi M, Bartoli E. Membranoproliferative glomerulonephritis associated with hepatitis C infection with no evidence of liver disease [Letter]. *JAMA* 1994;271:194.
345. Stehman-Breen C, Alpers C, Couser W, Willson R, Johnson R. Hepatitis C virus associated membranous glomerulonephritis. *Clin Nephrol* 1995;44:141–147.
346. Okada K, Takishita Y, Shimomura H, et al. Detection of hepatitis C virus core protein in the glomeruli of patients with membranous glomerulonephritis. *Clin Nephrol* 1996;45:71–76.
347. Gonzalo A, Navarro J, Bárcena R, Quereda C, Ortuno J. IgA nephropathy associated with hepatitis C virus infection [Letter]. *Nephron* 1995;69:354.
348. Roth D, Cirocco R, Zucker K, et al. *De novo* membranoproliferative glomerulonephritis in hepatitis C virus-infected renal allograft recipients. *Transplantation* 1995;59:1676–1682.
349. Gallay BJ, Alpers CE, Davis CL, Schultz MF, Johnson RJ. Glomerulonephritis in renal allografts associated with hepatitis C infection: a possible relationship with transplant glomerulopathy in two cases. *Am J Kidney Dis* 1995;26:662–667.
350. Burstein DM, Rodby RA. Membranoproliferative glomerulonephritis associated with hepatitis C virus infection. *J Am Soc Nephrol* 1993;4: 1288–1293.
351. Morales, JM, Fernandez-Zatarain G, Muñoz MA, et al. Clinical picture and outcome of allograft membranous glomerulonephritis in renal transplant patients with hepatitis C virus infection. *JASN,* 1995; 1106(abs).
352. Poynard T, Bedossa P, Chevallier M, et al. A comparison of three interferon alfa-2b regimens for the long-term treatment of chronic non-A, non-B hepatitis. Multicenter Study Group (see Comments). *N Engl J Med* 1995;332:1457–1462.
353. Casato M, Lagana B, Antonelli G, Dianzani F, Bonomo L. Long-term results of therapy with interferon-alpha for type II essential mixed cryoglobulinemia. *Blood* 1991;78:3142–3147.
354. Ferri C, Marzo E, Longombardo G, et al. Interferon-alpha in mixed cryoglobulinemia patients: a randomized, crossover-controlled trial. *Blood* 1993;81:1132–1136.
355. Misiani R, Bellavita P, Fenili D, et al. Interferon alfa-2a therapy in cryoglobulinemia associated with hepatitis C virus (see Comments). *N Engl J Med* 1994;330:751–756.
356. Dammacco F, Sansonno D, Han JH, et al. Natural interferon-alpha versus its combination with 6-methyl-prednisolone in the therapy of type II mixed cryoglobulinemia: a long-term, randomized, controlled study. *Blood* 1994;84:3336–3343.
357. Yamabe H, Johnson RJ, Gretch DR, et al. Membranoproliferative glomerulonephritis associated with hepatitis C virus infection responsive to interferon-alpha. *Am J Kidney Dis* 1995;25:67–69.
358. Jouet P, Roudot Thoraval F, Dhumeaux D, Métreau JM. Comparative efficacy of interferon alfa in cirrhotic and noncirrhotic patients with non-A, non-B, C hepatitis. Le Groupe Francais pour l'étude du Traitement des Hépatites Chroniques NANB/C. *Gastroenterology* 1994;106:686–690.
359. De Vecchi A, Montagnino G, Pozzi C, Tarantino A, Locatelli F, Ponticelli C. Intravenous methylprednisolone pulse therapy in essential mixed cryoglobulinemia nephropathy. *Clin Nephrol* 1983;19:221–227.
360. Quigg RJ, Brathwaite M, Gardner DF, Gretch DR, Ruddy S. Successful cyclophosphamide treatment of cryoglobulinemic membranoproliferative glomerulonephritis associated with hepatitis C virus infection. *Am J Kidney Dis* 1995;25:798–800.
361. Fong TL, Valinluck B, Govindarajan S, Charboneau F, Adkins RH, Redeker AG. Short-term prednisone therapy affects aminotransferase activity and hepatitis C virus RNA levels in chronic hepatitis C. *Gastroenterology* 1994;107:196–199.
362. Gretch DR, Bacchi CE, Corey L, et al. Persistent hepatitis C virus infection after liver transplantation: clinical and virological features. *Hepatology* 1995;22:1–9.
363. Richardson W, Colvin R, Cheeseman S, et al. Glomerulopathy associated with cytomegalovirus viremia in renal allografts. *N Engl J Med* 1981;305:57–63.
364. Herrera G, Alexander R, Cooley C, et al. Cytomegalovirus glomerulopathy: a controversial lesion. *Kidney Int* 1986;29:725–733.
365. Gregory M, Hammond M, Brewer E. Renal deposition of cytomegalovirus antigen in immunoglobulin-A nephropathy. *Lancet* 1988;1:11–14.
366. Waldo F, Britt W, Tomana M, Julian B, Mestecky J. Non-specific mesangial staining with antibodies against cytomegalovirus in immunoglobulin-A nephropathy. *Lancet* 1989;1:129–131.
367. Park J, Song J, Yang W, Kim S, Kim Y, Hong C. Cytomegalovirus is not specifically associated with immunoglobulin A nephropathy. *J Am Soc Nephrol* 1994;4:1623–1626.
368. Ozawa T, Stewart J. Immune-complex glomerulonephritis associated with cytomegalovirus infection. *Am J Clin Pathol* 1979;72: 103–107.
369. Beneck D, Greco M, Feiner H. Glomerulonephritis in congenital cytomegalic inclusion disease. *Hum Pathol* 1986;17:1054–1059.
370. Zikos D, Grewal K, Craig K, Cheng J-C, Peterson D, Fisher K. Nephrotic syndrome and acute renal failure associated with hepatitis A virus infection. *Am J Gastroenterol* 1995;90:295–298.
371. Barsoum R. Schistosomal glomerulopathies. *Kidney Int* 1993;44:1–12.
372. Lambertucci J, Godoy P, Neves J, Bambirra E, das Dores Ferreira M. Glomerulonephritis in *Salmonella-Schistosoma mansoni* association. *Am J Trop Med Hyg* 1988;30:97–102.
373. Sobh M, Moustafa F, El-Housseini F, Basta M, Deelder A, Ghoniem M. Schistosomal specific nephropathy leading to end-stage renal failure. *Kidney Int* 1987;31:1006–1011.
374. Martinelli R, Noblat A, Brito E, Rocha H. *Schistosoma mansoni*-induced mesangiocapillary glomerulonephritis: influence of therapy. *Kidney Int* 1989;35:1227–1233.
375. Sobh M, Moustafa F, Sally S, Deelder A, Ghoniem M. Effect of anti-schistosomal treatment on schistosomal-specific nephropathy. *Nephrol Dial Transplant* 1988;3:744–751.
376. Azevedo L, de Paula F, Ianhez L, Saldanha L, Sabbaga E. Renal transplantation and schistosomiasis mansoni. *Transplantation* 1987; 44:795–798.
377. Eknoyan G, Dillman R. Renal complications of infectious diseases. *Med Clin North Am* 1978;52:979–1003.
378. Chugh K, Sakhuja V. Glomerular diseases in the tropics. *Am J Nephrol* 1990;10:437–450.
379. White R. Quartan malarial nephrotic syndrome. *Nephron* 1973;11: 147–162.
380. Morel-Maroger L, Saimot A, Sloper J, et al. "Tropical nephropathy"

and "tropical extramembranous glomerulonephritis" of unknown aetiology in Senegal. *Br Med J* 1975;1:541–546.
381. Abdurrahman M, Aikhionbare H, Babaoye F, Sathiakumar N, Narayana P. Clinicopathological features of childhood nephrotic syndrome in northern Nigeria. *Q J Med* 1990;75:563–576.
382. Shahin B, Papadopoulou Z, Jenis E. Congenital nephrotic syndrome associated with congenital toxoplasmosis. *J Pediatr* 1974;85:336–370.
383. Disdier P, Harle J-R, Weiller P-J. Cryoglobulinemia and hepatitis C infection. *Lancet* 1991;338:1151–1152.
384. Ferri C, Greco F, Longombardo G, et al. Antibodies to hepatitis C virus in patients with mixed cryoglobulinemia. *Arthritis Rheum* 1991; 34:1606–1610.
385. Ferri C, Greco F, Longombardo G, et al. Antibodies against hepatitis C virus in mixed cryoglobulinemia patients. *Infection* 1991;19:417–420.
386. Casato M, Pucillo L, Lagana B, Taliani G, Goffredo F, Bonomo L. Cryoglobulinaemia and hepatitis C virus. *Lancet* 1991;337:1047–1048.
387. Galli M, Monti G, Monteverde A, et al. Hepatitis C virus and mixed cryoglobulinaemias. *Lancet* 1992;339:989.
388. Pechere-Bertschi A, Perrin L, de Saussure P, Widmann J, Giostra E, Schifferli J. Hepatitis C: a possible etiology for cryoglobulinaemia type II. *Clin Exp Immunol* 1992;89:419–422.
389. Bichard P, Ounanian A, Girard M, et al. High prevalence of hepatitis C virus RNA in the supernatant and the cryoprecipitate of patients with essential and secondary type II mixed cryoglobulinemia. *J Hepatol* 1994;21:53–63.
390. Cacoub P, Fabiani F, Musset L, et al. Mixed cryoglobulinemia and hepatitis C virus. *Am J Med* 1994;96:124–132.

Immunologic Renal Diseases,
edited by E. G. Neilson and W. G. Couser.
Lippincott-Raven Publishers, Philadelphia © 1997.

CHAPTER 42

Immunoglobulin A Nephropathy

Leendert A. van Es

Immunoglobulin (Ig)A nephropathy is the most common type of glomerulonephritis in large parts of the world (1). It is characterized by the deposition of IgA in the mesangial area of the glomeruli. The histology may vary from mild mesangial proliferation to severe crescentic glomerulonephritis. Clinically it is characterized by asymptomatic hematuria, followed several years later by proteinuria, hypertension, and reduction of the glomerular filtration rate (GFR). Deposits of IgA in the wall of extrarenal vessels may occur, but the presence of leukocytoclastic vasculitis is more suggestive for anaphylactoid purpura or Schönlein-Henoch syndrome. Mesangial deposition of IgA also may occur in systemic lupus erythematosus and in alcoholic liver disease; in order to establish the diagnosis of IgA nephropathy, these conditions should be excluded.

IgA nephropathy was first described by Berger (2) after the introduction of the immunofluorescence technique in the mid-1950s. The disease was discovered relatively late because hematuria without any other renal manifestations was not interpreted as a major clinical problem. The disease received more attention in the early 1980s when long-term follow-up data illustrated that most patients with IgA nephropathy have a slow indolent course to terminal renal failure (1). It subsequently became clear that the low prevalence of IgA nephropathy in certain parts of the world could be attributed to a restrictive policy with regard to renal biopsies in this disease (3). Because no effective therapy is yet known, most clinicians in the United States feel that taking a renal biopsy of a patient with isolated hematuria represents an aggressive diagnostic procedure without therapeutic consequences. For this reason IgA nephropathy has been studied more extensively in areas where renal biopsies are performed more regularly, such as in Europe and Asia (Table 1). When it was realized that IgA nephropathy is the most common type of glomerulonephritis, at least in more affluent parts of the world (1), the scientific interest in IgA nephropathy gained considerable momentum. The progress made in the past decade has not only provided more insight into the pathogenesis of the disease, but it also may foster a perspective that will lead to new therapeutic approaches.

IgA nephropathy has been reported to be associated with other diseases such as ankylosing spondylitis (4), celiac disease (5), dermatitis herpetiformis (6), and many other conditions (Table 2). It is not known what the common denominator is among these diseases that could explain the development of IgA nephropathy. When no other diseases are present, the diagnosis of primary IgA nephropathy or Berger's disease is established.

HISTOPATHOLOGY

The glomerular lesions described in renal biopsy samples of patients with IgA nephropathy can vary from mild mesangial or local and segmental intracapillary proliferation or mesangioproliferative glomerulonephritis to moderate or severe intra- and extracapillary proliferative lesions, including crescent formation (7).

Biopsy samples taken at an early stage of the disease with mild mesangial lesions show few polymorphonuclear cells and mononuclear cells in the glomeruli (8). However, when the glomerular lesions in the mesangium and capillaries are more severe, numerous mononuclear cells can be found in the mesangium and in Bowman's space (9). The number of macrophages in the glomeruli correlates with the presence of crescents and proteinuria (10). The crescents usually are not circumferential. In crescentic IgA nephropathy, not only macrophages, but T cells can be detected in the glomeruli. On the basis of the elevated expression of the receptor for interleukin-2 (IL-2), it is assumed that these lymphocytes are activated. Biopsy samples with crescentic IgA nephropathy show

L.A. van Es: Department of Nephrology, Leiden University Hospital, Leiden, The Netherlands.

TABLE 1. *Prevalence of IgA nephropathy*

Country	Percentage of glomerulonephritis		Percentage of biopsy samples	
	Average	Range	Average	Range
Singapore	51.6	47–56.2	44.2	33.7–52
Japan	41.2	30–46	26.3	11.9–35
Australia	29.5	18–41	12	12
United States	12.3	9.5–17.5	3.5	1.5–6.0
Canada	8.4	8.4	4.9	4.5–9.5
Finland	24	24	17.4	14–20.8
United Kingdom	24.3	18.1–31	10.5	4–16.8
France	27.8	20–49	15.4	7.8–20
Italy	26.9	17.5–45	13.3	13.3

Modified with permission (17).

more activated T-lymphocytes than are found in noncrescentic biopsy samples (9).

When IgA nephropathy progresses, tubulointerstitial changes develop. Mononuclear cells appear in the interstitium. These cells consist of macrophages and CD4- or CD8-positive lymphocytes (9). These data suggest that lymphocytes and macrophages may play a role in the pathogenesis of the glomerular and tubulointerstitial changes. Biopsy samples taken in more advanced stages of the disease are characterized by infiltration by mononuclear cells, tubular atrophy, and interstitial fibrosis, leading to widening of the interstitial space. The width of the cortical interstitium correlates with the serum creatinine level (7).

TABLE 2. *Diseases reported in association with IgA nephropathy*

Diseases
Rheumatic diseases
Ankylosing spondylitis
Rheumatoid arthritis
Gastrointestinal diseases
Celiac disease
Ulcerative colitis
Crohn's disease
Hepatic diseases
Hepatic cirrhosis
Alcoholic liver disease
Dermatologic diseases
Reiter's syndrome
Dermatitis herpetiformis
Psoriasis
Neoplastic diseases
Mycosis fungoides
Sézary syndrome
Bronchial carcinoma
Laryngeal carcinoma
IgA monoclonal gammopathy
Unclassified
Idiopathic pulmonary hemosiderosis
Retroperitoneal sclerosis
Sarcoidosis
Properdine deficiency
Diabetes

Immunofluorescence studies have shown that IgG and C3 are most commonly found in association with IgA. Biopsy samples with moderate to severe glomerular lesions do not show a higher percentage of IgG deposition than do biopsy samples with mild or minimal glomerular changes (11). IgM also can be present but is less common than IgG (12). C3 is frequently accompanied by properdin. However, complement components of the classical pathway are uncommon. The IgA deposits consist mainly of the IgA1 subclass with predominance of the light chain. Although J chain also may be associated with IgM, the presence of J chain strongly suggest that at least part of the IgA deposits if not all consist of polymeric IgA1 (pIgA1) (13). These deposits are frequently accompanied by components of the alternative pathway and the terminal sequence of the membrane attack complex (14).

Ultrastructurally all biopsy samples show deposits in the mesangium. By immunoelectron microscopy, IgA, IgG, IgM, and C3 can be detected between mesangial cells (15). Occasionally smaller masses of IgA and C3 can be observed along the peripheral glomerular capillary loops, the tubular basement membrane and within the interstitial matrix (15). The IgA deposits found in the capillary loops are usually localized in a subendothelial position, but they also can be intramembranous or subepithelial (1,12). Thinning and splitting of the lamina densa can be seen occasionally.

CLINICAL PRESENTATION

Patients with IgA nephropathy are usually young men who have asymptomatic microscopic hematuria (Table 3).

TABLE 3. *Clinical features of IgA nephropathy at presentation*

Clinical feature		Prevalence (%) Mean	Range
Age		30.4 yr	19–42 yr
Male/female ratio		2.16	1.1–10.3
Loin pain		31%	7–37%
Family history		11%	3–20%
Microscopic hematuria		87.5%	53–100%
Macroscopic hematuria		42.7%	5–87%
Infection-related exacerbations		40.7%	10–69%
Proteinuria	1–3 g/24 h	46.8%	18–81%
	>3 g/24 h	10.8%	0–38%
Hypertension		25.2%	7–52%
Reduced GFR		20.7%	5–38%

Modified with permission (17).

About 40% have recurrent macroscopic hematuria frequently preceded 1 or 2 days earlier by infections. Upper airway infections occur most frequently, but other infections also have been implicated, including urinary tract infections and mastitis (16). Loin pain can be present at presentation in about 30% of cases. A family history of glomerulonephritis or IgA nephropathy occurs in a minority of cases. Mild proteinuria is not uncommon, whereas heavy proteinuria is only present in a few cases. Proteinuria frequently antedates hypertension and the insidious but progressive loss of renal function (17).

Natural History of the Disease

Spontaneous remission has been documented in children and in adults. Of the 38% of Japanese children who were in clinical remission, very few had histological lesions in the repeat biopsy specimen (18). Clinical remission also may occur in 6% to 12% of adults with IgA nephropathy, but without histological improvement (17,19).

Patients with recurrent attacks of macroscopic hematuria frequently have an upper airway infection or other mucosal infections 1 or 2 days earlier (19). The urinary sediment of these patients also may show leukocyturia with a negative urine culture (17). Macroscopic hematuria occurs more often in children than in adults (1). Its prevalence varies with geographical areas: lower in Asia and Northern Europe and higher in Southern Europe and Australia (1,19). The long-term prognosis of children and adults with infection-related and recurrent macroscopic hematuria is more favorable (1,19,20). Patients with macroscopic hematuria and a significant increase of their serum creatinine frequently have intra- and extracapillary lesions with crescent formation in their biopsy samples (21). Patients can even develop acute renal failure either on the basis of crescentic glomerulonephritis or on the basis of renal tubular obstruction by red blood cell casts (22).

In the majority of patients, the disease has an indolent course manifested by chronic or intermittent microscopic hematuria. Because it may remain undetected for many years, it is difficult to establish the onset of the disease. It has been detected by periodic screening of Japanese school children at a young age, but in European studies it is usually detected in adults in their twenties or thirties (1). When biopsy samples of adults are compared with biopsy samples of children, the prevalence of tubulointerstitial changes is not higher, suggesting that not all cases of IgA nephropathy start at an early age.

In the course of IgA nephropathy, attacks of gross hematuria become less frequent. The majority of patients have persistent microscopic hematuria. The level of proteinuria, severity of hypertension, and degree of microscopic hematuria are indicators of progression of the disease, manifested by progressive loss of GFR (Table 4). It is obvious that when GFR is reduced at presentation less kidney function is left until terminal renal failure develops. The persistence of hyaline casts was recently reported as a prognostic indicator (17). The initially mild proteinuria may progress to heavy proteinuria in the nephrotic range. It frequently precedes the development of hypertension and the reduction of GFR (23,24).

TABLE 4. *Clinical and histological features associated with progression of IgA nephropathy*

Clinical features
The degree of proteinuria
Hypertension
Reduced GFR at presentation
The severity of microscopic hematuria
Persistence of hyaline casts
Histological features
The extent of global and segmental glomerulosclerosis
Crescent formation
Capsular adhesions
Tubular atrophy
Interstitial inflammation
Interstitial fibrosis
Blood vessel thickening
Immunological features
Density and mesangiocapillary
Deposition of IgA and C3

The extent of segmental and global sclerosis together with capsular adhesions are indicators of a progressive course (Table 4). The biopsy samples of children going into remission or going into a progressive course did not differ in their clinical presentation or the severity of the renal lesions in their initial biopsy samples (18). The two groups did not differ in the frequency of crescents or the degree of mesangial hypercellularity. However, an increase of mesangial matrix was usually seen in the follow-up biopsy samples of patients with persistent hematuria and proteinuria and not in biopsy samples of patients in clinical remission. Other studies have found a correlation between crescent formation and an adverse outcome. The progression in IgA nephropathy correlates with the degree of tubulointerstitial damage, such as tubular atrophy, interstitial infiltration by macrophages and T-lymphocytes, and interstitial fibrosis (7,8,25).

Hypertrophy and hyperplasia of intima and media of intrarenal arteries and arterioles, together with hyalinosis, have been observed in biopsy samples of patients without hypertension (18,26). These observations suggest that the vascular changes are not caused by hypertension but that systemic hypertension may be the consequence of these vascular changes. Recent studies have shown that low dosages of angiotensin-converting enzyme (ACE) inhibitors can reverse the proteinuria as well as the tubulointerstitial and vascular changes without influencing the level of the systemic blood pressure, suggesting that angioten-

TABLE 5. *Actuarial renal survival in patients with IgA nephropathy*

	Renal survival (%)[a]	
	Mean	Range
5 yr	94	83–100
10 yr	86.4	78–94
15 yr	77.4	71–88
20 yr	70	50–83

[a]Percentage of renal survival obtained from 22 reports and reviewed by Ibels and Györy (17).

sin II (Ang II) may play a role in the development of tubulointerstitial and vascular lesions.

Several studies have shown that both the intensity of deposition of IgA and C3 in the mesangium as well as the extension of this deposition in the direction of the glomerular capillary wall correlate with a progressive course of the disease (1). Children in clinical and histological remission have a significant diminution of IgA deposition. Multivariate analysis showed an independent unfavorable effect of combined mesangial and capillary deposition of IgM on renal outcome (17). However, the mesangial deposition of IgM and C3 possibly could be due to such deposits occurring in association with sclerotic lesions in the glomeruli.

IgA nephropathy was initially considered to be a benign disease. When 20-year follow-up data became available it was noted that every year a consistent percentage of this population develops terminal renal failure. About 7% to 10% of patients on chronic hemodialysis programs have IgA nephropathy as their original renal disease (27). Calculated from the first renal symptom, about 1.5% of patients with IgA nephropathy need dialysis each year (17). When calculated from the time of biopsy, about 1.3% of patients develop terminal renal failure each year (Table 5). These calculations cannot be applied to individual patients. Some patients have a rapid course, and others progress slowly to renal failure.

Geographical Differences

The geographical differences are heavily influenced by the accessibility of medical care and the biopsy policy. Despite these confounding factors, some striking differences have been reported. The incidence and prevalence in Japan and probably other Asian countries is high compared with the estimated incidence and prevalence in Europe (Table 1). The incidence in American Indians is the highest reported until now (28). The incidence in African Americans is low. The factors responsible for these geographical and racial differences are not known. They could be environmental, genetic, or both.

Genetic Predisposition

In an extensive family study in the United States, 60% of patients from eastern Kentucky were related to at least one other patient. Environmental factors such as occupation, types of residence, or food were excluded. This may suggest a genetic predisposition in the members of this pedigree (29). Several studies have reported the occurrence of IgA nephropathy in first-degree relatives (30, 31). However, in about 90% of the cases IgA nephropathy is a sporadic disease (Table 3).

The development of IgA nephropathy has been linked to various polymorphic genetic systems encoded within the human leukocyte antigen (HLA) major histocompatibility complex (MHC), such as the class I and class II HLA molecules, the complement components C2, C4, and factor B (class III), and tumor necrosis factor (32,33). When linkage is established, it usually is expressed as relative risk (RR). However, it should be noted that when an individual has a susceptibility gene with an RR of 5, his risk of acquiring the disease may increase, but the contribution of this gene to the pathogenesis of the disease still remains small.

IgA nephropathy has been associated with several phenotypes of the HLA MHC. However, these associations may differ widely among geographical areas. Disease association with HLA-B12 has been reported in the United States, whereas association with HLA-B35 has been reported in France, Australia, and the United States (Table 6). The association with HLA-DR4 was found in France and Japan and with HLA-DR1 in England. Other studies from Germany, The Netherlands, Japan, France, Italy, the United States, England, Finland, and Hungary did not disclose associations with HLA allotypes (33). HLA-B35 and HLA-DR4 also have been implicated in a more rapid progression of the disease.

The complement components C4 and factor B (Bf) are encoded within the MHC. An association of IgA nephro-

TABLE 6. *Association of IgA nephropathy with HLA phenotypes*

		Prevalence %	
HLA phenotype	Country	Patients	Controls
Class I			
HLA-B12	United States	59	20
HLA-B35	France	48	18
	United States	46	23
Class II			
HLA-DR1	England	49	24
HLA-DR4	France	49	19
	Japan	66	29
Class III			
C4	United States	18	4
BfFF	Germany	10	0

pathy was found with a homozygous C4 null phenotype and the Bf FF phenotype. A significant excess of the C3FF phenotype was found in a German and Dutch population (34). The disease also has been associated with the polymorphism of the heavy-chain switch region. A significant increase in the 7.4-kb Sα1 phenotype was observed in patients with IgA nephropathy (35). Recently an interesting association was found between a more rapid decline of renal function and the DD genotype of ACE (36).

ETIOLOGY

The onset or exacerbation of IgA nephropathy is frequently preceded by a respiratory tract infection a few days earlier (19). Infections at other locations also have been implicated (16,19). IgA nephropathy has been described as a complication of infections with *Campylobacter jejuni* (37), *Yersinia enterocolitica* (38), and *Mycoplasma pneumoniae* (39) (Table 7). Except in individual cases, no specific bacterial infection has been found to be associated with the development of IgA nephropathy. Several viruses have been implicated in the etiology of this disease. Extensive virological investigation for adenovirus, coxsackievirus, varicella zoster virus, cytomegalovirus, or Epstein-Barr virus in tonsils, renal tissue, and mouthwashings yielded no positive results (40). Hepatitis B and C do not seem to play any role (41).

IgA nephropathy also has been linked to sensitivity to specific food components. IgA nephropathy has been reported to be associated with ankylosing spondylitis (4) celiac disease (5), and dermatitis herpetiformis (6). Withdrawal of gluten from the diet of this selected group of patients resulted in both immunological and clinical improvement (42). It was shown in a large series of Italian patients that IgA antigliadin antibodies occur in only 3% of patients with IgA nephropathy. These patients had mucosal atrophy and reacted favorably on a gluten-free diet with respect to their IgA nephropathy (43). These data suggest that IgA nephropathy may occur as a complication of celiac disease, but in the majority of patients with IgA nephropathy, gluten sensitivity does not seem to play a pathogenetic role. IgA antibodies to other food components such as bovine serum albumin, ovalbumin, and lactoglobulin also have been detected in the sera of patients with IgA nephropathy (44). Compared with healthy controls, the IgA antibody titer directed against bovine gamma-globulin, beta-lactoglobulin, chicken gamma-globulin, ovalbumin, pig gamma-globulin, soy flower extract, or surface protein of *Streptococcus mutans* did not differ (45). Deposits of soy been and casein antigens could not be demonstrated in the glomeruli of Japanese patients (46). The results of these studies suggest that IgA nephropathy may not be just one disease but the common response of the mucosal immune system to various antigens.

TABLE 7. *Antigens presumed to be involved in the pathogenesis of IgA nephropathy*

Exogenous antigens	Endogenous antigens	Antigen Independent
Bacterial	Mesangial	Fibronectin
Yersinia	Endothelial	Fcα receptors
Campylobacter	Nuclear	
Mycoplasma	Cytoplasmic	
	IgG	
Viral		
Adenovirus		
Coxsackie		
Varicella zoster		
Cytomegalovirus		
Epstein-Barr		
Food		
Gliadin		
BSA		
Ovalbumin		
Casein		
Soy proteins		
Rice proteins		

PATHOGENESIS

The predominance of IgA in the mesangium strongly suggests that these deposits are the consequence of an immune response initiated at a mucosal surface. The association of recurrent macroscopic hematuria with infections of the upper respiratory tract suggests further that the IgA immune response is induced by microbial antigens. However, in the majority of patients no specific microbial strain or antigen has until now been implicated. Interestingly, the IgA deposited in the mesangium belongs almost exclusively to the IgA1 subclass. Three explanations could be given for the selective mesangial deposition of IgA1. First, the B-lymphocytes stimulated at a particular mucosal site have a predilection to produce IgA1 antibodies. The IgA subclass distribution varies with different mucosal locations (Table 8). Secondly, the

TABLE 8. *Subclass distribution of IgA plasma cells at various mucosal locations*

Mucosal location	IgA1 (%)	IgA2 (%)
Respiratory tract	85	15
Lacrimal	65	35
Mammary	65	35
Salivary	55	45
Duodenal	80	20
Jejunal	65	35
Ileal	55	45
Colonic	35	65

responsible antigen induces preferentially an IgA1 response as is known for proteins, whereas carbohydrates preferentially induce an IgA2 response. However, after vaccination with viral antigens both IgA1 and IgA2 responses can be observed. The third possibility is that patients with IgA nephropathy have a selective hyperresponsiveness for IgA1 responses. It is not possible to choose between these possibilities on the basis of the currently available data.

Macromolecular IgA in the Circulation

A pivotal observation with regard to the pathogenesis of IgA nephropathy is the high recurrence of mesangial IgA deposits in kidneys transplanted into recipients who had IgA nephropathy as their original disease (47). On the other hand, kidneys from patients with IgA nephropathy transplanted into recipients who originally did not have IgA nephropathy show spontaneous recovery (48). These clinical observations strongly suggest that a circulating factor in patients with IgA nephropathy is responsible for mesangial deposition of IgA. It is not known what this factor is. It can be circulating IgA-containing immune complexes or IgA polymers. The finding of extrarenal IgA deposits (49) is consistent with such a mechanism. Another possibility would be that circulating IgA antibodies react with antigens, receptors, or any other molecules on the surface of the mesangial cell. It is even conceivable that the hypothetical binding structure on the mesangial cell surface is more easily induced in patients with IgA nephropathy than in healthy individuals. It should be noted that the IgA deposits frequently recur but that clinical manifestations of IgA nephropathy in renal allografts are uncommon. It is assumed that the immunosuppressive regimen in transplant recipients prevents the full development of an inflammatory reaction after deposition of IgA has occurred in the mesangium.

The presence of macromolecular IgA in the circulation of patients with IgA nephropathy was first documented by sucrose density gradient ultracentrifugation of sera from patients with this disease (50). In 73% of patients, macromolecular IgA was found varying in size between 300 and 1,000 kDa. Because this IgA could bind to secretary component (SC), it probably represented pIgA or complexes of pIgA and antigen. Control subjects and patients with IgA nephropathy with mucosal infections both respond with increases in serum concentrations of pIgA, but in patients with IgA nephropathy the pIgA levels rise higher and persist longer (51). Episodes of macroscopic hematuria are associated in children with elevated levels of pIgA (52) and IgA-containing immune complexes (53). During infection-related relapses of macroscopic hematuria, children have more IgA-bearing B-lymphocytes in their circulation that produce more pIgA than is seen in control children with infections (52).

TABLE 9. *The prevalence of IgA complexes demonstrated by various assays*

Assay	% of patients positive
IgA Raji cell	50
	68
IgA conglutinin	40
pIgA Raji	62
Anti-IgA inhibition	77
Platelet aggregation	69

Reviewed by Feehally (54).

The presence of elevated serum levels of pIgA during relapses does not exclude the simultaneous presence of IgA immune complexes in the circulation. Because the antigen involved in the pathogenesis of IgA nephropathy is not known, the distinction between pure pIgA and pIgA-containing immune complexes cannot be made easily. Several antigen-independent techniques have been developed to demonstrate the presence of IgA complexes in sera of patients with IgA nephropathy (54). The prevalence of IgA complexes varies in different studies between 50% and 77% (Table 9). In contrast to the IgA complexes found in patients with anaphylactoid purpura, the macromolecular IgA in sera of patients with IgA nephropathy is not easily precipitated in 3% polyethylene glycol, suggesting a smaller molecular makeup than is found in anaphylactoid purpura (22). The fact that results of the Raji cell and Conglutinin tests are positive suggests that the detected IgA material was able to activate the complement system.

Elevated Levels of Serum IgA

Concentrations of serum IgA are elevated in about half of the patients (55). Increased levels of serum IgA in diseases associated with IgA nephropathy such as ankylosing spondylitis are well known, but IgA serum levels are also elevated in primary IgA nephropathy. This increase is only significant for the IgA1 subclass (55). Whether the serum concentrations of pIgA or pIgA1 are higher than in controls is still controversial. Studies have reported elevated pIgA as well as no increase of pIgA. The controversy could be explained by the clinical condition of the patient. Half of the patients with an episode of macroscopic hematuria have elevated pIgA, whereas none of the patients had this during a quiescent phase of the disease (52).

The increase in serum IgA could be the result of either decreased elimination or increased synthesis. Studies on the elimination of IgA in rodents have little relevance to humans because rodents have predominantly pIgA in their circulation and SC receptors on the sinusoidal side of their hepatocytes. In humans IgA is also eliminated by the liver, but humans have no or very few SC receptors on their hepatocytes. Human hepatocytes have asialoglyprotein receptors, which bind to desialylated galactosyl residues of the oligosacharide side chains of the IgA molecule. After endocytosis the receptor ligand is dissociated and IgA is degraded in the lysosomal compartment of the hepatocyte (56). Kuppfer cells have receptors for the Fc part of IgG and IgA, so called Fcγ and Fcα receptors. In addition these cells have so-called CRI or C3b receptors. Kuppfer cells play an important role in the clearance of IgA immune complexes in experimental animals. However, Kupffer cell depletion in experimental animals does not affect the clearance rate of complexes due to compensatory Fc receptor–mediated mechanisms (57). Few studies have been performed in human IgA nephropathy. Using radiolabeled IgA–IgG aggregates, a slower clearance rate was found in patients with IgA nephropathy than in controls (58).

Increased synthesis of IgA in patients was found after parenteral immunization. After subcutaneous vaccination with inactivated mumps virus or tetanus toxoid, significantly higher IgA antibody titers were found than in controls (59,60). In another study specific IgA responses against tetanus toxoid were found to be similar in patients and controls, but patients produced more pIgA antibodies and the pIgA response lasted longer (61). Higher IgA antibody responses also were found after intramuscular vaccination with inactivated influenza virus (62) and after oral vaccination with attenuated polio virus (63,64). These antigens probably represent recall antigens. The increased production of influenza-specific IgA antibodies was significantly higher only for IgA1 antibodies and not for IgA2, IgG, or IgM. Elevated production of monomeric and pIgA was found in the bone marrow of patients with IgA nephropathy (65). The connection between the mucosal immune system and the bone marrow, the so-called mucosa–bone marrow axis, is not based on the overflow of IgA antibodies from the mucosa into the vascular compartment but is probably based on traffic of either antigen-presenting cells or antigen-specific lymphocytes from the mucosa to the bone marrow. This mucosa–bone marrow axis has been confirmed by challenging healthy individuals intranasally with the cholera toxin B subunit (CTB). A significant positive correlation was found between plasma IgA anti-CTB antibodies and specific IgA1 antibody–forming cells in the bone marrow (66). Instead of high plasma responses after parenteral immunization with a recall antigen, a low or absent response was seen when patients were challenged intranasally with the neoantigen CTB. In contrast to controls, patients with IgA nephropathy did not develop an IgA anti-CTB response in the intranasal washes and a significantly lower IgA responses by their peripheral blood mononuclear cells, lower IgA anti-CTB plasma levels, and a lower IgA anti-CTB response in their bone marrow (66). These patients apparently have a defective mucosal response after intranasal challenge with a neoantigen, and they may need a more frequent and/or prolonged antigenic challenge before they can develop an effective mucosal (memory) response. As a consequence of the recurrent mucosal exposure to antigen, IgA production in the bone marrow becomes elevated, as do IgA plasma levels.

Formation of Mesangial Deposits

It has been suggested that the high levels of serum IgA in themselves could be responsible for mesangial IgA deposition. Although serum IgA levels are frequently elevated in IgA nephropathy, it does not occur in all patients. The rare occurrence of IgA nephropathy in patients with acquired immunodeficiency syndrome (AIDS) strongly argues against high serum IgA levels as a pathogenetic factor because these levels are significantly higher in patients with AIDS than in patients with IgA nephropathy (67).

Because results of the IgA complex assays were not positive in all patients with IgA nephropathy, hypotheses other than that involving the deposition of circulating IgA immune complexes in the mesangium have been proposed. In one theory, circulating IgA antibodies react with antigens either planted on the surface of the mesangial cell or intrinsically expressed by the mesangial cell (Table 7). Sera of patients with IgA nephropathy have been tested by immunofluorescence microscopy and by fluorescence-activated cell sorting. No IgA antimesangial antibodies were detected. Antibodies directed against umbilical vein endothelium were found in the sera of some patients. The prevalence of specific IgA and IgG antibodies in these patients varies between 15% and 35% (68,69). Autoantibodies directed against nuclear antigens, histone, and myeloperoxidase occur in a minority of patients. False-positive results due to the presence of IgA rheumatoid factor have not been sufficiently excluded (70). The involvement of microbial and dietary antigens has been suggested in case reports, but such involvement has not been demonstrated in larger series. Another theory has suggested that IgA is not bound to the mesangium by its antigenic specificity but by its carbohydrate composition, giving it affinity to the fibronectin matrix in the mesangium (71). This theory is not supported by other studies (67). Results of studies of the carbohydrate composition of IgA in sera of patients with IgA nephropathy suggest that the O-linked carbohydrates in the hinge region contain less terminal galactose. This would reduce the affinity of this IgA for mesangial cells instead of increasing it. Another possibility could be that mesangial cells in patients with IgA nephropathy have a high affinity for pIgA via specific Fcα receptors. Such a receptor is present on the mesangial cell (72). Its role in deposit formation is not yet clear.

Inflammatory Reaction in the Glomerulus

The acute initial phase of the disease is characterized by mesangial proliferation. Few monocytes are present unless the intra- and extracapillary inflammation is severe enough to lead to crescent formation (73). Crescents are frequently found during relapses characterized by macroscopic hematuria and reduction of GFR (21). Biopsy samples taken during relapses show more monocytes and T cells than do biopsy samples of patients with IgA nephropathy without crescents (73). During relapse these mononuclear cells express IL-2 receptors as a sign of activition. Polymorphonuclear leukocytes occur in very low numbers.

Several mediator systems have been implicated in the inflammatory process in the glomeruli. In analogy to models of experimental nephritis, complement activation has been studied in human biopsy samples. C3 and properdin are found at the same location as the IgA deposits in 75% to 100% of the cases (74). The presence of the membrane attack complex in the deposits correlates with disease activity (14). On the other hand, C9 does not seem to be essential because IgA nephropathy also occurs in patients with congenital C9 deficiency (75). Components of the classical pathway are found in fewer than 10% of cases, suggesting that C3 and the membrane attack complex are activated by the alternative pathway. When activation of complement by IgA is discussed, it is frequently stated that IgA is a poor activator of complement. Studies observing poor complement activation have used xenogeneic combinations of complement components and antibodies (22). When homologous proteins are used, IgA activates the alternative pathway on a molar basis as effectively as IgG activates the classical pathway (76).

TABLE 10. *Induction of cytokine production by mesangial cells in vitro*

Stimulus	Expression and/or production	Species
pIgA	IL-1	Human
IgA ICx	IL-6	Rat
IL-1	IL-6	Human
IL-1	IL-8	Human
TNF-α	IL-6	Human
IFN-γ	HLA class II	Human
IFN-γ	PDGF	Human
IFN-γ	PDGF receptors	Human
Ang II	IL-6	Mouse
Ang II	TGF-β	Rat
Ang II	Endothelin-1	Human
Thrombin	Endothelin-1	Human
TGF-β	Endothelin-1	Human
PDGF	Endothelin-1	Human
TNF-α	Endothelin-1	Human

Proliferative Response in the Glomerulus

This stage of the disease is characterized by proliferation of mesangial cells. Recent findings on the induction of cytokine production by mesangial cells (Table 10) raise the possibility that the proliferative response of the mesangium might be the result of local cytokine production (Table 10). IgA–immune complexes and pIgA induce the activation of mesangial cells (77). In contrast to monomeric IgA, pIgA binds efficiently to mesangial cells. This binding is not influenced by fibronectin or asialofetuin. By Scatchard plot analysis, these IgA receptors have a density of 7×10^6 per cell and an affinity of $1.4 \times 10^6\ M^{-1}$. The IgA–immune complexes and pIgA induce IL-6 production by mesangial cells in a dose-dependent fashion (77).

Activated mesangial cells produce monocyte chemotactic protein-1 (MCP-1), which attracts monocytes and T-lymphocytes but not polymorphonuclear leukocytes (78). The influx of monocytes can be responsible for the release of IL-1, IL-6, and tumor necrosis factor-α (TNF-α). IL-1 and TNF-α can induce the expression of adhesion molecules in endothelial cells (Fig. 1). The expression of intracellular adhesion molecule-1 (ICAM-1) in the glomerular capillaries of patients with IgA nephropathy correlates with the severity of the glomerular lesions (79). Once mesangial cells are activated by these cytokines, they start to produce IL-1, IL-6, platelet-derived growth factor (PDGF), and transforming growth factor-β (TGF-β) (Table 10). These and other cytokines have a proliferative effect on mesangial cells in vitro (80). The production of IL-6 and TGF-β also can be induced by Ang II (81). TGF-β is a potent inducer of endothelin-1 in mesangial and endothelial cells (82) (Table 10).

In renal biopsy samples of patients with IgA nephropathy, messenger RNA (mRNA) for IL-1, IL-6, TNF-α, and PDGF B chain can readily be demonstrated in monocytes and macrophages by in situ hybridization (83,84). Weaker staining can be observed in mesangial, tubular, and endothelial cells (84,85). IL-1 and IL-6 stimulates the proliferation of mesangial cells in vitro (86). It is not clear whether IL-6 has the same effect in vivo. The correlation that was observed between the level of IL-6 excretion in the urine and the severity of the glomerular lesions in IgA nephropathy suggests that IL-6 also may play an important role in vivo (87). Interferon-γ serum levels in patients with IgA nephropathy correlates with the glomerular expression of HLA class II molecules (88). Mesangial cells express mRNA for both the A and the B chain of PDGF. In IgA nephropathy the glomeruli show increased expression of PDGF and PDGF receptors (84). PDGF released by platelets, monocytes, and mesangial cells may stimulate mesangial cells to proliferate. These observations strongly suggest that the mesangial proliferation seen in the chronic stage of IgA nephropathy is the result of local production of cytokines by monocytes/macrophages, T-lymphocytes, and mesangial cells.

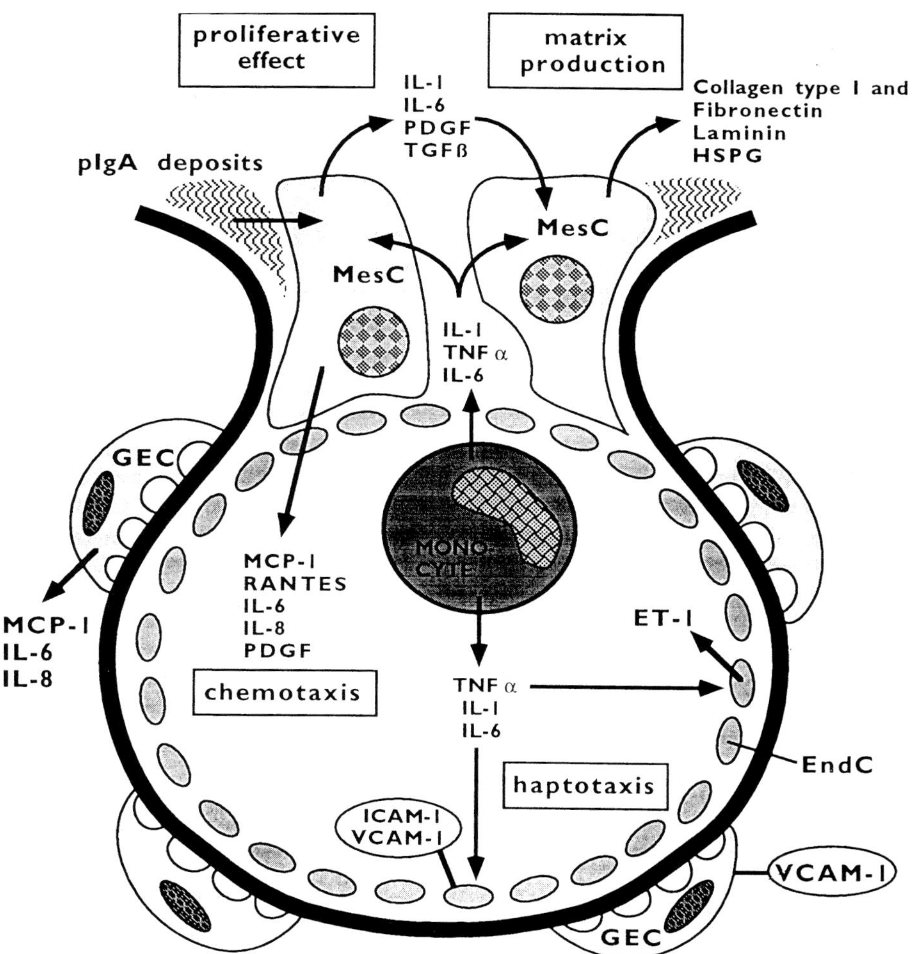

FIG. 1. Glomerular capillary loop demonstrating local cytokine production by recruited monocytes, mesangial cells (MesC), endothelial cells (End C), and glomerular epithelial cells (GEC).

Development of Glomerulosclerosis and Interstitial Fibrosis

Repeat biopsies in patients with IgA nephropathy have shown that kidneys with interstitial infiltrate and fibrosis progress to terminal renal failure (1). A positive correlation of glomerulosclerosis with progression of the disease would be expected but is less well established. It is puzzling to most investigators how glomerular abnormalities can lead to tubular atrophy, interstitial infiltrate, and fibrosis. For many years these changes were explained by glomerular ischemia and obsolescence resulting in functional deterioration of the downstream nephron, or so-called nephron loss. With the discovery of cytokine production by mesangial, tubular, and endothelial cells of the kidneys, new concepts have been proposed to explain the tubulointerstitial abnormalities that develop as a result of glomerular pathology. Cytokines produced by recruited cells such as monocytes and T-lymphocytes or produced by intrinsic cells in the glomeruli could reach the tubulointerstitium either by glomerular filtration or by transportation via the postglomerular capillaries. These cytokines may exert not only their effector functions in the tubulointerstitium, but they also stimulate the production of cytokines by renal tubules (Table 11). Proximal tubular epithelial cells produce MCP-1 (89), IL-6 (90), IL-8(91), TNF-α (92), and TGF-β (93). The intensity of macrophage infiltration in the interstitium correlates with the tubular staining of MCP-1 in biopsy samples of patients with IgA nephropathy (94). MCP-1 is not the only chemotactic factor produced by renal tubules. Osteopontin, IL-6, and RANTES are also chemoattractants that are produced by renal tubules. After lymphocytes and macrophages have been attracted to the interstitium, these cells may then stimulate cytokine production by tubular cells (Table 11). Another important stimulant of cytokine production is Ang II (95). It is not only a growth factor for smooth muscle cells, but also for mesangial cells and tubular epithelial cells. Mesangial cells have AT1 receptors for Ang II. In vitro, Ang II stimulates the proliferation of mesangial cells, which is inhibited by prostaglandin E1 and atrial natriuretic peptide.

TABLE 11. *Cytokine production by tubular epithelial cells in vitro*

Stimulus	Expression and/or production	Species
IL-1α	TNF-α	Human
TNF-α	MCP-1	Human
IL-1α	MCP-1	
IL-1α	IL-6	Human
IL-1α	IL-8	Human
TNF-α	ICAM-1	
TNF-α	HLA class II	Human
bFGF	TGF-β	Human
bFGF	PDGF-β	
Ang II	TGF-β	Rat
Ang II	Endothelin-1	Rabbit

Ang II also induces the synthesis of collagen type I by mesangial cells (96). ACE inhibitors prevent the development of glomerulosclerosis and interstitial fibrosis in several animal models. This effect is independent of the hemodynamic effects of ACE I.

Proximal tubular epithelial cells are able to produce a whole array of cytokines (Table 11) after stimulation by IL-1α, TNF-α, and IL-6. These cytokines are produced by monocytes and macrophages but also can be produced by tubular epithelial cells. Ang II is an autocrine as well as a paracrine cytokine. Renal tubular epithelial cells express the mRNA for all the components of the renin-angiotensin system (97), including angiotensinogen, renin, converting enzyme and the AT1 and AT2 receptors. Ang II stimulates the production of TGF-β by tubular epithelial cells (98). PDGF and TGF-β together with basic fibroblast growth factor (bFGF) are strong stimulants for fibroblasts (99–101) to produce matrix components. However, it is not clear which cells are responsible for the process of fibrosis. Glomerulosclerosis is caused by matrix production of mesangial cells. The matrix components deposited in the interstitium can be produced not only by fibroblasts (100) but also by renal tubular epithelial cells. These cells are of mesenchymal origin and may transdifferentiate into matrix-producing cells (101). After matrix components such as collagen type I, III, IV, and V, as well as lamininin and fibronectin have been secreted, they are deposited and rearranged to form fibrils, which ultimately lead to fibrosis and shrinkage of the renal cortex. The dominant role of Ang II in this process offers the opportunity to interfere in this fibrogenic process.

TREATMENT OF IgA NEPHROPATHY

The treatment of patients with IgA nephropathy with high-dose corticosteroids and azathioprine generally has not been accepted, except in cases presenting as rapidly progressive glomerulonephritis characterized histologically by necrotizing capillaritis and crescent formation (102). However, the majority of cases have an indolent course. In view of the hazards of aggressive immunosuppression, such treatment probably does not yield better results than no treatment at all (103). However, several studies have shown that immunosuppressive treatment for 2 or 3 months may result in a better prognosis after several years (104). Intervention in the inflammatory reactions and the subsequent cytokine cascade in the kidney could explain these long-term effects of immunosuppressive treatment. Therefore, the use of high-dose corticosteroids should be restricted to patients with histologically active signs of glomerulonephritis.

Patients with a more or less stable renal function, with or without proteinuria or hypertension, preferably are treated with ACE inhibition (105). Even when hypertension is not present, ACE inhibition is recommended on the basis of its beneficial effects on the production of cytokines and matrix components. Several studies have shown that ACE inhibition reduces urinary protein excretion in patients with IgA nephropathy (106) and preserves renal function. Interestingly, the deterioration of renal function correlates in untreated patients with the DD allotype of ACE (107). Patients in this category benefit the most from ACE inhibition (108). The use of intravenous immunoglobulins is still in an experimental stage (109). The use of fish oil has been reported to be beneficial in IgA nephropathy (110), but this has not been confirmed.

When renal failure develops and dialysis is required, the high risk of recurrence of IgA nephropathy in the transplanted kidney should not be a contraindication for transplantation. The IgA deposits may recur, but overt disease characterized by hematuria and/or proteinuria is uncommon. Whether the disease recurs more easily in kidneys donated by a living related donor is still controversial.

It is likely that the secondary prevention of renal failure in patients with IgA nephropathy is now within reach. When patients are treated at an early stage with inhibitors of fibrogenic cytokines, IgA nephropathy may continue to exist, but it may no longer lead to renal failure.

ACKNOWLEDGMENTS

The secretarial support of Mrs. E.C. Sierat-van der Steen and the pictorial skills of Mrs. M.A. van Dijk are greatly appreciated.

REFERENCES

1. D'Amico G. The commonest glomerulonephritis in the world: IgA Nephropathy. *Q J Med* 1987;245:709–727.
2. Berger J. IgA glomerular deposits in renal disease. *Transplant Proc* 1969;1:939–944.
3. Power DA, Muirhead N, Simpson JG, et al. IgA nephropathy is not a rare disease in the United Kingdom. *Nephron* 1985;40:180–184.

4. Ann Chen, Yat-Sen Ho, Yen-Chang Tu, Shan-Der Shieh, Han-Wen Hung, Chun-Tei Chou. Immunoglobulin a nephropathy and ankylosing spondylitis. *Nephron* 1988;49:313–318.
5. Pasternack A, Collin P, Mustonen J, et al. Glomerular IgA deposits in patients with celiac disease. *Clin Nephrol* 1990;34:56–60.
6. Pape JF, Melbye OJ, Oystese B, Brodwall EK. Glomerulonephritis in dermatitis herpetiformis. *Acta Med Scand* 1978;203:445–448.
7. Mackensen-Haen S, Eissele R, Bohle A. Contribution on the correlation between morphometric parameters gained from the renal cortex and renal function in IgA nephritis. *Lab Invest* 1988;59:239–244.
8. Alexopoulos E, Seron D, Hartley RB, Nolasco F, Cameron JS. The role of interstitial infiltrates in IgA nephropathy: a study with monoclonal antibodies. *Nephrol Dial Transplant* 1989;4:187–195.
9. Hai-Ling Li, Hancock WW, Dowling JP, Atkins RC. Activated (IL-2R+) intraglomerular mononuclear cells in crescentic glomerulonephritis. *Kidney Int* 1991;39:793–798.
10. Arima S, Nakayama M, Naito M, Sato T, Takahashi K. Significance of mononuclear phagocytes in IgA nephropathy. *Kidney Int* 1991;39: 684–692.
11. Gärtner HV, Hönlein F, Traub U, Bohle A. IgA-nephropathy (IgA-IgG-nephropathy/IgA-nephritis)—a disease entity? *Virchows Arch [A]* 1979;385:1–27.
12. Rodicio JL. Idiopathic IgA nephropathy. *Kidney Int* 1984;25:717–729.
13. Valentijn RM, Radl J, Haaijman JJ, et al. Circulating and mesangial secretory component–binding IgA-1 in primary IgA nephropathy. *Kidney Int* 1984;26:760–766.
14. Rauterberg EW, Lieberknecht HM, Wingen AM, Ritz E. Complement membrane attack (MAC) in idiopathic IgA-glomerulonephritis. *Kidney Int* 1987;31:820–829.
15. Dysart NK, Sisson S, Vernier RL. Immunoelectron microscopy of IgA nephropathy. *Clin Immunol immunopathol* 1983;29:254–270.
16. Thomas M, Ibels LS, Abbot N. IgA nephropathy associated with mastitis and haematuria. *Br Med J* 1985;291:867–868.
17. Ibels LS, Györy AZ. IgA nephropathy: analysis of the natural history, important factors in the progression of renal disease, and a review of the literature. *Medicine* 1994;73:79–102.
18. Yoshikawa N, Iijima K, Matsuyama S, et al. Repeat renal biopsy in children with IgA nephropathy. *Clin Nephrol* 1990;33:160–167.
19. Nicholls KM, Fairley KF, Dowling JP, Kincaid-Smith P. The clinical course of mesangial IgA associated nephropathy in adults. *Q J Med* 1984;210:227–250.
20. Suzuki S, Sata H, Kobayashi H, et al. Comparative study of IgA nephropathy with acute and insidious onset. *Am J Nephrol* 1992;12: 22–28.
21. Bennett WM, Kincaid-Smith P. Macroscopic hematuria in mesangial IgA nephropathy: correlation with glomerular crescents and renal dysfunction. *Kidney Int* 1983;23:393–400.
22. Van Es LA. Pathogenesis of IgA nephropathy. *Kidney Int* 1992;41: 1720–1729.
23. Neelakantappa K, Gallo GR, Baldwin DS. Proteinuria in IgA nephropathy. *Kidney Int* 1988;33:716–721.
24. Okada H, Suzuki H, Konishi K, Sakaguchi H, Saruta T. Histological alterations in renal specimens as indicators of prognosis of IgA nephropathy. *Clin Nephrol* 1992;37:235–238.
25. Alamartine E, Sabatier JC, Guerin C, Berliet JM, Berthoux F. Prognostic factors in mesangial IgA glomerulonephritis: an extensive study with univariate and multivariate analyses. *Am J Kidney Dis* 1991;18:12–19.
26. Clarkson AR, Seymour AE, Thompson AJ, Haynes WDG, Chan YL, Jackson B. IgA nephropathy, a syndrome of uniform morphology, diverse clinical features and uncertain prognosis. *Clin Nephrol* 1977; 8:459.
27. Clarkson AR, Woodroffe AJ, Bannister KM, Lomax-Smith JD, Aarons I. The syndrome of IgA nephropathy. *Clin Nephrol* 1984;21:7–14.
28. Hoy WE, Hughson MD, Smith SM, Megill DM. Mesangial proliferative glomerulonephritis in Southwestern American Indians. *Am J Kidney Dis* 1993;21:486–496.
29. Julian BA, Quiggins PA, Thompson JS, Woodford SY, Cleason K, Wyatt RJ. Familial IgA nephropathy. Evidence of an inherited mechanism of disease. *N Engl J Med* 1985;312:202–208.
30. Schena FP, Scivittaro V, Ranieri E, et al. Abnormalities of the IgA immune system in members of unrelated pedigrees from patients with IgA nephropathy. *Clin Exp Immunol* 1993;92:139–144.
31. Egido J, Julian BA, Wyatt RJ. Genetic factors in primary IgA nephropathy. *Nephrol Dial Transplant* 1987;2:134–142.
32. Medcraft J, Hitman GA, Sachs JA, Whichelow CE, Raafat I, Moore RH. Autoimmune renal disease and tumour necrosis factor gene polymorphism. *Clin Nephrol* 1993;40:63–68.
33. Lévy M, Lesavre P. Genetic factors in IgA nephropathy (Berger's disease). *Adv Nephrol* 1992;21:23–49.
34. Rambausek MH, Waldherr R, Ritz E. Immunogenetic findings in glomerulonephritis. *Kidney Int* 1993;43:S3–8.
35. Demaine AG, Rambausek M, Knight JF, Williams DG, Welsh KI, Ritz E. Relation of mesangial IgA glomerulonephritis to polymorphism of immunoglobulin heavy chain switch region. *J Clin Invest* 1988;81:611–614.
36. Hunley TE, Julian BA, Phillips JA III, et al. Angiotensin converting enzyme gene polymorphism: potential silencer motif and impact on progression in IgA nephropathy. *Kidney Int* 1996;49:571–577.
37. Carter JE, Cimolai N. IgA nephropathy associated with *Campylobacter jejuni* enteritis. *Nephron* 1991;58:101–102.
38. Friedberg M, Denneberg T, Brun C, Hannover Larsen J, Larsen S. Glomerulonephritis in infections with *Yersinia* enterocolitica O-serotype 3. *Acta Med Scand* 1981;209:103–110.
39. Kanayama Y, Shiota K, Kotumi K, et al. Mycoplasma pneumoniae pneumonia associated with IgA nephropathy. *Scand J Infect Dis* 1982;14:231–233.
40. Kunimoto M, Hayashi Y, Kuki K, et al. Analysis of viral infection in patients with IgA nephropathy. *Acta Otolaryngol* 1993;508:11–18.
41. Ström EH, Dürmüller U, Gudat F, Mihatsch MJ. Hepatitis C virus plays no role in the pathogenesis of immunoglobulin A nephropathy in liver cirrhosis. *Nephron* 1994;67:370.
42. Coppo R, Roccatello D, Amore A, et al. Effects of a gluten-free diet in primary IgA nephropathy. *Clin Nephrol* 1990;33:72–86.
43. Fornasieri A, Sinico RA, Maldifassi P, Bernasconi P, Vegni M, D'Amico G. IgA–antigliadin antibodies in IgA mesangial nephropathy (Berger's disease). *Br Med J* 1987;295:78–80.
44. Rostoker G, Petit-Phar M, Delprato S, et al. Mucosal immunity in primary glomerulonephritis: II. Study of the serum IgA subclass repertoire to food and airborne antigens. *Nephron* 1991;59:561–566.
45. Russell MW, Mestecky J, Julian BA, Galla JH. IgA-associated renal diseases: antibodies to environmental antigens in sera and deposition of immunoglobulins and antigens in glomeruli. *J Clin Immunol* 1986; 6:74–86.
46. Murakami T, Kawakami H. Questionable role of soy protein in childhood IgA nephropathy. *Nephron* 1993;64:395–398.
47. Odum J, Peh CA, Clarkson AR, et al. Recurrent mesangial IgA nephritis following renal transplantation. *Nephrol Dial Transplant* 1994;9:309–312.
48. Sanfilippo F, Croker BP, Bollinger RR. Fate of four cadaveric donor renal allografts with mesangial IgA deposits. *Transplantation* 1982; 33:370–376.
49. Baart de la Faille-Kuyper EH, Kater L, Kuijten RH, et al. Occurrence of vascular IgA deposits in clinically normal skin of patients with renal disease. *Kidney Int* 1976;9:424–429.
50. Lopez Trascasa M, Egido J, Sancho J, Hernando L. IgA glomerulonephritis (Berger's disease): evidence of high serum levels of polymeric IgA. *Clin Exp Immunol* 1980;42:247–254.
51. Jones CL, Powell HR, Kincaid-Smith P, Roberton DM. Polymeric IgA and immune complex concentrations in IgA-related renal disease. *Kidney Int* 1990;38:323–331.
52. Freehally J, Beattie TJ, Brenchley PEC, Coupes BM, Mallick NP, Postlethwaite RJ. Sequential study of the IgA system in relapsing IgA nephropathy. *Kidney Int* 1986;30:924–931.
53. Davin JC, Foidart JB, Mahieu PR. Relation between biological IgA abnormalities and mesangial IgA deposits in isolated hematuria in childhood. *Clin Nephrol* 1987;28:73–80.
54. Feehally J. Immune mechanisms in glomerular IgA deposition. *Nephrol Dial Transplant* 1988;3:361–378.
55. Van den Wall Bake AWL, Daha MR, Van der Ark A, Hiemstra PS, Radl J, Van Es LA. Serum levels and in vitro production of IgA subclasses in patients with primary IgA nephropathy. *Clin Exp Immunol* 1988;74:115–120.
56. Schwartz AL, Rup D. Biosynthesis of the human asialoglycoprotein receptor. *J Biol Chem* 1983;258:11249–11255.
57. Bogers WMJM, Stad RK, Janssen DJ, et al. Kupffer cell depletion in vivo results in preferential elimination of IgG aggregates and immune complexes via specific Fc receptors on rat liver endothelial cells. *Clin Exp Immunol* 1991;85:128–136.
58. Roccatello D, Picciotto G, Ropolo R, et al. Kinetics and fate of

IgA–IgG aggregates as a model of naturally occurring immune complexes in IgA nephropathy. *Lab Invest* 1992;66:86–95.
59. Pasternack A, Mustonen J, Leinikki P. Humoral immune response in patients with IgA and IgM glomerulonephritis. *Clin Exp Immunol* 1986;63:228–233.
60. Fortune F, Courteau M, Williams DG, Lehner T. T and B cell responses following subcutaneous immunization with tetanus toxoid in IgA nephropathy. *Clin Exp Immunol* 1992;88:62–67.
61. Layward L, Allen AC, Harper SJ, Hattersley JM, Feehally J. Increased and prolonged production of specific polymeric IgA after systemic immunization with tetanus toxoid in IgA nephropathy. *Clin Exp Immunol* 1992,88:394–398.
62. Van den Wall Bake AWL, Beyer WEP, Evers-Schouten JH, et al. Humoral immune response to influenza vaccination in patients with primary immunoglobulin a nephropathy. *J Clin Invest* 1989;84:1070–1075.
63. Leinikki PO, Mustonen J, Pasternack A. Immune response to oral polio vaccine in patients with IgA glomerulonephritis. *Clin Exp Immunol* 1987;68:33–38.
64. Waldo FB, Cochran AM. Systemic immune response to oral polio immunization in patients with IgA nephropathy. *J Clin Lab Immunol* 1989;28:109–114.
65. Van den Wall Bake AWL, Daha MR, Haaijman JJ, Radl J, Van der Ark A, Van Es LA. Elevated production of polymeric and monomeric IgA1 by the bone marrow in IgA nephropathy. *Kidney Int* 1989;35:1400–1404.
66. De Fijter JW, Eijgenraam JW, Braam CA, et al. Deficient IgA, immune response to nasal cholera toxin subunit B in primary IgA nephropathy. *Kidney Int* 1996 (in press).
67. Van den Wall Bake AWL, Kirk KA, Gay RE, Switalski LM, Julian A, Jackson S, Gay S, Mestecky J. Binding of serum immunoglobulins to collagens in IgA nephropathy and HIV infection. *Kidney Int* 1992;42:374–382.
68. O'Donoghue DJ, Darvill A, Ballardie FW. Mesangial cell autoantigens in immunoglobulin A nephropathy and Henoch-Schönlein purpura. *J Clin Invest* 1991;88:1522–1530.
69. Wang MX, Walker RG, Kincaid-Smith P. Clinicopathologic associations of anti-endothelial cell antibodies in immunoglobulin A nephropathy and lupus nephritis. *Am J Kidney Dis* 1993;22:378–386.
70. Sinico RA, Tadros M, Radice A, et al. Lack of IgA antineutrophil cytoplasmic antibodies in Henoch-Schönlein purpura and IgA nephropathy. *Clin Immunol Immunopathol* 1994;73:19–26.
71. Cederholm B, Wieslander J, Bygren P, Heinegard D. Circulating complexes containing IgA and fibronectin in patients with primary IgA nephropathy. *Proc Natl Acad Sci U S A* 1988;85:4865–4868.
72. Gomez-Querrero C, Gonzalez E, Egido J. Evidence for a specific IgA receptor in rat and human mesangial cells. *J Immunol* 1993;151:7172–7181.
73. Hai-Ling Li, Hancock WW, Hook DH, Dowling JP, Atkins RC. Mononuclear cell activation and decreased renal function in IgA nephropathy with crescents. *Kidney Int* 1990;37:1552–1556.
74. Wyatt RJ. The complement system in IgA nephropathy and Henoch-Schönlein purpura: functional and genetic aspects. *Contrib Nephrol* 1993;104:82–91.
75. Yoshioka K, Takemura T, Akano N, et al. IgA nephropathy in patients with congenital C9 deficiency. *Kidney Int* 1992;42:1253–1258.
76. Rits M, Hiemstra PS, Bazin H, Van Es LA, Vaerman JP, Daha MR. Activation of rat complement by soluble and insoluble rat IgA immune complexes. *Eur J Immunol* 1988;18:1873–1880.
77. Van den Dobbelsteen MEA, Van der Woude FJ, Schroeijers WEM, Van den Wall Bake AWL, Van Es LA, Daha MR. Binding of dimeric and polymeric IgA to rat renal mesangial cells enhances the release of interleukin 6. *Kidney Int* 1994;46:512–519.
78. Rovin BH, Yoshimura T, Tan L. Cytokine-induced production of monocyte chemoattractant protein-1 by cultured human mesangial cells. *J Immunol* 1992;148:2148–2153.
79. Tomino Y, Ohmuro H, Kuramoto T, et al. Expression of intercellular adhesion molecule-1 and infiltration of lymphocytes in glomeruli of patients with IgA nephropathy. *Nephron* 1994;67:302–307.
80. Floege J, Eng E, Young BA, Johnson RJ. Factors involved in the regulation of mesangial cell proliferation in vitro and in vivo. *Kidney Int* 1993;43(suppl):47–54.
81. Wolf G, Zahner R, Schroeder R, Stahl AK. Transforming growth factor beta mediates the angiotensin-II–induced stimulation of collagen type IV synthesis in cultured murine proximal tubular cells. *Nephrol Dial Transplant* 1996;11:263–269.
82. Kohno M, Horio T, Ikeda M, et al. Angiotensin II stimulates endothelin-1 secretion in cultured rat mesangial cells. *Kidney Int* 1992;42:860–866.
83. Yoshioka K, Takemura T, Murakami K, et al. Transforming growth factor-β protein and mRNA in glomeruli in normal and diseased human kidneys. *Lab Invest* 1993;68:154–163.
84. Gesualdo L, Pinzani M, Floriano JJ, et al. Platelet-derived growth factor expression in mesangial proliferative glomerulonephritis. *Lab Invest* 1991;65:160–167.
85. Yoshioka K, Takemura T, Murakami K, et al. In situ expression of cytokines in IgA nephritis. *Kidney Int* 1993;44:825–833.
86. Ruef C, Budde K, Lacy J, et al. Interleukin 6 is an autocrine growth factor for mesangial cells. *Kidney Int* 1990;38:249–257.
87. Dohi K, Iwano M, Muraguchi A, et al. *Clin Nephrol* 1991;35;1–5.
88. Yokoyama K, et al. Intraglomerular expression of MHC class II and Ki-67 antigens and serum γ-interferon levels in IgA nephropathy. *Nephron* 1992;62:169–175.
89. Prodjosudjadi W, Gerritsma JSJ, Klar-Mohamad N, et al. Production and cytokine-mediated regulation of monocyte chemoattractant protein-1 by human proximal tubular epithelial cells. *Kidney Int* 1995;48:1477–1486.
90. Boswell RN, Yard BA, Schrama E, Van Es LA, Daha MR, Van der Woude FJ. Interleukin 6 production by proximal tubular epithelial cells in vitro: analysis of the effects of interleukin 1α (IL-1α) and other cytokines. *Nephrol Dial Transplant* 1994;9:599–606.
91. Gerritsma JSJ, Hiemstra PS, Gerritsen AF, et al. Regulation and production in vitro of interleukin-8 by human proximal tubular epithelial cells. *Clin Exp Immunol* 1996;103:289–294.
92. Yard BA, Daha MR, Kooymans-Couthino M, et al. IL-1α stimulated TNFα production by cultured human proximal tubular epithelial cells. *Kidney Int* 1992;42:383–389.
93. Tikkanen I, Uhlenius N, Tikkanen T, et al. Increased renal expression of cytokines and growth factors induced by DOCA–NaCl treatment in Heymann nephritis. *Nephrol Dial Transplan* 1995;10:2192–2198.
94. Prodjosudjadi W, Gerritsma JSJ, Van Es LA, Daha MR, Bruijn JA. Monocyte chemoattractant protein-1 in normal and diseased human kidneys: an immunohistochemical analysis. *Clin Nephrol* 1995;44:148–155.
95. Mariyama T, Fujiwara Y, Kaneko T, Xia C, Imai E, Kamada T, Ueda N. Angiotensin II stimulates interleukin-6 release from cultured mouse mesangial cells. *J Am Soc Nephrol* 1995;6:95–101.
96. Wolf G, Neilson EG. Angiotensin II as a hypertrophogenic cytokine for proximal tubular cells. *Kidney Int* 1993;43:100–107.
97. Paul M, Wagner J, Dzau VJ. Gene expression of the renin–angiotensin system in human tissues. Quantitative analysis by the polymerase chain reaction. *J Clin Invest* 1993;91:2058–2064.
98. Pimentel JL, Sundell CL, Wang S, Kopp JB, Montero A, Martinez-Maldonado M. Role of angiotensin II in the expression and regulation of transforming growth factor-β in obstructive nephropathy. *Kidney Int* 1995;48:1233–1246.
99. Müller GA, Rodemann HP. Characterization of human renal fibroblasts in health and disease: I. Immunophenotyping of cultured tubular epithelial cells and fibroblasts derived from kidney with histologically proven interstitial fibrosis. *Am J Kidney Dis* 1991;17:680–683.
100. Goumenos DA, Brown CB, Shortland J, El Nahas AM. Myofibroblasts, predictors of progression of mesangial IgA nephropathy? *Nephrol Dial Transplant* 1994;9:1418–1425.
101. Kuncio GS, Neilson EG, Haverty T. Mechanisms of tubulointerstitial fibrosis. *Kidney Int* 1991;39:550–556.
102. Andreoli SP, Bergstein JM. Treatment of severe IgA nephropathy in children. *Pediatr Nephrol* 1989;3:248–253.
103. Clarkson AR, Woodroff AJ, Aarons IA, Thompson T. Therapeutic options in IgA nephropathy. *Am J Kidney Dis* 1988;12:443–448.
104. Kobayashi Y, Hiki Yoshiyuki, Fujii K, Kurokawa A, Tateno S. Moderately proteinuric IgA nephropathy: prognostic prediction of individual clinical courses and steroid therapy in progressive cases. *Nephron* 1989;53:250–256.
105. Cattran DC, Greenwood C, Ritchie S. Long-term benefits of angiotensin-converting enzyme inhibitor therapy in patients with severe

immunoglobulin A nephropathy: a comparison to patients receiving treatment with other antihypertensive agents and to patients receiving no therapy. *Am J Kidney Dis* 1994;23:247–254.
106. Maschio G, Cagnoli L, Claroni F, et al. ACE inhibition reduced proteinuria in normotensive patients with IgA nephropathy: a multicentre, randomized, placebo-controlled study. *Nephrol Dial Transplant* 1994;9:265–269.
107. Yorioka T, Suehiro T, Yasuoka N, Hashimoto K, Kawada M. Polymorphism of the angiotensin converting enzyme gene and clinical aspects of IgA nephropathy. *Clin Nephrol* 1995;44:80–85.
108. Yoshida H, Mitarai T, Kawamura T, et al. Role of the deletion of polymorphism of the angiotensin converting enzyme gene in the progression and therapeutic responsiveness of IgA nephropathy. *J Clin Invest* 1995;96:2162–2169.
109. Rostoker G, Desvaux-Belghiti D, Pilatte Y, et al. High-dose immunoglobulin therapy for severe IgA nephropathy and Henock-Schönlein Purpura. *Ann Intern Med* 1994;120:476–484.
110. Donadio JV, Bergstralh EJ, Offord KP, Spencer DC, Holley K. A controlled trial of fish oil in IgA nephropathy. *N Engl J Med* 1994;3:1194–1199.

Immunologic Renal Diseases,
edited by E. G. Neilson and W. G. Couser.
Lippincott-Raven Publishers, Philadelphia © 1997.

CHAPTER 43

Anti–Glomerular Basement Membrane Disease

Catherine M. Meyers, Raghuram Kalluri, and Eric G. Neilson

DEFINITION AND HISTORICAL PERSPECTIVE

Initial observations of coexistent glomerulonephritis and pulmonary hemorrhage were recorded in the autopsy findings of Ernest Goodpasture during the influenza pandemic of 1919 (1). One particular subject in this report, a febrile 18-year-old man, presented with upper respiratory complaints and soon developed massive hemoptysis and acute renal failure (1). Several similar cases were observed by other researchers in subsequent years and the eponym "Goodpasture's syndrome" was introduced to distinguish such cases of glomerulonephritis and pulmonary hemorrhage (2). A clearer understanding of pathogenic mechanisms of this autoimmune renal disease evolved over several decades, however, with recognition of anti–glomerular basement membrane (anti-GBM) antibodies in Goodpasture's syndrome in 1967, and recent identification of the target Goodpasture antigen expressed on mammalian basement membrane (3–5). As a result of these investigative milestones, diagnostic criteria of this disease have been significantly redefined (6). Anti-GBM antibody–mediated disease clearly represents a clinicopathologic entity with a wide spectrum of clinical manifestations (6–9). The current definition includes any patient with circulating or deposited anti-GBM antibodies and includes patients with isolated pulmonary involvement, combined pulmonary and renal disease (Goodpasture's syndrome), and individuals with rapidly progressive glomerulonephritis who lack hemoptysis (RPGN type I) (6–9).

Inasmuch as patients with Goodpasture's syndrome were initially designated on the basis of clinical presentation, many cases reported before the discovery of anti-GBM antibodies likely had other entities that produce pulmonary hemorrhage and glomerulonephritis (6). Indeed, recent assessment of the pathologic descriptions in Goodpasture's original report suggests that the findings in his index case are more consistent with systemic vasculitis than anti-GBM antibody–mediated disease (6).

C. M. Meyers, R. Kalluri, and E. G. Neilson: Department of Medicine, University of Pennsylvania School of Medicine, Renal-Electrolyte and Hypertension Division, Philadelphia, Pennsylvania 19104.

ETIOLOGY AND INCIDENCE

Anti-GBM antibody–mediated disease is an uncommon clinical entity that occurs with a worldwide distribution (10). Although the true incidence of this disorder is unknown, several hundred cases have been reported in the literature (11–14). Reported cases are typically idiopathic, but isolated sets of cases appear to be familial, occur after exposure to environmental agents, after viral infection, or as a complication of another form of glomerulonephritis (15–18). Early studies estimated that anti-GBM antibody–mediated disease comprised approximately 3% to 5% of all cases of glomerulonephritis, although current estimates suggest that the frequency is perhaps closer to 1% to 2% (19,20). Deposited anti-GBM antibodies are detected in approximately 20% of patients with rapidly progressive glomerulonephritis, 30% of which present with isolated renal involvement (9).

Anti-GBM antibody–mediated disease occurs primarily in whites, although it has been described in many different racial groups (10,14,21). In initial case reports, Goodpasture's syndrome afflicted primarily young white men (22,23). As a result of more definitive diagnostic criteria, however, and the wide availability of specific assays for detecting anti-GBM antibodies, recent studies indicate that all age groups and either gender can be affected (13,24–26). Isolated renal involvement in this disease tends to occur in slightly older patients with an even gender distribution (13,14,26). Overall, men still tend to predominate in many series, however, with the male to female ratios ranging from nearly 1:1 to 9:1 (10,

13,21,22). Most patients present during the second to fifth decades of life (21–23). The age range extends from childhood to the eighth decade of life, with a mean age of onset between 20 and 30 years (21–23,27). Anti-GBM antibody–mediated disease occurs at any time of year, although seasonal clusters have been described (14,28). These clusters perhaps result from various environmental triggers that demonstrate seasonal variation (10,14,28).

PATHOGENESIS AND PATHOPHYSIOLOGY

Experimental Models of Anti-GBM Antibody–Mediated Disease

Although the etiology of anti-GBM antibody–mediated disease has not been elucidated, experimental models have facilitated a better understanding of pathogenic mechanisms of this autoimmune renal disease (3,29,30). Early studies of immunization protocols using heterologous or homologous GBM preparations in complete Freund's adjuvant induced severe glomerulonephritis associated with endogenous linear immunoglobulin (Ig)G and complement deposition along the GBM (29). These initial observations of autoimmune nephritis were important because they clearly implicated pathogenic host immune responses that targeted the GBM (29). Passive transfer studies, using serum derived from animals with anti-GBM nephritis, suggested a role for circulating antibodies in mediating renal injury (30). However, induction of nephritis in primates by passive transfer of serum or renal eluates derived from diseased patients firmly established an important pathogenic role of anti-GBM antibodies in this disease (3).

Studies in experimental models also have demonstrated several mechanisms by which glomerular damage occurs in the setting of anti-GBM antibody–mediated disease (9). Anti-GBM antibodies can induce glomerular injury either as a direct effect of binding to the GBM or through activation of complement (31,32). Once activated, complement chemotactic factors may then attract effector cells such as neutrophils and macrophages (31, 33). These inflammatory cells have an established role in mediating experimental glomerulonephritis, primarily through the release of toxic metabolites (33–35). In addition, experimental evidence suggests that the terminal complement cascade complex, C5b-9 independently elicits severe glomerular capillary wall injury (31,36).

Cellular responses also may play a role in glomerular injury induced in this disease because cell-mediated immunity to GBM antigens has been described in Goodpasture's syndrome (37). Moreover, in the experimental literature, adoptive transfer of renal-derived T cells from diseased kidneys in some animals induces glomerulonephritis in naive recipients in the absence of antibody (38). Recent lymphocyte depletion studies in a model of autoimmune glomerulonephritis demonstrate dependence of GBM antigen-specific antibody responses on T-cell lymphocyte priming in susceptible animals (39). The potential therapeutic impact of understanding these T cell–mediated interactions is described in the treatment section of this chapter.

Elegant studies conducted by several investigators have recently identified and characterized the relevant Goodpasture antigen (4,40–42). Continued whole-animal analyses have demonstrated that immunization with Goodpasture antigen extracted from heterologous GBM induces full expression of Goodpasture's syndrome, including characteristic pulmonary and renal involvement (43). These unique reagents will likely provide new avenues of investigation that can better define critical epitope(s) of the target antigen as well as determinants of host susceptibility to this disease.

Goodpasture Antigen

Because early renal histopathologic observations in Goodpasture's syndrome correlated GBM antibody deposition with disease activity, subsequent decades of research focused on identifying and characterizing the target antigen of pathogenic circulating anti-GBM antibodies (44,45). Investigative efforts identified the primary target antigen as a component of type IV collagen and provided a detailed structural understanding of basement membrane collagen (4,40–42). This identification was established through rigorous immunochemical and molecular studies of solubilized constituents of basement membrane, predominantly type IV collagen (4,40–42).

Type IV collagen forms the backbone of basement membrane (Fig. 1A and B) and also serves as a scaffold for binding and alignment of other basement membrane constituents, such as laminin, fibronectin, heparin sulfate proteoglycan, and entactin (46–51). The structural building blocks, or monomers, of type IV collagen in basement membrane consist of three alpha chains that form a triple helix (Fig. 1C) (42,46–49,52,53). At least six genetically distinct alpha chains comprise type IV collagen (49). These chains include classical $\alpha1$ and $\alpha2$ chains, as well as more recently characterized $\alpha3$, $\alpha4$, $\alpha5$, and $\alpha6$ chains (49). Triple helical monomers possess three structural domains, the N-terminal 7S domain, a triple helical middle region, and a C-terminal globular noncollagenous (NC1) domain (Fig. 1B and C) (42, 46–49,52,53). Monomers assemble through NC1–NC1 interactions, forming dimers, and through 7S–7S interactions, forming tetramers, to generate a suprastructure (Fig. 1B). Such end-to-end interactions result in a hexameric NC1 region that contains six alpha chains derived from two triple helical monomers of the type IV collagen molecule (54).

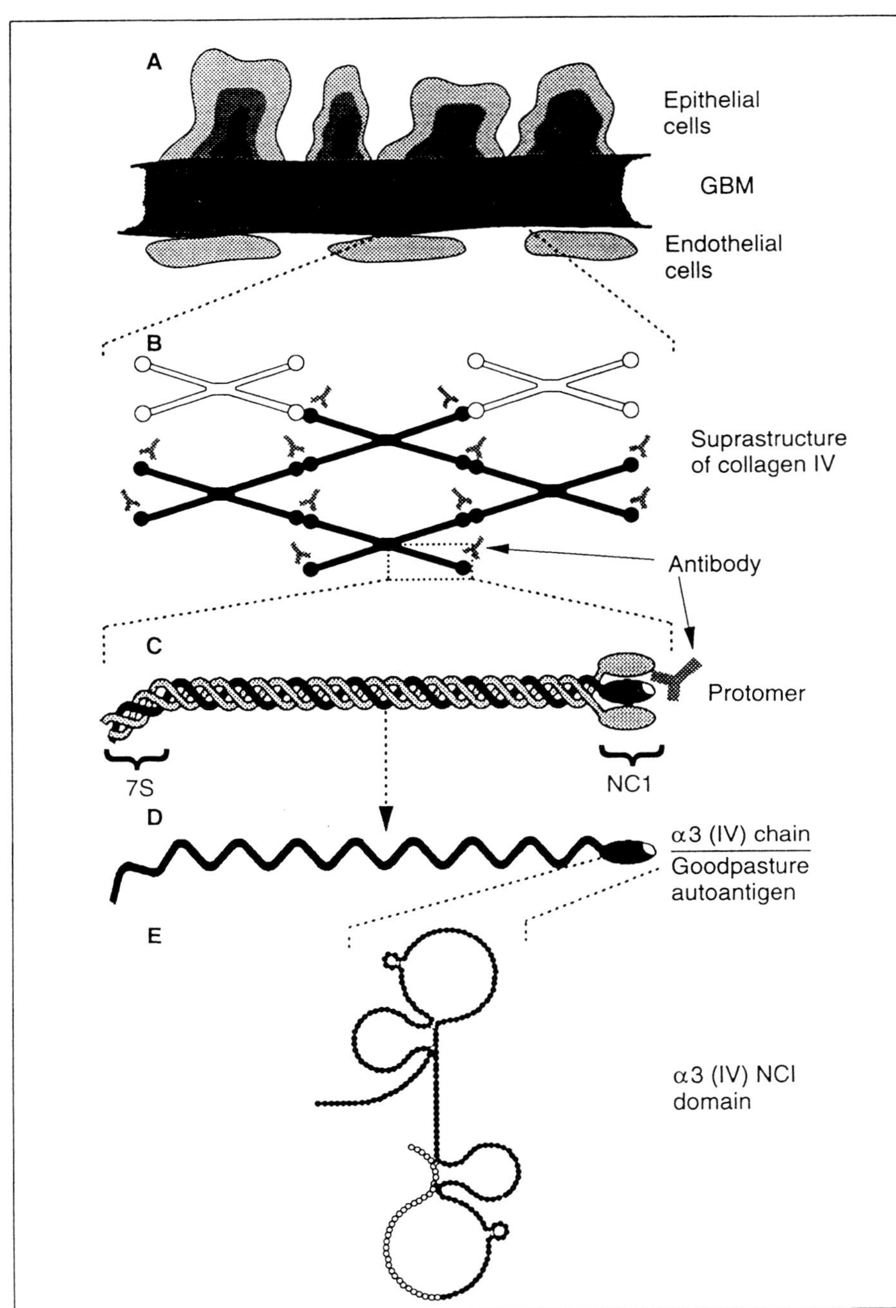

FIG. 1. Schematic illustration of the molecular structure of type IV Collagen and the Goodpasture antigen of GBM. **A:** The GBM is positioned between epithelial and endothelial cells. Type IV collagen is the target for the pathogenic autoantibodies in patients with anti-GBM antibody–mediated disease. **B:** Type IV collagen, the major protein constituent of GBM, exists as a supramolecular network. The dark area denotes triple helical molecules containing the Goodpasture antigen, α3(IV) chain. The light areas denote triple helical collagen molecules not containing the α3(IV) chain. The globular NC1 domain of type IV collagen and antibody localization site are represented by a circle and an arrow, respectively. **C:** Type IV collagen monomer with three alpha chains, derived from six genetically distinct alpha chains, in a triple helical conformation with C-terminal globular NC1 domains. The α3(IV) chain is shaded, with its NC1 domain binding autoantibody at a hypothetical binding site, shown in white. The 7S domain is located at the N-terminal. **D:** The complete α3(IV) chain, or Goodpasture antigen. **E:** Molecular structure of the NC1 domain with the intrachain disulfide pairing and the primary interaction site for antibodies, shown in white. Each dot represents one amino acid. Reprinted with permission (53).

Structural domains of type IV collagen can be excised from basement membrane by collagenase digestion, a biochemical attribute that facilitated identification of the Goodpasture antigen (49,54). Initial GBM collagenase digests yielded monomeric and dimeric components that reacted with anti-GBM antibodies isolated from patients with Goodpasture's syndrome (54–58). Subsequent work showed that these anti-GBM antibodies were directed against a monomeric subunit of the unique α3 chain of type IV [α3(IV)] collagen (Fig. 1D) (56). Further corroborative evidence implicating this GBM constituent in disease pathogenesis was obtained from in vitro expression systems of the human α3(IV) NC1 domain that demonstrated selective binding of translated products to pathogenic anti-GBM antibodies (59).

The α3 chain of type IV collagen is a polypeptide of 1,670 amino acids (60). The full-length translated polypeptide has a signal peptide of 28 amino acids, a 1,410-residue collagenous domain with a 14 residue N-terminal noncollagenous region, and a 232-residue NC1 region (60). The complete peptide sequence consists of 25 noncollagenous interruptions in the Gly-X-Y repeat and contains 24 cysteine residues (Fig. 1D and E) (60). This potential for multiple disulfide bond formation is likely relevant to the complex structural conformation of α3 within type IV collagen (60). The peptide sequence exhibits 45% to 70% homology with other alpha chains of type IV collagen, and its NC1 domain has 60% to 70% homology with the other alpha chain NC1 domains (49). Recent chromosome mapping localized the human gene to the q35-q37 region of chromosome 2 (61).

Although relevant epitopes of the Goodpasture antigen have not been fully characterized, secondary structure analysis of human α3(IV) NC1 domain shows several interesting features (Fig. 2) (59,62). Chou-Fasman algorithm analysis (Fig. 2C) predicts three antihelical regions, seven β-sheets, and 21 β-turns in the α3(IV) NC1 domain (63). Further examination of the α3(IV) NC1 peptide sequence shows 28 positively charged amino acids. Two major clusters of these basic amino acids are present in the N-terminal and C-terminal regions of the α3(IV) NC1 domain. One cluster lies within the N-terminal 26 amino acids from the triple helix-NC1 junction, which is 12 residues into the triple helix region and 14 residues into the NC1 region. The other cluster is within the last 36 amino acids of the C-terminal region. Local hydropathy plot analysis of the peptide sequence indicates four major hydrophilic regions within the α3 NC1 domain (Fig. 2A) that may be indicative of antigenic determinants (64). These hydrophilic segments correspond to the two clusters of basic amino acids in the peptide sequence. Antigenic index analysis, which combines information from

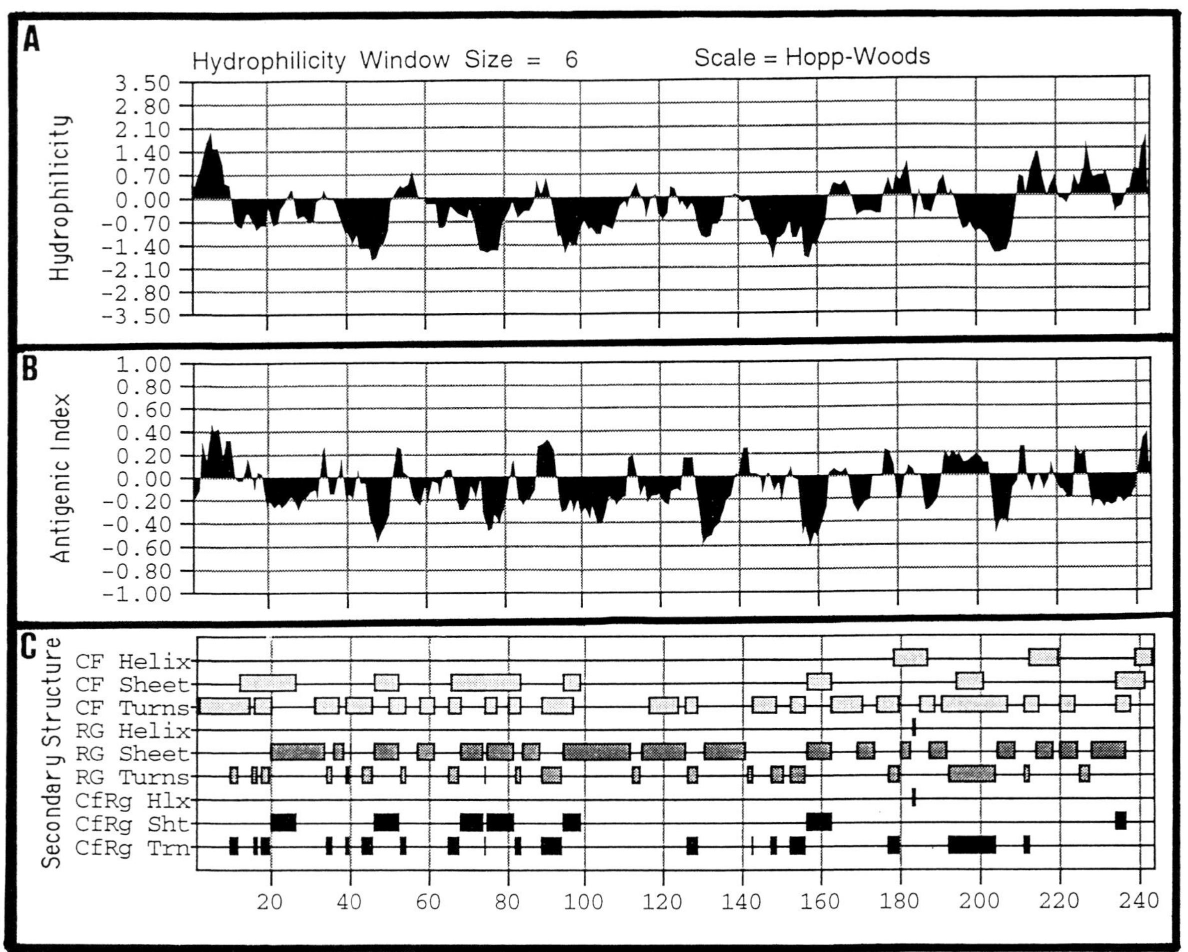

FIG. 2. Secondary structure analysis of the human α3(IV) NC1 domain. Complete NC1 domain and 12 amino acids of the triple helical region were included for these analyses. **A:** Hydrophilicity plot computed by the Hopp-Woods method, using a window of six amino acids (64). **B:** Antigenic index obtained by combining information from hydrophilicity, surface probability, and backbone flexibility predictions, as well as secondary structure predictions of Chou-Fasman and Robson-Garnier (65). The results produce a composite prediction of the surface contour of the α3(IV) NC1 domain. **C:** Secondary structure analysis using the Chou-Fasman (cf) and Robson-Garnier (rg) predictions. Use of both in one analysis to predict the secondary structure is denoted by cfrg (63,172,173).

secondary structure and local hydrophilicity predictions (Fig. 2B) also suggests prominent antigenicity in the terminal regions of the α3(IV) NC1 domain (65).

Recent reports have implicated two potential antibody-binding sites in the α3(IV) NC1 domain (66,67). Using a synthetic peptide strategy, a significant epitope was localized to the 36 C-terminal amino acid segment (Fig. 1E) (66). This is also the site of a distinctive hydrophilic amino acid cluster (Fig. 2A) (66). Based on regional hydrophilicity analysis and site-directed mutagenesis, a second proposed epitope is an 18–amino acid segment at the triple helix–NC1 junction of the α3(IV) NC1 domain (62,67). Structural analysis showed that the primary Goodpasture epitope is sequestered in α3-containing hexameric NC1 domains, but is exposed experimentally through dissociation with membrane denaturants (54). As discussed below, release of the relevant epitope from its immunologically privileged site, perhaps induced by various environmental agents or in appropriately susceptible hosts, may be a critical initiating event in anti-GBM antibody–mediated disease (68).

Despite the wide distribution of type IV collagen in parenchymal organs, Goodpasture antigen expression is relatively restricted (49). Recent studies indicate that α3 and α4 chains of type IV collagen are not ubiquitous basement membrane constituents (49). Immunofluorescence staining or immunoblotting with chain-specific antibodies demonstrates regional basement membrane localization of α3(IV) expression in kidney, lung, eye, aorta, choroid plexus, cochlea, and neuromuscular junctions (41,49,53,57,69–77). Similar monoclonal staining of human kidney detects predominantly GBM expression with minimal staining of distal tubular basement membrane (72). In view of the multiple organs that express α3(IV), however, the selective involvement of lung and kidney, and rarely the skin or eye, in anti-GBM antibody–mediated disease is particularly noteworthy (2,68, 78,79). Experimental evidence suggests that the lack of other α3(IV)-expressing organ involvement in anti-GBM antibody–mediated disease reflects either low-level α3(IV) chain expression or its immunologically privileged location within the basement membrane (80,81). Recent studies also show alternatively spliced α3(IV) transcripts, indicating tissue-specific expression of variant α3(IV) chains (67,82).

Important structural differences between GBM and alveolar basement membranes may explain why pulmonary hemorrhage develops in only a subset of patients with anti-GBM antibody–mediated disease (10). Although these basement membranes exhibit similar Goodpasture antigen distribution patterns, alveolar capillaries lack fenestrations typically present on glomeruli that impede large charged molecules such as antibodies (83). In the setting of alveolar endothelial injury, however, increased membrane permeability could facilitate pathogenic antibody access to relevant antigenic sites along the basement membrane (84). Support for this hypothesis is derived from clinical observations of patients with anti-GBM antibody–mediated disease (10). Such patients tend to develop severe pulmonary hemorrhage if afflicted with concurrent infection or fluid overload, or when administered high concentrations of oxygen and positive-pressure ventilation (85,86).

Disease Susceptibility

Factors that initiate anti-GBM antibody production in patients with anti-GBM antibody–mediated disease have not been clearly elucidated. Observations in the clinical literature suggest that this autoimmune disorder might be triggered by a variety of environmental exposures or infectious diseases (15,16). Because the Goodpasture antigen is sequestered within the type IV collagen molecule, such nonimmunologic damage to basement membrane could theoretically unmask the relevant epitope and initiate autoimmune events targeting basement membrane (49). Recent history of upper respiratory tract infection or flulike illness has been noted in 20% to 60% of reported cases (13,19, 21–23,27). An association between influenza infection and Goodpasture's syndrome has been documented by reports of disease clusters in defined geographic areas associated with influenza A2 outbreaks (16,28).

Environmental exposure to hydrocarbon solvents has been implicated as a precipitating event in some cases of Goodpasture's syndrome (15,87,88). History of exposure to a number of hydrocarbons such as organic solvents, hair-dressing solvents, paints, gasoline, and herbicides, has been reported in at least 30 cases in the literature (15, 87,88). Anecdotal reports of Goodpasture's syndrome also have been described after exposure to hard metal dust and chlorine gas, or D-penicillamine therapy in Wilson's disease (89–91). In this latter case, however, anti-GBM antibodies were not detected (91). In most published series of Goodpasture's syndrome, toxin exposure is recorded in fewer than 5% of affected individuals, although extensive historical information is generally not available in reported cases (13,19,21–23,27). Some investigators suggest that chemically mediated injury to the lung or renal parenchyma initiates a cascade of immunologic events that ultimately results in production of anti-GBM antibodies (68,88,92). Studies examining this hypothesis in the experimental setting show that although hydrocarbon exposure in animals induces glomerular injury, concurrent de novo production of anti-GBM antibodies is not observed (93,94).

Along similar lines, review of cigarette smoking habits in some series of anti-GBM antibody–mediated glomerulonephritis indicates a rather high incidence of tobacco smoking in patients with Goodpasture's syndrome (13, 95). Smokers with anti-GBM antibody–mediated disease appear to have a higher incidence of pulmonary hemorrhage in some studies, although their levels of circulating anti-GBM antibodies are similar to those of nonsmokers (13,95). It has been suggested that a tobacco-associated predisposition to pulmonary bleeding results from alterations in lung permeability effected by cigarette smoke (95). This smoke-induced increase in endothelial permeability may then alter the antigenicity of alveolar basement membrane, facilitating antibody production and its access to relevant basement membrane epitopes (20).

A genetic predisposition to anti-GBM antibody–mediated disease also has been suggested by the results of numerous studies (96–98). Early reports described cases of this disorder in identical twins and in familial clusters (96,97). Further analysis of major histocompatibility complex class II genes in affected individuals demonstrates an increased association of human leukocyte antigen (HLA)-DR2 in patients with Goodpasture's syndrome (98–100). Recent analysis of 53 patients with Goodpasture's syndrome showed a markedly increased frequency of DRw15, a subspecificity of DR2, in 76% of affected patients (101). This allelic determinant was detected in only 31% of control subjects (101). These observations implicate inheritance of specific immune response genes that may alter host susceptibility to anti-GBM antibody–mediated disease (101). One hypothesis suggests that infection or toxin-related Goodpasture's syndrome can occur in such autoimmune predisposed hosts, who may be less tolerant of organ-specific glycoproteins expressed in endogenous tissues (49,102).

Anti-GBM antibody–mediated disease also is observed as a consequence of renal transplantation (103). Isolated cases have been reported in transplant recipients with hereditary nephritis, such as Alport's syndrome, in which distinct morphologic abnormalities are present in native GBM (103,104). In X-linked Alport's syndrome, genetic mutations in the $\alpha5$ chain of type IV collagen result in absent or aberrant $\alpha5$ chain expression (105–107). Studies conducted recently suggest that $\alpha5$ chain abnormalities produce defective incorporation of the $\alpha3$ chain, or Goodpasture antigen, into type IV collagen of Alport GBM (108,109). This hypothesis is consistent with previous observations that show absent or reduced binding of Goodpasture anti-GBM antibodies to the Alport GBM (110,111). Renal transplantation with an intact, and antigenically distinct, GBM in such patients elicits an immune response targeting these neo-GBM antigens (103,104, 108). Although both circulating and deposited anti-GBM antibodies are frequently detected in transplant recipients with the Alport type of hereditary nephritis, anti-GBM antibody–mediated nephritis with allograft failure occurs in only 5% of recipients (112). Interestingly, post-transplant alloantibodies isolated from these patients with glomerulonephritis show predominant $\alpha3$ chain, or Goodpasture antigen, specificity (109). Factors that induce such injurious renal immune responses targeting the $\alpha3$ chain of basement membrane collagen in this small subset of Alport's syndrome recipients have not been delineated (109).

PATHOLOGY

Light Microscopy

Light microscopy findings in anti-GBM antibody–mediated renal disease show a spectrum of pathology, depending on the extent of disease at presentation (8,12,13, 113). Biopsies from patients with mild renal involvement and relatively normal renal function may exhibit normal histology or evidence of mild focal and segmental glomerular changes (12,13). These changes also may be associated with segmental necrosis and some epithelial crescent formation (12,19,21). Most commonly, crescent formation in seen in a significant portion of glomeruli, with circumferential cellular collections compressing glomerular tufts (Fig. 3A) (12,19,21). Silver stains typically exhibit destruction of the GBM, as well as of Bowman's capsule basement membrane (114). The composition of glomerular crescents depends on stage of disease at renal biopsy (115). If Bowman's capsule is intact, crescents are comprised predominantly of epithelial cells, although T-cell lymphocytes, monocytes, and polymorphonuclear leukocytes also can be seen (115). If the capsule is ruptured, monocytes and macrophages are frequently noted, as are some interstitial fibroblasts (115). These lesions do not usually involve endocapillary proliferation and may progress to global crescentic glomerulonephritis (115–117). Multinucleated giant cells have been noted in both glomerular and tubulointerstitial compartments (115–117). As previously described, anti-GBM antibody–mediated nephritis also can occur in the setting of other glomerular lesions, most notably membranous glomerulopathy (17).

In addition to the glomerular findings, tubulointerstitial inflammation of varying degree is generally apparent in renal biopsy samples (118). Tubulointerstitial changes are characterized by mononuclear cell infiltration and edema (118). These commonly associated tubulointerstitial changes are particularly evident in renal biopsy samples that demonstrate marked tubular basement membrane antibody deposition (118). Histologic evidence of renal vasculitis also has been reported in several series of anti-GBM antibody–mediated disease (119). More recent studies suggest that such individuals have coexistent antineutrophil cytoplasmic antibodies (ANCAs) (26,120, 121). The significance of vasculitis associated with anti-GBM antibody–mediated disease is discussed in the section on Differential Diagnosis in this chapter.

Inflammatory changes in glomerular crescents organize and become less cellular over several weeks to months (116,117). This process results in progressive

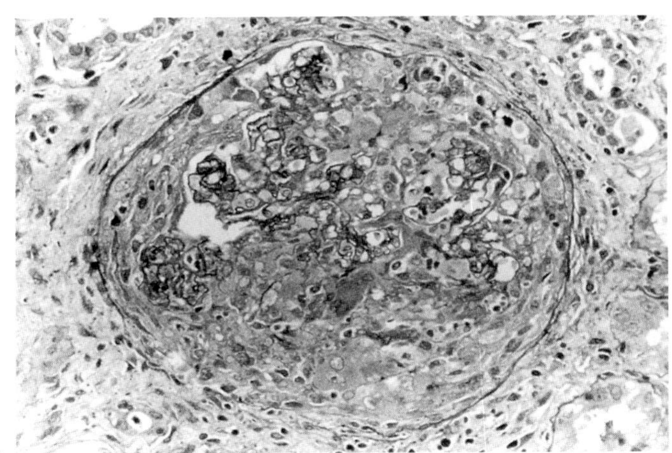
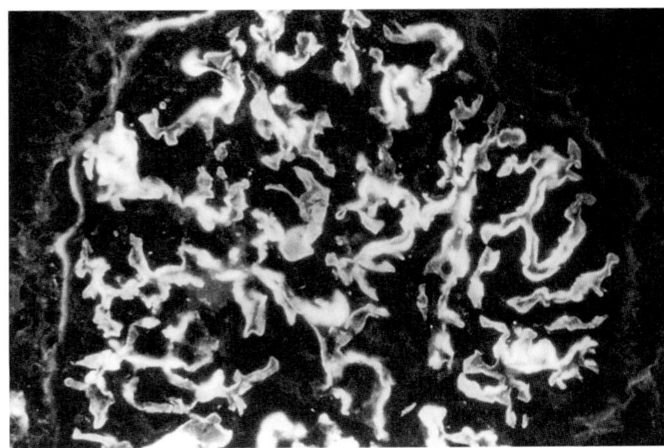

FIG. 3. A: Light microscopy findings of renal biopsy obtained from a patient with anti-GBM antibody–mediated disease (periodic acid-Schiff). The glomerulus shows mesangial hypertrophy, endocapillary proliferation, and crescent formation. Some tubulointerstitial infiltration and fibrosis are also apparent. **B:** Immunofluorescence staining of renal biopsy in anti-GBM antibody–mediated disease. The glomerular capillary loops and Bowman's capsule are outlined by a linear ribbonlike band of IgG. Photomicrographs courtesy of Dr. John E. Tomaszewski, Hospital of the University of Pennsylvania.

global glomerular sclerosis and fibrosis (116,117). On rare occasions, resolution of cellular crescents has been observed (122). With progressive disease, glomerular and tubulointerstitial changes result in global glomerulosclerosis with focal hyalinosis and interstitial fibrosis (116,117). Overall, these light microscopic findings are indistinguishable from other forms of crescentic glomerulonephritis that present with rapidly progressive renal failure (115–117). Further histologic and serologic evaluation is therefore indicated to establish a definitive diagnosis of anti-GBM antibody–mediated disease.

In the setting of pulmonary involvement, light microscopy findings typically show intra-alveolar hemorrhage and hemosiderin-laden macrophages, with evidence of alveolar septal widening (20,21,123). Inflammatory changes consistent with vasculitis, such as alveolar septal neutrophilic infiltration and edema also can be seen in patients presenting with an associated systemic vasculitis (124).

Electron Microscopy

Ultrastructural changes of anti-GBM-antibody–mediated renal disease consist predominantly of capillary subendothelial space widening (114). Immunoelectron microscopy indicates that this is the site of anti-GBM antibody binding (125). Segmental capillary endothelial cell detachment and luminal fibrin deposition also have been described (21,23). In addition, gaps also are noted in both the glomerular and Bowman's capsule basement membrane and may be widespread (21,23,125). It is likely that such basement membrane disruptions facilitate migration of relevant immune cells and fibroblasts into Bowman's space (19,114,117). Other associated defects include endothelial cell hypertrophy and hyperplasia, as well as epithelial foot process obliteration (21). Electron-dense deposits are not characteristic of anti-GBM antibody–mediated disease but have been reported (126). Electron microscopy of affected lung tissue typically demonstrate nonspecific findings such as type I and type II pneumocyte hyperplasia with basement membrane thickening (20,21,123).

Immunofluorescence

Immunofluorescence studies are of particular diagnostic importance in anti-GBM antibody–mediated disease (3,19,27,118,127). Linear ribbonlike deposition of IgG along the GBM is characteristic of this disease (Fig. 3B) (3,19,27,118,127). Most commonly, both circulating and deposited anti-GBM antibodies are IgG1, although other subclasses have been noted (128,129). IgA and IgM deposits also have been reported, albeit less commonly (128–130). Segmental or granular C3 deposits are observed in approximately 50% to 80% of reported cases, particularly in the setting of coexistent membranous nephropathy or in severely damaged glomeruli (19,21). IgG and C3 deposits also may be seen on distal tubules (20). C1q deposits are uncommon, although fibrin-related antigens frequently are detected within crescents, Bowman's space, or affected tubules (129,131).

Pulmonary biopsies have demonstrated similar linear or segmental linear antibody deposits along alveolar capillary basement membranes (130,132). These deposits can be focal in nature and, like the renal lesions, associated with C3 and fibrin deposition (130,132). Lung biopsy findings are frequently nonspecific, however, even in patients with pulmonary hemorrhage and high circulating anti-GBM antibody titers (130,132). Because renal immunofluorescence staining is generally positive in anti-GBM antibody–mediated disease, even in the absence of clinical or biochemical evidence of renal dysfunction, renal biopsy remains the diagnostic procedure of choice in this disorder (7,8,113,133).

CLINICAL MANIFESTATIONS AND LABORATORY FEATURES

Clinical Presentation

Patients with anti-GBM antibody–mediated disease present with a spectrum of clinical manifestations, depending on the extent of pulmonary and/or renal involvement (13,19,21–23,27). Table 1 lists the most commonly associated clinical manifestations of Goodpasture's syndrome compiled from six published series (13,19,21–23, 27). Hemoptysis is the most common presenting feature in Goodpasture's syndrome, occurring in 72% to 94% of reported cases (13,19,21–23,27). Moreover, isolated pulmonary involvement with episodes of hemoptysis precede the development of glomerulonephritis by several months to years in 50% to 80% of cases (13,19,21–23, 27). Pulmonary bleeding varies extensively in intensity, from mild episodes to life-threatening hemorrhage and is accompanied by dyspnea in 44% to 72% of cases or cough in 18% to 41% of cases. Constitutional symptoms of fatigue and weakness, nausea and vomiting, and weight loss also have been reported (13,19,21–23,27). Presentation with chest pain, gross hematuria, or fever and chills is not uncommon (13,19,21–23,27). Of note, 19% to 59% of patients in these published series relate a history of recent upper respiratory tract infection or flu-like illness before the onset of Goodpasture's syndrome (13,19,21–23,27). Atypical presentations of Goodpasture's syndrome with renal vein thrombosis, as well as central nervous system abnormalities, have been reported (14,134).

TABLE 1. *Clinical manifestations of Goodpasture's syndrome*

	Incidence (%)[a]
Symptoms	
Hemoptysis	72–94
Dyspnea	44–72
Cough	18–41
Prior flu or URI	19–59
Chills/fever	15–64
Fatigue/weakness	11–66
Chest pain	10–41
Gross hematuria	10–45
Nausea/vomiting	9–41
Weight loss	7–44
Signs	
Pallor	51–90
Rales/rhonchi	37–56
Peripheral edema	6–33
Mild/moderate hypertension	4–73
Funduscopic changes	0–33
Skin rash	0–22
Hepatosplenomegaly	0–20

[a]Incidence of findings compiled from data in published series (13,19,21–23,27) and derived from 189 patient presentations.

Physical examination at presentation commonly shows pallor, likely resulting from concurrent anemia in 51–90% of reported patients (Table 1) (13,19,21–23,27). Lung examination is generally abnormal in 37% to 56% of cases (13,19,21–23,27). Peripheral edema is observed in 6% to 33% of cases, as is mild to moderate hypertension (13,19,21–23,27). However, marked elevation of systemic blood pressure is atypical of anti-GBM antibody–mediated disease (14). It is more likely to occur in the setting of pre-existing hypertension or volume overload in acute renal failure (14, 20). Cutaneous and funduscopic abnormalities also have been reported, as has evidence of hepatosplenomegaly (13,19,21–23,27,79,135).

Radiologic Findings

Abnormal chest radiograph findings, noted in 79% to 100% of reported cases, likely result from alveolar hemorrhage, but coexistent pneumonia, atelectasis, or pulmonary edema in hospitalized patients is commonly observed (10,13,19,21–23,27). More typical yet nonspecific findings in Goodpasture's syndrome consist of diffuse alveolar filling that spares apices and bases (136). In an acute pulmonary hemorrhage, dense bilateral infiltrates appear with airspace consolidation (136,137). Recurrent episodes of bleeding can result in interstitial fibrosis and a persistent reticular pattern on chest radiography (137). Further thoracic imaging with computed tomography (CT) and magnetic resonance imaging are of limited utility, although CT scanning may be helpful in delineating a focus of hemoptysis (10).

Laboratory Studies

Commonly reported laboratory abnormalities in patients with anti-GBM antibody–mediated disease are listed in Table 2. Anemia is almost universal, reported in 78% to 100% of cases (13,19,21–23). Marked decreases in hemoglobin at presentation are generally out of proportion to the degree of pulmonary bleeding or renal insufficiency (13,19,21–23). In Goodpasture's syndrome, a microcytic–hypochromic iron deficiency anemia is most common, whereas in isolated anti-GBM antibody–mediated nephritis, a microangiopathic hemolytic anemia

TABLE 2. *Common laboratory abnormalities in Goodpasture's syndrome*

Laboratory abnormalities	Incidence (%)[a]
Anemia (Hgb ≤ 10.5 g)	78–100
Azotemia	55–90
Proteinuria	56–100
Hematuria	78–100
Pyuria	36–71
Cylinderuria	55–59
Abnormal chest radiograph (infiltrates)	79–100

[a]Incidence of findings compiled from data in published series (13,19,21–23) and derived from 178 patient presentations.

can be seen (27). A moderate leukocytosis also may be present (21). Patients present with functional renal impairment and azotemia in 50% to 90% of cases. Urinary studies show proteinuria in 56% to 100% of patients, although nephrotic range proteinuria is uncommon (13,19,21–23). Hematuria also has been reported in 78% to 100% of cases, with a significant incidence of pyuria and cylinderuria (13,19,21–23).

Detection of either circulating or deposited anti-GBM antibodies is essential for diagnosing this disorder (3,19, 27,118,127). Like deposited antibodies, circulating anti-GBM antibodies are most commonly IgG1, but rare circulating IgA antibodies have been reported (128). Circulating anti-GBM antibody levels do not correlate well with disease severity in most studies, although serial anti-GBM antibody titers are routinely obtained to monitor therapeutic response (12,14,19,27). Antibody titers are generally highest at presentation, and decline thereafter, even in untreated patients (19).

Before the identification of Goodpasture antigen, anti-GBM antibody screening was conducted by indirect immunofluorescence staining of primate or human kidney sections (19,21,27). Current diagnostic testing uses more sensitive and specific solid-phase assays such as radioimmunoassays, enzyme-linked immunosorbent assays, and immunoblotting (20). Most commercially available assays detect only IgG anti-GBM antibodies (138). As pathogenic anti-GBM antibodies bind to the α3(IV) NC1 domain, assays using purified intact type IV collagen derived from mammalian kidney, purified NC1 domain of type IV collagen, recombinant α3 NC1 domain, or purified M2 subunit of the NC1 domain have a specificity of greater than 98% for anti-GBM antibody–mediated disease. Assays using collagenase-digested human GBM as substrate are less specific (138).

Other non-Goodpasture anti-GBM antibodies also have been detected in patients with anti-GBM antibody–mediated disease (139–141). In addition, such anti-GBM antibodies are occasionally associated with other glomerulopathies and isolated nonrenal diseases (142–144). Studies indicate that they bind other GBM components such as laminin, entactin, and the 7S domain of type IV collagen (142–144). Their potential pathogenic role in these diseases has not been elucidated, although they may represent a secondary antibody response targeting antigens exposed on damaged basement membranes (58).

DIFFERENTIAL DIAGNOSIS

Considerable overlap of clinical manifestations exists with anti-GBM antibody–mediated disease and other disorders that induce pulmonary and/or renal disease (145, 146). Clinical reports of the last several decades highlight the wide spectrum of pathology associated with anti-GBM antibodies, from mild isolated pulmonary or renal involvement to severe combined pulmonary and renal failure (145,146). Diagnostic testing for circulating or deposited anti-GBM antibodies should therefore be performed in the clinical setting of unexplained hemoptysis, rapidly progressive glomerulonephritis, or glomerulonephritis with pulmonary hemorrhage (145,146). Serologic and histologic analyses are crucial for establishing a definitive diagnosis in a timely fashion (10). This is particularly important for anti-GBM antibody–mediated disease because studies indicate that early therapeutic intervention is critical for preserving renal function (12,14).

Concomitant glomerulonephritis and pulmonary hemorrhage are most frequently caused by pauci-immune glomerulonephritis and pulmonary vasculitis associated with ANCA, although anti-GBM antibody–mediated disease and immune-complex disease frequently have similar clinical presentations (6). Table 3 illustrates the serologic differentiation of these three broad diagnostic categories (6,138). As shown in Table 3, other relevant serologic studies in anti-GBM antibody–mediated disease, such as anti-DNA antibodies, anti-nuclear antibodies (ANA), and complement levels, are normal (6,138, 145,146). Results of serologic studies for antistreptolysin-O titers, rheumatoid factor, and cryoglobulin are also negative (6,138,145,146).

Recent studies suggest that 10% to 30% of anti-GBM–positive sera are also positive for ANCA, a serologic marker for systemic vasculitis (26,120,121,147,148). This observation is not surprising because the associa-

TABLE 3. *Serologic evaluation of glomerulonephritis and pulmonary hemorrhage*

Serology	Anti-GBM disease	ANCA-related disease	Immune-complex disease
Anti-GBM antibodies	+	−	−
Anti-DNA antibodies, ANA	−	−	+
Low complement (C3, C4)	−	−	+
ANCA	±	+	−

tion of anti-GBM antibody–mediated disease and vasculitis has been well-documented in the literature, even before the identification of ANCA (119,149–151). Indeed, several case reports have demonstrated concurrent or sequential anti-GBM antibody–mediated disease with several distinct morphologic forms of vasculitis (10,119,149–151). Although ANCA-associated anti-GBM disease has been reported in multiple small series, interpretation of clinical findings is hampered by the limited number of affected patients, as well as by the lack of standardized serologic screening methods (26,120,121,147,148). Future serologic studies, using more standardized assays, will likely address these issues. A spectrum of ANCA specificities have been reported in these patients, and other serology results, such as for ANA, anti-DNA antibodies, rheumatoid factor, and cryoglobulins, are typically negative (26,120, 121,147,148). Patients with both ANCA and anti-GBM antibodies appear to have a higher incidence of renal and extrarenal vasculitis (26,120,121,147,148). It is unclear whether these double-antibody–positive patients have different clinical responses or prognoses from those with single anti-GBM antibody positivity (26,120,121,147, 148). It is noteworthy that recorded relapses of anti-GBM antibody–mediated disease have been associated with ANCA positivity in the absence of circulating anti-GBM antibodies (120,147,152).

Renal biopsy plays a major role in diagnosing anti-GBM antibody–mediated disease, particularly if the results of serum studies are delayed or negative (145, 146). However, false-positive results with kidney biopsy have been reported in diabetic nephropathy and sporadically in other forms of glomerulonephritis (153,154). Occasionally in renal biopsy samples with fulminant destructive glomerulonephritis, the typical linear pattern of antibody deposition is disrupted and a more granular antibody deposition pattern is apparent (145,146,153). Because such biopsy patterns are more suggestive of immune-complex disease, detection of circulating anti-GBM antibodies in these cases is especially useful (145,146,153).

TREATMENT

During the past two decades, remarkable improvement in published morbidity and mortality statistics are apparent in clinical studies of anti-GBM antibody–mediated disease (12,13,22). Early studies reported 96% mortality in afflicted patients, with most patients succumbing to massive hemoptysis or renal failure (22). Treatment regimens included either supportive measures alone or in combination with steroids and/or cytotoxic agents (22). In addition, bilateral nephrectomy was advocated in some centers to control life-threatening pulmonary hemorrhage (19). More recent studies of anti-GBM antibody–mediated disease report less than 10% mortality (12–14). The apparent marked improvement in patient outcome in this disease has likely resulted from two distinct events (9). One factor relates to improvement in general medical care in the past two decades for acute renal failure or lung hemorrhage (9). In addition, widespread availability of rapid and definitive diagnostic testing for anti-GBM antibodies has permitted early diagnosis of milder forms of the disease (9). Clinical studies suggest that these early lesions are more amenable to therapeutic intervention and on occasion may remit spontaneously (12,14,87,155).

Because anti-GBM disease is an uncommon clinical entity, few controlled studies evaluating treatment protocols have been conducted. Although a variety of treatment regimens are described in the literature, current treatment recommendations in most centers manage patients aggressively with steroids, cytotoxic reagents, and plasma exchange (9,10,12–14). The relatively recent therapeutic addition of plasma exchange is worthy of further comment. The initial rationale for adding plasmapheresis therapy was based on its ability to rapidly clear circulating factors, such as antibodies, in view of the firmly established pathogenic role of anti-GBM antibodies in this disease (156). With the wide availability of extracorporeal circulation technology, numerous centers have reported marked improvements in patient outcome with its combined use in treatment protocols (27,156–159). A particularly striking effect on lung hemorrhage and renal failure, if caught early, has been reported by one group that treated many such patients (159). Although there is a tendency for patients treated with plasmapheresis to do better, data from controlled studies is limited by small patient numbers, and the null hypothesis probably could withstand a more rigorous test (160,161).

Current treatment recommendations for anti-GBM antibody–mediated disease vary, depending on disease severity at presentation, initial response to therapy, and institutional bias (9,10,160). In general, plasmapheresis, with 3- to 4-L exchanges using plasma as the replacement fluid, is performed either daily or on alternate days, with serial measurement of anti-GBM antibodies (9,10,160). Exchanges are continued until anti-GBM antibodies are no longer detected, at times requiring 2–3 weeks of therapy (9,10,160). In addition to anti-GBM antibody removal with plasma exchange, administered glucocorticoids and cytotoxic agents inhibit further antibody production. Prednisone (1 mg/kg/day) and cyclophosphamide (2–3 mg/kg/day) or azathioprine (1–2 mg/kg/day) are given, with appropriate dose adjustments for leukopenia or thrombocytopenia (14). Immunosuppressive therapy should be maintained for approximately 8 weeks, then tapered in accordance with clinical response (9,14). Therapy is most effective in patients treated early in the course of their disease (12,14). Other anecdotal treatment regimens that have had some success include cyclosporine therapy and extracorporeal immunoadsorption of IgG with staphylococcal protein A (162,163).

Although mortality statistics have improved, outcome for renal function in patients with anti-GBM antibody–mediated disease remains poor (12–14,27). Despite the success of medical therapy in reducing circulating anti-GBM antibodies, more specific therapies that target injurious renal immune responses are not currently available. Recent studies in experimental models of anti-GBM antibody–mediated disease are investigating the utility of antibody therapy targeting activated mononuclear cells in diseased animals (164,165). Administration of monoclonal antibodies recognizing adhesion molecules, such as intercellular adhesion molecule-1 and lymphocyte function-associated antigen 1, markedly abrogates histologic expression of disease, even if administered after onset of disease (164). Of note, early circulating and deposited antibody responses in treated animals are not significantly different from those in untreated animals, despite the marked reduction in renal inflammation and functional impairment (164). In other studies, treatment with a soluble chimeric cytotoxic T lymphocyte antigen 4 (CTLA-4) fusion protein (CTLA4Ig), which blocks T cell–dependent antibody responses and prolongs allograft survival in vivo, also has shown disease-protective effects of this compound in anti-GBM antibody–mediated disease (165). Further delineation of relevant determinants of such immune cell interactions in this disease may provide new therapeutic options for human autoimmune glomerulonephritis (164,165).

PROGNOSIS

As previously stated, overall mortality in anti-GBM antibody–mediated disease has dropped precipitously in the past two decades, from 96% in 1964 to 7–11% in recent years (12,13,22). The incidence of end-stage renal disease remains high, however, with 40% to 70% of affected patients requiring transplantation or chronic dialysis (12–14,27). In general the outlook for recovery of renal function is poor unless treatment is instituted early in the course of disease (12–14,27). Patients most likely to respond to therapy are neither oliguric nor dialysis-dependent and have serum creatinine levels of less that 6 to 7 mg/dl (12–14,27,145). Rapidly progressive loss of renal function and oligoanuria are particularly ominous prognostic features (12–14,27,145). Renal biopsy findings such as 50% to 100% glomerular involvement with circumferential crescent formation, severe tubular atrophy and interstitial fibrosis, extensive glomerular fibrosis, and organization of crescents also portend a grim prognosis for renal function (12–14,27,145).

Continued follow-up of patients treated for anti-GBM antibody–mediated disease is also important because occasional relapses and late recurrence have been reported (159,166,167). In general this occurs several months to years after the initial episode and involves the lung or kidney, or both organs simultaneously (86,159, 166,167). Interestingly, circulating anti-GBM antibody titers often are not elevated during disease relapse (159, 166,167). Therapeutic intervention with immunosuppression, at times with plasma exchange, has been successful in some reported cases (159,166).

Patients that develop end-stage renal disease as a result of anti-GBM antibody–mediated disease generally are considered excellent candidates for renal transplantation (10,153). Because persistent anti-GBM antibodies are likely to produce recurrent disease in the allograft, transplantation is routinely delayed until anti-GBM antibodies are no longer detectable (10,168,169). Recurrent linear immune deposits have been observed in some patients, without apparent impact on allograft function (170).

A recent study evaluating long-term pulmonary complications in patients with anti-GBM antibody–mediated disease showed a significant reduction in effective gas exchange (single breath carbon monoxide transfer factor corrected for alveolar volume, KCO) in eight patients who sustained pulmonary hemorrhage during their disease, compared with controls matched for age as well as degree and duration of renal disease (171). However, results of other pulmonary function studies and exercise testing were not different between the two groups (171). Although these findings suggest residual interstitial pulmonary fibrosis in long-term survivors, significant lung disease generally has not been observed in patients with renal failure resulting from anti-GBM antibody–mediated disease (10,171).

ACKNOWLEDGMENTS

This work was supported in part by the American Heart Association Clinician-Scientist Award (91-409), the National Kidney Foundation of the Delaware Valley, the Lupus Foundation of America, Inc., and the Margaret Q. Landenberger Research Foundation (to C.M.M.); and by grants DK-30280, DK-07006, DK-41268, and DK-45191 from the National Institutes of Health (to E.G.N.).

REFERENCES

1. Goodpasture EW. The significance of certain pulmonary lesions in relation to the etiology of influenza. *Am J Med* 1919;158:863–870.
2. Stanton MC, Tange JD. Goodpasture's syndrome: pulmonary hemorrhage associated with glomerulonephritis. *Aust Ann Med* 1958;7:132–144.
3. Lerner RA, Glassock RJ, Dixon FJ. The role of anti-glomerular basement membrane antibody in the pathogenesis of human glomerulonephritis. *J Exp Med* 1967;126:989–1004.
4. Wieslander J, Barr JF, Butkowski RJ, et al. Goodpasture antigen of the glomerular basement membrane: localization to noncollagenous

regions of type IV collagen. *Proc Natl Acad Sci U S A* 1984;81:3838–3842.

5. Kalluri R, Wilson CB, Weber M, et al. Identification of the α3(IV) chain of type IV collagen as the common autoantigen in anti-basement membrane disease and Goodpasture syndrome. *J Am Soc Nephrol* 1995;6:1178–1185.
6. Jones DA, Jennette JC, Falk RJ. Goodpasture's syndrome revisited. A new perspective on glomerulonephritis and alveolar hemorrhage. *N C Med J* 1990;51:411–415.
7. Harrity P, Gilbert-Barness E, Cabalka A, Hong R, Zimmerman J. Isolated pulmonary Goodpasture syndrome. *Pediatr Pathol* 1991;11: 635–646.
8. Knoll G, Rabin E, Burns BF. Antiglomerular basement membrane antibody–mediated nephritis with normal pulmonary and renal function. A case report and review of the literature. *Am J Nephrol* 1993; 13:494–496.
9. Couser WG. Rapidly progressive glomerulonephritis: classification, pathogenetic mechanisms, and therapy. *Am J Kidney Dis* 1988;11: 449–464.
10. Kelly PT, Haponik EF. Goodpasture syndrome: molecular and clinical advances. *Medicine* 1994;73:171–185.
11. Keller F, Nekarda H. Fatal relapse in Goodpasture's syndrome 3 years after plasma exchange. *Respiration* 1985;48:62–66.
12. Merkel R, Pullin O, Marx M, Netzer KO, Weber M. Course and prognosis of anti-basement membrane antibody (anti-BM-Ab)-mediated disease: report of 35 cases. *Nephrol Dial Transplant* 1994;9:372–376.
13. Herody M, Bobrie G, Gouarin C, Grunfeld JP, Noel LH. Anti-GBM disease: predictive value of clinical, histological and serological data. *Clin Nephrol* 1993;40:249–255.
14. Savage COS, Pusey CD, Bowman C, Rees AJ, Lockwood CM. Antiglomerular basement membrane antibody mediated disease in the British Isles 1980–4. *Br Med J* 1986;292:301–304.
15. Bombassei GJ, Kaplan AA. The association between hydrocarbon exposure and anti-glomerular basement membrane antibody–mediated disease (Goodpasture's syndrome). *Am J Ind Med* 1992;21:141–153.
16. Wilson CB, Smith RC. Goodpasture's syndrome associated with Influenza A2 virus infection. *Ann Intern Med* 1972;76:91–94.
17. Pettersson E, Tornroth T, Miettinen A. Simultaneous anti-glomerular basement membrane and membranous glomerulonephritis: case report and literature review. *Immunol Immunopathol* 1984;31:171–179.
18. Deodhar HA, Marshall RJ, Sivathondan Y, Barnes JN. Recurrence of Goodpasture's syndrome associated with mesangiocapillary glomerulonephritis. *Nephrol Dial Transplant* 1994;9:72–75.
19. Wilson CB, Dixon FJ. Anti-glomerular basement membrane antibody-induced glomerulonephritis. *Kidney Int* 1973;3:74–89.
20. Rees AJ, Lockwood CM. Antiglomerular basement membrane antibody–mediated nephritis. In: Schrier RW, Gottschalk CW, eds. *Diseases of the kidney*. Boston: Little, Brown; 1988:2091–2126.
21. Teague CA, Doak PB, Simpson IJ, Rainer SP, Herdson PB. Goodpasture's syndrome: an analysis of 29 cases. *Kidney Int* 1978;13:492–504.
22. Benoit FL, Rulon DB, Theil GB, Doolan PD, Watten RH. Goodpasture's syndrome. A clinicopathologic entity. *Am J Med* 1964;37:424–444.
23. Proskey AJ, Weatherbee L, Easterling RE, Greene JA, Weller MM. Goodpasture's syndrome. A report of five cases and review of the literature. *Am J Med* 1969;48:162–173.
24. Volpi A, Battini G, Conte F, et al. Acute renal failure in elderly due to Goodpasture's syndrome [Letter]. *Nephron* 1991;57:381–2.
25. Yankowitz J, Kuller JA, Thomas RL. Pregnancy complicated by Goodpasture syndrome. *Obstet Gynecol* 1992;79:806–808.
26. Bonsib SM, Goeken JA, Kemp JD, Chandran P, Shadur C, Wilson L. Coexistent antineutrophil cytoplasmic antibody and antiglomerular basement-membrane antibody associated disease—report of 6 cases. *Mod Pathol* 1993;6:526–530.
27. Briggs WA, Johnson JP, Teichman S, Yeager HC, Wilson CB. Antiglomerular basement membrane antibody–mediated glomerulonephritis and Goodpasture's syndrome. *Medicine* 1979;58: 348–361.
28. Perez GO, Bjornsson S, Ross AH, Amato J, Rothfield N. A mini-epidemic of Goodpasture's syndrome. *Nephron* 1974;13:161–173.
29. Steblay RW. Glomerulonephritis induced in monkeys by injections of heterologous glomerular basement membranes and Freund's adjuvant. *Nature* 1963;197:1173–1176.
30. Lerner RA, Dixon FJ. Transfer of ovine experimental allergic glomerulonephritis (EAG) with serum. *J Exp Med* 1966;124: 431–442.
31. Couser WG, Baker PJ, Adler S. Complement and the direct mediation of immune glomerular injury: a new perspective. *Kidney Int* 1985;28: 879–890.
32. Couser WG, Darby C, Salant DJ, Adler S, Stilmant MM, Lowenstein LM. Anti-GBM antibody-induced proteinuria in isolated perfused rat kidney. *Am J Physiol* 1985;249:F241–F250.
33. Sindrey M, Naish P. The mediation of the localization of polymorphonuclear leukocytes in glomeruli during the autologous phase of nephrotoxic nephritis. *Clin Exp Immunol* 1979;35:350–355.
34. Shah SV, Baricos WH, Basci A. Degradation of human glomerular basement membrane by stimulated neutrophils. *J Clin Invest* 1987;79: 25–31.
35. Holdsworth SR, Neale TJ. Macrophage-induced glomerular injury. Cell transfer studies in passive autologous anti-glomerular basement membrane antibody-initiated experimental glomerulonephritis. *Lab Invest* 1984;51:172–180.
36. Groggel GC, Salant DJ, Darby C, Rennke HG, Couser WG. Role of the terminal complement pathway in the heterologous phase of anti-glomerular basement membrane nephritis in the rabbit. *Kidney Int* 1985;27:643–651.
37. Mahieu P, Dardenne M, Bach J. Detection of humoral and cell-mediated immunity to kidney basement membranes in human renal diseases. *Am J Med* 1972;53:185–192.
38. Bolton WK, Chandra M, Tyson TM, Kirkpatrick PR, Sadovnic MJ, Sturgill BC. Transfer of experimental glomerulonephritis in chickens by mononuclear cells. *Kidney Int*1988;34:598–610.
39. Reynolds J, Sallie BA, Syrganis C, Pusey CD. The role of T-helper lymphocytes in priming for experimental autoimmune glomerulonephritis in the BN rat. *J Autoimmun* 1993;6:571–585.
40. Morrison KE, Mariyama M, Yang-Feng TL, Reeders ST. Sequence and localization of a partial cDNA encoding the human α3 chain of type IV collagen. *Am J Hum Genet* 1991;49:545–554.
41. Kleppel MM, Michael AF, Fish AJ. Antibody specificity of human glomerular basement membrane type IV collagen NC1 subunits: species variation in subunit composition. *J Biol Chem* 1986;261: 16547–16552.
42. Butkowski RJ, Shen GQ, Wieslander J, Michael AF, Fish AJ. Characterization of type IV collagen NC1 monomers and Goodpasture antigen in human renal basement membranes. *J Lab Clin Med* 1990;115: 365–373.
43. Kalluri R, Gattone V H Jr, Noelken ME, Hudson BG. The α3(IV) chain of type IV collagen induces autoimmune Goodpasture syndrome. *Proc Natl Acad Sci U S A* 1994;91:6201–6205.
44. Scheer RL, Grossman MA. Immune aspects of the glomerulonephritis associated with pulmonary hemorrhage. *Ann Intern Med* 1964;60: 1009–1021.
45. Sturgill BC, Westervelt FB. Immunofluorescence studies in a case of Goodpasture's syndrome. *JAMA* 1965;194:914–916.
46. Timpl R, Oberbaumer I, von der Mark H, et al. Structure and biology of the globular domain of basement membrane collagen type IV. *Ann N Y Acad Sci* 1985;460:58–72.
47. Timpl R, Dziadek M. Structure, development and molecular pathology of basement membranes. *Int Rev Exp Pathol* 1986;29:1–11.
48. Timpl R. Structure and biological activities of basement membrane proteins. *Eur J Biochem* 1989;180:487–502.
49. Hudson BG, Reeders ST, Tryggvason K. Type IV collagen: structure, gene organization, and role in human diseases. Molecular basis of Goodpasture and Alport syndromes and diffuse leiomyomatosis. *J Biol Chem* 1993;268:26033–26036.
50. Yurchenco PD, Tsilibary EC, Charonis AS, Furthmayr H. Models for the self-assembly of basement membrane. *J Histochem Cytochem* 1986;34:93–102.
51. Yurchenco PD, Ruben GC. Basement membrane structure in situ: evidence for lateral associations in the type IV collagen network. *J Cell Biol* 1987;105:2559–2568.
52. Timpl R, Wiedemann H, Van Veldon V, Furthmayr H, Kuhn K. A network model for the organization of type IV collagen molecules in basement membranes. *Eur J Biochem* 1981;120:203–211.
53. Hudson BG, Kalluri R, Gunwar S, Noelken ME, Mariyama M, Reeders ST. Molecular characteristics of the Goodpasture autoantigen. *Kidney Int* 1993;43:135–139.

54. Wieslander J, Langeveld J, Butkowski R, Jodlowski M, Noelken M, Hudson BG. Physical and immunochemical studies of the globular domain of type IV collagen: cryptic properties of the Goodpasture antigen. *J Biol Chem* 1985;260:8564–8570.
55. Butkowski RJ, Wieslander J, Wisdom BJ, Barr JF, Noelken ME, Hudson BG. Properties of the globular domain of type IV collagen and its relationship to the Goodpasture antigen. *J Biol Chem* 1985; 260:3739–3747.
56. Butkowski RJ, Langeveld JP, Wieslander J, Hamilton J, Hudson BG. Localization of the Goodpasture epitope to a novel chain of basement membrane collagen. *J Biol Chem* 1987;262:7874–7877.
57. Gunwar S, Ballester F, Kalluri R, et al. Glomerular basement membrane. Identification of dimeric subunits of the noncollagenous domain (hexamer) of collagen IV and the Goodpasture antigen. *J Biol Chem* 1991;266:15318–15324.
58. Hudson BG, Wieslander J, Wisdom BJJ, Noelken ME. Goodpasture syndrome: molecular architecture and function of basement membrane antigen [erratum *Lab Invest* 1989;61:690]. *Lab Invest* 1989;61: 256–269.
59. Neilson EG, Kalluri R, Sun MJ, et al. Specificity of Goodpasture autoantibodies for the recombinant noncollagenous domains of human type IV collagen. *J Biol Chem* 1993;268:8402–8405.
60. Mariyama M, Leinonen A, Mochizuki T, Tryggvason K, Reeders ST. Complete primary structure of the human α3(IV) collagen chain: coexpression of the α3(IV) and α4(IV) collagen chains in human tissues. *J Biol Chem* 1994;269:23013–23017.
61. Mariyama M, Zheng K, Yang TTL, Reeders ST. Colocalization of the genes for the α3(IV) and α4(IV) chains of type IV collagen to chromosome 2 bands q35-37. *Genomics* 1992;13:809–813.
62. Kalluri R, Sun MJ, Hudson BG, Neilson EG. The Goodpasture autoantigen—Structural delineation of 2 immunologically privileged epitopes on alpha-3(IV) chain of type-IV collagen. *J Biol Chem* 1996; 271:9062–9068.
63. Chou PY, Fasman GD. Conformational parameters for amino acids in helical, beta sheet and random coil regions calculated from proteins. *Biochemistry* 1985;13:211–222.
64. Hopp TP, Woods KR. Prediction of protein antigenic determinants from amino acid sequences. *Proc Natl Acad Sci U S A* 1981;78:3824–3828.
65. Jameson BA, Wolf H. The antigenic index: a novel algorithm, for predicting antigenic determinants. *Comput Appl Biosci* 1988;4:181–186.
66. Kalluri R, Gunwar S, Reeders ST, et al. Goodpasture syndrome: localization of the epitope for the autoantibodies to the carboxyl-terminal region of the α3(IV) chain of basement membrane collagen. *J Biol Chem* 1991;266:24018–24024.
67. Quinones S, Bernal D, Garcia SM, Elena SF, Saus J. Exon/intron structure of the human alpha 3(IV) gene encompassing the Goodpasture antigen (alpha 3(IV)NC1). Identification of a potentially antigenic region at the triple helix/NC1 domain junction. *J Biol Chem* 1992;267:19780–19784.
68. Hudson BG, Kalluri R, Tryggvason K. Pathology of glomerular basement membrane nephropathy. *Curr Opin Nephrol Hypertens* 1994;3: 334–339.
69. Turner N, Forstova J, Rees A, Pusey CD, Mason PJ. Production and characterization of recombinant Goodpasture antigen in insect cells. *J Biol Chem* 1994;269:17141–17145.
70. Kleppel MM, Santi PA, Cameron JD, Wieslander J, Michael AF. Human tissue distribution of novel basement membrane collagen. *Am J Pathol* 1989;134:813–825.
71. Kleppel MM, Fan WW, Cheong HH, Michael AF. Evidence for separate networks of classical and novel membrane collagen: characterization of α3(IV)-Alport antigen heterodimer. *J Biol Chem* 1992;267: 4137–4142.
72. Butkowski RJ, Wieslander J, Kleppel M, Michael AF, Fish AJ. Basement membrane collagen in the kidney: regional localization of novel chains related to collagen IV. *Kidney Int* 1989;35:1195–1202.
73. Reddy GK, Gunwar S, Kalluri R, Hudson BG, Noelken ME. Structure and composition of type IV collagen of bovine aorta. *Biochim Biophys Acta* 1993;1157:241–251.
74. Gunwar S, Noelken ME, Hudson BG. Properties of the collagenous domain of the alpha 3(IV) chain, the Goodpasture antigen, of lens basement membrane collagen. Selective cleavage of alpha (IV) chains with retention of their triple helical structure and noncollagenous domain. *J Biol Chem* 1991;266:14088–14094.
75. Sanes JR, Engavall E, Butkowski R, Hunter DD. Molecular heterogeneity of basal laminae: Isoforms of laminin and collagen IV at the neuromuscular junction and elsewhere. *J Cell Biol* 1990;111:1685–1699.
76. Savage COS, Pusey CD, Kershaw MJ, et al. The Goodpasture antigen in Alport's syndrome: studies with a monoclonal antibody. *Kidney Int* 1986;30:107–112.
77. Weber M, Pullig O, Kohler H. Distribution of Goodpasture antigens within various human basement membranes. *Nephrol Dial Transplant* 1990;5:87–93.
78. Ross JB, Cohen AD, Ghose T. Goodpasture's syndrome associated with skin involvement. *Arch Dermatol* 1985;121:1441–1444.
79. Rowe PA, Mansfield DC, Dutton GN. Ophthalmic feature of fourteen cases of Goodpasture's syndrome. *Nephron* 1994;68:52–56.
80. Derry CJ, Pusey CD. Tissue-specific distribution of the Goodpasture antigen demonstrated by 2-D electrophoresis and Western blotting. *Nephrol Dial Transplant* 1994;9:355–361.
81. Weber M, Pullig O. Different immunologic properties of the globular NC1 domain of collagen type IV isolated from various human basement membranes. *Eur J Clin Invest* 1992;22:138–146.
82. Feng L, Xia Y, Tang WW, Wilson CB. Alternative splicing of the NC1 domain of the human α3(IV) collagen gene: differential expression of mRNA transcripts that predict three protein variants with distinct carboxyl regions. *J Biol Chem* 1994;269:2342–2348.
83. Salant DJ. Immunopathogenesis of crescentic glomerulonephritis and lung purpura. *Kidney Int* 1987;32:408–425.
84. Jennings L, Roholt OA, Pressman D, Blau M, Andres GA, Brentjens JR. Experimental anti-alveolar basement membrane antibody mediated pneumonitis. *J Immunol* 1981;127:129–134.
85. Bowley NB, Steiner RE, Chin WS. The chest x-ray in antiglomerular antibody disease (Goodpasture's syndrome). *Clin Radiol* 1979;30: 419–429.
86. Rees AJ, Lockwood CM, Peters DK. Enhanced allergic tissue injury in Goodpasture's syndrome by intercurrent bacterial infection. *Br Med J* 1977;2:723–726.
87. Bernis P, Hamels J, Quoidbach A, Mhieu P, Bouvy P. Remission of Goodpasture's syndrome after withdrawal of an unusual toxic. *Clin Nephrol* 1985;23:312–317.
88. Stevenson A, Yaqoob M, Mason H, Pai P, Bell GM. Biochemical markers of basement membrane disturbances and occupational exposure to hydrocarbons and mixed solvents. *Q J Med* 1995;88:23–28.
89. Lechleitner P, Defregger M, Lhotta K, Totsch M, Fend F. Goodpasture's syndrome. Unusual presentation after exposure to hard metal dust. *Chest* 1993;103:956–957.
90. Siebels M, Andrassy K, Ritz E. Provocation of pulmonary haemorrhage in Goodpasture syndrome by chlorine gas. *Nephrol Dial Transplant* 1993;8:189.
91. Sternlieb I, Bennett B, Scheinberg IH. D-Penicillamine-induced Goodpasture's syndrome in Wilson's disease. *Ann Intern Med* 1975; 82:673–676.
92. Wilson CB. Immunologic diseases of the lung and kidney (Goodpasture's syndrome). In: Fishman AP, eds. *Pulmonary diseases and disorders*. 2nd ed. New York: McGraw-Hill; 1988:675–682.
93. Harman JW. Chronic glomerulonephritis and the nephrotic syndrome induced in rats with N,N′diacetylbenzidine. *J Pathol* 1971;104:107–127.
94. Klavis G, Drommer W. Goodpasture-syndrom und benzineinwirkung. *Arch Toxicol* 1970;26:40–55.
95. Donaghy M, Rees AJ. Cigarette smoking and lung hemorrhage in glomerulonephritis caused by autoantibodies to glomerular basement membrane. *Lancet* 1983;2:1390–1392.
96. D'Apice AJF, Kincaid-Smith P, Becker GJ, Loughhead MG, Freeman JW, Sands JM. Goodpasture's syndrome in identical twins. *Ann Intern Med* 1978;88:61–62.
97. Gossain VV, Gerstein AR, Janes AW. Goodpasture's syndrome: a familial occurrence. *Am Rev Respir Dis* 1972;105:621–624.
98. Rees AJ, Peters DK, Amos N, Welch KI, Batchelor JR. The influence of HLA-linked genes on the severity of anti-GBM antibody–mediated nephritis. *Kidney Int* 1984;26:444–450.
99. Huey B, McCormick K, Capper J, et al. Associations of HLA-DR and HLA-DQ types with anti-GBM nephritis by sequence-specific oligonucleotide probe hybridization. *Kidney Int* 1993;44:307–312.
100. Dunckley H, Chapman JR, Burke J, et al. HLA-DR and -DQ genotyping in anti-GBM disease. *Dis Markers* 1991;9:249–256.

101. Burns AP, Fisher M, Li P, Pusey CD, Rees AJ. Molecular analysis of HLA class II genes in Goodpasture's disease. *Q J Med* 1995;88:93–100.
102. Rees AJ. The immunogenetics of glomerulonephritis. *Kidney Int* 1994;45:377–383.
103. Shah B, First RM, Mendoza NC, Clyne DH, Alexander JW, Weiss MA. Alport's syndrome: risk of glomerulonephritis induced by anti-glomerular-basement membrane antibody after renal transplantation. *Nephron* 1988;50:34–38.
104. Kashtan CE, Butkowski RJ, Kleppel MM, Roy First M, Michael AF. Posttransplant anti-glomerular basement membrane nephritis in related males with Alport syndrome. *J Lab Clin Med* 1990;116:508–515.
105. Netzer K-O, Renders L, Zhou J, Pullig O, Tryggvason K, Weber M. Deletions of the *COL4A5* gene in patients with Alport syndrome. *Kidney Int* 1992;42:1336–1344.
106. Barker DF, Hostikka SL, Zhou J, et al. Identification of mutations in the *COL4A5* collagen gene in Alport syndrome. *Science* 1990;248:1224–1226.
107. Tryggvason K, Zhou J, Hostikka SL, Shows TB. Molecular genetics of Alport syndrome. *Kidney Int* 1993;43:38–44.
108. Hudson BG, Kalluri R, Gunwar S, et al. The pathogenesis of Alport syndrome involves type IV collagen molecules containing the alpha 3(IV) chain: evidence from anti-GBM nephritis after renal transplantation. *Kidney Int* 1992;42:179–187.
109. Kalluri R, Weber M, Netzer KO, Sun MJ, Neilson EG, Hudson BG. *COL4A5* gene deletion and production of post-transplant anti-alpha 3(IV) collagen alloantibodies in Alport syndrome. *Kidney Int* 1994; 45:721–726.
110. Kleppel MM, Kashtan C, Santi PA, Wieslander J, Michael AF. Distribution of familial nephritis antigen in normal tissue and renal basement membranes of patients with homozygous and heterozygous Alport familial nephritis. Relationship of familial nephritis and Goodpasture antigens to novel collagen chains and type IV collagen. *Lab Invest* 1989;61:278–289.
111. Kashtan C, Fish AJ, Kleppel M, Yoshioka K, Michael AF. Nephritogenic antigen determinants in epidermal and renal basement membrane of kindreds with Alport-type familial nephritis. *J Clin Invest* 1986;78:1035–1044.
112. Peten E, Pirson Y, Cosyns JP, et al. Outcome of thirty patients with Alport's syndrome after renal transplantation. *Transplantation* 1991; 52:823–826.
113. Bell DD, Moffatt SL, Singer M, Munt PW. Antibasement membrane antibody disease without clinical evidence of renal disease. *Am Rev Respir Dis* 1990;142:234–237.
114. Stejskal J, Pirani CL, Okada M, Mandelanakis N, Pollak VE. Discontinuities (gaps) of the glomerular capillary wall and basement membrane in renal disease. *Lab Invest* 1973;28:149–169.
115. Boucher A, Droz D, Adafer E, Noel L-H. Relationship between the integrity of Bowman's capsule and the composition of cellular crescents in human crescentic glomerulonephritis. *Lab Invest* 1987;56:526–534.
116. Morita T, Suzuki Y, Churg J. Structure and development of the glomerular crescent. *Am J Pathol* 1973;72:349–356.
117. Min KW, Gyorkey F, Gyorkey P, Yium JJ, Eknoyan G. The morphogenesis of glomerular crescents in rapidly progressive glomerulonephritis. *Kidney Int* 1974;5:47–56.
118. Andres G, Brentjens J, Kohli R, et al. Histology of human tubulointerstitial nephritis associated with antibodies in renal basement membranes. *Kidney Int* 1978;13:480–491.
119. Wu M-J, Rajaram R, Shelp WD. Vasculitis in Goodpasture's syndrome. *Arch Pathol Lab Med* 1980;104:300–307.
120. O'Donoghue DJ, Short CD, Brenchley PE, Lawler W, Ballardie FW. Sequential development of systemic vasculitis with anti-neutrophil cytoplasmic antibodies complicating anti-glomerular basement membrane disease. *Clin Nephrol* 1989;32:251–255.
121. Weber MF, Andrassy K, Pullig O, Koderisch J, Netzer K. Antineutrophil-cytoplasmic antibodies and antiglomerular basement membrane antibodies in Goodpasture's syndrome and in Wegener's granulomatosis. *J Am Soc Nephrol* 1992;2:1227–1234.
122. Hinglais N, Garcia-Torres R, Kleinknecht D. Long-term prognosis in acute glomerulonephritis. The predictive value of early clinical and pathologic features observed in 65 patients. *Am J Med* 1974;56:52–56.
123. Botting AJ, Brown AL, Diveritie MB. The pulmonary lesion in a patient with Goodpasture's syndrome as studied with the electron microscope. *Am J Clin Pathol* 1964;42:387–394.
124. Lombard CM, Colby TV, Elliott CG. Surgical pathology of the lung in anti-basement membrane antibody-associated Goodpasture's syndrome. *Hum Pathol* 1989;20:445–451.
125. Bonsib SM. Glomerular basement membrane discontinuities. *Am J Pathol* 1985;119:357–366.
126. Savage JA, Dowling J, Kincaid-Smith P. Superimposed glomerular immune complexes in anti-glomerular basement membrane disease. *Am J Kidney Dis* 1989;14:145–150.
127. Olsen S, Petersen VP, Hansen ES. Immunofluorescent studies of extracapillary glomerulonephritis. *Acta Pathol Microbiol Scand* 1974;249S:20–31.
128. Segelmark M, Butkowski R, Wieslander J. Antigen restriction and IgG subclasses among anti-GBM autoantibodies. *Nephrol Dial Transplant* 1990;5:991–996.
129. McPhaul JJ, Dixon FJ. Characterization of immunoglobulin G anti-glomerular basement membrane antibodies elicited from kidneys of patients with glomerulonephritis: II. IgG subtypes and in vitro complement fixation. *J Immunol* 1971;107:678–682.
130. Border WA, Baehler RW, Bhathena D, Glassock RJ. IgA anti-basement membrane nephritis with pulmonary hemorrhage. *Ann Intern Med* 1979;91:21–25.
131. Hoyer J, Michael AF, Hoyer L. Immunofluorescent localization of antihemophilic factor antigen and fibrinogen in human renal disease. *J Clin Invest* 1974;53:1375–1381.
132. Koffler D, Sandson J, Carr R, Kinkel HG. Immunologic studies concerning the pulmonary lesions in Goodpasture's syndrome. *Am J Pathol* 1969;54:293–301.
133. Lamriben L, Kourilsky O, Mougenot B, Ronco P, Sraer JD. Goodpasture's syndrome with asymptomatic renal involvement. Disappearance of antiglomerular basement membrane antibodies deposits after treatment. *Nephrol Dial Transplant* 1993;8:1267–1269.
134. Gottehrer A, Reynolds SD, Libys JJ, Stapleton RB, Heffner JE. Renal vein thrombosis. Initial manifestation of Goodpasture's syndrome. *Chest* 1991;99:239–40.
135. Hoscheit AM, Austin JK, Jones WL. Nonrhegmatogenous retinal detachment in Goodpasture's syndrome: a case report and discussion of the clinicopathologic entity. *J Am Optom Assoc* 1993;64:563–567.
136. Muller NL, Miller RR. Diffuse pulmonary hemorrhage. *Radiol Clin North Am* 1991;29:965–971.
137. Sybers RG, Sybers JL, Dickie HA, Paul LW. Roentgenographic aspects of hemorrhagic pulmonary-renal disease (Goodpasture's syndrome). *Am J Roentgenol* 1965;94:674–680.
138. Foster MH. Serologic evaluation of the renal patient. In: Jacobson HR, Striker GE, Klahr S, eds. *The principles and practice of nephrology*. 2nd ed. Philadelphia: BC Decker; 1995:71–85.
139. Kefalides NA, Ohno N, Wilson CB. Heterogeneity of antibodies in Goodpasture syndrome reacting with type IV collagen. *Kidney Int* 1993;43:85–93.
140. Hellmark T, Johansson C, Wieslander J. Characterization of anti-GBM antibodies involved in Goodpasture's syndrome. *Kidney Int* 1994;46:823–829.
141. Johansson C, Butkowski R, Swedenborg P, Alm P, Wieslander J. Characterization of a non-Goodpasture autoantibody to type IV collagen. *Nephrol Dial Transplant* 1993;8:1205–1210.
142. Bygren P, Cederholm B, Heinegard D, Wieslander J. Non-Goodpasture anti-GBM antibodies in patients with glomerulonephritis. *Nephrol Dial Transplant* 1989;4:254–261.
143. Kefalides NA, Pegg MT, Ohno N, Poon-King T, Zabriskie J, Fillit H. Antibodies to basement membrane collagen and to laminin are present in sera from patients with poststreptococcal glomerulonephritis. *J Exp Med* 1986;163:588–602.
144. Savige JA, Baker C, Gallicchio M, Varigos G. Circulating anti-glomerular basement membrane antibodies in coeliac disease and epidermolysis bullosa acquisita. *Aust N Z J Med* 1991;21:867–70.
145. Glassock RJ, Adler SG, Ward HJ, Cohen AH. Primary glomerular diseases. In: Brenner BM, Rector FC, eds. *The kidney*. 4th ed. Philadelphia: WB Saunders; 1991:1182–1279.
146. Glassock RJ, Adler SG, Ward HJ, Cohen AH. Secondary glomerular diseases. In: Brenner BM, Rector FC, eds. *The kidney*. 4th ed. Philadelphia: WB Saunders; 1991:1280–1368.

147. Jayne DRW, Marshall PD, Jones SJ, Lockwood CM. Autoantibodies to GBM and neutrophil cytoplasm in rapidly progressive glomerulonephritis. *Kidney Int* 1990;37:965–970.
148. Bosch X, Mirapeix E, Font J, et al. Prognostic implication of anti-neutrophil cytoplasmic autoantibodies with myeloperoxidase specificity in anti-glomerular basement membrane disease. *Clin Nephrol* 1991;36:107–113.
149. Wahls TL, Bonsib SM, Schuster VL. Coexistent Wegener's granulomatosis and anti-glomerular basement membrane disease. *Hum Pathol* 1987;18:205–211.
150. Komadina KH, Houk RW, Vicks SL, Desrosier KF, Ridley DJ, Boswell RN. Goodpasture's syndrome associated with pulmonary eosinophilic vasculitis. *J Rheumatol* 1988;15:1298–1301.
151. Dean SE, Saba SR, Ramirez G. Systemic vasculitis in Goodpasture's syndrome. *South Med J* 1991;84:1387–1390.
152. Vanhille P, Noel LH, Reumaux D, Fleury D, Lemaitre V, Gobert P. Late emergence of systemic vasculitis with anti-neutrophil cytoplasmic antibodies in a dialyzed patient with anti-glomerular basement glomerulonephritis. *Clin Nephrol* 1990;33:257–258.
153. Couser WG. Goodpasture's Syndrome. In: Jacobson HR, Striker GE, Klahr S, eds. *The principles and practice of nephrology*. 2nd ed. Philadelphia: BC Decker; 1995:139–143.
154. Westberg NG, Michael AF. Immunohistopathology of diabetic glomerulonephritis. *Diabetes* 1972;21:163–174.
155. Maxwell DR, Ozawa T, Nielsen RL, Luft FC. Spontaneous recovery from rapidly progressive glomerulonephritis. *Br Med J* 1979;2:643–646.
156. Lockwood CM, Boulton-Jones JM, Lowenthal RM, Simpson IJ, Peters DK, Wilson CB. Recovery from Goodpasture's syndrome after immunosuppressive treatment and plasmapheresis. *Br Med J* 1975;2: 252–254.
157. Erickson JB, Kurtz SB, Donadio JV, Helly KE, Wilson CB, Pineda AA. Use of combined plasmapheresis and immunosuppression in the treatment of Goodpasture's syndrome. *Mayo Clin Proc* 1979;54: 714–720.
158. Johnson JP, Whitman W, Briggs WA, Wilson CB. Plasmapheresis and immunosuppressive agents in antibasement membrane antibody-induced Goodpasture's syndrome. *Am J Med* 1978;64: 354–359.
159. Peters DK, Rees AJ, Lockwood CM, Pusey CD. Treatment and prognosis in antibasement membrane antibody mediated nephritis. *Transplant Proc* 1982;3:513–521.
160. Simpson IJ, Doak PB, Williams LC, et al. Plasma exchange in Goodpasture's syndrome. *Am J Nephrol* 1982;2:301–311.
161. Johnson JP, Moore J, Austin HA, Balow JE, Antonovcych TT, Wilson CB. Therapy of anti-glomerular basement membrane antibody disease: analysis of prognostic significance of clinical, pathologic factors. *Medicine* 1985;64:219–227.
162. Bygren P, Freiburghaus C, Lindholm T. Goodpasture's syndrome treated with staphylococcal protein A immunoadsorption. *Lancet* 1985;2:1295–1296.
163. Querin S, Schurch W, Beaulieu R. Ciclosporin in Goodpasture's syndrome. *Nephron* 1992;60:355–359.
164. Nishikawa K, Guo YJ, Miyasaka M, et al. Antibodies to intercellular adhesion molecule 1/lymphocyte function-associated antigen 1 prevent crescent formation in rat autoimmune glomerulonephritis. *J Exp Med* 1993;177:667–677.
165. Nishikawa K, Linsley PS, Collins AB, Stamenkovic I, McCluskey RT, Andres G. Effect of CTLA-4 chimeric protein on rat autoimmune anti-glomerular basement membrane glomerulonephritis. *Eur J Immunol* 1994;24:1249–1254.
166. Wu MJ, Moorthy AV, Beirne GJ. Relapse in antiglomerular basement membrane antibody mediated crescentic glomerulonephritis. *Clin Nephrol* 1980;13:97–102.
167. Dahlberg PJ, Kurtz SB, Donadio JV. Recurrent Goodpasture's syndrome. *Mayo Clin Proc* 1978;53:533–537.
168. Almkvist RD, Buckalew VM, Hirszel P. Recurrence of anti-glomerular basement membrane antibody mediated glomerulonephritis in an isograft. *Clin Immunol Immunopathol* 1981;18:54–61.
169. Couser WG, Wallace H, Monaco AP, Lewis EJ. Successful renal transplantation in patients with circulating antibody to glomerular basement membrane: report of two cases. *Clin Nephrol* 1973;1:381–383.
170. Bergrem H, Jervell J, Brodwall EK, Flatmark A, Mellbye O. Goodpasture's syndrome: a report of seven patients including long-term follow-up of three who received a kidney transplant. *Am J Med* 1980; 68:54–58.
171. Conlon PJ Jr, Walshe JJ, Daly C, et al. Antiglomerular basement membrane disease: the long-term pulmonary outcome. *Am J Kidney Dis* 1994;23:794–796.
172. Garnier J, Osguthorpe DJ, Robson B. Analysis of the accuracy and implications of simple methods for predicting the secondary structure of globular proteins. *J Mol Biol* 1978;120:97–120.
173. Robson B, Suzuke E. Conformational properties of amino acid residues in globular proteins. *J Mol Biol* 1976;107:327–356.

Immunologic Renal Diseases,
edited by E. G. Neilson and W. G. Couser.
Lippincott-Raven Publishers, Philadelphia © 1997

CHAPTER 44

Minimal-Change Nephrotic Syndrome

Kevin E.C. Meyers, Dean A. Kujubu, and Bernard S. Kaplan

Basham noted in 1858 (1) that

> A large amount of fresh matter has been added confirmatory of the object . . . that a careful examination and record of the microscopic appearances of the sediment in albuminous urine may at all times be accepted as a truthful interpretation of the advance or recession of the renal disorder. . . . Upon one point the author has seen reason to modify the opinion formerly expressed, that a state of inflammatory engorgement is universally the primary or antecedent stage of every form of morbis Brightii . . . it is believed that the absence of this symptom will be found chiefly in that form of the disease which produces the so-called waxy kidney. . . .

Although there is little debate about the definition of the nephrotic syndrome (NS), it is more difficult to define minimal-change nephrotic syndrome (MCNS). NS is characterized by edema, proteinuria, hypoalbuminemia, and hyperlipidemia. The designation "minimal-change" derives from histopathologic findings, but few patients with presumed MCNS are subjected to biopsy; furthermore, an objective description of "minimal" is difficult. Therefore, the terms "steroid-sensitive" and "steroid-responsive" NS are often used to denote MCNS. However, these terms are not synonymous because not all patients with minimal changes respond to steroids and not all of those who respond have minimal changes. A babble of other terms—lipoid nephrosis, minimal-lesion NS, and "nil" lesion disease—add to the confusion. MCNS occurs mainly in children, but also in adults. Patients present with edema, often after an ill-defined "upper respiratory tract infection", usually without gross hematuria, hypertension, or azotemia. MCNS usually responds to steroid treatment, tends to run a relapsing and remitting course, and rarely progresses to end-stage renal failure. In MCNS the glomerular changes are effacement and retraction of podocyte foot processes as seen by electron microscopy. There is no increase in mesangial cells, no matrix expansion, and no immune deposits (2). Most patients with MCNS and some with focal segmental glomerulosclerosis (FSGS) have steroid-sensitive (responsive) NS. Some patients diagnosed clinically with MCNS have increased numbers of immunoreactive T cells and monocytes in the mesangium. These are said to have mesangial "proliferation," follow a relatively benign course, and have variable responses to steroids (3,4). A small subset of patients with a clinical diagnosis of MCNS have mesangial deposits of immunoglobulin (Ig)M and a similar course and prognosis to MCNS (5–7). MCNS also can be defined in terms of response to steroids: steroid responsive, frequently relapsing, steroid dependent, and steroid resistant. FSGS can present ab initio with features of MCNS, or in some cases can occur later in the course of MCNS. Differentiating between MCNS and FSGS can be difficult because biopsy samples may not be obtained from the corticomedullary junction (8). Therefore, some patients diagnosed at first biopsy with MCNS may be thought to have FSGS at second biopsy (9). However, most patients with FSGS are unresponsive to steroid therapy, tend to present at an older age, are often hypertensive and azotemic, and have a worse outcome (10). Definitions of remission, relapse, and steroid responses are shown in Table 1 (11–16).

K.E.C. Meyers, D.A. Kujubu, and B.S. Kaplan: Division of Nephrology, Department of Medicine, The Children's Hospital of Philadelphia, and Renal, Electrolyte and Hypertension Division, University of Pennsylvania and Veterans Administration Hospital, Philadelphia, Pennsylvania 19104.

EPIDEMIOLOGY

The overall incidence of MCNS is two to seven per 100,000 population, and the prevalence in children under 16 years of age is 15 per 100,000 (17,18). MCNS occurs predominantly in children 2 to 8 years of age, with a peak incidence at 3 years of age (19). It is uncommon in children under 12 months of age and rare in children under 6 months of age and can occur at any time in adulthood (20,21). Boys are twice as commonly affected as girls (22), but the sex ratio is equal in adults (23). In the United

TABLE 1. *Definitions*

Remission	Negative or trace urine on Dipstix tests for at least 3 days (11)
Relapse	2+ proteinuria for 3 days in a person previously negative (11,12)
Frequent relapser	Two relapses within 6 mo or three relapses in 1 yr (13–15)
Steroid responsive	Disappearance of proteinuria within 8 wk of starting corticosteroids (11)
Steroid resistance	Failure to induce remission in 8 wk using conventional doses of corticosteroids (15,16)
Steroid dependence	A relapse while trying to wean from steroids or within two weeks of discontinuing steroids

Kingdom (24,25) and South Africa (26,27) the incidence is much greater in white and East Asian than in black children. The incidence of MCNS in families is 3.35% (28). Siblings are affected more often than a parent and child. The presentation and course are similar within families (29).

Many agents and conditions are associated with MCNS, but there are no definite causes (30–54) (Table 2). The most convincing associations are with nonsteroidal anti-inflammatory drugs (NSAIDs) (34), lithium (35,36), and Hodgkin's disease (43). MCNS is mainly associated with Hodgkin's lymphoma (55–57). Onset of NS may herald an underlying malignancy (47,58), and the NS may remit with treatment of the tumor and relapse with its recurrence (58,59). Many pharmacologic agents are also associated with MCNS, but causality is unproven (Table 2).

Allergens are implicated in the pathogenesis of MCNS (40,60,61). There is a higher prevalence of atopy (asthma and eczema) in patients with MCNS and their first degree relatives than in the general population (62,63). The increased number of relapses in spring and fall is additional circumstantial evidence for an allergenic cause or trigger of MCNS (38,60). Food allergies are suggested as causes (40,64). In a case-controlled trial, patients with MCNS had decreased proteinuria on an elemental diet. Milk challenge decreased serum C3, and proteinuria recurred (65). Adult patients with MCNS desensitized against specific allergens relapsed on re-exposure to the allergen (41,64). The significance of elevated serum IgE levels (66) and glomerular IgE deposits (67) is undetermined (68,69).

TABLE 2. *Possible causes of MCNS*

Drugs	Gold (30), penicillamine (31), ampicillin (32), mercury (33), nonsteroidal anti-inflammatory agents (34), lithium (35,36), trimethadone, paramethadone (37)
Allergies	Pollen (38), milk (39), pork (40), house dust (41), bee stings (42)
Tumors	Hodgkin's disease (43), and non-Hodgkin's disease (44), Kimura disease (45), renal oncocytoma (46), embryonal cell tumors (44), bronchogenic carcinoma (47)
Infections	Viral (48), schistosomiasis (49), Guillain-Barré syndrome (50)
Skin disorders	Dermatitis herpetiformis (51), melorheostosis (52), contact dermatitis (53)
Myasthenia gravis (54)	

Weak evidence links MCNS with the major histocompatability complex (62,70–82) (Table 3). Making sense of reported findings is difficult because of inconstant associations that may reflect different ethnic or racial backgrounds. Sample sizes differ, there are differences between children and adults, and some haplotypes paradoxically appear to confer protection.

PATHOGENESIS

Immunopathophysiology

Although the association with an atopic diathesis and specific antigenic challenges suggests an immunologic basis, the pathogenesis of MCNS is obscure (83). Shaloub proposed that MCNS is caused by a circulating glomerulotoxic lymphokine produced by aberrant T-cell repertoires (84). This hypothesis was based on the observations that MCNS often remits with measles, that patients are prone to pneumococcal infections, that they respond to cyclophosphamide and corticosteroids, and that there is an association with Hodgkin's disease (84). The ability of cyclosporine A (CsA), a relatively selective immunosuppressive agent for T cells, to maintain patients in remission lends credence to this hypothesis. None of the many immunologic abnormalities in MCNS (Table 4) cause the syndrome.

Humoral Immunity

Patients are prone to infections in part because of decreased serum IgG and IgA levels. Urinary losses of IgG and abnormalities in B-cell production and maturation in the presence of altered CD4+ T-cell regulation (85) account for the decrement in IgG levels. In contrast, IgM and IgE levels are elevated. Decreased serum IgG and IgA and increased IgM levels during relapse normalize during remission. IgG levels may remain low years after remission (86). In vitro studies suggest that B cells from patients with MCNS show impaired immunoglobulin synthesis in response to antigens (85). Moreover, MCNS patients often have lower titers of circulating anti-

TABLE 3. *Associations between MCNS and HLA type*

HLA	Haplotype	Country	Reference
Associations			
HLA I			
	B12	England	62,70
	B8	Ireland	71
	B27	France	72
	A1,B8	Germany	73
HLA II			
	DR7	Australia	74
	DR7	France	75
	DR7	Spain	76
	DR8	Japan	77
	DQw2	Japan	77
	DQw2	United States	78
No specific associations			
HLA III		United States	78
HLA III		Canada	79
Extended haplotypes			
	8, -DR3, -DR7	Germany	80
	A1, -B8, -DR3, -Dw52, and -SC051, and B44, -DR7, -DRw53, and -FC31	United States	78
No association in children			
HLA I, II, III		Japan	81
Confer protection			
DR2, DR4 found less frequently in MCNS			76,82

bodies to streptococcal and pneumococcal antigens than equally nephrotic patients with other glomerular lesions (87). Suboptimal responses to hepatitis B vaccine are observed in MCNS (88). Complement activation and immune complex formation do not have a role in the pathogenesis of MCNS. However, decreased alternate complement factors B and D levels (89,90) and circulating immune complexes (91) are observed in MCNS.

Cellular Immunity

There is decreased skin reactivity to common antigens known to induce delayed-type hypersensitivity responses. Reactivity returns when the patients enter remission. Most studies were unable to demonstrate significant changes in total lymphocyte number, T- and B-cell distributions, or T-cell subsets in nephrotic patients versus patients in remission, although some patients have an increase in circulating CD8+ T cells (92). During relapse, T cells show signs of activation, with increased expression of interleukin (IL)-2 receptor, CD69, and transferrin receptor. Increased production of IL-1 and IL-2 are reported (93). These changes may not be specific to MCNS (94).

T cells were detected in the glomeruli of patients with MCNS compared with glomeruli of normals (95). The significance of infiltrating T cells remains suspect in MCNS but may be important in MCNS associated with NSAID use, where a marked interstitial infiltrate of T cells is observed. The implication is that the activated T cells in the interstitium elaborate cytokines that enhance glomerular permeability. T cells from patients with MCNS demonstrate a decrease in mitogen-stimulated proliferation in vitro. This immune hyporesponsiveness is not specific for MCNS, but is characteristic of the nephrotic state. Some have implicated an overactive T-suppressor cell activity (96). Plasma factors from MCNS patients suppress mitogen-stimulated lymphocyte proliferation, which is not observed when the same lymphocytes are incubated in normal plasma (97). Although hyperlipidemic plasma itself may inhibit mitogen-induced proliferation, other humoral factors are implicated. One factor, soluble immune response suppressor (SIRS), was found in steroid-responsive but not steroid-

TABLE 4. *Immunologic abnormalities in MCNS*

Defective opsonization
Decreased alternate complement factors B and D
Circulating immune complexes
Abnormal humoral immunity
Decreased immunoglobulin production
Altered immunoglobulin levels
Decreased titers of specific antibodies
Abnormal cell-mediated immunity
Decreased delayed hypersensitivity reactions
Decreased proliferative responses to mitogens
Suppressor lymphokines
Increased suppressor cell activity

resistant nephrotic patients. Produced by CD8+ cells, SIRS is a 100- to 150-kDa multimeric complex capable of suppressing T-cell responses to antigens and B cell–mediated immunoglobulin production. Its production can be inhibited by corticosteroids. SIRS is neither specific for MCNS nor does it cause increased glomerular permeability when injected into animals (98).

Other Humoral Factors

Much work has focused on identifying humoral factors that may be responsible for enhanced glomerular permeability because of the absence of histologic evidence for glomerular inflammation and the spontaneous resolution of proteinuria after treatment of lymphoma (Table 5). Many cytokines, including interleukins, tumor necrosis factor (TNF), and interferon, were investigated. In some reports, elevated levels were found in MCNS (99–101). It is unclear how specific these finding are. Other investigators have sought to identify novel factors whose expression parallels disease activity. Vascular permeability factor (VPF), identified as a substance produced by mitogen-stimulated mononuclear cells from patients with MCNS, causes increased capillary permeability when injected intradermally into guinea pigs (Miles bioassay). Mononuclear cells from patients in remission produced lower amounts of VPF. VPF is not specific for MCNS. Moreover, when injected into rats, the resultant proteinuria did not correlate with the results of the Miles bioassay (102–104).

Vascular endothelial growth factors (VEGF), a family of related proteins produced by tumor cells, are mitogenic for endothelial cells in vitro and angiogenic in vivo (105). VEGF elicits a positive response using the Miles bioassay and was detected in glomerular epithelial cells of normal kidneys. VEGF induces proteinuria when injected into animals (106).

Conditioned media from mitogen-stimulated mononuclear cells from MCNS patients stimulate sulfate turnover in isolated kidney slices (107). Because sulfated molecules, such as heparan sulfate proteoglycan, are abundant in the glomerular basement membrane and may be responsible for its charge barrier, substances that stimulate their sulfation status may influence glomerular permeability. A 29-kDa protein fraction was characterized. This activity is not present in conditioned media taken from MCNS patients in remission (108). It has not been determined whether this causes proteinuria in animals. T-cell hybridomas generated glomerular permeability factor (GPF) from lymphocytes from MCNS patients (109). Conditioned media from the hybridomas induced proteinuria and foot process effacement when injected into rats. GPF is between 60 and 160 kDA and is distinct from IL-1, IL-2, IL-4, IL-6, TNF-α, and TNF-β. The specificity of GPF for MCNS has not been determined.

TABLE 5. *Putative circulating factors in MCNS*

Factor	Source
Vascular permeability factor (VPF)	Media from stimulated MCNS lymphocytes
Vascular endothelial growth factor (VEGF)	Tumor cells, macrophages
Glomerular permeability factor (GPF)	Media from T-cell hybridomas
Soluble immune response substance (SIRS)	Sera from patients with MCNS
Sulfate turnover factor	Media from stimulated MCNS lymphocytes
IL-8	Sera from patients with MCNS

Glomerular Pathophysiology

Glomerular capillary walls are high-capacity ultrafiltration membranes with low resistance to water flow and size- and charge-selective filtration barriers that effectively impede the passage of proteins (110). Clinical observations led to studies demonstrating restrictive transport of polyanions and facilitated filtration of polycations across the glomerular capillary wall (111,112). These studies suggested that the normal anionic charge barrier is perturbed in MCNS by as much as 50% (113). This was corroborated with anionic markers in immunohistochemical and electron microscopy studies, which demonstrated decreased capillary loop staining in MCNS (114). Sialic acid staining of glomeruli from MCNS is decreased compared with glomeruli from patients with nonglomerular renal disease (115). Charge selectivity is mainly due to the presence of highly sulfated sialoglycoproteins, such as heparan sulfate proteoglycan, in the glomerular basement membrane and on the surface of endothelial and visceral epithelial cells. The charge barrier is primarily responsible for the relative impermeability of the glomerular basement membrane to anionic albumin despite its relatively small molecular size. Alterations in glomerular basement membrane charge may be due to enzymes elaborated by mononuclear cells that digest heparan sulfate proteoglycan (116). Indeed, increased urinary glycosaminoglycans and heparan sulfate excretion are found in patients with glomerular diseases. Glycosaminoglycan excretion, normalized for creatinine, decreases with remission. Alternatively, the glomerular anionic charge barrier may be neutralized by circulating highly cationic substances. Highly cationic substances were isolated from plasma and urine of patients with MCNS (117). These substances were not characterized.

Depletion of the glomerular anionic charge barrier may be responsible for the effacement of foot processes in MCNS. Infusion of cationic substances, such as protamine, in animals results in foot process effacement, which is reversible by heparin (118). Foot process effacement is not specific for MCNS but is seen in any condition with proteinuria. Studies using noncharged, inert polymers with known molecular radii have demonstrated that size selectivity is also impaired (118) (Fig. 1). The size barrier is due to the presence of a continuous log normal distribution of molecular pores and a parallel population of larger shuntlike pores (119,120). In glomeruli from MCNS patients in relapse, molecular pore density and radii are reduced but the shunt pore pathway is increased in comparison with normals (121) (Fig. 2). Foot process effacement may account for the observed decrease in pore density.

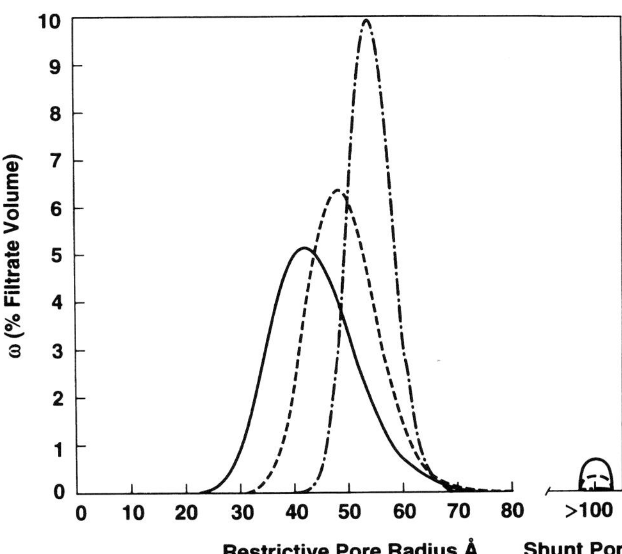

FIG. 2. Glomerular pore size distribution in nephrotic (____) or the remission stage (---) of MCNS is compared with that of healthy controls (_._._) The fraction of filtrate volume permeating the pores (in parentheses) is plotted as a function of the pore radius. The pores of the shunt pathway are dimensionless but calculated to exceed 8.0 nm radius. Reprinted with permission (121).

CLINICAL FEATURES

The patient looks miserable and complains of fatigue and general malaise. Edema, the most frequent presenting finding, can be insidious or rapid and is usually first apparent around the eyes in the mornings. It is frequently misdiagnosed as "an allergy" and is often treated inappropriately with antihistaminics. In the early stages the severity and extent of edema fluctuates. During the day periorbital swelling decreases and ankle swelling becomes more apparent. The patient has a bloated, waxy appearance. There is increasing swelling of the sacral region, genitalia, and abdomen. Severe edema may lead to breakdown of skin and infection. Ascites and/or pleural effusions may cause tachypnea or dyspnea. Ascites also causes a markedly protuberant abdomen and, in some cases, umbilical and inguinal hernias. Appetite is reduced, the patient complains of colicky abdominal pain, and there can be diarrhea or bulky stools. Abdominal pain may be the result of edema of the intestinal wall or primary peritonitis. Gastric irritation or pancreatitis must be considered if the patient is taking steroids. Volume status is assessed by interpreting the pulse rate, state of hydration, and orthostatic changes in blood pressure. Chronic hypoproteinemia can soften ear cartilage and produce lusterless hair and a white transverse band in nail beds. Mild hypertension occurs in most edematous patients before steroid therapy (78% of adults and 95% of children) (122). Hypertension may be a pressor response to volume depletion, and blood pressure can return to normal with volume expansion. The hypertension is attributed mainly to hypervolemia or loss of antihypertensive substance(s) in the urine. Hypertensive encephalopathy is uncommon and is associated with steroid treatment (123). Urine output is decreased and the urine is foamy and concentrated. Gross hematuria is unusual.

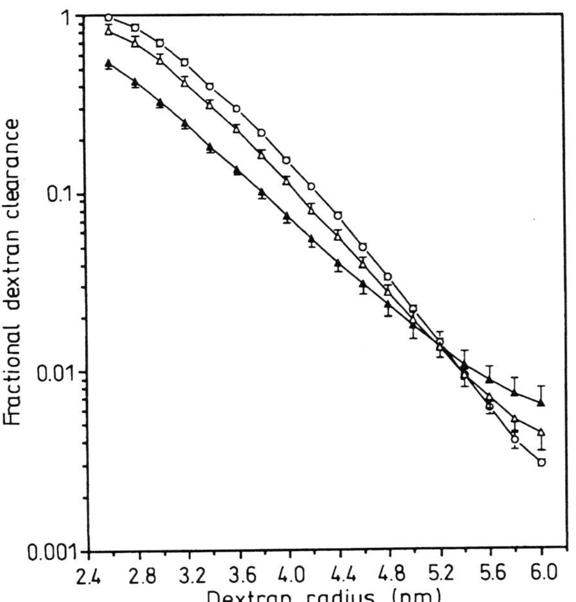

FIG. 1. Dextran sieving profiles in the nephrotic (▲) or remission stages (△) of MCNS compared with healthy controls (○). Reprinted with permission (121).

LABORATORY FINDINGS

The numerous laboratory perturbations are the consequences of large urinary losses of albumin (and other proteins), as well as of compensatory mechanisms (e.g., sodium and water retention). Complications (e.g., hypercoagulability) are secondary to these losses and compensations.

The serum albumin concentration is usually less than 2.5 g/dl. There is no correlation among the values for serum albumin, urine protein excretion, and severity of edema. However, edema becomes obvious when the serum albumin concentration decreases to less than 2.0 g/dl. Hyperlipidemia occurs during episodes of MCNS and persists in remission after steroids are stopped. There is a complex array of lipid derangements (Table 6).

The serum sodium concentration is often decreased as a result of free water retention or, less often, because of prolonged sodium restriction or acquired adrenal insufficiency. Factitious hyponatremia due to hyperlipidemia is less common with newer laboratory methods. Thrombocytosis can spuriously elevate serum potassium levels by in vitro release of potassium (124). Serum calcium concentrations are decreased as a consequence of hypoalbuminemia and urinary losses of 25-hydroxychole-calciferol binding protein. Serum creatinine concentration and blood urea nitrogen (BUN) are transiently increased at presentation in a third of children. The hematocrit is often increased as a result of intravascular volume depletion, and the white cell count and differential are normal. It is unclear why the platelet count may be increased to as high as 1,000,000/ml. The erythrocyte sedimentation rate is markedly elevated.

Protein excretion in the urine is normally less than 4 mg/m2/h in children (125). Normal adults excrete less than 150 mg/24 h. Urine protein is measured by the Dipstix method and by the protein/creatinine ratio (Uprot/Ucreat) in an early morning sample. Protein measurement in a 24-h urine collection is the standard, but the collection is difficult to do in incontinent children, collection errors are frequent, there is an inherant time delay, and it is difficult to do at home. The Dipstix test, based on tetrabromophenol blue colorimetry, detects albumin and is less sensitive to low molecular weight (MW) proteins, immunoglobulins, and Bence-Jones protein. Errors arise if the effect of dilution of the urine is ignored and therefore is best done on a concentrated early morning specimen. In MCNS the Dipstix measurement is 4+ (>2,000 mg/dl) and the Uprot/Ucreat ratio is above 1.0. The total protein excretion is approximately 0.63 multiplied by the Uprot/Ucreat (126). The selectivity index of proteinuria is rarely used to differentiate MCNS from other types of NS (127). Selectivity is determined by comparing the clearance of IgG (MW 170,000) to transferrin (MW 88,000). A ratio of less that 0.1 is termed selective proteinuria and implies that smaller MW macromolecules are preferentially filtered compared with larger molecules. Ratios higher that 0.2 imply major disruption of the glomerular size barrier with leakage of large MW proteins. In children, highly selective proteinuria is characteristic of MCNS. In adults, the index is of less value because there is overlap with other causes of NS. Although not specifically an index of glomerular permeability, elevated urinary excretion of retinol-binding protein and β2-microglobulin was observed in patients with steroid-resistant NS compared with steroid-sensitive patients (128). Increased urinary excretion of both molecules, which are markers of proximal tubular damage, suggest significant parenchymal injury that is less likely to respond to corticosteroids. Microscopic hematuria (more than three to five red blood cells per high-power field or urine Dipstix result of greater than trace for blood) is detected at diagnosis in 23% of children with MCNS (129).

TABLE 6. *Lipid, lipoprotein, and apoprotein abnormalities*

Lipid moiety	Increased	Decreased	Unchanged
Plasma lipids	Cholesterol		Free fatty acids
	Triglyceride Phospholipid		
Lipoproteins	LDL, VLDL, HDL3, LP(a)	HDL2	
Apoproteins	B, CII, E, CIII/CII ratio		AI, AII

Reprinted with permission (175).

Pathogenesis of Metabolic Derangements

There is no animal model of MCNS. Studies of proximal tubular mechanisms in the puromycin of aminonucleoside model must be interpreted with caution because it is unclear to what extent this toxin injures renal tubule cells.

The serum albumin concentration is the result of a balance between the rate of hepatic synthesis of albumin and the rate of catabolism plus the quantities lost in urine and stool. In MCNS, there is increased filtration of albumin. It is inferred that substantial quantities of filtered albumin are reabsorbed and catabolized by proximal tubule cells because the rate of synthesis should exceed the amount of albumin lost in the urine (3–5 g/day) and the small amounts lost in stool. Normally the liver is able to increase albumin production by 300%, and about 12 g/day are synthesized in response to decreased hepatic sinusoidal oncotic pressure (OP) and viscosity (130). In NS the fractional rate of renal albumin catabolism is increased but the absolute rate of catabolism is reduced (131). However, the liver cannot increase the rate of albumin synthesis sufficiently to match the urinary losses and increased catabolism, in part because of inadequate protein intake (132).

Edema is the result of an abnormal collection of fluid in interstitial tissues, but the mechanisms underlying the production and maintenance of nephrotic edema are not fully understood. The nephrotic state is dynamic, and different results are obtained because not all studies are conducted at similar stages of disease. Hypoalbuminemia per se may not be the crucial factor because edema does not occur in congenital analbuminemia (133) nor in all cases of NS. In MCNS, edema occurs when the serum albumin concentration decreases to less than 2.0 g/dl, and ascites and pleural effusions develop below a level of 1.5 g/dl (134). There is scanty evidence for an alteration in Starling forces in the development of edema. In fact, tissue albumin content during the recovery phase of NS is decreased (135), and extracellular fluid volume expansion should enhance natriuresis (136–138). However, according to the traditional view of edema formation, hypoalbuminemia lowers plasma OP and thereby favors fluid transudation into interstitial spaces; the resulting hypovolemia is a signal for the kidneys to retain salt and water. However, most patients with NS have normal or increased blood volume (139–143), although reduced blood volume (the underfilled circulation) was found in 7% to 38% of patients with NS (144,145). These differences may be due to the markers and methods used for measuring blood volume, the types of NS, ages of patients, and the patients' positions during the studies. Furthermore, conflicting results of increased and decreased natriuresis are obtained when renal sodium excretion is measured after blood volume expansion with hyperoncotic albumin or during head-out-of-water immersion (146–148).

Although the results of initial studies suggested that the glomerular filtration rate (GFR) in patients with MCNS was markedly increased, they relied mainly on creatinine clearances. It is now known that proteinuria stimulates creatinine secretion in the renal tubule, thereby elevating estimates of GFR based on creatinine clearance. GFR is actually slightly diminished, and in patients with volume depletion may be 20% to 30% of normal. A reduction in intravascular volume results in a decrease in intraglomerular hydraulic pressure, activation of vasoconstrictor mechanisms, and increased efferent arteriolar constriction in an effort to maintain GFR. A more pronounced decrease in the intravascular volume may reduce the glomerular capillary ultrafiltration coefficient (Kf).

Renal salt and water excretion are impaired in NS (149–155), but the mechanisms and tubular sites where sodium is reabsorbed remain undetermined. Antinatriuresis appears to be due to changes in the distal tubule or collecting duct (149,156–159), but the exact site of sodium retention may depend on the intravascular volume status. Volume depletion may cause enhanced proximal tubular sodium retention for restoration of intravascular volume and GFR. In circumstances in which plasma volume is normal or increased, sodium reabsorption may occur in the more distal part of the nephron (149,156–158). Despite demonstrating an appropriate increase in circulating atrial natriuretic factor (ANP) levels in response to volume expansion, urinary excretion of cyclic guanosine monophosphate (cGMP), an index of the renal actions of ANP, is blunted in nephrotic animals, suggesting that they have a relative ANP resistance (155). The observed ANP resistance may be due to heightened activity of a cGMP phosphodiesterase that metabolizes intracellular cGMP, inhibiting its ability to stimulate sodium reabsorption in inner medullary collecting duct cells (160).

Hypoalbuminemia lowers plasma OP, which favors transudation of fluid into interstitial spaces. Resulting hypovolemia signals the kidneys to retain salt and water. This view of the primacy of hypoalbuminemia/hypovolemia, termed the "underfill" hypothesis, was challenged by the inability to confirm a reduced blood or plasma volume in these patients. Some nephrotic patients have an elevated plasma volume status, suggesting to some investigators that salt and water retention is not secondary to intravascular volume depletion but rather is a primary abnormality of the kidneys in inappropriately reabsorbing salt and water ("overflow" hypothesis). Although these two hypotheses appear to be mutually exclusive, it is likely that in the wide spectrum of patients with MCNS, features of both underfill and overflow may be operative.

Increased plasma renin activity (PRA) and plasma aldosterone are found more frequently in MCNS than in other forms of NS (139,161–165). The vasoconstrictor (high PRA) and overflow (low PRA) hypotheses (144) have not been confirmed (164). PRA activity correlates inversely with plasma albumin concentration but does not correlate with sodium excretion, GFR, or blood volume. Angiotensin-converting enzyme inhibitors (ACEIs) do not induce natriuresis (166). Tubular sensitivity to aldosterone may be enhanced because spiranolactone increases sodium excretion (167).

Noradrenaline is elevated in MCNS in relapse and is normalized by albumin infusion and head-out-of-water immersion (147,148,161,168). Noradrenaline may enhance sodium reabsorption by stimulating proximal tubular sodium reabsorption independently of hemodynamic changes by stimulating renin release and by efferent arteriolar vasoconstiction to increase the filtraton fraction and proximal tubular sodium reabsorption. Argenine vasopressin (AVP) levels are increased during edema formation and return to basal levels in remission (161). The stimulus for AVP release is related to effective circulating blood volume and is nonosmotic (161). AVP may contribute to impaired water excretion in MCNS. Renal prostaglandins are activated during edema accumulation. The inhibition of prostaglandin synthesis in NS by NSAIDs may decrease the GFR (169–172).

Albumin infusion produces a fivefold increase in ANP and a decrease in vasoconstrictors (AVP, noradrenaline, PRA). The albumin-induced changes in sodium and water correlate with ANP levels and GFR but not with aldosterone or serum sodium (148).

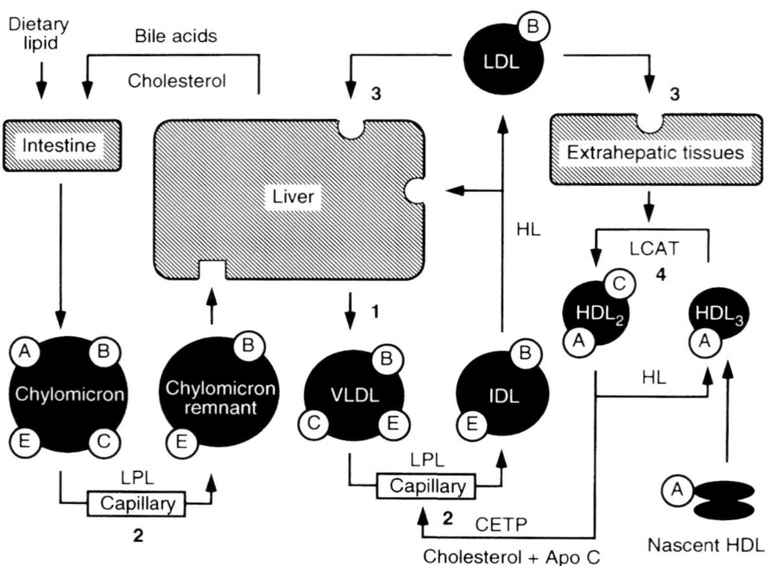

FIG. 3. Normal lipoprotein metabolism and abnormalities in NS. In NS, hepatic VLDL production is increased (1), leading to increased circulating levels of VLDL, IDL, and LDL. This is compounded by defective catabolism of these particles in the peripheral circulation as a result of reduced LPL (2) activity. In addition, receptor-mediated uptake of LDL particles may be inpaired (3). HDL maturation is inhibited as a result of diminished L.CAT activity (4). These defects in the HDL pathway are likely to contribute to impaired catabolism of triglyceride-rich lipoproteins. Reprinted with permission (175).

Hyperlipidemia (Fig. 3) is the result of increased hepatic synthesis of beta lipoprotein as a result of loss of high-density lipoprotein (HDL) cholesterol and an unidentified substance in the urine (131), as well as decreased portal vein OP (173). Hypercholesterolemia is always a component of MCNS, whereas hyperlipidemia occurs with profound reductions in serum albumin concentrations. Nephrotic hyperlipidemia is Frederickson types IIa, IIb, and V (174). There is increased hepatic lipoprotein and apoprotein synthesis and reduced peripheral clearance of lipoproteins (175). Nephrotic patients usually have increased low-density lipoprotein (LDL) and very low density lipoprotein (VLDL) and sometimes increased intermediate-density lipoproteins (IDLs). HDLs have abnormal lipid and apoprotein composition. HDL levels are normal or decreased because they are low MW substances and when lost in the urine produce lipiduria (176). Maturation of HDLs cannot occur because of reduced lecithin:cholesterol acetyltransferase (L.CAT) activity. Lysolecithin, which normally binds to albumin, inhibits L.CAT. L.CAT is also lost in the urine. Reduction in L.CAT activity results in less esterified cholesterol with less cholesterol transported by HDLs, as well as increased free cholesterol, which in turn reduces lipoprotein lipase (LPL) activity. The HDL/LDL ratios are reduced (176,177). The composition of LDL and VLDL is altered with an increase in amount of esterified and unesterified cholesterol. There is also an increase in the triglyceride to protein ratio in chylomicrons and VLDLs (178). Cholesterol synthesis is increased. The serum concentration is inversely related to albumin and OP (171) and correlates with renal albumin clearance (131). Hydroxymethylgluteryl CoA, the rate-limiting enzyme in cholesterol synthesis, is induced. Albumin or dextran infusions increase OP and transiently lower cholesterol levels (179,180). Serum cholesterol levels gradually normalize with remission of MCNS. Increased triglyceride production is inconstant. Apoprotein A, B, and E synthesis is increased, as shown by increased levels of messenger RNA for these proteins in experimental nephrosis (181,182). The peripheral clearance of chylomicrons, VLDLs, IDLs, and LDLs is reduced, and conversion of VLDLs to LDLs is defective (178,183). LPL activity is decreased because of increased inhibitors (free fatty acids) and reduced activators (glycosaminoglycans, Apo CII) (173,184–186).

The many coagulation abnormalities (Table 7) do not correlate directly with a risk for thrombosis. There is increased in vitro platelet aggregability and adhesion (187,188), in vivo deposition of fibrin, thrombin activation, and decreased fibrinolysis. Steroid treatment may enhance the tendency to thrombosis before remission occurs (189), but thrombi also occur in the absence of steroid treatment.

Serum total calcium levels are decreased in proportion to the degree of hypoalbuminemia. For every 1 g/dl decrease in serum albumin concentration, the serum calcium level decreases by 0.2 mg/dl. Some patients have low serum ionized calcium concentrations out of proportion to the degree of hypoalbuminemia and may have increased parathyroid hormone (PTH) levels and bone disease (190,191). Vitamin-D binding protein (DBP), which transports 25-hydroxy-cholecalciferol, is lost in the urine (192,193), and plasma levels of 1,25-dihydroxycholecalciferol are normal or decreased (193,194). Bone disease in MCNS therefore may be related to perturbations in the vitamin D–PTH axis and also to age of onset, duration of illness, frequency of relapses and use of corticosteroids (195,196). Serum

TABLE 7. *Coagulation abnormalities*

- Increased in vitro platelet aggregability
  - Hypoalbuminemia
    - Increased free arachidonic acid
    - Increased thromboxane A2
  - Increased LDL
  - Reduced platelet negative surface charges
  - Increased binding of vWF to glycoprotein Ib
  - Increased beta-thromboglobulin–sensitive marker of platelet activation
- Increased platelet adhesion
- Thrombocytosis
- Reduced erythrocyte deformability
- Increased von Willebrand factor
- Increased plasma viscosity
  - Hyperfibrinogenemia
- Volume depletion
- Lysolecithin-enriched LDL impairs nitric oxide production
  - Nitric oxide inhibits platelet adhesion
- Fibrin deposition
  - Increased fibrinopeptide A levels
  - Increased high molecular weight fibrin complexes
- Increased thrombin formation
  - Less effective thrombin inhibition
  - Antithrombin 3 deficiency (serum albumin <2.0 g/dl
- Increased alpha 2-macroglobulin; total antithrombolytic activity normal or increased
- Increased protein C and protein S
- Reduced free protein S
- Functional protein C deficiency may be present
- Decreased fibrinolysis
  - Decreased plasminogen
  - Increased alpha 2-antiplasmin prevents plasmin-fibrin binding
  - Reduced plasminogen–fibrin binding
  - Albumin is a cofactor for plasminogen–fibrin binding
  - Lipoprotein a (Lpa) may be a competitive inhibitor of plasminogen–fibrin binding
  - Lpa may inhibit the fibrin-dependent enhancement of plasminogen activation by tissue plasminogen activator (t-PA)

thyroid-binding globulin (TBG), thyroxine (T4), triiodothyronine (T3), and thyroid-stimulating hormone (TSH) are usually normal in adults with NS, and they are euthyroid, despite urinary losses of TBG, T4, and T3 (197,198). Greater losses of TBG and T4 occur in children, their serum TBG and T4 concentrations are low, and TSH levels are high, but they do not have hypothyroidism (199–201).

Increased urinary loss of trace metal–binding proteins, ceruloplasmin and transferrin, result in low levels of blood copper and iron. Iron-resistant microcytic hypochromic anemia may occur as a consequence of decreased erythrocyte copper (202,203). Serum zinc levels may be low as a result of losses in urine and low albumin levels because two thirds of circulatig zinc is bound to albumin (204). Zinc deficiency may contribute to growth retardation, immune dysfunction and delayed wound healing. It is unclear how much protein is wasted via the intestine as a result of malabsorption or lymphangiectasia because of methodologic problems (205–208).

COMPLICATIONS

As Barness et al. reported in 1950 (19),

> Few diseases tax the resources of the practitioner so extensively as the NS. He must be a combination of infectious disease expert, nutritionalist, physiologist, and psychiatrist for the patient and, above all, guide councellor and friend to the parents, who have to live day in and day out, for two or three years with a child who eats poorly and often has periods of irritability or depression, who frequently vomits or has diarrhea, whose appearance may become grotesque at times, and who may become desperately sick with peritonitis and bacteraemia at any moment. On the other hand, the satisfaction of seeing a patient restored to normal health after several years of edema is well worth the time and patience required.

MCNS induces a great deal of anxiety in patients and parents because of uncertain etiology, high likelihood of recurrence, fear of end-stage renal failure, and loathing of corticosteroids.

Patients with MCNS are at increased risk for measles (209), varicella (210), and primary peritonitis with encapsulated organisms (S. pneumoniae) (211,212). Factors that increase the risk of infections are low serum immunoglobulin levels (213), defective cell-mediated immunity (92), inadequate opsonization caused by loss of alternate pathway complement factors B and D (89,90, 214), immunosupressive therapy (215), and ascites. Edema and malnutrition may split the skin and thereby predispose patients to cellulitis.

Venous (216) and arterial (217) thromboses occur less often in adults (8.5–44%) (216) than in children (1.8–5%) with MCNS (218,219). Arterial thrombosis is found in half the children presenting with thromboembolic disease and can result in amputation, hemiplegia and mesenteric infarction (217). Subclinical pulmonary emboli were found in 28% of children with NS by radionucleotide perfusion studies (220). The cause of NS has a role in the development of renal vein thrombosis (RVT) because the highest incidence is in adults with membranous nephropathy (216,221). Acute onset of RVT is heralded by flank pain, macroscopic hematuria, mild hypertension, and mild azotemia. Treatment is with intravenous heparin followed by coumadin. Thrombolytic agents produce faster and more complete clot resolution, with a lower incidence of rethrombosis (222–224). Chronic RVT is usually asymptomatic. Ultrasonography shows a small kidney and renal venography shows collateral vessels. Renal venography is indicated if there is rapid unexplained deterioration in renal function, acute flank pain, macroscopic hematuria, pleuritic chest pain, or other symptoms suggestive of thromoembolism.

This uncommon complication of MCNS may occur as a result of severe intravascular volume depletion, bilateral renal vein thrombosis, pyelonephritis, or pharmacologic agents (225). Acute tubular necrosis is rare in children (226). Acute renal failure usually responds to agressive therapy with diuretics (227) or steroids (228) but may require dialysis. Recovery is usually complete.

There is no evidence for a causal association between MCNS and ischemic heart disease (229–232) despite hyperlipidemia, hypercoaguability, platelet hyperaggregation, corticosteroids, and hypertension. On the other hand, normal or increased HDL levels in MCNS may ameliorate the effects of hyperlipidemia (233). There are few reports of atherosclerosis and ischemic heart disease in children with MCNS (234–237).

Prolonged high-dose steroid therapy (238) and loss of DBP result in osteopenia. Decreased circulating active vitamin D metabolites result in decreased gastrointestinal calcium absorption, low serum ionized calcium, high PTH concentrations, and reduced urinary calcium excretion. The elevated PTH levels and deficiency of active vitamin D metabolites produce changes in bone structure (190) without clinical bone disease (196). This important complication can be caused by corticosteroid treatment, poor nutrition, reduced intake, decreased intestinal absorption, and increased protein losses from intestine and kidneys.

FSGS is a complication in a small percentage of patients who have had a definite response to corticosteroid therapy (239). Chronic renal failure never occurs in patients with MCNS unless they have developed FSGS (240).

PATHOLOGY

Light Microscopy

Glomeruli look normal or nearly so by light microscopy. The problem lies in the definition of normality. This applies especially to mild degrees of mesangial expansion, proliferation, and glomerulosclerosis. The mesangium is considered normal if there are two or fewer cells, expanded if there are three cells, and proliferative if there are four or more cells (241). These criteria may not be applicable to all age groups. Mesangial proliferation in the context of MCNS may not be a discrete entity, although these patients are more likely to be steroid resistant (242,243).

During normal development, up to 15% of glomeruli in outer cortical segments undergo spontaneous global sclerosis. The clinical course of patients with global sclerosis is similar to that of MCNS. However, the presence of a single glomerulus with FSGS portends a more severe prognosis, with steroid resistance and progressive azotemia.

Immunofluorescent and Electron Microscopy

Immunofluorescent staining is usually negative for immunoglobulins and complement. Mesangial IgM (5) or IgA (244) deposits are seen in a minority of patients who may have mesangial expansion and are often steroid dependent. Scanning electron microscopy shows effacement and retraction of epithelial foot processes. This reversible phenomenon occurs in association with proteinuria, is not specific for MCNS, and can persist for months after cessation of proteinuria (245).

MANAGEMENT

General Management

The objectives of treatment are to induce a remission as soon as possible to reduce the complications of untreated NS, to minimize medication side effects, and to provide psychosocial support (246). At presentation the patient is admitted to hospital for treatment, counseling, and education. Pertinent information is provided and repeated at follow-up visits. Parents and patients are taught how to monitor the condition. An illustrative booklet is invaluable. The potential side effects of steroids (mood, behavior, appetite changes, weight gain, acne, growth delay, hypertension, hair changes) are explained in detail.

Hypovolemia must be anticipated in patients who are markedly edematous, in those with diarrhea or vomiting, and when diuretics have been used. Hypovolemia is corrected with infusions of saline, plasma, or 5% albumin. A sodium-restricted diet of 1–2 g/24 h reduces edema formation and minimizes the risk of hypertension while on steroids. Intake of protein should be in keeping with the recommended daily allowance. A high-protein diet increases the glomerular filtration rate, increases albumin production, and augments albumin excretion without raising the serum albumin level (247). Low-protein diets reduce albuminuria but can cause malnutrition (248). Steroids increase the appetite. Calorie intake must therefore be controlled to reduce the likelihood of obesity (249). Restriction of sodium intake can help to reduce edema formation, but diuretics may be needed in some cases. Higher than expected doses of diuretics may be needed to effect salt and water removal because secreted diuretic molecules may bind to urinary albumin, rendering them ineffective inhibitors of specific transport processes in the nephron. In addition, there may be cellular resistance to diuretic action in NS. Considerable caution must be exercised because once a diuresis is effected, it is easy to induce hypovolemia and worsening azotemia. Massive edema can be treated with loop diuretics in combination with albumin infusions to maintain intravascular volume status. Dietary manipulation and drug therapy may reduce the risk of cardiovascular complications, especially when there are risk factors for ischemic heart disease (250).

Angiotensin-Converting Enzyme Inhibitors and NSAIDs

These have been used in patients with refractory proteinuria who failed to respond to other therapies. ACEIs block the local production of antiogensin II, which presumably contributes to the permselectivity defect in NS. NSAIDs induce a decrease in GFR, decreasing the amount of protein filtered, and affect the size-selective properties of the glomerular capillary wall. NSAIDs must be used with caution in patients with NS because their use may precipitate acute renal failure. Desensitization, disodium chromoglycate, and an oligoantigenic diet are ineffective.

Infections and Immunization

A PPD (purified protein derivative) must be placed before starting treatment with steroids. If a patient who has not had varicella or has no serum antibody titers to varicella is exposed while on a high dose of prednisone (>20 mg/m2) or an alkylating agent, varicella zoster immune globulin should be given if exposure occurred during the previous 96 h. The dose is 125 U/10 kg body weight to a maximum of 625 U. Patients who develop varicella or shingles are treated with acyclovir if they are on high doses of steroids or on an alkylating agent. If exposure to measles occurs, the patient's immune status is checked, quarantine measures are instituted, and gammaglobulin is administered. Patients with suspected peritonitis are treated with penicillin and an aminoglycoside or cephalosporin. This regimen is continued until culture results are available. If gram-positive diploccoci are identified in peritoneal fluid, penicillin is sufficient. Cellulitis is managed in the same way.

It has been suggested, without any evidence, that vaccinations or inoculations may precipitate a relapse. Decisions to immunize should not be influenced by this issue alone. Children treated with high-dose daily prednisone (>20 mg/m2) or alkylating agents should not be given live vaccinations, and live polio vaccine should not be given to siblings and household contacts. Pneumococcal and hemophilus vaccine should be given to adults and to children >2 years of age with MCNS when they are off steroids. Although antibody levels to S. pneumoniae are initially adequate, about 50% of patients do not maintain a protective antibody level a year later (251).

There are no criteria for use of intravenous immunoglobulin. Recommendations include IgG levels under 600 mg/dl in adults (213), low natural antibody levels, poor response to vaccine, and no protective antibody against the infecting organism.

Glucocorticoids

Corticosteroids (prednisone and prednisolone) remain the treatment of choice for MCNS despite their side effects and their inability to cure the condition.

Children

An initial high daily dose of steroids is required to achieve remission (Fig. 4) (240). A modified International Study of Kidney Disease in Children (ISKDC) regimen is prednisone in a dose of 60 mg/m2 for 4 weeks followed by 40 mg/m2 every second morning for another 4 weeks (252). The median time from starting treatment to remission is 2 weeks; by the end of 8 weeks, 95% are in remission.

1. Initial episode
Prednisolone 60 mg/mg^2/day (maximum 80 mg/day)
until remission, followed by
40 mg/m^2 (maximum 60 mg/day) on alternate days for 4 weeks

↓

2. First two relapses
Prednisolone 60 mg/mg^2/day (maximum 80 mg/day)
until remission, followed by
40 mg/m^2 (maximum 60 mg/day) on alternate days for 4 weeks

↓

3. Frequent relapser
Maintenance prednisolone 0·1–0·5 mg/kg/alternate days for
3–6 months, then reduce

↓

4. Relapse on prednisolone
>0·5 mg/kg/alternate days
Levamisole 2·5 mg/kg/alternate days for 4–12 months

↓

5. Relapse on prednisolone
>0·5 mg/kg/alternate days
and
Steroid side effects or risk factors
or
Relapse on prednisolone
>1·0 mg/kg/alternate days

Cyclosphosphamide 3 mg/kg/day for 8 weeks

↓

6. Post-cyclosphosphamide relapses
As 2–3 above

↓

7. Relapse on prednisolone
>0·5 mg/kg/alternate days

↓

Cyclosporin 5 mg/kg/day for one year

↓

8. Relapse post-cyclosporin
?

FIG. 4. A suggested management scheme for children with probable MCNS. Reprinted with permission (240).

There are other regimens. For example, prednisone is given in a dose of 2 mg/kg ideal body weight (to a maximum of 80 mg/day) or 60 mg/m2/day until the urine is protein free for 3 days (240). The child is considered steroid resistant if there is no response by 4 weeks. Once in remission, the dose is reduced to 40 mg/m2 every second morning for 4 weeks. Yet another regimen consists of a longer initial course of steroid therapy of 6 weeks (253,254). This may have the advantage of inducing a more prolonged initial remission but may cause more side effects. Urine should be checked for albumin every morning by Dipstix testing until it is established that the patient has entered into remission.

Relapses are common, and cannot be predicted reliably. About 80% of patients relapse at least once, 50% have frequent relapses but remain steroid responsive, and the remainder become steroid dependent (255,256). Relapses become less frequent in children as they grow older, and the majority "outgrow" the condition after puberty. Steroid dependence and resistance are more common in patients who relapse within 3 months of the first remission.

The first three relapses are managed in the same way as the first episode. Once the dose of steroids required to maintain a remission is established, patients who are frequent relapsers are given prednisone every second morning for 6 months in a dose of 0.1 to 0.5 mg/kg, and the dose is gradually tapered.

Adults

Because up to 40% of adults may undergo spontaneous remission, mildly affected patients who are asymptomatic can be treated with a low-sodium diet and a diuretic. If the MCNS persists, prednisone is given in a dose of 60 to 80 mg/day or 100 to 120 mg on alternate days. The remission rate is 60% at 8 weeks and 80% after 28 weeks of daily steroid therapy (257). Adults may require 10 to 16 weeks of daily steroid therapy to enter remission. Adults treated for 2 to 3 months on daily steroids have more relapses than those given alternate-day prednisone for 1 year so that those on daily steroids receive a greater cumulative steroid dose (258). Gradual tapering may help to prevent relapses that may be associated with reduced endogenous steroid production. Resistance as defined by failure to respond to 16 weeks of steroid therapy occurs in 10% to 15% of adults and increases with age. Repeated relapses are best managed with additional courses of steroids.

Alkylating Agents

Alkylating agents can induce prolonged remissions but are used judiciously because of potential side effects. The peripheral blood counts must be monitored regularly because of transient leukopenia. The drug is stopped transiently if the white cell count decreases to less than 4,000/ml. The risk of gonadal toxicity is greatest in postpubertal males. Azoospermia may occur after a cumulative dose of 300 mg/kg for cyclophosphamide (259) and 10 mg/kg for chlorambucil (260). Doses of cyclophosphamide of 2.5 mg/kg/day for 8 to 12 weeks infrequently cause alopecia or hemorrhagic cystitis. Leukemia is an uncommon complication (261,262). Patients are at risk for developing disseminated varicella while on an alkylating agent if they have not previously had varicella. Less frequent complications are nausea, anorexia, and hyperpigmentation. An additional complication of chlorambucil is seizures. There is no evidence that chlorambucil is more effective than cyclophosphamide.

The indications for using cyclophosphamide in children are frequent relapses while on more than 1 mg/kg of prednisone every other day or serious steroid-induced side effects. Cyclophosphamide is used in adults to treat frequently relapsing and steroid-resistant MCNS. The longer the course of therapy, the greater the likelihood of prolonged remission and side effects. A short course has little benefit: one third of children with frequently relapsing NS remain in remission after 1 year if given cyclophosphamide for less than 6 weeks, whereas two thirds remain in remission for more than 2 years after 12 weeks of therapy (263). Remission is not as well maintained with steroid-dependent NS (SDNS) (264). The current practice is to prescribe 2.5 to 3 mg/kg for an 8-week period after remission is induced with steroids; after cyclophosphamide is started, steroid doses are tapered gradually and are stopped 4 to 6 weeks after the course of cyclophosphamide is completed.

Cyclosporine A

CsA is used to treat SDNS if there are serious side effects of steroids and failure to respond to cyclophosphamide. Biopsy should be performed before starting and after completing CsA because of its propensity to cause interstitial fibrosis. Contraindications to CsA treatment are renal insufficiency, severe hypertension, and chronic tubulointerstitial changes. CsA is stopped if there is no response by 4 months. The plasma creatinine, blood pressure, and serum CsA levels must be monitored regularly. The dose is reduced if the serum creatinine concentration increases by more than 30% above the basal level. The maintenance dose is the lowest effective dose. The results of treatment with CsA in SDNS are shown in Table 8. CsA can be tapered and stopped after 1 to 2 years to see if the patient remains in remission. Most patients relapse when CsA is tapered or stopped, and they tend to respond less well to a second course of CsA (239). Some patients can be treated successfully with a combination of CsA and alternate-day steroid therapy. CsA is less effective in the treatment of steroid-resistant NS (Table 8).

TABLE 8. *Results of cyclosporine therapy*

	No. of patients	Complete remission n	Complete remission %
Steroid-dependent nephrotic syndrome			
Children	160	127	79
Adults	33	25	76
Steroid-resistant nephrotic syndrome			
Children	60	12	20
Adults	49	6	12

The most serious side effects of CsA are acute and chronic renal insufficiency. The dose must be reduced if the serum creatinine concentration increases to more than 30% above the baseline level, and it must be discontinued if the creatinine level continues to increase. Other side effects are gum hypertrophy, hirsutism, tremor, seizures, and hypertension. Azathioprine, levamisole, quinalones, mizoribine, sodium chromoglycate, and immunoglobulin infusions are not effective treatments of MCNS.

OUTCOME

Antibiotics have substantially reduced the mortality rate in MCNS, and corticosteroid therapy induces remissions and prevents relapses. Few children die from complications of MCNS or of its treatment. The prognosis in adults over 60 years of age is not as good (257,265). Deaths are caused by thrombosis, sepsis, oligoanuria, and cardiovascular disease. The tendency to relapse declines with age in children and adults. In children who present before 6 years of age, the incidence of relapses beyond 18 years of age is 5.5%. Adults may relapse over decades but tend to do so less frequently.

REFERENCES

1. Basham WR. *On dropsy connected with disease of the kidneys (morbus brightii), and on some other diseases of those organs, associated with albuminous and purulent urine.* 2nd edition. London: John Churchill, 1862:vii.
2. International Study of Kidney Disease in Children. Nephrotic syndrome in children: prediction of histopathology from clinical and laboratory characteristics at time of diagnosis. *Kidney Int* 1978;13: 159–165.
3. Bhasin HK, Abuelo JG, Nayak R, Esparza AR. Mesangial proliferative glomerulonephritis. *Lab Invest* 1978;39:21–29.
4. Waldherr R, Gubler MC, Levy M, Broyer M, Habib R. The significance of pure diffuse mesangial proliferation idiopathic nephrotic syndrome. *Clin Nephrol* 1978;10:171–179.
5. Ji-Yun Y, Melvin T, Sibley R, Michael A. No evidence for a specific IgM in mesangial proliferation of idiopathic nephrotic syndrome. *Kidney Int* 1984;25:100–106.
6. Vilches AR, Turner DR, Cameroon JS, Ogg CS, Chantler C, Williams DG. Significance of mesangial IgM deposition in "minimal change" nephrotic syndrome. *Kidney Int* 1982;46:10.
7. Mampaoo F, Gonzalo A, Teruel J, et al. Mesangial deposits of IgM in patients with the nephrotic syndrome. *Clin Nephrol* 1981;16:230–234.
8. Rich AR. A hitherto undescribed vulnerability of the juxtamedullary glomeruli in lipoid nephrosis. *Bull Johns Hopkins Hosp* 1957;100: 173–186.
9. Hayslett JP, Krasser LS, Bensch KG, et al. Progression of "lipid nephrosis" to renal insufficiency. *N Engl J Med* 1969;281:181–187.
10. Korbet SM, Schwartz MM, Lewis E. Primary focal segmental glomerulosclerosis: clinical course and response to therapy. *Am J Kidney Dis* 1994;23:773–783.
11. International Study of Kidney Disease in Children. Early identification of frequent relapsers among children with minimal change nephrotic syndrome. *J Pediatr* 1982;101:514–518.
12. Tranin EB, Boichis H, Spitzer A, et al. Late nonresponsiveness to steroids in children with minimal change nephrotic syndrome. *J Paediatr* 1975;87:519–523.
13. International Study of Kidney Disease in Children. Prospective controlled trial of cyclophosphamide therapy in children with the nephrotic syndrome. *Lancet* 1974;2:423–427.
14. Williams SA, Makker SP, Ingelfinger JR, et al. Long term evaluation of chlorambucil plus prednisone in the ideopathic nephrotic syndrome of childhood. *N Engl J Med* 1980;302:929–933.
15. McEnery PT, Strife CF. Nephrotic syndrome in childhood: Management and treatment in patients with minimal change disease, mesangial proliferation, or focal glomerulosclerosis. *Pediatr Clin North Am* 1982;89:875–894.
16. International Study of Kidney Disease in Children. Primary nephrotic syndrome in children; clinical significance of histopathologic variants of minimal change and of diffuse mesangial hypercellularity. *Kidney Int* 1981;20:765–771.
17. Schlesinger ER, Sultz HA, Mosher WE, Feldman JC. The nephrotic syndrome. Its incidence and implications for the community. *Am J Dis Child* 1968;116:623–632.
18. Rothenberg MB, Heymann W. The incidence of the nephrotic syndrome in children. *Pediatrics* 1957;19:446–452.
19. Barness LA, Moll GH, Janeway CA. Nephrotic syndrome I. Natural history of the disease. *Pediatrics* 1950;5:486–503.
20. Zech P, Colon S, Pointet P, et al. The nephrotic syndrome in adults aged over 60. Etiology, evolution and treatment of 76 cases. *Clin Nephrol* 1982;17:232.
21. Khokhar N, Akavaran NR, Quinones EM. Lipoid nephrosis in the elderly. *South Med J* 1980;73:790.
22. Galan E. Nephrosis in children. *Am J Dis Child* 1949;77:328–349.
23. Cameron JS, Turner DR, Ogg CS, et al. The nephrotic syndrome in adults with "minimal change glomerular lesion". *Q J Med* 1974;43: 461–488.
24. Sharples PM, Poulton J, White RHR. Steroid nephrotic syndrome is more common in Asians. *Arch Dis Child* 1985;60:1014–1017.
25. Feehally J, Kendell NP, Swift PGF, Walls J. High incidence of minimal change nephrotic syndrome in Asians. *Arch Dis Child* 1985;60: 1018–1020.
26. Coovadia HM, Adhikari M, Morel-Maroger L. Clinico-pathological features of the nephrotic syndrome in South African children. *Q J Med* 1979;48:77–91.
27. Meyers KEC, Thomson PD, Jacobs DWC, Kala UK. Peadiatric nephrology experience. Johannesburg and Baragwanath Hospitals, 1982–1988 inclusive. *Kidney Int* 1991;39:361.
28. White RHR. The familial nephrotic syndrome I. A European survey. *Clin Nephrol* 1973;1:215–219.
29. Moncreiff MW, White RHR, Glasgow E, et al. The familial nephrotic syndrome II. A clinicopathological study. *Clin Nephrol* 1973;1: 220–229.
30. Francis KL, Jenis EH, Jensen GH, et al. Gold-associated nephropathy. *Arch Pathol Lab Med* 1984;108:234.
31. Falck HM, Tornroth T, Kock B, et al. Fatal renal vasculitis and minimal change glomerulonephritis complicating treatment with penicillamine. *Acta Med Scand* 1979;205:133.
32. Rennke HG, Roos PC, Wall SG. Drug-induced interstitial nephritis with heavy glomerular proteinuria. *N Engl J Med* 1980;302:691.
33. Agner E, Henning J. Mercury poisoning and nephrotic syndrome in two young siblings. *Lancet* 1978;28:951.
34. Feinfeld DA, Olesnicky L, Pirani CL, et al. Nephrotic syndrome associated with use of the nonsteroidal anti-inflammatory drugs. *Nephron* 1984;37:174–179.
35. Wood IK, Parmelee DX, Foreman JW. Lithium-Induced nephrotic syndrome. *Am J Psychiatry* 1989;146:84–87.
36. Alexander F, Martin J. Nephrotic syndrome associated with lithium therapy. *Clin Nephrol* 1981;15:267–271.
37. Heymann W. Nephrotic syndrome after use of trimethadione and paramethadione in petit mal. *JAMA* 1967;202:127.
38. Hardwicke J, Soothill JF, Squire JR, Holti G. Nephrotic syndrome and pollen sensitivity. *Lancet* 1959;1:500–502.
39. Sandberg DH, McIntosh RM, Berstein CW, et al. Severe steroid-responsive nephrosis associated with hypersensitivity. *Lancet* 1977;1: 388–391.
40. Howanietz H, Lubec G. Idiopathic nephrotic syndrome, treated with steroids for five years, found to be allergic reaction to pork. *Lancet* 1984;2:450.
41. Laurent J, Lagrue G, Belghiti D, et al. Is house dust allergen a possible causal factor for relapse in lipoid nephrosis? *Allergy* 1984;38: 231–235.
42. Rytland DA. Onset of the nephrotic syndrome during a reaction to bee-sting. *Stanford Med Bull* 1955;13:224–233.

43. Moorthy AV, Zimmerman SW, Burkholder PM. Nephrotic syndrome in Hodgkin's disease: evidence for pathogenesis alternative to immune complex deposition. *Am J Med* 1976;61:471–447.
44. Eagen JW, Lewis EJ. Glomerulopathies of neoplasia. *Kidney Int* 1977;11:297–306.
45. Matsuda O, Makiguchi K, Ishibashi K et al. Long term effect of steroid treatment on nephrotic syndrome associated with Kimura's disease and a review of the literature. *Clin Nephrol* 1992;37:119–123.
46. Forland M, Bannayan GA. Minimal change lesion nephrotic syndrome with renal oncocytoma. *Am J Med* 1983;75:715.
47. Moorthy AV. Minimal change glomerular disease: a paraneoplatic syndrome in two patients with with bronchogenic carcinoma. *Am J Kidney Dis* 1983;3:58.
48. Grupe WE. Childhood nephrotic syndrome: clinical associations and response to therapy. *Postgrad Med* 1979;65:229–236.
49. Magalhaes-Filho AG, Barbosa AV, Ferreira TC. Glomerulonephrities in schistosomiasis with mesangial IgM deposits. *Mem Inst Oswaldo Cruz* 1981;76:181.
50. Froelich CJ, Searles RP, Davis LE, et al. A case of Guillain-Barré syndrome with immunologic abnormality. *Ann Intern Med* 1980;93: 563.
51. Gaboardi F, Perletti L, Combie M, et al. Dermatitis herpetiformis and nephrotic syndrome. *Clin Nephrol* 1983;20:49.
52. Roger D, Bonnetblance JM, Leroux-Robert C. Melorheostosis with associated minimal change nephrotic syndrome, mesenteric fibromatosis and capillary hemangiomas. *Dermatology* 1994;188: 166–168.
53. Rytand DA. Fatal anuria, the nephrotic syndrome and glomerulonephritis as sequels of the dermatitis of poison oak. *Am J Med* 1948; 5:548–560.
54. McDonald P, Kalra PA, Coward RA. Thymoma and minimal change glomerulonephritis. *Nephrol Dial Transplant* 1992;7:357–359.
55. Kaplan BS, Klassen J, Gault MH. Glomerular injury in patients with neoplasia. In: Creger WP, Coggins CH, Hancock EW, eds. *Ann Rev Med* 1976,117–125.
56. Peces R, Sanchez L, Gorostidi M, Alvarez J. Minimal change nephrotic syndrome associated with Hodgkins lymphoma. *Nephrol Dial Transplant* 1991;69:155–158.
57. Plager J, Stutzman L. Acute nephrotic syndrome as a manifestation of active Hodgkin's disease. *Am J Med* 1971;50:56–66.
58. Moorthy AV, Zimmerman SW, Burkholder PM. Nephrotic syndrome in Hodgkin's disease. *Am J Med* 1976;61:471–477.
59. Sherman RL, Susin M, Weksler ME. Lipoid nephrosis in Hodgkin's disease. *Am J Med* 1972;52:699–702.
60. Reeves WG, Cameron JS, Johanson SGO, et al. Seasonal nephrotic syndrome. Description and immunological findings. *Clin Allergy* 1975;5:121–137.
61. Richards W, Olson D, Church JA. Improvement of idiopathic nephrotic syndrome following allergy therapy. *Ann Allergy* 1977;39: 322–333.
62. Thomson PD, Barratt TM, Stokes CR, Turner MW, Soothill JF. HLA antigens and atopic features in steroid-responsive nephrotic syndrome of childhood. *Lancet* 1976;2:765–768.
63. Meadow SR, Sarsfield JK, Scott DG, et al. Steroid-responsive nephrotic syndrome and allergy: immunological studies. *Arch Dis Child* 1981;56:509–516.
64. Lagrue G, Laurent J. Allergy and lipoid nephrosis. *Adv Nephrol* 1983; 12:151–175.
65. Sandberg DH, McIntosh RM, Bernstein CW, et al. Severe steroid-responsive nephrosis asociated with hypersensivity. *Lancet* 1977;1: 388–391.
66. Groshong T, Mendelson L, Mendoza S, et al. Serum IgE in patients with minimal change nephrotic syndrome. *J Pediatr* 1973;83:76–77.
67. Gerber MA, Paronetto F. IgE in glomeruli of patients with nephrotic syndrome. *Lancet* 1971;1097–1099.
68. Roy LP, Westberg LP, Michael AF. Nephrotic syndrome—no evidence for a role of IgE. *Clin Exp Immunol* 1973;13:553–559.
69. Schulte-Wisserman H, Gortz W, Straub E. IgE in patients with glomerulonephritis and minimal-change nephrotic syndrome. *Eur J Pediatr* 1979;131:105.
70. Trompeter RS, Barratt TM, Kay R, Turner MW, Soothill JF. HLA, atopy and cyclophosphamide in steroid-responsive nephrotic syndrome. *Kidney Int* 1980;17:113–117.
71. O'Regan D, O'Callaghan U, Dundon S, Reen DJ. HLA antigens and steroid responsive nephrotic syndrome of childhood. *Tissue Antigens* 1980;16:147–151.
72. Cambon-Thomson A, Bouisson F, Abbai M, et al. HLA et Bf dans le syndrome nephrotique de l'enfant: differences entre les formes corticosensibles et corticorisistantes. *Pathol Biol* 1986;34:725–730.
73. Noss G, Bachman HJ, Obling H. Association of minimal change nephrotic syndrome (MCNS) with HLA-B8 and B-13. *Clin Nephrol* 1981;15:172–174.
74. Alfiler CA, Roy LP, Doran T, et al. HLA DRw7 and steroid-responsive nephrotic syndrome of childhood. *Clin Nephrol* 1980;14:71–74.
75. De Mouzon-Cambon A, Bouissou F, Dutau G, et al. HLA-DR7 in children with idiopathic nephrotic syndrome: correlation with atopy. *Tissue Antigens* 1981;17:518–524.
76. Nunez-Roldan A, Villechenous E, Fernandez-Andrade C, et al. Increased HLA-DR7 and decreased DR2 in steroid-responsive nephrotic syndrome. *N Engl J Med* 1982;306:366–367.
77. Kobayashi Y, Chen X-M, Hiki Y, et al. Association of HLA-DRw8 and DQw3 with minimal change nephrotic syndrome in Japanese adults. *Kidney Int* 1985;28:193–197.
78. Lagueruela CC, Bruettner TL, Cole BR, Kissane JM, Robson AM. HLA extended haplotypes in steroid-sensitive nephrotic syndrome of childhood. *Kidney Int* 1990;38:145–150.
79. McClean RH, Ruley EJ, Tina K, Medani C. Increased frequency of silent C4A allele (C4*Q0) of the fourth component of complement in the ideopathic nephrotic syndrome [Abstract]. *Kidney Int* 1988;33: 165.
80. Ruder H, Scharer K, Oplez G, et al. Human leucocyte antigens in ideopathic nephrotic syndrome in children. *Pediatr Nephrol* 1990;4: 478–481.
81. Jin DK, Kohasaka Tanaka M, Abe J, Kobayashi N. Human leucocyte antigens in childhood ideopathic nephrotic syndrome. *Acta Paediatr Jpn* 1991;33:709–713.
82. Clarke AGB, Vaughan RW, Stephens HAF, Chantler C, Williams DG, Welsh KI. Genes encoding the beta chains of HLA-DR7 and DQw2 define major susceptibility determinants for ideopathic nephrotic syndrome. *Kidney Int* 1990;38:145–150.
83. Pirotzky E, Hieblot C, Benveniste J, et al. Basophil sensitisation in ideopathic nephrotic syndrome. *Lancet* 1982;1:358–361.
84. Shalhoub RJ. Pathogenesis of lipoid nephrosis: a disorder of T-cell function. *Lancet* 1974;2:556–560.
85. Lin CY, Chen CH, Lee PP. In vitro B-lymphocyte switch disturbance from IgG into IgM mesangial nephropathy. *Pediatr Nephrol* 1989;3: 254–258.
86. Meadow SR, Sarsfield JK, Scott DG, Rajah SM. Steroid-responsive nephrotic syndrome and allergy: immunological studies. *Arch Dis Child* 1981;56:217–254.
87. Lange K, Ahmed U Seligson G, Grover A. Depression of endostreptosin, streptolysin O, and streptozyme antibodies in patients with ideopathic nephrosis with and without nephrotic syndrome. *Clin Nephrol* 1981;15:279–285.
88. La Manna A, Polito C, Foglia AC, et al. Reduced response to HBV vaccination in boys with steroid sensitive nephrotic syndrome. *Pediatr Nephrol* 1992;6:251–253.
89. McLean R, Forsgren A, Bjorksten B, Kim Y, Quie P, Michael A. Decreased serum factor B concentration associated with decreased opsonization of *Escherichia coli* in the ideopathic nephrotic syndrome. *Pediatr Res* 1977;11:910–916.
90. Ballow M, Kennedy T, Gaudio K, Siegel N, McLean RT. Serum hemolytic factor D factor values in children with steroid-responsive ideopathic nephrotic syndrome. *J Pediatr* 1982;100:192–196.
91. Cairns S, London R, Mallick. Circulating immune complexes in ideopathic glomerular disease. *Kidney Int* 1982;21:507–512.
92. Fiser RT, Arnold WE, Charlton RK, Steele RW, Childress SH, Shirkey B. T-lymphocyte subsets in nephrotic syndrome. *Kidney Int* 1991;40:913–916.
93. Mandreoli M, Beltrandi F, Casadei-Maldini M, et al. Lymphocyte release of soluable IL-2 receptors in patients with minimal change nephropathy. *Clin Nephrol* 1992;37:177–182.
94. Jordan SC, Querfeld U, Toyoda M, Prehn J. Serum interleukin-2 levels in a patient with focal glomerulosclerosis. *Pediatr Nephrol* 1990; 4:166–168.
95. Nagata K, Platt JL, Michael AF. Interstitial and glomerular immune cell populations in ideopathic nephrotic syndrome. *Kidney Int* 1984; 25:88–93.

96. Matsumoto K, Osakabe K, Harada M, Hatano M. Impaired cell-mediated immunity in lipoid nephrosis. *Nephron* 1981;29:190–194.
97. Mallick NP, Williams RJ, Waddell CC, Taunton OD, Twomey JJ. Inhibition of lymphoproliferation by hyperlipoproteinemic plasma. *J Clin Invest* 1976;58:950–954.
98. Schnaper HW. A regulatory system for soluable immune response supressor production in steroid-responsive nephrotic syndrome. *Kidney Int* 1990;38:151–159.
99. Saxena S, Mittal R, Andal A. Pattern of interleukins in minimal-change nephrotic syndrome. *Nephron* 1993;65:56–61.
100. Garin E, Blanchard D, Matsushima K, Djeu J. IL-8 production by peripheral blood mononuclear cells in nephrotic patients. *Kidney Int* 1994;45:1311–1317.
101. Suranyi M, Quiza C, Gausch A, Newton L, Myers B. Cytokine level in patients with the nephrotic syndrome. *Kidney Int* 1990;37:445.
102. Sobel A, Heslan JM, Branellec A, Lagrue G. Vascular permiability factor produced by lymphocytes of patients with nephrotic syndrome. *Adv Nephrol* 1981;10:315–332.
103. Tanaka R, Yoshikawa N, Nakamura H, Ito H. Infusion of peripheral blood mononuclear cell products from nephrotic children increases albuminuria in rats. *Nephron* 1989;60:35–41.
104. Maruyama K, Tomizawa S, Shimabukuro N, et al. Effect of supernatants derived from T lymphocyte cultures in minimal change nephrotic syndrome on rat kidney capillaries. *Nephron* 1989;51: 73–76.
105. Ferrara N, Houck K, Jakeman L, Leung DW. Molecular and biological properties of the vascular endothelial growth factor family of proteins. *Endocrin Rev* 1992;13:18–32.
106. Iijma K, Yoshikawa N, Connolly DT, Nakamura H. Human mesangial cells and peripheral blood mononuclear cells produce vascular permiability factor. *Kidney Int* 1993;44:959–966.
107. Garin EH, Boggs KP. Effect of supernatants from nephrotic peripheral blood mononuclear cells on 35-sulphate incorporation in rat glomerular basement membrane. *Pediatr Res* 1985;19:836–840.
108. Garin EH. Effect of prednisone on nephrotic peripheral blood mononuclear cell mediated increase in ^{35}sulphate uptake in rat glomerular basement membrane. *Nephron* 1989;53:268–272.
109. Koyama A, Fujisaki M, Kobayashi M, Igarashi M, Narita M. A glomerular permiability factor produced by human T-cell hybridomas. *Kidney Int* 1991;40:453–460.
110. Rennke HG, Venkatachalam MA. Glomerular permiability of macromolecules: effect of molecular configuration on the fractional clearance of uncharged dextran and neutral horseradish peroxidase in the rat. *J Clin Invest* 1979;63:713–717.
111. Bertolatus JA, Hunsicker LG. Glomerular sieving of anionic and neutral bovine albumins in proteinuric rats. *Kidney Int* 1985;28:467–476.
112. Rennke HG, Patel Y, Venkatachalam MA. Glomerular filtration of proteins: clearance of anionic, neutral and cationic horseradish peroxidase in the rat kidney. *Kidney Int* 1978;19:3254–3328.
113. Bridges C, Myers B, Brenner B, Deen W. Glomerular charge alterations in human minimal change nephropathy. *Kidney Int* 182;22: 677–684.
114. Carrie B, Salyer W, Myers B. Minimal change nephropathy: an electrochemical disorder of the glomerular membrane. *Am J Med* 1981: 70;262–267.
115. Blau E, Haas J. Glomerular sialic acid and proteinuria in human renal disease. *Lab Invest* 1973;28:477–481.
116. Sewell R, Brenchley P, Mallick N. Human mononuclear cells contain an endoglycosidase specific for hepran sulphate glycosaminoglycan demonstrable with the use of a specific solid-phase metabolically radiolabelled substrate. *Biochem J* 1989;264:777–783.
117. Levine M, Gascione P, Turner MW, Barratt TM. A highly cationic protein in the plasma and urine of children with steroid-responsive nephrotic syndrome. *Kidney Int* 1989;36:867–877.
118. Vahaskari VM, Root ER, Germuth FG, Robson AM. Glomerular charge and urinary protein excretion: effects of systemic and intrarenal polycation infusion in the rat. *Kidney Int* 1982;22: 127–135.
119. Deen WM, Bridges CR, Brenner BM, Myers BD. Heteroporous model of glomerular size selectivity: application to normal and nephrotic humans. *Am J Physiol* 1985;249F:374–389.
120. Oliver JD III, Anderson S, Troy JL, Brenner BM, Deen WM. Determination of glomerular size selectivity in the normal rat with Ficoll. *J Am Soc Nephrol* 1992;3:214–228.
121. Myers B, Gausch A. Mechanisms of proteinuria in nephrotic humans. *Pediatr Nephrol* 1994;8:107–112.
122. Kuster S, Mehls O, Seidel C, Ritz E. Blood pressure in minimal change and other types of nephrotic syndrome. *Am J Nephrol* 1990; 10:76–80.
123. Assadi FK, Lansky LL, John EG, Helgason CM, Tan WS. Acute hypertensive encephalopathy in minimal change nephrotic syndrome. *Child Nephrol Urol* 1990;10:96–99.
124. Graber M, Subramani K, Corish D, Schwab A. Thrombocytosis elevates serum potassium. *Am J Kidney Dis* 1988;12:116–120.
125. Barratt TM. Renal disorders. In: Clayton BE, Round JM, eds. *Chemical pathology and the sick child.* Oxford, England: Scientific Publications; 1984:120–149.
126. Abitol C, Zilleruelo G, Freundlich M, et al. Quantitation of proteiuria with urine protein/creatinine ratios and random testing with dipstix in nephrotic children. *J Pediatr* 1990;116:243–247.
127. Blainy JD, Brewer DB, Hardwicke J, et al. The nephrotic syndrome. Diagnosis by renal biopsy and biochemical and immunological analyses related to the response to steroid therapy. *Q J Med* 1960;29: 235–256.
128. Sesso R, Santos AP, Nishida SK, et al. Prediction of steroid responsiveness in the idiopathic nephrotic syndrome using urinary retinol-binding protein and beta-2-microglobulin. *Ann Intern Med* 1992;116: 905–909.
129. International Study of Kidney Disease in Children. Nephrotic syndrome: predicition of histopathology from clinical and laboratory characteristics at time of diagnosis. *Kidney Int* 1978;13:159–165.
130. Appel G. Lipid abnormalities in renal disease. *Kidney Int* 1991;39: 169–183.
131. Kaysen GA, Gambertoglio J, Felts J, Hutchison FN. Albumin synthesis, albuminuria and hyperlipidemia in nephrotic patients. *Kidney Int* 1987;31:1368–1376.
132. Kaysen GA, Jones H, Martin V, Hutchison FN. Albumin synthesis, albuminuria and hyperlipemia in nephrotic rats. *J Clin Invest* 1989; 83:1623–1629.
133. Bennhold H, Klaus D, Scheinlen PG. Volume regulation and renal function in analbuminemia. *Lancet* 1960;2:1169–1170.
134. Kaloyanides GJ. Edema. In: Massary SG, Glassock RJ, eds. *Textbook of nephrology.* Baltimore: Williams & Wilkins; 1983:430–440.
135. Koomans HA, Kortland W, Geers AB, Dorhout Mees EJ. Lowered protein content of tissue fluid in patients with the nephrotic syndrome: observations during disease and recovery. *Nephron* 1985; 40:391–395.
136. Seifter JL, Skorecki KL, Stivelmen JG, Haupert G, Brenner BM. Control of extracellular fluid volume and pathophysiology of edema formation. In: Brenner BM, Rector FL, eds. *The kidney.* Philadelphia: WB Saunders; 1986:343–384.
137. Zweifach BW. Capillary filtration and mechanisms of edema formation. *Pflugers Arch* 1972;336(suppl):81–85.
138. Zilleruelo G, Strauss J. Management of nephrotic edema. In: Stauss J, ed. *Hypertension, fluid-electrolytes and tubulopathies in pediatric nephrology.* The Hague: Martinus Nijhoff; 1982:189–205.
134. Eisenberg S. Blood volume in persons with the nephrotic syndrome. *Am J Med Sci* 1968;255:320–326.
140. Geers AB, Koomans HA, Boer P, Dorhout Mees EJ. Plasma volume (PV) measurments in patients with nephrotic syndrome (NS): a methodological study on the labelled albumin method. *Kidney Int* 1983:23;123.
141. Geers AB, Koomans HA, Dorhout Mees EJ. Plasma and blood volumes in patients with the nephrotic syndrome. *Nephron* 1984;38: 170–173.
142. Dorhout Mees EJ, Roos JC, Boer P, Yoe OH, Simatupang TA. Observation on edema formation in the nephrotic syndrome in adults with minimal lesions. *Am J Med* 1978;67:378–384.
143. Dorhout Mees EJ, Geers AB, Koomans HA. Blood volume and sodium retention in the nephrotic syndrome. A controversial pathophysiological concept. *Nephron* 1984;39:201–211.
144. Meltzer JI, Keim HJ, Largh JH, Sealey JE, Jan K-M, Chien S. Nephrotic syndrome: vasoconstriction and hypervolemic types indicated by renin-sodium profiling. *Ann Intern Med* 1979;91:688–696.
145. Garnett ES, Webber CE. Changes in blood-volume produced by treatment of the nephrotic syndrome. *Lancet* 1967;2:798–799.
146. Krishna GG, Danovitch GM. Effects of water immersion and renal function in the nephrotic syndrome. *Kidney Int* 1982;21:395–401.

147. Rascher W, Tulassay T, Seyberth HW, Himbert U, Lang U, Scharer K. Diuretic and hormonal response to head-out of water immersion in nephrotic syndrome. *J Pediatr* 1986;109:609–614.
148. Tulassy T, Rascher W, Lang RE, Seyberth HW, Scharer K. Atrial natriuretic peptide and other vacoactive hormones in nephrotic syndrome. *Kidney Int* 1987;31:1391–1395.
149. Ichikawa I, Rennke HG, Hoyer JR, Badr KF, Schor N, Troy JL. Role for internal mechanisms in the impaired salt excretion of experimental nephrotic syndrome. *J Clin Invest* 1983;71:91–103.
150. Brown EA, Markandu N, Sagnella GA, Jones BE, MacGregor GA. Sodium retention in nephrotic syndrome is due to an intrarenal defect: evidence from steroid-induced remission. *Nephron* 1985;39:290–295.
151. Koomans HA, Boer WH, Dorhout Mees EJ. Renal function during recovery from minimal lesion nephrotic syndrome. *Nephron* 1987;47:173–178.
152. Geers AB, Koomans HA, Roos JC, Boer P, Dorhout Mees EJ. Functional relationships in the nephrotic syndrome. *Kidney Int* 1984;26:324–330.
153. Shapiro MD, Nicholls KM, Groves BM, Schrier RW. Role of glomerular filtration rate in the impaired sodium and water excretion of patients with nephrotic syndrome. *Am J Kidney Dis* 1986;8:81–87.
154. Bohman SO, Jaremko G, Bohlin AB, Berg U. Foot process fusion and glomerular filtration rate in minimal change nephrotic syndrome. *Kidney Int* 1984;25:696–700.
155. Valentin J-P, Qui C, Muldowney WP, Ying WZ, Gardner DG, Humphreys MH. Cellular basis for blunted volume expansion natriuresis in experimental nephrotic syndrome. *J Clin Invest* 1992;90:1302–1312.
156. Grausz H, Lieberman R, Early LE. Effect of plasma albumin on sodium reabsorption in patients with nephrotic syndrome. *Kidney Int* 1972;1:47–54.
157. Bernard DB, Alexander EA, Couser WG, Levinski NG. Renal sodium retention during volume expansion in experimental nephrotic syndrome. *Kidney Int* 1978;14:478–485.
158. Baeyer H, van Liew JB, Klassen J, Boylan JW, Manz N, Muir P. Filtration of protein in the anti-glomerular basement nephrotic rat: a micropuncture study. *Kidney Int* 1976;10:425–437.
159. Bohlin AB, Berg U. Renal sodium handling in minimal change nephrotic syndrome. *Arch Dis Child* 1984;59:825–830.
160. Humphreys MH. Mechanisms and management of nephrotic edema. *Kidney Int* 1994;45:266–281.
161. Rascher W, Tulassay T. Hormonal regulation of water metabolism in children with nephrotic syndrome. *Kidney Int* 1987;32(suppl):83–89.
162. Medina A, Davies DL, Brown JJ, et al. A study of the renin-angiotensin system in the nephrotic syndrome. *Nephron* 1974;12:233–240.
163. Chonko AM, Bay W, Stein JH, Ferris TF. The role of renin and aldosterone in the salt retention of edema. *Am J Med* 1977;63:881–889.
164. Ammenti A, Muller-Weifel DE, Scharer K, Vecsei P. Mineralocorticoids in the nephrotic syndrome of children. *Clin Nephrol* 1980;14:238–245.
165. Kumagai H, Onoyama K, Iseki K, Omae T. Role of renin angiotensin aldosterone in minimal change nephrotic syndrome. *Clin Nephrol* 1985;23:229–235.
166. Brown EA, Markandu ND, Sagnella GA, Squires M, Jones BE, MacGregor GA. Evidence that some mechanism other than the renin system causes sodium retention in nephrotic syndrome. *Lancet* 1982;2:1237–1239.
162. Shapiro M, Hasbargen J, Cosby R, Yee B, Schrier R. Role of aldosterone in the Na retention of patients with nephrotic syndrome. *Kidney Int* 1986;29:203.
168. Kelsch RC, Light GS, Oliver WJ. The effect of albumin infusion upon plasma norepinephrine concentration in nephrotic children. *J Lab Clin Med* 1972;79:516–525.
169. Schlondorff D, Ardailou R. Prostaglandins and other arachidonic acid metabolites in the kidney. *Kidney Int* 1986;29:108–119.
170. Clive DM, Stoff JS. Renal symptoms associated with nonsteroidal antiinflammatory drugs. *N Engl J Med* 1984;310:564–572.
171. Donker AJM, Brentjens JRH, van der Hem GK, Arisz L. Treatment of the nephrotic syndrome with indomethacin. *Nephron* 1978;22:374–381.
172. Millet GU, Ruilope LM, Alcasar JM, et al. Participation of renal prostaglandins in the nephrotic syndrome. *Kidney Int* 1983;23:555.
173. Appel BG, Valeria A, Appel AS, Blum C. The hyperlipidemia of the nephrotic syndrome. *Am J Med* 1989;87:45N–50N.
174. Newmark SR, Anderson CF, Donadio JV, et al. Lipoprotein profiles in adult nephrotics. *Mayo Clin Proc* 1975;50:359–364.
175. Wheeler DC, Bernard D. Lipid abnormalities in the nephrotic syndrome: causes, consequences, and treatment. *Am J Kidney Dis* 1994;23:331–346.
176. Short CD, Durrington PN, Mallick NP, Hunt LP, Tetlow L, Ishola M. Serum and urinary high-density lipoproteins in glomerular disease with proteinuria. *Kidney Int* 1986;29:1224–1228.
177. Appel GB, Blum CB, Chien S, Kunis CL, Appel AS. The hyperlipidemia of the nephrotic syndrome. Relation to plasma albumin concentration, oncotic pressure, and viscosity. *N Engl J Med* 1985;312:1544–1548.
178. Kaysen GA. Hyperlipidemia of the nephrotic syndrome. *Kidney Int* 1991;39(suppl):8–15.
179. Baxter JH, Goodman HC, Allen JC. Effects of infusions of serum albumin on serum lipids and lipoproteins in nephrosis. *J Clin Invest* 1961;49:490–498.
180. Allen JC, Baxter JH, Goodman HC. Effects on dextran polyvinylpyrrolidone and gamma globulin on the hyperlipidemia of experimental nephrosis. *J Clin Invest* 1961;40:499–508.
181. Marsh JB. Lipoprotein metabolism in experimental nephrosis. *J Lipid Res* 1984;25:1619–1623.
182. Marshall JF, Apostolopoulos JJ, Brack CM, Howlett GJ. Regulation of apolipoprotein gene expression and plasma high density lipoprotein composition in experimental nephrosis. *Biochem Biophys Acta* 1990;1042:271–279.
183. Attman P-O, Alaupovic P. Pathogenesis of hyperlipidemia in the nephrotic syndrome. *Am J Nephrol* 1990;10:69–75.
184. Garber DW, Gottlieb BA, Marsh JB, Sparks CE. Catabolism of very low density lipoproteins in experimental nephrosis. *J Clin Invest* 1984;74:1375–1383.
185. Staprans I, Garon SJ, Hopper J, Felts JM. Characterization of glycosaminoglycans in urine from patients with nephrotic syndrome and control subjects and their effects on lipoprotein lipase. *Biochem Biophys Acta* 1981;678:414–422.
186. Ohta T, Matsunda I. Lipid and apolipoprotein levels in patients with nephrotic syndrome. *Clin Chim Acta* 1981;117:133–134.
187. Bennett A, Cameron JS. Platelet hyperaggregability in the nephrotic syndrome which is not dependent on arachidonic acid and serum albumin concentration. *Clin Nephrol* 1987;27:182–188.
188. Machleidt C, Mettang T, Starz E, Weber J, Risler T, Kuhlmann U. Multifactorial genesis of enhanced platelet aggregability in patients with nephrotic syndrome. *Kidney Int* 1989;36:1119–1124.
189. Ueda N. Effect of corticosteroids on some hemostatic parameters in children with minimal change nephrotic syndrome. *Nephron* 1990;56:374–378.
190. Goldstein DA, Haldimann B, Sherman D, Norman AW, Massry SG. Vitamin D metabolities and calcium metabolism in patients with nephrotic syndrome and normal renal function. *J Clin Endocrinol Metab* 1981;52:116–121.
191. Freundlich M, Bourgoignie JJ, Zilleruelo G, et al. Calcium and vitamin D metabolism in children with nephrotic syndrome. *J Pediatr* 1986;108:383–387.
192. Alon U, Chan JCM. Calcium and vitamin D homeostasis in the nephrotic syndrome: current status. *Nephron* 1984;36:1–4.
193. Auwerx J, DeKeyser L, Touillon R, De Moor P. Decreased free 1,25-dihydroxycholecalciferol index in patients with nephrotic syndrome. *Nephron* 1986;42:231–235.
194. Sato KA, Gary RW, Lemann J. Urinary excretion of 25-hydroxyvitamin D in health and nephrotic syndrome. *J Lab Clin Med* 1980;69:325–330.
195. Malluche HH, Goldstein DA, Massry SG. Osteomalacia and hyperparathyroid bone disease in patients with nephrotic syndrome. *J Clin Invest* 1979;64:494–500.
196. Korkor A, Schwartz J, Bergfeld M, et al. Absence of metabolic bone disease in adults patients with the nephrotic syndrome and normal renal function. *J Clin Endocrinol Metab* 1983;56:496–500.
197. Afrasiabi MA, Vaziri ND, Gwinup G, et al. Thyroid function studies in the nephrotic syndrome. *Ann Intern Med* 1979;90:335–338.
198. Gavin LA, McMahon FA, Castle JN, Cavalieri RR. Alterations in serum hormones and serum thyroxine-binding globulin in patients with nephrosis. *J Clin Endocrinol Metab* 1978;46:125–130.

199. Etling N, Fouque F. Effect of prednisone on serum and urinary thyroid hormone levels in children during the nephrotic syndrome. *Helv Paediatr Acta* 1982;37:257–265.
200. Ito S, Kano K, Ando T, Ichimura T. Thyroid function in children with nephrotic syndrome. *Pediatr Nephrol* 1994;8:412–415.
201. Fonseca V, Thomas M, Sweny P. Can urinary thyroid hormone loss cause hypothyroidism? *Lancet* 1991;38:475–476.
202. Hancock DE, Onstad JW, Wolf PL. Transferrin loss into the urine with hypochromic, microcytic anemia. *Am J Clin Pathol* 1976;65: 73–78.
203. Cartwright GE, Gubler CJ, Wintrobe MM. Studies on copper metabolism. XI. Copper and iron metabolism in the nephrotic syndrome. *J Clin Invest* 1954;33:865–872.
204. Perrone L, Gialanella G, Giordano V, La Manna A, Moro R, Ditoro R. Impaired zinc metabolic status in children affected by idiopathic nephrotic syndrome. *Eur J Pediatr* 1990;149:438–440.
205. Gordon RS. Exudative enteropathy. Abnormal permiability of the gastrointestinal tract demonstrable with labelled polyvinylpyrrolidine. *Lancet* 1959;1:325–330.
206. Jensen H, Jarnum S, Hart Hansen JP. Gastrointestinal protein loss and intestinal function in the nephrotic syndrome. *Nephron* 1966;3: 209–220.
207. Nussle D, Royer P. Pertes Digestives de proteines et syndrome nephrotiques de l'enfant. Etude avec la 131-I-albumine et la 125-g-globuline. In: *Protides of the biological fluids.* Amsterdam: Elsevier; 1964;12:220–223.
208. Salazar De Sousa J, Cunha GA, Araujo J. Association of nephrotic syndrome with intestinal lymphangiectasia. *Arch Dis Child* 1968;42: 245–248.
209. Meadow SR, Weller RO. Fatal systemic measles in a child receiving cyclophosphamide for nephrotic syndrome. *Lancet* 1969;25:876–878.
210. Close GC, Houston JB. Fatal haemorrhagic chickenpox in a child on long term steroids. *Lancet* 1981;2:480.
211. Krensky AM, Inglefinger JR, Grupe WE. Peritonitis in childhood nephrotic syndrome. *Am J Dis Child* 1982;136:732–736.
212. Rubin HN, Blau EB, Michaels RH. Hemophilus and pneumoccal peritonitis in children with nephrotic syndrome. *Pediatrics* 1975;56: 598–601.
213. Ogi M, Yokoyama H, Tomosugi N, et al. Risk factors for infection and immunoglobulin replacement therapy in adult nephrotic syndrome. *Am J Kidney Dis* 1994;24:427–436.
214. Strife FC, Jackson EC, Forristal J, West CD. Effect of the nephrotic syndrome on the concentration of serum compliment components. *Am J Kidney Dis* 1986;8:37–42.
215. Butler WT, Rossen RD. Effects of corticosteroids on immunity in man. *J Clin Invest* 1973;52:2629–2640.
216. Llach F, Papper S, Massry SG. Hypercoagulability, renal vein thrombosis and other thrombotic complications of the nephrotic syndrome. *Kidney Int* 1985;28:429–439.
217. Sullivan MJ III, Hough DR, Agodoa LCY. Peripheral arterial thrombosis due to the nephrotic syndrome. *South Med J* 1983;76: 1011–1016.
218. Mehls O, Andrassy K, Koderisch J, Herzog U, Ritz E. Hemostasis and thromboembolism in children with nephrotic syndrome. Differences from adults. *J Pediatr* 1987;110:862–867.
219. Egli F, Eliminger P, Stalder G. Thromboembolism in the nephrotic syndrome. *Pediatr Res* 1974;8:903.
220. Hoyer PF, Gonda S, Barthels M, Krohn HP, Brodehl J. Thromboembolic complication in children with nephrotic syndrome risk and incidence. *Acta Paediatr Scand* 1986;75:804–810.
221. Llach F, Papper S, Massry SG. The clinical spectrum of renal vein thrombosis: acute and chronic. *Am J Med* 1980;69:819–827.
222. Burrow CR, Walker WG, Bell WR, Gatewood OB. Streptokinase salvage of renal function after vein thrombosis. *Ann Intern Med* 1984; 100:237–238.
223. Crowley JP, Matarese RA, Quvedo SF, Garella S. Fibrinolytic therapy for bilateral renal vein thrombosis. *Arch Intern Med* 1984;144: 159–160.
224. Rowe JM, Rasmussen RL, Mader SL, et al. Successful thrombolytic therapy in two patients with renal vein thrombosis. *Am J Med* 1984; 77:111–114.
225. Jennette JC, Falk RJ. Adult minimal change glomerulopathy with acute renal failure. *Am J Kidney Dis* 1990;16:432–437.
226. Sakarcan A, Timmons C, Seikaly MG. Reversible acute renal failure in children with primary nephrotic syndrome. *J Pediatr* 1994;125: 723–727.
227. Lowenstein J, Schacht RG, Baldwin DS. Renal failure in minimal change nephrotic syndrome. *Am J Med* 1981;70:227–233.
228. Hulter HN, Bonner EL Jr. Lipoid nephrosis appearing as acute oliguric renal failure. *Arch Intern Med* 1980;140:403–405.
229. Alexander JH, Schapel GJ, Edwards DG. Increased incidence of coronary heart disease associated with combined elevation of serum triglyceride and cholesterol concentration in the nephrotic syndrome in man. *Med J Aust* 1974;2:119–122.
230. Gilboa N. Incidence of coronary heart-disease associated with nephrotic syndrome. *Med J Aust* 1976;1:207–208.
231. Kallen RJ, Byrnes RK, Aronson AJ, et al. Premature coronary atherosclerosis in a 5-year old with corticosteroid-refactory nephrotic syndrome. *Am J Dis Child* 1977;131:976–970.
232. Ordenez JD, Hiatt RA, Killebrew EJ, Fireman BH. The increased risk of coronary heart disease associated with nephrotic syndrome. *Kidney Int* 1992;44:638–642.
233. Wass VJ, Jarrett RJ, Chilvers C, et al. Does the nephrotic syndrome increase the risk of cardiovascular disease. *Lancet* 1979;2:664–667.
234. Gofman JW, Jones HB, Lindgren FT, Lyon TP, Elliot HA, Strisower B. Blood lipids and human atherosclerosis. *Circulation* 1950;2:161–178.
235. Schwartz H, Kohn JL. Lipoid nephrosis. A clinical and pathological study based on 15 years observation with special reference to prognosis. *Am J Dis Child* 1935;49:579–593.
236. Kallen RJ, Brynes RK, Aronson AJ, Lichtig C, Spargo BH. Premature coronary atherosclerosis in a 5-year old with corticosteroid-refractory nephrotic syndrome. *Am J Dis Child* 1977;131:976–980.
237. Nigond J, Grolleau-Raoux R. Thrombose carotidienne et infarctus du myocarde au cours d'un syndrome nephrotique. *Arch Mal Coeur* 1990;83:105–108.
238. Chesney RF, Hamstra A, Rose P, et al. Vitamin D and parathyroid hormone status in children with the nephrotic syndrome and chronic mild glomerulonephrids. *Int J Pediatr Nephrol* 1984;5:1.
239. Hulton SA, Neuhaus TJ, Dillon MJ, Barratt TM. Long-term cyclosporin A treatment of minimal-change nephrotc syndrome of childhood. *Pediatr Nephrol* 1994;8:401–403.
240. Consensus statement on management and audit potential for steroid responsive nephrotic syndrome. *Arch Dis Child* 1994;70:151–157.
241. International Study of Kidney Disease in Children. Primary nephrotic syndrome in children; clinical significance of histopathologic variants of minimal change and of diffuse mesangial hypercellularity. *Kidney Int* 1981;20:765–771.
242. Pardo V, Resigo I, Zillerullo G, et al. The clinical signifcance of mesangial IgM deposits and mesangial hypercellularity in minimal change nephrotic syndrome. *Am J Kidney Dis* 1984;3:264–269.
243. Allen WR, Travis LB, Cavallo T, et al. Immune deposits and mesangial hypercellularity in minimal change nephrotic syndrome: clinical relevance. *J Pediatr* 1982;100:188.
242. Choi J, Jeong HJ, Lee HY, Kim PK, Lee JS, Han DS. Significance of mesangial IgA deposition in minimal change nephrotic syndrome: a study of 60 cases. *Yonsei Med J* 1990;31:258–263.
245. Farquhar MG, Vernier RL, Good RA. An electron microscope study of the glomerulus in nephrosis, glomerulonephritis, and lupus erythematosus. *J Exp Med* 1957;106:649–660.
246. Brodehl J, Krohn HP, Ehrich JH. The treatment of minimal change nephrotic syndrome (lipoid nephrosis). Cooperative studies of the Arbeitsgemeinschaft fur Padiatrische Nephrol (APN). *Klin Paediatr* 1982;194:162.
247. Al-Bander H, Kaysen GA. Ineffectiveness of dietary protein augmentation in the management of the nephrotic syndrome. *Pediatr Nephrol* 1991;5:482–486.
248. Feehally J, Baker F, Walls J. Dietary manipulation in experimental nephrotic syndrome. *Nephron* 1988;50:247–252.
249. Rees L, Greene SA, Adlord P, et al. Growth and endocrine function in steroid sensitive nephrotic syndrome. *Arch Dis Child* 1988;63: 484–490.
250. D'Amico G, Gentile MG. Pharmacological and dietary treatment of lipid abnormalities in nephrotic patients. *Kidney Int* 1991;39(suppl): 56–69.
251. Spika JS, Halsey NA, Lee CT, et al. Decline of vaccine induced antipneumococcal antibody in children with nephrotic syndrome. *Am J Kidney Dis* 1986;7:466–470.

252. Abeitsgemeinschaft fur Padiatrische Nephrologie. Alternate-day vs intermittent prednisone in frequently relapsing nephrotic syndrome. *Lancet* 1979;1:401–403.
253. Broedehl J. Conventional therapy for ideopathic nephrotic syndrome. *Clin Nephrol* 1991;35(suppl):8–15.
254. Choonara IA, Heney D, Meadow SR. Low dose prednisolone in nephrotic syndrome. *Arch Dis Child* 1989;64:610–612.
255. Lewis MA, Baildom EM, Davis N, Houston IB, Postlethwaite RJ. Nephrotic syndrome: from toddlers to twenties. *Lancet* 1989;1: 255–259.
256. Koskimies O. Long-term outlook of primary nephrotic syndrome. *Arch Dis Child* 1982;57:544–548.
257. Noloasco F, Cameron JS, Heywood EF, et al. Adult-onset minimal-change nephrotic syndrome: a long-term follow-up. *Kidney Int* 1986; 29:1215–1223.
258. Simon P, Meyrier A. One year alternate day dosage, corticosteroid therapy reduces rate of further relapses in adults with minimal change nephrosis. *Kidney Int* 1989;35:201.
259. Bogdanovic R, Banicevic M, Cvoric A. Testicular function following cyclophosphomide treatment for childhood nephrotic syndrome: long-term follow-up study. *Pediatr Nephrol* 1990;4:451–454.
260. Guesry P, Lenoir G, Broyer M. Gonadal effects of chlorambucil given to prepubertal boys for nephrotic syndrome. *J Pediatr* 1978;92: 299–303.
261. Palmer RG, Dore CJ, Denman M. Cyclophosphamide induces more chromosomal damage than chlorambucil with connective tissue diseases. *Q J Med* 1986;228:395–400.
262. Grunwald H, Rosner F. Acute leukemia and immunosupressive drug use: a review of patients undergoing immunosupressive therapy for non-neoplastic diseases. *Arch Intern Med* 1979;139:461–466.
263. Abeitsgemeinschaft fur Padiatrische Nephrologie. Cyclophosphamide treatment of steroid dependent nephrotic syndrome: comparison with eight week with 12 week course. *Arch Dis Child* 1987;62; 1102–1106.
264. Abeitsgemeinschaft fur Padiatrische Nephrologie. Effect of cytoxic drugs in frequently relapsing nephrotic syndrome with and without steroid dependence. *N Engl J Med* 1982;306:451–454.
265. Coggins CH. Minimal change nephrosis in adults. 1981 Proceedings of the 8th International Congress of Nephrology, Athens. Basel: Karger; 1981:334–336.

Immunologic Renal Diseases,
edited by E. G. Neilson and W. G. Couser.
Lippincott-Raven Publishers, Philadelphia © 1997.

CHAPTER 45

Mesangioproliferative Disease

Hai Yan Wang and Yi Pu Chen

DEFINITION AND HISTORICAL PERSPECTIVE

Mesangial proliferative glomerulonephritis (MsPGN) is a pathomorphologic entity defined by light microscopy. It was first reported in children by Churg et al. in 1970 (1) and subsequently noted in adults by Morel-Maroger et al. in 1972 (2) and by Hayslett et al. in 1973 (3). In 1977 MsPGN was formally classified as one of the distinct pathological patterns of primary glomerulonephritis by the World Health Organization (4).

MsPGN is characterized by diffuse mesangial cell proliferation and/or mesangial matrix expansion with normal glomerular capillary walls. It is important to appreciate that several secondary glomerular diseases such as lupus nephritis, Schönlein-Henoch purpura nephritis, and some other primary glomerular diseases such as immunoglobulin (Ig)A nephropathy all may have prominent mesangial proliferation and/or expansion (Table 1). MsPGN in this chapter has been defined as a primary glomerular disease with mesangial cell proliferation and/or mesangial matrix expansion but without dominant IgA mesangial deposits or evidence of systemic disease such as systemic lupus erythematosus (SLE).

Most of the patients with MsPGN in Western countries have dominant IgM mesangial deposits (5–7). In China, however, the dominant immunoglobulin deposited in mesangium in most cases is IgG (8–10).

ETIOLOGY AND INCIDENCE

MsPGN is a relatively uncommon glomerular disease in Europe and North America, where it is found in only 2% to 10% of patients with primary nephrotic syndrome (1,11,12). However, MsPGN accounts for a higher proportion of patients with primary glomerular diseases, especially idiopathic nephrotic syndrome, in many countries of Asia, including Singapore (13–15), Japan (16,17), Thailand (18,19), India (20–23), Malaysia (24), Indonesia (25), and Saudi Arabia (26,27). In China MsPGN is one of the most common causes of glomerulonephritis. According to several large series of renal biopsies from northern (8,9,28–30), eastern (31,32), and southern (10) parts of China, MsPGN accounted for about a third of primary glomerular diseases and up to 50% of cases of primary nephrotic syndrome. In Australia, although MsPGN represented 31% of patients with primary glomerular diseases, it was seen in only 3% of patients with primary nephrotic syndrome (33).

The geographic distribution of MsPGN suggests that occurrence of this disease is probably related to genetic factors. This theory is supported by the fact that the incidence of MsPGN in Native American populations is much higher than in white populations in the United States (34,35). Nevertheless, there are insufficient data to draw any definite conclusions about the linkage between MsPGN and human leukocyte antigen because only a small number of patients have been tested (36–38).

The higher incidence of MsPGN in some countries is probably related to environmental factors as well, especially infections (8,9,18,20,27,28). In China we found that about 40% of cases with MsPGN had a prodromal upper respiratory tract infection (8,9). In India, Date et al. (20) noted that the decreasing prevalence of streptococcal infections between 1972 and 1987 was associated with a decreasing incidence of MsPGN. Recently we detected hepatitis C virus (HCV) messenger RNA (mRNA) in the renal biopsy specimens in three patients with MsPGN, which suggests that there may be an association between HCV infection and MsPGN (see Chapter 41) (39). However, Hoy et al. (34) were unable to incriminate either streptococcal or viral infection in Native Americans with MsPGN. If MsPGN is an infection-related immune-mediated disease, as seems likely, its pathogenetic mechanisms remain to be discovered.

H. Yan Wang and Y. Pu Chen: Division of Nephrology, The First Hospital, Beijing Medical University, Beijing, Peoples Republic of China.

TABLE 1. *Classification of diseases similar to MsPGN*

Primary glomerular diseases
IgA nephropathy
Resolving postinfectious glomerulonephritis
Secondary glomerular diseases
SLE
Schönlein-Henoch purpura
Rheumatoid arthritis
Liver cirrhosis
Diabetes mellitus[a]
Alport's syndrome

[a] Mesangial matrix expansion as principal change.

PATHOGENESIS

Like most forms of primary glomerulonephritis, MsPGN is probably an immune-mediated inflammatory disease.

The presence of diffuse granular immunoglobulin and complement deposits in the mesangium suggests an immune complex pathogenesis of MsPGN. In animal models MsPGN has been induced by chronic serum sickness (40–42), which indicates that circulating immune complex trapping in glomeruli is a possible pathogenic mechanism of MsPGN. If the circulating immune complexes (CICs) are of sufficient size and contain high-affinity antibody, especially when mesangial clearing function and systemic mononuclear phagocyte system function are damaged, the CICs may deposit in the mesangium and induce MsPGN (see Chapter 14). MsPGN also can be induced in rats by anti-Thy1 antibody (ATS model) (43–45) or by lens cularis hemagglutinin (LCH) and its antibody (anti-LCH model) (46). These two animal models demonstrate that in situ immune complex formation in glomeruli is another potential pathogenic mechanism in MsPGN. In the ATS model, antibody reacts with a fixed antigen expressed on the mesangial cell membrane, whereas in the LCH model the exogenous antigen LCH is first planted in glomeruli and then combines with its specific antibody locally to form immune complexes in situ. In addition, cell-mediated immunity also may play a role in the pathogenesis of MsPGN (47–49). Thus, in MsPGN it is likely that several immune pathogenetic mechanisms are responsible for the glomerular injury in different settings.

In most of the experimental animal models mentioned above, IgG, not IgM, is the principal immunoglobulin deposited in the mesangium (41,43–46). However, in the chronic serum sickness model in cats reported by Bishop et al. (42), abundant IgM mesangial deposits were seen with IgG. Whether the different immunoglobulin deposits reflect different pathogenic mechanisms remains to be elucidated. With regard to IgM deposits, some investigators believe these to be a nonspecific finding, which is probably the consequence of altered mesangial function (11,50–52). Others believe that these deposits have a pathogenic role and are involved in some way in the initiation of the disease process (6,7,53). In addition, the mechanism of mesangial proliferation in the absence of imunoglobulin deposition is unknown. It also should be noted that in some patients the disease occurs without detectable immunoglobulin deposition in the mesangium, suggesting a role for nonimmunoglobulin mediators such as cell-mediated reactions or cytokines in this process.

The glomerular injury that occurs in MsPGN is a consequence of inflammation induced by the immune mechanisms described above. Many inflammatory mediators released by activated resident kidney cells, including mesangial cells, as well as by cells migrating into the kidney, can stimulate and activate mesangial cells (54). After activation, mesangial cells undergo phenotypic changes, including proliferation, expression of α-smooth muscle actin and production of extracellular matrix components (54a). Subsequently, mesangial cells release various inflammatory mediators, including autocrine growth factors such as interleukin (IL)-1, IL-6, platelet-derived growth factor (PDGF), basic fibroblast growth factor (bFGF), and transforming growth factor-β (TGF-β), and overproduce extracellular matrix (55–62). Thus, in MsPGN, mesangial cells are not only targets of injury but are also active and direct cellular mediators of glomerular damage (55) and probably play a central role in mediating inflammation and sclerosis of glomeruli in this disease.

These mediators, which participate in glomerular inflammatory reactions, and the response of mesangial cells to these mediators have been discussed in detail in Sections III and IV in this book, particularly Chapters 20 and 29. Here, we review only briefly observations on animal models or patients. In the ATS model of MsPGN, an upregulation in mesangial cell expression of IL-1 mRNA (63), PDGF A and B chain mRNA (64–66), PDGF-β receptor mRNA and protein (65,66), TGF-B mRNA and protein (63,67), and bFGF mRNA and protein (68) has been found, and an amelioration of mesangial lesions in glomeruli by anti-PDGF antibody (69) or by anti–TGF-β antibody (70,71) also has been observed. In patients with MsPGN, including IgA nephropathy and non-IgA nephropathy (which are not separated in most reports), an enhanced expression of IL-6 mRNA and protein (72–76), PDGF B chain mRNA (77,78), PDGF-β receptor protein (78,79), and TGF-β mRNA and protein (80) in glomeruli has been found, and a hyperexcretion of urinary IL-6 (72–74) and endothelin-1 (ET-1) (81) also occurs. Although multiple mediators that result in glomerular injury have been identified in MsPGN, it is also clear that glomeruli with this lesion can heal and return to normal architecture (54a). The process of resolution of glomerular injury in MsPGN likely involves several mechanisms, including upregulation of antiproliferative factors (81a,81b), apoptosis (81c), and capillary repair through angiogenesis (81d). The factors that determine whether the disease will resolve or progress in individual cases have not been defined.

PATHOLOGY

Light Microscopy

MsPGN is characterized by varying degrees of mesangial hypercellularity and a concomitant increase in mesangial matrix, usually affecting all lobules of all glomeruli to a similar degree (6,11,33,82,83). The glomerular capillary walls are normal (6,11,82,83). When Masson's trichrome stain is used, discrete fuchsinophilic deposits, which are not as large as those in IgA nephropathy, are sometimes identified in the mesangium and paramesangium (11,33). In the early stages of the disease, glomerular capillary lumens are patent, and tubular, interstitial, and vascular lesions are absent.

However, when the disease progresses, the glomerular capillary lumens are narrowed by the extrusion of highly expanded mesangial matrix (8). Segmental sclerosis, hyalinosis, and capsular adhesions are present in some glomeruli (8,11,33). When segmental sclerotic lesions occur, some investigators (33), including ourselves (8), regard it as a separate lesion superimposed on the basic pathologic pattern, but others (84,85) believe it is a stage in the transition of pathologic features from MsPGN to focal and segmental sclerosis (FSGS), which may be a variant of classic FSGS (86) (see Chapter 44). In this stage of the disease, focal interstitial infiltration of inflammatory cells and fibrosis with focal tubular atrophy are often observed (8,10,87). Hyalinosis in arteriolar walls also may be seen (11).

Several semiquantitative grading systems have been used to assess severity and prognosis in MsPGN. Some of them are based on mesangial hypercellularity: 1+, three cell nuclei per mesangial area; 2+, four cell nuclei per mesangial area; 3+, five or more cell nuclei per mesangial area (82,87,88). Others evaluate degrees of expansion of mesangial matrix: 1+, mild mesangial matrix expansion with widely patent capillary lumens (Fig. 1); 2+, moderate mesangial matrix expansion with marrowed lumens in fewer than 50% of capillary loops (Fig. 2); 3+, severe mesangial matrix expansion with narrowed or obliterated lumens in more than 50% of capillary loops (Fig. 3) (8). In grade 3+, segmental sclerotic lesions are sometimes superimposed on mesangial proliferation. Many investigators have observed that there is a good correlation between the semiquantitatively measured pathologic grades and clinical findings in patients, including renal function and response to therapy (8,87,88).

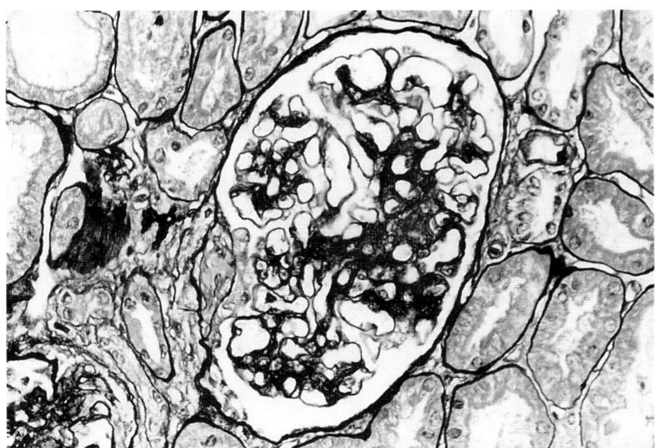

FIG. 2. MsPGN grade 2+. Moderate mesangial matrix expansion with narrowed lumens in <50% of capillary loops (PAS, original magnification ×400).

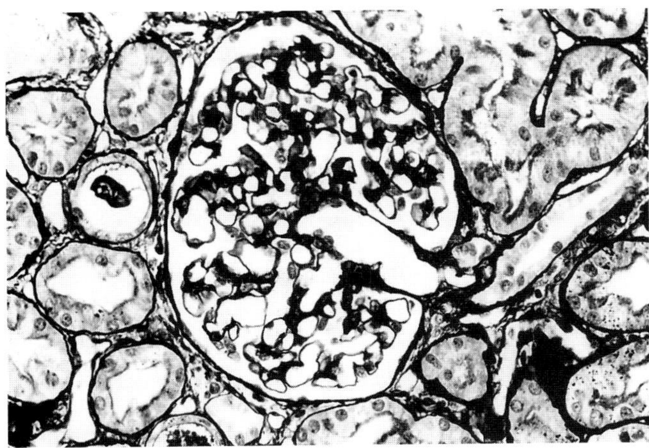

FIG. 1. MsPGN grade 1+. Mild mesangial matrix expansion with widely patent capillary lumens [periodic acid-Schiff (PAS), original magnification ×400].

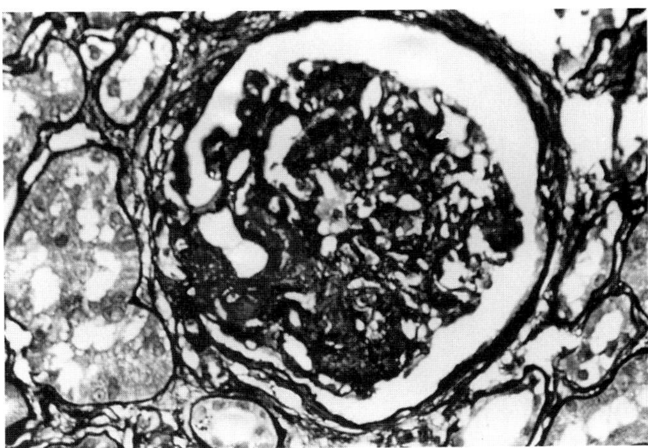

FIG. 3. MsPGN grade 3+. Severe mesangial matrix expansion with narrowed or obliterated lumens in >50% of capillary loops (PAS, original magnification ×400)

Immunofluorescence Microscopy

There are four patterns of immunofluorescent findings in MsPGN:

1. Dominant IgM deposits with or without C3. This is the most common type in Western countries (11), but in China it only accounts for 21% to 29% of MsPGN (8–10,31).
2. Dominant IgG deposits with or without C3 (Fig. 4). This is the most common finding in China and makes up about 60% of MsPGN (8,10), but it is uncommon in Western countries (11), except in African-American patients (89).
3. C3 deposits alone. This pattern occurs in 7% to 19% of MsPGN (8,90,91). The immune deposits mentioned above are all present in a granular pattern in the mesangium and sometimes simultaneously on adjacent capillary walls.
4. Negative immunofluorescence. The proportion of patients with no immunoglobulin deposition in MsPGN has been reported to be anywhere from 3% to 27% in different studies (8,10,11,82,91).

In 1978 MsPGN with dominant mesangial IgM deposits was termed "IgM" mesangial nephropathy" independently by two groups (6,7). However, the existence of IgM nephropathy as a separate disease entity and the prognostic significance of mesangial IgM deposits have been debated. Some investigators believe that mesangial IgM deposits are a marker of more severe disease, with a poor response to steroids and often progression to renal failure (6,7,53,92–106). However, others have not confirmed this hypothesis and believe instead that IgM deposits in the mesangium do not indicate a distinct clinicopathologic entity (20,50-52,85,90,106–117).

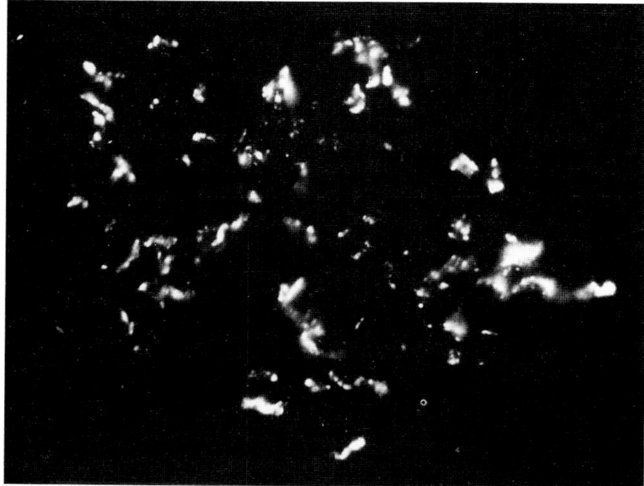

FIG. 4. MsPGN. Mesangial IgG deposits (original magnification ×500).

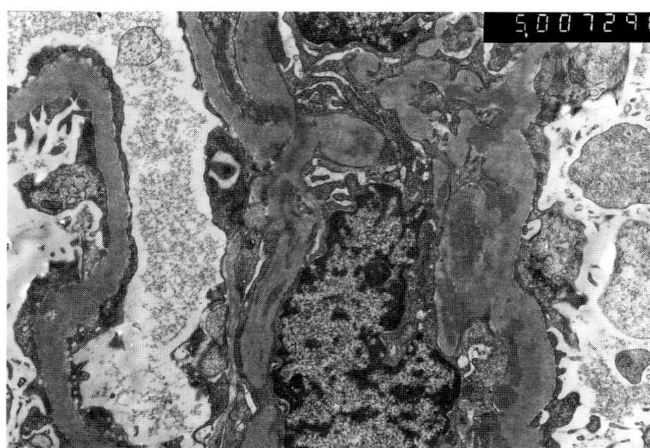

FIG. 5. MsPGN. Enlarged mesangium with small mesangial electron dense deposits (original magnification ×5,000).

Electron Microscopy

In addition to mesangial cells and matrix, electron-dense deposits can be observed in the mesangium in 20% to 50% of biopsy samples in MsPGN (Fig. 5) (8,10,11, 106,118). Thus, in this disease, immunofluorescence is probably a more sensitive technique for identifying immune deposits than is electron microscopy. Subendothelial or intramembranous electron-dense deposits on the capillary walls also are identified occasionally (6,118, 119). The deposits in MsPGN usually are not as large or conspicuous as in IgA nephropathy (11). Some of them seem to be typical electron-dense immune complex deposits, but others are ill-defined homogeneous dark condensates that also may be seen in minimal-change disease (MCD), even when immunofluorescence findings are negative (120). What these latter deposits mean remains to be elucidated. On the other hand, in many biopsy samples no electron-dense deposits can be detected even if immunofluorescence is positive (8,90,97). In patients with massive proteinuria, diffuse swelling and effacement of foot processes of epithelial cells are often observed as well.

CLINICAL MANIFESTATIONS AND LABORATORY FEATURES

Although MsPGN may occur at any age, it usually is found in older children and young adults (6,8,10,120). The male:female ratio is about 1.5:1 to 2.3:1 (8,10,12,82, 118,121). The onset of this disease is frequently insidious without antecedent upper respiratory infection in most cases reported in Western countries (6,34,120), but in China prodromal upper respiratory infection occurs in about 40% of patients with MsPGN (8,9).

The clinical presentation of MsPGN is varied, but four entities can be defined: asymptomatic proteinuria, isolated hematuria, proteinuria with hematuria, and nephrotic syndrome. Microscopic hematuria is present in most patients (60–70%) (8,10,12,21,30,82,118,122), and in less than one third of patients (15–30%) gross hematuria is also noted (8,9,12,31,82,121). Hypertension is usually mild and present in 20% to 40% of patients (8,11,21,30, 82,118,120,121). At the time of diagnosis, impaired renal function may be observed in 10% to 25% of patients (8, 36,82,118,120,121). Renal insufficiency and hypertension often occur in the patients with severe pathologic lesions (8,121).

Some studies have compared data on clinical manifestations in MsPGN and IgA nephropathy. It has been noted that the incidence of nephrotic syndrome in MsPGN is 1.5 to 3.0 times more common than in IgA nephropathy (9, 10,30,31), but conversely, the incidence of gross hematuria in MsPGN is less than in IgA nephropathy (9,30, 31,91,22).

Elevated serum IgM levels have been reported in over 30% of patients with IgM nephropathy (36,101,102,120). Decreased serum IgG levels are sometimes present in patients with nephrotic syndrome (120). Complement components in the serum are always normal, and conventional serologic tests are normal or negative (6,10,12,118, 120). The red blood cells in the urine are dysmorphic in patients with MsPGN hematuria (123).

DIFFERENTIAL DIAGNOSIS

MsPGN should be differentiated from other nephritic glomerular diseases with similar clinical features.

IgA Nephropathy

Although mesangial proliferation in IgA nephropathy is similar to that in MsPGN (124–126), the fuchsinophilic mesangial deposits seen with Masson's trichrome stain by light microscopy and the electron-dense deposits by electron microscopy in IgA nephropathy are more conspicuous than in MsPGN (see Chapter 42) (11,33). Clinically, in comparison with MsPGN, nephrotic syndrome is relatively uncommon, but hematuria, especially gross hematuria, is more often observed in IgA nephropathy (125–128). Both a short latent period between prodromal infection and the onset of gross hematuria (several hours to 3 days) and a raised serum IgA level suggest the diagnosis of IgA nephropathy (125,126). Immunofluorescence examination of the kidney biopsy sample can definitively differentiate IgA nephropathy from MsPGN by the demonstration of typical mesangial IgA deposits.

Resolving Postinfectious Glomerulonephritis

Mesangial proliferation with mesangial deposits of immunoglobulin (especially dominant IgG) and/or C3 are the pathomorphologic features of resolving postinfectious glomerulonephritis (see Chapter 41) (33,120). Therefore, MsPGN, especially with a prodromal upper respiratory infection and dominant IgG mesangial deposits, should be distinguished from resolving postinfectious glomerulonephritis. A careful review of the clinical course will may provide the best way to differentiate between these two diseases. In resolving postinfectious glomerulonephritis, a history of acute onset of disease after a prodromal upper respiratory infection with a latent period ranging from 7 to 21 days, as well as a history of a typical clinical presentation of acute nephritic syndrome with low serum C3 levels (during the first 8 weeks of the disease) and an elevated anti-streptolysin O (ASO) or streptozyme titer in serum should permit the diagnosis to be made (120).

Minimal-Change Disease

In patients with nephrotic syndrome, mild MsPGN should be distinguished from MCD (see Chapter 44). The important differences between these two diseases have been summarized in Table 2. Sometimes, the differentiating between them is difficult, especially when MCD has a mild prominence of mesangial cells and MsPGN has no definite electron-dense deposits. In this situation, the best way to distinguish between these two diseases is by immunofluorescence microscopy. Similarly, some patients with nephrotic syndrome, mesangial cell proliferation,

TABLE 2. *Differentiation between mild MsPGN and MCD in nephrotic patients*

	MsPGN	MCD
Clinical manifestations		
Age	Older children, young adults	Young children
Proportion of hematuria	Higher	Lower
Pathologic manifestations		
Light microscopy	Mild, but definite cell proliferation and matrix expansion	Nearly normal
Immunofluorescence	Mesangial deposits	Negative
Electron microscopy	Mesangial electron dense deposits in 20–50% of cases	No immune deposits

and sclerotic lesions may represent a stage in the spectrum of glomerular response to the mechanisms that cause minimal-change nephrotic syndrome (84,105,118, 120). It is likely that lesions such as IgM nephropathy (6,7) and C1q nephropathy (90,91,91a) are variants of MsPGN. Actually, many investigators find that the response of nephrotic syndrome to therapy is similar in these two diseases. Therefore, differentiating between them may not be required clinically (8,9).

Focal Glomerular Sclerosis

The differentiation between MsPGN and FGS is difficult in part because MsPGN in some patients may represent a transition between minimal-change nephrotic syndrome and FGS, or a more severe form of minimal change nephrotic syndrome leading to FGS (see Chapter 44 (84,105,115,120). In most patients with MsPGN, there is a greater prominence of nephritic rather than nephrotic features, and the lesions of FGS are absent from the biopsy sample, which shows predominantly mesangial cell proliferation and matrix expansion without sclerosis. However, there are some patients who present with idiopathic nephrotic syndrome, mesangial cell proliferation on the biopsy sample, and lesions of FGS as well. Whether these patients represent a severe form of MsPGN on which the lesion of FGS is superimposed (8,33) or simply a variant of classical FGS with more prominent mesangial cell proliferation and deposits (84–86) is not clear and will remain unresolved until the pathogenetic mechanisms of these two diseases are changed.

MsPGN in Systemic Diseases

Some patients with systemic diseases (such as SLE and Schönlein-Henoch purpura) have secondary renal disease with the same morphologic features as MsPGN by light microscopy (83,120). It is not difficult to differentiate these from primary MsPGN on the basis of multisystem manifestations, specific serum serologic tests, and immunopathologic features of the kidney lesion.

TREATMENT

For patients with asymptomatic proteinuria, isolated hematuria, or non-nephrotic proteinuria with hematuria and normal renal function, no effective therapeutic maneuvers can be recommended and treatment is only supportive. Upper respiratory infections should be prevented, hypertension controlled, and patients followed on a regular basis.

For patients with nephrotic syndrome or nephrotic range proteinuria, a more aggressive approach to therapy has been recommended. However, to date no randomized controlled trials have been conducted to document the safety and efficacy of any particular form of therapy.

In nephrotic patients with mild pathologic lesions and well-preserved renal function, a therapeutic regimen similar to that used in MCD nephrotic syndrome can be tried (see Chapter 44) (8,10,11,120). The newly diagnosed patients may be initially treated by oral prednisone or prednisolone alone (1.0 mg/kg/day for 8–12 weeks, then gradually taper dose), but the patients in whom steroid resistance, steroid dependence, or relapse has occurred should be treated with a combination of steroids with cytotoxic agents, such as cyclophosphamide (2.0 mg/kg/day for 8–12 weeks), chlorambucil (0.15–0.2 mg/kg/day for 8–12 weeks), or azathioprine. Among these, cyclophosphamide is often preferred in adults. The effect of combined steroid and cytotoxic drug therapy in inducing remission of nephrotic syndrome is generally better than that of steroids alone (12,53,84,107,129).

In the nephrotic patients with severe pathologic lesions, even if renal function is still preserved, combined therapy with steroids and cytotoxic agents could be considered at the outset but usually has little beneficial effect.

Cyclosporine (4–5 mg/kg/day for 3–6 months) has been used in a few patients with MsPGN in whom nephrotic syndrome was resistant to steroids and cytotoxic agents, but at present, no conclusions can be drawn regarding its efficacy because only a small number of patients have been so treated (130–134).

Two Chinese traditional medicines that have definite effects on nephrotic syndrome and have been widely used in China should be briefly mentioned. *Tripterygium wilfordii,* an anti-inflammatory and immunomodulatory drug, may effectively reduce glomerular immune deposits (135,136), repair the glomerular charge barrier (135,137,138), improve renal histologic changes (135, 139), including mesangial cell proliferation (135,140), and, consequently, reduce proteinuria in various animal models (135–141). In patients, including those with MsPGN, an effect on reducing proteinuria and inducing remission of nephrotic syndrome also has been suggested in several studies (135,139,140,142). *Astragalus* and *Angelica,* which increase albumin synthesis (143,144) and regulate albumin mRNA expression in the liver (145–147), also can sometimes increase serum albumin levels, reduce edema, and improve the general condition both in animal models (143–146,148) and in patients (147).

In patients with MsPGN, the response of nephrotic syndrome to steroids and cytotoxic agents depends on the severity of pathologic lesions by light microscopy. Our data in 1987 (8) showed that the rate of complete remission in mild MsPGN was 73%, in severe MsPGN 0% ($p < 0.01$); the rate of no response in mild MsPGN was only 7%, and in severe MsPGN 80% ($p < 0.05$). In addition, the therapeutic results with steroids and cytotoxic agents on nephrotic syndrome in mild MsPGN are similar to those in MCD as well as in IgA nephropathy with mild mesangial proliferation in China. Our study in 1990 (9) showed that percentages of clinical remission were 79% in mild MsPGN, 82% in MCD, and 77% in IgA nephropathy ($p > 0.05$). These data suggest that the results of light microscopy, as well as immunofluorescence, are especially important in predicting the response of nephrotic syndrome to therapy in patients with MsPGN.

PROGNOSIS

The long-term outcome of patients with MsPGN has not been well defined. Saito et al. (149) reported that the survival rate at 10 and 20 years after apparent onset of disease was 88% and 72%, respectively. In the series reported by O'Donoghue et al. (121), the renal survival rate was 80% at 5 years and 64% at 10 years.

Patients with isolated hematuria, or with low-grade proteinuria (<1.0 g/24 h) with or without accompanying hematuria, usually have a benign course, maintaining normal renal function for a prolonged period of time. However, a minority may develop a spontaneous remission or, conversely, worsen (12,104). Worsening may be heralded by an increase in proteinuria and/or appearance of hypertension.

In patients with nephrotic syndrome or nephrotic range proteinuria, patients with a good response to therapy may have a more favorable outcome, although they also may undergo multiple relapses (120,150); another subset of patients who are steroid-resistant or steroid-dependent have a poorer prognosis and gradually develop progressive loss of renal function, culminating in end-stage renal failure (93,98,151).

The following clinical and pathomorphologic features identified at the time of renal biopsy may indicate a worse prognosis in MsPGN: persistent heavy proteinuria, hypertension, reduced glomerular filtration rate, highly expanded mesangial matrix, pronounced mesangial hypercellularity, superimposed segmental sclerosis, high proportion of globally sclerotic glomeruli, and severe tubulointerstitial lesions (interstitial inflammation and fibrosis, tubular atrophy) (8,10,21,33,121,149,151–154). The significance of hematuria in determining prognosis is controversial.

Pregnancy in female patients with MsPGN is generally well tolerated, but if the patients have pre-existing hypertension and/or severe vascular lesions in the kidney, fetal and maternal complications of pregnancy may occur more frequently (155).

The recurrence of MsPGN in the transplanted kidney, to our knowledge, has not been reported. However, Streigel et al. (156) found that if the native kidney showed FSGS with generalized mesangial proliferation, the recurrence rate of FSGS in the transplanted kidney was 70%, but if only FSGS was present, the recurrence rate was 12%.

REFERENCES

1. Churg J, Habib R, White RHR. Pathology of the nephrotic syndrome in children. A report for the international study of kidney diseases in children. *Lancet* 1970;1:1299–1302.
2. Morel-Maroger L, Leathem A, Richet G. Glomerular abnormalities in non-systemic diseases. *Am J Med* 1972;53:170–184.
3. Hayslett JP, Kashgarian M, Bensch KG, Spargo BH, Freedman LR, Epstein FH. Clinicopathological correlations in the nephrotic syndrome due to primary renal disease. *Medicine (Baltimore)* 1973;52:93–120.
4. Sakakuti H. Classification of glomerular diseases by World Health Organization. *Jpn J Nephrol* 1979;21:349–355.
5. Van de Putte LBA, de la Riviere GB, van Breda Vriesman PJC. Recurrent or persistent hematuria. *N Engl J Med* 1974;290:1165–1170.
6. Bhasin HK, Abuelo JG, Nayak R, Esparza AR. Mesangial proliferative glomerulonephritis. *Lab Invest* 1978;39:21–29.
7. Cohen AH, Border WA, Glassock RJ. Nephrotic syndrome with glomerular mesangial IgM deposits. *Lab Invest* 1978;38:610–619.
8. Chen YP, Wang HY, Zou WZ. Non-IgA mesangial proliferative glomerulonephritis. Clinical and pathological analysis of 77 cases. *Chin Med J [Engl]* 1989;102:510–515.
9. Chen YP, Wang HY, Zou WZ, Geng L. IgA nephropathy (IgAN) and non-IgA nephropathy (non-IgAN) in mesangial proliferative glomerulonephritis (MsPGN) [Abstract]. Abstracts, 11th International Congress of Nephrology, Tokyo, 1990:338A.
10. Li YJ, Hu LF, Ye RG, Huang WC. Diagnosis and treatment of adult primary mesangial proliferative glomerulonephritis. *Chin J Nephrol [Chin]* 1990;6:137–141.
11. Cohen AH, Adler SG. Mesangial proliferative glomerulonephritis. In: Massry SG, Glassock RJ, eds. *Textbook of nephrology*. 3rd ed. Vol 1. Baltimore: Williams & Wilkins; 1995:739–742.
12. Brown EA, Upadhyaya K, Hayslett JP, Kashgarian M, Siegel NJ. The clinical course of mesangial proliferative glomerulonephritis. *Medicine (Baltimore)* 1979;58:295–303.
13. Woo KT, Chiange GS, Edmondson RP, et al. Glomerulonephritis in Singapore: an overview. *Ann Acad Med Singapore* 1986;15:20–31.
14. Yap HK, Murugasu B, Saw AH, et al. Patterns of glomerulonephritis in Singapore children—a renal biopsy perspective. *Ann Acad Med Singapore* 1989;18:35–39.
15. Lim CH, Woo KT. Glomerulonephritis in Singapore. In: Zhang JH, Du XH, Liu ZH, Li LS, eds. *Nephrology. Proceedings of 4th Asian–Pacific Congress of Nephrology*. Beijing: International Academic Publishers; 1991:167–176.
16. Hisano S, Ueda K. Asymptomatic haematuria and proteinuria: renal pathology and clinical outcome in 54 children. *Pediatr Nephrol* 1989; 3:229–234.
17. Sato H, Saito T, Furuyama T, Yoshinaga K. Histologic studies on the nephrotic syndrome in the elderly. *Tohoku J Exp Med* 1987;153:259–264.
18. Kirdpon S, Vuttivirojana A, Kovitangkoon K, Poolsawat SS. The primary nephrotic syndrome in children and histopathologic study. *J Med Assoc Thai* 1989;72(suppl 1):26–31.
19. Kashemsant C, Sritubtim W, Tapaneya-Olarn W, Boonpucknavig V, Boonpuchnavig S. The primary nephrotic syndrome in children at Ramathibodi Hospital: clinical and clinicopathological study. *J Med Assoc Thai* 1989;72(suppl 1):18–25.
20. Date A, Jeyaseelan L, Brahmadathan KN. Changing pattern of primary glomerulonephritis in a south Indian hospital. *Trans R Soc Trop Med Hyg* 1989;83:419–420.
21. Andal A, Saxena S, Chellani HK, Sharma S. Pure mesangial proliferative glomerulonephritis. A clinicomorphologic analysis and its possible role in morphologic transition of minimal change lesion. *Nephron* 1989;51:314–319.
22. Malhotra KK, Bhuyan UN, Srivastava RN, Dash SC, Ahlawat DS. Spectrum of glomerulonephritis in India. In: Zhang JH, Du XH, Liu ZH, Li LS, eds. *Nephrology. Proceedings of the 4th Asian–Pacific*

Congress of Nephrology. Beijing: International Academic Publishers; 1991:177–196.
23. Johny KV, Date A. Spectrum of renal diseases in India—based on percutaneous renal biopsies. *Ann Acad Med Singapore* 1975;2(suppl):44.
24. Prathap K, Looi LM. Morphological patterns of glomerular disease in renal biopsies from 1000 Malaysian patients. *Ann Acad Med Singapore* 1982;11:52–56.
25. Markum MS, Rahardjo JP, Oesman R, Sidabutar RP. Light microscopic examination of glomerulonephritis in General Hospital in Jakarta. *Ann Acad Med Singapore* 1975;2(suppl):17–19.
26. Abdurrahman MB, Elidrissy ATH, Shipkey FH, al Rasheed S, al Mugeiren M. Clinicopathological feature of childhood nephrotic syndrome in Saudi Arabia. *Ann Trop Paediatr* 1990;10:125–132.
27. Mattoo TK, Mahmood MA, al Harbi SM. Nephrotic syndrome in Saudi children. Clinicopathological study of 150 cases. *Pediatr Nephrol* 1990;4:517–519.
28. Wang H, Cheng H, Zou W, Chen Y, Huang H, Chen X. Adult primary nephrotic syndrome (NS) and symptomless proteinuria/haematuria in a Chinese medical center is associated with a high incidence of prodromal infections [Abstract]. Abstracts, 10th International Congress of Nephrology, London, 1987:101A.
29. Huang QY, Li XW, Zhang JY, Wang XN, Duan L, Bi ZQ. Clinicopathological studies in 165 cases of nephrotic syndrome. *Beijing Med J [Chin]* 1989;6:321–324.
30. Liu YH, Zhou W, Gong W, Zheng HG. The clinical pathological observation of adult primary nephrotic syndrome in 147 cases. *Chin J Nephrol [Chin]* 1994;10:163–165.
31. Li L, Li LS, Chen HP, et al. Primary glomerulonephritis in China. Analysis of 1001 cases. *Chin Med J [Chin]* 1989;102:159–164.
32. Lin Sy, Ying WZ, Sun YW, et al. Renal diseases in east China. Analysis based on 688 biopsied cases. *Chin J Nephrol [Chin]* 1988;4: 331–335.
33. Kincaid-Smith P, Whitworth JA. *The kidney. A clinico-pathological study*. 2nd ed. Oxford: Blackwell Scientific; 1987:45–47, 101–104.
34. Hoy HE, Smith SM, Hughson MD, Megill DM. Mesangial proliferative glomerulonephritis in southwestern American Indians. *Transplant Proc* 1989;21:3909–3912.
35. Hoy HE, Hughson MD, Smith SM, Megill DM. Mesangial proliferative glomerulonephritis in southwestern American Indians. *Am J Kidney Dis* 1993;21:486–496.
36. Helin H, Munstonen J, Pasternack A, Antonen J. IgM-associated glomerulonephritis. *Nephron* 1982;31:11–16.
37. Scolari F, Scaini P, Savoldi S, et al. Familial IgM mesangial nephropathy: a morphologic and immunogenetic study of three pedigrees. *Am J Nephrol* 1990;10:261–268.
38. Chen XM, Bai LQ, Zhou ZL, Wang JG. HLA-DR gene frequencies in adult nephrotic syndrome patients with non-IgA mesangial proliferative glomerulonephritis. *Chin J Nephrol [Chin]* 1995;11:110–101.
39. Wang HY, Yin X, Wang L, Liu FH. Hepatitis C virus (HCV) and glomerulonephritis—a screening of 736 cases. (Abst.) *Kidney Int* 1995; 48:626.
40. Dixon FJ, Feldman JD, Vasquez JJ. Experimental glomerulonephritis. *J Exp Med* 1961;113:899–920.
41. Zhang YK, Wang HY, Wang SX, et al. The modification of mesangial proliferative glomerulonephritis induced by chronic serum sickness in rabbits. *Chin J Nephrol [Chin]* 1986;2:2–4.
42. Bishop SA, Stokes CR, Lucke VM. Experimental proliferative glomerulonephritis in the cat. *J Comp Pathol* 1992;106:49–60.
43. Bagchus WM, Hoedmaeker Ph J, Rozing J, Bakker WW. Glomerulonephritis induced by monoclonal anti-thy 1.1 antibodies. A sequential histological and ultrastructural study in the rat. *Lab Invest* 1986;55: 680–687.
44. Yamamoto T, Wilson CB, Complement dependence of antibody-induced mesangial cell injury in the rat. *J Immunol* 1987;138: 3758–3765.
45. Yamamoto T, Wilson CB. Quantitative and qualitative studies of antibody-induced mesangial cell damage in the rat. *Kidney Int* 1987;32: 514–525.
46. Sekiyama S, Yoshida F, Yuzawa Y, et al. Mesangial proliferative glomerulonephritis induced in rats by a lentil lectin and its antibodies. *J Lab Clin Med* 1993;121:71–82.
47. Hori Y, Takamoto T, Nishida H, Ishizaki T, Yokoyama MM, Nomura G. Studies of cell-mediated immunity in mesangial proliferative glomerulonephritis—IgA nephropathy and non-IgA nephropathy [in Japanese]. *Jpn J Nephrol* 1989;31:723–733.
48. Carcia del Moral R, Gomez-Morales M, Cortes V, et al. Mononuclear cell subsets in IgM mesangial proliferative glomerulonephritis. *Nephron* 1993;65:215–222.
49. Toyabe S, Iwanaga T. An ultrastructural study of proliferative nephritis induced experimentally by a monoclonal antibody against mesangial cells: replacement of mesangial cells by cells of the monocyte–macrophage system. *Virchows Arch [B]* 1992;61:397–407.
50. Michael AF, Keane WF, Raij L, Vernier RL, Mauer SM. The glomerular mesangium. *Kidney Int* 1980;17:141–154.
51. Yang JY, Melvin T, Sibley R, Michael AF. No evidence for a specific role of IgM in mesangial proliferation of idiopathic nephrotic syndrome. *Kidney Int* 1984;25:100–106.
52. Vilches AR, Turner Dr, Cameron JS, Ogg CS, Chantler C, William DG. Significance of mesangial IgM deposition in "minimal change" nephrotic syndrome. *Lab Invest* 1982;46:10–15.
53. Tejani A, Nicastri AD. Mesangial IgM nephropathy. *Nephron* 1983; 35:1–5.
54. Atkins RC. Mesangial cells and their interactions. In: Zhang JH, Du XH, Liu ZH, Li LS, eds. *Nephrology. Proceedings of the 4th Asian–Pacific Congress of Nephrology*. Beijing: International Academic Publishers, 1991:91–98.
54a. Johnson RJ. Nephrology forum: the glomerular response to injury. Mechanisms of progression and resolution. *Kidney Int* 1994;45: 1769–1782.
55. Jordan SC, Jennette JC, Neale TJ, Yap HK, Blifeld C, Hanevold C. The glomerular diseases. In: Gonick HC, ed. *Current nephrology*. Vol 14. St Louis: Mosby Year Book; 1991:165–166.
56. Lovett DH, Szamel H, Ryan JL, Sterzel RB, Gemsa D, Resch K. Interleukin 1 and the glomerular mesangium. I. Purification and characterization of a mesangium cell–derived autogrowth factor. *J Immunol* 1986;136:3700–3705.
57. Ruef C, Budde K, Lacy J, et al. Interleukin-6 is an autocrine growth factor for mesangial cells. *Kidney Int* 1990;38:249–257.
58. Coleman DL, Ruef C. Interleukin-6: an autocrine regulator of mesangial cell growth. *Kidney Int* 1992;41:607–606.
59. Abboud HE, Poptic E, DiCorleto PE. Production of platelet-derived growth factor–like protein by rat mesangial cells in culture. *J Clin Invest* 1987;80:675–683.
60. Shultz PJ, DiCorleto PE, Silver BJ, Abboud HE. Mesangial cells express PDGF mRNAs and proliferation in response PDGF. *Am J Physiol* 1988;255:F674–F684.
61. Ziyadeh FN, Chen Y, Davila A, Goldfarb S, Wolf G. Self limited stimulation of mesangial cell growth in high glucose: autocrine activation of TGF-β reduces proliferation but increases mesangial matrix [Abstract]. *J Am Soc Nephrol* 1991;2:304.
62. Sterzel RB, Schulze-Lohoff E, Marx M. Cytokines and mesangial cells. *Kidney Int* 1993;43(suppl 39):26–31.
63. Wang HY, Zhao ZH. The effect of IL-1 and TGF-β in progressive mesangial proliferative glomerulonephritis [in Chinese]. *J Beijing Med Univ* 1992;24:292–294.
64. Yoshimura A, Gordon K, Alpers CE, et al. Demonstration of PDGF β-chain mRNA in glomeruli in mesangial proliferative nephritis by in situ hybridization. *Kidney Int* 1991;40:470–476.
65. Iida H, Seifer R, Alpers CE, et al. Platelet-derived growth factor (PDGF) and PDGF receptor are induced in mesangial proliferative nephritis in the rat. *Proc Natl Acad Sci U S A* 1991;88:6560–6564.
66. Johnson R, Iida H, Yoshimura A, Floege J, Bowen-Pope DF. Platelet-derived growth factor: a potentially important cytokine in glomerular disease. *Kidney Int* 1992;41:590–594.
67. Okuda S, Languino LR, Ruoslahti E, Bordor WA. Elevated expression of transforming growth factor-β and proteoglycan production in experimental glomerulonephritis. *J Clin Invest* 1990;86:543–462.
68. Floege J, Eng E, Lindner V, et al. Rat glomerular mesangial cells synthesize basic fibroblast growth factor. Release, upregulated synthesis, and mitogenicity in mesangial proliferative glomerulonephritis. *J Clin Invest* 1992;90:2362–2369.
69. Johnson RJ, Raines EW, Floege J, et al. Inhibition of mesangial cell proliferation and matrix expansion in glomerulonephritis in the rat by antibody to platelet-derived growth factor. *J Exp Med* 1992;175: 1413–1416.
70. Border WA, Okuda S, Languino LR, Sporn MB, Ruoslahti E. Suppression of experimental glomerulonephritis by antiserum against transforming growth factor. *Nature* 1990;346:371–374.
71. Border Wa, Noble NA, Yamamoto T, Tomooka S, Kagami S. Antagonists of transforming growth factor-β: a novel approach to

treatment of glomerulonephritis and prevention of glomerulosclerosis. *Kidney Int* 1992;41:566–570.
72. Horii Y, Muraguchi A, Iwano M, et al. Involvement of IL-6 in mesangial proliferative glomerulonephritis. *J Immunol* 1989;143:3949–3955.
73. Horii Y, Iwano M, Hirata E, et al. Role of interleukin-6 in the proliferative glomerulonephritis. *Kidney Int* 1993;43(suppl 39):71–75.
74. Coleman DL, Ruef C. Interleukin-6: an autocrine regulator of mesangial cell growth. *Kidney Int* 1992;41:604–606.
75. Dohi K, Iwano M, Horri Y. Interleukin-(IL-6) [in Japanese]. *Jpn J Clin Med* 1992;50:2916–2920.
76. Fukatsu A, Matsho S, Tamai H, Sakamoto N, Matsuda T, Hirano T. Distribution of interleukin-6 in normal and diseased human kidney. *Lab Invest* 1991;65:61–66.
77. Gesualdo L, Pinzani M, Floriano JJ, et al. Platelet-derived growth factor expression in mesangial proliferative glomerulonephritis. *Lab Invest* 1991;65:160–167.
78. Gesualdo L, Ranieri E, Pannarale G, Paolo SD, Schena FP. Platelet-derived growth factor and proliferative glomerulonephritis. *Kidney Int* 1993;43(suppl 39):86–89.
79. Fellström B, Klareskog L, Heldin CH, et al. Platelet-derived growth factor receptors in the kidney—upregulated expression in inflammation. *Kidney Int* 1989;36:1099–1102.
80. Yoshioka K, Takemura T, Murakami K, et al. Transforming growth factor-beta protein and mRNA in glomeruli in normal and diseased human kidney. *Lab Invest* 1993;68:154–163.
81. Roccatello D, Mosso R, Ferro M, et al. Urinary endothelin in glomerulonephritis patients with normal renal function. *Clin Nephrol* 1994; 41:323–330.
81a. Eng E, Floege J, Young BA, Couser WG, Johnson RJ. Does extracellular matrix expansion in glomerular disease require mesnagial cell proliferation? *Kidney Int* 1994;45(suppl):45–48.
81b. Pichler RH, Bassuk JA, Hugo C, et al. SPARC is expressed by mesangial cells in experimental mesangial proliferative nephritis and inhibits PDGF-mediated mesangial cell proliferation in vitro. *Am J Pathol* 1996;148:1153–1169.
81c. Baker AJ, Mooney A, Hughes H, et al. Mesangial cell apoptosis: a homeostatic mechanism operating in resolution of mesangial proliferative nephritis in vivo and induced by growth factor deprivation in vivo. *J Clin Invest* 1994;94:2105–2116.
81d. Iruela-Arispe L, Gordon K, Hugo C, et al. Participation of glomerular endothelial cells in the capillary repair of glomerulonephritis. *JASN* 1995;147:1715–1727.
82. Yang JY, Bai KM, Cui XL, Zhao JL, Liu JC, Zou WZ. Mesangial proliferative glomerulonephritis in children: a clinical and pathological study in 39 cases [in Chinese]. *Clin J Nephrol* 1989;5:204–207.
83. Churg J, Sobin LH. Renal disease. *Classification and atlas of glomerular diseases*. Tokyo: Igaku-Shoin; 1982:67–82, 127–165.
84. Tejani A. Relapsing nephrotic syndrome. *Nephron* 1987;45:81–85.
85. Hirszel P, Yamase HT, Carney WR, et al. Mesangial proliferative glomerulonephritis with IgM deposits. Clinicopathologic analysis and evidence for morphologic transitions. *Nephron* 1984;38:100–108.
86. D'Agati V. The many masks of focal segmental glomerulosclerosis. *Kidney Int* 1994;46:1223–1241.
87. A report of the Southwest Pediatric Nephrology Study Group. Childhood nephrotic syndrome associated with diffuse mesangial hypercellularity. *Kidney Int* 1983;24:87–94.
88. Murphy WM, Jukkola AF, Roy S. Nephrotic syndrome with mesangial-cell proliferations in children—a distinct entity? *Am Soc Clin Pathol* 1979;72:42–27.
89. Vehaskari VM, Robson AM. The nephrotic syndrome in children. *Ann Pediatr* 1981;10:42.
90. Habib R, Girardin E, Gagnadoux, MF, Hiuglais N, Levy M, Broyer M. Immunopathological findings in idiopathic nephrosis: clinical significance of glomerular "immune deposits." *Pediatric Nephrol* 1988; 2:402–408.
91. Migone L, Olivetti G, Allegri L, Dall'Aglio P. Mesangioproliferative glomerulonephritis. *Clin Nephrol* 1980;13:219–230.
91a. Ginesta JC, Almirall J, Torras A, Darnell A, Revert L. Long-evolution of patients with isolated C3 mesangioglomerulonephritis. *Clin Nephrol* 1995;43:221–225.
92. Allen WR, Travis LB, Cavallo T, Brouhard BH, Cunningham RJ. Immune deposits and mesangial hypercellularity in minimal change nephrotic syndrome: clinical relevance. *J Pediatr* 1982;100:188–191.
93. Cohen AH, Border WA. Mesangial proliferative glomerulonephritis. *Semin Nephrol* 1982;2:228–240.
94. Lawler W, Williams G, Trapey P, Mallick NP. IgM associated primary diffuse mesangial proliferative glomerulonephritis. *J Clin Pathol* 1980;33:1029–1038.
95. Jennett JC. Evolution of mesangial IgM nephropathy into focal segmental glomerulonephritis. *Am J Nephrol* 1981;1:222.
96. Kobayashi Y, Shigematsu H, Tateno S, Hiki Y. Nephrotic syndrome with diffuse mesangial IgM deposits. *Act Pathol Jpn* 1982;32:307–317.
97. Kipolovic J, Shvil Y, Pomeranz A, Ron N, Rubinger D, Oren R. IgM nephropathy: morphological study related to clinical findings. *Am J Nephrol* 1987;7:275–280.
98. Cavallo T, Johnson MP. Immunopathologic study of minimal-change glomerular disease with mesangial IgM deposits. *Nephron* 1981;27: 281–284.
99. Trachtman H, Carrol F, Phadke K, et al. Paucity of minimal-change lesion in children with early frequently relapsing steroid-responsive nephrotic syndrome. *Am J Nephrol* 1987;7:13–17.
100. Gurumurthy K, Tejani A, Nicastri Ad. Mesangial IgM nephropathy in children [Abstract]. *Kidney Int* 1983;23:125.
101. Zhang JH, Li LS, Chen HP, Zhang X. Mesangial IgM nephropathy [in Chinese]. *Chin Intern Med* 1984;23:141–144.
102. Li XW, Huang QY, Bi ZQ, et al. The IgM nephropathy and minimal change nephrotic syndrome in adults: clinico-pathological study [in Chinese]. *Chin J Nephrol* 1993;9:78–79.
103. Saha H, Mustoneu J, Pasternak A, Halin H. Clinical follow-up of 54 patients with IgM-nephropathy. *Am J Nephrol* 1989;9:124–128.
104. Abdurrahman MB, el Idrissy AT, Hafeez MA, Wright EA, Omar SA. Renal biopsy in Saudi children with nephrotic syndrome not responsive to corticosteroid: a preliminary report. *Trop Geogr Med* 1986;38: 141–145.
105. Habib R, Churg J, Bernstein J, et al. Minimal change disease, mesangial proliferative glomerulonephritis and focal sclerosis: individual entities or a spectrum of disease? In: Robinson RR, ed. *Nephrology*. New York: Springer-Verlag; 1984:634–644.
106. Papadopoulo ZL, Jenis EH, Tina LU, Novello AC, Jose PA, Calcagno PL. Chronic relapsing minimal change nephrotic syndrome with or without mesangial deposits: long-term follow up. *Int J Pediatr Nephrol* 1982;3:179–186.
107. Hsu HC, Chen WY, Lin GJ, et al. Clinical and immunopathologic study of mesangial IgM nephropathy: report of four cases. *Histopathology* 1984;8:435.
108. Pardo V, Riesgol, Zillernelo G, Strauss J. The clinical significance of mesangial IgM deposits and mesangial hypercellularity in minimal-change nephrotic syndrome. *Am J Kidney Dis* 1984;3:264–269.
109. Cattran D, Rance P, Cardella C, et al. Two variants of IgM nephropathy? [Abstract]. *Kidney Int* 1983;23:193.
110. Bhuyan UN, Srivastava RN. Incidence and significance of IgM mesangial deposits in relapsing idiopathic nephrotic syndrome of childhood. *Indian J Med Res* 1987;86:53–60.
111. Vangelist A, Frasca G, Biagini G, Bonomini V. Long term study of mesangial proliferative glomerulonephritis with IgM deposits. *Proc Eur Dial Transplant Assoc* 1981;18:503–506.
112. Gonzalo A, Mamposa F, Gallego N, Quereda C, Fierro C, Ortuno J. Clinical significance of IgM mesangial deposits in the nephrotic syndrome. *Nephron* 1985;41:246–249.
113. Vilche AR, Cameron JS. Mesangial deposits: is it a distinct pathological entity? *Am J Nephrol* 1988;8:346.
114. Murphy MJ, Bailey RR, McGiven AR. Is there an IgM nephropathy? *Aust N Z J Med* 1983;13:35.
115. Ma HH, Zhuang ZQ, Xie XA, Shao YZ. The clinical and pathological study of IgM nephropathy and minimal change disease nephrotic syndrome in children [in Chinese]. *Chin J Nephrol* 1994;10:8–11.
116. Vilches AR, Cameron JS, Turner DR. Minimal-change disease with mesangial IgM deposits. *N Engl J Med* 1980;303:1480.
117. Mampaso F, Gonzalo A, Teruel J, et al. Mesangial deposits of IgM in patients with the nephrotic syndrome. *Clin Nephrol* 1981;16:230–234.
118. Waldherr R, Gubler ME, Levy M, et al. The significance of pure diffuse mesangial proliferation in idiopathic nephrotic syndrome. *Clin Nephrol* 1978;10:171–179.
119. Mampaso F, Leyva-Cobian F, Marinez-Montero JG, et al. Mesangial proliferative glomerulonephritis with unusual intramembranous granular dense deposits. *Clin Nephrol* 1983;19:92–98.
120. Glassok RJ, Adler SG, Ward HJ, Cohen AH. Primary glomerular diseases. In: Brenner MB, Rector FC, eds. *The kidney*. Vol 1. 4th ed. Philadelphia: WB Saunders; 1991:1184–1192, 1223–1233.

121. O'Donoghue DJ, Lawler W, Hunt LP, Acheson EJ, Mallick NP. IgM-associated primary diffuse mesangial proliferative glomerulonephritis: natural history and prognostic indicators. *Q J Med* 1991; 79:333–350.
122. Kanai T, Kawamura T, Takazoe K, et al. Mesangial proliferative glomerulonephritis—non-IgA nephropathy [in Japanese]. *Jpn J Clin Med* 1986;46:1262–1268.
123. Li JZ, Chen YP, Bi ZQ, Bao YH, Shen YJ. Utilization of phase contrast microscopy for differentiating sources of hematuria [in Chinese]. *Chin J Intern Med* 1984;25:688–691.
124. Berger J. IgA glomerular deposits in renal disease. *Transplant Proc* 1969;1:934–944.
125. Schena FP. IgA nephropathies. In: Cameron JS, Davidson AM, eds. *Oxford text book of clinical nephrology.* Vol 1. New York: Oxford University Press; 1992:339–369.
126. Bi ZQ, Chen YP, Li XW, et al. Clinical and pathological analysis of 40 cases of IgA nephropathy [in Chinese]. *Chin J Intern Med* 1984; 23:136–140.
127. Chen YP, Wang HY, Zhou XJ, et al. IgA nephropathy with massive proteinuria: response to corticosteroid therapy [in Chinese]. *Chin J Intern Med* 1986;24:278–281.
128. Li LS, Liu ZH, Tao K, Nicholls K, Kincaid-Smith P. IgA nephrology in Chinese and Australian patients: a comparison between clinical and pathological features [in Chinese]. *Natl Med J China* 1991;71:153–155.
129. Mattoo TK. Kidney biopsy prior to cyclophosphamide therapy in primary nephrotic syndrome. *Pediatr Nephrol* 1991;5:617–619.
130. Ponticelli C, Rivolta E. Cyclosporine in nephrotic syndrome. *Transplant Proc* 1988;20(suppl 4):253–258.
131. Tejani A, Gonzalez R, Rajpoot D, Sharma R, Pomrantz A. A randomized trial of cyclosporine with low-dose prednisone compared with high-dose prednisone in nephrotic syndrome. *Transplant Proc* 1988; 20(suppl 4):262–264.
132. Zietse R, Wenting GJ, Karmer P, Schalekamp MADH, Weimer W. Fractional excretion of protein: a marker of the efficacy of cyclosporine A treatment in nephrotic syndrome. *Transplant Proc* 1988;20 (suppl 4):280–284.
133. Pan ZB, Huang LJ, Liu ZR, Liu J, Li FS. Short period effectivity of cylcosporine A on treating 5 cases with nephrotic syndrome [in Chinese]. *Chin J Nephrol* 1988;4:351–352.
134. Lou TQ, Yin PD, Li XP, Jiang D. Cyclosporine A treatment in primary nephrotic syndrome with steroid-resistance [in Chinese]. *Chin J Nephrol* 1991;7:168–170.
135. Li LS, Liu ZH. *Tripterygium wilfordii* (T.W.): a new lead in treating glomerular disease. In: Zhang JH, Du XH, Liu ZH, Li LS, eds. *Nephrology. Proceedings of the 4th Asian–Pacific congress of nephrology.* Beijing: International Academic Publishers; 1991:459–467.
136. Chen XM, Yu LF, Zhang CJ, Chen ZY, Li LS. Suppressive effect of *Trypterygium wilfordii* on the glomerular immune deposits in passive Heymann nephritis [in Chinese]. *Chin J Nephrol* 1990;6:10–12.
137. Wang HY, Li JZ, Zhu SL, Yu H, Mao SF, Zhang MH. The effect of *Tripterygil wilfordii, Astragali,* and *Angelicae* on permselectivity of glomerular capillary wall in aminonucleotide nephrosis [in Chinese]. *Natl Med J China* 1988;68:513–515.
138. Mao SF, Li JZ, Zhu SL, Yu H, Zhang MH, Wang HY. The effect of *Tripterygil wilfordii, Astragali,* and *Angelicae* on permselectivity of glomerular capillary wall in aminonucleotied nephrosis [Abstract]. Abstracts, 11th International Congress of Nephrology, Tokyo, 1990: 349A.
139. Li SL, Zhang X, Chen HP, et al. Clinical and experimental studies on the effect of *Tripterygium wilfordii* Hook in the treatment of nephritis [in Chinese]. *Natl Med J China* 1982;62:581–582.
140. Huang WC, Yin PD, Huang XP, Sun D, Li SM. Effects of cyclosporine A and *Tripterygium wilfordii* on glomerulonephritis: an experimental and clinical study [Abstract]. Abstracts, 4th Asian–Pacific Congress of Nephrology, Beijing, 1990:181.
141. Hu MC, Jiang XY. The reduction of proteinuria by *Tripterygium wilfordii* Hook F. in rats with daunomycin nephrosis: the role of a scavenger of free radical [Abstract]. Abstracts, 4th Asian–Pacific Congress of Nephrology, Beijing, 1990:194.
142. Li LS, Zhang X, Chen GY, Ji DX, Bao ZD. The clinical study of *Tripterygium wilfordii* Hook in the treatment of glomerulonephritis [in Chinese]. *Chin J Intern Med* 1981;20:216–220.
143. Gu J, Pan JS. the roles of *Astragali* and *Angelica* (A&A) on the protein metabolism in nephrotic rats [Abstract]. *Kidney Int* 1992;42:505.
144. Gu J, Pan JS, Cao H. The roles of *Astragali* and *Angelica* (A&A) on the protein metabolism in nephrotic rats [in Chinese]. *Chin J Nephrol* 1992;8:226.
145. Li LY, Wang HY, Zhu SL, Pan JS. Albumin mRNA study of hepatic protein synthesis in nephrotic syndrome rats treated with Chinese herbs. *Kidney Int* 1992;42:505.
146. Li LY, Wang HY, Zhu SL, Pan JS. Hepatic albumin's mRNA in nephrotic syndrome rats treated with Chinese herbs [in Chinese]. *Natl Med J China* 1995;75:276–279.
147. Li LY, Yu H, Pan JS, Wang HY. The study of protein metabolism on nephrotic patients with therapy of Chinese herbs [in Chinese]. *Chin J Intern Med* 1995;34:670.
148. Zhang YK, Wang HY, Wang SX, et al. The effect of Chinese medical herbs *Astragalus membranaceous* and *Angelica sinensis* on three kinds of experimental nephritis [in Chinese]. *Chin J Intern Med* 1986;25:222–225.
149. Saito T, Sato H, Kinoshita Y, Seino J, Furuyama T, Yoshinaga K. Prognosis of chronic glomerulonephritis—study on renal survival ratio of mesangial proliferative glomerulonephritis and membranoproliferative glomerulonephritis [in Japanese]. *Jpn J Nephrol* 1990; 32:959–965.
150. Siegel NJ, Gaudio KM, Krassner LS, McDonald BM, Anderson FP, Kashgarian M. Steroid-dependent nephrotic syndrome in children: histopathology and relapse after cyclophosphamide treatment. *Kidney Int* 1981;19:454–459.
151. Aubert J, Humain L, Chatelaut F, de Torrente A. IgM-associated mesangial proliferative glomerulonephritis and focal and segmental hyalinosis with nephrotic syndrome. *Am J Nephrol* 1985;5:449.
152. Dohi K, Nakamoto Y, Ishikawa H. Mesangial proliferative glomerulonephritis. Natural history and effects of dextran sulfate. *Jpn J Med* 1987;26:50–57.
153. Katafuchi R, Takebayashi S, Taguchi T, Harada T. Structural–functional correlation in serial biopsies from patients with glomerulonephritis. *Clin Nephrol* 1987;28:169–173.
154. Garcia del Moral R, Lazaro-Damas A, Gomez-Morales M, et al. Histopathologic factors with prognostic significance in mesangial proliferative glomerulonephritis. *Med Clin (Barc)* 1989;92:608–611.
155. Packham DK, North RA, Fairley KF, et al. Pregnancy in women with diffuse mesangial proliferative glomerulonephritis. *Clin Nephrol* 1988;29:193–198.
156. Striegel JE, Sibley RK, Fryd DS, Mauer SM. Recurrence of focal segmental sclerosis in children following renal transplantation. *Kidney Int* 1986;30(suppl 19):44–50.

Immunologic Renal Diseases,
edited by E. G. Neilson and W. G. Couser.
Lippincott-Raven Publishers, Philadelphia © 1997.

CHAPTER 46

Focal Segmental Glomerulosclerosis

H. William Schnaper

INTRODUCTION

In 1957, Rich (1) reported a series of autopsy specimens from patients whose initial clinical findings were similar to those of *minimal-change nephrotic syndrome* (MCNS), but who showed strikingly different histopathology. Similar to MCNS, there was no apparent inflammation of the glomerulus; but, unlike MCNS, the glomeruli showed extensive matrix accumulation and structural collapse. The abnormalities occurred to varying degrees in different glomeruli and usually affected only a segment of each glomerulus. Thus, it was termed *focal segmental glomerulosclerosis* (FSGS). Although other names have been used to describe this lesion, including focal and segmental glomerulosclerosis with hyalinosis, focal sclerosing glomerulonephritis, and focal sclerosing glomerulopathy, FSGS is now largely accepted as the correct appellation.

The events that lead to the development of FSGS are uncertain. The pathologic processes that are involved appear to be identical to those that mediate progressive loss of glomerular function in a wide range of other renal disorders (see chapter 33). Yet FSGS appears to be a disease entity that arises de novo, often accompanied by the nephrotic syndrome. Although this chapter is intended to consider the primary or idiopathic lesion known as FSGS, studies elucidating the process of glomerulosclerosis in other diseases will be considered when they might provide insight relevant to the pathogenesis of the primary lesion.

ETIOLOGY OF FSGS

FSGS presents with varied clinical manifestations. This strongly suggests that, rather than representing a single entity, the histopathologic findings of FSGS result from a common pathway of responses to a variety of stimuli. The nature of these stimuli is not well understood. In examining how the pathologic findings develop, it is helpful to consider that there are three forms of glomerulosclerosis. The first is primary FSGS. Patients with primary FSGS have no apparent underlying cause of their pathology and are therefore considered to have "idiopathic" disease. Most of these patients have overt nephrosis and may be categorized as having a form of idiopathic nephrotic syndrome (INS) (2). INS also includes patients with MCNS or mild mesangial hypercellularity. The incidence of FSGS in patients with nephrosis has varied from under 10% to >40% in individual studies (3), which may reflect age, ethnicity, or other characteristics of the patient population. As the presenting symptoms may differ among different patients, varying clinical courses and outcomes also suggest that distinct mechanisms may underlie different cases of FSGS.

In addition to the cases of INS that prove to be FSGS on biopsy, other cases of glomerulosclerosis are secondary to or associated with known diseases or clinical conditions. A list of diseases associated with FSGS is presented in Table 1. These include disorders that may involve the presence of foreign material in the circulation such as heroin nephropathy; alterations in glomerular hemodynamics such as are seen in oligomeganephronia, obesity, or preeclampsia; abnormal activation of cell function such as is likely to occur in human immunodeficiency virus infection; genetic disorders such as familial dysautonomia; and reactive or inflammatory disease such as would occur with reflux nephropathy, malignancy, or schistosomiasis. In many of these underlying conditions, focal sclerosis appears to result from an event related to a specific stimulus. These stimuli may provide some insight into potential causes of glomerulosclerosis. For example, glomerulosclerosis accompanies aging, suggesting that the glomerulus is particularly susceptible to the sclerotic process that generally occurs with age. An asso-

H. W. Schnaper: Department of Pediatrics, Northwestern University Medical School, Chicago, Illinois 60611.

TABLE 1. *Diseases associated with focal segmental glomerulosclerosis*

Idiopathic (primary) focal segmental glomerulosclerosis
Secondary glomerulosclerosis
Drugs
Analgesics (4)
Heroin (5)
Reflux/obstructive nephropathy (6)
Loss of renal mass/hyperfiltration
Unilateral renal agenesis (7)
Oligomeganephronia (8)
Segmental hypoplasia (9)
Obesity (10,11)
Preeclampsia (12)
Human immunodeficiency virus (13)
Diabetes mellitus
Human (rare) (14)
Hereditary disorders
Glycogen storage disease (type I)
Familial dysautonomia (15)
Spondyloepiphyseal dysplasia (16)
Sickle cell disease (17)
Aging (18)
Malignancy (19,20)
Transplantation
Recurrence (21)
De novo (22)
Miscellaneous
Radiation nephritis
Schistosomiasis (23)
Tuberculosis (24)
Infantile spasms (25)
Glomerular diseases
Alport
Post-streptococcal (26)
Membranous (27)
Other progressive renal diseases

Adapted from references 2, 9, and 28, and references noted in the list.

ciation with use of analgesics or with diabetes mellitus suggests that alterations in cell metabolism may influence the amount of matrix deposited in the kidney.

A third category of patients has another, underlying renal lesion. In these patients, the primary diagnosis is not focal sclerosis, yet there is evidence of segmental matrix accumulation and structural collapse consistent with the diagnosis of FSGS. This finding ominously suggests current or impending progressive glomerular loss, and raises the possibility that one final common pathway of nephron loss in chronic disease involves the same pathogenetic events that are involved in "primary" FSGS. Thus, progress in understanding the mechanism by which FSGS occurs in the absence of other apparent renal diseases may be useful for understanding general mechanisms of progression to end-stage renal disease. Conversely, insight regarding the influence of these underlying causes on the development of glomerulosclerosis may suggest cellular pathways that are activated in primary FSGS.

Heredity and FSGS

Several reports support the notion that there is a genetic predisposition to develop FSGS. There are at least 14 sibling pairs or triads with focal sclerosis reported in the literature (29–34). In several cases, two or three siblings developed proteinuria within several months of each other and subsequently proved to have FSGS on renal biopsy, suggesting a genetic predisposition leading to a common response to an identical stimulus. In one case, the sib pair was HLA identical, suggesting an immunogenetic predisposition. However, HLA typing of patients with FSGS has failed to yield consistent results. Glicklich and colleagues (35) found that both blacks and whites of all ages with FSGS had an increased incidence of HLA-DR4 (RR = 5.2 for blacks and 5.8 for whites), with the association being even stronger in adults (>18 years of age). HLA-A28 was associated with FSGS in black patients only. In a preliminary report by another group, HLA-B8, which has been associated with minimal-change disease (36–38), was also associated with FSGS in children (39). FSGS has been linked to HLA-DRw8 in nephrotic children of Hispanic origin (31,40), and B8 combined with DR3 and DR7 in German children (41). HLA-Bw53 was increased in black male adult patients with FSGS secondary to heroin nephropathy (42). In contrast, other studies have found no association (43–45). These discrepancies may reflect the fact that the studies were undertaken in different locations with populations of different ethnicities.

The HLA-typing results suggest that a genetic predisposition to glomerulosclerosis exists, but that it is multifactorial and inheritance is not clearly associated with a particular immunogenetic locus. More general, diffuse patterns of inheritance are reflected by specific racial patterns of incidence and severity. In a study of the North American Pediatric Registry of Transplants, black and Hispanic children accounted for 23% of all renal transplants performed, but for 38% of those performed for FSGS. In a single center, black and Hispanic children with nephrotic syndrome were found to be more likely to have FSGS; their initial serum creatinine and cholesterol concentrations were higher and their disease more often and more rapidly progressed to renal failure (46).

The likelihood of developing glomerulosclerosis as a secondary lesion also seems to have a hereditary component. Several groups have developed evidence that there is a genetic predisposition to develop renal failure. In Pima Indians with type-II diabetes mellitus, the likelihood of proteinuria in a patient increases with increasing frequency of proteinuria in parents. Moreover, the likelihood of a male diabetic presenting with an increased serum creatinine increases markedly if a parent has an increased creatinine (47). Although these results may simply indicate that severity of diabetes shows familial clustering, they also suggest that, given similar severity of the diabetes, there is familial clustering of severity of renal involvement.

Studies of first-degree relatives of patients receiving end-stage renal disease (ESRD) care indicate that African-Americans show similar clustering. Whereas 37% of such patients with type-II diabetes had a first-, second-, or third-degree relative receiving ESRD care, only 7% of a control population of type-II diabetics had relatives with severe renal disease (48). In general, African-American ESRD patients are more likely than white ESRD patients to have a relative receiving end-stage care (49). Interestingly, when patients with presumed hypertensive kidney disease were evaluated, a significant percentage of the relatives with renal failure proved to have causes other than hypertension for their kidney disease (50). These results suggest that, regardless of the potential stimulus for renal disease, some families show a predisposition for progression to renal failure. This predisposition may be attributable to racial differences in glomerular size or number (51). Although such a predisposition is not equivalent to FSGS, the fact that glomerulosclerosis is a common mechanism of progression of glomerular disease in diabetes mellitus and hypertension raises the possibility that certain groups show a genetic tendency to respond to an insult with glomerulosclerosis.

HISTOPATHOLOGY OF FSGS

The classic histopathology of FSGS, reported by Rich, appears first at the corticomedullary junction, although not all studies have confirmed this observation (52). The lesion subsequently progresses into the outer cortex. As a consequence, a more superficial renal biopsy early in the disease course might miss the lesion. The pathologic abnormalities affect only some glomeruli (focal) with only part of the glomerular tuft involved (segmental). On light microscopy, there is a segmental pattern of increased mesangial matrix accumulation. The associated glomerular capillary loops may be collapsed, with accumulation of acellular hyaline subendothelial deposits (Fig. 1). These appear to be composed of basement membranes and associated mesangial matrix, and often are adherent to the Bowman capsule (53). Within a single glomerulus, the lesion typically starts in the hilar region, spreading outward from the afferent arteriole or mesangial stalk, progressing into the tuft. Immunofluorescence microscopy often demonstrates immunoglobulin (Ig)-M and C3 deposits in a granular pattern. Unaffected glomerular areas may reveal IgM and C3 in a mesangial distribution. IgG usually is not present, although both IgG and IgA have been reported to be present in some cases (54). Electron microscopy shows diffuse epithelial cell foot-process fusion that affects nonsclerotic areas of the glomerulus. Paramesangial and subendothelial, finely granular electron-dense deposits may be seen. Four components may contribute to the development of the typical sclerotic lesion: glomerular basement membranes, mesangial matrix, collapsed vascular structures, and fibrous scar derived from interstitial collagen and related scar tissue components (55).

Nonglomerular findings may be present, even in primary FSGS, particularly with progressive disease. Tubular atrophy is often accompanied by interstitial inflammatory infiltrates, with the degree of inflammation being far greater than that seen in glomerulus (56). The number of tubules present may decrease due to "tubular dropout" from nephron loss, causing the appearance of a high concentration of glomeruli on low-power microscopy. With severe progression, interstitial fibrosis is seen. In addition, many of the glomeruli may become totally (globally) scarred. This sign of late glomerular involvement must be distinguished from the presence of an occasional, globally sclerosed glomerulus in otherwise normal kidneys (57).

Variations from Classic Histopathology

In a recent study (58), the percentage of involved glomerular tufts in a single biopsy section was significantly greater in adults than in children. Moreover, when the biopsy specimens were studied more completely by serial section, the number of tufts per glomerulus that were involved in both children and adults greatly increased. This suggests that patchy involvement within a single tuft may accentuate the apparently segmental nature of the lesion. To a large degree, the extent of segmental involvement reflects both the severity and duration of the lesion; however, variations in this finding may also reflect the etiology of the sclerosis.

Initially, it was postulated that the eosinophilic, hyaline deposits in some cases of FSGS, often adherent to the Bowman capsule, are a discrete lesion that identifies a subset of patients with a greater likelihood of progression to chronic renal insufficiency (59). However, this finding is now generally considered to be a part of the standard histopathology. Of greater significance may be differences from the usual centrifugal pattern of progression within the glomerulus. The perihilar origin of the matrix accumulation is less apparent in some forms of FSGS, particularly that associated with human immunodeficiency virus (HIV) nephropathy (13). Recently, a similar "collapsing glomerulopathy" has been described in the absence of evidence for HIV infection. In both HIV nephropathy and collapsing glomerulopathy, the dispersed distribution of the lesion causes it to appear to be less segmental (Fig. 2). The prognosis for the idiopathic form of collapsing glomerulopathy appears to be worse than that for typical FSGS (60).

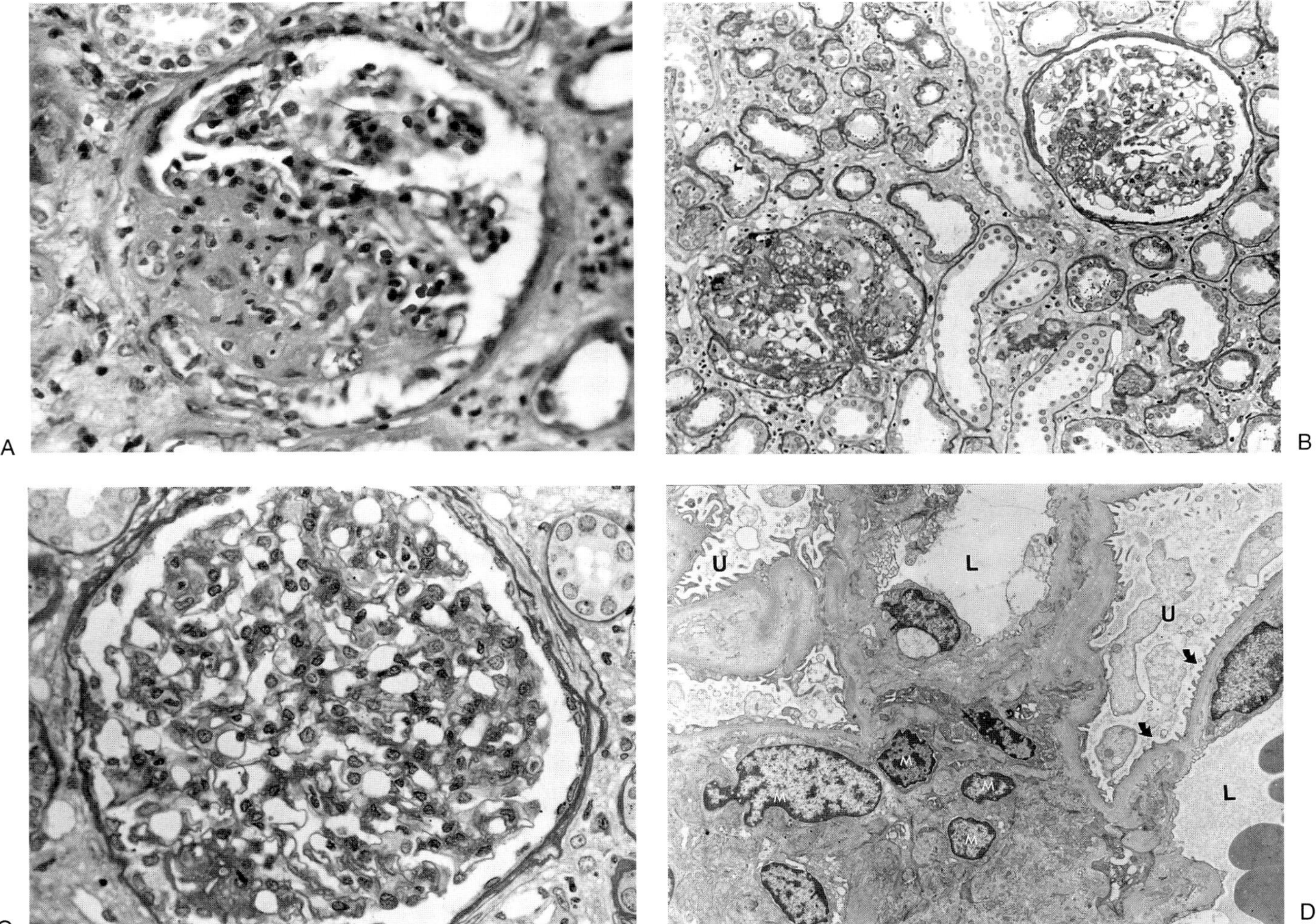

FIG. 1. Histopathology of glomerulosclerosis. **A:** A partially sclerosed glomerulus. Note the hilar distribution of the sclerosis with adherence to the Bowman capsule. Half of the glomerulus is relatively normal in appearance, demonstrating the segmental nature of the lesion. **B:** Adjacent glomeruli showing marked differences in degree of involvement, demonstrating the focal nature of the lesion. **C:** A glomerulus showing mesangial hypercellularity. **D:** An electron micrograph showing matrix accumulation in the bottom portion *(left and center)* of the micrograph, and an increased number of mesangial cells (nuclei marked). L, capillary lumen; U, urinary space. The *arrowheads* in the *upper right* show fusion of epithelial foot processes, with more normal podocyte architecture shown in the *upper left-hand corner* of the micrograph. Photographs provided by Dr. Wei Hsueh, Children's Memorial Hospital, Chicago, IL.

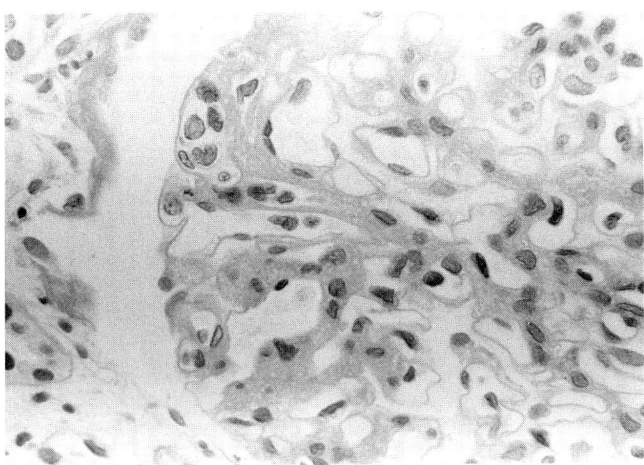

FIG. 2. Histopathology of a glomerulus from a patient with HIV-associated nephropathy. The matrix accumulation does not show the characteristic segmental appearance of idiopathic focal segmental glomerulosclerosis. Photograph provided by Dr. Paul Kimmel, George Washington University, Washington, DC.

Relationship Among Histopathologic Variants of Primary Nephrotic Syndrome (MCNS, FSGS, and Mesangial Proliferation)

INS may present without any significant glomerular histopathology (MCNS); it may show typical FSGS; or MCNS or FSGS may both be accompanied by mesangial cell proliferation. It is unclear whether these represent a spectrum of clinical findings resulting from the same underlying disease process or different diseases. According to the first view, patients with MCNS have the most benign form of the disease, while those with rapidly progressing FSGS represent the most malignant variant. Certainly, the initial clinical presentation of primary nephrotic syndrome in patients with either MCNS or FSGS may be the same. In support of the hypothesis that FSGS and MCNS are part of a continuous spectrum, some cases of MCNS are steroid resistant, whereas some cases of FSGS are steroid responsive (61). In contrast, the marked difference between MCNS and FSGS in percentage of patients responding to steroid therapy, as well as the higher frequency of chronic renal failure in the latter, support the notion that these represent two distinct disease entities (62).

As an alternative, idiopathic FSGS could represent a progressive form of glomerulosclerosis superimposed on MCNS, just as it is superimposed on other glomerular lesions. There are documented cases in which apparent MCNS developed into FSGS (63–66). Although this suggests that MCNS and FSGS are parts of a spectrum of disease, in some cases FSGS may have been missed in the early biopsies either because of a sampling error or because no juxtamedullary glomeruli were obtained. Further, increasing degrees of sclerosis on initial biopsy are associated with increasing likelihood of developing renal failure, again suggesting that the sclerotic process is simply a visible manifestation of the process by which some patients with primary nephrotic syndrome develop renal insufficiency (67). However, some cases of FSGS present without nephrotic syndrome or with only a very brief period of nephrotic symptoms.

The presence or absence of mesangial proliferative changes must also be taken into account in the relationship between MCNS and FSGS. Mild mesangial proliferation may represent a specific entity, a reactive response, or a transitional form between uncomplicated MCNS and FSGS (68). Both MCNS and FSGS may occur with or without mesangial proliferation. Rather than reflecting a different disease entity, mesangial proliferation could simply indicate a less common and perhaps less benign systemic response to the disease process. This would explain the observation that mesangial proliferation has been found to be an indicator of relatively poor outcome (69). Alternatively, mesangial proliferative disease might have histopathologic and physiologic elements similar to MCNS, but be a different disease, as indicated by its relative resistance to steroid therapy and the increased risk of azotemia (70). Habib and colleagues (71,72) have suggested that MCNS, FSGS, and diffuse mesangial proliferation represent variations of primary nephrotic syndrome, which may be found alone or in combination. Until the pathogenesis of each of these lesions is delineated, this issue will remain the subject of considerable debate.

PATHOPHYSIOLOGY OF FSGS

The pathogenesis of human FSGS is poorly understood. As stated previously, there are three clinical paradigms for the development of focal sclerotic changes in the glomerulus. In the first, FSGS is a primary manifestation of renal disease, with or without the presence of nephrotic syndrome. Second, systemic diseases such as diabetes mellitus may have glomerular manifestations in the kidney (14). Third, focal sclerotic changes can appear as a supervening finding in other renal diseases such as membranous nephropathy (27). It is not clear how many cases are truly "primary" because it is difficult to distinguish pathogenetically between primary lesions and those with unknown proximate causes. However, it is likely that the mechanisms involved in the generation and progression of sclerosis will prove to be similar; here data generated for one of the three clinical paradigms will be considered relevant to all.

Animal Models of FSGS

Four types of animal models have been developed that reflect some aspect of FSGS: models in which a direct insult to the kidney leads to sclerosis, "indirect" models wherein altered systemic physiology leads to the development of sclerosis, genetic models in which the glomerulosclerosis occurs "spontaneously" without requiring any additional manipulation of the animal by the investigator, and transgenic models. Although these models are not necessarily analogous to human FSGS, each provides information relevant to the physiologic determinants of sclerosis. They are described briefly here, and information gleaned from these models is considered in subsequent sections.

Direct Manipulations of the Kidney Leading to Focal Sclerosis

These include insults that increase the filtered load of the nephron, and those that alter either the metabolism of the kidney cells, their ability to retard the passage of macromolecules, or both. A classic model of progressive kidney disease results from overload proteinuria (73). Animals given repeated intraperitoneal injections of heterologous serum albumin develop massive proteinuria that includes both native and parenterally administered protein. Initially, there is no change in glomerular filtration rate (GFR). Markedly elevated transcapillary albumin transport leads to acute, reversible degenerative changes of glomerular epithelial cells, with development of large pore defects in the glomerular basement membrane (74). Subsequently, more complex changes may lead to sclerosis.

Another model involving nephron "overload" is subtotal renal ablation. Rats subjected to uninephrectomy undergo a compensatory increase in single-nephron (SN) GFR in the remaining nephrons (75). Removal of the right kidney and occlusion of two of the three extrarenal arterial branches to the left kidney causes progressive sclerosis in the remaining nephrons (76). This 5/6-nephrectomy model may be similar to certain forms of progressive human renal disease because hyperfiltration in remnant nephrons leads to proteinuria in humans (77).

A frequently used model of reversible matrix expansion is anti-thymocyte (Thy-1) nephritis (78). Rodents given antibody developed against a thymic antigen develop mesangial cell apoptosis and mesangiolysis, mesangial proliferation and hypercellularity, and proteinuria. These events lead to transient mesangial accumulation of matrix.

A fourth model involves a biochemical insult to the glomeruli in rats treated with adriamycin or with puromycin aminonucleoside (PAN) (79). Because the drugs are administered to the entire kidney, the nephrons are diffusely and relatively homogeneously affected (80). Unlike overload proteinuria, in PAN nephrosis there is associated loss of glomerular polyanion (81), a likely event in FSGS (82). Sclerosis occurs after a time delay, varying with the dose and frequency of exposure. This raises the possibility that the sclerotic changes result indirectly from the effects of proteinuria or from reduced nephron function, rather than being caused directly by the drugs themselves.

Alteration of Animal Physiology

Investigators have manipulated animals to cause them to become diabetic, hyperlipidemic, or hypertensive. Rats, mice, and hamsters have been made diabetic by administration of streptozotocin. These animals eventually develop focal sclerosis (83–85), even after administration of insulin to mitigate the severity of hyperglycemia. Rats (86) or guinea pigs (87) fed a high-cholesterol diet develop hypercholesterolemia and focal glomerulosclerosis. This model is particularly relevant in view of the potential contribution of the lipid abnormalities in nephrotic syndrome to progression of renal disease (see below). Several of these models, especially those involving genetically determined systemic hypertension, are considered in the next section.

Genetically Determined Abnormalities Leading to Glomerulosclerosis in Animals

These models include many of the systemic findings that are associated with secondary FSGS in humans: hypertension, obesity, hypercholesterolemia, diabetes mellitus, and aging. In humans, hypertension per se does not cause true glomerulosclerosis, but rather renal arteriolar sclerosis. In rats, however, hypertension is associated with development of a sclerotic lesion in the glomerulus. This suggests that at least certain strains have a different physiologic response to hypertension in the kidney, perhaps through a genetic mechanism similar to those suggested by familial clustering of secondary renal disease in humans. Hypertensive rat models include the spontaneously hypertensive rat (SHR) (88) and the Dahl salt-sensitive rat (89). Male Wistar rats develop a lesion identical to FSGS by 12 months of age (90). Fawn-hooded rats develop hypertension, proteinuria, and glomerulosclerosis at an early age (91). Preliminary reports indicate that a "renal failure" gene has been identified on chromosome 1 in these rats. Sclerosis and proteinuria both map to the locus; systemic hypertension also maps to rat chromosome 1 but at a location 40 cM away from the newly defined locus (92).

Several rodent models of obesity develop glomerulosclerosis. Notable among these is the obese Zucker rat. In these rats, severe obesity and hyperlipidemia are followed by proteinuria and FSGS (93). Obese Zucker rats have been determined to have polyunsaturated fatty-acid deficiency (94).

Transgenic Models of Glomerulosclerosis

FSGS models that have been developed include animals transgenic for a portion of HIV DNA (95) and mice overexpressing growth hormone (96). Although one of the effects of growth hormone is to stimulate insulinlike growth factor (IGF) production, IGF-1 transgenic animals do not develop sclerosis (96). In a model in which mice are transgenic for the viral SV40 large T antigen, associated with increased cellular proliferation, glomerular size increase was accompanied by sclerosis; this suggested that regulation of growth within the glomerulus is important in the development of FSGS (97). Mice transgenic for interleukin (IL) 6 may develop FSGS (98). Simultaneous, site-directed mutagenesis of the *fyn* and *yes* tyrosine kinase genes causes the mice to be born with degenerative renal disease resulting in segmental glomerulosclerosis (99). In another model, mice homozygous for a transgenic retrovirus develop focal sclerosis. Because all of the affected animals have a common insertion point for the proviral DNA, the insertion may have interrupted expression of a gene responsible for normal glomerular morphogenesis or function (100). The ablated gene, known as *mpv-17*, has subsequently been determined to encode for a peroxisomal protein producing reactive oxygen species (101). Although a role for this gene in the pathogenesis of FSGS remains to be determined, "rescue" of these animals by replacing the interrupted gene abrogates the development of FSGS (102).

Physiologic Conditions That May Contribute to the Development of Sclerosis

These conditions include systemic and intraglomerular hypertension, hyperfiltration (nephron overload), hyperlipidemia, coagulopathy, and inflammation.

Glomerular Hemodynamics

In humans, administration of the nonsteroidal anti-inflammatory agent, meclofenamate, slowed progression of recurrent FSGS in renal transplant recipients, presumably by altering renal hemodynamics (103). The association of systemic hypertension and vascular disease with glomerulosclerosis in an hereditary animal model (104) also implicates hemodynamic factors. Age-related glomerulosclerosis in male Wistar rats is ameliorated by a low-sodium diet (90). Glomerular capillary hypertension may have a more specific impact than systemic hypertension. In fawn-hooded rats, the degree of glomerular hypertension correlates with glomerulosclerosis (91). Glomerular hypertension also appears to be important in progression of scarring in several rat models (105–107). In experiments comparing normotensive and hypertensive diabetic rats, glomerular capillary hydrostatic pressure (P_{GC}) was found to be similar and the two groups of rats had similar degrees of glomerular sclerosis. Nonetheless, drugs intended to reduce systemic blood pressure decreased the extent of sclerotic changes in both the normotensive and hypertensive strains (108). These results suggests that both P_{GC} and systemic blood pressure affect the sclerotic process.

Increased Nephron Load

Glomerular capillary hypertension increases filtration surface area and the net driving force for ultrafiltration, increasing the passage of macromolecules across the glomerular filter. This increased filtration may be a critical factor in sclerosis. The severity of proteinuria and of glomerulosclerosis correlate in PAN nephrosis (79). Protamine, which enhances albuminuria, exacerbates the development and progression of disease in this model (109). Further, a high-protein diet, with its concomitant increase in SNGFR and P_{GC}, accelerates nephron loss in rats with 5/6 nephrectomy (110), whereas a low-protein diet prevents sclerosis in adriamycin-treated rats (111). In humans, although uninephrectomy occasionally has been associated with FSGS (112), long-term follow-up studies of sizable populations of adults (113) or children (114) who have undergone nephrectomy have not detected progressive renal impairment. This is consistent with the failure of uninephrectomy alone to cause glomerulosclerosis in most models, indicating that hyperfiltration must be severe to cause sclerosis by itself. In contrast, lesser degrees of hyperfiltration may be synergistic with other sclerogenic events. Uninephrectomy causes sclerosis in hypertensive SHR and WKY rats (115) or rats treated with anti-mesangial-cell antibodies. One potential explanation for conflicting data emphasizing the roles of either hyperfiltration or increased P_{GC} is that there are two phases in the development of the lesion, only one of which is hypertension-mediated (116).

It also is important to consider whether hyperfiltration itself causes sclerosis or whether it initiates another process. A likely mediating event involves the hypertrophy that accompanies nephron overload. Patients with apparent MCNS who subsequently develop FSGS show an increased glomerular tuft area in their initial biopsy specimens (65). This relationship also holds for early FSGS compared with MCNS (117). In another study, patients with INS who were refractory to therapy also had glomerular enlargement (118); it is not clear whether long-term follow-up of these refractory patients might subsequently demonstrate development of FSGS. The relative contribution of hypertrophy versus hyperfiltration to FSGS is addressed in an animal model in which rats underwent left 2/3 nephrectomy and right ureteral diversion into the peritoneal cavity (as opposed to right nephrectomy). The extent of glomerulosclerosis in remnant (left) kidney glomeruli was less than in comparable animals that had undergone right nephrectomy instead of diversion. Because the animals undergoing the ureteral diversion had similar SNGFR and P_{GC} to those undergoing nephrectomy, these results strongly suggest that a hypertrophic signal after the nephrectomy stimulated the development of glomerulosclerosis (119). Similarly, deep cortical glomeruli showed a special sensitivity to the development of sclerosis in very young rats subjected to subtotal nephrectomy, despite the fact that superficial cortical nephrons showed a much greater compensatory response in SNGFR (120). This finding, consistent with the histopathologic progression of FSGS in children from the corticomedullary junction toward the peripheral cortex, supports a predominant role for hypertrophy, rather than the initiating stimulus of hyperfiltration, in the pathogenesis of the sclerotic lesion.

Lipid-Mediated Injury

Lipid nephrotoxicity (121) may affect both the development and progression of FSGS. Many patients with FSGS manifest the lipid abnormalities that are part of the nephrotic syndrome. A role for lipid-mediated injury is supported by the similarity of the FSGS lesion to that of atherosclerosis (122). Mesangial cells take up and metabolize lipid in hyperlipidemic states (123). Further, PAN nephrosis is exacerbated by dietary cholesterol supplementation (124). Conversely, treatment of hyperlipidemia with probucol ameliorates development of FSGS in PAN nephrosis (125). It has been suggested that, by increasing renal vascular resistance, hypercholesterolemia contributes to increased P_{GC} (126). Certainly, drugs that lower glomerular vascular resistance ameliorate the progression of lipid-mediated renal disease in obese Zucker rats (127). But it is likely that lipids affect glomerular cell function more directly as well. In biopsies of patients with various renal diseases, only patients with FSGS showed a high incidence of glomerular foam cells being present (128). Lipid mediators may stimulate immune mechanisms in FSGS (129), even in the absence of classically "immune" stimuli (130). They also could act directly on glomerular cells, inducing production of growth factors and prostanoids that stimulate matrix overproduction, mesangial cell proliferation, vasoconstriction, and coagulation (129). For example, low-density lipoprotein stimulates fibronectin synthesis by cultured mesangial cells (131).

Hypercoagulability

Nephrotic syndrome is a hypercoagulable state, and coagulation may also contribute to the development of FSGS or to its progression to end-stage renal failure. Fibrin has been found both in sclerosed and in nonsclerosed segments of glomeruli in FSGS (81). Furthermore, treatment with anticoagulants both reverses coagulation abnormalities and improves outcome in patients and experimental animals with progressive glomerulopathies that are associated with glomerular sclerosis (132,133). Observations have suggested, however, that the effect of one anticoagulant, heparin, may be as an inhibitor of growth of mesangial cell proliferation and matrix production after injury, rather than as an anticoagulant (134). The inciting event for the coagulation changes might be visceral epithelial cell injury, which results from protein overload (9). Fibrin deposition would then lead to sclerotic changes, a process that could become self-perpetuating (135).

Inflammation

Because of the lack of significant immunoglobulin deposits and the absence of a massive cellular infiltrate in the glomerulus, FSGS has not been regarded as a classically immune-mediated renal disease. However, as our understanding of immune processes and our ability to detect immune responses have become more refined, a likely role has emerged for the immune system in disease pathogenesis. A relatively overlooked influence of successful dietary manipulation of progressive glomerular disease is its effect on immune function (136). Mononuclear cells infiltrate the glomerulus in FSGS, with a slight predominance of CD8+ (effector) T cells. In contrast, the interstitium contains more CD4+ cells (137). Further, in FSGS, frozen sections show increased mesangial cell expression of intercellular adhesion molecule 1 (138). In rat uninephrectomy/PAN-induced FSGS, infiltrating lymphocytes and macrophages were noted throughout the disease course, and inhibition of cellular immunity with corticosteroids ameliorated the lesion (139). Thus, the glomerular lesion in FSGS shows evidence of being immune mediated.

At the same time, inflammation plays a major role in the progressive interstitial fibrosis of FSGS and other forms of progressive renal disease (140,141). This may reflect the immunostimulatory effect of overload proteinuria (142). Tubulointerstitial reactions may be generated by specific filtered moieties such as iron-generated free radicals (143), or by the release of inflammatory fatty acids (144) or lipid mediators (145) filtered through the glomerulus while bound to plasma albumin. Thus, the immune system plays a significant role both in the development of glomerulosclerosis and in the progression of this lesion toward renal insufficiency.

MECHANISMS OF GLOMERULAR MATRIX ACCUMULATION AND STRUCTURAL COLLAPSE

Each of the physiologic abnormalities just discussed contributes to the development of glomerulosclerosis. In response to these stimulating events, the glomerulus undergoes a series of changes in cell function that generate the histopathologic picture of FSGS. These changes can be considered as a final common pathway leading to matrix accumulation and structural collapse.

Matrix Accumulation in FSGS

The extracellular matrix (ECM) in the glomerulus is found largely in the capillary loops and in the mesangium. The capillary loop ECM is comprised of the basement membranes secreted by the endothelial cells and the visceral epithelial cells; this probably accounts for its trilaminar structure. The most abundant constituent is type-IV collagen (146), with considerable laminin (147) and lesser amounts of entactin (nidogen) (148) and heparan sulfate proteoglycans (HSPGs). The highly anionic HSPG component is much more abundant in the glomerular basement membrane than in other vascular basement membranes, accounting in part for the unique sieving characteristics of the glomerular filter; it may be decreased in human diabetic nephropathy (149). The other major location of ECM in the glomerulus is the mesangial stalk. Although this matrix does not form a true basement membrane, its components are similar to those of the capillary wall ECM, differing in the presence of additional fibronectin and biglycan. Other components of the glomerular ECM include thrombospondin and chondroitin sulfate proteoglycans (146). Expression of mRNA for all of these proteins is high during renal development (150) but decreases to much lower levels at renal maturity. Fibronectin may be derived from the plasma (151) or from infiltrating cells, but also may be produced locally within the glomerulus (152).

In glomerular matrix expansion, the accumulating proteins may represent either an increased amount of normal constituents of the glomerular matrix or the presence of matrix proteins not normally found in the glomerulus, such as interstitial collagen (particularly type III collagen) and decorin, a small, nonaggregating proteoglycan (153). This pattern of expression may represent a "de-differentiation" of the glomerular cells because this altered matrix composition is similar to that found in the embryonic renal interstitial mesenchyme (154). In FSGS, type-IV collagen appears to accumulate largely in the mesangium, whereas type III collagen appears largely in the periglomerular synechiae (155). Thus, this disease does not represent a generalized process by which all cells are injured and react by producing a uniform scar tissue. In fact, in different renal diseases, different proteins accumulate. Fibronectin synthesis is increased in glomeruli isolated from 5/6-nephrectomy SHR rats (156). In human (157) and animal (158) models of diabetes, there are conflicting results, but the general impression is that there is mesangial accumulation of laminin, fibronectin, and type IV and type V collagen. Diabetes may also include alterations in the type of individual collagen chains involved in forming the collagen IV trimer because some models show increased α_3(IV) and α_4(IV), but less α_1(IV) and α_2(IV), being expressed. Conversely, steady-state glomerular levels of mRNA for α_1(IV) (159), as well as laminin B_1 (160) have been reported to be increased in diabetic mice. In PAN nephrosis, expression of mRNA for type IV collagen is increased (161). In human glomerulosclerosis, expression of mRNA for α_2(IV) collagen is increased (162). Together, these studies support the hypothesis that increased production of ECM proteins, especially laminin and collagens, plays an important role in FSGS and other progressive glomerular diseases.

ECM accumulation also may result from decreased degradation of ECM or from an alteration in the net balance between synthesis and degradation (163). Thus, the rate of turnover is important in determining the amount of ECM that is present (164,165). The role of matrix degradation has only recently become a focus of investigation. Two major pathways provide the specific machinery to degrade matrix proteins [see my review (163)]. The matrix metalloproteinases (MMPs) are a family of neutral, zinc-containing, calcium-dependent proteases that are secreted as proenzymes and catalytically activated. They are regulated post-translationally by a family of inhibitors, the tissue inhibitors of metalloproteinases. Although their substrate specificities overlap, each of the MMPs shows preferential efficiency for degrading specific ECM proteins. The other major matrix-degrading system, the plasminogen activator (PA)/plasmin pathway, involves a cascade of serine proteases that are important in fibrinolysis. Along with the MMP stromelysin, they participate in laminin degradation. The PAs, too, are activated proteolytically, and their activity is inhibited by the PA inhibitors, or PAIs. It is not clear whether under physiologic conditions the PA/plasmin system directly degrades laminin (166) or acts indirectly by initiating a cascade of MMP-mediated degradation (167). These enzymes and inhibitors are produced in varying degrees by cultured cells of mesangial (167), endothelial (168,169), and epithelial (170) origin.

The matrix-degrading enzymes and their inhibitors are produced in murine (171) and human (172) glomeruli, indicating that they could play a role in normal and abnormal glomerular matrix homeostasis. Although it is possible that these enzymes play a significant role in mediating acute glomerular injury, it is probable that much of the proteolytic damage in acute injury is mediated by products of infiltrating cells. In several animal models, it appears likely that the role of ECM proteases is to prevent or resolve matrix accumulation. For example, in the self-limited model of glomerular matrix expansion initiated by administration of anti-Thy-1 antibody, mRNA for gelatinase A (a basement membrane collagenase) (173) and PA activity (174) both peak at 5–7 days, a time when the matrix accumulation is beginning to resolve. This suggests that increased glomerular protease activity plays a role in resolution of matrix accumulation. A variety of more chronic models of glomerulosclerosis also have implicated abnormal matrix degradation (decreased protease production or activity, or increased production of protease inhibitors). Decreased total matrix protease activity has been found in glomeruli of rats with adriamycin nephropathy (175), streptozotocin diabetic nephropathy (176), and aging (177). In PAN-induced FSGS, decreased glomerular expression of mRNA for MMPs accompanies increased expression of mRNA for ECM proteins (178). These findings further support a role for ECM proteases in preventing glomerular matrix accumulation.

Cellular Responses to Sclerogenic Stimuli

Although altered net matrix turnover in FSGS appears certain, the mechanisms involved in this process are less clear. Given that hypertrophy appears to be important in sclerosis, it is likely that systemic hormonal regulators of cell growth, local mediators such as arachidonic metabolites, and cytokines or growth factors that mediate inflammatory responses will be involved in glomerular matrix accumulation. Mice transgenic for growth hormone manifest glomerulosclerosis (96). Additional genes, such as those for ECM, are activated in these models (179). Conversely, growth-hormone-deficient mice show resistance to the development of glomerulosclerosis after subtotal nephrectomy (180) or streptozotocin administration (181). IGF-1 activates mesangial cells to proliferate and secrete collagen in vitro (182). Further, receptors for IGF-1 are increased in diabetic mouse mesangial cells (183). These results invoke a role for abnormal growth-factor-mediated regulation of glomerular cells in disease.

Arachidonic acid metabolites may be produced after local stimuli or may result from systemic derangements that provide more substrate for local production. Thromboxane induces expression of mRNA for laminin, fibronectin, and type-IV collagen by mesangial cells (184). Inhibition of thromboxane synthesis retards progression of renal disease after either subtotal nephrectomy (185) or injection of anti-mesangial-cell antibodies (186).

Cytokines and growth factors, produced by cells intrinsic to the glomerulus or derived from infiltrating immune cells (187), may also mediate the development of focal sclerosis. IL-1 (188), epidermal growth factor (189), and IL-6 (190), each of which promotes mesangial cell proliferation in vivo or in vitro, may also stimulate matrix synthesis (191). Increased glomerular synthesis of tumor necrosis factor (TNF) α and IL-1 has been found in streptozotocin-induced diabetic nephropathy (192). Anti-platelet-derived growth factor (PDGF) antibodies block the increased proliferation observed when mesangial cells are exposed to the stimulatory effects of advanced glycosylation end products similar to those produced in diabetes (193). Intravenous infusion into rats of PDGF, or to a lesser extent, of basic fibroblast growth factor (bFGF), causes increased proliferation and some degree of mesangial expansion, but does not cause proteinuria (194). This finding suggests that the effect of PDGF and bFGF as mitogens or sclerogenic agents does not require the presence of proteinuria; the events causing proteinuria either lead to production of these cytokines or are the result of a distinct mechanism.

Perhaps the most widely studied cytokine or growth factor in the pathogenesis of matrix accumulation is transforming growth factor (TGF)-β. This growth factor mediates mesangial expansion in anti-Thy-1 glomerulonephritis (195). In human disease, TGF-β_1 has also been detected in the mesangium in IgA nephritis (196), diabetic glomerulosclerosis (197), and FSGS (198). In vivo transfection by direct gene infusion into the kidney also results in matrix accumulation (199). Further, inhibition of TGF-β activity decreases the enhancement of matrix production when cultured mesangial cells are exposed to advanced glycosylation end products (193). In Thy-1 nephritis, TGF-β is associated temporally with downregulation of PA activity and increased PAI-1 production (174). In addition, TGF-β directly stimulates PAI-1 production by mesangial cells (174). In contrast, this growth factor increases expression of gelatinase A (200), the major glomerular protease for degrading type IV collagen. Nonetheless, it is noteworthy that glomerular staining for TGF-β is increased in patients with diseases associated with matrix accumulation (196) and patients with FSGS have increased urinary excretion of TGF-β (201). These data strongly support a central role for TGF-β in glomerular matrix accumulation.

However, TGF-β does not by itself account for all cases of matrix expansion. In an in vitro model of "aging" mesangial cells, characterized by increasing matrix production and decreased ECM protease activity, TGF-β_1 did not accelerate assumption of the sclerotic phenotype by the cultured mesangial cells (202). Further, fawn-hooded rats treated with angiotensin-converting enzyme (ACE) inhibition show persistent glomerular staining with anti-TGF-β antibodies, but do not show sclerotic progression (203). This raises the possibility that angiotensin II is a mediator of hypertrophy and matrix expansion. Increased ACE activity is found in type-II diabetic patients who have proteinuria (204). In animal models, angiotensin is an important mediator of cardiac hypertrophy (205). In the glomerulus, angiotensin II stimulates mesangial cell contractility (206) and prostaglandin E_2 synthesis (207) This peptide enhances mesangial cell growth and synthesis of fibronectin (208), type-I collagen (209), and biglycan (210). In PAN-induced glomerular hypertrophy and sclerosis, ACE inhibition did not appreciably affect P_{GC} but did decrease sclerosis (80).

Because converting enzyme inhibition is more effective than other forms of antihypertensive therapy in abrogating glomerulosclerosis (211), perhaps the mechanism of this therapy is to block growth-factor-like effects rather than hemodynamic effects of angiotensin II. In addition, angiotensin may stimulate TGF-β synthesis (210). Although it is not clear whether effects of TGF-β or angiotensin II occur later in the sclerogenic pathway, it is likely that the two hormones, produced by multiple sources, have synergistic effects.

Abnormal glomerular cell function may reflect abnormalities intrinsic to the cell as well as responses triggered by mediators produced by other cells. In PAN nephrosis, mesangial cells in sclerotic glomeruli retain more colloidal carbon than do mesangial cells from nonsclerotic glomeruli (212). In the age-related glomerulosclerosis model of the Milan rat, cultured mesangial cells from affected rats show increased rates of growth compared with cells from normal controls (213). Glomeruli undergoing hypertrophy also express mRNA for protooncogenes associated with progression through the cell cycle (214). Some treatments directed toward altering systemic physiologic processes also may have direct modulatory effects on glomerular cell behavior. For example, the HMG–CoA-reductase inhibitor, lovastatin, which decreases plasma cholesterol concentrations by inhibiting hepatic cholesterol synthesis, has direct inhibitory effects on mesangial cell proliferation in the absence of elevated ambient lipid concentrations (215). Moreover, the salient effect of heparin on disease progression after subtotal nephrectomy, which is independent of glomerular hemodynamics (216), likely reflects a biologic effect of heparin on glomerular cells rather than an anticoagulant effect (217).

The response of glomerular cells to different stimuli may become more sclerogenic as the disease progresses. Normal cell–matrix interactions are critical to maintaining appropriately differentiated cell status (218); the nature of the cellular response to various signals depends in part upon cell attachment to matrix, binding of cell surface receptors for matrix proteins, and consequent determination of cell shape and activation of signal transduction mechanisms (219). Because the characteristics of the matrix will change as the sclerosis progresses, the nature of the cell–matrix interactions also is likely to change. Thus, the process of sclerosis will be sustaining, amplifying, and accelerating.

Figure 3 shows how a variety of physiologic processes associated with FSGS produce stimuli that lead to production of specific growth factors. Each of these in turn activates a variety of cellular reactions that initiate sclerosis. These events then cause further alterations in cell function that serve to perpetuate and amplify the sclerotic process.

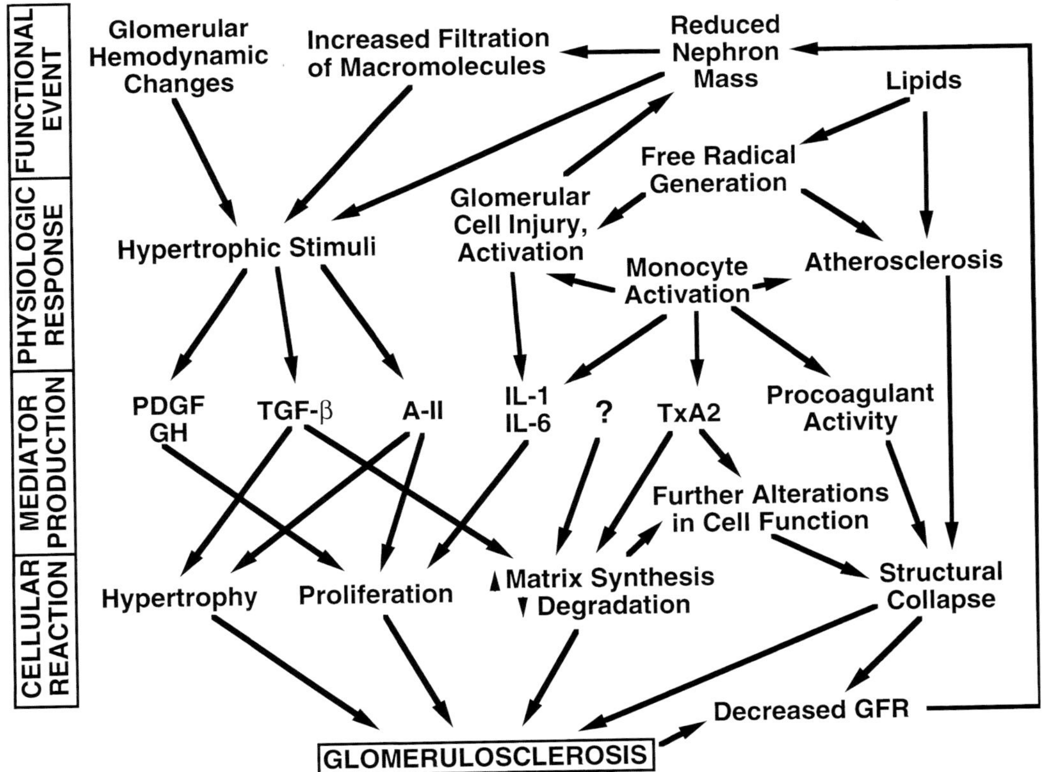

FIG. 3. Interaction among various factors involved in the pathogenesis of glomerulosclerosis.

CLINICAL ASPECTS OF FSGS

Presentation

Patients with FSGS can be categorized based on the presence or absence of nephrotic syndrome at presentation. Those who are nephrotic usually have the classic findings of albuminuria, hypoproteinemia, edema, and hypercholesterolemia (2). In three pediatric studies, 35 (20%) of 171 children with FSGS did not have nephrosis (220–222). The likelihood of adults presenting without nephrosis appears to be somewhat higher (9). However, the incidence of nephrotic syndrome in FSGS is difficult to determine accurately because some studies describe referral populations. Moreover, in older studies, where screening may have been performed less routinely and renal biopsy for relatively minor urinary abnormalities less aggressively pursued, nephrotic patients may have been more likely to be biopsied. Goldszer et al. suggest that the incidence of some sort of sclerotic lesion in biopsies performed to determine the basis of asymptomatic hematuria or proteinuria may be as high as 30–50% (9). Conversely, the incidence of FSGS in nephrotic children undergoing biopsy is 8–27% (223,224) and in nephrotic adults is only slightly higher (9).

Patients may present with FSGS at any age. In one study, the peak incidence for presentation in children occurred at 2–3 years of age. Interestingly, in this study, all of the children <3 years of age were male, accounting entirely for the male predominance found in the study (221). Although other studies have also cited a preponderance of male cases of FSGS, this is not universally true. Further, it is not clear whether such a preponderance might reflect the influence of other factors such as hypertension, atherosclerosis, or aging on the sclerotic process.

Although individual patients with MCNS or FSGS cannot be differentiated solely on the basis of clinical findings, nephrotic patients with FSGS are slightly more likely to present with hypertension, elevated serum creatinine concentration, and/or hematuria (222,225–228). In one study comparing children and adults with FSGS, children were less likely to be hypertensive or azotemic at the time of presentation than were adults (226). In adults, hypertension resulting from FSGS should be distinguished from the possibility of primary hypertension causing renal disease (48). This is especially important in African-American patients; as suggested by the familial clustering of renal diseases referred to previously, apparent hypertensive nephrosclerosis may prove to be FSGS on renal biopsy (229).

A renal biopsy is recommended in most nephrotic patients at presentation. Exceptions include some patients with other diseases that are likely to cause nephrosis, such as hepatitis B or HIV infection, or children aged 18 months to 6 years, in whom a therapeutic trial of corticosteroids is usually indicated. An alternative viewpoint is that, even in adults, a therapeutic trial of steroids may be as diagnostically useful as a biopsy (230).

Laboratory Findings

Urinalysis

The amount of proteinuria detected is a function of filtered load, fractional excretion, and fractional catabolism. Thus, although patients will usually have 3+ to 4+ dipstick proteinuria (>300 mg/dL), a patient with longstanding proteinuria and profound hypoalbuminemia (<1 g/dL) may have such a low filtered load of albumin that the protein content of the urine is relatively low. On the other hand, patients receiving parenteral albumin supplementation will spill most of it in the urine, markedly raising the daily urine protein excretion. In general, it is most useful to approximate the fixed urine protein by measuring protein excretion as a function of time or by determining the urine protein–creatinine ratio in nonazotemic patients. A normal ratio is <0.2 and a nephrotic-range result is usually considered to be >3.5 (231). In children, the quantity of proteinuria is often greater in FSGS than in MCNS (221).

The cause of proteinuria in FSGS remains a subject of some debate. Classically, MCNS has been considered to be a disorder of charge selectivity (232) because permselectivity curves show decreased fractional clearance of smaller macromolecules in MCNS (233) and proteinuria is selective for albumin. Proteinuria is generally felt to be less selective in FSGS, and permselectivity curves show both decreased clearance of smaller macromolecules and increased clearance of very large macromolecules (234). Nonetheless, at least one study has indicated that glomerular polyanion is reduced in FSGS as well as in MCNS (82). Moreover, it has been suggested that a combination of decreased pore radius and loss of electrostatic hindrance to filtration of anionic macromolecules is the basis of altered handling of proteins in both MCNS and FSGS (235).

The urinary sediment may show hematuria in up to 40% of cases. In uncomplicated nephrosis, the urine specific gravity should be elevated because of the nephrotic patient's tendency to retain fluid (2) and the presence of large amounts of additional solute (protein) in the urine. A low urine specific gravity may be of no significance but, if indicative of a urine concentrating defect, suggests the presence of tubulointerstitial disease, a sign of progressive renal involvement. Glycosuria (236) or the presence of *N*-acetyl-β-D-glucosaminidase or amino aciduria (237) also are potential signs of tubular dysfunction that suggest the presence of FSGS and the likelihood of disease progression. This possibility should be distinguished from Fanconi syndrome, which may present with proteinuria from the failure to reabsorb albumin from the glomerular filtrate.

Serum Chemistries

These depend upon the patient's presentation. Patients who are not nephrotic, and who present with isolated hematuria or proteinuria, may have no biochemical abnormalities of the serum or plasma. Nephrotic patients have hypoalbuminemia, and sometimes hypoproteinemia as well. Serum cholesterol is elevated. As the duration of nephrotic symptoms increases, plasma triglyceride concentrations also rise. The serum sodium may falsely appear to be low because of the dilutional effect of plasma lipids; the correct value can be determined from the sodium content of ultracentrifuged serum. True hyponatremia may reflect excessive antidiuretic hormone (238) or the dilutional effect of excess fluid intake in the face of sodium restriction and/or diuretics. Patients with or without nephrotic symptoms may have elevated serum urea nitrogen and creatinine values. If the patients are not nephrotic, these values reflect true impairment of glomerular filtration. Any patient with primary nephrotic syndrome, with or without FSGS, may manifest elevation of the serum urea nitrogen disproportionate to elevation of the serum creatinine because of decreased renal perfusion (2). Occasionally, nephrotic patients may develop reversible renal failure (239) secondary to intrarenal edema and disruption of the usual physical forces that maintain the GFR (240).

Serum IgG may be decreased in FSGS due to urinary losses. Individual serum complement components may be lost in the urine (241), but serologic evidence of complement consumption from renal inflammation is extremely rare.

TREATMENT OF FSGS

The broad spectrum of presentations and severity in FSGS make analysis of treatment difficult. At one time, it was felt that this disease had a uniformly negative outcome. However, this does not appear to be entirely true (see below). For this reason, aggressive treatment may be indicated unless side effects obviate its potential benefits. Treatment can be divided into therapy designed to address potential immune/inflammatory aspects of disease pathogenesis, symptomatic therapy, and treatments directed toward ameliorating disease progression by interrupting the physiologic events that have been associated with progression.

Treatments Directed Against Immune Dysfunction

Corticosteroid Therapy

Although FSGS is less responsive to steroids than is MCNS, some nephrotic patients with FSGS enter remission after steroid treatment. Treatment with at least 60 mg/day has been required for up to 9 months before some patients have responded. Even partial response to treatment using steroids, with or without alkylating agents, has stabilized renal function in 50% of nephrotic adults with FSGS (242).

At least half of patients, however, do not respond to conventional oral corticosteroids. Alternative therapeutic approaches have been sought. Children with prednisone-resistant FSGS have been treated with methylprednisolone boluses (30 mg/kg to a maximum of 1,000 mg) given intravenously every other day for six doses, followed by the same dose weekly for 10 weeks, with similar boluses thereafter on a tapering schedule. This was supplemented by oral prednisone, 2 mg/kg every other day, and some patients also received alkylating agents. Of 23 children treated, 12 entered remission, six had decreased proteinuria, and four remained nephrotic (243). Only one child developed renal failure (244). This treatment may lead to significant steroid-induced side effects, including the possibility of fatal infection (245), and it was found by others to be less efficacious when used in modified form (246). However, this aggressive use of corticosteroids yields a markedly improved response rate compared with other steroid protocols in children.

Alkylating/Cytotoxic Agents

Although only a minority of FSGS patients who are unresponsive to steroids will respond to alkylating agents (247), a report reviewing other studies found a significant increase in remission rate for patients receiving prednisone plus alkylating agents compared with patients receiving no treatment at all (248). Thus, despite the risks, a trial of cytotoxic therapy may be worth considering in selected patients. Only two of seven patients who had not responded to less aggressive forms of therapy benefited from the use of vincristine (249).

Children with FSGS may have a better response to treatment with cytotoxic drugs. A summary of nine series involving children (3) indicates that 57 (23%) of 247 children with FSGS were steroid responsive. Seventy unresponsive patients were treated with cytotoxic drugs, of whom 21 (30%) responded. Although 31% of the entire population responded to some sort of therapeutic intervention, only 20% of all the patients remained in remission by the time the studies were terminated. It was not possible to determine how many of these children presented with FSGS and nephrotic syndrome and how many were found to have this lesion only when they became steroid resistant after having had previous episodes of steroid-responsive nephrotic syndrome. These latter children usually prove resistant to all forms of treatment, including the use of cyclophosphamide (250). Although it has been reported that chlorambucil may be effective (251), this has not been evaluated in a prospective, controlled trial.

Cyclosporine and Macrolides

In a study of high-risk (black and Hispanic), unresponsive pediatric patients, very high doses of cyclosporine were used. Because cyclosporine is lipophilic, the higher doses were intended to counteract the effects of hyperlipidemia in these patients. Both proteinuria and the rate of disease progression were ameliorated (252). In contrast, in a study of 36 adults with INS, 14 of 36 patients had FSGS before initiation of cyclosporine therapy, 5.5 mg/kg/day. On repeat biopsy an average of 19.6 months later, FSGS was found in seven of the 22 patients with apparent MCNS on the initial biopsy, as well as in all 14 of the patients who had had FSGS previously. Unlike the patients with MCNS, the mean serum creatinine in the FSGS patients rose significantly. This was accounted for not by cyclosporine toxicity, but by progression of the glomerular FSGS lesion (253), suggesting that cyclosporine might exacerbate a tendency for glomerulosclerosis to develop or progress. Conflicting results reported with cyclosporine treatment may reflect differences in patient age or race; prospective, controlled studies would provide a more factual context for evaluating the efficacy of cyclosporine. FK-506 has been used in a small number of steroid-resistant nephrotics, including some with FSGS. The drug helped to control the level of proteinuria in some cases (254).

Symptomatic Treatment of Nephrotic Syndrome

Diuretics

In general, patients with nephrotic syndrome who are in a salt-retaining phase of their disease are somewhat less responsive to diuretics than are other patients with similar total-body water content. Although the explanation of this observation is the subject of some controversy, FSGS patients generally function as if their intravascular volume or effective arterial blood volume is decreased (2). There may be decreased glomerular perfusion with lowered distal tubular sodium delivery, interfering with diuretic effectiveness. Nonetheless, loop diuretics in conventional dosages are effective in most patients. In addition, metolazone or chlorthalidone are extremely effective singly or in combination with pure loop diuretics; caution should be employed in using diuretics so that excessive intravascular volume depletion does not lead to vascular collapse.

In patients with morbid edema, intravenous albumin may be an effective adjunct to diuretic therapy. The indications for such treatment include severe ascites with the potential for peritonitis, respiratory embarrassment from large pleural effusions, severe scrotal or vulval edema with potential for tissue breakdown, or other threatening complications. In addition, albumin infusion may be of diagnostic utility in patients who initially present with prolonged anuria due to avid sodium reabsorption. Intravenous 25% albumin, 1 g/kg up to 50 g, may be given; this should be followed by intravenous furosemide, 1 mg/kg up to 40 mg. Potential side effects of this treatment are severe and include the induction of hypertensive crisis or pulmonary edema. For this reason, it is recommended to begin with half the optimal albumin dose. An alternative means to induce diuresis or maintain steady fluid removal is by a continuous infusion of albumin. Repeated albumin infusions may delay remission in steroid-responsive nephrotic patients (255); in steroid-resistant patients, ongoing loss of albumin from the vascular space may ultimately expand the extravascular volume, worsening edema and decreasing the driving force for glomerular filtration. Therefore, regular use of albumin to maintain vascular volume and urine output is not recommended in most patients with FSGS.

Dietary Restriction of Sodium and Water

Nephrotic patients often appear to be in a sodium-retaining state and would benefit from limitation of sodium intake to ≤1,000 mg/day. Water intake can be restricted to ongoing urine output plus insensible losses. If this is not practical, adherence to a prescription approximating the sum of these two numbers will help to prevent increasing fluid retention.

Antihypertensive Therapy

This should be provided as needed to maintain acceptable levels of blood pressure. Before initiating treatment for high blood pressure, the patient should be evaluated for orthostasis and evidence of good tissue perfusion to rule out the possibility that hypertension represents a renin-mediated response to intravascular volume depletion. Use of antihypertensive agents to prevent or ameliorate disease progression is considered below.

Antibiotics or Vaccines

Infectious complications are a significant potential problem in nephrotic syndrome. Any sign of infection, such as fever, respiratory symptoms, severe abdominal pain, or localized swelling or tenderness, should be aggressively evaluated and, if appropriate, empiric antibiotic therapy should be initiated. Prophylactic antibiotics such as oral penicillin, 250 mg twice daily, are indicated for patients who have had repeated serious bacterial infections, but are not totally effective. Patients appear particularly susceptible to pneumococcal infections. In children, polyvalent pneumococcal vaccine and immunization against *Haemophilus influenzae* are recommended (256), although the efficacy of these vaccines may be suboptimal in patients who are losing immunoglobulin and opsonizing factors in the urine (257).

Treatment of Other Aspects of the Nephrotic State

Prolonged albuminuria depletes an important intravascular carrier protein. Other proteins may be lost as well. These should be considered in treating nephrotic patients. For example, vitamin-D-binding protein is lost in the urine, with concomitant loss of 25-OH-D. Patients with chronic nephrosis have profoundly decreased bone mineralization (258). For this reason, blood ionized calcium should be evaluated in patients with FSGS, and 25-OH-D supplementation should be considered. Thyroid-binding globulin is lost in the nephrotic urine; although patients with FSGS may therefore have low thyroid hormone levels, they are usually clinically euthyroid (259). The effects of loss of albumin as a carrier protein should also be considered when evaluating dosages and measured levels of drugs that are normally bound to plasma albumin in significant proportions, such as digoxin and anticonvulsants.

Treatments Directed at Physiologic Events Implicated in the Pathogenesis of Glomerulosclerosis

Antihypertensive Agents

In the diabetic rat, captopril therapy and combined therapy with reserpine, hydralazine, and hydrochlorthiazide were equally effective at lowering blood pressure. The initial pathologic findings were similar, but the triple-therapy regimen only delayed development of glomerulosclerosis. Protection was better in the captopril group in the short and longer terms, at least in part because the P_{GC} eventually rose despite the triple therapy. It did not rise in the captopril-treated rats (260). Similar results were obtained in rats subjected to subtotal nephrectomy and treated with enalapril (105). In humans, controlled trials indicate that ACE inhibitors in type I (261) and type II (262) diabetes are effective in reducing the relative risk of progressive renal failure in diabetic nephropathy. At least for this condition, such therapy is now recommended in high-risk individuals (263). Meta-analysis of published studies suggests that similar treatment also may be effective in other renal diseases (264).

Therapeutic Manipulations Intended to Reduce Hyperfiltration

If glomerulosclerosis is the result of increased permeability to macromolecules (hyperfiltration), decreasing the driving force for filtration should therefore improve outcome. In an uncontrolled pilot study, the nonsteroidal anti-inflammatory agent, meclofenamate, was found to reduce urine protein excretion by 40% without decreasing the total effective GFR in more than half of the 30 steroid-resistant nephrotic adults studied, 16 of whom had FSGS (265). In view of the potential renal toxicity of nonsteroidals, especially in volume-depleted patients such as nephrotics on diuretics (266), the effect of long-term use of this class of drugs remains to be determined. An alternative approach is restriction of dietary protein intake. This treatment, which reduces the filtered load of protein, ameliorates glomerular damage in progressive glomerulosclerosis in rats (111). It has been reported to be effective in slowing the rate of disease progression in humans (267), although subsequent studies found this to be true only under certain conditions (268). Although the mechanism of effect of decreased dietary protein intake is likely to involve altered glomerular perfusion and hyperfiltration, a role of calorie reduction in severely restricted diets cannot be excluded (269). Dietary protein restriction leads to general downregulation of expression of various mRNAs involved in ECM turnover in PAN nephrosis (178) and of genes related to the renin–angiotensin system in rats (270), suggesting that diet may also have direct effects on cell function as well as modulating hemodynamics. Dietary protein restriction also decreases plasma renin activity in humans (271). Thus, antihypertensive therapy or dietary restriction may be beneficial because of amelioration of glomerular hypertension because of effects on urinary filtration of protein, or via modulation of growth factors or cytokines (106,272). In view of studies showing beneficial effects, these treatment strategies may be useful in selected patients. However, the utility of chronic protein restriction in children should be weighed against the need to have adequate nutrition for growth.

Lipid-Lowering Agents

In nephrotic patients, elevated lipid levels may initiate or exacerbate the development of atherosclerotic cardiovascular disease. Moreover, in view of the likelihood that lipid-mediated damage is a participant in disease progression, decreasing plasma lipids may help to retard sclerosis. Low-density lipoprotein apheresis led to stabilization of function in a 15-year-old boy with rapidly progressing FSGS; this stabilization was subsequently maintained with pravastatin (273). Lipid-lowering agents are effective for reducing plasma cholesterol in nephrotic patients, especially HMG–CoA-reductase inhibitors (274). In obese Zucker rats, lovastatin delays progression of renal disease (275). Dietary supplementation with polyunsaturated fatty acids improves outcome in obese Zucker rats (276) or after subtotal nephrectomy in normal rats (277). It is noteworthy that lovastatin also enhances glomerular protease activity, suggesting that hyperlipidemia impairs normal ECM turnover (278).

Anticoagulant Therapy

Children with FSGS who were unresponsive to prednisone and cyclophosphamide were given prednisone plus dipyridamole or aspirin as a platelet inhibitor, with or without systemic anticoagulants. Platelet half-life was increased and proteinuria was decreased. Creatinine clearance was better preserved over time with use of platelet antagonists compared with controls (133). As discussed above, the effect of at least some anticoagulants may be through biologic effects beyond the coagulation system. Alternatively, use of antiplatelet agents is advocated by some clinicians to prevent venous thrombosis. Coagulopathy is most likely to pose a problem in patients who are intravascularly volume depleted. However, a review of the literature indicates that acute thrombotic events are much less common in FSGS than they are in membranous nephropathy (2). Thus, use of anticoagulants in FSGS patients should be reserved for those at highest risk for thrombotic events.

Therapeutic Approach to Patients

From the foregoing discussion, it is apparent that the approach to pediatric and adult patients is different. In general, pediatric nephrologists have tended to be more aggressive in treating FSGS. If a patient is not nephrotic and has normal renal function, there is no clear indication for a specific therapy. Like children, nephrotic adults may benefit from an extended trial of corticosteroids, up to 60–80 mg/day, because a majority of untreated patients will almost certainly reach renal failure. At most, however, ~50% of nephrotic adults will benefit from such treatment, and its potential benefit should be weighed against the ability to tolerate steroid toxicity. Symptomatic treatment should include judicious use of diuretics. ACE inhibitors may decrease proteinuria and retard disease progression, although the benefits of such therapy have been proven in large, controlled trials only in diabetics. Dietary protein restriction requires compliance with severe limitations in intake that may be difficult to achieve; because the efficacy of this intervention have not been proven in FSGS, its implementation should be considered only as a last resort.

In children, aggressive treatment is the most widely used approach. Most pediatric patients will have received oral prednisone for some time before undergoing renal biopsy. The recent success in treating some children with high-dose boluses of methylprednisolone is promising. Such treatment has significant side effects in children and is probably excessively toxic for older adults. Cyclosporine, widely reported to lack efficacy and perhaps even exacerbate FSGS in adults, has been used successfully in some children. Addressing the effectiveness of specific treatments requires studying a large number of patients in a controlled study. In pediatric patients, this would mandate a multicenter, controlled trial. Until the practical problems inherent to such studies can be overcome, the decision to use a specific therapy remains a matter of clinical judgment.

CLINICAL COURSE AND OUTCOME

Clinical Patterns in FSGS

As discussed previously, patients with FSGS may or may not have overt nephrotic symptoms. At least some nephrotic patients appear to have a more aggressive disease, with a rapid course that results in loss of renal function within 2–3 years. In contrast, those without nephrosis generally fare better. In one study of American adult patients, 92% of nonnephrotic patients with FSGS had renal survival after 10 years, whereas only 57% of nephrotic patients had renal survival (242). In a study of Japanese pediatric patients, however, symptoms at presentation did not affect outcome (222). Response to treatment also helps to predict outcome. In children, three types of patients have been defined: those who are steroid responsive, those who are initially steroid responsive but subsequently (usually within 18 months of presentation) become steroid resistant, and those who never respond to steroids. Whereas patients in the first group usually have a favorable prognosis, the other groups showed a high incidence of progression to renal insufficiency (279). A subgroup of patients has been defined that are young, severely nephrotic, and hypertensive, have nonselective proteinuria, and progress rapidly; a vascular component may be involved in these patients (62).

Complications of FSGS

Infection

Peritonitis is a particularly common in nephrotic syndrome in children (280), with some patients experiencing repeated episodes. It usually occurs in the presence of massive ascites. The most common infecting organism remains *Streptococcus pneumoniae*, which is found in approximately half of the cases (280); *Escherichia coli* is cultured in a further 25%; other organisms, including *Haemophilus influenzae*, also may be found. Other frequent infections include sepsis and pneumonia. Adults appear to show increased susceptibility to infection as well; when severe, this tendency may be mitigated by intravenous immunoglobulin replacement (281).

Complications of Treatment

The most common complications observed in patients with nephrotic syndrome may be iatrogenic. Steroid-induced side effects include infection, obesity, osteopenia, hirsutism, striae, and pseudotumor cerebri. Hypertension may occur but is seen less frequently if patients adhere to a sodium-restricted diet. Children who have received high doses of steroids for protracted periods of time show growth retardation; catch-up growth often occurs when steroid therapy is discontinued (282). Corticosteroid-induced cataracts have been found in a high percentage of children (283) but rarely impair visual acuity. The complications of alkylating agents include lymphopenia, bone-marrow suppression, seizures (associated with chlorambucil), and bladder toxicity (with cyclophosphamide), and potential long-term effects such as gonadal dysfunction or susceptibility to cancer. The long-term effects can be reduced by limiting the dosage and duration of cytotoxic therapy (2).

Thrombotic Phenomena

The incidence of thrombotic events is 1.8% in nephrotic children (284) and as high as 26% in adults (285). Thrombosis is especially common in the renal vein, where the blood is hemoconcentrated and where circulating inhibitors of coagulation may have been lost in the urine. Although thrombosis is more common in other forms of glomerular disease such as membranous nephropathy, patients with FSGS who are nephrotic do have a tendency toward thrombotic diathesis.

Complications of Pregnancy

Patients with FSGS show a high incidence of severe complications of pregnancy, including spontaneous abortion, stillbirth, and neonatal death (286). In addition, preeclampsia has been implicated rarely in FSGS (12). It is unclear whether this usually reversible lesion, which was distinguished from subclinical disease that might become manifest during pregnancy, is identical to the lesion of idiopathic FSGS.

Deaths in Patients with FSGS

In an older report on long-term outcome of treating nephrotic children, deaths from steroid-responsive disease were rare. In contrast, 20% of steroid-unresponsive patients, most of whom had FSGS, died (287). Many of the deaths were from infection, suggesting that aggressive efforts to induce remission may have led to profound immunosuppression. Other nonrenal causes of death that may be encountered include thromboembolic phenomena, hemorrhagic pancreatitis (224), and hypovolemic shock.

Prognosis

The outcome in FSGS is usually linked to the issue of response to treatment. A review of the literature regarding adult patients found that only five of 76 steroid-responsive patients but 46 of 100 steroid-unresponsive patients required ESRD therapy, although the length of follow-up varied among the studies (288). In a follow-up study ranging from 7 to 217 months, the Southwest Pediatric Nephrology Study Group reported that 21% of children with FSGS developed ESRD, another 23% had reduced GFR, and 37% had persistent proteinuria only; 11% were in remission and 8% were lost to follow-up (221). In a recently published retrospective study of adult patients, all patients who showed at least decreased proteinuria in response to prednisone had renal function 10 years later. In contrast unresponsive patients and untreated patients had similar (40%) 10-year renal survival.

Certain characteristics on renal biopsy may help to identify FSGS patients who will have progressive disease and a poor outcome. These include the presence of crescents (289), interstitial infiltrates (221,225), or mesangial hypercellularity (68,69,72,290). For example, in a group of FSGS patients followed for 1–10 years, 10 of 13 who had mesangial accentuation and proliferation in nonsclerotic portions of the glomeruli had values for GFR reduced to <90 mL/min/1.73 m^2; four of these patients had advanced renal failure. In contrast, none of the 11 patients without mesangial involvement had a similar reduction in renal function (69). Not all studies agree with this conclusion. It has been suggested that most patients with FSGS will develop mesangial hypercellularity at some stage in their disease course and that this pathologic abnormality does not correlate with prognosis (221). A better predictor of poor outcome is interstitial fibrosis (221,222,242). Tubulointerstitial involvement remains the most ominous prognostic indicator.

Because identical biopsy findings may have different outcomes, additional prognostic information can be gleaned from the patients' clinical findings. For example, presentation with nephrotic syndrome may suggest a more progressive lesion, although patients in whom nephrotic syndrome develops after proteinuria of considerable duration may have a more indolent form of the disease (242,291). Although the more indolent form of the disease may progress to renal failure (292), patients with early appearance of FSGS more frequently follow a rapid downhill course (291). In contrast, patients who develop late-onset FSGS are classically less responsive to steroids (250), again suggesting two distinct disease mechanisms yielding a common histopathologic finding. Other clinical indicators of a poor prognosis include hypertension and male sex (225).

Transplantation

Recurrence of FSGS is an accepted hazard in renal transplants (21,293). Habib and Kleinknecht found recurrence of FSGS in 26 of 229 transplant patients (224). In another report, a high percentage of patients who developed ESRD within 3 years of diagnosis of FSGS also experienced recurrence in their transplanted kidneys. Half of these patients lost the graft secondary to recurrent disease (294). The lesion appears to begin with focal segmental epithelial proliferation, followed by later scarring (295). Massive proteinuria may begin within the first 24 h after transplantation. The association of recurrence with the aggressive form of FSGS would again suggest that the rapidly progressive form represents a disease caused by a systemic factor, whereas the more indolent form may be a distinct entity resulting from damage induced by prolonged proteinuria. Further evidence for a circulating factor related to some forms of FSGS is provided by Savin and colleagues, who have found that sera from certain FSGS patients induce a marked change in albumin permeability of isolated rat glomeruli. The presence of this activity in patient serum corresponds with rapid recurrence of proteinuria and development of FSGS in the transplanted kidney (296).

The recurrence of nephrotic syndrome after renal transplantation is particularly difficult to treat. Anecdotal data suggest that plasmapheresis, in some cases with intensified immunosuppression, is effective in a number of patients (296,297). Other researchers have found that adsorption of patient plasma with a protein-A–Sepharose column similarly causes a decrease in urinary protein excretion. Although the column is most often used to remove IgG from plasma, initial characterization of the activity suggests that it is not an immunoglobulin (298).

CONCLUSION

FSGS is a pathologic diagnosis that describes the physical result of a series of events by which previously normal glomeruli undergo matrix accumulation and structural collapse. In some cases, it is idiopathic; in others, it represents a reaction to systemic disease or the result of other renal diseases. Different clinical outcomes are consistent with the existence of an heterogeneous group of diseases that have the common pathologic finding of FSGS. A special role for the immune system in both primary and secondary FSGS is suggested by emerging understanding of the role of lymphocytes and macrophages in FSGS, and by the fact that the best treatments for these disease are steroids, alkylating agents, and immunosuppressive agents directed against immune function. These therapies are not optimal, however. More specific treatments are likely to be derived from improved understanding of the underlying cellular mechanisms involved.

ACKNOWLEDGMENTS

This work was supported by grants DK51724 from the National Institute of Diabetes, Digestive and Kidney Diseases and HL49362 from the National Heart, Lung and Blood Institute.

REFERENCES

1. Rich AR. A hitherto undescribed vulnerability of the juxtamedullary glomeruli in lipoid nephrosis. *Bull Johns Hopkins Hosp* 1957;100:173–80.
2. Schnaper HW, Robson AM. Nephrotic syndrome: minimal change disease, focal glomerulosclerosis and related disorders. In: Schrier RW, Gottschalk CW, eds. *Diseases of the kidney.* 5th ed. Boston: Little, Brown, 1992:1731–84.
3. Melvin T, Sibley R, Michael AF. Nephrotic syndrome. In: Tune BM, Mendoza SA, eds. *Contemporary issues in nephrology: pediatric nephrology.* New York: Churchill Livingstone, 1984:191–230.
4. Nanra RS, Stuart-Taylor J, DeLeon AH, White KH. Analgesic nephropathy: etiology, clinical syndrome, and clinicopathologic correlations in Australia. *Kidney Int* 1978;13:79–92.
5. Cunningham EE, Brentjens JR, Zielezny MA, Andres GA, Venuto RC. Heroin nephropathy: a clinicopathologic and epidemiology study. *Am J Med* 1980;68:47–53.
6. Warshaw BL, Edelbrock HH, Ettinger RB, et al. Progression to end-stage renal disease in children with obstructive uropathy. *J Pediatr* 1982;100:183–7.
7. Kiprov DD, Colvin RB, McCluskey RT. Focal and segmental glomerulosclerosis and proteinuria associated with unilateral renal agenesis. *Lab Invest* 1982;46:275–81.
8. Bernstein J. Renal hypoplasia and dysplasia. In: Edelmann CM, ed. *Pediatric kidney disease.* Boston: Little, Brown, 1978:541–56.
9. Goldszer RC, Sweet J, Cotran RS. Focal segmental glomerulosclerosis. *Annu Rev Med* 1984;35:429–49.
10. Jennette JC, Charles L, Grubb W. Glomerulomegaly and focal segmental glomerulosclerosis associated with sleep-apnea syndrome. *Am J Kidney Dis* 1987;10:470–2.
11. Verani RA. Obesity-associated focal segmental glomerulosclerosis: pathological features of the lesion and relationship with cardiomegaly and hyperlipidemia. *Am J Kidney Dis* 1992;20:629–34.
12. Nagai Y, Arai H, Washazara Y, et al. FSGS-like lesions in pre-eclampsia. *Clin Nephrol* 1991;36:134–40.
13. D'Agati V, Suh J-I, Carbone L, Cheng J-T, Appel G. Pathology of HIV-associated nephropathy: a detailed morphologic and comparative study. *Kidney Int* 1989;35:1358–70.
14. Mauer SM, Bilous RW, Ellis E, Harris R, Steffes MW. Some lessons from the studies of renal biopsies in patients with insulin-dependent diabetes mellitus. *J Diabetic Complications* 1988;2:197–202.
15. Pearson J, Gallo G, Gluck M, Axelrod F. Renal disease in familial dysautonomia. *Kidney Int* 1980;17:102–12.
16. Bogdanovic R, Komar P, Cvoric A, et al. Focal glomerular sclerosis and nephrotic syndrome in spondyloepiphyseal dysplasia. *Nephron* 1994;66:219–24.
17. Verani RR, Conley SB. Sickle cell glomerulopathy with focal segmental glomerulosclerosis. *Child Nephrol Urol* 1991;11:206–8.
18. Anderson SA, Brenner BM. Effects of aging on the renal glomerulus. *Am J Med* 1986;80:435–42.
19. Eagen JW, Lewis EJ. Glomerulopathies of neoplasia. *Kidney Int* 1977;11:297–306.
20. Watson A, Stachura I, Fragola J, Bourke E. Focal segmental glomerulosclerosis in Hodgkin's disease. *Am J Nephrol* 1983;3:228–32.

21. Lewis EJ. Recurrent focal sclerosis after renal transplantation. *Kidney Int* 1982;22:315–23.
22. Cheigh JS, Mouradian J, Soliman M, et al. Focal segmental glomerulosclerosis in renal transplants. *Am J Kidney Dis* 1983;2:449–55.
23. Martinelli R, Perira LJC, Brito E, Rocha H. Clinical course of focal segmental glomerulosclerosis associated with hepatosplenic schistosomiasis mansoni. *Nephron* 1995;69:131–4.
24. Kala U, Milner LS, Jacobs DJ, Thomson PD. Impact of tuberculosis in children with idiopathic nephrotic syndrome. *Pediatr Nephrol* 1993;7:392–5.
25. Joh K, Usui N, Aizawa S, et al. Focal segmental glomerulosclerosis associated with infantile spasms in five mentally retarded children: a morphological analysis on mesangiolysis. *Am J Kidney Dis* 1991;17: 569–77.
26. Baldwin DS. Chronic glomerulonephritis: nonimmunologic mechanisms of progressive glomerular damage. *Kidney Int* 1982;21:109–20.
27. Lee HS, Koh HI. Nature of progressive glomerulosclerosis in human membranous nephropathy. *Clin Nephrol* 1993;39:7–16.
28. Glasssock RJ, Adler SG, Ward HJ, Cohen AH. Primary glomerular diseases. In: Brenner BM, Rector FC, eds. *The kidney.* Philadelphia: WB Saunders, 1991:1182–279.
29. Chandra M, Mouradian J, Hoyer FR. Familial nephrotic syndrome and focal segmental glomerulosclerosis. *J Pediatr* 1981;98:556–60.
30. Bader PL, Grove J, Trygstad CW, et al. Familial nephrotic syndrome. *Am J Med* 1974;56:34–43.
31. McCurdy FA, Butera PJ, Wilson M. The familial occurrence of focal segmental glomerular sclerosis. *Am J Kidney Dis* 1987;10:467–9.
32. Moncrieff MW, White RHR, Glasgow EF, Winterborn MH, Cameron JS, Ogg CS. The familial nephrotic syndrome. II. A clinicopathologic study. *Clin Nephrol* 1973;1:220–9.
33. Kim P-K, Pai K-S, Hwang CH, Park MS, Jeong HJ, Choi IJ. Familial nephrotic syndrome and HLA-DR5. *Child Nephrol Urol* 1991;11:55–60.
34. Trainin EB, Gomez-Leon G. HLA identity in siblings with focal glomerulosclerosis. *Int J Pediatr Nephrol* 1983;4:59–60.
35. Glicklich D, Haskell L, Senitzer D, Weiss RA. Possible genetic predisposition to idiopathic focal segmental glomerulosclerosis. *Am J Kidney Dis* 1988;12:26–30.
36. Lagueruela CC, Buettner TL, Cole BR, Kissane JM, Robson AM. HLA extended haplotypes in steroid-sensitive nephrotic syndrome of childhood. *Kidney Int* 1990;38:145–50.
37. Noss G, Bachmann HJ, Olbing H. Association of minimal change nephrotic syndrome (MCNS) with HLA-B8 and B-13. *Clin Nephrol* 1981;15:172–4.
38. O'Regan D, O'Callaghan U, Dundon S, Reen DJ. HLA antigens and steroid responsive nephrotic syndrome of childhood. *Tissue Antigens* 1980;16:147–51.
39. Lenhard V, Muller-Wiefel DE, Dippell J, Schroder D, Seidel S, Scharer K. HLA in minimal change nephrotic syndrome and focal segmental glomerulosclerosis. *Pediatr Res* 1980;14:1003A.
40. Tejani A, Nicastri A, Phadke K, et al. Familial focal segmental glomerulosclerosis. *Int J Pediatr Nephrol* 1983;4:231–4.
41. Ruder H, Scharer K, Opelz G, et al. Human leukocyte antigens in idiopathic nephrotic syndrome in children. *Pediatr Nephrol* 1990;4: 478–81.
42. Haskell LP, Glicklich D, Senitzer D. HLA associations in heroin-associated nephropathy. *Am J Kidney Dis* 1988;12:45–50.
43. Komori K, Nose Y, Inouye H, et al. Immunogenetical study in patients with chronic glomerulonephritis. *Tokai J Exp Clin Med* 1983; 8:135–48.
44. Noel LH, Descamps B, Jungers P, et al. HLA antigens in three types of glomerulonephritis. *Clin Immunol Immunopathol* 1983;10:19–23.
45. Freedman BI, Spray BJ, Heise ER. HLA associations in IgA nephropathy and focal and segmental glomerulosclerosis. *Am J Kidney Dis* 1994;23:352–7.
46. Ingulli E, Tejani A. Racial differences in the incidence and renal outcome of idiopathic focal segmental glomerulosclerosis in children. *Pediatr Nephrol* 1991;5:393–7.
47. Pettitt DJ, Saad MF, Bennett PH, Nelson RG, Knowler WC. Familial predisposition to renal disease in two generations of Pima Indians with type-2 (non-insulin-dependent) diabetes mellitus. *Diabetologia* 1990;33:438–43.
48. Freedman BI, Isakander SS, Appel RG. The link between hypertension and nephrosis. *Am J Kidney Dis* 1995;25:207–21.
49. Spray BJ, Atassi NG, Tuttle AB, Freedman BI. Familial risk, age at onset, and cause of end-stage renal disease in white Americans. *J Am Soc Nephrol* 1995;5:1806–10.
50. Bergman SM, Key BO, Rostand SG, Warnock DG. Familial characteristics of African Americans with H-ESRD in Jefferson County, AL. *J Am Soc Nephrol* 1994;5:325(abst).
51. Pesce C, Schmidt K, Fogo A, et al. Glomerular size and the incidence of renal disease in African Americans and Caucasians. *J Nephrol* 1994;7:355–8.
52. Gubler M-C, Broyer M, Habib R. Signification des lesions de sclerose/hyalinose segmentaire et focal (S/HSF) dans la nephrose. In: *Proceedings of the eighth international congress of nephrology.* Basel: Karger, 1978:437.
53. Habib R. Focal glomerulosclerosis. *Kidney Int* 1973;4:355–61.
54. Morel-Maroger L, Leathem A, Richet G. Glomerular abnormalities in non-systemic diseases: relationship between findings by light microscopy and immunofluorescence in 433 renal biopsy specimens. *Am J Med* 1972;53:170–84.
55. Thoenes W, Rumpelt HJ. The obsolescent renal glomerulus: collapse, sclerosis, hyalinosis, fibrosis. *Virchows Arch [A]* 1977;377:1–15.
56. Churg J, Habib R, White RHR. Pathology of the nephrotic syndrome in children: a report for the International Study of Kidney Disease in Children. *Lancet* 1970;1:1299–302.
57. Ellis D, Kapur S, Antonovych T, Salcedo JR. Focal glomerulosclerosis in children: correlation of histology with prognosis. *J Pediatr* 1978;93:762–8.
58. Fogo A, Glick AD, Horn SL, Horn RG. Is focal segmental glomerulosclerosis really focal? Distribution of lesions in adults and children. *Kidney Int* 1995;47:1690–6.
59. Hyman LR, Burkholder PM. Focal sclerosing glomerulonephropathy with segmental hyalinosis: a clinicopathologic analysis. *Lab Invest* 1973;28:533–44.
60. Detwiler RK, Falk RJ, Hogan SL, Jennette JC. Collapsing glomerulopathy: a clinically and pathologically distinct variant of focal segmental glomerulosclerosis. *Kidney Int* 1994;45:1416–24.
61. Siegel NJ, Kashgarian M, Spargo BH, Hayslett JP. Minimal change and focal sclerotic lesions in lipoid nephrosis. *Nephron* 1974;13:125–37.
62. Brown CB, Cameron JS, Turner DR, et al. Focal segmental glomerulosclerosis with rapid decline in renal function ("malignant FSGS"). *Clin Nephrol* 1978;10:51–61.
63. Artinano M, Etheridge WB, Stroehlein KB, Barcenas CG. Progression of minimal-change glomerulopathy to focal glomerulosclerosis in a patient with fenprofen nephropathy. *Am J Nephrol* 1986;6:353–7.
64. Hayslett JP, Krasser LS, Bensch KG, Kashgarian M, Epstein FH. Progression of "lipid nephrosis" to renal insufficiency. *N Engl J Med* 1969;281:181–7.
65. Fogo A, Hawkins EP, Berry PL, et al. Glomerular hypertrophy in minimal change disease predicts subsequent progression to focal glomerular sclerosis. *Kidney Int* 1990;38:115–23.
66. Trainin EB, Gomez-Leon G. Development of renal insufficiency after long-standing steroid-responsive nephrotic syndrome. *Int J Pediatr Nephrol* 1982;3:55–8.
67. Lichtig C, Ben-Izhak O, On A, Levy J, Allon U. Childhood minimal change disease and focal segmental glomerulosclerosis: a continuous spectrum of disease. *Am J Nephrol* 1991;11:325–31.
68. Hirszel P, Yamase HT, Carney WR, et al. Mesangial proliferative glomerulonephritis with IgM deposits: clinicopathologic analysis and evidence for morphologic transitions. *Nephron* 1984;38:100–8.
69. Schoeneman MJ, Bennett B, Greifer I. The natural history of focal segmental glomerulosclerosis with and without hypercellularity in children. *Clin Nephrol* 1978;9:45–54.
70. Border WA. Distinguishing minimal change disease from mesangial disorders. *Kidney Int* 1988;34:419–34.
71. Rosen S, Galvanek E, Levy M, Habib R. Glomerular disease. *Hum Pathol* 1981;12:964–77.
72. Waldherr R, Gubler MC, Levy M, Broyer M, Habib R. The significance of pure diffuse mesangial proliferation in idiopathic nephrotic syndrome. *Clin Nephrol* 1978;10:171–9.
73. Roy LP, Vernier RL, Michael AF. Effect of protein-load proteinuria on glomerular polyanion. *Proc Soc Exp Biol Med* 1972;141:870–4.
74. Weening JJ, van Guldener C, Daha MR, Klar N, van der Wal A, Prins FA. The pathophysiology of protein-overload proteinuria. *Am J Pathol* 1987;129:64–73.

75. Deen WM, Maddox DA, Robertson CR, Brenner BM. Dynamics of glomerular ultrafiltration in the rat. VII. Response to reduced renal mass. *Am J Physiol* 1974;227:556–62.
76. Olson JL, Hostetter TH, Rennke HG, Brenner BM, Venkatachalam MA. Altered glomerular permselectivity and progressive sclerosis following extreme ablation of renal mass. *Kidney Int* 1982;22:112–26.
77. Robson AM, Mor J, Root ER, et al. Mechanism of proteinuria in non-glomerular renal disease. *Kidney Int* 1979;16:416–29.
78. Bagchus WM, Jeunink MF, Elema JD. The mesangium in anti-Thy1 nephritis: influx of macrophages, mesangial cell hypercellularity, and macromolecular accumulation. *Am J Pathol* 1990;137:215–23.
79. Glasser RJ, Velosa JA, Michael AF. Experimental model of focal sclerosis. I. Relationship to protein excretion in aminonucleoside nephrosis. *Lab Invest* 1977;36:519–26.
80. Fogo A, Yoshida Y, Glick AD, Homma T, Ichikawa I. Serial micropuncture analysis of glomerular function in two rat models of glomerulosclerosis. *J Clin Invest* 1988;82:322–30.
81. Velosa JA, Glasser RJ, Nevins TE, Michael AF. Experimental model of focal sclerosis. II. Correlation with immunopathologic changes, macromolecular kinetics and polyanion loss. *Lab Invest* 1977;36: 527–34.
82. Kitano Y, Yoshikawa N, Nakamura H. Glomerular anionic sites in minimal change nephrotic syndrome and focal segmental glomerulosclerosis. *Clin Nephrol* 1993;40:199–204.
83. Makino H, Yamasaki Y, Hironaka K, Ota Z. Glomerular extracellular matrices in rat diabetic glomerulopathy by scanning electron microscopy. *Virchows Arch [B]* 1992;62:19–24.
84. Yong LC, Bleasel AF. Pathological changes in streptozotocin induced diabetes mellitus in the rat. *Exp Pathol* 1986;30:97–107.
85. Han JS, Doi K. Morphometric study on the renal glomeruli of streptozotocin (SZ)-induced diabetic APA hamsters. *Histol Histopathol* 1992;7:549–54.
86. Tolins JP, Stone BG, Raij L. Interactions of hypercholesterolemia and hypertension in initiation of glomerular injury. *Kidney Int* 1992;41: 1254–61.
87. Al-Shebeb T, Frohlich J, Magil AB. Glomerular disease in hypercholesterolemic guinea pigs: a pathogenetic study. *Kidney Int* 1988;33: 498–507.
88. Raij L, Azar S, Keane WF. Role of hypertension in progressive glomerular immune injury. *Hypertension* 1985;7:398–404.
89. Raij L, Azar S, Keane W. Mesangial immune injury, hypertension and progressive glomerular damage in Dahl rats. *Kidney Int* 1984;26: 137–43.
90. Elema JD, Arends A. Focal and segmental glomerular hyalinosis and sclerosis in the rat. *Lab Invest* 1975;33:554–61.
91. Simons JL, Provoost AP, Anderson S, et al. Pathogenesis of glomerular injury in the fawn-hooded rat: early glomerular capillary hypertension predicts glomerular sclerosis. *J Am Soc Nephrol* 1993;3:1775–82.
92. Brown DM, Provoost AP, Daly MJ, Lander ES, Jacob HJ. Genetic identification of *RF-1*, a gene responsible for renal failure in the fawn-hooded rat. *J Am Soc Nephrol* 1994;5:618(abst).
93. Kamanna VS, Kirschenbaum MA. Association between very-low-density lipoprotein and glomerular injury in obese Zucker rats. *Am J Nephrol* 1993;13:53–58.
94. Kasiske BL, O'Donnell MP, Lee H, Kim Y, Keane WF. Impact of dietary fatty acid supplementation in obese Zucker rats. *Kidney Int* 1991;39:1125–34.
95. Kopp JB, Klotman ME, Adler SH, et al. Progressive glomerulosclerosis and enhanced renal accumulation of basement membrane components in mice transgenic for human immunodeficiency virus type 1 genes. *Proc Natl Acad Sci USA* 1992;89:1577–81.
96. Doi T, Striker LJ, Quaife C, et al. Progressive glomerulosclerosis develops in transgenic mice expressing growth hormone and growth hormone releasing factor but not in those expressing insulinlike growth factor-1. *Am J Pathol* 1988;131:398–403.
97. MacKay K, Striker LJ, Stauffer JW, Agodoa LY, Striker GE. Relationship of glomerular hypertrophy and sclerosis: studies in SV-40 transgenic mice. *Kidney Int* 1990;37:741–8.
98. Suematsu S, Matsuda T, Aozasa K, et al. IgG1 plasmacytosis in interleukin 6 transgenic mice. *Proc Natl Acad Sci USA* 1989;86:7547–51.
99. Stein PL, Vogel H, Soriano P. Combined deficiencies of Src, Fyn, and Yes tyrosine kinases in mutant mice. *Genes Dev* 1994;8:1997–2007.
100. Weiher H, Noda T, Gray DA, Sharpe AH, Jaenisch R. Transgenic mouse model of kidney disease: insertional inactivation of ubiquitously expressed gene leads to nephrotic syndrome. *Cell* 1990;62: 425–34.
101. Zwacka RM, Reuter A, Pfaff E, et al. The glomerulosclerosis gene *Mpv17* encodes a peroxisomal protein producing reactive oxygen species. *EMBO J* 1994;13:5129–34.
102. Schenkel J, Zwacka RM, Rutenberg C, Reuter A, Waldherr R, Weiher H. Functional rescue of the glomerulosclerosis phenotype Mpv17 mice by transgenesis with the human Mpv17 analogue. *Kidney Int* 1995;48:80–4.
103. Torres VE, Velosa JA, Holley KE, Frohnert PP, Zincke H, Sterioff, S. Meclofenamate treatment of recurrent idiopathic nephrotic syndrome with focal segmental glomerulosclerosis after renal transplant. *Mayo Clin Proc* 1984;59:146–52.
104. Abramowsky CR, Aikawa M, Swinehart GL, Snadjar RM. Spontaneous nephrotic syndrome in a genetic rat model. *Am J Pathol* 1984; 117:400–8.
105. Anderson S, Meyer TW, Rennke HG, Brenner BM. Control of glomerular hypertension limits glomerular injury in rats with reduced renal mass. *J Clin Invest* 1985;76:612–9.
106. Remuzzi A, Puntorieri S, Battaglia C, Bertani T, Remuzzi G. Angiotensin converting enzyme inhibition ameliorates glomerular filtration of macromolecules and water and lessens glomerular injury in the rat. *J Clin Invest* 1990;85:541–9.
107. Garcia DL, Rennke HG, Brenner BM, Anderson S. Chronic glucocorticoid therapy amplifies glomerular injury in rats with renal ablation. *J Clin Invest* 1987;80:867–74.
108. Bank N, Klose R, Aynedjian HS, Nguyen D, Sablay LB. Evidence against increased glomerular pressure initiating diabetic nephropathy. *Kidney Int* 1987;31:898–905.
109. Saito T, Sumithran E, Glasgow EF, Atkins RC. The enhancement of aminonucleoside nephrosis by the co-administration of protamine. *Kidney Int* 1987;32:691–9.
110. Kenner CH, Evan AP, Blomgren P, Aronoff GR, Luft FC. Effect of protein intake on renal function and structure in partially nephrectomized rats. *Kidney Int* 1985;27:739–50.
111. Remuzzi G, Zoja C, Remuzzi A, et al. Low-protein diet prevents glomerular damage in adriamycin-treated rats. *Kidney Int* 1985;28:21–7.
112. Zucchelli P, Cagnoli L, Casanova S, Donini U, Pasquali S. Focal glomerulosclerosis in patients with unilateral nephrectomy. *Kidney Int* 1983;24:649–55.
113. Narkun-Burgess DM, Nolan CR, Norman JE, Page WF, Miller PL, Meyer TM. Forty-five year follow-up after uninephrectomy. *Kidney Int* 1993;43:1110–5.
114. Baudoin P, Provoost AP, Molenaar JC. Renal function up to 50 years after unilateral nephrectomy in childhood. *Am J Kidney Dis* 1993;21: 603–11.
115. Dworkin LD, Feiner HD. Glomerular injury in uninephrectomized spontaneously hypertensive rats: a consequence of glomerular capillary hypertension. *J Clin Invest* 1986;77:797–809.
116. Anderson S, Diamond JR, Karnovsky MJ, Brenner BM. Mechanisms underlying transition from acute glomerular injury to late glomerular sclerosis in a rat model of nephrotic syndrome. *J Clin Invest* 1988;82: 1757–68.
117. Suzuki J, Yoshikawa N, Nakamura H. A quantitative analysis of the glomeruli in focal segmental glomerulosclerosis. *Pediatr Nephrol* 1994;8:416–9.
118. Nyberg E, Bohman SO, Berg U. Glomerular volume and renal function in children with different types of the nephrotic syndrome. *Pediatr Nephrol* 1994;8:285–9.
119. Yoshida Y, Fogo A, Ichikawa I. Glomerular hemodynamic changes vs. hypertrophy in experimental glomerular sclerosis. *Kidney Int* 1989;35:654–60.
120. Ikoma M, Yoshioka T, Ichikawa I, Fogo A. Mechanism of the unique susceptibility of deep cortical glomeruli of maturing kidneys to severe focal glomerular sclerosis. *Pediatr Res* 1990;28:270–6.
121. Moorehead JF, Wheeler DC, Varghese Z. Glomerular structures and lipids in progressive renal disease. *Am J Med* 1989;87:5.12N–20N.
122. Avram MM. Similarities between glomerular sclerosis and atherosclerosis in human renal biopsy specimens: a role for lipoprotein glomerulopathy. *Am J Med* 1989;87:5.39N–43N.
123. Schlondorff D. Cellular mechanisms of lipid injury in the glomerulus. *Am J Kidney Dis* 1993;22:72–82.

124. Diamond JR, Karnovsky MJ. Exacerbation of chronic aminonucleoside nephrosis by dietary cholesterol supplementation. *Kidney Int* 1987;32:671–7.
125. Hirano T, Morohoshi T. Treatment of hyperlipidemia with probucol suppresses the development of focal and segmental glomerulosclerosis in chronic aminonucleoside nephrosis. *Nephron* 1992;60:443–7.
126. Anderson S, King AJ, Brenner BM. Hypercholesterolemia and glomerular injury: an alternative viewpoint. *Am J Med* 1989;87:5.34N–8N.
127. Schmitz PG, O'Donnell MP, Kasiske BL, Katz SA, Keane WF. Renal injury in obese Zucker rats: glomerular hemodynamic alterations and effects of enalapril. *Am J Physiol* 1992;263:F496–502.
128. Schonholzer KW, Waldron M, Magil AB. Intraglomerular foam cells and human focal glomerulosclerosis. *Nephron* 1992;62:130–6.
129. Kees-Folts D, Diamond JR. Relationship between hyperlipidemia, lipid mediators and progressive glomerulosclerosis in the nephrotic syndrome. *Am J Nephrol* 1993;13:365–75.
130. van Goor H, Fidler V, Weening JJ, Grond J. Determinants of focal and segmental glomerulosclerosis in the rat after renal ablation: evidence for involvement of macrophages and lipids. *Lab Invest* 1991; 64:754–65.
131. Studer RK, Craven PA, De Rubertis FR. Low-density lipoprotein stimulation of mesangial cell fibronectin synthesis: role of protein kinase C and transforming growth factor-beta. *J Lab Clin Med* 1995; 125:86–95.
132. Purkerson ML, Joist JH, Greenberg JM, Kay D, Hoffsten PE, Klahr S. Inhibition by anticoagulant drugs of the progressive hypertension and uremia associated with renal infarction in rats. *Thromb Res* 1982;26: 227–40.
133. Futrakul P. A new therapeutic approach to nephrotic syndrome associated with focal segmental glomerulosclerosis. *Int J Pediatr Nephrol* 1980;1:18–21.
134. Floege J, Eng E, Young BA, Couser WG, Johnson RJ. Heparin suppresses mesangial cell proliferation and matrix expansion in experimental mesangioproliferative glomerulonephritis. *Kidney Int* 1993; 43:369–80.
135. Cameron JS. Mechanisms of progression in glomerulonephritis. *Proc Eur Dial Transplant Assoc* 1983;19:617–26.
136. Diamond JR. Effects of dietary interventions on glomerular pathophysiology. *Am J Physiol* 1990;258:F1–8.
137. Markovic-Lipkovski J, Muller CA, Risler T, Bohle A, Muller GA. Mononuclear leukocytes, expression of HLA class II antigens and intercellular adhesion molecule 1 in focal segmental glomerulosclerosis. *Nephron* 1991;59:286–93.
138. Dal Canton A, Fuiano G, Sepe V, Caglioti A, Ferrone S. Mesangial expression of intercellular adhesion molecule-1 in primary glomerulosclerosis. *Kidney Int* 1992;41:951–5.
139. Saito T, Atkins RC. Contribution of mononuclear leukocytes to the progression of experimental focal glomerular sclerosis. *Kidney Int* 1990;37:1076–83.
140. Eddy AA. Experimental insights into the tubulointerstitial disease accompanying primary glomerular lesions. *J Am Soc Nephrol* 1994;5: 1273–87.
141. Schreiner GF, Harris KGP, Purkerson ML, Klahr S. Immunological aspects of acute ureteral obstruction: immune cell infiltrate in the kidney. *Kidney Int* 1988;34:487–93.
142. Eddy AA. Interstitial nephritis induced by protein-overload proteinuria. *Am J Pathol* 1989;135:719–33.
143. Cooper MA, Buddington B, Miller NL, Alfrey AC. Urinary iron speciation in nephrotic syndrome. *Am J Kidney Dis* 1995;25:314–9.
144. Thomas ME, Schreiner GF. Contribution of proteinuria to progressive renal injury: consequences of tubular uptake of fatty acid bearing albumin. *Am J Nephrol* 1993;13:385–98.
145. Kees-Folts D, Sadow JL, Schreiner GF. Tubular catabolism of albumin is associated with the release of an inflammatory lipid. *Kidney Int* 1994;45:1697–709.
146. Timpl R. Recent advances in the biochemistry of glomerular basement membrane. *Kidney Int* 1986;30:293–8.
147. Yurchenco PD, Schnittny JC. Molecular architecture of basement membranes. *FASEB J* 1990;4:1577–90.
148. Katz A, Fish AJ, Kleppel MM, Hagen SG, Michael AF, Butkowski RJ. Renal entactin (nidogen): isolation, characterization and tissue distribution. *Kidney Int* 1991;40:643–53.
149. Taamsma JT, van den Born J, Bruijn JA, et al. Expression of glomerular extracellular matrix components in human diabetic nephropathy: decrease of heparan sulphate in the glomerular basement membrane. *Diabetologia* 1994;37:313–20.
150. Mounier F, Foidart J-M, Gubler M-C. Distribution of extracellular matrix glycoproteins during normal development of human kidney. *Lab Invest* 1986;54:394–401.
151. Yoneyama T, Nagase M, Ikeya M, Hishida A, Honda N. Intraglomerular fibronectin in rat experimental glomerulonephritis. *Virchows Arch [B]* 1992;62:179–88.
152. Mosquera JA. Increased production of fibronectin by glomerular cultures from rats with nephrotoxic serum nephritis: macrophages induce fibronectin production in cultured mesangial cells. *Lab Invest* 1993; 68:406–12.
153. Brazy PC, Kopp JB, Klotman PE. Glomerulosclerosis and progressive renal disease. In: Keane WF, ed. *Lipids and renal disease.* New York: Churchill-Livingstone, 1991:11–35.
154. Foidart J-M, Foidart JB, Mahieu PR. Synthesis of collagen and fibronectin by glomerular cells in culture. *Renal Physiol* 1980;3:183–92.
155. Striker LM-M, Killen PD, Chi E, Striker GE. The composition of glomerulosclerosis. I. Studies in focal sclerosis, crescentic glomerulonephritis, and membranoproliferative glomerulonephritis. *Lab Invest* 1984;51:181–92.
156. Okuda S, Kanai H, Tamaki K, Onoyama K, Fujishima M. Synthesis of fibronectin by isolated glomeruli from nephrectomized hypertensive rats. *Nephron* 1992;61:456–63.
157. Kim Y, Kleppel MM, Butkowski R, Mauer SM, Weislander J, Michael AF. Differential expression of basement membrane collagen chains in diabetic nephropathy. *Am J Pathol* 1991;138:413–20.
158. Abrass CK, Peterson CV, Raugi GJ. Phenotypic expression of collagen types in mesangial matrix of diabetic and nondiabetic rats. *Diabetes* 1988;37:1695–702.
159. Ledbetter SE, Copeland EJ, Noonan D, Vogelli G, Hassell JR. Altered steady-state mRNA levels of basement membrane proteins in diabetic mouse kidneys and thromboxane synthase inhibition. *Diabetes* 1990;39:196–203.
160. Poulsom R, Kurkinen M, Prockop D, Boot-Handford RP. Increased steady-state levels of laminin B_1 mRNA in kidneys of long-term streptozotocin-diabetic rats. *J Biol Chem* 1988;263:10,072–6.
161. Nakamura T, Ebihara I, Fukui M, Tomino Y, Koide H. Effects of methylprednisolone on glomerular and medullary mRNA levels for extracellular matrices in puromycin aminonucleoside nephrosis. *Kidney Int* 1991;40:874–81.
162. Peten EP, Striker LJ, Caropme MA, Elliot SJ, Yang C-W, Striker GE. The contribution of increased collagen synthesis to human glomerulosclerosis: a quantitative analysis of α2IV collagen mRNA expression by competitive polymerase chain reaction. *J Exp Med* 1992;176: 1571–6.
163. Schnaper HW. Balance between matrix synthesis and degradation: a determinant of glomerulosclerosis. *Pediatr Nephrol* 1995;9:104–11.
164. Davies M, Martin J, Thomas GT, Lovett DH. Proteinases and glomerular matrix turnover. *Kidney Int* 1992;41:671–8.
165. Couchman JR, Beavan LA, McCarthy KJ. Glomerular matrix: synthesis, turnover and role in mesangial expansion. *Kidney Int* 1994;45: 328–35.
166. Liotta LA, Goldfarb RH, Terranova VP. Cleavage of laminin by thrombin and plasmin: alpha thrombin selectively cleaves the beta chain of laminin. *Thromb Res* 1981;21:663–73.
167. Baricos WH, Cortez SL, El-Dahr SS, Schnaper HW. ECM degradation by cultured human mesangial cells is mediated by a PA/plasmin/ MMP-2 cascade. *Kidney Int* 1995;47:1039–47.
168. Louise CB, Obrig TG. Human renal microvascular endothelial cells as a potential target in the development of the hemolytic uremic syndrome as related to fibrinolysis factor expression in vitro. *Microvasc Res* 1994;47:377–87.
169. Schnaper HW, Grant DS, Stetler-Stevenson WG, et al. Type IV collagenases and TIMPs modulate endothelial cell morphogenesis in vitro. *J Cell Physiol* 1993;156:235–46.
170. Knowlden J, Martin J, Davies M, Williams JD. Metalloproteinase generation by human glomerular epithelial cells. *Kidney Int* 1995;47: 1682–9.
171. Carome MA, Striker LJ, Peten EP, et al. Assessment of 72-kilodalton gelatinase and TIMP-1 gene expression in normal and sclerotic murine glomeruli. *J Am Soc Nephrol* 1994;5:1391–9.

172. Carome MA, Striker LJ, Peten EP, et al. Human glomeruli express TIMP-1 mRNA and TIMP-2 protein and mRNA. *Am J Physiol* 1993; 264:F923–9.
173. Lovett DH, Johnson RJ, Marti H-P, Martin J, Davies M, Couser WG. Structural characterization of the mesangial cell type IV collagenase and enhanced expression in a model of immune complex-mediated glomerulonephritis. *Am J Pathol* 1992;141:85–98.
174. Tomooka S, Border WA, Marshall BC, Noble NA. Glomerular matrix accumulation is linked to inhibition of the plasmin protease system. *Kidney Int* 1992;42:1462–9.
175. Paczek L, Teschner M, Schaefer RM, Kovar J, Romen W, Heidland A. Intraglomerular proteinases activity in adriamycin-induced nephropathy. *Nephron* 1992;60:81–6.
176. Teschner M, Schaefer RM, Paczek L, Heidland A. Effect of renal disease on glomerular proteinases. *Miner Electrolyte Metab* 1992;18: 92–6.
177. Reckelhoff JF, Baylis C. Glomerular metalloprotease activity in the aging rat: inverse correlation with injury. *J Am Soc Nephrol* 1993;3: 1835–8.
178. Nakamura T, Fukui M, Ebihara I, Tomino Y, Koide H. Low protein diet blunts the rise in glomerular gene expression in focal glomerulosclerosis. *Kidney Int* 1994;45:1593–605.
179. Peten EP, Yang C-W, Striker GE, Striker LJ. Gene activation in glomerulosclerosis: a role for growth-promoting hormones. *Kidney Int* 1994;45:S48–50.
180. Yoshida H, Mitarai T, Kitamura M, et al. The effect of selective growth hormone defect in the progression of glomerulosclerosis. *Am J Kidney Dis* 1994;23:302–12.
181. Chen NY, Chen WY, Bellush L, et al. Effects of streptozotocin treatment in growth hormone and growth hormone antagonist transgenic mice. *Endocrinology* 1995;136:660–7.
182. Feld SM, Hirschberg R, Artishevsky A, Nast C, Adler SG. Insulin-like growth factor I induces mesangial proliferation and increases mRNA and secretion of collagen. *Kidney Int* 1995;48:45–51.
183. Oemar BS, Foellmer HG, Hodgdon-Anandant L, Rosenzweig SA. Regulation of insulin-like growth factor receptors in diabetic mesangial cells. *J Biol Chem* 1991;266:2369–72.
184. Bruggeman LA, Horigan EA, Horikoshi S, Ray PE, Klotman PE. Thromboxane stimulates synthesis of extracellular matrix proteins in vitro. *Am J Physiol* 1991;261:F488–94.
185. Purkerson ML, Joist JH, Yates J, Valdes A, Morrison A, Klahr S. Inhibition of thromboxane synthesis ameliorates the progressive kidney disease of rats with subtotal renal ablation. *Proc Natl Acad Sci USA* 1985;82:193–7.
186. Stahl RAK, Thaiss F, Wenzel U, Schoeppe W, Helmchen U. A rat model of progressive chronic glomerular sclerosis: the role of thromboxane inhibition. *J Am Soc Nephrol* 1992;2:1568–77.
187. Nikolic-Paterson D, Lan HY, Hill PA, Atkins RC. Macrophages in renal injury. *Kidney Int* 1994;45(Suppl):S79–82.
188. Lovett DH, Martin M, Bursten S, Szamel M, Gemsa D, Resch K. Interleukin 1 and the glomerular mesangium. III. IL-1-dependent stimulation of mesangial cell protein kinase activity. *Kidney Int* 1988; 34:26–35.
189. Iida H, Seifert R, Alpers CE, et al. Platelet-derived growth factor (PDGF) and PDGF receptor are induced in mesangial proliferative nephritis in the rat. *Proc Natl Acad Sci USA* 1991;88:6560–4.
190. Ruef C, Budde K, Lacy J, et al. Interleukin 6 is an autocrine growth factor for mesangial cells. *Kidney Int* 1990;38:249–57.
191. Fogo A, Ichikawa I. Evidence for the central role of glomerular growth promoters in the development of sclerosis. *Semin Nephrol* 1989;9:329–42.
192. Hasegawa G, Nakano K, Sawada M, et al. Possible role of tumor necrosis factor and interleukin-1 in diabetic nephropathy. *Kidney Int* 1991;40:1007–12.
193. Throckmorton DC, Brogden AP, Min B, Rasmussen H, Kashgrian M. PDGF and TGF-β mediate collagen production by mesangial cells exposed to advanced glycosylation end products. *Kidney Int* 1995;48: 111–7.
194. Floege J, Eng E, Toung BA, et al. Infusion of platelet-derived growth factor or basic fibroblast growth factor induces selective glomerular mesangial cell proliferation and matrix accumulation in rats. *J Clin Invest* 1993;92:2952–62.
195. Okuda S, Languino LR, Ruoslahti E, Border WA. Elevated expression of transforming growth factor-β and proteoglycan production in experimental glomerulonephritis: possible role in expansion of extracellular matrix. *J Clin Invest* 1990;86:453–62.
196. Yoshioka K, Takemura T, Murakami K, et al. Transforming growth factor-β protein and mRNA in glomeruli in normal and diseased human kidneys. *Lab Invest* 1993;68:154–63.
197. Yamamoto T, Noble NA, Miller DE, Border WA. Sustained expression of TGF-beta 1 underlies development of progressive kidney fibrosis. *Kidney Int* 1994;45:916–27.
198. Yoshioka K, Takemura T, Tohda M, et al. Glomerular localization of type III collagen in human kidney disease. *Kidney Int* 1989;35: 1203–11.
199. Isaka Y, Fujiwara Y, Ueda N, Kaneda Y, Kamada T, Imai E. Glomerulosclerosis induced by in vivo transfection of transforming growth factor-β or platelet-derived growth factor gene into the rat kidney. *J Clin Invest* 1993;92:2597–601.
200. Marti HP, Lee L, Kashgarian M, Lovett DH. Transforming growth factor-β_1 stimulates glomerular mesangial cell synthesis of the 72-kd type IV collagenase. *Am J Pathol* 1994;144:82–94.
201. Kanai H, Mitsuhashi H, Ono K, Yano S, Naruse T. Increased excretion of urinary transforming growth factor beta in patients with focal glomerulosclerosis. *Nephron* 1994;66:391–5.
202. Schnaper HW, Kopp JB, Stetler-Stevenson WG, Bruggeman LA, Klotman PE, Kleinman HK. Regulation of TIMP-2 splice variants is independent of TGF-β in cultured glomerular mesangial cells. *J Am Soc Nephrol* 1993;3:664(abst).
203. DeHeer E, Verseput GH, Van der Wal AM, Bruijn JA, Provoost AP. Dissociation of persistent glomerular expression of TGFβ_1 and progression of renal disease in the lisinopril-treated fawn-hooded rat. *J Am Soc Nephrol* 1994;5:804(abst).
204. Ninomiya Y, Arakawa M. Serum angiotensin converting enzyme activity in type 2 (non-insulin-dependent) diabetic patients with chronic glomerulonephritis. *Diabetes Res* 1989;11:121–4.
205. Sen S, Tarazi RC, Bumpus FM. Effect of converting enzyme inhibitor (SQ14,225) on myocardial hypertrophy in spontaneously hypertensive rats. *Hypertension* 1980;2:169–76.
206. Dworkin LD, Ichikawa I, Brenner BM. Hormonal modulation of glomerular function. *Am J Physiol* 1983;244:F95–104.
207. Scharschmidt LA, Dunn MJ. Prostaglandin synthesis by rat glomerular mesangial cells in culture: effects of angiotensin II and arginine vasopressin. *J Clin Invest* 1983;71:1756–64.
208. Ray PE, Bruggeman LA, Horikoshi S, Aguilera G, Klotman PE. Angiotensin II stimulates human fetal mesangial cell proliferation and fibronectin biosynthesis by binding to AT1 receptors. *Kidney Int* 1994;45:177–84.
209. Wolf G, Haberstroh U, Neilson EG. Angiotensin II stimulates the proliferation and biosynthesis of type I collagen in cultured murine mesangial cells. *Am J Physiol* 1992;140:95–107.
210. Kagami S, Border WA, Miller DE, Noble NA. Angiotensin II stimulates extracellular matrix protein synthesis through induction of transforming growth factor-beta expression in rat glomerular mesangial cells. *J Clin Invest* 1994;93:2431–7.
211. Anderson S, Rennke HG, Brenner BM. Therapeutic advantage of converting enzyme inhibitors in arresting progressive renal disease associated with systemic hypertension in the rat. *J Clin Invest* 1986; 77:1993–2000.
212. Grond J, Koudstaal J, Elema JD. Mesangial function and glomerular sclerosis in rats with aminonucleoside nephrosis. *Kidney Int* 1985;27: 405–10.
213. Pugliese F, Ferrario RG, Ciavolella A, et al. Growth abnormalities in cultured mesangial cells from rats with spontaneous glomerulosclerosis. *Kidney Int* 1995;47:106–13.
214. Nakamura T, Ebihara I, Tomino Y, Koide H, Kikuchi K, Koiso K. Gene expression of growth-related proteins and ECM constituents in response to unilateral nephrectomy. *Am J Physiol* 1992;262:F389–96.
215. O'Donnell MP, Kasiske BL, Kim Y, Atluru D, Keane WF. Lovastatin inhibits proliferation of rat mesangial cells. *J Clin Invest* 1993;91:83–7.
216. Ichikawa I, Yoshida Y, Fogo A, Purkerson ML, Klahr S. Effect of heparin on the glomerular structure and function of remnant nephrons. *Kidney Int* 1988;34:638–44.
217. Purkerson ML, Tollefsen DM, Klahr S. N-sulfated/acetylated heparin ameliorates the progression of renal disease in rats with subtotal renal ablation. *J Clin Invest* 1988;81:69–74.
218. Schnaper HW, Kleinman HK. Regulation of cell function by extracellular matrix. *Pediatr Nephrol* 1992;7:96–104.

219. Ingber DE, Folkman J. Mechanicochemical switching between growth and differentiation during fibroblast growth factor-stimulated angiogenesis in vitro: role of extracellular matrix. *J Cell Biol* 1989; 109:317–30.
220. Habib R, Gubler MC. Focal sclerosing glomerulonephritis. In: Kincaid-Smith P, Matthew TH, Becker EL, eds. *Glomerulonephritis.* New York: Wiley, 1973:263–78.
221. Southwest Pediatric Nephrology Study Group. Focal segmental glomerulosclerosis in children with idiopathic nephrotic syndrome in children: a report of the Southwest Pediatric Nephrology Study Group. *Kidney Int* 1985;27:442–9.
222. Yoshikawa N, Ito H, Akamatsu R, et al. Focal segmental glomerulosclerosis with and without nephrotic syndrome in children. *J Pediatr* 1986;109:65–70.
223. International Study of Kidney Disease in Children. Nephrotic syndrome in children: prediction of histopathology from clinical and laboratory characteristics at time of diagnosis. *Kidney Int* 1978;13:159–65.
224. Habib R, Kleinknecht C. The primary nephrotic syndrome in childhood: classification and clinicopathologic study of 406 cases. In: Somers SC, ed. *Pathology annual.* New York: Appleton-Century Crofts, 1971:417–74.
225. Wehrmann M, Bohle A, Held H, Schumm G, Kendziorra H, Pressler H. Long-term prognosis of focal sclerosing glomerulonephritis: an analysis of 250 cases with particular regard to tubulointerstitial changes. *Clin Nephrol* 1990;33:115–22.
226. Newman WJ, Tisher CC, McCoy RC, et al. Focal glomerular sclerosis: contrasting clinical patterns in children and adults. *Medicine (Baltimore)* 1978;55:67–87.
227. Cameron JS, Turner DR, Ogg CS, Chantler C, Williams DG. The long-term prognosis of patients with focal segmental glomerulosclerosis. *Clin Nephrol* 1978;10:213–8.
228. Banfi G, Moriggi M, Sabadini E, Fellin G, D'Amico G, Ponticelli C. The impact of prolonged immunosuppression on the outcome of idiopathic focal-segmental glomerulosclerosis with nephrotic syndrome in adults: a collaborative retrospective study. *Clin Nephrol* 1991;36:53–9.
229. Freedman BI, Iskander SS, Buckalew VM, Burkart JM, Appel RG. Renal biopsy findings in presumed hypertensive nephrosclerosis. *Am J Nephrol* 1994;14:90–4.
230. Lau J, Levey AS, Kassirer JP, Pauker SG. Idiopathic nephrotic syndrome in a 53 year old woman: is a kidney biopsy necessary? *Med Decis Making* 1982;2:497–519.
231. Ginsberg JM, Chang BS, Matarese RA, Garella S. Use of single voided urine samples to estimate quantitative proteinuria. *N Engl J Med* 1983;309:1543–6.
232. Carrie BJ, Salyer WR, Myers BD. Minimal change nephropathy: an electrochemical disorder of the glomerular membranes. *Am J Med* 1981;70:262–8.
233. Robson AM, Cole BR. Pathologic and functional correlations in the glomerulopathies. In: Cummings NB, Michael AF, Wilson CB, eds. *Immune mechanisms in renal disease.* New York: Plenum, 1982: 109–127.
234. Guasch A, Hashimoto H, Sibley RK, Deen WM, Myers BD. Glomerular dysfunction in nephrotic humans with minimal changes or focal glomerulosclerosis. *Am J Physiol* 1991;260:F728–37.
235. Winetz JA, Robertson CR, Golbetz HV, Carrie BJ, Salyer WR, Myers BD. The nature of the glomerular injury in minimal change and focal sclerosing glomerulopathies. *Am J Kidney Dis* 1981;1:91–8.
236. McVicar M, Exeni R, Susin M. Nephrotic syndrome and multiple tubular defects in children: an early sign of focal segmental glomerulosclerosis. 1980;97:918–22.
237. Panchenko EL, Chesney RW, Roy S, Budreau AM, Boehm KA. The differential diagnostic value of urinary enzyme and amino acid excretion in children with nephrotic syndrome. *Pediatr Nephrol* 1994;8: 142–7.
238. Pedersen EB, Danielsen H, Sorenson SS, Jesperson B. Renal water excretion before and after remission of nephrotic syndrome: relationship between free water clearance and kidney function, arginine vasopressin, angiotensin II and aldosterone in plasma before and after water loading. *Clin Sci* 1986;71:97–104.
239. Lowenstein J, Schacht RG, Baldwin DS. Renal failure in minimal change nephrotic syndrome. *Am J Med* 1981;70:227–33.
240. Ichikawa I, Rennke HG, Hoyer JR, et al. Role for intrarenal mechanisms in the impaired salt excretion of experimental nephrotic syndrome. *J Clin Invest* 1983;71:91–103.
241. Strife CF, Jackson EC, Forristal J, West CD. Effect of the nephrotic syndrome on the concentration of serum complement components. *Am J Kidney Dis* 1986;8:37–42.
242. Rydel JJ, Korbet SM, Borok RZ, Schwartz MM. Focal segmental glomerulosclerosis in adults: presentation, course and response to treatment. *Am J Kidney Dis* 1995;25:534–42.
243. Griswold WR, Tune BM, Reznik VM, et al. Treatment of childhood prednisone-resistant nephrotic syndrome and focal segmental glomerulosclerosis with intravenous methylprednisolone and oral alkylating agents. *Nephron* 1987;46:73–7.
244. Mendoza SA, Reznik VM, Griswold WR, Krensky AM, Yorgin PD, Tune BM. Treatment of steroid-resistant focal segmental glomerulosclerosis with pulse methylprednisolone and alkylating agents. *Pediatr Nephrol* 1990;4:303–7.
245. Murphy JL, Kano HL, Chenaille PJ, Makker SP. Fatal *Pneumocystis* pneumonia in a child treated for focal segmental glomerulosclerosis. *Pediatr Nephrol* 1993;7:444–5.
246. Waldo FB, Benfield MR, Kohaut EC. Methylprednisolone treatment of patients with steroid-resistant nephrotic syndrome. *Pediatr Nephrol* 1992;6:503–5.
247. Maggiore Q, Martorano C. Immunosuppressive therapy in primary glomerulonephritides. *Contrib Nephrol* 1982;34:55–63.
248. Ponticelli C, Banfi G, Imbasciati E, Tarantino A. Immunosuppressive therapy in primary glomerulonephritis. *Contrib Nephrol* 1982;34: 33–54.
249. Almeida MP, Almeida HA, Rosa FC. Vincristine in steroid-resistant nephrotic syndrome. *Pediatr Nephrol* 1994;8:79–80.
250. International Study of Kidney Disease in Children. A controlled therapeutic trial of cyclophosphamide plus prednisone vs. prednisone alone in children with focal segmental glomerulonephritis. *Pediatr Res* 1980;14:1006(abst).
251. Baluarte HJ, Gruskin AB, Polinsky MS, et al. Chlorambucil therapy in the nephrotic syndrome. In: Gruskin AB, Norman M, eds. *Pediatric nephrology.* Boston: Martinus Nijhoff, 1981:423–429.
252. Ingulli E, Baqi N, Ahmad H, Moazami S, Tejani A. Aggressive, long-term cyclosporine therapy for steroid-resistant focal segmental glomerulosclerosis. *J Am Soc Nephrol* 1995;5:1820–5.
253. Meyrier A, Noel L, Auriche P, Callard P. Long-term renal tolerance of cyclosporin A treatment in the adult idiopathic nephrotic syndrome. *Kidney Int* 1994;45:1446–56.
254. McCauley J, Shapiro R, Ellis D, et al. Pilot trial of FK 506 in the management of steroid-resistant nephrotic syndrome. *Nephrol Dial Transplant* 1993;8:1286–90.
255. Yoshimura A, Ideura T, Iwasaki S, et al. Aggravation of minimal change nephrotic syndrome by administration of human albumin. *Clin Nephrol* 1992;37:109–14.
256. Steele RW. Current status of vaccines and immune globulins in children with renal disease. *Pediatr Nephrol* 1994;8:7–10.
257. Moore DH, Shackelford PG, Robson AM, Rose GM. Recurrent pneumococcal sepsis and defective opsonization after pneumococcal capsular polysaccharide vaccine in a child with nephrotic syndrome. *J Pediatr* 1980;96:882–5.
258. Tessitore N, Bonucci E, D'Angelo A, et al. Bone histology and calcium metabolism in patients with nephrotic syndrome and normal or reduced renal function. *Nephron* 1984;37:153–9.
259. Afrasiabi MA, Vaziri ND, Gwinup G, et al. Thyroid function studies in the nephrotic syndrome. *Ann Intern Med* 1979;90:335–8.
260. Anderson S, Rennke HG, Garcia DL, Brenner BM. Short and long term effects of antihypertensive therapy in the diabetic rat. *Kidney Int* 1989;36:526–36.
261. Lewis EJ, Hunsicker LG, Bain RP, Rohde RD. The effect of angiotensin-converting-enzyme inhibition on diabetic nephropathy: the Collaborative Study Group. *N Engl J Med* 1993;329:1456–62.
262. Neilsen FS, Rossing P, Gall MA, Skott P, Smidt UM, Parving HH. Impact of lisinopril and atenolol on kidney function in hypertensive subjects with diabetic nephropathy. *Diabetes* 1994;43:1108–13.
263. Bennett PH, Haffner S, Kasiske BL, et al. Screening and management of microalbuminuria in patients with diabetes mellitus: recommendations to the Scientific Advisory Board of the National Kidney Foundation from an ad hoc committee of the Council on Diabetes Mellitus of the National Kidney Foundation. *Am J Kidney Dis* 1995;25:107–12.
264. Kasiske BL, Kalil RS, Ma JZ, Liao M, Keane WF. Effect of antihypertensive therapy on the kidney in patients with diabetes: a meta-regression analysis. *Ann Intern Med* 1993;118:129–38.

265. Velosa JA, Torres VE, Donadio JV, Wagoner RD, Holley KE, Offord KP. Treatment of severe nephrotic syndrome with meclofenamate: an uncontrolled pilot study. *Mayo Clin Proc* 1985;60:586–92.
266. Brezin JH, Katz SM, Schwartz AB, Chinitz JL. Reversible renal failure and nephrotic syndrome associated with non-steroidal anti-inflammatory drugs. *N Engl J Med* 1979;301:1271–3.
267. Ihle BU, Becker GJ, Whitworth JA, Charlwood RA, Kincaid-Smith PS. The effect of protein restriction on the progression of renal insufficiency. *N Engl J Med* 1989;321:1773–7.
268. Klahr S, Levey AS, Beck CJ, et al. The effects of dietary protein restriction and blood-pressure control on the progression of chronic renal disease: modification of Diet in Renal Disease Study Group. *N Engl J Med* 1994;330:877–84.
269. Tapp DC, Wortham WG, Addison JF, Hammonds DN, Barnes JL, Venkatachalam MA. Food restriction retards body growth and prevents end-stage renal pathology in remnant kidneys of rats regardless of protein intake. *Lab Invest* 1989;60:184–95.
270. Correa-Rotter R, Hostetter TH, Rosenberg ME. Effect of dietary protein on renin and angiotensin gene expression after renal ablation. *Am J Physiol* 1992;262:F631–8.
271. Salahudeen AK, Hostetter TH, Raatz SK, Rosenberg ME. Effects of dietary protein in patients with chronic renal transplant rejection. *Kidney Int* 1992;41:183–90.
272. de Jong PE, Anderson S, de Zeeuw D. Glomerular preload and afterload reduction as a tool to lower urinary protein leakage: will such treatments also help to improve renal function outcome? *J Am Soc Nephrol* 1993;3:1333–41.
273. Hattori M, Ito K, Kawaguchi H, Tanaka T, Kubota R, Khono M. Treatment with a combination of low-density lipoprotein apheresis and pravastatin of a patient with drug-resistant nephrotic syndrome due to focal segmental glomerulosclerosis. *Pediatr Nephrol* 1993;7:196–8.
274. Aguilar-Salinas CA, Barrett PHR, Kelber J, Delmez J, Schonfeld G. Physiologic mechanisms of action of lovastatin in nephrotic syndrome. *J Lipid Res* 1995;36:188–99.
275. O'Donnell MP, Kasiske BL, Kim Y, Schmitz PG, Keane WF. Lovastatin retards the progression of established glomerular disease in obese Zucker rats. *Am J Kidney Dis* 1993;22:83–9.
276. Wheeler DC, Nair DR, Persaud JW, et al. Effects of dietary fatty acids in an animal model of focal glomerulosclerosis. *Kidney Int* 1991;39:930–7.
277. Ingram AJ, Parbtani A, Clark WF, et al. Effects of flaxseed and flaxseed oil diets in a rat–5/6 renal ablation model. *Am J Kidney Dis* 1995;25:320–9.
278. Teschner M, Paczek L, Schaefer L, Bahner U, Heidland A, Schaefer RM. Lovastatin ameliorates depressed intraglomerular proteolytic activities in experimental nephrotic syndrome. *Res Exp Med* 1994;194:349–56.
279. Arbus GS, Poucell S, Bacheyie GS, Baumal R. Focal segmental glomerulosclerosis with idiopathic nephrotic syndrome: three types of clinical response. *J Pediatr* 1982;101:40–5.
280. Krensky AM, Inglefinger JR, Grupe WE. Peritonitis in childhood nephrotic syndrome. *Am J Dis Child.* 1982;136:732–6.
281. Ogi M, Yokoyama H, Tomosugi N, et al. Risk factors for infection and immunoglobulin replacement therapy in adult nephrotic syndrome. *Am J Kidney Dis* 1994;24:427–36.
282. Fleisher DS, McCrory WW, Rapoport M. The effects of intermittent doses of adrenocortical steroids on the statural growth of nephrotic children. *J Pediatr* 1960;57:192.
283. Brockelbank JT, Harcourt RB, Meadow SR. Corticosteroid-induced cataracts in idiopathic nephrotic syndrome. *Arch Dis Child* 1982;53:30.
284. Egli F, Eiminger P, Stalder G. Thromboembolism in the nephrotic syndrome. *Pediatr Res* 1974;8:903.
285. Llach FH. Hypercoagulability, renal vein thrombosis, and thrombotic complications of nephrotic syndrome. *Kidney Int* 1985;28:429–39.
286. Cameron JS, Hicks J. Pregnancy in patients with pre-existing glomerular disease. *Contrib Nephrol* 1984;37:149–56.
287. International Study of Kidney Disease in Children. Minimal change nephrotic syndrome in children: deaths during the first 5 to 15 years' observation. *Pediatrics* 1984;73:497–501.
288. Agarwal SK, Dash SC, Tiwari SC, Bhuyan UN. Idiopathic adult focal segmental glomerulosclerosis: a clinicopathological study and response to steroids. *Nephron* 1993;63:161–71.
289. Ramirez F, Travis LB, Cunningham RJ, et al. Focal segmental glomerulosclerosis, crescent, and rapidly progressive renal failure. *Int J Pediatr Nephrol* 1982;3:175–8.
290. Mongeau JG, Corneille L, Robitaille P, O'Regan S, Pelletier M. Primary nephrosis in childhood associated with focal glomerulosclerosis: is long-term prognosis that severe? *Kidney Int* 1981;20:743–6.
291. Kashgarian M, Hayslett JP, Seigel NJ. Lipoid nephrosis and focal sclerosis: distinct entities or spectrum of disease. *Nephron* 1974;13:105–8.
292. Nash MA, Bakare MA, D'Agati V, Pirani CL. Late development of chronic renal failure in steroid-responsive nephrotic syndrome. *J Pediatr* 1982;101:411–4.
293. Malekzadeh MH, Heuser ET, Ettinger RB, et al. Focal glomerulosclerosis and renal transplantation. *J Pediatr* 1979;95:249–54.
294. Pinto J, Lacerda G, Cameron JS, Turner DR, Bewick M, Ogg CS. Recurrence of focal segmental glomerulosclerosis in renal allografts. *Transplantation* 1981;32:83–9.
295. Korbet SM, Schwartz MM, Lewis EJ. Recurrent nephrotic syndrome in renal allografts. *Am J Kidney Dis* 1988;11:270–6.
296. Savin VJ, Sharma R, Sharma M, et al. Circulating factor in recurrent focal segmental glomerular sclerosis. *N Engl J Med* 1996;334:878–83.
297. Cochat P, Kassir A, Colon S, et al. Recurrent nephrotic syndrome after transplantation: early treatment with plasmaphaeresis and cyclophosphamide. *Pediatr Nephrol* 1993;7:50–4.
298. Dantal J, Bigot E, Bogers W, et al. Effect of plasma protein adsorption on protein excretion in kidney-transplant recipients with recurrent nephrotic syndrome. *N Engl J Med* 1994;330:7–14.

Immunologic Renal Diseases,
edited by E. G. Neilson and W. G. Couser.
Lippincott-Raven Publishers, Philadelphia © 1997.

CHAPTER 47

Membranous Nephropathy

William G. Couser and Charles E. Alpers

INTRODUCTION

Membranous nephropathy (MN) is a glomerular disease characterized by predominantly, or exclusively, subepithelial immune-complex deposits associated with an increase in urine protein excretion, usually resulting in nephrotic syndrome (1–3). The disease causes <5% of nephrotic syndrome in children, ~25% in adults and, in patients over 50, ~35%, the most frequent cause of nephrotic syndrome in this age group (1–3). Although the term membranous glomerulonephritis has been in use for much of this century to describe a variety of glomerular lesions, the entity currently recognized as MN was not clearly defined until the 1950s. Jones utilized a silver methenamine stain to identify the capillary wall thickening as consequent to basement membrane expansion and to describe the presence of many "short silver positive projections of club or mushroom shape" or subepithelial "spikes," which are a diagnostic feature of the disease by light microscopy (4). Churg and Grishman, as well as Jones, noted that periodic acid–Schiff (PAS) and silver-negative areas between the spikes contributed to the capillary wall thickening and that glomerular cellularity in MN was not usually increased (5). The application of electron microscopy to the study of human renal biopsy specimens in the early 1960s revealed the characteristic appearance of multiple electron-dense deposits on the outer surface of the capillary wall beneath the epithelial cells (6,7). These were recognized as immune deposits by Mellors and Ortega, who reported the diffuse, finely granular staining for immunoglobulin G (IgG) in a subepithelial distribution that is now regarded as pathognomonic of MN (8). Thus, MN is a pathologic diagnosis made when the glomerulus exhibits diffuse subepithelial immune deposits without associated glomerular hypercellularity. Depending on the severity and duration of disease, subepithelial spikes, generalized thickening of basement membrane, sclerosis, and interstitial changes may also be present (see the section on *pathology*) (1–3).

MN is a lesion that may occur in the absence of any extrarenal or systemic disease (idiopathic MN) or may be seen as a feature of a number of other diseases, particularly autoimmune diseases such as systemic lupus erythematosus (SLE), chronic viral infections due to hepatitis-B virus (HBV) and C (HCV), exposure to certain drugs, and solid tumors (see Table 1). The idiopathic form of MN is believed to be an autoimmune disease probably mediated by antibodies to antigenic determinants expressed exclusively on the glomerular epithelial cell (GEC) (1). Whether the lesion, when it occurs in association with other disease processes, has a similar autoimmune mechanism triggered by stimuli such as viruses or drugs, or rather reflects a different immune process involving exogenous antigens, has not been established. The clinical consequence of subepithelial immune-deposit formation is an increase in urine protein excretion that results in nephrotic syndrome in ~80% of patients and slowly progressive renal disease in ~30–40% (1–3).

PATHOGENESIS AND PATHOPHYSIOLOGY

The pathogenesis of MN in humans is not known. Because of its association with other autoimmune diseases, such as SLE and diabetes, as well as the remarkable similarity of the human lesion to the rat model of Heymann nephritis mediated by antibodies to the GEC, the disease is likely to be autoimmune in nature (1). Current understanding of the events that lead to loss of tolerance and to the development of an autoimmune response are reviewed in detail in Chapter 6. Etiologic agents that have been identified in some cases of human MN are listed in Table 1 and include both HBV and HCV, drugs such as gold, penicillamine, captopril, porcine insulin, and nonsteroidal anti-

W. G. Couser: Department of Medicine, University of Washington, Seattle, Washington 98195.
C. E. Alpers: Department of Pathology, University of Washington, Seattle, Washington 98195.

TABLE 1. *Conditions and agents associated with membranous nephropathy*

Immune diseases
Systemic lupus erythematosus (165–175,327)
Rheumatoid arthritis (328–330)
Diabetes mellitus (160,164,331)
Hashimoto disease (18,19)
Graves disease (332,333)
Mixed connective tissue disease (334)
Sjögren syndrome (335,336)
Primary biliary cirrhosis (337,338)
Bullous pemphigoid (339,340)
Small bowel enteropathy syndrome (341–343)
Dermatitis herpetiformis (344,345)
Ankylosing spondylitis (346)
Graft-versus-host disease (347,349)
Guillain–Barre syndrome (361,362)
Infectious or parasitic diseases
Hepatitis B (182,183,350–352)
Hepatitis C (184–186)
Syphilis (353,354)
Filariasis (355)
Hydatid disease (356,357)
Schistosomiasis (358)
Malaria (359)
Leprosy (360)
Drugs and toxins
Gold (363–365)
Mercury (365,366)
Penicillamine (367)
Captopril (368,369)
NSAIDs (370,371)
Formaldehyde (372)
Hydrocarbons (373,374)
Bucillamine (375,376)
Miscellaneous
Tumors (189–194)
Sarcoidosis (377)
Renal transplantation (198–206)
Sickle cell disease (378)
Kimura disease (379)
Angiofollicular lymph node hyperplasia (380–382)

Listing excludes conditions where only a single case has been reported or where lesions were atypical of membranous nephropathy.
NSAIDs, nonsteriodal anti-inflammatory drugs.
Adapted from Rosen et al. (2).

inflammatory agents, as well as exposure to toxins, including hydrocarbons and formaldehyde. In ~75% of cases, however, no etiologic agent can be identified.

Immunogenetics

Regardless of what triggers the aberrant B-cell response that results in subepithelial immune-deposit formation in MN, there is increasing evidence that this response is HLA linked (see also Chapter 5). Thus, there is a threefold increase in relative risk for MN in patients of several races with HLA-DR3, and associations with HLA-B8 and B18 have been reported as well (9–11). One study also noted an increased prevalence of HLA-DR5 as well as DR3 in patients with MN and end-stage renal disease, suggesting that DR5 may relate to risk of progression (11). Another study has reported an increased incidence of the allotype BfF1 associated with HLA-B18 and DR3 (12). In Japanese patients, MN appears to be associated with HLA-DR2 (13), and Caucasians and Japanese patients share in the deletion of C4a that is found on the HLA-B8-DR2 haplotype (14).

Potential Pathogenic Antigens

Central to understanding the pathogenesis of human MN is identification of the antigen against which the subepithelial deposits of IgG in this disease are directed (15). Since antibodies in the circulation may be depleted by glomerular deposition, only intermittently present or irrelevant to the development of glomerular deposits, this requires careful study of IgG eluted without denaturation from fresh human tissue of patients with typical early MN and careful comparison with simultaneously obtained serum samples. Because of the paucity of suitable tissue available for examination, virtually no such studies have been completed to date. One preliminary report describes antibody in the eluate reactive with an antigen of uncertain origin localized in the immune deposits but not in normal glomeruli (16). Another approach is to identify the (presumably pathogenetic) antigen that is present in the deposits. Many reports have appeared identifying presumed antigens in glomerular deposits in patients with MN, including DNA (17), thyroglobulin (18,19), tumor-associated antigens (20,21), renal tubular epithelial antigens (22,23), and HBV proteins (24,25). However, localization of such proteins in a damaged glomerulus does not necessarily confirm a pathogenic role, no studies have established that the antibody deposits in glomeruli were reactive with these antigens, and the reports are often of individual, sometimes atypical, patients. Thus, the existing data on the pathogenesis of human MN do not establish what antigens and antibodies constitute the subepithelial deposits.

Mechanisms of Deposit Formation

With regard to mechanisms of subepithelial immune-deposit formation, these have been extensively reviewed elsewhere (26–28) and are discussed in detail in this book in Chapter 14. Three possibilities exist. The deposits could represent the passive glomerular trapping of preformed immune complexes derived from the circulation. This possibility is suggested by studies of chronic serum sickness induced in rabbits by repeated administration of a foreign protein, bovine serum albumin (29,30) (see also Chapter 35). Animals maintained in persistent antigen excess, or with very low avidity antibodies, developed predominantly subepithelial deposits of antigen and antibody that were presumed to represent the passive trapping of preformed, low molecular weight, soluble immune complexes (30–32). However, subsequent studies have generally failed to establish that preformed immune complexes could localize intact in a subepithelial distribution [reviewed by Couser and Salant (27)] unless they are either very small and strongly positively charged (properties not characteristic of circulating immune complexes in vivo) (33) or first localized on the proximal side of the glomerular filtration barrier before dissociating and presumably re-forming locally in a subepithelial distribution (34). Moreover, while the predominant site of deposit formation can be manipulated by altering complex size and charge, preformed immune complexes usually localize in detectable amounts in mesangial and subendothelial sites (28), whereas deposit formation in idiopathic MN is exclusively subepithelial (6,7). Finally, elevated levels of circulating immune complexes are only rarely detected in idiopathic MN (35,36).

Subsequent studies have shown that subepithelial immune-complex deposits can be induced much more readily by mechanisms of in situ immune-deposit formation in which either the antigen (37) or antibody (38), usually modified to have a strong positive charge, is localized first by binding to glomerular anionic sites followed by local interaction with the other component of the complex. This mechanism has certainly not been excluded in human MN. However, like circulating immune-complex trapping, deposits involving exogenous antigens usually develop in several different sites, the charge modification required is out of the physiologic range, and the process demands a continuous supply of relatively large amounts of antigen that could not be easily accounted for in the human disease. It now seems probable, though, that subepithelial immune deposits in chronic bovine serum albumin sickness may result in large part from such local mechanisms as opposed to mesangial and subendothelial deposits, which can be more confidently attributed to circulating complex trapping (27,28).

The third possibility, and in the authors' opinion the most likely, is the that the deposits manifest their unique and restricted pattern of localization in MN because they represent antibody reactive with an antigen that also exhibits a similarly restricted site of expression—that is, a component of the pedicel of the GEC. A number of such molecules capable of inducing subepithelial deposits have been identified and are discussed in more detail by Dr. Kerjaschki in Chapter 9, as well as in Chapters 17 and 31. A major point in favor of this hypothesis is the fact that a glomerular lesion indistinguishable from idiopathic MN in humans can be induced in rats by this mechanism. Thus, immunization of rats with an antigenic preparation derived from proximal tubular brush-border (Fx1A) results in the development over several weeks of exclusively subepithelial deposits of IgG, C3, and C5b-9 that closely simulate the human lesion (active Heymann nephritis autologous immune-complex nephropathy) (39, 40). These deposits also cause proteinuria and nephrotic syndrome with no accompanying hypercellularity (39, 40). Studies have clearly established that the mechanism by which subepithelial deposits develop in Heymann nephritis is through the direct binding of circulating IgG antibody to antigenic epitopes expressed on the membrane of the GEC (41–44) (see Chapter 9). The principal antigen in Heymann nephritis is gp330, now called megalin—an endogenous renal antigen present in clathrin-coated pits along the side and base of the podocyte foot processes (and in microvilli in the proximal tubular brush border) (44–46). Megalin, with a molecular weight of 516,715, contains all of the characteristic motifs of members of the low-density-lipoprotein receptor gene family and functions as a receptor for multiple ligands, including polybasic drugs (44,47). In addition to megalin, a more recently identified receptor-associated protein (RAP) that binds to megalin has also been shown to be a target antigen in Heymann nephritis (44,48). Megalin and RAP together are now referred to as the Heymann nephritis antigenic complex (HNAC), and both contain antigenic epitopes capable of independently inducing subepithelial immune-deposit formation. Once antigen–antibody interaction occurs on the GEC membrane, the locally formed immune complexes are patched and capped by the GEC in a process dependent on an intact GEC cytoskeleton (49–51). They are then shed from the cell surface where they lodge beneath the GEC and bind to the glomerular basement membrane (GBM) (52). At this site, they are relatively resistant to proteolysis and may persist for months without further deposit formation before slowly resolving (53–55). During this phase, the deposits may become surrounded by extensions of basement membrane assuming an intramembranous position in later stages of the disease (2). Although attempts to demonstrate circulating or deposited antibody reactive with gp330 in human disease have thus far been negative (56–59), antibody to RAP has not been looked for, and it is likely multiple other molecules with similar distribution and function on the GEC could serve as potential antigenic targets but have not been identified or characterized.

Although antibodies to the several antigenic determinants in the HNAC are sufficient to induce subepithelial immune deposits that mimic those seen in human MN, they are not sufficient by themselves to cause proteinuria, and other antibodies appear to be required (60,61). Recently, glycolipid-specific antibodies have been identified in antisera to Fx1A used to induce Heymann nephritis passively that appear to contribute to immune-complex formation and to be essential for complement activation and development of proteinuria (62).

Mediation of Injury

Based on experimental studies, the most important mediator of glomerular injury in MN is complement. The requirement for complement activation to cause glomerular injury (as measured by an increase in urine protein excretion) was first established by Salant, Couser, and colleagues in 1980 utilizing the passive Heymann nephritis (PHN) model in which the membranous lesion is induced by injection of antibody to Fx1A and nephrotic-range proteinuria develops within 5 days (63). An initial observation was that nephritogenic quantities of antibody deposited in glomeruli were unable to cause any increase in protein excretion in the absence of complement activation (63). The absence of any infiltration of glomeruli by inflammatory cells in PHN (and human MN) suggested that the complement effect did not involve generation of chemotactic factors such as C5a, the only nephritogenic function of complement identified at that time, but rather represented a new role for the complement system in mediating tissue injury (64). Subsequent studies have confirmed the lack of neutrophil involvement (64–66) and have established that the nephritogenic effect of complement in experimental MN is caused by the C5b-9 membrane-attack complex (66–69) (see also Chapter 18). Thus, proteinuria in the intact animal model of PHN (and in MN induced by exogenous antigens) is abolished by selective depletion of C6 (66,67). Proteinuria induced by anti-Fx1A in the isolated perfused kidney is prevented if serum deficient in C6 or C8 is used (68), and the increase in albumin permeability induced in the isolated glomerulus by anti-Fx1A antibody does not occur if C6 or C7 are not available (69). A pathologic role for the C5b-9 complex in MN is consistent with the observations of prominent deposition of several terminal complement components as well as neoantigens of the C5b-9 complex in subepithelial deposits in both active and passive Heymann nephritis (70,71) and also in human MN (72). Although S protein, or vitronectin, is also present in these deposits, suggesting that some C5b-9 complexes may be inactive (73), freeze-fracture studies of the GEC in PHN have clearly demonstrated membrane insertion of active C5b-9 complexes into the GEC (74). Following membrane insertion, the C5b-9 complex is internalized by the cell, where it is transported in multivesicular bodies to the surface of the cell facing the urinary space and exocytosed into the urine (74). This process occurs quickly, in contrast to disposal of antigen–antibody complexes, which are shed from the cell, bind to GBM, and persist for months. Exocytosis of C5b-9 results in increased urinary excretion of C5b-9, which is detectable only when active deposit formation and complement activation leading to C5b-9 insertion into GEC are occurring (75,76). That a similar process occurs in human MN is suggested by the observation from several laboratories that urinary C5b-9 excretion is increased in MN (77–80), particularly in early and active disease where deposit formation is most likely to be ongoing (77,78).

The mechanism by which sublytic C5b-9 insertion into the membrane of the GEC causes glomerular injury sufficient to produce nephrotic syndrome is thought to involve activation of the GEC to induce local production of potential inflammatory mediators that act directly on the underlying GBM (1,27). Sublytic amounts of C5b-9 stimulate production of a variety of inflammatory mediators by glomerular cells, including eicosanoids, cytokines such as tumor necrosis factor (TNF), growth factors including interleukin 1 and interleukin 6, reactive oxygen species, and extracellular matrix components (81–83). With regard to MN, experimental studies in the Heymann models document a complement-dependent increase in oxidant production by the GEC in vivo following C5b-9 attack (84), and modification of type-IV collagen in GBM by malondialdehyde indicating lipid peroxidation, a marker of oxidant injury (85). Moreover, expression of injury is substantially reduced by antioxidant therapy (85,86). However, a similar increase in production of the GEC-derived protease MMP-9 has also been documented prior to the onset of proteinuria in experimental MN (87), and it is likely that the damage to GBM that leads to increased protein filtration is mediated by both oxidants and proteases. In addition to direct GBM damage from GEC-derived mediators produced in response to C5b-9, detachment of GEC from GBM due to mechanical displacement by subepithelial deposits (88) or interference with cell–matrix interaction involving integrins may also be involved (89) (see also Chapter 31).

Consequences of Antibody-Complement-Mediated Injury in Membranous Nephropathy

The nature of the barrier defect in MN induced by antibody and complement has been explored in both experimental and clinical settings. Ultrastructural tracer studies demonstrate increased GBM permeability to large molecular weight proteins most apparent in areas of GEC detachment (90,91). Scanning electron microscopy of acellular glomeruli in MN reveals multiple circular craters (rather than pores) on the subepithelial surface whose sides later extend to assume a reticular configuration and then form bridges to encase the deposits (2).

Physiologic studies utilizing glomerular micropuncture and clearance measurements of differently sized and charged molecules document loss of both the size and charge selective filtration barrier in MN with protein leakage occurring through a population of relatively large "pores" (92–94). The decline in glomerular filtration rate (GFR) that develops over time in many patients with MN appears to reflect both the thickening of GBM as well as a marked reduction in epithelial slit pores due to podocyte swelling and broadening leading to an overall reduction in glomerular ultrafiltration coefficient and consequently GFR (92–94). It is likely that the extra glomerular interstitial changes with inflammation and fibrosis also contribute to the decline in GFR (95,96).

The mechanisms that underlie the development of capillary wall thickening and spikes in MN are incompletely understood. In early experimental MN, there is increased glomerular mRNA for type-I collagen and for the novel α3, 4, and 5 chains of type-IV collagen (97–99). Immunohistochemical studies document an increase in novel type-IV collagen chains and s laminin (97–99). In human MN, laminin B2 is a major component of GBM spikes (100,101), and novel chains of type-IV collagen (α3 [IV] and α4 [IV]) as well as nidogen and fibronectin increase on the subepithelial surface of the GBM (101). In more advanced disease, an increase in α1 [IV] is also present but in a more subendothelial distribution suggesting derivation from endothelial rather than epithelial cells (101). Hansch et al. have reported a marked increase in type-IV collagen production by GEC following sublytic C5b-9 attack (83), but others have not found collagen or laminin protein synthesis or mRNA to increase following antibody- and complement-induced GEC injury (98). Recent studies document a marked increase in the transforming growth factor (TGF) β_2 isoform in GEC in experimental MN as well as upregulation of TGFβ receptors on the GEC (102). Thus, C5b-9 may contribute to accumulation of extracellular matrix beneath GEC through selective modulation of TGFβ isoforms and receptors leading to overproduction of matrix components.

PATHOLOGY

The primary pathologic manifestations of MN are the result of the initial formation and accumulation of immune complexes on the subepithelial side of glomerular capillary walls and the resulting responses of the visceral epithelial cells and capillary basement membranes to this process. A series of stages of this process based primarily on ultrastructural appearances have been described, most notably by Ehrenreich and Churg, that depict a morphologic continuum comprising the initial deposition of complexes, responses of basement membrane synthesis that result in the surrounding and incorporation of the complexes into the basement membranes, and subsequent digestion of the deposits and basement membrane remodeling (103). It has also been recognized, in part based on elegant studies by Törnroth and colleagues, that while this continuum is conceptually useful to understand the varied capillary wall abnormalities that may be encountered in MN, an individual MN lesion need not necessarily evolve/progress through each of these stages in an orderly and predictable fashion as part of its natural history (104–106). Therefore, even as each of these morphologic stages of MN are described, an important caveat to bear in mind is that it is possible to proceed from some stages of immune-complex formation to resolution of the lesion without necessarily passing through intermediate stages. A second caveat is that the time frame of progression through any of the morphologic stages may vary considerably from individual to individual, and even glomerulus to glomerulus within the same individual. A third and perhaps the most important caveat is that it has not been possible to demonstrate meaningful, reliable clinical correlations (that is, functional alterations such as degree of proteinuria, prognostic outcomes, or response to therapy) that are based on classification of renal biopsy specimens demonstrating MN into any of these morphologic stages.

Light Microscopy

The most consistent abnormality in MN detectable by light microscopy is diffuse thickening of the peripheral capillary walls. In some cases of MN, however, basement membrane thickening may not be present and the glomerulus may appear entirely normal by this modality (Fig. 1). In such cases, the pathologic lesions of MN can be identified only by the characteristic features revealed by immunofluorescence or electron microscopy. This histologic appearance has been found to correspond to either "early" lesions (type-1 lesions in the ultrastructural schema of Ehrenreich and Churg) in which the deposits are small and there is little, if any, basement membrane response, or, alternately, to nearly resolved lesions. The more usual finding in cases of MN is homogeneous capillary wall thickening as manifest in hematoxylin–eosin (H&E)-stained or PAS-stained tissue sections (Fig. 2A). In these cases, abnormalities pathognomonic of MN are

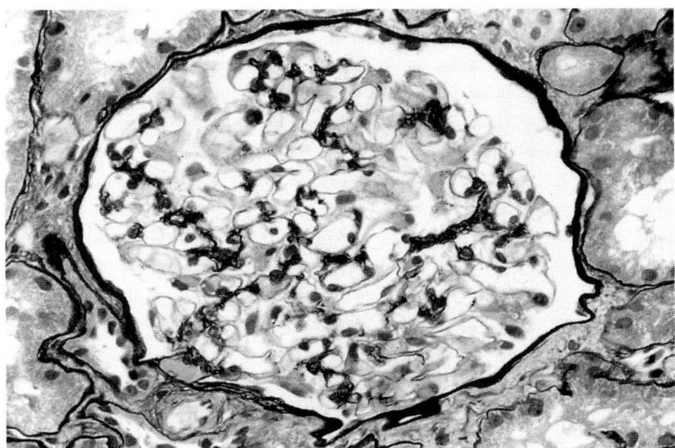

FIG. 1. Glomerulus with normal morphology and delicate basement membranes that proved to have stage-I membranous nephropathy by immunofluorescence and ultrastructural studies (see Fig. 5). Silver methenamine, original magnification, ×400.

A

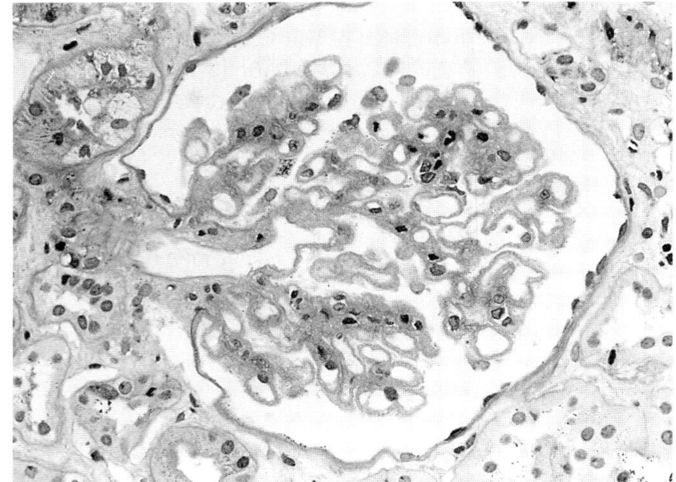

B

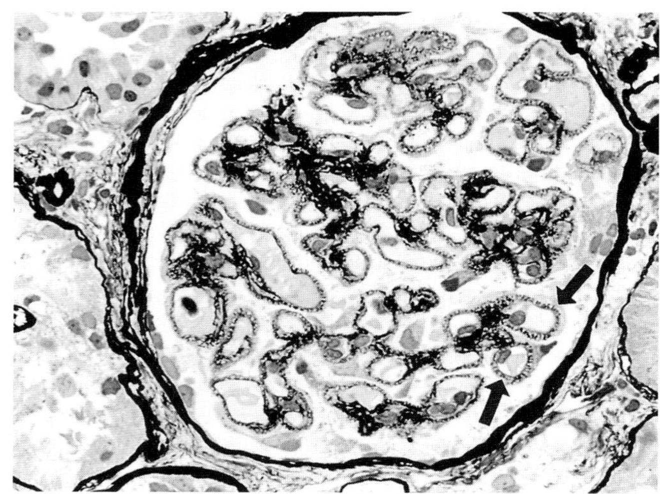

FIG. 2. A: Glomerulus with a more advanced stage of membranous nephropathy, showing diffuse thickening of capillary walls and the absence of cell proliferation or prominent inflammatory cell infiltration. Periodic-acid–Schiff, original magnification, ×400. **B:** Glomerulus from the same biopsy, stained with the silver methenamine reagents. The capillary walls show numerous "spikes" (*arrows*) of matrix material extending out from the original basement membranes toward the urinary space. The space between the spikes is occupied by immune complexes which do not bind silver methenamine. Original magnification, ×400.

demonstrable by histochemical stains that extend the information obtainable by H&E and PAS stains, as the latter generally do not enable discrimination between capillary wall thickening due to accumulated immune deposits extrinsic to the basement membrane and that due to increased basement membrane matrix. Tissue sections stained with silver methenamine or similar dyes that preferentially bind to basement membrane matrix but not immune complexes usually will reveal characteristic projections of the basement membrane, termed *spikes*, which have a perpendicular orientation to the capillary wall and point out toward the urinary space (Fig. 2B). As revealed by electron microscopy (see below), such spikes correspond to basement membrane synthesized in response to the formation of immune complexes on the external surface of the capillary wall. The unstained spaces between the projecting spikes of basement membrane are occupied by the immune complexes and entrapped elements of epithelial cell foot processes, materials that ordinarily do not bind to silver methenamine reagents. If the immune deposits become progressively incorporated into the capillary basement membranes, the appearance of the membranes will also change. They will continue to appear uniformly thickened in H&E- and PAS-stained tissue preparations, but silver-stained sections may reveal thickened capillary walls demonstrating rarefaction, or areas of lucency that are extensive and may give rise to a chainlike appearance of the capillary wall. Later stages in the disease process may result in irregularly thickened and remodeled basement membranes without lucency or evidence of persistent immune complexes, or may result in apparently normal remodeled capillary walls (107,108).

Although not a primary component of the disease process, other compartments of the glomerulus can be injured. The mesangium, not a site of immune-complex deposition in idiopathic MN, most often is without histologic abnormality. If mesangial proliferative changes are present and are associated with immune-complex deposition, usually this is evidence of lupus membranous nephritis (109). However, it has been increasingly recognized in many cases of membranous glomerulonephritis that glomeruli may be involved by focal and segmental glomerulosclerosis (FSGS) (110–112). This process, involving the mesangium, glomerular capillary structures, and glomerular epithelium, is morphologically indistinguishable from patterns of injury in idiopathic FSGS and has been encountered in 22% and 43% of patients in two recent large single institutional series of MN cases (111,112). It remains unknown whether the FSGS observed in the setting of MN is in some way a consequence of the MN lesion directly or a secondary event dependent on altered physiologic parameters such as glomerular blood pressures and flows and/or feedback mechanisms from the tubulointerstitium, or is mediated by factors independent of the MN process. Glomerular hypertrophy, which has been implicated in the pathogenesis of FSGS in other settings (see Chapter 33), has been identified as a feature of MN associated with FSGS compared with nonsclerotic MN cases in one study by Wakai and Magil (111). This observation could not be corroborated, though, in two series of MN reported by Lee and Koh (112) and Newbold et al. (113), who found no overall increase in glomerular size in patients with MN with or without FSGS. The clinical evidence obtained from these studies indicates that patients with concurrent MN and FSGS have a worse long-term prognosis and are less likely to respond to therapeutic interventions.

It has long been accepted that MN is distinguished from other immune-complex-mediated glomerulonephridites by the absence of a prominent component of cell proliferation as identified by counts of cell nuclei or mitoses. A study that measured glomerular cell proliferation in human renal biopsies using immunohistochemical detection of a protein (the proliferating cell nuclear antigen) whose expression is upregulated as proliferating cells traverse the cell cycle has confirmed the low levels of proliferation in all glomerular cell compartments in a small number of MN cases in contrast to other immune-complex-mediated glomerulonephridites (114). Cell activation is another phenotypic feature of injury that, to date, in the glomerulus has been generally identified by upregulated expression of α-smooth muscle actin by mesangial cells (114). In experimental MN, increased GEC expression of secreted protein acidic and rich in cysteine (SPARC) and desmin appears to mark GEC activation with SPARC apparently specific for C5b-9-mediated injury (115). Although currently there are no similar markers of injury that have been recognized for human visceral epithelial cells, the cell type most involved in the MN injury process, there is now evidence that upregulated production of the cytokine TNFα by these cells is a feature of MN (116). Studies by Neale et al. have demonstrated that upregulated TNFα expression is specific for membranous nephropathy as compared with other glomerulopathies (116). Accordingly, if substantiated by other studies, expressions of SPARC, desmin, and TNFα may serve as markers of injured visceral epithelial cells in MN. Since a functional role for these molecules in any form of glomerular injury has not yet been established, the pathophysiologic significance of this expression remains to be determined.

One other noteworthy difference between MN and other glomerulonephridites mediated by immune-complex formation in the capillary walls, such as acute postinfectious glomerulonephritis, membranoproliferative glomerulonephritis (MPGN), and the diffuse proliferative glomerulonephritis of SLE, is that these other entities typically involve concurrent injury to the mesangium and diffuse glomerular injury mediated by influxing leukocytes and platelets. MN is noteworthy for the absence of prominent intraglomerular accumulation of leukocytes. There is experimental evidence to support the idea that these differences in recruitment of neutrophils, mononuclear leukocytes, and platelets into glomerular capillaries are in part attributable to site of the immune-complex deposition in the capillary walls (117). Disease processes in which subendothelial immune complexes are common or may occur as part of the natural history of the lesion may be more able to transmit signals to hematopoietic cells in the circulation, most likely through focal fixation and activation of complement or upregulated expression of endothelial leukocyte adhesion molecules. Such signals are likely to be relatively inaccessible from complexes localized exclusively to distal and intramembranous locations in the capillary walls. The absence of a glomerular population of activated leukocytes may also explain the absence of cell proliferation and mesangial cell activation in MN, as the requisite stimuli to initiate these processes may be of leukocyte origin (118).

There is also an increasingly substantive body of evidence that the long-term functional impairment that may occur in patients with MN correlates with morphologic evidence of chronic tubulointerstitial injury (96,119–121). Such injury, manifest as interstitial fibrosis and tubular atrophy, also has been correlated to a lesser extent with the glomerular sclerosing injury just described. The mechanisms for the tubulointerstitial injury in cases of MN or other glomerulopathies remain unknown, but there is some experimental evidence to suggest that such interstitial events can be the consequence of activity of mediator molecules produced in the course of primary glomerular injury (122).

Immunofluorescence Microscopy

The immunofluorescence pattern in MN is a characteristic easily recognizable one of fine granular deposits of IgG and complement components located diffusely along all glomerular capillary walls (Fig. 3) (123–127). Early deposits are small and may appear almost continuous at low power but become larger and more discrete as the disease becomes more chronic. The deposits stain uniformly for IgG, often with a predominance of the IgG_4 subclass (127–129), although in de novo MN following transplantation IgG_1 and IgG_2 are more prominent (130). Staining for IgA and IgM is minimal in idiopathic MN, and the presence of strong staining for these immunoglobulins is very suggestive of SLE (2,3,131,132). C3 is also frequently present in the deposits. Most studies have found ~50% of patients positive for C3 (129,133, 134), although results are variable, and some authors have reported no detectable C3 staining (129,135). Most likely this reflects specificity of the commercial antibodies used. Anti-C3 antisera directed at C3c, the specificity of most commercial antihuman C3 antibodies, detect a breakdown product of C3b that is cleared very rapidly after formation and therefore reflects active, ongoing immune-deposit formation with complement activation (136). However, antibodies specific for C3d detect a covalently bound and persistent fragment of C3 that is present experimentally long after complement activation ceases (136). Thus, only a fraction of patients will be positive for C3 when only anti-C3c antibody is used, and patients who exhibit staining for C3c tend to have more severe disease (137). Staining for C3 using anti-C3c probably identifies patients with active disease, but staining for C3d is positive in most patients regardless of disease activity (137). Deposition of C5b-9 is

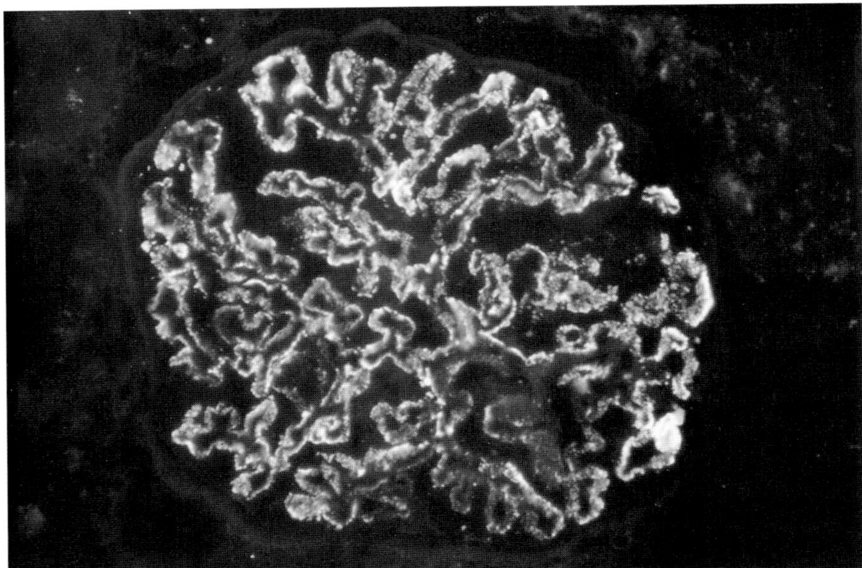

FIG. 3. Typical pattern of immunoglobulin G (IgG) deposition in membranous nephropathy as detected by immunofluorescence microscopy. There are widespread discrete, granular deposits of IgG localized to the peripheral capillary walls. Fluorescein-conjugated goat–antihuman C5b-9, original magnification, ×400.

also demonstrable in most cases of MN (Fig. 4) in a pattern similar to IgG and consistent with the hypothesis that C5b-9 mediates proteinuria in this disease (1,64). S protein is also usually present (73). Staining for C3 and C5b-9 is generally more pronounced than staining for C1q, C4, and C2, suggesting that complement activation in MN may occur primarily through the alternate rather than the classic complement pathway (72,138). Although a variety of other proteins and potential antigens have been demonstrated in selected patients, none of these antibodies are widely available or of documented clinical utility.

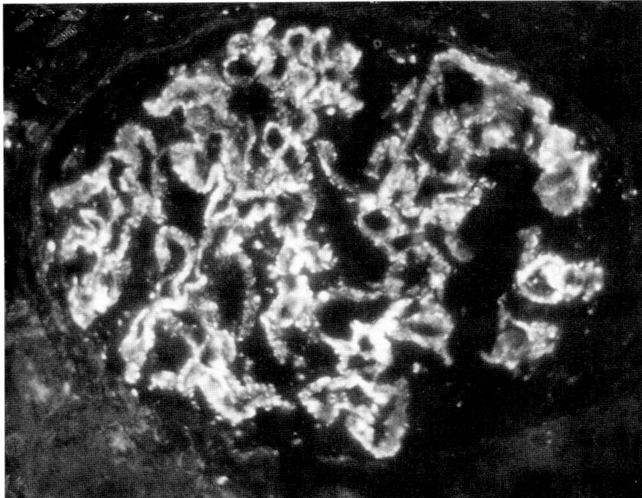

FIG. 4. Granular deposits of C5b-9 in membranous nephropathy as revealed by immunofluorescence microscopy. The distribution of deposits in peripheral capillary walls is identical to that found for immunoglobulin G as illustrated in Fig. 3. Fluorescein-conjugated goat–antihuman C5b-9, original magnification, ×400.

Electron Microscopy

The ultrastructural (by transmission electron microscopy) classification of MN, according to the widely accepted schema of Ehrenreich and Churg, divides cases into four groups (103). As originally conceived, these categories described four evolutionary stages (I, early; II, fully developed; III, advanced; and IV, late) of the disease process that corresponded to duration of disease (103). Some investigators have added a fifth stage to this schema—that of fully resolved injury with apparently normal, remodeled basement membranes. The stages do not have specific biologic correlates, but are useful depictions of what is in fact a morphologic continuum without sharp distinction.

In stage I, MN is characterized by the presence of homogeneous or finely granular electron-dense deposits on the subepithelial surface of the glomerular basement membrane (Fig. 5). The deposits tend to be small, and their distribution can vary widely, ranging from few or no deposits in a given capillary loop to widespread clusters of deposits that may even appear confluent. Characteristic of this stage is the absence of a prominent basement membrane response, although scanning electron microscopy of acellular preparations of the GBMs may demonstrate small craters even at this stage of disease (137,138). Visceral epithelial cell foot processes that overly these deposits are invariably effaced (Fig. 5), although they may be preserved in portions of the capillary loops uninvolved by immune-complex deposition.

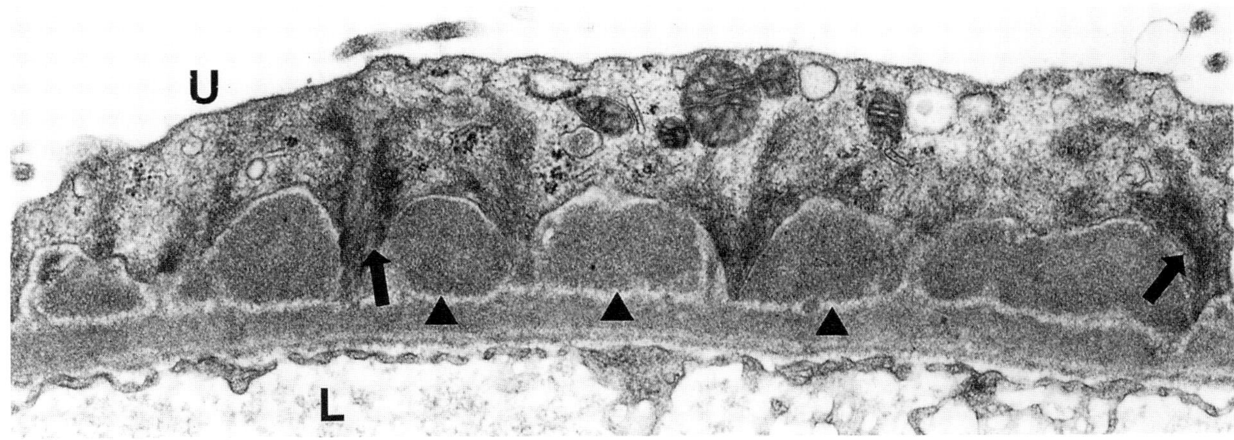

FIG. 5. Ultrastructural appearance of stage-I membranous nephropathy (same as in Fig. 1). The glomerular capillary basement membrane trilaminar architecture and fenestrated endothelium are unchanged, while numerous discrete electron-dense deposits (*arrowheads*) are present on the subepithelial surface of the basement membrane. The overlying visceral epithelial cells demonstrate effacement of the foot processes and show condensation of actin filaments within the cytoplasm near the immune deposits (*arrows*). *L,* capillary lumen; *U,* urinary space. ×27,000.

The corresponding histologic appearance of stage-I lesions is that of normal glomeruli or glomeruli with only slight thickening of capillary walls.

Stage-II MN is characterized by features of basement membrane response to the immune deposits (Fig. 6). At this stage, projections of basement membrane material, expanding outward from the lamina densa, can be identified that separate and appear even to surround many of the immune deposits. These projections correspond to the spikes identifiable on silver-methenamine-stained histologic sections. In some cases, the deposits (as well as entrapped cellular elements of the visceral epithelial cells), appear to indent the basement membrane, and this corresponds to the deeper craterlike changes in the basement membranes revealed by scanning electron microscopy (103,137,138). Other alterations of the architecture of the basement membranes are generally not identified at this stage. The overlying epithelial cells continue to demonstrate widespread foot-process effacement (Fig. 6).

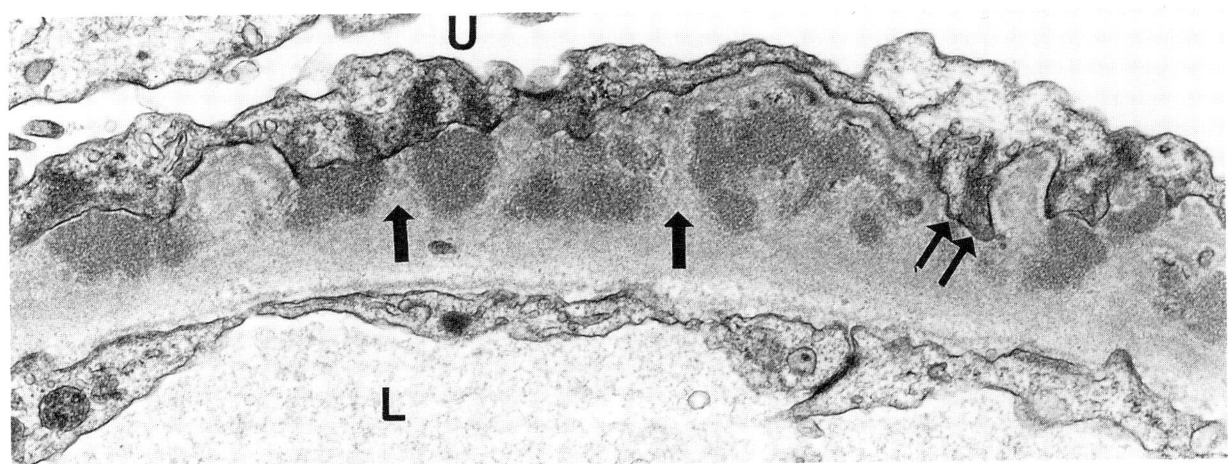

FIG. 6. Ultrastructural appearance of stage-II (approaching stage-III) membranous nephropathy. The electron-dense immune deposits are separated by "spikes" of basement membrane material (*arrows*), which focally appear to surround and cover the deposits (*center*). Such a process eventually may lead to incorporation of the deposits into the original basement membrane (stage III), which is still intact in this case. Overlying epithelial cells again demonstrate effacement of foot process, as well as foci of possible eventual entrapment of cytoplasmic processes between spikes or basement membrane material (*double arrows*). *L,* capillary lumen; *U,* urinary space. ×27,000.

Stage-III MN is characterized by more prominent and elongated spikes of basement membrane material that frequently surround the immune deposits and may even cover them. Although deposits are still generally well demarcated from the lamina densa of the basement membrane, the new accumulations of basement membrane material result in an appearance where the deposits now seem to be becoming progressively incorporated into a thickening capillary wall. The deposits in this stage vary in appearance. They may show extensive variation in size. Many retain the granular electron-dense appearance of earlier stages, whereas others may become progressively electron lucent, a feature that has been interpreted to indicate digestion of the deposits as well as a reparative response of the basement membrane. Capillary walls may also demonstrate zonal areas of lucency and layering of basement membrane material, similar to the lamininations of basement membrane that may be seen in hereditary nephritis of the Alport type (2).

In stage-IV disease, the basement membranes are considerably altered. They are thickened, and the normal trilayer (lamina rara interna, lamina densa, and lamina rara externa) structure is frequently indistinct. Extensive incorporation of deposits, demonstrating all degrees of electron lucency, into the basement membrane may be seen, while at other times the deposits may assume an electron density similar to that of the basement membrane and be relatively inapparent. Evidence of spikes is relatively infrequent. Also enmeshed within the thickened basement membrane may be ill-defined threadlike, fibrillar, and vesicular particles, which are residual debris from cellular elements—almost certainly those of visceral epithelial cells—that were entrapped in the course of the MN injury (see Fig. 6). These basement membranes correspond to thickened capillary walls with irregular rarefactions and lucencies seen in silver-methenamine-stained histologic preparations.

In end-stage MN, features of global glomerular obsolescence with capillary collapse, capsular adhesions, and collagenizaton of the urinary space are encountered, similar to any morphologically advanced form of renal injury resulting from any of a multitude of primary etiologies.

CLINICAL MANIFESTATIONS, LABORATORY FEATURES, AND ASSOCIATED DISEASES

Clinical Manifestations of Idiopathic Membranous Nephropathy

The idiopathic form of MN is almost always insidious in onset, with the development of peripheral edema the most common presenting complaint (139,140). Although the disease occurs in children (140), it is more commonly seen in patients over 30, with a median age of ~40 (123, 139,141–153). Most studies suggest two peaks of age distribution: one between 30 and 40 and a second around 50–60 years of age (139,143,153). MN is more common in men than women by about a 2–3:1 ratio (2,3,141–153). It is likely that the disease develops over a long latent or prodromal period, probably weeks or months, during which glomerular deposits are developing but urinary protein excretion is not sufficiently increased to cause symptoms (40,104–106). This period is asymptomatic and usually without any obvious inciting event. Patients come to medical attention because of proteinuria (~20%) or edema secondary to nephrotic syndrome (80%) (149–153). Proteinuria in idiopathic MN is usually in the 5- to 10-g/day range, lower than usually seen in minimal-change nephrotic syndrome, but values of >20 g/day can occur. The proteinuria, as documented by studies of glomerular barrier function, is usually nonselective (92–94). Urine protein excretion in MN may be quite variable day to day, with fluctuations reflecting changes in protein intake, posture, exercise, and hemodynamic variables more than activity or progression of disease (150,151). Microscopic hematuria may be seen in up to 50% of adults (139,152,153–158) and most children (158). Macroscopic hematuria is rare. Unlike most of the acute inflammatory glomerular diseases, hypertension is not a common feature of early MN but may occur in up to 30% of patients (141–145,153–159). Renal function is usually well preserved in early MN with nephrotic-range proteinuria commonly preceding any significant fall in GFR by weeks or months, particularly when reductions in GFR due to prerenal factors are eliminated (119,139, 141–143,153–155,159,161–163). Reduced GFR is present in <20% of patients initially, and uremia is very uncommon at presentation.

In addition to these clinical features of idiopathic MN, there are several associated conditions of clinical significance to consider early in the course of MN. Some of these are mentioned in Table 1, which lists secondary causes of MN.

Membranous Lupus Nephritis

The clinical and morphologic features of lupus nephritis are reviewed in more detail in Chapter 48. About 15–20% of patients with lupus nephritis have a class-V lesion with predominantly or exclusively subepithelial deposits and a disease very similar clinically and morphologically to idiopathic MN (165–167). Often these patients are young women with normal serologic findings who develop evidence of SLE at only a later time (165–175). Occasionally, typical class-IV, or diffuse proliferative, SLE will transform after aggressive therapy into a predominantly membranous lesion (176). Immunologically, patients with membranous lupus nephritis appear to represent a distinct group different both clinically and serologically from patients with diffuse proliferative lupus nephritis. They have lower levels of anti-DNA antibody, 25–50% have negative antinuclear antibody test results, and the antibody they do have is often of very low avidity (176–178). A renal biopsy specimen may be indistinguishable from that of idiopathic MN, but the diagnosis of SLE is strongly suggested by the presence of staining for IgA and IgM as well as IgG (129), by the presence of mesangial as well as subepithelial immune-complex deposits, sometimes with some mesangial cell proliferation, or by the presence of tubuloreticular structures (which are induced by α-interferon) in glomerular endothelial cells (109). As in idiopathic MN, patients with lupus MN generally present with nephrotic syndrome and may maintain well-preserved renal function for long periods (165,166,168–171). Also, as in idiopathic MN, the incidence of renal vein thrombosis is increased (179) (see below). Long-term kidney survival in pure lupus MN is good, exceeding 85% at 10 years, but survival declines with increasing signs of inflammation in the biopsy specimens or if the initial serum creatinine is elevated (180,180a). The natural history is not well defined and, in several series, patients have been treated with steroids and immunosuppressive agents utilizing protocols similar to those employed for diffuse proliferative lupus nephritis (181) (see Chapter 48). Although these protocols often use pulse cyclophosphamide, it is noteworthy that pulse cyclophosphamide does not appear to be useful in idiopathic MN (181a) and should be used with caution in lupus MN.

Membranous Nephropathy and Hepatitis B

The association between the chronic carrier state for HBV and MN is well established (182,350–352). The association is strongest in boys, where >80% of cases of MN worldwide are HBV positive (182). In the United States, ~20% of children with MN are positive for HBV (183). In adults, the incidence of HBV in patients with MN is as high as 30–40% in Asia but generally <1% in the United States (182). The clinical features, pathology, and treatment of HBV MN are considered in more detail in Chapter 41.

Membranous Nephropathy and Hepatitis C

Although HCV infection is characteristically associated with MPGN (see Chapter 41), several patients with HCV and MN have been reported (184–186). Unlike MPGN, HCV MN is usually not associated with cryoglobulins, rheumatoid factor, or hypocomplementemia (184). The pathogenesis of the lesion and why it differs from the lesion in HCV-associated MPGN is unknown.

Presumably the glomerular immune deposits result from formation of immune complexes containing HCV antigens as postulated for HBV-associated MN (see above) or represent the consequences of an autoimmune response induced by the HCV (187,188). Little is known of the long-term course and response to therapy of such patients. However, treatment with steroids or immunosuppressive agents would seem unwise as they may increase viral titers and lead to chronic active hepatitis. Preliminary data on the use of α-interferon therapy have been encouraging, with some patients experiencing significant reductions in proteinuria and improvement in renal function, usually in association with a reduction in viremia (184).

Cancer and Membranous Nephropathy

A third associated condition to be excluded is the presence of an occult malignancy. Up to 10% of all patients in some series with apparently idiopathic MN have had an associated malignancy (189), although the overall incidence is probably closer to 1–2% (189a). This figure rises to ~20% in patients over 60 (190–194). Although a wide variety of cancers have been reported in patients with MN, the best established associations are with cancer of the gastrointestinal tract, lung, and breast (reviewed in references 189a and 190–194). The reason for the association between cancer and MN is unknown. In some patients, tumor-specific antigens, including carcinoembryonic antigen, have been detected in glomerular deposits (20,21) and antibodies to tumor antigens may be present in the circulation (21). The subepithelial deposits in such patients may represent in situ formation of immune-complex deposits containing tumor antigens, antibody reactivity with tumor-related antigens shared with the GEC, or simply an increased incidence of two conditions that both occur in patients with poor humoral immune responses (195,196) but are causally unrelated. Whatever the mechanism, the nephrotic syndrome sometimes precedes clinical manifestations of the tumor by 12–18 months, mandating a careful search for occult malignancy in older patients with MN, for up to 50% harbor a tumor (197). There are reports of resolution of nephrotic syndrome after tumor removal (191–194), although this does not always occur (21). There are no data on the response of tumor-related MN to steroid or immunosuppressive therapy.

De Novo Membranous Nephropathy in Renal Allografts

Although recurrent glomerulonephritis in renal allografts is a well-recognized feature of several glomerular diseases, including MN (see below), MN is unique among glomerular diseases in presenting de novo as a disease of the allograft in patients whose original disease was not MN (198–206). In several series, de novo MN has been the underlying disease in up to 30% of transplant patients who develop nephrotic syndrome (199–207) and is second only to transplant glomerulopathy as a cause of nephrotic syndrome in transplants (208,209). No clinical features have been identified that predispose transplant patients to develop de novo MN, although those who do develop the disease appear to have HLA phenotypes similar to those associated with increased risk for idiopathic MN (210). The onset of the disease is slower than the onset of recurrent MN, averaging ~2 years after transplant, with a range of 4 months to several years (211–213). The prevalence of the disease increases with the life of the allograft, and de novo MN may be present in up to 20% of grafts 16 or more years after transplantation (198). All patients exhibit proteinuria, and ~60% are nephrotic. As in idiopathic MN, the incidence of thrombosis in the allograft renal vein is increased (202–204).

The pathogenesis of de novo MN is unknown but is presumably analogous to that of idiopathic MN. Serologic studies have identified an increased prevalence of small, preformed immune complexes, cationic IgG spectra types, and antibodies to brush-border or tubular epithelial antigens compared with other transplant patients (210), but the pathogenetic significance of these findings is unclear. Others have suggested the deposits result from low-avidity antibodies made by immunosuppressed patients to several major histocompatibility complex–determined antigens (211,212). Most studies suggest that de novo MN does not have a significant effect on allograft survival, and the graft loss in such patients is usually a consequence of rejection (198). The incidence of the disease has not been reduced by the use of cyclosporine for transplant immunosuppression, and there is no therapy of established benefit for this disorder.

Renal Vein Thrombosis in Membranous Nephropathy

There is a significant incidence of renal vein thrombosis in all forms of MN (160,197,213–215). There is no evidence that renal vein thrombosis causes MN, but it appears to develop more commonly in MN of any etiology than it does in other nephrotic diseases of comparable severity (160). The incidence of renal vein thrombosis in a carefully studied population of 100 Chinese patients with idiopathic MN who underwent prospective renal venography was 46% (216), a figure similar to that from retrospective studies in the United States (217,218). Risk factors include albumin levels below 2.0–2.5 g/dL, vigorous diuretic therapy, and bed rest (216). Patients with renal vein thrombosis do not have any more severe or progressive disease than those without, but are presumably at increased risk of developing thromboembolic complications and may be candidates for prophylactic anticoagulation (see the section on *treatment* below) (219).

Membranous Nephropathy and Rapidly Progressive Glomerulonephritis

Although uncommon, it is now well established that some patients with idiopathic MN develop a superimposed, rapidly progressive crescentic glomerulonephritis with nephritic features and abrupt loss of renal function (220–224) (see also Chapter 43). Many of these patients have had documented anti-GBM antibody as a cause of the rapidly progressive glomerulonephritis (220,222, 223). The usual sequence has been superimposition of acute anti-GBM nephritis on the course of chronic slowly progressive MN, but in some patients the two diseases have been detected simultaneously (223–227). Documentation of anti-GBM antibody requires a positive serum assay, since early immunofluorescence staining for IgG in MN can assume an almost linear configuration (2,3). The reason for this association is unclear. MN may somehow expose GBM antigens, resulting in stimulation of production of anti-GBM antibody, although antiglomerular antibodies are not commonly seen in other glomerular diseases. Alternatively, if the pathogenesis of MN is autoimmune, such patients may simply suffer from immune dysregulation that predisposes them to develop other autoimmune collagen–vascular diseases. Support for this hypothesis comes from the observation that animals injected with mercuric chloride often develop both MN and anti-GBM antibody-mediated glomerulonephritis (228,229) (see Chapter 35). When anti-GBM nephritis complicates MN, treatment should be initiated with cytotoxic drugs and plasma exchange as recommended for uncomplicated anti-GBM nephritis (see Chapter 43).

Laboratory Findings

The laboratory manifestations of idiopathic MN are those of idiopathic nephrotic syndrome of any etiology, including hypoalbuminemia, hyperlipidemia, and lipiduria (160) (see also Chapter 37). Studies to exclude secondary forms of the disease should be done, including determination of antinuclear antibody and C3 levels, tests for HBV and HCV, and screening for tumor markers such as prostate-specific antigen, carcinoembryonic antigen, and parathyroid hormone related protein (PTHrp) in older patients. No available routine laboratory tests identify the idiopathic form of MN. In these patients, all serologic parameters are normal. Despite the evidence for a pathogenic role for complement in this disease, circulating complement levels including C3, C4, and CH50, are generally normal (unless SLE is present) (2,3). Circulating immune-complex assays are often negative as well

(35,36). At an experimental level, it has been demonstrated that C5b-9-mediated injury to the GEC as occurs in experimental MN is accompanied by an increase in urinary excretion of C5b-9 that is not seen in other immune glomerular diseases and closely parallels the formation of new subepithelial deposits or disease activity (75–80). Presumably this reflects transport of newly inserted C5b-9 complexes by the GEC with exocytosis into the urinary space (74). In humans, considerable C5b-9 formation occurs in postglomerular proteinuric urine (77,230). By some assays, no increase in urinary C5b-9 excretion is seen in MN compared with other nephrotic disorders unless the measurement corrects for excretion of native complement components (77). However, when C5b-9 excretion is factored by excretion of C5, a significant increase in urinary C5b-9 excretion is present in patients with early idiopathic and lupus-associated MN (77), particularly when studied early in the course of the disease. This finding may represent a useful approach to assessing disease activity and determining the likelihood of progression and the need for immunosuppressive therapy as well as the response to it (78–80). In a recent study, 12 of 17 patients with persistent elevated urinary excretion of C5b-9 had progressive disease compared with only two of 18 patients whose urinary C5b-9 excretion ceased (80). However, the laboratory study that is most needed in this disease is an assay for the antibody in the circulation that is forming subepithelial deposits in glomeruli. Until this is identified, laboratory studies of patients with idiopathic MN are of no specific diagnostic or prognostic value.

DIFFERENTIAL DIAGNOSIS

The differential diagnosis of idiopathic MN is the differential diagnosis of idiopathic nephrotic syndrome and includes the primary renal diseases such as minimal-change nephrotic syndrome (Chapter 44), focal glomerulosclerosis (Chapter 46), and MPGN types I and II (Chapters 41 and 51), as well as secondary renal lesions such as diabetes and amyloid (Chapter 52). Appropriate serologic evaluation of such patients should include determination of antinuclear antibody and complement levels, tests for HBV and HCV, and assessment of HIV status (see also Chapter 37). However, there are no clinical or laboratory features that permit a diagnosis of MN without obtaining a renal biopsy specimen. Statistically, the disease is rare in children or patients under 30, whereas minimal-change nephrotic syndrome is common, and MN is the commonest cause of idiopathic nephrotic syndrome in patients over 50 (2,3,231). Mean urine protein excretion is usually <10 g in idiopathic MN, whereas higher values are usually seen in minimal-change nephrotic syndrome and focal sclerosis, but substantial overlap does occur (2,3). Hypertension is more common in focal sclerosis than in MN (2,3). However, despite suggestions that all patients with idiopathic nephrotic syndrome be subjected to empiric steroid therapy without undergoing a diagnostic renal biopsy (232), it is the authors' conviction that appropriate evaluation and treatment of such patients confers benefits that outweigh the small risks incurred with a percutaneous renal biopsy in experienced hands (see Chapter 37).

The finding of MN on biopsy does obligate the clinician to exclude treatable secondary causes such as lupus, HBV or HCV, and malignancy. These disorders can generally be confidently excluded by appropriate clinical and serologic evaluation, leading to a diagnosis of idiopathic MN by their exclusion.

COURSE AND PROGNOSIS

It is essential to approaching the question of therapy in MN to understand the natural history and prognosis of this disease when it is not treated. At the outset, it must be recognized that the disease is an insidious one in which the underlying immune pathogenetic mechanism is probably operative for weeks or months before the patient comes to medical attention. Another point that deserves emphasis is that the glomerular lesion in MN, at least as it is studied experimentally, also resolves very slowly, even if the glomerular deposition of antibody is halted completely. Thus, nephrotic kidneys from rats with typical stage-II to III MN transplanted into syngeneic normal hosts continue to display subepithelial immune deposits for several months and continue to excrete nephrotic-range proteinuria for even longer (53–55) despite cessation of urinary C5b-9 excretion and hence of ongoing immune-deposit formation (55). Thus, the clinical course of MN is dissociated from the immunopathologic events that produce it in both its early and its later stages. Since only the clinical parameters such as proteinuria and renal function can be measured in humans, our understanding of the natural history of the underlying disease process in MN is very incomplete.

When MN is induced by a drug such as penicillamine, resolution always follows discontinuation of the drug but may take 2–3 years (mean, 9–12 months) (232a). Several studies have addressed the natural history of untreated idiopathic MN (141–144,233–246). In children, a spontaneous remission of proteinuria occurs in >50% within 5 years, and 10-year renal survival is >90% (119,140,158, 233–246). Most women, and children under 10, will experience a spontaneous remission, and disease-specific therapy is rarely indicated (148,158,236). In adults, considerably more variability has been reported, but the prognosis is clearly worse than in children. Possible outcomes include spontaneous remission, persistent non-nephrotic proteinuria, persistent nephrotic syndrome, and death or dialysis. The approximate prevalence of these outcomes at various times after diagnosis is depicted in Fig. 7. The frequency of spontaneous complete remission is ~25% (144,145,152), usually in 3–5 years, and another 20–25% have partial remissions with persistent non-nephrotic proteinuria and usually a stable GFR (150–152). Nephrotic-range proteinuria may recur in 15–30% of patients who enter remission (142,143,237,247), and half of these also enter spontaneous remission (237). The long-term course in patients who achieve a partial remission, or who retain normal renal function 5 or more years after diagnosis, is quite good (3). In the 50% of patients with persistent nephrotic syndrome, the chances of developing progressive renal disease are significantly higher. Figures from multiple centers suggest that 25–40% of these patients will die or undergo dialysis in 5 years and >50% (or 25% of the total number of patients with MN) by 10 years (143,145,146,149,155,161,245,248). In patients who do develop progressive disease, the mean time to doubling of serum creatinine is ~30 months (238). However, there is a subset of patients with MN who progress much more rapidly developing end-stage renal disease within 3 years (malignant MN) (144). These latter patients are at significant risk of developing recurrent MN in renal allografts (see below).

As only a minority of patients with MN will develop progressive renal disease, considerable effort has been made to identify factors that can mark that subset and predict a progressive course in order to select patients for aggressive therapy (see below). Those factors that are accepted to impact adversely on outcome in MN are listed in Table 2. Age is one such factor. The usually benign course in young children is cited above. In one study, eight of nine patients with MN who were >60 years old had a progressive course (238). Most series also suggest that gender is another predictive variable, with males much more likely to progress than females (146, 147,149,163,250–252). The level of renal function at the time of diagnosis is also predictive. Patients who have lost GFR already are more likely to continue to lose it than are patients with normal GFRs (143,146,147,154, 158–161,250,253). The likelihood of progression in patients with an initially elevated creatinine may be up to 70% compared with <20% in patients with normal function at the outset (161). Proteinuria is a fourth major predictive factor. Nephrotic syndrome is associated with at least a two- to threefold increased risk of progression compared with nonnephrotic proteinuria (147,161) and, in some studies, renal failure has been reported only in patients who were nephrotic at the time of diagnosis (235). Although absolute correlations between the amount of proteinuria and the rate of progression have not been clearly established in MN, most authors agree that proteinuria of >10 g/day, particularly in males, confers a higher risk of progression (2,3,147). Hypertension is a fifth variable that clearly accelerates progression in MN as it does in most other glomerular diseases (143, 154,159,248,251,254). Systolic pressures of >135 mm Hg have been reported to increase the risk of subsequent renal failure by as much as threefold (253). Biopsy findings are also useful prognostic indicators. Complete remission occurs predominantly in patients with stage-I or II disease, and progression is rare (143,154,235,255). As in most glomerular diseases, there is a good correlation between the extent of tubulointerstitial and vascular disease on biopsy and ultimate outcome(157,248,251, 253,255), and some have found tubulointerstitial changes to be, with serum creatine, a powerful predictor of outcome (251).

Several other variables have also been suggested to have an adverse impact on prognosis in addition to those just discussed but are less well established as risk factors in long-term studies. These include immunogenetic fac-

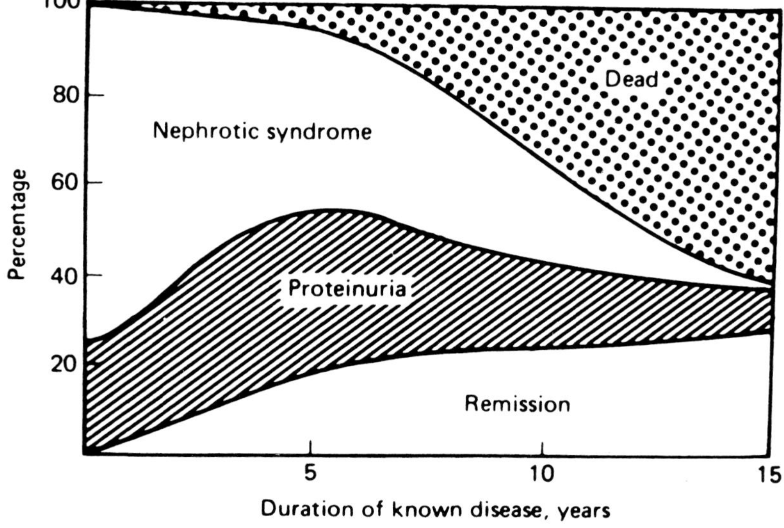

FIG. 7. Distribution of clinical outcomes in membranous nephropathy over a period of 15 years (from ref. 150).

TABLE 2. *Indicators of a poor prognosis in membranous nephropathy*

Advanced age
Male
Reduced renal function (at onset or within 5 years)
Nephrotic-range proteinuria (at onset or persistent)
Hypertension
Tubulointerstitial/vascular lesions
HLA-B18 Drw3, BfF1 DR5
Persistently elevated urinary C5b-9 excretion
? Poorly selected proteinuria
? Duration of disease
? Advanced stage of glomerular lesions
? Presence of glomerulosclerosis
? Cholesterol >260 mg/d[2]

Adapted from Rosen et al. (2).

tors (11), poorly selective proteinuria, hyperlipidemia (256), duration of disease, and the presence of focal sclerotic lesions on biopsy (111–113).

THERAPY

It must be stated at the outset that therapy of MN remains an area of controversy in immune renal disease (257–261). Experienced and well-respected clinicians have made recommendations ranging from no therapy for most patients (144) to prolonged, intensive therapy with pulse steroids and cytotoxic drugs for most patients (262). Because the disease is relatively common, a number of well-conducted prospective studies have been reported. However, many factors complicate interpretation of such studies. In the United States, most centers do not see the numbers of patients required for valid clinical studies of a disease like MN, and multicenter trials are necessary. Only a minority of patients with MN progress, making the number of patients required for study even larger. The multiple factors that influence prognosis (see above) are often not equally distributed between groups. Other factors that are not even measured, such as HLA typing, are likely important determinants of prognosis but are not controlled for. Progression, when it does occur, is usually very slow, necessitating many years of follow-up to detect differences between groups, a requirement often precluded by cost and logistical problems. The prognosis of most glomerular diseases has changed with time, making concurrent controls essential. Finally, the clinical outcome variables measured, primarily proteinuria and serum creatinine, are only indirect reflections of the disease process, which may be totally abrogated by treatment without any functional changes resulting for several months.

With these provisos in mind, the following summarizes the authors' interpretation of the most useful existing literature on treatment of MN without attempting to include all published articles (which exceed 300).

Non-Disease-Specific Therapy

A number of measures are now available that can reduce proteinuria in most glomerular disorders without the toxic side effects of steroid and immunosuppressive therapy. In most cases, a reduction in proteinuria improves prognosis and, when disease-specific therapy is needed, may also improve the likelihood of a response to such therapy (although this has not been proven). Several nonspecific forms of therapy for proteinuria deserve consideration in the management of all patients with nephrotic-range proteinuria caused by MN. Data from the Modification of Diet in Renal Disease study of protein restriction in progressive renal disease suggest a renal protective effect of moderate protein restriction (0.8 g/kg ideal body weight per day) on loss of GFR in proteinuric patients (263). *Protein restriction* alone may reduce proteinuria by 15–25% without known deleterious effects (264), and many studies suggest a direct relationship between the level of protein excretion and progression in glomerular diseases, including MN (265). A second approach is to use low doses of long-acting *angiotensin-converting enzyme (ACE) inhibitors* to decrease proteinuria. Several small, noncontrolled studies have suggested that ACE inhibitor therapy can reduce protein excretion by an average of ~35% in most patients with early MN without a significant reduction in blood pressure or GFR (264,266–270). The maximal benefit of these agents may require several weeks to develop, and the effects last for weeks after the drugs are discontinued, suggesting effects on mediators other than circulating ACE (271). Preliminary results suggest that this effect correlates with a reduced rate of loss of GFR (271,272), a benefit already established in other glomerular diseases (273). A third nonspecific therapy utilizes *nonsteroidal anti-inflammatory agents* to reduce proteinuria. Drugs such as indomethacin or meclofenamate often reduce urine protein excretion by 30–50%, an effect due in part to a reduction in GFR consequent to prostaglandin inhibition but apparently also due in part to restoration of glomerular-size selective function as well (274–277). Finally, several studies have reported additive effects of combining ACE inhibitors and nonsteroidal anti-inflammatory agents in treatment resulting in reductions of ≥50% in total urinary protein excretion (278). However, these results were generally obtained at the expense of a significant, albeit usually reversible, decrease in GFR, which is of uncertain long-term significance.

Other manifestations of nephrotic syndrome in patients with MN deserve consideration for therapy as well. The incidence of renal vein thrombosis has been variously estimated at 15–40% in nephrotic patients with MN (214–218,279,280), and the incidence of peripheral thrombosis and thromboembolism is significant (3). Risk is highest in patients with >10 g of proteinuria per day and serum albumin of <2.0 g/dL, and in patients treated intensively with diurectics or placed at bed rest (216–218). Anticoagulation is mandatory if such events occur. However, recent decision analysis studies indicate that the use of prophylactic oral anticoagulation in nephrotic patients is effective with the prevention of fatal embolic events outweighing the (minimal) risk of significant bleeding (219). Another issue is treatment of hyperlipidemia in nephrotic patients. In patients with persistent nephrotic syndrome and serum cholesterol levels exceeding 220 mg/dL, or elevated high-density-lipoprotein–low-density lipoprotein ratios, use of an HMG-CoA reductase inhibitor is probably indicated, as these lipid abnormalities are associated with an increased risk of coronary disease (281) and may contribute to progression (282). Although these agents can reduce total cholesterol, low-density lipoprotein and apolipoprotein B by 30–40% (283–285), elevated levels of lipoprotein a are usually not reduced (286), and the long-term effects of such therapy on atherosclerotic disease or renal disease progression have not been established.

Disease-Specific Therapy

The drugs most commonly employed to treat the underlying disease process in MN have been corticosteroids. Although a well-designed U.S. collaborative study suggested that treatment with alternate-day steroids for 8 weeks slowed progression of MN (249), the placebo-treated control group had an outcome worse than the anticipated natural history based on other studies, thus casting doubts on the conclusions. Two subsequent trials using steroids alone in similar doses have not demonstrated any significant beneficial effects in treated patients compared with controls (250,287). Based on these studies, current thinking is that treatment of MN with conventional doses of oral prednisone alone is not useful. It should be noted, though, that in the U.S. Collaborative Study, a small group of patients did enter remission during, or shortly after, oral steroid therapy (although they may have done so spontaneously) (249). Other studies have suggested that higher doses, or more prolonged courses, of oral steroid therapy may be beneficial (288,289). Short courses of intravenous (IV) pulse methylprednisolone have also been reported to stabilize deteriorating renal function in idiopathic MN, but long-term follow-up data are not available (290). Despite these caveats, in the authors' judgment, current evidence does not provide good justification for treating idiopathic MN with oral steroids alone.

Another treatment approach that has been widely used and extensively studied is the use of cytotoxic drugs, usually combined with steroids, in MN. A number of noncontrolled observations have suggested a significant benefit from cytotoxic drugs in MN (252,254,291). The largest and most recent controlled studies of cytotoxic drug therapy in MN are those by Ponticelli and colleagues in Italy, who have used a protocol employing three doses of methylprednisolone, 1.0 g IV, followed by oral prednisone (0.4–0.5 mg/kg/day) for 1 month, alternating with oral chlorambucil (0.2 mg/kg/day) for 1 month, with 6 months of total treatment. After 5 years of follow-up, almost 50% of the control group had worsening renal function compared with 10% of treated patients, and four of 39 control patients were on dialysis versus only one of 42 treated patients (252). At 10 years, the treated group continued to fare better with about a twofold higher incidence of complete and partial remissions and only 8% of patients dead or on dialysis compared with 40% of controls (292). Moreover, no long-term complications of therapy were noted. In a separate study, the benefits of this program appear to relate to the chlorambucil rather than to the methylprednisolone component of the regimen (293). When the Italian trials using chlorambucil are subjected to decision analysis using an average 40-year-old patient with MN, quality-adjusted life expectancy was reduced by 11 years with supportive therapy alone, 6 years with methylprednisolone alone, and only 4 years with methylprednisolone and chlorambucil therapy (294). Despite these impressive results, however, the Ponticelli regimen has not been universally accepted as the treatment of choice for MN. Some have not reproduced the results (295), and many have experienced significant problems with leukopenia and infectious complications, even at reduced chlorambucil doses, and particularly in patients with renal insufficiency (296–299). Moreover, the Ponticelli program has not been clearly shown to have a favorable risk–benefit ratio when employed only in that subset of patients with high risk of progression, although noncontrolled reports in this regard are encouraging (300).

Several studies have addressed the question of whether steroids and cytotoxic drugs are useful in that subset of patients with MN at high risk of progression—usually those with some documented loss of GFR and persistent nephrotic syndrome (289–291,301–304). Although most of these have reported beneficial results, the studies are generally small, with limited follow-up. One study from the Netherlands compared the alternate-month methylprednisolone/prednisone and chlorambucil regimen of Ponticelli (with a slightly lower dose of chlorambucil) with monthly pulses of methylprednisolone and cyclophosphamide in 18 patients with deteriorating renal function (305). After a mean follow-up of 15 months, four of nine chlorambucil-treated patients had stable or improved renal function, and only one was on dialysis, compared with only one patient with improved GFR in the cyclophosphamide-treated group and four on dialysis. However, four patients in the chlorambucil group had leukopenia or infectious complications, whereas no complications were noted in the cyclophosphamide-treated group (305). A similarly high incidence of side effects with marginal benefit has been reported by others treating progressive MN with chlorambucil (306). Some have advocated use of daily low-dose prednisone on chlorambucil months in order to minimize these effects (307).

Because of these concerns about side effects of chlorambucil, as well as data suggesting that cyclophosphamide may be a more effective immunosuppressive agent (308), and also the greater familiarity acquired with the use of this drug in treating lupus nephritis, cyclophosphamide has often been the cytotoxic drug of choice in treating MN, particularly in the United States. The reported experience with oral cyclophosphamide has also been favorable, although it has not been subjected to good controlled studies. In one noncontrolled study of 10 patients with documented progressive disease, mild renal insufficiency, and persistent nephrotic syndrome, treatment with alternate-day prednisone and daily cyclophosphamide (100 mg) for 1 year led to improved renal function in nine of 10 treated patients, with a mean urinary protein excretion that fell from 11.9 g to 2.3 g/day (302). Eight of these patients remained stable for periods of 12–42 months. In another small controlled study, 1 year of prednisone and oral cyclophosphamide therapy seemed to protect renal function with only one of nine treated patients on dialysis in 5 years, compared with 10 of 17 in a control group (303). Of interest is that a well-controlled study comparing 6 months of steroids and IV pulse cyclophosphamide with steroids alone showed no beneficial effect of IV cyclophosphamide (181), results similar to anecdotal reports by others (305). Attempts have been made to resolve the question of the efficacy of cytotoxic drug therapy in MN by subjecting the available literature to meta-analysis (309,310). Using various criteria for inclusion of studies, it was concluded that cytotoxic drug therapy is beneficial in reducing proteinuria in MN but that data on preservation of renal function were insufficient for analysis.

Two points emerge from the above discussion. One is that the need remains for a good prospective, controlled, long-term study of the utility of oral cytotoxic drug therapy in patients with MN at high risk of progression. Secondly, the benefits of cytotoxic drug therapy, while probably real, are accompanied by significant risk of toxicity and are of insufficient magnitude to be easily established or to be recommended with great enthusiasm to patients. Therefore, the search continues for other more effective and less toxic alternatives.

One such alternative that has generated significant enthusiasm in the recent past is the use of low-dose cyclosporin A (CSA) to treat MN. A number of noncontrolled, short-term trials of low-dose CSA (4–5 mg/kg) in MN have been reported (311–315). Most report that low-dose CSA can induce complete or partial remission in ~60–70% of patients without significant loss of renal function, but the relapse rate after ≤4 months of treatment has been relatively high. Longer periods of therapy appear to result in fewer relapses (315). In a recent prospective controlled study, Cattran et al. compared CSA (3.5 mg/kg/day) with placebo in 17 patients with persistent nephrotic syndrome and deteriorating renal function caused by MN. After 12 months of therapy with CSA, proteinuria was reduced 31% in the treated group versus 14% in controls, and the rate of deterioration in renal function slowed 88% in treated patients versus 23% in controls (316). At 2 years, six of eight placebo-treated patients had lost >70% of renal function, whereas only 25% of treated patients had a similar outcome. Six of eight CSA-treated patients maintained improved renal function and reduced proteinuria at a mean follow-up period of 21 months (316). However, the CSA-treated group had more problems with hypertension and transient increases in serum creatinine than did controls. CSA appears to reduce proteinuria by a direct effect on the glomerular barrier to protein filtration rather than by reducing GFR (317). Reports of its effect on glomerular deposits are conflicting, with one report demonstrating reduced deposits in treated patients (318) and one suggesting no effect (319). Thus, currently available data, albeit minimal, do suggest that low-dose CSA is useful in reducing proteinuria and preserving renal function in patients with progressive MN.

Another newer therapy with promising results in MN is IV immunoglobulin. Anecdotal reports of repeated administration of IV immunoglobulin for extended periods of time suggest that this treatment may reduce proteinuria and stabilize renal function in some patients with relatively severe disease (320). However, no controlled study of this therapy has yet been reported.

Finally, recent experimental studies document a marked decrease in proteinuria in experimental MN in animals treated with probucol, an antioxidant and inhibitor of lipid peroxidation (85). Anecdotal reports from the same group suggest that probucol may also be effective in some patients with MN resistant to other forms of therapy.

With the above in mind, our approach to the treatment of MN is as follows. Treatment with steroids and cytotoxic drugs is reserved for patients with persistent nephrotic syndrome and/or evidence of progressive disease. Patients with symptomatic proteinuria or nephrotic syndrome and a normal creatinine clearance are initially placed on nonspecific therapy to reduce protein excretion, including dietary protein restriction (0.8 g/kg/day) and a long-acting ACE inhibitor such as enalopril or lisinopril with dose adjusted until an effect on blood pressure is seen. If urine protein excretion is not reduced by 50% in 3 months, renal function is well maintained, and serum potassium is normal, a further reduction in protein excretion may be achieved by the addition of a nonsteroidal anti-inflammatory agent such as indomethacin 50–100 mg three times per day. If patients have, or develop, evidence of progressive disease in the form of a decline in GFR, or if a patient has persistent proteinuria in excess of 8 g/day for >6 months, disease-specific therapy is probably indicated, particularly in male patients. Further precision in selecting patients at high risk for progression and therefore candidates for therapy may be achieved using formulae that incorporate variables such as duration of persistent proteinuria, initial creatinine clearance, and rate of change in GFR (321). It is rare for children or female patients to meet these criteria, and most treatment candidates are older men. At present, we prefer to initiate specific therapy with steroids and cytotoxic drugs rather than CSA because of greater experience with these regimens and the greater possibility of inducing a long-term remission. We utilize oral steroids because most reports of cytotoxic drug therapy include steroids and because of their potential role in moderating some side effects of cytotoxic drug therapy (307). We use prednisone, 0.5 mg/kg/day, given on alternate days for 6 months. Steroids are combined with oral cyclophosphamide, 1–2 mg/kg/day, for 6 months with appropriate monitoring of white blood cell counts. Adequate hydration, including fluid intake at night, is emphasized to reduce bladder toxicity, particularly if substantial renal impairment is present. In the authors' judgment, there is no evidence that therapy is safe or effective if the creatinine clearance is <30 mL/min. Patients who experience complete or partial remissions are taken off therapy at 6 months and retreated if a relapse occurs. In patients who do not respond to therapy, have contraindications to steroids or immunosuppression, or who do not tolerate these drugs, treatment is switched to CSA, 4 mg/kg/day for 12 months. CSA dosage may be reduced if evidence of drug-induced decrease in renal function occurs. Patients with evidence of thrombotic disease and/or persistent proteinuria of >10 g/day with serum albumins of <2.0 g/dL are also treated prophylactically with oral coumadin and, if serum cholesterol is >220 mg/dL, lovostatin or pravastatin is added to control lipid levels.

PROGNOSIS

The prognosis of idiopathic MN untreated and treated with steroids and immunosuppressive drugs has been discussed extensively above. Despite aggressive therapy, however, 10–20% of patients will go on to end-stage renal disease, and MN accounts for ~4% of glomerular diseases leading to renal failure (322). Because de novo MN is a rather common event leading to nephrotic syndrome in the transplant patient, the exact incidence of recurrent MN has been difficult to determine, but it is probably ~10% (211,323). Patients at most risk of recurrence are those with the most active, aggressive disease. Most recurrences are in patients whose original disease progressed to renal failure in ≤3 years (324). There is also evidence that the recurrence rate is higher in well-matched, living-related donor kidneys (211,212,323–325). As in native kidneys, MN in renal transplants is associated with an increased incidence of renal vein thrombosis (326). The recurrence of subepithelial deposits has been reported as early as 8 days following transplantation (208), but the mean interval from transplantation to development of nephrotic syndrome is ~10 months (range, 1 month to 2 years) (209). This contrasts with de novo MN, which appears an average of 21 months after transplantation (range, 4 months to 6 years) (see above) (209,213). The effect of recurrent MN on the prognosis of the allograft is not well established. Over 50% of such grafts have failed, but the contribution of rejection to this outcome is difficult to separate from the contribution of recurrence. Most studies do not suggest any beneficial effect of additional immunosuppression on the recurrent glomerular lesion (202).

REFERENCES

1. Abrass C, Couser W. Pathogenesis of membranous nephropathy. *Annu Rev Med* 1988;39:517–30.
2. Rosen S, Törnroth T, Bernard D. Membranous glomerulonephritis. In: Tisher CC, Brenner BM, eds. *Renal pathology: with clinical and functional correlations.* 2nd ed. Philadelphia: JB Lippincott, 1994:258–93.
3. Glassock RJ, Cohen AH, Adler SG. Primary glomerular diseases. In: Brenner BM, ed. *The kidney.* 5th ed. Philadelphia: WB Saunders, 1996:1392–497.
4. Jones D. Nephrotic glomerulonephritis. *Am J Pathol* 1957;33:313–30.
5. Churg J, Grishman E. Subacute and chronic glomerulonephritis: histopathologic study by means of thin sections. *Am J Pathol* 1957;33:622–3.
6. Movat H, McGregor D. The fine structure of the glomerulus in membranous glomerulonephritis (lipoid nephrosis) in adults. *Am J Clin Pathol* 1959;32:109–27.
7. Spargo B, Arnold J. Glomerular extrinsic membranous deposit with the nephrotic syndrome. *Ann NY Acad Sci* 1960;86:1043–963.
8. Mellors RC, Ortega LG. Analytical pathology. III. New observations on the pathogenesis of glomerulonephritis, lipid nephrosis, periarteritis nodosa and secondary amyloidosis. *Am J Pathol* 1956;32:445–9.
9. Klouda P, Manos J, Acheson EJ, et al. Strong association between idiopathic membranous nephropathy and HLA-DRW3. *Lancet* 1979;2:770–1.
10. Berthoux F, Laurent B, LePetit J, et al. Immunogenetics and immunopathology of human primary membranous glomerulonephritis: HLA-A, B, DR antigens—functional activity of splenic macrophage Fc-receptor and peripheral blood T-lymphocyte subpopulations. Clin Nephrol 1984;22:15–20.
11. Freedman B, Spray F, Dunston G, Heise E. HLA associations in end-stage renal disease due to membranous glomerulonephritis: HLA-DR3 associations with progressive renal injury. *Am J Kidney Dis* 1994;23:797–802.
12. Dyer PA, Klouda PT, Harris R, Mallick NP. Properdin factor B alleles in patients with idiopathic membranous nephropathy. *Tissue Antigens* 1980;15:505–7.
13. Hiki Y, Kobayashi Y, Itoh I, Kashiwagi N. Strong association of HLA-DR2 and MT1 with idiopathic membranous nephropathy in Japan. *Kidney Int* 1984;25:953–7.
14. Muller G, Muller C. Immunogenetics of glomerulonephritis. *Clin Invest* 1993;71:822–4.
15. Couser WG. Research opportunities and future directions in glomerular disease. *Semin Nephrol* 1993;13:457–71.
16. Roberts ID, McGuire J, Short CD, Brenchley PEC. Immunohistochemical detection of a glomerular antigen in human membranous nephropathy. *J Am Soc Nephrol* 1985;6:882(abst).
17. Andres GA, Accinni L, Beister SM, et al. Localization of fluorescence-labelled anti-nucleotide antibodies in glomeruli of patients with active systemic lupus erythematosus nephritis. *J* Clin Invest 1970;49:2106–18.

18. Jordan S, Johnston W, Bergstein J. Immune complex glomerulonephritis mediated by thyroid antigens. *Arch Pathol Lab Med* 1978; 102:530–3.
19. O'Regan S, Fong J, Kaplan B, De Chadarevian J-P, Lapointe N, Drummond K. Thyroid antigen–antibody nephritis. *Clin Immunol Immunopathol* 1976;6:341–6.
20. Costanza M, Pinn V, Schwartz R, et al. Carcinoembryonic antigen–antibody complexes in a patient with colonic carcinoma and nephrotic syndrome. *N Engl J Med* 1973;289:520–3.
21. Couser W, Wagonfeld J, Spargo B, Lewis E. Glomerular deposition of tumor antigen in membranous nephropathy associated with colonic carcinoma. *Am J Med* 1974;57:962–70.
22. Douglas M, Rabideau D, Schwartz M, Lewis EJ. Evidence of autologous immune complex nephritis. *N Engl J Med* 1981;305:1326–9.
23. Zanetti M, Mandet C, Duboust A, Bedrossian J, Bariety J. Demonstration of a passive Heymann nephritis-like mechanism in a human kidney transplant. Clin Nephrol 1981;15:272–7.
24. Hirose H, Udo K, Kojima M, et al. Deposition of hepatitis B e antigen in membranous glomerulonephritis: identification by $F(ab)_2$ fragments of monoclonal antibody. *Kidney Int* 1984;26:338–41.
25. Collins A, Bhan A, Dienstag J, et al. Hepatitis B immune complex glomerulonephritis: simultaneous glomerular deposition of hepatitis B surface and e antigens. *Clin Immunopathol* 1983;26:137–53.
26. Couser W. Mechanisms of glomerular injury in immune-complex disease [Nephrology forum]. *Kidney Int* 1985;28:569–83.
27. Couser W, Salant D. In-situ immune complex formation and glomerular injury [Editorial review]. *Kidney Int* 1980;17:1–13.
28. Couser WG. In situ formation of immune complexes and the role of complement activation in glomerulonephritis. *Clin Immunol Allergy* 1986;6:267–86.
29. Germuth FJ, Rodriguez E. The relationships between the chemical nature of the antigen, antigen dosage, rate of antibody synthesis and the occurrence of arteritis and glomerulonephritis in experimental hypersensitivity. *Johns Hopkins Med J* 1957;101:149–69.
30. Dixon F, Feldman J, Vasquez J. Experimental glomerulonephritis: the pathogenesis of a laboratory model resembling the spectrum of human glomerulonephritis. *J Exp Med* 1961;113:899–920.
31. Dixon F, Vasquez JJ, Weigel W, Cochrane C. Pathogenesis of serum sickness. *Arch Pathol* 1958;68:18–28.
32. Germuth FJ, Rodriguez E. Immune complex deposit and anti-basement membrane disease. In: Immunopathology of the renal glomerulus. Boston: Little, Brown, 1973.
33. Gallo G, Caulin-Glaser T, Lamm M. Charge of circulating immune complexes as a factor in glomerular basement membrane localization in mice. *J* Clin Invest 1981;67:1305–13.
34. Caulin-Glaser T, Gallo G, Lamm M. Non-dissociating cationic immune complexes can deposit in glomerular basement membrane. *J Exp Med* 1983;158:1561–72.
35. Cairns S, London A, Mallick N. Circulating immune complexes in idiopathic glomerular disease. *Kidney Int* 1982;21:507–12.
36. Ooi Y, Ooi B, Pollak V. Relationship of levels of circulating immune complexes to histologic patterns of nephritis: a comparative study of membranous glomerulonephropathy and diffuse proliferative glomerulonephritis. *J Lab Clin Med* 1977;90:891–8.
37. Oite T, Batsford S, Mihatsch M, Takamiya H, Vogt A. Quantitative studies of in-situ immune complex glomerulonephritis in the rat induced by planted cationized antigen. *J Exp Med* 1982;155:460–74.
38. Agodoa L, Gauthier V, Mannik M. Antibody localization in the glomerular basement membrane may precede in-situ immune deposit formation in rat glomeruli. *J Immunol* 1985;134:880–4.
39. Heymann W, Hackel D, Harwood S, Wilson S, Hunter J. Production of the nephrotic syndrome in rats by Freund's adjuvants and rat kidney suspensions. *Proc Soc Exp Biol Med* 1959;100:660–4.
40. Couser W, Stilmant M, Darby C. Autologous immune complex nephropathy. I. Sequential study of immune complex deposition, ultrastructural changes, proteinuria and alterations in glomerular sialoprotein. *Lab Invest* 1976;34:23–30.
41. Van Damme B, Fleuren G, Bakker W, Vernier R, Hoedemaeker P. Experimental glomerulonephritis in the rat induced by antibodies directed against tubular antigens. IV. Fixed glomerular antigens in the pathogenesis of heterologous immune complex glomerulonephritis. *Lab Invest* 1978;38:502–10.
42. Couser W, Steinmuller D, Stilmant M, Salant D, Lowenstein L. Experimental glomerulonephritis in the isolated perfused rat kidney. *J* Clin Invest 1978;62:1275–87.
43. Cavallo T. Membranous nephropathy: insights from Heymann nephritis [Commentary]. *Am J Pathol* 1994;144:651–8.
44. Farquhar M, Saito A, Kerjaschki D, Orlando R. The Heymann nephritis antigenic complex: megalin (gp330) and RAP. *J Am Soc Nephrol* 1995;6:35–47.
45. Kerjaschki D, Farquhar M. The pathogenic antigen of Heymann nephritis is a membrane glycoprotein of the renal proximal tubule brush border. *Proc Natl Acad Sci USA* 1982;79:5557–61.
46. Kerjaschki D, Farquhar M. Immunocytochemical localization of the Heymann nephritis antigen (gp330) in glomerular epithelial cells of normal Lewis rats. *J Exp Med* 1983;157:667–86.
47. Farquhar MLG. The unfolding story of megalin (gp330): now recognized as a drug receptor [Editorial review].*J* Clin Invest 1995;96: 1404–13.
48. Orlando R, Kerjaschki D, Farquhar M. Megalin (gp330) possesses antigenic epitopes capable of inducing passive Heymann nephritis independent of the nephritogenic epitope in RAP. *J Am Soc Nephrol* 1995;6:61–7.
49. Matsuo S, Caldwell P, Brentjens J, Andres G. "In vivo" interaction of antibodies with cell surface antigens: a mechanism responsible for "in situ" formation of immune deposits in the zona pellucida of rabbit oocytes. *J* Clin Invest 1985;75:1369–80.
50. Camussi G, Brentjens JR, Noble B, et al. Antibody-induced redistribution of Heymann antigen on the surface of cultured visceral epithelial cells: possible role in the pathogenesis of Heymann glomerulonephritis. *J Immunol* 1985;135:2409–16.
51. Kerjaschki D, Miettinen A, Farquhar MG. Initial events in the formation of immune deposits in passive Heymann nephritis. *J Exp Med* 1987;166:109–28.
52. Kerjaschki D, Miettinen A, Farquhar M. Initial events in the formation of immune deposits in passive Heymann nephritis: gp330–anti-gp330 immune complexes form in epithelial coated pits and rapidly become attached to the glomerular basement membrane. *J Exp Med* 1987;166:109–28.
53. Lewis EJ, Bolton WK, Spargo BA, Stuart FP. Persistent proteinuria in the rat with Heymann nephritis. *Clin Res* 1972;20:763(abst).
54. Makker SP, Kanalas JJ. Course of transplanted Heymann nephritis kidney in normal host: implications for mechanism of proteinuria in membranous glomerulonephropathy. *J Immunol* 1989;142:3406–10.
55. Pruchno C, Burns M, Schulze M, et al. Urinary excretion of the C5b-9 membrane attack complex of complement is a marker of immune disease activity in autologous immune complex nephritis. *Am J Pathol* 1991;138:203–11.
56. Whitworth J, Leibowitz S, Kennedy M, et al. Absence of glomerular renal tubular epithelial antigen in membranous glomerulonephritis. Clin Nephrol 1976;5:159–62.
57. Zager R, Couser W, Andrews B, Bolton W, Pohl M. Membranous nephropathy: a radioimmunologic search for anti-tubular epithelial antibodies and circulating immune complexes. *Nephron* 1979;24:10–6.
58. Thorpe K, Cavallo T. Renal tubule brush border antigens: failure to confirm a pathogenetic role in human membranous glomerulonephritis. *J Clin Lab Immunol* 1980;3:125–7.
59. Collins A, Andres G, McCluskey R. Lack of evidence for a role of renal tubular antigen in human membranous glomerulonephritis. *Nephron* 1981;27:297–301.
60. Kerjaschki D, Horvat R, Binder S, et al. Identification of a 400-kD protein in the brush borders of human kidney tubules that is similar to gp330, the nephritogenic antigen of rat Heymann nephritis. *Am J Pathol* 1987;129:183–91.
61. Pietromonaco S, Kerjaschki D, Binder S, Ullrich R, Farquhar M. Molecular cloning of a major pathogenetic domain of the Heymann nephritis antigen gp330. *Proc Natl Acad Sci USA* 1990;87:1811–5.
62. Susani M, Schulze M, Exner M, Kerjaschki D. Antibodies to glycolipids activate complement and promote proteinuria in passive Heymann nephritis. *Am J Pathol* 1994;144:807–19.
63. Salant D, Belok S, Madaio M, Couser W. A new role for complement in experimental membranous nephropathy in rats. *J* Clin Invest 1980;66:1339–50.
64. Couser W, Baker P, Adler S. Complement and the direct mediation of immune glomerular injury [Editorial review]. *Kidney Int* 1985;28: 879–900.
65. Adler S, Salant DJ, Dittmer JE, Rennke HG, Madaio MP, Couser WG. Mediation of proteinuria in membranous nephropathy due to a planted glomerular antigen. *Kidney Int* 1983;23:807–15.
66. Baker P, Ochi R, Schulze M, Johnson R, Campbell C, Couser W.

Depletion of C6 prevents development of proteinuria in experimental membranous nephropathy in rats. *Am J Pathol* 1989;135:185–94.
67. Couser WG, Ochi RF, Baker PJ, Johnson RJ, Schulze M, Campbell C. Depletion of C6 reduces proteinuria in a model of membranous nephropathy induced with a non-glomerular antigen. *J Am Soc Nephrol* 1991;2:894–901.
68. Cybulsky A, Quigg R, Salant D. The membrane attack complex in complement-mediated glomerular epithelial cell injury: formation and stability of C5b-9 and C5b-7 in rat membranous nephropathy. *J Immunol* 1986;137:1511–6.
69. Savin V, Johnson R, Couser W. C5b-9 increases albumin permeability of isolated glomeruli in vitro. *Kidney Int* 1994;46:382–7.
70. Adler S, Baker P, Pritzl P, Couser W. Presence of terminal complement components in complement-dependent experimental glomerulonephritis. *Kidney Int* 1984;26:830–7.
71. Perkinson DT, Baker PJ, Couser WGC, Johnson RJ, Adler S. Membrane attack complex deposition in experimental glomerular injury. *Am J Pathol* 1985;120:121–8.
72. Falk R, Dalmasso A, Kim Y, et al. Neoantigen of the polymerized ninth component of complement: characterization of a monoclonal antibody and immunohistochemical localization in renal disease. *Clin Invest* 1981;72:560–73.
73. Falk R, Podack E, Dalmasso A, Jennette J. Localization of S protein and its relationship to the membrane attack complex of complement in renal tissue. *Am J Pathol* 1987;127:182–90.
74. Kerjaschki D, Schulze M, Binder S, et al. Transcellular transport and membrane insertion of the C5b-9 membrane attack complex of complement by glomerular epithelial cells in experimental membranous nephropathy. *J Immunol* 1989;143:546–52.
75. Schulze M, Baker P, Perkinson D, et al. Increased urinary excretion of C5b-9 distinguishes passive Heymann nephritis in the rat. *Kidney Int* 1989;35:60–8.
76. Pruchno C, Burns M, Schulze M, et al. Urinary excretion of the C5b-9 membrane attack complex of complement is a marker of immune disease activity in autologous immune complex nephritis. *Am J Pathol* 1991;138:203–11.
77. Schulze M, Donadio J, Pruchno C, et al. Elevated urinary excretion of the C5b-9 complex in membranous nephropathy. *Kidney Int* 1991; 40:533–8.
78. Brenchley P, Coupes B, Short C, O'Donoghue D, Ballardie F, Mallick N. Urinary C3dg and C5b-9 indicate active immune disease in human membranous nephropathy. *Kidney Int* 1992;41:933–7.
79. Coupes B, Kon S, Brenchley P, Short C, Mallick N. Temporal relationship between urinary C5b-9 and C3dg and clinical parameters in human membranous nephropathy. *Nephrol Dial Transplant* 1993;8:397–401.
80. Kon S, Coupes B, Short C, et al. Urinary C5b-9 excretion and clinical course in idiopathic human membranous nephropathy. *Kidney Int* 1995;48:1953–8.
81. Hansch G, Schieren G, Wagner C, Schonermark M. Immune damage to the mesangium: antibody- and complement-mediated stimulation and destruction of mesangial cells. *J Am Soc Nephrol* 1992;2: S139–43.
82. Schönermark M, Deppisch R, Riedasch G, Rother K, Hänsch GM. Induction of mediator release from human glomerular mesangial cells by the terminal complement components C5b-9. *Int Arch Allergy Appl Immunol* 1991;96:331–7.
83. Torbohm I, Schönermark M, Wingen A-M, Berger B, Rother K, Hänsch GM. C5b-8 and C5b-9 modulate the collagen release of human glomerular epithelial cells. *Kidney Int* 1990;37:1098–104.
84. Yamamoto K, Gewurz H. Isolation, characterization and identification of a modified form of C5b-9 consisting in three polypeptide chains. *J Immunol* 1978;120:2008–15.
85. Neale T, Ojha P, Exner M, et al. Proteinuria in passive Heymann nephritis is associated with lipid peroxidation and formation of adducts on type IV collagen. *J Clin Invest* 1994;94:1577–84.
86. Shah SV. Evidence suggesting a role for hydroxyl radical in passive Heymann nephritis. Am J Physiol 1988;254:F337–44.
87. McMillan J, Riordan JW, Couser WG, Pollock AS, Lovett DH. Characterization of a glomerular epithelial cell metalloproteinase as matrix metalloproteinase-9 with enhanced expression in a model of membranous nephropathy. *J Clin Invest* 1996;97:1094–101.
88. Leenaerts PL, Hall BM, Van Damme BJ, Daha MR, Vanrenterghem YF. Active Heymann nephritis in complement component C6 deficient rats. *Kidney Int* 1995;47:1604–14.
89. Adler S. Integrin receptors in the glomerulus: potential role in glomerular injury. *Am J Physiol* 1992;262:697–704.
90. Schneeberger E, Grupe W. The ultrastructure of the glomerular slit diaphragm in autologous immune complex nephritis. *Lab Invest* 1976;34:298–308.
91. Schneeberger E, O'Brien M, Grupe W. Altered glomerular permeability in Munich–Wistar rats with autologous immune complex nephritis. *Lab Invest* 1979;40:227–36.
92. Shemesh O, Ross J, Deen W, Grant G, Myers B. Nature of the glomerular capillary injury in human membranous glomerulopathy. *J Clin Invest* 1986;77:868–77.
93. Guasch A, Sibley R, Huie P, Myers B. Extent and course of glomerular injury in human membranous glomerulopathy. *Am J Physiol* 1992; 263:F1034–43.
94. Guasch A, Deen W, Myers B. Charge selectivity of the glomerular filtration barrier in healthy and nephrotic humans. *J Clin Invest* 1993; 92:2274–82.
95. Wehrmann M, Bohle A, Bogenschutze O, et al. Long-term prognosis of idiopathic membranous glomerulonephritis: an analysis of 334 cases with regard to tubulo-interstitial changes. *Clin Nephrol* 1989;31: 67–76.
96. Magil A. Tubulointerstitial lesions in human membranous glomerulonephritis: relationship to proteinuria. *Am J Kidney Dis* 1995;25: 375–9.
97. Minto AW, Fogel MA, Natori Y, et al. Expression of type 1 collagen mRNA in glomeruli of rats with passive Heymann nephritis. *Kidney Int* 1993;43:121–7.
98. Floege J, Johnson RJ, Gordon K, et al. Altered glomerular extracellular matrix synthesis and gene expression in experimental membranous nephropathy: studies in two models and cultured glomerular epithelial cells. *Kidney Int* 1992;42:573–85.
99. Minot AWM, Killen PD, Funabiki K, Bergijk E, Salant DJ. Increased abundance of α4 type IV collagen mRNA in passive Heymann nephritis (PHN): role of complement. *J Am Soc Nephrol* 1995; 6:902(abst).
100. Fukatsu A, Matsuo S, Killen P, Martin G, Andres G, Brentjens J. The glomerular distribution of type IV collagen and laminin in human membranous glomerulonephritis. *Hum Pathol* 1988;19:64–8.
101. Kim Y, Butkokwski R, Burke B, et al. Differential expression of basement membrane collagen in membranous nephropathy. *Am J Pathol* 1991;139:1381–8.
102. Shankland S, Pippin J, Pichler R, et al. Differential expression of transforming growth factor-β isoforms and receptors in experimental membranous nephropathy. *Kidney Int* 1996;50:116–124.
103. Ehrenreich T, Churg J. Pathology of membranous nephropathy. *Pathol Annu* 1968;3:145–86.
104. Törnroth T, Skrifvars B. The development and resolution of glomerular basement membrane changes associated with subepithelial immune deposits. *Am J Pathol* 1975;79:219–36.
105. Törnroth T, Tallqvist G, Pasternack A, Linder E. Nonprogressive, histologically mild membranous glomerulonephritis appearing in all evolutionary phases as histologically "early" membranous glomerulonephritis. *Kidney Int* 1978;14:511–21.
106. Törnroth T, Honkanen E, Pettersson E. The evolution of membranous glomerulonephritis reconsidered: new insights from a study on relapsing disease. *Clin Nephrol* 1987;28:107–17.
107. Noel LH, Zanetti M, Droz D, Barbanel C. Long-term prognosis of idiopathic membranous glomerulonephritis. *Am J Med* 1979;66:82–90.
108. Zucchelli P, Cagnoli L, Pasquali S, Casanova S, Donini U. Clinical and morphologic evolution of idiopathic membranous nephropathy. *Clin Nephrol* 1986;25:282–8.
109. Jennette JC, Iskandar SS, Dalldorf FG. Pathologic differentiation between lupus and non-lupus membranous glomerulopathy. *Kidney Int* 1983;24:377–85.
110. Van Damme B, Tardanico R, Vanrenterghem Y, Desmet V. Adhesions, focal sclerosis, protein crescents, and capsular lesions in membranous nephropathy. *J Pathol* 1990;161:47–56.
111. Wakai S, Magil AB. Focal glomerulosclerosis in idiopathic membranous glomerulonephritis. *Kidney Int* 1992;41:428–34.
112. Lee HS, Koh HI. Nature of progressive glomerulosclerosis in human membranous nephropathy. *Clin Nephrol* 1993;39:7–15.
113. Newbold KM, Howie AJ, Koram A, Adu D, Michael J. Assessment of glomerular size in renal biopsies including minimal change nephropathy and single kidneys. *J Pathol* 1990;160:255–8.

114. Alpers CE, Hudkins KL, Gown AM, Johnson RJ. Enhanced expression of "muscle-specific" actin in glomerulonephritis. *Kidney Int* 1992;41:1134–42.
115. Floege J, Alpers CE, Sage EH, et al. Markers of complement-dependent and complement-independent glomerular visceral epithelial cell injury in vivo: expression of antiadhesive proteins and cytoskeletal changes. *Lab Invest* 1992;67:486–96.
116. Neale TJ, Ruger BM, Macaulay H, et al. Tumor necrosis factor-alpha is expressed by glomerular visceral epithelial cells in human membranous nephropathy. *Am J Pathol* 1995;146:1444–54.
117. Salant DJ, Adler S, Darby C, et al. Influence of antigen distribution on the mediation of immunological glomerular injury. *Kidney Int* 1985;27:938–50.
118. Johnson RJ, Alpers CE, Pruchno C, et al. Mechanisms and kinetics for platelet and neutrophil localization in immune complex nephritis. *Kidney Int* 1989;36:780–9.
119. Ramzy MH, Cameron JS, Turner DR, Neild GH, Ogg CS, Hicks J. The long-term outcome of idiopathic membranous nephropathy. *Clin Nephrol* 1981;16:13–9.
120. Wehrmann M, Bohle A, Bogenschütz O, et al. Long-term prognosis of chronic idiopathic membranous glomerulonephritis. *Clin Nephrol* 1989;31:67–76.
121. Couser WG, Johnson RJ. Mechanisms of progressive renal disease in glomerulonephritis. Am J Kidney Dis 1994;23:193–198.
122. Pichler R, Giachelli C, Young B, Alpers CE, Couser WG, Johnson RJ. The pathogenesis of tubulointerstitial disease associated with glomerulonephritis: the glomerular cytokine theory. *Miner Electrolyte Metab* 1995;21:317–27.
123. Rosen S. Membranous glomerulonephritis: current status. *Hum Pathol* 1971;22:209–31.
124. Harrison DJ, Thomson D, MacDonald MK. Membranous glomerulonephritis. *J Clin Pathol* 1986;39:167–77.
125. Olbing HJ, Greifer I, Bennett BP, et al. Idiopathic membranous nephropathy in children. *Kidney Int* 1973;3:381–90.
126. Gartner HV, Watanabe T, Ott V, et al. Correlations between morphologic and clinical features in idiopathic perimembranous glomerulonephritis: a study on 403 renal biopsies of 367 patients. *Curr Top Pathol* 1977;65:1–29.
127. Bannister KM, Howarth GS, Clarkson AR, Woodroffe AJ. Glomerular IgG subclass distribution in human glomerulonephritis. *Clin Nephrol* 1983;19:161–5.
128. Doi T, Mayumi M, Kanatsu K, Suehireo F, Hamashima Y. Distribution of IgG subclasses in membranous nephropathy. *Clin Exp Immunol* 1984;58:57–62.
129. Roberts JL, Wyatt RJ, Schwartz MM, Lewis EJ. Differential characteristics of immune-bound antibodies in diffuse proliferative and membranous forms of lupus glomerulonephritis. *Clin Immunol Immunopathol* 1983;29:223–41.
130. Noel L-H, Aucouturier P, Monteiro RC, Preud'Homme JL, Lesavre P. Glomerular and serum immunoglobulin G subclasses in membranous nephropathy and anti-glomerular basement membrane nephritis. *Clin Immunol Immunopathol* 1988;46:186–94.
131. Jennette J, Iskandar S, Dalldorf FG. Pathologic differentiation between lupus and non lupus membranous glomerulopathy. *Kidney Int* 1983;24:377–85.
132. The Southwest Pediatric Nephrology Study Group: Comparison of idiopathic and systemic lupus erythematosus-associated membranous glomerulonephropathy in children. Am J Kidney Dis 1986;7:115–24.
133. Jennette JC, Iskandar SS, Daldord FG. Pathologic differentiation between lupus and nonlupus membranous glomerulopathy. *Kidney Int* 1983;24:377–85.
134. Bariety J, Druet PH, Lagrue G, Samarcq P, Milliez P. Les glomerulopathies "extra-membraneusus" (G.E.M): étude morphologique en microscopie optique, électronique et en immunofluorescence. *Pathol Biol (Paris)* 1970;18:5–32.
135. Pierides AM, Malasit P, Morley AR, Wilkinson R, Uldall PR, Kerr DNS. Idiopathic membranous nephropathy. *Q J Med* 1977;46:163–77.
136. Schulze M, Pruchno CJ, Burns M, Baker PJ, Johnson RJ, Couser WG. Glomerular C3c localization indicates ongoing immune deposit formation and complement activation in experimental glomerulonephritis. *Am J Pathol* 1993;142:179–87
137. Doi T, Kanatsu K, Nagai H, Suehiro F, Kuwahara T, Hamashima Y. Demonstration of C3d deposits in membranous nephropathy. *Nephron* 1984;37:323–35.
138. Quigg RJ, Cybulsky AV, Salant DJ. Effect of nephritogenic antibody on complement regulation in cultured rat glomerular epithelial cells. *J Immunol* 1991;147:838–45.
139. Gartner H, Fischbach H, Wehner H, et al. Comparison of clinical and morphological features of peri-(epi-extra)membranous glomerulonephritis. *Nephron* 1974;13:288–301.
140. Habib R, Kleinknecht C, Gubler M-C. Extramembranous glomerulonephritis in children: report of 50 cases. *J Pediatr* 1973;82:754–66.
141. Noel L, Zanetti M, Droz D, Barbanel C. Long-term prognosis of idiopathic membranous glomerulonephritis: study of 116 untreated patients. *Am J Med* 1979;66:82–90.
142. Row P, Cameron J, Turner D, et al. Membranous nephropathy: long-term follow-up and association with neoplasia. *Q J Med* 1975;44: 215–21.
143. Mallick N, Short C, Manos J. Clinical membranous nephropathy. *Nephron* 1983;34:209–19.
144. Donadio J, Torres V, Velosa J, et al. Idiopathic membranous nephropathy: the natural history of untreated patients. *Kidney Int* 1988;33:708–15.
145. Murphy B, Fairley K, Kincaid-Smith P. Idiopathic membranous glomerulonephritis: long-term follow-up in 139 cases. *Clin Nephrol* 1988;30:175–81.
146. Ehrenreich T, Porush J, Churg J, et al. Treatment of idiopathic membranous nephropathy. *N Engl J Med* 1976;295:741–6.
147. Hopper JJ, Trew P, Biava C. Membranous nephropathy: its relative benignity in women. *Nephron* 1981;29:18–24.
148. Couser WG. Glomerular disorders. In: Wyngaarden JB, Smith LH Jr, eds. *Cecil textbook of medicine.* 19th ed. Philadelphia: WB Saunders, 1992:551–68.
149. Zucchelli P, Cagnoli L, Pasquali C. Clinical and morphologic evolution of idiopathic membranous nephropathy. *Clin Nephrol* 1986;25: 282–8.
150. Cameron J. Pathogenesis and treatment of membranous nephropathy. *Kidney Int* 1979;15:88–103.
151. Coggins C, Frommer J, Glassock R. Membranous nephropathy. *Semin Nephrol* 1982;2:264–72.
152. Mallick N, Short C, Manos J. Clinical membranous nephropathy. *Nephron* 1983;34:209–19.
153. Gluck M, Gallo G, Lowenstein J. Membranous glomerulonephritis. *Ann Intern Med* 1973;78:1–12.
154. Honkanen E. Survival in idiopathic membranous glomerulonephritis. *Clin Nephrol* 1986;25:122–8.
155. Couser WG. Pathogenesis and theoretical basis for treatment of membranous nephropathy. *Nephrology* 1988;2:701–13.
156. Erwin D, Donadio JJ, Holley K. The clinical course of idiopathic membranous nephropathy. *Mayo Clin Proc* 1973;48:697–712.
157. Pierides A, Malasit P, Morley A, Wilkinson R, Uldall P, Kerr D. Idiopathic membranous nephropathy. *Q J Med* 1977;46:163–77.
158. Trainin E, Boichis H, Spitzer A, Greifer I. Idiopathic membranous nephropathy: clinical course in children. *NY State J Med* 1976;76: 357–60.
159. Franklin W, Jennings R, Earle D. Membranous glomerulonephritis: long-term serial observations on clinical course and morphology. *Kidney Int* 1973;4:36–56.
160. Bernard D. Extrarenal complications of the nephrotic syndrome. *Kidney Int* 1988;33:1184–202.
161. Kida H, Asamoto T, Yoloyama H, Tomosugi N, Hattori N. Long-term prognosis of membranous nephropathy. *Clin Nephrol* 1986;25: 64–9.
162. Forland M, Spargo B. Clinicopathological correlations in idiopathic nephrotic syndrome with membranous nephropathy. *Nephron* 1969;6: 498–525.
163. Pearl M, Burch R, Carvajal E, McCracken B, Wood H, Sternberg W. Nephrotic syndrome: a clinical and pathological study. *Arch Intern Med* 1963;112:130–40.
164. Warms P, Rosenbaum B, Michelis M. Idiopathic membranous glomerulonephritis occurring with diabetes mellitus. *Arch Intern Med* 1973;132:735.
165. Appel GB, Silva FG, Pirani CL, et al. Renal involvement in systemic lupus erythematosus (SLE): a study of 56 patients emphasizing histologic classification. *Medicine (Baltimore)* 1978;57:371–410.
166. Baldwin DS, Gluck MC, Lowenstein J, et al. Lupus nephritis: clinical course as related to morphologic forms and their transitions. *Am J Med* 1977;62:12–30.

167. Hill GS, Hinglais N, Tron F, et al. Systemic lupus erythematosus: morphologic correlations with immunologic and clinical data at the time of biopsy. *Am J Med* 1978;64:61–79.
168. Baldwin DS, Lowenstein J, Rothfield NF, et al. The clinical course of the proliferative and membranous forms of lupus nephritis. *Ann Intern Med* 1970;73:929–42.
169. Zweiman B, Kornblum J, Cornog J, et al. The prognosis of lupus nephritis: role of clinico-pathologic correlations. *Ann Intern Med* 1968;69:441–62.
170. Dujovne I, Pollak VE, Pirani CL, et al. The distribution and character of glomerular deposits in systemic lupus erythematosus. *Kidney Int* 1972;2:33–50.
171. Donadio JV Jr, Burgess JH, Holley KE. Membranous lupus nephropathy: a clinicopathologic study. *Medicine (Baltimore)* 1977;5 6:527–36.
172. Libit SA, Burke B, Michael AF, et al. Extramembranous glomerulonephritis in childhood: relationship to systemic lupus erythematosus. *J Pediatr* 1976;88:394–402.
173. Kallen RJ, Lee S-K, Aronson AJ, et al. Idiopathic membranous glomerulopathy preceding the emergence of systemic lupus erythematosus in two children. *J Pediatr* 1977;90:72–6.
174. Agnello V. The immunopathogenesis of lupus nephritis. *Adv Nephrol* 1976;6:119–35.
175. Appel GB, William GS, Meltzer JJ, et al. Renal vein thrombosis, nephrotic syndrome, and systemic lupus erythematosus: an association in four cases. *Ann Intern Med* 1976;85:310–7.
176. Lentz RD, Michael AF, Friend PS. Membranous transformation of lupus nephritis. *Clin Immunol Immunopathol* 1981;19:131–8.
177. Friend PS, Kim Y, Michael AF, et al. Pathogenesis of membranous nephropathy in systemic lupus erythematosus: possible role of non-precipitating DNA antibody. *BMJ* 1977;1:25.
178. Friend PS, Michael AF. Hypothesis: immunologic rationale for the therapy of membranous lupus nephropathy. *Clin Immunol Immunopathol* 1978;10:35–40.
179. Appel GB, Williams GS, Meltzer JI, Pirani CL. Renal vein thrombosis, nephrotic syndrome, and systemic lupus erythematosus: an association in four cases. *Ann Intern Med* 1976;85:310–7.
180. Pasquali S, Banfi G, Zucchelli A, Moroni G, Ponticelli C, Zucchelli P. Lupus membranous nephropathy: long-term outcome. *Clin Nephrol* 1993;39:175–82.
180a. Sloan RP, Korbet SM, Schwartz MM, Borok RZ. Long-term outcome in systemic lupus erythematosus membranous glomerulonephritis. *J Am Soc Nephrol* 1996;7:299–305.
181. Balow JE, Boumpas DT, Fessler BJ, Austin HA III. Management of lupus nephritis. *Kidney Int* 1996;49:S88–92.
181a. Falk RJ, Hogan SL, Muller KE, Jennette JC. Treatment of progressive membranous glomerulopathy: a randomized trial comparing cyclophosphamide and corticosteroids with corticosteroids alone. *Ann Intern Med* 1992;116:438.
182. Johnson RJ, Couser WG. Hepatitis B infection and renal disease: clinical, immunopathogenetic and therapeutic considerations. *Kidney Int* 1990;37:663–76.
183. Southwest Pediatric Nephrology Study Group. Hepatitis B surface antigenemia in North American children with membranous glomerulonephropathy. *J Pediatr* 1985;106:571–7.
184. Stehmann-Breen C, Alpers CE, Couser WG, Willson R, Johnson RJ. Hepatitis C virus associated membranous glomerulonephritis. *Clin Nephrol* 1995;44:141–7.
185. Rollino C, Roccatello D, Giachina O, Basolo B, Piccoli G. Hepatitis C virus infection and membranous glomerulonephritis. *Nephron* 1991;59:319–20.
186. Davda R, Peterson J, Weiner R, Croker B, Lau J. Membranous glomerulonephritis in association with hepatitis C virus infection. Am J Kidney Dis 1993;22:452–5.
187. Pawlotsky JM, Yahia MB, Andre C, et al. Immunological disorders in C virus chronic active hepatitis: a prospective case–control study. *Hepatology* 1994;19:841–8.
188. Warny M, Branard R, Cornu C, Tomasi JP, Geubel AP. Anti-neutrophil antibodies in chronic hepatitis and the effect of alpha-interferon therapy. *J Hepatol* 1993;17:294–300.
189. Lee J, Yamauchi H, Hopper JJ. The association of cancer and nephrotic syndrome. *Ann Intern Med* 1966;64:41–51.
189a. Burstein DM, Korbet SM, Schwartz MM. Membranous glomerulonephritis and malignancy. Am J Kidney Dis 1993;22:5–17.
190. Norris S. Paraneoplastic glomerulopathies. *Semin Nephrol* 1993;13:258–72.
191. Fer M, McKinney T, Richardson R, Hande K, Oldham R, Greco F. Cancer and the kidney: renal complications of neoplasms. *Am J Med* 1981;71:704–18.
192. Eagen J, Lewis E. Glomerulopathies of neoplasia. *Kidney Int* 1977; 11:297–306.
193. Alpers C, Cotran R. Neoplasia and glomerular injury. *Kidney Int* 1986;30:465–73.
194. Costanza M, Pinn V, Schwartz R, et al. Carcinoembryonic antigen–antibody complexes in a patient with colonic carcinoma and nephrotic syndrome. *N Engl J Med* 1973;289:520–3.
195. Ooi BS, Ooi YM, Hsu A, Hurtubise PE. Diminished synthesis of immunoglobulin by peripheral lymphocytes of patients with idiopathic membranous glomerulonephropathy. *J Clin Invest* 1980;65: 789–97.
196. Friend PS, Michael AF. Hypothesis: immunologic rationale for the therapy of membranous lupus nephropathy. *Clin Immunol Immunopathol* 1978;10:35–40.
197. Zech P, Colon S, Pointer P. The nephrotic syndrome in adults aged over 60: etiology, evolution and treatment of 76 cases. *Clin Nephrol* 1982;17:232–6.
198. Schwarz A, Krause P-H, Offermann G, Keller F. Impact of de novo membranous glomerulonephritis on the clinical course after kidney transplantation. *Transplantation* 1994;58:650–4.
199. Mathew TH. Recurrence of disease following renal transplantation. Am J Kidney Dis 1988;12:85–96.
200. Berger BE, Vincenti F, Biava C, Amend WJ, Feduska N, Salvatierra O. De novo and recurrent membranous glomerulopathy following kidney transplantation. *Transplantation* 1983;35:315–9.
201. Charpentier B, Levy M. Groupe Cooperatif de Transplantation de L'Ile de France. De novo membranous glomerulonephritis in renal allografts: Report of 19 cases in 1550 transplant recipients. *Nefrologie* 1982;3:158–166.
202. First MR, Mendoza N, Maryniak RK, Weiss MA. Membranous glomerulopathy following kidney transplantation. *Transplantation* 1984;38:603–7.
203. Antignac C, Hinglais N, Gubler M-C, Gagnadoux M-F, Broyer M, Habib R. De novo membranous glomerulonephritis in renal allografts in children. *Clin Nephrol* 1988;30:1–7.
204. Truong L, Gelfand J, D'Agati V, et al. De novo membranous glomerulopathy in renal allografts: a report of ten cases and review of the literature. *Am J Kidney Dis* 1989;14:131–44.
205. Steinmuller DR, Stilmant MM, Idelson BA, et al. De novo development of membranous nephropathy in cadaver renal allografts. *Clin Nephrol* 1978;9:210–8.
206. Schwarz A, Krause P-H, Offermann G, Keller F. Recurrent and de novo renal disease after kidney transplantation with or without cyclosporine A. *Am J Kidney Dis* 1991;17:524–31.
207. Michielsen P. Recurrence of the original disease: does this influence renal graft failure? *Kidney Int* 1995;48:S79–84.
208. Mathew TH. Recurrence of disease following renal transplantation. *Am J Kidney Dis* 1988;12:85–96.
209. Mathew T. Nephrotic syndrome patients in transplanted kidneys. In: Cameron J, Glassock R, Whelton A, eds. *The nephrotic syndrome.* New York: Marcel Dekker, 1988.
210. Ward HJ, Koyle MA. Immunopathologic features of de novo membranous nephropathy in renal allografts. *Transplantation* 1988;45:524–9.
211. Cameron JS, Williams DG. Glomerulonephritis. In: Holborow E, Reeves W, eds. *Immunology in medicine.* Orlando, FL: Academic, 1983:285–97.
212. Beaujean MA, Bouillenne C. Glomerulonephritis due to transplant rejection affecting a patient's own kidneys [Letter]. *Clin Nephrol* 1983;8:487.
213. Churg J, Grishman E, Goldstein M, Yunis S, Porush J. Idiopathic nephrotic syndrome in adults: a study and classification based on renal biopsies. *N Engl J Med* 1965;272:165–74.
214. Trew P, Biava C, Jacobs R, Hopper JJ. Renal vein thrombosis in membranous glomerulonephropathy: incidence and association. *Medicine (Baltimore)* 1978;57:69–82.
215. Llach F, Arieff A, Massry S. Renal vein thrombosis and nephrotic syndrome: a prospective study of 36 adult patients. *Ann Intern Med* 1975;83:a–14.

216. Wang H, Cheng H, Liu Y, Peng B, Zon W, Wang S. A prospective study of renal vein thrombosis in nephrotic syndrome. *Kidney Int* 1996 (in press).
217. Llach F, ed. *Renal vein thrombosis.* Mount Kisco, NY: Futura, 1983.
218. Llach F. Hypercoagulability, renal vein thrombosis and other thrombotic complications of nephrotic syndrome. *Kidney Int* 1985;28: 429–39.
219. Sarasin F, Schifferli J. Prophylactic oral anticoagulation in nephrotic patients with idiopathic membranous nephropathy. *Kidney Int* 1994; 45:578–85.
220. Klassen J, Elwood C, Grossberg AL, et al. Evolution of membranous nephropathy into anti-glomerular-basement-membrane glomerulonephritis. *N Engl J Med* 1974;290:1340–4.
221. Nicholson GD, Amin UF, Alleyne GAO. Membranous glomerulonephropathy with crescents. *Clin Nephrol* 1975;5:197–201.
222. Moorthy AV, Zimmerman SW, Burkholder PM, Harrington AR. Association of crescentic glomerulonephritis with membranous glomerulonephropathy: a report of three cases. *Clin Nephrol* 1976;6: 319–25.
223. Pettersson E, Törnroth T, Miettinen A. Simultaneous anti-glomerular basement membrane and membranous glomerulonephritis: case report and literature review. *Clin Immunol Immunopathol* 1984;31: 171–80.
224. Abreo K, Abreo F, Mitchell B, et al. Idiopathic crescentic membranous glomerulonephritis. Am J Kidney Dis 1986;8:257–61.
225. Pasternack A, Törnroth T, Linder E. Evidence of both anti-GBM and immune complex mediated pathogenesis in the initial phase of Goodpasture's syndrome. *Clin Nephrol* 1978;9:77–85.
226. Sharon Z, Rohde RD, Lewis EJ. Report of a case of Goodpasture's syndrome with unusual immunohistology and antibody reactivity. *Clin Immunol Immunopathol* 1981;18:402–14.
227. Tomaszewski M-M, Hassell LH, Moore J, Antonovych TT. Goodpasture's syndrome: local and diffuse deposition of antibody in glomerular basement membrane [Case Report]. *Clin Nephrol* 1983;20:44–8.
228. Roman-Franco AA, Turiello M, Albini B, Ossi E, Milgrom F, Andres G. Anti-basement membrane antibodies and antigen antibody complexes in rabbits injected with mercuric chloride. *Clin Immunol Immunopathol* 1978;9:464–81.
229. Druet P, Druet E, Potdevin F, Sapin C. Immune type glomerulonephritis induced by $HgCl_2$ in the Brown Norway rat. *Ann Immunol (Paris)* 1978;129:777–92.
230. Ogrodowski J, Hebert L, Sedmak D, Cosio F, Tamerius J, Kolb W. Measurement of SC5b-9 in urine in patients with the nephrotic syndrome. *Kidney Int* 1991;40:1141–7.
231. Genchi R, Korbet S, Schwartz M. The prevalence of glomerular lesions in nephrotic adults. In: Abstracts of the International Congress of Nephrology. Madrid, Spain (July). 1995:261(abst).
232. Levey A, Lau J, Pauker SG, Kassirer JP. Idiopathic nephrotic syndrome: puncturing the biopsy myth. *Ann Intern Med* 1987;107: 697–713.
232a. Hall CL, Fothergill CA, Blackwell HM, et al. The natural course of gold nephropathy: long term study of 21 patients. *BMJ* 1987;295: 745–54.
233. Tu W-H, Petitti D, Biava C, et al. Membranous nephropathy: predictors of terminal renal failure. *Nephron* 1984;36:118–24.
234. Latham P, Poncell S, Koresaar A, et al. Idiopathic membranous glomerulopathy in Canadian children: a clinicopathologic study. *J Pediatr* 1982;101:682–5.
235. Ramirez F, Brouhard B, Travis L, Ellis E. Idiopathic membranous nephropathy in children. *J Pediatr* 1982;101:677–81.
236. Hopper JJ, Trew P, Biava C. Membranous nephropathy: its relative benignity in women. *Nephron* 1981;29:18–24.
237. Manos J, Short C, Acheson E, et al. Relapsing idiopathic membranous nephropathy. Clin Nephrol 1982;18:286–90.
238. Davison A, Cameron J, Kerr D, et al. The natural history of renal function in untreated idiopathic membranous glomerulonephritis in adults. *Clin Nephrol* 1984;22:61–7.
239. Kida H, Asamoto T, Yokoyama H, et al. Long-term prognosis of membranous glomerulonephritis. *Clin Nephrol* 1986;25:64–9.
240. Honkanen E. Survival in idiopathic membranous glomerulonephritis. Clin Nephrol 1986;25:122–8.
241. MacTier R, Boulton-Jones J, Payton C, McLay A. The natural history of membranous nephropathy in the west of Scotland. *Q J Med* 1986;60:793–802.
242. Zucchelli P, Ponticelli C, Cagnoli L, et al. Prognostic value of T lymphocyte subset ratio in idiopathic membranous nephropathy. *Am J Nephrol* 1988;8:15–20.
243. Törnroth T, Honkanen E, Pettersson E. The evolution of membranous glomerulo-nephritis reconsidered: new insights from a study on relapsing disease. Clin Nephrol 1987;28:107–17.
244. Ponticelli C. Prognosis and treatment of membranous nephopathy. *Kidney Int* 1986;29:927–40.
245. Schieppati A, Mosconi L, Perna A, et al. Prognosis of untreated patients with idiopathic membranous nephropathy. *N Engl J Med* 1993;329:85–9.
246. Johnson RG, Couser WG. Membranous nephropathy. In: Bayless TM, Brain MC, Cherniak RM, eds. *Current therapy in internal medicine 1984–1985.* Philadelphia: BC Decker, 1984:1140–3.
247. Manos J, Short C, Acheson E, et al. Relapsing idiopathic membranous nephropathy. Clin Nephrol 1982;18:286–90.
248. Pollak V, Rosen S, Pirani C, Muehrcke R, Kark R. Natural history of lipoid nephrosis and of membranous glomerulonephritis. *Ann Intern Med* 1968;69:1171–96.
249. Collaborative Study of the Adult Idiopathic Nephrotic Syndrome. A controlled study of short-term prednisone treatment in adults with membranous nephropathy. *N Engl J Med* 1979;301:1301–6.
250. Cameron J, Healy M, Adu D. The Medical Research Council trial of short-term high-dose alternate-day prednisolone in idiopathic membranous nephropathy with nephrotic syndrome in adults. *Q J Med* 1990;74:133–56.
251. Wehrmann M, Bohle A, Bogenschutz O, et al. Long-term prognosis of chronic idiopathic membranous glomerulonephritis: an analysis of 334 cases with particular regard to tubulo-interstitial changes. *Clin Nephrol* 1989;31:67–76.
252. Ponticelli C, Zucchelli P, Passerini P, et al. A randomized trial of methylprednisolone and chlorambucil in idiopathic membranous nephropathy. *N Engl J Med* 1989;320:8–13.
253. Tu W-H, Petitti D, Biava C, Tulunay O, Hopper JJ. Membranous nephropathy: predictors of terminal renal failure. *Nephron* 1984;36: 118–24.
254. Suki W, Chavez A. Membranous nephropathy: response to steroids and immunosuppression. *Am J Nephrol* 1981;1:11–6.
255. Ponticelli C. Prognosis and treatment of membranous nephropathy. *Kidney Int* 1986;29:927–40.
256. Toth T, Takebayashi S. Factors contributing to the outcome in 100 adult patients with idiopathic membranous glomerulonephritis. *Int Urol Nephrol* 1994;26:93–106.
257. Glassock R. The therapy of idiopathic membranous glomerulonephritis. *Semin Nephrol* 1991;11:138–47.
258. Relman A. What have we learned about the treatment of idiopathic membranous nephropathy with steroids [Editorial]? *N Engl J Med* 1989;320:248–50.
259. Cameron J. Membranous nephropathy: still a treatment dilemma [Editorial]. *N Engl J Med* 1992;327:638–9.
260. Lewis E. Idiopathic membranous nephropathy: to treat or not to treat [Editorial]? *N Engl J Med* 1993;329:127–9.
261. Remuzzi G, Schieppati A, Garattini S. Treatment of idiopathic membranous glomerulopathy. *Curr Opin Nephrol Hypertens* 1994;3: 155–63.
262. Ponticelli C, Passerini P. Perspectives in clinical nephrology: treatment of the nephrotic syndrome associated with primary glomerulonephritis. *Kidney Int* 1994;46:595–604.
263. Klahr S, Levey A, Beck G, et al. The effects of dietary protein restriction and blood-pressure control on the progression of chronic renal disease. *N Engl J Med* 1994;330:877–84.
264. Rostoker G, Maadi A, Remy P, Lang P, Lagrue G, Weil B. Low-dose angiotensin-converting-enzyme inhibitor captopril to reduce proteinuria in adult idiopathic membranous nephropathy: a prospective study of long-term treatment. *Nephrol Dial Transplant* 1995;10:25–9.
265. Remuzzi G, Bertani T. Is glomerulosclerosis a consequence of altered glomerular permeability to macromolecules? *Kidney Int* 1990;38: 384–94.
266. Rostoker G. Idiopathic membranous nephropathy: new therapeutic trends. *Eur J Med* 1993;2:106–16.
267. Gansevoort RT, Heeg J, Vriesendorp R, et al. Antiproteinuric drugs in patients with idiopathic membranous glomerulopathy. *Nephrol Dial Transplant* 1992;11:91–6.
268. De Zeeuw D, Heeg J, Stelwagen T, et al. Mechanism of the antipro-

teinuric effect of angiotensin-converting enzyme inhibition. *Contrib Nephrol* 1990;83:160–3.
269. Thomas D, Hillis A, Coles G, et al. Enalapril treats the proteinuria of membranous glomerulonephritis without detriment to systemic or renal hemodynamics. Am J Kidney Dis 1991;18:38–43.
270. Praga M, Hernandez E, Montoyo C, et al. Long-term beneficial effects of angiotensin-converting enzyme inhibition in patients with nephrotic proteinuria. Am J Kidney Dis 1992;20:240–8.
271. Gansevoort RT, de Zeeuw D, de Jong PE. Long-term benefits of the antiproteinuric effect of angiotensin-converting enzyme inhibition in nondiabetic renal disease. Am J Kidney Dis 1993;22:202–6.
272. Praga M, Hern'andez E, Montoyo C, Andr'es A, Ruilope LM, Rodicio JL. Long-term beneficial effects of angiotensin-converting enzyme inhibition in patients with nephrotic proteinuria. Am J Kidney Dis 1992;20:240–8.
273. Lewis EJ, Hunsicker LG, Bain RP, Rohde RD. The effect of angiotensin-converting-enzyme inhibition on diabetic nephropathy. *N Engl J Med* 1993;329:1456–62.
274. Remuzzi A, Remuzzi G. The effects of nonsteroidal anti-inflammatory drugs on glomerular filtration of proteins and their therapeutic utility. *Semin Nephrol* 1995;15:236–43.
275. Neugarten J, Kozin A, Cook K. Effect of indomethacin on glomerular permselectivity and hemodynamics in nephrotoxic serum nephritis. *Kidney Int* 1989;36:51–6.
276. Golbetz H, Black V, Shemesh O, Myers BD. Mechanism of the antiproteinuric effect of indomethacin in nephrotic humans. *Am J Physiol* 1989;256:F44–51.
277. Gansevoort RT, Heeg JE, Vriesendorp R, de Zeeuw D, de Jong PE. Antiproteinuric drugs in patients with idiopathic membranous glomerulopathy. *Nephrol Dial Transplant* 1992;1:91–6.
278. Heeg JE, de Jong PE, de Zeeuw D. Additive antiproteinuric effect of angiotensin-converting enzyme inhibition and non-steroidal anti-inflammatory drug therapy: a clue to the mechanism of action. *Clin Sci* 1991;81:367–72.
279. Bellomo R, Wood C, Wagner I, et al. Idiopathic membranous nephropathy in an Australian population: the incidence of thromboembolism and its impact on the natural history [Letter]. *Nephron* 1993;63:240–1.
280. Bellomo R, Atkins RC. Membranous nephropathy and thromboembolism: is prophylactic anticoagulation warranted [Editorial]? *Nephron* 1993;63:249–54.
281. Radhakrishnan J, Appel AS, Valeri A, Appel GB. The nephrotic syndrome, lipids, and risk factors for cardiovascular disease. Am J Kidney Dis 1993;22:135–42.
282. Spitalewitz S, Porush JG, Cattran D, Wright N. Treatment of hyperlipidemia in the nephrotic syndrome: the effects of pravastatin therapy. Am J Kidney Dis 1993;22:143–50.
283. Chan PC, Robinson JD, Yeung WC, Cheng IK, Yeung HW, Tsang MT. Lovastatin in glomerulonephritis patients with hyperlipidaemia and heavy proteinuria. *Nephrol Dial Transplant* 1992;7:93–9.
284. Rabelink AJ, Hen'e RJ, Erkelens DW, Joles JA, Koomans HA. Effects of simvastatin and cholestyramine on lipoprotein profile in hyperlipidaemia of nephrotic syndrome. *Lancet* 1988;2:1335–8.
285. Massy ZA, Ma JZ, Louis TA, Kasiske BL. Lipid-lowering therapy in patients with renal disease. *Kidney Int* 1995;48:188–98.
286. Wanner C, Bohler J, Eckardt HG, Wieland H, Schollmeyer P. Effects of simvastatin on lipoprotein (a) and lipoprotein composition in patients with nephrotic syndrome. Clin Nephrol 1994;41:138–43.
287. Cattran DC, Delmore T, Roscoe J, et al. A randomized controlled trial of prednisone in patients with idiopathic membranous nephropathy. *N Engl J Med* 1989;320:210–5.
288. Hopper J Jr. Membranous glomerulonephritis. *Ann Intern Med* 1973; 79:285–7.
289. Bolton WK, Atuk NO, Sturgill BC, Westervelt FB Jr. Therapy of the idiopathic nephrotic syndrome with alternate day steroids. *Am J Med* 1977;62:60–70.
290. Short CD, Solomon LR, Gokal R, Mallick NP. Methylprednisolone in patients with membranous nephropathy and declining renal function. *Q J Med* 1987;65:929–40.
291. Ehrenreich T, Porush JG, Churg J, et al. Treatment of idiopathic membranous nephropathy. *N Engl J Med* 1976;295:741–6.
292. Ponticelli C, Zuchelli P, Passerini P, et al. A 10-year follow-up of a randomized study with methylprednisolone and chlorambucil in membranous nephropathy. *Kidney Int* 1995;48:1600–4.
293. Ponticelli C, Zucchelli P, Passerini P, Cesana B. Methylprednisolone plus chlorambucil as compared with methylprednisolone alone for the treatment of idiopathic membranous nephropathy. *N Engl J Med* 1992;327:599–603.
294. Piccoli A, Pillon L, Passerini P, Ponticelli C. Therapy for idiopathic membranous nephropathy: tailoring the choice by decision analysis. *Kidney Int* 1994;45:1193–202.
295. Vosnides G, Edipidis K, Sotsiou F, Papadakis G, Siakotos M, Lemoniatou H. Poor response of idiopathic membranous glomerulonephritis to alternate courses of steroids and chlorambucil. *Nephrol Dial Transplant* 1986;1:75(abst).
296. Mathieson PW, Turner AN, Maidment CG, Evans DJ, Rees AJ. Prednisolone and chlorambucil treatment in idiopathic membranous nephropathy with deteriorating renal function. *Lancet* 1988;2:869–72.
297. Mathieson P, Maidment C, Rees A. Immunosuppression for membranous nephropathy [Letter]. *Lancet* 1989;1:211.
298. Warwick G, Boulton-Jones JM. Immunosuppression for membranous nephropathy [Letter]. *Lancet* 1988;2:1361.
299. Wetzels J, Hoitsma A, Koene R. Immunosuppression for membranous nephropathy [Letter]. *Lancet* 1989;1:211.
300. Brunkhorst R, Wrenger E, Koch KM. Low-dose prednisolone/chlorambucil therapy in patients with severe membranous glomerulonephritis. *Clin Invest* 1994;72:277–82.
301. West ML, Jindal KK, Bear RA, Goldstein MB. A controlled trial of cyclophosphamide in patients with membranous glomerulonephritis. *Kidney Int* 1987;32:579–84.
302. Bruns FJ, Adler S, Fraley DS, Segel DP. Sustained remission of membranous glomerulonephritis after cyclophosphamide and prednisone. *Ann Intern Med* 1991;114:725–30.
303. Jindal K, West M, Bear R, Goldstein M. Long-term benefits of therapy with cyclophosphamide and prednisone in patients with membranous glomerulonephritis and impaired renal function. Am J Kidney Dis 1992;19:1:61–7.
304. Williams PS, Bone JM. Immunosuppression can arrest progressive renal failure due to idiopathic membranous glomerulonephritis. *Nephrol Dial Transplant* 1989;4:3:181–6.
305. Reichert LJ, Huysmans FT, Assmann K, Koene RA, Wetzels JF. Preserving renal function in patients with membranous nephropathy: daily oral chlorambucil compared with intermittent monthly pulses of cyclophosphamide. *Ann Intern Med* 1994;121:328–33.
306. Warwick G, Boulton-Jones J. Immunosuppression for membranous nephropathy [Letter]. *Lancet* 1988;2:1361.
307. Hebert LA. Therapy of membranous nephropathy: what to do after the (meta)analyses [Editorial]. *J Am Soc Nephrol* 1995;5:8:1543–5.
308. Hebert L. The primary glomerulopathies. In: Rakel RE, ed. *Conn's current therapy*. Philadelphia: WB Saunders, 1995;609–620.
309. Imperiale TF, Goldfarb S, Berns JS. Are cytotoxic agents beneficial in idiopathic membranous nephropathy? A meta-analysis of the controlled trials. *J Am Soc Nephrol* 1995;5:1553–8.
310. Hogan S, Muller K, Jennette J, Falk R. Treatment of idiopathic membranous glomerulopathy (IMG): a pooled analysis. *J Am Soc Nephrol* 1993;4:277(abst).
311. Zietse R, Wenting GJ, Kramer P, Schalekamp MA, Weimar W. Fractional excretion of protein: a marker of the efficacy of cyclosporine A treatment in nephrotic syndrome. *Transplant Proc* 1988;20:3:280–4.
312. DeSanto NG, Capodicasa G, Giordano C. Treatment of idiopathic membranous nephropathy unresponsive to methylprednisolone and chlorambucil with cyclosporin. *Am J Nephrol* 1987;7:74–6.
313. Rostoker G, Belghiti D, Ben Maadi A, et al. Long-term cyclosporin A therapy for severe idiopathic membranous nephropathy. *Nephron* 1993;63:335–41.
314. Guasch A, Suranyi M, Newton L, Hall BM, Myers BD. Short-term responsiveness of membranous glomerulopathy to cyclosporine. Am J Kidney Dis 1992;20:472–81.
315. Rostoker G, Belghiti D, Ben Maadi A, et al. Long-term cyclosporin A therapy for severe idiopathic membranous nephropathy. *Nephron* 1993;63:335–41.
316. Cattran DC, Greenwood C, Ritchie S, et al. A controlled trial of cyclosporine in patients with progressive membranous nephropathy. *Kidney Int* 1995;47:1130–5.
317. Ambalavana S, Fauvel J-P, Sibley R, Myers B. Mechanism of the antiproteinuric effect of cyclosporine in membranous nephropathy. *J Am Soc Nephrol* 1996;290–298.
318. Radhakrishnan J, Kunis CL, V DA, Appel GB. Cyclosporine treat-

ment of lupus membranous nephropathy. Clin Nephrol 1994;42: 147–54.
319. Ambalavanan S, Fauvel J-P, Sibley RK, Myers BD. Mechanism of the antiproteinuric effect of cyclosporine in membranous nephropathy. *J Am Soc Nephrol* 1996;7:290–8.
320. Palla R, Cirami C, Panichi V, Bianchi AM, Parrini M, Grazi G. Intravenous immunoglobulin therapy of membranous nephropathy: efficacy and safety. Clin Nephrol 1991;35:98–104.
321. Pei Y, Cattran D, Greenwood C. Predicting chronic renal insufficiency in idiopathic membranous glomerulonephritis. *Kidney Int* 1992;42:960–6.
322. Disney A. *Tenth report of the Australia and New Zealand Combined Dialysis and Transplant Registry (ANZDATA).* Adelaide, South Australia: Queen Elizabeth Hospital, 1986.
323. Mathew TH. Recurrence of disease following renal transplantation. Am J Kidney Dis 1988;12:85–96.
324. Lieberthal W, Bernard DB, Donohoe JF, Stilmant MM, Couser WG. Rapid recurrence of membranous nephropathy in a related allograft. Clin Nephrol 1979;12:222–8.
325. Obermiller LE, Hoy WE, Eversole M, Sterling WA. Recurrent membranous glomerulonephritis in two renal transplants. *Transplantation* 1985;40:100–2.
326. First MR, Mendoza N, Maryniak RK, Weiss MA. Membranous glomerulopathy following kidney transplantation: association with renal vein thrombosis in two of nine cases. *Transplantation* 1984;38: 603–7.
327. Adler SG, Johnson K, Louie JS, Liebling MR, Cohen AH. Lupus membranous glomerulonephritis: different prognostic subgroups obscured by imprecise histologic classifications. *Mod Pathol* 1990;3: 186–91.
328. Samuels B, Lee JC, Engleman EP, Hopper J Jr. Membranous nephropathy in patients with rheumatoid arthritis: relationship to gold therapy. *Medicine (Baltimore)* 1978;57:319–27.
329. Figueroa JE, Waxman J. Membranous nephropathy in rheumatoid arthritis. *South Med J* 1982;75:480–2.
330. Schwartzberg M, Burnstein SL, Calabro JJ, Jacobs JB. The development of membranous glomerulonephritis in a patient with rheumatoid arthritis and Sjögren's syndrome. *J Rheumatol* 1979;6:65–70.
331. Furuta T, Seino J, Saito T, et al. Insulin deposits in membranous nephropathy associated with diabetes mellitus. Clin Nephrol 1992;37: 65–9.
332. Weber JP Jr, Cawley LP. Membranous glomerulonephropathy: thyroid antigen–antibody immune complex MGN. *J Kans Med Soc* 1981; 82:397–9.
333. Horvath F Jr, Teague P, Gaffney EF, Mars DR, Fuller TJ. Thyroid antigen associated immune complex glomerulonephritis in Graves' disease. *Am J Med* 1979;67:901–4.
334. Kobayashi S, Nagase M, Kimura M, Ohyama K, Ikeya M, Honda N. Renal involvement in mixed connective tissue disease. Clin Nephrol 1981;5:282–9.
335. Moutsopoulos HM, Balow JE, Lawley TJ, Stahl NI, Antonovych TT, Chused TM. Immune complex glomerulonephritis in sicca syndrome. *Am J Med* 1978;64:955–60.
336. Bonet Sol J, Teixid'o Planas J, Costa Pinel B, Mayayo Artal E, Carrera M. Sjögren's syndrome and membranous glomerulonephritis. *Rev Clin Esp* 1985;177:191–3.
337. Rai GS, Hamlyn AN, Dahl MG, Morley AR, Wilkinson R. Primary biliary cirrhosis, cutaneous capillaritis, and IgM-associated membranous glomerulonephritis. *BMJ* 1977;1:817.
338. Reitsma DJ, Gratama S, Vroom TM. Clinical remission of membranous glomerulonephritis in primary biliary cirrhosis with cutaneous vasculitis. *BMJ* 1984;288:27–8.
339. Singhal PC, Scharschmidt LA. Membranous nephropathy associated with primary biliary cirrhosis and bullous pemphigoid. *Ann Allergy* 1985;55:484–5.
340. Esterly NB, Gotoff SP, Lolekha S, et al. Bullous pemphigoid and membranous glomerulonephropathy in a child. *J Pediatr* 1973;83: 466–70.
341. Ellis D, Fisher SE, Smith WI Jr, Jaffe R. Familial occurrence of renal and intestinal disease associated with tissue autoantibodies. *Am J Dis Child* 1982;136:323–6.
342. Martini A, Scotta MS, Notarangelo LD, Maggiore G, Guarnaccia S, De Giacomo C. Membranous glomerulopathy and chronic small-intestinal enteropathy associated with autoantibodies directed against renal tubular basement membrane and the cytoplasm of intestinal epithelial cells. *Acta Paediatr Scand* 1983;72:931–4.
343. Colletti RB, Guillot AP, Rosen S, et al. Autoimmune enteropathy and nephropathy with circulating anti-epithelial cell antibodies. *J Pediatr* 1991;118:858–64.
344. Tan CY, Davies MG, Marks R. Co-existing dermatitis herpetiformis and membranous glomerulonephritis. *Clin Exp Dermatol* 1980;5: 177–9.
345. Combs RC, Hazelrigg DE. Dermatitis herpetiformis and membranous glomerulonephritis. *Cutis* 1980;25:660–1.
346. Botey A, Torras A, Revert L. Membranous nephropathy in ankylosing spondylitis [Letter]. *Nephron* 1981;29:203.
347. Hiesse C, Goldschmidt E, Santelli G, Charpentier B, Machover D, Fries D. Membranous nephropathy in a bone marrow transplant recipient. Am J Kidney Dis 1988;11:188–91.
348. Muller GA, Muller CA, Markovic Lipkowski J, et al. Membranous nephropathy after bone marrow transplantation in ciclosporin treatment [Letter]. *Nephron* 1989;51:555–6.
349. Barbara JA, Thomas AC, Smith PS, Gillis D, Ho JO, Woodroffe AJ. Membranous nephropathy with graft-versus-host disease in a bone marrow transplant recipient. Clin Nephrol 1992;37:115–8.
350. Lai KN, Li PK, Lui SF, et al. Membranous nephropathy related to hepatitis B virus in adults. *N Engl J Med* 1991;324:1457–63.
351. Lai KN, Lai FM. Clinical features and the natural course of hepatitis B virus-related glomerulopathy in adults. *Kidney Int Suppl* 1991;35: S40–5.
352. Yoshikawa N, Ito H, Yamada Y, et al. Membranous glomerulonephritis associated with hepatitis B antigen in children: a comparison with idiopathic membranous glomerulonephritis. Clin Nephrol 1985;23:28–34.
353. O'Regan S, Fong JS, de Chaddar'evian JP, Rishikof JR, Drummond KN. Treponemal antigens in congenital and acquired syphilitic nephritis: demonstration by immunofluorescence studies. *Ann Intern Med* 1976;85:325–7.
354. Sanchez Bayle M, Ecija JL, Estepa R, Cambronero MJ, Martinez MA. Incidence of glomerulonephritis in congenital syphilis. Clin Nephrol 1983;20:27–31.
355. Ngu JL, Chatelanat F, Leke R, Ndumbe P, Youmbissi J. Nephropathy in Cameroon: evidence for filarial derived immune-complex pathogenesis in some cases. Clin Nephrol 1985;24:128–34.
356. Sal A, Sobrini B, Guisantes J, et al. Membranous glomerulonephritis secondary to hydatid disease. *Am J Med* 1981;70:311–5.
357. Vialtel P, Chenais F, Desgeorges P, Couderc P, Micouin C, Cordonnier D. Membranous nephropathy associated with hydatid disease [Letter]. *N Engl J Med* 1981;304:610–1.
358. Andrade ZA, Rocha H. Schistosomal glomerulopathy. *Kidney Int* 1979;16:23–9.
359. Hendrickise RG, Adeniyi A. Quartan malarial nephrotic syndrome in children. *Kidney Int* 1979;16:67–74.
360. Grover S, Bobhate SK, Chaubey BS. Renal abnormality in leprosy. *Lepr India* 1983;55:286–91.
361. Haslitt J. Membranous glomerulopathy associated with Landry–Guillian–Barre syndrome [Letter]. Am J Kidney Dis 1987;9:445.
362. Murphy BF, Gonzales MF, Ebeling P, Fairley KF, Kincaid-Smith P. Membranous glomerulonephritis and Landry–Guillain–Barre syndrome. Am J Kidney Dis 1986;8:267–70.
363. Törnroth T, Skrifvars B. Gold nephropathy prototype of membranous glomerulonephritis. *Am J Pathol* 1974;75:573–90.
364. Törnroth T, Skrifvars B. The development and resolution of glomerular basement membrane changes associated with subepithelial immune deposits. *Am J Pathol* 1975;79:219–36.
365. Gartner HV. Drug-associated nephropathy. I. Glomerular lesions. *Curr Top Pathol* 1980;69:143–81.
366. Tubbs RR, Gephardt GN, McMahon JT, et al. Membranous glomerulonephritis associated with industrial mercury exposure: study of pathogenetic mechanisms. *Am* J Clin Pathol 1982;77:409–13.
367. Dische FE, Swinson DR, Hamilton EB, Parsons V. Immunopathology of penicillamine-induced glomerular disease. *J Rheumatol* 1984;11:584–5.
368. Hoorntje SJ, Kallenberg CG, Weening JJ, Donker AJ, The TH, Hoedemaeker PJ. Immune-complex glomerulopathy in patients treated with captopril. *Lancet* 1980;1:1212–5.
369. Textor SC, Gephardt GN, Bravo EL, et al. Membranous glomerulopathy associated with captopril therapy. *Am J Med* 1983;74:705–12.
370. Cledes J, Gentric A, Briere J, Leroy JP. Extramembranous glomeru-

lonephritis (EMGN) during treatment with diclofenac. *Nephrologie* 1988;9:283.
371. Radford MG Jr, Holley KE, Grande JP, et al. Membranous glomerulonephropathy associated with the use of non-steroidal anti-inflammatory drugs. *J Am Soc Nephrol* 1994;5:359(abst).
372. Breysse P, Couser WG, Alpers CE, Nelson K, Gaur L, Johnson RJ. Membranous nephropathy and formaldehyde exposure. *Ann Intern Med* 1994;120:396–7.
373. Ehrenreich T. Renal disease from exposure to solvents. *Ann Clin Lab Sci* 1977;7:6–16.
374. Harrison DJ, Thomson D, MacDonald MK. Membranous glomerulonephritis. *J Clin Pathol* 1986;39:167–77.
375. Baba N, Nomura T, Sakemi T, Uchida M, Watanabe T. Membranous glomerulonephritis probably related to bucillamine therapy in two patients with rheumatoid arthritis. *Nippon Jinzo Gakkai Shi* 1991;33:629–34.
376. Kawano M, Nomura H, Iwainaka Y, et al. Bucillamine-associated membranous nephropathy in a patient with rheumatoid arthritis. *Nippon Jinzo Gakkai Shi* 1990;32:817–21.
377. Taylor RG, Fisher C, Hoffbrand BI. Sarcoidosis and membranous glomerulonephritis: a significant association. *BMJ* 1982;284:1297–8.
378. Kleinknecht C, Levy M, Gagnadoux MF, Habib R. Membranous glomerulonephritis with extra-renal disorders in children. *Medicine (Baltimore)* 1979;58:219–28.
379. Akosa AB, Sherif A, Maidment CG. Kimura's disease and membranous nephropathy. *Nephron* 1991;58:472–4.
380. Sonkodi S, Jarmay K, Korom I, et al. Angiolymphoid hyperplasia associated with membranous nephropathy. *Orv Hetil* 1984;125:1573–6.
381. Weisenburger DD. Membranous nephropathy: its association with multicentric angiofollicular lymph node hyperplasia. *Arch Pathol Lab Med* 1979;103:591–4.
382. Ruggieri G, Barsotti P, Coppola G, et al. Membranous nephropathy associated with giant lymph node hyperplasia: a case report with histological and ultrastructural studies. *Am J Nephrol* 1990;10:323–8.

C. Secondary Glomerular Diseases

Immunologic Renal Diseases,
edited by E. G. Neilson and W. G. Couser.
Lippincott-Raven Publishers, Philadelphia © 1997.

CHAPTER 48

Systemic Lupus Erythematosus

J. Stewart Cameron

DEFINITION AND HISTORICAL PERSPECTIVE

Lupus nephritis is by no means a common disorder. However, apart from its intrinsic interest and the insights the disease may give us about the immune system, its importance to practicing nephrologists is that it is a serious but usually treatable disease. Those looking after patients with lupus enter a contract that has no finite term. In many cases, the physician will determine, by his or her management during the early phases, what future the individual may expect.

The term *lupus* (Latin: *wolf*) has been used for many centuries in medicine to denote any skin condition in which one component was ulceration and eating away of the tissue. Rudolf Virchow (1) noted its use as early as the 13th and 16th centuries by Rogerius and Paracelsus, and Talbott (2) has reviewed the history of lupus in detail. Two dermatologists who played a part in the history of nephrology, Willan and Rayer, together with Thomas Bateman, separated lupus erythematodes from other forms of lupus in the early 19th century, and in 1833 Cazenave, following a suggestion by Biett, introduced the term *lupus erythémateux*. Moritz Kaposi of Vienna was the first to note that the condition could be systemic, with possible pleuropericarditis, neurologic problems, and coma complicating the condition, which could result in death; his paper published with Hebra was translated almost immediately into English (3) and became more widely known. Although Brooke in 1895 noted albuminuria in lupus (4), it was the writings of Sir William Osler in the 1890s that led to widespread recognition of visceral involvement, including renal disease (5). Important early papers in the study of renal disease in lupus were those by Keith and Rowntree in 1922 (6) and by Baehr and colleagues in 1935 (7), in which the postmortem histopathology of lupus nephritis was first described. However the modern definition of lupus nephritis awaited the seminal papers by Klemperer et al. (8) in 1941, again on postmortem results, and the amazingly complete description by Muehrcke and colleagues of renal biopsy specimen appearances in 1957 (9).

A "false positive" Wasserman reaction in patients with lupus was noted as early as 1922 by Gennerich (10). In 1948, Hargraves and his colleagues reported phagocytosis of nuclear material in bone-marrow preparations from patients with lupus (11), and in 1957 several workers (12,13) almost at the same time described antibodies directed against DNA, which have become an essential part of the definition of lupus. A year later, Bielschowsky and colleagues (14) noted that New Zealand black/white (NZB/W) cross F_1 mice developed a disease resembling lupus. Comparison and studies of these and other animal models of lupus have yielded major insights into its pathogenesis.

Definitions of Lupus

Thus, today lupus is defined by its clinical picture, together with antibodies directed against one or more nuclear components. It is best regarded as a *syndrome*, in which a number of different immunologic events may lead to a similar final common pathway and thus a similar clinical picture; it is not yet clear whether these represent different aspects of a single disease, but any subsets that can be identified have large overlaps with other subsets. The criteria of the American College of Rheumatology (ACR) (15), revised in 1982, have been applied widely for the diagnosis of lupus, although they were introduced to differentiate the disease from other closely related clinical conditions (Table 1). The presence of four or more of the major criteria is usually taken as establishing the diagnosis with ~96% sensitivity and specificity. It is

J. S. Cameron: United Medical and Dental Schools of Guy's and St. Thomas Hospitals, London SE1 9RT, United Kingdom.

TABLE 1. *The American College of Rheumatology (ACR) criteria for the diagnosis of lupus, revised 1982*

Criterion	Definition
1. Malar rash	Fixed erythema, flat or raised, over the malar eminences, tending to spare the nasolabial folds
2. Discoid rash	Erythematous raised patches with adherent keratotic scaling and follicular plugging; atrophic scarring may occur in older lesions
3. Photosensitivity	Skin rash as a result of unusual reaction to sunlight, by patient history or physician observation
4. Oral ulcers	Oral or nasopharyngeal ulceration, usually painless, observed by a physician
5. Arthritis	Nonerosive arthritis involving two or more peripheral joints, characterized by tenderness, swelling, or effusion
6. Serositis	(a) Pleuritis: convincing history of pleuritic pain or rub heard by a physician or evidence of pleural effusion *or* (b) Pericarditis: documented by ECG or rub or evidence of pericardial effusion
7. Renal disorder	(a) Persistent proteinuria >5 g/day or $>3+$ if quantitation is not performed *or* (b) Cellular casts: may be red cell, hemoglobin granular, tubular, or mixed
8. Neurologic disorder	(a) Seizures: in the absence of offending drugs or known metabolic derangements, for example, uremia, ketoacidosis, or electrolyte imbalance *or* (b) Psychosis: in the absence of offending drugs or known metabolic derangements, for example, uremia, ketoacidosis, or electrolyte imbalance
9. Hematologic disorder	(a) Hemolytic anemia: with reticulocytosis *or* (b) Leukopenia: $<4{,}000/\text{mm}^3$ on two or more occasions *or* (c) Lymphopenia: $<1{,}500/\text{mm}^3$ on two or more occasions *or* (d) Thrombocytopenia: $<100{,}000/\text{mm}^3$ in the absence of offending drugs
10. Immunologic disorder	(a) Positive lupus erythematosus cell preparation *or* (b) Anti-DNA: antibody to DNA in abnormal titer *or* (c) Anti-Sm: presence of antibody to Smith nuclear antigen *or* (d) False-positive serologic test for syphilis known to be positive for at least 6 months and confirmed by *Treponema pallidum* immobilization or fluorescent treponemal antibody absorption test
11. Antinuclear antibody	An abnormal titer of antinuclear antibody by immunofluorescence or an equivalent assay at any point in time and in the absence of drugs known to be associated with "drug-induced lupus" syndrome

The proposed classification is based on 11 criteria. For the purpose of identifying patients in clinical studies, a person shall be said to have systemic lupus erythematosus if any four or more than 11 criteria are present, serially or simultaneously, during any interval of observation. From Tan et al. (15).

important to remember that, with time, patients who initially do not satisfy the criteria may do so later, and that repeated assessment is necessary. For example, some patients begin with what appears to be single organ involvement—arthritis, nephritis (usually membranous or mesangiocapillary), or thrombocytopenia, often without serologic evidence of lupus—but later develop a full clinical and immunologic picture (16,17).

One of the crucial features for the diagnosis is the presence of antinuclear antibodies of particular specificities (18,19). Those against double-stranded DNA, and the Smith (sm) antigen are particularly useful (Table 2) because they are strongly associated with the presence of nephritis. The former is almost a sine qua non for the diagnosis of lupus, whereas the latter is highly specific, but present only in 15–50% of patients with nephritis, more in Afro-Caribbean patients than in Caucasians. Also, treatment may rapidly eliminate anti–double-stranded DNA (dsDNA) antibodies from the circulation, whereas the positivity on the fluorescent antinuclear antibody (FANA) test remains. Despite much study of the various patterns of FANA (diffuse, speckled, and so on), the reliability of these patterns in distinguishing lupus from other antinuclear-factor-positive diseases is very low, and they have fallen out of use, although a homogeneous pattern is most characteristic of lupus.

Defining "typical" or "core" patients with undoubted lupus by the presence of four or more American College of Rheumatology (ACR) criteria and a positive antinuclear factor and/or dsDNA antibodies excludes a considerable number of patients who belong to the lupus "family"of diseases, but do not satisfy the ARA criteria. These patients are in practice as important to recognize and to treat as those with "classic" lupus. Even today, there is no satisfactory terminology for such patients: "lupoid," "lupuslike," "antinuclear-factor-negative lupus," and "fringe lupus" have all been used. Most patients with a clinical lupus syndrome but a negative FANA have low titers of anti-Ro antibody; this subset of patients rarely has significant renal disease (20). The importance of this group of patients, apart from problems as to how to manage them, has increased recently with the realization that this group has a

TABLE 2. *Immunologic abnormalities in lupus*

Clinical
High incidence of infection
Enlarged spleen and lymph nodes
Immunologic
Immune complexes present
Immune complexes in circulation and tissues
Cryoglobulinemia
Low serum complement (CH50, C4 > C3)
Loss of CR1 receptors from red cells
Defective clearance by C3b and Fc phagocytosis
Resting B-cell overactivity
Hypergammaglobulinemia
Autoantibodies against nuclear antigens
High titers of antiviral antibodies
Autoantibodies against lymphocytes, immunoglobulin G, clotting factors, red cells, white cells, platelets, etc.
Poor response to B-cell mitogens
Poor antibody response to new antigens
Altered T-cell function
Lymphopenia
Low production of interleukin 2
High circulating interleukin-2 receptors
Depressed generation of CD8+ve cytotoxic/suppressor T cells
Low thymic factor(s)
Poor T-cell response to lectins
Poor induction of tolerance
Etc.

high incidence of antiphospholipid antibodies and associated thromboses (21) and abortions (see below), as well as inherited complement deficiencies (22,23).

ETIOLOGY AND INCIDENCE

The Origins of Autoimmunity

Our understanding of how autoimmunity and the lupus syndrome may arise remains incomplete, and the topic is dealt with in detail in Chapter 6. The reader can consult also the comprehensive text of Schonfeld and Isenberg (24) for an introduction to a vast, and often confusing, literature. A more recent review is that by Walport (25). A recent hypothesis suggests that pressures of infections in the environment, particularly tuberculosis, have led to the appearance of individuals with a propensity to generate Th1 cells, some of which may be autoreactive (26). In lupus, there is a state of generalized autoimmunity in which autoantibodies directed against a variety of self-components are present. This contrasts sharply with organ-specific autoimmunity such as found in myasthenia gravis and anti–glomerular basement membrane nephritis (see Chapter 43), in which clearly pathogenic autoantibodies are directed against a single self-epitope; in generalized autoimmunity, the role of the autoantibodies is, in contrast, unclear.

Genetics

A multigenic component to the etiology of lupus (27,28) is suggested by the fact that a *familial incidence* of lupus may be found, and is particularly common in children with lupus, at ~12–15% of cases (29,30). Many healthy *family members* of patients with lupus show antinuclear and other autoantibodies (29–31), and review of monozygotic twins, one of whom had lupus, gives a 25% concordance (32). Only rather weak *MHC* (major histocompatibility complex) *associations* have been noted in human lupus nephritis (31–34) or with various specific autoantibodies, the strongest being C4A or C4B null (31). Low production of tumor necrosis factor [coded within the MHC (35)] is associated in both murine and human lupus with greater susceptibility to the disease. Other candidate genes have been examined for associations with susceptibility to lupus, including the interleukin-1 receptor antagonist, immunoglobulin (Ig) gamma-marker allotypes, T-cell receptor genes, and drug hydroxylation, but none have yet been described that appear autonomous and not to depend on linkage disequilibrium with known associations. It is interesting that lupus appears to be rare in west Africa (see below), whereas it is relatively common in descendants of West Africans in the Caribbean, North America, and Europe; this could of course be explained by genetic admixture as well as by environmental factors.

Immunodeficiency

A proportion of patients lupus have *inherited immunodeficiencies*. Both *inherited deficiencies of complement components* (22,23), C1 esterase inhibitor deficiency and acquired deficiency of C3 from nephritic factors (see Chapters 18,51), have been found to be associated also with lupus, so deficiency of functional complement rather than a genetic linkage appears most likely with an inability to clear organisms and/or immune aggregates as a secondary result. In these individuals, lupus is usually mild and precocious in onset (36) and often antinuclear factor and DNA binding negative with anti-ENA antibodies. In C1 esterase inhibitor deficiency, the angioedema may precede the lupus. Most of these patients do well, although some deaths have been recorded (23). A deficiency of the *complement receptor*, CR1, has been described also and has been suggested to be inherited (37), but the evidence now points to it being acquired or acquired (38).

IgA deficiency is associated with lupus nephritis more often than would be expected by chance (39). These individuals are prone to a variety of sinopulmonary and gastrointestinal infections, so the relationship seems to be with greater antigenic stimulation of a susceptible subject. Defective Fc receptor function has been implicated also and is MHC linked (40).

Environmental Factors

This is perhaps the least understood aspect of lupus; the subject has been well reviewed by Mongey and Hess (41). The earliest hypotheses for the pathogenesis of lupus suggested that it was the result of an *infection* such as tuberculosis, and infections have been sought repeatedly without success. In particular, since their description, *retroviruses* have been thought to be candidates for the provocation of the lupus syndrome. Until now, though, there is no convincing evidence of their participation in the human disease, although there is an increased incidence of positive antinuclear tests in spouses of patients with lupus (42) and in laboratory workers who handle lupus sera (43).

Some *medicines* and *chemicals* such as hydralazine, procainamide, and a growing list of rare drugs are well known to be able to precipitate a lupus syndrome that, however, rarely affects the kidney and, when it does, the disease is normally mild. Risks for hydralazine-induced lupus have been determined and three genetic factors (femaleness, slow acetylator status, and the possession of the MHC antigen HLA-DR4) plus the environmental factor (hydralazine in a dose of >200 mg/24 h) account for 98% of the risk of developing lupus (44). However, acetylator status does not appear to affect susceptibility to idiopathic lupus. In susceptible strains of rats such as the Brown Norway, *mercuric chloride* induces a state of autoimmunity, although the syndrome does not resemble lupus clinically.

Immunologic Abnormalities in Lupus

These are summarized in Table 2; the likely primary events are either polyclonal hyperactivity of the B-cell system, defects of T-cell autoregulation, or both. The problem is to know how these come about. Several main hypotheses are available at present, all or some of which may operate and perhaps account for the variability of the syndrome and its outcomes (24,45). The *first hypothesis* is that not all autoreactive T cells undergo apoptosis and die in the thymus, but may persist into adult life in a state of suppression, with the emergence of clones of autoreactive cells and antibodies and tissue damage if this suppression fails. Although it is true that autoreactive cells and antibodies are common, especially in aged individuals, these antibodies are usually of IgM isotype, of low avidity, arise from germline encoded genes, and are of little or no pathologic significance. However, the possibility remains that high-avidity IgG antibodies might arise by a failure of suppression of these normal events.

A *second hypothesis* is that presentation of (perhaps altered) self-antigen to a mature immune system is capable of inducing germline mutations (46) that result in the production of new autoantibodies, which again are not adequately suppressed. Thus, autoimmunity could result as an antigen-driven, T-cell-dependent phenomenon. A crucial question requiring answer in this model is exactly what antigens are responsible for driving the T-cell response. Histone-derived peptides, transcription factors, and Ig idiopeptides have been considered. A variant of this hypothesis is that a viral or even a bacterial peptide might be the driving antigen: this requires that some autoantigens contain sequences that are similar or identical to those on the invading organisms against which the appropriate antibodies are induced, with which they cross-react (47): so-called antigenic mimicry. For example, anti-Sm antibody cross-reacts with the p24 *gag* protein of retroviruses (48). If idiopeptides were responsible, then B cells would be the presenting cell.

A *third hypothesis* is that rather than being a T-cell disorder, the initial problem is a nonspecific polyclonal stimulation of B cells perhaps via superantigens (49), which again fails to be suppressed and whose repertoire includes pathogenic autoantibodies. Recently, the *lpr* gene in the MRL mouse was identified as the APO-1/*fas* receptor (50–52) whose engagement leads to apoptosis; homozygosity for both this and the *gld* (generalized lymphoproliferative gene) leads to a failure of apoptosis, lymphoproliferation and autoantibody production with a lupus syndrome. However, search for analogous mutations of the APO-1/*fas* gene in human lupus has not been successful, and apoptosis seems to be greater than normal in human lupus, not less (53,54). The whole topic of autoreactivity is discussed in detail in Chapter 6.

Incidence and Prevalence (55,56)

The overall *prevalence* of lupus in the United States has varied in different studies from 15 (55,57) to 51 (56, 58) per 100,000 individuals, with an average of ~40/100,000. The prevalence is highest in black females (~200 per 100,000) population. In countries with a predominantly Caucasian population, prevalence varies from 12 and 27.8 (59) (England) to 39 (Sweden) (60) per 100,000 (55,59). A number of studies have examined the *incidence* of lupus, giving figures varying from 1.8 to 7.6 new cases per 100,000 per year. As for the prevalence data, incidence figures for black females were 25 times greater than for white males (0.3–0.4 vs 8–11) and 3–4 times greater for black females than white females. The incidence peaked in black women either from 15 to 44 or 25 to 34 years of age, but surprisingly in Sweden the incidence was highest in the oldest age group, 45–64 years (60). An intriguing aspect of the increased incidence of lupus among American and almost certainly Afro-Caribbean blacks is the relative rarity of lupus in their descendants of their progenitors in west Africa (61), although it is a little more common in east, south central, and southern Africa. Data for Orientals are conflicting: in

Hawaii, Serdula and Rhoads (62) and Maskarinec and Katz (63) found more than twice the prevalence of lupus among Orientals than Caucasians, but Fessel (58) noted no difference in San Francisco, and other studies have noted a relatively low prevalence in mainland China, Taiwan, and Japan (55). On the other hand, lupus seems to be extremely common in the relatively small populations of both Singapore and Hong Kong, although no epidemiologic data have been published.

Mortality data from the United States provide a similar picture, with figures from one to two deaths per million per year for white males,up to 10–20 for black females (55). Again, in the important study by Lopez-Acuna et al. (64) of >11,000 deaths attributed to lupus in the United States from 1968 to 1978, mortality for blacks peaked at 30–60 years, whereas for Caucasians the peak mortality was at >75 years of age. There was a modest decrease during the period studied, an important point because several studies have suggested an increasing incidence of lupus. Kaslow (65) examined data from 12 U.S. states with major oriental populations and noted three times as many deaths among blacks and twice as many among orientals as Europeans. Incidence is much lower in *children*. Lévy and colleagues (66) studied a racially mixed but predominantly Caucasian population in Paris and its environs and found an incidence of 0.22 cases/year among 10^5 children younger than 16 (95% confidence interval, 0.15–0.30), girls showing 0.36 cases and boys 0.08 cases per year.

Gender and Age

All the above data emphasize that *gender* is the major risk factor for the development of lupus. The female–male ratio rises from 2:1 in prepubertal children up to 4.5:1 throughout older childhood and adolescence (Table 3) to the 8–12:1 reported in series of adult-onset patients, falling back to 2:1 in the patients over 60 years of age. These data are in accord with the data from murine models of lupus that a female phenotype and specifically estrogens are precipitating factors in the emergence of clinical lupus, whereas androgens protect (see below). An onset of lupus before puberty is distinctly rare, although onsets in the first and second (66–68) years of life have been recorded. In male patients, the age distribution is the mirror image of female patients, either prepubertal or in middle age.

PATHOGENESIS AND PATHOPHYSIOLOGY

Animal Models of Lupus Nephritis (69)

Besides the NZB/W F_1 mouse (14), other strains susceptible to lupus have been described, including the MRL-*lpr* BXSB. These animal models have permitted a fruitful dialogue between the human experience and the animal models in understanding especially the genetics, but also the pathogenesis and treatment, of the disease. Both the NZB/W and MRL mice have as a primary defect events leading to B-cell proliferation, including defects in the *fas*/APO-1–ligand system (50–54), but increased B-cell proliferation may be only one route to generalized autoimmunity in humans. In mice, the disease is transmissible by bone marrow into irradiated recipients. The genetics are complicated: disease susceptibility genes, disease protective genes, disease accelerator genes, and genes determining individual manifestations have all been described. Environmental factors such as the Gross, lymphocytic choriomeningitis, or lactate dehydrogenase viruses have been noted. Spontaneous lupus has been reported also in a variety of other animals, particularly dogs, but also guinea pigs, hamsters, pigs, cats, and monkeys.

In addition, lupus can be provoked in mice by injecting cross-reactive isotypes, such as 16/6, very interestingly by injecting autoantibodies against DNA or phospholipid, by inducing graft-versus-host disease, and in rabbits by injecting peptides derived from the Sm antigen. (69) These various spontaneous and induced models point again to the many routes by which the syndromes known under the collective label of "lupus" can be induced and support the

TABLE 3. *Distribution of histologic patterns in patients with lupus nephritis*

WHO biopsy specimen class	Description	Guy's 1970–89 161 patients (233)	Collected children, 365 patients (139)	Seven adult series, 534 patients (353)	Donadio et al., 439 patients (354)	GISNEL, 539 patients (235)
I	Minimal change	1	6	0.5	0.2	0
II	Mesangial proliferative	12	19	25	22	7
III	Focal proliferative	15	23	19	35	12
IV	Diffuse proliferative	59	43	41	27	45
V	Membranous	16	9	15	15	14
VI	Glomerulosclerosis	0	1	1.5	0.7	0

GISNEL, Gruppo Italiano per lo Studio della Nefrite Lupica: 6% of the GISNEL series were allocated as "mixed."

idea that the human disease is likely both to be multifactorial and to involve different routes of pathogenesis and should be considered as a syndrome.

Genesis of Renal Injury in Lupus Nephritis: Possible Role of Immune Complexes and Autoantibodies

Renal injury is dealt with in detail in Sections III and IV of this book and is only summarized here in relation to lupus specifically. In lupus, much attention has focused on the possible roles in determining tissue damage of circulating immune aggregates on the one hand (70) and on antinuclear antibodies on the other. It now seems likely, however, that they play only a relatively minor role in the pathogenesis of the disease. Deficiencies in the handling of foreign material have been described also, perhaps inherited in association with the MHC haplotype HLA-A1-B8-DR3 (34) and perhaps also worsened by "saturation" of the monocyte–phagocytic system by immune aggregates (71), either free in the circulation or fixed to CR1 receptors stripped from erythrocytes.

Immune Aggregates

Immune aggregates are certainly present at sites of injury in glomeruli and in the tubules also in 60–65% of cases (72,73), as are complement components. Whether these are derived from circulating complexes or from in situ combination of antigen and antibody, is at present impossible to say. It has been assumed that the DNA–anti-DNA antibody system, so characteristic of lupus, must necessarily have a role in pathogenesis. However, it has proved difficult to show this: first, the system is, in vivo, in extreme antibody excess in the plasma, and circulating single-stranded DNA (ssDNA) and dsDNA concentrations are extremely low, usually present as DNA–histone complexes (nucleosomes) (74). It is now clear that one of the major immunogens in lupus is not DNA itself, or histone, but epitopes present only on the DNA–histone complex of the *nucleosome* (75), or even quaternary antigens on chromatin itself (76). Even if there are dsDNA–anti-dsDNA–histone complexes in the circulation, they are present only in tiny amounts (77,78). Anti-dsDNA antibody has been eluted together with dsDNA from nephritic kidneys (79), but the mere presence of antibody does not prove it to be damaging, and these now classic experiments need repeating (80). DNA has been demonstrated in immune aggregates (81) in the kidney also, but again its quantitative role is not clear.

Autoantibodies

One of the cardinal features of lupus is the synthesis and circulation of autoantibodies directed against nucleic acids and proteins concerned with intracellular transcriptional and translational machinery: the main targets are nucleosomes (DNA–histone), small nuclear ribonucleoproteins, and small cytoplasmic ribonucleoproteins. Autoantibodies are usually multiple. Patients with lupus nephritis usually show antibodies directed against dsDNA, Sm, and C1q (see Table 8). Evidence in humans that autoantibodies may be pathogenic derives from induction of a lupuslike disease in newborns associated with transplacental transfer of autoantibody. However, this occurs in a minority of newborns of mothers with lupus (<5%), and nephritis is never part of this syndrome. Unethical experiments infusing sera from lupus patients into patients with terminal disease, done 30 years ago, produced no effects (82). Only in experimental models is there direct evidence that anti-ssDNA or anti-dsDNA antibodies may be directly pathogenic, penetrating cells and causing proteinuria (83–85), and this has been shown also for human monoclonal anti-DNA antibodies (86).

However, the fixation of these antibodies to the kidney, both matrix and cells, now appears a much more complicated affair than as preformed immune aggregates with DNA (87–92). In some instances, dsDNA–anti-dsDNA antibody complexes fix to DNA receptors on cells, including endothelial cells (91–93); in others, histones appear to mediate binding to both matrix and cells (89,90,94–97), and histones are present at sites of immune aggregates in murine (96) and human lupus kidneys, but not in primary glomerulonephritis. Mesangial cells react with DNA nucleosomes (98) and take them up. Histone binding of DNA–anti-DNA complexes may account also for a major part of the apparent cross-reactivity of "anti-DNA" antibodies, especially monoclonal antibodies (99–102), and for reports of binding of anti-DNA antibodies to cell surface antigens (103). The role for apparent cross-reactivity of anti-dsDNA antibodies to proteins, if there is one, is not clear yet.

Effector Mechanisms of Renal Injury

There is no reason to believe that the effector mechanisms of renal damage (complement, polymorphs, monocytes, cytokines, eicosanoids, and so on) are different in lupus from other forms of primary nephritis, which have been reviewed elsewhere (104) and in sections 3 and 4 of this book. In recent years, as with primary glomerulonephritis, attention has turned to the tubules and *interstitium* as the major sites of injury determining outlook in lupus nephritis (72,105,106). The interstitial cellular infiltrate in lupus differs somewhat from the usual mix of CD4-positive T-helper lymphocytes and monocytes seen in primary glomerulonephritis in that there is quite frequently an excess of CD8-positive cytotoxic T lymphocytes in lupus—in 16 of 29 patients in our own study (72).

Differential Immunologic Findings in Patients With and Without Nephritis

This point has been examined by numerous investigators in an attempt to answer the question of why only some patients with lupus develop clinically evident nephritis. Those with nephritis usually show antibodies directed against dsDNA as well as ssDNA and do not have high titers of anti-Ro and anti-LA (see Table 8). In addition, those with nephritis have more avidly complement-binding anti-DNA antibodies (107), immune complexes that activate complement more avidly (108), higher-avidity anti-DNA antibodies (78), and higher-avidity anti-DNA antibodies in proliferative than membranous nephritis (109). The possible role of antibody charge has been discussed also, cationic antibodies having been suggested as more pathogenic (110).

RENAL HISTOLOGIC FINDINGS

Most nephrologists (but not all rheumatologists!) regard the presence of urinary or renal functional abnormalities as a strong, usually overriding indication for renal biopsy, although this view is not universally held (111). The value of the extra information obtained has been determined (112–114) and, in my opinion, the procedure is worthwhile in all cases with abnormal urine, especially in influencing initial treatment (see below).

There is a huge literature on the histology of the kidney in lupus nephritis (115–119). The overriding characteristic of this form of nephritis is its variability, between patients, within biopsy specimens, and even within glomeruli. In many biopsies, it can be difficult, because of this variability, to decide where in the spectrum a particular specimen should be classified, unless it is very severe or very mild. In the last decade, attention has reverted to the idea, proposed some years ago by Morel-Maroger et al. (120) and by Pirani and Salinas Madrigal (121), of histologic *activity* of disease versus scarring (*chronicity*) in renal biopsy specimens, and Austin and colleagues (122) have popularized a scoring system and global index involving both glomeruli and tubules to generate a numeric assessment of the specimens. Others, though, have been unable to replicate its utility (123).

In this context, the widely accepted classification of the World Health Organization (WHO) (117) must be viewed somewhat skeptically. At best, this description allows a general level of severity to be judged. Class III (focal proliferative nephritis) is a particular source of difficulties (118). Nevertheless, of patients biopsied in renal units, there is a remarkable homogeneity in the proportion of patients allocated to each class and, in untreated patients, WHO class was a powerful determinant of outcome. As we shall see, this is no longer true if patients with more severe nephritis are given more active treatment: in almost all series, more than half show WHO class III (focal proliferative) or IV (diffuse proliferative) nephritis, severe forms that most clinicians would treat vigorously. The proportion of class V (membranous) biopsy specimens is about the same in all series, 10–15% (Table 2). The various classes have been described in detail (115–119), but a brief description follows.

Class I biopsy specimens (Fig. 1A) are rare, especially in series based in renal units. Nevertheless, one may occasionally see patients with several grams of proteinuria per day who show no more than tiny mesangial aggregates of immunoglobulin and complement, with essentially normal glomeruli on light microscopy.

Class II (Fig. 1B,C) accounts for ~20% of patients. The only lesion is a diffuse expansion and proliferation of the mesangium with immune aggregates on both electron and immunohistologic examination. The capillary walls are more or less normal and free of immune aggregates. There are usually no tubulointerstitial lesions.

Class III (Fig. 1D,E) presents problems, because it can range from occasional focal and segmental necrotic or proliferative lesions, usually containing the nuclear dusting of degenerating apoptotic resident and infiltrating cells, often capped by a tiny crescent, to a quite diffuse presence of severe segmental lesions affecting the majority of glomeruli. On immunohistology and electron microscopy, capillary wall immune aggregates usually are present focally as well as diffuse mesangial deposits. In areas of activity, hyaline "thrombi" may be seen. (Fig. 2) Tubulointerstitial damage and focal interstitial infiltrates are usual and a powerful guide to prognosis. In most series, 30–40% of patients will show class III nephritis.

Class IV (Fig. 1F–H) is the single commonest type of biopsy specimen appearance in almost all series, accounting for 40–60% of cases. It differs little from class III except that virtually all glomeruli are affected, the lesions are more active and destructive, and small crescents are frequent. There are always areas, sometimes extensive, of subendothelial immune aggregates on electron microscopy and immunohistology, and usually areas of membranous appearance mixed in with these. Hyaline "thrombi" (Fig. 2) are present within many of the glomerular capillary loops (124). A few percent show appearances on optical microscopy and immunohistology that are identical to primary mesangiocapillary glomerulonephritis type I. There is a varying degree of glomerulosclerosis, and tubulointerstitial lesions, both active and scarring, are almost always present. Some patients show diffuse circumferential extracapillary proliferation, but true crescentic nephritis is rare in lupus. Even rarer, although mentioned in every text, are the amorphous masses of nuclear debris called *hematoxophil* bodies.

Class V, membranous nephropathy (Fig. 1I,J), is almost identical to the idiopathic form, with extracapillary immune aggregates separated by "spikes" of basement-membrane-like material, but almost always shows

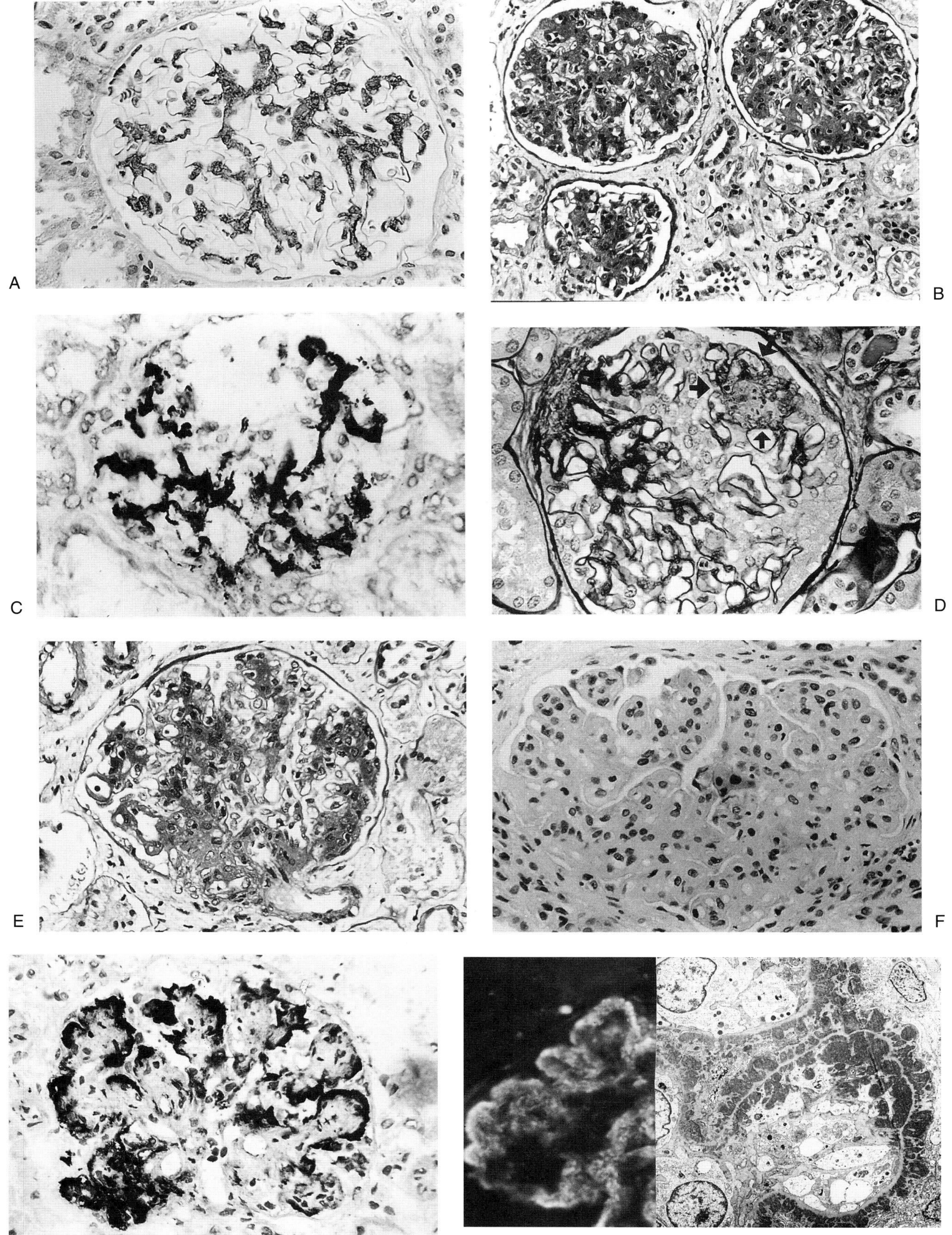
A
B
C
D
E
F
G
H

in addition mesangial deposits, which distinguishes it from primary membranous disease. Often the interstitium is normal, but 10–15% of patients may show tubular atrophy and fibrosis. Lupus membranous nephritis differs in several respects from idiopathic membranous nephritis: the immune aggregates are more irregular in size and distribution, there are almost always some mesangial deposits present, and immunohistology may show a "full house" of immunoglobulin and complement components. Aggregates of immunoglobulin and complement may be present in the tubular basement membranes as well.

Table 2 summarizes the frequency of these different histopathologic patterns in one cohort of our own series and in the literature on adults and children. The proportions are remarkably consistent between different series from various parts of the world (North America, the Far East, and Europe) and in patients at different ages.

On *immunohistology*, IgG is almost always the dominant immunoglobulin, IgG1 and IgG3 being especially prevalent, but a few patients show predominant IgA or IgM. Early complement components such as C4 and especially C1q are usually present along with C3. The finding of positivity for all three isotypes of immunoglobulin together with C3, C4, and C1q is called a "*full house*," which is present in about one quarter of patients with lupus and almost never in nonlupus disease. It is thus almost specific, but insensitive, as a method of diagnosing lupus histologically. Other immune reactants such as complement components B, C5b-9, properdin, and β1H are present also in many patients. Fibrin, sometimes accompanied by cross-linked fibrin, is often pre-

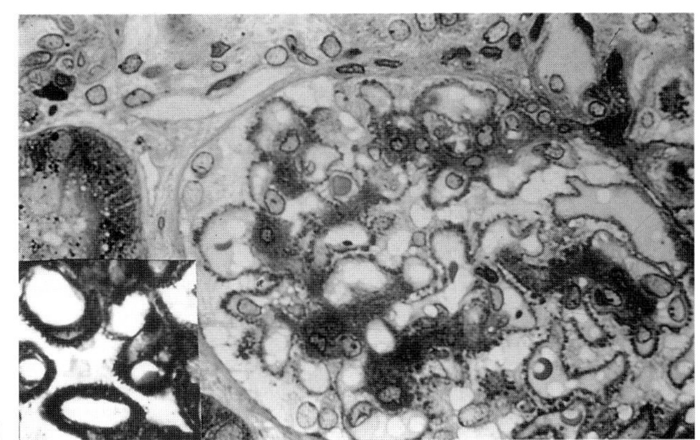
I

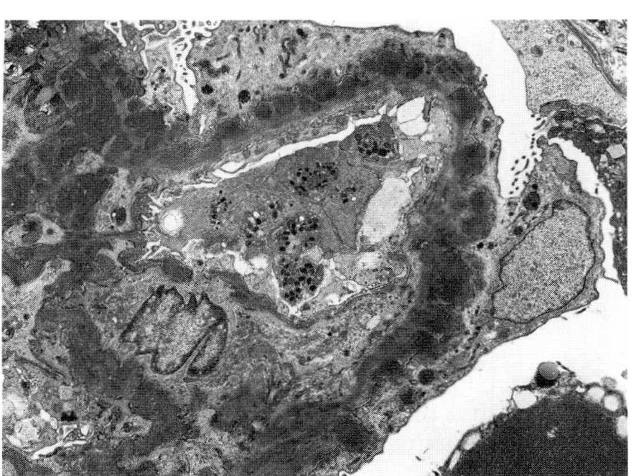
J

FIG. 1. The WHO classification of lupus glomerulonephritis. **A:** WHO class I lupus nephritis: the tuft is normal on optical microscopy, but the immunoperoxidase-conjugated antibody staining reveals extensive C1q (associated with IgG and C3) throughout the mesangial areas. **B:** WHO class II lupus nephritis (minimal changes): the mesangium is expanded, but there is little extracellularity of the tuft. Periodic acid–Schiff. **C:** WHO class II lupus nephritis (mesangial proliferative): the mesangium is shown by immunoperoxidase-conjugated antibodies to contain extensive deposits of IgG; however, there are no aggregates in the peripheral capillary walls of the tuft. **D:** WHO class III lupus nephritis (focal proliferative): in the top right of the glomerulus is an area of focal necrosis (*arrows*) surrounded by a degree of epithelial cell proliferation; this is mild example of class III nephritis. Silver methenamine/hematoxylin–eosin. **E:** A more severe example of WHO class III lupus nephritis: numerous areas of the tuft are affected by segmental capillary wall thickening, mesangial expansion, and cellular proliferation and infiltration. Periodic acid–Schiff. **F:** WHO class IV nephritis (diffuse proliferative): the tuft is enlarged by both an increase in matrix and an excess of cells, and capillary walls are thickened irregularly; the process affects the whole glomerulus. Hematoxylin–eosin. **G:** WHO class IV nephritis: immunoperoxidase conjugated antibody staining reveals dense aggregates of IgG along the peripheral capillary walls in a very irregular pattern. **H:** WHO class IV nephritis: (*left*) using a fluorescent-conjugated antibody against C3, the granular immune aggregates along the capillary wall are seen, and (*right*) electron microscopy reveals that these are present as dark masses at both subendothelial and subepithelial sites, with the capillary basement membrane between. **I:** WHO class V nephritis (membranous): a 1-μm plastic-embedded toluidine-blue-stained preparation reveals that the predominant aggregates are along the outside of the capillary wall. Inset: (*bottom left*) a silver methenamine preparation shows the typical "spikes" of basement membrane material (predominantly laminin) protruding into the subepithelial area; note that in the main picture there are abundant mesangial aggregates, as well as those along the capillary wall. **J:** WHO class V nephritis: electron microscopy shows the very irregular dark immune aggregates along the external surface and within the capillary wall.

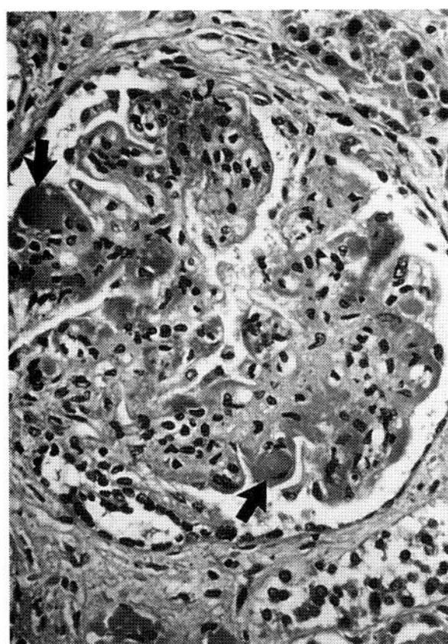

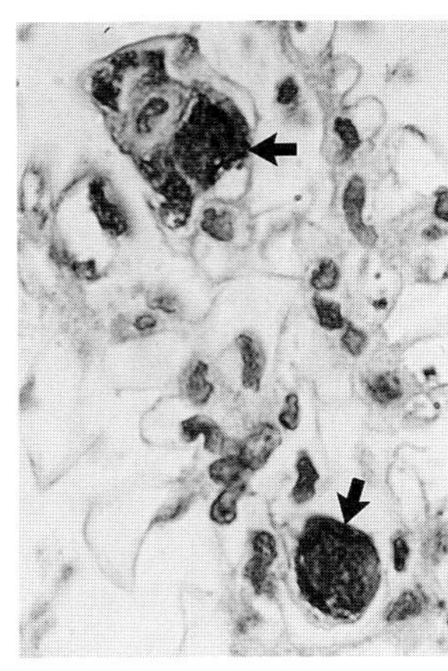

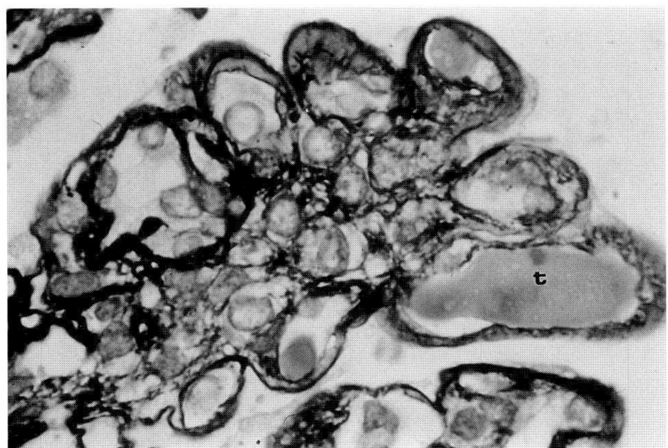

FIG. 2. *Top left:* Glomerular capillary "thrombi" (*arrow*) in a biopsy specimen showing class IV glomerulonephritis. *Top right:* Stained with a monoclonal antibody directed against platelet membrane antigens, the thrombi are shown to contain platelets as well as immunoglobulins, that is, they do have some characteristics of thrombi. Bottom: A higher power, which shows double contouring and immune aggregates in the capillary wall as well as a major "thrombus" (*T*). These lesions are usually seen in class IV specimens, but may be found also in active areas of class III specimens.

sent in class IV biopsy specimens but is rare in other classes (125).

Tubulointerstitial Nephritis

In ~50% of patients with nephritis, less in those with class II and up to three quarters of those with class IV, immune aggregates are present in the tubular basement membrane (72,73) (Fig. 3). They do not correlate with the density or composition of the interstitial infiltrate (Fig. 4), except for the presence of natural killer cells (72). In some patients, linear tubular immunofluorescence is seen, suggestive of anti–tubular basement membrane antibodies (126). The infiltrate is mainly T lymphocytes and monocytes, with only a few B cells, plasma cells, and natural killer cells. Among the T lymphocytes, both CD4-positive helper cells and CD8-positive cytotoxic cells are present. In contrast to primary glomerulonephritis, but similar to rejecting allografts, the numbers of CD8+ve cells exceed the number of CD4+ve cells in many patients. Active infiltration and invasion of tubules (*tubulitis*) is frequently seen in active disease. In more chronic disease (Fig. 4), the interstitium is expanded with a variable amount of collagen. In a few patients, an acute tubulointerstitial nephritis is seen in the absence of glomerular disease (127) and may present as acute renal failure.

Intrarenal Vessels

Although attention had been paid to glomeruli, tubules, and interstitium, only in recent years has attention been focused also on the intrarenal vessels in lupus nephritis (128–130). Vascular immune aggregates, hyaline and noninflammatory necrotizing lesions, true vasculitis with lymphocytic and monocyte infiltration of the vessel wall, and, more rarely, intrarenal arteriolar thrombi may all be seen. All are signs of a poor prognosis (see below) and thus are important to recognize. Some patients show the full clinical picture of a hemolytic–uremic syndrome, hematologically and histologically (131). We were able to show a correlation between the presence of antiphospholipid antibodies and intraglomerular thrombi (132), but others were not (133).

Amyloidosis and Other Glomerular Appearances

Only a handful of cases of amyloidosis have been reported (134,135) in association with lupus, which is in agreement with the fact that acute-phase proteins such as amyloid A and C-reactive protein do not increase during acute flares of activity in lupus, unlike almost every other inflammatory disease except ulcerative colitis. Dense-deposit disease (136) and pauci-immune necrotizing glomerulitis (137) have been reported in a setting of lupus in some patients.

Clinicopathologic Correlations

Clinical Features

Correlation of pathology with clinical features has been attempted by many authors. Whereas more severe histologic forms of nephritis have more severe clinical manifestations (122,138) and even though correlations are present, renal histology cannot be predicted with any certainty from the clinical picture (Fig. 5). For example, although not surprisingly patients with class IV biopsy specimens are significantly more frequently nephrotic, hypertensive, and show reduced renal function, these do not enable prediction of histology, even between class I/II, V, and IV,

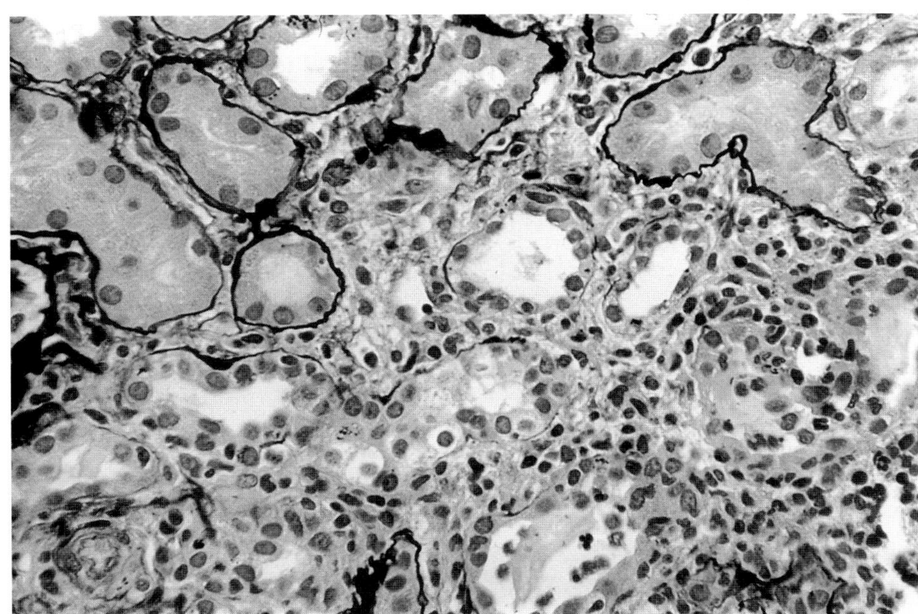

FIG. 3 Interstitial infiltrate of lupus nephritis invading and destroying tubules ("tubulitis"). The tubular basement membrane, stained black with silver, is digested in the lower half of the figure, and lymphocytes and macrophages invade the tubules.

whereas class III is particularly variable in presentation (138). Thus, of 82 patients studied in our own series with lupus nephritis and a full nephrotic syndrome seen during the period 1970–1989 (Fig. 5), 34 (42%) showed class IV, 30 (37%) class III, 10 (12%) class V, and 8 (10%) class II; 16 other class IV patients were not nephrotic. Similarly, 54 of 109 were hypertensive, but only 39 of these showed class IV biopsy specimens, and 17 class IV patients were normotensive. Renal function is perhaps the best clinical guide: glomerular filtration rate (GFR) (measured by a single injection isotopic method) averaged 39 ± 33 mL/min/1.73m^2 in 51 class IV patients, 91 ± 35 in 19 class V patients, and 87 ± 27 in 30 class II patients. Patients with class V biopsy specimens often show nephrotic range proteinuria, but normal renal function. Interstitial changes correlate well with GFR at the time of biopsy, both cells (72) and interstitial volume (139,140), as well as with outcome, which is discussed below.

Serologic Studies

By the time a renal biopsy is done, the patient will almost certainly have received some immunosuppres-

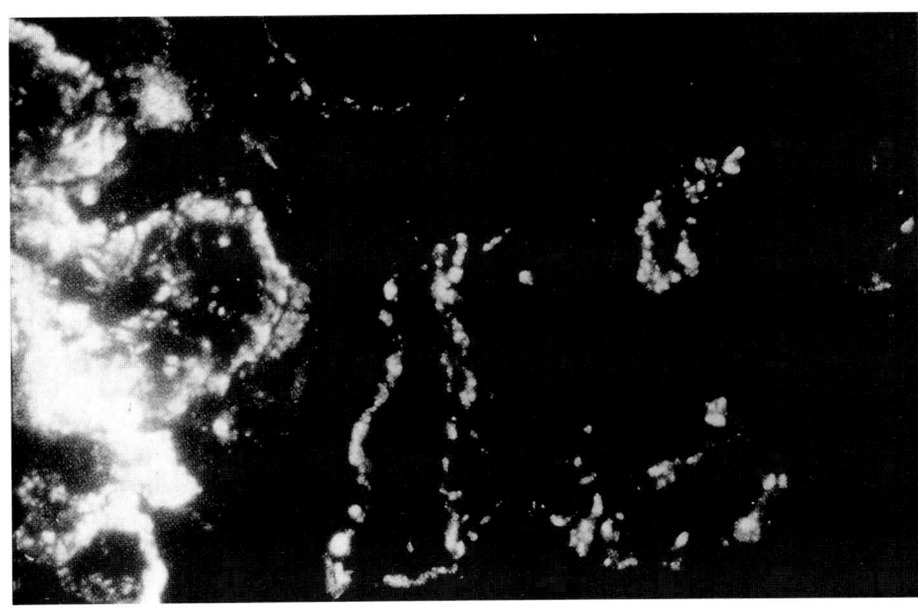

FIG. 4. Immune aggregates (C3) in the tubular basement membranes (*TBM*) (*right*) as well as within the glomerulus (*left*) as demonstrated by fluorescein-conjugated antisera. Such TBM aggregates are common in lupus nephritis, being found in 60–65% of biopsy specimens overall, and with increasing frequency from class II (20%) through class IV (75%).

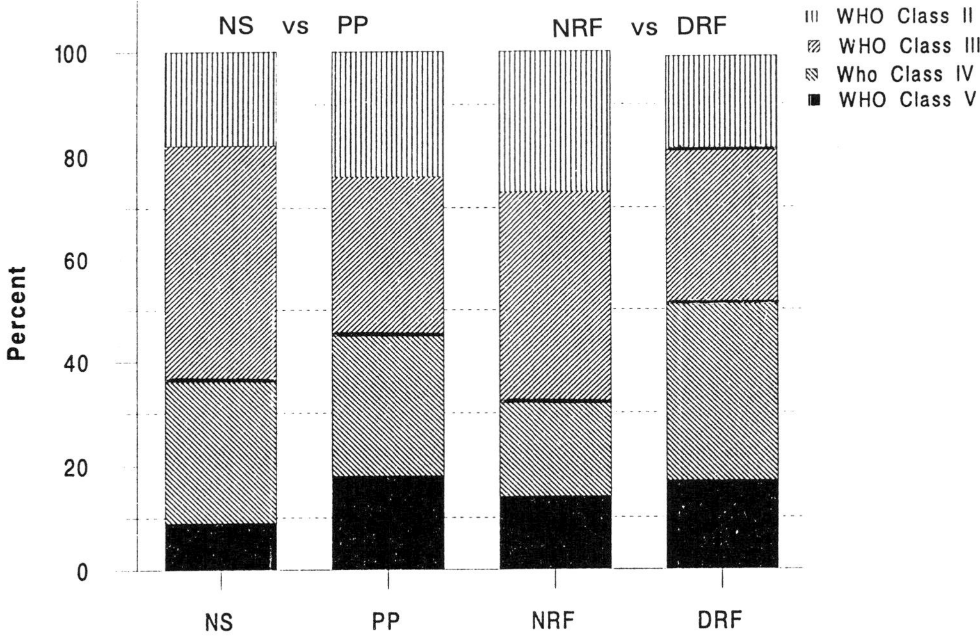

FIG. 5. Clinicopathologic correlations between patients with (left) nephrotic syndrome (NS) or proteinuria (PP), and (right) normal or diminished renal function (NRF/DRF), and WHO class of renal biopsy specimen. Although there are significant correlations at <0.05 level between these two sets of parameters, in terms of predicting the specimen appearance the clinical picture is almost useless.

sive treatment that will alter the serologic results. Titers of dsDNA antibody were similar in our own patients in all histologic groups in our own data (Fig. 6), as in a number of other studies (138), but Hill et al. (140) and Appel et al. (140a), in adults, and Klein et al. (141), in children, noted higher titers in grade-IV biopsy specimens. Again, our own data showed no difference between complement levels in different grades, although those with grade-IV specimens tended to have lower C3 and C4 concentrations, as in Klein's study (141). After all, patients without any renal disease at all may show extremely high dsDNA-binding levels and very low complement concentrations.

CLINICAL MANIFESTATIONS AND LABORATORY FEATURES

Organ Involvement

The clinical manifestations of lupus are Protean, but a number of symptoms and signs, and combinations of these, are particularly common. The Eurolupus project has published recently an analysis of 1,000 patients seen mostly in rheumatology clinics (142), and Wallace (143) reviews some of the literature up to 1993 on a thousand more. Note that the Eurolupus data is derived from rheumatology clinics, and nephropathy was present in only 16% of patients at onset and 39% during evolution.

Fries and Holman (144) make the point that patients with nephritis tend to have more alopecia and oral ulceration, but have less arthritis and facial rash or Raynaud phenomenon, and Schaller (145) points out also that childhood lupus is more often acute in onset than in adults. Although renal signs and symptoms may be present in half of the adults and more than three quarters of children at onset, this is rarely the dominant initial complaint. Serious renal disease usually evolves later (see below). The initial complaints are often nonspecific, three quarters of patients showing fever and malaise without weight loss.

A *rash* (146) was present in half the Eurolupus patients and three quarters of the collected series, usually the well-known "butterfly" rash on the face; *livedo reticularis* may be seen on exposed areas (147) in 5% of patients at onset and in 15% later in the course. Occasionally, the rash is purpuric, suggesting vasculitis, with alterations in the nailbed capillaries, and sometimes ulcerating lesions or vasculitic lesions, especially around the ankles. Discoid lupus is not common in patients with lupus nephritis, but photosensitivity is common. Some degree of *hairfall* is common, amounting to patchy alopecia in a few; *oral ulceration* is a presenting feature in 10% of patients.

The *arthralgia* (148) of lupus is common, occurring in three quarters of patients, almost never deforming, although this can occur (149). Nevertheless, an initial diagnosis of "rheumatoid arthritis" is often made clini-

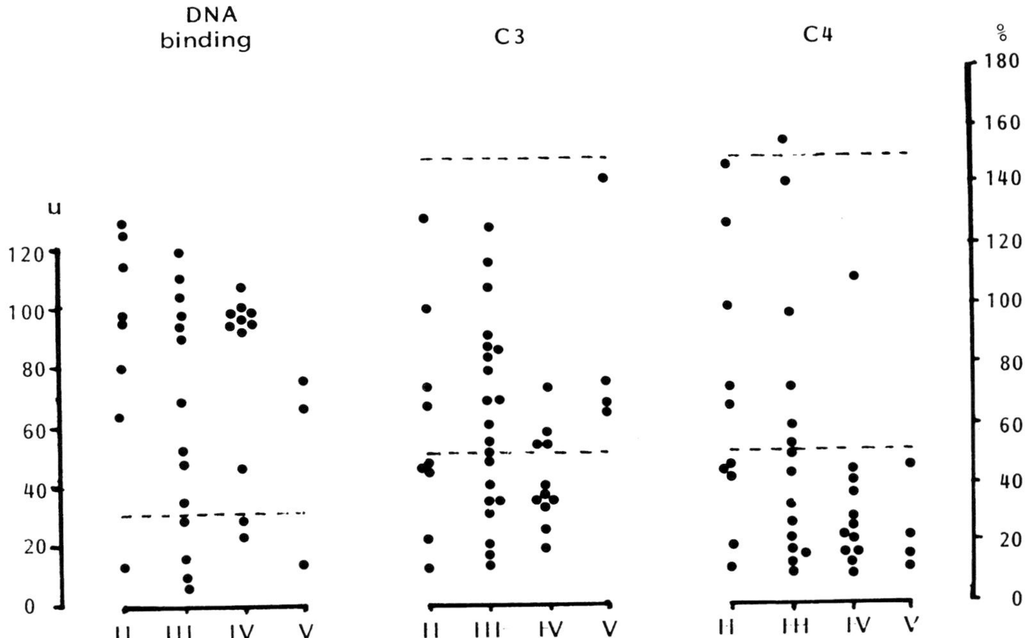

FIG. 6. Correlations between WHO class and (*left*) binding of double-stranded DNA in vitro by sera, and (*right*) plasma C3 and C4 concentrations in percent normal. Normal ranges are indicated by the *dotted lines*. It can be seen that there is only scant correlation between the biopsy specimen class and the serologic parameters, although there is a tendency for patients with class IV specimens to have lower C3 and C4 concentrations J. S. Cameron, unpublished data.

cally. Usually several joints are affected at once, often in the hands, but with almost any joint being a possible target; some *myalgia* is common in untreated patients at onset, often accompanied by weakness, but a diagnosis of *myositis* is rare.

Pleuritis and *pericarditis* (150–152) affect ~40% of patients sooner or later, usually with pain, but sometimes with symptomless effusions, most easily diagnosed on echocardiography. *Myocarditis* with heart failure occurs, but is rare. *Endocarditis* of the Libman–Sachs type (150–152) has been associated recently with the presence of antiphospholipid antibodies (153,154) and is difficult to diagnose except on echocardiography, which should be a routine investigation. Systolic murmurs are of course common in patients with acute lupus in the presence of anemia, fever, and tachycardia; diastolic murmurs are (as always) more frequently sinister. *Pulmonary hypertension* in lupus (155) may be the result of multiple pulmonary emboli in association with antiphospholipid antibody, sometimes with vena caval thrombosis (156). However, it is associated clinically with Raynaud phenomenon in about three quarters of cases (155) and may represent a similar phenomenon in the lung. Treatment is ineffective and the outlook poor: heart–lung transplantation is possible in some cases.

During the acute phase, as well as infections, *acute pulmonary hemorrhage* can be seen (157) that may be fatal, as in one of our own patients, but early treatment with intravenous methylprednisolone appears to be effective in reversing it. Abramson and colleagues (158) have emphasized the frequency (27%) of *acute reversible hypoxemia* in young adults with acute lupus, which usually responds to treatment; its pathogenesis is unclear. Treatment of chronic *fibrosing alveolitis*, a well-recognized feature of lupus, is unsatisfactory and often progressive (159).

Splenomegaly and *lymphadenopathy* (160) are present in about one quarter to one third of patients with lupus. However, the subset of patients with this presentation together with fever and weight loss rather rarely develop nephritis, especially severe nephritis, so this presentation is less often seen in patients referred to renal units.

Neuropsychiatric involvement (161–163) is present at an obvious clinical level in about one third of patients (162,164), although it may be a presenting feature (165,166) in ~12% of patients and can be an isolated feature to begin with. It is an important source of morbidity and mortality and is often present to some degree in patients with severe lupus nephritis (164a). Sensitive tests such as cerebral blood-flow measurement (162, 167), positron-emission tomography (164), and magnetic resonance imaging (162,166) may show abnormalities additional to those revealed even by computed axial tomography, but whose significance is not yet clear

(167). Minor degrees of mood disorder and behavior are common, but difficult to interpret in the setting of an acute and disturbing illness (162,163). These, especially if associated with persistent headache (sometimes but not always of migrainous type), may be the prodrome of serious overt neuropsychiatric disorder. The pathogenesis of neuropsychiatric lupus remains uncertain, but antineuronal antibodies and cerebral vascular lesions associated with an antiphospholipid antibody (see below) appear may be responsible for the diffuse and focal infarctive patterns, respectively.

Diagnosis of neuropsychiatric lupus can be difficult. *Chorea* may be seen, especially in children with neurologic lupus (168), sometimes in association with antiphospholipid antibody (169). In addition, cranial nerve palsies—for example, ophthalmoplegias, fits, and hemiparesis—in addition to coma and frank psychosis (160) or brainstem lesions (170) are found. If the patient is already on immunosuppression, infections may mimic acute cerebral lupus, and there is always worry that corticosteroids may be responsible. In practice, this is extremely rare, and it is usually safe to assume that lupus, and not the steroids, is the villain if infection can be excluded. The C-reactive protein level may help distinguish central nervous system infections from active lupus (171,172), and cerebrospinal fluid findings will exclude meningitis. Various immunologic tests have been proposed, especially on the cerebrospinal fluid, but none is proven yet (162,163).

Clinical hematologic abnormalities are common (160): many patients show a *normochromic normocytic anemia* at presentation, and some patients present with purpura, not from associated vasculitis but from *thrombocytopenia*. Overt *thrombosis* is rare at onset, but its appearance (173) should of course prompt a search for antiphospholipid antibodies (see the section on *laboratory investigations*).

Gastrointestinal (174) and *hepatic* (175,176) *abnormalities* are relatively rare, although bowel upsets are often reported, nausea is common, and at autopsy bowel infiltration with inflammatory cells is common (177). Some patients suffer major vasculitic lesions in the bowel (153,177).

Raynaud phenomenon is common in young adults with lupus, affecting 20–30% and often preceding the clinical onset of other manifestations of disease. In some patients, it is very severe, with loss of digital tissue, as in scleroderma. Patients with renal disease rarely have severe Raynaud phenomenon, however, and overall it is a favorable feature in terms of survival (178).

Renal Manifestations of Lupus

Usually ~30–50% of unselected patients with lupus are reported to have abnormalities of urine tests or renal function early in their course (179–181), and up to 60% of adults and 80% of children may develop overt renal abnormalities later. Data on mode of onset in relation to histology in one cohort of our own series from 1980 to 1989 are presented in Table 4: the dominant feature of renal lupus is *proteinuria*, present in almost every patient, often sufficient to be associated with some degree of *edema*, that is, with a nephrotic syndrome, present in about half of lupus patients with nephritis (182,183) (Table 4). It has been suggested that *hypercholesterolemia* is less common or absent in lupus patients with a nephrotic syndrome (184), but later studies (185) (including our own unpublished

TABLE 4. *A: Renal manifestations of adults with systemic lupus at presentation of renal disease*

Renal presentation	All		WHO biopsy specimen class IV	
	n	%	n	%
Nephrotic syndrome	30	37	18	38
Asymptomatic urinary abnormality	30	37	11	23
Rapidly progressive renal failure	20[a]	24	17[a]	35
Acute nephrotic syndrome	2	2	2	4
Total	82	100%	48	100%

[a]Seven of the patients had proteinuria in the nephrotic range.
From Mc'Ligeyo and J. S. Cameron et al., unpublished data from patients presenting 1980–89 at Guy's Hospital.

B: Presentation of children with lupus nephritis, collected from the literature (139)

n	NS <3 g	Prot <3 g/24 h	Hematuria		BPraised	GFR < 80/ P_{creat}raised	ARF
			Macro	Micro			
208	114 55%	89 43%	4 1.4%	125/159 79%	48/121 40%	103 50%	3 1.4%

NS, nephrotic syndrome; Prot, proteinuria; BPraised, blood pressure >2 SD above normal for age; P_{creat}raised, plasma creatinine of >125 μmol/L; GFR, glomerular filtration rate *or* creatinine clearance of <80 mL/min; ARF, acute renal failure requiring dialysis.
For details of sources, see Cameron (139).

data) do not support this suggestion. Although persistent *microscopic hematuria* was common, it was never found in isolation. At presentation, 20–50% of patients were assessed as *hypertensive*, although these data are necessarily "soft" given the nature and diversity of age, technique, and normal ranges, but surprisingly this was not more common in those with nephritis; when the different histologic grades of nephritis are examined, however, as expected those with more severe nephritis were more commonly hypertensive (class II, 17%; and class IV, 55%) (182,183). Over half of our patients had *reduced renal function* at diagnosis, as judged by a reduced GFR or increased plasma creatinine. Some patients present in *acute renal failure* (186) as in our own series, but this is rare. In one third of unselected patients (18,144), the urinary sediment contains *granular casts*, often containing red cells, as well as red cells in excess of normal, depending on the severity of the nephritis.

Renal Tubular Dysfunction

This is disturbed, not surprisingly in view of both tubular basement membrane immune aggregates and interstitial nephritis. In a high proportion of patients (187,188), urinary excretion of light chains and β_2-microglobulin are both increased. Recently, hyperkalemic renal tubular acidosis has been emphasized (189,190), and the hyperkalemia may a problem.

Laboratory Investigations of Lupus Nephritis

Again a useful source of information is the Eurolupus data (142).

Hematology

Hematologic abnormalities in lupus are frequent. *Anemia* of moderate degree is common, but a positive test for anti–red cell antibodies can be obtained in a minority of patients with lupus, and severe hemolytic anemias are not often seen. *Leukopenia* is common also, and half have a white cell count of $< 5000/\mu L$, whereas *thrombocytopenia* is less common, being found in one quarter of patients.

The leukopenia presumably results from anti–white cell antibodies, although these are rarely sought specifically, but the origins of the thrombocytopenia are complicated (191), resulting from accelerated destruction after binding of antiplatelet antibody, sequestration of platelets in the kidneys, and lysis and/or phagocytosis of circulating platelets by reaction of both antiphospholipid antibodies and immune complexes, including dsDNA–anti-dsDNA complexes, with circulating platelets.

A number of abnormalities of hemostasis besides those involving platelets may be present. *True lupus anticoagulants* may be present in the form of antibodies directed against factors leading to fibrin formation, such as factors VIII and IX, but also less commonly factors XI and XII. These lead to clinical bleeding as well as prolongation of clotting times.

Antiphospholipid Antibodies and the "Lupus Anticoagulant"

However, it is the misnamed "lupus anticoagulant" activity based on the presence of antiphospholipid antibodies that has received most attention in recent years. These antibodies prolong phospholipid-dependent coagulation studies in vitro, but in vivo are associated with thrombosis; we have reviewed this topic in detail previously (192). The mechanisms by which these antibodies interfere with the coagulation studies in vitro is clear; what promotes thrombosis in vivo remains a mystery, although a central role for thrombomodulin–protein-C activity seems likely.

In a series of 76 adults and children with lupus nephritis studied in our own clinic, 43% of patients (132) had antiphospholipid antibodies, whereas, in the study by Shergy et al. (193), the proportion was 29%. In our study (192), in which all patients had clinically evident lupus nephritis, the only association with thrombosis was of intraglomerular capillary thrombi with IgG isotype antibodies, and IgA isotype antibodies with thrombocytopenia. Only eight patients had peripheral thrombotic episodes, however, and these did not correlate with IgG antibody, as they have in other much larger rheumatology-based surveys (194). The possible associations of antiphospholipid antibodies with cardiac manifestations (153,154) and with neurologic disease (195) have been mentioned already. It is important to note that despite the in vitro prolongation of clotting times, it is safe to perform needle biopsies in the presence of antiphospholipid antibodies, whereas, in contrast, a prolongation of kaolin-cephalin (clotting) time (KCT) that reverses on mixing with normal plasma is the result of a true anticoagulant and will require cover with fresh-frozen plasma (124).

Immunologic Tests and the Diagnosis of Lupus

Few clinicians would be happy to make a diagnosis of lupus without some *antinuclear antibodies* in the serum, preferably directed against dsDNA (15,196–198). Thus, almost 100% of patients in published series (see Table 5) have positive tests; that this does not represent the whole picture as seen in clinical practice has been mentioned already. Usually, "lupuslike" patients with negative antinuclear antibody tests show little or no renal disease (20), although there are exceptions (20) and >80% of these "fringe" patients usually have antiphospholipid antibodies (G. Frampton, unpublished observations).

TABLE 5. *A: Autoantibodies to nuclear antigens in autoimmune diseases*

Double-stranded DNA (dsDNA)	Nucleus	Native DNA
Single-stranded DNA (ssDNA)	Nucleus	Denatured DNA
Histones	Nucleus	Forms core around which dsDNA "wraps"; classes are H1, H2A, H2B, H3, and H4
Centromere	Nucleus	Localized to region of condensing metaphase chromosomes; consists of three proteins 17, 80, and 140 kD
Smith (Sm)	Nucleus	Complex polypeptide consisting of various proteins, including B8 (29 kD), B (28 kD), D (16 kD), D8 (15.5 kD), E (12 kD), F (11 kD), and G (9.4 kD), combined with small nuclear RNAs (designated U1, U2, U4, U5, and U6); involved in mRNA splicing
Nuclear ribonucleoprotein (nRNP or U1 RNP)	Nucleus	Proteins of 70, 33(A), and 22(C) kD; involved in mRNA splicing
Ro/SSA	Nucleus/cytoplasm	Ribonucleoprotein: exists in two major forms, 60- and 52-kD proteins complexed with Y1–Y5 RNAs
La/SSB	Nucleus/cytoplasm	Ribonucleoprotein: 48-kD ubiquitous nuclear protein thought to function as an RNA polymerase-14 transcription factor
Jo-1	Cytoplasm	50-kD protein, tRNA histidyl synthetase
Scl-70	Nucleus	100-kD native protein and 70-kD degradation product DNA topoisomerase 1
Heat-shock protein (Hsp90)	Cytoplasm/cell surface	90-kD protein that plays an important physiologic role in "guarding" steroid hormone receptors, until displaced by the hormones themselves

B: Autoantibodies in lupus

Autoantibodies	Frequency (%)	Specificity (diagnostic marker)	Association with disease activity	Clinical subsets
Anti-dsDNA	40–90	High	+	Renal lupus
Anti-ssDNA	70	Low	-	—
Antihistone	70	Low	-	Drug-induced lupus
Anti-Sm	5–30	High	-	—
Anti-U1-RNP	25–35	Low	-	No generally agreed disease association
Anti-SSA/Ro	35	Low	-	Neonatal lupus, ANA -negative systemic lupus erythematosus, subcutaneous lupus erythematosus, lupuslike syndrome with homozygous C2 + C4 deficiency, photosensitive skin rash, interstitial pneumonitis
Anti-SSB/La	15	Low	-	Neonatal lupus, mild disease with Sjögren syndrome
Antiribosomal P protein	25–35	Low	-	Neuropsychiatric disease, particularly psychosis, but claimed controversial
Anti-Hsp90	25	Low	-	Renal disease and low C3
Antiphospholipid	25–50	Low-	-	"Antiphospholipid syndrome"
Anti-RA33	20–40	Low	-	Erosive arthropathy and lack of dermatologic involvement

The rate of positivity depends not only on the population studied, but on the technique used. The three most common assays used to detect anti-dsDNA antibodies are the classic Farr assay, which detects only high-avidity antibodies; the enzyme-linked immunosorbent assay, which picks up also low-avidity antibodies; and the slide *Crithidia lucilae* kinetoplast test, which again detects a wide range of antibodies (197). Correlations with the appearance or presence of systemic lupus, and the presence and severity of nephritis, are best with high-avidity antibodies in the Farr assay (199), so this test is preferable in renal units, but, for screening diagnosis, the enzyme-linked immunosorbent assay has advantages because it will detect positives in many FANA-positive patients in whom the Farr assay is negative and who do have lupus.

Anti-Sm antibodies are almost entirely specific for lupus, but are found only in ~30% of patients and thus have a very low sensitivity. They are usually detected by immunodiffusion assays (198).

Immune complexes can be detected in the serum of the majority of patients with or without lupus (200) by one of the 40 or so tests available, especially those patients with nephritis, and the titer in general rises and falls with indices of clinical activity. Their utility in diagnosis is minimal, however, because so many other conditions show immune complexes of varying biologic activity.

Hypocomplementemia is found at presentation in more than three quarters of untreated patients with lupus (142,201), again in a greater proportion of those with evident nephritis (179). The concentration of C4 and C1q tends to be more depressed than C3, which almost never occurs in idiopathic mesangiocapillary nephritis (although this pattern is common also in essential cryoglobulinemia) or acute glomerulonephritis, suggesting complement activation via the classic pathway. However, concentrations of properdin and factor B are depressed also, with activation of the alternative pathway (202), which is always recruited through generation of fresh C3b by the classic pathway. The C5b-" complex is found in the circulation in increased amounts also (203). Hypocomplementemia was more common in younger subjects than in adults, along with raised anti-dsDNA binding.

DIFFERENTIAL DIAGNOSIS (204)

The commonest other diagnoses made in patients who were, in fact, suffering from lupus were *rheumatic fever*, *rheumatoid arthritis*, and *hemolytic anemia*. Overall, ~50% of patients with lupus are initially suspected of having a disease other than lupus. As noted above, the presence of four or more of the ARA criteria (15) has a 96% sensitivity and specificity when applied to a population of patients seen in rheumatology clinics. These criteria, as already pointed out, have been used widely in situations outside their initial remit, although they do provide security in scientific studies that one is dealing with "typical" patients. The problem is that in the real world of ward and clinic, many patients fall outside this exclusive definition, but still need management and treatment.

Differentiation from *rheumatic fever* is relatively easy, but in a child with chorea is not so easy. Nephritis has been reported in a minority of patients with *mixed connective tissue disease*; the differential diagnosis can be difficult clinically, but analysis of the antinuclear antibody for the anti-Ro and anti-La antibodies and the absence of anti-dsDNA antibodies should make the diagnosis clear. *Rheumatoid arthritis* does not of course show systemic features, but on occasion proteinuria will be induced by one of the drugs used in its treatment and cause problems in diagnosis; in addition, rather rarely there may be associated glomerulonephritis, sometimes proliferative but also membranous in pattern. Some of these patients go on to develop full clinical and immunologic lupus. The presence of erosions and a deforming arthritis makes lupus very unlikely, but does not exclude it. *Henoch–Schönlein purpura* is much commoner in childhood than lupus, and on occasion differentiation may be difficult: the rash of lupus may be purpuric and can affect the lower limbs only, and a few patients with lupus may have predominant IgA in their renal biopsy specimens with raised serum IgA concentrations. Lupus may on occasion be complicated by a *vasculitis* that causes difficulties of diagnosis with other forms of vasculitis. The presence of anti-dsDNA antibodies and a positive FANA is of course crucial, but interpretation of antineutrophil cytoplasmic antibodies (ANCAs; see Chapter 49) is difficult in the presence of antinuclear antibodies and may be interpreted as a positive P-ANCA (205). On histology, however, the finding of major multiple immunoglobulin deposition together with complement in the affected glomeruli, and a proliferative/membranous pattern rather than a necrotizing glomerulitis, should cause no difficulty.

TREATMENT OF LUPUS NEPHRITIS

The evaluation of treatment in lupus nephritis presents peculiar difficulties because it is a disease in which the main characteristic is that each patient's pattern of disease, spontaneous evolution, and response to treatment differs. This means that the usual tools of enquiry, such as the prospective randomized controlled trial, are blunt instruments with which to explore possible benefits from therapy. The effect of extrarenal lupus on outlook may be a major one.

As I have emphasized previously (206), in the treatment of lupus nephritis we are dealing with two quite distinct therapeutic problems. The first is the *induction treatment* of severe acute life-threatening disease, often affecting many systems and usually near the onset of the disease; here the threat of the disease is paramount. The second is the *maintenance treatment* and long-term management of chronic, more or less indolent disease, during which protection from the side effects of treatment becomes more and more important. The effects of a facially disfiguring disease, predominantly of girls and young women, in a society that overvalues appearance, the impact of chronic ill health and treatment on the patient and family, and the management of some forms of extrarenal lupus all require attention. Finally, the problems of compliance with disfiguring treatments are familiar to all physicians and may have an impact on our approach to treatment.

The Role of Renal Biopsy in Determining Treatment

Almost all physicians [see Albert et al. (207) for the contrary view] feel that lupus nephritis of all types requires treatment with corticosteroids and that thereby prognosis is improved; we (182,206,208,209) and others (210–212) have summarized the evidence for this statement elsewhere. However, it is important to emphasize that no trial directly comparing, prospectively, a corticosteroid-treated group with one not so treated has ever been performed (207); nor, given present beliefs, is one likely to be performed. In this respect, the data of Ropes (213) are of great interest: she studied 68 patients with lupus and proteinuria who were left untreated, and in 16 (28%) the proteinuria became intermittent or disappeared. Despite all of the many well-known side effects of corticosteroid treatment, most physicians have felt the price worth paying, at least in the short and medium terms.

One crucial point is what role renal biopsy specimen appearances should play in determining treatment. The majority view (182,210,214) has been that initial biopsy in those with urinary abnormalities allows definition of different patterns of histopathology, of varying severity, which enables more appropriate treatment; occasional voices of dissent, though, are heard (111,215). In most patients with absent or trivial urinary abnormalities, the specimen appearances will be bland (216), the outlook good (217), and treatment unnecessary; although Leehey et al. (218) have argued the contrary view. Whether treatment with corticosteroids at this point might prevent subsequent evolution of severe disease, and how often this happens, has never been tested. There is equally little evidence that early treatment of those with minor but definite urinary abnormalities, but normal renal function and mild histopathologic appearances (mesangial nephritis only, WHO class II), alters subsequent evolution (219). Nor is the evidence clear on whether the outcome of membranous nephropathy (WHO class V) (220–222) improves following treatment, although most clinicians would treat patients with this pattern. Nevertheless, a proportion of such patients will evolve, usually slowly, into renal failure.

Therefore, it is in those groups with focal proliferative nephritis of varying severity (WHO class III) or severe diffuse proliferative glomerulonephritis (WHO class IV) that corticosteroids seem to have the most to offer. Although no prospective trials have been conducted to determine whether maximum benefit is obtained by "tailoring" the treatment to the histology in this way, it is difficult to argue with the successful improvement in outlook described in the next section.

The Acute Phase: Induction Treatment

High-Dose Oral Corticosteroids and Intravenous Methylprednisolone

Because of the knowledge of the pathogenesis of lupus outlined above, following early work, treatment was usually begun with high doses of oral corticosteroids alone (223–225), with major success in quelling activity of the disease, but a heavy penalty in terms of side effects. The action of these drugs is summarized in Chapter 39.

More recently, since 1975 (226) intravenous (I.V.) "pulses" or "boluses" of very high doses of methylprednisolone have become a usual part of initial treatment (227–229), mimicking the successful use of similar treatment in transplant rejection in the early 1970s. The reasons for using this type of treatment are not secure, although now better evidence supports the original justification by Cathcart et al. (226)—namely, the resemblance between the interstitial infiltrate of lupus nephritis and that of allograft rejection (72,73). An immediate dramatic lymphopenia is usually obtained. This treatment has been used extensively in adults with lupus [see Cameron (206) for a review] and for treatment of severe extrarenal lupus. The only controlled trial reported so far mainly concerned adult patients with nonrenal lupus (230), and small numbers did not allow secure conclusions.

From 1980 to 1990 we used IV methylprednisolone to treat 43 of a total of 82 patients with lupus nephritis, 32 of whom had class IV biopsy results. Improvement was seen in almost three quarters of the patients, a result consonant with those reported elsewhere (227–229), although results in cerebral lupus have been disappointing (230). In our own series, only six of 11 patients with severe cerebral lupus improved during or immediately after this treatment. It is difficult to say whether these results are better in cost–benefit analysis than could be obtained with conventional high-dose oral steroids. However, it is the impression of many clinicians that the advantage of I.V. methylprednisolone backed up by low oral dosages of prednisolone from the start is that it has fewer side effects, particularly on facial appearance. This is of course provided that the course is limited to (at the most) two courses of 3 days' I.V. administration of 0.5–1.0 g methylprednisolone. Certainly, no one has suggested that results obtained using the I.V. route are *worse* than those following oral steroids; trials in allograft rejection have shown no difference in outcome, and 0.4, 0.5, and 0.6 g had the same effect as 1.0 g I.V. Side effects described following I.V. injection of high doses of corticosteroids include cardiac arrhythmias (231) or even cardiac arrest if they are injected through central venous lines, and unpleasant flushing sensations. Acute hypertension may be seen (232) and very occasionally acute psychosis. All of these complications seem to be commoner in children and adolescents with lupus.

Cytotoxic Agents in the Acute Phase

The pharmacology and toxicity of these compounds is reviewed in Chapter 39. There has been controversy about whether the addition of cytotoxic agents such as azathioprine/6-mercaptopurine, nitrogen mustard, cyclophosphamide, or chlorambucil confers short- or long-term benefit (206,233). Donadio and Glassock (234) examined this subject exhaustively and concluded that there is no good evidence that the addition of cytotoxic agents, whether in the acute or both the acute and the chronic phases, improves outlook. Another major collaborative retrospective series (235), involving 700 patients, suggested the same conclusion. Nevertheless, most physicians use cytotoxic agents in both the acute and the maintenance phases of lupus nephritis. During the 1980s, we used a cytotoxic agent in 69 of 82 patients with lupus nephritis presenting to our service. Why is this? After early anecdotal descriptions, the 1970s saw the publication of a number of controlled trials using either cyclophosphamide or azathioprine together with prednisolone, compared with prednisolone alone [see Cameron (206,236,237) for a review]. The results individually were equivocal, but not all the patients studied had overt renal disease, follow-up was short, and very mixed patients were grouped together. It is impossible to distinguish effects specifically relating to the use of cytotoxic agents in the acute phase per se, because no studies have been published in which they were used only in the acute phase, contrasted with a group treated with prednisolone alone.

Taking all the trials of acute and chronic treatment together, however, the death rate among all the controls was more than double that in all the test groups (33 vs 15) (206), and a more recent formal meta-analysis of these trials (237) came down unequivocally in favor of an extra clinical benefit of cytotoxic agents. In addition, a crucial observation is that the long-term follow-up of the National Institutes of Health (NIH) trials has shown a better histologic appearance at 10–15 years in those groups treated with a cytotoxic agent than in those treated with prednisolone alone (238) (Fig. 7), although it was not possible to distinguish in this analysis a difference between the various drugs used (azathioprine versus various forms of cyclophosphamide) or the route of administration (oral versus I.V.). Data in the azathioprine-treated patients, in this analysis, did not differ statistically from data for the prednisolone-treated group, but the confidence intervals in these studies are very large because the various groups treated included only 18–30 patients.

Only the group treated with I.V. cyclophosphamide showed improved survival in contrast to a group of (partially historic) controls treated only with prednisolone (239,240), but again there was no difference between those treated with either oral or I.V. cyclophosphamide and with azathioprine (Fig. 8). Steinberg and Steinberg (240) also point to the fact that differences in outcome did not become apparent until more than 5 years' follow-up had been achieved. These important topics are discussed further in the section on *maintenance treatment* below. The bladder toxicity of cyclophosphamide (241) is well known, together with its general oncogenic potential (242) and its gonadal toxicity after only a few months of administration, especially in male patients and in children (243). Therefore, most clinicians, if they wish to use the drug, will now use daily oral cyclophosphamide only during the acute phases of the disease for no more than 8–12 weeks. One 23-year-old woman treated by us with cyclophosphamide for 2½ years in the late 1960s developed a bladder carcinoma after 14 years of follow-up, and another has premalignant changes in her bladder. Carcinoma of the bladder has been reported also after long-term treatment using long-term oral cyclophosphamide for Wegener granulomatosis (244). However, the toxicity on the bladder of an 8- to 12-week course appears to be negligible, judging from the many patients treated in this fashion for minimal change disease (see Chapter 44). Nevertheless, the strategy of large doses of

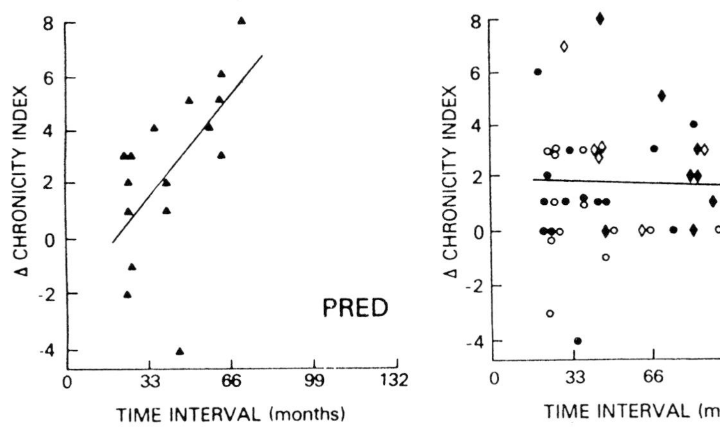

FIG. 7. Combined analyses from a number of trials, conducted at the National Institutes of Health, of prednisone plus cytotoxic agents versus prednisone alone (238). Data are shown for the change in chronicity index (glomerular and interstitial fibrosis plus sclerosis) in individual patients, as shown by repeat biopsies 24–132 months apart. On the *left*, data from patients receiving prednisone alone show a steady increase in the chronicity index, whereas on the *right* there is an insignificant change in chronicity index during the period of study in those receiving a cytotoxic agent in addition. Various cytotoxic therapies were given, including intravenous and oral cyclophosphamide, oral azathioprine, and oral azathioprine plus cyclophosphamide; there was no difference in the data between any of these groups. From Balow et al. (238), with permission.

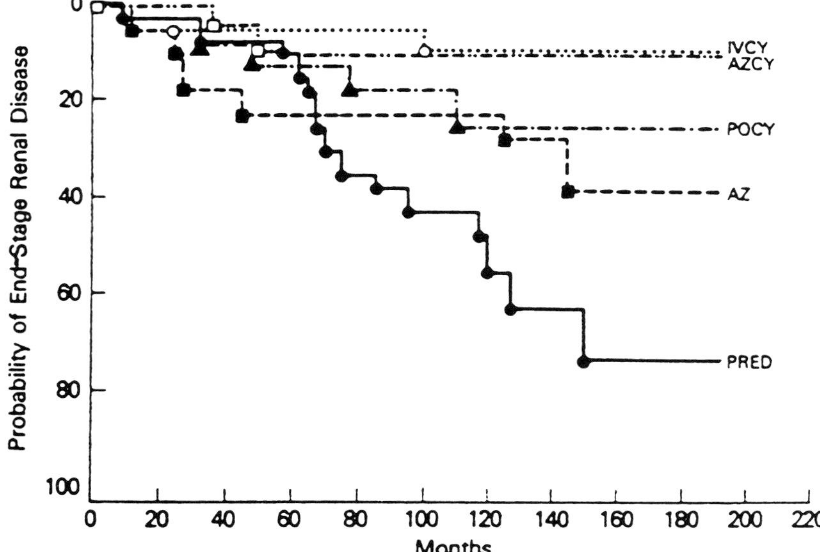

FIG. 8. Renal survival of patients in the various trials conducted at the National Institutes of Health (240). The control groups receiving only prednisolone have been pooled for contrast with those in the individual trials receiving cytotoxic agents in addition. IVCY, intravenous boluses of cyclophosphamide; AZCY, oral cyclophosphamide plus oral azathioprine; POCY, oral cyclophosphamide; AZ, oral azathioprine; PRED, prednisolone only. Note the rather small numbers in each test group, and that the lines are indistinguishable up to 60 months following entry. Only the data from the IVCY differ at the 0.05 level from those for prednisolone alone, but equally (as with the histologic data reviewed in Fig. 10) there is no significant difference between data from any of the groups given a cytotoxic agent. From Steinberg and Steinberg (240), with permission.

I.V. cyclophosphamide during both the acute and the chronic phases of the disease has been advocated strongly, principally by the NIH group and as a result a large number of uncontrolled studies, usually on small numbers of patients have been published. Although this technique avoids bladder toxicity, the effects on the gonads and general oncogenicity remain, and sterilization and leukemia have both been recorded. These are all effects seen with longer-term treatment, however, and are discussed below.

Cyclophosphamide or other mustards, by whichever route, do have the advantage for the induction phase of treatment in that it is a much more powerful inhibitor of B cells than is azathioprine (see Chapter 39), and the resynthesis of autoantibodies is reduced to normal levels rapidly and efficiently. Thus, a number of clinicians, now including our unit, prefer it for induction therapy. The question of whether I.V. administration is necessary or desirable during the acute phase remains unanswered, as does whether it is the better drug for long-term maintenance, which is discussed below.

Plasma Exchange

Although there is an obvious rationale for plasma exchange in lupus, it must be said straight away that the role of plasma exchange in acute severe lupus nephritis, if there is one, has yet to be defined [see Cameron (206) and Wallace (245) for reviews]. Most workers have assumed that concomitant immunosuppression should be given to avoid "rebound" antibody synthesis when exchange ceases, which makes interpretation difficult.

Recent strong advocates of plasma exchange have been the group of Kincaid-Smith (246), who suggested that 11 of 12 patients with severe lupus nephritis had some recovery of renal function, and during the 1980s we used plasma exchange in 25 of 82 patients, 20 (of 48) of whom showed class IV renal biopsy results. We, Kincaid-Smith, and others have used a relatively intensive course of exchange, one plasma volume daily for 7–10 days. However, using a more modest regimen of thrice weekly exchange, Lewis and colleagues could show no benefit over conventional combined cytotoxic and corticosteroid therapy in >80 patients with class IV glomerulonephritis (247). Wei et al. (248) also treated stable patients with plasma exchange and mild disease, but for only 2 weeks, so few if any conclusions could be drawn despite the blinded design of their study, which showed no difference between controls and test patients. Whether more intensive exchange might achieve benefit will require a further expensive and prolonged trial. Plasma exchange synchronized with I.V. cyclophosphamide has been employed also with short-term favorable results (249,250); as usual, it is not clear which component, or whether the combination of both, might achieve benefit, but trials (251) are nearing completion. There is an impression that plasma exchange may have a role in the treatment of severe neuropsychiatric lupus, although controlled data are lacking. It has often been employed, as in our own unit, in patients apparently resistant to other treatments, with improvement in some. However, a delayed effect of the previous intense immunosuppression cannot be excluded.

The adverse effects of plasma exchange are difficult to distinguish from those of the concomitant immunosuppression: infection is the principal hazard (252,253) [although Pohl et al. (254) noted no extra risks for infection following plasma exchange per se in the interhospital-controlled study] and citrate toxicity is another. The procedure is safer through peripheral access than through central venous catheters.

Initial Treatment in Practice

How, therefore, should one begin treatment for a patient showing severe proliferative lupus nephritis with reduction in GFR and a nephrotic syndrome? *Prednisolone* remains the principal treatment, and despite lack of evidence of extra benefit of IV methylprednisolone, we prefer this to tapering high-dose oral corticosteroids, against a background of a maintenance dose from the beginning of 7.5–15 mg/24 h of prednisolone. More than one course of three I.V. doses may be needed, but no more than three such courses should be used. Despite a lack of evidence as to what dose is adequate, we still use 1 g for each bolus, but almost certainly 0.5 g would be adequate. This alone should suffice in nephritis of WHO classes I, II, and V.

In more severe nephritis (WHO classes III and IV), there is much in favor of *cyclophosphamide* as the cytotoxic agent of choice in the acute phase (Chapter 39) and, during the past 6 years, we have moved to using it routinely in the acute phase by the oral route. Should one use, in addition to prednisolone, *intravenous* cyclophosphamide in the acute phase of the disease as advocated by the NIH group? Undoubtedly, this treatment has become popular in the acute phase of lupus, often being used in doses lower than those recommended by the NIH (see the discussion of *maintenance treatment* below), but it does not seem logical to use a drug I.V. that was specifically developed for oral use (see Chapter 39), when one of its active principles (nitrogen mustard) is available as well. The drug has to be extensively metabolized before it is active, so (unlike with methylprednisolone) there is no immediate effect. Since the patient is usually in the hospital at this point, compliance should not be an issue. We, in contrast, have tended during the last 5 years to use 8–12 weeks of *oral cyclophosphamide* 3 mg/kg ideal body weight for height, reduced to 2 or even 1 mg/kg/24 h in the presence of renal insufficiency, as induction therapy. This regimen is almost devoid of side effects and does not involve the induction of leukopenia as the I.V. regimen does, with attendant risks of infection.

There are no firm indications for *plasma exchange* in acute lupus, but we and many other units use it on a daily basis for at least a week when control is not obtained by the previous regimens, including two courses of high-dose I.V. methylprednisolone and cyclophosphamide by one route or another, or in severe neuropsychiatric lupus, which often responds poorly to conventional treatments.

Intravenous γ-globulin is discussed below, since its use remains experimental.

Maintenance Treatment of the Chronic Phase

Usually, the acute disease will be under control after 12 weeks or less, although some patients may have a stormy course and require several rounds of I.V. methylprednisolone. Once the disease is relatively quiescent clinically and immunologically, however, the question of maintenance treatment arises. This is when treatment is most difficult, and most difficult to evaluate (206). The balance of benefit between strategies to avoid relapses or smoldering disease activity, and the many side effects of the drugs, is poorly evaluated despite a number of controlled trials and a huge amount of anecdotal information.

Corticosteroids

Corticosteroids have been, and remain, the backbone of treatment in the maintenance phase; no studies of other treatments without prednisolone have been attempted. In this phase, we must try to avoid the many side effects of long-term corticosteroids, which limits dosage to 5–15 mg/24 h. No formal comparisons of daily and alternate-day double-dosage regimens (255) and daily regimens have been done in patients with lupus, but data from transplanted children or those with idiopathic nephrotic syndromes show only modest effects of improved growth, despite evidence of powerful benefit on the hypothalamic–pituitary–adrenal axis. Nevertheless, many pediatricians use such alternate-day regimens in the chronic phase of treatment without seeing relapses, and they have been used occasionally in adults in an attempt to minimize toxicity (255). Monthly pulses of methylprednisolone have also been used (256), but again the toxicity and benefits of this regimen have never been investigated.

Cytotoxic Agents

The arguments for and against the use of cytotoxic agents have been discussed above in consideration of the acute phase (233–237). At the moment, most interest and discussion centers around the optimum use of regimens involving I.V. cyclophosphamide, but in my view there is, as yet, no good evidence that this regimen is that which offers the best cost–benefit ratio in the long term.

Cyclophosphamide

The use of oral cyclophosphamide for longer than ~12 weeks should be avoided, because of bladder and other toxicity (233,234,239,243,257). Therefore, regular monthly and then bimonthly IV cyclophosphamide has been advocated (238–240,258–261), and results in medium (239) and long terms (240,262) (Fig. 8) are statistically superior to those obtainable with prednisolone alone. Sclerosis in the kidney with time is also retarded by the use of cytotoxic agents (Fig. 7), but again there was no difference between data for those patients treated with a variety of agents in addition to corticosteroids (239).

However, it has become evident that the IV cyclophosphamide regimen, like prolonged daily oral treatment, carries a considerable risk of gonadal damage, with late menarche and early menopause a regular finding in a dose- and age-dependent fashion and older recipients showing greater toxicity (263). This may be a particularly important point in the many transpubertal children with lupus, who probably tolerate the treatment better. This same dose- and age-dependent toxicity has been reported in groups given long-term oral cyclophosphamide (257). Gonadal damage could in theory be limited by giving the pulse timed so that a developing follicle is not present, but apart from complicating the regimen there is no evidence as yet that this is effective. An added disadvantage is that, in older adolescent or adult patients, pregnancy can not be contemplated during such treatment, although it may be possible at a later date for those who do not become sterile. What the oncogenic risk of such regimens may be, or what the effect may be on germline mutations, will not be evident for many years. The oncogenic potential of the drug, apart from that in the bladder, remains whatever route of administration is used, and at least one case of development of acute leukemia following this regimen has already been reported (264). A major additional advantage of this regimen, however, is that in noncompliant teenagers it permits low corticosteroid dosage, with acceptable effects on appearance, and the treatment can be observed to have entered the patient—not a minor point in city center practice! The regimen recommended by the NIH regularly produces leukopenia and, as just discussed, carries some gonadal toxicity. It is by no means secure that this regimen is the optimum way to use the drug by the IV route, but other regimens have been examined so far in an anecdotal fashion (265).

Azathioprine

In the initial NIH trials (238,239), although the histologic and clinical results using azathioprine in addition to corticosteroids did not differ statistically at 10 years from the results in the groups treated with prednisolone alone, there was in addition no difference between the azathioprine data and those obtained using the pulse cyclophosphamide, because small numbers of patients resulted in the confidence limits on all of these data being very wide (Fig. 8). Azathioprine in doses of 2–2.5 mg/kg/24 h has proved remarkably safe in the very long term (266,267), although higher doses will of course induce leukopenia. Previously we used this agent during the acute phase of the disease (206), as did Ponticelli and colleagues (268) and Esdaile et al. (269); more recently, we have transferred patients to this drug after only 8–12 weeks of induction with oral cyclophosphamide, as outlined in the previous section on acute disease. There is evidence that the addition of azathioprine does not increase the incidence of infection (267) (which mostly depends on the dosage of steroids). One beneficial effect of azathioprine (and cyclophosphamide) is that use of these drugs almost certainly has a steroid-sparing effect. In addition, withdrawal of azathioprine without change in steroid dosage may lead to relapse (270). Also, despite worrying data in rodents, in humans, azathioprine does not seem to carry such a large oncogenic potential as mustardlike drugs, although a small risk is undoubtedly present (271,272). In a disease of young women, pregnancy during maintenance azathioprine can be encouraged and is safe. Azathioprine has been alleged to cause pancreatitis (273), and despite rare reports of intrahepatic cholestasis, it seems that in humans (274) hepatotoxicity is minimal; we have seen only one certain case in 2,000 renal transplants and none in lupus.

Certainly, in lupus nephritis long-term results as good or better than the best obtainable with cyclophosphamide, by whatever route, can be achieved by initial IV methylprednisolone followed by combined azathioprine and corticosteroids (233,268,269) (Fig. 9). Whether initial use of cyclophosphamide, orally or IV, brings extra benefit over azathioprine is as yet unknown, since no trial comparing these two regimens has been done, although one has begun in the Netherlands.

Chlorambucil and Methotrexate

Chlorambucil has been advocated as maintenance treatment also (275,276), but has been little used for lupus; it has never been subjected to any controlled trials, and its gonadal effects and oncogenic potential are, if anything, greater than those of cyclophosphamide (277). More recently, low-dose weekly *methotrexate* has been suggested, as in rheumatoid arthritis, for maintenance treatment, with beneficial results even in resistant patients (278,279). However, few patients reported to date have had any clinical nephritis, so its effects (if any) on lupus nephritis are unknown.

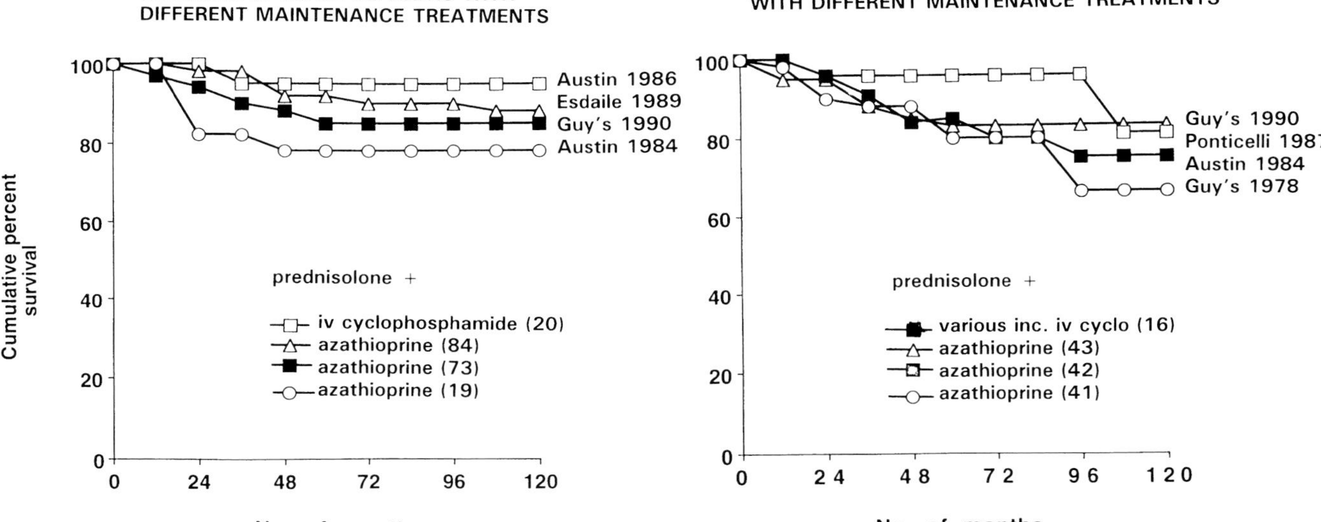

FIG. 9. *Left:* Renal survival in lupus nephritis in four series of patients treated with azathioprine (214,233,239) and the National Institutes of Health (NIH) trial data (239) for patients treated with intravenous cyclophosphamide; there is no statistical difference in the outcomes. *Right:* Renal survival in patients with WHO class IV lupus nephritis treated with azathioprine (233,268,441) compared with NIH data for intravenous cyclophosphamide (214); there is no statistical difference in the outcomes.

Cyclosporine

Cyclosporine might be expected to benefit patients with lupus because of its powerful effect on helper T-cell clonal expansion through inhibition of interleukin-2 synthesis (see Chapter 39). After favorable results in mice with lupus (280), trials were begun in the human disease. Only a small amount of data have been published formally (281–282) together with some abstracts (283,284) despite widespread use, and the relative silence in the literature, despite some years of interest, suggest that in general the results have not been overwhelmingly good.

Meyrier (285) collected and summarized the published and unpublished results in 35 patients, mostly acute, up to 1991. The dosage used was 2–9 (mean, 5) mg/kg/24 h to avoid nephrotoxicity. Only a few patients showed a strong response [see, for example, Le François et al. (283)], but rebound following withdrawal of treatment in some seems to confirm an effect. There was no effect in reducing anti-dsDNA antibody. In general, it did not appear to be useful in acute lupus, but can have a role in the maintenance phase as a steroid-sparing agent and to reduce proteinuria in major nephrotic syndromes.

Tacrolimus (FK 506) has been shown to reduce proteinuria and prolong life in NZB/W and MRL/*lpr* mice (286); to date, its use has not been reported in human lupus. It seems to have similar nephrotoxicity to cyclosporine, however.

Plasma Exchange

Studying patients already on chronic maintenance immunosuppression, Clark and colleagues (287) addressed the question of what the effect of regular long-term plasma exchange might be on steroid dosages in an unblinded trial and found that a reduction in dosage was possible without relapses. In two of our patients who could not tolerate cytotoxic agents, we have used regular exchanges, with objective evidence of improvement in cerebral lupus in one.

Intravenous γ-Globulin

Because a decade's experience suggests that I.V. γ-globulin preparations are effective in reversing idiopathic thrombocytopenia (288), it has been used also in small series of patients with lupus (289–291), including advanced disease (292). Lin et al. (293) treated six children with lupus nephritis resistant to corticosteroids and cyclophosphamide and suggest that their renal disease improved both clinically and histologically. Schifferli et al. (294) warn that a transient decline in renal function may follow its use in nephrotic patients. A major problem is that preparations of I.V. γ-globulin differ in their properties, and even within one manufacturer's product there may be differences between batches. How I.V. γ-globulin might act is speculative, but modification of anti-idiotype networks by the anti-idiotypic antibodies in the preparation is the most usual explanation offered. However, recently Oravec and colleagues (295) showed that Sandoglobulin™ inhibited thromboxane A_2 and endothelin production by cultured endothelial cells, but not prostaglandin I_2, so the latter's action may be more complex.

Total Lymphoid Irradiation

The results of short-term (296,297) and longer-term (298) follow-ups in a group of patients with severe resistant lupus given total lymphoid irradiation, on the model of that used for Hodgkin disease and more recently for transplantation, have been encouraging, with minimal requirements for immunosuppression subsequently, but again the use of this technique on prepubertal or transpubertal patients raises extra worries. Nevertheless, again it seems likely that this approach will be explored further in selected adults or in patients who cannot or will not take medicines long term.

The Maintenance Phase: Summing Up

Thus, it is my opinion that the addition of a cytotoxic agent to the maintenance treatment regimen for severe lupus nephritis *does* have advantages, but that the physician must choose the agent and route of administration based on inadequate information. The difference in the various regimens is only in their greater or lesser morbidity in the short or the long term, and it is on this that their utility must be judged. My own feeling is that cyclophosphamide in the acute phase may have advantages, but the route of administration may be irrelevant and, in the long term, any extra benefit of IV monthly pulse cyclophosphamide over azathioprine has yet to be demonstrated, whereas the IV cyclophosphamide regimen is definitely more gonadotoxic and teratogenic than azathioprine maintenance. Therefore, I prefer to use azathioprine as the first line of maintenance treatment from 12 weeks onward, reserving IV cyclophosphamide for noncompliant patients and for those few who continue to deteriorate during azathioprine treatment. We have used IV γ-globulin only in a few resistant patients with treatment-related toxicity. As others have observed, some patients appear to go into remission, but relapse is frequent.

Serologic Tests and Treatment

The value (or lack of value) of immunologic tests in guiding such treatment has been debated extensively. A number of authors have suggested that in the maintenance phase of treatment, or off all treatment, levels of anti-dsDNA antibody are associated with subsequent relapses (299–301). Although this may be generally true, a number of patients maintain elevated levels for years without relapse, and there is a fine balance between undertreatment and overtreatment. In our opinion, the main value of DNA-binding levels is that *normal* values usually permit safe reduction of steroid dosage during the chronic phase (302). Similar conclusions can be reached about complement concentrations during the acute phase in severe renal disease: clinical and biochemical data are almost always sufficient.

Can We Stop Treatment in Lupus?

The goal of long-term management in patients with lupus nephritis is suppression of disease with minimum side effects of treatment. This balance is not easily achieved, but close attention to the details of individual patients can improve performance, despite lack of real measures of disease activity. Judicious use of repeat biopsies may suggest whether a slow decline in renal function and proteinuria is the result of active glomerulonephritis or of secondary sclerosis, which at the moment we seem powerless to arrest. Normal results from immunologic tests are a help in this distinction, but we remain convinced that in selected patients a repeat biopsy is useful.

Nevertheless, it is becoming clear that—although we have seen patients have severe renal relapse 22 and 28 years after onset of disease when treatment is reduced—after 3, 5, and 10 years or more, treatment can be stopped altogether even in some patients with very severe lupus at onset because their disease has apparently "burnt out" (268,303,304), although a proportion may relapse. How best can we judge when and in whom this can be done? At the moment, our own policy is not to consider stopping treatment until ~4–5 years have elapsed, often more. This is based on previous experience of frequent relapses in patients whose treatment was stopped earlier. We examine the stability of renal function using GFR measurements, the normality or abnormality of the urine, complement concentrations, and DNA antibody titers, and often perform another renal biopsy. Proteinuria at this stage does not always indicate activity of disease, but may be a concomitant of previously induced glomerulosclerosis. Nevertheless, absence of clinical proteinuria is reassuring. Only if all tests suggest quiescent disease would we start by removing the concomitant cytotoxic agent (if in use) and then, some months later, cautiously and slowly reduce the dosage of corticosteroids over several months, meanwhile watching all parameters. Despite this caution, sadly one may be rewarded by a relapse some weeks or months after stopping treatment, even following years of disease quiescence.

Other Treatments for Lupus Nephritis

A number of other treatments have been used for lupus with or without nephritis, without making a major impact on clinical practice; these are summarized briefly here.

Anticoagulants and Antiplatelet Agents

There is strong evidence that hemostatic mechanisms, both platelet (191) and fibrin mediated (305), are active in lupus nephritis, and suggestions have been made that antithrombin (306,307), antiplatelet (191,308), or fibrinolytic (309–312) agents might be of use in treating the condition, especially when glomerular capillary thrombi are present in the kidney (124). The major evidence of platelet activation, which I have summarized elsewhere (191), strongly points to a possible role for antiplatelet agents in treatment of lupus nephritis. Even in the presence of corticosteroids, however, it *is* safe to treat with acetylsalicylate 75 mg/24 h or an equivalent dose 2–3 times a week. *Ancrod* defibrinates the patient effectively with a surprising lack of side effects, and Pollak's group has reported excellent long-term results even in severe progressive nephritis (309–312). This treatment deserves further evaluation, especially in resistant nephritis.

Indomethacin

This has also been used in lupus (307), but in view of the fall in GFR in lupus nephritis when using all nonsteroid anti-inflammatory drugs (313), and their potential for inducing interstitial nephritis (314), this has not proved popular. Perhaps, more selective antiprostaglandin therapy with thromboxane synthetase inhibitors or thromboxane receptor antagonists will prove useful (315); it is too early to judge.

Antimalarials

There is no strong evidence that these are effective in lupus nephritis, either alone or as an agent to reduce steroid dosage (18). We have found that disfiguring cutaneous lesions already resistant to oral corticosteroids are almost always resistant to chloroquine.

T-Cell Modulation

Levamisole, frentizole, and isoprinosine have been advocated [see Shearn (184) for a review] but are no longer used because of side effects and lack of effect.

Prostaglandins and Dietary Fat

Administration of the ω-3 unsaturated acids eicosapentanoic acid (EPA) and docosohexanoic acid shifts prostaglandin production from the 2 to the 3 series. [e.g. TXA_3 instead of TAX_2] EPA has been shown to protect mice from lupus nephritis, with a reduction in anti-dsDNA antibody titers, whereas a high-tallow (saturated) diet accelerates the disease. Kincaid-Smith and her group (316) and Clark and colleagues (317) have studied the effects of EPA in human lupus with favorable short-term effects on hematuria (316), blood fats (317), and hemostatic parameters (317). Anti-dsDNA titers were not affected, however. Some of these effects are particularly attractive in view of the excessive and accelerated vascular disease reported in young women with lupus (318), which forms a major late morbidity and mortality (319) (see below). Westberg and Tarkowski (320) saw no difference in clinical parameters after 6 months of treatment, but Walton et al. (321) in their blind controlled trial showed an effect on parameters of disease activity in relatively mild lupus.

Extracorporeal Removal of Antibody

Several attempts at removal of anti-dsDNA antibody by using extracorporeal immunoabsorbent circuits have been made in small numbers of patients (322–325). Although improvement in these patients was claimed to follow from the immunoabsorption, it is impossible to determine whether this would have occurred from the concomitant immunosuppression alone.

Androgens

The strong association of lupus with female gender and reproductive years, together with the animal evidence of protection by androgens, led to treatment with various androgenic compounds; but with the possible exception of danazol, no benefit has been noted [see Cameron (206) for a review].

Treatment of Lupus Nephritis: The Future

Clearly present treatments for lupus, although successful, are quite unsatisfactory because of side effects. A number of new immunosuppressive drugs used in transplantation may hold promise for treatment of autoimmune disease (326), as may leflunomide (327) and 2-chlorodeoxyadenosine (328). However, these agents remain nonspecific.

Work in murine lupus has shown that monoclonal antibodies directed against dsDNA (307), anti-dsDNA antibodies (329), anti-idiotypic antibodies (330), CD4 T-helper cells (331), MHC class II antigens involved in antigen presentation (332,333), and the interleukin-2 receptor CD25 (334) are all capable of inhibiting lupus. Anti-CD4 antibodies have been used clinically in humans to treat rheumatoid arthritis, and a few patients with lupus (335). These monoclonals are best "humanized" for long-term use (336). Other strategies are available to block any of these reactions, such as ligand homologues, receptor homologues, and soluble forms of soluble receptors.

Toxic agents such as ricin or diphtheria toxin may be spliced to either ligands (337,338) or antibodies (339, 340), enabling destruction of the cell after endocytosis of the antibody and its cell surface target.

Blocking the binding of ligands that lead to the "second signal" during antigen presentation is an attractive strategy in both organ transplantation and the treatment of autoimmunity. The multiplicity of these ligands (intracellular adhesion molecule 1–lymphocyte-function-associated antigen 1, CD28–B7, MHC–CD4, and so on) suggests that such a strategy will not be easy, but it appears that the pair of the immunoglobulin superfamily molecule B7 on the antigen-presenting cell and the 44-kD glycoprotein CD28 on the T cell is of particular importance (341). Soluble chimeric analogues of CD28 that can bind to B7 have been synthesized (CTLA4Ig) and look promising as blocking agents in vivo (342).

In addition, peptides derived from (or mimicking) the CD4 T-cell receptor could block presentation and switch off the immune response (343,344). Peptides derived from the HLA molecules themselves can be used in a similar fashion (345). Attempts at oral desensitization have been made in both rheumatoid arthritis (346) and multiple sclerosis (347), and this approach could prove fruitful in lupus also—provided we feel confident that, for example, nucleosomes are the target we should exploit. Finally, there remains the option of removing the autoreactive stem cells altogether by marrow ablation and replacing them with normal stem cells (348).

TABLE 6. *Survival of patients with severe diffuse lupus nephritis (WHO class IV) in different periods*

Date of publication	Reference	Authors	5-year actuarial survival (%)
1957	9	Muehrcke et al.	10[a]
1964	223	Pollak et al.	25
1970	374	Baldwin et al.	23
1971	180	Estes and Christian	25
1973	439	Striker et al.	76
1973	440	Nanra and Kincaid-Smith	78
1976	120	Morel-Maroger et al.	78
1979	441	Cameron et al.	78
1986	239	Austin et al.	83
1987	268	Ponticelli et al.	97
1987	367	Leaker et al.	74[b]
1989	269	Esdaile et al.	87
1991	—	Mc'Ligeyo et al.	82
1991	442	McLaughlin et al.	74
1992	235	GISNEL[c]	85

[a]Two-year survival.
[b]Class IVb only.
[c]Gruppo Italiano per lo Studio della Nefrite Lupica.

These series are not strictly comparable because different starting points have been taken in some series (onset of lupus/onset of nephritis), and some report patient rather than renal survival. Also, the small numbers in all of these individual series mean that the confidence limits for all of these figures are large. However, the trend is so strong as to overcome all of these objections.

CLINICAL COURSE AND PROGNOSIS

The clinical course of lupus can no longer be considered separately from treatment, because there is no doubt that the outlook for patients with lupus has improved enormously in recent years (206) (Table 6): 30 or more years ago, almost no patients with severe grade-IV nephritis survived more than 1 or 2 years (9); this has been transformed into 10-year survivals approaching 90%. The only statement that can be made with certainty about the course of lupus, treated or untreated, is that it is capricious. As already noted, most patients presenting with lupus nephritis have relatively active disease; in a few unfortunates, this continues with involvement of more and more organ systems until the patient dies.

In most patients today, however, there is a gratifying response to early treatment, a return of well-being and of lupus test results to within normal limits, improvement in renal function and decrease in proteinuria, and relatively quiescent disease thereafter, usually under continuing immunosuppression, which can be tapered out eventually without further relapse. A third pattern is the patient in this quiescent state who suddenly has a relapse, sometimes with an identifiable precipitating event, sometimes not. In some patients, the pattern of relapse is constant, for example, with thrombocytopenia in every relapse; in others, completely new phenomena may appear "out of the blue" and present new and urgent problems of management.

Because lupus is a multisystem disease, the outlook does not of course depend only on what happens to renal function, especially now that this is treatable by dialysis and transplantation. Also, many accessory factors, such as the socioeconomic circumstances of the family (210, 349,350) and the comprehension of treatment goals, may be more important than purely biologic phenomena and in the real world are crucial in determining outlook in this complicated disorder with effective, but sometimes incomprehensible, treatment that must be carried out over many years, even when the patient feels and is apparently well. Measures to deal with these problems may be as important (or even more important) as specific treatments in determining survival, and measures to deal with them should be attempted (351).

Outcome in Relation to Clinical Data

Naturally, clinical data have been examined by many authors for clues to prognosis (182,235,349–370). An *age at onset* of >55 years has been suggested by several series (122,353,354) to be a determinant of prognosis, since lupus is often a milder disease in relatively older patients. This was not borne out, though, by the large series of Wallace et al. (349), who found the same survival in patients with onset at greater or less than 50 years of age. Nor did age at onset affect the outcome in the very large collected series (>1,000 patients) of Ginzler et al. (355) or the analysis by Swaak et al. (352).

The outcome of lupus in *childhood* has been the subject of some controversy, which I have reviewed in detail elsewhere (139,335,359). In our own series of 80 patients with onset of lupus nephritis under the age of 20 years, 5- and 10-year estimates of renal survival were 85% and 82%, and in the data from Minneapolis (360) on 70 childhood onset cases, the figures were 85% and 81%. However, many other series have reported poorer survival among children than among adults (349). Esdaile et al. (269) performed a Cox analysis on 87 patients and noted no difference in renal failure or renal death among those above and below 24 years of age at onset, which agreed with the findings of Austin et al. (122). In general, there seems to be little difference in the survival of adults and children or adolescents with lupus nephritis when other factors are considered (122,355,361), although some authors such as Ginzler and Schorn (210) have interpreted essentially the same data in the opposite fashion, suggesting that children still do worse than adults. Certainly, the difference, if any, is not major.

Gender has been studied as a prognostic factor by several authors. Male patients, of course, form only a small minority of patients with lupus, which makes comparison difficult except in the largest series. Wallace et al. (349), Austin et al. (122), and Swaak et al. (362) all found that men did worse than women, whereas Esdaile et al. (269) suggested in their Cox analysis a higher rate of renal failure among males, but no difference in nonrenal deaths. In contrast, Ginzler et al. (355), using a stepwise linear regression model, found no difference in their large collected series. Tejani et al. (363) and other pediatricians (364) have suggested a poorer outcome for boys, especially those with a prepubertal onset, but the numbers are small and other confusing factors such as race (see the next paragraph) are difficult to correct for.

Race is an obvious target for analysis, since the incidence and prevalence of lupus is so much higher in blacks and Orientals compared with Caucasians (55–59, 62), although even within Caucasian groups the incidence seems to be highest in those with an origin in the Indian subcontinent. Many authors, ourselves included, found no difference in outcome comparing black and Caucasian patients (182,212,286,361,364). The issue is complicated by the fact that black Americans differ in so many ways from Caucasians, particularly in socioeconomic status (351,354,365,366). Ginzler et al. (355) and Austin et al. (356,357) did, however, find a poorer outcome for blacks in their large studies. Tejani et al. (363) suggested that black children with an onset before puberty form a particularly high-risk group. Gordon et al. (366), examining national mortality from lupus in the United States, again suggested a higher mortality among black females than white.

Ginzler et al. (355) also examined the *clinical severity of nephritis* as a predictor of outcome. Despite the undoubted fact that many patients with initially severe disease may have a favorable outcome, a *raised plasma creatinine* at onset in this and several other studies (354,356,358) was strongly associated with a poor outcome. Leaker et al. (367), though, saw no difference. The magnitude of proteinuria or the presence of a nephrotic syndrome is more controversial: we (182), Wallace et al. (349), and the Gruppo Italiano (235) noted no difference in outcome among those with nephrotic range or lesser degrees of proteinuria in univariate analyses. However, Esdaile et al. (269), Appel et al. (368), and Donadio et al. (354) found poorer survival among their nephrotic patients, in Appel's data particularly among those with persistent nephrotic syndrome.

Hypertension—at least severe hypertension—is not as commonly present in lupus nephritis at apparent onset as in some other forms of glomerulopathy [for example, 10 of 87 in the study by Esdaile et al. (269); see also Budman and Steinberg (369)], and was not examined as a prognostic factor in either of two of the largest studies cited above (360,355); nor is it mentioned in the majority of follow-up studies. Esdaile et al. (269) did not find any association between outcome and high blood pressure itself, but only with comorbid conditions; the Gruppo Italiano (235), Ward and Studenski (370), and Donadio et al. (354), however, showed a poorer survival among their hypertensive subgroup. Of course, in almost all patients, if hypertension is present at outset or appears later, it is usually treated vigorously. Nevertheless, it is interesting that, unlike IgA nephropathy for example, high blood pressure does not seem to be a powerful predictor of a poor outcome in lupus nephritis.

Esdaile et al. (269) found, as Ginzler et al. (355) had previously, that the total *number of ARA criteria* for the diagnosis of lupus present at onset was a useful index of a poorer outcome. Swaak et al. (362) noted a poorer prognosis among those with increasing number of clinical relapses, but this was in a population predominantly not under heavy immunosuppression.

Indices of clinical activity of the lupus itself have been examined in a number of studies [see Esdaile et al. (269) and Fries et al. (361) for discussion], many of which either do not deal with lupus nephritis or do not specify how many of the group studied had nephritis and are therefore of little use for our present purpose.

Prognosis in Relation to Immunologic Tests

It is clear that at any time point, including presentation, there are correlations between immunologic tests such as complement concentrations and levels of circulating anti-dsDNA antibody, and the severity of the clinical picture, judged in a variety of ways (200,301, 371–373). Their clinical utility in predicting outcome is small, however. When a group exclusively consisting of patients with nephritis is examined, thrombocytopenia, hypocomplementemia and a raised DNA binding at onset all predicted poor outcome also in Esdaile's (269) analysis. Austin et al. (356) also found hypocomplementemia to be predictive of a poor prognosis, together with anemia, which was a risk factor also in Donadio's analysis (354).

Prognosis in Relation to Renal Histologic Features

Pattern of Glomerular Disease

At a histologic level, a considerable body of data is available. The WHO classification (117,119), which includes a category of sclerosing glomerulopathy (120,182), has been the most studied. However, as indicated above, although in the past considerable differences in outcome between milder and more severe forms were found (182,223,374), many recent reports, including our own data (Fig. 10), find no or little difference in outcome

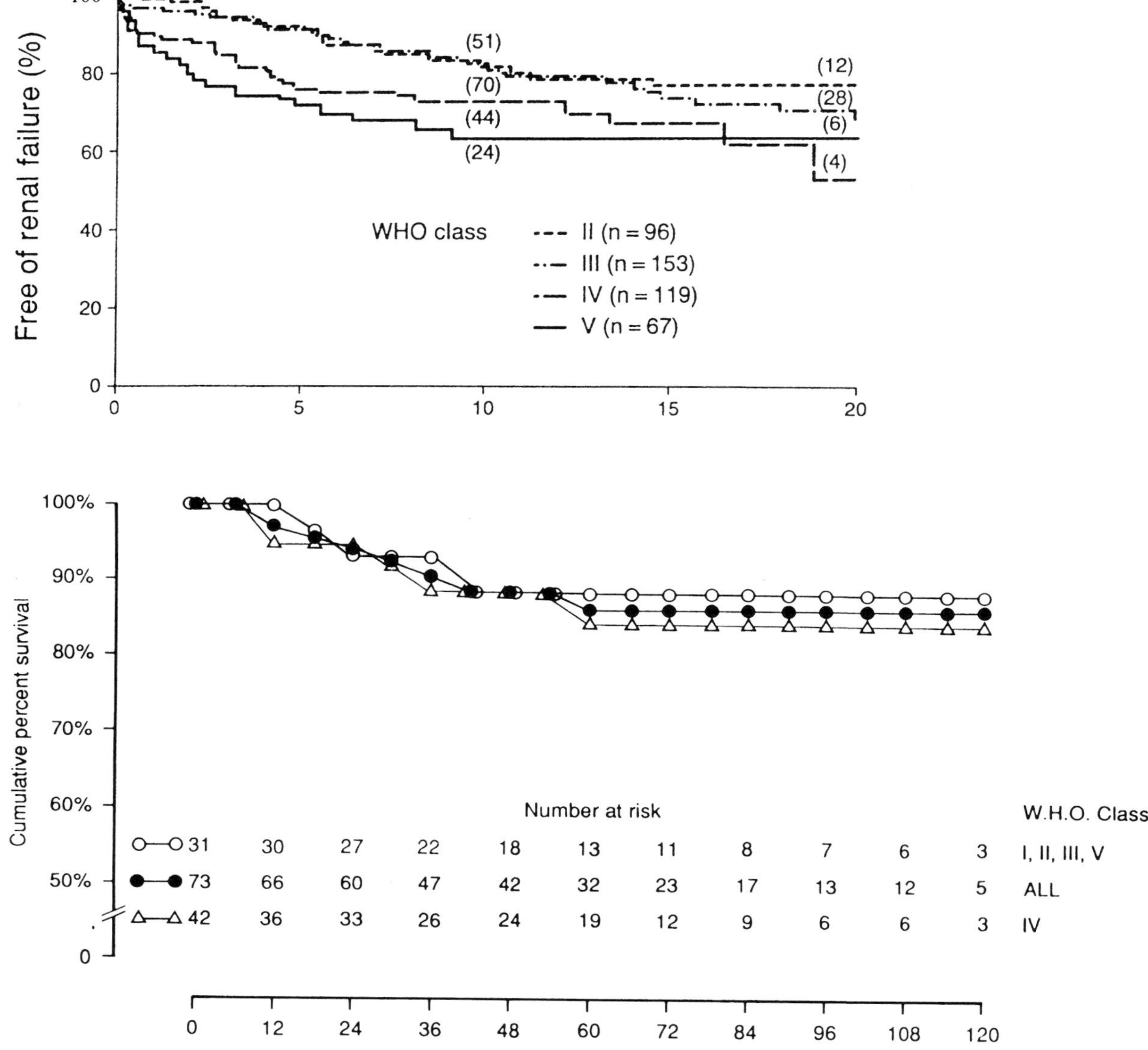

FIG. 10. Two sets of data of renal outcome in relation to WHO histology class. The *top* presents very long-term data from Donadio et al. (354) demonstrating that class IV and class V patients do worse than those with class II and class III. Our own data for the 1980–1989 cohort (*bottom*) show no difference at all over the first 10 years.

between different WHO classes in treated patients (233, 235,286,337). In contrast, Appel et al. (376), in a rather small study (56 patients studied, 1976–1986), noted a better survival in those with class II (mesangial) nephritis compared with the other histologic classes, and the 1984 article by Austin et al. (214) also reported a poorer survival in those with class IV nephritis, as did Nossent et al. (112) and the recent much larger analysis by the GISNEL group (235). Donadio et al. (354), in the largest single-center long-term experience, used a Cox proportional hazards method (Fig. 10). Although WHO class was just significant in univariate analysis ($p = 0.04$), this significance disappeared in the multivariate analysis. All authors (182,211,354,372,374) are agreed, though, that patients showing WHO class V pattern, that is, membranous nephropathy, almost always run an indolent course, although renal failure occurs in a minority (220–222, 375).

A particular problem exists with regard to patients classified as having WHO class III appearances: focal proliferative glomerulonephritis. A very diverse outcome has been reported for such individuals (118, 123,376,377), which illustrates the great variation in severity within this group, to the point where division into IIIa (less severe focal nephritis) and IIIb (more severe) has been recommended. As noted above, this lack of differentiation in outcome by WHO class has largely come about by an improvement in the survival of those with more severe disease, so that this now resembles that of milder forms of lupus nephritis, which remains essentially unchanged. In turn, this is presumably—although not certainly (237–240)—the result of therapeutic decisions to treat those patients with more severe histologic appearances more aggressively.

Individual Elements of Histology

Analyses have been performed also to assess the predictive value of individual elements of the histologic picture. Two observations appear to show some reliability in predicting a poor outcome. The first of these is *extensive subendothelial deposits*, especially if they persist in repeated biopsies (112–114,378,379). The value of this observation may now be vitiated in the majority of patients by aggressive treatment of such a histologic appearance. Still of value, though, are *tubulointerstitial changes*, which were noted by Muehrcke et al. (9) as long ago as their classic report of 1957. These changes point to a poor prognosis in a number of studies (72,269,357, 380,381). Magil et al. (381) found that the number of nonspecific esterase-positive cells (macrophages) correlated with outcome, and we (72) have shown, using monoclonal antibodies to phenotype the interstitial cells, correlations between both the numbers of infiltrating monocytes and T cells and the subsequent GFRs (Fig. 11). *Crescents* also have been related to a poorer prognosis (357,382), as in other forms of nephritis, but very extensive crescentic disease is relatively uncommon in lupus. Vascular lesions within the biopsy specimen (128–130, 383) and *intraglomerular capillary thrombi* (124) have been associated with unfavorable outcomes also, although the latter observation has been contested (133,367).

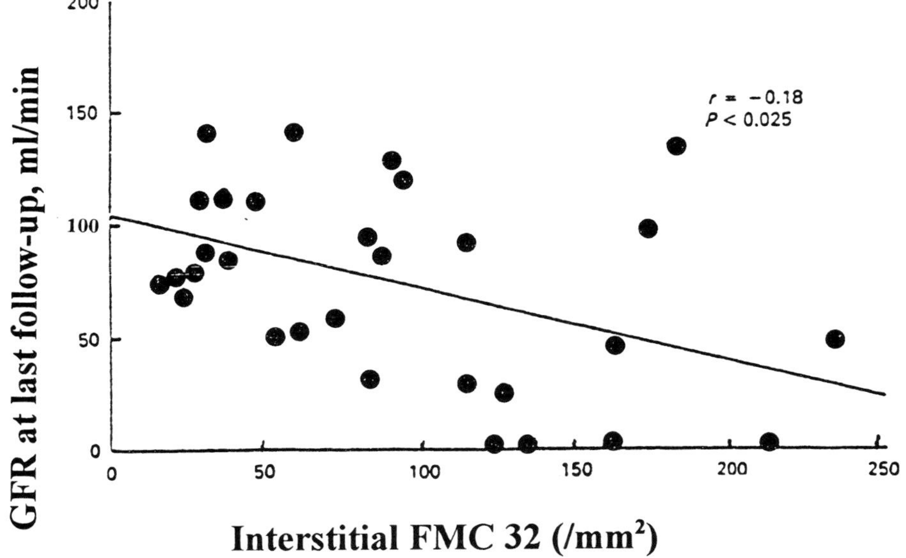

FIG. 11. Relationship between the number of macrophages (monoclonal antibody FMC32+ve cells) and the GFR measured a mean of 5.5 yeas later. From Alexopoulos et al. [72].

Transformation of Histologic Appearances

Initial reports emphasized the distinction between appearances (10,121,374). However, longer-term study and serial biopsies showed that, in many instances, transformations of WHO classes is quite frequent (Table 7) (115,360,384–386). A particularly common transformation is one from class IV diffuse proliferative glomerulonephritis to a predominant membranous (class V) pattern under successful treatment. As renal function improves, proteinuria may become massive under these circumstances.

Activity/Chronicity Indexes

Because of dissatisfaction with the data obtained by considering the morphologic pattern of the nephritis, which is in any case very variable between and within glomeruli in lupus nephritis, an alternative approach has gained support: that of assessing the histologic *activity* of the nephritis, on the one hand, and its apparent *chronicity*, on the other, as judged by the extent of sclerosis. This approach was pioneered by Pirani and Salinas-Madrigal (121), Morel-Maroger (120), and others in the 1960s and 1970s, but became popular after Austin et al. published a report (122) describing the calculation of activity and chronicity indices using data from both glomeruli and interstitium in either case. This approach enabled these workers (122) to identify clear groups of high and low risk for a poor outcome, and also permitted therapeutic decisions especially about when and when not to use aggressive treatment. These data were supported by the analyses by Magil et al. (381), Esdaile et al. (269), and Nossent et al. (112), a high chronicity index being in general the best predictor of subsequent renal failure; but several other authors have found poor or absent association of outcome with either index or combinations of them (123,362,368), although the follow-up in the study by Schwartz et al. (123) was only 2 years.

Additional Value of Renal Biopsy Data

Finally, the additional value for predicting outcome of the information from renal biopsies over that available from clinical studies has been examined by several authors (113,114,116,122,269,381) using different multivariate models and different sets of data. Fries et al. (361) and others suggested that there was only minimal extra value in the analysis of renal biopsy specimens in lupus nephritis when using then what approximates to the WHO classification now. Whiting-O'Keefe and colleagues (113,114) came to less pessimistic conclusions, although only the degree of sclerosis and the presence/absence of subendothelial deposits seemed of any great value. Austin et al. (122) suggested more positively that, not only did the WHO classification of biopsy data add useful information, but the chronicity index was an even better predictor of outcome. Magil et al. (381) came to similar positive conclusions in their model, but later Esdaile et al. (269) found no biopsy information that added to the clinical predictions. The value of biopsy in directing more aggressive—and possibly more successful—therapeutic strategies is almost impossible to evaluate, but certainly this behavior interfered to a major extent with any or all of the analyses just discussed.

Inapparent Renal Disease in Lupus

A number of authors have noted that patients without clinical manifestations of nephritis have, in renal biopsy specimens, changes in their glomeruli amounting to glomerular disease. There have been few follow-up studies on such patients, but the study by Leehey et al. (218) showed that the majority of patients remain without clinical nephritis for some years, although even severe diffuse proliferative patterns may be observed in some. It is equally obvious, though, that all patients with clinically evident nephritis must go through a period of absent or

TABLE 7. *Transformation of renal biopsy specimen appearances in subsequent renal biopsies in patients with lupus*

WHO class	Description	Number	Number rebiopsied	Final pathologic classification				
				I	II	III	IV	V
I	Minimal	17	6	1	3	1	—	1
II	Mesangial	16[a]	6	—	2	1	3	—
III	Focal proliferative	14[b]	8	2	1	1	4	—
IV	Diffuse proliferative	13[c]	13	—	4	3	6	—
V	Membranous	5[d]	5	—	—	—	1	4
	Total	65	38	3	10	6	14	5

[a]One interval biopsy revealed focal, final biopsy diffuse.
[b]One interval biopsy revealed mesangial, final biopsy normal.
[c]One patient, interval biopsies mesangial, final biopsy diffuse. One patient, two interval biopsies focal, final biopsy diffuse. One patient, interval biopsy mesangial, final biopsy focal.
[d]One patient, interval biopsy focal, final biopsy diffuse.
Data from Platt et al. 1982 (360).

occult disease before this becomes evident; how many of these patients have disease that runs a subclinical course for a prolonged period is not known.

Final Outcome and Mortality in Lupus Nephritis

Overall mortality has improved dramatically during the 1970s, and survival is now up to 80% or even 90% at 5–10 years in most large series (233,235,239,254,262, 268,269,354,362,367) (Table 6) with a loss of the previously observed large differences in survival between various histologic classes (182,223,374), as noted above.

The most *recent status* of the 1980–1989 cohort of our series after a median follow-up of 7 years (range, 1–14 years) (Table 8) shows encouraging results compared with 20 years ago. It should be noted that only four patients (5%) are in full remission off all treatment, and only 47 (63%) have normal renal function; 10 have plasma creatinine concentrations ranging from 141 to 622 μmol/L already; will the conditions of the other 28 with persisting proteinuria evolve eventually into renal failure? We have seen relapses as late as 22, 25, and 28 years following onset after planned or accidental reductions in immunosuppression, with significant loss of renal function. The report by Moroni and colleagues (387) is more encouraging: of 34 patients who had actually completed 10 years of follow-up, six had died, three were on end-stage treatment, six had raised plasma creatinines (three with proteinuria), six had minor proteinuria with normal function, and 15 were in complete remission; 11 patients (32%) had been off all treatment for a mean of 7.5 years. There are surprisingly few data on the longer-term status of patients with lupus nephritis in relation to treatment: How commonly is it possible to attain stable remission after discontinuing all therapy? Is there a difference between patients treated with cyclophosphamide or azathioprine in this respect?

Entry into end-stage renal failure remains the principal cause of "death" among lupus patients with evident nephritis (Table 9). Although the great majority of these patients survive (see below), a distressing number do actually die after being taken on to dialysis, or following transplantation, infections being the main cause of death in this group. Two of 12 deaths in our group of patients occurred after they had started treatment for end-stage renal disease (ESRD), both in the early phases, one of pulmonary hemorrhage on dialysis and the other of sepsis complicated by thrombosis following transplantation.

The *causes of death* among lupus patients, of course, are much more varied than in other forms of primary glomerulonephritis confined to the kidney in young adults in whom renal failure is the dominant cause. Table 9 compares proximate causes of death reported among children (total, 136 deaths) (139) and in three large adult series (322,388,389) in which causes of nearly 400 deaths were analyzed, and in the large single-center study by Donadio et al. (354). It must be remembered that the data in this table cover a considerable time span, and that they may not reflect contemporary events—particularly in relation to treatment-related deaths, such as those due to sepsis. It must not be forgotten also that, in many instances, the circumstances of death were complicated, with several factors involved, but with only the major factor being noted in Table 9. The follow-up in Donadio's series was much longer than in the other two sets of data, and this is reflected in the increased incidence of cardiovascular deaths and malignancies.

Infection was, perhaps not surprisingly, the commonest cause of death overall in 46 (36.5 %) of 126 children and in 104 (31%) of 333 adults, and extrarenal lupus of the central nervous system or lung was prominent. Similar data are available from other series (233,319,332,333,353). An excess of accelerated *cardiovascular mortality*, particularly from myocardial ischemia in long-term survivors, is disturbing (319,354,390,391). In Donadio's series (354), this was the single commonest cause of death (48% of 100 deaths in which a cause could be determined) and was a common cause of death among our own patients (319), major coronary artery disease being present in many during their 30s; one boy died of a myocardial infarct of

TABLE 8. *Most recent status of patients with lupus nephritis presenting 1980–89 (3–13 years of follow-up)*

WHO biopsy specimen class	n	Complete[a] remission	Proteinuria and normal function	Proteinuria and impaired function	End-stage renal disease	Number of deaths	Causes of death			
							Sepsis		Renal failure	
I	1	0	0	0	1	0	—	—	—	—
II	8	3	2	2	0	1	—	—	1	—
III	11	6	3	0	1	1	1	—	—	—
IV	47	12	11	12	6	6	3	1	1	1
V	13	3	7	2	1	0	—	—	—	—
Total	80	24	23	16	9[b]	8	4	1	2	1

[a]Of 24 patients, 20 were still receiving immunosuppressive treatment.
[b]Four of these patients are dead from causes unrelated to their lupus nephritis.
Unpublished data from S.Mc'Ligeyo and J. S. Cameron.

TABLE 9. *Causes of death in children and adults with lupus nephritis*

Main cause of death	Children[a]	Adults[b]	Donadio et al. (354)
Renal failure[c]	48 (38%)	94 (28%)	15 (16%)
Infections	46 (37%)	104 (31%)	16 (17%)
Active lupus, other organs	21 (17%)	42 (13%)	9 (9%)
CNS	8	25	—
Lung	4	6	5
Heart	3	9	—
Gut	1	2	4
Liver	1	0	—
Other	4	0	—
Cardiovascular (not lupus)	2 (1.6%)	12 (4%)	45 (48%)
Pulmonary embolus	2 (1.6%)	9 (3%)	—
Pulmonary hypertension	2 (1.6%)	0	—
Unrelated causes	0	20 (6%)	—
Other and unknown	5 (4%)	52 (16%)	59
Malignancy			9 (10%)
Total number of deaths	126	333	153

[a]See Cameron (139) for details.

[b]From Karsh et al. (389), Rosner et al. (388), and Wallace and Hahn (18).

[c]Renal failure has been taken to equal "death" for the purposes of this analysis, whereas in practice most patients are treated by dialysis and/or transplantation. Some have in fact died, but it is impossible to derive exactly how many in several of the series reported here. In the data from Donadio et al. (354), actual death only is recorded.

The adult data, and some of the papers included in the pediatric analysis, include patients without evident lupus nephritis.

severe widespread atheroma at the age of only 19 while waiting to join our ESRD program. The pathogenesis of these late vascular lesions is not clear, but corticosteroid treatment, hyperlipidemia, and immune complexes may all play a part, since interactions between immune complexes and hyperlipidemia to accelerate atheroma formation are well described (392,393) in experimental animals.

Complications of Lupus and Its Treatment

It is best to consider the complications of the primary disease, lupus, together with those of current treatment, because in so many instances these are additive (for example, infections, vascular complications, osteonecrosis, and thrombosis). As the survival of patients with lupus has improved, so the long-term morbidity of the disease and its treatment have become more and more important (381).

Sepsis

If ESRD is excluded and only actual death considered, then, as just noted, *sepsis* is *the* commonest cause of death (394). This vulnerability to infection arises principally from treatment with immunosuppressive drugs and is proportional to the corticosteroid dosage (267); in this study, the addition of azathioprine made no difference. However, patients with lupus already have deficient immune systems, and infections are more common in untreated lupus (395,396), although this tendency is made much worse by treatment.

Herpes zoster is particularly common in younger patients (360), localized in many but with dissemination in one child of 18 with fatal results. Nagasawa et al. (397) also noted a high incidence of zoster in their adult patients: 40 of 92 individuals. Early treatment with acyclovir of all cases of zoster as soon as they appear, before any signs of dissemination are evident, should prevent avoidable tragedies. We have seen zoster meningitis in one patient successfully treated, albeit late.

Pyogenic meningitis can be a major problem and resulted in the deaths of two of our patients (one with pneumococcal and one *n. meningitidis*). *Cryptococcus* may present in this fashion and should always be looked for in the cerebrospinal fluid of any lupus patients with meningitis. The C-reactive protein concentration is useful (but not specific) in distinguishing relapse of lupus from infection, since there is some (usually minor) increase with exacerbations of disease (172,173).

Bacterial endocarditis is rare but also presents problems (398). The difficulty is, of course, that a number of patients with lupus will show thrombotic vegetations on echocardiography that relate to antiphospholipid antibodies (153,154) rather than to infection. Problems also arise in patients *presenting* with culture-negative endocarditis and a positive antinuclear factor. This may occur as a nonspecific result of polyclonal activation in persistent bacteremia, or alternatively the lupus may present with a thrombotic endocarditis. Obviously, it is wise when in doubt to treat for bacterial endocarditis with a full course of antibiotics.

In patients reported by Ginzler et al. from a large collaborative study comprising 665 patient-years of follow-up (267), only 12 episodes of zoster were seen, a much lower incidence than in children, but the data of Nagasawa et al. (397) cited above must be recalled. Urinary tract infections were common—72 episodes in 63 patients—and 15 cases of severe oral candidiasis were noted.

Thromboses

Thromboses complicate the course of lupus with some frequency: ~12% of patients (370). Apart from the antiphospholipid antibody already discussed (132,192, 193–195), other risk factors are present (191,399), including depressed release of plasminogen activator (400,401) and possibly also antagonists of plasmin, decreased plasma concentration of free protein S (399), and raised von Willebrand factor levels (401). Finally, monocyte-derived procoagulant activity is increased in lupus (402). On top of all this, if a patient with lupus develops a nephrotic syndrome, in addition to all the thrombogenic stimuli of lupus will be added the thrombogenic potential of the alterations in platelet function and plasma coagulation factors seen in nephrotics (403).

Thrombosis may affect almost any vessel in the body, but venous thromboses form the great majority, unless an antiphospholipid antibody is present; then, arterial thromboses may be seen more frequently (194,195), with cerebral thrombosis being particularly common, but even the aorta may be involved. We have seen an adolescent boy who thrombosed his inferior vena cava (173,404), and pulmonary embolism is common, perhaps causes pulmonary hypertension (155). Renal venous thrombosis is common in lupus patients, including bilateral thrombosis (173,404,405). A number of patients with a mixed picture of lupus and a hemolytic–uremic syndrome or thrombotic thrombocytopenic purpura have been described (131,4 06,407); such patients may suffer acute renal failure and have in general a poor prognosis.

Ischemic Necrosis of Bone

This is a common complication, being present in 28 of 172 patients in the study by Weiner and Abeles (408), and may affect also pediatric patients, having been found in 19 of 70 children in another study (360). In our own pediatric series, however (206), only three of the first 50 children and adolescents developed this complication, and only two of 32 developed it in the study by Lacks and White (409). The pathogenesis is not clear; it may present in patients who have never received corticosteroids, and Nagasawa and colleagues (410) speculate that yet again a thrombotic pathology dependent on antiphospholipid antibody may underlie ischemic necrosis in some patients. Nevertheless, their patients with this complication had received a greater dose of prednisolone than those without, and other studies (408,411) conclude that total dosage of corticosteroids is the predominant event.

The femoral head is the commonest site of involvement in adult series (408,412), but in the pediatric series reported by Bergstein et al. (413) the commonest site was the femoral condyle. Almost any other bone may be involved, the next most frequent being the humeral head, the border of the scapula, and the carpus or tarsus; in many unfortunate patients, multiple sites (up to five of six) may be involved. Since >50% of patients with one hip affected will develop the disease bilaterally (412), management of the first hip must be planned with the other in mind. The long-term future of joint replacements in such young patients has not yet been explored fully.

Accelerated Atherogenesis

With improvements in survival of patients with lupus, this has emerged as a major problem. Vascular disease is a major cause of later mortality (319,390,391). Myocardial infarcts have been reported in very young patients (414), in the absence of vasculitis, and we have seen this in several 10- to 20-year-old patients. Possible risk factors for atheroma in patients with lupus include corticosteroid treatment (415). However, interaction between hyperlipidemia (416) and immune complexes remains a worrying possibility (392,393). Of patients with lupus, 20–40% are hypertensive (235,269,353,369), even children (417), and in a minority all of the risks of uremia, dialysis, and transplantation are added.

Neoplasia

The incidence is increased in populations of patients with lupus compared with controls, even though the absolute incidence remains low. Two risk factors are the basic immune dysregulation present in lupus and the added effect of chronic immunosuppression, which is well known to induce some forms of neoplasia in other situations—for example, following transplantation. Either might be mediated by direct damage to chromosomes or by facilitation of oncogenic viruses. Lymphomas, which may be found at an intracerebral site (272), as in allograft recipients, seem to be the principal form of tumor noted in patients with lupus (418). The apparent induction period may be weeks to many years; some patients present with lymphoma *before* the clinical onset of lupus. In the study of adults by Lewis et al. (419), six of 18 tumors in 484 women with lupus were carcinoma of the cervix, compared with only one lymphoma. None had received any cytotoxic therapy, although all had received corticosteroids. It is interesting that no deaths from neoplasms were noted in the collected series summarized in Table 9, although among the adults some of the "other" causes were neoplasms, unrelated to therapy in most cases. In Donadio's long-term follow-up (354), only nine deaths were from neoplasia among 153 recorded. Even this low incidence probably represents and increased risk, however, remembering the young average age of lupus patients (mean, 33.5 ± 14 years at onset in Donadio's series).

Growth Retardation in Children

This is inevitable in children and adolescents treated long term with corticosteroids, reaching 12 of 32 in the study by Lacks and White (409); but surprisingly, in view of a wealth of data on corticosteroid-treated children with asthma, nephrotic syndrome, juvenile rheumatoid arthritis, and after transplantation, there seems to be little information on the terminal height achieved by children with lupus, and such studies are needed. Certainly, all clinics are aware of stunted young adults, particularly those with an onset of lupus before puberty. Possibly young women (the majority in this group) tolerate the social and psychological consequences of growth retardation better than young males, but this has not been studied. We have studied the growth of 15 children with lupus nephritis treated for a minimum of 2 years with corticosteroids (M. Greco et al., unpublished data) and, at the end of 2–10 years of treatment, height was more than 2 SD below expected in six of 13, and >3 SD in four of 13. The height of three children, however, was above the 50th centile, the main correlation being with the number of days on daily corticosteroids, which emphasizes the need to use alternate-day corticosteroids wherever possible.

Other Complications

Pancreatitis is a rare but well-known complication of treated lupus and has caused the deaths of lupus patients (360). The lupus itself, the corticosteroid therapy, and maybe also azathioprine (252) are all capable of inducing the disease. *Cataracts* are frequent after years of prednisolone treatment [10 (31%) of 32 (409) and 14 (20%) of 70 in other series (360)], but are usually symptomless, although occasionally lens removal and replacement may be necessary. This is safe even in the presence of immunosuppression. *Gastrointestinal hemorrhage* may be caused by either vasculitis of the bowel or corticosteroid-induced ulceration. The latter is much more common, but both occasionally cause death.

Steroid-induced diabetes mellitus has, hardly surprisingly, been described, although infrequently. *Raised intracranial pressure* (420) may appear and complicate yet further neurologic and psychiatric assessment. *Proximal myopathy* is underdiagnosed (421), and osteopenia and vertebral collapse may be seen. A *Cushingoid appearance* and *hirsutism* are common and a major disincentive for adolescent girls to take their steroids, so that compliance in this group of patients is poor, leading on occasion to major relapses with complications from untreated disease.

Side effects of cytotoxic drugs are discussed in Chapter 39. Apart from facilitation of infection and induction of malignancy, these center around the problems of corticosteroid side effects, which we have just discussed, and *marrow depression* with the use of cytotoxic agents. Azathioprine induces a macrocytosis before anemia becomes evident, and evaluation of iron status by the mean corpuscular volume is impossible. Cyclophosphamide usually induces a lymphopenia before a total leukopenia becomes evident, which is useful in monitoring. With conventional brief courses of oral therapy, bladder toxicity is not a problem, but minor hairfall may occur. The effects of long-term IV "pulse" cyclophosphamide were discussed above in the analysis of profit and loss of cytotoxic therapy for lupus nephritis.

End-Stage Renal Disease, Dialysis, and Transplantation

Today only a few patients enter end-stage renal failure, forming only ~1–2% of all patients in ESRD in the United States and in Europe (422). Arce-Salinas et al. (423) examined risk factors for ESRD in a long-term follow-up study and noted that male gender, clinical activity index, crescents, and interstitial changes were the major determinants, compared with case controls. The management of patients with lupus in ESRD may present special problems, however. Whereas it is true that many patients will have inactive disease by the time they enter end-stage renal failure 5–20 years after onset (424–427), another group of patients enter irreversible renal failure quite rapidly and may have active disease and a higher mortality (428–430).

One characteristic is that, along with those suffering ESRD from vasculitis or hemolytic–uremic syndromes, patients in ESRD from lupus nephritis frequently recover enough renal function to come off dialysis, at last for a period of months or years (401), and in some cases indefinitely. Thus, one should not rush to use transplantation in lupus patients in ESRD, but consider 1 or 2 years on dialysis first. The amount of irreversible sclerosis and active inflammation in a renal biopsy specimen may help to determine the reversibility of the renal disease. Some patients will continue to require immunosuppression after they have entered ESRD (428,429); usually prednisolone alone will suffice. Nevertheless, survival of lupus patients on dialysis compares favorably with that of other primary renal diseases (422–430).

Regular Dialysis Treatment

Patients with lupus have a particular problem in maintaining patent vascular access for dialysis and often suffer multiple thromboses (431). This is related in some cases to antiphospholipid antibodies, but in other patients a thrombotic tendency that relates to endothelial dysfunction is present. In addition, some patients have Raynaud phenomenon with poor peripheral perfusion, and veins may be small and difficult to use for successful arteriovenous fistulae. Otherwise, patients with lupus make good candidates for dialysis, whether continuous ambulatory peritoneal dialysis or hemodialysis.

Transplantation

Transplantation in lupus can be performed with only a few extra precautions, compared with other recipients. First, cross-matching donors with lupus patients may be difficult because, as well as transfusion, pregnancy, or allograft-induced alloantibodies, the sera of many patients with lupus who have never been pregnant or had a transfusion or transplantation may contain antilymphocyte antibodies (432,433). The majority of these are of IgM isotype and low affinity and react with the common leukocyte CD45 antigen (432). These are little problems, since pretreatment of the serum with dithiothreitol removes them by dissociating the disulfide bonds of the IgM. However, some similar antibodies are cytotoxic, may be of IgG isotype as well, and will thus register in conventional cross-matches. Their target antigens, though, even if they include MHC antigens, are not allospecific.

Second, as in dialysis, thrombosis may be a problem after transplantation, especially in patients with antiphospholipid antibodies. Radha Krishnan and colleagues (433) noted that four patients of eight with lupus who had antiphospholipid antibodies had thrombotic episodes following transplantation, versus none in five who did not. Both renal arterial and venous thromboses have been noted as well as thromboses in more conventional sites. Thus, it is worth considering anticoagulation in patients with circulating antiphospholipid antibodies of IgG isotype in high titers. Activity of lupus, not surprisingly, falls from levels found on dialysis to very low levels (434), presumably because of the immunosuppressive drugs used to avert rejection.

An obvious worry is the possibility of recurrent lupus nephritis in the allograft, especially in the presence of active disease, but the striking feature of transplantation in lupus remains the very low rate of recurrence in lupus nephritis (422–432), even in some patients with active disease at the time of transplantation. The incidence seems to be about 1:100 cases or less, and even in those in whom recurrence has been clearly identified, usually it has been of little clinical significance and almost never a cause of graft loss (435,436). This could be telling us that the kidney itself must have some determinant that allows the appearance of nephritis, and that is missing from the allografted kidney. It is not clear why the incidence of recurrence should be relatively higher in some series (437,438), and it is notable in the report by Nyberg et al. (437) that, although electron-dense immune aggregates were present in glomeruli of allografts, in no case was IgG—the hallmark of lupus nephritis—detected, the predominant immunoglobulin in all cases being IgM.

Immunosuppression usually does not need to be modified in patients with lupus, although cyclosporine monotherapy is best avoided because this drug is not a powerful suppressant of lupus and relapse has been described using this drug (408). There is no difference in the number and severity of rejections in recipients with lupus and, with current immunosuppressive regimens, there seems to be no higher incidence of infections.

REFERENCES

1. Virchow R. Historical note on lupus [in German). *Arch Pathol Anat* 1865;32:139–43.
2. Talbott JH. Historical background of discoid and systemic lupus erythematosus. In: Wallace DJ, Hahn BH, eds. *Dubois' lupus erythematosus Philadelphia: Lea and Febiger, 1993:3–10.*
3. Kaposi M. New reports on knowledge of lupus erythematosus [in German). *Arch Dermatol Syph* 1872;4:36–8. See also Hebra F, Kaposi M. *On diseases of the skin, including the exanthemata.* Tay W, trans; Hilton Fagge C, ed. London: New Sydenham Society, 1886–1890 and 1874.
4. Brooke HG. Lupus erythematosus and tuberculosis. *Br J Dermatol* 1895;7:73–7.
5. Osler W. On the visceral manifestations of the erythema group of skin diseases. *Am J Med Sci* 1904;127:1–23.
6. Keith NM, Rowntree LG. Study of renal complications of disseminated lupus erythematosus: report of four cases. *Trans Assoc Am Physicians* 1922;37:487–502.
7. Baehr G, Klemperer P, Schifrin A. Diffuse disease of the peripheral circulation usually associated with lupus erythematosus. *Trans Assoc Am Physicians* 1935;50:139–55.
8. Klemperer P, Pollack AD, Baehr G. Pathology and disseminated lupus erythematosus. *Arch Pathol* 1941;32:569–631.
9. Muehrcke RC, Kark RM, Pirani CL, Pollak VE. Lupus nephritis: a clinical and pathological study based on renal biopsies. *Medicine (Baltimore)* 1957;36:1–146.
10. Gennerich W. The present state of the lupus erythematosus question [in German). *Arch Dermatol Syph* 1922;138:403–10.
11. Hargraves MM, Richmond H, Morton R. Presentation of 2 bone marrow elements: "tart" cell and "LE" cell. *Proc Staff Meet Mayo Clin* 1948;23:25–8.
12. Friou GJ. The significance of the lupus globulin–nucleoprotein reaction. *Ann Intern Med* 1958;49:866–74.
13. Seligmann M. Demonstration in the blood of patients with disseminated lupus erythematosus: a substance determining a precipitation reaction with desoxyribonucleic acid. *C R Acad Sci (Paris)* 1957; 244:243–5.
14. Bielschowsky M, Helyer BJ, Howie JB. Spontaneous haemolytic anaemia in mice of the NZB/B1 strain. *Proc Univ Otago Med School (NZ)* 1959;37:9–11.
15. Tan EM, Cohen AS, Fries JF, et al. The 1982 revised criteria for the classification of systemic lupus erythematosus. *Arthritis Rheum* 1982;25:1271–77.
16. Cairns SA, Acheson EJ, Corbett CL, et al. The delayed appearance of an antinuclear factor and the diagnosis of systemic lupus erythematosus in glomerulonephritis. *Postgrad Med J* 1979;55:723–7.
17. Adu D, Williams DG, Taube D, et al. Late onset systemic lupus erythematosus and lupus-like disease in patients with apparent idiopathic glomerulonephritis. *Q J Med* 1983;52:471–87.
18. Wallace DJ, Hahn BH, eds. Section 4: Autoantibodies. In: *Dubois' lupus erythematosus.* Philadelphia: Lea and Febiger, 1993:181–276.

19. Worrall J, Snaith ML, Batchelor R, Isenberg DA. SLE: a rheumatological view. *Q J Med* 1990;275:319–30.
20. Fessel WJ. ANF negative lupus systemic lupus erythematosus. *Am J Med* 1978;64:80–6.
21. Scolari F, Savoldi S, Costantino E. Antiphospholipid syndrome and glomerular thrombosis in the absence of overt lupus nephritis. *Nephrol Dialysis Transplant* 1993;8:1274–6.
22. Agnello V. Complement deficiency states. *Medicine (Baltimore)* 1978;57:1–23.
23. Roberts JL, Schwartz MM, Lewis EJ. Hereditary C2 deficiency and systemic lupus erythematosus associated with severe glomerulonephritis. *Clin Exp Immunol* 1978;31:328–38.
24. Schonfeld Y, Isenberg DA. *The mosaic of autoimmunity.* Amsterdam: Elsevier, 1989.
25. Walport MJ. The pathogenesis of systemic lupus. In: Cameron JS, Davison AM, Grünfked J-P, Kerr DNS, Ritz E, eds. *Oxford textbook of clinical nephrology.* 2nd ed. New York: Oxford University Press, 1996 (in press).
26. Jones DEJ, Bassendine MF. Infection, evolution and autoimmunity: a hypothesis. *Q J Med* 1995;88:919–25.
27. Lewkonia RM. The clinical genetics of lupus. *Lupus* 1992;1:55–62.
28. Arnett FC. The genetic basis of lupus erythematosus. In: Wallace DJ, Hahn BH, eds. *Dubois' lupus erythematosus.* Philadelphia: Lea and Febiger, 1993:13–36.
29. Arnett FC, Schulman LE. Studies in familial systemic lupus erythematosus. *Medicine (Baltimore)* 1976;55:313–22.
30. Miles S, Isenberg D. A review of serological abnormalities in relatives of SLE patients. *Lupus* 1993;2:145–50.
31. Fielder AHL, Walport MJ, Batchelor JR, et al. Family studies of the major histocompatibility complex in patients with systemic lupus erythematosus: importance of null alleles of C4A and C4B in determining disease susceptibility. *BMJ* 1983;286:425–8.
32. Deapen D, Escalante A, Wienreb L, et al. A revised estimate of twin concordance in systemic lupus erythematosus. *Arthritis Rheum* 1992; 35:311–8.
33. Fronek Z, Timmerman LA, Alper CA, et al. Major histocompatibility complex associations with systemic lupus erythematosus. *Am J Med* 1988;85(Suppl 6A):42–4.
34. Reveille JD, Schrohenloher RE, Acton RT, Barger BO. DNA analysis of HLA-DR and DQ genes in American blacks with systemic lupus erythematosus. *Arthritis Rheum* 1989;32:1243–51.
35. Jacob CO. Tumor necrosis factor α in autoimmunity: pretty girl or old witch? *Immunol Today* 1992;13:122–5.
36. Clemenceau S, Castellano F, de Oca MM, Kaplan C, Danon F, Levy M. C4 null alleles in childhood onset systemic lupus erythematosus: is there any relationship with renal disease? *Pediatr Nephrol* 1990; 4:207–12.
37. Wilson JG, Fearon DT. Altered expression of complement receptors as a pathogenetic factor in systemic lupus erythematosus. *Arthritis Rheum* 1984;27:1321–8.
38. Walport M, Ng YC, Lachmann PJ. Erythrocytes transfused into patients with SLE and haemolytic anaemia lose complement receptor type 1 from their cell surface. *Clin Exp Immunol* 1987;69:501–7.
39. Yewdall V, Cameron JS, Nathan AW, et al. Systemic lupus erythematosus and IgA deficiency. *J Clin Lab Immunol* 1983;10:13–8.
40. Lawley TJ, Hall RP, Fauci AS, et al. Defective Fc receptor functions associated with the haplotype HLA-A1-B8-DRw3 haplotype. *N Engl J Med* 1981;304:185–92.
41. Mongey A-B, Hess EV. The potential role of environmental agents in systemic lupus erythematosus and associated disorders. In: Wallace DJ, Hahn BH, eds. *Dubois' lupus erythematosus.* Philadelphia: Lea and Febiger, 1993:37–48.
42. Lowenstein MB, et al. *Family study of systemic lupus erythematosus.* Arthritis Rheum 1977;20:1293–303.
43. de Horatius RJ, et al. Lymphocytotoxic antibodies in laboratory personnel exposed to SLE sera [Letter]. *Lancet* 1979;2:1141.
44. Batchelor JR, Welsh KI, Mansilla R, et al. Hydralazine-induced systemic lupus erythematosus: influence of HLA-DR and sex on susceptibility. *Lancet* 1983;1:1107–9.
45. Steinberg AD, Krieg AM, Gourley MF, Klinman DM. Theoretical and experimental approaches to generalized autoimmunity. *Immunol Rev* 1990;118:129–63.
46. Diamond B, Katz JB, Paul E, Aranow C, Lustgarten D, Scharff MD. The role of somatic mutation in the pathogenic anti-DNA response. *Annu Rev Immunol* 1992;10:731–57.
47. Talal N, Garry RF, Schur PH, et al. A conserved idiotype and antibodies to retroviral protein. *J Clin Invest* 1990;85:1866–71.
48. Zack DJ, Yamamoto K, Wong AL, Stempiak M, French C, Weisbart RH. DNA mimics a self-protein that may be a target for some anti-DNA antibodies in systemic lupus erythematosus. *J Immunol* 1995; 54:1987–94.
49. Drake CG, Kotzin BL. Superantigens: biology, immunology and potential role in disease. *J Clin Immunol* 1992;12:149–62.
50. Cohen PL, Eisenberg RA. The *lpr* and *gld* genes in systemic lupus erythematosus: life and death in the *fas* lane. *Immunol Today* 1992; 13:427–8.
51. Rose LM, Latchman DS, Eisenberg DA. Bcl-2 and Fas: molecules which influence apoptosis—a possible role in SLE? *Autoimmunity* 1994;17:271–8.
52. Elkon KB. Apoptosis and SLE. *Lupus* 1994;3:1–2.
53. Elkon KB. Apoptosis in SLE: too little or too much? *Clin Exp Rheumatol* 1994;12:1553–9.
54. Mysler E, Bini P, Ramos P, Friedman SM, Krammer PH, Elkon KB. The apoptosis 1/Fas protein in human systemic lupus erythematosus. *J Clin Invest* 1994;93:1029–34.
55. Hochberg MC. The epidemiology of systemic lupus erythematosus. In: Wallace DJ, Hahn BH, eds. *Dubois' lupus erythematosus.* Philadelphia: Lea and Febiger, 1993:49–57.
56. Citera G, Wilson WA. Ethnic and geographic perspectives in SLE. *Lupus* 1993;2:351–3.
57. Siegel M, Lee SL. The epidemiology of systemic lupus erythematosus. *Semin Arthritis Rheum* 1973;3:1–54.
58. Fessel WJ. Systemic lupus erythematosus in the community: incidence, prevalence, outcome, and first symptoms—the high prevalence in black women. *Arch Intern Med* 1974;134:1027–35.
59. Johnson AE, Gordon C, Palmer RG, Bacon PA. The prevalence and incidence of systemic lupus erythematosus in Birmingham, England: relationship to ethnicity and country of birth. *Arthritis Rheum* 1995; 38:551–8.
60. Nived O, Sturfelt G, Wollheim F. Systemic lupus erythematosus in an adult population in Southern Sweden: incidence, prevalence, and validity of the ARA revised classification criteria. *Br J Rheumatol* 1985;24:147–54.
61. Symmons DPM. Lupus around the world: frequency of lupus in people of African origin. *Lupus* 1995;4:176–8.
62. Serdula MK, Rhoads GG. Frequency of systemic lupus erythematosus in different ethnic groups in Hawaii. *Arthritis Rheum* 1979;22: 328–33.
63. Maskarinec G, Katz AR. Prevalence of systemic lupus erythematosus in Hawaii: is there a difference between ethnic groups? *Hawaii Med J* 1995;54:406–9.
64. Lopez-Acuna D, Hochberg MC, Gittelsohn AM. Mortality from discoid and systemic lupus erythematosus in the United States 1968–78. *Arthritis Rheum* 1982;25(Suppl):S80.
65. Kaslow RA. High rate of death caused by systemic lupus erythematosus among US residents of Asian descent. *Arthritis Rheum* 1982;25: 414–6.
66. Lévy M, Montes de Oca M, Babron MC. Lupus érythemateux disséminé chez l'enfant: Étude collaborative en région parisienne. In: *Journées Parisiennes Pédiatrie Paris: Flammarion, 1989:52–8.*
67. Grossman J, Schwartz RH, Callerame ML, Condemi JI. Systemic lupus erythematosus in a one year old child. *Am J Dis Child* 1975; 129:123–5.
68. Lehman TJA, McCurdy DK, Bernstein BH, King KK, Hanson V. Systemic lupus erythematosus in the first decade of life. *Pediatrics* 1989;83:235–9.
69. Hahn BH. Animal models of systemic lupus erythematosus. In: Wallace DJ, Hahn BH, eds. *Dubois' lupus erythematosus.* Philadelphia: Lea and Febiger, 1993:157–77.
70. Koffler D, Agnello V, Thoburn R, Kunkel MG. SLE, the prototype of immune complex nephritis in man. *J Exp Med* 1971;134:169S–79S.
71. Davies KA, Peters AM, Beynon HLC, Walport MJ. Immune complex processing in patients with systemic lupus erythematosus: in vivo imaging and clearance studies. *J Clin Invest* 1992;90:2075–83.
72. Alexopoulos E, Cameron JS, Hartley BH. Lupus nephritis: correlation of interstitial cells with glomerular function. *Kidney Int* 1990; 37:100–9.
73. Brentjens JR, Sepulveda M, Baliah T, et al. Interstitial immune complex nephritis in patients with systemic lupus erythematosus. *Kidney Int* 1975;7:342–50.

74. Rumore PM, Steinman CR. Endogenous circulating DNA in systemic lupus erythematosus: occurrence as multimeric complexes bound to histone. *J Clin Invest* 1990;86:69–74.
75. Mohan C, Adams S, Stanik V, Datta SK. Nucleosome: a major immunogen for pathogenic autoantibody-inducing T cells of lupus. *J Exp Med* 1993;177:1367–81.
76. Burlingame RW, Boey ML, Starkebaum G, Rubin RL. The central role of chromatin in autoimmune responses to histones and DNA in systemic lupus erythematosus. *J Clin Invest* 1994;94:184–92.
77. Adu D, Dobson J, Williams DG. DNA–anti-DNA circulating complexes in the nephritis of systemic lupus erythematosus. *Clin Exp Immunol* 1981;43:605–14.
78. Koffler D, Agnello V, Kunkel HG. Polynucleotide immune complexes in the serum and glomeruli of patients with systemic lupus erythematosus. *Am J Pathol* 1974;74:109–22.
79. Winfield JB, Faiferman I, Koffler D. Avidity of anti-DNA antibodies in serum and IgG glomerular eluates from patients with systemic lupus erythematosus. *J Clin Invest* 1977;59:90–6.
80. Sasaki T, Hatekayama A, Shibata S, et al. Heterogeneity of immune complex derived anti-DNA antibodies associated with lupus nephritis. *Kidney Int* 1991;39:746–53.
81. Mailinde D, Londoño I, Russo P, Bendayan M. Ultrastructural localization of DNA in immune deposits of human lupus nephritis. *Am J Pathol* 1993;143:304–11.
82. Marmont AM. The transfusion of active LE plasma into nonlupus recipients, with a note on the LE cell. *Proc Natl Acad Sci USA* 1965;124:838–51.
83. Foster MH, Cixman B, Madaio MP. Biology of disease: nephritogenic autoantibodies in systemic lupus erythematosus—immunochemical properties, mechanisms of immune deposition, and genetic origins. *Lab Invest* 1993;69:494–507.
84. Raz E, Brezis M, Rosenmann E, Eilat D. Anti-DNA antibodies bind directly to renal antigens and induce kidney dysfunction in the isolated perfused rat kidney. *J Immunol* 1989;142:3076–82.
85. Vlahakos D, Foster MH, Ucci AA, et al. Murine monoclonal anti-DNA antibodies penetrate cells, bind to nuclei, and induce glomerular proliferation and proteinuria in vivo. *J Am Soc Nephrol* 1992;2:1345–54.
86. Ehrenstein MR, Katz DR, Griffiths MH, et al. Human IgG anti-DNA antibodies deposit in kidneys and induce proteinuria in SCID mice. *Kidney Int* 1995;48:705–11.
87. Termaat R-M, Assmann KJM, Dijkman H, et al. Anti-DNA antibodies can bind to the glomerulus via two distinct mechanisms. *Kidney Int* 1992;42:1363–71.
88. Chan TM, Frampton G, Staines N, Hobby P, Perry GJ, Cameron JS. Different mechanisms by which monoclonal anti-DNA antibodies bind to human endothelial cells and glomerular mesangial cells. *Clin Exp Immunol* 1992;88:68–74.
89. Kramers C, Hyikema MN, van Bruggen MCJ, et al. Anti-nucleosome antibodies complexed to nucleosomal antigens show anti-DNA reactivity and bind to rat glomerular basement membrane in vivo. *J Clin Invest* 1994;94:568–77.
90. Tax WJM, Kramers C, van Bruggen MCJ, Berden JMH. Apoptosis, nucleosomes, and nephritis in systemic lupus erythematosus. *Kidney Int* 1995;48:666–73.
91. Frampton G, Hobby P, Morgan A, Staines NA, Cameron JS. A role for DNA in anti-DNA antibodies binding to endothelial cells. *J Autoimmun* 1991;4:463–78.
92. Lake HA, Morgan A, Henderson B, Staines NA. A key role for fibronectin in the sequential binding of native dsDNA and monoclonal anti-DNA antibodies to components of the extracellular matrix: its possible significance in glomerulonephritis. *Immunology* 1985;54:389–95.
93. Chan TM, Frampton G, Cameron JS. Identification of DNA-binding proteins on the endothelial cell plasma membrane. *Clin Exp Immunol* 1993;91:110–4.
94. Schmiedeke T, Stoeckl F, Weber R, Sugisaki Y, Batsford S, Vogt A. Histones have high affinity for the glomerular basement membrane: relevance for immune complex formation in lupus nephritis. *J Exp Med* 1989;169:1879–94.
95. Schmiedke T, Stoeckl F, Muller S, et al. Glomerular immune deposits in murine models may contain histones. *Clin Exp Immunol* 1992;90:453–8.
96. Stockl F, Muller S, Batsford S, et al. A role for histones and ubiquitin in lupus nephritis? *Clin Nephrol* 1994;41:10–7.
97. Kramers K, Hylkema M, Termaat R-M, Brinkman K, Smeenk R, Berden J. Histones in lupus nephritis. *Exp Nephrol* 1993;1:224–8.
98. Coritsidis GN, Beers PC, Rumore PM. Glomerular uptake of nucleosomes: evidence for receptor-mediated mesangial binding. *Kidney Int* 1995;47:1258–65.
99. Lafer EM, Rauch H, Andrezejewski C, et al. Polyspecific monoclonal lupus autoantibodies reactive with both polynucleotides and phospholipids. *J Exp Med* 1981;153:897–909.
100. Faaber P, Truus TPM, Van de Putte LBA, Capel PJA, Berden JHN. Cross-reactivity of human and murine anti-DNA antibodies with heparan sulfate. *J Clin Invest* 1986;77:1824–30.
101. Brinkman K, Termaat RM, de Jong J, van den Brink HG, Berden JHM, Smeenk RJT. Cross-reactive binding patterns of monoclonal antibodies to DNA are often caused by DNA/anti-DNA immune complexes. *Res Immunol* 1989;140:595–612.
102. Rubin RL, Theofilopoulos AN. Monoclonal autoantibodies reacting with multiple structurally related and unrelated macromolecules. *Int Rev Immunol* 1988;3:71–8.
103. Jacob L, Tron F, Bach JF, Louvard D. A monoclonal anti-DNA antibody also binds to cell surface protein(s). *Proc Natl Acad Sci USA* 1984;81:3842–5.
104. Couser WG, Salant DJ, Madaio MP, Adler S, Groggel GC. Factors influencing glomerular and tubulointerstitial patterns of injury in SLE. *Am J Kidney Dis* 1982;2(Suppl 1):126–34.
105. Cameron JS. Tubular and interstitial factors in the progression of glomerulonephritis. *Pediatr Nephrol* 1992;6:292–303.
106. D'Agati VD, Appel GB, Estes D, Knowles DM II, Pirani CL. Monoclonal antibody identification of infiltrating mononuclear leukocytes in lupus nephritis. *Kidney Int* 1986;30:573–81.
107. Sontheimer RD, Gilliam JN. DNA antibody class, subclass, and complement fixation in systemic lupus erythematosus with and without nephritis. *Clin Immunol Immunopathol* 1978;10:459–67.
108. Roberts JL, Wyatt RJ, Schwartz MM, et al. Differential characteristics of immune bound antibodies in diffuse proliferative and membranous forms of lupus glomerulonephritis. *Clin Immunol Immunopathol* 1983;29:223–31.
109. Friend PS, Kim Y, Michael AF, Donadio JV. Pathogenesis of membranous nephropathy in systemic lupus erythematosus: possible role of non-precipitating DNA antibody. *BMJ* 1977;1:25.
110. Suzuki N, Harada T, Mizushima Y, Sakane T. Possible pathogenic role of cationic anti-DNA antibodies in the development of nephritis in patients with systemic lupus erythematosus. *J Immunol* 1993;151:1128–36.
111. Malleson PN. The role of the renal biopsy in childhood onset systemic lupus erythematosus: a viewpoint. *Clin Exp Rheumatol* 1989;7:563–6.
112. Nossent HC, Henzen-Logmans SC, Vroom TM, Berden JHM, Swaak TJG. Contribution of renal biopsy data in predicting outcome in lupus nephritis. *Arthritis Rheum* 1990;33:970–6.
113. Whiting-O'Keefe Q, Henke JE, Shearn MA, Hopper J Jr, Biava CG, Epstein WV. The information content from renal biopsy in systemic lupus erythematosus. *Ann Intern Med* 1982;96:718–23.
114. Whiting-O'Keefe Q, Riccardi PJ, Henke JE, Shearn MA, Hopper J Jr, Epstein WV. Recognition of information in renal biopsies of patients with lupus nephritis. *Ann Intern Med* 1982;96:723–7.
115. Baldwin DS. Clinical usefulness of the morphological classification of lupus nephritis. *Am J Kidney Dis* 1982;2:142–9.
116. Schwartz MM. The role of renal biopsy in the management of lupus nephritis. *Semin Nephrol* 1985;5:255–63.
117. Churg J, Bernstein J, Glassock RJ. *Renal disease:* classification and atlas of glomerular diseases 2nd ed. New York: Igaku Shoin, 1995.
118. Lewis EJ, Kawala K, Schwartz MM. Histologic features that correlate with the prognosis of patients with lupus nephritis. *Am J Kidney Dis* 1987;10:192–7.
119. Kashgarian M. Lupus nephritis: lessons from the path lab. *Kidney Int* 1994;45:928–38.
120. Morel-Maroger L, Mery JPh, Droz D, et al. The course of lupus nephritis: contribution of serial renal biopsies. *Adv Nephrol* 1976;6:79–86.
121. Pirani CL, Salinas-Madrigal L. Evaluation of percutaneous renal biopsy. In: Sommers SC, ed. *Pathology annual*; vol 3. New York: Appleton Century Crofts, 1968;249–54.
122. Austin HA III, Muenz LR, Joyce KM, et al. Prognostic factors in lupus nephritis: contribution of renal histologic data. *Am J Med* 1983;75:382–91.
123. Schwartz MM, Bernstein J, Hill GS, Holley K, Phillips EA, and the Lupus Nephritis Study Group. Predictive value of renal pathology

in diffuse proliferative glomerulonephritis. *Kidney Int* 1989;36: 891–6.
124. Kant KS, Pollak VE, Weiss MA, Glueck HI, Miller MA, Hess EV. Glomerular thrombosis in systemic lupus erythematosus: prevalence and significance. *Medicine (Baltimore)* 1981;60:71–86.
125. McCutcheon J, Evans B, D'Cruz DP, Hughes GRV, Davies DR. Fibrin deposition in SLE glomerulonephritis. *Lupus* 1993;2:99–103.
126. Makker SP. Tubular basement membrane antibody-induced interstitial nephritis in systemic lupus erythematosus. *Am J Med* 1980;69: 949–52.
127. Gur H, Koplovic Y, Gross DJ. Chronic predominant interstitial nephritis in a patients with systemic lupus erythematosus: a follow-up of three years and review of the literature. *Ann Rheum Dis* 1987;46: 617–23.
128. Tsumagari T, Fukumoto S, Kinjo M, Tanaka K. Incidence and significance of intrarenal vasculopathies in patients with systemic lupus erythematosus. *Hum Pathol* 1984;16:43–9.
129. Banfi G, Bertani T, Boeri V, et al. Renal vascular lesions as a marker of poor prognosis in patients with lupus nephritis. *Am J Kidney Dis* 1991;18:240–8.
130. Appel GB, Pirani CL, D'Agati V. Renal vascular complications of systemic lupus erythematosus. *J Am Soc Nephrol* 1994;4:1499–515.
131. Fox DA, Faix JD, Coblyn J, Fraser J, Smith B, Weinblatt ME. Thrombotic thrombocytopenic purpura and systemic lupus erythematosus. *Ann Rheum Dis* 1986;45:319–22.
132. Frampton G, Hicks J, Cameron JS. Significance of anti-phospholipid antibodies in patients with lupus nephritis. *Kidney Int* 1991;39: 1225–331.
133. Miranda JM, Garcia-Torres R, Jara LJ, et al. Renal biopsy in systemic lupus erythematosus: significance of glomerular thrombosis—analysis of 108 cases. *Lupus* 1994;3:25–9.
134. Huston DP, McAdam KPWJ, Balow JE, et al. Amyloidosis in systemic lupus erythematosus. *Am J Med* 1981;70:320–3.
135. Orellana C, Collado A, Hernandez MV, Font J, Del Olmo JA, Muñoz-Gomez J. When does amyloidosis complicate systemic lupus erythematosus? *Lupus* 1995;4:415–7.
136. Friedman AC, Chesney RW, Oberley TU, et al. Clinical systemic lupus erythematosus with dense deposit disease. *Int J Pediatr Nephrol* 1983;4:171–5.
137. Akhtar M, Al-Dalaan A, El-Ramahi KM. Pauci-immune necrotizing lupus nephritis: report of two cases. *Am J Kidney Dis* 1994;23:320–5.
138. Sinniah R, Feng PH. Lupus nephritis: correlation between light, electron microscopic and immunofluorescent findings and renal function. *Clin Nephrol* 1987;16:3340–51.
139. Cameron JS. Lupus nephritis in childhood and adolescence. *Pediatr Nephrol* 1994;8:230–49.
140. Hill GS, Hinglais N, Torn F, Bach J-F. Systemic lupus erythematosus: morphologic correlations with immunologic and clinical data at the time of biopsy. *Am J Med* 1978;64:61–79.
141. Klein MH, Thorner PS, Yoon S-J, Poucell S, Baumal R. Determination of circulating immune complexes, C3 and C4 complement components and anti-DNA antibody in different classes of lupus nephritis. *Int J Pediatr Nephrol* 1984;5:75–82.
142. Cervera R, Khamashta M, Font J, et al. Systemic lupus erythematosus: clinical and immunologic patterns of disease expression in a cohort of 1000 patients. *Medicine (Baltimore)* 1993;72:113–24.
143. Wallace DJ. The clinical presentation of SLE. In: Wallace DJ, Hahn BH, eds. *Dubois' lupus erythematosus Philadelphia: Lea and Febiger, 1993:317–21.*
144. Fries JF, Holman HR. Systemic lupus erythematosus: *a clinical analysis.* Philadelphia: WB Saunders, 1975.
145. Schaller J. Lupus in childhood. *Clin Rheum Dis* 1982;8:219–28.
146. Wallace DJ. Cutaneous manifestations of SLE. In: Wallace DJ, Hahn BH, eds. *Dubois' lupus erythematosus.* Philadelphia: Lea and Febiger, 1993:356–69.
147. Desser KB, Sartiano GP, Cooper JL. *Lupus livedo and cutaneous infarction.* Angiology 1969;20:261.
148. Wallace DJ. The musculoskeletal system. In: Wallace DJ, Hahn BH, eds. *Dubois' lupus erythematosus Philadelphia: Lea and Febiger, 1993:322–31.*
149. Bywaters EGL. Jaccoud's syndrome: a sequel to the joint involvement of systemic lupus erythematosus. *Clin Rheum Dis* 1975;1: 125–48.
150. Quismorio FP. Cardiac abnormalities in systemic lupus erythematosus. In: Wallace DJ, Hahn BH, eds. *Dubois' lupus erythematosus.* Philadelphia: Lea and Febiger, 1993:332–42.
151. Quismorio FP. Pulmonary manifestations. In: Wallace DJ, Hahn BH, eds. *Dubois' lupus erythematosus Philadelphia: Lea and Febiger,* 1993:343–55.
152. Nihoyannopoulos P, Gomez PM, Joshi J, Loizou S, Walport MJ, Oakley C. Cardiac abnormalities in systemic lupus erythematosus. *Circulation* 1990;82:369–75.
153. Galve E, Candell-Riera J, Pigrau C, Permaeyer-Miralda G, Garcia-del Castillo H, Soler-Soler J. Prevalence, morphologic types and evolution of cardiac valvular disease in systemic lupus erythematosus. *N Engl J Med* 1988;319:817–23.
154. Leung W-H, Wing K-L, Lau C-P, Wong C-K, Liu H-W. Association between antiphospholipid antibodies and cardiac abnormalities in patients with systemic lupus erythematosus. *Am J Med* 1990;89:411–9.
155. Horn CA. Pulmonary hypertension and auto-immune disease. *Chest* 1993;104:279–80.
156. Asherson RA, Oakley C. Pulmonary hypertension and systemic lupus erythematosus. *J Rheumatol* 1986;13:1–5.
157. Schwab EP, Schumacher HR Jr, Freundlich B, Callegari PE. Pulmonary hemorrhage in systemic lupus erythematosus. *Semin Arthritis Rheum* 1993;23:8–15.
158. Abramson SB, Dobro J, Eberle M, et al. Acute reversible hypoxemia in systemic lupus erythematosus. *Ann Intern Med* 1991;114:941–7.
159. Weinrib L, Sharma OP, Quismorio FP Jr. A long-term study of interstitial lung disease in systemic lupus erythematosus. *Semin Arthritis Rheum* 1990;20:48–56.
160. Qismorio FP. Hemic and lymphatic abnormalities in SLE. In: Wallace DJ, Hahn BH, eds. *Dubois' lupus erythematosus.* Philadelphia: Lea and Febiger, 1993:418–30.
161. Van Dam AP. Diagnosis and pathogenesis of CNS lupus. *Rheumatol Int* 1991;11:1–11.
162. Wallace DJ, Metzger AL. Systemic lupus erythematosus and the nervous system. In: Wallace DJ, Hahn BH, eds. *Dubois' lupus erythematosus Philadelphia: Lea and Febiger, 1993:370–85.*
163. West SG. Neuropsychiatric lupus. *Rheum Dis Clin North Am* 1994; 20:129–58.
164. Rubbert A, Miarienhagen J, Pirner K, et al. Single-photon emission computed tomography analysis of cerebral blood flow in the evaluation of central nervous system involvement in systemic lupus erythematosus. *Arthritis Rheum* 1993;36:1253–62.
164a. Ginsburg KS, Wright EA, Larson MG, et al. A controlled study of the prevalence of cognitive dysfunction in randomly selected patients with systemic lupus erythematosus. *Arthritis Rheum* 1992;35:776–82.
165. Lim L, Ron MA, Ormerod IEC, et al. Psychiatric and neurological manifestations in systemic lupus erythematosus. *Q J Med* 1988;66: 27–38.
166. Kent DL, Haynor DR, Longstreth WT Jr, Larson EB. The clinical efficacy of magnetic resonance imaging in neuroimaging. *Ann Intern Med* 1994;120:856–71.
167. Holman BL. Functional imaging in systemic lupus erythematosus: an accurate indicator of central nervous system involvement? *Arthritis Rheum* 1993;36:1193–5.
168. Herd JK, Mehdi M, Uzendoski DM, Saldivar VA. Chorea associated with systemic lupus erythematosus: report of 2 cases and review of the literature. *Pediatrics* 1978;61:308–13.
169. Khamashta MA, Gil A, Anciones B, et al. Chorea in systemic lupus erythematosus: association with antiphospholipid antibodies. *Ann Rheum Dis* 1988;47:681–3.
170. McAbee GN, Barasch ES. Resolving MRI lesions in lupus erythematosus selectively involving the brainstem. *Pediatr Neurol* 1990;61: 186–9.
171. Becker GJ, Waldburger M, Hughes GRV, Pepys M. Value of serum C-reactive protein measurement in the investigation of fever in systemic lupus erythematosus. *Ann Rheum Dis* 1980;39:50–2.
172. Honig S, Gorevic, Weissmann G. C-reactive protein in systemic lupus erythematosus. *Arthritis Rheum* 1977;20:1065–70.
173. Mintz G, Acevedo-Vasquez E, Guterriez-Espinosa G, Avelar-Garnica F. Renal vein thrombosis and inferior vena cava thrombosis in systemic lupus erythematosus. *Arthritis Rheum* 1984;27:539–44.
174. Nadorra RL, Nakazato Y, Landing BH. Pathologic features of gastrointestinal tract lesions in childhood onset systemic lupus erythematosus: study of 26 patients with review of the literature. *Pediatr Pathol* 1987;7:245–59.

175. Runyon BA, La Breque DR, Anuras S. The spectrum of liver disease in systemic lupus erythematosus: report of 33 histologically-proved cases and review of the literature. *Am J Med* 1980;60:187–94.
176. Miller MH, Urowitz MB, Gladman DD, Blendis LM. The liver in systemic lupus erythematosus. *Q J Med* 1984;53:401–9.
177. Laing TJ. Gastrointestinal vasculitis and pneumatosis intestinalis due to systemic lupus erythematosus: successful treatment with pulse intravenous cyclophosphamide. *Am J Med* 1988;85:555–8.
178. Dimant J, Ginzler E, Schlesinger M, et al. The clinical significance of Raynaud's phenomenon in systemic lupus erythematosus. *Arthritis Rheum* 1979;22:815–9.
179. Kellum RE, Haserick JR. Systemic lupus erythematosus: a statistical evaluation of mortality based upon a consecutive series of 299 patients. *Arch Intern Med* 1964;113:200–7.
180. Estes D, Christian CL. The natural history of systemic lupus erythematosus by prospective analysis. *Medicine (Baltimore)* 1971;50:85–95.
181. Harvey AM, Schulman LE, Tumulty A, Conley, Schonrich EH. Systemic lupus erythematosus: review of the literature and clinical analysis of 138 cases. *Medicine (Baltimore)* 1954;33:291–437.
182. Adu D, Cameron JS. Lupus nephritis. *Clin Rheum Dis* 1982;8: 153–83.
183. Baldwin DS, Gluck MC, Lowenstein J, Gallo GR. Clinical course as related to the morphologic forms and their transitions. *Am J Med* 1977;62:12–30.
184. Shearn MA. Normocholesterolemic nephrotic syndrome of systemic lupus erythematosus. *Am J Med* 1965;36:250–61.
185. Groggel GC, Cheung AK, Ellis-Benigni K, Wilson DE. Treatment of nephrotic hyperlipoproteinemia with gemfibrozil. *Kidney Int* 1989; 36:266–71.
186. Phadke K, Trachtman H, Nicastri A, Chen CK, Tejani A. Acute renal failure as the initial manifestation of systemic lupus erythematosus in children. *J Pediatr* 1984;105:38–41.
187. Kozeny GA, Barr W, Bansal VK, et al. Occurrence of renal tubular dysfunction in lupus nephritis. *Arch Intern Med* 1987;147:891–5.
188. Yeung CK, Wong KL, Ng RP, Ng WL. Tubular dysfunction in systemic lupus erythematosus. *Nephron* 1984;36:84–8.
189. Dreyling KW, Wanner C, Schollmeyer P. Control of hyperkalemia with fluorocortisone in a patient with systemic lupus erythematosus. *Clin Nephrol* 1990;33:179–83.
190. Lee FO, Quismorio FP, Troum OM, Anderson PW, Do YS, Hsueh WA. Mechanisms of hyperkalemia in systemic lupus erythematosus. *Arch Intern Med* 1989;148:397–401.
191. Cameron JS. The platelet in renal disease. In: Page CF, ed. *Platelets in health and disease.* Oxford: Blackwell, 1991:228–60.
192. Cameron JS, Frampton G. The "antiphospholipid syndrome" and the "lupus anticoagulant." *Pediatr Nephrol* 1990;4:662–78.
193. Shergy WJ, Kredich DW, Pisetsky DS. The relationship of anticardiolipin antibody to disease manifestations in pediatric systemic lupus erythematosus. *J Rheumatol* 1988;15:1389–94.
194. Alarcon-Segovia D, Delezé M, Oria CV, et al. Antiphospholipid antibodies and the antiphospholipid syndrome in systemic lupus erythematosus: a prospective study of 500 consecutive patients. *Medicine (Baltimore)* 1990;68:353–65.
195. Asherson RA, Khamashta MA, Gil A, et al. Cerebrovascular disease and antiphospholipid antibodies in systemic lupus erythematosus, lupus-like disorders and the primary antiphospholipid syndrome. *Am J Med* 1991;86:391–9.
196. Ward MM, Pisetsky DS, Christensen VD. Anti–double stranded DNA antibody assays in SLE: correlation of longitudinal antibody measurements. *J Rheumatol* 1990;17:220–4.
197. Reeves WH, Satoh M, Wang J, Chou C-H, Ajmani AK. Antibodies to DNA, DNA-binding proteins, and histones. *Rheum Dis Clin North Am* 1994;20:1–28.
198. Hahn BH, Tsao BP. Antibodies to DNA. In: Wallace DJ, Hahn BH eds. *Dubois' lupus erythematosus.* Philadelphia: Lea and Febiger, 1993:195–201.
199. Swaak T, Smeenk R. Detection of anti-dsDNA as a diagnostic tool: a prospective study in 441 non-systemic lupus erythematosus patients with anti-dsDNA antibody (anti-dsDNA). *Ann Rheum Dis* 1985;44: 245–51.
200. Klein MH, Thorner PS, Yoon S-J, Poucell S, Baumal R. Determination of circulating immune complexes, C3 and C4 complement components and anti-DNA antibody in different classes of lupus nephritis. *Int J Pediatr Nephrol* 1984;5:75–82.
201. Porcel JM, Vergani D. Complement and lupus: old concepts and new directions. *Lupus* 1992;1:343–9.
202. Kerr LD, Adelberg BR, Schulman P, Spiera H. Factor B activation products in patients with systemic lupus erythematosus. *Arthritis Rheum* 1989;32:1406–13.
203. Falk RJ, Dalmasso AP, Kim Y, Lam S, Michael A. Radioimmunoassay of the attack complex of complement in serum from patients with systemic lupus erythematosus. *N Engl J Med* 1985;312:1594–9.
204. Wallace DJ. Differential diagnosis and disease associations. In: Wallace DJ, Hahn BH, eds. *Dubois' lupus erythematosus.* Philadelphia: Lea and Febiger, 1993:473–84.
205. Schnabel A, Csernok E, Isenberg DA, Mrowka C, Gross WL. Antineutrophil cytoplasmic antibodies in systemic lupus erythematosus. Prevalence, specificities and clinical significance. *Arthritis Rheum* 1995;38:633–7.
206. Cameron JS. The treatment of lupus nephritis. *Pediatr Nephrol* 1989; 3:350–62.
207. Albert DA, Hadler NM, Ropes MW. Does corticosteroid therapy affect the survival of patients with systemic lupus erythematosus? *Arthritis Rheum* 1979;22:945–53.
208. Cameron JS. The nephritis of systemic lupus erythematosus. In: Kincaid-Smith P, D'Apice AJP, Atkins RC, eds. *Progress in glomerulonephritis.* New York: John Wiley, 1979:387–423.
209. Cameron JS. The treatment of immunologically mediated renal disease. In: Zabriskie J, Fillit H, Villareal H, Becker EL, eds. Clinical immunology of the kidney. New York: John Wiley, 1983:407–40.
210. Ginzler EM, Schorn K. Outcome and prognosis in systemic lupus erythematosus. *Rheum Dis Clin North Am* 1988;14:67–78.
211. Pollak VE, Dosekun AK. Evaluation of treatment in lupus nephritis: effect of prednisone. *Am J Kidney Dis* 1982;2(Suppl 1):170–7.
212. Urman JD, Rothfield NF. Corticosteroid treatment in systemic lupus erythematosus: survival studies. *JAMA* 1977;238:2272–6.
213. Ropes MW. Observations on the natural history of disseminated lupus erythematosus. *Medicine (Baltimore)* 1964;43:387–91.
214. Austin HA III, Muenz LR, Joyce KM, Antonovych TT, Balow JE. Diffuse proliferative lupus nephritis: identification of specific pathologic features affecting outcome. *Kidney Int* 1984;25:689–95.
215. Fries JF, Porta J, Liang MH. Marginal benefit of renal biopsy in systemic lupus erythematosus. *Arch Intern Med* 1978;138:1386–9.
216. Hollcraft RM, Dubois EL, Lundberg GD, et al. Renal change in systemic lupus erythematosus with normal renal function. *J Rheumatol* 1976;3:251–61.
217. O'Dell JR, Hays RC, Guggenheim SJ, Steigerwald JC. Systemic lupus erythematosus without clinical renal abnormalities: renal biopsy findings and clinical course. *Ann Rheum Dis* 1985;44:415–9.
218. Leehey DJ, Katz AI, Azaran AH, Aronson AJ, Spargo BH. Silent diffuse lupus nephritis: long term follow-up. *Am J Kidney Dis* 1982; 2(Suppl 1):188–96.
219. Esdaile JM, Abrahamowicz M, Mackenzie T, Hayslett JP, Kashgarain M. Time-dependent long-term prediction in lupus nephritis. *Arthritis Rheum* 1994;37:359–68.
220. Donadio JV, Burgess JH, Holley KE. Membranous lupus nephropathy: a clinicopathologic study. *Medicine (Baltimore)* 1977;56:527–36.
221. Wang F, Looi LM. Systemic lupus erythematosus with membranous nephropathy in Malaysian patients. *Q J Med* 1984;53:209–26.
222. Pasquali S, Banfi G, Zucchelli A, Moroni G, Ponticelli C, Zucchelli P. Lupus membranous nephropathy: long-term outcome. *Clin Nephrol* 1993;39:175–82.
223. Pollak VE, Pirani CL, Schwartz FD. The natural history of the renal manifestations of systemic lupus erythematosus. *J Lab Clin Med* 1964; 64:537–50.
224. Harvey A McG, Shulman E, Tumulty AP, Lockard Conley C, Schoenreich EH. Systemic lupus erythematosus: review of the literature and clinical analysis of 138 cases. *Medicine (Baltimore)* 1954;33:291–437.
225. Smith FG, Witman N, Latta H. Lupus glomerulonephritis: the effect of large doses of corticosteroids on renal function and renal lesions in children. *Am J Dis Child* 1965;110:302–8.
226. Cathcart ES, Idelson BA, Scheinberg MA, Couser WG. Beneficial effects of methylprednisolone "pulse" therapy in diffuse proliferative nephritis. *Lancet* 1974;1:163–66.
227. Kimberly RP, Lockshin MD, Sherman RL, McDougal JS, Inman RD, Christian CL. High-dose intravenous methylprednisolone pulse therapy in systemic lupus erythematosus. *Am J Med* 1981;70:817–22.
228. Ponticelli C, Zucchelli P, Banfi G, et al. Treatment of proliferative

lupus nephritis by intravenous high-dose methylprednislone. *Q J Med* 1982;51:16–24.
229. Isenberg DA, Morrow WJW, Snaith MC. Methylprednisolone pulse therapy in the treatment of systemic lupus erythematosus. *Ann Rheum Dis* 1982;41:347–51.
230. Mackworth Young CG, David J, Morgan SH, Hughes GRV. A double blind, placebo controlled trial of intravenous methylprednisolone in systemic lupus erythematosus. *Ann Rheum Dis* 1988; 47:496–502.
231. Ueda N, Yoshikawa T, Chihara M, Kawaguchi S, Niinomi Y, Yasaki T. Atrial fibrillation following methylprednisolone pulse therapy. *Pediatr Nephrol* 1988;2:29–31.
232. Bettinelli A, Paterlini G, Mazzucchi E, Giani M. Seizures and transient blindness following intravenous pulse methylprednisolone in children with primary glomerulonephritis. *Child Urol Nephrol* 1991; 11:41–3.
233. Cameron JS. What is the role of long-term cytotoxic agents in the treatment of lupus nephritis? *J Nephrol* 1993;6:172–6.
234. Donadio JV, Glassock RJ. Immunosuppressive drug therapy in lupus nephritis. *Am J Kidney Dis* 1993;21:239–50.
235. Gruppo Italiano per lo Studio della Nefrite Lupica (GISNEL). Lupus nephritis: prognostic factors and probability of maintaining life-supporting renal function 10 years after the diagnosis. *Am J Kidney Dis* 1992;19:473–9.
236. Wagner L. Immunosuppressive agents in lupus nephritis: a critical analysis. *Medicine (Baltimore)* 1976;55:239–50.
237. Felson DT, Anderson J. Evidence for the superiority of immunosuppressive drugs and prednisone over prednisone alone in lupus nephritis. *N Engl J Med* 1984;311:1528–33.
238. Balow JE, Austin HA, Muenz LR, et al. Effect of treatment on the evolution of renal abnormalities in lupus nephritis. *N Engl J Med* 1984;311:491–5.
239. Austin HA III, Klippel JH, Balow JE, et al. Therapy of lupus nephritis: controlled trial of prednisone and cytotoxic drugs. *N Engl J Med* 1986;314:614–9.
240. Steinberg AD, Steinberg SC. Long-term preservation of renal function in patients with lupus nephritis receiving treatment that includes cyclophosphamide versus those treated with prednisolone alone. *Arthritis Rheum* 1991;34:945–50.
241. Wall RL, Clausen KP. Carcinoma of the urinary bladder in patients receiving cyclophosphamide. *N Engl J Med* 1975;293:271–3.
242. Grunwald H, Rosner F. Acute leukemia and immunosuppressive drug therapy for non-neoplastic diseases. *Arch Intern Med* 1979;139: 461–6.
243. Trompeter RS, Evans PR, Barratt TM. Gonadal function in boys with steroid-responsive nephrotic syndrome treated with cyclophosphamide for short periods. *Lancet* 1981;1:1177–9.
244. Stilwell TJ, Benson RC, de Remee RA, McDonald TJ, Weiland LH. Cyclophosphamide induced bladder toxicity in Wegener's granulomatosis. *Arthritis Rheum* 1988;31:465–70.
245. Wallace DJ. Plasmapheresis in lupus. *Lupus* 1993;2:141–3.
246. Leaker BR, Becker GJ, Dowling JP, Kincaid-Smith P. Rapid improvement in severe lupus glomerular lesions following intensive plasma exchange associated with immunosuppression. *Clin Nephrol* 1986;25:236–44.
247. Lewis EJ, Hunsicker LG, Lan S-P, Rohde RD, Lachin JM, for the Lupus Nephritis Collaborative Study Group. A controlled trial of plasmapheresis therapy in severe lupus nephritis. *N Engl J Med* 1992; 326:1373–9.
248. Wei N, Klippel JH, Huston DP, et al. Randomized trial of plasma exchange in mild systemic lupus erythematosus. *Lancet* 1983;1:17–21.
249. Dau PC, Callahan J, Parker R, Golbus J. Immunologic effects of plasmapheresis synchronized with pulse cyclophosphamide in systemic lupus erythematosus. J Rheumatol 1991;18:270–6.
250. Schroeder JO, Euler HH, Loffler H. Synchronization of plasmapheresis and pulse cyclophosphamide in severe systemic lupus erythematosus. *Ann Intern Med* 1987;107:344–6.
251. Euler HH, Schroeder JO, Zeuner RA, Teske E. A randomized trial of plasmapheresis and subsequent pulse cyclophosphamide in severe lupus: design of the LPSG trial. *Int J Artif Organs* 1991;14: 639–46.
252. Cohen J, Pinching AJ, Rees AJ, Peters DK. Infection and immunosuppression: a study of the infective complications of 75 patients with immunologically-mediated disease. *Q J Med* 1982;51:1–15.
253. Wing EJ, Bruns FJ, Fraley DS, Segel DP, Adler S. Infectious complications with plasmapheresis in rapidly progressive glomerulonephritis. *JAMA* 1980;244:2423–6.
254. Pohl MA, Lan S-P, Berl T, and the Lupus Nephritis Collaborative Study Group. Plasmapheresis does not increase the risk for infection in immunosuppressed patients with severe lupus nephritis. *Ann Intern Med* 1991;114:924–9.
255. Ackerman GL. Alternate day steroid therapy in lupus nephritis. *Ann Intern Med* 1970;72:511–9.
256. Liebling MR, McLaughlin K, Boonsue S, Kasdin J, Barnett EV. Monthly pulses of methylprednisolone in SLE nephritis. J Rheumatol 1982;9:543–8.
257. Wang CL, Wang F, Bosco JJ. Ovarian failure in oral cyclophosphamide treatment for systemic lupus erythematosus. *Lupus* 1995;4: 11–4.
258. Balow JE. Treatment and monitoring of patients with lupus nephritis. *Nephrol Dial Transplant* 1990;5(Suppl 1):58–9.
259. McCune WJ, Golbus J, Zeldes W, Bohlke P, Dunne R, Fox DA. Clinical and immunologic effects of monthly administration of cyclophosphamide in severe systemic lupus erythematosus. *N Engl J Med* 1988; 318:1323–31.
260. Lehman TJA, Sherry DD, Wagner-Weiner L, et al. Intermittent intravenous cyclophosphamide therapy for lupus nephritis. *J Pediatr* 1989;114:1055–60.
261. Belmont HM, Storch M, Buyon J, Abramson S. New York University/Hospital for Joint Diseases experience with intravenous cyclophosphamide treatment: efficacy in steroid unresponsive lupus nephritis. *Lupus* 1995;4:104–8.
262. Boumpas DT, Austin HA III, Vaughan EM, et al. Controlled trial of pulse methylprednisolone versus two regimens of pulse cyclophosphamide in severe lupus nephritis. *Lancet* 1992;340:741–5.
263. Boumpas DT, Austin HA III, Vaughan EM, Yarboro CH, Klippel JH, Balow JE. Risk for sustained amenorrhea in patients with systemic lupus erythematosus receiving intermittent pulse cyclophosphamide therapy. *Ann Intern Med* 1993;119:366–9.
264. Gibbons RB, Westerman E. Acute nonlymphocytic leukemia following short term, intermittent intravenous cyclophosphamide treatment of lupus nephritis. *Arthritis Rheum* 1988;31:1552–4.
265. Houssiau FA, D'Cruz DP, Haga H-J, Hughes GRV. Short course of weekly low-dose intravenous pulse cyclophosphamide in the treatment of lupus nephritis: a preliminary study. *Lupus* 1991;1:31–5.
266. Ginzler E, Sharon E, Diamond H, Kaplan D. Long-term maintenance therapy with azathioprine in systemic lupus erythematosus. *Arthritis Rheum* 1975;18:27–34.
267. Ginzler E, Diamond H, Kaplan D, Weiner M, Schlesinger M, Seleznick M. Computer analysis of factors influencing frequency of infection in systemic lupus erythematosus. *Arthritis Rheum* 1978;21:37–44.
268. Ponticelli C, Zucchelli P, Moroni G, Cagnoli L, Banfi G, Pasquali S. Long-term prognosis of diffuse lupus nephritis. *Clin Nephrol* 1987; 28:263–71.
269. Esdaile JM, Levinton C, Federgreen W, Hayslett JP, Kachgarian M. The clinical and renal biopsy predictors of long-term outcome in lupus nephritis: a study of 87 patients and review of the literature. *Q J Med* 1989;72:779–833.
270. Sharon E, Kaplan D, Diamond HS. Exacerbation of systemic lupus erythematosus after withdrawal of azathioprine therapy. *N Engl J Med* 1973;288:122–4.
271. Kinlen LJ, Sheil AGR, Peto J, Doll R. Collaborative United Kingdom–Australasian study of cancer in patients treated with immunosuppression. *BMJ* 1979;2:1461–6.
272. Lipsmeyer EA. Development of malignant cerebral lymphoma in a patient with systemic lupus erythematosus treated with immunosuppression. *Arthritis Rheum* 1972;15:183–6.
273. Nogueira JH, Freedman MA. Acute pancreatitis as a complication of Imuran therapy in regional enteritis. *Gastroenterology* 1972;62: 1040–1.
274. Sparberg M, Simon N, del Greco F. Intrahepatic cholestasis due to azathioprine. *Gastroenterology* 1969;57:439–41.
275. Epstein WV, Grausz H. Favorable outcome in diffuse proliferative glomerulonephritis of systemic lupus erythematosus. *Arthritis Rheum* 1974;17:129–42.
276. Snaith ML, Holt JM, Oliver DO, Dunhill MO, Halley W, Stephenson AC. Treatment of patients with systemic lupus erythematosus including nephritis with chlorambucil. *BMJ* 1973;2:197–201.

277. Cameron JS. Chlorambucil and leukemia [Letter]. *N Engl J Med* 1977;296:1055.
278. LeBlanc BAEW, Dagenais P, Urowitz MB, Gladman DD. Methotrexate in systemic lupus erythematosus. *J Rheumatol* 1994;21: 836–8.
279. Wilson K, Abeles M. A two year open-ended trial of methotrexate in systemic lupus erythematosus. *J Rheumatol* 1994;21:1640–7.
280. Israel-Biet D, Noel L-H, Bach MA, Dardenne M, Bach JF. Marked reduction of DNA antibody and glomerulopathy in thymulin or cyclosporin A–treated (NZB × NZW) mice. *Clin Exp Immunol* 1983;54: 359–65.
281. Favre H, Miescher PA, Huang YP, Chatelanat F, Mihatsch MJ. Ciclosporin (sic) in the treatment of lupus nephritis. *Am J Nephrol* 1989;9(Suppl 1):57–60.
282. Feutren G, Querin S, Noel LH, et al. Effects of cyclosporine in severe systemic lupus erythematosus. *J Pediatr* 1987;111:1063–8.
283. Le Francois N, Deleix P, Laville M, Zech P, Traeger J. Treatment of lupus nephritis with cyclosporin A: a patient with a 1 year follow-up. *Kidney Int* 1984;26:225(abst).
284. Bonomo L, Caccavo D, Lagana B, Amoroso A, Mitterhofer AP. Treatment with cyclosporin of SLE: results of long-term follow-up. *Lupus* 1995;4(Suppl 2):113(abst).
285. Meyrier A. Treatment of glomerular disease with cyclosporin A. *Nephrol Dial Transplant* 1989;4:923–31.
286. Takabayashi K, Koike T, Kurasawa K, et al. Effect of FK-506, a novel immunosuppressive drug, on murine systemic lupus erythematosus. *Clin Immunol Immunopathol* 1989;51:110–7.
287. Clark WF, Lindsay RM, Ulan RA, Cordy PE, Linton AL. Chronic plasma exchange therapy in SLE nephritis. *Clin Nephrol* 1981;16: 20–3.
288. Schwartz SA. Intravenous immunoglobulin (IVIG) for the therapy of autoimmune disorders. *J Clin Immunol* 1990;10:81–9.
289. Jordan SC. Intravenous γ globulin therapy in systemic lupus erythematosus and immune complex disease. *Clin Immunol Immunopathol* 1989;53(Suppl):S164–9.
290. Abdou NI, Yesnosky P, Chou A, Suenaga R, Mitamura K, Evans M. Intravenous human immunoglobulin (IVIg) therapy in active SLE: a twelve month in vivo and in vitro study. *Lupus* 1995;4(Suppl 2): 111(abst).
291. Monova D, Belovzhedov N. High dose immunoglobulin G (IVIG) in lupus glomerulonephritis (LGN). *Lupus* 1995;4(Suppl 2):112(abst).
292. Becker BN, Fuchs H, Hakim R. Intravenous immune globulin in the treatment of patients with systemic lupus erythematosus and end-stage renal disease. *J Am Soc Nephrol* 1995;5:1745–50.
293. Lin C-Y, Hsu H-C, Chiang H. Improvement in histological and immunological change in steroid and immunosuppressive drug-resistant lupus nephritis by high-dose intravenous gamma globulin. *Nephron* 1989;53:303–10.
294. Schifferli J, Leski M, Favre H, Imbach P, Nydegger U, Davies K. High dose intravenous IgG treatment and renal function. *Lancet* 1991;337:457–8.
295. Oravec S, Ronda N, Carayon A, Milliez J, Kazatchkine MD, Hornych A. Normal human polyspecific immunoglobulin G (intravenous immunoglobulin) modulates endothelial cell function in vitro. *Nephrol Dial Transplant* 1995;10:796–800.
296. Strober S, Field E, Hoppe RT, et al. Treatment of intractable lupus nephritis with total lymphoid irradiation. *Ann Intern Med* 1985;102: 450–8.
297. Strober S. Total lymphoid irradiation in alloimmunity and autoimmunity. *J Pediatr* 1987;111:1051–5.
298. Strober S, Farinas MC, Field EH, et al. Lupus nephritis after total lymphoid irradiation: persistent improvement and reduction in steroid dosage. *Ann Intern Med* 1987;197:689–91.
299. Lloyd W, Schur PH. Immune complexes, complement and anti-DNA in exacerbations of systemic lupus erythematosus (SLE). *Medicine (Baltimore)* 1981;60:208–17.
300. Appel AE, Sablay JB, Golden RA, Barland P, Grayzel AI, Bank N. The effect of normalization of serum complement and anti-DNA antibody on the course of lupus nephritis: a two year prospective study. *Am J Med* 1978;64:278–83.
301. Swaak AJ, Aarden LA, Statius Van Eps LW, et al. Anti-dsDNA and complement profiles as prognostic guides in systemic lupus erythematosus. *Arthritis Rheum* 1979;22:226–35.
302. Cameron JS, Lessof MH, Ogg CS, Williams BD, Williams DG. Disease activity in the nephritis of systemic lupus erythematosus in relation to serum complement concentration, DNA-binding capacity and precipitating anti-DNA antibody. *Clin Exp Immunol* 1976;25: 418–27.
303. Ponticelli C, Moroni G, Banfi G, Ponticelli C. Discontinuation of therapy in diffuse proliferative lupus nephritis [Letter]. *Am J Med* 1988;85:275.
304. Tozman ECS, Urowitz MB, Gladman DD. Prolonged complete remission in previously severe SLE. *Ann Rheum Dis* 1982;41:39–40.
305. Remuzzi G, Rossi E, eds. *Haemostasis and renal disease.* London: Butterworths, 1988.
306. Cade R, Spooner G, Schlein G, et al. Comparison of azathioprine, prednisolone and heparin alone or combined in treating lupus nephritis. *Nephron* 1973;10:37–56.
307. Conte J, Mignon-Conte M, Suc J-M. Réflexions critiques sur le traitement de la néphropathie lupique: Étude comparée de l'action des corticoïdes, de l'association indomethacine–anti-paludéen de synthese, et de l'heparine. *J Urol Nephrol* 1973;4–5:333–50.
308. Parbtani A, Frampton G, Kasai N, Yewdall V, Cameron JS. Platelet and plasma serotonin concentrations in glomerulonephritis. III. The nephritis of systemic lupus erythematosus. *Clin Nephrol* 1980;14: 164–72.
309. Dosekun AK, Pollak VE, Glas-Greenwalt P, et al. Ancrod in systemic lupus erythematosus with thrombosis: clinical and fibrinolytic effect. *Arch Intern Med* 1984;144:37–42.
310. Kant KS, Pollak VE, Dosekun AK, Glas-Greenwalt P, Weiss MA, Glueck R. Lupus nephritis with thrombosis and abnormal fibrinolysis: effect of ancrod. *J Lab Clin Med* 1982;105:77–88.
311. Kim S, Wadwha NK, Kant KS, et al. Fibrinolysis in glomerulonephritis treated with ancrod: renal functional, immunologic and histopathologic effects. *Q J Med* 1988;69:879–95.
312. Hariharan S, Pollak VE, Kant KS, Weiss MA, Wadhwa NK. Diffuse proliferative lupus nephritis: long-term observations in patients treated with ancrod. *Clin Nephrol* 1990;34:61–9.
313. Kimberly RP, Gill JR, Bowden RE, Keiser HR, Plotz PH. Elevated urinary prostaglandins and the effects of aspirin in lupus erythematosus. *Ann Intern Med* 1978;89:336–41.
314. Bender WL, Whelton A, Beschorner WE, Darwish MO, Hall-Craggs M, Solez K. Interstitial nephritis, proteinuria, and renal failure caused by non-steroidal anti-inflammatory drugs: immunologic characterization of the inflammatory infiltrate. *Am J Med* 1984;76: 1006–12.
315. Pierucci A, Simonetti BM, Pecci G, et al. Improvement of renal function with selective thromboxane antagonism in lupus nephritis. *N Engl J Med* 1989;320:421–5.
316. Leaker B, Quist R, Salehi N, Kincaid-Smith PS. The effect of eicosapentanoic acid on active lupus nephritis. *Kidney Int* 1986;30: 629(abst).
317. Clark WF, Parbtani A, Huff MW, Reid B, Holub BJ, Falardeau P. Omega-3 fatty acid dietary supplementation in patients with systemic lupus erythematosus (SLE). *Kidney Int* 1989;36:653–60.
318. Haider YS, Roberts WC. Coronary arterial disease in systemic lupus erythematosus. *Am J Med* 1981;70:775–81.
319. Correia P, Cameron JS, Lian JD, et al. Why do patients with lupus nephritis die? *BMJ* 1989;290:126–31.
320. Westberg G, Tarkowski A. Effect of maxEPA in patients with SLE. *Scand* J Rheumatol 1990;19:137–43.
321. Walton AJE, Snaith ML, Locniskar M, Cumberland AG, Morrow WJW, Isenberg DA. Dietary fish oil and the severity of symptoms in patients with systemic lupus erythematosus. *Ann Rheum Dis* 1991;50: 463–6.
322. El-Habib R, Laville M, Traeger J. Specific adsorption of circulating antibodies by extracorporeal plasma perfusions over antigen coated collagen flat membranes: applications to systemic lupus erythematosus. *J Clin Lab Immunol* 1984;15:111–7.
323. Palmer A, Gjorstrup P, Severn A, Welsh K, Taube D. Treatment of systemic lupus erythematosus by extracorporeal immunoadsorption [Letter]. *Lancet* 1988;2:272.
324. Terman DS, Buffaloe G, Mattioli C, et al. Extracorporeal immunoadsorption: initial experiences in human systemic lupus erythematosus. *Lancet* 1979;2:824–7.
325. Gaubitz M, Schmitz-Linneweber B, Perniok A, Fischer R, Schneider M. IG-immunoabsorption in SLE: first experiences. *Lupus* 1995; 4(Suppl 2):113(abst).

326. First MR. Renal transplantation for the nephrologist: new immunosuppressive drugs. *Am J Kidney Dis* 1992;19:3–9.
327. Bartlett RR. An introduction to leflunomide. *Agents Actions* 1994;41: ix–xiv [Special conference issue].
328. Saven A, Piro LD. 2-Chlorodeoxyadenosine: a newer purine analog active in the treatment of indolent lymphoid malignancies. *Ann Intern Med* 1994;37:551–8.
329. Hahn B, Ebling FM. Suppression of NZB/NZW murine nephritis by administration of a syngeneic monoclonal antibody to DNA. *J Clin Invest* 1981;71:1728–36.
330. Hahn BH, Ebling FM. Suppression of murine lupus nephritis by administration of an anti-idiotypic antibody to anti-DNA. *J Immunol* 1984;132:187–90.
331. Wofsy D, Seaman WE. Reversal of advanced murine lupus in NZB/NZW F_1 mice with monoclonal antibody to L3T4. *J Immunol* 1987;138:3247–53.
332. Adelman NE, Watling DL, McDevitt HO. Treatment of (NZB × NZW) F_1 disease with anti I-A monoclonal antibodies. *J Exp Med* 1983;158:1350–5.
333. Vladitiu AO. Treatment of autoimmune diseases with antibodies to class II major histocompatibility complex antigens. *Clin Immunol Immunopathol* 1991;61:1–17.
334. Kelley VE, Gaulton GN, Hattori M, Ikegami H, Eisenbarth G, Strom TB. Anti-interleukin 2 receptor antibody suppresses murine diabetic insulitis and lupus nephritis. *J Immunol* 1988;140:59–61.
335. Hiepe F, Brink I, Thiele B, Burmester G-R, Volk H-D, Emmrich F. Treatment of severe systemic lupus erythematosus (SLE) with monoclonal anti-CD4 antibodies (MAX.165H). *Lupus* 1995;4(Suppl 2): 99(abst).
336. Winter G, Milstein C. Man-made antibodies. *Nature* 1991;349: 293–9.
337. Kelley VE, Bacha P, Pankewycz O, Nichols JC, Murphy JR, Strom TB. Interleukin 2–diphtheria toxin fusion protein can abolish cell-mediated immunity in vivo. *Proc Natl Acad Sci USA* 1988;85: 3980–4.
338. Lederboum-Glaski H, FitzGerald D, Chaudhary V, Adhya S, Pastan I. Cytotoxic activity of an interleukin 2–*Pseudomonas* exotoxin chimeric protein produced in *Escherichia coli*. *Proc Natl Acad Sci USA* 1988;85:1922–6.
339. Pankewycz O, Strom TB, Kelley VE. Therapeutic strategies using monoclonal antibodies in autoimmune disease. *Curr Opin Immunol* 1989;1:757–63.
340. Stafford FJ, Fleisher TA, Lee G, et al. A pilot study of anti-CD5 ricin A chain conjugate in systemic lupus erythematosus. *J Rheumatol* 1994;21:2068–70.
341. June CH, Bluestone JA, Nadler LM, Thampson CB. The B7 and CD28 receptor families. *Immunol Today* 1994;15:321–31.
342. Perico N, Imberti O, Bontempelli M, Remuzzi G. Toward novel anti-rejection strategies: in vivo immunosuppressive properties of CTLA4Ig. *Kidney Int* 1995;47:241–6.
343. Adorini L, Barnaba V, Bona C, et al. New perspectives on immunointervention in autoimmune diseases. *Immunol Today* 1990;11:383–6.
344. Kingsley G, Panayi G, Lanchbury J. Immunotherapy of rheumatic diseases: practice and prospects. *Immunol Today* 1991;12:177–9.
345. Sayegh MH, Khoury SJ, Hancock WW, Weiner HL, Carpenter CB. Induction of immunity and oral tolerance with polymorphic class II MHC allopeptides in the rat. *Proc Natl Acad Sci USA* 1992;89: 7762–6.
346. Trentham DE, Dynesius-Trentham RA, Orav EJ, et al. Oral administration of type II collagen improves rheumatoid arthritis. *Science* 1993;261:1727–30.
347. Weiner HL, Mackin GA, Matsui M, et al. Double-blind trial of oral tolerization with myelin antigen in multiple sclerosis. *Science* 1993; 259:1321–4.
348. Marmont AM. Immune ablation with stem-cell rescue: a possible cure for systemic lupus erythematosus. *Lupus* 1993;2:151–6.
349. Wallace DJ, Podell T, Weiner J, Klinenberg JR, Forouzeh S, Dubois EL. Systemic lupus erythematosus–survival patterns: experience with 609 patients. *JAMA* 1981;245:934–8.
350. Studenski S, Allen NB, Caldwell DS, Rice JR, Pilisson RP. Survival in systemic lupus erythematosus: a multivariate analysis of demographic factors. *Arthritis Rheum* 1987;301:326–32.
351. Liang MH, Partridge AJ, Daltroy LH, Straaton KV, Galper SR, Holman HR. Strategies for reducing excess morbidity and mortality in blacks with systemic lupus erythematosus. *Arthritis Rheum* 1991;34: 1187–96.
352. Swaak AJG, Nossent JC, Smeenk RJT. Prognostic factors in systemic lupus erythematosus. *Rheumatol Int* 1990;11:127–32.
353. Golbus J, McCune WJ. Systemic lupus erythematosus: classification, prognosis, immunopathogenesis and treatment. *Rheum* Dis *Clin North Am* 1994;20:213–42.
354. Donadio JV Jr, Hart GM, Bergstralh EJ, Holley KE. Prognostic determinants in lupus nephritis: a long-term clinicopathologic study. *Lupus* 1995;4:109–15.
355. Ginzler, EM, Diamond HS, Weiner M, et al. A multicentre study of outcome in systemic lupus erythematosus. I. Entry variables as predictors of prognosis. *Arthritis Rheum* 1982;25:601–11.
356. Austin HA III, Boumpas DT, Vaughan EM, Balow JE. Predicting outcome in severe lupus nephritis: contribution of clinical and histological data. *Kidney Int* 1994;45:544–50.
357. Austin HA III, Boumpas DT, Vaughan EM, Balow JE. High-risk features of lupus nephritis: importance of race and clinical and histological features in 166 patients. *Nephrol Dial Transplant* 1995;10: 1620–8.
358. Ballou SP, Khan MA, Kushner I. Clinical features of systemic lupus erythematosus: differences related to race and age of onset. *Arthritis Rheum* 1982;25:55–60.
359. Cameron JS. Nephritis of systemic lupus erythematosus. In: Edelmann CE, Spitzer A, Travis LB, Meadow R, eds. *Pediatric nephrology*. 2nd ed. Boston: Little Brown, 1993:1407–65.
360. Platt JL, Burke BA, Fish AJ, Kim Y, Michael AF. Systemic lupus erythematosus in the first two decades of life. *Am J Kidney Dis* 1982;2(Suppl 1):212–22.
361. Fries JF, Weyl S, Holman HR. Estimating prognosis in systemic lupus erythematosus. *Am J Med* 1974;57:561–5.
362. Swaak AJG, Nossent JC, Bronsfeld W, et al. Systemic lupus erythematosus. I. Outcome and survival: Dutch experience with 110 patients studied prospectively. *Ann Rheum Dis* 1989;48:447–54.
363. Tejani A, Nicastri AD, Chen C-K, Fikrig S, Gurumurthy K. Lupus nephritis in black and Hispanic children. *Am J Dis Child* 1983;137: 481–3.
364. Celermajer DS, Thorner PS, Baumal R, Arbus GS. Sex differences in childhood lupus nephritis. *Am J Dis Child* 1984;138:586–8.
365. Petri M, Perez-Gutthann S, Longenecker JG, Hochberg M. Morbidity of systemic lupus erythematosus: role of race and socioeconomic status. *Am J Med* 1991;91:345–53.
366. Gordon MF, Stolley PD, Schinnar K. Trends in recent systemic lupus erythematosus mortality rates. *Arthritis Rheum* 1981;24:762–9.
367. Leaker B, Fairley KF, Dowling J, Kincaid-Smith P. Lupus nephritis: clinical and pathological correlation. *Q J Med* 1987:62:163–79.
368. Appel GB, Cohen DJ, Pirani CL, Melzer JI, Estes D. Long term follow up of patients with lupus nephritis: a study based on the classification of the World Health Organization. *Am J Med* 1987;83: 877–85.
369. Budman DR, Steinberg AD. Hypertension and renal disease in systemic lupus erythematosus. *Arch Intern Med* 1976;136:1003–7.
370. Ward MM, Studenski S. Clinical prognostic factors in lupus nephritis. *Arch Intern Med* 1992;152:2082–8.
371. Spronk PE, Limburg PC, Kallenberg CGM. Review: serological markers of disease activity in systemic lupus erythematosus. *Lupus* 1995;4:86–94.
372. Hecht B, Siegel N, Adler M, et al. Prognostic indices in lupus nephritis. *Medicine (Baltimore)* 1976;55:163–81.
373. Valentijn RM, van Overhagen H, Hazevoet HM, et al. The value of complement and immune complex determinations in monitoring disease activity in patients with systemic lupus erythematosus. *Arthritis Rheum* 1985;28:904–13.
374. Baldwin DS, Lowenstein J, Rothfield NF, Gallo G, McCluskey RT. The clinical course of the proliferative and membranous forms of lupus nephritis. *Ann Intern Med* 1970;73:924–9.
375. Lentz RD, Michael AF, Friend PF. Membranous transformation of lupus nephritis. *Clin Immunol Immunopathol* 1981;19:131–8.
376. Appel GB, Silva FG, Pirani CL, et al. Renal involvement in systemic lupus erythematosus (SLE): a study of 56 patients emphasizing histologic classification. *Medicine (Baltimore)* 1978;57:371–410.
377. Grishman E, Churg J. Focal segmental lupus nephritis. *Clin Nephrol* 1982;17:5–13.
378. Dujovne I, Pollak VE, Pirani CL, Dillard MG. The distribution and

character of glomerular deposits in systemic lupus erythematosus. *Kidney Int* 1972;2:33–50.
379. Tateno S, Kobayashi Y, Shigematsu H, Hiki Y. Study of lupus nephritis: its classification and the significance of subendothelial deposits. *Q J Med* 1983;52:311–31.
380. Park MH, D'Agati V, Appel GB, Pirani CL. Tubulo-interstitial disease in lupus nephritis: relation to immune deposits, interstitial inflammation, glomerular changes, renal function, and prognosis. *Nephron* 1986;44:309–19.
381. Magil AB, Puterman ML, Ballon HS, et al. Prognostic factors in diffuse proliferative lupus glomerulonephritis. *Kidney Int* 1988;34:511–7.
382. Yeung CK, Wong KL, Wong WC, et al. Crescentic lupus glomerulonephritis. *Clin Nephrol* 1984;21:251–8.
383. Bhuyan UN, Malaviya AN, Dash SC, et al. Prognostic significance of renal angiitis in systemic lupus erythematosus (SLE). *Clin Nephrol* 1983;20:109–13.
384. Ginzler EM, Nicastri AD, Chen CK, et al. Progression of mesangial and focal to diffuse lupus nephritis. *N Engl J Med* 1974;291:693–6.
385. Soon Lee H, Mujais SH, Kasinath BS, et al. Course of renal pathology in patients with systemic lupus erythematosus. *Am J Med* 1984;77:612–20.
386. Zimmerman SW, Jenkins PG, Shelp WD, et al. Progression from minimal or focal to diffuse proliferative lupus nephritis. *Lab Invest* 1978;32:665–72.
387. Moroni G, Banfi G, Ponticelli C. Clinical status of patients after 10 years of lupus nephritis. *Q J Med* 1992;84:681–9.
388. Rosner S, Ginzler EM, Diamond HS, et al. A multicenter study of outcome in systemic lupus erythematosus. II. Causes of death. *Arthritis Rheum* 1982;25:612–7.
389. Karsh J, Klippel JH, Balow JE, Decker JL. Mortality in lupus nephritis. *Arthritis Rheum* 1979;22:274–769.
390. Urowitz MB, Bookman HAM, Kowhler BE, et al. The bimodal mortality pattern of systemic lupus erythematosus. *Am J Med* 1976;60: 221–5.
391. Rubin LA, Urowitz MB, Gladman DD. Mortality in systemic lupus erythematosus: the bimodal pattern revisited. *Q J Med* 1985;55: 87–98.
392. Minick CR, Murphy GE, Campbell WG. Experimental induction of atherosclerosis by the synergy of allergic injury to arteries and a lipid-rich diet. 1. Effect of repeated injections of horse serum in rabbits fed a dietary cholesterol supplement. *J Exp Med* 1966;124: 635–52.
393. Fernandes G, Alonso DR, Tanaka T, Thaler HT, Yunis EJ, Good RA. Influence of diet on vascular lesions in autoimmune prone B/W mice. *Proc Natl Acad Sci USA* 1983;80:874–7.
394. Wallace DJ. Infection in systemic lupus erythematosus. In: Wallace DJ, Hahn BH, eds. *Dubois' systemic lupus erythematosus.* Philadelphia: Lea and Febiger, 1993:454–6.
395. Staples PJ, Gerding DN, Decker JL, Gordon RS. Incidence of infection in systemic lupus erythematosus. *Arthritis Rheum* 1974;17:1–10.
396. Nived O, Sturfelt G, Wollheim F. Systemic lupus erythematosus and infection: a controlled and prospective study including epidemiological data. *Q J Med* 1985;55:271–87.
397. Nagasawa K, Yamauchi Y, Tada Y, Kusaba T, Niho Y, Yoshikawa H. High incidence of herpes zoster in patients with systemic lupus erythematosus: an immunological analysis. *Ann Rheum Dis* 1990;49: 630–3.
398. Lehman TJA, Palmeri ST, Hastings C, Klippel JH, Plotz PH. Bacterial endocarditis complicating systemic lupus erythematosus. *J Rheumatol* 1983;10:655–8.
399. Haselaar P, Derksen RHWM, Blokzijl L, et al. Risk factors for thrombosis in lupus patients. *Ann Rheum Dis* 1989;48:933–40.
400. Angles-Cano E, Sultan Y, Clavel J. Predisposing factors to thrombosis in systemic lupus erythematosus: possible relation to endothelial cell damage. *J Lab Clin Med* 1979;94:312–23.
401. Byron MA, Allington MJ, Chapel HM, Mowat AG, Cederholm-Williams S. Indications of vascular cell endothelial cell dysfunction in systemic lupus erythematosus. *Ann Rheum Dis* 1987;46:741–5.
402. Cole EH, Schulman J, Urowitz M, Keystone E, Williams C, Levy GA. Monocyte procoagulant activity in glomerulonephritis associated with systemic lupus erythematosus. *J Clin Invest* 1985;75: 861–8.
403. Cameron JS. Coagulation and thromboembolic complications in the nephrotic syndrome. *Adv Nephrol* 1984;23:75–114.
404. Appel GB, Williams GS, Melzer JI, Pirani CL. Renal vein thrombosis, nephrotic syndrome and systemic lupus erythematosus. *Ann Intern Med* 1976;85:310–7.
405. Ogg CS, Cameron JS, Maisey MN, et al. Renal vein thrombosis in the nephrotic syndrome. In: Schreiner GE, Winchester RJ, eds. *Controversies in nephrology.* New York: Masson, 1982:160–8.
406. Gelfand J, Truong L, Stern L, Pirani CL, Appel GB. Thrombotic thrombocytopenic purpura syndrome in systemic lupus erythematosus: treatment with plasma exchange. *Am J Kidney Dis* 1985;6: 154–60.
407. Itoh Y, Sekine H, Hosono O, et al. Thrombotic thrombocytopenic purpura in two patients with systemic lupus erythematosus: clinical significance of antiplatelet antibodies. *Clin Immunol Immunopathol* 1990;57:125–36.
408. Weiner ES, Abeles M. Aseptic necrosis and gluco-corticosteroids in systemic lupus erythematosus: a reevaluation. *J Rheumatol* 1989;16: 604–8.
409. Lacks S, White P. Morbidity associated with childhood systemic lupus erythematosus. *J Rheumatol* 1990;17:941–5.
410. Nagasawa K, Ishii Y, Mayumi T, et al. Avascular necrosis of bone in systemic lupus erythematosus: possible role of haemostatic abnormalities. *Ann Rheum Dis* 1989;48:672–6.
411. Felson DT, Anderson JJ. A cross study evaluation of association between steroid dose and bolus steroids and avascular necrosis of bone. *Lancet* 1987;1:902–6.
412. Zizic TM, Hungerford DS, Stevens MB. Ischemic bone necrosis in systemic lupus erythematosus. I. Early diagnosis of ischemic necrosis of bone. *Medicine (Baltimore)* 1980;59:134–42. II. The treatment of ischemic necrosis of bone in systemic lupus erythematosus. *Medicine (Baltimore)* 1908;59:143–8.
413. Bergstein JM, Wiens C, Fish AJ, Vernier RL, Michael A. Avascular necrosis of bone in systemic lupus erythematosus. *J Pediatr* 1974;85: 31–5.
414. Ishikawa S, Segar WE, Gilbert EF, Burkholder PM, Levy JM, Visekul C. Myocardial infarct in a child with systemic lupus erythematosus. *Am J Dis Child* 1978;132:696–9.
415. Bulkley HB, Roberts WC. The heart in systemic lupus erythematosus and the changes induced in it by corticosteroid therapy. *Am J Med* 1975;58:243–64.
416. Ilowite NT, Samual P, Ginzler E, Jacobson MS. Dyslipoproteinemia in pediatric systemic lupus erythematosus. *Arthritis Rheum* 1988;31: 859–63.
417. Ostrov BE, Min W, Eichenfeld AH, Goldsmith DP, Kaplan B, Athreya BH. Hypertension in children with systemic lupus erythematosus. *Semin Arthritis Rheum* 1989;19:90–8.
418. Canoso JJ, Cohen AS. Malignancy in a series of 70 patients with systemic lupus erythematosus. *Arthritis Rheum* 1974;17:383–90.
419. Lewis RB, Castor CW, Knisley RE, Bole GG. Frequency of neoplasia in systemic lupus erythematosus and rheumatoid arthritis. *Arthritis Rheum* 1976;19:1256–60.
420. Carlow TJ, Glaser JS. Pseudotumor cerebri syndrome in systemic lupus erythematosus. *JAMA* 1974;228:197–200.
421. Askari A, Vignos PJ, Moskowitz RW. Steroid myopathy in connective tissue diseases. *Am J Med* 1976;61:485–92.
422. Rodby RA. Management of the systemic lupus erythematosus patient with end-stage renal disease. *Semin Dial* 1989;2:180–5.
423. Arce-Salinas CA, Villa AR, Martínez-Rueda JO. Factors associated with chronic renal failure in 121 patients with diffuse proliferative lupus nephritis: a case–control study. *Lupus* 1995;4:197–203.
424. Cheigh JS, Kim H, Stenzel KH, et al. End stage renal disease in systemic lupus erythematosus: long term follow-up on the prognosis of patients and the evolution of lupus activity. *Am J Kidney Dis* 1990;16:189–95.
425. Coplon NS, Diskin CJ, Petersen J, et al. The long-term clinical course of systemic lupus erythematosus in end-stage renal disease. *N Engl J Med* 1981;308:186–90.
426. Krishnan G, Thaker L, Angstadt JD, Capelli JP. Multicenter analysis of renal allograft survival in lupus patients. *Transplant Proc* 1991;23:1755–6.
427. Brown CD, Rao TKS, Maxey W, Butt KMH, Friedman EA. Regression of clinical and immunological expression of systemic lupus erythematosus consequent to development of uremia. *Kidney Int* 1979; 16:884(abst).
428. Correia P, Cameron JS, Ogg CS, Williams DG, Bewick M, Hicks JA.

End-stage renal failure in systemic lupus erythematosus with nephritis. *Clin Nephrol* 1984;22:293–302.

429. Kimberly RP, Lockshin MD, Sherman RL, Mouradian J, Saal S. Reversible "end-stage" lupus nephritis. *Am J Med* 1983;74:361–8.
430. Nossent HC, Swaak TJG, Berden JHM, and the Dutch Working Party on Systemic Lupus Erythematosus. Analysis of disease activity in 55 patients with end-stage renal failure treated with hemodialysis or continuous ambulatory peritoneal dialysis. *Am J Med* 1990;89: 169–74.
431. Jarrett MP, Santhanam S, Del Greco F. The clinical course of end-stage renal disease in systemic lupus erythematosus. *Arch Intern Med* 1983;143:1353–6.
432. Winfield JB, Fernstein P, Czyczyk J, Wang E, Marchalonis J. Antibodies to CD45 and other cell membrane antigens in systemic lupus erythematosus. *Springer Semin Immunopathol* 1994;16:201–10.
433. Nossent HC, Swaak TJG, Berden JHM. Renal transplantation in systemic lupus erythematosus [Letter]. *Ann Intern Med* 1991;114:991.
434. Radhakrishnan J, Williams GS, Appel GB, Cohen DJ. Renal transplantation in anticardiolipin antibody-positive lupus erythematosus patients. *Am J Kidney Dis* 1994;23:286–9.
435. Nossent HC, Swaak TJG, Berden JHM, and the Dutch Working Party on SLE. Systemic lupus erythematosus after renal transplantation: patients and graft survival and disease activity. *Ann Intern Med* 1991;114:183–8.
436. Ward LA, Jelveh Z, Feinfeld DA. Recurrent membranous lupus nephritis after renal transplantation: a case report and review of the literature. *Am J Kidney Dis* 1994;23:326–9.
437. Nyberg G, Blohmé I, Persson H, Olausson M, Svalander C. Recurrence of SLE in transplanted kidneys: a follow-up transplant biopsy study. *Nephrol Dial Transplant* 1992;7:1116–23.
438. Roth D, Fernandez J, Diaz A, et al. Recurrence of lupus nephritis following renal transplantation. *J Am Soc Nephrol* 1992;3:878(abst).
439. Striker GE, Kelly MR, Quadracci LJ, Scribner BH. The course of lupus nephritis: a clinicopathological correlation of fifty patients. In: Kincaid-Smith P, Mathew TH, Becker EL, eds. *Glomerulonephritis New York: John Wiley, 1973:1141–66.*
440. Nanra RS, Kincaid-Smith P. *Lupus nephritis: clinical course in relationship to treatment.* In: Kincaid-Smith E, Mathew TH, Becker EL, eds. *Glomerulonephritis* New York: John Wiley, 1973:1193–210.
441. Cameron JS, Turner DR, Ogg CS, et al. Systemic lupus nephritis: a long-term study. *Q J Med* 1979;48:1–24.
442. McLaughlin J, Bombardier C, Farewell VT, Gladman DD, Urowitz MB. Kidney biopsy in systemic lupus erythematosus. II. Survival analyses according to biopsy results. *Arthritis Rheum* 1991;34:1268–73.

Immunologic Renal Diseases,
edited by E. G. Neilson and W. G. Couser.
Lippincott-Raven Publishers, Philadelphia © 1997.

CHAPTER 49

Renal Vasculitis

Ronald J. Falk and J. Charles Jennette

DEFINITIONS AND HISTORICAL PERSPECTIVE

In 1866, Kussmaul and Maier described two patients with periarteritis nodosa, one of whom had glomerulonephritis (1). In 1903, Ferrari first used the term polyarteritis acuta nodosa instead of periarteritis nodosa to describe the transmural, rather than perivascular, nature of the lesions (2). It was not until 1948 that glomerulonephritis was described as a frequent occurrence in patients with arteritis (3). First Klinger in 1931 (4) and then Wegener in 1936 (5) described a granulomatous variant of small vessel vasculitis that now bears the name Wegener granulomatosis. In 1952, Zeek and her associates differentiated necrotizing vasculitis into clinical and pathologic categories, including a form of small vessel vasculitis that she called "hypersensitivity angiitis" (6). This form of vasculitis differed from periarteritis nodosa, which is a form of necrotizing vasculitis confined to arteries but not affecting lungs or glomeruli.

In 1954, Godman and Churg provided the first detailed description of what is now called *Wegener* granulomatosis. They described a triad of upper and lower respiratory tract granulomatous inflammation, systemic vasculitis, and necrotizing glomerulonephritis (7). Godman and Churg realized that from a pathologic perspective, Wegener granulomatosis, Churg–Strauss syndrome, and what they call microscopic periarteritis had shared pathologic features. Classic polyarteritis nodosa differed from these three diseases by having the vasculitis confined to arteries. Unfortunately, the insights of Godman and Churg were forgotten for decades. In 1993, an international consensus conference was held in Chapel Hill, North Carolina, resulting in the Chapel Hill Consensus Conference for Nomenclature of Systemic Vasculitis (8). The definitions adopted for Wegener granulomatosis, Churg–Strauss syndrome, and microscopic polyangiitis (that is, Zeek's hypersensitivity angiitis and Godman and Churg's microscopic periarteritis) were very similar to those proposed by Godman and Churg in 1954. The terms and definitions of vasculitis adopted by this consensus conference are listed in Table 1, with predominant distributions of renovascular injury shown in Fig. 1. In this scheme, large vessel vasculitides are separated from medium-sized and small vessel vasculitides. Giant cell arteritis and Takayasu arteritis rarely involve the kidney, except for occasional impairment of renal artery perfusion, and are characterized by granulomatous inflammation of the aorta and its major branches. Giant cell and Takayasu arteritis are separated largely on the basis of age, that is, giant cell arteritis in older and Takayasu arteritis in younger patients. Medium-sized vessel vasculitides, including classic polyarteritis nodosa and Kawasaki disease, involve necrotizing inflammation of arteries but without glomerulonephritis or vasculitis in arterioles, capillaries, or venules. Kawasaki disease usually occurs in children and is associated with mucocutaneous lymph node syndrome. Polyarteritis nodosa affects the kidneys more often than does Kawasaki disease. Both diseases injure the kidneys by causing arterial occlusion or rupture resulting in infarction or hemorrhage, respectively (9).

Small vessel vasculitides differ from large and medium-sized vasculitides in that they involve vessels other than arteries, including frequent involvement of glomerular capillaries. Immunopathologic categorization of small vessel vasculitides is afforded by the results of indirect immunofluorescence microscopic findings of immune-complex-mediated lesions versus the absence or paucity of immune deposits. The term *pauci-immune necrotizing vasculitis* or *glomerulonephritis* indicates the relative paucity of immunoglobulin deposition when compared with immune-complex disease or antiglomeru-

R. J. Falk: Department of Medicine, University of North Carolina School of Medicine, Chapel Hill, North Carolina 27599.

J. C. Jennette: Department of Pathology, University of North Carolina School of Medicine, Chapel Hill, North Carolina 27599.

TABLE 1. *Names and definitions of vasculitis adopted by the Chapel Hill Consensus Conference on the Nomenclature of Systemic Vasculitis*

Large vessel vasculitis[a]	
Giant cell (temporal arteritis)	Granulomatous arteritis of the aorta and its major branches, with a predilection for the extracranial branches of the carotid artery. *Often involves the temporal artery. Usually occurs in patients older than 50 and often is associated with polymyalgia rheumatica.*
Takayasu arteritis	Granulomatous inflammation of the aorta and its major branches. *Usually occurs in patients younger than 50.*
Medium-sized vessel vasculitis[a]	
Polyarteritis nodosa (classic polyarteritis nodosa)	Necrotizing inflammation of medium-sized or small arteries without glomerulonephritis or vasculitis in arterioles, capillaries, or venules.
Kawasaki disease	Arteritis involving large, medium-sized, and small arteries and associated with mucocutaneous lymph node syndrome. *Coronary arteries are often involved. Aorta and veins may be involved. Usually occurs in children.*
Small vessel vasculitis[a]	
Wegener granulomatosis[b,c]	Granulomatous inflammation involving the respiratory tract and necrotizing vasculitis affecting small to medium-sized vessels (for example, capillaries, venules, arterioles, and arteries). *Necrotizing glomerulonephritis is common.*
Churg–Strauss syndrome[b,c]	Eosinophil-rich and granulomatous inflammation involving the respiratory tract and necrotizing vasculitis affecting small to medium-sized vessels and associated with asthma and blood eosinophilia.
Microscopic polyangiitis (microscopic polyarteritis)[b,c]	Necrotizing vasculitis with few or no immune deposits affecting small vessels (capillaries, venules, or arterioles). *Necrotizing arteritis involving small and medium-sized arteries may be present. Necrotizing glomerulonephritis is very common. Pulmonary capillaritis often occurs.*
Henoch–Schönlein purpura[c]	Vasculitis with immunoglobulin-A-dominant immune deposits affecting small vessels (capillaries, venules, or arterioles). *It typically involves the skin, gut, and glomeruli and is associated with arthralgias or arthritis.*
Essential cryoglobulinemic vasculitis[c]	Vasculitis with cryoglobulin immune deposits affecting small vessels (capillaries, venules, or arterioles), and associated with cryoglobulins in serum. *Skin and glomeruli are often involved.*
Cutaneous leukocytoclastic angiitis	Isolated cutaneous leukocytoclastic angiitis without systemic vasculitis or glomerulonephritis.

[a] Large artery refers to the aorta and the largest branches directed toward major body regions (for example, to the extremities and the head and neck); medium-sized artery refers to the main visceral arteries (for example, renal, hepatic, coronary, and mesenteric arteries); and small artery refers to the distal arterial radicals that connect with arterioles (for example, renal arcuate and interlobular arteries). Note that some small and large vessel vasculitides may involve medium-sized arteries, but large and medium-sized vessel vasculitides do not involve vessels smaller than arteries.

[b] Strongly associated with antineutrophil cytoplasmic autoantibodies.

[c] May be accompanied by glomerulonephritis and can manifest as nephritis or pulmonary–renal vasculitic syndrome.

Modified from Jennette et al. (8).

lar basement membrane (anti-GBM) disease (10). Wegener granulomatosis, Churg–Strauss syndrome, and microscopic polyangiitis are diseases characterized as pauci-immune forms of vasculitis, whereas the immune-complex small vessel vasculitides include Henoch–Schönlein purpura, cryoglobulinemic vasculitis, rheumatoid vasculitis, lupus vasculitis, and serum sickness vasculitis. Wegener granulomatosis is separated from microscopic polyangiitis on the basis of granulomatous inflammation involving the respiratory tract. Churg–Strauss syndrome is characterized by eosinophilia, eosinophil-rich granulomatous inflammation of the respiratory tract, and a history of asthma. Of the pauci-immune small vessel vasculitides, Wegener granulomatosis and microscopic polyangiitis frequently cause severe renal disease, primarily because of severe glomerulonephritis, whereas Churg–Strauss syndrome only occasionally causes substantial renal disease.

This chapter focuses on the pauci-immune vasculitides because immune-complex vasculitides, such as cryoglobulinemic vasculitis (Chapter 41) and Henoch–Schönlein purpura (Chapter 50), and anti-GBM disease (Chapter 43) are discussed in detail in other chapters.

INCIDENCE AND EPIDEMIOLOGY

It is difficult to ascertain the incidence of vasculitis in the general population, because it depends on the population studied. Studies based on a small number of patients

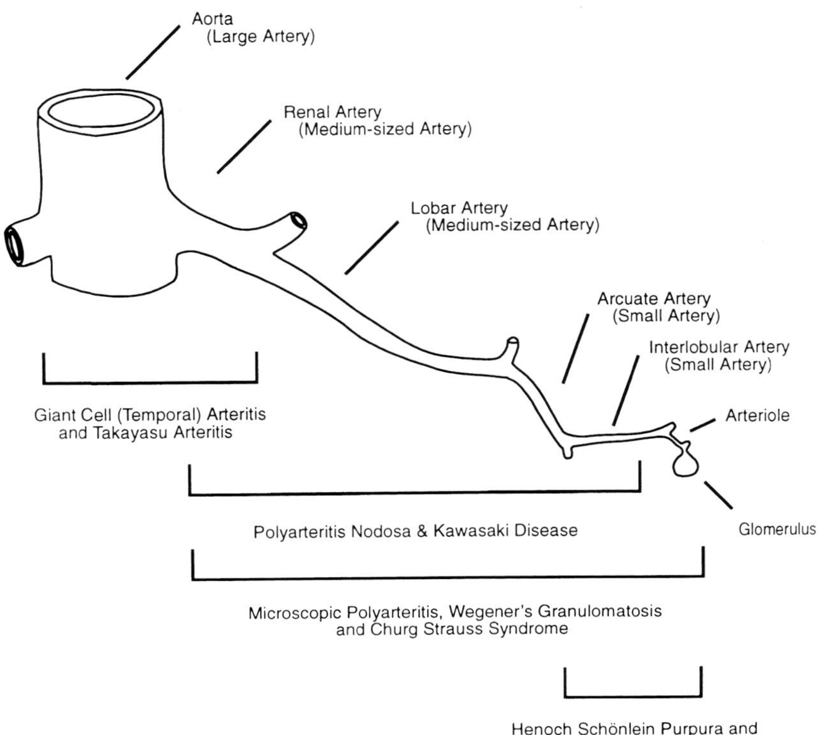

FIG. 1. Predominant distribution of renal vascular involvement by systemic vasculitides. Note that medium-sized renal arteries can be affected by large, medium-sized, and small vessel vasculitides, but arterioles and glomeruli are affected by small vessel vasculitides alone based on the definitions in Table 1. Reprinted with permission from Jennette et al. (8).

have suggested an annual incidence of 10 per million in a study from a district general hospital from 1972 to 1980 (11). Subsequent estimates of the combined incidence of Wegener granulomatosis and microscopic polyangiitis in the United Kingdom were only 1.5 per million between 1980 to 1986, with an increase to 6.1 per million from 1987 to 1989 (12). The overall incidence of systemic vasculitis excluding giant cell arteritis from 1988 to 1994 was 42 per million, a fourfold increase over previous estimates.

The incidence of pauci-immune necrotizing crescentic glomerulonephritis is more readily determined among patients with renal disease. The first description of rapidly progressive glomerulonephritis without immune deposits as a separate disease entity was provided by Couser, Bolton, and associates in 1979 (58). This entity is the most common cause of rapidly progressive glomerulonephritis when compared with immune-complex or anti-GBM disease (13,58). Most patients with pauci-immune crescentic glomerulonephritis have clinical or pathologic evidence of systemic vasculitis. This observation has led some to consider this form of glomerulonephritis to be renal vasculitis when there is no evidence for systemic vasculitis. When vasculitis is found in the biopsy specimen, the pauci-immune category of glomerulonephritis is found in 84% of cases.

To date, very little is known about the epidemiology and genetics of necrotizing glomerulonephritis and systemic vasculitis. Silica has been suggested as an occupational exposure that increases the risk of Wegener granulomatosis (14). This finding has been corroborated by Gregorini et al., who have suggested that renal damage occurs more frequently in silica-exposed patients (15). Necrotizing glomerulonephritis is found in patients who ingest pharmaceutical agents, such as propylthiouracil (16), hydralazine (17,18), or penicillamine (19). The mechanism by which these agents result in vascular inflammation, as well as the incidence of the problem, have yet to be determined.

Little is known about the genotype of patients with necrotizing vasculitis (20). In two different centers in Europe, there appears to be a decreased frequency of HLA-DR13 in patients with Wegener granulomatosis and a significant decrease in frequency of HLA-DR6 when compared with control (21). The decrease in HLA-DR6 is probably a consequence of a decreased frequency of DR13. In contrast, DR14 frequency was similar in the vasculitic and control populations.

SEROLOGIC STUDIES

Substantial advances have been made in the serologic analysis of patients with necrotizing vasculitis. In 1982, Davies et al. reported eight patients with antineutrophil autoantibodies associated with necrotizing glomerulonephritis (22). These eight patients had been exposed to an arbovirus that may have predisposed them to renal injury. Since then, substantial work has demonstrated the serologic importance of antineutrophil cytoplasmic autoantibodies (ANCAs) (23–25). ANCAs react not only with neutrophils but also with monocytes (26). Two ANCA patterns, determined by indirect immunofluorescence microscopy, are observed on ethanol-fixed normal human neutrophils. They are a cytoplasmic staining pattern (C-ANCA) with central accentuation of the immunofluorescence and a perinuclear staining pattern (P-ANCA) (Fig. 2). The majority of C-ANCAs react with a shrine proteinase called *proteinase 3* (Jr) found within the neutrophil azurophilic granules (27–30). Some C-ANCAs (~10–20%) react with other neutrophil antigens. PR3 is a 29-kD serine proteinase and is primarily a glycoprotein. Molecular cloning analysis indicates identity with P29b and myeloblastin (31). Recent investigation of another azurophilic granule constituent known as bactericidal permeability-increasing factor (BPI) suggests that some C-ANCAs react with BPI (32). The reactivity with BPI, however, is relatively nonspecific in that it is also found in patients with other nonnecrotizing glomerular diseases and in patients with nonspecific inflammatory processes (33).

The other major ANCA subtype is P-ANCA. P-ANCAs react with myeloperoxidase (MPO) in >90% of patients with necrotizing vasculitis cases (24,34,35). MPO is a microbicidal enzyme found in azurophilic granules of neutrophils and in lysosomes of monocytes. MPO is a member of the peroxidase multichain family, which also includes lactoperoxidase, thyroperoxidase, and eosinophil peroxidase. This multigene family is highly conserved among mammalian species, with homology shared at the nucleotide and amino acid sequence. These enzymes share structural features and similar catalytic mechanisms (36,37). P-ANCAs that do not react with MPO are found in ulcerative colitis, primary sclerosing cholangitis, and Felty syndrome (38–40). The specificity of these ANCAs are, for the most part, unknown. Several minor specificities for P-ANCAs have been elucidated, including elastase and lactoferrin primarily observed in patients with lupus erythematosus (41,42). Antielastase and antilactoferrin antibodies are uncommon in patients with necrotizing vasculitis (43, 44). Some P-ANCA sera do react with azurosidin (a serine proteinase) (45), but the frequency of reactivity to azurosidin is low and is also found in patients with nonarteritic inflammatory diseases (33).

Serologic testing for ANCAs is now available throughout most of the world. The most common assay is still indirect immunofluorescence microscopy. Antigen-specific assays are gaining increasing importance, especially to detect and quantify MPO ANCA and PR3 ANCA.

The autoantibody response to MPO and proteinase appears to be directed toward conformational epitopes (46,47). MPO ANCAs react with intact MPO, an interaction abrogated by thermal denaturation of MPO into heavy- and light-chain subunits. Fusion proteins created from the random insertion of 100- to 300-base-pair fragments of MPO cDNA into an expression system reveals that most MPO-ANCA sera react with a restricted number of epitopes found either in the heavy chain and spanning two anti-parallel-helixes or in the junction between the heavy and light chains. Similarly, PR3 ANCA appears to react with a conformational epitope that is easily destroyed by denaturation. Several regions of the PR3 molecule appear to be epitopes for PR3 ANCA (48).

Virtually nothing is known about those factors responsible for the generation and perpetuation of the ANCA autoimmune response (see Chapter 13). The idiotypic response of patients with ANCA has been carefully

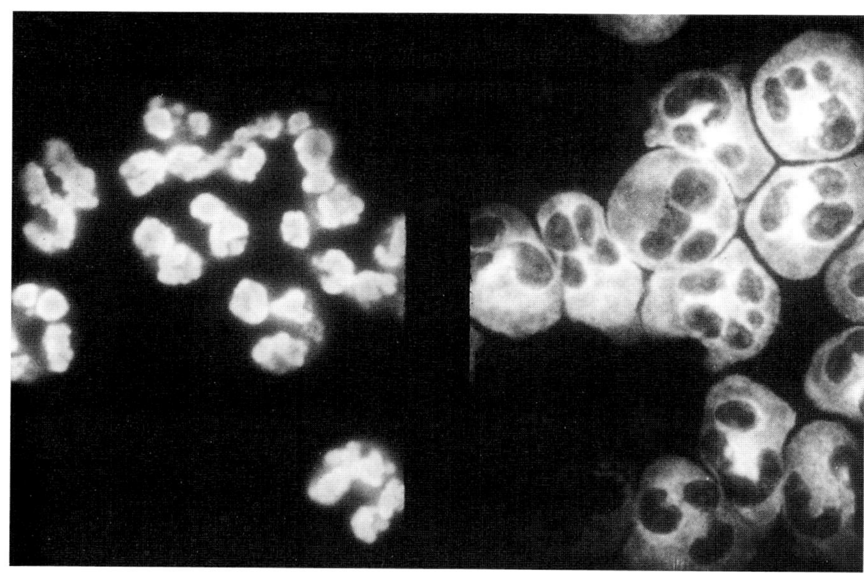

FIG. 2. By indirect immunofluorescence microscopy, antineutrophil cytoplasmic autoantibodies (ANCAs) have either **(A)** perinuclear staining pattern (P-ANCA) or **(B)** cytoplasmic staining pattern (C-ANCA). Reprinted with permission from Jennette and Falk (13).

investigated and appears to be relatively restricted (49, 50). The clonality of the MPO ANCA has been examined using both isoelectric focusing and the development of a murine monoclonal anti-idiotype antibodies (49). Of ANCA-positive patients, 69% had two or fewer ANCA clonotypes to MPO, whereas 31% had more than two clonotypes. Clonality was stable over the course of the disease and was shared among unrelated patients. The sharing of similar idiotypes was proven by the development of a murine monoclonal anti-idiotype antibody that was able to extract MPO ANCA from the proband's plasma and from thee other MPO-ANCA patients, but not from control antibody preparations. The demonstration of shared idiotypy suggests a restricted number of autoreactive epitopes of the MPO molecule or that MPO-ANCA antibodies are encoded by germline genes. These data are corroborated by the observation that there are common or public anti-idiotypes in pooled intravenous immunoglobulin preparations (50).

SEROLOGIC CORRELATION WITH DISEASE

ANCAs are found in >90% of patients with Wegener granulomatosis (23–25,51). PR3 ANCAs are more commonly associated with the granulomatous inflammation found in Wegener granulomatosis, although PR3 ANCAs also are found in patients with microscopic polyangiitis and renal-limited necrotizing glomerulonephritis without evidence of systemic disease (52). MPO ANCAs are more commonly found in patients with microscopic polyangiitis and in patients with necrotizing crescentic glomerulonephritis without evidence of systemic vasculitis (52,53). While it was previously thought that MPO ANCAs were only rarely found in patients with Wegener granulomatosis, a recent European collaborative trial has confirmed that as many as 20% of patients with Wegener granulomatosis have MPO ANCAs whereas PR3 ANCAs are found in 80% of these patients (54). Asthma and peripheral eosinophilia are typically present in patients with the Churg–Strauss syndrome with granulomatous inflammation of the respiratory tract and necrotizing glomerulonephritis. These individuals usually have MPO ANCAs (55). Thus, although there is a general association of ANCA specificity and disease phenotype, it is difficult to use the ANCA subtype to differentiate between different categories of necrotizing vasculitis (56,57).

Enzyme-linked immunosorbent assays or radioimmunoassays using purified antigens to detect ANCAs have an approximate sensitivity and specificity of 95%. Despite this high sensitivity and specificity, the positive predictive value of the test depends on the study population. In patients with appropriate clinical evidence for Wegener granulomatosis, systemic vasculitis, or rapidly progressive glomerulonephritis, the positive predictive value is >90%. The positive predictive value in patients with any evidence for acute nephritis (for example, hematuria and proteinuria with no renal insufficiency) is only 50%, whereas there is virtually no positive predictive value for the test when used in a generalized hospital population. Thus, ANCA testing is most useful in the setting of a clinical and/or pathologic finding consistent with a systemic vasculitis.

PATHOLOGY OF PAUCI-IMMUNE NECROTIZED SMALL VESSEL VASCULITIS AND PAUCI-IMMUNE NECROTIZING AND CRESCENTIC GLOMERULONEPHRITIS (FIG. 3)

The shared pathologic feature in all categories of pauci-immune small vessel vasculitis is segmental fibrinoid necrosis of vessels, often with neutrophil infiltration and/or leukocytoclasia in acute lesions. This necrotizing injury can affect many different types of vessels in many different tissues resulting in many different clinical manifestations (10). Although small and medium-sized arteries may be affected, capillaries (for example, glomerular and alveolar), venules, and arterioles are more frequent targets. Necrotizing glomerulonephritis with crescents is a common manifestation of pauci-immune small vessel vasculitis. Pauci-immune necrotizing glomerulonephritis is characterized by segmental fibrinoid necrosis and crescent formation (24,58,59). Immunofluorescence microscopy differentiates pauci-immune from immune-complex-mediated and anti-GBM disease. In contrast to the immune-complex-mediated crescentic glomerular diseases, there is little glomerular hypercellularity (for example, a proliferative response). The GBM is frequently disrupted or fragmented in areas of necrosis, as is the Bowman capsule. The disruption of the Bowman capsule may be accompanied by periglomerular multinucleated giant cells. The necrotizing lesions can be global and diffuse but usually are focal and segmental. Crescent formation is common. When areas of necrotizing injury scar, a focal sclerosing pattern is observed that must be differentiated from primary idiopathic focal segmental glomerulosclerosis. Chronic changes are manifest by fibrous crescents and chronic interstitial nephritis and fibrosis in nephron segments whose glomeruli have been damaged. Outside of the glomerulus, segmental necrotizing vascular injury is found in the walls of venules, capillaries, arterioles, and even arteries. An interesting renal vasculitic variant is that of vascular inflammation of the medullary vasa recta resulting in a hemorrhagic medullary interstitial nephritis.

In Wegener granulomatosis, granulomatous inflammation is found in the upper or lower respiratory tract with accompanying necrotizing vasculitis marked by areas of fibrinoid necrosis with infiltrates of primarily neutrophils in acute lesions or, in older lesions, mononuclear leukocytes. Granulomatous inflammation may occur without

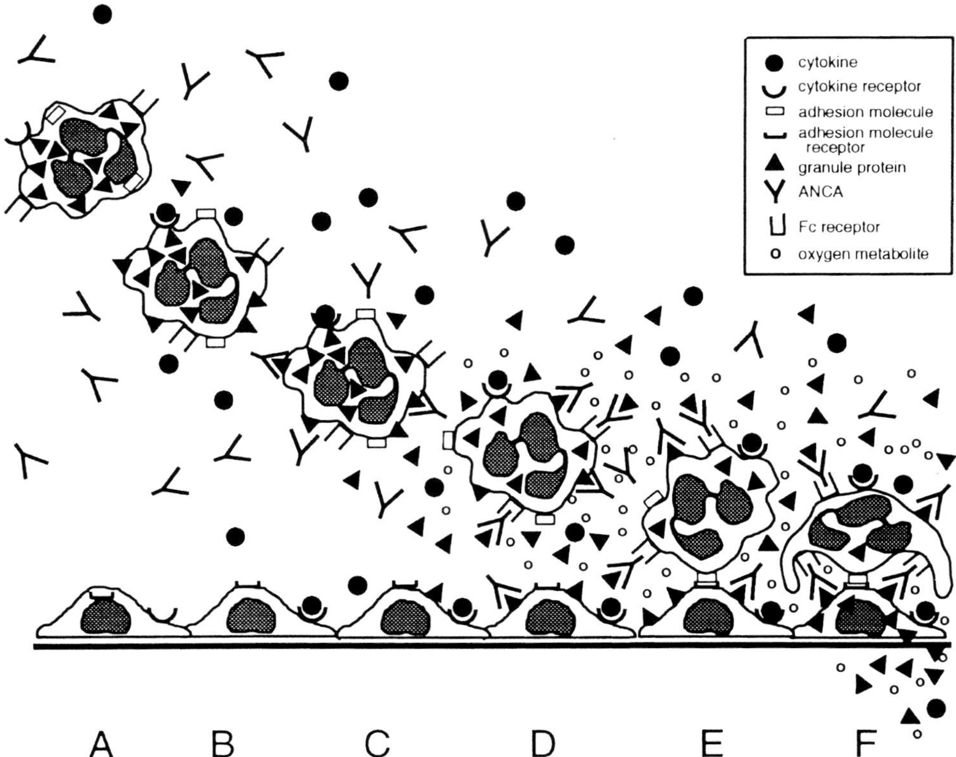

FIG. 3. A possible sequence of events resulting in antineutrophil cytoplasmic autoantibody (ANCA) vasculitis based on in vitro observations. **A:** Circulating quiescent neutrophils contain cytoplasmic ANCA targets, including myeloperoxidase (MPO) and proteinase 3 (PR3) that are not accessible to interact with ANCAs. **B:** Priming of neutrophils with cytokines results in expression of ANCA target antigens on the cell surface. **C:** ANCAs bind to target antigens at the cell surface. **D:** Neutrophils are activated by Fc-independent and Fc-dependent events resulting in the release of toxic oxygen metabolites and degranulation of enzymes. **E:** Neutrophils adhere to endothelial cells via adhesion molecules and ligands. **F:** Additional activation occurs via interaction with ANCAs bound to antigens on endothelial cells, and endothelial cells and other vascular tissues are injured by the inflammatory events. Reprinted with permission from Jennette and Falk (67).

overt vasculitis especially in the respiratory tract. The granulomas in Wegener granulomatosis have been described by Fienberg et al. as loose granulomas with multinucleated giant cells and palisading leukocytes (60). These granulomas are dissimilar from the compact granulomas of sarcoid or tuberculosis. Outside the respiratory tract, the vascular inflammation of Wegener granulomatosis is identical to that of microscopic polyangiitis.

Microscopic polyangiitis, sometimes called microscopic polyarteritis, is defined as necrotizing vasculitis, with few or no immune deposits, affecting small vessels (capillaries, venules, or arterioles) (10,52,61). Necrotizing arteritis involving small and medium-sized arteries may also be present in the form of aneurysmal dilatation of medium-sized arteries in the setting of coexistent capillaritis or venulitis included under the definition of microscopic polyangiitis (see Fig. 1). It is important to note that many patients with microscopic polyangiitis have involvement of arteritis, venules, and capillaries, but not arteries. In such patients, the term microscopic polyarteritis is not appropriate. Necrotizing glomerulonephritis is very common in this condition, as is pulmonary capillaritis. In the acute phase of this lesion, the injury is characterized histologically by fibrinoid necrosis and neutrophil infiltration, occasionally with a thrombotic process. Neutrophils typically undergo karyorrhexis (leukocytoclasia). In all of these lesions, the chronic picture is that of a mononuclear leukocyte infiltration with fibrosis. The glomerular lesions of microscopic polyangiitis, Wegener granulomatosis, and Churg–Strauss syndrome are pathologically identical and are all characterized by segmental fibrinoid necrosis and crescent formation.

Churg–Strauss syndrome is defined by the presence of granulomatous inflammation and vasculitis in patients with a history of asthma and eosinophilia (62,63). The histologic lesions are often eosinophil rich, yet the necrotizing vasculitis and glomerulonephritis of this syndrome are identical in histology in microscopic polyangiitis or Wegener granulomatosis. Infiltrating eosinophils also are found in patients with Wegener granulomatosis and microscopic polyangiitis, but tend to be more conspicuous in patients with Churg–Strauss syndrome. From a clinical perspective, the nephritis in Churg–Strauss syndrome is much less prominent and the pulmonary lesions are more noticeable.

MEDIUM-SIZED VASCULITIDES

Necrotizing arteritis can be produced not only by microscopic polyangiitis, Wegener granulomatosis, and Churg–Strauss syndrome, but also by polyarteritis nodosa and Kawasaki disease. Classic polyarteritis nodosa is an uncommon form of vasculitis according to definitions agreed upon in the Chapel Hill Nomenclature Consensus Conference: that is, necrotizing vasculitis involving arteries alone and not capillaries or venules. This arteritis is characterized by a segmental fibrinoid necrosis. The arterial lesions of polyarteritis nodosa and microscopic polyangiitis are indistinguishable on histologic examination. The necrotizing injury to the medium-sized vessel walls results in aneurysm formation seen on radiographic studies. The clinical features of this disease are that of pain, hypertension, and/or massive intraperitoneal hemorrhage as a consequence of rupture of an aneurysm. By definition, glomerulonephritis or tubulointerstitial nephritis is not found in classic polyarteritis nodosa (64–66). Especially in Europe, classic polyarteritis nodosa is associated with antibodies to hepatitis B (64).

Kawasaki disease, another medium-sized vasculitis, is also known as the cutaneous lymph node syndrome and is typically found in children (9). This disease involves coronary arteries far more often than other forms of vasculitis. The renal artery is involved in one-fourth of patients. There is evidence for both aneurysm dilatation as well as stenosis. The progressive combination of acute edema and infiltration by neutrophils and monocytes results in progressive arterial scarring with stenosis and aneurysm formation. The clinical process is manifest by fever, lymphadenopathy, and mucocutaneous inflammation. A useful differential diagnostic observation is that polyarteritis nodosa and Kawasaki disease are ANCA negative, whereas microscopic polyangiitis and Wegener granulomatosis are ANCA positive.

PATHOGENESIS OF SMALL VESSEL VASCULITIS

ANCAs Are Pathogenic: The Hypothesis

The pathogenesis of necrotizing small vessel vasculitis and glomerulonephritis is still not known. The pauci-immune necrotizing and crescentic vascular diseases are marked by the absence or paucity of immune-complex deposition and, as such, it is difficult to implicate classic mechanisms of immune-complex-mediated damage. There is no evidence that immune complexes are deposited from the circulation or that there is an antigen deposited within the part of the vessel wall that subsequently elicits an antibody response. What is it, then, that results in the activation of leukocytes, their interaction with the endothelium, margination, and subsequent penetration through the vascular wall? Since the necrotizing vasculitides are marked by the accumulation of polymorphonuclear leukocytes in the early phase of the disease, it is interesting to speculate that neutrophils are drawn to the endothelium by factors other than immune deposits.

At least three different hypotheses relate ANCAs to the pathogenesis of vasculitis. Substantial in vitro data suggest that both MPO ANCAs and PR3 ANCAs activate normal human polymorphonuclear leukocytes (67–69) (Fig. 4). This interaction results in a respiratory burst and degranulation of primary and secondary granule constituents (69,70). Interestingly, the interaction of antibodies with many antigens contained within neutrophil azurophilic granules appears to result in neutrophil activation; that is, in addition to MPO ANCAs and PR3 ANCAs, antibodies to BPI, azurosidin, and elastase, among others, also activate neutrophils when these cells have been primed with a cytokine (71). Because ANCA antigens are found within the primary granule, it is necessary for these granule constituents to be expressed on the surface of the neutrophils for an antibody–antigen interaction. Indeed, under the influence of cytokines such as tumor necrosis factor α (TNF-α) or peptides such as formyl-methionine, ANCA antigens are rapidly translocated to the polymorphonuclear leukocyte cell surface (69,72,73). The expression of these proteins occurs within seconds and allows for antibody–antigen interaction. Interestingly, in patients with active Wegener glomerulonephritis, ANCA antigens are found more commonly on the surface of cells in vivo than in disease remission or in control populations (73). These in vivo observations lend credence to the possibility that ANCA antigens are made available for antibody binding.

Whether neutrophil activation is a consequence of ANCA binding to Fc-receptor-IIα engagement or due to the binding of the Fab$'_2$ portion of ANCA has been carefully analyzed and is the subject of substantial controversy. Several investigators have suggested that the Fab$'_2$ portion of the molecule can activate cytokine-primed neutrophils (69,74), whereas others suggest that the Fc portion of the molecule is more important (75,76). While ANCA-associated Fc-receptor-IIα receptor engagement certainly occurs, blockade of this receptor with specific antibody inhibits ANCA-induced neutrophil activation by $<30\%$ (77). Carefully prepared Fab$'_2$ fragments are able to induce neutrophil activation, whereas the Fab fragment alone does not. Neutrophils can be activated by Fab portions of either PR3 ANCAs or MPO ANCAs that are cross-linked. Curiously, Fab$'_2$ fragments are capable of inducing a superoxide production to a greater extent

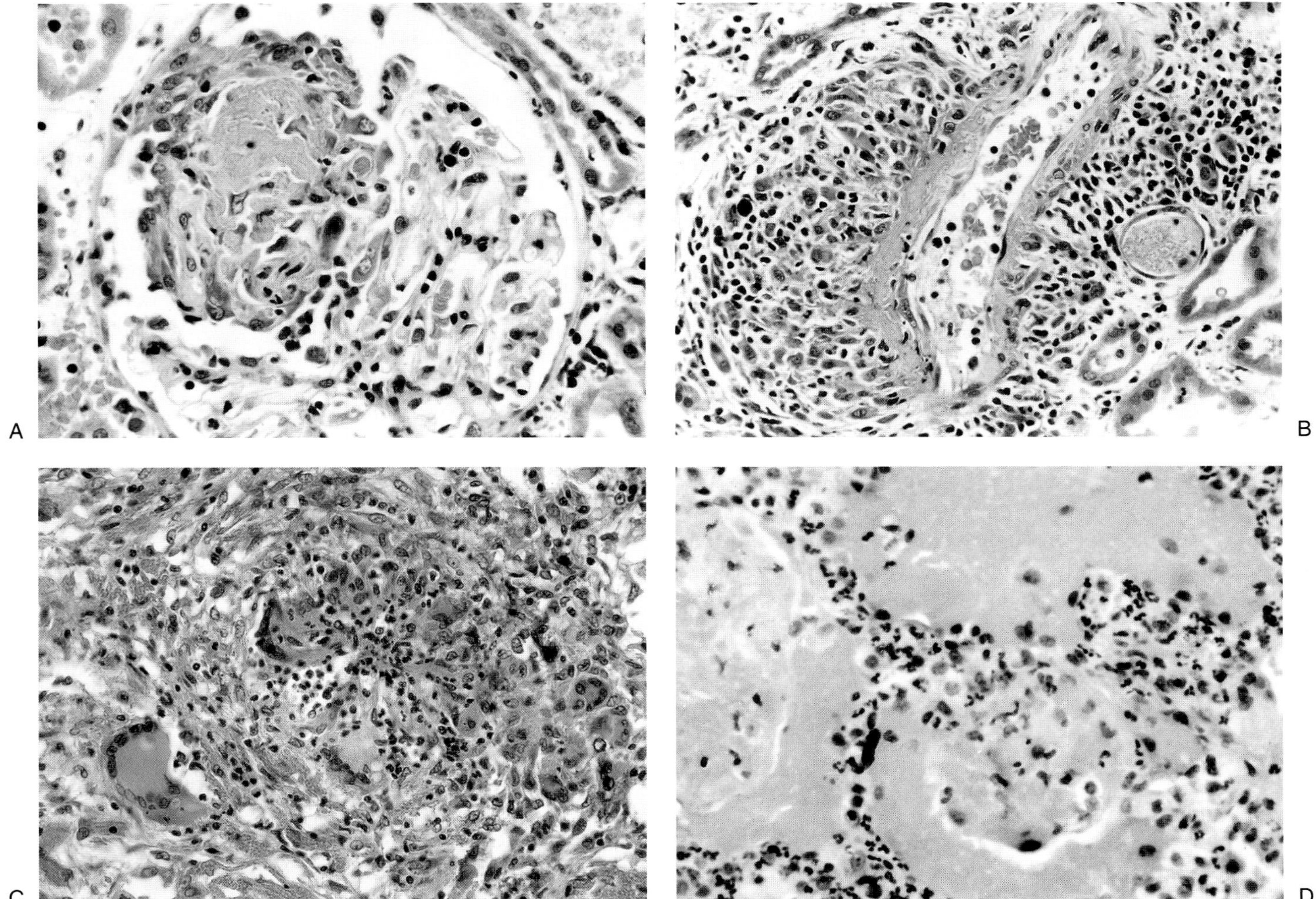

FIG. 4. A: Glomerulus with segmental fibrinoid necrosis and slight crescent formation. **B:** Small artery with segmental fibrinoid necrosis and adjacent inflammatory cell infiltration. **C:** Necrotizing granulomatous inflammation in the lung with scattered multinucleated giant cells. **D:** Pulmonary alveolar capillaritis with intra-alveolar hemorrhage. Note the numerous neutrophils in the alveolar septa. Reprinted with permission from Jennette and Falk (13).

than is the intact molecule. The cause of this phenomenon is not clear, but may be due to the presence of naturally occurring anti-Fab′$_2$ molecules in the circulation of patients with autoimmune diseases.

Upon ANCA-induced neutrophil activation, neutrophils are capable of interacting with and damaging endothelial cells in culture (78,79). This interaction occurs via the CD11/CD18 integrin pathway, resulting in endothelial cell damage (80). In an in vivo model of dermal vascular permeability in rats, ANCA-induced neutrophil activation resulted in increased albumin permeability as well as the accumulation of leukocytes. However, no histologic damage was evident in these dermal vessels (81).

An alternative theory for the pathogenic mechanism of ANCA-induced endothelial damage suggests that ANCA antigens are planted along the endothelium at the time of neutrophil activation. These antigens are able to interact with antibody in a manner analogous to a planted antigen with in situ immune-complex formation. Because the surfaces of endothelial cells are anionic, cationic proteins such as MPO and PR3 can bind to their surfaces and can be recognized by ANCAs. This hypothesis has gained credence from studies using rats preimmunized with human ANCA antigens. PR3 or MPO is perfused into the renal artery along with hydrogen peroxide and other granule enzymes, resulting in glomerulonephritis (82, 83). Much controversy exists as to whether this is a model of immune-complex disease or parallels the human pauci-immune condition. Brouwer et al. contend that, in this model, immune complexes disappear over the course of 10 days, depending upon the strain of animal used (82,83). Yang et al. have countered this observation by demonstrating that immune complexes persist for up to 10 days, and the degree of injury in the glomerulus closely corresponds to the degree of immunofluorescence localization of immunoglobulins (84). It comes as no surprise that planting an antigen along the GBM in a previously immunized animal would result in immune-complex formation.

A third possible pathogenic role for ANCAs stems from the observations that PR3 may be expressed by cytokine-treated human umbilical vein endothelial cells (85). If these cells are capable of producing ANCA antigens themselves during intense inflammatory stimulation, then ANCAs could bind to endogenous endothelial antigens, resulting in an immune-complex disease or direct antibody-dependent cell cytotoxicity (86,87). Even these observations have been challenged, as other investigators have not found PR3 mRNA in endothelium (88).

If PR3 is not endogenously made by endothelium, it is possible that PR3 released by the neutrophil activation could cause direct endothelial damage. PR3 causes detachment and cytolysis of human endothelial cells (89) and induces endothelial cells to produce interleukin 8, (90). PR3 and elastase, but not MPO, induce endothelial apoptosis in both a time- and dose-dependent fashion (91).

No single pathogenic hypothesis has led to the development of an animal model. More than one of these hypothetical pathogenic pathways might be occurring congruently.

Antiendothelial Cells

Antiendothelial cell antibodies (AECAs) have been found in the circulation of patients with systemic vasculitis, especially in Kawasaki disease (92). Whether AECAs in Kawasaki disease are pathogenic has been recently called into question. Nash et al. (93) observed that AECAs were present in a proportion of Kawasaki disease patients, as well as febrile controls, and that there were no differences in the presence of AECAs with or without coronary artery aneurysms. Similar controversy surrounds the issue of whether AECAs are found in patients with pauci-immune necrotizing vasculitis (94). Whereas AECAs have different reactivities from ANCAs (95), there is very little evidence for AECAs in either microscopic polyangiitis or Wegener granulomatosis (96). One may conjecture that some AECAs may be a consequence of the in vitro interaction of antibodies to PR3 with human umbilical vein endothelial cells (97). Alternatively, an AECA has been proposed that shares epitopes of autoantibodies that react with a lysosomal membrane glycoprotein H-LAMP-2 in neutrophil granulocytes (that is, an ANCA) and to a similar membrane protein on glomerular endothelial cells (98). This intriguing possibility raises the speculation that ANCAs may cross-react with endothelial cells and this cross-reactivity causes endothelial cell damage.

The α_1-Antitrypsin Story

α_1-Antitrypsin is the natural inhibitor of PR3, and the elastalytic effects of PR3 activity on endothelial cells and other tissue elements might be enhanced in the setting of α_1-antitrypsin deficiency. α_1-Antitrypsin is complexed to PR3 even during isolation of PR3 (99). Several reports now suggest that severe α_1-antitrypsin deficiency is associated with C-ANCAs and Wegener granulomatosis and necrotizing glomerulonephritis (100–102). The absolute amount of α_1-antitrypsin may not be as important as the phenotype of the deficiency; for example, severe α_1-antitrypsin PiZ is found in patients with ANCA-associated disease substantially more often than in controls (101). There does appear to be a strong link between the α_1-antitrypsin PiZ allele and Wegener granulomatosis (103).

Interestingly, PR3 ANCAs bind to and interfere with neutrophil PR3 activity (104,105). Thus, in some ways, PR3 ANCAs behave in the same fashion as α_1-antitrypsin. One may conjecture that the presence of these antibodies would actually decrease any proteolytic effect of PR3 and thereby decrease its inflammatory potential. As of yet, it is not clear how to reconcile the observation that ANCA-associated diseases are found more frequently in the presence of α_1-antitrypsin deficiency and the observation that PR3 ANCAs also bind to the catalytic site of PR3. The development of anti-PR3 antibodies might be related to the increased propensity of unbound or uninhibited PR3 to stimulate autoantibody formation.

THE ROLE OF T CELLS

Wegener granulomatosis is characterized by granulomatous inflammation with a large mononuclear leukocyte infiltrate containing monocytes, macrophages, and CD4-positive T cells (106). Nonetheless, the target antigen of these T cells has not been elucidated. An increase in the levels of soluble interleukin-2 receptors preceding relapse has been reported in patients with Wegener granulomatosis (107,108). Lymphocytes isolated from patients with Wegener granulomatosis proliferate in response to crude neutrophil abstracts that contain PR3 (109,110). Specific assays to detect T-cell proliferation to PR3 and MPO in patients with Wegener granulomatosis have generally not been revealing. Proliferation induced by mitogens and recall antigens did not differ between patients and controls (111); however, patients with Wegener granulomatosis who were positive for PR3 ANCAs did respond more strongly to PR3 than to MPO and had higher responses to PR3 when compared with controls. Patients with MPO ANCAs did not have a similar proliferative response to MPO (112).

The roll of T cells in the pathogenesis of vascular inflammation has been explored using an animal model of mercuric-chloride-induced leukocytoclastic vasculitis.

Anti-MPO antibodies are found in Brown Norway rats that develop intestinal vasculitis 24 h after treatment. A role of T cells in the pathogenesis of early (day 4) and peak (day 17) vasculitis wants studied using a murine anti-rat T-cell receptor monoclonal antibody (113). Although this antibody completely inhibited T-cell function, it had no impact on mercuric-chloride-induced vasculitis at day 4, but did prevent it at day 17. Thus, in this model, early vasculitis may be independent of T cells (during the neutrophil dominant phase) whereas peak vasculitis is a T-cell-dependent process.

Animal Models

Several potential animal models of systemic vasculitis have been studied in which ANCAs are found (114). To date, all of these animal models fall short of replicating human pauci-immune necrotizing and crescentic glomerulonephritis or necrotizing vasculitis. As noted in the preceding section, MPO ANCAs are found in the mercuric chloride Brown Norway model of vasculitis, although in this model there is substantial polyclonal B cell activation resulting in the production of multiple autoantibodies (115). These rats develop substantial gastrointestinal vasculitis, yet it is still a matter of speculation as to whether ANCAs are pathogenetically related to the vascular inflammation.

The MRL-*lpr*/*lpr3* mouse model has been used to study ANCAs as well (116). In these mice, a systemic vasculitis developed and there were antibodies to MPO in their circulation. No proof exists that ANCAs caused the vasculitic inflammation. Monoclonal antibodies to MPO from these mice are largely polyreactive (117), yet, in a preliminary study by Harper et al. (118), one of these anti-MPO monoclonals was transferable to control mice, which developed vasculitis. These intriguing results need to be confirmed. A similar mouse strain that develops a spontaneous crescentic glomerulonephritis and vasculitis is the SCG/Kinjoh strain (119). These mice have antibodies to MPO, and the murine monoclonal antibodies can be derived from these mice that are specific for MPO. Attempts at passively transferring the disease with these antibodies have proven to be unsuccessful.

Another mouse model has been developed by Schoenfeld et al. (120,121). Mice were immunized with PR3-ANCA immunoglobulin from a patient with fulminant Wegener granulomatosis. After a 6-week interval, these mice formed both anti-idiotype antibodies (Ab1) as well as murine PR3 ANCAs (Ab2) presumably through the idiotypic network. A perivascular lymphocytic infiltrate and microabscesses were found in the lungs without evidence of granulomatous inflammation. The perivascular lymphocytic infiltration is dissimilar from necrotizing vasculitis; nonetheless, this model does suggest that the anti-idiotypic network may be capable of generating ANCAs.

CLINICAL STUDIES

Demographics

The population of patients with ANCA-associated necrotizing vasculitis has a mean age of 54 years (122), although patients as young as 2 and as old as 90 may be afflicted with this condition. The disease process is more common in Caucasians than in African-Americans, with a ratio of 7:1. Males and females are equally affected. Limited observations suggest that the ANCA-associated disease process in northern latitudes more often produces the phenotype of Wegener granulomatosis, whereas the phenotypic expression in warmer climates is more often that of microscopic polyangiitis and renal-limited necrotizing glomerulonephritis.

The initial disease onset is heralded by a flulike illness manifest by a migratory asymmetric polyarthropathy and myalgias. Frank arthritis with sinovitis is found in only 10% of patients. Fever, anorexia, and malaise are typical with the onset of the disease, which is more common in winter and early spring (122).

Clinical Features of Renal Disease

The signs and symptoms of ANCA vasculitis are extremely varied because many organs may be affected. Renal dysfunction caused by glomerulonephritis is a major feature in many patients. The typical presentation of a patient with necrotizing and crescentic glomerulonephritis is that of a rapidly progressive glomerulonephritis (53,122–125). The median serum creatinine in a series of 130 patients was 4.5 mg/dL. Hematuria is invariably present with dysmorphic red blood cells found on urinalysis as well as red cell casts. Proteinuria ranges from as low as 0.7 g to as high as 21 g (52). Most patients, however, tend to have only mild to moderate amounts of proteinuria with a mean level of 2.7 g/24 h. Although the presentation of rapidly progressive glomerulonephritis is common, some patients have very focal necrotizing lesions that manifest as asymptomatic hematuria with minimal amounts of proteinuria; other patients have a course typical of an acute nephritis. Some patients only present to medical care at the time of end-stage renal disease. It is in these individuals that a very indolent clinical course has been followed. The majority of patients with necrotizing glomerulonephritis have hypertension and, at times, hypertension that is difficult to control.

Diseases of the Respiratory Tract

Fully half of all patients with pauci-immune necrotizing glomerulonephritis have a pulmonary–renal vasculitic syndrome (52,53,122,126,127). The pulmonary process may vary from fleeting infiltrates and mild cough to life-threatening pulmonary hemorrhage. Patients with the syndrome of microscopic polyangiitis typically have a capillaritis on biopsy that results in hemoptysis and alveolar infiltrates on chest radiography. The infiltrates may be localized or diffuse, involving one or both lungs, and wax and wane over the course of days to weeks. All too often, prior to diagnosis of pulmonary vasculitis, patients have been treated with antibiotics with the presumption that the infiltrates are due to a bacterial process (128). Granulomatous inflammation usually appears on chest roentgenogram as nodules and cavities. Smaller lesions are best seen on fine-cut computed tomography.

The most worrisome complication of pulmonary–renal vasculitic syndromes is life-threatening pulmonary hemorrhage (127,129). Of patients with necrotizing glomerulonephritis, 10% have massive pulmonary hemorrhage that has a 50% mortality rate (53). Pulmonary hemorrhage is usually preceded by a history of intermittent hemoptysis, but at times explosive bleeding occurs resembling that of anti-GBM antibody-mediated Goodpasture syndrome (see Chapter 43).

In addition to the acute manifestations of pulmonary vasculitis, chronic pulmonary conditions have emerged in association with ANCAs, such as chronic interstitial pulmonary fibrosis and bronchiolitis obliterans. Some patients with end-stage renal disease have pulmonary fibrosis of uncertain etiology and then develop acute alveolar capillaritis during a relapse of ANCA-associated vasculitis.

Upper respiratory tract symptoms include bloody sinusitis and may involve an individual sinus or be manifest by pansinusitis (130). Necrotizing lesions of the nose are typically present in patients with Wegener granulomatosis, but are also found in patients with microscopic polyangiitis (52). Biopsy of these tissues is frequently nondiagnostic with acute and chronic inflammation, but occasionally necrotizing vascular inflammation is found. The classic saddle-nose deformity of patients with Wegener granulomatosis is unusual and is a consequence of inflammatory destruction of cartilage in the nose (131, 132). Blockage of eustacian tubes with granulomatous inflammation leads to serous otitis media with bacterial superinfections complicating the treatment process. Hearing loss is unfortunately all too common. Careful evaluation by ear, nose, and throat surgeons using fiberoptic visualization of the entire pharynx and posterior pharynx is essential to view the upper respiratory tract adequately and to biopsy appropriate lesions.

One of the most problematic areas of respiratory tract involvement is tracheal stenosis, usually in the subglottic region (133). Airways are blocked by unilateral or bilateral edema and inflammation often followed by fibrosis. These lesions tend to respond to treatment, but are a frequent source of stridor and dyspnea.

Other Organ Systems (Table 2)

A variety of vasculitic processes can cause concurrent renal and dermal disease (that is, renal–dermal syndrome), including systemic lupus erythematosus (SLE), Henoch–Schönlein purpura, cryoglobulinemia, and ANCA vasculitis (134,135). The clinical manifestations of dermal vasculitis are numerous. The most classic lesion is palpable purpura, usually on the lower extremities or on the hands, that waxes and wanes. More serious lesions are ulcers, which may be shallow or, when bigger vessels are involved, larger necrotizing lesions may occur. Ulcers may begin with papules or nodules that then ulcerate in their center. It is frequently difficult to ascertain whether a chronic ulcer is a consequence of untreated vasculitis or of secondary infection (136,137). Urticaria is more common than is usually appreciated.

Gastrointestinal manifestations of systemic vasculitis have been underreported. Fully one third of patients with ANCA necrotizing glomerulonephritis have gastrointestinal symptoms that most typically manifest as nonhealing gastric or peptic ulcers (52,138). Vasculitic lesions can sometimes be demonstrated by endoscopic biopsy, yet typically a presumptive diagnosis is made clinically by the favorable response to corticosteroid therapy. Vasculitis in the pancreas results in pancreatitis with abdominal pain. Widespread vasculitic lesions in the small and large intestines cause gastrointestinal bleeding and melena, yet the most dreaded complication of gastrointestinal vasculitis is perforation of a viscus with polymicrobial peritonitis and sepsis. The liver is rarely involved with necrotizing vasculitis (139). Autoimmune hepatitis and sclerosing cholangitis, however, are associated with a type of P-ANCA that is not specific for MPO (140).

The neurologic manifestations of necrotizing vasculitis are usually peripheral neuropathy with mononeuritis multiplex (138,141). Several peripheral nerves may be

TABLE 2. *Organ involvement*[a]

Organ system involvement	Number of patients	% of patients	MPA	NCGN
Total number of patients	107		69	38
Renal	107	100	69	38
Pulmonary	38	36	38	0
Upper respiratory tract	14	13	14	0
Musculoskeletal	10	9	10	0
Neurologic	9	8	9	0
Gastrointestinal	6	6	6	0
Cutaneous	13	12	13	0
Ocular	2	2	2	0

[a]MPA, microscopic polyangiitis; NCGN, necrotizing crescentic glomerulonephritis.

Reprinted with permission from Nachman et al. (52).

affected at any given time or sequentially. Nerve conduction velocities are typically abnormal, and sural nerve biopsies are useful to pinpoint the diagnosis if no histologic confirmation of a vasculitis is found elsewhere. Sural nerve biopsies are only useful if there are positive nerve conduction velocities. Rarely do patients with small vessel vasculitis have central nervous system findings. When they do, seizures are the most common manifestation. Severe hypertension or uremia must be excluded as a cause of central nervous system dysfunction. Magnetic resonance imaging findings are usually unremarkable, although nonspecific gadolinium-enhancing lesions can be observed in a diffuse pattern. Arteritis of the carotid arteries is an uncommon, but reported, complication of ANCA vasculitis (142).

Lesions of the eye are common in patients with ANCA vasculitis. Red eyes are usually the consequence of iritis and/or uveitis or sclerokeratitis (143–145). ALthough this process may be present subclinically, careful ophthalmologic examination is frequently revealing. Rarely, optic neuritis is a consequence of vascular inflammation (146).

Reproductive organs are occasionally affected, with testicular pain or prostatitis. Testicular pain is usually unilateral and can be severe.

Coronary artery disease is an uncommon manifestation of ANCA vasculitis, unlike Kawasaki disease in children in which coronary artery aneurysms are a predominant feature of the vasculitic component of the disease (147). In the generally elderly population with ANCA vasculitis, it is difficult to ascertain whether anginal-like symptoms are a consequence of atherosclerotic disease or of small vessel vasculitis. In a series of our patients (52), six died of myocardial infarction during complete remission, but four died during the active part of their disease. In these four individuals, it was difficult to prove that a myocardial infarction was attributable to vasculitis, because each patient had preexisting atherosclerotic disease.

Laboratory Findings in Patients with ANCA Vasculitis

In addition to ANCA studies, other serologic studies are of interest: 10–20% of patients will have a positive ANA, although only rare individuals will have a positive double-stranded DNA. Complement levels, that is C3 and C4, and total hemolytic complement levels are normal, as are measurements of cryoglobulins and rheumatoid factor. During disease activity, sedimentation rate and CRP level are elevated. Both the CRP level and the sedimentation rate are only approximate correlates of disease activity and may be adjunctive tests in following disease remission and relapse. Results of liver function tests are usually normal. An elevated amylase and lipase, coupled with abdominal pain, should prompt the clinician to consider the possibility of pancreatic involvement with a vasculitic process.

Differential Diagnosis

Necrotizing and crescentic glomerulonephritis may be mimicked by several other aggressive glomerular diseases. Certainly, lupus nephritis or anti-GBM disease present with a rapidly progressive glomerular disease. The problem is made more complex by the observation that ~20% of patients with anti-GBM disease with serologic evidence for anti-GBM antibodies and linear staining along the GBM also have a positive ANCA (148–150). In those individuals with evidence for anti-GBM disease, the presence of a positive ANCA increases the likelihood of a small vessel vasculitis in organs other than the kidneys and lungs. Patients with SLE may have a positive ANCA, although the P-ANCA pattern detected by indirect immunofluorescence microscopy is usually confounded by ANA. Some lupus patients do have MPO ANCAs or elastase/lactoferrin ANCAs, although the significance of these is not certain (15,41,42,151).

Pulmonary–renal vasculitic syndromes are caused by anti-GBM disease, ANCA vasculitis, and by some immune-complex vasculitides, especially severe SLE. Serologic tests and renal histology help to differentiate among these possibilities. A difficult differential diagnosis occurs in patients with ANCA-positive glomerulonephritis who develop pulmonary infiltrates without hemoptysis. A concomitant infection (especially tuberculosis or a fungal process) or an infection caused by immunosuppressive therapy must be considered. Bronchoscopic findings include or exclude an infection. Trans-scopic open-lung biopsies are useful in elucidating whether pulmonary lesions are infectious in origin or due to a necrotizing capillaritis or granulomatous inflammation. Infections of the upper respiratory tract may be difficult to differentiate from acute vasculitic inflammation. Fiber-optic transillumination of the upper airways with biopsy of affected tissues is necessary to include or exclude vascular inflammation.

Substantial confusion exists in differentiating between Henoch–Schönlein purpura and ANCA-associated renal–dermal vasculitic syndromes. The clinical syndrome of palpable purpura, hematuria, and red blood cell casts is frequently diagnosed as Henoch–Schönlein purpura, even when there is no evidence for immunoglobulin-A (IgA) deposition on skin biopsy. The age of a patient who has purpura and nephritis is useful for predicting the likelihood of Henoch–Schönlein purpura versus ANCA vasculitis. More than 80% of preadolescent children with renal–dermal vasculitic syndrome will have Henoch–Schönlein purpura, whereas >80% of adults over 60 years of age will have ANCA vasculitis. While IgA-ANCAs have been considered in Henoch–Schönlein purpura, their detection may be laboratory artifact (152). Renal biopsy allows for the differentiation of a proliferative IgA-dominant form of glomerulonephritis from pauci-immune necrotizing and crescentic glomerulonephritis. Since the treatment strategies are different for Henoch–

Schönlein purpura and in ANCA-associated pauci-immune crescentic glomerulonephritis, the differential diagnosis is critical.

Cryoglobulinemic vasculitis with nephritis and purpura, and SLE with nephritis and purpura, present in a similar fashion as ANCAs and dermal disease. The presence of a cryoglobulin in the serum is an important differentiator between ANCAs and cryoglobulinemic diseases (153). Cryoglobulinemia typically has a depressed C4, C3, and total hemolytic complement. Hypocomplementemia, positive ANA or double-stranded DNA suggest a diagnosis of SLE. For the most part, ANCA vasculitis has normal levels of C3, C4, and CH50.

Nonvasculitic vasculopathies that can mimic vasculitis include thrombotic microangiopathies and atheroembolization. Renal biopsy or biopsy of affected vessels in other tissues enables the pathologic diagnosis of these diseases.

Treatment

Immunosuppressive therapy is the mainstay of treatment for necrotizing and crescentic ANCA glomerulonephritis and systemic ANCA vasculitis (52,55,154,155). With anti-inflammatory or immunosuppressive agents, the therapy must be tailored to the size of the patient, especially with respect to body surface area. Protocol prescriptions for the care of patients with systemic vasculitis need to recognize that each individual responds differently to prednisone, cyclophosphamide, or azathioprine. Oral corticosteroids alone, once the mainstay of therapy, are not sufficient by themselves for controlling glomerular inflammation or systemic manifestations or severe vasculitis. Moreover, the risk of relapse in patients treated with oral corticosteroids when compared with intravenous or oral cyclophosphamide therapy is threefold greater than in cyclophosphamide-treated patients (52).

A typical form of therapy for necrotizing and crescentic ANCA glomerulonephritis begins with pulse methylprednisolone. The exact dose of pulse Medrol (methylprednisolone) has decreased over time from the initial recommendations of 30 mg/kg to the more typical 15-mg/kg dose (58,58a). A dose of 7 mg/kg given on 3 consecutive days is probably equally efficacious (52). Oral corticosteroids are usually given at a dose of 1 mg/kg for the first month, followed by alternate-day therapy. Alternate-day therapy is decreased by, for instance, 10 mg/week. Once the patient is on 60 mg of prednisone for a day alternating with no prednisone on the following day, the prednisone dose may again be dropped by 10/week until the corticosteroid therapy is terminated. Patients remain on corticosteroids for only 3–4 months. During this time, oral or intravenous cyclophosphamide is prescribed. Oral cyclophosphamide is typically given at a dose of 2 mg/kg/day, with the dose adjusted based on the leukocyte count obtained every 2 weeks (156,157). The leukocyte count must be carefully monitored while the patient is on tapering doses of prednisone, because the cyclophosphamide dose must be adjusted downward as the prednisone dose is decreased (158). One of the major problems associated with long-term oral cyclophosphamide therapy is that the effective dose may not be achieved as a consequence of bone-marrow suppression or bladder toxicity. Intravenous cyclophosphamide given on a monthly basis for at least the first 6 months is an alternative form of therapy (52,122). The dosage is initiated at 500 mg/$M^{2)}$ and adjusted on the basis of the 2-week leukocyte nadir. The target leukocyte count is between 3,000 and 5,000 cells/M^3. If tolerated, the dose is sequentially adjusted upward, first to 750 mg/M^2 and then up to 1 g/M^2 if the leukocyte nadir has not been appropriately decreased.

The optimum length of therapy for either oral or intravenous cyclophosphamide has not been determined. Initial therapy for Wegener granulomatosis often has been continued for as long as 2 years (158), although treatment for 6–12 months may have comparable results.

The side effects of intravenous versus oral cyclophosphamide appear to be different. Hemorrhagic cystitis is found in <10% of patients who remain adequately hydrated on oral cyclophosphamide. With intravenous cyclophosphamide, hemorrhagic cystitis is extremely uncommon. Infections, both minor and major, are a consequence of either form of therapy. Because the total dose of cyclophosphamide with oral medications amounts to roughly three times that given with intravenous cyclophosphamide, it is no surprise that the rate of infection with intravenous cyclophosphamide is typically one-third of that in oral cyclophosphamide-treated patients. The issue of long-term malignancy, especially transitional cell carcinoma of the bladder and lymphoma, remains a devastating fear for patients treated with an alkylating agent (159). In the long-term study of Wegener granulomatosis conducted by the National Institutes of Health, 15% of patients developed a transitional cell carcinoma of the bladder (160). Whether the same frequency will occur in patients treated with intravenous cyclophosphamide has yet to be determined. An additional complication of either form of cyclophosphamide is gonadal toxicity. This is more common in patients who are perimenopausal or over the age of 35. Cyclophosphamide is not as much of a danger in adolescents who have not undergone puberty. Whether leuprolite acetate serves to protect ovarian function during the course of intravenous cyclophosphamide therapy remains a subject of investigation.

Alternative Treatment Strategies

Because of the complications of cyclophosphamide therapy, alternative strategies have been proposed. In the United Kingdom, oral cyclophosphamide is only continued for 3 months and then azathioprine at a dose of 2 mg/kg is administered and continued for an indefinite period (154,161).

Recently, Hoffman et al. have suggested that methotrexate is a useful therapy for systemic vasculitis (162). Although corticosteroids and methotrexate have yet to be compared in a prospective trial with cyclophosphamide, fewer side effects are associated with this approach. Unfortunately, methotrexate is not useful in patients with serum creatinine of >2 mg/dL prior to the onset of therapy, because of the risk of substantial side effects.

Several prospective trials have been conducted with plasma exchange and rapidly progressive glomerulonephritis and systemic vasculitis (163–165a). There does not appear to be any benefit with this form of therapy, except in patients who are dialysis dependent at the onset of therapy (165). In this study, pulse methylprednisolone was not used, and thus it is not clear whether plasmapheresis has an additional beneficial effect in steroid-treated patients. Without documented evidence of efficacy, most investigators regard plasmapheresis as useful only in patients with life-threatening pulmonary hemorrhage.

Pooled intravenous γ-globulin contains anti-idiotypes for both MPO and PR3 ANCAs (50). Pooled intravenous γ-globulin therapy has been tried with reported success in an anecdotal fashion for induction therapy as well as in those patients resistant to cyclophosphamide therapy (166–168). The efficacy of this approach has yet to be proven in a controlled fashion.

Trimethoprin–sulfamethoxazole has been touted as beneficial in the treatment of Wegener granulomatosis with local–regional involvement in the upper airways or the lungs (169). A brief trial of trimethoprin–sulfamethoxazole may be warranted to treat nasal vasculitic inflammation.

Treatment Resistance

Treatment resistance is defined as the progressive decline in renal function with the persistence of an active urine sediment, or persistence or new appearance of any extrarenal manifestation of vasculitis despite immunosuppressive therapy (52). Using this definition, the majority of patients with resistant renal disease arrive at the time of diagnosis with an elevated serum creatinine, glomerulosclerosis, and interstitial fibrosis on renal biopsy, and rapidly require dialysis. These patients are at or near end-stage disease. Additional aggressive immunosuppressive therapy will not result in recovery of life-sustaining renal function.

A more troubling group of patients are those who have an explosive clinical picture with pulmonary hemorrhage and a rapidly rising serum creatinine. These patients have an extremely high mortality rate, so immunosuppressive therapy must begin promptly, including plasmapheresis or pulse Medrol and the use of intravenous or oral cyclophosphamide. Since death from this disease may occur in days to weeks, prompt diagnosis and the earliest institution of aggressive therapy are warranted.

A third category of patients with resistant disease are those in whom intravenous or oral cyclophosphamide has been administered, but who have never responded to this drug with a lowering of the white blood count to between 3,000 and 5,000 cells/M^3. In these patients, higher amounts of oral or intravenous cyclophosphamide, or more frequent dosing at every 2 or even every 3 weeks, may be necessary to bring the disease process into remission. Patients resistant to oral cyclophosphamide are usually resistant to intravenous cyclophosphamide.

A very small group of patients [three (2.5%) of 121] are truly resistant to standard immunosuppressive therapy. These individuals begin with low serum creatinine values and have a progressive course despite adequate doses of corticosteroids and intravenous or oral cyclophosphamide. The therapy of this group of patients is currently under investigation. Alternative treatments include pooled intravenous γ-globulin or, if this fails, the use of humanized antibodies to anti-CD4 and anti-CD52 (monoclonal antilymphocyte antibodies) (170).

ANCA Titers and Disease

The value of ANCA serologic testing during management of patients with ANCA vasculitis and clinical course is still a matter of discussion (171,172). There is but a single prospective study examining the prevention of relapse using ANCA titers to dictate immunosuppressive therapy that demonstrated fewer episodes of clinical relapse (173). Serologic testing using enzyme-linked immunosorbent assays with purified MPO or PR3 suggests that ANCA titers correlate with disease activity (174). In general, ANCA titer increases during exacerbation and decreases during disease quiescence, although there are numerous exceptions to this general statement. In some patients, ANCA titers remain elevated despite disease quiescence, or ANCA titers may rise for months before there is any evidence of clinical disease activity. A rapid rise in ANCA titer, however, most likely signifies recurrence of disease activity. When ANCA-positive patients no longer have detectable ANCAs and then develop a renewed ANCA response, clinical relapse is likely to occur. Nevertheless, most clinicians would not treat a patient on the basis of a serologic abnormality, but rather would rely on recognized signs or symptoms of the disease relapse.

Renal Prognosis

Several statistical analyses have been applied to populations of patients with necrotizing glomerulonephritis

TABLE 3. *Predictors of disease-related death*[a]

Predictor	Relative risk of death[b]	95% Confidence interval	p
Pulmonary hemorrhage (present versus absent)	8.64	(3.36, 22.19)	0.0002
Any pulmonary symptoms (present versus absent)	2.36	(0.80, 6.95)	0.16
Disease category (MPA versus NCGN alone)	1.68	(0.48, 5.82)	0.61
ANCA pattern (C-ANCA versus P-ANCA)	3.78	(1.22, 11.70)	0.031
Race (African American versus Caucasian)	2.41	(0.75, 7.77)	0.34
Treatment (cyclophosphamide versus corticosteroids alone)	0.18	(0.05, 0.66)	0.012

ANCA, antineutrophil cytoplasmic autoantibody (C, cytoplasmic staining pattern; P, perinuclear staining pattern); MPA, microscopic polyangiitis; NCGN, necrotizing crescentic glomerulonephritis.

Reprinted with permission from Hogan et al. (53).

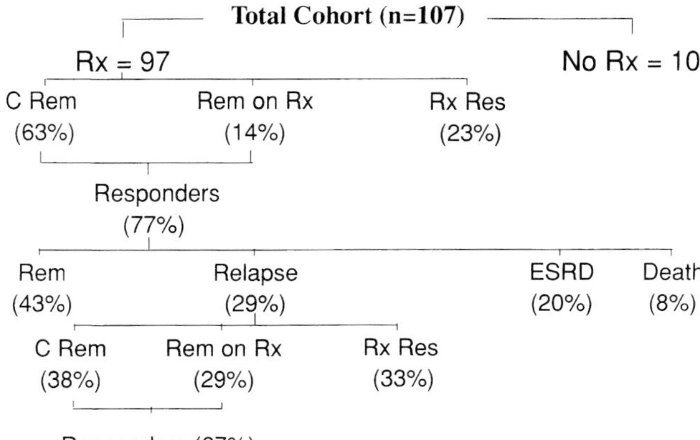

FIG. 5. The response to treatment and outcome of the 107 eligible patients with microscopic polyaniitis (MPA) and necrotizing crescentic glomerulonephritis (NCGN). Rx, treatment; C Rem, complete remission; Rem on Rx, remission on therapy; Rx Res, treatment resistant; ESRD, end-stage renal disease. Reprinted with permission from Nachman et al. (52).

and systemic vasculitis (53,175,176). Several variables, including the serum creatinine, renal biopsy finding (especially tubulointerstitial nephritis), and even an elevated white blood count, have been proposed as prognostic markers. A recent multivariate analysis suggested that the entry serum creatinine was the most important long-term predictor of renal function when variables such as age, pathology indices, microscopic polyangiitis versus renal-limited necrotizing glomerulonephritis, or pulmonary versus no pulmonary findings were measured (53) (Table 3). African-American patients have a much poorer prognosis than Caucasians, even though African-Americans are only rarely affected by this disease. Of all of the pathology indices, interstitial fibrosis on renal biopsy proved to be an important independent risk factor in individuals with an entry creatinine of <3 mg/dL. When serum creatinines were >4.5 mg/dL, however, tubulointerstitial sclerosis by itself was no longer a predictor, whereas the entry serum creatinine continued to be a poor prognostic variable.

Relapses

Even though treatment using oral corticosteroids with either intravenous or oral cyclophosphamide result in complete long-term remission in 70–75% of patients, relapse occurs in ≥25% within a mean of 18 months after therapy is stopped (52) (Fig. 5). Relapse during therapy should raise the question of the adequacy of therapy vis-à-vis the target leukocyte count and compliance with therapy. Relapse typically occurs in the same organ system that was initially affected, although new organ systems are occasionally involved. Relapses in the lung tend to occur in exactly the same locus as the original injury, as does relapse in the upper respiratory tract. It is possible that relapse may be triggered by concomitant viral or bacterial infection, especially episodes of flulike illness. Patients should be offered influenza vaccines to decrease the possibility of recrudescence as a consequence of influenza during winter months. *Staphylococcus aureus* nasal carriage has been associated with an increased risk of relapse (177). In a recent prospective randomized control trial, cotrimazol was shown to decrease the risk of nasal relapse, but did not alter the risk of relapse in the lung or the kidney (178).

Treatment of Dialysis-Dependent Patients

Approximately 20% of patients will need medical attention requiring dialysis at the time of diagnosis and, of these, approximately half will come off dialysis with aggressive therapy within 4–8 weeks. Immunosuppressive therapy after this period increases the risk–benefit ratio, as there is little hope for restoration of renal function. Although the majority of patients who can discontinue dialysis will have a slow decline in their renal function, the dialysis-free interval may last for up to 3 years. Patients should participate in the decision as to whether this dialysis-free interval is worth the risk of 2–3 months of high-dose immunosuppressive therapy.

Transplantation

Recurrence of glomerulonephritis or vasculitis after renal transplantation has been reported, albeit in a very small number of patients (179–183). Recurrences are not confined to the kidney, as there are well-reported cases of recurrence of Wegener granulomatosis with tracheal stenosis (184) or with pulmonary disease, including granulomatous inflammation as well as pulmonary hemorrhage from capillaritis (182).

One of the most perplexing questions confronting clinicians regards the ANCA titer status prior to renal transplantation. To date, there are no good longitudinal data to suggest whether or not the ANCA titer must normalize prior to renal transplantation. In general, however, renal transplantation should be avoided in those patients in whom there is clinical evidence of active vasculitis, in a patient with persistently negative ANCA titers who becomes ANCA positive, or in the setting of a rapidly rising ANCA titer.

REFERENCES

1. Kussmaul A, Maier R. Ueber eine bisher Nicht beschriebene eigenthümniche arteriener Krankung (Periarteritis Nodosa) die mit Morbis Birghtii und rapid fortschreitender allgemeiner, Muskellähmung einhergeht. *Dtsch Arch Klin Med* 1866;1:484.
2. Ferrari E. Ueber Polyarteriitis Acuta Nodosa (sogenannte Periarteritis Nodosa) und ihre Beziehungen zur Polymyositis und Polyneuritis Acuta. *Beitr Pathol Anat* 1903;34:350–86.
3. Davson J, Ball J, Platt R. The kidney in periarteritis nodosa. *Q J Med* 1948;17:175–202.
4. Klinger N. Grenzformen der periarteritis nodosa. *Frankfurt Z Pathol* 1931;42:455–80.
5. Wegener F. Ueber generalisierte, septische Gefaserkrankungen. *Verh Dtsch Pathol Ges* 1936;29:202–9.
6. Zeek PM. Periarteritis nodosa: a critical review. *Am J Clin Pathol* 1952;22:777.
7. Godman GC, Churg J. Wegener's granulomatosis: pathology and review of the literature. *Arch Pathol* 1954;58:533–53.
8. Jennette JC, Falk RJ, Andrassy K, et al. Nomenclature of systemic vasculitides: proposal of an international consensus conference. *Arthritis Rheum* 1994;37:187–92.
9. Shackelford PG, Strauss AW. Kawasaki syndrome. *N Engl J Med* 1991;324:1664–6.
10. Jennette JC, Wilkman AS, Falk RJ. Anti-neutrophil cytoplasmic autoantibody-associated glomerulonephritis and vasculitis. *Am J Pathol* 1989;135:921–30.
11. Scott DG, Bacon PA, Elliott PJ, Tribe CR, Wallington TB. Systemic vasculitis in a district general hospital 1972–1980: clinical and laboratory features, classification and prognosis of 80 cases. *Q J Med* 1982;51:292–311.
12. Scott D, Watts R. Classification and epidemology of systemic vasculitis. *Br J Rheumatol* 1994;33:897–900.
13. Jennette JC, Falk RJ. Antineutrophil cytoplasmic autoantibodies and associated diseases: a review. *Am J Kidney Dis* 1990;15:517–29.
14. Nuyts G, Van Vlem E, De Vos A, et al. Wegener granulomatosis is associated to exposure to silicon compounds: a case–control study. *Nephrol Dial Transplant* 1995;10:1–4.
15. Gregorini G, Ferioli A, Donato F, et al. Association between silica exposure and necrotizing crescentic glomerulonephritis with p-ANCA and anti-MPO antibodies: a hospital-based case–control study. *Adv Exp Med Biol* 1993;336:435–40.
16. Dolman KM, Gans RO, Vervaat TJ, et al. Vasculitis and antineutrophil cytoplasmic autoantibodies associated with propylthiouracil therapy. *Lancet* 1993;342:651–2.
17. Nassberger L, Sjoholm AG, Jonsson H, Sturfelt G, Akesson A. Autoantibodies against neutrophil cytoplasm components in systemic lupus erythematosus and in hydralazine-induced lupus. *Clin Exp Immunol* 1990;81:380–3.
18. Westburg G, Johansson AC, Nassberger L, Sjoholm A, Bjorck S. Rising titers of IgG anti-MPO in patients with healed necrotizing glomerulonephritis caused by hydralazine. In: *Third International Workshop on ANCA* 1990 (Abstr).
19. Devogelaer JP, Pirson Y, Vandenbroucke JM, Cosyns JP, Brichard S, Nagant de Deuxchaisnes C. D-penicillamine induced crescentic glomerulonephritis: report and review of the literature. *J Rheumatol* 1987;14:1036–41.
20. Spencer SJ, Burns A, Gaskin G, Pusey CD, Rees AJ. HLA class II specificities in vasculitis with antibodies to neutrophil cytoplasmic antigens. *Kidney Int* 1992;41:1059–63.
21. Hagen EC SC, D'Amaro J. Decreased frequency of HLA-DR13DR6 in Wegener's granulomatosis. *Kidney Int* 1995;48:801–5.
22. Davies DJ, Moran JE, Niall JF, Ryan GB. Segmental necrotising glomerulonephritis with antineutrophil antibody: possible arbovirus aetiology. *BMJ* 1982;285:606.
23. Van der Woude FJ, Rasmussen N, Lobatto S, et al. Autoantibodies against neutrophils and monocytes: tool for diagnosis and marker of disease activity in Wegener's granulomatosis. *Lancet* 1985;1:425–9.
24. Falk RJ, Jennette JC. Anti-neutrophil cytoplasmic autoantibodies with specificity for myeloperoxidase in patients with systemic vasculitis and idiopathic necrotizing and crescentic glomerulonephritis. *N Engl J Med* 1988;318:1651–7.
25. Hagen EC, Ballieux BE, van Es LA, Daha MR, van der Woude FJ. Antineutrophil cytoplasmic autoantibodies: a review of the antigens involved, the assays, and the clinical and possible pathogenetic consequences. *Blood* 1993;81:1996–2002.
26. Charles LA, Falk RJ, Jennette JC. Reactivity of antineutrophil cytoplasmic autoantibodies with mononuclear phagocytes. *J Leukoc Biol* 1992;51:65–8.
27. Niles JL, Pan GL, Collins AB, et al. Antigen-specific radioimmunoassays for anti-neutrophil cytoplasmic antibodies in the diagnosis of rapidly progressive glomerulonephritis. *J Am Soc Nephrol* 1991;2: 27–36.
28. Rao NV, Wehner NG, Marshall BC, Gray WR, Gray BH, Hoidal JR. Characterization of proteinase-3 (PR-3), a neutrophil serine proteinase: structural and functional properties. *J Biol Chem* 1991;266: 9540–8.
29. Ludemann J, Utecht B, Gross WL. Anti-neutrophil cytoplasm antibodies in Wegener's granulomatosis recognize an elastinolytic enzyme. *J Exp Med* 1990;171:357–62.
30. Jennette JC, Hoidal JR, Falk RJ. Specificity of anti-neutrophil cytoplasmic autoantibodies for proteinase 3 [Letter; comment]. *Blood* 1990;75:2263–4.
31. Jenne DE, Tschopp J, Ludemann J, Utecht B, Gross WL. Wegener's autoantigen decoded [Letter]. *Nature* 1990;346:520.
32. Zhao MH, Jones SJ, Lockwood CM. Bactericidal/permeability-increasing protein (BPI) is an important antigen for anti-neutrophil cytoplasmic autoantibodies (ANCA) in vasculitis. *Clin Exp Immunol* 1995;99:49–56.
33. Yang JJ, Tuttle R, Falk RJ, Jennette JC. Frequency of anti-bactericidal/permeability-increasing protein (BPI) and anti-azurocidin in patients with renal disease. *Clin Exp Immunol* 1996 (in press).
34. Sinico RA, Gregorini G, Radice A, et al. Clinical significance of autoantibodies to myeloperoxidase in vasculitic syndromes. *Contrib Nephrol* 1991;94:31–7.
35. Cohen Tervaert JW, Goldschmeding R, Elema JD, et al. Autoantibodies against myeloid lysosomal enzymes in crescentic glomerulonephritis. *Kidney Int* 1990;37:799–806.
36. Ten RM, Pease LR, McKean DJ, Bell MP, Gleich GJ. Molecular cloning of the human eosinophil peroxidase: evidence for the existence of a peroxidase multigene family. *J Exp Med* 1989;169: 1757–69.
37. Klebanoff SJ. Oxygen metabolism and the toxic properties of phagocytes. *Ann Intern Med* 1980;93:480–9.
38. Mulder AHL, Broekroelofs J, Horst G, Limburg PC, Nelis GF, Kallenberg CGM. Anti-neutrophil cytoplasmic antibodies (ANCA) in inflammatory bowl disease: characterization and clinical correlates. *Clin Exp Immunol* 1994;95:490–7.
39. Coremans IE, Hagen EC, van der Voort EA, van der Woude FJ, Daha

MR, Breedveld FC. Autoantibodies to neutrophil cytoplasmic enzymes in Felty's syndrome. *Clin Exp Rheumatol* 1993;11:255–62.
40. Jennette JC, Falk RJ. Antineutrophil cytoplasmic autoantibodies in inflammatory bowel disease. *Am J Clin Pathol* 1993;99:221–3.
41. Cambridge G, Wallace H, Bernstein RM, Leaker B. Autoantibodies to myeloperoxidase in idiopathic and drug-induced systemic lupus erythematosus and vasculitis. *Br J Rheumatol* 1994;33:109–14.
42. Schnabel A, Csernok E, Isenberg DA, Mrowka C, Gross WL. Antineutrophil cytoplasmic antibodies in systemic lupus erythematosus: prevalence, specificities, and clinical significance. *Arthritis Rheum* 1995;38:633–7.
43. Coremans IE, Hagen EC, Daha MR, et al. Antilactoferrin antibodies in patients with rheumatoid arthritis are associated with vasculitis. *Arthritis Rheum* 1992;35:1466–75.
44. Cohen Tervaert JW, Mulder L, Stegeman C, et al. Occurrence of autoantibodies to human leucocyte elastase in Wegener's granulomatosis and other inflammatory disorders. *Ann Rheum Dis* 1993;52:115–20.
45. Wilde CG, Snable JL, Griffith JE, Scott RW. Characterization of two azurophil granule proteases with active-site homology to neutrophil elastase. *J Biol Chem* 1990;265:2038–41.
46. Falk RJ, Becker M, Terrell R, Jennette JC. Anti-myeloperoxidase autoantibodies react with native but not denatured myeloperoxidase. *Clin Exp Immunol* 1992;89:274–8.
47. Roberts DE, Peebles C, Curd JG, Tan EM, Rubin RL. Autoantibodies to native myeloperoxidase in patients with pulmonary hemorrhage and acute renal failure. *J Clin Immunol* 1991;11:389–97.
48. Royal MO, Reisner HM, Jennette JC, Falk RJ. Mapping immunodominant epitopes of myeloperoxidase. *Clin Exp Immunol* 1995;101 (Suppl 1):36(abst).
49. Nachman PH, Reisner HM, Yang JJ, Jennette JC, Falk RJ. Shared idiotypy among patients with myeloperoxidase–ANCA-associated glomerulonephritis and vasculitis. *Lab Invest* 1996;
50. Jayne DR, Esnault VL, Lockwood CM. Anti-idiotype antibodies to anti-myeloperoxidase autoantibodies in patients with systemic vasculitis. *J Autoimmun* 1993;6:221–6.
51. Kallenberg CGM, Brouwer E, Weening JJ, Cohen Tervaert JW. Antineutrophil cytoplasmic antibodies: current diagnostic and pathophysiological potential. *Kidney Int* 1994;46:1–15.
52. Nachman PH, Hogan SL, Jennette JC, Falk RJ. Treatment response and relapse in ANCA-associated microscopic polyangiitis and glomerulonephritis. *J Am Soc Nephrol* 1996;7:33–9.
53. Hogan SL, Nachman PH, Wilkman AS, Jennette JC, Falk RJ, and the Glomerular Disease Collaborative Network. Prognostic markers in patients with ANCA-associated microscopic polyangiitis and glomerulonephritis. *J Am Soc Nephrol* 1996;7:23–32.
54. Hagen EC. Development and standardization of solid-phase assays for the detection of antineutrophil cytoplasmic antibodies (ANCA) for clinical application: report of a large clinical evaluation study. *Clin Exp Immunol* 1995;101(Suppl 1):29.
55. Cohen P, Guillevin L, Baril L, Lhote F, Noel LH, Lesavre P. Persistence of antineutrophil cytoplasmic antibodies (ANCA) in asymptomatic patients with systemic polyarteritis nodosa or Churg–Strauss syndrome: follow-up of 53 patients. *Clin Exp Rheumatol* 1995;13: 193–8.
56. Falk RJ, Jennette JC. A nephrological view of the classification of vasculitis [Review]. *Adv Exp Med Biol* 1993;336:197–208.
57. Cohen Tervaert JW, Elema JD, Kallenberg CG. Clinical and histopathological association of 29kD-ANCA and MPO-ANCA. *APMIS Suppl* 1990;19:35.
58. Stilmant MM, Bolton WK, Sturgill BC, Schmitt GW, Couser WG. Crescentic glomerulonephritis without immune deposits: clinicopathologic features. *Kidney Int* 1979;15:184–95.
58a. Bolton WK, Couser WG. Pulse intravenous methylprednisolone therapy of acute crescentic rapidly progressive glomerulonephritis. *Am J Med* 1979;66:495–502.
59. Jennette JC, Falk RJ. The pathology of vasculitis involving the kidney. *Am J Kidney Dis* 1994;24:130–41.
60. Fienberg R, Mark EJ, Goodman M, McCluskey RT, Niles JL. Correlation of antineutrophil cytoplasmic antibodies with the extrarenal histopathology of Wegener's (pathergic) granulomatosis and related forms of vasculitis. *Hum Pathol* 1993;24:160–8.
61. Savage CO, Winearls CG, Evans DJ, Rees AJ, Lockwood CM. Microscopic polyarteritis: presentation, pathology and prognosis. *Q J Med* 1985;56:467–83.
62. Churg J. Nomenclature of vasculitic syndromes: a historical perspective. *Am J Kidney Dis* 1991;18:148–53.
63. Specks U, DeRemee RA. Granulomatous vasculitis: Wegener's granulomatosis and Churg–Strauss syndrome. *Rheum Dis Clin North Am* 1990;16:377–97.
64. Guillevin L, Lhote F, Jarrousse B, et al. Polyarteritis nodosa related to hepatitis B virus: a retrospective study of 66 patients [Review]. *Ann Med Interne (Paris)* 1992;143(Suppl 1):63–74.
65. Guillevin L, Visser H, Noel LH, et al. Antineutrophil cytoplasm antibodies in systemic polyarteritis nodosa with and without hepatitis B virus infection and Churg–Strauss syndrome: 62 patients. *J Rheumatol* 1993;20:1345–9.
66. Godeau P, Guillevin L, Bletry O, Wechsler B. Periarteritis nodosa associated with hepatitis B virus: 42 cases [in French; author's translation]. *Nouv Presse Med* 1981;10:1289–92.
67. Jennette JC, Falk RJ. Pathogenic potential of anti-neutrophil cytoplasmic autoantibodies. *Lab Invest* 1994;70:135–7.
68. Keogan MT, Esnault VL, Green AJ, Lockwood CM, Brown DL. Activation of normal neutrophils by anti-neutrophil cytoplasm antibodies. *Clin Exp Immunol* 1992;90:228–34.
69. Falk RJ, Terrell RS, Charles LA, Jennette JC. Anti-neutrophil cytoplasmic autoantibodies induce neutrophils to degranulate and produce oxygen radicals in vitro. *Proc Natl Acad Sci U S A* 1990;87:4115–9.
70. Brouwer E, Huitema MG, Mulder AH, et al. Neutrophil activation in vitro and in vivo in Wegener's granulomatosis. *Kidney Int* 1944;45: 1120–31.
71. Charles LA, Caldas ML, Falk RJ, Terrell RS, Jennette JC. Antibodies against granule proteins activate neutrophils in vitro. *J Leukoc Biol* 1991;50:539–46.
72. Caldas ML, Charles LA, Falk RJ, Jennette JC. Immunoelectron microscopic documentation of the translocation of proteins reactive with ANCA to neutrophil cell surfaces during neutrophil activation. In: *Third International Workshop on ANCA* 1990(abst).
73. Csernok E, Ernst M, Schmitt W, Bainton DF, Gross WL. Activated neutrophils express proteinase 3 on their plasma membrane in vitro and in vivo. *Clin Exp Immunol* 1994;95:244–50.
74. Zhao MH, Lockwood CM. Anti-F(ab)$_2$ autoantibodies in systemic vasculitis. *Clin Exp Immunol* 1993;93(Suppl 1):23(abst).
75. Porges AJ, Redecha PB, Kimberly WT, Csernok E, Gross WL, Kimberly RP. Anti-neutrophil cytoplasmic antibodies engage and activate human neutrophils via FcgammaRIIa. *J Immunol* 1994;153:1271–80.
76. Mulder AH, Heeringa P, Brouwer E, Limburg PC, Kallenberg CG. Activation of granulocytes by anti-neutrophil cytoplasmic antibodies (ANCA): a Fc gamma RII-dependent process. *Clin Exp Immunol* 1994;98:270–8.
77. Kettritz R, Jennette J, Falk R. Anti-neutrophil cytoplasmic autoantibodies (ANCA) trigger superoxide release of human neutrophils by cross-linking their target antigens. *J Am Soc Nephrol* 1995;6:835 (Abstr).
78. Ewert BH, Jennette JC, Falk RJ. Anti-myeloperoxidase antibodies stimulate neutrophils to damage human endothelial cells. *Kidney Int* 1992;41:375–83.
79. Savage CO, Pottinger BE, Gaskin G, Pusey CD, Pearson JD. Autoantibodies developing to myeloperoxidase and proteinase 3 in systemic vasculitis stimulate neutrophil cytotoxicity towards cultured endothelial cells. *Am J Pathol* 1992;141:335–42.
80. Ewert BH BM, Jennette JC. Anti-myeloperoxidase antibodies (aMPO) stimulate neutrophils to adhere to cultured human endothelial cells utilizing the beta-2-integrin CD11/18. *J Am Soc Nephrol* 1992;3:585(abst).
81. Kiser MA, Falk JC. Effects of antibodies to myeloperoxidase (aMPO) on vascular permeability and neutrophil accumulation in vivo. *J Am Soc Nephrol* 1992;3:599(abst).
82. Brouwer E, Huitema MG, Klok PA, et al. Anti-myeloperoxidase-associated proliferative glomerulonephritis: an animal model. *J Exp Med* 1993;177:905–14.
83. Brouwer E, Klok PA, Huitema MG, Limburg PC, Weening JJ, Kallenberg CGM. Strain differences in immune responsiveness between Brown Norway and Lewis rats: implications for the animal model of anti-myeloperoxidase associated glomerulonephritis. *Cell* 1994.
84. Yang JJ, Jennette JC, Falk RJ. Immune complex glomerulonephritis is induced in rats immunized with heterologous myeloperoxidase. *Clin Exp Immunol* 1994;97:466–73.
85. Mayet WJ, Csernok E, Szymkowiak C, Gross WL, Meyer zum

Buschenfelde KH. Human endothelial cells express proteinase 3, the target antigen of anticytoplasmic antibodies in Wegener's granulomatosis. *Blood* 1993;82:1221–9.

86. Mayet WJ, Schwarting A, Meyer zum Buschenfelde KH. Cytotoxic effects of antibodies to proteinase 3 (C-ANCA) on human endothelial cells. *Clin Exp Immunol* 1994;97:458–65.
87. Ballieux BE, Zondervan KT, Kievit P, et al. Binding of proteinase 3 and myeloperoxidase to endothelial cells: ANCA-mediated endothelial damage through ADCC? *Clin Exp Immunol* 1994;97:52–60.
88. King WJ, Adu D, Daha MR, et al. Endothelial cells and renal epithelial cells do not express the Wegener's autoantigen, proteinase 3. *Clin Exp Immunol* 1995;102:98–105.
89. Ballieux BE, Hiemstra PS, Klar-Mohamad N, et al. Detachment and cytolysis of human endothelial cells by proteinase 3. *Eur J Immunol* 1994;24:3211–5.
90. Berger S, Seelen M, Hiemstra P, et al. Proteinase 3 (PR3), the major autoantigen of Wegener's granulomatosis (WG), enhances IL-8 production by human endothelial cells (HUVEC) in vitro. *J Am Soc Nephrol* 1995;6:822.
91. Yang J, Kettritz R, Falk R, Jennette J, Gaido M. Induction of endothelial cell apoptosis by proteinase 3 (PR3). *J Am Soc Nephrol* 1995;6: 858(abst).
92. Leung DY, Geha RS, Newburger JW, et al. Two monokines, interleukin 1 and tumor necrosis factor, render cultured vascular endothelial cells susceptible to lysis by antibodies circulating during Kawasaki syndrome. *J Exp Med* 1986;164:1958–72.
93. Nash M, Shah V, Dillon M. ANCA and AECA are not increased in acute Kawasaki disease, a childhood vasculitis. *Clin Exp Immunol* 1995;101:64(abst).
94. Chan TM, Frampton G, Jayne DR, Perry GJ, Lockwood CM, Cameron JS. Clinical significance of anti-endothelial cell antibodies in systemic vasculitis: a longitudinal study comparing anti-endothelial cell antibodies and anti-neutrophil cytoplasm antibodies. *Am J Kidney Dis* 1993;22:387–92.
95. Savage CO, Pottinger BE, Gaskin G, Lockwood CM, Pusey CD, Pearson JD. Vascular damage in Wegener's granulomatosis and microscopic polyarteritis: presence of anti-endothelial cell antibodies and their relation to anti-neutrophil cytoplasm antibodies. *Clin Exp Immunol* 1991;85:14–9.
96. Varagunam M, Nwosu Z, Adu D, et al. Little evidence for anti-endothelial cell antibodies in microscopic polyarteritis and Wegener's granulomatosis. *Nephrol Dial Transplant* 1993;8:113–7.
97. Mayet WJ, Hermann EM, Csernok E, Gross WL, Meyer zum Buschenfelde KH. In vitro interactions of c-ANCA (antibodies to proteinase 3) with human endothelial cells. *Adv Exp Med Biol* 1993; 336:109–13.
98. Kain R, Matsui K, Exner M, et al. A novel class of autoantigens of anti-neutrophil cytoplasmic antibodies in necrotizing and crescentic glomerulonephritis: the lysosomal membrane glycoprotein h-lamp-2 in neutrophil granulocytes and a related membrane protein in glomerular endothelial cells. *J Exp Med* 1995;181:585–97.
99. Ballieux BE, Hagen EC, van der Keur C, et al. Isolation of a protein complex from purulent sputum consisting of proteinase-3 and alpha 1-antitrypsin reactive with antineutrophil cytoplasmic antibodies. *J Immunol Methods* 1993;159:63–70.
100. Dolman KM, Stegeman CA, van de Wiel BA, et al. Relevance of classic anti-neutrophil cytoplasmic autoantibody (C-ANCA)-mediated inhibition of proteinase 3–alpha 1-antitrypsin complexation to disease activity in Wegener's granulomatosis. *Clin Exp Immunol* 1993; 93:405–10.
101. Esnault VL, Testa A, Audrain M, et al. Alpha 1-antitrypsin genetic polymorphism in ANCA-positive systemic vasculitis. *Kidney Int* 1993; 43:1329–32.
102. Gronhagen Riska C, Teppo AM, Honkanen E, Ikaheimo R. Alpha-1-antitrypsin, CRP and interleukin-6 in ANCA-positive vasculitis. *Adv Exp Med Biol* 1993;336:337–40.
103. Elzouki AN, Wieslander M. Strong link between the alpha 1-antitrypsin PiZ allele and Wegener's granulomatosis. *J Intern Med* 1994; 236:543–8.
104. Van de Wiel BA, Dolman KM, van der Meer-Gerritsen CH, Hack CE, von dem Borne AE, Goldschmeding R. Interference of Wegener's granulomatosis autoantibodies with neutrophil proteinase 3 activity. *Clin Exp Immunol* 1992;90:409–14.
105. Daouk GH, Palsson R, Arnaout MA. Inhibition of proteinase 3 by ANCA and its correlation with disease activity in Wegener's granulomatosis. *Kidney Int* 1995;47:1528–36.
106. Brouwer E, Cohen Tervaert JW, Weening JJ, Kallenberg CG. Immunohistopathology of renal biopsies in Wegener's granulomatosis: clues to its pathogenesis? *Am J Kidney Dis* 1991;18:205.
107. Schmitt WH, Heesen C, Csernok E, Rautman A, Gross WL. Elevated serum levels of soluble interleukin-2 receptor in patients with Wegener's granulomatosis: association with disease activity. *Arthritis Rheum* 1992;35:1088–96.
108. Stegeman CA, Cohen Tervaert JW, Huitema MG, Kallenberg CG. Serum markers of T cell activation in relapses of Wegener's granulomatosis. *Clin Exp Immunol* 1993;91:415–20.
109. Van der Woude FJ, van Es LA, Daha MR. The role of the c-ANCA antigen in the pathogenesis of Wegener's granulomatosis: a hypothesis based on both humoral and cellular mechanisms. *Neth J Med* 1990;36:169–71.
110. Petersen J, Rasmussen N, Szpirt W, Hermann E, Mayet W. T lymphocyte proliferation to neutrophil cytoplasmic antigen(s) in Wegener's granulomatosis. In: *Third International Workshop on ANCA* 1990 (abst).
111. Brouwer E, Stegeman CA, Huitema MG, Limburg PC, Kallenberg CG. T cell reactivity to proteinase 3 and myeloperoxidase in patients with Wegener's granulomatosis (WG). *Clin Exp Immunol* 1994;98: 448–53.
112. Ballieux BE, van der Burg SH, Hagen EC, van der Woude FJ, Melief CJ, Daha MR. Cell-mediated autoimmunity in patients with Wegener's granulomatosis (WG). *Clin Exp Immunol* 1995;100:186–93.
113. Mathieson PW, Lockwood CM, Oliveira DB. T and B cell responses to neutrophil cytoplasmic antigens in systemic vasculitis. *Clin Immunol Immunopathol* 1992;63:135–41.
114. Kettritz R, Yang JJ, Kinjoh K, Jennette JC, Falk RJ. Animal models in ANCA–vasculitis (Review). *Clin Exp Immunol* 1995;101(Suppl 1) 12–5.
115. Mathieson PW, Thiru S, Oliveira DBG. Mercuric chloride-treated brown Norway rats develop widespread tissue injury including necrotizing vasculitis. *Lab Invest* 1992;67:121–9.
116. Mathieson PW, Qasim FJ, Esnautl VL, Oliveira DB. Animal models of systemic vasculitis. *J Autoimmun* 1993;6:251–64.
117. Harper JM, Lockwood CM, Cooke A. Anti-neutrophil cytoplasm antibodies in MRL-*lpr*/*lpr* mice. *Clin Exp Immunol* 1993;93(Suppl 1): 22.
118. Harper MC, Milstein C, Cooke A. Pathogenic anti-MPO antibody in MRL/*lpr* mice. *Clin Exp Immunol* 1995;101(Suppl 1):54(abst).
119. Kinjoh K, Kyogoku M, Good RA. Genetic selection for crescent formation yields mouse strain with rapidly progressive glomerulonephritis and small vessel vasculitis. *Proc Natl Acad Sci U S A* 1993;90: 3413–7.
120. Blank M, Tomer Y, Stein M, et al. Immunization with anti-neutrophil cytoplasmic antibody (ANCA) induces the production of mouse ANCA and perivascular lymphocyte infiltration. *Clin Exp Immunol* 1995;102:120–30.
121. Tomer Y, Gilburd B, Blank M, et al. Characterization of biologically active antineutrophil cytoplasmic antibodies induced in mice.: pathogenetic role in experimental vasculitis. *Arthritis Rheum* 1995;38: 1375–81.
122. Falk RJ, Hogan S, Carey TS, Jennette JC. Clinical course of anti-neutrophil cytoplasmic autoantibody-associated glomerulonephritis and systemic vasculitis: the Glomerular Disease Collaborative Network. *Ann Intern Med* 1990;113:656–63.
123. Pusey CD, Gaskin G. Disease associations with anti-neutrophil cytoplasmic antibodies. *Adv Exp Med Biol* 1993;336:145–55.
124. Andrassy K, Koderisch A. Wegener's granulomatosus with renal involvement: patient survival and correlations between initial renal function, renal histology, therapy and renal outcome. *Clin Nephrol* 1994;
125. Sizeland PC, Bailey RR, Lynn KL, Robson RA. Wegener's granulomatosus with renal involvement: a 14 year experience. *NZ Med J* 1990;103:366–7.
126. Thomas DM, Moore R, Donovan K, Wheeler DC, Esnault VL, Lockwood CM. Pulmonary–renal syndrome in association with anti-GBM and IgM ANCA. *Lancet* 1992;339:1304.
127. Bosch X, Lopez-Soto A, Mirapiex E. Antineutrophil cytoplasmic autoantibody-associated alveolar capillaritis in patients presenting with pulmonary hemorrhage. *Arch Pathol Lab Med* 1994;118:517–8.

128. Li PK, Lai FM, Ko GT, Lai KN. Microscopic polyarteritis presenting with chest infections and acute appendicitis. *Aust NZ J Med* 1992;22: 56–9.
129. Jayne DR, Jones SJ, Severn A, Shaunak S, Murphy J, Lockwood CM. Severe pulmonary hemorrhage and systemic vasculitis in association with circulating anti-neutrophil cytoplasm antibodies of IgM class only. *Clin Nephrol* 1989;32:101–6.
130. Davenport A, Lock RJ, Wallington TB. Clinical relevance of testing for antineutrophil cytoplasm antibodies (ANCA) with a standard indirect immunofluorescence ANCA test in patients with upper or lower respiratory tract symptoms. *Thorax* 1994;49:213–7.
131. Vartiainen E, Nuutinen J. Head and neck manifestations of Wegener's granulomatosis. *Ear Nose Throat J* 1992;71:423–4.
132. Andrassy K, Rasmussen N. Treatment of granulomatous disorders of the nose and paranasal sinuses (Review). *Rhinology* 1989;27:221–30.
133. Hoare TJ, Jayne D, Rhys Evans P, Croft CB, Howard DJ. Wegener's granulomatosis, subglottic stenosis and antineutrophil cytoplasm antibodies. *J Laryngol Otol* 1989;103:1187–91.
134. Jennette CJ, Milling DM, Falk RJ. Vasculitis affecting the skin: a review [Editorial]. *Arch Dermatol* 1994;130:899–906.
135. Burrows NP, Lockwood CM. Antineutrophil cytoplasmic antibodies and their relevance to the dermatologist (Review). *Br J Dermatol* 1995;132:173–81.
136. Daoud MS, Gibson LE, DeRemee RA, Specks U, el-Azhary RA, Su WP. Cutaneous Wegener's granulomatosis: clinical, histopathologic, and immunopathologic features of thirty patients. *J Am Acad Dermatol* 1994;31:605–12.
137. Nakabayashi I, Yoshizawa N, Kubota T, et al. ANCA associated vasculitis allergica cutis (VAC) and mild proliferative necrotizing glomerulonephritis. *Clin Nephrol* 1993;40:265–9.
138. SK, Fleming KA, Chapman TW. Prevalence of anti-neutrophil antibody in primary sclerosing cholangitis and ulcerative colitis using an alkaline phosphatase technique. *Gut* 1992;33:1370–5.
139. Grcerska L, Polenakovic M. Fibrinoid necrosis of the liver in a patient with ANCA-associated crescentic glomerulonephritis (GN) during pregnancy [Letter]. *Clin Nephrol* 1995;43:278–9.
140. Mulder AH, Horst G, Haagsma EB, Limburg PC, Kleibeuker JH, Kallenberg CG. Prevalence and characterization of neutrophil cytoplasmic antibodies in autoimmune liver diseases. *Hepatology* 1993; 17:411–7.
141. Moore PM, Fauci AS. Neurologic manifestations of systemic vasculitis: a retrospective and prospective study of the clinicopathologic features and responses to therapy in 25 patients. *Am J Med* 1981;71: 517–24.
142. Logar D, Rozman B, Vizjak A, Ferluga D, Mulder AH, Kallenberg CG. Arteritis of both carotid arteries in a patient with focal, crescentic glomerulonephritis and anti-neutrophil cytoplasmic autoantibodies. *Br J Rheumatol* 1994;33:167–9.
143. Florine CW, Dwyer M, Holland EJ. Wegener's granulomatosis presenting with sclerokeratitis diagnosed by antineutrophil cytoplasmic autoantibodies (ANCA). *Surv Ophthalmol* 1993;37:373–6.
144. Kaufman AH, Niles JL, Foster CS. ANCA test in ophthalmic inflammatory disease [Review]. *Int Ophthalmol Clin* 1994;34:215–27.
145. Hagen EC, van de Vijver Reenalda H, de Keizer RJ, et al. Uveitis and anti-neutrophil cytoplasmic antibodies. *Clin Exp Immunol* 1994;95: 56–9.
146. Belden CJ, Hamed LM, Mancuso AA. Bilateral isolated retrobulbar optic neuropathy in limited Wegener's granulomatosis. *J Clin Neuro-ophthalmol* 1993;13:119–23.
147. Parrillo JE, Fauci AS. Necrotizing vasculitis, coronary angiitis, and the cardiologist. *Am Heart J* 1980;99:547–54.
148. Jayne DR, Marshall PD, Jones SJ, Lockwood CM. Autoantibodies to GBM and neutrophil cytoplasm in rapidly progressive glomerulonephritis. *Kidney Int* 1990;37:965–70.
149. Short AK, Esnault VL, Lockwood CM. Anti-neutrophil cytoplasmic antibodies and anti-glomerular basement membrane antibodies: two coexisting distinct autoreactivities detectable in patients with rapidly progressive glomerulonephritis. *Am J Kidney Dis* 1995;26:439–45.
150. Bygren P, Rasmussen N, Isaksson B, Wieslander J. Anti-neutrophil cytoplasm antibodies, anti-GBM antibodies and anti-dsDNA antibodies in glomerulonephritis. *Eur J Clin Invest* 1992;22:783–92.
151. Pauzner R, Urowitz M, Gladman D, Gough J. Antineutrophil cytoplasmic antibodies in systemic lupus erythematosus. *J Rheumatol* 1994; 21:1670–3.
152. Sinico RA, Tadros M, Radice A, et al. Lack of IgA antineutrophil cytoplasmic antibodies in Henoch–Schönlein purpura and IgA nephropathy. *Clin Immunol Immunopathol* 1994;73:19–26.
153. D'Amico G, Colasanti G, Ferrario F, Sinico RA. Renal involvement in essential mixed cryoglobulinemia. *Kidney Int* 1989;35:1004–14.
154. Pusey CD, Gaskin G, Rees AJ. Treatment of primary systemic vasculitis. *APMIS Suppl* 1990;19:48–50.
155. Briedigkeit L, Ulmer M, Gobel U, Natusch R, Reinhold Keller E, Gross WL. Treatment of Wegener's granulomatosus. *Adv Exp Med Biol* 1993;336:491–5.
156. Fauci AS, Katz P, Haynes BF, Wolff SM. Cyclophosphamide therapy of severe systemic necrotizing vasculitis. *N Engl J Med* 1979;301: 235–8.
157. Fauci AS, Haynes B, Katz P. The spectrum of vasculitis: clinical, pathologic, immunologic and therapeutic considerations. *Ann Intern Med* 1978;89:660–76.
158. Hoffman GS, Leavitt GS. Wegener's granulomatosis: an analysis of 158 patients. *Ann Intern Med* 1992;116:488–98.
159. Choy DS, Gearhart RP, Gould WJ, Sauer J, Jacobson L, Rosenthal B. Development of multiple carcinomas in a long term survivor of Wegener's granulomatosus treated with immunosuppressive drugs. *NY State J Med* 1989;89:680–2.
160. Tarlar-Williams C, Hijazi Y, Walther M, et al. Cyclophosphamide-induced cystitis and bladder cancer in patients with Wegener granulomatosis. *Ann Intern Med* 1996;124:477–84.
161. Gaskin G, Savage CO, Ryan JJ, et al. Anti-neutrophil cytoplasmic antibodies and disease activity during long-term follow-up of 70 patients with systemic vasculitis. *Nephrol Dial Transplant* 1991;6: 689–94.
162. Hoffman GS, Leavitt RY, Kerr GS, Fauci AS. The treatment of Wegener's granulomatosis with glucocorticoids and methotrexate. *Arthritis Rheum* 1992;35:1322–9.
163. Rifle G, Dechelette E. Treatment of rapidly progressive glomerulonephritis by plasma exchange and methylprednisolone pulses: a prospective randomized trial of cyclophosphamide—interim analysis: the French Cooperative Group. *Prog Clin Biol Res* 1990;337:263–7.
164. Frasca GM, Zoumparidis NG, Borgnino LC, Neri L, Vangelista A, Bonomini V. Plasma exchange treatment in rapidly progressive glomerulonephritis associated with anti-neutrophil cytoplasmic autoantibodies. *Int J Artif Organs* 1992;15:181–4.
165. Pusey CD, Rees AJ, Evans DJ, Peters DK, Lockwood CM. Plasma exchange in focal necrotizing glomerulonephritis without anti-GBM antibodies. *Kidney Int* 1991;40:757–63.
165a. Glockner WM, Sieberth HG, Wichmann HE, et al. Plasma exchange and immunosuppression in rapidly progressive glomerulonephritis. *Clin Nephrol* 1988;29:1–8.
166. Jayne DR, Davies MJ, Fox CJ, Black CM, Lockwood CM. Treatment of systemic vasculitis with pooled intravenous immunoglobulin. *Lancet* 1991;337:1137–9.
167. Tuso P, Moudgil A, Hay J, et al. Treatment of antineutrophil cytoplasmic autoantibody-positive systemic vasculitis and glomerulonephritis with pooled intravenous gammaglobulin. *Am J Kidney Dis* 1992;20:504–8.
168. Richter C, Schnabel A, Csernok E, Reinhold-Keller E, Gross WL. Treatment of Wegener's granulomatosis with intravenous immunoglobulin. *Adv Exp Med Biol* 1993;336:487–9.
169. Leavitt RY, Hoffman GS, Fauci AS. The role of trimethoprim/sulfamethoxazole in the treatment of Wegener's granulomatosis. *Arthritis Rheum* 1988;31:1073–4.
170. Mathieson PW, Cobbold SP, Hale G, et al. Monoclonal-antibody therapy in systemic vasculitis. *N Engl J Med* 1990;323:250–4.
171. Cohen Tervaert JW, van der Woude FJ, Fauci AS, et al. Association between active Wegener's granulomatosis and anticytoplasmic antibodies. *Arch Intern Med* 1989;149:2461–5.
172. Kerr GS, Hallahan TA. Limited prognostic value of changes in anti-neutrophil cytoplasmic antibody titers in patients with Wegener's granulomatosus. *Adv Exp Med Biol* 1993;336:389–92.
173. Cohen Tervaert JW, Huitema MG, Hene RJ, et al. Prevention of relapses in Wegener's granulomatosis by treatment based on antineutrophil cytoplasmic antibody titre. *Lancet* 1990;336:709–11.
174. DeOliveira J, Gaskin G, Dash A, Rees AJ, Pusey CD. Relationship between disease activity and anti-neutrophil cytoplasmic antibody concentration in long-term management of systemic vasculitis. *Am J Kidney Dis* 1995;25:380–9.

175. Dupre Goudable C, Modesto O. In Wegener's granulomatosus initial renal biopsy predicts response to treatment better than peak plasma creatinine. *Contrib Nephrol* 1991;94:181–5.
176. Briedigkeit L, Kettritz R, Gobel U, Natusch R. Prognostic factors in Wegener's granulomatosis. *Postgrad Med J* 1993;69:856–61.
177. Stegeman CA, Tervaert JW, Sluiter WJ, Manson WL, de Jong PE, Kallenberg CG. Association of chronic nasal carriage of *Staphylococcus aureus* and higher relapse rates in Wegener granulomatosis [see comments]. *Ann Intern Med* 1994;120:12–7.
178. Stegeman CA, Tervaert JW, de John PE, Kallenberg CGM. Prevention of relapses of Wegener's granulomatosis by treatment with trimethoprin–sulfamethoxazole: a multi-center placebo controlled trial in 81 patients. *Clin Exp Immunol* 1995;101:44.
179. Steinman TI, Jaffe BF, Monaco AP, Wolff SM, Fauci AS. Recurrence of Wegener's granulomatosis after kidney transplantation: successful re-induction of remission with cyclophosphamide. *Am J Surg Pathol* 1980;4:191–6.
180. Grotz W, Wanner C, Rother E, Schollmeyer P. Clinical course of patients with antineutrophil cytoplasm antibody positive vasculitis after kidney transplantation. *Nephron* 1995;69:234–6.
181. Yang CW, Kim YS, Kim SY, Bang BK. Renal transplantation of ANCA-positive idiopathic crescentic glomerulonephritis: two-year follow-up [Letter]. *Clin Nephrol* 1994;42:209.
182. Rosenstein ED, Ribot S, Ventresca E, Kramer N. Recurrence of Wegener's granulomatosis following renal transplantation [Review]. *Br J Rheumatol* 1994;33:869–71.
183. Morin MP, Thervet E, Legendre C, Page B, Kreis H, Noel LH. Successful kidney transplantation in a patient with microscopic polyarteritis and positive ANCA [Letter]. *Nephrol Dial Transplant* 1993; 8:287–8.
184. Boubenider SA, Akhtar M, Alfurayh O, Algazlan S, Taibah K, Qunibi W. Late recurrence of Wegener's granulomatosis presenting as tracheal stenosis in a renal transplant patient [Review]. *Clin Transplant* 1994;8:5–9.

Immunologic Renal Diseases,
edited by E. G. Neilson and W. G. Couser.
Lippincott-Raven Publishers, Philadelphia © 1997.

CHAPTER 50

Henoch–Schönlein Purpura

Norishige Yoshikawa

DEFINITION AND HISTORICAL PERSPECTIVE

Henoch–Schönlein purpura is a clinical syndrome and a mutisystem disorder affecting predominantly the skin, joints, gastrointestinal tract, and kidneys, although other organs are rarely involved (1,2). All features are not necessarily present in every case.

In 1801, Heberden (3) described a 5-year-old boy with abdominal pain, vomiting, melena, joint pains, and petechial hemorrhages on his legs, and whose urine was "tinged with blood." In 1837, Schönlein (4) first described the condition that he called "peliosis rheumatica," purpura rheumatica, in which arthralgia was associated with purpura. In 1868, Henoch (5) described the gastrointestinal manifestations of purpura rheumatica and, 30 years later, he referred to nephritis as a complication (6). Osler (7) attributed the symptoms to anaphylaxis, and the term "anaphylactoid purpura," introduced by Frank (8), remains popular in the United States (9), whereas most European and Japanese writers favor the eponymous title. Other terms used include "purpura rhumatoide" (10) and "Schönlein–Henoch syndrome" (11–13), the latter acknowledging historical precedence. However, "Henoch–Schönlein purpura" remains popular, as well as being traditional, and is used in this chapter.

ETIOLOGY AND INCIDENCE

The etiology of Henoch–Schönlein purpura remains obscure. The illness is preceded by upper respiratory infection in 30–50% of patients (14,15), but evidence of a streptococcal etiology has not been substantiated (14–17). No causative agent is apparent in the majority of patients. Other infections implicated in a few children include varicella (14), measles (12), rubella (14), adenovirus (18), hepatitis A (19) and B (20), *Yersinia* (21), *Shigella* (22), mycoplasma pneumonia (23), and staphylococcal septicemia (24), but without acceptable evidence of a causal relationship. Henoch–Schönlein purpura has been also reported to follow smallpox and influenza vaccination (25,26), insect bites (27), exposure to cold (28), and trauma (29). In adult patients, Henoch–Schönlein purpura has been reported in association with human immunodeficiency virus infection (30), Behçet disease (31), uveitis (32), squamous cell carcinoma (33), and rheumatoid arthritis (34).

Henoch–Schönlein purpura is observed mainly in children, but adults may also be affected (35–37). It is rare in children under 2 years of age and has a peak incidence around 4–5 years of age, followed by a gradual decline toward adolescence. The larger childhood series indicate a slight male preponderance (14,15,38,39). The annual incidence estimated by Nielsen (40) in Denmark and by Stewart and associates (41) in Ireland were 14 and 13.5 cases per 100,000 children, respectively. Forty years ago, Henoch–Schönlein purpura was less than half as common as post-streptococcal nephritis in the United Kingdom (42), but whereas the latter is now uncommon in developed countries, the incidence of Henoch–Schönlein purpura seems to have remained stable. There is a significant seasonal variation in incidence, with a peak during winter (15,17,35). Although Henoch–Schönlein purpura has a wide geographic distribution, there is appreciable variation. Recent clinical reports based on large numbers of patients have originated mostly from Europe [United Kingdom (14,43–45), France (15), and Finland (46)] and Asia [Japan (17,38) and Singapore (36)], and the condition appears to be less common in North America and Africa. These differences may be both environmental and racial, since Henoch–Schönlein purpura is rare in blacks in the southern United States (47,48) and in Indians (49).

A familial incidence of Henoch–Schönlein purpura is rare (14,50), suggesting that genetic factors are not of major etiologic significance. There appears to be no asso-

N. Yoshikawa: Department of Pediatrics, Kobe University School of Medicine, Kobe 650, Japan.

ciation between HLA antigens (51) or immunoglobulin heavy-chain switch region gene (52) and Henoch–Schönlein purpura.

The proportion of patients with renal involvement has been reported to be 20–100% (14,17,35,53–57). These variations may depend on the method of detection of nephritis (13). In many of the early studies, serial routine urinalysis was not used, and transient microscopic hematuria was probably missed. Two studies in which routine urinalysis was carried out on all Henoch–Schönlein purpura hospital admissions reported renal involvement in 41% (55) and 61% (17), respectively.

PATHOGENESIS AND PATHOPHYSIOLOGY

Although the pathogenesis of Henoch–Schönlein purpura remains uncertain, there is substantial evidence that it is an immune-complex-mediated disease. Granular electron-dense deposits are observed in the glomerular mesangial areas by electron microscopy and confirmed as containing immunoglobulin (Ig) A and C3 by immunofluorescence microscopy. Circulating IgA immune complexes have been detected by several different specific assays, often associated with IgG immune complex (58–61). Many immunologic abnormalities that may lead to the formation of IgA immune complex have been reported in patients with Henoch–Schönlein purpura. Mesangial IgA deposits recur frequently in allografted kidneys in patients with Henoch–Schönlein purpura (62–64), and this evidence indicates that the mesangial IgA must be of host origin. Moreover, glomerular IgA deposits associated with histologic lesions similar to those of human Henoch–Schönlein purpura nephritis can be induced in laboratory animals by passive administration of preformed polymeric IgA–concanavalin-A complex (65).

The Nature of IgA Deposits

The most prominent finding in the glomeruli of renal biopsy specimens from patients with Henoch–Schönlein purpura nephritis is mesangial IgA deposition. IgA is the second most common immunoglobulin and contributes to immunity at the level of the external secretory system. IgA exists in monomeric and polymeric forms. Monomeric IgA represents ~90% of the serum IgA and is produced mainly by the circulating lymphocytes and plasma cells in the spleen and bone marrow. Polymeric IgA is produced mostly by lymphocytes and plasma cells in the gastrointestinal and respiratory tracts, where it is synthesized as monomers and then secreted as dimers linked by the J chain, which is also produced within the plasma cells. During the passage of dimeric IgA molecules through the mucosal epithelium toward the external lumen, the secretory component is attached through specific noncovalent interactions; this component appears to protect the dimeric IgA from the proteolytic enzymes present in the external secretions. IgA has two subclasses: IgA1 and IgA2. About 90% of serum is composed of IgA1, whereas IgA2 is mostly derived from the local mucosa of the gastrointestinal and respiratory tracts (66). Both IgA1 and IgA2 are produced in the mucosae. Most investigators have indicated that IgA1 is the predominant subclass present in the glomeruli from patients with Henoch–Schönlein purpura nephritis (67–70). J chain, independent of IgM, has also been identified in the mesangium in patients with Henoch–Schönlein purpura nephritis (67,71). Secretory component is not present in the mesangial deposits (69). Although the capacity of the mesangial deposits to bind secretory component has not been examined in Henoch–Schönlein purpura nephritis, immunofluorescence studies of renal biopsy sections from patients with IgA nephropathy have indicated that secretory component binds to the mesangial areas in vitro (72). These observations suggest that the mesangial IgA deposits in Henoch–Schönlein purpura nephritis are polymeric.

A number of studies have suggested that the alternative complement pathway has a pathogenetic role in Henoch–Schönlein purpura. This hypothesis is consistent with the typical immunohistologic demonstration of C3 and properdin in a pattern and distribution similar to that of IgA in the glomeruli, often in the absence of C1q and C4 (15,36, 73). The detection of the membrane-attack complex of complement further supports the pathogenetic role of complement activation in this disease (74). Activation of the alternative complement pathway is observed in patients with Henoch–Schönlein purpura nephritis (75,76), and increased serum terminal complement complex has been reported in the active phase of disease (77). However, there is no direct evidence that the activation is mediated by IgA deposits in the glomeruli, and the mediator as well as the pathophysiologic significance of this complement activation remain to be determined.

Because IgA is the main immunoglobulin directed against antigens (viral and bacterial) in the exocrine system, and because of the frequent association between upper respiratory tract infection and the development of Henoch–Schönlein purpura, it has been suggested that certain viral or bacterial infections may lead to Henoch–Schönlein purpura and that IgA may act as the antibody to viral or bacterial antigens. Little effort has been directed toward the search for antigens and for the antibody specificity of the mesangial IgA in Henoch–Schönlein purpura. Emancipator reported the development of gut lesions, purpura, glomerular lesions, and hematuria in a bacterial polysaccharide model induced in mice, and suggested that Henoch–Schönlein purpura could be an expression of an antigen-dependent process (78). With regard to antibody specificity, IgA eluted from cryostat sections of Henoch–Schönlein purpura nephritis biopsies has been reported to react with mesangial areas of their own and other Henoch–Schönlein purpura nephritis patients' biopsy specimens (79,80).

In conclusion, the immunochemical nature of the mesangial deposits in Henoch–Schönlein purpura nephritis is consistent with antigen–polymeric IgA complexes predominantly of A1 subclass, and perhaps multispecific for ubiquitous mucosally derived antigens.

The IgA Immune System

The finding of an increased serum IgA level was first reported in Japanese children with Henoch–Schönlein purpura by Tanaka and associates (81). There is now general agreement that serum levels of IgA are increased in half of the patients with Henoch–Schönlein purpura during acute illness (15,82,83). Serum IgA levels return to normal as the acute illness resolves. In addition to the increased levels of serum IgA, various types of autoantibodies of the IgA class have been recognized. These autoantibodies include IgA-rheumatoid factor (84–86), IgA antineutrophil cytoplasmic antibody (87,88), IgA anti-IgG antibody (89), and IgA anticardiolipin antibody (90). The presence of IgA-rheumatoid factors has been related to disease activity (39). IgA immune complexes are also frequently detected (58–61). Coppo et al. (91) noted a higher prevalence of immune complexes during acute disease. Levinsky and Barratt (58) found that immune complexes also contained IgG and only the IgG-containing immune complexes were nephritogenic in Henoch–Schönlein purpura. Codeposition of IgG in the mesangium and the presence of circulating IgG-containing immune complexes suggested that IgG immune complexes might play an important role in the renal damage (92). Not all patients with Henoch–Schönlein purpura have circulating immune complexes. There are at least two explanations for the absence of circulating immune complexes (13). These patients might have immune complexes only intermittently or formation of mesangial IgA deposits in patients without circulating immune complexes might be due to in situ formation of the immune complex directly in the mesangium. O'Donoghue and associates (93) demonstrated autoantibody binding specifically to glomerular antigen(s) present on the mesangial cell and found only in IgA nephropathy and Henoch–Schönlein purpura. Circulating IgA–fibronectin aggregates, macromolecules aggregated on a nonimmune basis, have been demonstrated in patients with Henoch–Schönlein purpura (94,95). The presence of fibronectin in the circulating aggregates may play an important role in the preferential deposition of nephritogenic IgA-containing immune complexes in the mesangium (94).

An increased number of circulating IgA-producing lymphocytes have been found during the acute phase of disease (96–98), but not when the disease is clinically inactive (98,99). IgA production is highly T cell dependent, and the increased production in Henoch–Schönlein purpura indicates altered T-cell function. Casanueva et al. (99) noted the existence of persistent abnormalities in the cellular immune mechanisms regulating the immunoglobulin synthesis (impaired T-cell suppressor activity) in IgA nephropathy, but not in Henoch–Schönlein purpura. Defective clearance of immune complexes from the circulation may also be important, but this seems more likely to be a consequence rather than the cause of the increased immune-complex load (100).

Mechanisms of Glomerular Injury

Mechanisms by which IgA mesangial deposits create glomerular injury in Henoch–Schönlein purpura nephritis are still unknown. It is not clear how the IgA deposits lead to glomerular injury. The nonphlogistic nature of IgA (101) and the occurrence of mesangial deposits of IgA alone in celiac disease without evidence of nephritis (102) or in hepatobiliary diseases, with only minor urinary abnormality, suggests that IgA per se is not noxious to the glomerulus (78) and other mechanisms may be involved in glomerular injury in Henoch–Schönlein purpura nephritis (93). Accumulating evidence supports the importance of complement activation in renal injury in Henoch–Schönlein purpura nephritis (75,76). The membrane-attack complex of complement C5b-9 has been recognized as an important mediator of glomerulonephritis. IgG is an efficient activator of complement (103), but the interaction between IgA and the complement system remains controversial (104). Colten and Bienerstock (105) have shown that monomeric IgA does not activate complement. In contrast, Hiemstra et al. (106) have reported that IgA1 fragments can activate the alternative pathway of complement. Emancipator et al. (107) demonstrated the absence of urinary abnormalities and the mild or equivocal histologic changes induced by IgA deposition alone in contrast to the microscopic hematuria and glomerulonephritis observed when IgG and C3 are codeposited with IgA immune complexes in mice.

The roles of platelets (108), coagulation factors (109, 110), and vasoactive prostanoids (111,112) in glomerular injury have been discussed but remain unclear.

The roles of cytokines and growth factors in glomerular injury have been demonstrated. Horii et al. (113) and Ruef et al. (114) demonstrated that interleukin (IL) 6 may be an autocrine growth factor responsible for proliferation of mesangial cells. In IL-6 transgenic mice (115), the mesangial proliferation is associated with heavy proteinuria and a polyclonal increase in immunoglobulins. In these studies, antibody to human IL-6 diminished mesangial cell proliferation and improved renal function. Thus, abnormally regulated production of IL-6 either by mesangial cells or by infiltrating T cells may be responsible for the mesangial cell proliferation in IgA-associated glomerulonephritis, including Henoch–Schönlein purpura nephritis (116). Takemura et al. (117) demonstrated IL-1, IL-6, and tumor necrosis factor α mRNA in monocyte-macrophages infiltrating the glomeruli, but rarely in mesangial cells in patients with Henoch–Schönlein purpura nephritis. These findings suggest that infiltrating monocyte-macrophages, rather than resident mesangial cells, are the major source of inflammatory cytokines in human Henoch–Schönlein purpura nephritis.

PATHOLOGY

The pathology of the extrarenal vasculitis has been reviewed elsewhere (1) and is not discussed in this chapter. The renal lesions have been extensively described previously (11,14,15,17,38,43–46,118–121).

Light Microscopy

Although various glomerular changes are observed on light microscopy of renal biopsy specimens, there are two basic types of glomerular lesions: mesangial proliferation and epithelial crescent formation. Typically, both lesions are seen to coexist (Fig. 1). Mesangial proliferation is caused by combinations of hypercellularity and increase in matrix, causing varying degrees of mesangial expansion. This abnormality varies considerably in severity and may be either diffuse, affecting at least 80% of glomeruli, or focal and segmental. The commonest appearance is that of diffuse but mild mesangial proliferation with focal accentuation, particularly in lobules affected by epithelial crescents.

When proliferation is severe, polymorphonuclear leukocytes and mononuclear cells may infiltrate the glomerular tufts, though not as severely as is seen typically in post-streptococcal nephritis. Using monoclonal antibodies, Nolasco et al. (122) found an increase in total leukocytes and monocytes/macrophages and both the CD4 and the CD8 T-cells subsets in Henoch–Schönlein purpura nephritis. Yoshioka et al. (123) found increase in monocytes/macrophages, as well as intraglomerular deposition of cross-linked fibrin in a degree proportional to the number of mononuclear cells. Severe mesangial proliferation may also be associated with mesangial interposition in which cell and matrix migrate into the capillary walls, between the basement membrane and endothelial cytoplasm, giving the capillary walls a "double contour" appearance on silver staining. Mesangial interposition is only rarely diffuse in Henoch–Schönlein purpura nephritis, when it may superficially mimic the appearance of mesangiocapillary (membranoproliferative) glomerulonephritis (15). Occasionally, lobules, particularly those underlying crescents, may also become necrotic, as indicated by the presence of nuclear debris and eosinophilic material, although others may rarely undergo mesangiolysis, with aneurysmal capillary dilation.

In epithelial crescents, the proliferating visceral and parietal epithelial cells cause adhesion between the glomerular tuft and the Bowman capsule, thereby obliterating the urinary space. Crescents vary in size from small segmental ones affecting one or two lobules to the circumferential type. Larger cellular crescents characteristically show "pseudotubule" formation in which the cells are recognized locally to form cannulae. During the acute phase, crescents are predominantly cellular and may contain fibrin. Later, they become fibrous. At the point of adhesion, the glomerular capillaries will eventually become

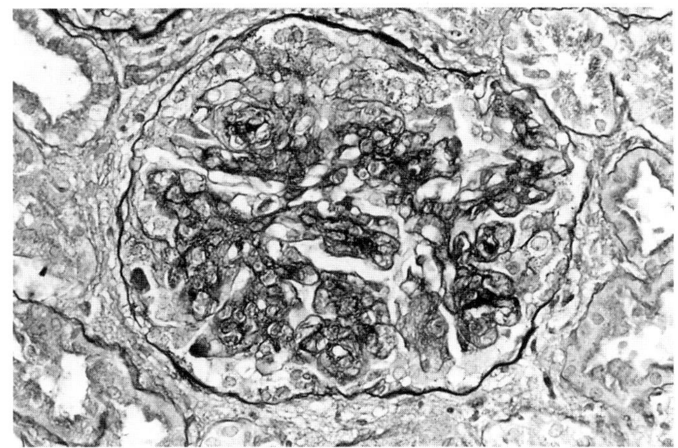
A

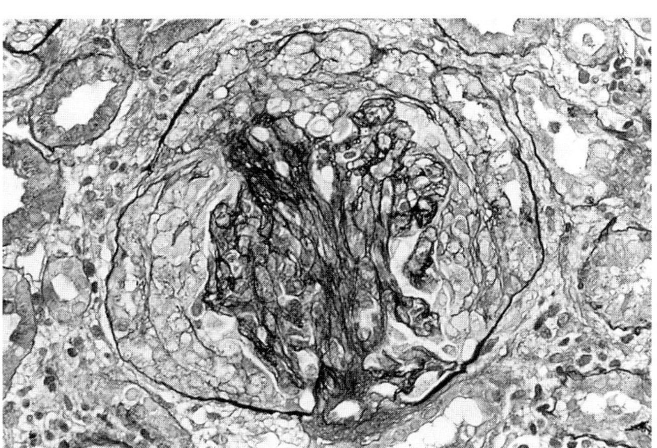
B

FIG. 1. A: A glomerulus from a patient with Henoch–Schönlein purpura nephritis: there is a moderate increase of mesangial cellularity and matrix, and a fibrocellular crescent. Periodic acid–Schiff, ×600. **B:** A glomerulus from a patient with Henoch–Schönlein purpura nephritis: a circumferential crescent is evident. Periodic acid–Schiff, ×600.

obliterated by sclerosis, and whereas a small crescent will leave no more than a segmental scar, a circumferential one will cause global sclerosis. Typically, a biopsy specimen shows a mixture of predominantly small and, occasionally, large crescents, but rarely a high proportion of glomeruli may be affected by circumferential crescents, resulting in severely compromised renal function and rapid progression to end-stage renal failure. Changes observed in repeat renal biopsies suggest that small crescent may be capable of resolution without fibrosis. Small adhesions are frequently seen between the tuft and the Bowman capsule, in the absence of true crescent formation.

Tubulointerstitial changes such as tubular atrophy and interstitial fibrosis that may be observed are secondary to the glomerular lesions and generally commensurate with their severity. Isolated foci of tubular atrophy may be seen with moderate glomerulonephritis, but, in severe, crescentic nephritis, it is usually more extensive and associated with widespread interstitial edema and cellular infiltration, which may later progress to fibrosis.

Inflammatory changes affecting the renal arterioles are rare in Henoch–Schönlein purpura. Levy et al. (15) reported occasionally finding arteriolar necrosis in two of 100 biopsy specimens investigated, and perivascular cellular infiltration was absent. There is only one report of exudative vasculitis, with intramural and perivascular leukocytic infiltration, affecting an extraglomerular arteriole in an adult suffering from apparently typical Henoch–Schönlein purpura (124).

Because the mesangial proliferation usually resolves without causing to permanent damage, the morphologic severity of Henoch–Schönlein purpura nephritis is best assessed by the extent of glomerular involvement with crescents and segmental lesions, including necrosis and sclerosis. The classification used most is that evolved by the pathologists of the International Study of Kidney Disease in Children (38,43,44):

I. Minimal glomerular abnormalities
II. Pure mesangial proliferation
III. Minor glomerular abnormalities or mesangial proliferation, with crescents/segmental lesions (sclerosis, adhesions, thrombosis, necrosis) in <50% glomeruli
IV. As III but with crescents/segmental lesions in 50–75% glomeruli
V. As III but with crescents/segmental lesions in >75% glomeruli
VI. Membranoproliferative-like lesion

Each of the severity grades is based on the percentage of glomeruli showing crescents and segmental lesions and is further subdivided according to whether the mesangial proliferation is (a) focal and segmental or (b) diffuse. The clinicopathologic correlations of this classification have been effectively tested in follow-up studies (14, 38,43–45). However, it should be noted that grade VI, the rare membranoproliferative-like lesion, does not denote the most severe type; its severity is best assessed according to the frequency of crescent formation and sclerosis.

Immunofluorescence Microscopy

The characteristic immunopathologic pattern of Henoch–Schönlein purpura nephritis is the presence of IgA in the glomerular mesangium (Fig. 2). There are also deposits of IgG and/or IgM with the same staining pattern as IgA, usually with lesser intensity and frequency. In our series (38), mesangial IgA deposits were associated with IgG in 35% of patients and IgM in 33%. C3 was observed in a similar distribution pattern in 60%, although it was usually less intense than IgA. However, the early classic complement components—C4 and C1q—are usually absent (15,36). Properdin often occurs in the same distribution as C3 (15,73). Fibrin(ogen)-related antigens are found in more than two-thirds of patients (15,118) and are thought to be one of the injurious agents in the glomeruli. Although, in most patients, IgA is present only in the mesangial regions, in ~10% of patients it is also observed in the peripheral capillary walls. Such peripheral capillary wall deposits, whether documented by immunofluorescence or electron microscopy, have been associated with more severe clinical manifestations and a poor renal outcome (44).

Electron Microscopy

Electron-microscopic abnormalities are mainly observed in the mesangium, which is variably enlarged by a combination of increased cytoplasm and matrix. Electron-dense deposits in the mesangium are the most constant and prominent feature and are seen in almost all

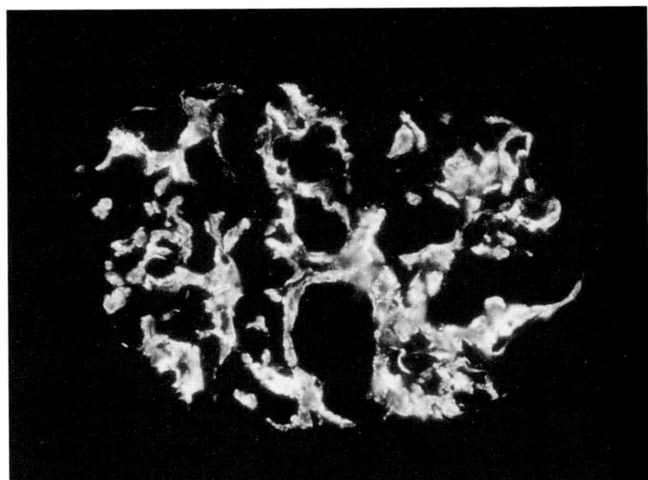

FIG. 2. Immunofluorescence micrograph showing mesangial IgA deposits from a patient with Henoch–Schönlein purpura nephritis. ×600.

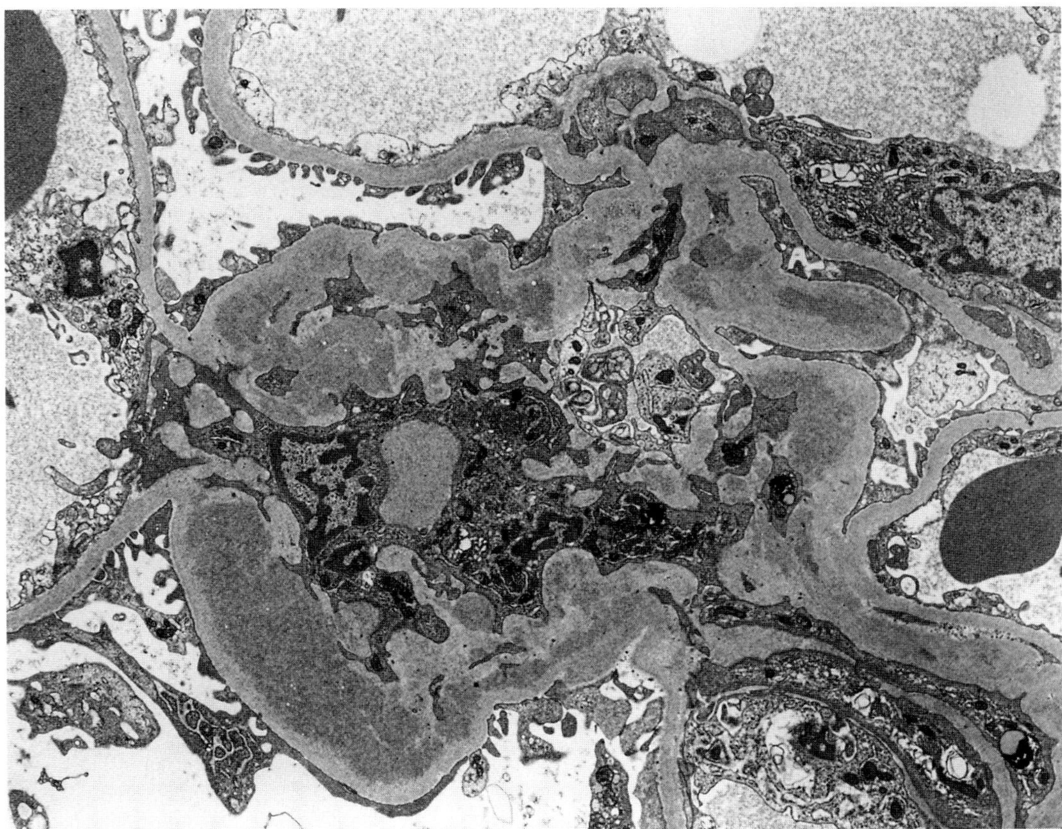

FIG. 3. Electron micrograph showing numerous electron-dense deposits in the mesangium. ×5,000.

patients (44). They are granular masses situated immediately beneath the lamina densa in the perimesangial region and expanded mesangium (Fig. 3). The size and extent of mesangial deposits vary from patient to patient. Peripheral glomerular capillary wall deposits are also found in the subendothelial and subepithelial regions. Immunoelectron microscopy confirmed that these deposits contain predominantly IgA, with smaller amounts of C3 and IgG (121). This technique also demonstrated IgA in the lamina densa immediately beneath subepithelial deposits, suggesting that immune complexes may be transported through the basement membrane. Subendothelial deposits occur most frequently in the capillary wall adjacent to the mesangium, although they are also observed in the peripheral part of the loop. Subepithelial deposits are also frequently found. They are generally small, flat, and localized to a few capillary loops; the humps typical of acute post-streptococcal glomerulonephritis are never observed. We (44) found a positive correlation between a poor outcome and the presence of subepithelial dense deposits. "Lysis" of the glomerular basement membrane is also seen quite frequently in children with Henoch–Schönlein purpura nephritis (120). In affected areas of the glomerular capillary walls, the lamina densa is thin and irregular, and the epithelial aspect of the glomerular basement membrane shows irregular segments of low electron density with an expanded "washed out" appearance. Lysis was mainly observed adjacent to subepithelial deposits and was associated with the presence of polymorphonuclear leukocytes in the capillary lumen and occasionally in direct contact with the basement membrane, suggesting that polymorphs may play a part in mediating the lysis. This particular lesion correlated with the severity of mesangial proliferation, the frequency of crescents, and a poor outcome. The epithelial foot processes are generally well preserved, but diffuse foot-process effacement may be seen in patients with the nephrotic syndrome.

Repeat Renal Biopsy

Niaudet et al. (125) demonstrated a good correlation between the histologic changes with time and both the clinical status and outcome of the patients. Patients who improved showed resolution of mesangial proliferation and the transition of previous crescents to small fibrous adhesions, in addition to a reduced number of affected glomeruli. In most patients who improved, IgA deposits were diminished considerably and, in a few, deposits had disappeared. In contrast, patients with active nephritis usually showed continuing proliferation, although fibrous crescents and segmental sclerosis affected a similar proportion of glomeruli. Patients progressing to end-stage renal failure showed mainly fibrotic glomeruli and severe tubulointerstitial lesions.

CLINICAL MANIFESTATIONS AND LABORATORY FEATURES

Extrarenal Manifestations

The extrarenal manifestations of Henoch–Schönlein purpura are characteristic and may occur in any order and any time over a period of several days or weeks.

Skin

Typically, the skin lesion begins with erythematous macules, some of which develop into slightly raised urticarial papules, which soon become purpuric. The eruption is of symmetric distribution, affecting predominantly the extensor surfaces of the lower legs and forearms, and the buttocks, but sparing the trunk. Purpura may occasionally affect the earlobes, nose, and external genitalia, but in typical mild cases is confined to the ankles. In older children, purpura may be the sole cutaneous manifestation whereas, in preschool children, urticaria may occur without purpura, although localized edema of the dorsum of hands and feet, face, and scalp may be seen (12,126). As the primary lesions fade, new crops of purpura commonly recur up to 3 months from onset and occasionally much longer (14,15,35), and sometimes associated with the recurrence of abdominal and joint symptoms.

Joints

About 70% of children (14,15,126) exhibit joint involvement, and joint symptoms may be the initial manifestation. Joint involvement mainly affects the knees, ankles, elbows, and wrists. This consists of arthralgia and periarticular edema, without the overlying erythema, tenderness, or joint effusions; it is transient and leaves no residual damage.

Gastrointestinal Tract

Gastrointestinal manifestations occur in 50–70% of all affected children (126), but the incidence rises to >90% in those who have renal involvement (14,15). The commonest symptom is abdominal colic, often severe and accompanied by vomiting, although melena occurs in half the cases (126). Occasionally, a mass may be palpable in the upper abdomen, suggesting intussusception, and when the abdominal symptoms precede the other manifestations, laparotomy is sometimes considered necessary (14). Intussusception secondary to severe purpura of the bowel is common in older children (13). A protein-losing enteropathy has been reported (127,128), possibly accounting for the occasional observation of hypoalbuminemic edema in the absence of heavy proteinuria. Vasculitic lesions have been reported in many other organs, but with extreme rarity (1).

Renal Manifestations

Renal manifestations occur at any time. The first urinary abnormality is usually noticed after other symptoms, but hematuria sometimes may be the initial feature. In 80% of children with a urinary abnormality, the first abnormality is detected within 4 weeks of onset of the illness. In most of the remainder, the urine abnormality develops within the next 8 weeks (10). Recurrences of renal manifestations are common and appear to be particularly so in those in whom severe renal damage develops. The relapses may occur at the time of an upper respiratory tract infection. There are no correlations between the severity of extrarenal manifestations and the severity of renal manifestations.

Although the clinical presentation of Henoch–Schönlein purpura nephritis is varied, ranging from asymptomatic urinary abnormalities to acute renal failure, four basic pathophysiologic disturbances can generally be identified at onset: hematuria, proteinuria, hypertension, and impaired renal function. Individually or in combination, they make up the various syndromes of Henoch–Schönlein purpura nephritis as follows:

1. Microscopic hematuria, transient or persistent
2. Macroscopic hematuria, initial or recurrent
3. Persistent heavy proteinuria (usually with microscopic hematuria)
4. Nephritic syndrome
5. Nephrotic syndrome
6. Mixed nephritic–nephrotic syndrome

Minimal renal involvement may cause no more than transient microscopic hematuria, detectable only by routine urinalysis during the acute illness. The illness also presents with initial macroscopic hematuria, usually lasting for a few days but occasionally up to several weeks, followed by microscopic hematuria that may persist for months or years. Macroscopic hematuria usually gives rise to transient heavy proteinuria. Persistence of heavy proteinuria of ≥1 g/day/m^2 body surface area with microscopic hematuria usually signifies nephritis of moderate severity. In these cases, the blood pressure and renal function are usually normal. Impaired renal function may sometimes be detected only by routine determination of the plasma creatinine level, but it more often occurs together with macroscopic hematuria as an acute nephritic syndrome associated with combinations of hypervolemia, oliguria, and hypertension (14). Massive proteinuria may lead to nephrotic syndrome (serum albumin, <25 g/L), with pitting edema of the face and ankles, and sometimes ascites. The most severe clinical presentation is a mixed nephritic–nephrotic syndrome in which hematuria, hypertension, and renal function impairment are combined with proteinuria and hypoalbuminemic edema (14).

Laboratory Features

There are no specific laboratory findings for Henoch–Schönlein purpura. In typical patients in whom the diagnosis is beyond doubt, the little investigation that is required is mainly directed toward assessing the extent of renal involvement. If purpura is absent but has been suggested by the patient's recent history, the feces should be tested for occult blood, the finding of which would support a diagnosis of Henoch–Schönlein purpura. If there is any doubt about the etiology of the purpura, a full blood count and coagulation screen should be performed. Clotting factor XIII, a fibrin-stabilizing factor, is significantly decreased in children with Henoch–Schönlein purpura. Although serum IgA level is raised in a significant proportion of cases of Henoch–Schönlein purpura, investigating it in individual patients does not contribute to management.

In every case of Henoch–Schönlein purpura, the urine should be routinely tested for blood and protein at onset and at least weekly until systemic signs have resolved in order not to overlook a mild nephritis. If urinary abnormalities are found, proteinuria should be quantified. The serum total protein and albumin levels should also be measured routinely. The serum creatinine level should be measured routinely to estimate renal function and, if necessary, the glomerular filtration rate should be determined.

Clinicopathologic Correlations

Renal biopsy is rarely needed for diagnosis, but is used to assess the severity of glomerulonephritis. It is required only in patients in whom the initial presentation is severe (nephritic and/or nephrotic) or in whom heavy proteinuria persists for >1 month. The more severe the clinical presentation is, the higher is the percentage of glomeruli affected by crescents and segmental lesions. Our findings (14,38,43,45), summarized in Table 1, demonstrate that (a) patients with initial macroscopic and/or persistent microscopic hematuria who do not have persisting heavy proteinuria have glomerular lesions of grade III or less; (b) those with a nephritic or nephrotic onset, or persistent heavy proteinuria, have a 10–20% chance of grade-IV to V lesions; (c) a mixed nephritic–nephrotic presentation carries a 60% risk of grade-IV to V lesions; and (d) the majority of grade-I to III lesions resolve, whereas an increasing proportion of grade-IV to V lesions do not.

TABLE 1. *Clinicopathologic correlations in Henoch–Schönlein purpura nephritis*

Clinical presentation	Biopsy grades	Approximate risk of renal failure (%)
Macroscopic/microscopic hematuria, and proteinuria minimal or absent	I–II, rarely III	<5
Hematuria and persistent heavy proteinuria	I–IV	15
Acute nephritic syndrome	II–IV	15
Nephrotic syndrome	II–IV, rarely I or V	40
Nephritic–nephrotic syndrome	II–V, mostly V	>50

From White and Yoshikawa (2), with permission.

DIFFERENTIAL DIAGNOSIS

The distribution of the rash and the accompanying gastrointestinal and articular lesions is usually so characteristic that the diagnosis is not in doubt. Difficulty may rarely arise when the skin eruption consists entirely of urticarial lesions without purpura. Although it is not feasible to diagnose Henoch–Schönlein purpura in the absence of cutaneous manifestations, there is anecdotal evidence that it occurs, albeit rarely (1). Hypoalbuminemic edema is occasionally observed in the absence of heavy proteinuria and may be caused by a protein-losing enteropathy (127). Quantitative assessment of proteinuria is therefore essential.

In older children and adults, the combination of joint symptoms and purpura makes it necessary to consider systemic lupus erythematosus and polyarteritis nodosa as alternative diagnoses (35). The light-microscopic findings of glomeruli in patients with systemic lupus erythematosus and those with Henoch–Schönlein purpura nephritis are similar and may be indistinguishable. In systemic lupus erythematosus, however, glomerular IgA deposits, when present, are less prominent than IgG deposits, and C1q deposits are almost always present. Antinuclear antibodies are usually absent in patients with Henoch–Schönlein purpura nephritis. The differential diagnosis between Henoch-Schönlein purpura nephritis and the microscopic form of polyarteritis nodosa is difficult. Mesangial IgA deposits are absent in polyarteritis nodosa. Therefore, the diagnosis of the microscopic form of polyarteritis nodosa should be considered in any patients with clinical signs of Henoch–Schönlein purpura if mesangial IgA deposits are not demonstrated (13).

Relationship with IgA Nephropathy

The relationship between IgA nephropathy and Henoch–Schönlein purpura nephritis is complex. The morphologic and immunopathologic features are similar in the two conditions (13,129), which are characterized by various degrees of focal or diffuse mesangial proliferation, the diffuse deposition of IgA in the mesangium, and electron-dense deposits in the mesangium. Elevated serum IgA levels are found in both IgA nephropathy and Henoch–Schönlein purpura nephritis, and IgA-containing circulating immune complexes have been demonstrated in both conditions. The two disorders have been reported to coexist in different members of the same family (48,130), including a pair of monozygotic twins who developed them simultaneously following a well-documented adenovirus infection (18), and to affect the same patient at different times (131). It has been suggested that the two conditions are variants of the same process and that IgA nephropathy is Henoch–Schönlein purpura nephritis without the rash (13,18,132). Although there are similarities in their pathologic and immunologic features, the clinical courses of the two conditions are different and the pathogenesis is not clear. Our study (38) suggests that Henoch–Schönlein purpura nephritis is an acute disease and glomerular lesion is nonprogressive after the onset, so prognosis is associated with the severity of glomerular change at the onset. In contrast, IgA nephropathy is a chronic, slowly progressive glomerular lesion, which may lead eventually to chronic renal failure, whatever the presentation. It is therefore reasonable that IgA nephropathy and Henoch–Schönlein purpura nephritis are treated as different clinicopathologic entities until pathogeneses of the two conditions are better understood.

TREATMENT

In mild cases, no treatment is required, provided that the urine is adequately monitored, and ambulatory care may suffice. Indeed, the prolonged bed rest that was customary in the past occasionally led to complications such as femoral vein thrombosis and psychosocial problems (14). Although severe abdominal pain and vomiting are self-limiting, resolution can be hastened by the administration of steroids (133). Utani et al. (134) reported that factor-XIII concentrate replacement resolved severe abdominal symptoms in adults with Henoch–Schönlein purpura associated with a decreased level of factor-XIII activity.

The initial treatment of the renal manifestations will depend on their nature and severity. The hypertension that accompanies an acute nephritic syndrome probably depends on sodium and water retention, and usually is transient. Modest dietary salt and water restriction, together with a loop diuretic, may be sufficient, but if hypertension persists or an encephalopathy is imminent, more aggressive antihypertensive therapy will be needed. When the renal lesion presents as a nephrotic syndrome, salt and water restriction will again be needed, but because of hypovolemia, diuretics must be given with caution. However, hypoalbuminemia is rarely as severe in Henoch–Schönlein purpura nephritis as it is in the idiopathic nephrotic syndrome, and the need to administer intravenous albumin is exceptional.

At present, there is no treatment of proven value for Henoch–Schönlein purpura nephritis, although some regimens have been proposed and tested, with controversial results. These include (a) glucocorticoids and/or immunosuppressive drugs to manipulate the abnormal immune response and (b) plasma exchange to remove circulating IgA immune complexes. Preliminary observations, made 30 years ago, suggested that corticosteroids afforded no benefit (135), and subsequent studies confirmed this (14, 15,43). Habib et al. (13) described the beneficial role of methylprednisolone pulse therapy in the treatment of severe Henoch–Schönlein purpura nephritis. We used methylprednisolone pulse therapy in seven children who had acute renal insufficiency, but six progressed to chronic renal failure (136). A recent prospective study (137) demonstrated that early administration of prednisone could prevent the development of nephritis in children with Henoch–Schönlein purpura. However, Saulsbury (138) showed that early corticosteroid therapy did not prevent the development of nephritis in children with Henoch–Schönlein purpura in a retrospective study. Immunosuppressive agents tried include azathioprine (14,135), cyclophosphamide (14,15), and chlorambucil (15), and although some successes were claimed initially on the basis of partial or complete remission, the natural history of the renal lesion was not at that time fully appreciated. An uncontrolled trial of combined steroids, immunosuppressive, and anticoagulant therapy in rapidly progressive glomerulonephritis of various causes, including Henoch–Schönlein purpura nephritis, suggested that deterioration of renal function could be retarded or occasionally halted, provided that the patient was not already severely oliguric (139). We used prednisolone, cyclophosphamide, and anticoagulant drugs to treat seven children who had acute renal insufficiency: five completely recovered and only one progressed to chronic renal failure (136). Plasma exchange combined with glucocorticoids and immunosuppressive drugs is probably of value in patients with rapidly progressive crescentic disease, but full recovery remains unlikely (140–142).

PROGNOSIS

The long-term morbidity and mortality of Henoch–Schönlein purpura are almost exclusively attributable to renal disease. Several centers have reported the correlation of both clinical presentation and renal morphology with outcome (10,14,17,43,45,120). In our experience, of 122 children with renal involvement (38), 14 (11%) were found to be in established chronic renal failure or to have died as a result, and a further seven patients (6%) had active disease. However, these patients were selected for investigation because of their renal involvement, and the overall prognosis of Henoch–Schönlein purpura is better appreciated from two large series in which the conditions of patients both with or without nephritis were followed up, giving estimated incidences of end-stage renal failure of 2% (46) and 5% (17).

The results of follow-up studies demonstrate that absolute conclusions regarding the prognostic value of the clinical presentation for individual patients are not possible. It is clear, however, that those children who present with slight proteinuria and/or hematuria have an excellent prognosis and that patients who present with persistent heavy proteinuria, acute nephritic syndrome, and/or nephrotic syndrome are at risk of developing chronic renal failure. The 23-year follow-up study by Goldstein et al. (45) indicated that ~15% of patients with a nephritic onset or persistent heavy proteinuria, 40% of those with a nephrotic presentation, and <50% of those with a mixed nephritic–nephrotic onset have ongoing urinary abnormalities, and that many of these patients ultimately develop renal failure (Table 1).

The proportion of glomeruli with crescents or segmental lesions (sclerosis, adhesions, thrombosis, or necrosis) seems to be the most important prognostic indicator. The larger the number of glomeruli affected by crescents or segmental lesions, the poorer the prognosis is. The relationship between histologic grade and outcome in our 122 children with Henoch–Schönlein purpura nephritis who were biopsied and whose conditions were followed for at least 2 years is summarized in Table 2, which demonstrates a progressively worsening outcome with increasing histologic severity, as judged by the percentage of patients in each grade showing either active disease or chronic renal failure: 0% for grade I, 4% for grade II, 9% for grade III, 33% for grade IV, and 83% for grade V. Of the 72 patients who completely recovered, 67 had <50% of their glomeruli affected by crescents or segmental lesions. In contrast, of the 13 patients who developed chronic renal failure, 12 had >50% of their glomeruli affected by crescents or segmental lesions.

TABLE 2. *Relationship between biopsy grade and outcome in Henoch–Schönlein purpura nephritis*

Biopsy grade	No. of patients	Normal urine	Slight proteinuria and/or hematuria	Heavy proteinuria	Renal failure
I	22	14	8		
II	22	15	6	1	
III	53	38	10	4	1
IV	12	5	3	1	3
V	12		2	1	9
Total	121	72	29	7	13

Goldstein et al. (45) observed that 17 of 78 of the patients traced, whose initial progress was assessed by Meadow et al. (14) two years after onset, showed clinical deterioration at their final reassessment >19 years later. It is of interest that seven of these patients had apparently completely recovered after a follow-up of 10 years. Moreover, in women, 16 (36%) of the 44 successful pregnancies were complicated by hypertension, persistent proteinuria, or both. The late development of hypertension and proteinuria after a period of normality, and the pregnancy proteinuria, together with the progressive decline in renal function that may follow initial improvement, are consistent with a sequence of glomerular hyperfiltration followed by secondary glomerulosclerosis (143), when glomerular destruction due to the original disease has been extensive. Since most subjects found by Goldstein et al. (45) to have residual abnormalities were asymptomatic, it follows that children who have Henoch–Schönlein purpura nephritis with a severe clinical onset or biopsy grade require almost indefinite follow-up.

Recurrence in the Renal Allograft

In Henoch–Schönlein purpura nephritis, clinical recurrence in the renal allografts is rare, but the recurrence of the mesangial IgA deposits with lack of symptoms is frequent (13,62–64,144). Recurrent disease appears to be strongly associated with living related donor transplantation. The significance of this is unclear, but the association of disease recurrence with living related donor transplantation may imply a genetic predisposition. In the report by Hasegawa et al. (64), there were nine histologic recurrences among 12 living related donor grafts, five of them associated with clinical manifestations. In contrast, clinical recurrence was not observed in five cadaveric grafts, and four of these showed no IgA deposits on biopsy. Habib et al. (13) observed asymptomatic IgA deposits in 11 of the 13 cadaveric grafts, but only one of 13 patients developed a disease related to recurrence. In the light of these findings, it can be argued that, although there is no contraindication to cadaveric transplantation, living related donor allografts should be avoided.

REFERENCES

1. White RHR. Henoch–Schönlein purpura. In: Churg A, Churg J, eds. *Systemic vasculitides.* New York: Igaku-Shin, 1991:203–17.
2. White RHR, Yoshikawa N. Henoch–Schönlein nephritis. In: Holliday MA, Barratt TM, Avner ED, eds. *Pediatric nephrology.* Baltimore: Williams and Wilkins, 1993:729–38.
3. Heberden W. *Commentarii di morboriana:* historia et curatione. London: Payne, 1801.

4. Schönlein JL. *Allgemeine und specielle pathologie und therapie*; vol 2. 3rd ed. Herisau: Literatur-Comptoir, 1837:48.
5. Henoch EH. Verhandlungen arztlicher Gesellschaffen. *Berl Klin Wochenschr* 1868;5:517.
6. Henoch EH. *Vorlesungen über Kinderkrankheiten.* 8th ed. Berlin: Hirschwalt, 1895.
7. Osler W. Visceral lesions of purpura and allied conditions. *BMJ* 1914;1:517–25.
8. Frank E. Die essentielle Thrombopenie. *Berl Klin Wochenschr* 1915; 52:454–8.
9. Bunchman TE, Mauer SM, Sibly RK, Vernier RL. Anaphylactoid purpura: characteristics of 16 patients who progressed to renal failure. *Pediatr Nephrol* 1988;2:393–7.
10. Levy M, Broyer M, Arsan A, et al. Glomérulonéphrites du purpura rhumatoide chez l'enfant: histoire naturelle et étude immunopathologique. *Adv* Nephrol Necker 1976;6:174–226.
11. Meadow SR. Schönlein–Henoch syndrome. In: Edelmann CM Jr, ed. *Pediatric Kidney Disease.* 2nd ed. Boston: Little, Brown, 1992: 1525–33.
12. Gairdner D. Schönlein–Henoch syndrome. *Q J Med* 1948;17:95–122.
13. Habib R, Niaudet P, Levy M. Schönlein–Henoch purpura nephritis and IgA nephropathy. In: Tisher C, Brenner B, eds. *Renal pathology:* with clinical and functional correlations. 2nd ed. Philadelphia: JB Lippincott, 1994:472–523.
14. Meadow SR, Glasgow EF, White RH, Moncrieff MW, Cameron JS, Ogg CS. Schönlein–Henoch nephritis. *Q J Med* 1972;41:241–58.
15. Levy M, Broyer M, Arsan A, Levy BD, Habib R. Anaphylactoid purpura nephritis in childhood: natural history and immunopathology. *Adv Nephrol Necker Hosp* 1976;6:183–228.
16. Ayoub EM, Hoyer J. Anaphylactoid purpura: streptococcal antibody titers and beta1c-globulin levels. *J Pediatr* 1969;75:193–201.
17. Kobayashi O, Wada H, Okawa K, Takeyama I. Schönlein–Henoch's syndrome in children. *Contrib Nephrol* 1977;4:48–71.
18. Meadow SR, Scott DG. Berger disease: Henoch–Schönlein syndrome without the rash. *J Pediatr* 1985;106:27–32.
19. Garty BZ, Danon YL, Nitzan M. Schoenlein–Henoch purpura associated with hepatitis A infection [Letter]. *Am J Dis Child* 1985;139.
20. Maggiore G, Martini A, Grifeo S, De GC, Scotta MS. Hepatitis B virus infection and Schönlein–Henoch purpura. *Am J Dis Child* 1984; 138:681–2.
21. Rasmussen NH. Henoch–Schönlein purpura after yersiniosis [Letter]. *Arch Dis Child* 1982;57:322–3.
22. Roza M, Galbe M, Gonzalez BC, Fernandez M, Miguell MA. Henoch–Schoenlein purpura after shigellosis [Letter]. *Clin Nephrol* 1983;20:269.
23. Liew SW, Kessel I. Mycoplasmal pneumonia preceding Henoch–Schönlein purpura [Letter]. *Arch Dis Child* 1974;49:912–3.
24. Alwar AJ. Schönlein–Henoch syndrome: a case report and literature review. *East Afr Med J* 1982;59:357–60.
25. Jimenez EL, Dorrington HJ. Vaccination and Henoch–Schoenlein purpura [Letter]. *N Engl J Med* 1968;279:1171.
26. Patel U, Bradley JR, Hamilton DV. Henoch–Schönlein purpura after influenza vaccination. *Br Med J Clin Res Educ* 1988;296:1800.
27. Burke D, Jellinek J. Nearly fatal case of Schönlein–Henoch syndrome following insect bite. *Am J Dis Child* 1954;88:772–4.
28. Rogers PW, Bunn SJ, Kurtzman NA, White MG. Schönlein–Henoch syndrome associated with exposure to cold. *Arch Intern Med* 1971; 128:782–6.
29. Talbot D, Craig R, Falconer S, Tomson D, Milne DD. Henoch–Schönlein purpura secondary to trauma [Letter]. *Arch Dis Child* 1988;63:1114–5.
30. Kimmel PL, Phillips TM, Ferreira CA, Farkas ST, Abraham AA, Garrett CT. Idiotypic IgA nephropathy in patients with human immunodeficiency virus infection [Brief report; see comments]. *N Engl J Med* 1992;327:702–6.
31. Furukawa T, Hisao O, Furuta S, Shigematsu H. Henoch–Schönlein purpura with nephritis in a patient with Behçet's disease. *Am J Kidney Dis* 1989;13:497–500.
32. Yamabe H, Ozawa K, Fukushi K, et al. IgA nephropathy and Henoch–Schönlein purpura nephritis with anterior uveitis. *Nephron* 1988;50:368–70.
33. Caims S, Mallick N, Lawler W, Williams G. Squamous cell carcinoma of bronchus presenting with Henoch–Schönlein purpura. *BMJ* 1978;2:474–5.
34. Mitsuhashi H, Mitsuhashi M, Tsukada Y, Yano S, Naruse T. Henoch–Schönlein purpura in rheumatoid arthritis. *J Rheumatol* 1994;21:1138–40.
35. Cream JJ, Gumpel JM, Peachey RD. Schönlein–Henoch purpura in the adult: a study of 77 adults with anaphylactoid or Schönlein–Henoch purpura. *Q J Med* 1970;39:461–84.
36. Sinniah R, Feng PH, Chen BT. Henoch–Schoenlein syndrome: a clinical and morphological study of renal biopsies. *Clin Nephrol* 1978;9: 219–28.
37. Fogazzi GB, Pasquali S, Moriggi M, et al. Long-term outcome of Schönlein–Henoch nephritis in the adult. *Clin Nephrol* 1989;31:60–6.
38. Yoshikawa N, Ito H, Yoshiya K, et al. Henoch–Schoenlein nephritis and IgA nephropathy in children: a comparison of clinical course. *Clin Nephrol* 1987;27:233–7.
39. Knight JF. The rheumatic poison: a survey of some published investigations of the immunopathogenesis of Henoch–Schönlein purpura. *Pediatr Nephrol* 1990;4:533–41.
40. Nielsen HE. Epidemiology of Schönlein–Henoch purpura. *Acta Paediatr Scand* 1988;77:125–31.
41. Stewart M, Savage JM, Bell B, McCord B. Long term renal prognosis of Henoch–Schönlein purpura in an unselected childhood population. *Eur J Pediatr* 1988;147:113–5.
42. Lewis I. The Henoch–Schönlein syndrome (anaphylactoid purpura) compared with certain features of nephritis and rheumatism. *Arch Dis Child* 1955;30:212–6.
43. Counahan R, Winterborn MH, White RH, et al. Prognosis of Henoch–Schönlein nephritis in children. *BMJ* 1977;2:11–4.
44. Yoshikawa N, White RH, Cameron AH. Prognostic significance of the glomerular changes in Henoch–Schoenlein nephritis. *Clin Nephrol* 1981;16:223–9.
45. Goldstein AR, White RH, Akuse R, Chantler C. Long-term follow-up of childhood Henoch–Schönlein nephritis. *Lancet* 1992;339:280–2.
46. Koskimies O, Mir S, Rapola J, Vilska J. Henoch–Schönlein nephritis: long-term prognosis of unselected patients. *Arch Dis Child* 1981;56: 482–4.
47. Galla J, Kohaut E, Alexander R, Mestecky J. Racial differences in the prevalence of IgA-associated nephropathies. *Lancet* 1984;ii:522.
48. Levy M. Do genetic factors play a role in Berger's disease? *Pediatr Nephrol* 1987;1:447–54.
49. Bhuyan UN, Tiwari SC, Malaviya AN, Srivastava RN, Dash SC, Malhotra KK. Immunopathology & prognosis in Henoch–Schönlein glomerulonephritis. *Indian J Med Res* 1986;83:33–40.
50. Farley TA, Gillespie S, Rasoulpour M, Tolentino N, Hadler JL, Hurwitz E. Epidemiology of a cluster of Henoch–Schönlein purpura [See comments]. *Am J Dis Child* 1989;143:798–803.
51. Ostergaard JR, Storm K, Lamm LU. Lack of association between HLA and Schoenlein–Henoch purpura. *Tissue Antigens* 1990;35:234–5.
52. Jin DK, Kohsaka T, Kobayashi N. The polymorphism of the immunoglobulin heavy chain switch region gene in IgA nephropathy, Henoch–Schönlein nephritis and idiopathic nephrotic syndrome. *Pediatr Nephrol* 1993;7:449–51.
53. Philpott M. The Schönlein–Henoch syndrome in childhood with particular reference to the occurrence of nephritis. *Arch Dis Child* 1952; 27:480–1.
54. Derham R, Rogerson M. The Schönlein–Henoch syndrome in childhood with particular reference to renal sequelae. *Arch Dis Child* 1956;31:364–8.
55. Koskimies O, Rapola J, Savilahti E, Vilska J. Renal involvement in Schönlein–Henoch purpura. *Acta Paediatr Scand* 1974;63:357–63.
56. Ilan Y, Naparstek Y. Schönlein–Henoch syndrome in adults and children. *Semin Arthritis Rheum* 1991;21:103–9.
57. Zurowska AM, Wrzolkowa T, Uszycka KM. Henoch–Schönlein nephritis in children: a clinicopathological study. *Int J Pediatr Nephrol* 1985;6:183–8.
58. Levinsky RJ, Barratt TM. IgA immune complexes in Henoch–Schönlein purpura. *Lancet* 1979;2:1100–3.
59. Kauffmann RH, Herrmann WA, Meyer CJ, Daha MR, Van EL. Circulating IgA-immune complexes in Henoch–Schönlein purpura: a longitudinal study of their relationship to disease activity and vascular deposition of IgA. *Am J Med* 1980;69:859–66.
60. Coppo R, Basolo B, Martina G, et al. Circulating immune complexes containing IgA, IgG and IgM in patients with primary IgA nephropathy and with Henoch–Schoenlein nephritis: correlation with clinical and histologic signs of activity. *Clin Nephrol* 1982;18:230–9.
61. Feehally J. Immune mechanisms in glomerular IgA deposition. *Nephrol Dial Transplant* 1988;3:361–78.

62. Baliah T, Kim KH, Anthone S, Anthone R, Montes M, Andres GA. Recurrence of Henoch–Schönlein purpura glomerulonephritis in transplanted kidneys. *Transplantation* 1974;18:343–6.
63. Nast CC, Ward HJ, Koyle MA, Cohen AH. Recurrent Henoch–Schönlein purpura following renal transplantation. *Am J Kidney Dis* 1987;9:39–43.
64. Hasegawa A, Kawamura T, Ito H, et al. Fate of renal grafts with recurrent Henoch–Schönlein purpura nephritis in children. *Transplant Proc* 1989;21:2130–3.
65. Davin JC, Dechenne C, Lombet J, Rentier B, Foidart JB, Mahieu PR. Acute experimental glomerulonephritis induced by the glomerular deposition of circulating polymeric IgA–concanavalin A complexes. *Virchows Arch [A]* 1989;415:7–20.
66. Silva F, Hogg R. IgA nephropathy. In: Tisher C, Brenner B, eds. *Renal pathology:* with clinical and functional correlations. Philadelphia: JB Lippincott, 1989:434–93.
67. Conley ME, Cooper MD, Michael AF. Selective deposition of immunoglobulin A1 in immunoglobulin A nephropathy, anaphylactoid purpura nephritis, and systemic lupus erythematosus. *J Clin Invest* 1980; 66:1432–6.
68. Tomino Y, Endoh M, Suga T, et al. Prevalence of IgA1 deposits in Henoch–Schoenlein purpura (HSP) nephritis. *Tokai J Exp Clin Med* 1982;7:527–32.
69. Rajaraman S, Goldblum RM, Cavallo T. IgA-associated glomerulonephritides: a study with monoclonal antibodies. *Clin Immunol Immunopathol* 1986;39:514–22.
70. Russell MW, Mestecky J, Julian BA, Galla JH. IgA-associated renal diseases: antibodies to environmental antigens in sera and deposition of immunoglobulins and antigens in glomeruli. *J Clin Immunol* 1986; 6:74–86.
71. Egido J, Sancho J, Mampaso F, et al. A possible common pathogenesis of the mesangial IgA glomerulonephritis in patients with Berger's disease and Schönlein–Henoch syndrome. *Proc Eur Dial Transplant Assoc* 1980;17:660–6.
72. Bene M, Faure G, Duheille J. IgA nephropathy: characterization of the polymeric nature of mesangial deposits by in vitro binding of free secretory component. *Clin Exp Immunol* 1982;47:527–34.
73. Evans DJ, Williams DG, Peters DK, et al. Glomerular deposition of properdin in Henoch–Schönlein syndrome and idiopathic focal nephritis. *BMJ* 1973;3:326–8.
74. Kawana S, Shen GH, Kobayashi Y, Nishiyama S. Membrane attack complex of complement in Henoch–Schönlein purpura skin and nephritis. *Arch Dermatol Res* 1990;282:183–7.
75. Garcia FM, Martin A, Chantler C, Williams DG. Serum complement components in Henoch–Schönlein purpura. *Arch Dis Child* 1978;53: 417–9.
76. Petersen S, Taaning E, Soderstrom T, et al. Immunoglobulin and complement studies in children with Schönlein–Henoch syndrome and other vasculitic diseases. *Acta Paediatr Scand* 1991;80:1037–43.
77. Kawana S, Nishiyama S. Serum SC5b-9 (terminal complement complex) level, a sensitive indicator of disease activity in patients with Henoch–Schönlein purpura. *Dermatology* 1992;184:171–6.
78. Emancipator SN. Immunoregulatory factors in the pathogenesis of IgA nephropathy [Clinical conference]. *Kidney Int* 1990;38:1216–29.
79. Tomino Y, Sakai H, Endoh M, et al. Cross-reactivity of eluted antibodies from renal tissues of patients with Henoch–Schönlein purpura nephritis and IgA nephropathy. *Am J Nephrol* 1983;3:315–8.
80. Tomino Y, Endoh M, Miura M, Nomoto Y, Sakai H. Immunopathological similarities between IgA nephropathy and Henoch–Schoenlein purpura (HSP) nephritis. *Acta Pathol Jpn* 1983;33:113–22.
81. Tanaka M, Fuzisawa S, Okuda R. Anaphylactoid purpura in childhood: III. Follow-up study of serum levels of immunoglobulins. *Ann Paediatr Jpn* 1969;15:19–26.
82. Trygstad CW, Stiehm ER. Elevated serum IgA globulin in anaphylactoid purpura. *Pediatrics* 1971;47:1023–8.
83. Simila S, Kouvalainen K, Lanning M. Serum immunoglobulin levels in the course of anaphylactoid purpura in children. *Acta Paediatr Scand* 1977;66:537–40.
84. Saulsbury FT. The role of IgA1 rheumatoid factor in the formation of IgA-containing immune complexes in Henoch–Schönlein purpura. *J Clin Lab Immunol* 1987;23:123–7.
85. Saulsbury FT. IgA rheumatoid factor in Henoch–Schönlein purpura. *J Pediatr* 1986;108:71–6.
86. Saulsbury FT. Heavy and light chain composition of serum IgA and IgA rheumatoid factor in Henoch–Schönlein purpura. *Arthritis Rheum* 1992;35:1377–80.
87. Saulsbury FT, Kirkpatrick PR, Bolton WK. IgA antineutrophil cytoplasmic antibody in Henoch–Schönlein purpura. *Am J Nephrol* 1991; 11:295–300.
88. Ronda N, Esnault VL, Layward L, et al. Antineutrophil cytoplasm antibodies (ANCA) of IgA isotype in adult Henoch–Schönlein purpura. *Clin Exp Immunol* 1994;95:49–55.
89. Blanco QA, Blanco C, Alvarez J, Solis P, Conde F, Gomez S. Anti-immunoglobulin antibodies in children with Schönlein–Henoch syndrome: absence of serum anti-IgA antibodies. *Eur J Pediatr* 1994; 153:103–6.
90. Burden A, Gibson I, Roger R, Tillman D. IgA anticardiolipin antibodies associated with Henoch–Schönlein purpura. *J Am Acad Dermatol* 1994;31:857–60.
91. Coppo R, Basolo B, Piccoli G, et al. IgA1 and IgA2 immune complexes in primary IgA nephropathy and Henoch–Schönlein nephritis. *Clin Exp Immunol* 1984;57:583–90.
92. Waldo F, Cochran A. Mixed IgA–IgG aggregates as a model of immune complexes in IgA nephropathy. *J Immunol* 1989;142:3841–6.
93. O'Donoghue DJ, Darvill A, Ballardie FW. Mesangial cell autoantigens in immunoglobulin A nephropathy and Henoch–Schönlein purpura. *J Clin Invest* 1991;88:1522–30.
94. Jennette JC, Wieslander J, Tuttle R, Falk RJ. Serum IgA–fibronectin aggregates in patients with IgA nephropathy and Henoch–Schönlein purpura: diagnostic value and pathogenic implications—the Glomerular Disease Collaborative Network. *Am J Kidney Dis* 1991;18: 466–71.
95. Cederholm B, Linne T, Wieslander J, Bygren P, Heinegard D. Fibronectin–immunoglobulin complexes in the early course of IgA and Henoch–Schönlein nephritis. *Pediatr Nephrol* 1991;5:200–4.
96. Kuno SH, Sakai H, Nomoto Y, Takakura I, Kimura M. Increase of IgA-bearing peripheral blood lymphocytes in children with Henoch–Schoenlein purpura. *Pediatrics* 1979;64:918–22.
97. Casanueva B, Rodriguez VV, Merino J, Arias M, Garcia FM. Increased IgA-producing cells in the blood of patients with active Henoch–Schönlein purpura. *Arthritis Rheum* 1983;26:854–60.
98. Casanueva B, Rodriguez VV, Luceno A. Circulating IgA producing cells in the differential diagnosis of Henoch–Schönlein purpura. *J Rheumatol* 1988;15:1229–33.
99. Casanueva B, Rodriguez VV, Farinas MC, Vallo A, Rodriguez SJ. Autologous mixed lymphocyte reaction and T-cell suppressor activity in patients with Henoch–Schönlein purpura and IgA nephropathy. *Nephron* 1990;54:224–8.
100. Woodroffe A. Summary of the pathogenesis of IgA nephropathy. In: Clarkson A, ed. *IgA nephropathy.* Boston: Martinus Nijhoff, 1987: 204–13.
101. Pfaffenboch G, Lamm M, Gigli I. Activation of the guinea pig alternative complement pathway by mouse IgA immune complexes. *J Exp Med* 1982;155:231–247.
102. Pasternack A, Collin P, Mustonen J, et al. Glomerular IgA deposits in patients with celiac disease. *Clin Nephrol* 1990;34:56–60.
103. Ratnoff W, Fearon D, Austen K. The role of antibody in the activation of the alternative complement pathway. *Springer Semin Immunopathol* 1983;6:361–84.
104. Kilian M, Mestecky J, Russell M. Defense mechanisms involving Fc-dependent functions of immunoglobulin A and their subversion by bacterial immunoglobulin A proteases. *Microbiol Rev* 1988;52:296–318.
105. Colten H, Bienerstock J. Lack of C3 activation through the classical or alternative pathway by human secretory IgA anti–blood group A antibody. *Adv Exp Med* 1976;45:305–12.
106. Hiemstra P, Biewenga J, Gorter A, et al. Activation of complement by human serum IgA, secretory IgA and IgA1 fragments. *Mol Immunol* 1988;25:527–33.
107. Emancipator SN, Ovary Z, Lamm ME. The role of mesangial complement in the hematuria of experimental IgA nephropathy. *Lab Invest* 1987;57:269–76.
108. Boros G, Gofman L, Samsik J, Nagy J, Hamori A, Deak G. Blood coagulation abnormalities in the Schönlein–Henoch syndrome in adults. *Acta Med Acad Sci Hung* 1979;36:151–66.
109. Fukui H, Kamitsuji H, Nagao T, et al. Clinical evaluation of a pasteurized factor XIII concentrate administration in Henoch–Schönlein purpura: Japanese Pediatric Group. *Thromb Res* 1989;56:667–75.

110. Kamitsuji H, Tani K, Yasui M, et al. Activity of blood coagulation factor XIII as a prognostic indicator in patients with Henoch–Schönlein purpura: efficacy of factor XIII substitution. *Eur J Pediatr* 1987; 146:519–23.
111. Túri S, Nagy J, Haszon I, Havass Z, Nemeth M, Bereczki C. Plasma factors influencing PGI_2-like activity in patients with IgA nephropathy and Schönlein–Henoch purpura. *Pediatr Nephrol* 1989;3: 61–7.
112. Tonshoff B, Momper R, Schweer H, Scharer K, Seyberth HW. Increased biosynthesis of vasoactive prostanoids in Schönlein–Henoch purpura. *Pediatr Res* 1992;32:137–40.
113. Horii Y, Muraguchi A, Iwano M, et al. Involvement of IL-6 in mesangial proliferative glomerulonephritis. *J Immunol* 1989;143: 3949–55.
114. Ruef C, Budde K, Lacy J, et al. Interleukin 6 is an autocrine growth factor for mesangial cells. *Kidney Int* 1990;38:249–57.
115. Horii Y, Iwano M, Suematsu S, et al. Interleukin-6 and mesangial proliferation: generation and characterization of IL-6 transgenic mice. In: Sakai H, Sakai O, Nomoto Y, eds. *Pathogenesis of IgA nephropathy.* Tokyo: Harcourt Brace Jovanovich Japan, 1990:127–43.
116. Clarkson A, Woodroffe A, Aarons I. IgA nephropathy and Henoch–Schönlein purpura. In: Schrier R, Gottschalk C, eds. *Diseases of the kidney.* Boston: Little, Brown, 1993:1839–64.
117. Takemura T, Yoshioka K, Murakami K, et al. Cellular localization of inflammatory cytokines in human glomerulonephritis. *Virchows Arch* 1994;424:459–64.
118. Heaton JM, Turner DR, Cameron JS. Localization of glomerular "deposits" in Henoch–Schönlein nephritis. *Histopathology* 1977;1: 93–104.
119. Hurley RM, Drummond KN. Anaphylactoid purpura nephritis: clinicopathological correlations. *J Pediatr* 1972;81:904–11.
120. Yoshikawa N, Yoshiara S, Yoshiya K, Matsuo T, Okada S. Lysis of the glomerular basement membrane in children with IgA nephropathy and Henoch–Schönlein nephritis. *J Pathol* 1986;150:119–26.
121. Yoshiara S, Yoshikawa N, Matsuo T. Immunoelectron microscopic study of childhood IgA nephropathy and Henoch–Schönlein nephritis. *Virchows Arch [A]* 1987;412:95–102.
122. Nolasco F, Cameron J, Hartley B. Intraglomerular T cells and monocytes in nephritis: study with monoclonal antibodies. *Kidney Int* 1987;31:1160–6.
123. Yoshioka K, Takemura T, Aya N, Akano N, Miyamoto H, Maki S. Monocyte infiltration and cross-linked fibrin deposition in IgA nephritis and Henoch–Schoenlein purpura nephritis. *Clin Nephrol* 1989;32:107–12.
124. Falls WJ, Ford KL, Ashworth CT, Carter NW. Renal vasculitis in a nonfatal case of Henoch–Schönlein purpura. *Ann Intern Med* 1966; 64:1276–80.
125. Niaudet P, Levy M, Broyer M, Habib R. Clinicopathologic correlations in severe forms of Henoch–Schönlein purpura nephritis based on repeat biopsies. *Contrib Nephrol* 1984;40:250–4.
126. Allen D, Diamond L, Howell D. Anaphylactoid purpura in children (Schönlein–Henoch syndrome). *Am J Dis Child* 1960;99:833–54.
127. Jones NF, Creamer B, Gimlette TM. Hypoproteinaemia in anaphylactoid purpura. *BMJ* 1966;2:1166–8.
128. Reif S, Jain A, Santiago J, Rossi T. Protein losing enteropathy as a manifestation of Henoch–Schönlein purpura. *Acta Paediatr Scand* 1991;80:482–5.
129. Yoshikawa N, White R. IgA nephropathy. In: Holliday M, Barratt T, Avner E, eds. *Pediatric nephrology.* Baltimore: Williams and Wilkins, 1993:719–28.
130. Montoliu J, Lens XM, Torras A, Revert L. Henoch–Schönlein purpura and IgA nephropathy in father and son. *Nephron* 1990;54:77–9.
131. Hughes FJ, Wolfish NM, McLaine PN. Henoch–Schönlein syndrome and IgA nephropathy: a case report suggesting a common pathogenesis. *Pediatr Nephrol* 1988;2:389–92.
132. Weiss JH, Bhathena DB, Curtis JJ, Lucas BA, Luke RG. A possible relationship between Henoch–Schönlein syndrome and IgA nephropathy (Berger's disease): an illustrative case. *Nephron* 1978;22: 582–91.
133. Rosenblum ND, Winter HS. Steroid effects on the course of abdominal pain in children with Henoch–Schönlein purpura. *Pediatrics* 1987;79:1018–21.
134. Utani A, Ohta M, Shinya A, et al. Successful treatment of adult Henoch–Schönlein purpura with factor XIII concentrate. *J Am Acad Dermatol* 1991;24:438–42.
135. White R, Cameron J, Trounce J. Immunosuppressive therapy in steroid-resistant proliferative glomerulonephritis accompanied by the nephrotic syndrome. *BMJ* 1966;2:853–60.
136. Yoshikawa N, Ito H, Matsuo T. Henoch–Schönlein nephritis: prognostic factors. In: Brodehl J, Ehrich H, eds. *Paediatric nephrology.* Berlin: Springer-Verlag, 1984:226–9.
137. Mollica F, Li VS, Garozzo R, Russo G. Effectiveness of early prednisone treatment in preventing the development of nephropathy in anaphylactoid purpura. *Eur J Pediatr* 1992;151:140–4.
138. Saulsbury FT. Corticosteroid therapy does not prevent nephritis in Henoch–Schönlein purpura. *Pediatr Nephrol* 1993;7:69–71.
139. Brown CB, Wilson D, Turner D, et al. Combined immunosuppression and anticoagulation in rapidly progressive glomerulonephritis. *Lancet* 1974;2:1166–72.
140. Kauffmann RH, Houwert DA. Plasmapheresis in rapidly progressive Henoch–Schoenlein glomerulonephritis and the effect on circulating IgA immune complexes. *Clin Nephrol* 1981;16:155–60.
141. Camerone G, Garelli S, Valbonesi M, Mosconi L. Plasma exchange treatment in a patient with severe Schoenlein–Henoch purpura). *Minerva Med* 1982;73:1185–7.
142. Coppo R, Basolo B, Roccatello D, Piccoli G. Plasma exchange in primary IgA nephropathy and Henoch–Schönlein syndrome nephritis. *Plasma Ther* 1985;6:705–23.
143. Brenner B. Hemodynamically mediated glomerular injury and the progressive nature of kidney disease. *Kidney Int* 1983;23:647–55.
144. Meulders Q, Pirson Y, Cosyns JP, Squifflet JP, van Ypersele de Strihou C. Course of Henoch–Schönlein nephritis after renal transplantation: report on ten patients and review of the literature. *Transplantation* 1994;58:1179–86.

Immunologic Renal Diseases,
edited by E. G. Neilson and W. G. Couser.
Lippincott-Raven Publishers, Philadelphia © 1997.

CHAPTER 51

Idiopathic Membranoproliferative Glomerulonephritis

Robert B. Miller, Clifford E. Kashtan, Barbara A. Burke, and Youngki Kim

INTRODUCTION

Membranoproliferative glomerulonephritis (MPGN) is a chronic, progressive form of GN that occurs primarily in older children and young adults. It is characterized by a distinctive glomerular morphology under the light microscope, in which endocapillary proliferation and glomerular capillary wall thickening produce diffusely enlarged and lobulated glomerular tufts. Membranoproliferative glomerulonephritis was originally recognized as a chronic GN associated with persistent hypocomplementemia by West et al. (1) and Gotoff et al. (2). Subsequent observations have indicated that persistent hypocomplementemia is commonly but not universally observed in patients with MPGN (3,4).

Membranoproliferative glomerulonephritis is a light-microscopic description, and glomerular lesions resembling MPGN are seen in a variety of disorders. In most instances, the clinical and laboratory features allow differentiation between primary and secondary MPGN. In this chapter, only the primary, idiopathic form of MPGN is discussed.

Three types of idiopathic MPGN have been recognized on the basis of ultrastructural findings (Table 1). These appear to be separate disease entities, with differences in pathogenesis, natural history, and response to therapy, although MPGN type III is considered by some to be a variant of MPGN type I (5–7). In this chapter, MPGN types I and III are treated as separate disease entities.

Membranoproliferative glomerulonephritis has been reported to lead to end-stage renal disease (ESRD) in up to 88% of untreated patients (8). The United States Renal Data System (USRDS) reported between 1988 and 1991 that cases of MPGN (type not specified) represented 0.4% of all patients starting therapy for ESRD (9). The North American Pediatric Renal Transplant Cooperative Study (NAPTRCS) reported that 2.9% of patients receiving dialysis during 1992 had ESRD resulting from MPGN I or II (III was not mentioned) (10). Membranoproliferative glomerulonephritis has been found in 1–2% of renal biopsy specimens from children and adults (11–16). Although the USRDS (9) noted a slight male preponderance, numerous other studies have not found a difference in numbers of male and female patients (1,8, 12,17–29). The USRDS and other studies (1,8,9,12, 17–29) have noted that MPGN is rarely reported in groups other than Caucasians, raising the possibility of a predilection by race (30).

CLINICAL PRESENTATION AND COURSE

The clinical manifestations of the three types of MPGN are quite similar, making meaningful clinical distinctions between them difficult. Membranoproliferative glomerulonephritis is primarily a disease of children and young adults, with the age of onset usually between 6 and 30 years (12,29,31–34). Types I and III occur primarily in older children and adults (12,29,33,34). Patients with type II tend to be younger at onset than those with type I (27,31).

Examination of patients with MPGN I usually reveals microscopic hematuria, asymptomatic proteinuria, or both (13,23,29) (Table 1). Proteinuria is the usual presenting

R. B. Miller: Department of Pediatrics, University of Minnesota, Minneapolis, Minnesota 55455.

C. E. Kashtan: Department of Pediatrics, University of Minnesota, Minneapolis, Minnesota 55455.

B. A. Burke: Department of Laboratory Medicine and Pathology, University of Minnesota, Minneapolis, Minnesota 55455.

Y. Kim: Departments of Pediatrics and Laboratory Medicine and Pathology, University of Minnesota, Minneapolis, Minnesota 55455.

TABLE 1. *Comparison of typical MPGN types I, II, and III[a]*

Finding	Type I	Type II	Type III
Clinical			
Acute nephritic episode	Uncommon	Common	Uncommon
Nephrotic syndrome	Common	Common	Common
Hematuria	Common	Common	Common
Hypertension	Common	Common	Common
Recurrence in transplanted kidneys	Occasional	Usual	Unknown
Morphologic			
Subendothelial deposits	Present	Absent[b]	Present
Subepithelial deposits	Absent[b]	Present	Present
Intramembranous dense deposits	Absent	Present	Absent
C3 mesangial rings and railroad tracks	Absent	Present	Absent
Complement			
C3	Normal or reduced	Reduced	Reduced
C1 and C4	Normal or reduced	Normal	Normal
C5	Normal or reduced	Normal	Reduced
NF_t	Absent[b]	Absent	Present
NF_a	Absent[b]	Present	Absent[b]

NF_t: $C3NeF_{I/III}$, auto-antibody to C3/C5 convertase $[(C3b)_nBbP]$; NF_a: $C3NeF_{II}$, auto-antibody to C3 convertase (C3bBb).

[a]Except for the morphologic findings described, significant overlap between the three types may exist.

[b]May be present in some patients.

symptom in MPGN III (23,33–35), whereas hematuria, gross or microscopic, is variably present at onset (24,34,36). In contrast, the onset of MPGN II is frequently associated with acute nephritic episodes, characterized by oliguria, edema, hematuria, hypertension, and acute renal insufficiency (27,37). Rarely, cases of MPGN I and III present with acute nephritic episodes (7,13,23,32–34) (Table 1). A history of infections, especially upper respiratory infections, preceding the onset of symptoms is often elucidated in patients with MPGN. Elevated streptococcal antibody titers are occasionally found (13,23,38), but a pathologic link between streptococcal infections and MPGN has not been established. Acute nephritic episodes caused by MPGN may be difficult to distinguish from post-streptococcal glomerulonephritis on clinical grounds alone (see Chapter 47). Gross hematuria is rarely seen after the first year of disease in all types of MPGN (24,29).

Whereas proteinuria is usually present during the course of MPGN, the development of nephrotic syndrome is much more variable (Table 1). Nephrotic syndrome may spontaneously remit during the course of MPGN I (29). Although nephrotic syndrome may develop in up to 80% of patients with MPGN II (21,39), it rarely develops in patients with MPGN III (24,36,40). Hypertension develops in 50–80% of patients with MPGN (31,36,40) (Table 1). Progression to ESRD occurs in 50% of untreated patients by 11 years (5,29), with renal insufficiency developing in another third. Risk factors present at onset of disease that correlate with progression to ESRD include renal insufficiency (11,23,29,41,42), hypertension (11,23,24,29,31, 36,41), and nephrotic syndrome (4,23,29,37,39). The disease of patients in whom nephrotic syndrome never develops is unlikely to progress to ESRD (29,43,44).

COMPLEMENT ABNORMALITIES

The Classic and Alternative Pathways

The complement system consists of classic and alternative pathways (45,46,47) (Fig. 1). The role of complement in renal disease is discussed extensively in Chapter 17. The classic pathway, which is composed of 11 serum proteins (C1q, C1r, C1s, C2–9), is activated by immune complexes or aggregates of IgG and IgM. There are at least four serum proteins in the alternative pathway, which includes factors B and D as well as properdin. The alternative pathway bypasses the early components of the classic pathway (C1, C2, C4), entering the complement cascade at the level of C3 with the subsequent activation of C5–9, and is activated by IgA aggregates or complex polysaccharides such as zymosan and endotoxin (47–49).

Initiation of the classic pathway begins with the fixation of C1 by activators, leading to the activation of C4 and C2 and generation of C3 convertase (C4b2a) of the classic pathway. In the alternative pathway, factor B and factor D interact with C3b, which is generated by activation of either pathway or by the ongoing interaction of factor B, factor D, and C3. This interaction leads to the generation of C3 convertase of the alternative pathway (C3bBb). C3 convertase of either the classic or alternative pathway cleaves C3 into two fragments, C3a and C3b, with the subsequent activation of C5–9 (47,48).

The activity of C3bBb is controlled by two plasma inhibitory proteins, factor I and factor H. Factor I inactivates C3b to C3bi. Factor H displaces Bb from C3bBb, making the C3b molecule vulnerable to the action of factor I. Properdin (P) is not essential for the initiation

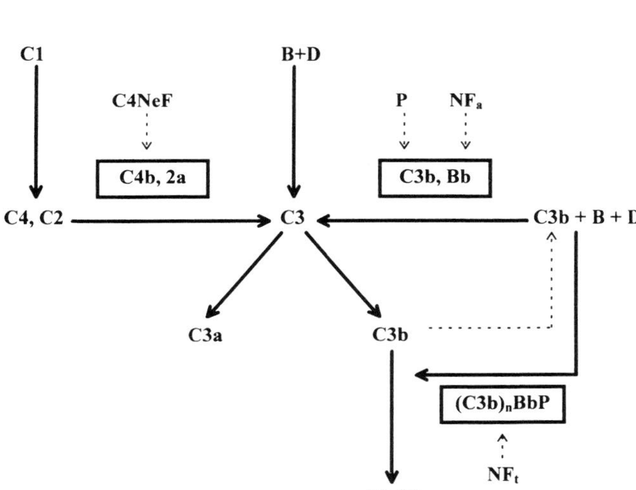

FIG. 1. Simplified scheme of the classic and alternative pathways.

of the alternative pathway, but by stabilizing C3bBb it plays an important role in amplification of the system (47,48).

Serum Complement Levels in Membranoproliferative Glomerulonephritis

Serum concentrations of C3 are low in 50–65% of patients with MPGN I at diagnosis (4,29,50–53) (Table 1). Serial determinations of C3 usually reveal fluctuating levels, with most patients exhibiting low C3 levels at some time during the course of the disease (29,50–53). Additionally, serum levels of early (C1q, C4, and C2) and terminal (C5, C6, C7, and/or C9) components of the classic pathway, as well as alternative pathway components, are frequently decreased (51, 52,54).

In MPGN II, the serum concentrations of C3 remain persistently low in almost all patients (12,29,50–53) (Table 1). Occasional patients remain normocomplementemic throughout the course of the disease. In contrast to MPGN I, serum concentrations of early (C1q, C4, C2) and terminal components (C5–9) of the classic pathway are normal in MPGN II. Serum levels of factor B and properdin are usually normal (52), a pattern very similar to that seen in partial lipodystrophy (55).

Serum levels of C3 are also decreased in most patients with MPGN III (Table 1). Patients with severely depressed C3 levels have low C5 and properdin levels (52). C6, C7, and C9 levels are reduced in 75% of patients with MPGN III. Of those patients with moderately depressed C3 levels, only 50% have low C5 and properdin levels, and levels of C6, C7, and C9 are normal (52).

Nephritic Factors

The presence of circulating C3 nephritic factors (56,57) is another anomaly of the complement system in patients with MPGN. C3 nephritic factors are auto-antibodies of the IgG class. Three distinct C3 nephritic factors have been identified to date. NF_a, also known as $C3NeF_{II}$ (58), stabilizes the alternative pathway C3 convertase (C3bBb) by protecting the complex from inactivation by factor H. The activity of NF_a is properdin-independent and heat-insensitive (59,60). This allows rapid, continuous fluid-phase C3 breakdown via the C3b amplification loop, with little effect on the terminal complement components (47,52,61–65). Although both properdin and NF_a bind to and stabilize C3bBb, the effect of properdin is reversible by the action of factor H, whereas that of NF_a is not, allowing NF_a to activate the alternative pathway continuously. NF_a is found in 81% of patients with MPGN II (59) and 60–70% of patients with partial lipodystrophy (55). It is present infrequently in MPGN I (50,51,54,59,66).

NF_t, also known as *C3NeF:P* or $C3NeF_{I/III}$, is a properdin-dependent and heat-sensitive factor that slowly converts C3 and activates terminal complement components (59,60,67,68). The ability of NF_t to activate C3 and terminal complement components and its functional dependence on properdin imply that it stabilizes properdin-bound C3/C5 convertase of the alternative pathway [$(C3b)_n$BbP] (59). NF_t has been found in 20–30% of patients with MPGN I and 78% of patients with MPGN III (59,67).

A third nephritic factor, C4NeF, is an auto-antibody directed against the classic pathway C3 convertase (C4b2a) complex. C4NeF has been described in MPGN I in combination with C3bBb-stabilizing factor, which presumably is NF_t (69).

The different complement profiles in the various types of MPGN most likely reflect the differences in the mode of complement activation. Thus, in MPGN I complement is activated via the classical and alternative pathways by immune complexes and NF_t and NF_a in a minority of patients. In MPGN II and III complement is activated via the alternative pathway by NF_a and NF_t respectively (52,70).

Yamada et al. (71) recently demonstrated the ability of peripheral blood mononuclear cells (PBMC) from a patient with partial lipodystrophy to produce NF_a. Hiramatsu et al. (72) also demonstrated production of NF_a by immortalized lymphocytes from a patient with MPGN II, but not by PBMC from a patient with MPGN I. However, the production of NF_a is not specific to patients with MPGN. Mitogen-stimulated PMBC from normal infants and adults also possess the capacity to make NF_a (73,74).

Complement Synthesis in MPGN

Metabolic studies employing radiolabeled C3 have shown a decreased C3 synthetic rate in MPGN (75–77). Furthermore, Colten et al. (78) demonstrated decreased synthesis of C3 in short-term cultures of liver biopsy material from patients with MPGN, compared with cultures of material from patients with other hypocomplementemic renal diseases and from normal subjects. Thus, the hypocomplementemia of MPGN may reflect both increased consumption and decreased synthesis of complement components, as shown by Charlesworth et al. (79). However, despite the marked abnormalities of the complement system, there is no correlation between the serum levels of NF_a, NF_t, or complement and the clinical activity or progression of MPGN (3,80–83).

PATHOGENESIS

The pathogenesis of MPGN is not well understood. Membranoproliferative glomerulopathy has been associated with a number of complement-deficient states, including partial lipodystrophy (55) and genetic deficiency of C1q (55), C2 (54,84–86), C3 (87,88), C6 (87, 88), C7 (87), C8 (87), factor B (87), factor H (89,90), and C1 esterase inhibitor (91). Peters and Williams (92) and Miller and Nussenzweig (93) postulated that complement depletion represents an immune deficiency state that predisposes to infection and immune complex formation. An equally plausible explanation for the development of MPGN is that complement deficiency or depletion or both influence the in vivo fate of immune complexes by impairing their solubilization and disaggregation (94–98) (see Chapters 1 through 3). The role of activation of the alternative complement pathway in the pathogenesis of MPGN is uncertain. The presence of NF_a and NF_t in MPGN and the occurrence of MPGN in factor H-deficient humans and animals suggest that unregulated generation of C3 convertase of the alternative pathway may cause or predispose to the development of MPGN (89,90). In experimental models, however, prolonged hypocomplementemia induced by the chronic administration of zymosan (99) or cobra venom factor (CoVF) (100) has failed to produce GN. Furthermore, patients with partial lipodystrophy may have circulating NF_a and hypocomplementemia without having renal disease (55,68), and placental transfer of maternal NF_a does not cause renal disease (101). These observations suggest that systemic complement activation and resultant hypocomplementemia are not injurious to the kidneys *per se*.

The available evidence suggests that MPGN I is mediated by glomerular deposition of immune complexes. Clinical evidence includes (a) demonstration of immunoproteins in the kidney by immunofluorescence; (b) the presence of circulating immune complexes and cryoglobulins in serum (102–107); and (c) the occurrence of GN morphologically similar to MPGN I in immune complex diseases such as systemic lupus erythematosus (108), chronic bacteremia (31,42,109,110), and chronic hepatitis C infection. Indeed, a significant portion of adult patients with type I MPGN (20% in the United States and up to 60% in northern Japan) appear to have the disease as a consequence of chronic hepatitis C infection (110a, b,c). (The entity of hepatitis C nephropathy is covered in more detail in Chapter 41.) Kuriyama (111) was able to produce renal lesions similar to those in MPGN I by repeated injections of egg albumin. In this model of chronic serum sickness, MPGN developed in animals that produced precipitating antibody of high avidity, whereas membranous nephropathy (MN) developed in those with nonprecipitating antibody of low avidity. The clinical, morphologic, and serologic similarities between MPGN I and GN associated with certain defined infections (e.g., shunt nephritis and hepatitis B and C nephritis) suggest a common pathogenesis resulting from chronic exposure to an infectious antigen. In this context, a number of different antigens, yet to be defined, might be responsible for MPGN I.

Immune complexes may also play a role in MPGN II and III, as evidenced by the demonstration of circulating immune complexes (102–106) and glomerular deposition of immunoproteins (51) in patients with these diseases. However, the composition of the dense deposits in MPGN II remains mysterious. Galle and Mahieu (112) showed that the biochemical composition of MPGN II glomerular basement membrane (GBM) is similar to that of normal GBM, except for increased sialic acid and decreased cystine content. On the basis of this finding, they suggested that the dense deposits may represent the accumulation of a biochemically modified glycoprotein component of normal basement membrane. However, the dense deposits do not react with antibodies against known extracellular matrix components, including type 4 collagen, laminin, fibronectin, or nidogen (113 and Y. Kim, *unpublished observations*). The dense deposits are highly osmiophilic by electron microscopy and can be extracted with lipid solvents, suggesting that they are rich in unsaturated fatty acids, a feature that is not characteristic of the known glycoprotein constituents of GBM (114).

The frequent recurrence of MPGN II in the transplanted kidney (see below) is compelling evidence that a systemic factor plays a crucial role in its pathogenesis. However, there is no evidence that the dense deposits of MPGN II are composed of circulating proteins. Antisera against immunoglobulins do not react with the deposits, and antibodies to C3 bind to the surface of the deposit but not within the deposit (see below). Thioflavin T, which reacts with amyloid proteins, stains dense deposits intensely (115). However, the dense deposits do not react with antisera against the amyloid proteins SAA and SAP (Y. Kim, *unpublished observations*).

Immune complexes may be the initial pathogenetic factors in all types of MPGN, and the dense deposits of MPGN II may reflect a unique host response to this immunologic stimulus. On the other hand, the dense deposits may represent a novel protein or a host protein that has lost its antigenic determinants and is no longer recognizable by immunohistologic techniques. Although MPGN II is included within the spectrum of MPGN, these characteristic dense deposits, which regularly recur in the transplanted kidney, establish MPGN II as being unique among forms of MPGN. Establishing the identity of the dense deposit material will be critical in obtaining a full understanding of the pathogenesis of MPGN II.

The histologic hallmarks of MPGN are mesangial cell proliferation and mesangial matrix increase, but the factors involved in these mesangial alterations have not been identified. In experimental anti-Thy-1 mesangial proliferative GN, both platelet-derived growth factor (PDGF) and basic fibroblast growth factor (bFBG) have been implicated in mesangial cell proliferation and extracellular matrix accumulation (116–118) (see Chapter 19). More recently, the membrane attack complex of complement (C5b–9) has been shown to play a pivotal role in mesangial cell proliferation and matrix expansion in this model (119) (see Chapter 17). In cultured mesangial cells, a sublytic concentration of C5b–9 stimulates the synthesis of cytokines such as interleukin 1, which can in turn increase the synthesis of PDGF (120). Because C5b–9 has previously been shown to be present together with C3 in glomeruli affected with both MPGN I and II (121,122), it is quite plausible that C5b–9 may play a similar role in the pathogenesis of MPGN.

PATHOLOGY

Membranoproliferative Glomerulonephritis Type I (Fig. 2)

Light Microscopy

Light microscopy reveals diffuse mesangial cellular proliferation and increased mesangial matrix. The glomerular involvement may occasionally be focal, especially in early stages of the disease (123). The glomerular tufts are diffusely enlarged and lobulated, with mean glomerular volumes three times those of normal individuals (19). The fraction of glomerular volume occupied by mesangium is increased twofold (19). Interposition of mesangial cytoplasm between GBM and endothelium causes the glomerular capillary walls to appear thickened

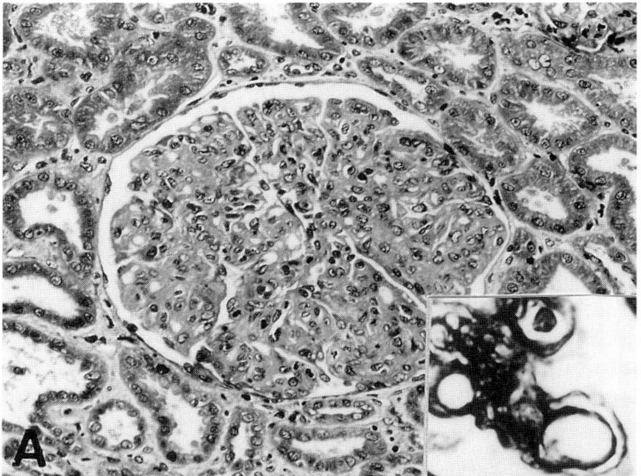

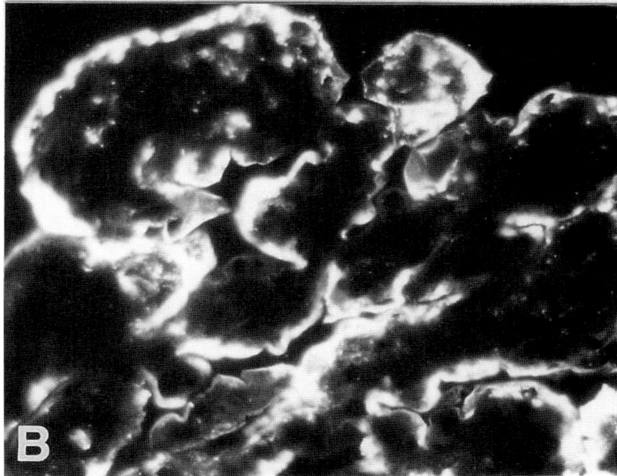

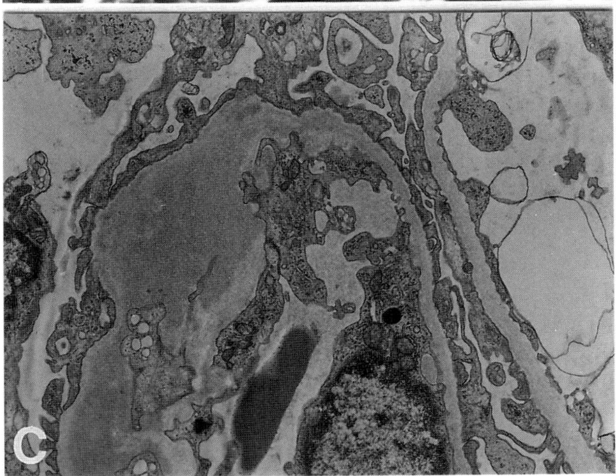

FIG. 2. MPGN I. **A:** Light microscopy shows an enlarged glomerulus with increased mesangial cellularity and matrix. *Insert* demonstrates splitting of glomerular capillary walls. H&E, ×150. **B:** Immunofluorescence microscopy shows granular deposition of C3 along the GBM in a peripheral lobular distribution and to a lesser extent in the mesangium. ×450. **C:** Electron microscopy of a portion of a glomerulus shows normal GBM. Note the subendothelial electron-dense deposits. ×6500.

(124). However, by periodic acid–Schiff (PAS) or silver staining the GBM is of normal thickness. The splitting of the glomerular capillary walls that is typical of MPGN results from PAS staining of GBM on either side of the interposed mesangial cytoplasm. Neutrophils may be seen in increased numbers in glomeruli. Epithelial crescents may also be present and are usually indicative of a poor prognosis (5,6,29,125). Renal functional disturbances correlate with mesangial expansion and especially mesangial cellular proliferation (19). Tubular atrophy and interstitial fibrosis are typical of advanced MPGN I. Tubulointerstitial changes are inversely correlated with creatinine clearance in MPGN (6,19,126).

Electron Microscopy

Ultrastructural evaluation of the GBM reveals normal thickness. New basement membrane-like material is found beneath the endothelium in association with fine, granular, electron-dense deposits. Between these two layers of GBM are varying amounts of mesangial cytoplasm, giving rise to the characteristic GBM splitting (or "tram track"). Mesangial deposits are typically observed, and humplike subepithelial deposits may occasionally be present (20,23,127). When MPGN results from hepatitis C, deposits may exhibit the characteristics of cryoglobulins (110a,b,c).

Immunofluroescence Microscopy

Immunofluorescence microscopy invariably reveals C3 and properdin deposition in the mesangium and along peripheral glomerular capillary walls in a subendothelial location. IgG, IgA, and IgM may also be found in these locations, but in lesser frequency and intensity than C3. C1q and C4 are also variably found in patients with MPGN I (20,23,55,127–129).

Membranoproliferative Glomerulonephritis Type II (Fig. 3)

Light Microscopy

The glomerular capillary walls exhibit irregular but generally extensive thickening. Mild to moderate diffuse mesangial cellular proliferation, with or without mesangial matrix increase, results in lobular accentuation. Marked eosinophilic and refractile ribbonlike thickening of the glomerular capillary walls is characteristic, which frequently compromises the patency of the glomerular capillaries. Segmental thickening of tubular basement membranes and Bowman's capsule is not unusual (20,23).

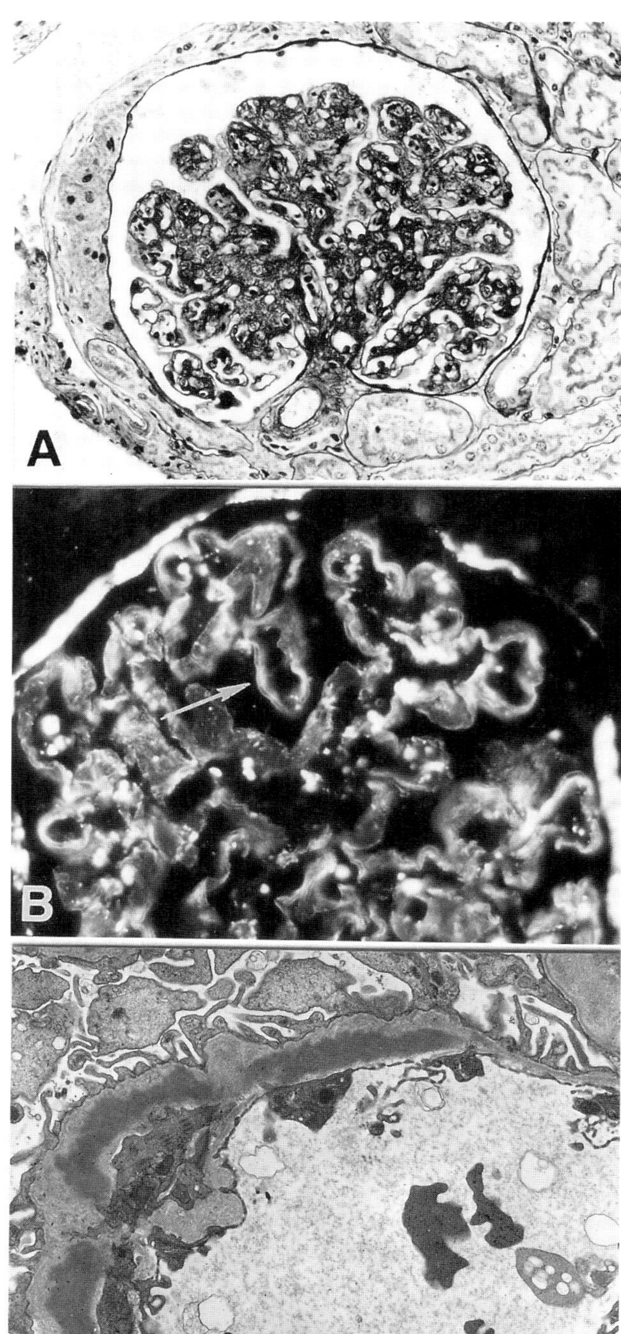

FIG. 3. MPGN II. **A:** Light microscopy shows thickening of the GBM caused by the presence of dense-deposit material. Note that the mesangial changes are less prominent than in MPGN I. PAS, ×150. **B:** Immunofluorescence microscopy shows C3 "railroad tracks" (*arrow*). ×450. **C:** Electron microscopy shows thick, ribbonlike dense deposits occupying the GBM. ×6500.

Circumferential epithelial crescents are variably present (27). Interstitial changes including fibrosis and chronic inflammation are focal initially, and later become generalized. Thickening of arteriolar basement membranes is generally inconspicuous by light microscopy; intimal and, to a lesser degree, medial proliferation parallels interstitial changes in severity (21,130).

Electron Microscopy

The characteristic lesion is thickening of the GBM secondary to a homogeneous and strongly electron-dense (i.e., dense deposit) material within the lamina densa and mesangium. These deposits correspond to the eosinophilic and refractile ribbonlike deposits seen by light microscopy. The dense deposits may be linear, fusiform, or globular. The amounts of deposits vary from capillary loop to capillary loop. On occasion, the dense deposits are focally distributed and are discovered only after a meticulous search (123). Mesangial interposition is also evident, although it is usually less extensive than that observed in MPGN I. Dense deposits are also found focally in Bowman's capsule and in tubular basement membranes (12,21,44,51,130).

Immunofluorescence Microscopy

By immunofluorescence, a specific finding in all patients with MPGN II is the presence of C3 along the margins of the dense deposits, giving a double linear appearance ("railroad tracks") to the glomerular capillary walls. C3 is also present within the mesangium outlining circular dense deposits ("mesangial rings"). These C3 railroad tracks and mesangial rings also contain properdin and C4, but not immunoglobulins (12,21,44,51, 128,130). Therefore, by electron and immunofluorescence microscopy, the dense deposits in MPGN II appear to be different from the granular immune deposits observed in MPGN I and other forms of GN. However, granular deposits of immunoproteins similar to those observed in MPGN I may also be seen in MPGN II, but IgG and the early complement components are infrequently found and the deposition of immunoproteins is quantitatively less.

Extrarenal Dense Deposits

Dense-deposit material similar to GBM deposits was found in the eye of a patient with MPGN II at autopsy (131). The deposit was present in the basement membrane of the ciliary epithelium and throughout the extent of the inner collagenous layer of Bruch's membrane, with both linear thickening and focal deposition resembling drusen. Numerous other studies have demonstrated funduscopic abnormalities in patients with MPGN II (132–136), including massive drusenlike deposits and mottled pigmentation as well as extensive hyperfluorescence on fluorescein angiography. The number and size of these lesions appear to increase in direct relationship to the duration of the renal disease (134). The etiology of these deposits is unknown, but their formation may represent a breakdown of the blood-retina barrier (133). Some patients also demonstrate subretinal neovascularization, usually in the region of the macula, as a late complication. This neovascularization has been associated with visual loss caused by bleeding, exudation, and subsequent scar formation (134). The development of central serous retinopathy has been observed (137).

Dense deposits have been observed in sinusoidal basement membranes of the spleen (15), but not in the brain, heart, liver, lung, adrenals, or pancreas (14). Extrarenal deposits have not been described in patients with MPGN I or III.

Membranoproliferative Glomerulonephritis Type III (Fig. 4)

Light Microscopy

The prevailing characteristic is widespread but irregular glomerular capillary wall thickening, caused by the accumulation of deposits in the GBM. Single glomerular capillary loops may assume a hump-backed appearance associated with segmental formation of "spikes" of new GBM material. The true character of the GBM lesion becomes evident with methenamine silver stain, which reveals irregular thickening of capillary loops with interruption of the basement membrane (33,34,138). Depending on the extent of deposition, short or long segments of the capillary walls lose their original staining properties, becoming increasingly silver-negative and thickened. This type of thickening tends to be lucent rather than dense, and bumpy rather than linear in character. The mesangial regions may be prominent by silver stain. There is a variable increase in lobulation, mesangial hypercellularity, and mesangial matrix by PAS staining, but this tends to be less severe than in MPGN I (7,33).

Electron Microscopy

The glomerular capillary wall deposits are irregularly shaped, moderately dense, and fairly uniform in composition. With silver impregnation, the position of the deposits in the basement membrane is irregular and not characteristic. Subendothelial and subepithelial deposits are widespread and frequently contiguous with each other. These membrane-spanning deposits, in combination with replication and disruption of the lamina densa, give the basement membrane a fenestrated appearance.

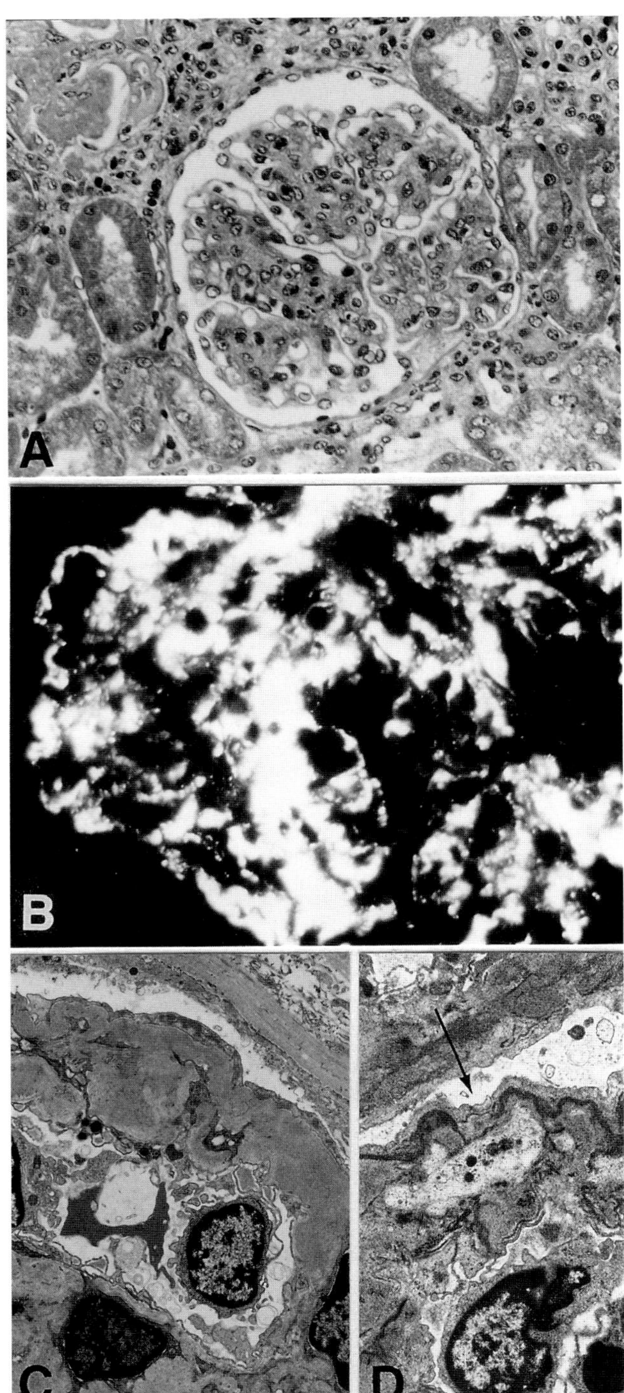

FIG. 4. MPGN III. **A**: Light microscopy shows widespread but irregular glomerular capillary wall thickening. H&E, ×150. **B:** Immunofluorescence microscopy shows diffuse granular C3 staining of the glomerular capillary walls and mesangium. ×350. **C:** Electron microscopy reveals irregular electron-dense deposits throughout the GBM (intramembranous and subendothelial). ×2800. **D:** Electron microscopy with silver impregnation staining shows disruption of the GBM (*arrow*). ×2800.

Some subepithelial deposits, however, are not in continuity with the subendothelial deposits, and appear as humps. The deposits are frequently segmentally distributed, with affected capillary loops adjacent to loops with little alteration. The presence of deposits within the mesangium is common. Mesangial interposition is, however, variable (33,34,40).

Immunofluorescence Microscopy

The main immunohistochemical finding is abundant granular C3 and properdin staining, predominantly within the glomerular capillary walls. C3 is also found within the mesangium, with greater frequency than in MPGN I. IgG, IgM, and IgA are found in only a minority of biopsy specimens, and staining for these components does not correspond with C3 distribution (7,40).

TREATMENT

The treatment of patients with MPGN remains an unsettled issue. The current mainstay of treatment is corticosteroids. Alternate-day steroid therapy has been the most extensively investigated form of treatment in pediatric patients with MPGN. McEnery (28) has reported the results of alternate-day prednisone therapy in 76 patients (MPGN I, 43%; MPGN II, 22%; MPGN III, 34%) who received 1.5 to 2 mg/kg as a single dose on alternate days, with a gradual reduction to 0.4 to 1 mg/kg. Cumulative renal survival, calculated from the date of initiation of the prednisone regimen, was 75% in the tenth year, and 59% in the twentieth year of treatment (28). Serial biopsies in successfully treated patients showed decreased mesangial interposition, increased patency of capillary lumina, and thinner capillary walls associated with maintenance of normal renal function, reduction in proteinuria, and increased plasma protein levels (139). Those patients treated within 1 year of presentation demonstrated improved histopathology, manifested by more open capillary loops and decreased mesangial matrix, compared with those in whom initiation of treatment occurred after 1 year. Glomerular sclerosis developed at an annual average rate of 3.5% for 2 to 3 years after start of therapy. Renal biopsy results demonstrated that by 4.5 years after start of therapy, no further sclerosis was noted if the patient did not experience a relapse (140). There was, however, no difference in renal survival between patients treated within 1 year of disease onset and more than 1 year after disease onset (28). McEnery and McAdams (141) also described six patients with MPGN II treated with alternate-day prednisone. These patients exhibited reduced mesangial proliferation and increased capillary patency on follow-up biopsies, and the location of the dense deposits changed from the lamina densa to the lamina rara interna.

Ford et al. (142) described 19 patients with MPGN I who were stratified into four groups based on creatinine clearance and proteinuria. Initial corticosteroid dosage ranged from 20 mg every other day to 30 mg/kg each day intravenously for 3 days consecutively. Therapy was then decreased based on the patient's clinical status and was continued for a mean duration of 38 ± 3 months. Hypertension was present at diagnosis in 13, and developed in 5 during therapy. Follow-up renal biopsies revealed decreased glomerular inflammatory activity in 88% of patients. The mean creatinine clearance after therapy was 126 ± 5 mL/min/1.73 m^2, with 8 patients having normal results of urinalysis. These authors concluded that early therapy with a limited course of corticosteroids and control of associated hypertension may forestall progressive renal insufficiency in MPGN I. Bergstein and Andreoli (25) also reported that alternate-day steroid therapy improved the renal survival of patients with MPGN I.

The International Study of Kidney Disease in Children (8) conducted a prospective randomized trial of alternate-day prednisone therapy in 80 children with idiopathic MPGN (42 MPGN I, 14 MPGN II, 17 MPGN III, 7 non-typable). Forty-seven patients received prednisone and 33 received placebo. The treatment regimen consisted of prednisone 40 mg/m^2, maximum 60 mg, given in a single dose in the morning every other day for 5 years. Follow up at 10 years by Kaplan-Meier analysis showed 61% of patients receiving prednisone were stable, without treatment failure or renal failure, compared with only 12% of patients receiving placebo. When patients with MPGN I and III were combined because of concern about delineation of the two groups, 33% of the prednisone group were treatment failures, whereas 58% of placebo-treated patients were treatment failures. The number of patients with MPGN II was not sufficient to elucidate a difference between the treatment and placebo groups. Although this study demonstrated overall differences between treated and untreated patients, the efficacy of therapy in each type of MPGN could not be determined.

Somers et al. (44) found no differences in renal survival between treated and untreated children with MPGN who were not nephrotic. Although this study was retrospective and not randomized, the results suggest that MPGN patients without nephrotic syndrome or hypertension may not require therapy.

Other treatment regimens for MPGN have demonstrated variable results. Regimens utilizing cyclophosphamide, dipyridamole, warfarin, and heparin resulted in improved renal survival in some studies (143,144), but not in others (5,21,31). Tiller et al. (145) and Cattran et al. (146) reported that anticoagulant therapy combined with cyclophosphamide was of no benefit and was associated with a high drop-out rate because of toxicity. Donadio et al. (147) initially observed a beneficial effect of aspirin and dipyridamole therapy in patients with MPGN, but the 10-year renal survival rates were not statistically different in treated and untreated patients (148).

Although there is no universally accepted treatment regimen for MPGN, patients with hypertension, renal insufficiency, or significant proteinuria are at risk for progression to ESRD, and alternate-day prednisone therapy should be strongly considered. All patients, even if not receiving therapy, require frequent evaluation for reduction in renal function or the onset of hypertension. In those patients in whom significant proteinuria or renal insufficiency develops, consideration should be given to initiating alternate-day prednisone therapy. Control of hypertension is imperative to allay further renal damage. Currently, we consider discontinuing alternate-day prednisone therapy after 2 years if renal function and blood pressure have normalized, proteinuria is minimal, and hematuria has resolved. A repeat renal biopsy may be useful in guiding decisions to alter therapy.

TRANSPLANTATION

Transplantation for patients with MPGN who proceed to ESRD may be complicated by recurrence of the disease in the renal allograft. Recurrence of MPGN I has been reported in 6–70% of allografts (149–152). Unfortunately, the diagnosis of recurrence in some of the grafts was based solely on clinical grounds, without pathologic confirmation. The diagnosis of recurrent MPGN I requires the presence of typical immunofluorescence and electron microscopic findings, because the glomerular lesions of chronic transplant nephropathy and MPGN are impossible to distinguish by light microscopy alone (152). Graft failure from recurrent disease has been described in 6–20% of patients with MPGN I, and has been variably associated with persistent posttransplant hypocomplementemia (150,151).

Histologic recurrence of MPGN II occurs almost invariably in renal allografts. Clinically evident disease, as manifested by hematuria, proteinuria, nephrotic syndrome, or allograft failure, has appeared in from none to 60% of the patients, depending on the series (21,39,114, 153–155). Clinical recurrence has not been correlated with hypocomplementemia, nephritic factor activity, or evidence of recurrence in a previous graft (153–154). The development of nephrotic syndrome in the allograft is frequently associated with ultimate allograft failure (153).

Acknowledgment

We express our appreciation to Marie-Claire Gubler, M.D., for her assistance in providing MPGN III illustrations, and to Ms. Kathy Divine for her assistance in preparing the illustrations.

REFERENCES

1. West CD, McAdams AJ, McConville JM, Davis NC, Holland NH. Hypocomplementemic and normocomplementemic persistent (chronic) glomerulonephritis: clinical and pathologic characteristics. *J Pediatr* 1965;67:1089–1112.
2. Gotoff SP, Fellers FX, Vawter GF, Janeway CA, Rosen FS. The beta 1C globulin in childhood nephrotic syndrome. Laboratory diagnosis of progressive glomerulonephritis. *N Engl J Med* 1965;273:524–529.
3. West CD, McAdams AJ. Serum β1C globulin levels in persistent glomerulonephritis with low serum complement: variability unrelated to clinical course. *Nephron* 1970;7:193–202.
4. Cameron JS, Ogg CS, White RHR, Glasgow EF. The clinical features and prognosis of patients with normocomplementemic mesangio-capillary glomerulonephritis. *Clin Nephrol* 1973;1:8–13.
5. Cameron JS, Turner DR, Heaton J, et al. Idiopathic mesangiocapillary glomerulonephritis. *Am J Med* 1983;74:175–192.
6. Taguchi T, Bohle A. Evalution of change with time of glomerular morphology in membranoproliferative glomerulonephritis: a serial biopsy study of 33 cases. *Clin Nephrol* 1989;6:297–306.
7. Jackson EC, McAdams AJ, Strife CF, Forristal J, Welch TR, West CD. Differences between membranoproliferative glomerulonephritis types I and III in clinical presentation, glomerular morphology, and complement perturbation. *Am J Kidney Dis* 1987;9:115–120.
8. Tarshish P, Bernstein J, Tobin JN, Edelmann CM Jr. Treatment of mesangiocapillary glomerulonephritis with alternate-day prednisone—a report of the International Study of Kidney Disease in Children. *Pediatr Nephrol* 1992;6:123–130.
9. US Renal Data System. *1994 Annual Data Report*. Bethesda, MD: National Institues of Health, National Institute of Diabetes and Digestive and Kidney Diseases; July 1994.
10. Avner ED, Chavers B, Sullivan EK, Tejani A. Renal transplantation and chronic dialysis in children and adolescents: the 1993 annual report of the North American Pediatric Renal Transplant Cooperative Study. *Pediatr Nephrol* 1995:9:61–73.
11. Schmitt H, Bohle A, Reineke T, Mayer-Eichberger D, Vogt W. Long-term prognosis of membranoproliferative glomerulonephritis type I. *Nephron* 1990;55:242–250.
12. Habib R, Gubler MC, Loirat C, Maiz HB, Levy M. Dense deposit disease: a variant of membranoproliferative glomerulonephritis. *Kidney Int* 1975;7:204–215.
13. Antoine B, Faye C. The clinical course associated with dense deposits in the kidney basement membranes. *Kidney Int* 1972;1:420–427.
14. Thorner P, Baumal R. Extraglomerular dense deposits in dense deposit disease. *Arch Pathol Lab Med* 1982;106:628–631.
15. Ormos J, Magori A, Sonkodi S, Streitmann K. Type 2 membranoproliferative glomerulonephritis with electron-dense basement membrane alterations in the spleen. *Arch Pathol Lab Med* 1979;103:265–266.
16. Droz D, Zanetti M, Noel LH, Leibowitch J. Dense deposits disease. *Nephron* 1977;19:1–11.
17. Warady BA, Guggenheim SJ, Sedman A, Lum GM. Prednisone therapy of membranoproliferative glomerulonephritis in children. *J Pediatr* 1985;107:702–707.
18. Chapman SJ, Cameron JS, Chantler C, Turner D. Treatment of mesangiocapillary glomerulonephritis in children with combined immunosuppression and anticoagulation. *Arch Dis Child* 1980;55:446–451.
19. Hattori M, Kim Y, Steffes MW, Mauer SM. Structural-functional relationships in type I mesangiocapillary glomerulonephritis. *Kidney Int* 1993;23:381–386.
20. Kim Y, Michael AF. Idiopathic membranoproliferative glomerulonephritis. *Annu Rev Med* 1980;31:273–288.
21. Lamb V, Tisher CC, McCoy RC, Robinson RR. Membranoproliferative glomerulonephritis with dense intramembranous alterations. A clinicopathologic study. *Lab Invest* 1977;36:607–617.
22. Herdman RC, Pickering RJ, Michael AF, Vernier RL, Fish AJ, Gewurz H, Good RA. Chronic glomerulonepritis associated with low serum complement activity (chronic hypocomplementemic glomerulonephritis). *Medicine* 1970;49:207–226.
23. Levy M, Gubler MC, Habib R. New concepts on membranoproliferative glomerulonephritis. In: Kincaid-Smith P, d'Apice AJF, Atkins RC, eds. *Progress in Glomerulonephritis*. New York: John Wiley; 1979:177–207.
24. Iitaka K, Ishidate T, Hojo M, Kuwao S, Kasai N, Sakai T. Idiopathic membranoproliferative glomerulonephritis in Japanese children. *Pediatr Nephrol* 1995;9:272–277.
25. Bergstein JM, Andreoli SP. Response of type I membranoproliferative glomerulonephritis to pulse methylprednisolone and alternate-day prednisone therapy. *Pediatr Nephrol* 1995;9:268–271.
26. Vargas R, Thomson KJ, Wilson D, et al. Mesangiocapillary glomerulonephritis with dense "deposits" in the basement membranes of the kidney. *Clin Nephrol* 1976;5:73–82.
27. Southwest Pediatric Nephrology Study Group. Dense deposit disease in children: prognostic value of clinical and pathologic indicators. *Am J Kidney Dis* 1985;6:161–169.
28. McEnery PT. Membranoproliferative glomerulonephritis: the Cincinnati experience—cumulative renal survival from 1957 to 1989. *J Pediatr* 1990;116:S109–114.
29. Habib R, Kleinknecht C, Gubler MC, Levy M. Idiopathic membranoproliferative glomerulonephritis in children. Report of 105 cases. *Clin Nephrol* 1973;1:194–214.
30. Berry PL, McEnery PT, McAdams AJ, West CD. Membranoproliferative glomerulonephritis in two sibships. *Clin Nephrol* 1981;16: 101–106.
31. Davis AE, Schneeberger EE, Grupe WE, McCluskey RT. Membranoproliferative glomerulonephritis (MPGN type I) and dense deposit disease (DDD) in children. *Clin Nephrol* 1978;9:184–193.
32. McEnery PT, Coutinho MJ. Membranoproliferative glomerulonephritis. In: Holliday MA, Barratt TM, Avner ED, eds. *Pediatric Nephrology*. Baltimore: Williams and Wilkins; 1994:739–753.
33. Strife CF, McEnery PT, McAdams AJ, West CD. Membranoproliferative glomerulonephritis with disruption of the glomerular basement membrane. *Clin Nephrol* 1977;7:65–72.
34. Anders D, Argicola B, Sippel M, Thoenes W. Basement membrane changes in membranoproliferative glomerulonephritis. *Virchows Arch A Pathol Anat Histopathol* 1977;376:1–19.
35. Kashtan CE, Burke B, Burch G, Gustav Fisker S, Kim Y. Dense intramembranous deposit disease: a clinical comparison of histological subtypes. *Clin Nephrol* 1990;33:1–6.
36. Burkholder PM, Marchand A, Krueger RP. Mixed membranous and proliferative glomerulonephritis. *Lab Invest* 1970;23:459–479.
37. Klein M, Poucell S, Arbus GS, McGraw M, Rance CP, Yoon SJ, Baumal R. Characteristics of a benign subtype of dense deposit disease: comparison with the progressive form of this disease. *Clin Nephrol* 1983;20:163–171.
38. Jenis EH, Sandler P, Hill GS, Knieser MR, Jensen GE, Roskes SD. Glomerulonephritis with basement membrane dense deposits. *Arch Pathol* 1974;97:84–91.
39. Bennett WM, Fassett RG, Walker RG, Fairley KF, d'Apice AJF, Kincaid-Smith P. Mesangiocapillary glomerulonephritis type II (dense-deposit disease): clinical features of progressive disease. *Am J Kidney Dis* 1989;13:469–476.
40. Strife CF, Jackson EC, McAdams AJ. Type III membranoproliferative glomerulonephritis: long-term clinical and morphologic evaluation. *Clin Nephrol* 1984;21:323–334.
41. Coutinho M, McEnery PT. Membranoproliferative glomerulonephritis (MPGN)—experience with discontinuation of prednisone therapy and identification of factors correlating with outcome. *J Am Soc Nephrol* 1992;3:309(abst).
42. Donadio JV Jr, Slack TK, Holley KE, Ilstrup DM. Idiopathic membranoproliferative (mesangiocapillary) glomerulonephritis. *Mayo Clin Proc* 1979;54:141–150.
43. Cameron JS, Glasgow EF, Ogg CS, White RHR. Membranoproliferative glomerulonephritis and persistent hypocomplementaemia. *Br Med J* 1970;4:7–14.
44. Somers M, Kertesz S, Rosen S, Herrin J, Colvin R, Palacios de Carreta N, Kim M. Non-nephrotic children with membranoproliferative glomerulonephritis: are steroids indicated? *Pediatr Nephrol* 1995;9: 140–144.
45. Fearon DT, Austen KF. The alternative pathway of complement—a system for host resistance to microbial infection. *N Engl J Med* 1980; 303:259–263.
46. Muller-Eberhard HJ. Complement. *Annu Rev Biochem* 1975;44: 697–724.
47. Peters DK. Complement and membranoproliferative glomerulonephritis. In: Kincaid-Smith P, d'Apice AJF, Atkins RC, eds. *Progress in Glomerulonephritis*. New York: John Wiley; 1979: 77–89.

48. McLean RH. Complement and glomerulonephritis—an update. *Pediatr Nephrol* 1993;7:226–232.
49. Hyman LR, Jenis EH, Hill GS, Zimmerman SW, Burkholder PM. Alternate C3 pathway activation in pneumococcal glomerulonephritis. *Am J Med* 1975;58:810–814.
50. Kim Y, Vernier RL, Fish AJ, Michael AF. Immunofluorescence studies of dense deposit disease. *Lab Invest* 1979;40:474–480.
51. Ooi YM, Vallota EH, West CD. Classical complement pathway activation in membranoproliferative glomerulonephritis. *Kidney Int* 1976;9:46–53.
52. Varade WS, Forristal J, West CD. Patterns of complement activation in idiopathic membranoproliferative glomerulonephritis types I, II, and III. *Am J Kidney Dis* 1990;26:196–206.
53. Habib R, Loirat C, Gubler MC, Levy M. Morphology and serum complement levels in membranoproliferative glomerulonephritis. *Adv Nephrol Necker Hosp* 1974;4:109–136.
54. Levy M, Gubler MC, Sich M, Beziau A, Habib R. Immunopathology of membranoproliferative glomerulonephritis with subendothelial deposits (type I MPGN). *Clin Immunol Immunopathol* 1978;10:477–492.
55. Sissons JGP, West RJ, Fallows J, Williams DG, Boucher BJ, Amos N, Peters DK. The complement abnormalities of lipodystrophy. *N Engl J Med* 1976;294:461–465.
56. Spitzer RE, Vallota EH, Forristal J, Sudora E, Stitzel A, Davis NC, West CD. Serum C3 lytic system in patients with glomerulonephritis. *Science* 1969;164:436–437.
57. Vallota EH, Gotze O, Speigelberg HL, Forristal J, West CD, Muller-Eberhard HJ. A serum factor in chronic hypocomplementemic nephritis distinct from immunoglobulins and activating the alternative pathway of complement. *J Exp Med* 1974;139:1249–1261.
58. Strife CF, Prada AL, Clardy CW, Jackson E, Forristal J. Autoantibody to complement neoantigens in membranoproliferative glomerulonephritis. *J Pediatr* 1990;116:S98–102.
59. Clardy CW, Forristal J, Strife CF, West CD. A properdin dependent nephritic factor slowly activating C3, C5, and C9 in membranoproliferative glomerulonephrits, types I and III. *Clin Immunol Immunopathol* 1989;50:333–347.
60. Ohi H, Tanuma Y. Does nephritic factor relate to the disease activity in hypocomplementemic membranoproliferative glomerulonephritis? *Nephron* 1992;62:116.
61. Austen KF. Homeostasis of effector systems which can also be recruited for immunologic reactions. *J Immunol* 1978;121:793–805.
62. Daha MR, Austen KF, Fearon DT. Heterogeneity, polypeptide chain composition and antigenic reactivity of C3 nephritic factor. *J Immunol* 1978;120:1389–1394.
63. Daha MR, Fearon DT, Austen KF. C3 nephritic factor (C3NeF): stabilization of fluid phase and cell bound alternative pathway convertase. *J Immunol* 1976;116:1–7.
64. Davis AE, Ziegler JB, Gelfand EW, Rosen FS, Alper CA. Heterogeneity of nephritic factor and its identification as an immunoglobulin. *Proc Natl Acad Sci U S A* 1977;74:3980–3983.
65. Scott DM, Amos N, Sissons JGP, Lachmann PH, Peters DK. The immuoglobulin nature of nephritic factor (NeF). *Clin Exp Immunol* 1978;32:12–24.
66. Williams DG, Peters DK, Fallows J, Petrie A, Kourilsky O, Morel-Maroger L, Cameron JS. Studies of serum complement in the hypocomplementemic nephritides. *Clin Exp Immunol* 1974;18:391–405.
67. Power DA, Ng YC, Simpson JG. Familial incidence of C3 nephritic factor, partial lipodystrophy and membranoproliferative glomerulonephritis. *Q J Med* 1990;75:387–398.
68. Tanuma Y, Ohi J, Hatano M. Two types of C3 nephritic factor: properdin-dependent C3NeF and properdin-independent C3NeF. *Clin Immunol Immunopathol* 1990;56:226–238.
69. Tanuma Y, Ohi H, Watanabe S, Seki M, Hatano M. C3 nephritic factor and C4 nephritic factor in the serum of two patients with hypocomplementaemic membranoproliferative glomerulonephritis. *Clin Exp Immunol* 1989;76:82–85.
70. West CD. Idiopathic membranoproliferative glomerulonephritis in childhood. *Pediatr Nephrol* 1992;6:96–103.
71. Yamada A, Ohi J, Okano K, Watanabe S, Seki M, Hotano M, Koitabashi Y. Production of C3 nephritic factor by cultured lymphocytes derived from a patient with partial lipodystrophy. *J Clin Lab Immunol* 1988;27:35–37.
72. Hiramatsu M, Balow JE, Tsokos GC. Production of nephritic factor of alternative complement pathway by EBV-transformed B cell lines derived from a patient with membranoproliferative glomerulonephritis. *J Immunol* 1986;136:4451–4455.
73. Spitzer RE, Stitzel AE, Tsokos GC. Production of IgG and IgM autoantibody to the alternative pathway C3 convertase in normal individuals and patients with membranoproliferative glomerulonephritis. *Clin Immunol Immunopathol* 1990;57:10–18.
74. Spitzer RE, Stitzel AE, Tsokos GC. Evidence that production of autoantibody to the alternative pathway C3 convertase is a normal physiologic event. *J Pediatr* 1990;116:S103–108.
75. Alpers CA, Rosen FS, Watson L. Studies of the in vivo behavior of human C3 in normal subjects and patients. *J Clin Invest* 1967;46:2021–2034.
76. Peters DK, Martin A, Weinstein A, Cameron JS, Barratt TM, Ogg CS, Lachmann PJ. Complement studies in membranoproliferative glomerulonephritis. *Clin Exp Immunol* 1972;11:311–320.
77. Ruddy S, Carpenter CB, Chin KW, et al. Human complement metabolism: an analysis of 144 studies. *Medicine* 1975;54:165–178.
78. Colten HR, Levey RH, Rosen FS, Alpers CA. Decreased synthesis of C3 in membranoproliferative glomerulonephritis. *J Clin Invest* 1973;52:20a(abst).
79. Charlesworth JA, Williams DG, Sherington E, Lachmann PJ, Peters DK. Metabolic studies of the third component of complement and the glycine-rich beta glycoprotein in patients with hypocomplementemia. *J Clin Invest* 1974;53:1578–1587.
80. Holland NH, Bennett NM. Hypocomplementemic (membranoproliferative) glomerulonephritis. *Am J Dis Child* 1972;123:439–445.
81. West CD. Pathogenesis and approaches to therapy of membranoproliferative glomerulonephritis. *Kidney Int* 1976;9:1–7.
82. Jones DB. Membranoproliferative glomerulonephritis: one or many diseases? *Arch Pathol Lab Med* 1977;101:457–461.
83. Vallota EH, Forristal J, Davis NC, West CD. The C3 nephritic factor and membranoproliferative nephritis: correlation of serum levels of the nephritic factor with C3 levels, with therapy, and with progression of the disease. *J Pediatr* 1972;80:947–959.
84. Kim Y, Friend PS, Dresner IG, Yunis EJ, Michael AF. Inherited deficiency of the 2nd component of complent: its occurrence with membranoproliferative glomerulonephritis. *Am J Med* 1977;62:765–771.
85. Loirat C, Levy M, Peltier AP, Broyer M, Checoury A, Mathieu H. Deficiency of the 2nd component of complement: its occurrence with membranoproliferative glomerulonephritis. *Arch Pathol Lab Med* 1980;104:467–472.
86. Sobel AT, Moisy M, Hirbec G, et al. Hereditary C2 deficiency associated with non-systemic glomerulonephritis. *Clin Nephrol* 1979;12:132–136.
87. Coleman TH, Forristal J, Kosaka T, West CD. Inherited complement component deficiencies in membranoproliferative glomerulonephritis. *Kidney Int* 1983;24:681–690.
88. Coleman TH, Forristal J, West CD. Hereditary C6 deficiency in membranoproliferative glomerulonephritis (MPGN) type I. *Pediat Res* 1979;13:446(abst).
89. West CD. Nephritic factors predispose to chronic glomerulonephritis. *Am J Kidney Dis* 1994;21:956–963.
90. Levy M, Halbwachs-Mecarelli L, Gubler MC, et al. H deficiency in two brothers with atypical intramembranous deposit disease. *Kidney Int* 1986;30:949–956.
91. Peters DK, Lachmann PJ. Immunity deficiency in pathogenesis of glomerulonephritis. *Lancet* 1974;1:58–60.
92. Peters DK, Williams DG. Complement and mesangiocapillary glomerulonephritis: role of complement deficiency in the pathogenesis of nephritis. *Nephron* 1974;3:189–197.
93. Miller GW, Nussenzweig V. The new complement function: solubilization of antigen-antibody aggregates. *Proc Natl Acad Sci U S A* 1975;72:418–422.
94. Takahashi M, Tack BF, Nussenzweig V. Requirements for the solubilization of immune aggregates by complement. Assembly of a factor B-dependent C3-convertase on the immune complexes. *J Exp Med* 1977;145:86–100.
95. Takahashi M, Czop J, Ferreira A, Nussenzweig V. Mechanism of solubilization of immune aggregates by complement. Implications for immunopathology. *Transplant Rev* 1976;32:121–139.
96. Takahashi M, Takahashi S, Brade V, Nussenzweig V. Requirements

for the solubilization of immune aggregates by complement. The role of the classical pathway. *J Clin Invest* 1978;62:349–358.
97. Bartolotti SR, Peters DK. Complement fixation in acute serum sickness: assembly of glomerular-bound C3-convertase. *Clin Exp Immunol* 1979;37:391–398.
98. Digeon M, Laver M, Riza J, Black JF. Detection of circulating immune complexes in human sera by simplified assays with polyethylene glycol. *J Immunol Methods* 1977;16:165–183.
99. Verroust PJ, Wilson CB, Dixon FJ. Lack of nephritogenicity of systemic activation of the alternative complement pathway. *Kidney Int* 1974;6:157–169.
100. Simpson IJ, Moran J, Evans DJ, Peters DK. Prolonged complement activation in mice. *Kidney Int* 1978;13:467–471.
101. Kim Y, Shvil Y, Michael AF. Hypocomplementemia in a newborn infant caused by a placental transfer of C3 nephritic factor. *J Pediatr* 1978;92:88–90.
102. Ooi YM, Vallota EH, West CD. Serum immune complexes in membranoproliferative and other glomerulonephritides. *Kidney Int* 1977; 11:275–283.
103. Meyer O, Descamps B. Detection of soluble immune complexes by the technique of ADCC inhibition in human diseases. *J Clin Lab Immunol* 1979;2:311–318.
104. Stuhlinger WD, Verroust PJ, Morel-Maroger L. Detection of circulating soluble immune complexes in patients with various renal diseases. *Immunology* 1978;400:43–47.
105. Woodroffe AJ, Border WA, Theofilopoulos AN, Gotze O, Glassock RJ, Dixon FJ, Wilson CB. Detection of circulating immune complexes in patients with glomerulonephritis. *Kidney Int* 1977;12: 268–278.
106. Border WA. Immune complex detection in glomerular diseases. *Nephron* 1979;24:105–113.
107. Williams DG, Garcia-Fuentes M, Losito A. Cryoglobulinemia in mesangiocapillary glomerulonephritis. *Seventh International Congress on Nephrology*. Montreal, Canada, June 18–23, 1978:G-11 (abst).
108. Hill GS, Hinglais N, Tron F, Bach JF. Systemic lupus erythematosus. Morphologic correlations with immunologic and clinical data at the time of biopsy. *Am J Med* 1978;64:61–79.
109. Black JA, Challacombe DN, Ockende BG. Nephrotic syndrome associated with bacteremia after shunt operations for hydrocephalus. *Lancet* 1965;2:921–924.
110. Dobrin RS, Day NK, Quie PG, Moore HL, Vernier RL, Michael AF, Fish AJ. The role of complement, immunoglobulin and bacterial antigen in coagulase-negative staphylococcal shunt nephritis. *Am J Med* 1975;59:660–673.
110a. Johnson RJ, Gretch DR, Yamabe H, et al. Membranoproliferative glomerulonephritis associated with hepatitis C virus infection (see Comments). *N Engl J Med* 1993;328:465–470.
110b. Misiani R, Bellavita P, Fenili D, et al. Hepatitis C virus infection in patients with essential mixed cryoglobulinemia. *Ann Intern Med* 1992;117:573–577.
110c. Yamabe H, Johnson RJ, Gretch DR, et al. Hepatitis C virus infection and membranoproliferative glomerulonephritis in Japan. *J Am Soc Nephrol* 1995;6:220–223.
111. Kuriyama T. Chronic glomerulonephritis induced by prolonged immunization in the rabbit. *Lab Invest* 1973;28:224–235.
112. Galle P, Mahieu P. Electron dense alterations of kidney basement membranes. A renal lesion specific of a systemic disease. *Am J Med* 1975;58:749–764.
113. Kashtan CE, Kim Y. Distribution of the α1 and α2 chains of collagen IV and of collagens V and VI in Alport syndrome. *Kidney Int* 1992; 42:115–126.
114. Muda AO, Barsotti P, Marinozzi V. Ultrastructural histochemical investigations of "dense deposit disease." Pathogenetic approach to a special type of mesangiocapillary glomerulonephritis. *Virchows Arch A Pathol Anat Histopathol* 1988;413:529–537.
115. Churg J, Duffy JL, Bernstein J. Identification of dense deposit disease. A report for the International Study of Kidney Diseases in Children. *Arch Pathol Lab Med* 1979;103:67–72.
116. Iida H, Seifert R, Alpers CE, et al. Platelet-derived growth factor (PDGF) and PDGF receptor are induced in mesangial proliferative nephritis in the rat. *Proc Natl Acad Sci U S A* 1991;88:6560–6564.
117. Floege J, Eng E, Lindner V, Alpers CE, Young BA, Reidy MA, Johnson RJ. Rat glomerular mesangial cells synthesize basic fibroblast growth factor. Release, upregulated synthesis, and mitogenicity in mesangial proliferative glomerulonephritis. *J Clin Invest* 1992;90: 2362–2369.
118. Floege J, Eng E, Young BA, Alpers CE, Barrett TB, Bowen-Pope DF, Johnson RJ. Infusion of platelet-derived growth factor or basic fibroblast growth factor induces selective glomerular mesangial cell proliferation and matrix accumulation in rats. *J Clin Invest* 1993;92: 2952–2962.
119. Brandt J, Pippen J, Schulze M, et al. Role of the complement membrane attack complex (C5b-9) in mediating experimental mesangioproliferative glomerulonephritis. *Kidney Int* 1996;49:335–343.
120. Schonermark M, Deppisch R, Riedasch G, Rother K, Hansch GM. Induction of mediator release from human glomerular mesangial cells by the terminal complement components C5b-9. *Int Arch Allergy Appl Immunol* 1991;96:331–337.
121. Falk RJ, Dalmasso AP, Kim Y, Tsai CH, Scheinman JI, Gewurz H, Michael AF. Neoantigen in the polymerized ninth component of complement. *J Clin Invest* 1983;72:560–573.
122. Hinglais N, Kazatchkine MD, Bhakdi S, Appay MD, Mandet C, Grossetete J, Bariety J. Immunohistochemical study of the C5b-9 complex of complement in human kidneys. *Kidney Int* 1986;30: 399–410.
123. Strife CF, McAdams AJ, West CD. Membranoproliferative glomerulonephritis characterized by focal, segmental proliferative lesions. *Clin Nephrol* 1982;18:9–16.
124. Mandalenakis N, Mendoza N, Pirani CL, Pollak VE. Lobular glomerulonephritis and membranoproliferative glomerulonephritis. A clinical and pathologic study based on renal biopsies. *Medicine* 1971; 50:319–355.
125. D'Amico G, Ferrario F. Mesangiocapillary glomerulonephritis. *J Am Soc Nephrol* 1992;2:S159–S166.
126. Bohle A, Bader R, Grund KE, Mackensen S, Neunhoeffer J. Serum creatinine concentration and renal interstitial volume. Analysis of correlations in endocapillary (acute) glomerulonephritis and in moderately severe mesangioproliferative glomerulonephritis. *Virchows Arch A Pathol Anat Histopathol* 1977;375:87–96.
127. Donadio JV Jr, Holley KE. Membranoproliferative glomerulonephritis. *Semin Nephrol* 1982;2:214–227.
128. Davis BK, Cavallo T. Membranoproliferative glomerulonephritis: localization of early components of complement in glomerular deposits. *Am J Pathol* 1976;84:283–298.
129. Barbiano di Belgiojoso G, Tarantino A, Bazzi C, Colasanti G, Guerra L, Durante A. Immunofluorescence patterns in chronic membranoproliferative glomerulonephritis (MPGN). *Clin Nephrol* 1976; 303–310.
130. Sibley RK, Kim Y. Dense intramembranous deposit disease: new pathologic features. *Kidney Int* 1984;25:660–670.
131. Duvall-Young J, MacDonald MK, McKechni NM. Fundus changes in (type II) mesangiocapillary glomerulonephritis simulating drusen: a histopathological report. *Br J Ophthalmol* 1989;73:297–302.
132. Duvall-Young J, Short CD, Raines MF, Gokal R, Lawler W. Fundus changes in mesangiocapillary glomerulonephritis type II: clinical and fluorescein angiographic findings. *Br J Ophthalmol* 1989;73:900–906.
133. Raines MF, Duvall-Young J, Short CD. Fundus changes in mesangiocapillary glomerulonephritis type II: vitreous fluorophotometry. *Br J Ophthalmol* 1989;73:907–910.
134. Leys A, Proesmans W, Van Damme-Lombaerts R, Van Damme B. Specific eye fundus lesions in type II membranoproliferative glomerulonephritis. *Pediatr Nephrol* 1991;5:189–192.
135. Beaumont P. Fundus changes in mesangiocapillary glomerulonephritis. *Br J Ophthalmol* 1989;73:932.
136. Michielse B, Leys A, Van Damme B, Missotten L. Fundus changes in chronic membranoproliferative glomerulonephritis type II. *Doc Ophthalmol* 1991;76:219–229.
137. Ulbig MR, Riordan-Eva P, Holz FG, Rees HC, Hamilton PA. Membranoproliferative glomerulonephritis type II associated with central serous retinopathy. *Am J Ophthalmol* 1993;116:410–413.
138. Anders D, Thoenes W. Basement membrane changes in membranoproliferative glomerulonephritis. *Virchows Arch A Pathol Anat Histopathol* 1975;369:87–109.
139. McEnery PT, McAdams AJ, West CD. Membranoproliferative glomerulonephritis: improved survival with alternate day prednisone therapy. *Clin Nephrol* 1980;13:117–124.
140. McEnery PT, McAdams AJ, West CD. The effect of prednisone in a

high-dose, alternate-day regimen on the natural history of idiopathic membranoproliferative glomerulonephritis. *Medicine* 1986;64: 401–424.

141. McEnery PT, McAdams AJ. Regression of membranoproliferative glomerulonephritis type II (dense deposit disease): observation in six children. *Am J Kidney Dis* 1988;12:138–146.
142. Ford DM, Briscoe DM, Shanley PF, Lum GM. Childhood membranoproliferative glomerulonephritis type I: limited steroid therapy. *Kidney Int* 1992;41:1606–1612.
143. Kincaid-Smith P. The natural history and treatment of mesangiocapillary glomerulonephritis. In: Kincaid-Smith P, Mathew TH, Becker EL, eds. *Glomerulonephritis: Morphology, Natural History and Treatment*. New York: John Wiley; 1973:591–609.
144. Chapman SJ, Cameron JS, Chantler C, Turner D. Treatment of mesangiocapillary glomerulonephritis in children with combined immunosuppression and anticoagulation. *Arch Dis Child* 1980;55:446–451.
145. Tiller DJ, Clarkson AR, Matthew T, et al. A prospective randomized trial in the use of cyclophosphamide, dipyridamole, and warfarin in membranous and mesangiocapillary glomerulonephritis. In: Zurukzoglu W, Papadimitriou M, Pyrpasotoulos M, Sion M, Zamboulis C, eds. *Proceedings of the 8th International Congress of Nephrology. Advances in Basic and Clinical Nephrology*. Athens: Karger; 1981:345.
146. Cattran DC, Cardella CJ, Roscoe JM, Charron RC, Rance PC, Ritchie SM, Corey PN. Results of a controlled drug trial in membranoproliferative glomerulonephritis. *Kidney Int* 1985;27:436–441.
147. Donadio JV Jr, Anderson DR, Mitchell JC III, Holley KE, Ilstrup DM, Fuster V, Chesboro JH. Membranoproliferative glomerulonephritis: a prospective clinical trial of platelet inhibitor therapy. *N Engl J Med* 1984;310:1421–1426.
148. Donadio JV, Offord KP. Reassessment of treatment results in membranoproliferative glomerulonephritis with emphasis on life-table analysis. *Am J Kidney Dis* 1989;14:445–451.
149. Broyer M, Gagnadoux MF, Guest G, Buerto D, Niaudet P, Habib R, Busson M. Kidney transplantation in children: results of 383 grafts performed at Enfants Malades Hôpital from 1973 to 1984. *Adv Nephrol Necker Hosp* 1987;16:307–333.
150. Cameron JS. Glomerulonephritis in renal transplants. *Transplantation* 1982;34:535–538.
151. Hamburger J, Crosnier J, Noel LH. Recurrent glomerulonephritis after renal transplantation. *Annu Rev Med* 1978;29:67–72.
152. Cameron JS, Turner DR. Recurrent glomerulonephritis in allografted kidneys. *Clin Nephrol* 1977;7:47–54.
153. Eddy A, Sibley R, Mauer SM, Kim Y. Renal allograft failure due to recurrent dense intramembranous deposit disease. *Clin Nephrol* 1984; 21:305–313.
154. Beaufils J, Gubler MC, Karam J, Gluckman JC, Legrain M, Kuss R. Dense deposit disease: long-term follow-up of three cases of recurrence after transplantation. *Clin Nephrol* 1977;7:31–37.
155. Curtis JJ, Wyatt RJ, Bhathena D, Lucas BA, Holland NH, Luke RG, Forristal J. Renal transplantation for patients with type I and type II membranoproliferative glomerulonephritis. Serial complement and nephritic factor measurements and the problem of recurrence of disease. *Am J Med* 1979;66:216–225.

Immunologic Renal Diseases,
edited by E. G. Neilson and W. G. Couser.
Lippincott-Raven Publishers, Philadelphia © 1997.

CHAPTER 52

Amyloidosis and the Dysproteinemias

Melvin M. Schwartz and Stephen M. Korbet

INTRODUCTION

Amyloidosis and the dysproteinemias comprise a spectrum of diseases with a common pathogenesis related to renal deposition of immunoglobulin-derived material. They are discussed under the headings of amyloidosis, paraproteinemias, cryoglobulinemias, and immunotactoid glomerulopathy.

AMYLOIDOSIS

Definition

Amyloidosis is the rubric for diseases characterized by extracellular accumulation of protein polymers and defined by their histochemical and ultrastructural appearance. The protein polymers share a tertiary structure that confers their staining characteristics and stability under physiologic conditions (1). Progressive interstitial accumulation causes organ dysfunction and symptoms.

Historical Perspective

Amyloidosis was named by Virchow for the color reaction, typical of starch, that followed the application of iodine and sulfuric acid to gross specimens (2). This interpretation was controversial for he was aware of studies suggesting a protein composition. Amyloidosis has been classified by its clinical associations and sites of deposition (3), but the current classification (4) is based upon the biochemistry of the deposits. The type of amyloid of concern in this chapter is designated AL for immunoglobulin light-chain-derived amyloid, and it occurs in primary (no associated disease process), myeloma-associated, and tumor-forming amyloidosis.

The ordered structure of amyloid was anticipated by morphologic studies. When Congo-red-stained amyloid is polarized, it exhibits a characteristic apple-green birefringence (Fig. 1), and as the filters are moved through crossover, different areas exhibit the green color (dichroism) (5,6). This implied regularity of structure was reflected by the ultrastructural demonstration of amyloid fibrils (Fig. 2) (7). These features are common to all types of amyloid and pure preparations of fibrils (1). X-ray crystallography demonstrated that the fibrils were composed of polypeptide chains oriented perpendicular to the long axis of the fibril in a twisted β-pleated sheet (1). Thus, the tertiary structure of amyloid is reflected by its ultrastructural appearance and determines its histochemical specificity.

Etiology and Incidence

Amyloidosis was found in only 0.7% of 11,586 autopsies performed at one hospital from 1961 to 1970 (8). The etiology of amyloidosis is related to its clinical associations (9), including multiple myeloma (10) and chronic inflammatory diseases (11), but in the United States the majority of amyloidosis is primary (12). The incidence of amyloidosis related to plasma cell dyscrasias has not changed, but the etiology of secondary amyloidosis has shifted from chronic suppurative infections to the rheumatic diseases.

Pathogenesis

Amyloid is composed of circulating protein precursors (1). In AL amyloid, the major protein component is an homogeneous intact immunoglobulin light chain or a light-chain fragment containing the N-terminal, variable

M. M. Schwartz and S. M. Korbet: Department of Pathology and Section of Nephrology, Department of Medicine, Rush Medical College, Chicago, Illinois 60612.

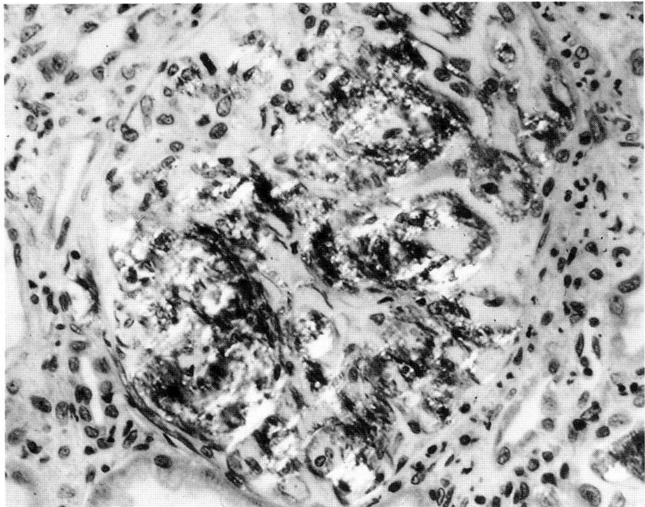

FIG. 1. Glomerular amyloid deposits stained with Congo red and polarized. The amyloid deposits are seen birefringent areas interspersed with nonbirefringent Congo-red–stained areas. Congo red, ×300.

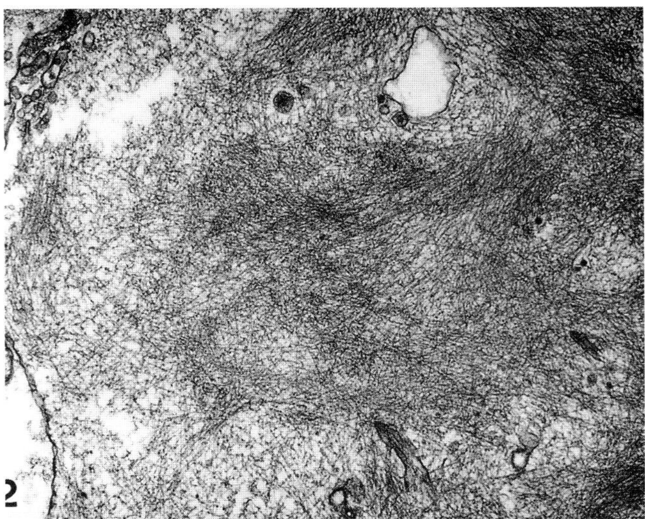

FIG. 2. Ultrastructural appearance of glomerular mesangial deposits of amyloid. Amyloid is seen as randomly arranged extracellular nonbranching fibrils measuring ~10 nm in diameter. Uranyl acetate and lead citrate, ×70,000.

(V_L) portion (13,14). However, not all light chains are amyloidogenic (1,15–18). Consistent loss of amino acids from the C-terminal end of light chains (19) implies a role for proteolysis in fibrillogenesis (1), and high local concentrations of precursor protein as well as destabilizing, fibrillogenic point mutations may also be involved.

The association between multiple myeloma and amyloid (1,20,21) suggests that production of abnormal light-chain sequences underlies fibrillogenesis, and various amino acid substitutions and deletions in amyloidogenic light chains have been demonstrated (1,22). Amino acid substitutions, occurring at structurally critical portions of V_L, have been used to create mutant V_L in an *Escherichia coli*-expression system. The resulting V_L aggregates to form AL fibrils under conditions in which the wild-type V_L remains soluble. Studies in secondary, anyloid A (AA) (23–29) and hereditary amyloidosis (30–32) also support a molecular basis for fibrillogenesis.

Amyloid fibrils are associated with other proteins, including amyloid P, glycosaminoglycans, proteoglycans, fibronectin, and apolipoprotein E (33–35). These proteins may participate in fibrillogenesis (36). However, in vitro fibrillogenesis requires only pure preparations of V_L (37), which suggests that the other proteins are neither necessary for the initiation of fibrillogenesis nor for stabilization of β-pleated sheets. Thus, amyloidogenic proteins contain sequences that form b-pleated sheets when they are altered by proteolysis, mutational changes that predispose one to proteolysis, or point mutations, deletions, or structural modifications that alter the molecular structure without proteolysis (38).

Pathology

The kidneys may be enlarged in amyloidosis (39,40), and the amount of amyloid is inversely proportional to renal size (40). Amyloid is eosinophilic, acellular, and weakly periodic-acid–Schiff (PAS) positive (5,6). Its affinity for Congo red dye and birefringence under polarized light distinguishes it from other hyaline materials.

The distinction among the different fibril (4) types is usually accomplished by clinicopathologic correlation because the pattern of renal involvement in primary (39) and secondary (41) amyloidosis is indistinguishable (42–44). Histologic (45,46) and immunochemical (19,47–49) methods are available for distinguishing between AA and AL amyloid.

Renal amyloid (50,51) is almost always present in the glomeruli and blood vessels (43,44). Tubular involvement and interstitial involvement are less frequent, but when they occur, the medullary interstitium and vasa recta are more frequently involved than the cortex (21,42, 44). The initial glomerular deposits are in the mesangium (40,42–44). As the deposits extend into the subendothelium (40) and infiltrate and replace the basal lamina, focal fraying, loss of argyrophilia (40,44), and breaks (42) in the basement membrane occur. Subepithelial deposits form silver-positive spikes (40) in ~50% of the biopsies studied by light microscopy (42), leading to confusion with membranous glomerulonephritis (51).

Antisera specific for immunoglobulin heavy chains, complement components, and fibrinogen stain amyloid with variable and sometimes confusing results (21,51, 52). Staining appears to be specific, but inconsistent and present in both primary and secondary forms. The immune reactants are not part of the amyloid fibril, and their mechanism of association and pathologic implications remain unknown.

All amyloid fibrils form randomly arranged, thin, rigid, nonbranching fibrils by electron microscopy (53,54). They vary from 50 to 300 Å in diameter (53,54), averaging between 90 and 110 Å, and measuring up to 14,000 Å in length. The fibrils are seen in the same sites identified by light microscopy (21,42,44,52,53,55–59).

Clinical Manifestations and Laboratory Features

In 99% of cases, the patients are older than 40 years, and 64% are men (10). Multiple myeloma is present in 21% of patients with amyloidosis, but the separation of myeloma-associated AL from a nonmalignant plasma cell dyscrasia is not always possible (60). Fatigue and weight loss are the commonest presenting features, but most signs and symptoms result from renal and cardiac involvement (12).

Proteinuria is present in >80% of patients with primary amyloidosis and is associated with the nephrotic syndrome in 37% (10). In patients with myeloma-associated amyloidosis (AL), proteinuria may result exclusively from light-chain excretion. While 65% of these patients have Bence Jones proteinuria, only 39% have albuminuria. In contrast, patients with primary amyloidosis without myeloma have Bence Jones proteinuria in 8% and albuminuria in 82% of cases (10). At presentation, renal insufficiency is already present in up to 47% of patients (51).

The demonstration and characterization of a monoclonal serum or urine protein are critical in the diagnosis of AL amyloidosis (61). In >80%, a monoclonal protein is identified in either the urine or serum by immunoelectrophoresis (10). In patients with the nephrotic syndrome, a monoclonal protein will be identified 94% of the time (12). In 20% of amyloid patients, the monoclonal protein consists of only free light chains, and these are most often λ (62). Patients in whom a monoclonal protein is not identified are less likely to have renal involvement.

The diagnosis of AL is based on histologic features, and biopsy of an involved tissue is critical. As a result of its systemic nature, several procedures have been evaluated. Aspiration of abdominal fat has yielded positive results in 72–84% of patients with systemic amyloidosis (12,63,64). Kyle and Gertz (12) suggest that fat aspiration be the initial diagnostic procedure in the evaluation of AL. Indirect evidence of amyloidosis has been demonstrated with the use of radiopharmaceuticals (65,66). Recently, radiolabeled human serum amyloid P has demonstrated uptake into one or more sites in patients with biopsy-proven amyloid (67). The greatest utility of these tests may be in targeting sites for biopsy and monitoring the progression or regression of amyloid deposits in therapeutic trials.

Prognosis and Treatment

The median survival in AL patients with the nephrotic syndrome is 18 months (68). Even though the degree of proteinuria does not correlate with survival, the presence of free light chains portends a poor prognosis particularly in patients with λ light chains in the urine. A significantly poorer prognosis is also seen in patients with renal insufficiency, with a median survival of 14.9 months in contrast to 25.6 months for patients with normal renal function.

The treatment of AL has focused on inhibiting the production of the paraprotein with the use of cytotoxic regimens that often include prednisone and melphalan. In patients with the nephrotic syndrome, a response to melphalan and prednisone has been associated with a reduction or complete resolution of proteinuria and improvement in renal function (69–71). Unfortunately, <30% of patients respond (11). The prognosis of responders is significantly better, with a median survival of 89 months, with 78% surviving 5 years. Thus, a trial of therapy is strongly recommended.

Therapies with colchicine (71,72), recombinant interferon α–2 (73) and α-tocopherol (vitamin E) (74) have been attempted, but they have not been effective in achieving regression or improving survival. End stage renal disease (ESRD) is one of the major complications of amyloidosis. Although amyloidosis accounts for <0.5% of ESRD in the United States, the 1-year mortality rate is one of the highest (75). On dialysis, the median survival is 8.2 months (62). Peritoneal dialysis may create less hemodynamic stress in patients with cardiomyopathy (76), but survival is not significantly different from those on hemodialysis (62).

Fewer than 1% of patients with ESRD are considered for renal transplantation (75,77), and >90% of those have secondary amyloidosis (78). The experience with transplantation in AL is extremely limited. If chemotherapy improves life expectancy in AL amyloidosis, nephrologists may reconsider these patients for transplantation.

DYSPROTEINEMIAS

The dysproteinemias (plasma cell dyscrasias) are characterized by proliferation of a single clone of immunoglobulin-producing cells that produce a monoclonal immunoglobulin and/or immunoglobulin fragment (paraprotein) seen by immunoelectrophoresis of the urine and\ or serum proteins as an homogeneous peak or "spike." The different forms of renal pathology seen in the dysproteinemias are caused by the renal deposition of the immunoglobulin product.

Historical Perspective, Incidence, and Definition of Diseases

Henry Bence Jones in 1847 noted an abnormal protein in the urine of a patient with multiple myeloma (79). Multiple myeloma is a clonal neoplasm of malignant plasma cells, and virtually all patients have a paraprotein in the serum and/or urine. To distinguish patients with multiple myeloma from patients with other paraproteinemias and benign monoclonal gammopathy (80,81), the diagnosis requires a combination of histologic, serologic, and radiographic features (82). A spectrum of renal pathology (83) is associated with multiple myeloma and other benign and malignant hematolymphoid proliferations (84,85), including amyloidosis (as just discussed), myeloma cast nephropathy with and without Fanconi syndrome, renal disease associated with benign monoclonal gammopathy, monoclonal immunoglobulin deposition disease (MIDD), and Waldenström macroglobulinemia.

Myeloma kidney or cast nephropathy results from the formation of tubular casts containing light chains. Renal involvement in benign monoclonal gammopathy is unusual and is limited to isolated reports of glomerulonephritis. MIDD has both glomerular and tubular lesions related to nonamyloid tissue deposits of the monoclonal immunoglobulin. Autopsies on consecutive patients with multiple myeloma demonstrated amyloidosis in 10%, cast nephropathy in 30%, and MIDD in three of 57 patients (86,87). Cast nephropathy is seen at biopsy in 63–86% of patients with multiple myeloma (88–90). Waldenström macroglobulinemia is a rare condition with infrequent renal involvement caused by a monoclonal proliferation of "plasmacytoid" lymphocytes producing a monoclonal immunoglobulin (Ig) M (91,92). AL amyloidosis, which occurs in <5% of patients with monoclonal IgM (93), is the most common clinical form of renal involvement in Waldenström macroglobulinemia.

Pathogenesis of Dysproteinemias

The pathogenesis of the renal lesions in the dysproteinemias relates to the properties of the paraproteins. The pathogenicity of light chains in multiple myeloma is contrasted with light chains in normal individuals and in patients with myeloma without renal involvement (81,94, 95) that are removed from the circulation by the kidney without causing renal damage (96,97). These clinical observations are supported by experimental studies in which morphologic and functional defects seen in patients have been reproduced in animals following exposure to paraproteins (95,98–100).

Structural changes in immunoglobulin molecules may affect their pathogenicity by causing abnormal glomerular filtration, nephrotoxicity, and immune-mediated inflammation. The isoelectric point (pI) (5–7) and the tendency of Bence Jones proteins to undergo homotypic aggregation (18–22,33) may alter glomerular filtration. High molecular weight polymers and proteins with a low pI will not readily pass the glomerular filter and will tend to remain in the circulation and deposit in tissue. In Waldenström macroglobulinemia, the size of the molecule produced and homotypic aggregation in MIDD may explain the lack of renal involvement in the former and tissue deposition in the latter. In contrast, monomeric and dimeric Bence Jones proteins with an high pI will pass the glomerular filter in large amounts with the potential to cause tubular pathology. In general, patients with paraproteinemias either present with cast nephropathy or tissue deposits of nonamyloid paraproteins, but not both. The basis for this dichotomy is at least partly due to the effect of pI and homotypic aggregation upon glomerular permeability of paraproteins.

There is abundant circumstantial evidence linking the presence of Bence Jones proteinuria with decreased renal function and acute renal failure [reviewed by Silva et al. (101)]. It may be directly toxic to the renal tubules, and Tamm–Horsfall protein (102,103), which is an invariable component of myeloma casts, may be involved (90,99, 100,104–109). The destructive interstitial nephritis that accompanies cast nephropathy has been attributed to rupture of obstructed tubules with release of tubular contents (110) and the recruitment of inflammatory mediators (111). Crystals are seen in the casts and within tubular epithelial cells in some patients with cast nephropathy and in approximately one-half the patients with Fanconi syndrome associated with Bence Jones proteinuria (112). The properties of these crystal-forming Bence Jones proteins (109,113) suggest that they exert their effect by interfering with tubular function (96,97) after they are taken into tubular lysosomes and partially digested (109,113,114).

Immunoglobulin aggregates or complexes of immunoglobulin and rheumatoid factor with anti-immunoglobulin activity can behave as immune complexes and activate complement. This mechanism underlies the glomerulonephritis seen in benign monoclonal gammopathy and cryoglobulinemia.

Pathology of Myeloma Cast Nephropathy

The casts are dense, frequently lamellated and fractured, and they increase in size with time (5). They are surrounded by macrophages, giant cells (5,101,115–117), and a destructive interstitial nephritis (115) (Fig. 3). The casts and the tubular epithelial cells may contain rhomboid or needle-shaped crystals (118,119). Patients with cast nephropathy do not have systemic amyloidosis (101), but the casts (101,115,120), interstitium, and blood vessels may contain amyloid (5). The casts most commonly contain λ light chains (3,101,115,121), and immu-

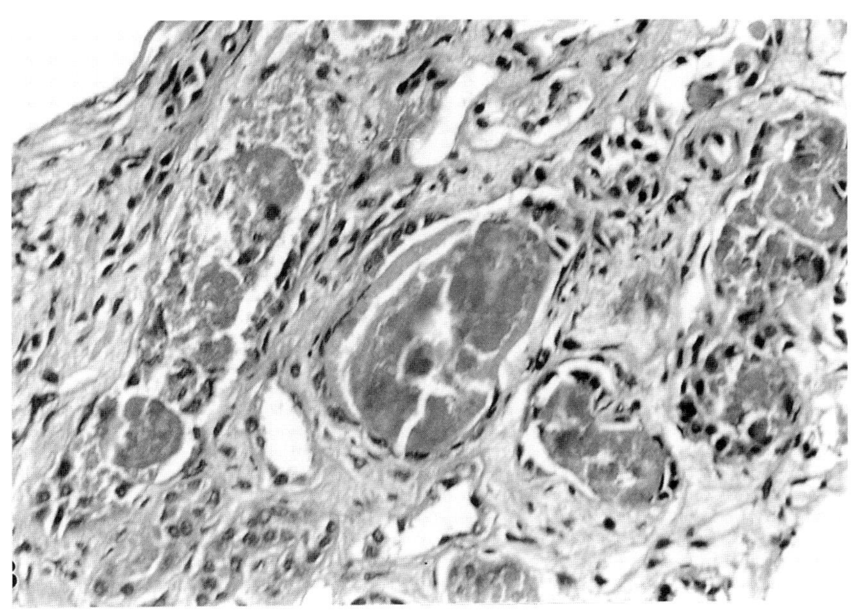

FIG. 3. Myeloma kidney (cast nephropathy). The tubules are atrophic and contain dense, refractile, fractured casts. The associated interstitium is fibrotic. Hematoxylin–eosin, ×250.

noglobulins and serum proteins (101,102,116,121–123) may be present. Plasma cell infiltrates are seen in 10% of the cases (124). When light-chain deposition disease and amyloidosis are excluded, multiple myeloma has mild glomerular changes and inconsistent glomerular immune deposits (115,125,126).

The extent of cast formation parallels the degree of interstitial fibrosis and tubular atrophy, and tubular rupture does not occur in the absence of casts (115). Despite the role of casts in the pathogenesis of the tubulointerstitial lesion, renal function correlates with interstitial fibrosis and tubular atrophy (101,115,126) and not with cast formation (101).

Clinical Manifestations and Laboratory Features of Multiple Myeloma

Multiple myeloma rarely occurs in young adults, with 98% occurring in patients >40 years of age. Clinical and laboratory features at presentation include bone pain (66%), anemia (60–80%), hypercalcemia (30–45%), hyperuricemia (40–60%), and a palpable liver (21%) (81, 124). Proteinuria is observed in >80–90% of cases and is the nephrotic range in 25% (94). Renal tubular dysfunction is observed in some resulting in abnormalities in acidification and concentration and in the Fanconi syndrome (94). Immunoelectrophoresis demonstrates a monoclonal heavy chain in the serum in >80% of cases, but in 8% only free monoclonal light chains are found (81). Immunoelectrophoresis of the urine demonstrates monoclonal light chains in 80% of cases with κ accounting for 58% (81). Fewer than 1% of patients with multiple myeloma have no evidence of a paraprotein when both serum and urine are evaluated.

One of the most serious complications of multiple myeloma is renal insufficiency, which is present in 50–70% of patients at presentation with a serum creatinine >2 mg/dL in 30–40% (81,94,124,127,128). Multiple myeloma may present as idiopathic acute renal failure with no serologic or clinical evidence of a paraproteinemia, and the diagnosis is made at renal biopsy and confirmed on bone marrow (129,130).

Acute renal failure in multiple myeloma may be precipitated by dehydration, hypercalcemia, and an acidic urine (90,100,131,132). Furosemide or radiocontrast material, which may promote cast formation by causing volume contraction, and nonsteroidal anti-inflammatory agents, which may be independent factors in cast formation, should be used cautiously or avoided (90,100). The initial treatment of renal failure includes decreasing light-chain production and creating a renal tubular environment less conducive to cast formation.

Prognosis and Treatment

The median survival in myeloma patients is 20–30 months, with a 5 year survival of 18–27% (81,128,133). The most common cause of death is renal failure (15–20%). In patients with renal failure, the median survival is <4 months (90,124,127,128). Thus, aggressive treatment is required in this setting. To decrease the production of light chains, alkylating agents (melphalan) in combination with prednisone are standard therapy. In addition, hydration (2–3 L/day), alkalinization of the urine, and correction of hypercalcemia are initiated. Experimentally, colchicine and reducing agents have been shown to prevent cast formation, but these observations have not been confirmed clinically (100).

Renal failure is acute in >75% of myeloma patients at presentation, and it is reversible with therapy in >50% (88,90). This results in survivals which are similar to that in myeloma patients without renal failure (12–20 months) (90,134). For patients requiring dialysis, recovery of renal function sufficient to discontinue dialysis has been observed in up to 38% of cases, but may take >3 months (90,128,135,136). Factors that predicted a favorable response to therapy included previously normal or only mild renal insufficiency, evidence for precipitating factors, and early, aggressive treatment (88).

Plasmapheresis results in dramatic reduction in paraprotein concentration and improvement in renal function in myeloma patients with significant renal insufficiency or ESRD, but has not consistently shown an improvement in survival over patients treated with chemotherapy and forced diuresis alone (88,137,138). In a recent controlled trial, however, the 1-year survival was 66% in patients treated with plasma exchange compared with 28% in the control patients (139). It has been claimed that peritoneal dialysis may also be efficacious in the removal of light chains, but it does not appear to be as efficient as plasmapheresis (138).

Even with aggressive treatment, progression to ESRD may occur in up to 64% of myeloma patients (89). Multiple myeloma, however, accounts for only 1.1% of all new ESRD patients (77). On chronic dialysis, survival up to 20 months has been reported (89), with a median survival of 7.5–13 months (77,137,140). The survival on dialysis depends on response to chemotherapy, with responders surviving 47 months from diagnosis (37 months on dialysis) as compared with 17 months for nonresponders (12 months on dialysis) (141). Both hemodialysis and peritoneal dialysis have been used in myeloma patients with ESRD and appear to be equally effective (140,142–144). A major cause of morbidity in dialysis patients is sepsis (145,146). For patients on peritoneal dialysis, high peritonitis rates of one episode per 5.6 patient-months have been observed and may significantly effect the success of this therapy (141).

Renal transplantation is generally not considered in patients with multiple myeloma, because of their extremely poor prognosis. There are reports of stable myeloma patients in whom cadaveric renal transplants resulted in long-term survival (>12 months) with no recurrence of myeloma kidney (134,147,148). Thus, for patients without extrarenal manifestations of myeloma for >1 year, transplantation may prove to be an alternative to dialysis.

Pathology of Monoclonal Immunoglobulin Deposition Disease

MIDD is defined by the demonstration of immunoglobulin chains in the kidneys and other viscera that do not take up Congo red and do not have an organized ultrastructure (149). First recognized as isolated deposits of κ light chains (70% of cases), examples of λ light-chain (20% of cases), light- and heavy-chain (<10% of cases), and isolated heavy-chain deposits now define the spectrum of this entity (109). Since first described in 1976 (150), >150 cases have been reported (19), and light-chain deposition disease is the most common. However, the histologic and ultrastructural pathologic features are similar and are presented together.

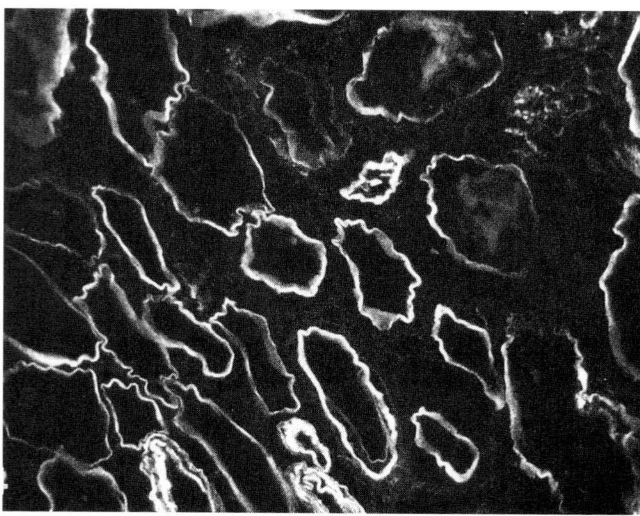

FIG. 4. Tubular immunofluorescence in monoclonal immunoglobulin deposition disease (κ glomerulopathy). The tubular basement membranes stain intensely with antiserum directed against κ light chain (λ light chains and heavy-chain determinants were negative). ×300.

In MIDD, the principal clinical feature is glomerular proteinuria (see below), but the commonest histologic finding and the defining immunochemical features are seen in the renal tubules (19,149,151–153). There is bright, retractile, PAS-positive, Congo-red-negative, ribbonlike thickening of the tubular basement membranes, most prominent in the medulla. The tubular epithelium may remain well-preserved despite extensive basement membrane changes. Similar deposits may be seen surrounding the vasa recta and lying free in the medullary interstitium. They form electron-dense, punctate deposits on the external (interstitial) side of the basal lamina, with no evidence of fibril formation (152,154). The tubular basement membrane deposits are smooth and linear by fluorescence microscopy (Fig. 4). These are either κ or λ, with a κ to λ ratio of 4:1 (19,152). Complement is rarely present, and amyloid P is absent (19).

Nodular glomerulosclerosis, resembling diabetic glomerular disease, is present in 60% of cases (149). The glomeruli have multiple, acellular, PAS-positive, nonargyrophilic, Congo-red-negative nodules that compress the capillaries, which may be thickened (Fig. 5). There are inconstant electron-dense, subendothelial, granular,

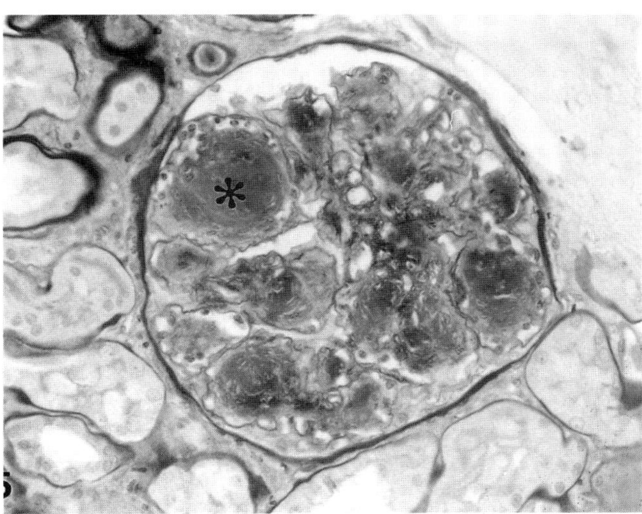

FIG. 5. Nodular glomerular sclerosis in monoclonal immunoglobulin deposition disease. The glomerular lesion resembles diabetic glomerular sclerosis, but the diagnosis depends upon the characteristic tubular immunopathology (see Fig. 4). Periodic acid–Schiff, ×220.

punctate deposits that may diffusely infiltrate the basal lamina. Although the glomeruli may contain linear deposits of monotypic immunoglobulin light and\or heavy chains, the finding is inconsistent, and the demonstration of typical tubular immunopathology remains the premier diagnostic feature of this disease.

Clinical Manifestations and Laboratory Features

MIDD is a disease of adults >40 years old. Renal involvement is a presenting feature in essentially all patients. Proteinuria is present in >90% of cases and in the nephrotic range in 28–53% (152,153,155). Renal insufficiency is a presenting feature in >85% and rapidly deteriorates to ESRD.

MIDD, like amyloidosis, is a systemic infiltrative disorder that can involve essentially any major organ and cause dysfunction. In the majority of patients, a monoclonal protein is identified in either the serum, urine, or both, but in 20–35% no monoclonal immunoglobulin is present (149,153). However, biosynthetic studies of the bone marrow in a number of these patients have demonstrated excess production of the paraprotein (152–154). MIDD commonly occurs in patients with lymphoplasmacytic disorders such as multiple myeloma, but 30–60% of cases have no evidence of hematologic malignancy at presentation (152,153,155).

Prognosis and Treatment

Patient survival at 1 and 5 years is 89% and 70%, respectively, and renal survival at 1 and 5 years is 67% and 37%, respectively (155). Treatment is with melphalan and prednisone (155). Untreated patients with renal involvement progress to ESRD within 2–23 months (152). With therapy, 60–80% of patients with a creatinine <4 mg/dL will have improvement or stabilization of their renal function (152,155). For patients with creatinines >4 mg/dL, >80% progress to ESRD despite therapy (155). Thus, early identification and treatment of patients with MIDD may significantly alter the course of renal disease.

Renal transplantation has been successfully performed in patients with MIDD who were in remission with no other major organ involvement, but disease recurs in >50% and may lead to graft loss (153,155–159).

CRYOGLOBULINEMIC GLOMERULONEPHRITIS

Cryoglobulins are proteins that precipitate from properly collected and cooled serum (5). Three categories are described (160): type-1 cryoglobulins are isolated monoclonal immunoglobulins and types 2 and 3 are mixed cryoglobulins in which one immunoglobulin acts as an antibody (rheumatoid factor) against polyclonal IgG. The antiglobulin activity is a mononclonal immunoglobulin in type 2 (>90% IgMκ) and a polyclonal immunoglobulin in type 3. In type-2 cryoglobulinemia, a characteristic pattern of glomerulonephritis develops that is called cryoglobulinemic glomerulonephritis (161). Type-1 cryoglobulinemias are usually associated with hematologic malignancies (5,160), and rarely have renal involvement. The mixed cryoglobulinemias, which account for 60–75% of the total (160,162), have many underlying diseases (160,162,163), which are discussed under specific diseases. However, 30% have no associated disease (29,160, 162,164), and Melzer et al. (165) named the association of mixed cryoglobulinemia of unknown etiology presenting with purpura, weakness arthralgia, and glomerular lesions essential mixed cryoglobulinemia (EMC). Since 1991, serologic studies have demonstrated an association between EMC and hepatitis-C virus (HCV) antibodies and HCV RNA (166–170). The prevalence of HCV RNA approaches 100% in EMC patients with glomerulonephritis (166). D'Amico and colleagues postulate that HCV is involved in all types of mixed cryoglobulinemia and suggest that EMC no longer exists as a discrete entity (166, 171,172). The association of EMC, hepatitis virus, and cryoglobulinemia is covered in detail in chapter 41.

IMMUNOTACTOID GLOMERULONEPHRITIS

Definition and Historical Perspective

Immunotactoid glomerulopathy (ITG) is a primary glomerular disease that is defined by organized ultrastructural deposits of immunoglobulin (173). Other

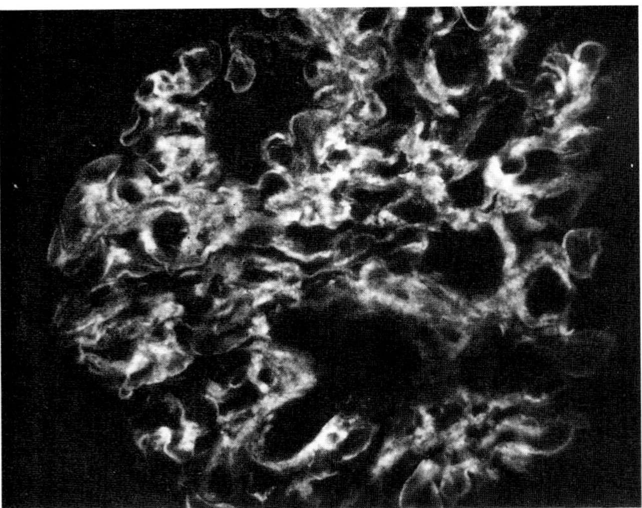

FIG. 6. Immunotactoid glomerulopathy by immunofluorescence microscopy. There are diffuse mesangial and focal paramesangial and glomerular basement membrane deposits. Goat–anti-human immunoglobulin G, ×330.

names have been used that emphasize the fibrillar structure and histochemistry of the deposits, but they ignore the immunoglobulin content of the fibrils (Fig. 6) (173).

The fibrils are 18–22 nm in diameter (range, 10–49 nm), which is approximately twice the diameter of amyloid fibrils, but within the range of other forms of fibrillary glomerular deposits (Fig. 7) (173–175). The morphology of the deposits is variable, with most arranged randomly as they infiltrate the glomerulus. In a few cases, larger fibrils are tightly packed into highly organized parallel arrays, reminiscent of the paracrystalline structures seen in some cases of paraproteinemia and cryoglobulinemia (174). These ultrastructural differences have suggested that the smaller (18–22 nm) randomly arranged fibers be called fibrillary glomerulonephritis while reserving the diagnosis of ITG for cases with the larger parallel fibrils (176–178). The rational for this dichotomy is that the larger fibrils are allegedly associated with hematolymphoid neoplasms, and the deposits have a higher prevalence of monoclonality. However, neither neoplasia nor monoclonality is consistently observed in either group (179). Since the clinical presentation and course of these two groups are the same and there is no specific therapy for either, ITG is diagnosed in all patients with organized glomerular immune deposits after exclusion of other diseases associated with organized glomerular immune deposits (174).

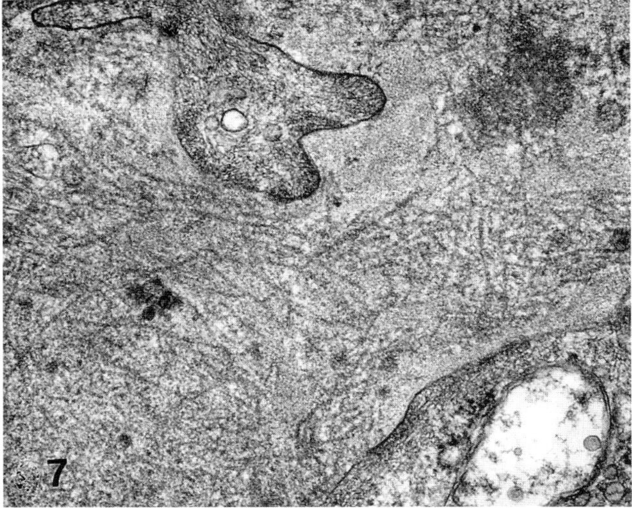

FIG. 7. Immunotactoid glomerulopathy, electron microscopy of mesangial deposits. The deposits resolve into nonbranching, randomly arrange microfibrils that average 21 nanometers in diameter. Uranyl acetate and lead citrate, ×95,000.

Etiology and Incidence

Immunotactoid glomerulopathy has been identified with increasing frequency since its description in 1977 (180), and there are now >150 cases in the literature (173). Its etiology is unknown, but by analogy to AL amyloidosis and the dysproteinemias, the immunoglobulin precursors must be produced by bone-marrow-derived plasma cells or B lymphocytes but in undetectable amounts. The deposits in ITG may represent either immune complexes with restricted antigenic specificity or abnormal monoclonal serum proteins (173), and glomerular filtration creates an environment that is favorable for their local deposition. The prolonged, indolent course that is consistent with gradual accumulation of deposits, and the paucity of extrarenal (181,182) and extraglomerular deposits in ITG (173), are consistent with this hypothesis.

Pathogenesis and Pathophysiology

Renal pathology and dysfunction in ITG are caused by the glomerular deposition and accumulation of deposits without destructive inflammatory lesions. The pathogenesis of renal dysfunction is analogous to amyloidosis where fibrils initially interfere with glomerular capillary wall function, causing proteinuria, but further accumulation leads to atrophy of parenchymal cells and glomerular obsolescence (54).

The constant association with complement suggests that immunotactoids have immune-complex-like features, but the absence of hypocomplementemia (see below) and proliferation makes this interpretation problematic (5). In a few cases, the deposits are monoclonal immunoglobulins, suggesting a pathogenetic mechanism akin to MIDD. There is no further support for either mechanism, but the findings imply that, like amyloidosis, ITG represents the final immunopathologic expression of several pathogenetic mechanisms.

Pathology

The pathology of ITG is almost exclusively glomerular, and it reflects the location in the mesangium and the glomerular capillary wall of immunotactoids (5,173, 174). In all cases, the mesangium is expanded by PAS-positive, Congo-red-negative material with associated mild mesangial hypercellularity (183). In addition, the glomerular capillary walls may be thickened and, with the silver stain, spikes, holes, and double contours are seen. Cellular and fibrocellular crescents are reported, but glomerular necrosis is unusual (184).

Immunoglobulins and complement localize to the mesangium and capillary walls at the same sites as the immunotactoids visualized by electron microscopy (173,174). Immunogold electron microscopy demonstrates heavy chains, light chains, complement, and amyloid P exclusively in the fibrils (185,186). The deposits contain equal amounts of κ and λ light chains in 75% of the cases, and in the remainder the deposits are monoclonal.

TABLE 1. *Classification of the fibrillary glomerulopathies*

Amyloid (Congo red positive)
AL amyloid
Primary
Multiple myeloma
Tumor-forming amyloid
AA amyloid
Rheumatic diseases
Chronic suppurative and granulomatous inflammation
Tumors
Mediterranean fever
Familial amyloidosis
Nonamyloid (Congo red negative)
Immunoglobulin-derived fibrils
Cryoglobulinemias
Mixed essential
Multiple myeloma
Chronic lymphocytic leukemia
Monoclonal gammopathies
"Benign"
Multiple myeloma
Monoclonal immunoglobulin deposition disease
Chronic lymphocytic leukemia
Systemic lupus erythematosus
Immunotactoid (fibrillary) glomerulopathy
Non-immunoglobulin-derived fibrils
Diabetes mellitus
Others

Clinical Manifestations and Laboratory Features

Patients with ITG range in age from 10 to 80 years, with an average age of 44 years at presentation (173), and 60% are men. Proteinuria is the presenting finding in all patients (0.3–26 g/24 h), with the nephrotic syndrome in >60%. Renal insufficiency (45%), microscopic hematuria (66%), and hypertension (78%) are also commonly seen at presentation. By definition, these patients do not have cryoglobulinemia, a paraproteinemia, or systemic lupus erythematosus even though up to 19% have been reported to have positive antinuclear antibodies (usually in low titer and/or in a speckled pattern) (175,177). Patients with evidence of these features should be categorized appropriately and not diagnosed as having ITG.

Immunotactoid glomerulopathy does not appear to represent a systemic disease. To date, extrarenal involvement has only been described in two patients (181,182). Furthermore, patients with ITG do not have clinical symptoms or evidence of multisystem involvement. With follow-up, patients have not been reported to have developed clinical or serologic evidence of a systemic disease or a dysproteinemia. Thus, ITG is best classified as a primary glomerular process distinct from the other immunoglobulin-derived fibrillary glomerulopathies (Table 1) (174). The disorders included in this classification are defined histochemically, with amyloid, possibly the best known, being defined by its positive reaction with Congo red stain.

Prognosis and Treatment

Patients with ITG have a progressive course of renal failure leading to ESRD over 4 years (173,177). This is similar to other primary glomerulopathies but is distinct from that of the other fibrillary glomerulopathies that experience a more rapid decline to ESRD (174). Since ITG appears to be an immune-mediated lesion, one might expect a favorable response to a trial of immunotherapy, but the reported therapeutic experience in ITG is limited. The response to therapy with steroids alone, steroids with cytotoxic agents, and steroids with plasmapheresis is <10% (184,187,188).

Features at presentation that are associated with a poor renal prognosis are hypertension, nephrotic proteinuria, and renal insufficiency (173,175). Even though detailed analyses have been reported, there is little information on the prognostic significance of the various pathologic features of ITG. In our experience, those patients with more extensive glomerular involvement have a worse prognosis (175).

The overall survival in patients with ITG is quite good as one might expect in patients with a primary glomerulopathy. The survival at 1 year is 100%, with >80% of patients alive at 5 years. As a result, renal transplantation should be a treatment consideration in ITG patients with ESRD. To date, renal transplantation has been reported in four patients followed from 2 to 6 years (173,184,189). ITG recurred in two patients after 21 and 60 months, leading to loss of the transplant in one patient 3 years later. Thus, transplantation appears to be a viable option for patients with ITG.

REFERENCES

1. Glenner GG. Amyloid deposits and amyloidosis: the β-fibrilloses. *N Engl J Med* 1980;302:1283–92.
2. Virchow R. Amyloid degeneration. In: *Cellular pathology as based upon physiological and pathological histology* [Translated from the second edition of the original by Frank Chance, B.A., M.B. Cantab.]. London: John Churchill, 1860:409–27.
3. Reiman HA, Koucky RF, Eklund CM. Primary amyloidosis limited to tissue of mesodermal origin. *Am J Pathol* 1935;11:977–88.
4. Anonymous. Nomenclature of amyloid and amyloidosis: WHO–IUIS Nomenclature Sub-Committee. *Bull World Health Organ* 1993;71: 105–12.
5. Hill GS. Dysproteinemias, amyloidosis, and immunotactoid glomerulopathy. In: Heptinstall RH, ed. *Pathology of the kidney.* Boston: Little, Brown, 1992:1631–713.
6. Morel-Maroger Striker LJ, Preud'homme J-L, D'Amico G, Striker GE. Monoclonal gammopathies, mixed cryoglobulinemias, and lymphomas. In: Tisher CC, Brenner BM, eds. *Renal pathology with clinical and functional correlations.* Philadelphia: JB Lippincott, 1994: 1442–90.
7. Cohen AS, Calkins E. A light and electron microscopic study of human and experimental amyloid disease of the kidneys. *Arthritis Rheum* 1959;2:70–71.
8. Thornton C. Amyloid disease: an autopsy review of the decades 1937–46 and 1961–70. *Ulster Med J* 1983;52:31.
9. Ivanyi B. Frequency of light chain deposition nephropathy relative to renal amyloidosis and Bence Jones cast nephropathy in a necropsy study of patients with myeloma. *Arch Pathol Lab Med* 1990;114: 986–7.
10. Kyle RA, Greipp PR. Amyloidosis (AL): clinical and laboratory features in 229 cases. *Mayo Clin Proc* 1983;58:665–83.
11. Gertz MA, Kyle RA, Greipp PR. Response rates and survival in primary systemic amyloidosis. *Blood* 1991;77:257–62.
12. Kyle RA, Gertz MA. Systemic amyloidosis [Review]. *Crit Rev Oncol Hematol* 1990;10:49–87.
13. Glenner GG, Harada M, Isersky C, Cuatrecasas P, Page D, Keiser H. Human amyloid protein: diversity and uniformity. *Biochem Biophys Res Commun* 1970;41:1013–9.
14. Harada M, Isersky C, Cuatrecasas P, et al. Human amyloid protein chemical variability and homogeneity. *J Histochem Cytochem* 1971; 19:1–15.
15. Levo Y, Pick AI, Frohlichman R. Predominance of lambda-type Bence Jones proteins in patients with amyloidosis and plasma cell dyscrasia. In: Wegelius O, Pasternack A, eds. *Amyloidosis.* New York: Academic, 1976:291–8.
16. Ozaki S, Abe M, Wolfenbarger D, Weiss DT, Solomon A. Preferential expression of human lambda-light-chain variable-region subgroups in multiple myeloma, AL amyloidosis, and Waldenström's macroglobulinemia. *Clin Immunol Immunopathol* 1994;71:183–9.
17. Sletten K, Husby G, Natvig JB. N-terminal amino acid sequence of amyloid fibril protein AR, prototype of a new lambda-variable subgroup, V lambda V. *Scand J Immunol* 1974;3:833–6.
18. Skinner M, Benson MD, Cohen AS. Amyloid fibril protein related to immunoglobulin lambda-chains. *J Immunol* 1975;114:1433–5.
19. Gallo G, Picken M, Buxbaum J, Frangione B. The spectrum of monoclonal immunoglobulin deposition disease associated with immunocytic dyscrasias. *Semin Hematol* 1989;26:234–45.
20. Osserman EF. Amyloidosis: tissue proteinosis—gammaloidosis. *Ann Intern Med* 1961;55:1033–6.
21. Thoenes W, Schneider H-M. Human glomerular amyloidosis—with special regard to proteinuria and amyloidogenesis. *Klin Wochenschr* 1980;58:667–80.
22. Aucouturier P, Khamlichi AA, Preud'homme JL, Bauwens M, Touchard G, Cogne M. Complementary DNA sequence of human amyloidogenic immunoglobulin light-chain precursors. *Biochem J* 1992;285:149–52.
23. Benditt EP, Eriksen N, Hermodson MA, Ericsson LH. The major proteins of human and monkey amyloid substance: common properties including unusual N-terminal amino acid sequences. *FEBS Lett* 1971; 19:169–73.
24. Ein D, Kimura S, Terry WD, Magnotta J, Glenner GG. Amino acid sequence of an amyloid fibril protein of unknown origin. *J Biol Chem* 1972;247:5653–5.
25. Levin M, Franklin EC, Frangione B, Pras M. The amino acid sequence of a major nonimmunoglobulin component of some amyloid fibrils. *J Clin Invest* 1972;51:2773–6.
26. Husby G, Sletten K, Michaelsen TE, Natvig JB. Alternative non-immunoglobulin origin of amyloid fibrils. *Nature* 1972;238:187.
27. Bausserman LL, Herbert PN, McAdam KP. Heterogeneity of human serum amyloid A proteins. *J Exp Med* 1980;152:641–56.
28. Eriksen N, Benditt EP. Isolation and characterization of the amyloid-related apoprotein (SAA) from human high density lipoprotein. *Proc Natl Acad Sci USA* 1980;77:6860–4.
29. Gorevic PC, Levo Y, Frangione B, Franklin EC. Polymorphism of tissue and serum amyloid A (AA and SAA) proteins in the mouse. *J Immunol* 1978;121:138–40.
30. Jacobson DR, Buxbaum JN. Genetic aspects of amyloidosis [Review]. *Adv Hum Genet* 1991;20:69–123.
31. Uemichi T, Liepnieks JJ, Benson MD. Hereditary renal amyloidosis with a novel variant fibrinogen. *J Clin Invest* 1994;93:731–6.
32. Zalin AM, Jones S, Fitch NJ, Ramsden DB. Familial nephropathic non-neuropathic amyloidosis: clinical features, immunohistochemistry and chemistry. *Q J Med* 1991;81:945–56.
33. Husby G, Stenstad T, Magnus JH, Sletten K, Nordvag BY, Marhaug G. Interaction between circulating amyloid fibril protein precursors and extracellular tissue matrix components in the pathogenesis of systemic amyloidosis. *Clin Immunol Immunopathol* 1994;70:2–9.
34. Westermark GT, Norling B, Westermark P. Fibronectin and basement membrane components in renal amyloid deposits in patients with primary and secondary amyloidosis. *Clin Exp Immunol* 1991;86:150–6.
35. Gallo G, Wisniewski T, Choi-Miura NH, Ghiso J, Frangione B. Potential role of apolipoprotein-E in fibrillogenesis. *Am J Pathol* 1994;145:526–30.
36. Jarrett JT, Lansbury PT Jr. Amyloid fibril formation requires a chemically discriminating nucleation event: studies of an amyloidogenic sequence from the bacterial protein OsmB. *Biochemistry* 1992;31: 12,345–52.
37. Glenner GG, Ein D, Eanes ED, Bladen HA, Terry W, Page DL. Creation of "amyloid" fibrils from Bence Jones proteins in vitro. *Science* 1971;174:712–4.
38. Buxbaum J. Mechanisms of disease: monoclonal immunoglobulin deposition—amyloidosis, light chain deposition disease, and light and heavy chain deposition disease [Review]. *Hematol Oncol Clin North Am* 1992;6:323–46.
39. Symmers WS. Primary amyloidosis: a review. *J Clin Pathol* 1956;9: 187–211.
40. Bell ET. Amyloid disease of the kidneys. *Am J Pathol* 1933;9:185–204.
41. Heptinstall RH, Joekes AM. Renal amyloid: a report on 11 cases proven by renal biopsy. *Ann Rheum Dis* 1960;19:126–34.
42. Dikman SH, Churg J, Kahn T. Morphologic and clinical correlates in renal amyloidosis. *Hum Pathol* 1981;12:160–9.
43. Nakamoto Y, Hamanaka S, Akihama T, Miura AB, Uesaka Y. Renal involvement patterns of amyloid nephropathy: a comparison with diabetic nephropathy. *Clin Nephrol* 1984;22:188–94.
44. Watanabe T, Saniter T. Morphological and clinical features of renal amyloidosis. *Virchows Arch [A]* 1975;366:125–35.
45. van Rijswijk MH, van Heusden CW. The potassium permanganate method: a reliable method for differentiating amyloid AA from other forms of amyloid in routine laboratory practice. *Am J Pathol* 1979;97: 43–58.
46. Watanabe S, Jaffe E, Pollock S, Sipe J, Glenner G. Amyloid AA protein: cellular distribution and appearance. *Am J Clin Pathol* 1977;67: 540–4.
47. Gallo GR, Feiner HD, Chuba JV, Beneck D, Marion P, Cohen DH. Characterization of tissue amyloid by immunofluorescence microscopy. *Clin Immunol Immunopathol* 1986;39:479–90.
48. Fujihara S, Balow JE, Costa JC, Glenner GG. Identification and classification of amyloid in formalin-fixed, paraffin-embedded tissue sections by the unlabeled immunoperoxidase method. *Lab Invest* 1980; 43:358–65.

49. van de Kaa CA, Hol PR, Huber J, Linke RP, Kooiker CJ, Gruys E. Diagnosis of the type of amyloid in paraffin wax embedded tissue sections using antisera against human and animal amyloid proteins. *Virchows Arch [A]* 1986;408:649–64.
50. Magnus-Levy A. Bence-Jones-Eiweiss und Amyloid. *Z Klin Med* 1931;116:510–31.
51. Ogg CS, Cameron JS, Williams DG, Turner DR. Presentation and course of primary amyloidosis of the kidney. *Clin Nephrol* 1981;15: 9–13.
52. Nolting SF, Campbell WC Jr. Subepithelial argyrophilic spicular structures in renal amyloidosis: an aid in diagnosis—pathogenic considerations. *Hum Pathol* 1981;12:724–34.
53. Shirahama T, Cohen AS. Fine structure of the glomerulus in human and experimental renal amyloidosis. *Am J Pathol* 1967;51:869–911.
54. Cohen AS, Calkins E. Electron microscopic observations on a fibrous component in amyloid of diverse origins. *Nature* 1959;183:1202–3.
55. Jones BA, Shapiro HS, Rosenberg BF, Bernstein J. Minimal renal amyloidosis with nephrotic syndrome. *Arch Pathol Lab Med* 1986; 110:889–92.
56. Ansell ID, Joekes AM. Spicular arrangement of amyloid in renal biopsy. *J Clin Pathol* 1972;25:1056–62.
57. Moorthy AV, Burkholder PM. Unusual appearance of amyloid in renal biopsy specimen. *Arch Pathol Lab Med* 1977;101:664–5.
58. Shiiki H, Shimokama T, Yoshikawa Y, Onoyama K, Morimatsu M, Watanabe T. Perimembranous-type renal amyloidosis: a peculiar form of AL amyloidosis. *Nephron* 1989;53:27–32.
59. Gise Hv, Christ H, Bohle A. Early glomerular lesions in amyloidosis: electron microscopic findings. *Virchows Arch [A]* 1981;390: 259–72.
60. Gertz MA, Kyle RA. Primary systemic amyloidosis: a diagnostic primer [Review]. *Mayo Clin Proc* 1989;64:1505–19.
61. Isobe T, Osserman EF. Patterns of amyloidosis and their association with plasma-cell dyscrasia, monoclonal immunoglobulins and Bence Jones proteins. *N Engl J Med* 1974;290:473–7.
62. Gertz MA, Kyle RA, O'Fallon WM. Dialysis support of patients with primary systemic amyloidosis: a study of 211 patients. *Arch Intern Med* 1992;152:2245–50.
63. Duston MA, Skinner M, Shirahama T, Cohen AS. Diagnosis of amyloidosis by abdominal fat aspiration: analysis of four years' experence. *Am J Med* 1987;82:412–4.
64. Gertz MA, Li CY, Shirahama T, Kyle RA. Utility of subcutaneous fat aspiration for the diagnosis of systemic amyloidosis (immunoglobulin light chain). *Arch Intern Med* 1988;148:929–33.
65. Gertz MA, Brown ML, Hauser MF, Kyle RA. Utility of gallium imaging of the kidneys in diagnosing primary amyloid nephrotic syndrome. *J Nucl Med* 1990;31:292–5.
66. Lee VW, Skinner M, Cohen AS, Ngai S, Peng TT. Renal amyloidosis: evaluation by gallium imaging. *Clin Nucl Med* 1986;11:642–6.
67. Hawkins PN, Lavender JP, Pepys MB. Evaluation of systemic amyloidosis by scintigraphy with ^{123}I-labeled serum amyloid P component. *N Engl J Med* 1990;323:508–13.
68. Gertz MA, Kyle RA. Prognostic value of urinary protein in primary systemic amyloidosis (AL). *Am J Clin Pathol* 1990;94:313–7.
69. Bradstock K, Clancy R, Uther J, Basten A, Richards J. The successful treatment of primary amyloidosis with intermittent chemotherapy. *Aust NZ J Med* 1978;8:176–9.
70. Cohen HJ, Lessin LS, Hallal J, Burkholder P. Resolution of primary amyloidosis during chemotherapy: studies in a patient with nephrotic syndrome. *Ann Intern Med* 1975;82:466–73.
71. Benson MD. Treatment of AL amyloidosis with melphalan, prednisone, and colchicine. *Arthritis Rheum* 1986;29:683–7.
72. Cohen AS, Rubinow A, Anderson JJ, et al. Survival of patients with primary (AL) amyloidosis: colchicine-treated cases from 1976 to 1983 compared with cases seen in previous years (1961 to 1973). *Am J Med* 1987;82:1182–90.
73. Gertz MA, Kyle RA. Phase II trial of recombinant interferon alpha-2 in the treatment of primary systemic amyloidosis. *Am J Hematol* 1993;44:125–8.
74. Gertz MA, Kyle RA. Phase II trial of alpha-tocopherol (vitamin E) in the treatment of primary systemic amyloidosis. *Am J Hematol* 1990; 34:55–8.
75. United States Renal Data System. Incidence and causes of treated ESRD. *Am J Kidney Dis* 1993;22(Suppl 2):30–7.
76. Browning MJ, Banks RA, Harrison P, et al. Continuous ambulatory peritoneal dialysis in systemic amyloidosis and end-stage renal disease. *J R Soc Med* 1984;77:189–92.
77. Port FK, Nissenson AR. Outcome of end-stage renal disease in patients with rare causes of renal failure. II. Renal or systemic neoplasms. *Q J Med* 1989;73:1161–5.
78. Pasternack A, Ahonen J, Kuhlback B. Renal transplantation in 45 patients with amyloidosis. *Transplantation* 1986;42:598–601.
79. Jones HB. Papers on chemical pathology: prefaced by the Gulstonian Lectures, read at the Royal College of Physicians, 1847. *Lancet* 1847; 2:88–92.
80. Kyle RA. Monoclonal gammopathy of undetermined significance [Review]. *Blood Rev* 1994;8:135–41.
81. Kyle RA. Multiple myeloma: review of 869 cases. *Mayo Clin Proc* 1975;50:29–40.
82. Kyle RA. Monoclonal proteins and renal disease [Review]. *Annu Rev Med* 1994;45:71–7.
83. Touchard G. Renal biopsy in multiple myeloma and in other monoclonal immunoglobulin-producing diseases. *Ann Med Interne (Paris)* 1992;143(Suppl 1):80–3.
84. Moulin B, Ronco PM, Mougenot B, Francois A, Fillastre JP, Mignon F. Glomerulonephritis in chronic lymphocytic leukemia and related B-cell lymphomas. *Kidney Int* 1992;42:127–35.
85. Touchard G, Bauwens M, Preud'homme JL. Glomerulopathies in monoclonal dysglobulinemias [in French]. *Rev Prat* 1991;41:2459–63.
86. Schubert GE. Myeloma kidney. I. Incidence of pathological–anatomical findings [Author trans] [in German]. *Klin Wochenschr* 1974;52: 763–70.
87. Ivanyi B, Varga G, Nagy J, Berkessy S, Keresztury S. Light chain deposition nephropathy in necropsy material. *Zentralbl Pathol* 1991; 137:366–71.
88. Ganeval D, Rabian C, Guérin V, Pertuiset P, Landias P, Jungers P. Treatment of multiple myeloma with renal involvement. *Adv Nephrol Necker Hosp* 1992;21:347–70.
89. Innes A, Cuthbert RJ, Russell NH, Morgan AG, Burden RP. Intensive treatment of renal failure in patients with myeloma. *Clin Lab Haematol* 1994;16:149–56.
90. Rota S, Mougenot B, Baudouin B, et al. Multiple myeloma and severe renal failure: a clinicopathologic study of outcome and prognosis in 34 patients. *Medicine (Baltimore)* 1987;66:126–37.
91. Lindstrom FD, Hed J, Enestrom S. Renal pathology of Waldenström's macroglobulinaemia with monoclonal antiglomerular antibodies and nephrotic syndrome. *Clin Exp Immunol* 1980;41:196–204.
92. Morel-Maroger L, Basch A, Danon F, Verroust P, Richet G. Pathology of the kidney in Waldenström's macroglobulinemia: study of sixteen cases. *N Engl J Med* 1970;283:123–9.
93. Krajny M, Pruzanski W. Waldenström's macroglobulinemia: review of 45 cases. *Can Med Assoc J* 1976;114:899–905.
94. De Fronzo RA, Cooke CR, Wright JR, Humphrey RL. Renal function in patients with multiple myeloma. *Medicine (Baltimore)* 1978;57: 151–66.
95. Solomon A, Weiss DT, Kattine AA. Nephrotoxic potential of Bence Jones proteins. *N Engl J Med* 1991;324:1845–51.
96. Maack T. Renal handling of low molecular weight proteins. *Am J Med* 1975;58:57–64.
97. Wochner RD, Strober W, Waldmann TA. The role of the kidney in the catabolism of Bence Jones proteins and immunoglobulin fragments. *J Exp Med* 1967;126:207–21.
98. Smolens P, Venkatachalam MA, Stein JH. Myeloma kidney cast nephropathy in a rat model of multiple myeloma. *Kidney Int* 1983;24: 192–204.
99. Clyne DH, Pesce AJ, Thompson RE. Nephrotoxicity of Bence Jones proteins in the rat: importance of the protein isoelectric point. *Kidney Int* 1979;16:345–52.
100. Sanders PW, Booker BB. Pathobiology of cast nephropathy from human Bence Jones proteins. *J Clin Invest* 1992;89:630–9.
101. Silva FG, Pirani CL, Mesa-Tejada R, Williams GS. The kidney in plasma cell dyscrasias: a review and a clinicopathologic study of 50 patients. In: Fenoglio CE, Wolff M, eds. *Progress in surgical pathology*. New York: Masson, 1982:131–76.
102. Hoyer JR, Seiler MW. Pathophysiology of Tamm–Horsfall protein. *Kidney Int* 1979;16:279–89.
103. Kumar S, Muchmore A. Tamm–Horsfall protein: uromodulin (1950–1990). *Kidney Int* 1990;37:1395–401.

104. Melcion C, Mougenot B, Baudouin B, et al. Renal failure in myeloma: relationship with isoelectric point of immunoglobulin light chains. *Clin Nephrol* 1984;22:138–43.
105. Johns EA, Turner R, Cooper EH, Maclennan IC. Isoelectric points of urinary light chains in myelomatosis: analysis in relation to nephrotoxicity. *J Clin Pathol* 1986;39:833–7.
106. Huang ZQ, Kirk KA, Connelly KG, Sanders PW. Bence Jones proteins bind to a common peptide segment of Tamm–Horsfall glycoprotein to promote heterotypic aggregation. *J Clin Invest* 1993;92:2975–83.
107. Sanders PW, Herrera GA, Chen A, Booker BB, Galla JH. Differential nephrotoxicity of low molecular weight proteins including Bence Jones proteins in the perfused rat nephron in vivo. *J Clin Invest* 1988; 82:2086–96.
108. Sanders PW, Booker BB, Bishop JB, Cheung HC. Mechanisms of intranephronal proteinaceous cast formation by low molecular weight proteins. *J Clin Invest* 1990;85:570–6.
109. Ronco PM, Mougenot B, Touchard G, Preud'homme J-L, Aucouturier P. Renal involvement in hematological disorders: monoclonal immunoglobulins and nephropathy. *Curr Opin Nephrol Hypertens* 1995;4:130–8.
110. Thomas DB, Davies M, Williams JD. Release of gelatinase and superoxide from human mononuclear phagocytes in response to particulate Tamm Horsfall protein. *Am J Pathol* 1993;142:249–60.
111. Thomas DB, Davies M, Peters JR, Williams JD. Tamm Horsfall protein binds to a single class of carbohydrate specific receptors on human neutrophils. *Kidney Int* 1993;44:423–9.
112. Maldonado JE, Velosa JA, Kyle RA, Wagoner RD, Holley KE, Salassa RM. Fanconi syndrome in adults: a manifestation of a latent form of myeloma. *Am J Med* 1975;58:354–64.
113. Aucouturier P, Bauwens M, Khamlichi AA, et al. Monoclonal Ig L chain and L chain V domain fragment crystallization in myeloma-associated Fanconi's syndrome. *J Immunol* 1993;150(8 Pt 1):3561–8.
114. Leboulleux M, Lelongt B, Mougenot B, et al. Protease resistance and binding of Ig light chains in myeloma-associated tubulopathies. *Kidney Int* 1995;48:72–9.
115. Hill GS, Morel-Maroger L, Mery JP, Brouet JC, Mignon F. Renal lesions in multiple myeloma: their relationship to associated protein abnormalities. *Am J Kidney Dis* 1983;2:423–38.
116. Cohen AH, Border WA. Myeloma kidney: an immunomorphogenetic study of renal biopsies. *Lab Invest* 1980;42:248–56.
117. Alpers CE, Magil AB, Gown AM. Macrophage origin of the multinucleated cells of myeloma cast nephropathy. *Am J Clin Pathol* 1989; 92:662–5.
118. Maldonado JE, Velosa JA, Kyle RA, Wagoner RD, Holley JE, Salassa RM. Fanconi syndrome in adults: a manifestation of a late form of myeloma. *Am J Med* 1958;58:354–64.
119. Silva FG, Meyrier A, Morel-Maroger L, Pirani CL. Proliferative glomerulopathy in multiple myeloma. *J Pathol* 1980;130:229–36.
120. Limas C, Wright JR, Matsuzaki M, Calkins E. Amyloidosis and multiple myeloma: a reevaluation using a control population. *Am J Med* 1973;54:166–73.
121. Levi DF, Williams RC Jr, Lindstrom FD. Immunofluorescent studies of the myeloma kidney with special reference to light chain disease. *Am J Med* 1968;44:922–33.
122. Smith JF, Van Hegan RI, Esnouf MP, Ross BD. Characteristics of renal handling of human immunoglobulin light chain by the perfused rat kidney. *Clin Sci (Colch)* 1979;57:113–20.
123. Mackenzie MR, Wuepper KD, Jordan G, Fudenberg HH. Rapid renal failure in a case of multiple myeloma: the role of Bence Jones proteins. *Clin Exp Immunol* 1968;3:593–601.
124. Kapadia SB. Multiple myeloma: a clinicopathologic study of 62 consecutively autopsied cases. *Medicine (Baltimore)* 1980;59:380–92.
125. Olsen S. Mesangial thickening and nodular glomerular sclerosis in diabetes mellitus and other diseases. *Acta Pathol Microbiol Scand [A]* 1972;233:203–16.
126. Stekhoven JH, van Haelst UJ. Unusual findings in the human renal glomerulus in multiple myeloma: a light- and electron-microscopic study. *Virchows Arch [B]* 1971;9:311–21.
127. Bernstein SP, Humes HD. Reversible renal insufficiency in multiple myeloma. *Arch Intern Med* 1982;147:2083–6.
128. Rayner HC, Haynes AP, Thompson JR, Russell N, Fletcher J. Perspectives in multiple myeloma: survival, prognostic factors and disease complications in a single center between 1975 and 1988. *Q J Med [New Ser]* 1991;79:517–25.
129. Border WA, Cohen AH. Renal biopsy diagnosis of clinically silent multiple myeloma. *Ann Intern Med* 1980;93:43–6.
130. Stone MJ, Frenkel EP. The clinical spectrum of light chain myeloma: a study 35 patients with special reference to the occurrence of amyloidosis. *Am J Med* 1975;58:601–18.
131. Sanders PW. Pathogensis and treatment of myeloma kidney. *J Lab Clin Med* 1994;124:484–8.
132. Sanders PW, Herrera GA. Monoclonal immunoglobulin light chain–related renal diseases. *Semin Nephrol* 1993;13:324–41.
133. Kyle RA, Beard CM, O'Fallen WM, Kurland LT. Incidence of multiple myeloma in Olmsted County, Minnesota: 1978 through 1990, with a review of the trend since 1945. *J Clin Oncol* 1994;12:1577–83.
134. Bear RA, Cole EH, Lang A, Johnson M. Treatment of acute renal failure due to myeloma kidney. *Can Med Assoc J* 1980;123:750–3.
135. Pichette V, Querin S, Desmeules M, Ethier J, Copleston P. Renal function recovery in end-stage renal disease. *Am J Kidney Dis* 1993; 22:398–402.
136. Burke JR Jr, Flis R, Lasker N, Simenhoff M. Malignant lymphoma with "myeloma kidney" acute renal failure. *Am J Med* 1976;60:1055–60.
137. Johnson WJ, Kyle RA, Pineda AA, O'Brien PC, Holley KE. Treatment of renal failure associated with multiple myeloma. *Arch Intern Med* 1990;150:863–9.
138. Montemurro NE, Di Maggio A, Strippoli P, et al. Combined dialysis and plasma-exchange in acute renal failure. *Biomater Artif Cells Immobil Biotechnol* 1993;21:283–7.
139. Zucchelli P, Pasquali S, Cagnoli L, Ferrari G. Controlled plasma exchange trial in acute renal failure due to multiple myeloma. *Kidney Int* 1988;33:1175–80.
140. Iggo N, Palmer AB, Severn A, et al. Chronic dialysis in patients with multiple myeloma and renal failure: a worthwhile treatment [See comments]. *Q J Med* 1989;73:903–10.
141. Korzets A, Tam F, Russell G, Feehally J, Walls J. The role of continuous ambulatory peritoneal dialysis in end-stage renal failure due to multiple myeloma. *Am J Kidney Dis* 1990;16:216–23.
142. Molby L, Hansen HH, Jensen EL. Development and treatment of renal insufficiency in multiple myeloma [Review] [in Danish]. *Ugeskr Laeger* 1994;156:4343–7.
143. Uriu K, Kaizu K, Abe R, et al. A case of multiple myeloma treated with long-term peritoneal dialysis [in Japanese]. *Sangyo Ika Daigaku Zasshi* 1984;6:391–6.
144. Tapson JS, Mansy H, Wilkinson R. End-stage renal failure due to multiple myeloma: poor survival on peritoneal dialysis. *Int J Artif Organs* 1988;11:39–42.
145. Duvic C, Viron B, Michel C, Mignon F. End-stage chronic renal failure in myeloma: results of dialysis [in French]. *Rev Med Interne* 1993;14:792–8.
146. Kihara M, Ikeda Y, Shibata K, Masumori S, Ebira H. Maintenance hemodialysis in IgD-lambda-type multiple myeloma associated with severe renal failure [in Japanese]. *Nippon Jinzo Gakkai Shi* 1994;36: 177–81.
147. Spence RK, Hill GS, Goldwein MI, Grossman RA, Barker CF, Perloff LJ. Renal transplantation for end-stage myeloma kidney: report of a patient with long-term survival. *Arch Surg* 1979;114:950–2.
148. Humphrey RL, Wright JR, Zachary JB, Sterioff S, De Fronzo RA. Renal transplantation in multiple myeloma: a case report. *Ann Intern Med* 1975;83:651–3.
149. Preud'homme JL, Aucouturier P, Striker L, et al. Monoclonal immunoglobulin deposition disease (Randall type): relationship with structural abnormalities of immunoglobulin chains. *Kidney Int* 1994;46: 965–72.
150. Randall RE, Williamson WC Jr, Mullinax F, Tung MY, Still WJ. Manifestations of systemic light chain deposition [Review]. *Am J Med* 1976;60:293–9.
151. Calkins E, Cohen AS. Diagnosis of amyloidosis. *Bull Rheum Dis* 1960;10:215–218.
152. Ganeval D, Noel LH, Preud'homme JL, Droz D, Grunfeld JP. Light-chain deposition disease: its relation with AL-type amyloidosis. *Kidney Int* 1984;26:1–9.
153. Buxbaum JN, Chuba JV, Hellman GC, Solomon A, Gallo GR. Monoclonal immunoglobulin deposition disease: light chain and light and heavy chain deposition diseases and their relation to light chain amyloidosis—clinical features, immunopathology, and molecular analysis. *Ann Intern Med* 1990;112:455–64.

154. Gallo GR, Feiner HD, Katz LA, et al. Nodular glomerulopathy associated with nonamyloidotic kappa light chain deposits and excess immunoglobulin light chain synthesis. *Am J Pathol* 1980;99:621–44.
155. Heilman RL, Velosa JA, Holley KE, Offord KP, Kyle RA. Long-term follow-up and response to chemotherapy in patients with light-chain deposition disease. *Am J Kidney Dis* 1992;20:34–41.
156. Lin JJ, Miller F, Waltzer W, Kaskel FJ, Arbeit L. Recurrence of immunoglobulin A-kappa crystalline deposition disease after kidney transplantation. *Am J Kidney Dis* 1995;25:75–8.
157. Alpers CE, Tu W-H, Hopper J, Biava CG. Single light chain subclass (kappa chain) immunoglobulin deposition in glomerulonephritis. *Hum Pathol* 1985;16:294–304.
158. Gerlag PGG, Koene RAP, Berden HM. Renal transplantation in light chain nephropathy: case report and review of the literature. *Clin Nephrol* 1986;25:101–4.
159. Alpers CE, Marchioro TL, Johnson RJ. Monoclonal immunoglobulin deposition disease in a renal allograft: probable recurrent disease in a patient without myeloma. *Am J Kidney Dis* 1989;13:418–23.
160. Brouet JC, Clauvel JP, Danon F, Klein M, Seligmann M. Biologic and clinical significance of cryoglobulins: a report of 86 cases. *Am J Med* 1974;57:775–88.
161. Monga G, Mazzucco G, Coppo R, Piccoli G, Coda R. Glomerular findings in mixed IgG–IgM cryoglobulinemia: light, electron microscopic, immunofluorescence and histochemical correlations. *Virchows Arch [B]* 1976;20:185–96.
162. Gorevic PD, Kassab HJ, Levo Y, et al. Mixed cryoglobulinemia: clinical aspects and long-term follow-up of 40 patients [Review]. *Am J Med* 1980;69:287–308.
163. Enzenauer RJ, Arend WP, Emlen JW. Mixed cryoglobulinemia associated with chronic Q-fever. *J Rheumatol* 1991;18:76–8.
164. D'Amico G, Colasanti G, Ferrario F, Sinico RA. Renal involvement in essential mixed cryoglobulinemia. *Kidney Int* 1989;35:1004–14.
165. Meltzer M, Franklin EC, Elias K, McCluskey RT, Cooper N. Cryoglobulinemia: a clinical and laboratory study. II. Cryoglobulins with rheumatoid factor activity. *Am J Med* 1966;40:837–56.
166. D'Amico G, Fornasieri A. Cryoglobulinemic glomerulonephritis: a membranoproliferative glomerulonephritis induced by hepatitis C virus [Review]. *Am J Kidney Dis* 1995;25:361–9.
167. Pawlotsky JM, Roudot-Thoraval F, Simmonds P, et al. Extrahepatic immunologic manifestations in chronic hepatitis C and hepatitis C virus serotypes. *Ann Intern Med* 1995;122:169–73.
168. Bichard P, Ounanian A, Girard M, et al. High prevalence of hepatitis C virus RNA in the supernatant and the cryoprecipitate of patients with essential and secondary type II mixed cryoglobulinemia. *J Hepatol* 1994;21:58–63.
169. Agnello V, Chung RT, Kaplan LM. A role for hepatitis C virus infection in type II cryoglobulinemia [See comments]. *N Engl J Med* 1992; 327:1490–5.
170. Miescher PA, Huang YP, Izui S. Type II cryoglobulinemia [Review]. *Semin Hematol* 1995;32:80–5.
171. Misiani R, Bellavita P, Fenili D, et al. Hepatitis C virus infection in patients with essential mixed cryoglobulinemia. *Ann Intern Med* 1992;117:573–7.
172. Schifferli JA, French LE, Tissot J-D. Hepatitis C virus infection, cryoglobulinemia, and glomerulonephritis. *Adv Nephrol Necker Hosp* 1995;24:107–29.
173. Korbet SM, Schwartz MM, Lewis EJ. Immunotactoid glomerulopathy [Review]. *Am J Kidney Dis* 1991;17:247–57.
174. Korbet SM, Schwartz MM, Lewis EJ. The fibrillary glomerulopathies [Review]. *Am J Kidney Dis* 1994;23:751–65.
175. Korbet SM, Schwartz MM, Rosenberg BF, Sibley RK, Lewis EJ. Immunotactoid glomerulopathy. *Medicine (Baltimore)* 1985;64:228–43.
176. Fogo A, Qureshi N, Horn RG. Morphologic and clinical features of fibrillary glomerulonephritis versus immunotactoid glomerulopathy. *Am J Kidney Dis* 1993;22:367–77.
177. Iskandar SS, Falk RJ, Jennette JC. Clinical and pathologic features of fibrillary glomerulonephritis. *Kidney Int* 1992;42:1401–7.
178. Alpers CE. Immunotactoid (microtubular) glomerulopathy: an entity distinct from fibrillary glomerulonephritis? *Am J Kidney Dis* 1992;19: 185–91.
179. Schwartz MM. Immunotactoid glomerulopathy: the case for Occam's razor [Editorial; comment]. *Am J Kidney Dis* 1993;22:446–7.
180. Rosenmann E, Eliakim M. Nephrotic syndrome associated with amyloid-like glomerular deposits. *Nephron* 1977;18:301–8.
181. Ozawa K, Yamabe H, Fukushi K, et al. Case report of amyloidosis-like glomerulopathy with hepatic involvement. *Nephron* 1991;58:347–50.
182. Masson RG, Rennke HG, Gottlieb MN. Pulmonary hemorrhage in a patient with fibrillary glomerulonephritis. *N Engl J Med* 1992;326: 36–9.
183. Duffy JL, Khurana E, Susin M, Gomez-Leon G, Churg J. Fibrillary renal deposits and nephritis. *Am J Pathol* 1983;113:279–90.
184. Alpers CE, Rennke HG, Hopper J Jr, Biava CG. Fibrillary glomerulonephritis: an entity with unusual immunofluorescence features. *Kidney Int* 1987;31:781–9.
185. Casanova S, Donini U, Zucchelli P, Mazzucco G, Monga G, Linke RP. Immunohistochemical distinction between amyloidosis and fibrillar glomerulopathy. *Am J Clin Pathol* 1992;97:787–95.
186. Yang GC, Nieto R, Stachura I, Gallo GR. Ultrastructural immunohistochemical localization of polyclonal IgG, C3, and amyloid P component on the Congo red–negative amyloid-like fibrils of fibrillary glomerulopathy. *Am J Pathol* 1992;141:409–19.
187. Schifferli JA, Merot Y, Chatelanat F. Immunotactoid glomerulopathy with leucocytoclastic skin vasculitis and hypocomplementemia: a case report. *Clin Nephrol* 1987;27:151–5.
188. Schwartz MM, Lewis EJ. The quarterly case: nephrotic syndrome in a middle-aged man. *Ultrastruct Pathol* 1980;1:575–82.
189. Korbet SM, Rosenberg BF, Schwartz MM, Lewis EJ. Course of renal transplantation in immunotactoid glomerulopathy. *Am J Med* 1990; 89:91–5.

Immunologic Renal Diseases,
edited by E. G. Neilson and W. G. Couser.
Lippincott-Raven Publishers, Philadelphia © 1997.

CHAPTER 53

Hemolytic Uremic Syndrome and Thrombotic Thrombocytopenic Purpura

John R. Brandt and Ellis D. Avner

DEFINITION AND HISTORICAL BACKGROUND

The hemolytic uremic syndrome (HUS) and thrombotic thrombocytopenic purpura (TTP) comprise a heterogeneous group of disorders characterized by small-vessel vasculopathy. Thrombotic thrombocytopenic purpura was initially described by Moschcowitz in 1928 and named by Singer in 1947 (1). Later, Baehr, Symmers, and others described the histopathologic features (2–4) that Symmers called thrombotic microangiopathy (TMA). TTP is characterized by the clinical pentad of fever, thrombocytopenia, microangiopathic anemia, neurologic abnormalities, and renal abnormalities (1,5,6). HUS was first described by Gasser in 1955 and has since become recognized as one of the leading causes of acute renal failure in children (7). It is characterized by the clinical triad of thrombocytopenia, microangiopathic anemia (Fig. 1), and acute renal insufficiency (7,8). Between 1958 and 1960, Habib described the characteristic renal pathologic findings of the renal arterioles and glomerular vessels in childhood HUS and noted their similarity to the lesions of TMA described in TTP (3,9–12)

The history of these diseases is marked by a persistent confusion about the relationship between the two entities. Although the underlying vascular pathologic lesions are similar in HUS and TTP, the distribution of lesions and the ensuing clinical manifestations result in distinct syndromes. In their classical manifestations they are clearly defined clinicopathologic entities. But many cases do not adhere to the classical descriptions. Clinical findings overlap and diverge from these classic syndromes, resulting in a steadily expanding array of names: TTP, HUS, HUS/TTP, typical HUS, atypical HUS, etc. There are probably multiple etiologic precipitants of TMA, and a particular patient's clinical presentation is likely the result of an interaction of etiologic and host factors. The differentiation between HUS and TTP rests with the clinical milieu in which these lesions are observed rather than with any significant difference in histology or distribution of lesions.

HUS/TTP is a vasculopathy. It is likely that these two clinical entities represent overlapping clinical syndromes of a single pathologic entity. At the same time, it is likely that there are a variety of pathophysiologic mechanisms that can lead to the TMA of HUS/TTP. Evidence suggests that damage to the endothelial cell layer of the blood vessels leads to localized thrombosis, consumption of platelets, and structural damage to erythrocytes as they negotiate these localized areas of thrombosis. In HUS the primary vascular bed affected is the renal microvasculature, and clinical symptoms are predominantly those of renal insufficiency. In TTP this process classically predominates in the central nervous system; therefore, neurologic findings are prominant. It is important to remember that in either syndrome TMA can involve multiple vascular beds leading to a wide range of clinical symptoms.

The importance of classifying patients into categories of disease lies in the prognostic and therapeutic implications of these categories. Individuals with a TTP-like syndrome benefit from plasma therapy. Those with classical HUS appear do well with only supportive care.

CLASSIFICATION AND ETIOLOGY

HUS is divided into two broad categories. Diarrhea-associated (D+ or typical) HUS and non–diarrhea-associated (D- or atypical) HUS (13). The distinction is impor-

J. R. Brandt: Children's Hospital and Medical Center, Department of Pediatrics, University of Washington, Seattle, Washington 98105.

E. D. Avner: Department of Pediatrics, Rainbow Babies and Children's Hospital, Cleveland, Ohio 44106.

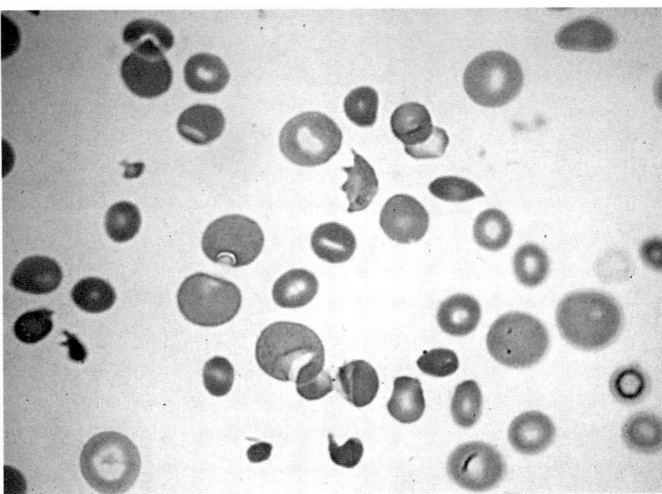

FIG. 1. Peripheral smear showing microangiopathic hemolysis.

tant because of marked discrepancies in acute course, mortality, and prognosis between the two forms. Typical HUS follows a gastrointestinal prodrome of acute infectious, usually bloody, diarrhea, almost always caused by *Escherichia coli* O157:H7 (14,15). Typical HUS (a) occurs mostly in young children between the ages of 6 months and 4 years; (b) predominantly involves the hematopoietic system and kidneys; (c) has a comparatively low mortality rate; (d) resolves within 1 to 2 weeks with a relatively low rate of chronic sequelae; and (e) almost never recurs (13,16). In contrast, atypical HUS (a) is often insidious in onset; (b) follows a nondiarrheal illness or has no prodrome; (c) is associated with a high mortality rate; (d) is characterized by a high incidence of extrarenal involvement, especially neurologic abnormalities, and is associated with a high incidence of chronic sequelae; and (e) is much more likely to recur (13,17). We prefer the terms *typical* and *atypical HUS.* A significant proportion of *E. coli* O157:H7–associated HUS presents without the prodromal diarrhea (18). Therefore, the absence of diarrhea may not always indicate the presence of atypical HUS.

Atypical HUS appears to be more closely related, clinically and prognostically, to TTP than to typical HUS. Both atypical HUS and TTP tend to follow a chronic, sometimes relapsing course, and has a high mortality rate: about 50% without plasmapheresis and 5% to 10% with plasmapheresis in TTP (6,19) and about 25% (without plasmapheresis) in atypical HUS (20). The pathologic lesion in TTP is identical to that in HUS (16). Interestingly, TTP has been seen after hemorrhagic colitis (21). TTP has been associated with many of the same factors known to trigger HUS, including *E. coli* O157:H7 infections, oral contraceptives, pregnancy and the postpartum state, chemotherapy agents, transplantation, drugs of abuse, and infectious agents, including human immunodeficiency virus (HIV). Etiologic factors associated with HUS/TTP are summarized in Table 1.

TABLE 1. *Etiology of HUS/TTP*

Etiology of HUS/TTP	Reference (HUS/TTP)
Infectious	
Strong association:	
Verotoxigeni *E. coli* O157:H7	15,32,33,39,261, 262,263/264
Shigella dysenteraie	265–267/
Streptococcus pneumoniae	83,86,268/
Weak association:	
Campylobacter	269,270/271
Yersinia	272,273/
Aeromonas	274,275/
Echovirus	276/
Varicella	277/
Salmonella typhaie	278/
Microtabes	279/
HIV	280/43
Drugs	
Mitomycin, bleomycin, vincristine	281,282,283/
Cisplatinum	282/
"Crack" cocaine	284/
Quinine	98,285,286/
Ticlopidine	/287,288
Transplantation drugs:	
Cyclosporine	214,289/290
FK506 (tacrolimus)	/291
OKT3	292/
Pregnancy	178,186,293,294/53,54
Oral contraceptives	295,296/297
Malignancy	298–300/
Hereditary	301,302/183,303–307
Inborn errors of vitamin B12 metabolism	308–310/
Intrinsic renal disease	311–315/
Autoimmune disease	
Kawasaki	316/
Scleroderma	317,318
SLE	319,320/321

INCIDENCE AND EPIDEMIOLOGY

HUS occurs throughout the world in an epidemic pattern (14,15). A few areas seem to have endemic HUS with yearly outbreaks; this occurs in Argentina, Holland, South Africa, and the west coast of the United States. The incidence of HUS appears to have increased in many, but not all, locales since its initial description in 1955 (15). In King County, Washington, the incidence in children under the age of 15 years increased from 0.6 per 100,000 in the early 1970s to 1.74 per 100,000 between 1980 and 1985 (22). In Minnesota, the incidence in children under 18 years of age increased from 0.5 to 2.0 cases per 100,000 between 1979 and 1988 (23). Reported cases of

HUS also have increased in the United Kingdom during the 1980s (24,25), and in The Netherlands there was a tenfold increase in HUS between 1965 and 1982 (26). In contrast, in Salt Lake City no sustained increase in incidence (average incidence 1.42 per 100,000) was seen between 1971 and 1990n (27). Some of the reported increase may be due to increased recognition of HUS and reporting bias, but in King County, Washington, the severity of the patient's illness on admission did not differ between the periods studied. The incidence for all children overall is currently one to two per 100,000 children. The incidence in young children is higher, with incidences as high as 7.1 in 100,000 under age 2 years (23,28–30). The incidence of HUS/TTP in adults is not well studied, and often the distinction between HUS and TTP is difficult to determine because of the large clinical overlap in symptoms. One study showed an incidence of TTP in Minnesota of 0.1 per 100,000 per year (31) .

The majority of cases of HUS are associated with contamination of food with verotoxin producing enterohemorrhagic *E. coli* (VTEC), principally *E. coli* O157:H7 (14,15). Waterborne and person-to-person transmission also has been documented (14,15). The major resevoirs for VTEC are beef and dairy cattle, in which *E. coli* 0157:H7 is carried asymptomaticaly in the gastrointesinal tract. *E. coli* 0157:H7 from the animal's intestinal tract contaminates beef or milk during processing (14). The attack rate for hemorrhagic colitis after ingestion of VTEC depends on host susceptibility, with infants and the elderly having higher attack rates. In population-based studies, attack rates range from 0.6 to 2.6 cases per 1,000 exposed individuals (32–34). In case control studies of day care–associated outbreaks, attack rates of 22% to 67% have been reported (35–37). A contaminated community water supply outbreak had an attack rate of 6.7% (38), and an outbreak in a nursing home showed an attack rate of 33% in the elderly residents (39). The rate of secondary transmission of *E. coli* O157:H7 in daycare or household contacts is 7% to 10% (33,40). Of those who develop hemorrhagic colitis, 8% to 10% go on to develop HUS (14,41).

There does not appear to be any gender preference for HUS. TTP is more common in women than in men, with a 3:2 incidence ratio (5,6,19,42–44). HUS appears to be more common in whites than in other racial groups in some areas (45,46) but not in other areas (23,28,47,48). TTP does not appear to have any strong racial bias (19, 43,49,50). *E. coli* O157:H7 infections are much more common in children of all ages than in adults, although the elderly are at an increased risk compared with other adults (34,39,40,51). In the Northern hemisphere there is a clear seasonal variation in the diarrhea-associated form of HUS, with most cases occurring in the summer months and the fewest in winter (34,52).

Non–VTEC-associated (atypical) HUS occurs in a sporadic manner and has multiple etiologic precipitants. Likewise, the epidemiology of TTP is poorly understood. The majority of cases are sporadic and not clearly associated with any identifiable etiologic precipitant. The most common single TTP-associated conditions are pregnancy and the post-partum state, which may account in part for the relative preponderance of female patients with TTP (42,53,54). Up to 10% of cases are seen in association with collagen vascular diseases (42). Recently a significant number of cases have been seen in association with HIV infections (43).

PATHOLOGY OF HUS AND TTP

The characteristic histopathologic lesion that characterizes HUS (9) and TTP (3,4) is TMA (Fig. 2). TMA is thought to be initiated by endothelial injury, which is followed by local intravascular platelet thrombosis, which obstructs blood vessels with platelet–fibrin thrombi and leads to shearing and fragmentation of red blood cells and ischemic tissue injury (Fig. 2A). The condition is notable for the absence of any evidence of cellular infiltrate or underlying vasculitis.

The kidneys bear the brunt of the injury in HUS. Three morphologic variants of HUS are seen, based on the predominant histology: (a) glomerular TMA, (b) cortical necrosis, and (c) arterial TMA . In samples of glomerular TMA subjected to biopsy early in the disease course, there is swelling of endothelial cells and widening of the subendothelial space of glomerular capillaries. This represents endothelial detachment from the underlying basement membrane and gives a double-contour appearance to the capillary wall. The vascular lumen is partially or totally obstructed by fragmented erythrocytes, fibrin, and platelets, and the subendothelial space is filled with fibrinlike material, lipids, and pale fluffy substances of undetermined composition (Fig. 2A and D). The mesangial cells may be swollen but are not increased in number, and mesangiolysis is seen rarely (Fig. 2B) (10,55). Small crescents may occasionally be present (56). Preglomerular arteriolar lesions are always seen, but the glomerular pathology predominates (9,10). Immunofluorescence shows fibrinogen in the glomeruli (9,10). In rare cases scattered granular deposits of C3, immunoglobulin (Ig)G, and/or IgM may be found in the glomerular vessels (57–59). In samples of glomerular TMA subjected to biopsy late in the disease course, affected glomeruli show segmental or global sclerosis (56).

In arteriolar TMA, the renal arterioles and occasionally interlobular arteries are predominatly involved (10,59, 60) (Fig. 2C). Arterial TMA is characterized by swelling of arteriolar endothelial cells and narrowing or obstruction of the vessel lumen (10). Fibrinoid necrosis, in which fibrin infiltrates the vascular wall, may be seen in severe cases (56). In some cases the arterial wall may take on the appearance of intimal thickening commonly seen in TTP

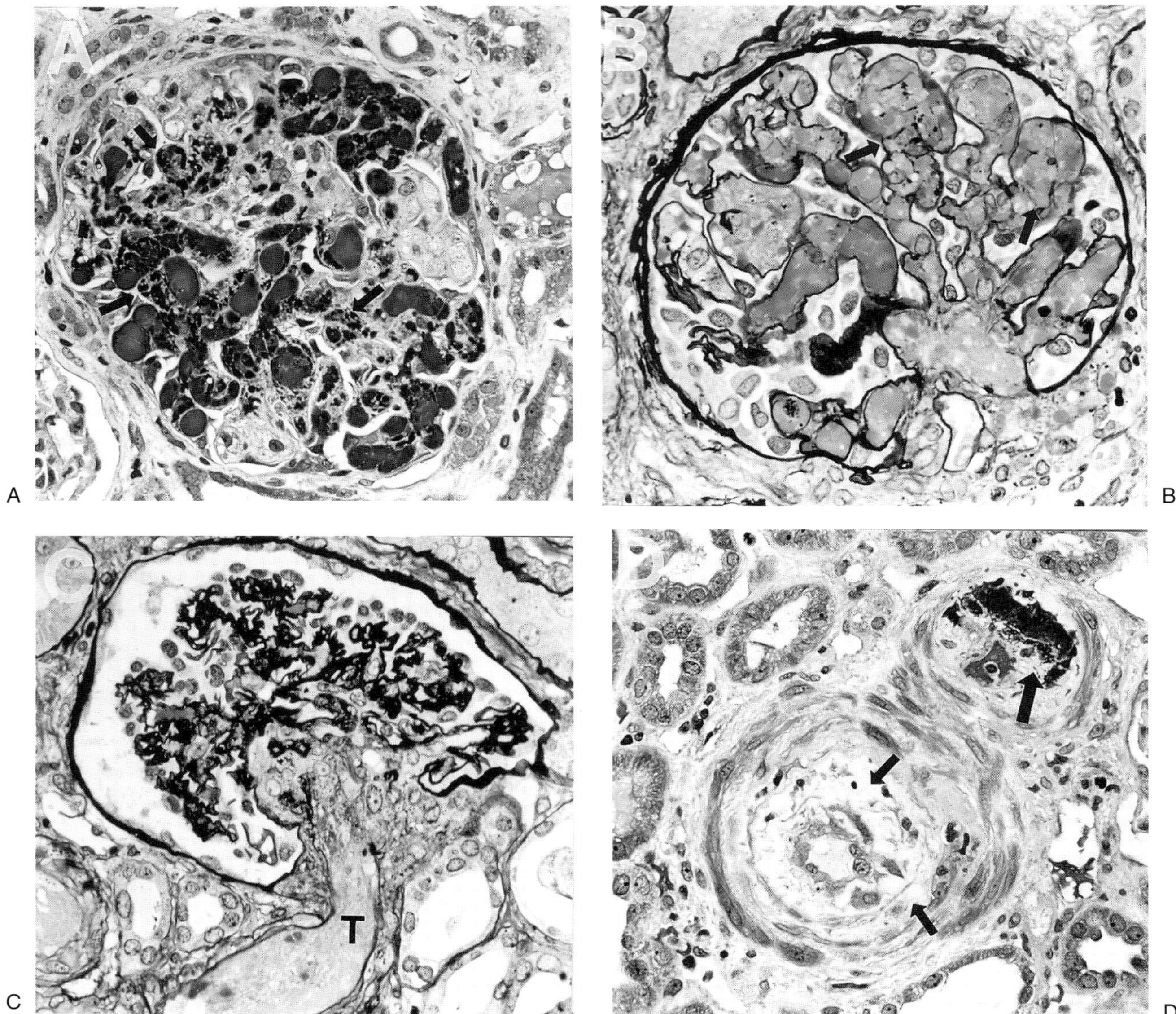

FIG. 2. Pathologic manifestations of hemolytic uremic syndrome (HUS). **A:** Glomerulus with widespread intracapillary thromboses demonstrating numerous red blood cell fragments (arrows) associated with these thrombi. Adjacent tubules show features of acute tubular injury. Trichrome stain. **B:** Glomerulus with widespread intracapillary thromboses, but also demonstrating mesangiolysis as indicated by the disruption and disappearance of the usual silver staining mesangial matrix (arrows). Silver methenamine stain. **C:** Glomerulus with thrombus (T) occluding the hilar arteriole. With this obstruction to normal blood flow, the glomerulus exhibits ischemic injury characterized by wrinkling of basement membranes, collapse of hypoperfused capillaries, and shrinkage of the glomerular tuft. Silver methenamine stain. **D:** Interlobular arteries demonstrating the characteristic mucinous intimal swelling of HUS (small arrows) and the focal presence of arterial thrombosis with accumulation of fibrin and red blood cell fragmentation (large arrow). Trichrome stain. (Photomicrographs kindly provided by Dr. Charles E. Alpers, Department of Pathology, University of Washington, Seattle, WA).

but also seen at times in pre-eclampsia, malignant hypertension, renal vascular rejection, and scleroderma (10, 56). Aneurysmal dilatation of arterioles and glomeruloid structures common in TTP are occasionally seen (56). Glomeruli show typical glomerular TMA lesions or shrinking of the glomerular tuft due to ischemic injury (56) (Fig. 2C). Tubules are often atrophic with hyaline casts and red cells (56).

With cortical necrosis the lesion may be patchy or diffuse, and noninfarcted portions of the cortex contain glomerular and arteriolar TMAs, but normal interlobular arteries (9,10).

The pattern of cortical necrosis is predominantly seen in infants, and prognosis is related to the degree of necrosis. Glomerular TMA is most common in young children, and disease severity and prognosis are related to the proportion of affected glomeruli. Patients with HUS with only glomerular TMA have a better prognosis than do those with arteriolar TMA or cortical necrosis (61). However, in up to 10% of adult cases of HUS, the only renal histopathology seen on biopsy is acute tubular necrosis (62). In addition to renal involvement, identical lesions of enothelial swelling, microthrombi, and necrosis can be seen in many organs. TMA in the heart, lungs, brain, pancreas, liver, and colon all have been described (59).

TTP is characterized by the widely disseminated TMA lesions in the small arteries, arterioles, and capillaries, especially at the arteriocapillary junctions. The lesions tend to be more widely distributed than those of HUS. The most commonly involved organs are the brain, heart, kidneys, pancreas, adrenal gland, and spleen (3,4,6,11). Microaneurysm formation is common (3,63). Proliferation of cells, presumably of endothelial origin, in the arteriolar wall may lead to structures that resemble glomeruli, called glomeruloid structures (2,64). Significant proliferation of endothelial and myointimal cells is more prominent than in HUS. Glomerular findings are typically much less pronounced than in HUS. Microthrombi similar to that seen in the arterioles are seen, but swelling and proliferation of capillary walls are uncommon. Glomerular sclerosis may be seen (56). Tubular damage and chronic interstitial inflammation or fibrosis is variable (56). Immunofluorescence findings show fibrin in the thrombi of arterioles and glomerular capillaries (65). Platelets are seen in nonrenal tissue (66–68) but rarely in the kidney (56). Rarely, IgG and C3 are found in glomeruli (65,69). As with HUS, there is a marked absence of any evidence of underlying vasculitis.

Thrombotic microangiopathic lesions are also observed with malignant hypertension, cyclosporine nephrotoxicity, renal vascular transplant rejection, and scleroderma. These entities can usually be differentiated from HUS/TTP on clinical grounds.

PATHOPHYSIOLOGY OF HUS AND TTP

The fundamental pathogenic mechanisms of TMA in HUS and TTP are still poorly understood, and it is probable that there are several mechanisms that may initiate TMA. Histopathologic studies suggest that endothelial cell injury followed by localized intravascular thrombosis is the sentinel pathologic event in HUS and TTP, but the precise manner by which this is initiated is unclear. The fluid state of the blood is maintained by a delicate balance of procoagulant factors in the plasma and platelets and anticoagulant factors produced in the endothelial cell. Theories of pathogenesis of HUS/TTP center around three possible processes: (a) direct endothelial injury disrupting the anticoagulant properties of the vessel wall, (b) the abnormal presence of a platelet-aggregating substance, and (c) the lack of a platelet aggregation inhibitor.

Direct Endothelial Injury

Cytotoxin

Bacterial agents that are known to precipitate HUS are also known to cause endothelial cell injury. The cytotoxin found in *Shigella dysenteriae* type I and *E. coli* 0157:H7 has been shown to be cytotoxic for human endothelial cells in culture (70). This toxin is referred to as a shigalike toxin (SLT) or, alternatively, as a verotoxin because of its cytotoxicity in vero cell lines. *E. coli* that elaborate this toxin are known as verotoxigenic *E. Coli* (VTEC). This toxin is composed of an A and several B subunits. The B subunit binds to the the disaccharide galactose alpha-1-4 galactose in the terminal trisaccharide sequence of globotriosyl ceramide (Gb3), a cell surface receptor found on human endothelial cells. It also binds to the erythrocyte P_1 antigen (71). After binding, the A subunit is internalized and binds to the 60S subunit of the ribosome, halting protein transcription and leading to cell death (72). Rabbits injected with VTEC develop TMA lesions in the brain, lungs, cecum, and cerebellum, but not in the kidney (73,74). The disribution of pathologic lesions parallel the distribution of Gb3 receptors in this species (74). Human renal endothelial cells appear to have many Gb3 receptors (75). There is evidence that Gb3 receptors may be upregulated by lipopolysaccharide, present both in *S. dysenteraie* and *E. coli* O157:H7 (75). The cytokines interleukin-1 and tumor necrosis factor (released by activated macrophages and posssibly mesangial cells) also upregulate Gb3 receptor concentrations in human endothelial cells (75,76). However, Gb3 concentrations in human renal tissue are lower in children than in adults, in marked contrast to the distribution of VTEC-mediated disease, indicating that receptor availability alone cannot explain the age distribution of HUS (77).

It has been postulated that binding to the erythrocyte P_1 antigen, a pentosyl ceramide molecule (which has a terminal alpha 1–4 galactose ceramide identical to Gb3) may be protective by binding free cytotoxin and decreasing endothelial cell binding. Individuals with high expressions of erythrocyte P1 antigen may therefore be at decreased risk of HUS from SLT (71,78,79).

HUS also occurs after neuraminidase-producing pneumococcal infection. Bacterial neuraminidase is capable of cleaving sialic acid residues from the surface of endothelial cells, red blood cells, and platelets exposing the Thomsen-Freidenreich antigen(T-antigen) (80–85). Anti–Thomsen-Freidenreich IgM can cause agglutination of platelets and red blood cells. Use of IgM containing blood products may aggravate the disease (86). These patients, in contrast to all other forms of HUS/TTP, may have a positive Coombs test (13,85).

Neutrophils

Neutrophils also have been implicated in the pathogenesis of endothelial injury in HUS. Tumor necrosis factor and interleukin 1, which are released from endotoxin-activated leukocytes, can potentiate the effects of shigatoxin on endothelial cells (75,76). Children with HUS and elevated peripheral white blood cell counts had poorer outcomes in some studies (23,87–90). White blood cells from children with D+ HUS have increased adherence to endothelial cells, and patients' neutrophils have been shown to induce endothelial injury (91). Increased concentrations of interleukin-8, an activator of neutrophils, and neutrophil elastase, a marker of neutrophil activation, have been demonstrated in the plasma of children with typical HUS (92–94). Although these findings suggest a role for neutrophil activation in endothelial injury in HUS, it is unclear whether neutrophil activation precedes or follows initial endothelial injury.

Immunoglobulins

Immunologic mediators of endothelial injury may play a role in HUS/TTP. Complement-fixing IgG and IgM capable of lysing cultured human umbilical vein endothelial cells have been identified in the sera of some children with acute HUS (95) and some patients with TTP (96). In TTP, IgG-related immune injury to endothelial cells and platelets has been documented (97). The association of TTP with autoimmune disorders such as systemic lupus erythematosis (SLE), scleroderma, and rheumatoid arthritis suggests a possible role for immune complexes in TTP. Quinine-dependent antibodies that react with endothelial cells, platelets, neutrophils, T cells, or erythrocytes have been reported in patients with quinine-associated HUS/TTP (98–100). However, despite such circumstantial evidence, no specific endothelial cell antigen has been identified in HUS or TTP, and therapuetic trials using anti-immunoglobulin therapy have been disappointing (101–103).

Prostacyclin

Prostacyclin (PGI_2) is a potent inhibitor of platelet aggregation synthesized by endothelial cells (104) that is normally released after platelet adherence to exposed sub-endothelial basement membrane components (105). PGI_2 is important in limiting thrombus formation locally at the site of endothelial injury. Deficient bioavailabilty of serum PGI_2 has been documented in some patients with familial HUS (106–108) and idiopathic TTP (109,110). Urinary 6-keto-PGF1-alpha, a PGI_2 metabolite, has been found to be reduced in the acute phase, and increased during remission, in HUS (111). However, others have found increased levels of PGI_2 metabolites (112,113), and the ability of serum from HUS/TTP patients to stimulate PGI_2 activity in vitro is diminished in some (107,114–116), but not all (117,118), patients with adult and atypical childhood forms of HUS. Although PGI_2 defects are less common in typical HUS, VTEC-mediated cell injury of vascular endothelium is accompanied by decreased PGI_2 synthesis (119). Despite this evidence of a deficiency in bioavailability of PGI_2 in some patients with HUS/TTP, PGI_2 infusion studies have demonstrated no clinically significant effects in TTP (120,121) or HUS (122).

Presence of a Platelet Aggregation Potentiator

Platelets

Platelet aggregation is an important step in the development of TMA lesions in HUS and TTP. In TTP and HUS, platelet survival is short and fibrinogen turnover normal or slightly elevated, suggesting consumption of platelets in the absence of disseminated intravascular coagulation (123,124). In children with HUS, a characteristic pattern of impaired platelet function is seen. In vitro, their platelets fail to aggregate normally in response to proaggregating agents, and morphologically the platelets are degranulated and in an exhausted state (123). During recovery, platelet-aggregating ability normalizes despite the persistence of uremia in some patients (125,126). Plasma from some TTP patients agglutinate autologous and homologous platelets (97,127).

These findings indicate that intravascular platelet activation occurs during acute HUS/TTP and is the probable cause of thrombocytopenia. Initiating factors for this aggregation remain obscure. Whether platelet aggregation is a primary pathogenic event that is followed by endothelial injury or is a result of endothelial injury is unknown.

von Willebrand Factor

Abnormal von Willebrand factor (vWF) is another candidate for initiating TMA in HUS/TTP. Von Willebrand factor is the carrier protein for procoagulant factor VIII, which agglutinates platelets and is required for platelet adhesion to subendothelial collagen (128). Abnormalities of vWF have been documented in chronic relapsing TTP (129,130) and HUS (131,132) which may predispose toward platelet aggregation. Unusually large vWF multimers that predispose toward platelet aggregation were found in some patients with TTP during remissions but were missing during the active phase of a relapse (129,130,133). These unusually large vWF multimers may be present due to a deficiency of the normal processing of the large vWF multimers made by endothelial cells before release. Unusually large vWF multimers could predispose toward episodes of microvascular thrombosis by binding and activating platelets on exposed subendothelial surfaces. In patients with recurrent TTP, these unusually large vWF multimers are noted during remissions but disappear during acute relapses (129,130,133). This finding suggest that TTP patients may be predisposed to episodes of microvascular thrombosis due to the presence of these unusually large vWF multimers. Clearance of the multimers could be due to agglutination with platelets, decreased synthesis from damaged endothelial cells, or accelerated catabolism due to increased release of plasminogen activator from endothelial cells or other proteases from platelets, leukocytes, or other cells (134).

However, in one study heterologous anti-vWF antibodies did not prevent platelet agglutination in TTP plasma (135). In some patients with HUS, other abnormalities in vWf were found during acute episodes that resolve after the episode, these abnormalities were distinct from those seen in chronic relapsing TTP. Despite the variety of evidence, it is unknown at this time whether the abnormalities of vWf seen in TTP and HUS are a cause or a consequence of endothelial injury (129, 131,132,136,137)

Thromboxane A2

A potent platelet proaggregatory factor, thromboxane A2 (TXA_2), is normally released by platelets in response to endothelial injury (138). TXA_2 appears to be increased in the kidney of patients in the acute phase of HUS (139). This increase in TXA_2 combined with the deficiency in the bioavailability of the platelet aggregation inhibitor, PGI_2, may one of the factors that tips the balance toward platelet aggregation in some patients with HUS.

Tissue Plasminogen Activator

Tissue plasminogen activator (t-PA) is a factor normally synthesized and released by endothelial cells and platelets. Plasminogen activator is important in fibrinolysis, the process by which fibrin clot formation is controlled and ultimately resolved. Both HUS and TTP are characterized by a shortened platelet survival time but a normal or a slightly elevated fibrinogen turnover rate, indicating a low level of fibrinolysis in the presence of ongoing thrombus formation (124,140,141). In children with HUS, a circulating plasminogen activator inhibitor (PAI-1) has been described and is hypothesized to inhibit normal fibrinolysis (142). In patients with TTP, t-PA activity was shown to be low, and t-PA inhibitors were significantly elevated in plasma (143). It has been conjectured that t-PA inhibitors could be synthesized by rapidly proliferating endothelial cells in HUS or TTP lesions and may bind and inactivate circulating t-PA and impair fibrinolysis. Bergstein found that removal of PAI-1 by peritoneal dialysis was associated with improved renal outcome in childhood HUS (142).

Absence of a Platelet Aggregation Inhibitor

In some adults with TTP, a platelet-aggregating factor is inhibited by normal plasma or by the patient's plasma during remission but not the patient's plasma in the acute phase of TTP (97,144,145). These findings suggest that TTP plasma contains a platelet-aggregating factor that is inhibited by a factor in normal plasma or that normal plasma has a platelet aggregation inhibitor, which is lost in some patients with TTP. The identity of this factor remains a mystery. Some evidence suggests that it may be an immunoglobulin, and other studies suggest that it is not (134). Platelet-aggregating activity also has been noted in children with HUS (146,147).

CLINICAL MANIFESTATIONS

Hemolytic Uremic Syndrome

The clinical course of typical HUS is characterized by the sudden onset of acute renal insufficiency in conjuction with a microangiopathic anemia, and thrombocytopenia (7,60). Children usually present with decreased urine output after an episode of bloody diarrhea, caused by *E. coli* O157:H7. They rapidly develop varying degrees of renal insufficiency that may require fluid and electrolyte management, control of hypertension, or dialysis. Although patients with severe disease often require blood and platelet transfusions, the severity of hemolysis or thrombocytopenia bears no direct relationship to the severity, length, or outcome of the renal disease. In addition, patients may develop clinical or histopathologic evidence of dysfunction in any organ system. The most common extrarenal sites of involvement include the brain, lungs, heart, pancreas, and cecum (59,148,149). Active disease typically resolves over 1 to 2 weeks, and a majority of patients recover completely. Those with severe ischemic injury to organs may have permanent sequelae, most commonly renal.

Urine protein excretion in the acute phase of HUS is typically 1 to 2 g/24 h but may be in the nephrotic range (150), Renaud found that 90% of patients with atypical HUS but no patients with typical HUS had marked proteinuria, 48% in the nephrotic range (151). Sodium is often low at presentation and urate often increased due to red cell lysis (150). Patients with typical HUS are often normotensive at presentation due to fluid depletion from diarrhea and vomiting, whereas patients with atypical

HUS are often hypertensive at presentation. Hypertension is often secondary to fluid overload. The role of the renin-angiotensin system in HUS-related hypertension is unclear; results of some studies have shown that hypertension is independent of the renin level (152,153), whereas others have suggested a renin-dependent mechanism for hypertension (154,155).

Thrombotic Thrombocytopenia Purpura

TTP is classically defined as the clinical pentad of fever, thrombocytopenia, neurologic abnormalities, renal abnormalities, and microangiopathic hemolytic anemia. The classic pentad is found in 34% to 77% of patients at presentation, whereas the triad of fever, neurologic abnormalities, and renal abnormalities is present in 52% to 100% (5,19,31,43,156–158). Neurologic abnormalities are often subtle at presentation. Mental status changes and headache are the most common findings (5,6,43, 157). Knowing the serum lactate dehydrogenase (LDH) level may be helpful in diagnosis. Thompson found that serum LDH was elevated in 43 of 44 patients, with a median level of 1,200 U/L. TTP is more common in women by approximately a 3:2 ratio (5,6,31,43,44,156). TTP is most common in the third decade of life but may be seen at any age (49) and the common association of TTP with pregnancy may be responsible, in part, for this age distribution (54).

With the advent of early intervention in TTP, attempts have been made to simplify diagnostic criteria to allow early detection of disease. Recent studies have suggested that only the presence of microangiopathic anemia and thrombocytopenia are required for diagnosis (Table 2) (43,44,159). At entry into a recent prospective trial of plasmapheresis on 102 patients with TTP, 24% had fever, 59% renal disease, 63% neurologic abnormalities, and 100% thrombocytopenia and microangiopathic anemia (43). Other common presenting symptoms are hemorrhage/purpura (38–78%) (5,43,44,49,157), fatigue (25–29%) (5,6,49), and gastrointestinal complaints (14–24%) (5,6,49).

Hemorrhagic symptoms are common at presentation, occurring in 38% to 78% of patients with TTP (5,6,43,49, 157,159). They are secondary to thrombocytopenia and typically consist of epistaxis, hematuria, gastrointestinal bleeding, or menorrhagia. More severe hemorrhagic symptoms can develop at any time and include subarachnoid hemorrhage, ovarian rupture, and hemoptysis (43). Occasionally, patients with severe multisystem disease develop disseminated intravascular coagulopathy (DIC), but this is uncommon at presentation.

Neurologic findings remain the pre-eminent clinical sign of TTP, both at presentation and during the disease course, despite improvements in early diagnosis and treatment. Neurologic abnormalities are observed in 60% to 100% of patients with TTP at presentation (Table 2) and in almost all patients at some point during the course of the disease (6,31,42–44,49,156,157,160,161). The most common neurologic findings at presentation are headache in 18% to 35% of patients (49,157), mental status changes in 43% to 50% (43,49,157), paresis in 15% to 46% (43,49,157), coma in 0% to 4% (43,49,157), seizures in 10% to 20% (43,49,157), and visual problems in 2% to 6% (43,49). Fluctuating neurologic status is the hallmark of TTP, presumably due to widespread microvascular thrombosis of the cerebral vasculature (162). During the disease course the percentages of patients with the most common neurologic findings are headache in 24% to 50% (5,6,49,160), mental status changes in 15% to 80% (5,6,49,160), visual changes in 8% to 15% (5,6,31,49,160), seizure in 16% to 41% (5,6,31,49,160),

TABLE 2. *Presenting features of TTP (% of patients with findings)*

Study	Year	n	Fever	Neurologic dysfunction	Anemia	Low platelets	Renal dysfunction (abnormal urine/azotemia)	Triad[a]	Pentad[b]
Amorosi	1966	16	81	60	88	93	88/55	NR	NR
Petit	1980	38	87	100	100	100	82/18	100	NR
Kennedy	1980	48	60	71	98	100	95/65	NR	NR
Cuttner	1980	20		95	90	90	95/50	95	55
Ridolfi	1981	25	88	NR	96	NR	92/76	52	40
Rose	1987	38	37	94	86	95	NR/73	94	37
Rock	1991	102	24	63	100	100	52[c]	63	NR
Thompson	1992	41	61	78	100	100	NR/44	78	34
Hayward	1994	52	58	61	100	100	NR	NR	NR

NR, not reported
[a] Fever, hemolytic anemia, and low platelets.
[b] Fever, hemolytic anemia, low platelets, neurologic dysfunction, and renal dysfunction.
[c] Details of renal dysfunction not reported.

paresis in 8% to 41% (5,6,31,49,160), and coma in 20% to 39% (5,6,31,49,160).

Abdominal pain may be pronounced in some patients with TTP (5,6,163). Like the abdominal pain seen in childhood HUS, it can be severe enough to lead to exploratory laparotomy (23,72). Thompson noted significant abdominal pain in 12 of 44 consecutive patients with TTP with no evidence of pancreatitis or other identifiable pathology (43). This pain may be due to ischemic bowel secondary to TMA involvement of the colon or small intestine, which has been noted in childhood HUS (59,164).

Pregnancy-Related HUS/TTP

The triad of microangiopathic anemia, acute renal failure, and thrombocytopenia in pregnancy or the postpartum state may occur in three entities: TTP, HUS, and severe eclampsia with the HELLP syndrome (hemolysis with red cell fragmentation, elevated liver enzymes, and low platelet count) (165). Because of overlap in clinical symptoms, it can be difficult to differentiate these entities. TMA is a rare but serious event in pregnancy. The incidence is unknown. Acute renal failure necessitating dialysis occurs in approximately one in 10,000 pregnancies (166) and HUS/TTP accounts for only a small percentage of these (167–170). The clinical history and time of onset are important in making the diagnosis. Preeclampsia is usually preceded by hypertension and typically occurs in the third trimester or within 1 to 2 days of parturition. It is more common in primigravidas. Thrombocytopenia occurs in 15% to 50% of women with preeclampsia (171). Both pre-eclampsia and HELLP are associated with abnormalities of clotting and some degree of consumptive coagulopathy (54,171), not typically seen in HUS/TTP. A depressed antithrombin III level is seen in HELLP but not HUS/TTP and can help differentiate pre-eclampsia/HELLP from TTP or HUS (54,172,173). Renal failure is uncommon with uncomplicated preeclampsia unless significant hypotension develops.

In the HELLP syndrome, 80% to 90% of patients present with malaise, right upper quadrant or epigastric pain, and nausea (167). Like simple pre-eclampsia, HELLP occurs primarily in the third trimester of pregnancy or soon after delivery. HELLP is more common in multiparous women. By definition, all patients have microangiopathic anemia, thrombocytopenia, and elevated liver enzymes. Approximately 50% have some decrease in renal function, and 10% have acute renal failure (167, 171). The absence of fever and abnormalities of clotting and aminotransferases helps differentiate it from classic HUS or TTP.

TTP more commonly occurs earlier in gestation, with mild renal involvement but with fever and prominant hematologic and neurologic findings (54,167). Weiner reviewed 65 cases of pregnancy-related TTP over 23 years and found that 89% occurred prenatally at an average gestational age of 23.5 weeks (54). Fetal thrombocytopenia is not seen, suggesting that if a causative factor exists in the maternal plasma it does not cross the placenta (54).

The etiology of HUS/TTP in pregnancy is elusive. Prodromal infections have been documented in isolated cases of postpartum HUS (174–177), as have antiphospholipid antibodies (178). Ergot derivatives and estrogens used during delivery or postpartum have been implicated (179). A genetic predisposition to HUS/TTP has been implicated in several cases (180–184). Pregnancy-associated HUS typically occurs after delivery, 2 to 30 days postpartum, and may follow either an uneventful pregnancy or pre-eclampsia (171), although it rarely has been reported during pregnancy (185,186) or after ectopic pregnancies (187,188). Thrombocytopenia may precede the development of anemia, and a prolonged bleeding time may precede the decrease in platelets. Like other forms of HUS/TTP, clotting tests, including PT/PTT, fibrin split products, and antithrombin III are normal. On renal biopsy, HUS/TTP can be differentiated from pre-eclampsia by the prescence of subendothelial fibrin deposits in the arterioles in HUS/TTP. In pre-eclampsia the renal biopsy typically shows swollen glomerular endothelial cells (endotheliosis) without evidence of the subendothelial fibrin deposition seen in HUS/TTP (189).

DIFFERENTIAL DIAGNOSIS

The finding of microangiopathic anemia, thrombocytopenia, and acute renal failure with or without neurologic abnormalities should be considered as presumptive evidence of HUS/TTP. However, several other possible disorders must be kept in mind (Table 3). Severe pre-eclampsia, malignant hypertension, SLE, systemic scleroderma, acute bacterial endocarditis, and DIC all may show the classic clinical triad of HUS: acute renal failure (ARF), decreased platelets, and microangiopathic anemia. ARF and thrombocytopenia also may be seen in bilateral renal vein thrombosis. ARF associated with cutaneous purpura may be seen in DIC or Schönlein-Henoch purpura. Thrombocytopenia and microangiopathic anemia may be seen in Evan syndrome (idiopathic thrombocyto-penic purpura and autoimmune hemolytic anemia). Giant hemangiomas may lead to platelet sequestration. Solitary microangiopathic anemia may be a sign of metastatic cancer, especially gastric carcinoma (190). Paroxysmal nocturnal hemoglobinuria with thrombotic complications is also a diagnostic consideration in cases of unexplained hemolysis with renal abnormalities and low platelets (191,192). In high-risk populations, HUS/TTP may be the presenting illness in HIV infection (43) (see Chapter 54). Acute hemorrhagic fever and renal syndrome (HFRS), characterized by a febrile illness that

TABLE 3. *Differential diagnosis of HUS/TTP*

Diagnosis	Hemolytic anemia	Low platelets	Renal findings	Neurologic dysfunction	Fever	Differential features
HUS	+	+	+	+/–	+/–	
TTP	+	+	+	+	+	
DIC	+	+	+/–	+/–	+/–	Coagulopathy/ purpuric rash
Hemorrhagic fever and renal syndrome	+[a]	+	+	+	+	Coagulopathy/rash
Schönlein-Henoch purpura	–	–	+/–	–	+/–	Purpuric rash
Malignant hypertension	+	+	+/–	+/–	–	HTN history
HELLP	+	+	+/–	+	–	Preeclampsia
ABE	+	+	+/–	–	–	Heart murmur
SLE/scleroderma	+/–	=/–	+/–	+/–	+/–	Positive serology
Evan's syndrome	+	+	–	–	–	Coomb's test positive
HIV with HUS/TTP	+	+	+	+/–	+/–	Serology
Bilateral RVT	+	+	+	–	–	Renal ultrasound
Malignancy	+/–	+/–	+/–	+/–	+/–	
PNH	+	+	+	–	–	Positive cryoglobulin

+, usually present; –, not usually present; +/–, may be be present or absent; ABE, acute bacterial endocarditis; RVT, renal vein thrombosis; PNH, paroxysmal hemoglobinuria; Evan's syndrome, immune thrombocytopenia and hemolytic anemia.
[a] Nonhemolytic.

leads to oliguria, thrombocytopenia, and a nonhemolytic anemia, also should be considered in areas where HFRS is endemic (193).

TREATMENT OF HUS AND TTP

Because the pathogenic factor(s) responsible for HUS/TTP have not been elucidated, therapy has been directed toward correcting the physiologic aberrations observed in patients. Currently, treatment for HUS/TTP falls into several categories: symptomatic treatment alone, anticoagulant/antiplatelet agents, plasma therapies, immune mediators, and miscellaneous treatments. In TTP, plasmapheresis is clearly the most efficacious therapy. In HUS no therapy has been convincingly demonstrated to be superior to supportive care alone. However, because most treatment series in HUS have included both typical and atypical forms of the disease, there is a concern that the good outcomes seen with patients with typical *E. coli* O157:H7–associated HUS (95% of cases) may mask any effect of therapy on the poor outcome of patients with atypical HUS. One recent study suggests that plasmapheresis offers benefit in atypical HUS (20).

Controlled studies in HUS using the antithrombolytic agents heparin (194,195), urokinase (196), dipyridamole (195,197), and streptokinase (198) to block or limit procoagulant activity have shown no definitive benefit. The use of glucocorticoids (199) and gammaglobulin (101) in uncontrolled studies to block immune-mediated mechanisms likewise have shown no benefit in HUS. In TTP, isolated reports of success have been described using gammaglobulin (200). Glucocorticoids, although widely used, have not been shown to be efficacious in controlled studies independent of other therapies.

Plasma Therapy

Over the past 15 years plasma exchange has emerged as the primary treatment for TTP. In 1980 Bukowski reviewed the literature on the treatment of TTP and found that overall about 76% of patients responded to plasma exchange. Other studies have confirmed the role of plasma exchange in adult HUS/TTP. In pregnancy-associated TTP, Weiner found 68% maternal mortality without plasma therapy and none when plasma therapy was used (54). In a retrospective study of patients with TTP treated with plasma exchange or exchange transfusion (whole blood exchange), a significantly higher response rate was seen with plasma exchange (160). Byrnes (201) had shown that plasma infusion alone may be beneficial, but Rock et al. showed in a controlled, randomized trial a significant improvement in 6 months of survival in patients treated with plasmapheresis compared with plasma infusions (44). All patients also received antiplatelet therapy. Both plasmapheresis and plasma infusion therapy result in a significant improvement in survival over supportive treatment alone (44). Bell et al. showed in an uncontrolled clinical trial that plasma exchange with plasmapheresis was superior to corticosteroid treatment, plasma infusion alone, or antiplatelet agents (19). Hayward et al. reviewed 67 episodes in 52 patients in Toronto between 1977 and 1988. All patients and all but two episodes were treated with plasma therapy as well as various other therapies, including aspirin (90%), dipyridamole

(96%), steroids (63%), vincristine (4%), immune globulin (4%), danazol (8%), dextran (3%), and splenectomy (33%). They found 92% overall survival and no statistically significant benefit from any therapy added to plasma exchange (42).

Because of the rapidity with which hematologic and neurologic findings may advance in TTP (44,49,163, 202), it is important to initiate plasma exchange as soon as the diagnosis has been made. Hematologic abnormalities usually resolve within 1 to 2 weeks. Neurologic abnormalities often respond quickly, resolving in hours or days with successful treatment (43,203). In most studies plasma exchange volumes are 1 to 2 plasma volumes (40–80 ml/kg) with fresh-frozen plasma used as replacement fluid (44,163,202,204–206). Higher exchange volumes are associated with re-exchange of already infused plasma. The serum LDH may be followed to guide therapy. One study suggested a postexchange LDH of less than 400 U as a marker of adequate exchange (163). LDH levels higher that 400 U postexchange indicate a need for higher exchange volumes, and a rapid increase in postexchange LDH indicates a need for continued aggressive therapy (19,207). Daily plasma exchange should be continued until neurologic abnormalities have resolved, and the platelet and LDH levels are normal for several days. Plasma exchange is continued every other day and then less frequently for 2 to 4 weeks (207). Relapses are most common in the month after stopping therapy and usually respond to plasma exchange or in some cases plasma infusion alone (205,208). In cases in which inadequate treatment response is achieved or prolonged plasma exchange therapy is required (>4 weeks), the use of large plasma volumes or cryosupernatant plasma or the addition of one of the alternative treatment modalities discussed below should be considered.

In childhood HUS, results of plasma therapy trials have been inconclusive. Loirat et al. looked prospectively at 79 children with HUS and found less cortical necrosis on renal biopsy samples taken within 1 month of the onset of illness in patients treated with plasma infusions versus supportive care only. However, there was no effect on clinical outcome at 1 year (122). Gianviti et al. looked retrospectively at plasma exchange in children with HUS who were at high risk for severe sequelae. He found no statistically significant effect of plasma exchange on glomerular filtration rate (GFR) at 1 year follow-up. However, no patient in the plasma exchange group (of 11) had a GFR of less than 60 ml/min/1.73 m^2 at follow-up, whereas 49% (nine of 22) in the untreated group did. End-stage renal disease was present at 1 year follow-up in 18% of patients in the supportive care group and none of the plasma exchange patients (209). Neither study differentiated typical from atypical HUS cases. In atypical childhood HUS, Fitzpatrick found 56% mortality in patients treated before the availability of plasma exchange versus no mortality in 11 patients treated with plasma exchange (seven also recieved PGI_2) (20). In the Canadian Apheresis Study Group's randomized prospective trial of plasma exchange versus plasma infusion in TTP, all patients received aspirin and dipyridamole and were then randomized to receive plasma infusions or plasmaphereis. At 6 month follow-up plasma exchange was associated with 78% survival and 78% success rate (measured by improvement in platelet count and stability or improvement of neurologic status) versus 50% survival and 31% treatment success in the plasma infusion group (44).

The treatment of HUS/TTP in pregnancy is, like other forms of these syndromes, plasma therapy with dialysis if indicated. Pre-eclampsia and HELLP syndrome are best managed by delivery of the infant.

Interpretation of studies in childhood HUS is complicated by a lack of differentiation between typical and atypical HUS. Clinical studies in the past decade suggest that the outcome of typical HUS is favorable with only dialysis and supportive treatment (210,211) but that atypical HUS is associated with a high morbidity rate (20). The advent of effective peritoneal and hemodialysis for young children with acute renal failure since the 1970s has done more to improve outcomes in childhood HUS than any other interventional therapy. Still, reports of improvement in atypical HUS with plasma exchange or plasmapheresis (20,212–215) and the clinical similarities between atypical HUS and TTP suggest that these entities may be closely related and prognostically different from typical HUS. Atypical HUS, like TTP, responds favorably to plasma therapy (20). Additional controlled studies are required to determine whether plasma therapy has a role in the treatment of typical childhood HUS.

Corticosteroids

Glucocorticoid therapy has been used for many years in TTP to decrease splenic platelet sequestration, diminish red blood cell damage, or improve vascular integrity. Bukowski reviewed the therapy of TTP in 1981, before the widespread use of plasma therapies, and found only a 10% success rate with glucocorticoids alone (216). This was of some value given the 95% death rate associated with TTP before 1966 (6). More commonly, glucocorticoids have been used in combination with other treatment modalities. In Bell's study of 108 patients with HUS/TTP, 54 were initially treated with only corticosteroids. Fifty-five percent of patients assigned to corticosteroids alone responded, and this group was less likely to relapse than were those in the plasmapheresis/corticosteroids group (19). Forty-four percent of those initially started on corticosteroids failed to respond, and plasma therapy was added (19). One uncontrolled trial in children with HUS showed no substantial benefit from corticosteroid use (217). However, despite their widely accepted addition to many therapeutic regimens, including plasma therapy, the use of glucocorticoids in TTP is not supported by a large body of data.

Antiplatelet Agents

Despite evidence that platelet aggregation is involved in the pathogenesis of HUS/TTP, the use of antiplatelet agents to decrease the degree of TMA has been disappointing. Aspirin, dipyridamole, heparin, dextran, and sulfinpyrazone have been used in combination with steroids, plasmapheresis, or splenectomy (218–220). Few studies have looked at antiplatelet therapy alone. In the era before plasmapheresis, several studies suggested an improvement in survival of TTP with aspirin and dipyridamole (216,221–223). However, in both the Canadian apheresis study and a retrospective study of 108 patients with TTP, outcome was independent of aspirin and dipyridamole use (19,44,159). These agents increase the risk of bleeding in patients who are already at high risk given their thrombocytopenia. In the absence of clear evidence of efficacy, these agents should be withheld unless patients are unresponsive to plasma therapy. PGI_2 infusions have been reported to be effective in some patients with TTP (224,225), but other reports suggest no effect (120,226).

In childhood HUS, controlled studies using heparin (194), heparin/dipyridamole (195), and urokinase/heparin (196) have failed to show any therapeutic benefit. Similarly, uncontrolled reports using aspirin with dipyridamole (227), or dipyridamole and heparin (228) have been disappointing. Likewise, PGI_2 infusion has shown no definitive benifit in children with HUS (229,230).

Immunoglobulin

Intravenous gammaglobulin has been used with some success in isolated reports of patients with TTP, usually after failure of other treatments (231–234). The rationale for its use is based on the finding of platelet-agglutinating activity, which could be inhibited by normal IgG (97,147, 235). Isolated reports of success with intravenous immunoglobulin (IVIG) in TTP (200,232,236) have not been followed by any reported trials or controlled studies in TTP. In children with HUS, trials of IVIG showed no benefit in terms of either platelet counts or patient outcome (101,199).

Miscellaneous Treatments

Treatment of TTP with vincristine in patients unresponsive to plasma therapy (237–239) has been reported. Strong evidence of a therapuetic effect is lacking.

Splenectomy has been used in patients with TTP to decrease splenic sequestration of platelets and red cells. Several reports have suggested that it may improve outcome in TTP, but in most instances it has been used in combination with other therapies (157,240,241). Liu found that splenectomy in combination with glucocorticoids and dextran infusions may be beneficial in patients who fail to respond to plasmapheresis (242).

Platelet Transfusions

Because active HUS/TTP is associated with widespread deposition of microvascular platelet thrombi, there is concern that platelet transfusions may fuel the thrombotic process and increase the risk of ischemic tissue injury. There have been reports of increased morbidity after platelet transfusions (19,243). Because of the risk of hemorrhagic complications with severe thrombocytopenia, platelet transfusions are appropriate only in patients with active bleeding, during invasive procedures, or with severe thrombocytopenia (platelet count of $<10,000/mm^3$).

Blood Transfusions

Blood transfusions are often required for symptomatic anemia. Packed red blood cells, filtered to avoid anti–human leukocyte antigen antibody formation, should be used to keep the hematocrit above 20% to 25%. Correcting the hematocrit to normal is often futile in the face of ongoing hemolysis and may increase the risk of significant hypertension. After resolution of the disease, the hematocrit returns to normal over 2 to 6 months. Folate supplementation may be helpful during this period because of the depletion of folate stores during the period of active hemolysis when the bone marrow is rapidly producing new erythrocytes. In *Pneumococcus*-associated HUS, IgM containing blood products may worsen the disease through IgM-mediated endothelial cell injury and should be avoided if possible (86).

Dialysis and Symptomatic Therapy

Children with typical HUS appear to do as well with dialysis and symptomatic therapy as with any of the above mentioned interventions, but those with atypical HUS do poorly (20,151) and may benefit from plasma therapy. Symptomatic therapy includes strict fluid and electrolyte management with dialysis therapy as indicated. Early institution of dialysis is associated with improved outcome (244,245). Hypertension not related to fluid overload is primarily renin mediated and often can be controlled with a calcium channel blocker, hydralazine, or beta-blockers. Angiotensin-converting enzyme inhibitors' effects on intraglomerular blood flow can theoretically lead to further injury of glomeruli with marginal blood flow and should be used with caution in the acute phase of disease. Anticonvulsant therapy should be used for seizures. Enteral or parenteral nutrition for patients unable or disinterested in eating is of paramount importance to avoid the complications of malnutrition and to promote repair of injured tissue. Insulin and/or bowel rest is necessary if diabetes mellitus or pancreatitis develops, and attention to the risk of ischemic colitis is imperative in patients with HUS (164). Medication dosages should be adjusted for the degree of renal failure present. Potential nephrotoxins should be avoided if possible.

PROGNOSIS

Mortality in adult TTP/HUS has been remarkably reduced with the onset of plasma exchange. Before plasma exchange, mortality was typically 95% (6). In the past 10 years there has been an almost complete reversal of outcome, with 90% surviving the acute illness (19,44). The elderly are at higher risk for poor outcomes (246).

Pregnancy-related TTP/HUS places both the mother and fetus at risk, although outcome has improved with the advent of plasma exchange. Weiner found 75% of TTP-associated pregnancies led to maternal (44%) and/or fetal/infant death (73%) (54). Growth retardation was common, but treatment decreased its incidence if started before placental infarcts had occurred (54). Plasma therapy significantly improves the maternal and fetal outcome, with maternal mortality reported at 68% (19 of 28) without and 0% (none of 17) with plasma therapy (54). Hayward found 11% mortality in nine cases of pregnancy-related HUS/TTP treated with plasma exchange (42). Because the majority of pregnancy-associated HUS occurs postpartum, fetal loss is uncommon. Of the nine cases of antenatal HUS reviewed by Weiner, four were diagnosed on the day of delivery.

Relapses occur in approximately 30% of patients with idiopathic TTP (19,42,156,163,205). Most relapses occur within a few months of the initial episode. Bell found that 84% of relapses occurred within 1 month of diagnosis and 97% within 2 months (19), and Hayward found in a review of 52 cases over 12 years that 60% of relapses occurred within 2 months (42). However relapses may occasionally occur many years after initial diagnosis (156,205). Patients with TTP who are refractory to plasmapheresis in their initial presentation are at a high risk of death and often fail to respond to other therapies (42, 156,247,248). Permanent sequelae from TTP occur in a minority of patients. Neurologic sequelae have been seen in approximately 13% to 17% of survivors (42,156,248). Renal sequelae are probably less common. Rose found no permanent renal sequelae in 30 survivors of TTP (156), and Bell reported no residual organ damage in 98 survivors during 1 year of follow-up (19). However, Hayward reported that four of 48 adult survivors of HUS/TTP were dialysis dependent and five had mild renal impairment (42) .

The outcome in childhood HUS appears to fall into two distinct categories based on whether the child had typical *E. coli* O157:H7–associated HUS or atypical HUS. In typical childhood HUS, the outcome is generally good. The mortality rate in the past 10 years for typical childhood HUS has ranged from 0% to 8% (29,87,211,249). In contrast, atypical childhood HUS carries a mortality risk of 25% (20). Fitzpatrick recently reviewed 20 consecutive cases of atypical HUS seen over 20 years in London. Nine cases occurred before their adoption of plasma exchange for atypical HUS cases. Of these nine patients, there were four deaths (44%), two cases of residual end-stage renal disease, one case of residual nephropathy, and one relapsing case. In the group of 11 patients treated with plasma exchange, there were one late death (9%) and 10 relapses (20). In Fitzparick's series, 30% of children had neurologic involvement at presentation, and four (67%) of these children died, three in the acute phase and one during a relapse (20). Renaud et al. described the courses and outcomes of 42 consecutive children over the age of 3 years with childhood HUS in Paris over 35 years. In the 21 patients with atypical HUS, the mortality rate was 32% versus 10% in those with typical HUS. Residual nephropathy developed in 77% of survivors of atypical HUS versus 17% of those with typical HUS. Relapses occurred in 69% of patients with atypical HUS and 0% in those with typical HUS (151).

Long-term outcome in typical HUS is generally more favorable, but 17% to 39% experience long-term impairment; about 3% to 16% with end-state renal disease, 1% to 16% with chronic renal insufficiency, 0% to 20% with hypertension, 15% to 31% with proteinuria, and 2% to 28% with mild depressions of measured GFR (29,87,211,250). Some patients presented with decreased renal function after an asymptomatic interval of several years (29). Permanent neurologic sequalae was noted by Siegler (29) in only one of five children who experienced strokes in the acute phase of typical HUS in a long-term follow-up of 74 patients with typical childhood HUS.

Transplantation outcome in childhood HUS is good, with graft survival similar to that seen for other diseases (249,251–255). Graft survival appears higher if an interval of at least 1 year after HUS elapses before transplantation (249,252). Because of a concern about recurrent TMA in transplant patients after cyclosporine use, cyclosporine is often withheld from these patients (256,257). However, it is unclear whether the risk of recurrence of HUS exceeds the risk of graft failure without cyclosporine. A review of over 4,500 first renal grafts in the European Dialysis and Transplant Registry showed a low incidence of recurrence of HUS (258). Miller found that recurrence is more common in transplant recipients with atypical HUS than in those with typical childhood HUS (254), but overall graft survival was greater in transplant recipients treated with cyclosporine than in those not treated with cyclosporine (251,252).

Lifelong follow-up is certainly required in these patients. Patients with apparent full recovery may present with HTN, proteinuria, or progressive renal insufficiency 10 to 20 years after a single episode of childhood HUS (259). The reason for this is unclear but is thought to be due to progressive glomerulosclerosis after the loss of a significant percentage of functioning glomeruli during the acute phase of illness. Serum creatinine levels are poor indicators of mild levels of renal insufficiency. Therefore, creatinine-independent measures of renal function, such as iothalamate or DTPA (47,260), should be used to monitor these patients over time.

REFERENCES

1. Singer K, Bornstein F, Wile S. Thrombotic thrombocytopenic purpura. Hemorrhagic diathesis with generalized platelet thromboses. *Blood* 1947;2:542.
2. Baehr G, Klemperer P, Schifrin A. An acute febrile anemia and thrombocytopenic purpura with diffuse platelet thromboses of capillaries and arterioles. *Trans Assoc Am Physiol* 1936;51:43.
3. Symmers V. Thrombotic microangiopathic haemolytic anaemia (thrombotic microangiopathy). *Br Med J* 1952;2:897.
4. Gore I. Disseminted arteriolar and capillary platelet thrombosis: a morphologic study of its pathogenesis. *Am J Pathol* 1950;26: 155–167.
5. Ridolfi RL, Bell WR. Thrombotic thrombocytopenic purpura. Report of 25 cases and review of the literature. *Medicine (Balt)* 1981;60: 413–428.
6. Amorosi E, Ultman JE. Thrombotic thrombocytopenic purpura: report of 16 cases and review of the literature. *Medicine* 1966;45:139.
7. Gasser C, Gautier E, Steck A, Siebermann RE, Oescslin R. Hamolytischuramische Syndrome: Bilaterale Nierenrindennekrosen bie akuten erworbenen hamolytischen Anamien. *Schweiz Med Wochenschr* 1955;85:905–909.
8. Gianantonio CA, et al. The hemolytic-uremic syndrome. Renal status of 76 patients at long-term follow-up. *J Pediatr* 1968;72:757–65.
9. Habib R, Mathieu H, Royer P. Maladie thrombotique arteriole-capillaire du rein chez l'enfant. *Rev Fr Et Clin Biol* 1958;3:891–895.
10. Habib R. Pathology of the hemolytic uremic syndrome. In: Kaplan B, Trompeter J, Moake J, eds. *Hemolytic uremic syndrome and thrombotic thrombocytopenic purpura.* New York: Marcel Dekker; 1992: 315–353.
11. Moschcowitz E. Hyaline thrombosis of the terminal arterioles and capillaries: a hitherto undescribed disease. *Proc N Y Pathol Soc* 1924; 24:21–24.
12. Royer P, Habib R, Mathieu H. La microangiopathie thrombotique du rein chez l'enfant. *Ann Pediatr (Paris)* 1960;36:572–587.
13. Kaplan B, The hemolytic uremic syndromes (HUS). *AKF Nephrol Lett* 1992;9:29–36.
14. Griffin PM, et al. Illnesses associated with *Escherichia coli* 0157:H7 infections. A broad clinical spectrum. *Ann Intern Med* 1988;109: 705–12.
15. Griffin PM, Tauxe RV. The epidemiology of infections caused by *Escherichia coli* O157:H7, other enterohemorrhagic *E. coli*, and the associated hemolytic uremic syndrome. *Epidemiol Rev* 1991;13:60–98.
16. Kwaan HC. Clinicopathologic features of thrombotic thrombocytopenic purpura. *Semin Hematol* 1987;24:71–81.
17. Fitzpatrick MM, et al. Atypical (non–diarrhea-associated) hemolytic-uremic syndrome in childhood. *J Pediatr* 1993;122:532–537.
18. Gianviti A, et al. Haemolytic-uremic syndrome (HUS) in children: clinical features and outcome of cases positive and negative for verotoxin producing *E. coli* infection (VTEC) [Abstract]. *JASN* 1994; 5:393.
19. Bell WR, et al. Improved survival in thrombotic thrombocytopenic purpura–hemolytic uremic syndrome. Clinical experience in 108 patients. *N Engl J Med* 1991;325:398–403.
20. Fitzpatrick MM, et al. Atypical (non–diarrhea-associated) hemolytic-uremic syndrome in childhood. *J Pediatr* 1993;122:532–537.
21. Kovacs MJ, et al. Thrombotic thrombocytopenic purpura following hemorrhagic colitis due to *Escherichia coli* 0157:H7. *Am J Med* 1990; 88:177–179.
22. Tarr PI, et al. The increasing incidence of the hemolytic-uremic syndrome in King County, Washington: lack of evidence for ascertainment bias. *Am J Epidemiol* 1989;129:582–586.
23. Martin DL, et al. The epidemiology and clinical aspects of the hemolytic uremic syndrome in Minnesota. *N Engl J Med* 1990;323: 1161–1167.
24. British Paediatric Association–Communicable Disease Surveillance Centre surveillance of haemolytic uraemic syndrome 1983–4. *Br Med J Clin Res Ed* 1986;292:115–7.
25. Haemolytic uraemic syndrome. British paediatric surveillance unit/ CDSC surveillance scheme. *Commun Dis Rep Wkly Ed* 1990;21:1.
26. Van Weiringen PM, Monnens LAH, Schretlen EDAM. Haemolytic-uraemic syndrome. *Arch Dis Child* 1974;49:432–437.
27. Siegler RL. Spectrum of extrarenal involvement in postdiarrheal hemolytic-uremic syndrome. *J Pediatr* 1994;125:511–518.
28. Tarr PI, Hickman RO. Hemolytic uremic syndrome epidemiology: a population-based study in King County, Washington, 1971 to 1980. *Pediatrics* 1987;80:41–45.
29. Siegler RL, et al. A 20-year population-based study of postdiarrheal hemolytic uremic syndrome in Utah. *Pediatrics* 1994;94:35–40.
30. Rowe PC, et al. Epidemiology of hemolytic-uremic syndrome in Canadian children from 1986 to 1988. The Canadian Pediatric Kidney Disease Reference Centre. *J Pediatr* 1991;119:218–224.
31. Petitt RM. Thrombotic thrombocytopenic purpura: a thirty year review. *Semin Thromb Hemost* 1980;6:350–355.
32. Riley L, et al. Hemorrhagic colitis associated with a rare *Escherichia* serotype. *N Engl J Med* 1983;308:681–685.
33. Bell BP, et al. A multistate outbreak of *Escherichia coli* O157:H7–associated bloody diarrhea and hemolytic uremic syndrome from hamburgers. The Washington experience. *JAMA* 1994;272:1349–1353.
34. Ostroff SM, Kobayashi JM, Lewis JH. Infections with *Escherichia coli* O157:H7 in Washington State. The first year of statewide disease surveillance. *JAMA* 1989;262:355–359.
35. Report from the PHLS Communicable Disease Surveillance Centre. *Br Med J Clin Res Ed* 1987;295:1545–1546.
36. Belongia EA, et al. An outbreak of *Escherichia coli* O157:H7 colitis associated with consumption of precooked meat patties. *J Infect Dis* 1991;164:338–343.
37. Spika JS, et al. Hemolytic uremic syndrome and diarrhea associated with *Escherichia coli* 0157:H7 in a day care center. *J Pediatr* 1986; 109:287–291.
38. Swerdlow DL, et al. A waterborne outbreak in Missouri of *Escherichia coli* O157:H7 associated with bloody diarrhea and death. *Ann Intern Med* 1992;117:812–819.
39. Carter AO, et al. A severe outbreak of *Escherichia coli* O157:H7–associated hemorrhagic colitis in a nursing home. *N Engl J Med* 1987; 317:1496–1500.
40. Salmon L, Smith R. How common is *Escherichia coli* O157 and where is it coming from? Total population surveillance in Wales 1990–1993 [Abstract]. Presented at VTEC 94: 2nd international symposium and workshop on verocytotoxin (shiga-like toxin)–producing *Escherichia coli* infections, 1994, Bergamo, Italy.
41. Rowe P, et al. Collaborative cohort study of the risk of HUS after *E. coli* O157:H7 infection. Presented at the 2nd international symposium and workshop on Verocytotoxin (Shiga-like toxin)–producing *Escherichia coli* infections, 1994, Bergamo, Italy.
42. Hayward CP, et al. Treatment outcomes in patients with adult thrombotic thrombocytopenic purpura–hemolytic uremic syndrome. *Arch Intern Med* 1994;154:982–987.
43. Thompson CE, et al. Thrombotic microangiopathies in the 1980s: clinical features, response to treatment, and the impact of the human response to treatment, and the impact of the human immunodeficiency virus epidemic. *Blood* 1992;80:1890–1895.

44. Rock GA, et al. Comparison of plasma exchange with plasma infusion in the treatment of thrombotic thrombocytopenic purpura. Canadian Apheresis Study Group. *N Engl J Med* 1991;325:393–397.
45. Jernigan SM, Waldo FB. Racial incidence of hemolytic uremic syndrome. *Pediatr Nephrol* 1994;8:545–547.
46. Kibel MA, Barnard PJ. The haemolytic-uraemic syndrome: a surveyin South Africa. *South Afr Med J* 1968;42:692–698.
47. Brandt JR, et al. *Escherichia coli* O 157:H7–associated hemolytic uremic syndrome after ingestion of contaminated hamburgers. *J Pediatr* 1994;125:519–526.
48. Rogers MF, et al. Hemolytic-uremic syndrome—an outbreak in Sacramento, California. *West J Med* 1986;144:169–173.
49. Kennedy SS, Zacharski LR, Beck JR. Thrombotic thrombocytopenic purpura: analysis of 48 unselected cases. *Semin Thromb Hemost* 1980;6:341–349.
50. Shepard K, et al. Thrombotic thrombocytopenic purpura treated with plasma exchange or exchange transfusions. *West J Med* 1991;154: 410–413.
51. MacDonald K, et al. *Escherichia coli* O157:H7, an emerging gastrointestinal pathogen. *JAMA* 1988;259:3567–3570.
52. Pai C, et al. Epidemiology of sporadic diarrhea due to verocytotoxin-producing *Escherichia coli*; a two year prospective study. *J Infect Dis* 1988;157:1054–1057.
53. Remuzzi G, et al. Thrombotic thrombocytopenic purpura—a deficiency of plasma factors regulating platelet–vessel–wall interaction? [Letter]. *N Engl J Med* 1978;299:311.
54. Weiner CP. Thrombotic microangiopathy in pregnancy and the postpartum period. *Semin Hematol* 1987;24:119–129.
55. Shigematsu H, et al. Mesangial involvement in hemolytic-uremic syndrome. A light and electron microscopic study. *Am J Pathol* 1976; 85:349–362.
56. Heptinstall R. Hemolytic uremic syndrome, thrombotic thrombocytopenic purpura, and systemic sclerosis (systemic scleroderma). In: Heptinstall R, ed. *Pathology of the kidney*. Boston: Little, Brown; 1992:1163–1233.
57. Gonzalo A, et al. Hemolytic uremic syndrome with hypocomplementemia and deposits of IgM and C3 in the involved renal tissue. *Clin Nephrol* 1981;16:193–199.
58. McCoy RC, Abramowsky CR, Krueger R. The hemolytic uremic syndrome, with positive immunofluorescence studies. *J Pediatr* 1974;85: 170–174.
59. Argyle JC, et al. A clinicopathological study of 24 children with hemolytic uremic syndrome. A report of the Southwest Pediatric Nephrology Study Group. *Pediatr Nephrol* 1990;4:52–58.
60. Gianantonio CA, et al. The hemolytic-uremic syndrome. *Nephron* 1973;11:174–192.
61. Loirat C, et al. Hemolytic-uremic syndrome in the child. *Adv Nephrol Necker Hosp* 1993;22:141–168.
62. Inninger R, de Oliveira V, Bohle A. Correlation of structure and function in haemolytic uraemic syndrome. In: *Xth International Congress of Nephrology*. London: Alden Press; 1987.
63. Orbison JL. Morphology of thrombotic thrombocytopenic purpura with demonstrations of aneurysms. *Am J Pathol* 1952;28:129.
64. Macwhinney JBJ, et al. Thrombotic thrombocytopenic purpura in childhood. *Blood* 1962;19:181.
65. Feldman JD, et al. The vascular pathology of thrombotic thrombocytopenic purpura. An immunohistochemical and ultrastructural study. *Lab Invest* 1966;15:927–946.
66. Neame PB, et al. Thrombotic thrombocytopenic purpura: report of a case with disseminated intravascular platelet aggregation. *Blood* 1973;42:805–814.
67. Saracco SM, Farhi DC. Splenic pathology in thrombotic thrombocytopenic purpura. *Am J Surg Pathol* 1990;14:223–229.
68. Berkowitz LR, Dalldorf FG, Blatt PM. Thrombotic thrombocytopenic purpura: a pathology review. *JAMA* 1979;241:1709–1710.
69. Kwaan HC. The pathogenesis of thrombotic thrombocytopenic purpura. *Semin Thromb Hemost* 1979;5:184–198.
70. Obrig TG, et al. Direct cytotoxic action of Shiga toxin on human vascular endothelial cells. *Infect Immun* 1988;56:2373–2378.
71. Taylor CM, et al. The expression of blood group P1 in post-enteropathic haemolytic uraemic syndrome. *Pediatr Nephrol* 1990;4:59–61.
72. Milford DV, Taylor CM. New insights into the haemolytic uraemic syndromes. *Arch Dis Child* 1990;65:713–715.
73. Richardson SE, et al. Experimental verocytotoxemia in rabbits. *Infect Immun* 1992;60:4154–4167.
74. Zoja C, et al. Verotoxin glycolipid receptors determine the localization of microangiopathic process in rabbits given verotoxin-1. *J Lab Clin Med* 1992;120:229–238.
75. Obrig TG, et al. Endothelial heterogeneity in Shiga toxin receptors and responses. *J Biol Chem* 1993;268:15484–15488.
76. Van de Kar NC, Monnens LA, Van Hinsbergh VW. Tumor necrosis factor and interleukin 1 induced expression of the glycolipid verotoxin receptor in human endothelial cells. Implications for the pathogenesis of the haemolytic uraemic syndrome. *Behring Inst Mitt* 1993; 93:202–209.
77. Boyd B, Lingwood C. Verotoxin receptor glycolipid in human renal tissue [erratum *Nephron* 1989;51:582]. *Nephron* 1989;51:207–210.
78. Bitzan M, et al. Evidence that verotoxins (Shiga-like toxins) from *Escherichia coli* bind to P blood group antigens of human erythrocytes in vitro. *Infect Immun* 1994;62:3337–3347.
79. Moake JL. Haemolytic-uraemic syndrome: basic science. *Lancet* 1994;343:393–397.
80. Feld L, et al. Pneumococcal pneumonia and hemolytic uremic syndrome. *Pediatr Infect Dis* 1987;6:693–695.
81. McGraw M, et al. Haemolytic uraemic syndrome and the Thomsen Freidenreich antigen. *Pediatr Nephrol* 1989;3:135–139.
82. Novak RW, Martin CR, Orsini EN. Hemolytic-uremic syndrome and T-cryptantigen exposure by neuraminidase-producing pneumococci: an emerging problem? *Pediatr Pathol* 1983;1:409–413.
83. Myers KA, Marrie TJ. Thrombotic microangiopathy associated with *Streptococcus pneumoniae* bacteremia: case report and review. *Clin Infect Dis* 1993;17:1037–1040.
84. Poschmann A, et al. [Neuraminidase induced hemolytic anemia. Experimental and clinical observations (author's translation)]. *Monatsschr Kinderheilkd* 1976;124:15–24.
85. Eber SW, et al. [Hemolytic-uremic syndrome in pneumococcal meningitis and infection. Importance of T-transformation (translation)]. *Monatsschr Kinderheilkd* 1993;141:219–222.
86. Erickson LC, et al. *Streptococcus pneumoniae*–induced hemolytic uremic syndrome: a case for early diagnosis. *Pediatr Nephrol* 1994;8: 211–213.
87. Coad NA, et al. Changes in the postenteropathic form of the hemolytic uremic syndrome in children. *Clin Nephrol* 1991;35:10–16.
88. Fitzpatrick MM, Dillon MJ. Current views on aetiology and management of haemolytic uraemic syndrome. *Postgrad Med J* 1991;67: 707–709.
89. Milford DV, et al. Prognostic markers in diarrhoea-associated haemolytic-uraemic syndrome: initial neutrophil count, human neutrophil elastase and von Willebrand factor antigen. *Nephrol Dial Transplant* 1991;6:232–237.
90. Walters MD, et al. The polymorphonuclear leucocyte count in childhood haemolytic uraemic syndrome. *Pediatr Nephrol* 1989;3:130–134.
91. Forsyth KD, et al. Neutrophil-mediated endothelial injury in haemolytic uraemic syndrome. *Lancet* 1989;2:411–414.
92. Fitzpatrick MM, et al. Interleukin-8 and polymorphoneutrophil leucocyte activation in hemolytic uremic syndrome of childhood. *Kidney Int* 1992;42:951–956.
93. Fitzpatrick MM, et al. Neutrophil activation in the haemolytic uraemic syndrome: free and complexed elastase in plasma. *Pediatr Nephrol* 1992;6:50–53.
94. Milford D, et al. Neutrophil elastases and haemolytic uraemic syndrome [Letter]. *Lancet* 1989;2:1153.
95. Leung DY, et al. Lytic anti-endothelial cell antibodies in haemolytic-uraemic syndrome. *Lancet* 1988;2:183–186.
96. Foster PA, Anderson JC. Effects of plasma from patients with thrombotic thrombocytopenic purpura (TTP) on cultured human endothelial cells. *Blood* 1979;54:240a.
97. Burns ER, Zucker FD. Pathologic effects of plasma from patients with thrombotic thrombocytopenic purpura on platelets and cultured vascular endothelial cells. *Blood* 1982;60:1030–1037.
98. Gottschall JL, et al. Quinine-induced immune thrombocytopenia associated with hemolytic uremic syndrome: a new clinical entity. *Blood* 1991;77:306–310.
99. Stroncek DF, et al. Characterization of multiple quinine-dependent antibodies in a patient with episodic hemolytic uremic syndrome and immune agranulocytosis. *Blood* 1992;80:241–248.

100. Neahring BJ, et al. Anti-endothelial cell (EC) antibodies in plasma of patients with quinine-induced hemolytic uremic syndrome (HUS) [Abstract]. *Blood* 1992;80:53.
101. Robson WL, et al. The use of intravenous gammaglobulin in the treatment of typical hemolytic uremic syndrome. *Pediatr Nephrol* 1991;5: 289–292.
102. Durand JM, et al. Ineffectiveness of high-dose intravenous gammaglobulin infusion in thrombotic thrombocytopenic purpura [Letter]. *Am J Hematol* 1993;42:234.
103. Kondo H. Effect of intravenous gammaglobulin infusion on recurrent episodes of thrombotic thrombocytopenic purpura (TTP) [Letter]. *Eur J Haematol* 1993;50:55–56.
104. Moncada S. Prostacyclin and thromboxane A2 in the regulation of platelet–vascular interactions In: Remuzzi G, Mecca G, de Gaetano G, eds. *Hemostasis, prostaglandins, and renal disease*. New York: Raven; 1980:175–180.
105. French J. Atherosclerosis in relation to the structure and function of the arterial intima, with special reference to the endothelium. *Rev Exp Pathol* 1966;5:253–353.
106. Remuzzi G, et al. Familial deficiency of a plasma factor stimulating prostacyclin activity. *Thromb Res* 1979;16:517–525.
107. Turi S, et al. Disturbances of prostacyclin metabolism with hemolytic uremic syndrome in first degree relatives. *Clin Nephrol* 1986;25: 193–198.
108. Wu KK, et al. Serum prostacyclin binding defects in thrombotic thrombocytopenic purpura. *J Clin Invest* 1985;75:168–174.
109. Machin SJ, et al. A plasma factor inhibiting prostacyclin-like activity in thrombotic thrombocytopenic purpura. *Acta Haematol* 1982;67: 8–12.
110. Chen YC, et al. Accelerated prostacyclin degradation in the thrombotic thrombocytopenic purpura. *Lancet* 1981;2:267–269.
111. Noris M, et al. Renal prostacyclin biosynthesis is reduced in children with hemolytic-uremic syndrome in the context of systemic platelet activation. *Am J Kidney Dis* 1992;20:144–149.
112. Stuart M, Spitzer R, Coppe D. Prostanoids in hemolytic uremic syndrome. *J Pediatr* 1985;106:936–939.
113. Hautekeete ML, et al. 6-keto-PGF1 alpha levels and prostacyclin therapy in 2 adult patients with hemolytic-uremic syndrome. *Clin Nephrol* 1986;26:157–159.
114. Jorgensen KA, Pedersen RS. Familial deficiency of prostacyclin production stimulating factor in the hemolytic uremic syndrome of childhood. *Thromb Res* 1981;21:311–315.
115. Wiles PG, et al. Inherited plasma factor deficiency in haemolytic-uraemic syndrome [Letter]. *Lancet* 1981;1:1105–1106.
116. Remuzzi G, et al. Haemolytic-uraemic syndrome: deficiency of plasma factor(s) regulating prostacyclin activity? *Lancet* 1978;2: 871–872.
117. Rizzoni G, et al. Plasma infusion for hemolytic-uremic syndrome in children: results of a multicenter controlled trial. *J Pediatr* 1988;112: 284–290.
118. Schlegel N, et al. Childhood hemolytic uremic syndrome. Absence of deficiency of plasma prostacyclin stimulating activity. *J Pediatr* 1987;111:71–77.
119. Karch H, et al. Purified verotoxin of *Escherichia coli* O157:H7 decreases prostacyclin synthesis by endothelial cells. *Microb Pathogen* 1988;5:2373–2378.
120. Budd GT, et al. Prostacyclin therapy of thrombotic thrombocytopenic purpura [Letter]. *Lancet* 1980;2:915.
121. Johnson JE, et al. Ineffective epoprostenol therapy for thrombotic thrombocytopenic purpura. JAMA 1983;250:3089–3091.
122. Loirat C, et al. Treatment of the childhood haemolytic uraemic syndrome with plasma. A multicentre randomized controlled trial. The French Society of Paediatric Nephrology. *Pediatr Nephrol* 1988;2: 279–285.
123. Katz J, et al. Platelet, erythrocyte, and fibrinogen kinetics in the hemolytic uremic syndrome of infancy. *J Pediatr* 1973;83:739–748.
124. Berberich FR, et al. Thrombotic thrombocytopenic purpura. Three cases with platelet and fibrinogen survival studies. *J Pediatr* 1974;84: 503–509.
125. Fong JS, Kaplan BS. Impairment of platelet aggregation in hemolytic uremic syndrome: evidence for platelet "exhaustion." *Blood* 1982;60: 564–570.
126. Walters MD, et al. Intravascular platelet activation in the hemolytic uremic syndrome. *Kidney Int* 1988;33:107–115.
127. Lian EC, et al. Presence of a platelet aggregating factor in the plasma of patients with thrombotic thrombocytopenic purpura (TTP) and its inhibition by normal plasma. *Blood* 1979;53:333–338.
128. Hoyer L. The factor VIII complex: structure and function. *Blood* 1981;58:1–13.
129. Moake JL, et al. Unusually large plasma factor VIII:von Willebrand factor multimers in chronic relapsing thrombotic thrombocytopenic purpura. *N Engl J Med* 1982;307:1432–1435.
130. Rowe JM, et al. Thrombotic thrombocytopenic purpura: recovery after splenectomy associated with persistence of abnormally large von Willebrand factor multimers. *Am J Hematol* 1985;20:161–168.
131. Rose PE, et al. Abnormalities of factor VIII related protein multimers in the haemolytic uraemic syndrome. *Arch Dis Child* 1984;59: 1135–1140.
132. Moake JL, et al. Abnormal VIII: von Willebrand factor patterns in the plasma of patients with the hemolytic-uremic syndrome. *Blood* 1984; 64:592–598.
133. Miura M, et al. Efficacy of several plasma components in a boy with chronic relapsing thrombocytopenia and hemolytic anemia who responds repeatedly to normal plamsa infusions. *Am J Hematol* 1984; 17:307–319.
134. Lian EC. Pathogenesis of thrombotic thrombocytopenic purpura. *Semin Hematol* 1987;24:82–100.
135. Lian E, Siddiqui F. Investigation of the role of von Willebrand factor in thrompocytopenic purpura. *Blood* 1986;66:1219–1221.
136. Rose PE, et al. Factor VIII von Willebrand protein in haemolytic uraemic syndrome and systemic vasculitides. Lancet 1990;335: 500–502.
137. Heimsworth M, Sherbotie J, Kaplan B. Abnormal factor VIII: von willebrand (VIII:Wb) multimers in patients with hemolytic uremic syndrome (HUS) or thrombotic thrombocytopenic purpura (TTP) may predict thrombotic episodes [Abstract]. *Pediatr Nephrol* 1989;3: C182.
138. Hamberg M, et al. Isolation and structure of two prostaglandin endoperoxidases that cause platelet aggregation. *Proc Natl Acad Sci U S A* 1971;66:1231–1234.
139. Tonshoff B, et al. Increased thromboxane biosynthesis in childhood hemolytic uremic syndrome. *Kidney Int* 1990;37:1134–1141.
140. Harker LA, Slichter SJ. Platelet and fibrinogen consumption in man. *N Engl J Med* 1972;287:999–1005.
141. Kwaan HC. Role of fibrinolysis in thrombotic thrombocytopenic purpura. *Semin Hematol* 1987;24:101–109.
142. Bergstein JM, Riley M, Bang NU. Role of plasminogen-activator inhibitor type 1 in the pathogenesis and outcome of the hemolytic uremic syndrome. *N Engl J Med* 1992;327:755–759.
143. Glas GP, et al. Fibrinolysis in health and disease: abnormal levels of plasminogen activator, plasminogen activator inhibitor, and protein C in thrombotic thrombocytopenic purpura. *J Lab Clin Med* 1986;108: 415–422.
144. Brandt J, Kennedy M, Senhauser D. Platelet aggregating factor in thrombotic thrombocytopenic purpura. *Lancet* 1979;2:463–464.
145. Bukowski RM, King JW, Hewlett JS. Plasmapheresis in the treatment of thrombotic thrombocytopenic purpura. *Blood* 1977;50:413–417.
146. Loirat C, et al. Platelet aggregating activity in hemolytic uremic syndrome [Abstract]. *Pediatr Nephrol* 1989;3:C182.
147. Monnens L, et al. Platelet aggregating factor in the epidemic form of hemolytic-uremic syndrome in childhood. *Clin Nephrol* 1985;24: 135–137.
148. Robson WL, Leung AK, Kaplan BS, Hemolytic-uremic syndrome. *Curr Probl Pediatr* 1993;23:16–33.
149. Upadhyaya K, et al. The importance of nonrenal involvement in hemolytic-uremic syndrome. *Pediatrics* 1980;65:115–120.
150. Neild GH. Haemolytic-uraemic syndrome in practice [erratum *Lancet* 1994;343:552]. *Lancet* 1994;343:398–401.
151. Renaud C, et al. Haemolytic uraemic syndrome: prognostic factors in children over 3 years of age. *Pediatr Nephrol* 1995;9:24–29.
152. Proesmans W, et al. Plasma renin activity in haemolytic uraemic syndrome. *Pediatr Nephrol* 1994;8:444–446.
153. Grunfeld B, et al. Systemic hypertension and plasma renin activity in children with the hemolytic-uremic syndrome. *Int J Pediatr Nephrol* 1982;3:211–214.
154. Habib R, Gagnadoux MF, Broyer M. [Hemolytic-uremic syndrome in children and arterial hypertension (translation)]. *Arch Mal Coeur Vaiss* 1981;73:37–43.

155. Powell HR, et al. Plasma renin activity in acute poststreptococcal glomerulonephritis and the haemolytic-uraemic syndrome. *Arch Dis Child* 1974;49:802–807.
156. Rose M, Eldor A. High incidence of relapses in thrombotic thrombocytopenic purpura. Clinical study of 38 patients. *Am J Med* 1987;83: 437–444.
157. Cuttner J. Thrombotic thrombocytopenic purpura: a ten-year experience. *Blood* 1980;56:302–306.
158. Myers TJ. Treatment of thrombotic thrombocytopenic purpura with combined exchange plasmapheresis and anti-platelet agents. *Semin Thromb Hemost* 1981;7:37–42.
159. Rock G, et al. Thrombotic thrombocytopenic purpura: outcome in 24 patients with renal impairment treated with plasma exchange. Canadian Apheresis Study Group. *Transfusion* 1992;32:710–714.
160. Shepard KV, et al. Thrombotic thrombocytopenic purpura treated with plasma exchange or exchange transfusions. *West J Med* 1991; 154:410–413.
161. Silverstein A. Thrombotic thrombocytopenic purpura. The initial neurologic manifestations. *Arch Neurol* 1968;18:358–362.
162. O'Brien JL, Sibley WA. Neurological manifestations of thrombotic thrombocytopenia purpura. *Neurology* 1958;8:55–63.
163. Taft EG. Advances in the treatment of TTP. *Prog Clin Biol Res* 1990; 337:151–155.
164. Tapper D, et al. Lessons learned in the management of hemolytic uremic syndrome in children. *J Pediatr Surg* 1995;30:158–163.
165. Pritchard J, et al. Intravascular hemolysis, thrombocytopenia, and other hematolgic abnormalities associated with severe toxemia of pregnancy. *N Engl J Med* 1954;250:89–98.
166. Krane N. Acute renal failure in pregnancy. *Arch Intern Med* 1988; 148:2347–2357.
167. Saltiel C, et al. Hemolytic uremic syndrome in association with pregnancy. In: Kaplan B, Trompeter R, Moake J, eds. *Hemolytic uremic syndrome and thrombotic thrombocytopenia purpura*. New York: Marcel Dekker; 1992:241–254.
168. Alexopoulos E, et al. Acute renal failure in pregnancy. *Renal Failure* 1993;15:609–613.
169. Chugh KS, et al. Acute renal cortical necrosis—a study of 113 patients. *Renal Failure* 1994;16:37–47.
170. Grunfeld JP, Pertuiset N. Acute renal failure in pregnancy: 1987. *Am J Kidney Dis* 1987;9:359–362.
171. McCrae K, Samuels P, Schreiber A. Pregnancy-associated thrombocytopenia: pathogenesis and management. *J Am Soc Hematol* 1992; 80:2697–2714.
172. Byrnes JJ, Moake JL. Thrombotic thrombocytopenic purpura and the haemolytic-uraemic syndrome: evolving concepts of pathogenesis and therapy. *Clin Haematol* 1986;15:413–442.
173. Weiner C. The clinical spectrum of preeclampsia. *Am J Kidney Dis* 1987;9:312–316.
174. Coratelli P, Buongiorno E, Passavanti G. Endotoxemia in hemolytic uremic syndrome. *Nephron* 1988;50:365–367.
175. Bollaert PE, et al. Hemorrhagic colitis with *Streptococcus pyogenes* preceding hemolytic uremic syndrome during early pregnancy [Letter]. *Nephron* 1989;52:103–104.
176. Steele BT, et al. Post-partum haemolytic-uremic syndrome and verotoxin-producing *Escherichia coli* [Letter]. *Lancet* 1984;1:511.
177. Churg J, et al. Hemolytic uremic syndrome as a cause of postpartum renal failure. *Am J Obstet Gynecol* 1970;108:253–261.
178. Kniaz D, et al. Postpartum hemolytic uremic syndrome associated with antiphospholipid antibodies. A case report and review of the literature. *Am J Nephrol* 1992;12:126–133.
179. Stratta P, et al. Postpartum hemolytic uremic syndrome (HUS) following beta-orthoestradiol benzoate and dimethylergonovine therapies. *Biol Res Pregnancy* 1986;7:171–175.
180. Wiznitzer A, et al. Familial occurrence of thrombotic thrombocytopenia purpura in two sisters during pregnancy. *Am J Obstet Gynecol* 1992;166:20.
181. Pirson Y, et al. Hemolytic uremic syndrome in three adult siblings: a familial study and evolution. *Clin Nephrol* 1987;28:250–255.
182. Fuchs WE, et al. Thrombotic thrombocytopenic purpura. Occurrence two years apart during late pregnancy in two sisters. *JAMA* 1976;235: 2126–2127.
183. Bergstein J, et al. Hemolytic-uremic syndrome in adult sisters. *Transplantation* 1974;17:487–490.
184. Alqadah F, Zebeib MA, Awidi AS. Thrombotic thrombocytopenic purpura associated with pregnancy in two sisters. *Postgrad Med J* 1993;69:229–231.
185. Jacobs P, Dubovsky DW. Haemolytic-uraemic syndrome during the first trimester of pregnancy. Case report. *Br J Obstet Gynaecol* 1983; 90:578–580.
186. Nissenson AR, Krumlovsky FA, del Greco F. Postpartum hemolytic uremic syndrome. Late recovery after prolonged maintenance dialysis. *JAMA* 1979;242:173–175.
187. Judlin P, et al. [Uremic-hemolytic syndrome occurring in extra-uterine pregnancy. Apropos of a case]. *Rev Fr Gynecol Obstet* 1988;83: 557–559.
188. Creasy GW, Morgan J. Hemolytic uremic syndrome after ectopic pregnancy: postectopic nephrosclerosis. *Obstet Gynecol* 1987;69: 448–449.
189. Spargo B, McCartney CP, Winemuller R. Glomerular capillary endotheliosis in toxemia of pregnancy. *Arch Pathol Lab Med* 1959;68: 593–599.
190. Murgo A. Thrombotic microangiopathy in the cancer patient including those induced by chemotherapuetic agents. *Semin Hematol* 1987; 24:161–177.
191. Rietschel RL, et al. Skin lesions in paroxysmal nocturnal hemoglobinuria. *Arch Dermatol* 1978;114:560–563.
192. Kletzel M, Arnold WC, Berry DH. Paroxysmal nocturnal hemoglobinuria presenting as recurrent hemolytic uremic syndrome. *Clin Pediatr Phila* 1987;26:319–320.
193. Niklasson BS. Haemorrhagic fever with renal syndrome, virological and epidemiological aspects. *Pediatr Nephrol* 1992;6:201–204.
194. Vitacco M, Sanchez AJ, Gianantonio CA. Heparin therapy in the hemolytic-uremic syndrome. *J Pediatr* 1973;83:271–275.
195. Proesmans W, et al. Antithrombolytic therapy in childhood haemolytic uraemic syndrome: a randomized prospective study. In: *Sixth international symposium of paediatric nephrology*. Hannover, Germany: Springer-Verlag; 1984.
196. Loirat C, et al. [Treatment of childhood hemolytic-uremic syndrome with urokinase. Cooperative controlled trial (translation)]. *Arch Fr Pediatr* 1984;41:15–19.
197. Van Damme-Lombaerts R, et al. Heparin plus dipyridamole in childhood hemolytic-uremic syndrome: a randomized prospective study. *J Pediatr* 1988;113:913–918.
198. Monnens L, et al. Treatment of the hemolytic-uremic syndrome. Comparison of the results of heparin treatment with the results of streptokinase treatment. *Helv Paediatr Acta* 1978;33:321–328.
199. Sheth KJ, Gill JC, Leichter HE, High-dose intravenous gamma globulin infusions in hemolytic-uremic syndrome: a preliminary report. *Am J Dis Child* 1990;144:268–270.
200. Wong P, Itoh K, Yoshida S. Treatment of thrombotic thrombocytopenic purpura with intravenous gamma globulin [Letter]. *N Engl J Med* 1986;314;385–386.
201. Byrnes JJ, Khurana M. Treatment of thrombotic thrombocytopenic purpura with plasma. *N Engl J Med* 1977;297:1386–1389.
202. Roberts AW, Gillett EA, Fleming SJ. Hemolytic uremic syndrome/thrombotic thrombocytopenic purpura: outcome with plasma exchange. *J Clin Apheresis* 1991;6:150–154.
203. Vianelli N, et al. Prompt plasma-exchange treatment and coma reversibility in two patients with thrombotic thrombocytopenic purpura. *Haematologica* 1991;76:72–74.
204. Pisciotto P, et al. Treatment of thrombotic thrombocytopenic purpura. Evaluation of plasma exchange and review of the literature. *Vox Sang* 1983;45:185–196.
205. Onundarson PT, et al. Response to plasma exchange and splenectomy in thrombotic thrombocytopenic purpura. A 10-year experience at a single institution. *Arch Intern Med* 1992;152:791–796.
206. Blitzer JB, et al. Thrombotic thrombocytopenic purpura: treatment with plasmapheresis. *Am J Hematol* 1987;24:329–339.
207. George J, El Harake M. Thrombocytopenia due to enhanced platelet destruction by nonimmunologic mechanisms. In: Beutler, et al., eds. *Williams hematology*. New York: McGraw-Hill; 1995:1290–1315.
208. Bell W. Thrombotic thrombocytopenic purpura [Clinical Conference]. *JAMA* 1991;265:91–93.
209. Gianviti A, et al. Plasma exchange in children with hemolytic-uremic syndrome at risk of poor outcome. *Am J Kidney Dis* 1993;22:264–266.
210. Milford DV, White RH, Taylor CM. Prognostic significance of proteinuria one year after onset of diarrhea-associated hemolytic-uremic syndrome. *J Pediatr* 1991;118:191–194.

211. Fitzpatrick MM, et al. Long term renal outcome of childhood haemolytic uraemic syndrome. *Br Med J* 1991;303:489–492.
212. Feldhoff CM, et al. Plasma exchanges in frequently recurrent hemolytic-uremic syndrome in a child. *Int J Pediatr Nephrol* 1983;4: 239–242.
213. Misiani R, et al. Haemolytic uraemic syndrome: therapeutic effect of plasma infusion. *Br Med J Clin Res Ed* 1982;285:1304–1306.
214. Venkat KK, et al. Reversal of cyclosporine-associated hemolytic-uremic syndrome by plasma exchange with fresh-frozen plasma replacement in renal transplant recipients. *Transplant Proc* 1991; 23:1256–1257.
215. Brichard B, et al. Plasma infusion as treatment for 33 children with haemolytic uraemic syndrome: a good therapy? *Acta Clin Belg* 1993; 48:156–163.
216. Bukowski RM, et al. Therapy of thrombotic thrombocytopenic purpura: an overview. *Semin Thromb Hemost* 1981;7:1–8.
217. Lieberman E. Hemolytic-uremic syndrome. *J Pediatr* 1972;80:1–16.
218. Birgens H, Ernst P, Hansen MS. Thrombotic thrombocytopenic purpura: treatment with a combination of antiplatelet drugs. *Acta Med Scand* 1979;205:437–439.
219. Gundlach WJ, Tarnasky R. Thrombotic thrombocytopenic purpura. Remission following treatment with aspirin and dipyridamole. *Minn Med* 1977;60:20–21.
220. Marmont AM, et al. Thrombotic thrombocytopenic purpura successfully treated with a combination of dipyridamole and aspirin. *Haematologica* 1980;65:222–231.
221. Ponticelli C, et al. Hemolytic uremic syndrome in adults. *Arch Intern Med* 1980;140:353–357.
222. del Zoppo GJ, et al. Antiplatelet therapy in thrombotic thrombocytopenic purpura. *Semin Hematol* 1987;24:130–139.
223. Zacharski LR, Walworth C, McIntyre OR, Antiplatelet therapy for thrombotic thrombocytopenic purpura. *N Engl J Med* 1971;285: 408–409.
224. Tardy B, et al. Intravenous prostacyclin in thrombotic thrombocytopenic purpura: case report and review of the literature. *J Intern Med* 1991;230:279–282.
225. Fitzgerald GA, et al. Intravenous prostacyclin in thrombotic thrombocytopenic purpura. *Ann Intern Med* 1981;95:319–322.
226. Hensby CN, et al. Prostacyclin deficiency in thrombotic thrombocytopenic purpura [Letter]. *Lancet* 1979;2:748.
227. O'Regan S, et al. Aspirin and dipyridamole therapy in the hemolytic-uremic syndrome. *J Pediatr* 1980;97:473–476.
228. Arenson EBJ, August CS. Preliminary report: treatment of the hemolytic-uremic syndrome with aspirin and dipyridamole. *J Pediatr* 1975;86:957–961.
229. Beattie TJ, et al. Plasmapheresis in the haemolytic-uraemic syndrome in children. *Br Med J Clin Res Ed* 1981;282:1667–1668.
230. Defreyn G, et al. Abnormal prostacyclin metabolism in the hemolytic uremic syndrome: equivocal effect of prostacyclin infusions. *Clin Nephrol* 1982;18:43–49.
231. Chin D, et al. Treatment of thrombotic thrombocytopenic purpura with intravenous gammaglobulin [Letter]. *Transfusion* 1987;27:115–116.
232. Finn NG, Wang JC, Hong KJ. High-dose intravenous gamma-immunoglobulin infusion in the treatment of thrombotic thrombocytopenic purpura. *Arch Intern Med* 1987;147:2165–2167.
233. Kolodziej M. Case report: high-dose intravenous immunoglobulin as therapy for thrombotic thrombocytopenic purpura. *Am J Med Sci* 1993;305:101–102.
234. Raniele DP, Opsahl JA, Kjellstrand CM. Should intravenous immunoglobulin G be first-line treatment for acute thrombotic thrombocytopenic purpura? Case report and review of the literature. *Am J Kidney Dis* 1991;18:264–268.
235. Lian EC, et al. Inhibition of platelet-aggregating activity in thrombotic thrombocytopenic purpura plasma by normal adult immunoglobulin G. *J Clin Invest* 1984;73:548–555.
236. Viero P, et al. Thrombotic thrombocytopenic purpura and high-dose immunoglobulin treatment [Letter]. *Ann Intern Med* 1986;104:282.
237. Levin M, Grunwald HW. Use of vincristine in refractory thrombotic thrombocytopenic purpura. *Acta Haematol* 1991;85:37–40.
238. Welborn JL, Emrick P, Acevedo M. Rapid improvement of thrombotic thrombocytopenic purpura with vincristine and plasmapheresis. *Am J Hematol* 1990;35:18–21.
239. O'Connor NT, Bruce JP, Hill LF. Vincristine therapy for thrombotic thrombocytopenic purpura. *Am J Hematol* 1992;39:234–236.
240. Rutkow IM. Thrombotic thrombocytopenic purpura (TTP) and splenectomy: a current appraisal. *Ann Surg* 1978;188:701–705.
241. Reynolds PM, et al. Thrombotic thrombocytopenic purpura-remission following splenectomy. Report of a case and review of the literature. *Am J Med* 1976;61:439–447.
242. Liu ET, Linker CA, Shuman MA. Management of treatment failures in thrombotic thrombocytopenic purpura. *Am J Hematol* 1986;23: 347–361.
243. Harkness DR, et al. Hazard of platelet transfusion in thrombotic thrombocytopenic purpura. *JAMA* 1981;246:1931–1933.
244. Trompeter RS, et al. Haemolytic-uraemic syndrome: an analysis of prognostic features. *Arch Dis Child* 1983;58:101–105.
245. Kaplan BS, et al. An analysis of the results of therapy in 67 cases of the hemolytic-uremic syndrome. *J Pediatr* 1971;78:420–425.
246. Knupp CL. Thrombotic thrombocytopenic purpura in older patients. *J Am Geriatr Soc* 1988;36:331–338.
247. McCarthy L, Kotylo P, Lister K. Plasma exchange and thrombotic thrombocytopenic purpura, the Indiana University Medical Center experience. *Prog Clin Biol Res* 1990;337:115–117.
248. Ben YD, et al. Permanent neurological complications in patients with thrombotic thrombocytopenic purpura. *Am J Hematol* 1988;29: 74–78.
249. Gagnadoux MF, Habib R, Broyer M. Outcome of renal transplantation in 34 cases of childhood hemolytic-uremic syndrome and the role of cyclosporine. *Transplant Proc* 1994;26:269–270.
250. Gagnadoux M, et al. Long-term (15–25 years) prognosis of childhood hemolytic-uremic syndrome (HUS) [Abstract]. *J Am Soc Nephrol* 1993;4(3):275.
251. Bassani CE, et al. Renal transplantation in patients with classical haemolytic-uraemic syndrome. *Pediatr Nephrol* 1991;5:607–611.
252. Eijgenraam FJ, et al. Renal transplantation in 20 children with hemolytic-uremic syndrome. *Clin Nephrol* 1990;33:87–93.
253. Repetto H, et al. Renal transplantation in children with idiopathic "classic" hemolytic uremic syndrome (idioHUS) [Abstract]. *Pediatr Nephrol* 1989;3:C185.
254. Miller R, et al. Recurrence (R) of hemolytic uremic syndrome in renal allografts: a single center report [Abstract]. *J Am Soc Nephrol* 1994;5: 1024.
255. McEnery PT, et al. Renal transplantation in children and adolescents: the 1992 annual report of the North American Pediatric Renal Transplant Cooperative Study. *Pediatr Nephrol* 1993;7:711–720.
256. Chavers BM, et al. De novo hemolytic uremic syndrome following renal transplantation. *Pediatr Nephrol* 1990;4:62–64.
257. Van Buren D, et al. De novo hemolytic uremic syndrome in renal transplant recipients immunosuppressed with cyclosporine. *Surgery* 1984;98:54–62.
258. Broyer M, Selwood N, Brunner F. Recurrence of primary renal disease on kidney graft: a European pediatric experience. *J Am Soc Nephrol* 1992;2(suppl):2557.
259. Siegler RL, et al. Long-term outcome and prognostic indicators in the hemolytic-uremic syndrome. *J Pediatr* 1991;118:195–200.
260. O'Regan S, et al. Hemolytic uremic syndrome: glomerular filtration rate, 6 to 11 years later measured by 99m TcDPTA plasma slope clearance. *Clin Nephrol* 1989;32:217–220.
261. Karmali MA, et al. Sporadic cases of haemolytic-uraemic syndrome associated with faecal cytotoxin and cytotoxin-producing Escherichia coli in stools. *Lancet* 1983;1:619–620.
262. Pickering LK, Obrig TG, Stapleton FB. Hemolytic-uremic syndrome and enterohemorrhagic Escherichia coli. *Pediatr Infect Dis J* 1994; 13:459–475.
263. Lopez EL, et al. Hemolytic uremic syndrome and diarrhea in Argentine children: the role of Shiga-like toxins. *J Infect Dis* 1989;160: 469–475.
264. Thrombotic thrombocytopenic purpura associated with *Escherichia coli* O157:H7—Washington. *MMWR* 1986;35:549–551.
265. Khoshoo K, et al. Haemolytic uraemic syndrome associated with *Salmonella* dysentery. *Acta Pediatr Scand* 1988;77:604–605.
266. Butler T, et al. Risk factors for development of hemolytic uremic syndrome during shigellosis. *J Pediatr* 1987;110:894–897.
267. Koster F, et al. Hemolytic-uremic syndrome after shigellosis. Relation to endotoxemia and circulating immune complexes. *N Engl J Med* 1978;298:927–933.
268. Alon U, Adler S, Chan J. Hemolytic uremic syndrome associated with *Streptococcus pneumoniae*. *Am J Dis Child* 1984;138:496–499.

269. Chamovitz BN, et al. *Campylobacter jejuni*–associated hemolytic-uremic syndrome in a mother and daughter. *Pediatrics* 1983;71: 253–256.
270. Delans RJ, et al. Hemolytic uremic syndrome after *Campylobacter*-induced diarrhea in an adult. *Arch Intern Med* 1984;144:1074–1076.
271. Morton AR, et al. *Campylobacter* induced thrombotic thrombocytopenic purpura [Letter]. *Lancet* 1985;2:1133–1134.
272. Tsukahara H, et al. Haemolytic uraemic syndrome associated with *Yersinia enterocolitica* infection. *Pediatr Nephrol* 1988;2:309–311.
273. Prober CG, Tune B, Hoder L. *Yersinia* pseudotuberculosis septicemia. *Am J Dis Child* 1979;133:623–624.
274. San JVH, and Pickett DA. *Aeromonas*-associated gastroenteritis in children. *Pediatr Infect Dis J* 1988;7:53–57.
275. Bogdanovi'c R, et al. Haemolytic-uraemic syndrome associated with *Aeromonas hydrophila* enterocolitis. *Pediatr Nephrol* 1991;5: 293–295.
276. O'Regan S, et al. The hemolytic uremic syndrome associated with ECHO 22 infection. *Clin Pediatr Phila* 1980;19:125–127.
277. Sharman VL, Goodwin FJ. Hemolytic uremic syndrome following chicken pox. *Clin Nephrol* 1980;14:49–51.
278. Baker NM, et al. Haemolytic-uraemic syndrome in typhoid fever. *Br Med J* 1974;2:84–87.
279. Mettler NE. Isolation of a microtatobiote from patients with hemolytic-uremic syndrome and thrombotic thrombocytopenic purpura and from mites in the United States. *N Engl J Med* 1969;281: 1023–1027.
280. Chauveau D, et al. Hemolytic uremic syndrome (HUS) and thrombotic thrombocytopenic purpura (TTP) in seven HIV patients. *J Am Soc Nephrol* 1994;5:389.
281. Murgo AJ. Thrombotic microangiopathy in the cancer patient including those induced by chemotherapeutic agents. *Semin Hematol* 1987; 24:161–177.
282. Gardner G, Mesler D, Gitelman HJ. Hemolytic uremic syndrome following cisplatin, bleomycin, and vincristine chemotherapy: a report of a case and a review of the literature. *Renal Failure* 1989;11:133–137.
283. Valavaara R, Nordman E. Renal complications of mitomycin C therapy with special reference to total dose. *Cancer* 1985;55:47–50.
284. Tumlin JA, Sands JM, Someren A. Hemolytic-uremic syndrome following "crack" cocaine inhalation. *Am J Med Sci* 1990;299:366–371.
285. Stroncek DF, et al. Characterization of multiple quinine-dependent antibodies in a patient with episodic hemolytic uremic syndrome and immune agranulocytosis. *Blood* 1992;80:241–248.
286. Maguire RB, Stroneck DF, Campbell AC. Recurrent pancytopenia, coagulopathy, and renal failure associated with multiple quinidine-dependent antibodies. *Ann Intern Med* 1993;119:215–217.
287. Ellie E, et al. Thrombotic thrombocytopenic purpura associated with ticlopidine [Letter]. *Stroke* 1992;23:922–923.
288. Page Y, et al. Thrombotic thrombocytopenic purpura related to ticlopidine. *Lancet* 1991;337:774–776.
289. Beaufils H, et al. Hemolytic uremic syndrome in patients with Behcet's disease treated with cyclosporin A: report of 2 cases. *Clin Nephrol* 1990;34:157–162.
290. Atkinson K, et al. Cyclosporin A associated nephrotoxicity in the first 100 days after allogeneic bone marrow transplantation: three distinct syndromes. *Br J Haematol* 1983;54:59–67.
291. Holman MJ, et al. FK506-associated thrombotic thrombocytopenic purpura. *Transplantation* 1993;55:205–206.
292. Abramowicz D, et al. Induction of thrombosis within renal grafts by high-dose prophylactic OKT3. *Lancet* 1992;339:777.
293. Strauss RG, Alexander RW. Postpartum hemolytic uremic syndrome. *Obstet Gynecol* 1976;47:169–173.
294. Segonds A, et al. Postpartum hemolytic uremic syndrome: a study of three cases with a review of the literature. *Clin Nephrol* 1979;12: 229–242.
295. Brown CB, et al. Haemolytic uraemic syndrome in women taking oral contraceptives. *Lancet* 1973;1:1479–1481.
296. Hauglustaine D, et al. Recurrent hemolytic uremic syndrome during oral contraception. *Clin Nephrol* 1981;15:148–153.
297. Holdrinet RS, de Pauw BE, Haanen C. Hormonal dependent thrombotic thrombocytopenic purpura (TTP). *Scand J Haematol* 1983;30: 250–256.
298. Koree S, et al. treatment of cancer associated hemolytic uremic syndrome with staphylococcal protein A immunoperfusion. *J Clin Oncol* 1986;4:210–215.
299. Laffay D, et al. Chronic glomerular microangiiopathy and metastatic carcinoma. *Hum Pathol* 1979;10:433.
300. Lesesne JB, et al. Cancer-associated hemolytic-uremic syndrome: analysis of 85 cases from a national registry. *J Clin Oncol* 1989;7: 781–789.
301. Kaplan BS, Chesney RW, Drummond KN. Hemolytic uremic syndrome in families. *N Engl J Med* 1975;292:1090–1093.
302. Cledes J, Perrichot R. Familial hemolytic uremic syndrome (fHUS): a retrospective study [Abstract]. *J Am Soc Nephrol* 1994;5:390.
303. Elias M, et al. Thrombotic thrombocytopenic purpura and haemolytic uraemic syndrome in three siblings. *Arch Dis Child* 1988;63: 644–646.
304. Hagge WW, et al. Hemolytic-uremic syndrome in two siblings. *N Engl J Med* 1967;277:138–139.
305. Hellman RM, Jackson DV, Buss DH. Thrombotic thrombocytopenic purpura and hemolytic-uremic syndrome in HLA-identical siblings. *Ann Intern Med* 1980;93:283–284.
306. Kirchner KA, et al. Hereditary thrombotic thrombocytopenic purpura: microangiopathic hemolytic anemia, thrombocytopenia, and renal insufficiency occurring in consecutive generations. *Nephron* 1982;30:28–30.
307. Kaplan B, Kaplan P. Hemolytic uremic syndrome in families. In: Kaplan B, Trompeter R, Moake J, eds. *Hemolytic uremic syndrome and thrombotic thrombocytopenia purpura*. New York: Marcel Dekker; 1992:213–225.
308. Chenel C, et al. [Neonatal hemolytic-uremic syndrome, methylmalonic aciduria and homocystinuria caused by intracellular vitamin B 12 deficiency. Value of etiological diagnosis (translation)]. *Arch Fr Pediatr* 1993;50:749–754.
309. Geraghty MT, et al. Cobalamin C defect associated with hemolytic-uremic syndrome. *J Pediatr* 1992;120:934–937.
310. Russo P, et al. A congenital anomaly of vitamin B12 metabolism: a study of three cases. *Hum Pathol* 1992;23:504–512.
311. Siegler RL, Brewer ED, Pysher TJ. Hemolytic uremic syndrome associated with glomerular disease. *Am J Kidney Dis* 1989;13: 144–147.
312. Siebels M, et al. Hemolytic uremic syndrome complicating postinfectious glomerulonephritis in an adult. *Am J Kidney Dis* 1995;25: 336–339.
313. Krensky AM, et al. Hemolytic uremic syndrome and crescentic glomerulonephritis complicating childhood nephrosis. *Clin Nephrol* 1983;19:99–106.
314. Dische FE, Culliford EJ, Parsons V. Haemolytic uraemic syndrome and idiopathic membranous glomerulonephritis. *Br Med J* 1978;1: 1112–1113.
315. Date A, et al. The pattern of medical renal disease in children in a south Indian hospital. *Ann Trop Paediatr* 1984;4:207–211.
316. Ferriero DM, Wolfsdorf JI. Hemolytic uremic syndrome associated with Kawasaki disease. *Pediatrics* 1981;68:405–406.
317. Meyrier A, et al. Hemolytic-uremic syndrome with anticardiolipin antibodies revealing paraneoplastic systemic scleroderma. *Nephron* 1991;59:493–496.
318. Ricker DM, Sharma HM, Nahman NSJ. Acute renal failure with glomerular thrombosis in a patient with chronic scleroderma. *Am J Kidney Dis* 1989;14:524–526.
319. Asherson RA, Cervera R, Font J. Multiorgan thrombotic disorders in systemic lupus erythematosus: a common link? *Lupus* 1992;1: 199–203.
320. Asherson RA, Khamashta MA, Hughes GR. Lupus, thrombotic thrombocytopenic purpura, and antiphospholipid antibodies [Letter]. *Ann Neurol* 1989;25:312–313.
321. Banfi G, et al. Renal vascular lesions as a marker of poor prognosis in patients with lupus nephritis. Gruppo Italiano per lo Studio della Nefrite Lupica (GISNEL). *Am J Kidney Dis* 1991;18:240–248.

Immunologic Renal Diseases,
edited by E. G. Neilson and W. G. Couser.
Lippincott-Raven Publishers, Philadelphia © 1997.

CHAPTER 54

Clinical and Immunopathogenic Aspects of Human Immunodeficiency Virus–Associated Renal Diseases

Paul L. Kimmel

DEFINITION AND HISTORICAL PERSPECTIVE

The beginning of the human immunodeficiency virus (HIV) epidemic was marked by efforts to establish the epidemiology of the acquired immunodeficiency syndrome (AIDS), identify the risk factors associated with its occurrence, and clarify its pathogenesis. Salient features characterizing the illness included constitutional symptoms, lymphadenopathy and neurologic disorders, impairment of both the cellular and humoral arms of the immune system, and the presence of the opportunistic infections and malignancies that defined the syndrome. The link between AIDS and renal disease was first made by investigators at the State University of New York Downstate Medical Center in Brooklyn, who described a series of patients with AIDS and focal segmental glomerulosclerosis (FGS) (1). The investigators suggested that these patients, for the most part, had not used illicit drugs and had no other known risk factors for the development of kidney disease. They termed the entity AIDS-associated nephropathy. Shortly thereafter, reports from the University of Miami School of Medicine confirmed the presence of renal disease in patients with AIDS but broadened the clinical and histologic spectrum of the nephropathy, including both mesangial hyperplasia and FGS (2). Such findings were confirmed by other groups (3,4). However, other early series reported the presence of a heterogeneous set of renal diseases in patients with AIDS (5,6), which suggested that the nephropathies encountered in such patients might be nonspecific and related to risk factors associated with its pathogenesis, such as intravenous drug use or the superinfections that characterize AIDS, or iatrogenic causes, such as the medications used to treat the syndrome and its complications. Other investigators disputed whether the relationships between AIDS and renal disease were indeed causal, suggesting that they might be only epiphenomenal, or more related to the genetic background of affected patients (7,8). The identification of HIV as the causative agent of AIDS has aided nephrologists in understanding the pathogenesis of many of the heterogeneous renal diseases associated with the viral illness. Several nephrologic syndromes have been associated with HIV infection, including fluid and electrolyte disorders, urinary abnormalities, nephritic and nephrotic syndrome, and acute and chronic renal failure. For the purposes of this chapter, the renal diseases intimately associated with HIV infection can be categorized as HIV-associated nephropathies. These consist of the classic HIV-associated nephropathy, manifested pathologically by FGS (HIVFGS), immune complex renal diseases associated with HIV infection (HIVICD) and HIV-associated thrombotic thrombocytopenic purpura and hemolytic uremic syndrome (HIV-TTP/HUS).

P. L. Kimmel: Division of Renal Diseases and Hypertension, Department of Medicine, George Washington University Medical Center, Washington, D.C. 20037.

ETIOLOGY AND INCIDENCE

HIV infection may be complicated by proteinuria in approximately 6% to 10% of patients (9). Almost half of the patients with AIDS in an outpatient setting demonstrated greater than 2 g proteinuria/24 h and 9% had greater than 3 g/24 h (2). Similarly, among inpatients, approximately half had proteinuria and one third had urinary protein excretion greater than 2 g/24 h (3). These data may reflect the patient demographics of the particular urban medical centers and the case definition of AIDS used in early studies. In another study of HIV-infected patients without clinical renal disease, approximately one third of patients, regardless of stage of disease, race, or gender, had glomerular permeability or renal tubular reabsorptive defects (10). Glomerular and tubular abnormalities in HIV-infected patients were similar in quality and magnitude to those of a control group of hospitalized, febrile patients without a history of HIV infection or renal disease, suggesting that fever or abnormal cytokine regulation, perhaps as a result of opportunistic or HIV infection, may have been associated with the pathogenesis of the renal abnormalities.

Clinical nephropathy may occur in patients at any stage of HIV infection and is associated with the risk factors for HIV infection (9). Whether specific risk factors, such as intravenous drug use, are etiologically or disproportionately associated with the development of nephropathy remains controversial (9). However, renal complications affect specific subsets of the population (9,11–14), suggesting that a host response or genetic component may be associated with the incidence and pathogenesis of the disease. Chronic renal disease has been reported disproportionately in black male patients in the United States (9,11–14) and in black patients in France (9,15). Factors linked to socioeconomic status also may be related to disease pathogenesis (14).

The prevalence of HIV-infected patients treated in dialysis units in the United States has plateaued at approximately 1% to 2% of the population (16). However, in urban areas where HIV infection is epidemic, such as New York City, Miami, and Washington, D.C., the prevalence of HIV-infected patients treated in dialysis units, the majority of whom have a form of HIV-associated renal disease, may range from 7% to 30% (17–19). The survival of such patients is limited compared with the general end-stage renal disease (ESRD) population (9,17,19). In a small epidemiologic survey, the prevalence of human immunodeficiency viremia was greater in HIV-infected patients with renal disease compared with those without nephropathy (20). The renal disease in this study might have been a result of HIV infection, or the viremia might have been a consequence of further immunosuppression secondary to renal disease.

HIVFGS is the most common chronic renal disease whose pathogenesis is intimately associated with HIV infection in adults. HIVICD is much less common, perhaps in part because such patients are often not evaluated using renal biopsy. However, depending on clinical criteria for the performance of renal biopsy, one quarter to more than a third of patients with HIV infection and nephrotic-range proteinuria may have HIVICD (15,21, 22). HIV-associated thrombotic microangiopathy may be less common, but over 70 cases of TTP and at least 15 cases of HUS have been reported in patients with HIV infection (23). The majority of patients with HIVFGS and HIVICD have been of African descent. However, all patients with HIV-associated immunoglobulin A nephropathy (HIVIgAN) reported to date have been white or Hispanic (24). Most patients with HIVIgAN are homosexual men, although the disease also has been reported in boys. Most patients with HIV-TTP/HUS have been men, with perhaps a higher proportion of white patients affected than black or Hispanic men (23), possibly reflecting the epidemiology of HIV infection in the general population.

PATHOGENESIS AND PATHOPHYSIOLOGY

Although the pathogenesis of the renal diseases associated with HIV infection is only incompletely understood, findings in these disorders are likely to provide insight into the pathophysiology of other, more common renal diseases. Interestingly, as outlined above, HIV-infected patients with renal disease, in the presence or absence of ESRD, are more likely to have infective viremia than HIV-infected patients without renal failure (20). This may represent a causal relationship or, alternatively, is a result of decreased viral clearance concomitant with further impairment in immune regulation in HIV-infected patients with kidney disease. The host response to chronic HIV infection includes continued antibody synthesis, abnormal cell-mediated immune responses, and cellular antiviral responses, all of which may affect renal pathologic outcomes. An immunologic response to HIV infection may culminate in HIVFGS, immune complex glomerulonephritis, or HIV-TTP/HUS. A range of pathologic renal outcomes, as a result of the interplay of viral factors, genetic background, and host responses, is analogous to the spectrum of kidney diseases noted in patients with hepatitis B virus infection (22).

HIVFGS

The pathogenesis of FGS in HIV-infected patients is unknown. This disorder in uninfected patients is thought to be related in part to disordered regulation and coordination of renal matrix production and degradation (25–27). After the original reports of FGS in patients with HIV infection, a recurrent criticism attempting to dissociate the renal disease from the viral illness suggested that the nephropathy was related to risk factors for HIV infection such as intravenous drug use. Several lines of evidence suggest that the renal disease is intimately linked with the pathogenesis of the viral infection. Connor et al. (28) and others (29–31) demonstrated HIVFGS in infants and children of HIV-infected mothers. Dickie et al. (32) and Kopp et al. (33), as well as others (34), have demonstrated renal disease resembling HIVFGS in mice transgenic for HIV, implicating a direct role of HIV peptides and renal cellular responses in the pathogenesis of HIVFGS (34). Renal disease, including histologic changes consistent with human FGS (35) and interstitial nephritis (36), has been reported in primates infected with simian immunodeficiency virus (SIV), a genetically distinct lentivirus closely related to HIV-1 and HIV-2 (34). Proviral SIV DNA is detected in widespread tissue distribution in the majority of animals with advanced disease. SIV gene expression, or the presence of SIV proteins in renal tissue, might contribute to the pathogenesis of nephropathy in these studies (34). Finally, feline immunodeficency virus infection also has been associated with the development of renal disease resembling FGS in approximately 9% of infected cats (34). Such data suggest that the risk factors for developing AIDS are not crucial to the development of nephropathy but (a) do highlight the role of viral processes in the pathogenesis of renal disease and (b) are consistent with the interaction of host factors and genetic predisposition determining the extent and type of kidney disease.

The great majority of HIV-infected patients with renal disease also show the presence of HIV genome in the kidney (21,37). However, the presence of HIV genome in autopsy tissue of patients without renal abnormalities also has been demonstrated (21). Because HIV genome appears to be present ubiquitously in renal tissue of HIV-infected patients with and without nephropathy, it is clear that the presence of HIV DNA in the kidney does not determine the type of renal disease, nor is it alone sufficient to induce nephropathy. Therefore, triggering and facilitating mechanisms are likely associated with mechanisms that cause nephropathy (21). Understanding the pathogenesis of such renal disease and nature of such mechanisms is essential in developing preventive or ameliorative strategies. Some of these possible factors are outlined below.

Immune Cell Infiltration in Renal Tissue

Both HIVFGS and HIVICD are characterized by dense interstitial immune cell infiltration (1–4,9,12,13,22,38), which aids in the identification of its HIV-associated nature (38). The majority of patients with HIVFGS have a prominent interstitial infiltrate of macrophages and lymphocytes (primarily T cells) (4,39). The proportion of interstitial macrophages is higher in HIVFGS compared with HIVICD, whereas interstitial tissue from patients with HIVFGS has a lower percentage of B cells than does HIVFGS (39). These data constitute a remarkable finding in a disease characterized by peripheral T-helper cell depletion. What mediates T-cellular infiltration into renal tissue in HIV-associated nephropathies is unknown. Infiltrating immune cells can enhance nephropathogenic processes in tissue by secreting growth factors, cytokines, and chemokines (40–43), and macrophages serve as antigen-presenting cells. Chemokines (chemoattractive cytokines) (43) may play a role in mediating renal tissue damage by infiltrating lymphocytes and mononuclear cells. The cell-mediated response may be modulated because of the abnormal immunoregulation seen in patients with HIV infection. Lymphocytes and macrophages of HIV-infected patients are infected with the virus (9,44,45). HIV peptides modulate T-cell function (45–47), which might alter immune effector cell biology in renal tissue. The differential proportion of immune cells could be a result of different chemokine profiles in renal tissue in different nephropathies caused by the same virus, reflecting different pathologic processes that attract different cell types to the locus of injury. Alternatively, infiltration of different immune cells in renal tissue may result in the expression of different renal diseases. Infected and uninfected immune cells in renal tissue could have profound effects on the development of glomerular sclerosis and interstitial fibrogenesis (48).

Cytokines and Growth Factors in the Pathogenesis of Nephropathy

Cytokines and growth factors may effect the pathogenesis of HIVFGS in at least two ways: direct effects on renal cells and effects on the HIV life cycle. A recent study demonstrated increased proliferation of mesangial cells exposed to pooled sera from HIV-infected donors compared with control sera, suggesting that circulating factors in patients with HIV infection might adversely affect renal cell biologic responses (49). Interferons (IFNs) are expressed by immune cells in response to viral infections (50). IFN-α induces the tubular reticular structures that are characteristic of HIVFGS in lymphoid tissue in vitro (51,52) and has been proposed as a marker of progression of HIV infection (53). IFN-τ, a product of T-lymphocytes, has antiproliferative and protein synthetic effects on mesangial cells (54,55). Treatment with IFNs has been associated with reversible nephropathy, including interstitial nephritis and glomerulonephritis (56–58). We recently showed increased levels of IFN-α in renal glomerular and interstitial tissue in HIVFGS compared with idiopathic FGS and control tissue (59). Such local cytokine and growth factor dysregulation may contribute to the development of fibrosis and sclerogenesis (60).

A role for cytokines and growth factors in the activation of latent HIV-1 virus also has been suggested (44, 61). Cytokines and growth factors induce proliferation and matrix synthesis by mesangial cells (62). Basic fibroblast growth factor is overexpressed in renal tissue from an HIV transgenic murine model of HIV nephropathy (63), as it is in Kaposi's sarcoma (64). Transforming growth factor-β (TGF-β) is a bifunctional regulator of mesangial cell growth (65), but generally has antiproliferative effects, and results in increased net synthesis and decreased degradation of extracellular matrix (66). Because macrophages and lymphocytes produce TGF-β, their presence in the kidney may be related to sclerogenesis (65,66). Elevated TGF-β levels in plasma and tissues have been reported in patients with AIDS (67). Preliminary studies indicate that higher levels of tissue cytokines, chemokines, and TGF-β are present in HIVFGS compared with idiopathic FGS, detected by immunochemical methods (59,68). Mesangial cells transfected with HIV-1 long terminal repeat (LTR) sequences, exposed to TGF-β, had increased levels of HIV-1 LTR expression in in vitro conditions compared with cells exposed to other cytokines and growth factors (including platelet-derived growth factor) (69), indicating that TGF-β specifically might increase HIV replication in renal tissue.

Role of Renal HIV Infection

The role of renal HIV infection in the pathogenesis of nephropathy is unclear. Injury to glomerular epithelial cells may play a primary role in the pathogenesis of idiopathic FGS (25–27). Preliminary evidence suggests that renal tubular epithelial, glomerular epithelial cells, and mesangial cells can be infected by HIV (9,37,70). Glomerular epithelial cells undergo characteristic morphologic changes that may contribute to the "collapsing glomerulosclerosis" of HIVFGS (25–27,38). In addition, glomerular and tubular epithelial cells have been shown to harbor HIV nucleic acid by in situ hybridization (37) and polymerase chain reaction (PCR) techniques (21). However, the ability of glomerular epithelial and mesangial cells to be infected with HIV in vitro is controversial (70,71). HIV gene products are present intracellularly in glomerular tissue from human renal biopsy samples of HIV-infected patients with renal disease (22,72), but conclusive evidence of productive infection of renal cells in humans has not yet been demonstrated.

Nephropathogenic Effects of HIV-1 Proteins

Possible roles for HIV structural and regulatory proteins in the pathogenesis of nephropathy have been described (73,74). Recombinant glycoprotein (gp)120 is cytotoxic, causing death of astrocytes in human brain cultures in vitro (75) and inducing cellular IFN-α and -τ, tumor necrosis factor-α, IgG, interleukin (IL)-1, and IL-6 production (76,77). The HIV-1 *trans*-activator protein Tat variably stimulates or inhibits cell proliferation depending on the experimental system studied (47,78). Tat protein stimulates production of TGF-β1 by macrophages (79) and has specific effects on immune cell function (47,80). HIV gp120 protein can modulate the function of immune cells and induce apoptosis (45,81). HIV peptides also may modulate renal cellular function, leading to the expression of disease. HIV gp120 decreased mesangial cellular gelatinase activity in an in vitro model (82), which could be an important factor in the decreased matrix degradation and rapid development of glomerulosclerosis encountered in HIVFGS. Renal cells could be exposed to relatively high levels of such HIV peptides as a result of renal infection or because of their presence in the circulation and to subsequent concentration as a result of glomerular filtration and tubular reabsorption. Glycoprotein 120 increases TGF-β messenger RNA expression, coupled with decreased mesangial cell proliferation in vitro, consistent with a physiologic effect of TGF-β (83). Because TGF-β has been associated with sclerotic responses, increased renal cellular expression of TGF-β, as a result of renal infection or exposure to circulating HIV peptides, might be a mechanism for the pathogenesis of virally induced FGS. Increased numbers of apoptotic cells have been noted in tubules in tissue from patients with HIVFGS compared with idiopathic FGS (84). It is possible that apoptosis contributes to the development of nephropathy in HIV-infected patients. Other HIV peptides may have pathogenic effects on renal cells, increasing production of matrix components and effecting cellular responses, including cytokine, growth factor, and adhesion molecule synthesis (73,74). Finally, HIVFGS is characterized by increased tissue levels of immunoreactants, including IFN-τ receptor protein and nonpolymorphic major histocompatibility complex class II protein (59,74). The pres-

TABLE 1. *Pathogenic factors in HIV-associated renal diseases*

Immune cell infiltration in renal tissue
HIVFGS
HIVICD
HIVIgAN
Cytokines and growth factors
TGF-β
Chemokines
Others
Role of renal HIV infection
Cytotoxic and other effects of HIV-1 proteins
gp120
Tat
Others
Antigen presentation
IFN-α and -τ
HIV peptides
Immune cells
Host factors
Age
Gender
Ethnic background
Tissue type
Immunologic responsiveness
Socioeconomic status/access to care

ence of such proteins in renal tissue characterized by high levels of HIV proteins suggests local immune activation, with the potential to respond to presentation of non-self peptides, perhaps of HIV origin.

All the mechanisms outlined above may be involved in the rapidly progressive renal failure, characterized pathologically by FGS, seen in patients with HIV infection (Table 1). Theoretically, high circulating and local cytokine and growth factor levels, found in patients with HIV infection or AIDS, might induce increased matrix production by HIV-infected or uninfected glomerular epithelial, endothelial, and mesangial cells. Mesangial cell TGF-β production, possibly concomitant to mesangial cell HIV infection, might act in an autocrine fashion. Such increased cytokine levels might induce increased mesangial cell growth and matrix production, leading to a vicious cycle of cytokine-induced cellular proliferation and matrix production, leading to renal insufficiency, and further cytokine-induced dysfunction (69,74). Such an inexorably developing spiral is consistent with the rapid progression to global sclerosis and ESRD seen in patients with HIV infection and nephropathy.

HIVICD

Membranoproliferative and diffuse proliferative glomerulonephritis, and membranous nephropathy, diseases often associated with immune pathogenic mechanisms, have been reported in patients with HIV infection (5,6,9,12,13,15,21,22,24,30,37,58,72,85–88). In several studies of HIV-infected patients with nephrotic range proteinuria, more than a quarter had glomerulonephritis (15,21,22,30). The relationship of these different renal diseases to the underlying HIV infection has been unclear. Three main types of clinically distinguishable HIVICD may be delineated: HIV-associated immune glomerulonephritis (HIVGN), a mixed sclerotic-immune complex nephropathy (15), and HIVIgAN (22,24,87,89–94). The mixed lesion may represent a later stage of glomerulonephritis, or the two diseases may have different pathogenic determinants. Studies to address these hypotheses have not yet been performed but will include the serial biopsy of patients with mild lesions.

Circulating immune complexes (CICs), often identifiable as HIV related, are common in HIV-infected patients at all stages of the disease (22,95,96). CICs composed of immunoglobulins, characteristically IgG or IgA, reactive with specific HIV antigens such as p24, gp41, and gp120, are present, and identical complexes may be eluted in higher titer from renal tissue of patients with HIVICD. We studied four black male HIV-infected patients with renal failure and proteinuria who had proliferative glomerulonephritis, renal insufficiency, and proteinuria (72). One had a clinical constellation consistent with postinfectious glomerulonephritis, with mild renal insufficiency. The other three had evidence of glomerulosclerosis and interstitial fibrosis, in addition to glomerular inflammation and electron microscopic evidence of deposits in the mesangium and glomerular capillaries, consistent with a mixed type of HIVGN. CICs were isolated in all four, composed of IgA–p24, IgG–gp120, and IgG–p24. Identical complexes were eluted from renal tissue in three of the cases. Eluted antibodies reacted with the HIV antigens isolated from the

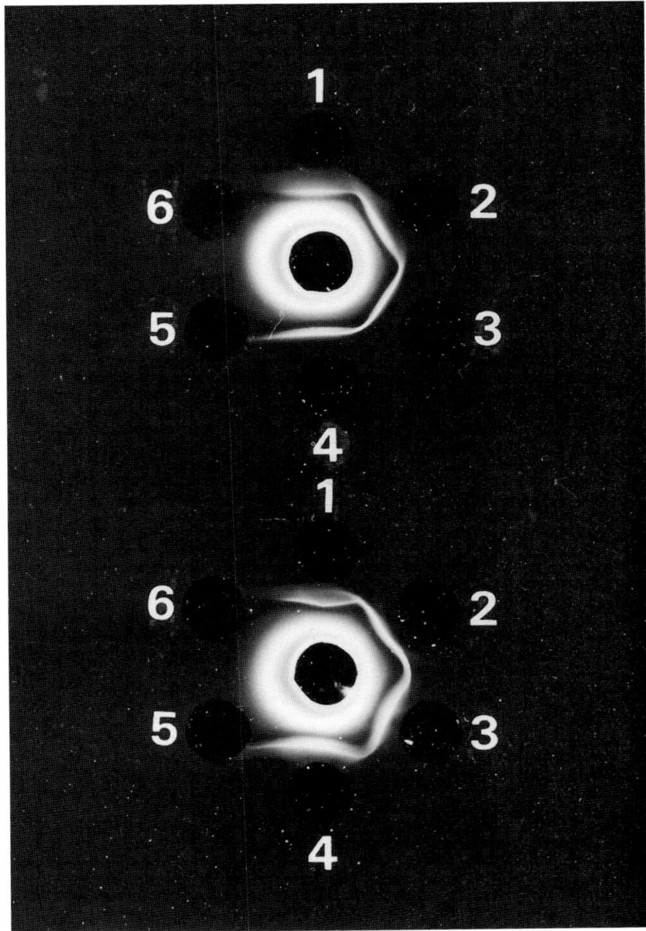

FIG. 1. This double-immunodiffusion study depicts a CIC and the eluate of the deposited renal immunoreactants isolated from a patient with HIV infection and glomerulonephritis. IgM antibody from the CIC was placed in the upper central well, whereas IgM antibody from the eluate was placed in the central well of the lower panel. HIV p24 from the eluate, from the CIC, and from the urine and recombinant HIV p24 were placed in peripheral wells 1–4, respectively. Recombinant HIV gp41 and human serum albumin in peripheral wells 5 and 6 served as controls for viral and human antigens. The study demonstrated that immunoreactivity of the antibodies with antigen from the CIC, from the renal eluate, from the urine, and with the recombinant HIV peptide was specific. The similarity of the two immunodiffusion studies established the identity of the CIC and the eluate immunoreactants.

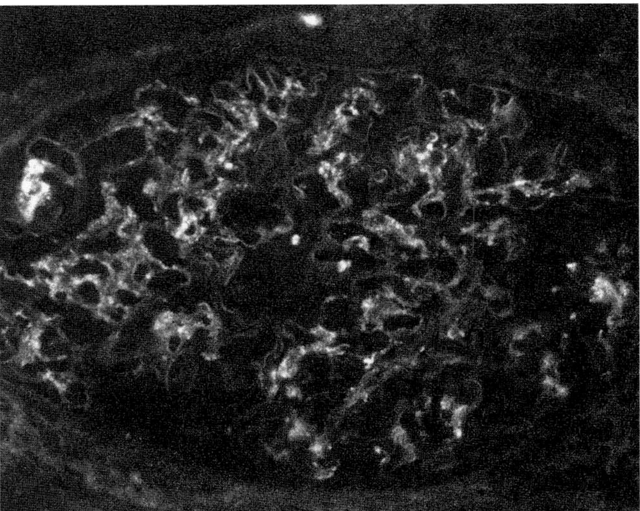

FIG. 2. Immunofluorescence photomicrograph of IgG staining in a granular mesangial and scanty peripheral distribution in a glomerulus from a patient with HIV-associated immune complex glomerulonephritis. A similar pattern of HIV p24 antigen was detected in an acid-eluted glomerulus by laser-enhanced fluorescence micrography (original magnification ×300). Reprinted with permission (72).

TABLE 2. *Possible pathogenic mechanisms of inflammatory and sclerotic renal disease in HIV infection*

1. Classic immune complex disease
   - A. Circulating viral antigens/host antiviral antibody
   - B. Circulating endogenous antigens induced by viral changes in shed membrane proteins/host antibody
2. In situ immune mediated mechanisms of nephropathogenesis
   - A. Viral antigen deposited in renal tissue
     - i. Vral antigen binds to renal cell, initiating host humoral or cell-mediated immune response
   - B. Viral gene expression in renal tissue
     - i. Viral antigen binds to renal cell, initiating host humoral or cell-mediated immune response
     - ii. Usurpation of cell machinery
       - a. Viral proteins may cause cell death by apoptosis or other mechanisms, or cause cell dysfunction
       - b. Increased propensity to the development of circulating or in situ immune pathogenic mechanisms
       - c. Virally induced abnormal host cell proteins cause induction of genetic responses leading to increased matrix synthesis, and/or decreased degradation, including upregulation of cytokine, chemokine, growth factor, or adhesion molecule production, which may result in nephropathy

CICs (Fig. 1). Direct immunofluorescence in glomerular tissue showed the presence of immunoglobulin (Fig. 2) and intracellular glomerular and particularly mesangial HIV antigens, identified by laser enhanced microscopy (72). PCR techniques confirmed the presence of HIV genome in all four biopsy samples (72). Such data are consistent with circulating immune complex mechanisms of the pathogenesis of glomerulonephritis (97–100) (Table 2). However, the finding of HIV gene products in renal tissue also raises the possibility that in situ mechanisms of immune complex nephropathy (Table 2) are involved in the pathogenesis of the renal disease.

Cryoglobulinemia has been reported in patients with HIV infection, but its role in mediating renal disease is unclear (101–103). Antibodies synthesized in response to retroviral infection may form cryoprecipitable complexes. However, vasculitis and cryoglobulinemia appear to be relatively rare compared with the prevalence of both HIV infection and HIV-associated renal diseases (88). It is also frequently difficult, in the absence of intensive immunochemical analysis, to assess whether the cryoglobulinemia is associated with HIV or other coexistent infections. The role of concurrent infection with hepatitis B virus, hepatitis C virus, and other viral infections in the pathogenesis of renal disease in patients with HIV infection has not been assessed adequately (88).

The pathogenesis of HIVICD is largely unknown. The majority of patients with HIVICD demonstrated the presence of proviral HIV DNA in tubular and glomerular cells of biopsy samples and autopsy tissue by PCR (21, 22,72,92) and in vitro DNA hybridization techniques (37). Such renal tissue markers are also present in renal tissue from patients with AIDS without clinically obvious renal disease (21,22,37). Therefore, the potential role of cellular incorporation of HIV gene products in the development of renal disease by in situ or cell-mediated mechanisms, contrasted with circulating immune mechanisms (Table 2), is unknown (22,72,92,88,99,100). The development of glomerulonephritis may be dependent on the renal parenchymal incorporation of HIV antigens, although renal cellular HIV infection may be an insufficient condition for disease expression. It is possible that renal cellular viral infection itself, by the expression of viral antigens or synthesis or alteration of renal cellular proteins, leads to subsequent attachment of circulating anti-HIV antibodies or anti-HIV antibody/HIV peptide complexes to an implanted or transformed antigen (22, 72,99,100) (Table 2). Alternatively, such findings may be the result of deposition of CICs in renal tissue, which subsequently initiate an inflammatory response (22,72, 97–100). Analysis of pathologic tissue cannot differentiate definitively between these two pathogenic mechanisms. In addition, the binding of host antibody to endogenous shed circulating antigens or tissue antigens induced by viral infection may account for the failure to detect viral antigens in renal tissue of patients with HIV-induced, immune-mediated renal disease. Finally, cell-mediated immune responses may amplify inflammatory and sclerogenic responses induced by circulating or in situ immune-mediated initiating mechanisms (Table 2).

Similarly, the role of genetic and host responses may be crucial in determining renal pathologic outcomes (Table 1). It is possible that certain specific immune responses, perhaps related to particular modes of antigen presentation or specific CICs, are more likely to provoke an ongoing renal inflammatory response. Physicochemical properties of immune complexes, such as their composition, size, charge, antigen:antibody ratio, binding affinities, complement-binding and -activating capacity, and circulating and tissue concentrations, have been implicated in influencing pathologic outcome (22,99, 100). HIV-infected children may be at relatively high risk for developing HIVGN (30). Finally, the role of concurrent or intercurrent viral infection in affecting renal responses remains to be determined.

In one HIV-infected patient treated with IFN-α who developed proteinuria, an IFN-α–IgG complex was noted in the circulation and in higher titer in renal eluates of tissue showing findings of membranoproliferative glomerulonephritis and immune complex tubular disease (58). Disordered immunoregulation as a result of the HIV infection, or treatment with IFN, or a combination of the two may have affected the response to the CIC or may have altered the tissue response, culminating in nephropathy.

Because HIVGN is characterized by a dense interstitial infiltrate (15,21,22,39,72,92), immune cell infiltration in renal tissue may be important in its pathogenesis. Because different interstitial cell populations characterize HIVFGS and HIVGN, the immune cell population also may have an important effect on histologic outcome. Alternatively, different pathogenic processes may elicit different infiltrating cells. Cytokines and growth factors, which are products of immune cells, also may enhance or modify nephropathogenic events, including inflammation and the development of fibrosis (Table 2). As outlined above, patients treated with IFNs have developed a variety of different nephropathies, including glomerulonephritis (57,58). IFNs are expressed both in response to viral infections and in some autoimmune diseases (50) and may enhance nephropathogenic processes at the tissue level (22). In addition, HIV-1 proteins have cytotoxic and other effects on renal cells that could enhance nephropathogenicity, as described above. Glycoprotein 120, as outlined above, is cytotoxic and induces changes in cytokine and growth factor expression. HIV-1 Tat protein has variable stimulatory or inhibitory effects on cell proliferation (47,78). Glycoprotein 120 and gp120–anti-gp120 antigen–antibody complexes are immunomodulatory (45,77,81). Therefore, HIV peptides and antibodies directed against them may modulate renal cellular function, leading to or enhancing inflammatory renal disease.

HIVIgAN

Pathogenic mechanisms in HIVIgAN are probably similar to those thought important in the development of IgA nephropathy in the absence of underlying viral infection (104,105). Indeed, viral infections have been implicated in the pathogenesis of IgA nephropathy before the HIV epidemic (104). CICs containing IgA have been implicated in the pathogenesis of the renal disease in patients with HIVIgAN, as in patients with IgAN in the absence of viral infection (104,105). IgA antibodies directed against HIV antigens are part of the early response to HIV infection (106–110). Circulating antigen–antibody complexes containing IgA are frequently present in HIV-infected patients. A substantial proportion of the polyclonal immunoglobulin response in HIV-infected patients is composed of IgA, and IgA-containing immune complexes are frequently found in patients with HIV infection and AIDS (106–110). These immune responses may partially explain the prevalence of IgAN seen in HIV-infected patients. IgA rheumatoid factors are common in patients with IgAN, and defects in immunoregulation have been implicated in the pathogenesis of IgAN in the absence of HIV infection (104,105). Rather than being the chance association of two unrelated diseases, it appears that the renal disease is intimately associated with the viral infection.

One report of an autopsy survey suggested that IgA deposition is uncommon in renal tissue of HIV-infected subjects (111). Such data and the common findings of circulating IgA immune complexes in the presence of a disease characterized by polyclonal gammopathy emphasize that other factors must be important in the pathogenesis of clinically apparent nephropathy. Katz et al. (93) evaluated three white homosexual men and a Hispanic boy with HIVIgAN. All patients had CICs composed of immunoglobulins, including IgA reactive with several HIV antigens, and IgA rheumatoid factors (93). Our studies in two patients with HIVIgAN (92) demonstrated the presence of CICs containing anti-HIV antibodies complexed with idiotypic IgA antibodies. Immunochemical analysis of these complexes showed that the complexed IgAs expressed selective binding to papain-digested Fab fragments of IgG anti-HIV gp41 (case 1) or chymotrypsin-digested monomers of IgM anti-HIV p24 (case 2) antibodies, but were unable to inhibit specific antigen binding in either case. These findings indicated that the complexed IgAs were idiotypic, rather than merely rheumatoid factors, reacting with common idiotypes expressed on the hypervariable regions of the target immunoglobulins. Identical immune complexes could be eluted from tissue subjected to biopsy in higher concentration than in the circulating immune complex. The IgA anti-immunoglobulin response in both patients was specific for immunoglobulin type and for immunoglobulin reactivity with specific HIV antigens in each individual patient. The anti-HIV antigen response also was specific for both viral peptide and patient. In one patient, the immune complex was cryoprecipitable. In addition, HIV gene sequences were amplified by PCR from renal tissue from both patients with HIVIgAN, as demonstrated in patients with HIVFGS and HIVICD. Such data are consistent with findings in IgAN in uninfected populations, suggesting immune mediation and a genetic predisposition to a particular pathologic outcome (104,105). In addition, these data are consistent with an in situ immune- (as well as a CIC-) mediated pathogenesis of nephropathy. However, the specific factors mediating nephropathogenicity in these selected patients are unknown.

HIV-TTP/HUS

The pathogenesis of HIV-TTP/HUS is unknown. In uninfected patients, a variety of etiologic factors have been identified, including bacterial infections (particularly with verocytotoxin-producing *Escherichia coli* O157:H7); drugs such as cyclosporine, mitomycin, and bleomycin; and coexistent illnesses such as neoplasms, systemic lupus erythematosus, and scleroderma (23). The contribution of such factors to the pathogenesis of HIV-TTP/HUS is unclear, but endothelial injury, deficiency of inhibitors of platelet aggregation, and abnormalities in the coagulation cascade have all been implicated. The clinical findings in HIV-TTP/HUS are thought to result, in part, from the capillary and arteriolar deposition of platelet-fibrin thrombi in end organs such as the brain and kidneys. HIV peptides such as p24 may be important pathogenic factors, perhaps because of their cytopathic effects (112) or as a result of changes engendered after infection of endothelial cells.

PATHOLOGY

HIVFGS

Classic HIVFGS has characteristic glomerular, tubular, and interstitial changes and is marked by the presence of ultrastructural changes in endothelial cells (1–4,12,13,38). Grossly, kidneys may be enlarged (9,12,113–115). Mesangial hyperplasia may be an early stage of the nephropathy (9). Glomerular capillary wall collapse of varying severity is often noted (Fig. 3). Lipid-containing macrophages are found within glomerular capillaries. Glomerular visceral epithelial cells are hyperplastic and hypertrophic and may contain vacuoles and protein droplets. Capillary lumina are narrowed and in late stages may be obliterated by segmental or diffuse and global increases in mesangial matrix. Obsolescent glomeruli can be seen in cases associated with renal insufficiency. Tubular cells often exhibit degenerative changes and necrosis. Flattening and simplification of tubular epithelial cells may be noted with loss of nuclei, and in proximal cells brush border staining may be noted.

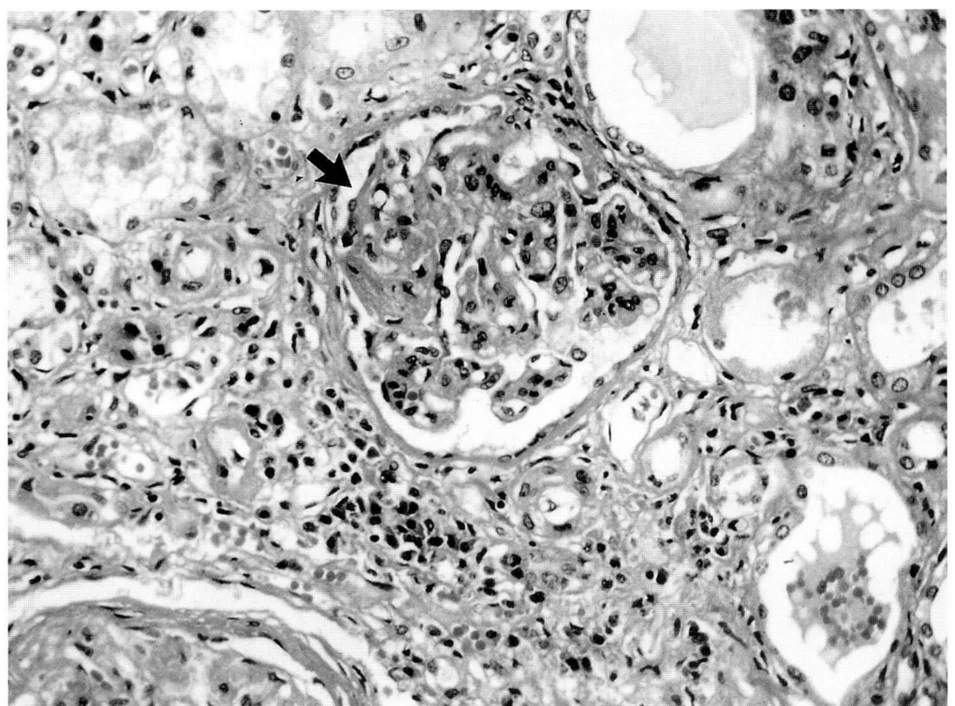

FIG. 3. Light microscopy of renal tissue from a patient with HIVFGS, showing segmental collapse and consolidation of tuft (arrow). There is an interstitial lymphoplasmacytic infiltrate. Focal tubular atrophy and tubular dilatation are present. Proteinaceous material is present within dilated tubules (original magnification ×160).

Microcystic tubular dilatation is a hallmark of the disease. The interstitium is characterized by an immune cell infiltrate composed of mononuclear cells, primarily macrophages and T-lymphocytes (4,38), in approximately equal numbers (39). There is a relative paucity of B-lymphocytes compared with T-lymphocytes (39). Interstitial edema and fibrosis are often present. Arteries and arterioles are usually normal. Immunofluorescence microscopy often shows IgM and C3 in segmental or mesangial lesions, but C1 deposition also may be encountered. Electron microscopy shows glomerular epithelial cell foot process effacement, wrinkling and folding of the glomerular basement membrane, and segmental glomerular collapse (9,114). Occasionally, electron-dense deposits are encountered within the mesangium. Tubular reticular structures, probably induced by IFN-α (52,115), are commonly appreciated in the cytoplasm of glomerular and peritubular capillary endothelial cells (Fig. 4). However, these are not pathognomonic because they may be seen in patients with lupus and, rarely, in those with heroin nephropathy (8). Cylindrical confronting cisternae (also known as test-tube and ring-shaped forms) (116–118) may be noted in tubular and interstitial cells. These ultrastructural features are thought to represent stacks of closely apposed membranes (115). Nuclear bodies, although not specifically associated with HIVFGS, may be noted in interstitial, tubular, endothelial, and glomerular visceral epithelial cells (115).

Although the individual features of HIVFGS are not specific, the combination of glomerular collapse with epithelial cell abnormalities, segmental increased mesangial matrix, microcystic tubular dilatation and dense interstitial infiltrate on light microscopy, and abundant tubular reticular structures on electron microscopy is distinctive

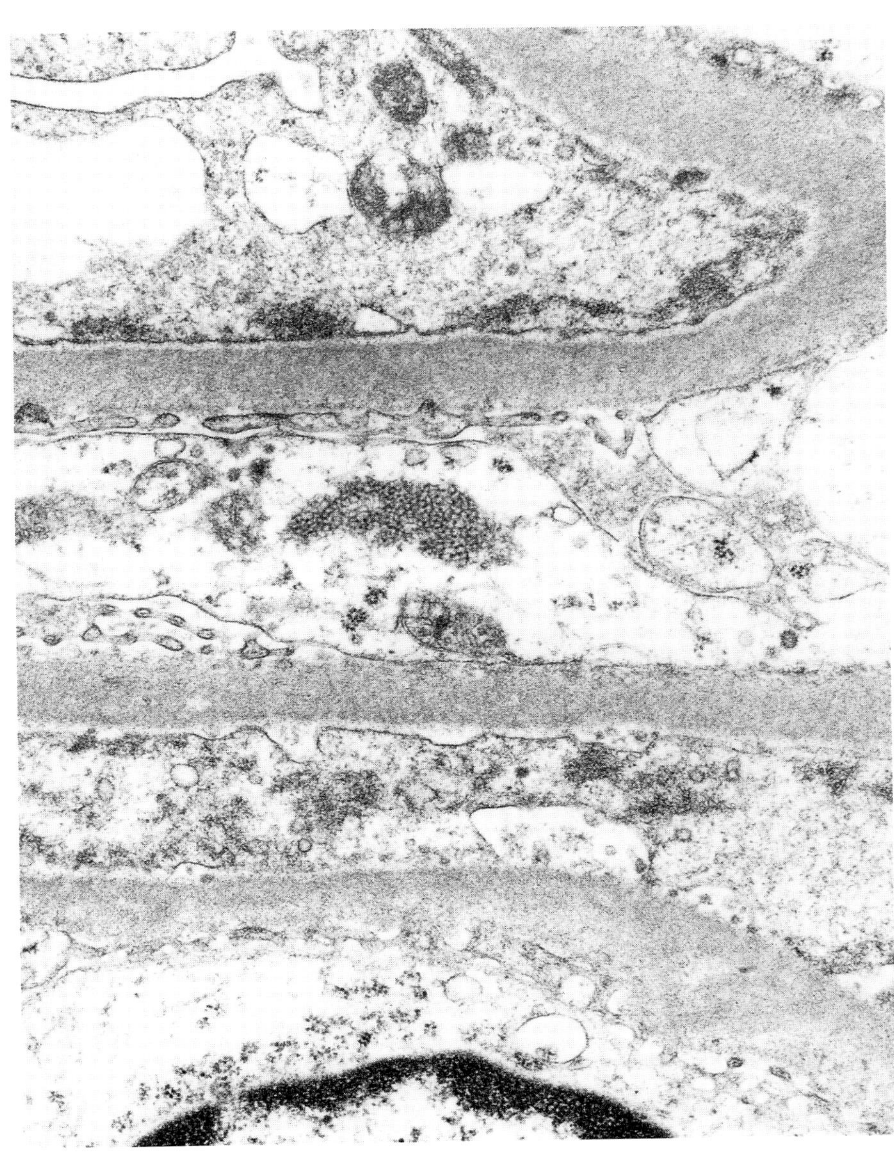

FIG. 4. This electron micrograph shows typical tubular reticular structures within an endothelial cell from a renal biopsy performed in a patient with HIV-associated renal disease (original magnification ×31,200).

and highly characteristic of HIVFGS. Several different groups of investigators (4,38,114,116–118) have emphasized the specific nature of the combination of these pathologic findings of glomerular, tubular, and interstitial abnormalities, as well as the importance of ultrastructural abnormalities in establishing the pathologic diagnosis. Indeed, findings of such a "pan-nephropathy" often prompts the pathologist to request the serologic data from the clinician, if not previously provided.

HIVICD

The pathology of HIVICD is variable, and has been described previously (22,88). Nochy et al. (15) described several subtypes of HIVGN, including a diffuse exudative endocapillary proliferative form they termed *postinfectious*. A second type resembles lupus nephritis, with diffuse endocapillary proliferative changes, wire loops, hyaline thrombi in capillary lumina, and mesangial, intracapillary, and subepithelial deposits of immunoglobulin, C3, and C1q. Finally, these investigators delineated a mixed type of glomerulonephritis with features of both FGS and ICD. In a series of patients with well-characterized HIVGN (22,72), a spectrum of pathologic changes, including variable degrees of mesangial expansion, segmental and diffuse increase of mesangial cells and matrix, and segmental or diffuse proliferation of glomerular tufts has been noted (22,72,88). Increased cellularity with lobular transformation, segmental condensation or simplification of glomerular tufts, and segmental or global proliferative and sclerosing changes may be appreciated. Glomerular visceral epithelial cells were often prominent, and fibrocellular crescents were frequently present. Microcystic tubular dilatation and atrophy, as well as interstitial fibrosis or edema, were often noted. Biopsy samples were characterized by interstitial infiltration with mononuclear cells, primarily lymphocytes and to a lesser extent macrophages. There was a relatively increased proportion of interstitial B-lymphocytes, rather than T-lymphocytes, compared with HIVFGS (39). Occasional interstitial plasma cells, polymorphonuclear leukocytes, and eosinophils may be noted. Infiltrating cells may rarely disrupt the tubular basement membrane.

Immunofluorescence microscopy demonstrated intramembranous and mesangial deposits of immunoglobulins (including variable amounts of IgA, IgM, IgG) and complement (C3, C4, and C1q) (72). Electron microscopy usually showed subendothelial, intramembranous, and mesangial electron-dense deposits. Electron-dense deposits were found within mesangial cells, and glomerular capillaries occasionally exhibited subepithelial and subendothelial deposits (Fig. 5). Foot processes of visceral epithelial cells were approximated. Tubular reticular structures can be detected in endothelial cells.

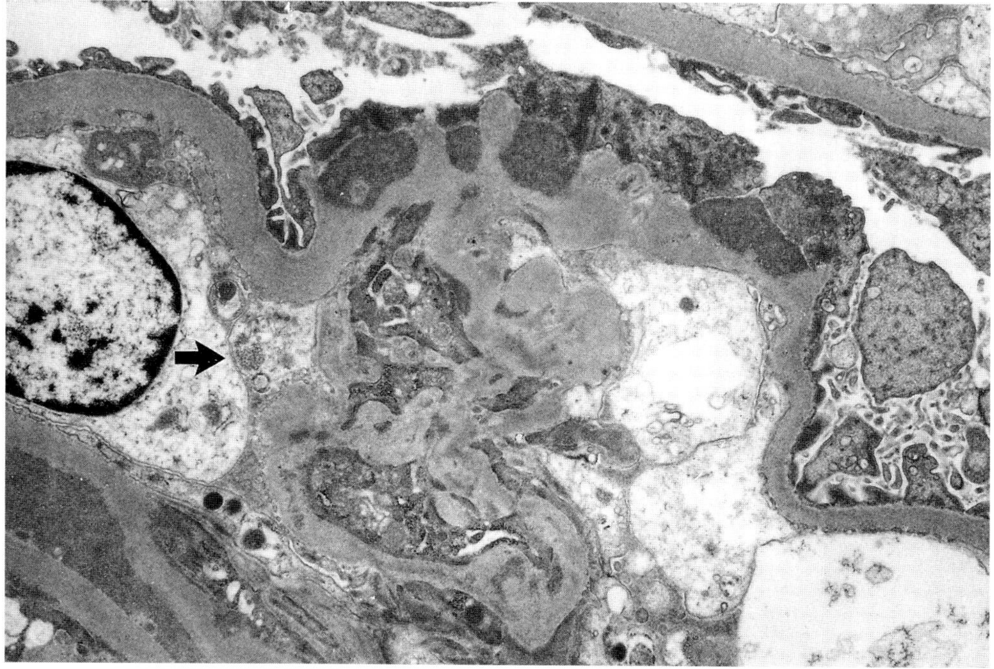

FIG. 5. Electron microscopy of a renal biopsy sample from a patient with HIV-associated immune complex glomerulonephritis. The patient had low-grade proteinuria and slight diminution in creatinine clearance. Prominent, subepithelial electron-dense deposits of variable size may be appreciated, as may smaller mesangial deposits (original magnification ×18,000). Tubular reticular structures are seen in the cytoplasm (arrow). Reprinted with permission (72).

HIVIgAN

The pathology of HIVIgAN also has been described previously (22,88). Light microscopy usually shows diffuse or segmental increase in mesangial matrix, with segmental proliferative changes. Rarely, thrombi are seen in glomerular capillaries, and areas of segmental sclerosis may be noted. Occasionally fibrocellular crescents are seen (88,91–93). IgA, by definition, is the predominant immunoglobulin in the mesangium and in glomerular capillary walls, along with C3, IgM, and less often IgG. Electron microscopy shows increased mesangial matrix with mesangial and peripheral intramembranous and/or subepithelial electron-dense deposits. Tubular reticular structures may be noted in glomerular endothelial cells. Nuclear bodies may be seen in interstitial cells (93).

HIV-TTP/HUS

The pathologic findings in HIV-TTP/HUS are similar to those encountered in patients in the absence of HIV infection (23). Platelet and fibrin thrombi are found in glomerular capillaries, renal arterioles, and interlobular arteries. Arteriolar intimal edema, endothelial cell swelling, fibrinoid necrosis, and onion skin lesions may be present. Immunofluorescence staining has demonstrated fibrin and fibrinogen deposits in arterioles, as well as deposition of fibrinogen, C1q, C3, C4, IgA, IgM, and kappa and lambda light chains in glomeruli (23,119–121). Electron microscopy demonstrates separation of glomerular capillary endothelial cells from basement membrane by granular material. Glomerular tufts may be collapsed. Ischemic wrinkling and focal denudation of the basement membrane may be appreciated (23,120–123). Such findings are nonspecific and may typically be seen in FGS. Tubular reticular structures may be noted in endothelial cell cytoplasm (23,120,121,123).

CLINICAL MANIFESTATIONS AND LABORATORY FEATURES

HIVFGS

Renal function may diminish from relatively normal to very low levels, necessitating treatment for ESRD, over a period of weeks to months (9,12,13,124). This rapid progression of disease is not characteristic of other renal diseases in which glomerulosclerosis is seen, such as diabetic and heroin-associated nephropathy. A small percentage of patients may have a relatively more insidious course of progressive renal insufficiency. This may relate to earlier detection, differences in underlying pathology (mesangial hyperplasia vs. sclerotic and collapsing lesions), differences in treatment or other poorly understood factors. There are almost no data regarding serial analyses of histology in patients in whom a diagnosis of HIV-associated mesangial proliferation, hyperplasia, or HIVFGS has been made (4,9,125). Normal or enlarged echogenic kidneys are characteristic of HIVFGS.

Hypertension is uncommon in patients, even in the face of severe diminution in glomerular filtration rate (9, 12,126,127). The reasons for this are unknown, but the presence of coexisting gastrointestinal disorders, malnutrition, and anorexia may limit solute load and extracellular volume. Alternatively, autonomic neuropathy may be important in interfering with appropriate vasoconstrictive responses in HIV-infected patients, particularly in advanced stages of the illness. Nephrotic-range proteinuria is usually associated with HIVFGS, yet hypercholesterolemia is relatively uncommon (124,127). Hypoalbuminemia is common and may be severe, although edema appears to be relatively uncommon, perhaps for reasons similar to those underlying the relative rarity of hypertension in this population. Serum complement levels are usually within the normal range (127). The clinicopathologic features of HIVFGS and other renal syndromes associated with HIV infection are outlined in Table 3.

HIVICD

HIVGN (22,72) is characterized by the triad of proliferative glomerulonephritis, renal insufficiency, and proteinuria. The level of renal insufficiency and proteinuria is variable. Nephrotic-range proteinuria, often to high levels, and progression to ESRD are not uncommon. However, hematuria is not an invariable finding. Red blood cell and granular casts are variably present on urinalysis. Renal insufficiency and hypocomplementemia to a variable degree are encountered. Patients with HIVICD may have mild hypertension, in contrast with those with HIVFGS. It appears, from the small number of cases studied, that the stage of HIV infection is not related to the occurrence of disease (22,72).

HIVIgAN

Patients usually have hematuria and variable levels of proteinuria, sometimes in the nephrotic range. Red cell casts are usually noted. Renal insufficiency is common, but is often stable and can improve. Serum IgA levels are increased, but, as noted above, this is a common finding in HIV-infected patients in the absence of renal disease. Occasional patients have hypertension.

The low reported prevalence of IgAN in HIV-infected patients may be related to a true low incidence of the disease (22,24,88,92), perhaps related to individual host responses and genetic background in infected patients (22,24,92,104). Alternatively, the low prevalence may reflect the reluctance to perform renal biopsies in patients with urinary abnormalities and mild renal insufficiency,

TABLE 3. *Clinical renal syndromes in HIV-infected patients*

Renal disease	Demographics	Stage of HIV infection	Progression	Clinical presentation	Pathology
HIVFGS	Predominantly black; children and adults	Variable	Rapid	Nephrotic syndrome; azotemia	Glomerular capillary collapse, hypertrophy and hyperplasia of glomerular epithelial cells; segmental or diffuse increase in messangial matrix; microcystic tubular dilatation, tubular simplification, flattening necrosis and degeneration; interstitial immune cell infiltrate of lymphocytes and macrophages; TRS
HIVIgA	White and Hispanic; children and adults	Early	Slow	Proteinuria; hematuria; mild renal insufficiency; rheumatoid factor; hypocomplementemia	Focal or diffuse messangial proliferation; focal proliferative glomerulonephritis; crescentic glomerulonephritis; TRS
HIVICD	Black/white; children and adults	Variable	Variable	Proteinuria, variable from low grade to nephrotic range; variable renal insufficiency from mild to advanced chronic renal failure; occasional patients with hypocomplementemia	Postinfectious, lupuslike and mixed inflammatory–sclerotic; mesangial expansion and variable proliferative and sclerosing changes; microcystic tubular dilatation and interstitial inflammation; TRS
HIV TTP/ HUS	White/black/ Hispanic	Variable	Variable; renal failure more common in HUS	Microangiopathic hemolytic anemia, proteinuria and hematuria; variable thrombocytopenia, renal insufficiency, and neurologic abnormalities	Platelet and fibrin thrombi in glomerular capillaries and renal arterioles; fibrinoid necrosis; acute tubular necrosis; TRS

TRS, tubular reticular structures.

in the absence of perceived effective treatment, and in the presence of an underlying disease thought to be more related to survival than the complicating nephropathy (88,92).

HIV-TTP/HUS

The clinical features of HIV-TTP/HUS are similar to those encountered in patients in the absence of HIV infection (23). The distinction between HUS and TTP is somewhat arbitrary, and differentiation between the two entities may be difficult. These syndromes may be thought of as comprising a spectrum of disorders rather than two different diseases. A diarrheal prodrome, the presence of concurrent or pre-existing bacterial enteritis, severe hemolysis with relatively well-preserved platelet count, and severe renal insufficiency may favor a clinical diagnosis of HIV-associated HUS, whereas neurologic abnormalities and profound thrombocytopenia in the absence of severe hemolysis and marked renal insufficiency is more typical of TTP. Nonspecific complaints such as fever and headache may be seen in association with gastrointestinal symptoms such as abdominal pain, nausea, vomiting, and diarrhea. Symptoms referrable to the hematologic disorders, such as abnormal bruising and bleeding, skin manifestations such as petechiae, and neurologic symptoms such as paresthesias, visual disturbances, change in mental status, and seizures, also may be seen in such patients. Physical findings include fever, petechiae and ecchymoses, lymphadenopathy, hepatomegaly and splenomegaly, focal neurologic deficits, stupor, and coma. Laboratory abnormalities include Coombs negative hemolytic anemia and signs of microangiopathic hemolytic anemia seen on peripheral smear (such as schistocytes, nucleated red blood cells, and spherocytes). Thrombocytopenia, more usual and severe in TTP compared with HUS, is common. Lactate dehydrogenase levels are frequently elevated, but prothrombin and partial thromboplastin times are typically in the normal range. Urinalysis usually shows proteinuria, hematuria, and granular casts. Variable levels of renal insufficiency are present. Nephrotic-range proteinuria is relatively uncommon. The clinical course may be rapid and explosive (23).

DIFFERENTIAL DIAGNOSIS

Glomerular diseases may occur in HIV-infected patients that are unrelated to the viral infection, related to coinfections, or reflect the immune dysregulation seen in HIV infection (12,21,22,128). Clinical findings and urinalysis often do not provide sufficient discrimination to predict histology. In patients with nephrotic-range proteinuria, renal disease secondary to hepatitis B infection should be considered (86,129), especially because the coinfection rate of HBV and HIV is extremely high. Likewise, glomerulopathies related to syphilitic infection and amyloidosis should be considered as well in patients with HIV infection (9,12). Several patients with coexistent long-standing diabetes mellitus and HIV infection, with nephrotic range proteinuria and abnormal renal function, had diabetic nephropathy rather than a renal disease obviously associated with HIV infection (21,22). Finally, we recently studied an HIV-infected patient treated with IFN-α who developed IFN-α–IgG immune complex membranoproliferative glomerulonephritis, demonstrating that glomerulonephritis in HIV-infected patients may be secondary to a host response to treatment (58).

Renal biopsy is therefore important in determining the histologic diagnosis in patients with HIV infection and renal disease, including those who present with nephrotic-range proteinuria (21,22,72,86,128). Examination of renal tissue is the only definitive way to diagnose HIVFGS and HIVICD. In order to make a definitive diagnosis of HIVGN, renal biopsy must show histologic evidence of glomerular inflammation, with immunofluorescent microscopy confirming deposition of immunoglobulin and complement and electron microscopy demonstrating mesangial or capillary deposits (22,72,99,100) (Figs. 2 and 5). More precise diagnosis may be achieved by identifying HIV protein–immunoglobulin complexes in glomerular capillaries or the mesangium in higher titer than in the circulation, although such studies are often primarily research techniques (22,72).

HIV-TTP/HUS may be considered a "great masquerader." Disseminated intravascular coagulation, HIV-associated immune thrombocytopenia, combinations of drug toxicities, neurologic disorders, and renal dysfunction of various etiologies may all mimic presentations of HIV-TTP/HUS (23). The classic findings of fever, renal dysfunction, thrombocytopenia, and neurologic disease are sufficiently common in HIV-infected patients that a high index of suspicion and confirmation of the diagnosis by examination of the peripheral smear are critical in establishing a diagnosis. Diagnosis of HIV-associated thrombotic microangiopathies is important because instituting therapy expeditiously may be crucial in attaining optimal patient outcomes.

TREATMENT AND PROGNOSIS

HIVFGS

Patients with mesangial disease may have a better prognosis (9,124) compared with those with classic HIVFGS, but this issue has not been studied rigorously. Children also may have a less aggressive course of progressive renal insufficiency (130), but in those children who manifest HIV-associated renal diseases, diagnosis is made at a mean of 3 to 4 years of age, and the level of diagnostic evaluation and follow-up investigation may be quite different from that in the adult population. Although there have been anecdotal reports of improvement in renal function and outcome in patients treated with antiretroviral drugs, there is no established, effective therapy for HIVFGS. The role of antiretroviral therapy in the treatment of HIVFGS, while perhaps beneficial, has not been assessed in a randomized, controlled trial (131–135).

Appel and Neill (136) reported steroid-induced remission of laboratory signs of nephrotic syndrome in a patient with HIV and hepatitis B virus infections. The histology was consistent with IgM nephropathy and did not show interstitial immune cell infiltration, and ultrastructural markers of HIV-associated renal diseases were not noted. Therefore, the relationship of the renal disease to HIV infection in this patient is unknown. Four patients with HIVFGS, renal insufficiency, and proteinuria treated with glucocorticoids showed improvement in renal function in an uncontrolled trial (137). Two of the four patients developed opportunistic infections during treatment. In a recent update, Smith and coworkers showed reduced proteinuria and diminution in level of serum creatinine with corticosteroid therapy in an uncontrolled trial in 20 patients with HIVFGS (138). Seventeen of the patients had HIVFGS demonstrated on renal biopsy, and three were presumed to have the disease. The patients were treated with 60 mg of prednisone a day for a two-to-eleven-week course, while the glucocorticoid was tapered. Serum creatinine levels fell in 17 patients, and proteinuria improved in 12 of the 13 patients tested. Complications were relatively common but severe: new opportunistic infection in six patients, steroid-induced psychosis in two patients, and one patient had upper gastrointestinal bleeding. We have tried therapy with glucocorticoids in selected patients with HIVFGS without success. Quantitation of relative risks and benefits of such therapy await the performance of larger, well-controlled treatment trials, stratifying for stage of viral illness, treatment with antiretroviral drugs and other potential confounding medications, histologic parameters and entry level of urinary protein excretion and renal function.

Angiotensin-converting enzyme inhibitors (ACEIs) have been shown to be beneficial therapy in several different renal and glomerular diseases. A temporally associated decrease in urinary protein excretion has been documented in a patient with HIVFGS, treated with fosinopril, an angiotensin converting enzyme inhibitor, but an effect on renal function, and prolongation of course to ESRD was not noted (139). Captopril, another ACEI, was recently demonstrated to be associated with increased length of time before death or initiation of

ESRD therapy in a nonrandomized, case control study (140). Nine patients with HIVFGS treated with 6.25 to 25 mg captopril three times daily were matched by age, race, gender, CD4 count, and serum creatinine concentration with nine control patients not treated with ACEIs. Mean renal survival was enhanced in the captopril group compared with patients not treated with an ACEI. Two patients we treated have had relatively little change in mild renal insufficiency for as long as a year and a half to two years. A randomized, double-blinded, placebo-controlled trial stratified for risk, host, renal function, viral and treatment factors will determine if ACEIs are safe and effective treatment for HIVFGS, and whether this therapy is superior to treatment with glucocorticoids.

Until more definitive studies are available, it is the practice at George Washington University Medical Center to ensure that the patient with HIVFGS is treated with antiretroviral drugs, if appropriate. Steroid therapy may be used, but the clinician must monitor the patient closely for the development of side effects and superinfections. The risk:benefit ratio associated with the use of angiotensin-converting enzyme inhibitors appears to be low, and they have been used at George Washington in patients with hypertension and to treat patients with excessively high urinary protein excretion and edema.

Although initial reports suggested that the course of patients with AIDS and ESRD who were treated with renal replacement therapy was dismal (1,141), these data were largely collected during the period before HIV testing. HIV-infected patients with ESRD have been treated with hemodialysis and continuous ambulatory peritoneal dialysis. Their survival seems to be linked primarily to the patients' stage of the underlying viral illness when ESRD therapy is initiated rather than to the severity or type of renal disease (17,19,142,143). Mean survival of a year to a year and a half has been reported in HIV-infected patients with ESRD who had not yet developed AIDS (17,19,139,142). Currently the role of renal transplantation in the treatment of patients with HIVFGS is unclear. The role of medically prescribed immunosuppression in mediating graft and patient survival in patients with HIV infection who have undergone renal transplantation is unknown (12,143). Although several patients with HIV infection and renal disease have been treated with renal transplantation (12,143), because of diminished life expectancy and fear of immunosuppressive complications, particularly increased susceptibility to opportunistic infections, in most transplantation programs HIV-infected patients are given a relatively low priority for receiving cadaveric organs (143).

HIV-ICD

Prognosis may depend, in part, on renal functional status and histologic findings. All patients we evaluated with findings of mixed disease progressed to ESRD (22). Another patient with mild urinary abnormalities and well-preserved renal function had relatively stable renal function for almost 2 years, whereas the viral illness progressed. Antiretroviral therapy had been instituted in some patients with HIVICD, without obvious effect. Its role in the treatment of HIVGN must be studied rigorously. The role of therapy with glucocorticoids in improving the course of HIVGN is also unknown, although anecdotal reports have shown limited efficacy. Such therapies also need to be evaluated in proper clinical trials. There have been no controlled trials of specific treatment interventions in patients with HIV-ICD.

HIV-IgAN

Jindal et al. treated a patient with renal insufficiency and IgAN with glucocorticoids before the diagnosis of the concurrent HIV infection (91). The level of circulating creatinine decreased, suggesting that a beneficial clinical response may have been related to this treatment. However, most patients have had mild, nonprogressive renal insufficiency (22,24,92). The effects of glucocorticoid and antiretroviral therapy on the natural history of the disease are unknown and have not been evaluated in controlled trials.

HIV-TTP/HUS

Patients with HIV infection who develop thrombotic microangiopathies have a poor prognosis. Approximately a third of patients died in the acute phase of illness, despite the institution of aggressive therapeutic regimens (23). Longer term survival is also poor. Plasma infusion and plasmapheresis have been used as the mainstays of therapy. Glucocorticoids, vincristine, infusion of immunoglobulins, and less well studied therapies have been used with variable outcomes (23). Complete or partial remissions have been reported in the majority of patients, but relapses and patients refractory to therapy are common. The role of antiretroviral therapy in such patients is unknown. Because of the relative rarity of this clinical entity, there is an understandable paucity of controlled trials of appropriate therapies. It is the practice at George Washington University Medical Center to treat patients with HIV-TTP/HUS with antiretroviral drugs, glucocorticoids, and plasmapheresis.

REFERENCES

1. Rao TKS, Filippone EJ, Nicastri AD, Landesman SH, Frank E, Chen CK, Friedman EA. Associated focal and segmental glomerulosclerosis in the acquired immunodeficiency syndrome. *N Engl J Med* 1984; 310:669–673.
2. Pardo V, Aldana M, Colton RM, et al. Glomerular lesions in the

acquired immunodeficiency syndrome. *Ann Intern Med* 1984;101: 429–434.
3. Soni A, Agarwal A, Chander P, et al. Evidence for an HIV-related nephropathy: a clinicopathological study. *Clin Nephrol* 1989;31: 12–17.
4. D'Agati V, Cheng JI, Carbone L, Cheng JT, Appel G. The pathology of HIV-nephropathy: a detailed morphologic and comparative study. *Kidney Int* 1989;35:1358–1370.
5. Gardenswartz MH, Lerner CW, Seligson GR, et al. Renal disease in patients with AIDS: a clinicopathologic study. *Clin Nephrol* 1984;21: 197–204.
6. Vaziri ND, Barbari A, Licorish K, Cesario T, Gupta S. Spectrum of renal abnormalities in acquired immunodeficiency syndrome. *J Natl Med Assoc* 1985;77:369–375.
7. Brunkhorst R, Brunkhorst U, Eisenbach GM, Schedel I, Deicher H, Koch KM. Lack of clinical evidence for a specific HIV-associated glomerulopathy in 203 patients with HIV infection. *Nephrol Dial Transplant* 1992;7:87–92.
8. Humphreys MH. Human immunodeficiency virus–associated nephropathy. East is east and west is west? *Arch Intern Med* 1990;150: 253–255.
9. Bourgoignie JJ. Renal complications of human immunodeficiency virus type I. *Kidney Int* 1990;37:1571–1584.
10. Kimmel PL, Umana WO, Bosch JP. Abnormal urinary protein excretion in HIV infected patients. *Clin Nephrol* 1993;39:17–21, 1993.
11. Bourgoignie JJ, Ortiz-Interiano C, Green DF, Roth D. Race, a co-factor in HIV-1 associated nephropathy. *Transplant Proc* 1989;21:3899–3901.
12. Glassock RJ, Cohen AH, Danovitch G, Parsa P. HIV infection and the kidney. *Ann Intern Med* 1990;112:35–49.
13. Seney FD Jr, Burns DK, Silva FG. AIDS and the kidney. *Am J Kidney Dis* 1990;16:1–13.
14. Cantor ES, Kimmel PL, Bosch JP. Effect of race on the expression of AIDS associated nephropathy. *Arch Intern Med* 1991;151:125–128.
15. Nochy D, Glotz D, Dosquet P, et al. Renal disease associated with HIV infection: a multicentric study of 60 patients from Paris hospitals. *Nephrol Dial Transplant* 1993;8:11–19.
16. Alter MJ, Favero MS, Moyer LA, Blend LA. National surveillance of dialysis associated diseases in the US. *ASAIO Trans* 1990;37:97–108.
17. Ortiz C, Meneses R, Jaffe D, Fernandez JA, Perez G, Bourgoignie JJ. Outcome of patients with human immunodeficiency virus on maintenance hemodialysis. *Kidney Int* 1988;34:248–253.
18. Reiser IW, Shapiro WB, Porush JG. Incidence and epidemiology of HIV infection in 320 patients treated in an inner city hemodialysis center. *Am J Kidney Dis* 1990;15:26–31.
19. Kimmel PL, Umana WO, Simmens SJ, Watson J, Bosch JP. Continuous ambulatory peritoneal dialysis and survival of HIV infected patients with ESRD. *Kidney Int* 1993;44:373–378.
20. Kimmel PL, VedBrat SS, Pierce P, et al. Prevalence of viremia in HIV-infected patients with renal disease. *Arch Intern Med* 1995;155: 1578–1585.
21. Kimmel PL, Ferreira-Centeno A, Farkas-Szallasi T, Abraham A, Garrett CT. Viral DNA in microdissected renal biopsies of HIV infected patients with nephrotic syndrome. *Kidney Int* 1993;43:1347–1352.
22. Kimmel PL, Phillips TM. Immune complex glomerulonephritis associated with HIV infection. In: Kimmel PL, Berns JS, Stein JH, eds. *Renal and urologic aspects of HIV infection.* New York: Churchill Livingstone; 1995:77–110.
23. Berns JS. Hemolytic uremic syndrome and thrombotic thrombocytopenic purpura associated with HIV infection. In: Kimmel PL, Berns JS, Stein JH, eds. *Renal and urologic aspects of HIV infection.* New York: Churchill Livingstone; 1995:111–134.
24. Bourgoignie JJ, Pardo V. HIV-associated nephropathies. *N Engl J Med* 1992;327:729–730.
25. Rennke HG, Klein PS. Pathogenesis and significance of non-primary focal and segmental glomerulosclerosis. *Am J Kidney Dis* 1989;13: 443–456.
26. Schwartz MM, Korbet SM. Primary focal segmental glomerulosclerosis. *Am J Kidney Dis* 1993;22:874–883.
27. D'Agati V. The many masks of focal glomerulosclerosis. *Kidney Int* 1994;46:1223–1241.
28. Connor E, Gupta S, Joshi V, et al. Acquired immunodeficiency syndrome associated renal disease in children. *J Pediatr* 1988;113: 39–44.
29. Rousseau E, Russo P, Lapointe N, O'Regan S. Renal complications of acquired immunodeficiency syndrome in children. *Am J Kidney Dis* 1988;11:48–50.
30. Strauss J, Abitbol C, Zilleruelo G, et al. Renal disease in children with the acquired immunodeficiency syndrome. *N Engl J Med* 1989;321: 625–630.
31. Ingulli E, Tejani A, Fikrig S, Nicastri A, Chen CK, Pomrantz A. Nephrotic syndrome associated with acquired immunodeficiency syndrome in children. *J Pediatr* 1991;119:710–716.
32. Dickie P, Felser M, Eckhaus M, et al. HIV-associated nephropathy in transgenic mice expressing HIV-1 genes. *Virology* 1991;185:109–119.
33. Kopp JB, Klotman ME, Adler SH, et al. Progressive glomerulosclerosis and enhanced renal accumulation of basement membrane components in mice transgenic for human immunodeficiency type 1 genes. *Proc Natl Acad Sci U S A* 1992;89:1577–1581.
34. Kopp JB, Klotman PE. Animal models of lentivirus-associated renal disease. In: Kimmel PL, Berns JS, Stein JH, eds. *Renal and urologic aspects of HIV infection.* New York: Churchill Livingstone; 1995: 381–404.
35. Baskerville A, Ramsay A, Cranage MP, et al. Histopathological changes in simian immunodeficiency virus infection. *J Pathol* 1990; 162:67–75.
36. Hirsch VM, Zack PM, Vogel AP, Johnson PR. Simian immunodeficiency virus infection of macaques: end-stage disease is characterized by widespread distribution of proviral DNA in tissues. *J Infect Dis* 1991;163:976–988.
37. Cohen AH, Sun NCJ, Shapsak P, Imagawa DT. Demonstration of HIV in renal epithelium in HIV-associated nephropathy. *Mod Pathol* 1989;2:125–128.
38. Cohen AH, Nast CC. HIV-associated nephropathy. A unique combined glomerular, tubular and interstitial lesion. *Mod Pathol* 1988;1: 87–97.
39. Bodi I, Abraham AA, Kimmel PL. Macrophages in HIV-associated kidney diseases. *Am J Kidney Dis* 1994;24:762–767.
40. Main IW, Nikolic-Paterson DJ, Atkins RC. T cells and macrophages and their role in renal injury. *Semin Nephrol* 1992;12:395–407.
41. Schreiner GF. Role of macrophages in glomerular injury. *Semin Nephrol* 1991;11:268–275.
42. Cattell V. Macrophages in acute glomerular inflammation. *Kidney Int* 1994;45:945–952.
43. Miller MD, Krangel MS. Biology and biochemistry of the chemokines: a family of chemotactic and inflammatory cytokines. *Crit Rev Immunol* 1992;12:17–46.
44. Greene WC. Molecular biology of HIV type I infection. *N Engl J Med* 1991;324: 308–317.
45. Pantaleo G, Graziosi C, Fauci AS. New concepts in the pathogenesis of HIV infection. *N Engl J Med* 1993;328:327–335.
46. Ammar A, Sahraoui Y, Tsapis A, Bertoli A-M, Jasmin C, Georgoulias V. HIV-infected adherent cell inhibitory factor (p29) inhibits normal T cell proliferation through decreased expression of high affinity IL-2 receptors and production of IL-2. *J Clin Invest* 1992;90:8–14.
47. Viscidi RP, Mayur K, Lederman HM, Frankel AD. Inhibition of antigen-induced lymphocyte proliferation by Tat protein from HIV-1. *Science* 1989;246:1606–1608.
48. Strutz F, Neilson EG. The role of lymphocytes in the progression of interstitial disease. *Kidney Int* 1994;45(suppl):45:106–110.
49. Mattana J, Abramovici M, Singhal PC. Effects of human immunodeficiency virus sera and macrophage supernatants on mesangial cell proliferation and matrix synthesis. *Am J Pathol* 1993;143:814–822.
50. Schattner A. Interferons and autoimmunity. *Am J Med Sci* 1988;295: 532–544.
51. Bockus D, Remington F, Luu J, Bean M, Hammar S. Induction of cylindrical confronting cisternae in Daudi lymphoblastoid cells by recombinant alpha-interferon. *Hum Pathol* 1988;19:78–82.
52. Rich SA. De novo synthesis and secretion of a 36-kD protein by cells that form lupus inclusions in response to α-interferon. *J Clin Invest* 1995;95:219–226.
53. Eyster ME, Goedert JJ, Poon M, Preble OT. Acid-labile alpha interferon: a possible preclinical marker for AIDS in hemophilia. *N Engl J Med* 1983;309:583–586.
54. Kakizaki Y, Kraft N, Atkins RC. Differential control of mesangial cell proliferation by interferon gamma. *Clin Exp Immunol* 1991;85: 157–163.

55. Martin M, Schwinzer R, Schellekens H, Resch K. Glomerular mesangial cells in local inflammation. Induction of expression of MHC class II antigens by interferon-gamma. *J Immunol* 1989;142:1887–1894.
56. Averbusch SD, Austin HA, Sherwin SA, Antonovych T, Bunn PA, Longo DL. Acute interstitial nephritis with the nephrotic syndrome following recombinant leukocyte a interferon therapy for mycosis fungoides. *N Engl J Med* 1984;310:32–34.
57. Lederer E, Truong L. Unusual glomerular lesion in a patient receiving long-term interferon alpha. *Am J Kidney Dis* 1992;20:516–518.
58. Kimmel PL, Abraham AA, Phillips TM. Membranoproliferative glomerulonephritis in a patient treated with interferon alpha for HIV infection. *Am J Kidney Dis* 1994;24:858–863.
59. Phillips TM, Kimmel PL. High-performance capillary electropheretic analysis of inflammatory citokines in human biopsies. *J Chromatogr* 1994;656:259–266.
60. Kuncio GS, Neilson EG, Haverty T. Mechanisms of tubulointerstitial fibrosis. *Kidney Int* 1991;39:550–556.
61. Bednarik DP, Folks TM. Mechanism of HIV-1 latency. *AIDS* 1992;6: 3–16.
62. Kujubu DA, Fine LG. Polypeptide growth factors and renal disease. *Am J Kidney Dis* 1989;14:61–73.
63. Ray PE, Bruggeman L, Weeks B, et al. bFGF low affinity receptors in the pathogenesis of human immunodeficiency virus associated nephropathy in transgenic mice. *Kidney Int* 1994;46:759–772.
64. Ensoli B, Barillari G, Gallo RC. Cytokines and growth factors in the pathogenesis of AIDS-associated Kaposi's sarcoma. *Immunol Rev* 1992;127:147–155.
65. Sharma K, Ziyadeh F. The transforming growth factor-β system and the kidney. *Semin Nephrol* 1993;13:116–128.
66. Border WA, Ruoslahti E. Transforming growth factor-β in disease: the dark side of tissue repair. *J Clin Invest* 1992;90:1–7.
67. Allen JB, Wong HL, Guyre PM, Simon GL, Wahl SM. Association of circulating receptor FCYRIII+ monocytes in AIDS patients with elevated TGF-β levels. *J Clin Invest* 1991;87:1773–1779.
68. Bodi I, Kimmel PL, Abraham AA, Sporn MB, Klotman PE, Kopp JB. Increased TGF-β expression in HIV-associated nephropathy. *J Am Soc Nephrol* 1993;4:461.
69. Shukla RR, Kumar A, Kimmel PL. Transforming growth factor-β increases the expression of HIV-1 gene in transfected human mesangial cells. *Kidney Int* 1993;44:1022–1029.
70. Green DF, Resnick L, Bourgoignie JJ. HIV infects glomerular endothelial and mesangial, but not epithelial cells in vitro. *Kidney Int* 1992;41:956–960.
71. Alpers CE, McClure J, Bursten SL. Human mesangial cells are resistant to productive infection by multiple strains of human immunodeficiency virus types 1 and 2. *Am J Kidney Dis* 1992;19:126–130.
72. Kimmel PL, Phillips TM, Ferreira-Centeno A, Farkas-Szallasi T, Abraham AA, Garrett CT. HIV-associated immune mediated renal disease. *Kidney Int* 1993;44:1022–1029.
73. Rappaport J, Kopp JB, Klotman PE. Host virus interactions and the molecular regulation of HIV-1: role in the pathogenesis of HIV-associated nephropathy. *Kidney Int* 1994;46:16–27.
74. Shukla RR, Kimmel PL, Kumar A. Molecular biology of HIV-1 and kidney disease. In: Kimmel PL, Berns JS, Stein JH, eds. *Renal and urologic aspects of HIV infection.* New York: Churchill Livingstone; 1995:77–110.
75. Pullium L, West D, Haigword N, Swanson NRA. HIV-1 envelope gp120 alters astrocytes in human brain cultures. *AIDS Res Hum Retrovir* 1993;9:439–444.
76. Capobianchi MR, Ameglio F, Fei P, et al. Coordinate induction of INF α and τ by recombinant HIV-1 glycoprotein 120. *AIDS Res Hum Retrovir* 1993;9:957–962.
77. Capobianchi MR, Ankel H, Ameglio F, Paganelli R, Pizzoli PM, Dianzani F. Recombinant gp120 of HIV is a potent interferon inducer. *AIDS Res Hum Retrovir* 1992;8:575–579.
78. Ensoli B, Barillari G, Zaki RC, Wong-Stall F. Tat protein of HIV-1 stimulates growth of cells derived from Kaposi sarcoma lesions of AIDS patients. *Nature* 1990;345:84–86.
79. Zauli G, Re MC, Davis B, et al. Tat protein stimulates production of TGF-β1 by bone marrow macrophages: potential mechanism for HIV-1–induced hematopoietic suppression. *Blood* 1992;80:3036–3043.
80. Buonaguro L, Barillari G, Chang HK, et al. Effects of HIV-1 Tat protein on the expression of inflammatory cytokines. *J Virol* 1992;66: 7159–7167.
81. Banda NK, Bernier J, Kurahara DK, et al. Cross-linking CD4 by HIV gp120 primes T cells for activation-induced apoptosis. *J Exp Med* 1992;176:1099–1106.
82. Singhal PC. Human immunodeficiency virus-1 gp120 and gp160 envelope proteins modulate mesangial cell gelatinolytic activity. *Am J Pathol* 1995;147:25–32.
83. Shukla RR, Kumar A, Kimmel PL. Effect of HIV-1 gp120 on TGF-β gene expression in human mesangial cells. *J Am Soc Nephrol* 1994;5: 702.
84. Bodi I, Abraham AA, Kimmel PL. Apoptosis in human immunodeficiency virus–associated nephropathy. *Am J Kidney Dis* 1995;26:286–291.
85. Kenneth KK, Factor SM. Membranoproliferative glomerulonephritis and plexogenic pulmonary arteriopathy in a homosexual man with acquired immunodeficiency syndrome. *Hum Pathol* 1987;18:1293–1296.
86. Guerra IL, Abraham AA, Kimmel PL, Sabnis SG, Antonovych TT. Nephrotic syndrome associated with chronic persistent hepatitis B in an HIV antibody positive patient. *Am J Kidney Dis* 1987;10:385–388.
87. Ortiz-Butcher C. The spectrum of kidney diseases in patients with human immunodeficiency virus infection. *Curr Opin Nephrol Hypertens* 1993;2:355–364.
88. Kimmel PL, Moore J Jr. Viral glomerulonephritis. In: Schrier RW, Gottschalk CW, eds. *Diseases of the kidney.* 6th ed. Boston: Little, Brown; 1997:1595–1618.
89. Kenouch S, Delahousse M, Mery J-P, Nochy D. Mesangial IgA deposits in two patients with AIDS related complex. *Nephron* 1990; 54:338–340.
90. Trachtman H, Gauthier B, Vinograd A, Valderrama E. IgA nephropathy in a child with human immunodeficiency virus type 1 infection. *Pediatr Nephrol* 1991;5:724–726.
91. Jindal KK, Trillo A, Bishop G, Hirch D, Cohen A. Crescentic IgA nephropathy as a manifestation of human immunodeficiency virus infection. *Am J Nephrol* 1991;11:147–150.
92. Kimmel PL, Phillips TM, Ferreira-Centeno A, Farkas-Szallasi T, Abraham AA, Garrett CT. Idiotypic IgA nephropathy in patients with HIV infection. *N Engl J Med* 1992;327:702–706.
93. Katz A, Bargman JM, Miller DC, Guo J-W, Ghali VS, Schoeneman MJ. IgA nephritis in HIV-positive patients: a new HIV-associated nephropathy? *Clin Nephrol* 1992;38:61–68.
94. Schoeneman MJ, Ghali V, Lieberman K, Reisman L. IgA nephritis in a child with human immunodeficiency virus: a unique form of human immunodeficiency virus-associated nephropathy? *Pediatr Nephrol* 1992;6:46–49.
95. Morrow WJW, Wharton M, Stricker R, Levy JA. Circulating immune complexes in patients with the acquired immunodeficiency syndrome contain the AIDS-associated retrovirus. *Clin Immunol Immunopathol* 1986;40:515–524.
96. McDougal JS, Kennedy MS, Nicholson JKA, et al. Antibody response to human immunodeficiency virus in homosexual men. *J Clin Invest* 1987;80:316–324.
97. Couser WG. Mechanisms of glomerular injury in immune-complex disease. *Kidney Int* 1985;28:569–583.
98. Couser WG. Mediation of immune glomerular injury. *J Am Soc Nephrol* 1990;1:13–29.
99. Glassock RJ. Immune complex-induced glomerular injury in viral diseases: an overview. *Kidney Int* 1991;40(suppl):35:5–7.
100. Wilson CB. The renal response to immunologic injury. In Brenner BM, Rector FC, eds. *The kidney.* 4th ed. Philadelphia: WB Saunders; 1991:1062–1181.
101. Taillan B, Garnier G, Pesce A, et al. Cryoglobulinemia related to hepatitis C virus infection in patients with the human immunodeficiency virus infection [Letter]. *Clin Exp Rheumatol* 1993;11:350.
102. Stricker RB, Sanders KA, Owen WF, Kiprov DD, Miller RG. Mononeuritis multiplex associated with cryoglobulinemia in HIV infection. *Neurology* 1992;42:2103–2105.
103. Gherardi R, Belec L, Mhiri C, et al. The spectrum of vasculitis in human immunodeficiency virus–infected patients. *Arthritis Rheum* 1993;36:1164–1174.
104. Emancipator SN. Immunoregulatory factors in the pathogenesis of IgA nephropathy. *Kidney Int* 1990;38:388–392.
105. Galla JH. IgA nephropathy. *Kidney Int* 1995;47:377–387.
106. Fling J, Fischer JR, Boswell RN, Reid MJ. The relationship of serum IgA concentration to human immunodeficiency virus infection: a cross-

sectional study of HIV-positive individuals detected by screening in the United States Air Force. *J Allergy Clin Immunol* 1988;82:965–970.

107. Procaccia S, Lazzarin A, Colucci A, et al. IgM, IgG and IgA rheumatoid factors and circulating immune complexes in patients with AIDS and AIDS related complex with serological abnormalities. *Clin Exp Immunol* 1987;67:236–244.
108. Jackson S, Dawson LM, Kotler DP. IgA1 is the major immunoglobulin component of immune complexes in the acquired immunodeficiency syndrome. *Clin Immunol* 1988;8:64–68.
109. Jackson S, Tarkowski A, Collins JE, et al. Occurrence of polymeric IgA1 rheumatoid factor in the acquired immunodeficiency syndrome. *Clin Immunol* 1988;8:390–396.
110. Lightfoote MM, Folks TM, Redfield R, Gold J, Sell K. Circulating IgA immune compexes in AIDS. *Immunol Invest* 1985;14:341–345.
111. Bene M-C, Canton P, Amiel C, May T, Faure G. Absence of mesangial IgA in AIDS: a postmortem study. *Nephron* 1991;58:240–241.
112. Del Arco A, Martinez MA, Pena JM, et al. Thrombotic thrombocytopenic purpura associated with human immunodeficiency virus infection: demonstration of p24 antigen in endothelial cells. *Clin Infect Dis* 1993;17:360–363.
113. Pardo V, Meneses R, Ossa L, Jaffe DJ, Strauss J, Roth D, Bourgoignie JJ. AIDS-related glomerulopathy: occurrence in specific risk groups. *Kidney Int* 1987;31:1167–1173.
114. Bourgoignie JJ, Pardo V. The nephropathology in human immunodeficiency virus (HIV-1) infection. *Kidney Int* 1991;35(suppl):19–23.
115. Cohen A. Renal pathology of HIV-associated nephropathy. In: Kimmel PL, Berns JS, Stein JH, eds. *Renal and urologic aspects of HIV* infection. New York: Churchill Livingstone; 1995:155–180.
116. Chander P, Soni A, Suri A, Bhagwat R, Yoo J, Treser G. Renal ultrastructural markers in AIDS-associated nephropathy. *Am J Pathol* 1987;126:513–526.
117. Chander P, Agarwal A, Soni A, Kim K, Treser G. Renal cytomembranous inclusions in idiopathic renal disease as predicitve markers for the acquired immunodeficiency syndrome. *Hum Pathol* 1988;19: 1060–1064.
118. Alpers CE, Harawi S, Rennke HG. Focal glomerulosclerosis with tubuloreticular inclusions: a possible predictive value for acquired immunodeficiency syndrome. *Am J Kidney Dis* 1988;12:240–242.
119. Charasse C, Michelet C, Le Tulzo Y, et al. Thrombotic thrombocytopenic purpura with the acquired immunodeficiency syndrome: a pathologically documented case report. *Am J Kidney Dis* 1991;17: 80–82.
120. Berns JS, Tomaszewski JE. Hemolytic uremic syndrome and thrombotic thrombocytopenic purpura associated with human immunodeficiency virus infection and the acquired immunodeficiency syndrome. In: Kaplan BS, Trompeter RS, Moake JL, eds. *Hemolytic uremic syndrome and thrombotic thrombocytopenic purpura.* New York: Marcel Dekker, 1992:299.
121. Francois A, Dhib M, Dubois D, Fillastre JP, Hemet J. Thrombotic microangiopathy as the first manifestation of HIV infection. *Clin Nephrol* 1993;39:352–354.
122. Segal GH, Tubbs RR, Ratliff NB, Miller ML, Longworth DL. Thrombotic thrombocytopenic purpura in a patient with AIDS. *Cleve Clin J Med* 1990;57:360–366.
123. Frem GJ, Rennke HG, Sayegh MH. Late renal allograft failure secondary to thrombotic microangiopathy–human immunodeficiency virus nephropathy. *J Am Soc Nephrol* 1994;4:1643–1648.
124. Langs C, Gallo GR, Schacht RG, Sidhu G, Baldwin DS. Rapid renal failure in AIDS-associated focal glomerulosclerosis. *Arch Intern Med* 1990;150:287–292.
125. Pardo V, Wetli CV, Strauss J, Bourgoignie JJ. The renal complications of drug abuse and human immunodeficiency virus. In: Tischer C, Brenner BM, eds. *Pathology of the kidney.* 2nd ed. New York: Williams & Wilkins; 1994:390–418.
126. Bourgoignie JJ, Meneses R, Ortiz C, Jaffe D, Pardo V. The clinical spectrum of renal disease associated with human immunodeficiency virus. *Am J Kidney Dis* 1988;12:131–137.
127. Bourgoignie JJ. Glomerulosclerosis associated with HIV infection. In: Kimmel PL, Berns JS, Stein JH, eds. *Renal and urologic aspects of HIV infection.* New York: Churchill Livingstone; 1995:59–75.
128. Korbet SM, Schwartz MM. Human immunodeficiency virus infection and nephrotic syndrome. *Am J Kidney Dis* 1992;20:97–103.
129. Schectman JM, Kimmel PL. Remission of hepatitis B–associated membranous glomerulonephritis in human immunodeficiency virus infection. *Am J Kidney Dis* 1989;17:716–718.
130. Pardo V, Strauss J, Abitbol C, Zilleruelo G. Renal disease in children with HIV infection. In: Kimmel PL, Berns JS, Stein JH, eds. *Renal and urologic aspects of HIV infection.* New York: Churchill Livingstone; 1995:135–154.
131. Babut-Gay ML, Echard M, Kleinknecht D, Meyrier A. Zidovudine and nephropathy with HIV infection [Letter]. *Ann Intern Med* 1989; 111:856–857.
132. Cook PP, Appel RG. Prolonged clinical improvement in HIV-associated nephropathy with zidovudine therapy [Letter]. *J Am Soc Nephrol* 1990;1:842.
133. Lam M, Park MC. HIV-associated nephropathy—beneficial effect of zidovudine therapy. *N Engl J Med* 1990;323:1775–1776. (letter).
134. Michel C, Dosquet P, Ronco P, Mougenot B, Viron B, Mignon F. Nephropathy associated with infection by human immunodeficiency virus: a report on eleven cases including 6 treated with zidovudine. *Nephron* 1992;62:434–440.
135. Ifudu O, Rao TKS, Tan CC, Fleischman H, Chirgwin K, Friedman EA. Zidovudine is beneficial in human immunodeficiency virus associated nephropathy. *Am J Nephrol* 1995;15:217–221.
136. Appel RG, Neill J. A steroid-responsive nephrotic syndrome in a patient with human immunodeficiency virus infection. *Ann Intern Med* 1990;113:892–893.
137. Smith MC, Pawar R, Carey JT, et al. Effect of corticosteroid therapy on human immunodeficiency virus-associated nephropathy. *Am J Med* 1994;97:145–151.
138. Smith MC, Austen JL, Carey JT, et al. Prednisone improves renal function and proteinuria in human immunodeficiency virus-associated nephropathy. *Am J Med* 1996;101:41–48.
139. Burns GC, Matute R, Onyema D, Davis I, Toth I. Response to inhibition of angiotensin converting enzyme in human immunodeficiency virus associated nephropathy: a case report. *Am J Kidney Dis* 1994; 23:441–443.
140. Kimmel PL, Mishkin GJ, Umana WO. Captopril and renal survival in patients with HIV associated nephropathy. *Am J Kidney Dis* 1996;28: 202–208.
141. Rao TKS, Friedman EA, Nicastri AD. The types of renal diseases in the acquired immunodeficiency syndrome. *N Engl J Med* 1987;316: 1062–1068.
142. Feinfeld DA, Kaplan R, Dressler R, Lynn RI. Survival of human immunodeficiency virus–infected patients on maintenance hemodialysis. *Clin Nephrol* 1989;32:221–224.
143. Vijayvargiya R, Bosch JP. Dialysis and transplantation in patients with HIV infection. In: Kimmel PL, Berns JS, Stein JH, eds. *Renal and urologic aspects of HIV infection.* New York: Churchill Livingstone; 1995:253–277.

Immunologic Renal Diseases,
edited by E. G. Neilson and W. G. Couser.
Lippincott-Raven Publishers, Philadelphia © 1997.

CHAPTER 55

Recurrent and De Novo Glomerular Disease in Renal Transplants

J. Andrew Bertolatus and Lawrence G. Hunsicker

DEFINITION AND HISTORICAL PERSPECTIVE

Immunologically mediated glomerular disease occurs in transplanted kidneys in at least three recognized circumstances: First, a patient with loss of native-kidney function due to immune-mediated glomerulopathy may have persistence of systemic factors (so-called nephritogenic environment) after transplantation, leading to recurrence of original disease. Second, glomerulopathies may occur de novo in the transplanted kidney by mechanisms that remain to be defined, perhaps as a manifestation of the alloimmune response to foreign antigens present on the graft. Although de novo disease is most clearly demonstrated in patients with nonimmunologic forms of native-kidney disease, the appearance of a histologic form of disease known to be distinct from that of a patient's original disorder can also be observed. Third, subclinical or mild glomerular disease may be present rarely in the donor kidney at the time of transplantation.

The problem of recurrent glomerular disease in the transplanted kidney is as old as the practice of clinical transplantation. In fact, as Merrill stated in a 1969 review of this topic (1), "the development of glomerulonephritis and subsequent renal failure in the first successful human kidney transplant between identical twins was a striking and discouraging complication." Original reports and reviews from this early era of transplantation stressed the frequency and severity of recurrent disease. Particularly striking was the very high incidence of graft loss (~60%) attributed to recurrent disease in the first large report on human renal isografts, transplanted between identical twins (2). Several explanations were advanced for the frequency of recurrence, including lack of immunosuppression, early transplantation in patients with apparently active acute proliferative glomerular disease, and the relatively long period of risk for recurrence, because of the lack of graft loss due to acute rejection. Recurrent disease seemed to be less frequent in allografts than in isografts (1,3), an observation that was generally attributed to use of nonspecific immunosuppression for rejection prophylaxis and perhaps to the fact that the post-transplantation outcome of these patients was much more heavily influenced by rejection than by recurrent disease. Experience with allografts also indicated that individuals whose original disease was nonimmunologic in nature could develop clinical and histologic evidence of immune glomerular disease, leading to recognition of de novo glomerulopathies in transplanted kidneys.

Initial experimental studies on the pathogenesis of immunologic renal diseases pointed toward two mechanisms of glomerulonephritis: the production of antikidney (primarily antiglomerular basement membrane) antibodies, and renal trapping of circulating preformed immune complexes comprised of antibody and endogenous or exogenous antigens. It was recognized that either of these mechanisms could persist in the recipient after native nephrectomy and transplantation, and that these mechanisms of renal injury could lead to recurrent disease. The observation of recurrent disease in clinical transplantation was viewed as a confirmation of the existence of a nephritogenic environment in the recipient and proved that glomerular disease was often the result of a systemic process not limited solely to the kidney, even in the "primary" glomerular diseases.

During the first 10 years or so of the development of clinical transplantation in humans, investigators began asking questions about recurrent disease that still serve

J. A. Bertolatus and L. G. Hunsicker: Department of Internal Medicine, University of Iowa, Iowa City, Iowa 52242.

as a useful framework for clinicians discussing this topic today:

What is the incidence of recurrent original disease in transplanted kidneys?

What is the impact of recurrent disease on the clinical utility of transplantation in specific patients? How often does recurrent disease cause premature graft loss, as opposed to recurrence that is recognized histologically but of little functional consequence?

How is the incidence of disease recurrence influenced by histocompatibility matching? Are certain diseases more likely to recur in well-matched grafts, particularly in living-donor grafts? How does the use of specific immunosuppressive strategies influence the incidence of recurrent disease? Would more specific transplant immunosuppression, or induction of tolerance to donor antigens, actually increase the likelihood of recurrent disease because of the absence of suppression of nephritogenic responses directed against the recipient's self-antigens?

What is the optimal timing of transplantation in patients with immunologic glomerular disorders? Should a period of dialysis be interposed before transplantation and, if so, how long should this period be? Are there markers of disease that can be used to ascertain the safety of transplantation in these patients?

How should recurrent (or de novo) glomerular disease in the transplant patient be treated?

It will be evident that the additional experience of the last 20 years or so has provided more insight into many of these questions, but there is considerable uncertainty remaining about others.

This topic has been the subject of a number of recent comprehensive reviews (4–8).

INCIDENCE

The incidence of recurrent glomerular disease remains somewhat uncertain primarily because of several limitations of the available data. First, biopsy documentation of the original renal disease is often lacking, in large part because many patients present with renal failure advanced beyond the point where a biopsy has any clinical utility. Removal of the end-stage native kidneys is no longer routine, and histologic examination of nephrectomy specimens is often inconclusive as to original disease. Second, assessments of rates of recurrent disease may underestimate the true rates of functionally significant late recurrences because few transplant programs uniformly perform biopsies on every failing graft or even on every graft with strong clinical evidence of glomerular disease, such as proteinuria or hematuria. Many of these instances of late graft failure are simply attributed to "chronic rejection." On the other hand, the relative frequent performance of graft biopsies for diagnosis of rejection, especially in the first year after transplantation, may often lead to accidental demonstration of histologic recurrences of disease that have little or no clinical significance. This tends to bias literature reports toward histologic recurrence data, which is of considerable interest from the standpoint of immunologic mechanisms, but perhaps less critical in guiding clinical practice and in advising prospective transplant recipients. Finally, it is sometimes difficult to differentiate between morphologic manifestations of immune injury arising because of alloimmunity or due to long-standing hemodynamically mediated injury, from similar evidences of injury due to recurrent disease. This is discussed in greater detail in the section on *transplant glomerulopathy*.

Published estimates of the frequency of recurrent disease have come from two types of reports. The first category is that of pathology-based, single-center reports, usually based on a review of all graft biopsies showing evidence of glomerular disease during a defined period of time (9–15); a larger number of single-center reports focus on recurrence of specific diseases. Those cases of allograft glomerular disease occurring in recipients whose original disease was definitively diagnosed (usually by biopsy) are then used to estimate the frequency of recurrence. The major strength of these single-center reports is that they are more likely to be based on a complete survey of a transplant population during a specific time period and also on a more consistent approach to diagnosis of both original and recurrent disease. These reports usually identify histologic recurrences as well as clinically significant recurrences, including graft losses due to recurrence.

In addition to the single-center reports, a small number of transplant registries or surveys have attempted to obtain a more comprehensive view of the problem of recurrent disease in adult (8) and especially in pediatric (16–18) transplant recipients. These reports rely on accurate reporting of data from participating centers and suffer from a lack of information on primary disease in a high proportion of cases. Only data regarding graft losses are presented, without any estimates of the frequency of histologic or clinical recurrence. The larger North American and European transplant registries do not contain consistent, verified information on primary disease, especially with respect to glomerulonephritis. For example, in recent reports on the effects of primary renal disease from the United Network for Organ Sharing (UNOS) Kidney Transplant Registry (19,20), the second largest diagnostic category of disease causing end-stage renal disease (ESRD) after diabetes mellitus was "chronic glomerulonephritis," accounting for ~25% of total registry entries with any information on primary disease. In addition, there is no consistent determination of causes of graft failure. Despite these limitations, the information regarding primary disease that is available in the UNOS registry provides at least a rough estimate of the numbers of patients with specific primary diseases undergoing renal transplantation (19–21). The insight into the more global impact of these diseases on graft survival gained from this perspective can be useful in balancing the more negative perspective present in case reports and smaller series.

From these various sources, the following picture of the problem of disease recurrence emerges: The rate of recurrence, particularly as defined by histology, varies widely from 1% to 30% of allografts and is much higher for certain immunologic renal diseases than others. The rate of graft *loss* from recurrent disease is much lower than the rate of recurrence per se, occurring in only 1–2% of all transplanted kidneys and accounting for ~5% of all graft failures. The problem of disease recurrence is more significant in pediatric recipients, primarily because of the relatively high proportion of cases of renal failure due to focal segmental glomerular sclerosis in this population (Table 1).

RECURRENT PRIMARY GLOMERULAR DISEASES (TABLE 1)

Focal Segmental Glomerular Sclerosis (FSGS)

In 1972, Hoyer et al. described the recurrence of nephrotic syndrome in transplant patients whose original disease was FSGS (22). Since that time, it has become clear that FSGS is the most clinically significant form of recurrent disease, constituting a major problem in the management of patients with this form of primary kidney disease. Based on a large number of single-center reports and registry surveys describing the course of >400 patients receiving kidney transplants (23–34), the incidence of recurrent disease appears to be ~30%. The most common presentation is the development of heavy, often nephrotic-range, proteinuria within the first year after transplantation and often within days to weeks. In the largest study, the median time to recurrence was 14 days (34).

The specific etiology of the recurrent disease, like that of the primary disorder, remains unknown. The rapid recurrence of disease after transplantation points toward a circulating mediator that persists despite immunosuppression, a concept supported by observations that the plasma (35) or plasma fractions (36) from patients with recurrent FSGS can cause proteinuria in rats and can alter the albumin permeability of normal glomeruli in vitro (37). Although testing of patient sera on normal glomeruli has provided some preliminary information on the nature of the putative factor (36,38), precise identification has not been accomplished.

Diagnosis is usually established by graft biopsy performed for investigation of proteinuria or graft dysfunction. Histologic features of recurrent FSGS are considered to be identical to those of the native-kidney disease, with segmental sclerotic lesions involving glomeruli in a focal distribution. On electron-microscopic examination,

TABLE 1. *Recurrence of primary immunologic glomerular disorders*

Type	Recurrence, %[a]	Graft loss, %[b]	Clinical presentation	Specific comments
Focal segmental glomerular sclerosis	30%	10–15%	Nephrotic syndrome (often within first year after transplant)	Recurrence rate 50–80% in retransplants after first recurrence; may respond to plasmapheresis
Membranoproliferative glomerulonephritis (type I)	38–64%	4–8%	Proteinuria, hematuria	—
Membranoproliferative glomerulonephritis (type II: dense-deposit disease)	~100%	10%	Microhematuria, proteinuria; often clinically silent	Measurements of C3 or C3 nephritic factor not useful
Membranous nephropathy	7–26%	5–10%	Nephrotic syndrome, slowly progressive graft dysfunction	Should screen for hepatitis-B-virus infection
Immunoglobulin-A nephropathy	50%	≤10%	Microhematuria, proteinuria, progressive graft dysfunction	Incidence of significant graft recurrences may increase with time
Anti-GBM disease	Rare	Rare	Acute glomerulonephritis	Recurrence unlikely if transplantation delayed until anti-GBM antibodies are absent
Idiopathic rapidly progressive	Rare, ~1–2%	Rare but reported	Acute glomerulonephritis	—

[a]Includes histologic and clinically significant recurrences.
[b]Refers to percent of total number of patients transplanted for end-stage renal disease due to specific primary disorder.
GBM, glomerular basement membrane.

the predominant feature is foot-process effacement. Because it is now well recognized that focal glomerular sclerosis is a common pathologic feature in many renal disorders, the problem in differential diagnosis is to distinguish "secondary" glomerular sclerosis in a renal allograft from a recurrence of the primary form of the disease; usually, this distinction can be made based on a knowledge of the clinical course and biopsy findings associated with the patient's original renal disease. Cheigh and co-workers addressed this problem by identifying all allograft biopsy or nephrectomy specimens with focal glomerular sclerosis in a 3-year period (27). Focal sclerotic lesions were identified in 18 (16%) of 154 sampled grafts. Six cases were identified as recurrent FSGS, while the other 12 were felt to represent de novo FSGS in patients with other primary renal diseases. Histologically, those with de novo FSGS had a significantly greater degree of obliterative arteriopathy attributed to chronic vascular rejection, leading to the hypothesis that the de novo form of FSGS may be related to glomerular ischemia or perhaps to compensatory changes in glomeruli of a graft with reduced numbers of functioning nephrons. Clinically, patients with de novo FSGS had a somewhat later onset of disease, and had nephrotic proteinuria less often, than those with recurrent FSGS.

Many investigators have focused their analyses of recurrent FSGS on identification of risk factors that predict a higher than average likelihood of disease recurrence. Table 2 summarizes the risk-factor information contained in the three largest, most recently published series (31,33–34). Most authors agree that the strongest predictor of recurrent disease is the recurrence of FSGS in a previous allograft, with a likelihood of recurrence in the second graft being as high as 80% (33). The outlook for a successful second transplant is particularly poor in patients who develop rapid onset of nephrotic syndrome and loss of graft function after a first transplant. Patients with recurrent disease who experience prolonged graft function from a first allograft are still at high risk of disease recurrence in a subsequent graft, but are less likely to have early graft failure; a second transplant has more utility in this subgroup of patients.

TABLE 2. *Risk factors for recurrent focal segmental glomerulosclerosis (FSGS)*[a]

Risk factors identified as significant in all three studies[a]
Recurrence of FSGS in a previous graft
White or Hispanic recipient (compared with African-American)
Rapid course of original FSGS[b]
Risk factors with significant but not unanimous support
Mesangial proliferation in original FSGS biopsy specimen[c]
Age of recipient (young child versus adolescent or adult)
Factors not predictive of recurrence
Immunosuppression without cyclosporine
Use of living related kidney donor
Increased level of cadaver donor matching

[a]Analysis based primarily on the three largest reported series (31,33–34); ~270 grafts.

[b]Significant factor in two studies (33–34); trend toward significance in a third (31).

[c]Evaluated only in two (31,34) of the three largest reports.

There is also good agreement that a rapid "malignant" course of the original disease, characterized by severe nephrotic syndrome and a short interval between FSGS diagnosis and ESRD, is predictive of recurrence. An accelerated course of the primary disease was a significant risk factor in two of the three largest studies, with a trend toward significance observed in the third (Table 2). In addition, two of these three studies identified a two- to threefold higher rate of recurrence in white or Hispanic patients as compared with blacks (Table 2). The third study did not address the issue of ethnicity.

There is less agreement regarding two other potential risk factors for recurrence: recipient age and the presence of mesangial proliferation on the original biopsy showing FSGS in the native kidneys. It has been observed that the recurrence rate is lower in adults and adolescents than in younger children (31,33). However, in the North American pediatric registry (34), which has no data on adults, there was no difference between adolescents and younger children in the fraction of patients developing recurrent FSGS.

Several additional potential risk factors for recurrence suggested by earlier, smaller studies are not supported by the more recent, larger analyses (Table 2). At one time, it was advanced that use of a living related donor, or perhaps a well-matched cadaveric donor, predisposed patients to FSGS recurrence; at present, the best evidence does not support this contention. In addition, the accumulated experience available to date suggests the use of cyclosporine has not reduced the frequency of recurrence in FSGS patients.

Recurrent disease clearly has a substantial impact on the prognosis of patients with FSGS who undergo transplantation. The rate of graft failure attributable to recurrent disease is estimated at 20–50% of grafts with recurrent disease or ~6–15% of all grafts in FSGS patients, if the recurrence rate is 30%. In a recent UNOS review of the impact of primary disease on transplant outcomes, FSGS was one of the few diseases associated with a significant reduction in estimated half-life of graft function (5½ years for FSGS patients, as compared with 9 years for all cadaveric recipients) (19).

The high rate of clinically significant recurrence has led some transplant programs to recommend that FSGS patients not receive a living-donor transplant, particularly if they have risk factors for recurrence (39). However, this strategy will unnecessarily deny the benefits of living-donor transplantation to some patients in order to benefit a few. It now appears unlikely that the incidence of recurrence is higher with living donors. Perhaps the most informative data are those of the North American

Pediatric Registry, showing that graft survival over the first 2–3 years is ~10% higher in FSGS patients receiving live-donor kidneys, an increment similar to that observed in transplant recipients in general (34) (Fig. 1). If use of a living donor is contemplated for an FSGS patients, it is imperative that the donor be counseled about the risk of recurrent disease so that this information can be incorporated into the donor's decision-making process.

Treatment of recurrent FSGS has remained problematic. As mentioned, the use of cyclosporine immunosuppression has not had a significant impact on the frequency of recurrence. Although some have argued for use of higher cyclosporine doses in FSGS patients with recurrent disease (40), there has not been a consistent recommendation for this approach. Several reports have documented that patients with recurrent FSGS, like other nephrotics, will have a reduction in proteinuria during treatment with nonsteroidal anti-inflammatory agents (41–43) or angiotenson-II-converting inhibitor therapy (33); however, the long-term impact of these therapies on preservation of graft function remains uncertain. The most promising therapies for recurrent FSGS center on the removal of the putative circulating factor by plasmapheresis (37,44) or immunoabsorption (36). Either of these approaches has the ability to induce a remission of proteinuria during extracorporeal therapy in most patients. The impact on the long-term outcome is less clear. With respect to plasmapheresis, a number of individuals treated early in the course of recurrence appeared to have a sustained remission lasting up to 2 years (37). Interestingly, pheresis therapy was associated with a marked reduction in the ability of patient sera to cause increased albumin permeability of isolated normal glomeruli (37), suggesting that removal of a circulating factor was the mechanism for the observed therapeutic benefit. Paralleling these results, the material eluted from immunoadsorption columns used to treat recurrent FSGS patients caused increased protein excretion in rats (36).

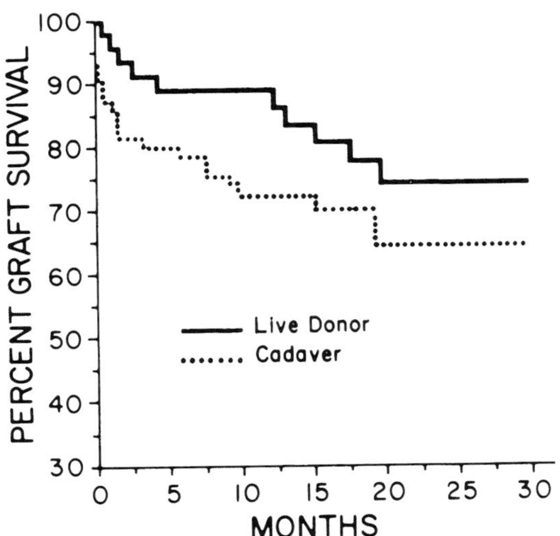

FIG. 1. Graft survival in patients with renal failure due to focal segmental granulosclerosis according to donor type. Data are from the North American Pediatric Renal Transplant Cooperative Study. Reprinted with permission from Tejani and Stablein (34).

Membranoproliferative Glomerulonephritis (MPGN) Type I

Recurrence of MPGN type I (MPGN with subendothelial dense deposits) in transplanted kidneys has been clearly documented (8–9,12,15,16), especially in cases in which disease has recurred in more than one allograft in a single recipient (9,15,45,46). Almost all authors comment on the fact that diagnosis of recurrent MPGN is hampered by the morphologic similarities between this process and transplant glomerulopathy, a more common entity felt to represent a glomerular manifestation of chronic rejection (see below). Biopsy features that seem to point toward recurrent MPGN include the presence of crescents, subepithelial deposits or "humps," and extensive C3 deposition (8).

In the larger reported series, the incidence of histologic recurrence is in the range of 38–64% (9,11,15), with a much lower incidence (4–8%) of graft loss secondary to recurrence (8,16). The majority of patients with histologic recurrence will have proteinuria and hematuria, though many have stable renal function for many years. There are no significant clinical predictors of recurrence, other than perhaps an aggressive course of the original disease, typically seen in conjunction with glomerular crescents on biopsy examination.

Johnson et al. have recently reported an association between hepatitis-C virus (HCV) infection and MPGN in the native kidneys (47). It is not presently known what fraction of patients with native-kidney MGPN, previously considered "idiopathic," is attributable to HCV or whether HCV-related MPGN will recur in allografts. As the occurrence of de novo MPGN in HCV-infected transplant patients whose original disease was not MPGN has now been reported (48), it seems quite likely that some cases of recurrent MPGN are also related to HCV. In view of the prevalence of HCV infection in the ESRD and transplant recipient populations, it would seem prudent to evaluate the HCV status of all patients with recurrent MPGN.

Membranoproliferative Glomerulonephritis (Type II: Dense-Deposit Disease)

MPGN type II, or dense-deposit disease, is distinguished from MPGN type I by the presence on electron-microscopic examination of distinctive, ribbonlike electron-dense deposits within the glomerular basement membrane. MPGN type II is typically seen in association with hypocomplementemia (depressed serum C3 levels) and the presence of an autoantibody (C3 nephritic factor, or NEF) that binds to C3 convertase and abnormally prolongs its persistence in serum. In contrast to MPGN type I, the dense-deposit lesions are unique and unlikely to be confused with any other pathologic process in the transplanted kidney. There is good agreement in the literature that the histologic recurrence rate is quite high, approaching 100% (9,15,49–54). The dense deposits have been observed as early as 20 days after transplantation (15).

Although the rate of recurrence detected by biopsy is high, the frequency of clinical consequences attributed to the presence of the dense deposits is much lower, perhaps only 10% (9,15,49–54). Many patients have no urinary abnormalities, whereas others may have microhematuria and low-grade proteinuria with stable graft function. Only one fairly small single-center study has suggested that the rate of graft loss from recurrent disease is high (55).

Serial measurements of C3 levels or of C3NEF appear to have no utility in judging the risk of recurrence or in following the patient's condition after transplantation (53,56). Patients with no complement abnormalities before transplantation have been observed to develop recurrent disease. After transplantation, C3 levels usually return to normal, and C3NEF disappears, even in patients with recurrence (53,56).

Membranous Nephropathy (MN)

Membranous nephropathy (MN) is a common cause of nephrotic syndrome in adults, accounting for ~20% of cases (57). The disease tends to occur in older patients. Spontaneous remissions are relatively common, and those whose disease does not remit often have a very slowly progressive course, even in the absence of therapy (58,59). As a result, individuals with ESRD from MN are only a small percentage of recipients in most transplant programs, accounting for <5% of renal transplantations performed in individuals with glomerular disorders (8).

Recurrent MN in the transplanted kidney is well documented (4,6,50–57), though many of the reports include only a small number of patients. Although one early series reported a recurrence rate of 57% (4), more recent large series indicate a recurrence rate of 7–26% (55–57). In the Australia–New Zealand registry, there were no documented recurrences in 120 patients transplanted who had MN (8); it seems likely that the lower estimates of the frequency of recurrence (<10%) are correct.

The usual presentation of individuals with MN recurrence has been proteinuria, which usually progresses to the nephrotic range. As with native-kidney MN, renal function is either stable or only slowly lost, so that the course of graft survival may not be much different from that observed for cadaver allografts in general (57).

Estimation of the frequency of disease recurrence is made somewhat more difficult by the observation that ~4–5% of individuals whose original renal disease is clearly not due to MN develop de novo MN (discussed later in this chapter) in the allograft. Because relatively few individuals with MN undergo transplantation and the recurrence rate is low, it should follow that in any transplant series most cases of allograft MN will represent de novo disease. For example, of 18 cases of allograft MN identified in the University of Iowa transplant program over an 8-year period, three grafts (in two patients) developed recurrent disease, while 13 cases were clearly de novo disease and two others were indeterminate (J. A. Bertolatus, unpublished observations). Other series of allograft MN agree that de novo MN is much more common than recurrent disease, with a ratio of de novo–recurrent disease of 4:1 (55,56).

The frequency of de novo disease raises an interesting question: Does MN in the allograft of a patient with ESRD caused by native-kidney MN represent recurrence or does it represent de novo MN mediated by the mechanism responsible for this disorder in those whose renal failure was not caused by MN? There is some evidence to support the existence of true MN recurrence [summarized by Mathew (8)]. The rate of recurrence (10%) is higher than the incidence of de novo disease (2–5%). In addition, the interval between transplantation and development of proteinuria is shorter in patients thought to have recurrence, and recurrence in MN patients seems to be more frequent in those patients whose original disease followed an aggressive course.

Evaluation of the transplant patient with MN should include testing for evidence of hepatitis-B virus (HBV) infection. Chronic HBV infection is associated with MN and accounts for a significant proportion of MN cases in the Asian population (58). Although the proportion of allograft MN associated with HBV infection is not well established because data on HBV status are not provided by most reports, one group reported that one of five patients with recurrent MN was positive for HBV surface antigen (57).

No specific therapy for allograft MN can be recommended as effective at present. Addition of high doses of steroids to the baseline immunosuppressive regimen is probably not helpful (56).

Immunoglobulin-A (IgA) Nephropathy

IgA nephropathy (IgAN) is considered to be the most common primary glomerulopathy in the world (58,59). The native-kidney form of the disease is typically characterized by episodes of flank pain and gross hematuria. Hypertension, nephrotic proteinuria, and decreased renal function at the time of diagnosis are recognized as predictors of eventual renal insufficiency (60). A minority of patients will experience rapid deterioration in renal function; these patients usually have glomerular crescents on renal biopsy. Most patients appear to follow a relatively benign course at least in the intermediate term, with renal survival of ≥80% after 10-year follow-up (59,60). However, when multiple studies of IgAN are compared, there is a tendency for the reported frequency of ESRD to increase with the duration of follow-up, suggesting that the fraction of IgAN patients eventually developing ESRD after >10 years may be somewhat higher than has been generally believed (59). In the UNOS renal transplant registry, IgAN was identified as the primary disease for 2% of renal transplant recipients (21).

Berger and co-workers, who first described IgAN in the native kidneys, were also the first to report the recurrence of IgA deposition in the renal allograft (61). The experience of this group has been updated several times over the past 20 years (62,63) and now includes 32 renal transplantations in IgAN patients (63) with protocol biopsies performed periodically after grafting regardless of clinical course. Mesangial IgA deposition was observed in 53% of the allografts, suggesting that histologic recurrence of IgAN is quite common. This estimate of the frequency of histologic recurrence has been corroborated in a number of other reports (11,15). Biopsy diagnosis of recurrent IgAN is based on immunofluorescence microscopy, using the same criteria as applied to the native kidneys (61–63), with the hallmark being mesangial deposition of IgA, quantitatively greater than or equal to deposition of other immunoglobulins. Recurrent IgAN must be distinguished from transmission of donor disease (64–67) and possibly from de novo IgAN (14).

The clinical significance of recurrent IgAN has generally been considered to be minimal, without a major impact on graft function and graft outcome. In the UNOS registry, graft survival for the 508 IgAN patients is actually significantly longer than that of recipients with other primary diseases (Fig. 2), which argues strongly against a markedly negative impact of recurrent disease, despite its relatively frequent occurrence (19). However, more detailed analysis of recent series indicates that recurrent IgAN is not always benign. In one of the largest single-center reports, recurrent IgA deposits were seen in 17 (60%) of 29 of biopsied grafts (out of a total of 51 grafts in patients with IgAN) (68). These patients fell into three groups based on clinical course. Three patients had no clinical evidence of disease; urinalysis, glomerular morphology by light microscopy, and renal function were all normal. Six patients had microhematuria and mesangial expansion, but stable renal function. Five patients (~10% of the entire IgAN group) had mesangial proliferation, heavy proteinuria, and progressive renal insufficiency. It is interesting that the proportion of patients with progressive disease (~10%) was quite similar to the percentage of native-kidney IgAN patients who developed renal failure after 10 years (59,60). In addition, this study showed

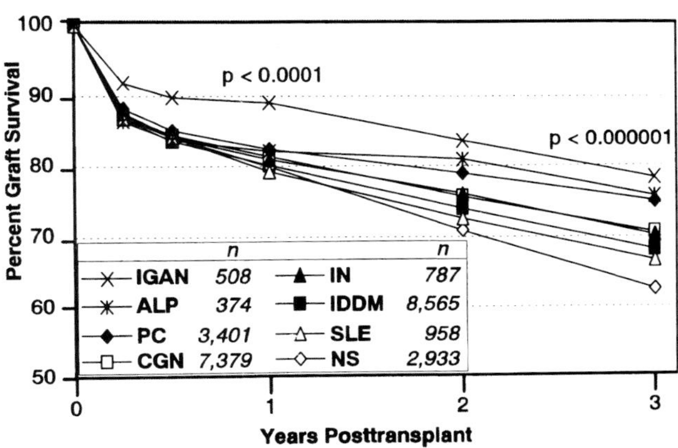

FIG. 2. Graft survival after renal transplantation in patients with different primary renal disorders. IGAN, IgA nephropathy; ALP, Alport syndrome; PC, polycystic renal disease; CGN, chronic glomerulonephritis; IN, interstitial nephritis; IDDM; insulin-dependent diabetes mellitus; SLE, systemic lupus erythematosus; NS, nephrosclerosis. The p values indicate that there are significant differences between the groups at 1 and 3 years, but do not refer to specific between-group comparisons. Data are from UNOS Kidney Transplant Registry. Reprinted with permission from Hirata and Terasaki (19).

a correlation between cumulative frequency of histologic recurrence and length of time after biopsy. If one extrapolates from the data on native-kidney IgAN (59,60), the impact of IgAN on renal function may also increase slowly but steadily with time. Short-term stability of renal function (as reflected in 1- to 3-year graft survival rates) does not mean that recurrent IgA deposition is totally benign over longer periods. From a practical standpoint, however, the average half-life of graft function for all cadaver kidneys, regardless of primary kidney disease, is ~9 years (21). A recurrent disease that takes 9 years or longer to cause significant loss of graft function will obviously not have much impact on transplantation success, at least as reflected in aggregate data (15).

A number of possible predictors for recurrence of clinically significant recurrences of IgAN have been examined. The only one that is broadly supported by the reported experience is the presence of crescentic disease, and a rapidly progressive clinical course, in the original kidney presentation (8,64,69). Some authors have suggested that recurrence is also more likely in living-related-donor grafts, particularly those from haploidentical donors (64,69). Other reports do not support this contention (70), and even in a series demonstrating a higher frequency of recurrence in recipients of living-donor kidneys, the only individual with a clinically significant recurrence after a living-donor transplant had the crescentic form of the disease (69). The UNOS registry data indicate that IgAN patients who receive living-donor grafts have an increment in graft survival compared with cadaveric kidney recipients similar to that observed for transplant recipients in general (21), so a major negative impact of living-donor transplantation in IgAN is unlikely. In general, living-donor transplantation can be offered to IgAN patients without major reservations, with one possible exception—the presence of the crescentic form of IgAN in the original kidneys. These patients probably have a higher risk of clinically significant recurrence so that, at a minimum, careful donor and recipient counseling is mandatory. Brensilver et al. (64) describe an individual with crescentic IgAN who lost two sequential living-related-donor grafts to aggressive recurrent IgAN. One graft had IgA deposition demonstrated at the time of transplantation, leading to the conclusion that the donor probably had subclinical IgAN. The other graft was presumably lost to recipient disease alone, as no deposits were present at transplantation. This report indicates the existence of inherited predisposition to IgAN and the need for very careful screening of living donors when the recipient has IgAN.

If IgA deposition in a renal graft can be clinically silent, it should not be surprising that IgA deposits will occasionally be present in kidneys from living and cadaveric donors, and literature reports indicate that this has occurred (64–67). Interestingly, it has been documented that the deposits may disappear with time after transplantation of these kidneys into patients with other forms of kidney disease, indicating that IgAN is a systemic disorder and that IgA deposition probably has to be an ongoing process for a long period of time to lead to chronic renal damage.

At present, no therapy has been proven effective for the occasional patient judged to be losing graft function from recurrent IgAN. The Mayo Collaborative Nephrology Group recently reported that fish-oil therapy slowed progression of IgAN in native-kidney disease (71). Although this study did not include kidney transplant patients, the relatively benign nature of the treatment would make it reasonable to apply it to patients with a histologic or clinical picture suggesting graft dysfunction secondary to recurrent IgAN.

Antiglomerular Basement Membrane (Anti-GBM) Disease

In 1973, when Wilson and Dixon reviewed their experience with 63 patients who had glomerulonephritis associated with circulating anti-GBM antibodies, they documented the histologic recurrence of linear anti-GBM staining in ~55% of the 34 patients undergoing renal transplantation (72). Graft failure attributable to recurrent disease occurred in at least seven cases, which understandably led to considerable caution in the transplantation in these patients. Over the years since this series was presented, the largely anecdotal reported experience with this relatively rare immunologic disorder has established several facts (73–75). Although the risk of recurrent disease is lessened by delaying transplantation until assays for circulating anti-GBM antibodies are negative, there have been recurrences in patients with negative assays (72). This has generally been attributed to the insensitivity of the older immunoassay methods used for detection (72), so it is possible that use of the modern solid-phase assays for detection of these antibodies will reduce the likelihood of false negatives. On the other hand, some patients with positive tests for circulating anti-GBM antibodies have had successful transplants (74,75), and many patients with histologic recurrence have few or no clinical manifestations (71).

At present, most transplant programs appear to follow the practice of delaying transplantation until assays for anti-GBM antibodies are negative. Mathew, in his recent review (8), notes that reports of significant recurrences of anti-GBM disease have become virtually nonexistent in recent years. The Australia–New Zealand registry had only two recorded graft losses from anti-GBM disease among 89 patients who underwent transplantation for this disorder (8). In the UNOS registry, graft survival for the ~230 patients with the diagnosis of Goodpasture syndrome was no different from that for the overall group (21). Taken together, these observations suggest that, with current precautions, transplantation in anti-GBM-mediated renal disease leads to acceptable outcomes.

Idiopathic Rapidly Progressive Glomerulonephritis (RPGN)

Many cases of crescentic glomerulonephritis will be associated with evidence of other immunopathogenetic mechanisms such as IgAN, anti-GBM disease, or vasculitis. Those cases that cannot be classified as any other glomerular or systemic disorder are typically referred to as "idiopathic RPGN." Recurrence of this entity in transplanted kidney has been reported (9–11,76), but is generally considered to be rare. The best available estimate probably comes from the Australia–New Zealand registry, which records only two graft losses recognized as having been caused by recurrent disease out of 127 patients undergoing renal transplantation for RPGN-induced renal failure (8).

RECURRENT SECONDARY GLOMERULAR DISEASES (TABLE 3)

Systemic Lupus Erythematosus (SLE)

Prior to 1975, the presence of SLE as the cause of renal failure was regarded as a contraindication to renal transplantation (77). This conclusion was based on the poor overall prognosis for SLE patients as evidenced by short-

TABLE 3. *Recurrence of systemic immune disorders involving the kidney*

Type	Recurrence, %	Graft loss, %	Clinical presentation	Specific comments
Systemic lupus	1[a]–50%[b]	Low, ~1%	Hematuria, proteinuria	Serologic studies not predictive of recurrence; most centers delay transplantation 6–12 months after active disease
HUS/TTP	5%	5%	Thrombotic microangiopathy	Avoid oral contraceptives; recurrences not prevented with tacrolimus
Henoch–Schönlein purpura	35%	11%	Hematuria, proteinuria; often clinically silent	
Wegener granulomatosis	Reported but rare		Usually nonrenal disease more significant	Should not use cyclophosphamide primarily, but useful for renal/nonrenal recurrence; ANCA testing not useful
Amyloidosis	25%	Uncommon	Proteinuria with stable graft function	Extrarenal disease usually determines survival
Progressive systemic sclerosis	Uncommon	Uncommon	Vasculitic lesions in kidney	—

[a]Clinical recurrence rate.
[b]Histologic recurrence rate, with protocol biopsies.
ANCA, neutrophil cytoplasmic antibody; HUS/TTP, hemolytic uremic syndrome/thrombotic thrombocytopenic purpura.

ened survival on dialysis (78) and fear of recurrence in the graft (77). Because SLE is a multisystem disorder typically associated with the presence of circulating autoantibodies, the introduction of a new kidney into this presumably nephritogenic milieu might reasonably be predicted to lead to a high incidence of recurrent disease. In 1975, however, a report from the Advisory Committee to the National Institutes of Health/American College of Surgeons Transplant Registry indicated that, at least in the short term (1–2 years), patient and graft survival in SLE patients were comparable to the results observed in non-SLE patients (79). Since that time, the transplant community has accumulated considerable experience with SLE patients, as demonstrated by the fact that >1,200 transplant recipients identified as having renal failure from SLE have been reported to the UNOS registry since 1987 (20,21). The UNOS data indicate that 1- and 3-year graft survival in SLE patients is similar to the rate for the registry group as a whole.

The registry data are supplemented by a number of more detailed single-center analyses of experience with SLE patients, which support the contention that the results of transplantation in this group are generally good (80–86). There are a number of anecdotal reports of recurrent disease causing severe graft injury or troublesome nonrenal disease manifestations. As with other forms of renal disease, reports that emphasize histologic recurrence or include "surveillance" biopsies of kidneys with no clinical evidence of graft dysfunction have shown a higher incidence of recurrent disease, up to 50% in one series (86). On the other hand, two large studies including a total of 54 grafts in SLE patients identified no case of recurrent disease (80,81). The consensus is that the frequency of clinically significant recurrence is on the order of 1% (Table 3) (8). The low frequency of recurrence of this systemic disorder has been attributed to various factors, including the "burning out" of disease activity when ESRD develops, the immunosuppressive effects of uremia, and the antirejection immunosuppressive regimen (8).

Although the experience described above indicates that individuals with SLE should clearly be considered as renal transplant candidates, the timing of transplantation continues to be a significant unresolved issue. Most authors recommend a waiting period of 6–12 months on dialysis before transplantation, which may allow further "burning out" of the immunopathogenetic mechanisms responsible for renal injury (8). Literature support for this recommendation can be found in a study in which longer pretransplantation dialysis times were associated with a higher likelihood of good graft function (82), but this has not been observed uniformly (80). Serologic studies such as those of antinuclear antibodies, antibodies to double-stranded DNA, and complement component levels are of little or no help in determining the timing of transplantation. Many patients with abnormal serologic results have a benign post-transplantation course (80–82), whereas others have been described as having histologic recurrence of SLE in the graft with normal serologic results (86). In addition, any attempt to use serologic data for timing of transplantation in SLE is confounded by the observation that 29% and 22% of patients continue to have serologic evidence of disease activity after 5 or 10 years of ESRD, respectively, despite having a very low incidence of clinical activity of SLE (6.5% and 0% at 5 and 10 years, respectively) (81).

Thrombotic Microangiopathies: Hemolytic Uremic Syndrome (HUS)/Thrombotic Thrombocytopenic Purpura (TTP)

Hemolytic uremic syndrome is responsible for ~5% of cases of childhood ESRD (17) and a lower proportion of cases in adults. Collating the major series of HUS recurrence in transplanted kidneys identifies a total of 17 cases of graft loss due to recurrent disease out of a total of 306 patients, mostly children, who underwent transplantation for this disorder, a 5% rate of graft loss due to recurrence (Table 3) (8,16,17,87–90). The range of reported rates of recurrence is very broad, from ≤1% in a large European pediatric registry report (16) to as high as 40% in a single-center report (87), with no apparent reason for the variability. HUS differs from most other recurrent renal diseases in that, although clinically mild recurrences have occasionally been observed, most recurrences are severe and very likely to lead to graft loss. It is worth noting that, in the UNOS registry, HUS is one of the few primary diseases associated with 1- and 3-year graft survival significantly lower (by ~10%) than those of recipients with other diseases, regardless of donor source (19,20). The presentation is similar to that of the original disease, with onset of a microangiopathic hemolytic anemia, evidence of red cell fragmentation, and thrombocytopenia, typically within the first few days or weeks after transplantation (Table 3). Pathologically, the hallmark is deposition of fibrin microthrombi in the glomeruli. The only predisposing factors mentioned in the literature as being associated with a higher risk of recurrence are renal transplantation very soon after active HUS, familial HUS (which may be associated with a specific defect in antithrombotic mechanisms), and recurrence of HUS in a previous renal graft. Many reports mention the occasional patient who has lost two or even three sequential renal grafts to recurrent HUS. In one case, oral contraceptive therapy triggered a relatively late recurrence of HUS in a patient whose original disease had also been associated with similar treatment (91), suggesting that this form of birth control should be avoided or used with great caution in these patients (Table 3).

Recognition of recurrent HUS may be hampered by the fact that cyclosporine can induce an identical syndrome in transplant patients with non-HUS primary renal disease (92) or even in recipients of nonrenal transplants such as liver or bone marrow. Cyclosporine may cause an increase in thrombotic events in transplant recipients (93), perhaps by inhibiting the production of vasodilatory prostaglandins by vascular endothelium (94). Given these observations, it is not surprising that there has been some controversy about whether cyclosporine should be avoided in patients with HUS, because use of this drug might increase the chance of recurrence. In our opinion, given the benefit of cyclosporine in achieving and maintaining higher rates of graft function, and the relatively low overall rate of recurrence in the reported experience, it is not advisable to eliminate cyclosporine. The recipient should be monitored closely for evidence of recurrent HUS by using the peripheral blood smear, platelet count, bilirubin, and lactate-dehydrogenase level. If evidence of HUS develops, consideration should be given to discontinuing cyclosporine temporarily or at least to reducing the cyclosporine dose.

Recurrent HUS has been treated with the modalities employed in the native-kidney disease, including antiplatelet drugs, plasmapheresis, plasma infusion, and administration of prostaglandins, with no consistent results. Despite reports of improvement in cyclosporine-induced HUS after switching to tacrolimus (FK506), the frequency of recurrent disease is not significantly less in patients receiving primary tacrolimus immunosuppression (90).

In contrast to HUS, the less common microangiopathic disorder TTP affects primarily adult patients. In one small series of five adult patients who underwent transplantation because of TTP-associated renal failure, there was no instance of recurrent disease (95).

Henoch–Schönlein Purpura (HSP)

HSP is a systemic vasculitis involving skin, joints, gastrointestinal tract, and kidney. The renal lesion of HSP is morphologically identical to that of IgAN, though the tendency of HSP-associated glomerulonephritis to cause progressive renal disease is probably greater than is typical in IgAN, especially in adults. HSP is an uncommon cause of renal failure in the transplant-recipient population, with only ~125 patients in the UNOS registry data base (21). Estimates of the frequency and clinical significance of recurrent HSP can be obtained from two single-center reports (96,97) with a total of 25 patients undergoing transplantation for renal disease due to HSP. The overall recurrence rate after at least 5 years of follow-up was 35%, with a risk of graft loss due to HSP of 11% (Table 3). As in the case of IgAN, there is an increase in the cumulative recurrence rate with time after transplantation (97).

Approximately 60% of individuals with histologic recurrence have no clinical evidence of renal disease. The others will have microhematuria and/or proteinuria and, in some cases, progressive renal dysfunction.

Interestingly, there is no striking correlation between recurrence of systemic disease, primarily as manifested by purpura, and renal recurrence. Some patients develop purpura without any evidence of renal disease, and only about half of the patients with renal recurrence have purpura (97).

It seems reasonable to delay transplantation in HSP until systemic disease is in remission and especially until purpura is resolved. Some authors have advocated a delay of 1 year after resolution of purpura, but several patients have had recurrent disease after delays of 18–37 months (97).

Wegener Granulomatosis (WG)

WG is recorded as the cause of renal failure in only 170 transplant recipients in the latest UNOS registry report covering 1987–1994 (21). These patients had 1- and 3-year graft survival rates comparable to those of other transplant recipients, indicating that the rate of significant renal recurrence is probably low. Although case reports document that recurrent disease can occur (98–103), the frequency is too low to enable an accurate assessment of the risk (Table 3). Recent reviews of the post-transplant course of WG patients suggest that reactivation of nonrenal disease is more important clinically than recurrence of renal disease (Table 3) (100,103). Antineutrophil cytoplasmic antibodies (ANCAs) have been recognized as a serologic marker for WG, with a variable relationship to disease activity. Although it makes sense to defer transplantation until clinically significant disease activity is minimal, there is no need to await disappearance of ANCAs. A recent series of 20 WG transplant recipients demonstrated good overall outcomes despite a positive ANCA titer in 8 of 12 patients tested at the time of transplantation (102).

Cyclophosphamide is the mainstay of WG therapy and has been effective in inducing remission of recurrent disease in transplant patients (Table 3) (98). This has led some authors to recommend routine inclusion of cyclophosphamide in the immunosuppressive regimen of these patients (98). However, given the low frequency of recurrence and the substantial morbidity associated with long-term cyclophosphamide therapy, it is preferable to reserve cytotoxic therapy for actual recurrences of WG.

Amyloidosis

Based on two fairly large single-center reports (104,105) and a comprehensive review including a larger number of case reports and small series (106), the histologic recurrence rate of amyloidosis is ~25% (Table 3). This appears to apply to both primary (AL) and secondary (AA) amyloidosis. However, most patients reported to have recurrent amyloidosis in the renal graft have not had proteinuria, and graft loss attributable to this process is even more uncommon (106). The clinical picture is often dominated by progression of extrarenal disease (Table 3). Premature death from nonrenal complications, and not graft loss, is the most probable explanation for the reduction in graft survival noted in the ~80 patients with amyloidosis reported to the UNOS registry (21). In addition to recurrent disease, there has also been at least one report of de novo secondary amyloidosis occurring in a transplanted kidney (106).

In the specific instance of amyloidosis associated with familial Mediterranean fever, colchicine therapy has been mentioned as reducing the likelihood of recurrence in the transplanted kidney (107–111).

Progressive Systemic Sclerosis (PSS) (Scleroderma)

The number of individuals with PSS-associated renal failure undergoing renal transplantation is small, with only 40 cases reported to the UNOS registry from 1987 to 1994 (21). Although there have been reports of disease recurrence (112–114), the vascular lesions of PSS in the kidney resemble those of chronic vascular rejection, leading some authors to question whether recurrence can be documented by histology alone (8). In one case, PSS-associated autoantibodies could be eluted from a failed renal graft, providing some additional support that PSS can recur (114). However, the published experience is simply too small to permit any meaningful statement about the risk or clinical significance of recurrent PSS (Table 3).

DE NOVO IMMUNOLOGIC DISORDERS (TABLE 4)

Transplant Glomerulopathy (TGP)

In most reported series of transplant recipients undergoing biopsy evaluation for proteinuria (115–121), the most common diagnosis is TGP (122), also referred to as allograft glomerulopathy (123). This process accounts for 20–30% of cases of persistent proteinuria in transplant patients, which gives an overall incidence of 2–9% of all renal graft recipients (115–119). The usual clinical presentation is the development of abnormal proteinuria (>1 g/day) that is often in, or progresses to, the nephrotic range, usually in conjunction with graft dysfunction. On light microscopy, the most important finding is glomerular GBM reduplication similar to MPGN, which is the lesion most easily confused with TGP (120). Immunofluorescence findings are usually minimal, with at most weakly positive staining for IgM and C3 (120). Electron microscopy does not typically show the large subendothelial electron-dense deposits seen in MPGN. Rather, the most characteristic electron-microscopic finding is a change described as electron-lucent thickening of the

TABLE 4. *De novo immunologic glomerular disorders in the renal allograft*

Type	Frequency, %	Graft loss, %	Clinical presentation	Specific comments
Membranous nephropathy	2%	?	Proteinuria, often nephrotic; on average 4–5 years after transplant, slowly progressive graft dysfunction	Often associated with biopsy findings of chronic rejection
HCV-associated MPGN	5%	?	Proteinuria >1 g/day	—
Anti-GBM disease in Alport syndrome	3–4%	75%[a]	Hematuria, proteinuria; linear GBM staining by immunofluorescence microscopy	Risk factors: male gender, deafness, renal failure at age <30, prior recurrence, large gene deletion(?)
Transplant glomerulopathy	2–9%	100%[b]	Proteinuria, often nephrotic; often with biopsy evidence of chronic rejection	—

[a]Rate of graft loss in those with anti-GBM disease.
[b]Rate of graft loss within 6–12 months after diagnosis of transplant glomerulopathy.
GBM, glomerular basement membrane; HCV, hepatitis-C virus; MPGN, membranoproliferative glomerulonephritis.

lamina rara interna of the GBM (120) (Fig. 3). Some authors have described a progression of changes from an early or "evolving" TGP, characterized by endothelial and mesangial cell swelling, to a later "advanced" stage in which GBM reduplication and mesangial cell interposition are seen (124).

While the etiology of TGP is unknown, most authors consider this lesion to represent a glomerular form of chronic vascular rejection, which is often present in biopsy specimens with TGP (120,121). TGP may occasionally be present concurrently with other de novo or recurrent glomerulopathies (120) (Fig. 3).

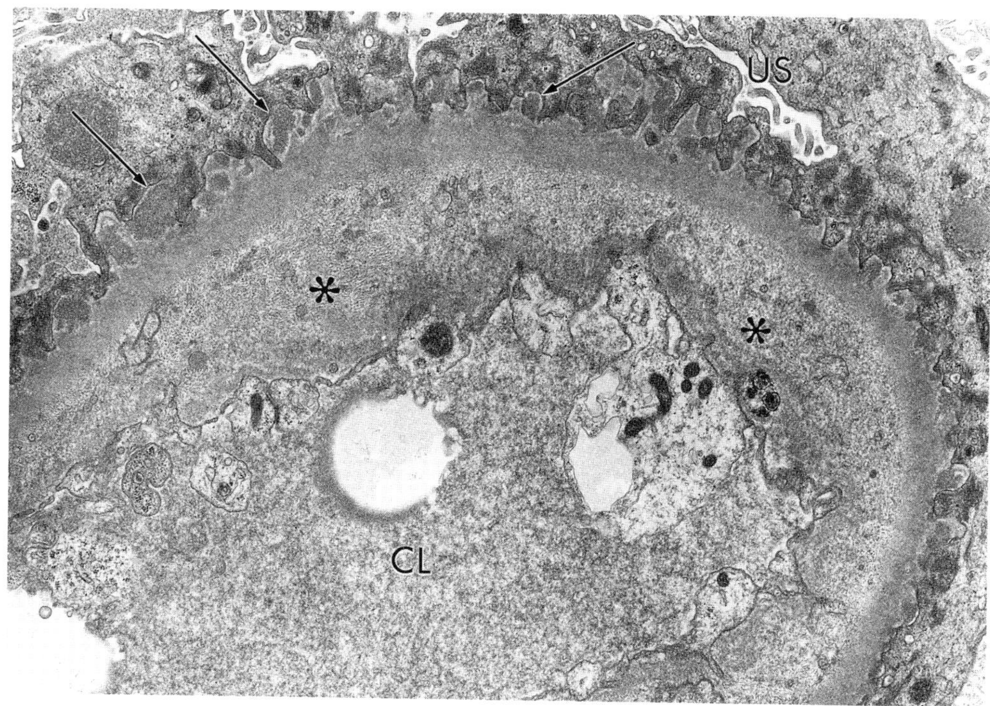

FIG. 3. Electron micrograph of renal transplant biopsy specimen from a patient with de novo membranous nephropathy and transplant glomerulopathy that demonstrate subepithelial electron-dense deposits (*arrows*) and subendothelial lucency (). CL, capillary lumen; US, urinary space. Original magnification, ×13,200. Photomicrograph provided by Dr. Donna Lager, Department of Pathology, University of Iowa College of Medicine, Iowa City, IA, U.S.A.

The finding of TGP implies a poor prognosis for continued graft function, perhaps because of the strong association with vascular rejection. In most series, most grafts with TGP are nonfunctional within 6–12 months after diagnosis (117–121).

De Novo Membranous Nephropathy

MN is the second most common de novo glomerulopathy, leading to clinically significant manifestations in ~2% of renal transplant recipients (55,56,125–130) and observed histologically in as many as 9% of allografts when protocol biopsies are routinely performed (Table 4) (131). Because native-kidney MN is the cause of renal failure in only ~1% of transplant recipients (57), and MN recurs in at most 20% of allografts, it follows that most cases of allograft MN represent de novo disease (55,56).

The usual presentation is that of abnormal proteinuria, typically of nephrotic degree, occurring on average 4–5 years after successful transplantation (Table 4). Diagnosis is made by allograft biopsy. In addition to the subepithelial deposits typical of MN, findings of acute cellular rejection or chronic rejection are commonly noted (129,130), though it is not certain that the frequency of these findings is higher than expected for allografts biopsied relatively late after transplantation (Fig. 3 and Table 4). No clinical predictors for the development of de novo MN have been identified. It is not associated with either higher or lower than average degrees of donor–recipient histocompatibility matching. The incidence is not lower in cyclosporine-treated recipients, as compared with those immunosuppressed with azathioprine and prednisone (128,130). The "recurrence" of de novo MN in second or subsequent regrafts in patients losing a first graft after diagnosis of de novo MN has been documented (132,133), raising the question of whether specific host factors might predispose certain individuals to the development of this form of graft injury (133). However, it is not yet clear that development of de novo MN in a first graft is a significant risk factor for recurrence of the problem in later grafts. In one large adult series (130), a few patients who developed de novo MN in second grafts had no history of proteinuria or biopsy findings of MN in a first graft. In addition, eight patients with de novo MN received second grafts that showed no evidence of MN during a follow-up period averaging >4 years. On the other hand, in a large pediatric series that described of a group of 55 recipients of second allograft recipients, the four cases of de novo MN identified were all in patients who had developed MN in their first grafts (133).

The pathogenesis of de novo MN remains unknown. In one large series, two of 21 patients with de novo MN were positive for HBV surface antigen, while five were HCV positive and two had antibodies to human immunodeficiency virus (130). While the association between MN and HBV is well recognized, the pathogenetic role of the other viruses in MN is uncertain. The relatively common presence of findings of acute or chronic rejection in biopsy specimens demonstrating de novo MN has suggested to several investigators that de novo MN might represent a morphologic form of chronic rejection that develops in a subset of patients and therefore might be related to the humoral response to alloantigens. In Heymann nephritis, the animal model most commonly employed to study MN, the subepithelial deposits develop as a consequence of in situ formation of immune complexes between a glycoprotein antigen on the base of the glomerular epithelial cells and circulating antibodies that react with this antigen. Immunochemical studies performed on sera from de novo MN patients indicate that some of these individuals probably have small, cationic circulating immune complexes that would be predicted to deposit in a subepithelial location (134). However, these immunopathologic and immunochemical studies have not yet identified the nature of the antigen–antibody system responsible for de novo MN.

Most recent series suggest that the impact of de novo MN on overall post-transplant graft survival is relatively small, owing to the late onset of the problem and to the fact that even after MN is diagnosed many grafts continue to function for years (129,130). Several reports mention that treatment with high-dose steroids had no impact on proteinuria or course of renal function (55,130), though this form of treatment has not been systematically studied. The efficacy of cytotoxic agents has not been tested in allograft MN in protocols similar to those used for native-kidney MN (135,136). The relatively late onset of de novo MN, coupled with the benign course experienced by many patients, suggests that maintenance of adequate immunosuppression, and retransplantation when necessary, are probably the best strategies for dealing with de novo MN at present. Even if second or subsequent allografts are at higher risk for de novo MN, the impact on expected graft survival is not severe enough to justify avoidance of retransplantation.

De Novo Membranoproliferative Glomerulonephritis and Hepatitis-C Infection

Since the development of antibody testing for detection of HCV infection, it has become apparent that ~10–25% of renal transplant recipients are infected with this virus (137–139), reflecting the high prevalence of this infection in the ESRD population on dialysis (140) and the transmission of HCV via kidneys obtained from HCV-infected donors, estimated to represent 2% of the U.S. donor pool (138,141,142). A recent report documents that the association between HCV infection and a form of glomerulonephritis with MPGN morphology extends to the renal allograft (48). Roth and co-workers found biopsy evidence of MPGN in five of 98 HCV-infected transplant recipients. Patients from the HCV-infected cohort were selected for biopsy because of proteinuria of >1 g/day (Table 4). Of the eight proteinuric patient, three had biopsy findings of chronic rejection, while the other five had MPGN. Immunochemical studies on the sera of these patients were consistent with the presence of immune complexes containing HCV. A more complete assessment of the clinical impact of these interesting observations will require further analysis and longer follow-up. Although all of the patients had nephrotic-range proteinuria, it is worth noting that all five had serum creatinine values of <2.0 mg/dL, and three of the five were already >5 years after transplantation. Patients with native-kidney glomerular disease in association with HCV infection have been reported to have decreased proteinuria, with no improvement in renal function, during treatment with α-interferon (143). However, the fear of provoking rejection with this immunomodulatory drug continues to limit its use in organ-transplant recipients, even those with HCV-related liver disease.

Anti-GBM Disease in Alport Syndrome

In 1982, McCoy and co-workers demonstrated the presence of anti-GBM antibodies in the circulation and the renal allograft of a patient with renal failure caused by Alport syndrome (144). In addition, it was noted that sera from patients with anti-GBM disease usually did not react with the basement membranes of in kidneys from Alport patients (144). Since that time, studies of post-transplantation anti-GBM sera obtained from Alport-syndrome patients have played an important role in delineating the molecular basis for this type of hereditary nephritis, which was recently summarized in a comprehensive review by Kashtan and Michael (145). The majority of cases of hereditary nephritis of the Alport type result from mutations in the COL4A5 gene, which encodes the α5(IV) collagen polypeptide chain, one of several types of collagen α chain normally present in basement membrane collagen (146). Even though the mutation is present in the COL4A5 gene, the GBM of Alport patients typically also lacks several other α chains [α3(IV) and α4(IV)] normally present in GBM, presumably because the α5(IV) chain is needed for normal stabilization and retention of these other α chains in basement membrane (Table 4). The mutations associated with Alport syndrome differ from kindred to kindred. It is estimated that ~80% of cases involve point mutations (with no particular tendency to occur at a mutation "hot spot" in the gene), whereas the others are due to gene rearrangements causing deletions of large segments of the gene (145).

The autoantibodies that develop after transplantation of a normal kidney into some Alport patients have been characterized as having one of two specificities. In one group of patients, the antibodies bind to a domain of α5(IV) collagen, which is absent from the patients' native kidneys because of the defective gene. In others, the antibody response is directed against α3(IV) or α4(IV) collagen epitopes. In either group, the Alport patient probably forms autoantibodies after transplantation of a kidney with normal collagen α chains in the basement membranes because of a failure to develop tolerance to the absent collagen α chains owing to their absence during maturation of the immune system (Table 4).

Based on literature reports, it is estimated that the frequency of anti-GBM antibody formation in Alport patients after kidney transplantation is ~3–4% (145, 147–152). The usual presentation is hematuria and rising creatinine, developing most often within the first year after the transplant (Table 4). Immunofluorescence examination of allograft biopsy tissue shows linear deposition of IgG (Table 4). Light microscopic findings may be normal in some patients (152), while those with more clinically significant disease will typically have a crescentic nephritis. Assays for circulating anti-GBM antibodies may find that some are present, though not all patients with linear GBM immunostaining have detectable circulating antibodies (150). Graft loss has been reported to occur in as many as 76% of cases (145), though some patients with linear IgG deposits have little or no clinical allograft dysfunction (147,150,152).

Kashtan and Michael summarize several risk factors for development of anti-GBM disease in the Alport patient undergoing renal transplantation (145). Almost all (~90%) of the reported cases have occurred in males, even though a considerable number of females with Alport syndrome have undergone renal transplantation (Table 4). Therefore, if the incidence of anti-GBM disease is expressed for male Alport patients undergoing transplantation, the figure rises to 5–7%. All of the patients with anti-GBM disease have been deaf, and most have had renal failure before age 30 (Table 4). If a first graft is lost to anti-GBM antibody production, the incidence of recurrence after retransplantation is very high, even after several years of delay and even if there are no detectable circulating anti-GBM antibodies between transplants. There is some evidence that anti-GBM antibodies develop in Alport patients with certain specific genetic defects in the COL4A5 gene, particularly those associated with large deletions (153). This would be consistent with reports of occurrence of anti-GBM nephritis in more than one patient from within the same kindred (154,155) and perhaps might explain the other phenotypic characteristics of the subset of Alport patients with anti-GBM disease, such as the nearly uniform presence of deafness.

Although post-transplantation anti-GBM disease in Alport patients is an important scientific and clinical problem, the existence of this complication should not be used to discourage Alport patients from undergoing primary renal transplantation. If anything, overall outcomes in this patient group are superior to those of the transplant-recipient population in general, perhaps owing to the young age and generally good overall health of these individuals (19,21). Recognition of this relatively uncommon problem is important for several reasons. First, anti-GBM disease must be considered in the evaluation of hematuria, proteinuria, or graft dysfunction in Alport transplant recipients, because clinically significant anti-GBM disease with crescentic nephritis may respond to therapy with pheresis or cytotoxic agents. Second, the occurrence of anti-GBM disease in one member of a kindred should lead to heightened surveillance for this problem in other family members. Finally, although the Alport population in general experiences good outcomes after renal transplantation, significant recurrences after retransplantation in patients who develop anti-GBM nephritis in a first graft are so common that further transplants should be undertaken with a clear understanding of the high risk of failure. In the future, it is possible that genetic studies will enable accurate identification of those Alport patients at risk for post-transplantation anti-GBM disease.

PROTEINURIA AND THE NEPHROTIC SYNDROME IN RENAL TRANSPLANT RECIPIENTS

Based on several large series in the literature (115–119), ~11–28% of transplant recipients develop persistent abnormal proteinuria, defined as protein excretion in of >1 g (115,118,119) or 2 g (117) per day, for ≥6 months. Transient proteinuria, lasting ≤ 6 months, is most commonly observed in association with acute rejection episodes and is not predictive of poor graft survival.

In these series, graft biopsies of patients with persistent proteinuria most commonly demonstrate chronic rejection, often with TGP, accounting for ~60% of the total group. Most of the remaining biopsies show allograft glomerulonephritis, with approximately equal numbers of cases judged to represent recurrent or de novo processes.

A common question that arises in the management of renal transplant recipients with proteinuria, with or without concomitant reduction in graft function, is whether a biopsy is needed for a histopathologic diagnosis. Since at present there are no effective therapies for the common causes of proteinuria observed in most series, it is unlikely that biopsy diagnosis will alter the therapeutic approach to the patient. For example, switching patients with proteinuria and chronic rejection to tacrolimus-based immunosuppression has not been helpful and is perhaps even detrimental (156,157). However, a biopsy could be recommended in a few situations. If recurrent focal segmental glomerulosclerosis is suspected, it is important to document the recurrence histologically because these individuals may respond to therapy with plasmapheresis and because of the implications for retransplantation in the future. Recurrence of anti-GBM disease, WG, or vasculitis in the graft, though uncommon, might respond to therapy with cytotoxic agents or plasmapheresis. Patients known to have had these diseases as the cause of their original renal failure should probably undergo biopsy, especially if they have hematuria in addition to proteinuria and abnormal graft function. If the patient's original renal disease is unknown or never substantiated by renal biopsy, a graft biopsy could conceivably provide information on the primary diagnosis that might be of use in managing the patient's graft dysfunction or in counseling the recipient about future transplants if the current graft fails.

In view of the relationship between HBV and HCV and proteinuric disorders of the transplanted kidney discussed earlier in this chapter, all renal transplant patients with significant proteinuria should undergo serologic evaluation for infection with these viruses and biochemical assessment of liver function.

Several studies in renal transplant patients demonstrate that use of angiotensin-II-converting enzyme (ACE) inhibitors causes an acute reduction in proteinuria that is sustained at least for a matter of weeks (158–160). Although the decreased protein excretion may be helpful in managing the symptoms related to the nephrotic syndrome, no reports as yet have confirmed that ACE inhibitor therapy is associated with prolongation of renal allograft function. Dietary protein restriction in patients with chronic graft dysfunction can also decrease proteinuria and produce short-term changes in renal hemodynamics that are associated with renal protection (161). As with ACE inhibitors, however, there have so far been no long term studies demonstrating a clinically useful preservation of graft survival with dietary protein restriction.

CONCLUSION

Based on the information reviewed in this chapter, many of the questions posed in the introduction can be answered. The incidence of clinically significant disease recurrence, leading to graft dysfunction and early graft loss, is low, probably in the range of 1–2% of all renal transplants. Histologically demonstrated recurrences are much more common and may have important implications about mechanisms of disease, though these recurrences should generally not be given as much weight in assessing the utility of transplantation in particular renal disorders. There is little evidence to indicate that use of well-matched cadaveric or living-donor grafts leads to a higher incidence of recurrent disease. Use of cyclosporine or tacrolimus has not led to a marked decrease in the problem of disease recurrence; whether newer immunosuppressive agents such as mycophenolate mofetil will alter recurrence rates remains to be seen.

In patients with focal segmental glomerular sclerosis or hemolytic uremic syndrome, recurrent disease is a major problem that can lead to early graft loss in a significant proportion of patients. Even in these disorders, we would agree with the recently published guidelines of the Patient Care and Education Committee of the American Society of Transplant Physicians (162), which emphasize the role of patient and donor counseling about the risks of recurrent disease, as opposed to routine avoidance of transplantation in specific renal diseases.

Acknowledgment

We thank Dr. Donna Lager, Department of Pathology, University of Iowa College of Medicine, for permission to use Fig. 3.

REFERENCES

1. Merrill JP. Glomerulonephritis in renal transplants. *Transplant Proc* 1969;1:994–1004.
2. Glassock RJ, Feldman D, Reynolds ES, Dammin GJ, Merrill JP. Human renal isografts: a clinical and pathologic analysis. *Medicine (Baltimore)* 1968;47:411–54.
3. Hamburger J, Crosnier J, Dormont J. Observations in patients with a well tolerated homotransplanted kidney. *Ann NY Acad Sci* 1964;120: 558–77.
4. Ramos EL, Tisher CC. Recurrent diseases in the kidney transplant. *Am J Kidney Dis* 1994;24:142–54.
5. Mathew TH. Recurrence of disease following renal transplantation. *Am J Kidney Dis* 1988;12:85–96.
6. Cameron JS. Recurrent primary disease and de novo nephritis following renal transplantation. *Pediatr Nephrol* 1991;5:412–21.
7. Cameron JS. Recurrent renal disease after renal transplantation. *Curr Opin Nephrol Hypertens* 1994;3:602–7.
8. Mathew TH. Recurrent disease after renal transplantation. *Transplant Rev* 1991;5:31–45.
9. Morzycka M, Croker BP, Seigler HF, Tisher CC. Evaluation of recurrent glomerulonephritis in kidney allografts. *Am J Med* 1982;72: 588–98.
10. Hamburger J, Crosnier J, Noel L. Recurrent glomerulonephritis after renal transplantation. *Annu Rev Med* 1978;29:67–72.
11. O'Meara Y, Green A, Carmody M, et al. Recurrent glomerulonephritis in renal transplants: fourteen years' experience. *Nephrol Dial Transplant* 1989;4:730–4.
12. Mathew TH, Mathews DC, Hobbs JB, Kincaid-Smith P. Glomerular lesions after renal transplantation. *Am J Med* 1975;59:177–90.
13. Honkanen E, Tornroth T, Pettersson E, Kulhback B. Glomerulonephritis in renal allografts: results of 18 years of transplantations. *Clin Nephrol* 1984;21:210–9.
14. Neumayer H-H, Kienbaum M, Graf S, Schreiber M, Mann JFE, Luft FC. Prevalence and long-term outcome of glomerulonephritis in renal allografts. *Am J Kidney Dis* 1993;22:320–5.
15. Habib R, Antignac C, Hinglais N, Gagnadoux M-F, Broyer M. Glomerular lesions in the transplanted kidney in children. *Am J Kidney Dis* 1987;10:198–207.
16. Broyer M, Selwood N, Brunner F. Recurrence of primary renal disease on kidney graft: a European pediatric experience. *J Am Soc Nephrol* 1992;2(Suppl 3):S255–7.
17. Alexander SR, Arbus GS, Butt KMH, et al. The 1989 report of the North American Pediatric Renal Transplant Cooperative Study. *Pediatr Nephrol* 1990;4:542–53.
18. Stablein DM, Tejani A. Five-year patient and graft survival in North American children: a report of the North American Pediatric Renal Transplant Cooperative Study. *Kidney Int* 1993;44(Suppl 43):S16–21.
19. Hirata M, Terasaki PI. The long-term effect of primary disease on cadaver-donor renal transplant recipients. In: Terasaki PI, Cecka JM, eds. *Clinical transplants 1993.* Los Angeles: UCLA Tissue Typing Laboratory, 1994:485–98.
20. Katznelson S, McClelland J, Cecka JM. Primary disease effects and associations. In: Terasaki PI, Cecka JM, eds. *Clinical transplants 1994.* Los Angeles: UCLA Tissue Typing Laboratory, 1995:1–18.
21. Cecka JM, Terasaki PI. The UNOS scientific renal transplant registry. In: Terasaki PI, Cecka JM, eds. *Clinical transplants 1994.* Los Angeles: UCLA Tissue Typing Laboratory, 1995:1–18.
22. Hoyer JR, Raij L, Vernier RL, Simmons RL, Najarian JS, Michael AF. Recurrence of idiopathic nephrotic syndrome after renal transplantation. *Lancet* 1972;2:343–48.
23. Malekzadeh MH, Heuser ET, Ettenger RB, et al. Focal glomerulosclerosis and renal transplantation. *J Pediatr* 1979;95:249–54.
24. Leumann EP, Briner J, Donckerwolcke RA, Kuijten R, Largiader F. Recurrence of focal segmental glomerulosclerosis in the transplanted kidney. *Nephron* 1980;25:65–71.
25. Maizel SE, Sibley RK, Horstman JP, Kjellstrand CM, Simmons RL. Incidence and significance of recurrent focal segmental glomerulosclerosis in renal allograft recipients. *Transplantation* 1981;32: 512–26.
26. Pinto J, Lacerda G, Cameron JS, Turner DR, Bewick M, Ogg CS. Recurrence of focal segmental glomerulosclerosis in renal allografts. *Transplantation* 1981;32:83–9.
27. Cheigh JS, Mouradian J, Soliman M, et al. Focal segmental glomerulosclerosis in renal transplants. *Am J Kidney Dis* 1983;2:449–55.
28. Axelsen RA, Seymour AE, Mathew TH, Fisher G, Canny A, Pascoe V. Recurrent focal glomerulosclerosis in renal transplants. *Clin Nephrol* 1984;21:110–4.
29. Vincenti F, Biava C, Tomlanovitch S, et al. Inability of cyclosporine to completely prevent the recurrence of focal glomerulosclerosis after kidney transplantation. *Transplantation* 1989;47:595–8.
30. Banfi G, Colturi C, Montagnino G, Ponticelli C. The recurrence of focal segmental glomerulosclerosis in kidney transplant recipients treated with cyclosporine. *Transplantation* 1990;50:594–6.
31. Senggutuvan P, Cameron JS, Hartley RB, et al. Recurrence of focal segmental glomerulosclerosis in transplanted kidneys: analysis of incidence and risk factors in 59 allografts. *Pediatr Nephrol* 1990;4: 21–8.
32. Ingulli E, Tejani A. Incidence, treatment, and outcome of recurrent focal segmental glomerulosclerosis posttransplantation in 42 allografts in children: a single center experience. *Transplantation* 1991; 51:401–5.
33. Artero M, Biava C, Amend W, Tomlanovich S, Vincenti F. Recurrent focal glomerulosclerosis: natural history and response to therapy. *Am J Med* 1992;92:375–83.
34. Tejani A, Stablein DH. Recurrence of focal segmental glomerulosclerosis posttransplantation: a special report of the North American Pediatric Renal Transplant Cooperative Study. *J Am Soc Nephrol* 1992;2 (Suppl 3):S258–63.
35. Zimmerman SW. Increased urinary protein excretion in the rat produced by serum from a patient with recurrent focal glomerular sclerosis after renal transplantation. *Clin Nephrol* 1984;22:32–8.
36. Dantal J, Bigot E, Bogers W, et al. Effect of plasma protein adsorption on protein excretion in kidney-transplant recipients with recurrent nephrotic syndrome. *N Engl J Med* 1994;330:7–14.
37. Artero ML, Sharma R, Savin VJ, Vincenti F. Plasmapheresis reduces proteinuria and serum capacity to injure glomeruli in patients with recurrent focal glomerulosclerosis. *Am J Kidney Dis* 1994;23:574–81.
38. Savin VJ, Chonko AM, Sharma R, Gunwar S, Sharma M. Factor present in serum of patients with minimal change nephrotic syndrome or focal sclerosing glomerulopathy causes an immediate increase in glomerular protein permeability in vitro. *J Am Soc Nephrol* 1990;1: 567(abst).
39. Stephanian E, Matas A, Mauer SM, et al. Recurrence of disease in patients retransplanted for focal segmental glomerulosclerosis. *Transplantation* 1992;53:755–7.
40. Ingulli E, Tejani A, Butt KMH, Rajpoot A, Ettenger RB. High dose cyclosporine therapy in recurrent nephrotic syndrome following renal transplantation. *Transplantation* 1990;49:219–21.
41. Torres VE, Velosa JA, Holley KE, Frohnert PP. Meclofenamate treat-

ment of recurrent idiopathic nephrotic syndrome with focal segmental glomerulosclerosis after renal transplantation. *Mayo Clin Proc* 1984; 59:146–52.

42. Regester RF, Goldman MH. Meclofenamate treatment of posttransplant nephrotic syndrome. *Transplant Proc* 1991;23:1789–90.
43. Kooijmans-Coutinho MF, Tegzess AM, Bruijn JA, Florijn KW, Van Es LA, Van der Woude FJ. Indomethacin treatment of recurrent nephrotic syndrome and focal segmental glomerulosclerosis after renal transplantation. *Pediatr Nephrol* 1993;8:469–73.
44. Dantal J, Baatard R, Hourmant M, Cantarovich D, Buzelin F, Soulillou JP. Recurrent nephrotic syndrome following renal transplantation in patients with focal glomerulosclerosis: a one-center study of plasma exchange effects. *Transplantation* 1991;52:827–31.
45. Zimmerman SW, Hyman LR, Vehling DT, et al. Recurrent membrano-proliferative glomerulonephritis with glomerular properdin deposition in allografts. *Ann Intern Med* 1976;80:169–75.
46. Glicklich D, Matas AJ, Sablay LB, et al. Recurrent membranoproliferative glomerulonephritis type I in successive renal transplants. *Am J Nephrol* 1987;7:143–9.
47. Johnson RJ, Gretch DR, Yamabe H, et al. Membranoproliferative glomerulonephritis associated with hepatitis C virus infection. *N Engl J Med* 1993;328:465–70.
48. Roth D, Cirocco R, Zucker K, et al. De novo membranoproliferative glomerulonephritis in hepatitis C virus–infected renal allograft recipients. *Transplantation* 1995;59:1676–82.
49. Droz D, Nabarra B, Noel LH, Leibowitch J, Crosnier J. Recurrence of dense deposits in transplanted kidneys. I. Sequential survey of the lesions. *Kidney Int* 1979;15:386–95.
50. McLean RH, Geiger H, Burke B, et al. Recurrence of membranoproliferative glomerulonephritis following kidney transplantation: serum complement component studies. *Am J Med* 1976;60:60–72.
51. Turner DR, Cameron JS, Bewick M, et al. Transplantation in mesangiocapillary glomerulonephritis with intramembranous dense "deposits": recurrence of disease. *Kidney Int* 1976;9:439–48.
52. Lamb V, Tisher CC, McCoy RC, Robinson RR. Membranoproliferative glomerulonephritis with dense intramembranous alterations: a clinicopathologic study. *Lab Invest* 1977;36:607–17.
53. Curtis JJ, Wyatt RJ, Bhathena D, Lucas BA, Holland NH, Luke RG. Renal transplantation for patients with type I and type II membranoproliferative glomerulonephritis: serial complement and nephritic factor measurements and the problem of recurrence of disease. *Am J Med* 1979;66:216–25.
54. Beaufils H, Gubler MC, Karam J, Gluckman JC, Legrain M, Kuss R. Dense deposit disease: long term follow-up of three cases of recurrence. *Clin Nephrol* 1977;7:31–7.
55. Eddy A, Sibley R, Mauer SM, Kim Y. Renal allograft failure due to recurrent dense intramembranous deposit disease. *Clin Nephrol* 1984; 21:305–13.
56. Leibowitch J, Halbwachs L, Wattel S, Gaillard MH, Droz D. Recurrence of dense deposits in transplanted kidney. II. Serum complement and nephritic factor profiles. *Kidney Int* 1979;15:396–403.
57. Austin HA, Antonovych TT, MacKay K, Boumpas DT, Balow JE. Membranous nephropathy. *Ann Intern Med* 1992;116:672–82.
58. Donadio JV, Torres VE, Velosa JA, et al. Idiopathic membranous nephropathy: the natural history of untreated patients. *Kidney Int* 1988;33:708–15.
59. Schieppati A, Mosconi L, Perna A, et al. Prognosis of untreated patients with idiopathic membranous nephropathy. *N Engl J Med* 1993;329: 85–9.
60. Briner J, Binswanger U, Largiader F. Recurrent and de novo membranous glomerulonephritis in renal cadaver allotransplants. *Clin Nephrol* 1980;13:189–96.
51. Innes A, Woodrow G, Boyd SM, Beckingham IJ, Morgan AG. Recurrent membranous nephropathy in successive renal transplants. *Nephrol Dial Transplant* 1994;9:323–5.
52. Lieberthal W, Bernard DB, Donohoe JF, Stilmant MM, Couser WG. Rapid recurrence of membranous nephropathy in a related allograft. *Clin Nephrol* 1979;12:222–8.
53. Rubin RJ, Pinn VW, Barnes BA, Harrington JT. Recurrent idiopathic membranous glomerulonephritis. *Transplantation* 1977;24:4–9.
54. Dische FE, Herbertson BM, Melcher DH, Morley AR. Membranous glomerulonephritis in transplant kidneys: recurrent or de novo disease in four patients. *Clin Nephrol* 1981;15:154–63.
55. Monga G, Mazzucco G, Basolo B, et al. Membranous glomerulonephritis in transplanted kidneys: morphologic investigation on 256 renal allografts. *Mod Pathol* 1993;6:249–58.
56. Berger BE, Vincenti F, Biava C, Amend WJ, Feduska N, Salvatierra O. De novo and recurrent membranous glomerulopathy following kidney transplantation. *Transplantation* 1983;35:315–9.
57. Couchoud C, Pouteil-Noble C, Colon S, Touraine J-L. Recurrence of membranous nephropathy after renal transplantation. *Transplantation* 1995;59:1275–9.
58. Lai KN, Li PKT, Lui SF, et al. Membranous nephropathy related to hepatitis B virus in adults. *N Engl J Med* 1991;324:1457–63.
59. Schena FP. A retrospective analysis of the natural history of primary IgA nephropathy worldwide. *Am J Med* 1990;89:209–15.
60. D'Amico G. Influence of clinical and histological features on actuarial renal survival in adult patients with idiopathic IgA nephropathy, membranous nephropathy, and membranoproliferative glomerulonephritis: survey of the recent literature. *Am J Kidney Dis* 1992;20: 315–23.
61. Berger J, Janeva H, Nabarra B, et al. Recurrence of mesangial deposition of IgA nephropathy after renal transplantation. *Kidney Int* 1975; 7:232–41.
62. Berger J, Noel LH, Nabarra B. Recurrence of mesangial IgA nephropathy after renal transplantation. *Contrib Nephrol* 1984;40:195–7.
63. Berger J. Recurrence of IgA nephropathy in renal allografts. *Am J Kidney Dis* 1988;12:371–2.
64. Brensilver JM, Mallat S, Scholes J, McCabe R. Recurrent IgA nephropathy in living-related donor transplantation: recurrence or transmission of familial disease? *Am J Kidney Dis* 1988;12:147–51.
65. Sanfilippo F, Croker PB, Bollinger RR. Fate of four cadaveric renal allografts with mesangial IgA deposits. *Transplantation* 1982;33: 370–76.
66. Silva FG, Chander P, Pirani C, et al. Disappearance of glomerular mesangial IgA deposits after renal allograft transplantation. *Transplantation* 1982;33:214–16.
67. Suganuma T, Morozumi K, Satoh A, et al. Studies of IgA nephropathy in renal transplantation. *Transplant Proc* 1989;21:2123.
68. Odum J, Peh CA, Clarkson AR, et al. Recurrent mesangial IgA nephritis following renal transplantation. *Nephrol Dial Transplant* 1994;9:309–12.
69. Bachman U, Biava C, Amend W, et al. The clinical course of IgA-nephropathy and Henoch–Schönlein purpura following renal transplantation. *Transplantation* 1986;42:511–5.
70. Frohnert PP, Velosa JA, Donadio JV, Sterioff S. Renal transplantation in IgA nephropathy: the effect of HLA matching on recurrence of primary disease. *Transplant Proc* 1994;26:1892.
71. Donadio JV, Bergstralh EJ, Offord KP, Spencer DC, Holley KE. A controlled trial of fish oil in IgA nephropathy. *N Engl J Med* 1994; 331:1194–9.
72. Wilson CB, Dixon FJ. Anti-glomerular basement membrane antibody-induced glomerulonephritis. *Kidney Int* 1973;3:74–89.
73. Bergrem H, Jervell J, Brodwall EK, Flatmark A, Mellbye O. Goodpasture's syndrome: a report of seven patients including long-term follow-up of three who received a kidney transplant. *Am J Med* 1980; 68:54–8.
74. Cove-Smith JR, McLeod AA, Blamey RW, Knapp MS, Reeves WG, Wilson CB. Transplantation, immunosuppression and plasmapheresis in Goodpasture's syndrome. *Clin Nephrol* 1978;9:126–8.
75. Couser WG, Wallace A, Monaco AP, Lewis EJ. Successful renal transplantation in patients with circulating antibody to glomerular basement membrane: report of two cases. *Clin Nephrol* 1973;1:381–8.
76. Turney JH, Adu D, Michael J, et al. Recurrent crescentic glomerulonephritis in renal transplant recipient treated with cyclosporin [Letter]. *Lancet* 1985;1:1104.
77. Buda JA, Lattes CG, Grant JP, et al. Feasibility of renal transplantation in systemic lupus erythematosus. *Surg Forum* 1970;21:252–4.
78. Kimberly RP, Lockshin MD, Sherman RL, Beary JF, Mouradian J, Cheigh JS. End stage lupus nephritis: clinical course to and outcome on dialysis—experience with 39 patients. *Medicine (Baltimore)* 1981; 60:277–87.
79. Advisory Committee to the Renal Transplant Registry. Renal transplantation in congenital and metabolic diseases. *JAMA* 1975;232: 148–53.
80. Bumgardner GL, Mauer SM, Payne W, et al. Single-center 1–15-year results of renal transplantation in patients with systemic lupus erythematosus. *Transplantation* 1988;46:703–9.

81. Cheigh JS, Kim H, Stenzel KH, et al. Systemic lupus erythematosus in patients with end-stage renal disease: long-term follow-up on the prognosis of patients and the evolution of lupus activity. *Am J Kidney Dis* 1990;16:189–95.
82. Roth D, Milgrom M, Esquenazi V, Straus J, Zilleruelo G, Miller J. Renal transplantation in systemic lupus erythematosus: one center's experience. *Am J Nephrol* 1987;7:367–74.
83. Rivera M, Marcen R, Pascual J, Naya MT, Orofino L, Ortuno J. Kidney transplantation in systemic lupus erythematosus nephritis: a one center experience. *Nephron* 1990;56:148–51.
84. Amend WJC, Vincenti F, Feduska N, et al. Recurrent systemic lupus erythematosus involving renal allografts. *Ann Intern Med* 1981;94: 444–8.
85. Ward LA, Jelveh Z, Feinfeld DA. Recurrent membranous lupus nephritis after renal transplantation: a case report and review of the literature. *Am J Kidney Dis* 1994;23:326–9.
86. Nyberg G, Blohme I, Persson H, Olausson M, Svalander C. Recurrence of SLE in transplanted kidneys: a follow-up transplant biopsy study. *Nephrol Dial Transplant* 1992;7:1116–23.
87. Hebert D, Kim EM, Sibley RK, Mauer MS. Post-transplantation outcome of patients with hemolytic–uremic syndrome: update. *Pediatr Nephrol* 1991;5:162–7.
88. Bassani CE, Ferraris J, Gianantonio CA, Ruiz S, Ramirez J. Renal transplantation in patients with classical haemolytic–uraemic syndrome. *Pediatr Nephrol* 1991;5:607–11.
89. Eijgenraam FJ, Donckerwolcke RA, Monnens LA, Proesmans W, Wolff ED, Van Damme B. Renal transplantation in 20 children with hemolytic–uremic syndrome. *Clin Nephrol* 1990;33:87–93.
90. Scantlebury VP, Shapiro R, McCauley J, et al. Renal transplantation under cyclosporine and FK 506 for hemolytic uremic syndrome. *Transplant Proc* 1995;27:842–3.
91. Hauglustaine D, Van Damme B, Vanrenterghem Y, Michielsen P. Recurrent hemolytic uremic syndrome during oral contraception. *Clin Nephrol* 1981;15:148–53.
92. Sommer BG, Innes JT, Whitehurst RM, Sharma HM, Ferguson RM. Cyclosporine-associated renal arteriopathy resulting in loss of allograft function. *Am J Surg* 1985;149:756–64.
93. Vanrenterghem Y, Roels L, Lerut T, et al. Thromboembolic complications and haemostatic changes in cyclosporin-treated cadaveric kidney allograft recipients. *Lancet* 1985;1:999–1002.
94. Neild GH, Rocchi G, Imberti L, et al. Effect of cyclosporin A on prostacyclin synthesis by vascular tissue. *Thromb Res* 1983;32:373–9.
95. Arias-Rodrigues M, Sraer J-D, Kourilsky O, et al. Renal transplantation and immunological abnormalities in thrombotic microangiopathy of adults. *Transplantation* 1977;23:360–5.
96. Hasegawa A, Kawamura T, Ito H, et al. Fate of renal grafts with recurrent Henoch–Schönlein purpura nephritis in children. *Transplant Proc* 1989;21:2130–3.
97. Meulders Q, Pirson Y, Cosyns J-P, Squifflet J-P, Van Ypersele de Strihou C. Course of Henoch–Schönlein nephritis after renal transplantation. *Transplantation* 1994;58:1179–86.
98. Steinman TI, Jaffe B, Monaco AP, Wolff SM, Fauci AS. Recurrence of Wegener's granulomatosis after kidney transplantation: successful re-induction of remission with cyclophosphamide. *Am J Med* 1980; 68:458–60.
99. Kuross S, Davin T, Kjellstrand CM. Wegener's granulomatosis with severe renal failure: clinical course and results of dialysis and transplantation. *Clin Nephrol* 1981;16:172–80.
100. Tzardis PJ, Gruessner RWG, Matas AJ, et al. Long-term follow-up of renal transplantation for Wegener's disease. *Clin Transplant* 1990;4: 108–11.
101. Lowance DC, Vosatka K, Whelchel J, et al. Recurrent Wegener's granulomatosis. *Am J Med* 1992;92:573–5.
102. Schmitt WH, Haubitz M, Mistry N, Brunkhorst R, Erbsloh-Moller B, Gross WL. Renal transplantation in Wegener's granulomatosis. *Lancet* 1993;342:860.
103. Rich LM, Piering WF. Ureteral stenosis due to recurrent Wegener's granulomatosis after kidney transplantation. *J Am Soc Nephrol* 1994; 4:1516–21.
104. Pasternack A, Ahonen J, Kuhlback B. Renal transplantation in 45 patients with amyloidosis. *Transplantation* 1986;42:598–601.
105. Hartmann A, Holdaas H, Fauchald P, et al. Fifteen years' experience with renal transplantation in systemic amyloidosis. *Transpl Int* 1992; 5:15–8.
106. Harrison KL, Alpers CE, Davis CL. De novo amyloidosis in a renal allograft: a case report and review of the literature. *Am J Kidney Dis* 1993;22:468–76.
107. Zemer D, Pras M, Sohar E, Gafni J. Colchicine in familial Mediterranean fever. *N Engl J Med* 1976;294:170–1.
108. Ravid M, Robson M, Kedar I. Prolonged colchicine treatment in four patients with amyloidosis. *Ann Intern Med* 1977;87:568–70.
109. Skrinskas G, Bear RA, Magil A, Lee KY. Colchicine therapy for nephrotic syndrome due to familial Mediterranean fever. *Can Med Assoc J* 1977;117:1416–7.
110. Zemer D, Mordechai P, Sohar E, Modal M, Cabili S, Gafni J. Colchicine in the prevention and treatment of the amyloidosis of familial Mediterranean fever. *N Engl J Med* 1986;314:1001–5.
111. Zemer D, Livneh A, Danon YL, Pras M, Sohar E. Long-term colchicine treatment in children with familial Mediterranean fever. *Arthritis Rheum* 1991;34:973–7.
112. Merino GE, Sutherland DE, Kjellstrand CM, Simmons RL, Najarian JS. Renal transplantation for progressive systemic sclerosis with renal failure: case report and review of previous experience. *Am J Surg* 1977;133:745–9.
113. Woodhall PB, McCoy RC, Gunnells JC, Seigler HF. Apparent recurrence of progressive systemic sclerosis in a renal allograft. *JAMA* 1976;236:1032–4.
114. McCoy RC, Tisher CC, Pepe PF, Cleveland LA. The kidney in progressive systemic sclerosis: immunohistochemical and antibody elution studies. *Lab Invest* 1976;35:124–31.
115. Bear RA, Aprile M, Sweet J, Cole EH. Proteinuria in renal transplant recipients: incidence, cause, prognostic importance. *Transplant Proc* 1988;20:1235–6.
116. Castelao AM, Grino JM, Seron D, et al. Pathological differential diagnostics of proteinuria and late failure after renal transplantation. *Transplant Proc* 1992;24:110–2.
117. First MR, Vaidya PN, Maryniak RK, et al. Proteinuria following renal transplantation: correlation with histopathology and outcome. *Transplantation* 1984;38:607–12.
118. Vathsala A, Verani R, Schoenberg L, et al. Proteinuria in cyclosporine-treated renal transplant recipients. *Transplantation* 1990;49: 35–41.
119. Kim HC, Park SB, Lee SH, Park KK, Park CH, Cho WH. Proteinuria in renal transplant recipients: incidence, cause and prognostic importance. *Transplant Proc* 1994;26:2134–5.
120. Briner J. Transplant glomerulopathy. *Appl Pathol* 1987;5:82–7.
121. Habib R, Zurowska A, Hinglais N, et al. A specific glomerular lesion of the graft: allograft glomerulopathy. *Kidney Int* 1993;44(Suppl 42): S104–11.
122. Zollinger HU, Moppert J, Thiel G, Rohr HP. Morphology and pathogenesis of glomerulopathy in cadaver kidney allografts treated with antilymphocyte globulin. *Curr Top Pathol* 1973;57:1–48.
123. Cameron JS, Turner DR. Recurrent glomerulonephritis in allografted kidneys. *Clin Nephrol* 1977;7:47–54.
124. Maryniak RK, First MR, Weiss MA. Transplant glomerulopathy: evolution of morphologically distinct changes. *Kidney Int* 1985;27: 799–806.
125. Cosyns J-P, Pirson Y, Squifflet J-P, et al. De novo membranous nephropathy in human renal allografts: report of nine patients. *Kidney Int* 1982;22:177–83.
126. Levy M, Charpentier B, et al. De novo membranous glomerulonephritis in renal allografts: report of 19 cases in 1550 transplant recipients. *Transplant Proc* 1983;15:1099–102.
127. Antignac C, Hinglais N, Gubler M-C, Gagnadoux M-F, Broyer M, Habib R. De novo membranous glomerulonephritis in renal allografts in children. *Clin Nephrol* 1988;30:1–7.
128. Montagnino G, Colturi C, Banfi G, Aroldi A, Tarantino A, Ponticelli C. Membranous nephropathy in cyclosporine-treated renal transplant recipients. *Transplantation* 1989;47:725–7.
129. Truong L, Gelfand J, D'Agati V, et al. De novo membranous glomerulonephropathy in renal allografts: a report of ten cases and review of the literature. *Am J Kidney Dis* 1989;14:131–44.
130. Schwarz A, Krause P-H, Offermann G, Keller F. Impact of de novo membranous glomerulonephritis on the clinical course after kidney transplantation. *Transplantation* 1994;58:650–4.
131. Habib R, Antignac C, Hinglais N, Gagnadoux M-F, Broyer M. Glomerular lesions in the transplanted kidney in children. *Am J Kidney Dis* 1987;10:198–207.

132. Cosyns J-P, Pirson Y, Van Ypersele de Strihou C, Alexandre GPJ. Recurrence of de novo graft membranous glomerulonephritis. *Nephron* 1981;29:142–5.
133. Heidet L, Gagnadoux M-F, Beziau A, Niaudet P, Broyer M, Habib R. Recurrence of de novo membranous glomerulonephritis on renal grafts. *Clin Nephrol* 1994;41:314–8.
134. Ward HJ, Koyle MA. Immunopathologic features of de novo membranous nephropathy in renal allografts. *Transplantation* 1988;45: 524–9.
135. Ponticelli C, Zucchelli P, Passerini P, et al. A randomized trial of methylprednisolone and chlorambucil in idiopathic membranous nephropathy. *N Engl J Med* 1989;320:8–13.
136. Jindal K, West M, Bear R, Goldstein M. Long-term benefits of therapy with cyclophosphamide and prednisone in patients with membranous glomerulonephritis and impaired renal function. *Am J Kidney Dis* 1992;19:61–67.
137. Stempel CA, Lake J, Kuo G, Vincenti F. Hepatitis C: its prevalence in end-stage renal failure patients and clinical course after kidney transplantation. *Transplantation* 1993;55:273–6.
138. Pereira BJG, Milford EL, Kirkman RL, et al. Prevalence of hepatitis C virus RNA in organ donors positive for hepatitis C antibody and in the recipients of their organs. *N Engl J Med* 1992;327:910–15.
139. Roth D, Zucker K, Cirocco R, et al. The impact of hepatitis C virus infection on renal allograft recipients. *Kidney Int* 1994;45:238–44.
140. Simon N, Courouce A-M, Lemarrec N, Trepo C, Ducamp S. A twelve year natural history of hepatitis C virus infection in hemodialyzed patients. *Kidney Int* 1994;46:504–11.
141. Pereira BJG, Milford EL, Kirkman RL, Levey AS. Transmission of hepatitis C virus by organ transplantation. *N Engl J Med* 1991;325: 454–60.
142. Pereira BJG, Wright TL, Schmid CH, et al. Screening and confirmatory testing of cadaver organ donors for hepatitis C virus infection: a U.S. National Collaborative Study. *Kidney Int* 1994;46:886–92.
143. Johnson RJ, Gretch DR, Couser WG, et al. Hepatitis C virus–associated glomerulonephritis: effect of α-interferon therapy. *Kidney Int* 1994;46:1700–4.
144. McCoy RC, Johnson HK, Stone WJ, Wilson CB. Absence of nephritogenic GBM antigen(s) in some patients with hereditary nephritis. *Kidney Int* 1982;21:642–52.
145. Kashtan CE, Michael AF. Alport syndrome: from bedside to genome to bedside. *Am J Kidney Dis* 1993;22:627–40.
146. Barker DF, Hostikka SL, Zhou J, et al. Identification of mutations in the COL4A5 collagen gene in Alport syndrome. *Science* 1990;248: 1224–7.
147. Peten E, Pirson Y, Coysns J-P, et al. Outcome of thirty patients with Alport's syndrome after renal transplantation. *Transplantation* 1991; 52:823–6.
148. Goldman M, Depierreux M, De Pauw L, et al. Failure of two subsequent renal grafts by anti-GBM glomerulonephritis in Alport's syndrome: case report and review of the literature. *Transpl Int* 1990;3: 82–5.
149. Milliner DS, Pierides AM, Holley KE. Renal transplantation in Alport's syndrome: anti-glomerular basement membrane glomerulonephritis in the allograft. *Mayo Clin Proc* 1982;57:35–43.
150. Querin S, Noel L-H, Grunfeld J-P, et al. Linear glomerular IgG fixation in renal allografts: incidence and significance in Alport's syndrome. *Clin Nephrol* 1986;25:134–40.
151. Shah B, First MR, Mendoza NC, Clyne DH, Alexander JW, Weiss MA. Alport's syndrome: risk of glomerulonephritis induced by anti-glomerular-basement-membrane antibody after renal transplantation. *Nephron* 1988;50:34–8.
152. Gobel J, Olbricht CJ, Offner G, et al. Kidney transplantation in Alport's syndrome: long-term outcome and allograft anti-GBM nephritis. *Clin Nephrol* 1992;38:299–304.
153. Ding J, Zhou J, Tryggvason K, Kashtan CE. COL4A5 deletions in three patients with Alport syndrome and posttransplant antiglomerular basement membrane nephritis. *J Am Soc Nephrol* 1994;5:161–8.
154. Kashtan C, Butkowski R, Kleppel M, First M, Michael A. Posttransplant anti-glomerular basement membrane nephritis in related males with Alport syndrome. *J Lab Clin Med* 1990;116:508–15.
155. Helderman JH. The case of the two disparate diseases: a medical mystery. *Am J Nephrol* 1991;11:157–63.
156. McCauley J, Shapiro R, Scantlebury V, et al. FK 506 in the management of transplant-related nephrotic syndrome and steroid-resistant nephrotic syndrome. *Transplant Proc* 1991;23:3354–6.
157. McCauley J, Shapiro R, Jordan M, et al. FK 506 in the management of nephrotic syndrome after renal transplantation. *Transplant Proc* 1993;25:1351–4.
158. Traindl O, Falger S, Reading S, et al. The effects of lisinopril on renal function in proteinuric renal transplant recipients. *Transplantation* 1993;55:1309–13.
159. Rell K, Linde J, Morzycka-Michalik M, Gaciong Z, Lao M. Effect of enalapril on proteinuria after kidney transplantation. *Transpl Int* 1993;6:213–7.
160. Morales JM, Andrews A, Montoyo C, et al. Effect of captopril, an angiotensin converting enzyme inhibitor, on the massive proteinuria due to chronic rejection after renal transplantation: a prospective study. *Transplant Proc* 1992;24:92–3.
161. Salahudeen AK, Hostetter TH, Raatz SK, Rosenberg ME. Effects of dietary protein in patients with chronic renal transplant rejection. *Kidney Int* 1992;41:183–90.
162. Kasiske BL, Ramos EL, Gaston RS, et al. The evaluation of renal transplant candidates: clinical practice guidelines. *J Am Soc Nephrol* 1995;6:1–33.

D. Interstitial Nephritis

Immunologic Renal Diseases,
edited by E. G. Neilson and W. G. Couser.
Lippincott-Raven Publishers, Philadelphia © 1997.

CHAPTER 56

Acute Interstitial Nephritis

Gerald B. Appel

DEFINITION AND HISTORICAL PERSPECTIVE

Acute interstitial nephritis (AIN), also called acute *tubulointerstitial nephritis*, is a form of inflammatory renal disease in which the parenchymal damage is predominantly localized to the tubules and the area between them rather than to the glomeruli or the vasculature (1–6). Although AIN may have diverse etiologies, the majority of cases are related to medications and infectious agents, either by direct invasion or as a remote effect. Acute bacterial pyelonephritis with direct invasion of the kidney by the organisms will not be considered here. Infrequently, patients may have idiopathic AIN, either as an isolated renal disease or as part of a group of syndromes of unknown etiology but with distinct clinical presentations. All forms of AIN are characterized by interstitial edema with patchy tubular damage and tubulitis, as well as focal interstitial infiltrates. The clinical manifestations, although varied, are typically those of acute renal insufficiency and renal failure or of tubular dysfunction due to the renal involvement. Due to the acute nature of the process, if appropriate treatment is instituted promptly, the disease is potentially reversible and need not result in severe permanent renal dysfunction.

Historically, the first description of AIN is often attributed to W.T. Councilman in 1898 (7), who examined the kidneys of 42 cases, mostly children, who had died of scarlet fever or diphtheria. He described the lesions as "an acute inflammation of the kidney characterized by cellular and fluid exudation in the interstitial tissue, accompanied by, but not dependent on, degeneration of the epithelium: the exudate is not purulent in character and the lesions may be both diffuse and focal."

Councilman was not the first to note such changes, but he did recognize that the kidneys were sterile and proposed that "soluble" substances were exerting a chemotactic role. Many reports in the preantibiotic era confirmed the findings of Councilman. Medication-related nephrotoxicity was recognized with the sulfonamides and early antimicrobial therapy. By the 1960s, the classic clinical picture and pathology of penicillin-related AIN was defined. Over time, with better antimicrobial therapy of the infectious etiologies of AIN and with wider use of medications capable of producing AIN, medication-related AIN has become the most common pattern of AIN. Several unique clinical presentations, such as seen with nonsteroidal antiinflammatory drugs (NSAIDs), have been described. As recently as 1972, there was debate as to the existence of idiopathic AIN that was related neither to infections nor drugs (8). Several clinical variants of this so-called idiopathic AIN have become well recognized and better defined.

INCIDENCE AND ETIOLOGY

The true incidence of AIN is unknown for several reasons. Biopsy is required for a firm diagnosis because the clinical manifestations, although suggestive at times, are not diagnostic. Mild cases may be overlooked or attributed to other forms of reversible medication-related renal disease. For example, some patients with mild AIN due to drugs such as trimethoprim sulfamethoxazole or cimetidine (Tagamet) may have his renal dysfunction attributed to interference with creatinine secretion by these agents. Once the drug has been discontinued, other clinical features of AIN will no longer appear. On the other hand, some severely ill patients are too sick to undergo renal biopsy, and the AIN may be attributed to other forms of acute renal failure associated with similar clinical features, such as rapidly progressive glomerulonephritis and cholesterol emboli. The incidence also will vary depending on the population studied (9–11). In Finnish military recruits, 174 of 314,000 had persistent proteinuria or

Director of Clinical Nephrology, Columbia-Presbyterian Medical Center, New York, New York 10032.

hematuria leading to a renal biopsy (9). Of these, only two—0.7 per 100,000—had interstitial nephritis, while in an autopsy series AIN was found in 1% of 25,000 autopsies. A second autopsy series found AIN with cellular infiltrates in 87 of 7,980 cases, for a similar incidence of about 1% (11). In large unselected series of patients biopsied, between 1% and 2% of patients have had AIN (10,11). However, this rises to 11–15% of biopsies performed in patients with acute renal failure (12,13). An even higher percentage of patients with normal-sized kidneys and acute renal failure have been shown on biopsy to have AIN (14). Clearly, most patients with functional or prerenal azotemia and classic acute tubular necrosis do not come to renal biopsy. At Columbia Presbyterian Medical Center, of X biopsy specimens analyzed over a 2-year period, the vast majority of nontransplant biopsy specimens were in patients with glomerular diseases, but X% of those with tubulointerstitial disease had AIN as their primary diagnosis. The most common etiologies of AIN may be divided as follows:

1. Those related to use of medications
2. Those related to infectious agents
3. Those associated with systemic disease or glomerular diseases
4. Idiopathic disease

In each category, there are a number of important subgroups (see Table 1).

Of the major causes of AIN, if one excludes direct infection of the kidney, such as with acute bacterial pyelonephritis, medication-related AIN is currently by far the most commonly reported (2,4,5,15). Drug-related AIN has been reported with overuse of more than 75 different medications. In the literature, antibiotics of the β-lactam class, penicillins and cephalosporins, were particularly common offending agents (16–19). In part, this relates to the common use of these drugs in seriously ill patients in whom a severe renal reaction is not easily overlooked, and it may relate to the particularly high incidence of AIN seen with one specific agent of this class, methicillin. The literature contains over 100 cases of AIN attributed to methicillin, a semisynthetic penicillin no longer available, but only about a dozen cases of true penicillin-related AIN (15–19). AIN has also been noted with many other penicillins and cephalosporin antibiotics, including both second- and third-generation cephalosporins (2,19). Among the other antimicrobials that have produced AIN, many have been in individual patients or in poorly documented cases. However, the sulfonamides, rifampin, and the quinolones have all produce a convincing number of cases with strong clinical suspicion or histologic confirmation of AIN. Two antiviral agents, acyclovir (Zovirax) and foscarnet (Foscavir), can also produce tubulointerstitial damage, although this may be more similar to acute tubular necrosis than to interstitial nephritis (20–22). Diuretics of a number of classes, including thiazides, the loop diuretic furosemide (Lasix), and triamterene (Dyazide, Dyrenium, Maxzine) have been incriminated in producing AIN. The incidence of diuretic-related AIN is very small when compared with the large numbers of patients with reversible renal dysfunction due to volume depletion associated with diuretic use. Nonsteroidal agents from every chemical class may produce AIN (23,24). The clinical pattern most often produced is unique in that this is the only class of medications in which the AIN and acute renal failure are typically accompanied by the nephrotic syndrome (NS) and the histologic picture of minimal change disease. Finally, of the more than 25 other drugs that have been documented to produce AIN, only a few have produced more than isolated cases. The more frequent offenders include allopurinol (Zyloprim), diphenylhydantoin (Dilantin), sulfinpyrazone (Anturane), and cimetidine (2–6).

TABLE 1. *Etiologies of acute interstitial nephritis*

Medication-related AIN
AIN associated with infections
Direct invasion of the kidney
Remote infection
Idiopathic AIN
AIN associated with glomerular and systemic diseases

A number of infectious agents has been associated with renal dysfunction. The organisms may produce parenchymal damage, either through direct invasion of the kidney or by indirect relation to a systemic process producing AIN. This chapter will not discuss the acute pyelonephritis associated with direct infections of the kidney. However, for some infectious etiologies of interstitial renal damage, it is unclear whether actual parenchymal tissue invasion has occurred. Even when there are organisms in the parenchyma, it is unclear how their presence relates to the inflammatory renal process. Moreover, it is likely that some cases of antibiotic-associated AIN are truly related to the underlying infection rather than to the medications. AIN associated with remote or systemic infections has been caused by bacteria, parasites, and viruses (see Table 2). Bacterial infections associated with AIN include those due to both gram-positive and gram-negative organisms, as well as to mycoplasmal species. In the preantibiotic era, scarlet fever and diphtheria were the infections most commonly associated with the finding of AIN at autopsy (7).

Although infection-associated AIN has dramatically decreased in the modern era, in some series, between 20% and 50% of cases of AIN in children have been related to streptococcal infections (25). Other bacterial organisms, including *Brucella, Legionella, Yersinia, Mycobacterium leprae*, and *mycoplasma* have all been associated with AIN in isolated cases (26–32). Parasitic infections with Leishmanial species have been associated with AIN (33,34). An autopsy and biopsy study of Brazilian patients

TABLE 2. *Medications associated with AIN*

β-Lactam antibiotics
Methicillin*
Penicillin
Ampicillin
Flucloxacillin
Oxacillin
Nafcillin
Carbenicillin
Amoxicillin
Mezlocillin
Cephalothin
Cephalexin
Cephradine
Cephaloridine
Cefotaxime
Cefoxitin
Cefaclor
Other antimicrobials
Sulfonamides*
Trimethoprim-sulfamethoxazole*
Rifampin*
Polymixin
Tetracyclines
Vancomycin
Isoniazid
Chloramphenicol
Ethambutol
Minocycline
Erythromycin
Para-aminosalicyclic acid
Ciprofloxacin
Norfloxacin
Piromidic acid
Spiramycin
Nonsteroidal antiinflammatory agents
Ketoprofen*
Fenoprofen*
Indomethacin
Ibuprofen
Benoxaprofen
Phenazone
Mefanamic acid
Tolmetin
Diflunisol
Zomepirac
Piroxicam
Diclofenac
Surprofen
Diuretics
Thiazides
Furosemide
Ethacrynic acid
Chlorthalidone
Triamterene

TABLE 2. *(continued.)*

Other medications
Phenindione*
Glafenin*
Diphenylhydantoin*
Cimetidine*
Sulfinpyrazone*
Allopurinol*
Carbamazepine
Clofibrate
Azathioprine
Aspirin
Phenylpropanolamine
Aldomet
Phenobarbital
Leukocyte interferon A
Haldol
Coumadin
Tofranil
Diazepam
Valproic acid
Chlorprothixene
Captopril
Propanolol
Amphetamines
Doxepin
Quinine
Ranitidine

*Medication frequently associated with AIN

with Kala-azar due to visceral leishmaniasis showed 21 patients with renal failure to have AIN (32). Rare cases of AIN associated with *Toxoplasmosis gondii* infection have been reported (35). Of the viral lesions, most cases relate to EB virus and measles (36,37). In early reports of AIN, scarlet fever, diphtheria, and measles were commonly associated with AIN, while varicella, influenza, and polio were not. An immune complex glomerulonephritis has been noted in infectious mononucleosis, and an interstitial nephritis may accompany this or occur independently. How often this occurs is unknown but many cases may be subclinical. In 1–2% of cases of severe mononucleosis, acute renal insufficiency may occur (36,37). This has been associated with biopsy-documented AIN in several cases. Indeed, renal biopsies of patients with infectious mononucleosis without clinical renal findings have demonstrated the histologic findings of AIN. An acute inflammatory reaction typical of AIN has been found in up to one third of biopsied patients with Kawasaki's disease (38). In infection with human immunodeficiency virus, much attention has been focused on the glomerular lesion of collapsing focal sclerosis. Nevertheless, prominent tubulointerstitial infiltrates are very common in HIV nephropathy. It is unclear how they relate to glomerular lesions in pathogenesis and in terms of the progression to renal failure (39). Likewise, although a number of viral agents have been cultured from renal tissue during acute infections, it is unclear to what extent direct tissue damage as opposed to remote effects play a role in the pathogenesis of the renal disease. This is true for bacterial infections such as leptospirosis, mycobacterial infections, rickettsial infections, and infections due to many viruses including herpes viruses, CMV, hantavirus, polomavirus, and adenovirus.

AIN induced through different pathogenetic mechanisms has also been noted with a number of primary glomerulopathies and systemic diseases (2,6). AIN with anti-TBM antibodies along with glomerular damage induced by anti-GBM antibodies occurs in a number of glomerulonephritides, including Goodpasture's syndrome, membranous nephropathy, and familial nephritis. The AIN may be associated with immune complex deposits along the TBM in systemic lupus, membranoproliferative glomerulonephritis, and mixed cryoglobulinemia. In SLE interstitial damage may occur along with the glomerular involvement or, more rarely, as an isolated occurrence. AIN may also be a significant component of sarcoidosis and Sjogren's syndrome. Idiopathic AIN is defined by the occurrence of this pattern of renal damage in the absence of a clear etiologic inciting factor or associated disease (8,10,41). Thus, it requires a process of exclusion to rule out associated drug reactions, infections, or known systemic disease. Several distinct clinical and histopathologic patterns have been described that may have entirely different pathogenetic mechanisms.

PATHOGENESIS AND PATHOPHYSIOLOGY

Despite evidence for the involvement of a number of causal mechanisms, the pathogenesis of even the most common forms of AIN is complex remains to be defined (1,2,5,6). For example, why some medications produce this lesions far more frequently than do others of the same chemical class remains unclear. Although all agents of the b-lactam group can produce AIN, why is methicillin the number one offender (15)? It does not appear to relate to the extent of serum protein binding, to the route of excretion by renal tubular secretion, or to the presence of infection being treated by methicillin, as none of these features are unique to methicillin among the β-lactam antibiotics. Indeed, patients receiving methicillin prophylactically before open-heart surgery without active infection have developed this renal lesion (42). The rate of AIN cases has also been much higher with methicillin than with other penicillins or cephalosporins in the same setting. Likewise, it is unclear why an individual develops AIN at one specific time in response to a given drug they may have taken previously or for prolonged periods of time. Many patients have received NSAIDs for prolonged periods of time before they develop the adverse renal reaction of AIN (43,44). In medication-related AIN there is good clinical evidence for immune-mediated reactions (1,2,5,6). Only a small number of patients taking the drugs are afflicted, and the reaction is not dose-related. The presence of hypersensitivity features such as rash, fever, eosinophilia, and eosinophiluria point to an allergic-immune response (1—3,5,6). On histopathologic study, the nature of the cellular inflammatory infiltrates, as well as occasional cases with suggestive immunofluorescence or electron microscopic evidence of an immune reaction, support one of several immunologic mechanisms. Moreover, the recurrence shortly after rechallenge with the same or a similar drug also suggests an immune mechanisms (45–47).

Although there is no direct animal model of drug-induced AIN, many experimental models of tubulointerstitial nephritis suggest potential immunologic mechanisms of damage (see Chapter XXX) (1). As the kidney is usually the predominant organ involved in AIN, it is tempting to relate the initiation of AIN to the kidney's role as an excretory organ for many drugs (1,2,5,6,47). The initial step may occur through the binding of drug hapten to kidney structural protein, either tubular or interstitial. Most medications are small drugs capable of only a weak immunologic response. However, they may serve as haptens that can bind to other proteins and become immunogenic. Thus, in certain settings, filtered or secreted drugs become bound to kidney structural proteins. In the case of penicillin the benzyl-penicilloyl hapten and in the case of methicillin, the dimethoxyphenypenicilloyl hapten have been localized, bound to kidney structural proteins along the tubular basement membranes (16,47–50). This, by itself, is not adequate to produce AIN, as these haptens have been found bound to structural interstitial renal tissue of patients receiving these drugs without developing AIN (51). However, under given circumstances, and perhaps under certain genetic predisposition, the drug–protein conjugate may initiate one of several immune responses leading to full-blown AIN (1).

Subsequently, in some cases, a humoral response with development of anti-TBM antibodies to combined drug hapten and kidney protein may damage the kidney. Several patients with drug-induced AIN have had evidence of circulating anti-TBM antibodies (47,48,50,52,57). Sera from several patients with anti-TBM antibodies have reacted to a glycoprotein derived from collagen-solubilized human renal tissue. Others have had circulating antibodies that bound to proximal tubule brush border antigens (53). On immunofluorescence microscopy, a number of patients with AIN have had linear deposits of immunoglobulin or complement localized along the TBMs (16–18,42,46,47,54–57). Moreover, complement levels have at times been depressed in some patients with AIN (15,52).

IgE levels have been found to be increased in a number of patients with AIN (58,59). Interstitial inflammatory infiltrates have also at times been documented to reveal IgE containing plasma cells (60). The precise role of these antibody producing cells is unclear.

Nevertheless, the above evidence for a humoral response producing AIN is found in only a very small fraction of the patients. Majority have neither circulating anti-

TBM antibodies, depressed complement levels, nor evidence of immune deposits by immunofluorescence or electron microscopy. These findings, combined with the prominent cellular interstitial infiltrates with large numbers of lymphocytes and macrophages, have suggested a cell-mediated reaction (1,6). In several patients, a delayed hypersensitivity reaction to intradermal drug injection has been documented (16,48). Moreover, in AIN associated with NSAIDs, the presence of minimal change NS also suggests a cell-mediated lymphokine-directed reaction (23,43,44). Using monoclonal antibodies to analyze the interstitial inflammatory infiltrates in cases of AIN, a predominance of T lymphocytes over B lymphocytes has been noted (61–63). Among the T cell subsets, the ratio of cytotoxic-suppressor cell population to the helper-inducer T cell population has been variable (61–63). However, the percentage of each cell subtype has not been statistically different from that in patients with AIN due to β-lactam drugs (T4:T8 ratio 1). Thus, though a role for cell-mediated reactions is suggested by these data, the exact mechanisms of tissue injury remain to be defined. Eosinophils are found in the biopsies of many patients with AIN. They may be drawn into the inflammatory reaction by eosinophilic chemotactic factors and may contribute to the reaction by the release of proteases, leukotrienes, superoxide radicals, and peroxidases (1).

The etiology of the acute renal failure and reduction in the glomerular filtration rate in AIN is probably directly related to the inflammation of the interstitial compartment as the severity of the AIN often correlates with the severity and diffuse nature of the inflammatory infiltrates (64). Interstitial edema may cause elevated intratubular pressures, as can intratubular obstruction due to sloughed intraluminal cells. This may surpass the ultrafiltration pressure in the glomerular capillaries and cause the decrease in glomerular filtration rate (GFR). Whether components of tubular back-leak across damaged epithelium, renal vasoconstriction, or tubuloglomerular feedback play a role in this form of acute renal failure is unclear (64). The cellular inflammatory infiltrates also are likely to play a key role in the tubular dysfunction prominent in some cases of AIN. This may be due to direct structural damage from cellular infiltration and "tubulitis" or from release of mediators of inflammation from invading cells damaging normal tubular cell function.

PATHOLOGY

The typical pathologic feature of drug-related AIN on light microscopy consists of patchy to diffuse inflammatory interstitial infiltrates associated with edema and focal tubular damage (Fig. 1) (1,6,15,16). In general, glomerular and vascular compartments are spared. The infiltrate is usually focal in nature, involves the corticomedullary junction and cortex sparing the medulla, and is composed of lymphocytes, monocyte/macrophages, plasma cells, and a variable number of eosinophils (Fig. 2). Eosinophilic infiltrates can be entirely absent, although they typically compose from 2% to 10% of the infiltrating cells (17,59,65). In

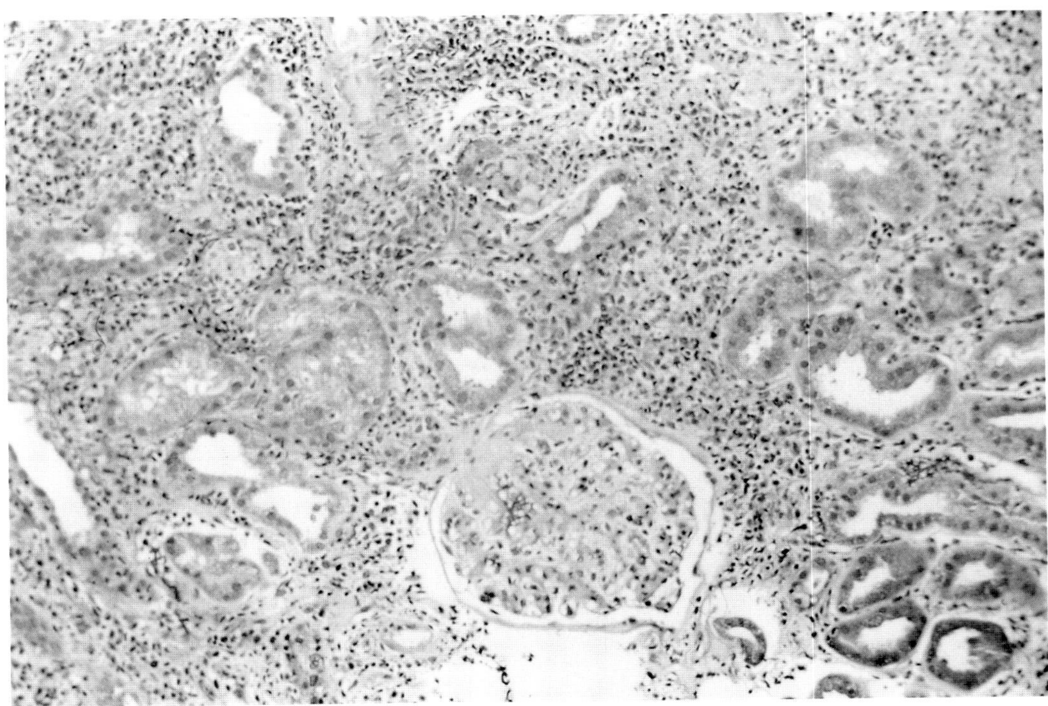

FIG. 1. Acute interstitial inflammatory infiltrate and edema separates tubules and glomeruli.

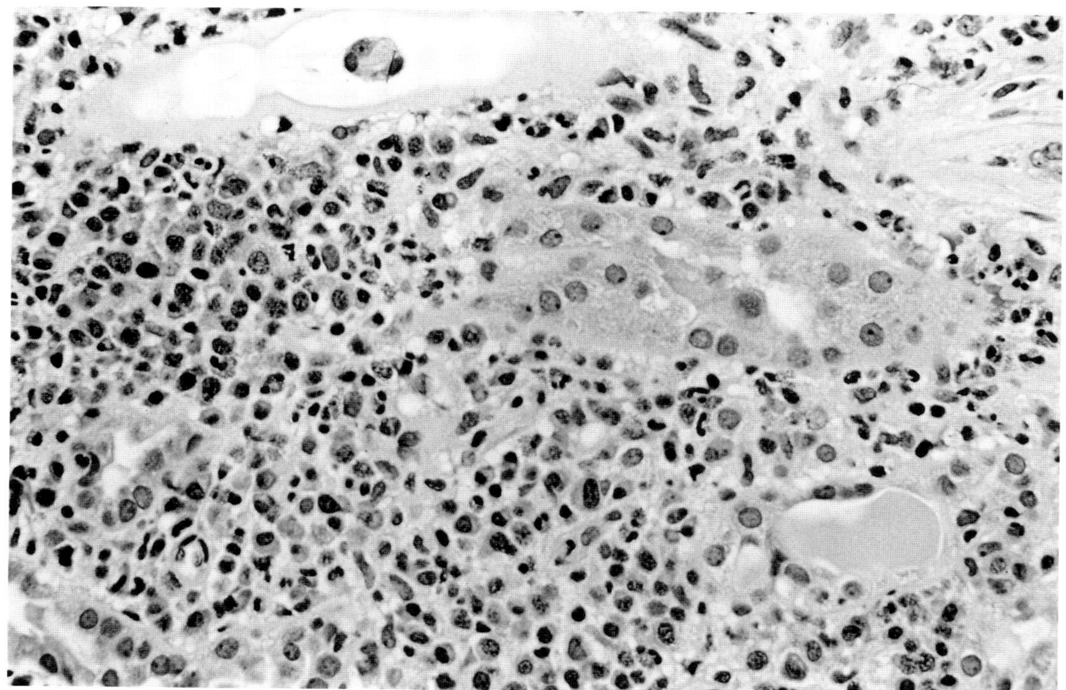

FIG. 2. Inflammatory infiltrate in acute interstitial nephritis composed of mononuclear cells, lymphocytes, and eosinophiles with prominent bilobed nuclei.

some cases, the macrophages have an epithelioid character and lead to true granuloma formation (Fig. 3) (55,66,67). A characteristic lesion of AIN is invasion of the tubules by lymphocytes and other cells—so-called tubulitis (Fig. 4) (59). This finding and the presence of focal tubular necrosis rather than extensive necrosis favors the diagnosis of interstitial nephritis over that of acute tubular necrosis. The distal nephron is involved by tubulitis more commonly than is the proximal nephron in most biopsied cases studied by lectin or immunohistochemical study.

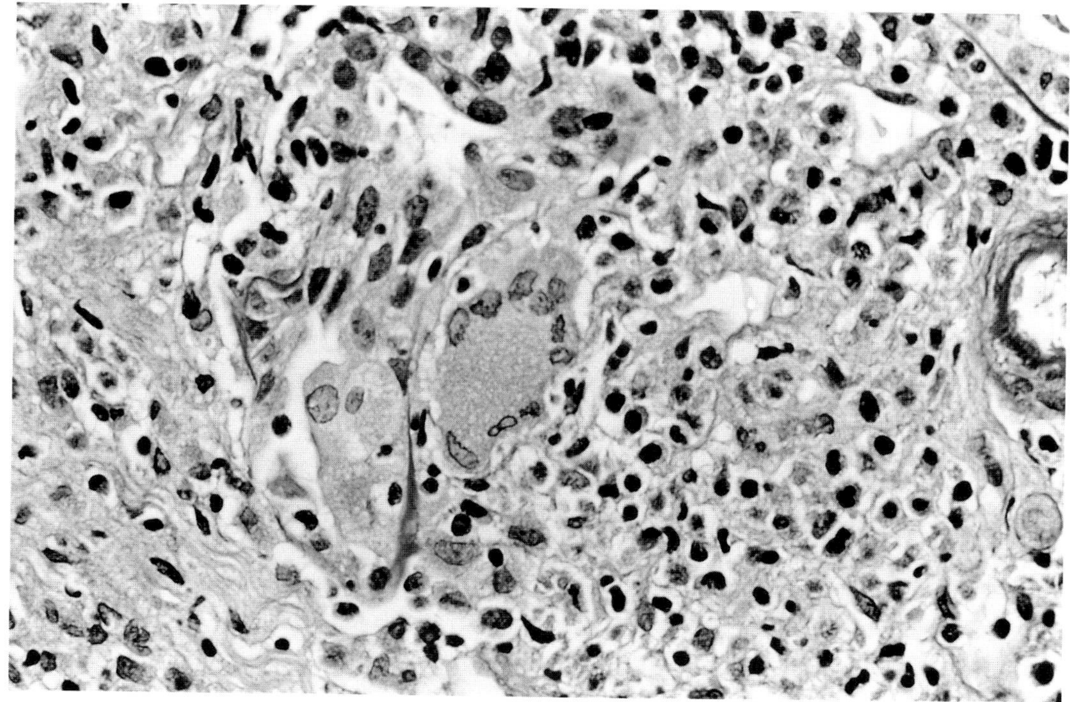

FIG. 3. Multinucleated giant cells in inflammatory infiltrate in drug-related AIN.

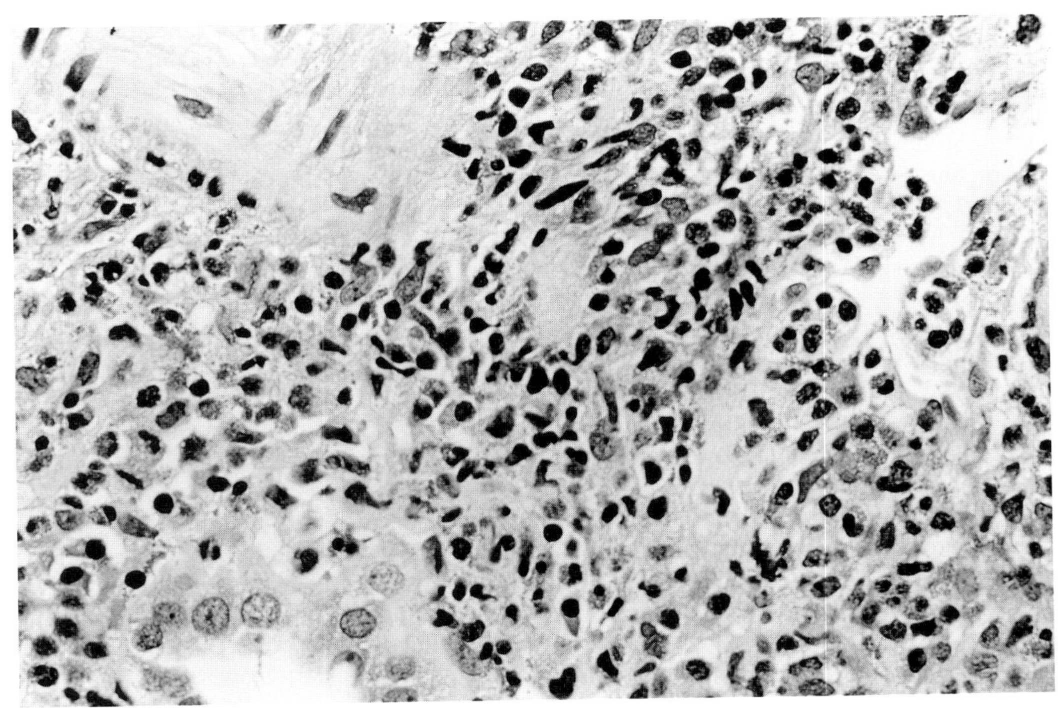

FIG. 4. Tubulitis with inflammatory cells infiltrating between the tubular cell lining the tubular basement membranes.

By immunofluorescence microscopy, in most cases, neither complement components nor immunoglobulins are found within the interstitium (15,16,55). In less than 20% of reported cases, linear staining along the tubular basement membranes has been noted (15,47). It is likely that this is an overestimate as such cases are more dramatic histopathologically and have a firmer diagnosis leading to greater reporting frequency. Likewise, occasional cases have had granular immunofluorescence for IgG along the TBMs. By electron microscopy, most of the changes are found to relate to tubular injury and infiltration by inflammatory cells (68). Only in rare cases have electron-dense deposits been found along the TBMs (54).

While NSAIDs may produce functional acute renal failure due to prostaglandin inhibition and several other patterns of renal injury, they can produce a unique pattern of AIN (see later) (23,24,43,44,). Here, the acute inflammatory infiltrate in most cases is characterized by fewer eosinophils and more plasma cells (44). The most striking clinical finding is the NS. In all but a few cases, the histopathology has been that of minimal change nephrotic syndrome, with normal glomeruli detected by light microscopy and immunofluorescence, and effacement of the foot processes found on electron microscopy (23,24,43,44). Only rare cases have been associated with either focal sclerosis or membranous nephropathy (69–71). In AIN associated with infections, the classic initial description of Councilman (7) is still accurate. There are interstitial edema and a focal cellular infiltrate composed of plasma cells, and lymphocytes with rare eosinophils or neutrophils. In certain infection-associated cases of AIN, such as secondary to Legionnaire disease, neutrophils may be more prominent (28,29). Tubulitis may also be present.

In AIN associated with systemic or glomerular disease, the pathology of the interstitium varies with the specific disease and the presumed pathogenesis (3,6). In all cases, a patchy interstitial inflammatory infiltrate is common. In patients with anti-TBM antibodies, bright linear immunofluorescence staining for IgG and, rarely, other immunoglubulins are found along the TBMs. C3 and other complement components are variably found. In diseases with immune complex damage such as SLE, the immunofluorescence may show granular deposits of immunoglobulin and complement along the TBMs, and electron microscopy often confirms the presence of electron-dense immune type deposits. Similar findings may be present in mixed cryoglobulinemia and in Sjogren's syndrome, although in the latter interstitial lymphocytic infiltration without immune deposits are more common. Finally, a granulomatous interstitial nephritis is found in up to 20% of patients with sarcoid at autopsy.

In the patients with idiopathic AIN with or without associated uveitis or bone marrow granulomata, the renal pathology usually shows inflammatory infiltrates of eosinophils, lymphocytes, and plasma cells (41). The percentage of each cell type is variable, and often proximal tubular cell damage predominates. Occasionally, renal granulomas have been noted on biopsy in these patients.

CLINICAL MANIFESTATIONS AND LABORATORY FINDINGS

Despite the many medications incriminated as causing AIN, the β-lactam antibiotics, the penicillins, and the cephalosporins remain among the foremost offenders. These drugs have been reported in the literature to cause several hundred cases of AIN, and the clinical features, laboratory findings, and course of the disease are well defined (15,16,18,52).

Penicillin-induced AIN occurs in all decades of life. Whereas occurence in men have predominated by a 3:1 ratio, this predominance likely reflects a higher percentage of mens treated with the antistaphylococcal drug methicillin rather than any true sex predilection (15). The dose of the β–lactam antibiotic has usually not been excessive; however, the duration of therapy is often prolonged, with over three-fourths of patients receiving over 10 days of therapy and over a third receiving greater than 20 days of therapy (15).

The clinical features of penicillin-associated AIN include the hypersensitivity triad of rash (30–50%), secondary fever (75–80%), and peripheral blood eosinophilia (80%) (16–18,58). However, less than a third of patients have the complete triad of rash, fever, and eosinophilia at the time renal function starts to decrease (15). The rash, maculopapular or morbilliform on the torso and extremities, is a classic drug eruption. Secondary fever spikes, after defervescence from the original febrile episode occurring with the infectious disease, often occur 2–3 weeks into the course of the antibiotic therapy. Less common features associated with AIN include loin pain, arthralgia, lymphadenopathy, and other systemic organ involvement, e.g., hepatitis.

Mild proteinuria and pyuria are common urinary findings. Nephrotic range proteinuria and red blood cell count cast are uncommon in this nonglomerular disease and can usually be explained by incidental concomitant glomerular pathology (1,2,5,72). With the exception of the NSAIDs, only rarely has glomerular pathology been attributed to the offending drug producing the AIN (73–75). Hematuria, a cardinal feature of penicillin-associated AIN, is present in over 90% of cases. Gross hematuria is found in up to one third of patients. Eosinophiles in the urinary sediment is a frequent and a helpful diagnostic finding (17). In one study, all nine patients with methicillin AIN had eosinophiluria noted by Wright stain, whereas none of 43 other patients with acute renal failure of diverse causes had this finding (17). Another study showed that 10 of 11 patients with AIN had eosinophiluria, as opposed to none of 30 patients with ATN, none of 10 with acute pyelonephritis, and only 1 of 15 with acute cystitis (76). The Hansel stain was positive in 10 of 11 cases of AIN versus a positive Wright stain in only two of eleven cases in this study. Although the exact sensitivity and specificity of eosinophiluria in diagnosing AIN remains unclear at present, a recent study suggests that eosinophiluria of over 5% of the total urinary leukocytes to be strongly suggestive of AIN (65). However, some degree of eosinophiluria has also been noted in up to 40% of patients with rapidly progressive glomerulonephritis and in an even higher percentage of patients with acute prostatitis (65). There is no good correlation between the degree of eosinophilia in the peripheral blood and the degree of eosinophiluria.

Radiographic and ultrasonographic examination of the kidneys in AIN typically shows them to be of normal size or enlarged (45,58). The urinary sodium and the fractional excretion of sodium have been elevated (>60 mEq/L and >1%) in a number of studies but have been reported to be reduced in others (77). Gallium scanning has been suggested as a screening test to distinguish drug-induced AIN from renal failure due to acute tubular necrosis (58). In one study, all 11 patients with drug-related AIN had intense diffuse bilateral uptake of the gallium nuclide. This was found in less than 10% of patients with a variety of other renal disorders and in no patient with ATN (58). However, the value of this test is unclear as positive reports have been noted in acute bacterial pyelonephritis, acute glomerulonephritis, and even in several patients with minimal change NS (58,78–80).

A number of other classes of medications other than the β–lactam antibiotics may produce AIN with either typical or atypical features. Sulfonamides, although long known to produce acute renal failure through intratubular crystallization and obstruction, can clearly cause classic AIN with the full hypersensitivity triad (2,4–6,15). The widely used antimicrobial combination of trimethoprim-sulfamethoxazole can also produce this form of renal damage. Rifampin (Rifadin, Rifamate, Rifater, Rimactane) may be associated with a unique pattern of AIN (81–83). In over 60 patients receiving either intermittent (2–3 times per week) or discontinuous therapy, on rechallenge with rifampin there is the sudden onset of fever, flank pain, hematuria, and acute renal failure. Rifampin-related AIN may also be associated with myalgia, hemolysis, and thrombocytopenia. Histopathology ranges from classic AIN to a picture indistinguishable from acute tubular necrosis. It is clearly wise to avoid the intermittent or discontinuous use of this drug. Recently, two new unusual features in a case of rifampin-related AIN have been noted—its occurrence during continuous therapy and the presence of nephrotic range proteinuria. This case is the exception, however, rather than the typical case (73).

A number of other antimicrobials producing AIN infrequently or in a less well documented fashion is listed in Table 1. Several recent reports of AIN associated with use of the quinolone antibiotics have been reported (84,85). It is unclear whether these cases with ciprofloxacin, norfloxacin, etc. are just sporadic or are the harbinger of many cases to come as these drugs are used more widely.

Diuretics, including the thiazides and chlorthalidone (Combipres, Tenoretic, Thalitone, Atenolol, Clonidine, Hygroton, Regroton, Demi-Regroton), furosemide, ethacrynic acid (Endecrin), and ticrynafen have all been well documented to cause AIN (86). However, this is a rare occurrence, reported in less than 30 cases, despite the millions of courses of diuretics used. When diuretic-induced renal dysfunction is associated with true AIN, it often has occurred in patients with prior renal disease (the NS, hypertension), and patients have presented with the classic hypersensitivity features of rash, fever, and eosinophilia.

The NSAIDs may produce salt and water retention, decreased renal blood flow and GFR, and hyperkalemia associated with hyporenin hypoaldosteronism, all perhaps due to inhibition of prostaglandins (23,44). They also can cause AIN with a number of unique features (23,24,43,44). The population developing AIN is usually in the older age group (50s to 80s), despite many young patients receiving these drugs. Patients typically have a prolonged exposure to the drugs (months to years) before developing AIN (44). The hypersensitivity features of rash, fever, and eosinophilia are uncommon, as are hematuria and eosinophiluria (23). This is true even when AIN with interstitial eosinophilia is found on renal biopsy. Finally, AIN caused by the NSAIDs has frequently been associated with minimal change NS. The drug-induced nature of this lesion is clear: minimal change is reported in all but a few cases, despite the fact that this pattern comprises less than 20% of idiopathic nephrotic syndrome in the adult age group (24,43). The onset of the NS coincides with the onset of the acute renal failure from AIN. The NS and AIN usually remit together several weeks after discontinuing the NSAIDs, regardless of whether steroid therapy is given. In isolated cases, nonsteroidal agents have been associated with the NS due to focal sclerosis and membranous nephropathy (9,70,71).

Two drugs not used in the US, the analgesic glafenin and the anticoagulant phenindione, have been associated with numerous cases of well-documented AIN (25). Anticonvulsants of a number of different chemical structures, including diphenylhydantoin, phenobarbital (Arco-Lase, Bellatal, Bellergal-S, Donnatal, Quadrinal, Mudrane, Rexatal, Solfoton), and carbamazepine (Atretol, Tegretol) have all been associated with renal failure related to AIN. Some patients have had, in addition to the classic hypersensitivity triad, lymphadenopathy and evidence of glomerular damage or vasculitis. Likewise, allopurinol may produce AIN in association with glomerular damage and vasculitis (88). The widely used drug cimetidine has caused this pattern of renal failure, as has the uricosuric, antiplatelet agent sulfinpyrazone. Several recent reports deal with ranitidine (Zantac)-induced AIN. Again, it is unclear whether these are isolated cases or early reports of an increasing number of such cases. The pattern is again that of classic AIN. Regardless of the offending medication and clinical presentation, the majority of patients have nonoliguric renal failure and never have less than 400 cc of urine volume per day (15). Renal failure leading to dialysis occurs in up to 25% of patients. The renal failure typically initially improves rapidly over days to weeks, with cessation of drug treatment or immunosuppressive therapy. There is then more gradual further improvement over a longer period of time.

While acute nonoliguric renal failure is the most common finding in drug-related AIN, several other clinical and laboratory features may occasionally dominate a given patient's presentation. Tubular dysfunction may be noted by prominent hyperkalemia, hyperchloremic metabolic nonaninon gap acidosis; and, occasionally, findings of proximal tubular dysfunction such as bicarbonaturia, hypophosphatemia, hypouricemia, glycosuria, and aminoaciduria (5,49,89,90). Rare patients have had prominent hypokalemia and hypomagnesemia due to renal tubular wasting of these ions (91).

The most common clinical manifestation of interstitial nephritis associated with infection is progressive renal insufficiency. The renal failure may be oliguric or nonoliguric and typically remits as the infection is adequately treated.

Idiopathic AIN has been reported most frequently in adolescent females, although it may occur in both sexes at any age (8,10,41,92). Some patients may present with renal failure without any hypersensitivity features. Some have isolated eosinophilia with the renal dysfunction and others have fever, weight loss, and uveitis-iritis occurring before or during the episode of renal failure. Other clinical findings in individual cases include hypergammaglobulinemia, positive tests for rheumatoid factor, elevated sedimentation rates, and tubular defects leading to glycosuria and aminoaciduria. Granulomatous lesions have been found in the bone marrow of some of these patients. The renal failure is typically nonoliguric and may remit spontaneously, especially in young females. In adults, the disease is more likely to be progressive without treatment.

DIFFERENTIAL DIAGNOSIS

A renal biopsy is required to establish the diagnosis of AIN. In the absence of a biopsy, many renal diseases with similar presentations of either acute renal failure or of tubular defects may be mistaken for AIN. As the list of medications associated with AIN has grown, many patients developing acute renal failure of the acute tubular necrosis type will be on drugs that could potentially produce AIN. The findings of rash, fever, and eosinophilia are helpful in leading to a correct diagnosis of AIN. Likewise, microscopic hematuria on urinalysis or gross hematuria are both typical in AIN but uncommon in ATN, where the urinary sediment usually reveals granular or tubular epithelial cell casts. The presence of urinary eosinophilia is perhaps the best clinical differential finding. In several series of patients, almost all with AIN had urinary eosinophilia, whereas no patient with ATN had this urinary finding (17). Urinary eosinophiluria may not correlate with the degree of pyuria or peripheral blood eosinophilia. In those patients, however, with greater than 5% eosinophiluria, the diagnosis is most often AIN (65).

Other diseases with prominent acute renal failure may mimic AIN. Idiopathic rapidly progressive glomerulonephritis, polyarteritis nodosa, and other systemic vasculitides may be associated with acute renal failure, fever, rash, and urinary eosinophilia. The urinary sediment in these patients is typically that of an active glomerulonephritis with not only erythrocytes but erythrocyte casts as well. Many of these patients will be seropositive for antineutrophil cytoplasmic antibodies helping to establish the diagnosis. Proteinuria is also usually lower in patients with AIN than in those with vasculitis and glomerular lesions.

Patients with cholesterol emboli may present with progressive renal failure, fever, petechial rash, and eosinophilia (93) . A history or clinical findings of atherosclerotic disease or vascular or angiographic procedures is helpful. Fundoscopic examination to check for cholesterol emboli in retinal vessels (Hollenhorst plaques) or biopsy of involved skin may also establish the diagnosis. In all of the above disorders, any tubular dysfunction is secondary to the glomerular damage or to the acute change in glomerular filtration rate. In AIN, a hyperchloremic metabolic acidosis may be present early in the course of the disease, as may other tubular defects.

Patients on diuretics often experience a decrease in GFR with volume contraction. In the absence of rash, fever, and eosinophilia, this form of renal dysfunction is far more common than is AIN. In patients taking nonsteroidal agents, acute renal failure due to prostaglandin inhibition is usually not associated with urinary sediment changes or with the hypersensitivity triad of rash, fever, and eosinophilia. It also is not associated with heavy proteinuria seen so commonly in patients with nonsteroidal-associated AIN with minimal change NS.

Some patients with clinical or laboratory features suggestive of AIN are too ill to undergo renal biopsy to establish the diagnosis. In many such patients, the potential offending medications are merely withdrawn. If resolution of the renal dysfunction occurs, a presumptive diagnosis of AIN is made. Although recurrence with rechallenge with the drug would solidify the diagnosis, this is obviously neither ethical nor clinically prudent. In a similar fashion, in some patients with milder renal dysfunction with suggestive clinical features of AIN, it is easier and safer to discontinue all potentially offending medications and to follow the course of the patient. Resolution of the clinical and laboratory findings are taken as presumptive evidence of AIN.

TREATMENT

The treatment of AIN consists of three areas of intervention: (a) correction of the inciting event when possible; (b) provision of supportive care during the phase of acute renal dysfunction; and (c) use of corticosteroids and other immunosuppression in select patients (1,2,5,94). In cases of suspected or documented medication-induced AIN, the offending medication should be withdrawn. Congeners and cross-reacting medications of similar structure or class should be avoided.

Exacerbations of β-lactam-related AIN have been documented when patients with methicillin AIN were rechallenged with either nafcillin or cephalothin (45,46,52). In the case of NSAIDs, all drugs of this group, regardless of differences in chemical structure, must be avoided. In most cases of medication-related AIN, there will be reversal of the acute renal dysfunction with cessation of use of the offending drugs. In patients with nonsteroidal AIN associated with the NS, patients typically experience remission of both the renal failure and their heavy proteinuria. In some critically ill patients in which it is unclear which drug is the offending medication, it may be necessary to withdraw or substitute several medications simultaneously to be certain the offending agent is removed.

In patients with AIN associated with systemic infections, treatment of the underlying infection usually results in resolution of the AIN. Indeed, the declining incidence of this form of AIN in the modern era has been ascribed to the widespread use of antibiotics. In patients with idiopathic AIN, the inciting agent is, by definition, unknown, and therapy is directed at supportive care and immunosuppressive therapy. Supportive care in patients with AIN includes management of electrolyte balance, acid-base status, and volume regulation as in all patients with acute renal failure. Because many patients with AIN have nonoliguric acute renal failure, management of the renal failure may be easier than in patients with classic oliguric ischemic ATN. Dialysis should be instituted before the appearance of uremic complications. In oliguric patients, this is generally when the blood urea nitrogen (BUN) approaches 100 mg/dL or the plasma creatinine reaches 8–10 mg/dL; in clinically stable patients without oliguria, dialysis may often be delayed longer, awaiting return of renal function. Most patients recover enough function to discontinue dialysis after several weeks of supportive care (15,95). However, isolated patients have required several months of dialytic support before recovery of renal function.

Most therapeutic trials of immunosuppressive therapy in AIN have used corticosteroids (1,2,94). The goals of such therapy have been twofold: to promote more rapid recovery from the initial renal failure and to prevent or ameliorate chronic residual structural and functional damage to the kidney. Both isolated case reports and uncontrolled series on the use of corticosteroids to treat medication-related AIN have reported dramatic improvements in renal function coincident with the use of the steroids. Likewise, some retrospective series of patients have shown improved GFR and less damage on repeat renal biopsy in corticosteroid-treated patients (10,95). There are, however, no randomized controlled trials in medication-related AIN to document the value of corticosteroids, either in reversing the renal failure or in preventing chronic residual renal damage.

A study of patients with methicillin-related AIN and severe renal failure compared a 10-day course of high-dose prednisone (Deltasone, Prednicen, Sterapred) (average daily dose 60 mg/day) in eight patients to no steroid therapy in a comparable group of patients (17). The group treated with corticosteroids fared better with a lower mean final serum creatinine (1.4 mg/dL vs. 1.9 mg/dL), a shorter duration of acute renal failure, and a greater percentage of patients (75% vs. 33%) whose renal function returned to premethicillin baseline.

This study was, however, not randomized nor blinded in any fashion. A second uncontrolled therapeutic trial in medication-related AIN treated seven patients with severe acute renal failure (six of seven required dialysis) with high-dose daily intravenous prednisolone ((Prelone) (500–1,000 mg) for several days (46). A diuresis and fall in serum creatinine occurred within 72 hours in each patient.

Another study retrospectively reviewed the effect of high-dose daily prednisone (40–80 mg daily for 4–6 weeks) versus no corticosteroid therapy in patients with medication-related AIN due to a variety of drugs (10). There was no difference in the duration of acute renal failure requiring supportive therapy. However, the prednisone-treated group had a statistically lower serum creatinine at 8 weeks than did the untreated group. Several retrospective studies have shown that patients treated with steroids have a more rapid decline in the serum creatinine and improved GFR at long-term follow-up 9–30 months later than did comparable groups of patients who did not receive steroid treatment (10,95).

In patients with documented AIN, our approach is to use steroids for those patients with rapidly progressive renal dysfunction, more diffuse lesions on renal biopsy, and with those approaching dialysis (94). We have chosen not expose those patients with mild dysfunction in whom the GFR appears to improve with only discontinuation of the offending drug to the risks of steroid therapy. We have used a number of regimens successfully, including: prednisone at 60 mg daily for 4–6 weeks, alternate-day prednisone (120 mg every other day) for a similar time period, or 1–3 pulses of IV methylprednisolone (500–1,000 mg), followed by prednisone daily or every other day. Steroid therapy has also been used successfully to treat both the acute renal failure and minimal change NS seen with the use of NSAIDs. Some cases with severe prolonged acute renal failure have experienced dramatic improvement after institution of corticosteroids. It is still unclear, however, what percent of patients require steroid treatment as most patients experience a spontaneous recovery from both the NS and the acute renal failure after the nonsteroidal agent is discontinued.

From these studies there is suggestive, but hardly conclusive, data that in some cases the short-term use of corticosteroids can hasten the recovery of acute renal failure and that this treatment may lead to improved residual renal function. The risk of therapy with any immunosuppressive drug must be weighed carefully against the potential benefits of such therapy. Because most patients with medication-related AIN recover function by merely discontinuing the offending medications, it is often judicious to reserve corticosteroids for those patients with severe acute renal failure requiring dialysis who do not appear to be improving despite discontinuation of the offending drugs. Oral or intravenous cyclophosphamide (Cytoxan, NEOSAR), cyclosporine (Neoral, Sandimmune), and other immunosuppressive drugs have been used only in isolated anecdotal cases of medication-related AIN. They should still be regarded as experimental and reserved for only refractory patients in whom other therapy has failed and the benefits of these potentially hazardous treatments appear to outweigh the risks of therapy.

Most patients with AIN associated with remote infections recover renal function with treatment of their underlying systemic infectious disease. The risks of exacerbating the basic infection with immunosuppressives must be weighed against any benefits of corticosteroid therapy. On the other hand, many cases of idiopathic AIN have been treated successfully with corticosteroids. Adolescent females often have spontaneous remissions of their renal dysfunction, whereas adults often require corticosteroid therapy for improvement. Although there are no controlled studies, a short trial of pulse steroids or high-dose corticosteroids is reasonable in progressive cases as there is no inciting medication to discontinue or infection to treat.

PROGNOSIS

Medication-related AIN is usually a self-limited disease, once the offending drug has been discontinued. Almost all patients recover from the acute renal failure and are able to discontinue dialytic support. Of the 17% of patients who required dialytic support in a review of 156 courses of b-lactam-induced AIN, there were only four deaths as a result of renal failure (15). As in many other forms of acute renal failure, the time to recovery of renal function is variable, ranging from days to several months. Prolonged dialytic support does not preclude major recovery of renal function. Several studies have reviewed factors predictive of a poor prognosis for recovery of the acute renal failure in medication-related AIN (10,95). These include severity of the initial acute renal failure (i.e., persistent acute renal failure), more diffuse histologic damage, and the presence of granulomatous interstitial damage on renal biopsy. Long-term residual renal dysfunction is more likely in patients with lack of early rapid improvement of their GFR, in the elderly, and in patients with more severe and diffuse histologic damage (10,18,95). In patients with AIN related to the use of NSAIDs, most will have a remission of both the acute renal failure and the NS within several weeks of discontinuing the drug (43). Some patients have had persistent renal failure or nephrotic range proteinuria for many months (43). In contrast to idiopathic minimal change NS in adults, relapses of NSAID-related NS are extremely rare. Other unusual occurrences include the progression to end-stage renal disease and the appearance of focal segmental glomerulosclerosis on repeat biopsy in rare cases.

Repeat biopsies in patients with medication-related AIN often show interstitial fibrosis and some glomerulosclerosis, despite apparent good recovery of renal function, as measured by the serum creatinine. It is likely that many of these patients have suffered an irreversible loss of functional renal tissue or renal "reserve" (10,95). In some studies, greater long-term histologic damage has been documented on renal biopsy in certain patients, including older patients, those with more severe initial renal failure, those with a slower recovery of renal function, those with greater histologic damage on initial biopsy, and those not treated with corticosteroids (10,18,95). The long-term significance of this loss of functional tissue and GFR has not yet been determined in terms of morbidity or ultimate progression to end-stage renal disease.

The renal prognosis of patients with AIN associated with systemic infections is good, as long as the patient recovers from the infectious process. Residual renal dysfunction rarely requires dialysis or supportive measures. Children with idiopathic AIN typically experience complete recovery of renal function, either spontaneously or with steroid therapy. This is especially true of those with the syndrome of AIN associated with uveitis. Repeat biopsies have often shown total resolution of the inflammatory infiltrates, and only rarely is there significant residual fibrosis. It is unclear whether adults fare as well and whether corticosteroid therapy is necessary for good recovery of long-term function in this population.

REFERENCES

1. Neilson EG. Pathogenesis and therapy of interstitial nephritis. *Kidney Int* 1989;35:1257–1270.
2. Appel GB. Acute interstitial nephritis. In: HR Jacobson, GE Striker, S Klahr, eds. *The Principles and Practice of Nephrology*. Philadelphia: BC Decker, Inc., 1991;356–368.
3. Andres GA, McCluskey RT. Tubular and interstitial renal disease due to immunologic mechanisms. *Kidney Int* 1975;7:271–289.
4. Ten RM, Torres VE, Milliner DS, et al. Acute interstitial nephritis: immunologic and clinical aspects. *Mayo Clin Proc* 1988;63:921.
5. Cameron JS. Allergic interstitial nephritis: clinical features and pathogenesis. *Q J Med* 1988;66:97.
6. Colvin RB, Fang LST. Interstitial nephritis. In: CC Tisher, BM Brenner, eds. *Renal Pathology*. New York: JB Lippincott, 1994;723–768.
7. Councilman WT. Acute interstitial nephritis. *J Exp Med* 1898;3: 393–420.
8. Chazan JA. Garella S, Esparza A. Acute interstitial nephritis: a distinct clinicopathologic entity. *Nephron* 1972;9:10–26.
9. Pettersson E, von Bonsdorff M, Tornroth T, Lindholm H. Nephritis among young Finnish men. *Clin Nephrol* 1984;22:217–222.
10. Laberke HG, Bohle A. Acute interstitial nephritis: correlations between clinical and morphological findings. *Clin Nephrol* 1980;14: 263–273.
11. Zollinger HU, Mihatsch MJ. Renal pathology. In: *Biopsy*, vol 1. Berlin: Springer-Verlag, 1978;407–410.
12. Richet G, Sraer JD, Kourilsky O, Kanfer A, Mignon F, Whitworth J, Morel-Maroger L. La ponction biopsie renale dans les insuffisances renales aigues. *Ann Med Int* 1978;129:445–447.
13. Wilson DB, Turner DR, Cameron JS, Ogg CS, Brown CB, Chantler C. Value of renal biopsy in acute intrinsic renal failure. *Br Med J* 1976;2:459–461.
14. Farrington K, Levison DA, Greenwood RN, Cattell WR, Baker LR. Renal biopsy in patients with unexplained renal impairment and normal kidney size. *Q J Med* 1989;70:221–233.
15. Appel GB, Neu HC. Acute interstitial nephritis due to beta lactam antibiotics. In: Fillastre JP, Whelton A, Tulkens P, eds. *Antibiotic Nephrotoxicity*. France: INSERM, 1982.
16. Baldwin DS, Levine BB, McCluskey RT, Gallo GR. Renal failure and interstitial nephritis due to penicillin and methicillin. *N Engl J Med* 1968;279:1245–1252.
17. Galpin JE, Shinaberger JH, Stanley TM, et al. Acute interstitial nephritis due to methicillin. *Am J Med* 1978;65:756–765.
18. Ditlove J, Weidman P, Sernstien M, Massry SG. Methicillin nephritis. *Medicine* 1977;56:483–491.
19. Revert L, Montoliu J. Acute interstitial nephritis. *Semin Nephrol* 1988;8:82–88.
20. Deray G, Martinez F, Katlma C, et al. Foscarnet nephrotoxicity: mechanisms, incidence, and prevention. *Am J Nephrol* 1989;9:316.
21. Cacoub P, Deray G, Baumalou A. Acute renal failure induced by foscarnet: four cases. *Clin Nephrol* 1988;29:315.
22. Sawyer MH, Webb DE, Balow J, Strauss SE. Acyclovir induced renal failure: clinical course and renal histology. *Am J Med* 1988;84:1067.
23. Clive DM, Stoff JS. Renal syndromes associated with nonsteroidal antiinflammatory drugs. *N Engl J Med* 1984;310:563–572.
24. Abraham PA, Keane WF. Glomerular and interstitial disease induced by nonsteroidal anti-inflammatory drugs. *Am J Nephrol* 1984;4:1–6.
25. Ellis D, Fried WA, Yunis EJ, Blau EB. Acute interstitial nephritis in children: A report of 13 cases and review of the literature. *Pediatrics* 1981;67:862–870.
26. Dunea G, Kark RM, Lannigan R, Dalessio D, Muehrcke RC. Brucella nephritis. *Ann Int Med* 1969;70:783–790.
27. Fattah HA, Khuffash FA. Reversible renal failure in a child with Brucellosis. *Ann Trop Paediatr* 1984;4:247–250.
28. Poulter N, Gabriel R, Porter GA, Bartlett CC, Kershaw M, McKendrick GD, Venkataraman R. Acute interstitial nephritis complicating Legionnaire's disease. *Clin Nephrol* 1981;15:216–220.
29. Shah A, Check F, Baskin S, Reyman T, Manard R. Legionnaire's disease and acute renal failure: case report and review. *Clin Infect Dis* 1992;14:204–207.
30. Iijima K, Yoshikawa N, Sato K, Matsuo T. Acute interstitial nephritis associated with *Yersinia pseudotuberculosis* infection. *Am J Nephrol* 1989;9:236–240.
31. Okada K, Yano I, Kagami S, Funai M, Kawahito S, Okamoto T, Imagawa A, Kuroda Y. Acute tubulointerstitial nephritis associated with *Yersinia pseudotuberculosis* infection. *Clin Nephrol* 1991;35: 105–109.
32. Pasternack A, Helin H, Vantinnen T, Jarventie G, Vesikari T. Acute tubulointerstitial nephritis in a patient with *Mycoplasma pneumoniae* infection. *Scand J Infect* 1979;11:85–87.
33. Duarte MI, Silva MR, Goto H, Nicodemo EL, Amato NV. Interstitial

nephritis in human kala azar. *Trans R Soc Trop Med Hyg* 1983;77: 531–537.
34. Carvaca F, Munoz A, Pizarro JL, de Saantamaria AJ, Fernandez-Alonso J. Acute renal failure in visceral leishmaniasis. *Am J Nephrol* 1991;11:350–352.
35. Guignard JP, Torrado A. Interstitial nephritis and toxoplasmosis in a 10-year-old child. *J Peds* 1974;84:381–382.
36. Woodroffe AJ, Row PA, Meadows R, Lawrence JR. Nephritis is infectious mononucleosis. *Q J Med* 1974;43:451–460.
37. Kopolovic J, Pinkus G, Rosen S. Interstitial nephritis in infectious mononucleosis. *Am J Kidney Dis* 1988;12:76–77.
38. Amano S, Hazama F, Kubagawa H, Tasaka K, Haebara H, Hamashima Y. General pathology of Kawasaki's disease. *Acta Pathol Jpn* 1980;30:681–694.
39. D'Agati V, Suh JI, Carbone L, Appel GB. Pathology of HIV nephropathy: a detailed morphologic and comparative study. *Kidney Int* 1989;35:1358–1370.
40. Spital A, Panner BJ, Sterns RH. Acute idiopathic tubulointerstitial nephritis: report of two cases and review of the literature. *Am J Kidney Dis* 1987;9:71–78.
41. Appel GB, Kunis CL. Acute tubulointerstitial nephritis. In: RS Cotran, BM Brenner, JH Stein, eds. *Contemporary Issues in Nephrology*, vol 10. New York: Churchill Livingstone, 1983;151–187.
42. Olsen S, Asklund M. Interstitial nephritis with acute renal failure following cardiac surgery and treatment with methicillin. *Acta Med Scand* 1976;199:305–310.
43. Feinfeld DA, Olesnicky L, Pirani CL, Appel GB. Nephrotic syndrome associated with use of the nonsteroidal anti-inflammatory drug. *Nephron* 1984;37:174–179.
44. Pirani CL, Valeri A, D'Agati V, Appel GB. Renal toxicity of nonsteroidal anti-inflammatory drugs. *Contrib Nephrol* 1987;35:159–175.
45. Saltessi D, Pussey CD, Rainford DJ. Recurrent acute renal failure due to antibiotic induced interstitial nephritis. *Br Med J* 1979;1:1182–1183.
46. Pussey CD, Saltissi D, Bloodworth L, et al. Drug associated acute interstitial nephritis: clinical and pathological features and the response to high dose steroid therapy. *Q J Med* 1983;52:194–211.
47. Sanjad SA, Haddad GG, Nassar VH, Nephropathy an underestimated complication of methicillin therapy. *J Peds* 1974;84:873–877.
48. Kleinknecht D, Kanfer A, Morel-Maroger L, Mery JP. Immunologically mediated drug induced acute renal failure. *Contrib Nephrol* 1978;10:42–52.
48. Border WA, Lehman DH, Egan JD, Sass HJ, Glode JE, Wilson CD. Anti-tubular basement membrane antibodies in methicillin associated interstitial nephritis. *N Engl J Med* 1974;291:381–384.
49. Cogan MC, Arieff AI. Sodium wasting, acidosis, and hyperkalemia induced by methicillin interstitial nephritis. *Am J Med* 1978;64: 500–507.
50. Silverstien RL, Eigenbrodt EH, McPhaul JJ Jr. Interstitial nephritis caused by methicillin. *Am J Clin Pathol* 1980;76:316–321.
51. Colvin RB, Burton JR, Hyslop NE, Spitz L, Lichtenstein NS. Penicillin associated interstitial nephritis. *Ann Int Med* 1974;81:404.
52. Nolan CM, Abernathy RS. Nephropathy associated with methicillin therapy. *Arch Int Med* 1977;137:997–1000.
53. Clayman MD, Michaud L, Brentjens J, et al. Isolation of the target antigen of human anti-TBM associated interstitial nephritis. *J Clin Invest* 1986;77:1143–1147.
54. Appel GB, Garvey G, Silva F, Francke E, Neu C. Neu HC, Weissman J. Acute interstitial nephritis due to amoxicillin therapy. *Nephron* 1981;27:313–315.
55. Mignon F, Mery JP, Mougenot B, Ronco P, Roland J, Morel-Maroger L. Granulomatous interstitial nephritis. *Adv Nephrol* 1984;13: 219–245.
56. Milman N. Acute interstitial nephritis during treatment with penicillin and cephalothin. *Acta Med Scand* 1978;203:227–230.
57. Lehman DH, Wilson CB, Dixon FJ. Extraglomerular immunoglobulin deposits in human nephritis. *Am J Med* 1975;58:765–796.
58. Linton AL, Clark WF, Driedger AA, et al. Acute interstitial nephritis due to drugs. *Ann Int Med* 1980;93:735–741.
59. Ooi BS, Jao W, First MR, Mancilla R, Pollak VE. Acute interstitial nephritis: a clinical and pathological study based on renal biopsies. *Am J Med* 1975;59:614–628.
60. Farrup P, Christensen E. IgE containing plasma cells in acute interstitial nephropathy. *Lancet* 1974;2:718.
61. Boucher A, Droz D, Adafer E, Noel L-H. Characterization of mononuclear cell subsets in renal cellular interstitial infiltrates. *Kidney Int* 1986;29:1043–1049.
62. Bender WL, Whelton N, Beschorner WE, Darwish MD, Hall-Craggs M, Solez K. Interstitial nephritis, proteinuria and renal failure caused by nonsteroidal anti-inflammatory drugs. *Am J Med* 1984;76:1006–1012.
63. D'Agati VD, Theise, ND, Pirani CL, Knowles DM, Appel GB. Interstitial nephritis related to nonsteroidal anti-inflammatory agents and beta-lactam antibiotics. A comparative study of the interstitial infiltrates using monoclonal antibodies. *Mod Pathol* 1989;2: 390–396.
64. Fried T. Acute interstitial nephritis: Why do the kidneys fail? *Postgrad Med* 1993;93:105–120.
65. Corwin HL, Korbet SM, Schwartz MM. Clinical correlates of eosinophiluria. *Arch Int Med* 1985;145:1099.
66. Vanhille P, Kleinknecht D, Morel-Maroger L, Kanfer A, Lemaitre V, Mery JP, Callard P, Dracon M, Leaderich J. Drug induced granulomatous interstitial nephritis. *Proc Eur Dial Transplant Assoc* 1983;20:646–649.
67. Schwarz A, Krause PH, Keller F, Offermann G, Mihatsch MJ. Granulomatous interstitial nephritis after nonsteroidal anti-inflammatory drugs. *Am J Nephrol* 1988;8:410–416.
68. Olsen TS, Wassef NF, Olsen HS, Hansen HE. Ultrastructure of the kidney in acute interstitial nephritis. *Ultrastruct Pathol* 1986;10: 1–16.
69. Campistol JM, Galfre J, Botey A, et al. Reversible membranous nephritis associated with diclofenac. *Nephrol Dial Transplant* 1989; 4:393.
70. Tattersall J, Greenwood R, Farrington K. Membranous nephropathy associated with diclofenac [letter]. *Postgrad Med* 1989;68:392.
71. Radford MG Jr, Holley KE, Grande JP, et al. Membranous glomerulopathy associated with the use of nonsteroidal antiinflammatory drugs [abst]. *J Am Soc Nephrol* 1994;5:359.
72. Siegala JF, Biava CG, Hulter HN. Red blood cell casts in acute interstitial nephritis. *Arch Int Med* 1988;138:1419–1421.
73. Neugarten J, Gallo GR, Baldwin DS. Rifampin induced nephrotic syndrome and acute interstitial nephritis. *Am J Nephrol* 1983;3:38.
74. Averbach SD, Austin HA, Sherwin SA, et al. Acute interstitial nephritis with the nephrotic syndrome following recombinant leukocyte A interferon therapy for mycosis fungoides. *N Engl J Med* 1984; 310:32.
75. Gaughan WJ, Sheth VR, Francos GC, Michael HJ, Burke JF. Ranitidine-induced acute interstitial nephritis with epithelial cell foot process fusion. *Am J Kidney Dis* 1993;22:337–340.
76. Nolan CR, Anger MS, Kelleher SP. Eosinophiluria, a new method of detection and definition of clinical spectrum. *N Engl J Med* 1986;315: 1516–1519.
77. Lins RL, Verpooten GA, de Clerck DS, de Broe ME. Urinary indices in acute interstitial nephritis. *Clin Nephrol* 1986;26:131–133.
78. Wood BC, Sharma JN, Germann DR, et al. Gallium citrate 67 imaging in noninfectious interstitial nephritis. *Arch Int Med* 1978;138: 1665–1666.
79. Linton AL, Richmond JM, Clark WF et al. Gallium 67 scintigraphy in the diagnosis of acute renal failure. *Clin Nephrol* 1985;24:84.
80. Graham GD, Lundy MM, Moreno AJ. Failure of gallium 67 scintigraphy to identify reliably noninfectious interstitial nephritis: concise communication. *J Nucl Med* 1983;24:568.
81. Nessi R, Benoldi GL, Redaelli B, Filippo GS. Acute renal failure after rifampin: a case report and survey of the literature. *Nephron* 1976;16:148.
82. Flynn Ct, Rainford DJ, Hope E. Acute renal failure and rifampicin: danger of unsuspected intermittent dosage. *Br Med J* 1974;2:482.
83. Poole G, Stradling P, Worledge S,. Potentially serious side effects of high-dose twice-weekly rifampicin. *Br Med J* 1971;3:343–347.
84. Lo WK, Rolston KV, Rubenstien EB, Bodey GP. Ciprofloxacin-induced nephrotoxicity in patients with cancer. *Arch Int Med* 1993;153:1258.
85. Allon M, Lopez EJ, Min KW. Acute Renal failure due to ciprofloxacin. *Arch Int Med* 1990;150:2187.
86. Lyons H, Pinn VW, Cortell S, et al. Allergic interstitial nephritis causing reversible renal failure in four patients with idiopathic nephrotic syndrome. *N Engl J Med* 1973;288:124–128.
87. Warren GV, Korbet S, Schwartz MM, Lewis EJ. Minimal change glomerulopathy associated with nonsteroidal antiinflammatory drugs. *Am J Kidney Dis* 1989;13:127.

88. Grussendorf M, Andrassy K, Wladherr R, Ritz E. Systemic hypersensitivity to allopurinol with acute interstitial nephritis. *Am J Nephrol* 1981;1:105–109.
89. Neelakantappa K, Gallo GR, Lowenstein J. Ranitidine associated interstitial nephritis and Fanconi syndrome. *Am J Kidney Dis* 1993; 22:333–334.
90. Cogan MG. Tubulointerstitial nephropathies: a pathophysiologic approach. *West J Med* 1980;132:134–142.
91. Braden GL, Germain MJ, Fitzgibbons JP. Impaired potassium and magnesium homeostasis in acute interstitial nephritis. *Nephron* 1985; 41:273–278.
92. Levy M, Guesry P, Loirat C, Dommergues JP, Nivat H, Habib R. Immunologically mediated tubulointerstitial nephritis in children. *Contrib Nephrol* 1979;16:132–140.
93. Wilson DM, Salazar TL, Farkouh ME. Eosinophiluria in atheroembolic disease. *Am J Med* 1991;91:186–189.
94. Appel G, Levine M. Acute interstitial nephritis. In: A Fauci, M Lichtenstein, eds. *Current Therapy in Allergy, Immunology, and Rheumatology*. 1988.
95. Kida H, Abet, Tonosugi N, Koshino Y, Yokoyama H, Mattori N. Prediction of the long term outcome in acute interstitial nephritis. *Clin Nephrol* 1984;22:55–60.

Subject Index

Subject Index

H

Q

R

W

X

Y

Z